Textbook of
BASIC NURSING

Caroline Bunker Rosdahl, RN-C, BSN, MA

Staff Nurse
Hennepin County Medical Center
Minneapolis, Minnesota

Formerly Associate Education Specialist
University of Minnesota School of Nursing
Minneapolis, Minnesota

Assistant Director Emeritus
Anoka-Hennepin Technical College
Anoka, Minnesota

Instructor, Vocational-Technical Education
University of Minnesota
Minneapolis/St. Paul, Minnesota

Mary T. Kowalski, RN, BA, BSN, MSN

Professor and Director of Nursing and Health Careers
Cerro Coso Community College
Ridgecrest, California

◆ LIPPINCOTT WILLIAMS & WILKINS

A **Wolters Kluwer** Company

Philadelphia • Baltimore • New York • London
Buenos Aires • Hong Kong • Sydney • Tokyo

Acquisitions Editor: Lisa Stead
Development Editor: Joe Morita
Production Editor: Nicole Walz
Senior Production Editor: Sandra Cherrey Scheinin
Senior Production Manager: Helen Ewan
Art Director: Carolyn O'Brien
Illustration Coordinator: Brett MacNaughton
Cover Design: M.W. Design, Inc.
Manufacturing Manager: William Alberti
Indexer: Michael Ferreira
Compositor: Circle Graphics
Printer: Quebecor

Edition 8

Library of Congress Cataloging-in-Publication Data

Textbook of basic nursing / [edited by] Caroline Bunker Rosdahl, Mary Kowalski.—8th ed.
   p. cm.
  Includes bibliographical references and index.
  ISBN 0-7817-3429-0 (alk. paper)
   1. Practical nursing. I. Rosdahl, Caroline Bunker. II. Kowalski, Mary.

RT62 .R58 2002
610.73—dc21

2002034026

Care has been taken to confirm the accuracy of the information presented and to describe generally accepted practices. However, the authors, editors, and publisher are not responsible for errors or omissions or for any consequences from application of the information in this book and make no warranty, express or implied, with respect to the content of the publication.

The authors, editors, and publisher have exerted every effort to ensure that drug selection and dosage set forth in this text are in accordance with the current recommendations and practice at the time of publication. However, in view of ongoing research, changes in government regulations, and the constant flow of information relating to drug therapy and drug reactions, the reader is urged to check the package insert for each drug for any change in indications and dosage and for added warnings and precautions. This is particularly important when the recommended agent is a new or infrequently employed drug.

Some drugs and medical devices presented in this publication have Food and Drug Administration (FDA) clearance for limited use in restricted research settings. It is the responsibility of the health care provider to ascertain the FDA status of each drug or device planned for use in his or her clinical practice.

No endorsement of specific actions of LPN/LVNs in violation of state statutes or Board of Nursing rules was intended or implied in this book. Each nurse must assume the responsibility to practice within the rules and guidelines of the state and of the healthcare area within which he or she is employed.

This 8th Edition of my book, my life's work, is dedicated to:

Emily Paige Malcolm Rosdahl

and

Bailey Katrina Bunker Rosdahl

You are my legacy to the world!

Caroline Bunker Rosdahl

I wish to dedicate this book to Caroline Bunker Rosdahl who has devoted astronomical numbers of hours to the education of nurses. A nurse, an educator, and an author, Caroline has assisted countless students to become successful practical/vocational nurses. She has been the soul of this textbook for more than 30 years.

Mary T. Kowalski

Section Editors, Contributors, Consultants, Reviewers

SECTION EDITORS

Vicki Earnest, RN, MS
Chair Allied Health
Health, Math, and Science
Community College of Denver
Denver, Colorado
CHAPTERS 74–92

Marjorie L. Roark, RN, BSN, Med
Nurse Educator
Professional Development
The University of Chicago Hospitals
Chicago, Illinois
CHAPTERS 33–63

NCLEX-STYLE QUESTIONS WRITER

Lazette Nowicki, RN, MSN
Nursing Assistant Professor
Allied Health
Sacramento City College
Sacramento, California

CONTRIBUTORS

Martha J. Baird, RN, CNM, NP, MSN
Director of Education
Women's Health Care Nurse Practitioner Program
Harbor-UCLA Research and Education Institute
Los Angeles, California
CHAPTERS 64–66

Mary Jancaric Dierich, RN, MSN, C-NP, CURN
Nurse Practitioner
Urologic Surgery
University of Minnesota
Minneapolis, Minnesota
CHAPTER 88

Deborah A. Fulton, RN, CNP, MS
Nurse Practitioner/Advance Practice Nurse
Hennepin County Medical Center
Minneapolis, Minnesota
CHAPTERS 47, 93, 94

Stacy Glass, RN, BA
Clinical Nurse Specialist
The Center for Men's Health & Infertility—Urology
University of Minnesota
Minneapolis, Minnesota
CHAPTER 89

Jennifer Johnson, RN, BSN, MSN, c
Professor of Nursing
Allied Health
Bakersfield College
Bakersfield, California
CHAPTERS 9–14

Laurie Kaudewitz, BSN, MSN, RN-c
Assistant Professor
Family Community Nursing
East Tennessee State University
Johnson City, Tennessee
CHAPTERS 67–69

Celesta Kirk, RN, CS, MA, MSN, FNP
Associate Professor, College of Nursing
Dept. of Family–Community Nursing
East Tennessee State University
Johnson City, Tennessee
CHAPTERS 71–73

Barbara D. Klaus, RN, MSN, ANP
Adult Nurse Practitioner, HIV
Department: Infectious Disease Section
VA Medical Center: ID Section
Denver, Colorado
CHAPTER 84

Betsy Manchester, MN, RNP, OCN
Nursing Faculty
University of Phoenix and LACC District
Palmdale, California
CHAPTER 70

Judith L. Miller, RN, MS
Clinical Assessment Associate
The Peer Review Organization of New Jersey
East Brunswick, New Jersey
CHAPTERS 95, 96, 98

Patricia A. Mullen, MSN, CNS, CCRN
Instructor
Department of Nursing
Regis University School of Healthcare Professions
Denver, Colorado
CHAPTERS 75 and 87

Patricia Reder, RN
Nurse Case Manager
Case Management
Innovative Care Management
Clackamas, Oregon
CHAPTERS 80, 85, 86

Kathleen Ricco, RN, BSN, CRNH
Hospice Nurse and Nursing Instructor
Cerro Coso Community College
Ridgecrest, California
CHAPTER 99

Rosemary L. Rosdahl, RPh, BS
Pharmacist and Owner, Watertown Pharmacy
Watertown, Minnesota
CHAPTER 62

Diane Shantz

Kathleen Sodergren, RN, PhD, BSN, MSN
Clinical Nurse Specialist—Breast Cancer
Oncology Department
Mercy/Unity Hospitals
Coon Rapids and Fridley, Minnesota
CHAPTER 90

Patricia Vincent
Diabetes Educator
Sage Community Health Center
Ridgecrest, California
CHAPTERS 30–32

Lisa Wehner, MSN
Associate Professor
Nursing and Allied Health
State University of New York at Delhi
Delhi, New York
CHAPTERS 15–26

Mary E. Zaccagnini, RN, MS, AOCN
Clinical Nurse Specialist
Oncology Department
University of Minnesota
Minneapolis, Minnesota
CHAPTERS 71 and 82

CHAPTER CONSULTANTS

Mary Ellis Goode, RN, BS, MEd
Parish Nurse
Bethel Methodist Church
Mound, Minnesota
Consultant on Parish Nursing
CHAPTER 101

Patricia Rusca, RN
Visiting Nurse Association of Central Jersey
Red Bank, New Jersey
Consultant on Prospective Payment System
CHAPTER 98

Janina Stephens, RN-C, CRN
Visiting Nurse Association of Central Jersey
Red Bank, New Jersey
Consultant on Rehabilitation
CHAPTER 96

Eileen Toughill, NPC, PhD
Continence Specialist
Consultant on Rehabilitation
CHAPTER 96

INDEPENDENT CONSULTANTS

Maryann Foley, RN, BSN
Nursing Clinical Consultant
Flourton, Pennsylvania

Marilee LeBon, BA
Developmental Editor
Mountaintop, Pennsylvania

REVIEWERS

Debra Aucoin-Ratcliff, MA
Programs Director
Northern California Training Institute
Rocklin, California

Ruth Ann Benfield, RN, Med, MSN, CRNP
Professor
Nursing Department
Montgomery County Community College
Blue Bell, Pennsylvania

Valerie J. Benedix, RN, BSN
Nursing Instructor
Nursing Department
Clovis Community College
Clovis, New Mexico

Joanne Carlson, MS, APRN
Nursing Coordinator
Nursing Department
Ogden Weber Applied Technology College
Layton, Utah

Mary Ann Cosgarea, RN, BSN, BA
Coordinator/Nurse Administrator
Portage Lakes Career Center
W. Howard Nicol School of Practical Nursing
Cuyahoga Falls, Ohio

Sybil Damon, RN, PhD
Academic Dean
West Coast University
Los Angeles, California

Patricia A. Dickman, RN, BA
Nursing Instructor
BM Spur School of Practical Nursing

Laurie Fontenot, RN, C
Department Head
Health Occupations (PN, MA, NA)
Louisiana Technical College
T. H. Harris Campus
Opelousas, Louisiana

Sandra Handelman, AS, BSN, MS
Clinical Instructor
Nursing Department
South University
Boynton Beach, Florida

Kenn Hazell, MSN, ARNP
Staff Nurse
Emergency/Trauma Department
Broward General Medical Center
Ft. Lauderdale, Florida

Perpetua McDonald, RN, BSN
Nursing Instructor
Practical Nursing
St. Paul Technical College
St. Paul, Minnesota

Joanne Neihardt, RN, MSN, CS, NP
Faculty
Health Careers
Kirtland Community College
Roscommon, Michigan

Kathy A. Nicely, RN, BSN
Instructor
Level I Med-Surg Adults, Pharmacology
Great Oaks School of Practical Nursing
Cincinnati, Ohio

Johnnie Nichols, LVN, ADN, BSN
Nursing Instructor
Vocational Nursing
Panola College
Carthage, Texas

Mabel Smith-Duffus
Director
Port St. Lucie School of Practical Nursing
Port St. Lucie, Florida

Darlyn Weikel, RNC, MSN
Associate Professor
Health Sciences (Nursing: ADN/PN)
North Central State College
Mansfield, Ohio

The *Textbook of Basic Nursing,* Edition 8, evolves from the previous successful editions of this classic nursing textbook. Traditionally, this textbook has been an integral part of the education of many practical/vocational nurses, and will be no less so in the 21st century. Edition 8 has been thoroughly revised, updated, and many comprehensive changes designed to encourage and assist nursing students in their programs have been made. Program directors will find this text to be responsive to the needs of both students and instructors.

Material is presented in a number of ways, allowing each student to learn in his or her preferred/optimum learning style. Each student can learn by *reading, performing* (skills), *seeing* (pictures, boxes, diagrams), and by applying gained knowledge to critical thinking exercises.

SUMMARY OF TEXTBOOK FEATURES

- Student-friendly; manageable reading level
- Flexible to suit the instructor's needs
- Cost effective for the student, instructor, and nursing programs
- General-to-specific and simple-to-complex in the development of chapters
- Full-color figures and drawings that illustrate, demonstrate, and highlight important concepts
- Numerous tables and boxes that summarize, emphasize, and organize important topics
- Key learning concepts and nursing alerts emphasized throughout
- Comprehensive, covering all content areas of the NCLEX-PN
- Healthcare trends, concerns, and lifestyle considerations of the 21st century included
- Sociocultural and ethnic considerations emphasized
- Mathematics concepts reviewed
- Pharmacology concepts and medication classifications presented
- Medication administration theory and techniques presented and illustrated
- Medication boxes summarize common medications for specific conditions, diseases, and disorders
- Age-related concerns presented, as well as integrated throughout text
- Basic Nursing Procedures detailed
- Nursing Skills Guidelines summarized

- Nursing Process integrated with conditions, diseases, and disorders
- Nursing Care Plans developed using NANDA terminology and the Nursing Process
- CD-ROM focusing on the care of a diabetic patient who develops chronic wounds as a result of the disease. This interactive program encourages independent decision-making and critical thinking skills, and it implements the Nursing Process.
- NANDA diagnoses relating to specific diseases or disorders presented
- Nursing considerations and interventions relating to specific topics presented
- Life cycle stages and changes specified, as well as integrated throughout text
- Specific topics (eg, nutrition, disease processes, health maintenance and prevention, and sociocultural concepts) integrated throughout the text
- Maslow's Hierarchy, Erikson's Life Span Stages, Kübler-Ross' Stages of Death and Dying, and other important theorists presented and integrated into content areas
- Learning objectives highlight important concepts of chapters
- Terminology highlighted and defined
- Acronyms and abbreviations delineated
- NCLEX-PN examination-type questions given in each chapter, as well as in ancillary materials
- Critical thinking exercises presented in each chapter
- Client and Family Teaching boxes highlight important teaching concepts
- Comprehensive chapter on the history of nursing
- Websites and other computer-related topics included
- Ancillary package to enhance learning includes the following:
  - Student Self-Study CD-ROM (located in back of text)
  - Student Workbook
  - Procedure (Skills) Checklist
  - Instructors' Manual and Testbank

One of the main features of this text is that it closely mirrors the educational guidelines established by the National Council of State Boards of Nursing for the Licensing Examination for Practical/Vocational Nurses (NCLEX-PN). The table at the end of this Preface lists the test plan for the NCLEX-PN and shows where the NCLEX-PN content is found in this text. Also summarized in the table are the many NCLEX-PN content areas that are integrated throughout the text.

The Textbook of Basic Nursing is designed to be student-friendly. Numerous full-color photographs and drawings are found throughout the text. The figures and drawings highlight important points, illustrate nursing procedures, and create visual representations of concepts discussed in the text. The reading level is designed to be understandable to the maximum number of students, including those for whom English is a second language. Key **English-to-Spanish** phrases are included in Appendix A.

There also is a CD-ROM included at the back of the text that contains pronunciations for all of the New Terminology and Glossary terms in the book. Students can click on each term to hear the correct pronunciation. This tool will be helpful to students learning unfamiliar medical terms and to ESL and foreign students.

Included are numerous **Client Care Concepts,** such as the activities of daily living, as well as the more advanced needs related to specific diagnostic tests, conditions, diseases, and disorders. **Nursing Procedures** present step-by-step instructions with many full-color illustrations; rationales are included to support the understanding of these steps. **Nursing Skill Guidelines** are summaries of important concepts, teaching, skills performance, or nursing considerations. Special **life span considerations** are integrated throughout.

Learning objectives, introduced for the first time ever in an earlier edition of this text, have become a standard in all nursing texts. These objectives are important guidelines for students and faculty. As a teaching and learning tool, the objectives are developed to highlight the important subjects of each chapter. Expanded terminology sections in each chapter highlight the key words and present new and significant **terminology** relevant to each chapter. Medical terminology, including prefixes, suffixes, and root words, is also contained in Appendix D.

Nursing and all healthcare fields are filled with **abbreviations and acronyms.** Each chapter of this text has delineated the abbreviations and acronyms that are important to the understanding of the language of medicine and nursing. The acronyms are used and defined in the text, as well as in Appendix B.

When studying content and preparing for examinations, a suggestion for students would be to start by addressing the learning objectives and learning the medical terminology and acronyms. Relating this terminology to the **critical thinking concepts** and **nursing considerations** of the learning objectives will promote student learning and enhance retention of subject matter for each chapter.

A **glossary of terms** is highly advantageous to the novice nurse. A comprehensive glossary is found in the back of this book. Also in Appendix C is a list of the most **common laboratory tests,** as well as normal values.

Instructors will appreciate the logical design and simple format. This text is comprehensive and relevant to practical/vocational nursing course content. General healthcare issues in the beginning sections of the book lead to the more complex and specific healthcare issues in later units. **Legal and ethical issues, confidentiality,** and the **holistic care** of client and fam-

ily are common topics presented in specific chapters as well as integrated throughout the text. Emphasis is placed on specific **ethnic, cultural, and religious factors** related to healthcare and its delivery.

The essential concepts of **anatomy and physiology** are developed in the unit on structure and function. The units related to **pediatric nursing** and **adult medical-surgical nursing** are presented in the same order as are the chapters in the body structure and function unit. Pertinent pathophysiology of diseases and disorders, as contrasted to the normal, is presented along with nursing considerations relevant to these problems.

In addition to the specific content areas of anatomy and physiology and adult medical-surgical nursing, this text also includes comprehensive chapters on **nutrition, diet and diet therapy,** and **cultural considerations. Maternity-obstetrics, newborn care, pediatrics,** and **geriatrics** are thoroughly discussed. The special topics of **psychiatric** nursing and **substance abuse** nursing are also presented in comprehensive chapters.

Pharmacology and **medication administration** are presented in separate chapters, as well as specific medications being integrated into medical-surgical and specific skills chapters. Conditions, diseases, and disorders are organized into units dedicated to maternity-obstetric, neonatal, pediatric, mature adult, and geriatric nursing.

New and expanded chapters in this edition address nursing in sites other than the acute care hospital. These community settings are providing employment for growing numbers of practical/vocational nurses. Separate chapters are included in **extended care, rehabilitation** nursing, **ambulatory** healthcare, **home care,** and **hospice** nursing.

The **graduating nurse** obtains valuable information in the final unit of the book relating to employment opportunities in many of these areas, as well as in **acute care settings.** A separate chapter on **job-seeking** skills is included. Components of **teamwork, leadership,** and **supervision** are emphasized in specific chapters, as well as integrated throughout the text.

The content is well developed, while maintaining educational concepts relevant to the practical/vocational nurse. The functional task-based aspects of practical/vocational nursing are integrated with the need for the complexities of critical thinking.

Supplemental texts to cover NCLEX-PN content areas are not required. Thus, *Textbook of Basic Nursing,* Edition 8, is *cost effective* for the individual student, as well as efficient for nursing programs and individual instructors.

Programs differ in their order of presentation of content material. *Textbook of Basic Nursing,* Edition 8, is adaptable and capable of being individualized for each school's curriculum. Rarely does a program start with chapter one and go consecutively chapter-by-chapter to the end of the text. With the organization of *Textbook of Basic Nursing,* the instructor will be able to smoothly transition from one topic to another.

Within chapters the reader will find cross-references to similar or common topics. A student can refer to other chapters within this text for additional, supplemental information on specific topics. Cross-referencing also helps to minimize repetition of subject matter. An instructor has flexibility in the presentation of content, but also can be assured that the student will have access to various aspects of related topics. The cohesiveness of related topics can be adapted to each instructor's or program's needs.

Numerous Website addresses, comprehensive resources, and a current bibliography also add to the advantages of this text for students and instructors. These resources are presented in one general location to facilitate further research into nursing and healthcare issues.

The goal of the state boards of nursing and the National Council is to ensure healthcare protection for the public and to provide measures of the competencies necessary for entry-level practical/vocational nursing across the United States and its territories, as well as Canada and other English-speaking countries. The goal of this textbook is to provide the student with the educational tools needed to achieve success on the NCLEX-PN and to safely practice nursing as an LPN/LVN. Best wishes to students and instructors as you use this textbook!

Caroline Bunker Rosdahl
Mary T. Kowalski

OVERVIEW OF THE APRIL 2002 TEST PLAN FOR THE NCLEX-PN EXAMINATION*	RELATED CONTENT IN *TEXTBOOK OF BASIC NURSING*	
A. Safe, Effective Care Environment **The practical/vocational nurse provides nursing care and collaborates with others to enhance the care delivery setting and to protect clients, significant others, and other healthcare personnel through:**	**Units**	**Integrated Concepts**
1. Coordinated Care The practical/vocational nurse collaborates with other healthcare team members to facilitate effective client care *Related content includes, but is not limited to:* Advance Directives Advocacy Client Care Assignments Client Rights Confidentiality Concepts of Management and Supervision Consultation With Members of the Healthcare Team Continuity of Care Continuous Quality Improvement Establishing Priorities Ethical Practice Healthcare Delivery System Incident/Irregular Occurrence/Variance Reports Informed Consent Legal Responsibilities Referral Processes Resource Management 2. Safety and Infection Control The practical/vocational nurse protects clients and healthcare personnel from environmental hazards. *Related content includes, but is not limited to:* Accident/Error Prevention Disaster Planning First Aid Handling Hazardous and Infectious Materials Medical and Surgical Asepsis Microbiology Standard (Universal) and Other Precautions Use of Client Safety Device	Unit I The Nature of Nursing Unit II Personal and Environmental Health Unit VI The Nursing Process Unit VII Safety in the Health Care Facility Unit VIII Client Care Unit XVI The Transition to Practicing Nurse	• Assessment and Data Collection • NANDA Diagnoses • Planning and Goal Setting • Implementations and Nursing Considerations • Evaluations • Sample Nursing Care Plans • Maslow's Hierarchy of Needs • Erikson's Life Span Stages • Kübler-Ross Stages • Cultural and Ethnic Considerations • Community Healthcare • Key Nursing Concepts • Nursing Alerts
B. Health Promotion and Maintenance **The practical/vocational nurse provides and assists in directing nursing care, and promotes and maintains health through incorporating knowledge of the following areas:**		
3. Growth and Development Through the Life Span The practical/vocational nurse assists the client and significant others during the normal expected stages of growth and development from conception through advanced old age. *Related content includes, but is not limited to:* Aging Process Ante/Intra/Postpartum and Newborn Development Stages and Transitions Expected Body Image Changes Family Interaction Patterns Family Planning Human Sexuality 4. Prevention and Early Detection of Disease The practical/vocational nurse provides client care related to prevention and early detection of health problems. *Related content includes, but is not limited to:* Data-Collection Techniques Disease Prevention Health Promotion Programs Health Screening Immunizations Lifestyle Choices	Unit II Personal and Environmental Health Unit III Development Throughout the Life Cycle Unit VI The Nursing Process Unit VII Safety in the Healthcare Facility Unit X Maternal and Newborn Nursing	Life Cycle Considerations and Concerns: • Fetus and Newborn • Pediatrics • Adult • Maternity • Geriatrics • Psychiatric • Family Development • Client and Family Teaching • Key Concepts • Nursing Alerts • Anatomy and Physiology • Basic Human Needs • Public Health Concepts

OVERVIEW OF THE APRIL 2002 TEST PLAN FOR THE NCLEX-PN EXAMINATION*	RELATED CONTENT IN TEXTBOOK OF BASIC NURSING	
C. Psychosocial Integrity The practical/vocational nurse provides nursing care that promotes and supports the emotional, mental, and social well-being of the client and significant others in the following areas:	**Units**	**Integrated Concepts**

5. Coping and Adaptation The practical/vocational nurse promotes the ability of the client and/or significant others to cope, adapt, and/or problem-solve situations related to illnesses, disabilities, and stressful events. *Related content includes, but is not limited to:* Behavior Management Sensory/Perceptual Alterations Coping Mechanisms Situational Role Changes End-of-Life Issues Stress Management Grief and Loss Support Systems Mental Health Concepts Therapeutic Communication Religious and Spiritual Unexpected Body Image Influences on Health Changes 6. Psychosocial Adaptation The practical/vocational nurse participates in recognizing and providing care for clients with maladaptive behavior and assists with behavior management of the client with acute and/or chronic mental illness and cognitive psychosocial disturbances. *Related content includes, but is not limited to:* Abuse and Neglect Mental Illness Concepts Behavioral Interventions Suicide Prevention Chemical Dependency Therapeutic Environment Crisis Intervention Use of Client Safety Devices	Unit XI Pediatric Nursing Unit XIII Gerontological Nursing Unit XIV Mental Health Nursing	Life Cycle Considerations & Concerns: • Fetus and Newborn • Pediatrics • Adult • Maternity • Geriatrics • Psychiatric • Substance Abuse • Community Healthcare • Client and Family Teaching • Cultural Considerations
D. Physiologic Integrity The practical/vocational nurse promotes physical health and well-being by providing care and comfort, reducing client risk potential, and assisting to manage the client's health alterations.		
7. Basic Care and Comfort The practical/vocational nurse provides comfort and assistance in the performance of activities of daily living. *Related content includes, but is not limited to:* Assistive Devices Nutrition and Oral Hydration Elimination Palliative Care Mobility/Immobility Personal Hygiene Non-pharmacologic Pain Rest and Sleep Interventions 8. Pharmacologic Therapies The practical/vocational nurse provides care related to the administration of medications and monitors clients receiving parenteral therapies. *Related content includes, but is not limited to:* Adverse Effects Pharmacologic Actions Drug Interactions Pharmacologic Agents Expected Effects Side Effects Medication Administration	Unit IV Structure and Function Unit V Nutrition and Diet Therapy Unit VII Safety in the Healthcare Facility Unit VIII Client Care Unit IX Pharmacology and Administration of Medications Unit X Maternal and Newborn Nursing Unit XI Pediatric Nursing Unit XII Adult Care Nursing Unit XIII Gerontological Nursing Unit XV Nursing in a Variety of Settings	Nursing Considerations Related to • Maternity • Fetus and Newborn • Pediatrics • Young Adult • Mature Adult • Geriatrics • Psychiatric • End-of-Life Care • Medication Boxes • Safety • First Aid • Rehabilitation

OVERVIEW OF THE APRIL 2002 TEST PLAN FOR THE NCLEX-PN EXAMINATION*	RELATED CONTENT IN *TEXTBOOK OF BASIC NURSING*	
D. Physiologic Integrity (*Continued*)	**Units**	**Integrated Concepts**

9. Reduction of Risk Potential
    The practical/vocational nurse reduces the client's potential for developing complications or health problems related to treatments, procedures, or existing conditions.
        Related content includes, but is not limited to:
 	
Diagnostic Tests
Laboratory Values
Potential for Alterations
  in Body Systems
 	
Potential Complications of
  Diagnostic Tests, Procedures,
  Surgery, and Health
  Alterations
Therapeutic Procedures
 	
10. Physiologic Adaptation
    The practical/vocational nurse participates in providing care to clients with acute, chronic or life-threatening physical health conditions.
        Related content includes, but is not limited to:
 	
Alterations in Body Systems
Basic Physiology
Fluid and Electrolyte
  Imbalances
Medical Emergencies
 	
Radiation Therapy
Respiratory Care
Unexpected Response to
  Therapies
		• Nutritional Concepts
		• Key Concepts
		• Nursing Alerts
		• Cultural
		  Considerations
		• Disease and Disorders
		• Nursing
		  Procedures
		• Nursing Skill
		  Guidelines

*Source:
National Council of State Boards of Nursing, Inc.
676 N. St. Clair Street, Suite 550
Chicago, IL 60611-2921
http://www.nscbn.org

Acknowledgements

Nursing educators have always had a unique and formidable job. They must provide the ladder of the science of nursing knowledge and integrate the latticework of the art of nursing. The authors of *Textbook of Basic Nursing,* Edition 8, are extremely grateful to the many contributors from across the nation. Each contributor has dedicated hours researching content, writing text, and checking details.

Special thanks go to Joe Morita, Managing Editor, and Sandra Cherrey Scheinin, Senior Production Editor, both from Lippincott Williams & Wilkins. They inherited an enormous task in the middle. You showed great organizational and delegational skills in creating an integrated whole out of chaos. Your vision of the completed project, your thoroughness, and your patience are much appreciated.

Caroline Bunker Rosdahl and Mary T. Kowalski

Some of the special people who have helped me include:

- Marge Roark Lofgreen, who worked on sections of the book and gave me moral support. You are a good friend.
- Maryann Foley, who edited large sections of the book and helped write portions of chapters at the last minute. And Marilee LeBon, who also edited large sections of manuscript and who showed great patience and perseverance in writing and rewriting of specific sections, particularly body structure and function. You both showed great attention to detail. This is most unusual and very much appreciated.
- Mary Kowalski, who stepped in as co-author, not realizing what a huge job it would be. You hung in there and did an excellent job. Thanks.
- My family and friends, who showed great patience, love, and helpfulness during this process. John Gray and Hennepin County Medical Center, who allowed me to schedule my work hours around the book schedule. And my three bands, which provided me with needed recreation and diversion.

In memory of my parents, Frank and Pearl Bunker.

Caroline Bunker Rosdahl

Many individuals have guided my career in nursing and in nursing education. Diane Neville, Chriss Benvenuti, Sybil Damon, and I have shared many experiences as nurses, directors, and teachers. We have seen the nursing profession change, develop, decline, and resurge in the last 25 years. The student vocational nurses at Cerro Coso Community College and I have greatly benefited from the hard work and dedication of many individuals including Pat Knapik, Pat Duran, and June Wasserman. Barbara Boullear and Kathy Ricco are fantastic people and great instructors who represent the standards of the profession and promote the education of nurses. Many thanks to these individuals for all of their efforts in behalf of nursing.

In Memory of Kathy Rose and Anabel.

Mary T. Kowalski

Contents

Unit V
NUTRITION AND DIET THERAPY

PART *B*
Nursing Care Skills

Unit VI
THE NURSING PROCESS

Unit VII
SAFETY IN THE HEALTHCARE FACILITY

PART 6
Nursing Throughout the Life Cycle

Unit X
MATERNAL AND NEWBORN NURSING

Unit XI
PEDIATRIC NURSING

Unit XII
ADULT CARE NURSING

Unit XIII
GERONTOLOGICAL NURSING

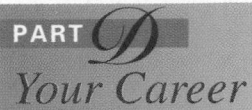

PART D
Your Career

Summary of Special Displays

NURSING CARE GUIDELINES

Foundations of Nursing

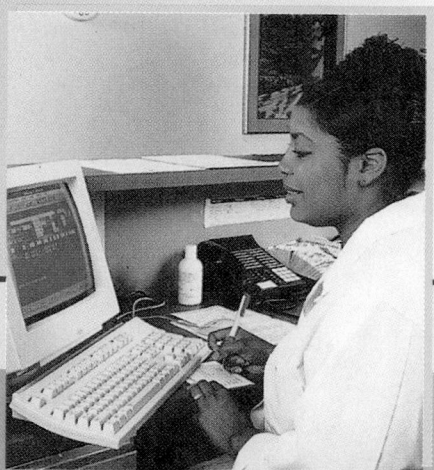

Unit I

THE NATURE OF NURSING

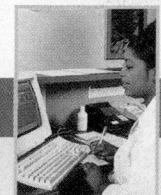

1

The Origins of Nursing

LEARNING OBJECTIVES

1. Explain how certain events in ancient and medieval times influenced the development of contemporary nursing.
2. Discuss Florence Nightingale's influence on modern nursing practice.
3. List at least ten of Florence Nightingale's nursing principles that are still practiced today.
4. Identify important individuals who contributed to the development of nursing in the United States.
5. Name some pioneer nursing schools in the United States.
6. List important milestones in the history of practical nursing education.
7. Explain war-related developments in nursing.
8. Discuss current trends that are expected to influence the nursing profession in the 21st century.
9. Describe the importance of nursing insignia, uniforms, and the nursing school pin.

NEW TERMINOLOGY

caduceus
Hippocratic oath
holistic healthcare

insignia
Nightingale lamp

You have chosen to be a nurse. The word *nurse* derives from the Latin word meaning *to nourish*. You are embarking on a career that combines scientific principles, technical skills, and personal compassion. Although people have been performing many nursing skills for centuries, nursing in its present form began to emerge only in the 19th century. Contemporary nursing continues to evolve as society and its healthcare needs and expectations change. Nursing must continue to adapt to meet society's goals and to provide needed services in the changing world.

Nursing is a practical and noble profession. It provides a stable career in the ever-changing world of healthcare, with plenty of career options.

Individual attributes required to be a nurse include a strong sense of responsibility and the highest standards of integrity. Personal conviction and flexibility are necessary foundations of a nurse. A nurse must be well educated, and integrate the art and the science of working with people.

NURSING'S HERITAGE

A detailed history of nursing is beyond the scope of this book. All nurses should become familiar with some important people and developments in the history of nursing.

Early Influences

In ancient times, people often attributed illness to punishment for sins or to possession by evil spirits. Most primitive tribes had a medicine man, or shaman, who performed rituals using various plants, herbs, and other materials, to heal the sick. Many tribal rituals included dances, chants, and special costumes and masks. Some groups used human or animal sacrifices. Women had various roles in ancient health practices, depending on the culture and social customs. Women were often involved with assisting in childbirth.

Care of the sick is discussed in the Bible, the Talmud, and other ancient texts. Centers in India and Babylonia provided care for the sick before the time of Christ. By 500 BC, the advanced Greek civilization had begun to acknowledge causes of disease other than punishment by God or demonic possession. Based on mythical figures, the **caduceus** and the staff of Aesculapius are the modern symbols of medicine (Fig 1-1). The Greeks began to establish centers, sometimes called hostels or hospitals, for care of the sick and injured. They used warm and mineral baths, massage, and other forms of therapy that female priestesses sometimes administered. Pregnant women or people with an incurable illness were not admitted to these hostels.

The Influence of Hippocrates

One of the early outstanding figures in medicine was Hippocrates, born in 460 BC on the Greek island of Kos. Hippocrates is the acknowledged "Father of Medicine." Hippocrates denounced the idea of mystical influence on disease. He was also the first person to propose concepts such as physical assessment, medical ethics, client-centered care, and systematic observation and reporting. By emphasizing the importance of caring for the whole person (**holistic healthcare**), he helped to lay the groundwork for nursing and medicine. Contemporary healthcare practitioners preserve the principles of Hippocrates. Typically, a physician will repeat the **Hippocratic oath** when graduating from a school of medicine. The Florence Nightingale pledge and Practical Nurses' pledge are based on this oath.

Early medical educators helped to solidify the need for practitioners to be well-educated individuals. Physicians were eventually required to obtain a university degree as a doctor of medicine (MD). Specialized healthcare education and training became standard as scientific knowledge increased. Modern medicine has multiple medical and surgical specializations; for instance, the client can be described as having heart and lung diseases, or injury and trauma.

Relatively unchanged from the beginning is the concept that a nurse must be aware of the whole client. The holistic approach translates into the nurse's attentiveness to a client's personal needs from various perspectives. The nurse is aware of the client's emotions, lifestyles, physical changes, spiritual needs, and individual challenges. Nursing is unique in this approach to healthcare.

The Roman Matrons

The first recorded history of nursing begins with Biblical women who cared for the sick and injured. Many were in the religious life. For instance, Phoebe, mentioned in the Epistle

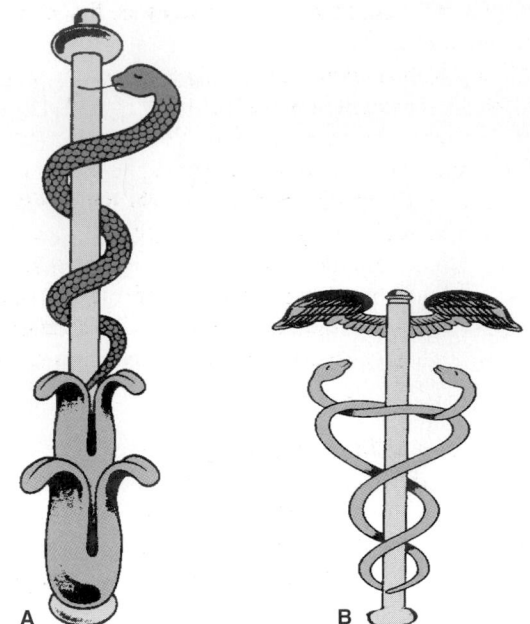

FIGURE 1-1. Symbols of medicine. (**A**) Aesculapius, a mythical Greek god of healing and son of Apollo, had many followers who used massage and exercise to treat patients. This god is also believed to have used the magical powers of a yellow, nonpoisonous serpent to lick the wounds of surgical patients. Aesculapius was often pictured holding the serpent wrapped around his staff or wand; this staff is a symbol of medicine. (**B**) Another medical symbol is the caduceus, the staff of the Roman god Mercury, shown as a winged staff with two serpents wrapped around it.

to the Romans (about 58 AD), is known as the first deaconess and visiting nurse.

Fabiola, a Roman woman, is credited with influencing and paying for the construction of the first free hospital in Rome in 390 AD. Another Roman woman, Saint Marcella, converted her beautiful home into a monastery, where she taught nursing skills. She is considered the first nursing educator. Saint Paula is credited with establishing inns and hospitals to care for pilgrims traveling to Jerusalem. She is said to be the first person to teach the philosophy that nursing is an art rather than a service. Saint Helena, the mother of the Roman Emperor Constantine, is credited with establishing the first gerontological facility, or home for the aged.

Monastic and Military Nursing Orders

Beginning in the first century, several monastic orders were established to care for the sick. Sometimes, the monastery itself became the refuge for the sick; in other cases, members of a religious order founded a hospital. Both men and women of religious orders performed nursing care.

During the Crusades (1096–1291), female religious orders in northern Europe were nearly eliminated. Male military personnel, such as the Knights Hospitalers of St. John in Jerusalem, conducted most nursing care. Because these military men were required to defend the hospital as well as care for the sick, they wore suits of armor under their religious habits. The symbol for this order was the Maltese Cross, which later became the symbol of the Nightingale School. This symbol was the forerunner of nursing school pins worn today.

The Reformation

In the 1500s, during the European religious movement called the Reformation, many monasteries closed and the work of women in religious orders nearly ended. Until the 1800s, the few women who cared for the sick were prisoners or prostitutes. Nursing was considered the most menial of all tasks, and the least desirable. This period is called the *dark ages of nursing.*

Fliedner in Kaiserswerth

In 1836, Pastor Theodor Fliedner established the Kaiserswerth School for Nursing in his parish in Kaiserswerth, Germany. It was one of the first formally established schools of nursing in the world. Out of it grew the Lutheran Order of Deaconesses, which Fliedner directed. Its most famous student was Florence Nightingale.

By the late 1800s, many schools for trained nurses existed throughout Europe. The status of nursing began to improve and many women, including members of religious orders, once again became involved in nursing care.

Florence Nightingale

Even during the days when nursing was considered menial and undesirable, some women continued to care for the sick. Probably the most famous was Florence Nightingale (Fig. 1-2).

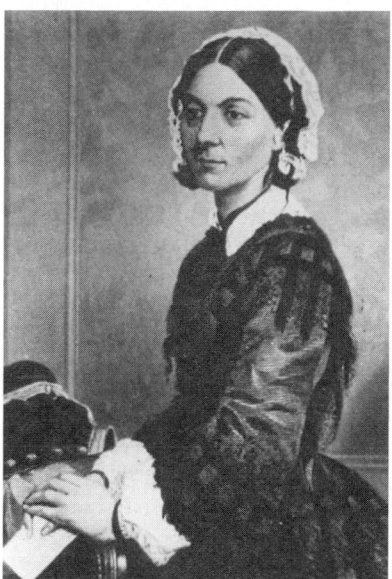

FIGURE 1-2. Florence Nightingale. (Photo courtesy of the Center for the Study of the History of Nursing.)

Most nurses before her time received almost no training. Not until she graduated from Kaiserswerth and began to teach her concepts did nursing become a respected profession.

Nightingale was born in Italy in 1820 to wealthy English parents. When she was still very young, her parents returned to England. In 1844, an American doctor visited the family, and Nightingale asked him if entering the field of nursing would be appropriate for her. The reply from Dr. Samuel Gridley Howe has become a classic quotation. He said:

> My dear Miss Florence, it would be unusual (for you to enter nursing), and in England whatever is unusual is apt to be thought unsuitable; but I say to you, go forward, if you have a vocation for that way of life; act up to your aspiration and you will find that there is never anything unbecoming or unladylike in doing your duty for the good of others. Choose your path, go on with it, wherever it may lead you, and God be with you![1]

In 1851, Nightingale entered the Deaconess School in Kaiserswerth. She was 31 years old, and her family and friends were strongly opposed to her becoming a nurse. After her graduation in 1853, she became superintendent of a charity hospital for governesses. She trained her attendants on the job and greatly improved the quality of care. In 1854, the Crimean War began. Nightingale gained fame during this conflict. She entered the battlefield near Scutari, Turkey with 38 other nurses and cared for the sick and injured. The nurses had few supplies and little outside support. Nonetheless, Nightingale insisted on establishing sanitary conditions and providing quality nursing care, which immediately reduced the mortality rate. Her persistence made her famous and she and her nurses were greatly admired. Her dedicated service both during the day and at night, when she and her nurses made their rounds carrying oil lamps, created a public image of the lady with the lamp. In time the **Nightingale lamp** or the "Lamp of Learning" (Fig 1-3) became a symbol of nursing and nursing education. Today,

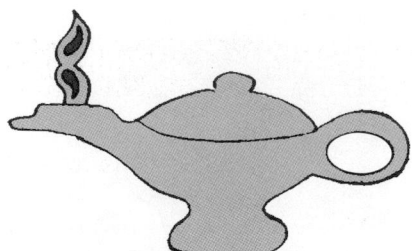

FIGURE 1-3. The "Nightingale lamp" (also known as the "Lamp of Nursing" or the "Lamp of Learning") is an insignia of nursing and nursing education. The lamp represents the warmth of caring. The light of the lamp symbolizes the striving for excellence. The oil represents the energy and commitment of the nurse to heal others.

many schools of nursing display a model of the lamp or a picture of Florence Nightingale carrying a lamp.

Nightingale's Definition of Nursing

Nightingale had definite and progressive ideas about nursing. Her definition of nursing, published in 1859, is still important today. She said, "Nature alone cures. Surgery removes the bullet out of the limb, which is an obstruction to cure, but nature heals the wounds . . . Medicine assists nature to remove the obstruction, but does nothing more. And what nursing has to do in either case, is to put the patient in the best condition for nature to act upon him."[1]

The Nightingale School

Building on the respect she had established in the Crimean War, Nightingale opened the first nursing school outside a hospital in 1860. The nursing course was 1 year in length and included both classroom and clinical experience, a major innovation at that time. Students gained clinical experience at St. Thomas Hospital in London. Because it was financially independent, the school emphasized learning, rather than service to the hospital. Some principles of the Nightingale School for Nurses are still taught today:

- Cleanliness is vital to recovery.
- The sick person is an individual with individual needs.
- Nursing is an art and a science.
- Nurses should spend their time caring for others, not cleaning.
- Prevention is better than cure.
- The nurse must work as a member of a team.
- The nurse must use discretion, but must follow the physician's orders.
- Self-discipline and self-evaluation are important.
- A good nursing program encourages a nurse's individual development.
- The nurse should be healthy in mind and body.
- Teaching is part of nursing.
- Nursing is a specialty.
- A nurse does not graduate, but continues to learn throughout his or her career.
- Nursing curricula should include both theoretical knowledge and practical experience.

The Nightingale School included other innovations:

- Establishment of a nurses' residence
- Entrance examinations and academic and personal requirements, including a character reference
- Records of each student's progress—later known as the "Nightingale plan," a model for current nursing programs
- Records of employment of students after graduation, or a formal register—the beginnings of nursing practice standards

NURSING IN THE UNITED STATES

Nursing in the colonial United States was primarily a family matter, with mothers caring for their own families or neighbors helping each other. Throughout the 19th and 20th centuries, historical and nursing developments interacted to build the foundation of modern nursing practice. The establishment and growth of a system of nursing education is the most important development that has shaped today's nursing. Box 1-1 lists important milestones in the development of nursing in both the United States and Canada.

The First Nursing Schools

The influence of Florence Nightingale and the Kaiserswerth school extended to the United States when Pastor Fliedner came to Pittsburgh, PA with four nurse–deaconesses. In 1849, he became involved with the Pittsburgh Infirmary, the first Protestant hospital in the United States. Today it is called Passavant Hospital. The four deaconesses trained other nurses and started the movement to educate American nurses. The Pittsburgh Infirmary was the first real school of nursing in the United States, although limited training existed in other hospitals in New York and Pennsylvania before 1849.

In 1873, three nursing programs based on the Nightingale plan were formally established: Bellevue Hospital School of Nursing in New York; Connecticut Training School in New Haven; and Boston Training School at Massachusetts General Hospital.

Notable American Nurses

With the onset of the Civil War (1861–1865), the public need for nurses became more evident. In 1861, the Union Army appointed Dorothea Lynde Dix (1802–1887) Superintendent of Female Nurses. Her job was to recruit volunteer nurses to treat men injured in the war. Dix is especially remembered for her campaign against the inhumane treatment of the mentally ill. One of Dix's volunteers was Louisa May Alcott (author of *Little Women*). Another was Clara Barton (1821–1912), who in 1881 founded the organization now known as the American Red Cross.

Melinda Ann (Linda) Richards (1841–1930) was the first trained nurse in the United States. She graduated in the early 1870s and organized the school of nursing at Massachusetts General Hospital, then called the Boston Training School.

Isabel Hampton Robb (1860–1910) was the founder of the school of nursing at Johns Hopkins University. She is credited with founding two national nursing organizations, one in 1911,

➤➤ BOX 1-1

MILESTONES IN MODERN NURSING IN THE UNITED STATES AND CANADA

1849	Pittsburgh Infirmary begins training nurses in America.
1861	Dorothea Dix is appointed Superintendent of Female Nurses of the Union Army in the American Civil War.
1872–1873	Women's Hospital (Philadelphia), Bellevue Hospital School of Nursing (New York), Connecticut Training School (New Haven), and Boston Training School are founded.
1873	Melinda Richards becomes the first trained nurse in the United States.
	Howard University established an 18-month program for black students. The school was transferred to Freedman Hospital the next year.
1879	Mary Eliza Mahoney is the first black graduate nurse in the United States.
1881–1882	Clara Barton founds the American branch of the Red Cross.
1892	The New York YMCA founds the Ballard School of Practical Nursing.
1893	Lillian Wald and Mary Brewster found the first Visiting Nurse Service.
1894	Isabel Robb and Lavinia Dock found the American Society of Superintendents of Training Schools of Nursing (later, Education Committee of National League for Nursing).
1897	Nurses' Associated Alumnae of the United States and Canada organizes (later, part of American Nurses Association [ANA]).
1899	International Council of Nurses (ICN) organizes.
1900	Isabel Robb founds the *American Journal of Nursing.*
early 1900s	Mary Breckinridge establishes a nurse midwife school.
1901	Congress establishes the U.S. Army Nurse Corps.
1903	The states of North Carolina, New York, New Jersey, and Virginia pass nursing licensure laws.
1905	*Canadian Nurse* first publishes (in both French and English).
1907	Thompson Practical Nursing School is founded in Brattleboro, Vermont; Mary A. Nutting and Isabel Robb establish the first college-based nursing program (Teacher's College–Columbia University).
1908	American Red Cross starts home nursing classes; Congress establishes the Navy Nurse Corps; National Association of Colored Graduate Nurses is founded.
1909	University of Minnesota becomes the first school to continuously educate nurses at the university level.
1914	Mississippi becomes the first state to license practical nurses.
1917	Smith-Hughes Vocational Education Act passes, enabling federal funding for practical nursing education.
1918	The Household Nursing Association School of Attendant Nursing in Boston and the National League for Nursing Education are founded.
1919	Ethyl Johns establishes the first baccalaureate program in the British Empire in Vancouver, BC; Minneapolis Vocational School establishes the first vocational school–based PN program.
1930	Arizona establishes a nursing program for Native American women.
1938	New York becomes the first state to mandate licensure of practical nurses.
1939	Graduate School of Midwifery is established in Kentucky.
1940	ANA establishes "Male Nurses' Section"; six states offer option for PN licensure.
1941	Association of Practical Nurse Schools is founded in Chicago (later NAPNES).
1942	U.S. Office of Education establishes national curriculum for practical nurses.
1943	President Franklin Roosevelt signs bill for the U.S. Cadet Nurse Corps (operates until 1945).
1947	University of Minnesota establishes experimental four-quarter practical nursing program in collegiate setting (operates until 1967); U.S. Office of Education publishes *Practical Nursing, an Analysis of the Practical Nurse Occupation with Suggestions for Organization of Training Programs.*
1949	Lillian Kuster founds National Federation of LPNs (NFLPN); U.S. Air Force Nurse Corps organizes.
1950	National practical nursing curriculum develops; LPN licensure becomes available in many states; all states now use the State Board Test Pool Examination for licensure; several organizations combine to create National League for Nursing (NLN).
1951	NAPNES publishes *Journal of Practical Nursing;* National Association of Colored Graduate Nurses dissolves, and ANA admits these nurses.

(continued)

➤➤ BOX 1-1

MILESTONES IN MODERN NURSING IN THE UNITED STATES AND CANADA (CONTINUED)

1952	First 2-year associate degree program for educating RNs opens in the United States (Teacher's College–Columbia University).	1973	*Textbook of Basic Nursing,* 2nd edition, is first to delineate behavioral/learning objectives for students; ANA begins certifying nurses in specialty practice.
1953	National Student Nurses' Association (NSNA) is founded.	1976	Health Occupations Students of America (HOSA) is founded in Oklahoma.
1954	Nearly 300 practical nursing programs exist; U.S. Army gives first male nurse rank equal to female nurses; male nurses are allowed to join Nurse Corps.	1979	NLN publishes entry-level competencies of graduates of PN/VN programs.
1955	All states now have laws to license practical nurses.	1983	Congress establishes Medicare reimbursement on basis of Diagnosis-Related Groups (DRGs).
1959	U.S. Department of Health, Education, and Welfare publishes *Guides for Developing Curricula for Education of Practical Nurses* by Dorothea Orem.	1989	American Medical Association (AMA) proposes 9-month program for Registered Care Technologists, which is prevented by major opposition from nursing.
1961	NLN begins offering accreditation for PN programs.	1994	First computerized examination, NCLEX, is given for nursing licensure.
1966	NLN accredits the first PN program—the Chicago Public School Practical Nursing Program.	1996	National certification in long-term care becomes available to LPN/LVNs.
1971	National Black Nurses' Association is founded; Lucille Kinlein is first nurse to function as independent practitioner.		

which eventually emerged as the American Nurses Association (originally called the Alumnae Association). She and Lavinia Lloyd Dock (1858–1956) founded the American Society of Superintendents of Training Schools of Nursing in 1894, which in 1903 evolved into the Education Committee of the National League for Nursing. Robb wrote one of the earliest nursing textbooks, *Materia Medica for Nurses,* and co-authored a four-volume *History of Nursing.* Robb also founded the *American Journal of Nursing.* She introduced charting and nurse licensure to improve continuity of care. She also initiated the idea of graduate nursing study in the late 1800s.

Lillian Wald (1867–1940) is considered the founder of American public health nursing. She is best known for founding the Henry Street Settlement Visiting Nurse Society (VNS) in New York City in 1893. The Henry Street Settlement was a neighborhood nursing service that became a model for similar programs in the United States and other countries. Wald also convinced New York City schools to have a nurse on duty during school hours. She persuaded President Theodore Roosevelt to create a Federal Children's Bureau, and insisted that nursing education occur in institutions of higher learning.

Mary E. Mahoney (1845–1926) promoted fair treatment of African Americans in healthcare. She was the first African American graduate nurse, and promoted integration and better working conditions for minority healthcare workers in Boston.

Mary Breckinridge (1881–1965) was a pioneer as a visiting nurse–midwife to the mountain people of Kentucky in the early 1900s, often making her rounds on horseback. She also started one of the first midwifery schools in the United States.

Collegiate Nursing Education

In 1907, Mary Adelaide Nutting (1858–1947) and Isabel Robb were instrumental in establishing the first college-based nursing program at Teachers College of Columbia University. Nutting thus became the first nurse to be on a university staff. She was also instrumental in founding the International Council of Nurses.

In 1909, the University of Minnesota established the first continuous program to educate nurses at the university level, with an enrollment of four students. Isabel Robb strongly influenced the organization of this program, which is considered the beginning of nursing as a profession. This program, however, did not lead to a bachelor's degree until 1919, when several other schools had also initiated college- and university-based nursing programs.

The History of Practical Nursing Education

Practical nursing, also called vocational nursing, has existed for many years. Women often cared for others and called themselves practical nurses. Not until the 1890s, however, was formal education in practical nursing available.

Pioneer Schools

Curricula in all of the early practical nursing schools included child care, cooking, and light housekeeping, in addition to care of the sick at home. Hospital care was not necessarily included.

Ballard School.   In 1892, the Young Women's Christian Association (YWCA) opened the first practical nursing school in the United States in Brooklyn, New York. Later, it was named the Ballard School because Lucinda Ballard provided the funding. Practical nursing (attendant nursing) was one of several courses offered to women. This program was a 3-month course to train women in simple nursing care, emphasizing care of infants and children, older adults, and the disabled in their own homes. The Ballard School closed in 1949 because of YWCA reorganization.

Thompson Practical Nursing School.   Thomas Thompson, a wealthy man who lived in Vermont during the Civil War, learned that women were making shirts for the army at only a dollar a dozen. In his will, he left money to help them. Richard Bradley, his executor, was a public-spirited man and determined that the local citizens needed nursing service. In 1907, he used some of Thompson's money to establish the Thompson Practical Nursing School in Brattleboro. This school still exists today.

Household Nursing School.   In Boston, a group of women wanted to provide nursing care in the home for people who were sick. They called on Bradley for advice, and he encouraged them to follow Brattleboro's example. In 1918, the Household Nursing Association School of Attendant Nursing opened. The school was later renamed the Shepard-Gill School of Practical Nursing in honor of Katherine Shepard Dodge, the first director, and Helen Z. Gill, her associate and successor. This school operated until 1984.

In all, 36 practical nursing schools opened during the first half of the 20th century in the United States. Between 1948 and 1954, 260 additional programs had opened. Today, more than 1,300 practical nursing programs exist in the United States.

American Red Cross Training

In 1908, the American Red Cross began offering home nursing education to teach lay women appropriate nursing care for illnesses within their own families. Jane Delano (1862–1919) was an Army nurse who was instrumental in this movement. Chapter 7 discusses the Red Cross in more detail.

Practical Nursing in Vocational and Community Colleges

In the early part of the 20th century, nursing schools—training both practical nurses and registered nurses—were traditionally located in or affiliated with hospitals. In 1917, the U.S. Congress passed the Smith-Hughes Act, the funds from which gave impetus to vocational-technical and public education. In 1919, the first vocational school-based nursing program opened in Minneapolis at Minneapolis Vocational High School. Today, the majority of practical nursing and associate's-degree nursing programs are located in vocational education settings or in community colleges.

Other Milestones in Practical Nursing Education

The Association of Practical Nurse Schools was founded in 1941. It was later renamed the National Association of Practical Nurse Education and Service.

In 1914, Mississippi became the first state to designate licensed practical nurses (LPNs). By 1955, all states had laws to license practical nurses. The first state to have mandatory licensure for LPNs to practice was New York. Chapter 2 discusses permissive and mandatory licensure more fully.

During World War II, people realized that nurses needed a consistent curriculum. In 1942, the U.S. Office of Education planned and advocated the first practical nursing curriculum for the entire country.

In 1966, the Chicago Public School system's program was the first practical nursing program to be accredited by the National League for Nursing (NLN).

Nursing During Wartime

Nursing during wartime has long been important. From Florence Nightingale in the Crimea to the American Civil War, Spanish–American War, Korea, Vietnam and continuing into Desert Storm in the 1990s, nurses have always played a vital role.

World War I marked the first emergency training of nurses. The Army School of Nursing was established; Annie W. Goodrich (1876–1955) wrote the curriculum. Hundreds of women were trained in this abbreviated program; however, nearly all of them left nursing and returned to homemaking after the war's end in 1918.

The U.S. Cadet Nurse Corps was established during World War II, with Lucile Petry Leone (1902–1999) as Director. More than 14,000 volunteer nurses graduated in about 2 years. Originally, the plan was to draft nurses into the Army. A major opponent to this idea was Katherine J. Densford (1890–1978), Director of the School of Nursing at the University of Minnesota. She promised to train expanded numbers of nurses in a short time, if the government abandoned the nurse draft. Because of Densford's efforts, the student population at Minnesota multiplied by five in a matter of weeks; more than 1,200 cadets graduated from that school alone.

World War II also marked the first time that men as well as women were actively recruited into nursing. Male nurses were not given equal rank to female nurses in the Armed Forces, however, until 1954. By the war's end in 1945, the world had changed. Many cadet nurses remained in the field, especially in the military. This employment gave many women a measure of independence that they had not previously known. After this time, emphasis was placed on improved graduate education for nurses. Nurses also began to assume a broader, more responsible role—a trend that continues today.

Current Nursing Trends

As you will note from your reading and from studying Box 1-1, nursing evolved rapidly in the 20th century. Many factors influenced trends that are expected to continue in the 21st century. This book has been written with these trends in mind:

Higher client acuity in hospital and long-term settings: Because of limitations on payment for healthcare, hospital stays are markedly shorter than they were just 10 years ago. Clients in all healthcare facilities are more acutely ill than in years past. Long-term care facilities also find clients with highly acute conditions because of the growth of home care for those with more manageable conditions. Such developments require nurses working in all care areas to have higher levels of skill, additional education, and more specialization.

Shift to community-based care: Most clients now receive healthcare outside acute care settings. For example, a great deal of surgery is now done on an outpatient basis; many clients receive care for chronic or long-term conditions at home; and community clinics provide primary healthcare for many clients. Thus, today's nursing is delivered in a much wider range of settings than in the past.

Technology: Nurses, clients, and family members often must learn to operate highly sophisticated equipment to manage conditions in the home. This equipment makes accuracy in diagnosis and treatment possible. The teaching role of nursing is emphasized to a greater extent.

Social factors: Many clients are homeless, unemployed, or underemployed. Many people have no health insurance. Devastating diseases, such as acquired immunodeficiency syndrome (AIDS) or tuberculosis, are becoming more prevalent. These factors create a need for more healthcare in the public sector.

Lifestyle factors and greater life expectancy: Today's society and the healthcare industry emphasize prevention of disease, healthy lifestyles, and wellness programs. Many people are living much longer and are more active and healthy into their later years than in past generations. Greater life expectancy is causing huge growth in the areas of extended, long-term, and home care. This growth will require larger numbers of nurses to work in such fields.

Changes in nursing education: Today's nursing programs emphasize education over service to clinical sites. They identify specific objectives (outcomes) for students. An earlier edition of this textbook was the first to identify learning objectives in practical nursing. Many LPN/LVNs are returning to school to become registered nurses, and many "career ladder" programs are available.

Autonomy: The women's movement has influenced nurses, many of whom are women, to be more assertive and independent. Today's nursing role is more collaborative, rather than nurses being subservient to physicians. Primary care, previously delivered only by physicians, is now being delivered by advanced practice nurses as well.

NURSING INSIGNIA

An **insignia** is a distinguishing badge of authority or honor. The symbolism dates back to the 16th century in Europe, when only a nobleman could wear a coat of arms. Later this privilege was expanded to include members of guilds (craftsmen).

Certain types of training schools, including religious nursing orders, were also given the privilege. Until recently, female nurses wore nursing caps and all nurses were awarded a school pin at graduation. Some schools also had distinguishing capes. The "Nightingale lamp," "Lamp of Nursing," or "Lamp of Learning" remains a standard of nursing insignia (Fig. 1-3).

Nursing Uniforms

Even though nurses in today's healthcare facilities usually do not wear traditional white uniforms or nursing caps, looking professional is important. Clients usually feel more comfortable when nurses are easily identifiable and distinguishable from other staff. For example, a name tag is required whenever you give nursing care, no matter where you are employed.

The Nursing School Pin

You may receive a nursing pin at graduation that symbolizes your school of nursing. Early nursing symbols were usually religious in nature. Today, many nursing school pins bear some religious symbol, such as a cross (based on the Maltese Cross) or a Star of David, even though the school may not be directly affiliated with a religious organization. The Nightingale lamp is also a common component of the nursing pin.

☛ KEY CONCEPT

Remember that as you embark on your nursing career, you continue nursing's history and heritage.

➤ STUDENT SYNTHESIS

Key Points

- Medicine men and women and religious orders cared for the sick in early times.
- Florence Nightingale contributed a great deal to the development of contemporary nursing.
- Establishment of nursing schools in the United States began in the late 19th century.
- The first practical nursing school in the United States opened in 1892 in New York.
- Nursing during the First and Second World Wars contributed to the profession's and to women's evolving roles in society.
- Many current societal and healthcare trends are influencing the nursing profession, including higher levels of client acuity in hospital settings, more community-based care, technological advances, changing lifestyles, greater life expectancy, changing nursing education, and more nursing autonomy.
- Nursing insignia, such as those found on nursing school pins, often symbolize nursing's history and heritage.

Critical Thinking Exercises

1. Explain how the changing role of women in society helped contribute to the changing role of nursing.
2. Determine why established standards of nursing practice and education are so important to the development of nursing as a respected profession.
3. A friend interested in nursing asks you about the profession's history and its place in today's society. How would you answer your friend? What developments and milestones would you highlight?

NCLEX-Style Review Questions

1. Florence Nightingale opened the first school of nursing outside a hospital that stressed:
   a. Cleanliness
   b. Discipline
   c. Learning
   d. Service to the hospital
2. Which of the following was the first practical nursing school in the United States?
   a. Ballard School
   b. Household Nursing School
   c. Kaiserswerth School
   d. Thompson Practical Nursing School
3. Which of the following trends are expected to influence nursing in the 21st century?
   a. Autonomy of nurses
   b. Higher client acuity
   c. Increased hospital based care
   d. Shorter life expectancy of clients

Reference

1. Nightingale, F. (1992). *Notes on nursing: What it is and what it is not* (Commemorative Edition 1859). Philadelphia: Lippincott.

CHAPTER

2

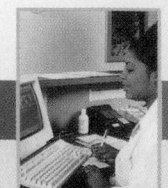

Beginning Your Nursing Career

LEARNING OBJECTIVES

1. Compare the education and level of practice between registered and practical nurses.
2. Explain the various types of educational programs that lead to licensure.
3. Identify at least one of the standards of the National Federation of Licensed Practical Nurses in relationship to each of the following: education, legal status, and practice.
4. Differentiate between permissive and mandatory licensure.
5. Discuss the reasons for a nurse to seek licensure.
6. Identify the importance of the nurse's pledge.
7. Explain the importance of nursing theory and how a theoretical framework helps nurses in their learning, understanding, and practice.
8. List the roles of today's nurse, briefly explaining each one.
9. Discuss the importance of nurses projecting a professional image.
10. Describe nursing organizations, their membership requirements, and benefits.

NEW TERMINOLOGY

accreditation
advanced practice nurse
approval
licensure
mandatory licensure

nurse practice act
permissive licensure
practical nurse
theoretical framework

ACRONYMS

AALPN	HOSA	NFLPN
AJN	ICN	NLN
ANA	LPN/LVN	PACE
ANCC	NAPNES	RN
CHAP	NCLEX	

Nursing provides service to help people meet the daily needs of life when they have difficulty satisfying these needs on their own. As students, nurses bring certain knowledge, skills, attitudes, and abilities to their nursing program. They will develop skills and knowledge in school. Their ability to act independently will depend on your professional background, motivation, and work environment. Defining all the specific roles of a nurse is difficult because these roles constantly change. Factors that influence nursing activity include new discoveries in the biomedical field, development of new healthcare knowledge, changes in patterns of health services and payment, and the relationships among healthcare team members.

This chapter discusses various programs for nursing education, approval and accreditation, licensure, a code of ethics, the role and image of the nurse, and nursing organizations. Chapter 3 examines information about the healthcare system, and Chapter 6 discusses the concepts of health and wellness.

HEALTHCARE: A MULTIDISCIPLINARY APPROACH

The sophisticated healthcare system of the 21st century requires many trained individuals working together in a complex healthcare system (Table 2-1). Many contemporary healthcare positions originated as functions of either the physician or the nurse. For example, the duties of a hospital dietitian and the physical therapist started as functions of nursing. As knowledge of nursing and medicine grew, several segments of healthcare became their own professions. Healthcare has a tremendous variety of specialties and subspecialties. All healthcare positions have unique educational requirements.

To achieve licensure as a medical doctor, an individual starts with a minimum of 4 years of undergraduate study. Their education continues with 4 years of medical school, after which the graduate doctor must take a licensure exam prior to practicing. As a new doctor of medicine, the physician who wishes to specialize must continue his or her education as a resident,

■■■ TABLE 2-1 ⬧ ALLIED HEALTH PROFESSIONALS

Chiropractor—Manipulates the musculoskeletal system and spine to relieve symptoms

Dental Hygienist—Trained and licensed to work with a dentist by providing preventive care

Dietitian—Trained nutritionist who addresses dietary needs associated with illness

Electrocardiograph Technician—Assists with the performance of diagnostic procedures for cardiac electrical activity

Electroencephalograph Technician—Assists with the diagnostic procedures for brain wave activity

Emergency Medical Technician—Trained in techniques of administering emergency care enroute to trauma centers

Histologist—Studies cells and tissues for diagnosis

Infection Control Officer—Identifies situations at risk for transmission of infection and implements preventive measures

Laboratory Technician—Trained in performance of laboratory diagnostic procedures

Medical Assistant (Administrative or Clinical)—Assists the physician in the front and/or back medical office, clinic, or other medical settings

Medical Secretary—Trained in secretarial sciences with an emphasis on medical applications

Medical Transcriptionist—Trained in secretarial sciences to make typed records of dictated medical information

Nuclear Medical Technician—Specializes in diagnostic procedures using nuclear devices

Occupational Therapist—Evaluates and plans programs to relieve disorders that interfere with activities

Paramedic—Trained in advanced rescue and emergency procedures

Pharmacist—Prepares and dispenses medications by the physician's order

Phlebotomist—Trained to perform venipunctures

Physical Therapist—Plans and conducts rehabilitation procedures to relieve musculoskeletal disorders

Psychologist—Trained in methods of psychological assessment and treatment

Radiographer—Works with a radiologist or physician to operate radiologic equipment for diagnosis and treatment

Respiratory Therapist—Trained to preserve or improve respiratory function

Risk Manager—Identifies and corrects potential high-risk situations within the healthcare field

Social Worker—Trained to evaluate and correct social, emotional, and environmental problems associated with the medical profession

Speech Therapist—Treats and prevents speech and language disorders

Surgical Technician or Technologist—Assists doctors and nurses in the operating room

Unit Clerk—Performs the administrative duties in a hospital patient care unit

Hosley, J., Jones, S., & Molle-Matthews, E. (1997). *Textbook for medical assistants.* Philadelphia: Lippincott-Raven.

which requires another 2 to 6 years of study. These years can be followed by additional years of advanced study. The physician is responsible for diagnosing and treating clients. In this role, the physician often acts as a team leader (Fig 2-1).

TYPES OF NURSING PROGRAMS

Nurses are an important part of the healthcare team. Four basic types of educational programs lead to a credential in nursing (Table 2-2). Three programs allow the graduate to take the licensure examination and to become a registered nurse (**RN**). The fourth, a practical or vocational nursing program, allows the graduate to take the licensure examination and to become a licensed **practical nurse** (**LPN**) or a licensed vocational nurse (**LVN**).

Registered Nurses

Registered nurses spend from 2 to 4 years learning their profession. In addition, they may have special training that allows them to practice public health nursing or to specialize in fields such as surgery. RNs are responsible for care of the acutely ill; teaching professional and practical nursing students; managing personnel; and taking charge in various healthcare settings. RNs also perform many duties that only physicians performed 30 years ago. For example, the RN may be first assistant in surgery. RNs may continue their education to become nurse anesthetists, nurse midwives, or advanced practice nurses.

Basic Education
Three basic types of education lead to the RN license:

1. A student attends a 2-year program at a community or junior college and receives an associate's degree (AD) in nursing. This AD-RN is educated primarily as a bedside nurse and is sometimes called a *technical nurse*. In some states, some nursing groups are advocating different licensure for RNs who graduate from AD programs, as opposed to graduates of 4-year programs.
2. The 3-year program was formerly sponsored by and based in a hospital. Most of today's 3-year programs, however, are affiliated with community and state colleges that grant college credits. Some states no longer have 3-year programs.

3. The 4-year program in a college or university leads to a baccalaureate, or bachelor's degree in nursing. The graduate of this program may enter graduate school to study for an advanced master's or doctorate degree. Most of these programs aim to prepare professional nurses who will be teachers or administrators or who will assume other leadership positions. Many bachelor's graduates become certified as public health nurses and work in community health.

Some community colleges have programs that admit only LPNs. The LPN is usually required to take general education courses before admission. Then, with approximately one additional year of education, an LPN becomes eligible to take the licensure examination and become an RN. This program leads to an associate's degree.

Advanced Nursing Credentials
Several types of advanced certification are available to RNs. The American Nurses Credentialing Center (**ANCC**) of the American Nurses Association (ANA) grants a total of 27 advanced certificates.

Generalist nursing certificates require a bachelor's degree and an examination. These certificates are available in 14 specialties including psychiatric-mental health, medical-surgical, gerontologic, perinatal, maternal-child, pediatrics, general practice, continuing education, and community health.

A clinical nurse specialist certificate is available in five areas of nursing: psychiatric-mental health–adult, psychiatric-mental health–child, medical-surgical, gerontologic, and community health.

An **advanced practice nurse,** formerly called the nurse practitioner, is an RN, usually with a master's degree, who has specialized in a particular field. In addition to the RN license, the state issues a license to practice, or the state's Nurse Practice Act grants authority to practice. The ANCC certifies advanced practice nurses in adult nursing, family practice, gerontology, pediatrics, and school nursing. Advanced practice nurses assess clients, assist in the diagnosis and treatment of illness, and, in many states, are authorized to prescribe medications. Nurses with other additional educational preparation, such as midwives and anesthetists, are described later in this book.

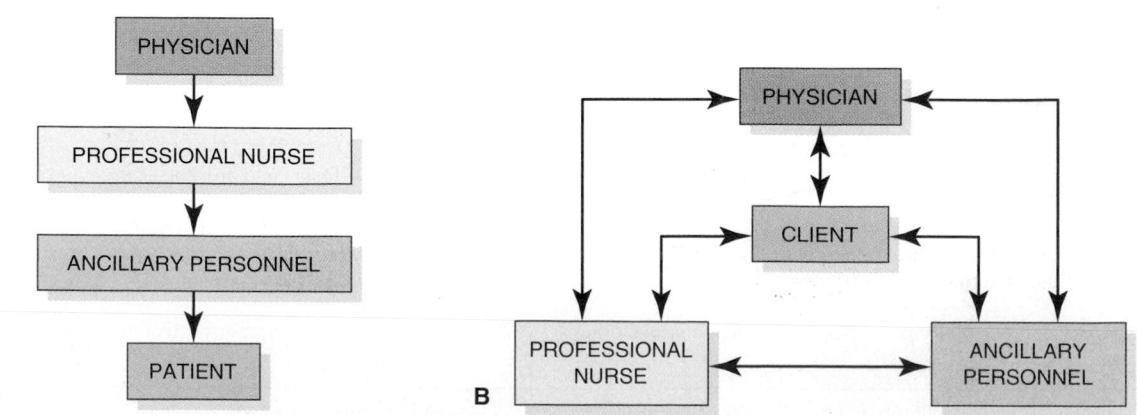

FIGURE 2-1. Traditional (**A**) and contemporary (**B**) views of healthcare practice.

▪▪▪ TABLE 2-2 Nursing Practice and Educational Levels

Classification	Functions and Role	Educational Requirements
(Certified) Nurses Aide (CNA) Unlicensed Assistive Personnel (UAP)	Provides basic nursing care of clients in a long-term care facility. Works under the supervision of a LVN, RN, or MD. In some facilities, the "aide" is referred to as Unlicensed Assistive Personnel.	2 months to 6 months Educational requirements may differ between the CNA and the UAP.
Licensed Practical/ Vocational Nurse (LPN/LVN)	Provides nursing care in long-term and acute care facilities. May also work in physician offices and clinic settings. Works under the supervision of a RN or MD.	1 to 2 years
Registered Nurse (RN)	Provides direct and indirect nursing care, supervision, and leadership in a wide variety of healthcare settings	2 to 4 years Associates Degree (AD) or Bachelor's Degree (BS or BA) or Master's Degree (MS or MA)
Advance Practice Nurse or Nurse Practitioner (NP)	An RN who receives additional training in a specialized field such as pediatrics, maternity, geriatrics, family practice, or mental health	RN with a master's degree plus additional and specific education and internship in the field of specialty

Practical Nurses/Vocational Nurses

Practical or vocational nurses are licensed under specific state laws (**Nurse Practice Acts**) to care for clients in various settings in the same manner as is the RN. The term vocational nurse is used in Texas and California in place of practical nurse. Generally, the LPN/LVN works under the direct or indirect supervision of an RN or physician. The functions and responsibilities of the practical/vocational nurse and the registered nurse often coincide. Many LPN/LVNs supervise nursing assistants or aides.

Do not confuse the position of the individual who is called a nurse's aide, nursing assistant, certified nursing assistant (CNA), or unlicensed assistive personnel (UAP) with the LPN/LVN or RN. While the aide may receive a certification by the state when completing a nurse aide training course, this individual is not licensed, and therefore, not regulated, by a state nurse practice act. A nursing assistant, aide, or UAP is a person who is taught via on-the-job training or in short-term programs to help clients and residents meet the needs of daily living, such as hygiene and dressing.

Current functions of the LPN/LVN include providing bedside care, doing wound care, administering prescribed medications, monitoring client status, and reporting reactions to medications or treatments to the RN or physician. Individual states or healthcare agencies may limit the practical/vocational nurse's care of intravenous lines, complex treatment and medication regimens, and functions related to primary or complex healthcare assessment of clients.

Box 2-1 presents standards of nursing practice of LPN/LVNs promoted by the National Association for Practical Nurse Education and Service, an association for the representation of LPN/LVNs. Another association, the National Federation of Licensed Practical Nurses lists its standards of practice for the practical/vocational nurse in Box 2-2. These two major agencies are discussed later in this chapter.

According to the Bureau of Labor Statistics *Occupation Outlook Handbook* for 2002-2003, most practical/vocational

➤➤ BOX 2-1

STANDARDS OF PRACTICE FOR LPNs/LVNs

The LPN/LVN provides individual and family-centered nursing care in the following ways:

- Using appropriate knowledge, skills, and abilities
- Using principles of the nursing process to meet specific client needs in diversified healthcare settings
- Maintaining appropriate written documentation and using effective communication skills with clients, family, significant others, and members of the healthcare team
- Executing principles of crisis intervention to maintain safety
- Providing appropriate education to clients, family, and significant others to promote health, facilitate rehabilitation, and maintain wellness
- Serving as an advocate to protect client rights

The LPN/LVN fulfills his or her professional responsibilities in the following ways:

- Applying the ethical principles underlying the profession of nursing
- Following legal requirements
- Following the policies and procedures of the employing facility
- Cooperating and collaborating with all members of the healthcare team to meet the needs of family-centered nursing care
- Assuming accountability for his/her nursing actions
- Seeking educational opportunities to improve knowledge and skills

National Association for Practical Nurse Education and Service. (2000). *Standards of practice and code of ethics for licensed practical/vocational nurses.* Silver Spring, MD: Author.

from a nursing program, a student nurse must meet the minimum standards of the approved nursing program.

Licensure of Nurses

Licensing laws, often referred to as **Nurse Practice Acts,** protect the public from unqualified workers and establish standards for the profession or occupation. Licensing laws establish a minimum level of requirements for competence and practice. Obtaining **licensure** helps the public determine the difference between a qualified and an unqualified worker.

The first licensure laws for nursing were passed in 1903 in North Carolina, New York, Virginia, and New Jersey. The first LPN law was passed in Mississippi in 1914. In 1940, fewer than 10 states had LPN laws, but by 1955 all states had LPN laws. Every state and the District of Columbia, Puerto Rico, Guam, American Samoa, the Virgin Islands, the Canadian provinces, and the North Mariana Islands now have licensing laws for both RNs and LPNs.

Any student who has graduated from an approved nursing program is eligible to take an exam provided by the National Council of State Boards of Nursing. The exam is called the National Council Licensure Examination (**NCLEX**). The NCLEX-RN is the licensing exam for Registered Nurses. The NCLEX-PN is for licensed practical/vocational nurses. After successful completion of the NCLEX and prior to receiving a license, the Boards of Nursing of each state may require licensing fees, fingerprints, and documentation from nursing programs.

Licensing laws vary from state to state. For instance, in some states it is illegal for any nurse to practice nursing for pay without a license. This regulation is called **mandatory licensure.** Most states now have laws mandating licensure of both LPNs and RNs. The mandatory law usually protects the functions of the nurse, as well as the use of the title. In other words, if a state has a mandatory licensure law, a nurse cannot perform the functions designated as exclusive to nursing without proper licensure in that state. Chapter 4 discusses further aspects of licensure and the legal issues surrounding it.

In some states only RNs are affected. In other states, the law does not forbid practicing nursing without a license, but does forbid using the title Registered Nurse or Licensed Practical Nurse if the nurse does not have a license. This practice is called **permissive licensure.**

☛ KEY CONCEPT

Licensure establishes a minimum level of competence for nursing. It ensures that a licensed nurse meets a basic level of excellence in practice and knowledge.

THE NURSE'S PLEDGE

All nurses are expected to practice ethically, conducting themselves appropriately as members of a specific group. As a nurse, you also accept responsibilities within the role delineated by licensure. Chapter 4 is devoted to a discussion of the legal and ethical aspects of nursing.

Many ethical principles are reflected in the Nurse's Pledge, which many students recite at graduation. Even if the pledge is not part of your graduation ceremony, it should serve as a guide for nursing practice. RNs recite the Florence Nightingale Pledge, and LPNs recite the Practical Nurse's Pledge (Box 2-3). The basic philosophy of nursing care espoused in both pledges is the same. Notice the similarity between them.

THEORIES OF NURSING

As a science, nursing is based on the theory of what it is, what nurses do, and why. Nursing is a unique discipline and is separate from medicine. It has its own body of knowledge on which delivery of care is based.

Nursing programs usually base their curricula on one or more nursing theories. Such theories provide a skeleton on which to hang knowledge. This theoretical framework gives you and other students a basis for forming a personal

➤➤ BOX 2-3

NURSING PLEDGES

Florence Nightingale Pledge

I solemnly pledge myself before God and in the presence of this assembly: To pass my life in purity and to practice my profession faithfully.

I will abstain from whatever is deleterious and mischievous, and will not take or knowingly administer any harmful drug.

I will do all in my power to maintain and elevate the standards of my profession, and will hold in confidence all personal matters committed to my keeping, and all family affairs coming to my knowledge in the practice of my profession.

With loyalty will I endeavor to aid the physician in his work, and devote myself to the welfare of those committed to my care.

The Practical Nurse's Pledge

Before God and those assembled here, I solemnly pledge:

To adhere to the code of ethics of the nursing profession.

To cooperate faithfully with the other members of the nursing team and to carry out faithfully and to the best of my ability the instructions of the physician or the nurse who may be assigned to supervise my work.

I will not do anything evil or malicious and I will not knowingly give any harmful drug or assist in malpractice.

I will not reveal any confidential information that may come to my knowledge in the course of my work.

And I pledge myself to do all in my power to raise the standards and the prestige of practical nursing.

May my life be devoted to service, and to the high ideals of the nursing profession.

philosophy of nursing. It also helps you to systematically develop problem-solving skills. A **theoretical framework** provides a reason and a purpose for nursing actions. Other factors also involved in nursing actions include ethics, safety, confidentiality, and culture. The theoretical framework on which this book is based is that of meeting basic human needs.

Throughout this book, you will learn ways to perform nursing procedures. You will also be presented with *rationales,* or reasons for these actions. These rationales are based on nursing's knowledge base. After you graduate and become more experienced, you will realize that more than one correct way exists to perform particular procedures. You must always follow the nursing protocols of the healthcare facility in which you are employed.

Nursing theories are often expressed in relationship to factors such as mind, body, spirit, and emotions. Most theories also include a definition of health. Be sure to consider all these factors when delivering nursing care so that you provide holistic care—care of the whole person. Among the many nursing theories are those of Florence Nightingale, Virginia Henderson, Dorothea Orem, Sister Callista Roy, and Betty Neuman. Table 2-3 outlines the general concepts related to these theories.

ROLES AND RESPONSIBILITIES OF THE NURSE

Today's nurse functions in a number of roles. As a nurse, you have a responsibility to maintain your own health. You also will need to project a professional image to your clients, their families, and the general public. Doing so will help others have confidence in your nursing abilities.

Contemporary Nursing Roles

Nurses are respected as a healthcare resource in the community. Examine the following roles of the nurse (Fig. 2-2). As you progress through your nursing program, you may be able to think of other roles that nurses assume in their practice. For example:

The nurse is a care provider. Nurses help each person achieve the maximum level of wellness possible. In some cases, clients will achieve total wellness; in others, compromises must be made.

The nurse is an advocate. Nurses serve this important role by ensuring that clients receive necessary care, and by intervening when necessary. Nurses help clients understand their rights and responsibilities. They explain details about procedures, so clients are able to give informed consent.

The nurse is a communicator. The nurse documents client care and the client's response. Professional nurses write care plans with input from other healthcare staff members—much of the staff uses this important plan. Nurses record information in daily flow sheets, or nursing notes. They record medications and treatments. They communicate with other healthcare team members in daily reports and team meetings, to maintain continuity of care.

TABLE 2-3 Theories of Nursing

Theorist	Model	Concepts
Florence Nightingale (1859)	Natural-Healing	Nature alone cures. Nursing assists the person to an improved condition for nature to take its course. Health is "freedom from disease."
Virginia Henderson (1955)	Independent-Functioning	Mind and body are one. Nursing's role is to assist clients to perform functions they would perform unaided if they had the necessary strength, will, or knowledge. Functions vital to health are the ability to breathe normally, eat/drink adequately, eliminate wastes, move/position oneself, sleep, dress, maintain body temperature, maintain hygiene, and keep the skin intact. Safety, communication, worship, work, recreation, and learning are individualized. Health is the ability to function independently.
Dorothea Orem (1958)	Self-Care	Building on Maslow's "Hierarchy of Human Needs" (see Chap. 5), nursing assists clients to meet self-care needs necessary to maintain life, health, and well-being. Health is the ability to meet self-care needs, which are physiologic, psychological, and sociologic.
Sister Callista Roy (1964)	Adaptation	An individual's state of health/illness moves back and forth on a continuum (see Chap. 6). Nursing focuses on the body, mind, spirit, and emotion and focuses on holistic healing, rather than curing. Each person's health status fluctuates, because humans are constantly interacting in a dynamic (changing) environment.
Betty Neuman (1972)	Systems	Humans deal with forces in both internal and external environments. The goal of the whole person is stability and harmony. Health is "relative" in terms of psychological, sociocultural, developmental, and physiologic factors.

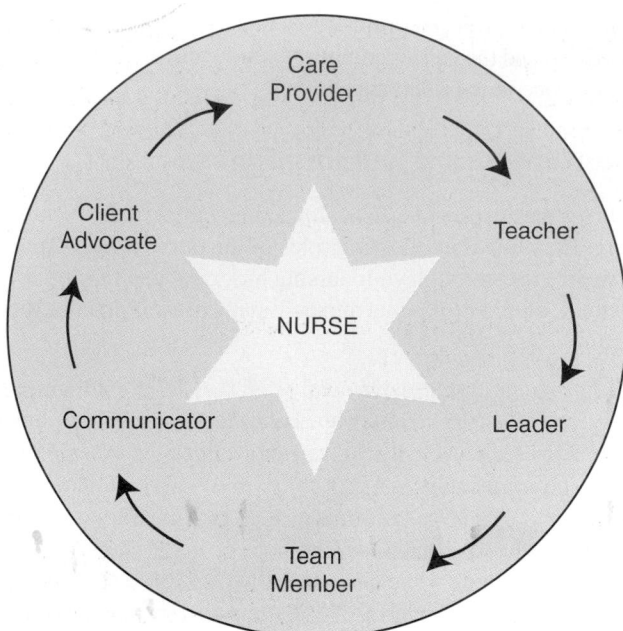

FIGURE 2-2. The roles of the nurse include, but are not limited to, care provider, communicator, teacher, advocate, leader, and team member.

The nurse is a team member. Nurses work cooperatively with other healthcare professionals to provide the best care possible.

The nurse is a teacher. Professional nurses write teaching plans and assist people in preventing illness and injury before they occur. Other members of the healthcare team assist with teaching as well. Together, the healthcare team teaches clients and families about illness, surgical procedures, performed tests, and home care. Clients learn about medications, when and how to take them, expected side effects, and possible adverse reactions. During childbirth, many nurses teach prenatal classes and assist with labor and delivery, providing encouragement and support. Later, they often teach new mothers important self-care as well as care measures for the new baby.

The nurse is a leader. Nurses must work with clients to motivate them to achieve important goals. Leadership is power, and nurses can use their skills to direct that power for improvement, not only in their clients' health, but in the facilities in which they work, the community, and for the entire healthcare system.

☛ KEY CONCEPT

Always practice nursing ethically. When you recite your pledge at graduation, you are promising to abide by this code.

The Nurse's Image

Today's society is filled with information about leading a healthier lifestyle. Many people are working to change their behaviors to restore or maintain good health.

As a nursing student and as a nurse, you need to project a professional image. Remember that you represent not only yourself to the public, but also your school, the healthcare facility for which you work, and the entire healthcare system.

Your nursing program will give you specific guidelines to follow regarding style of dress and grooming when you conduct clinical nursing practice. Box 2-4 identifies some general considerations to help you project the image of the nurse. Remember that many of the measures listed in Box 2-4 are important not only to project a professional image, but also to maintain maximum levels of safety, hygiene, and protection for you and your clients.

Today's Nursing Student

Many of today's nursing students are returning to school after several years outside education. You may be one of these adult learners, who has entered a nursing program with the additional responsibilities of a home, family, and outside job. Adult learners may need to master new skills in addition to learning their nursing skills. For example, some adult learners have not

➤➤ BOX 2-4

PROJECTING THE IMAGE OF A NURSE

- Follow general practices of good grooming and hygiene: bathe/shower daily, use deodorant, brush teeth, avoid bad breath (especially if you smoke).
- Keep hair clean, pulled away from the face, and off the neck.
- Wear a minimum of jewelry—it can harbor microorganisms and could injure a client.
- Clients may act out—protect yourself by keeping your hair short or pinned up, and avoiding large earrings, neckties, and necklaces.
- Keep moustaches and beards neatly trimmed.
- Avoid aftershave, cologne, and perfume. Clients may be allergic to them.
- Use a minimum of makeup. Nail polish is not recommended.
- Wash hands often. Make sure fingernails are short and clean. Clip hangnails.
- Cover cuts or open wounds for your protection.
- Wear washable clothes/uniforms and sweaters.
- Wear pants long enough to reach your shoe tops.
- Keep skirts long and loose enough so you can bend and lift without embarrassment.
- Wear safe and comfortable shoes. Most facilities do not allow sandals or clogs.
- Always wear your name tag—it is part of your uniform.
- Follow guidelines in Chapter 6 for maintaining optimum health.
- Follow any additional guidelines specified by your school or clinical facility.

worked much with computers, e-mail, or the Internet. All students, and especially those with multiple responsibilities, must plan a schedule that provides ample time for classes, household duties, studying, work, family, and personal time. Managing all of these responsibilities will be a challenge, but the rewards can be great.

NURSING ORGANIZATIONS

Nursing organizations provide educational programs and professional publications. They often participate in collective bargaining for nurses. Nursing organizations allow members to keep up to date with trends in nursing and to discuss them with their peers. Professional organizations also monitor healthcare laws and regulations and establish standards of care. Nurses should recognize the importance of belonging to the appropriate organization.

Organizations participate in establishing national policies. For example, controversy exists over the educational qualifications for different levels of nursing. Only by being a member of your appropriate nursing organization can you keep informed of changes and trends.

National Organizations

National Association for Practical Nurse Education and Service

The National Association for Practical Nurse Education and Service (**NAPNES**) was the first national nursing organization to concentrate all its efforts on the development and improvement of practical nursing education, together with advancing the interests of PNs themselves. It was organized in 1941 as the Association of Practical Nurse Schools, with 20 members.

NAPNES has three types of membership:

Individual: Open to RNs who are instructors and directors of practical nursing schools; LPNs; representatives of hospital, health, and education groups; and citizens interested in helping practical nursing grow and improve

Per capita: Open to members of state practical nursing associations voting a per capita assessment of dues

Future/student: Open to students in approved practical nursing schools on a divided payment basis while they are in the school; full membership is continued for a year after graduation at no extra cost

NAPNES has the following purposes:

* To further the cause and image of practical nursing
* To improve practical nursing education
* To provide continuing education for PNs

The NAPNES national office answers inquiries about practical nursing. NAPNES sends consultants to state or other groups to establish practical nursing programs. It publishes helpful booklets and other materials, including a newsletter, *NAPNES Forum,* and the *Journal of Practical Nursing.* NAPNES also publishes the *Declaration of Functions of the*

Licensed Practical/Vocational Nurse, which is updated regularly. NAPNES has helped PNs to organize their own state associations, and every year it holds a convention with special sessions for both practicing PNs and students. NAPNES provides scholarships for students, as well as low-cost insurance programs for students and graduates. NAPNES also offers certification programs for LPNs in pharmacology and long-term care.

National Federation of Licensed Practical Nurses, Inc.

Organized in 1949 in New York State, the National Federation of Licensed Practical Nurses (**NFLPN**) is the professional organization providing leadership for nearly one million LPNs and LVNs and students in the United States and Canada. It bases membership on a three-tier concept of local, state, and national enrollment, which consists of LPNs, LVNs, and PN/VN students. Affiliate membership has also been established to allow membership for those who have an interest in the work of the NFLPN, but who are neither LPNs/LVNs nor nursing students. Affiliate members receive all communications and may attend all meetings; however, they cannot vote or hold office. NFLPN has members in every state in the United States and in many Canadian provinces.

NFLPN has the following purposes:

* To foster high standards of nursing education and practice so that the best nursing care will be available
* To encourage continuing education as a priority for the purpose of personal growth and improved client care
* To achieve recognition for LPNs and LVNs and to advocate their effective utilization in every type of healthcare facility
* To interpret the role and function of the LPN and LVN for the public to win greater understanding and appreciation of the contribution of practical/vocational nursing to the healthcare system
* To represent practical/vocational nursing through relationships with other groups that share the common goal of improved care
* To serve as the central source of information regarding what is new and changing in nursing education and practice (2001).

NFLPN holds an annual convention to discuss matters involving practical nursing. At this convention, the organization sets its policies and makes recommendations to constituent state organizations. The national office serves as a resource to members. The organization strongly urges members to attend continuing education programs at the national convention and in local communities.

NFLPN publishes a bimonthly newsletter, *NFLPN Update,* which reports on national NFLPN activities and news from constituent states. It also offers: reviews of books and new products, articles of professional and personal interest, industry trends, career information, legislative notes, coming events, and continuing education opportunities. NFLPN is also involved in legislation through relationships with regulatory agencies. In this way policymakers can better identify the role of practical/vocational nursing in healthcare. NFLPN also sponsors legislative conferences for its members. Rather than having its own accreditation process, NFLPN supports the accreditation services of the National League for Nursing.

American Association of Licensed Practical Nurses

This organization is smaller than NAPNES and NFLPN with affiliates in about 16 states. The American Association of Licensed Practical Nurses (**AALPN**) is concerned primarily with education and legislation. In some states, AALPN participates in the collective bargaining process. The organization recently worked with the Joint Commission on Accreditation of Healthcare Organizations to help develop their policy statement, which specifically identifies the LPN/LVN as part of the healthcare team. The statement also says that the LPN/LVN can supervise the work of others in certain situations.

National League for Nursing and Community Health Accreditation Program

Founded in 1952, the National League for Nursing and Community Health Accreditation Program (**NLN-CHAP**) is an organization whose members are interested in furthering nursing and nursing education. NLN-CHAP is open to individuals, such as RNs and LPNs, and to institutions, such as nursing programs and hospitals.

NLN-CHAP has various departments, among them the Council of Practical Nursing Programs (CPNP), which was originally established in 1961. Through its Department of Evaluation, NLN-CHAP has developed a number of tests widely used by nursing schools. Among the tests that practical nursing schools use are an entrance test called the Pre-Admission and Classification Examination (**PACE**) and several achievement tests. PACE, which consists of aptitude and achievement sections, is used as a qualification for entrance to some nursing programs. The achievement tests are given to determine how well a student is doing after admission to the program. These tests focus on pharmacology, maternal-child nursing, medical-surgical nursing, and psychiatric principles. Other tests are available for programs that prepare students for RN licensure. Most of the NLN tests follow the format of NCLEX licensing examinations. Taking these tests helps prepare nurses for the NCLEX-RN or NCLEX-PN.

One of the most important functions of NLN-CHAP is the voluntary accreditation of nursing programs, at both the RN and LPN levels. Accreditation signifies that a program meets or exceeds the minimum approval requirements of the state in which it is located. NLN-CHAP has many useful publications, among them its monthly publication, *Nursing and HealthCare*. NLN-CHAP is also the accrediting body for community-based healthcare organizations.

Health Occupations Students of America

Organized in 1976, Health Occupations Students of America (**HOSA**) is a vocational organization specifically designed for students in secondary and postsecondary health occupations, including nursing. By 1997, HOSA membership had grown to over 70,000. HOSA sponsors local, state, and national conventions and contests to assist students in improving their knowledge and skills and to provide opportunities to meet students from other schools and healthcare disciplines.

American Nurses Association

The American Nurses Association (**ANA**) is an organization whose membership is composed of RNs. ANA often sponsors workshops for nurses. It publishes several periodicals and a great deal of literature. ANA's most widely circulated journal is the *American Journal of Nursing* (**AJN**). ANA considers itself the official voice for professional nursing in the United States. It assists with collective bargaining in many states.

State Affiliates of National Organizations

The national nursing associations usually have state affiliates, and sometimes, local chapters. This gives all nurses the opportunity to attend meetings and become active in the nursing organization of their choice. Most national organizations also have student affiliates, so you can begin your professional membership as a student.

State organizations often publish newsletters of local interest. Sometimes scholarships, continuing education, and other services are available to members.

☛ KEY CONCEPT

All nursing students and graduates should belong to an organization, so they will have a voice in the future of the profession.

International Nursing Organizations

Nursing organizations are also found at the international level. Perhaps the best known is the International Council of Nurses (**ICN**), with headquarters in Switzerland. ANA also has an International Nursing Center (INC). International organizations work to expand nursing services, to improve the quality and availability of care in developing countries, to improve the overall quality of nursing education throughout the world, and to encourage young adults to pursue the career of nursing worldwide. Many nurses from other countries come to the United States and Canada for advanced education, some under the auspices of the ICN, or the INC of the ANA.

➤ STUDENT SYNTHESIS

Key Points

- Differences exist in the education and level of nursing practice between RNs and PNs.
- Several types of nursing education lead to licensure as a registered nurse or as a practical/vocational nurse.
- Only graduates of state-, commonwealth-, territory-, or province-approved schools of nursing are eligible to take the licensure examination.

- Most states have mandatory licensure laws for nurses. Nurse licensure is available in all states, territories, and Canadian provinces.
- Nurses promise to practice ethically when they recite pledges at graduation.
- Many nursing programs base their curricula on nursing theories. These theoretical frameworks provide reasons and purposes for nursing actions.
- The nurse assumes many roles. Many responsibilities accompany the title of "nurse."
- Projecting a professional image is important. Such an image helps nurses to properly represent their school, place of employment, and the healthcare industry. Moreover, it serves to protect and to maintain safety for clients and nurses themselves.
- Nursing organizations set standards of practice for RNs and LPNs. A primary nursing responsibility is to be familiar with these standards.
- Nursing organizations assist in continuing education and collective bargaining. Additionally, they offer a forum for discussion of nursing issues with peers.

Critical Thinking Exercises

1. Discuss the difference in the roles, practices, and functions of the physician, the LPN and the RN. If you started your nursing career as a nurse's aide, describe your experiences working with nurses.
2. Interview class members and have them relate an experience in healthcare. What events are significant in the individual's past medical history and how did the members of the healthcare team affect the individual's perspective of the experience?
3. A nursing student in your group tells you that she cheated on an examination yesterday. What would you do and why? How does your response relate to nursing practice?

4. Ask your instructor for a copy of your program's "Philosophy and Objectives." Compare and contrast them with your own personal standards and philosophy of nursing. Do you find similarities? Differences?

NCLEX-Style Review Questions

1. Which of the following is a function of the LPN/LVN?
   a. Is in charge in various healthcare settings
   b. Directs nurses and other people who work in hospitals
   c. Provides direct patient care
   d. Teaches professional and practical nursing students
2. Practice standards for the LPN/LVN include which of the following?
   a. Is not responsible for direct patient care; the RN is responsible
   b. Functions with other healthcare team members in promoting health
   c. Functions at the level of independent practitioner
   d. Independently formulates nursing diagnoses
3. Which national organization strives to achieve recognition and adequate utilization for LPN's/LVN's?
   a. ANA
   b. HOSA
   c. NAPNES
   d. NFLPN

References

1. National Association for Practical Nurse Education and Service. (2000). *Licensed practical nursing: The work of the caregiver.* Silver Spring, MD: Author.
2. National Federation of Licensed Practical Nurses, Inc. (revised 2001). *Nursing practice standards for the licensed practical/vocational nurse* (rev.). Garner, NC: Author.

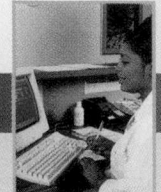

CHAPTER

3

The Healthcare Delivery System

LEARNING OBJECTIVES

1. Discuss at least three trends and challenges of healthcare in the 21st century. Relate these changes to the needs of nurses, healthcare practitioners, and the consumers of healthcare (clients).
2. Define and discuss at least three differences between acute care and extended care facilities.
3. Identify at least two types of healthcare services provided in each type of healthcare facility.
4. Identify at least three services available to meet the healthcare needs of the community.
5. State at least two functions of a school nurse and an industrial nurse.
6. State at least two functions of JCAHO. Relate these functions to nursing standards of care.
7. Define the term quality assurance and state its function in healthcare facilities.
8. Explain the role of the client representative, advocate, or ombudsperson.
9. Describe at least six methods of payment for healthcare services.
10. Determine the role of complementary or holistic care in the delivery of healthcare.
11. Identify at least three negative impacts of consumer fraud on public wellness.

NEW TERMINOLOGY

acuity	incentive programs
capitation fee	managed care
case management	Medicaid
chain-of-command	Medicare
client	outcome-based care
complementary healthcare	patient
co-pay	prospective payment
holistic healthcare	quality assurance
home healthcare	telehealth
hospice	third-party payment

ACRONYMS

CQI	ICU	PPO
DRG	JCAHO	RUG
ECF	NLN	SNF
HMO	OSHA	SSDI
ICF	POS	UAP

This textbook primarily addresses nursing in the context of a healthcare facility that cares for the very ill, or a facility that has services that provide long-term or extended care. Throughout the book you will note references to specific nursing situations such as geriatrics, pediatrics, or home health.

Your school of nursing may provide clinical experiences in acute care and long-term care, as well as supplemental clinical experiences in ambulatory care settings such as clinics or home care. Field trips to specialty areas may be available, eg, dialysis units, burn units, or rehabilitation centers.

This chapter discusses concepts related to basic healthcare service in the United States. The student and the consumer need to be aware of different types of healthcare facilities and payment plans, as well as the common types of healthcare services.

Your student nursing experiences are individual and unique. It is the responsibility of the student to achieve the maximum benefits from each experience.

☞ KEY CONCEPT

Remember: The principles of excellent nursing care are universal.

HEALTHCARE TRENDS IN THE 21ST CENTURY

Healthcare continues to change dramatically. The **National League for Nursing (NLN)** has identified ten trends to watch in this century (Box 3-1). Changes include an emphasis on wellness and individuals assuming more responsibility for their own health. Technology will continue to influence healthcare in direct and indirect ways. The cost of healthcare technology also remains a major consideration. The use of technology in healthcare will provide new avenues of diagnosis, treatment, and nursing care. Chapters 6 and 7 provide additional information in the areas of wellness and community health.

Prior to the 1980s, healthcare was primarily the concern of physicians who treated patients during times of illness. Preventive care, such as cardiac screening or cardiac rehabilitation, was not considered until after a problem developed. Enormous amounts of money are needed to care for patients with existing health problems. Additionally, the quality of life for individuals who are ill has lifestyle and financial consequences.

Research into the rising costs of healthcare revealed that many patient and financial needs could be met by preventive care. Patients needed better health education with ongoing screening and monitoring of illness. Additionally, the focus of many aspects of health and healthcare could and should be the responsibility of the patient.

Preventive care can literally prevent health problems before they develop. The benefits of remaining healthy were also extremely cost effective. The trend evolved to prevent illness and accidents, as often as possible, before they occur.

Starting in the 1980s, the concept of **managed care** or **case management** was implemented to halt rapidly rising medical costs and to increase efficiency in care delivery. **Man-**

> ▶ ▶ BOX 3-1

NLN TEN TRENDS TO WATCH

Transformations taking place in nursing and nursing education have been driven by major socioeconomic factors, as well as by developments in healthcare delivery and professional issues unique to nursing. Here are 10 trends to watch, described in terms of their impact on nursing education.

1. Changing Demographics and Increasing Diversity
2. The Technological Explosion
3. Globalization of the World's Economy and Society
4. The Era of the Educated Consumer, Alternative Therapies and Genomics, and Palliative Care
5. Shift to Population-Based Care and the Increasing Complexity of Patient Care
6. The Cost of healthcare and the Challenge of Managed Care
7. Impact of Health Policy and Regulation
8. The Growing Need for Interdisciplinary Education for Collaborative Practice
9. The Current Nursing Shortage/Opportunities for Lifelong Learning and Workforce Development
10. Significant Advances in Nursing Science and Research

Source: Heller, B. R., Oros, M. T., & Durney-Crowley, J. The future of nursing education: ten trends to watch (3/17/01). http://www.nln.org/nlnjournal/infotrends.htm

aged care is a plan for continual monitoring and maintenance of an individual's health. It promotes wellness-focused care and preventive medicine. Although the **patient,** who now is being called a **client,** remains an individual, the managed care organization can standardize goals for clients with similar disorders. The client can be treated on an individual case-by-case basis, but a group of individuals with the same disorder can have similar goals or plans.

☞ KEY CONCEPT

Because healthcare recipients are involved in the management of their own health, they are often referred to as clients, rather than as patients. Client implies active participation in the choice of the (healthcare) service. The client makes decisions regarding health.

The term patient implies a relatively passive acceptance of health services and providers, or cases in which the individual is unable to make decisions about his or her own care.

In this text, the term client is used.

Managed care plans are called many names including *critical pathways, care maps, clinical pathways,* or *standard nursing care plans.* These plans identify desired outcomes and timelines. Healthcare professionals must follow such plans to receive full reimbursement for services from third-party payers.

Health maintenance organizations (HMOs) are examples of managed care systems. HMOs emphasize disease prevention and health promotion. Their goal is to avoid health problems by preventing conditions that could become more serious (and more costly). Clients are often treated on an outpatient basis, and hospitalizations are minimized. HMOs will be discussed in more detail later in this chapter.

Trends that differentiate HMOs from "traditional" healthcare have evolved. In the 21st century, healthcare may involve discussion among the healthcare practitioner (eg, physician), an insurance provider who agrees to pay for the treatment or therapy, and the client.

The role of the nurse is being redefined to meet the challenges of managed care and reimbursement regulations. In some cases, **unlicensed assistive personnel (UAPs)** are being hired to administer nursing care. This practice is becoming more common across the country and is often a subject of controversy. The standards of education for UAPs are generally much less stringent than the educational requirements for a licensed nurse.

As a result of financial constraints and the influence of managed care plans, clients may have treatment outside a hospital, such as in a wound-care treatment center or a rehabilitation center. Clients can be admitted to the hospital, have a surgical procedure performed, and be discharged in the same day.

To be admitted to an acute care facility, the client must meet a minimum level or need for healthcare services known as **acuity.** Clients admitted to acute care facilities have high levels of acuity. Thus the person receiving care in the hospital is often more critically ill than in the past. Hospitalizations are of shorter duration and—as a result—the client is often discharged while he or she still needs healthcare services.

As a result of specific changes in the delivery of healthcare services, extended care facilities (ECFs) and **home healthcare** services have restructured to meet the intermediate acuity needs of clients. In the recent past, ECFs were exclusively the "nursing home" or long-term care facility for the aging adult. Twenty-first century clients may be transitioned or transferred from one level of care (acuity) to another level of care. For example, a client may be discharged from an acute care hospital to be admitted into an extended care facility. At the ECF, the client may receive physical therapy and rehabilitation prior to being discharged to home. A client may be monitored at home by a home-health nurse. Employment for nurses in all of these areas is projected to increase in the future.

The myriad of changes in healthcare will continue to alter the role of nurses in the 21st century, whether they practice in acute/subacute, extended, community-based, or home care settings (which are discussed later in this chapter). Challenges of the 21st century include disparities in access to healthcare, inequities in access to healthcare insurance, and continued high-risk behaviors such as smoking. Chapter 6 discusses health indicators in more detail.

As the healthcare system and methods of payment develop and change in this century, so will nurses' responsibilities and the facilities in which they work. Nurses must continue to be involved in planning for future healthcare service. Teamwork will remain important, but the methods of collaboration will change. For example, the increasing use of UAPs as care partners and increasing responsibilities for licensed practical nurses will undoubtedly have profound effects on the delivery of healthcare.

Nursing plays a significant role in the attainment of client care outcomes. As a nurse, you will need to understand and to articulate the value of well-educated staff for the delivery of healthcare in the 21st century.

HEALTHCARE SETTINGS AND SERVICES

Acute Care Facilities

Acute Care Hospitals

Acute care hospitals are the most commonly known healthcare facility. Acute care implies that a client in the hospital has a serious condition that needs to be closely monitored by healthcare professionals, particularly nurses. Acute care facilities admit clients for short periods of time, usually only a matter of a few days. Clients are often very sick and need a great deal of nursing care. Box 3-2 summarizes services that are commonly found in acute care facilities.

Intensive Care Units

Intensive care units (ICUs) that care for the critically ill are found in acute care facilities. ICUs may specialize in medical, surgical, respiratory, coronary, burn, neonatal, and pediatric care areas. ICUs provide care for clients by specially trained

➤ ➤ BOX 3-2

SERVICES COMMONLY FOUND IN AN ACUTE CARE FACILITY

An Acute Care Facility May Have a Wide Variety of Services for the Healthcare Client

Administration
Admitting and Discharge
Ambulatory Care/Outpatient Surgery
Dietary
Emergency Care
Home Health
Intensive Care Unit
Laboratory
Medical Unit
Neonatal
Obstetrics/Gynecology
Pediatrics
Physical Therapy
Radiology
Respiratory Therapy
Surgical Unit
Telemetry Unit
Transitional Care/Step Down Units

nurses. Many ICUs use high-tech equipment and health status monitors.

Many hospitals have areas that are classified as *subacute care* or *step-down* units. A person may move to a subacute unit when the level of acuity of care has decreased. However, the client is not considered ready for discharge. A client may be transferred from an ICU to a step-down unit prior to being discharged from the hospital.

Most general hospitals provide "same-day" surgery, also known as *outpatient* or *ambulatory care centers.* In the past, nearly all surgical procedures required hospital admission. Economic issues forced the increase of surgeries performed on an outpatient basis. The client can return home the same day to recuperate. Outpatient treatment centers have become very popular because they save the client time and money. Day-surgery centers built by physician groups often compete with an acute care facility's outpatient department.

Specialized Hospitals

Specialized hospitals are facilities that admit only one type of client. Examples include government veteran hospitals, psychiatric, or pediatric hospitals. Specialized hospitals may also have units for medical, surgical, or intensive care. Other types of specialized hospitals include facilities for the developmentally or mentally disabled. Some facilities care for specific conditions such as head and spinal cord injuries or substance abuse.

Although its primary function is to provide healthcare, the hospital performs other functions. For example, your clinical facility has the added role of education, and many large hospitals, particularly those affiliated with a university, also play an important role in research.

With acute care facilities sending individuals home earlier to recover from surgery or illness, the need for home healthcare has increased. In some cases, nursing care is available 24 hours a day in the home. However, in most cases, the family and other lay caregivers need to take responsibility for some care. Nurses are vital in teaching individuals how to perform care in the home.

Home Healthcare

Home healthcare may be a service provided by an acute care facility, or it may be a service provided by an agency that specializes in healthcare (Fig 3-1).

☛ KEY CONCEPT

Many individuals prefer to be cared for at home. Home care is also less expensive than hospitalization. Individuals often have family or friends who can assist in their care. Home health nursing and hospice care have greatly enhanced the quality of healthcare available in the home.

Hospice

Hospice care specializes in the care of the terminally ill. This service also may be part of the services available from an acute care facility. Hospice care and home care share similar nursing objectives. However, they are two different specialty areas of

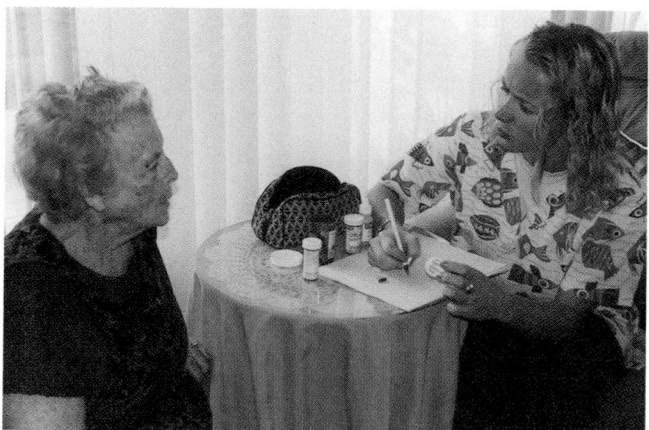

FIGURE 3-1. Taking time to teach clients about their medication and treatment program promotes interest and cooperation. Older adults who are actively involved in learning about their medication and treatment program and the expected effects may be more likely to adhere to the therapeutic regimen. (Smeltzer, S., Bare, B. [1999]. *Brunner and Suddarth's textbook of medical-surgical nursing* [9th ed. p. 42]. Philadelphia: Lippincott Williams & Wilkins.)

care provided to clients outside of hospitals. Chapter 99 discusses hospice care.

Healthcare services have recognized the need for respite care. Respite care provides part-time supervision of clients who have chronic conditions. Family or friends who are the primary caregivers for children and adults with serious, chronic medical conditions or mental illness need respite care. The client may be taken to a facility for part of the day. The client receives supervised care and has an opportunity for socialization outside the home. The caregiver has a chance to be relieved of the exhausting and constant responsibility and stress of caring for someone 24 hours a day.

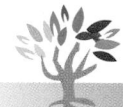

SPECIAL CONSIDERATIONS: THE LIFE SPAN

The frail or confused elderly may have difficulty managing at home without assistance. Nurses, discharge planners, and physicians work as a team to provide safe and adequate care to those individuals living at home. Home health agencies and social services can assist in discharge planning and make arrangements for home care or public health nursing visits.

Telehealth

Telehealth is a service that is relatively new and growing. The term telehealth refers to the ability to access a nurse or physician via telephone or computer audio/video link. Nurses can communicate and assist clients in numerous ways using distance communication modes. Frequent contact with clients helps to increase medication compliance and to recognize potential problems before they become acute problems. Thus unscheduled visits to the physician, the emergency room, and rehospitalization are decreased. Physicians use telehealth to contact other physicians or specialty facilities. Rural communities find the immediate contact with physician specialists a great asset in client care. This concept will be discussed in more detail later in this text.

Extended Care Facilities

Some facilities admit clients for longer periods of time than is common in acute care hospitals. These **extended care facilities (ECFs)** include nursing homes, inpatient rehabilitation centers, inpatient treatment centers for chemical dependency, and facilities for chronic mental healthcare. Some facilities are attached to a general hospital; others are free-standing. More emphasis is being placed on returning people to their homes or other community-based living facilities as quickly as possible. Thus, the population in long-term care facilities is changing.

The federal government divides nursing homes into two categories: a skilled nursing facility or an intermediate care facility. The **skilled nursing facility (SNF)** provides 24-hour nursing care under the supervision of a registered nurse (RN). The **intermediate care facility (ICF)** provides 24-hour service from nursing assistants under supervision of an LPN/LVN, with an RN as a consultant. Many rules and regulations apply to nursing homes. The employment opportunities for nurses continue to grow in this area.

Community Health Services

Community health services provide care for individuals and families within a specific area, such as a neighborhood, a small town, or a rural county. The costs of in-hospital medical care, along with governmental limits and regulations, have forced many people to be cared for in the community, rather than in a hospital.

One type of community health service is the public health service. Public Health Departments offer immunizations, well-baby checks, and treatment for specific diseases such as tuberculosis or sexually transmitted diseases (STDs).

Community health clinics offer low-cost healthcare services to the public. Prenatal and pediatric care, diabetic care, and general medical-surgical ambulatory care services may be offered by community health clinics. Chapter 7 discusses community health and community-based health services in more detail.

Independent living facilities may provide care for a small number of individuals in a house located in a community neighborhood. These facilities provide a stable, home-like environment for mentally challenged individuals, while still providing some degree of supervision.

Healthcare in School and Industry

Most school systems provide some healthcare services for students, particularly those with disabilities. A nurse may be on duty full-time, or divide time among several schools. In addi-

tion to assisting ill children or children in emergencies, the nurse provides preventive care by performing regular assessments, teaching, screening for common disorders, supervising the administration of immunizations and medications, and providing health counseling.

Children with special physical challenges receive more intensive nursing care, sometimes on a one-to-one basis. An increasing number of school systems operate or house school-based comprehensive clinics to provide total healthcare to students.

Industries in which machinery is operated usually employ a nurse for health promotion and interventions. Teaching is part of the nurse's responsibility, and prevention of accidents is a major goal. The industrial nurse often serves as liaison between the industry and the **Occupational Safety and Health Administration (OSHA).** OSHA is discussed in Chapter 7.

QUALITY ASSURANCE

Quality of care has become a major issue for both consumers and providers of healthcare. **Quality assurance** is defined as a pledge to the public that healthcare services will provide optimal achievable goals and maintain standard excellence in the services rendered.

Hospital Accreditation

Just as your nursing program can be accredited, a hospital or other healthcare facility also can be accredited. Accreditation implies that the facility has met rigid, minimum standards of service to the client and the community. The agency that assigns this recognition to hospitals is called the **Joint Commission for Accreditation of Healthcare Organizations (JCAHO).** Other facilities have similar accreditation processes.

JCAHO has established rigid standards for an ongoing quality assurance program in hospitals, as well as for community health centers, home care agencies, and various levels of extended care facilities. JCAHO requires objective and systematic monitoring and evaluation of the quality and appropriateness of client care. The quality assurance procedure requires healthcare facilities to identify what they mean by "quality" and to define their evaluation methods.

Components of Quality Care

Quality management requires that healthcare services be well-planned and delivered in a manner that ensures good care. Adequate staff and support services, such as nursing care, must be available.

Quality control and quality assurance focus on delivery of care. The process of care is important, as is the outcome. *Process* relates to how care is given. *Outcome* relates to the result, which is also known as **outcome-based care.**

Nurse accountability, which involves the delivery and accurate documentation of quality care, is vital. healthcare facilities and agencies have **contiguous (or continuous) quality improvement (CQI)** committees that monitor the quality of ongoing care.

Standards for Quality Assurance

Each healthcare facility establishes individual standards of quality to guide the nursing staff in providing care. In general, these standards include:

- *Standards of nursing practice:* Procedures used in the delivery of care, the hospital policy book, textbooks, and other references. Sometimes the term *nursing protocol* is used. Standards of nursing practice focus on the giver of care, the nurse, and on the nursing process (see Unit 6).
- *Standards of client/patient care:* Activities determined by client expectations or by personal standards of care. What did the client expect? How well did nursing care meet the client's expectations? Standards of client care focus on the recipient of care, the client. The client participates in developing the nursing care plan. (The "case manager" is responsible for making sure the client's care is planned and carried out appropriately.)
- *Standards of performance:* How well the nurse performs, as compared with a job description. How well you meet standards of performance as a nursing student will change as you progress through the program. As you become more experienced, you will be expected to provide more complex nursing care.

The *nursing audit* committee or CQI committee evaluates care given to clients. *Peer review* allows nurses to constructively critique each other.

Client Representatives or Advocates

Many hospitals have initiated the position of client (patient) representative, advocate, liaison, or ombudsperson. This person's role is to act as consumer advocate. As an advocate, the ombudsperson assists the client and family by resolving concerns or problems. The goal is to focus on client care, needs, and concerns, not the problems that may be encountered during the hospital admission.

Client representatives often help clients and their families find needed services. They listen and answer questions. Representatives can help families find housing, restaurants, parking, child care, or chaplain services. During hospitalization, clients have the right to contact their representatives if they have a problem or concern. Each individual is informed about and receives a copy of the Patient's Bill of Rights (see Chap. 4). In preparation for discharge, the advocate can make sure the family knows where to purchase needed supplies and medications. The nursing *case manager* has overall responsibility for the client's care. The *advocate* assists as needed.

ORGANIZATION AND OWNERSHIP OF HEALTHCARE FACILITIES

Hospital Organization

Hospitals are almost always governed by a board of directors or trustees, or in the case of a university hospital, by a board of regents. This board appoints the administrators of the hospital. The hospital administrator in turn develops an organizational structure. Box 3-3 lists some of the numerous administrative individuals who are necessary in a modern healthcare facility.

➤➤ BOX 3-3

ADMINISTRATIVE INDIVIDUALS IN A HEALTHCARE FACILITY

Each Healthcare Facility Requires Numerous Trained Individuals Working Together. The *Chain-of-Command* Binds the Hospital Team Members into Organized Units

Chief Executive Officer
Medical Staff and Services
Nursing Staff and Services
Financial Officer
Quality Assurance
Engineering and Maintenance
Environmental Services
Safety Officer
Medical Records
Purchasing
Dietician
Human Resources
Billing and Accounts
Infection Control
Education

It is important that the student and future employee learn the administrative structure of the each healthcare facility. All facilities follow a **chain-of-command** or organizational reporting system. It is critical that the nurse use the appropriate system for communication (ie, chain-of-command) with peers and supervisors. Figure 3-2 gives an overview of administrative organization in a typical healthcare facility.

☛ KEY CONCEPT

While you are in your nursing program, your chain-of-command begins with your instructor. Problems, concerns, or issues should first be directed to your immediate supervisor (instructor). Each program will have a designated chain-of-command for students to follow.

Teamwork is a critical component of healthcare. To provide care, members of the healthcare team collaborate in their assessments, planning, and delivery of care. Team members communicate with one another and with clients so that services are neither duplicated nor omitted. Their goal is to help clients maintain wellness. When they find problems, team members focus their energies on restoring clients to health. As a nurse or a nursing student, you are part of the team providing healthcare.

Hospital Ownership and Funding

In addition to types of clients served, healthcare facilities are classified in relation to ownership and funding structure. These lines are becoming blurred, as mergers occur between various types of hospitals.

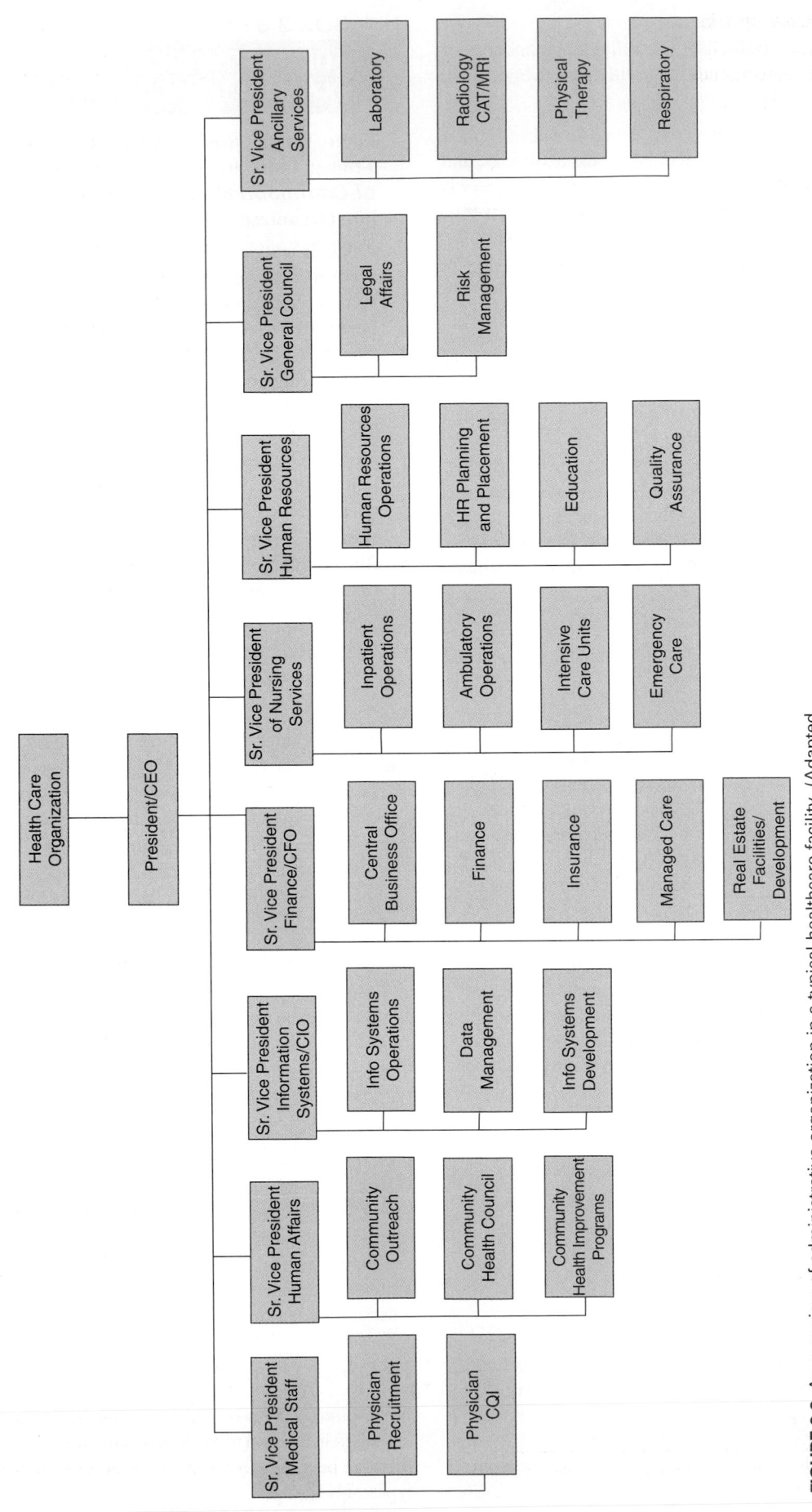

FIGURE 3-2. An overview of administrative organization in a typical healthcare facility. (Adapted from Baker, J., & Baker, R. [2000]. *healthcare finance* [p. 9]. Gaithersburg, MD: Aspen.)

Governmental Ownership

Governmental, public, or official hospitals are owned and operated by local, state, or federal units of government. These governmental agencies are also called *official* hospitals. They are nonprofit organizations. Table 3-1 provides some examples.

Private Ownership

Private or voluntary hospitals are owned and operated by individuals or by groups, such as churches, labor unions, and fraternal organizations. These hospitals may be established as for-profit or not-for-profit organizations.

For-Profit Versus Not-for-Profit

A further classification of hospitals relates to distribution of their profits:

- *Proprietary, investor-owned,* or *for-profit* hospitals are those in which profits are returned to shareholders. Very few such hospitals exist today. Many nursing homes, however, fall into this category.
- *Not-for-profit* hospitals constitute the majority of all hospitals. In the not-for-profit hospital, profits are returned to the funding agency, and are used for improvements to the facility, added equipment, and other related costs.

FINANCING HEALTHCARE

The costs of healthcare continue to be a concern. Various programs and legislation have evolved to address this issue. Societal, legal, and ethics issues influence the costs of healthcare (see Chap. 4).

The Health Planning and Resources Development Act of 1975 established legislation to govern the amount and types of facilities, services, and workers needed in each designated geographic area in the United States. It also aimed to prevent duplication of healthcare procedures and, ultimately, to reduce healthcare costs. The initial act of 1975 identified priorities, some of which have changed or expanded since then. These priorities continue to evolve.

Resources for the 21st century must include the following healthcare priorities:

- Primary care services for medically underserved populations, especially those in rural or economically depressed areas; establishment of satellite clinics in remote areas where transportation is difficult or impossible, such as the regional delivery system in Alaska
- Mobile services available in low-population areas, such as visits from mobile mammography, magnetic resonance imaging, or computed tomography scan units by truck/plane to these areas on a scheduled basis
- Multi-institutional systems for the coordination or consolidation of expensive or specialized health services (eg, obstetrics; pediatrics; emergency, intensive, and coronary care; radiation therapy)
- The development of institutions on a geographically integrated basis to prevent excessive duplication of services
- Multi-institutional arrangements for sharing support services (eg, purchasing and bookkeeping)
- Uniform cost accounting, simplified reimbursement, and utilization reporting systems
- Improved financial management procedures
- Cooperation and/or mergers of hospitals and other healthcare facilities, sometimes between private and public institutions
- Case management to oversee the administration and cost of healthcare services to individual clients
- Improvements in the quality and ongoing quality assessment of healthcare
- Promotion of the nursing profession as a career
- Use of advanced practice nurses as independent providers, in collaboration with physicians
- Training and increased use of assistants to physicians
- Use of complementary care methods, such as acupuncture and herbal medicine
- Additional and early services for pregnant women and at-risk children
- Group medical practices, HMOs, and other organized systems of healthcare delivery
- Special healthcare screenings, immunizations, walk-in clinics, feeding programs, and other services—for the homeless, recent immigrants from developing countries, and other high-risk populations
- Improved identification, screening, treatment, and management of the chronically chemically dependent population
- Disease prevention, including studies of nutritional and environmental factors and provision of preventive healthcare services
- Community-based care and services, rather than institutionalization, for populations such as the chronically and persistently mentally ill and the profoundly mentally retarded

■■■ TABLE 3-1 *T*YPES OF OWNERSHIP OF HEALTHCARE FACILITIES

Profit Oriented—Proprietary
  Individual
  Partnership
  Corporation

Nonprofit—Voluntary
  Church Associated (eg, Loma Linda University Medical Center)
  Private-School Associated
  Foundation Associated (eg, Shriner's Hospitals)

Nonprofit—Government
  Federal (eg, Veterans Administration)
  State (eg, university hospital)
  County (eg, city or county hospital)
  City (eg, city or county hospital)
  City-County (eg, city or county hospital)

Adapted from Baker, J., & Baker, R. (2000). *healthcare finance* (p. 7). Gaithersburg, MD: Aspen.

- Mainstreaming in school of children with physical, emotional, and mental challenges; provision of healthcare to these children as needed
- Consideration of cultural differences in the planning and delivery of healthcare
- Effective methods of educating the public concerning proper healthcare and the effective use of available services
- Additional research and development of medications and treatments for devastating diseases, such as AIDS

Methods of Payment

After World War II, most healthcare in the United States was provided by a fee-for-service system: a client went to a physician and paid for each service performed. To help families with limited funds to pay for the care of seriously ill persons, a **third-party payment** system developed. The third party is generally some sort of health insurance plan.

Various health insurance plans or third-party payment systems exist. The "traditional plans" and the "managed care plans" of third-party payment are summarized below. Table 3-2 compares general features of traditional and managed care services.

Private Insurance

An individual or a family purchases private health insurance. Its cost is high, and the insurance company often refuses to insure anyone who is considered a health risk. Therefore, many people cannot afford or are unable to obtain private insurance.

Group Insurance

Group insurance offers coverage for people who belong to a certain group. For example, many companies, institutions, and fraternal organizations offer members group insurance benefits. In this situation, the premium is fairly low, and usually people are insured without a physical examination. Group plans may exclude coverage for preexisting conditions and may require a waiting period before clients can receive services.

In either private or group insurance, coverage is available for medical bills, hospitalization, and other related services, such as surgery or laboratory tests. The insurance may cover care in a private clinic or an HMO. People may purchase coverage only for themselves, or they may purchase family coverage for members of the immediate family.

Many plans also offer insurance that pays a set amount if a person becomes unable to work due to illness or injury, known as long-term disability insurance.

Health Maintenance Organizations

Health Maintenance Organizations (HMOs) offer health services for a fixed monthly charge called a *premium.* Members prepay for healthcare services generally through payroll deductions, governmental agencies (eg, Medicare, Medicaid), or individual monthly fees. The fee or premium paid in advance to the HMO is called the **capitation fee** (also referred to as *capitated payment*). Members must use a physician within the HMO network. The physician uses medical services and specialty referrals that are provided by the HMO. Some HMOs have contracted healthcare facilities for their members.

Each plan will also have some type of additional financial obligation or predetermined **co-pay**, that is charged to the client at the time of each visit. Typical services provided to the client by the HMO are listed in Box 3-4.

Some HMOs provide dental and optical services, as well as medical and surgical services. The provider is responsible for

TABLE 3-2 Comparison of Three Types of Healthcare Plans

	Traditional Insurance	HMO Managed Care	PPO Managed Care
Choice of primary healthcare providers (eg, physicians, hospitals)	Personal selection of any healthcare provider (eg, physician, nurse practitioner, hospital)	Selection of healthcare provider within HMO network Use of healthcare provider outside of network is at member's own expense	Selection of healthcare provider within PPO network Use of healthcare provider outside of network is partially paid but at a higher expense
Choice of specialists	Personal selection of specialist Some insurance policies may require preapproval for physician or procedure	HMO primary physician approves specialist Use of specialist or procedures outside of network is at member's own expense	Selection of specialist within PPO network Use of specialist or procedure outside of network may be partially paid but at a higher expense
Additional costs (out-of-pocket costs)	Annual deductible of $100–$500 Possible co-pay responsibility of 20% of costs; limit on co-pay costs may apply Routine visits may not be covered	Co-pay for each visit and for prescription drugs Co-pay ranges widely ($5–$25) Generally no deductibles to pay Sometimes co-pay for hospital and emergency room visits (may be higher than office visit co-pay)	Co-pay for each visit and for prescription drugs Co-pay ranges widely ($5–$25) For use of provider outside of PPO network, member pays a deductible and then the plan may pay a percentage of the costs

Adapted from Children's Medical Center of Dallas. *Understanding the basics.*
Website: http://www.childrens.com/basics.htm

➤➤ BOX 3-4

TYPICAL SERVICES OF A MANAGED CARE SYSTEM

Services provided vary from plan to plan, and not all services may be available. Some services may be available at additional costs.

Dental exams and routine care
Diabetic care
Family planning and birth control
Health education, eg, anti-smoking, substance abuse
Home healthcare
Hospice care
Immunizations
Inpatient medical and surgical care
Laboratory and x-ray services
Long-term care
Prenatal, labor and delivery, and childbirth care
Prescription drugs
Routine checkup
Speech, hearing, and vision exams
Urgent care
Well-child care

managing the client in the most appropriate and cost-effective manner, to achieve desired outcomes.

Just like any individual, HMO members can elect to go to any physician or seek any medical service that is not part of the HMO network. However, the HMO will generally not pay for this service unless it is preapproved by the administrators of the plan. Emergency room visits may be approved at the time of the client's need.

Features and services of most HMOs include:

- *Group practice:* Several physicians and specialists practice together.
- *Prepayment:* A person or company pays a certain amount in advance (capitation fee) and then is entitled to whatever care is needed. Sometimes, the client pays a small added cost (**co-pay**) as well.
- *Prevention:* The emphasis is on preventing disease, rather than treating it after it develops.
- *Treatment:* When diseases or disorders occur, they are treated, but the HMO makes decisions as to the type of treatment.

Some states require that employees in large organizations be given a choice between group insurance and HMO membership.

Some employers have initiated **incentive programs** to encourage employees to practice healthy habits. They reward employees for smoking cessation, weight loss, and regular physical examinations. Employees are encouraged to be seen in an urgent care center for routine illnesses rather than the emergency room. Usually the co-pay is much higher in the emergency room if urgent care was available at the same time.

Preferred Provider Organizations

Similar to HMOs, **preferred provider organizations (PPOs)** are used to deliver healthcare within a "managed" system. PPOs are made up of groups of healthcare practitioners who contract with the PPO to provide services. They refer clients among their groups. They usually require that their clients receive healthcare services from a member of that group, unless a special exception is made.

PPO members may use any of the services of the PPO or they can elect to go outside of the PPO network for service. However, the cost of the service outside of the PPO network is generally higher. For example, a PPO may pay 90% of the cost of a visit to a PPO physician but only 70% of the cost to a physician who is not a PPO contracted physician.

Point of Service Plans

A **point of service (POS)** plan is similar to HMO and PPO plans, in that they are all types of managed care. The POS plan also contracts with physicians and other healthcare providers. The client is "managed" by a primary care doctor within the network of POS providers. In this plan, a client may seek care outside of the POS network but will pay a larger share of the healthcare costs. The percentage of cost outside of the POS varies. Often the lines that define a HMO, PPO, and POS are indistinguishable.

Medicare

Medicare, a federal health insurance program, is available to nearly everyone over age 65, no matter what their financial status is. The insured person contributes to monthly premiums. The hospital insurance portion of Medicare provides partial payment for inpatient care and for extended outpatient care or home care. Medicare has, in recent years, begun to pay for preventive care such as mammograms, Pap tests, and flu and pneumonia immunizations.

Medicare is also available to younger people receiving **Social Security Disability Insurance (SSDI)** payments. SSDI is a type of insurance program for employees who have become unable to work. SSDI is administered by the Social Security Administration (SSA). Both employees and employers pay into the SSDI fund, and it is reflected in the FICA tax on payroll deduction forms.

SSDI is not the same program as workers' compensation. To be qualified to receive SSDI, employees must be totally incapacitated from gainful employment for at least a year. Workers' compensation benefits may pay for partial disabilities, and the benefits may be for a shorter period of time.[1]

Medicaid

Medicaid is a joint effort of federal and state governments. The federal government has set up guidelines for Medicaid, but individual states design their own programs. Therefore, regulations, eligibility requirements, and benefits vary greatly among the 50 states.

Generally, Medicaid is for people over the age of 65, those who are blind or disabled, or those who are members of families receiving Aid to Families With Dependent Children. States are ensured access to preventive healthcare (prenatal care, immunizations, and health and developmental screening) for women, infants, and children through their Medicaid programs. Medicaid is a public health insurance program for which people must qualify. The program is tax supported; thus, people who receive Medicaid benefits do not pay monthly premiums.

Medicaid pays for inpatient and outpatient services, including physician or advanced practice nurse services; laboratory and x-ray services; and screening, diagnosis, and treatment for children. It also pays for home care services and family planning. Some states support services such as dental care and eye care, immunization clinics, well-child clinics, and various preventive medicine and rehabilitation programs. Most Medicaid programs are now structured as Medicaid care systems, although some services remain fee-for-service.

Medicaid-waiver programs, including those for the chronically disabled, older adults, and people with AIDS, facilitate the ability of these participants to remain at home and within the community. Medicaid often waivers some of the qualification criteria and regulations for these clients.

People who are eligible for Medicare and Medicaid can supplement one program with the other. Medicaid may pay expenses not covered by Medicare if a person is eligible for both programs.

☛ KEY CONCEPT

Both Medicare and Medicaid are undergoing constant changes. These changes tend to be more visible to the public when they occur along with changes in the presidency or legislature. Be aware of the impact of these changes on clients, their families, and healthcare institutions.

Prospective Payment

In 1983, an amendment to the federal Social Security legislation changed the delivery of healthcare. This amendment created a prospective payment system, originally only affecting Medicare payments, but later adopted by other third-party payers. **Prospective payment** is a reimbursement system in which a predetermined amount is allocated for treating individuals with specific diagnoses.

The type of payment and reimbursement that existed in years past was called *retrospective payment.* This system reimbursed all actual costs of providing care. Many people felt that these costs were excessive, which contributed to the development of the system of prospective payment.

Diagnosis-Related Groups
Prospective payment is based on categories called diagnosis-related groups (DRGs) for hospitals and for home care. The term used in nursing homes and ECFs is **resource utilization groups (RUGs).**

The DRG system of prospective payment is based on medical diagnoses. Under this system, a federal agency has predetermined how much it "should" cost to treat a certain condition in a particular area of the United States. In this system, each client is classified according to the particular diagnosis (eg, hip surgery, pneumonia, or heart attack). The costs for the client's care are based on federally determined standards for that diagnosis.

The amount paid to the healthcare facility is predetermined and is *without consideration of the actual costs of providing care to the client.* Thus, a hospital treating an individual with a serious illness or surgery will receive the same reimbursement whether the person is hospitalized for 5 days or for 25 days.

Because a pre-set or *prospective* amount of money is paid for each diagnosis, the healthcare facility loses money if an individual client's care costs more than average. The facility gains money, however, if a client's care costs less than the average.

At the beginning of the 1990s, healthcare in the United States was a big business, and one of the top three industries in the country. healthcare continues to be a big business, but the emphasis is shifting from inpatient to community-based care. With the implementation of DRGs, facilities must be run cost effectively or they will not survive. Not all states, however, continue to use DRGs. For example, in 1993 New Jersey deregulated, allowing the state to make more decisions itself.

Impact of Changes in Third-Party Payment

The evolving system of healthcare financing in the United States has greatly affected the delivery of healthcare. Changes include:

- Emphasis on wellness, disease prevention, and health promotion
- Greatly decreased length of hospital stays
- Use of hospitals for only the critically ill
- Higher levels of client acuity in nursing homes
- Fewer admissions for inpatient care
- Sicker people discharged from hospitals, needing more care at home
- Families taking more responsibility for care
- Need for more outpatient care because procedures formerly done in the hospital are done on an outpatient basis
- More community-based care and home care nursing
- More specialized care
- More diversified hospitals that rent medical equipment, provide home care, and have day-surgery centers and ECFs—in addition to providing inpatient care
- Decentralized administration
- Need for more cooperation among departments to maximize resources
- Mergers of several hospitals or nursing homes to form a large corporation
- More computers used for information processing
- Advertising and marketing of hospital services as hospitals compete for clients

- More concern for clients and their reactions to care
- Many small hospitals closing or changing their emphasis because they can no longer compete (eg, converting to nursing homes)

COMPLEMENTARY HEALTHCARE

Many people believe that means other than traditional Western medicine can cure diseases and help them to achieve optimum health. These methods and beliefs are known as alternative healthcare or **complementary healthcare.** Several such modalities are discussed below. They may be used alone or in conjunction with other therapies. Only qualified practitioners should be used. Some practitioners must be licensed to legally practice.

Chiropractic, Physical, and Occupational Therapy

Chiropractic manipulates the spinal column and joints to treat pain and certain disorders. This therapy is based on the structure and function of the body. Chiropractors believe that the relationships between the spinal column and nervous system are important. Chiropractic adjustments seek to achieve a balance between these systems.

Physical therapy (PT) and occupational therapy (OT) are forms of rehabilitation after disease or injury. They use exercise, heat, cold, electrical muscle stimulation, splinting, ultraviolet radiation, and massage to improve circulation and to strengthen and retrain muscles. Physical therapy is also important in the management of chronic disorders such as arthritis. Occupational therapy is important in teaching skills that will enable people to return to work, manage their homes, or care for themselves again.

Holistic Healthcare

Holistic healthcare was at the center of many beliefs and practices of ancient civilizations. Holism became accepted in North American healthcare within the last half of the 20th century. Holism is a philosophy that considers the "whole person," or the multidimensional aspects of the human being, to be in need of healthcare.

The person is seen as a complete and integrated unit. The individual is a physical, psychological, and spiritual being. However, each individual is more than the sum of these three concepts. The goal in integrated healthcare is to combine disciplines to meet the person's overall needs.

Wellness not only means absence of disease and the meeting of one's basic needs, but also includes avoidance of hazardous situations and the ability to cope with stress. Persons experiencing high-level wellness are better able to achieve personal growth and contentment, as well as the freedom to be creative.

Holistic healthcare refers to comprehensive and total care of a person by meeting his or her needs in all areas: physical, emotional, social, spiritual, and economic. Rather than defining health in terms of disease, **holistic healthcare** emphasizes wellness.

Holistic healthcare teaches that individuals can be in control of their own life and health, and that people can largely *determine* the quality of their life. Chapter 5 relates the concepts of holistic healthcare and wellness to Maslow's Hierarchy of Human Needs.

Clients have the right to be actively involved in their own care. Rather than passively following the physician's orders, clients should consider the physician's advice and make informed decisions about care they wish to receive. Clients also have the right to refuse care. Part of your nursing responsibility is to teach clients and to answer their questions. You will also teach clients ways to prevent disease and to improve their health.

Nurses and other healthcare professionals should provide holistic care in a supportive and positive fashion, to help clients maintain a self-image as a worthy human being. By sincerely caring about your clients and respecting their ways of life, you can strengthen their feelings of self-respect and dignity.

Herbalists and Vibrational Remedies

Herbalists promote health through the use of herbs and other plants (botanicals). In many cases the use of herbs is combined with a healthful diet, exercise, and other healthy practices. "Vibrational remedies" include flower essences and homeopathy.

Acupuncture and Acupressure

Acupuncture, a healing method originating from Chinese medicine, is based on *Chi*, which is believed to be the energy of life. Acupuncture views health and its functions as energy balance—and disease as imbalance—in the body. Acupuncture therapy includes the use of very fine needles inserted into specific energy points underneath the skin to balance the body's flow of energy.

The use of this procedure is increasing in Western culture and is becoming more accepted by traditional allopathic medicine. It allows the body to heal naturally and does not involve the use of drugs, although herbal extracts and vitamins may be used. Acupuncture is often combined with meditation and exercise. It can be used for health promotion, such as weight control or smoking cessation, as well as for healing.

Clients can learn acupressure (external pressure applied to the energy points) for pain and symptom control between acupuncture treatments. Physical therapy and chiropractic use many of the same energy and pressure points.

Relaxation and Imagery

Relaxation and imagery are becoming more common in many areas of healthcare. Therapeutic relaxation begins with the client sitting or lying in a comfortable position, with eyes gently closed and the body relaxed. The person breathes deeply and concentrates on systematically and progressively relaxing all the muscles in the body. The person may also visualize relaxing images such as clouds or colors. Hypnosis and self-hypnosis make use of relaxation techniques.

Imagery involves calling up mental pictures or events, usually after the client completely relaxes. Although the person can use any of the senses, the most common is visual imagery. Imagery is often used in cancer therapy. For example, clients visualize their cells as being big and strong and the cancer as being small and weak. Or, clients picture the cancer cells being destroyed by their own white blood cells or visualize themselves as being well and whole. Other practitioners teach clients to "love the cancer out of existence." Imagery is also used in pain and spasm control, weight reduction, and smoking cessation.

Meditation

Many religious groups practice meditation, which consists of deep personal thought and breath control. The meditating person can keep his or her eyes open or closed. A word or phrase (mantra) may be repeated to aid concentration. Meditation strives to "clear or still the mind" through the art of "quiet thinking." Those who meditate change their concentration from the external world to the internal world, bringing mindfulness to oneself. Meditation helps decrease anxiety and enables people to better cope with stress. People can meditate while doing any relaxing activity: sitting, gardening, knitting, or walking.

Therapeutic Touch

Therapeutic touch is a specific noninvasive modality that does not require entering the body or puncturing the skin. Therapeutic touch grew out of the holistic healthcare movement. It was developed by Dora Kunz and Dolores Krieger and is based on the ancient practice of "laying on of hands," although the skilled practitioner never actually touches the client. Therapeutic touch teaches that each person is surrounded by an energy field. This electromagnetic field can be detected by magnetic resonance imaging.

The practitioner first "centers" himself or herself, achieving a sense of peace or wholeness, and then assesses and maximizes the client's energy with the goal of *restoring harmony.* Should the practitioner sense that the client's energy flow is obstructed, depleted, or disordered, the practitioner tries to direct the client's energy to unblock and balance the areas of disturbed flow. Therapeutic touch aids relaxation, lowers muscle tension, and may decrease the client's need for medication. It is considered to be a healing meditation.

CONSUMER FRAUD

Unlike complementary healthcare methods, which are acceptable modalities used in place of or along with conventional Western methods, many fraudulent healthcare practices and treatments are on the market.

The public spends an estimated $25 billion per year on "sure cures" for every imaginable ailment. The result is that ill people run the risk of delaying vital treatment until it is too late. Cancer and arthritis "cures" are the most common frauds. So-called "cures" for AIDS and chronic fatigue are also on the rise.

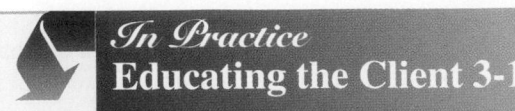

In Practice
Educating the Client 3-1

DETECTING FRAUDS

When teaching clients and families about consumer fraud, be sure to address the following concepts:

- Encourage people to develop their consumer awareness. Support groups are available for those who have been victims of fraud and for advocates of consumer rights. Help direct clients and families to such avenues if appropriate.
- Warn clients and families to suspect products, treatments, or methods with the following advertising claims:
  - "Special formula"
  - Supported by unrecognized "healthcare experts" or celebrities
  - Testimonials by those who have used the product ("It really works!!")
  - Attractive refund policy if not "completely satisfied"
- Discuss with clients their option to consult other qualified healthcare practitioners about their current treatment and prognosis (second opinion).
- Explain to clients that they have rights to information about their health and about any product or treatment measure that they use or are interested in pursuing.

Misleading the public (consumer fraud) is illegal. A great deal of money is at stake, so new schemes continue to develop. Why are so many people taken in by claims for a drug or other magic cure? People who are experiencing pain may be willing to try anything at any cost. Also, the general public often cannot tell the difference between true and false claims. As a nurse, you may be asked for your opinion about a questionable medical practice. Although people must make their own decisions, encourage them to find out all the facts before starting any untested healthcare measure.

➤ STUDENT SYNTHESIS

Key Points

- Many changes in the healthcare system in the 21st century will bring new and unknown challenges for nurses.
- Types of healthcare facilities include hospitals, which now primarily treat people with acute conditions; extended care facilities, where care is given for a longer time; and community services, which include outpatient care, walk-in care, home healthcare, and care in schools and industries.

Employment opportunities for nurses exist in all these areas.

- The Joint Commission for Accreditation of Healthcare Organizations establishes quality and appropriate care standards.
- Many hospitals have established the position of client advocate (representative, ombudsperson) to help the client and family adapt to hospitalization.
- Third-party payment has been the method of payment for healthcare in the United States for a number of years. A variety of organizations provide this service.
- Complementary healthcare will play an increasing role in the healthcare delivery system in the United States in the future. Holism is a philosophy that views the "whole person."

Critical Thinking Exercises

1. Relate Florence Nightingale's theory of nursing (see Chap. 2) to modalities such as therapeutic touch, meditation, and imagery.
2. Obtain a copy of a "critical pathway" or detailed nursing care plan from your healthcare facility. Analyze this document and its relationship to holistic healthcare.
3. Evaluate today's healthcare system and project forward about 25 years. How do you envision healthcare delivery? Relate your predictions to at least one theory of nursing, as presented in Chapter 2. Also relate your beliefs to the concept of holistic healthcare.

NCLEX-Style Review Questions

1. Current trends in the delivery of healthcare include which of the following?
   a. Preventing disease by education and screening
   b. Preventing clients from overusing doctors
   c. Treating all clients the same
   d. Treating the ill patient and the disease
2. Persons who are on Medicare:
   a. Do not pay any money to receive care
   b. Must have contributed to the plan during employment
   c. Pay monthly premiums
   d. Only receive immunizations
3. The goal of health maintenance organizations is to:
   a. Assist elderly persons
   b. Avoid health problems by prevention
   c. Maximize profit
   d. Provide care in the home

Reference

1. Physicians' Disability Services and Pds Disability Facts. *Fifteen key questions about disability benefits.* Website: http://www.disabilityfacts.com/faqs.html.

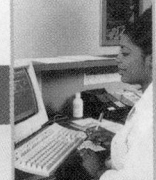

4

Legal and Ethical Aspects of Nursing

LEARNING OBJECTIVES

1. Define the following medical-legal terms: crime, felony, misdemeanor, liability, tort, negligence, malpractice, assault, battery, informed consent, libel, and slander.
2. Discuss the concept of false imprisonment and relate the discussion to your daily nursing practice.
3. Explain at least three implications for nurses for the issues of abandonment of care, invasion of privacy, and confidentiality.
4. State at least five special healthcare issues and relate them to nursing.
5. Define and discuss the purpose of a Nurse Practice Act.
6. State at least four components of a Nurse Practice Act.
7. State at least three functions of a State Board of Nursing.
8. State the purpose of the NCLEX-PN.
9. State at least eight common-sense precautions that nurses can take against lawsuits.
10. State at least two benefits and two limitations of the Good Samaritan Act.
11. Discuss at least four rationales for the concept of professional boundaries.
12. Define and discuss the three major types of advance directives.
13. State three types of persons who are vulnerable to deficient or harmful care.
14. Differentiate between biological death and brain death.
15. Define and discuss at least four ethical concepts that relate to nursing.
16. State at least three rights of healthcare clients and three responsibilities of healthcare clients.

NEW TERMINOLOGY

advance directive
assault
assisted suicide
battery
brain death
crime
endorsement
ethics
euthanasia
felony

Good Samaritan Act
informed consent
liability
libel
malpractice
misdemeanor
negligence
Nurse Practice Act
slander
tort

ACRONYMS

AHA	CPR	NCSBN
AMA	LPN/LVN	PSDA
CAT	NAHC	RN
CEH	NCLEX-PN	UNOS
CEU	NCLEX-RN	

Chapter 2 talked about standards of practice, the Nightingale Pledge, and the Practical Nurses' Pledge. Legal and ethical issues of nursing practice were introduced. This chapter further explores legal and ethical issues and relates them to the concepts of nursing and healthcare.

Laws are formal written rules of behavior that govern conduct and ensure the protection of citizens. **Ethics** refers to moral principles and values that guide human behaviors. Ethics and ethical standards evolve in cultures where there exist the concepts of right and wrong. The healthcare system combines the practice of medicine and nursing with a complex system of laws, societal beliefs, and cultural values.

The ethical standards of the healthcare profession and the laws of the United States and Canada are carefully designed to protect both you and those you serve. You are responsible for becoming familiar with these legal and ethical standards before caring for clients.

LEGAL ISSUES OF NURSING PRACTICE

In the course of your activities both as a student and later as a licensed nurse, you are held responsible for maintaining established standards of nursing care. You will encounter many situations involving legal responsibilities. In addition to avoiding those acts that all citizens know are illegal, you must not violate other important laws that are specific to healthcare.

For example, federal law requires that healthcare facilities keep records about the dispensing of narcotics. This law specifies that narcotics are to be given under the direction and supervision of a physician, osteopath, dentist, or veterinarian. In a hospital, all narcotics are kept double locked, and every dose or tablet must be accounted for. Violation of the Controlled Substances Act is a serious crime. Table 4-1 summarizes common sources of law and gives examples related to nursing and healthcare.

Legal Terminology

A **crime** is a wrong committed against a person or property or public good. A crime occurs when there is violation of a law.

In a crime, intention to do wrong is also present. Crimes may be misdemeanors or felonies.

A **felony** is a serious crime. Healthcare workers can be convicted of felonies for such offenses as falsification of medical records, insurance fraud, theft of narcotics, or practicing without a license.

A **misdemeanor** is a crime that is considered not as serious as a felony. A misdemeanor is still a serious charge and may be cause for revocation of a nursing license. Possession of controlled substances may be either a misdemeanor or a felony as defined by the local, state, or federal laws.

Liability is the legal responsibility for one's actions or failure to act appropriately. A crime may be the deliberate *commission* of a forbidden act or *omission* of an act required by law.

A nurse may be liable if a client receives the wrong medication and is harmed (an "act of commission"). Examples of other nursing *crimes of commission* would be participation in an illegal abortion, participation in **euthanasia** ("mercy killing"), and practicing nursing without a license or beyond the legal limits of your nursing practice.

A nurse also may be liable if a client did not receive a prescribed medication and was harmed (an "act of omission"). *Crimes of omission* include failure to perform a prescribed treatment, failing to report child or elder abuse, and failure to report a specified communicable disease or an animal bite.

A **tort** is an injury that occurred because of another person's intentional or unintentional actions or failure to act. The injury can be physical, emotional, or financial. A tort involves a breach of duty that one person owes another, such as the duty of a nurse to care for a client. Examples of intentional torts include assault, battery, false imprisonment, invasion of privacy, and defamation. The example of an unintentional tort is negligence. Malpractice is defined as professional negligence.

Negligence is defined as harm done to a client as a result of neglecting duties, procedures, or ordinary precautions. Negligence is one of the most common causes of lawsuits by clients of healthcare. Negligence describes the failure to act as a reasonable person would have acted in a similar situation. Negli-

■■■ TABLE 4-1 *C*OMMON SOURCES OF LAW

Type of Law	General Purpose	Example of Law
Constitutional Law	Law written as part of a local, state, or federal constitution	Protection of right to free speech
Statutory Law	Any law enacted by a legislative body	Creation of Nurse Practice Act
Administrative Law	Empowers agencies to create and enforce rules and regulations	Development of State Boards of Nursing
Criminal Law✓	Laws that define offenses that violate the public welfare	Prosecution of violation of provisions of Nurse Practice Act
Civil Law	Protects civil rights such as freedom from invasion of privacy and freedom from threats of injury	Healthcare client charges nurse with invasion of privacy and violation of confidentiality laws

gence takes into account your educational level and experience. Thus, negligence is balanced against what another nurse with similar education and experience would have done in a similar situation. A nurse can be found negligent and be sued for damages for any of the following reasons:

- Performing nursing procedures that have not been taught
- Failing to follow standard protocols as defined by the facility's policy and procedure manuals
- Failing to report defective or malfunctioning equipment
- Failing to meet established standards of safe care for clients
- Failing to prevent injury to clients, other employees, and visitors
- Failing to question a physician's order that seems incorrect

Malpractice is the improper, injurious, or faulty treatment of a client that results in illness or injury. Harm that results from a licensed person's actions or lack of actions can be called malpractice. A nurse commits malpractice when his or her conduct deviates from the normal or expected standard of behavior that would be performed by someone of similar education and experience in similar circumstances.

Healthcare professionals are held to higher standards than untrained individuals. Standards of practice are defined by the state's Nurse Practice Act, written agency policies and procedures, documented standards of care such as a nursing care plan, and the testimony of expert witnesses. Additional information regarding Nurse Practice Acts is found in the next section of this chapter.

Assault is a threat or an attempt to do bodily harm. Assault includes physical or verbal intimidation. A gesture that the client may perceive as a threat is an assault if the client believes that force or injury may follow. Telling the client that you are going to restrain him in bed if he tries to get out of bed without assistance is an assault.

Battery is physical contact with another person without that person's consent. Physical striking or beating is battery. Also considered to be battery may be the touching a person's body, clothing, chair, or bed. A charge of battery can be made even if the contact did not cause physical harm. Giving an injection that the client refuses is battery. Forcing the client to get out of bed can be considered both assault and battery. To protect nurses and other healthcare individuals from the charge of battery, clients sign a general permission for care and treatment. Prior to any special test, procedure, or surgery, clients sign another consent. Informed consent is discussed below.

Consent for care is provided by the individual, parent, or guardian if the client is a minor, mentally retarded, or mentally incompetent. In an emergency, the law assumes inferred consent. *Inferred consent* means that in life-threatening circumstances, the client would provide consent for care.

NURSING ALERT
The nursing student *never* serves as a witness to any legal papers or documents.

Informed consent means that tests, treatments, and medications have been explained to the person, as well as outcomes, possible complications, and alternative procedures. Before any person receives routine treatment, a specialized diagnostic procedure, an invasive procedure, special medical or surgical treatment, or experimental therapy, he or she must give informed consent. Usually, the physician explains the situation and obtains consent. The physician and all healthcare workers must be reasonably satisfied that the client understands what will be done and what the expected or adverse results are likely to be. All teaching must be documented.

☛ Key Concept

All teaching must be documented.

The client or a legal guardian must understand and sign the consent form before the performance of any procedure. In certain extreme emergencies, no one may be available to give consent. In such cases, procedures may be performed without specific written or verbal consent; however, each facility will have specific protocols that will need to be followed. For example, if an unconscious client is admitted to an emergency room and needs immediate surgical intervention before family can be located, some facilities allow for two physicians to sign an emergency consent. In some cases, a court order to administer treatment is obtained.

The person who will perform any procedure is ultimately responsible for obtaining consent. As a nurse, you must confirm that the signed consent is in a client's health record before performing any procedure. In cases of serious surgery or life-threatening procedures, physicians usually obtain consent. *Students do not obtain consent or witness consent forms.*

Nonconsensual physical contact may be required if the client is mentally ill, intoxicated, or endangering the safety of self or others. (Chapter 93 discusses care in the mental health unit.) Legal protection in this type of circumstance relies heavily on thorough documentation. It is critical for the healthcare provider to describe the behavior of the client that resulted in the use of force. The documentation should specify that the situation required the type of restraint that was used. Excessive force is never appropriate.

False imprisonment or restraint of movement may be charged in certain situations, such as the use of unnecessary restraints or solitary confinement. By law, a person cannot be restrained against his or her will unless the person has been convicted of a crime or a court order exists permitting restraint. False imprisonment may be a result of either physical or chemical limitations.

Libel and slander relate to personal integrity. **Libel** refers to a written statement or photograph that is false or damaging. Special precautions must be taken to avoid libel when using e-mail communications. The Internet and electronic communications have the potential of carrying personal conversations into the public domain.

Slander is the term given to malicious verbal statements that are false or injurious. Clearly, nurses must avoid untrue and unwise statements at all times. Slander can take the form of gossip and exaggerations, eg, "That nurse is lazy," "The supervisor doesn't know what she is doing," or "Doctor XYZ's patients always have complications." *Defamation* is an act that harms a person's reputation and good name.

Abandonment of care is a legal term that implies that a healthcare professional has prematurely stopped caring for a client. For example, if a client cannot safely be left alone, you may be found liable if the client under your care is injured while unsupervised. If a home care client has an infection or stops taking medications, you may be found liable if you fail to report this information in a timely manner. To avoid the charge of abandonment, you NEVER leave your employment or clinical assignment, even in an emergency, without proper notification being given to your supervisors.

Invasion of privacy and confidentiality are of critical legal and medical concern. The *right to privacy* means that a client has the right to expect that his or her property will be left alone. Healthcare individuals may be charged with trespassing, illegal search and seizure, or releasing private information (even if the information is true). Remember that you are violating the law if you give out any information about a client without his or her written consent. Also, prevent clients and visitors from seeing other clients' health records and private information. For example, be careful not to pull client information onto the computer screen where other clients can see it (Fig. 4-1).

Student nurses are often assigned research projects that contain a client's medical history and personal information. Rather than using client names or initials, it is more prudent to use code numbers. If lost or misplaced, even your scratch notes can be the basis for a breach of confidentiality lawsuit. ALWAYS protect the client's confidentiality.

Because confidentiality is so important, avoid gossip and preserve the privacy of your clients. Violation of confidential-

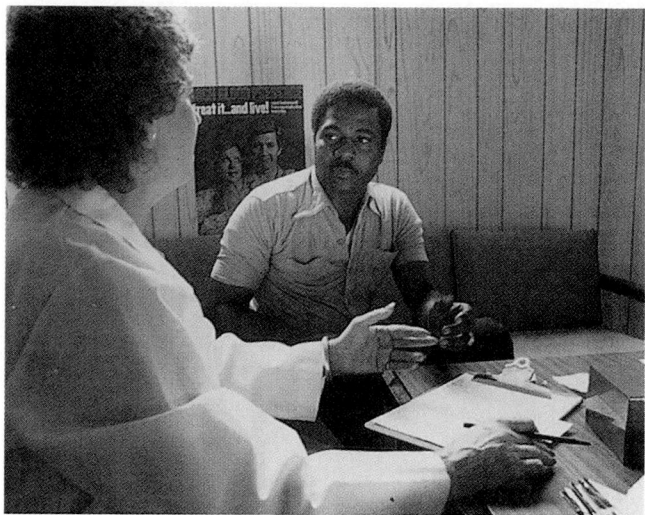

FIGURE 4-2. When interviewing clients, make sure to maintain privacy by waiting until visitors leave and closing doors. (Hosley, J. B., Jones, S. A., & Molle-Matthews, E. A. [1997]. *Lippincott's textbook for medical assistants,* [p. 295]. Philadelphia: Lippincott Williams & Wilkins.)

ity or misuse of the health record is a violation of privacy laws (Fig. 4-2). If a client requests anonymity, just acknowledging the person's hospitalization can be a violation of the law.

☞ KEY CONCEPT

Keep up to date on current legislation by reading nursing journals and attending continuing education classes. Ignorance of the law does not protect you from prosecution.

Special Healthcare Concerns

The laws relating to healthcare are many and varied. A basic understanding of laws that apply to nursing is essential so that you can make informed decisions about your practice. The following are common healthcare issues that have particular legal and sometimes ethical implications:

- *Duty to provide treatment.* The person's ability to pay should not determine whether he or she receives care. Laws regulate the rights of the person and of the healthcare facility.
- *Abortion and sterilization.* State laws differ as to what types of consents are required, who must be notified, and who must sign the consent. The length of gestation for a legal abortion also differs between states.
- *Experimentation.* Stringent regulations govern research studies using human beings. All participants in such studies must give informed consent.
- *Release from liability.* A person may leave the healthcare facility **against medical advice (AMA),** or may refuse treatment. Laws specify the extent of responsibility of the facility and of physicians and nurses.
- *Death in the hospice facility or during the hospice program at home.* When a person is expected to die (as in hospice), the laws relating to pronouncement of death are different from those in other situations.

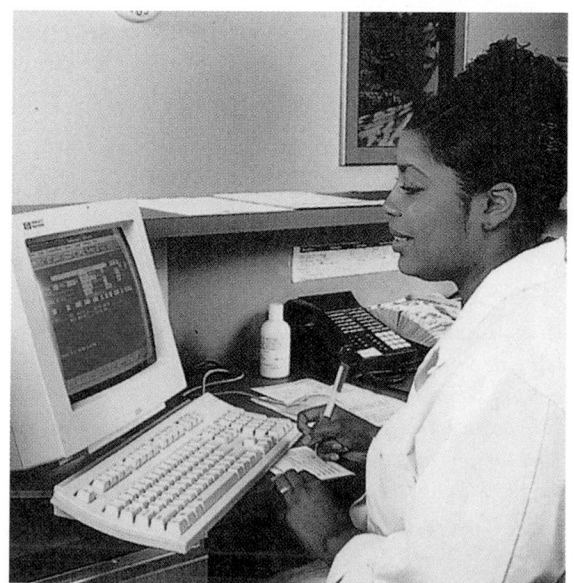

FIGURE 4-1. Computers are excellent tools for nurses but they can be a source of loss of confidentiality for the client. (Hosley, J. B., Jones, S. A., & Molle-Matthews, E. A. [1997]. *Lippincott's textbook for medical assistants,* [p. 157]. Philadelphia: Lippincott Williams & Wilkins.)

REGULATIONS OF NURSING PRACTICE

Legislation for the Practice of Nursing: The Nurse Practice Act

Nursing is a specific profession that has legal definitions as to scope or boundaries of practice. The laws for the practice of nursing are written by the legislature of each state or province. The law that defines and regulates the practice of nursing in the United States is called the **Nurse Practice Act.** In Canada it is called the Nurses (Registered) Act. These laws define the title of "nursing" and regulate the many aspects of the field of nursing.

In some areas a single Nurse Practice Act is written to include both registered and practical nurses. In other areas, licensed practical nursing and registered nursing have completely separate Nurse Practice Acts.

Only individuals who are regulated by Nurse Practice Acts can legally be called nurses. Certified Nurses Aides are not licensed personnel because they do not function under nurse practice legislation. However, many states require that they complete basic, minimal training by qualified instructors. When the training is complete, the individual may apply to the state for "certification." Currently, unlicensed assistive personnel (UAP) and medical assistants are not licensed personnel, and may or may not have any formal healthcare training.

State Boards of Nursing

The legislative power to initiate, regulate, and enforce the provisions of the Nurse Practice Act is delegated to a specific state agency often known as the State Board of Nursing. The state governor may appoint Board members but the criteria and credentials for Board members generally are written within the Nurse Practice Act. For example, in states with a single Board, the law usually requires that a specified number of **licensed practical/vocational nurses (LPN/LVNs)** be Board members, so that LPN/LVNs have a representative voice in affairs concerning them. The state nursing associations also make recommendations for Board appointments.

Boards are subject to legal parameters, but usually they have some leeway in interpreting aspects of the Nurse Practice Act. For example, the Board may define LPN/LVN limitations regarding working with intravenous lines and administering intravenous medications. The Boards work cooperatively with other regulating Boards, such as the Board of Medical Examiners and the Pharmacy Board. All state "Boards" may be part of one or more larger state agencies such as the Department of Consumer Affairs or the Department of Health Services.

Sometimes State Nursing Boards are known by other titles, such as the Board of Nurse Examiners. In the recent past, the State Boards of Nursing were responsible for the creation of the licensing exam (thus the name "Nurse Examiners"). However, the licensing exams today are written by the National Council of State Boards of Nursing, which will be discussed in more detail below.

Licensing laws vary from state to state in many respects. The goal of nurse planners is to establish uniform requirements so that a license issued in one state will be recognized in all states. A national nursing license has also been proposed.

The law or Nurse Practice Act in each state, province, or territory defines regulations for practical and registered nursing. Licensing and renewal fees generally provide revenue for the Boards.

The major concepts of the legislation of Nurse Practice Acts include:

- Definition of practical and registered nursing
- Nursing functions protected by the law
- Requirements for an approved school of nursing (eg, length of program, curricula, admission requirements)
- Establishment of requirements for licensure (eg, age, graduation from an approved course, criminal background screening checks)
- Process and procedures for becoming licensed in each state, territory, or province
- Procedures for maintaining licensure, including required continuing education
- Issuing and renewing nursing licenses
- Conditions under which a license may be suspended or revoked and conditions for reinstatement
- Procedures for transferring licenses from one state to another (interstate endorsement)

The facility in which you are employed has the right to limit the functions of a nurse. For example, a facility may state that only specially trained nurses may perform certain procedures—even if the Nurse Practice Act states that the nurse may legally do that procedure. However, a facility cannot allow a nurse to practice without a license or beyond the legal definitions of practice of that state.

Your employer may also require that you have additional education in specialized fields in order to work in that facility. Generally, training in **cardiopulmonary resuscitation (CPR)** is required by all clinical facilities. To work in specialty care units such as geriatrics, wound care, intensive care, or pediatric care, your employer may require that you complete additional nursing courses. These advanced courses are generally not part of your nursing program and are not listed as educational requirements by the Nurse Practice Act. Education in nursing is a life-long, continual process; a nurse never stops learning.

☛ KEY CONCEPT

- *Always practice within the limits of practical or registered nursing as you were taught.*
- *Use good common sense and judgment.*
- *Ask if you are unsure.*
- *Report any errors immediately.*
- *Report any defective equipment immediately.*

Cause for Revoking or Suspending a License

The Nurse Practice Act defines conditions under which a license can be revoked. Such conditions include drug or alcohol abuse, fraud, deceptive practices, criminal acts, previous disciplinary action, and gross or ordinary negligence. For example, telling an employer that you are a **registered nurse (RN)** if you are actually an LPN/LVN is a deceptive practice and is cause for revoking the LPN/LVN license.

The Licensing Exam: The NCLEX

After successful completion of your nursing program, and prior to being able to practice as a LPN/LVN or RN, your first responsibility is to pass either the **National Council Licensing Examination for Practical Nurses (NCLEX-PN)** or the **National Council Licensing Examination for Registered Nurses (NCLEX-RN).**

The **National Council of State Boards of Nursing (NCSBN)** is responsible for the NCLEX exams. It is the National Council's responsibility to provide the State Boards of Nursing with a valid and reliable exam that can demonstrate that a licensure candidate has passed the exam with minimal competence to perform safe and effective entry-level nursing care. The purpose of the NCLEX-PN is to separate candidates into two groups: those who can pass with minimal entry-level knowledge and those who cannot.

The NCLEX-PN and NCLEX-RN are used by all 50 states, the District of Columbia, and the U.S. territories of Guam, the Virgin Islands, American Samoa, Puerto Rico, and the Northern Marianna Islands. The NCLEX was first implemented in 1994 in a computerized form called **computerized adaptive testing (CAT).** Test questions are written by practicing clinical nurses and educators. Revisions to the CAT are made on a regular basis. Extensive surveys are conducted every three years to ensure that the test questions accurately reflect job tasks normally performed by the novice nurse. The NCLEX-PN has its most significant content areas in nursing process and client needs. Each of these two areas is further subdivided into specific subject areas. A further discussion of the NCLEX-PN plan is beyond the scope of this chapter.

Due to the nationwide utilization of the NCLEX, when a nurse moves from one state to another state, the nurse is not required to take another licensing exam. The nurse applies for licensure in the new state and may receive a license by the process of **endorsement.** Licensing fees and other fees may be required by the individual state and the nurse may need to file specific documentation in the new state. The situation is similar in Canada, except in Ontario.

After you become licensed, you will be required to renew that license at specified intervals. Many states require both LPN/LVNs and RNs to take courses that document that you are maintaining currency in nursing. Continuing education classes must meet specified criteria. The classes are allotted **continuing education units (CEUs)** or **continuing education hours (CEHs).** The numbers of required units or hours is dictated by your State Board of Nursing and are commonly mandated for license renewal. Some states specify what courses must be taken. For example, Minnesota requires a course in infection control; in New York, course content in child abuse is required for RN re-licensure. On satisfactory completion of these courses, you will receive a certificate. You will be required to maintain your own records of continuing education courses. Your records may be audited by your State Board of Nursing.

Legal Responsibilities in Nursing

Safeguards for the Nurse and Student

Although as a practical or vocational nurse you are likely to work under the direction of other nurses and physicians, you are personally liable for any harm a client suffers as a result of your own acts. Healthcare facilities may also be legally liable for their employees' acts of negligence. Legal actions involving negligent acts by a person engaged in a profession may become malpractice lawsuits.

Common-Sense Precautions

Follow Accepted Procedures.   Protect yourself from possible lawsuits by always performing procedures as taught and as outlined in the procedure manual of your healthcare facility. If these policies are incorrect or inadequate, work to improve them through the proper channels.

Be Competent in Your Practice.   You are always responsible for your own behavior. Refuse to perform procedures for which you have not been prepared. Ignorance is not a legal defense. Neither will lack of sleep or overwork be accepted as a legal reason for carelessness about safety measures or mistakes.

Ask for Assistance.   Always ask for help when you are unsure about how to perform a procedure. Do not assume responsibilities beyond those of your level. Admitting that you do not know how to perform a procedure is always better than attempting to do it and injuring someone. Also question any physician's order that you do not understand, cannot read, or in which you believe an error exists.

Document Well.   The importance of keeping exact records of all treatments and medications, as well as a record of a client's reactions and behavior, cannot be overemphasized. The health record is the written and legal evidence of treatment. The record is to reflect facts only, not personal judgments. *Careful* and *accurate* documentation is vital for each client's welfare and your own (Fig. 4-3). Chapter 37 discusses documentation in detail.

☞ KEY CONCEPT

Careful documentation is perhaps the most important thing you can do to protect yourself against an unjustified lawsuit. If you do not document a treatment or medication, legally the measure is considered not to have been done. You can be held accountable. Of course, you will be held accountable for performing an illegal or negligent act, whether or not you document it.

Do Not Give Legal Advice to Clients.   The laws governing personal and property rights of an individual are many and complex. Never attempt to advise a client on legal rights or financial matters. Encourage clients to confer with their families and to consult an attorney.

Do Not Accept Gifts.   Accepting gifts from clients is unwise for several reasons. Some clients are considered *vulnerable adults* (eg, mentally ill, retarded, or confused individuals). Exchange of gifts could compromise your professional

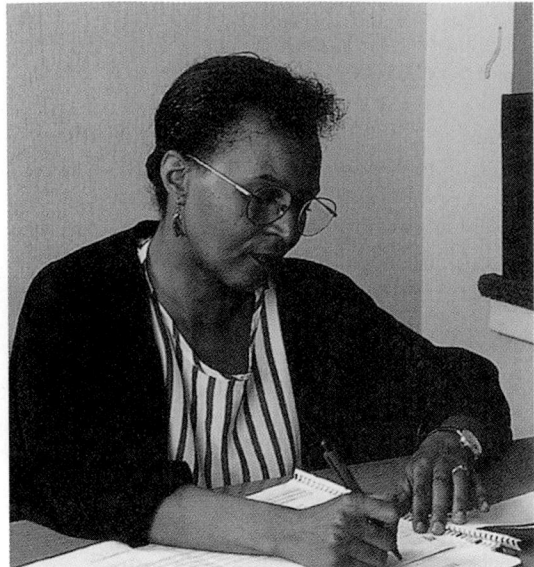

FIGURE 4-3. Careful documentation and reporting are nursing responsibilities and also help to maintain legal records. (Hosley, J. B., Jones, S. A., & Molle-Matthews, E. A. [1997]. *Lippincott's textbook for medical assistants,* [p. 205]. Philadelphia: Lippincott Williams & Wilkins.)

position, and you could be accused of coercing the client. Some clients may feel that by accepting a gift, you now "owe" them special care or services. Because determining appropriate gift acceptance is difficult, the safest measure is to accept no gifts. An exception to this rule would be in the event that a client wishes to give candy or flowers to all staff on a hospital unit to share.

Do Not Help a Client Prepare a Will. *Never* attempt to help a client prepare a will or any other legal document. The law has formal requirements a will must meet to make it valid. As a graduate, you may be asked to witness the signing of a will. After the death of a client, you and other witnesses may be asked to testify as to the mental competence of the testator or to other conditions prevailing at the time of execution of the will.

Consider a Malpractice Insurance Policy. Malpractice insurance is available through private insurance companies and sometimes through the healthcare facility or a professional organization. The wise nurse carries malpractice insurance. Even if you are found innocent of charges in a case, preparing a defense still costs money. Malpractice insurance will cover these charges if you have practiced within the limits of your job description and level of training. Healthcare facilities usually carry umbrella liability insurance that covers the facility if an employee is named in a legal action. This insurance does not always protect the individual nurse; thus, having your own insurance is also important. Many professional and technical personnel protect themselves from paying court-imposed settlements by carrying private malpractice insurance.

Obtain the services of a lawyer specializing in medical/nursing malpractice at the first sign that you are involved in an illegal or negligent act or that you may be named in a lawsuit. Notify your malpractice carrier immediately because it may

➤➤ **BOX 4-1**

EXAMPLES OF SITUATIONS IN WHICH NURSES CAN BE HELD LIABLE

- Burns, falls, incorrect medications
- Lack of common nursing judgment (eg, using an oral thermometer for a confused or out-of-control patient)
- Failure to follow the policies of the healthcare facility to protect the client and his or her belongings
- Allowing an unsafe condition to continue
- Damages that arise from violation of the client's rights
- Treatment without informed consent (can be considered assault and battery)
- Stories, information, or photographs given without consent
- Revelation of confidential information
- Assault of one client by another client

appoint an attorney for you. Insist on your legal rights. If you remember your limitations and practice within the scope of your education, you should have no difficulty with lawsuits and your clients will be safe. Box 4-1 gives examples of situations in which you may be held liable.

☛ KEY CONCEPT

Malpractice insurance covers nurses only when they act "as any prudent nurse would." In other words, if you deliberately commit an illegal act or are negligent beyond accidental errors, your malpractice insurance and that of your employer will probably not be valid.

Legal Concerns of Emergencies

In some states, the law requires any person who witnesses an automobile or other accident to give aid to persons injured in that accident. In most states, a person who has medical or nursing education is *required to assist,* if needed. In areas other than those to which this law applies, no person is legally obligated to render aid during an emergency. Each person who gives assistance should act as a reasonably prudent person would, within the limits of education and experience. Thus, as a nurse, you will be expected to render a higher level of emergency care than an untrained person. A law called the **Good Samaritan Act** is in effect in most states. This law protects you from liability if you give emergency care *within the limits of first aid* and if you act in a "reasonable and prudent manner."

Stay informed regarding legal issues surrounding all types of documentation.

Professional Boundaries

All healthcare personnel must maintain appropriate professional boundaries. Abstain from benefiting personally at the client's expense. Be sure to refrain from inappropriate involvement in the client's personal relationships. By doing so, you help to promote the client's independence. Remember the following important considerations:

Power versus vulnerability: You, as a nurse, have power in your position and access to private client information. Do not exploit this power.

Boundary crossings: Any questionable behavior should be brief, unintentional, and not repeated. Evaluate any such incidents immediately if they occur.

Boundary violations: Excessive personal disclosures or asking clients to keep secrets are examples. Such actions can cause clients distress and are inappropriate.

Professional sexual misconduct: Seductive, sexually demeaning, or harassing behavior is illegal and is a breach of the trust placed in you. Such misconduct constitutes just cause for dismissal from a job.

Remain helpful to clients without taking advantage of them. Your duty is to practice in the area of *therapeutic involvement.* Over-involvement includes boundary crossings and violations, and sexual misconduct. Under-involvement causes disinterest and client neglect.

Danger signals of over-involvement include excessive self-disclosure, defensiveness about the relationship, believing that only you can meet a particular client's needs, spending excessive time with one client, flirting, or overt sexual acts. Evaluating each interaction you have with clients is vital to ensure that the relationship is helpful and that you are not over- or under-involved. If you have questions, your nursing instructor or the facility's nursing supervisor can assist you.

ADVANCE DIRECTIVES

To preserve a client's rights, all healthcare workers need to be aware of the client's wishes regarding continuing, withholding, or withdrawing treatment in the event the person cannot make these decisions for himself or herself. An **advance directive** is a legal document in which a person either states choices for medical treatment or names someone to make treatment choices if he or she loses decision-making ability.

✚👁 NURSING ALERT

Competent adults must speak for themselves. Another person cannot decide to withhold treatment, as long as the client is able to make decisions. If the client cannot talk, other means of communication may be used. Such information must be carefully documented, witnessed, and signed. If the person is legally incompetent, the court may make decisions about care.

☛ KEY CONCEPT

If no documented evidence exists to the contrary, the healthcare team uses all means available to keep a person alive. Without a living will or other advance directive, a full "code" is called on all those who suffer a cardiac arrest, and full resuscitation efforts are made.

The federal government passed the **Patient Self-Determination Act (PSDA)** in 1991. This law requires all healthcare institutions to comply with the provisions of this act or to forfeit reimbursement from Medicare and other types of funding. This legislation mandates an individual's right to some sort of advance directive. The law *requires* that all adults admitted to any healthcare facility must be asked if they have an advance directive and given assistance if they desire more information. Box 4-2 describes the nurse's role in carrying out mandates of this legislation.

Three major types of advance directives exist:

- Living will
- Directives to physicians
- Durable power of attorney for healthcare

Living Will

A *living will* is a written and legally witnessed document (but can be executed without an attorney) that requests no extraordinary measures to be taken to save a person's life in the event of terminal illness. The living will goes into effect only if the person becomes unable to make his or her own decisions regarding care. The living will may indicate life-sustaining treatments that the person does or does not want used, and may specify comfort measures to be used or not used. Some form of living will legislation is in place throughout the United States. A great deal of controversy surrounds this issue. For example, in some states, living will legislation states that artificial nutrition and hydration must be maintained, even if the

---

➤➤ BOX 4-2

THE NURSE'S RESPONSIBILITY IN DETERMINATION OF ADVANCE DIRECTIVES

- Understand the different types of advance directives.
- Know specific advance directives that apply to certain areas (such as in mental health units).
- Obtain assistance if clients wish to change an advance directive, as their condition or desires change.
- Teach clients so they can make informed decisions.
- Inform clients that they have the right to refuse treatment or can refuse life-prolonging measures, but can still receive palliative care and pain control.

On admission, ask clients if they understand the concept of advance directives and the Patient Self-Determination Act. Make sure that clients know what a living will and durable power of attorney are. If the client wishes to initiate advance directives, provide proper assistance (often by referring client to another party). If the client already has a living will, be sure to place this information in the health record, notify the physician, and document appropriately. Copies of the living will must be on file in the healthcare facility or agency.

person has previously requested that no artificial means be used to sustain life. In addition, various states have slightly different formats for living wills and do not necessarily recognize documents written in another state. A living will does not automatically expire in a certain length of time. It is in effect until the individual changes or revokes it. If a person has a living will, a copy is kept on file in the healthcare facility. Physicians and nurses are bound by the person's wishes.

Directive to Physicians

A *directive to physicians* is another type of written document that can be useful for terminally ill adults who have no other person to name as their agent for making healthcare decisions. In this case, the person directs the physician to be his or her decision-maker. The physician must also agree, in writing, to accept this responsibility.

Durable Power of Attorney for Healthcare

In this written document, a client names another person to make healthcare decisions for him or her should the client become unable to do so. This designated person does not need to be a relative. Individuals should discuss *durable power of attorney* in advance with those they wish to designate as their decision-makers.

Mental Health Advance Declaration

In addition to the general advance declaration available to all persons, the *mental health advance declaration* establishes specific guidelines for psychiatric care. In this case, the mental health declaration specifies an individual's wishes concerning intrusive mental health treatment (such as electroconvulsive therapy and special types of medications called neuroleptics). Even if the person who refuses these treatments is committed as mentally ill or mentally ill and dangerous, these treatments may not be given without a specific court order.

VULNERABLE PERSONS

Children and some adults are considered vulnerable to deficient or harmful care. Reporting suspected child abuse or vulnerable adult abuse is mandatory in the United States and Canada. In addition, most states have laws protecting persons considered to be vulnerable, which includes almost any hospitalized individual. Laws protecting the vulnerable are particularly important for those who work with mentally ill, mentally retarded, or confused persons. Older people are often considered vulnerable adults. The law protects vulnerable persons from injury, abuse, or neglect while receiving care in the healthcare facility, nursing home, school, or their own home. Often, a person's isolation in his or her own home can increase the person's vulnerability. Families can also be charged with abuse under the vulnerable adult laws. (Chap. 98 discusses home care issues.)

LEGAL DEFINITIONS OF DEATH

Death is the permanent cessation of all vital functions, including those of the heart, lungs, and brain.[1] Death can be categorized as biological death or brain death. Laws and rules in the healthcare facility relate to the biological and physiological definitions of death.

☛ KEY CONCEPT

No uniform definition of clinical death *exists in the United States. Each state has slightly different criteria.*

Determination of Death

State laws still differ as to what constitutes death and how death is pronounced. The Uniform Determination of Death Act was recommended to the states for enactment in 1980; it suggested criteria for biological death and brain death. The diagnosis of death is a legal and ethical concern to healthcare providers. Before removal of organs or tissues for donation, especially when a person's vital processes are being maintained artificially, the wishes of the client and the family need to be in harmony with legal regulations.

Biological death is death due to natural causes. With today's advanced life support systems, the statutory definition of death needs criteria—other than the absence of breathing and heartbeat—to determine biologic death.

Brain death is the cessation of brain function. Brain death may also be known as *clinical death.* The physical body may be kept functioning for periods of time by artificial means; however, in brain death the brain has a lack of response to stimuli, lack of cephalic reflexes (see below), and absent stimulation to breathe. A client with the diagnosis of brain death may be considered a donor candidate for organ transplantation. Organ transplants are discussed in the latter portion of this chapter. Criteria for the diagnosis of brain death include the following:

- *Cessation of breathing* after artificial ventilation is discontinued (usually requires cessation for at least 3 minutes)
- *Cessation of heartbeat* without external stimuli
- *Unresponsiveness* to external stimuli
- *Complete absence of cephalic reflexes* (the lowest form of brain stem reflexes). Some states accept the absence of some cephalic reflexes.
- *Pupils fixed and dilated.* Some states accept pupils unresponsive to light but not necessarily dilated.
- *Irreversible cessation of all functions of the brain.* In some states, this includes all functions of the brain stem as well. This brain and brain stem function can be assessed by evaluation of reflexes. In some cases, one or more electroencephalograms are done to confirm the diagnosis of clinical death.

Exceptions

In all cases that may involve the determination of death, the following *exceptions* are identified:

- Marked hypothermia (core body temperature below 90°F [32.2°C], such as might follow a near-drowning episode)
- Severe depression of the central nervous system (CNS) after drug overdose with a CNS depressant, such as a barbiturate

Determination of clinical death is complex and controversial. Check the laws in your state.

ETHICAL STANDARDS OF HEALTHCARE

Ethics is defined as conduct appropriate for all members of a group. Chapter 2 gives standards of nursing practice. A code of ethics builds on these standards. Today, healthcare workers confront many ethical issues that have arisen as a result of increased knowledge and technology, changing demographic patterns, and consumer demands.

Prejudice, Personal Values, and Nursing

Each individual brings personal values to the healthcare system. These values include beliefs about such concepts as life and death, a higher power, who should receive healthcare and what kind of care, and complex issues such as abortion and euthanasia. Values are the culmination of heritage, culture, and one's family of origin, combined with life experiences. Values evolve as life situations change. A person's values may change when faced with illness, injury, and possible death. To be of optimum support to each client, you must undergo your own personal values clarification process.

☛ KEY CONCEPT

Be aware of your feelings and behavior. Always act in the client's best interests.

Consciously examining your own values, beliefs, and feelings about life and healthcare issues is helpful because it provides you with a frame of reference. Your beliefs may be different from those of your peers and clients. Prejudice in nursing is imposing your beliefs and value system onto others. When practicing nursing, your personal beliefs and those of your clients may be radically different. Remember, however, that you must also allow clients the freedom to formulate and to express their own values. *Do not impose your values on clients.*

Quality of Life

Quality of life is a complicated ethical issue. At what point does the healthcare team decide that a person should receive treatment or not? For example, not enough donated organs or specialized facilities are available to serve everyone who needs them. How then is the decision made as to who receives life-saving treatment and who does not? Healthcare ethics comes into play in such decisions.

Part of the discussion as to who receives treatment centers around the quality of life expected following treatment. Can

treatment measurably improve the quality of a person's life or life expectancy? Would others benefit more? Who decides on the quality of another person's life? Who makes the decision as to who lives and who dies? What determines quality of life? Some suggested criteria include ability to work, ability to physically function, chronological age, contributions to society, happiness or satisfaction with life, ability to care for oneself, and the person and family's opinions.

Nurses' Role Regarding Ethics

You are expected to practice ethically. Because of the intimate nature of nursing, you are often the first person to recognize that an ethical problem exists. You are responsible for bringing forth these issues and for participating in decision-making. Box 4-3 presents a code of ethics for nurses. Whether nursing practice occurs in the United States, Canada, or the international community, basic ideas remain the same.

➤➤ BOX 4-3

THE CODE OF ETHICS FOR LPN/LVNs

This Code, adopted by NFLPN/LVN in 1961 and most recently revised in 1996, "provides a motivation for establishing, maintaining, and elevation of professional standards. Each LP/VN, upon entering the profession, inherits the responsibility to adhere to the standards of ethical practice and conduct as set forth in this Code."

- Know the scope of maximum utilization of the LP/VN as specified by the Nursing Practice Act, and function within this scope.
- Safeguard the confidential information acquired from any source about the patient.
- Provide healthcare to all patients regardless of race, creed, cultural background, disease, or lifestyle.
- Refuse to give endorsement to the sale and promotion of commercial products or services.
- Uphold the highest standards in personal appearance, language, dress, and demeanor.
- Stay informed about issues affecting the practice of nursing and the delivery of healthcare and, when appropriate, participate in government and policy decisions.
- Accept the responsibility for safe nursing by keeping oneself mentally and physically fit and educationally prepared to practice.
- Accept responsibility for membership in (professional organizations) and participate in efforts to maintain the established standards of nursing practice and employment policies that lead to quality patient care.

National Federation of Licensed Practical Nurses, Inc. (1996). *Nursing practice standards for the licensed practical/vocational nurse* (rev.). Raleigh, NC: Author.

Ethical Issues in Treatment

Examples of some major issues in healthcare ethics are presented below. Some issues that were mentioned in the legal section of this chapter are also issues for ethical debate.

Organ Transplantation. Many organs are successfully transplanted from person to person. In some cases, as in heart transplant, the donor must be pronounced legally dead before the organ be can be removed. To keep the organ at its healthiest, however, it must be recovered at the moment the donor is pronounced clinically dead. In most cases, circulation and ventilation are artificially maintained until the organ is removed.

These situations involve such issues as defining clinical death and informed consent. Organ donation is a difficult decision for a family to make at such a traumatic time. A person can simplify matters in advance by designating that he or she wishes to be an organ donor on an organ donor card or a driver's license.

The **United Network of Organ Sharing (UNOS)** was established to ensure fairness in the receipt of donated organs. This computerized network links all procurement organizations and maintains a list of potential organ recipients. UNOS has established specific criteria to determine which recipient will be eligible to receive a donated organ. It is not possible to purchase an organ, nor is it possible to guarantee that a particular recipient will receive a donated organ (except in the case of a living related donor).

☞ Key Concept

Even if a person designates himself or herself as a "donor" on a driver's license, the next-of-kin usually must give permission after death. If you wish to be an organ donor, discuss your feelings with your family now.

Who Should Receive Treatment? Other factors may influence decisions to give or to withhold treatment. Who will pay for the treatment, which sometimes amounts to hundreds of thousands of dollars? Should treatment be given, even against the person's will? (If the healthcare team makes this decision, it is called *beneficence.* If the client makes the decision, it is termed *autonomy.*) Can a client legally refuse treatment? Under what circumstances does the client lose this right?

Refusal of Treatment. Usually a person gives permission for treatment; thus, refusal is seen as reversal of that permission. States debate the individual's right to refuse life-saving treatment. If any argument among family members or doubt on the part of the healthcare team exists, *treatment must be given* until the case is resolved in court. A court order must be obtained before treatment may be withheld or removed. (If a person refuses treatment and it is illegally given, however, this may constitute battery on the part of the healthcare team.)

The only time a person does not have the right to make the decision to refuse treatment is when the greater public interest would be in danger. For example, if a person has a communicable disease or is in immediate danger of harming self or others and refuses treatment, legal action may be taken.

Termination of Treatment. Termination of treatment, or withdrawal of treatment, involves the conscious decision to stop treatment once it has been started. The treatment may be withdrawn at the client's request or when the healthcare team determines brain death has occurred. Stopping treatment once it has begun is often more difficult legally than is withholding treatment altogether.

- *Withholding treatment.* Withholding treatment means denial of treatment or care because treatment has been deemed inappropriate, not enough of a particular treatment is available (as in donor kidneys or dialysis), or the client or family has refused it.
- *Euthanasia.* In the past, euthanasia was called "mercy killing." It meant the deliberate taking of a person's life to put the individual out of misery. This definition has been amended to include the withdrawal or withholding of treatment.

A great deal of discussion and controversy has occurred in recent years **about assisted suicide.** The laws surrounding this ethical problem differ among states.

The Ethics Committee

Healthcare facilities have ethics committees made up of healthcare professionals, chaplains, social workers, and others. The chief functions of the ethics committee are education, policy-making, case review, and consultation. These committees are important because they bring together a variety of healthcare workers from various disciplines. They are able to share ideas and concerns related to their field. Many nurses bring a unique voice to the committee because they act as an advocate for their clients (Fig 4-4).

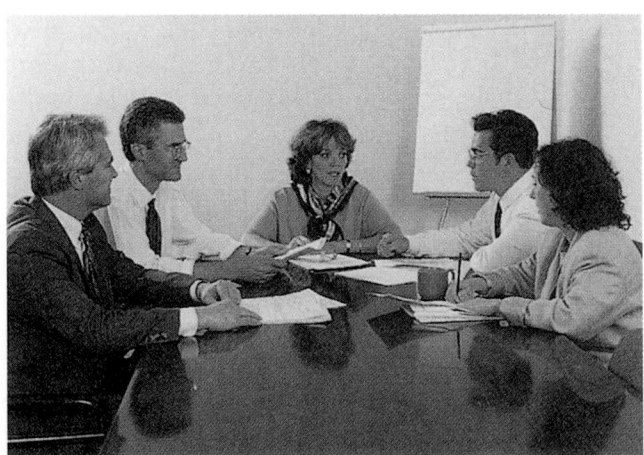

FIGURE 4-4. The Ethics Committee may comprise nurses, physicians, social workers, religious leaders, and community members. (Hosley, J. B., Jones, S. A., & Molle-Matthews, E. A. [1997]. *Lippincott's textbook for medical assistants,* [p. 23]. Philadelphia: Lippincott Williams & Wilkins.)

CLIENTS' RIGHTS AND RESPONSIBILITIES

Clients also have rights and responsibilities. The concept of clients' rights stem from the rise of the consumer movement. The public demands the right to quality care.

Clients' Rights

In 1972, the **American Hospital Association (AHA)** adopted *A Patient's Bill of Rights,* which states the rights of hospitalized individuals (Box 4-4). The AHA regularly updates this information, which serves as a basis for decision-making in hospital care. This bill of rights helps to ensure the concept of basic human rights and is widely accepted among healthcare providers.

☛ KEY CONCEPT
_____

Clients are active participants in their own healthcare.

Other groups have also formulated statements about rights of the health consumer, including the **American Medical Association (AMA)** and several nurses' associations. The **National Association for Home Care (NAHC)** has issued a Client Bill of Rights similar to that of the AHA. Local and national consumer groups constantly seek quality care and accountability in the healthcare facility. The client's right to confidentiality is always important (Box 4-5).

Clients' Responsibilities

The client is an active participant in formulating his or her care plan and making healthcare decisions. Thus, the client also has a responsibility to participate in and cooperate with care given. Certain cooperative actions can be expected from clients. Your duties as a nurse are to help your clients understand their responsibilities, teach them how to enhance their recovery process, and assist them to attain their greatest level of health and wellness. Reasonably request and expect the following of your clients:

➤➤ BOX 4-4

PATIENT/CLIENT'S BILL OF RIGHTS

The American Hospital Association first adopted *A Patient's Bill of Rights* in 1972, and revised it in 1992. Other organizations have created similar documents. The rights within such documents can be exercised on a patient's behalf by a designated individual if the patient lacks decision-making capacity, is legally incompetent, or is a minor. The intention of the bill of rights is to promote the interests and well-being of all clients in healthcare facilities. No facility can make a person waive his or her rights to be admitted. Patients/clients are expected to participate in their own care. Effectiveness of care depends in part on their fulfillment of certain responsibilities.

Patients/clients have the following rights:

- To receive considerate and respectful care
- To obtain relevant, current, and understandable information about diagnosis, treatment, and prognosis; to discuss and request information related to specific procedures and treatments, risks involved, possible length of recuperation, and medically reasonable alternatives
- To know the identity of caregivers, including students
- To know financial implications of treatment choices and available payment methods
- To make decisions about the plan of care
- To refuse recommended treatments or plans of care and the medical consequences (unless mandated by law) and, if refusing, to receive other appropriate care or transfer to another facility
- To have an advance directive or to designate a surrogate decision-maker

- To be advised of their rights under state law
- To have every consideration of privacy—all communications and records pertaining to their care will be treated as confidential (except in cases of suspected abuse or public health hazard)
- To review their medical records and have them explained (unless restricted by law)
- To expect the facility to respond reasonably to requests for appropriate and medically indicated care and services
- To expect evaluation, services, and referrals, as indicated by urgency of the case
- To be transferred to another safe and legal facility if needed; risks and benefits must be explained
- To be informed about business relationships among the healthcare facility, educational institutions, other providers, and third-party payers that may influence care
- To consent or to refuse to participate in research or human experimentation and to have such studies fully explained prior to consent; refusal must not alter care given
- To expect reasonable continuity of care and to be informed when care from the facility is no longer appropriate
- To be informed of healthcare facility policies and practices relating to care, treatment, and responsibilities
- To be informed of resources for resolving disputes, grievances, and conflicts
- To expect efficient and equitable care to be given to others and to the community

Adapted from: American Hospital Association. (1992). *A patient's bill of rights.* Chicago: Author

➤➤ BOX 4-5

RIGHT TO CONFIDENTIALITY

The client has the right to expect that his or her privacy will be protected. *Privacy* means that information is available to the client, but not to the public. Information collected may be used to provide effective care, to develop treatment guidelines, to determine ability to pay for care, to bill third-party payers, and to anonymously conduct research studies. The client may refuse to give information, but in this case, the quality of care may be limited by lack of information.

• To provide, to the best of their knowledge, accurate and complete information about matters relating to their health
• To be responsible for understanding their diagnosis/treatment
• To follow the recommended treatment plan
• To be responsible for their own actions if they refuse treatment, do not follow instructions, leave the healthcare facility, or terminate services against advice
• To report changes in their condition
• To keep appointments
• To meet financial obligations related to healthcare

☞ Key Concept

The nurse or physician also has the right to bring charges against a client for an unlawful act, such as a physical attack.

➤ STUDENT SYNTHESIS

Key Points

• You are legally and ethically bound to practice nursing within the rules and regulations of your Nursing Practice Act and within the laws of your state, territory, or province.
• Several types of advance directives allow individuals to plan ahead and to make decisions in advance about healthcare to be received if they become incapacitated.
• Individuals have the right to accept or to refuse treatment in most situations.
• You will encounter many ethical decisions in healthcare. Some of these require the assistance of an ethics committee.

Critical Thinking Exercises

1. Discuss how your personal values relate to your choice of nursing as a profession. Discuss how you think this will relate to your nursing practice in the future.
2. As you come on duty, you check your client's chart and notice that he received an injection of Demerol 100 mg at 2:00 pm and again at 3:30 pm today. Two different nurses administered these injections. Administration of the medication is ordered for every 4 hours.
   a. What actions would you take and why?
   b. What legal implications apply to this situation?
   c. Discuss this situation in relationship to the importance of documentation.
   d. Has a crime been committed? Why or why not?
3. You see a licensed nurse at the facility where you work take some money out of a coworker's backpack. What actions would you take and why? How does this scenario affect your coworker's nursing license? How could it affect your nursing license (if you were licensed at this time)?
4. You are working part-time in a hospital while you attend school. A client there is being discharged tomorrow and asks you on a date next Saturday. (Assume that you are single and find the client attractive.)
   a. What is your response? Why?
   b. What are the legal implications of dating a client?

NCLEX-Style Review Questions

1. What standard of care is the vocational nursing student held to when providing care normally performed by a licensed vocational nurse?
   a. The student is held to the same standard as the licensed vocational nurse.
   b. The student is held to the same standard as an unlicensed person.
   c. The student is not responsible for his or her actions; the nursing instructor is responsible.
   d. The student is not responsible for his or her actions.
2. Which of the following is the nurse's responsibility in obtaining informed consent?
   a. Ask the physician to complete the form.
   b. Confirm that the signed consent is in the chart prior to the procedure.
   c. Explain all risks, complications, and alternative treatment to the client.
   d. The nurse has no responsibility with informed consent.
3. Safeguards for the nurse and student nurse against litigation include:
   a. Ask for help only when absolutely necessary.
   b. Document briefly at the end of each shift.
   c. Follow accepted procedures.
   d. Try to keep up on current trends when time allows.

Reference

1. Venes, D., & Thomas, C. L. (Eds.) (2001). *Taber's cyclopedic medical dictionary* (19th ed.). Philadelphia: F. A. Davis.

Unit II

PERSONAL AND ENVIRONMENTAL HEALTH

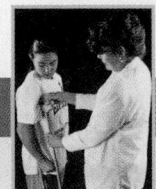

CHAPTER

5

Basic Human Needs

LEARNING OBJECTIVES

1. Describe and discuss the hierarchy of needs, from the simple to the complex, as developed by Maslow.
2. Define the term regression and explain at least two examples of regression.
3. List at least five physiologic needs of all people and animals.
4. List five examples of nursing activities that help an individual meet basic physiologic human needs.
5. List four examples of nursing activities that help an individual meet the needs of security and safety.
6. List two examples of nursing activities that help an individual obtain the goal of self-esteem.
7. List two examples of nursing activities that help an individual obtain the goal of self-actualization.
8. Address the basic and aesthetic needs of individuals who are homeless, or who have a terminal illness, or who have lost their jobs and source of income.
9. Relate at least three community or societal needs to the hierarchy of needs of an individual.

NEW TERMINOLOGY

aesthetic needs
hierarchy of needs
physiologic needs
primary needs
psychological needs
regression

secondary needs
self-actualized
self-esteem
social needs
survival needs

In 1943, psychologist Abraham H. Maslow described a theory of human needs, which identified simple basic needs in relation to the more complex, higher lever needs. These needs are common to all people regardless of age, sex, race, social class, and state of health (well or ill). Maslow asserted that people respond to needs and need satisfaction as whole and integrated beings.

Nursing has been defined as a helping relationship. As a nurse, you will help people to satisfy their basic needs and to reduce threats to this need fulfillment. Dorothea Orem's theory of nursing (see Chap. 2) and many nursing programs and textbooks are based on Maslow's theory of needs. This textbook incorporates Maslow's hierarchy of needs. Most types of nursing care are prioritized using the same hierarchy. This chapter summarizes human needs and explains their relationship to health and nursing care.

MASLOW'S HIERARCHY OF NEEDS

Maslow defined the basic needs of all people as a progression from simple physical needs (needed for survival) to more complex ones, called **aesthetic needs.** He called this progression a **hierarchy of needs.** On this hierarchy or ladder (Fig. 5-1), needs are ranked by their importance to the individual's survival.

A person must meet the needs at the foundation of the hierarchy before working toward meeting higher-level needs.

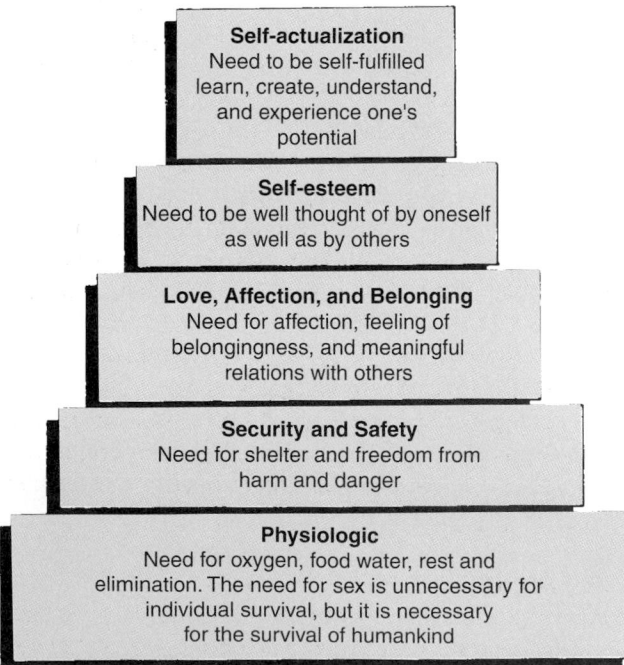

FIGURE 5-1. Hierarchy of needs. According to Maslow, basic physiologic needs, such as for food and water, must be met before a person can move on to higher-level needs, such as security and safety. Nursing is based on helping people to meet the needs they cannot meet by themselves because of age, illness, or injury.

Individuals must meet needs at the first level, such as oxygen and food, to survive.

After they meet their basic **survival needs,** people can progress to more complex needs such as safety, love, and self-esteem. For example, people who are hungry will not be concerned about cleanliness or learning until they are fed. Individuals in pain will not be concerned about personal appearance or relationships with others until pain is relieved. Those facing surgery will not be able to learn about the operation unless they feel safe and secure. **Regression,** or focusing on a lower-level need that has already been fulfilled, is common in illness or injury. For example, a client recovering from an illness will focus on physical and emotional energies on recovery (**physical needs**) before returning to employment (security).

NURSING'S RELATIONSHIP TO BASIC NEEDS

Illness or risk for illness occurs when people are unable to satisfy one or more of their basic needs independently. Much of your nursing career will center on assisting people to meet these needs. Nursing also involves helping people to avoid risks or threats to their basic human needs. You will be helping others to prevent complications before they begin.

Many situations will arise in which you will assist clients to meet their needs. You may feed an infant, provide full range of motion for a person who has had a stroke, give a tube feeding to a person who cannot swallow, bathe a person who is in a full body cast, or play with a child. You may encourage the recovering person to attend to personal care, visit with someone who is lonely or frightened, or arrange for a social worker or a member of the clergy to visit. This text discusses needs common to all people *and* individual needs that may be unique. Illness may modify a person's perception of his or her needs. As a result, the client's "need priority" may differ from what you would expect. Illness or injury may present a block or obstacle to the meeting of needs. Nursing tries to help remove those obstacles.

Meeting needs is a process; it is never static. In addition, needs are interrelated and some needs depend on others.

☛ KEY CONCEPT

Nursing is concerned with helping people meet their needs. Much of nursing deals with assisting clients to meet basic physiologic needs that they cannot meet independently.

In many cases, the nurse can determine the client's level of need satisfaction by looking at him or her. For example, the nurse can estimate oxygenation by looking for cyanosis (blueness of skin) and difficulty breathing. Listening to the client is also helpful. The client may tell the nurse that he or she is hungry, thirsty, or in pain.

☛ KEY CONCEPT

Basic needs are common to all people; thus, basic needs are universal. *Individuals of all cultures have basic needs; in other words, basic needs are* transcultural—*across all cultures. Needs can be satisfied or they can be blocked.*

OVERVIEW OF INDIVIDUAL NEEDS

Basic Physiologic Needs

First-level needs are called **physiologic needs,** survival needs, or primary needs. Without them, a person or animal will die. They take precedence over higher-level needs. Primary needs must be met to sustain life; **secondary needs** are met to give quality to life.

☛ KEY CONCEPT
_____

Primary needs must be met to maintain life. *Secondary needs* must be met to maintain quality of life.

Oxygen

Oxygen is the most essential of all basic survival needs. Without oxygen circulating in the bloodstream, a person will die in a matter of minutes. Oxygen is provided to the cells by maintaining an open airway and adequate circulation.

As a nurse, you will constantly evaluate the oxygenation status of your clients. Various situations can threaten the body's oxygen supply. For example, emphysema, asthma, paralysis, or secretions may make breathing difficult; circulation may be impaired, thus preventing oxygen from reaching the cells. Some breathing difficulties also have an emotional component.

Water and Fluids

Water is necessary to sustain life. The body can survive only a few days without water, although certain conditions may alter this length of time. For example, the person in a very hot climate needs more water and fluids to sustain life than the person in a cold climate. The fluids in the body must also be in balance, or homeostasis, to maintain health.

Examples of conditions in which individuals may require assistance to meet their fluid needs include unconsciousness, inability to swallow, and severe mental illness. If the kidneys do not function, the body may retain water in the tissues (edema) or the body may not have enough water (dehydration). The nurse can assist in these conditions by measuring intake and output, weighing the client daily, and observing intravenous infusion of fluids.

Food and Nutrients

Nutrients are necessary to maintain life, although the body can survive for several days or weeks without food. Poor nutritional habits, inability to chew or swallow, nausea and vomiting, food allergies, refusal to eat, and overeating pose threats to a client's nutritional status. The nurse helps by feeding the client monitoring calorie counts or maintaining alternative methods of nutrition such as tube feedings.

Elimination of Waste Products

Elimination of the body's waste products is essential for life and comfort. The body eliminates wastes in several ways. The lungs eliminate carbon dioxide and water; the skin eliminates water and sodium; the kidneys eliminate fluids and electro-lytes; the intestines discharge solid wastes and fluids. ι body should inappropriately allow wastes to accumulate, ma⸗ serious conditions can result.

A bowel obstruction, bladder cancer, kidney disease, and gallbladder disease disrupt normal elimination. Difficulty in breathing, poor circulation, acid–base imbalance, allergies, cuts, wounds, diabetes, and infection also hinder adequate elimination.

The nurse may help the client eliminate wastes by giving an enema, catheterizing the person, or assisting with dialysis. You may assist with surgery to eliminate a bowel obstruction and administer medications to relieve diarrhea or constipation. You may give oxygen to assist with breathing. You may inject insulin for the diabetic client to aid in proper carbohydrate metabolism.

Sleep and Rest

Sleep and rest are important in maintaining health. The amount of sleep that people need varies; factors such as pregnancy, age, and general health have an influence. The absence of sleep is not immediately life threatening, but can cause various disorders if allowed to continue. For example, sleep deprivation aggravates some forms of mental illness.

The nurse can assist clients to get enough sleep and rest by providing safe, comfortable, and quiet surroundings. Various treatments such as a soothing back rub, warm tub bath, warm milk, and certain medications can also promote sleep.

Activity and Exercise

Activity stimulates both the mind and body. Exercise helps maintain the body's structural integrity and health by enhancing circulation and respiration. Mobility is not necessary for survival, but some form of exercise is needed to maintain optimum health.

The nurse can assist the client to obtain needed exercise in many ways. Examples include encouraging a person to walk after surgery, teaching a client to walk with crutches, providing passive range of motion, and teaching the person in a cast to do exercises. Clients in nursing homes are encouraged to exercise, even if they are confined to wheelchairs. Physical therapists and nurses work together to assist clients with rehabilitation of injured bones and muscles. The person who is paralyzed from the waist down can do push-ups in bed and many other upper body exercises. Turning the immobilized person often helps to prevent lung problems, skin breakdown, circulatory problems, bowel obstruction, and pressure ulcers (bedsores).

Sexual Gratification

Sexual gratification is important; however, unlike other basic physiologic needs, sexual gratification may be sublimated. The need for sex is not vital to the survival of the individual, but it is vital to the survival of the species.

The nurse will need to be aware of sexuality issues when care is given. Perhaps an older male client is not comfortable with a younger male or female nurse. A client may also wish to discuss sexual problems with you. As part of the assessment, the nurse may learn that he client has concerns relating to sexual issues. For example, the client recovering from surgery may be concerned about the physical effects of sexual intercourse on a healing incision. Remember that age or physical disability usually does not eliminate a person's desire for sexual activity.

Security and Safety Needs

The second level of Maslow's hierarchy of needs relates to safety. At this level, there are both physical and **psychological needs** (Fig. 5-2).

Freedom from Harm
People must feel safe and secure, both physically and emotionally, before being comfortable enough to move on to meet other needs. They must feel free from harm, danger, and fear. Characteristics of safety include predictability, stability, and familiarity, as well as feeling safe and comfortable and trusting other people. Financial security is also a component of this need.

Safety adaptations are made for age, whether the person is old or very young. The person who is physically challenged often needs special adaptations. The nurse may assist in removing threats to safety from the client's environment. Examples include using proper handwashing techniques, preventing wound infections by using sterile dressings, using a night light, disabling the gas stove in the home of a person with Alzheimer's disease, and locking up poisons in the home to safeguard small children. The nurse can explain to clients their surgical procedure before surgery, as well as any other treatments or medications. Such discussion can help clients feel safer and can aid in postoperative recovery.

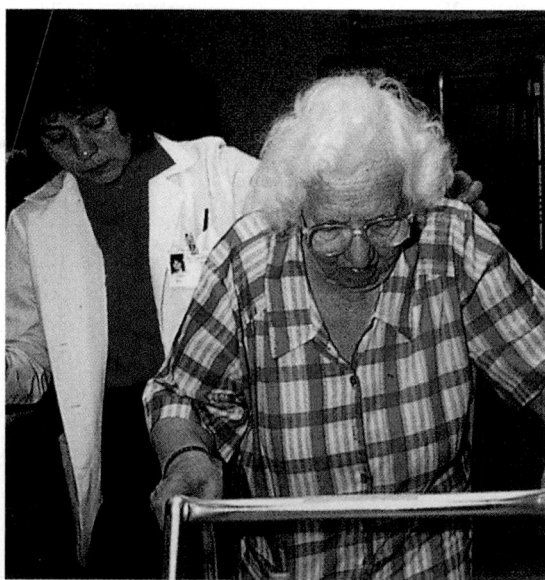

FIGURE 5-2. Security and safety needs can be met by helping the client ambulate using a walker. Notice how the nurse uses her body position and her arms to anticipate helping the client in case of loss of balance.

☛ KEY CONCEPT

Any type of abuse is a threat to the basic need for safety and security. If a person feels unsafe, he or she cannot pursue higher level needs.

Abuse.   Abuse within the home has always existed. Society is becoming less tolerant of all types of domestic abuse. Legal penalties for abuse are becoming more severe. Abuse may take the form of spousal or partner battering, child abuse, or rape by family members or others. Often, people find it difficult to escape from abusive situations for many reasons. Resources within the community can assist victims. The nurse is legally bound to report any suspected abuse in the clients. Remember that abuse also can occur in the healthcare facility. Abuse must be reported immediately.

✚⊙   **N u r s i n g   A l e r t**
If you, as a nurse, do not report suspected abuse, you could be subject to arrest and civil penalties.

Healthcare.   Consider higher-level coping skills in relationship to planned versus unplanned healthcare. People who are living in poverty, starving, homeless, or who feel unsafe are unable to plan ahead for healthcare. In addition, some people are disabled by mental illness or chronic abuse of drugs. In most cases, people in these situations become ill first and then seek healthcare. Such behaviors are concrete methods of dealing with illness, or emergency responses to the stimulus of illness (episodic healthcare). People in developing countries often have no access at all to healthcare. Their healthcare needs are unmet, thus shortening their life expectancy.

People in more comfortable situations are able to strive for wellness and prevention of illness (see Chap. 6). They experience a more abstract means of coping and of seeking healthcare. Abstract thinking and action require higher-level skills, including planning and being able to understand the consequences of being unprepared.

Shelter
The lack of adequate shelter may not always be life threatening, but will thwart the ability of a person to progress toward a higher level of needs. A person's shelter should provide the warmth necessary to maintain an adequate body temperature, in addition to helping the person feel safe.

A large number of Americans are homeless, including growing numbers of children. Often, healthcare providers are unaware that a client is homeless. Be alert when interviewing clients; a comprehensive evaluation is often needed to uncover this situation because the person may be embarrassed or ashamed.

The homeless person with children to care for faces great problems. Such individuals not only must find food and shelter for themselves, but for their children as well. Safety is an issue, because it is more difficult to protect themselves and their children at the same time. The children lack a sense of security because they do not know where they belong and often do not understand what is happening.

The homeless spend most of their energy trying to cope with daily life. They may travel great distances by foot to locate food and other necessities. They face the constant dangers of disease, frostbite, or physical harm from others. They often must move from place to place, sometimes to avoid the law or to fulfill time limits in shelters. Many homeless people carry all their belongings with them to avoid theft. With all of these contributing factors, these individuals have little emotional energy left to worry about meaningful relationships, belonging to a group, maintaining cleanliness, or going to school. No time exists to be creative. Finding a permanent job without an address or telephone is almost impossible, adding to despair and hopelessness. These people are often mired at the lower levels of the basic needs hierarchy.

Healthcare for the homeless is a problem that many areas are addressing. Some community health and public agencies have nursing services that provide outreach, health assessment, and health monitoring programs for individuals and families. For example, screening these individuals for tuberculosis and other communicable diseases and giving immunizations to the children are important both to the individual as well as to the health of the public.

Temperature Regulation

Several factors can threaten the body's need for temperature regulation, including excessive external heat or cold or a high internal fever in response to an infection. The human body functions within a relatively narrow survival range of temperatures. Core temperature survival ranges for the human body (under usual circumstances) are given below using equivalent values from the Celsius and Fahrenheit scales:

35°C to 41°C; "Normal oral temperature" = 37°C
95°F to 106°F; "Normal oral temperature" = 98.6°F

The body has mechanisms to assist in temporary regulation of body temperature. These mechanisms include shivering, goose flesh, and perspiration. The nurse will assist clients to meet the need for temperature regulation in cases such as a severe burn, a high fever, or exposure to extreme heat (heat stroke) or cold (hypothermia, frostbite) by monitoring the client's temperature and providing treatment for the effects of thermal damage.

Love, Affection, and Belonging

Societal Needs

Social needs are addressed in the third level of Maslow's hierarchy. The needs for love, affection, and belonging are fundamental human needs; however, people must meet survival and security needs before they can address social needs. Love and affection begin with bonding between the infant and mother at birth and must continue throughout life for a person to meet needs at this level. All people need to feel that they have meaningful relationships with others and that they belong to a group. People need the acceptance of their families and friends. The elderly person and the young person in society often have much in common in that they may not feel

a part of a group. They may feel that they are not useful or appreciated. Encouragement and assurance from loved ones can help to alleviate such anxieties.

When an ill or injured person is in a healthcare facility, he or she is often separated from friends and family. The person who is confined to home may also lack social contacts. Many people are very frightened and do not feel safe, especially when they are ill. The nurse can assist these people by encouraging visitors, cards, and telephone calls, and by visiting with the client whenever possible. Explain to the client's family that the person needs more reassurance and acceptance if he or she is disfigured or disabled in any way. Clients being cared for at home need social support, stimulation, and encouragement from nurses and their loved ones. Do not forget the universal need for diversion, recreation, and social interactions.

☛ KEY CONCEPT

A need at any given level of the hierarchy is more urgent to the person if the needs below it are satisfied. Thus, a person who is not preoccupied with obtaining oxygen and finding food will be able to be concerned with love and belonging.

Spiritual Needs

Many people believe in a higher power. This power takes many different forms, depending on one's religious background, ethnicity, and life experiences. The person who is ill or injured may find comfort in spirituality. The nurse can help clients to meet their spiritual needs by assisting them to worship services, by providing reading or video materials, or by contacting the client's clergy person or the chaplain of the healthcare facility.

Self-esteem Needs

The term **self-esteem** (self-image, self-respect) is related to the person's perception of self. Positive self-esteem is an appreciation of one's own personal worth. A person who feels that his or her contributions are appreciated (by family, friends, employers) is more likely to have self-confidence. People meet their esteem needs when they think well of themselves (through achievement, adequacy, competence) and are well thought of by others (through recognition, status, awards, prestige).

Those who are ill or injured or who undergo surgery may have altered levels of self-esteem. This scenario is often true in situations that change a client's appearance and lifestyle, such as amputation of a limb. Many women experience difficulty with their self-image after a hysterectomy or breast removal. As a nurse, you will be able to assist such individuals to regain positive self-esteem by encouraging independence, by rewarding progress, and by allowing them to perform as much self-care as possible. Observe these clients for symptoms of regression, depression, over-dependency, or a refusal to cooperate. Low self-esteem also directly relates to disorders such as chemical dependency. See Box 5-1 for examples of nursing interventions throughout the hierarchy of needs.

➤➤ BOX 5-1

HIERARCHY OF NEEDS AND NURSING INTERVENTIONS

Nursing actions and Maslow's hierarchy can take many forms. This box gives examples of nursing interventions that can assist a client to meet basic and aesthetic human needs. The hierarchy begins at the bottom and works upward.

Self-Actualization

Acknowledging the accomplishments of the individual.

Self-Esteem

Promoting positive self-image after surgery.
Encouraging an individual's progress in rehabilitation.
Providing an opportunity for bonding with a new infant.

Love, Affection, and Belonging

Allowing the client's family to visit while in the hospital.
Encouraging the family to participate in the care of the client.
Allowing religious leaders and friends to visit and perform religious rites.
Being sensitive to a client's particular needs as it relates to his or her role in society, eg, financial provider, caretaker of others, or person with a disability.

Security and Safety

Checking identification of client prior to administering medication.
Taking defective equipment from a client's environment and reporting the defect.
Monitoring the client's safety while in the shower, ambulating in the hall, or getting in or out of bed.
Performing a safety check in the home environment for a child or an elderly adult.
Reporting abuse to the proper authority.

Basic Physiologic Needs

Administering oxygen.
Assisting with feeding a client.
Assisting with hygiene and elimination.
Maintaining warmth for a newborn.

☛ KEY CONCEPT

There is danger that the needs of the nurse can influence the level of nursing care. Be careful not to let this endanger your client!

Self-actualization Needs

The **self-actualized** person has "reached his or her full potential." Thus, needs at this level are the highest-order needs. The self-actualized person is comfortable enough to plan ahead and to be creative. Great artists and musicians are often functioning in the self-actualized sphere. The person incorporates all levels to function as a self-actualized person. As with other

levels of Maslow's hierarchy, lower-level needs must first be satisfied before the person can work at self-actualization. Remember that people can function partially on this level, even though all other needs have not been met. Those who are comfortable with themselves and their place in the world have the emotional energy to plan, to learn, and to create.

The term *self-actualized* implies a fully functioning person. Maslow described this state as a "more comfortable relationship with reality." The self-actualized person is able to cope with life's situations, to deal with failure, and to be free of anxiety. This person has a sense of humor, is self-controlled, and is able to deal with stress in productive ways. Self-actualization can take the form of being a better person, obtaining an education, being a good parent, or learning to grow roses.

Many psychologists believe that people reach this level many times throughout life, yet very few people believe they have reached the peak of self-actualization permanently. An individual who has met his or her highest goal is most likely to continue to create new personal or professional goals. Thus, the process of becoming self-actualized continually flows as new goals are born, develop, and are achieved. As a nursing student, you are striving toward self-actualization as well, and you will continue to strive toward new achievements as your career develops (Fig. 5-3).

While in your nursing program, you would be wise to think about Maslow's hierarchy of needs. You will do much better in your nursing program if you do not have to worry about where you will live, whether or not you and your children are safe, or if you have enough money for food. Basic needs must be met first. When these primary needs are met, then the individual will have physical and psychological energy to reach the higher levels of the pyramid.

☛ KEY CONCEPT

Homelessness is a threat to the person's basic need for warmth, shelter, and safety. If a person is responsible for others, such as children, the threats multiply. The higher needs of self-esteem or aesthetics cannot be addressed at all.

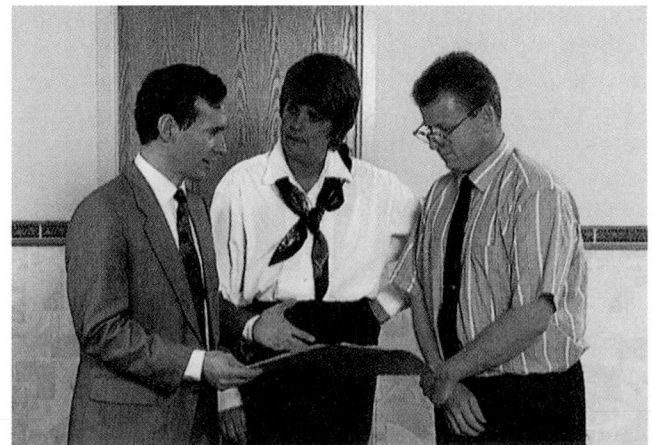

FIGURE 5-3. One way of achieving self-esteem is by having good working relationships with your peers. Self-actualization needs can be met by being allowed to succeed in personal endeavors.

FAMILY AND COMMUNITY NEEDS

The family unit has needs that must be met for life to run smoothly. The special needs of the family include developmental tasks and functions to meet the needs of its members. The highly functioning family also works toward common goals as a group. Chapter 9 describes family development in more detail. Needs are met in a variety of family structures.

The community has basic needs concerning the welfare of all its residents. Among these needs are public health measures (such as immunization programs), access to healthcare, maintenance services (such as water and electricity), environmental concerns (pollution), safety (police and highways), and emergency services (ambulances and paramedics). Chapter 7 discusses issues involving community health.

➤ STUDENT SYNTHESIS

Key Points

- Physiologic needs drive all human beings and animals.
- Human needs are thought of in progressive levels, known as a *hierarchy*.
- Psychological needs are at a higher level than physiologic needs.
- A person must meet lower-level needs before he or she can address higher-level needs.
- Illness or injury can interfere with a person's ability to meet basic needs.
- Illness or injury can also cause a person to regress to a lower level of functioning.
- Nursing can assist a person to meet needs or to eliminate potential threats to need satisfaction.
- Many factors, such as loss of income, illness, homelessness, and personal crises threaten basic human needs.
- Health is a continually fluctuating and fluid state of physiologic and psychological well-being.
- Relationships with others, including family and the community, are higher-level needs that can be addressed only after basic physiologic needs are met.

Critical Thinking Exercises

1. Describe how you are meeting your higher-level needs while you are a nursing student.
2. Reflect on a time when you were unable to pursue higher-level needs because one or more of your basic needs were not being satisfied. Examine ways you altered this situation to meet your needs.
3. Consider the care of a client who does not speak the same language as you. Discuss possible client needs that may be unmet. Determine any considerations for you to take to improve quality of care.
4. Using Maslow's hierarchy of needs, discuss possible unmet needs for the following: a person who has been evicted, a client in a nursing home with no immediate family, a mother of triplets, a person who has difficulty breathing, and a nursing student during exam week.

NCLEX-Style Review Questions

1. According to Maslow, which of the following needs would have priority for an individual?
   a. Be well thought of by others
   b. Experience one's potential
   c. Obtain food
   d. Protect against danger
2. Which of the following nursing actions would help a client meet security and safety needs?
   a. Assist client to eat
   b. Encourage client to walk after surgery
   c. Provide a soothing back rub
   d. Report signs of abuse
3. During an illness, it is not uncommon for a client to focus on a lower level of need. This is called:
   a. Aesthetic needs
   b. Regression
   c. Survival
   d. Secondary needs

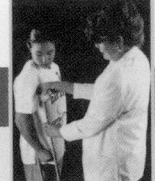

CHAPTER

6

Health and Wellness

LEARNING OBJECTIVES

1. State the World Health Organization's definition of health.
2. List five components of health and describe how each is attained.
3. Define and differentiate the terms morbidity and mortality.
4. Discuss at least four nursing implications related to the financing of healthcare.
5. State at least three preventive healthcare measures that have benefited American society.
6. Explain the wellness–illness continuum. Discuss the implications of acute and chronic illnesses as part of the continuum.
7. Relate the concept of wellness to Maslow's hierarchy of human needs.
8. Define and differentiate the terms lifestyle factor and risk factor.
9. State at least five lifestyle or risk factors that can directly affect health. Identify at least three nursing considerations for each factor.
10. List at least four sources of healthcare education and information.
11. Identify at least three health concerns of each of the following age groups: infants, children, adolescents and young adults, mature adults, and older adults. State at least four nursing implications related to each.
12. Identify at least nine categories of diseases or disorders that are deviations from wellness.

NEW TERMINOLOGY

acute illness	illness
benign	infection
carcinogenic	lifestyle factor
chronic illness	local
congenital disorders	malignant
contagious	metastasis
defense mechanisms	morbidity
disease	mortality
domestic violence	neoplastic
dysfunctional	organic disease
elder abuse	osteoporosis
etiology	preterm birth
functional disease	risk factor
health	stress
hereditary	systemic
homeostasis	wellness
hypertension	

ACRONYMS

CAD	MI	SIDS
CHD	MVA	STD
COPD	NCHS	WHO
CVA	PSA	

As a nurse, you will be a component of a complex healthcare system that involves local, state, national, and global health issues and trends. Nurses are affected directly and indirectly by these concerns.

Healthcare issues and trends are important concepts for society in general. As a student and later in your career, you must be aware of the broadest issues affecting healthcare, such as the complexities of healthcare finance. You should understand the factors that contribute to a healthy lifestyle and practice them. Risk factors of health need to be recognized. You will need to understand your client's changing healthcare concerns throughout his or her lifetime.

Nurses need to be able to answer questions on multiple topics accurately and to refer clients to appropriate resources when necessary. You will also serve as an example to clients, your family, and others.

HEALTH AND WELLNESS

The World Health Organization (**WHO**) was established by the United Nations in 1948 to improve worldwide health. Since then, WHO has promoted a global social conscience of healthcare and health reform. Box 6-1 summarizes the major achievements and future goals of WHO.

Health, according to WHO, is a state of complete physical, mental, and social well being, and not merely the absence of disease or infirmity.

Health is much more than physical well-being. Health includes the concepts of mind-body-spirit homeostasis. **Homeostasis** is the balance of all of the components of the human organism. Homeostasis implies continual adaptation to maintain a balance of sameness, that is to say, we must continuously adjust to our psychological, physical, and spiritual environment to maintain a balance.

Health influences everything in our lives. Our work, play, social, professional, and interpersonal relationships are influenced by our psychological, physical, and spiritual health. Health must be considered in its broadest, holistic sense, which includes the following components:

Physical health: Physical fitness, the body functioning at its best
Emotional health: Feelings and attitudes that make one comfortable with oneself
Psychological or *mental health:* A mind that grows and adjusts, is in control, and is free of serious stress
Social health: A sense of responsibility and caring for the health and welfare of others
Spiritual health: Inner peace and security, comfort with one's higher power, as one perceives it

Disease is a change in the structure or function of body tissues, biologic systems, or the human mind. **Illness** is the response to disease that involves a change in function. **Infection** is a change in the structure and function of body tissues caused by invasion from harmful microorganisms.

☞ KEY CONCEPT

*A person seeks professional healthcare when he or she is unable to meet needs without assistance. A person responds to threats to **wellness**; such threats may be potential, perceived, or actual.*

ENVIRONMENTAL HEALTH

Today's society confronts many problems that must be addressed in order to improve the overall health of the community. These include waterborne illnesses, lead poisoning, assorted air pollutants, radon poisoning, toxic chemicals, hazardous waste disposal, biological contamination, safe disposal of solid wastes, and food and drug safety. Chapter 7 discusses these and other environmental issues in more detail.

MORBIDITY AND MORTALITY

Morbidity refers to the number of people with an illness or disorder relative to a specific population. For example, influenza morbidity rates (percentage of persons with the disease) are released every year. Thus, the morbidity rates for influenza may be 25% of the older population in any particular year, but only 2% of the younger population for that same year.

Mortality refers to the chances of death associated with a particular illness or disorder. According to the National Center for Health Statistics (**NCHS**), the mortality rate of women dying from lung cancer increased 400% from 1960 to 1990. This increase in mortality is directly related to the increase in the number of women who started smoking during these years.

➤➤ BOX 6-1

THE ACCOMPLISHMENTS AND GOALS OF THE WORLD HEALTH ORGANIZATION

Health is a state of complete physical, mental, and social well-being and not merely the absence of disease or infirmity.

Achievements and Goals
• Eliminated smallpox
• Monitors mortality and morbidity of many diseases and disorders
• Sets standards for air, water, sanitation, and pharmaceutical preparations
• Performs field research and data collection
• Promotes social conscience and the advancement of health science throughout the world
• Eliminates polio, leprosy, iodine deficiencies, and many more area-specific infections
• Promotes health research and preventative medicine

Developed from material at the WHO Internet site: http://www.who.int/

The NCHS lists five leading causes of morbidity and mortality in the United States as follows:

- Heart disease, eg, coronary artery disease (**CAD**) and myocardial infarction (**MI**), also known as a heart attack
- Cancer
- Cerebrovascular accident (**CVA**) or stroke
- Chronic obstructive pulmonary disease (**COPD**)
- Unintentional injury

Detailed information is found at the NCHS Division of Data Services website, at http://www.cdc.gov/nchs.

Other leading causes of death include diabetes, chronic liver disease, suicide, occupational injuries, homicide, motor vehicle accidents (**MVA**), and HIV/AIDS. The morbidity and mortality rates vary from one age group to another. Lifestyle factors and risk factors influence the numbers of illnesses and deaths. Lifestyle and risk factors will be discussed later in this chapter.

Many morbidity and mortality rates could be decreased by effective preventive measures. Box 6-2 lists several informational health-related websites.

The Centers for Disease Control and Prevention (CDC) and the NCHS maintain an extensive and comprehensive Web site of information. Useful and interesting information is available on a wide range of health-related topics at http://www.cdc.gov/nchs.

FINANCES AND HEALTHCARE

The United States spends more on health than other industrialized countries. National healthcare expenditures exceed 1.15 trillion dollars a year, or about 14% of our total gross national product. Other industrialized countries spend only about 10%.[1]

Funding issues in healthcare are major concerns to clients and healthcare professionals. One factor is the willingness of the government to allocate funds to healthcare. The allocation of funds is often influenced by the political atmosphere and social priorities at that moment.

Without finances, the technical advances (such as the CT scanner seen in Figure 6-1) that occurred in industrialized countries in the late 20th century will not be able to continue. Premiums, including private and public insurance sources, for healthcare are affected. Actual costs of treatment to clients and healthcare providers are influenced by the practicality of financial support.

Countries that do not have financial resources have higher incidences of problems that could be cured or treated (eg, TB, HIV/AIDS). In our highly mobile global community, the health problems of our neighboring countries can and do become local health concerns.

Many individuals have lifetime, recurring problems that tend to worsen in severity over time. The costs of care for long-term or chronic illnesses such as diabetes and obstructive lung diseases, are huge. These costs are projected for the years 1995 to 2050 in Table 6-1.

➤➤ **BOX 6-2**

INFORMATIONAL WEBSITES FOR HEALTH AND HEALTHCARE

American Association of Diabetes Educators
http://www.aadenet.org

American Diabetes Association
http://www.diabetes.org

Centers for Disease Control and Prevention
http://www.cdc.gov/diabetes/
http://www.cdc.gov/nchs

Department of Veterans Affairs
http://www.va.gov/health/diabetes/

Health Resources and Services Administration
http://www.hrsa.dhhs.gov

Indian Health Service
http://www.ihs.gov

Juvenile Diabetes Foundation International
http://www.jdfcure.com

**National Diabetes Education Program:
A joint program of NIH & CDC**
http://ndep.nih.gov
http://www.cdc.gov/diabetes/projects/ndeps.htm

National Institute of Diabetes and Digestive and Kidney Disease of the National Institutes of Health
http://www.niddk.nih.gov

U.S. Department of Health and Human Services, Office of Minority Health
http://www.omrhc.gov

National Council of La Raza
http://www.nclr.org

Developed from material at http://www.cdc.gov/diabetes/pubs/facts/98.htm

Another lifetime, chronic illness is HIV/AIDS. The United States spends an excess of $10 billion per year on this one infection. More than half of this cost goes to medical care. Twenty percent of this money goes toward research, while 8% is used for education and prevention programs. Expensive and powerful drugs have decreased the mortality rates of AIDS in the United States. However, the morbidity rates, or rates of infection, remain steady at about 15,000 persons per day becoming infected worldwide.[1]

Healthcare trends are influenced by the current scientific knowledge of health. Examples include the knowledge of the negative effects of tobacco products and the positive effects of good nutrition. Health research has resulted in many changes in healthcare knowledge and delivery. Cures for chronic illnesses could result in more money being available for illness prevention in the future.

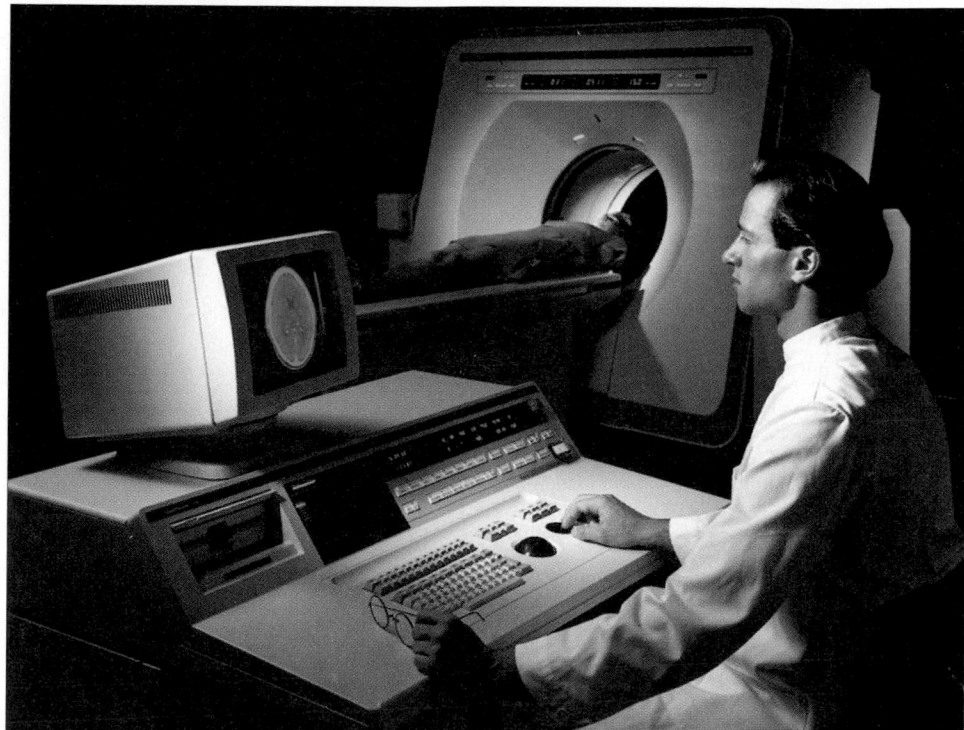

FIGURE 6-1. Computed tomography (CT) scanner. Healthcare technology has had many beneficial developments; however, they are often costly. (Cohen B., & Wood, D. [2000]. *Memmler's structure and function of the human body* [7th ed., p. 141]. Philadelphia: Lippincott Williams & Wilkins. Photo courtesy of Philips Medical Systems.)

Childhood immunizations represent a cost-effective and very efficient use of healthcare monies. The positive effects of childhood immunizations cannot be overstated. These advances were a result of combined financial and scientific resources, plus the relentless persistence of nurses, physicians, and other healthcare professionals.

PREVENTION AND HEALTHCARE

Today's healthcare system emphasizes prevention rather than treatment of disease. The WHO allocates funds, resources, and time to numerous prevention projects. The United States is stressing health and fitness on a nationwide scale.

This movement began in the early 1980s and has grown and expanded since then. healthcare providers, health insurance companies, life insurance companies, and numerous health-focused agencies (eg, American Diabetes Association, American Dietetic Association) have become heavily involved in the campaign for improved health. These groups encourage health-ier lifestyles through information campaigns designed to educate the public.

Prevention services, also called primary healthcare services, have had significant positive effects on healthcare issues such as prenatal care for mothers and infants, anti-smoking campaigns, and mammography for women. Secondary healthcare services provide individuals with specific medical or surgical therapies generally in acute care settings. Rehabilitation or tertiary services have greatly enhanced the level of health of clients with chronic illness or disability.

NHCS and CDC statistics clearly show that disparities in healthcare and preventive healthcare exist. Certain segments of the population, including low-income families, minority groups, and those facing physical disability and mental illness, encounter more difficulty in obtaining healthcare than others. These people are often unable to make lifestyle changes that could improve their health. Additionally, in order to benefit from preventive care, an individual must have physical and financial access to resources. These disparities are most evident in African American, Asian, Pan-Asian, and Hispanic

■■■ **TABLE 6-1** *E*STIMATED NUMBERS OF PEOPLE AND DIRECT MEDICAL COSTS FOR PEOPLE WITH CHRONIC CONDITIONS, SELECTED YEARS 1995–2050

	1995	2000	2005	2010	2020	2030	2040	2050
People	99 million	105 million	112 million	120 million	134 million	148 million	158 million	167 million
Dollar costs	$470 billion	$503 billion	$539 billion	$582 billion	$685 billion	$798 billion	$864 billion	$906 billion

Smeltzer, S., & Bare, B. (1999). *Brunner and Suddarth's textbook of medical-surgical nursing.* (9th ed., p. 111). Philadelphia: Lippincott Williams & Wilkins.

With permission from Robert Wood Johnson Foundation. (1996). *Chronic care in America: A 21st century challenge.* Princeton, NJ: Author.

communities. The United States must continue to focus on extending the benefits of good health to these and other vulnerable populations. Chapter 8 discusses race and ethnic diversity in more detail.

In the early 1990s, the United States Department of Health and Human Services published a report on present conditions and a comprehensive plan for future health improvement entitled *Healthy People 2000*. This report represents a strategy for significantly improving the health of the nation by preventing major chronic illnesses, injuries, and diseases. Personal responsibility is the key to good health.

The 21st century has new national goals with *Healthy People 2010*. Disease prevention and leading a healthy lifestyle are the nation's best chance at reducing the money spent each year to treat preventable illness and impairment. The individual, the community, and healthcare professionals are challenged to take specific steps to ensure good health and long life.

The health of the nation will be measured by looking at ten Leading Health Indicators. These indicators reflect major health concerns and public health issues in the United States. They are designed to motivate action and provide reliable data that reflect changes. Each indicator has one or more objectives or project goals (467 total goals) to be reached by the year 2010. The Leading Health Indicators are:

1. Physical Activity
2. Overweight and Obesity
3. Tobacco Use
4. Substance Abuse
5. Responsible Sexual Behavior
6. Mental Health
7. Injury and Violence
8. Environmental Quality
9. Immunization
10. Access to Healthcare

The data for all 467 *Healthy People 2010* objectives are updated quarterly on the National Center for Health Statistics' DATA2010 website. See http://www.health.gov/healthypeople/ LHI/1hiwhat.htm and http://www.health.gov/healthypeople/Data.

THE WELLNESS–ILLNESS CONTINUUM

Most people are not totally healthy or totally ill at any given time. An individual's daily state of health falls somewhere on a continuum from high-level wellness to death. Figure 6-2 illustrates the basic concept of the wellness–illness continuum. The state of wellness or illness fluctuates depending on the individual.

The following components contribute to a state of wellness:

• Good physical self-care
• Prevention of illness/injury
• Using one's full intellectual potential
• Expressing emotions and managing stress appropriately
• Comfortable and congenial interpersonal relationships

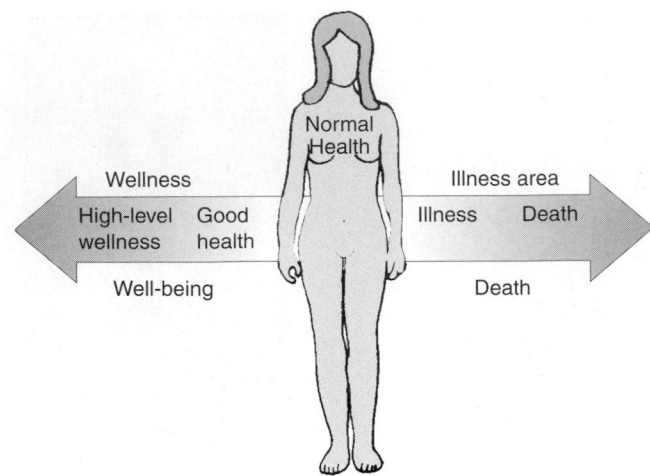

FIGURE 6-2. The wellness–illness continuum. Individuals function on a fluctuating continuum of health and illness.

• Concern about one's environment and conditions throughout the world

Acute illnesses are illnesses that interfere with the continuum for a short period of time. Acute illnesses generally develop suddenly and resolve within a specified period of time. The common cold is an acute illness. You may be ill for a few days, and then return to your normal state of health.

Chronic illnesses such as arthritis, asthma, or HIV/AIDS result in a long-term health disturbance. Individuals with chronic illnesses function within the wellness–illness continuum, but often are limited by their disorder.

A person may have an acute illness, a chronic illness, or both. It is very common for an individual with a chronic illness to become acutely ill. For example, a person might become acutely ill from a seasonal virus, or someone with a chronic illness may become unstable from an acute asthma attack. The elderly commonly have both acute and chronic illnesses. Figure 6-3 illustrates the possible fluctuations of acute and chronic illnesses.

Healthcare facilities are also known by the terms *acute care* or *long-term care*. Acute care hospitals provide short-term care for clients with serious illnesses. Long-term care facilities such as rehabilitation centers or skilled nursing facilities are responsible for the care of residents with chronic illness. Occasionally, a resident may become seriously ill and need to be transferred to an acute care facility.

Maslow's hierarchy relates to this continuum (see Chapter 5). If people find their needs blocked or threatened, they move toward the illness end of the continuum. When their basic needs are satisfied and they move toward self-actualization, they move toward the wellness end. The body adapts to change to maintain homeostasis. High-level wellness is called *optimum health*.

Remember that people may become self-actualized at any point on the health–illness continuum. If total absence of dis-

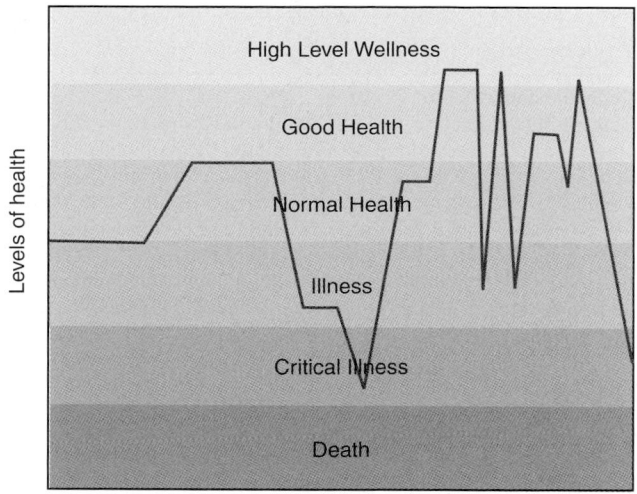

FIGURE 6-3. The wellness–illness continuum shows the different levels of health a person experiences over a lifetime. (Timby, B., Scherer, J., Smith, N. [1998]. *Introductory medical-surgical nursing* [7th ed., p. 4]. Philadelphia: Lippincott Williams & Wilkins.)

ease or disability is impossible, a person can adjust and accept this as a fact of life, and possibly, death.

LIFESTYLE AND RISK FACTORS

Lifestyle factors are patterns of living that we choose to follow, such as the amount and type of exercise performed by an individual. Nutrition, smoking, substance abuse, stress, and violence are also lifestyle factors an individual can control. These factors may also include risk factors. **Risk factors** may or may not be preventable. Smoking is a risk factor that is preventable. Our genetic makeup contains risk factors that we cannot control. Certain risk factors are related to our occupation, environment, or age.

Specific lifestyle factors can contribute dramatically to improvement of overall health and reduced deaths. These factors include the reduction or elimination of risk factors that are known to cause illness and injury. Table 6-2 summarizes areas of health promotion for some specific topics.

Physical Activity

Physical activity is recommended for all people. Moderate physical activity enhances energy, reduces stress, and provides relaxation. Physical activity is essential in the management of chronic conditions such as diabetes and arthritis. It helps in weight control and decreases the percentage of body fat. Exercise increases the activity and health of the cardiovascular system. It improves flexibility, muscle tone, strength, and stamina. It helps to increase the levels of good cholesterol in the blood. Exercise helps to prevent life-threatening conditions such as coronary heart disease (**CHD**), obesity, and cancer. Sleep and rest are also important to maintain health.

Recommendations for physical activity have changed in recent years. Today's recommendations are acceptable and

easy to accomplish. Every American adult should accumulate 30 minutes or more of moderate-intensity physical activity most days of the week. This activity does not have to be in the form of traditional exercises. It also does not have to be 30 minutes at one time, but can accumulate throughout the day (eg, three 10-minute walking sessions each day). Note that this level of exercise is for maintenance and prevention. Individuals who are striving to lose weight or to build strength will need more intense levels of activity. Taking the stairs instead of the elevator, parking at the far end of the parking lot, walking during lunch breaks, riding a bike, swimming, skiing, or playing tennis are examples of exercise.

A growing problem in the United Stated is inadequate exercise for children. Reasons include excessive television viewing and video-game playing, and reduced physical activity programs in schools. Family caregivers need to encourage exercise because it helps children to reach their best physical, mental, and spiritual potential.[1]

☛ KEY CONCEPT

Exercise helps to prevent osteoporosis and hypertension. It reduces stress, promotes weight loss, and improves heart health. Walking is exercise that almost anyone can do. It helps to prevent many disorders. A 30-minute walk each day reduces the risk of death from heart disease by 35%.

Nutrition

In recent years, a great deal of attention has been given to nutrition. The U.S. Surgeon General states that 70% of illnesses are related to nutrition. Poor nutrition contributes to congestive heart failure, cancer, obesity, and growth retardation in children. High sugar intake, pesticide use, fertilizer overuse, and food additives also contribute to disease. The major components of a healthy diet include reduced fat and sodium intake, adequate calcium intake, and increased intake of fiber and natural carbohydrates. Box 6-3 lists several recommendations for low-fat eating. Unit 5 covers nutrition and diet therapy.

Some programs to improve the American diet include nutrition education in schools, improved quality and choices in school lunches, worksite nutritional programs, and home-delivered meals for older adults. Primary care providers who educate and counsel clients on healthcare topics can provide additional help on nutritional issues, if needed. Laws now require labeling of food products, so consumers can be better informed. More reduced-fat foods are now available.

☛ KEY CONCEPT

Some situations in combination dramatically increase risks. For example, the combination of high cholesterol and hypertension increases the risk of coronary heart disease up to six times. Add smoking to that combination and the risk increases up to 20 times.

■■■ TABLE 6-2 *H*EALTH PROMOTION AND DISEASE PREVENTION MEASURES

Healthy Pregnancy

Pregnant women can avoid infant disorders with early prenatal care, avoidance of tobacco and alcohol, and by taking dietary supplements of folic acid. They should avoid contracting chickenpox and STDs, and should use caution with household chemicals and cat litter.

Childhood Injuries and Illnesses

Use baby monitors and gun locks, prevent poisoning, detect and treat parasites early, and follow immunization programs. Family caregivers can take first aid and parenting classes. Some health-care agencies provide discounts on items such as car seats, bike helmets, and gun locks; rentals of larger items are often available. Many states have very strict laws regarding use of safety devices, such as bike helmets and car seats for children under a certain age.

Dental Health

Regular preventive dental care is essential for all people, as are dietary measures to improve dental health (eg, adequate calcium and fresh fruits and vegetables). Regularly floss, and brush with fluoride toothpaste to prevent gum disease and tooth decay. In some cases, antibacterial rinses, sealants, and additional fluoride are recommended.

Vision Care

Preventive measures include regular checkups for early detection of glaucoma and cataracts, prescription of corrective lenses, safe management of contact lenses, use of adequate lighting, and correct eyelid care. The Occupational Safety and Health Administration (OSHA) requires eyewash stations in many industrial sites.

Heart Health

Prevention of heart attack includes a low-fat diet, regular exercise, maintenance of appropriate body weight, avoidance of tobacco, prevention of diabetes, stress management, and management of blood pressure and cholesterol.

Smoking

Smoking cessation programs stress reasons to quit smoking, and conditions aggravated or caused by tobacco use. They provide assistance to break the habit. Following the passage of Clean Indoor Air Laws, most healthcare facilities, worksites, and public buildings are smoke free. Restaurants have smoke-free areas and most airlines prohibit smoking, except under specific conditions. Laws restrict the sale of tobacco products to minors; advertising is regulated in an attempt to avoid exposure to persons under 18. The Great American Smoke Out day is held annually to encourage smoking cessation. Some insurance companies reward people who do not smoke.

Diabetes

Weight management and following dietary, exercise, and medication guidelines are crucial. Early detection is key to the prevention of related disorders and death.

Hypertension

Increase physical activity, reduce weight (a loss of 10 pounds can significantly decrease blood pressure), limit alcohol intake, and do not add extra salt to foods. Read food labels to determine sodium content. Be aware that certain foods, such as sea salt, brine, onion/garlic/seasoned salt, baking soda/powder, monosodium glutamate (MSG), and soy sauce contain high sodium levels. Eat a banana, orange, potato, or some watermelon daily; they are high in potassium. Take prescribed blood pressure medications and have regular checkups.

Cholesterol

Manage cholesterol by eating low-fat foods and increasing activity. For every 10% reduction in cholesterol, heart disease risk is lowered by 20%.

Cancer

Follow a low-fat diet with adequate fiber. Adhere to screening recommendations for specific cancers, avoid overexposure to the sun, and refrain from smoking.

Reproductive Health

Protective measures include education, safer sex practices, abstinence, monogamy, use of condoms, frequent checkups, and fertility control methods.

Osteoporosis

Eat foods high in calcium, including milk and dairy products. Vitamin D helps the body absorb calcium. Skim milk is better than whole milk because it is fat free and contains the same amount of calcium. Physical activity is also important.

Alcohol and Drugs

Programs are available to detect and to treat abuse and to educate children and adults. Excessive alcohol use can lead to high blood pressure and other disorders.

Eating Disorders

Education and detection programs are available for obesity, anorexia nervosa, and bulimia.

Mental Health

Manage stress. Recognize the symptoms of depression, anxiety, panic disorder, and seasonal affective disorder. Access suicide prevention and abuse hotlines and programs, if necessary.

Regular Physical Examinations and Self-Examinations

Adhere to recommendations for mammograms, breast and testicular self-exams, routine screening for cancer (phenolsulfonphthalein [PSP], occult blood in stool, proctoscopy), and screening for exposure to tuberculosis. Maintain immunizations throughout life.

Abstinence From Tobacco Products

Cigarette smoking is the single leading cause of preventable death in the United States. Yet, about 25% of the population smokes.[1] More than 4,000 substances, including highly addictive nicotine, are found in cigarette smoke. Many of these chemicals are known to cause cancer. Chemicals that cause cancer are called **carcinogenic.** Cancers caused or aggra-

vated by smoking are those of the lung, mouth, throat, esophagus, bladder, kidney, pancreas, and cervix.

Other medical conditions that result from smoking include heart disease and chronic respiratory diseases. Respiratory disorders include asthma, emphysema, bronchitis, pneumonia, and other acute and chronic respiratory disorders. Tobacco-related heart attack and stroke deaths surpass lung cancer deaths each year. More than 40% of all fatal heart attacks and

RECOMMENDATIONS FOR LOW-FAT EATING

- Eat low-fat sources of protein: fish, skinless poultry, lean red meat, or pork (trim fat).
- Cook with low-fat methods: broil, roast, grill, stir fry, or microwave.
- Make sandwiches with low-fat meats, and vegetable substitutions.
- Eat low-fat frozen dinners. Be sure to check sodium content first.
- Eat two to three servings of skim or 1% milk and low-fat yogurt daily. Limit cheese. Use low-fat or fat-free cheese, mayonnaise, and sour cream.
- Use a maximum of 2 to 3 tablespoons margarine, butter, mayonnaise, or oil daily. Use nonstick cookware/spray. Use vegetable oils low in saturated fat: canola, safflower, corn, soybean, sunflower, and olive. Choose fat-free sauces and dressings.
- Have at least six servings of bread, cereal, rice, pasta, potatoes, and cooked dried peas or beans daily. Eat low-fat crackers, cereals, and pasta sauce. Top potatoes with vegetables or low-fat yogurt. Add pasta, rice, and grains to soups.
- Be sure to eat at least five servings of fruit and vegetables daily. Use fruit for snacks and use fat-free dips. Try dried fruits. Microwave/steam vegetables; use herbs, not fat or salt, for flavoring. Eat fresh fruits and vegetables. Add vegetables to soups, casseroles, spaghetti, and sandwiches. Top cereals and ice milk with fruit. Drink fruit juice instead of soda pop.
- Have a maximum of four egg yolks per week; egg whites are not limited. Use egg substitutes.
- Limit foods with hidden fat, such as sweets and fried foods.
- Eat breakfast to increase metabolism and maintain energy.
- Eat a variety of foods and eat only when hungry.

strokes in people under age 65 are a result of smoking. Smoking one to four cigarettes per day doubles a person's chance of having a heart attack.[1]

Secondhand smoke also causes cardiovascular diseases, heart attacks and numerous respiratory problems. The chemicals found in smoke that a non-smoker breathes are more dangerous than the smoke that is inhaled by the smoker.[1] Secondhand smoke is especially damaging to the young, developing lung tissues of infants and children. Acute and chronic pulmonary problems occur early in the lives of children of smokers.

The highly addictive substance nicotine (found in cigarettes) makes platelets more sticky, which can injure heart arteries or form clots and cause a heart attack. Smoking contributes to heart disease because nicotine increases plaque buildup in arteries; it causes the insides of arteries to form rough, chapped places. Sticky cholesterol can attach there more easily and build up plaque, which can increase the chances of a heart attack.

Low-tar, filtered, and menthol cigarettes are just as dangerous as plain ones. Smokeless tobacco is also dangerous. Studies show it can cause cancers of the mouth, larynx, and esophagus and may contribute to stomach cancer.

Benefits of Smoking Cessation

Smoking cessation has an immediate effect on the improvement of health. Twenty minutes after a last cigarette, a person's blood pressure and pulse return to normal levels. In 8 hours, oxygen and carbon dioxide levels normalize. In one year, the excess risk of heart disease drops by half. In 15 years, a former smoker's risk of heart disease is the same as that of a nonsmoker. Even people who have already had a heart attack can help prevent another by not smoking. The health benefits of quitting smoking are much greater than the risks of weight gain that may occur.

☛ KEY CONCEPT
_____

Smoking one pack of cigarettes per day doubles a person's risk of heart attack and increases the risk of death from heart attack by 70%.

Tobacco Use and Pregnancy

Concerns abound for the child of the pregnant woman who smokes. Studies have shown that pregnant women who smoke less than one pack of cigarettes per day increase their chances of having a low birth weight baby by 53%. Women who smoke more than one pack per day increase these chances by up to 130%. Pregnant women who smoke also increase the chances of **preterm births** (born early, before the expected due date) and stillborn babies. The risk of sudden infant death syndrome (**SIDS**) doubles for children of mothers who smoked during pregnancy.[1]

Substance Abuse

Three out of every five Americans drink alcoholic beverages. Everyone who drinks alcohol is influenced to some extent. Therefore, each person has the potential of abusing alcohol. It is a mistake to think that only the stereotypical "alcoholic" abuses alcohol.[1]

The abuse of alcohol and other drugs contributes in many ways to decreased public health. Accidents and homicides are major causes of death. Alcohol and drugs often contribute to these events. In addition to accidents, alcohol abuse contributes to such disorders as cirrhosis of the liver, diverticulitis, and mental health conditions, such as depression and suicide.

Substance abuse also contributes to family strife, domestic violence, work absenteeism, and unemployment. Increased use of marijuana, cocaine, crack, heroin, and similar "street" drugs has become a major factor in the rising crime rate in the United States. Substance abuse also directly affects the health of the individual as well as the health of society.

Laws regulating substance use have become more stringent, but the appeal and habit-forming nature of many illegal drugs offset the effects of the laws in many cases. In addition, the huge amount of money to be made on drugs has rendered laws difficult to enforce. Chapter 94 describes chemical dependency treatment programs and the nurse's role in detoxification.

Stress

Stress is normal. It is the physical and mental wear-and-tear of life. **Stress** is a mental or physical tension exerted upon an individual's homeostasis. It is often associated with change. Some stress is beneficial, because it offers people a challenge that keeps them moving toward goals. Stress can also alert people to danger, helping them deal with emergencies. Sometimes, stress is harmful and can interfere with homeostasis.

Physical causative factors of stress include injury, diseases and disorders, and invasion of pathogens. Psychological factors include fear, anxiety, crisis, happiness, and change. Often the stress is not the actual physical or emotional event, but the stress is our *reaction* to the event. For example, getting married is a highly emotional event. The preparations for marriage cause stress. This type of stress can be energizing or damaging to the individual.

Cumulative stress leads to health problems. The individual may be able to adapt to a major change, such as moving to a new state or starting a nursing program. However, stress can be much greater, and can lead to physical and emotional dysfunction if additional change is added, such as a sudden loss of transportation. Individuals need to recognize that stress is insidious (sneaky) and often we do not recognize the symptoms until a crisis emerges.

Unmanaged stress causes or aggravates disorders such as overeating, mood swings, chronic diseases, chemical dependency, and use of tobacco. Stress manifests in many forms, such as physical symptoms (pain, frequent infections, fatigue) and emotional symptoms (the use of negative defense mechanisms). **Defense mechanisms** are internal stress reducers, even though they may not be truthful or effective ways of adapting to a stressful situation. Examples of such defense mechanisms include projection (blaming someone else) and denial. Lack of motivation and activity can also be stressful. This may occur when an individual retires.

Violence and Abuse

Domestic violence and abuse are probably among the fastest-growing public health problems in the United States today. This is violence that occurs in the home. Abuse by a male partner is the single largest cause of injury to women in the United States. Spousal abuse is becoming more com-

monly reported, with nearly 15 million cases reported per year. However, unreported cases could greatly increase the total numbers.[1]

Domestic abuse occurs at all racial, ethnic, and socioeconomic levels, although persons with higher levels of education and income may be better equipped to hide it. Some cultures permit violence to women as a prerogative of the male members.

Violence is a community and a nationwide concern. Violence in the workplace is becoming more common as stress levels increase. Violence in schools can start at elementary levels and continue through the educational system. Increasing numbers of gang members, and the use of drugs such as crack and crank cocaine, contribute greatly to rising violence—especially in young adults.

Rape and other sexual crimes are more frequently reported today than in the past. Many people suffer from the aftereffects of childhood sexual abuse several years later.

Homicide, usually weapon related, is growing as a cause of death for young adults. Also growing is the reported incidence of child homicide, abuse, and neglect.

Elder abuse and neglect are problems that promise to increase in the 21st century. This form of abuse occurs to the dependent and often frail elderly. Many times the abused or neglected senior is dependent on the care of one or more family members. Physical abuse, poor nutrition, lack of medical care, and emotional abuse such as threats are examples of elder abuse.

Baby-boomers are the large number of people born after World War II, in the years 1946–1964. As seen in Figure 6-4, baby-boomers in the 21st century have become mature adults and represent a bulky stratum of growing numbers of older Americans.

People are living longer and many do not have the resources to care for the side effects of aging. These seniors will be

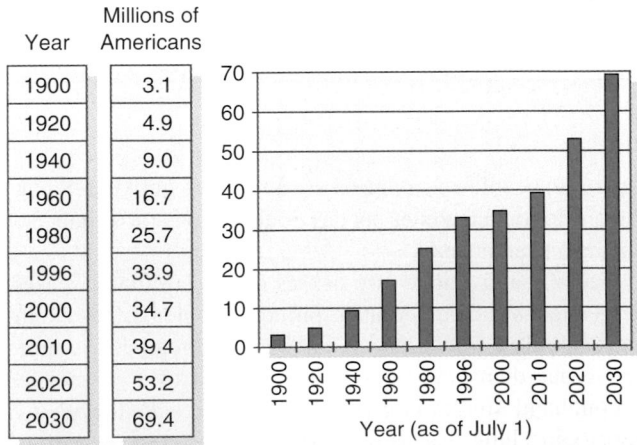

Year	Millions of Americans
1900	3.1
1920	4.9
1940	9.0
1960	16.7
1980	25.7
1996	33.9
2000	34.7
2010	39.4
2020	53.2
2030	69.4

FIGURE 6-4. A profile of Americans aged 65 years and older. This data is used to predict the health of millions of Americans aged 65 and older in the year 2030. (Based on data from the U.S. Bureau of the Census.) (Smeltzer, S., & Bare, B. [1999]. *Brunner and Suddarth's textbook of medical-surgical nursing* [9th ed., p. 149]. Philadelphia: Lippincott Williams & Wilkins.)

using the healthcare system in the early 21st century in large numbers, perhaps more than can be adequately cared for with current resources.

Abuse commonly occurs in families where personal and financial resources have been exhausted. In many cases, older adults may not be receiving the care they need. This is a form of neglect. The isolation of living alone or with relatives sometimes allows abuse to continue without detection or reporting. Chapter 91 discusses the needs of the elderly and the potential of elder abuse and neglect in more detail.

Conflict resolution and anger management programs attempt to reduce rates of violence. Your nursing responsibility is to report any cases of suspected abuse or violence. Victims of domestic violence can receive assistance at shelters, by using a telephone hotline, or through individual counseling. Local law enforcement and social service agencies are other available resources.

☛ Key Concept

Physical activity; having a well-balanced, low-fat diet; maintaining a healthy body weight; and not smoking can reduce the incidence of many disorders.

EDUCATION AND HEALTH PROMOTION

One way to combat society's health problems is through extensive education. Education can be the leading source of prevention of disease and disabilities. Numerous sources of information are available, for example:

- Formal courses in school (eg, mine safety)
- Informal courses (eg, prenatal and birth courses)
- Public service announcements and advertisements
- Informational flyers, brochures, and books
- Non-profit organizations (eg, American Cancer Society, American Lung Association)
- Healthcare providers
- Internet websites

✚👁 **N u r s i n g   A l e r t**

Web sites offer wonderful and easy access to hundreds of health-related information sites. However, use caution when gathering information. Not all sites use information based on truth and documented fact. Double check your resources and use sites that have reliable, professional, and current information. See Box 6-2 for Web addresses of several healthcare resource sites.

Individuals need to be aware of their risk and lifestyle factors. If your parents had high blood pressure (**hypertension**), then you may be at risk for this condition. Awareness of the potential problem helps you initiate measures to prevent the complications of hypertension. Education includes frequent monitoring of blood pressure, maintenance of an ideal weight, exercise, and compliance with a medication regimen.

Many schools and healthcare facilities offer classes that emphasize child development and effective parenting. All levels of schooling offer age-appropriate health education courses. Special programs are set up in worksites to educate employees on topics from the safe operation of equipment to the hazards of lifting heavy objects. Many of these educational resources are free. The courses are effective ways of educating individuals and preventing illness and injury. Thus, the employer or facility requires that all employees attend these courses. Acute and long-term healthcare facilities have voluntary and mandatory educational in-service programs for hospital staff.

Many insurance and pharmaceutical companies publish materials aimed at assisting people to live more healthy lives. Information is provided with all prescribed drugs. These companies also publish materials regarding selected disorders and their management, laboratory and other diagnostic tests, and surgical procedures. Such materials are often published in languages in addition to English to better serve target populations. They are also available on audiotape and videotape for persons who cannot read. Students should use caution with some materials, as they may be promotional to advertise the product.

Television programs and public service announcements emphasize healthier lifestyles. Many programs are targeted at selected populations, such as teenagers, maternal care, older adults, those living in poverty, and members of minority groups.

☛ Key Concept

If you understand the concepts of healthy living, you will be better able to teach your clients.

AGE-RELATED HEALTH CONCERNS

Health is a family concern. You are aware that if one person in the family has the common cold, then the rest of the family is more apt to get the virus also. Healthy habits are also contagious. Simple examples such as frequent handwashing educate others in the ways of prevention.

Avoidance of risk behaviors can be part of a family's healthy lifestyle. Children who see smoking in their home are more likely to develop the habit. Good eating habits become generational.

There are specific concerns related to each age group. Some of these concerns relate to avoidable risk and lifestyle factors.

Infants

According to the CDC and NCHS, the United States has lowered its infant mortality rate to 0.7% (7 newborns or infants out of 1000 die). This number is still too high, compared with other industrialized countries. In Native American, Hispanic, and African American populations, the infant mortality rate is higher than that of whites. The rate of infant mortality for African Americans is twice that for white Americans.

Low birth weight, congenital anomalies, SIDS, and respiratory distress syndrome are known to contribute to one half of all infant deaths.

Two major factors, the education level and the financial resources of the mother, influence mortality rates. Many women do not obtain prenatal care. The reasons include lack of available finances (even though prenatal care can be free or income adjusted), lack of transportation to the facility, and lack of interest in obtaining prenatal care. Infants and mothers who have prenatal care have a significantly decreased morbidity and mortality rate. If prenatal care is neglected, the infant often has an unhealthy beginning. A healthy infant has a much better chance of growing and developing into a fulfilled adult.

Children

The number one cause of death in young children in America is accidental injury. Asthma is the leading cause of illness in children and can be life threatening. Asthma is twice as prevalent in homes where smoking occurs. Asthma also is influenced by environmental conditions such as air pollution.[1]

The misuse of firearms has lead to an increase in mortality and morbidity of children and young adults. If a weapon is kept in the home, statistics show that a child is five times more likely to be injured or killed by a firearm. Death by firearm is the second leading cause of death for ages 10 to 24 and it is the third leading cause of death for ages 25 to 34.

Lack of exercise and physical play activities is a growing concern for the young. Obesity is present in at least one third of the young. Children who are overweight are much more likely to develop health risk factors (eg, coronary artery disease) in their youth, that will stay with them throughout their lifetimes.[1]

The great news is that major childhood infectious diseases are preventable. The six childhood scourges of the past have highly effective immunizations. Immunizations are available against measles, mumps, rubella, diphtheria, pertussis, and tetanus. Newer vaccines against hepatitis A and B, chicken pox, and the flu are also eliminating illness in children. Because of the effectiveness of modern immunization programs, infectious diseases are no longer the problem they were in the past. The public must remain alert to these potential killers because these diseases have not been eliminated. They can only be prevented with proper and complete immunizations.

Adolescents and Young Adults

Risk behaviors are more prevalent in adolescents and young adults. For example, one third of high school students smoke, compared with 25% of the general population. Substance abuse is another risk behavior common in adolescents and young adults.[1]

Specific lifestyle factors influence this age group. Peer pressure is stronger in this age group than in others. Additionally, this population has the lowest rate of utilization of healthcare, possibly due to the costs of healthcare; a high unemployment rate; and lack of healthcare insurance.

Motor Vehicle Accidents
Motor vehicle accidents are the leading causes of morbidity and mortality for ages 10 to 24. Young white men have the highest accident mortality rate, twice that of young African American men.

Firearms
Firearms and other weapons, such as knives, are the second leading cause of death for young adults. At least 10 young people a day die due to firearms. Death and injury related to firearms cost the United States about 20 billion dollars a year.[1]

Homicide is the second leading cause of death in adolescents and young adults. It is the number one cause of death among African American youth; this is six times higher than the rate for whites. The practice of carrying a weapon has been identified in about 30% of young males and about 6% of young females. Low socioeconomic status is the greatest risk factor for death by homicide.

Binge Drinking
Binge drinking is defined as having five or more alcoholic drinks in one day at least once per month. Weekend binge drinking is not uncommon in high school students and is very common in college students. Alcohol is not metabolized in young adults as efficiently as in older adults. Thus, the effects of alcohol consumption are often tragic. MVAs, violent acts, and suicides are often associated with alcohol consumption.

Suicide
Suicide is also a leading cause of death in this age group. It is the second-leading cause of death in whites. The African American suicide rate is half that of the white population. Households with firearms have five times the number of suicides compared with households without firearms. Suicide has increased 30% in the last decade, with 96% of these deaths due to gun use. Young women attempt suicide three times as often as men, but the rate of suicide completion in young women is much lower than that found in young men.[1]

Eating Disorders
Young women who begin dysfunctional eating habits often develop eating disorders between the ages of 12 and 25. Eating disorders include self-starvation, binging, purging, excessive exercise, and overuse of diuretics, laxatives, and diet pills. Chapters 72 and 87 discusses eating disorders in detail, as well as their treatment.

Sexual Health and Safe Sex
Sexual health and safe-sex concerns are a result of the peer pressure that exists for early sexual activity. Sexual activity involves consequences such as sexually transmitted diseases (STDs), pregnancy, and emotional distress. HIV/AIDS is the

fifth-leading cause of death between the ages of 25 and 44. This rate has increased significantly in teens and women, especially women of color. Ninety percent of HIV cases in this age group are transmitted by only two methods: heterosexual intercourse and sharing of contaminated needles and syringes.

The use of condoms is recommended for sexually active individuals, whether or not they use other fertility control measures. Condom use does not prevent all disease transmission. Therefore, the use of condoms is considered "safer" but not totally "safe" sex. The use of a dental dam is recommended for those who engage in oral sexual contact.

Abstinence is the only 100% effective way of preventing pregnancy, exposure to herpes, gonorrhea, syphilis, and other STDs. Teen pregnancy has decreased somewhat in the last decade of the 20th century. This trend is most likely a result of grassroots, local, state, and national educational efforts.

Some schools have peer support groups for students who have chosen to abstain from sex before marriage. Chapter 69 discusses sexuality and STDs in more detail.

Pregnancy

Pregnancy occurs most often to women in their twenties. The maternal and infant morbidity risks are significantly higher in teenage mothers and mothers over the age of 35. Prenatal care is imperative, especially with the higher risk pregnancies (see Table 6-2.) Unit 10 discusses pregnancy in detail.

Pregnant women who smoke or use cocaine, crack, heroin, marijuana, alcohol, or a number of other drugs, also put their babies at high risk. Use of crack or cocaine, even one time, can cause learning disabilities, preterm birth, low birth weight, fetal stroke, miscarriage, and stillbirth. Cocaine use increases the chance of preterm birth by 25%.

Pregnant women should maintain a healthy weight, eat a balanced diet (with special modifications), continue physical activity, avoid smoking, avoid alcohol, and avoid all medications (including over-the-counter drugs) without a physician's prescription.

Mature Adults

Heart Disease and Cancer

Heart disease and cancer rank as the top causes of adult deaths in the United States. At least 20% of Americans have heart disorders; a million people die each year from heart-related problems.

A full 25% of Americans have hypertension. In adults over the age of 70, the percentage rises to 64%. Hypertension can lead to stroke and heart attack. Kidney damage often results. The incidence of hypertension is equal in men and women, although it is more common in African Americans, especially men.

Many lifestyle factors increase the risk for hypertension. For example, women who take birth control pills and smoke, significantly increase their risk. Also contributing are a lack of physical activity, excess body weight, use of alcohol, and high salt (sodium) intake.

Diabetes Mellitus

Diabetes mellitus is increasing in all age groups, with an increase of about 600% in the last decade of the 20th century. Nearly 16 million people in the United States have diabetes mellitus. Many individuals have undiagnosed diabetes. Diabetes costs the United States about $100 billion dollars annually. One fourth of the money Medicare spends is for care of people with diabetes. Six percent of the total population has diabetes, with that number tripling to 18% for people over 65 years of age.[1]

Diabetes is the largest cause of kidney failure, blindness, and limb amputation in the United States. Clients with diabetes have two times the rate of cardiovascular disease and two to four times the numbers of CVAs. Hypertension is 60% to 70% more likely in diabetic clients. Each of these secondary chronic illnesses leads to further physical and mental deterioration.[1]

Diabetes is sometimes preventable and generally manageable, but not curable. The incidence of diabetes is higher in African Americans, Hispanic Americans, Native Americans, and Asian Americans. Race increases the risk, but nutrition, weight control, and lifestyle management can offset many of these risks. Preventive education is important.

Men's Health

Men's health issues include the number one and two killers, which are heart disease and cancer. Heart disease, including heart attack, kills 500,000 men each year in the United States. Cancer is three times more likely in males than in females. Prostate and lung cancer are the most common cancers in men.[1]

African American men are at highest risk of heart disease and hypertension, with a 47% higher rate than that found in white men. Lung diseases, suicides, and Alzheimer's disease are less common in African American than in white Americans.[1]

Men need to consider prevention of accidents, a leading cause of death in all male age groups. In adult men, accidents are the third leading cause of death (after heart disease and cancer). Men are 2.5 times more likely to die in motor vehicle accidents than women, especially men aged 15 to 24 (five times more likely).[1]

Men should be aware of prostate health. Benign prostatic enlargement is common and can be symptom free or cause difficulty in urination. Prostate cancer is the most common cancer found in American men, and is more common in African American men. Men at highest risk are those with obstructive urinary symptoms or an enlarged prostate, or those with a father or brother who died of prostate cancer before age 65. The prostate-specific antigen (**PSA**) test is used as a screening tool and to determine the effectiveness of treatment after cancer is diagnosed.

Men should also self-examine for testicular cancer. Each year testicular cancer is diagnosed in 7,100 men in the United States, most of whom are between the ages of 15 and 35. Careful observation for symptoms and regular examinations are the best preventive measures against prostate and testicular cancer.

Women's Health

Women's health issues include concerns related to reproduction and menopause. Maternal health is discussed in Unit 10. Menopause brings additional health challenges to women.

Osteoporosis (loss of bone density) is the most prevalent bone disease in the world and causes more than one million fractures of the hip, spine, and wrist yearly in the United States. At least 20% of older people with hip fractures do not survive more than a year. About one third of women over age 50 suffer spinal fracture, resulting in loss of height and a stooped appearance.[1]

After menopause, the loss of the estrogenic hormones speeds bone density loss, which affects 60% to 75% of all postmenopausal women. Women lose bone density and have twice as many fractures as men, especially if they are slender or underweight. The incidence of osteoporosis is higher in white and Asian American women than in other races.[1]

These factors also influence the incidence of various disorders. For example, cardiovascular disease affects 10% of women between ages 45 and 64; after age 65, the incidence rises to 25%. Cardiovascular disease causes 45% of deaths among all women and becomes the leading cause of death by age 65. The healthcare community is just coming to recognize the threat of heart disease to women.

Women who lack calcium are also at higher risk of developing osteoporosis. Lack of exercise is a contributing factor, as are smoking, family history of osteoporosis in mother or sister, and women who had their ovaries removed before age 50.

Cancer is a concern for women. Because of the increase of smoking in women, lung cancer now leads the mortality rate due to cancer in women. Breast and ovarian cancer are the second and third leading causes of cancer deaths in the United States.

Women need to protect themselves through regular checkups, including mammography (for breast cancer) and Pap tests (for cervical cancer). Studies have shown that mammograms detect early problems in 50% of all diagnosed breast cancer cases. For women at normal risk, a baseline mammogram is recommended at age 40 and every 1 to 2 years until age 50. After age 50, annual mammograms are recommended. For women at higher risk, the baseline mammogram is recommended between age 35 and 40, with followup in 1 year. After age 40, annual examinations are essential. All women should do breast self-examination monthly.

Older Adults

The major causes of death in the older population are heart disease, cancer, stroke, COPD, pneumonia, and influenza. Many chronic problems are also of concern because of their impact on the person's everyday life. These problems include arthritis, osteoporosis, incontinence, vision and hearing impairment, and dementia.

Suicide in older adults is more likely than for any other age group. Alzheimer's disease is among the 10 leading causes of death of those over 65 years of age.[1] Chapter 91 discusses aging in more detail.

CATEGORIES OF DEVIATION FROM WELLNESS

Disease

Diseases are classified in several ways. Usually, they are classified according to their **etiology** (cause), the body system that they affect, the extent of their involvement in the organ or body, or the way they are acquired. Classifying diseases according to cause is not always satisfactory, because the ultimate etiologies of many diseases are still unknown.

Organic and Functional Diseases

A disease is classified as organic or functional. **Organic disease** means that detectable structural change has occurred in one or more organs that also alters usual function. **Functional disease** is a disorder in which a structural cause cannot be identified. The person, however, experiences changes that affect his or her ability to conduct the usual activities of daily living. The person is said to be **dysfunctional** if he or she cannot perform usual activities.

Hereditary Disorders

One or both biologic parents may transmit a **hereditary** (genetic) disorder to an embryo, resulting in the child's physical impairment. For example, hemophilia (prolonged blood clotting time) is a hereditary disorder transmitted from mother to child. It appears mostly in male children because it is almost always carried on the X chromosome. The mother is the carrier and generally free of symptoms.

Congenital Disorders

Congenital disorders are also present at birth. Unlike hereditary disorders, however, they are not necessarily transmitted through genes. Congenital disorders may be genetic or may be caused by another unfavorable condition that affects normal fetal development. For example, herpesvirus in the mother can be transmitted through the placenta or during the birth process and can cause congenital defects. If a woman contracts rubella (German measles) during pregnancy, the disease may cause body abnormalities or defects in the infant. Consumption of alcohol or smoking by a pregnant woman can profoundly affect the fetus. Congenital heart disease and clubbed feet (deformities of bones in the feet) are examples of abnormal fetal development.

Infectious Diseases

A common cause of disease is invasion of the body by microorganisms, such as bacteria or viruses, or by animal parasites. This microscopic invasion is called an *infection*. Some infections are **local,** which means the area of invasion is limited to one area or organ. **Systemic** infections involve the whole body. Microorganisms that cause infections may or may not be **contagious,** which means the infection can be transferred from one person to another. Chapter 40 discusses microorganisms in more detail.

Deficiency Diseases

Deficiency diseases are disorders of nutrition that result from a lack of one or more dietary nutrients. For example, lack of vitamin C causes scurvy. A deficiency of several vitamins, or general malnutrition, is more common in the United States than is a single vitamin deficiency. If the body does not use nutrients properly (malabsorption syndrome), various disorders result. Deficiency diseases also may be seen in the immune system. An immunodeficiency syndrome caused by HIV/AIDS is often manifested in the body by infections, malignancies, and neurologic disease.

Metabolic Disorders

A disturbance of one or more of the endocrine glands causes metabolic disorders. Endocrine glands secrete hormones that regulate body processes (see Chap. 20). For example, the thyroid hormone affects the rate of metabolism for the entire body, and insulin deficiency results in diabetes mellitus. Dysfunction occurs from hypersecretion (too much) or hyposecretion (too little) of a hormone.

Neoplastic Diseases

The growth of abnormal tissue or tumors is called **neoplastic.** These growths can be benign or malignant. A **benign** tumor results from the growth of cells similar to the tissue in which it appears. A benign tumor is often surrounded by a capsule. Once removed, the tumor usually does not recur. It may be disfiguring, but it is not dangerous unless it crowds other structures or robs surrounding tissues of their blood supply. A **malignant** tumor (eg, cancer) is a wild and disorderly growth of cells that is unlike the tissue from which it arises. This cell growth robs normal tissues of nutrients. Malignant cells also tend to spread to other parts of the body, a process called **metastasis.**

Traumatic Injuries

Traumatic injuries are those injuries caused by external forces. Injuries incurred in automobile accidents and falls are examples. Mental trauma (eg, emotional distress) also falls under this category.

Occupational Disorders

Certain occupational groups are subject to conditions particular to their jobs. Construction workers constitute 20% of deaths due to occupational causes.[1] Agricultural workers and miners also have high rates of mortality.

Morbidity can also be related to occupational exposures. Employees who work around chemicals, radiation, and other hazardous materials are more likely to be susceptible to acute and chronic conditions. People working in noisy areas for prolonged periods must wear protective devices to prevent permanent hearing loss.

➤ STUDENT SYNTHESIS

Key Points

- Although many definitions of health exist, optimum health includes physical, emotional, mental, social, and spiritual well-being.
- The state of one's health is on a continuum and is dynamic, changing from day to day.
- The concept of high-level wellness relates to the higher level needs in Maslow's hierarchy.
- Lifestyle changes can have a major impact on health and wellness.
- The four most important wellness lifestyle factors are physical activity, healthy diet, maintenance of appropriate body weight, and not smoking.
- Some stress is beneficial, whereas too much stress can lead to physical and emotional disorders.
- Keys to changing behavior include health promotion, education, and community health awareness.
- Infant mortality remains a health concern in the United States.
- The major cause of death and disability in young children involves accidents.
- Accidents continue to be a major health concern for adolescents and young adults, along with homicide and suicide.
- Heart disease and cancer are the top causes of death in adults.
- The etiology of diseases and disorders may be organic, functional, hereditary, congenital, infectious, deficiency, metabolic, neoplastic, traumatic, or related to an occupation.

Critical Thinking Exercises

1. Based on the information provided in this chapter, give your own definition of health.
2. Describe "high-level wellness" in terms of your own lifestyle. What measures can you take to improve your own health?
3. A client does not understand what is meant by "health promotion." How would you explain it to the client? What measures would you stress to the person to optimize wellness?

4. Relate wellness and a healthy lifestyle to Maslow's hierarchy of needs.

NCLEX-Style Review Questions

1. The nurse understands that the probable effect of a client's choosing to continue to smoke cigarettes will be:
   a. Decreased risk for cancer
   b. Increased risk of heart disease and heart attack
   c. Increased risk of domestic violence
   d. Lowered heart rate and blood pressure
2. Today's healthcare system emphasizes:
   a. Disease prevention
   b. Mental health treatment
   c. Screening only for high risk clients
   d. Treatment of diseases
3. Health promotion and disease prevention measures include which of the following?
   a. Decreasing physical activity in persons with hypertension to lower blood pressure
   b. Helping clients with diabetes to manage their weight and follow dietary guidelines
   c. Instructing the client with a risk for cancer to follow a high-fat diet to decrease risk
   d. Informing the public that prevention of heart attack includes a low-protein diet

Reference

1. National Center for Health Statistics, Division of Data Services, 6525 Belcrest Road, Hyattsville, MD 20782-2003; (301) 458-4636; Website: http://www.cdc.gov/nchs/.

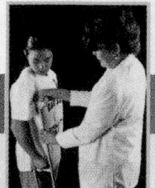

CHAPTER

7

Community Health

LEARNING OBJECTIVES

1. Define the term *community.* State the relationship of community to that of the health of a community. Identify at least four types of communities.
2. Identify the health-related functions of WHO and UNICEF.
3. State at least six achievements attributed to improvements in public health that resulted in an increase of lifespan in the 20th century.
4. Define and differentiate among the USPHS, the HHS, and the OPHS.
5. Discuss at least six functions of the HHS.
6. Identify at least four functions of the CDC.
7. Identify at least four functions of the FDA.
8. Discuss the purpose of the NIH and state the role of the NINR.
9. Identify at least four functions of OSHA.
10. Identify at least three functions of the Social Security Agency.
11. Identify the role and at least two functions of each of the following organizations: APHA, National Safety Council, the Red Cross, and the VNA.
12. Differentiate between organizations that are related to specific disorders and organizations promoting specific health goals.
13. Identify at least seven programs that are common to state healthcare services.
14. Discuss primary care and functions of the community health center.
15. Identify at least three causes of each of the following types of pollution: air, water, land, and noise.
16. Discuss the significance of plumbism, radiation, and biohazardous waste pollution.

NEW TERMINOLOGY

biohazardous
bionomics
community
community health
demography
ecology
plumbism

pollution
primary healthcare
radiation
radon
target population
worker's compensation

ACRONYMS

(*Note:* Each government agency has its own acronym and not all acronyms in this chapter are listed below.)

APHA	MUA	UNICEF
CDC	NAHCC	USDA
DOA	NHIC	USPHS
DOL	NIH	VNA
EPA	NINR	WHO
FDA	OPHS	WIC
FQHC	SSA	
HHS	UN	

A group of individuals who interact with each other for the mutual benefit of their common interests to support a sense of unity or belonging is a **community**. You are a member of many communities: Your family, school, place of employment, town or city, state or province, nation, and the world. Community can also refer to a smaller organization, such as a retirement home or a health maintenance organization.

Communities are studied as a part of **demography**, which is the study of populations. Demography examines the dynamic balances among population size, racial and ethnic distribution, economic opportunities, growth potential, and other indicators. Health concerns are based on a community's demographics as well as a nation's overall health and economy. World and national events influence state and local communities. The welfare and priorities of the individual are balanced against the needs and resources of a community.

Community health is the aggregate health of a population: a town, state, nation, or planet, for example. A community's health is continuously monitored using the 10 Leading Health Indicators, as discussed in Chapter 6. Health status is also monitored by statistics such as rates of birth, morbidity (illness), mortality (death), teen pregnancy, immunizations, sexually transmitted diseases, prevalence of infectious diseases, and prevalence of cancer.

Other factors influencing societal health include rates of crime, juvenile justice, and high school graduations. Poverty levels, population density, incidences of domestic violence, and adequate housing (rental and ownership) contribute to community health.

HEALTHCARE WORLDWIDE

Health promotion is a worldwide concern. The United Nations (**UN**) established the World Health Organization (**WHO**) in 1948. The guidelines established by the WHO have become international standards for sanitation, chemical safety, water purification, immunizations, and infectious diseases. Chapter 6 reviews the accomplishments and goals of this organization.

Hundreds of international healthcare and non–healthcare agencies are linked to the WHO. After events such as earthquakes, floods, or volcanic eruptions, a country may need extensive assistance to prevent starvation and widespread disease. The UN tailors specific programs to meet the needs that arise from natural disasters.

The WHO sends healthcare professionals to nations to combat diseases and disorders at both the community and the individual level. The infections of malaria, tuberculosis, HIV, and other diseases are major international health concerns. Women of childbearing age are of special concern. Public health officials are increasing their efforts to decrease smoking in other countries. The diseases associated with the high-fat, high-salt, and high-calorie intake of Western industrialized countries—such as cardiac disease and hypertension—are noted. Mental health issues are also addressed.

Another UN program, the United Nations Children's Fund (**UNICEF**), helps children, especially those in developing countries. Some of its goals include nutrition instruction, development of low-cost food supplements, support of general education, childhood immunization programs, procedures for supplying safe water, and infant rehydration programs.

HEALTHCARE ON THE NATIONAL LEVEL

United States Public Health Service

The United States Public Health Service (**USPHS**) celebrated its 200th birthday in 1998. Since 1798, it has had many responsibilities, including investigation and control of communicable diseases, protection from disease carried by immigrants, control of sanitation, prevention of disease spread through interstate commerce, and control of the manufacture and sale of biologic products.

The achievements of the USPHS are truly impressive. Life expectancy in the early 1900s was about 45 years. In the last decade of the 20th century, the lifespan of Americans had been lengthened by 30 years, to more than 75 years. Advances in public health contribute to 25 of these additional 30 years, according to the CDC. Eight of the most notable achievements include:

- Vaccinations
- Motor-vehicle safety
- Safer workplaces
- Control of infectious diseases
- Declines in deaths from coronary heart disease and stroke
- Safer and healthier foods
- Healthier mothers and babies
- Recognition of tobacco use as a health hazard

The USPHS is the forerunner of the U.S. Department of Health and Human Services (**HHS**). HHS was created by Congress and is one of the Executive Agencies of the U.S. President. Other Executive Agencies also have health-related functions. These cabinet-level offices include the Department of Agriculture (**USDA**) and the Department of Labor (**DOL**). The USPHS includes:

- Agencies of HHS
- Program offices
- Surgeon general
- Emergency preparedness
- Minority health
- Population affairs

The Office of Public Health and Science (**OPHS**) is an office that provides leadership and coordination across agencies of the USPHS and HHA. The National Health Information Center (**NHIC**) is a service of the OPHS that provides health information to both consumers and healthcare professionals. Some of the offices of the OPHS include:

- Office of the Surgeon General
- Office of Women's Health
- Office of Emergency Preparedness
- NHIC
- National Vaccine Program Office

- President's Council of Physical Fitness and Sports
- Office of Disease Prevention and Health Promotion (ODPHP)

Department of Health and Human Services

The Department of Health and Human Services is a highly versatile agency that has a myriad of responsibilities. The agencies that constitute the branches of HHS are listed below. Each of these programs provides a multitude of services. The student is encouraged to check the website of each agency for further information at http://www.hhs.gov/agencies/.

Administration for Children and Families (ACF): Provides services and assistance to needy children and families

Administration on Aging (AOA): Provides services to the elderly, promoting independence and providing home-delivered meals

Agency for Healthcare Research and Quality (AHRQ): Provides research designed to improve quality of healthcare, including information on costs and client safety

Agency for Toxic Substances and Disease Registry (ATSDR): Provides information, assessments, and educational training related to the U.S. Environmental Protection Agency's (**EPA**) national priorities list of hazardous substances and waste sites

Centers for Disease Control and Prevention (**CDC**): Provides health surveillance to monitor and prevent outbreaks of disease; guards against international disease transmission; maintains national health statistics; provides for immunization services; and supports research into disease and injury prevention

Centers for Medicare & Medicaid Services (CMS): Administers the Medicare and Medicaid programs and the Children's Health Insurance Program

Food and Drug Administration (**FDA**): Provides for the safety of foods and cosmetics, and the safety and effectiveness of pharmaceuticals, biological products, and medical devices

Health Resources and Services Administration (HRSA): Provides health resources for medically underserved populations such as migrant workers, the homeless, and residents of public housing; oversees the national organ transplantation system; provides services to decrease infant mortality, and to improve the health of children and of people with AIDS

Indian Health Service (IHS): Provides a network of hospitals, and health centers and stations for American Indians and Alaska Natives of 557 federally recognized tribes

National Institutes of Health (**NIH**): Provides for research projects in 27 separate institutes for thousands of health-related subjects

Substance Abuse and Mental Health Services Administration (SAMHSA): Provides services to improve the quality and availability of substance abuse prevention, addiction treatment, and mental health services

Three of the branches of HHS will be discussed in further detail: the CDC, the FDA, and the NIH. Box 7-1 provides numerous websites for Governmental Health Agencies.

☛ KEY CONCEPT

Health information is available from many sources. A referral service called the National Health Information Center (NHIC) provides health professionals and consumers with resource organizations. Their website is http://www.health.gov/nhic/.

Centers for Disease Control and Prevention

The mission of the CDC is to promote health and quality of life by preventing and controlling disease, injury, and disability.

➤➤ BOX 7-1

WEBSITES FOR GOVERNMENTAL HEALTH AGENCIES

- Administration for Children and Families: http://www.acf.dhhs.gov
- Agency for Healthcare Research and Quality: http://www.ahcpr.gov
- Agency for Toxic Substances and Disease Registry: http://www.atsdr.cdc.gov
- Centers for Disease Control and Prevention: http://www.cdc.gov
- Centers for Medicare & Medicaid Services (formerly Healthcare Financing Administration): http://www.cms.hhs.gov
- Department of Health and Human Services: http://www.hhs.gov
- Environmental Protection Agency: http://www.epa.gov
- Food and Drug Administration: http://www.fda.gov
- General Accounting Office (GAO): http://www.gao.gov
- Government Printing Office (GPO): http://www.gpo.gov
- Health Resources and Services Administration: http://www.hrsa.dhhs.gov
- Indian Health Service: http://www.ihs.gov
- Library of Congress: http://www.loc.gov
- National Highway Traffic Safety Administration: http://www.nhtsa.dot.gov
- National Institutes of Health: http://www.nih.gov
- National Library of Medicine: http://www.nlm.nih.gov
- Occupational Safety and Health Administration: http://www.osha-slc.gov/index.html
- Substance Abuse and Mental Health Services Administration: http://www.samhsa.gov
- USDA Office of Public Health and Science: http://www.fsis.usda.gov/OPHS/ophshome.htm
- White House: http://www.whitehouse.gov

This well-recognized agency is a major force in the protection of the health and safety of citizens. It also functions as an advocate for environmental health, health promotion, and education.

CDC national headquarters is located in Atlanta, Georgia, but it also has health departments in 47 states and employees in 45 countries. It works with 170 public health disciplines throughout the world to monitor health, detect and investigate health problems, conduct research to enhance prevention, promote healthy behaviors, and foster safe and healthy environments.

In conjunction with state and local health departments, the public is protected in numerous ways by the efforts of the CDC. A few roles of the CDC include:

- Investigating disease outbreaks at a local, national, or international level, such as the 2001 anthrax contamination of postal workers and others
- Providing current and accurate health-related information to the public
- Fostering cooperative relationships with national, state, and local organizations to combat dangerous environmental exposures, such as what might occur in the air, the water, and the workplace

The CDC is subdivided into organizational components based on expertise in healthcare areas, some of which include:

- National Center on Birth Defects and Developmental Disabilities
- National Center for Chronic Disease Prevention and Health Promotion
- National Center for Health Statistics
- National Center for HIV, STD, and TB Prevention
- National Center for Infectious Diseases
- National Center for Injury Prevention and Control
- National Immunization Program

Food and Drug Administration

The FDA's mission is to promote and protect public health by helping safe and effective products reach the market in a timely way, and by monitoring products for continued safety after they are in use. The FDA blends science and law to protect consumers.

The headquarters for the FDA is in greater Washington, D.C., but it also has 167 field offices. Employees perform inspections, surveillance, laboratory studies, and educate industrial and public sectors. The FDA does not develop or test products itself; it reviews the results of laboratory and clinical testing done by individual companies.

The FDA regulates food ingredients, complex medical and surgical devices, medications, and radiation-emitting products. FDA accomplishments include:

- Requiring that new drugs and complex medical devices (eg, cardiac pacemakers) be proven safe before they are put into a consumer market
- Establishing performance standards for products such as x-ray machines, mammography equipment, and microwave ovens

- Requiring safety practices in blood banking
- Requiring accurate, truthful, and useful labeling for prescription drugs, over-the-counter medications, foods, and dietary supplements
- Conducting scientific research and providing standards and guidelines to make regulatory decisions
- Requesting or requiring that manufacturers recall unsafe products

National Institutes of Health

The mission of the NIH is to uncover new knowledge that will lead to better health for everyone. There are 27 separate institutes or centers. These individual institutes are located in 75 buildings on more than 300 acres in Bethesda, MD. Box 7-2 lists the 27 Institutes. Each institute works in its specific field to accomplish the following goals:

- Conducting research on-site or through universities, medical schools, hospitals, or other research institutions
- Training research investigators
- Promoting improved sharing of medical information

A National Institute for Nursing Research (**NINR**) was established in 1993. The establishment of a separate Institute for Nursing Research is an important recognition of the uniqueness of the field of nursing. The NINR separates the funding for nursing research from other Institute research funding, such as medicine.

The NINR supports research and establishes a scientific basis for the care of individuals across the lifespan. The focus of nursing research is to discover ways to benefit clients. These areas include:

- Management of clients during illness and recovery
- Reduction of risks for disease and disability
- Promotion of needs for underserved, high-risk clients such as those with chronic illness and healthcare disparities
- Care for individuals at the end of life
- Promotion of the care of families within a community

Other Federal Agencies

Occupational Safety and Health Administration

Along with the HHS, the U.S. Department of Labor (DOL) is an Executive Agency of the federal government. Several subdivisions of the DOL gather information related to working conditions, occupational hazards, international child labor, and numerous other work-related issues.

The Occupational Safety and Health Administration (**OSHA**) is the subdivision of the DOL that works to prevent occupational injury and illness. OSHA's mission is to send every worker home whole and healthy every day. OSHA has affiliations with individual state agencies that focus on occupational health and safety. OSHA accomplishments include:

- Standards for safety and health protection in the workplace
- Standards for occupational exposure to blood-borne pathogens
- Standards published to protect construction workers

➤➤ BOX 7-2

NATIONAL INSTITUTES OF HEALTH RESEARCH INSTITUTES

The National Institutes of Health (NIH) comprises 27 separate research institutes. The NIH website has detailed information on each institute at its Web site, http://www.nih.gov/.

- Office of the Director (OD)
- National Cancer Institute (NCI)
- National Eye Institute (NEI)
- National Heart, Lung, and Blood Institute (NHLBI)
- National Human Genome Research Institute (NHGRI)
- National Institute on Aging (NIA)
- National Institute on Alcohol Abuse and Alcoholism (NIAAA)
- National Institute of Allergy and Infectious Diseases (NIAID)
- National Institute of Arthritis and Musculoskeletal and Skin Diseases (NIAMS)
- National Institute of Child Health and Human Development (NICHD)
- National Institute on Deafness and Other Communication Disorders (NIDCD)
- National Institute of Dental and Craniofacial Research (NIDCR)

- National Institute of Diabetes and Digestive and Kidney Diseases (NIDDK)
- National Institute on Drug Abuse (NIDA)
- National Institute of Environmental Health Sciences (NIEHS)
- National Institute of General Medical Sciences (NIGMS)
- National Institute of Mental Health (NIMH)
- National Institute of Neurological Disorders and Stroke (NINDS)
- National Institute of Nursing Research (NINR)
- National Library of Medicine (NLM)
- National Institute for Biomedical Imaging and Bioengineering (NIBIB)
- Warren Grant Magnuson Clinical Center (CC)
- Center for Information Technology (CIT)
- National Center for Complementary and Alternative Medicine (NCCAM)
- National Center for Research Resources (NCRR)
- National Center on Minority Health and Health Disparities (NCMHD)
- John E. Fogarty International Center (FIC)
- Center for Scientific Review (CSR)

Source: NIH Web site http://www.nih.gov/

- Ergonomic standards to prevent musculoskeletal disorders

Healthcare workers are directly affected every day by the blood-borne pathogen standard. This standard ensures the education and protection of all levels of healthcare workers, in all settings, regarding blood-borne pathogens, particularly hepatitis B and HIV. OSHA standards mandate that all healthcare agencies and facilities develop policies and procedures, as well as staff education programs. It also encourages immunization of healthcare workers against hepatitis B. Ultimately this standard serves to protect consumers as well.

Another subdivision of the DOL is the Bureau of Labor Statistics, which assists with worker's compensation. **Worker's compensation** provides financial compensation to a person who has been injured at work or who has contracted a disease that can be directly related to his or her job. The federal government supervises the program, and employers are required to contribute funds, based on the hazards of the particular occupation and the place of employment.

Social Security Administration

In 1995, the Social Security Administration (**SSA**) split from the HHS to become an independent agency. The SSA provides retirement income for many people and financial assistance for healthcare to special populations.

Persons over age 62 or 65, and those of any age with special disabilities or handicaps, may receive financial support from this agency, as well as from Medicare and Medicaid (see Chap. 3), which the SSA oversees. Regular Social Security benefits are also available to persons under age 62 as a result of the death, disability, or retirement of a parent or spouse.

USDA Women, Infants, and Children

The USDA is responsible for the control of insect- and animal-borne diseases, meat and other food inspections, and school lunch programs. The USDA is also the agency that administers the Special Supplemental Nutrition Program for Women, Infants, and Children (**WIC**). The goal of this program is to improve the health of pregnant women, new mothers, and their infants. Most states also have a Department of Agriculture (**DOA**).

Other Nationwide Organizations

American Public Health Association

Founded in 1872, the American Public Health Association (**APHA**) is the world's oldest and largest organization of public health professionals. Its goal is to provide leadership, influence policies, and establish public health priorities. APHA has the following priorities:

- Combining the knowledge of researchers, healthcare providers, administrators, and teachers
- Providing better personal and environmental health, **pollution** control, and smoke-free environments
- Assisting with chronic and infectious illnesses
- Providing professional education in public health

National Safety Council

The mission of the National Safety Council is to educate and influence society to adopt safety, health, and environmental policies, practices, and procedures that prevent and mitigate human suffering and economic losses arising from preventable causes.

The Council operates as a non-government organization to gather information regarding safety and health information in the United States. Founded in 1913, the Council started work in factories, construction sites, and other workplaces. It was later expanded to include highway, community, and recreational safety.

The national and state Councils promote safety by analyzing causes of accidents and suggesting preventive measures. They disseminate information about accident prevention in industry, in the home, and on public highways. For example, highway and traffic laws protect everyone by requiring inspection of motor vehicles, issuing driver's licenses, establishing speed regulations, and providing highway markings. All states now require seat belts and head rests as standard equipment in new motor vehicles.

The Council influences public opinion, attitudes, and behavior in other areas. Building and electrical codes require mandatory sprinkler systems, automatic alarm systems, emergency lighting, and regular inspections, which reduce fires, accidents, and health hazards. Educational programs and training help to convert the information gained by the Council into direct actions that affect community well-being.

The Red Cross

The International Red Cross and the Red Crescent Movement work worldwide to provide services that assist individuals, communities, and nations (see Special Considerations: Culture 7-1). These agencies work independently of governments and are apolitical. Their goals are to be nondiscriminatory, to assist the wounded of the battlefield, to protect life and health, and to ensure respect for the human being.

Founded by nurse Clara Barton in 1881, the American Red Cross is a humanitarian organization led by volunteers and guided by its Congressional Charter and the Fundamental Principles of the International Red Cross Movement. The American Red Cross added the function of providing disaster relief to the basic international charter of providing assistance to soldiers on a battlefield. The mission of the Red Cross is to provide help to victims of disaster and to help people prevent, prepare for, and respond to emergencies.

Although not a federal agency, the Red Cross provides national services. For example, local Red Cross chapters work with community health associations and public health departments to coordinate services during disasters. Well-known in the health service industry, the Red Cross manages blood banks and tissue donation services to recover skin, bone, heart valves, and other tissues for transplant. Services provided by the American Red Cross include:

> *Armed forces emergency services:* Communications, counseling, financial assistance
> *Biomedical services:* Blood, tissue, and plasma services in national testing laboratories
> *Community services:* Food and nutrition, homeless issues, and transportation
> *Health and safety services:* Swimming, youth programs, health and safety programs
> *International services:* Emergency disaster response, tracing individuals, and providing messages

Visiting Nurse Association

The Visiting Nurse Association (**VNA**) is a not-for-profit, community-based home care agency based nationwide. The VNA is an agency of the United Way charities. It provides care to any person regardless of his or her ability to pay. Services can also be billed to Medicare, Medicaid, and private insurance companies. VNAs collaborate with other health and social service agencies throughout the community, setting up health linkages and networks.

Health services may be provided in a person's home or in a senior residence, board-and-care home, or homeless shelter. Services may be therapeutic or preventive in nature. For example, a VNA may conduct tuberculin screening, immunizations for communicable diseases, or education programs about sexually transmitted diseases (STDs). Refer to Chapter 98. Direct care services provided by the VNA include:

- Skilled nursing
- Physical therapy
- Maternal and child care
- Medical social work
- Pain management
- Hospice
- Private duty nursing
- Enterostomal therapies
- IV and enteral therapies

Organizations Related to Specific Diseases

The American Cancer Society, the National Society for the Prevention of Blindness, the American Heart Association, the American Diabetes Association, the Cystic Fibrosis Foundation, the National Easter Seal Society–March of Dimes, and numerous other organizations fulfill the need for funding and education devoted to specific diseases. These national voluntary agencies often have state or regional affiliates.

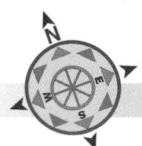

SPECIAL CONSIDERATIONS: CULTURE

The symbol of a red cross was adopted by the International Red Cross Movement as a symbol of neutrality. However, some societies view the Red Cross emblem as a religious symbol. In Islamic countries, the symbol of a Red Crescent is used. In Israel, a symbol of the Red Shield of David designates the function of the Movement.

In many cases, volunteer organizations sponsor activities or conduct fund drives to raise money for treatment or research relating to their particular area of interest. They may also receive some funding from campaigns such as those conducted by the United Way. Many organizations publish pamphlets, books, and audiovisual materials to educate the public. Clinics and physician's offices are often sources of free brochures, as depicted in Figure 7-1.

Voluntary health agencies include those that provide direct service and those that provide education and conduct fundraising. Voluntary organizations have a great impact because they appeal to public sentiment, and citizens participate in them directly.

Organizations that Promote Specific Health Goals

Some voluntary health agencies are concerned not with disease, but with the promotion of one aspect of health. For example, Planned Parenthood of America focuses on family planning and prevention of STDs. Their counselors, physicians, and nurses assist people by providing genetic counseling, abortion counseling, infertility examination, and birth control. They may also provide prenatal care. Another such organization, the La Leche League, advances maternal and newborn health by encouraging breastfeeding.

HEALTHCARE AT THE STATE LEVEL

State health laws must conform to federal laws, but states also have the right to make their own health laws, if necessary. Many state agencies are also affiliated with federal agencies such as OSHA. Sometimes funding for programs is derived from money received from both federal and state agencies, as is the case with Medicaid.

Typically, state healthcare services may be grouped into separate programs under a State Department of Health, or under broader umbrellas such as a Department of Consumer Affairs or a Department of Health and Human Services.

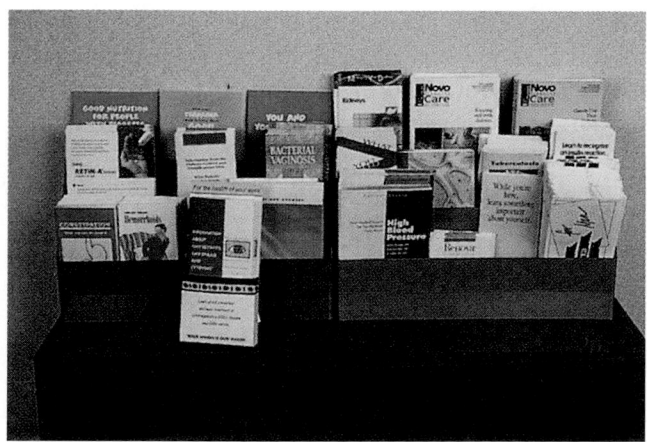

FIGURE 7-1. Clinics and physician's offices are often sources of free brochures. Check the reception area or ask the physician for free information. (Hosley, J. B., Jones, S. A., Molle-Matthews, E. A. [1997]. *Lippincott's textbook for medical assistants* [p. 105]. Philadelphia: Lippincott Williams & Wilkins.)

Regardless of the titles, the services that the states provide remain basically standard. However, the comprehensiveness of services in each state may differ widely. Programs or agencies on state levels address many specific healthcare concerns including:

- Aging
- Children's health
- Families in need
- Mental health
- Special populations, such as minorities and persons with disabilities (hearing and vision impaired, physical disabilities)
- Alcohol and substance abuse
- Environmental health
- Communicable diseases
- Safety and disability issues

In addition to services that are directly related to the healthcare of a community, state agencies provide certification and licensing requirements for healthcare professionals (nurse aides, nurses, and physicians). Additional regulatory agencies may be available for ancillary healthcare providers such as chiropractors, optometrists, midwives, pharmacists, or physical therapists.

State health departments serve as consultants to local health departments and exercise regulatory powers over them. State health departments often serve as surveyors to enforce federal health requirements, along with planning health requirements for their own jurisdictions.

HEALTHCARE AT THE LOCAL LEVEL

City, town, or county health departments focus on the health protection of persons within their jurisdiction. Usually the Department of Health operates under a Board of Health or Public Health Service. These departments carry out policies and regulations under the direction of a health officer. State regulations mandate requirements for health officer licensure; public health education is a prerequisite.

Health departments provide services dealing with conditions that affect all residents. Their personnel inspect places where food is sold, and the people who handle food. They check water and milk supplies, housing, and sewage and other waste disposal facilities. They monitor and control air quality. They may provide school health services and health education, community clinics, or hospital/nursing home care.

Public health and home care nursing services are often provided through city or regional health departments. Other services that local health departments may provide include occupational health services (to industries) and school nursing services. Additional healthcare settings and services are discussed in Chapter 3.

The Community Health Center

The local or regional health department often sponsors community-based healthcare, sometimes in the form of a community health center or family health center. Centers with similar functions may be referred to as *public health centers* and function under the state's public health department.

Community health centers usually belong to an organization called the National Association of healthcare Centers (**NAHCC**). These centers provide a wide range of services, including **primary healthcare,** which is family-focused healthcare that emphasizes health education and healthy lifestyles. The goal is to decrease the potential for illness and to provide early treatment if illness does occur. Thus, primary healthcare emphasizes health promotion and disease prevention (see Chap. 6).

Community health centers may provide healthcare services in locations where specific populations known as target populations are found. **Target populations** are subgroups in a community with unique or special healthcare needs, such as the homeless, the elderly, the young, migrant workers, or immigrants. When health centers are located near the target population, individuals have easier access to healthcare. Compared with traditional medical clinics, community-based healthcare is more cost effective, is less disruptive to the individual's lifestyle, and promotes better compliance with followup care.

Sites for community health centers vary. Some sites include housing projects, churches, schools, homeless shelters, or locations on major streets near bus lines or commuter train stations. Primary healthcare is also available in schools, neighborhood centers, day care centers, retirement communities, group homes for the mentally ill or mentally retarded, municipal buildings, homeless shelters, and battered women's shelters.

The community health center may provide testing for various disorders, including tuberculosis, STDs (including HIV), and lead poisoning. It provides immunizations and prenatal services.

Infants and older adults are served in wellness programs or through nursing care and preventive services provided in the home. Other services of the community health center include programs for special clients, such as those with AIDS, the homeless, migrant workers, and teen parents. The centers refer clients as necessary to other providers for further care.

The U.S. Public Health Service designates and monitors certain community health centers, called Federally Qualified healthcare (**FQHC**). FQHCs provide healthcare in parts of the United States identified as medically underserved areas (**MUA**). Bilingual staff members are present in many centers, to better serve the varied populations in the local service area.

Advanced practice nurses (nurse practitioners), working with physicians, often provide primary healthcare in community health centers. Available services include physical screenings, maternal and prenatal care, and specialized examinations for both men and women. A more complete discussion of community-based healthcare is found in Unit 15.

In some areas, local and state health departments no longer provide direct client services. These departments now refer clients to private providers through Medicaid, managed care programs, and contracted care with private physicians or clinics.

THE ENVIRONMENT

Humanity is only one part of a complex system that depends on the balance of life, growth, and death of all living organisms on the planet. This growing recognition has awakened many concerned citizens to the need to preserve this balance. The study of mutual relationships between living beings and their environment is called **ecology** or **bionomics.** The federal EPA was established in an attempt to control problems relating to the environment and its ecology.

Pollution

The task of maintaining ecologic balances to preserve safe air to breathe, water to drink, and food to eat is complicated. **Pollution** (contamination and impurity) severely compromises the ecologic balance. New sources of energy that will not pollute the air, the land, or water are being sought. As a nurse and member of the healthcare team, you will be called on to know about and to work for a healthy and safe environment.

Air Pollution
Air pollution is greatest in industrial areas. However, every community has some air pollution, even though it may have comparatively few industries. Pollution also tends to drift from cities to the nearby countryside and suburbs. For instance, Philadelphia's air pollution often drifts over its suburbs and southern New Jersey.

A great source of air pollution is exhaust from automobiles, although methods are being developed to alleviate this problem. In cities such as Denver and Los Angeles, atmospheric conditions, geography, fog, smoke, and automobile exhaust gases combine to produce smog. The harmful substances in this smog cannot blow away naturally because of the location of mountain ranges. Similar situations have developed in many other cities, particularly those surrounded by mountains. Some cities have alerts during which schoolchildren are not allowed to play outside and residents are warned about the dangers. Some larger cities of the Americas, such as Mexico City, have driving bans (when residents are allowed to drive their cars only on alternate days to decrease smog levels).

Air pollution is responsible for increases in respiratory infections, such as chronic bronchitis and emphysema. The incidence of asthma is increasing, especially in the young. Poor air quality, tobacco smoke, and numerous other pollutants are directly connected to asthma. Heavy pollution causes irritation of the eyes, nose, and throat and may have other serious health effects as yet unknown. Polluted air damages plant life, including farm crops. For example, many vineyards on the West Coast have been abandoned because smog adversely affected the growth of grapes. Pollution is also destructive to the materials that buildings are made of.

Indoor Pollution.   Pollution inside buildings is a growing concern. Persons who work in certain industrial environments must wear protective gear to prevent lung disorders. In addition, office buildings, hotels, and other public buildings are now tightly sealed, with air cooling, heating, and ventilation controlled mechanically. Such regulation may contribute to respiratory disorders such as asthma and sinusitis, particularly if the air is not exchanged often enough. Smoking is not allowed in many public buildings.

Furnaces or tuck-under garages may release carbon monoxide and other dangerous gases into a home's atmosphere. Homes should not be too tightly sealed, to avoid buildup of these gases. A carbon monoxide detector should be present in every home, along with a smoke detector.

Smoking.   Chapter 6 discusses the health risks of smoking at length. Studies have shown that the risks of some disorders are almost as great, if not greater, for the person who inhales secondhand smoke as for the person who actually smokes. This concern is of importance to all people, particularly families with small children, because secondhand smoke is likely to influence the development of disorders such as asthma and ear infections. Older adults who inhale secondhand smoke are particularly susceptible to pneumonia—a leading cause of death among senior citizens.

Many companies, healthcare facilities, schools, and other public buildings are now smoke free. Smoking is not allowed on commercial airline flights within the United States and on many international flights. Schools and healthcare facilities usually declare their buildings and grounds as totally nonsmoking premises; in many cases, this designation is mandated by law or by accrediting agencies. Most restaurants have nonsmoking areas, hotels have nonsmoking rooms, and smoke-free rental cars are available.

Water Pollution

Water pollution is a serious and increasing health hazard. Contaminated water transmits a number of diseases, including typhoid fever, dysentery, and infectious hepatitis. Water pollution not only affects people but is also a menace to recreation areas, wildlife, and fish. Each year, polluted water kills millions of fish and shellfish in the United States. The mercury level in water and seafood is particularly dangerous for pregnant women. Guidelines from public health officials establish amounts of seafood and fish from designated areas that can be eaten safely in a specified time.

Increasing demands on the national water supply make it necessary to reuse water, thereby requiring that wastewater be treated to make it safe for reuse. In many areas, this treatment is inadequate. Legislation now gives the USPHS authority and funds to establish water treatment projects. The federal government has also enacted legislation establishing sanitary sewer districts around many lakes and along rivers. In this manner, the quality of public waters will be maintained and improved.

Land Pollution

As the population grows, it produces more garbage and trash. Large cities are running out of places to dump their trash. People often do not want landfills or incinerators in their neighborhoods. In previous years, barges of trash and garbage were shipped to smaller nations or dumped into the ocean. More recently, the United States has become aware of its worldwide

responsibilities. Trash cannot continue to pollute foreign lands or the planet's largest natural resource, the oceans. As a result, most communities have developed recycling programs, well-managed landfills, and pollution-free incinerators.

A new danger exists regarding landfills. As land near cities becomes increasingly scarce, homes and other buildings are being built on old landfill sites. This practice has been proven to contribute to diseases (including cancer), particularly in children.

Radon is a chemical element that occurs in nature as a by-product of the disintegration of radium. It contributes to diseases, including lung cancer. Radon can collect in spaces that are poorly ventilated, such as caves. It can also seep into homes through cracks in the foundation or the basement floor. The more tightly sealed a home is, the greater the danger of radon exposure. Each home should be tested periodically for radon and appropriate measures taken to eliminate it.

Noise Pollution

Damage to the delicate structures of the ear is caused by loud noise or music. Chronic exposure to loud noise, such as loud music, poses the greatest hazard to hearing. Noise pollution also causes stress. Laws are in place to regulate noise. OSHA requires workers in occupations that are extremely noisy to wear ear protection. Recreational activities such as target shooting require ear protection.

Other Types of Pollution

Other situations contribute to pollution and endanger the environment. An oil spill can kill many fish and animals, and thus limit or contaminate food supplies. Insecticides and agricultural chemicals pose a threat to water and clean air. Workers may bring hazardous substances home on their clothing, thereby endangering the health of their family members. For example, in addition to causing cancer that may affect the workers themselves, asbestos particles on clothing contribute to chronic obstructive pulmonary disease in the families of workers.

Lead Poisoning (Plumbism).   Lead poisoning (**plumbism**) continues to be a significant public health problem. It causes serious mental and physical disabilities, particularly in young children. Many cities have programs to test children for lead poisoning and to remove leaded paint and lead pipes from older buildings. Lead can also be present in the soil, partially as a result of exhaust from cars that used leaded gasoline. Lead can also be found in newspaper print and old toys with chipped paint. Plumbism is discussed further in Chapter 73.

Radiation.   Citizens are concerned about **radiation** (ionizing waves of energy that penetrate objects). Many disputes between the public and power companies using nuclear fuel remain unresolved. One problem concerns the disposal of radioactive wastes. Repercussions from accidents in the 1980s at Three Mile Island in Pennsylvania and Chernobyl in the Ukraine continue to raise questions about the world's freedom from dangerous radiation.

Biohazardous Waste Disposal.   Proper and safe disposal of **biohazardous** medical wastes, which are infectious and harmful to humans or animals, is the responsibility of every institutional and individual healthcare provider. Policies and procedures dictate the processes by which the disposal of medical wastes should occur. These processes must meet the multiple-standard regulations of OSHA, the Department of Environmental Protection, and local and state health departments.

Nurses performing home care must be especially careful to dispose of medical waste properly and to teach clients and families correct disposal methods. Medical equipment companies can provide containers and bags for proper disposal of sharps and biohazardous materials.

☞ KEY CONCEPT

You are part of the world community. Participate in protecting the world you live in. Teach others to protect the environment as well.

➤ STUDENT SYNTHESIS

Key Points

- You are a member of many communities and should serve as an advocate and educator to protect those communities.
- Healthcare services are provided on international, national, state, and local levels.
- Federal agencies include the United States Public Health Service and the Department of Health and Human Services. These agencies have many branches and numerous programs.
- The blood-borne pathogen standard established by OSHA has significantly affected nursing procedures and delivery of services in healthcare facilities.
- The Social Security Administration supervises the Medicare and Medicaid programs.
- Voluntary health agencies may be set up to provide direct service, education, or fund-raising to combat a particular disease or for specific health concerns.
- Public and private agencies often work together to provide healthcare services.
- Many primary healthcare services are provided at community health centers. These services include examinations, health screening, immunizations, education, support groups, and illness care.

- Community health is concerned with environmental issues, including air, water, land, and noise pollution; plumbism; radiation; and biohazardous waste disposal.

Critical Thinking Exercises

1. Evaluate healthcare services provided in your community.
2. What types of pollution are a problem in your community? Discuss various ways that you can contribute to reducing the problem.
3. As a member of the healthcare industry, what special responsibilities do you feel you have toward the community? Are you responsible in special ways for the environment?

NCLEX-Style Review Questions

1. Which agency should the nurse notify regarding a client with infected rat bites who reports that the entire apartment complex is infected with rats?
   a. American Red Cross
   b. Department of Agriculture
   c. Food and Drug Administration
   d. Social Security Administration
2. The community health center in your area has hired you to assist with projects during the summer. You would expect that your duties might include:
   a. Arranging times for all families served by this center to come to the central office so that care can be given in one location
   b. Referring clients with suspected sexually transmitted disease to a hospital for screening
   c. Scheduling clients for visits to the emergency room to receive immunizations and prenatal care
   d. Working with clients in group homes for the mentally ill or mentally retarded, day care centers, or in school settings
3. Encouraging families to obtain and use a radon testing kit would help prevent disease related to:
   a. Air pollution
   b. Land pollution
   c. Noise pollution
   d. Water pollution

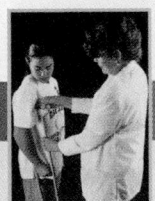

8

Transcultural Healthcare

LEARNING OBJECTIVES

1. Define and state the components of culture, subculture, race, minorities, and ethnicity.
2. Identify four major subcultural groups of your community, your state, and the United States.
3. Define and give examples of prejudice, ethnocentrism, and stereotyping.
4. Identify three barriers to providing culturally competent nursing care.
5. List at least eight nursing considerations that need to be considered as part of a cultural assessment.
6. Discuss at least two ways in which each of the following influence nursing care: values and beliefs, taboos and rituals, concepts of health and illness, language and communication, diet and nutrition, elimination, and death and dying.
7. Assess the importance of religious and spiritual beliefs for clients experiencing illness.
8. Compare and contrast the following belief systems: magicoreligious, scientific/biomedical, holistic medicine, yin–yang, and hot–cold.
9. Discuss the common philosophies of mental illness in at least three different cultures and state how these ideas affect nursing care.
10. Identify at least three important qualifications for a professional interpreter.
11. Discuss at least three cultural aspects of each of the following: personal space and touching, eye contact, diet and nutrition, elimination and concepts of death and dying. Relate these aspects to concepts of nursing care.

NEW TERMINOLOGY

beliefs
cultural diversity
cultural sensitivity
culture
curandero
ethnocentrism
ethnicity
ethnonursing
imam
karma
minister
minority
mullah
nirvana

norms
prejudice
priest
rabbi
race
rituals
stereotype
subculture
shaman
taboos
transcultural nursing
values
yin–yang

In the late 20th century, nurse and anthropologist Madeleine Leininger helped develop the concept that a client has physical, spiritual, psychological, and socioeconomic needs that exist in our complex, diverse world.

As a nurse, you are responsible for becoming acquainted with the predominant cultures in your community. Remember to view each person within a group as an individual and to provide care in a nonjudgmental way. Individuals identify with their cultural, ethnic, racial, and religious backgrounds to various degrees. The nurse must be aware of his or her own beliefs and be sensitive to the beliefs of others.

CULTURE AND ETHNICITY

Definitions of Culture

Culture is the accumulated learning for generational groups of individuals within structured or non-structured societies. Individuals experience a cultural heritage with others. It is a heritage that is learned through formal and informal experiences through the life cycle. Culture consists of the combined heritage of language and communication style, health beliefs and health practices, customs and rituals, and religious beliefs and practices. Culture is influenced by environment, expectations of society, and national origin.

☛ Key Concept

All cultural information in this book is general. These generalizations are used for descriptive purposes, but remember that not everyone in a particular group follows all the practices or shares the same beliefs and characteristics.

The way an individual behaves in social groups and as an individual within that group is also part of one's culture. An individual learns, evaluates, and behaves according to specified **values** within a culture. Cultural concepts and beliefs provide the blueprints or guides for determining one's personal and societal values, individual beliefs, and lifelong practices. A pattern of values, attitudes, social, political, economic, educational and other behaviors emerge from the learned culture and are shared in a defined group over time as an identifiable heritage. Box 8-1 presents some characteristics of culture.

Subcultures. **Subcultures** are groups within dominant cultures. Subcultures form because individuals share characteristics that belong to an identifiable group such as occupations (nurse, teacher, politician), religions (Islam, Methodist, Baptist), geographic origins (New Englander, Midwesterner, Californian), or age (infant, teenager, elderly). Nursing students also comprise a subculture because of the unique experiences and growth process that are universal components of all student nursing populations. Table 8-1 lists the major subcultures that exist in the United States. The term *American* is correctly used to define all persons living in North, Central, or South America.

Race. The term **race** is used to differentiate large groups of humankind that share common biological and sociological characteristics. *Race* implies genetic characteristics associated with having ancestors from a specific part of the world. Race

➤➤ BOX 8-1

CHARACTERISTICS OF CULTURE

- A *way of life* for a group of individuals
- The sum of *socially inherited* characteristics, handed down from generation to generation
- A group's *design for living*—socially transmitted assumptions about the physical and social world
- *Learned* from birth—socialization (not genetic)
- *Unique* to each ethnic group
- Shared by members of the same group (identity)
- *Complex* and all-encompassing
- Often an *unconscious process*
- An *adaptation* to various conditions (environmental, technical, available resources)
- *Dynamic* (always changing)

should not be confused with ethnicity or culture. Box 8-2 defines the federal standards of race. Racial mixing has blurred the *physical* characteristics of individuals. The nurse must be aware that obvious physical attributes, such as skin, hair, or eye color, are not accurate indicators of race. Genetic diseases are not limited to individuals who physically appear to be of a particular race.

Minorities within a population may be identified as subcultures. Physical and cultural characteristics of a group may differ from the predominant group of a particular region. African Americans, Latinos (or *Hispanics*), Asian Americans, and Native Americans are the four identified subcultures of the U.S., according to the Centers for Disease Control (CDC). Each group has specific and distinctive features and is also part of larger cultural groups. These groups can be divided into smaller groups; for example, Latinos include Mexicans, Puerto Ricans, Cubans, Guatemalans, and others. Minorities can also be identified according to religion, occupation, sexual orientation, or gender.

■■   **TABLE 8-1   *M*AJOR AMERICAN SUBCULTURAL GROUPS**

Subculture	Countries of Origin
African American	Africa, Haiti, Jamaica, West Indian Islands, Dominican Republic
Latino/Hispanic	Mexico, Puerto Rico, Cuba, South and Central America
Asian American	China, Japan, Korea, Philippines, Thailand, Indochina, Vietnam, Pacific Islands
Native American	North American Indian nation and tribes including Eskimos and Aleuts

Timby, B., K., Scherer, J., C., Smith, N., E. (1999). *Introductory medical-surgical nursing* (7th ed., p. 89). Philadelphia: Lippincott Williams & Wilkins.

➤ ➤ BOX 8-2

RACE AND HISPANIC ETHNICITY

The categories and definitions for race and ethnicity used in this text are consistent with the federal standards established by the Office of Management and Budget (OMB). The federal government considers *race* and *Hispanic ethnicity* to be two separate and distinct concepts.

The five *racial* categories are:

1. **American Indian or Alaskan Native** refers to people having origins in any of the original peoples of North and South America, including Central America, and who maintain tribal affiliation or community attachment.
2. **Asian** refers to people having origins in any of the original peoples of the Far East, Southeast Asia, or the Indian Subcontinent. It includes people who indicated their race or races as "Asian Indian," "Chinese," "Filipino," "Korean," "Japanese," "Vietnamese," or "Other Asian."
3. **Native Hawaiian and other Pacific Islander** refers to people having origins in any of the original people of Hawaii, Guam, Samoa, or other Pacific Islands.
4. **Black or African American** refers to people having origins in any of the Black racial groups of Africa, ~~Native Australians, Caribbean, S. Europe~~ (handwritten)
5. **White** refers to people having origins in any of the original peoples of Europe, the Middle East, or ~~North Africa~~.

Hispanics may be of any race. The OMB defines Hispanic or Latino as "a person of Cuban, Mexican, Puerto Rican, South or Central American, or other Spanish culture or origin regardless of race." The terms "Hispanic" and "Latino" are used interchangeably.

The six *racial/ethnic* categories are:

1. All Hispanic
2. Hispanic Black
3. Hispanic White
4. All Non-Hispanic
5. Non-Hispanic Black
6. Non-Hispanic White

Further information can be found at the following websites:

http://www.census.gov/population/www/socdemo/race.html

http://www.census.gov/population/www/socdemo/hispanic.html

Source: U.S. Census Bureau website www.census.gov/population/prod/2001pubs/c2kbrol-1.pdf, *Overview of race and Hispanic origin, 2000.* Issued March 2001.

The term **minority** can be misleading. For example, a Texas rancher in the skyscrapers of Manhattan can be seen as a minority. A Vietnamese immigrant can be part of the majority of a population in one geographic location, just as a descendent of early European settlers can be part of a minority in parts of the United States. Global shifts of multiple groups of individuals are continually revising cultures and subcultures and remaking majority and minority groups. This phenomenon is happening on all continents. The results of these shifts can be beneficial to society or may lead to fervent nationalism and hostility.

Cultures are not stagnant or unchanging. Economics and politics influence culture. The "American Dream" was built upon the cultural belief that a better lifestyle for youth is possible than that which occurred in our parents' or grandparents' lifetime. → nationality (handwritten)

Ethnicity is the common heritage shared by a specific culture. Now many people work hard to retain their cultural and ethnic identification. This is demonstrated in Scandinavian celebrations in the Midwest; Hispanic celebrations of Cinco de Mayo in the Southwest; traditional Mardi Gras celebrations in Louisiana; Native American pow wows; and Chinese New Year celebrations. Many ethnic groups celebrate special occasions, such as weddings, with traditional activities and foods. Some people strongly identify with their culture of origin and make an effort to pass traditions along to their children. Tacos and burritos are examples of types of food in the southwestern United States that are shared with other ethnic backgrounds. Cultures are often associated with religious beliefs, and religion may be a strong factor in a person's ethnicity.

Groups show ethnic pride in various ways. For example, a celebration of religious and cultural heritage is demonstrated by the St. Patrick's Day Parade in New York City. Some ethnic groups retain links to their country of origin by wearing specific items such as an Asian Indian sari, clothing with African patterns, or Native American jewelry.

Cultural Diversity

Cultures are becoming so interwoven and blended that specific identification of cultural groups is difficult. The mix of cultural groups in the United States changed in the 20th century. For example, the number of people who identify themselves as a minority in the U.S. census has increased. In 1970, the percentage of minorities was 12.5%; in 1990, it was approximately 25%. In the 2000 census, minorities such as Latino have surpassed the traditional majorities of ethnic Caucasians in several states. National projections predict that ethnic minority groups will compose 51% of the total U.S. population by the late 21st century.

Currently, the Hispanic community is the fastest-growing group in the United States and is projected to be the largest nonwhite group in the country by 2005. The Asian/Pacific Islander group is also expanding rapidly, with a 95% growth rate expected in the early 21st century. To date, as many as 150 different ethnic groups and more than 500 tribes of Native Americans have been identified in the United States.

In addition to expanding birth rates among specific ethnic groups, immigrants from many countries are entering the United States in large numbers. Both factors are influencing current population trends.

As you can see from the statistics and from your own experience, **cultural diversity** has become part of our world. Individuals will meet people of many ethnic groups both as citizens and as nurses. When a nurse cares for clients from her own culture, she will likely understand their language, values, and beliefs. When a nurse encounters clients from cultures that are unfamiliar, however, understanding and communication may become difficult. To be effective, the nurse must transcend cultural barriers and approach every client with patience, empathy, concern, and competence. A high level of self-awareness is also important. Before you can understand another person's culture, you must first understand and accept your own.

The American Nurses foundation and its affiliate, the American Nurses Association (ANA), promote nursing issues of cultural competency and ethnic diversity. In a 1991 position statement, the ANA identified the critical need for nurses to be aware of cultural variations of clients. Three concepts are important:

- Knowledge of cultural diversity is vital at all levels of nursing practice.
- Approaches to nursing practice that do not incorporate cultural sensitivity are ineffective.
- Knowledge about cultures and their impact on interactions with healthcare is essential for nurses.

Census and culture statistics can currently be found on two websites. These websites have valuable information for healthcare providers. Local, state, and countrywide information can be obtained. A nurse should be aware of the cultures, subcultures, ethnic groups, and races within the nurse's area of employment.

The National Center for Health Statistics maintains a comprehensive website with a large variety of health data relating to general and specific populations. The site can be found at *www.cdc.gov/nchs.* The Census 2000 website contains huge amounts of detailed information relating to population numbers and trends. Focus is given to the major U.S. subgroups. That site can be found at *www.census.gov/population/www/socdemo/race.html.*

Barriers to Culturally Competent Care

Prejudice is a belief based on preconceived notions about certain groups of people. Prejudices can be unfair, biased beliefs. Many people have been the victims of prejudice. Overweight individuals, homosexuals, racial groups, and others have been the victims of prejudice. Prejudice exists in subtler forms, an example being a fixed negative opinion against authority figures that some people harbor. Many individuals are prejudiced without realizing it. Consider that you may be prejudiced against men with beards, women in short skirts, individuals with high IQs, etc. Are you pre-judging others on the basis of personal appearance or a unique trait?

Ethnocentrism is the belief that one's own culture is the best and only acceptable way. It shows lack of cultural sensitivity. If a person is ethnocentric, he or she is unable to see the value in other cultures. As a nurse, seeing beyond your own particular ethnic/cultural group is important for effective communication and understanding.

The term **stereotype** refers to classifying or categorizing people, and believing that all those belonging to a certain group are alike. In the movies, the villain is often stereotyped as wearing the black hat while the hero wears the white hat. Stereotyping infers preconceived but often incorrect, negative notions. It is inappropriate to assign derogatory characteristics (such as lazy, dishonest, or stupid) to groups due to stereotyping. Additionally, individuals will always maintain some uniqueness within a group. People are all more alike than they are different.

Cultural Sensitivity

Cultural sensitivity is the understanding and tolerance of all cultures and lifestyles. It is crucial in the delivery of competent nursing care. Develop cultural sensitivity when working with individuals from every ethnic/cultural group. Cultural sensitivity allows the nurse to more accurately understand and to accept the behavior of others. Nurses are better able to deliver care, being sensitive to cultural factors involved in the client's health or illness.

No culture is better or worse than another. Additionally, cultures are ever changing; they evolve over many generations. Box 8-3 lists many nursing considerations that can be used as a part of cultural assessments.

CULTURALLY INFLUENCED COMPONENTS

Being a member of a cultural group means that certain components of that culture are common to many of its members. Common cultural components can be classified in terms of *values and beliefs, taboos and rituals,* concepts of *health and illness, language and communication, diet and nutrition* practices, *elimination* patterns, and attitudes toward *death and dying.* These factors are discussed throughout this text. Remember that you can learn much more about all aspects of ethnicity and culture than can be presented here. Three categories of cultural treatment, beliefs, and practices are summarized in Box 8-4.

Beliefs and Values

Each ethnic/cultural group has **beliefs,** or concepts the members believe to be true. Beliefs that an individual develops are ingrained by the age of 10 years old. Beliefs can be based on fact, fiction, or a combination of both. Beliefs can be difficult to change. A change in belief systems can be a milestone in an individual's life. The recognition of the reality or fantasy of Santa Claus usually denotes a change in a child's belief

➤➤ BOX 8-3   *Study*

TRANSCULTURAL NURSING CONSIDERATIONS AND CULTURAL ASSESSMENT

Transcultural nursing stresses that many subgroups exist within each culture. Not all members of a group share the same beliefs or traditions. Consider the following elements as you work with others:

- Your own cultural background; differences and similarities between you and the client
- Definition of health and illness accepted by an ethnic group
- Importance of religion, religious beliefs, and religious practices
- Concepts relating to causes of illness and injury
- Ethnic/folk medicine practices; the use of special clothing, amulets, or rituals
- Attitudes toward various types and models of healthcare, eg, holistic, biomedical, spiritual
- Relationships, responsibilities, and roles of men and women (decision-makers)
- Economic level of client/family (socioeconomic status)
- Environmental factors and related disorders (eg, poverty, lead poisoning)
- Verbal and nonverbal communication patterns (personal space, touching, eye contact)
- Language differences between healthcare staff and client/family
- Modesty, machismo, and concept of human body

- Reactions to pain, birth, and death
- Reactions to aging and care of the elderly
- Capacity of, resources for, and sources of support persons such as family, friends, or religious groups
- Attitudes about mental illness or retardation
- Food restrictions or preferences
- Attitudes about factors such as physical appearance, amputation, obesity; adaptation to prescribed therapeutic diets
- Group identity; importance and type of family structure, cohesiveness within the group; traditional roles of men and women
- "Visibility" of ethnic background (eg, African American, Asian American)
- Disorders specific to an ethnic group (eg, Tay-Sachs, sickle cell anemia)
- Attitudes about education, time, and authority
- Predominant occupations within the group; role models
- "Westernization" of younger members
- Number of people belonging to that group in the same geographic area as the healthcare facility
- Prejudices within a cultural group relating to other members of the same group; stereotypes of and prejudices against other particular groups
- Mixed families (mixed race, religion, or cultural background)

Adapted from Timby, B., K., Scherer, J., C., Smith, N., E. (1999). *Introductory medical-surgical nursing* (7th ed.). Philadelphia: Lippincott Williams & Wilkins.

---

system. Historical belief systems can change, leading to new beliefs, such as the change from a monarchy to a democracy.

A group lives by **values,** which shape how an individual perceives right or wrong and what is desirable or valuable. Values influence a person's responses to the world and to others. People's values define who they are, their identity, and their views of the world. Each person's values are unique and influence behavior and self-esteem. From values evolve **norms,** which become rules for behavior in a group. Society develops sanctions or laws that serve to enforce norms.

Nurses must recognize that different beliefs and values exist. The issues of life and death are value-laden concepts that affect nursing. For example, the decision to terminate life-support, to have an elective abortion, or to refuse blood products may be related to the client's cultural, ethnic, or religious beliefs and values. Even if the nurse does not agree with the decision, she must respect that individuals have the right and responsibility for their own beliefs and values.

☛ KEY CONCEPT

People are probably more tied to their cultural and ethnic beliefs when ill than when feeling well. Illness is stressful

and may lead individuals to revert to what is known and comfortable.

Taboos and Rituals

Every culture has **taboos** that its members cannot violate without discomfort and risk of separation from the group. Each culture also has **rituals,** which members are often required to practice for comfort, acceptance, and inclusion. Rituals are usually performed by individuals within a culture who maintain a high level of respect and authority among their peers. Native Americans use the arts of a **shaman** (medicine man). Latinos have **curanderos** (traditional lay persons) who assist a client with herbs and counseling. Moslims (Muslims) follow the guidance of a **mullah.** Christians have **ministers** or **priests,** and Jews have **rabbis.** A person may be more likely to consider taboos and to follow rituals when experiencing illness than when feeling well because of their cultural beliefs or values.

Often, taboos and rituals are associated with religious or spiritual services pertaining to healing, death, or dying. Nurses need to be aware that these are important components of the client's system of health beliefs. See Table 8-2 for more on traditional health beliefs and practices.

➤➤ BOX 8-4

THREE CATEGORIES OF CULTURALLY INFLUENCED TREATMENT, BELIEFS, AND PRACTICES

1. **Traditional Healers and Practices**
   - Clients from African American, Native American, and Hispanic cultures may use roots, potions, and herbs for treating illnesses. Native American Shamans, or Hispanic folk healers (**curandero** in Spanish) may see a client to administer herbs, at the client's request. Some people choose to wear herbs or an amulet around the neck. Do not remove such articles if at all possible.
   - Chinese and Filipino cultures often use massage, herbal medicine, and acupuncture.
   - Some groups wear copper bracelets as a preventive measure or cure for arthritis.
   - Elders may place their hands on the head of a Mormon who is ill or injured, to bring a healing blessing.
   - Approximately 80% of the world's people believe in mal ojo, the "evil eye." Families often put a bracelet or *amulet* on newborns to protect them. Even though this belief may not be firm, amulets may still be worn customarily. For example, in Greece, virtually everyone wears an amulet to ward off the evil eye.
   - Some people who practice Roman Catholicism or Greek Orthodoxy want a small statue of the Virgin Mary next to their bed and a Catholic medal or cloth scapular pinned to their clothing. Do not remove these articles during examinations or surgery unless absolutely necessary.
   - Some cultures customarily burn candles and keep bedside altars with statues of saints. Part of the Native American/Alaska Native culture and religion is the burning of certain plant substances, as well as the use of herbal medicine. Jewish people may wish to have a menorah (special candelabra) at the bedside. Clients may receive special permission to continue these cultural practices in the healthcare facility. (An electric version of the menorah is available if candles are not allowed.)
   - In Puerto Rican and many Native American and Hispanic cultures, medical doctors provide most healthcare, but naturalists and spiritualists also play an important role.

2. **Traditional Family Roles and Practices in Healthcare**
   - People of many cultures will supplement medicine prescribed by physicians with home remedies and herbal medicines. In other cases, they will buy prescribed medicines, but not use them. Discuss medication practices with clients, especially those with diabetes or other medication-dependent disorders, to ensure that they are using required insulin or other medication. Some people believe that diabetes will improve if they eat salty and sour foods, in combination with herbs.
   - In many cultures, the family is of utmost importance, providing clients with total economic, physical, and psychological support. Hospitalized Hispanic, Southeast Asian, East Indian, or Amish clients may have one or more family members remain with them at all times. People of these cultures (and others) may often have large numbers of visitors from several generations.
   - In many cultures, the immediate or extended family makes decisions about an individual's healthcare. The client may or may not have a say in decisions. For example, the role of women in East Indian, Pakistani, and Arab cultures is often to be subservient to men. A woman from these cultures may be more inclined to follow instructions from a male nurse or physician. Her husband or father may make all decisions for her.
   - Virginity and machismo play important cultural roles. A young woman who is a virgin may be reluctant to talk to or be examined by a male physician or nurse. Amish women and women of many East Indian, Asian, Muslim, and Hispanic groups are often uncomfortable receiving care from male physicians or nurses. East Indian and Amish women, in particular, often wish to wear their native dress, even in the hospital. Amish, Somalian, and many Arab women keep their heads covered. Some men are uneasy about being bathed by female nurses, especially if the nurses are young. They may prefer to wait until their wives or other family members visit to assist with baths and personal care.

3. **Traditional Group or Societal Practices**
   - In some cultures, such as Northern European, time and punctuality are very important. In other cultures, such as many Native American and Mexican American groups, schedules are more flexible. Be aware of this difference when scheduling appointments or giving care instructions.
   - Cultural groups react differently to pain. Some groups are stoic, whereas others tend to cry out with pain.
   - Many people, especially those who speak only limited English, try to be cooperative and agreeable. They will nod and say "yes" when you ask if they understand, even if they do not. Make sure that these clients can explain procedures and instructions, in their own words, back to you, to facilitate understanding.

■■ TABLE 8-2 ✐*T*RADITIONAL HEALTH BELIEFS AND PRACTICES

Cultural Group	Health Belief	Health Practices
Anglo-Americans	Illness is caused by infectious microorganisms, organ degeneration, and unhealthy lifestyles.	Physicians are consulted for diagnosis and treatment; nurses provide physical care.
African Americans	Supernatural forces can cause disease and influence recovery.	Individual and group prayer is used to speed recovery.
Asian Americans	Health is the result of a balance between *yin* and *yang* energy; illness results when equilibrium is disturbed.	Acupuncture, acupressure, food, and herbs are used to restore balance.
Latinos/Hispanics	Illness and misfortune occur as a punishment from God, referred to as *castigo de Dios,* or they are caused by an imbalance of "hot" or "cold" forces within the body.	Prayer and penance are performed to receive forgiveness; the services of lay practitioners who are believed to possess spiritual healing power are used; foods that are "hot" or "cold" are consumed to restore balance.
Native Americans	Illness occurs when the harmony of nature (Mother Earth) is disturbed.	A *shaman,* or medicine man, who has both spiritual and healing power, is consulted to restore harmony.

*As reported by the U.S. Census Bureau in 1990.

Timby, B., K., Scherer, J., C., Smith, N., E. (1999). *Introductory medical-surgical nursing* (7th ed., p. 92). Philadelphia: Lippincott Williams & Wilkins.

Health and Illness

Culture greatly influences an individual's concepts of health and illness. Such beliefs can affect a person's recovery from illness or injury. Each society has norms relating to the meaning of illness, how an ill person should behave, and what means should be used to assist him or her. Strive to accommodate each client's healthcare beliefs and practices (as long as they are safe), even if you do not fully understand or agree with them.

Health Belief Systems
Several health belief systems exist. Among these systems are:

Magicoreligious: The belief that supernatural forces dominate. For example, the Christian Scientist religion believes in healing by prayer alone. Many people believe we are influenced by spirits, gods, or demons. Some cultures believe fate decides life, in that things happen for a purpose designed by a higher spiritual being. It is often not necessary that the individual understand the event. Other groups believe that illness and adversity serve as punishment for sins. Some people believe that trouble or pain is God's will.

Scientific/biomedical: The belief that physical and biomedical processes can be studied and manipulated to control life. For example, the Shintoist religion believes that people are inherently good; illness is caused when the person comes into contact with pollutants. Western medicine often takes the approach that the body has individual body systems, eg, pulmonary, integumentary, endocrine, and so on. Therefore, specialists are hired to address the specific concerns of diseased or injured parts of the human body.

Holistic medicine: The belief that the forces of nature must be kept balanced. The holistic approach combines the physical, psychological, and spiritual health or illness of an individual. Health is defined in terms of the person's relationship with nature and the universe (wholeness). Life is considered as only one aspect of nature. From this belief system come holistic medicine, herbal medicine, and concepts of Mother Earth. Many Native Americans and Asians follow the holistic approach. Therapies such as chiropractic and acupuncture are based on this theory (see Chap. 3). Native Americans often follow three holistic concepts: *prevention, treatment,* and *health maintenance.*

Yin–yang and hot–cold theories: The belief that illness develops when life forces are out of balance. Many cultures believe in the **yin–yang** or hot–cold aspects of wellness and illness, as summarized in Box 8-5.

Many people also believe in a complex system of five basic energies/elements/substances in nature (wood, fire, earth, metal, water). This theory is an expansion of yin–yang and is also involved in the healing process. Many Filipino and Hispanic groups believe that heat, cold, wetness, and dryness must be balanced for health. Certain illnesses are considered hot or cold, wet or dry. Foods, activities, medications, and herbal substances, classified as hot or cold, are added or subtracted to bring about balance. Other ethnic groups that use parts of the yin–yang or hot–cold theories include Asian, African American, Arab, Muslim, and Caribbean peoples. An important point is that various ethnic groups have differing beliefs as to which illnesses and which treatments are hot or cold.

➤➤ BOX 8-5

YIN–YANG

Yin and yang represent "unified opposites" that are interrelated. A yin condition requires a yang treatment and vice versa. The forces of nature are balanced to provide harmony and homeostasis.

Yin	Yang
matter	energy
female	male
negative	positive
darkness/night	light/day
cold	warmth
emptiness	fullness
weak	strong
expansion	contraction
hypofunction	hyperfunction

The U.S. healthcare system is constantly evolving and incorporating elements from many different belief systems. Be aware of popular and folk practices among members of your community. By doing so, you will better appreciate the range of services available for use by clients. Chapter 3 introduces some complementary therapies, many of which are based on elements of the above systems.

Treatment and Healing Beliefs and Practices

Cultural/ethnic groups have many beliefs and practices for times of illness. Table 8-2 gives some generalizations designed to provide you with an overview of the wide variations and similarities. Caution should be observed with learning concepts of culture because it is possible to stereotype individuals based on perceived cultural generalizations. Clients are often happy to explain their beliefs to you, so you can better understand and care for them.

Attitudes Toward Mental Illness

Mental illness is not accepted in all cultures as a consequence of biological disease. Western medicine and psychiatry and their approaches to mental illness are based on the accepted findings of late 20th century science. The belief that chemical changes in the brain can cause mental disorders is a relatively new concept for many cultures. Some cultures consider mental disorders a disgrace to the individual and to the family.

In contrast to the biological, scientific approach of Western medicine is the belief in the spirit world. Science may consider a person's behavior to be abnormal or even psychotic if spirits, angels, or a deity is involved. Members of that culture may hear the spirits talking. Some individuals believe in a curse or "evil eye." Western medicine traditionally considers this type of belief a deviation, whereas it may be an accepted belief in that client's culture.

Some may consider behavior to be deviant because an individual chooses not to follow cultural norms, eg, length of hair, type of dress, type of lifestyle.

Statistically, a higher percentage of people from groups other than white are diagnosed as mentally ill in the United States. Poverty and the inability to obtain early medical care may contribute to these figures. Western medicine's current diagnostic tools may also be unable to interpret and to evaluate properly the thought processes and beliefs of persons from diverse cultures.

Language and Communication

The nurse and the clients may speak different languages. In addition, a person may speak the English language in everyday life, but may be uncomfortable trying to use medical terms in their second language. Also, many people find it difficult to speak in a second language when they are ill. Difficulties arise when no one is available to translate. Such situations may interfere with client care. Accurate interpretation of verbal and nonverbal communication is particularly important in an area such as the mental health unit, where these factors are integral to diagnosis and treatment.

☛ KEY CONCEPT

A great deal of communication takes place using nonverbal cues, hand signals, and pictures. Clients will be appreciative if you learn a few words in their language. Remember that a smile is understood in almost any language.

Ways to Facilitate Communication

Methods are available to facilitate transcultural communication. One of the most common is through the use of a professional interpreter. Box 8-6 gives some practical solutions to English language barriers. Following is a list of various ways to communicate:

Professional interpreter: If possible, obtain the services of a trained interpreter, either in person or by telephone. An interpreter can help set up a list of common terms or a photo board for routine requests. In addition to providing the client with comfort and safety, a trained interpreter often understands the culture of the person, as well as the language. The skilled interpreter can explain nonverbal cues, in addition to what the client says. The objective interpreter is an invaluable staff resource, as illustrated in Figure 8-1.

Family as interpreter: Sometimes, a family member or significant other can act as an interpreter. Having a member of the family translate may be inappropriate, however. Most importantly, it may compromise the client's confidentiality. Translations are often inaccurate because family members may be unfamiliar with healthcare terminology. They may unintentionally change the meaning of what is said or may omit information, not realizing the importance of every word.

➤➤ BOX 8-6

COMMUNICATING WITH NON–ENGLISH SPEAKING CLIENTS

When Clients Speak No English

- Learn a second language, especially one spoken by a large ethnic population serviced by the healthcare agency.
- Speak words or phrases in the client's language, even if it is not possible to carry on a conversation.
- Refer to an English/foreign language dictionary for bilingual vocabulary words; *Taber's Cyclopedic Medical Dictionary* contains medical words and phrases in Spanish, Italian, French, and German.
- Construct a loose-leaf folder or file cards with words in one or more languages spoken by clients in the community.
- Develop a list of employees or individuals to contact in the community who speak a second language and are willing to act as translators; in an extreme emergency, international telephone operators may be able to provide assistance.
- Select a translator who is the same gender as the client and approximately the same age, if possible.
- Look at the client, not the translator, when asking questions and listening to the client's response.

When English is a Second Language

- Determine if the client speaks or reads English, or both.
- Speak slowly, not loudly, using simple words and short sentences.
- Avoid using technical terms, slang, or phrases with a double or colloquial meaning like "Do you have to use the john?"
- Ask questions that can be answered by a "yes" or "no."
- Repeat the question without changing the words, if the client appears confused.
- Give the client sufficient time to process the question from English to the native language, and respond back in English.
- Rely heavily on nonverbal communication, and pantomime if necessary.
- Avoid displaying impatience.
- Ask the client to "read this line," to determine the client's ability to follow written instructions, which are provided in English.

Timby, B., K., Scherer, J., C., Smith, N., E. (1999). *Introductory medical-surgical nursing* (7th ed., p. 90). Philadelphia: Lippincott Williams & Wilkins.

Mistakes may also be intentional, to avoid embarrassment. Gender differences may increase translation difficulties. Men may not be comfortable discussing female problems or female anatomy, or vice versa.

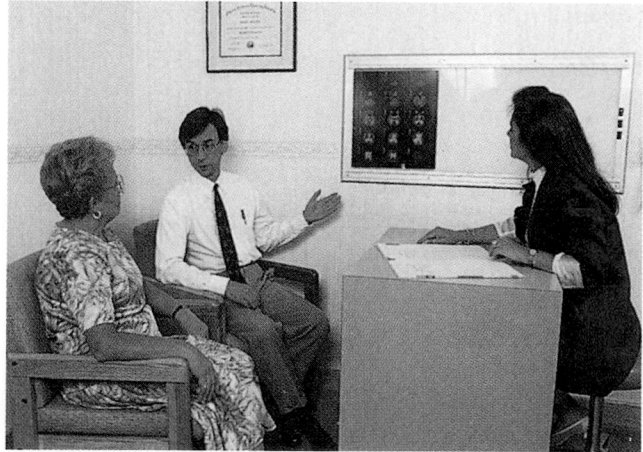

FIGURE 8-1. Interpreters are important components of the healthcare team. An interpreter used in healthcare settings should have several qualities: a) the interpreter should know and understand the nuances of medical language; b) the interpreter should know the formal, slang, and conversational levels of the language that he or she is interpreting; and c) the interpreter should be able to communicate without inferring judgment, bias, or personal opinions. (Hosley, J. B., Jones, S. A., & Molle-Matthews, E. A. [1997]. *Lippincott's textbook for medical assistants* [p. 65]. Philadelphia: Lippincott Williams & Wilkins.)

Nurse as interpreter: In some cases, a nurse or other healthcare worker is bilingual and can assist with translating; however, problems may arise. The bilingual healthcare worker may not know medical terminology in the native language and may not have time available to leave his or her own clients to translate for others.

Personal Space and Touching

Personal space refers to a person's comfort zone. Types of personal space include *intimate space* (reserved for close family members) and *personal space* (for contact with the general public). Americans, Canadians, and the British have the largest personal space zone of all cultures, requiring several feet for comfort. In many cultures, such as those of Latin America, Japan, and the Middle East, maintaining such a large space would be considered rejecting and insulting.

Touching is often culture related. Nurses must touch clients to perform treatments; however, they need to remain aware that taboos are also involved. For example, Europeans often pat children on the head as a sign of affection. In some Asian cultures, however, touching a child on the head is a sign of disrespect and is believed to cause illness. A safer approach is to touch children on the hand or arm when talking to or looking at them, but not to touch them on the head without permission.

Hispanic people and people from Mediterranean regions frequently touch each other. Both males and females may kiss each other when meeting, or hold hands while walking. When meeting clients, offer to shake hands, but do not be offended if they decline. Many cultures consider touching a member of the opposite sex or making the first move to offer the hand to a superior to be improper. For example, some Middle Eastern cultures teach that women may not touch any man other than their husbands.

A nurse may be in a particular dilemma if he or she needs to undress a client from particular cultures. For example, a young female nurse may ask an elderly gentleman to remove his shirt for an x-ray. The client may resist the request for two reasons. It may not be appropriate in his culture for a younger person to give commands to an older person. In addition, it may not be appropriate for a male to undress when requested by a stranger, especially if the stranger is female. If you were the nurse, what would you do?

Eye Contact

Eye contact can give important cues about clients. This action is culturally influenced. In most European-based cultures, direct eye contact is considered normal. If not part of the total body language, lack of eye contact in that culture may infer lack of respect, inattention, and avoidance of the truth.

In Native American, Arab, and some Southeast Asian cultures, members believe that looking a person in the eye during conversation is improper and impolite. It may also be interpreted as challenging or hostile. Some individuals may stare at the floor and hesitate before answering, a sign that they are concentrating on what is being said. Others are taught to respect their elders and authority figures. They often expect nurses to make eye contact with them, but do not reciprocate. The Muslim–Arab woman avoids eye contact, especially with men, as a sign of modesty. Facial expressions may be totally absent. Take care not to misinterpret these nonverbal cues. Consider the possibility of cultural influences.

Diet and Nutrition

Cultural eating rituals vary. In some cultures, women and men do not eat together or do not eat with children. In others, eating is a family event, and all family members eat together. Eating utensils vary from the knife, fork, and spoon of Western cultures to the chopsticks of many Asian cultures.

Some religions maintain strict dietary practices. For example, those who practice Orthodox Judaism and Islam follow Old Testament teachings. They do not eat pork and will not eat meat and dairy products together. They also keep separate dishes for these foods. People within the Islamic culture strictly observe religious holidays, keeping a long fast that is often followed by a large feast. In the Mormon and Seventh Day Adventist religions, diet also plays an important part. Most followers eliminate tea, coffee, alcohol, and strong spices. Some religious groups are vegetarians. Most ethnic groups have special food customs and rituals surrounding holidays and special events, such as weddings. Because nutri-

tion and dietary customs play such a large part in health and treatment of illness, a separate chapter (Chap. 31) is devoted to this subject.

Elimination

People of various cultures treat the elimination of bodily wastes (voiding and defecation) differently. Many cultures consider elimination to be a private function. Some people are unable to void or to use a bedpan or commode unless they have complete privacy, which may be difficult in a healthcare facility. Many people of Arab cultures consider the left hand dirty and use it only to clean themselves after elimination.

Death and Dying

Each cultural group has an attitude or series of beliefs about death and dying. Some cultural groups consider death a natural part of life that is not to be feared. For example, many Asian cultures consider death to be preordained, believing that when a person's time to die has come, nothing can stop it. Traditional Western culture tries to prevent death and to prolong life at all costs. Ways of mourning also differ. Some cultural groups believe that the person is happier or better off and rejoice; others cry and mourn loudly. In some cultures, survivors formally mourn for a designated period of time. Others isolate children from death, not allowing them to see a dead body. In some cultures, a pregnant woman is not allowed to see a dead body, fearing danger to the fetus. Many cultures forbid suicide. In some cultures, the person who commits suicide may not be allowed a funeral or traditional burial. Table 8-3 summarizes general cultural factors that affect client care.

RELIGIOUS/SPIRITUAL CUSTOMS AND TRADITIONS

Religion is a vital part of many people's lives. In the United States, 35,000 churches with 1,500 different identified sects exist. Because the nurse will be caring for people of different faiths, she should learn about major religious differences. By doing so, she will be better equipped to determine, with the help of her clients, sources of spiritual and religious support. Important points about several major religions are presented in this section.

Those who are injured or ill need reassurance, and they may talk to a nurse about their illness and spiritual beliefs. Respect their confidences. Maintain a nonjudgmental attitude. Suggest a visit from a spiritual leader, but do not contact such a person without first asking if the client wants such counsel.

☛ KEY CONCEPT

Even though members of a religious, ethnic, or cultural group may share similarities, each person is different. Remember not to stereotype individuals. All members of a group do not behave or believe alike.

■■■ TABLE 8-3 𝒞ULTURAL FACTORS THAT AFFECT CLIENT CARE

White Middle Class

Family
• Nuclear family is highly valued.
• Elderly family members may live in a nursing home when they can no longer care for themselves.

Folk and Traditional Healthcare
• Self-diagnosis of illnesses
• Use of over-the-counter drugs (especially vitamins and analgesics)
• Dieting (especially fad diets)
• Extensive use of exercise and exercise facilities

Values and Beliefs
• Youth is valued over age.
• Cleanliness
• Orderliness
• Attractiveness
• Individualism
• Achievement
• Punctuality

Common Health Problems
As a result of the high value placed on achievement:
• Cardiovascular diseases
• Gastrointestinal diseases
• Some forms of cancer
• Motor vehicle accidents
• Suicides
• Mental illness
• Chemical abuses

African American

Family
• Close and supportive extended-family relationships
• Develop strong kinship ties with nonblood relatives from church or organizational and social groups
• Family unity, loyalty, and cooperation are important
• Frequently matriarchal

Folk and Traditional Healthcare
• Varies extensively and may include spiritualists, herb doctors, root doctors, conjurers, skilled elder family members, voodoo, faith healing

Values and Beliefs
• Present oriented
• Members of the African American clergy are highly respected in the black community
• Frequently highly religious

Common Health Problems
• Hypertension (precise cause unknown, may be related to diet)
• Sickle cell anemia
• Skin disorders; inflammation of hair follicles, various types of dermatitis and excessive growth of scar tissue (keloids)
• Lactose enzyme deficiency resulting in poor toleration of milk products
• Higher rate of tuberculosis
• Diabetes mellitus
• Higher infant mortality rate than in the white population

Asian

Beliefs and practices vary, but most Asian cultures share some characteristics.

Family
• Welfare of the family is valued above the person.
• Extended families are common.
• A person's lineage (ancestors) is respected.
• Sharing among family members is expected.

Folk and Traditional Healthcare
• Theoretical basis is in Taoism, which seeks a balance in all things.
• Good health is achieved through the proper balance of yin (feminine, negative, dark, cold) and yang (masculine, positive, light, warm).
• An imbalance in energy is caused by an improper diet or strong emotions.
• Diseases and foods are classified as hot or cold and a proper balance between them will promote wellness (eg, treat a cold disease with hot foods).
• Many Asian healthcare systems use herbs, diet, and the application of hot or cold therapy. Also, many Asians believe

that there are points on the body that are located on the meridians or energy pathways. If the energy flow is out of balance, treatment of the pathways may be necessary to restore the energy equilibrium.
Acumassage—Technique of manipulating points along the energy pathways
Acupressure—Technique for compressing the energy pathway points
Acupuncture—Technique by which fine needles are inserted into the body at energy pathway points

Values and Beliefs
• Strong sense of self-respect and self-control
• High respect for age
• Respect for authority
• Respect for hard work
• Praise of self to others is considered poor manners.
• Strong emphasis on harmony and the avoidance of conflict

(continued)

■■■ **TABLE 8-3** *𝒞*ULTURAL FACTORS THAT AFFECT CLIENT CARE (CONTINUED)

Common Health Problems
- Tuberculosis
- Communicable diseases
- Malnutrition
- Suicide
- Various forms of mental illness
- Lactose enzyme deficiency

Hispanic, Mexican American

Family
- Familial role is important.
- *Compadrazgo:* Special bond between a child's parents and his or her grandparents
- Family is the primary unit of society.

Folk and Traditional Healthcare
- *Curanderas(os):* Frequently folk healers who base treatments on humoral pathology; basic functions of the body are controlled by four body fluids or "humors":
  Blood—hot and wet
  Yellow bile—hot and dry
  Black bile—cold and dry
  Phlegm—cold and wet
- The secret of good health is to balance hot and cold within the body; therefore, most foods, beverages, herbs, and medications are classified as hot (*caliente*) or cold (*fresco, frio*) (a cold disease will be cured with a hot treatment).

Values and Beliefs
- Respect is given according to age (older) and sex (male).
- Roman Catholic Church may be very influential.
- God gives health and allows illness for a reason; therefore, may perceive illness as a punishment from God. An illness of this type can be cured through atonement and forgiveness.

Common Health Problems
- Diabetes mellitus and its complications
- Poverty and resultant problems, such as poor nutrition, inadequate medical care, poor prenatal care
- Lactose enzyme deficiency

Hispanic, Puerto Rican

Since the Jones Act of 1917, all Puerto Ricans are American citizens.

Family
- *Compadrazgo*—same as in Mexican-American culture

Folk and Traditional Healthcare
- Similar to that of other Spanish-speaking cultures

Common Health Problems
- Parasitic diseases, such as dysentery, malaria, filariasis, and hookworms
- Lactose enzyme deficiency

Values and Beliefs
- Place a high value on safeguarding against group pressure to violate a person's integrity (may be difficult for Puerto Ricans to accept teamwork)
- Reticent about personal and family affairs (psychotherapy may be difficult to achieve at times because of this belief)
- Proper consideration should be given to cultural rituals such as shaking hands and standing up to greet and say goodbye to people.
- Time is a relative phenomenon; little attention is given to the exact time of day.
- *Ataques*—Culturally acceptable reaction to situations of extreme stress, characterized by hyperkinetic seizure activity

Native Americans

Each tribe's beliefs and practices vary to some degree.

Family
- Families are large and extended.
- Grandparents are official and symbolic leaders and decision makers.
- A child's namesake may assume equal parenting authority with biological parents.

Folk and Traditional Healthcare
- Medicine men (shaman) are frequently consulted.
- Heavy use of herbs and psychological treatments, ceremonies, fasting, meditation, heat, and massages

Common Health Problems
- Alcoholism
- Suicide
- Tuberculosis
- Malnutrition
- Communicable diseases
- Higher maternal and infant mortality rates than in most of the population
- Diabetes mellitus
- Hypertension
- Gallbladder disease

(continued)

■■■ **TABLE 8-3** *C*ULTURAL FACTORS THAT AFFECT CLIENT CARE (CONTINUED)

Values and Beliefs

• Present oriented. Taught to live in the present and not to be concerned about the future. This time consciousness emphasizes finishing current business before doing something else. • High respect for age • Great value is placed on working together and sharing resources.	• High respect is given to a person who gives to others. The accumulation of money and goods often is frowned on. • Some Native Americans practice the Peyotist religion in which the consumption of peyote, an intoxicating drug derived from mescal cacti, is part of the service. Peyote is legal if used for this purpose. It is classified as a hallucinogenic drug.

Taylor, C., Lillis, C., & LeMone, P. (1996). *Fundamentals of Nursing* (2nd ed., pp. 122–125). Philadelphia: Lippincott-Raven.

Hosley, J. B., Jones, S. A., Molle-Matthews E., A. (1997). *Lippincott's textbook for medical assistants* (pp. 62–64). Philadelphia: Lippincott Williams & Wilkins.

Christianity

Christians worship God and his son, Jesus Christ. Sunday is the major day of worship in most Christian sects. Easter (Christ's resurrection) and Christmas (Christ's birthday) are the most important holidays, but Christians also observe other holy days. Bible reading and prayer are important aspects of faith. Several rites exist within the Catholic Church, although the Roman Rite is the largest and most influential. Roman Catholics outnumber Protestants worldwide; however, the opposite is true in the United States. Box 8-7 discusses healthcare–related beliefs and practices of several Christian religions.

Judaism

The term *Jewish* refers to the total culture, religion, history, and philosophy of life shared by a group of people whose origins date back to the prophet Abraham. Their religious beliefs are called Judaism. Judaism is practiced at three major levels: Reform, Orthodox, and Conservative. Reform Jews are the most liberal in their beliefs; Orthodox Jews adhere strictly to their traditions; Conservatives fall in the middle. Within the Orthodox group are various branches, including a sect called Hasidism. Hasidic Jews live and work only within their own community and wear traditional clothing. Some of the strictest groups select only specific healthcare providers.

Within the Jewish faith, circumcision of male infants is considered a religious ceremony. The spiritual leader is called a rabbi. The Jewish day of worship, or Sabbath, is from sundown Friday to sundown Saturday. Other than the Sabbath, the most important Jewish holidays are Yom Kippur, Rosh Hashanah, and Passover. Elective procedures such as diagnostic tests are not performed on the Sabbath or holy days.

Kosher laws govern dietary practices for Orthodox Jews. This custom is often difficult for Jews to follow during illness. Although nonsectarian healthcare facilities do not prepare kosher meals, frozen kosher meals are available. The person's family can also bring in food. Not all Jews observe kosher dietary laws. Ask your clients and notify the dietary department accordingly. Practicing Jews generally do not eat pork or shellfish, even if they do not follow kosher laws otherwise.

Islam

Muslims (Moslems) are believers in Islam, the religion founded by Mohammed. Islam is one of the largest and fastest-growing religions in the world. Islam contains many divisions of varying strictness. Be sensitive to what type of Muslim a client is, because so many variations exist within the religion. Most Muslim groups in the United States are similar. They generally follow the teachings of the Koran, which influences diet, attitudes about women, and death. Muslims pray five times a day, facing Mecca. The Sabbath is Friday. Pork and alcohol are prohibited. Muslims do not believe in faith healing and do not baptize infants. In death, prescribed procedures for washing and shrouding the body are followed by the clergy person, also called the **imam.** Some African Americans who follow the basic teachings of the Koran are members of the Nation of Islam or are considered Black Muslims.

Eastern Religions

The number of people in the United States from China, Korea, Japan, India, and Southeast Asia is increasing. Many of these people practice various Asian religions, and numerous people of non-Asian descent are becoming followers as well. Asian religions have a great influence on Western medicine. North America is increasingly accepting of traditional Asian therapies, such as acupuncture, yoga, and biofeedback. Transcendental meditation influences hypnotherapy and relaxation practices.

Two main branches of the Buddhist religion exist, the northern (*Mahayana*) and southern (*Hinayana*). Based on the teachings of Gautama Buddha, Buddhists believe that hard work and right living enable people to attain **nirvana,** a state in which the soul no longer lives in a body and is free from desire and pain. On many holy days, Buddhists may decline surgery or other treatment. Baptism is performed after a child is mature. Life is preserved; life support is acceptable. If a Buddhist dies, the family will usually send for a Buddhist priest, who performs last rites and chanting rituals. Buddhists are often cremated.

➤➤ BOX 8-7

HEALTH BELIEFS OF CHRISTIAN RELIGIONS

Roman Catholic: During illness or an emergency, a Roman Catholic client may want a priest to hear confession and give communion. The priest may also say Mass (religious services) in the client's hospital, nursing home room, or in the home. At such times, provide privacy. A person may receive the sacrament of *anointing of the sick* (for comfort and consolation) many times; it is often given at communal services as well. (To prepare the client who is in bed, loosen the covers at the foot of the bed.) Once called *last rites,* this sacrament is now given regularly, not just in emergencies. If a Catholic person dies suddenly, this sacrament can be administered conditionally, within 2 hours after death. Infant baptism is mandatory for Catholics. A lay person can baptize in an emergency. Many Catholics wear a crucifix or have an amulet or scapular attached to their clothing. They should be allowed to wear such articles in the healthcare facility.

Orthodox: Teachings are similar to Roman Catholicism, but religious calendars differ.

Protestantism: The many denominations in the Protestant faith evolved from the Reformation of the 16th century. Protestant groups include Lutheran, Methodist, Episcopal, Baptist, and Congregational. Forms of worship vary from informal to highly ritualistic; basic beliefs are similar. Following the belief in the "priesthood of believers," many Protestant denominations permit baptism by a lay person in an emergency. Some Protestants believe in "faith healing" or healing by "laying on of hands." The ill person may wish to receive communion. Ask if the client would like you to contact the minister/pastor or a hospital chaplain.

Church of Jesus Christ of Latter Day Saints: This church, also known as the LDS or Mormon church, is growing rapidly worldwide. LDS members are often health-conscious and very devoted to family and church. Members of the priesthood are revered as healers; a bishop or elder is called on during illness. The LDS member is allowed to receive healthcare; however, extraordinary life support measures are evaluated individually. Although no specific healers or regular healing services are held, LDS members often believe in divine healing. No specific religious rite is needed if an infant dies, but baptism for the dead is important for adults, as is the person's genealogy. During illness, an LDS member may wish to use one of four books for spiritual healing: The King James Version of the Bible, Doctrine and Covenant, Pearl of Great Price, or The Book of Mormon. The LDS health code is The World of Wisdom. Adult Mormons wear a special undergarment (temple garment), which may be worn under a hospital gown, but which may also be removed at the individual's discretion. Mormons do not use alcohol, coffee, or tobacco.

Christian Science: Christian Scientists forbid surgery and many other forms of medical care, such as blood transfusions or taking medications. They view alcohol, coffee, and tobacco as drugs that are forbidden. They believe all illness stems from the mind and that appropriate mental processes can cure illness. Treatment consists of prayer and counsel for the ill person; certified practitioners perform healing. There is no formal clergy and no baptism. In the event of death, no last rites are performed. Autopsy is forbidden.

Seventh Day Adventist: Seventh Day Adventists believe that good health depends on an orderly life. They emphasize the holistic concept of health. Adventists do not use alcohol, coffee, tea, tobacco, and over-the-counter drugs and do not allow blood transfusions. They do not eat pork; many are vegetarian. In the event of death, there are no last rites. Communion or baptism by an elder may be desirable in serious illness, but infants are not baptized.

Jehovah's Witness: Jehovah's Witnesses believe that each person is a minister. Blood transfusions are prohibited and Witnesses will not eat anything that has ever contained blood. In the case of death, there are no last rites. Infants are never baptized.

Amish and Mennonite: The Amish ("plain people") lifestyle and traditions are closely tied to religion. Although variations exist among Amish groups, they share many common beliefs. Prayer is customary before meals and at bedtime. Women are very modest; most births are at home. If a man must be shaved, he loses ministerial rights until his beard regrows. Both men and women may object to a surgical prep. They may refuse to relinquish traditional clothing in acute care facilities. In case of death, established protocols are followed. Some groups allow embalming; others wash and dress the person and place them in the casket themselves. They most often do not smoke or drink. Contact with the outside world is discouraged, especially for children. Homes do not have electricity, television, radios, or telephones. Thus, contacting families in an emergency is difficult. Transportation is by horse and buggy, but in an emergency, modern conveniences may be used. Mennonites/Progressive Amish groups follow more modern practices. They may drive automobiles (dark color); electricity and modern farm machinery are allowed. Television and radios are discouraged, however. Nursing is accepted as a noble, helping profession.

Often considered the oldest religion in the world, Hinduism has many different divisions. U.S. Hindus generally follow a scripture (the *Vedas*) and believe that Brahman is the center and source of the universe. Reincarnation is a central belief. Life is governed by the law of **karma,** stating that rebirth (reincarnation) depends on behavior in life. Karma is also significant in promoting health or causing disease. The goal of life is to attain nirvana, as in Buddhism. Some Hindus believe in faith healing; others believe illness is punishment for sins. Hindus often do not eat meat, but the religion does not dictate this practice. Some religious practices are dictated by the caste system (hierarchy of society); others are based on race or skin color. There are many spiritualists in some Hindu sects.

Confucianists have a high appreciation of life. Their desire to keep the body from untimely death results in an emphasis on public health and preventive medicine. *Taoism* teaches that good health results from harmony of the universe with proper balancing of internal and external forces. Following Tao is to know and to live a natural life.

☛ KEY CONCEPT

No matter how different your beliefs might be from those of your clients, respect each person's values. Respond in a nonjudgmental manner.

IMPLEMENTING CULTURALLY COMPETENT CARE

This chapter has presented a great deal of information about various cultural, ethnic, and religious groups. Remember to consider all aspects of the total person. **Transcultural nursing** is defined as caring for clients while taking into consideration their religious and sociocultural backgrounds. Madeleine Leininger, the international leader in the field, has also called this *ethnic-sensitive nursing care* or **ethnonursing.** Many culturally related considerations and procedures are integrated throughout this text.

Cultural Influences on Individual Clients

Determine cultural influences that might impact the client's progress through the healthcare system. The registered nurse will perform a thorough nursing assessment that includes a cultural assessment. The nursing plan of care is written by the team with cultural assessment in mind. This assessment is one component in the information gathering and planning phases of the nursing process. The licensed practical nurse will assist in performing culturally competent nursing care, based on the nursing care plan. The client may be involved in the development of the plan. Client and family compliance with the plan of care depends largely on whether or not that plan is acceptable within the client's particular culture. Help to make sure that the client understands what is to be done and why. Figure 8-2 provides examples of common cultural concerns.

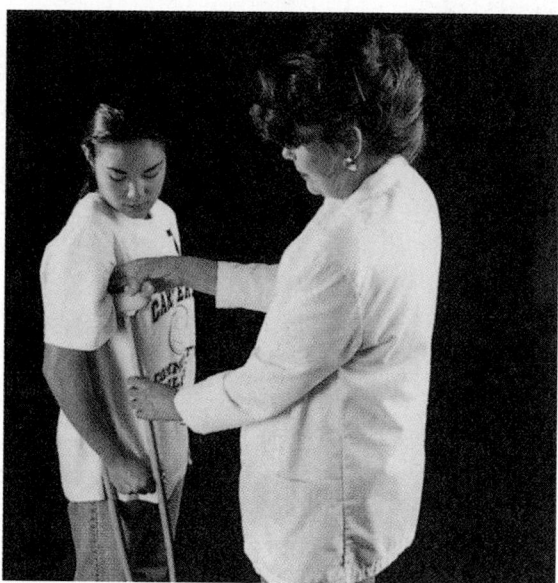

FIGURE 8-2. In the healthcare environment, nurses must communicate with clients of different ages, genders, races, and cultures. A nurse needs to remain sensitive to the needs of the client. In this example, imagine that the client being fitted for crutches has been told one of the following scenarios: a) she will not be able to go to the school prom; b) she will need to have her leg removed to save her life from the cancer in her leg; or c) she will not be able to lift her 2-year-old son until the injury is healed. Consider that there are differences in age, race, gender, or culture between the nurse and the client. How would these differences affect your approach to this client? (Hosley, J. B., Jones, S. A., & Molle-Matthews, E. A. [1997]. *Lippincott's textbook for medical assistants* [p. 543]. Philadelphia: Lippincott Williams & Wilkins.)

The Culturally Diverse Healthcare Team

As seen in Figure 8-3, cultural, ethnic, and racial mixtures within the healthcare team are common. The number of non-white nurses in the United States has increased, but not as quickly as the overall minority population. The critical shortage of registered nurses in the United States has led to increased recruiting of foreign-born and foreign-trained nurses. It may be difficult for foreign nurses to work in the United States because of differences in educational background, difficulties in becoming licensed, and language barriers.

All nurses bring cultural, ethnic, and religious backgrounds to nursing. Learn from cultural diversity, whether from clients or coworkers. Nurses should capitalize on and appreciate the heritage of all peoples, including their own.

➤ STUDENT SYNTHESIS
Key Points

- Many definitions are possible for *culture. Culture* refers to a shared set of beliefs and values among a specific group of people.
- Subculture, minorities, and ethnic and racial mixes are components of cultural heritage.

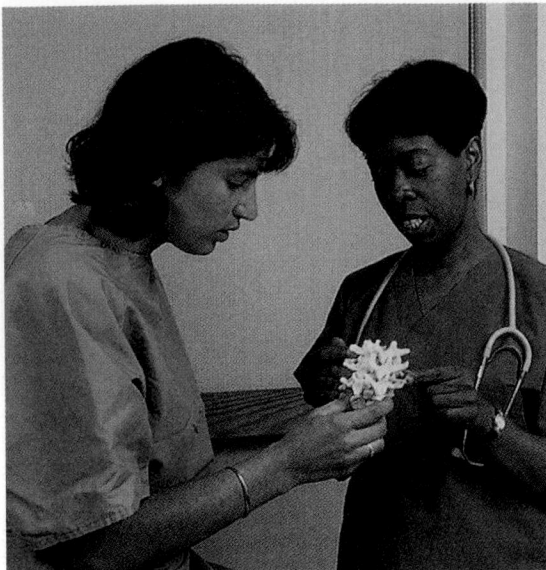

FIGURE 8-3. Within a culturally diverse healthcare system, communication is the key. Individuals communicate verbally, with the types of language that they use, with their body language, and with silence. Here, a nurse is communicating using a model of the spine. She uses lay terms for body parts and frequently asks the client to restate or explain what has been taught to her. (Hosley, J. B., Jones, S. A., & Molle-Matthews, E. A. [1997]. *Lippincott's textbook for medical assistants* [p. 505]. Philadelphia: Lippincott Williams & Wilkins.)

- The mix of ethnic groups in the United States changes continually.
- Prejudice, ethnocentrism, and stereotyping interfere with providing culturally sensitive nursing care.
- Many ethnic/cultural factors affect the delivery and acceptance of traditional Western healthcare.
- Many cultures subscribe to beliefs such as karma, yin–yang, spirits, or fate as causes and cures for illness.
- Cultural and religious traditions are not always followed by every member of a group.
- To facilitate communication and promote good nursing care, the nurse should be acquainted with the predominant cultural and religious groups within the community.
- The nurse may suggest a visit from a spiritual leader, but should not call one without first asking the client.
- Transcultural nursing is nursing that considers the religious and sociocultural backgrounds of all clients.

Critical Thinking Exercises

1. Consider the beliefs of at least three cultures regarding illness and health. How do they compare with your personal beliefs?
2. Your Chinese American client follows the yin–yang principle. Explain how this client's beliefs may affect your nursing care.
3. Assess ways in which you can help your Jewish client keep kosher in the healthcare facility.

Discuss similarities between kosher laws and dietary observances of other religions.

4. Reflect on and analyze an interaction that you consider inappropriate from a transcultural nursing viewpoint. What was inappropriate about the interaction? Why? Would your feelings change if the interaction had been between you and another person? Why or why not?
5. Quickly write your initial and immediate reactions to each of the following situations. Do not change or amend your initial answer after writing it. After you have responded to all the situations, evaluate and discuss your responses in terms of the transcultural nursing concepts presented in this chapter. How might any of these situations be modified to be more comfortable for the client, you, and the healthcare staff?
   - A Native American man wants to burn herbs in his room and wants to see a healer from his tribe while in the facility.
   - A lesbian is at your clinic for artificial insemination, accompanied by her female partner.
   - A Jehovah's Witness is seriously hemorrhaging and refuses to have a blood transfusion.
   - A man is accused of child abuse after performing religious healing rites that left scars on his child; the father is in the hospital for mental health evaluation to determine if he is competent to stand trial.
   - An Amish woman refuses to take off her customary clothing and put on a hospital gown before a diagnostic test.
   - A family from Somalia refuses to leave their child alone in the hospital.

NCLEX-Style Review Questions

1. When caring for a Muslim client, which dietary restrictions would you expect to see?
   a. Alcohol and caffeine
   b. Beef and pork
   c. Caffeine and fruit
   d. Pork and alcohol
2. Which action would be most appropriate when caring for a client whose health practices are different from the nurse's health practices?
   a. Ask the client to explain the practice.
   b. Ignore the practice and continue with care.
   c. Subtly ask family members about the practice.
   d. Watch the client and try to figure out the practice.
3. The nurse is caring for a client from an Asian culture. Which nursing action would be appropriate when caring for a child?
   a. Gently pat the child's head when talking to the child.
   b. Hug the child whenever entering the child's room.
   c. Never touch the child anywhere.
   d. Touch the child's hand or arm when looking at the child.

Unit III

DEVELOPMENT THROUGHOUT THE LIFE CYCLE

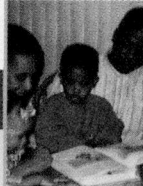

CHAPTER

9

The Family

LEARNING OBJECTIVES

1. Identify five universal characteristics of families.
2. Discuss the importance of parent–child and sibling relationships.
3. List the functions and tasks of families.
4. Describe various types of family structure.
5. Explain the influences of culture, ethnicity, and religion on the family.
6. Discuss the stages of the family life cycle and important milestones and tasks of these stages.
7. Identify common stressors on today's family.
8. Differentiate between effective and ineffective family coping patterns.

NEW TERMINOLOGY

binuclear family
cohabitation
communal family
commuter family
dual-career/dual-worker
   family
dysfunctional family
extended family
family

foster family
functional family
gay or lesbian family
nuclear dyad
nuclear family
reconstituted family
siblings
single-adult household
single-parent family

The family has traditionally been a central focus of nursing. As the basic unit of society, the family profoundly influences its individual members. All nursing care should involve the family. When giving care, nurses must consider the particular needs, circumstances, goals, and priorities of each family and the members within it. Thus, understanding concepts related to the family and its influence over individuals is essential for providing appropriate nursing care.

CHARACTERISTICS OF THE FAMILY

What is a family? This question may seem simple, but the answer constantly evolves, reflecting changes that occur within society. A family basically can be thought of as a group of two or more individuals who are related to each other by blood, marriage, or adoption and who usually live together. Historically, the meaning of family centers around childbearing and childrearing. These activities now encompass less than half of an adult's life prior to old age. Lower birth rates, longer life expectancy, the evolving role of women, divorce, and alternative lifestyles and living arrangements have influenced modern society's perceptions of family. A broader definition, which reflects societal changes of the 21st century, is that a **family** consists of two or more people who are joined together by bonds of sharing and emotional closeness, and who identify themselves as being part of that family.

☛ KEY CONCEPT

A client's family includes any person that he or she identifies as a family member.

Although every family is unique, families share five universal characteristics:

1. A family is a small social system.
2. A family performs certain basic functions.
3. A family has structure.
4. A family has its own cultural values and rules.
5. A family moves through stages in its life cycle.

The Family as a Social System

The family is a living social system. Although it is a basic unit of society, it is also complex. The family is a group of individuals who are interdependent; the choices and actions of one family member often influence other family members. For example, when one member of a family is ill, the entire family is affected. In another example, when a mother returns to full-time outside employment after several years of staying at home to care for children, ramifications abound for all members of the immediate, and perhaps the extended, family.

The roles people play within a family may be many and varied. One major relationship played out in a family is that of the parent–child relationship. Another is the relationship between siblings.

Parenting

Parenting is the ability of one or more people to help a child meet his or her needs and to guide that young person through developmental tasks. Parenting styles differ in each family. Some families are strict in discipline, whereas others are lenient or even indifferent. A person's own upbringing may guide his or her parenting style. Other parents learn their styles by watching role models or by following moral or religious teachings.

Parenting is an enormous responsibility and brings rewards and challenges. Although essential parental tasks include providing children with food, shelter, and safety, the ability to help children develop their own identity, self-confidence, and creativity is also of fundamental importance. The lack of adequate self-esteem may play a role in the development of problems later in life, including chemical dependency, eating disorders, and depression. You will often need to communicate to parents and other family caregivers the importance of encouraging their children and helping them to meet their needs. In Practice: Educating the Client 9-1 summarizes suggestions for helping families to build their children's self-esteem and independence.

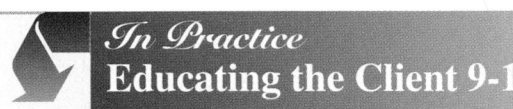
In Practice
Educating the Client 9-1

WAYS TO PROMOTE CHILDREN'S SELF-ESTEEM AND INDEPENDENCE

- Spend quality time with children, including playtime and instruction.
- Communicate with children, using eye contact and listening attentively to their questions and responses.
- Establish and maintain routines.
- Encourage children in their endeavors, and express pleasure, enthusiasm, and interest over their achievements and activities.
- Offer constructive criticism when necessary.
- Recognize the difference between normal incidents of misbehavior and continued patterns of behavioral problems.
- Adapt expectations to children's level of maturity and age group.
- Give children room to make their own decisions, while providing supportive guidance.
- Act as a role model for appropriate behaviors.
- Use discipline with logic and consistency.
- Apologize for mistakes but never apologize for fair punishments.
- Read to children.
- Tell children that they are loved and special, and reinforce these words with actions.

Siblings

Because of continued interaction over many years, **siblings** (brothers and sisters) exert powerful influences on one another. The sibling relationship is the first peer relationship that many people experience. It is long-standing, often lasting for six decades or more.

Siblings can fulfill many roles for each other: protector, supporter, comforter, teacher, social planner, friend, and disciplinarian (Fig. 9-1). Although siblings share many experiences, each one has a different perspective on those experiences. Birth order often plays a large role in shaping the experiences of siblings. For example, the firstborn in a family usually recalls experiences differently than the youngest child. Many other factors, including the time between each child's birth, are as influential on sibling relationships as birth position.

Family Functions and Tasks

The family is organized as a unit for the achievement of certain functions. Five basic family functions can be identified:

1. Providing for physical health
2. Providing for mental health
3. Socializing members
4. Reproducing
5. Providing economic well-being

The reproductive function is obviously significant for society because it is necessary for maintaining human life on Earth. Supporting individuals in their physical, emotional, economic, and social growth, however, is also vital to family and societal well-being.

The family performs many tasks that encompass these five functions and that are critical for survival and continuity. Notice how the essential family tasks relate to Maslow's hierarchy of basic human needs discussed in Chapter 5:

Provision for physical needs: Food, shelter, clothing, safety, healthcare

Allocation of resources: Careful planning and use of family money, material goods, space, and abilities

Division of labor: Assigning the workload, including responsibility for household income and household management

Socialization: Guiding toward acceptable standards of elimination, food intake, sexual drive, respect for others and their possessions, sense of spirituality

Reproduction, recruitment, and release: Bearing or adopting children, adding new members by marriage, and allowing members to leave

Maintenance of order: Providing interaction and communication opportunities, discipline, affection, sexual expression

Assistance with fitting into the larger society: Community, school, spiritual center, organizations

Maintenance of motivation and morale: Recognition, affection, encouragement, family loyalty, help in meeting crises, philosophy of life, spirituality

☛ KEY CONCEPT

The basic functions and tasks of the family focus on providing for physical health, providing for mental health, socializing its members, reproducing, and providing for economic well-being.

FAMILY STRUCTURE

Many different types of families exist in today's society, which is more tolerant of change than past generations. When working with clients, nurses will encounter many of these variations. No type of family structure is inherently better than another. Rather, it is the quality of interactions among individuals that dictates the family's ability to cope, adapt, and thrive. Although the family structures of clients may differ from the nurse's own personal experience, understanding and appreciating various family forms is critical for providing nonjudgmental and informed nursing care.

Many adults live alone in apartments or houses with no children involved. This is called a **single-adult household.** This scenario is common for young adults before entering into other types of family structures, or for older individuals who have lost a partner through separation, divorce, or death. Some people also make a lifetime commitment not to marry or to have children. Many single adults have extensive networks of friends and relatives on whom they rely for support and social interaction.

Nuclear Families

The most familiar family form is the **nuclear family:** a two-generation unit consisting of a husband, wife, and their immediate children—biologic, adopted, or both—living within one household (Fig. 9-2). In the past, the father in the nuclear family worked outside the home, while the wife stayed home to care for children. Because of changes in gender roles and rela-

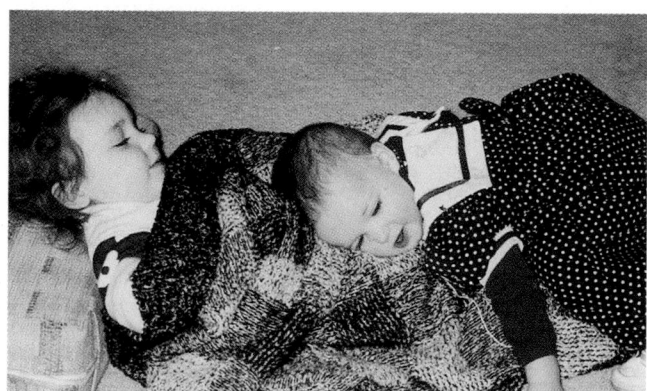

FIGURE 9-1. The sibling relationship is extremely influential. Siblings fulfill many roles for one another, including companion, teacher, and friend. (Craven, R. F., & Hirnle, C. J. [2000]. *Fundamentals of nursing: Human health and function* [3rd ed., p. 1269]. Philadelphia: Lippincott Williams & Wilkins.)

FIGURE 9-2. The nuclear family consists of a married man and woman with one or more children, living together in one household. (Craven, R. F., & Hirnle, C. J. [2000]. *Fundamentals of nursing: Human health and function* [3rd ed., p. 1252]. Philadelphia: Lippincott Williams & Wilkins.)

tionships, some fathers now remain at home to care for the household and children, while mothers provide most of the family income.

With the majority of mothers in all families working outside the home, family roles are more complex than ever. Outside employment for both partners in a family may necessitate careful structuring of household tasks. Nuclear families in which both parents work outside the home are referred to as **dual-career** or **dual-worker families.** Child-care arrangements often become a major issue for working parents. Couples with children may work different shifts or may stagger their work hours so that one parent is at home at all times to care for children. A common option for the dual-working family is to use daycare services.

A married couple that lives together without children is a **nuclear dyad.** Couples with no children, or couples with children who reside elsewhere, are examples of nuclear dyads.

In the **commuter family**, both adults are usually professionals. Often one has been transferred to another city, but the other prefers to remain with the present employment. Partners must commute a long distance, usually on weekends, to be together.

Extended Families

The **extended family** consists of the nuclear family and other related people, such as grandparents, aunts, uncles, and cousins. These family members may live together in one house, or in close proximity to one another. This type of family is also called a *kin network* or a *three-generation family.* Various members may share babysitting and disciplining of children. Members of the extended family may also influence parental decisions regarding childrearing.

The family in which grandparents assume responsibility for raising children is becoming increasingly common for a number of reasons. An adolescent parent who is in school or work

during the day may need the help of a parent. Some parents are unable to care for their children because of divorce, drug abuse, mental illness, or imprisonment. Although family involvement is an asset, older grandparents may have difficulties meeting basic needs for the family because of financial difficulties or illness.

Single-Parent Families

The **single-parent family** involves an adult head of the house with dependent children. The adult may be single as a result of separation, divorce, death, or never being married. Divorce and births to unmarried women have contributed to the shift from the two-parent family to the single-parent family. Current estimates by the Centers for Disease Control and Prevention (CDC) approximate that about one third of children in the United States are living in single-parent families.

Binuclear and Reconstituted Families

Divorce has contributed greatly to changes in common family situations. A **binuclear family** is one in which a separation or divorce of the adult partners occurs, but both parents continue to assume a high level of childrearing responsibilities. Joint custody arrangements are especially useful for binuclear families in which separated parents continue to live in close proximity to one another. Other custodial arrangements following a separation or divorce may require children to alternate households regularly, or to live with a noncustodial parent on weekends or over summer vacations. Adults who live without their children for extended periods often find that continually resuming and letting go of their hands-on parental role is especially challenging.

Many divorced adults remarry. If the newly married man and woman both have custody of their children from previous relationships, the two sets of children are placed together at a later stage in their lives, rather than being born into the situation. Such families are called *blended* or **reconstituted families.** These families may also include infants born into such an arrangement.

Alternative Families

The term **cohabitation** refers to unmarried individuals in a committed partnership living together, with or without children. People may live in cohabitation arrangements before, in between, or as an alternative to marriage.

Intimate partners of the same sex may live together or own property together. In this **gay or lesbian family,** one of the partners may have children from a previous relationship, or the couple may adopt children together. Artificial insemination is an option for lesbian couples who wish to raise children.

In a **communal family,** several people live together. They often strive to be self-sufficient and minimize contact with the outside society. Members share financial resources, work, and child-care responsibilities.

In a **foster family,** children live in temporary arrangements with paid caregivers. Theoretically, these children are meant to return to their family of origin when conditions permit, or to otherwise be placed for adoption. In some cases, the children remain in the foster home until adulthood.

INFLUENCE OF CULTURE, ETHNICITY, AND RELIGION

Families develop an internal culture. Members use their accumulated knowledge to interpret experiences and to define acceptable behaviors and actions. The actions of one family member may have significant effects on the family structure.

Each culture or ethnic group sets standards for its members (see Chap. 8). As people of a particular ethnic background move to the United States or Canada, they tend to live in communities of like-minded people. This network gives them support and helps them maintain their ethnic ideals. As families move into the general society (by relocation, or as young people attend a school or college outside the ethnic community), some of their ethnic ideals may change.

Traditionally, families married within their own ethnic, racial, or religious groups. Today, families with partners from different ethnic groups and racial heritages are more common. A family may represent two very different religious or spiritual groups. Each person brings into the family cultural factors reflecting his or her background. Adjustments must be made to acknowledge and accept each other's differences. Box 9-1 lists examples of cultural factors related to family.

FAMILY STAGES

In the following chapters, you will learn about developmental stages and tasks for individuals to achieve. The family also develops through various stages and tasks. Table 9-1 summarizes the important features of these stages, which revolve around the processes of childbirth and childrearing, and are most reflective of nuclear families. Other types of families may skip or overlap certain stages, or may never experience them.

Transitional Stage

The transitional stage refers to the period when single young adults (usually in their twenties or early thirties) are financially independent from their family of origin and live outside the family home. This stage has evolved as a norm in recent years as young adults delay marriage, often choosing to live alone or with others of a similar age first. During the transitional stage, individuals usually develop intimate relationships, perhaps leading to cohabitation or marriage. Men and women experience this stage differently, depending on their goals, which may be family and children, career success, or both.

Expanding Family Stage

In this stage, families are created, new members are added, and roles and relationships increase. This stage begins when an individual selects a partner with whom he or she makes a commitment, and ends when the first child leaves the home to begin his or her own transitional stage.

Establishment

Single adults move into the establishment phase when they choose a partner and set up a household. Establishing a household may or may not involve marriage. Building a mutually satisfying relationship, maintaining relations with extended family, and deciding whether or not to have children are developmental tasks associated with establishment. This phase often contains its own transitions, as individuals shift from living independently to learning to share and to maintain an interdependent relationship.

Childbearing

A family enters this phase with the birth or adoption of its first child. Seldom is a relationship as fulfilling as that of parent to child. No matter how an individual or couple may initially feel about a pregnancy, the arrival of a first child is usually an occasion of wonder and joy. Individuals, finished with waiting, are ready for their new role of parents. The transition to parenthood, however, is often difficult. Although new parents are now faced with childcare responsibilities, they also need to maintain a mutually satisfying relationship as a couple during this period.

An enormously important issue that dual-earner families must confront during this time is adequate childcare arrangements. Regardless of whether both parents work out of financial necessity or by choice, they need to develop and adjust to a plan that leaves young children in the care of another. Sometimes parents can arrange different work schedules for childcare purposes. Although children may benefit from always being with one parent or the other, the relationship between the adults often suffers because of inadequate time for each other.

➤➤ BOX 9-1

CULTURAL, ETHNIC, AND RELIGIOUS CONSIDERATIONS THAT INFLUENCE FAMILIES

- Choice of marriage partner (who chooses the spouse)
- Dating customs
- How many spouses a person may have
- Living arrangements
- Status of men and women
- Family decision-makers
- Roles of various family members
- Attitudes toward children
- Type of discipline
- Family disciplinarian
- Attitudes toward older adults in the family
- Choice of vocation or occupation
- How to deal with emotions: anger, grief, sadness, and so forth
- Attitudes toward education

■■■ **TABLE 9-1** *Stages of the Family Life Cycle and Associated Developmental Tasks*

Stage	Specific Tasks
Transitional	• Separating from one's family of origin • Developing intimate relationships • Establishing independence in work and finances
Expanding Family	
Establishment	• Building a mutually satisfying relationship • Incorporating spouse/partner into relationships with extended family • Setting up a household and delineating household responsibilities for each partner • Planning for own family
Childbearing	• Integrating an infant into the family • Maintaining a satisfying couple relationship • Expanding relationships with extended family by adding the parenting and grandparenting roles
Childrearing	• Meeting basic physical needs of all family members • Socializing children (peers, school, community) • Integrating new child members while meeting needs of other children • Maintaining a satisfying couple relationship
Contracting Family	
Child launching	• Releasing young adults to work, college, military service, and marriage with appropriate assistance • Adjusting the couple relationship as children leave the family home • Expanding the family circle with the marriage or relationships of children
Postparenting	• Assisting aging parents • Maintaining a healthy lifestyle • Continuing relationships with children and parents • Adjusting to retirement • Strengthening the couple relationship
Aging	• Finding a satisfactory living arrangement • Maintaining a satisfying couple relationship • Coping with the loss of a life partner • Keeping intergenerational family connections open • Accepting one's own mortality

Childrearing

Families in this phase include those with preschoolers, school-age children, and adolescents. Once children arrive, family life forever changes. The members of the family must continually adjust to one another.

Socialization of children is a major task of child-rearing. Along with peer relationships and school activities, parents should encourage participation in community activities. Family transportation may seem never-ending, as children are taken to and from their activities. Childrearing families often are pressured for time. Children's schedules must be considered as part of the family timetable. The parents' mealtimes and sleep patterns must change when children arrive. As children grow older, the scheduling of family members becomes more hectic. Arrangements first must be made for babysitters, then often for carpools and attendance at school functions. The adults' responsibilities and community contacts usually increase during this active time. However, adults must find time to encourage the growth tasks of all members of the family and combine them into a family design or plan (Fig. 9-3).

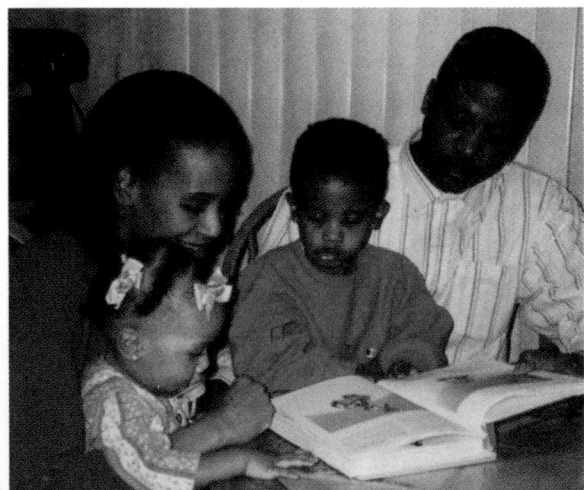

FIGURE 9-3. The family in the childrearing stage focuses much attention on socializing children, and on spending time communicating and sharing activity. (Craven, R. F., & Hirnle, C. J. [2000]. *Fundamentals of nursing: Human health and function* [3rd ed., p. 275]. Philadelphia: Lippincott Williams & Wilkins.)

At this point in the family cycle, communication is a developmental task for all members. Communication between partners, including sexual relations, may be sharply displaced as the family grows. Private conversation is difficult because children are omnipresent. Adults need to plan times when they can be alone together without children, to maintain a mutually gratifying relationship. They also need to encourage communication for the entire family and keep the channels open for children to share their daily experiences, thoughts, ambitions, and ideas.

Contracting Family Stage

During the contracting family stage, the family becomes smaller. Children who have grown into adults leave to begin lives and families of their own. Parents must adjust to new roles as individuals. A couple may begin to rediscover one another or to reevaluate their relationship and individual paths.

Child Launching

In this phase, the family has reached its maximum size. Child launching begins when the first child leaves home to live independently and ends when the last child leaves home. This phase represents the outcome of preparing children for adult life. As each child leaves home, the parental task is to reorganize the family from a home full of children, to a home again occupied only by adults. The length of this period varies. In past generations, adults were involved in childrearing until old age. With a longer life span and smaller families, parents may now launch children 20 years before they retire. In some families, children live at home until their thirties, or return to the family home after college—usually for financial reasons—lengthening the child-launching phase of the family. An important developmental task at this time is to accept and to appreciate, even if one does not always approve of, the differences in ideals, habits, and philosophies of the new generation.

Postparenting

This phase begins when the youngest child leaves the home and continues until the retirement or death of a partner. Once associated with middle years (approximately ages 40–60), this phase may occur later, as couples delay starting their families and adult children continue to live in the parental home. Many people find their middle years a comfortable and serene period. Fewer demands allow more time to enjoy life. Financial burdens related to children are fewer, and time for shared activities increases. Readjustment to a period in which children figure somewhat less prominently is necessary. Couples who share common goals and interests are likely to enjoy this period. An important task is maintaining relationships with aging parents and grown children. During this phase, individuals may take on a new role—grandparent. The middle-aged couple finds that the rewards of time allow both of them to come to terms with themselves and to gain satisfaction in opportunities still available. Planning for financial security in later years is essential. The expense of raising children has been lifted, and family income is usually at its peak.

☞ KEY CONCEPT

Adjustment to retirement may be difficult if careful financial planning is not done, or if hobbies and activities were not developed in earlier years.

Aging

As partners get older, they face several challenges. Many older adults decide to relocate. Deciding where to live is difficult for many older people. Often they have lived in the same home for 20 or 30 years or more. The place holds many memories, and it is hard to let go. Sometimes, the need for one partner to go to a nursing home makes the decision more difficult.

Fixed retirement income is insufficient for many people because of inflation. Even though costs go up, the pension stays the same. Many older people have saved what they once thought would be enough money to take care of themselves in their retirement years. Unfortunately, even one short illness can wipe out a modest savings account. Older adults then may be forced to sell their home or seek financial assistance.

As people get older, they may experience a decline in their physical faculties. A good sense of humor is probably the greatest asset in dealing with this deterioration. Older adults must get some sort of exercise, maintain an adequate diet, and get enough rest. Single adults may experience difficulty with proper nutritional habits. Individuals who lose a partner may not know how to cook, or may not want to bother to cook just for themselves. A regular physical examination is important to detect minor difficulties before they become major problems.

Older adults must accept death as another stage of life. They need to plan their legal affairs and to discuss finances for the future. If they have not yet made a will, they should do so now. Many people will live alone at least part of their lives because of divorce or death of a partner. Five times as many widowed women as widowed men are in the United States. Three reasons contribute to this disparity: women live longer than men; women tend to marry men who are older than they are; and widowed men are much more likely to remarry than widowed women.

STRESS AND FAMILY COPING

Every family encounters stress, which is inevitable but can be faced and handled appropriately. In addition to the normal changes, adaptations, and pressures of the family cycle, financial, physical, and emotional stresses may occur at any time. Often, stressors are interrelated, contribute to, and exacerbate one another.

Family stress is different from other types of stress because of the interdependent relationships that exist in families. When one member is under stress, the entire family is affected. Many families are able to develop socially acceptable means of dealing with stress. These **functional families** use ... cope, and often become stronger as a result of ... experience. Other families cannot cope. The res... stressors build, and coping systems disintegrate. Th... of family is called a **dysfunctional family** or *at*

Socioeconomic Stressors

Socioeconomic circumstances can greatly influence families. Income determines recreational pursuits. One family may be able to afford a vacation, whereas another family finds recreational opportunities in picnics and free community offerings. A family's income level often influences choices such as housing, education, daycare facilities, material goods, and nutrition.

Because of economic constraints, adults may have to work two jobs or several part-time jobs to provide for the family, which affects the amount of time they can spend with partners or children. Older siblings may be required to take on more household or babysitting responsibilities. Daycare may replace home care for children. In extended families, grandparents, aunts, or uncles may provide childcare. All these circumstances can place significant levels of stress on the entire family unit.

Poverty knows no boundaries. Families living in poverty face a variety of health and social problems, including homelessness, high rates of infant mortality, malnutrition, anemia, lead poisoning, high dropout rates from school, crime, and shortened life span. While the overall poverty rate dropped in 2000, about 31 million people in North America live in poverty, including the working poor, the homeless, migrant farm workers, residents of low-employment areas (including rural, mountain, and urban communities), and many older adults (about 10 percent). Women living alone or with their children represent a large percentage of people living in poverty (about 25 percent). The feminization of poverty may be attributed to changes in family structure. When a relationship breaks up, it is not uncommon to find that the man usually retains his income and status, while the woman and children enter a lower category of poor female-headed households. Further difficulties can arise when a parent fails to pay needed child support. Table 9-2 shows a graphic representation of poverty in the United States.

Divorce and Remarriage

A family's coping ability may be significantly compromised during a divorce. Adults who are facing separation from their partners—and a return to single life—may feel overwhelmed. They may become preoccupied with their own feelings, thereby limiting their ability to handle the situation effectively or to be strong for their children. The breakdown of the family system may require a restructuring of responsibilities, employment, childcare, and housing arrangements. Animosity between adults may expose children to uncontrolled emotions, arguments, anger, and depression.

Children may feel guilt and anxiety over their parents' divorce, believing the situation to be their fault. They may be unable to channel their conflicting emotions effectively. Their school performance may suffer, or they may engage in misbehavior. Even when a divorce is handled amicably, children may experience conflicts about their loyalties and may have difficulties making the transition from one household to another during visitation periods. Box 9-2 depicts some of the ues a family may face during the divorce process.

■■■ TABLE 9-2 *2*000 POVERTY STATISTICS FOR THE UNITED STATES

Family Type	Percentage
Female-householder families	25
Blacks	22
Hispanics	21
People under age 18	16
People living in the South	13
People over 65 years of age	10
Asian and Pacific Islanders	11
White, non-Hispanics	8

Note: Percentage will be more than 100 because some people fall into more than one category.

Source: U.S. Census Bureau website: http://www.census.gov, *Poverty in the United States 2000.*

Experts estimate that approximately 50% of all children whose parents divorce will experience another major life change within 3 years: remarriage. The arrival of a stepparent in the home presents additional stressors for children. Adapting to new rules of behavior, adjusting to a new person's habits, and sharing parents with new family members can cause resentment and anger. When families blend children, rivalries and competition for parental attention can lead to repeated conflicts.

Family Violence

The most common and least reported cases of violence in the United States are incidents of family violence. Abuse of children, partners, siblings, and older adults usually manifests

➤➤ **BOX 9-2**

FAMILY ISSUES IN THE DIVORCE PROCESS

- Relationships change, causing interpersonal conflict and tension.
- Former spouses must redefine their relationship with each other.
- Parental authority must be defined in an effort to maintain consistency in child-rearing decisions.
- Children may experience confusion and fear of abandonment by their parents.
- Financial support and visitation must be arranged.
- Parental conflict can lead to emotional problems in the child.
- From the child's perspective, loyalty conflicts may arise.
- All family members may experience the stages of the grieving process.

Emery, R., & Dillon, P. (1994). Conceptualizing the divorce process. *Family Relations, 43*(4), 374–380.

itself in physical, emotional, or sexual mistreatment, exploitation, and neglect. Other, less blatant forms of abusive behavior include interfering with another family member's outside social networks; misusing money and other resources; displaying inappropriate jealousy; monopolizing another person's time; and blocking a person from receiving needed healthcare. Cultural and economic pressures may contribute to such situations, because abused individuals may be afraid to expose the situation to outsiders, or may be financially or emotionally dependent on their abuser.

Abusive situations and other dysfunctional patterns of coping usually affect children the most. Children model their behaviors and develop their attitudes by watching the adults that they love and trust. Many children who were abused or who witnessed abuse in their families often grow up to be abusive as well, continuing a cycle of family violence. Chapter 71 discusses child abuse in more detail.

Addictions

The family in which one or more members have an addictive disorder face continual pressure and stress. Addictions may be in the form of drug or alcohol abuse, gambling disorders, sexual compulsions, or workaholism. In all such cases, the addiction begins to replace the family as a wellspring of support and a source for social interaction. The entire family suffers, as it begins to focus on ways to accommodate and incorporate the addictive behavior, while hiding it from those outside the family circle. Partners and children are often neglected, and financial resources often begin to dwindle as addicted individuals continue their behavior. Chapter 94 presents a detailed discussion of issues related to substance abuse and other addictions.

Acute or Chronic Illness

Illness can strike anyone at any time. Some illnesses are acute, while others become chronic. In either case, the family must deal with an enormous amount of pressure when one of its members faces illness. Financial issues may become a great concern, even if the family is fortunate enough to have good insurance coverage. Employment issues may need to be reconsidered, along with adjustments in schedules and social activities. Worry, anxiety, concern, and fear may be issues for the family witnessing a loved one's compromised or declining condition.

As a nurse, you are likely to work with many families who are dealing with acute and chronic illnesses. Throughout this book, you will find many strategies to help others pull together and deal effectively with such situations.

Effective and Ineffective Coping Strategies

Individuals and families respond to both everyday and more severe stressors in many ways. The response to major stressors can be depicted in two phases: adjustment and adaptation. During each phase, a family will employ different coping strategies. Box 9-3 highlights the two phases of a family's response to stress.

➤➤ BOX 9-3   914 513 284N

PHASES OF A FAMILY'S RESPONSE TO MAJOR STRESS

Adjustment Phase
1. The family tries to maintain the status quo with minimal disruption to the family unit.
2. The family may deny or ignore the stressor.
3. The family may remove the demands of the stressor.
4. The family may accept the demands created by the stressor.

Adaptation Phase
1. The family realizes that regaining stability will involve changes in the family structure.
2. Friends and community provide assistance with the problem-solving process during the stressful period.
3. Roles, rules, boundaries, and patterns of behavior within the family are altered as needed in order to regain stability.

➤ STUDENT SYNTHESIS

Key Points

- The family is the basic unit of society, but it is a complex unit.
- All nursing care should involve clients and their families.
- Although each family is unique, families share five universal characteristics: Every family is a small social system; has certain basic functions; has a structure; has its own cultural values and rules; and moves through stages in its life cycle.
- Roles and relationships within a family are many and varied; the primary ones include parent–child and sibling relationships.
- The functions and tasks of the family help individuals to meet their basic human needs.
- Although many different family structures exist, all can be efficient, supportive, and satisfying.
- Cultural, ethnic, and religious factors influence family outcomes.
- Family development progresses through predictable stages, with important developmental tasks.
- The family that can cope with stress is functional; families that cannot cope are dysfunctional or at risk.

Critical Thinking Exercises

1. This chapter presents the stages of family development, based primarily on the nuclear family. Consider how family structure might influence the family life cycle in the following situations:

a single-parent family; a family in which grand-parents are raising grandchildren; a blended family; and a binuclear family.

2. Sharon, a sophomore in high school, is pregnant with her first child. She lives with her mother (who works full-time), grandmother, and younger brother. Her parents have been divorced for several years, and she has limited contact with her father. Her boyfriend wants to help raise the child. Based on this information, identify potential stressors for Sharon and her family. Assess possible ways the family can best handle Sharon's pregnancy. What effects will the new baby have on the family's structure and stages?

3. Consider special needs for the following individuals and ways families can identify and meet those needs: children of a blended family; adopted children; older parents living with their grown children; a widow with no children; a single father; a gay couple considering adoption; and a couple who must live apart for 6 months because of employment considerations.

NCLEX-Style Review Questions

1. What is the most important etiological factor in developing a dysfunctional family?
   a. Large number of family members
   b. Lower income than neighbors
   c. Poor response to stressors
   d. Rural location of family

2. The establishment of a family, childbearing, and childrearing are part of which stage of the family cycle?
   a. Contracting family
   b. Expanding family
   c. Postparenting
   d. Transitional family

3. During the separation stage of divorce, developmental tasks include which of the following?
   a. Adapting to new living arrangements
   b. Counseling sessions with ex-spouse
   c. Parent-teacher counseling sessions
   d. Admitting failure of parental skills

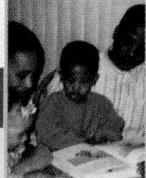

CHAPTER

10

Infancy and Childhood

LEARNING OBJECTIVES

1. List the characteristics and sequence of human growth and development.
2. Explain developmental regression.
3. Discuss Havighurst's theory of developmental tasks.
4. Describe Erikson's stages of psychosocial development, including the challenges and virtues of each stage.
5. Explain the four stages of human cognitive development as described by Piaget.
6. Describe the role of play in childhood development.
7. Discuss the importance of anticipatory guidance for caregivers as their children grow and progress to new developmental stages.
8. Discuss growth and development for infants, toddlers, preschoolers, and school-age children, highlighting key areas of concern.

NEW TERMINOLOGY

bonding
cephalocaudal
cognitive
development
enuresis
environment
growth
hereditary
infancy

interdependent
masturbation
newborn
object permanence
proximodistal
regression
stranger anxiety
toddler

The preceding chapter talked about the importance of the family: its functions, types, and stages. Individuals also move through stages. The study of individual growth and development begins with this chapter on infancy and childhood.

Chapter 5 discussed basic human needs. An understanding of these basic needs is necessary before you attempt to study growth and development across the life span. For example, infants require assistance to meet their most basic survival needs, such as food, water, and elimination. When these needs are met, toddlers begin to develop needs for safety, security, and socialization. As children become adolescents and eventually adults, they begin to meet their higher-level needs and to assist members of the younger generation in meeting these needs.

Children are a country's future—its citizens of tomorrow. As a nurse, you are likely to care for both healthy and sick children. Understanding normal patterns of growth and development is important. By knowing how most children can be expected to behave at particular stages, you will be better prepared to care for any child. An understanding of normal behavior is also necessary before you can recognize abnormal behavior. For example, it is helpful to know that regression may occur during illness. During **regression**, a child's behavior may go backward to that of an earlier stage of development.

GROWTH AND DEVELOPMENT

Growth and development, considered a single process, continues throughout childhood and into adulthood. **Growth** is defined as a change in body size and structure; **development** is a change in body function.

Concepts of Growth and Development

Growth and development occurs in an orderly sequence; a person must accomplish a simple developmental task before he or she can attempt another, more complex task. Most children are able to perform certain tasks at about the same age, although normal variations exist.

In relation to the body, the process of growth and development follows cephalocaudal and proximodistal directions (Fig. 10-1). **Cephalocaudal** means from head to tail; babies lift their heads before they sit up; they make sounds before they walk. **Proximodistal** means from the center to the outside; babies roll over before they grasp small objects.

Growth and development also progresses from simple to complex; the baby learns to sit before learning to walk, and to babble before learning to speak. Growth and development is inclusive and holistic, involving the entire child and family. Culture, ethnicity, and religion influence the process.

All aspects of growth and development are influenced by each other, or **interdependent.** For example, children cannot learn to control their bowel movements (development) until their muscles are strong enough (growth), and until they can understand what is expected of them (development). Consider the interdependent process of learning to walk:

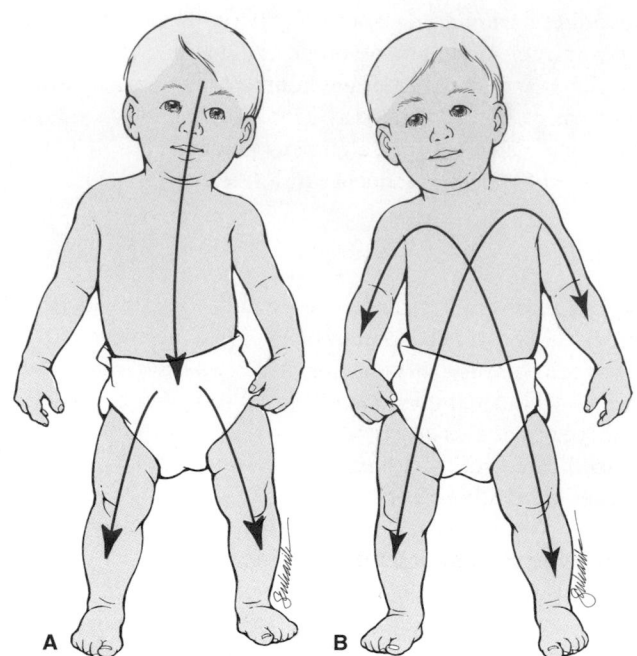

FIGURE 10-1. Principles of growth and development. (**A**) Cephalocaudal growth and development proceed from head to toe or tail. (**B**) Proximodistal growth and development proceed from the center outward.

- Walking is controlled by motor development.
- Motor development depends on normal bone and muscle growth.
- Normal growth depends on adequate food and energy.
- The nervous system exercises overall control over the process.
- Caregivers and loved ones provide the encouragement and emotional support needed for the child to progress.

☞ KEY CONCEPT

Growth is a change in body size and structure; development is a change in body function. The process of growth and development has the following characteristics:

- *Orderly sequence*
- *Simple to complex*
- *Cephalocaudal*
- *Inclusive*
- *Proximodistal*
- *Interdependent*

Influences on Growth and Development

Heredity and environment influence child growth and development. Discussions have persisted for years, and continue today, about which element has a stronger influence or whether they are of equal importance.

Hereditary characteristics are inherited from parents and are often called *genetic* factors. Skin color, eye color, and body build are examples of hereditary characteristics. **Environment** is the sum of all the conditions and factors surrounding the child. Housing, neighborhood, number of siblings, placement in sibling order, and amount of healthcare available are examples of environmental elements. A baby born into a large family may develop differently from one born into a small family. Religious practices, ethnicity, and location of birth also influence a child's development.

Growth and Development Theories

A number of theories can be used to understand, explain, and predict behavior in children and adults. No one theory covers the whole spectrum of behavior, so it is wise to consider each person from a combination of viewpoints. Three especially important theories are Robert Havighurst's theory of developmental tasks, Erik Erikson's psychosocial theory, and Jean Piaget's cognitive theory.

Havighurst: Developmental Tasks

Physical growth occurs without personal effort, but development is an active process in which the person must participate. Havighurst theorizes that each life stage has its own group of *developmental tasks* that a person must accomplish to become a mature, fully functioning individual. As a person perfects each task, he or she is prepared to take on the next task. Although every person must meet these tasks by himself or herself, the individual must receive support from family, friends, and teachers. Box 10-1 presents the developmental tasks of childhood for each stage.

Erikson: Psychosocial Development

Erikson's theory of human development focuses on the psychosocial and environmental aspects of personality as the person progresses from birth to death. Erikson stresses that each individual is the product of interactions among heredity, environment, and culture. He emphasizes that the rate of development varies. The main points of Erikson's theory are:

- Each stage of development contains a psychosocial *challenge* or critical period, during which the person must deal with a major life change. If the person fails to meet the challenge, he or she faces certain difficulty in achieving the next level of development. For example, infants who do not achieve a sense of trust that their needs will be met will have difficulty achieving autonomy as toddlers.
- In each stage of development, a *significant person or group* exerts a lasting influence on the ongoing development of the child. For example, the person who acts as family caregiver is most significant to the infant, whereas the peer group has greater influence on the adolescent.
- Similar to Havighurst's theory, the individual must *accomplish* certain tasks related to the psychosocial challenge of each particular stage. Children are able to perform these tasks with help from parents, siblings, and other important people.
- Certain virtues are appropriate for each developmental stage. *Virtues* are beneficial, challenging, and exciting characteristics that emerge as individuals successfully

> ➤ ➤ BOX 10-1

HAVIGHURST'S DEVELOPMENTAL TASKS OF CHILDHOOD

Birth to 24 Months (2 yrs)
- Learn to take solid food
- Learn to walk
- Learn to talk   1 yr. 6 mo. –

Toddler and Preschool (18 Months to 6 Years)
- Control processes of elimination
- Learn sex differences and modesty
- Get ready to read
- Begin to form the conscience—to know right from wrong
- Form concepts and be able to name them

Middle Childhood (6–12 Years)
- Learn to get along with age mates
- Learn fundamental skills of reading, writing, and figuring
- Perfect physical skills and games
- Develop a wholesome attitude about the self
- Identify with a masculine or feminine social role
- Develop conscience, morality, values
- Learn the difference between work and play
- Develop industry and a pleasure in competition with others
- Develop personal independence
- Develop attitudes toward groups and social institutions

accomplish the tasks of that developmental stage and thus successfully resolve the psychosocial challenge.

Table 10-1 summarizes these points as they relate to each particular stage of childhood.

Piaget: Cognitive Development

The term **cognitive** refers to knowledge, understanding, or perception. Thus, cognitive development is the development of the process of thinking. Piaget stated that cognitive development "is a continuous progression" beginning with the reflexes of the newborn, which are spontaneous and automatic. The infant progresses to acquired habits. The child then goes on to acquire knowledge and develop intelligence.

Cognitive development is cumulative; that is, what is learned is based on what has been known before. This theory is used in your nursing program. Information is presented to you in a progression from simple to complex. For example, you learn normal body structure and function and normal development before you study deviations from those parameters.

Piaget's four major levels of cognitive development are:

1. *Sensorimotor.* Up to age 2, children learn by touching, tasting, and feeling. They learn to control body movement. They develop an understanding of **object permanence,** the knowledge that an object seen in

■■■ TABLE 10-1 𝓔RIKSON'S THEORY OF PSYCHOSOCIAL DEVELOPMENT—CHILDHOOD

Concept	Infancy (1–12 months)	Toddlerhood (1–3 years)	Preschool (3–6 years)	School Age (6–12 years)
Challenge	Trust vs. mistrust	Autonomy vs. shame and doubt	Initiative vs. guilt	Industry vs. inferiority
Significant other	Family caregivers	Family	Family	School and neighborhood
Necessary accomplishment	Develop trust	Learn appropriate behaviors; learn right from wrong	Learn rules and regulations; establish independence	Learn to get along with others; learn school subjects
Virtues	Hope	Self-control; will-power	Direction; purpose	Self-esteem; competence
Ways to help the child succeed	Establish routines; satisfy basic needs	Set limits; let child make simple choices; encourage curiosity; give gentle guidance	Consistent discipline; explain things; praise	Manage sibling rivalry; give responsibility; recognize accomplishments away from home

a particular spot, but temporarily hidden from view under a blanket, continues to exist and will return to view when it is uncovered.

2. *Preoperational.* Children from ages 2 to 7 investigate and explore the environment and look at things from their own point of view.
3. *Concrete operations.* Between ages 7 through 11, children "internalize" actions and can perform them in the mind. Cognition at the concrete operations level exhibits the following characteristics:

    Reversibility: Children walk to school and know that by reversing the direction of the walk they can get home again.

    Seriation: Children can arrange things in a series, from big to little or in a numbered sequence.

    Conservation of matter: Children begin to understand quantities, weight, and volume. They recognize that 8 ounces of juice is the same amount whether it is in a can or a glass.
4. *Formal operations.* After age 12, children can think in the abstract. Complex problem-solving is included in this category.

Role of Play in Child Development

Play is important to child development. Children learn about the world through play. Experimentation, exploration, success, and failure are a part of maturation. Play with other children encourages peer cooperation, interaction, and sharing. It enhances fine and large muscle coordination and strengthens muscles.

Infant and toddler play is usually an interaction among children, the family, and simple toys. Children learn about people and objects by using all five senses. They repeatedly imitate the play and learn about their surroundings. The attention span of most infants and toddlers lasts about 5 to

10 minutes. Within limits, family caregivers may need to regularly change activities. As children get older and head into the preschool years, language becomes an important part of play. Caregivers begin to talk to children about toys and how to use them.

Solitary play occurs when children play alone with their own toys in the same area as others, but without interaction. Solitary play is most common during infancy. Toddlers exhibit parallel play, which occurs when two children play side-by-side with the same or similar toys but do not interact with each other or the other's toy (see Figure 10-2). Preschoolers begin to play directly with other children. Young school-aged children engage in cooperative and interactive play and may expand the playgroup from 2 or 3 children to an entire classroom. Older school-aged children play structured games with defined roles, rules, and ways to win. They learn to take turns, play fairly, and accept losses graciously.

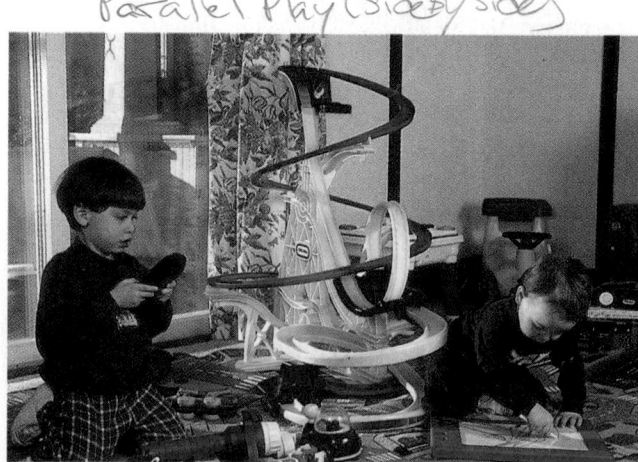

FIGURE 10-2. Toddlers show their growing interest in peers through parallel (side-by-side) play. (Craven, R. F., & Hirnle, C. J. [2000]. *Fundamentals of nursing: Human health and function* [3rd ed., p. 272]. Philadelphia: Lippincott Williams & Wilkins.)

Anticipatory Guidance

During each stage of childhood, behavioral and developmental issues will be of concern to family caregivers. Many families express worries that their children are not behaving like other children of a similar age. As a nurse, an important concept for you to communicate is that normal growth and development occur within a wide range. For example, one child may walk by age 1, yet another masters walking closer to age 2. Both children are developing normally. Be sure to emphasize to families the importance of recognizing each child's pace of development and natural abilities. By providing anticipatory guidance, you can alert concerned families to normal growth and development patterns and to common areas of concern for particular age groups. Safety education for all children is a high priority.

When they understand the stages of development, know behaviors to expect within certain ranges, and are aware of concerns and safety issues for children, most family caregivers enjoy watching the progress of their children. Adults who view changes in their children as signs of progress are usually happier and better equipped to help children become self-sufficient. Children's instinctive curiosity and physical growth carry them to new fields to conquer. The challenge of parenting is to help children develop in such a way that they maintain their eagerness to learn throughout their lives.

Sincere concern for their children's long-range development leads many people to find ways to improve understanding and family relationships. Many schools have parenting classes as a regular part of their adult education curriculum. Such knowledge and understanding does not eliminate the need for parental discipline and guidance, but enhances it and encourages mutual respect within the family. Understanding the needs and the problems of children can supply clues to more effective methods of control and discipline. It supports both adults and children in working toward their mutual goals of increased abilities, skills, self-knowledge, and self-discipline.

THE NEWBORN

A baby is called a **newborn** or *neonate* in the first 4 weeks. The newborn's reactions to internal and external stimuli help to shape the child physically, intellectually, emotionally, and socially. The newborn is extremely vulnerable, tender, and delicate. Both healthcare professionals and family caregivers must take many precautionary measures to help ensure the newborn's safety and ability to thrive. Chapters 66 and 68 discuss newborn care in more detail.

INFANCY: 1 TO 12 MONTHS

The period from 1 to 12 months of age is called **infancy.** During this stage, the person matures both physically and emotionally with greater speed than at any other time of the lifespan. Individual patterns of growth and development vary for each infant. A protective, loving environment in a nurturing,

responsive family contributes enormously to an infant's ability to thrive and adapt.

Physical Growth

During the first 3 months of life, infants gain about 0.9 kg (2 lb) per month and grow about 2.5 to 5.0 cm (1–2 in.). From 3 to 6 months, they gain about 0.45 kg (1 lb) per month. By the age of 6 months, most infants have doubled their birth weight. By the end of 1 year, they weigh about three times their birth weight. They have increased their birth height by about half, as well. Initially, most weight gain is fat, then muscle, and then bone density.

Teeth begin to erupt at 6 to 7 months of age. The first teeth to erupt generally are the two lower central incisors, followed by the four top central incisors. By age 1, most babies have six to eight teeth (Fig. 10-3). Because tooth eruption patterns vary greatly, however, family caregivers should not be alarmed if an infant does not follow the usual pattern.

The first teeth are known as deciduous teeth. The term *deciduous* literally means "falling off" or "subject to being shed." Like the leaves shed by deciduous trees, children eventually lose their deciduous or baby teeth, which the permanent teeth replace.

Psychosocial Development

Establishment of trust in primary caregivers is clearly the most important psychosocial *challenge* of infancy. Infants are helpless beings, entirely trusting others to meet their basic

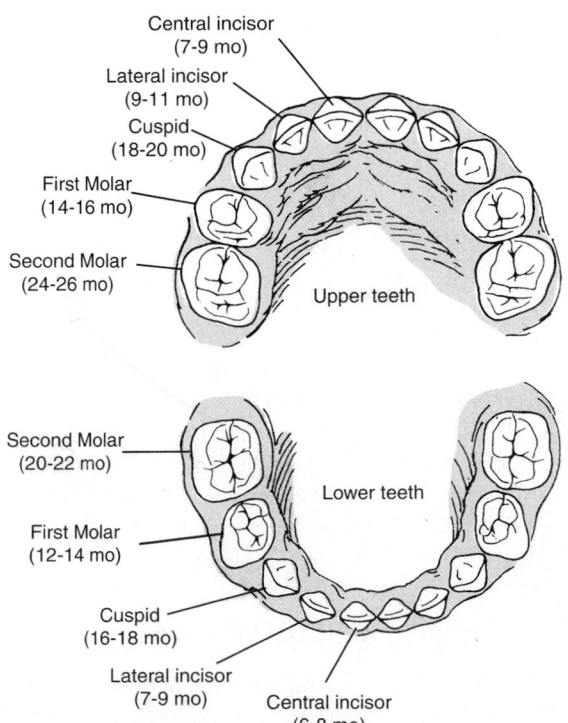

FIGURE 10-3. Approximate ages of eruption and locations of deciduous (baby) teeth.

needs. If trust is established, infants also achieve the *virtue* of this stage—hope (see Table 10-1). If trust is not established, the later challenges of autonomy and initiative will be delayed.

Changing Families and the Role of Caregivers

In the past, many women did not work outside the home and were mainly responsible for care of children. Although many women still assume primary responsibility for their babies, children in today's world often have a variety of caregivers. Many fathers are taking a more active role in spending time with their babies, feeding, changing, bathing, and playing with them. Some fathers are leaving their jobs or working from home to stay with their children, while mothers continue their careers outside the home. Many children are growing up in nontraditional circumstances, with grandparents, aunts and uncles, other relatives, and foster parents acting as the primary nurturers. Remember, however, that most mothers still carry the main responsibility for childcare. Many of these women are also the main providers for their families, adding to increased role expectations, family stressors, and a need for outside support systems.

Bonding

Bonding, which is the attachment to parents and other family caregivers, is of vital importance for infants. The feeling of love, nurturing, and connection to other people is one of the most important aspects of being human. Bonding between mother and child begins before birth. The process of attachment between mother and baby continues during infancy and truly begins to develop between father and child at this time. Skin-to-skin contact is important, because touch contributes to a baby's ability to thrive. Babies bond with others as well, whether they act in place of or in conjunction with parents. Attachment is an interactive process, relying on participation from both adult and baby to be successful. Attachment strengthens over time.

Accomplishing Tasks

Being totally dependent on others for care, infants must learn to develop trust: the feeling that caregivers will meet their needs. Needs of the infant include safety, holding, cuddling, feeding, stroking, and sucking (breast-feeding, bottle, pacifier). Infants are able to tolerate frustration in small amounts only. They expect their needs to be met immediately.

Family caregivers must assist infants in the establishment of a system of routines. This system should include items such as feeding, playtime, rest, and sleep. Routines help infants to establish feelings of trust, because they begin to learn what to expect.

Cognitive and Motor Development

The cognitive abilities and motor skills of infants are directly linked to their interactions with their families. During infancy, as throughout the entire lifespan, the rate of each infant's development varies, depending on his or her physical maturity and environmental factors.

1 to 3 Months

During the first 3 months of life, an infant's progress can be witnessed almost daily. When babies are 6 weeks old, they begin to make purposeful movements and stop crying when picked up; they are beginning to expect that someone will comfort them. As they become aware of their surroundings, babies smile, babble when spoken to, and follow lights within view. They turn their head toward sounds, and can differentiate between pleasant and unpleasant noises. They pay attention to their parents' voices. Although lack of head control is still marked, most babies can stare directly ahead for a short time by 8 weeks and may be able to focus their eyes on a light. Babies cry to signal needs, and stop crying when they are comforted and satisfied. These babies develop a preferred sleeping position. Although sleeping habits vary widely, these infants will probably sleep from 18 to 20 hours a day.

By 3 months, babies can reach for and grasp articles. They laugh, squeal, and look at objects for several seconds. They are able to turn over and can follow a moving object with their eyes. Between 2 and 3 months, infants develop a social smile and respond to pleasurable interactions with expressions of happiness. Their favorite sight is the human face.

4 to 8 Months

Between 4 and 8 months, babies learn to sit with support and begin to coo and babble, especially when someone talks to them. Their lacrimal glands (tear glands) have developed fully, and they shed tears. These babies usually sleep all night and take two or three naps during the day. They learn about the world by putting objects into their mouths, especially toes, and by touching various textures and shapes. The abilities to hold the head steady, recognize people, and hold their bottles begin to emerge. Babies start to splash in the bath and smile at their reflection in the mirror.

During this stage, babies can pull up to sitting, and sit for a short time without support. They turn over in bed without help, hold their bottles, and grab their own toes. If offered a new toy, these infants drop what they are holding to take the new toy, and pass the toy from hand to hand. They now play "peek-a-boo." They may get up on their knees and begin to rock forward and back in preparation for crawling. Babies can distinguish between good and bad voices, and will listen for tones of approval.

Some authorities feel that behavioral differences related to sex may be noted in infants aged 6 months; they observe that boys may begin to be more assertive and girls to be more passive. This issue is extremely controversial. Some researchers believe that sex roles are learned, whereas others believe that hereditary factors or differences in development of the endocrine system, particularly the hypothalamus gland, may be involved.

9 to 12 Months

As infants near completion of the first year, they have learned to crawl and can be very curious, exploring their world. Babies of this age respond when called by name, can copy movements, and know the meaning of the word "no." By 10 months, babies can usually pull up to standing while holding onto something, and can walk with both hands held. They then learn to walk around furniture and stand alone. At 1 year, most children can take a few steps alone. They can walk if someone else holds one hand.

One-year-olds hold their bottles and drink out of cups without difficulty. They have strong pincer grasps, and pick up small objects, such as raisins, from the table. They say two or three simple words, such as "baby" and "bye-bye." They laugh aloud. These babies imitate a variety of speech sounds, and begin to say "mama" and "dada," referring specifically to each. They love games such as simplified hide-and-seek. They distinguish between people they recognize and strangers, clinging to familiar persons and pulling away from strangers. Unfamiliar people, places, and events upset these babies and they resist. This **stranger anxiety** is seen between the ages of 9 and 15 months, with its peak at 12 months. It recurs during the toddler years.

Areas of Concern

Feedings
A variety of opinions exist concerning infant feeding. Breast milk or infant formula offers complete nutrition in the first year. Solid foods provide babies with necessary iron and vitamins, and the opportunity to learn to take food from a spoon, to chew, and to swallow. Some healthcare providers claim that infants should not have solids until 9 months to 1 year of age because their digestive tracts are immature. Others think that 6 months of age is the appropriate time to introduce babies to solids. Most providers agree that solids should not be introduced into the diet before infants reach 6 months of age.

Incorporating solids into the diet too early has been linked to food allergies. Research indicates that giving solids early does not help infants sleep all night. It is better for children and easier for family caregivers to start solids later, so that infants receive the proper balance of nutrients and can quickly progress to table foods.

Introduction of new foods follows a logical sequence. Iron-fortified infant cereal, mixed with breast milk or human milk substitute, is the suggested first solid. It should be given by spoon, not bottle. New foods should be added weekly, so caregivers can quickly identify food allergies and intolerances. Fruits and vegetables can be added slowly, with meats added after the first year. No matter at what age solids begin to be added to an infant's diet, caregivers should avoid including typically allergenic foods, such as dairy products, citrus fruits, tomatoes, chocolate, wheat, seafood, and eggs, until after age 1. Although formula or breast milk may still be used, many infants drink whole milk by age 1. Goat's milk may be a better alternative than cow's milk.

The feeding process is nurturing and pleasurable for infants. Babies grow and thrive when they receive affection, tactile stimulation, and a feeling of satiety (fullness) during feedings. Skin-to-skin contact and vocal responses from caregivers are important at these times. For breast-fed infants, bottle feedings are a convenient method for fathers and other family members to bond with infants and show them attention. Both breast-fed and bottle-fed babies need to be held closely, stroked, sung to, and rocked during feedings.

Bottle Mouth
Nursing bottle mouth is a serious dental condition that results when infants are placed in bed with a bottle of breast milk, formula, or juice that is propped on a blanket or towel. Erosion of tooth enamel, deep cavities, and tooth loss result from the prolonged contact of milk and juice sugars with emerging teeth. Lost primary teeth do not maintain space for the permanent teeth, which may erupt decayed. Nursing bottle mouth may affect appearance, chewing, eating habits, and speech development.

Weaning
Weaning, the change from feeding infants exclusively breast milk or formula to incorporating a variety of solid foods, should begin when babies can sit upright on their own, support their own head and neck, and grasp objects in their fingers and put them in their mouths. A cup can substitute for the breast or bottle. Feeding should start with cereal and pureed baby food given with a spoon.

Sucking
Infants need to develop their sucking reflexes. They will suck on their thumbs, fists, and fingers when they are not feeding. Sucking provides comfort and relieves tension and anxiety. Some babies use a pacifier for sucking when they are tired or fussy. Thumb-sucking may begin at around 3 or 4 months of age. Most infants pop everything into their mouth by the time they reach 7 months, and the thumb is a handy object.

Daycare
Daycare is a difficult decision that many parents must consider. Various options are available, including daycare centers, preschool learning centers, family daycare homes, or daycare providers (eg, nannies) in the home. Many states require childcare providers to be licensed and to meet certain requirements such as provider training, health and safety laws, and home or center inspection. Studies have supported the idea that children thrive in daycare centers where each child is given a high level of individualized attention. One of the most important factors for parents to consider when making the decision is the ratio of daycare personnel to children. Cost is also a factor. Safety is vital.

TODDLERHOOD: 1 TO 3 YEARS

The **toddler** phase encompasses approximately ages 1 to 3 years. Although physical growth is not as rapid as in infancy, toddlers make especially significant progress in their motor skills and their psychosocial and cognitive development. Toddlerhood is a period of great learning, and children's personalities begin to emerge more distinctly during these years. Growing independence, however, may lead to increased conflicts and difficulties with family caregivers.

Physical Growth

The slowed physical growth of toddlers is reflected by the fact that between 1 and 4 years of age, children usually gain only 1.8 to 2.7 kg (4–6 lb) annually and grow only about 5.0 to 7.6 cm (2–3 in.) per year. However, toddlers make great strides in their physical and motor skills. They fit simple objects into appropriate holes and build towers of two or three blocks. Most children have 20 deciduous teeth by age 2½ and readily self-feed table foods. Figure 10-3 shows approximate ages of eruption of deciduous teeth. They drink easily from a cup with a spout.

Psychosocial Development

The psychosocial *challenge* for this period is autonomy (independence) versus shame and doubt (see Table 10-1). The mobile toddler begins to establish independence by walking, self-feeding, playing, and speaking.

The *virtues* of the toddler stage are self-control and willpower, which evolve naturally as toddlers receive consistent discipline. Family members can foster the development of self-control and willpower by allowing toddlers to make simple choices, thereby reinforcing independence. This process also enhances the development of self-pride and the beginnings of positive self-esteem.

Cognitive and Motor Development

Intellectual and social development become more evident as toddlers grow physically. Children moving into toddlerhood have passed through several peak stages of accomplishment (*equilibrium*) and several stages of frustration (*disequilibrium*). Their growth rate slows, and social, physiologic, and psychological functions also advance at a slower rate. New skills continue to appear. For example, creeping 1-year-olds become dashing, climbing explorers at 15 months (Fig. 10-4). Peak periods of accomplishment, however, are farther apart.

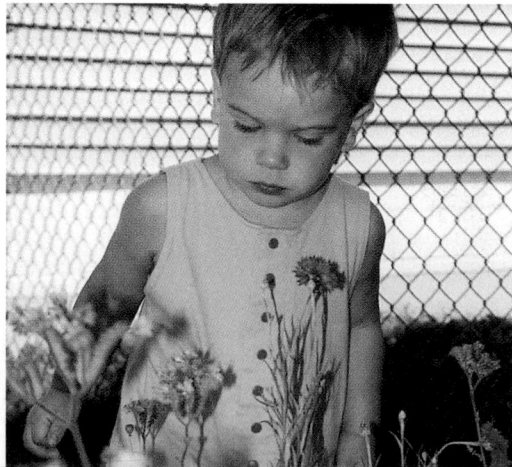

FIGURE 10-4. Toddlers enter a stage of autonomy, promoting exploration. (Taylor, C., Lillis, C., & LeMone, P. [2001]. *Fundamentals of nursing: The art and science of nursing care* [4th ed., p. 142]. Philadelphia: Lippincott Williams & Wilkins.)

Verbal skills improve. By age 1½, toddlers have a vocabulary of about 20 to 30 words, although they understand many more, as shown by their ability to follow directions. Social contacts begin to broaden, as toddlers share playtime with other children. Toddlers play next to their playmates rather than with them. This parallel play continues until social skills develop further.

By 18 months of age, children begin to sense that they can control certain aspects of their environment. They start to take advantage of their ability to exert control to the fullest. These toddlers may sometimes seem to take the greatest pleasure from always opposing others. They climb up the stairs without help but often crawl. Generally, these children cannot go down the stairs. They run on level ground, seldom fall, and pull along toys. They throw a ball to another person without falling and turn pages in a book two or three at a time. Eighteen-month-olds identify certain items in a book, and indicate their own nose, eyes, and ears.

As mid-toddlers learn to move with more sureness, they explore their surroundings with interest. Because these children are accident prone, definite limits are necessary. By age 2, neuromuscular coordination increases. Children now put on and take off simple items of clothing, such as slip-on shirts. They climb upstairs without crawling, and throw or kick a large ball. The tower of blocks they build is now five to seven blocks high, and most toddlers love to knock it over and set it up again. These toddlers string large beads, scribble with crayons, turn a doorknob, put on socks and pants, wash their hands, and turn book pages one at a time.

Typical 2-year-olds like riding toys. These children become frustrated with toys they cannot manage or with things they cannot do. Emotions are close to the surface—extremely happy or very sad. Children at this age love activity, noise, water, animals, and other people, as long as they get their own way. At the same time, they want acceptance from their families. Their favorite word is "no."

By age 3, toddlers begin to reach a stage of happy, conforming equilibrium. "No" changes to "yes," and routines become more flexible. Increased motor and language skills enable 3-year-olds to accomplish the developmental tasks required as they head into the preschool years.

Areas of Concern

Toilet Training

Toilet training is a major developmental accomplishment, and a learning process that requires patience and family encouragement. Toddlers are ready for toilet training when they sit comfortably on a toilet or potty without assistance, walk forward and backward, remove clothing with elastic bands, and stay dry for at least 2 hours. Behavioral changes before or after wetting or soiling indicate each child's emotional readiness, which usually emerges between 18 and 30 months of age. A child may be physically ready by 24 months, but not psychologically ready until age 3. Family members need to role model the behavior and respond to accidents with re-teaching, not punishment.

Bowel training is usually accomplished with less effort than bladder training, but this is not true for all children, especially boys. Some perfectly normal children still do not have total conscious control by 5 years of age. Most family caregivers are relieved to find that toilet training, barring occasional accidents, is well underway by 3 years of age. Accidents, however, are likely during illness, emotional upsets, or schedule changes.

Accident Prevention

Safety issues are important concerns for children of all ages. During the toddler stage, children begin to explore more often and with greater recklessness. They require constant supervision from family caregivers to prevent all sorts of accidents, ranging from minor scrapes and bruises to life-threatening tragedies. In fact, accidents are the leading cause of death for children between the ages of 1 and 4 years. Accidents involving motor vehicles top the list, followed by drowning, burning, poisoning, and falling.

Along with continual supervision, family caregivers can take many measures to prevent accidents for toddlers and older children as well (Fig. 10-5). Educating the Client 10-1 contains several tips for preventing minor problems and major catastrophes. Chapter 71 also discusses safety precautions for children.

Limit Setting

Although families should encourage the endless curiosity of toddlers, they must begin to establish limit setting for children during this stage. At this young age, simple, consistent guidance is important. Toddlers must know exactly what behaviors are expected and what behaviors are unacceptable. Such guidance enables toddlers to learn right from wrong. It also sets a pattern for later years, when rules and regulations evolve into discipline.

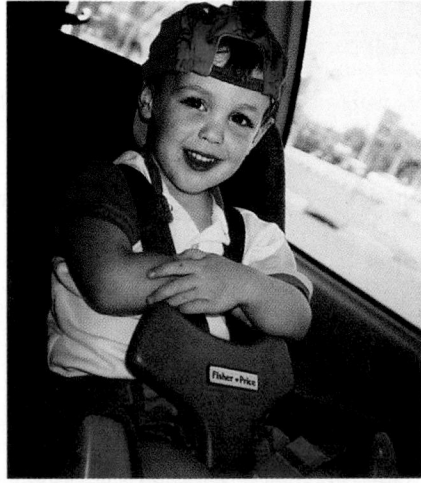

FIGURE 10-5. Safety considerations are of vital importance for all children. Child safety seats are an important measure in the prevention of injury or death from motor vehicle accidents. (Taylor, C., Lillis, C., & LeMone, P. [2001]. *Fundamentals of nursing: The art and science of nursing care* [4th ed., p. 142]. Philadelphia: Lippincott Williams & Wilkins.)

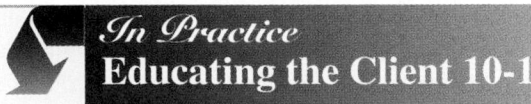

In Practice
Educating the Client 10-1

ACCIDENT PREVENTION FOR CHILDREN

Motor Vehicle
• Restrain child in a safety seat for all car trips.
• Place child in the back seat of the car, away from air bags.
• Closely supervise the child outdoors.
• Provide fenced-in play areas.
• Teach child to never run into street.

Drowning
• Supervise the child near all water—bathtubs, toilets, pools, sinks, small basins, and so forth. A small child can drown in a very small amount of water.
• Empty small pools after use. Fence in pools.
• Teach child not to run near bodies of water.

Fire and Burns
• Turn handles of pans toward center of stove.
• Keep child away from stoves, fire, matches, electrical cords, sockets, and so forth.
• Set hot water heater temperature at 120°–130°F.
• Test water temperature before immersion.
• Use safety covers on electrical outlets.

Falls
• Gate stairways; teach child to hold railings.
• Open windows from top. Use window guards.
• Move furniture away from upstairs windows.

Ingestion and Aspiration
• Avoid feeding the child nuts, grapes, popcorn, raisins, hard candy, lollipops.
• Childproof the home for coins, pins, balloons—especially near the crib.
• Teach child to not run with objects in the mouth and to not open things with teeth.

Poisoning
• Keep child-proof caps on toxic products.
• Store and lock all medications and vitamins, out of children's reach.
• Read labels carefully before using any drugs.
• Have emergency drugs like ipecac in the home.
• Keep poison control center number on all phones.
• Inspect homes you are visiting for safety hazards.

Ipecac — emetic, induce vomitting.

Thumb Sucking and the Security Blanket

Most dental authorities agree that thumb sucking can cause damage, especially during the eruption of baby teeth. The long-term effects of the habit depend on factors such as fre duration, and intensity. The more frequent the suc greater the percentage of time it is practice potential for permanent damage to mouth

Peer pressure may eventually embarrass children and cause thumb sucking to stop. Helping children to stop thumb sucking is difficult. Suggestions include:

- Substitute a pacifier for the thumb. Pacifiers are softer and less damaging to the teeth.
- Try to redirect behavior into other activities.
- Praise children when they avoid sucking the thumb for a period of time.
- Give these children a little extra attention: thumb sucking may reflect insecurity or loneliness.

Insecurity may also be expressed by the child's attraction to a blanket or stuffed toy. As they develop their own sense of security this object will be left behind. Some children who are ill, even when older, may gain comfort from a previously relinquished thumb, blanket, or stuffed toy.

Temper Tantrums

The "terrible twos" is a familiar term given to the temper tantrums that toddlers are apt to display during their second and third years (they are common for children between ages 18 months and 3 years). Tantrums are outbursts of anger and frustration. During a tantrum, toddlers may cry excessively, scream, throw themselves on the floor, hit, kick, bite, throw things, or hold their breath. Tantrums are more common when children are hungry, tired, frustrated, or feeling neglected.

Communicate to families that children are not throwing tantrums in an effort to deliberately misbehave. Tantrums usually result from feelings of frustration at being unable to express feelings and at a lack of control over day-to-day decisions. Family caregivers should attempt to ignore tantrums at home. They should avoid giving in to children's demands during these outbursts, because doing so can encourage future instances of such behavior. When children throw tantrums in public, they should be physically removed from the situation and alerted that such behavior is unacceptable. Family caregivers must discipline with love and confidence without getting caught up in the toddler's out-of-control emotions.

Sleep Habits and the Family Bed

Regular sleep restores energy, heals the body, and helps to organize the thoughts of the day. Most toddlers sleep 12 hours overnight and take naps during the day. Sometimes children resist sleep because they think that they are missing out on family activity. When overly tired, toddlers may actually have an extra burst of energy and want to run, jump, and play. Promoting regular sleep habits is essential. Bedtime rituals to relax a child include dimming the lights, reading a story, or singing a song while rubbing the child's back gently. Warm milk promotes relaxation and sleep because it contains the enzyme tyramine.

Some children fear darkness. Insisting on sleep at sleep times may be impossible occasionally; family caregivers may need to settle for children taking some quiet rest time alone instead.

Many family caregivers struggle with the decision to bring children into their bed when they cry in the middle of the night. authorities believe that this "family bed" prevents children from learning to fall asleep on their own, and leads to children exerting control over adults. Other authorities promote the idea of the family bed as comforting to the child. The alternative is allowing children to cry themselves to sleep, which may upset and disturb many families, leading to frustration and mistrust. Each family must resolve this dilemma for themselves according to the family caregivers' beliefs about childcare. What works for one family may not work for others.

Separation Anxiety

Like infants, toddlers may also display signs of anxiety when confronted with strangers or separated from the family for extended periods of time. This behavior usually peaks for toddlers at about 24 months. Upon separation from loved ones, children may cry, scream, lash out physically at others, and call for the missed person. This behavior is especially difficult when families must leave a child with a new babysitter. Separation, however, is necessary for proper emotional development and is a situation to which toddlers must adjust. Family caregivers must deal with toddlers firmly, providing reassurance that they will return and will not be gone for very long. Separation or stranger anxiety that continues past the age of 2 or is especially intense deserves evaluation by a healthcare professional.

PRESCHOOL: 3 TO 6 YEARS

Between the ages of 3 and 6, the preschool stage, children assume greater responsibility in their daily activities and exhibit more mature levels of interaction with others. Their enhanced ability to communicate gives pre-schoolers confidence, which contributes to their willingness to cooperate with caregivers and to express needs and frustrations. Curiosity is rampant and imagination is vivid during these years. Preschoolers pretend and experiment; however, they may exhibit aggressive behavior and develop minor fears due to enhanced levels of activity and imagination.

Physical Growth

Preschoolers weigh about 13.6 to 15.6 kg (30–35 lb) and are 76 to 91 cm (30–36 in.) tall. Although by age 3 children achieve about half of their eventual adult height, physical development slows. These children will probably gain less than 2.7 kg (6 lb) per year and about 7.6 cm (3 in.) annually until entering school. They exhibit a steadier walk than toddlers, because they are less top-heavy.

Psychosocial Development

The family unit functions as the primary relationship in the life of the preschooler. Individual independence continues to be important. Constant talking and questioning allow preschoolers to learn. Children begin to learn sexual roles through fantasies and games. They also become aware of, and are sometimes anxious about, body differences between males and females. According to Erikson, the *challenge* for preschoolers is to acquire initiative, the ability to take action without being told; otherwise, a sense of guilt will prevail. The *virtues* for this age group are direction and purpose (see Table 10-1).

Sigmund Freud termed this stage the *oedipal stage.* During these years, children focus attention and interest on the parent of the opposite sex. Children may feel competitive and jealous toward the same-sex parent; boys talk of marrying their mother, and girls of marrying their father. Because they still love their same-sex parent, these children may feel a sense of guilt or upset due to their conflicting emotions. Their repressed feelings may manifest themselves in nightmares, sudden phobias, or aggression toward other family members. Children may also copy the actions of their same-sex caregivers, as a way of resolving their feelings about them.

Generally, these children try hard to do what is expected and to be obedient and helpful. They are sensitive to social interactions, and scolding may easily hurt their feelings. Socially, preschoolers play with other children, as well as next to them. They make up simple games by age 3. They learn to share and wait their turn.

Play differences between boys and girls may develop. Some girls show a preference for quiet play, such as card games, dolls, and coloring. In contrast, some boys prefer rough and loud games; they play with trucks, balls, hammers, and other tools. Different ways that society expects girls and boys to act may cause such play differences, rather than biologic determinants. Remember, however, that not all boys or girls always exhibit behaviors considered typical of their sex. Many girls are athletic from an early age and enjoy cars, games, and sports. Similarly, boys may prefer reading, drawing, and coloring instead of rough-and-tumble activities. Families should encourage children to enjoy all sorts of activities, and promote fun and achievement in areas that interest children.

Cognitive and Motor Development

Motor skills become more refined by age 3. Most children now dress and undress almost completely, manage large buttons and zippers, form objects with clay, and draw recognizable forms, such as a square or a person. They climb up stairs, now alternating feet. They must put both feet on each step while coming down, jumping off the bottom step. They can stand on one foot and ride tricycles; they build towers with 9 or 10 blocks and can copy a circle on paper. Intellectually, development progresses to the point where children count to three or higher, identify objects in pictures, and tell which of several objects are alike. Their vocabulary numbers about 1,000 words, which 3-year-olds use in incessant talk. The ability to use words also reflects their growing ability to reason; these children ask questions constantly.

Three-year-olds have a great desire to be independent and to do things on their own. They can brush their teeth, although muscular coordination and judgment are not developed to the point where they can regularly perform this task properly. Parental supervision is essential. Three-year-olds can eat without assistance.

Play and growth activities of 3-year-olds proceed with ease and delight. Wants and the ability to carry out desires are well balanced—these children are pleased with themselves and

their playmates. They are friendly and willing to share. Their interest in words and in sharing thoughts and knowledge make 3-year-olds enjoyable and entertaining companions.

By age 4, preschoolers begin to look at a wider world, though it may extend only to the corner of the block, and they believe they can conquer it. Preserving some of this confidence while firmly controlling it may become difficult. Four-year-olds now have a speaking vocabulary of at least 2,000 words and probably count to 15 or 20. They can usually print part of their name and state their age and full name. When quarreling, boys of this age often engage in physical fighting, including hitting, kicking, and biting. Girls are more likely to yell at each other in their disagreements.

Many families will find that preschoolers are comfortable with themselves and their relationships with others by age 5. They are satisfied with the world of home and family. They know their full address and telephone number. Many may learn with computers. Many 5-year-olds live in a land of make-believe, with imaginary playmates and an imaginary family with fanciful names. The developmental tasks that they have mastered are sufficient for the moment.

Areas of Concern

Sibling Rivalry

Some preschoolers who are used to being the only child in a family must handle the arrival of a new and younger sibling. Or single or divorced parents may marry or remarry at this time, creating blended families. These situations require adjustment for all family members, but they may present special problems and stressors for preschoolers. Rivalry for parental attention may cause ongoing conflicts and unhappiness (Fig 10-6). The preschooler who must welcome a new baby into the family may feel jealous of the attention devoted to the new child and may begin to display regressive behavior (crawling instead of walking, soiling instead of using the potty, etc.). Children may fear that they are loved less than the

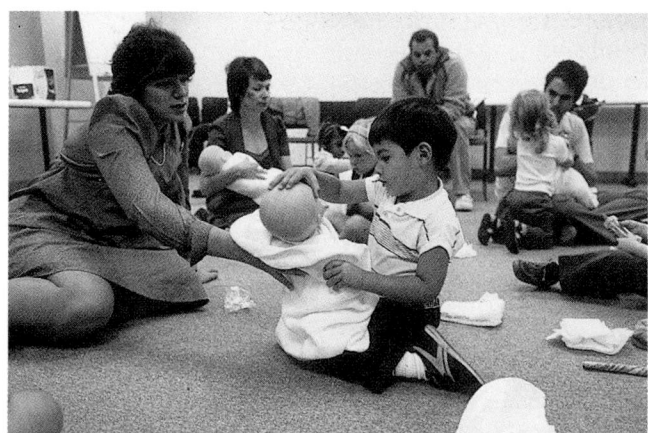

FIGURE 10-6. Sibling rivalry can be a problem throughout the lifespan. Toddlers and preschoolers who are preparing for younger siblings to join their families may benefit from sibling preparation classes. (Craven, R. F., & Hirnle, C. J. [2000]. *Fundamentals of nursing: Human health and function* [3rd ed., p. 1255] Philadelphia: Lippincott Williams & Wilkins.)

others. Families must cooperate to create a home that is fair to all children, yet encourages each person's individuality. Reassurances of love, amounts of attention that are appropriate to each child's stage and special needs, and encouragement of activities that involve the entire family help to diffuse sibling rivalry. Encourage families to understand that a preschooler's regressive or competitive behavior stems from conflicting emotions and new stressors. Individualized attention and interest in daily activities should assist the preschooler through the period of adjustment.

Phobias and Nightmares

Preschoolers are exposed to more of the world. As their thought processes, imaginations, and memories develop, they may experience fears and frightening dreams. Loud, rough animals can scare children, as can aggressive older children or displays of temper from adults. Images on television or in movies may also frighten young children. Preschoolers may suddenly become afraid of the dark. They may believe monsters or ghosts are hiding in their rooms.

Family members should try to minimize children's exposure to threatening elements and images. Providing reassurance, and discussing fears or nightmares, can help ease children's worries and may provide clues to underlying causes of the problem.

Masturbation

Children as young as 1 year, who like to touch and to handle things, may find that touching certain parts of the body gives them pleasant sensations. **Masturbation** is the term given to the handling and self-stimulation of the genital organs. A preschool child may find that handling the genitals relieves tensions arising from conflicts with others. Nothing is abnormal or shameful about this practice if children are taught that masturbation should be done in private but never in public. Shaming, threatening, or punishing children for masturbating may damage their later sexual expression. Happy, busy children are unlikely to seek frequent comfort in masturbation.

Enuresis

Enuresis, or bed-wetting, is more likely to occur in boys. In most cases, the underlying reason is physiologic or emotional immaturity. Waking the child during the night or restricting fluids between the evening meal and bedtime sometimes helps. Some children have an irritable bladder, a condition in which a small amount of urine in the bladder causes the desire to urinate. In this case, a physician may order a medication to decrease irritability. Children also can be taught to withhold the urine voluntarily during the daytime. This gradually distends the bladder, increasing its size and promoting retention.

SCHOOL AGE: 6 TO 10 YEARS

Achievements youngsters make during infancy, toddlerhood, and preschool prepare them for formal education. School-age children embark on a period of rapid learning, not only in the educational setting, but through increased encounters with

people outside the family circle, and expanded awareness of the world around them. As they complete this stage, children approach physical maturity and head into the emotional, social, and intellectual challenges of adolescence (see Chap. 11).

Physical Growth

As they approach age 6, children begin to lose their deciduous teeth. Permanent teeth usually start to erupt in the early school years. From the time children enter school, a slow, steady period of growth begins. School-age children gain about 2.3 to 3.2 kg (5–7 lb) and grow about 6.4 cm (2½ in.) a year until puberty (sexual maturity), at which time they experience a growth spurt. From age 6 or 7 until puberty, identifying an average growth rate becomes difficult, because variations among normal children are wide.

Psychosocial Development

During the school years, the significant person for children changes from the family to people from the school or neighborhood, such as teachers, schoolmates, or best friends. Independence is important. Learning to produce things (schoolwork, projects) takes precedence. These children explore their ever-expanding world and begin to collect pets, dolls, rocks, baseball cards, video games, books, and other objects.

The development of a sense of industry is the major psychosocial *challenge;* if school-age children do not attain this sense, a feeling of inferiority results. School-age children need recognition for their accomplishments, such as school achievements, cooperative participation in groups that stress skill development (Cub Scouts, Girl or Boy Scouts, 4-H), sports teams that stress physical prowess and fair play, and band or orchestra, which encourage musical talent. This recognition leads to a sense of belonging, and feelings of competence and self-worth, the *virtues* of this developmental stage.

Cognitive and Motor Development

Because school occupies so many waking hours, events there play a large part in the lives of school-age children. As they explore this new world beyond home, children become increasingly independent. Fitting in is very important to school success. Family is often ousted from first place. The saving grace is an eagerness to try new situations and an enthusiasm for learning and adventure. Additionally, children begin to learn that they must abide by rules, not only at home but in school and other outside settings as well. Encourage families to recognize that self-development and reaching out from the family are big steps forward.

Reasoning and conceptual powers expand. By age 6, most children can tell time and count to at least 40 or 50; typically, they recognize the letters of the alphabet, numbers from 1 to 10, and their own name. At 7, they produce all language sounds, use simple logic, and grasp basics of mathematics. Printing becomes clearer.

During the early school years, many children express the desire for a retreat of their own. Boys and girls of this age are aware of each other, but typically prefer not to play together. In fact, they are usually antagonistic and may fight and call each other unkind names. Classrooms of children may break up into several distinct playgroups. Friends begin to occupy an important place in their lives. The members of the clique usually share secrets, including a favorite hangout. Boys and girls may fight openly at times.

Between the ages of 8 and 10, children learn to write in cursive. By age 9, most children spend much of their time with friends, clubs, and groups. Despite evidence of self-reliance, children may begin to worry and complain about tasks that involve responsibility, such as schoolwork and home chores. At the completion of this stage, well-adjusted 10-year-olds are friendly and realistic, accepting themselves and life as it comes.

Areas of Concern

Sibling Rivalry

Sibling rivalry, the competition among brothers and sisters, may lead to jealousy, trauma, verbal arguments, and sometimes physical fights. This rivalry is natural; brothers and sisters compete, whether as preschoolers or as schoolchildren. Adults may become referees in an attempt to maintain a calm family atmosphere. To avoid being drawn into triangles, they must treat each child equally and fairly. As siblings progress through the school years, they should become responsible for resolving their own differences. Families should be aware of the inevitability of sibling rivalry, and adults should intervene only when absolutely necessary. However, adults must be sure to set definite ground rules for siblings (eg, no physical or emotional harm). In dealing with this issue, families can teach and learn the importance of mutual respect, forgiveness, and appreciation of individual talents.

Responsibilities

The school-age child should have some responsibilities in the home (Fig. 10-7). Responsibilities may be as simple as cleaning the bedroom, setting and clearing the table, washing

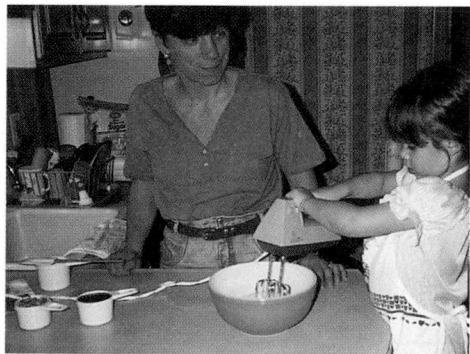

FIGURE 10-7. Assisting a parent helps a child develop a sense of belonging and accomplishment. (Taylor, C., Lillis, C., & LeMone, P. [2001]. *Fundamentals of nursing: The art and science of nursing care* [4th ed., p. 146]. Philadelphia: Lippincott Williams & Wilkins.)

dishes or loading the dishwasher, taking out the trash, or walking the family pet. These tasks allow the child to acquire a sense of responsibility (see Table 10-1).

Sex Education

A child's education regarding sexuality begins at birth. Children are socialized into gender roles and gradually learn to understand differences between males and females from their continued interactions with the world. Today's western societies focus continually on sex in its television programming, movies, songs, and clothing. Children are exposed to provocative material at earlier ages. Because of different rates of maturity, some girls start menstruating as early as age 9.

Controversy exists over the proper age at which to introduce children to some type of formal sex education. Many communities are working to integrate age-appropriate sexual education across the school curriculum. Family caregivers must realize the importance, however, of being able to explain sexual issues and questions to their children outside the classroom. Adults who feel uncomfortable or awkward talking to their school-age children about such matters should consider setting up a discussion between a healthcare provider or another reliable adult and the child. In this way children receive correct information from trusted individuals, rather than believing the often-inaccurate stories passed along from peers.

➤ STUDENT SYNTHESIS

Key Points

- Growth and development is an ongoing process throughout childhood.
- Growth and development progresses in a particular sequence (cephalocaudal: head to toe; and proximodistal: center outward).
- Theorists including Havighurst, Erikson, and Piaget have identified specific tasks to accomplish and stages to pass through to become a mature, fully functional person.
- Play is an important element of growth and development that helps prepare children for more mature levels of functioning.
- Nurses and other healthcare providers can give anticipatory guidance to help prepare family caregivers for the normal areas of concern that arise during each developmental stage.
- Infancy, which ends at age 1 year, is the period of fastest growth and development over the entire life span.
- Toddlerhood (1–3 years) is a time marked by exploration, growing independence, and conflicting emotions.
- Children during the preschool years (3–6 years) exhibit imagination, improved communication skills, and curiosity.

• School greatly influences children aged 6 to 10 as they branch away from the family home. They develop relationships with peers, participate in school and community activities, and learn more about the world around them.

Critical Thinking Exercises

1. Based on Erikson's psychosocial theory, discuss why children with parents who are too lenient or who are overprotective may experience difficulties with issues of trust and autonomy.
2. A mother who has just given birth to a newborn boy is facing difficulty with her 3-year-old daughter, Jill. Jill has been stealing and hiding the baby's toys, crawling around the house, and having emotional outbursts more often. Considering Jill's age and stage of development, explain what is happening and ways for Jill's mother to handle the situation.
3. Grace, who is 10 years old, lives with her father Joe, a single parent. She has not received much information about sex and body development from Joe because he feels very awkward discussing such issues with her. Grace has just started her first menstrual cycle. How can Joe handle the situation, ensuring that his daughter receives accurate information?

NCLEX-Style Review Questions

1. According to Havighurst, developmental tasks that must be accomplished by the toddler or preschool child include:
   a. Control of the process of elimination
   b. Learning to talk
   c. Learning to walk
   d. Perfecting physical skills and games
2. Concepts of growth and development include:
   a. Growth from complex to simple
   b. Growth in an orderly sequence
   c. Growth from outside to center
   d. Growth from tail to head
3. The leading cause of death in toddlerhood is:
   a. Accidental poisonings
   b. Burnings
   c. Drownings
   d. Motor vehicle accidents

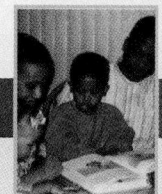

CHAPTER

11

Adolescence

LEARNING OBJECTIVES

1. Explain the term puberty and its relationship to adolescence.
2. Relate the theories of Havighurst, Erikson, and Piaget to adolescent growth and development.
3. Explain how skill development contributes to expanding cognition and decision-making.
4. Discuss the different stages of adolescence.
5. Describe the specific physical changes that occur between ages 11 and 20.
6. Discuss sexual development for boys and girls.
7. Identify the importance of relationships for adolescents.
8. Describe the cognitive, emotional, and moral development that occurs during adolescence.
9. Discuss appropriate discipline strategies for adolescents.
10. Design a plan for presenting information about human sexuality to adolescents.

NEW TERMINOLOGY

adolescence
menarche
nocturnal emission

peer group
preadolescence
puberty

Puberty (from the Latin word meaning *adult*) is the period when a person becomes able to reproduce sexually. **Adolescence** is the developmental period between puberty and maturity. It spans the ages between 11 and 20 years, after which a person enters early adulthood.

A rapid growth spurt marks adolescence, by the end of which individuals achieve adult height. Although tremendous physical growth occurs, emotional needs predominate during this period; adolescents spend much of their time searching for meaning in life and for a sense of identity. Adolescents are required to make critical choices that may help to determine the shape of their lives. Such choices include the use of alcohol and other substances, moral obligations and respect for others, school attendance, relationships (family, friends, and sexuality), education after high school, and career alternatives.

GROWTH AND DEVELOPMENT THEORIES

The theories of Havighurst, Erikson, and Piaget continue to apply to individuals as they enter the adolescent stage. All three theories stress the adolescent's burgeoning maturity and expanding abilities.

Havighurst: Developmental Tasks

According to Havighurst, the ultimate task of adolescence is to "grow up." Heredity and environment, the culture in which the individual lives, and the young person's own determination and self-perceptions all contribute to the success of his or her progress to maturity.

Although authorities define the components of achieving maturity in various ways, they generally agree on certain important steps. The tasks of adolescence ultimately involve achieving independence from parental domination and accepting individual responsibility for oneself (Box 11-1). An adolescent slowly becomes emancipated from parental ties by achieving intellectual, emotional, and economic independence. To initiate and maintain satisfactory interpersonal relations, adolescents must develop positive concepts of self-identity, self-respect, and self-control to carry them through to adulthood. They begin to expand their social obligations. To start

> ➤➤ BOX 11-1

> ### HAVIGHURST'S DEVELOPMENTAL TASKS OF ADOLESCENCE
>
> - Develop appropriate and mature relationships with peers of both sexes
> - Achieve emotional independence
> - Accept physique and use body effectively
> - Develop social roles of one's culture
> - Prepare for adult life and adult relationships
> - Prepare for career, education, and other pursuits
> - Acquire values and ethics; develop ideology
> - Behave in a socially acceptable way

making good independent decisions, maturing adolescents must recognize the purpose and consequences of their actions, and be willing to accept responsibility for both successes and failures.

Erikson: Psychosocial Development

The adolescent faces many difficult decisions during the teen years concerning the future and the adult world. What vocation should I choose? Should I go to college? Can I afford further education? Do the courses I am taking in high school meet the college's admission criteria? Should I join the military? Will I want to get married someday? Should I have a baby though I am not married? Should I live with my parents or move out? Erikson's theory of psychosocial development, presented in Chapter 10, continues for adolescence (Table 11-1). The major challenge of adolescence is the achievement of identity: Who am I? Where am I going? With whom? And, How am I going to get there? If this phase is not resolved, the result is role confusion.

The significant group for the adolescent is the **peer group,** which is made up of contemporaries, or a group of people with whom one associates (Fig. 11-1). The peer group is often more important than the family and can influence adolescents in many ways. Peer pressure to try cigarettes, alcohol, marijuana,

---

▪▪▪ TABLE 11-1 *E*RIKSON'S THEORY OF PSYCHOSOCIAL DEVELOPMENT—ADOLESCENCE

Concept	Adolescence
Challenge	Personal identity versus role confusion
Significant others	Peer group, opposite sex, family
Necessary accomplishments	Make life decisions; achieve personal identity; accept responsibility
Virtues	Independence; self-esteem; self-reliance; self-control; devotion; fidelity
Ways to help the adolescent succeed	Provide privacy; encourage activities; support decisions; allow independence; give recognition and acceptance; maintain a good family atmosphere; facilitate information gathering

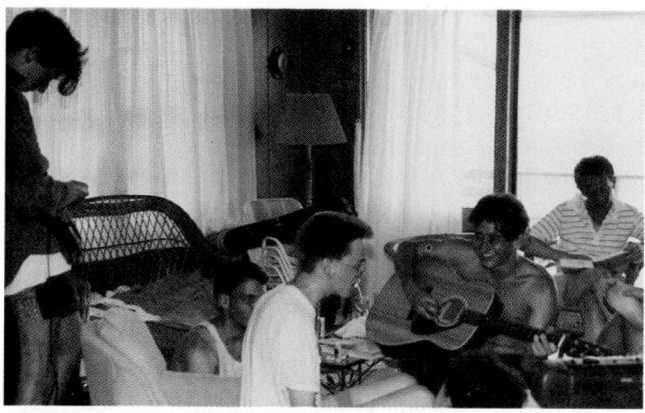

FIGURE 11-1. Throughout adolescence into young adulthood, peer relationships influence psychosocial development. (Craven, R. F., & Hirnle, C. J. [2000]. *Fundamentals of nursing: Human health and function* [3rd ed., p. 274]. Philadelphia: Lippincott Williams & Wilkins.)

or other drugs can be the first step to chemical dependency or substance abuse. The peer group can help to determine whether a young person gets good grades in school, joins the military, or buys a car.

Piaget: Cognitive Development

According to Piaget, the person from 12 to 15 years of age enters stage IV of cognitive development: formal operations. The adolescent thinks in the abstract and develops skills to participate in complex problem-solving.

Skill development is part of cognitive growth and is also preparation for the future. Skill development includes activities such as gymnastics, photography, writing, carpentry, auto mechanics, and dancing. Many skills developed during the teen years help adolescents make educational and career choices. Teens enhance their leadership and diplomatic abilities by participating in student government, debate, and other school programs. Plays, science competitions, choral groups, orchestra, and band are other avenues for young people to increase their intelligence, talent, sense of cooperation, and community spirit. Religious groups geared for teenagers often hold many activities that attempt to provide a sense of moral instruction as well. Sports often become a primary interest. Cooking may appeal to both girls and boys. Most of today's adolescents have never known life without computers, and may develop a keen interest in experimenting with them. Adult encouragement and guidance are needed for skill development.

ADOLESCENT GROWTH AND DEVELOPMENT

Adolescence can be divided into stages. The first stage can be called pubescence, preadolescence, or early adolescence. This stage usually lasts from ages 11 to 14, with girls often maturing faster. It is sometimes referred to as an "awkward stage," as the person teeters between childish and mature ways of appearing, thinking, and behaving. Middle adolescence lasts from ages 15 to 17. Individuals of these ages are most likely to exhibit behavior considered "typical" of the adolescent. The late adolescent stage lasts from ages 18 to 20. During this time, young people complete their transition into adulthood. The developmental changes of adolescence have prepared them to exhibit the independence and responsibility that have grown as they begin college life, join the military, or seek employment.

Characteristics of Developmental Stages

Early Adolescence (Ages 11–14)

During this period, also known as **preadolescence,** young people often waver between a desire for independence and trust from their families and silliness, playfulness, and a need for regular approval. Rebellion against authority figures, noisy and faultfinding quarrels with siblings, and evasion of household tasks can be sources of conflict. Patience is essential. As early adolescents attempt new undertakings to test independence and self-reliance, they need strong familial support and guidance. As they get older, adolescents become more controlled emotionally and better able to see situations in perspective. Psychological awareness and objectivity begin to broaden beyond the self to understand the feelings and behavior of others. A growing sense of humor helps to make family relationships more pleasant.

Because young adolescents are usually enthusiastic, they bring spirit and buoyancy to their undertakings. Involvement in extensive projects in school shows initiative and effort, and perhaps involves detailed computer use. However, this high initiative may get out of hand. Planned parties and social events require adult supervision to prevent boisterousness from ruining events.

As they head toward middle adolescence, young teenagers may display tendencies to seclusion and moodiness. Emerging reasoning leads to reflection on themselves and others and to assessment of new experiences. Appraisals of interaction between self and the world require a place and time, so young teenagers may begin to spend more time alone. Because both girls and boys have long associations with the mirror, they will use the mirror as a prop for role-playing and for testing and measuring themselves in imagined situations. A teenager's contemplation will naturally include an assessment of the family. As they develop their own perspective of family structure and roles, their criticisms and withdrawals often become a source of puzzlement and hurt to family members. The maturing adolescent takes frequent flights of independence, but has a strong need to return to the "nest" for guidance and encouragement.

By age 14, adolescents are becoming more accepting of other people, and more conscious of what makes their own personality unique from others. They may begin to develop better relationships with siblings, finding that they like their brothers and sisters more than they thought. "Talk, talk, talk" is many adults' version of this age. Some authorities state that verbalizing ideas is a true growth characteristic and a developmental achievement. Teenagers now show an increased natural ability in perceiving many sides of a situation. They are no longer frustrated by being unable to express or to verbalize ideas. They can say what they think, a task of maturity.

Middle Adolescence (Ages 15–17)

Introspection and fluctuations in self-assurance mark the middle adolescent years, which can baffle many families. Physical alterations, loud self-assertion, self-preoccupation, rapid shifts between dependent and independent attitudes, blithe spirit, and mood swings are challenges for even the most patient and supportive families. Teenagers are pulling away from childhood in a quest for self-reliance (see Table 11-1). Although they value the ability to depend on home and school, these teenagers need to counterbalance security with independence. Because they are searching for balance, immaturity frequently results in withdrawal, belligerence, or defiance. They may begin to believe that any advice from family caregivers is an effort to control them completely. Adolescents may seek guidance away from home.

By age 15 or 16, most adolescents begin to form some ideas about the future and to plan for more than present interests and activities. Vague ideas about courtship, marriage, career, and families of their own result in scrutiny of the family of origin. Family members may sometimes feel rejected because they fail to meet the perfectionist standards of observant middle teenagers.

Increased independence and interest in the opposite sex now cause many young people to take more responsibility for self-care and personal cleanliness. They like to choose their own clothing. Many adolescents of this age group seek part-time employment because a job provides money.

By the time they are about 17, most middle teenagers are beginning to exhibit true attitudes of maturity. In interpersonal relations, they show an interest in others and an awareness and acceptance of social responsibilities. As they head into late adolescence and young adulthood, they tend to have friendships with many people of both sexes.

Late Adolescence (Ages 18–20)

Older adolescents begin to grapple with everyday, mature issues. They move away from familiar people, places, and things. Graduation from high school leads many teens to colleges and universities far from home, where they become responsible for themselves. Those attending school who remain close to home or at home still find their social circles expanded and their intellectual horizons challenged, as they take courses of particular interest and importance to them. Some late teens enter the work force or join the military after finishing school. Branching into such worlds necessitates increased maturity and improved social and professional skills. During these years, moral questions and issues involving ethical decision-making gain relevance. Increased knowledge and awareness may lead to reflection and internal reevaluation. Exposure to different peoples and other ways of thinking may lead young people to question previously accepted values and ideas.

Relationships are usually important during these years. Young men and women may enjoy dating a variety of individuals. Long-term romantic relationships and friendships that lasted throughout high school may be tested or come to an end, as social circles expand and interests change. As teenagers move into the adult world and are expected to behave maturely, previously critical adolescents may come to appreciate and develop better relationships with parents and other family members.

Physical Growth

Physical changes characterize adolescence. Similar to the childhood periods of growth and development, outward signs of maturity vary. By age 13, most young people reach 90% of their adult height and have all their permanent teeth except the third molars or "wisdom teeth." They have at least tripled in height and gained 15 times their birth weight. During adolescence, the extremities lengthen, the hands and feet grow, and the hips, chest, and shoulders widen. Girls usually grow between 2 and 8 inches in height and boys 4 to 12 inches during adolescence.

Hormonal changes control growth and many other physical aspects. Increased glandular activity causes an increase in sweat and contributes to the development of body odors (though there are racial differences). Glandular changes also are partly responsible for the development of acne in some adolescents. Body hair grows in previously hairless areas: the pubic area, under the arms, and for boys, on the face and chest. Hair on other areas such as the arms and legs becomes thicker and coarser.

Alterations in body chemistry, developmental challenges, plus an ever-increasing capacity to consume food provide adolescents with a great supply of energy. By the time a person is approximately age 18, he or she has reached full height, reproductive organs are adult size, and secondary sex characteristics are pronounced.

Sexual Development

Development in Boys

Some boys at age 11 do not yet show the changes of puberty. Others have started to grow rapidly again, and yet others may already have a heavy or defined skeletal structure. Physical growth varies markedly in 12-year-old boys as well. The average boy shows some pubertal changes by the end of this year. The testicles and penis enlarge, and changes occur in the appearance of the scrotum. Pubic hair begins to appear. Spontaneous erections and occasional ejaculations without external cause may be confusing. Young boys should understand that the involuntary discharge of semen while sleeping (**nocturnal emission**) is a normal part of reproductive health. Other natural developments of puberty are a change in voice and the appearance of chin whiskers.

Most boys grow more at 14 than at any other age. A strong, muscular appearance and continued deepening of the voice add to the impression of maturity. Nocturnal emissions have begun for most boys by this age. By age 16, most young men are close to their adult height.

Development in Girls

Girls also show great variation in sexual development. The average 11-year-old girl has begun a period of rapid growth and shows signs of approaching sexual maturity. Breast and hip development may be noticeable during these years. Pubic hair starts to grow. By age 13, many girls have experienced **menarche,** the onset of menstruation. Early periods frequently are irregular, and normal cycles may not be established for a few years.

By age 14, many girls have the physical appearance of young women. Few grow in height after age 14. Breasts and other secondary sex characteristics are those of an adult. By age 16, the menstrual cycle has become regular and the young woman generally accepts menstruation as part of adult life.

Sexual Identity and Orientation

Sexual identity may be confusing. As adolescents struggle to understand themselves and begin to experiment, they may question their sexual preferences. Some people may develop a same-sex crush during this period or participate in homosexual activity. For many adolescents, these feelings and behaviors reflect a temporary, experimental stage that does not affect later heterosexuality.

Many gays and lesbians, however, first come to realize their sexual orientation during the teen years. Recognition that they are "different" from others can cause homosexual youths much confusion. Fear of rejection from their families, friends, and community may lead to suffering and unhappiness. In a period marked by the need for self-acceptance and a sense of belonging, gay and lesbian adolescents are at risk for alienation, doubt, and depression. In fact, homosexual youths account for 30% of all teen suicides each year.

Sex Education

Most adolescents are naturally curious about sex, sexuality, and changes in their bodies. If adults provide information with sensitivity, adolescents can form healthy sexual attitudes. If parents, teachers, and counselors do not give such information, adolescents will seek answers elsewhere. Unwholesome attitudes or incorrect beliefs may develop from information they receive from peers and older adolescents who appear to "know it all." The result may be premature and unsafe sexual activities.

Sexual activity at younger ages is increasing. Even though birth control is available, many young people fail or refuse to use it. In addition, the incidence of sexually transmitted diseases (STDs) is on the rise. Many adolescents who may fear pregnancy fail to recognize the risks of gonorrhea, syphilis, genital warts, and HIV/AIDS as well.

Most adolescents welcome sex education as necessary. Family caregivers and other trusted adults can help adolescents to establish reasonable boundaries and, at the same time, give accurate information. Adolescents need the opportunity to discuss with both peers and concerned adults the emotional conflicts involved with refusing and accepting sexual activity. Such discussions help them make better decisions. Sexually active adolescents need counseling about the use of condoms to help prevent STDs, and other forms of birth control to prevent pregnancy.

Nursing Alert

Adolescents must understand that all forms of birth control contain some risk of failure. Only abstinence is 100% effective against pregnancy and sexually transmitted diseases.

Psychosocial Development

The major task of adolescence is to form a sense of identity. Ironically, much of the person's sense of self during this time is defined by relationships with other people. Group conformity and "fitting in" with peers is of great importance to most adolescents. At the same time, outward expressions of rebellion against parents, teachers, and other authority figures are common.

Family Relationships

Family relationships may be delicate throughout adolescence. Attitudes toward younger siblings may alternate between protectiveness and annoyance. Attitudes toward family caregivers range from harsh criticism and displeasure to genuine understanding and great love. During adolescence, solid family relationships can influence lifetime interpersonal success because they foster self-esteem and respect for and from others. Respect from others is essential for adolescents to maintain psychological and emotional health. Such respect includes recognizing the need for self-assertion, privacy, information, acceptance, experimentation, and growth in all developmental areas.

Peer Relationships

During adolescence, close friendships and first romantic relationships become important factors in the development of a young person's identity as a future adult. These relationships also influence feelings of acceptance and belonging.

Friendship. Adolescence is a time of forming friendships, with members of both the same and opposite sexes. Social activities are usually with the same select groups of individuals. School cliques are common. Many adolescents also have one or two best friends of the same sex during these years, with whom they spend large amounts of time. These friendships are often important emotional preparation for more intimate and romantic relationships with others as the person matures.

Dating. Dating becomes a significant issue during these years (Fig. 11-2). Early teen dates usually consist of large groups of both boys and girls going to the mall or the movies. As adolescents get older, they begin to pair off into couples. Many people experience their first steady relationship during these years. First love brings many complicated feelings. A breakup with a first boyfriend or girlfriend can be extremely difficult for the adolescent to handle emotionally.

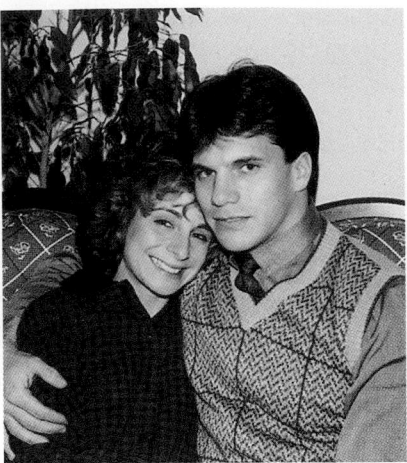

FIGURE 11-2. A primary developmental task of adolescence is to achieve new and more mature relationships. (Taylor, C., Lillis, C., & LeMone, P. [2001]. *Fundamentals of nursing: The art and science of nursing care* [4th ed., p. 149]. Philadelphia: Lippincott Williams & Wilkins.)

Peer Pressure and Risk Taking.   To define their identity, exert their independence, and "prove" to peers that they are maturing, adolescents may take significant risks with their health and well-being, school success, and relationships. Such risk-taking behavior includes noncompliance with a medical regimen, school truancy, sexual promiscuity, dangerous activities such as skydiving or car racing, drinking, and using drugs. Adolescents may not be fully knowledgeable of the possible consequences of their actions, or they may insist that they do not care. They are especially vulnerable to unsafe situations because of natural immaturity and the pressure for acceptance. Many adolescents feel a sense of immortality, assuming that nothing bad can happen to them. They are often competitive, with a desire to set themselves apart from the crowd.

Some adolescents who do not "fit" into a same-age peer group may seek the companionship of young adults who give them access to cars, alcohol, cigarettes, money, and mature relationships. The adolescent may come to depend on the older person's interest for a sense of security or identity. The young adult may take advantage of the adolescent's role confusion and social immaturity. The result may be even greater pressure for the adolescent to become involved in substance abuse, sexual promiscuity, and delinquency. Young adult men, for example, father a large number of teenage pregnancies, partly because of the dependent relationship and imbalance of power and maturity between an adolescent girl and a young adult man.

Families can help adolescents to overcome peer pressure by modeling safe habits and practices. They should promote a safe home environment where adolescents receive appropriate responses for their actions and assistance with finding alternative and satisfying recreation and relationships. Parents and older siblings should give information to adolescents about the hazards of risk taking, and positively reinforce appropriate practices. Attempting to make adolescents aware of the consequences of risk taking usually works better than exerting authority or using law enforcement and punitive measures. The goal is to make teenagers themselves part of the solution.

Food and Eating Habits

Adolescents have special nutritional needs that are important for optimum health (see Chap. 30). As a result of multiple activities and less adult supervision over meals, young people may indulge in a diet composed primarily of "junk food" that is high in fat, sugar, and empty calories. Recent studies have indicated that the number of overweight adolescents in this country is increasing. Poor dietary habits can also lead to problems as metabolism slows and young adults lead a more sedentary lifestyle. Bad nutritional habits at any age can lead to fatigue, unhealthy appearance, and susceptibility to illness.

Teenage boys normally have huge appetites. Many can eat large amounts of food without seeming to gain weight. Some boys lose or gain weight for a specific purpose. Some boys become concerned with achieving a muscular appearance, consuming protein drinks and spending time at a gym in an effort to "pump up." Or they may engage in dangerous weight loss practices to achieve a lower-than-normal body weight for sports such as wrestling.

Girls are often very concerned about appearance. They may fret continually that they are fat. Gaining just 2 or 3 pounds can make adolescent girls depressed or discouraged. Anorectic or bulimic patterns of eating may emerge during these years. Anorexia is marked by eating minimal amounts of food; bulimia is characterized by a pattern of binge eating, followed by induced vomiting or the use of laxatives. Chapters 72 and 87 discuss both disorders. Be aware that although most people who suffer from these problems are young women, teenage boys and young men sometimes are afflicted as well. Obesity for both sexes can also be a serious problem.

Areas of Concern

Adolescents develop physically and socially at various rates. As they take on more responsibilities, they may have special concerns that their families will share. As a nurse, you need to be prepared for questions related to these and other areas. Educating the Client 11-1 lists tips for providing guidance.

Communicate to families that a solid family life helps teenagers achieve a positive self-image. Young people are usually happiest when family relationships are based on mutual respect and affection. Mutual respect recognizes the adult's task to discipline the adolescent in an age-appropriate manner, and the adolescent's ability to adjust to changing discipline. The gradual path to independence demands the development of self-discipline. Most teenagers will agree that they desire firm disciplinary measures, imposed fairly according to their age and the nature of their misbehavior. Many experts on child behavior agree that strict "discipline for discipline's sake" only stirs rebellion and undermines self-respect.

Adults must remember that many fluctuations in adolescent behavior are a normal part of growing up. Adolescents are learning to make decisions and to assume responsibility for those decisions. Home support is invaluable. A home that acts as a base—for friendships and personal activities, family conferences for planning and problem-solving, wholesome companionship within the family, and acknowledged moral

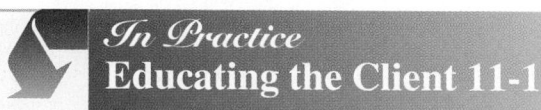

In Practice
Educating the Client 11-1

ADOLESCENT CONCERNS ABOUT GROWTH
AND DEVELOPMENT

- Development of healthy habits: cleanliness, balanced nutrition, sleep and rest, activity and exercise
- Safety measures with motor vehicles and bikes
- Importance of scholastic and skill achievement
- Importance and development of self-respect
- Selection of peers as friends
- Wise counseling about sex and sexuality
- Responsibilities resulting from sexual activity
- Problems that arise from substance use and abuse (cigarette smoking, alcohol, recreational drugs)

and ethical standards—furnishes guidelines for adolescents, who learn to respect and to live with themselves and others.

Adolescents who are loved, accorded a measure of freedom and responsibility, disciplined sensibly and respectfully, and encouraged to grow and to achieve personal identity, usually respond with love and respect for family. They enjoy family life and achieve a healthy, mature adulthood. The future family life of young people, when they raise their own children, will probably be patterned after these positive family experiences.

☛ KEY CONCEPT

Parents need help in accepting their "child" as an "adult."

➤ STUDENT SYNTHESIS

Key Points

- Adolescence is a turbulent time, marked by rapid physical growth and frequent emotional upheavals.
- Puberty is the time when a person matures sexually and becomes able to reproduce.
- The developmental tasks of adolescence involve the formation of a self-image, establishment of goals for the future, and building relationships with others.
- Skill development in adolescence helps teenagers to learn more and may influence future career and educational choices.
- Great variation exists in physical and emotional maturity among young people.
- Relationships with family and friends and dating contribute to the adolescent's self-perceptions and interpersonal skills.
- Solid family communication and relations help adolescents get through difficult challenges.
- Age-appropriate discipline is important for adolescents trying to withstand peer pressure.

- Sex education from trusted adults helps teenagers avoid mistakes based on misinformation.

Critical Thinking Exercises

1. Twelve-year-old George comes to the healthcare facility upset. He is the shortest boy in his class. While other boys have begun to show some facial hair, George is still waiting for his voice to change. Explain how you would address George's concerns. What information would you give him?

2. Paul is 15 years old and has been dating Julie for a few months. They are not sexually active, but many of their friends are. Paul is afraid to have sex, believing he and Julie are too young. He is becoming increasingly anxious, however, under the pressure and scrutiny of his friends. He is afraid to talk to his parents about the situation; however, when sorting the laundry, his mother found a condom in his pocket that a friend had given to him "just in case." Paul's mother consults you for healthcare advice. Based on your knowledge of peer pressure and adolescent sexuality, what advice would you provide Paul and his mom?

3. Darcy is 17 and a junior in high school. She's a popular teenager who is mature for her age. Recently, a friend's older brother, a college junior, has taken an interest in Darcy and asked her out on a date. Darcy is excited by the prospect of seeing an "older man," yet is worried about his expectations. What is your reaction to this situation? What questions might she have?

NCLEX-Style Review Questions

1. According to Havighurst, the primary task of adolescence is to:
   a. Achieve an identity
   b. Develop formal operations
   c. Form peer groups
   d. Grow up

2. Which of the following behaviors would the nurse expect to see during late adolescence?
   a. Dealing with everyday issues
   b. Introspection and fluctuations in self-assurance
   c. Rebellion against authority
   d. Seclusion and moodiness

3. Which strategy would be most effective when teaching adolescents about risk-taking behaviors?
   a. Allow peers to talk to each other about risk-taking behaviors
   b. Encourage adolescents to develop friendships with young adults
   c. Make the adolescent aware of the consequences of risk-taking behaviors
   d. Require the adolescent to promise not to engage in risk-taking behaviors

CHAPTER

12

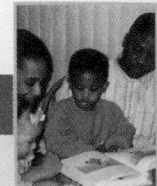

Early and Middle Adulthood

LEARNING OBJECTIVES

1. List Havighurst's developmental tasks for early and middle adulthood.
2. Describe Erikson's theory of psychosocial development as it applies to young and middle adults.
3. Compare Levinson's "individual life structure" theory with the theories of Havighurst and Erikson.
4. State Sheehy's "phases of adulthood."
5. Discuss the implications of life choices made during early adulthood.
6. Examine one aspect of life (eg, vocation, intimate relationships) and apply it across middle adulthood.

NEW TERMINOLOGY

generativity

intimacy

isolation

midlife transition

This chapter examines the development of the individual throughout early and middle adulthood. Remember that the process of growth and development is a continuum. Certain aspects of late adolescence and the beginning of adulthood are interrelated and may overlap. This is true for other stages of adulthood as well.

ADULT GROWTH AND DEVELOPMENT THEORIES

Although researchers have been more active in establishing theories of development in childhood and adolescence, theories do exist regarding development in adulthood. Havighurst's developmental tasks and Erikson's psychosocial theory can be applied to adults. This chapter also discusses two theories specific to adult growth and development proposed by Daniel Levinson and Gail Sheehy.

Havighurst: Developmental Tasks

From your knowledge of Havighurst in Chapters 10 and 11, you know that to become mature and fully functioning, a person must complete certain tasks during particular stages of development. Havighurst bases his developments tasks on learned behaviors that arise from biologic, psychological, and social origins during various stages of life. Mastering these tasks sets the stage for the person to accomplish more complex tasks. Box 12-1 lists the developmental tasks of early and middle adulthood. Note that the tasks of early adulthood center on relationships, career choices, and family establishment. Young

➤➤ BOX 12-1

HAVIGHURST'S DEVELOPMENTAL TASKS OF EARLY AND MIDDLE ADULTHOOD

Early Adulthood (20–40 Years of Age)
• Select a mate
• Learn to live with mate
• Start a family
• Raise children
• Manage a home
• Begin occupation
• Involve self in civic and religious group activities
• Form social groups

Middle Adulthood (40–65 Years of Age)
• Assist children to become responsible adults
• Achieve social and civic responsibility
• Attain satisfying career
• Develop leisure activities and hobbies appropriate to age
• Strengthen relationship with partner
• Accept and adjust to physical status of middle age
• Deal with and assist aging parents

adults spend much of their time learning to live and work with others and helping children meet their basic needs. Although relationships and careers continue to be important in middle adulthood, developmental tasks focus more on self-awareness and personal fulfillment. According to this theory, failure to complete the task of each stage may lead to failure in tasks at subsequent stages.

Erikson: Psychosocial Development

As discussed in Chapters 10 and 11, Erikson's theory examines the psychosocial development of various age groups. Table 12-1 shows his theory for early and middle adults.

Remember that Erikson focuses on the psychosocial challenges that individuals face in the various life stages. People must meet and master these challenges before moving successfully to the next stage. Like children and adolescents, adults continue to face challenges as sets of positive versus negative outcomes. As people mature, however, these challenges become choices over which adults exert control. Individuals are no longer simply confronted with a challenge to conquer. Rather, they consider issues, make value judgments, and directly affect outcomes. Consequences of decisions are thought out before choices are made, in contrast to the approach of young adults, who follow the "Do now, worry about the consequences later" motto. Additionally, adults can revise their choices as they continue throughout life.

Early Adulthood: Intimacy Versus Isolation
In early adulthood, people confront choices about their occupation, education, relationships, living environment, and independence. Young adults often work hard to achieve financial and emotional independence from their families of origin. They begin to establish life goals and values, although their attitudes may change later in life. Intimacy versus isolation is the challenge of this stage. Individuals choose to establish relationships with others (**intimacy**) or to remain detached (**isolation**) from others. Related choices include the following:

• Entering a serious relationship or remaining single
• Working in a people-oriented occupation (such as nursing) or in a quieter occupation (such as freelance work in one's home)

Middle Adulthood: Generativity Versus Stagnation
By the time individuals reach middle adulthood, they have chosen a lifestyle. As they get older, many changes to this lifestyle start to happen. Children who were a focus of concern and attention grow up and leave home. Plans for retirement from a longtime occupation or career path must be considered. Body processes change, and physical abilities start to slow and decline. Generativity versus stagnation is the challenge. The tasks of **generativity** occur when middle adults decide to pass on learning and share skills with younger generations. Adults who focus on individual pursuits and interests are considered to be in the phase of stagnation. Examples of opposite choices in this phase include:

■■■ TABLE 12-1 ℰRIKSON'S THEORY OF PSYCHOSOCIAL DEVELOPMENT— EARLY AND MIDDLE ADULTHOOD

Concept	Early Adulthood (20–40 Years)	Middle Adulthood (40–65 Years)
Challenge	Intimacy versus isolation	Generativity versus self-absorption
Necessary accomplishments	Choose relationship style; select occupation; build independence	Develop self; plan retirement; raise family; enhance relationships
Virtues	Affiliation; love	Production; caring; cooperation

- Climbing the corporate ladder and making a great deal of money, or developing the intellectual self by working on advanced degrees and reading extensively
- Spending time with a significant other, or pursuing solitary interests
- Learning new activities, or participating in known recreation for satisfaction

Levinson: Individual Life Structure

Daniel Levinson, a theorist of adult development, has formulated age-linked periods of adulthood (Table 12-2). He connects development with the ability to make successful transitions. During each period of development, the adult makes decisions that are built upon previous experiences. Transition between each phase is determined by the choices made. He theorizes that the interaction of three components forms life's patterns:

Self (values and motives)
Social and cultural aspects
Set of roles in which the individual is involved

When something changes in one of these components, a reorganization of the whole life structure occurs.

Sheehy: Phases of Adulthood

With the work of Erikson, Levinson, and others as background, Gail Sheehy has written extensively on adult development in *Passages* and *Pathfinders*. Her work has helped to expand and clarify the "phases of adulthood" (Table 12-3). Whereas Levinson based his theory largely on the experiences of adult men, Sheehy's portrait is more balanced and focuses greatly on women's views of adulthood.

☛ KEY CONCEPT

Erikson and other theorists stress that meeting developmental challenges depends on individual characteristics, support from society, and cultural influences. For example, establishing intimacy is a key challenge for young adults. Cultural patterns and societal expectations greatly influence romantic relationships and their forms.

■■■ TABLE 12-2 ℒEVINSON'S CLASSIFICATIONS OF ADULTHOOD

Age	Period	Transitions
18–22	Early adult transition	• Adult choices • Establishment of adult identity • Career choice • Intimate relationships • Personal goals
22–28	Getting into the adult world	• Balance of choices
28–33	30s transition	• Possible change of lifestyle • Marriage/partnership • Divorce • Change of career
33–39	Settling down	• Balance of choices
40–45	Midlife transition	• Reappraisal of goals and values • Self-identity • Renegotiation of relationships • Change of perspectives
45–65	Payoff years	• Balance of choices

Levinson, D. J. (1986). *The seasons of a man's life.* New York: Ballantine.

▪▪▪ TABLE 12-3 *𝒮*HEEHY'S PHASES OF EARLY AND MIDDLE ADULTHOOD			
Ages	**Phase**	**Decisions and Issues**	**Virtues**
20–30	"Trying Twenties"	• Leaving home • Building adult relationships • Seeking roots	• Exploration • Experimentation
30–40	"Catch Thirties"	• Establishing a new home • Focusing on career goals • Dealing with family issues • Channeling restlessness	• Energy
40s–50s	"Time of Renewal"	• Changing self-image • Handling midlife crises • Dealing with aging parents • Facing own mortality	• Experience

Adapted from Sheehy, G. (1984). *Passages: Predictable crises of adult life.* New York: Bantam.

DEVELOPMENT IN EARLY ADULTHOOD

The following section integrates concepts based on the above theories for early adulthood. Most adults go through all the following stages at some point. Keep in mind, however, that individual choices and circumstances are more influential than chronological age in determining patterns of development. When a developmental stage is not completed or all tasks are not accomplished, an individual will have to address the immediate issues before making the transition in the next phase. For example, a 29-year-old who is diagnosed with a chronic illness may need to re-evaluate his or her options for starting a family or making career choices.

20 to 30 Years

Leaving Home

An important decision that young adults make relates to leaving their home of origin. No one correct way exists, simply different ways. Some young people face financial problems that force them to return to their family homes temporarily. Leaving home can follow any of several patterns:

- A person leaves home and does not move back.
- A person stays at home until he or she is forced to leave by family members.
- A person leaves, returns, leaves, returns, and continues a cycle of moving in and out.
- A person leaves, but remains within close proximity to the family of origin by moving next door.

Choosing a Career

Occupational choices are closely tied to education. Both are related to the economic situation, goals, abilities, and interests of the individual. People of all ages should enjoy their work, believe they are doing the best with their abilities, and feel they are contributing to society. Sometimes, circumstances prevent individuals from following their dreams, and they are forced to make adjustments. Adaptability to such circumstances depends largely on how well adults made adjustments throughout childhood and adolescence. Many people have more than one interest and consider alternate choices with relative ease. Although independent decision-making is necessary, support from family and friends is also important.

Establishing an Adult Identification: Seeking Oneself

Sheehy describes the young person from ages 20 to 30 as seeking to establish roots. These adults often feel that they should do a particular thing with their lives. Families, peers, and surrounding cultural attitudes influence this for all people. Individuals face a dilemma when they feel that their choices can no longer be changed or that a decision settles an issue forever. For example, young people may fear a commitment to marriage with a longtime partner because it will limit their freedom. They may hesitate to embark on a specific career path, fearing that they will be forced to do that job forever.

Clearly, two opposing impulses are at work during this time. Young adults want to build a safe structure for the future, and have commitments and security. Yet, they also want to explore, experiment, and keep the structure flexible. An individual's ability to balance these opposing forces determines how easily and quickly he or she passes through this phase of provisional adulthood.

Establishing Adult Relationships

Those who live on a college campus in the late teen and early adult years are surrounded by similar-aged and like-minded individuals. As they move away from college and leave their families of origin, young adults may find themselves lonely. With time, they form new friendships and intimate relationships that provide support and understanding. Such relationships include coworkers, male and female housemates, intimate homosexual or heterosexual relationships, cohabitation, marriage, and religious orders. Some adults live with parents or other relatives for social support as well.

About 2,250,000 marriages occur annually in the United States, according to the Centers for Disease Control and Prevention (CDC). People decide to marry for various reasons. Some marry to escape life with their parents. Others marry because they feel it is expected of them. Men tend to marry in their late 20s, while women tend to marry in their mid 20s. Some people marry for protection, to be taken care of, or for prestige. Ideally, people marry because they find someone they love and with whom they want to spend their lives.

Couples in their twenties who live together often prefer to postpone marriage until after completing college, establishing a career, and building up adequate financial resources. Others do not want to commit to a long-term relationship until later in life, if at all. Some adults live together for the same reasons others marry—for protection, to share expenses, or to escape the parental home.

People in homosexual relationships face many of the same challenges. An additional challenge may include deciding on whether or not to make the nature of the relationship public knowledge. Couples may also face prejudices and discrimination that heterosexual couples will not have to encounter.

Starting a Family

In general, society still expects most adults to marry and to establish a family and home (Fig. 12-1). Many adults postpone marriage or childbirth until their thirties, preferring to establish careers and to become financially secure first. The rate of teenage pregnancies and unplanned pregnancies has decreased in the past 10 years.

Still, teenagers are often thrust into the responsibilities of parenthood before they are ready. Chapter 9 discusses various family structures and the growing number of single-parent families arising from divorce and out-of-wedlock births. Grandparents and other relatives sometimes play pivotal roles in such families.

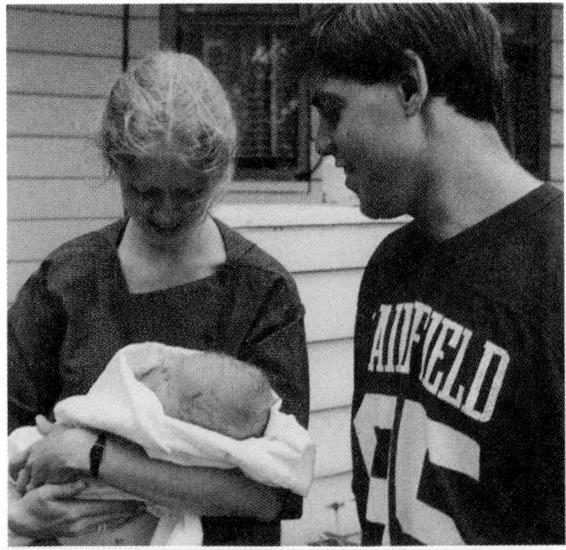

FIGURE 12-1. Starting and shaping a family are significant aspects of the young adult period. (Craven, R. F., & Hirnle, C. J. (2000). *Fundamentals of nursing: Human health and function* (3rd ed.). Philadelphia: Lippincott Williams & Wilkins.)

Historically, the roles of authority, provider, and protector of the family have been associated with the male. Yet many men in today's society are challenged to maintain these perceptions. More women are successfully entering the workforce and becoming provider, caregiver, and protector. As a result, the two-income family has had to adjust and redistribute family roles.

For many couples, division of labor includes sharing childcare responsibilities, enabling both mothers and fathers to develop close relationships with their children. Participation from both parents in household tasks and childrearing often contributes to a strong family unit.

Reappraising Commitments

As adults head into their thirties, restlessness, confusion, and doubt become common. Adults may find themselves asking, "Now that I am where I wanted to be, what do I want out of this life?" From about ages 28 to 32, individuals often make new choices and reappraise previous commitments. Adults who married young may question staying with their partners. They may consider a career change. These adults now realize that they can make their own decisions based on their own feelings and not the beliefs of others.

30 to 40 Years

Settling In

In their early thirties, adults begin to settle. Many adults now purchase a home. They are usually established in a career. They become more comfortable with their intimate and other adult relationships. Life becomes more rational and orderly.

Making Career Decisions

Career issues are important. A couple working different hours or shifts can develop difficulty with marital interaction time, family time, and child-rearing responsibilities in their relationship.

Those who desire upward mobility must follow the rules of the corporate culture. Companies may require individuals to transfer from one city to another. For dual-career families, conflicts may arise. For example, if one partner receives a desirable job offer in another state, the couple must choose to stay together with the present employment, to move and have the other partner seek a suitable job in the new state, or to live apart and have a commuting relationship.

Adults in their thirties may find themselves without a job as companies are taken over by bigger conglomerates, headquarters move to another city, and plants close. Some adults decide to embark on a new career path or to return to school. Changes in career status, either voluntary or because of economic needs, can place stress on couples and families. Individuals must engage the support and assistance of the entire family.

Addressing Women's Issues

Women in their thirties must make specific decisions related to childbearing. As their thirties advance, women realize that they must choose to have children now or it may soon be too late.

Career goals and motherhood can conflict. A woman in her thirties who has never married may feel pressured to find the right person with whom to have a baby because life is passing her by. Adoption and artificial insemination are options for single women. Women who choose to have babies outside a committed relationship face the responsibilities and challenges of single parenthood. Women in relationships who have delayed pregnancy may face difficult decisions about employment, child-care arrangements, and responsibilities.

Facing Transitions

Many changes occur as the adult approaches middle adulthood. Growing children spend more time away from home, and are more interested in being with their peers. Adults responsible for childrearing may experience feelings of loss and loneliness. They must find new interests. As the children leave home, the parents begin to examine their relationship. They may develop a new depth of intimacy or decide that they have lost their intimacy and decide to divorce. Career changes and transfers to other cities may make home life and intimacy less stable. Divorces may occur and related adjustments must be made. A divorced adult may face the challenges of dating and financial instability, as well as redefining the relationship with the ex-spouse.

DEVELOPMENT IN MIDDLE ADULTHOOD

The following section summarizes the main points of theories related to middle adulthood. Changing demographics are extending this period, as more people live into their eighties and nineties. This discussion considers middle adulthood to range from approximately ages 40 to 65. Depending on each individual's circumstances, the following activities may fall anywhere within that age span.

Addressing Midlife Transitions

The developmental task of middle adulthood is generativity versus self-absorption, as adults face **midlife transitions.** Images of significant others also change in middle adulthood. As they look at partners, siblings, and friends of similar ages, adults recognize that they too are getting older. Visualizing their own aging, however, may be difficult.

Individuals become concerned with guiding future generations. Middle adults have a great deal to offer in the way of experience and advice. They can view younger generations with a softer, less critical eye. Competition is less important than before. Middle adults cooperate with others in the workplace, particularly after age 50. They are productive and know how to complete tasks quickly, accurately, and efficiently. They base a great deal of creativity on experience.

Sometimes, adults entering midlife feel panicky. They may believe other people their age have achieved more and that they must do something creative or impressive before it is too late. Individuals with childrearing responsibilities wonder what they will do when children leave home. Some people at this stage are unable to accept aging and may feel frustrated and unful-

filled. They may feel that they have failed to achieve the goals of their youth. Theorists call these circumstances *midlife crisis* or *midlife transition.* A midlife transition can involve a sense of failure in the chosen profession, feelings of sexual inadequacy, fear of inevitable death, or frustration with aging parents or grown children. Sometimes, individuals feel an incredible desire to escape. They may act out temporarily in inappropriate or unexpected ways. Problems that may ensue if individuals fail to resolve this stage include brooding, physical illness, suicide, chemical dependency, and depression.

Adjusting to Role Changes

Self and family perceptions and roles begin to change during this stage. As children grow older, receive more education, and become better at sports than their parents, the realization begins to dawn on the entire family—children are turning into adults themselves.

Middle-aged adults often face the aging of their own parents. Arrangements may be necessary for placement in a nursing home or for home care. Even middle adults whose older parents maintain a high level of independence and functioning may need to provide some type of financial and emotional support. Roles are reversed, and former children become the responsible caretaker.

Sometimes people in their middle years are caught between caring for both aging parents and their own growing children. Personal needs and goals are often shoved aside. Such adults have been referred to as the *sandwich generation.* As the older adult population expands, and grown children remain or move back in with their families of origin, the sandwich generation will face difficult issues for longer periods.

Marital status sometimes changes in the middle years. Some individuals divorce, or spouses or significant others die. In either case, adults must adapt to new roles and expectations. Personal activities need to be incorporated into changing lifestyles. In even the most stable and long-lasting marriages, fluctuations are common. For example, a marriage that had previously been harmonious may have periods of communication difficulties, resulting in an increased number of arguments. As partners develop and confront their own issues, the relationship must accommodate their findings and decisions if it is to remain healthy.

Perceiving One's Own Mortality

As individuals approach age 50, death becomes more of a reality. Sometimes a relative or friend of the same age dies unexpectedly. Adults start to come to grips with their own mortality. They may become frightened by the prospect of death. Or they may experience a spiritual revival and become more comfortable with death's inevitability.

Re-establishing Equilibrium

As they head into their sixties, adults look forward to new challenges. They often accept life as it is. Equilibrium is re-established.

When adults are in their forties or fifties, their children often marry. As children move into their own homes and raise their own families, middle adults realize that life is becoming more peaceful. Grandchildren provide excitement and renewal (Fig. 12-2). As grandparents, many middle adults can spend more time with their grandchildren than they did with their own children. The passage of time and a different perspective help many adults to view grandchildren with more patience and a less critical eye than they had as young parents.

Planning for Retirement

Some companies now offer early retirement packages to employees; thus, some people leave the work force as early as age 50 or 55. In preparation for a productive and interesting retirement that may last for 25 years or more, adults should develop interests and hobbies in midlife.

Financial planning is an important component of retirement. The money available for pensions has declined in many companies, and many corporations offer no pension at all. Middle-aged adults need to plan their own retirement funds and investments. Large houses may be sold for simpler living arrangements. Individuals may look for part-time work and may consider relocating to warmer or more scenic environments. Many adults consider a return to school at this age, enrolling in colleges and universities.

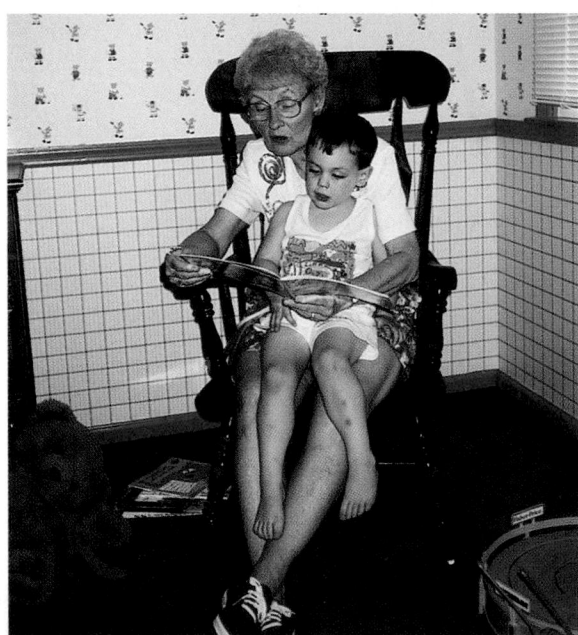

FIGURE 12-2. Grandchildren provide an interest and renewal for many middle aged adults. (Taylor, C., Lillis, C., & LeMone, P. [2001]. *Fundamentals of nursing: The art and science of nursing care* [4th ed., p. 122]. Philadelphia: Lippincott Williams & Wilkins.)

➜ STUDENT SYNTHESIS

Key Points

- Adults must meet certain developmental tasks to mature comfortably.
- Development continues throughout life and during adulthood; periods of stability alternate with periods of transition.
- Because many adults choose to live with other people, integrating individual goals into joint goals is often helpful.

Critical Thinking Exercises

1. Based on the developmental stages as outlined in this chapter, explain how a serious illness such as a heart attack can affect the achievement of developmental tasks for the following clients: a 35-year-old; a 45-year-old; a 55-year-old.
2. Describe how developmental stages for men and women may differ, based on gender roles in society.
3. Consider your own developmental stage. Which theorist best matches your ideas of development? What developmental task is the highest priority for you right now?

NCLEX-Style Review Questions

1. According to Erikson, a 30-year-old adult faces which psychosocial developmental challenge?
   a. Dealing with aging parents
   b. Generativity versus self-absorption
   c. Identifying a career
   d. Intimacy versus isolation
2. A 47-year-old adult expresses concerns of not achieving lifelong goals. The client displays increased alcohol intake and depression. The client is experiencing:
   a. A midlife crisis
   b. Failure to establish a career
   c. Isolation instead of intimacy
   d. Provisional adulthood
3. Women in their thirties face specific decisions related to:
   a. Career choices
   b. Childbearing
   c. Facing mortality
   d. Leaving home

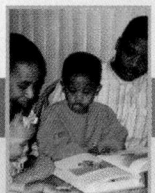

CHAPTER

13

Older Adulthood and Aging

LEARNING OBJECTIVES

1. Describe Havighurst's developmental tasks related to older adulthood.
2. Explain the psychosocial development of older adults as defined by Erikson.
3. Discuss Levinson's and Sheehy's perspectives on older adulthood.
4. Identify positive factors in the development of the aging person.
5. List stressors for older adults.
6. Identify implications for society related to the increasing numbers of older adults.
7. Explain at least five challenges for future health care related to changing demographics.

NEW TERMINOLOGY

ageism
gerontology

mortality
reminiscence

ACRONYM

AARP

Theorists have recently devoted more attention to the growth and development processes of older adults. The achievements, problems, and characteristics of older adulthood are as important as the milestones of earlier years.

Clients 65 years of age and older predominate in many of today's health care settings. The elderly account for 36% of acute care hospital admissions. Whether you practice nursing in a hospital, extended care facility, ambulatory clinic, or home, you are bound to interact with older people. Knowledge of normal aging processes enables you to help clients understand and adapt to normal changes in function. By knowing and recognizing normal changes that accompany aging, you are prepared to recognize abnormal, pathologic developments. Most older Americans have at least one chronic condition and many elderly people have multiple chronic conditions.[1]

DEVELOPMENTAL THEORIES OF OLDER ADULTHOOD

Development and maturation occur throughout older adulthood. The physical changes that begin in middle adulthood continue. These physical changes are interrelated with life circumstances and psychosocial development. Common physical changes include changes in vision, muscle strength, and reproductive functioning. Psychosocial development adapts as the individual learns to function within new limitations, eg, using glasses for reading and getting assistance with lifting objects.

Havighurst: Developmental Tasks

Similar to the previous life stages, Havighurst suggests that older adulthood has its own set of developmental tasks for individuals to accomplish. These tasks focus on necessary adjustments that arise from inevitable physical and social change associated with age. Box 13-1 summarizes Havighurst's developmental tasks of older adulthood.

➤ ➤ BOX 13-1

HAVIGHURST'S DEVELOPMENTAL TASKS OF OLDER ADULTHOOD

- Adjust to decreasing physical strength and declining health
- Adjust to retirement and fixed income
- Adjust to death of spouse or companion
- Establish social relationships with persons of same age and with younger persons
- Establish appropriate living arrangements
- Make arrangements for care, if needed
- Accept one's own mortality
- Find satisfaction in one's family
- Accept oneself as an aging person

Erikson: Psychosocial Development

Erikson has included older adulthood in his psychosocial theory of human development (Table 13-1). The psychosocial challenge for this developmental stage is ego integrity versus despair. Older adults can reflect on the events and decisions of their lives. Individuals achieve ego integrity when they sense that their lives have meaning and have been worthwhile. They are comfortable with past resolutions and do not regret past decisions. If older adults do not meet the challenges of aging, they are likely to feel that life is too short. Regrets and feelings of failure may envelop them. Individuals may have feelings of despair if they cannot accept that death is part of the normal life cycle.

Therapists use the concept of *life review* to help older clients avoid despair. By reviewing life's events, older adults can gain a new, more positive perspective on the conflicts of earlier stages. When working with older clients in health care practice, you can encourage **reminiscence.** Listening to older adults describe past joys and successes increases a person's satisfaction and self-esteem.

Levinson: Individual Life Structure

In Levinson's individual life structure theory, life after age 65 is a time for adults to find a new balance of involvement with society and the self. Older adulthood becomes an opportunity for choosing modes of living more freely than before. Adults are less interested in societal approval and are more concerned with using their own inner resources to the highest potential. This period is marked by life review. Successful transitions in this stage result in wisdom and stability.

Sheehy: Phases of Adulthood

Sheehy believes that older adults need to feel comfortable with life changes to attain the dignity that is part of aging. Like Levinson, Sheehy stresses that older adults have the opportunity to value themselves apart from the standards and agendas of others. Breaking out of unsatisfactory life patterns is impor-

■ ■ ■ **TABLE 13-1** *E*RIKSON'S THEORY OF PSYCHOSOCIAL DEVELOPMENT— OLDER ADULTHOOD

Concept	65 Years +
Challenge	Ego integrity versus despair
Necessary accomplishments	Balance choices; achieve stability; retire; evaluate life; accept life choices
Virtues	Renunciation; wisdom; dignity

tant at this time. Older people should not be afraid to change and grow. Wisdom is the special virtue of this stage of life.

☛ Key Concept

Tasks of older adulthood are important challenges for development. Remember that each older person, because of his or her life history, will experience aging uniquely.

DEVELOPMENT IN OLDER ADULTHOOD

Age is more than an accumulation of years. The aging process affects people in different ways. Some people age faster than others. Some people seem never to age. The various aspects of aging—physical, psychosocial, and spiritual—do not occur at the same rate for all individuals. Heredity, congenital conditions, altered use of nutrients by the body, changes in hormone production, electrolyte imbalance, physical demands, environment, lifestyle (eg, smoking and exercise), and lifetime nutritional habits contribute to the way individuals age. To fully adapt to aging and thrive in this new stage, older adults must confront many lifestyle changes. Special Considerations: The Life Span 13-1 summarizes such changes.

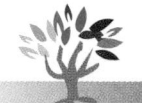 **Special Considerations: The Life Span**

Lifestyle Changes in the Older and Aging Population

• General change in physiologic, psychological, and sociologic functions and roles
• Change in some body functions and abilities
• Adaptation to chronic physical or emotional disorders
• Change in employee or employer role
• Greater amount of leisure time
• Reduction of income
• Change of residence
• Change in parenting roles (sometimes a reversal)
• Adaptation to loss of spouse or partner
• Development of coping mechanisms to deal with accumulated changes
• Adaptation to possible changes in sexuality
• Reevaluation of self-worth
• Maintenance of self-esteem and independence
• More time for meditation and contemplation of life
• Adaptation to prospect of death

The study of the aging process in all its dimensions (physical, psychological, economic, sociologic, and spiritual) is called **gerontology.** Gerontology—or geriatrics—is the study of the medical problems and care associated with older adults. Because gerontology is a more inclusive, holistic term, nurses who specialize in this type of care often prefer the term gerontologic nursing for their specialty.

Ageism refers to labeling and discriminating against older adults. It is prejudice based on chronological age. Ageism is seen in attitudes that depict older people as grumpy, rigid, or stingy. Ageism can occur in the provision of health care. Older persons may not receive standard diagnostic and therapeutic treatments that are given regularly to young or middle-aged clients. Attitudes of healthcare personnel may reflect ageism if they call older people names that suggest their age, such as "gramps." When providing nursing care, you should avoid the attitudes and behaviors of ageism to promote a better relationship with older adults.

Medical diagnosis is not the only factor that influences a person's level of independent functioning. For example, an older woman recovering from hip surgery may recover faster if she has interesting and worthwhile activities waiting for her. Because the physical, psychosocial, and spiritual dimensions of older adults are so interrelated, holistic nursing care is necessary.

Physical Changes

Many age-related changes are based on general physical alterations. The human body is changing from the time of conception until death. Changes in the body's ability to function at previous levels are normal. Optimal function for age is the goal. Remember that physical aging progresses at different rates throughout a person's cells, organs, and body systems. Additionally, the overall aging process varies from person to person. Normal changes related to aging often mean a greater vulnerability to disease and disability but are not in themselves pathologic. Older people can adapt to normal physical changes because they occur gradually. Scientists and healthcare providers are continually learning more about ways to limit disabilities and to promote optimum functioning in advancing years.

In Unit 4, each chapter covers a particular body system. These chapters conclude with the effects of aging on each particular system and a table that reviews such changes. For that reason, normal physical changes are not discussed here in detail, but are summarized in Box 13-2.

➤➤ BOX 13-2

MAJOR PHYSICAL CHANGES RELATED TO NORMAL AGING PROCESSES

• Decrease in functioning of organs
• Change in visual and auditory acuity
• Decreased reaction time
• Unsteady gait, decreased sense of balance
• Decrease in tactile sensations
• Stiff joints
• Increased emotional and physical losses
• Decreased capacity for recovery from injury or illness

Psychosocial Considerations

Older people usually want to remain independent for as long as possible. Independence does not necessarily mean living alone. However, it does mean retaining control over the major aspects of life. The three key elements of maintaining independence are health, financial stability, and social resources. Transportation opportunities are part of these concerns. A loss of functional ability may make self-care difficult. Financial losses may prevent the maintenance of living quarters. Other people may be unavailable for social support. Such factors place older adults in danger of losing their independence. Older individuals and their families can strive to promote independence in every area possible. See Special Considerations: Culture 13-1.

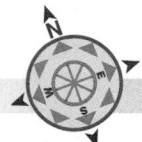

SPECIAL CONSIDERATIONS: CULTURE

Independence

Remember that in many cultural groups, it is considered unthinkable for older relatives to live alone or in nursing homes. In these situations, independence is linked with maintaining a pivotal role as part of an extended family.

Self-esteem accompanies independence. It involves accepting the aging process and one's life history and decisions. Often, older adulthood is a time for individuals to reflect on the events of their lives and to reinterpret them with the wisdom that comes with experience and understanding. Skilled and sympathetic listeners can foster this process and point out successes. Interest from other people, especially those from younger generations, can boost older people's self-esteem.

Participation in social activities is important for older adults. As they age, people usually must adjust their social activities. Individuals may enjoy spending time at one of the many social organizations that have arisen for senior citizens. The health and attitudes of a partner can strongly influence social decisions. A couple may want to spend more time together after retirement. If a partner becomes ill, the other person may have to assume full responsibility for cooking, cleaning, and other household activities.

At some point, individuals may have to give up driving, which is a major component of independence. The older person may live in an area that may be unsafe for walking alone, eliminating walking as a mode of transportation. Getting on and off a bus may be difficult. Taxicabs are expensive. This type of situation creates a need for assistance from others. As individuals need increasing help getting to grocery stores, banks, healthcare facilities, and places of worship, they become more dependent on support persons among their relatives and friends. Taking advantage of community resources will help lessen this dependence on family and friends.

Areas of Concern

The vast majority of older people are active, healthy adults. Sometimes, people mistakenly consider normal aging processes to be signs of illness. Physical and cognitive changes that occur with aging are normal and require adaptation. Coping skills and attitudes toward life will, in part, determine if individuals can accept the changes.

Some important areas of concern follow. Chapter 91 continues the discussion about serious areas of concern and nursing care for the aging person who needs assistance to meet daily needs.

Work, Retirement, and Activities

Older adults should realize that activity is necessary for life. They should choose and plan activities that will bring them joy and happiness. Some older people continue to work outside the home or do consulting from a home office. Others retire, travel, and spend time with spouses, grandchildren, and other loved ones. Participation in volunteer work is rewarding for many older individuals. Healthcare and social agencies depend on volunteers to supplement busy staff. Volunteerism can take many forms. Some older volunteers share their knowledge in museums and zoos as guides and teachers; some help babies and children feel the love of a caring person; others deliver meals to the homebound. These activities often fulfill the desire of older adults to feel needed and included, along with providing valued services for others.

Some individuals begin hobbies and activities before retirement that they can continue for many years (Fig. 13-1). All kinds of educational opportunities are open for older people. They may go back to school to complete a college or

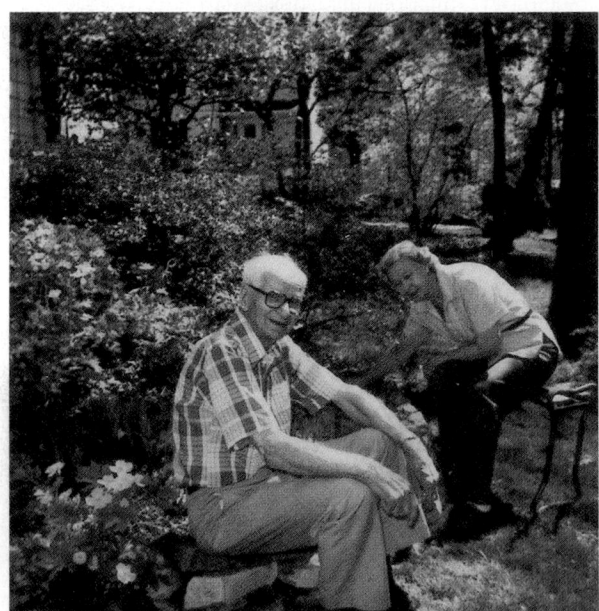

FIGURE 13-1. This couple, married 61 years, enjoys gardening together. They've found that they can continue most activities with only minor adjustments. (Taylor, C., Lillis, C., & LeMone, P. [2001]. *Fundamentals of nursing: The art and science of nursing care* [4th ed., p. 161]. Philadelphia: Lippincott Williams & Wilkins.)

graduate degree. They can pursue interests as diverse as art and music appreciation, acting, and computers. Banks offer courses on how to manage finances. The International Elderhostel program offers opportunities for travel and study with other older persons who share similar interests.

Finances and Poverty

Most people have to adjust to a fixed income after retirement. Usually, they have less money to spend than before. Simultaneously, clothing and commuting expenses may decrease. Older adults benefit from planning a budget before retirement so adjustments are easier. Living on a fixed income has made moving from homes in high-crime areas difficult for some older adults. Although they own their own homes, the value has decreased. Unfortunately, many lack the financial resources to move to safer, more secure neighborhoods.

Some older people have little or no income when a financially supportive spouse or family member dies. They may be separated from family and other persons who can help them. Many homeless people are older adults. Some older adults in the United States and Canada live in rural areas with limited social and health care facilities. In general, older minority groups are poorer than the overall population. The lack of financial resources with which to meet basic needs creates major stress for older adults.

Stress and Loss

Mental health problems may increase with age because physical and psychological stressors accumulate. Many stressors affect the aging population. Changes in physical, financial, and family dynamics are high stressors, eg, loss of spouse, retirement, or changes in vision. The ability to adapt to change is important. Individuals who try to adapt to stress as they did in the past may find that many of the options of youth are no longer available. People with fixed habits and attitudes may face difficulty adjusting to change. The accumulation of stressors can be stressful in itself. Dealing with one stress at a time is easier than having them occur rapidly or together. In some cases, escaping accumulated stress is impossible. For example, the loss of a spouse is traumatic in itself, but to lose a spouse who had been the major source of income and the supplier of transportation can become overwhelming. Adapting to stress and loss is a normal life cycle requirement of getting older.

Generally, older adults are less concerned with the opinions of others. Experience with past crises—not necessarily age—influences their response to stress. An active lifestyle helps older people to cope. Choosing and maintaining social and civic activities and functions appropriate to health, energy level, income, and personal interests can help individuals to thrive.

One word summarizes many stressors that older adults encounter: Loss. Losses can be subtle or catastrophic. They are often cumulative. The degree to which a loss becomes a stressor depends on a person's attitude toward it. For instance, one woman may easily accept the fact that her hair is graying and her skin is becoming wrinkled. Another woman may be very disturbed by these changes. Other areas with potential for loss include general appearance, physical ability, health condition, retirement, divorce, death of a spouse or other peers, and isolation from family.

Spirituality

As individuals age and pass through developmental stages, they often have an opportunity to explore the spiritual side of their nature and to re-examine spiritual needs. Although spirituality and religion are often thought of as connected, they are not necessarily the same thing. Taylor, Lillis, and LeMone define spirituality as "anything that pertains to a person's relationship with a nonmaterial life force or higher power"; religion, on the other hand, refers to an "organized system of beliefs about a higher power" often expressed in "forms of worship, spiritual practices, and codes of conduct."[2]

The principles and beliefs of religion and spirituality become important sources of personal solace. This finding may be due to the need for older people to understand death as it approaches. It may also be a part of achieving integrity. Those who have experienced a full life may be able to examine questions of a spiritual nature with more depth and objectivity than younger individuals.

☛ KEY CONCEPT

Some people do not adhere to a specific religion but fulfill their spiritual needs by having some quiet, private time to pray or to reflect. Ask clients if you can assist them in some way to meet such needs, and then respect their wishes.

Mortality

Death of spouses and peers causes older adults to reflect on their own death or **mortality.** Religious or spiritual beliefs may strongly influence their attitudes. People prepare for death in different ways. They may systematically talk about the past and be especially interested in sharing family history and experiences with their offspring. Some wish to take a life inventory. They may draw up a family tree, create a scrapbook, organize photograph albums, or create an audio- or videotape to share memories with grandchildren (Fig. 13-2). They may plan for

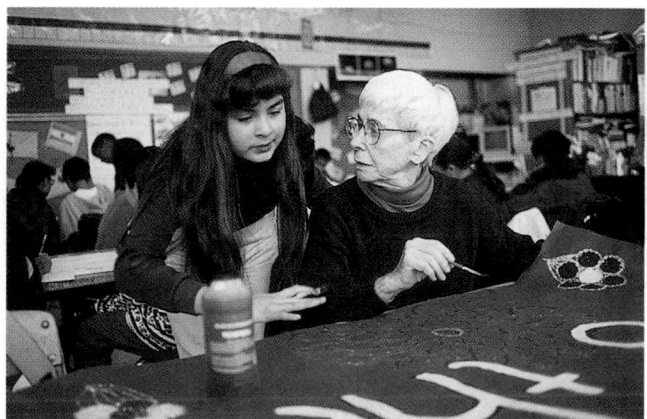

FIGURE 13-2. Social relationships provide an opportunity to share past experiences. (Taylor, C., Lillis, C., & LeMone, P. [2001]. *Fundamentals of nursing: The art and science of nursing care* [4th ed., p. 167]. Philadelphia: Lippincott Williams & Wilkins.)

their funeral, choosing music and scripture to be used. Funeral planning should not be considered morbid, but a part of a person's ability to maintain control over the organization of life.

DEMOGRAPHICS AND POPULATION TRENDS

Demographics is the study of characteristics and changes that cause balance in a population. Demographics related to the aging population is an important consideration for the industrial sector, housing, social agencies, and the health care system. Life expectancy continues to increase in the United States and Canada. The fastest growing segment of the population is that of persons 85 years and older. The number of people who are more than 100 years old is increasing and should continue to grow well into the 21st century. Estimates are that more than 100,000 Americans are over the age of 100.[3] A few key facts about the older population are listed in Special Considerations: The Life Span 13-2.

Because the number of "old-old" people (85 and over) is increasing so rapidly, research has not yet been able to keep up with their needs. An exciting research prospect is to define this period as a unique stage in life, with its own developmental tasks that build on—but are separate from—those of the age group 65 to 85 years.

The following issues related to the expanding older population are among the challenges for society to examine in the 21st century[3]:

- Consumers expect quality, convenient, and cost-effective services for older adults. Groups like the American Association of Retired Persons (**AARP**) and the Gray Panthers are likely to have significant political influence.
- Financial planning needs to begin in early adulthood to promote self-sufficiency and independence in old age.
- Urban transportation systems must assist older adults in maintaining social contacts and provide easier access to preventive health care facilities.
- More flexible working and retirement schedules, opportunities for volunteer work, and recognition of past contributions are necessary to maximize the resources within the older adult population.
- Fitness programs designed for older adults should promote better health in an effort to lower healthcare costs.
- Better nutrition in younger years benefits people as they age. Nutrition should play a greater role in preventive healthcare, restoration of health, and maintenance of optimal health throughout the life span.
- Counseling in the areas of health, psychosocial situations, and economic well-being must become standard practice.
- The legal and ethical issues of death and dying will continue to be part of the individual's and society's concerns.
- Better training of healthcare professionals in the areas of aging is necessary. Special focus is needed to address the physical changes in older men and women.

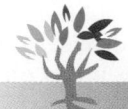

SPECIAL CONSIDERATIONS: THE LIFE SPAN

The Older Population and Society

- Many older people live on a fixed income, which represents a reduction in resources for them. Income is from savings, investments, and retirement.
- A majority rely on Social Security income, which was originally designed as a *supplement* to other income.
- Many older people continue to work full-time or part-time.
- Most older adults own their own homes; many do not move after retirement.
- Most older people live in urban areas. Trends in housing are toward group housing, shared housing, or retirement communities.
- Older minority populations are more likely to face health problems because they are more likely to live below the poverty level.
- Many healthcare professionals have only begun to recognize that women's healthcare needs differ from those of men of the same age.
- About one third of prescription medications are taken by seniors; often multiple drugs are taken by one person. Adverse drug reactions are more likely to occur in older adults.
- Health problems and disabilities increase with advancing age.
- Seven states contain 45% of the U.S. elderly population (California, New York, Florida, Illinois, Ohio, Pennsylvania, and Texas).
- Children of aging parents are frequently faced with responsibility for their parents. Some of these "children" are over 65 themselves.
- Men earn an average of twice the per capita annual income of women. Many widowed women are living at a much lower income level than they did when their spouse was alive.
- Among the aging population, women outnumber men. At age 65, the ratio is 3:1. At age 85, the ratio is 5:1.
- Nearly 80% of men at age 65 are married. Only 45% of women at age 65 are married; the majority are widows.

✂ STUDENT SYNTHESIS

Key Points

- The process of aging is a continuation of earlier development. Each person differs in the speed with which he or she ages, in adaptations made to aging, and in coping mechanisms.
- *Ageism* refers to discrimination against individuals as they grow older.

- Challenges for older people include remaining independent, maintaining self-esteem, finding outlets for energies and interests, developing a happy lifestyle within financial means, continuing positive relationships with others, meeting all basic human needs, and confronting mortality.
- Stress, loss, and poverty are significant concerns for older adults.
- Population trends are necessitating more research for adult development past age 85.
- Society must examine healthcare concerns related to the expanding older population.

Critical Thinking Exercises

1. John, a 70-year-old man, comes in for a regular checkup to the healthcare facility where you work. He is in good health. During the past few visits, he has made remarks indicating that he feels useless and his life is over. "My whole life has been a disappointment," he said sadly on his last visit. John's wife died about a year ago. His children live close by. Though he is lonely, he wants to maintain independence and "not be a burden" on them. Based on your learning from this chapter, how would you respond to John? How can you help him to achieve ego integrity? What suggestions would you give him to help him conquer loneliness?
2. Consider the lifestyle you hope to enjoy as an older adult. What measures can you take now to help ensure the possibility of such a lifestyle? Explain the importance of good nutritional practices and preventive healthcare measures in your plan.
3. Think about your reactions when you see older people in the grocery store, in the bank line, or driving in traffic ahead of you. Are any of your reactions examples of ageism? Are your ideas about the behavior of older people proven correct or incorrect most of the time? As a nurse, what measures can you take to avoid treating clients with prejudices based on age and other factors?

NCLEX-Style Review Questions

1. Prejudice based on chronological age by labeling and discriminating against older adults is known as:
   a. Acceptance
   b. Ageism
   c. Gerontology
   d. Mortality
2. According to Havighurst, developmental tasks for the older adult include:
   a. Adjusting to decreasing physical strength
   b. Reflecting on the events and decisions of their lives
   c. Reminiscence about past joys and successes
   d. Valuing the self apart from the standards of others
3. Changing demographics pose which of the following challenges for future healthcare practice?
   a. Ensuring all older adults are self-actualized
   b. Providing cosmetic surgery to a large number of people
   c. Providing quality, cost-effective services
   d. Valuing religion and spirituality

References

1. Administration on Aging. *Profile of older Americans 2000.* http://www.aoa.gov/aoa/stats/profile.
2. Taylor, C., Lillis, C., & LeMone, P. (2001). *Fundamentals of nursing: The art and science of nursing care* (4th ed., p. 818). Philadelphia: Lippincott Williams & Wilkins.
3. Eliopoulos, C. (2001). *Gerontological nursing* (5th ed.). Philadelphia: Lippincott Williams & Wilkins.

CHAPTER

14

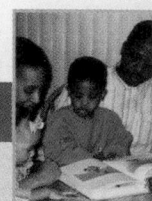

Death and Dying

LEARNING OBJECTIVES

1. Explain death's relationship to the process of growth and development.
2. Discuss how culture, ethnicity, and religion influence attitudes toward death.
3. Describe the ways in which spirituality can help individuals cope with death.
4. Define what is meant by terminal illness.
5. Identify the six stages of coping with impending death.
6. Differentiate between preparatory and reactive depression.
7. Explain ways in which the death of an individual affects the family unit and how families grieve.

NEW TERMINOLOGY

detachment
preparatory depression

reactive depression
terminal illness

Understanding death as a normal part of life is a fundamental concept. Despite great advances in technology, medicine cannot cure every illness, and science has yet to be able to stop the aging process. All people eventually deal with the death of a loved one. As humans age, they also must face their own impending mortality. As nurses work in the healthcare field, they are likely to find themselves caring for dying individuals in many situations, including acute care, in a hospice program, in a nursing home, or in a client's home. Chapter 59 discusses specific nursing care for dying individuals and their families.

Basic human needs are a priority for the dying person. Families have special needs as they deal with loss and grief. This chapter examines death as the final stage of growth and development.

DEATH

Death is part of life, an extension of birth. Everything that lives in this world will someday perish. Naturally, some people develop a fear of dying because what comes after death is unknown. When healthy and active, most people think of themselves as immortal. Although people can imagine others dying, they often have trouble imagining their own death.

Death is one of the most profound emotional experiences humans encounter. Because Western medicine and beliefs are based on preserving life, admitting that a person cannot be cured or revived is often difficult. Resolving feelings about the reality of death is a continuing challenge for many individuals.

☛ KEY CONCEPT

Death is a natural part of life. How you feel about it will influence how helpful you are to dying individuals and their families. Fear and anxiety are natural. By confronting your feelings and reaching out to support others in meeting death with dignity, you will become more comfortable with the concept of death.

Influences of Culture, Ethnicity, and Religion

Cultural, ethnic, and religious beliefs help to shape peoples' attitudes toward death. How one dies and how one responds to death vary greatly, depending on the cultural context. In many cultures, death is a social event with great meaning for the whole of society, whereas in others, death is considered a private, hidden occurrence. Some cultures celebrate when a person dies, believing that he or she is in a better place. Others mourn for extended periods. Some cultures view death as an intensely personal experience, with families keeping most of their emotions and feelings within a private circle. Other cultures grieve openly.

Religion also plays a large role in the client's and family's responses to death and dying. Many religions have specific laws regarding death, and ceremonies for commemorating the dead person's passage from life. Table 14-1 lists the approaches of various religions to death and dying.

■■■ TABLE 14-1 𝓡ELIGIOUS BELIEFS AND PRACTICES RELATED TO DEATH

Religion	Practices
Amish & Mennonite	Family cares for the body; funeral is often at home
Baptist	Prayer; communion; call pastor
Buddhist	Priest performs last rites and chanting rituals; cremation is common
Christian Science	Reader is called; no last rites; autopsy is forbidden
Episcopal	Prayer; communion; confession; sacrament of the sick
Friends (Quakers)	Individual communicates with God; no belief in afterlife
Greek Orthodox	Prayer; communion; sacrament of the sick; mandatory baptism
Hindu	Priest performs ritual of thread around neck or wrist, water is put in mouth; family cares for the body; cremation is common
Judaism	After death, a rabbi or designate cleanses the body
LDS/Mormon	Baptism required (adults); body is dressed in temple garments; call bishop/elder
Lutheran	Prayer; communion; call pastor
Muslim	Imam performs specific procedures for washing and shrouding body, with assistance of the family; body is buried facing Mecca
Pentecostal	Prayer; communion; call pastor
Presbyterian	Prayer; communion; call pastor
Roman Catholic	Prayer; sacrament of the sick; communion; mandatory baptism
Russian Orthodox	Prayer; communion; sacrament of the sick; mandatory baptism
Scientologist	Confession; visit with pastoral counselor
Seventh-Day Adventist	Baptism; communion
Unitarian	Prayer; cremation is common

Spirituality and Death

Death often forces people to consider profound questions: the meaning of life, the existence of the soul, and the possibility of an afterlife. Individuals faced with death, their close friends, and family often rely on a spiritual foundation to help them meet these challenging concepts. Spirituality takes several forms. Bernard and Schneider mention three levels of spiritual support for dying persons.[1] The first level is drawing strength from God. The second level is strength generated by prayer. The third level is strength from caring relationships with others. For those whose spirituality does not include beliefs rooted in organized religion, support may take the form of compassionate care and the acceptance of personal beliefs. For those whose spirituality includes an expression of a specific religious practice, the availability of rituals can bring comfort and support.

Consider the spiritual dimension of your clients' needs. You do not have to be a specialist or expert in this area to feel comfortable and competent. Meeting basic human needs is an expression of caring that dying individuals will appreciate, even if they can no longer communicate with you verbally. In other words, you honor the process of dying. Gifts that you can bring to clients and families are interaction, attention, and concern. A return benefit of this gift is a lessening of your fear of death.

Kübler-Ross's Stages of Dying

Most people hope death will occur naturally, after many enjoyable years of life and accomplishment. In such cases, death ensues well into a person's old age, without sickness or suffering for the individual or family. Unfortunately, not everyone is lucky enough to experience death this way. **Terminal illness** is a state in which an individual faces a medical condition that will end in death within a limited period. Chapter 99 examines hospice nursing, which specializes in the care of terminally ill individuals.

Dr. Elisabeth Kübler-Ross, among other authors, has described certain phases through which a person may pass in an attempt to cope with impending death. All terminally ill people pass through some of these stages, unless death is instantaneous or the person is unable to resolve conflicts. The family, to complete the grieving process, also may pass through the same basic stages. These stages can overlap, and a person can go back and forth from one stage to another.

Note that one of the important developmental tasks of older adulthood involves confronting one's impending mortality. Many older adults also pass through some of the stages of dying, as they face the realization that they will not live forever. A benefit of normal aging is being able to gradually adjust to the inevitability of death, rather than having to confront it with the immediacy of terminally ill individuals. Table 14-2 reviews the following steps in dealing with death.

Denial and Isolation

In this stage, the person does not believe that the diagnosis is correct: "This can't be happening to me." During this stage, he or she may seek advice from several doctors, hoping that one of them will offer a more acceptable prognosis.

Anger and Rage

In this stage, the person asks: "Why did this happen to me? Why now?" Often, the individual envies the person who is young and healthy; he or she may lash out at family members or healthcare personnel. Sometimes, the person facing terminal illness is young. When dealing with an individual who is facing terminal illness and seems angry, understand that the

person is behaving naturally. The anger that the person is expressing is due to the difficulty of the situation and not the actions of you or others who are trying to help. The person is rebelling against the feeling of sudden helplessness.

Bargaining and Developing Awareness

During this stage, which may be very short, an individual makes deals with God or with himself or herself: "If I live just 2 more weeks, I can see my son get married." When the bargained-for time has passed, the person may make another such bargain, in the hopes of postponing death indefinitely.

Depression

The person realizes that he or she is going to die and that nothing can be done to stop it. He or she may feel a severe sense of loss about leaving employment, spending money on healthcare bills, saying goodbye to children and other loved ones, and the greatest loss of all, leaving life itself.

Depression often involves two stages: verbal and nonverbal. During the verbal stage, also called **reactive depression,** the individual concentrates on past losses. Those experiencing reactive depression need reassurance and encouragement from others. Some people find comfort in writing the story of their lives.

Later, during the nonverbal stage, also called **preparatory depression,** a person realizes the impact of loss. During this phase, encouragement is not meaningful because individuals realize that they will be leaving behind everything they have known. They may wish to plan for life after death or for their family after they die, or they may daydream or sleep a great deal to escape reality. Other people can be most helpful by just being there. A touch of the hand or a kind word will be more helpful than meaningless chatter.

Acceptance and Peace

As an individual resolves emotional conflicts about death, he or she enters the stage of realization and acceptance of the inevitability of death. To reach this point, a person usually must have had time and assistance in working through the earlier stages. As dying persons resign themselves to death, they may seem devoid of all feeling. This time is particularly difficult for the family, who may interpret an individual's acceptance of death as a rejection of life and of them. The family must come to understand that the person will be unable to die comfortably unless the family helps the individual to give up everything associated with life. Although the dying person may be unable or unwilling to communicate, he or she usually will appreciate short visits or the presence of a family member.

☛ KEY CONCEPT

The stages of denial, anger, bargaining, depression, and acceptance are also followed during the client's adjustment to serious illness, stress (eg, divorce), and many other life events.

Detachment

The final stage of dying is **detachment,** when an individual gradually separates from the world so a two-way communica-

■■■ TABLE 14-2 ⨍TAGES OF DEALING WITH DEATH

Stage	Response	Suggestions for Helping the Person Cope
Denial and Isolation Shock, often followed by a feeling of isolation	"No, not me!"	Answer questions honestly. Allow person to talk to physician. Do not argue.
Anger and Rage Rage	"Why me?"	Listen. Do not take the client's anger personally. Do not get angry yourself.
Bargaining and Developing Awareness Guilt	"Yes me, but . . ." "If I could just live until . . ."	Try to assist in client's wishes. Encourage family support. Offer spiritual assistance from clergy or support groups.
Depression Grief (Verbal stage) (Nonverbal stage)	"Yes, me."	Be there. Listen. Offer counseling or social service assistance. Offer encouragement. Allow person to rest.
Acceptance and Peace Self-reliance	"My time is close, and it's OK."	Provide physical care. Be there. Keep room lighted. Support family members.
Detachment Decathexis	No communication	Continue to include person in conversation. Allow person to detach. Provide physical care. Try not to leave the individual alone. Support the family.

Based, for the most part, on the work of Dr. Elisabeth Kübler-Ross.

tion no longer exists with people around him or her. Because dying people may be unresponsive during this time, care from others (including nursing care) is primarily directed toward physical needs. Even if they do not respond, however, many people can still hear and understand what is being said (see Chap. 59).

☞ KEY CONCEPT

Examining Kübler-Ross's stages of grief can help you understand a person's reactions to terminal illness and loss. These stages explain the range of reactions that clients may express. However, never assume that a dying person should be in any one stage at a particular time. Dying persons work through their grief in their own ways, moving back and forth from one stage to another, and even skipping some stages. Your role is to be understanding and supportive.

Death's Impact on the Family

Often families with a member who is dying experience stress more keenly than the dying person does. They are coping with deep feelings of anticipated loss, but do not know how to approach their dying loved one. They want to relieve pain but they do not know what to do to help. Efforts to appear hopeful and cheerful may confuse the dying person because that is not his or her need at that time. Be aware that not all family members may be in the same stage as each other or as the client. Sometimes, the dying person who has achieved a sense of acceptance or detachment actually provides strength for family members who are having difficulties facing the impending loss.

☞ KEY CONCEPT

The family must realize that crying or sadness in front of dying loved ones is acceptable. Such behavior can be therapeutic, because otherwise the dying individual may feel that nobody cares.

Everyday problems confront a family when the death of a member occurs. Financial concerns may become an increasing source of worry. Arrangements for babysitting, transportation, and temporary housing for out-of-town visitors may need to be addressed. Funeral or commemorative services must be pre-

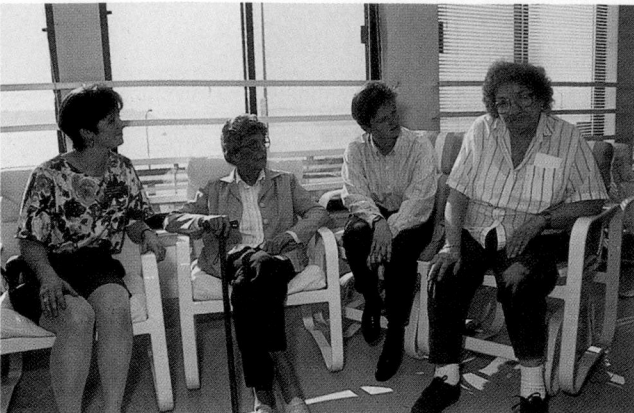

FIGURE 14-1. Support groups can help people work through their feelings of grief. (Craven, R. F., & Hirnle, C. J. [2000]. *Fundamentals of nursing: Human health and function* [3rd ed., p. 1287]. Philadelphia: Lippincott Williams & Wilkins.)

pared. The family must handle all these things at a time often marked by shock, loneliness, and sadness. Occasionally, the stress becomes difficult for families to handle, resulting in increased conflicts and outbursts of emotion. Families that pull together and avoid taking any unchanneled expressions of feeling personally are likely to cope best. Support from friends, neighbors, and coworkers can also be a tremendous help (Fig. 14-1).

Often, families question how to handle death when children are in the family. Although very young children may be unable to express their thoughts clearly, they do grieve and need to be part of the family's mourning. Adults should talk honestly and clearly with children about illness and death when it occurs. Children should be allowed to see the body or attend the funeral (or both) if they wish to do so. Children who are dying should be told the truth and be allowed to ask questions.

The process of dying has been compared to the process of labor. They are both parts of the same life journey. They both touch people in deep and lasting ways. Individuals and families who experience this process form bonds beyond those of the everyday world.

➜ STUDENT SYNTHESIS

Key Points

- Death is a normal part of the total life process.
- Culture, ethnicity, and religion influence attitudes toward death and the way people express grief and loss.
- Spirituality is an outlet that helps individuals to handle death and dying.
- Most people, if they do not die suddenly, pass through definite stages during the dying process. The ultimate goal is acceptance.
- Families who face the impending death of a member may endure enormous stress. They need encouragement to express their emotions.

- Family members and spouses need support following the death of a loved one.

Critical Thinking Exercises

1. You are working with a person who is terminally ill. Discuss what you might observe in each of Kübler-Ross's six stages of dying. How would you modify your behaviors and expectations for each of these stages?
2. Consider experiences that you have had with death among your family members or friends. Examine these experiences as closely as you can remember, and compare them with the stages that Kübler-Ross describes. What did others say that was helpful to you? Determine how you can build on your experiences to help others during your nursing career.
3. Describe how your spiritual beliefs would affect your responses in the following situations: a client who asks you to pray with him; a person who questions angrily why God allows her to suffer; an ill family member who asks you to help him to "end it all."

NCLEX-Style Review Questions

1. A client has been diagnosed with a terminal illness. The client states, "Why has this happened to me?" The client is in which stage of grieving?
   a. Acceptance
   b. Anger
   c. Bargaining
   d. Denial
2. Which action would be most appropriate to support the spiritual concerns of a terminally ill client who has not practiced a formal religion?
   a. Avoid talking to the client about this issue.
   b. Encourage the client to quickly join a religious group.
   c. Encourage the client to gain strength from caring relationships.
   d. Offer to pray with the client.
3. When a client is grieving, which of the following is a correct statement?
   a. The client may move back and forth from one stage to another.
   b. The client will move from one step to the next.
   c. The client should be forced to move quickly through stages to reach acceptance.
   d. The client should be forced to discuss his or her feelings.

Reference

1. Bernard, J., & Schneider, M. (1996). *The true work of dying: A practical and compassionate guide to easing the dying process.* New York: Avon Books.

Unit IV

STRUCTURE AND FUNCTION

CHAPTER

15

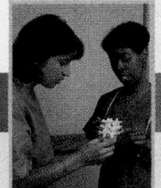

Organization of the Human Body

LEARNING OBJECTIVES

1. Define the term homeostasis and relate this to the study of anatomy and physiology.
2. Define and differentiate the terms chemistry, physics, and matter. State how these concepts relate to homeostasis.
3. State the three types of matter and the three states of matter.
4. Describe the basic organization of atoms, elements, compounds, and mixtures.
5. Explain the difference between a physical and a chemical change.
6. Break down the following words into the components of prefix, root, and suffix: intravenous, hepatitis, dysphagia.
7. Define and differentiate among anatomy, physiology, and pathophysiology.
8. Define and demonstrate the anatomical position.
9. Differentiate among the sagittal, transverse, and frontal planes.
10. Define the following terms relating to body direction: superior, inferior, anterior, posterior, proximal, distal, ventral, and dorsal.
11. Describe the four basic structural levels of the body. Differentiate among cells, tissues, organs, and systems.
12. Point out on a chart the basic structural elements of the human cell. Explain the functions of each structure.
13. Define contractility, conductivity, irritability, and reproduction as they relate to the human cell.
14. Differentiate between RNA and DNA.
15. Differentiate between mitosis and meiosis and define each.
16. List the four major types of tissue. Give an example of each.
17. List the major systems in the body, and state which organs make up each system.
18. State at least four nursing considerations related to cells, tissues, organs, and body systems.

NEW TERMINOLOGY

anabolism	meiosis
anatomic position	membrane
anatomy	metabolism
atom	mitosis
body cavity	mixture
catabolism	nucleus
cell	organ
cell membrane	pathophysiology
chemical change	physical change
chromosome	physiology
cilia	plane
compound	plasma membrane
cytoplasm	platelet
diaphragm	protoplasm
dorsal	quadrant
element	sagittal
enzyme	system
eponym	tissue
frontal	transverse
gene	ventral
homeostasis	viscera
medical terminology	

ACRONYMS

DNA	RBCs	RUQ
LLQ	RLQ	WBCs
LUQ	RNA	

The human body is a precisely structured arrangement of liquids, gases, and solids. The body is made up of atoms, molecules, and chemicals, and is approximately 60% water. Many chemical reactions occur in the body. These chemical reactions are organized and result in specific independent, yet interrelated, actions. These actions are essential for normal body function. Nurses must be knowledgeable about these concepts, because caring for clients involves looking at individual body systems and at how alterations in one system affect other systems. Most healthcare is interdisciplinary in nature. Individuals working in some disciplines, such as pharmacy or laboratory technology, use information related to the cellular, molecular, and chemical aspects of the body. Other individuals, including physicians, nurses, and therapists, focus more on body structures and specific functions of complete body systems. All healthcare professionals share a basic understanding of body structure and use common terminology when communicating with one another. This chapter introduces medical terminology, chemistry, and the science of anatomy and physiology.

CHEMISTRY AND LIFE

Before beginning any course in life science, a basic knowledge of chemistry and physics is important. *Chemistry* is the science concerned with the structure and composition of matter and the chemical reactions these substances produce. *Physics* is the science of the laws of matter and their interactions with energy.

Chemistry is the basis for **homeostasis,** the dynamic balance of anatomy and physiology. Homeostasis is the physical and emotional equilibrium (balance) a person strives to maintain. It depends on a person's cumulative chemical reactions, physical condition, and emotional status.

A simplified discussion of chemistry begins with the discussion of matter. *Matter* can be defined as anything that occupies space and has weight. The three kinds of matter are element, compound, and mixture. The three states of matter are solid, liquid, and gas.

Elements, Compounds, and Mixtures

All matter, living and nonliving, can be broken down into 92 natural and 20 man-made elements.[1] An **element** is a pure, simple chemical. Twenty-one different elements are found in the human body. All elements have specific letter abbreviations frequently used in healthcare settings. Seven elements make up approximately 99% of human body weight. These elements and their symbols are: carbon (C), hydrogen (H), oxygen (O), nitrogen (N), phosphorus (P), sulfur (S), and calcium (Ca). Elements found in very small amounts, but which are vital to human life, are: sodium (Na), chlorine (Cl), potassium (K), iron (Fe), and iodine (I). Other elements found in trace amounts include: fluorine (F), chromium (Cr), manganese (Mn), cobalt (Co), copper (Cu), zinc (Zn), selenium (Se), magnesium (Mg), and molybdenum (Mo).

An **atom** is the smallest part of any element. Atoms are composed of subatomic (smaller than an atom) particles or structures. The main subatomic particles are electrons, protons, and neutrons. Protons and neutrons are located in the **nucleus** (center) of the atom. Electrons whirl around the nucleus. An atom of one element differs from that of another element due to the arrangement of its subatomic particles. For instance, a hydrogen atom has one proton and one neutron forming the nucleus, with one electron whirling around it. An atom of oxygen has a nucleus comprising eight protons and eight neutrons, with eight electrons whirling around it (Fig. 15-1).

Atoms of one element are able to interact with atoms of another element. When atoms of two or more elements react chemically with one another, they form a variety of substances called **compounds.** In every compound, the elements combine in definite proportions. For example, the most common compound found on the surface of the earth and in the human body is *water.* Water forms when two hydrogen atoms combine with one oxygen atom. The two hydrogen atoms each have one electron and one proton. The oxygen atom has eight electrons and eight protons, which because of the specific electrical charge, can combine with only two hydrogen atoms. In chemical shorthand, water is expressed as H_2O (two parts hydrogen to one part oxygen).

Not all elements or compounds combine chemically when brought together. A **mixture** is a blend of two or more substances that have been mixed together without forming a new compound. Salt water (saline) is an example of a mixture. Both the salt and the water remain as separate compounds. Their chemical composition is not changed. They can be brought together in any proportion, and they can be easily separated.

Physical and Chemical Changes

Water has a definite chemical structure, H_2O. Normally it is a liquid. If you lower the temperature of the water so that it

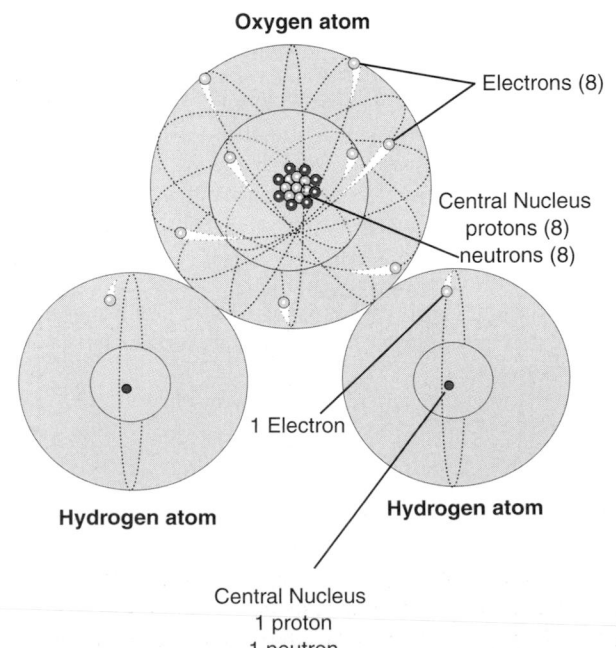

FIGURE 15-1. The compound water (H_2O). Note the structure of the oxygen and hydrogen atoms.

freezes, it changes to a solid (ice); if you raise the temperature of the water so that it boils, it becomes water vapor (steam, a gaseous state). The water has undergone a **physical change,** that is, a change in its outward properties. However, the chemical composition is still H₂O in any of the three states in which it occurs. Its chemical structure remains unchanged.

If you pass a direct electric current through a sample of water, however, a different change occurs. The water gradually disappears, because the electric current causes water to break down into its two invisible gaseous elements: hydrogen and oxygen. A **chemical change** has occurred. Familiar types of chemical changes are the processes of burning (combustion) and the rusting of iron (oxidation). In chemical reactions, substances change into other substances that no longer have the same chemical structures as before. Completely rusted iron no longer has the same characteristics as iron; burned wood is no longer wood, but ashes and gas.

☛ KEY CONCEPT

Physical change: Outward properties change, but chemical properties remain the same (eg, changes in temperature convert water into ice or steam).

Chemical change: One substance changes to another, or the compound breaks down into atoms of elements, and its energy is transferred (eg, an electric current breaks down water into hydrogen, oxygen, and heat).

MEDICAL TERMINOLOGY

To study body structure and function, an understanding of the vocabulary used in the healthcare field, commonly called **medical terminology,** is necessary. So much is involved in medical terminology that it can be regarded as a separate course of study.

Sources of Medical Terms

Learning the meaning of a medical term is easier when you know the original source of the word. Many medical terms have their roots in Greek or Latin words. Modern language is another source of medical words. Some terms are *acronyms,* words formed by combining letters of a word or phrase. For instance, MASH stands for mobile army surgical hospital. AIDS is an acronym for acquired immunodeficiency syndrome. Many acronyms used in healthcare are listed in Appendix B. **Eponyms** are words based on the names of people—for example, Parkinson's disease and Alzheimer's disease.

Parts of Words

Most medical terms consist of two or three parts: prefix, root, and suffix. The *prefix* is at the beginning of a word. Not all medical terms have a prefix. Appendix D lists prefixes and some roots with a dash after the letters (eg, intra-, hypo-, or sub-). The *root* of a word is the word's foundation. All medical terms have at least one root, which may begin the word. The *suffix* is the word's ending. Most medical words have a suffix.

Appendix D also lists suffixes with a dash before the letters (eg, -itis, -ic, or -pathy).

A combining vowel (usually o) joins a root to another root or to a suffix. For example, thermometer (therm = heat; meter = measuring device). Medical terminology texts list roots combined with a vowel; this form is known as the *combining form.* Examples of combining forms are hepat-o, oste-o, and neur-o.

Although the root is the core of the word, a prefix or suffix can totally change its meaning. A prefix introduces another thought or explains the root. For example, epigastric means "on the stomach," while hypogastric means "below the stomach." The suffix is added to clarify, to make a new word, or to change the meaning of the root. For example, tonsillitis means "inflammation of the tonsils," and tonsillectomy means "removal of the tonsils."

Prefixes, roots, and suffixes can be used in various combinations. Sometimes a word may be a combination of two or three roots and connecting vowels. For example, electrocardiogram breaks down to: a record (suffix: -gram) of electricity (root: electr-) of the heart (root: cardi-). Note the two uses of o as a combining vowel: joining two roots, and joining a root and suffix. Therefore, electrocardiogram means "a record of the electrical activity of the heart."

To simplify a medical term, first break it down into its components. Start with the suffix, then go to the prefix, and end with the root. For example, the following is a breakdown of the term intravenous:

-ous (suffix) means "pertaining to"
intra- (prefix) means "within"
ven (root) means "vein"

Thus, the word intravenous means "pertaining to within a vein." See Appendix D for a list of many prefixes, suffixes, and roots.

☛ KEY CONCEPT

Healthcare professionals use medical terminology to communicate assessment findings, diagnostic test results, and other pertinent information.

ANATOMY AND PHYSIOLOGY

The study of body structure is called **anatomy.** The study of how the body functions is called **physiology.** An understanding of the body requires knowledge of both the structures of the body and how these structures relate to and function with one another. An awareness of normal anatomy and physiology is important as a basis for understanding abnormal conditions, such as disease or injury. The study of disorders of functioning is called **pathophysiology.**

BODY DIRECTIONS

Now that medical terminology has been introduced, you are ready to apply these terms to body structure and function.

Several terms are used to designate areas and directions of the body. These terms help students to specify the location of an organ or system. They also help healthcare professionals to communicate with each other.

Anatomic Position

Medical texts present the body from a standard reference point known as **anatomic position.** The body is pictured standing erect with arms at the sides and palms turned forward (Fig. 15-2). When viewing anatomic pictures or diagrams, the right side of the body is on the left side of the drawing (the same as looking at a person facing you).

Body Planes

A body **plane** is an imaginary flat surface that divides the body into sections (see Fig. 15-2). The following are planes of the body:

Frontal (coronal plane): the vertical plane that passes through the body longitudinally from head to toe, dividing it into front and back parts

Sagittal: the vertical plane that passes through the body lengthwise and divides the body into right or left sides; the *midsagittal* plane passes through the midline from top to bottom, dividing the body into equal right and left halves

Transverse: the horizontal plane that passes through the body, dividing it into upper (superior) and lower

(inferior) parts; transverse planes may be imagined at any level

Body Positions

In addition to viewing the body in terms of planes, the body is also described by the relationship of one body part to another. These are termed *body positions* or *body directions* (Fig. 15-3). Body directions will assist you in describing the locations of organs or body positions during your nursing career. Table 15-1 lists and describes these body directions.

Body Cavities

A **body cavity** is a space within the body that contains internal organs (**viscera**). Within the body are two groups of cavities that contain various organs. They are the **dorsal** (posterior, back) and the **ventral** (anterior, front) cavities (Fig. 15-4). The dorsal cavity is subdivided into the cranial and spinal cavities. The ventral cavity is subdivided into the thoracic and abdominal cavities. The **diaphragm** is a large muscle that separates the ventral cavities. Often, the abdominal cavity is subdivided again into the abdominal and pelvic portions and is referred to as the abdominopelvic cavity. No specific anatomic division exists between the abdominal and pelvic areas. Table 15-2 lists the contents of each body cavity.

The abdominal cavity can be divided into more precise areas containing specific organs by two different methods. The first method divides the abdomen into four **quadrants,** using the umbilicus (navel) as a central crossing point for the hori-

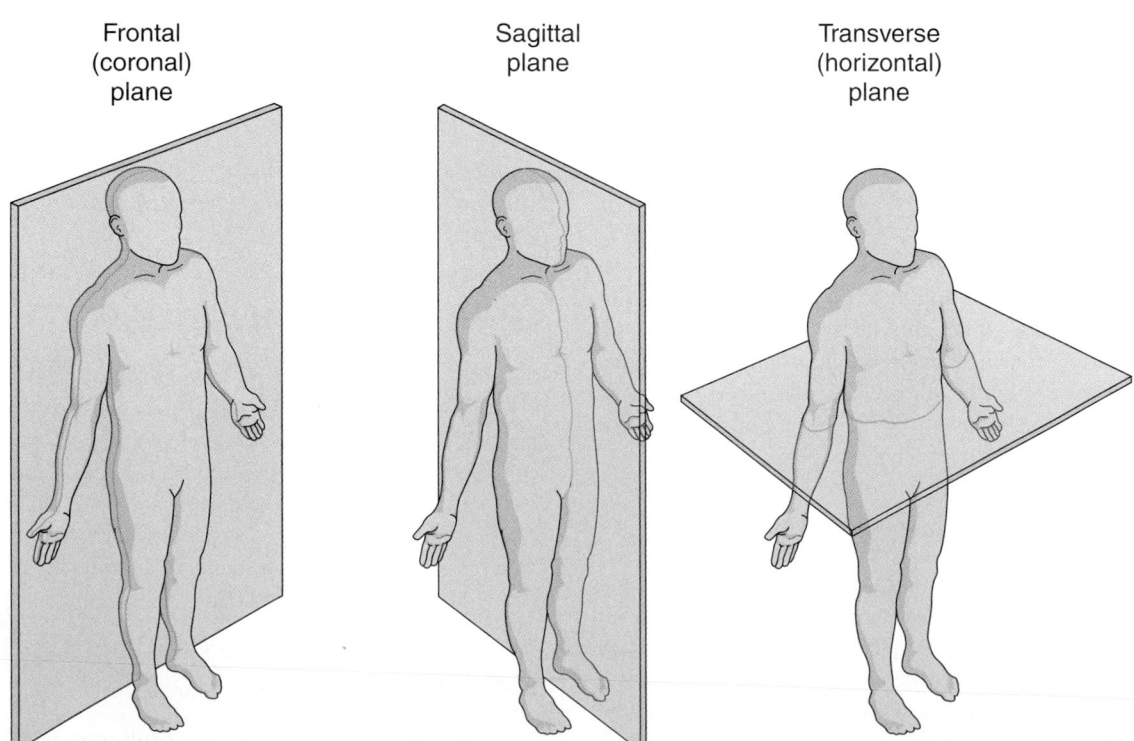

Frontal (coronal) plane   Sagittal plane   Transverse (horizontal) plane

FIGURE 15-2. Body planes. The body is shown here in anatomic position.

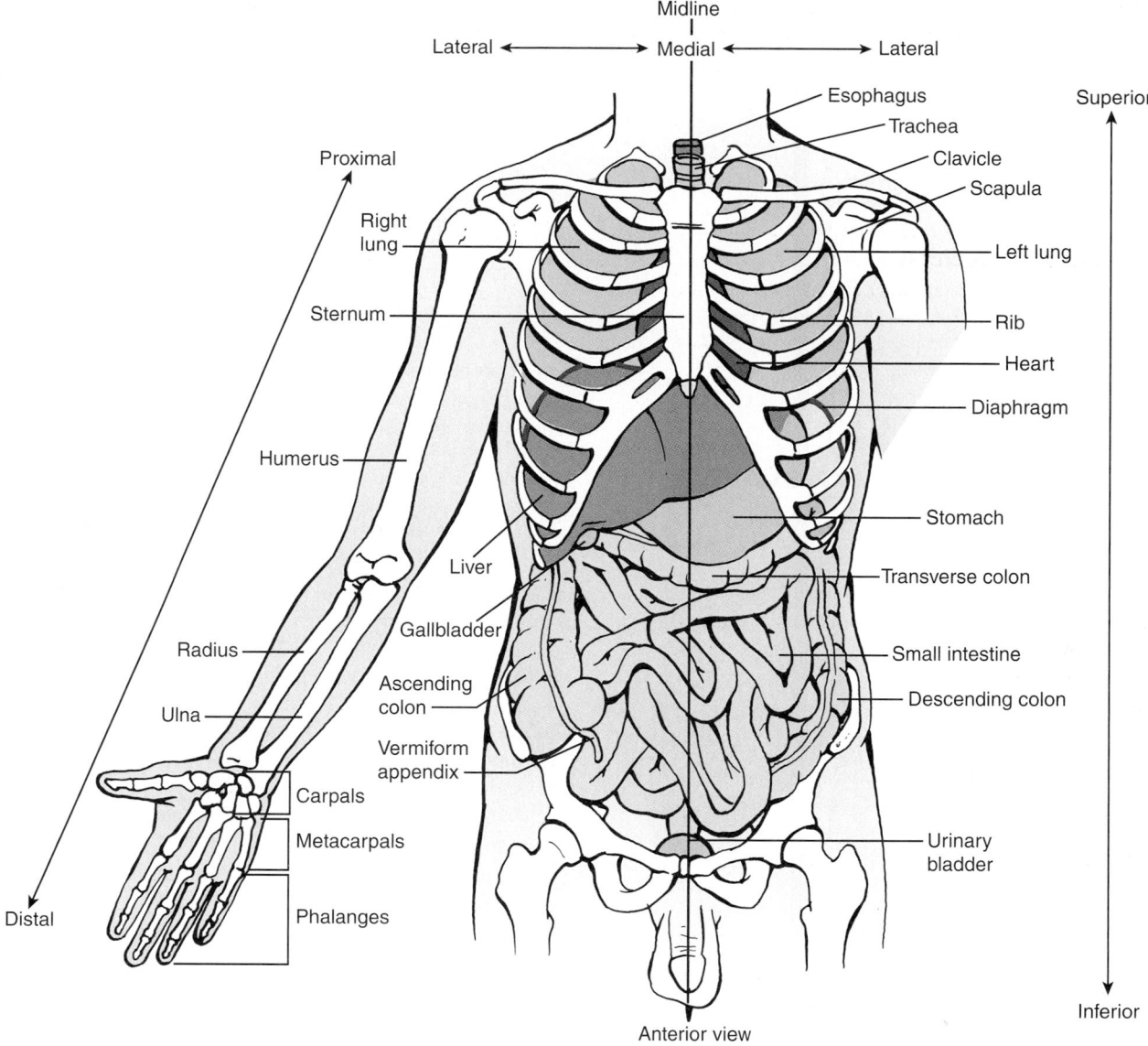

FIGURE 15-3. **(A)** Body directions assist in describing the location of organs or body positions. (*continued on next page*)

zontal and vertical dividing lines. The horizontal dividing line extends from side to side. The vertical dividing line extends from the tip of the xiphoid process to the mons pubis. These divisions result in the formation of four quadrants or rectangles referred to as the right upper quadrant (**RUQ**), right lower quadrant (**RLQ**), left upper quadrant (**LUQ**), and left lower quadrant (**LLQ**) (Fig. 15-5).

The second method uses the costal (rib) margins and pubic bones as horizontal dividing lines for three major regions. The central area above the costal margins is referred to as the epigastric (epi = above; gastr = stomach) region. The central area below the pubic bones is referred to as the hypogastric or suprapubic (on the pubis) region. The central area between these two dividing lines is referred to as the umbilical region. Corresponding lateral (side) regions are referred to as the left and right hypochondriac regions; left and right iliac regions; and between these, the left and right lumbar regions (Fig. 15-6).

STRUCTURAL LEVELS IN THE BODY

Four basic structural levels are found within the body:

Cells—the basic units
Tissues—made up of cells
Organs—made up of tissues
Systems—made up of organs

Cells

The **cell** is the basic unit of structure and function in all living things. Each cell is alive and carries out specific activities. The smallest forms of life, such as bacteria, are composed of a single cell. The human body, on the other hand, is made up of trillions of cells.

Although the human body has many different types of cells, all cells contain the same basic chemicals and similar struc-

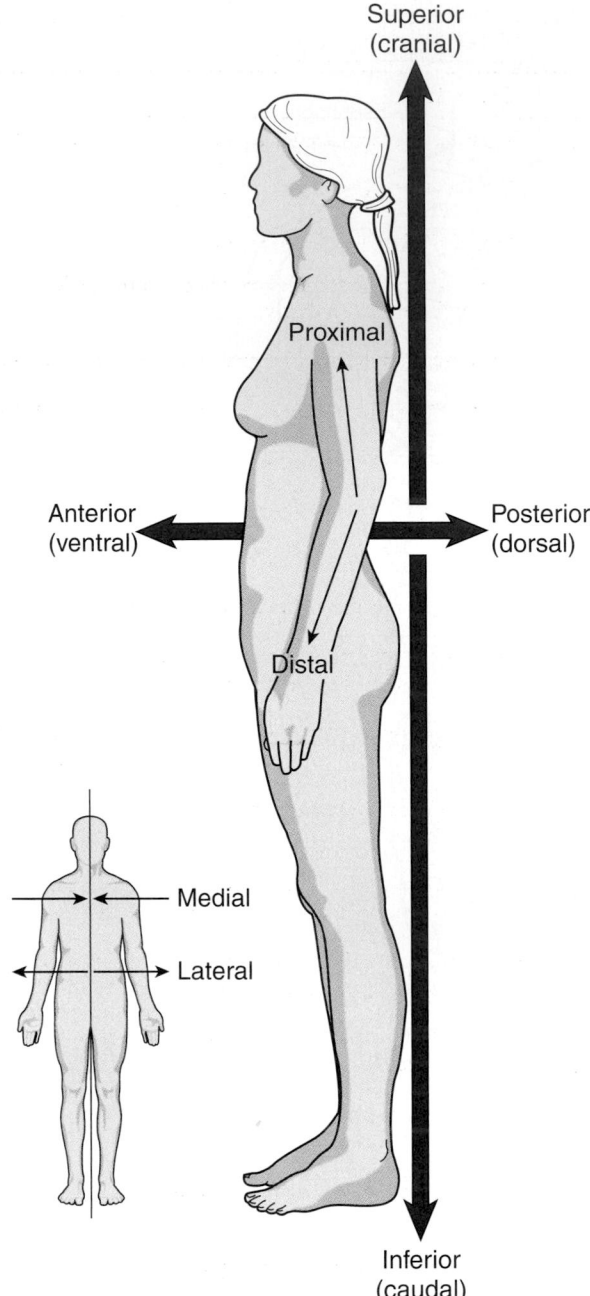

FIGURE 15-3. *Continued* (**B**) Directional terms.

tural features. Despite being the smallest living subunit of the human body, the cell functions as a member of a highly organized team.

☛ KEY CONCEPT

The cell is the basic unit of structure and function for all living things.

Special Properties

As team members, cells have become specialized in anatomic structure and physiologic function. Some cells have highly developed abilities for **metabolism**—the ability to process, obtain energy from, and create new products, using the chemicals found in foods. The two phases of metabolism are anabolism and catabolism. **Anabolism** is the building up, assimilation, or conversion of ingested substances. **Catabolism** is the process of breaking down, disintegrating, or tearing substances into simpler substances. By virtue of the breakdown of substances, particularly food, energy is released.

Cells have other specialized properties:

Contractility: Muscle cells can move or contract.
Conductivity: Nerve cells are specialized to send and receive impulses.
Irritability: Cells respond to stimuli.
Reproduction: Cells duplicate themselves.

The properties of metabolism, contractility, conductivity, irritability, and reproduction are present to some degree in all cells. However, an individual cell does not function independently. Rather, it develops specialties, interrelated with other cells. This teamwork permits the organism to have organization and adaptability, which is not possible in the single-cell microorganism.

☛ KEY CONCEPT

Cells have special abilities such as metabolism, contractility, conductivity, irritability, and reproduction.

Cellular Structure and Function

Cytology is the science that investigates the formation, structure, and function of cells. The study of various sample cells teaches a great deal about the general condition of an entire organism.

Cells are too small to be seen without a microscope, except for the egg cell (ovum), which is just visible to the naked eye. Human cells vary in shape, function, and size.

Cell shape may be round, spherical, rectangular, or irregular. Some cells change shape as they move, but each category of cells retains its shape; for example, nerve cells will always look like nerve cells.

Although cells have similar abilities, their functions are specialized. Nerve cells have filaments on their ends that carry or receive impulses. Muscle cells are long thin fibers that permit contraction and relaxation of the cell. A fat cell is large, with empty spaces suitable for storing lipids (fats).

Most cells vary in size from 1 to 100 microns or micrometers, abbreviated µ (1 micron = 1/25,000 of an inch. A micrometer, commonly referred to as a micron, is one millionth of a meter or one-thousandth of a millimeter). Ten to 1,000 cells fit on the head of a pin, depending on the cell.

Although minute in size, the complexity of cell structure is amazing. Collectively, all parts that make up a cell are called **protoplasm.** The cell parts can be divided into those found in the nucleus and those found in the cytoplasm. The cell's **nucleus** is its control center, responsible for reproduction and coordination of other cellular activities. The nucleus houses the chromosomes and the nucleolus. The **cytoplasm** is the area of the cell not located in the nucleus. The structures located in the cytoplasm are the mitochondria, the Golgi apparatus (or Golgi bodies), lysosomes, endoplasmic reticulum, ribosomes, and the centrosomes (which contain centrioles) (Tab. 15-3).

■■■ **TABLE 15-1** 𝓑ODY DIRECTIONS

Position	Definition	Examples
Superior	"Above" or in a higher position	The knee is superior to the toes but inferior to the femur.
Inferior	"Below" or in a lower position	The lips are inferior to the nose but superior to the chin.
Cranial	In or near the head	The brain is in the cranial cavity.
Caudal	Near the lower end of the body, (ie, near the end of the spine), "tail"	The buttocks, the muscles on which we sit, are located at the caudal end of the body.
Anterior or ventral	Toward the front or "belly" surface of the body	The nose is on the anterior, or ventral, surface of the head.
Posterior or dorsal	Toward the back of the body	The calf is on the posterior, or dorsal, surface of the leg.
Medial	Nearer the midline	The nose is medial to the eyes.
Lateral	Farther from the midline, toward the side	The ears are lateral to the nose.
Internal	Deeper within the body	The stomach is an internal body organ.
External	Toward the outer surface of the body	The skin covers the external surface of the body.
Proximal	Nearest the origin of a part	In the upper extremity (arm), the area above the elbow is proximal to the forearm below.
Distal	Farthest from the origin of a part	In the lower extremity (leg), the area below the knee is distal to the thigh.
Central	Situated at or pertaining to the center	The brain and the spinal cord are part of the central nervous system.
Peripheral	Situated at or pertaining to the outward part of a surface	The peripheral nerves go to body parts and return to the central nervous system.
Parietal	Pertaining to the sides or the walls of a cavity	The walls of the abdominal cavity are lined with a membrane called the parietal peritoneum.
Visceral	Pertaining to the organs within a cavity	The stomach and intestines are visceral organs in the abdominal cavity.
Supine	Lying with the face upward	A person lying on the dorsal surface of the body or (on the back) is supine.
Prone	Lying with the face downward	A person lying on the ventral surface, or the front of the body, is prone.
Deep	Away from the surface	The knife wound was deep in the abdomen.
Superficial	On or near the surface	The child had a superficial cut.

Inside the nucleus is a structure called the *nucleolus* (plural: nucleoli). The nucleolus is composed of protein, deoxyribonucleic acid (**DNA**), and ribonucleic acid (**RNA**). The nucleolus's function is not well understood, but it is involved in making ribosomes (minute granules that float free in the cytoplasm or are attached to the endoplasmic reticulum in cells that contain a high concentration of RNA). Ribosomes play an important role in protein synthesis.

The nucleus also contains chromosomes. **Chromosomes** are made up of DNA molecules that form genetic material called *genes*. **Genes** contain information about inherited characteristics. These genes are carried on the chromosomes in single file. The human cell has 46 chromosomes.

RNA is responsible for taking the genetic message from the DNA molecule and transporting this message to the ribosomes in the cytoplasm. The ribosomes then use this message to reproduce protein substances according to the specifications carried by the RNA. Therefore, DNA (Fig. 15-7) and RNA are key to the reproductive process. Cell reproduction will be discussed later in this chapter.

The **cell membrane** or **plasma membrane** surrounds the cell's outer boundary and is capable of selective permeability, meaning that it can regulate what enters and leaves the cell. (Chap. 17 addresses cellular transport, which is the movement of substances across membranes.) The nuclear membrane surrounds the nucleus. Some cells have cilia. **Cilia**

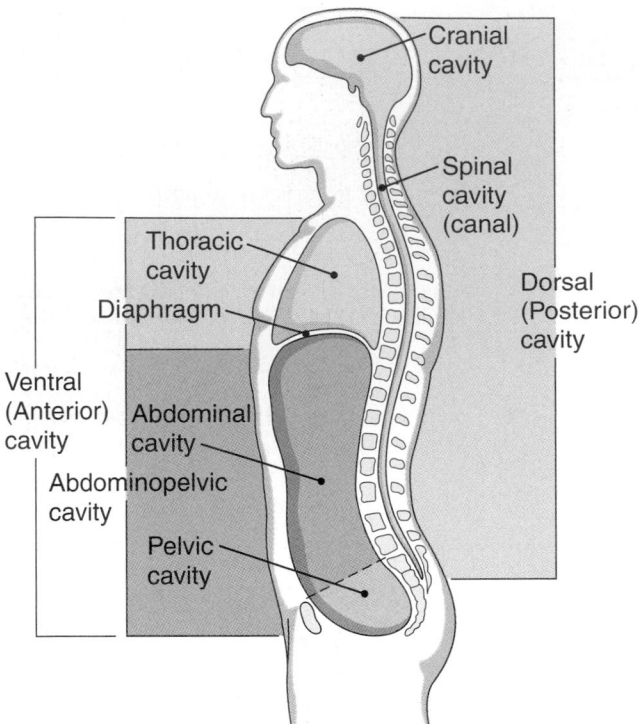

FIGURE 15-4. Side view of the body cavities.

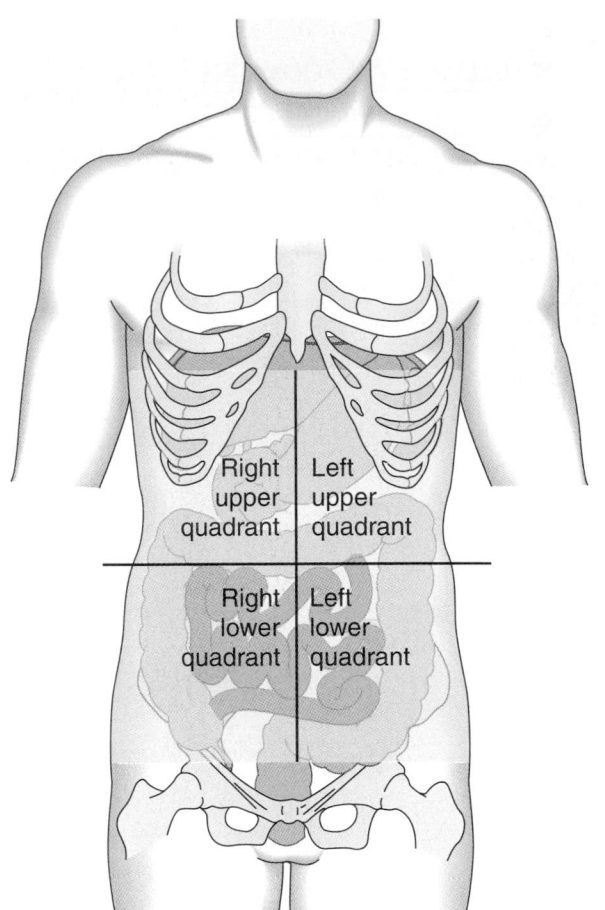

FIGURE 15-5. Quadrants of the abdomen, showing some of the organs within each quadrant.

are hairlike threads that sweep materials across the cell surface. To simplify the complex parts of the cell and the functions of these parts, it is useful to separate cell parts into those found in the nucleus and those found in the cytoplasm. Refer to Table 15-3 for functions of cellular parts and to Figure 15-8 for their locations.

TABLE 15-2 𝓑ODY CAVITIES AND THEIR CONTENTS

Cavity	Contents
Dorsal (Posterior) Cavity	
Cranial cavity	Brain
Vertebral cavity (spinal cavity)	Spinal cord
Ventral (Anterior) Cavity	
Thoracic cavity	Heart
Pericardial cavity	Each contains a lung
Two pleural cavities	Large blood vessels, trachea,
Mediastinum	esophagus, and thymus gland
Abdominal cavity (abdominopelvic cavity)	Stomach, most of the intestines, liver, gallbladder, pancreas,
Upper abdominal cavity	spleen, kidneys, adrenal glands, and ureter
Pelvic cavity	Urinary bladder, remaining part of intestines, rectum, and internal reproductive organs

Cell Reproduction

Mitosis.   Through a complicated process called **mitosis,** cells divide into two parts to reproduce themselves. Each of the daughter cells is an exact genetic duplicate of the original or "mother" cell. The body can be thought of as a group of cells, and mitosis is responsible for the body's growth, repair, and replacement of injured and dead tissues.

The amazing process of mitosis occurs as a result of a rearrangement of particles in the nucleus (Fig. 15-9). Briefly, two centrosomes (clusters of cytoplasm located near the nucleus) separate and are drawn toward opposite ends of the cell (*metaphase*). (The centrioles are organelles within the centrosomes. They play a vital role in organizing the parts of the cells called "spindles" during metaphase.) The nuclear membrane then disappears. The chromosomes split, and half of each chromosome moves toward each centrosome. The cell then begins to elongate, thinning in the middle with the plasma (cell) membrane following the same shape (*anaphase*). The cell finally splits into two parts, with half of the cytoplasm, nuclear material, and cell membrane in each new cell. Because of the genes, each new cell is identical to the original from which it was formed.

Mitosis is essential for the following:

- Growth of a single fertilized egg; after conception, the fertilized egg grows into trillions of cells

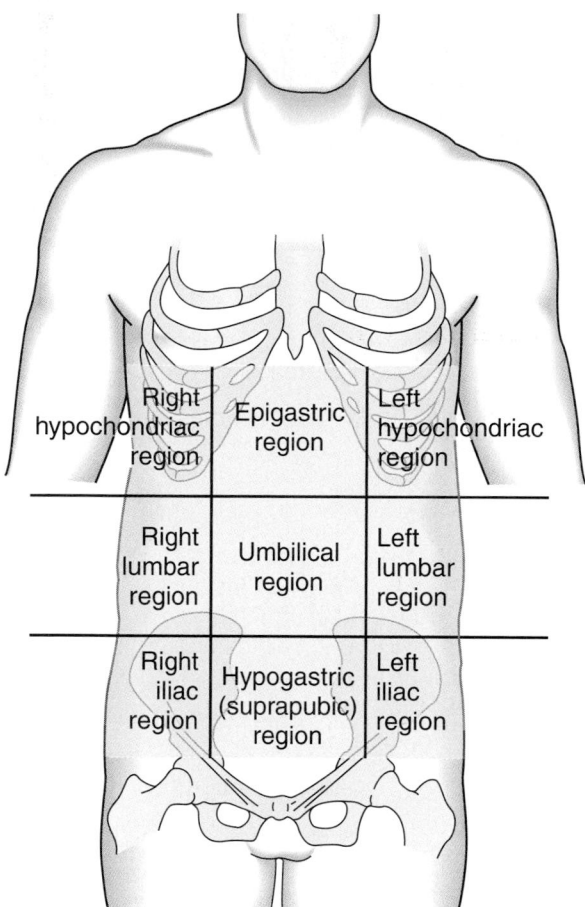

FIGURE 15-6. The nine regions of the abdomen.

■■■ TABLE 15-3 *Cellular Parts and Their Functions*

Part	Function
Parts Found in the Nucleus	
Chromosome	Carries genetic factors
Gene	Contains hereditary information found on the chromosome
Nucleoli	Globules that contain RNA and DNA
DNA	Stores and transfers genetic information
RNA	Chemical messenger that facilitates the duplication of genes by DNA
Parts Found in the Cytoplasm	
Mitochondria	Powerhouse of the cell: place where body actually makes energy
Golgi apparatus (Golgi body)	Synthesizes carbohydrates and packages substances for secretion from cell
Lysosomes	Sacs that contain digestive enzymes to destroy ingested materials, such as bacteria or damaged parts
Endoplasmic reticulum	Extensive network of tubules that serve as a passageway for material within the cell
Ribosomes	Site of protein synthesis: some are found in endoplasmic reticulum and some are free floating in cytoplasm
Centrosome	Plays role in cellular reproduction (mitosis)

- Repair of wounds by replacing damaged or dead cells
- Tumor formation in which abnormal cells, dividing by mitosis, result in more abnormal cells

Certain cells in the body are unable to reproduce in an adult. Muscle cells or neurons (nerve cells) that die lose their functions. Loss of muscle cells in the heart due to a heart attack may damage the heart so severely that it loses the ability to contract effectively. Destruction of spinal cord neurons results in paralysis and loss of sensation below the level of the injury.

Meiosis. Sperm cells and ova reproduce by meiosis, a more complex process of cell division. In **meiosis,** cell division produces eggs or sperm that contain half the total number (23) of chromosomes. Upon fertilization, the nuclei of an egg and a sperm cell fuse, forming a new organism that has the full complement of chromosomes (46 chromosomes).

Enzymes. **Enzymes** are one type of complex protein structure determined by DNA. (Enzymes do not enter into chemical compounds, but speed up chemical reactions.) Every one of the thousands of different chemical reactions that occur in the human body requires a specific enzyme to speed it up. DNA directs the formation of thousands of different proteins to meet the needs of enzyme production.

Proteins. Another task of DNA is the formation of other proteins that make up skin, muscle, blood vessels, and all internal organs. DNA builds the body's proteins from endless

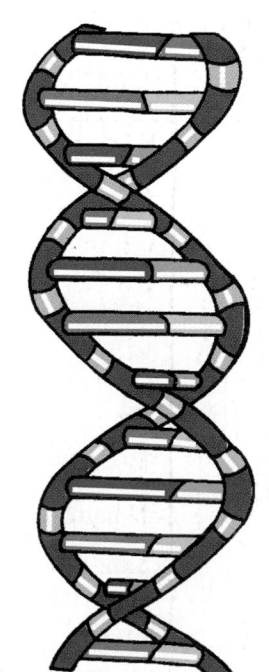

FIGURE 15-7. A DNA molecule.

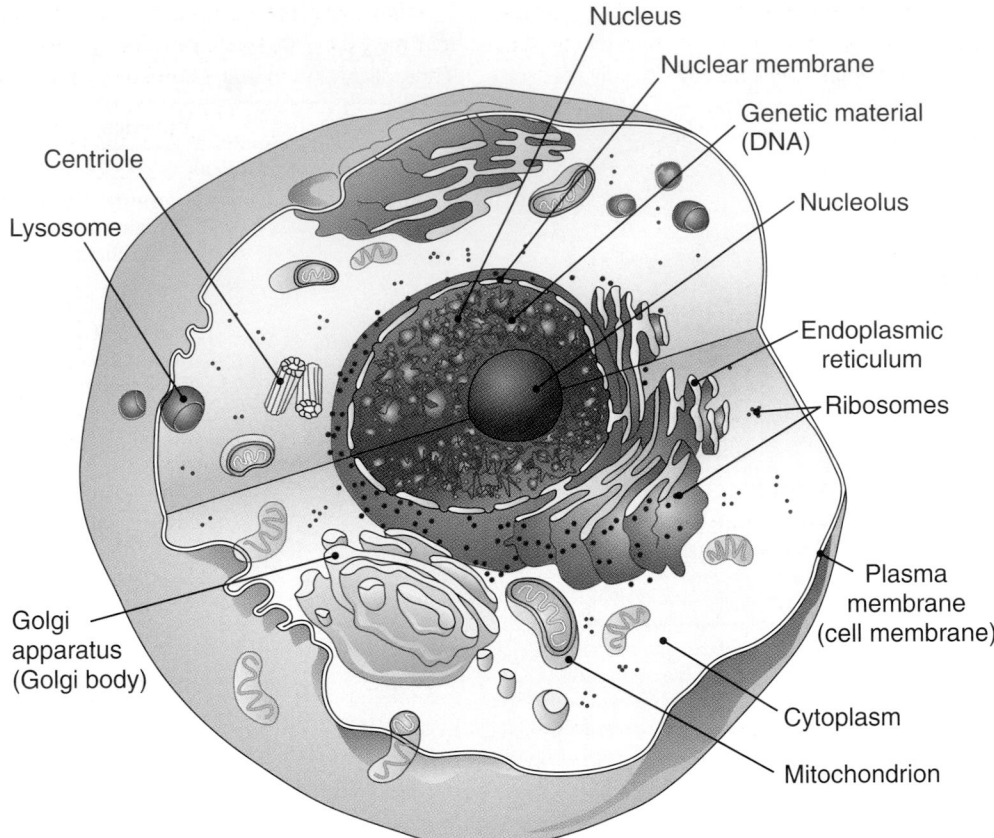

FIGURE 15-8. Diagram of a typical animal cell, showing the main organelles. The nucleus is the control center of the cell. The organelles (endoplasmic reticulum, mitochondria, Golgi bodies or Golgi apparatus, and lysosomes) in the cytoplasm are the functional substances. The plasma membrane is made up of lipids (fats) and proteins. Channels in the membrane are of vital importance in the transport of materials across the plasma membrane.

combinations of 20 amino acids. If all the coded DNA instructions found in one single cell were translated into English, they would fill more than 100 volumes of an encyclopedia.

☛ KEY CONCEPT

Enzymes are complex proteins that speed up chemical reactions.

Tissues

Cells of the same type and structure form **tissues,** each of which has a special function. The list below identifies the four principal types of human body tissues and their basic functions:

• *Epithelial tissue* protects body parts and produces secretions.

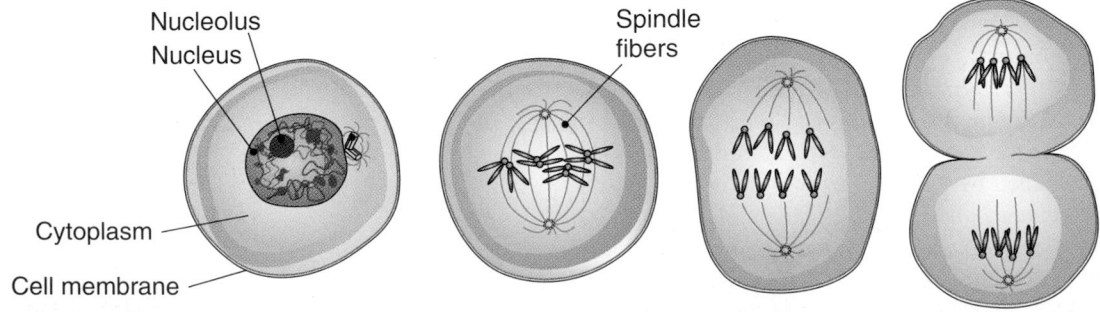

FIGURE 15-9. A simplified version of mitosis: The centrioles within the centrosome divide, the chromatin material of the nucleus changes into rod-shaped chromosomes, and two daughter cells form within the cell membrane. The daughter cells then split into two distinct cells that are identical to the original cell. The cell shown is for illustration purposes only. It is not a human cell, which has 46 chromosomes (23 pairs of chromosomes).

- *Connective tissue* anchors and supports other body structures. *Blood* is a special type of connective tissue that brings food and oxygen to the cells, and carries wastes away.
- *Muscle tissue* provides movement of the body.
- *Nerve tissue* conducts impulses to and from all parts of the body.

Epithelial Tissue

Functions.   The following are the main functions of epithelial tissue:

- Cover and protect all body surfaces, cavities, and lumina (hollow portions of blood vessels or body tubes)
- Absorb and secrete substances from the digestive tract
- Secrete substances from glands
- Provide filtration in the kidneys
- Form highly specialized epithelial tissues in the taste buds and nose
- Transport particles contained in mucus away from the lungs

Generally, epithelial tissue is *avascular* (without blood vessels). To receive nourishment, the tissue must receive nutrients from underlying tissue, such as connective tissue, through a process called *diffusion.*

In places where epithelium is subject to much destruction, the tissue is modified to provide greater protection. For example, calluses form on the bottom of the feet or on the palms of the hands to withstand greater wear and tear. Because the outer layers of epithelial cells are constantly being worn off at the body's surface, the underlying layers of epithelium are continually producing new cells. Therefore, epithelium is in a continuous state of regeneration.

Types.   Several types of cells make up epithelial tissue. Each type of cell has a characteristic shape and may be found in single or multiple layers (Fig. 15-10). The term *simple* is used for a single layer of cells. The term *stratified* means several layers of cells. For example, squamous (scaly) cells can be found in single layers, as in the alveoli (air sacs) of the lungs, or they can be stratified, as in the mouth and the esophagus.

Transitional epithelium is a type of stratified squamous epithelium. It has the ability to change shape. For example, it enables the bladder to fill and stretch without damaging its walls.

FIGURE 15-10. Types of epithelial tissue. (**A**) Simple squamous (basement membrane) tissue is found in the lungs. (**B**) Simple cuboidal tissue is found in the ovaries, thyroid, sweat glands, and salivary glands. (**C**) Simple columnar tissue is found in the stomach and intestines and in ducts of glands. (**D**) Pseudostratified columnar tissue (ciliated shown) is found in the mucous membranes of respiratory passages and eustachian tubes. It also exists in nonciliated form, which is found in the ducts of some glands, such as the parotid salivary gland and the male urethra. (**E**) Transitional tissue lines the urinary bladder. It varies in shape, depending on whether the bladder is full or empty; when full, the cells slide and stretch. (**F**) Stratified squamous tissue makes up the epidermis of the skin and the lining of the mouth, pharynx, ovaries, and vagina. Types of epithelial tissue *not shown* include stratified columnar, which is found in the epiglottis, parts of the pharynx and anal canal, and the male urethra; and simple ciliated columnar, which is found in the lining of bronchi, the nasal cavity, the oviducts, and in the lining of the uterus.

Ciliated epithelium is a type of columnar cell epithelium that has fine, hairlike extensions on its surface called *cilia.* The cilia move in waves and carry materials across the cell surface. In a very effective protective mechanism, specialized cilia sweep mucus with trapped dust and bacteria away from sterile areas, such as the lungs, toward nonsterile areas, such as the trachea and the mouth. Cilia are also found in the

A Simple squamous
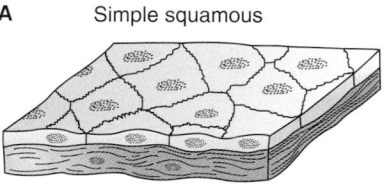

B Simple cuboidal
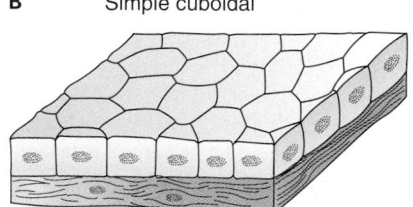

C Simple columnar
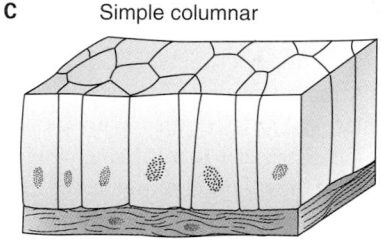

D Pseudostratified columnar ciliated
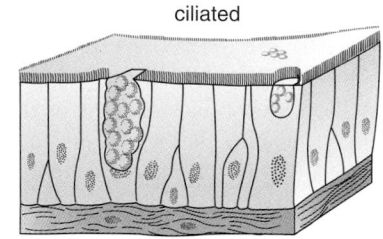

E Transitional
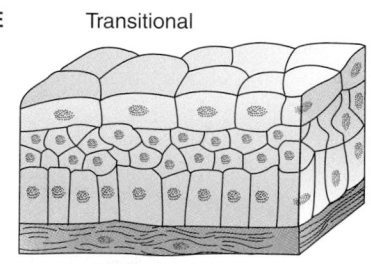

F Stratified squamous
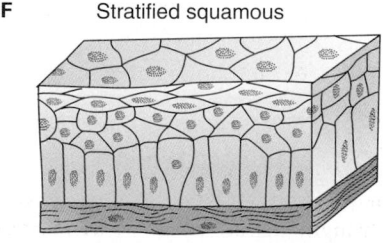

oviducts (uterine tubes) and help to move the ovum toward the uterus.

Epithelial cells shaped like goblets have the ability to form secretions. These cells are called *glands* and are discussed in Chapter 20.

Connective Tissue

The different types of connective tissue vary greatly in structure and function. The main functions of connective tissue are:

- Support, bind, or connect other tissues
- Provide nutrients to all body organs and remove waste
- Store vital nutrients, such as fat or calcium
- Provide protection for organs

The classification of connective tissues varies, but generally connective tissues are organized according to each specific *matrix* (type of structural network). Blood has a liquid matrix called plasma. Adipose connective tissue has a matrix of collagen fibers and adipose (fat) cells. Bone has a matrix of tightly packed cells that are rich in calcium.

Blood.   Blood is usually classified as a form of connective tissue because it has a matrix of specialized cells called *plasma,* the liquid portion of blood. The major formed elements of plasma are the three types of blood cells: erythrocytes (red blood cells or **RBCs**), leukocytes (white blood cells or **WBCs**), and thrombocytes (platelets). RBCs carry the oxygen and carbon dioxide needed for cellular respiration or the formation of energy. WBCs destroy pathogens and develop immunity to some diseases. **Platelets** are cell fragments that play a major role in the blood-clotting process.

Soft Connective Tissue.   The three types of soft connective tissue are areolar (loosely structured), fibrous (densely structured), and adipose (fatty).

Areolar tissue (loose connective tissue) is the most abundant connective tissue in the body. It resembles a packing material that holds things in place. It provides support for body parts and allows for some stretching in all directions. It is highly vascular, meaning that it contains numerous blood vessels; therefore, areolar tissue plays an important role in cell nutrition. It is perfectly suited for the diffusion of nutrients and waste materials across cell membranes (see Chap. 17). Areolar tissues are located where the body can intercept pathogens before they enter the bloodstream, such as just underneath the skin and beneath the epithelial tissue that lines the digestive and respiratory tracts.

Fibrous connective tissue is found where a need for flexible strength exists, such as in the dermis layer of the skin and in ligaments and tendons. (Ligaments connect bone to bone; tendons connect muscle to bone.) The blood supply to fibrous connective tissue is poor, which is the reason why it heals relatively slowly.

Elastic connective tissue can stretch to one and one-half times its original size. Like a rubber band, it snaps back to its original size. It is found in areas that are stretched on a regular basis, such as the large arteries, the larynx (voice box), the alveoli (air sacs), and the external ear.

Adipose tissue is fatty. It stores fats (lipids) as a food reserve and is found throughout the body. It serves as a padding to pro-

tect various body structures, such as the eyeballs and kidneys. It insulates against heat loss. Researchers have noted that most of our body's adipose tissue is formed prenatally (before birth) and during the first year of life. Although dieting and exercise may eliminate stored fat within the adipose tissue, the adipose tissue itself remains, waiting to be restocked with new energy stores (ie, new fat).

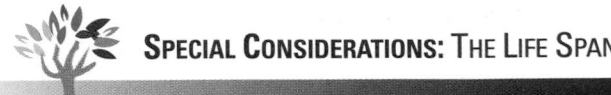

SPECIAL CONSIDERATIONS: THE LIFE SPAN

Adipose Tissue

Theorists have suggested that increased amounts of fats eaten during the child's first year of life will lead to an increase in adipose tissue, which may predispose a person to obesity in later years. This idea has not been proven, but many authorities hold it in high regard.

Hard Connective Tissue.   Hard connective tissue includes bone and cartilage. Bone is the hardest connective tissue. It gives the entire body structure, support, and mobility. Being well supplied with blood vessels (vascular), bone is also the site of numerous metabolic activities, such as the storage of calcium. Some bones contain red bone marrow, which produces RBCs.

Cartilage is tough, elastic tissue found between segments of the spinal cord (the vertebrae) and between the ends of the long bones. Cartilage gives shape to the nose, larynx, and external ear. Between bones, cartilage serves as a shock absorber and reduces friction between moving parts. (Most bones are first formed as one type of cartilage and later convert into bone through a process known as *ossification.*) Cartilage is poorly supplied with blood vessels; therefore, injured cartilaginous tissue heals slowly, if at all.

Muscle Tissue

Muscle tissues contain unique fibers that can contract (shorten) and relax, bringing about movement. Chemicals sent to the muscles from the nervous system supply the stimulus to contract.

Muscle tissue may be classified in several ways. It may be classified according to:

Function—skeletal, smooth, and cardiac
Appearance—striated (striped) and nonstriated
What controls its action—voluntary or involuntary (see Chap. 18)

Nerve Tissue

Nerve tissue is composed of neurons and neuroglia. *Neurons* are the actual working nerve cells that respond to stimuli. There are several types of neurons, but the two main types are the *sensory* (afferent) nerves and the *motor* (efferent) nerves. They send impulses to, and receive impulses from, all parts of the body (see Chap. 19).

Membranes

Membranes are sheets of epithelial or connective tissue that act together to cover surfaces, line surfaces, or separate organs or lobes (such as in the lungs). Some membranes produce secretions.

Epithelial membranes are subdivided into mucous and serous membranes. Connective tissue membranes are subdivided into skeletal and fascial membranes.

Epithelial Membranes. *Mucous* membranes are also known as *mucosa*. They line body cavities that open to the outside of the body. The mucus secreted by these membranes lubricates and protects against bacterial invasion and other foreign particles.

Serous membranes are also known as *serosa*. They line body cavities that do not open to the exterior. These membranes secrete serous fluid, which is thinner than mucus. It prevents friction when organs are in contact with one another. Serous membranes are divided into two layers: parietal and visceral. The *parietal* layer is the portion of the membrane attached to the wall of the body cavity; the *visceral* layer covers internal organs.

Connective Tissue Membranes. *Skeletal* membranes are connective tissue membranes that cover bones and cartilage. They act chiefly to support body structures. *Synovial* membrane is a type of skeletal membrane that lines freely moveable joint cavities, and secretes synovial fluid. (*Synovial fluid* is a lubricant that provides for the smoother motion of bone, reducing friction between the moving parts.)

Fascial membranes are sheets of tissues that hold organs in place. The superficial fascia is a layer that connects the skin to underlying structures. Deep fascia binds muscles to tendons to anchor bones, and separates muscles into functional groups.

Organs and Systems

An **organ** is a group of different types of tissues that form in a specific manner to perform a definite function (see Fig. 15-3A). For example, the heart is a combination of muscle, nerve, connective (blood), and epithelial tissues. Organs do not work independently but are associated with other organs. Organs have many functions.

Groups of organs are called **systems.** Each organ contributes its share to the function of the whole. Systems do specialized work in the body, but all systems depend on one another. An understanding of the structure and function of body systems is the basis for personal health habits and care of clients. Chapters 16 through 29 discuss the structure and function of body systems and their organs. See Table 15-4 for specific body systems and the components of each system.

It is important to remember that the organs and systems of the body are interdependent. That is, they depend on each other for proper functioning. In general, a malfunction of one system of the body often causes malfunctions in other systems as well. Disorders of the various body systems in adults are described and discussed in Unit 12. Disorders in children are discussed in Unit 11.

TABLE 15-4 ✎ *M*AJOR BODY SYSTEMS AND THEIR COMPONENTS

System	Components
Integumentary	Skin and its appendages, such as hair, nails, and sweat and oil glands
Musculoskeletal	Bones, joints, and muscles
Nervous	Brain, spinal cord, and nerves
Endocrine	Organs (thyroid, pituitary, adrenal, pancreas, ovary, testis) that produce hormones
Sensory	Organs (eyes, ears, tongue, nose, skin) that supply body with information
Cardiovascular	Organs (heart, blood vessels, and tissues) that transport blood to all parts of the body
Hematologic and lymphatic	Blood, its components (erythrocytes, leukocytes, platelets, and plasma), and lymphatic vessels
Immunologic	Specific blood cells and lymphatic organs
Respiratory	Lungs and passages leading to the lungs
Digestive	Organs (mouth, esophagus, stomach, intestines, liver, gallbladder, pancreas) involved in taking in and converting food to substances the body can use
Urinary	Organs (kidneys, ureter, bladder, and urethra) that rid the body of waste and water
Male reproductive	External sex organs and all related internal structures (penis, testes, vas deferens, epididymis)
Female reproductive	External sex organs and all related internal structures (vagina, oviducts, ovaries, uterus, vulva)

☛ KEY CONCEPT

The body operates as an integrated whole. The optimum functioning of one body system often depends on the functioning of other systems.

➤ STUDENT SYNTHESIS

Key Points

• The human body is made up of solids, liquids, and gases that function independently but are interrelated.

- The study of the human body can be subdivided into the studies of anatomy (structure), physiology (function), and pathophysiology (disorders of function).
- Medicine has developed a sophisticated system of describing anatomy and physiology called medical terminology. To assist the learner, much of this terminology can be broken down into prefixes, suffixes, and root words.
- The body is described in terms of superior, inferior, dorsal, and ventral directions. It is also described in terms of transverse, frontal, and sagittal planes, and specific cavities containing viscera.
- Homeostasis is the dynamic balance of an individual's physical and mental functioning.
- Substances are capable of undergoing physical changes in outward appearance or chemical changes with the transfer of energy and change in structure.
- The body can be described in terms of a single cell, which collaborates with similar cells in groups called tissues.
- Similar tissues, functioning as a group, constitute organs.
- Groups of organs make up body systems.
- Each cell is composed of many complex structures. Each structure has a specific duty that relates to the body as a whole.
- Cells have similar abilities, but have developed specialized functions. Some special abilities include metabolism, contractility, conductivity, and irritability.
- Genes, the controllers of heredity, are found on chromosomes.
- Body cells replicate (reproduce) through mitosis. Sex cells (eggs and sperm) replicate through meiosis.
- Human cells have 46 chromosomes.
- The body is made up of four basic kinds of tissue: epithelial, connective, muscle, and nerve.
- The body is organized according to systems (groups of organs) that work together to perform certain functions that contribute to the overall workings of the body.

Critical Thinking Exercises

1. Pick one body system and explain how its failure may affect other systems.

2. After listing the functions of the four types of body tissue, explain how these tissues complement each other.
3. A classmate is having trouble understanding the functions, structure, and properties of cells. How could you help your fellow student to better grasp these concepts?

NCLEX-Style Review Questions

1. Hepatitis means:
   a. Inflammation of the gallbladder
   b. Inflammation of the liver
   c. Removal of the gallbladder
   d. Removal of the liver
2. Which plane describes dividing the body into left and right sides?
   a. Coronal
   b. Frontal
   c. Midsagittal
   d. Transverse
3. Which of the following is an example of a compound found in the body?
   a. Calcium
   b. Nitrogen
   c. Phosphorous
   d. Water
4. Which part of the cell contains hereditary information?
   a. Gene
   b. Golgi apparatus
   c. Lysosomes
   d. Ribosomes
5. Which of the following is a function of connective tissue?
   a. Cover body surfaces
   b. Provide nutrients to all body organs
   c. Secrete substances from the digestive tract
   d. Transport particles contained in mucus away from the lungs

Reference

1. Cohen, B., & Wood, D. (2000). *Memmler's structure and function of the human body* (7th ed.). Philadelphia: Lippincott Williams & Wilkins.

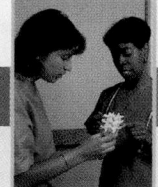

16

The Integumentary System

LEARNING OBJECTIVES

1. Describe the structures and main functions of the skin.
2. Describe the functions of keratin and melanin.
3. Identify the structures of a nail.
4. Compare and contrast the different functions of the sudoriferous glands and the sebaceous glands.
5. Define radiation, convection, evaporation, and conduction and give an example of each.
6. Explain the purpose of "goose bumps" or "goose flesh."
7. Discuss the skin's role in sensory awareness.
8. Name five changes that occur in aging skin.
9. Describe two ways to protect skin from damage.

NEW TERMINOLOGY

alopecia	hypodermis
carotene	integument
cerumen	keratin
ceruminal glands	melanin
collagen	radiation
conduction	sebaceous glands
convection	sebum
corium	skin turgor
dermis	squamous
desquamation	subcutaneous tissue
diaphoresis	sudoriferous glands
epidermis	thermoregulation
evaporation	transdermal
freckles	vitiligo
friable	

ACRONYMS

Hb or Hgb	SPF	UV

The skin and its accessory structures form the body's integumentary system. **Integument** means covering. Because skin covers the entire outside of the body, it is the body's largest organ. It is called an *organ* because it is composed of a variety of tissues, each of which has a specific purpose.

The skin contains several types of epithelial tissue that are partially responsible for the skin's protective and absorptive functions. Glands made of epithelial tissue provide secretions from the body's internal environment to the external world. Connective tissues attach skin to underlying muscle. Nervous tissue is integrated throughout the skin to help the body react to the world around it. Nerves are responsible for sensations of heat, cold, pain, touch, and pressure. In addition, the integumentary system depends on other tissues, organs, and systems. The skin and its accessory structures create a dynamic surface for communication between internal and external forces.

☞ KEY CONCEPT

The integumentary system is composed of the skin and its accessory structures: hair, nails, and glands. Integument *means* covering.

STRUCTURE AND FUNCTION

Primary functions of the integumentary system are protection, thermoregulation (temperature regulation), metabolism, sensation, and communication (Box 16-1). The skin produces substances that aid in protection and metabolism. Secreted oil acts as a waterproofing material, while protecting the skin from drying and cracking. Perspiration helps rid the body of waste products.

The skin has some absorptive powers. Scientists are learning how to use this mechanism to apply medications **transdermally** (through the skin). Certain skin cells are also important components of the immune system, which helps fight off foreign invaders (see Chap. 24).

Skin

Structurally, the skin is divided into two principal layers: the thin, superficial layer called the *epidermis* and the deep, thicker layer called the **dermis**. The **hypodermis** (commonly called the *subcutaneous tissue*) is not actually part of the skin, yet is discussed along with it because it anchors the skin to underlying tissues and organs. The epidermis makes up the skin's outer layer. Below the epidermis lies the dermis, which contains the important structures of hair, glands, blood vessels, and nerves. The hypodermis is a single layer of fat tissue below the dermis. It cushions, supports, nourishes, and insulates the skin (Fig 16-1).

The Epidermis

The **epidermis** is the outermost protective layer of the skin. It is composed of **squamous** (scaly) epithelium, stratified into several layers. The innermost layer of the epidermis is composed of living cells and is called the *stratum basale* (base) or *stratum germinativum,* indicating its role in germinating new cells. Here in the deepest level of the epidermis, mitosis (divi-

➤➤ BOX 16-1

FUNCTIONS OF THE INTEGUMENTARY SYSTEM

Protection
- Provides a physical barrier against microorganisms and foreign materials
- Helps prevent absorption of substances from outside the body
- Defends against many chemicals
- Protects against water loss or gain
- Protects underlying structures, such as fragile organs
- Protects against excessive sun exposure (ultraviolet rays)
- Cushions internal organs against trauma
- Produces secretions for protection and water regulation

Thermoregulation
- Controls body temperature by convection, evaporation, conduction, and radiation
- Helps body adjust to external changes in temperature
- Helps dissipate heat during exercise
- Produces shivering and "goose flesh" to keep body warm in cool temperatures
- Cools the body through evaporation

Metabolism
- Provides insulation (skin hairs, subcutaneous fat)
- Helps produce and use vitamin D
- Helps the body eliminate certain waste products
- Absorbs medication
- Provides storage of fat
- Contributes to changes in cardiac output and blood pressure

Sensation
- Perceives stimuli: heat, cold, pain, pressure, touch
- Provides social and sexual communication
- Allows for physical intimacy

Communication
- Communicates feelings and moods through facial expressions
- Portrays feelings of anger, embarrassment, or fear (eg, flushing, sweating, pallor)
- Communicates cultural and sexual differences through skin and hair color
- Portrays body image via skin's general appearance

sion and replication of cells) occurs. As these cells, known as *keratinocytes* (see Table 16-1), divide in the basal layer, they push older cells toward the body's surface. Thus, the living inner cells of the epidermis continually replace the outer cells. The replacement process takes between 2 and 4 weeks for the inner cells to totally replace the outer layer.

The outer layer, the *stratum corneum* or *horny layer,* provides a barrier against light, heat, bacteria, and chemicals. This layer contains all the dead cells from the layers below.

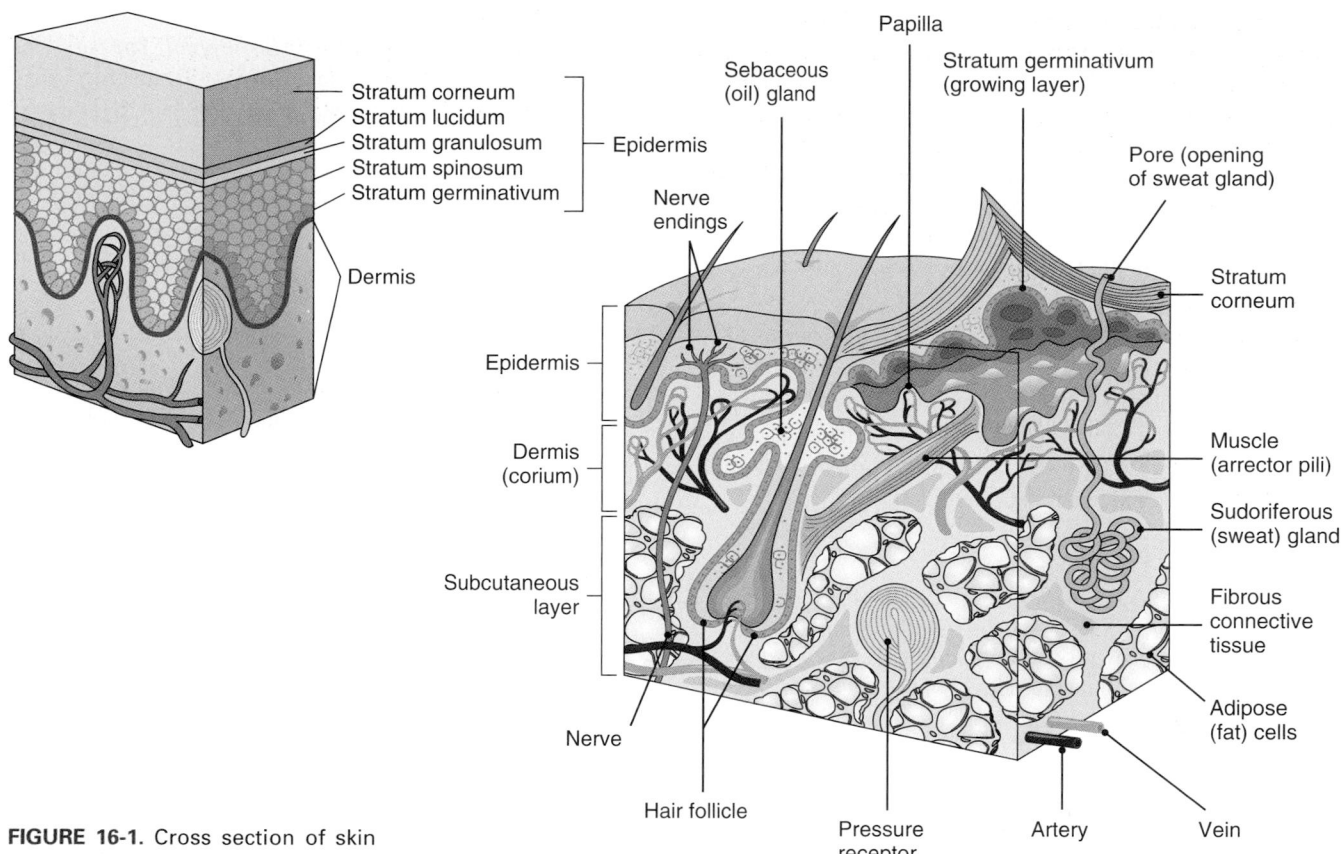

FIGURE 16-1. Cross section of skin structures.

These cells are rubbed off constantly through washing and friction. This process is called **desquamation.**

All that is left of the cells after desquamation is a protein called **keratin.** Keratin is the body's true protector. It creates a waterproof barrier. Most microorganisms cannot penetrate unbroken skin because of keratin.

☛ KEY CONCEPT

Damage through the base layer of the epidermis to the dermis (such as in a second- or third-degree burn) takes longer to heal because the damaged skin has lost its mitotic (reproductive) structures.

■■ TABLE 16-1 𝒫RINCIPAL CELLS OF THE EPIDERMIS

Type	Function
Keratinocyte	Produces keratin, which waterproofs and protects skin
Melanocyte	Produces the pigment melanin
Langerhans (also called *nonpigmented granular dendrocyte*)	Provides immune response
Merkel	Promotes sensation of touch

The epidermis has no nerves or blood supply. It does not receive direct nourishment from the circulatory system. Normally the epidermis and the dermis do not lie flat on one another. The dermis reaches up into the epidermis, causing ripples on the skin surface that are particularly visible on the tips of the fingers; here, this is known as fingerprints.

Sometimes friction causes a separation of the epidermis and dermis, leading to tissue fluid accumulation (blister). Areas of greater friction, such as the soles of the feet and the palms of the hands, cause the epidermis there to thicken and to develop calluses.

The Dermis

The **dermis,** also known as the **corium,** is the "true skin." It is the thickest skin layer, composed entirely of live cells. The dermis contains blood and lymph vessels, nerves, hair follicles, sweat (sudoriferous) glands, and oil (sebaceous) glands. The dermal layer nourishes and supports the ever-changing epidermis.

Several types of connective tissue are found in the dermis. One of these is **collagen** ("colla" means glue), a tough, resistant, and flexible fibrous protein. In youth, collagen is loose and elastic. Collagen hardens and loses elasticity with age.

The Subcutaneous Tissue

The **subcutaneous tissue** (or **hypodermis**) is the layer beneath the dermis and on top of the layer of muscle. Its purpose is to attach the epidermal and dermal layers to underlying

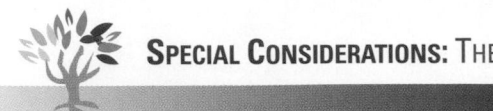

SPECIAL CONSIDERATIONS: THE LIFE SPAN

Wrinkling of Skin

Wrinkles occur due to the loss of collagen and elastic fibers in the skin. (Cigarette smoking has been linked to a more rapid destruction of these fibers, and can lead to the development of wrinkles at a younger age.)

organs. It specializes in the formation and storage of *lipocytes* (fat cells). Functionally, the subcutaneous tissue cushions and protects underlying areas. It also serves as a heat insulator. The amount of fat stored depends on the body region and an individual's age, sex, and nutritional state.

Skin Color

A combination of three pigments produces normal coloration of the skin: melanin, carotene, and hemoglobin.

Melanin is a brown-black pigment produced by *melanocytes,* found mostly in the basal layer of the epidermis. People of all races have the same number of melanocytes. Individual differences in skin color depend on the amount of pigment the melanocytes produce. The amount of melanin produced is a reflection of genetics and exposure to ultraviolet (**UV**) light. Melanin protects the body from the damaging effects of UV light. (*Albino* individuals are born without the ability to make melanin from the melanocytes. A true albino person has totally white hair and skin. This person's eyes look red because of the lack of pigment in the iris and because of the reflection of the blood vessels in the eyes.)

Freckles are patches of melanin clustered together. "Liver spots" (age spots) are also clusters of melanin, forming flat, brown-to-black freckle-like patches as a person ages. **Vitiligo** is a skin condition in which the melanocytes stop making melanin, causing distinct, localized areas of white.

Carotene is a yellowish pigment found in parts of the epidermis and dermis. Carotene is the precursor to vitamin A. It tends to be more abundant in the skin of Asian people.

Hemoglobin is a pigment found in red blood cells. Oxygen binds to the hemoglobin (**Hb, Hgb**) molecule and is carried by the red blood cells. The bright-red color of oxygenated blood flowing throughout the dermis gives a pinkish tone to the skin of light-skinned people.

Accessory Structures

The hair, nails, sebaceous (oil) glands, sudoriferous (sweat) glands, and ceruminal glands are the main accessory structures (appendages) of the skin.

Hair

Hair covers almost all the skin except for a few areas, such as the palms, soles, and penis. Dense hair covers the scalp, axilla, and pubis in adults. Male hormones may cause greater density of hair on men's entire bodies and influence their ability to grow facial and chest hair.

Hair is composed of keratinized cells. The visible, but dead, portion of hair above the skin is the *shaft.* The part lying below the skin is the *root.* Each hair grows from a tiny sac or bulb within a *hair follicle* (see Fig. 16-1). The dermal skin layer provides nutrients for growing hair in much the same manner as the epidermis receives nutrients. (Topical hair care products do not affect hair growth, only the general appearance of visible hair.) Hair grows slowly (approximately 1 mm every 3 days). Each follicle contains a single hair root, which, as long as it is alive, will continue to grow a hair. We all lose 25 to 100 hairs each day. Each hair lost is actually pushed out by the growth of a new hair.

Baldness (**alopecia**) is related to disease, high fever, emotional stress, surgery, pregnancy, starvation, chemotherapy, radiation, or hereditary factors. The male hormone, testosterone, contributes to male pattern baldness in men. Healthy women rarely become totally bald, although they may experience thinning hair with age.

Hair color is due to the type and amount of melanin in a layer of hair. The greater the amount of melanin, the darker the hair. Red hair is due to a pigment with an iron base (trichosiderin).

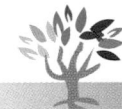

SPECIAL CONSIDERATIONS: THE LIFE SPAN

Melanin in Hair

As people age, they lose melanin, and their hair appears gray; with a total loss of melanin, hair appears white.

Surrounding each hair follicle are small, smooth muscles called the *arrector pili* (singular: *arrectores pilorum*). Stimulated by cold or fear, these involuntary muscles contract, making the hairs stand erect. This phenomenon gives the skin the appearance of "goose flesh" or "goose bumps." These erect hairs provide an "air cushion" for the skin—a protective, insulating body mechanism.

The primary function of hair is protection. Scalp hair protects against sunlight and insulates against cold. Eyelashes and eyebrows have the distinctive purpose of keeping dust particles and perspiration out of the eyes. Nostril hair protects against inhaling objects such as foreign particles or insects. Hair in the ear canal serves a similar purpose.

Clinically, hair can reveal several adverse conditions. A hair sample can reveal environmental exposure to heavy metals or other poisons much more accurately than a blood specimen. Hair texture can also reveal an individual's nutritional status. A hair sample yields DNA and therefore can be used for identification purposes.

Nails

Nails protect the sensitive tips of fingers and toes. They help a person grab and pick up objects. Nails are tightly packed cells of the stratum corneum of the epidermis. The parts of a fingernail, as depicted in Fig. 16-2, are keratinized dead cells.

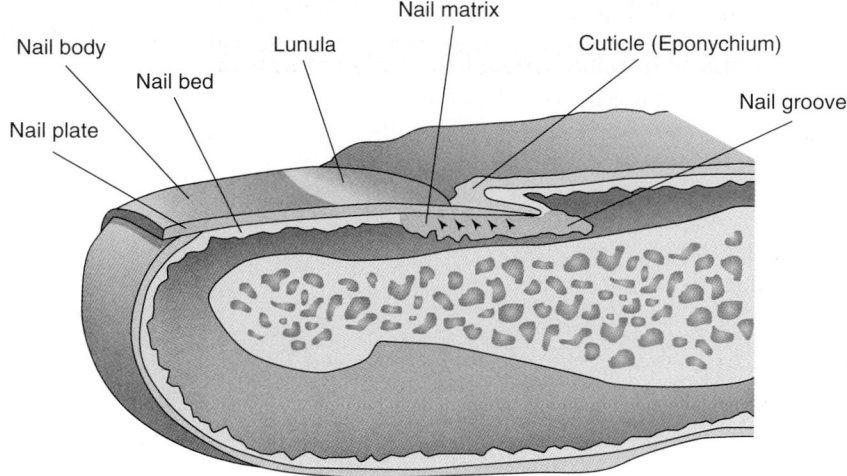

FIGURE 16-2. Parts of a fingernail. **Nail matrix:** Where nail growth occurs; part of nail groove. **Lunula:** White, half–moon shaped area at base of nail; white color is caused by air mixed with keratin. **Cuticle (eponychium):** Band of epidermis covering nail bed; called "hangnail" when it splits. **Nail bed:** Epidermis under the nail.

Nail growth occurs in the nail matrix. The new cells push the older cells away from the nail bed at a rate of approximately 1 millimeter per week. A fingernail lost through trauma takes about 3 to 5 months to regrow, and a toenail takes about 12 to 18 months to completely regrow. A nail will continue to regrow as long as the live cells in the nail bed remain undamaged.

Nails normally reflect a pinkish tone because of rich vascular areas in the fingers. When gentle pressure is applied and released, the nail becomes white but quickly returns to a pink color. Unhealthy nails may point to poor circulatory status and several nutritional deficiencies.

 N u r s i n g   A l e r t

Nail biting is often a nervous habit. Caution clients against nail biting because it can lead to skin infections.

SPECIAL CONSIDERATIONS: NUTRITION

Effects of Diet on Skin, Hair, and Nails

Healthy skin, hair, and nails depend on a well-balanced diet. Protein and vitamin deficiencies leave skin and hair dull, dry, and flaky. Minerals such as iron, copper, and zinc are necessary for the prevention of abnormal skin pigmentation and changes in hair and nails.[1] Starvation can cause excessive hair loss and nail deformities.

Sebaceous or Oil Glands

The **sebaceous glands** (oil glands) lie close to the hair follicles, into which they usually drain (see Fig. 16-1). **Sebum** is the oily secretion of these glands; it travels to the surface of the skin through the hair follicles. Sebum helps make the skin soft and the hair glossy. As a defense mechanism, sebum prevents drying of the skin, thereby protecting it from cracking. Cracked areas in the skin are an invitation to invasion by microorgan-

isms. Sebum also helps to waterproof the top layer of the epidermis (the *stratum corneum*).

The activity of the sebaceous glands increases at puberty. Sebum may trap bacteria in the skin's pores, causing inflamed or infected glands, commonly known as pimples or acne.

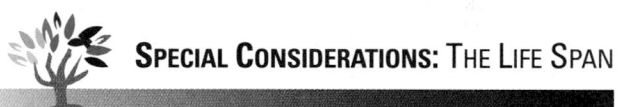 **SPECIAL CONSIDERATIONS:** THE LIFE SPAN

Sebaceous Glands

Aging decreases the activities of the sebaceous glands; therefore, older skin is transparent, more dry than youthful skin, and more fragile (**friable**). This occurrence is due to a flattening of the epidermal and dermal skin layers and a thinning of the dermal layers, which predisposes an older adult to skin tears. A decrease in glandular secretions also causes drying of the skin.

Sudoriferous or Sweat Glands

The **sudoriferous glands** (sweat glands) are located in the dermis. There are three types of glands: apocrine, eccrine, and mammary glands.

Apocrine sweat glands become active during puberty, secreting a milky sweat into the hair follicle. The apocrine glands are most numerous in the axillae, pubic region, areolae of the breasts, external ear canals, and eyelids. The nominal odor from these glands gives each person an individual scent. Skin surface bacteria cause the apocrine sweat to become odoriferous. A "cold sweat" occurs when emotional stressors, such as anxiety or fear, stimulate these glands.

The second type, *eccrine* sweat glands, are distributed widely over the body, but are especially numerous on the upper lip, forehead, back, palms, and soles. Eccrine glands secrete sweat into numerous ducts that empty into pores. One inch of skin contains approximately 3,000 sweat glands.

Perspiration (sweat) is nearly 100% water, with trace amounts of urea, uric acid, salts, and other elements. The primary function of perspiration is to assist in the regulation of body temperature by providing a cooling effect. Perspiration also moisturizes the skin's surface and excretes waste products through the skin's pores. In some disease states, the skin increases its capacity as an excretory organ, a noticeable clinical sign of pathology. (**Diaphoresis** refers to excessive perspiration.)

Mammary glands are a third, specialized type of sudoriferous gland. They secrete milk. Chapter 29 discusses these glands in greater detail.

Ceruminal Glands

Ceruminal glands are specialized glands found only in the skin of the external auditory meatus, a passage that leads into the ear. The function of these glands is to protect the tympanic membrane (eardrum), which is essential to hearing.

Cerumen (ear wax) that accumulates excessively may impair hearing and promote infection in the ear canal. The moisture content of cerumen varies somewhat among the races, and this may affect hearing acuity or the tendency toward ear infections.

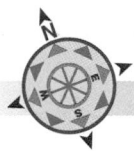

SPECIAL CONSIDERATIONS: CULTURE

Cerumen

Dry cerumen (gray, brittle, and flaky) occurs most often in Native Americans (84%), Alaska Natives, and people of Asian descent. The remaining 16% have wet cerumen. Wet cerumen (dark brown, moist, and sticky) occurs most often in African Americans (99%) and whites (97%). Do not confuse these differences with physical disorders. For example, flakes of cerumen can be mistaken for dry lesions of eczema or psoriasis.

SYSTEM PHYSIOLOGY

Although the integumentary system's functions are many, protection is by far the most important.

Protection

The skin and its accessory structures guard the body from noxious outside elements, preventing invasion into the internal environment. The skin further protects the body by retarding the loss of body fluid and by excreting waste products.

Thermoregulation

The integumentary system is also responsible for maintaining the body's internal temperature through a process called **thermoregulation.** The body's temperature must remain fairly constant for all other systems to function properly. The skin also helps the individual to experience the outside world through sensory awareness. The physiology of these two particular activities is discussed below.

Body temperature is an indicator of physiologic changes occurring in a person's body. One important nursing technique is how to measure accurate body temperature.

The body uses thermoregulation to regulate and to balance body temperature. The body loses heat through four processes: radiation, convection, evaporation, and conduction (Tab. 16-2). The body conserves heat through shivering and "goose flesh."

The sweat glands and the lungs are major factors in the thermoregulation of the body's internal temperature.

Mechanisms of Heat Loss

If the body becomes too warm, the dermal capillaries dilate (widen), and more blood flows to the skin surface. Because more blood is brought to the surface, body heat is lost to the surrounding air by radiation, convection, evaporation, or conduction.

Radiation.   People and animals give off infrared heat rays through **radiation.** A large percentage of a person's body heat is lost through the head, because it functions similar to a chimney.

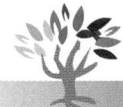

SPECIAL CONSIDERATIONS: THE LIFE SPAN

Heat Loss in Newborns

To prevent heat loss in the newborn, keep the infant away from drafts and place him or her in a temperature-regulated environment. Keep the infant dry and place a hat on the head.

Convection.   In **convection,** heat is transferred from a surface (the skin) to the surrounding gases (the air). For example, an air current (such as a fan) can move warm air away from the skin's surface. Convection results in the loss of body heat.

Evaporation.   Water on the body's surface can be perspiration (sweat) or water from an outside source, such as a shower. Water on the skin is lost by evaporation, which causes a cooling effect. **Evaporation** is the returning of water to the air through vapor. The body normally loses about 500 milliliters of water per day due to insensible (unnoticed) evaporation. Too much water loss can lead to dehydration.

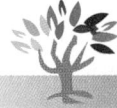

SPECIAL CONSIDERATIONS: THE LIFE SPAN

Heat Transfer in Infants

Infants are prone to heat loss, due to a large body surface area in proportion to their size. They are prone to loss through all four mechanisms of heat transfer, especially evaporation. This is particularly true immediately after birth.

■■■ TABLE 16-2 ⟋ℳECHANISMS OF HEAT TRANSFER

	Radiation	Convection	Evaporation	Conduction
Definition	The diffusion or dissemination of heat by electromagnetic waves	The dissemination of heat by motion between areas of unequal intensity	The conversion of a liquid to a vapor	The transfer of heat to another object during direct contact
Example	The body gives off waves of heat from uncovered surfaces.	An oscillating fan blows currents of cool air across the surface of a warm body.	Body fluid in the form of perspiration and insensible loss is vaporized from the skin.	The body transfers heat to an ice pack, causing the ice to melt.
Illustration				

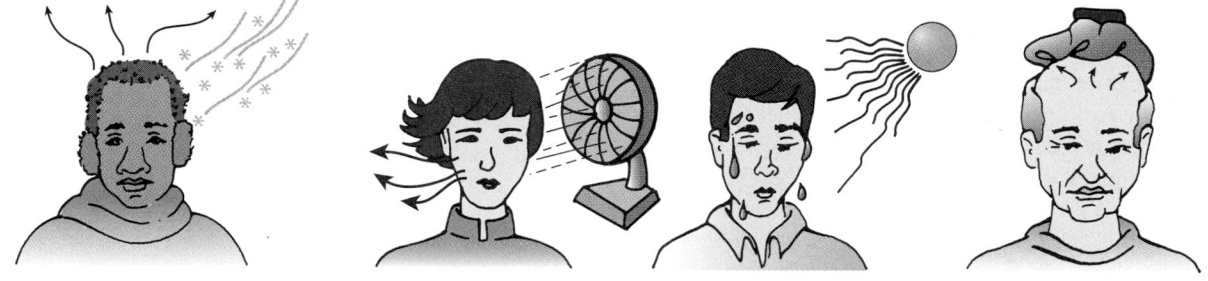

Taylor, C. (2001). *Fundamentals of nursing: The art and science of nursing care* (4th ed., p. 420). Philadelphia: Lippincott Williams & Wilkins.

Conduction. **Conduction** is the transfer of heat from one object to another by direct contact. It is the least important mechanism in the transfer of heat away from the body; however, within the body a large amount of heat is transmitted by conduction to the skin via the blood vessels. When the body comes in contact with a cooler object, the body transfers heat away from itself. For example, a cool cloth on the forehead or a tepid bath can help a person feel cooler on a hot day. Table 16-2 summarizes the mechanisms of heat transfer discussed here.

Mechanisms of Heat Production and Conservation

Blood vessel constriction, shivering, and "goose flesh" are thermoregulation processes that help to warm the body. When the body becomes too cool, dermal capillaries constrict (narrow), reducing the amount of heat lost through the skin. This constriction of superficial capillaries also causes the skin color to change from its normal color to a more pale color. The reflex action of shivering helps to produce added heat. As stated before, the *arrector pili* muscles contract and cause "goose bumps" to provide an insulating layer against cold.

 **Nursing Alert**

Vasoconstriction in the extremities can cause pallor (whiteness) and coolness of the skin. *Cyanosis* (red-blue coloring) is a condition due to hypoxia (lack of oxygen in the bloodstream) or hypothermia (severe decrease in body temperature).

SPECIAL CONSIDERATIONS: THE LIFE SPAN

Preventing Heat Loss in Infants

Very young infants do not have the ability to shiver to produce heat. Infants should be kept warm by adding clothing, particularly a hat, or external heat sources.

Metabolism. The skin insulates the body by heat-production mechanisms and with its subcutaneous fat located under the dermal layer. The more subcutaneous fat a person has, the better their ability to insulate the body. *Vasoconstriction* can occur when blood needs to be directed away from the periphery (that is, the skin) and moved toward the major organs of the body, such as the heart and brain, to maintain homeostasis (the regulation of blood pressure and cardiac output) in the body.

Vitamin D Production

The skin plays a role in the body's production of vitamin D from sunlight. Vitamin D is important for the growth and repair of bones, because it facilitates the absorption of calcium and phosphorous from the small intestine. Vitamin D is produced in the skin by sunlight (UV light); then, via enzymes in the body, it is changed into a substance known as *calcitrol.* Calcitrol plays a role in absorbing calcium from the body's gastrointestinal tract.

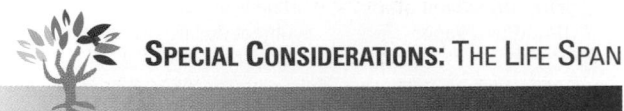

SPECIAL CONSIDERATIONS: THE LIFE SPAN

Vitamin D Deficiency

Lactase, the enzyme needed to break down the milk sugar lactose, decreases with advancing age, resulting in milk intolerance for some older adults. Decreased intake of irradiated milk accompanied by limited sun exposure (secondary to confined bed rest or nursing home living) doubles the risk of vitamin D deficiency in older adults. Bone loss (due to the inability to metabolize calcium) is one consequence of vitamin D deficiency.

Communication and Sensory Awareness

The skin receives stimuli from the outside world, providing a dynamic interaction between external and internal environments. Nerve endings in the dermis register pain and pleasure. The nerve receptors in the skin sense hot and cold and provide the original message to the brain. The body may react with a reflex response, for example by withdrawing the hand from a hot stove or a frozen piece of metal. (These unconscious reactions are discussed in later chapters.) This sensory awareness is part of the skin's protection of the body. The pain caused by other trauma creates bodily awareness in the same way.

The skin can also detect comfortable sensations. It registers the loving touch of a friend or family member. The skin and blood vessels are involved in foreplay, love making, and sexual response. Much of the communication between a newborn and its parents comes through the sense of touch. Nurses also use touch in therapeutic ways in the care of their clients.

Communication also occurs through facial movements and changes in skin color. For example, blushing usually changes the skin color to a redder or darker hue. Human differences also are displayed in how a person uses makeup on skin and polish on nail surfaces.

Disorders of the skin and other structures of the integumentary system are discussed in Chapter 74.

EFFECTS OF AGING ON THE INTEGUMENTARY SYSTEM

Table 16-3 summarizes the major effects of aging on the system. Normal changes are influenced by heredity, dietary habits, sun exposure, smoking, hydration level, and general health.

With age, skin tends to become dry and often appears scaly. It takes on a transparent or translucent appearance and, with the

■ ■ ■ TABLE 16-3 *Effects* OF AGING ON THE INTEGUMENTARY SYSTEM

Factors	Result	Nursing Implications
Melanin is either lost or migrates and clusters in the epidermal layer.	"Age spots" or "liver spots" result.	Reinforce self-esteem. Discuss available makeup.
Epidermal and dermal layers flatten.	Skin tends to tear ("fragile" or friable skin).	Assess for skin tears. Use caution in handling the older person.
Capillary bed in dermis becomes more friable (fragile)—blood can ooze into dermis.	Dark red patches in the skin (purpura) are commonly seen on arms of older adults.	Be careful when handling the arms of clients with purpura.
Capillaries leak small amounts of blood into tissues.	Petechiae occur (small red dots on skin).	Explain to the person that makeup may be used.
Individual may have loss of sensation and loss of abilities.	Person is unable to detect or treat cause of ulcerated areas; pressure ulcers may develop more quickly.	Inspect skin frequently, especially bony prominences, arms, and feet.
There is loss of elasticity in dermis, loss of subcutaneous layer of fat, and loss of collagen fibers.	Wrinkles. Decreased strength of skin layer.	Discourage smoking and exposure to the sun. Reinforce self-esteem.
Turgor is lost.	Wrinkles. "Tenting" on some areas can give false positive (for dehydration).	Avoid using areas of skin that normally develop wrinkles for assessing turgor. (Do not use back of hand; OK to use arm or leg.)
Some insulating function is lost with loss of subcutaneous fat.	Heat is lost more rapidly. The older person may be chilly.	Provide extra blankets or sweater. Avoid chilling during treatments.

(continued)

■■■ **TABLE 16-3** *E*FFECTS OF AGING ON THE INTEGUMENTARY SYSTEM (CONTINUED)

Factors	Result	Nursing Implications
Dermal layer thins.	Skin becomes transparent.	Explain to client.
Changes occur in hair distribution, influenced by heredity and other factors. General loss of body hair occurs.	Axillary, pubic, and scalp hair thins. Men may develop thicker hair in nose, ears, and eyebrows; hair on head becomes thinner.	Be careful when giving hair care. Excess hair in nose or ears may be clipped carefully.
Female hormones are lost.	Women may develop facial hair (hirsutism).	Assist in removal of facial hair. Prevent injury.
Nails grow more slowly and become thicker.	Nails, especially toenails, become thick and brittle.	Refer to podiatrist as needed.
The glands in the skin decrease their secretions.	Less perspiration and less oily skin than before causes skin to become very dry (may appear scaly).	Advise that daily shower or bath may not be needed (bath may dry skin more). Be sure skin is clean, because skin is more fragile and more subject to breakdown. Use lotion as needed.
Thermoregulation abilities are lost.	More susceptible to heatstroke.	Teach individual to avoid overheating. Observe in hot weather; encourage intake of adequate fluids.
Circulation is reduced.	Wound healing takes longer—old or damaged cells are not readily replaced.	Provide careful wound care. Prevent further injury. Refer to physician as needed.

loss of subcutaneous (under the skin) fat, the skin may sag and become wrinkled. **Skin turgor** (tone) is reduced; a pinched area does not return immediately into position. The glands in the skin decrease their secretions; therefore, the older person has less perspiration and less oily skin. Hair becomes coarser and increases in areas such as the nose, ears, and eyebrows. Male pattern baldness is common. Women may develop hirsutism (facial hair).

The skin of the older person is more fragile (**friable**) and more subject to breakdown than the skin of the young person. The skin loses its elasticity, partly because of impaired circulation. The loss of subcutaneous fat removes some of the skin's insulating function; heat is lost more rapidly. For this reason, older people often have difficulty keeping warm.

In general, aged skin becomes thinner, epidermal turnover decreases, and the number of protective cells diminishes. As a result, many older adults heal poorly and are at increased risk for pressure ulcers, fungal or viral skin infections, and skin cancer.

MAINTENANCE OF HEALTHY SKIN

The various functions of the skin (and related structures) make it a very important organ of the body. The skin requires nutrients and hydration to keep it functioning well. Eating a healthy diet and drinking plenty of fluids daily are practices that can assist the skin to remain healthy. Sun exposure can be a risk to the skin. Excess exposure can cause burns, premature aging of the skin, or skin cancer. In order to protect the skin, exposure to the sun should be limited by wearing long-sleeved clothing, hats, sunscreen with a **SPF** (sun protection factor) of at least 15, and staying in the shade as much as possible.

☛ KEY CONCEPT

Skin is the first line of defense against infection. Therefore, maintenance of skin integrity is a high priority.

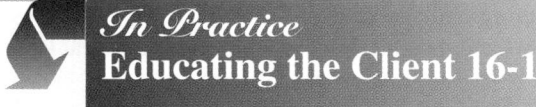 **N u r s i n g   A l e r t**
The use of sunscreens is not advisable for infants under 6 months of age.

In Practice
Educating the Client 16-1

SUNSCREENS

Sunscreens are used to protect the skin from the sun's UV rays. They can assist in prevention of skin cancers caused by sun exposure. Apply sunscreen thoroughly and evenly so there is complete coverage. Reapply after sweating or swimming. Remember, even if the SPF factor is high, there is a suggested limit to the amount of time that is recommended for a person to remain in the sun, to prevent the risk of sunburn. Always read the directions on the bottle of sunscreen and follow them exactly.

When using sunscreen, also consider allergies to the sunscreen ingredients and adverse reactions with certain medications. Sunscreens may cause problems for people with certain skin problems, such as skin cancer or lupus, or for people undergoing radiation or chemotherapy.

Virtually every tissue and organ in the body takes an active part in maintaining homeostasis. Body fluids, which are composed of water and the substances dissolved and suspended in it, form the environment of each body cell. The fluids move into and out of the cells, bringing with them enzymes, hormones, and nutrients, as well as removing waste products (the end products of metabolism). This continual movement of fluids is necessary for maintaining stable or constant conditions in the body's internal environment (homeostasis). This chapter reviews the importance of water and various electrolytes, and the main systems of fluid transport within the body.

HOMEOSTASIS

Homeostasis is the dynamic process through which the body maintains balance by constantly adjusting to internal and external stimuli. (Home/o means constant or sameness and the suffix -stasis means controlling; therefore, homeostasis means "controlling sameness.") The concept of homeostasis is the basis for understanding most physiologic processes.

For the body to maintain homeostasis, it must be able to sense minute (tiny) changes and react appropriately. To do so, the body has sensors and integrating centers that involve the cells of all the body's systems.

Negative and Positive Feedback

All components of the body constantly send tiny signals that cause responses. Simply stated, **feedback** is the relaying of information about a given condition to the appropriate organ or system.

Negative feedback occurs when the body reverses an original stimulus to regain physiologic balance (homeostasis). Body systems resist deviations, normally allowing for small variations only. Blood pressure control and maintenance of body temperature are examples of negative feedback systems. Illness interrupts negative feedback; healthcare measures attempt to restore negative feedback mechanisms. All nursing care aims at restoring and maintaining the individual's homeostasis or equilibrium (normal state) as much as possible.

In *positive feedback,* the body enhances or intensifies the original stimulus. The body senses deviations, but the feedback generally is not homeostatic. In fact, with positive feedback, the body responds by making the deviation greater. A normal example is a woman in labor. When labor begins, impulses are sent to stimulate the release of the hormone oxytocin, which then increases uterine contraction strength and frequency. In an abnormal condition, positive feedback systems can lead to greater instability and frequently lead to death.

Systems Involved in Feedback

The major systems involved in feedback are the nervous and endocrine systems, which are discussed in Chapters 19 and 20, respectively. Simply explained, the nervous system regulates homeostasis by sensing system deviations and sending nerve impulses to appropriate organs to restore balance. The endocrine system uses the release and action of hormones to maintain homeostasis.

☞ KEY CONCEPT

An individual must maintain internal homeostasis to maintain health.

BODY FLUIDS

Fluids make up a large portion of the body. Body fluids are composed of water and electrolytes (substances that dissolve in water).

Location of Fluids

Body fluids are divided between two main compartments: the intracellular fluid (**ICF**) and the extracellular fluid (**ECF**). ICF is the fluid inside the cells and constitutes about two thirds of the total body fluid in an adult. ECF is the fluid outside the cells and constitutes about one third of the total body fluid in an adult. Fluids continuously move between compartments (Fig. 17-1). The compartments contain slightly different components, and several homeostatic mechanisms work to maintain the correct balance of fluid to solid substances within each compartment.

Intracellular Fluid
ICF functions as a stabilizing agent for the parts of the cell. It helps to maintain cell shape. ICF also assists with the transport of nutrients across the cell membrane and in and out of the cell.

Extracellular Fluid
ECF appears mostly as *interstitial* (tissue) fluid and *intravascular* (within the blood vessels) fluid. **Interstitial** fluid is found between the cells. **Intravascular** fluid is the watery fluid of the blood known as *plasma.* Specialized ECFs, such as synovial fluid in the joint cavities, **CSF** (cerebral spinal fluid) in the brain and spinal cord, and aqueous fluid in the eyes are also present in the body. Some additional ECFs are located in the **GI** (gastrointestinal) tract, liver, biliary tracts, and lymphatic vessels.

The volume of ECF is the most important regulated aspect of body fluid balance. Without an adequate volume of ECF, the body cannot maintain normal blood pressure. A significant loss of ECF volume can drop blood pressure to a life-threatening point where cells can no longer function, due to a lack of oxygen and nutrients. This results in a condition known as *hypovolemic shock.* Too much ECF can place a person in a fluid overload state, leading to high blood pressure and risk for conditions such as congestive heart failure.

☞ KEY CONCEPT

ECF is the fluid that is most important in fluid balance.

The body monitors ECF volumes closely and sends messages to the brain, kidneys, and pituitary gland to maintain control. Primary mechanisms involved in regulation include: the actions of the thirst center in the hypothalamus; the release of antidiuretic hormone (**ADH**) from the pituitary gland; the

Backyard lawn   as compared to   Organism such as human body

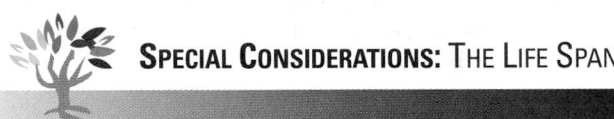

Extracellular Fluid

Soil

Interstitial or fluid within the tissues, eg, muscle tissue

Water source within soil

Intravascular fluid eg, fluid within plasma of capillaries

Intracellular Fluid

Seed

Intracellular fluid, eg, fluid within any cell of the body

FIGURE 17-1. Examples of fluid compartments. Fluid continually moves between compartments.

effects of the renin–angiotensin–aldosterone (**RAA**) system; and the release of the atrial natriuretic peptide (**ANP**) hormone by the heart (Fig. 17-2).

The Thirst Center. The thirst center in the hypothalamus stimulates or depresses the desire for a person to drink.

Antidiuretic Hormone. ADH is released from storage in the posterior pituitary gland as part of the negative feedback mechanism in response to conditions within the cardiovascular system. For example, ADH is released in response to low blood volume (as seen in low blood pressure) or in response to an increase in concentration of sodium in the intravascular fluid (blood plasma). ADH regulates the amount of water that the kidneys absorb. When ADH is released, the production of urine is decreased and water reabsorption in the kidney tubules is increased.

The RAA System. The RAA system is used to control fluid volume. When there is a decrease in blood volume, renin is released by the kidneys. The renin causes secretion of angiotensin I, which is converted to angiotensin II (by an enzyme) in the lungs. Angiotensin II causes constriction of the blood vessels to increase blood pressure, and the secretion of aldosterone. Aldosterone controls the reabsorption of sodium by the kidneys. Water "follows" sodium (or salt). This concept is explained later in this chapter.

Atrial Natriuretic Peptide. The heart can also play a role in correcting overload imbalances by releasing ANP from the right atrium. ANP promotes renal diuresis (kidney excretion) of sodium and water. Figure 17-2 illustrates fluid regulation in the body. These processes will be discussed further in Chapter 27.

Overhydration and Edema

Overhydration is an excess of water in the body. **Edema** is the excess accumulation of fluid in the interstitial (tissue) spaces. This fluid can also be called **third-space fluid.** Edema is due

SPECIAL CONSIDERATIONS: THE LIFE SPAN

Risk for Fluid Volume Deficit

Infants have considerably more body fluid by percentage than adults do, the majority of which is ECF. They are at an increased risk for fluid volume deficit because ECF is lost more easily than ICF. Also, immature kidney function places infants and young children at risk for alterations in fluid and electrolyte levels.

to a disruption of the filtration and osmotic forces of the body's circulating fluids. Some causes of edema include obstruction of venous blood or lymphatic return, increased capillary permeability or increased capillary pressure, external pressure (eg, tight binders or casts), and inflammatory reactions. A loss of the proteins in the plasma of the blood also leads to edema. Box 17-1 discusses some of the causes of edema.

Some edema may be local, such as in an injured ankle. Edema can also be systemic (throughout the body), which is symptomatic of other, more profound medical problems. Many conditions such as burns, kidney disease, congestive heart failure, or malignancies (cancer) can result in systemic edema. Treatment of edema is directed at treating the underlying cause. Diuretics are medications commonly given for systemic edema. (These medications increase the total loss of body fluids and salts via the kidneys.)

Some body fluids are not available for functional use. These are the extracellular fluids that have collected within the interstitial spaces in various parts of the body. Excess fluid accumulations in the interstitial spaces are often due to inflammatory conditions. Examples include pleural effusion (an accumulation

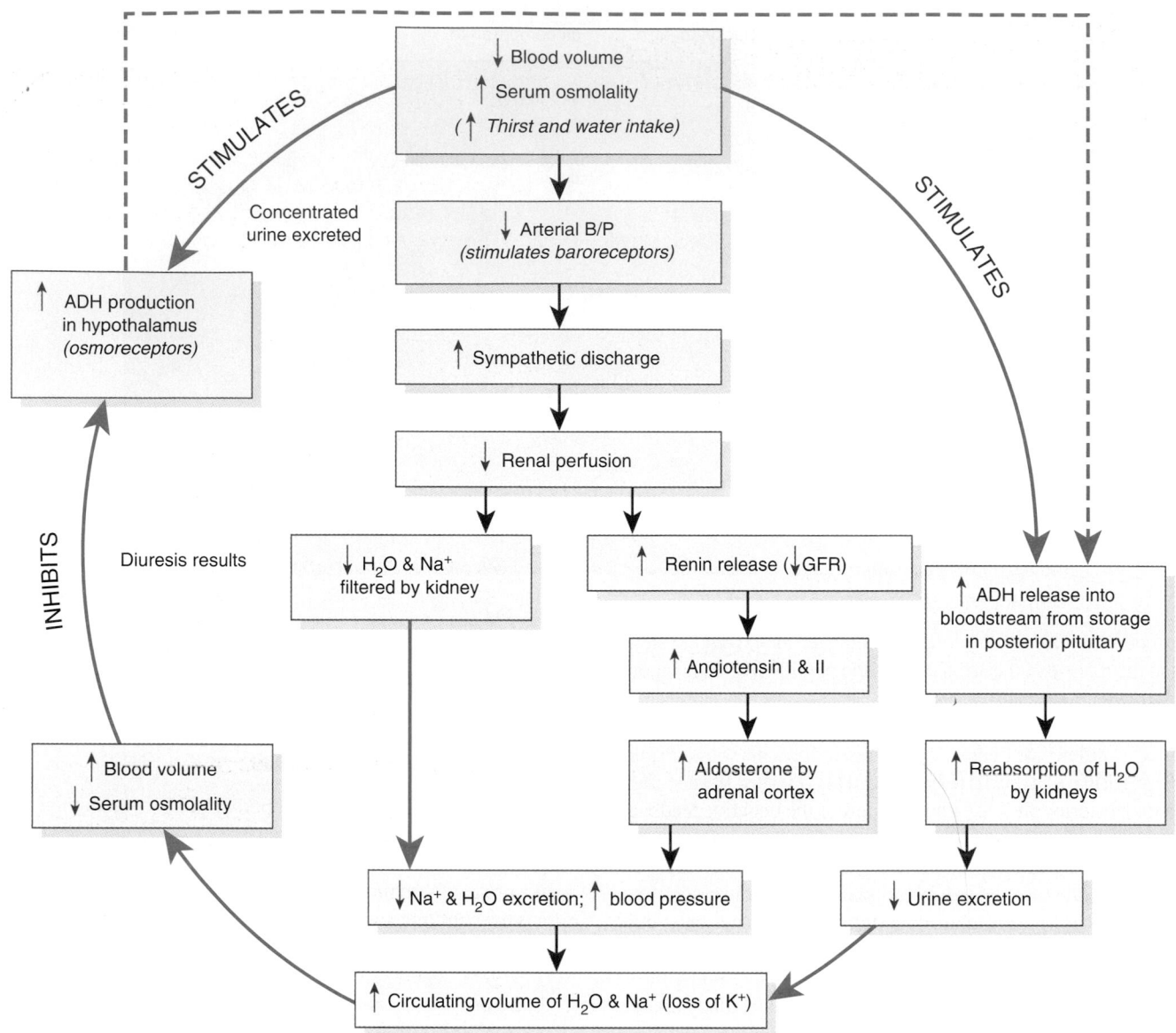

FIGURE 17-2. Fluid regulation cycle, including antidiuretic hormone (ADH) and the renin–angiotensin–aldosterone (RAA) system.

of fluid between the pleura of the lungs) or pericardial effusion (an accumulation of fluid within the pericardial sac around the heart). Disease processes, such as **ascites** (an excess amount of fluid in the peritoneal cavity) and **anasarca** (severe generalized edema), are also the result of abnormal fluid shifts. *Fluid volume excess* is the term often used as the descriptive nursing term in the nursing care plan for an excessive amount of intravascular and/or interstitial fluid.

Dehydration

Many disorders result in a deficiency of body water or an excessive loss of water from the body (**dehydration**). In dehydration, the body's output of water is greater than its intake. Dehydration can be associated with an increase in sodium or a disturbance of certain other electrolytes, such as potassium. Diarrhea, vomiting, inappropriate use of diuretics, decreased

fluid intake, excessive heat and sweating, fever, gastrointestinal suction, certain medications, and hemorrhage may contribute to dehydration. Certain diseases, such as diabetes (both mellitus and insipidus) and Addison's disease can also lead to dehydration.

Early in dehydration, the person feels thirsty and drinks more fluid. If the fluid intake cannot keep up with the fluid loss, dehydration increases in severity. The body compensates by reducing the urine output of the kidneys and shutting down sweating. Water moves from the intracellular fluid compartments into the intravascular fluids. If the dehydration is not corrected, the body tissues begin to dry out and malfunction. Brain cells are particularly susceptible to dehydration; a sign of severe dehydration is mental confusion. Untreated, this can progress to coma. Dehydration can also cause severe damage to organs such as the kidneys and liver, due to low blood pressure caused by reduced circulating blood volume. As in edema, treat-

CAUSES OF EDEMA

Increased Capillary Pressure
Arteriolar dilatation
    Allergic responses (eg, hives, angioneurotic edema)
    Inflammation
Venous obstruction
    Hepatic obstruction
    Heart failure
    Thrombophlebitis
Increased vascular volume
    Heart failure
    Increased levels of adrenocortical hormones
    Premenstrual sodium retention
    Pregnancy
    Environmental heat stress
Effects of gravity
    Prolonged standing

Decreased Colloidal Osmotic Pressure
Decreased production of plasma proteins
    Liver disease
    Starvation or severe protein deficiency
Increased loss of plasma proteins
    Protein-losing kidney diseases
    Extensive burns

Increased Capillary Permeability
Inflammation
Immune responses
Neoplastic disease
Tissue injury and burns

Obstruction of Lymphatic Flow
Infection or disease of the lymphatic structures
Surgical removal of lymph nodes

---

ment of dehydration is first directed at the underlying cause of the situation. Supplemental fluids and electrolytes are often administered.

The nursing terminology referring to dehydration is *fluid volume deficit.* Disorders related to fluid and electrolyte balance, including edema and dehydration, are discussed in more detail in Chapter 75.

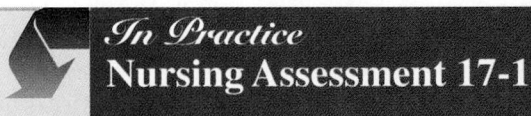

In Practice
Nursing Assessment 17-1

EARLY SYMPTOMS OF DEHYDRATION

Thirst is a primary indicator of hydration status. Therefore, assess your clients for thirst as an early symptom of dehydration.

Water

Water performs many significant functions in the human body. It provides an efficient medium for delivery of nutrients to the cells, and export of waste products from the cells. It helps to regulate many body processes and pressures. It protects and lubricates bodily materials. It is especially important in the regulation of blood pressure and fluid and electrolyte balance. Box 17-2 identifies these and other important functions of water.

☞ KEY CONCEPT

Water (H₂O) is vital to human life. The body cannot carry on most of its activities without it.

Water is of vital importance to the body and constitutes the greatest portion of body weight. Age, sex, and individual body structure cause variations in the percentage of total body water to total body weight. Children can be composed of more than 75% body water. Adult men are about 60% body water. Fat cells contain the least water of any cells in the body. Therefore, adult women have the lowest water content (about 50%), due to the presence of greater amounts of subcutaneous fat. Table 17-1 summarizes body water and its breakdown by individual and various water compartments.

Special Characteristics of Water

Certain properties of water make it important for body chemistry. Knowing the properties of water will aid your understanding of the rationale behind numerous nursing interventions.

- *A great difference in temperature is needed to bring about a physical change in water.* Water boils at 100°C (212°F) and freezes at 0°C (32°F). This temperature span is great enough to allow many physical reactions to occur that do not affect the chemical composition of the water

FUNCTIONS OF WATER

- Primary solvent within the body
- Primary compound in all body fluids
- Suspension agent
- Helps regulate body temperature, body pH, and fluid pressures inside and outside cells
- Assists or participates in chemical reactions
- May be end product of chemical reactions

Water in Solution with Other Substances
- Transports nutrients and oxygen to cells
- Transports waste products away from cells
- Acts as "bumper" to protect cells and organs
- Lubricates to prevent outer walls (parietal) from rubbing against inner walls (visceral) of organs
- Participates in maintenance of blood pressure
- Helps regulate acid–base and fluid–electrolyte balance

TABLE 17-1 WATER AS A PERCENTAGE OF BODY WEIGHT

Water Compartment	Infant (%)	Adult (%) Man	Adult (%) Woman	Elderly Person (%)
Extracellular				
Intravascular	4	4	5	5
Interstitial	25	11	10	15
Intracellular	48	45	35	25
Total body water	77	60	50	45

itself. Water can become a solid, a liquid, or a gas with only a temperature change. Water temperature, however, changes relatively slowly. Water can absorb much heat before increasing its temperature, or it can lose heat before decreasing its temperature. It needs heat to change from a liquid to a gas. The *evaporation* process (change from liquid to gas) removes heat from the body.

• *Water directly and indirectly participates in all chemical reactions that occur in the body.* Chemically, each water molecule (H_2O) is made up of two elements, hydrogen (2 atoms) and oxygen (1 atom). During metabolism, numerous chemical changes in the body separate water molecules into their component elements for use elsewhere. Hydrogen is the main component of the pH system of the body, which is discussed later in this chapter. *Oxidation* is the process through which the body uses oxygen to form needed new substances. Indirectly, water acts as the solution in which other chemicals ionize (dissociate). When substances change into ions, they become available to participate in other chemical reactions.

• *Water is a good solvent.* A **solvent** is a liquid (that dissolves solutes). A **solute** is the substance dissolved in a solvent. Many compounds, such as salts and sugars, dissolve easily in water. Nutrients and wastes are transported as solutes in water. Body water contains two main types of solutes: nonelectrolytes and electrolytes. Nonelectrolytes include proteins, glucose, carbon dioxide, oxygen, and organic acids. Electrolytes are solutes that generate an electrical charge when dissolved in water. They are discussed in the next section of this chapter.

• *Water functions as a suspension agent.* Many larger molecules, such as lipids and proteins, are easily suspended in water. These suspensions must be kept in motion, or the larger molecules will settle to the bottom. For example, red blood cells settle out of suspension unless kept in motion in the watery medium of blood. An individual's blood pressure partially depends on intravascular water as a suspension agent, with specific amounts of proteins, electrolytes, and minerals as solutes.

• *Water exerts pressure against the walls or vessels that contain it.* This pressure is known as *hydrostatic pressure* and occurs because water has weight and volume. The amount of pressure depends on the depth of the liquid. Regardless of the amount, water in a tall, thin container

exerts more hydrostatic pressure than water in a shallow container.

• Osmotic pressure is pressure that develops when a semipermeable membrane separates two solutions containing different concentrations of solutes. In other words, *the amount of solutes in water affects the pressure that the water can exert against surrounding membranes.* The greater the amount of solutes, the greater the amount of pressure. This principle is normally maintained within very narrow limits. Human body cells have an osmotic pressure nearly equal to that of the circulating fluid of the blood. Solutions exerting equal pressures on opposite sides of the membrane are said to be **isotonic.** Stronger solutions, compared to those on the opposing side of a membrane, are said to be **hypertonic.** Hypertonic solutions will cause blood cells to shrink because osmosis (discussed later) will draw fluid out of the cells. Weaker solutions, compared to an opposing solution, are called **hypotonic.** Hypotonic solutions cause blood cells to swell.

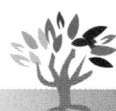 **SPECIAL CONSIDERATIONS:** THE LIFE SPAN

Risk for Fluid Volume Imbalances in Older Adults

Loss of thirst sensations in older adults leads to decreased consumption of fluids and therefore increased risk for fluid volume deficit. Cardiovascular and renal problems, along with nutritional habits, may cause sodium and water retention, leading to overload states.

Electrolytes

Electrolytes are active chemicals or elements within the body. An **electrolyte** is an element or a compound that will dissociate into ions (see discussion below) when dissolved in water. An ion is able to conduct a weak electric current.

Electrolytes are found in the form of inorganic salts, acids, and bases. They are found in all body fluids. Their concentrations, however, vary. Because electrolytes are active chemicals, their concentrations are measured according to their chemical activity, and expressed as milliequivalents (**mEq**).

Health professionals commonly see the results of electrolytes, as in an electrocardiogram. Electrodes on the surface of the body detect electrical currents produced by the action of the heart. These electrical events can be graphically visualized. Laboratory tests are also done to determine blood levels of various electrolytes. An excess or deficiency of certain key electrolytes can cause serious physical disorders.

Ions

Each chemical element has an electrical charge, either positive (+) or negative (−). An element may be able to connect or "bond" to another element. This bonding ability or attraction between chemicals is determined by the chemical and by its electrical charge.

Many elements gain or lose electrons that circle around them. An atom that has gained or lost one or more electrons is called an **ion** and has acquired an electrical charge. Ions are atoms or groups of atoms that are in search of a bonding partner. Some ions have the ability to bond with only one other ion; others can bond with two or more. This ability is expressed in terms of a positive ($^+$) or negative ($^-$) value and is called the *valence*. The valence would then be expressed as $^+$ or $^-$ and so forth. For example, sodium has a valence of $^+1$ (Na^+); sulfate has a valence of $^-2$ (SO_4^{--}). The number of plus or minus signs indicates the number of ions with which this particular ion is able to bind. Therefore, sodium (Na^+) can only bind with one negatively charged ion that has a valence of minus 1, such as chloride (Cl^-). This compound would then be **NaCl,** which is sodium chloride or common table salt.

A positively charged ion is known as a **cation.** A negatively charged ion is known as an **anion.** Examples of cations include sodium (**Na$^+$**), potassium (**K$^+$**), calcium (**Ca^{++}**), magnesium (**Mg^{++}**), iron (**Fe^{++}**), and hydrogen (**H$^+$**). Examples of anions include chloride (**Cl$^-$**), bicarbonate (**HCO$_3^-$**), sulfate (**SO$_4^{--}$**), and phosphate (**HPO$_4^{--}$**). (Use this memory helper for cation: (ca+ion). This will help you to remember the positive charge, thereby recalling which substances are cations and which are anions.)

The cation, because it has a positive charge, is attracted by a negatively charged ion. The anion, because it is negatively charged, is drawn toward the positive charge. In other words, opposites attract.

Ionization

The process of *ionization* involves the dissociation of compounds into their respective ions. The separation of chemical compounds into free-standing ions releases these chemicals for use in other chemical reactions. Ionization of the water molecule (**H$_2$O** or **HOH**) releases equal amounts of hydrogen ions (H^+) and hydroxyl ions (OH^-). Each of these two ions is now free to combine with another substance to form an acid, a base, or a salt. The ionization of table salt or sodium chloride (NaCl) will release a sodium ion (Na^+) and a chlorine ion (Cl^-). Each of these ions can recombine with other ions into new substances the body may need, such as the combination of hydrogen and chlorine, hydrochloric acid (**HCl**).

Important Electrolytes

The major intracellular electrolytes are potassium (K^+), magnesium (Mg^{++}), sulfate (SO_4^{++}), and phosphate (HPO_4^{--}). The major extracellular electrolytes are sodium (Na^+), chloride (Cl^-), calcium (Ca^{++}), and bicarbonate (HCO_3^-). Sodium is the most important extracellular cation. Chloride is the most important extracellular anion. These two ions combine to form sodium chloride or NaCl (ordinary table salt), which is one of the most common compounds in the body. Normal saline (**NS**) is a salt solution (0.9% NaCl) and is commonly administered IV (intravenously) to augment body fluids. NS is referred to as

isotonic because it has the same NaCl concentration as normal body fluids.

☞ KEY CONCEPT

Remember that NaCl (salt) is a compound; a chemical change has taken place to form it. Saline solution is a mixture *because it can be easily separated, without a chemical reaction. A* compound *combines elements in exact proportions, which are the same each time. A* mixture *can mix the components in different proportions. Therefore, a saline solution can be isotonic (0.9%), or it can be in any other proportion and still be a saline solution (such as the half-normal saline [0.45%] also commonly used in IV solutions).*

The most dominant cation intracellularly (inside the cells) is potassium (K^+). The most dominant anion is phosphate (HPO_4^{--}). ICF also contains sodium, but in much smaller amounts than outside the cell. The balance of intracellular potassium to extracellular sodium is an extremely important aspect of energy production.

The body needs all these electrolytes for normal functioning of nerves and muscles, developing the structures of the body cells, blood clotting, and coordinating the body's activities. Table 17-2 summarizes the functions of major electrolytes and the dietary sources needed to obtain them. Organs involved in the homeostatic mechanisms that maintain electrolyte balance include the kidneys and the adrenal, parathyroid, and thyroid glands. In the clinical setting, *electrolyte balance* refers to the maintenance of normal serum concentrations of electrolytes in the blood. Measuring the concentration of electrolytes in the ICF is difficult; therefore, serum concentrations (ECF: intravascular) are used to assess and to manage clients with imbalances. Table 17-3 provides normal serum electrolyte ranges for an adult. Chapter 75 describes disorders that occur when electrolytes are not within the normal range.

FLUID AND ELECTROLYTE TRANSPORT

Nutrients and oxygen must enter the cells of the body while waste products exit the body. During this exchange, substances must pass through various fluid compartments and cellular membranes (also known as plasma membranes). Each ion or molecule has its own specific way or ways in which it can be transported across membranes.

The cell membrane separates the intracellular environment from the extracellular environment. The composition of the intracellular environment differs from that outside the cell. These differences must be maintained for the cell (and consequently the organism) to survive. The membrane allows some molecules to pass through, while resisting or preventing others from entering (or leaving) the cell.

The ability of a membrane to allow molecules to pass through is known as **permeability.** Factors that affect permeability include:

- The size of the pores in the membrane
- The external and internal pressures exerted on the molecules (*osmotic pressure*)

TABLE 17-2 *M*AJOR FUNCTIONS AND FOOD SOURCES OF ELECTROLYTES

Electrolyte	Major Functions	Food Sources
Cations		
Sodium (Na$^+$)	Maintenance of osmotic pressure; thus, maintains body fluid balance Assists with normal functioning of neurons and muscle cells Essential for buffer system (acid–base balance)	Table salt, meat, dairy foods, eggs; many processed and preserved foods including bacon, pickles, and ketchup
Potassium (K$^+$)	Maintenance of osmotic pressure; thus, maintains body fluid balance Normal functioning of neurons and muscle cells, including the heart Essential for buffer system (acid–base balance)	Dry fruits, nuts, many vegetables, meat
Calcium (Ca^{++})	Assists with normal functioning of neurons and muscle cells, including the heart Maintenance of bones Essential for blood clotting	Milk and other dairy products, broccoli and other green leafy vegetables, sardines
Magnesium (Mg^{++})	Assists with normal functioning of neurons and muscle cells, including the heart Maintenance of bones	Green leafy vegetables, legumes, chocolate, peanut butter, whole grains
Anions		
Chloride (Cl$^-$)	Maintenance of osmotic pressure; thus, maintains body fluid balance Essential for buffer system (acid–base balance) Maintains acidity of gastric juice (stomach acid–HCl)	Cheese, milk, fish An excess of chloride ions is called *acidosis.*
Bicarbonate (HCO$_3$$^-$)	Maintenance of osmotic pressure; thus, maintains body fluid balance Essential for buffer system (acid–base balance)	Does not need to be specifically included in the diet. Excess bicarbonate ions can result from overuse of antacids, such as sodium bicarbonate (NaHCO$_3$, baking soda). The body also can lose acids as a result of illness. An excess of bicarbonate ions is called *alkalosis.*
Phosphate (HPO$_4$$^{--}$, PO$_4$)	Maintenance of bones Assists with normal functioning of nerves and muscle cells Assists with formation of ATP Assists with metabolism of nutrients	Whole grains, milk and other dairy foods, meat, fish, poultry

TABLE 17-3 *N*ORMAL SERUM ELECTROLYTE VALUES

Electrolyte	Serum Value
Cations	
Sodium (Na$^+$)	135–145 mEq/L
Potassium (K$^+$)	3.5–5.0 mEq/L
Calcium (Ca^{++})	4.3–5.3 mEq/L (8.9–10.1 mg/dL)
Magnesium (Mg^{++})	1.5–1.9 mEq/L (1.8–2.3 mg/dL)
Anions	
Chloride (Cl$^-$)	95–108 mEq/L
Bicarbonate (HCO$_3$$^-$)	22–26 mEq/L
Phosphate (HPO$_4$$^{--}$, H$_2PO_4$$^-$)	1.7–2.6 mEq/L (2.5–4.5 mg/dL)

Normal value ranges may vary slightly from laboratory to laboratory.

- The pressure of the fluid against the membrane (*hydrostatic pressure*)
- The electrical charges of the molecule, the plasma membrane, or the body fluid
- The solubility of the molecules
- The size of the molecules

Permeability of Membranes

Freely permeable membranes will allow almost any food or waste substance to pass through. Freely permeable walls allow easy transfer of fluid and substances from the intravascular fluid to the interstitial fluid. After the substances arrive in the interstitial fluid around the cells, they must still penetrate the cellular membrane to reach the ICF, where the majority of the body's work occurs.

The cellular membrane is selectively permeable, meaning that each cell's membrane allows only certain specific substances to pass through. Movement across the cellular membrane occurs in one of four ways:

- Molecules move through the cell membrane, including oxygen, carbon dioxide, and steroids.
- Substances pass through membrane channels. These channels are of various sizes and allow only a certain size range and electrical charge to traverse the membrane.
- Carrier molecules in the membrane assist substances across the barrier.
- A vesicle (membrane-bound sac) transports large molecules or whole cells across the plasma membrane.

Some molecules move passively through the membrane; thus, they do not require any energy output by the body. *Passive transport* mechanisms include diffusion, osmosis, and filtration. Another form of transport uses energy and requires assistance. It is called *active transport*. This type of transport is used when molecules are too large or too specialized to pass through membranes without assistance.

Passive Transport

Diffusion

Diffusion is the random movement of molecules from an area of higher concentration to an area of lower concentration. Atoms and molecules constantly move and bombard each other at random. The tendency of such movement is to equalize the number of molecules in any given area—the molecular equivalent of seeking homeostasis. If molecules are highly concentrated, they collide often and attempt to move to a place with fewer collisions. Diffusion means "to spread out." Following diffusion, equilibrium is reached, with no further exchange of molecules. The molecules continue to move, but the number in each area or on each side of a membrane stays the same. (Heat speeds up diffusion because heat makes molecules move faster.)

Diffusion commonly occurs in liquids and gases. For example, when liquid cream or powdered creamer is added to coffee it spreads out (diffuses). Smoke or perfume diffuses in a room.

Diffusion is the most important mechanism by which nutrients and wastes pass across the cell membrane. In the body, oxygen and carbon dioxide diffuse across the cell membranes of the alveoli in the lungs, as shown in Figure 17-3. When a person takes in a breath, more oxygen (O_2) molecules are drawn into the alveoli. They are pushed passively toward the pulmonary (lung) capillaries where the O_2 level is lower. Oxygen crosses the cell membrane out of the lungs and into the pulmonary capillaries. The oxygenated blood then passes into the pulmonary vein and from there is transported to various parts of the body. Carbon dioxide (CO_2) gas is exchanged in the same manner, except in the reverse direction because of the pressure. The designation "p" indicates the "power" or "potential" of oxygen or carbon dioxide (see Fig. 17-3).

Osmosis

Osmosis is the diffusion of water across a semipermeable membrane. Water molecules move passively from an area where they are higher in number (more dilute, with fewer solutes), to an area where they are lower in number (more concentrated, with more solutes). The homeostatic mechanism of osmosis equalizes the concentrations of solutes within the body. As seen in Figure 17-4, water moves from an area that has a *hypotonic solution* (a dilute solution with a fewer number of solutes) to an area that has a *hypertonic solution* (a concentrated solution with a greater number of solutes). If water from a less concentrated solution is moving into a red blood cell (RBC), the RBC becomes swollen, due to this influx of water. The reverse is then true. An RBC will shrink if it is losing water to a surrounding hypertonic solution (that is, a concentrated solution with a solute number higher than that found in the RBC).

Even though there are many types of solutes that may be in solution, a common one is salt. Therefore, when thinking about osmosis, think of salt as the solute and think about the phrase: "water follows salt." This will help you to remember which direction the water will move. So, osmosis can be thought of

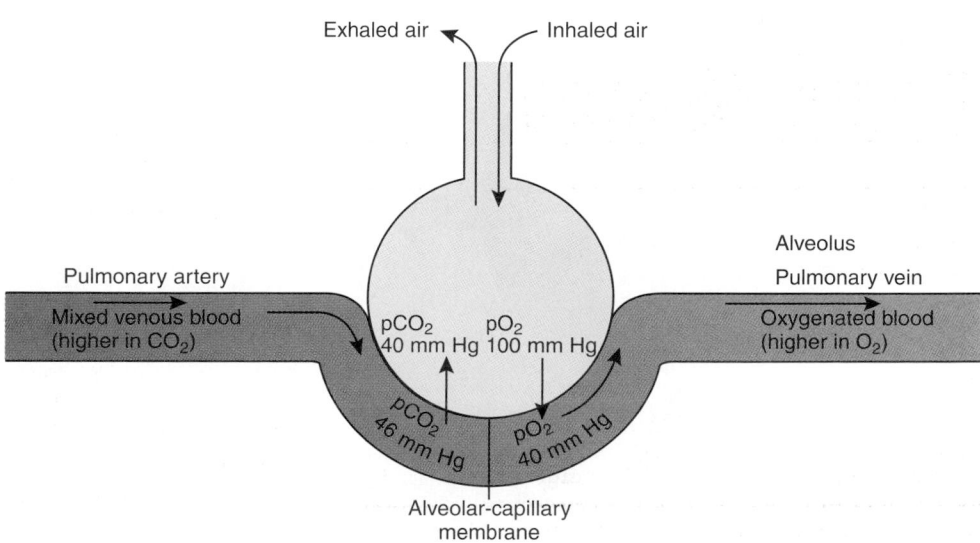

FIGURE 17-3. The process of diffusion showing gas exchange in the alveoli. Oxygen is transported across the alveolar-capillary membrane from the alveoli of the lungs to the capillaries, which contain unoxygenated blood. The carbon dioxide in the capillaries (area of greater concentration) moves into the alveoli (area of lesser concentration). This simple diffusion is an example of passive transport.

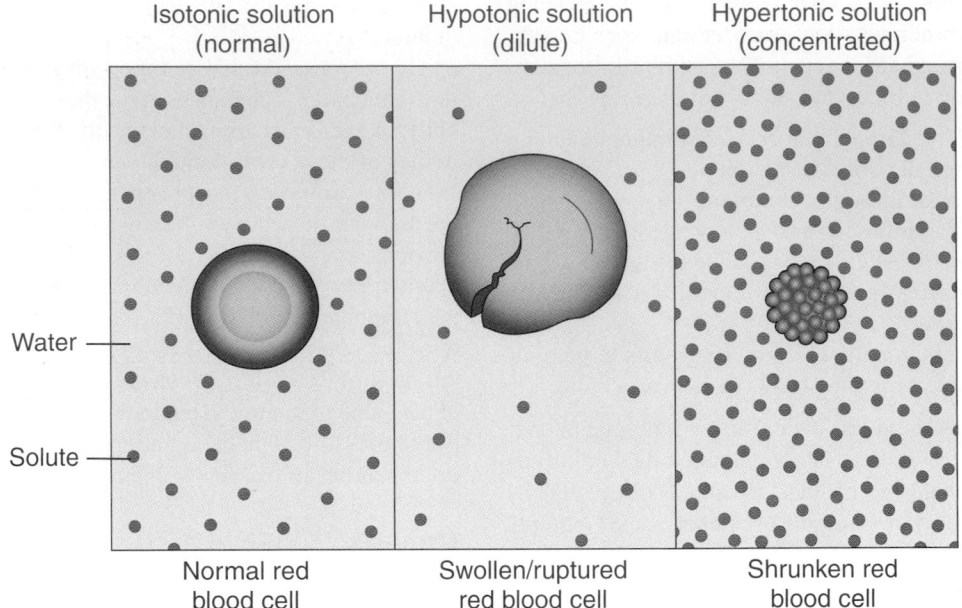

Isotonic solution
(normal)

Hypotonic solution
(dilute)

Hypertonic solution
(concentrated)

Water

Solute

Normal red
blood cell

Swollen/ruptured
red blood cell

Shrunken red
blood cell

FIGURE 17-4. Osmosis. Water moving through a red blood cell membrane in solutions with three different concentrations of solute. All these actions have the goal of equalizing the solute concentration on both sides of the cell membrane. *Left:* The isotonic (normal) solution has the same concentration as the cell, and the water moves into and out of the cell at the same rate. *Center:* The hypotonic (diluted) solution causes the cell to swell and eventually hemolyze (burst) because of the large amount of water moving into the cell. *Right:* The hypertonic (concentrated) solution draws water out of the cell, causing it to shrink.

as "pulling pressure," pulling the water into the concentrated solution.

Filtration

Filtration is the transport of water and dissolved materials through a membrane from an area of higher pressure to an area of lower pressure. Filtration requires mechanical pressure. Liquids and solutes are passed through holes in a membrane. The size of the holes and the differences in pressures (mechanical force) on each side determine the amount of filtration. Filtration can be thought of as a "pushing pressure," as it pushes water and solutes through a membrane from a higher pressure area to a lower pressure area. Figure 17-5 shows filtration through a vein (venule) and artery.

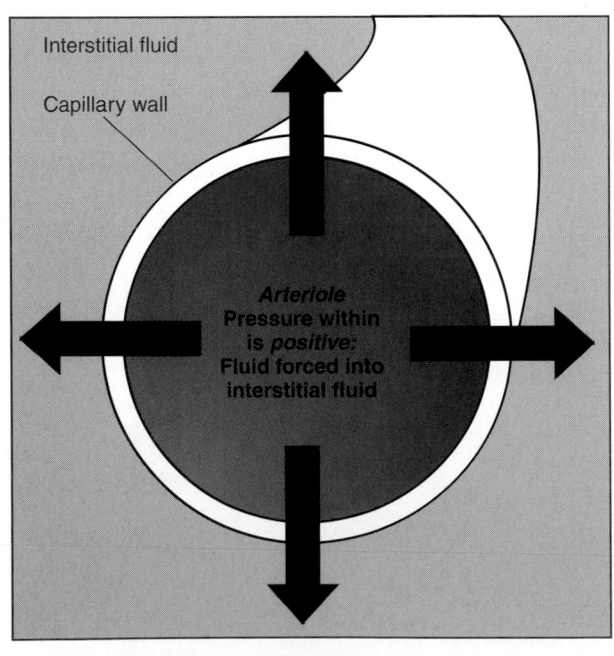

Interstitial fluid

Capillary wall

Arteriole
Pressure within
is *positive:*
Fluid forced into
interstitial fluid

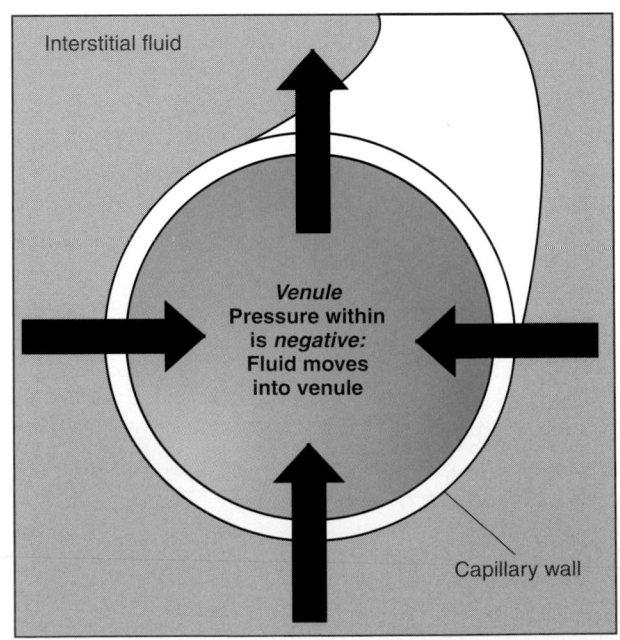

Interstitial fluid

Venule
Pressure within
is *negative:*
Fluid moves
into venule

Capillary wall

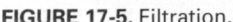

FIGURE 17-5. Filtration.

Filtration is common in the body. Blood pressure (a mechanical force) pushes water and small dissolved particles, such as sugars and salts, through the walls of the capillaries into the interstitial fluid. The larger blood cells and proteins are too large to be pushed through, and remain inside the capillaries.

Active Transport

Active transport mechanisms require energy expenditure in the form of adenosine triphosphate (ATP). Active transport processes can move solutes "uphill." Specific molecules outside a cell, even if they are fewer in number, can be assisted into the cell, where a greater concentration already exists.

The best example of active transport is the sodium–potassium pump. More sodium ions exist outside the cell than inside. The natural tendency would be for sodium to diffuse across the cellular membrane into the cell. If this process continued unchecked, however, the homeostatic mechanism (which governs nerve transmissions and muscle contractions) would go berserk. Active transport mechanisms figuratively "pump out" sodium ions from inside the cell, while transporting potassium into the cell.

Another example of active transport involves the transport of glucose and amino acids into the cells lining the small intestine. The intestinal cells use ATP to create this active transport, even if the movement of the solutes (glucose and amino acids) is from a higher to a lower concentration.

☛ KEY CONCEPT

If a transfer does not need energy, it is passive *transport.*
If a transfer requires energy, it is active *transport.*

FLUID AND ELECTROLYTE BALANCE

Fluid and electrolyte balance is vital for the proper functioning of all body systems. The body must maintain the correct proportion of fluids to solutes in each compartment.

The body compensates for imbalances immediately. For example, if excess carbon dioxide (CO_2) accumulates, a person breathes faster to take in more oxygen. If the respiratory system cannot handle the imbalance, chemical buffers attempt to achieve a balance. Additionally, the kidneys can adjust the pH of the ECF. Numerous hormones also act to influence fluid and electrolyte retention and excretion.

Electrolytes may be lost through vomiting, diarrhea, or hemorrhage, thus upsetting the body's fluid and electrolyte balance.

Water Intake and Output

The body conserves and reuses water as much as possible. The kidneys, and to some extent the intestines, continuously filter and recycle water. Each day, a person must take in approximately the same amount of fluid as he or she loses. The body can survive many days without food, but only a few days without water.

TABLE 17-4 *N*ORMAL WATER BALANCES (INTAKE AND OUTPUT)			
Intake		**Output**	
Source	*Amount*	*Source*	*Amount*
Liquids	1,300 mL	Urine	1,500 mL
Foods	1,000 mL	Skin*	600 mL
Metabolism	300 mL	Lungs*	300 mL
		Feces	200 mL
TOTAL	2,600 mL	*TOTAL*	2,600 mL

*Often referred to as "insensible water losses"

The term health professionals use to monitor fluid balance is *intake and output.* Accurate intake and output records are vital when caring for clients with fluid deficits or excesses. Table 17-4 gives sources and approximate amounts for human intake and output.

Intake refers to the water and other fluids that are taken into the body each day. Water is obtained from three sources: liquid intake (by mouth or by a method such as an IV), as a result of food metabolism, and as the end product of cellular respiration. The average adult takes in approximately 2,000 to 4,000 **mL** (milliliters) per day (a little more than 2 to 4 quarts).

To avoid an overload of water in the body, approximately the same amount that is taken into the body must be put out. Water output occurs normally through the kidneys, in sweat, as water vapor from the lungs, and in feces. Sweat may be sensible (visible, able to be sensed) or **insensible** (not perceptible to the senses) water loss.

Many factors influence water loss. For example, water output increases with exercise, fever, some medications, and certain diseases. Ill individuals may need more fluids because of excess drainage from wounds, vomiting, or bleeding. A fever can cause a person to use about four times the amount of fluids that he or she would need normally. *Diaphoresis* (profuse sweating) can cause considerable fluid loss. Each form of fluid loss will also alter the body's electrolyte concentrations.

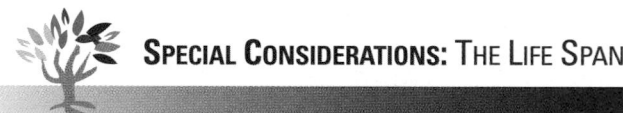

SPECIAL CONSIDERATIONS: THE LIFE SPAN

Adolescents are at risk for fluid and electrolyte imbalances due to excessive exercise, poor fluid intake during or after exercise, excessive use of salt and high-sodium soft drinks, and following fad diets or diets lacking important nutrients—especially iron and calcium.

ACID–BASE BALANCE

Acid–base balance is another important aspect of homeostasis. In the discussion on ionization, you learned that chemical compounds that break up into ions are called electrolytes and that these electrolytes can combine and recombine to form acids, bases, and salts. The body needs many salts to regulate its acid–base levels and to coordinate water balance. For example, it needs sodium to maintain the electrical potential across cell membranes and to maintain acid–base balance. Potassium acts within the cells in much the same way that sodium acts outside the cells. Chlorine plays a major role in acid–base balance due to its production of hydrochloric acid (HCl). Water contains the components of both an acid (the hydrogen ion or H^+) and a base (the hydroxyl ion or OH^-). Pure water is considered a neutral solution. A neutral solution contains equal parts of hydrogen and hydroxyl ions.

Acids, Bases, and Salts

An **acid** is one type of compound that contains the hydrogen ion (H^+). A **base** (also known as an *alkali*) is a compound that contains the hydroxyl ion (OH^-). A **salt** is created when the positive ions (usually a mineral) of a base replace the positive hydrogen ions of an acid. A salt is an electrolyte that is made up of a cation (other than a hydrogen ion) and an anion (other than a hydroxyl ion). For example, hydrochloric acid (HCl) can combine with the base sodium hydroxide (**NaOH**) to yield water and table salt. Thus, HCl + NaOH = HOH + NaCl. (Or an acid plus a base yields water and a salt.)

The body contains several important salts: sodium chloride (NaCl), potassium chloride (**KCl**), calcium chloride (**CaCl$_2$**), calcium carbonate (**CaCO$_3$**), calcium phosphate (**Ca$_3$[PO$_4$]$_2$**), and sodium sulfate (**Na$_2$SO$_4$**).

Potential of Hydrogen (pH)

The symbol **pH** refers to the potential or power (p) of hydrogen ion (H^+) concentration within a solution. The pH scale ranges from 0 to 14. Pure water, which is neutral, has a pH of 7. If the pH number is lower than 7, the solution is an acid. Some household acids include vinegar and lemon juice. Acids contain more hydrogen ions than bases. If the number is greater than 7, the solution is basic (or alkaline). The pH of ICF is approximately 6.8 to 7.0. Some household alkaline solutions

include baking soda, detergents and oven cleaners. Basic solutions contain more hydroxyl ions than acids.

Fluids open to the environment may be strongly acidic or alkaline and not harm the body. For example, lemon juice has a high acidity of two and sodium bicarbonate (baking soda) has a high alkalinity of 12; however, these substances do not harm the body. On the other hand, some substances either in the environment or in the body (such as HCl) could be harmful. Figure 17-6 shows the pH scale for body fluids.

☛ KEY CONCEPT

Low pH = high number of hydrogen ions; high pH = low number of hydrogen ions.

A change in the pH of a solution by one pH unit means a tenfold change in hydrogen ion concentration. For example, a substance with a pH of 5 contains 10 times more hydrogen ions than a substance with a pH of 6 (1 unit = 10^1). A pH of 5 means that a substance has 100 times more hydrogen ions than a substance with a pH of 7 (2 units = 10^2). Understanding the impact of changes in pH on the body is extremely important. For example, the pH of blood and lymph (ECF) is normally slightly alkaline, about 7.35 to 7.45. The body must maintain the slightly alkaline pH of blood within this narrow range, because a decrease or increase of only one pH unit will result in a chemical disaster. One of the body's normal negative feedback mechanisms is to continually correct the body's tendency to develop acidosis (too many hydrogen atoms) by returning the serum pH back into its alkaline state. The lungs and the kidneys are the organs of the body that are the most involved in H^+ regulation.

Buffers

Chemical reactions that occur constantly in the body release many acidic or basic ions. Because of the constant changes in this mixture, a buffering or stabilizing system must exist to prevent a pH imbalance. A **buffer** is a chemical system set up

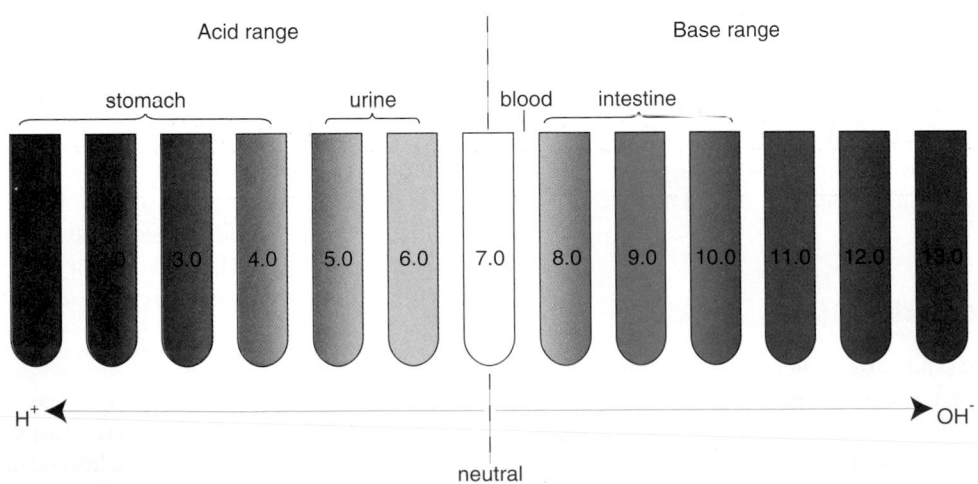

FIGURE 17-6. The pH scale measures degree of acidity (H^+ ion concentration) or alkalinity (OH^- ion concentration).

to resist changes, particularly in the level of hydrogen ions. Buffering reactions—which can occur in less than a second—constantly alter acids and bases on many levels, to maintain a correct ratio. The body has many buffer systems that are utilized in maintaining homeostasis. Some buffer systems use phosphates, proteins, and hemoglobin as part of their buffer systems. One of the major buffer systems is the bicarbonate buffer system that is discussed below.

The Bicarbonate Buffer System

Sodium bicarbonate ($NaHCO_3$, a weak base) and carbonic acid (H_2CO_3, a weak acid) are the body's major chemical buffers. Because of its tendency toward acidosis, the body has a greater need for sodium bicarbonate (a base). In fact, the body contains 20 times more sodium bicarbonate than carbonic acid.

Carbon Dioxide.   Chemical buffers are clinically significant, particularly in respiratory illnesses. Carbon dioxide (CO_2) is a potential acid because once dissolved in water, it becomes carbonic acid, which is abbreviated H_2CO_3 ($CO_2 + H_2O = H_2CO_3$). When CO_2 increases (as in a client with chronic obstructive pulmonary disease), the carbonic acid content also increases. The opposite can occur in hyperventilation states—where CO_2 decreases, resulting in a decrease of carbonic acid. Therefore, much of the acid in the body is controlled through the respiratory system, most specifically the lungs. The major acid controlled by the lungs is CO_2. The respiratory system can very rapidly compensate for too much acid or too little acid in the body by having the respiratory rate of the person increase or decrease, thereby altering the amount of CO_2 in the body. When you think about respiratory acidosis or alkalosis, think about the lungs and how they will work to compensate for imbalances, using the carbon dioxide (CO_2) dissolved in the blood.

Bicarbonate.   The kidneys regulate the bicarbonate level in the ECF by conserving or excreting bicarbonate ions from the renal tubules. Bicarbonate levels are important in maintaining the acid–base balance in the body. The bicarbonate ions (HCO_3^-) are basic (alkaline) components in the body, and the kidneys are one of the major factors in regulating the amount of base (bicarbonate) in the body. If there is too much

or too little base in the body, one way the body's metabolism can compensate for this disorder is by having the kidneys excrete more or fewer bicarbonate ions. When you think about acid–base balance in the body, think about the kidneys and how they might compensate for imbalances using bicarbonate ions. It is important to prevent severe acidosis or alkalosis.

☛ KEY CONCEPT

Consider:
Lungs–Acid–$CO_2 \rightarrow H_2CO_3$
Kidneys–Base–HCO_3^- ions

Major mechanisms to control acid–base balance:
• *Acid is excreted by the kidneys, mostly as ammonia*
• *pH buffers:*
  bicarbonate–base
  carbon dioxide–acid
• *Excretion of CO_2 (constantly produced by the cells)*

Measurement of Arterial Blood Gases.   Arterial blood gases (**ABGs**) are measured in a laboratory test to determine the extent of compensation by the buffer system. The pH level of a blood gas indicates if there is more acid or base in the blood. After that is done, the normal range for ABGs is used as a guide, and the determination of which area might have a disorder first is based upon whether the pH is acidic or alkaline (basic).

If it is determined that the pH is basic, the HCO_3^- level is considered next, because the kidneys are the organs where bicarbonate ion levels are regulated. If the pH is acidic, the $paCO_2$ (or pCO_2, the carbon dioxide content of arterial blood) is assessed, because the lungs are the site where the majority of acid is regulated. This will give you a beginning approach to ABG interpretation. Table 17-5 shows normal ABG values. Table 17-6 illustrates acidosis and alkalosis, in relationship to pH, CO_2, and HCO_3^- values. The distinction between metabolic and respiratory states is shown. To make blood gas values easier to remember, it is common to use the pH range of 7.35 to 7.45 and a $PaCO_2$ range of 35 to 45 as a guideline for students. Chapter 75 describes disorders in fluid balance in more detail.

▪▪▪ TABLE 17-5 𝒩ORMAL ARTERIAL BLOOD GAS VALUES

Abbreviation	Normal Range	Definition
pH	7.37–7.43	Reflects the hydrogen ion concentration in arterial blood Acidosis: <7.37 Alkalosis: >7.43
$PaCO_2$	36–44 mm Hg	Reflects partial pressure of carbon dioxide in arterial blood Hypocapnia: low partial pressure of carbon dioxide in arterial blood, <36 mm Hg Hypercapnia: high partial pressure of carbon dioxide in arterial blood, >44 mm Hg
PaO_2	80–100 mm Hg	Partial pressure of O_2 in arterial blood
HCO_3^-	22–26 mEq/L	Amount of bicarbonate in arterial blood

■■■ **TABLE 17-6** $\mathscr{A}$ **COMPARISON OF RESPIRATORY AND METABOLIC ACIDOSIS AND ALKALOSIS**

Acidosis			Alkalosis	
Respiratory	↓ pH ↑ CO_2	Normal serum pH 7.35–7.45	↑ pH ↓ CO_2	Respiratory
Metabolic	↓ pH ↓ HCO_3^-		↑ pH ↑ HCO_3^-	Metabolic

Note that the primary difference between respiratory conditions is a variation in pH that is influenced by changes in CO_2 levels. The primary difference between metabolic conditions is a variation in pH that is influenced by changes in bicarbonate ion concentration (HCO_3^-).

Source: M. Kowalski, using information from Porth, C. M. (1998). *Pathophysiology: Concepts of altered health states* (5th ed., p. 633). Philadelphia: Lippincott Williams & Wilkins.

Chapter 85 discusses respiratory disorders, which are often assessed in part by ABGs.

☛ KEY CONCEPT

The pH of the ECF must be maintained between 7.35 and 7.45 for health. Extremes (below 6.8 or above 7.8) are usually fatal.

EFFECTS OF AGING ON THE SYSTEM

Dehydration is a common and serious problem for older adults. Normally, the levels of electrolytes, acids, bases, and salts do not change as a person ages; however, in the older person, ICF levels decrease by about 8% because muscle tissue changes to adipose tissue. (Fat cells contain less water than muscle cells.) See Table 17-7.

As people age, their thirst sensation decreases; therefore, older people may be unaware of their need to consume fluids. Many medications cause fluid loss. Chronic diseases, such as renal failure, heart failure, or COPD, contribute to alterations in fluid and electrolyte and acid–base balance. Nutritional habits, exercise, and activity levels also influence body fluid levels.

Increased release of calcium from the bones to maintain normal serum calcium levels in older adults predisposes them to osteoporosis and an increased incidence of fractures from falls. Laxative abuse reduces gastrointestinal absorption of fluid and electrolytes.[1]

➤ **STUDENT SYNTHESIS**

Key Points

- Homeostasis is a state of dynamic equilibrium; the body constantly adjusts to external and internal stimuli.
- Feedback is the relaying of information to and from organ systems (especially the nervous and endocrine systems). Feedback keeps the body's functioning capacity within normal boundaries.
- The body has two main fluid compartments: intracellular (within the cells) and extracellular. Extracellular fluid is located in blood vessels (plasma) and in tissues (interstitial fluid).
- Homeostatic mechanisms involved in the regulation of ECF include the actions of the thirst center, antidiuretic hormone (ADH), renin-angiotensin-aldosterone system (RAA), and atrial natriuretic peptide (ANP).

■■■ **TABLE 17-7** $\mathscr{E}$ **FFECTS OF AGING ON FLUID AND ELECTROLYTE BALANCE**

Factor	Result	Nursing Implications
Intracellular fluid levels decrease; thirst sensation declines.	Dehydration is common.	Encourage intake of foods and fluids; regulate temperature control.
Muscle tissue turns to fat.	Older people may gain weight.	Encourage exercise, activity, and a balanced diet.
Many medications cause fluid loss.	Medications may contribute to dehydration.	Be sure that the person on certain medications drinks enough water.
Circulatory and renal disorders may cause fluid retention.	Edema may develop.	Monitor the client's sodium intake and blood pressure; encourage intake of foods with potassium; administer medications as ordered.

- Water acts as a solvent and as a suspension agent. It helps regulate body temperature, pH, and fluid pressures inside and outside the cell. It assists and participates in chemical reactions.
- Electrolytes are substances that dissociate in water into ions. Ions are electrically charged particles that circulate in the body fluids and take part in the body's chemical reactions.
- Normal saline (0.9% NaCl) is an isotonic solution. Stronger solutions are hypertonic; weaker solutions are hypotonic.
- Fluids are transported passively (without ATP energy), or actively (with ATP energy).
- A person's intake and output must be balanced to avoid a fluid deficit (dehydration) or a fluid excess (edema).
- The body has buffer systems that help to maintain the serum pH in the narrow range between 7.35 and 7.45 (or 7.37 and 7.43). Acids and bases are important components of this system.
- The body utilizes the lungs to maintain or excrete carbon dioxide and the kidneys to maintain or excrete bicarbonate as part of the buffer system used to regulate pH. Arterial blood gases are drawn to determine how well the body's acid–base balance is functioning.
- Minute fluid and electrolyte and acid–base changes occur constantly throughout the body, but the overall status in the healthy person is stability and equilibrium. To be healthy, a person's body must maintain this balance as much as possible.

Critical Thinking Exercises

1. Considering the importance of maintaining ECF volume in the body, identify how an excessive dietary intake of table salt can be dangerous.
2. Explain why a person who is suffering from heartburn or upset stomach may take an over-the-counter antacid for symptom relief without causing fluid and electrolyte imbalance.
3. Older adults are at increased risk for fluid and electrolyte imbalances, partially due to decreased thirst sensations. Discuss why extreme outdoor temperatures can place older adults at significant risk.

NCLEX-Style Review Questions

1. ECF is composed primarily of:
   a. Aqueous fluid and lymphatic fluid
   b. CSF and interstitial fluid
   c. Interstitial and intravascular fluid
   d. Vascular fluid and CSF
2. A chemical system set up to resist changes, particularly in the level of pH, is:
   a. A base
   b. A buffer
   c. A salt
   d. An acid
3. Water is moved across semipermeable membranes by the process of:
   a. Active transport
   b. Diffusion
   c. Filtration
   d. Osmosis
4. To balance water output, an average adult must have fluid intake of:
   a. 500–900 mL per day
   b. 1000–2000 mL per day
   c. 2000–4000 mL per day
   d. 4000–6000 mL per day
5. The primary organs involved in pH regulation are:
   a. Kidneys and lungs
   b. Heart and intestines
   c. Lungs and endocrine glands
   d. Skin and kidneys

Reference

1. Craven, R. F., & Hirnle, C. J. (2000). *Fundamentals of nursing: Human health and function* (3rd ed.). Philadelphia: Lippincott Williams & Wilkins.

CHAPTER

18

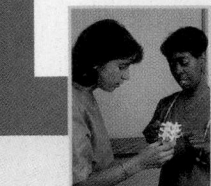

The Musculoskeletal System

LEARNING OBJECTIVES

1. List the four classifications of bones according to shape.
2. Locate and name the major bones of the body and their functions.
3. Explain the function of red bone marrow.
4. Name three types of joints and give an example of each.
5. Differentiate between the axial and appendicular skeletons.
6. List the five divisions of the vertebral column and the number of vertebrae in each division.
7. In the skills lab, locate and name the bones on a demonstration skeleton
8. Differentiate between an adult and an infant skull. Describe two functions of fontanels. Locate the anterior and posterior fontanel on a newborn.
9. Compare and contrast skeletal, smooth, and cardiac muscles and their functions.
10. Locate and name the major muscle groups in the body and indicate the actions of each muscle group.
11. State three factors that influence bone growth.
12. Explain the process by which muscles produce heat.
13. Explain the effects of overusing and underusing muscles.
14. Differentiate between tendons and ligaments.

NEW TERMINOLOGY

acetabulum
articulation
atrophy
bursa
calcaneus
carpal
cartilage
clavicle
coccyx
contractility
diaphysis
elasticity
epiphysis
extensibility
extension
femur
fibula
flexion
gait
hematopoiesis
humerus
ilium
intercostal muscle
irritability
isometric
isotonic
joint
ligament

malleolus
mandible
marrow
maxilla
muscle tone
ossification
osteoblast
osteoclast
osteocyte
patella
pelvis
periosteum
phalanx
pubic arch
radius
range of motion
reabsorption
sacrum
scapula
sinus
sternum
symphysis pubis
tendons
thorax
tibia
ulna
vertebral column

Most people take for granted the fact that their bodies produce all kinds of motion. By working in harmony, the various components of the body produce actions that allow independence and discovery. The musculoskeletal system includes the skeleton, joints, bursae, ligaments, muscles, and tendons. The skeleton provides the bony framework for the human body. The entire system works together to enable physical movement.

STRUCTURE AND FUNCTION

A systematic way to study the structure and function of the musculoskeletal system is to study the skeleton, the muscles, and how they work together. Although each component is distinct and unique, the system overall cannot function without each part working together. An examination of the structure and function of the musculoskeletal system must consider the skeleton, skeletal divisions, and the muscles.

THE SKELETON

The functions of the skeleton are support, protection, movement, hematopoiesis (blood formation), and storage (Box 18-1). Not only is the skeleton the framework of the body, but it is also living. Although the bone itself is hard and filled with calcium deposits, the cells of the bone are living organisms. Each bone is made up of several types of tissue; therefore, bones are considered organs.

Bones

The human body has 206 bones (Fig. 18-1). Bones, the marrow within certain bones, and the minerals with which bones

➤ ➤ BOX 18-1

FUNCTIONS OF THE SKELETON

Support
• Supports the body
• Provides framework for the body
• Gives shape to the body

Protection
• Protects vital organs
• Protects soft tissues

Movement
• Provides locomotion (walking, movement) by attachment of muscles, tendons, and ligaments

Hematopoiesis
• Produces red blood cells
• Produces white blood cells
• Produces platelets

Storage
• Provides calcium
• Provides phosphorus

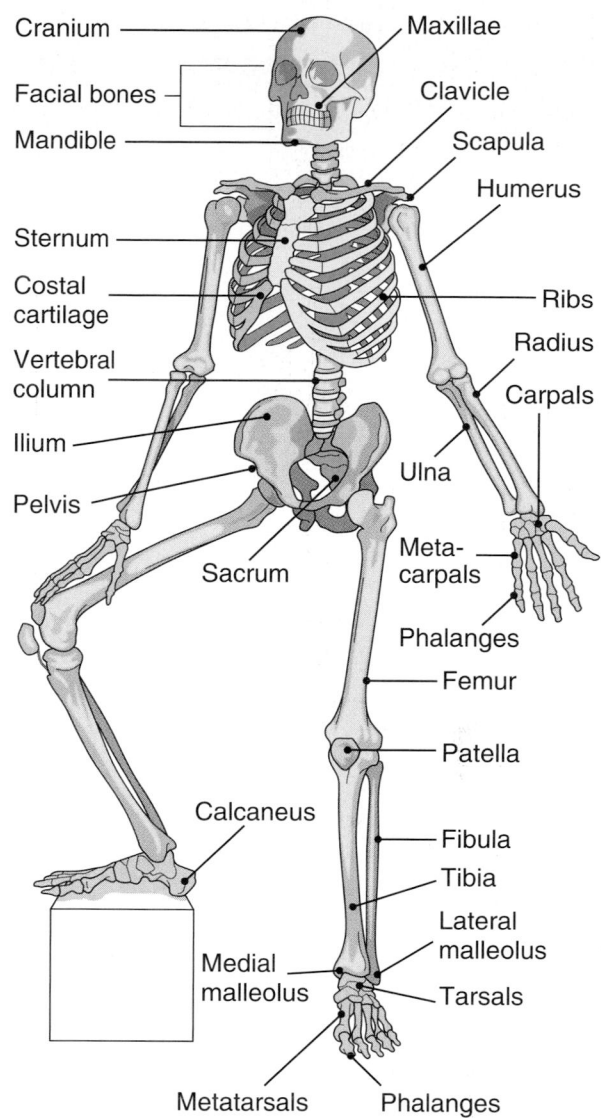

FIGURE 18-1. The skeleton.

are made (calcium and phosphorous) contribute to the homeostatic functioning of the body.

Classification
Bones are classified according to their shape: long, short, flat, or irregular. *Long bones* have an extended shape and provide the body with support and strength. *Short bones* are approximately cube shaped. *Flat bones* are shaped exactly as the name suggests, and provide broad surfaces for muscle attachments. *Irregular bones* are similar to short bones, but are irregular in shape. The irregular bone classification includes small, rounded bones called *sesamoid bones*. Sesamoid bones develop within joints and tendons. The patella (kneecap) is the largest sesamoid bone. Table 18-1 lists the classifications of bones, along with their functions and examples.

Structure
Bone tissue comes in two types. *Compact bone* is hard and dense. It composes the shaft of long bones and the outer layer of other bones. *Spongy bone* is composed of small bony plates.

TABLE 18-1 CLASSIFICATION OF BONES

Classification	Functions	Examples/Locations
Long	Act as levers; support frame	Arms, legs, femur, tibia, radius
Short	Facilitate movement; transfer forces	Wrists, ankles, feet
Flat	Serve as muscle attachment and for protection	Cranial, ribs, shoulder blades, hips
Irregular	For attachment of other structures or articulations	Facial, vertebrae, patella

of red blood cells, white blood cells, and platelets. This manufacturing process is called **hematopoiesis.**

The **periosteum** is a hard, fibrous connective tissue membrane that covers most of the outside of the bone. It merges with tendons and ligaments. The periosteum contains the blood vessels that supply oxygen and nutrients to the bone cells, keeping them alive. The blood cells also supply bone-building substances and minerals that harden the bone by filling the intercellular spaces.

Two types of osseous (bony) tissue are involved in construction of the long bones of the extremities. The **diaphysis,** or shaft of the long bone, is hard and compact. The end of the long bones, the **epiphysis,** is spongelike and is covered by a shell of harder bone (Fig. 18-2). The diaphysis and epiphysis do not fuse until full growth is achieved. The place where the diaphysis and epiphysis meet is called the *epiphyseal growth plate.*

Markings.   The contours of bones resemble the configuration of an interesting landscape with its hills and valleys. Hundreds of bone markings are found, with special characteristics that identify each type. A *facet* is a small plane or smooth area. The most commonly known facets are those of the spinal column. Each vertebra contains facets, which are the locations for articulation (a joint) with the heads of the ribs (Fig. 18-3).

It contains more spaces than compact bone. The hollow inner part of the bone is filled with a soft substance called **marrow.** Marrow comes in two forms: yellow and red. Yellow marrow (as seen in soup bones) is found in the central cavities of the long bones and is mostly fat. The red marrow is found in the ends of long bones, in the bodies of the vertebrae, and in flat bones. Red bone marrow is responsible for the manufacturing

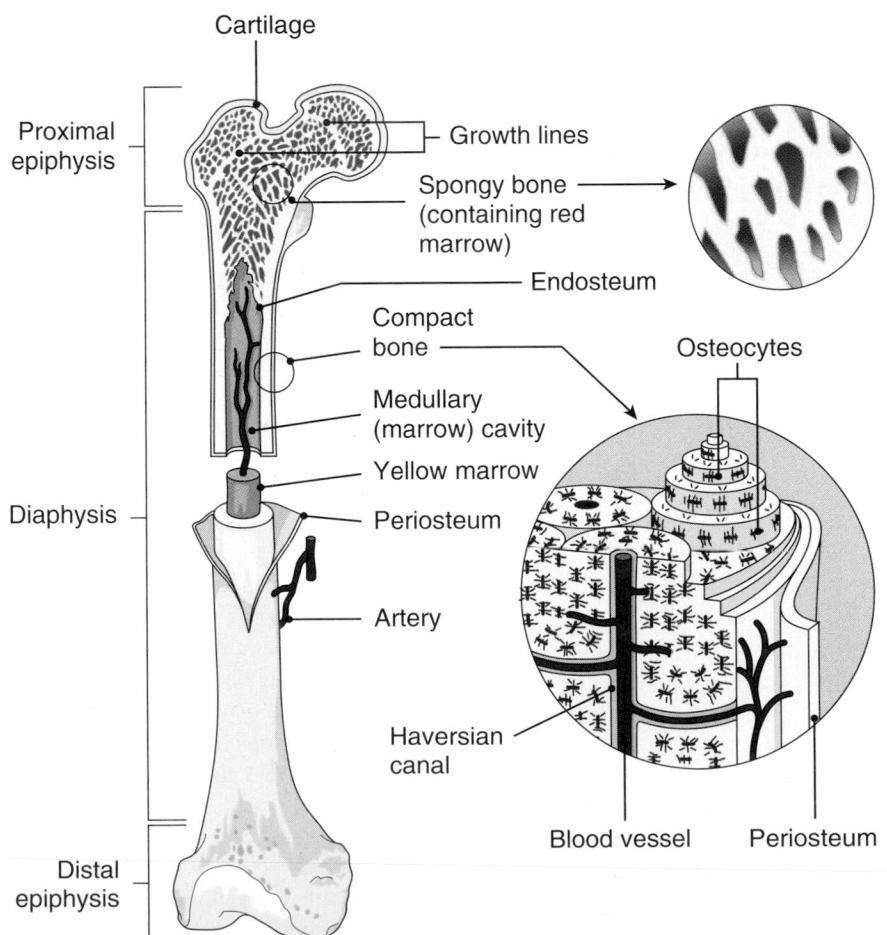

FIGURE 18-2. The structure of a long bone; the composition of compact bone.

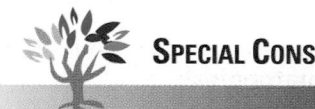

SPECIAL CONSIDERATIONS: THE LIFE SPAN

Damage to the Epiphyseal Growth Plate

Damage to the epiphyseal growth plate by trauma will cause cessation of growth in long bones and results in shortening of the limb involved. The younger the child is when an injury occurs, the greater the final deficit in length between the injured limb and the uninjured limb will be.

A *condyle* is a large, rounded projection, usually for articulation with another bone. A *tuberosity* is a large, elevated, knoblike projection, usually for muscle attachment. The tibia has condyles and tuberosities on both ends, where it articulates with the thigh and ankle bones and connects with muscles and tendons (see Fig. 18-1).

A flat projection or area is called a *plate*. The dental plate (dorsal or roof plate) makes up the roof of the mouth. The foot plate is the flat portion of the stapes, which is one of the tiny bones in the middle ear. The foot plate of the stapes contacts the oval window to conduct sound waves to the inner ear (see Figures 21-3 and 21-4).

Any prominence or projection of bone is called a *bony process*. A spine (spina) is a *sharp process;* a ridge or crest is a *thin* or *narrow process.* (A distinct border or ridge, usually on the superior aspect of a bone, is most commonly called a *crest.*) There are several commonly-known bony processes in the body. The great (greater) trochanter of the femur is a large bony process (Fig. 18-4). (The head of the femur is the rounded, knoblike end of the femur, a condyle. The head of the femur lies in the hip socket, the acetabulum. The head is separated from the trochanter by a slender region called the *neck.*) A familiar crest in the body is the iliac crest, which lies at the top of the ileum, or iliac bone (Fig. 18-5). Each bone of the vertebral column also contains several processes, including the spinous process and the transverse process (Fig. 18-6). The *pedicle* is another process that forms part of the vertebral arch of the vertebral column (see Fig. 18-3).

A *tubercle* is a small rounded knob or nodule, usually for the attachment of a tendon or ligament. One tubercle is shown in Figure 18-5 (this particular tubercle is the location of the attachment of the pubofemoral ligament).

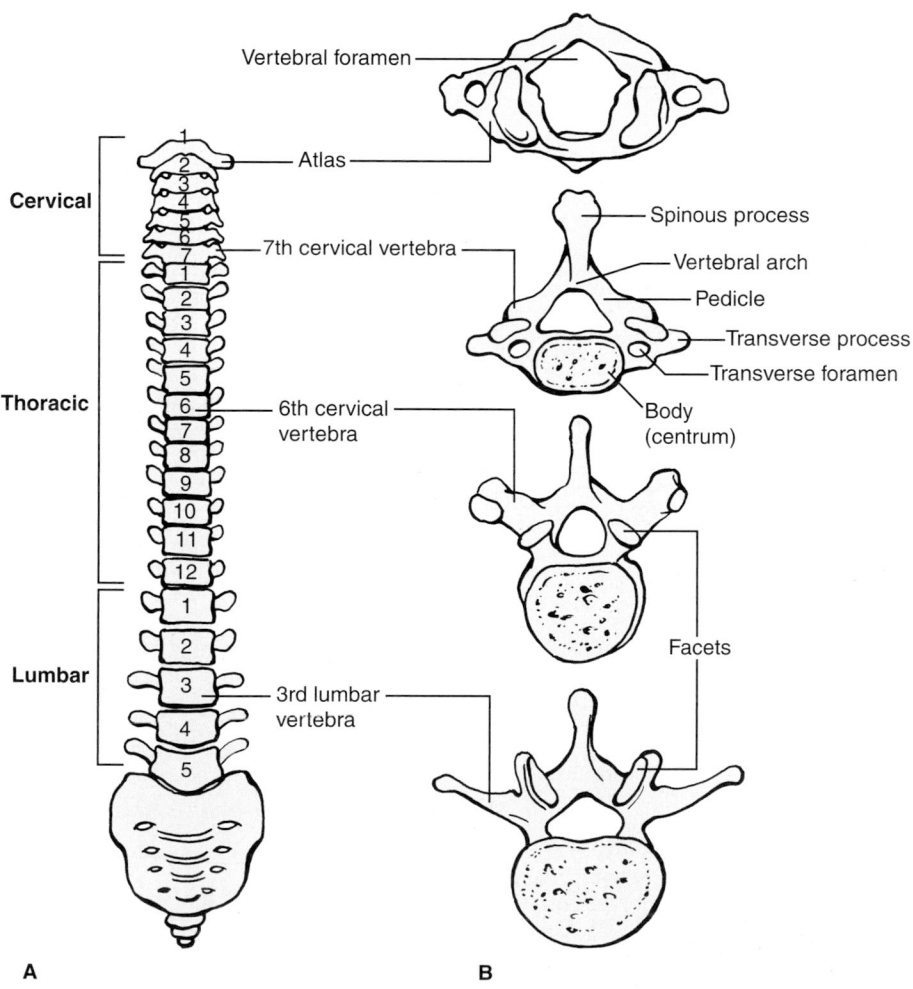

FIGURE 18-3. (A) Front view of the vertebral column. **(B)** Vertebrae from above. Note the cartilage between the vertebrae, called *intervertebral disks.*

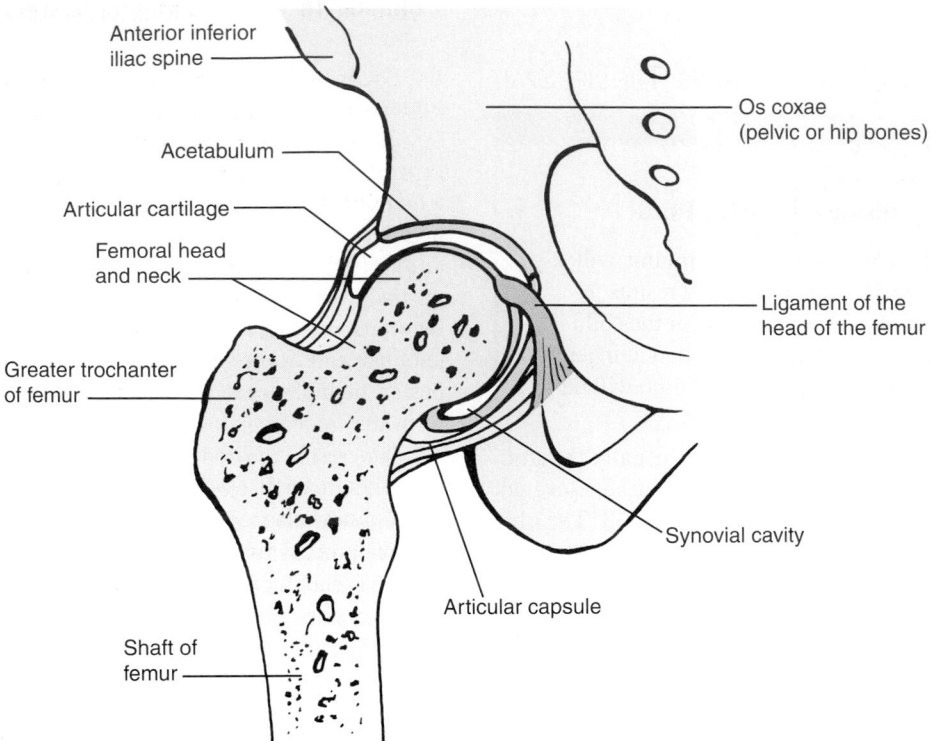

FIGURE 18-4. Hip joint. Section through right hip joint, showing insertion of head of femur into the acetabulum.

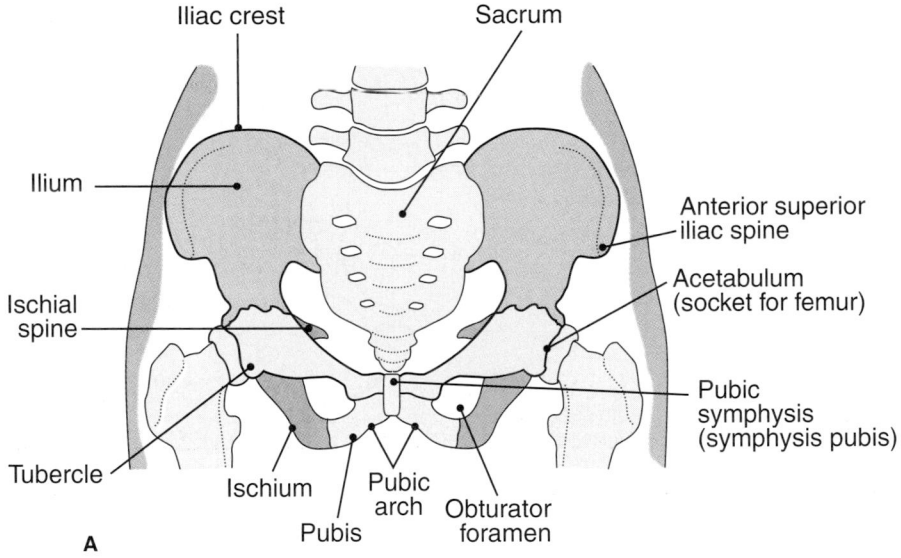

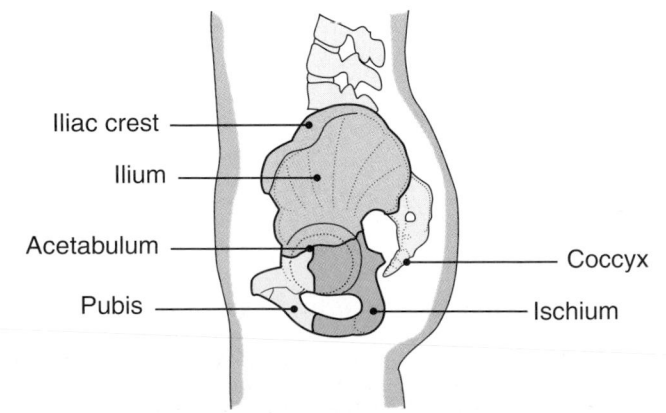

FIGURE 18-5. The pelvic bones. (**A**) Anterior view. (**B**) Lateral view.

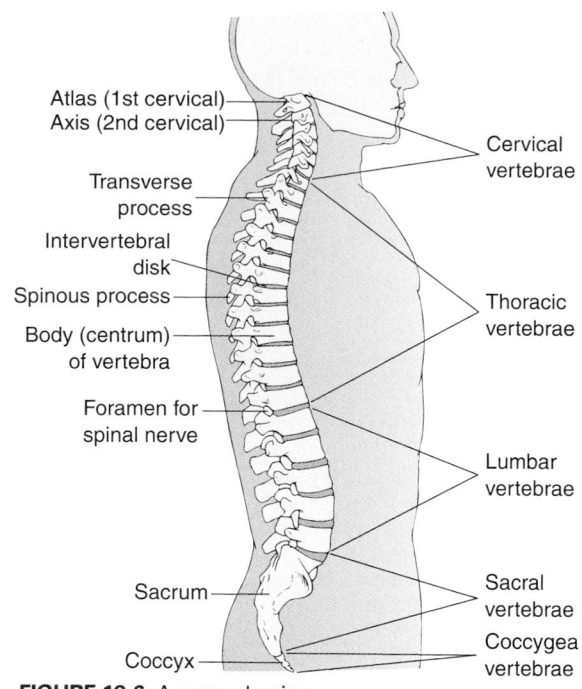

Atlas (1st cervical)
Axis (2nd cervical)
Cervical vertebrae
Transverse process
Intervertebral disk
Spinous process
Body (centrum) of vertebra
Thoracic vertebrae
Foramen for spinal nerve
Lumbar vertebrae
Sacrum
Sacral vertebrae
Coccygea vertebrae
Coccyx

FIGURE 18-6. A normal spine.

Open Areas. Openings (holes or open areas) also occur in bones. A hole through which blood vessels, ligaments, and nerves pass is called a *foramen* (plural: foramina). A long, tubelike hole is sometimes called a *canal.* Figure 18-3 shows the foramina of the spinal column. Note the *transverse foramen,* through which blood vessels and nerves pass, and the *vertebral foramen,* through which the spinal cord passes. Other important foramina and canals in the body provide passages for blood vessels and nerves. These include the *apical foramen,* an

opening in the root of each tooth; the *sciatic foramen* in the hip bone; *Alcock's canal* in the perineal area; the *carotid canal,* through which the carotid blood vessels pass into the cranium (head); and the *infraorbital canal* in the eye socket.

A **sinus** is a sponge-like air space within a bone, such as the paranasal sinuses within the skull bones (see Fig. 25-1). A dent, trench, or depression usually is called a *fossa* (plural: fossae). The *cranial* or *cerebral fossae* are depressions in which the brain rests. The olfactory bulb (for the sense of smell) lies in the *ethmoid fossa,* and the mandible (lower jaw bone) lies in the *mandibular* or *glenoid fossa.*

Joints

The points at which bones attach to each other are called **joints** or **articulations** (Table 18-2). Joints make hundreds of motions possible, because of the way the bones are attached. Joints are classified according to the degree of movement they permit:

- *Synarthroses* (*synarthrodial, fibrous,* or *fixed joints;* also called *sutural ligaments*) are immovable. The most familiar synarthroses are the joints between the bones of the skull (see Fig. 18-7). These joints are not firmly fixed in infants, but become fused by adulthood, as a result of the interlocking projections and by fibrous connective tissue growth. The joints of the skull are also called *sutures,* because they are so tightly bound or fused together. (A *syndesmosis* is a type of fibrous joint in which bones are united by fibrous connective tissue, forming an interosseous membrane or ligament. A *gomphosis* is a type of fibrous joint in which a conical process is inserted into a socket type of structure.)
- *Amphiarthroses* (*amphiarthrodial* or *cartilaginous joints*), such as those of the symphysis pubis or the articu-

▪▪▪ TABLE 18-2 *C*LASSIFICATION OF JOINTS

Type of Joint	Actions	Example
Synarthroses: immovable, fibrous	No motion	Bones of the skull fitted together with interlocking notches (in adults) (see Fig. 18-7)
Amphiarthroses: slightly movable, cartilaginous	Slight degree of motion or flexibility	Vertebral column (see Figs. 18-3 and 18-6) Symphysis pubis
Diarthroses: freely movable (synovial) Hinge joints	Motion like a door on hinges	Finger, elbow, and knee joints (see Fig. 18-8)
Ball-and-socket joints	Rotation	Shoulders and hips (see Fig. 18-8)
Pivot joints	Motion like that of turning a doorknob	Elbow (turn forearm) (see Fig. 18-8)
Gliding joints	Gliding motion	Wrist
Condyloid joints	Allow motions in two planes at right angles	Wrist, foot, hand
Saddle joints	Opposing surfaces are concavoconvex (fit together like two saddles with riding surfaces together); allow a wide range of movements	Thumb, vertebrae, ankle

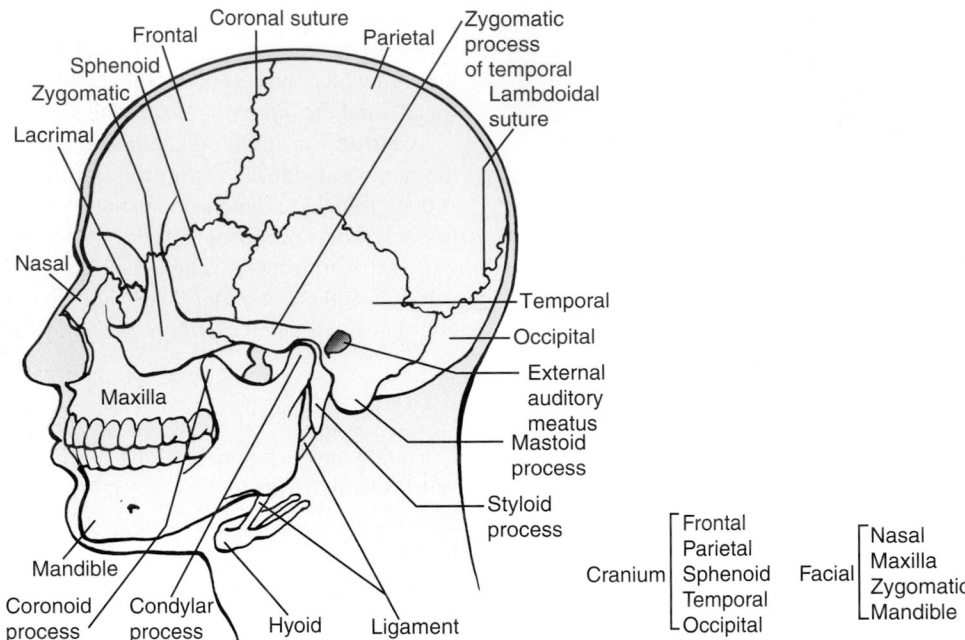

FIGURE 18-7. Bones of the adult skull.

lations between the ribs and the spinal column, are slightly movable (see Fig. 18-5). Their movement is very limited. Here, cartilage lies between the articulating bones. (A *synchrondosis* is a type of cartilaginous joint in which the cartilage is converted into bone by adulthood. An example is the coccyx [see Fig. 18-5]).

- *Diarthroses (synovial joints)* are freely movable, allowing movement in various directions. In addition to being present at the ends of the bones, these joints also contain ligaments and cartilage. The ligaments are tough fibers that bind bones together and are discussed below. A thin, smooth layer of articular cartilage covers and pads synovial joints, and an articular capsule encloses the ends of the bones. The capsules are lined with synovial membrane, which secretes *synovial fluid,* a lubricating material. Some synovial joints also contain *bursae,* fluid-filled sacs that cushion the movements of muscles and tendons (see Figs. 18-4 and 18-8).

Synovial joints.   Synovial joints are further classified according to their structure and range of movement. Types of synovial joints and examples include:

- *Hinge (ginglymus) joint* allows movement in only one plane, similar to the hinge of a door—as in the elbow and the finger joints between phalanges. (The jaw is a hinge joint, but it can also move slightly from side to side. The knee and ankle joints are hinge joints that allow some rotary movement as well.)
- *Ball-and-socket (spheroidal) joint* in which the rounded end of one bone moves within a cup-shaped depression in the other bone—as in the hip.
- *Pivot joint* in which one bone pivots or turns within a bony or cartilagenous ring—as in the atlas (first cervical

vertebra) and head rotating on the axis (second cervical vertebra).

- *Gliding (arthrodial, plane) joint* where the bones slide against each other– as in the intervertebral joints, and parts of the wrist and ankle joints.
- *Condyloid joint* where the oval-shaped head of one bone moves within the elliptical cavity in another, permitting all movements except axial rotation—as in the wrist (between the radius and the carpal bones) and at the base of the index finger (see Fig. 18-9).
- *Saddle joint* where movements can be shifted in several directions—as in the ankle and the base of the thumb.

An example of the hinge joint used to move the knee is shown in Fig. 18-8B. An example of a ball-and-socket joint is shown in Fig. 18-4.

Bursae.   **Bursae** (singular: bursa) are small, flat sacs lined with synovial membrane and filled with synovial fluid. They help ease movement, while reducing friction. Bursae are located around joints that are susceptible to pressure and trauma, such as the knee, shoulder, elbow, and hip.

Ligaments.   Strong fibrous bands called **ligaments** hold bones together. Some ligaments, known as *accessory ligaments,* do not move or stretch, but strengthen or support other ligaments to produce stability in the joint. Some ligaments connect bones to muscles or to cartilage. Ligaments also support internal organs and other structures. Many ligaments allow for great flexibility, stretching, and movement. A ligament is said to *arise* or originate in the bone or structure that is more stationary. It is said to *insert* into the bone that does most of the movement.

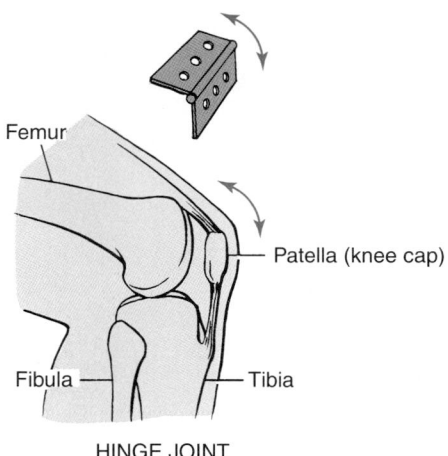

Femur

Patella (knee cap)

Fibula

Tibia

HINGE JOINT

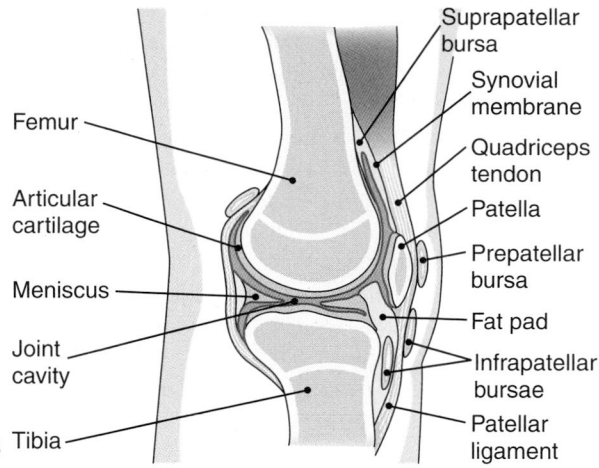

Suprapatellar bursa

Synovial membrane

Femur

Quadriceps tendon

Articular cartilage

Patella

Prepatellar bursa

Meniscus

Fat pad

Joint cavity

Infrapatellar bursae

B Tibia

Patellar ligament

FIGURE 18-8. *Continued* (**B**) The knee joint (sagittal section).

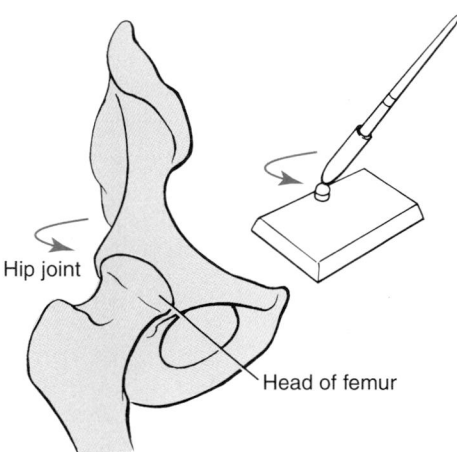

Hip joint

Head of femur

BALL - AND - SOCKET JOINT

There are hundreds of ligaments in the body. Common examples include:

- *arcuate ligament*—connects the diaphragm with the lowest ribs and first lumbar vertebrae
- *broad ligament* of uterus—a part of the peritoneum that supports the uterus, connecting the uterus and the pelvic wall
- *broad ligament* of liver (*falciform ligament*)—fold of peritoneum that helps attach the liver to the diaphragm, and also separates the right and left lobes of the liver
- *cruciate* ("cross-shaped") *ligaments* of knee—one anterior and one posterior—arise from the femur and attach to the tibia at the knee (frequent site of football injury)
- *Henle's ligament*—attaches rectus abdominus muscle to the pubic bone

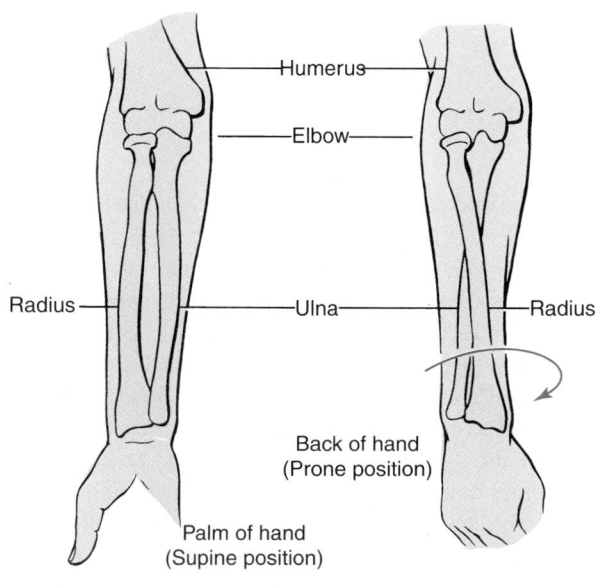

Humerus

Elbow

Radius

Ulna

Radius

Back of hand (Prone position)

Palm of hand (Supine position)

A PIVOT JOINT

FIGURE 18-8. (**A**) Some freely moveable joints. (*continued*)

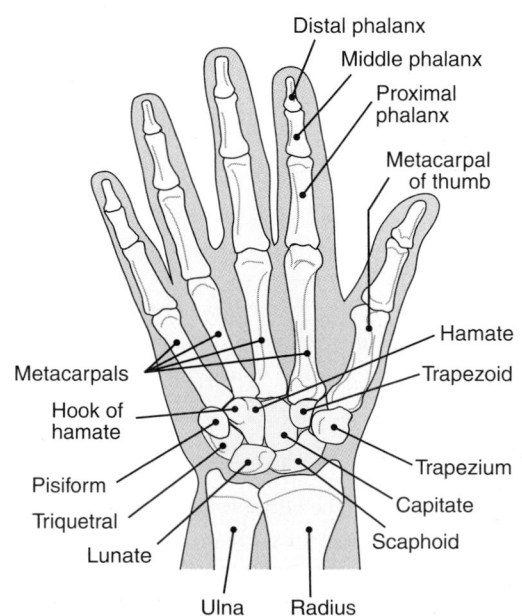

Distal phalanx

Middle phalanx

Proximal phalanx

Metacarpal of thumb

Hamate

Trapezoid

Metacarpals

Hook of hamate

Trapezium

Pisiform

Capitate

Triquetral

Scaphoid

Lunate

Ulna   Radius

FIGURE 18-9. Bones of the right hand, anterior (palmar) view.

- *inguinal ligament* (*Poupart's ligament*)—attaches anterior superior spine of ilium to spine of pubis
- *medial ligament*—large fan-shaped ligament on medial side of ankle
- *patellar ligament*—in the knee, attaches quadriceps femoris ("quads") to the patella and on down to the tibia (also called the *patellar tendon*)
- *periodontal ligament*—connective tissue surrounding roots of the teeth and holding them in place
- *pubofemoral ligament*—connects pubis and femur
- *rhomboid ligament*—connects cartilage of first rib to underside of clavicle
- *round ligament of femur*—broad ligament arising from acetabulum and inserting on head of femur

Cartilage.   **Cartilage** is a type of connective tissue organized into a system of fibers. *Articular cartilage* covers the ends of the long bones, such as in the knee or hip joint. It helps to reduce friction in the joints and to distribute weight evenly. Cartilage provides a slick surface for rotation (as in the wrist or ankle) and absorbs shocks and jars to the body (for example, between vertebrae).

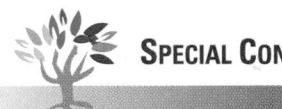 Special Considerations: The Life Span

Pliability of Bones

The bones of children are more pliable than those of adults because they contain a larger proportion of cartilage. You may find when working with children that their bones are more bendable for this reason.

Divisions of the Skeleton

The skeleton has two divisions: the axial skeleton and the appendicular skeleton. The *axial skeleton* contains the bones in the center or axis of the body. The *appendicular skeleton* contains the bones of the extremities and appendages of the body. Table 18-3 summarizes the major bones and divisions of the skeleton.

☞ Key Concept

The axial skeleton contains the bones in the center of the body such as the skull, vertebral column, and rib cage. The appendicular skeleton contains the bones of the extremities.

The Axial Skeleton

The bones of the skull, the vertebral column, and the thoracic (rib) cage make up the axial skeleton.

Skull.   Twenty-eight separate bones make up the skull (Table 18-4). The eight flat bones of the cranium protect the brain, eyes, and ears. The 14 facial bones are lightweight, irregularly shaped, and generally small. The three pairs of

TABLE 18-3 Divisions of the Adult Skeletal System	
Regions of the Skeleton	**Number of Bones**
Axial Skeleton	
Skull	
Cranium	8
Face	14
Hyoid	1
Auditory ossicles	6
Vertebral column	26
Thorax	
Sternum	1
Ribs	24
	Subtotal = 80
Appendicular Skeleton	
Pectoral (shoulder) girdles	
Clavicle	2
Scapula	2
Upper limbs (extremities)	
Humerus	2
Ulna	2
Radius	2
Carpals	16
Metacarpals	10
Phalanges	28
Pelvic (hip) girdle	
Hip, pelvic, or coxal bone	2
Lower limbs (extremities)	
Femur	2
Fibula	2
Tibia	2
Patella	2
Tarsals	14
Metatarsals	10
Phalanges	28
	Subtotal = 126
	Total = 206

bones of the middle ear (ossicles) are essential for hearing (see Chap. 21). Figure 18-7 illustrates the major bones of the skull. Thin fibrous membranes called *sutures* closely unite these bony surfaces. Sutures do not permit movement. The newborn's skull is different from an adult's skull. The newborn cranium has several membranes located between the cranial bones called *fontanels* (Fig. 18-10). These fontanels permit the skull of the infant to change shape as it passes through the vaginal canal, and allow growth of the infant's head.

The cranial and facial bones give the face its individual shape. Although the basic shape and arrangement of these bones are universal, subtle variations contribute to each person's unique face. There are two *maxillae* (singular: **maxilla**) that fuse to create the upper jawbone. The lower jawbone, the **mandible,** is the only movable facial bone. The mandible can move up and down, as well as forward (protraction) and backward (retraction).

TABLE 18-4 *THE 28 BONES OF THE ADULT SKULL*

Bones of the Cranium (8)

Two parietal: top and sides of head

One occipital: back and base of head

One frontal: forehead, roof of skull and nasal cavities

Two temporal: sides and base of skull (contain ear cavities); mastoid cells in tip

One sphenoid: center of base of skull

One ethmoid: roof of nasal cavity, base of cranium, upper part of nasal septum (also includes the paired and fused superior and middle conchae)

Bones of the Face (14)

Two nasal: bridge of nose

One vomer: divides nasal cavity, as part of nasal septum

Two inferior turbinates (conchae): in the nostrils

Two lacrimal (orbitals): front part of eye sockets

Two zygomatic: prominent part of cheeks; base of eye sockets

Two palate (palatines): back of hard palate

Two maxillae: upper jaw, front of hard palate

One mandible: lower jaw—only movable bone in skull

Auditory Ossicles (6) in the Ear

One pair malleus (hammer)

One pair incus (anvil)

One pair stapes (stirrup)

SPECIAL CONSIDERATIONS: THE LIFE SPAN

Fontanels

In newborns and infants, the skull bones are separated by spaces called fontanels. The anterior (front) fontanel is diamond-shaped and the posterior fontanel is triangular. Fontanels can be gently palpated on all healthy newborns.

A small horseshoe-shaped bone, the *hyoid,* lies just behind and below the mandible and directly above the larynx. The hyoid is not directly attached to any bone of the skull. Rather, it is attached by muscles and ligaments, and seems to float. Tongue muscles also are attached to the hyoid bone, to assist in swallowing. Four pairs of cavities or sinuses in the cranial bones make the skull lighter and enhance vocal sounds. The sinuses are named for the bones in which they lie: *frontal, ethmoid, sphenoid,* and *maxillary.* These sinuses are lined with a mucous membrane that is continuous with the nasal mucosa; the sinuses drain into the nasal cavity.

Vertebral Column. The **vertebral column,** or spine, holds the head, stiffens and supports the middle portion of the body, and provides attachments for the ribs and pelvic bones (see Fig. 18-6). The spine also protects the spinal cord, which passes from the brain down through the bony rings that make up the spinal canal (vertebral foramen). In children the vertebral column consists of 33 or 34 bones. Fusions of these bones occur during the process of growth and development. Therefore, the vertebral columns of most adults consist of 26 bones, or vertebrae.

The vertebrae are constructed on a common plane; each vertebra varies in its structure, but is designed to fit with the

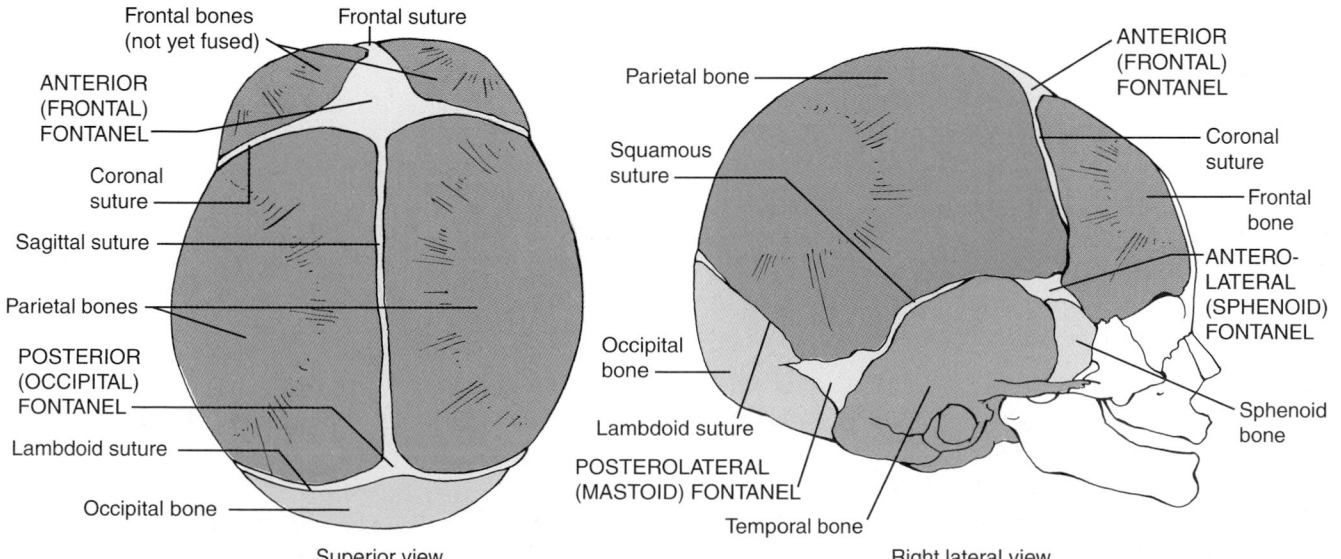

FIGURE 18-10. Fontanels of the skull at birth.

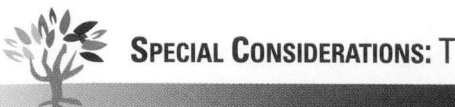

SPECIAL CONSIDERATIONS: THE LIFE SPAN

Spine Abnormalities

Scoliosis is an abnormal lateral (sideways) curvature of the spine. It occurs most commonly during adolescence and is more frequently found in girls than in boys. *Lordosis,* also known as "swayback," is an exaggeration of the normal lumbar spine curve in the small of the back. Assessment during routine health exams in children includes evaluation of the straightness of the spine or of abnormal curvatures of the spine (see Chapters 72 and 73). *Kyphosis,* commonly known as "widow's hump" or "humpback," may occur in aging and is more common in women (see Chapter 91).

vertebra beneath it (see Fig. 18-3). The top seven vertebrae are called the *cervical vertebrae* and are located in the neck. The first vertebra, or *atlas,* supports the skull. The second vertebra, or *axis,* has an especially wide surface so that the head can turn freely.

Directly below the cervical vertebrae are the 12 *thoracic vertebrae,* to which the ribs are attached. The next five vertebrae are the *lumbar vertebrae.* They are located in the small of the back. In adults, the *sacral vertebrae* are fused and are called the **sacrum.** The sacrum anchors the pelvis. The spinal column ends in a single bone in adults. This bone is the **coccyx,** commonly called the *tailbone.*

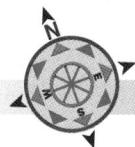

SPECIAL CONSIDERATIONS: CULTURE

Vertebrae

Most people have 26 vertebrae. Individuals from certain cultural groups may have fewer—11% of African American women have 23 vertebrae, and 12% of Alaska Natives and Native Americans have 25.

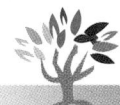

SPECIAL CONSIDERATIONS: THE LIFE SPAN

Sacral Vertebrae in Children

Children have 5 sacral vertebrae. These fuse to form the sacrum in the adult. Also in children, the last 4 vertebrae, the coccygeal vertebrae, are small and incomplete. These vertebrae later fuse to form the coccyx in the adult.

Rounded plates of cartilage called intervertebral disks separate the vertebrae anteriorly from one another. These disks

act as shock absorbers during walking, jumping, or falling. A "slipped" disk refers to an intervertebral disk that has shifted out of position. A "ruptured" disk occurs when pressure forces some less dense tissue sideways, causing a protrusion in the walls of the disk (like a squashed grape). Either of these situations can place pressure on a nerve, causing great discomfort.

On the inner side of each vertebra is a bony structure called the *arch,* which forms an opening, or spinal (vertebral) foramen, through which the spinal cord passes. Jutting from the arch are several fingerlike extensions, or processes, to which ligaments and tendons of the muscles of the back are anchored. The muscles, the ligaments, and the cartilage disks help to make the vertebral column strong, yet flexible. They enable the person to bend forward, backward, and side-to-side and to rotate the central portion of the body.

On each vertebra is an area where the ribs articulate with the vertebrae. This is called a *facet joint* (pronounced fah-set'). These joints are lined with cartilage, but may become misaligned. Many cases of back pain, particularly in the lower back, involve misalignment of these facet joints.

The normal spine has four curves that help to balance the body (see Fig. 18-6). Disease, injury, and poor posture distort these curves.

Thoracic (Rib) Cage.   The **thorax** (chest) is a cavity formed by 12 pairs of flat, narrowed bones called *ribs* (costae). These ribs make up the thoracic or rib cage. The ribs are arranged in pairs, 12 on each side. From their attachment to the spine at the back, the ribs curve out and to the front like barrel hoops. The relatively elastic cartilage on the ends of the ribs provides room for the chest and the abdomen to expand. The thoracic cage protects the heart, lungs, and the great thoracic blood vessels. It is also a supportive structure for the bones of the shoulder girdle. The floor of the thorax is the muscle called the *diaphragm.*

The first seven pairs of ribs, the "true ribs" or *vertebrosternal ribs,* are attached posteriorly to the thoracic vertebrae and anteriorly to the sternum. The next three pairs of ribs, the "false ribs" or *vertebrocostal ribs,* are also attached to the vertebrae posteriorly. However, they are joined only to each other anteriorly, via the costal cartilages. The last two pairs of ribs are also considered "false ribs." They are also known as "floating ribs" or *vertebral ribs,* because they are attached only posteriorly to the vertebrae and are not attached to each other.

The front boundary of the upper part of the thorax is the **sternum** or *breastbone,* a flat, sword-shaped bone in the middle of the chest opposite the thoracic vertebrae in the back. The sternum is made up of three sections. The *manubrium* is at the top; the *body* of the sternum is in the middle; and the *xiphoid process* projects out at the bottom (Fig. 18-11).

The Appendicular Skeleton

The appendicular skeleton is composed of the bones of the upper and lower extremities and the pelvic girdle (see Fig.18-1).

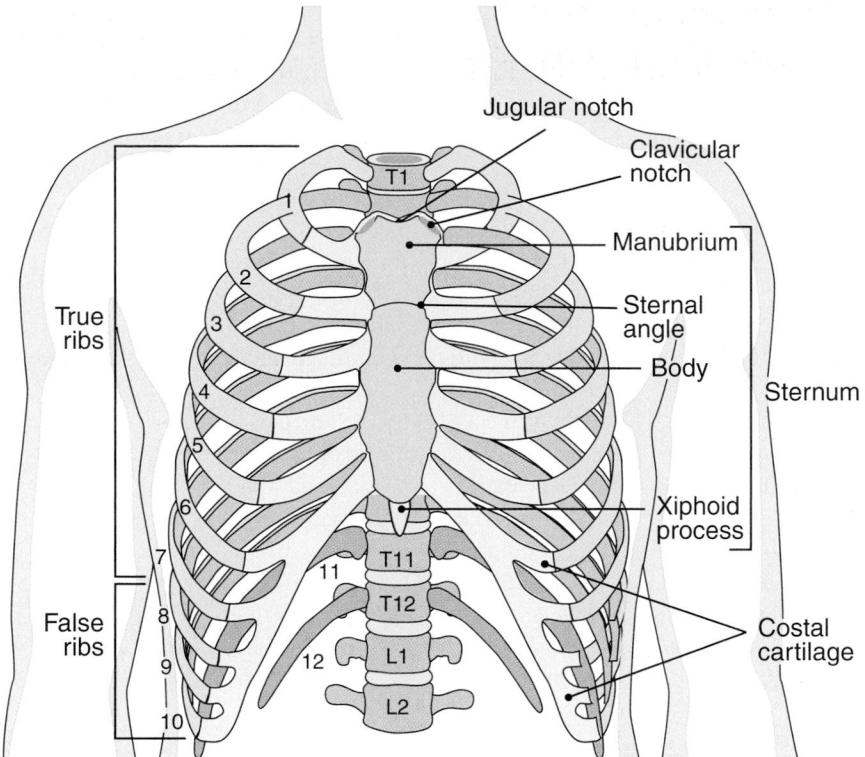

FIGURE 18-11. Bones of the thorax (anterior view). The first seven pairs of ribs are the true ribs; pairs 8 through 12 are the false ribs, of which the last two pairs are floating ribs.

Upper Extremities. The upper extremities include the shoulders and arms. Four bones form the *shoulder girdle,* which anchors the arms. Two long, thin bones, the **clavicles** (collar bones), are attached to the sternum and extend outward at a right angle to it on either side. Opposite the clavicles on each side of the back is a **scapula,** or shoulder blade. A scapula is a flat, triangular bone attached to the outer end of the clavicle on the skeleton. It attaches to the trunk of the body medially with the manubrium of the sternum. The structure of the scapula gives the body free movement of the shoulders and arms.

The **humerus** is the largest long bone found in the upper arm. The upper end is attached to the scapula, and the lower end meets the two forearm bones to form the elbow joint.

The forearm has two bones. The larger forearm bone, the **ulna,** has two hollows in its upper end. The lower end of the humerus fits into one of these depressions. The upper end of the smaller forearm bone, the radius, fits into the other. The **radius** lies beside the ulna and is attached to it at the upper end. Both the radius and the ulna are attached to the wrist bones to form the wrist joint (see Fig. 18-1). The arrangement of these bones allows the palm to be turned forward (*supine position, supination*) or backward (*prone position, pronation*). The radius and ulna move so freely with the wrist bones and each other that when the palm turns down, the radius crosses the ulna (see Fig. 18-8A).

More than 25% of the total number of bones in the human body are found in the hands and wrists. The many small bones in these areas allow for a great range of motion, such as twisting, bending, grasping, and squeezing. These bones enable human beings to perform such activities as playing musical instruments, writing, and picking up minute objects with the thumb and forefinger.

Figure 18-9 depicts the bones of the hand. The eight **carpal** bones, or wrist bones, are small and irregular bones that support the base of the palm. They are attached to the radius, the ulna, and the five long, slender, and slightly curved metacarpal bones that form the palm of the hand. The other ends of the metacarpal bones attach to the *phalanges,* or finger bones. Three phalanges are in each finger and two are in each thumb, with joints between each phalanx. (Any bone of either a finger or a toe is called a **phalanx.**)

Lower Extremities. The **femur** (thigh bone) is the upper bone of the leg. It is the body's longest and strongest bone and supports the weight of the upper body. The lower end of the femur is attached to the tibia of the lower leg at the knee joint. The upper end of the femur, described as the head (of the femur), is attached to the pelvic bone in a ball-and-socket joint, where its rounded head fits into a depression called the **acetabulum.** The head of the femur joins the shaft of the femur by a short length of bone called the *neck.* This area is a common site of fractures, particularly in older adults. Elevations on either side of the junction of the shaft and the neck are called the *trochanters* and serve as points of muscle attachment (see Fig. 18-4).

There are two bones in the lower leg: the tibia, or shin bone, and the fibula. The **tibia** is the weight-bearing long bone of the lower leg. The upper end of the tibia is attached to the lower end of the femur at the knee joint. A small bone, the **patella** (kneecap), which is buried in a tendon that passes over the joint, protects the front of the knee joint. The lower end of the tibia meets the bones of the ankle and the other bone of the lower leg, the fibula, to form the ankle joint.

The other bone in the lower leg, the **fibula,** is smaller than the tibia and is attached to the fibula at the upper end. The fibula is not a weight-bearing bone. It is not a part of the knee joint. The lower end of the fibula is involved in forming the ankle joint. There is a protrusion on the lower end of the tibia that can be felt on the medial side of the ankle. This is called the *medial malleolus.* There is another projection called the *lateral* (side) *malleolus* located where the distal end of the fibula meets the ankle bones (see Fig. 18-1).

The foot is constructed to support the weight of the entire body and at the same time to provide flexibility and resilience (Fig. 18-12). The seven *tarsal* bones of the ankle are compact and shaped irregularly; the largest of these bones (the **calcaneus**) is in the heel. The tarsal bones join the five *metatarsal* bones, or instep bones, to form two arches: the *longitudinal arch,* which extends from the heel to the toe; and the *transverse* or *metatarsal arch,* which extends across the foot. The weight of the body falls on these arches, and the many joints spring and give when a person walks. Weak muscles lessen this spring, and high spiky heels and poor posture upset the body balance, flattening the arches. The 14 bones of the toes, the *phalanges,* are attached to the metatarsals. The big toe has two phalanges; each of the other toes has three.

In general, the hands and feet are built alike, but the bones of the hands are finer and the joints are more numerous (29 bones are in the wrist and hand, and 26 are in the ankle and foot). The hands are designed for fine and flexible movements, and the feet are designed for support. Together, these bones account for about half the total number of bones in the body.

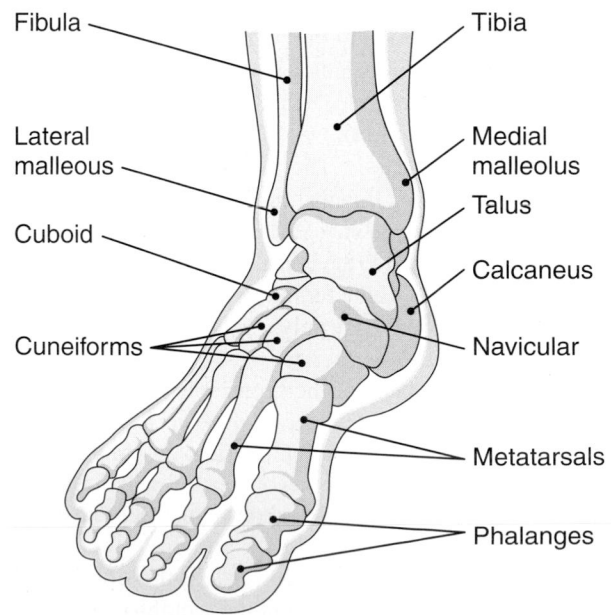

FIGURE 18-12. Bones of the right foot.

Fibula — Tibia
Lateral malleous — Medial malleolus
Cuboid — Talus
Cuneiforms — Calcaneus
— Navicular
— Metatarsals
— Phalanges

The Pelvic Girdle. Two large, irregularly shaped innominate *hip bones* (or *os coxae*) attach posteriorly to the sacrum (Fig. 18-5) to form the *pelvic girdle* or **pelvis.** The bones spread outward at the top and become narrow at their front lower edges. In the fetus, these bones develop as three separate bones known as the ilium, the ischium, and the pubis, which usually fuse by the time growth is completed. The age for normal completion of bone growth varies, from the late teens to the early twenties. The **ilium** is the upper flaring portion that one usually identifies as the hip bone. The *ischium* is the lower, stronger portion. The pubic bones meet in front and are joined by a pad of cartilage; this juncture is called the **symphysis pubis.**

Connected to the sacrum and the coccyx posteriorly, these bones form the *pelvic cavity,* which houses the urinary bladder, the rectum, and in women, the uterus and ovaries. In men, the prostate and some of the glands are contained within the pelvis. A woman's pelvis is larger and wider than a man's, which is nature's way of providing room for the development and vaginal delivery of the fetus. The angle of the pelvic opening (**pubic arch**) is less than a 90° angle in the man, and greater than a 90° angle in the woman.

THE MUSCLES

Functions of the skeleton include giving shape to the body and providing for mobility. Without the aid of muscles, the body would be as immobile as a classroom skeleton. Although the skeleton determines the size of the body's framework, muscle and fat determine a person's body shape. Functions of muscles are body movement, blood circulation, and heat production (Box 18-2).

Muscle Classification

Chapter 15 lists three types of muscle tissue: skeletal, smooth, and cardiac. Each type is also identified according to its appearance. Skeletal and cardiac muscles are *striated,* meaning that they consist of fibers marked by bands crossing them, which gives them a striped appearance. Smooth muscle is *nonstriated.* Muscles are further determined to be *voluntary* or *involuntary.* Table 18-5 presents the different muscle types.

Skeletal Muscles. *Skeletal muscles,* which control movements of the skeleton, are muscles under voluntary (conscious) control. They constitute approximately 40% of body weight. Their functions are locomotion, facial expression, and posture.

Smooth Muscles. *Smooth muscle* controls involuntary motions inside body organs (viscera). Smooth muscle is also known as *involuntary* or *visceral muscle.* Smooth muscle is responsible for propelling urine through the urinary tract, moving food along the digestive tract, dilating the pupils of the eyes, and dilating and contracting blood vessels to assist in blood circulation. Smooth muscles also respond to nervous stimulation in emergencies.

Cardiac Muscle. *Cardiac muscle* is the middle layer of the heart (myocardium). It is responsible for propelling blood

➤➤ BOX 18-2

FUNCTIONS OF MUSCLES

Voluntary Movement
• Enable walking, standing, sitting, and other movements
• Maintain body in upright position
• Participate in body balance

Involuntary Muscle Action
• Maintain heartbeat to pump blood
• Provide arterial blood flow
• Promote lymphatic and venous blood return to heart
• Dilate and contract blood vessels to control blood flow
• Maintain respiration
• Perform digestion processes
• Perform elimination processes
• Participate in reflexes
• Enable all other involuntary actions of body

Protection
• Protect body in emergency by reflex action
• Cover, surround, and protect internal organs (viscera)
• Support internal organs

Miscellaneous
• Produce heat
• Assist in maintaining stable body temperature (in shivering, "goose flesh," muscles give off heat)
• Provide shape to body

through the blood vessels. It works automatically; therefore, it is also an involuntary muscle.

☞ KEY CONCEPT

• *Skeletal muscle is responsible for locomotion, facial expression, and posture. These muscles are under voluntary control.*
• *Smooth muscle controls involuntary motion inside body organs.*
• *Cardiac muscle is involuntary and responsible for propelling blood through blood vessels.*

Structure of Skeletal Muscles

Skeletal muscles are considered organs. They possess multinucleated cells and a connective tissue framework. Muscles lie in sheets and cords beneath the skin and cover the bones. Each muscle fiber is comparable in size to a human hair and can hold about 1,000 times its own weight. Muscle fibers are wrapped together in bundles, and several bundles form a muscle.

Each muscle is covered by a sheath of connective tissue (*fascia*), which separates individual muscles or surrounds muscle groups, forming *compartments*. Most muscles attach one bone to another or extend from one part to another.

One end of the muscle, the *origin,* is relatively immobile. It is attached to the more stationary of the two bones needed for movement. The *insertion* is the part of the muscle that attaches to the bone that undergoes the greatest movement. The main

■■■ **TABLE 18-5** $\mathcal{C}$**OMPARISON OF THE DIFFERENT TYPES OF MUSCLE TISSUE**

	Smooth	Cardiac	Skeletal
Location	Wall of hollow organs, vessels, respiratory passageways	Wall of heart	Attached to bones
Cell characteristics	Tapered at each end, single nucleus, nonstriated	Branching networks, single nucleus, lightly striated	Long and cylindrical; multinucleated; heavily striated
Control	Involuntary	Involuntary	Voluntary
Action	Produces peristalsis; contracts and relaxes slowly; may sustain contraction; helps maintain blood pressure by regulating size of arteries	Pumps blood out of heart; self-excitatory but influenced by nervous system and hormones	Produces movement at joints; stimulated by nervous system; contracts and relaxes rapidly; produces heat through aerobic production of energy; assists in blood return to heart

part of the muscle is called the *belly*. The fibrous muscle tissue that covers bone is called *periosteum*. It is continuous with collagen fibers that form tendons and ligaments.

Tendons

The ends of fascia lengthen into tough cords called **tendons**. Tendons attach muscle to bones. The tendons have sheaths lined with a synovial membrane that permits a smooth, gliding movement.

To understand the anatomy of a muscle and its tendon, place the hand on the thick muscle at the calf. Some of the strongest muscles in the body are located here. Move the hand toward the ankle. As both the leg and the muscles become narrower, the tissues become tough, fibrous, and ropelike. This occurs because approximately halfway to the ankle, the muscle is attached to the *Achilles tendon,* which extends down to the heel.

Major Muscles of the Body

Table 18-6 lists the important body muscles, which are also identified in Figures 18-13 and 18-14.

Diaphragm and Intercostals

The *diaphragm* is one of the most vital muscles in the body. It is the dome-shaped muscle that forms the division between the thoracic and abdominal cavities. As the diaphragm contracts, it pulls downward, enlarging the thoracic cavity. The **intercostal muscles** are located between the ribs. When they contract, the thoracic cavity enlarges, both from side to side and from front to back.

The diaphragm and the intercostal muscles are the primary muscles of respiration. The contractions of the diaphragm and the intercostals work together to enlarge the chest space

■ ■ ■ TABLE 18-6 𝒯MPORTANT MUSCLES OF THE BODY

Muscle	Location*	Action	Notes
Neck and Shoulders			
Sternocleidomastoid	Side of neck	Helps keep head erect	If diseased or injured, head is permanently drawn to one side (torticollis).
Deltoid	Shoulder	Moves upper arm outward from body	Site for intramuscular injections
Arm and Anterior Chest			
Biceps	Front of upper arms	Flexes forearm	
Triceps	Posterior to biceps	Extends forearm	
Pectoralis major Pectoralis minor Serratus anterior	Anterior upper portion of chest Anterior chest, arising from ribs	Help to bring arms across chest	Known as "pecs"
Respiration			
Diaphragm (see Figures 25-1 and 25-4)	Between the abdominal and thoracic cavities	Assists in process of breathing	When diaphragm contracts, it moves downward, making chest cavity larger, forming a partial vacuum around lungs, and causing air to rush into them. When it relaxes, it pushes upward, and air is forced out of lungs.
Intercostal	Between the ribs	Helps to enlarge the chest cavity (side to side and back to front)	Same actions as above
Abdomen			
Internal oblique External oblique Transversus abdominis Rectus abdominis	Flat bands that stretch from ribs to pelvis, overlapping in layers from various angles	Support abdominal organs	An opening in muscle creates weakness where a hernia (rupture) may occur. Common is an inguinal hernia. Known as "abs"
Back and Posterior Chest			
Trapezius dorsi	Across back and posterior chest	Helps to lift shoulder	
Latissimus dorsi and other back muscles	Across back and posterior chest	Work in groups; help to stand erect, balance when heavy objects are carried, and turn or bend body; adduct upper arm	

(continued)

■■■ **TABLE 18-6** *I*MPORTANT MUSCLES OF THE BODY (CONTINUED)

Muscle	Location*	Action	Notes
Gluteal			
Gluteus maximus Gluteus medius Gluteus minimus	Form the buttocks	Help change from sitting to standing positions; help in walking	Gluteus medius used as site for intramuscular injections
Thigh and Lower Leg			

Quadriceps femoris group
  Rectus femoris
  Vastus lateralis
  Vastus intermedius
  Vastus medialis
	Anterior thigh	Extends leg and thigh	Rectus femoris and vastus lateralis used as site of intramuscular injection. Known as "quads"

Hamstring group
  Biceps femoris
  Semimembranosus
  Semitendinosus
	Posterior thigh	Flexes and extends leg and thigh	

Gracilis	Thigh	Flexes and adducts leg; adducts thigh	
Sartorius	Thigh	Flexes and rotates thigh and leg	Called "tailor's muscle" because it allows sitting in cross-legged position
Tibialis anterior	Anterior lower leg	Elevates and flexes foot	
Gastrocnemius	Calf	Flexes foot and leg	
Soleus	Calf	Extends and rotates foot	Give calf rounded appearance
Peroneus longus	Calf	Extends, abducts, and everts foot	
Achilles tendon	Attaches calf muscles to heel bone	Allows extension of foot and gives "spring" to walk	Term derived from Greek mythology
Head			
Orbicularis oculi	Head	Moves eyes and wrinkles forehead	Disorder may cause strabismus ("cross-eye")
Orbicularis oris	Head	Moves mouth and surrounding facial structures	
Masseter	Head	Assists in chewing by raising lower jaw	
Buccinator	Head	Moves fleshy portion of cheek for smiling	

*For placement of many of these muscles, see Figure 18-9.

and to form negative pressure within the thoracic cavity. This pressure causes atmospheric air to rush into the lungs, in an effort to equalize the pressure (see Chap. 17). Relaxation of these muscles causes the thoracic cavity to become smaller, thereby forcing air out of the lungs and into the atmosphere.

Muscles of the Hands and Feet
The muscles and tendons of the hands and feet are arranged in a slightly different manner from those of the rest of the body. Many bones, muscles, and tendons in the hands and feet are necessary to provide movement for these complex body parts. Because bulky muscles would make clumsy motions, the larger muscles used to move the hands and feet are located in the

forearms and the lower legs. For example, when you flex your fingers to clench your fist, you can feel the muscles move and tighten in your forearm. Other muscles begin at the wrist and extend into long, thin tendons that attach to the bones of the fingers. This placement permits accuracy and a variety of movements without great bulk.

SYSTEM PHYSIOLOGY
Formation of Bone Tissue

Bones are active, living organs that change greatly during a person's lifetime. The small, mostly cartilaginous bones of the

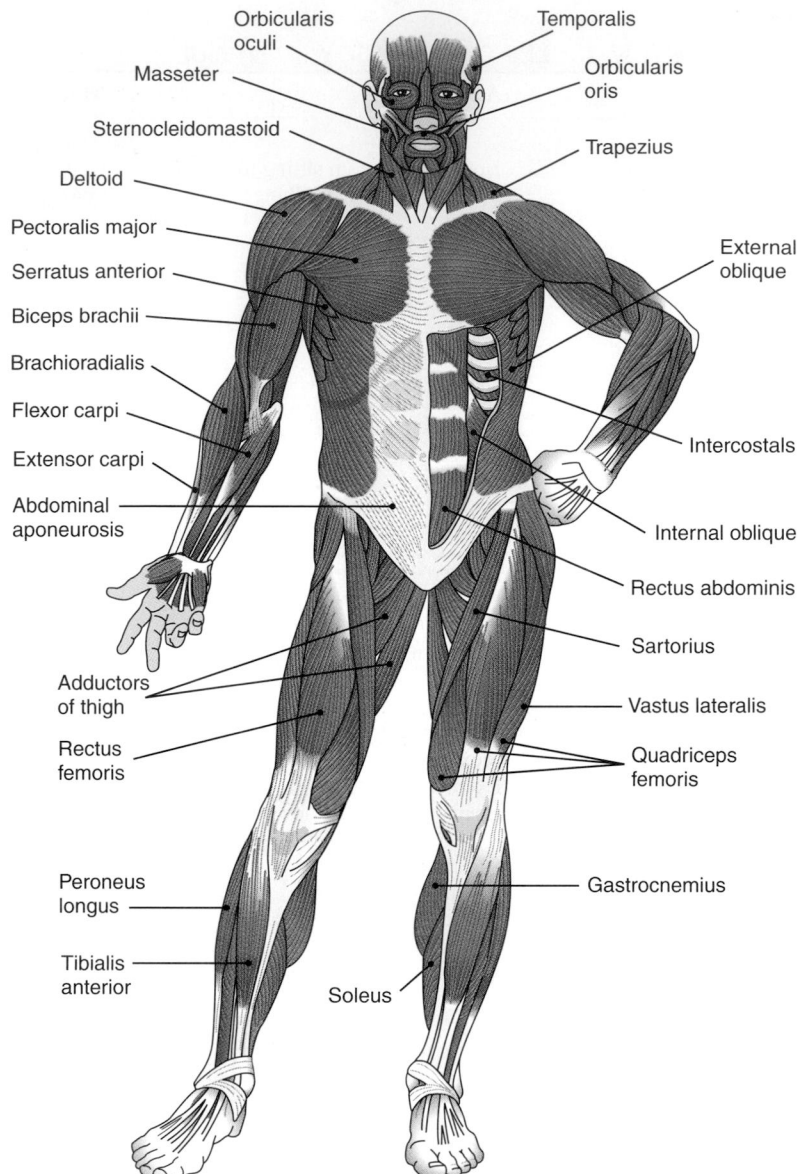

FIGURE 18-13. Muscles of the body, anterior view.

baby grow in diameter and length and continue to harden until growth is complete, usually between the ages of 18 and 21. Although bone structure and size alter primarily to accommodate growth, change also continues into later life, when the primary growth period is essentially over. Bone cells multiply rapidly in the growing years. When the growth spurts have stopped, new cells form only to replace dead or injured ones and to repair breaks. With age, bones become harder and more brittle, breaking more easily.

Although bone tissue hardens due to deposits of calcium and phosphorus, bones are made up of living cells. Bone-building cells are called **osteoblasts. Ossification** is the formation of bone by osteoblasts, and is the process by which bones become hardened, due to an increase in calcified tissue. Ossification progresses from the middle of the shaft outward. The hardened, mature bone cell is called an **osteocyte.** Other cells, the **osteoclasts,** assist in the resorption (or **reabsorption**) (act

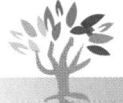

SPECIAL CONSIDERATIONS: Tʜᴇ Lɪꜰᴇ Sᴘᴀɴ

Bone Growth

Bone growth is rapid during infancy, steady in childhood, and has a rapid spurt in adolescents before the epiphyseal growth plate hardens and growth ceases.

of removal by absorption) or breakdown of bone. This process allows bones to grow and change shape. Bones continue building up and resorbing throughout life.

The following factors affect bone growth and maintenance:

• *Heredity:* genes

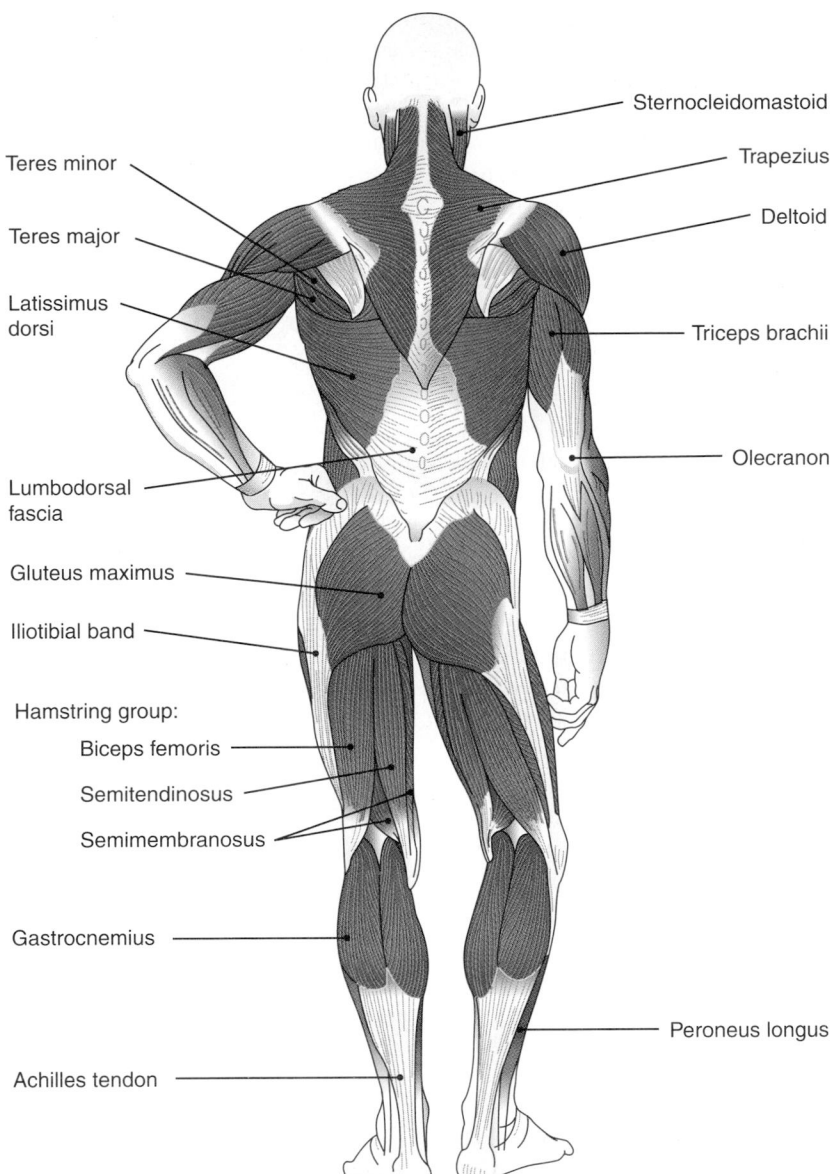

FIGURE 18-14. Muscles of the body, posterior view.

- *Nutrition:* protein, vitamins (A, D, C), and minerals (calcium, phosphorus) (see Chap. 30)
- *Exercise:* weight bearing (provides stress to strengthen bones)
- *Hormones:* affect rate of bone growth, calcium metabolism, energy production, and overall maintenance (see Chap. 20)

SPECIAL CONSIDERATIONS: NUTRITION

Lack of Vitamin D

Lack of vitamin D causes a bone malformation in children called *rickets* and in adults called *osteomalacia.*

Muscle Contractions

Some characteristics of muscle tissue are similar to those observed when stretching a heavy rubber band. Muscle tissue has the following special characteristics:

- **Contractility:** the ability to shorten and to become thicker
- **Extensibility:** the ability to stretch
- **Elasticity:** the ability to return to normal length after stretching
- **Irritability:** the ability to respond to a stimulus, often a nerve impulse that originates in the spinal cord and travels to a nerve

Muscles operate under an all-or-none principle. An individual muscle fiber cannot partially contract. If a stimulus is strong enough to cause contraction, each stimulated fiber will contract as much as it can. If the stimulus is not strong enough, the fiber will not contract at all. As you will learn in Chapter 19, the nervous system responds to the stimulus and directs muscle action. Muscles do not respond without stimuli.

Contraction and Relaxation

The elasticity of muscles allows them to work in pairs having opposite actions. When one muscle of the pair contracts, the other relaxes. A single muscle or a set of muscles, called the *prime mover,* initiates movement. When an opposite movement is to be made, another set of muscles called the *antagonist* takes over. Muscles that assist one another in movement are called *synergic* or *synergistic* muscles. When the elbow bends, the muscle in the upper arm contracts, hardens, and thickens as the muscle fibers shorten to raise the forearm (**flexion**). At the same time, the muscles on the back of the upper arm relax, lengthen, and pull against the front muscles. They will then pull the forearm straight (**extension**) in the opposing movement.

Power Source

Muscles need energy to move. Digested foods furnish carbon, hydrogen, and oxygen from which the body makes *glycogen* (sugar), a special form of stored glucose the body uses for fuel. The body also breaks down fatty acids for fuel. This fuel is called *adenosine triphosphate* (ATP). The blood brings oxygen and ATP, which react with one another (oxidation), to the muscle cells. The result of this oxidation process is energy and heat. Most of the body's heat originates from muscle activity. When muscles are very active, they draw on the reserve glycogen stored in their cells. When the body is cold, it uses the ability of muscles to produce heat rapidly by the automatic device of general muscle action (shivering). To produce a great amount of heat in an emergency, the body produces the more violent action of total body chilling.

Oxidation also produces the waste products of carbon dioxide and lactic acid. The blood carries carbon dioxide to the lungs, where it is removed in breathing. The urinary system and the sweat glands remove lactic acid from the body. Vigorous or prolonged muscle action produces such a large quantity of waste products, especially lactic acid, that the blood cannot carry it away fast enough. Some lactic acid thus accumulates in the muscle cells. Furthermore, skeletal muscles cannot remain in a contracted state for long periods of time without tiring. Gradually, due to a buildup of lactic acid and resultant lack of oxygen, a muscle becomes fatigued. Consequently, after exercise or prolonged use, muscles become achy and sore. A simple formula helps to summarize the action of muscles:

muscle cell + food and oxygen
↓
heat and energy
↓
by-products: lactic acid and carbon dioxide

Muscle Tone

Because human beings stand erect against the constant pull of gravity, many muscles in the body are constantly in a mild state of contraction to help maintain balance. Even relaxed muscles are ready to go into action if they are in good condition. This state of slight contraction and the ability to spring into action is called **muscle tone** (tonus). Physical exercise improves the tone of the muscles and increases their size. An idle muscle loses its tone and wastes away. If a person does not use certain muscles or uses them very little, the muscles become flabby and weak (atonic) and may **atrophy** (waste away).

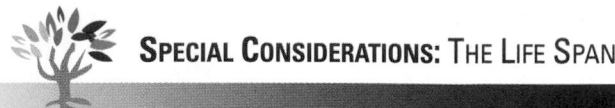

SPECIAL CONSIDERATIONS: THE LIFE SPAN

Retaining Muscle Tone

Children who sit in school all day need to have an opportunity for vigorous play after school. Their bodies need such stimulation to build and to maintain muscle tone.

Pressure on the nerves in muscles makes them sore. People who must often lie on their backs complain of aches and pains in these muscles. Strain or inactivity also affects them. For these reasons, a back rub can be comforting. When caring for a client with back pain, be sure to adjust the person's body to positions that do not cause strain. Change the position frequently, and support the person on his or her first time out of bed.

Nursing Alert
The client's position in bed should be the same *as if he or she were standing.* If this position is not ensured, the muscles may remain contracted because of the abnormal position *(contracture)*.

Isometric and Isotonic Contractions. Besides the constant muscle contractions that are considered muscle tone, two other types of contractions are important. **Isometric** contractions do not increase the length of a muscle, but do increase muscle tension. For example, if you push against an unmovable object or tense the muscles in your upper arm, your muscles tighten. This is an isometric contraction or exercise. Bedridden clients are encouraged to do isometric exercises, even if they cannot be out of bed.

Isotonic contractions shorten and thicken the muscle, causing movement. Exercises such as swimming, jogging, or bicycling are examples of isotonic exercises.

Rehabilitation. An injured or inactive muscle can be retrained to do its work. Except for the simplest movements, muscles work in groups. Therefore, retraining usually requires working more than one muscle. Today people are being helped to recover the use of injured or inactive muscles. Physicians often prescribe rehabilitation activities under the guidance of physical therapists and occupational therapists. Nurses may work under the direction of these specialists to help clients with selected exercises. Re-educating muscles is sometimes a long process. Improvement is likely to be so gradual that it is hardly noticeable from day to day. Clients often need encouragement to persevere.

Mobility

Purposeful coordinated movement of the body requires the integrated functioning of the skeleton, skeletal muscles, and nervous system. *Body mechanics* is the efficient use of the body as a machine (see Chap. 48).

Newborns are uncoordinated in their movements. Maturation of the central nervous system is necessary to prepare children to move purposefully. Babies are born with crawling and stepping reflexes that need to be developed in later infancy. The process of growth and development enables children to progress through certain stages. First they learn to sit up, then to crawl. They then learn to stand and to take steps with help. They begin to walk holding on to someone else's hand, and then walk without assistance. Children eventually progress to stair climbing, running, skipping, and hopping.

Increased mobility allows for increased independence. An adult **gait** pattern, or manner of walking, develops between ages 3 and 5. Infants have a wide-based gait. As children mature, the base narrows. They swing their arms in coordination. Stride and walking speed increase, and movements become smooth and graceful. Normal changes of aging cause the gait of older adults to widen again.

Range of motion (ROM) is the total amount of motion that a joint is capable of. ROM exercises are important for prevention and rehabilitation of musculoskeletal conditions (see Chaps. 47, 48, 76, and 96). Lack of mobility can result in changes in most organ systems. Some of the musculoskeletal changes include: decreased joint flexibility, decreased muscle tone and strength, and blood clots in the legs (as a result of muscle inactivity, which is needed to move the blood). Disorders of the musculoskeletal system are discussed in Chapter 76.

EFFECTS OF AGING ON THE SYSTEM

With aging, individuals gradually lose bone, as well as muscle strength and endurance. The muscle cells atrophy (a deterioration in size and function of cells) and fat cells replace them. Bone tissue does not replace itself as quickly as in younger years. Osteoporosis and fractures are common because of mineral loss from within the bone. Women are affected by osteoporosis more than men because of the loss of female hormones in menopause. Many older women take hormone replacements, vitamin D, and calcium supplements to help prevent osteoporosis. Joints commonly develop *osteoarthritis* (degenerative joint disease). Muscle aches and back pains are common due to the skeletal changes that cause conditions such as *kyphosis* (hunchback). Table 18-7 summarizes major effects of aging on the musculoskeletal system.

■■■ TABLE 18-7 *E*FFECTS OF AGING ON THE MUSCULOSKELETAL SYSTEM

Factor	Result	Nursing Implications
Bones		
Bone mass and strength is lost	Osteoporosis	Assess for fractures
Calcium is lost (greater in women)	Hunched posture (kyphosis: hump-back; lordosis: swayback) Back pain Brittle bones	Encourage vitamin D and calcium supplements Advise exercise to minimize bone loss Teach safety and prevention of falls Hormone replacement therapy often prescribed
Vertebral column shortens	Decrease in height (demineralization of bones)	
Joints		
Degeneration occurs in joints	Arthritis Osteoarthropathy Joint stiffness	Encourage person to increase mobility with active and passive range of motion exercises Hydrotherapy often helpful
Muscles		
Muscle cells are lost Muscle cells are replaced by fat Elasticity of fibers is lost	Loss of muscle strength Gain of fat tissue (and weight) Loss of flexibility Easy fatigability Resting tremors may occur	Give suggestions on how to carry daily items (eg, groceries) when it becomes more difficult Encourage person to control weight Suggest walking and swimming (good exercise for older adults); physical activity reduces loss of muscle, tissue, tone, and elasticity and increases flexibility Advise that exercise promotes psychologic stimulation Encourage proper nutrition, particularly adequate protein, vitamins, and minerals

The *nervous system* takes impressions and information from the outside world (external stimuli) and selectively stores this information in the memory for future reference and application. It also coordinates messages from internal body systems (internal stimuli), making it possible for the body to readjust constantly to changing internal and external environments. Consequently, the nervous system is the director of all body activities.

The nervous system is often likened to a telephone system. Through a network of wires, messages come into a central processor, where the necessary connections are made to send messages to the right places. Similarly, the nervous system is organized to bring messages into a center that relays them to certain body parts. The brain and spinal cord act as the central processor. The **nerves** are the wires that carry incoming and outgoing information.

No body system functions alone. The activities of various systems are interrelated, integrated, and coordinated by messages carried from one system to another. The nervous system is responsible for much of this communication. **Neurology** is the study of the nervous system.

STRUCTURE AND FUNCTION

The functions of the nervous system are communication and control (Box 19-1). To understand these functions, the nurse must first learn about the specialized cells of the nervous system (*neurons* and *neuroglia*), and the types of nerves that are made up of these cells.

▸▸ BOX 19-1

FUNCTIONS OF THE NERVOUS SYSTEM

Communication
• Monitors impressions and information from external stimuli
• Monitors information from internal stimuli
• Responds to danger, pain, and other situations
• Responds to internal and external changes
• Helps to maintain homeostasis
• Responds to conscious decisions and thoughts
• Coordinates processing of new learning

Control
• Directs all body activities
• Maintains blood pressure, respiration, and other vital functions
• Regulates body systems (in coordination with endocrine system)
• Coordinates reflex actions
• Controls instinctual behaviors
• Controls conscious movement and activities
• Stores unconscious thoughts

Cells of the Nervous System

The nervous system has two types of cells: the neuron (nerve cell) and the neuroglia. The **neuron** is the basic structural and functional cell of the nervous system. Neurons are specialized to respond to chemical and physical stimuli, and messages are conducted and transferred through them. The human brain regulates more than 10 billion neurons throughout the body at all times.

The number of **neuroglia** found in the body is five times greater than the number of neurons found in the body. Neuroglia support and connect nervous tissue, but do not transmit impulses.

Neurons

Neurons perform many functions. In the brain, they influence thinking, affect memory, and regulate other organs and glands. Although neurons are microscopic, they vary greatly in size and length.

A neuron is composed of three basic parts: one *cell body* and two *processes* (consisting of an *axon* and numerous *dendrites*). Figure 19-1 illustrates the structure of neurons.

Structure and Function. Each neuron has only one cell body, which contains the nucleus. Neurons do not divide and reproduce by mitosis like other cells of the body. After a nerve cell body is destroyed, it is gone forever. Protein synthesis occurs within the cell body in specialized organelles called *Nissl bodies (chromatophilic substance),* which are unique to the neuron. The cell body may be quite a distance from its axon or dendrites.

An **axon** is an extension that carries impulses away from the neuron cell body. An axon may be as short as a few millimeters, or it may be longer than a meter. It may be myelinated (covered in a protective layer), or it may be bare. This structural difference is important.

An axon surrounded by a **myelin sheath** (a fatty covering) is said to be *myelinated.* Myelinated axons conduct impulses more rapidly than unmyelinated axons. The myelin sheath electrically insulates one nerve cell from another. Without this sheath, these nerve cells would short circuit.

Dendrites are short, often highly branched extensions of the cell body. Dendrites receive impulses from the axons of other neurons and transmit these impulses toward the cell body. Dendrites respond to chemical messages sent across the synapse, which is the tiny space that separates neurons from each other.

A **synapse** is the junction, or space, between the axon of one neuron and the dendrites of the next. A nerve can transmit impulses in only one direction because of the location of neurotransmitters. A **neurotransmitter** is a chemical that an axon releases to allow nerve impulses to cross the synapse and therefore reach the dendrites. Cell bodies and dendrites do not have neurotransmitters. The receiving cell quickly inactivates the neurotransmitter with a specific opposing chemical to prevent continuous impulses. An example of a neurotransmitter is *acetylcholine,* which is inactivated by an enzyme called *cholinesterase. Dopamine, norepinephrine,* and *serotonin* are also neurotransmitters. These names may be familiar to you

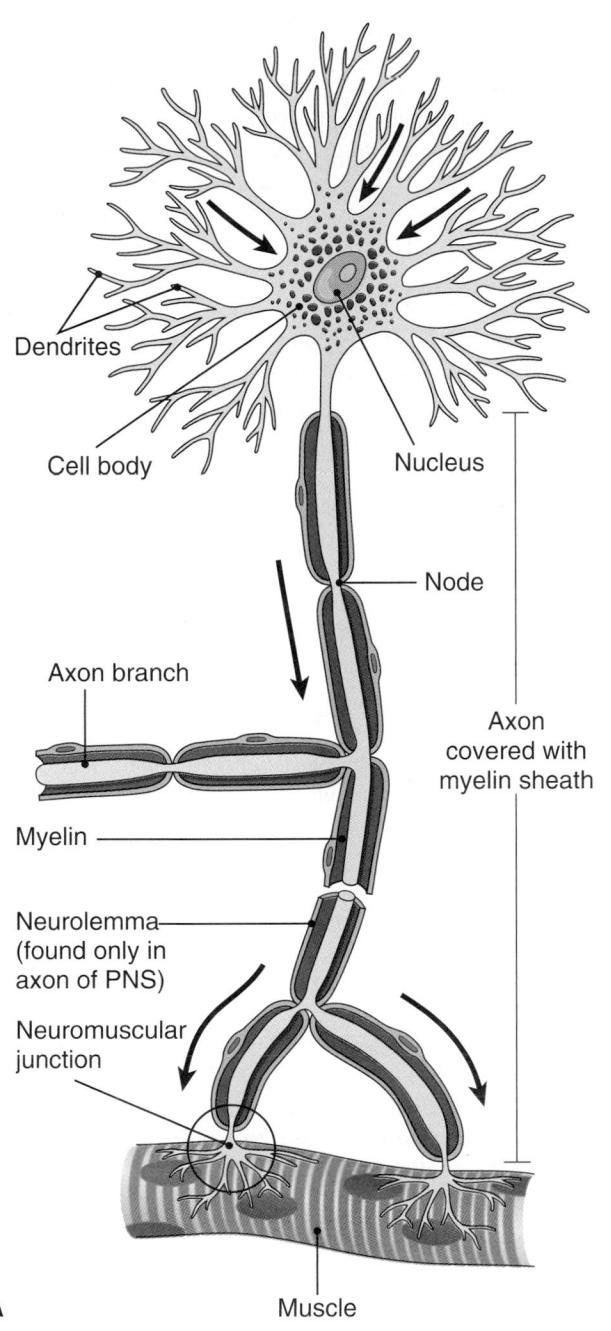

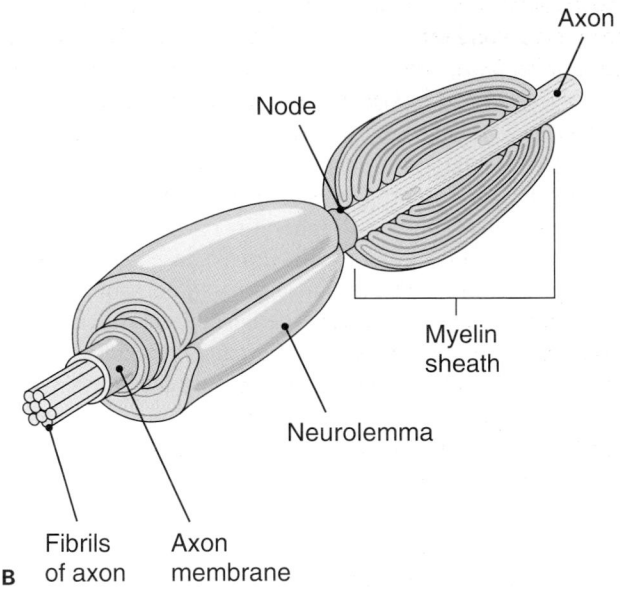

FIGURE 19-1. A motor neuron. (The break in the axon shows that the axon is longer than pictured.) The *arrows* show the direction of the nerve impulse. *Above right* is the formation of the myelin sheath. The outermost layer of the Schwann cell forms the *neurolemma*. Spaces between the cells are the *nodes*.

because many of their properties have been developed into useful pharmacological products.

Classification. Neurons can be classified according to their shape, but they are more commonly remembered by their functions: sensory neurons, motor neurons, or interneurons.

- Sensory (**afferent**) neurons receive and transmit messages *to the central nervous system* from all parts of the body.
- Motor (**efferent**) neurons receive and transmit messages *from the central nervous system* to all parts of the body.
- **Interneurons** (*connectory* or *association neurons* or *integrators*) can be thought of as a link between the two

other types of neurons. They are *interconnecting* neurons. Interneurons are located only within the central nervous system.

☞ KEY CONCEPT

The three types of neurons are sensory neurons, motor neurons, and interneurons.

Nerves. Sensory neurons make up *sensory nerves.* Motor neurons make up *motor nerves,* which alter muscle activity and cause glands to secrete. Both sensory and motor neurons make up what are known as *mixed nerves,* which are further discussed later in this chapter.

Neuroglia

Neuroglia (**glial cells**) are much more numerous than neurons. They can multiply to fill spaces that have been previously occupied by neurons. Some brain tumors are called *gliomas* because they are caused by the rapid growth of glial cells. There are four types of neuroglia in the central nervous system: astrocytes, oligodendrocytes, microglia, and ependymal cells. The two types of neuroglia in the peripheral nervous system are the neurolemmocytes and Schwann cells. These types of cells help form the blood–brain barrier, the cerebrospinal fluid, and the myelin sheath. They also obtain nutrients (specifically glucose) for the neurons, and support and protect the central and peripheral nervous systems in various other ways.

DIVISIONS OF THE NERVOUS SYSTEM

The nervous system is divided into two major parts: the central nervous system and the peripheral nervous system. The central nervous system consists of the brain and the spinal cord. The peripheral nervous system consists of the cranial nerves, spinal nerves, and the autonomic (or automatic) nervous system. The divisions and subdivisions of the human nervous system are discussed in the following sections.

Central Nervous System

The central nervous system (**CNS**) is made up of the brain, the spinal cord, and accessory structures. The *spinal cord* functions as a major pathway to carry information between the body and the brain. The *brain* is responsible for interpreting this information and for directing body responses.

The Brain

The human brain is composed of approximately 100 billion neurons and innumerable synapses. It weighs approximately 1.36 kilograms (3 lb), which is about 2% of the body's weight. However, the brain uses approximately 20% of the body's circulating blood flow (about 750 mL/min). The brain has an extensive and specialized vascular supply. It has a higher metabolic rate than the rest of the body, and this rate remains constant during physical or mental exercise. The brain must have a constant flow of oxygen and nutrients, especially glucose. A failure of blood flow for as few as 10 seconds will result in unconsciousness. The brain is particularly sensitive to toxins and drugs.

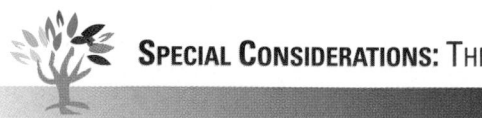

SPECIAL CONSIDERATIONS: THE LIFE SPAN

Infant Blood–Brain Barrier

Infants have an immature blood–brain barrier. This allows substances to pass into the brain of an infant that would not normally enter an adult's brain.

Although the brain has many parts, it functions as an integrated whole. Box 19-2 summarizes the components and functions of the brain.

Cerebrum.   Eighty percent of the brain's volume is the **cerebrum** (Fig. 19-2), which fills the upper part of the cranium (skull cavity). The cerebrum is divided into two *layers* and two *halves (hemispheres)*. Each portion of the cerebrum has individualized functions. All the portions, however, are integrated, and many areas overlap.

Cerebral Cortex. The adjective *cerebral* pertains to the unique human abilities of learning, intelligent reasoning, and judgment. The *cerebral cortex* is the outside layer of the brain. It is made of soft *gray matter*, mostly nerve cell bodies. The cortex is wrinkled and folded back on itself many times. These folds are called *convolutions* or *gyri* (singular: *gyrus*). The crevices between the folds are called *fissures* or *sulci* (singular: *sulcus*). Because of the folds, the cortex has a large surface area and therefore contains millions of neurons.

The cerebral cortex is divided into four lobes. These lobes are named after the overlying cranial bones: frontal, parietal, temporal, and occipital. These special centers in the cerebrum enable humans to associate impressions and information, which becomes knowledge.

- The **frontal lobe** is larger in humans than in all other animals. It controls the areas for *written* and *motor speech* (see Fig. 19-2). It is largely responsible for the ability of humans to achieve higher levels of mental functioning, including conception, judgment, speech, and communication. The *frontal lobe* is involved with motor functions that direct body movements.
- The *sensory area* is located in the **parietal lobe.** This area interprets sensations such as touch, temperature, and pain, which are received from the skin. Spatial ability (the ability to recognize shapes and sizes) is also located in this area.
- The **temporal lobe** controls the sensations of hearing, auditory interpretation, and smell. The *auditory* areas both receive and interpret transmissions.
- Visual transmissions and interpretation occur in the *visual* areas of the **occipital lobe.** These areas direct a person's visual experiences.

White Matter. The interior of the brain consists of *white matter*. It lies under the cerebral cortex. Billions of synapses between axons and dendrites are located here. This area is white because of the myelinated axons that connect the lobes of the cerebrum to each other and to all other parts of the brain.

Cerebral Hemispheres. The right hemisphere of the brain controls the muscles of and receives sensory information from the left side of the body. The left hemisphere controls the muscles of and receives sensory information from the right side. This phenomenon is a result of **decussation** (crossing) of the nerve tracts within the brain's medulla. Figure 19-2 shows some functional areas of the cerebrum. The two hemispheres of the brain process information differently. The right side is associated with spatial perception, pictures, art, and musical ability. The left hemisphere is connected with analytic and verbal skills (eg, reading and writing, words, symbols, mathematics, and speech) and walking.

The *corpus callosum* is a band of approximately 200 million neurons located deep within the brain. It connects the right and left cerebral hemispheres. The corpus callosum allows one

➤➤ BOX 19-2

COMPONENTS OF THE BRAIN AND THEIR FUNCTIONS

Cerebrum: center of conscious thought and higher mental functioning.

Cerebral cortex: gray matter (nerve cell bodies); outer layers of cerebrum; has convolutions (grooves) and elevations (gyri) that increase brain's surface area

Inner portion of brain

White matter: location of billions of connections due to presence of dendrites and myelinated axons

Lobes

Frontal: location of higher mental processes (intelligence, motivation, mood, aggression, planning); site for verbal communication and voluntary control of skeletal muscles

Parietal: location of skin, taste, and muscle sensations; speech center; forms words to express thoughts and emotions; interprets textures and shapes

Temporal: location of sense and smell and auditory interpretation; stores auditory and visual experiences; forms thoughts that precede speech

Occipital: location of eye movements; integrates visual experiences

Hemispheres: longitudinal fissure divides brain into two halves

Corpus callosum: connects hemispheres internally

Diencephalon: interbrain located between the cerebral hemispheres and brain stem

Thalamus: consolidates sensory input; influences mood and body movements; is associated with strong emotions

Hypothalamus: center for temperature regulation, hunger, peristalsis, thirst, sex, and sleep–wake cycle; controls heart rate and blood vessel diameter; influences pituitary gland secretions; controls muscles of swallowing, shivering, and urine release

Limbic system: consists of the hippocampus and the reticular formation; responsible for learning, long-term memory, wakefulness, and sleep

Cerebellum: second-largest part of the brain; location of involuntary movement, coordination, muscle tone, posture, and equilibrium

Brain stem: connects cerebral hemispheres with spinal cord

Midbrain: located at top of brain stem; acts as visual and auditory reflex center; righting reflex located here

Pons (bridge): carries messages between cerebrum and medulla; acts as respiratory center to produce normal breathing patterns

Medulla: located at floor of skull; connects the brain to the spinal cord; vital for life; descending nerve tracts from brain cross here to opposite side; contains centers for many body functions (cardiac, vasomotor, and respiratory center; swallowing, coughing, and sneezing reflexes)

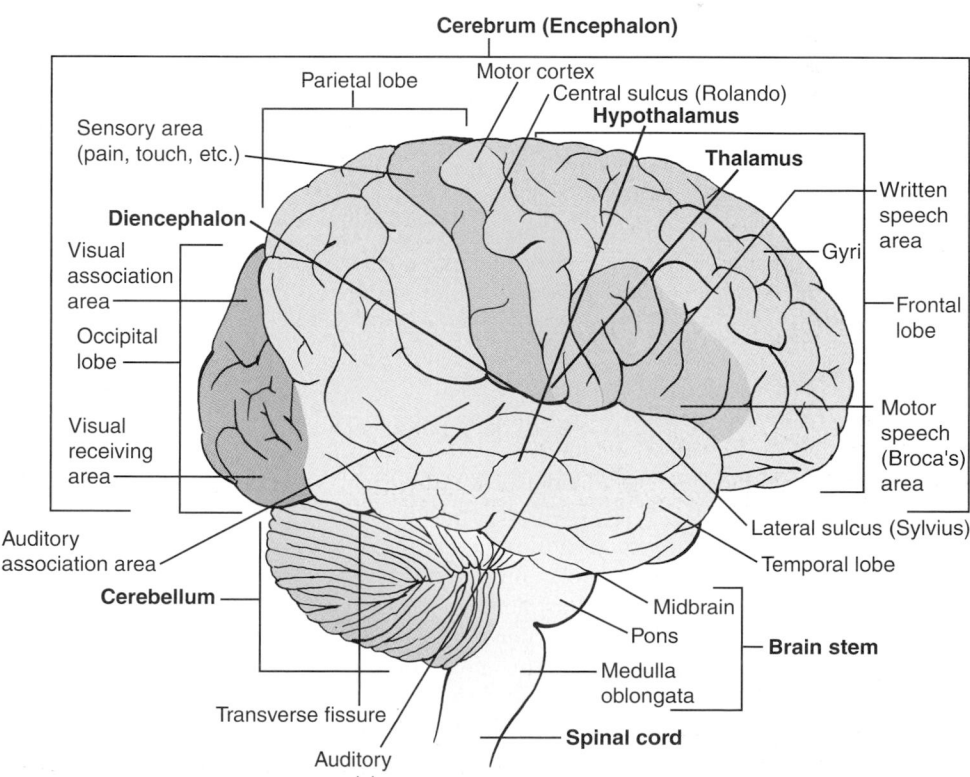

FIGURE 19-2. The human brain, showing the lobes and sulci (fissures) of the cerebrum as well as the cerebellum. Major functional areas also are indicated.

cerebral hemisphere to share information with the other. If this structure is severed, the right hand will literally not know what the left hand is doing.

☞ KEY CONCEPT

Individuals who have had a cerebrovascular accident (eg, stroke) affecting one brain hemisphere show symptoms (eg, paralysis) on the opposite side of the body. A left-sided stroke is common; in this case, the right side of the body may be paralyzed.

Thalamus.   The **thalamus** is located in the *diencephalon* portion of the brain, between the hemispheres and brain stem. It lies just superior to the hypothalamus. It is a relay station between the cutaneous (skin) receptors and the cerebral cortex for all sensory impulses, except smell. The thalamus integrates sensations so that a person can perceive a whole experience and not just individual impulses. For example, touching a snowball produces sensations of cold, pressure, texture, and shape. The thalamus integrates all of these sensations to present the whole picture. The thalamus also has some crude awareness of pain. It may suppress unimportant sensations to permit the cerebrum to concentrate on important aspects of daily activities.

Hypothalamus.   Although small, the **hypothalamus** is vital to human functioning. It is located below the thalamus in the diencephalon portion of the brain. Most functions of the hypothalamus relate directly or indirectly to the regulation of visceral activities. The hypothalamus has a role in increasing or decreasing bodily functions, and it regulates the release of hormones from the pituitary gland (which regulates many of the body's hormones) (see Chap. 20). These functions include regulation of body temperature, water balance, sleep, appetite, and emotions.

Limbic System.   The **limbic system** is located between the cerebrum and the inner brain. It is largely responsible for maintaining a person's level of awareness. The limbic system includes the hippocampus and the reticular formation. The *hippocampus* functions in learning and long-term memory. The *reticular formation* has a role in sensory input coming into the cerebral cortex. It also governs wakefulness and sleep, through a portion of the reticular formation called the reticular activating system (**RAS**). This system is affected by environmental stimuli via the eyes and ears, which activate the RAS to assist a person in awakening and in maintaining alertness.

Cerebellum.   The **cerebellum** is the second-largest part of the brain (see Fig. 19-2). Its functions are concerned with movement: muscle tone, coordination, and equilibrium. It coordinates the action of voluntary muscles and adjusts to impulses from the proprioceptors within muscles, joints, and sense organs. (*Proprioceptors* relay information about balance and body position.) The adjustments made in the cerebellum help a person to maintain balance when walking, to make graceful movements, to throw a ball, or to go inline skating.

Brain Stem.   The **brain stem** connects the cerebral hemispheres with the spinal cord. It includes the midbrain, the pons, and the medulla (see Fig. 19-2).

The **midbrain** is located at the very top of the brain stem and functions as an important reflex center. Visual and auditory reflexes are integrated here. When you turn your head to locate a sound, you are using the midbrain. The *righting reflex*, or the ability to keep the head upright and to maintain balance, is also located here.

The word "pons" means "bridge." The term reflects the fact that the **pons** contains nerve tracts that carry messages between the cerebrum and the medulla. The pons has respiratory centers that work with the medulla to produce a normal breathing pattern.

The **medulla** (also known as *medulla oblongata*) lies just below the pons and rests on the floor of the skull. It is continuous with, but not part of, the spinal cord. Nerve tracts that descend from the brain cross to the opposite side here. The medulla contains centers for many vital body functions, including the *cardiac center* (regulates heart rate), *vasomotor center* (regulates the diameter of blood vessels, thereby regulating blood pressure), and *respiratory center* (regulates breathing). Other activities of the medulla are concerned with reflexes, such as swallowing, coughing, and sneezing. Because the medulla is responsible for regulating so many vital body processes, any injury to the occipital bone at the base of the skull can be instantly fatal because of its proximity to the medulla.

The Spinal Cord

The **spinal cord** is a long mass of nerve cells and fibers extending through a central canal from the medulla to the approximate level of the first or second lumbar vertebra (see Chap. 18). Its position within the vertebral column helps to protect the spinal cord from shocks and injuries. This protection is essential because the nerve fibers of the spinal cord cannot regenerate after an injury.

The spinal cord has two main functions: to conduct impulses to and from the brain and to act as a *reflex center*. The reflex center in the cord receives and sends messages through the nerve fibers. This "circle" is known as a **reflex arc** (Fig. 19-3). The reflex center acts as a substation for messages and relieves the brain of routine work. Some nerve fibers in the cord are sensory; that is, they carry messages to the brain. Other nerve tracts are motor, carrying messages away from the brain.

☞ KEY CONCEPT

The nerve fibers of the spinal cord cannot regenerate after an injury.

Accessory Structures

The three major accessory structures of the central nervous system are the meninges, cerebrospinal fluid, and ventricles.

Meninges.   The brain and the spinal cord (that is, the CNS) are covered with three protective membranes called the **meninges** (Figure 19-4). The *dura mater,* the outer layer, is a tough fibrous covering that adheres to the bones of the skull. The middle layer is a delicate web of tissue called the *arachnoid.* The *pia mater,* the inner layer, lies closely over the brain and spinal cord. It is thin and vascular, containing many blood vessels that bring oxygen to nourish the nervous tissue.

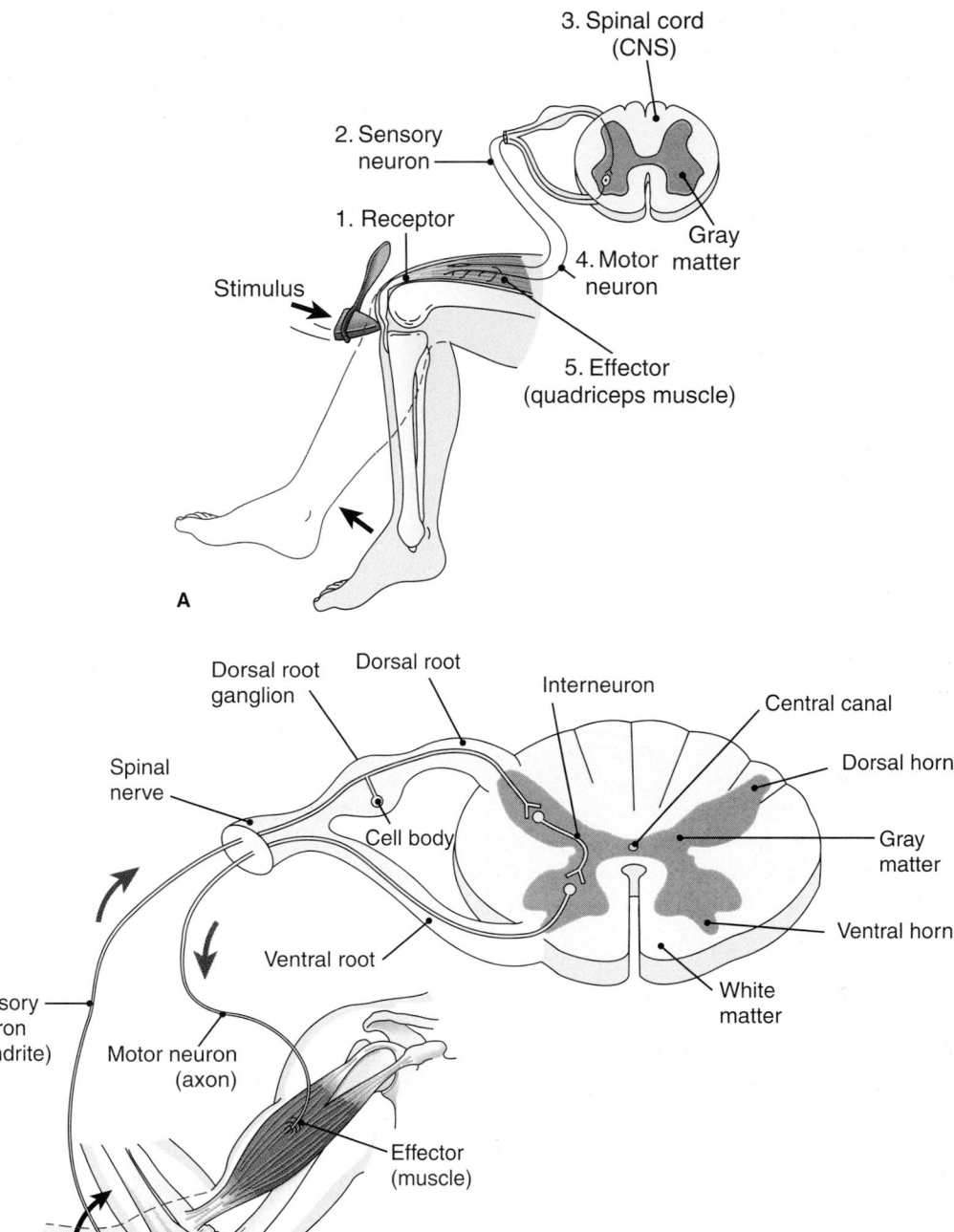

FIGURE 19-3. Reflex arcs, showing pathways of impulses in response to a stimulus. (**A**) The cross-section of the spinal cord shows the simplest reflex, the patellar (knee-jerk) reflex, which involves only sensory and motor neurons. (**B**) The response to a painful stimulus, such as a flame, also involves a central neuron. This is a three-neuron reflex arc.

The space between the arachnoid membrane and the pia mater is the *subarachnoid space.* The subarachnoid space contains cerebrospinal fluid, the tissue fluid of the CNS.

☞ KEY CONCEPT

Head trauma can result in intracranial bleeds with blood accumulating under specific meninges: under the dura matter (subdural), or under the arachnoid (subarachnoid).

Cerebrospinal Fluid.   Cerebrospinal fluid (**CSF**) is a lymph-like fluid that forms a protective cushion around and within the CNS (Box 19-3). CSF allows the brain to "float" within the cranial vault, which changes the effective weight of the brain from about 1,500 grams to about 50 grams. The CSF removes cellular waste from nerve tissue and lessens damage caused on impact by spreading out the force of trauma. It is produced in specialized capillary

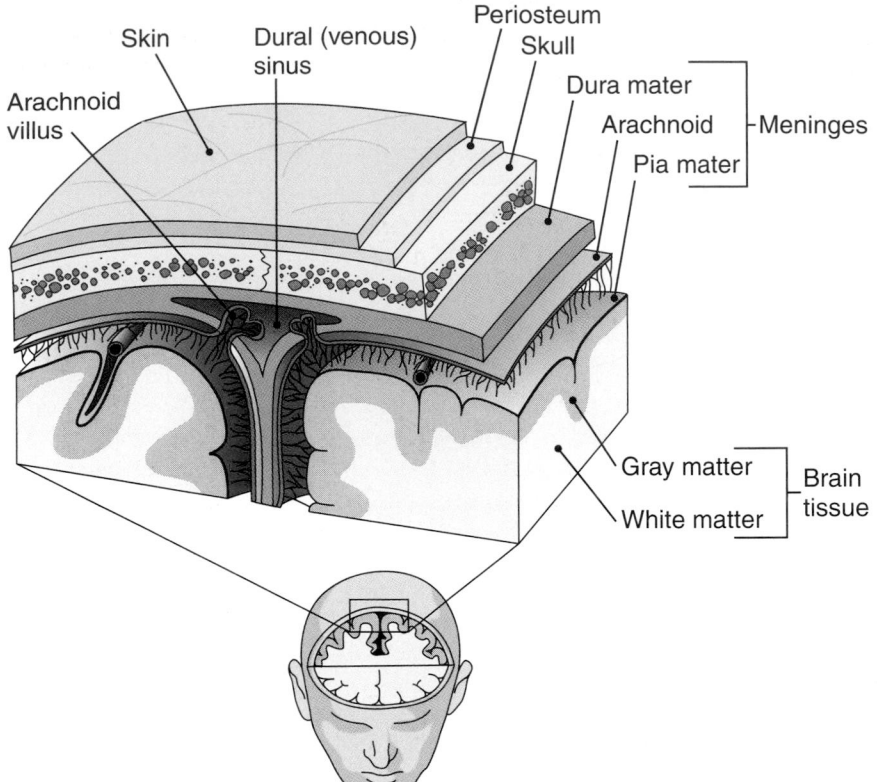

FIGURE 19-4. Frontal (coronal) section of the top of the head, showing meninges and related parts.

networks (the *choroid plexuses*) in the ventricles of the brain. About 800 milliliters are produced each day, although only 150 to 200 milliliters circulate at any one time. Arachnoid villi reabsorb some CSF into the blood, where it becomes blood plasma again.

A physician may withdraw a small amount of CSF through the space between two vertebrae. This procedure is called a *lumbar puncture* or *spinal tap*. Laboratory studies of CSF can reveal bleeding into the CNS and infections of the brain or its meninges. A lumbar puncture can also introduce medications such as antibiotics or anesthetics into the CSF, and can measure CSF pressure.

➤➤ BOX 19-3

FUNCTIONS OF CEREBROSPINAL FLUID

- Acts as shock absorber for the brain and spinal cord
- Carries nutrients to the brain
- Carries wastes away from the brain
- Keeps the brain and spinal cord moist, thus preventing friction
- Can be tested to determine the presence of some diseases
- Can be used to transmit medications

Nursing Alert

The pressure of the cerebrospinal fluid (CSF) reflects the pressure of the fluid in and around the brain (intracranial pressure [ICP]). Increased ICP can be a sign of a serious disorder, such as bleeding within the brain; brain tumors; swelling of the brain as a result of trauma; hydrocephalus; or an infection within the CNS.

Ventricles.   Deep within the brain are four **ventricles,** or cavities. These are lined with ependymal cells. They also contain many blood vessels from the pia mater, which make up the choroid plexuses. The choroid plexuses produce CSF, which fills the ventricles.

In Practice
Nursing Assessment 19-1

HEAD TRAUMA

If a client has a head trauma and fluid is noted leaking from the ears or nose, this fluid should be tested for glucose. Glucose is present in the cerebrospinal fluid (CSF). If the test is positive for glucose, notify a healthcare provider immediately because the fluid is most likely CSF. Leaking CSF is a serious danger signal.

Nursing Alert

The skull is a rigid container that contains brain tissue, CSF, and blood. The volume of these components determines the intracranial pressure (ICP). A large increase in any of these factors can increase ICP. This can cause brain hypoxia, herniation of the brain (brain contents being pushed through an opening), or death.

Peripheral Nervous System

The peripheral nervous system (**PNS**) is made up of two nerve groups: cranial nerves and spinal nerves. The terms *cranial* and *spinal* indicate that the nerves begin either in the brain or in the spinal cord. The nerves of the PNS are sensory, motor, or mixed, depending on which direction(s) nerve impulses are conducted.

The autonomic nervous system and its subdivisions (discussed later in this section) are also classified as part of the PNS.

Cranial Nerves

The 12 pairs of **cranial nerves** attach directly to the brain. Most of the cranial nerves carry impulses to and from the brain and various structures around the head. One pair, however, acts on the organs of the thorax and the abdomen.

Cranial nerves are given Roman numerals, and numbered in the order in which they originate in the brain (from front to back). Table 19-1 lists cranial nerves and their functions. A common mnemonic used to remember the twelve cranial nerves is: On Old Olympus, Towering Top A Finn And German View Some Hops. However, note that the *acoustic* nerve (A) is now called the vestibulocochlear nerve. The *spinal accessory* nerve (S) is now just called the accessory nerve.

To remember the classification of functions of these nerves, use the mnemonic: Some Say Marry Money But My Brother Says Bad Business Marry Money. The S represents *sensory* nerves, M stands for *motor* nerves, and B means that the corresponding nerve has *both* sensory and motor functions (also known as a *mixed nerve*). The oculomotor, trochlear, abducens, accessory, and hypoglossal are actually mixed nerves; however, they are primarily motor. Therefore, this mnemonic reflects these nerves' primary function (motor).

Although all of the cranial nerves are important, one nerve deserves special attention. The **vagus nerve** (cranial nerve X) serves a much larger portion of the body than the others. It affects many body functions that are beyond conscious control. Branches of the vagus innervate muscles of the pharynx, larynx, respiratory tract, heart, esophagus, and parts of the abdominal viscera. Therefore, the vagus nerve has reflex control of heart rate, sneezing, hunger, secretions from glands in the stomach, and constrictions within the respiratory tract. It is also involved in sympathetic and parasympathetic responses. For this reason, it is called "the wanderer."

The gross functioning of most of the cranial nerves can be assessed with simple actions, such as asking the client to move or clench the jaw (cranial nerve V: mandibular branch of the trigeminal nerve). See In Practice: Nursing Assessment 47-1 in Chapter 47 for more examples of cranial nerve assessments.

Spinal Nerves

The 31 pairs of **spinal nerves** attach to the spinal cord. Each group of spinal nerves is named for its corresponding part of the spinal cord: cervical (8 pairs), thoracic (12 pairs), lumbar (5 pairs), sacral (5 pairs), and coccygeal (1 pair). Each spinal nerve contains a dorsal (posterior) root, which receives sensory information, and a ventral (anterior) root, which carries motor impulses to muscles and glands. A group of spinal nerves forms a **plexus** (plural: plexuses). Examples of plexuses include the cervical plexus, where the phrenic nerve (which controls the diaphragm) arises; the brachial plexus, where the nerves to the upper arms (such as the radial and ulnar nerves) arise; the lumbosacral plexus, from which the sciatic nerve arises; and the pudendal plexus, from which nerves to the perineum arise. An injury to any of the plexuses could cause nerve damage resulting in weakness, numbness, or diminished movement. The cervical plexus and phrenic nerve have an important role in respiration. If the cervical plexus is damaged above the area of the phrenic nerve, respiratory arrest will occur. These nerves carry impulses such as temperature, touch, pain, muscle tone, and balance. They also transport motor impulses to the skeletal muscles. In some situations, physicians prescribe medication to block these nerves to reduce pain or discomfort.

☛ KEY CONCEPT

Spinal Nerves
Cervical: 8 pairs: cervical plexus—phrenic nerves—diaphragm
Thoracic: 12 pairs
Lumbar: 5 pairs: lumbosacral plexus—sciatic nerve
Sacral: 5 pairs
Coccygeal: 1 pair

Spinal Cord Injuries. Injury to the spinal cord causes swelling, which can result in temporary paralysis. If the spinal cord is cut through completely (*transection*), paralysis below the level of injury is permanent. Paralysis occurs when nerve impulses are interrupted and can no longer reach the spinal nerves and brain. Damage is permanent because the spinal cord cannot regenerate itself. If the injury is close to where the brain and the spinal cord connect, damage to the respiratory center can result in death. Further discussion of brain and nervous system disorders is contained in Chapter 77.

Autonomic Nervous System

The autonomic nervous system (**ANS**) is composed of portions of the CNS and PNS. It is generally classified under the PNS; however the ANS is highly specialized. The ANS functions independently and without conscious effort. It innervates organs that are not usually under voluntary control, particularly cardiac muscle, smooth (visceral) muscles, and glands. The ANS contains *visceral motor neurons* to these three areas. Figure 19-5 illustrates the ANS and the organs it influences. The body's ability to maintain homeostasis is largely due to the ANS.

The ANS has two divisions: sympathetic and parasympathetic. As shown in Figure 19-5, stimuli to the illustrated structures originate in both divisions, but they often function

■■■ **TABLE 19-1** *T*HE CRANIAL NERVES AND THEIR FUNCTIONS

Number	Name	Main Function	Distribution
I	**O**lfactory	Smell (**S**ensory)	Nasal mucous membrane
II	**O**ptic	Vision (**S**ensory)	Retina
III	**O**culomotor	Eye movements (**M**otor)	Most ocular muscles
IV	**T**rochlear (smallest cranial nerves)	Voluntary eye movements (**M**otor)	Superior oblique muscle of eye
V	**T**rigeminal (largest cranial nerves)	Sensations of head and face; movement of mandible (**B**oth)	Skin of face; tongue; teeth; muscles of mastication (chewing)
	Ophthalmic branch	Sensations from front of head and face, eye sockets, and upper nose (Sensory)	
	Maxillary branch	Sensations from nose, mouth, and upper jaw, cheek, and upper lip (Sensory)	
	Mandibular branch	Sensations of tongue, lower teeth, chin (Both)	
VI	**A**bducent (Abducens)	Eye movements (**M**otor)	Lateral rectus muscle of eye
VII	**F**acial	Taste; facial expressions (**B**oth)	Muscles of expression; taste buds
VIII	Vestibulocochlear (**A**coustic) Cochlear division	Hearing and balance Conduct impulses related to hearing (**S**ensory)	Internal auditory meatus
	Vestibular division	Conduct impulses related to equilibrium (balance) (Sensory)	Inner ear
IX	**G**lossopharyngeal	Controls swallowing; gives information on pressure and oxygen tension of blood (**B**oth)	Pharynx, posterior third of tongue, parotid
X	**V**agus ("wanderer") (The only cranial nerve not restricted to head and neck)	Somatic motor function; parasympathetic functions; speech (**B**oth)	Pharynx, larynx, heart, lungs, esophagus, stomach, abdominal viscera
XI	Accessory (**S**pinal accessory)	Rotation of head; raising of shoulder (**M**otor)	Arising from medulla and spinal cord
XII	**H**ypoglossal	Movement of tongue (**M**otor)	Intrinsic muscle of tongue

Mnemonic	Cranial Nerve	Mnemonic	Main Function
On	I Olfactory	Some	Sensory
Old	II Optic	Say	Sensory
Olympus	III Oculomotor	Marry	Motor
Towering	IV Trochlear	Money	Motor
Top	V Trigeminal	But	Both
A	VI Abducens	My	Motor
Finn	VII Facial	Brother	Both
And	VIII (Acoustic) Vestibulocochlear	Says	Sensory
German	IX Glossopharyngeal	Bad	Both
View	X Vagus	Business	Both
Some	XI (Spinal) Accessory	Marry	Motor
Hops	XII Hypoglossal	Money	Motor

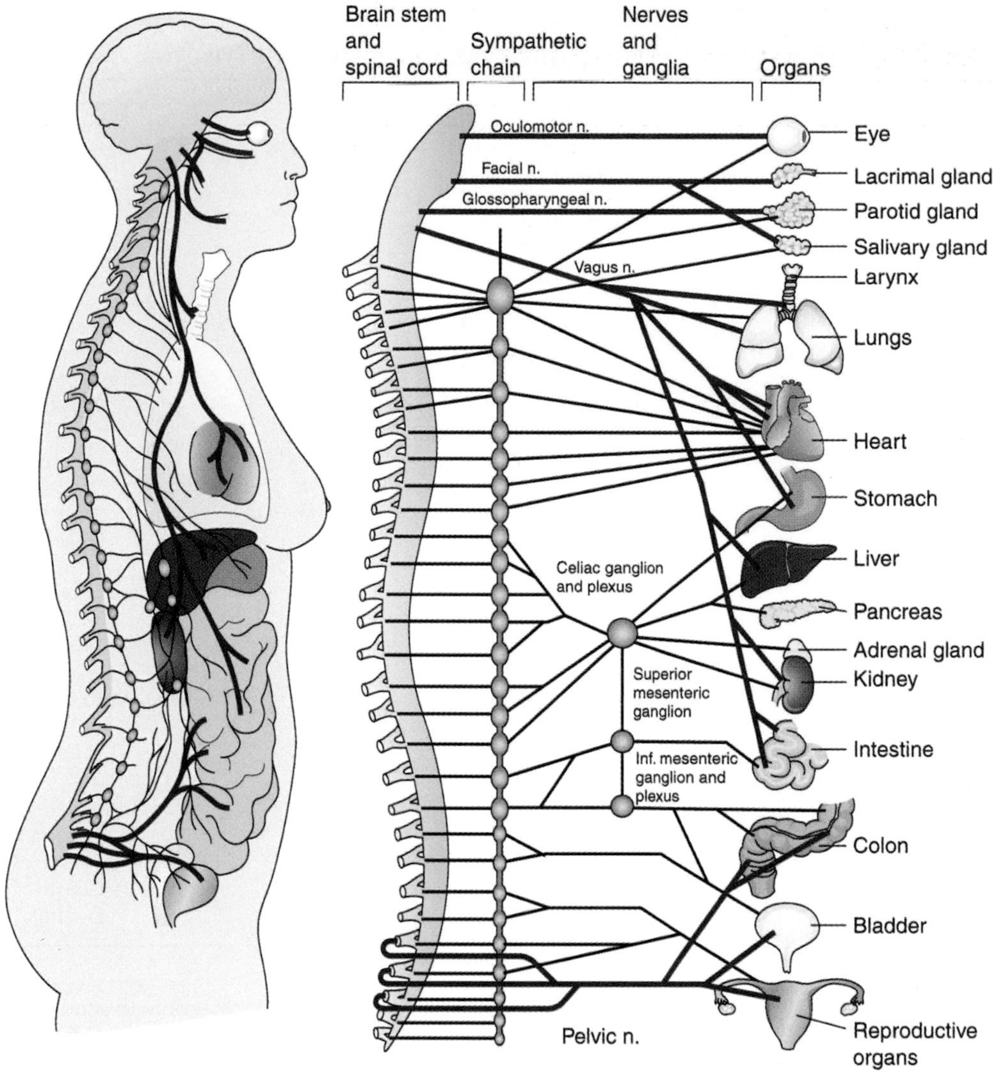

FIGURE 19-5. Anatomy of the autonomic nervous system. The purple lines represent the parasympathetic nervous system (craniosacral division). The black lines represent the sympathetic nervous system (thoracolumbar division).

in opposition to each other. For instance, sympathetic nerves increase heart rate and dilate the pupil of the eye; parasympathetic nerves slow heart rate and constrict the pupil. Table 19-2 summarizes the effects of both divisions of the ANS on selected organs.

Many chemicals are produced by the ANS, simulating drugs that work in a similar manner as the autonomic nerves. Simply stated, some drugs "turn on" or mimic either the sympathetic or parasympathetic nervous system. Other drugs "turn off" or "lyse" the sympathetic or parasympathetic subdivisions of the ANS.

Sympathetic Division
The **sympathetic** division of the ANS produces a response that prepares individuals for an emergency, extreme stress, or danger. This "fight or flight" response readies people to defend themselves or to flee from danger. During an emergency, the heart beats faster and the breathing rate increases. The skin becomes pale, secondary to the diversion of blood flow away from the skin. Blood flow also decreases to structures such as

the external genitalia and the abdominal organs. Thus, body processes such as digestion slow or stop, allowing more blood to flow to the more vital organs: the brain, the lungs, and the large muscles that move the body during an emergency. Involuntary defecation or urination can occur.

Obviously, the body can sustain an emergency awareness for only a limited time. The homeostatic mechanism that balances the sympathetic nervous system (**SNS**) is the parasympathetic nervous system.

☛ Key Concept

The sympathetic nervous system prepares the body for "fight or flight." It acts "in sympathy" with an emergency.

Parasympathetic Division
The **parasympathetic** division of the ANS is its predominant aspect. The parasympathetic division generally produces responses that are the normal functions of the body while it is at rest or not under unusual or extreme stress. The effects are often opposite to the effects of the sympathetic division. Unlike

■ ■ ■ **TABLE 19-2** $\mathscr{E}$**FFECTS OF THE SYMPATHETIC AND PARASYMPATHETIC SYSTEMS ON SELECTED ORGANS**

Effector	Sympathetic System	Parasympathetic System
Pupils of eye	Dilation	Constriction
Sweat glands	Stimulation	None
Digestive glands	Inhibition	Stimulation
Heart	Increased rate and strength of beat	Decreased rate and strength of beat
Bronchi of lungs	Dilation	Constriction
Muscles of digestive system	Decreased contraction	Increased contraction (peristalsis)
Kidneys	Decreased activity	None
Urinary bladder	Relaxation	Contraction and emptying
Liver	Increased release of glucose	None
Penis	Ejaculation	Erection
Adrenal medulla	Stimulation	None
Blood vessels to		
Skeletal muscles	Dilation	Constriction
Skin	Constriction	None
Respiratory system	Dilation	Constriction
Digestive organs	Constriction	Dilation

the sympathetic division, however, the parasympathetic system does not normally activate in a way that affects the body overall. For example, it can decrease the body's heart rate without affecting other organs.

To return to homeostasis after a "fight or flight" episode, the parasympathetic nerves return the heart rate to normal, resume digestive processes, and restore blood flow to the skin, abdominal organs, and genitalia. Previously normal patterns of defecation and urination return.

☛ Key Concept

The ANS functions independently, without conscious effort, to innervate cardiac muscle, smooth visceral muscle, and glands. It has two divisions: the sympathetic and parasympathetic. The sympathetic division prepares a person for an emergency. The parasympathetic division maintains normal body functions and returns the person's body back to normal after a stressful situation.

SYSTEM PHYSIOLOGY

Transmission of Nerve Impulses

Messages from one part of the body to another can take several possible nerve pathways. The body is thrifty in its use of the body's resources and in its patterns of automatic activities. As

a rule, it uses the quickest route to send a message. The body builds patterns (reflexes) and habits by using the same nerve pathways repeatedly. The same kind of message tends to follow the same path every time. Repeated motions become more or less automatic.

Action Potential

A neuron receives electrical and chemical impulses, which make it possible for the neuron to transfer a stimulus from one area of the body to another and to elicit a response. The *electrical impulse* is due to the positive and negative charges of electrolytes (see Chap. 15).

At rest, the cell membrane of a neuron contains an electrical charge. Ions are concentrated outside the membrane. A stimulus, or *nerve impulse,* causes an organized, rapid exchange of sodium and potassium ions across the cell membrane. These ions spread like an electric current along the membrane. This action is called the **action potential.** An action potential takes only milliseconds (tiny fractions of a second). As a result, many neurons can transmit impulses at over several meters per second.

At the synapse, neurotransmitters act chemically to transfer an impulse from the axon of one neuron to the dendrites of another. This needed adjustment causes a reversal of the first cell's polarity (electrical charge), back to its original state. Therefore, as quickly as the polarity occurs, it reverses itself to bring the cell back to its resting state. This alternating depolarization and repolarization moves as a wave along the length of the neuron and becomes a transmitted message.

The All-or-None Law
Either a nerve impulse is transmitted across a particular synapse or it is not. There are no exceptions. Because an impulse cannot be partially transmitted, this law is known as the *all-or-none* response of nerve tissue.

Electroencephalogram
An electroencephalogram (**EEG**) is a visual record of the electrical activity of millions of neurons in the form of various waves within the brain. Brain wave activity is often examined to diagnose neurologic problems. In many states, cessation of brain wave activity has become a legal consideration in the confirmation of biological death.

Actions of Three Types of Neurons
Sensory Neurons.   The sensory neurons (neurons of sensation) are also known as *afferent* neurons because they carry impulses *to* the brain or spinal cord from the periphery of the body by means of receptors. **Receptors** are end organs that initially receive stimuli from outside and within the body (Fig. 19-6).

Receptors are usually classified in three ways. *Exteroceptors* (related to the external environment) are involved in touch, cutaneous (skin) pain, heat, cold, smell, vision, and hearing.

Proprioceptors carry sensations of position and balance, or movement of the body in space. *Interoceptors* (related to the body's internal environment) respond to changes in the internal organs (viscera), such as visceral pain, hunger, or thirst.

After the receptors have picked up an impulse, fibers of the sensory neurons carry the sensation to the CNS. Here, the interneurons analyze and distribute the impulses. Some interneurons act as integrators, and the impulse is carried to a motor neuron.

Motor Neurons.   If the body requires action after receiving a stimulus, the CNS sends an impulse by the fibers of the motor neurons to a muscle or a gland to cause the proper response. Motor neurons are also called *efferent* neurons because they carry impulses *away* from the CNS. The structures that carry out activity are called **effectors.** Effector neurons are classified as somatic-voluntary or visceral- involuntary.

To understand the difference between these types of effector neurons, consider an insect bite. A sensory neuron makes the initial sting known to the brain. The brain interprets the sensation. It sends a message via *somatic-voluntary* neurons to the appropriate muscles. A person manifests a response by slapping the insect away. This action is *voluntary,* in that it can be controlled. An example of a *visceral-involuntary* response is the peristaltic movement of food through the digestive system. Such movement is not under a person's voluntary control; rather it depends on the nervous system's ability to process information and to relay appropriate messages.

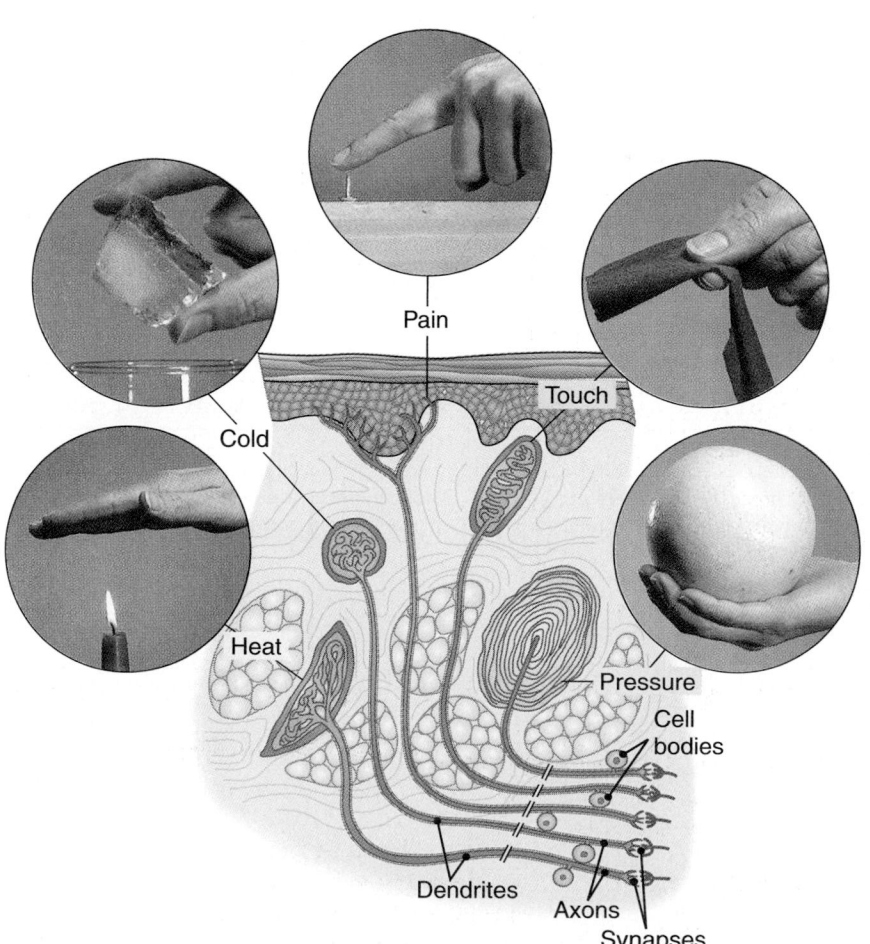

FIGURE 19-6. The receptors (exteroceptors) in the skin receive stimuli related to temperature, pain, touch, and pressure. The cell bodies and synapses, which are located in the dorsal root ganglia and spinal cord, are included in this drawing to suggest the continuity of sensory pathways from the skin to the central nervous system. The neurons in this case are sensory (afferent) neurons.

Interneurons.   Neurons that serve to integrate signals between the neurons of various parts of the CNS are called *interneurons.* Interneurons are found only in the CNS (see Fig. 19-3B). They carry out or integrate sensory or motor impulses. They assist with thinking, learning, and memory. They can be thought of as a link between the two other types of neurons.

Reflexes

A **reflex** is an automatic or involuntary response to a stimulus; therefore, a reflex occurs without conscious thought. Reflexes are homeostatic; that is, they attempt to maintain homeostasis. They move the body from danger, keep the body from falling, and maintain a relatively constant blood pressure, pH, and level of water reabsorption. The different types of reflexes vary in complexity.

☛ KEY CONCEPT

A reflex is an involuntary response to a stimulus. Reflexes work to maintain homeostasis in the body.

Reflexes do not operate as isolated parts of the nervous system. Reflexes are integrated into the CNS as a reflex arc; therefore, the brain may inhibit or exaggerate a reflex when it receives a stimulus. For example, a person reflexively blinks the eyes when danger approaches, but after the brain realizes the danger, the person acts as a whole unit and moves the body away.

Other examples of reflexes include constriction of the pupil of the eye when it is exposed to light, the automatic increase in heart rate when the body senses a lowering of blood pressure, and the patellar (knee-jerk) reflex that occurs when an examiner taps the patellar tendon just below the kneecap. Deep-tendon reflexes are often tested as part of a clinical assessment to see if the nervous system is functioning properly. Figure 19-3 illus-trates some simple reflexes. The nurse requires additional inservice education to be competent in testing reflexes.

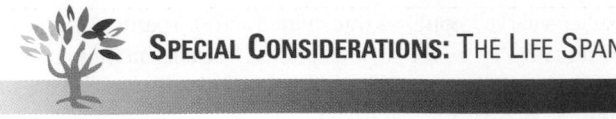

SPECIAL CONSIDERATIONS: THE LIFE SPAN

Reflexes

Infants and small children also have slower reflexes due to the immaturity of their nervous system. The myelin sheathing is still forming during infancy; therefore an infant's response to stimuli is not as rapid as an older child's or an adult's.

EFFECTS OF AGING ON THE SYSTEM

Intelligence, memory, the capacity to learn, and personality do not normally change as a person ages. Genetics, environmental conditions, physical changes resulting from disease processes, and psychological stressors are more likely than the aging process to influence such factors. A person's ability to adapt is usually limited more by one's physical body than by mental functioning. Table 19-3 outlines the effects of aging on the nervous system.

Generally, nerve cells cannot reproduce themselves. Damage to brain cells may result in the permanent loss of some or all mental functions. Common causes of loss of mental function in older people include cerebrovascular accidents, such as stroke; conditions such as Alzheimer's disease; and conditions related to atherosclerosis ("hardening of the arteries"). In addition, trauma, drugs, and degenerative disorders can cause irreversible organic brain damage in people of all ages.

■■■ **TABLE 19-3** ℰFFECTS OF AGING ON THE NERVOUS SYSTEM

Factor	Result	Nursing Implications
Thought processes and ability to learn or reason should be retained.	Thought process, reasoning, or learning changes are not normal.	Treat older adults as normal, intelligent people. Evaluate any changes in personality or thought processes. If underlying pathology exists, understand the disease and its progression.
Sleep patterns may change; however, amount of sleep needed often is relatively unchanged. Less rapid eye movement (dream) sleep occurs.	Person feels less rested; wakefulness periods at night are common. Older individuals may start using sleeping aids.	Watch for behavioral changes caused by prescription and over-the-counter drugs. Be aware of client's stressors; clinical depression secondary to cumulative losses is common. Encourage exercise during the day and eating a light meal in the evening. Reassure client that shorter periods of sleep are common. Caution against excess use of sleep aids.

(continued)

■■■ TABLE 19-3 *𝓔*FFECTS OF AGING ON THE NERVOUS SYSTEM (CONTINUED)

Factor	Result	Nursing Implications
Number of neurons decreases.	Person exhibits decrease in voluntary movements.	Allow for longer response time.
Rate and spread of nerve transmission decreases.	Persons may be startled more easily. Reflexes may be slowed. Decision-making may be slower.	Prevent accidents. Teach safe driving and defensive driving techniques.
Thermoregulation abilities often are reduced.	Older adults are more prone to heat stroke or effects of cold. Skin may remain pink, even if client is cold (may not become pale or blue).	Increase layers of clothing in all weather. Tell client foot protection is important because of decreased sensation and slowed circulation.
Some short-term memory loss is normal.	Person may be disoriented as to time and date.	Reorient client as needed.
Long-term memory usually is good.		Initiate opportunities to reminisce because reminiscing is beneficial.
Motor skills are affected by physiologic changes in other systems.	Person may lack dexterity. Falls are often common.	Encourage maintenance of abilities by daily exercise (walking is excellent). Encourage use of cane or walker for stability if needed. Remove obstacles, such as scatter rugs, to prevent falls. Provide adequate lighting.

Safety and *preventive measures* are priorities for teaching when working with older adults. Loss of equilibrium and changes in proprioception (spatial awareness) can contribute to falling. Herpes zoster (shingles) is a painful inflammation of nerve endings that often affects older people.

Older adults who exhibit signs of confusion need to be evaluated to target the cause of confusion and to determine if it is treatable. Sometimes electrolyte imbalances, hypoxia, small strokes, drugs, pain, stress, or anemia result in confusion. Confusion related to such factors is usually reversible. True dementia (such as in Alzheimer's disease) is irreversible (see Chap. 92).

➡ STUDENT SYNTHESIS

Key Points

- The primary functions of the nervous system are communication and control.
- The two types of cells of the nervous system are the neuron and the neuroglia.
- A neuron consists of a cell body, axon, and dendrites.
- The functions of the neuroglia are to protect and support the CNS and PNS.
- The central nervous system consists of the brain, spinal cord, and accessory structures.
- The four cerebral lobes—frontal, parietal, temporal, and occipital—are located in both hemispheres of the brain. The frontal lobe is responsible for higher mental processes. The parietal lobe is responsible for speech and some sensory input. The temporal lobe is responsible for smell, hearing, and some memory. The occipital lobe is responsible for vision.
- The thalamus is responsible for integration of strong sensations into a total.
- The hypothalamus regulates many body functions such as temperature, thirst, hunger, urination, swallowing, and the sleep–wake cycle.
- The cerebellum is responsible for muscle control.
- The brain stem is made up of the midbrain, pons, and medulla. The midbrain functions as a reflex center. The pons contains nerve tracts and carries messages between the cerebrum and medulla. The pons is also responsible for respiration. The medulla contains centers for vital body functions such as heart rate, vasomotor tone, and respirations.
- The two functions of the spinal cord include conducting impulses to and from the brain and acting as a reflex center.
- The three meninges include the dura mater, the arachnoid, and the pia mater.
- Twelve pairs of cranial nerves arise from the brain. Most of these convey impulses to and from the brain and the structures of the head.

- The spinal nerves are attached to the spinal cord. They are divided into 8 cervical pairs, 12 thoracic pairs, 5 lumbar pairs, 5 sacral pairs, and 1 coccygeal pair.
- The autonomic nervous system is divided into the sympathetic and parasympathetic divisions. The sympathetic system prepares individuals for emergencies. The parasympathetic system maintains body functions under normal conditions.
- The three types of neurons are sensory (afferent), motor (efferent), and interneurons (integrators). Sensory neurons carry information to the brain. Motor neurons carry information away from the brain. Interneurons respond to viscera.

Critical Thinking Exercises

1. Discuss how an injury to each of the following areas of the brain might manifest itself in an individual: frontal lobe, parietal lobe, temporal lobe, and occipital lobe. Differentiate between these in terms of signs and symptoms and if they occur on the right side versus the left side of the brain.
2. Explain why a person who suffers an injury to the spinal cord that results in physical paralysis can still retain brain functioning, but a person who suffers a brain injury may experience limited or no movement.

NCLEX-Style Review Questions

1. The accessory nerve, cranial nerve XI, is responsible for:
   a. Eye movements
   b. Rotation of the head
   c. Sensations of the head
   d. Somatic motor function
2. The three parts of a neuron are the:
   a. Axon, dendrite, and cell body
   b. Synapse, acetylcholine, and gyri
   c. Convolutions, dendrite, and cell body
   d. Bridge, gyri, and axon
3. The function of the area in the brain known as white matter is to:
   a. Control wakefulness and sleep
   b. Increase the brain's surface area
   c. Influence mood and body movements
   d. Make connections between the brain's two hemispheres
4. The autonomic nervous system is composed of the:
   a. Parasympathetic and sympathetic nervous systems
   b. Peripheral and central nervous systems
   c. Sympathetic and central nervous systems
   d. Brain and spinal cord
5. The function of the cerebrum is:
   a. To act as a respiratory center
   b. To aid in establishing sleep–wake patterns
   c. To control higher mental functioning
   d. To store information in long-term memory

20

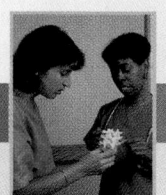

The Endocrine System

LEARNING OBJECTIVES

1. Differentiate between exocrine and endocrine glands.
2. Name three general functions of the endocrine system. List at least two specific actions related to each major function.
3. Describe the relationship between the hypothalamus and the pituitary gland.
4. Name and state the functions of the hormones released by the anterior, middle, and posterior divisions of the pituitary gland.
5. Describe the actions of the hormones responsible for calcium balance.
6. Describe the relationships between the "releasing" hormones and the "inhibiting" hormones.
7. Describe the hormones involved in "fight or flight," and give three examples of their effects and body responses during an emergency.
8. Explain the functions of the thyroid hormones.
9. On a chart, locate the adrenal glands and describe the functions of the mineralocorticoids and the glucocorticoids.
10. Discuss the location of insulin secretion and explain how insulin and glucagon regulate blood sugar levels.
11. Identify a medical condition in which the client lacks adequate insulin production.
12. Identify the major hormones secreted by the thymus. Briefly identify its relationship to the body's immune response.
13. Identify the glands of reproduction in both males and females. Identify the sex hormones they produce and state the normal effects of these hormones.
14. List at least three hormones secreted by non-endocrine glands or organs, and state the function of each of these hormones.
15. Discuss negative and positive feedback as they relate to the endocrine system.
16. Describe two functions of prostaglandins.
17. Describe four effects of aging on the endocrine system.

NEW TERMINOLOGY

adenohypophysis	hormone
adrenal gland	hypothalamus
β endorphin	insulin
corticosteroid	islets of Langerhans
endocrine gland	mineralocorticoid
erythropoietin	neurohypophysis
exocrine gland	parathyroid
gland	pineal gland
glucagon	pituitary gland
glucocorticoid	prostaglandin
goiter	thymus
gonadotropin	thyroid gland

ACRONYMS

ACTH	GRH	PRH
ANf	HCG	PRL
ANP	hGH	PTH
CRH	ICSH	T_3
FSH	LH	T_4
GH	LT	TRH
GHIH	MIF	TSH
GHRH	MSH	
GnRH	PIH	

The *endocrine system* comprises a group of glands located in various parts of the body. A **gland** is a group of specialized cells that secrete a substance (in this case, hormones) in response to signals. The glands themselves neither need nor use the hormones they produce.

Two major types of glands exist in the body: endocrine and exocrine. Some glands, however, can perform both endocrine and exocrine functions. Table 20-1 compares endocrine and exocrine glands.

Endocrine glands secrete hormones directly into the bloodstream. These hormones are primarily regulatory in function and act on remote tissues (called *target tissues*). The major portion of this chapter discusses endocrine glands.

Exocrine glands secrete substances into ducts that open onto the body's external or internal surface. The exocrine glands usually secrete substances that serve a protective or functional purpose. Exocrine glands include sweat glands, mammary glands, mucous membranes, salivary glands, and lacrimal (tear) glands. Examples of exocrine secretions are sweat, milk, bile, tears, and pancreatic fluid.

Hormones are chemical regulators that integrate and coordinate body activities. They speed up or slow down the activities of entire body organs or systems. Some hormones affect the rate of various activities of individual cells. Hormones also affect one another. Too much or too little of a particular hormone interferes with or counteracts the actions of other hormones. The blood transports hormones.

Hormones may be produced in response to nervous stimulation, the level of specific substances in the blood, or other hormones. This chapter discusses specific hormones and the glands that secrete them.

STRUCTURE AND FUNCTION

The endocrine system provides a network for the regulation and integration of all body cells, organs, and systems. The main functions of the endocrine system are regulation of growth, maturation, metabolism, and reproduction. Box 20-1 summarizes these functions.

The glands of the endocrine system include the pituitary, thyroid, parathyroid, adrenal, and pineal. In addition, several organs that are not exclusively endocrine glands also contain cells that secrete hormones. Four such organs are the hypothalamus, gonads, pancreas, and thymus. Figure 20-1 illustrates the shapes and locations of specific endocrine structures. In addition, specialized hormones are secreted in such diverse organs of the body as the gastrointestinal tract, the kidneys, and

the heart. The following sections describe the more specific locations of these glands and organs; the hormones they produce; and hormonal actions.

☛ KEY CONCEPT
***

Functions of the endocrine system include regulation of growth and maturation, metabolism, and reproduction.

Pituitary Gland

The **pituitary gland,** also called the *hypophysis,* is about the size of a pea. It is located in a saddle-shaped hollow in the sphenoid bone called the *sella turcica.* (The sphenoid bone is located at the base of the brain's frontal lobe.) Two parts make up the pituitary gland: the anterior and posterior lobes. These lobes are sometimes classified as two separate glands because their functions and embryonic development are very different.

Role of the Hypothalamus

In the past, theorists believed that the pituitary itself secreted the hormones needed for all vital body functions. However, research has shown that the "pituitary hormones" are either secreted by—or their secretion is directly controlled by—the hypothalamus.

The **hypothalamus** is a tiny but complex portion of the brain, which is attached to the pituitary by means of the infundibular (hypophyseal) stalk. The hypothalamus is considered the "master controller" or the "master gland." Specialized cells in the hypothalamus release hormones that either inhibit release or promote release of other hormones from the anterior lobe of the pituitary. These hypothalamus hormones are described as *releasing hormones* or *inhibiting hormones* (Table 20-2). Figure 20-2 illustrates the role of the hypothalamus in regard to the pituitary gland; the secretion of pituitary hormones; and the organs affected by pituitary hormones. Chapter 19 discusses non-endocrine functions of the hypothalamus.

Anterior Lobe

The anterior lobe of the pituitary, also called the **adenohypophysis,** releases several hormones (see Table 20-3). Many of these hormones are called *glycoproteins* because they are made of carbohydrates and proteins. The hypothalamus controls the adenohypophysis; therefore, neural commands release these hormones. Five of these hormones (the tropic hormones) control the growth, development, and proper functioning of other endocrine glands.

■■■ TABLE 20-1 𝒞OMPARISON OF ENDOCRINE AND EXOCRINE GLANDS

Gland	Definition	Action	Functions of Secretions	Examples
Endocrine	Ductless glands; glands of internal secretion	Secrete hormones into circulation	Regulatory	Insulin, ACTH
Exocrine	Secrete into a duct; glands of external secretion	Secrete substances directly into duct or body opening	Protective, functional	Digestive juices, tears, sweat

➤➤ BOX 20-1

FUNCTIONS OF THE ENDOCRINE SYSTEM

Growth and Maturation
- Regulates growth
- Regulates body's response to stress

Metabolism
- Regulates metabolism
- Regulates absorption of nutrients
- Regulates use of glucose in cellular respiration
- Maintains body pH by maintaining fluid and electrolyte concentrations

Reproduction
- Produces sexual characteristics
- Controls reproductive processes
- Activates lactation

Tropic Hormones.   Corticotropin-releasing hormone (**CRH**) from the hypothalamus causes the release of adrenocorticotropic hormone (**ACTH** or *corticotropin*) from the anterior lobe of the pituitary gland. ACTH stimulates the adrenal cortex to produce glucocorticoids—such as cortisol—which are vital in metabolizing carbohydrates. ACTH also has melanocyte-stimulating properties that can increase skin pigmentation.

Thyrotropin-releasing hormone (**TRH**) from the hypothalamus causes the release of thyroid-stimulating hormone (**TSH** or *thyrotropin*) from the pituitary. TSH stimulates the thyroid gland to produce and to secrete thyroxine (T_4) and triiodothyronine (T_3) (discussed later in this chapter). The hypothalamus also functions to inhibit TSH, by releasing growth hormone inhibiting hormone (**GHIH**).

The hormone known as growth hormone (**GH**), human growth hormone (**hGH**), or *somatotropin* is produced by and released from the anterior pituitary. This hormone is stimulated by the release of growth hormone releasing hormone (**GRH** or **GHRH**) by the hypothalamus. GH stimulates growth in all body tissues. It assists with the movement of amino acids into tissue cells and the transformation of amino acids into proteins that the body needs. It aids in the release of fatty acids from adipose (fat) tissue so that they can be used for energy. GH helps to regulate blood nutrient levels after eating and during periods of fasting. When sufficient amount of GH has been released, the hypothalamus secretes GHIH (discussed in the previous paragraph) to inhibit further release of growth hormone.

Gonadotropin-releasing hormone (**GnRH**) causes the anterior pituitary to secrete two hormones called **gonadotropins** that stimulate the sex glands (gonads) in the body. These two gonadotropic hormones are follicle-stimulating hormone and luteinizing hormone:

- Follicle-stimulating hormone (**FSH**) stimulates the growth and secretion of ovarian follicles in women and the production of sperm in men.

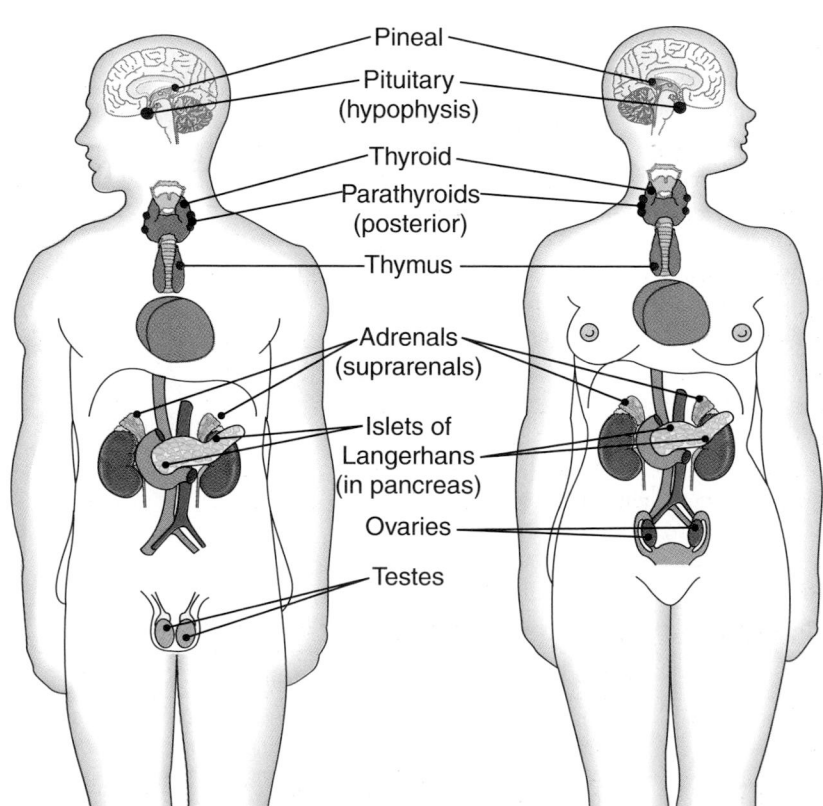

FIGURE 20-1. Location of the major endocrine glands in the body.

■■■ **TABLE 20-2** *H*YPOTHALAMUS HORMONES AFFECTING HORMONE SECRETION FROM THE PITUITARY GLAND

Releasing Hormones (Stimulating Hormones) From Hypothalamus	Inhibiting Hormones From Hypothalamus	Pituitary Hormones Stimulated or Inhibited
Corticotropin-releasing hormone (CRH)	Melanocyte-inhibiting factor (MIF)	Adrenocorticotropic hormone (ACTH) Melanocyte-stimulating hormone (MSH)
Growth hormone releasing hormone (GRH or GHRH)	Growth hormone inhibiting hormone (GHIH) or somatostatin	Growth hormone (GH) or human growth hormone (hGH) or somatotropin
Thyrotropin-releasing hormone (TRH)	Growth hormone inhibiting hormone (GHIH) or somatostatin	Thyroid-stimulating hormone (TSH) or thyrotropin
Prolactin-releasing hormone (PRH)	Prolactin-inhibiting hormone (PIH)	Prolactin (PRL)
Gonadotropin-releasing hormone (GnRH)		Interstitial cell-stimulating hormone (ICSH) in men or luteinizing hormone (LH) in women Follicle-stimulating hormone (FSH)

• Luteinizing hormone (**LH**) in women stimulates ovulation and the formulation of the corpus luteum. In men, LH is called interstitial cell-stimulating hormone (**ICSH**). ICSH influences the secretion of testosterone and other sex hormones from specialized areas in the testes. LH/ICSH and FSH are known as *gonadotropic* hormones because they influence the gonads (the reproductive organs).

Beta Endorphins.   Other hormones chemically similar to ACTH are the **β-endorphins.** These hormones have the same effects as opiate drugs, such as morphine. (As a matter of fact, the term *endorphin* was coined by combining the words *endogenous* [within the body] and *morphine.*) Stress and exercise produce the stimuli for release of endorphins.

Prolactin.   Prolactin (**PRL**), stimulated by prolactin-releasing hormone (**PRH**), is a hormone secreted by the anterior lobe of the pituitary that stimulates milk production in women following pregnancy. Men secrete PRL as well; however, its function in men is not yet understood. Inhibition of prolactin occurs due to the hypothalamus' secretion of prolactin-inhibiting hormone (**PIH**).

Middle Lobe

Some texts identify a middle lobe of the pituitary. The most important hormone secreted there is melanocyte-stimulating hormone (**MSH**), which is stimulated by CRH from the hypothalamus. MSH influences skin pigmentation and is chemically similar to ACTH (produced in the anterior lobe). The hypothalamus *inhibits* secretion of MSH by secreting melanocyte-inhibiting factor (**MIF**).

Posterior Lobe

The posterior lobe of the pituitary, also called the **neurohypophysis,** is actually an outgrowth of the hypothalamus and is embryonically derived from the nervous system. The hypothalamus and pituitary gland are in close proximity to each other. The two posterior-lobe pituitary hormones, oxytocin and vasopressin, are secreted *in the hypothalamus* by neurosecretory cells, and then *released* by the neurohypophysis (see Fig. 20-2).

Oxytocin stimulates the uterus to contract during delivery and helps to keep it contracted after delivery (to prevent hemorrhage). It also stimulates the release of milk from a new mother's breasts.

Vasopressin or *antidiuretic hormone* (ADH) functions in several ways. It stimulates contraction of blood vessels to raise blood pressure; affects the uterus; and influences reabsorption (resorption) of water by the kidney tubules. Table 20-3 describes the actions of these two hormones. Chapter 27 describes the process of water reabsorption by the kidneys.

☛ KEY CONCEPT

Although there are subtle differences in the definitions of reabsorption (the term used in this book) and resorption, these terms are often used interchangeably to mean the reuse of materials such as proteins, glucose, and electrolytes to restore essential components to the body. An example of this process is the selective reabsorption of extracellular fluid in the tubules of the kidney.

Thyroid Gland

The **thyroid gland,** the largest of the endocrine glands, lies in front of the neck, just below the larynx, with a wing (lobe) on either side of the trachea (Fig. 20-3). The thyroid secretes two hormones: thyroxine (T_4) and triiodothyronine (T_3). These hormones are synthesized in the thyroid gland from iodine. More T_4 (90%) is found in the blood, compared to T_3 (10%). It is believed that T_4 is converted to T_3 before it can work in the body. These hormones regulate body metabolism, controlling

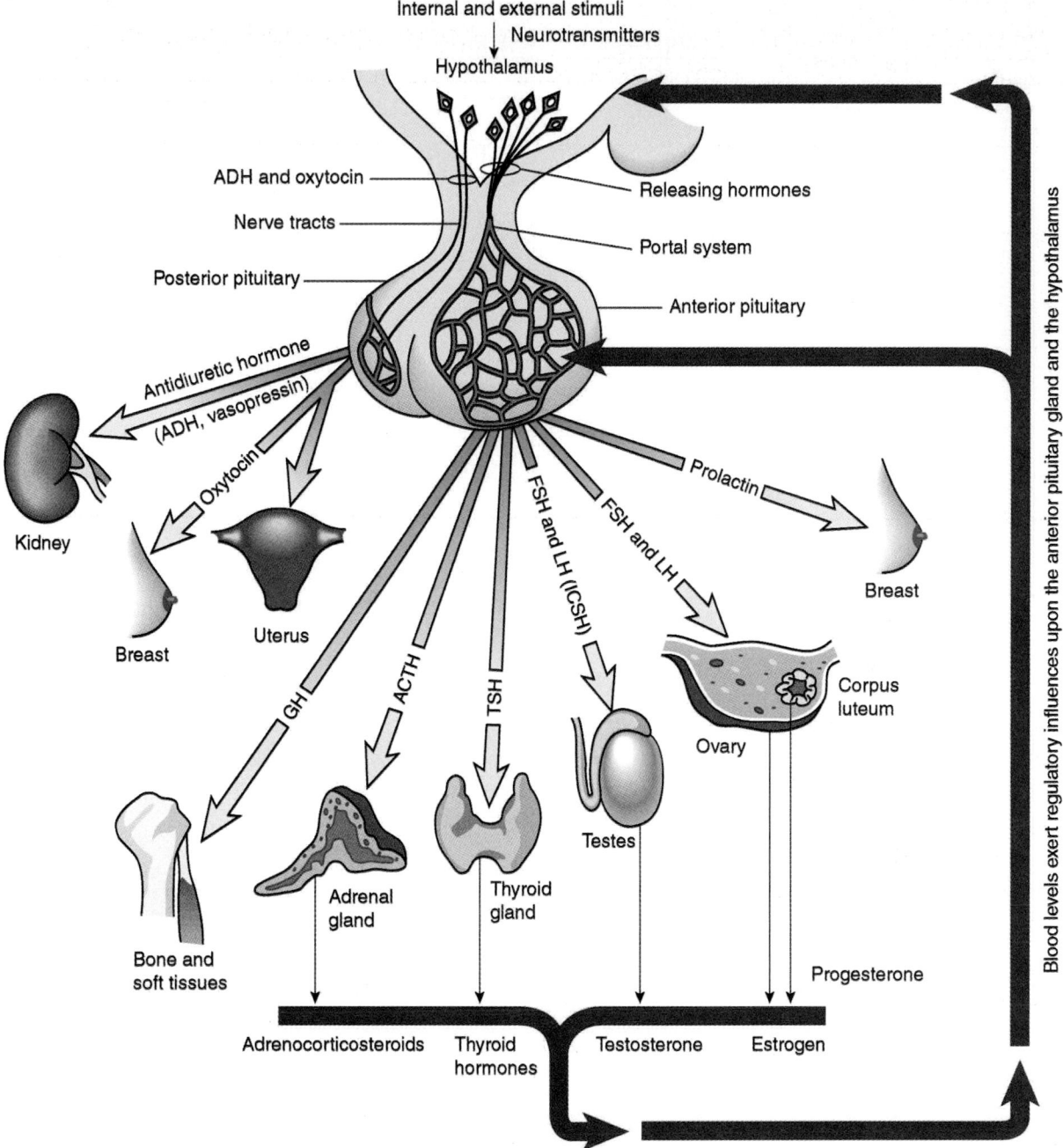

FIGURE 20-2. The pituitary gland, the relationship of the hypothalamus to pituitary action, and the hormones secreted by the anterior, middle, and posterior pituitary lobes.

the rate at which cells do their work. The thyroid removes iodine from the blood to make T$_4$; a person's diet must supply this iodine.

If there is insufficient dietary intake of iodine, a disorder called a **goiter** (an enlarged thyroid gland) may result. Goiter occurs due to a lack of iodine in the body, which causes low levels of thyroid hormones in the body. As a result, the hypothalamus secretes a hormone called thyroid-stimulating hormone (TSH). When excess TSH is secreted, it causes the thyroid gland to enlarge.

Another hormone the thyroid secretes is called *calcitonin* or *thyrocalcitonin.* It is involved in the maintenance of the body's

calcium levels. When circulating calcium levels are high, calcitonin responds by promoting increased storage of calcium in bones and increased renal excretion of calcium, resulting in lowered serum calcium levels.

Parathyroids

The **parathyroids** are small glands, each about the size of a pea, that lie on either side of the undersurface of the thyroid gland (see Fig. 20-3). Usually, there are four, in two pairs; despite their relatively small size, the parathyroids are essential to health and to life itself.

■■■ TABLE 20-3 *I*MPORTANT SECRETIONS OF THE ENDOCRINE SYSTEM

Gland/Organ	Hormone(s) Secreted/Released	Actions
Pituitary		
Anterior lobe (adenohypophysis)	Adrenocorticotropic hormone (ACTH)	Stimulates adrenal cortex to produce cortisol; can stimulate melanocytes
	β-Endorphins	Produces analgesia
	Growth hormone (GH or hGH), somatotropic hormone	Controls bone and tissue growth and regulates metabolism
	Thyroid-stimulating hormone (TSH)	Regulates thyroid hormone
	Follicle-stimulating hormone (FSH)	Stimulates growth and secretion of eggs in ovaries (female) and sperm in testes (male)
	Luteinizing hormone (LH) (females)	Helps control ovulation and menstruation; important in sustaining pregnancy
	Interstitial cell-stimulating hormone (ICSH) (males)	Stimulates secretion of male hormones
	Prolactin, lactogenic hormone (PRL)	Stimulates mammary glands to produce milk
Middle lobe	Melanocyte-stimulating hormone (MSH)	Increases skin pigmentation
Posterior lobe (neurohypophysis)	Oxytocin	Causes uterine contractions; stimulates milk production
	Vasopressin (ADH)	Raises blood pressure; promotes water reabsorption in kidney tubules: influences uterus
Thyroid	Thyroxine (T_4) Triiodothyronine (T_3)	Regulate body metabolism (require iodine) and growth and development Stimulates calcium to leave plasma and allows it to enter bones
	Calcitonin (thyrocalcitonin)	Calcitonin (CT) speeds calcium absorption from blood; promotes calcium deposit in bone; inhibits osteoclasts, thereby promoting bone formation Stimulates bone to release or reabsorb calcium and enter blood; regulates phosphorous balance; assists in reabsorption of magnesium
Parathyroid	Parathormone/Parathyroid hormone (PTH)	Promotes formation of calcitrol and assists in release of calcium, magnesium, and phosphorous into blood
Adrenals (Suprarenals)		
Adrenal medulla	Catecholamines Epinephrine (adrenaline) Norepinephrine	Mimic actions of the sympathetic nervous system, adapt to stress; cause many body processes to speed up, especially in an emergency
Adrenal cortex	Corticosteroids/corticoids Mineralocorticoids Glucocorticoids	Regulate electrolyte levels in extracellular fluid Influence glucose, amino acid, and fat synthesis in metabolism; decrease inflammatory responses
	Sex hormones Androgens (males) Estrogens and progestins (females) (progesteron is the primary progestin)	Produce male sex characteristics Produce female sex characteristics
Gonads		
Testes (male)	Testosterone	Develops male sex characteristics (also influenced by androgens)
Ovaries (female)	Estrogen and progestins	Regulate female sex characteristics, functions, and menstruation
Pancreas		
Alpha cells (islets)	Glucagon	Speeds glycogenolysis; raises blood sugar
Beta cells (islets)	Insulin	Enables cells to use glucose; lowers blood sugar
Delta cells (islets)	Somatostatin	Inhibits release of insulin and glucagon

(continued)

■■■ **TABLE 20-3** *I*MPORTANT SECRETIONS OF THE ENDOCRINE SYSTEM (CONTINUED)

Gland/Organ	Hormone(s) Secreted	Actions
F cells (islets)	Pancreatic polypeptide	Inhibits secretion of somatostatin and pancreatic digestive enzymes
Thymus	Thymosin (thymic hormone)	Stimulates production of T cells for cellular immunity
Pineal	Melatonin	Regulates sleep–wake cycles; may play a role in influencing reproductive processes

SPECIAL CONSIDERATIONS: NUTRITION

Iodine food sources include shellfish and iodized salt. A lack of iodine in the body could cause a decrease in thyroid function over a period of time. Common symptoms a healthcare provider could see in a client with decreased thyroid function are fatigue, weight gain, and complaints of being cold. Goiter is often a later consequence of insufficient iodine.

The parathyroids secrete a hormone, *parathormone* or *parathyroid hormone* (**PTH**), that regulates the amounts of calcium and phosphorus in the blood, which in turn affect nerve and muscle irritability. When the blood calcium level is too low, parathormone is secreted. This secretion increases the number and size of osteoclasts (large cells associated with reabsorption of bone). Therefore, parathormone causes calcium to leave the bones. PTH also enhances reabsorption of calcium and magnesium, and excretion of phosphorus in the kidneys.

PTH has an additional effect on the kidneys in that it promotes the formation of *calcitriol,* a hormone synthesized from vitamin D. Calcitriol increases the rate of calcium, magnesium, and phosphorus absorption from the gastrointestinal tract into the blood. Therefore, PTH has the opposite action to calcitonin.

Adrenal Glands

The two **adrenal glands,** also known as the *suprarenal glands,* sit like hats, one atop each kidney (see Fig. 20-1). Like the pituitary gland, the adrenal glands each have two parts; each part produces different hormones.

Adrenal Medulla

The central portion of the adrenal gland, called the *medulla,* secretes hormones called *catecholamines,* which are made from amino acids. Epinephrine and norepinephrine are the two catecholamines. *Epinephrine* (adrenaline) constitutes about 80%

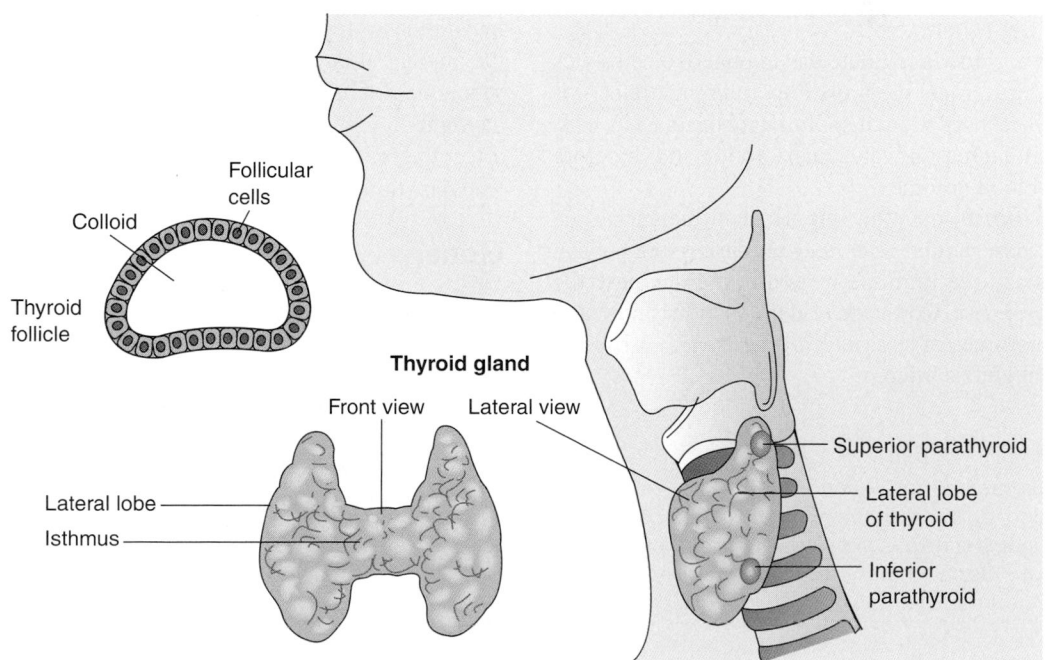

FIGURE 20-3. The thyroid gland and the follicular structure. A lateral view of a parathyroid gland is also shown.

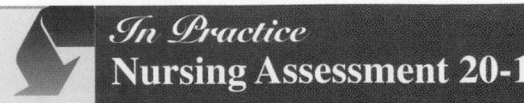

TETANY

A client with a deficiency of calcium will usually have muscle twitching and spasms, and possibly convulsions. These signs are called *tetany.*

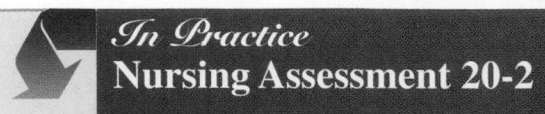

GLUCOCORTICOIDS

Look for the classic signs of "moon face" or "buffalo hump" in clients taking glucocorticoids. These signs are a result of redistribution of fat in the body, giving the client an appearance of being overweight or obese. They include a round face ("moon face"), a large abdomen, and a hump on the person's back ("buffalo hump").

of the medulla's total secretion. Its actions are to make the heart beat faster, contract blood vessels, raise blood pressure, and increase muscle power by causing the liver to release glucose for energy. The hormone *norepinephrine* has some—but not all—the actions of epinephrine.

These two hormones from the adrenal medulla mimic the action of the sympathetic nervous system. However, the adrenal medulla is not necessary for life, because the sympathetic nervous system can take over its activities. These hormones are active in emergencies; fright, anger, love, and grief stimulate them. They are said to prepare people for "fight or flight." The functions of the medulla are important because they help individuals adapt to stress.

☞ KEY CONCEPT

Epinephrine and norepinephrine are major catecholamines and are involved in "fight or flight."

Adrenal Cortex

The outer part of the adrenals, the cortex, secretes many compounds called **corticosteroids** or *corticoids.* Three types of corticosteroids exist: mineralocorticoids, glucocorticoids, and the sex hormones (androgens and estrogens). All these compounds derive from cholesterol.

Mineralocorticoids regulate the amount of electrolytes in the body. Aldosterone, the most important mineralocorticoid, stimulates reabsorption of sodium into the plasma. This action results in increased water reabsorption and therefore an increase in blood volume.

Glucocorticoids have an important influence on the synthesis of glucose, amino acids, and fats during metabolism. They also depress the immune response and decrease the inflammatory response. Corticosteroid production is normally increased during times of stress. *Hydrocortisone (cortisol)* is the predominant glucocorticoid.

✚👁 Nursing Alert

Clients taking glucocorticoids take longer to become healed, and may have a decreased response to infections due to the drug's anti-inflammatory response. Therefore, consider a small rise in temperature a significant finding in these clients.

The sex hormones of the adrenal cortex (*androgens, estrogens,* and *progestins*) supplement the sex hormones of the gonads. The adrenals primarily produce androgens, with only minute amounts of estrogen and progesterone secretion. Table 20-3 identifies selected steroids and their functions.

Pineal Gland

The **pineal gland** (pineal body) is a small, cone-shaped structure located at the top portion of the brain's third ventricle (see Fig. 20-1). It produces *melatonin* in a way not completely understood, but somehow related to the amount of exposure to environmental light. Melatonin is thought to participate in the maintenance of the sleep–wake cycle. In sunlight, sympathetic nerve fibers release norepinephrine, which inhibits the secretion of melatonin and results in wakefulness. In darkness, the lack of norepinephrine stimulates the secretion of melatonin, resulting in sleepiness.

Melatonin or another pineal hormone may also regulate the release of substances from the hypothalamus that stimulate and affect the secretion of gonadotropin. Therefore, the pineal gland may influence reproductive functions. Theorists speculate that the amount of daylight animals receive regulates their pineal secretions, influencing their breeding seasons. The effect of daylight on humans is not well understood, but is believed to affect the brain and to influence the rate of gonad (ovary and testis) maturation.

Gonads

The *gonads* are the glands of reproduction: the testes of the male and the ovaries of the female (see Fig. 20-1). In addition to producing sperm, the testes produce *testosterone,* the male sex hormone. Other steroid hormones produce masculinizing effects; as a group, they are called *androgens.* The ovaries produce *estrogen* and *progesterone,* which, in addition to regulating female sex characteristics, are responsible for menstruation. Chapters 28 and 29 describe the actions of the sex-related hormones in more detail.

Pancreas

The *pancreas* lies behind the stomach, between the duodenum and the spleen. It is both an endocrine and an exocrine gland.

As an exocrine gland, it releases digestive enzymes into the duct system leading to the small intestine (see Chap. 26).

The endocrine portion of the pancreas exists in the one to two million small islands (*islets*) scattered throughout its body and tail. Within these islets, called the **islets of Langerhans** (pancreatic islets), are special types of cells that secrete pancreatic hormones. These cells are known as alpha, beta, delta, and F cells. The types of hormones secreted are: glucagon, insulin, somatostatin, and pancreatic polypeptide (see Table 20-3).

Approximately 20% of the cells in the islets of Langerhans are *alpha cells.* Alpha cells secrete the hormone **glucagon,** which acts in opposition to insulin. (Glucagon raises blood sugar; insulin lowers blood sugar.) Glucagon is needed to break down glycogen (stored sugar) into glucose, a process called *glycogenolysis.* It also stimulates the breakdown of fats and proteins for conversion in the liver into additional glucose. This conversion of excess amino acids and fatty acids into glycogen, which is later released as glucose, is called *gluconeogenesis.*

Approximately 70% of the islet cells are *beta cells.* They secrete the hormone **insulin,** which is a protein substance. Insulin is the key regulator of carbohydrate, protein, and fat metabolism and storage. The primary function of insulin is to control the blood's glucose level. Insulin accomplishes this task in several ways, as listed in Box 20-2. The actions of insulin and related disorders are discussed further in Chapter 78.

Approximately 5% of the cells within the islets are *delta cells.* Delta cells secrete *somatostatin,* which is "identical to the growth hormone inhibiting hormone (GHIH) secreted by the hypothalamus."[1] Somatostatin inhibits the release of insulin and glucagon. The way this control mechanism operates is unknown.

The remaining 5% of the islet cells are *F cells.* F cells secrete *pancreatic polypeptide,* which inhibits the secretion of somatostatin and pancreatic digestive enzymes.

> ➤➤ BOX 20-2

> ### ACTIONS OF INSULIN TO CONTROL GLUCOSE LEVEL
>
> - The major stimulus for synthesis and secretion of insulin is an elevated blood glucose level.
> - Insulin increases the cell membrane's permeability to glucose. After it is in the cell, glucose is used in cellular respiration to produce energy.
> - Insulin stimulates the liver to convert extra glucose into glycogen (*glycogenesis*), and helps the liver and muscles to store glycogen. Glycogen is stored as body sugar, commonly referred to as *animal starch.*
> - Insulin increases the transfer of amino acids across muscle membranes for synthesis into proteins.
> - Insulin speeds fatty acid synthesis (*lipogenesis*) for fat storage.
> - Insulin slows *glycogenolysis* (glycogen breakdown) and *gluconeogenesis* (formation of glucose from noncarbohydrate sources).

☞ Key Concept

Insulin is a hormone needed to transport glucose into cells for cells to function. If there is a lack of insulin or if the insulin is not working as it should, an increased blood glucose level will result. A condition known as diabetes mellitus results when there is a disturbance in the oxidation or utilization of glucose (usually the result of a malfunction of the beta cells of the pancreas). Because insulin is necessary for adequate functioning of the body, medical intervention is necessary to manage diabetes mellitus.

Thymus

The **thymus** lies behind the sternum (breast bone). In infants and children, the thymus is relatively large. After puberty, the thymus becomes smaller, but little is known of the long-term effects of this phenomenon.

The thymus produces *thymosin* (thymic hormone), a protein that stimulates production of small lymphocytes called *T cells* (also called *T lymphocytes, T helper cells,* or *thymus-dependent cells*). The thymus also secretes other hormones believed to assist in the maturation of T cells. T cells are essential for the development of cellular immunity and the body's response to invading organisms. If the T-cell count of a person is diminished, that person would have a diminished ability to fight off attacking pathogens. This type of diminished immune response may be seen in the person with AIDS (acquired immunodeficiency syndrome) or in the client undergoing cancer chemotherapy. Additional information about T cells is discussed in Chapter 24. HIV and AIDS are detailed in Chapter 84.

Other Sites That Secrete Hormones

Gastrointestinal Tract

The *stomach* wall secretes a hormone called *gastrin,* which stimulates the gastric glands to secrete gastric juice. The lining of the upper part of the small intestine secretes hormones (*pancreozymin, secretin*) that stimulate the pancreas to release pancreatic juice, and another hormone that regulates the release of bile from the gallbladder and causes the gallbladder to contract (*cholecystokinin*). These hormones will be discussed further in Chapter 26.

Placenta

The placenta is also a temporary endocrine gland, secreting hormones that help a woman to maintain a pregnancy. These hormones include estrogen, progesterone, and human chorionic gonadotropin (**HCG**). Estrogen and progesterone will be discussed further in Chapter 29. Pregnancy is discussed in Chapter 64.

☞ Key Concept

The presence of high levels of HCG in a woman's body provides the basis for the commonly used tests to determine pregnancy.

EFFECTS OF AGING ON THE SYSTEM

Table 21-3 summarizes the effects of aging on the sensory system.

Eye and Vision Changes

Presbyopia.   The lens of the eye becomes less elastic with aging, and often is not able to accommodate well enough to see close objects. Reading material must be held at arm's length for it not to seem blurry. In some cases, a book may need to be held so far away to make the letters clear that they are no longer identifiable.

Presbyopia is a gradual loss of the function of accommodation and usually begins between the ages of 40 and 45. Presbyopia usually results in farsightedness. A person can be provided with eyeglasses called bifocals or trifocals that will correct the situation. *Bifocals* have two different types of lenses in the eyeglasses. The top lens is formulated to permit a person to see items far away. The bottom section of the lens is created to see near items clearly. *Trifocals* are formulated in the same manner, except that there are three sections of the lens, one for viewing objects at a distance, one for viewing objects in the intermediate viewing area, and one for viewing objects up close.

Other Visual Disorders.   As people get older, they need more light to read because the pupil is no longer able to dilate fully and therefore cannot let in enough light.

Loss of visual acuity may also occur if debris (waste material) builds up within the eye. This process may occur at any time, but is more common in older people because of extended exposure over the years to the sun's ultraviolet rays.

The slowing of all body secretions may affect the lacrimal glands, and may lead to extraordinarily dry eyes. Older adults may use artificial tears, in the form of eye drops, to help provide moisture and lubrication to the eyes.

Clouding of the lens may occur at any age. The cloudy or opaque lens that results is called a *cataract*. It most often occurs by later middle age. When visual changes interfere with daily living or quality of life, the cataract is surgically removed and an artificial lens is implanted.

Ptosis, a paralytic drooping of the upper eyelid, may occur as a result of the normal aging process or because of continued eye strain over many years. Severe ptosis that interferes with vision can be surgically corrected.

Ear and Hearing Changes

Many older people experience a degenerative loss of hearing, called **presbycusis,** which often begins at about age 60. The most common cause of presbycusis is deterioration of the cochlear structures. This specific difficulty is most often a result of the loss of hair cells in the organ of Corti. Usually the loss is most noticeable when responding to certain sound frequencies, particularly higher frequencies.

■■■ TABLE 21-3 *E*FFECTS OF AGING ON THE SENSORY SYSTEM

Factor	Result	Nursing Implications
Vision/Eye Changes		
Lens accommodation decreases.	Presbyopia	Advise a vision check for corrective lenses.
Depth perception decreases.	More light needed Difficulty judging the height of curbs and steps Falls common	Encourage use of hand rails, canes, and walkers. Advise to avoid fast moves or turns. Make client aware of dangers.
Peripheral vision decreases.	Driving may be dangerous	Encourage a defensive driving class. Avoid standing at client's side.
Ability to react to darkness and to bright light decreases; night vision decreases.	Takes longer for eyes to adjust when entering a dark room or bright sunlight	Advise use of a night light. Advise person to avoid night driving if possible.
Color perception decreases.	Difficulty discerning hues of blue, green, and violet	Use yellow, red, and black for signs.
A grayish white ring (arcus senilis) forms around the iris.	May lower self-esteem and body image	Enhance client's self-esteem.
Tear formation decreases.	Dry, itchy eyes More prone to infections	Advise about medication ("artificial tears"). Advise against rubbing eyes.
Fluid circulation in eye decreases.	Increased risk for glaucoma	Encourage regular visual exams, including intraocular pressure measurement.

(continued)

■■■ **TABLE 21-3** *E*FFECTS OF AGING ON THE SENSORY SYSTEM (CONTINUED)

Factor	Result	Nursing Implications
Hearing/Ear Changes		
Numerous functional and structural changes occur in ear components.	Presbycusis Progressive hearing loss Loss of perception of high pitch, sound location, tracking sounds, normal conversation	Discuss hearing aid evaluation. Person may benefit from "helper" dog or special telephone volume controls. Face person when talking to him or her. Speak clearly but not too loudly. Advise against driving if hearing is compromised.
	Increased incidence of vertigo, dizziness, and tinnitus	Tell client to use hand rails and to avoid sudden movements.
Structural changes affect balance and equilibrium.	Increased incidence of falls Dizziness on change of position	Advise the use of hand rails. Advise person to change positions slowly.
Increased buildup of cerumen.	Hearing loss	Suggest frequent ear examinations.
Taste Changes		
Taste sensation decreases.	Decreased appetite May try to compensate by increasing salt and sugar intake, aggravating conditions such as hypertension and diabetes	Monitor nutritional status. Teach proper nutrition.
	Risk for consuming spoiled foods	Teach client to check expiration dates on containers.
Smell Changes		
Smell perception decreases.	May not smell smoke or poisonous substances (eg, gas leak)	Teach client to install smoke detectors and preventive safety measures.
Tactile Changes		
Efficiency and the number of sensory nerve endings (all sensations affected) decrease.	Stronger stimuli are needed for person to perceive sensations. Pain associated with some conditions may differ.	Monitor client's overall condition. Do not ignore complaints.

Other causes of impaired hearing in older people include:

- An injury or illness earlier in life (diabetes, otitis media, Meniere's syndrome)
- Fusing of the ossicles in the middle ear, impairing their ability to vibrate freely
- Bone formation around the oval window
- Decalcification of skull bone, impairing bone conduction of sound
- Decreased cochlear function
- A disorder in the nerve pathway that carries sound impulses to the brain
- A disorder in the area of the brain where the impulses are received, which interferes with interpretation of sound impulses
- Presbycusis (progressive hearing loss in aging)
- Lifelong exposure to loud noises, damaging the eardrum or structures of the inner ear
- Excess cerumen (ear wax)
- Certain medications: quinine, aminoglycosides (ie, gentamicin, streptomycin), aspirin, loop diuretics (for example, furosemide [Lasix])

A hearing aid may help many older people with these and other hearing problems (see Chap. 79).

Changes in Other Senses

The senses of smell and taste gradually become less keen as a person ages. These changes result from loss of nerve function, which interferes with the transmission of the sensations to the brain. Another factor relates to the taste buds. Connective tissue cells gradually replace the taste buds as the person ages. By age 75, estimates are that the person has approximately only 40% of the taste buds that were functioning at age 30. With the loss of the sense of taste, the person does not feel as hungry and may need to be encouraged to eat even when not hungry. He or she may also use salt and spices excessively to compensate for the loss of sensation in the tastebuds.

The vocal cords of the older person may simply "wear out," making speech difficult or impossible. The person is able to whisper at first, but may lose that ability as the condition progresses. The voice may deepen, due to thickening and loss of mobility of the vocal cords.

➤ STUDENT SYNTHESIS

Key Points

- The five senses are seeing, hearing, tasting, smelling, and touching.
- The eye is the organ of vision. It has many protective mechanisms. Light rays travel through several structures of the eye before focusing on the retina.
- The eyeball has three major layers of tissue: sclera and cornea, choroid layer, and retina.
- Several cranial nerves are involved in vision.
- Three sets of extraocular muscles control eye movements.
- The three parts of the ear are the external, the middle, and the inner ear.
- The external ear is responsible for protecting the internal structures of the ear from foreign substances and for catching and carrying sound waves to the middle ear. The middle ear is responsible for the transmission of sound. The inner ear is responsible for transmitting sound waves and information about body position to the brain.
- The semicircular canals of the inner ear are responsible for balance.
- Taste buds are responsible for the perceptions of sweet, salty, sour, and bitter.
- Receptors for the sense of smell are located in the upper nasal cavity (olfactory receptors).
- Receptors for the sense of touch are called tactile receptors and are located throughout most areas of the body.
- Proprioceptors are located in muscles, tendons, and joints.
- Referred pain is perceived in a place other than where it originates.
- The temporal, parietal, occipital, and cerebellar areas of the brain are responsible for interpreting sensory stimuli. The temporal lobe is responsible for interpreting sounds via the vestibulocochlear nerve from the inner ear. The parietal and temporal lobes are responsible for interpreting taste. The occipital lobe receives visual information via the optic nerve from the eye. The cerebellum is responsible for maintaining equilibrium and coordination.

Critical Thinking Exercises

1. What anatomic structure of the eye does a contact lens come in contact with? Why is meticulous care necessary to prevent infection or irritation to that structure?
2. Referring to Table 21-1, explain how injury to each of the listed cranial nerves would affect vision.
3. Explain why your ears plug in an airplane, especially when you have a cold.
4. Explain to a client why taking a sour liquid medication through a straw helps to minimize the unpleasant taste.

NCLEX-Style Review Questions

1. The purpose of the choroid layer of the eye is to:
   a. Allow light to be transmitted through it
   b. Bring oxygen and nutrients to the eye
   c. Give color to the eye
   d. Provide the receptors to allow for vision
2. The function of the lens is to:
   a. Allow binocular vision
   b. Lubricate the eye
   c. Refract light rays
   d. Sense color
3. Which structure separates the external ear and middle ear?
   a. External auditory meatus
   b. Ossicles
   c. Oval window
   d. Tympanic membrane
4. The function of the semicircular canals is to:
   a. Maintain balance while the body is moving
   b. Provide information regarding if the body is at rest
   c. Reflexively contract at sudden, loud noises
   d. Transmit sound waves to the brain
5. Hearing loss in older adults is most noticeable:
   a. At very high frequencies
   b. By the age of 40
   c. In the evening
   d. When in a quiet environment

Reference

1. Tortora, G. J., & Grabowski, S. R. (1996). *Principles of anatomy and physiology* (8th ed.). New York: HarperCollins.

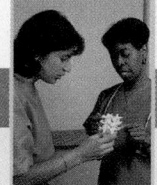

The Cardiovascular System

LEARNING OBJECTIVES

1. Differentiate between the endocardium, myocardium, epicardium, and pericardium.
2. Describe the chambers of the heart and locate them on an anatomical model. State and locate on an anatomical model the vessels that enter and exit these chambers.
3. Define and describe the function of the atrioventricular valves, semilunar valves, chordae tendineae, and papillary muscles.
4. On a chart or model, trace the path of blood through both sides of the heart, and define this path using correct terminology.
5. List, locate, and describe the structure and function of the coronary arteries that supply the heart tissue (myocardium) with blood. Explain the purpose of collateral circulation.
6. Compare and contrast the structure of arteries, capillaries, and veins, and describe the function of each.
7. Describe the path of an electrical impulse through the conduction system of the heart. Describe the purpose of this electrical activity.
8. Explain what creates the normal heart sounds, S_1 and S_2, and note where each of these sounds is best heard.
9. Define cardiac output and describe the factors that regulate it.
10. Define blood pressure and differentiate between systolic and diastolic pressures.
11. Identify major factors that affect the regulation of blood pressure.
12. State four changes in the cardiovascular system caused by aging. Discuss selected nursing implications for each.

NEW TERMINOLOGY

afterload
aorta
aortic valve
apex
atria
bicuspid valve
collateral circulation
coronary sinus
diastole
endocardium
epicardium
ischemia
microcirculation

mitral valve
myocardium
pericardial fluid
pericardium
preload
pulmonic valve
pulse
pulse pressure
semilunar valve
septum
systole
tricuspid valve

ACRONYMS

AV	LCA	S_2
BP	LCX	SA node
CO	LMCA	sBP
CO_2	MI	SV
dBP	O_2	SVC
HR	PDA	SVR
IVC	RCA	
LAD	S_1	

The *cardiovascular system* is designed for transportation and communication throughout all parts of the body. In approximately one minute, a drop of blood travels through the right side of the heart, the lungs, the left side of the heart, and the systemic circulation, completing its circuit by returning to the right side of the heart. In this brief time, the cells located at the tips of the toes and fingers receive oxygen (O_2) from the lungs, and nutrients from the intestines. They simultaneously send carbon dioxide (CO_2) and other wastes to be excreted. The cardiovascular system plays a vital role in this process.

STRUCTURE AND FUNCTION

The cardiovascular system is composed of the heart and blood vessels. Its functions include pumping blood and transporting gases, nutrients, and wastes (Box 22-1).

HEART

The *heart* is a strong, muscular pump about the size of a doubled-up fist. It weighs less than one pound (approximately 250 to 310 g). It lies in the thoracic cavity in the mediastinal space (behind the sternum and between the lungs). The heart is shaped like an irregular and slightly flattened cone. The inferior (lower) point is the **apex,** which is formed by the tip of the left ventricle. The *apical pulse* is counted here. The wide superior (top) margin, called the *base,* lies opposite the apex and is formed mostly by the left atrium.

The heart wall has three layers: endocardium, myocardium, and epicardium (Fig. 22-1).

- The **endocardium** (inner heart) is a membrane lining the heart's interior wall.
- Thick, strong muscles make up the **myocardium** (*myo* = muscle), the middle and thickest layer. Cardiac muscle (see Chap. 18) is a unique type of *involuntary* muscle with striated cells.
- The **epicardium** (*epi* = upon) is the thin outer layer of the cardiac wall (also called the visceral layer of the serous pericardium).

➤➤ BOX 22-1

FUNCTIONS OF THE CARDIOVASCULAR SYSTEM

Functions of The Heart
Pumping Action
- Pumps blood to body and lungs
- Receives blood from body and lungs
- Influences blood pressure

Functions of The Blood Vessels
Transportation
- Provide channels through which blood and lymph travel
- Provide areas (capillaries) where transfer of gases, nutrients, fluids, electrolytes, and wastes can occur

The **pericardium** (*pericardial sac*) is a sac that surrounds and protects the heart. It is also made up of three layers:

- The *epicardium* portion of the heart wall also makes up the pericardium's visceral layer and adheres to the heart's surface.
- The parietal layer is the *inner serous pericardium.*
- The space between the visceral and parietal layers is called the *pericardial space* or *cavity.* It houses a small amount of fluid called **pericardial fluid** that acts as a lubricant and reduces friction between the layers as the heart contracts and relaxes.
- The outermost layer is called the *fibrous pericardium,* which anchors the heart in the mediastinum and prevents overfilling.

Heart Chambers and Valves

A complete muscular wall called the **septum** divides the heart into right and left sides. The two sides are completely separated, with no communication from right to left. Each side is a separate pump.

Chambers
The interior of the heart is divided into four chambers (see Fig. 22-1).

Atria.   The two upper chambers are the right and left **atria** (singular: atrium). These thin-walled, low-pressure chambers are receiving centers for blood.

Ventricles.   The two lower chambers are the right and left *ventricles.* Ventricles are high-pressure chambers because they pump blood out of the heart. The left ventricle must contract with sufficient force to send blood to the entire body; therefore, its muscle walls are thickest and its internal pressures are highest. The right ventricle needs only to pump blood into the low-pressure lungs, and therefore is a thinner-walled chamber.

☛ KEY CONCEPT

The left ventricle is the thickest chamber of the heart. It pumps blood out to the rest of the body.

Valves
As each heart chamber contracts, it pushes blood either into a ventricle or out of the heart to the lungs or body. The cardiac valves are one-way flaps of tissue that open and close in response to pressure changes within the chambers. These unidirectional valves allow blood to flow in one direction only, preventing backflow.

Atrioventricular Valves.   The atrioventricular (**AV**) valves lie between the atria and ventricles. The valve between the right atrium and the right ventricle is called the **tricuspid valve,** because it is formed of three flaps (cusps) of tissue. The valve between the left atrium and the left ventricle is called the **mitral valve (bicuspid valve)** because it has only two flaps of tissue. The tissue flaps attach to tendon-like strands called *chordae tendineae.* These strands are then anchored to papillary muscles located on the inner surface of the ventricles.

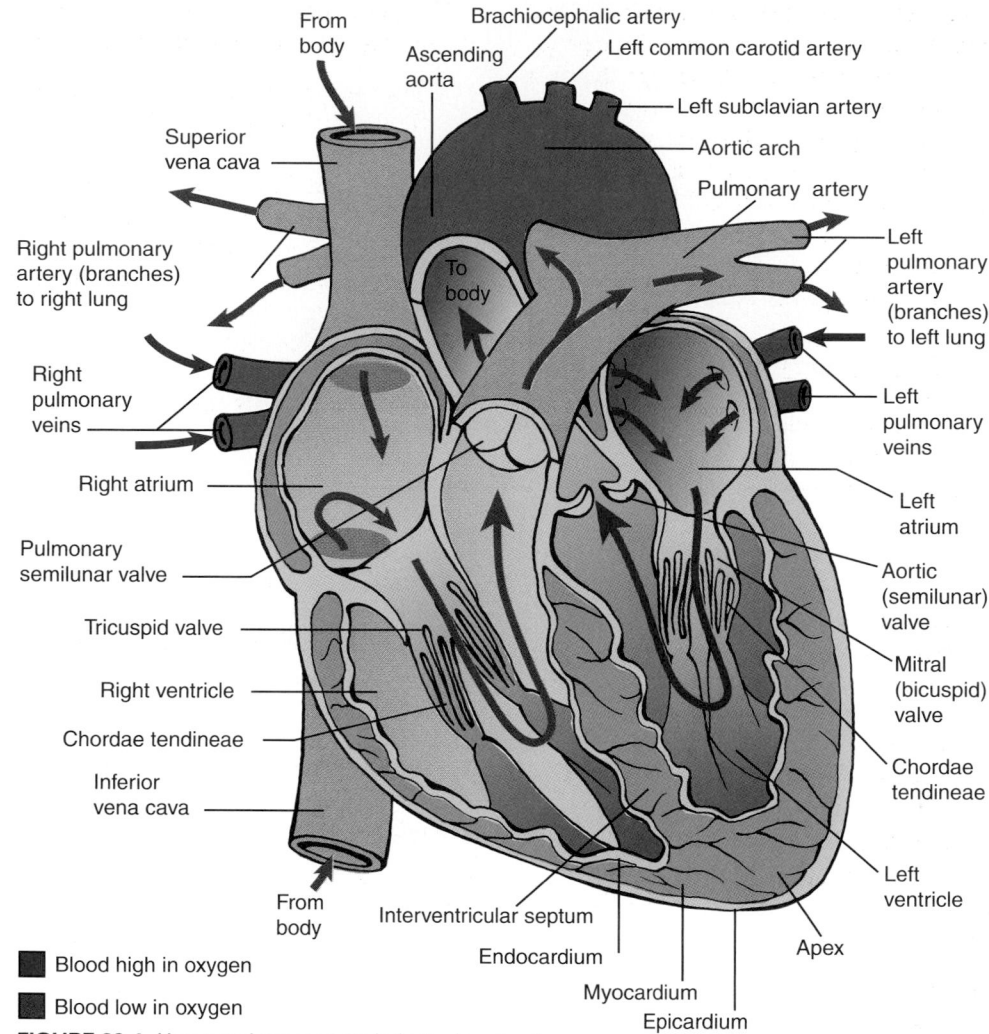

FIGURE 22-1. Heart and great vessels (anterior view).

Blood flows from the atria to the ventricles through open AV valves when pressure in the ventricles is lower than pressure in the atria. During this time, the papillary muscles and chordae tendineae relax. As the ventricles contract, increased pressure causes the AV valves to close. The papillary muscles also contract at this time, tightening the chordae tendineae, to prevent the valve cusps from everting (turning inside-out). If the AV valves, chordae tendineae, or papillary muscles become damaged, backflow of blood (*regurgitation*) into the atria can occur with ventricular contraction.

Overflow Valves.   Each ventricle empties through a valve with three crescent-shaped (half-moon) cusps. These valves are called the **semilunar valves.** The pulmonary semilunar valve separates the right ventricle from the pulmonary artery and is called the **pulmonic valve.** The **aortic valve** separates the left ventricle from the aorta, the body's largest artery. Increased ventricular pressure, as when the ventricles contract, opens the semilunar valves. As the ventricles relax, blood begins to flow backward toward the ventricles. Blood fills the semilunar cusps and causes the valves to close. Therefore, the semilunar valves prevent backflow from their respective arteries into their ventricles.

Route of Blood Flow Through the Heart

Figure 22-1 illustrates the pathway for normal blood flow through the heart's chambers and valves. The right atrium receives *deoxygenated* blood from the superior and inferior vena cava and the coronary sinus. Blood then passes through the tricuspid valve into the right ventricle. It moves on through the pulmonic valve during ventricular contraction to enter the pulmonary artery and lungs, where it receives oxygen.

Oxygenated blood then returns to the left atrium via the pulmonary veins. It travels through the mitral valve and into the left ventricle. During ventricular contraction, the blood from this chamber exits through the aortic valve into the aorta and out to the systemic circulation (Figure 22-2). Chapter 23 presents further discussion related to pulmonic and systemic circulation, and describes the make up of the blood in more detail. Chapter 25 describes gas transfer in and out of blood vessels.

☛ KEY CONCEPT
_____

The pulmonary arteries are the only arteries in the body that carry deoxygenated blood. The pulmonary veins are the only veins that carry oxygenated blood.

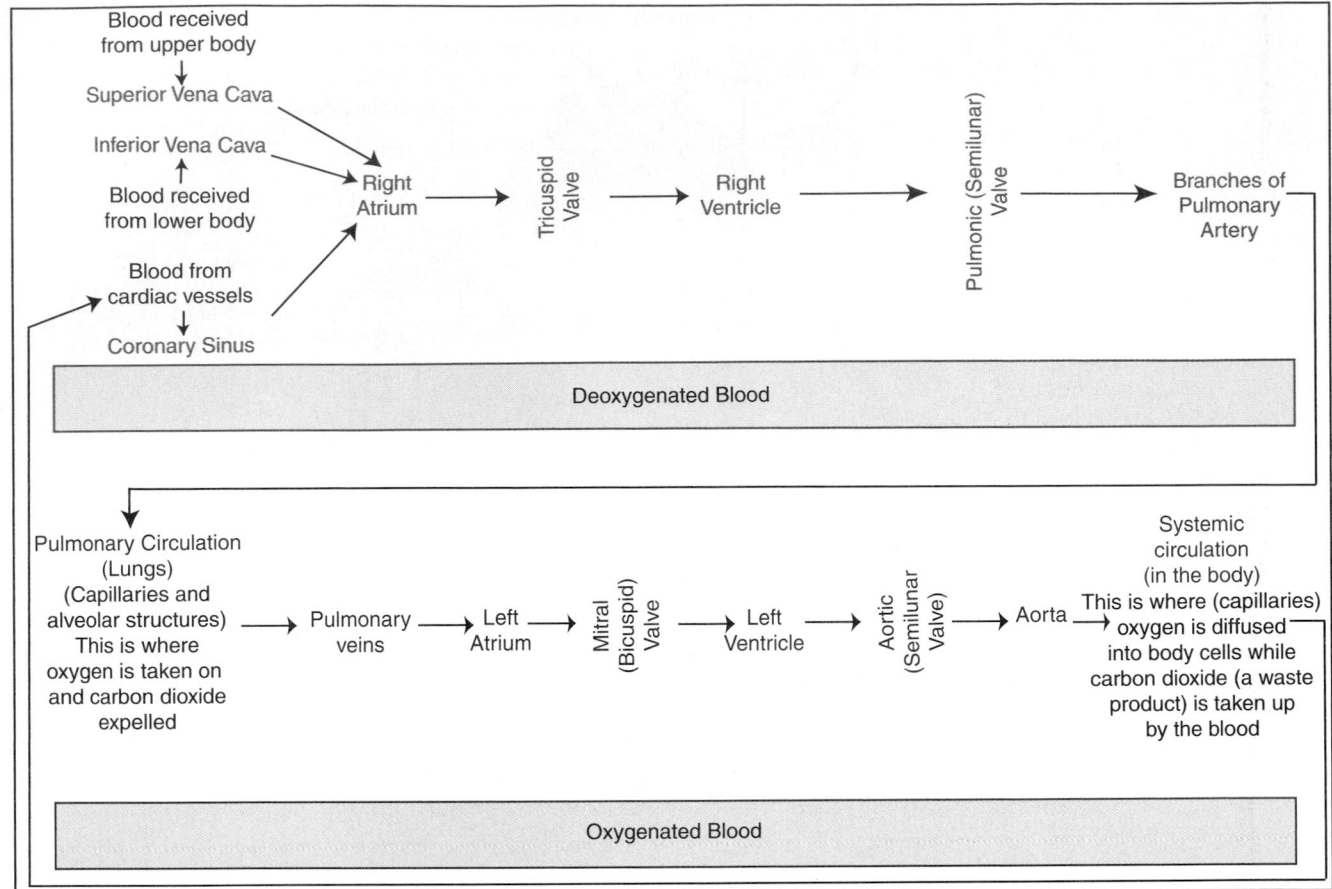

FIGURE 22-2. The circle of blood flow in the body.

Blood Vessels of the Heart

Coronary Arteries

The heart muscle must have its own blood supply because the heart tissue absorbs none of the blood that flows through its chambers. Therefore, two *coronary arteries* (right and left) branch off the ascending aorta to provide blood to the heart muscle (Fig. 22-3). Their openings (or orifices) lie behind two cusps of the aortic valve. They receive their blood supply during ventricular relaxation, when the valves are closed. The right and left coronary arteries extend over the heart's surface and divide into smaller branches that penetrate the myocardium to supply heart tissue with oxygen and nourishment. They are called the *coronary* arteries because they fit over the heart like a crown (*corona*). Their patterns and branches vary among individuals more than any other part of the cardiac anatomy.

Left Coronary Artery. The left coronary artery (**LCA**), also known as the left main coronary artery (**LMCA**), passes along the left atrium and divides into two branches: the anterior interventricular branch or left anterior descending artery (**LAD**) and the left circumflex artery (**LCX**).

The LAD descends along the anterior intraventricular groove to provide blood to most of the ventricular septum and the anterior portion of the left ventricle. The LAD and its branches also supply blood to the anterior papillary mus-

cles, the apex of the left ventricle, and the right and left bundle branches.

The LCX extends around the left side of the heart, along the groove between the left atrium and the left ventricle, to supply blood to the left atrium and the lateral and posterior portions of the left ventricle. It supplies blood to the sinoatrial (SA) node in approximately 40% of the population and to the AV node in approximately 10% of the population.

Right Coronary Artery. The right coronary artery (**RCA**) branches out along the right AV groove to supply blood to the right atrium and right ventricle. It also provides blood to the SA node in approximately 60% of the population and to the AV node in 90% of the population.

The main branch of the RCA that supplies the right side of the heart is called the *marginal branch*. In most people, a second branch travels down the posterior intraventricular septum to supply blood to the posterior septum, the inferior and posterior portions of the left ventricle, and the posterior left papillary muscle. This branch is called the posterior descending artery (**PDA**). In some people the PDA comes off the LCX to supply blood to these areas. This arrangement is known as "left coronary dominance."

Collateral Circulation. An important factor in heart physiology is that the large coronary arteries join in very few places. Consequently, if one of these arteries becomes plugged, the blood has no way to detour. A blockage of these arteries

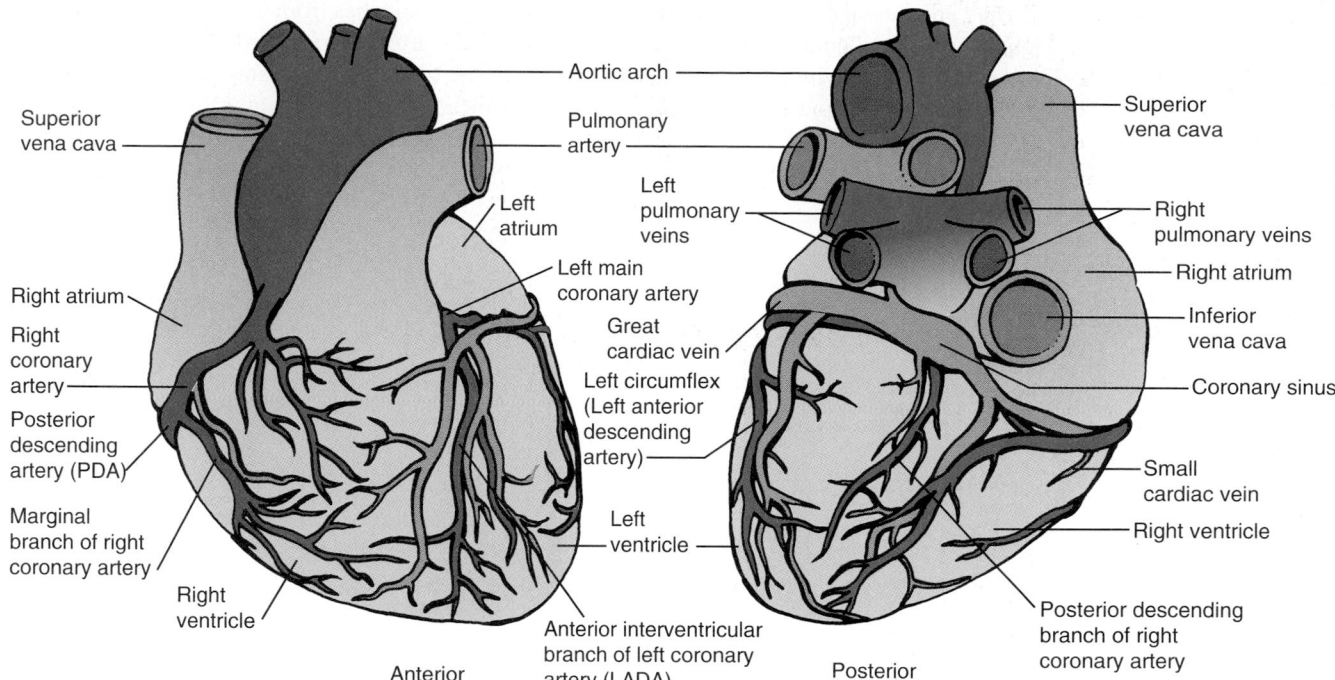

FIGURE 22-3. Coronary arteries and cardiac veins. *Left,* Anterior view, *Right,* Posterior view. It is important to note that coronary circulation patterns vary among people.

causes either myocardial insufficiency **ischemia** (reversible cell injury due to decreased blood and oxygen supply), or myocardial infarction (**MI**), which is a localized area of dead tissue caused by a lack of blood supply. Over time, **collateral circulation** may help to supply blood to "at risk" tissue. Collateral circulation occurs when two vessels that nourish the same area interconnect. Very small interconnections are normally found among microscopic branches of the coronary arteries throughout the heart. When coronary obstruction occurs gradually (as with atherosclerosis), these vessels can enlarge to nourish the endangered heart muscle.

Coronary Veins

The coronary arteries drain into capillaries in the myocardium, where delivery of oxygen and nutrients occurs, along with waste removal. Blood then leaves the capillaries and most of it enters the venous system via two main veins. These two principal vessels are the *great cardiac vein,* which drains blood from the anterior surface of the heart, and the *middle cardiac vein,* which drains the heart's posterior surface. These vessels transport blood into an opening called the **coronary sinus,** which returns the blood to the right atrium (see Fig. 22-2).

SYSTEMIC BLOOD VESSELS

Blood is carried through the body in a set of tubes or *blood vessels:* arteries, capillaries, and veins. The arteries carry blood *away* from the heart, the capillaries serve as "in-between" channels, and the veins carry blood *toward* the heart.

SPECIAL CONSIDERATIONS: THE LIFE SPAN

Physiologic Differences and Coronary Heart Disease

Anatomic and physiologic differences can make coronary heart disease potentially a more dangerous threat for women than men. Women's hearts are on the average 10% smaller than men's hearts, with corresponding smaller coronary arteries. Smaller vessel size leads to decreased perfusion (circulation), especially in the presence of atherosclerosis. Clots can form more easily in women's coronary arteries due to higher fibrinogen levels and greater fibrinolytic activity with advancing age. Increased clot formation, coupled with decreased coronary artery size, can increase the risk of vessel occlusion. Also, some hormonal influences are believed to be linked to birth control pills.

☛ KEY CONCEPT

Arteries carry blood away *from the heart. Veins carry blood* toward *the heart (except in the pulmonary circuit).*

Arteries and Arterioles

Arteries are elastic and smooth (involuntary) muscular tubes that, with the exception of the pulmonary artery, carry oxygenated blood to body cells. They are known as "resistance vessels" that can support high pressures and hold large volumes of blood. Table 22-1 lists major arteries, which are also illustrated in Figure 22-4. The largest artery, the **aorta,** is divided into the *ascending aorta, aortic arch, thoracic aorta,* and *abdominal aorta.* From the aorta, the arteries branch into smaller vessels, like branches from the central trunk of a tree. The smallest of the arteries are called *arterioles.* Arterioles contain less elastic tissue and more smooth muscle than arteries. Constriction and dilation of the arterioles regulates blood pressure and flow. By changing vessel diameter, the volume of blood supplied to the tissues increases or decreases.

■■■ TABLE 22-1 *M*AJOR ARTERIES

Name	Distribution
Branches of the Ascending Aorta	
Left and right coronary arteries	Heart muscle
Branches of the Aortic Arch	
Brachiocephalic (innominate) branches into	
Right subclavian	Right upper extremity
Right common carotid	Right side of head and neck
Left common carotid	Left side of head and neck
Left subclavian	Left upper extremity
Each subclavian artery extends into	
Axillary	Axilla
Brachial	Arm proper
Radial	Thumb side of forearm and wrist
Ulnar	Medial side of hand
Branches of the Thoracic Aorta	
Bronchial	Lungs
Esophageal	Esophagus
Intercostals	Muscles and other structures of chest wall
Superior phrenic	Posterior and superior surfaces of diaphragm
Branches of Abdominal Aorta	
Celiac trunk branches into	
Left gastric	Stomach
Splenic	Spleen
Hepatic	Liver
Superior mesenteric	Small intestine and first half of large intestine
Inferior mesenteric	Second half of large intestine
Phrenic	Diaphragm
Suprarenal (adrenal)	Adrenal glands
Renal	Kidneys
Ovarian (female) or testicular (male; formerly spermatic arteries)	Sex glands
Lumbar	Musculature of the abdominal wall
Common iliac branches into internal iliac	Pelvic muscles, bladder, rectum, prostate, reproductive organs
External iliac branches into	
Femoral	Thigh
Popliteal	Knee
Tibial	Leg, ankle, heel
Dorsalis pedis	Foot

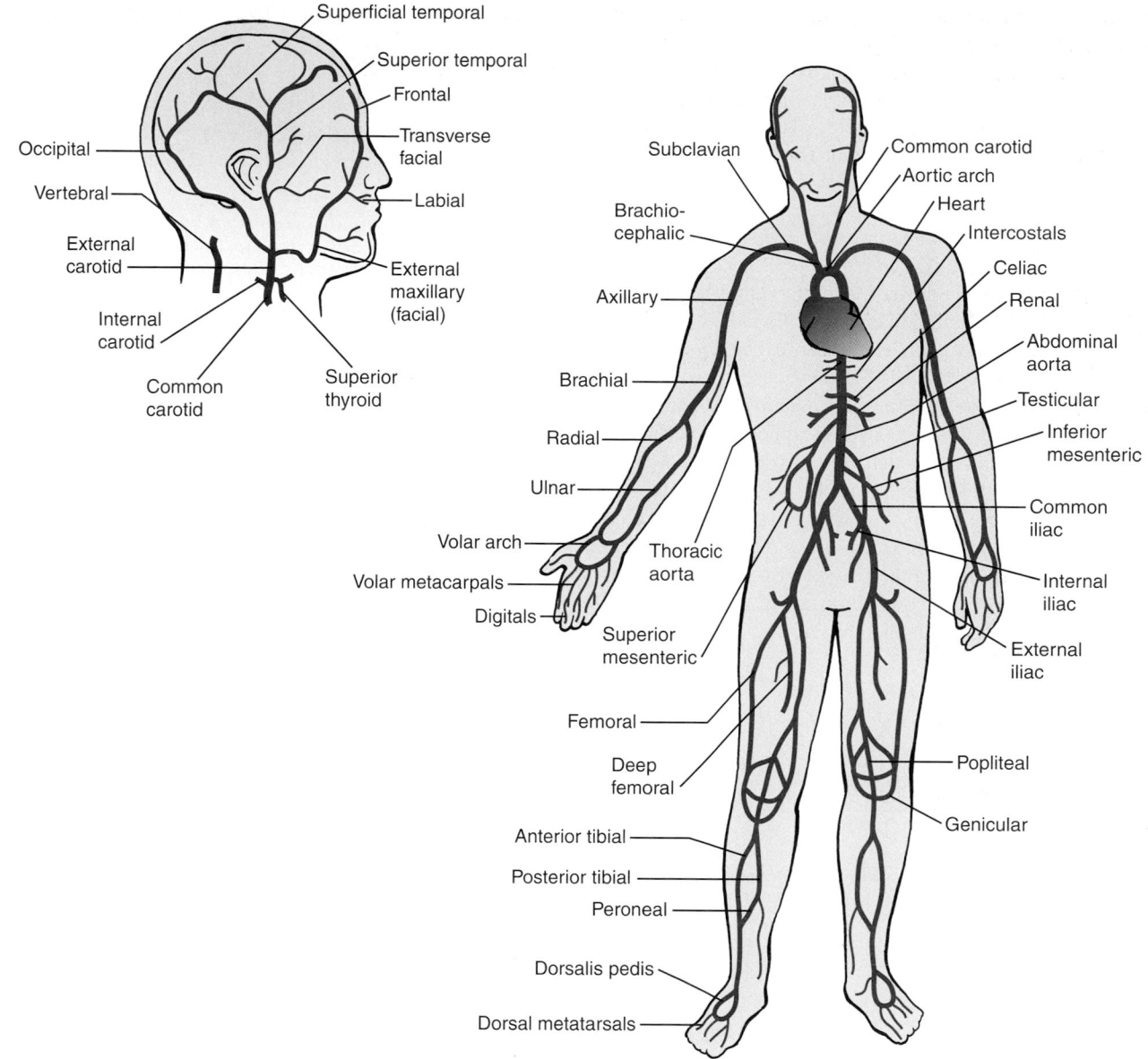

FIGURE 22-4. Principal systemic arteries. The arterial system carries blood away from the heart. Major pressure points (pulse points) are used to count the pulse or to stop hemorrhage.

Capillaries

From the arterioles, blood flows into the smallest vessels of all, *capillaries.* Blood flow through the capillaries is known as **microcirculation.** Capillaries are so small that the tiny red blood cells must pass through them in single file. (One estimate of the total length of blood vessels in the body is 60,000 miles. Capillaries make up most of this length.) In the capillaries, blood flows slowly, allowing time for oxygen and nutrients to leave the blood vessels and to enter body tissues. Chapter 17 discusses transport of nutrients, salts, gases, and wastes across the cell membrane and through the capillary wall. Exchanges through the capillary wall are due to diffusion and filtration. The relatively high osmotic pressure of albumin (a plasma protein) within capillaries pulls interstitial fluid into them. The fluid that is pulled back into capillaries contains cellular waste products now on their way to the kidneys for excretion.

(*Ecchymotic* areas [black and blue marks] result from ruptured capillaries.)

Veins and Venules

At the same time that blood is delivering materials to cells, it is picking up waste products. From the capillaries, the blood starts back toward the heart through *venules,* the smallest veins. The branches of the veins grow larger and fewer as they near the heart, until finally the blood reaches the *superior vena cava* (**SVC**) and *inferior vena cava* (**IVC**) (plural: cavae). These two large veins return blood to the right atrium. The SVC returns blood from the head, neck, and arms, and the IVC returns blood from the lower body. Venous blood is dark red because the oxygen has been replaced with carbon dioxide and other wastes. (*An exception occurs within the pulmonary veins, which carry oxy-*

genated blood to the left atrium.) Table 22-2 lists major veins, which are illustrated in Fig. 22-5.

Venous Blood Return. Venous valves contribute to efficient venous blood flow from the extremities, and permit blood to flow in one direction only. Also contributing to venous return is the location of veins (between skeletal muscles). Muscle contractions squeeze blood toward the heart. Because of its slow journey through the capillaries, blood loses its original force from heart contractions by the time it reaches the veins. Therefore, veins do not pulsate. When a vein is cut, the muscles in the wall constrict, and blood flows in a steady stream rather than pulsating like arterial blood.

Systemic veins and venules are also called "blood reservoirs" or "capacitance vessels." They house approximately 60% of the body's blood volume at rest, and have the capacity to store more blood when needed. Healthcare professionals often administer medications that promote *venodilation,* which results in an increased storage capacity of the veins, thereby decreasing the volume of blood returning to a failing heart. The venous "reservoir" system also serves as a depot for blood that can quickly be diverted to other vessels if needed. For example, the *vasoconstriction* (contraction) of veins helps to compensate for blood loss during hemorrhage.

SYSTEM PHYSIOLOGY

Cardiac Conduction

Special bundles of unique tissue in the heart transmit and coordinate electrical impulses to stimulate the heart to beat (Fig. 22-6). The first of these bundles is embedded in the wall of the right atrium at the junction of the SVC. It is called the *sinoatrial node* (**SA node** or *sinus node*), which is considered the heart's "pacemaker." Normal heartbeat originates in the SA node, typically at a rate of 60 to 100 beats per minute. The normal sinus impulse is transmitted over the heart via specialized fibers known as the *conduction system.* These impulses stimulate the heart's chambers to contract. The SA node sets the pace, and the rest of the heart follows its bidding. This swift message is first sent out over the internodal pathways to the muscular tissue of the atria, which causes the atria to contract.

☛ KEY CONCEPT

The SA node is the "pacemaker" of the heart. The person with a poorly functioning SA node usually requires the implant of an electronic pacemaker.

■■■ **TABLE 22-2** 𝓜AJOR VEINS

Name	Drainage Areas
Superficial Veins	
Cephalic, basilic, median cubital	Hand, forearm, elbow
Saphenous	Lower extremities
Temporal	Skull
Deep Veins	
Axillary, brachial, subclavian	Arms
Radial, ulnar	Hands
Femoral, popliteal, tibial	Thigh, knee, and leg
Iliac, internal and external	Pelvis and legs
Jugular	Face and neck
Brachiocephalic	Union of subclavian and jugular veins
Superior Vena Cava	Upper half of body; formed by union of both brachiocephalic veins
Azygos vein	Chest wall into superior vena cava
Inferior Vena Cava	Lower half of body; begins with union of two common iliac veins
Receives venous blood from	
Iliac veins	Pelvis and legs
Lumbar veins	Dorsal part of trunk and spinal cord
Testicular/ovarian veins	Sex organs
Renal veins	Kidneys
Suprarenal veins	Adrenal glands
Hepatic veins	Liver
Hepatic Portal Vein	Abdominal organs to the liver
Receives venous blood from	
Mesenteric veins	Intestines
Splenic vein	Spleen
Gastric vein	Stomach
Pancreatic vein	Pancreas

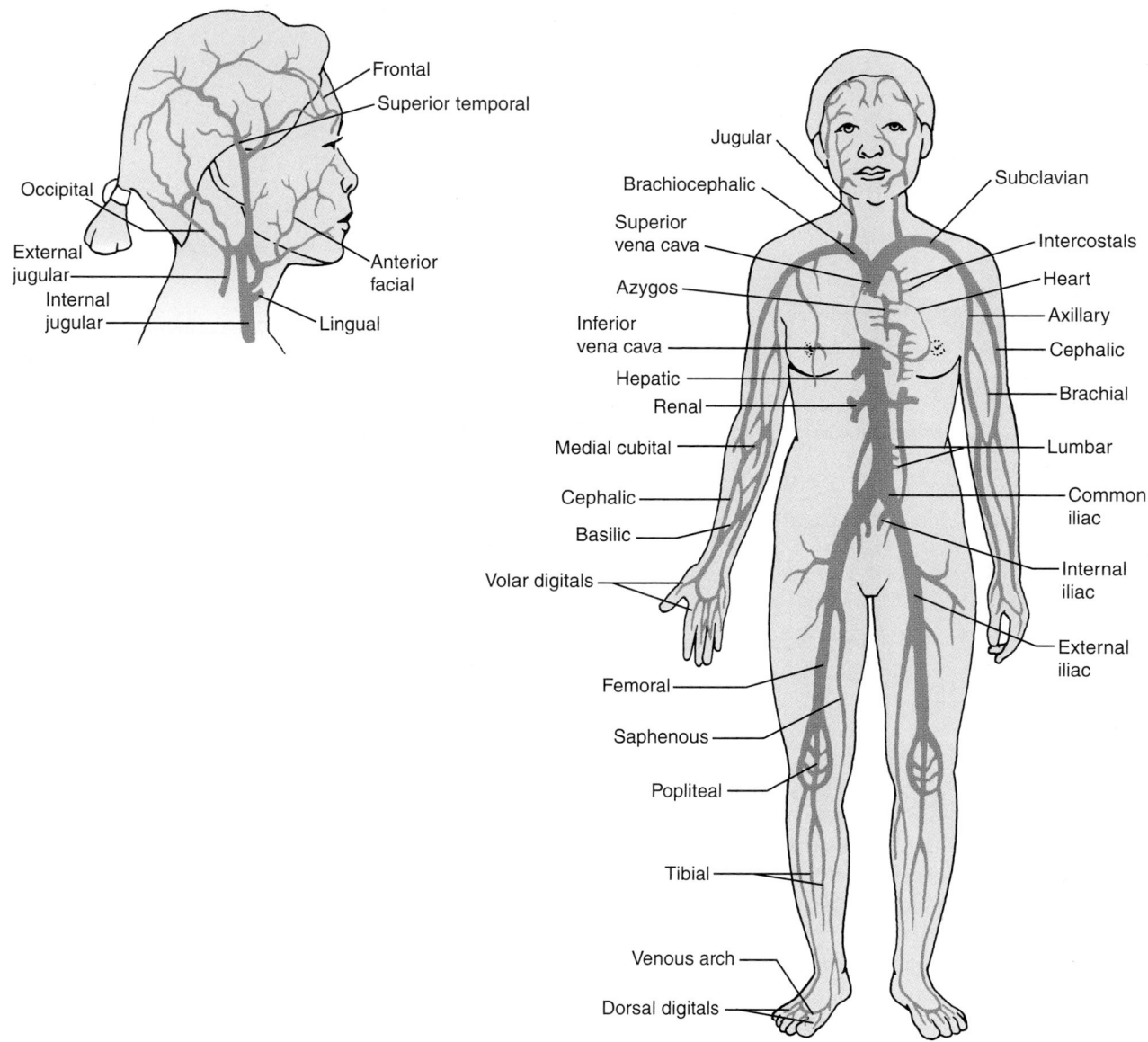

FIGURE 22-5. Principal systemic veins. The veins carry blood toward the heart.

The next bundle, the *atrioventricular node* (*AV node*), is found in the lower part of the right atrium near the ventricle. The AV node picks up the message like a receiving station, and holds onto it until the atria have contracted and emptied blood into the ventricles. When the ventricles are ready to receive the impulse, the AV node transmits it through the *bundle of His* (pronounced *hiss*) (AV bundle) and down the interventricular septum to the *right* and *left bundle branches*. From there, the fibers penetrate the ventricular muscle and terminate in the *Purkinje fibers*. When the Purkinje fibers pick up the message, they stimulate the ventricles to contract. The heart then rests for a short period and begins the process all over again.

☛ KEY CONCEPT

The electrical activity of the heart must occur before the mechanical, or pumping, activity of the heart can respond with a heartbeat.

Should the SA node fail to fire an impulse, escape beats from other pacemaker cells within the AV node or ventricles will take over to keep the heart beating. When this occurs, the heartbeat becomes slower. If the SA node and AV node fail to fire an impulse, the ventricles must fire an impulse in order to maintain a heart rate. The ventricles will only contract at a rate of 20 to 40 beats per minute if this occurs, so be aware that a heart rate this slow might not support life. If the ventricles do not fire an impulse, cardiac arrest will occur.

☛ KEY CONCEPT

Conduction System of the Heart
• *SA (sinoatrial) node (pacemaker)*
• *AV (atrioventricular) node*
• *Bundle of His (AV bundle)*
• *Right and left bundle branches*
• *Purkinje fibers to muscles of ventricles*

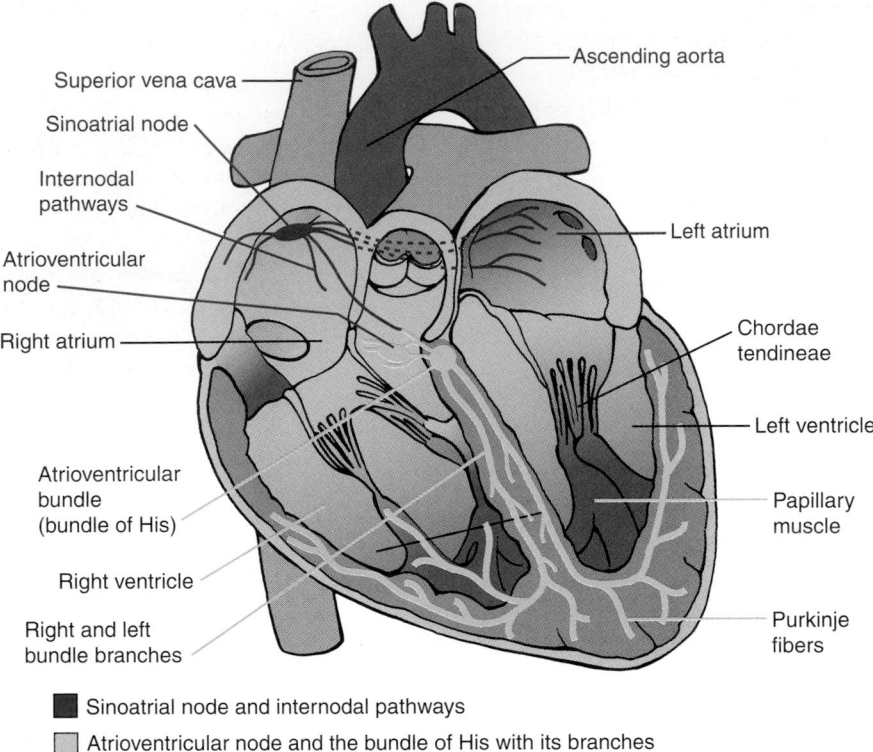

Sinoatrial node and internodal pathways

Atrioventricular node and the bundle of His with its branches

FIGURE 22-6. The conduction system of the heart.

The heart has several features that combine to regulate its rate. Cardiac muscles have automaticity: the ability to contract spontaneously and regularly (without neural input) because the cardiac cells can generate their own electrical impulse by themselves. If the heart cannot be regulated by the body any longer, then other interventions such as medications or pacemaker insertion would be required to reestablish homeostasis.

To maintain homeostasis in individual situations, such as in an emergency, the autonomic nerves send input from cardiac centers in the brain's medulla to the heart. These cardiac centers have both accelerating and braking devices. Together, they permit an accurate and delicate control of heart rate in response to internal and external stimuli.

Cardiac Cycle

In less than one second, both atria contract as both ventricles relax. Immediately after this, both ventricles contract as both atria relax. This process is considered one *cardiac cycle* or one heartbeat. This sequence of dual contractions, the atria followed by the ventricles, is called **systole.** Systole takes up one third of the cardiac cycle.

Atrial relaxation, followed by ventricular relaxation, is called **diastole.** Diastole takes up two thirds of the cardiac cycle, allowing time for the chambers to adequately fill with blood. One cardiac cycle is made up of systole of the atria and ventricles and diastole of the atria and ventricles. These contraction and relaxation processes occur almost simultaneously on the left and right sides of the heart.

☛ KEY CONCEPT

The contraction that pumps the blood from the heart is called systole, *and the period when the heart relaxes is called* diastole. *The heart is actually in systole twice, once for the atria and once for the ventricles. Additionally, both the atria and ventricles have periods of diastole. If the terms* systole *and* diastole *are used without specific reference to either atria or ventricles, they usually imply the contraction and relaxation of the ventricles.*

Heart Sounds

Events in the cardiac cycle produce sounds that can be auscultated (heard) with a stethoscope. These sounds include normal heart sounds, and might also include abnormal heart sounds.

Normal Heart Sounds. The first normal heart sound (S_1) is called the "lub" and is produced by closure of the AV valves when the ventricles contract. The second heart sound (S_2) is called the "dub" or "dup" and is produced by the closure of the semilunar valves when the ventricles relax. Hence, S_1 occurs at the beginning of systole and S_2 occurs at the beginning of diastole. The first sound is loudest and longest. It can be heard over all the pericardium, but is usually loudest at the apex of the heart. S_2 is more easily heard at the base of the heart.

Abnormal Heart Sounds. Abnormal heart sounds, sometimes called *extra sounds,* are described as *gallops, rubs,* and *murmurs.* The third (S_3) or fourth (S_4) heart sounds, known as "gallop" sounds, occur when ventricular filling creates audible vibrations during a normally silent diastolic phase. "Rub" sounds may be heard when the layers of the pericardium rub together due to inflammation, as in pericarditis. *Murmurs* are extra heart sounds resulting from turbulent blood flow through the heart's chambers and valves. A *heart murmur* may be clinically significant, especially if related to a structural defect in the heart valves or in the walls separating the heart's chambers. In adults, murmurs are most typically due to narrowing (*stenosis*) of a valve or to blood regurgitating through a valve that does not close properly. Many children and 10% of adults have nonpathologic murmurs, called "functional murmurs."

Pulse

Arterial walls are strong and elastic. They expand as the heart pumps blood to the body. This rhythmic expansion is the **pulse.** The pulse can be felt where arteries are close to the surface. Pulse assessment locations are named for the artery in each area: radial (wrist), carotid (neck), popliteal (back of knee), femoral (groin), tibial (ankle), pedal (foot), axillary (armpit), and temporal (temple). These points are called *pressure points* or *pulse points.* (See Figure 43-2 in Chapter 43.)

Cardiac Output

Cardiac output (**CO**) is the amount of blood that the ventricles pump out in 1 minute. In the resting adult, the normal amount is between 4 and 6 liters. The stroke volume (**SV**) is the volume of blood ejected with each heartbeat. When calculating the CO, multiply the SV by the number of beats per minute or heart rate (**HR**). Therefore, any changes in the amount of blood that leaves the heart, or changes in a client's heart rate, will affect his or her cardiac output. Increases in SV or HR will result in increased CO. This increase can occur during exercise to increase blood volume to the rest of the body. *Low* cardiac output can result in decreased blood supply to the body and therefore, decreased oxygen and nutrients to the cells.

The formula for calculating cardiac output is:

$$CO = SV \times HR$$

Factors Affecting Ventricular Resistance

To adapt to the body's metabolic needs, the heart can alter its CO. In addition, the autonomic nervous system can influence HR. For example, in a dangerous situation, the heart rate increases. This increases the cardiac output.

Factors called *preload* and *afterload* can affect SV. **Preload** is the amount of pressure or "stretching force" against the ventricular wall at end-diastole (maximum relaxation of the heart). When more blood volume is returned to the ventricles, the muscle fibers in the ventricles stretch to accommodate the excess. *Starling's law* states that the greater the stretch, the greater the following force of contraction. The greater the contraction, the more volume ejected, resulting in increased SV.

Afterload is the amount of pressure or resistance the ventricles must overcome to empty their contents. A decrease in this resistance would make it easier for the ventricles to empty, resulting again in an increase in SV.

Norepinephrine and epinephrine, which are released by the sympathetic nervous system, also improve the ability of the ventricles to overcome resistance and to empty their contents, by increasing the strength of contractions.

Blood Pressure

Blood pressure (**BP**), a function of CO and *systemic vascular resistance* (resistance in the blood vessels of the body), is the force that blood exerts against the walls of blood vessels. Systolic blood pressure (**sBP**), determined in part by CO, is the pressure exerted against the vessel walls during ventricular systole. Diastolic blood pressure (**dBP**) is the pressure exerted during ventricular diastole (relaxation). The difference between systolic and diastolic pressure is called **pulse pressure.**

☛ KEY CONCEPT

When you measure blood pressure, you record the systolic (contraction) pressure and the diastolic (relaxation) pressure of the blood within the arteries.

Systemic vascular resistance (**SVR**) or *total peripheral resistance* is the force opposing the movement of blood through the blood vessels. SVR primarily affects diastolic blood pressure. SVR is typically thought of as "vasomotor tone." This means that blood vessels can change (increase or decrease) their diameter (*constriction* or *dilation*) depending upon the needs of the body. BP is the highest as blood leaves the left ventricle to start its journey through the aorta. The differences in BP as blood flows through the systemic circulation are necessary for filtration of nutrients through capillaries.

☛ KEY CONCEPT

Blood flows from high pressure to low pressure.

Blood Pressure Regulation. Many factors other than the force and rate of the pumping heart help to maintain or to regulate BP. Regulating systems include the nervous, endocrine, cardiovascular, and urinary systems. Factors affecting BP are those that affect CO, SVR, or both. These factors may include the amount and contents of circulating blood; elasticity and ability of smooth muscles in arterial walls to dilate and to constrict; plaque buildup on arterial walls; kidney functioning; and hormones. Scientists also believe that diet, physical and emotional status, smoking, and heredity influence BP.

EFFECTS OF AGING ON THE SYSTEM

The cardiovascular system shows structural and functional losses associated with aging (Table 22-3). Pinpointing normal physiologic changes is difficult, however, because lifestyle and habits contribute greatly to the continuing health of the system. Heredity, hormones, and stress levels also influence normal changes.

As individuals get older, their systolic blood pressure often rises due to stiffening of the large arteries. This stiffening is the result of calcification of vessel walls (arteriosclerosis or "hard-

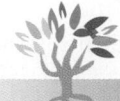

SPECIAL CONSIDERATIONS: THE LIFE SPAN

Factors Influencing the Cardiovascular System

Patient-Controlled Lifestyle Factors

- Amount, type and regularity of exercise
- Quality of rest and sleep
- Weight, in relation to optimal weight
- Stress factors
- Salt intake
- Fat intake and cholesterol levels
- Carbohydrate intake
- Medication compliance
- Oral contraceptive use
- Smoking and smokeless tobacco use
- Use of street drugs
- Anorexia/bulimia and other eating disorders

Other Factors

- Diabetes
- Hypertension
- Other chronic illnesses
- Lung disorders
- Heredity/genetics
- Kidney disorders
- Decreased blood clotting time
- Water retention/edema
- Systemic infection
- Hemorrhage
- Disorders of the blood and lymph, including hemophilia, leukemia, sickle cell disease, lupus erythematosus, anemia
- Streptococcal infections
- Electrolyte imbalance
- Sex (males and postmenopausal females = higher risk)

ening of the arteries"). Other blood vessels also become less elastic. These developments depend partially on genetic factors and current lifestyle. The left ventricular wall thickens to accommodate vascular stiffening, and the myocardial fibers themselves become less elastic or *distensible*. Heart valves also undergo calcification and lipid accumulation, resulting in valve *stenosis* (narrowing or contraction). The aortic valve is usually more involved than the mitral valve.

The number of pacemaker cells in the SA node decreases, increasing the likelihood of sinus node dysfunction. A concurrent decrease in bundle of His (AV bundle) fibers also contributes to increased incidence of heart block. Supraventricular and ventricular *ectopic* (extra) heartbeats increase with age, and should not automatically be considered an indicator of disease.

As a result of aging, the heart is not as able to cope with exercise as in youth. It is able to function adequately under normal circumstances, however. Keep in mind that life-

style habits play a major role in the development of cardiovascular diseases, especially atherosclerosis or plaque buildup in the blood vessels. This buildup narrows the arteries and slows blood flow. Lifestyle habits contribute to the development of long-term atherosclerosis. These habits, coupled with physiologic changes due to aging, may certainly explain why such a high incidence of heart disease is found in older adults.

➤ STUDENT SYNTHESIS

Key Points

- The cardiovascular system consists of the heart and the blood vessels.
- The heart is a strong, muscular pump that lies between the lungs in the mediastinum.
- The heart wall has three layers: endocardium, myocardium, and epicardium. The epicardium is also considered to be the *innermost layer* of the pericardium that surrounds the heart to cushion and protect it.
- The septum divides the heart into right and left halves. The heart is further divided into four chambers: two superior atria and two inferior ventricles.
- The valves of the heart allow unidirectional blood flow through the heart.
- The principal arteries that supply the heart muscle itself with blood are the right and left coronary arteries.
- Arteries, capillaries, and veins carry blood through the body.
- The conduction system of the heart consists of unique tissue specializing in the formation, transmission, and coordination of electrical impulses that stimulate the heart to beat.
- The normal "pacemaker" of the heart is the SA node.
- A cardiac cycle normally lasts less than 1 second and consists of the contraction (systole) and relaxation (diastole) of both atria, followed by both ventricles.
- Events in the cardiac cycle create normal, and sometimes extra, heart sounds.
- Cardiac output is the amount of blood the ventricles pump out in 1 minute. The formula for calculating cardiac output is $CO = SV$ (stroke volume) $\times HR$ (heart rate). Normally, cardiac output equals 4 to 6 liters per minute.
- Blood pressure is the force exerted by the blood against the walls of the blood vessels. Systolic blood pressure is the force during ventricular contraction. Diastolic blood pressure is the force during ventricular relaxation.
- The nervous, endocrine, cardiovascular, and urinary systems work together to regulate blood pressure.

■■■ **TABLE 22-3** $\mathscr{E}$**FFECTS OF AGING ON THE CARDIOVASCULAR SYSTEM**

Component of the Cardiovascular System	Change	Result	Nursing Implications
Blood vessels	Increased rigidity of vessels from decreased elasticity	Increased BP LV Hypertrophy (dilation of the left ventricle)	Advise to decrease fat intake and reduce sodium intake. Assess client on multiple medications for hypotension (low BP), including antihypertensive and diuretic medications.
	Dilation of blood vessels due to weakening	Risk for varicose vein formation	Prevent venous stasis and pressure ulcers.
Heart, valves, and conduction system	Fibrosis in the conduction system and heart Calcification of the valves Increased size of myocardium and atria Decreased cardiac output	Changes on electrocardiogram (ECG) Bradycardia (decreased HR) and/or irregular heart rate Fatigue Signs/symptoms of heart failure are possible Abnormal heart sounds	Pace activities to provide for rest periods. Teach client how to take own pulse rate and to recognize client's own "normal" pulse rate. Teach what to do in case of dizziness.
Cells	Ability of cells to absorb oxygen decreases	Heart rate takes longer to return to normal after exercise	Encourage rest periods.
Receptor (baroreceptor) responses in the arteries	Decreased sensitivity to stimuli	Dizziness, fainting possible, postural hypotension can occur	Teach client to get up and move slowly. Teach client what to do in case of dizziness. Assess all medications the client is taking, including antihypertensive and diuretic medications. Assess electrolyte levels.

• Separating normal physiologic changes of the cardio-vascular system in older adults is difficult because changes are often interrelated with heredity, lifestyle habits, and coexisting diseases or disorders.

Critical Thinking Exercises

1. Explain why a client with coronary artery disease is at high risk for developing a venous disorder.
2. Discuss the ways that you think electrolyte and acid–base imbalances would affect the cardio-vascular system. Give a rationale for your answer.
3. Based on your knowledge of cardiovascular anatomy and physiology, identify some reasons why the following factors could adversely affect cardiovascular functioning: high levels of stress, smoking, lack of exercise, poor diet.

NCLEX-Style Review Questions

1. The tricuspid valve is located between the:
   a. Left atrium and left ventricle
   b. Left ventricle and aorta
   c. Right atrium and right ventricle
   d. Right ventricle and pulmonary artery
2. Exchange of nutrients, salts, gases, and wastes across capillary walls occurs by:
   a. Diffusion and filtration
   b. Osmosis and filtration
   c. Pinocytosis and diffusion
   d. Pinocytosis and osmosis
3. The normal adult heart rate is set by the:
   a. Atrioventricular node
   b. Purkinje fibers
   c. Septum
   d. Sinoatrial node

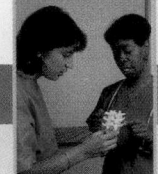

CHAPTER

23

The Hematologic and Lymphatic Systems

LEARNING OBJECTIVES

1. Describe the principal functions of the blood and its mechanisms to maintain homeostasis.
2. Identify the four plasma proteins and their chief functions.
3. Outline the structure and function of the red blood cells, white blood cells, and platelets.
4. Discuss the importance of chemotaxis and phagocytosis in fighting invading organisms.
5. Describe the mechanism of blood clotting.
6. Identify the four blood groups and explain Rh. Discuss what components contribute to the color of blood.
7. Name the universal blood transfusion recipient and the universal donor. Explain why they are so named.
8. Describe lymphatic circulation and the filtration role of the lymph nodes.
9. Describe the circle of Willis and the blood–brain barrier, and state their functions.
10. Explain where blood from the digestive organs and spleen travels before returning to the heart.
11. Describe what occurs, regarding the blood, in the digestive organs and spleen.
12. Discuss at least three normal changes in the hematologic and lymphatic systems caused by aging.

NEW TERMINOLOGY

agglutination	lymph
albumin	lymph node
anastamose	lymphocyte
coagulation	monocyte
crossmatching	phagocytosis
embolus	plasma
endocytosis	platelet
erythrocyte	prothrombin
fibrin	Rh factor
fibrinogen	spleen
globulin	thrombin
hematopoiesis	thrombocyte
hemorrhage	thrombus
hemostasis	tonsil
leukocyte	

ACRONYMS

BBB	MABP	Rh–
Hb	RBC	WBC
Hgb	Rh+	

The hematologic system consists of the components of the blood (ie, plasma and formed elements) and the bone marrow, the primary organ that manufactures blood cells. The lymphatic system consists of the lymphatic vessels and tissues. Other organs and structures, such as the spleen, liver, and kidneys, also perform specific functions related to these systems.

STRUCTURE AND FUNCTION

The *hematologic system* has three general functions: transportation, regulation, and protection. These functions involve removal of hematologic waste products, delivery of nutrients and oxygen to cells, blood volume regulation, blood cell and antibody production, and blood coagulation. The *lymphatic system* transports dietary fats to the blood, drains interstitial fluid, helps protect the body from infection, and provides immunity. It also returns any excess proteins that may escape from the blood vessels to the systemic circulation. Box 23-1 lists the functions of the hematologic and lymphatic systems.

☛ KEY CONCEPT

The hematologic and lymphatic systems have transportation and protective functions in the body. Also, blood functions in regulatory processes in the body, and lymph functions in the manufacture of formed elements and the absorption and storage of substances in the body.

BLOOD

Blood is a versatile vascular fluid that is heavier, thicker, and more viscous than water. Although it is a liquid, it has an adhesive quality that contributes to its ability to form solid clots. The primary objective of blood is to maintain a constant environment for the rest of the body's tissues. It maintains this homeostasis via its viscosity (thickness), its ability to carry dissolved substances, and its ability to move to all body parts. Blood is responsible for the transportation of oxygen, carbon dioxide, nutrients, heat, waste products, and hormones to and from the cells. It also helps regulate pH, body temperature, and cellular water content. It contributes to protection from blood loss and foreign body invasion.

Blood is considered a connective tissue because almost all of it is made of cells that share many characteristics with other connective tissues in terms of origin and development.[1] It differs from other connective tissues, however, in that its cells are not fixed, but move freely in the liquid portion of the blood known as *plasma.*

Hematopoiesis (hemopoiesis) refers to the production and maturation of blood cells. The red bone marrow manufactures all blood cells, or "formed elements" in blood. Other tissues, such as tissues of the lymph nodes, spleen, and thymus, contribute to additional production and maturation of agranular white blood cells.

Blood is composed of both plasma and formed elements. It is carried through a closed system of vessels pumped by the

➤➤ **BOX 23-1**

FUNCTIONS OF THE HEMATOLOGIC AND LYMPHATIC SYSTEMS

Blood
Transportation
- Transports oxygen to body cells and carbon dioxide away from body cells
- Exchanges oxygen for carbon dioxide at cellular level
- Transports water, nutrients, and other needed substances, such as salts (electrolytes) and vitamins, to body cells
- Aids in body heat transfer
- Transports waste products from cells to sites from which they are released (eg, kidney removes excess water, electrolytes, and urea; liver removes bile pigments and drugs)
- Transports hormones from sites of origin to organs they affect
- Transports enzymes

Regulation
- Contributes to regulation of body temperature
- Assists in maintenance of acid–base balance
- Assists in maintenance of fluid–electrolyte balance

Protection
- Fights disease and infection (leukocytes)
- Promotes clotting of blood (platelets and specialized factors)
- Provides immunity due to antibodies and antitoxins (specialized cells)

Lymph
Transportation
- Carries fluid away from tissues
- Carries wastes away from tissues

Absorption
- Absorbs fats and transports fats to blood (lacteals)
- Stores blood (spleen)
- Destroys worn-out erythrocytes

Protection
- Filters waste products out of blood
- Filters foreign substances out of blood (including dead blood cells, bacteria, smoke by-products, cancer cells)
- Destroys bacteria
- Participates in antibody production to fight foreign invasion

Manufacture
- Manufactures lymphocytes and monocytes
- Manufactures erythrocytes (spleen in fetus)

heart (see Chap. 22). The volume of circulating blood differs with individual body size; however, the average adult body contains approximately 4 to 6 liters.

☛ KEY CONCEPT

Blood is composed of plasma and formed elements.

Plasma

Blood **plasma** is the fluid portion of circulating blood. It constitutes 55% of blood volume. Plasma is 90% water. Its remaining 10% consists primarily of plasma proteins, but it also includes salts (electrolytes), nutrients, nitrogenous waste products, gases, hormones, and enzymes.

The salts contained in the plasma are sodium (Na^+), calcium (Ca^+), potassium (K^+), and magnesium (Mg^{++}). The plasma also contains ions of other elements in the form of bicarbonates, sulfates, chlorides, and phosphates (see Chap. 17). Plasma absorbs these salts from food for use by body cells. The maintenance of these salts within the plasma controls the chemical and acid-base balance of the blood, and contributes to the entire body's chemical and fluid balance.

Plasma Proteins

Four groups of plasma proteins are manufactured in the liver. **Albumin** is the largest group, accounting for 60% to 80% of plasma proteins. Its important function is to provide thickness to the circulating blood volume, thus providing osmotic pressure. (Osmotic pressure draws water from surrounding tissue fluid into capillaries. Therefore, osmotic pressure maintains fluid volume and blood pressure.) Loss of albumin can result in dramatic fluid shifts, edema, hypotension, and even death. (These concepts are explained in Chapter 17.) **Fibrinogen** and **prothrombin** are two other plasma proteins; both are essential for blood clotting.

Globulin is the fourth type of plasma protein. Two types of globulin (alpha and beta) are made in the liver and act as carriers for molecules, such as fats. Gamma globulins (immunoglobulins [Ig]) are antibodies. Antibodies are materials that are synthesized by the body in response to antigens (foreign invaders), thus providing us with immunity against infection and disease (see Chap. 24).

☛ KEY CONCEPT

Albumin, the largest group of plasma proteins, helps maintain blood pressure and circulating fluid volume. The three other circulatory plasma proteins are fibrogen, prothrombin, and globulin.

Formed Elements

The remaining 45% of blood volume consists of formed elements. These elements are red blood cells (**RBCs**), white blood cells (**WBCs**), and platelets. Figure 23-1 illustrates the various types of WBCs and RBCs.

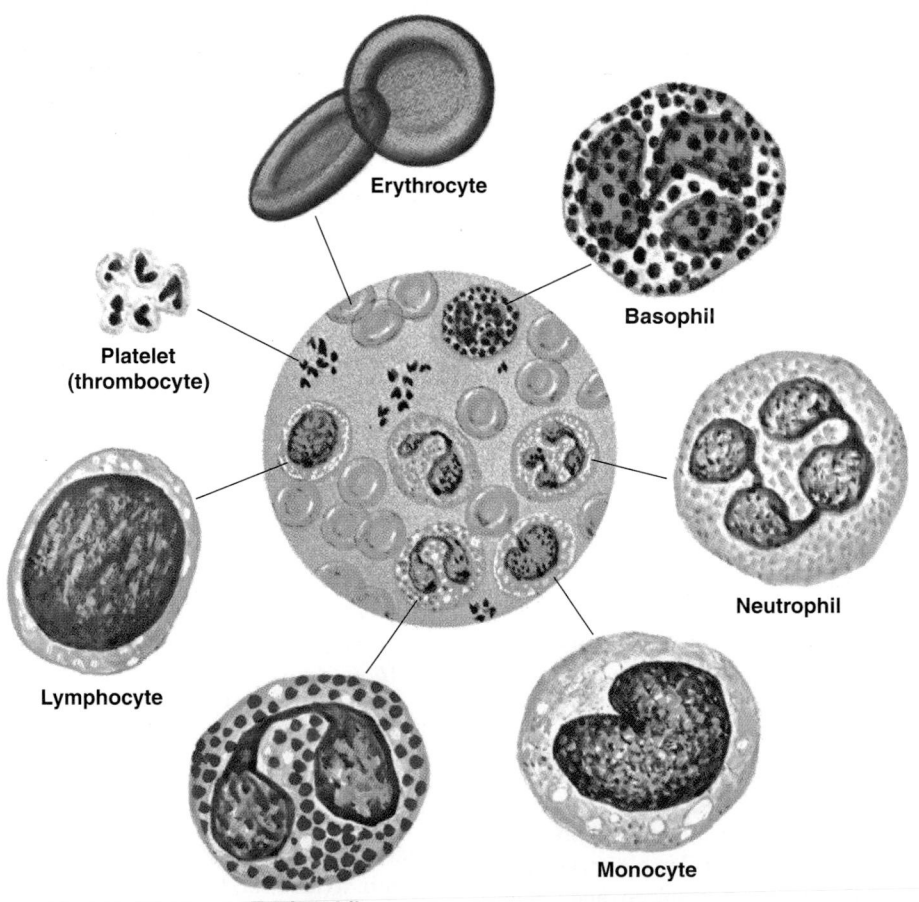

FIGURE 23-1. Normal types of blood cells. Erythrocytes are the red blood cells. The other cells shown are white blood cells (leukocytes). Granulocytes (granular leukocytes) consist of the neutrophils, the basophils, and the eosinophils. Agranulocytes (agranular leukocytes) consist of the monocytes and lymphocytes. Also shown are platelets (thrombocytes).

Red Blood Cells

RBCs, also called **erythrocytes** (erythro = red; cyte = cell), are flattened, biconcave disks. (*Biconcave* means that both sides of the element are thinner in the center than at the edges.) When RBCs mature, they have no nucleus.

Erythrocytes are the most numerous of the blood cells. About 25 trillion RBCs are found in the body. Approximately 3,000 RBCs could be placed side by side within a 1-inch space. They are made from stem cells in red bone marrow. The RBCs are fragile and wear out quickly. The liver and the spleen destroy old, used RBCs. The life of an individual RBC is about 120 days.

Each RBC contains molecules of the compound hemoglobin (**Hgb** or **Hb**). Hemoglobin is composed of the iron-containing pigment *heme* and a protein, *globin.* (Iron is the pigment that makes RBCs appear red.) As blood passes through the lungs, the iron in hemoglobin picks up oxygen in a loose chemical combination. When hemoglobin is saturated with oxygen, the blood is bright red. As blood circulates through the capillaries, the hemoglobin gives its oxygen to various cells of the body and picks up their carbon dioxide. The deoxygenated blood is much darker in color.

☛ Key Concept

Iron in the hemoglobin picks up oxygen in the lungs. This oxygen is exchanged for carbon dioxide at the cellular level.

White Blood Cells

WBCs, also known as **leukocytes** (*leuko* means white; *cyte* means cell), defend the body against disease organisms, toxins, and irritants. They differ greatly from RBCs. WBCs contain nuclei and can move independently in an ameboid fashion. WBCs also assist in repairing damaged tissues. Sometimes they die during this activity and collect with bacteria to form pus.

There are two types of WBCs: granular and agranular.

Granular Leukocytes (Granulocytes).   These are divided into three subgroups: basophils, eosinophils, and neutrophils.

- *Basophils* are involved in allergic and inflammatory reactions. These cells contain heparin (an anticoagulant), and histamine. Histamine is a chemical that is released when there is a foreign invader in the body, along with other substances in the basophil. These substances cause an inflammatory or a hypersensitivity reaction in the body, resulting in vasodilation and edema, itching, and possibly bronchial constriction. These signs and symptoms are the result of an allergic or inflammatory response.
- *Eosinophils* are characterized by a speckled or grainy cytoplasm and survive only about 12 hours to 3 days. They increase in number during allergic reactions and parasitic infections, and are believed to release chemicals to assist the body in detoxifying foreign proteins or engulfing and devouring invaders (**phagocytosis** or **endocytosis**). Eosinophils may also have a role in decreasing the release of chemical mediators during allergic reactions.

- *Neutrophils* are the most numerous of WBCs. These can also be called *polymorphonuclear (PMNs)* or *segmented* neutrophils (*segs*). Neutrophils are considered to be first in the line of defense against bacteria. Because of their ability to move away from blood vessels, neutrophils can move directly to sites of infection. They push or squeeze through the capillary wall and rush to the threatened spot. They find their way to foreign or damaged tissues by their attraction to certain chemical substances (*chemotaxis*). They are colorless unless they are stained to be visible under the microscope. The neutrophils increase in number, and engulf and devour invaders (*phagocytosis* or *endocytosis*). Neutrophils increase in number during bacterial infections, burns, or inflammation. Because they have a short lifespan (approximately 10 hours), they need to be replaced frequently. When an infection occurs, more neutrophils are released from the bone marrow. When the demand for these granulocytes is very high, the bone marrow releases immature neutrophils called *bands*. When looking at WBC counts, an increased number of bands signifies an infection. This increase in bands may also be described as a "shift to the left." Figure 23-2 illustrates phagocytosis.

Agranular Leukocytes (Agranulocytes).   These are divided into two subgroups: monocytes and lymphocytes. Under normal conditions, agranular lymphocytes are functional for about 100 to 300 days. They are produced in the lymphatic tissue of the spleen, lymph nodes, and thymus, and in the hemopoietic tissues in red bone marrow.

- **Monocytes** are transformed into *macrophages,* which are phagocytic cells. These WBCs play a role in acute and chronic inflammatory processes. A high monocyte count may be due to a viral or fungal infection, tuberculosis, or chronic diseases.
- **Lymphocytes** can be differentiated into various types. The most important of these are *B lymphocytes (B cells)* and *T lymphocytes (T cells).* These lymphocytes play an important role in the immune response and are discussed in greater detail in Chapter 24. Lymphocytes increase in number during infectious processes that might be caused by viral infections or immune diseases.

☛ Key Concept

Granular leukocytes:
- *Basophils—involved in the inflammatory process and allergic reactions*
- *Eosinophils—involved in allergic reactions and parasitic infections*
- *Neutrophils—involved in phagocytosis; defense against bacteria*

Agranular leukocytes:
- *Monocytes—transformed into macrophages; involved in phagocytosis*
- *Lymphocytes—involved in immune responses*

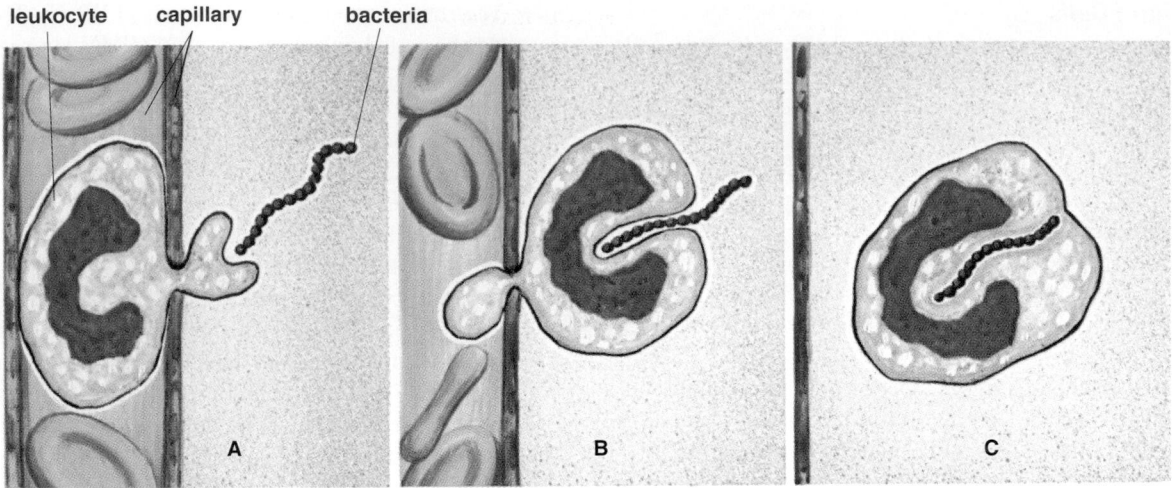

leukocyte   capillary   bacteria

endothelial cell

FIGURE 23-2. Phagocytosis. (**A**) Leukocytes squeeze out of blood vessels and rush to the site of an invading organism. (**B**) When foreign matter (such as bacteria or dead tissue) comes in contact with the cell membrane of the neutrophil, the cell membrane surrounds and pinches off the area, leaving the membrane intact. (**C**) Consequently, the engulfed material is enclosed in a membranous vesicle within the neutrophil, where enzymes within the cell destroy the foreign material.

Platelets

Platelets, also called **thrombocytes** (*thrombo* means clot; *cyte* means cell), are the smallest of blood's formed elements. They are not whole cells, but rather are fragments of larger cells. They lack nuclei but are capable of ameboid movement. They are formed in red bone marrow. Platelets are essential for blood clotting.

Blood Clotting and Hemorrhage

Hemostasis refers to the cessation of bleeding. When damage or rupture occurs to blood vessels, the hemostatic response must be quick and carefully controlled to stop blood loss. This hemostatic initial response includes vascular spasm (vasoconstriction), platelet plug formation, and blood clotting (that is, the **coagulation** process that forms a fibrin clot).[2] (Remember: homeostatis means balance or stability.)

Clotting

Blood clotting protects the body from losing vital plasma fluid and blood cells by sealing off broken blood vessels. Without this action, individuals would not survive even minor cuts and wounds. The process of clot formation involves a number of complex activities within the blood, some of which are not totally understood. Figure 23-3 illustrates the clotting mechanism.

When tissue is injured, platelets break down and cause the release of a chemical, *thromboplastin,* which interacts with certain protein factors and calcium ions to form *prothrombin activator.* This activator then reacts with additional calcium ions to convert the plasma protein *prothrombin* to **thrombin.** Thrombin then converts the soluble plasma protein *fibrinogen* into insoluble threads of **fibrin.** The threads of fibrin form a net to entrap RBCs and platelets to form a clot. This clot acts like a plug in a hole, and tends to draw injured edges together. As the clot shrinks, a clear yellow liquid called *serum* is squeezed

out. Serum is like plasma except that fibrinogen and other clotting elements needed in the coagulation process are no longer present. Coagulation is a complicated mechanism that cannot occur if any necessary elements are missing. Vitamin K is necessary for the formation of prothrombin and other clotting factors. (Bacteria in the colon produce most vitamin K.)

A **thrombus** is a stationary clot. An **embolus** is a clot that circulates. Both of these clots can lead to death if they plug arteries to the heart, lungs, or brain. Several medications are available to treat blood clots and are discussed in Unit 9.

☛ KEY CONCEPT

The initial response to a disruption in a blood vessel includes vascular spasm (vasospasm), platelet plug formation, and the coagulation process that forms a fibrin clot. Platelets, calcium ions, and vitamin K are important elements in this complex coagulation process.

Hemorrhage

The literal definition of **hemorrhage** is escape of blood from blood vessels; however, hemorrhage is usually thought of as the loss of a considerable amount of blood. A cut or torn blood vessel allows blood to escape. Hemostatic mechanisms, such as clotting, are beneficial in preventing hemorrhage in smaller vessels, but extensive hemorrhage from larger vessels requires medical intervention.[3] Extensive or severe hemorrhage is serious, because the body can lose so much fluid and oxygen-carrying RBCs that death may result. Inability to clot in extensive hemorrhage may be due to a variety of factors: force behind the flow of blood, size of the wound, volume of blood lost, or a deficiency in any of the coagulant substances. Severe hemorrhage is treated with blood replacement, using blood from another person. This replacement of blood is called a *transfusion.*

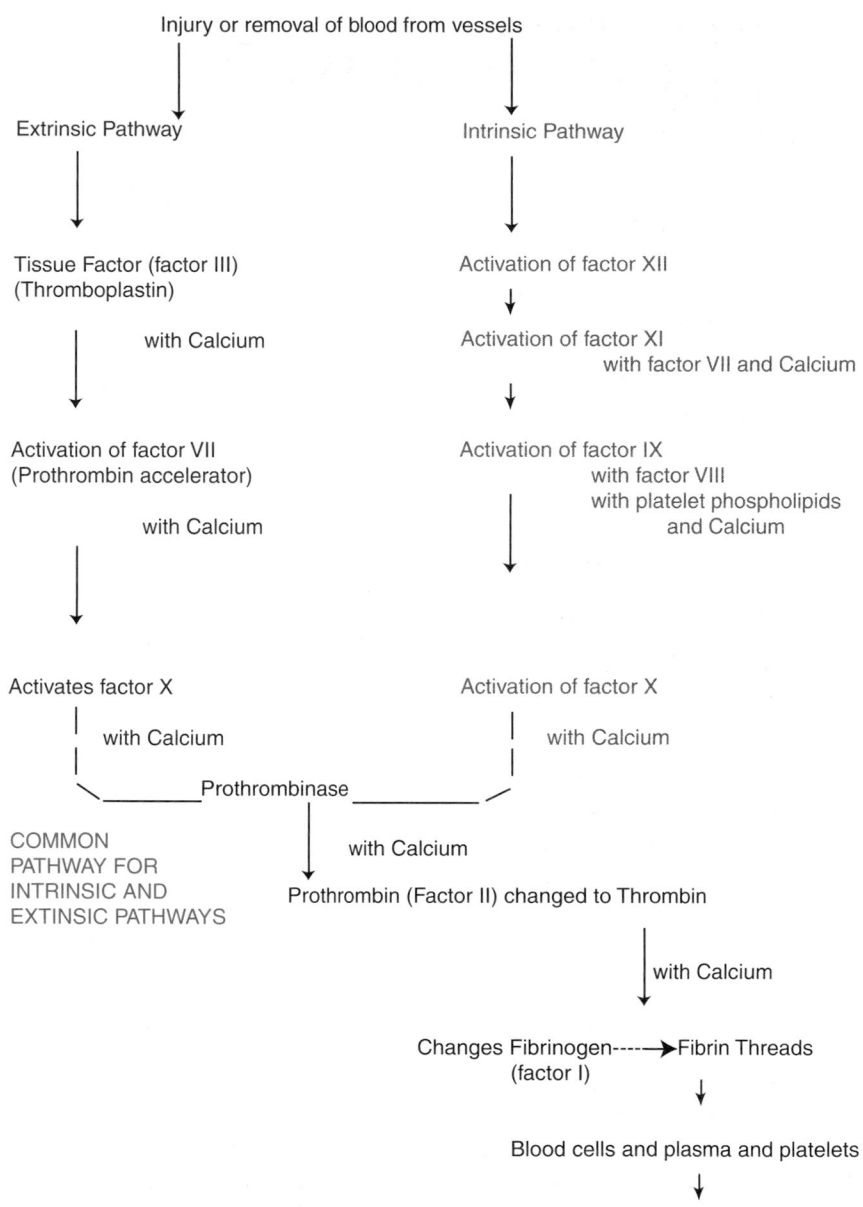

FIGURE 23-3. Final steps in the formation of a blood clot. Adapted from: Cohen, B. & Wood, D. (2000). *Memmler's structure and function of the human body* (7th ed., p. 187). Philadelphia: Lippincott Williams & Wilkins.

☞ KEY CONCEPT

Often, more blood is lost from a torn or nicked blood vessel than from a vessel that is cleanly cut through. The muscles in a blood vessel contract as a protective measure. If these muscles are cut unevenly, they cannot effectively close the blood vessel.

Hemorrhage from an artery comes in spurts. Hemorrhage from a vein comes in a steady flow.

Blood Groups

Blood falls into one of four groups: A, B, AB, and O (Table 23-1). These blood types are inherited (genetic) combinations of antigens and antibodies found on the membranes of RBCs. **Crossmatching** is a laboratory test of donor and recipient cells to check for **agglutination** (clumping of cells). If an

incompatible type of blood is given to a person, a fatal transfusion reaction may result.

Except for blood types, no differences exist in the blood of healthy people of different races or genders. Blood does not carry or transmit mental, emotional, or physical characteristics.

Rh Factors

Just like a blood group, **Rh factors** are also inherited antigens. (The Rh system is named after the Rhesus monkey used in early experiments.) Of the several types of antigens that may be found on the surface of RBCs, more than 40 are loosely connected to the Rh system. The most commonly found Rh factor and the one most likely to cause a transfusion reaction is abbreviated D (Duffy). Blood is tested for the presence of D antigen.

If a person's blood contains D factor, the person is said to be Rh-positive (**Rh+** or D+); if this factor is absent, the person is Rh-negative (**Rh−**). The percentage of Rh-negative

TABLE 23-1 𝓑LOOD GROUPS AND COMPATIBILITIES

Blood Group	Percent of Population	Antigen on Erythrocytes	Antibody in Plasma	Can Donate Red Blood Cells to	Can Receive Red Blood Cells From
A	41%	A	Anti-B (reacts against B antigen)	A or AB	A or O
B	10%	B	Anti-A (reacts against A antigen)	B or AB	B or O
AB	4%	A and B	None	AB	A, B, AB, or O*
O	45%	None	Anti-A and Anti-B (reacts against both A and B factors)	A, B, AB, or O†	O

*Blood group AB is known as the universal recipient because people of this group may receive red blood cells from donors of any ABO group in an extreme emergency.

†Blood group O is known as the universal donor, because these red blood cells may be given to people of any ABO group in an extreme emergency.

people is lower within some races; approximately 2% to 7% of African Americans and 1% of Asians and Native Americans are Rh-negative, while more than 10% of Caucasians are Rh-negative.

When an Rh-negative person receives Rh-positive blood, he or she develops antibodies that could cause a severe reaction to subsequent blood transfusions. This can also occur in an Rh-positive pregnancy in an Rh-negative mother. (Unit 10 discusses in more detail the Rh factor and its effects on pregnancy.)

LYMPH

The lymphatic system is related to, yet separate from, the hematologic system. Body cells normally are bathed in tissue fluid. Some of this fluid drains into blood capillaries and flows directly to the veins. Another group of vessels, called *lymphatic vessels,* also drains this fluid. The lymphatic vessels begin as a network of tiny closed-ended lymphatic capillaries in spaces between cells. These capillaries are slightly larger than blood capillaries, and have a unique structure that allows interstitial fluid to flow into them but not out. The excess fluid and certain other waste products that collect here form the thin, watery, colorless liquid known as **lymph.** Because lymph originally derives from plasma, its composition is much the same, except that lymph is lower in protein content. Specialized lymphatic capillaries called *lacteals* absorb digested fats and fat-soluble vitamins in the small intestine. Figure 23-4 depicts the lymphatic system.

Movement of Lymph

Lymphatic vessels are thin-walled vessels with one-way valves that prevent backflow of lymph fluid. These vessels are located both superficially (near the skin surface) and deeper in the body. Most lymphatic vessels are located near the venous system and are named according to their body location. An example of this would be *femoral* lymphatic vessels that are located in the thighs. Lymphatic vessels carrying fluid eventually form a network of vessels in specific areas of the body. These areas are called *regional nodes.* After the fluid moves through the

nodes, it is transported by other lymphatic vessels to either the right lymphatic duct or the thoracic duct.

Lymph fluid is propelled through the body by rhythmic contractions. These contractions occur due to changes in abdominal and thoracic pressure during breathing, and also due to skeletal muscle contractions that promote the return of venous blood—and subsequently lymphatic fluid—to the heart.

Lymph Nodes and Nodules

Small bundles of special lymphoid tissue termed **lymph nodes** are situated in clusters along the lymphatic vessels. Many of these nodes appear in the neck (*cervical*), groin (*inguinal*), and armpits (*axillary*) (see Fig. 23-4). Before lymph reaches the veins, it passes through these nodes. A capsule of connective tissue covers each node. Each node is densely packed with lymphocytes.

Lymph nodes perform several vital functions. The most important is that of filtration. The "swollen glands" that may appear in a person's cervical, inguinal, and axillary regions during illness are really lymph nodes at work. They are trying to filter and destroy pathogens. The nodes have enlarged as their macrophages (phagocytic cells) eat and destroy invaders. When palpated, these enlarged, nonmalignant nodes are soft and tender. They may become quite painful.

Lymph nodules are small masses of nonencapsulated lymphatic tissues that stand guard in all mucous membranes. Because membranes line cavities that open to the external environment, nodules are in strategic locations to filter substances that enter the body. Mucous membranes line the respiratory, gastrointestinal, urinary, and reproductive tracts. Some areas of lymph nodules or tissues have special names: for example, Peyer's patches, which are found in the small intestine.

Lymph Nodes and Cancer

Cancer cells can travel from their primary site of invasion to distant sites by way of the lymph nodes. Lymph nodes may either function to filter out cancer cells or may inadvertently spread cancer to other body sites. For this reason, when cancer surgery is performed, the lymph nodes in the area are also tested. If no cancer cells are present in adjoining lymph nodes,

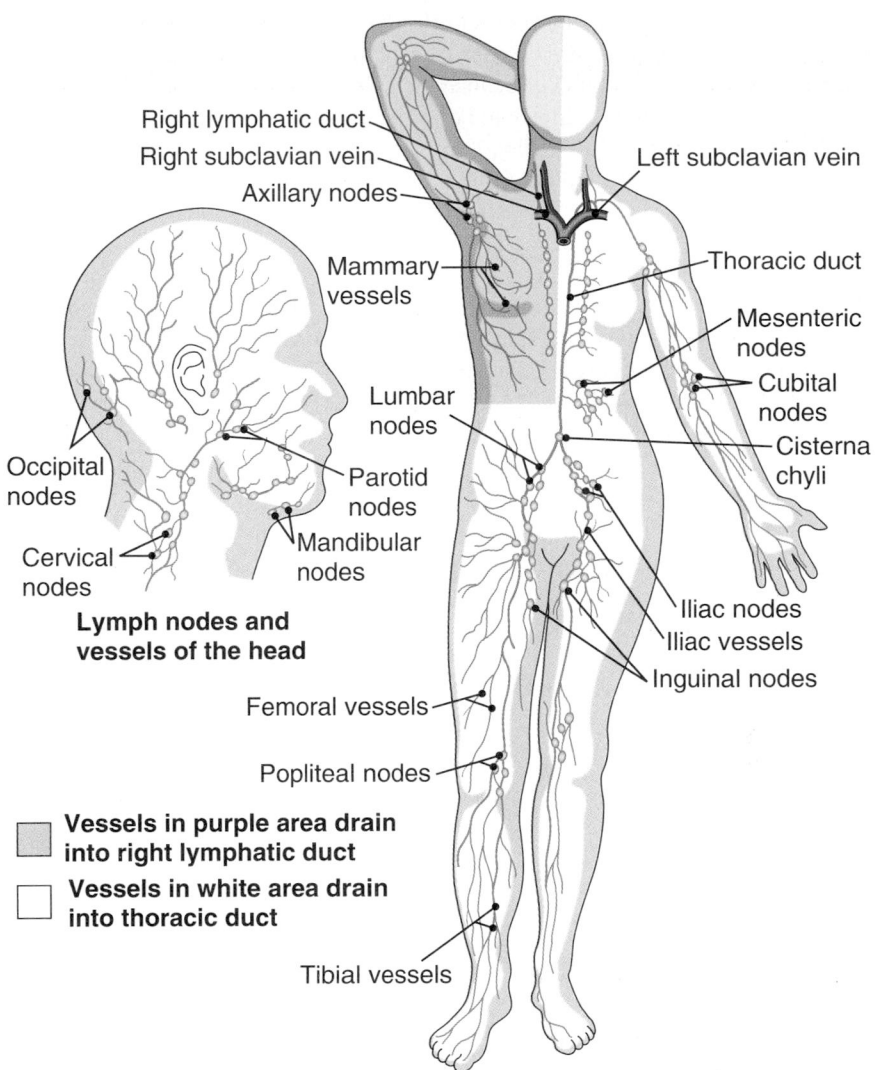

Right lymphatic duct
Right subclavian vein
Axillary nodes
Mammary vessels
Left subclavian vein
Thoracic duct
Mesenteric nodes
Cubital nodes
Cisterna chyli
Lumbar nodes
Occipital nodes
Parotid nodes
Mandibular nodes
Cervical nodes
Iliac nodes
Iliac vessels
Inguinal nodes
Femoral vessels
Popliteal nodes
Tibial vessels

Lymph nodes and vessels of the head

☐ **Vessels in purple area drain into right lymphatic duct**

☐ **Vessels in white area drain into thoracic duct**

FIGURE 23-4. The lymphatic system.

the cancer was most likely localized to its original site. If the cancer is found in the lymph nodes, it is said to be *spreading* or *metastasized.* In some cases, the adjoining lymph nodes are removed during surgery. Removal may be a precautionary measure, or may be necessary because the nodes already contain cancer cells. Palpable cancerous lymph nodes may be enlarged and, unlike nodes fighting infection, feel firm and nontender.

☞ KEY CONCEPT

Lymph nodes function to filter and destroy pathogens. Swollen glands are a sign of the lymph nodes trying to rid the body of these pathogens. Lymph nodes may also be invaded by cancer cells, and may actually serve as reservoirs from which the cancer cells are spread throughout the body. This is why lymph nodes are often removed along with a cancerous (malignant) tumor.

Lymphatic Organs

The lymphatic organs are the tonsils, spleen, and thymus. They are masses of lymphatic tissue with somewhat different func-

tions than those of the lymph vessels or nodes. The tonsils and spleen are designed to filter tissue fluid, although not necessarily lymph. The thymus plays a more active role in the development of the immune system, and is discussed in greater detail in Chapter 24.

Tonsils
Tonsils form a ring of lymphatic tissue around the pharynx. This tissue forms a protective barrier for substances entering the oral and respiratory passages. The tonsils may become so loaded with bacteria that removal (tonsillectomy) is advisable. A slight enlargement, however, is not an indication for surgery.

Spleen
The **spleen** is an organ containing lymphoid tissue designed to filter blood. It is a somewhat flattened, dark purple organ about 6 inches (15.24 cm) long and 3 inches (7.62 cm) wide.[1] It is located directly below the diaphragm, above the left kidney, and behind the stomach.

The spleen has several functions. In the fetus, the spleen (along with the liver) has a role in blood cell formation (later on, this role is taken over by the red bone marrow). In an adult, the spleen destroys old RBCs and forms *bilirubin* from the hemoglobin in RBCs. It acts as a reservoir for blood, which can be released to the body quickly in an emergency such as a hemorrhage. The spleen also filters and destroys pathogens and other foreign materials in the blood. Specially treated B lymphocytes that produce antibodies against foreign antigens, and T lymphocytes that attach to invading viruses or foreign entities, are contained in the spleen. Both of these types of lymphocytes have an active role in the immune system of the body (see Chap. 24). The spleen also contains monocytes, which become macrophages in the spleen to fight infection by the mechanism of phagocytosis. All of these agranulocytes help the body fight infection in different ways.

Although its functions are important, the spleen can be removed without ill effects. A person without a spleen, however, is more susceptible to some bacterial infections, such as pneumonia and meningitis. After the spleen is removed, the liver, bone marrow, and lymph nodes assume some of the spleen's functions.

☞ KEY CONCEPT

The spleen destroys old RBCs, filters and destroys pathogens, manufactures lymphocytes and monocytes, and is a reservoir for blood.

SYSTEM PHYSIOLOGY

Blood Circulation

Blood flows in a circuitous route throughout the entire body. The blood vessels, subdivided into two *circuits* (pulmonary and systemic), together with the four chambers of the heart, form the closed system for the flow of blood (see Chapter 22).

Pulmonary Circulation

The phase of circulation in which blood is pumped through the lungs to get rid of waste products (particularly CO_2) and to pick up a supply of oxygen (O_2) is called *pulmonary circulation.* Blood in the general (systemic) circulation returns to the *right atrium* of the heart. It passes into the *right ventricle* and then into the *pulmonary artery* (the only artery in the body that carries unoxygenated blood). The blood continues to capillaries in the lungs where carbon dioxide, carried in hemoglobin, is exchanged for oxygen from the lungs. Small veins collect the blood from the lung capillaries. These veins combine eventually into four *pulmonary veins,* which pour oxygenated blood into the *left atrium* of the heart. (The pulmonary veins are the only veins that carry oxygenated blood.) Figure 23-5 illustrates pulmonary circulation.

Systemic Circulation

From the left atrium, the oxygenated blood enters the *left ventricle.* The left ventricle pumps the blood out of the left side of the heart into the general circulation or *systemic circulation.* Its purpose is to carry blood, and therefore nutrients and oxygen, to body cells and to return with accumulated waste products. As blood leaves the left ventricle, it surges into the largest artery

of the body, the *aorta.* The aorta is further divided into the *ascending aorta, aortic arch, thoracic aorta,* and *abdominal aorta,* which is divided into smaller arteries. The blood travels through smaller and smaller arterial branches. From the smallest arteries, the *arterioles,* the blood enters the capillaries, where oxygen and food are exchanged for waste products. The blood begins its journey back to the heart from capillaries to *venules,* then to larger *veins,* and finally through the *inferior* and *superior vena cava* (plural: cavae) to the right atrium, thereby completing the circuitous route.

Hepatic–Portal Circulation. The hepatic–portal circulation is a subdivision of systemic circulation. It is an efficient detour in the pathway of venous return, directed at transporting raw materials in the form of carbohydrates, fats, and proteins from the digestive organs and the spleen to the liver.

The hepatic–portal circulation is unique because it begins and ends with capillaries (Fig. 23-6). The capillaries from the stomach, intestine, spleen, and pancreas empty into veins. These veins drain into a common vessel, the *portal vein,* which leads into the liver.

In the liver, blood again enters capillaries, called *sinusoids.* Here, the liver extracts appropriate materials and chemically modifies them. The liver synthesizes, stores, detoxifies, regulates, and transforms these raw materials into useful substances that the entire body needs. The useful substances and the blood then empty into the *hepatic vein.* The hepatic vein leads to the *inferior vena cava.* Chapter 26 describes digestion and the functions of the liver in more detail.

Cerebral Circulation

Circulation to the brain is vital in maintaining life and the ability to function. Anteriorly, one branch of the *common carotid artery* is the *internal carotid artery.* The internal carotid **anastamoses** (connects) with the circle of Willis (see below), thus providing oxygenated blood to the brain.

Oxygenated blood also arrives at the brain by another route. The *right vertebral artery* and *left vertebral artery* branch off from the *subclavian artery* at the posterior aspect of the brain. These two vertebral arteries join at the brain stem and create the *basilar artery.* From here, blood is transported to the circle of Willis.

The *circle of Willis (cerebral arterial circle)* is formed by the *anterior communicating artery, posterior communicating artery, anterior cerebral artery, posterior cerebral artery,* and *internal carotid artery.*[4] Figure 23-7 shows the arteries that supply the brain, including the arteries of the circle of Willis. All of these arteries supply different areas of the brain with blood. Blood returns to the heart via venous sinuses that transport blood to the internal jugular veins and back to the heart.

Cerebral blood flow is 10% to 15% of the total cardiac output. One factor that impacts blood flow is blood pressure. To maintain adequate *cerebral perfusion* (blood flow to the brain), the mean arterial blood pressure (**MABP**) is calculated, based upon the relationship of the sBP and the dBP. The brain requires a continuous flow of blood because it requires a constant supply of oxygen and nutrients (specifically glucose) to survive. The brain does not have the ability to create a collateral circulation, as does the heart in some cases.

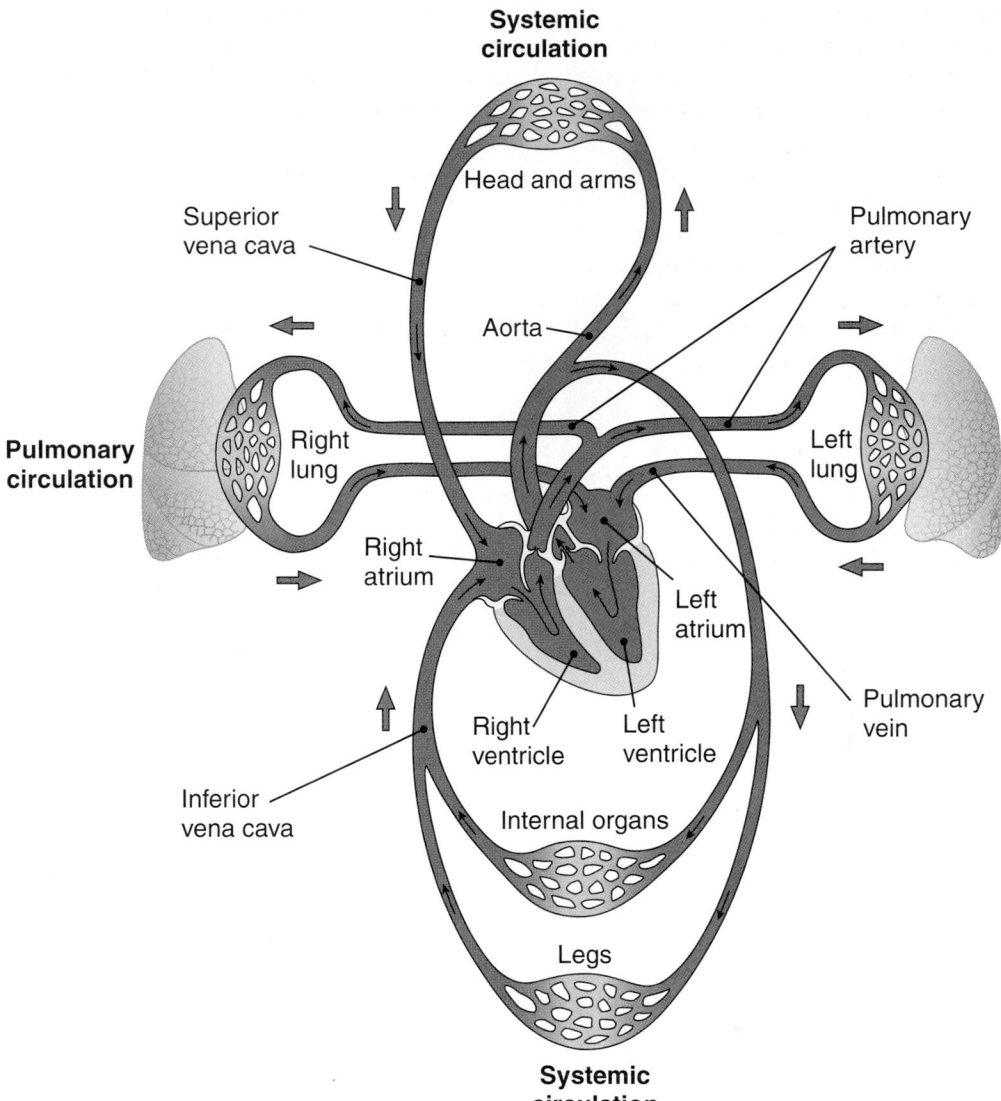

FIGURE 23-5. The heart is a double pump. The *pulmonary circuit* carries blood to the lungs to be oxygenated; the *systemic circuit* carries blood to all other parts of the body.

The circle of Willis is important because it allows blood to continue to flow in the brain if there is a blockage in one of the arteries that supplies the circle of Willis. An *embolus* is a clot that can lodge in an artery, thereby causing a blockage. In the brain, the *middle cerebral artery* branch is the most likely location for emboli.[2] A disruption of blood flow for any reason, for even a short period of time, can cause unconsciousness. Brain damage can occur if the disruption lasts for more than a few minutes (due to brain cell death).

Blood–Brain Barrier.   The blood–brain barrier (**BBB**) is an "adaptation of the circulation" that protects the brain. Specialized cells in brain capillaries allow only certain substances from the blood to enter the brain.[1] Capillaries in the brain are less permeable and much tighter than other capillaries in the body. Also, specialized brain neuroglia called *astrocytes* assist in creating selective permeability in the brain.

☞ KEY CONCEPT

The blood–brain barrier works to protect the brain from harmful substances.

Lymphatic Circulation

Lymph only carries fluid *away* from tissues. It does not have a pumping system of its own. Its circulation depends on the movement of skeletal muscles. Muscular contractions and pressure changes that the thoracic cavity produces during respiration also assist with lymph circulation.

The lymph from the upper right quadrant of the body drains into the *right lymphatic duct*. The remainder of the body's lymph drains into the left lymphatic duct, commonly known as the *thoracic duct*. The right lymphatic duct and the thoracic duct then drain into the *left subclavian vein* at the base of the neck, where lymph mixes with blood plasma and becomes part of the general circulation.

Lymph enters lymph nodes through several *afferent* ("bringing toward") lymph vessels. The lymph nodes filter out dangerous substances (such as cancer cells and bacteria), dead RBCs, and foreign matter (eg, smoke by-products) that become trapped in the nodes. The lymph then continues to flow away from the node through one or two *efferent* ("taking away") lymph vessels into the bloodstream. Plasma cells and lympho-

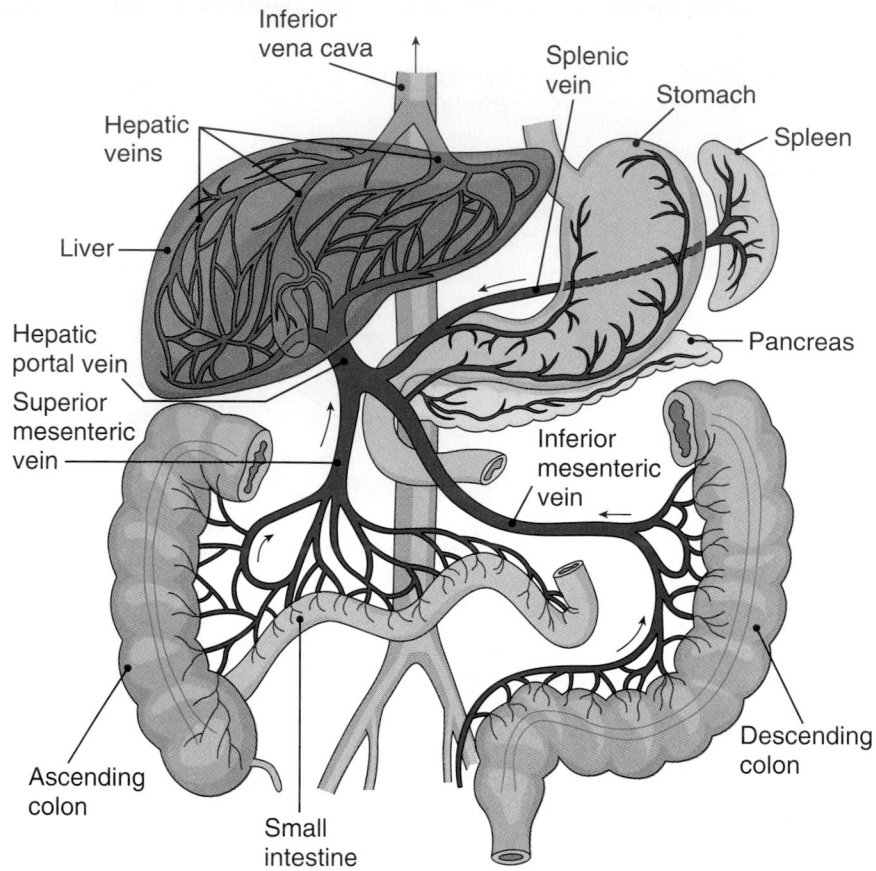

Inferior
vena cava

Splenic
vein

Stomach

Spleen

Hepatic
veins

Liver

Pancreas

Hepatic
portal vein

Superior
mesenteric
vein

Inferior
mesenteric
vein

Ascending
colon

Descending
colon

Small
intestine

FIGURE 23-6. Hepatic–portal circulation.

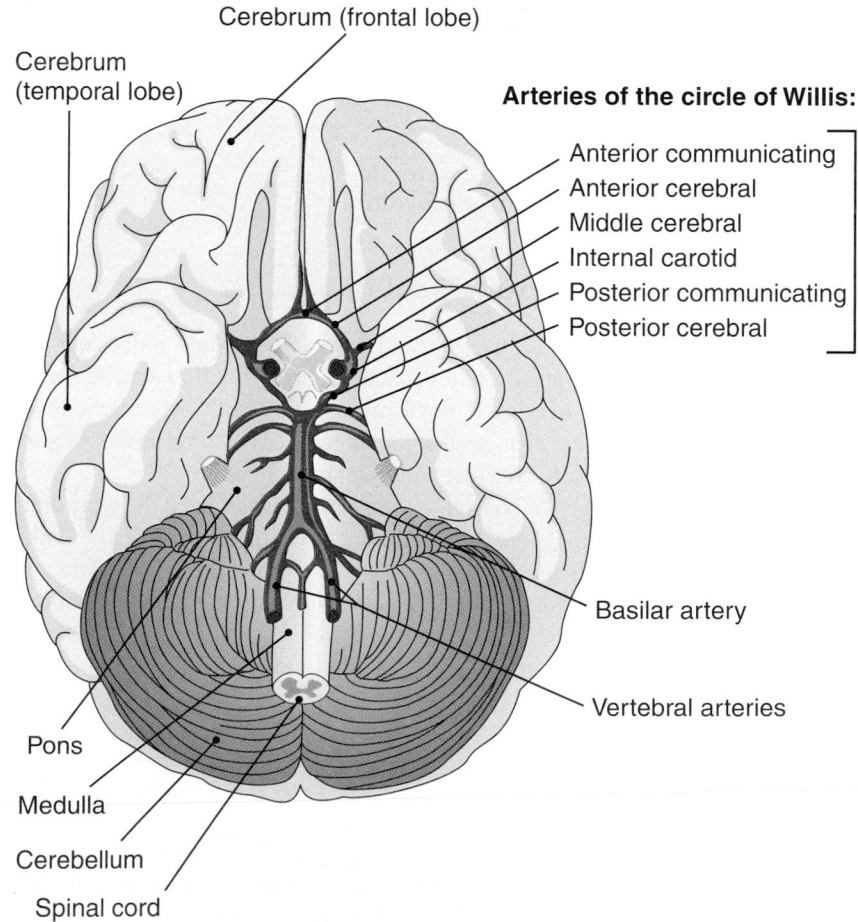

Cerebrum (frontal lobe)

Cerebrum
(temporal lobe)

Arteries of the circle of Willis:

Anterior communicating
Anterior cerebral
Middle cerebral
Internal carotid
Posterior communicating
Posterior cerebral

Basilar artery

Vertebral arteries

Pons

Medulla

Cerebellum

Spinal cord

FIGURE 23-7. Arteries that supply the brain, viewed from behind. The arteries that make up the circle of Willis are shown in the center of the brain.

cytes that have reproduced within a lymph node can also be added to lymph for transportation to the blood.

Disorders of the blood and lymph can be quickly life-threatening. Chapter 80 discusses heart and blood vessel disorders; Chapter 81 describes blood and lymph disorders; and Chapter 82 discusses cancer, which is often spread via the lymphatic system.

EFFECTS OF AGING ON THE SYSTEM

In the older adult, hematopoiesis may decline due to a loss of active bone marrow. Alterations in tissue oxygenation may therefore occur, especially during periods of stress, due to ineffective RBC production. The number of platelets in older adults may also slightly decrease, although fibrinogen levels and coagulation factors may increase. WBC production itself typically shows no real change. However, age-related changes in organs of the immune system can result in altered antigen-antibody responses and increased incidence of infection. Blood volume is reduced in older adults, due to decreased muscle mass and metabolic rate. The range for albumin also drops. Table 23-2 presents the effects of aging on these systems.

➛ STUDENT SYNTHESIS

Key Points

- Blood is composed of plasma and formed elements.
- The functions of the hematologic system are transportation, regulation, and protection.
- The major elements of the blood are RBCs, WBCs, and platelets.
- Hematopoiesis, the formation of blood cells, originates in stem cells in red bone marrow.
- Plasma is 90% water. The remaining 10% is composed of proteins, salts, nutrients, wastes, gases, hormones, and enzymes.
- Erythrocytes, or RBCs, are the most numerous of the blood cells. Each RBC contains hemoglobin, which is responsible for carrying oxygen.

- All WBCs fight infection. Each of the five types (basophil, eosinophil, neutrophil, lymphocyte, monocyte) has different mechanisms to combat invaders.
- Platelets and numerous clotting factors must react in sequence before clotting can occur.
- Hemorrhage is usually thought of as the loss of a considerable amount of blood. Hemostasis refers to the stoppage of bleeding.
- The ABO and Rh blood groups are inherited combinations of antigens and antibodies.
- Lymph tissues filter blood, destroy pathogens, and develop antibodies against antigens.
- Lymphatic organs include the tonsils, spleen, and thymus.
- The pulmonary circulation allows blood to be oxygenated for distribution in the systemic circulation.
- The largest circulatory route is the systemic circulation, which transports oxygen, nutrients, and wastes to and from all body cells.
- Several arteries come together in the brain to form the circle of Willis. This arterial circle helps to maintain and protect cerebral blood flow to the brain.
- The blood–brain barrier selectively determines what substances will enter the brain from the blood. Its purpose is to prevent harmful substances from entering the brain.
- The hepatic–portal circulation moves venous blood from the abdominal organs (GI system, pancreas, spleen) to the liver via the portal vein. The blood travels through the liver where it can undergo a variety of changes before entering the hepatic vein and then the inferior vena cava that will transport blood back to the heart.
- The lymph system drains interstitial fluid into lymphatic vessels, which empty into the veins.

Critical Thinking Exercises

1. Explain how blood, interstitial fluid, and lymph are related to the maintenance of homeostasis.

■■■ **TABLE 23-2** 𝓔**FFECTS OF AGING ON THE HEMATOLOGIC AND LYMPHATIC SYSTEMS**

Factor	Result	Nursing Implications
Stem cells and marrow reserves decrease	Increased vulnerability to problems with clotting, oxygen transport, and fighting infection Decreased blood volume	Assess the aging adult for a weakened ability to compensate for illness.
Hemoglobin levels decrease	May be secondary to decreased intake of iron-rich foods	Assess for evidence of gastrointestinal bleeding before concluding that anemia is due to aging. Ensure adequate dietary intake of iron-rich foods.
Leukocyte production decreases	Less of a response to infection; may feel less pain	Monitor closely for early signs of infection (eg, increased fatigue, anorexia, or mental confusion) because the body may not show fever or elevated leukocyte count.

2. Explain why you think some people choose to have some of their own blood removed and stored for possible future use in an emergency.
3. Discuss how inhalation promotes or inhibits the flow of lymphatic fluid.

NCLEX-Style Review Questions

1. Which of the following helps maintain circulating blood volume?
   a. Albumin
   b. Fibrin
   c. Globin
   d. Thrombin
2. Which blood group is known as the universal donor?
   a. A
   b. AB
   c. B
   d. O

3. Effects of aging include which of following?
   a. Bone marrow reserves increase
   b. Hemoglobin levels decrease
   c. Leukocyte production increases
   d. Vulnerability to infection decreases

References

1. Cohen, B., & Wood, D. (2000). *Memmler's structure and function of the human body* (7th ed.). Philadelphia: Lippincott Williams & Wilkins.
2. Porth, C. (2002). *Pathophysiology: Concepts of altered health states* (6th ed.). Philadelphia: Lippincott Williams & Wilkins.
3. Tortora, G. J., & Grabowski, S. R. (1996). *Principles of anatomy and physiology* (8th ed.). New York: Harper Collins.
4. Smeltzer, S. C. & Bare, B. G. (2000). *Brunner and Suddarth's textbook of medical-surgical nursing* (9th ed.). Philadelphia: Lippincott Williams & Wilkins.

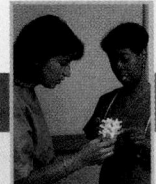

CHAPTER

24

The Immune System

LEARNING OBJECTIVES

1. Describe lymphocytes, their functions, and where they are produced.
2. Differentiate between B cells and T cells (lymphocytes).
3. Name the five categories of antibodies and describe two nursing implications related to a lack of or decrease in antibody production.
4. Differentiate between nonspecific and specific immunity.
5. Differentiate between naturally acquired active and passive immunity and artificially acquired active and passive immunity. Give an example of each type.
6. Describe the process of antibody-mediated immunity.
7. Explain how the "lock-and-key" concept applies to the antigen–antibody complex.
8. List the three mechanisms antibodies use to destroy antigens.
9. Describe two effects of aging on the immune system.

NEW TERMINOLOGY

acquired immunity
antibody-mediated
  immunity
artificially acquired
  immunity
B cells/B lymphocytes
cell-mediated immunity
complement fixation
cytokine
gamma globulin
humoral immunity

immunity
immunization
inborn immunity
macrophage
naturally acquired immunity
nonspecific immunity
specific immunity
T cells/T lymphocytes
thymus
vaccine

ACRONYMS

Ab
Ag

Ig

IgG

The human body must always protect itself against foreign invasion. A complex defense system is in place to counterattack such invasions. The immune system in humans consists of nonspecific defense responses (eg, phagocytosis) and specific immune responses (eg, humoral and cell-mediated immunity). **Immunity** is the body's ability to recognize and destroy specific pathogens and to prevent infectious diseases. When the immune system is compromised, immunodeficiency diseases may occur. When the immune system is overreactive, disorders such as allergies and autoimmune disorders may result.[1]

STRUCTURE AND FUNCTION

The body's *immune system* includes the *bone marrow, lymphoid organs,* and the *mononuclear phagocyte system* (also called the *reticuloendothelial system*). Primary functions of the immune system include defense, homeostasis, and surveillance. Box 24-1 describes these functions. Figure 24-1 shows the specific organs and tissues involved in the immune system.

BONE MARROW AND LYMPHOCYTE PRODUCTION

The cells in the bone marrow are capable of developing into any of three types of blood cells: erythrocytes (red blood cells or RBCs), leukocytes (white blood cells or WBCs), or thrombocytes (platelets).

WBCs defend the body against disease organisms, toxins, and irritants. The two types of WBCs are granular (neutrophils,

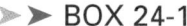

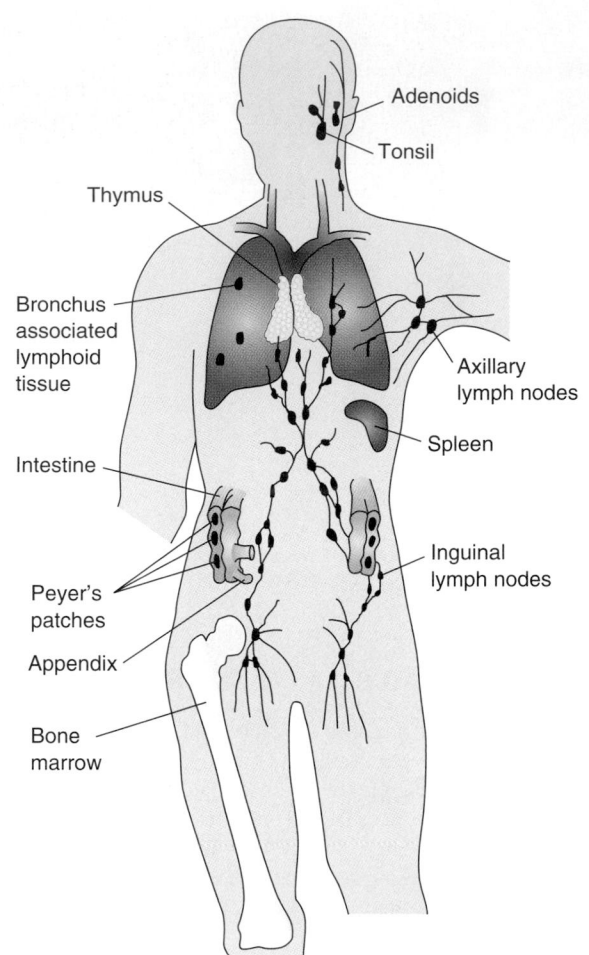

FIGURE 24-1. Central and peripheral lymphoid organs and tissues.

➤➤ **BOX 24-1**

FUNCTIONS OF THE IMMUNE SYSTEM

Defense
• Resists invasion by foreign microorganisms, including viruses and intracellular parasites
• Attacks some pathogens directly
• Attacks foreign antigens—usually proteins (including transplanted organs)
• Helps body to fight cancer cells
• Produces antibodies and immunoglobulins
• Produces inflammatory response
• Produces memory cells

Homeostasis
• Digests and removes damaged cellular substances
• Kills diseased cells (especially those infected with viruses)

Surveillance
• Recognizes and destroys cellular mutations
• Recognizes and destroys foreign cells
• Monitors for presence of antigens

basophils, and eosinophils) and agranular (monocytes and lymphocytes). This chapter focuses on lymphocytes.

• Lymphocytes are the "cornerstone" of the immune system; they alone have the ability to recognize foreign substances in the body.
• Differentiation of lymphocytes into special lymphocytes called **B cells** (**B lymphocytes**) and **T cells (T lymphocytes)** must occur before detection of foreign invaders begins. T lymphocytes help to protect against viral infections, and can detect and destroy some cancer cells. B lymphocytes develop into cells that produce antibodies (plasma cells).

Figure 24-2 illustrates the development of immune system cells.

☛ KEY CONCEPT

Lymphocytes formed in the bone marrow and lymphatic tissues are able to transform into specialized cells called B cells and T cells. B cells provide humoral immunity by reacting to the presence of antigens to produce antibodies. These antibodies then target antigens for destruction. T cells, which proliferate at the direction of thymic hormones, attack infected cells and provide cell-mediated immunity.

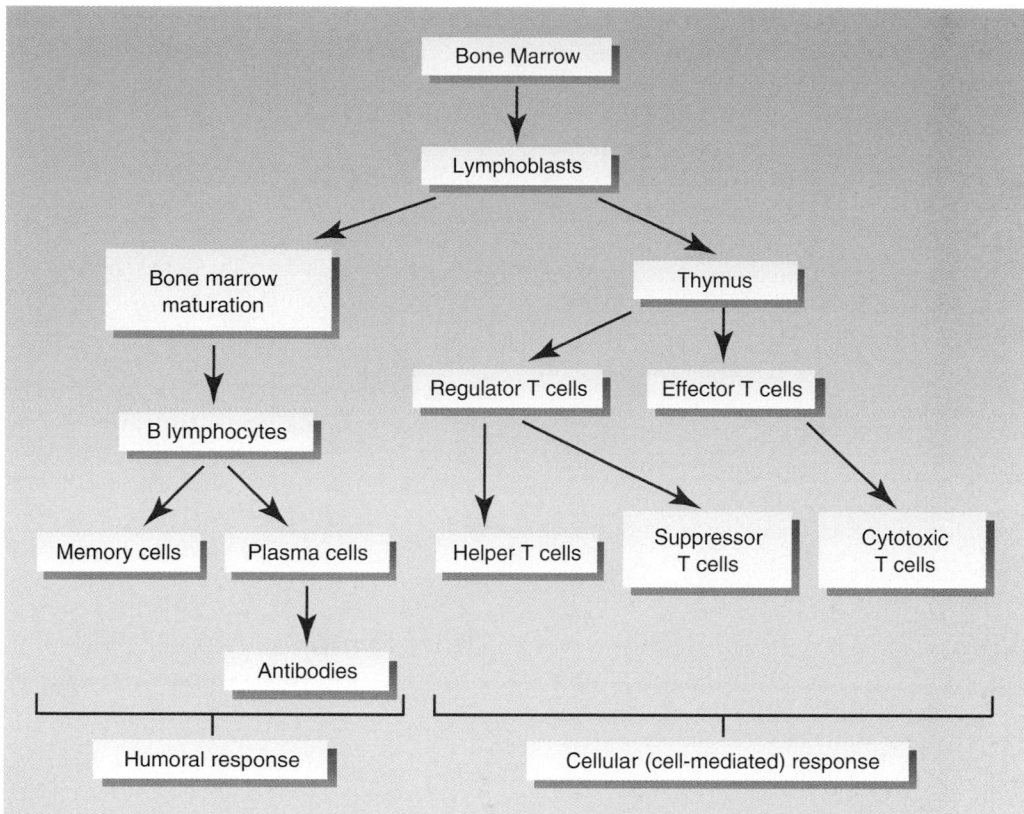

FIGURE 24-2. Development of the cells of the immune system.

B Lymphocytes

Stem cells in the bone marrow are responsible not only for the production of B lymphocytes, but also for their maturation. After they mature, B cells can become activated in the blood and produce antibodies. Exposure to an antigen in the bloodstream activates B cells to enlarge and to multiply rapidly to produce colonies of clones, although B cells do not respond to all pathogens. Most of these clones become plasma cells, which produce specific antibodies to circulate in the blood. These antibodies provide the form of immunity called **humoral immunity** (*humoral*=body fluid). In the process of humoral immunity, **macrophages** (large cells) engulf and destroy antigens after antibodies have identified them for destruction.

Those clones that do not become plasma cells remain in the body as *memory cells*. On repeated exposure to an antigen, the memory cells are ready to produce antibodies immediately. This "immunologic memory" makes a person immune to reinfection with a disease after he or she has had it.[2] Unfortunately this is not true for all diseases.

☛ KEY CONCEPT

The second exposure to an antigen can cause a quicker and more dramatic response than the first because of "immunologic memory." The first exposure will have a more delayed reaction because it takes some time to form the antibodies to the antigen. Antibodies are ready for the second exposure and quickly act.

B lymphocytes are found predominantly in organized lymphoid tissues, such as the spleen. They constitute only about 10% to 20% of the circulating lymphocytes in the tissues and the blood. Even fewer B cells are found in the lymph.[3]

Antigens and Antibodies

Antigens.   An antigen (**Ag**) is any foreign substance or molecule entering the body that stimulates an immune response (the activity of B or T lymphocytes). Most antigens are large protein molecules found on the surface of foreign organisms, RBCs, or tissue cells; on pollen; and in toxins and foods. Some carbohydrates and lipids also act as antigens.[2]

Antibodies.   An antibody (**Ab**) is a protein substance that the body produces in response to an antigen. *B lymphocytes* are responsible for antibody production. All antibodies are contained in a portion of the blood plasma called the *gamma globulin fraction.* Therefore, antibodies are commonly called **gamma globulins** or immunoglobulins (**IgG** or **Ig**).[2]   The five basic groups of immunoglobulins are:

- *IgM:* Stimulates complement activity. This is the antibody produced upon initial exposure to an antigen (such as after a first tetanus vaccination). IgM is abundant in the blood, but is not usually present in organs and tissues. It is not transferred across the placenta.
- *IgG:* Protects the fetus before birth against antitoxins, viruses, and bacteria. (It is the only antibody transferred from mother to fetus across the placenta.) IgG is the

most common antibody and is produced upon second and future exposures to an antigen (eg, after a tetanus booster). It is present in the blood (intravascular) and in the tissues (extravascular). IgG (often called gamma globulin) is the main component of commercial immunoglobulin.

- *IgA:* Protects mucosal surfaces. The major component of secretions such as saliva, tears, and bronchial fluids, IgA is transported across mucous membranes. It is important in the defense against invasion of microbes via the nose, eyes, lungs, and intestines. IgA is found in blood, as well as in GI and mucosal secretions. It is also found in breast milk.
- *IgE:* Responsible for immediate-type allergic reactions, including latex allergies. Although this antibody causes problems in developed countries, it is helpful in the developing world in fighting against parasitic infections, such as river blindness.
- *IgD:* Believed to function as an antigen receptor. It is present in the blood in very small amounts.

Each *antigen* (foreign invader) stimulates the production of its own specific *antibody.* The body can make about 1 million individual antibodies. Antibodies do not destroy antigens, but label antigens for destruction.

☛ KEY CONCEPT

IgG is the most abundant immunoglobulin found in the blood. Maternal IgG crosses to the fetus via the placenta, thereby transferring immunity to the fetus for the first few months of a newborn's life.

Nursing Alert

Latex allergies may be due to an IgE mediated reaction. Latex allergies can occur due to contact with the skin or mucous membrane, or inhalation. Persons exposed may have signs of urticaria (hives), dermatitis (usually of the hands), asthma, or severe anaphylaxis.

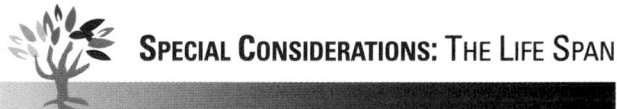 **SPECIAL CONSIDERATIONS: THE LIFE SPAN**

Children with spina bifida are exposed to latex during frequent urinary catheterizations and operations. This places them at high risk (18%–60%) for latex allergies.[5]

T Lymphocytes

Some immature stem cells produced in the bone marrow migrate to the thymus gland to become T cells (thymus-derived lymphocytes). T cells make up the remaining 80% to 90% of lymphocytes found in the circulating blood. While in the thymus, T cells proliferate and become sensitized (capable of

combining with specific foreign antigens). T lymphocytes produce an immunity called **cell-mediated immunity.**

T lymphocytes are generally responsible for fighting cancer cells, viruses, and intracellular parasites. They function in the body to differentiate between "self" and "non-self." Usually this is helpful in fighting off foreign pathogens. However, this function can also become a problem, because T cells are responsible for tissue and organ rejection after transplants. This is due to the fact that the T cells recognize these tissues as "non-self" and work to eliminate them. (Specific anti-rejection medications must be given to neutralize this rejection response in the recipient.)

Several types of T lymphocytes exist, each of which has its own function. For a T cell to react with a specific antigen, the antigen must first be presented to the T cell on the surface of a macrophage. Macrophages, when combined with T cells, release substances called *interleukins,* which stimulate T-cell growth.[2] Table 24-1 identifies the types and associated functions of the B lymphocytes and T lymphocytes.

Other Lymphocytes

A *natural killer cell* is slightly larger than a B or a T cell. These natural killer cells kill certain microbes and cancer cells. They are called *natural* because they do not require the maturation and "education" of B cells and T cells, but are ready to target specific cells as soon as they are produced. They also secrete some cytokines.

Cytokines

Cytokines are proteins that act as messengers to help regulate some of the functions of the lymphocytes and macrophages during the process of immune response. Some cytokines are given by injection to treat specific diseases.

A number of cytokines that have been identified are:

- *interferon-alpha:* used to treat certain cancers, such as hairy cell leukemia
- *interferon-beta:* believed to be helpful in multiple sclerosis
- *interleukin-1:* produced by macrophages, mobilizes T lymphocytes
- *interleukin-2:* produced by T cells, stimulates production of interferon. Used to treat many solid cancers, such as malignant melanoma and kidney cancer. (Also has adverse effects)
- *interleukin-3:* required for differentiation of certain T cells
- *interleukin-8:* guides neutrophils to the source of an antigen
- *interleukin-12:* stimulates natural killer cells
- *granulocyte colony-stimulating factor:* used to help increase neutrophils in clients who are undergoing chemotherapy

LYMPHOID ORGANS

Primary (Central) Lymphoid Organs

Along with the bone marrow, the **thymus** is considered a *central* or *primary* lymphoid organ. This small gland weighs

▪▪▪ TABLE 24-1 *Lymphocytes Involved in Immune Responses*

Cell Type	Function	Type of Immune Response
B cell	Produces antibodies or immunoglobulins (IgA, IgD, IgE, IgG, IgM)	Humoral
T cell		Cellular
Helper T_4	Attacks foreign invaders (antigens) directly Initiates and augments inflammatory response	
Helper T_1	Increases activated cytotoxic T cells	
Helper T_2	Increases B-cell antibody production	
Suppressor T	Suppresses the immune response	
Memory T	Remembers contact with an antigen and on subsequent exposures mounts an immune response	
Cytotoxic T (killer T)	Lyses cells infected with virus; plays a role in graft rejection	
Non-T or B lymphocytes		Nonspecific
Null cells	Destroys antigens already coated with antibody	
Natural killer (NK) (granular lymphocyte)	Defends against microorganisms and some types of malignant cells; produces cytokines	

Smeltzer, S. C., & Bare, B. G. (2001). *Brunner & Suddarth's textbook of medical-surgical nursing* (9th ed., p. 1338.). Philadelphia: Lippincott Williams & Wilkins.

1 ounce at most. It is located in the mediastinum of the upper chest. The thymus is most active early in life and begins to atrophy (shrink and die) at puberty. T lymphocytes must mature in the thymus gland before they can perform their immune functions. The thymus produces hormones called *thymosin, thymic humoral factor (THF), thymic factor (TF),* and *thymopoietin.* These hormones promote the proliferation and maturation of T cells in the thymus and other lymphoid tissues throughout the body.

Peripheral (Secondary) Lymphoid Organs

The *peripheral* or *secondary* lymphoid organs of the immune system include the lymphoid structures scattered in the submucosal layers of the respiratory, gastrointestinal, and genitourinary tracts; the lymph nodes; and the spleen. The defense functions of these organs are primarily related to the filtration of tissue fluid or lymph for foreign particles and external microorganisms.

THE MONONUCLEAR PHAGOCYTE SYSTEM

The *mononuclear phagocyte system,* or *reticuloendothelial system,* consists of specialized cells throughout the body that can ingest foreign particulate matter. These cells begin as monocytes and transform into macrophages (*phagocytic* or *endocytic* cells) after entering other tissues via the bloodstream. This system is concerned with the destruction of worn-out blood cells, bacteria, cancer cells, and other foreign substances that are dangerous to the body. Some macrophages have special names, such as *Kupffer cells* in the liver sinusoids, and *dust cells* in the lungs.

Mononuclear phagocytes play a very important role in both nonspecific and specific immunity. In specific immunity they are responsible for capturing (via phagocytosis), processing, and presenting the antigen to the lymphocytes for destruction. The macrophage-bound antigen, when presented to the B or T lymphocyte, triggers the humoral or cell-mediated immune response.[4]

SYSTEM PHYSIOLOGY

Nonspecific Defense Mechanisms

The body possesses several defense systems. *Nonspecific defense mechanisms* (sometimes called **nonspecific immunity**) fight against a variety of foreign invaders. The following are several of the body's nonspecific defense mechanisms:

- The *skin* provides a physical barrier and secretes enzymes that kill or reduce the virulence of bacteria.
- *Tears* dilute and wash away irritating substances and microbes.
- *Neutrophils* and *monocytes* ingest and destroy bacteria and toxins and remove cellular debris.
- *Interferon* is a protein made by several types of cells that inhibits virus production and infection.

- *Fever* intensifies the effects of interferons, inhibits the growth of some microbes, and speeds up body reactions aiding in tissue repair.
- The respiratory tract contains *cilia* and *macrophages* (phagocytic cells) in its mucous membrane lining that trap and remove microbes and dust.
- The stomach contains *hydrochloric acid,* which destroys pathogens.
- *Vomiting, defecation,* and *urination* expel microbes from the body along with the normal waste products.

Specific Defense Mechanisms

Specific defense mechanisms (**specific immunity**) are considered the final line of defense against disease. Specific defense mechanisms are able to recognize and to respond to specific substances. *Humoral* and *cell-mediated immunity* are considered specific defense mechanisms because they act against particular harmful substances. Specific immunity can be classified into two main categories: inborn and acquired.

Inborn Immunity

Inborn immunity refers to immunity that is inherited or genetic. This inherited or innate immunity may be common to all members of a species (eg, humans have specific immunity to many diseases of animals). Inborn immunity may also be common to a specific population, sex, race, or to an individual person.

Acquired Immunity

Acquired immunity is attained through natural or artificial sources. Both *naturally* and *artificially* acquired immunity can be attained either *actively* or *passively* (Figure 24-3).

Naturally Acquired Immunity. **Naturally acquired immunity** occurs when a person is not deliberately exposed to a causative agent. This immunity can occur both *actively* and *passively*.

Naturally Acquired Active Immunity. *Naturally acquired active immunity* results when a child is exposed to, and develops, a disease (eg, measles or chickenpox) and subsequently builds up antibodies (immunity) to infections that are caused by the same organism. Individuals can also develop acquired immunity during their lives as they are exposed to disease-causing organisms. They do not necessarily have to become ill with the disease; they just build up immunity slowly. In other words, acquired immunity is built on lifetime exposures. Remember that the body manufactures not only cells that target the infecting antigen, but also memory cells. Each time the person is exposed to the disease, the memory cells activate a response that produces antibodies to the offending antigen. Usually, the response is faster with each exposure, as the "memory" increases. Naturally acquired active immunity can last a few years or for a lifetime.

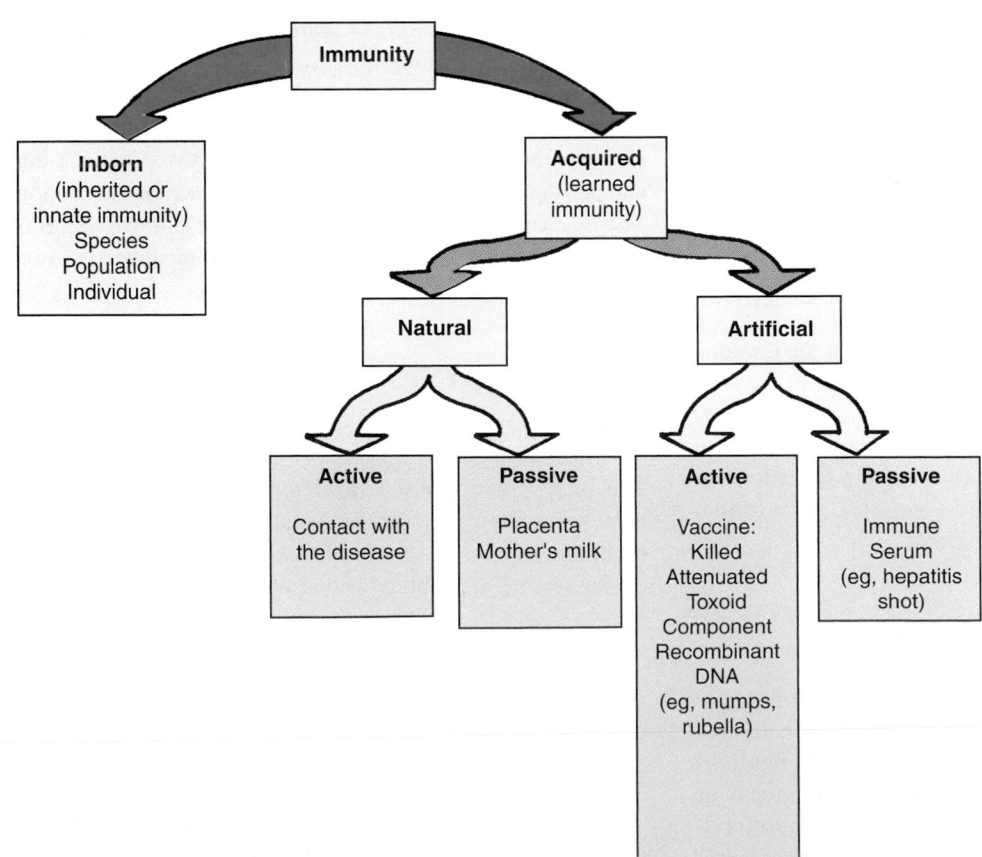

FIGURE 24-3. Types of specific immunity.

☛ Key Concept

Exposure to disease-causing organisms during one's life stimulates the process of acquired immunity.

Naturally Acquired Passive Immunity. *Naturally acquired passive immunity* occurs between mothers and their infants. Immunity is transferred from mother to fetus during pregnancy via the placental circulation exchange. If the baby is breast-fed, the baby also receives protection after birth through the mother's breast milk. Naturally acquired passive immunity can last up to six months of age, when the infant's own immune system begins to take over.

Artificially Acquired Immunity.   **Artificially acquired immunity** occurs when a person is deliberately exposed to a causative agent. Artificially acquired immunity can also be acquired through *active* or *passive* means.

Artificially Acquired Active Immunity. *Artificially acquired active immunity* occurs through an injection of the causative agent (antigen) into the person's system. This is called *vaccination, inoculation,* or **immunization**; the substance injected is called a **vaccine**. The causative agent is diluted to reduce its virulence (strength) so that the recipient will form antibodies without becoming ill. (The presence of the antigen causes antibody formation in the person's body.) Examples of vaccines are those for pertussis (whooping cough), influenza, measles (rubeola), German measles (rubella), and mumps. Many healthcare workers are immunized for hepatitis B. Tetanus is an example of an immunization that can be either active or passive. The active form is given as a tetanus booster, and causes the person to form his or her own antibodies against tetanus.

Artificially Acquired Passive Immunity. *Artificially acquired passive immunity* occurs with the injection of ready-made antibodies into a person's system. These antibodies were produced by another individual's immune system. An example of this type of immunity is the immunization for rabies. This immunization contains ready-made anti-rabies antibodies and is given in the event of a bite by a rabid animal. This immunization is also usually required if the animal cannot be located and tested. Tetanus toxoid can also be given in the passive form if a person has become ill with the disease of tetanus.

Another type of artificially acquired passive immunity is instituted with the injection of immunoglobulin IgG (gamma globulin). This immunization is given after disease exposure and results in only short-term immunity.

Antigen–Antibody Reaction

Antigen–antibody reactions begin with the B lymphocytes, whose job is to produce humoral immunity. *Humoral immunity* is the body's resistance to circulating disease-producing antigens and bacteria. B cells become plasma cells, and then work to produce antibodies.

Antibody-mediated immunity changes an antigen, rendering it harmless to the body. The antibody accomplishes this task by binding to an antigen, forming an antigen–antibody complex. This binding can be compared to a "lock-and-key" mechanism. In the same way that keys are cut individually to fit a particular lock and no other, an antibody forms in response to a specific antigen. The patterns on the membrane surface of the antigen and antibody fit together with the same discrimination with which a key fits into a lock. The match must be perfect.

After attaching to the antigen, the antibody uses one of several mechanisms to disarm the antigen. The antibody can neutralize the antigen's toxins. Or, the antibody can cause harmful cells to clump together so that macrophages and phagocytes can destroy them. (Antibodies promote or enhance phagocytosis by helping phagocytes attach to the cells they will destroy.)

Another mechanism for antigen destruction is called **complement fixation.** A *complement* is a group of proteins normally present, but inactive, in the blood. These complements help in the attack on invading antigens. Complements become active when exposed to the altered cellular shape caused by the antigen–antibody complex. When activated, complements cause the formation of highly specialized antigen–antibody complexes that target specific cells. These newly formed complexes cause holes to develop in cell membranes. Sodium and water flow into the cells, causing them to burst open and be destroyed.

Immune system disorders are being identified more frequently today and are believed to be the cause of many other—as yet unidentified—disorders. Chapter 82 describes cancer, which many researchers believe has an immune component. Chapters 83 and 84 describe some of the more common immune and autoimmune disorders.

☛ Key Concept

Immune response:

• *Recognition (of antigen) via antigen processing: Mostly by macrophages. Antigens ingested, broken up, packaged, carried to the surface of cell membrane, and assigned to T-cell receptor.*
• *Mobilization (of immune system): Cytokines released, other lymphocytes activated, natural killer cells stimulated to secrete interferon. Interleukin-8 acts as signal to guide neutrophils to antigen (chemotaxis).*
• *Attack (killing or eliminating microbes): By macrophages, neutrophils, and natural killer cells. If invading microbe cannot be eliminated, it can be encapsulated or imprisoned by special cells (granuloma); eg, granuloma (tubercle) encloses the bacteria that causes tuberculosis rendering it unable to cause the illness.*

Autoimmune reaction: Malfunctioning or misinterpretation by immune system of body's own tissues. (Examples: rheumatoid arthritis, scleroderma, myasthenia gravis, pernicious anemia.)

Immunodeficiency disorders: Immune system is compromised and does not function adequately to prevent infections (most widely known is AIDS).

EFFECTS OF AGING ON THE SYSTEM

Older adults have fewer T cells and B cells. The T cells and B cells that remain function poorly as stem cells. Consequently, the immune system of the older adult acts with a slower, muted

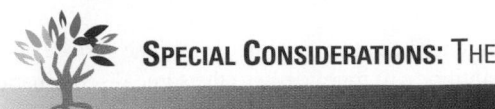

SPECIAL CONSIDERATIONS: THE LIFE SPAN

Infections frequently manifest themselves in older adults as a change in mental status. The cardiovascular system cannot keep up with the increased metabolic demands that an unrecognized infection imposes. The result is cerebral hypoxia or "delirium." Because of this atypical presentation, older adults are susceptible to developing bacteremia (bacteria in the blood) that, if untreated, can quickly progress to septic shock.

inflammatory process and response to infection. Older adults usually have a baseline body temperature lower than 98.6° Fahrenheit. Therefore, they do not always have a febrile response to infection (Table 24-2). (Fever helps kill microorganisms.)

➤ STUDENT SYNTHESIS

Key Points

- Immunity is the specific resistance to disease that involves the production of a specific lymphocyte or antibody against a specific antigen.
- Both B cells and T cells derive from stem cells in the bone marrow.
- B cells go on to mature in the bone marrow, whereas T cells complete their maturation and develop immunocompetence in the thymus gland.
- Antigens are substances (usually proteins) the immune system recognizes as foreign.
- An antibody is a protein that reacts specifically with the antigen that triggers its production.
- Humoral immunity refers to destruction of antigens by antibodies.

- Immunity can be inborn or acquired. Both naturally and artificially acquired immunity can be actively or passively acquired.
- Cell-mediated immunity refers to destruction of antigens by T cells.
- Exposure to disease-causing organisms over one's lifetime stimulates the process of acquired immunity.
- Humoral or antibody–mediated immunity protects the body against circulating disease-producing antigens and bacteria.
- Antibodies use several mechanisms to destroy antigens: neutralizing toxins, facilitating phagocytosis, imprisoning invader cells (granuloma), and complement fixation.

Critical Thinking Exercises

1. Disease-producing organisms are all around you. Brainstorm as to how these organisms could contaminate the food supply. What widespread effects could such an occurrence have on a population?
2. The mother of a newborn visits your healthcare facility. She has been reading some information about vaccines, but does not understand how they work or why they are so important. How would you address this issue? What information and explanations would you give to the mother to promote her understanding?
3. Based on the information above, what advantages in terms of immunity might an infant who is breast-fed have over an infant who is formula-fed?
4. Describe the relationship between immunity and the medical condition, AIDS.

NCLEX-Style Review Questions

1. Which of the following cells have the ability to recognize foreign substances in the body?
   a. Erythrocytes
   b. Lymphocytes
   c. Platelets
   d. Plasma cells

TABLE 24-2 ℰFFECTS OF AGING ON THE IMMUNE SYSTEM

Factor	Result	Nursing Implications
Numbers of T cells and B cells decrease.	Immune system reacts more slowly. Increased incidence of tumors Greater susceptibility to infections	Assess regularly for signs of infection.
Baseline body temperature is lower.	Absence of febrile response to infection	Observe clients closely for clinical signs or symptoms of infection. Offer blankets and keep room warm. *Change* in temperature is often more significant than actual temperature.

2. Which immunoglobulin is found in the blood as well as in the tissues?
   a. IgA
   b. IgE
   c. IgG
   d. IgM
3. After an individual has been exposed to and developed a disease, which type of immunity will prevent the individual from having the disease with subsequent exposure to the disease?
   a. Naturally acquired active immunity
   b. Artificially acquired immunity
   c. Inborn immunity
   d. Naturally acquired passive immunity

References

1. Porth, C. (2002). *Pathophysiology concepts of altered health states* (6th ed.). Philadelphia: Lippincott Williams & Wilkins.
2. Cohen, B., & Wood, D. (2000). *Memmler's structure and function of the human body* (7th ed.). Philadelphia: Lippincott Williams & Wilkins.
3. Burrell, L. O., Gerlach, M. J. & Pless, B. S. (1997). *Adult nursing: Acute and community care* (2nd ed.). Stamford, CT: Appleton & Lange.
4. Lewis, S. M., Collier, I. C., & Heitkemper, M. M. (1996). *Medical-surgical nursing: Assessment and management of clinical problems* (4th ed.). St. Louis: Mosby-Year Book.
5. McKinney, E. S., Ashwill, J. W., Murray, S. S., et al. (2000). *Maternal-child nursing*. Philadelphia: Lippincott Williams & Wilkins.

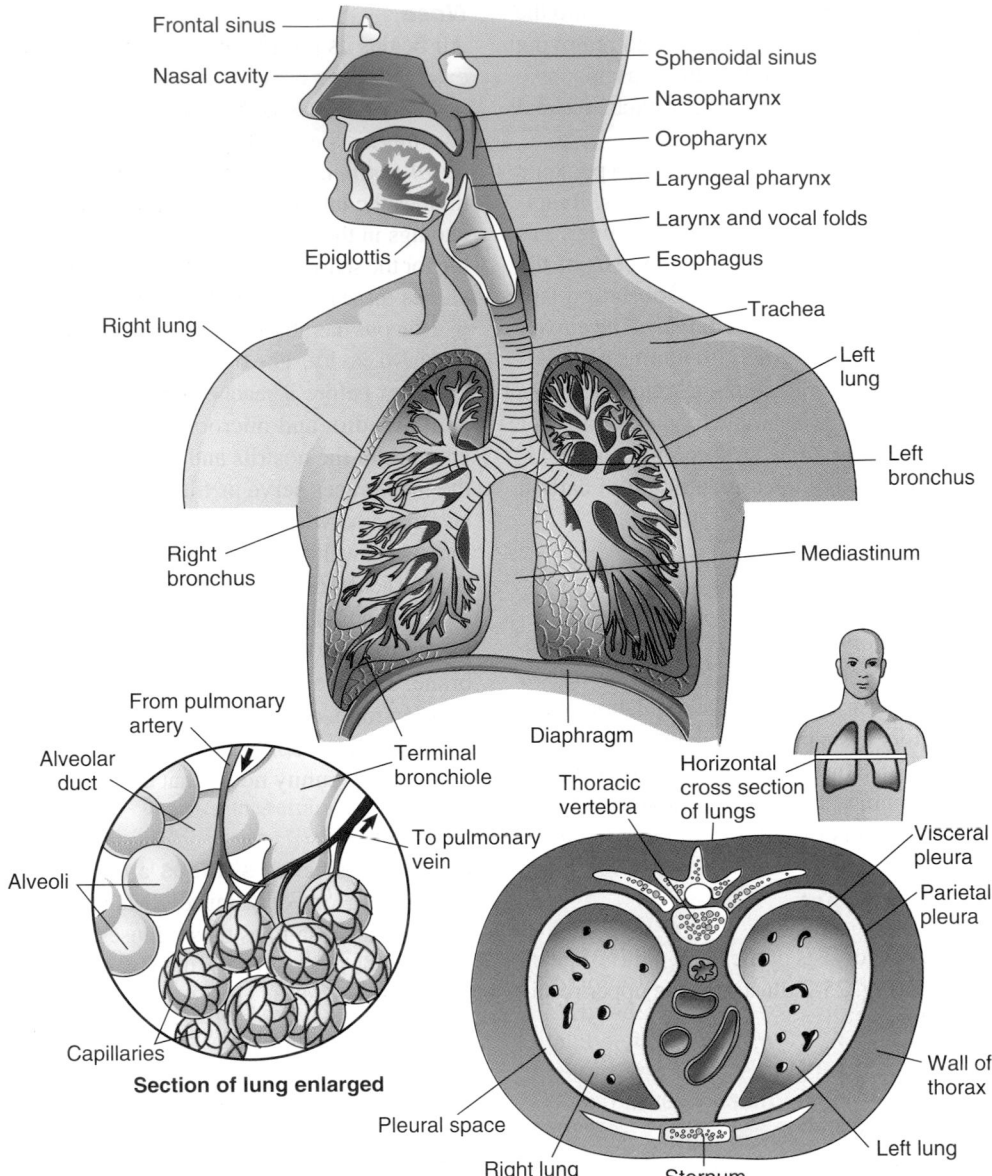

FIGURE 25-1. The respiratory system. *Top,* upper respiratory structures and the structures of the thorax. *Bottom* (left), an enlarged section of the lung and (right) a horizontal cross section of both lungs.

eign invaders (along with the tonsils). Enlargement of the adenoids can cause snoring or obstruction of the upper airway. Only rarely does an adult have adenoids; when an individual approaches adulthood, the adenoids usually atrophy (waste away). During the act of swallowing, the soft palate and uvula elevate to block the nasal cavity, preventing food from entering the respiratory system. The **auditory** (eustachian) **tubes** connect the nasopharynx with the middle ear. These **eustachian tubes** permit air to enter or to leave the middle ear cavities, permitting proper functioning of the tympanic membranes (eardrums).

Oropharynx.   The **oropharynx** is the part of the pharynx extending from the uvula to the epiglottis. Commonly called the "throat," the oropharynx carries food to the esophagus and air to the trachea. Two sets of tonsils are in the oropharynx: the two *palatine tonsils* are located posteriorly, on each

side of the oral cavity, and the *lingual tonsils* are located at the base of the tongue. The palatine tonsils are the ones commonly removed during a tonsillectomy. These two sets of tonsils encircle the throat and have a role in the immune system (in addition to the adenoids). Their function is to destroy foreign substances that are inhaled or ingested.[1]

Laryngopharynx.   The **laryngopharynx** is the lowest portion of the pharynx. It extends from the epiglottis to the openings of the larynx and esophagus. The division of the laryngopharynx provides separate passageways for food and air.

Larynx (Voice Box)

From the pharynx, air passes into the **larynx,** a boxlike structure made of cartilages held together by ligaments. The function of these cartilages is to keep the airway open at all times.

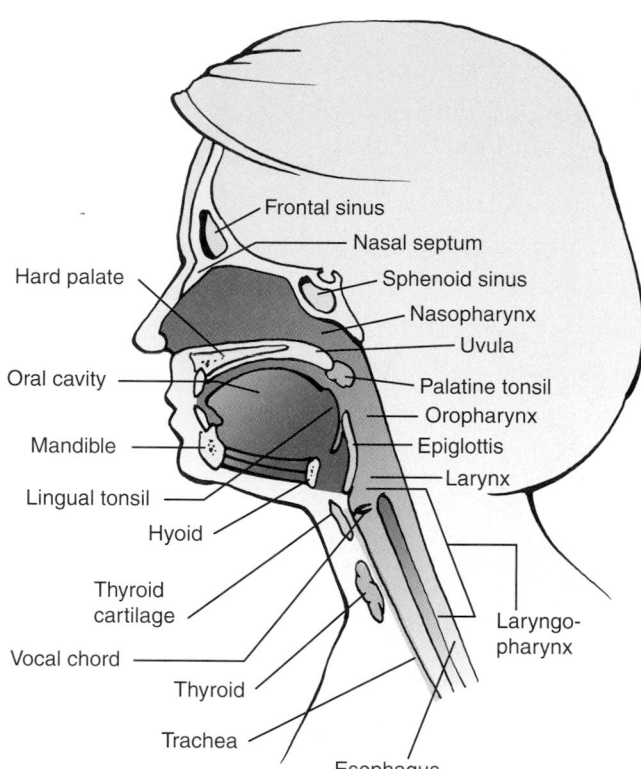

Frontal sinus
Nasal septum
Sphenoid sinus
Hard palate
Nasopharynx
Uvula
Oral cavity
Palatine tonsil
Oropharynx
Mandible
Epiglottis
Larynx
Lingual tonsil
Hyoid
Thyroid
cartilage
Laryngo-
pharynx
Vocal chord
Thyroid
Trachea
Esophagus

FIGURE 25-2. Anatomy of the upper respiratory tract.

(The largest and most prominent cartilage is the *thyroid cartilage,* commonly known as the "Adam's apple.") The larynx is located in the midline of the neck.

> ### Nursing Alert
> In the event of a blocked airway, a *tracheotomy* may be needed. This is an artificial opening, either temporary or permanent, in the trachea.

The larynx serves as an air passageway between the pharynx and the trachea. Although the pharynx acts as a dual passageway for air and food, only air is allowed to pass into the larynx. A lid or cover of cartilage called the **epiglottis** ("trap door cartilage") guards the entrance to the larynx. The epiglottis automatically closes when you swallow, preventing food from entering the lower respiratory passage. The *glottis* is the opening on either side of the vocal cords. If a portion of food accidentally becomes lodged in the larynx, coughing can usually dislodge it. If not, the air passage may be blocked; such a blockage can be fatal unless proper emergency treatment is given. (You will, no doubt, be taking a course in obstructed airway and cardiopulmonary resuscitation, if you have not already done so.)

Vocal Cords.   Within the larynx are the **vocal cords,** two triangle-shaped membranous folds that extend from front to back. As air leaves the lungs and passes over the vocal cords, the cords vibrate, and the vibration produces sound. The size of the vocal cords and the larynx varies, accounting for the difference in people's voices. A man has a larger larynx—

and therefore a deeper voice—than most women. Your voice becomes louder and stronger when you rapidly force out a lot of air.

Trachea (Windpipe)

Air passes from the larynx into the **trachea,** a tube approximately 4.5 inches (11 cm) long and 1 inch in diameter in adults. It consists of cartilage and connective tissue, and extends from the lower end of the larynx into the chest cavity behind the heart. Immediately posterior to the larynx and the trachea is the tube called the *esophagus,* which transports food from the pharynx to the stomach (see Chap. 26). The trachea's horseshoe-shaped cartilaginous rings provide sufficient rigidity to keep it open at all times for air to pass through. The rings are flexible enough, however, to permit bending of the neck.

Ciliated mucous membrane lines the trachea. As in the nose, mucus in the trachea traps inhaled foreign particles, which the waves of cilia carry out of the respiratory tract through the pharynx.

Lower Respiratory Tract

Figure 25-3 illustrates the lower respiratory tract. It consists of the bronchi and lungs.

Bronchi

As the trachea enters the chest cavity, it divides into two smaller tubes called the **bronchi.** There is an indented area, called the *hilum,* where each bronchus enters the lung and branches off. The arteries, veins, bronchi, and nerves enter the lungs at the hilum as well. One (primary) bronchus enters each lung. The right bronchus is shorter and wider than the left bronchus, which makes it a more common site for aspiration of foreign objects.

> ### Nursing Alert
> Because the right bronchus is shorter and wider than the left, it is more easily accessible. Therefore, the right bronchus is more susceptible to aspiration of fluids or foreign objects.

The Tracheobronchial Tree.   Each bronchus continues to divide into smaller branches to form what commonly is called the *bronchial tree* or *tracheobronchial tree.* This bronchial tree spreads throughout the lung tissue. As the bronchi become smaller, their walls become thinner, the amount of cartilage decreases, and they become known as **bronchioles.** The bronchi and bronchioles continue to be lined with ciliated mucous membrane. The bronchioles branch first into **alveolar ducts,** which look like stems, and end in many **alveolar sacs,** which look like clusters of grapes (see Fig. 25-1). Each lung contains millions of alveoli. These microscopic "balloons" give the lungs their spongy appearance. The walls of the alveoli are composed of a single layer of cells and are lined with a chemical called **surfactant,** which helps to prevent the alveolar walls from collapsing between breaths.

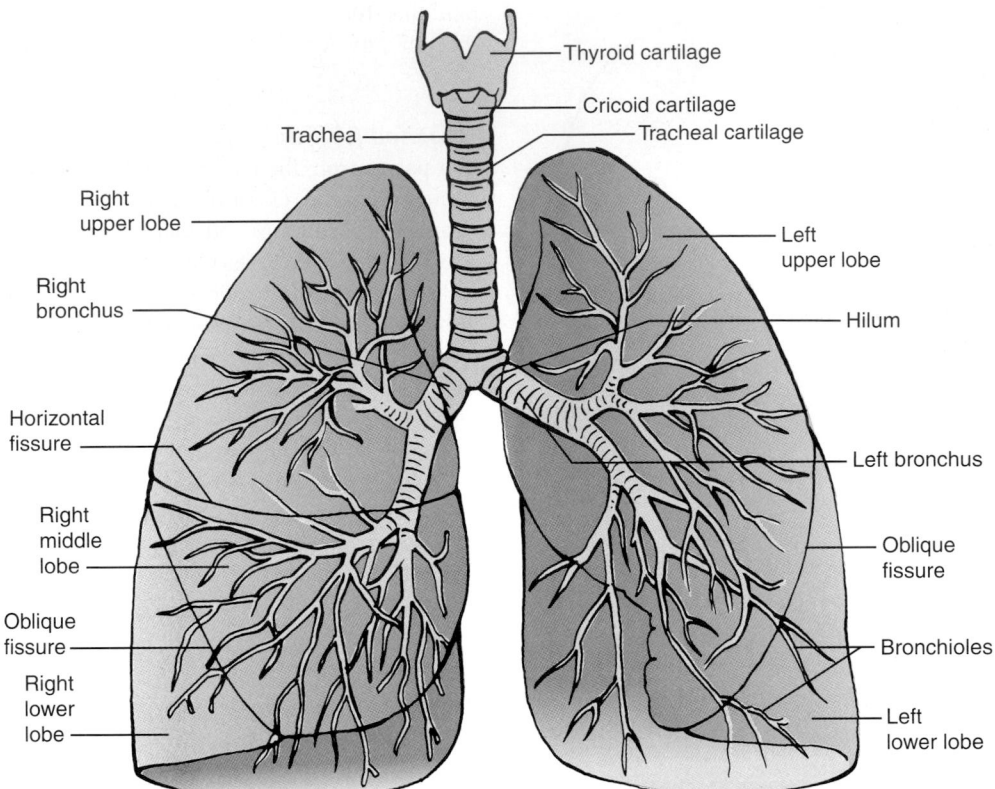

FIGURE 25-3. The lower respiratory tract. The lungs consist of five lobes. The right lung has three lobes (upper, middle, lower); the left has two (upper and lower). The lobes are further subdivided by fissures. The bronchial tree inflates with air to fill the lobes.

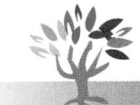 **SPECIAL CONSIDERATIONS:** THE LIFE SPAN

Surfactant

Surfactant does not form until after the seventh gestational month. Premature newborns may have insufficient surfactant, which results in collapse of the alveoli. A newborn with this problem (called *hyaline membrane disease*) must exert tremendous energy to breathe. As a result, the infant may die due to fatigue of the respiratory muscles and inadequate ventilation. Mechanical ventilation and derived (synthetic) surfactant are used until the newborn can produce his or her own surfactant.

Surfactant.   *Surfactant* is a substance secreted by the great alveolar cells (type II cells) of the lungs, and is a mixture of phospholipids (a special type of fat that also contains phosphorus). The main phospholipids in surfactant are lecithin and sphingomyelin. The surfactant in the lungs acts to break up the surface tension in the pulmonary (lung) fluids, much like laundry detergent breaks up dirt particles. This reduces friction and preserves the elastic property of lung tissue, thus preventing collapse of the alveolar walls between breaths.

Lungs

Humans have two cone-shaped **lungs** that fill the chest cavity. They are the stations where blood picks up oxygen and drops off its load of carbon dioxide. The top of each triangular cone is called the *apex*. The lower, wide portion that fits over the diaphragm is called the *base*. The lungs are spongy tissue filled with alveoli, nerves, and blood and lymph vessels. They are separated by the heart, the large blood vessels, the esophagus, and other contents of the **mediastinum,** the area lying between the lungs in the thorax (chest).

The lungs are divided into sections called *lobes*. The right lung has three lobes, and the left has two (see Fig. 25-3).

Pleura.   The lower respiratory tract contains a smooth double-layered sac of serous membrane called **pleura** (see Fig. 25-1). One layer covers the lungs (the **visceral pleura**), and the outer layer (the **parietal pleura**) lines the chest cavity. Their surfaces are in constant contact and are moist, because they secrete serous lubricating fluid. The pleura allow the lungs to move without causing pain or friction against the chest wall. The space between the two layers of the pleura is called the **pleural cavity** or **pleural space.** A vacuum normally exists within this space.

Nursing Alert

Pleurisy is an inflammation of the pleura caused by infection, injury, or tumor. In addition, air or fluid accumulation in the pleural space can cause partial or total lung collapse.

SYSTEM PHYSIOLOGY

Breathing

Ventilation (breathing) is the mechanical process of respiration that moves air to and from the alveoli. Ventilation is divided into inhalation and exhalation. Breathing air in is called *inhalation* or **inspiration;** breathing out is called *exhalation* or **expiration.** Adults usually average between 14 and 20 respirations per minute; the rate is much higher in children. Normal respiration is called **eupnea;** difficult breathing is known as **dyspnea.**

Normal breathing occurs as a result of nervous stimulation of the respiratory center in the brain's medulla. Because the lungs cannot move by themselves, the actions of the muscles surrounding them inflate and deflate them. The medulla sends impulses to the diaphragm and the intercostal muscles. The **diaphragm** is a dome-shaped muscle separating the thoracic and abdominal cavities. It contracts and flattens to increase chest space and create a vacuum (Fig. 25-4). The **intercostal muscles** are located between the ribs; they contract to lift and spread the ribs during inhalation, adding to the vacuum.

The actual movement of air from the external to the internal environment occurs as a result of differences in existing

> **Nursing Alert**
> Any interruption in the closed chest can be immediately life-threatening, because it disrupts the vacuum necessary for inspiration. Therefore, a puncture wound or other opening into the chest must be immediately closed, to prevent death.

pressures between the atmosphere and the chest cavity. A partial vacuum exists internally. On inspiration, the chest cavity increases in size. Air goes into the lungs when the *intrathoracic* (within the thoracic cavity) *pressure* is below that of the surrounding atmosphere (*subatmospheric pressure*).

Expiration is a passive process. On expiration, the muscles of the chest wall and lungs relax. Movements of the diaphragm and the intercostal muscles cause the volume of the thoracic cavity to become smaller. Air rushes out when the pressures within the thoracic cavity rise above that of the atmosphere. In addition, the reduced size of the thoracic cavity forces the air out.

Regulation of Respirations

The medulla's respiratory center automatically controls the depth and rate of respirations without requiring a person's

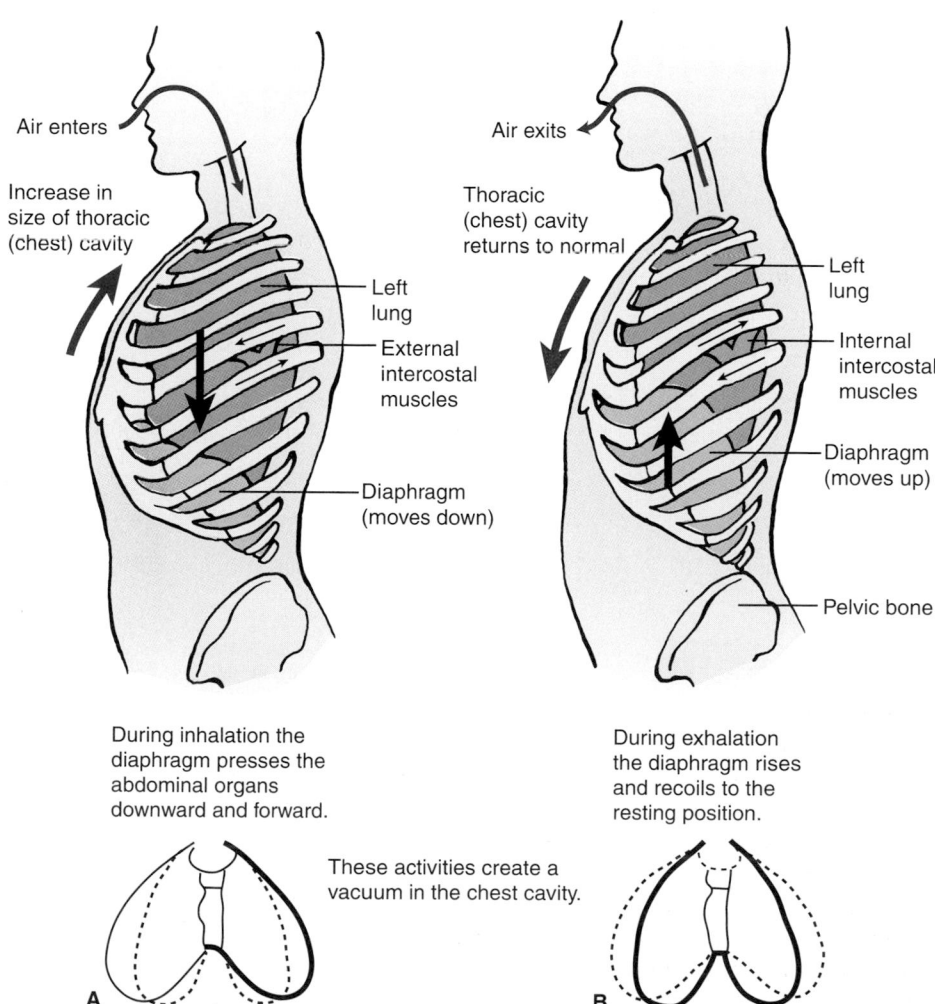

FIGURE 25-4. Pulmonary ventilation. **(A)** Inhalation (inspiration). **(B)** Exhalation (expiration).

conscious thought. The pons has centers that work with the medulla to produce a normal breathing rhythm. The cerebral cortex allows some voluntary control over breathing when talking, singing, eating, or changing the rate of breathing. You can even stop breathing for a minute or two by holding your breath. The medulla, however, will take over control eventually.

Chemoreceptors in the medulla stimulate the muscles of respiration primarily in response to changes in carbon dioxide levels. Therefore, carbon dioxide—not oxygen—is the major regulator of respiration.

☞ KEY CONCEPT

A low blood level of carbon dioxide is the major stimulus for breathing in healthy adults.

Lung Volumes and Capacities

Lung capacity varies with sex, size, physical condition, and age. Pulmonary diseases and other diseases that limit expansion of the chest cavity greatly influence a person's comfort and ability to survive. The ability of the lungs and thorax to expand also influences lung volumes and capacities. Table 25-1 contains key terms, descriptions, and normal values for a healthy male adult. (The values for women are 20% to 25% lower.)

Internal (Tissue) and External (Pulmonary) Respiration

The two types of respiration are external and internal. The exchange of oxygen (O_2) for carbon dioxide (CO_2) *within the alveoli of the lungs* is called **external respiration** (*pulmonary respiration*) because it is the part of the respiratory cycle involved with the external environment. After oxygen is brought into the body, it attaches to hemoglobin for transport to tissues and cells. The exchange of oxygen (O_2) for carbon dioxide (CO_2) *within the cells* is called **internal respiration** or **cellular respiration** (*cell breathing*). An increase in carbon dioxide levels stimulates respiration. Carbon dioxide and water are the waste products of respiration. Some water is excreted as waste; some is recycled for use in the body.

▪▪▪ TABLE 25-1 *L*UNG VOLUMES AND LUNG CAPACITIES

Term	Symbol	Description	Normal Value*	Significance
Lung Volumes				
Tidal volume	V_T or TV	The volume of air inhaled and exhaled with each breath	500 mL or 5–10 mL/kg	The tidal volume may not vary, even with severe disease.
Inspiratory reserve volume	IRV	The maximum volume of air that can be inhaled after a normal inhalation	3000 mL	A sigh takes advantage of the IRV potential.
Expiratory reserve volume	ERV	The maximum volume of air that can be exhaled forcibly after a normal exhalation	1100 mL	Expiratory reserve volume is decreased in restrictive disorders, such as obesity, ascites, pregnancy.
Residual volume	RV	The volume of air remaining in the lungs after a maximum exhalation	1200 mL	Residual volume may be increased in obstructive disease.
Lung Capacities				
Vital capacity	VC	The maximum volume of air exhaled from the point of maximum inspiration VC = TV + IRV + ERV	4600 mL	A decrease in vital capacity may be found in neuromuscular disease, generalized fatigue, atelectasis, pulmonary edema, and COPD.
Inspiratory capacity	IC	The maximum volume of air inhaled after normal expiration IC = TV + IRV	3500 mL	A decrease in inspiratory capacity may indicate restrictive disease.
Functional residual capacity	FRC	The volume of air remaining in the lungs after a normal expiration FRC = ERV + RV	2300 mL	Functional residual capacity may be increased in COPD and decreased in ARDS.
Total lung capacity	TLC	The volume of air in the lungs after a maximum inspiration TLC = TV + IRV + ERV + RV	5800 mL	Total lung capacity may be decreased in restrictive disease (atelectasis, pneumonia) and increased in COPD.

*Values for healthy men; women are 20%–25% less.

COPD, chronic obstructive pulmonary disease; ARDS, acute respiratory distress syndrome.

Smeltzer, S. C., & Bare, B. G. (2001). *Brunner and Suddarth's textbook of medical-surgical nursing* (9th ed., p. 379). Philadelphia: Lippincott Williams & Wilkins.

☞ KEY CONCEPT

Respiration *is the exchange of gases between a person's external environment and internal cells.*

External respiration *is gas exchange at the lung level.* Internal respiration *is gas exchange at the cellular level.*

Gas Exchange

Chapters 22 and 23 introduce the concept of pulmonary circulation. Unoxygenated blood from the right ventricle of the heart flows into the pulmonary artery. The blood continues to capillaries in the lungs where an exchange of gases (oxygen and carbon dioxide) occurs via diffusion through the alveoli. The walls of the alveoli are one cell-layer thick, and are surrounded by equally thin capillaries. When oxygen enters the lungs, it travels through the walls of the alveoli into capillaries. At the capillary level, oxygen diffuses into the capillaries and is bound to hemoglobin (in red blood cells) in capillary blood. Small veins collect the now-oxygenated blood from the lung capillaries. These veins combine eventually into four pulmonary veins, which pour oxygenated blood into the left atrium. The blood in the left atrium will travel through the left ventricle and through the aorta out to the rest of the body. This oxygenated blood then travels to tissues where the oxygen–hemoglobin bond is broken easily and oxygen is released into tissues. At the same time that oxygen is diffusing from the alveoli into the capillaries, the capillaries are transferring carbon dioxide (received from body tissues) into the alveoli. Carbon dioxide is a waste product of metabolism (or from the work that the body is performing) and is transported to pulmonary capillaries in three main forms: dissolution in plasma; in combination with proteins; or by formation into bicarbonate (HCO_3^-) ions in the blood. During exhalation, this carbon dioxide is released from the lungs into the air. This cycle then begins again.

✚👁 **N u r s i n g   A l e r t**
Many factors can cause a decrease in gas exchange, including immobility, thoracic/pulmonary surgery, or pneumonia. Encouraging frequent coughing and deep breathing exercises should assist in improving oxygen delivery to the lungs and tissues. Supplemental oxygen may also be ordered to improve arterial oxygen levels.

Regulation of Acid–Base Balance

The primary function of the respiratory system is the exchange of gases. Another important function is the regulation of the pH of all body fluids. The respiratory and renal systems interact to maintain homeostasis (see Chap. 17).

Carbon dioxide can alter pH, because it reacts with water to form carbonic acid (H_2CO_3). Carbonic acid can break down to form H^+ and HCO_3^- (hydrogen ion and bicarbonate ion). These ions are important to the buffer system (and the respiratory process is part of the buffer system), which helps the body maintain proper pH levels (see Chap. 17). The hydrogen ion often combines to form acids, such as hydrochloric acid (HCl). The bicarbonate ion often combines to form basic compounds, which counteract acids. One such base compound is sodium carbonate ($NaHCO_3$), which, outside the body, is known as baking soda.

☞ KEY CONCEPT

The respiratory system is the major mechanism for excretion and elimination of carbon dioxide (CO_2) from the body. (CO_2 is constantly being produced by the body as a by-product of metabolism.)

If a person has a breathing disorder, carbon dioxide can build up in the body, dangerously lowering the blood pH. This condition, called respiratory acidosis, *can be caused by disorders such as emphysema, severe pneumonia, asthma, and pulmonary edema. Untreated, respiratory acidosis is life-threatening. Too little CO_2 in the blood is called* respiratory alkalosis, *and is most commonly caused by hyperventilation (excessively rapid, deep breathing).*

Respiratory Reflexes

Coughing and sneezing are protective reflexes needed to dislodge materials from the respiratory passages. The bronchi and trachea have sensory receptors that initiate a cough, in response to foreign particles or irritating substances. The sneezing reflex is similar to coughing, except that the source of irritation is in the nasal passages.

Yawning is another respiratory reflex. Theorists conjecture that yawning is a response to a lack of oxygen or an accumulation of carbon dioxide. (No one knows why yawning is contagious.) Yawning also equalizes pressure between the middle ear and the outside atmosphere, helping a person to maintain balance.

Respiratory disorders are very common. They are aggravated by such things as pollutants in the air and cigarette smoking. Chapter 85 describes respiratory disorders in more detail and Chapter 86 outlines the steps in administering supplemental oxygen.

☞ KEY CONCEPT

Coughing, sneezing, and yawning are protective respiratory reflexes.

✚👁 **N u r s i n g   A l e r t**
Smoking can decrease the efficiency of the respiratory system. Nicotine causes a decrease in bronchial diameter, constriction of blood vessels, a decrease in ciliary function (which assists in moving foreign particles out of the respiratory tract), and can destroy lung tissue itself over time. These factors can all result in a decrease in gas exchange. In addition, many tobacco products contain substances (such as tars) that can build up in the lungs.

EFFECTS OF AGING ON THE SYSTEM

The organs of the respiratory system lose their elasticity with age. Table 25-2 summarizes major effects of aging on the respiratory system. The chest walls become stiffer, and the lungs cannot expand as much; therefore, less air is exchanged with

■■■ **TABLE 25-2** ℰFFECTS OF AGING ON THE RESPIRATORY SYSTEM

Factor	Result	Nursing Implications
Functional capacity decreases because of: • Increased rigidity of thorax and diaphragm • Decreased numbers of alveoli and diffusion ability • Decreased strength in breathing and coughing	More energy needed to breathe Less ability to compensate for respiratory needs in stress or illness Hypoventilation can lead to respiratory problems and pneumonia May develop dyspnea (shortness of breath) with exertion Morning cough common (decreased ability to eliminate secretions)	Encourage good ventilation with daily exercise such as walking. Advise older person to avoid contact with children or others with respiratory tract infections. Advise client to see physician early if symptoms occur. Encourage changing position slowly to avoid orthostatic vital sign changes. Advise to change position at least every 2 hours.
The size of the chest wall decreases as a result of kyphosis and osteoporosis.	Difficulty breathing deeply	Help client know his or her own ability.
Immobility is common	Pneumonia is a threat	Encourage moving, coughing, and deep breathing.

each breath. The ratio of the pressures of oxygen and carbon dioxide in the lungs may change, causing difficulties in blood oxygenation and exchange of oxygen for carbon dioxide at the cellular level.

The changes of aging can also make the older person more susceptible to respiratory disorders, such as pneumonia. This susceptibility occurs not only as a result of decreased elasticity of the lungs and bronchioles, but also because of decreased ciliary action and the decreased secretion of mucus in respiratory tract linings.

➥ STUDENT SYNTHESIS

Key Points

- The pathway for external breathing is nose → pharynx → larynx → trachea → bronchi → bronchioles → alveoli (where oxygen is exchanged for carbon dioxide).
- The pathway for oxygen distribution and carbon dioxide return (internal breathing) is alveoli → capillaries (hemoglobin combines with oxygen) → cells → capillaries (carbon dioxide exchange) → alveoli. The deoxygenated blood moves to the lungs via the general circulation and the pulmonary circuit. In the alveoli of the lungs, carbon dioxide is exchanged for oxygen and CO_2 is exhaled.
- The pharynx is divided into three areas: nasopharynx, oropharynx, and laryngopharynx.
- The trachea and esophagus are both located in the pharynx. The epiglottis is a protective flap that covers the trachea during swallowing to prevent foreign matter from entering the respiratory system.
- The pleura has two layers. One layer covers the lung and the other layer lines the chest wall. Serous fluid secreted by the pleura enables the lungs to move without pain or friction.

- External respiration is the exchange of gases (oxygen and carbon dioxide) at the lung level. Internal respiration is the exchange of gas at the cellular level.
- The various lung volumes and capacities describe the volume of air in the lungs (or left in the lungs) in relation to inspiration or expiration. These amounts can vary depending upon the sex and size of the client and upon existing respiratory disorders.
- Nasal hair, mucus, and cilia are protective structures of the respiratory system. Sneezing, coughing, and yawning are protective reflexes of the respiratory system.

Critical Thinking Exercises

1. Alterations in systems other than the respiratory system can affect the process of breathing and gas exchange. List the systems that may be involved, and describe the types of alterations that might cause such problems.
2. Based on the information in this chapter, explain why you think a person with a cold sometimes experiences changes in his or her voice.
3. Explain the relationship between aerobic exercise and optimum pulmonary functioning. (Feel free to research articles on the Internet to find support for your answer.)
4. Define each of the following acronyms. Discuss a possible medical cause and two nursing implications for each:
   decreased ERV
   decreased TLC
   increased FRC
   decreased FRC
   increased RV

NCLEX-Style Review Questions

1. The major regulator or respiration is:
   a. Carbon dioxide
   b. Lung capacity
   c. Muscle activity
   d. Oxygen
2. Which area of the respiratory system is more susceptible to aspiration?
   a. Alveoli
   b. Bronchioles
   c. Left bronchus
   d. Right bronchus

3. The functional unit of the respiratory system is the:
   a. Airway
   b. Alveolus
   c. Bronchus
   d. Trachea

Reference

1. Tortora, G. J., & Grabowski, S. R. (1996). Principles of anatomy and physiology (8th ed.). New York: HarperCollins.

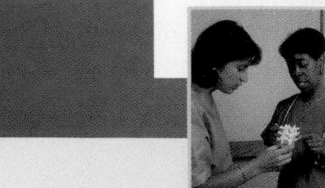

The Digestive System

LEARNING OBJECTIVES

1. On a chart, trace the digestive pathway, naming the major organs of the gastrointestinal (GI) tract and the function of each.
2. Define the following terms and processes: mastication, deglutition, and peristalsis.
3. Explain the actions of hydrochloric acid (HCl), gastrin, intrinsic factor, cholecystokinin, and pancreatic juice in the process of digestion.
4. Describe two functions of the pancreas and gallbladder as they relate to digestion.
5. Describe four functions of the liver.
6. Describe the physiology of digestion and absorption, including how carbohydrates, fats, and proteins are absorbed in the small intestine.
7. Identify and describe two major categories of metabolism.
8. Explain how the large intestine changes its contents into fecal material.
9. Describe three effects of aging on the digestive system.

NEW TERMINOLOGY

absorption	ingestion
alimentary canal	jejunum
appendix	lacteal
bile	liver
bolus	mastication
cardiac sphincter	micelle
cecum	oral cavity
chyme	peristalsis
colon	peritoneum
defecation	pyloric sphincter
deglutition	pylorus
dentin	rectum
digestion	rugae
duodenum	saliva
dysphagia	salivation
emesis	sphincter
esophagus	tongue
feces	vermiform appendix
gallbladder	villi
gingiva	

ACRONYMS

ATP	CHO	LES

The body needs a constant supply of energy to perform its many tasks. You breathe, your heart beats, you talk, you laugh, and you move around. You can do all these things because your digestive system converts the food you eat into fuel for your body's energy demands.

The breakdown of food into usable materials for energy is called **digestion**. During digestion, food that is eaten is broken down into smaller elements. The process of transferring these food elements into the circulation for transport is called **absorption**. After absorption, the elements are carried to the body's cells to be used for energy. The physiology of digestion and absorption is discussed near the end of this chapter. The efficient food-processing machine responsible for digestion and absorption is called the digestive tract. It is also called the **alimentary canal**, *gastrointestinal (GI) tract*, and *GI system.*

The GI tract or canal is like a tube, approximately 30 feet (9.1 m) long; it runs through your body and is open to the outside at both ends (mouth and anus) (Fig. 26-1). The entire GI tract is lined with mucous membrane. Food travels through the GI tract in about 24 to 36 hours. The actions of the digestive system are subject to control by the nervous system. The endocrine system also plays a major part in the functioning of the GI system.

☛ KEY CONCEPT

Because the GI tract is open to the outside, and because you introduce non-sterile material into it (food), it is not considered sterile.

Elements that are broken down by digestion to provide fuel for the body are called *nutrients*. These nutrients are carbohydrates, proteins, and fats. They are made of carbon, hydrogen, and oxygen; proteins also contain nitrogen. Chapter 30 discusses the important role of these nutrients.

STRUCTURE AND FUNCTION

Figure 26-1 shows the major organs of the digestive system. Follow this illustration as you learn about the various functions of each organ.

The main function of the overall digestive system (Box 26-1) is to break down food into simpler forms that the circulatory vessels can carry and pass through the cell membranes to the cells. The cells then use these food molecules or nutrients for energy and to build, maintain, and repair body tissues.

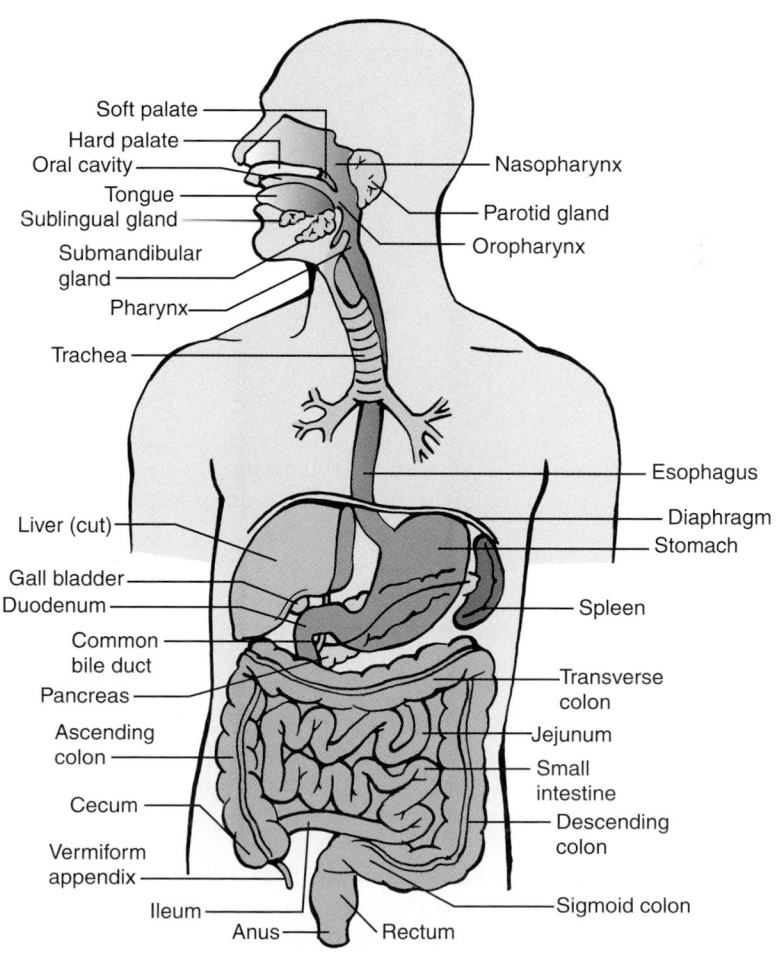

FIGURE 26-1. The digestive system.

➤➤ **BOX 26-1**

FUNCTIONS OF THE DIGESTIVE SYSTEM

Food Processing and Storage
- Breaks down food into smaller particles (mechanical digestion).
- Converts food into substances that can be absorbed (chemical digestion)
- Moves food materials through the gastrointestinal tract (peristalsis)
- Stores nutrients until needed

Manufacture
- Manufactures enzymes, hydrochloric acid, intrinsic factor, mucus, and other materials to assist in digestion
- Manufactures regulatory hormones in stomach
- Manufactures vitamin K and some B-complex vitamins in large intestine

Absorption
- Provides absorption of nutrients, mainly from small intestine, into capillaries

Reabsorption and Elimination
- Reabsorbs water for reuse by the body
- Reabsorbs minerals and vitamins
- Forms feces from remaining waste products
- Produces defecation

Mouth

The mouth is also called the **oral cavity.** Food is taken into the body through the mouth, where digestion begins. The teeth cut, chop, and grind food so that food particles become smaller and more of their surface can be exposed to the actions of digestive juices and enzymes. The mouth's chief digestive functions are to receive food via **ingestion** (to take in), to prepare food for digestion, and to begin the digestion of starch.

Palate

The roof of the mouth is made up of the hard and soft palates. The *hard palate* is close to the front of the mouth and is composed of the palatine bones and parts of the maxillary bones. The *soft palate* is mostly muscle tissue. It separates the mouth from the nasopharynx, which is the area of the pharynx behind the nose. The soft palate is shaped like an arch in the back of the mouth, and opens onto the oropharynx, the area of the pharynx behind the mouth. The structure that can be seen suspended in the back of the open mouth is the *uvula*. The *tongue* covers the floor of the mouth. The walls of the mouth cavity are the *cheeks* and the *teeth*.

Salivary Glands

Three pairs of salivary glands pour 1 to 1.5 liters of saliva into the mouth each day. The names of these glands indicate their locations: *sublingual* (under the tongue), *parotid* (cheek), and *submandibular* (under the lower jaw). The salivary glands are

exocrine glands because their secretions are not directly released into the circulation, but are released into the oral cavity. **Saliva** is a thin, watery fluid that contains *ptyalin,* also called *salivary amylase.* It also contains water, mucus, and salts. The nervous system controls the secretion of saliva (**salivation**).

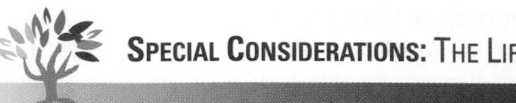

SPECIAL CONSIDERATIONS: THE LIFE SPAN

Prolapsed Glands

Prolapse of the submandibular glands may occur in older adults and could be mistaken for a tumor. Unlike tumors, however, these drooping submandibular glands feel soft and are seen on both sides of the neck.[1]

Saliva moistens food particles and makes food easier to swallow. Through the action of ptyalin, saliva begins to break down starch into smaller sugar molecules. Saliva helps prevent oral infections because it contains *lysozymes* (bacteriocidal enzymes) and immunoglobulins (IgA). The pH of saliva is normally between 6 and 7. Saliva also assists with speech and taste.

Teeth

The teeth are set in spaces or *sockets* in the upper and lower jaw bones: the *maxilla* and *mandible.* Humans have two sets of teeth: the *deciduous* ("falling out") or baby teeth, and a *permanent* or adult set (Fig. 26-2). A baby's deciduous teeth usually

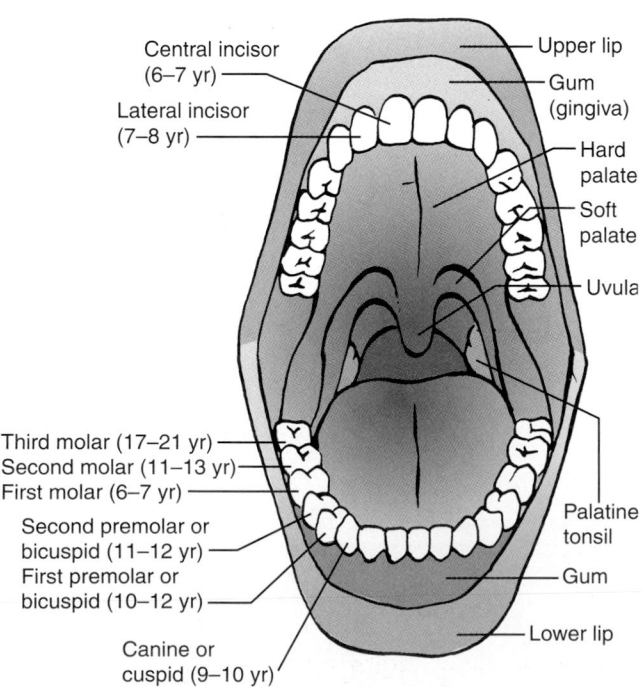

FIGURE 26-2. The mouth, showing the teeth and tonsils. Approximate ages for eruption of permanent teeth are shown.

begin to erupt between 6 and 8 months of age, and the 20 teeth are usually complete by 30 months of age (see Fig. 10-3 in Chap. 10). At the age of about 6 years, children's permanent teeth begin to appear. As the permanent teeth grow in, they push out the deciduous teeth, replace them, and fill in the spaces in the jaw. The permanent set has 32 teeth. The chief function of teeth is to break food into small particles, which is accomplished through **mastication,** or the act of chewing.

Types and Locations

The teeth are named and located as follows:

- The *incisors* are the front teeth. They cut and tear food.
- The *canines* or *cuspids* are the side teeth. They hold and tear food.
- The *bicuspids (premolars)* and the *molars* crush and grind food.
- The last permanent teeth, the *wisdom teeth,* sometimes do not appear before adulthood. They are located in the far back of the mouth. If a person's jaws are small and jaw space limited, the wisdom teeth may not have room to erupt and may become *impacted* in the tissue. Impacted wisdom teeth may require surgical removal.

Parts

A tooth has three parts: crown, neck, and root. The *crown* is the enamel-covered part of the tooth visible in the mouth. (Tooth enamel is the hardest structure in the body.) The tooth narrows into a *neck* at the gumline. (The *gum* is also known as the **gingiva.**) The *root* of the tooth is in the bony socket. A substance called *cement* (or *cementum*) covers the root. Beneath the enamel and the cement is a hard bonelike substance called **dentin,** which is the bulk of tooth material. The tooth's center is the *pulp cavity.* The *pulp* contains many nerve endings and blood vessels, which enter through the roots (via the root canal) from the tooth sockets. The teeth are embedded in and nourished by bone. See Figure 26-3 for a diagram of a tooth.

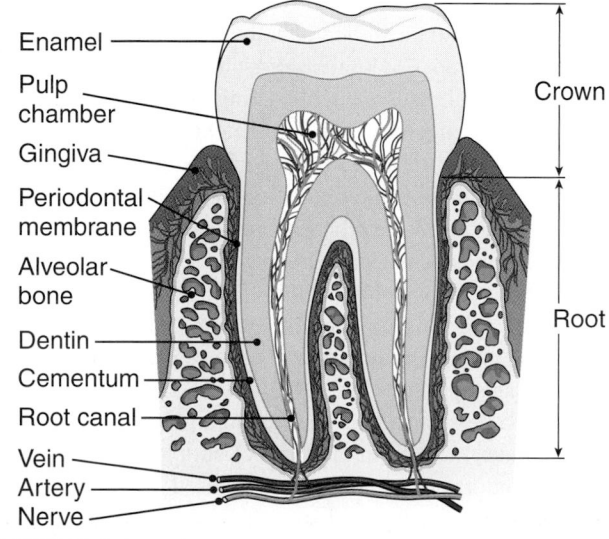

Enamel
Pulp chamber
Gingiva
Periodontal membrane
Alveolar bone
Dentin
Cementum
Root canal
Vein
Artery
Nerve

Crown
Root

FIGURE 26-3. A tooth.

☞ KEY CONCEPT

When tooth decay is so advanced that it permanently damages the pulp, a root canal procedure or removal of the tooth (extraction) is required.

Tongue

The **tongue** is a tough skeletal muscle covered with mucous membrane. It is attached to four bones: the mandible, two temporal bones, and the hyoid. On the bottom of the tongue is a fold of mucous membrane called the *frenulum.* This structure helps to attach the tongue to the floor of the mouth.

☞ KEY CONCEPT

In some cases, the frenulum is short or too tightly attached. This makes speech difficult, and the person is said to be "tongue-tied." This situation can be surgically corrected.

The tongue has several functions. It senses the temperature and the texture of food. It mixes food with saliva, and moves food into position to be chewed. The voluntary movement of the tongue begins the swallowing process, called **deglutition,** by pushing food into the pharynx, the next portion of the digestive tube.

The upper surface of the tongue appears rough because of visible indentations (*fissures*) and projections (*papillae*). The taste buds are microscopic nipple-like projections located on the sides of the papillae. They are specialized nerve endings that allow detection of various flavors. Chapter 21 discusses the structures of the tongue and the location of taste buds.

The taste buds distinguish among flavors. Although all types of taste buds are found on most areas of the tongue, they are concentrated as follows: salty (tip and sides of the tongue), bitter (back of the tongue), sweet (tip of tongue), and sour (sides of tongue). Alkaline and metallic flavors are sometimes considered distinct flavors as well. Remember that a person's ability to taste food also depends on the sense of smell. Smoking decreases both taste and smell.

Pharynx

The tongue lifts the ball of food that has mixed with saliva. This ball is called a **bolus,** meaning *lump.* The initial swallowing of food is a voluntary action. The tongue pushes the bolus into the muscular tube behind the mouth called the *pharynx,* where the movement of food becomes involuntary. (The epiglottis covers the larynx and prevents food from entering the respiratory tract.) Contractions of the pharynx continue the act of swallowing, and push food into the muscular *esophagus.* The pharynx is lined with mucous membrane. Smooth or involuntary muscles pass food along by waves of contractions called **peristalsis,** an alternating relaxation and contraction of muscles that sends food through the digestive tube.

☞ KEY CONCEPT

*The medical term for difficulty in swallowing is **dysphagia**.*

Esophagus

The **esophagus,** or *gullet,* is approximately 10 inches (25.4 cm) in length; it extends from the pharynx into the neck and thorax and, through an opening in the diaphragm, to the stomach. It is also lined with mucous membrane. The role of the esophagus in digestion is to serve as a passageway. A muscle located between the esophagus and the stomach is called the **cardiac sphincter** or *lower esophageal sphincter* (**LES**). Sometimes this muscle is called the *gastroesophageal sphincter.* This sphincter guards the opening of the stomach by preventing food from reentering into the esophagus. A **sphincter** is a circular muscle. As waves of peristalsis push food through the lower esophagus, the cardiac sphincter or LES opens (allowing food to enter) and closes (to keep food in the stomach).

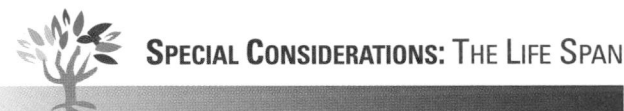

Nursing Alert

- If the lower esophageal sphincter (LES) does not relax as it should, food can be prevented from entering the stomach. This condition is known as *achalasia.*
- If the lower esophageal sphincter (LES) does not close adequately, the contents of the stomach can reenter the esophagus. The stomach contents contain gastric juices that are acidic. When these substances reenter the esophagus, a burning sensation can result. This condition is known as *heartburn.* If this reflux of acid continues, it can lead to esophageal or gastric (stomach) ulcers. *Acid reflux* can sometimes be successfully treated with medications and specific lifestyle changes.

SPECIAL CONSIDERATIONS: THE LIFE SPAN

The GI system is immature in an infant. Therefore, regurgitation ("spitting-up") of feedings (breast milk or formula) is common. This immaturity gradually improves and usually resolves around 3 months of age.

Stomach

The stomach is a muscular, collapsible pouch or sac capable of being greatly distended (expanded). It is located in the upper left side of the abdominal cavity, and receives its blood supply from the celiac artery. The rounded portion above the level of the cardiac sphincter, containing the opening from the esophagus, is called the *fundus.* The central and largest portion is called the *body;* the lower narrow portion, which attaches to the small intestine, is called the **pylorus.** The **pyloric sphincter** controls the opening between the stomach and the duodenal portion of the small intestine. (The prefix referring to the stomach is *gastr[o]-.*)

The strong walls of the stomach consist of three layers of smooth muscle: a circular layer, a longitudinal layer (muscle

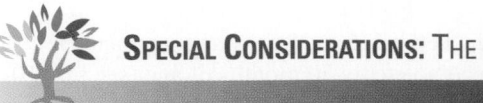

SPECIAL CONSIDERATIONS: THE LIFE SPAN

In infants, projectile vomiting (vomiting with great force) can be a sign of *pyloric stenosis* (a narrowing of the pyloric sphincter).

fibers going the long way), and an oblique layer (muscle fibers on a slant or an angle). This spread of muscles in all directions allows much motion for stirring and churning food and breaking it into small particles. When the stomach is empty, it collapses and lies in folds called **rugae.** These rugae allow the stomach to distend greatly when food is eaten. Figure 26-4 shows the stomach and a portion of the duodenum.

In the stomach, all foods mix with gastric juices and churn until they are in a semi-liquid form called **chyme.** This process usually takes 3 to 5 hours. Peristalsis of the stomach's smooth muscles normally moves food toward the pyloric outlet. The pyloric sphincter at the lower opening of the stomach contracts to keep the food in the stomach until it is thoroughly mixed. The sphincter then relaxes to let peristaltic waves push food in small amounts into the small intestine.

If the stomach is irritated or too full, sometimes the direction of the waves of peristalsis reverses and forces material back into the lower end of the esophagus. Reverse peristalsis within the stomach, combined with contractions of abdominal muscles and the diaphragm, forces food back through the esophagus and out through the mouth, causing vomiting (**emesis**).

Small Intestine

The small intestine is the longest part of the digestive tract, approximately 20 feet (6.1 m) long and 1.5 inches (3.81 cm) in diameter. It lies coiled on itself in the abdominal cavity. This allows the organ to fit in the abdominal cavity. It is about 18 feet longer than the large intestine, which follows it. (The prefix referring to the intestines is *enter[o]-.*) The small intestine is divided into the *duodenum,* the *jejunum,* and the *ileum.* Food elements move from the stomach through the three divisions of the small intestine while being altered by a variety of secretions and enzymes. The movement of these substances through the small intestine is by peristalsis, rhythmic waves that cause contraction and relaxation of smooth muscle.

Most of the digestive processes occur in the small intestine. Intestinal glands here secrete enzymes for the digestion of all foods. These enzymes are proteins that act as *catalysts,* promoting and speeding up chemical reactions, but not actually undergoing changes themselves. The intestinal enzymes break carbohydrates, proteins, and fats into materials that the cells can use. To be absorbed by the blood and lymph capillaries, carbohydrates must be in the form of simple sugars: glucose, fructose, and galactose. Before being used by the body, proteins must also be digested into their simplest state; amino acids and fats must be converted to fatty acids and glycerol.

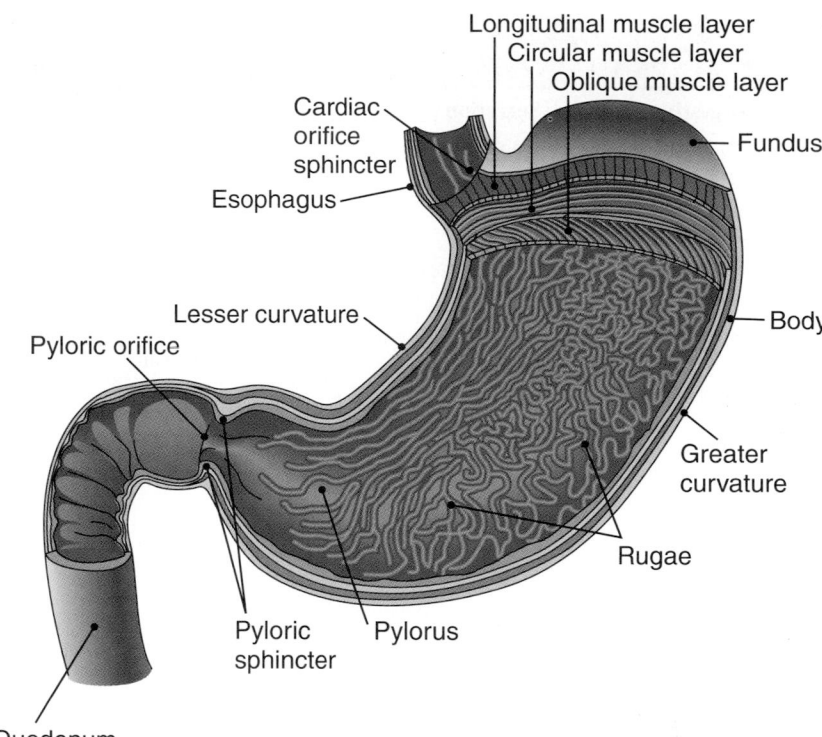

FIGURE 26-4. Longitudinal section of the stomach and a portion of the duodenum. Rugae and the three muscular layers are shown.

☞ KEY CONCEPT

Very few chemical reactions in the body can occur without catalysts. Each enzyme facilities specific chemical reactions.

The small intestine has numerous secretions, not just enzymes. *Mucus* lubricates and protects the intestinal wall lining from the highly acidic chyme and digestive enzymes. *Cholecystokinin* is a secreted hormone that stimulates the pancreas to secrete pancreatic juice, and the gallbladder to contract, resulting in the release of bile. *Secretin* is another hormone that influences the secretion of pancreatic juice by the pancreas. This juice contains bicarbonate ions (HCO_3^-). Sodium bicar-

bonate ($NaHCO_3$), a chemical compound formed by the sodium ion (Na^+) and the bicarbonate ion (HCO_3^-), is a basic (alkali) substance in the body. It helps to neutralize the very acidic chyme (Table 26-1).

Duodenum

The first portion of the small intestine is the 10- to 12-inch C-shaped **duodenum** (see Fig. 26-4). The duodenal wall contains specialized cells and glands designed to secrete mucus. This mucus protects the small intestine from the strongly acidic chyme, which enters from the stomach. As chyme enters the duodenum, more digestive juices are added. **Bile,** a greenish brown liquid manufactured by the liver and stored in the gall-

■■ **TABLE 26-1** 𝓔**NZYMES AND THEIR ACTIONS**

Area of Digestive System	Secretion	Enzyme	Action
Mouth			
Salivary glands	Saliva (also contains water, mucus, and salts)	Salivary amylase (ptyalin)	Begins to break down starch (CHO) into simpler carbohydrates, such as dextrin Assists swallowing Softens and lubricates food Dissolves some food components
Stomach			
Stomach lining	Mucus		Protects lining
	Mucin		Strongly stimulates secretion of gastric acid (HCl) and pepsin
Specialized cells of pyloric glands	Gastrin (regulatory hormone)		Weakly stimulates secretion of pancreatic enzymes and contraction of gallbladder

(continued)

■■■ **TABLE 26-1** ℰ**NZYMES AND THEIR ACTIONS (CONTINUED)**

Area of Digestive System	Secretion	Enzyme	Action
Parietal cells	Hydrochloric acid (HCl)		Hydrolyzes some CHO into glucose and fructose Destroys microorganisms Changes pepsinogen to pepsin
	Intrinsic factor		Needed for absorption of vitamin B_{12}, which is needed for development of RBCs
Chief cells	Pepsinogen	Pepsin	Begins digestion of proteins into polypeptides
	Gastric lipase	Lipase	Begins digestion of fats by breaking down triglycerides (very little occurs in stomach); acts only on emulsified fats
Kidney (juxtaglomerular cells)		Renin	Regulates blood pressure
Liver	Bile		Emulsifies fats stored in gallbladder
Pancreas Acinar cells (exocrine function)	Pancreatic juice	Amylase Lipase Trypsin Chymotrypsin Carboxypeptidase Bicarbonate ions	Act in small intestine to digest proteins, carbohydrates, and fats Helps neutralize chyme Provides proper pH for enzymes
Pancreas (endocrine function)	Insulin (hormone) Glucagon (hormone)		Enables cells to use glucose Elevates blood sugar levels
Small Intestine Duodenum and jejunum	Cholecystokinin (hormone secreted in response to presence of fat) Secretin (hormone)		Activates gallbladder to release bile Stimulates pancreas to secrete pancreatic juice Inhibits stomach digestion Stimulates secretion of bicarbonate ions from pancreas
	Receives bile *from* gallbladder		Breaks fats into tiny droplets (emulsification)
	Receives pancreatic juice *from* pancreas	Pancreatic protease (trypsin)	Split proteins into amino acids
		Chymotrypsin	More complex proteins broken down in intestine and at brush border
		Carboxypeptidase	Stimulates release of water and HCO_3^- from pancreas
		Pancreatic amylase (and intestinal amylase)	Converts complex CHO into maltose and isomaltose
		Pancreatic lipase	Breaks down emulsified fat into fatty acids, glycerol, and mono-glycerides
		Intestinal lipase	Completes digestion of mono-glycerides
		Sucrase	Breaks sucrose into fructose and glucose
Intestinal wall mucosa		Maltase	Breaks maltose into glucose
		Lactase	Breaks lactose into galactose and glucose
		Amylase	Converts CHO to maltose
		Protein enzymes (peptidases)	Assist in digestion of proteins

The
the live
known
manufa
join to
it flow
the gal

As
activat
gallbla
up wit
comm
then er
(a sma
(see F

Panc
The p
6 inch
26-5).
exocri
insuli
sugar
pancro
The ao

• A
• ‐
• I

Mo
and a
help t
tion to
atic ju
ions (
HCO
zyme
Pa
atic d
quate

Peri
The ‖
cover
organ
betw
that ‖
mese
Som
omer
behir
allov
natir

SY:
Pro

For
ken

bladder, pours in through the *common bile duct* to emulsify fats in preparation for further digestive action.

Jejunum and Ileum
Chyme travels through the remaining portions of the small intestine, the **jejunum** (about 8 ft long), and the *ileum* (about 11 ft long). (The word *jejunum* derives from a Latin word meaning "fasting intestine"; it has been so named because, when dissected, the jejunum is almost always empty. The word ileum means "flank" or "groin.") The entire small intestine is lined with mucous membrane. Numerous lymph nodules are in the ileum, both solitary and grouped. Those grouped together are called *aggregated lymphatic follicles* or *Peyer's patches.*

A sphincter-like muscle, located where the large and small intestines meet, acts as a valve to prevent backflow of material to the small intestine; it also regulates the forward flow. This muscle is called the *ileocecal valve,* from the names of the two joining parts: the *ileum* of the small intestine and the *cecum* of the large intestine.

Large Intestine
The large intestine, like the remainder of the GI tract, is lined with mucous membrane. The large intestine is much wider than the small intestine (its diameter is approximately 2.5 inches, or 6.35 cm), but it is only about 5 feet (1.5 m) long. It does not coil, but lies in folds, and is divided into different areas called the *cecum, colon,* and *rectum.* Water reabsorption is the large intestine's main function. Intestinal bacteria function to inhibit the growth of pathogens in the large intestine and some produce vitamin K, which is necessary for blood clotting. Absorption of vitamins and minerals and the formation of feces are also functions of the large intestine.

Cecum and Appendix
The first portion of the large intestine is the **cecum,** a blind pouch about 2 to 3 inches (5 to 7.6 cm) long. A small finger-like projection of the cecum is the **vermiform** (worm-shaped) **appendix,** also known simply as the **appendix,** which has no known function. (The word *appendix* derives from the Latin word meaning "appendage.") It has the same lymphoid tissue as tonsils and like the tonsils, it frequently becomes infected, a condition called *appendicitis.* (It is prone to infection because fecal material that enters cannot always drain out.) The cecum and appendix are located in the right lower quadrant of the abdominal cavity (see Fig. 26-1).

Colon
The next and longest portion of the large intestine is the **colon,** a continuous tube divided into three parts, which take their names from the course they follow. The *ascending* (going up) *colon* travels up the right side of the abdominal cavity; the *transverse* (going across) *colon* crosses to the left side in the upper part of the cavity; the *descending* (going down) *colon* goes down the left side into the pelvis. The next and last portion, which is called the *sigmoid* (*sigma* is the Greek letter S) *colon,* ends at the rectum. Figure 26-1 illustrates the colon.

Rectum and Anus
The **rectum** is about 5 inches (12.7 cm) in length and terminates at the anal canal, which is the terminal (end) portion of the large intestine and is about 1 to 1.5 inches long (2.54 to 3.8 cm). Its opening to the outside (*anus*) is guarded by internal and external sphincter muscles. The external sphincter is under a person's control and can be consciously contracted and relaxed.

☛ KEY CONCEPT

The pathway of food materials through the body is as follows: mouth → pharynx → esophagus → (cardiac sphincter) → stomach → (pyloric sphincter) → small intestine (duodenum → jejunum → ileum) → (ileocecal valve) → large intestine (cecum → colon: ascending, transverse, descending, sigmoid → rectum) → anus.

Accessory Organs
Accessory organs of the digestive system include the liver, gallbladder, pancreas, and peritoneum. Figure 26-5 shows the accessory organs of digestion.

Liver
The **liver** is the body's largest glandular organ and lies just below the diaphragm in the upper right quadrant of the abdominal cavity (see Fig. 26-5). It receives its blood supply from the hepatic artery and is divided into two major and two minor lobes. (The prefix referring to the liver is *hepat[o]-.*) In humans, the liver weighs about 3 pounds (1.36 kg) and resembles calf liver in color and texture.

The liver plays such an important part in overall bodily functions that one cannot live long if it is severely diseased or injured. Only the brain is capable of more functions than the liver. Some of the liver's main functions include:

- Absorption of bilirubin from the destruction of old RBCs
- Detoxification of blood (removal of toxins or poisons)
- Storage of fat-soluble vitamins (vitamins A, D, E, K) and iron
- Formation of vitamin A; storage of vitamin B complex
- Formation of plasma proteins (albumin, prothrombin, globulins)
- Synthesis of urea, which is a waste product from proteins
- Storage of glucose in a form called *glycogen*
- Synthesis of clotting factors (fibrinogen; prothrombin; factors V, VII, IX, X)
- Formation of triglycerides and cholesterol
- Secretion of bile
- Secretion of heparin (anticoagulant)
- Synthesis of immunoglobulins
- Breaking down of fats
- Storage of fat and carbohydrates
- Regulation of amino acids
- Production of body heat
- Storage of minerals

TABLE 27-2 *Effects of Aging on the Urinary System (Continued)*

Factor	Result	Nursing Implications
The bladder lining becomes fibrotic, and muscles weaken in the ureters and bladder.	Decreases capacity of bladder to about 200 mL, causing urinary frequency and incontinence Loss of muscle tone, causing bladder to retain urine because it cannot empty completely; loss of tone, causing nocturia or incontinence	Allow for frequent bathroom visits. Make available devices or pads to absorb leaks for ambulatory clients. Watch for bladder infection and urinary retention. Allow 3 h between administration of last evening fluids and bedtime. Do not use evening fluids that stimulate voiding (eg, coffee, tea, colas, alcohol). Make bathroom and bedroom safe for nighttime visits—move obstacles, keep a night light on.
Cancer or benign hypertrophy of the prostate is common in men.	Frequent urge to void Retention of urine Sexual dysfunction	Encourage frequent testicular self-exam. Encourage medical evaluation.
Pelvic muscles weaken and relax in women due to decreased levels of estrogen and perinatal trauma from childbirth	Incontinence Uterine or bladder prolapse Bladder infections common	Instruct in pelvic exercises. Do not use incontinence pads for clients confined to bed (to prevent pressure ulcers). Offer bedpan or assist client to bathroom q2h. Provide adult incontinence pads for ambulatory clients. Assess symptoms of bladder infections. Teach proper feminine hygiene.

products (urea, creatinine, and uric acid). Drugs may reach toxic levels in the kidneys because they are not adequately filtered. Secretion and removal of substances such as ammonia are not as efficient. The threshold for glucose decreases, and higher blood sugar levels may be noted.

The bladder of the older adult has a smaller capacity; therefore, *urinary frequency* (inability to wait) and **nocturia** (waking up to void at night) are common. The bladder muscles become weaker, leading to *urinary retention* (abnormal holding), dribbling, and *stress incontinence* (involuntary voiding on actions such as sneezing or coughing). Incontinence may need medical evaluation. Enlargement of the prostate (see Chap. 28) may also cause urinary difficulties in older men.

Chapter 88 describes urinary disorders in more detail. Chapter 89 describes male urinary disorders in conjunction with the discussion of reproductive disorders.

➜ STUDENT SYNTHESIS

Key Points

- The urinary system eliminates wastes, controls water volume, regulates electrolyte levels, maintains pH balance, activates vitamin D, secretes renin and erythropoietin, and helps to regulate blood pressure.
- The kidneys lie behind the peritoneum (they are retroperitoneal).
- Nephrons are the functional units of kidneys. Nephrons formulate urine; the rest of the urinary system expels it.
- Nephrons consist of renal corpuscles (glomerulus, Bowman's capsule) and renal tubules (proximal convoluted tubule, loop of Henle, distal convoluted tubule).
- Urine is 95% water and 5% solutes (salts, nitrogenous waste products, metabolites, hormones, toxins).
- Urine is formed by three processes: glomerular filtration, tubular reabsorption, and tubular secretion. In addition, ADH assists in the regulation of water balance in the kidneys to maintain the body's homeostasis.
- Micturition (voiding) is the release of urine; involuntary voiding is called urinary incontinence.
- As the body ages, the number of functional nephrons decreases.

Critical Thinking Exercises

1. Based on the discussion of anatomy in this chapter, explain whether you believe men or women have a higher incidence of urinary tract infections. Give reasons for your answer.
2. Annie, a 65-year-old woman, comes to the health-care facility concerned. She has noticed that she is

waking up during the night to urinate. A few times she has been unable to control her bladder. What information would you give Annie to address her concerns?
3. Discuss why an adequate intake of water is essential to proper functioning of the urinary system.

NCLEX-Style Review Questions

1. Which two hormones does the kidney produce?
   a. Antidiuretic hormone and atrial natriuretic peptide
   b. Atrial natriuretic peptide and erythropoietin
   c. Erythropoietin and aldosterone
   d. Renin and erythropoietin

2. How much urine is excreted daily?
   a. 250–400 mL
   b. 500 mL
   c. 1,000–1,500 mL
   d. 2,000 mL
3. Due to smaller bladder capacity, older adults frequently experience:
   a. Micturition
   b. Nocturia
   c. Stasis
   d. Tubular resorption

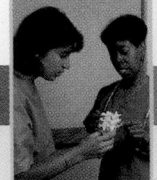

CHAPTER

28

The Male Reproductive System

LEARNING OBJECTIVES

1. Name the three major classifications of hormones that influence the male reproductive system and state their functions.
2. Identify the testes, penis, and scrotum of the male reproductive system and discuss their functions.
3. Discuss the role of the epididymis, ductus deferens, and ejaculatory duct in the male reproductive system.
4. Describe how sperm migrate through the reproductive system.
5. Describe the components of ejaculatory fluid and their sources.
6. Explain how ejaculatory fluid is deposited into the vagina for reproductive purposes.
7. State two effects of aging on the male reproductive system.

NEW TERMINOLOGY

androgen
bulbourethral (Cowper's) gland
circumcision
climacteric
copulation
ductus deferens
ejaculation
epididymis
erection
foreskin
gamete
glans penis
gonad

interstitial cells
nocturnal emission
orgasm
penis
perineum
prostate
puberty
scrotum
semen
seminal vesicle
seminiferous tubule
spermatozoa
testes
testosterone

The previous systems you have studied in this unit have focused on sustaining the individual. The *reproductive systems* work distinctly to continue the species and to pass genetic information from parents to child. Unlike other body systems that are generally similar for both sexes, the reproductive system in adult males is very different from that in women. This chapter examines the male reproductive system. Chapter 29 discusses the female reproductive system.

Sexual reproduction involves the combined effort of both internal organs and external structures. Keep in mind that sexual reproduction is a dependent process that involves the reproductive systems of both the man and the woman.

STRUCTURE AND FUNCTION

The organs of the male reproductive system function to produce and transport sperm (Box 28-1). Keep in mind that a man's reproductive capacity is directly associated with sexual excitement, penile erection, and ejaculation. A woman's ability to reproduce does not depend on sexual excitement because conception can occur through mechanical means (eg, artificial insemination). Sexual pleasure, however, is equally important for both men and women.

The *male reproductive system* consists of the testes, ductal system, scrotum, penis, and accessory glands. *Internal structures* include the testes (produce sperm), ducts (transport sperm), and the glands (produce secretions). The *external structures* of the male reproductive system are the penis and the scrotum. The area between the scrotum and the anus is called the **perineum.** Fig. 28-1 illustrates the male reproductive structures.

Testes

The paired **testes** (singular: testis) are also known as the *testicles.* They produce **spermatozoa** (sperm cells) and secrete sex hormones. (The combining forms for testis in medical terms are orcho/o, orchi/o, and orchid/o.)

In the adult man, the testes are two almond-shaped glands, one on each side of the scrotum (described later in this chapter). The testes are small, approximately 1.5 to 2 inches (3.7 to 5 cm) long, and 1 inch (2.5 cm) wide and thick. Tissue layers,

➤ BOX 28-1

FUNCTIONS OF THE MALE REPRODUCTIVE SYSTEM

Development of Sexual Characteristics
• Secretes hormones that initiate puberty
• Maintains specific male characteristics
• Secretes mucus, spermatic fluid, and other substances

Reproduction
• Produces sperm
• Passes genetic information to infants
• Participates in copulation and fertilization

one of which partitions the testis into 250 to 300 wedge-shaped lobules, cover each testis. Each lobule contains the functional units of the testis, which are called the **seminiferous tubules.** Each seminiferous tubule is tightly convoluted. The combined length of a man's seminiferous tubules is about half a mile! Within these tubules, the sperm cells are produced and mature. Between the tubules are small clusters of specialized endocrine cells, called **interstitial cells,** which secrete *testosterone* and other *androgens* (male hormones). These cells lining the tubules produce sperm also.

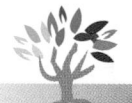

SPECIAL CONSIDERATIONS: THE LIFE SPAN

Nocturnal Emissions

Pubescent boys may experience penile erection and spontaneous ejaculation of semen during sleep. These **nocturnal emissions** are normal and are thought to be caused by hormonal changes.

The Ductal System

The male reproductive organs have a system of ducts that store and transport sperm from the testicles to the urethra. These ducts include the paired epididymides (singular: **epididymis**), the ductus deferentia (singular: ductus deferens), and the ejaculatory ducts.

Epididymis

The *epididymis* (plural: epididymides) is a long, comma-shaped organ attached to the posterior surface of the testis. This tightly coiled tube is approximately 20 feet (6 m) long, but is so tiny that it can barely be seen with the naked eye. Within the epididymis, millions of sperm cells are in their final stages of maturation. Sperm cells are unable to fertilize an egg unless they mature in the epididymis. Smooth muscles propel sperm into the ductus deferens.

Ductus Deferens

The sperm continue their journey through a tube called the *vas deferens* or **ductus deferens** (plural: ductus deferentia), which is about 18 inches (45 cm) long. It transports sperm from the epididymis to the ejaculatory duct. The ductus deferens passes upwards posterior to the testis, then through the inguinal canal, which lies in the muscles of the abdominal wall. The ductus then enters the abdominal cavity and continues over the top and down the posterior surface of the urinary bladder, into the pelvic cavity. Peristaltic contractions propel sperm cells through the ductus. Each ductus deferens joins a duct from the seminal vesicles. These ducts, together with blood vessels, lymphatic vessels, nerves, and connective tissue coverings, make up the *spermatic cord.* The spermatic cord is covered with connective tissue.

The spermatic cord passes through an opening in the muscular abdominal wall called the *inguinal canal.* Normally the

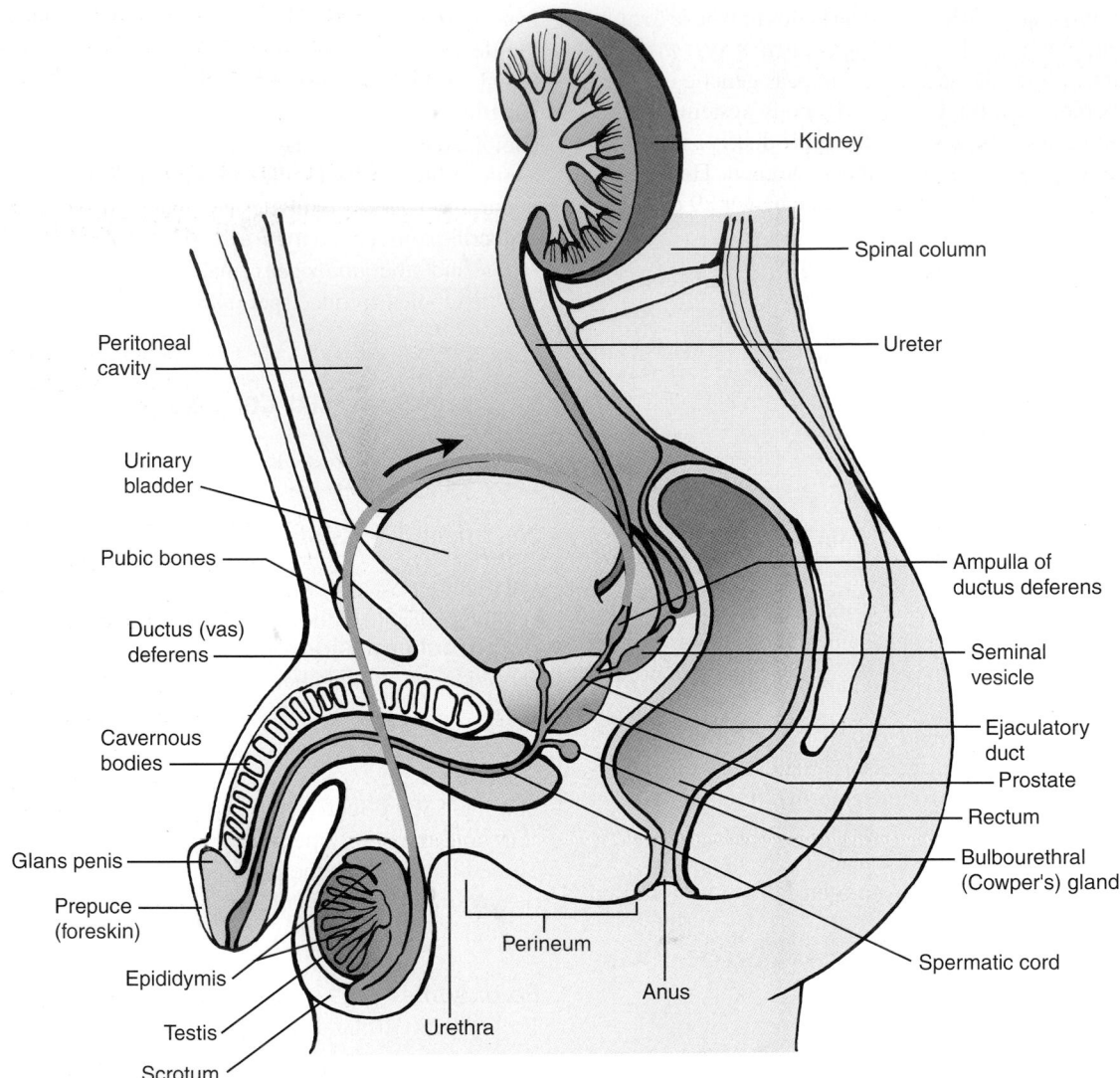

FIGURE 28-1. Organs of the male reproductive system, showing one testis. The *arrow* indicates the course of sperm cells through the duct system.

inguinal canal firmly encloses the spermatic cord as it passes through the abdominal wall. It is a weak spot, however, and a common site for herniation in men (*inguinal hernia*). It is also the site where the testicles descend into the scrotum before birth.

☛ KEY CONCEPT

It is the two vas deferens *or* ductus deferentia *which are ligated (tied) and cut in the male sterilization procedure, called* vasectomy. *This operation does not affect erection or ejaculation.*

Ejaculatory Ducts

The *ejaculatory ducts* are about 1 inch (2 cm) long. Each one originates where the ampulla of the ductus deferens joins the duct from the seminal vesicle (see Fig. 28-1). The ejaculatory ducts empty into the urethra. The ejaculatory ducts also receive

secretions from the prostate gland. (The semen, mixed with various secretions, is called ejaculatory fluid.)

Scrotum

The testes are enclosed in a saclike structure called the **scrotum,** which is suspended behind the base of the penis. The scrotum supports and protects the testes. The external appearance of the scrotum varies, depending on environmental conditions and the contraction of its attached muscles. The muscles involuntarily contract and bring the testicles closer to the body as external temperature lowers. Temperature of the testes (35° C or 95° F) is lower than internal body temperature. This temperature is maintained to facilitate sperm production.

Penis

The **penis** is a cylindrical organ located immediately in front of the scrotum. It is composed of three masses of cavernous

Nursing Alert

Exposure to increased temperature over a period of time can impair *spermatogenesis* (sperm production) in the testes. It is also thought that wearing tight-fitting undergarments might contribute to infertility and decreased numbers of sperm, due to the close contact of the scrotum with the rest of the body.

(erectile) tissue, each of which contains smooth muscle, connective tissue, and blood sinuses (large vascular channels). When blood flow through these sinuses is minimal, the penis is soft and flaccid. At the time of sexual excitement, blood fills the sinuses and the penis becomes firm and erect. The firm penis is called an **erection.** The erect penis is capable of penetrating the vagina to deposit sperm.

The smooth cap of the penis is called the **glans penis** and is covered by a fold of loose skin that forms the hoodlike **foreskin** (*prepuce*). Surgical removal of this foreskin, called **circumcision,** is sometimes performed on male babies (see Chap. 66).

The urethra within the penis serves as a common passageway for both the urinary and reproductive systems. (Urine and ejaculatory fluid do not pass through the urethra simultaneously.) An involuntary sphincter located at the base of the bladder automatically inhibits micturition during semen ejaculation.[1]

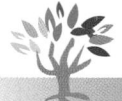

SPECIAL CONSIDERATIONS: THE LIFE SPAN

Undescended Testes

Undescended testes (*cryptorchidism*) can occur in infants. This is a situation in which the testes do not move down into the scrotal sac. It occurs more often in premature infants, but can occur in up to 4% of term infants. Undescended testes can increase the temperature in the testes, which could result in decreased sperm production. Therefore, documentation of the presence of undescended or descended testes is important for all male infants.

Accessory Glands

Seminal Vesicles

The two **seminal vesicles** are convoluted, sac-shaped glands about 2 inches (5 cm) long, which are located posterior to the urinary bladder. They secrete a sticky, alkaline, yellowish substance, called **semen,** which serves as a fluid medium for sperm. Seminal vesicles secrete about 60% of all of a man's semen. The secretion contains many nutrients, citric acid, coagulation proteins, and prostaglandins.

Prostate Gland

The **prostate** is a doughnut-shaped muscular gland lying just below the bladder. It surrounds the neck of the urethra as the urethra emerges from the bladder (see Fig. 28-1). The glandu-

lar tissue adds an alkaline secretion to semen, which increases sperm motility. The muscular portion of the prostate contracts during ejaculation to expel semen from the urethra.

SPECIAL CONSIDERATIONS: THE LIFE SPAN

Prostate Removal

Some men are unable to have an erection or to ejaculate after prostate removal because of tissue damage or because too much muscle tissue had to be removed.

Bulbourethral Glands

The **bulbourethral (Cowper's) glands** are located below the prostate glands. They are approximately the size of a pea and secrete an alkaline mucus into tiny ducts, which empty into the urethra. This mucus coats the urethra to neutralize the pH of urine residue; it also lubricates the penis.

Sperm survive better in an alkaline medium than in an acid medium. Alkalinity helps maintain sperm motility. A woman's vagina is acidic because of its normal flora (natural bacterial population). The alkaline environment of seminal fluid helps to neutralize the acidic vaginal pH and to maintain sperm motility.

HORMONAL INFLUENCES

The male reproductive system develops during childhood and adolescence. It does not become functional until hormones act on it during **puberty** (or *pubescence*), the stage of life during which the reproductive organs become fully functional (see Chap. 11). In boys, puberty occurs around 12 to 16 years of age, although variations exist.

Hormones from the hypothalamus, the pituitary gland, and the gonads influence the reproductive system. Before puberty (*prepubescence*), the blood concentration of **androgens** (male hormones) and *estrogens* (female hormones) are the same in every person. When a boy reaches puberty, the hypothalamus stimulates the secretion of both interstitial cell-stimulating hormone (ICSH) and follicle-stimulating hormone (FSH) from the anterior pituitary (see Chap. 20). As a result, the organs of the reproductive system (genitals) begin to function, and secondary sex characteristics appear. ICSH and FSH are gonadotropic hormones. In the man, these hormones have two main effects:

- They stimulate the **gonads** (sex glands) to secrete hormones.
- FSH stimulates the formation of sperm.

The major androgen is **testosterone.** ICHS stimulates the production of testosterone. During puberty, male glandular development becomes very active. The pubescent boy begins to develop a beard, and pubic and axillary hair. He notices an increase in hair growth all over his body. Musculature develops. His body becomes broader in the shoulders and remains narrow in the hips. His voice deepens. These are called *secondary sexual characteristics.* Testosterone also maintains the functioning of male accessory organs and stimulates protein anabolism. As a result, a man has larger and stronger musculature than a woman.

SYSTEM PHYSIOLOGY

Sperm Cells and Spermatogenesis

Beginning when a male is around 13 years old, and continuing throughout life, the male gonads, stimulated by testosterone, form sperm cells. The sperm cell is the male **gamete,** one of two cells that must unite to initiate development of a new individual. This formation of mature and functional spermatozoa is called *spermatogenesis.* Normal spermatogenesis does not occur if the testes are too warm or too cold (above or below 35° C [95° F]).

> ### Nursing Alert
>
> Certain illnesses, notably mumps, can cause reproductive difficulties in males. About one third of males who contract mumps after puberty develop *orchitis* (inflammation of the testes). This often results in sterility, emphasizing the need for immunization of infants against mumps.

The stem cells of sperm cell development are called *spermatogonia.* Spermatogonia divide by mitosis and then meiosis to form *spermatocytes* (see Chap. 15). The next form is called *spermatids,* which eventually develop into *spermatozoa.* The testes produce millions of spermatozoa each day. It takes about 2 months for sperm cells to mature until they are stored in the ductus deferens.

Sperm cells are highly specialized and are made up of several divisions (Fig. 28-2). The *head* contains 23 chromosomes. The tip of the head, the *acrosome,* contains enzymes that can dissolve the tough cell wall of the ovum (the female sex cell). The *body* (middle piece) contains mitochondria, which provide the energy necessary for locomotion. The whiplike *tail* is a flagellum that propels the sperm with a lashing motion.

After sperm and semen combine in the ejaculatory duct, semen (now also known as *ejaculatory fluid*) contains about 60 to 100 million sperm cells per milliliter. Semen with a sperm count of less than 10 to 20 million per milliliter may have difficulty fertilizing an ovum.

The amount of semen each man ejaculates (expels from the body) varies from 2 to 5 milliliters. After ejaculation into a woman's vagina, a sperm can survive up to 3 days. Of the average 250 million sperm cells ejaculated, only about 100 survive to contact the ovum in the oviduct. Under normal conditions, only one sperm fertilizes the ovum.

☛ KEY CONCEPT
_____

Sperm have 23 chromosomes. Sperm can live for a maximum of three days after ejaculation.

Copulation

Sexual intercourse or sexual union between a man and a woman is called **copulation,** *intercourse,* or *coitus.* The man inserts his erect penis into the vaginal canal and deposits semen containing sperm when he ejaculates.

The male sex act is a complex series of reflexes consisting of several components: erection, secretion, emission, and ejaculation. *Erection* occurs when nervous impulses from the spinal cord and brain cause vasodilation of the arteries of the penis. When the arteries dilate, venous return is obstructed and the cavernous tissue in the penis becomes engorged with blood. (Inability to achieve erection is called *impotence.*) *Secretions* from the male glands lubricate the passageway for semen. Emission is the accumulation of sperm cells and secretions in the urethra. **Ejaculation** is the forceful expulsion of semen from the ejaculatory ducts, through the urethra. **Orgasm** is the physical and emotional, pleasurable sensation that occurs at the climax of sexual intercourse; in men it is accompanied by the ejaculation of semen.

Disorders of the male reproductive system are discussed in Chapter 89. Sexually transmitted disorders are described in Chapter 69.

EFFECTS OF AGING ON THE SYSTEM

As men age, they may experience changes (sometimes called *andropause* or male **climacteric**) but at a much slower rate than women (Table 28-1). No sharp demarcation of beginning or end of sexual activity or reproductive ability is found in the male reproductive system. Men never stop producing sperm, but their rate of sperm production decreases because their level of testosterone secretion declines with age. Men also may gain weight and become more prone to atherosclerosis and osteoporosis. Many men experience benign or malignant hypertrophy (enlarging) of the prostate gland. Prostate hypertrophy may cause difficulty in urination, retention of urine, incontinence, or inability to have an erection.

Head cap-acrosome
(contains special enzymes
to penetrate wall of ovum)

Tail (provides
locomotion)

Head (23 chromosomes)

Body (contains
mitochondria for energy)

Neck

About 60 micrometers (without tail)

The ovum is approximately 120 micrometers with tail.
FIGURE 28-2. A human sperm cell.

▪▪▪ TABLE 28-1 *E*FFECTS OF AGING ON THE MALE REPRODUCTIVE SYSTEM

Factor	Result	Nursing Implications
Testosterone levels decrease.	Degeneration of testicles Decrease in sperm production Difficulty in achieving and maintaining an erection Frequency of erection decreases Prostate gland enlarges—may be benign or malignant; may have difficulty voiding	Educate client that these changes are normal. Refer client to counseling, if needed. Encourage testicular self-examination. Encourage medical examination to catch early prostate cancer.
Fibrosis, sclerosis, and vascular changes occur in penis.	Difficulty achieving or maintaining erection	Encourage medical examination. Refer client to counseling, if needed.

➥ STUDENT SYNTHESIS

Key Points

- Internal organs of the male reproductive system include the testes (containing the seminiferous tubules), ducts, and glands (seminal vesicles, prostate, bulbourethral).
- External structures of the male reproductive system include the scrotum and penis.
- The ducts of the male reproductive system include the epididymis, ductus deferens, and ejaculatory duct. Sperm mature in the epididymis, travel through the ductus deferens, and join other secretions in the ejaculatory duct before exiting the body.
- The scrotum is a sac that supports and protects the testes.
- The penis serves as a common passageway for both the urinary and reproductive systems.
- The male reproductive system is under the influence of hormones from the hypothalamus, pituitary, and gonads.
- Male hormones are called androgens. Testosterone is the major male androgen.
- In men, gonadotropic hormones stimulate the formation of sperm and the secretion of hormones from the sex glands.
- Ejaculatory fluid contains semen from the seminal vesicles, sperm from the vas deferens, alkaline secretions from the prostate, and mucus from the bulbourethral glands.
- Sperm cells are called spermatozoa and are stored in the ductus deferens.
- During copulation, the penis becomes firm in order to penetrate the vagina. The urethra within the penis serves as a passageway for sperm and semen during ejaculation. (No urine is able to pass during sexual intercourse.)

Critical Thinking Exercises

1. Sperm cannot survive in conditions that are too warm or too cold. Discuss circumstances in which a man's sperm count might be lowered.
2. A 50-year-old man comes to the facility where you work. He is marrying a woman of childbearing age. The couple plans to try to have a baby. The man is worried about his chances for conception due to his age. What information would you give this man?

NCLEX-Style Review Questions

1. The internal structures of the male reproductive system include:
   a. Glans penis
   b. Penis
   c. Scrotum
   d. Testes
2. During cold temperatures, the muscles of the scrotum:
   a. Contract
   b. Relax
   c. Shiver
   d. Spasm
3. The prostate gland adds an alkaline secretion to semen to:
   a. Ensure semen is the same pH as the vagina
   b. Increase sperm motility
   c. Promote sperm growth
   d. Provide nutrients and prostaglandins

Reference

1. Cohen, B., & Wood, D. (2000). *Memmler's structure and function of the human body* (7th ed.). Philadelphia: Lippincott Williams & Wilkins.

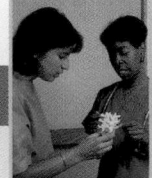

CHAPTER

29

The Female Reproductive System

LEARNING OBJECTIVES

1. Name the major hormones that influence the female reproductive system.
2. Describe the functions of the ovaries, uterus, clitoris, and vagina.
3. Explain the role of the mammary glands in the reproductive process.
4. Describe the functions of LH, FSH, and progesterone in the female reproductive system.
5. Discuss the process of oocyte maturation and ovulation.
6. List the three phases of the ovarian cycle and describe what occurs during each phase.
7. List the three phases of the uterine cycle and explain what occurs during each phase.
8. Discuss menopause and the physical changes that accompany it.
9. Identify two effects of the aging process on the female reproductive system other than menopause, and list the nursing implications for each effect.

NEW TERMINOLOGY

Bartholin's gland	menstruation
cervix	mons pubis
clitoris	oocyte
endometrium	ova
estrogen	ovary
fallopian tube	oviduct
fimbriae	ovulation
gonadotropic hormone	perineum
hymen	progesterone
labia majora	uterus
labia minora	vagina
mammary gland	vulva
menarche	zygote
menopause	

ACRONYMS

ERT	HRT

The male and female reproductive systems are responsible for the continuation of the human species. The male system produces sperm, and the female system is responsible for producing eggs, or ova. Sperm can fertilize these ova, thereby beginning the reproductive process. The female reproductive system also has an amazing added function of providing an environment necessary for the growth and development of a fetus (a developing infant in the uterus).

Although men begin to produce sperm during puberty and continue to do so for the rest of their lives, a woman's reproductive capacity is limited, beginning with the first menstrual period and ending during menopause. The menstrual cycle is extremely important in understanding the female reproductive system. It is explained in detail later in this chapter.

STRUCTURE AND FUNCTION

The *female reproductive system* consists of the ovaries, oviducts, uterus, vagina, and external genital structures. The *internal organs*—the single uterus, the vagina, and the paired ovaries—are located within the pelvis between the urinary blad-der and the rectum. These structures are held in place by a group of ligaments, the most conspicuous of which is the *broad ligament*. The *external structures* consist of components of the vulva. The *mammary glands* (breasts) are also considered female reproductive organs. Figures 29-1 and 29-2 illustrate the female reproductive system. Box 29-1 reviews its primary functions.

REPRODUCTIVE ORGANS

Ovaries

The gonads (sex organs) in women are the **ovaries.** The ovaries produce female gametes or **ova** (singular: ovum) and secrete female sex hormones (estrogens). Although several estrogens exist (the primary one is estradiol), the entire classification **estrogen** commonly refers to female sex hormones collectively as a single hormone.

The ovaries are two almond-shaped glands, each about 1.5 inches (3.8 cm) in length, located within the brim of the pelvis, one on either side of the uterus (see Fig. 29-1). (The combining form relating to ovary is oophor/o-.)

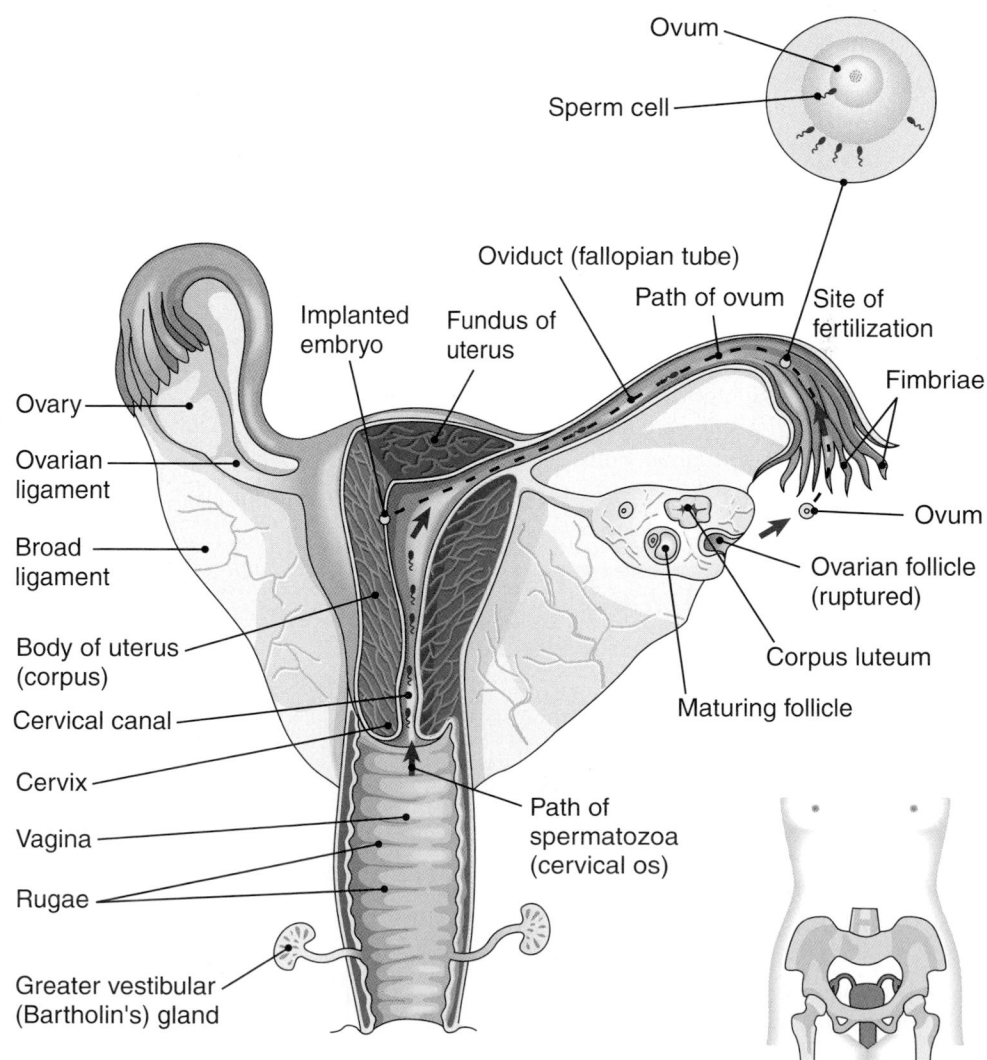

FIGURE 29-1. The female reproductive system (interior view).

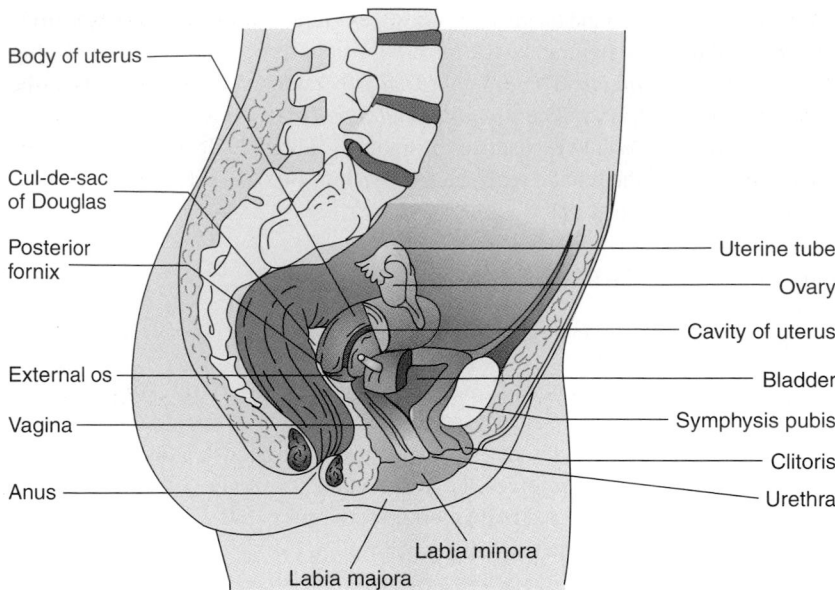

FIGURE 29-2. The female reproductive organs, as seen in sagittal section.

(Labels in figure:)
Body of uterus
Cul-de-sac of Douglas
Posterior fornix
External os
Vagina
Anus
Labia majora
Labia minora
Uterine tube
Ovary
Cavity of uterus
Bladder
Symphysis pubis
Clitoris
Urethra

Oviducts

Sometimes called *uterine tubes* or *ovarian tubes,* the **oviducts** or **fallopian tubes** are the passageway for the ovum between the ovary and the uterus (see Fig. 29-1). The oviducts are 4 to 5 inches (10–12.5 cm) long. One oviduct is located on each side of the uterus; each is associated with one ovary.

As the ovum bursts from the ovary into the pelvic cavity, the oviduct catches it in structures called **fimbriae.** Fimbriae are the fringe-like ends of the oviducts. Cilia on the inner surfaces of the fimbriae, and on the lining of the oviducts, help move the ovum toward the uterus. Smooth muscles of the oviducts contract in peristaltic waves, which also helps to propel the ovum. The inner layer of the oviducts contains mucous-secreting cells that assist in transporting the ovum, and may also provide nutrients for the ovum as it travels in the oviducts.

Fertilization of the ovum (the meeting of the sperm and the ovum) normally occurs about midway in the oviduct. The

➤➤ BOX 29-1

FUNCTIONS OF THE FEMALE REPRODUCTIVE SYSTEM

Development of Sexual Characteristics
• Secrete hormones that initiate puberty
• Maintain specific female sexual characteristics
• Secrete mucus, vaginal fluids, and other substances

Reproduction
• Produce ova
• Pass genetic information to infant
• Participate in copulation and fertilization
• Maintain and nourish fetus until birth

Infant Nourishment
• Produce breast milk

fertilized ovum is called a **zygote.** The zygote travels to the uterus, where it becomes embedded in the uterine lining in preparation for growth into a new individual (see Chap. 64). If fertilization does not occur, the ovum dissolves.

Because no closed connection exists between the ovary and the oviduct, it is possible for the ovum to "escape" into the abdominal cavity.

✚👁 Nursing Alert

An *ectopic* (outside the uterus) pregnancy is an emergency situation, endangering the life of the mother. In an ectopic pregnancy, the ovum becomes fertilized and enters the abdominal cavity or becomes lodged in the oviduct (see Chap. 67).

☞ KEY CONCEPT

Fertilization occurs in the outer one-third portion of the uterine tube (the oviduct). It is the oviduct or uterine tube that is ligated (tied) and cut in the sterilization procedure called tubal ligation.

Uterus

The **uterus** is a hollow, muscular, upside-down-pear–shaped organ in the center of the pelvic cavity above and behind the urinary bladder (see Fig. 29-2). The uterus is considered to be the major female sex organ, even though the gonads are the ovaries. The nonpregnant uterus is about 3 inches (7.5 cm) long, 2 inches (5 cm) wide, and 1 inch (2.5 cm) thick. It is also called the *womb.* The zygote matures into a full-term fetus in the uterus. The uterus normally is tipped forward (*anteverted*), but in some women it is tipped posteriorly (*retroverted*). Although it is movable, the uterus is held in position by strong structures, the *broad* and the *round ligaments.* During pregnancy, the uterus increases its size about 16 times (from about

60 g to about 950 g); its capacity increases from about 2.5 milliliters to 5,000 milliliters. After a term pregnancy, the uterus shrinks considerably, but it never returns to its original size.

Figure 29-1 shows the parts of the uterus. The *fundus* is the round upper surface; the oviducts enter here. The body (*corpus*) is the broad, large central portion. The **cervix** is the narrow lower end, which opens into the vagina. The external *cervical os* (mouth of the cervix) is the opening. It can be visualized during a vaginal examination. The normal size of the cervical os is about the diameter of the graphite in a pencil. The nonpregnant cervix feels like the end of a nose. (The combining form for terms regarding the uterus is hystero/o-.)

The uterus has three layers: serous, muscular, and mucous. The *serous* (outer) *layer* is called the *perimetrium* and is a fold of the peritoneum. The *muscular layer* is called the *myometrium;* it is the smooth muscle that increases in size during pregnancy and contracts during labor and delivery. The *mucous layer* is the **endometrium,** which forms the maternal portion of the placenta during pregnancy.

The uterus receives the fertilized ovum and provides housing and nourishment for a fetus. At the end of gestation, the uterus expels the fetus (*delivery*). Pregnancy, labor, and delivery are discussed in Unit 10.

Vagina

The cervix projects into a muscular canal, which is about 4 inches (10 cm) long and is called the **vagina** (see Fig. 29-1). The vagina's superior, domed portion has deep recesses, called the *fornices* (singular: fornix), around where the cervix extends into the vagina. Glandular secretions from the mucous membrane lining its walls moisten the vagina. The mucus is acidic and retards microbial growth. (The alkaline semen can temporarily neutralize the vagina's acidic environment.) *Rugae* are expandable folds within the vaginal walls that accommodate insertion of the penis and passage of the fetus during childbirth. The vagina's functions are to receive sperm, to provide an exit for menstrual flow, and to serve as the birth canal.

The **hymen** is a thin mucous membrane over the vaginal opening. It may close the vaginal orifice completely, or it may be absent from birth. More commonly it has one or more perforations. A woman can injure the hymen in various ways (eg, during normal exercise, by using tampons, or during the first sexual intercourse). The presence or absence of a hymen is not a reliable indicator of a woman's virginity.

External Genitalia

The external genitalia are collectively called the **vulva** (*pudendum*). The vulva include the vestibule and its surrounding structures. The *vestibule* contains the openings of the urethra, the vagina, and the Bartholin's glands (see Fig. 29-1). The external structures include the mons pubis, labia majora, labia minora, clitoris, and prepuce (Fig. 29-3).

The **mons pubis** is a fatty pad over the symphysis pubis (see Fig. 29-3). Posterior to the mons pubis extend two rounded folds of skin called the **labia majora** (*labia majus*). After puberty, the mons pubis and the labia majora are covered with coarse pubic hair. A thin pair of skin folds medial to the labia majora are the **labia minora** (*labia minus*), which unite just above the clitoris to form the *prepuce*. The labia minora skin folds can be spread apart or "opened" to expose the vestibule floor. The vestibule floor contains **Bartholin's glands** (vestibular glands), which lubricate the vagina. If the openings of the Bartholin's glands become obstructed, Bartholin cysts can result.

The **clitoris** is a small erectile structure that responds to sexual stimulation. The structure of the clitoris is similar to the structure of the penis. Both become engorged with blood as a result of sexual excitement, and stimulation of either structure often leads to orgasm.

The female (obstetrical) **perineum** is the space between the vaginal orifice and the anus. It is made up of strong muscles that act as sling-like supports for pelvic organs.

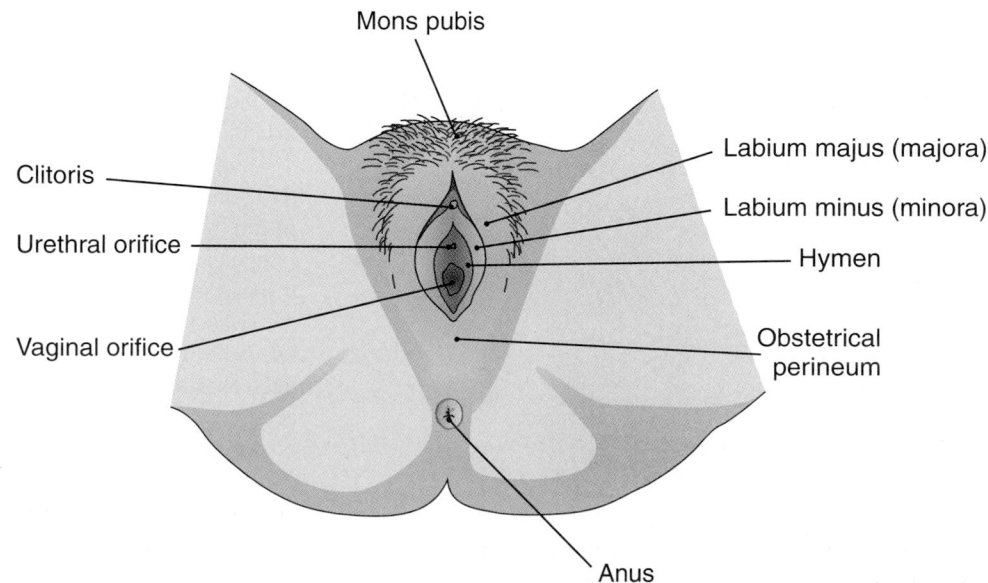

FIGURE 29-3. The external female genitalia, seen from below. The area lying between the orifice of the vagina and the anus is the obstetric *perineum.* Note the location of the urinary orifice (meatus).

Mons pubis

Clitoris

Urethral orifice

Vaginal orifice

Labium majus (majora)

Labium minus (minora)

Hymen

Obstetrical perineum

Anus

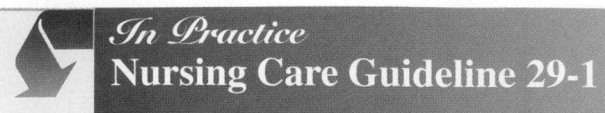

In Practice
Nursing Care Guideline 29-1

EPISIOTOMY

During childbirth, the skin and muscles of the perineum area may be torn. To prevent such tearing, an incision called an *episiotomy* is often made. A clean, straight incision heals better than an irregular skin and muscle tear. Slow stretching of the perineum during delivery may prevent tearing and make an episiotomy unnecessary.

BREASTS

The breasts are not direct reproductive organs; however, they are hormonally influenced and are directly linked to the reproductive process, providing nutrition for babies following childbirth. Before puberty, breast structure in boys and girls is similar. Both have rudimentary glandular systems. With the onset of puberty, *estrogens* and *progesterone* in girls lead to breast enlargement. Both boys and girls may have some breast sensitivity in early puberty. Boys may even develop slight swellings, but symptoms disappear quickly.

The **mammary glands** are modified sweat glands (Fig. 29-4). They are located in the breasts, anterior to the *pectoralis major* muscles. Hormones (*prolactin* and *oxytocin*) stimulate them to produce and to release milk after childbirth. Each breast is divided into 15 to 20 *lobes* of glandular tissue, covered by adipose (fat) tissue, which gives the breast its shape. The lobes are made up of *lobules,* which consist of milk-secreting cells in glandular alveoli. From the alveoli, small *lactiferous ducts* converge toward each nipple like the spokes of a wheel. Each lactiferous duct forms a small reservoir for milk.

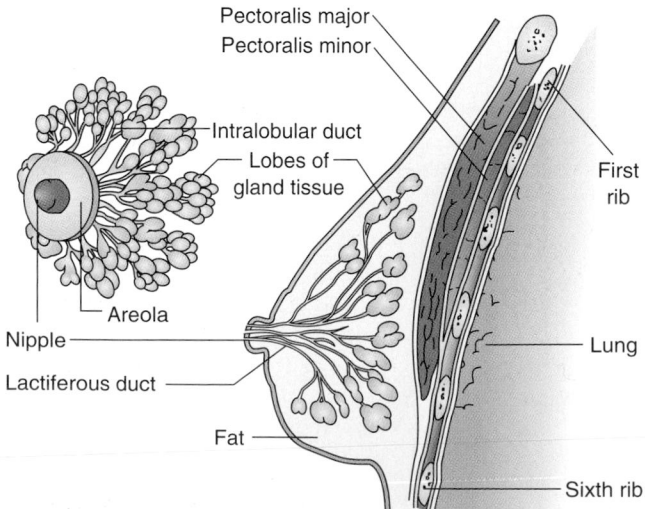

FIGURE 29-4. The breast, showing the glandular tissue and ducts of the mammary glands.

The structures of the breast include the nipple, the areola, and the areolar glands. The *nipple* is a circular projection containing some erectile tissue. It is surrounded by the pigmented *areola. Areolar glands,* which are close to the skin's surface, make the areola appear rough. The secretions of the areolar glands keep the nipples from drying out. The breasts enlarge during pregnancy as a result of stimulation by *estrogen* and *progesterone.* The areolae become more heavily pigmented and do not totally return to their previous color after pregnancy.

HORMONAL INFLUENCES

The hypothalamus, the pituitary gland, and the gonads all contribute to the hormonal regulation of the female reproductive system. Remember that before puberty, androgens (male hormones) and estrogens (female hormones) are at the same levels in both boys and girls.

The hypothalamus stimulates the secretion of the **gonadotropic hormones,** which include luteinizing hormone (LH) and follicle-stimulating hormone (FSH) in women. The main effects of LH and FSH include stimulating the formation of ova, and stimulating the secretion of hormones from the sex organs. Gonadotropic hormones also stimulate the development of female sexual characteristics. The ovaries begin to secrete *estrogens.* The estrogens include estradiol, estriol, and estrone. After puberty, the corpus luteum of the ovary produces another hormone, **progesterone,** which functions primarily during pregnancy.

The pubescent girl exhibits many changes as a result of estrogen production. The characteristic feminine contour appears, breast tissue develops, and unique fatty deposits appear. The glands become active, and hair appears in the pubic and axillary areas. Although voice changes are not as marked as those in a boy, the voice does deepen and mature in tone and quality. As the glands of reproduction become active, menstruation occurs. All of these female secondary sex characteristics depend on the secretion of *estrogen* and *progesterone.*

SYSTEM PHYSIOLOGY
Egg Cells and Oogenesis

All the *ova* (egg cells) that an individual woman will produce in her lifetime are present as **oocytes** at her birth. Each oocyte develops in different stages throughout a woman's life. About 5 to 7 million of them begin as *oogonia* in the female fetus' fourth to fifth gestational month. Before birth, most oogonia (singular: oogonium) either degenerate or begin meiosis. At the start of meiosis, the oogonium is called a *primary oocyte.* A newborn girl has about 2 million primary oocytes. Then, between birth and puberty, the number of these primary oocytes decreases to 300,000 to 400,000—of these, only 300 to 400 eventually develop into mature egg cells.

At puberty, hormones stimulate the primary follicle to continue its development and to become a *secondary follicle.* The secondary follicle enlarges and forms a bump on the ovary. When the secondary follicle matures, it is called the *graafian follicle.* From the time of puberty until menstruation ceases during menopause, at approximately monthly intervals, a mature graafian follicle ruptures the surface of the ovary. Now known as the *ovum,* it is expelled into the pelvic cavity near the oviduct (which leads to the uterus). This ovum will live up to 24 hours before it begins to degenerate, unless it is fertilized by a sperm.

Menstrual Cycle

The *menstrual cycle* is actually two interrelated continuous cycles: the *ovarian cycle* and the *uterine cycle* (Fig. 29-5). The anterior pituitary gland releases secretions that control both cycles. These changes occur in sexually mature, non-pregnant women and culminate in menstruation. **Menstruation** is the flow of blood and other materials from the uterus through the vagina.

The first menstrual period is called **menarche** and marks the onset of puberty. This rhythmical series of changes then occurs about every 28 days. This process is referred to as a *menstrual period, menses,* or *period.* Great variation occurs, however, among women and also within one woman's month-to-month cycle.

Menstrual cycles continue as long as ovarian hormones stimulate the uterine lining. Between 40 and 55 years of age, the ovaries become less active, because they no longer respond to FSH. Thus, eggs no longer mature, and the ovaries stop producing estrogens. This decrease in ovarian function occurs gradually. The result is the inability to become pregnant and **menopause** (cessation of menstruation). Menopause, a normal process, sometimes occurs abruptly. Usually it is so gradual that the woman's body adjusts without much difficulty. Because many hormonal changes are involved, however, menopausal women may experience some unpleasant symptoms, such as headaches, irritability, insomnia, anxiety, or depression. One of the most common symptoms is the sensation of heat (*hot flashes*). Hormonal imbalances affect the diameter of blood vessels, causing their abrupt dilation or contraction. External indicators of menopause include a tendency to gain weight; thinning of hair; growth of hair on the upper lip; and dry, itchy skin.

☞ KEY CONCEPT

The onset of menopause can begin as early as 35 to 40 years of age. It is defined as the permanent cessation of menses for more than a year.

Ovarian Cycle

During the ovarian cycle, the ovum matures and is expelled from the ovary into the oviduct. While this is happening, the maturation of another ovum is withheld until the next cycle. The three phases of the ovarian cycle are the *follicular phase, ovulation,* and the *luteal phase* (see Fig. 29-5). Table 29-1 discusses the hormones and phases of the ovarian cycle.

Follicular Phase.   The *follicular phase* lasts from about day 4 to about day 14. During this time, under the influence of FSH, several follicles begin to ripen and the ovum within each begins to mature. One follicle will become dominant; it is called the *graafian follicle.* The other follicles stop growing.

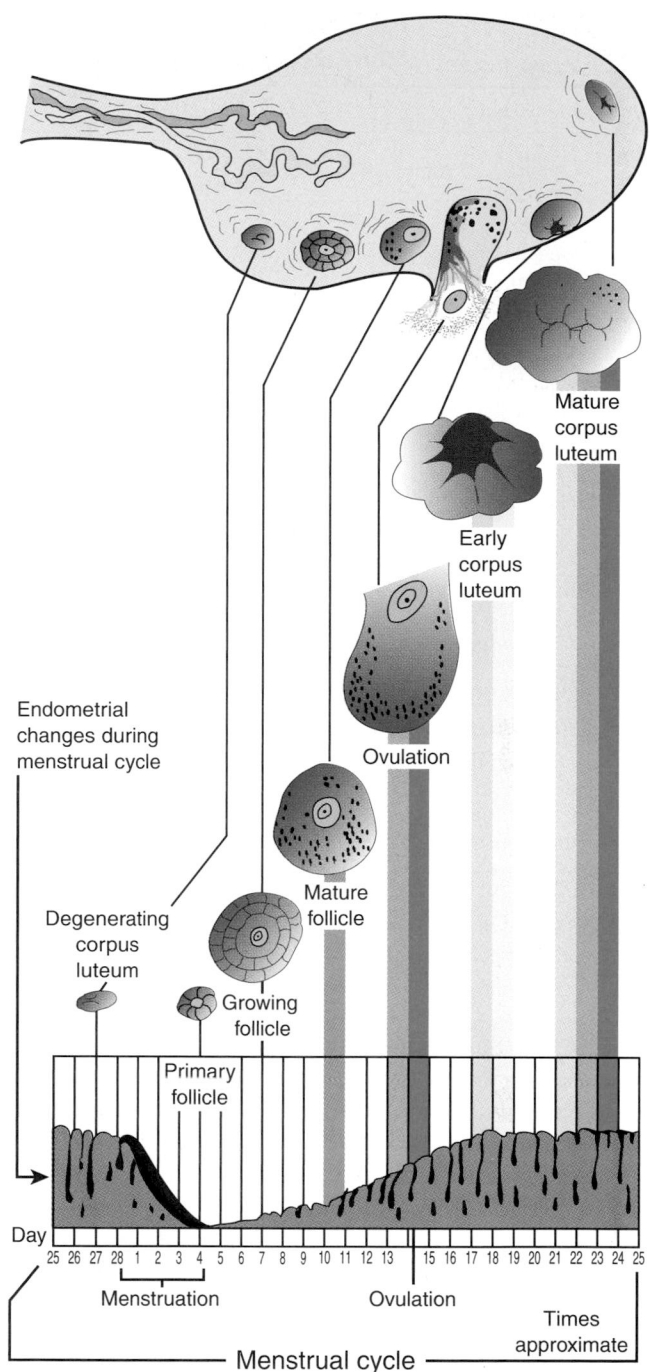

FIGURE 29-5. One menstrual cycle, and the corresponding changes in the endometrium.

Ovulation.   About day 14, a surge of hormones causes the ovum to burst through the ovary. This act is called **ovulation.** It usually occurs in the middle of the 28-day menstrual cycle (about 14 days before the onset of the next menses). Some fertility control and enhancement methods are based on calculation of the time of ovulation.

☞ KEY CONCEPT

Some women experience sharp pains or cramps when ovulation occurs. This is known as mittelschmerz (meaning "middle pain" in German).

■■■ **TABLE 29-1** *H*ORMONAL CHANGES DURING THE MENSTRUAL CYCLE

Phase	Menstrual	Follicular	Ovulation	Luteal	Premenstrual
Days*	1 2 3 4 5 6 7 8	9 10 11 12 13 14	15 16 17 18 19	20 21 22 23 24 25	26 27 28 1 2
Ovary	Degenerating corpus luteum; beginning follicular development	Growth and maturation of follicle	Ovulation	Active corpus luteum	Degenerating corpus luteum
Estrogen Production	Low	Increasing	High	Declining, then a secondary rise	Decreasing
Progesterone Production	None	Low	Low	Increasing	Decreasing
FSH Production	Increasing	High, then declining	Low	Low	Increasing
LH Production	Low	Low, then increasing	High	High	Decreasing
Endometrium	Degeneration and shedding of superficial layer. Coiled arteries dilate, then constrict again.	Reorganization and proliferation of superficial layer	Continued growth	Active secretion and glandular dilation; highly vascular; edematous	Vasoconstriction of coiled arteries; beginning degeneration

*Times approximate

Smeltzer, S. C., & Bare, B. G. (2001). *Brunner and Suddarth's textbook of medical-surgical nursing* (9th ed., p. 1195). Philadelphia: Lippincott Williams & Wilkins.

Luteal Phase. During the *luteal phase,* the empty, ruptured graafian follicle becomes the *corpus luteum* and begins to secrete *progesterone* and *estrogen.* These hormones cause the endometrium to become greatly thickened and vascular (engorged). If the ovum is fertilized, it becomes embedded in the *endometrium* (the endometrial lining of the uterus) and becomes a fetus. If the ovum is not fertilized, the secretion of progesterone decreases, and the corpus luteum begins to decline. Levels of FSH start to rise on about day 2 to begin preparation for the next cycle.

Uterine Cycle

The endometrium of the uterus has a similar cycle (see Fig. 29-5). It is called the *uterine cycle* or *endometrial cycle.* This process prepares the uterus for implantation of an ovum (egg). The uterine cycle is controlled by the ovarian cycle, and will vary depending upon whether or not fertilization of the ovum occurs. The three phases of the uterine cycle are the *proliferative phase,* the *secretory phase,* and the *menstrual (menstruation) phase.*

Proliferative (Buildup) Phase. While the ovarian follicles are producing increased amounts of estrogen, the endometrium prepares for possible fertilization. The endometrium thickens from about day 4 to about day 14, as shown at the bottom of Figure 29-5.

Secretory Phase. As the endometrium prepares for implantation of the fertilized ovum, pronounced endometrial growth occurs. If fertilization does not occur, the corpus luteum degenerates and hormonal levels fall. Withdrawal of hormones causes the endometrial cells to change, and menstruation begins.

Menstruation. The sloughing off of the endometrium causes *menstruation.* Menstruation averages 3 to 5 days but may last 2 to 8 days. During menstruation, FSH levels rise and several ovarian follicles begin to develop again. Thus begins the next endometrial cycle. Hormonal changes during menstruation are shown in Table 29-1.

☛ KEY CONCEPT

Maturation of an ovum occurs during the ovarian cycle; growth of the lining (endometrium) of the uterus occurs during the uterine cycle. Together, these cycles are known as the menstrual cycle.

The changes that take place if the ovum is fertilized and pregnancy is established are described and illustrated in Chapter 64. Disorders of the female reproductive system are discussed in Chapter 90. Sexually transmitted disorders are described in Chapter 69.

■■■ **TABLE 29-2** *E*FFECTS OF AGING ON THE WOMAN'S REPRODUCTIVE SYSTEM

Factor	Result	Nursing Implications
Ovaries stop producing estrogen and progesterone.	Inability to become pregnant Cessation of menstruation—woman may have hot flashes, headaches, dizziness, or heart palpitations May need estrogen replacement therapy (ERT). Uterus and ovaries get smaller. Vagina shortens and thins. Vaginal secretions decrease. Breasts get smaller and softer. Hair thins on scalp, axillae, and external genitalia. Hair grows on upper lip. Muscles of upper arms and legs get flabby. Weight gain around midline occurs. Skin dries.	Watch for signs of depression. Refer for medical evaluation. Refer for counseling, if needed. Counsel client to use water-soluble lubricant, if needed for comfort. Advise client to wear a good support bra. Discuss removal by electrolysis or waxing. Educate client about an exercise program. Discuss need for fewer calories to maintain weight. Stress exercise. Advise client to use a lotion or moisturizer.
Estrogen production is deficient.	Increase in atherosclerosis; thus, increase in heart disease Osteoporosis increases; bones become subject to fractures as they become brittle.	Educate client about a low-fat, low-salt diet. Encourage an exercise program. Educate about increased calcium intake. Encourage exercise and weight maintenance. Refer for physical examination and possible estrogen therapy.

Female Sexual Response

Female neural pathways involved in controlling the sexual response are the same as those found in the male. During sexual excitement, the erectile tissues within the clitoris and around the vaginal opening become engorged with blood. The vestibular glands secrete mucus before and during coitus (sexual intercourse). If the clitoris is stimulated with sufficient intensity and duration, the woman will feel the physical and psychological release of orgasm. The nipples of the breasts also contain erectile tissues that respond to sexual excitement and orgasm. Unlike a man, a woman can experience successive orgasms with minimal rest.

EFFECTS OF AGING ON THE SYSTEM

Female climacteric is called *menopause* (discussed previously). Several physical conditions are associated with loss of estrogen. Vascular disease and heart disease are less common in premenopausal women than in men. After menopause, the rate of heart disease between men and women is about equal. *Osteoporosis* is a condition in which bones become brittle and porous and fracture more easily. This condition is more common in women, and worsens when hormones are absent. Estrogen replacement therapy (**ERT**) or hormone replacement therapy (**HRT**) may be prescribed to lessen menopausal symptoms.

Older women may also suffer from urinary incontinence, the result of aging and childbirth trauma. Breast tissue may become smaller and more pendulous (sagging) as muscles relax and are replaced by fat. Loss of muscle tone causes external genital structures to sag; the vagina shortens and becomes less elastic. Intercourse may become painful (*dyspareunia*) as the vaginal mucosal wall becomes thinner and vaginal secretions decrease. The uterus may fall (*prolapse*) into the vagina. In addition, the older woman is more prone to vaginal infections. Changes in sexual response are relatively minor and are usually related to physical changes in the vagina. Table 29-2 lists the effects of aging on the woman's reproductive system.

➤ **STUDENT SYNTHESIS**

Key Points

- The internal organs of the female reproductive system include the ovaries, oviducts, uterus, and vagina.
- The external organs of the female reproductive system are the vulva and breasts.
- The egg cell is called an oocyte. Maturation begins in the fourth or fifth month of a female fetus' gestation and ends with menopause. A mature oocyte is called an ovum.
- Fertilization of the ovum occurs in the fallopian tube or oviduct. A fertilized ovum is called a zygote and becomes embedded in the uterine lining.
- The mammary glands function to produce and to release milk after childbirth.
- Hormones from the hypothalamus, anterior pituitary gland, and the gonads influence the female reproductive system.

- Female hormones are called estrogens.
- In women, gonadotropic hormones stimulate the formation of ova and the secretion of hormones from the sex organs.
- Menarche is the first menstrual period and marks the onset of puberty.
- Menstruation is the monthly flow of blood and other materials from the uterus.
- Menopause is the time when menstrual periods cease and the woman can no longer reproduce.
- The three phases of the ovarian cycle are the follicular phase, ovulation, and the luteal phase.
- The three phases of the uterine cycle are the proliferative phase, the secretory phase, and menstruation.

Critical Thinking Exercises

1. Explain why a 32-year-old woman who had her uterus and ovaries removed might want to consider hormone replacement therapy.
2. Janie, a 12-year-old girl, is experiencing her first menstrual period. Her mother brings her to the health-care facility for you to explain the physical process that is occurring. What information would you give Janie? How would you explain menstruation to her?

NCLEX-Style Review Questions

1. The mucus in the vagina is normally acidic to:
   a. Help sperm reach the uterus
   b. Provide lubrication
   c. Retard microbial growth
   d. Stimulate menstruation
2. Fertilization of the ovum normally occurs in the:
   a. Uterine tube
   b. Ovary
   c. Uterus
   d. Vagina
3. Estrogen replacement therapy is given to women in menopause to:
   a. Decrease menopausal symptoms
   b. Increase the woman's sex drive
   c. Minimize the aging process
   d. Treat depression

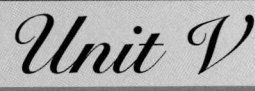

Unit V

NUTRITION AND DIET THERAPY

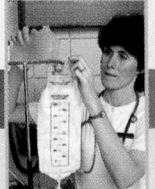

CHAPTER

30

Basic Nutrition

LEARNING OBJECTIVES

1. Define nutrition and explain three functions of each of the six classes of major nutrients.
2. List the major dietary sources of carbohydrates and differentiate among monosaccharides, disaccharides, and polysaccharides.
3. Differentiate between saturated and unsaturated fatty acids. Explain cholesterol, LDL, and HDL.
4. Define amino acid. Differentiate between complete and incomplete proteins.
5. Explain the body's need for water and describe at least four functions of water.
6. List six major minerals and four trace minerals and state their functions.
7. Name the fat-soluble and water-soluble vitamins and list their main functions and food sources.
8. Identify the components of the Food Guide Pyramid and note the servings allotted for each part of the pyramid.
9. Discuss BMI, obesity, and malnutrition and how they relate to a healthy diet.
10. Identify at least three special nutritional considerations related to infancy, childhood, adolescence, early and middle adulthood, and the elderly.

NEW TERMINOLOGY

amino acid
beriberi
cholesterol
disaccharide
essential nutrient
glycogen
hydrogenated
hyperglycemia
hypoglycemia
lipid
macronutrient
malnutrition
micronutrient
mineral

monosaccharide
nutrient
nutrient density
nutrition
pellagra
phytochemical
polysaccharide
protein
rickets
saturated fat
scurvy
trans-fat
triglyceride

ACRONYMS

AI	HCl	PKU
BMI	HDL	RBC
CHO	HFCS	RDA
DRI	IBW	REE
EAR	kcal or C	UL
FDA	LDL	USDA
GDM	PCM	USP

Food is vital to life. Humans eat to stay alive and to be healthy. In fact, food is one of the most important items in Maslow's hierarchy of human needs (see Chap. 5). Food is also enjoyable and brings pleasure to life.

Nutrition is the study of nutrients and how the body utilizes the nutrients in food. Nutrition has a great impact on human well-being, behavior, and the environment.

The science of nutrition continues to evolve as our understanding of its role has shifted from simply preventing dietary deficiencies to reducing the risk of chronic diseases, including osteoporosis, cancer, and heart disease. For instance, before the Nutrition Labeling and Education Act of 1993, food labels were required to list the B vitamins thiamine, riboflavin, and niacin because deficiencies in these nutrients were once common. Today, current public health concerns are reflected in the order in which mandatory dietary components must appear on food labels: total calories, calories from fat, total fat, saturated fat, cholesterol, and sodium. Listing the B vitamins is now optional.

Results from many research studies have indicated that nutrients and other compounds found in food may increase optimal health and even prevent specific health problems. New discoveries about previously unidentified components in plant foods, known as **phytochemicals**, suggest that thousands of naturally occurring chemicals in foods may help protect against disease. Future recommendations for daily nutrient intakes will likely be made from the perspective of optimizing health, rather than simply preventing deficiencies.

This chapter begins with the concept of basic nutrition, and information about the functions and sources of nutrients. Nutrient digestion is included where appropriate. Using this knowledge as a foundation, characteristics of a healthy diet are presented and common nutritional problems are discussed. The chapter concludes with a discussion of nutritional concerns across the life span.

☛ KEY CONCEPT

No one food provides all nutrients. Eating a balanced and varied diet is the only way to provide the body with all necessary nutrients.

NUTRIENTS

Nutrients are substances needed for growth, maintenance, and repair of the body. The body can make some nutrients if adequate amounts of necessary precursors (building blocks) are available. **Essential nutrients** are those that a person must obtain through food because the body cannot make them in sufficient quantities to meet its needs. The six classes of nutrients are carbohydrate, fat, protein, water, minerals, and vitamins. Carbohydrate, fat, and protein provide energy and are called **macronutrients.** Vitamins and minerals regulate body processes and are called **micronutrients.** Water is necessary for virtually every body function (see Chap. 17). A guide to daily food choices and recommended serving sizes is depicted in Figure 30-1 and Box 30-1. The Food Guide Pyramid is discussed later in this chapter.

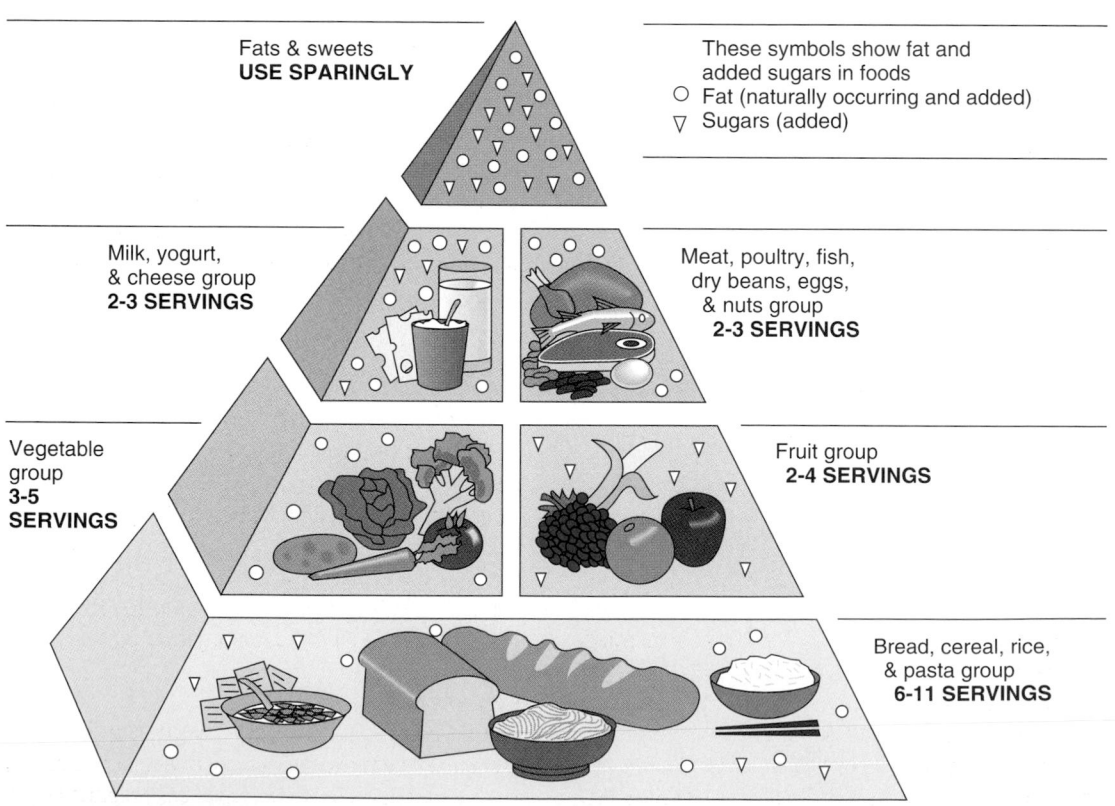

FIGURE 30-1. The Food Guide Pyramid.

➢➢ BOX 30-1

SERVING SIZES

What Counts as a Serving?

Bread, Cereal, Rice, and Pasta Group
(Grains Group)—whole grain and refined
• 1 slice of bread
• About 1 cup of ready-to-eat cereal
• ½ cup of cooked cereal, rice, or pasta

Vegetable Group
• 1 cup of raw leafy vegetables
• ½ cup of other vegetables—cooked or raw
• ¾ cup of vegetable juice

Fruit Group
• 1 medium apple, banana, orange, pear
• ½ cup of chopped, cooked, or canned fruit
• ¾ cup of fruit juice

Milk, Yogurt, and Cheese Group (Milk Group)*
• 1 cup of milk† or yogurt†
• 1½ ounces of natural cheese† (such as cheddar)
• 2 ounces of processed cheese† (such as American)

Meat, Poultry, Fish, Dry Beans, Eggs, and Nuts Group
(Meat and Beans Group)
• 2–3 ounces of cooked lean meat, poultry, or fish
• ½ cup of cooked dry beans# or ½ cup of tofu counts as 1 ounce of lean meat
• 2½-ounce soyburger or 1 egg counts as 1 ounce of lean meat
• 2 tablespoons of peanut butter or ⅓ cup of nuts counts as 1 ounce of meat

---

Note: Many of the serving sizes given above are smaller than those on the Nutrition Facts Label. For example, 1 serving of cooked cereal, rice, or pasta is 1 cup for the label but only ½ cup for the pyramid.
*This includes lactose-free and lactose-reduced milk products. One cup of soy-based beverage with added calcium is an option for those who prefer a non-dairy source of calcium.
†Choose fat-free or reduced-fat dairy products most often.
#Dry beans, peas, and lentils can be counted as servings in either the meat and beans group or the vegetable group. As a vegetable, ½ cup of cooked, dry beans counts as 1 serving. As a meat substitute, 1 cup of cooked, dry beans counts as 1 serving (2 ounces of meat).
Source: United States Department of Agriculture and United States Department of Health and Human Services. (2000). *Nutrition and your health: Dietary guidelines for Americans* (5th ed.). Website: http://www.health.gov/dietaryguidelines/dga2000.

Dietary Reference Intakes

In 1941, the Food and Nutrition Board of the National Academy of Sciences published the first Recommended Dietary Allowances (RDAs) that set a standard for the intake of specific nutrients to meet the needs of healthy Americans. Continued research has shown that the RDA levels have limited value and are often misrepresented and misused. The focus of RDAs has traditionally been the prevention of deficiency disorders. The Food and Nutrition Board of the National Academy of Sciences changed its approach to setting nutrient reference levels. The study of nutrition has expanded to include the role of nutrients in preventing chronic diseases.

A combination of experts in several food and nutrition organizations had instituted an expanded system called the Dietary Reference Intakes (**DRIs**). This system includes four standards that list reference intake levels of essential nutrients for most healthy population groups. The DRIs consist of Recommended Dietary Allowances, Adequate Intake, Tolerable Upper Intake Level, and Estimated Average Requirement. These standards are described below.

Recommended Dietary Allowances (**RDAs**): Recommendations for average daily dietary intake level that is sufficient to meet the nutrient requirement of nearly all healthy individuals (97% to 98%) in a particular life stage and gender group.

Adequate Intake (**AI**): Recommended nutrient intake that is assumed to be adequate. It is based on observed or estimated nutrient intake by a group (or groups) of healthy people and is used when an RDA cannot be determined.

Tolerable Upper Intake Level (**UL**): The highest level of daily nutrient intake that is likely to pose no risk of adverse health effects for almost all individuals in the general population.

Estimated Average Requirement (**EAR**): A daily nutrient intake value that is estimated to meet the requirement of half the healthy individuals in a life stage and gender group.

Kilocalories and Energy

The unit of measurement that specifies the heat energy in a particular amount of food is called a kilocalorie (**kcal** or **C**). A *kilocalorie* is defined as the amount of heat required to raise the temperature of 1 kilogram of water 1° Celsius. The caloric value of foods can be determined in the laboratory. In this process, the heat that is given off by the burning of the test food raises the temperature of a known amount of water. The calorie values of energy nutrients follow:

• 1 gram carbohydrate yields 4 C
• 1 gram fat yields 9 C
• 1 gram protein yields 4 C

Calorie charts stating the number of kilocalories in an average serving of various foods are available without cost from a number of sources. The National Dairy Council has published many excellent booklets that can be obtained from local dairy councils. The U.S. Government Printing Office is also a good source of nutrition information. Fast-food restaurants will provide kilocalorie charts upon request.

Requirements

From a nutrition standpoint, calories are synonymous with energy. The amount of energy (calories) a healthy individual needs depends on his or her age, sex, weight, body composition, and activity level. The energy requirements of an individual are the total calories needed to maintain body processes, or resting energy expenditure (**REE**). For most adults, REE accounts for most of the energy used in a typical day. REE is higher for men than for women because men have more muscle mass; likewise, younger adults have a higher REE than older adults because people lose muscle mass as they age. Growth, pregnancy, lactation, and fever increase REE.

In adults, activity typically accounts for 25% to 30% of total energy used. The actual amount of energy used for physical activity depends on the duration and intensity of the activity. For instance, people at desk jobs need fewer kilocalories than laborers, who use their muscles a great deal. Also, heavier people use more energy than lighter people when performing the same activity because they move a greater amount of weight.

Empty Calories

The term *empty calories* is an imprecise term applied to foods that supply calories with few or no nutrients. Examples of empty calorie foods are candy, soft drinks, alcohol, and sugar. Empty calorie foods can contribute to nutrient deficiencies if they take the place of other nutrient-rich foods, such as substituting soft drinks for milk or alcohol for food. Although not considered a nutrient, one gram of alcohol provides 7 C.

Enzymes and Digestion

Thousands of chemical reactions occur daily in the body. Without enzymes, these reactions would take much more time and use excessive energy. *Enzymes* are biologic catalysts made of proteins. With the exception of pepsin and trypsin, all enzymes end in the suffix -ase. Each enzyme has a specific three-dimensional form that works only with matching shapes of other chemicals in a lock-and-key manner; each enzyme will catalyze only one specific reaction. Enzymes temporarily bond with the other chemicals until they form a new compound, at which point the enzyme is released. Several factors affect enzyme action. For example, each enzyme works best in a particular pH and temperature. Temperatures greater than 106° Fahrenheit destroy most enzymes; thus, the body generally cannot survive sustained high temperatures.

A major area of enzyme action is digestion. The salivary glands in the mouth make enzymes that begin starch digestion. Enzymes found in pancreatic secretions and in the intestinal-wall brush border villi break food into particles that can be absorbed. More information about enzymes is included in the following discussions of specific nutrients.

Carbohydrates

Carbohydrates (**CHO**) are made of carbon, hydrogen, and oxygen, and are classified as either simple or complex, based on the number of sugar molecules present. The major function of carbohydrates is to provide energy. Carbohydrates are the most widely used energy source in the world. For the people of many countries, 80% of their total daily calories come from complex carbohydrates. All carbohydrates, with the exception of fiber, provide 4 C per gram. (Fiber is not truly digested, and there-fore provides no energy.) The simple carbohydrate *glucose* is the body's major source of energy.

Another important function of carbohydrates is the ability to spare protein. If inadequate carbohydrate is available, however, the body burns protein for energy. This protein comes from food and from the body's own muscle tissue. Therefore, in cases of inadequate carbohydrate and protein intake, not only would muscle wasting occur, but adequate protein would not be available for the repair of body tissues.

All plant foods, except plant oils (like corn, soy, and olive), contain carbohydrates. Milk is the only non-plant source of carbohydrate. Rich sources of carbohydrate include breads and cereals, legumes and dried beans, fruits, and vegetables. Sugar and "sweets" also provide non-complex carbohydrates. Table 30-1 summarizes facts about carbohydrates.

Digestion

Digestion of carbohydrates begins in the mouth. In this process, the action of salivary amylase or ptyalin, enzymes present in saliva, begins breaking down starch into smaller carbohydrates, known as dextrin. No enzymatic digestion of carbohydrates occurs in the stomach, but some carbohydrates may be hydrolyzed into units of glucose and fructose when subjected to the stomach's hydrochloric acid.

In the small intestine, an enzyme from the pancreas, called pancreatic amylase, converts complex carbohydrates into maltose, a disaccharide (double sugar). In the intestinal wall, the enzymes sucrase, maltase, and lactase are available to complete the digestion process. The end products of carbohydrate digestion—glucose, fructose, and galactose—are absorbed through the intestinal mucosa. The liver converts fructose and galactose to glucose, which can be used for immediate energy or stored in the liver and muscle as glycogen. Glucose that remains after energy and glycogen needs are met is converted to fat and stored. The only form of sugar that the body can use is glucose.

Fiber in the diet is acted on by digestive enzymes but passes out of the body virtually undigested.

Simple Carbohydrates

Monosaccharides and **disaccharides** contain one (mono-) or two (di-) sugar (-saccharide) molecules; they are classified as *simple carbohydrates* or *simple sugars*. Simple carbohydrates may or may not taste sweet. Glucose, fructose, and galactose are monosaccharides. Sucrose, lactose, and maltose are disaccharides.

Monosaccharides.   *Glucose,* also called *blood sugar, dextrose,* or *grape sugar,* is the most commonly occurring sugar in the body. Terms such as **hyperglycemia,** which means abnormally high blood sugar, or **hypoglycemia,** which means abnormally low blood sugar, refer to the blood's level of glucose. The body must change other forms of sugar into glucose before it can use these sugars. Sources of natural glucose are honey, fruits, and some vegetables.

Fructose, also called *levulose* or *fruit sugar,* is the sweetest simple sugar and is found naturally in honey, fruits, and saps. Commercial forms of fructose, namely crystalline fructose and

■■■ **TABLE 30-1** ⨍UMMARY OF CARBOHYDRATES, FATS, AND PROTEINS

Nutrient	RDAs	Sources	Functions
Carbohydrate	None set; suggested intake 45%–55% of total calories; minimum amount needed to prevent ketosis is about 100 g	• Bread and cereal • Pasta and rice • Potato, lima beans, corn • Dried beans and peas • Fruits, vegetables, milk • Sugar, syrup, jelly, jam, honey	• Major source of energy (glucose) • Provides fiber • Spares protein • Excess is stored as fat
Fat	None set; suggested intake less than 30% of total calories; need small amount to carry fat-soluble vitamins and to perform other functions (about 15–20 g)	• Butter and cream • Salad oils and dressings • Cooking and table fats • Fat in meats • Olives, avocados • Fried foods	• Supplies large amount of energy in a small amount of food; excess stored as fat • Conserves body heat • Helps keep skin healthy by supplying essential fatty acids • Carries vitamins A, D, E, and K • Important in structure of nerve tissue; protects and insulates body parts
Protein	Adult: 44–56 g Child: 23–34 g Infant: 2–2.2 g/kg body weight Pregnancy: 60 g Lactation: 65 g	• Meat, fish, poultry, eggs • Milk and cheese • Dried beans and peas • Peanut butter and nuts • Fortified bread and cereals	• Builds and repairs all tissues • Helps build blood and forms antibodies to fight infections • Supplies energy; excess stored as fat • Assists in acid–base and fluid balance

high-fructose corn syrup (**HFCS**), are widely used in sweetened processed foods and soft drinks.

Galactose is not usually found free in nature, but it is found combined with glucose in the disaccharide lactose (milk sugar). Few other significant sources of galactose exist.

Disaccharides. *Sucrose,* commonly known as table sugar, is composed of fructose and glucose. It is the most common sweetener in the diet, and is used on the table and in cooking. Although it goes by many different names (*crystallized sugar, raw sugar, turbinado sugar, brown sugar, powdered sugar, molasses*), no caloric or nutritional difference exists among its many forms. Sources of sucrose are sugar beets, sugar cane, maple syrup, and some fruits.

Lactose is the sugar found in milk. It is neither as soluble nor as sweet as sucrose. It is not found in plants; it is formed only in the mammary glands. The enzyme lactase splits lactose into galactose and glucose. Most infants can tolerate lactose, but many adults cannot. If a person lacks the enzyme lactase, bloating, gas, and diarrhea can occur when milk products are ingested. This condition, known as *lactose intolerance,* is different from an actual milk allergy caused by an immune reaction to protein in milk. Many people with lactose intolerance can tolerate hard cheese, yogurt, and lactase-containing milk, although individual tolerances vary greatly. Commercial products are available over-the-counter that provide the enzymes needed to digest lactose.

Maltose is not found freely in food but is produced as an intermediate in starch digestion. It is also produced through the process of malting (malted milk) and brewing (beer). Because it is readily soluble and easily changed into glucose, it is often used in infant formulas in the form of maltodextrin.

Sugar has been blamed for causing obesity, diabetes, heart disease, and hyperactivity in children. Modern research, however, has contradicted these claims, and evidence suggests that sugar is not an independent risk factor for any particular disease. Sugar, like other fermentable carbohydrates, can increase a person's risk of dental cavities. Sugar is considered "empty-calorie" food since it contains no nutrients (honey contains some trace nutrients), and its consumption often displaces nutrient-dense foods in the diet. Box 30-2 provides the student with several tips on eating fewer sugars.

➤➤ BOX 30-2

TIPS FOR EATING LESS SUGAR

- **Replace soft drinks with 100% fruit juice or low-fat milk.** Total calorie intake may not change significantly, but the intake of vitamins, minerals, and phytochemicals will increase. It is the total package that is important, not just the amount of calories.
- **Rely on natural sugars in fruit to satisfy a "sweet tooth."** Besides being less concentrated in sugars than candy, cookies, pastries, and cakes, fruits boost nutrient and fiber intake.
- **Cut sugar in home-baked products, if possible.** Although in some foods reducing the amount of sugar does not appreciably alter taste or other qualities, in others it can be disastrous. For instance, because sugar in jams and jellies inhibits the growth of mold, less sugar results in a product that supports mold growth.

Adapted from: Dudek, S. (2001). *Nutrition essentials for nursing practice* (4th ed., p. 38). Philadelphia: Lippincott Williams & Wilkins.

Complex Carbohydrates

Complex carbohydrates or **polysaccharides** are made of long chains of many sugar molecules arranged in such a way that they do not taste sweet. They are usually insoluble in water. Starch, dextrin, glycogen, and fiber are complex carbohydrates.

Starch.   *Starch* is the form of carbohydrate stored in plants and is the chief source of carbohydrates in the diet. Starch is made up of many glucose units linked together. The main sources of starch are grains, roots, bulbs, legumes, tubers, and seeds (Fig. 30-2). Starch grains are encased in a tough covering that is broken down in the process of digestion. Cooking starch-containing foods speeds up their digestion because enzymes in saliva can act on cooked starch, but have little effect on raw starch. Starch must be broken down into glucose before the body can use it.

Dextrin.   *Dextrin* is formed as an intermediate in starch digestion by the action of enzymes or heat (eg, cooking and

toasting). Dextrin is a gummy material that forms as a part of starch's digestive process.

Glycogen.   **Glycogen** is not a significant form of carbohydrate in the diet, but it is the body's storage form of carbohydrate. After the body meets its energy needs, the liver and muscle cells convert excess glucose to glycogen and store it for later use. On average, adult glycogen storage is limited to slightly more than 1 pound. Athletes may practice *carbohydrate loading* to maximize their glycogen storage for long-distance events.

Dietary Fiber.   *Dietary fiber,* commonly known as *roughage,* is a group name for the portion of plants resistant to digestion by human enzymes. Although they are not truly digested, some types of fiber are broken down by colonic bacteria to produce fatty acids and gas. Most plant foods are composed of various amounts and types of both water-insoluble and water-soluble fiber.

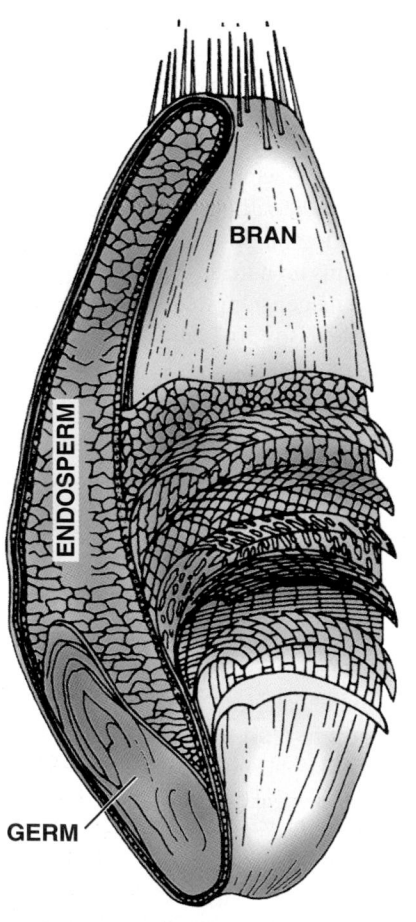

COMPONENT	RICHEST IN:
BRAN	Fiber Vitamin B$_6$ Pantothenic acid Niacin Selenium
GERM	Fat Thiamine Vitamin E Potassium Phosphorus Iron Selenium
ENDOSPERM	Protein Starch

Whole grains and flours contain the entire grain, or seed, which includes the endosperm portion plus the following components:

- The **bran**, or outer layer, which is rich in B vitamins and fiber. Technically, bran cereals are not truly whole-grain products, because the endosperm and germ are missing, but they are a concentrated source of fiber. Bran can be derived from wheat, oats, corn, or rice.
- The **germ**, the small embryo or sprouting portion of the seed. Some B vitamins, minerals, and some protein are found in the germ. Because the germ also contains fat, it is usually not included in flours, because fat limits the keeping quality of flours. Technically, wheat germ is not a whole grain because the bran and endosperm portions are removed.

FIGURE 30-2. A whole wheat kernel. The compartments of the whole wheat kernel are the bran, the germ, and the endosperm. Adapted from Dudek, S. (2001). *Nutrition essentials for nursing practice* (4th ed.). Philadelphia: Lippincott Williams & Wilkins.

Cellulose, lignin, and some hemicelluloses are the framework of plants and are water insoluble (cannot be broken down with water). They are most abundant in wheat bran and other whole-grain bread and cereals. The skin, stalks, leaves, and pulp of vegetables and the skin and pulp of fruits are all good fiber sources. Insoluble fiber holds water, increases stool bulk, decreases transit time of food through the intestines, and helps prevent constipation.

Pectin, gums, mucilages, and some hemicelluloses are water-soluble fibers that absorb water to form a gel. They slow gastric emptying time, improve glucose tolerance in people with diabetes, and bind bile acids (which helps lower high cholesterol levels). Water-soluble fibers are found in oats, legumes, apples, and citrus fruits.

Dietary fiber plays a role in preventing constipation, lowering serum glucose and cholesterol levels, and possibly aiding in weight reduction by promoting a feeling of fullness. Experts recommend that Americans eat more fiber of all types, increasing total daily intake to at least 20 to 35 grams. People can obtain this amount of fiber each day by eating at least five servings of fruits and vegetables, and at least six servings of breads and cereals that are identified as good or excellent sources of fiber.

Fats (Lipids)

Fats or **lipids** give flavor and texture to food. Fat is a concentrated energy source that the body can easily store. Most fat in food is in the form of **triglycerides,** which are composed of three fatty acids (tri-) and one glycerol (-glyceride). Like carbohydrates, triglycerides are made of carbon, hydrogen, and oxygen. The body also stores fat in the form of triglycerides, which it can make in the liver from an excess of carbohydrate, protein, and fat.

The major function of fat is to provide energy. Fat provides 9 C per gram: more than twice the calories of carbohydrate or protein. At rest, fat normally supplies about 40% of the body's energy needs. Fat also carries fat-soluble vitamins in the body and provides essential fatty acids that play a role in cholesterol metabolism. It helps maintain the function and integrity of capillaries and cell membranes, and is a precursor of the hormones known as *prostaglandins* and the phospholipids in cell membranes. Fat cushions major organs to protect them from injury and insulates the body from extreme temperatures. Dietary fat provides *satiety* (satisfaction), because fat leaves the stomach more slowly than carbohydrate or protein.

Fat comes from animals and plant oils. Fat that can be easily identified in foods that appear fatty, such as ground meat and butter, is known as *visible fat.* Fat hidden in foods that do not appear fatty, such as milk, cheese, egg yolks, nuts, desserts, and meat that is marbled with fat, is called *invisible fat.* Table 30-1 summarizes information about fats.

Digestion

Because fats do not dissolve in water, no fat digestion occurs in the mouth and very little occurs in the stomach. When fat reaches the small intestine, bile released from the gallbladder breaks the fat into tiny droplets. In the small intestine, pancreatic lipase breaks down these droplets of emulsified fat into fatty acids, glycerol, and monoglycerides. Once inside the mucosal cells of the small intestine, intestinal lipase completes the digestion of monoglycerides into fatty acids and glycerol. Most fatty acids are absorbed via the lymph system; only glycerol and certain fatty acids can be absorbed directly into the bloodstream.

Fatty Acids

Based on the number of double bonds between carbon atoms, fatty acids are classified as either *saturated* (no double bonds) or *unsaturated* (one or more double bonds). There are two types of unsaturated fatty acids, *monounsaturated* (one double bond) or *polyunsaturated* (two or more double bonds). Most food fats contain all three types of fatty acids; the type present in the greatest proportion determines whether a food is considered unsaturated or saturated.

Saturated Fatty Acids. Generally, foods that are high in **saturated fat** content are solid at room temperature because they already contain their full complement of hydrogen. Except for the fat found in poultry and many fish, all animal fats are high in saturated fat. Coconut, palm, and palm kernel oils are the only plant sources naturally high in saturated fat. Because a high saturated fat intake raises serum cholesterol levels, Americans are advised to lower their intake of total fat and saturated fat.

A recently recognized type of fatty acid called **trans-fat** is created when a polyunsaturated fatty acid, such as vegetable oil, is hydrogenated to make it solid at room temperature (as in margarine). In this process, known as *hydrogenation,* manufacturers add hydrogen to liquid oils—such as corn, cottonseed, soybean, and coconut oils—to make them more stable and to decrease the chance of rancidity. The degree of hydrogenation determines the saturation and firmness of the resultant product. **Hydrogenated** fats have fewer essential fatty acids than the original oil, because the unsaturated fat content is lowered. Additionally, trans-fat acids are associated with adversely altering serum levels of some specialized proteins called *lipoproteins.* Lipoproteins are discussed later in this chapter.

Unsaturated Fatty Acids. Unsaturated fatty acids are capable of adding more hydrogen to their molecular structure, because one or more double bonds exist between carbon atoms. Unsaturated fats tend to be soft or liquid at room temperature, and are susceptible to rancidity when exposed to light and oxygen over a long period. Poultry, freshwater fish, and all plant oils (except coconut, palm, and palm kernel oils) are high in unsaturated fat. Olive, canola, and peanut oils are high in monounsaturated fats. Safflower, sunflower, soybean, and corn oils are rich sources of polyunsaturated fats. Both monounsaturated and polyunsaturated fats help lower blood cholesterol levels when used in place of saturated fats. See Figure 30-3.

Linoleic acid and linolenic acid are polyunsaturated fatty acids considered essential fatty acids because people lack the enzymes needed to synthesize them. Because arachidonic acid is made from linoleic acid, arachidonic acid becomes an essential fatty acid when linoleic acid intake is deficient. Each essential fatty acid has a distinct role in cell structure and

Generally, unsaturated fats have the following characteristics:
  • They are soft or liquid at room temperature.
  • They have low melting points—the more double bonds in fatty acid, the lower the melting point. For instance, soft margarine (high in unsaturated fatty acids) melts quicker than butter (lower in unsaturated fatty acids).

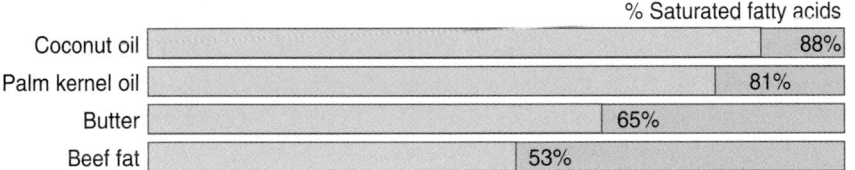

Monounsaturated fats and oils

% Monounsaturated fatty acids

Olive oil	71%
Canola oil	53%
Peanut oil	49%
Soft margarine	47%
Chicken, turkey	42%

Polyunsaturated fats and oils

% Polyunsaturated fatty acids

Safflower oil	75%
Sunflower oil	64%
Soybean oil	58%
Corn oil	55%

Saturated fats and oils

% Saturated fatty acids

Coconut oil	88%
Palm kernel oil	81%
Butter	65%
Beef fat	53%

FIGURE 30-3. Unsaturated fat. All food fats contain a mixture of saturated, monounsaturated, and polyunsaturated fatty acids. This figure shows the predominate types of fatty acids in selected fats and oils. Adapted from Dudek, S. (2001). *Nutrition essentials for nursing practice* (4th ed.). Philadelphia: Lippincott Williams & Wilkins.

function and is important in normal development. Vegetable oils, leafy vegetables, meat, and fatty fish are sources of essential fatty acids. Because dietary sources are common and the body stores them, essential fatty acid deficiency is extremely rare. Infants given formulas deficient in linoleic acid and hospitalized clients receiving prolonged lipid-free parenteral nutrition are the only groups at risk for fatty acid deficiency. A fatty acid deficiency causes, among other symptoms, a rash or dermatitis.

Cholesterol
Cholesterol is a member of a large group of compounds called *sterols*. Cholesterol is found only in animal tissues, and the body needs it to produce hormones, vitamin D, and bile acids. Cholesterol is a component of all cell membranes and also a major part of brain and nerve tissue. The body makes cholesterol from metabolites produced during the metabolism of energy. On average, the body makes more than twice the amount of cholesterol consumed in the average American diet. Foods high in cholesterol include organ meats (such as liver, kidneys, and brains) and egg yolk. Lesser amounts of cholesterol are found in whole milk products and meats.

Cholesterol is transported by lipoprotein molecules, which are found in the blood. High-density lipoproteins (**HDL**), the "good cholesterol," function to transport cholesterol from the tissues back to the liver, and in doing so, help lower serum cholesterol levels and the risk of heart disease. HDL levels can be increased by exercise, weight loss, smoking cessation, and moderate alcohol consumption. Low-density lipoproteins (**LDL**), the "bad cholesterol," transport cholesterol from the liver to the tissues. They are implicated in the development of atherosclerosis and coronary artery disease. A diet that is high in saturated fat increases serum LDL levels. Theorists believe that the ratio between these HDL and LDL levels is more significant for assessing health risk than is total cholesterol count. Trans-fat acids are known to increase serum levels of LDL, while decreasing serum levels of HDL.

Protein

Protein is the foundation of every body cell and is the only nutrient that builds and repairs tissue. In the absence of dietary protein, the body begins to use protein from the bloodstream, muscles, and organs to carry on daily activities. Every major organ, except the brain, will shrink during a prolonged dietary deficiency of protein. Proteins are made up of **amino acids,** which consist of carbon, hydrogen, oxygen, and nitrogen. Some amino acids also contain phosphorus, sulfur, cobalt, and iron. A small pool of amino acids is stored throughout the body for use in building proteins.

Proteins produce and repair all major body constituents. They are needed for the formation of muscles, connective tissue, glands, organs, skin, and blood clotting factors. Every cell in the body contains some protein. Proteins also help maintain the body's fluid balance; blood proteins called *albumins* and *globulins* help keep intracellular and extracellular fluids where they belong. If a person has a low protein intake, fluid balance may not be controlled, and edema may develop in the lower extremities. Another important function of protein is its contribution to the body's acid–base balance (see Chap. 17).

Hormones such as *thyroid hormone* and *insulin* are made from protein; all enzymes are proteins. *Antibodies* are also made from protein; therefore, proteins are a key component of the body's immune system (see Chap. 24). Proteins can be converted to glucose and burned for energy. The protein that remains after the body's protein needs are met may be converted to triglycerides in the liver and stored as fat. The body cannot store excess protein as protein.

Protein comes from both animal and plant sources (see Table 30-1).

Digestion
Chemical digestion of protein starts in the stomach. An enzyme (pepsin) breaks down the basic structure of the protein into polypeptides. In the small intestine, pancreatic juices containing enzymes (eg, pancreatic protease [or trypsin] and chymotrypsin) split some of the proteins into amino acids. These amino acids are absorbed directly into the blood and used by the body.

The remaining *dipeptides* (two amino acids linked together) and *tripeptides* (three amino acids linked together) are further broken down into amino acids in the intestine and at the brush border villi of the intestinal walls.

Amino Acids
Proteins are complex molecules composed of at least 100 individual units known as *amino acids*. The variations in physical characteristics and functions of individual proteins are due to the difference in the amounts and types of individual amino acids present, and the order in which they are arranged.

Of the 22 known amino acids, nine are considered essential because the body cannot make them at a rate sufficient to meet its needs for growth and maintenance. Therefore, they must be supplied by the diet. The essential amino acids are valine, leucine, isoleucine, phenylalanine, threonine, methionine, lysine, tryptophan, and histidine.

The body can synthesize nonessential amino acids if the diet contains enough nitrogen and energy. Nonessential amino acids are no less important than essential amino acids, but a dietary intake of them is unnecessary. The more common nonessential amino acids are alanine, cystine, glutamine, glycine, and serine.

☞ KEY CONCEPT

Essential and nonessential amino acids are needed to maintain life and normal growth; essential amino acids must be consumed through the diet.

Complete and Incomplete Proteins
"Complete" and "incomplete" are simplistic, imprecise terms used to indicate the quality of a protein. *Complete proteins,* or *high-quality proteins,* provide all essential amino acids in sufficient quantities and proportions for growth and maintenance. All animal proteins except gelatin are complete proteins. Some plant proteins, such as processed soy protein, are also complete. *Incomplete proteins* lack sufficient amounts of one or more essential amino acids. Plant proteins are generally considered incomplete, although the actual quality of protein varies considerably among different plant sources. Fortunately, different plants are missing different essential amino acids. By eating a variety of plant proteins over the course of the day, a person can obtain all essential amino acids.

Water

With the exception of oxygen, nothing is more essential to life than water. Human beings can survive for weeks without food but only days without water.

Chapter 17 noted that about 60% of an adult's body weight and up to 80% of an infant's body weight is water. It also stated that an adult loses about 2.5 quarts (2.37 liters) of water per day by perspiring, urinating, and exhaling. To maintain fluid balance in body cells, lost fluid must be replaced. Food provides some fluid, but it must be supplemented by drinking water and other liquids. Most authorities agree that the average adult needs 6 to 8 glasses of fluid per day.

Water composes a large percentage of cellular makeup. Blood distributes nutrients to the cells; water is one of blood's essential components. Water is the solvent in which vital chemical changes occur in the body, and it is also necessary for controlling body temperature. No organ of the body can function without water. Water is so necessary to life that nature has provided human beings with an inborn warning device: thirst is our strongest appetite.

Minerals

Minerals are vital for building bones and teeth. They help maintain muscle tone, regulate body processes, and maintain acid–base balance. Table 30-2 summarizes information on minerals. The body absorbs some minerals more readily than others, and foods vary considerably in the amount of minerals they contain. Some minerals are lost in cooking, and some are lost in body wastes.

Electrolytes
Electrolytes consist of minerals in the form of salts, acids, and bases. A more detailed discussion of electrolytes may be found in Chapter 17. Sodium (Na^+), potassium (K^+), chloride (Cl^-), and magnesium (Mg^+) work together in a close electrolyte relationship, and have many similar functions. They are essential for maintaining the osmotic pressure balance between a cell and its surrounding fluids, for helping to maintain normal acid–base balance, and for normal nerve and muscle functioning.

▪▪▪ TABLE 30-2 𝒮UMMARY OF MAJOR MINERALS

Mineral and Sources	Functions	Deficiency/Toxicity Signs and Symptoms
Calcium (Ca) **Adult AI** 19–50 yr: 1000 mg 51+ yr: 1200 mg **Adult UL:** 2.5 g/d • Milk and milk products, fortified orange juice, green leafy vegetables, small fish with bones, legumes	Bone and teeth formation and maintenance, blood clotting, nerve transmission, muscle contraction and relaxation, cell membrane permeability, blood pressure	*Deficiency* Children: impaired growth Adults: osteoporosis *Toxicity* Constipation, increased risk of renal stone formation, impaired absorption of iron and other minerals
Chloride (Cl) **Adult Estimated Minimum Requirement:** 750 mg • ¼ tsp salt = 750 mg Cl • Same sources as sodium	Fluid and electrolyte balance, component of hydrochloric acid in stomach	*Deficiency* Rare; may occur secondary to chronic diarrhea or vomiting and certain renal disorders *Toxicity* Vomiting, hypertension in chloride-sensitive people

Magnesium (Mg)
 Adult RDA
 Men:
    19–30 yr: 400 mg
    31+ yr: 420 mg
 Women:
    19–30 yr: 310 mg
    31+ yr: 320 mg
 Adult UL: 350 mg/d from supplements only (does not include intake from food and water)
 • Green leafy vegetables, nuts, legumes, whole grains, seafood, chocolate, cocoa
	Bone formation, nerve transmission, smooth muscle relaxation, protein synthesis, CHO metabolism, enzyme activity	*Deficiency*
		 Weakness, confusion. Growth failure in children. Severe deficiency: convulsions, hallucinations, tetany
		
		 Toxicity
		 Rare; nausea, vomiting, low blood pressure

Phosphorus (P) **Adult RDA** Men and women: 700 mg **Adult UL:** To age 70: 4 g/d 70+ yr: 3 g/d • All animal products (meat, poultry, eggs, milk), bread, ready-to-eat cereal	Bone and teeth formation and maintenance, acid–base balance, energy metabolism, cell membrane structure, regulation of hormone and coenzyme activity	*Deficiency* Rare; weakness and bone pain *Toxicity* Low blood calcium
Potassium (K) **Adult Estimated Minimum Requirement:** 2000 mg • Fruits and vegetables, legumes, whole grains, milk, meats, coffee	Fluid and electrolyte balance, acid–base balance, nerve impulse transmission, catalyst for many metabolic reactions, involved in skeletal and cardiac muscle activity	*Deficiency* Muscular weakness, paralysis, anorexia, confusion (occurs with dehydration) *Toxicity* (from supplements/drugs) Muscular weakness, vomiting
Sodium (Na) **Adult Estimated Minimum Requirement:** 500 mg • ¼ tsp salt = 500 mg Na • 75% of Na intake is from processed foods: canned soups, meats, vegetables; convenience and restaurant foods; pizza; processed meats	Fluid and electrolyte balance, acid–base balance, maintains muscle irritability, regulates cell membrane permeability and nerve impulse transmission	*Deficiency* Rare except with chronic diarrhea or vomiting and renal disorders; nausea, dizziness, muscle cramps *Toxicity* Excess is normally excreted. Impaired excretion (eg, secondary to renal disorders) causes edema and acute hypertension

(continued)

■■■ TABLE 30-2 ⨍UMMARY OF MAJOR MINERALS (CONTINUED)

Mineral and Sources	Functions	Deficiency/Toxicity Signs and Symptoms
Sulfur (S) No recommended intake • All protein foods (meat, poultry, fish, eggs, milk, legumes, nuts)	Component of disulfide bridges in proteins; component of biotin, thiamine, and insulin	*Deficiency* Unknown *Toxicity* In animals, excessive intake of sulfur-containing amino acids impairs growth

Adapted from Dudek, S. (2001). *Nutrition essentials for nursing practice* (4th ed., pp. 139 & 142). Philadelphia: Lippincott Williams & Wilkins.

Sodium

Sodium (Na) is the major ion in extracellular fluids. The body's actual requirement for sodium is very small; most North Americans consume many times more sodium (table salt) than necessary. Usually, the greater a person's sodium intake, the greater the amount of sodium he or she excretes in the urine. Some individuals retain sodium, which can result in edema and hypertension. Because research shows that populations who have a high intake of sodium are at greater risk for hypertension and cardiovascular disease, individuals should choose a diet moderate in salt and sodium. High sodium intake may also increase the risk of osteoporosis by promoting increased urinary calcium excretion. Although meat, milk, and some vegetables provide sodium, approximately 75% of consumed sodium in the United States comes from processed and convenience or "fast" foods.

Potassium

Potassium (K) is the major ion in intracellular fluid (fluid inside the cells). Potassium is widespread in foods and is especially abundant in fruit (bananas particularly), bran, fresh meats, and many vegetables. Salt substitutes often contain potassium in place of sodium. People are advised to eat more fruits and vegetables to boost their potassium intake, which may help reduce blood pressure.

Chloride

Chloride (Cl) is needed for the production of hydrochloric acid in the stomach. It is also one of the ions involved in the body's complex buffering system. Most chloride in the average Western diet comes from salt (60% of salt is chloride).

Magnesium

Magnesium (Mg) has many functions, including bone formation and maintenance of homeostasis. Magnesium combines with calcium and phosphorus in the bones (50% to 60% of the body's magnesium is in the bones). Magnesium is also an activator of enzymes and is involved with RNA in protein synthesis.

Calcium

Calcium (Ca) is the mineral most likely to be deficient in a typical adult diet. Calcium makes up about 2% of the adult human body; 99% of the body's calcium is in the bones and teeth. It also has other important uses such as keeping the body fluids balanced, helping blood clot, and regulating heart and other muscle activity and nerve responses. Normal blood levels of calcium are maintained (even when calcium intake is inadequate) through the action of hormones. These hormones influence calcium absorption, urinary calcium excretion, and the movement of calcium into and out of bones. Because bone gives up calcium at its own expense when calcium intake is inadequate, a chronic calcium deficiency increases the risk of *osteoporosis* (thinning of the bone). Altered blood calcium levels occur secondary to other disorders or from hormonal abnormalities, not from a dietary deficiency.

The best sources of dietary calcium are milk, yogurt, hard cheese, and calcium-fortified orange juice. The vitamin D and lactose content of milk also promotes calcium absorption. Good sources of calcium include calcium-fortified cereals, kale, broccoli, and canned salmon with bones. The most recent DRI for calcium was increased to 1000 to 1200 milligrams for most adults to maximize bone density and to reduce the risk of osteoporosis for women and men.

If normal dietary intake does not supply the DRI, supplementation may be indicated. Calcium carbonate is an excellent form of calcium for people up to the age of 50. Calcium citrate is a more readily absorbable form of calcium due to decreased release of hydrochloric acid (**HCl**) in the stomach, and is recommended for people over the age of 50.

Phosphorus

Every body cell contains phosphorus (P), which accounts for about 1% of adult body weight. Eighty percent of the phosphorus in the human body is found in the bones and teeth. Phosphorus has more functions than any other mineral in the body. It helps the cells use carbohydrates, fats, and proteins, and regulates acid–base balance. It is also important for normal nerve and muscle functioning. Almost all foods contain phosphorus, especially those rich in protein (meat, fish, poultry, nuts, legumes, milk, and milk products).

Trace Minerals

Some minerals are present in, and needed by, the body in very small amounts; they are nevertheless important in body processes. These minerals are called *trace minerals*. Table 30-3 summarizes some of the trace minerals utilized by the body.

■■ TABLE 30-3 ⨍UMMARY OF TRACE MINERALS

Mineral and Sources	Functions	Deficiency/Toxicity Signs and Symptoms
Iron (Fe) **Adult RDA** Men: 10 mg Women (19–50 yr): 15 mg (51+ yr): 10 mg • Beef liver, red meats, clams, tofu, legumes, fortified cereals, bread	Oxygen transport via hemoglobin and myoglobin; constituent of enzyme systems	*Deficiency* Lowered immunity, decreased work capacity, weakness, fatigue, itchy skin, pale nailbeds and eye membranes, impaired wound healing, intolerance to cold temperatures *Toxicity* Increased risk of infections, lethargy, joint disease, hair loss, organ damage, enlarged liver, amenorrhea, impotence Accidental poisoning in children causes death
Zinc (Zn) **Adult RDA** Men: 15 mg Women: 12 mg • Meat, poultry, fish, egg yolks, legumes, whole grains, milk	Tissue growth and wound healing; sexual maturation and reproduction; constituent of many enzymes in energy and nucleic acid metabolism; immune function; vitamin A transport; taste perception; associated with insulin	*Deficiency* Abnormal glucose tolerance, growth retardation, impaired wound healing, impaired sense of smell, weight loss, diarrhea, nausea, night blindness, delayed onset of puberty, anorexia, irritability, low sperm count *Toxicity* Anemia, elevated LDL, lowered HDL, diarrhea, vomiting, impaired calcium absorption, fever, renal failure, muscle pain, dizziness, reproductive failure
Iodine (I) **Adult RDA** 150 µg • Iodized salt, seafood, bread, dairy products	Component of thyroid hormones that regulate growth, development, and metabolic rate	*Deficiency* Goiter, weight gain, lethargy During pregnancy may cause severe and irreversible mental and physical retardation (cretinism) *Toxicity* Enlarged thyroid gland
Selenium (Se) **Adult RDA** Men and women: 55 µg **Adult UL:** 400 µg/d • Seafood, liver, kidney, other meats • Grains grown in selenium-rich soil	Works as an antioxidant with vitamin E	*Deficiency* Heart disease *Toxicity* Nausea, vomiting, abdominal pain, diarrhea, hair and nail changes, nerve damage, fatigue
Copper (Cu) **Adult Estimated Safe and Adequate Intake:** 1.5–3.0 mg • Organ meats, seafood, nuts, seeds	Used in the production of hemoglobin; component of several enzymes; used in energy metabolism	*Deficiency* Rare; anemia, bone abnormalities *Toxicity* Vomiting, diarrhea
Manganese (Mn) **Adult Estimated Safe and Adequate Intake:** 2.0–5.0 mg • Widely distributed in foods. Best sources are whole grains, tea, pineapple, kale, strawberries	Component of enzymes involved in fat synthesis, growth, reproduction, and blood clotting	*Deficiency* Rare *Toxicity* Rare; nervous system disorders
Fluoride (Fl) **Adult AI:** Men: 3.8 mg Women: 3.1 mg • Fluoridated water, water that naturally contains fluoride, tea	Formation and maintenance of tooth enamel, promotes resistance to dental decay; role in bone formation and integrity	*Deficiency* Susceptibility to dental decay; may increase risk of osteoporosis *Toxicity* Fluorosis (mottling of teeth), nausea, vomiting, diarrhea, chest pain, itching

(continued)

TABLE 30-3 *S*UMMARY OF TRACE MINERALS (CONTINUED)

Mineral and Sources	Functions	Deficiency/Toxicity Signs and Symptoms
Chromium (Cr) *Adult Estimated Safe and Adequate Intake:* 50–200 µg • Meat, whole grains, nuts, cheese	Cofactor for insulin	*Deficiency* Insulin resistance, impaired glucose tolerance *Toxicity* Dietary toxicity unknown Occupational exposure to chromium dust damages skin and kidneys
Molybdenum (Mo) *Adult Estimated Safe and Adequate Intake:* 75–250 µg • Milk, legumes, bread, grains	Component of many enzymes; works with riboflavin to incorporate iron into hemoglobin	*Deficiency* Unknown *Toxicity* Occupational exposure to molybdenum dust causes gout-like symptoms

Adapted from Dudek, S. (2001). *Nutrition essentials for nursing practice* (4th ed., pp. 146–147). Philadelphia: Lippincott Williams & Wilkins.

Iron. Iron (Fe) is an essential part of every body cell and is also a constituent of hemoglobin (Hgb), a substance in the red blood cells (**RBCs**) that carries oxygen. The body is thrifty with its supply of iron, and continually reuses it by salvaging the iron from worn-out RBCs. Young children, teenagers, and women require more iron than do men. Iron-deficient anemia is the most common deficiency disorder in the United States.

Iodine. Iodine (I) is needed for production of the hormone thyroxine, and is essential for normal thyroid gland functioning. Some parts of the United States, especially areas near the Great Lakes and the Rocky Mountains, have almost no iodine in the soil; consequently, food products from these regions contain no natural sources of iodine. Goiter, an enlargement of the thyroid gland, was common in these areas prior to the use of iodized salt, which has virtually eliminated goiter in the United States.

Other Trace Minerals. Other trace minerals include chromium (Cr), which plays a role in the function of insulin; copper (Cu), which helps form hemoglobin; and zinc (Zn), which is important in producing hormones and RNA, and which can enhance or depress the immune system depending on whether intake exceeds or fails to meet requirements. Selenium (Se) is a component of an antioxidant and is being studied for its role in cancer prevention. The following trace minerals may be essential for humans in very small amounts: arsenic, boron, bromine, cadmium, fluorine, lead, lithium, manganese, molybdenum, nickel, silicon, tin, and vanadium. Recent DRI levels were published for some of these minerals (see Table 30-3).

Vitamins

"Vita" is the Latin word for "life." The word "vitamin" signifies the importance of vitamins to humans. *Vitamins* comprise carbon, oxygen, hydrogen, and sometimes nitrogen or other elements. When first discovered, vitamins were given alphabetical names such as vitamin A, vitamin B, and so on. Research has shown that vitamins belong to groups. Because they are organic substances, vitamins can be converted to other forms and are susceptible to oxidation and destruction. They may also be precursors to other chemicals. As a result of the increasing awareness of individual vitamins, vitamins are more accurately referred to by a group name or a specific name such as "ascorbic acid" for Vitamin C. Table 30-4 and Table 30-5 contain both common and specific names of most known vitamins.

Small amounts of vitamins are necessary to help regulate body processes, including synthesizing body compounds like bone and blood, and extracting energy from carbohydrates, fat, and protein. Most vitamins work in the form of a coenzyme that promotes the action of enzymes. Without vitamins, thousands of chemical reactions cannot occur. The body, with a few exceptions, cannot produce vitamins; therefore, vitamins are an essential component of a healthy diet. Box 30-3 provides some general principles related to vitamins.

Foods are the natural sources of vitamins and should supply daily vitamin needs. Foods differ greatly in the amount and number of vitamins they contain. Table 30-4 and Table 30-5 identify the major vitamins, their sources, their functions, and deficiency disorders that occur when the body does not get enough of a particular nutrient.

Vitamins are available in commercial, over-the-counter forms. Some vitamins are available by prescription, because physicians may want to prescribe high dosages for certain marked deficiencies. Vitamins vary in their solubility, which influences how they are absorbed, transported through the blood, stored, and excreted. Vitamins with the United States Pharmacopoeia (**USP**) seal on the label are guaranteed to meet set purity and solubility standards.

☞ KEY CONCEPT

A, D, E, and K are fat-soluble vitamins; C and B-complex are water-soluble vitamins.

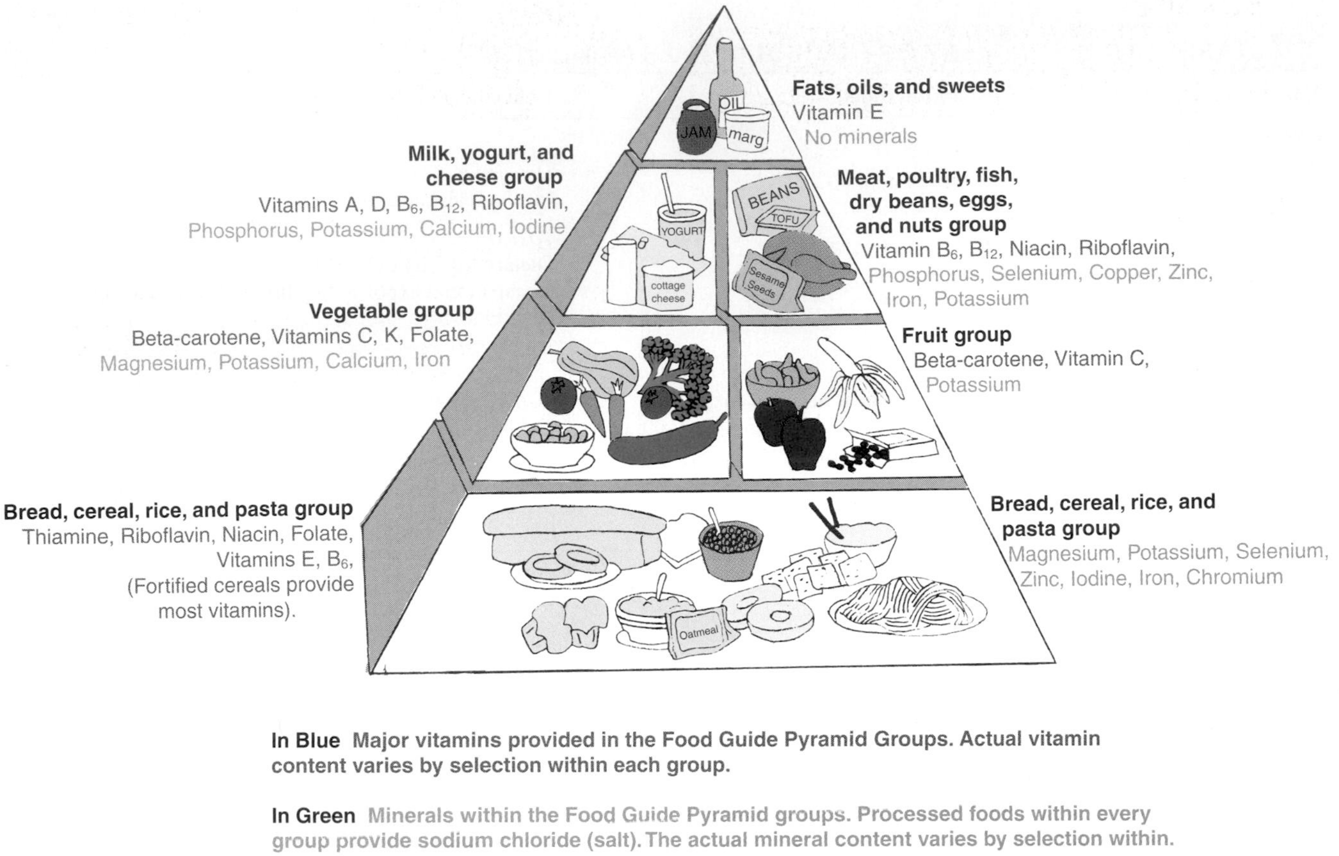

FIGURE 30-4. Major vitamins and minerals in foods of the Food Guide Pyramid. Adapted from Dudek, S. (2001). *Nutrition essentials for nursing practice* (4th ed.). Philadelphia: Lippincott Williams & Wilkins.

Many healthy individuals choose to take commercial vitamins as a safeguard against less-than-optimal food choices. Those who take supplements should select a balanced multivitamin that does not exceed the UL for any nutrient. See In Practice: Educating the Client 30-1 for more information about vitamin supplements.

Fat-soluble Vitamins

Fat-soluble vitamins (see Table 30-4) are absorbed into the lymphatic circulation with fat and must attach to a protein carrier to be transported through the blood. The body stores fat-soluble vitamins primarily in the liver and in fat tissue. Because they are stored, deficiency symptoms are slow to develop. Vitamins A and D are toxic when consumed in excess of need over a prolonged period. Cooking does not easily destroy fat-soluble vitamins.

Vitamin A. *Retinol* or vitamin A is a group of related substances that promote growth, sustain normal vision, support normal reproduction, and maintain healthy skin and mucous membranes (thereby increasing the body's resistance to infection). Preformed vitamin A is found only in animal sources, such as liver, butter, and egg yolk; fortified milk is also a good source. Carotene is a precursor of vitamin A; that is, the body converts carotene to vitamin A, but not quickly enough to be toxic. Excellent food sources of carotene are deep orange and deep green fruits and vegetables, such as sweet potatoes, win-

ter squash, carrots, broccoli, spinach, green leafy vegetables, and cantaloupe.

Vitamin D. *Calciferol* or vitamin D is a group of sterols essential in regulating the body's use of calcium and phosphorus. A marked deficiency of vitamin D hampers growth and affects bone hardness. This deficiency causes a childhood condition known as **rickets,** in which the bones do not harden as they should, but instead bend into deformed positions, such as bowlegs. Pregnant and lactating women must provide themselves with enough vitamin D to prevent rickets from developing in the child, and to preserve their own bones and teeth. Sunlight on the skin plays a role in the conversion of vitamin D to its active form, as does the functioning of the liver and kidneys. The best food sources of vitamin D are fish liver oils and fortified milk.

Groups at the highest risk for vitamin D deficiency are totally breast-fed infants, vegetarians who consume no dairy products (see Chap. 31), and people who get little sunshine (such as institutionalized or homebound individuals). Secondary vitamin D deficiency can occur in people with liver disease, kidney disease, or fat malabsorption syndromes. Because excess vitamin D is toxic, vitamin D should be supplemented only with physician approval.

Vitamin E. *Alpha-tocopherol* or vitamin E is sometimes called the "reproductive vitamin" or the "anti-sterility vitamin"

➤➤ BOX 30-3

GENERAL PRINCIPLES RELATED TO VITAMINS

- Some vitamins are lost by exposure to air or during food storage. Fresh foods retain most vitamins when properly stored. Frozen foods are second, although their vitamin C content may be higher than that of improperly handled fresh food. Canned foods are third. (Canned foods should be processed carefully and not stored too long.)
- Some vitamins are fat soluble and are stored in the body in this form. The diet must include enough fat to carry an adequate supply of these vitamins (15–20 g).
- Some vitamins are water soluble. Cook foods in a small amount of water and use the cooking water, if possible, in gravies, sauces, and soups.
- High temperatures destroy vitamins. Do not overcook food, and serve it at once.
- In some foods, the highest concentration of vitamins is in the portion likely to be thrown away, such as the outer leaves of lettuce and vegetable peels.
- A clinical condition called *hypervitaminosis* can occur as a result of an excess of a particular vitamin or vitamins. Hypervitaminosis occurs almost exclusively from supplement use, not from dietary intake.

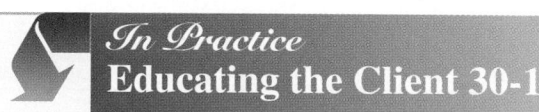

In Practice
Educating the Client 30-1

VITAMINS

Encourage people who take vitamin supplements to consider the following:

- *Freshness:* Vitamin pills can lose their potency over time, especially when stored in a bathroom medicine cabinet. Look for pills with an expiration date on the label. Do not use after the expired date.
- *Price:* In most cases, cost has little to do with vitamin quality.
- Supplements should provide no more than 100% Daily Value, because more is not necessarily better, and in some instances, is toxic.
- Supplements should contain no unnecessary ingredients. The average diet supplies enough biotin, pantothenic acid, phosphorus, iodine, and chloride. Trace minerals, such as nickel, silicon, and boron may be unnecessary. Sugar in vitamins is safe, because the small amount contained within a vitamin pill is not harmful.

because it was originally found to be a necessary component for reproduction in animals. However, no evidence supports the concept that vitamin E has an effect on human reproduction or sexual function. Although the role of vitamin E is not fully understood, it has been proven to be a powerful antioxidant. In this role, it protects vitamins A and C, as well as some fatty acids and phospholipids in the cell membrane, from destruction by oxidation. Vitamin E deficiency is rare, except in malabsorption disorders, such as cystic fibrosis and pancreatic disorders. Vitamin E is found in plant fat and vegetable oils, products made with vegetable oils (such as margarine and shortening), wheat germ, nuts, and green leafy vegetables.

Vitamin K. *Menadione* or vitamin K is essential in the formation of prothrombin and at least five other proteins that

■■■ **TABLE 30-4** *S*UMMARY OF FAT-SOLUBLE VITAMINS

Vitamin and Sources	Functions	Deficiency/Toxicity Signs and Symptoms
Vitamin A (Retinol) ***Adult RDA*** Men: 1000 µg RE* Women: 800 µg RE • Retinol: Liver, milk, butter, cheese, cream, egg yolk, fortified milk, margarine, and ready-to-eat cereals • Carotenoids: Spinach, collards, kale, mustard greens, broccoli, carrots, peaches, pumpkin, red peppers, sweet potatoes, winter squash *RE = retinol equivalents 1 RE = 1 µg retinol or 6 µg β carotene	The formation of visual purple, which enables the eye to adapt to dim light Normal growth and development of bones and teeth Formation and maintenance of mucosal epithelium to maintain healthy functioning of skin and membranes, hair, gums, and various glands Important role in immune function	*Deficiency* Night blindness, or the slow recovery of vision after flashes of bright light at night Bone growth ceases; bone shape changes; enamel-forming cells in the teeth malfunction; teeth crack and tend to decay Skin becomes dry, scaly, rough, and cracked; keratinization or hyperkeratosis develops; mucous membrane cells flatten and harden: Eyes become dry (xerosis); irreversible drying and hardening of the cornea can result in blindness Decreased saliva secretion → difficulty chewing, swallowing → anorexia Decreased mucous secretion of the stomach and intestines → impaired digestion and absorption → diarrhea, increased excretion of nutrients Susceptibility to respiratory, urinary tract, and vaginal infections increases

(continued)

■■■ **TABLE 30-4** *SUMMARY OF FAT-SOLUBLE VITAMINS (CONTINUED)*

Vitamin and Sources	Functions	Deficiency/Toxicity Signs and Symptoms
		Toxicity Headaches, vomiting, double vision, hair loss, bone abnormalities, liver damage Can cause birth defects during pregnancy
Vitamin D (calciferol) ***Adult AI**** Men and Women: 5 µg/d to age 50 10 µg/d ages 51–70 15 µg/d over age 70 ***Adult UL:*** 50 µg/d • Sunlight on the skin • Liver, fatty fish, egg yolks, fortified milk, ready-to-eat cereals, and margarine *In the absence of sunlight and as cholecalciferol. 1 µg cholecalciferol = 40 IU vitamin D	Maintains serum calcium concentrations by: Stimulating GI absorption Stimulating the release of calcium from the bones Stimulating calcium reabsorption from the kidneys	*Deficiency* Rickets (in infants and children) Retarded bone growth Bone malformations (bowed legs) Enlargement of ends of long bones (knock-knees) Deformities of the ribs (bowed, with beads or knobs) Delayed closing of the fontanel → rapid enlargement of the head Decreased serum calcium and/or phosphorus Malformed teeth; decayed teeth Protrusion of the abdomen related to relaxation of the abdominal muscles Increased secretion of parathyroid hormone Osteomalacia (in adults) Softening of the bones → deformities, pain, and easy fracture Decreased serum calcium and/or phosphorus, increased alkaline phosphatase Involuntary muscle twitching and spasms *Toxicity* Kidney stones, irreversible kidney damage, muscle and bone weakness, excessive bleeding, loss of appetite, headache, excessive thirst, calcification of soft tissues (blood vessels, kidneys, heart, lungs), death
Vitamin E (tocopherol) ***Adult RDA*** Men and Women: 15 mg*/d ***Adult UL:*** 1000 mg/d • Vegetable oils, margarine, salad dressing, other foods made with vegetable oil, nuts, seeds, wheat germ *As α tocopherol	Acts as an antioxidant to protect vitamin A and PUFA from being destroyed Protects cell membranes	*Deficiency* Increased RBC hemolysis In infants, anemia, edema, and skin lesions *Toxicity* Relatively nontoxic High doses enhance action of anticoagulant medications
Vitamin K (menadione) ***Adult RDA*** Men: 80 µg Women: 65 µg • Bacterial synthesis, green leafy vegetables, liver, milk, vegetables of the cabbage family	Synthesis of blood-clotting proteins and a bone protein that regulates blood calcium	*Deficiency* Hemorrhaging *Toxicity* No symptoms have been observed from excessive vitamin K

Adapted from Dudek, S. (2001). *Nutrition essentials for nursing practice* (4th ed., pp. 107–109). Philadelphia: Lippincott Williams & Wilkins.

are required for the clotting of blood. Because vitamin K is found in a variety of foods, the average diet supplies an adequate amount. Good sources are liver, egg yolk, cauliflower, cabbage, spinach, and other green leafy vegetables. Intestinal bacteria synthesize vitamin K in insufficient quantities to meet the total vitamin K requirement. The limited amount the body stores is found in the liver. A dietary deficiency is unlikely. Intake of foods that contain high amounts of vitamin K should

be limited when taking anticoagulants such as warfarin. Signs of hemorrhaging may be due to a vitamin K deficiency, which is treated in adults with either oral or intramuscular administration of vitamin K.

Water-soluble vitamins

Water-soluble vitamins (see Table 30-5) include vitamins C and B complex. They are absorbed directly through the intesti-

■■■ **TABLE 30-5** 𝒮UMMARY OF WATER-SOLUBLE VITAMINS

Vitamin and Sources	Functions	Deficiency/Toxicity Signs and Symptoms
Thiamine (Vitamin B₁) **Adult RDA** Men: 1.2 mg/d Women: 1.1 mg/d • Whole grain and enriched breads and cereals; liver, legumes, nuts	Coenzyme in energy metabolism Promotes normal appetite and nervous system functioning	*Deficiency* Beriberi Mental confusion Fatigue Peripheral paralysis Muscle weakness and wasting Painful calf muscles Anorexia Edema Enlarged heart Sudden death from heart failure *Toxicity* No toxicity symptoms reported
Riboflavin (Vitamin B₂) **Adult RDA** Men: 1.3 mg/d Women: 1.1 mg/d • Milk and other dairy products; whole grain and enriched breads and cereals; eggs, meat, green leafy vegetables	Coenzyme in energy metabolism Aids in the conversion of tryptophan into niacin	*Deficiency* Ariboflavinosis Dermatitis Cheilosis Glossitis Photophobia Reddening of the cornea *Toxicity* No toxicity symptoms reported
Niacin (Vitamin B₃) **Adult RDA*** Men: 16 mg/d Women: 14 mg/d **Adult UL:** 35 mg/d • All protein foods; whole grain and enriched breads and cereals *As niacin equivalents (NE) 1 mg niacin = 60 mg tryptophan	Coenzyme in energy metabolism Promotes normal nervous system functioning	*Deficiency* Pellagra: 4 (Ds) Dermatitis (bilateral and symmetrical) and glossitis Diarrhea Dementia, irritability, mental confusion → psychosis Death, if untreated *Toxicity* (from supplements/drugs) Flushing, liver damage, gastric ulcers, low blood pressure, diarrhea, nausea, vomiting
Pyridoxine (Vitamin B₆) **Adult RDA** Men: 1.3 mg/d to age 50 1.7 mg/d after 50 Women: 1.3 mg/d to age 50 1.5 mg/d after 50 **Adult UL:** 100 mg/d • Meats, fish, poultry, legumes, fruits, green leafy vegetables, whole grains, nuts	Coenzyme in amino acid and fatty acid metabolism Helps convert tryptophan to niacin Helps produce insulin, hemoglobin, myelin sheaths, and antibodies	*Deficiency* Dermatitis, cheilosis, glossitis, abnormal brain wave pattern, convulsions, and anemia *Toxicity* Depression, fatigue, irritability, headaches; sensory neuropathy characteristic
Folate/Folic acid (Vitamin B₉) **Adult RDA*** Men and women: 400 µg/d **Adult UL:** 1,000 µg/d (applies to forms obtained from food, supplements, or combination) • Leafy vegetables, legumes, seeds, liver, orange juice, some fruits; breads, cereals, and other grains are fortified with folic acid	Coenzymes in DNA synthesis— therefore vital for new cell synthesis and the transmission of inherited characteristics	*Deficiency* Glossitis, diarrhea, macrocytic anemia, depression, mental confusion, fainting, fatigue *Toxicity* Too much can mask B₁₂ deficiency

*As dietary folate equivalent (DFE) 1 DFE = 1 µg food folate = 0.6 µg folic acid (from fortified food or supplement) consumed with food = 0.5 µg synthetic (supplemental) folic acid taken on an empty stomach

(continued)

■■■ **TABLE 30-5** ⨏UMMARY OF WATER-SOLUBLE VITAMINS (CONTINUED)

Vitamin and Sources	Functions	Deficiency/Toxicity Signs and Symptoms
Cobalamin (Vitamin B₁₂)		
Adult RDA	Coenzyme in the synthesis of new cells	*Deficiency*
Men and women: 2.4 µg/d (people over 50 should meet their RDA mainly by consuming foods forti- fied with vitamin B₁₂ or a supple- ment containing vitamin B₁₂) • Animal products: meat, fish, poultry, shellfish, milk, dairy products, eggs • Some fortified foods	Activates folate Maintains nerve cells Helps metabolize some fatty acids and amino acids	GI changes: glossitis, anorexia, indigestion, recurring diarrhea or constipation, and weight loss Macrocytic anemia: pallor, dyspnea, weakness, fatigue, and palpitations Neurologic changes: paresthesia of the hands and feet, decreased sense of position, poor muscle coordination, poor memory, irritability, depression, paranoia, delirium, and hallucinations *Toxicity* No toxicity symptoms reported
Pantothenic Acid		
Adult AI	Part of coenzyme A used in energy metabolism	*Deficiency* Rare; general failure of all body systems
Men and women: 5 mg/d • Widespread in foods • Meat, poultry, fish, whole grain cereals, and legumes are among best sources		*Toxicity* No toxicity symptoms reported, although large doses may cause diarrhea
Biotin (Vitamin H)		
Adult AI	Coenzyme in energy metabolism, fatty acid synthesis, amino acid metabolism, and glycogen formation	*Deficiency* Rare; anorexia, fatigue, depression, dry skin, heart abnor- malities
Men and women: 30 µg/d • Widespread in foods • Eggs, liver, yeast breads, and cereals are among best choices • Synthesized by GI flora		*Toxicity* No toxicity symptoms reported
Ascorbic acid (Vitamin C)		
Adult RDA	Collagen synthesis Antioxidant Promotes iron absorption Involved in the metabolism of certain amino acids Thyroxin synthesis Immune system functioning	*Deficiency* Bleeding gums, pinpoint hemorrhages under the skin Scurvy
Men: 90 mg/d Women: 75 mg/d **Adult UL:** 2 g/d • Citrus fruits and juices, peppers, broccoli, cauliflower, Brussels sprouts, cantaloupe, kiwifruit, mustard greens, strawberries, tomatoes		Hemorrhaging Muscle degeneration Skin changes Delayed wound healing: reopening of old wounds Softening of the bones → malformations, pain, easy fractures Soft, loose teeth Anemia Increased susceptibility to infection Hysteria and depression *Toxicity* Diarrhea, abdominal cramps, nausea, headache, insomnia, fatigue, hot flashes, aggravation of gout symptoms

Adapted from Dudek, S. (2001). *Nutrition essentials for nursing practice* (4th ed., pp. 113–115). Philadelphia: Lippincott Williams & Wilkins.

nal walls into the bloodstream. They are also easily absorbed and excreted in urine when consumed in excess. Water-soluble vitamins are considered non-toxic because the body generally does not store them. Deficiencies develop more quickly with them than with fat-soluble vitamins because water-soluble vitamins are not readily stored and are excreted rapidly. Food, light, heat, acids, and alkaline solutions can easily destroy water-soluble vitamins.

Vitamin C.   Vitamin C is probably equally well known by its chemical name, *ascorbic acid.* Over the years, experts

have recognized its many functions, but continue to discover further uses. One of the functions of vitamin C in vital body processes is to aid in the formation of collagen, the most impor- tant protein in connective tissue. By holding cells together, col- lagen contributes to healthy tissue and to the proper functioning of blood vessels, skin, gums, bones, joints, and muscles— essentially, all body tissues and organs. Vitamin C is also in- volved in reactions involving numerous other compounds, such as folic acid, histamine, neurotransmitters, bile acids, leuko- cytes, and corticosteroids. Vitamin C enhances the absorption of the form of iron that is predominate in plants, and is an effective antioxidant. Individuals who have had surgery or who have suffered extensive burns frequently receive large supplemental doses of ascorbic acid; it is essential to wound healing.

The classic disease of vitamin C deficiency, **scurvy,** is rare in the United States. Symptoms of scurvy include bleeding gums, loose teeth, sore and stiff joints, tiny hemorrhages, and great weight loss. Lesser vitamin C deficiencies affect health by causing listlessness, irritability, and lowered resistance to disease.

Vitamin C is probably the most unstable of all the vitamins. Exposure to air, drying, heating, and storing destroy it. As an acid, it survives longer in acidic surroundings; therefore, baking soda (the alkali, sodium bicarbonate) should not be added to food sources of vitamin C during cooking. Tomatoes retain vitamin C better than other vegetables because they contain acid. Freezing fruits and vegetables helps to preserve their vitamin C content, but they should be used immediately after thawing. Carefully canned fruits and vegetables also retain this vitamin because air is excluded during the canning process.

Because vitamin C is destroyed by heat and is water soluble, cooking should be done in as little water as possible, and overcooking should be avoided. Many raw fruits and vegetables, especially citrus fruits, are high in vitamin C. For instance, one cup of orange juice provides more than the RDA for vitamin C. Research has yet to confirm Linus Pauling's theory that vitamin C can prevent or cure the common cold. Because of its antioxidant properties, vitamin C may play an important role in cancer prevention. However, some studies have shown that mega-doses of vitamin C may increase the resistance of cancer cells to chemotherapy treatment. Doses greater than the DRI may increase the risk of kidney stones in some people.

Populations at risk for vitamin C deficiency include people who do not eat fruits and vegetables, alcoholics, and people of low socioeconomic status. Smokers require extra vitamin C because nicotine inhibits its absorption.

Vitamin B Complex.   The B complex vitamins are generally known as thiamine, riboflavin, niacin, folate or folic acid, cobalamin, pyridoxine, biotin, and pantothenic acid. Most B complex vitamins have numbers such as B_1, B_{12}, etc. However, the trend is to identify the vitamin by its proper name in lieu of a number (see Table 30-5).

The following B complex vitamins are all widely distributed in foods. Although each one is chemically distinct, they share many similar functions, dietary sources, and deficiency symptoms.

Thiamine (B_1): Thiamine promotes general body efficiency. It plays a role in growth, cell metabolism, appetite, neurologic functioning, RNA and DNA formation, and normal muscle tone in cardiac and digestive tissues. As part of a coenzyme, thiamine is essential for the metabolism of carbohydrate and certain amino acids. Signs of a deficiency of thiamine are poor appetite, fatigue, irritability, general lethargy, nausea, vomiting, loss of weight and strength, depression, mental confusion, and poor intestinal tone. A severe deficiency causes **beriberi,** a disease of the nervous system that leads to paralysis and death from heart failure.

The best food sources of thiamine are pork, whole-grain and enriched breads and cereals, legumes, peas, organ meats, and dried yeast.

The body does not store thiamine to any great extent. Thiamine is lost during cooking, especially when cooking is prolonged or at high temperatures. Alkalis also destroy thiamine. In the United States, thiamine deficiency occurs most frequently in persons who abuse alcohol, because they "waste" thiamine in the metabolism of alcohol. A thiamine supplement is usually prescribed for these clients.

Riboflavin (B_2): Riboflavin functions primarily as a component of two coenzymes that catalyze many reactions, including the metabolism of carbohydrate, fat, and protein. It is essential for growth. Riboflavin deficiency is rare in the United States; people at the greatest risk for deficiency are those who take in large amounts of alcohol, older adults, people on low-calorie diets, and people with malabsorption syndromes. Signs of a riboflavin deficiency include *cheilosis* (cracking and sores at the corners of the mouth), *glossitis* (inflammation of the tongue, with a smooth texture and purplish-red color), and *stomatitis* (inflammation of the lining of the mouth). The body does not store riboflavin to any extent; therefore, a person's diet must provide a steady supply.

Riboflavin is available in a wide variety of foods, but only in small quantities. The best sources are milk and milk products, meat, poultry, fish, and whole-grain or enriched breads and cereals. Exposure of riboflavin to light while in solution destroys it.

Niacin (B_3): Niacin exists as *nicotinic acid* and *nicotinamide.* It plays a vital role in the release of energy from carbohydrate, fat, and protein. It is also needed for the production of fatty acids, cholesterol, and steroid hormones.

The best sources of niacin are lean meat, liver, kidney, yeast, peanut butter, whole-grain and enriched products, and dried peas and beans. Niacin is not readily destroyed by heat, light, acids, or alkalis. The body stores only a small amount of niacin.

A marked niacin deficiency leads to the disease **pellagra.** The mucous membranes of the mouth and digestive tract become red and inflamed, and lesions appear on the skin. Symptoms of severe deficiency progress through the four Ds: dermatitis, diarrhea, dementia, and death. A lesser deficiency brings on these same symptoms in a milder form.

Niacin deficiency is rare, except in persons who abuse alcohol. Physicians sometimes prescribe nicotinic acid in gram quantities to help lower blood cholesterol levels; however, side effects are common. These possible side effects include flushing of the skin, hot flashes, headache, hypotension, tachycardia, hypoglycemia, and liver damage.

Folate/folic acid (B_9): Folate is the group name for this B complex vitamin. Folate plays a major role in the synthesis of DNA and RNA, and in the formation of red and white blood cells. Folic acid is the form of folate used in vitamin supplements. It is also involved in the synthesis of certain enzymes and in amino acid metabolism. Folate is available in many foods. Excellent sources include enriched cereals, liver, organ meats, milk, eggs, asparagus, broccoli, green leafy vegetables, dried peas and beans, and orange juice. Cereals and breads are now required by the Food and Drug Administration (**FDA**) to be fortified with folic acid.

Deficiency results in megaloblastic (macrocytic) anemia, glossitis, diarrhea, poor growth, impaired nerve function, and increased risk of heart attack. Intake of high amounts of folate masks vitamin B_{12} deficiency (*pernicious anemia*), which, when left untreated, can cause irreversible neurologic damage or death. Folic acid deficiency is common in all parts of the world. In the United States, folic acid deficiency is most common among older adults, pregnant women, alcoholics, fad dieters, and women taking oral contraceptives. A folate supplement is usually prescribed for these individuals. New research has proven that folate, given before conception and during early pregnancy, helps prevent neural tube defects, such as spina bifida.

Cobalamin (B_{12}): Cobalamin is a family of compounds, all of which contain cobalt. It is important in folate metabolism and in blood cell formation. It is also involved in maintaining the myelin sheath covering certain nerves. Cobalamin and folate are needed to activate each other.

For the intestine to absorb vitamin B_{12}, intrinsic factor must be present. *Intrinsic factor* is a protein-containing compound the stomach produces in the presence of hydrochloric acid. Conditions that impair the secretion of intrinsic factor, such as gastric surgery or gastric cancer, cause B_{12} malabsorption and pernicious anemia, an anemia characterized by abnormal RBCs known as *megaloblasts*. Vitamin B_{12} deficiency in the United States is due to impaired absorption, not an inadequate dietary intake.

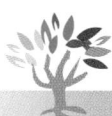

SPECIAL CONSIDERATIONS: THE LIFE SPAN

Cobalamin (Vitamin B_{12})

Older adults are at risk of cobalamin (B_{12}) deficiency because of a high prevalence of atrophic gastritis related to aging. People with atrophic gastritis are unable to adequately absorb vitamin B_{12} from food, but are able to absorb vitamin B_{12} from vitamin pills. Thus, oral supplements, not injections as previously thought, may be needed to prevent vitamin B_{12} deficiency in older people.

Vitamin B_{12} deficiency leads to anemia, neurologic symptoms, increased risk of heart attack, and other general-

ized symptoms. Because the body stores vitamin B_{12}, it may take years for symptoms to develop.

Vitamin B_{12} is found exclusively in animal sources; therefore, pure vegetarians who consume no animal products are at risk of vitamin B_{12} deficiency. Bacteria in the small intestine may produce small amounts of absorbable vitamin B_{12}.

Pyridoxine (B_6): Vitamin B_6 is a family of compounds: *pyridoxal, pyridoxine,* and *pyridoxamine.* The general name is pyridoxine. Vitamin B_6 is needed for enzyme activity in the metabolism of protein, carbohydrate, and fat. It is especially important in protein metabolism. Other functions include forming heme for hemoglobin, metabolizing neurotransmitters, synthesizing myelin sheaths, and maintaining cellular immunity.

Rich sources of vitamin B_6 are meat, fish, poultry, and eggs. Whole-wheat products, nuts, and oats are also good sources. Most diets contain adequate amounts of vitamin B_6. Current research has shown that vitamin B_6 is ineffective in the treatment of premenstrual syndrome.

A deficiency of vitamin B_6 is most likely to occur secondary to malabsorption syndromes, alcoholism, or certain drug therapies, and is most likely to develop in people with multiple B vitamin deficiencies. Symptoms may include retarded growth, confusion, headaches, and seizures. A deficiency of vitamin B_6 may also increase the risk of heart attack. Large quantities of vitamin B_6 taken for months or years can cause neurologic problems, such as difficulty walking, numbness of the feet and hands, clumsiness, and nerve degeneration. Symptoms gradually improve after the vitamin is discontinued.

Biotin: Biotin (rarely seen as vitamin H) is essential in the functioning of many enzymes. It acts as a coenzyme in the metabolism of carbohydrate and fat, and aids in the removal of certain nitrogen groups from amino acids.

Biotin is found in almost all foods. Liver, egg yolks, soy flour, cereals, and yeast are the best sources of biotin.

Biotin deficiency is rare except when a person consumes large amounts of raw egg whites. A substance in the egg white, avidin, binds biotin and keeps it from being absorbed.

Pantothenic Acid: Pantothenic acid is involved in a number of metabolic processes in humans, especially in the metabolism of protein, carbohydrates, and fats. Because of its central role in energy metabolism, it is vital to all energy-requiring body processes. The average diet supplies a sufficient amount; no RDA has been established. The word pantothenic means "widespread," and pantothenic acid is found in many foods. Good sources include liver, organ meats, egg yolk, dried peas and beans, broccoli, whole grains, lean meats, and poultry.

A HEALTHY DIET

A healthy diet is one that provides an adequate amount of each essential nutrient needed to support growth and development, perform physical activity, and maintain health. In addition to meeting physiologic requirements, diet is also used to satisfy a variety of personal, social, and cultural needs. These factors must be considered in diet planning (see Chap. 32). The diets of all individuals must consist of foods that are easily attainable and affordable. People can use an infinite variety and combination of foods to form a healthy diet. The current philosophy is that no good foods or bad foods exist, and that all foods can be enjoyed in moderation.

Although ensuring that the diet provides enough nutrients is important, of greater concern for most Americans today is avoiding dietary excesses, particularly of calories, fat, cholesterol, and sodium, which are associated with the development of several chronic diseases. Many Americans can achieve risk reduction by implementing dietary and lifestyle changes.

How can you choose a diet that provides sufficient amounts of essential nutrients, but not excessive amounts of others, and help your clients do the same? Where is the line between adequate nutrition and "over" nutrition? As a nurse, you are often in a position to promote wellness by counseling clients and their families on the "why" and "how to" of food choices. Today's most important nutritional concepts are *variety, moderation,* and *balance.*

Dietary Guidelines for Americans

The purpose of *Dietary Guidelines for Americans,* now in its fifth edition, is to provide the healthy public over age 2 with practical and positive suggestions for choosing a diet that meets nutritional requirements, supports activity, and reduces the risk of chronic disease. These guidelines are not intended as a diet prescription for specific individuals, but serve as a starting point from which people can plan healthy diets (Table 30-6).

Because eating is one of life's greatest pleasures, the *Guidelines* emphasize variety, flexibility, and enjoyment. They focus on the total diet, not individual foods to avoid, and stress the importance of physical activity in health.

The Food Guide Pyramid

The United States Department of Agriculture (**USDA**) introduced the Food Guide Pyramid (see Fig. 30-1 and Box 30-1) in 1992. This pyramid is recognized as the official food guide for the United States. It is a complex graphic designed to illustrate the *Dietary Guidelines for Americans,* although it does not address sodium, weight control, and alcohol use. The pyra-

---

■■■ **TABLE 30-6** *D*IETARY GUIDELINES FOR AMERICANS AND ADVICE FOR TODAY

Guideline	Advice for Today
Eat a variety of foods. *Rationale:* No single food supplies all 40-plus essential nutrients in amounts needed. Variety also helps reduce the risk of nutrient toxicity and accidental contamination.	Enjoy eating a variety of foods. Get the many nutrients your body needs by choosing among the varied foods you enjoy from these groups: grain products, vegetables, fruits, milk and milk products, protein-rich plant foods (beans, nuts), and protein-rich animal foods (lean meat, poultry, fish, and eggs). Remember to choose lean and low-fat foods and beverages most often. Many foods you eat contain servings from more than one food group. For example, soups and stews may contain meat, beans, noodles, and vegetables.
Balance the foods you eat with physical activity—maintain or improve your weight. *Rationale:* Excess weight increases the risk of numerous chronic diseases, such as hypertension, heart disease, and diabetes.	Try to maintain your body weight by balancing what you eat with physical activity. If you are sedentary, try to become more active. If you are already very active, try to continue the same level of activity as you age. More physical activity is better than less, and any is better than none. If your weight is not in the healthy range, try to reduce health risks through better eating and exercise habits. Take steps to keep your weight within the healthy range (neither too high nor too low). Have children's heights and weights checked regularly by a health professional.
Choose a diet with plenty of grain products, vegetables, and fruits. *Rationale:* Plant foods provide fiber, complex carbohydrates, vitamins, minerals, and other substances important for good health. They are also generally low in fat.	Eat more grain products (breads, cereals, pasta, and rice), vegetables, and fruits. Eat dry beans, lentils, and peas more often. Increase your fiber intake by eating more of a variety of whole grains, whole grain products, dry beans, fiber-rich vegetables and fruits such as carrots, corn, peas, pears, and berries.
Choose a diet low in fat, saturated fat, and cholesterol. *Rationale:* High-fat diets increase the risk of obesity, heart disease, and certain types of cancer.	To reduce your intake of fat, saturated fat, and cholesterol, follow these recommendations, as illustrated in the Food Guide Pyramid, which apply to diets consumed over several days and not to single meals or foods. • Use fats and oils sparingly. • Use the Nutrition Facts Label to help you choose foods lower in fat, saturated fat, and cholesterol. • Eat plenty of grain products, vegetables, and fruits. • Choose low-fat milk products, lean meats, fish, poultry, beans, and peas to get essential nutrients without substantially increasing calorie and saturated fat intakes.

(continued)

▪▪▪ TABLE 30-6 *𝒟*ɪᴇᴛᴀʀʏ **GUIDELINES FOR AMERICANS AND ADVICE FOR TODAY (CONTINUED)**

Guideline	Advice for Today
Choose a diet moderate in sugars. *Rationale:* Foods high in added sugar are often "empty calories." Both sugars and starches promote tooth decay.	Use sugars in moderation—or sparingly if your calorie needs are low. Avoid excessive snacking, brush with a fluoride toothpaste, and floss your teeth regularly. Read the Nutrition Facts Label on foods you buy. The food label lists the content of total carbohydrate and sugars, as well as calories.
Choose a diet that is moderate in salt and sodium. *Rationale:* A high salt intake is associated with higher blood pressure.	Fresh fruits and vegetables have very little sodium. The food groups in the Food Guide Pyramid include some foods that are high in sodium and other foods that have very little sodium, or that can be prepared in ways that add flavor without adding salt. Read the Nutrition Facts Label to compare and help identify foods lower in sodium within each group. Use herbs and spices to flavor food. Try to choose forms of foods that you frequently consume that are lower in sodium and salt.
If you drink alcoholic beverages, do so sensibly and in moderation. *Rationale:* Current evidence suggests that moderate drinking is associated with a lower risk for coronary heart disease in some individuals. However, higher levels of alcohol intake raise the risk for high blood pressure, stroke, heart disease, certain cancers, accidents, violence, suicides, birth defects, and overall mortality (deaths). Too much alcohol may cause cirrhosis of the liver, inflammation of the pancreas, and damage to the brain and heart.	• If you drink alcoholic beverages, do so sensibly and in moderation. • Limit intake to one drink per day for women or two per day for men, and take with meals to slow alcohol absorption. • Avoid drinking before or when driving or whenever it puts you or others at risk.

Source: United States Department of Agriculture and United States Department of Health and Human Services. (2000). *Nutrition and your health: Dietary guidelines for Americans* (5th ed.). Website: http://www.health.gov/ dietaryguidelines/dga2000.

mid shape conveys the fundamental concepts of moderation and balance. Unlike previous food guides, the pyramid suggests a range of daily servings from each major food group (to avoid excesses), not a minimum daily requirement (to avoid deficiencies). The lower end of each range is intended for people who consume about 1,600 calories daily; the upper end of each range is suggested for a 2,800-calorie diet. Table 30-7 summarizes the recommended servings per day.

The pyramid is divided into five major food groups. The USDA recommends that the bottom three sections of the pyramid—plant-based foods: starch (the bread, cereal, rice, and pasta group), vegetables, and fruit—serve as the founda-

▪▪▪ TABLE 30-7 *ℛ*ᴇᴄᴏᴍᴍᴇɴᴅᴇᴅ **SERVINGS PER DAY**

Food group	Children ages 2 to 6 years, women, some older adults (about 1,600 calories)	Older children, teen girls, active women, most men (about 2,200 calories)	Teen boys, active men (about 2,800 calories)
Bread, Cereal, Rice, and Pasta Group (Grains Group)—especially whole grains	6	9	11
Vegetable Group	3	4	5
Fruit Group	2	3	4
Milk, Yogurt, and Cheese Group (Milk Group)—preferably fat free or low fat	2 or 3*	2 or 3*	2 or 3*
Meat, Poultry, Fish, Dry Beans, Eggs, and Nuts Group (Meat and Beans Group)—preferably lean or low fat	2, for a total of 5 ounces	2, for a total of 6 ounces	3, for a total of 7 ounces

*The number of servings depends on your age. Older children and teenagers (ages 9 to 18 years) and adults over the age of 50 need 3 servings daily. Others need 2 servings daily. During pregnancy and lactation, the recommended number of milk group servings is the same as for nonpregnant women.

Adapted from U.S. Department of Agriculture, Center for Nutrition Policy and Promotion. (1996). *The Food Guide Pyramid.* Home and Garden Bulletin No. 252.

tion of a healthy diet. The apex of the pyramid (fats, oils, and sweets) are not major food groups, so no foods are pictured there. The USDA recommends that people consume items from the apex sparingly.

When using the pyramid as a teaching tool, you must stress that each group provides some nutrients, but no group supplies adequate amounts of all essential nutrients. People should eat some foods from each group daily. Because not all foods within a group are nutritionally equivalent, people should also select different foods from within each group. For instance, within the meat group, pork is a rich source of thiamine, but most other items are not. Likewise, red meats are high in saturated fat, but skinless poultry is not.

Diet Planning

In the hospital or other healthcare facility, a dietitian will most likely plan menus. As a nurse, you will need to understand dietary requirements to teach clients effectively. Emphasize foods with **nutrient density;** that is, foods that provide significant amounts of key nutrients per volume consumed. Nutrient density becomes increasingly important for those with diminished appetites due to nausea, pain, inactivity, boredom, or anxiety. For instance, hospitalized individuals often have increased protein requirements to promote healing. Encouraging clients with high protein requirements to consume all their meat and milk is far more effective for their healing processes than stressing the need to eat all their mashed potatoes and carrots.

At the same time, keeping meals interesting is important. Food and mealtimes take on much greater significance in a healthcare setting, and are often the highlight of the client's day. Food is also one area of care over which clients can "vent" their frustrations and feelings of helplessness. So although nutrient density is important from a medical standpoint, eating less nutritious foods may sometimes be important on an emotional level.

Nutritional Problems

The nutritional problems of most Americans are not due to deficiencies of single nutrients but to overconsumption of nutrients. The 1998 report of the *Top Leading Causes of Death* released by the Centers for Disease Control (CDC), revealed that, of the 10 leading causes of death, four are associated with dietary excesses and imbalances:

Coronary artery disease
Certain types of cancer
Cerebral vascular accident (stroke)
Diabetes mellitus

Overnutrition also contributes to such conditions as hypertension, osteoporosis, dental caries (decay), gastrointestinal diseases, and obesity. Although no one can say for certain exactly what proportion of these disorders is due to diet, evidence suggests that a diet high in calories, fat (especially saturated fat), cholesterol, and sodium, but low in complex carbohydrates and fiber, contributes significantly to the high rates of chronic diseases among many North Americans.

Health and Body Weight

Body Weight Assessment.   In the past, Ideal Body Weight (**IBW**) was used to describe optimal weight for optimal health. A general guideline for IBW for women and men is as follows:

> *For adult women:* Allow 100 pounds for 5 feet of height; add 5 pounds for each additional inch.
> *For adult men:* Allow 106 pounds for 5 feet of height; add 6 pounds for each additional inch.

The total may be adjusted upward or downward by 10% to account for individual differences in body frame size. Although this method has been accepted as a standard, other individual differences may render this method inappropriate for determining an individual's ideal body weight. Newer standards for weight replace "ideal" with "healthy" because "ideal" is difficult to define. "Healthy" weights are listed as a range for any given height, to account for differences in body composition among individuals that may affect weight without adversely affecting health. For instance, two people of the same height may have the same amount of fat tissue, but one may weigh more because of greater muscle mass and bone density.

While IBW continues to be used in many clinical settings, the newer Body Mass Index (**BMI**) is being used more frequently. The fifth edition of *Dietary Guidelines for Americans* recommends the use of BMI and waist measurement to evaluate the body weight of adults.

BMI measures weight in relation to height. Defined as weight in kilograms divided by height in meters squared, BMI allows comparison of weights among people of differing heights. Nomograms have eliminated the need to perform calculations; BMI can be simply obtained, by plotting weight against height (see Figure 30-5). Weight is broken down into 4 classifications: Healthy weight BMI: 18.5 to 24.9; Overweight BMI: 25 to 30; Obese BMI: 30 to 40; Very Obese BMI: >40. However, some people may be above their "healthy weight" according to their BMI, but not be "overweight." For instance, neither IBW nor BMI takes into account the body composition of people who are muscular (eg, athletes) or who have greater bone density, and therefore may weigh more than their "healthy weight."

To increase the accuracy of weight classification, the waist measurement may be used in conjunction with BMI as recommended in *Dietary Guidelines for Americans*. This method is based on the premise that health risks increase as waist measurement increases. A waist measurement of greater than 35 inches for women, or greater than 40 inches for men, indicates a greater risk of health problems—even if BMI is within the healthy weight parameters.

Overweight and Obesity.   The percentage of Americans who fall into the "overweight" and "obese" categories has increased dramatically over the past two decades and is now considered to be at epidemic levels. Overweight individuals are individuals who weigh 10% to 20% more than the "ideal" weight per height. However, an individual who has large muscle mass can be overweight without being obese. Currently, over 51% of the population in the United States is overweight.

Height*   **BMI (Body Mass Index)**

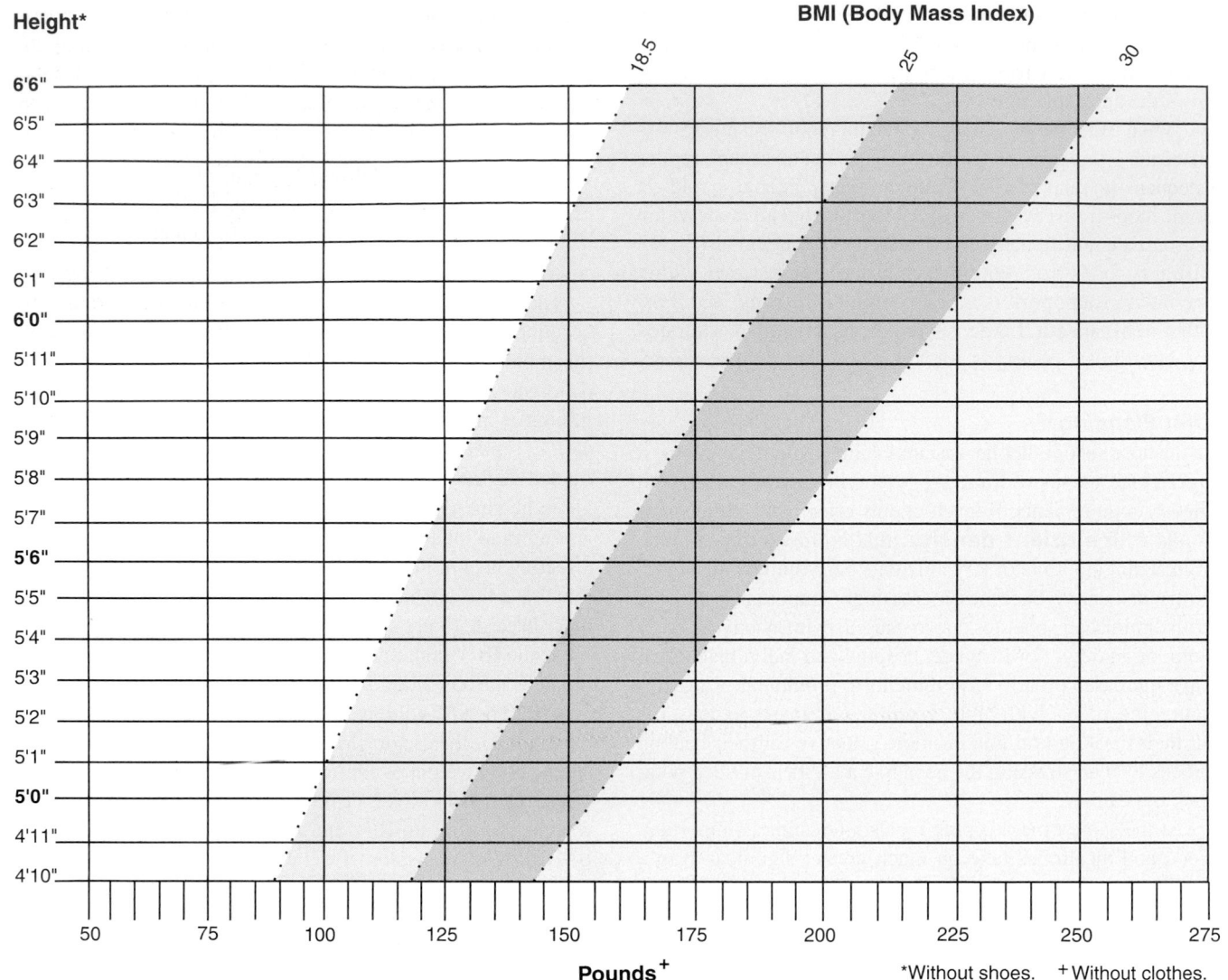

Body mass index (BMI) measures weight in relation to height. The BMI ranges shown above are for adults. They are not exact ranges of healthy and unhealthy weights. However, they show that health risk increases at higher levels of overweight and obesity. Even within the healthy BMI range, weight gains can carry health risks for adults.

Directions: Find your weight on the bottom of the graph. Go straight up from that point until you come to the line that matches your height. Then look to find your weight group.

    Healthy Weight BMI from 18.5 up to 25 refers to healthy weight.
    Overweight BMI from 25 up to 30 refers to overweight.
    Obese BMI 30 or higher refers to obesity. Obese persons are also overweight.

Source: Report of the Dietary Guidelines Advisory Committee on the Dietary Guidelines for Americans (2000, p.3).

FIGURE 30-5. Body mass index and healthy weight.

Obesity refers to an excessive amount of fat on the body. A woman is obese if she has body fat greater than 33%; obesity for men is body fat greater than 25%. Overweight or obese people do not necessarily consume adequate amounts of all nutrients, even though they may overeat.

Malnutrition
Malnutrition literally means "bad nutrition." Too much or too little of one or more nutrients may cause poor nutrition; however, malnutrition most commonly refers to *under*nutri-

tion. Inadequate food intake may cause malnutrition, or it may occur secondary to alterations in digestion, absorption, or metabolism of nutrients.

Although certain population groups are at risk for vitamin and mineral deficiencies (eg, alcoholics, adolescent girls, pregnant and lactating women, people of low socioeconomic status, and people with certain chronic diseases), severe deficiencies are rare in the United States. The prevalence of mild deficiencies, which may not produce obvious physical symptoms but can be detected through blood analysis, varies among nutrients. Ironically, hospitalized clients are at risk for protein-calorie malnutrition (**PCM**), which is seen in diets that are low in calories and protein, and can prolong hospitalization, delay wound healing, and lower resistance to infection.

NUTRITION ACROSS THE LIFE SPAN

Eating a balanced diet throughout life is the basis of good health. Because cultural and family background often influences diet, educating women during pregnancy and family caregivers during childrearing years has the potential to have a positive impact on the nutritional health of future generations.

Pregnancy

Women who consume an adequate diet during pregnancy provide the fetus, placenta, and maternal tissues with the nutrients necessary for growth and development. A good diet cannot guarantee a successful pregnancy, but it can optimize the chance of delivering a healthy full-term infant. Although the requirements for almost all nutrients increase during pregnancy, adequate intake of protein, iron, calcium, vitamin D, and folic acid is especially important. Calorie needs actually increase by only 300 C per day during the second and third trimesters, and not at all during the first trimester, if pre-pregnancy weight is adequate. Therefore, nutrient density is necessary to avoid overeating. Most physicians prescribe prenatal vitamin and mineral supplements. See Tables 30-2 through 30-7 and Chapter 64 for specific dietary recommendations.

Pregnant women with a family history of diabetes are at increased risk for developing gestational diabetes mellitus (**GDM**). All women should be screened for GDM between weeks 24 and 28 of their pregnancy. If a woman tests positive for GDM, she must be monitored closely, and she should see a dietitian to be placed on a special diet to control her blood sugars. GDM places the baby at higher risk for pre- and postnatal complications. Women who are diagnosed with GDM are at high risk for developing type 2 diabetes later in life. Achieving a healthy body weight after pregnancy lowers this risk.

Infancy

The first year of life is marked by the most rapid growth outside the mother's womb. Infants double their birth weight in 6 months and triple it in a year. This rapid growth explains an infant's high use of energy.

The American Academy of Pediatrics recommends exclusive breastfeeding for the first 5 to 6 months of life. Breast milk provides all essential nutrients in optimal amounts and in a form that the infant can easily tolerate and digest, without artificial colorings, flavorings, or preservatives. Overfeeding is unlikely. Breastfeeding is associated with a significant decrease in the incidence and duration of both gastrointestinal and nongastrointestinal infections, and it protects against food allergies. Breastfeeding may also decrease the risk of certain chronic diseases later in life, such as type 2 diabetes and Crohn's disease.

Formula feeding is an acceptable alternative if breastfeeding is contraindicated or the mother is unable or unwilling to breastfeed. Infant formulas designed to resemble breast milk provide comparable nutritional benefits, although they lack some of the unique qualities of breast milk. Formula does not contain docosahexenaeoic, a fatty acid present in human breast milk that promotes cognitive brain development. Cow's milk and whey-adjusted formulas are available for full-term infants; formulas made from soy isolates or casein may be given to infants intolerant to routine formulas. A variety of formulas are also available for infants with special needs, such as premature infants and infants with specific metabolic disorders like phenylketonuria (**PKU**) (see Chap. 71). Because cow's milk is a poor source of iron, may cause intestinal bleeding, and provides unsuitably high levels of protein, phosphorus, and electrolytes, it should not be given until after the age of 1 year. Whole milk should be used between ages 1 and 2 years.

Feeding infants on demand (when they are hungry) is preferable. If an infant is hungry, cries, and is then fed and satisfied, the caregiver creates a sense of trust and prevents frustration. Taking time to hold the infant while feeding is important, even if using a bottle. Mealtime should be pleasurable and comforting, because infants react to their caregivers' emotions.

Generally, infants are not developmentally ready for solid foods until 6 months of age. Iron-fortified infant rice cereal is recommended as the first solid food because it is unlikely to cause an allergic reaction (it is *hypoallergenic*). Caregivers should introduce plain new foods one at a time for 5 to 7 days; if the infant is allergic, the caregiver can easily identify the offending food. As the intake of solid food increases, the intake of breast milk or formula should decrease to avoid displacing the intake of other nutrient-rich foods. By 12 months of age, milk intake should total 16 to 24 ounces per day, all by cup. Because of the risk of botulism, infants should not be given honey until after the age of 1 year.

Supplement use for infants is controversial. From birth to age 6 months, breast-fed infants may be given supplemental fluoride and vitamin D, with iron added after 4 months of age. Formula-fed infants may be given iron if the formula is not fortified, and fluoride if the local water supply is not fluoridated. Infants usually do not need supplements during the second 6 months of life, if they are fed iron-fortified infant cereal and their diet is adequate in vitamins C and D. High-risk infants may be given a multivitamin or multimineral supplement.

Childhood

Caregivers with healthy eating habits set a good nutritional example for children. Permanent eating habits usually develop during childhood.

☞ KEY CONCEPT

Children should not be forced to eat. Usually children eat as much as needed.

Appetite fluctuates widely because of erratic growth patterns. Children should be allowed to eat to satisfy hunger. Generally, for young children a serving size equals 1 tablespoon of food per year of age; thus the serving size for a 2-year-old child is 2 tablespoons. Offering seconds is better than overwhelming the child with too much food. Young children eat an average of five to seven times a day; well-planned snacks can significantly contribute to total nutrient intake.

A child's food preferences may change. Small amounts of new foods can be introduced with familiar favorites. Adults should encourage children to taste new foods, but respect their individual likes and dislikes. It is not important if children refuse to eat a particular food (eg, squash), as long as they have a reasonable intake from each of the major food groups. Small children usually prefer mildly flavored foods and finger foods.

Children should not be required to clean their plates but should stop eating when they are no longer hungry. Nutritious desserts, pudding, fruit, and low-fat yogurt should be part of the meal, not bribes or rewards for eating other foods. To decrease the risk of choking in young children, supervised eating and avoidance of foods that most often cause choking (eg, hot dogs, candy, nuts, grapes, popcorn, celery, and tough meat) are necessary.

Minimizing distractions and noise promotes enjoyable meals. Family caregivers should eat with children, allowing 20 to 30 minutes per meal. Food should never be used to reward, punish, bribe, or convey love. Occasional table accidents should be expected. A high chair, infant seat, booster chair, or child's table and chairs next to the adult's table may encourage eating and make children more comfortable. Children should be encouraged to participate in food preparation and clean-up.

SPECIAL CONSIDERATIONS: NUTRITION

Children and Fat

Fat is an important energy source for children because they have small stomachs and high energy needs. Children, especially those under 2 years old, need some fat in their diets. Children between the ages of 1 and 2 years should consume whole milk. Children over 2 years should drink low-fat milk. Failure to thrive has been seen in children whose families are overly concerned about avoiding obesity in children and therefore severely restrict fat in the child's diet.

Common nutritional problems during childhood are iron deficiency anemia and obesity. Dietary changes, combined with prescribed supplements, can usually correct anemia. Obesity is harder to treat. Although obese infants do not necessarily grow up to be fat adults, an overweight 5-year-old may be on the road to lifelong weight problems. Childhood obesity has increased dramatically in recent years and has been linked to a sedentary lifestyle, which includes long hours of television viewing and playing computer games. Treatment for childhood obesity is not food restriction, but changes in dietary practices (eg, less junk food and fast food, and smaller servings) and an increase in physical activity.

Adolescence

A period of rapid growth, accompanied by an enormous appetite, characterizes the adolescent years. The teenager needs extra food to meet the needs of growth and body development. Enjoyment, along with peer and social pressures, often influences adolescent food choices more than nutritional and health considerations. Snacking may constitute 30% or more of an adolescent's total calorie intake each day. Unfortunately, snacks are often high in fat, sugar, or sodium. Adolescents must be encouraged to select nutritious snacks. Meal skipping—especially breakfast—is a common nutritional concern, as is the frequent use of fast foods. Eating disorders are described in Chapter 72.

☛ KEY CONCEPT

Caregivers of adolescents need to be alert to disorders such as obesity, anorexia, and bulimia and should seek appropriate assistance for these disorders as soon as possible.

Caregivers should allow adolescents to make choices. Sometimes, the foods they choose are not very harmful. A slice of cold pizza for breakfast is better than no breakfast at all. Generally, nagging is ineffective.

Iron deficiency anemia may be a problem for girls after the onset of menses, and in boys during their growth spurt. Iron deficiency anemia can lead to fatigue and decreased ability to concentrate and to learn. Although an iron-rich diet can help to prevent iron deficiency, it usually cannot treat iron-deficiency anemia after it is established. Iron supplements are then used in conjunction with diet. See In Practice: Educating the Client 30-2 for more information about iron deficiency.

Early and Middle Adulthood

During this period, calorie requirements may decrease because the person is no longer growing and is less active. Using the Food Guide Pyramid and choosing a wide variety of foods will add interest to menu planning.

☛ KEY CONCEPT

Good nutritional habits should be practiced throughout a lifetime. Education is the cornerstone to good nutrition; good nutrition is the cornerstone to good health.

Beginning in young adulthood, muscle and bone mass declines and the proportion of fat increases, resulting in a decrease in REE. Physical activity may also decline. These two factors result in a decrease in calorie requirements. Being overweight can become a problem during this stage of life. It can be managed by carefully following the Food Guide Pyramid and developing an active exercise program. The need for most

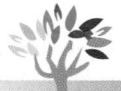

In Practice
Educating the Client 30-2

IRON

Iron deficiency is the most common nutritional deficiency in the United States. Groups at risk are infants under age 2, adolescents, menstruating women, older adults, minorities, and people with low incomes. Preventive measures are maximizing iron intake and iron absorption. Dietary components do not affect the absorption of heme iron (mainly in meat), but greatly affect the absorption of nonheme iron (mainly in plants).

Measures to prevent iron deficiency include the following:

• Choosing iron-fortified cereals over non-fortified varieties
• Using whole-grain products
• Cooking in iron pots whenever possible
• Consuming a rich source of ascorbic acid (vitamin C) like orange juice or tomatoes at every meal
Rationale: Ascorbic acid enhances absorption of iron.
• Eating meat with every meal, if possible.
• Avoiding coffee and tea immediately before and after meals (both interfere with iron absorption)
• Avoid taking calcium and iron supplements at the same time
Rationale: Calcium interferes with the absorption of iron.

Calcium and Osteoporosis

Estrogen-deficient osteoporosis, a disease characterized by a decrease in total bone mass and deterioration of bone tissue, affects women. Although symptoms may not appear until old age, osteoporosis begins to develop much earlier in life. Although an adequate calcium intake is important throughout life, many researchers believe that the biggest impact on preventing osteoporosis is made between 4 and 20 years of age, when calcium retention in girls is at its peak.

Consuming an adequate calcium intake before and after puberty helps maximize peak bone mass, which is the greatest amount of bone mass an individual will ever have. Then, after the age of 35 when bone loss exceeds bone gain, the body is better equipped to withstand the loss without adverse side effects. Unfortunately, few women consume the current RDA for calcium. Many women feel they do not want to add the extra calories in milk to their diet. Without milk or milk products in the diet, calcium needs are unlikely to be met. Encourage women to drink skim milk, to use skim milk yogurt for dessert, and to use calcium-fortified orange juice and calcium supplements, all excellent sources of calcium that the body absorbs well. Other types of osteoporosis affect men.

Calcium supplements should be considered in people above 35 years of age. There are several types of calcium supplements, each with advantages and indications for use.

other nutrients, with the exception of iron, stays the same or increases in late adulthood. Thus, nutrient density is important to avoid overeating.

Older Adulthood and Aging

Throughout the life cycle, nutrition significantly affects health and the quality of life. Studies show that a lifetime of good eating habits promotes health maintenance in old age. Poor lifelong eating habits contribute to many degenerative disorders associated with aging, such as diabetes, osteoporosis, hypertension, and atherosclerosis.

As a group, older adults are at risk for nutritional problems because of physiologic, economic, and psychosocial changes. Some nutrient requirements, such for as vitamin B_{12}, become greater with age due to decreased ability to absorb nutrients. Data on the nutritional requirements of older adults over the age of 70 have been included as a separate group in the current DRIs. Previously, the oldest age category was 51+ years. As people continue to live longer, this age group may need to be broken down further, for a 70-year-old versus a 95-year-old individual.

Many factors can negatively affect the food intake of older people. Difficulty chewing, which is related to loss of teeth and periodontal disease, places many individuals at risk of poor

intake. Changes in taste and smell cause food to be less flavorful and less enjoyable. Social isolation, impaired mobility, and depression are other factors that may influence food intake. Many older adults are economically deprived; the lower the income, the greater the likelihood the diet will be inadequate. Also, multiple and chronic use of medications can impair intake by altering appetite, the ability to taste, or nutrient digestion, absorption, or utilization.

Constipation is common among older individuals. It is related to decreased abdominal muscle tone, decreased physical activity, and inadequate fluid and fiber intake. Constipation is also a common side effect of many drugs. Wheat bran and fresh fruits and vegetables (if chewing is not impaired) may help alleviate constipation. A decreased thirst sensation makes older adults more prone to dehydration; they should be encouraged to drink even if they do not feel thirsty. As with younger people, variety, balance, and moderation are the keys to a good diet. Empty-calorie foods should be limited. Small frequent meals may help maximize intake if appetite is impaired. Assistive devices are available for people whose physical impairments make eating or preparing food difficult.

Depression, common among the older population, can have a negative impact on eating behavior and may lead to malnutrition. Individuals who live alone or in long-term care facilities are at especially high risk. Positive socialization can improve their emotional state and food intake. Congregate dining programs provide a hot, balanced midday meal and the opportunity to socialize at low or no cost. Nurses working in long-term care facilities can have a tremendous impact on the emotional and physical well-being of these vulnerable individuals by providing them with compassionate and quality care.

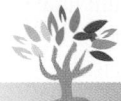 SPECIAL CONSIDERATIONS: THE LIFE SPAN

Salts and Sugar

Older adults may have a decreased ability to differentiate tastes, especially salts and sugars. Some adults compensate for this loss by increasing their intake of salts and sugar, which can be detrimental to their health. Too much salt can promote hypertension. Too much sugar can lead to weight gain and the effect of obesity.

➤ STUDENT SYNTHESIS

Key Points

- Essential nutrients (carbohydrates, fat, protein, water, minerals, and vitamins) provide energy, build and repair tissues, and regulate body processes.
- Kilocalories or calories provide the body with needed energy.
- Carbohydrates provide energy, fiber, and sweetness. They spare protein.
- Fats supply energy, essential fatty acids, satiety, and flavor. They carry fat-soluble vitamins, protect organs, and regulate body temperature.
- Proteins repair and build body tissues, contribute to fluid and acid–base balance, form hormones and enzymes, and provide immune functions.
- Fat-soluble vitamins are vitamins A, D, E, and K; water-soluble vitamins are vitamin C and B complex.
- In healthy people, vitamins and minerals should not be supplemented in excess of the DRIs.
- The key concepts in diet planning are variety, balance, and moderation.
- Four of the 10 leading causes of death are related to an over-consumption of nutrients.
- No one food or food group can supply all necessary nutrients.

- Calcium, iron, and protein are important nutrients in the diets of infants, children, adolescents, and pregnant and lactating women.
- Nutritional needs and patterns of intake vary with age.

Critical Thinking Exercises

1. Demonstrate an understanding of the Food Guide Pyramid by planning a day's diet for yourself.
2. Consider the nutritional problems of Americans as they relate to leading causes of death. Would you recommend a low-fat diet to someone whose weight and cholesterol levels are normal?
3. Explain why you, as a nurse, should be familiar with nutrition and nutrients for yourself and your clients.
4. Describe the dietary challenges faced by the homeless person. How can this person be assisted?

NCLEX-Style Review Questions

1. The purpose of the Food Guide Pyramid is to:
   a. Emphasize foods' nutrient density
   b. Help people control weight and limit sodium intake
   c. Illustrate the *Dietary Guidelines for Americans*
   d. Indicate bad and good foods
2. Fat-soluble vitamins include:
   a. A, D, E, and K
   b. B complex, D, and K
   c. C and B complex
   d. K, C, and thiamine
3. Which of the following are good sources of carbohydrates?
   a. Butter and cream
   b. Salad oils and dressings
   c. Fish and eggs
   d. Pasta and rice
4. Which of the following minerals is essential in forming and maintaining bones?
   a. Calcium
   b. Copper
   c. Iron
   d. Magnesium
5. Older adults are at risk for nutritional problems because of:
   a. Diarrhea associated with aging
   b. Difficulty chewing related to loss of teeth
   c. Enhanced sense of smell
   d. Enhanced absorption related to use of medications

CHAPTER

31

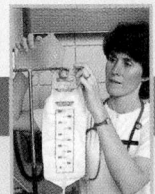

Transcultural and Social Aspects of Nutrition

LEARNING OBJECTIVES

1. Explain the influence of geographical regions on food choices.
2. Identify common dietary practices of several ethnic groups.
3. Identify at least three dietary practices related to each of the following religions: Islam, Judaism, Mormon, and Roman Catholicism.
4. Name the four general types of vegetarian diets and identify what types of foods are eaten within each type of diet.
5. Describe how the lacto-ovo vegetarian can meet protein needs.
6. Relate the following factors to food choice: financial status, emotional state, social and physical factors, and ethnic heritage.

NEW TERMINOLOGY

kosher
soul food
tofu
tortillas

vegan
vegetarian

Cultural background influences eating patterns. Ethnic heritage and religious beliefs often determine what people eat and how they prepare food. Because eating supplies food for the soul as well as the body, the science of nutrition is also an art. Although many Americans believe what they eat affects their health, nutritional considerations have a lesser impact on most people's food choices than do personal food preferences and aversions influenced by region, ethnic heritage, religious beliefs, and other sociocultural factors. Ignoring the significance of these factors in a client's food choices can undermine diet planning and nutritional counseling. This chapter explores how these factors may influence a client's food choices and the type of nutritional care the nurse may need to consider. Cultural, ethnic, and religious practices in general are discussed in Chapter 8.

Remember that you can help clients to meet their nutritional needs through a seemingly infinite variety and combination of foods. Many types of "diets" and foods can promote good health. Realizing the emotional value that some foods have for an individual is extremely important.

REGIONAL PREFERENCES

Various regions of the United States have developed unique eating patterns, which is a result—in part—of the availability of certain foods. These customs began before economic, safe, and quick transport of foods from one part of the country to another was possible. For example, people in the South tend to eat more fresh fruits and vegetables than do people in the North. Another influence on regional food patterns is the presence of many people with the same ethnic background in a concentrated geographic area. For example, many large cities have Scandinavian smorgasbords and Chinese restaurants. Grocery stores in many states offer many ethnic foods that may be purchased by a variety of cultural groups. Regional dietary customs have become much less defined in recent years due to the growing influence of fast-food chains, rapid transportation systems, and relocation of people to other areas.

☞ KEY CONCEPT

The nurse cannot change the dietary beliefs of clients. However, you can help clients to adjust their diet within their belief structures.

ETHNIC HERITAGE

Culture affects the way a person thinks, feels, and behaves. It also influences eating habits. Food preferences may become particularly important during illness. When illness necessitates dietary changes, healthcare professionals should attempt to integrate the person's ethnic and religious food preferences as much as possible. Understanding these preferences will enable you to assist clients in reaching optimum nutritional health. Chapter 8 discusses transcultural healthcare and ethnic considerations.

When people first immigrate to North America, they usually continue to eat their native foods as long as they can buy or grow the ingredients. Eventually, they may adopt Western food habits. The second generation, especially, adapts to local foods and habits; they may observe traditional customs only on special occasions and holidays. With food changes, many people develop "Western" diseases. Box 31-1 lists how ethnic diets may affect health and illness.

The following sections identify and describe cultural groups with significant representation in the United States; Table 31-1

➤ BOX 31-1

ETHNIC DIETS AND THEIR RELATIONSHIP TO HEALTH AND ILLNESS

- People of all ethnic groups have a source of starch or carbohydrate (eg, pasta, potatoes, bread, rice).
- Low intake of milk and dairy products may predispose individuals to bone disorders, such as rickets or osteoporosis.
- Lactose intolerance in many people of a given race or ethnic group is reflected in their limited use of dairy products. Individuals with lactose intolerance must meet their calcium needs through other foods.
- High sodium (salt) intake is often a factor in hypertension and cardiac disease.
- High caloric intake often causes people in certain cultural groups to be overweight. Obesity is a status symbol in some cultures.
- Intake of high amounts of fried foods and fats may predispose people to atherosclerosis, gallbladder disease, and obesity.
- Long cooking of vegetables causes a loss of water-soluble vitamins.
- High sugar intake may predispose individuals to dental caries or diabetes. A high sugar intake can increase the risk of nutrient deficiencies if empty-calorie foods (eg, soft drinks) take the place of nutritious foods (eg, skim milk). High intake of empty calories also increases the risk of obesity.
- Many people find comfort in traditional ethnic foods when ill, even if they do not follow these traditions when well.
- The family or client may insist on following religious or cultural practices during illness.
- Some cultural groups ascribe certain foods as "hot" or "cold" according to properties unrelated to temperature. Individuals within these groups may eat specific foods to combat certain illnesses that are "hot" or "cold."
- Some cultural groups believe that specific foods cause illness. They believe other foods may cure or prevent illness.
- Food provided in a healthcare facility may be unacceptable to some people because it violates a cultural or religious practice. In some cases, the ill person is exempt from following religious food practices during illness.

Group	Staples	Nutritional Concerns
Black (African) Americans	Fish; chicken; all parts of the pig (chops, ribs, ham, bacon, sausage, salt pork, jowls, neck bones, ham hocks, chitterlings [lining of intestine], feet, tail, ears); greens (mustard, dandelion, turnip) often cooked with fatty meat; stewed okra; corn; tomatoes; sweet potatoes and squash may be made into pies; grits; rice; yams; biscuits, corn-bread; high intake of sweets, including sweetened beverages	Diet is high in fat (fatty meats, fried foods), sodium (salted meats), and sugar. Diet may be inadequate in calcium and vitamin D.
Hispanic Americans		
Mexican	Many varieties of beans; steamed rice; corn products such as tortillas made from lime-soaked cornmeal; chili peppers; stewed tomatoes and tomato puree; potatoes; meat and sausages; fish; poultry; eggs; milk custards and bread puddings; lard; sweet chocolate and coffee drinks; cakes; pastries	Hot and cold foods should be balanced. Most vegetables are cooked so long that they lose most of their nutritional value. Diet is high in fiber and starch. Lard is frequently added during food preparation. Because milk, green leafy vegetables, and fruit intakes are low, diet may be inadequate in calcium, iron, vitamin A, and vitamin C. Obesity is common.
Cuban	Stews and casseroles flavored with sage, parsley, bay leaf, thyme, cinnamon, curry, capers, onion, cloves, garlic, saffron; soup served daily. Fried foods, especially fish, poultry, eggs; rice; many varieties of beans	Fruit and vegetables are not eaten regularly. Main meal is usually served at lunch.
Puerto Rican	Steamed white rice; many bean varieties; eggs (omelettes) are frequently the main dish; wheat breads; starchy fruits and vegetables, such as cassavas, yams, breadfruit, plantains, and green bananas; green peppers; tomatoes; garlic; dried, salted fish; salt pork, bacon; lard; olive oil; sugar; jams and jellies, sweet pastries; sugared fruit juices; cafe con leche (coffee and hot milk)	Limited use of meats; most food is cooked for long periods or fried. Malt beer is believed to be nutritious and may be given to children and breastfeeding mothers. Diet provides almost all essential nutrients, but may be low in calcium.
Asian Americans		
Chinese	Rice and rice gruel; wheat noodles; corn; green vegetables, especially from the cabbage family; squashes; cucumbers; eggplant; leafy vegetables; various shoots, including bamboo, mung, and soy; sweet potatoes; radishes; onions; peas and pods; mushrooms; roots; many local, seasonal vegetables; pickled vegetables; sea vegetables; plums; peaches; tangerines; kumquats and other citrus fruits; litchis; longans; mangoes; papayas; pomegranates; soybean products such as tofu (soybean curd), soy sauces, bean noodles, and soy milk; small portions of pork, chicken, duck, lamb; sugar as seasoning	Yin (negative)–yang (positive) concept of balancing intake; moderation is valued. Obesity is rare. Regional differences in food choices exist. Rice symbolizes life and fertility. Raw vegetables are rarely served. Diet is high in fiber and many nutrients, is low in fat, and may be low in protein; is often high in sodium.
Japanese	Rice; vegetables; pickled vegetables; soy as miso (soup), tofu, bean paste, and soy sauce; fruits; salads; fish with bones; sugar as seasoning; sea vegetables; seafood; ginseng; green tea; fruit for dessert	Common preparation methods include broiling, steaming, boiling, and stir-frying. Meat portions are small. Milk is rarely used by adults. Diet is low in fat, rich in nutrients, high in sodium.
Southeast Asian	Rice (in large quantities) is eaten at every meal; rice noodles, rice sticks, rice papers; fish; soybean products; wide variety of fruits and vegetables; soft drinks and sweets	Milk is rarely used after childhood. Familiar fruits and vegetables may not be available or affordable in the United States.
Middle Eastern	Lamb and goat; bread; rice; beans; lentils; yogurt; feta cheese; olives; tomatoes; olive oil	Calcium and protein intake may be inadequate. A meal is not considered well prepared unless a large quantity of fat has been added.
Native American	*Southeast:* corn; cornmeal; coontie (flour from a palmlike plant); fried breads; swamp cabbage (now illegal to harvest); pumpkins, squashes; papayas; alligator; snake; wild hog; duck; fish; shellfish *Northeast:* blueberries; cranberries; beans; corn; pumpkins; fish; lobster; wild game; maple syrup *Midwest:* bison; beans; corn; melons; squash; tomatoes *Southeast:* corn (many colors and varieties); beans; squash; pumpkins; chili peppers; melons; pine nuts; cactus *Northeast and Alaska:* salmon; caviar; other fish; otter; seal; whale; bear; elk; other game; wild fruits; acorns (and other wild nuts); wild greens	Food has great religious and social significance. Corn is a status food for most tribes. Milk is seldom used; calcium intake is usually low. Diets on some reservations are considered poor. High rate of obesity.

highlights dietary staples for each. In this discussion related to ethnic heritage, generalizations are made. Not all members of a group observe these particular practices. Habits of some members of each particular group are described, and much blending of cultures occurs.

Black Americans

Black Americans comprise many different cultural groups. Their food habits may be based on West Indian, African, or regional American influences. Black Americans who have been in the United States for several generations usually share local meal patterns.

Eating patterns reflect those of the country from which a person originated. Those who have emigrated from the Caribbean may rely on the staple rice and bean combination. They may consume cooked starchy tubers such as cassava, yams, and plantains, and tropical fruits such as mango and papaya.

Soul food refers to both cooking style (fried, barbecue) and particular foods (eg, black-eyed peas, collard greens) that blacks and whites in the southeastern United States commonly eat. Although people living in other areas may be unfamiliar with soul food, many who move from the South continue to prefer it.

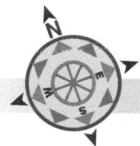

SPECIAL CONSIDERATIONS: CULTURE

Hypertension

Hypertension is common in African Americans, especially men, and in Asian Americans who use a great deal of salt and monosodium glutamate.

Hypertension, obesity, and diabetes are common health problems for black Americans. Alterations in diet (specifically reducing the high intake of sodium, fat, and sugar) may help prevent these chronic diseases. Because lactose intolerance is common, calcium and vitamin D intake may be inadequate if milk products are avoided.

Hispanic Americans

Hispanic people represent the fastest-growing segment of the United States population. They are a varied group, speaking over 21 different dialects of Spanish and other languages. Their food habits vary as well. The Hispanic American population is a mixture of Mexican, Cuban, and Puerto Rican individuals. Other Hispanic Americans are mostly from Central and South America.

Throughout Latin America, foods are believed to be either "hot" or "cold," although neither term refers to a food's actual temperature. Many Hispanic Americans believe that a balance of hot and cold is needed to maintain health. Although this theory may affect food choices during illness, it is difficult to

predict exactly how, because no rigid guidelines classify foods or illnesses as hot or cold.

Mexican

Mexican Americans often serve **tortillas** with all meals, along with rice and refried beans. Tortillas made from corn and treated with lime water are an important source of calcium, and therefore are more nutritious than flour tortillas (which are becoming more common). Meats are usually marinated or heavily spiced, and are often chopped or ground. Chorizo, a Mexican sausage, is a popular food choice. Most Mexican foods are fried. Adults use limited amounts of milk and milk products, except in popular sweet baked desserts. Mexican Americans also enjoy sweetened beverages, such as hot chocolate, cafe con leche (coffee with milk), and carbonated drinks. They often consume beer with meals. Incidences of obesity and diabetes are high. A Food Guide Pyramid with popular Mexican fare appears in Figure 31-1.

Cuban

Cuban Americans reflect a predominantly Spanish influence in their cooking styles. They use rice and beans extensively, and serve meat as income allows. Adults use limited amounts of milk; therefore, calcium levels may be deficient. Food is not as highly spiced as in some other Hispanic cultures. Fried foods are popular. The main meal is served at noon.

Puerto Rican

Although dietary practices are changing rapidly among younger people, the traditional Puerto Rican diet is important, especially during illness. Breakfast and lunch are light, with dinner served late. (Hospitalized clients may require adaptation of meal schedules.) The traditional diet consists of rice, beans, salted codfish, and "viandas" (root vegetables, green cooking bananas [plantains], and breadfruit). Some clients may refuse to eat hospital food. A dietary consultation and permission for the family to bring all food from home can be helpful. Soup made from homegrown chicken is seen as healing food. Foods considered "hot" in the stomach cannot be eaten during certain illnesses. ("Hot" does not imply temperature; it refers to reactions in the stomach.) Women do not eat "sour" foods during menses, pregnancy, or immediately after childbirth.

Asian Americans

Asian Americans represent a diverse group of more than 30 cultures. Rice is the staple food for many cultures. Asian food influences come from China, the Philippines, Japan, Korea, India, and the Southeast Asian peninsula.

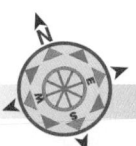

SPECIAL CONSIDERATIONS: CULTURE

Lactose Intolerance

Lactose intolerance is more common in African Americans, American Indians, and Asians than in whites.

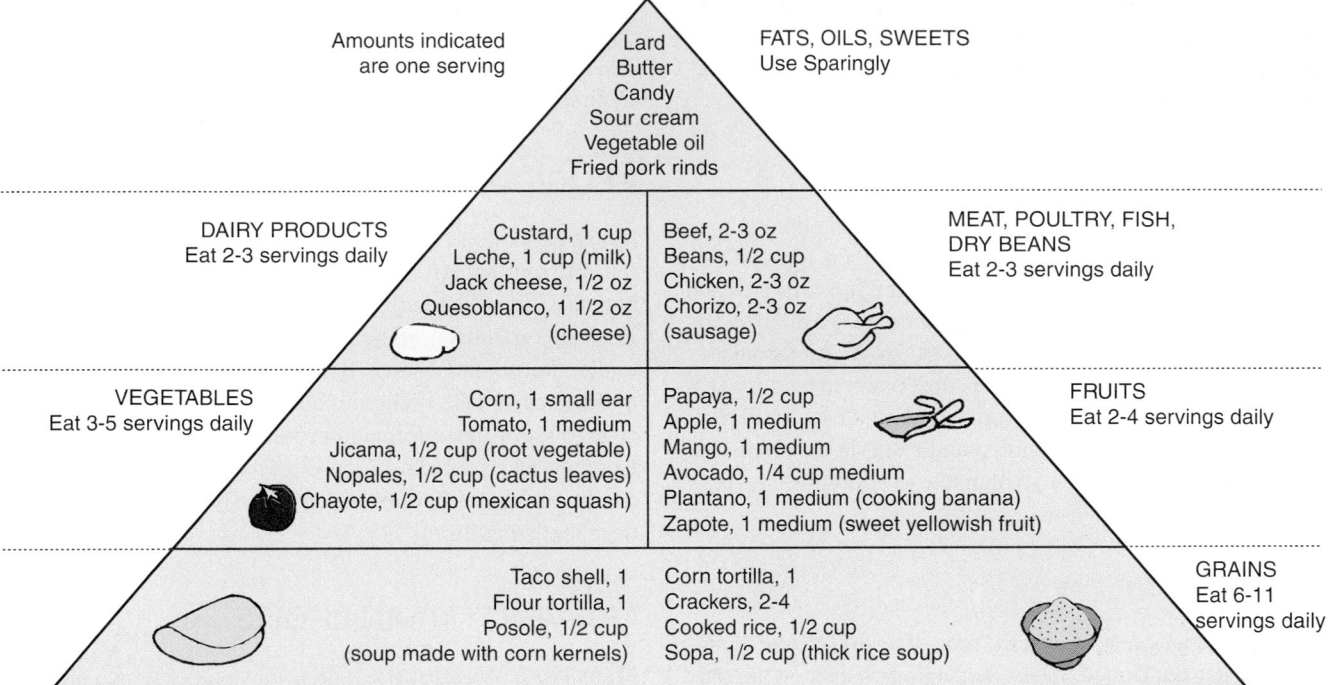

Amounts indicated are one serving

Lard / Butter / Candy / Sour cream / Vegetable oil / Fried pork rinds

FATS, OILS, SWEETS
Use Sparingly

DAIRY PRODUCTS
Eat 2-3 servings daily

Custard, 1 cup
Leche, 1 cup (milk)
Jack cheese, 1/2 oz
Quesoblanco, 1 1/2 oz
(cheese)

Beef, 2-3 oz
Beans, 1/2 cup
Chicken, 2-3 oz
Chorizo, 2-3 oz
(sausage)

MEAT, POULTRY, FISH,
DRY BEANS
Eat 2-3 servings daily

VEGETABLES
Eat 3-5 servings daily

Corn, 1 small ear
Tomato, 1 medium
Jicama, 1/2 cup (root vegetable)
Nopales, 1/2 cup (cactus leaves)
Chayote, 1/2 cup (mexican squash)

Papaya, 1/2 cup
Apple, 1 medium
Mango, 1 medium
Avocado, 1/4 cup medium
Plantano, 1 medium (cooking banana)
Zapote, 1 medium (sweet yellowish fruit)

FRUITS
Eat 2-4 servings daily

Taco shell, 1
Flour tortilla, 1
Posole, 1/2 cup
(soup made with corn kernels)

Corn tortilla, 1
Crackers, 2-4
Cooked rice, 1/2 cup
Sopa, 1/2 cup (thick rice soup)

GRAINS
Eat 6-11
servings daily

FIGURE 31-1. Food Guide Pyramid with popular Mexican fare. (Reprinted with permission from the American Dietetic Association.)

Chinese

Chinese eating habits and cooking techniques vary by geographic region. Of the five regions, Cantonese (southern China) is the style of choice of most Chinese Americans living in the United States. Some Chinese believe in the theory of **yin–yang.** Yin conditions are treated with Yang foods, and vice-versa, to achieve a balance between positive and negative energy. (see Chap. 8).

The Chinese diet is low in fat and high in starch. Chinese Americans use meats more as a condiment than as an entrée—therefore, quantities are small. Dinner may not have a main course. Stir-frying and other quick cooking methods are most common; ovens are rarely used. Food preparation is generally more time consuming than is the actual cooking. Some adults dislike milk and cheese; therefore, lactose intolerance is common. Limiting sodium is difficult because of the extensive use of soy sauce and other high-sodium seasonings.

Japanese

Japanese Americans carefully prepare food and enjoy it for its simplicity, purity, and beauty. The arrangement of food, color contrast, and shape are important elements of meals, which are light and use little animal fat. A good protein and calcium source is **tofu** (soybean curd). Japanese use many vegetables (including seaweed, bamboo shoots, and bean sprouts). Commonly, their meals contain fish, soup, fresh or pickled vegetables, and tea. Breakfast usually consists of a bowl of rice gruel. As is the case with Chinese Americans, limiting sodium is difficult because of the extensive use of soy sauce and monosodium glutamate. Lactose intolerance is common.

Southeast Asian

Cooking styles differ among regions in Cambodia, Vietnam, and Laos due to the variety of cultures influencing each area. The influence of India on Cambodian cooking is evidenced by the abundance of dishes with curry. Chinese and French culinary influences are seen in Vietnam. Individuals tend not to adhere to formal mealtimes; family members may serve themselves over a 1- to 3-hour period. The most important meal is at midday.

Cambodian Americans use plates, forks, and spoons, but consider knives at the table to be barbaric. Raw vegetable salads are common, as are pungent sauces with meats and fish. Cambodians rarely snack between meals, and hot water is the beverage of choice.

The diet of Vietnamese Americans consists of poultry and cheaper cuts of pork, with beef used on rare occasions. Fermented fish (high in sodium) is often used to make a sauce that is added to almost every cooked dish. Rice is served separately, not mixed with other foods. Tea is the most common beverage. Stir-frying is common, and food is quite spicy.

Laotian cooking is similar to Cambodian, except food is more highly spiced, often with lemon grass and curries of pepper and coriander. The eating utensils are the same as those used by Cambodians; however, eating with the fingers is common. Meals rely on fresh ingredients or long cooking times. Bananas and other fruits are commonly eaten. Coffee and tea are the beverages of choice.

Chinese and Japanese cultures heavily influence Korean food. Rice, often mixed with other grains or red beans, is served at every meal. Food is well seasoned, and all three meals are relatively the same size. Seafood accounts for the majority of animal protein, and may be eaten raw, steamed, or salted and dried. Beef is a favorite food choice. Korea's "dairy products" are bean curd and soymilk.

Middle Eastern Americans

Middle Eastern American cultural groups are less diverse than those previously discussed, as a result of their long history of conquest. Traditions do vary, but staples are similar. Each mouthful of food is eaten with a bite of bread. Vegetables and legumes are often the entree; all forms of pork are customarily forbidden. Women are considered subservient to men, and eat only after the men and children are fed, even if they are ill. Traditional food beliefs are common and result in maternal-fetal malnutrition, which leads to a high rate of stillbirths, low birth weight infants, and maternal deaths.

Native Americans

Dietary practices vary among the more than 300 Native American tribes in the United States, depending on their geographic location and the availability of food. Several chronic disorders are common, including obesity and diabetes. Many Native

Americans are lactose intolerant, and their diets may be calcium deficient. Deficiencies of riboflavin and vitamins A and C are also common. Native Americans use many spices, including green chili (which contains vitamin C).

RELIGIOUS BELIEFS

Many people eat specific foods in certain combinations or refrain from eating certain foods because of their religious beliefs. Cultural and religious practices are often intertwined. Box 31-2 identifies some major religious customs relating to diet. Particularly when ill, individuals are often unwilling to deviate from their religious dietary customs. The nurse will need to know this information when caring for clients. Foods that must be prepared using special equipment or under certain conditions can usually be ordered in advance or prepared by the client's family.

THE VEGETARIAN CHOICE

Many types of **vegetarian** diets exist, all of which have the common characteristic of being based mainly on plant foods. Four types of vegetarians exist:

➤➤ BOX 31-2

DIETARY PRACTICES BASED ON RELIGIOUS BELIEF

Jewish
Due to differences in interpretation, Jews vary in how strictly they follow dietary laws. Reform Jews practice minimal observance of general dietary laws. Conservative Jews may follow dietary laws only at home. Orthodox Jews adhere strictly to dietary laws. **Kosher** eating demands the following:
- Separate dishes, pans, and silverware are used to prepare and to serve meat and dairy foods.
- Meat and dairy may not be eaten at the same meal.
- Meats must be slaughtered by a ritual method and only the front quarter of the animal may be eaten.
- Some parts of beef, veal, lamb, mutton, goat, venison, chicken, turkey, goose, and pheasant are eaten.
- Pork products, rabbit, shellfish, and scavenger fish are not allowed.
- Food must be prepared ahead of time for the Sabbath, which is sundown Friday to sundown Saturday.
- Certain days of fasting are observed, but a rabbi may excuse older or ill clients.

Church of Jesus Christ of Latter Day Saints (Mormon)
Mormons use no stimulants (eg, coffee, tea, or caffeine-containing carbonated beverages) and no alcoholic beverages. Members observe "fast offerings," giving up two meals on the first Sunday of each month. (Money saved is used to feed the poor.) Mormons live by a health code and the Word of Wisdom; they are to preserve their bodies and

maintain the best possible health. Meat is eaten sparingly and "in season" (winter).

Roman Catholic
Dietary and fasting regulations are mostly voluntary. Some Catholics abstain from eating meat on Fridays. Those aged 14 to 59 must fast and abstain from meat on Fridays during Lent. Ash Wednesday and Good Friday are observed as days of fast and abstinence (a priest may excuse older or ill adults). Catholics do not eat or drink (except water) for 1 hour before taking Holy Communion.

Seventh Day Adventist
Seventh Day Adventists are often lacto-ovo vegetarians or vegans. They use no stimulants (coffee, tobacco) and avoid pork, shellfish, and alcohol. In-between meal snacking is discouraged.

Hindu
Hindus believe that all life forms are sacred because they might be the reincarnation of an ancestor. Most Hindus are lacto-ovo vegetarians, and they do not use alcohol. Coffee, tea, and chocolate are widely used.

Islam (Muslim)
In Islam, dietary laws are similar to Jewish kosher laws. In addition, no alcoholic beverages are allowed, but tea is permitted. Muslims fast for a month each year, avoiding food from dawn until after dark. Foods considered healthy are honey, dates, milk, meat, seafood, and olive oil.

- **Vegans** are strict vegetarians and exclude all animal products (meat, fish, poultry, eggs, milk, and dairy products) from their diet.
- *Lacto-vegetarians* eat plant foods, plus dairy products (no eggs). Figure 31-2 shows a Food Guide Pyramid with food choices for lacto vegetarians.
- *Ovo-vegetarians* eat plant foods, plus eggs (no dairy products).
- *Lacto-ovo-vegetarians* eat plant foods, dairy products, and eggs.

Even among these broad classifications, variations are found in the extent to which vegetarians avoid animal products. For instance, some people call themselves vegetarians just because they do not eat red meat. Vegetarianism is gaining popularity in the United States. More frequently, people declare they are "mostly" vegetarian, usually meaning that they are mostly lacto-ovo vegetarian, with meat products included in their diet from once per week to once per day.

Benefits of the Vegetarian Choice

People choose a vegetarian diet for a variety of reasons: religious, ecological, economic, philosophical, or ethical. Potential health benefits are another consideration. Compared to non-vegetarians, vegetarians have lower rates of coronary artery disease, hypertension, non–insulin-dependent diabetes, and obesity. Studies have shown that Seventh Day Adventist vegetarians have lower mortality rates from colon cancer than the general population. Vegetarian diets may also offer some protection against both lung and breast cancers. In Practice: Educating the Client 31-1 gives recommendations for a balanced vegetarian diet.

Balancing the Vegetarian Diet

Many people mistakenly assume that consuming an adequate protein intake is impossible if they exclude animal products from their diet. They may think that they must give special attention to combining ("complementing") plant proteins at each meal, to ensure that all essential amino acids are present at the same time. In truth, plant sources of protein alone can provide sufficient amounts of essential and nonessential amino acids, if calorie intake is adequate and the types of plant proteins eaten are reasonably varied over the course of the day.

Although vegetarians often consume less protein than non-vegetarians, most vegetarian diets meet or exceed the Dietary Recommended Intakes (DRIs) for protein. Vegetarians who include some type of animal product in their diet are likely to

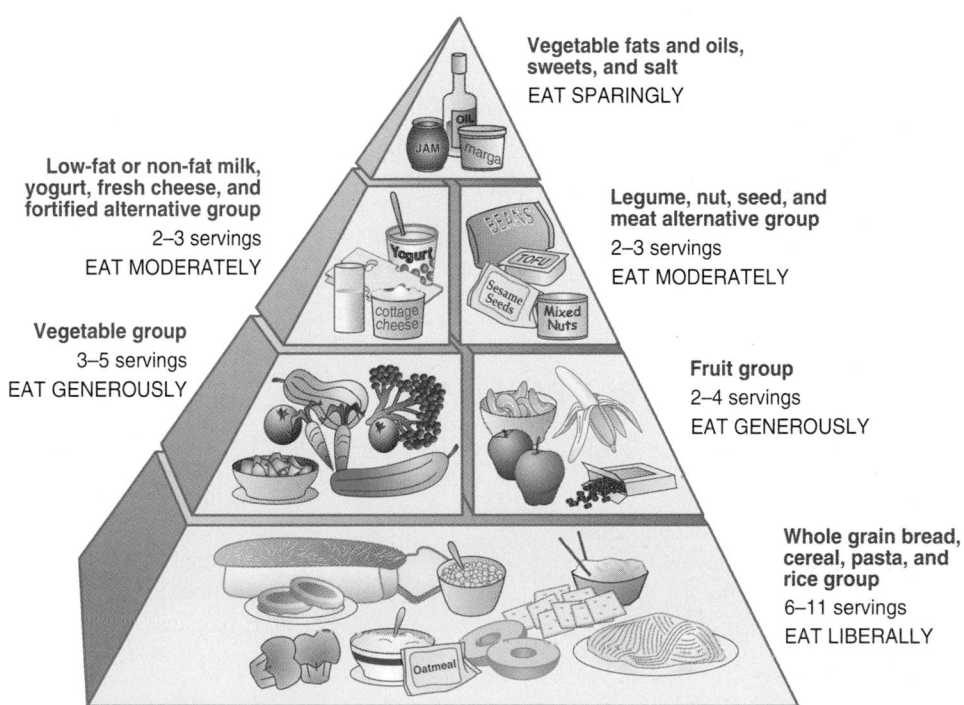

FIGURE 31-2. Lacto-vegetarian Food Guide Pyramid. Adapted from Dudek, S. (2001). *Nutrition essentials for nursing practice,* (4th ed.). Philadelphia: Lippincott Williams & Wilkins.

Vegetable fats and oils, sweets, and salt
EAT SPARINGLY

Low-fat or non-fat milk, yogurt, fresh cheese, and fortified alternative group
2–3 servings
EAT MODERATELY

Legume, nut, seed, and meat alternative group
2–3 servings
EAT MODERATELY

Vegetable group
3–5 servings
EAT GENEROUSLY

Fruit group
2–4 servings
EAT GENEROUSLY

Whole grain bread, cereal, pasta, and rice group
6–11 servings
EAT LIBERALLY

Internet Addresses for Information on Vegetarian Diets

North American Vegetarian Society
www.cyberveg.org/navs

Vegetarian Resource Group
www.vrg.org

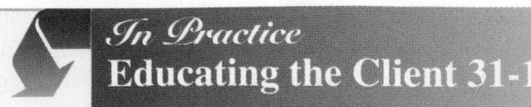

In Practice
Educating the Client 31-1

A BALANCED VEGETARIAN DIET

Include the following recommendations when teaching about vegetarian diets:

- Eat a wide variety of foods—the greater the variety, the greater the probability of attaining an adequate diet.
- Be sure to eat enough calories.
- Limit foods with low nutritive value. Avoid empty calories and alcohol.
- Use whole-grain products rather than refined foods, or choose fortified or enriched cereals.
- Include a food rich in vitamin C with every meal. Vitamin C enhances iron absorption.
- If milk and milk products are included in the diet, choose low-fat or non-fat varieties.
- Limit egg yolks to no more than four per week.
- Vegans need a reliable source of vitamin B_{12}: fortified breakfast cereal, fortified soy beverages, or a supplement. If sunlight exposure is limited, a vitamin D supplement may be needed as well.

consume an adequate amount of each nutrient, as long as they meet their calorie needs. Pure vegans (no animal products) need a reliable source of cobalamin (vitamin B_{12})—such as vitamin supplements or fortified foods like some breakfast cereals, soy beverages, and some brands of nutritional yeast. (Vitamin B_{12} is found naturally only in animal products.) If their exposure to sunlight is limited, vegetarians may require supplements of vitamin D. Calcium, iron, and zinc intake is usually adequate (even for children) when the diet is varied and contains adequate calories. A food guide for vegetarians appears in Table 31-2.

OTHER SOCIOCULTURAL FACTORS

The following factors influence people and their eating patterns:

- Social aspects of eating
- Emotional attitudes about food
- Food fads and fallacies
- Economic conditions
- Physical status

Social Factors

Most people prefer to eat with others, rather than alone, and are probably used to eating their meals with family or coworkers. When people are admitted to a healthcare facility, they may suddenly find themselves alone in a room with a dinner tray.

▪▪▪ TABLE 31-2 $\mathcal{F}$OOD GUIDE PYRAMID FOR VEGETARIAN MEAL PLANNING

Fats, Oils, and Sweets
Use sparingly
Candy, butter, margarine, salad dressing, cooking oil

Milk, Yogurt, and Cheese Group
0–3 servings daily*
   Milk—1 cup
   Yogurt—1 cup
   Natural cheese—1½ oz
Vegetarians who choose not to use milk, yogurt, or cheese need to select other food sources rich in calcium.

Dry Beans, Nuts, Seeds, Eggs, and Meat Substitutes Group
2–3 servings daily
   Soy milk—1 cup
   Cooked dry beans or peas—½ cup
   1 egg or 2 egg whites
   Nuts or seeds—2 Tbsp
   Tofu or tempeh—¼ cup
   Peanut butter—2 Tbsp

Vegetable Group
3–5 servings daily
   Cooked or chopped raw vegetables—½ cup
   Raw leafy vegetables—1 cup

Fruit Group
2–4 servings daily
   Juice—¾ cup
   Dried fruit—¼ cup
   Chopped, raw fruit—½ cup
   Canned fruit—½ cup
   1 medium-size piece of fruit, such as banana, apple, or orange

Bread, Cereal, Rice, and Pasta Group
6–11 servings daily
   Bread—1 slice
   Ready-to-eat—1 oz
   Cooked cereal—½ cup
   Cooked rice, pasta, or other grains—½ cup
   Bagel—½

Source: 1997 American Dietetic Association Position Paper on Vegetarianism—The Vegetarian Resource Group: http://www.vrg.org/nutrition/adapaper.htm.

They may have limited input regarding what foods they are served. Illness and feelings of loneliness often result in poor nutritional intake (see also Chapter 32). The following are some guidelines to provide a sense of social involvement for clients during meals:

- Visit the client for a few minutes.
- Allow two clients to eat together.
- In a double room, open the curtain.
- Let clients meet in a common lounge for meals.
- Encourage family members to visit at mealtime.
- Turn on the television or radio.
- Place flowers nearby.

- Encourage the client to telephone home and talk with family members while eating.

Emotional Factors

Emotional factors influence nutritional behavior and total health. These factors may affect the eating patterns of the client in a healthcare facility. Food may become a reward. Purees of certain foods may be considered "for babies." A client may feel guilty for not eating all the food on the tray or may overeat just because the food is there. Clients who are sad, lonely, or depressed may overeat or refuse to eat.

Food Fads and Fallacies

From quick weight-loss schemes to home remedies for almost any ailment, food fads are big business in the United States. Sometimes, the claims behind food fads directly oppose scientific understanding of nutrition and health. Other claims capitalize on legitimate studies to exploit public interest. Either way, wasted money is only one consequence of following food fads. Direct toxicity, and failure to seek legitimate healthcare, are other possible outcomes that can significantly affect health.

The best protection against food frauds is to become a better-educated consumer. The *Dietary Guidelines for Americans* and the Food Guide Pyramid provide an excellent foundation for basic nutritional principles and advice. In Practice: Educating the Client 31-2 gives pointers for the nurse to help clients evaluate a food fad or quick weight-loss scheme. Clients with specific concerns about food fads, or who may be at risk for health problems because of them, should be directed to a dietitian.

Economic Conditions

A family's financial status may influence a person's eating habits. Food is relatively inexpensive in the United States. More affluent people tend to eat at restaurants more often. They generally consume more vegetables and fruits, but also eat more fat due to a higher intake of cheese, meat, fish, and poultry. Diets higher in fat are associated with heart disease, cancer, and other disorders. When income rises, people tend to eat fewer eggs, rice, and beans. People with lower incomes may skip meals. The homeless or "street people" may beg or look through trash for food.

Physical Condition

Clients experiencing illness may not be well or strong enough to eat. When caring for clients who are not strong enough to eat

✚◎ N u r s i n g   A l e r t
If you encounter a client who does not have enough money for food, initiate a referral for the client to social services.

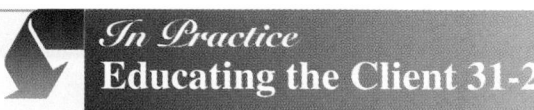

In Practice
Educating the Client 31-2

FOOD FADS AND FALLACIES

Fad diets and quick weight-loss schemes add up to a multimillion-dollar industry in the United States. Credentials are blurred, claims are exaggerated, and the consumer is bewildered. Because fad diets are often here today and gone tomorrow, it's hard to keep up with what's hot and what's not. Advise clients to look for the following criteria before they jump on the latest diet bandwagon:

- The plan is realistic and flexible, not a collection of rigid menus, a one-size-fits-all approach, or "must-have" food combinations.
- It suggests consultation with a doctor.
- The plan uses food, not pills or potions, to meet nutritional requirements.
- It uses food from each of the major food groups, not eliminating any as "bad," unhealthy, or dangerous. The number of servings recommended from each food group compares with the suggestions in the Food Guide Pyramid.
- It adequately supplies all nutrients.
- It is founded on sound nutritional principles, not unsubstantiated claims.
- It recommends exercise.
- It does not promote more than 1 to 2 lb of weight loss per week (greater amounts equate with loss of lean tissue and water, not true loss of fat, which is the actual goal).
- It is safe . . . indefinitely. There are no time limits for discontinuation of the diet.
- It allows nutritious snacking.
- It emphasizes portion control.
- It recognizes the importance of behavior modification for long-term success.
- It offers a maintenance plan.
- It is reasonably priced.

on their own, the nurse must take time to feed them. Feeding is an excellent time to make a physical and psychological assessment of the client. Consider absence of teeth, ill-fitting dentures, or difficulty swallowing when planning meals. When nutritional needs are increased, such as after major surgery to promote healing, obtaining an adequate amount of nutrients to treat acute illness takes precedence over following a low-fat or low-calorie diet for chronic disease prevention. Malnutrition is common among those with AIDS; therefore, increased calorie and protein intake is required to replenish losses. Other diet modifications may be necessary to alleviate symptoms or complications, such as limiting fat for malabsorption, increasing fluid for diarrhea or fever, and providing small frequent meals for anorexia or fatigue.

Full Liquid Diet.   If a full liquid diet is to be used for a long time, nutritional supplements (eg, Ensure, Glucerna) should be added. Be aware of any side effects of these supplements, such as diarrhea, constipation, gas, and bloating.

Soft Diet

A **soft diet** may vary from one facility to another. The terminology is sometimes nebulous, and the nurse must often clarify the physician's order regarding which type of soft diet is ordered. Knowing the rationale or purpose of the diet will help differentiate which type of soft diet is needed: regular, digestive, or mechanical.

One form of soft diet is the *digestive soft diet.* It is a nutritionally adequate diet that is low in fiber, connective tissue, and fat. Gas-forming foods are eliminated and mild seasonings are used. In the post-surgical client, this diet acts as a transition between a liquid diet and the full or general diet. In the digestive soft diet, the physician may order modifications to the soft diet that eliminate some listed foods (see Table 32-1).

☞ Key Concept

The progression of diets should be: clear liquid, full liquid, soft, regular diet. A client's diet should progress as soon as possible to ensure an adequate nutritional intake and to increase the client's sense of well-being.

The *mechanical soft diet,* or dental soft diet, is used for the person who has difficulty chewing or swallowing, such as a client who is **edentulous** (without teeth), has oral problems, or has had a cerebrovascular accident. It is also a nutritionally adequate diet and meats, fruits, and vegetables may be chopped, ground, or pureed, depending on the client's ability to chew and swallow. If necessary, the diet may be ordered as a pureed, mechanical soft diet.

High-Fiber Diet

A high-fiber diet has an increased amount of both insoluble and soluble fiber. *Insoluble fiber* helps increase stool bulk and stimulates peristalsis. *Soluble fiber* helps lower the serum cholesterol level and improves glucose tolerance in diabetes. A high-fiber diet is often ordered as part of the treatment for constipation and diverticulosis. Potential problems with a high-fiber diet are cramping, diarrhea, and gas, especially if fiber is added to a diet too quickly or in excessive amounts. To achieve a high-fiber diet, foods high in fiber are substituted for those low in fiber. Increased fluid intake is important to following a high-fiber diet. Box 32-3 lists good sources of fiber.

Low-Residue Diet

The **low-residue diet** is composed of foods that the body can absorb completely, so that little residue is left for the formation of feces. This diet is also called a *fiber-controlled diet.* It may be prescribed for severe diarrhea, colitis, diverticulitis, other gastrointestinal disorders, intestinal obstruction, and before and after intestinal surgery. This diet may be inadequate in iron, calcium, and some vitamins and minerals because of limited

> ➤ **BOX 32-3**

SOURCES OF FIBER

Rich in Insoluble Fiber
- Wheat and corn bran
- Whole wheat breads and cereals
- Brown rice
- Bananas
- Cauliflower
- Nuts
- Lentils
- Green beans
- Green peas

Rich in Soluble Fiber
- Citrus fruits
- Pectin

Rich in Both Insoluble and Soluble Fiber
- Oat bran
- Barley
- Navy beans
- Kidney beans
- Apples
- Broccoli
- Carrots

food choices and over-processing of fruits and vegetables. Suitable foods on the low-residue diet include:

- Ground and well-cooked meats, chicken, and fish
- Seafood
- Eggs (not fried) and mild cheese
- Fruit and vegetable juices without pulp
- Pureed or strained vegetables
- Canned fruit and firm bananas
- White rice, plain noodles, plain pasta, and potatoes
- Refined white or seedless rye breads and crackers
- 2 cups of milk or the equivalent (eg, yogurt)
- Bouillon, broth, strained, or cream soups made from allowed foods
- Plain desserts in moderation

Foods to be avoided on the low-residue diet include:

- Whole-grain breads and whole-grain cereals
- Nuts, seeds, coconut, and anything containing them
- Potato skins, peanut butter, and popcorn
- Whole-grain pasta and wild or brown rice
- Raw vegetables and gas-producing vegetables
- All other fresh fruits and all dried fruits
- Tough, fibrous meats and dried peas and beans
- Spicy foods

Bland Diet

The bland diet has often been prescribed for those with ulcers, esophagitis, gastroesophageal reflux disease (**GERD**) or heartburn, gastritis, hiatal hernia, or other disorders of the gastrointestinal tract. The goal of this diet is to limit foods that stimulate the production of gastric acid. The impact of a bland diet may or may not be effective in treating a digestive disorder. Many prescriptions and over-the-counter medications are currently available to treat and/or cure GERD and stomach ulcers.

The following foods should be avoided on the bland diet:

- Alcohol
- Caffeine (including chocolate and cola drinks) and decaffeinated coffee and tea
- Red and black pepper
- Chili powder
- Fried foods and foods high in fat
- Peppermint and spearmint oils

Individuals following a bland diet should be encouraged to avoid other foods that may cause them discomfort, because intolerances are often individual. Instruct clients not to lie down for an hour after meals; to maintain ideal weight; and to eat smaller, more frequent meals. If they smoke, advise them to cut down or stop. Discourage milk-based diets—the stomach must secrete additional gastric acid to help neutralize milk's alkaline nature.

Energy Value Modifications

Diets modified for energy include high- and low-calorie diets.

High-Calorie Diet
Underweight occurs frequently in persons with prolonged illness. Symptoms such as lack of appetite, vomiting, diarrhea, and high fever can cause severe weight loss. A high-calorie diet may also be used for hyperthyroidism, undernutrition, and general malnutrition. The person who has been severely burned needs a large amount of protein to rebuild lost tissue, and carbohydrate to spare protein. A high-calorie diet generally contains over 3,000 calories and 130 grams protein.

The successful high-calorie diet accounts for individual food preferences and eating habits. The high-calorie diet is high in protein, carbohydrate, fat, vitamins, and minerals. Clients with a depressed appetite may need smaller and more frequent meals. Unless a definite reason exists for excluding solid foods, clients are allowed to have solids if they can chew and digest them easily.

Low-Calorie Diet
A low-calorie diet is used to promote weight loss in those with, or at risk for, complications related to obesity. Because research indicates that a high-fat diet, not excess calories alone, contributes to obesity, a low-fat, low-calorie diet may be the best way to achieve weight loss. The Diabetic Exchange Lists for Meal Planning are often used to plan weight-loss diets. These lists are explained in the next section of this chapter.

Fad diets are dangerous because they are almost always unbalanced. A balanced reducing diet provides enough calories to supply body needs, while allowing for a safe weight reduction of 1 to 2 pounds per week. (One pound of body fat is equivalent to 3,500 calories; to lose 1 lb of fat per week, a person needs to reduce daily calorie intake by 500. A 1,000-calorie decrease per day is needed to lose 2 lb/wk, which is a drastic reduction in intake. Experts advise limiting weight loss to no more than 2 lb/wk.) For some guidelines for a low-calorie diet, see In Practice: Educating the Client 32-1.

Nutrient Modifications

The modification of certain nutrients is necessary for some conditions. Your knowledge of the nutrients contained in various foods will help you to explain these diets to your clients. Diets may be altered in their content of carbohydrate, fat, protein, minerals, or electrolytes.

Carbohydrate-Controlled Diets
Diabetic Diet. The goals of diabetes mellitus treatment are to maintain blood sugar and fat levels as near to normal as possible, and to prevent or delay the onset of complications. Nutrition therapy is the cornerstone of diabetes management, regardless of the affected person's weight, blood glucose levels, or use of medications. The one-size-fits-all approach to diet planning has been discarded, for a more liberal approach that focuses on consistency in the amount of carbohydrate consumed, rather than the need to avoid simple sugars. New guidelines for diabetes management stress the importance of individualizing the diet according to the individual's assessment data, treatment goals, and need for exercise.

The **carbohydrate-controlled diet** may be based on the Diabetic Exchange Lists for Meal Planning or Carbohydrate Counting. Although both methods are used, Carbohydrate Counting has become increasingly popular with the advent of the Nutrition Facts Label on most food products.

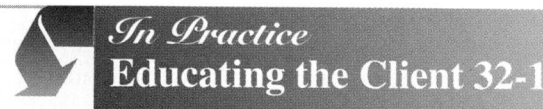

In Practice
Educating the Client 32-1

LOW-CALORIE DIET

To decrease calorie intake, encourage clients and families to practice the following dietary habits:

- Eat slowly and concentrate on the smell, taste, and texture of food.
- Eat a variety of foods that are low in calories and high in nutrients—check the Nutrition Facts labels on packaged foods.
- Eat less fat and fewer high-fat foods.
- Eat smaller portions and limit second helpings of foods high in fat and calories.
- Eat more fruits and vegetables that do not have added fat or sugar.
- Eat pasta, rice, breads, and cereals without added fats and sugars used in preparation or at the table.
- Eat fewer sugars and sweets (eg, candy, cookies, cake, soda).
- Drink less or no alcohol.

The American Diabetes Association and the American Dietetic Association devised the exchange lists and update them as they gain further knowledge about nutrients and diabetes. The lists place foods into three groups, which are subdivided into exchange lists. The Carbohydrate Group contains the following exchanges: starch, fruit, milk, other carbohydrates, and vegetables. The Meat and Meat Substitute Group contains four lists grouped according to fat content (very lean, lean, medium fat, high fat). The Fat Group contains the Fat Exchange List. Exchange Lists are also helpful in planning other diet modifications.

A serving of each exchange is assigned a value for calories, protein, carbohydrate, and fat. Serving sizes may vary (to standardize the amount of each nutrient per exchange). This system provides the client with a simplified meal plan and a wide variety of foods from which to choose. The client's physician or dietitian sets up an individualized diet containing specified numbers of each exchange for meals and snacks.

The Carbohydrate Counting method is based upon counting grams of carbohydrate in all foods and beverages consumed. A client is given an allowance of carbohydrate grams that is to be consumed evenly throughout a day. Clients can track carbohydrate grams by using the Nutrition Facts label on food products, and books that list the carbohydrate content of foods.

Usually, the physician orders a specific calorie-level diet. Most people with type I diabetes are of normal weight or underweight, and therefore, their calorie level should be sufficient to maintain weight or to gain weight as needed. Eighty percent to 90% of clients with type II diabetes are obese. Low-calorie diets and weight loss can lower their blood glucose and fat levels and improve insulin action. Unfortunately, these clients seldom achieve long-term weight loss. Older residents of extended care facilities may follow a more liberal diet that simply limits the use of sugar and high-fat foods.

Clients with diabetes do not need special foods. Clients should eat foods in their natural form (whole fruits instead of juices, brown rice instead of white) to increase fiber intake. Fiber helps regulate blood glucose levels by slowing gastric (stomach) emptying time. Concentrated sweets (sugar, honey, molasses, jams, jellies, and desserts) are no longer prohibited, but they must be counted to maintain consistent carbohydrate intake. Also, because they provide few nutrients except calories, they should be limited if weight loss is desired. Alcohol should be used only with a physician's approval because it can cause hypoglycemic reactions, especially when combined with diabetes medication. Individualizing the diet according to the client's likes and dislikes and usual pattern of intake improves the chance of long-term compliance. Encourage the client to follow the treatment plan to minimize the possibility of complications.

Lactose-Restricted Diet.   People with *lactose intolerance* lack sufficient amounts of the enzyme *lactase,* which is needed to digest the sugar (lactose) in dairy products. As a result, they develop cramping, gas, and diarrhea after ingesting lactose. Because individual tolerance to lactose varies greatly, and lactose intolerance secondary to various gastrointestinal disorders may be temporary, these clients should be urged to include small amounts of milk in their diets to determine their level of tolerance. Often, individuals who are unable to tolerate a glass of milk between meals can tolerate yogurt, aged cheeses, lactose-reduced milk, or milk consumed with food. Milk in cooked breads and other foods is omitted for clients with severe lactose intolerance. Lactose-free milk and over-the-counter medications such as Lactaid may be helpful for lactose-intolerant clients.

High- and Low-Fat Diets

Fat-Controlled Diet.   A **fat-controlled diet** is often the first step in treating individuals with elevated blood lipids or fats (**hyperlipidemia**). These clients may have a high cholesterol level, a high triglyceride level, or both. Untreated hyperlipidemia can contribute to coronary heart disease, which often has such serious consequences as heart attack, stroke, or death. Heredity or improper diet may cause hyperlipidemia or it may have a secondary cause, such as diabetes mellitus, hypothyroidism, nephrotic syndrome, or renal failure. In secondary hyperlipidemia, the primary goal is to treat the underlying disease.

The diet for hyperlipidemia is altered in both the total amount of fat and the type of fat provided. The initial diet (Step One Diet) consists of less than 30% of total calories from fat, with less than 10% of this from saturated fat. Monounsaturated fats should provide at least 10% of total calories, and cholesterol intake should be limited to 300 milligrams per day. Carbohydrates should account for about 50% to 55% of calories, with most of that percentage coming from complex carbohydrates, such as whole grains and legumes. Overweight individuals should also lose weight. Diets of clients with hyperlipidemia may have calorie restrictions as well.

If the Step One Diet fails to achieve blood lipid level goals, the diet may advance to the Step Two level, which is more restrictive in saturated fat and cholesterol.

Low-Fat Diet.   Low-fat diets are used for clients with malabsorption syndromes because fat aggravates diarrhea and promotes nutrient losses. In these cases, total fat is limited to 25 to 50 grams per day, depending on the severity of symptoms. The type of fat is not modified. Low-fat diets may also be prescribed for those with pancreatic and gallbladder diseases.

High-Fat Diet.   High-fat diets are prescribed for children with seizure disorders, when anticonvulsant drugs and a balanced diet have failed to control seizures. This **ketogenic diet** is extremely low in carbohydrates and is sometimes as high as 80% to 90% fat. This diet is difficult to follow, and must be supplemented with vitamins and minerals. It may lose its effectiveness over time.

Protein-Controlled Diets

High-Protein Diet.   A high-protein diet encompasses a range of protein intakes that vary from 1.2 grams of protein per kilogram of body weight to 5.0 grams per kilogram of body weight, depending on the severity of depletion and causative factors. Protein requirements increase whenever metabolism increases or when tissue needs to be replaced, such as following burns, major trauma, surgery, multiple fractures, hepatitis, and sepsis. Malabsorption syndromes that waste protein, such as diseases of the gastrointestinal tract, and the acute phases of inflammatory bowel disease and celiac disease, also elevate protein needs. Protein-losing hemodialysis and peritoneal dialysis patients are treated with a high-protein diet. Clients on dialysis must limit dairy products due to the high phosphorus and potassium content.

Sources of high-quality protein (ie, protein that contains all the essential amino acids) include eggs (highest quality), meats, poultry, fish, cheeses, and milk. Commercial liquid protein supplements often boost protein intake. To ensure that protein is used for protein synthesis and not for energy needs, a high-protein diet should also be high in carbohydrates.

Protein-Restricted Diet. Kidney and liver disorders are treated with a controlled-protein diet. The amount of protein allowed may be based on the client's weight (eg, 0.6 to 0.8 g/kg body weight), or may be ordered as a total amount per day (eg, 40 or 60 g). Again, to ensure that dietary protein is used for protein needs, not energy requirements, non-protein calorie intake should be high. Most protein should be of high quality and should be spread evenly over the day's meals. Other restrictions, such as sodium and fluid, may also be necessary. Because a low-protein diet differs dramatically from the typical American diet, long-term compliance is difficult for many to achieve.

Gluten-Restricted Diet. Celiac disease, a hereditary disorder, is a malabsorption syndrome caused by sensitivity to *gluten,* a protein found in wheat, rye, oats, and barley. A portion of gluten (gliadin) causes the intestinal villi to atrophy and flatten, which severely reduces the absorptive surface of the intestines and impairs brush-border enzyme activity. Consequently, the absorption of many nutrients is impaired. Permanent elimination of gluten from the diet quickly and almost completely reverses the intestinal changes, although lactose intolerance may persist. Some other clients may need restricted gluten. The gluten-restricted diet eliminates many foods, including numerous breads and cereals, beer, ale, commercial chocolate milk, malted milk, cakes, cookies, commercial salad dressing (gluten is a stabilizer), and meat substitutes, such as textured protein products. Breads, cereals, and desserts made with rice, rice flour, corn, cornmeal, potato flour, arrowroot, soybean flour, and tapioca are acceptable. Special gluten-free products are commercially available, but they tend to be expensive.

Diets With Controlled Minerals and Electrolytes

Sodium-Controlled Diets. The sodium-controlled diet has different levels of restriction, depending on the client's disease and the amount of edema present. *Edema* is an excess accumulation of water and salts in tissues, especially in the lower extremities, which can sometimes be controlled by limiting sodium intake. A sodium-controlled diet is often prescribed for those with cardiac, vascular, and some kidney diseases. Box 32-4 lists substances to avoid in sodium-restricted diets.

A *mild sodium restriction* of 3,000 to 4,000 milligrams per day is also known as a *no added salt* diet. A limited amount

➤➤ BOX 32-4

DIETARY SUBSTANCES TO AVOID OR OMIT IN SODIUM RESTRICTION*

Examples are given in parentheses.
- Table salt
- Vegetable salts (onion, celery, garlic salt); vegetable flakes (parsley, celery)
- Any smoked, processed, or cured meat or fish (ham, smoked fish, bacon, corned beef, cold cuts, frankfurters, sausage, tongue, salt pork, chipped beef, anchovies, pickled herring)
- Meat extracts, bouillon cubes, meat sauces
- Salty foods (potato chips, popcorn)
- Prepared condiments (relish, Worcestershire sauce, steak sauces, catsup, pickles, mustard, olives, soy sauce)
- Prepackaged frozen foods, packaged sauce mixes, packaged gravy mix, soup mix; frozen peas and lima beans
- Prepackaged noodle, rice, or potato dishes
- Canned soups, chili, beef stews
- Prepared flour mixes (coating for frying chicken or fish)
- Packaged baking mixes (cake mix, frosting, pancakes)
- Frozen fish fillets and shellfish, except oysters
- Sauerkraut
- Canned meats, canned vegetables, ready-made spaghetti sauces
- Butter, cheeses, peanut butter

*Some foods are permissible if prepared without salt. Consult the label for dietary information.

Nursing Alert
Minerals and electrolytes are critical components of the body's natural chemistry. Caution must be used when restricting these important substances.

of salt is allowed in cooking, but no salt is added at the table. Overtly salty foods, such as canned soups, beef stew, chili, pickles, olives, potato chips, soy sauce, and cured meats are discouraged. This diet is used when a person suffers from mild hypertension and stable kidney or heart disease.

A *moderate sodium restriction* of 1,000 to 2,000 milligrams per day is used in cases of severe edema, hypertension, and heart disease. This diet omits the foods listed in Box 32-4. Salt is not used in cooking or at the table. Milk and milk products are limited to the equivalent of 2 cups of milk daily, and the use of regular bread may be restricted.

Strict and *severe sodium restrictions* of 500 and 250 milligrams per day, respectively, are unpalatable and hard to follow. They are only used in severe conditions and for short periods (usually only in a hospital setting). These diets eliminate virtually all foods with added salt and allow only limited quantities of meat, milk, and regular bread. The use of distilled water may be necessary.

Salt substitutes are available, but should only be used with a physician's approval. Salt substitutes often contain other electrolytes, such as potassium, which may also be restricted (especially in individuals with kidney disease). Clients may use sodium-free blends of herbs and spices in place of salt to season foods.

The diet for clients with acute heart disease is sometimes divided into five or six small meals daily. Gas-forming foods, foods that are hard to chew or swallow, and stimulants such as coffee and tea should be avoided. The overweight cardiac or hypertensive individual is usually also on a calorie-controlled diet, because extra weight adds to the burden on the heart. These clients should be encouraged to quit smoking and to avoid alcohol.

Calcium- or Phosphorus-Modified Diets.   A high calcium intake is indicated for both the prevention and treatment of osteoporosis. Excellent sources of calcium include milk, yogurt, and cheese. A low-phosphorus diet may be indicated for the person with kidney failure. Because protein foods are high in phosphorus, pre-dialysis clients suffering from renal disorders *and* following a low-protein diet are automatically restricting their phosphorus.

Potassium-Modified Diet.   A high-potassium diet is given to clients who are taking diuretics. Diuretics flush excess salt and water out of the body, but also cause a loss of potassium. Potassium is widespread in the diet; excellent sources include milk, fresh or dried fruits (especially bananas), fresh vegetables, dried peas and beans, whole-grain bread and cereals, fruit juices such as orange and prune, sunflower seeds, watermelon, nuts, molasses, cocoa beans, fresh fish, beef, ham, and poultry. Potassium intake may be limited during end-stage renal failure.

Diets Modified by Serving Size

Often, small frequent feedings help maximize food intake in clients with high nutritional needs or **anorexia** (loss of appetite or refusal to eat). Clients who have recently undergone gastric surgery can usually tolerate frequent small meals. Six small feedings are common, although the number can vary. Any diet can be divided into six meals. Liquid supplements often replace one or more meals because they are nutritionally dense, are easily consumed, and tend to leave the stomach quickly, making them less likely to interfere with the next meal.

Diets Modified for Allergens

Sometimes people have an allergic reaction to certain food substances. This reaction is caused by an autoimmune response to specific proteins called *allergens* in these foods. Allergies to milk, eggs, chocolate, grains, peanuts, and specific fruits are common. Although fruits are not considered protein foods, they contain trace amounts of protein that can cause an allergic reaction. When necessary, these foods are eliminated from the diet. Depending upon the number of allergens and how widespread they are in the diet, vitamin and mineral supple-

ments may be necessary to ensure a nutritionally adequate intake.

☛ KEY CONCEPT

The optimal modified diet in theory may not be practical for an individual in either the home or clinical setting. The practicality of a diet depends on the person's prognosis, level of intelligence and motivation, support systems, financial status, religious or ethnic background, and co-existing medical conditions.

NUTRITIONAL SUPPORT

Nutritional support is instituted when a person is unable to meet nutritional needs orally. Nutritional support can be short- or long-term. Hospitals often discharge clients who are still receiving nutritional support. Tube feedings are sometimes maintained indefinitely. Nutritional support includes tube feedings, total parenteral nutrition, and administration of intravenous fluids. See Chapter 87 for additional information.

Tube Feedings

A **tube feeding** is a means of providing liquid nourishment through a tube into the gastrointestinal (GI) tract. Tube feedings may also be called *enteral feedings* because they involve the GI tract. This type of feeding may be necessary in certain conditions that prohibit the person from taking adequate oral nourishment. Examples include loss of consciousness, inability to swallow, esophageal or gastric cancer or trauma, oral trauma, mouth surgery, or anorexia. Those suffering from conditions with increased nutritional requirements, such as burns, infection, surgery, or fractures, may also need supplemental nutrition. In some cases, tube feeding is necessary to supply or to maintain adequate nutritional status. A client with any type of enteral tube feeding *must* have a functioning GI tract (see In Practice: Nursing Procedure 32-1).

Types of Formulas

The liquid formulas for tube feedings contain adequate amounts of protein, fat, carbohydrate, vitamins, and minerals to maintain good nutrition. Routine formulas generally provide about 1 calorie per milliliter. They are lactose free, low in residue, and 14% to 16% protein. Routine formulas are also available in high-calorie, high-protein, and high-fiber varieties. Specialized formulas marketed specifically for stress, renal failure, liver failure, diabetes, AIDS, and other disorders are available.

A dietitian can help the physician to choose the right formula for an individual. Ready-mixed formulas are available in cans; powdered formulas are also available. Table foods pureed in a blender are often used in the home. Major considerations in choosing a formula are the type and amount of formula and the amount of extra water needed. The cost of different formulas varies.

Placement Sites

Sites of access to the gastrointestinal tract may differ. If the tube is passed through the client's nose and into the stomach, it is called a nasogastric tube (**NG tube**). This method is un-

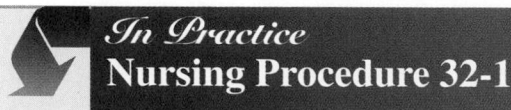

INSERTING A NASOGASTRIC (NG) TUBE (NASOGASTRIC INTUBATION)

Supplies and Equipment

Occasionally, two people may be needed for insertion. One person assists the client with positioning, holding the glass of water (if allowed), and encouragement.

Gloves
Nasogastric tube
Water-soluble substance (K-Y jelly)
Protective towel covering for client
Emesis basin
Tape for marking placement and securing tube
Glass of water (if allowed)
Straw for glass of water
Stethoscope
60 mL catheter tip syringe
Rubber band and safety pin
Suction equipment or tube feeding equipment

Steps

1. Gather equipment and supplies.
2. Check the physician's order and determine the type, size, and purpose of the NG tube.
   RATIONALE: *If the physician did not order a specific size, it is generally acceptable to insert a size 16 or 18 French, which are standard adult sizes. Sizes suitable for children vary from a very small size 5 French for children to size 12 French for older children. Larger NG (size 20 to 30 French) or enteric tubes such as an Ewald tube (which is used for gastric lavage of toxins) and the Cantor tube or Miller-Abbot tube may require insertion by a physician. The Cantor and Miller-Abbot tubes are quite large and have mercury, air, or fluid-filled bags attached to the distal end of the tube. The purpose of the bag is to advance the tube with peristaltic waves, with the therapeutic intent of breaking up intestinal blockages.*
3. Check the client's identification band. *Rationale: Be sure that the procedure is being done on the correct client, with the appropriate type of tube.*
4. Obtain NG suction equipment or NG tube feeding equipment as required.
   RATIONALE: *The physician may order a specific type of NG tube such as a Levin for short-term use for gavage or lavage; or a Salem sump with its two lumens, generally used for lavage and gastric suctioning; or a silicone type tube used for long-term placement for tube feedings.*
5. Set up tube-feeding equipment or suction equipment and test to make sure it functions properly.
   RATIONALE: *Be sure that the equipment is functioning properly and is at the right rate of flow or strength of suction, prior to using it on the client.*

6. Instruct the client in the procedure and assess his or her capability of cooperating with the procedure.
   RATIONALE: *It is not advisable to explain the procedure too far in advance, as the client's anxiety about the procedure may interfere with its success. It is important that the client relax, swallow, and cooperate during the procedure.*
7. Wash your hands. Put on gloves.
   RATIONALE: *Clean, not sterile, technique is necessary because the GI tract is not sterile.*
8. Position client in full Fowler's position if possible. Place a clean towel over the client's chest as a bib-type protection.
9. Measure the length of the tube that will be needed to reach the stomach.
10. With a damp washcloth, wipe the client's face and nose. Do not use soap. It may be necessary to wipe the outside of the nose with an alcohol wipe. Be sure to cover the eyes with a small, dry towel or washcloth when wiping down the exterior of the nose with an alcohol wipe.
    RATIONALE: *The NG tube will stay more secure if taped on a clean, non-oily nose. If the nose has been cleaned with an alcohol wipe, the tape will stay more secure and the tube will not move in the throat—causing gagging or discomfort later.*
11. Protect the eyes from any alcohol fumes from the alcohol wipe by briefly covering them with a cloth.
12. Ask the client if he or she has difficulty breathing out of one nares. You may test for nares obstructions by closing one nostril and then the other and asking the client to breathe through the nose for each attempt. If the client has difficulty breathing out of one nares, try to insert the NG tube in that nares and not the other.
    RATIONALE: *Many individuals have nasal obstructions or blocked nasal passages. After the procedure, the client may breathe more comfortably if the "good" nares remains patent. The blocked nasal passage may not be totally occluded and thus still be able to pass a NG tube. It may be necessary to use the more patent nares for insertion.*
13. Put on gloves and apply water-soluble lubricant to 4 to 8 inches of the tube.
    RATIONALE: *The tube slides in more easily if well-lubricated. The mucosa is less likely to be*

(continued)

In Practice
Nursing Procedure 32-1 (*Continued*)

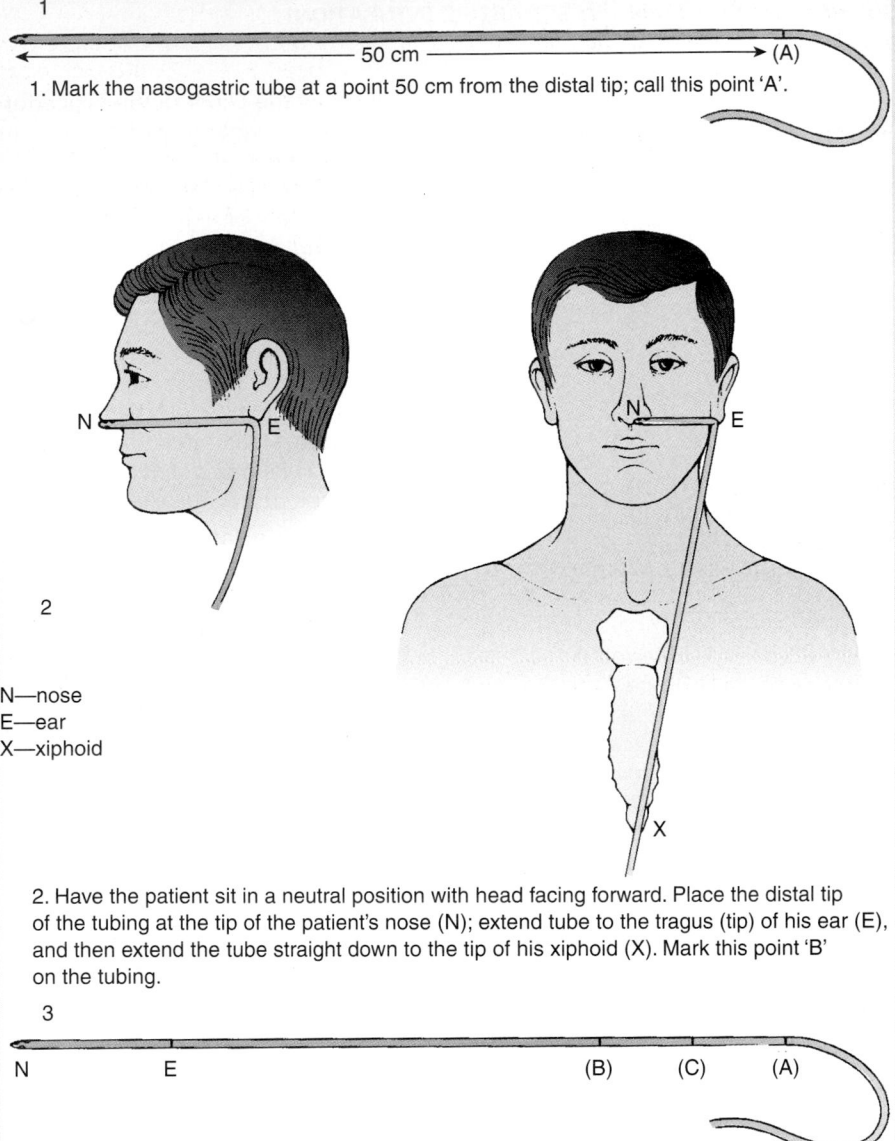

1. Mark the nasogastric tube at a point 50 cm from the distal tip; call this point 'A'.

N—nose
E—ear
X—xiphoid

2. Have the patient sit in a neutral position with head facing forward. Place the distal tip of the tubing at the tip of the patient's nose (N); extend tube to the tragus (tip) of his ear (E), and then extend the tube straight down to the tip of his xiphoid (X). Mark this point 'B' on the tubing.

3. To locate point C on the tube, find the midpoint between points A and B. The nasogastric tube is passed to point C to ensure optimum placement in the stomach.

Measuring length of nasogastric tube for placement into stomach

damaged during insertion. The physician may numb the nose and nasopharynx with a numbing solution to ease client comfort and suppress the gag reflex. Sometimes, having the client hold ice chips in the mouth for a few minutes prior to the procedure can also have a numbing effect that can minimize the gag reflex.

14. With the client sitting up, flex the head forward. Tilt the tip of the nose upward and insert the tube gently into the nose to as far as the back of the throat. Guide the tube straight back.

15. When the tube reaches the nasopharynx, stop briefly and have the client lower his or her head slightly.

16. Ask the client to swallow as the tube is advanced. Advance the tube several times as the client swallows until the correct marked position on the tube is reached.
    RATIONALE: *Flexing the head aids in the anatomical insertion of the tube. The tube is less likely to pass into the trachea. When the client swallows, the tube has a better chance of passing into the stomach instead of the trachea. Stimulating the*

In Practice
Nursing Procedure 32-1 (*Continued*)

gag reflex is normal, but swallowing while gently advancing the tube will minimize the gag reflex.

17. If coughing, persistent gagging, cyanosis, or dyspnea occur, remove the tube immediately.
RATIONALE: *The tube may be in the trachea.*

18. If obstruction is felt, pull out the tube and try the other nares.

19. Encourage the client to breathe through his or her mouth.

20. Have the client or the assistant hold the glass of water with the straw. Keep an emesis basin and tissues handy.

21. Insert the tube as far as the pre-marked insertion point. Place a temporary piece of tape across the nose and tube.
RATIONALE: *In this way, you can check for placement before securing the tube. If you do not secure the tube prior to checking for placement, the tube may move out of position.*

22. Check the back of the client's throat to make sure that the tube is not curled in the back of the throat.

23. Check the tube for correct placement by at least two and preferably three of the following methods:

A. Aspirate stomach contents. Stomach aspirate will appear cloudy, green, tan, off-white, bloody, or brown. It is not always possible to visually distinguish between stomach and respiratory aspirates.
Special note: The small diameters of some NG tubes makes aspiration problematic. The tubes themselves collapse when suction is applied via the syringe. Thus, contents cannot be aspirated.

B. Check pH of aspirate. Measuring the pH of stomach aspirate is considered more accurate than visual inspection. Stomach aspirate generally has a pH range of 0 to 4, commonly less than 4. The aspirate of respiratory contents is generally more alkaline, with a pH of 7 or more.

C. Inject 30 mL of air into the stomach and listen with the stethoscope for the "whoosh" of air into the stomach. The small diameter of some NG tubes may make it difficult to hear air entering the stomach.

D. Confirm by x-ray placement. X-ray visualization is the only method that is considered positive.

24. Once stomach placement has been confirmed, tape the tube using your prepared tape strips or a commercial NG securing tape.

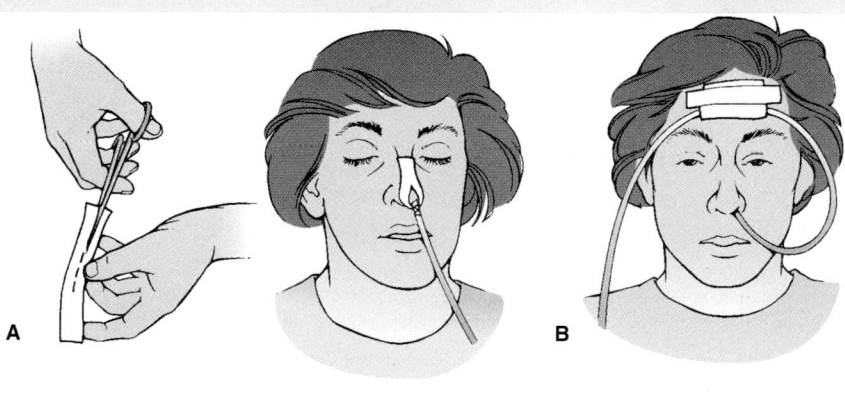
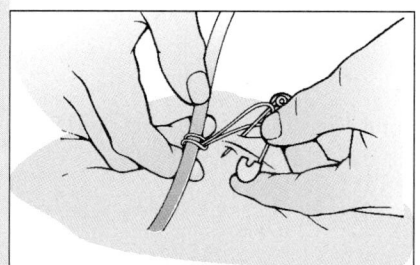
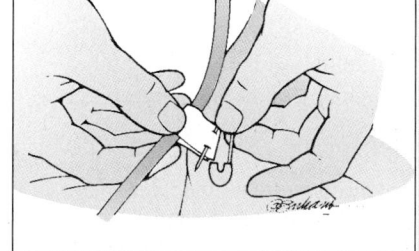

Securing nasogastric and nasoenteric tubes. (**A**) The nasogastric tube is secured to the nose with tape to prevent injury to the nasopharyngeal passages; the cheek may also be used. (**B**) Tape is placed on the forehead and the nasoenteric tube is taped to it; thereby allowing the tube to be advanced until the desired placement is achieved. (**C,D**) Secure tubing to the client's gown with either an elastic band or tape attached to a safety pin to prevent tension on the line during movement.

(*continued*)

In Practice
Nursing Procedure 32-1 (*Continued*)

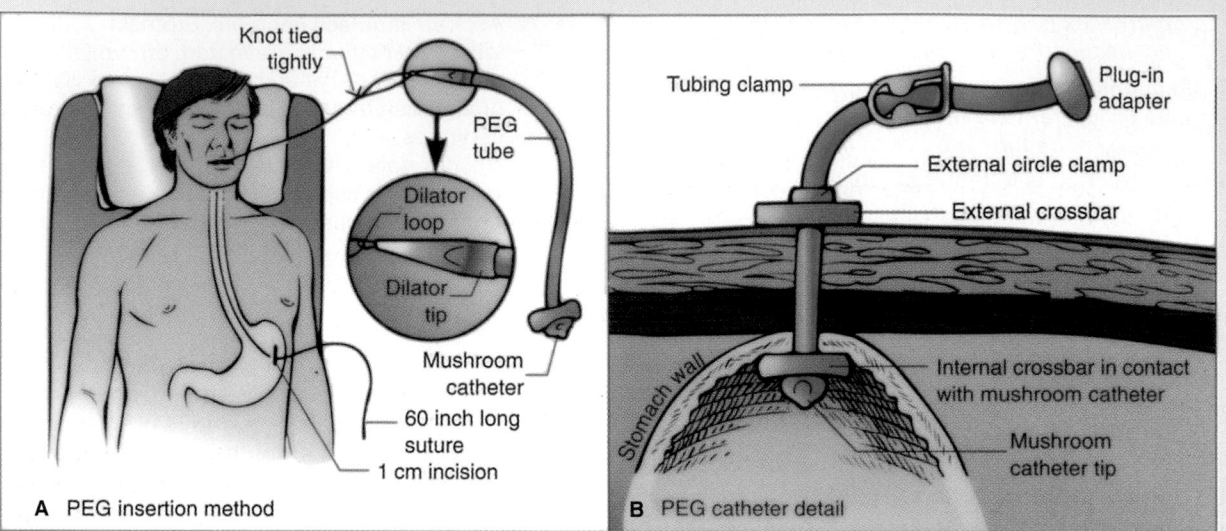

Knot tied tightly

PEG tube

Dilator loop

Dilator tip

Mushroom catheter

60 inch long suture

1 cm incision

A PEG insertion method

Tubing clamp

Plug-in adapter

External circle clamp

External crossbar

Stomach wall

Internal crossbar in contact with mushroom catheter

Mushroom catheter tip

B PEG catheter detail

(**A**) Percutaneous endoscopic gastrostomy (PEG). (**B**) A detail of the abdomen and the PEG tube, showing catheter fixation.

25. Clean the client's environment and position the client for comfort.

26. To prevent aspiration of stomach contents during NG tube feedings, the head of the bed must remain elevated at 30 degrees or more at all times.

27. Chart the procedure stating the date, time, type and size of NG tube used, left or right nares used, amount and type of aspirate, suction or feeding started, and client response to the procedure also recorded. It is not uncommon to have slight bleeding from irritation of the mucosa in the nose. Any trauma or difficulty during the procedure needs to be charted, documented, and observed.

28. After the procedure, chart and monitor the type of suction used and the amount of suction, eg, *#16 Fr Levin tube inserted right nares with minimal difficulty and set to low intermittent suction at 25 mmHg per Gomco.* During each shift, monitor and record the suction in mmHg and the amount and type of aspirate.

29. Institute monitoring of intake and output (I & O).

30. Always confirm placement of the NG tube prior to insertion of medications, application of suction, or instillation of tube feedings.
    RATIONALE: *It is possible for the tube to become dislodged between treatments.*

Adapted from: Smeltzer, S. C. & Bare, B. G. (2000). *Textbook of medical-surgical nursing* (9th ed., p. 838). Philadelphia: Lippincott Williams & Wilkins and Ellis, J. R., Nowlis, E. A., & Bentz, P. M. (1996). *Modules of basic nursing skills, volume II* (6th ed., pp. 263–266). Philadelphia: Lippincott Williams & Wilkins.

comfortable, and is not used for long-term administration. A tube called a gastrostomy tube (**G tube**) may be placed directly into the stomach through the abdominal wall, or a jejunal tube (**J tube**) may be inserted into the jejunum of the small intestine.

Tubes and Terminology

The name that is given to an enteral tube feeding device may be derived from a particular device, the type of procedure used, or the placement of the tube. The following are common types of tubes:

- *Nasogastric:* through the nose into the stomach
- *Percutaneous:* percutaneous endoscopic gastrostomy (**PEG**): placed through the skin
- *Endoscopic:* placed with an instrument called an *endoscope*

- *Gastrostomy:* inserted into the stomach
- *Button feeding device:* a small silicone device used in place of a gastrostomy tube

Each tube has its own equipment, but the means of formula instillation is similar for all types of tubes.

The PEG tube extends 12 to 15 inches beyond the skin, and has a cap covering the end. A short crosspiece (bolster) is placed near the opening through the skin (**stoma**). The nurse must note on the tube the level at which the tube enters the skin, and report any change immediately.

A button may replace the PEG-type G tube, especially if long-term administration is anticipated. The function of the button is the same as for the PEG tube; however, the button is level with the skin. It is less cumbersome, and more difficult for the confused or agitated adult client or the child to pull out.

Nursing Considerations

In Practice: Nursing Procedure 32-2 outlines steps in tube feeding. The nurse is also responsible for washing or replacing the feeding bag, as per hospital policy, and documenting care.

Clients receiving tube feedings may continue to eat or drink by mouth, if the physician allows. The client may need an extra water ("free water") allowance, administered with or in-between feedings. Water is especially important if the person has a fever, or if signs of inadequate hydration develop. Document findings and alert the physician if untoward signs develop: dry mouth, poor skin turgor (tone), complaints of thirst, illness, fever, or physical complaints (see In Practice: Educating the Client 32-2).

Table 32-2 summarizes problems in tube feeding and nursing actions to be taken.

Intravenous Therapy

Intravenous (**IV**) therapy or *parenteral therapy* involves injecting into a vein any number of sterile solutions that the body needs, including drugs and electrolytes. Simple IV solutions, infused through a peripheral vein, contain water with low concentrations of dextrose, electrolytes, or both. IV solutions are used on a short-term basis to restore or maintain fluid and electrolyte balance. Because it is nutritionally inadequate, simple IV therapy is not used for more than a few days without some sort of supplementation. Parenteral nutrition is used when the client cannot take sufficient amounts of nutrients via the enteral route (GI tract). These clients include those with severe burns or a disorder of the GI tract (eg, surgical removal of parts of the GI tract) that may inhibit absorption of nutrients.

Total and Peripheral Parenteral Nutrition

Total parenteral nutrition (**TPN**) is a specifically formulated and calculated solution that is nutritionally complete to meet a specific individual's needs. Sometimes TPN is called *hyperalimentation*, although this term is not completely accurate.

Total parenteral nutrition is used when the gastrointestinal tract is functioning improperly, such as in stomach cancer, or when a person has multiple trauma, severe infection, burns, or multi-organ failure. TPN is infused directly into the blood circulation and bypasses the digestive tract. Several types

---

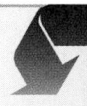

In Practice
Nursing Procedure 32-2

ADMINISTERING A TUBE FEEDING
Supplies and Equipment

Gloves
Feeding pump (optional)
Clamp (optional)
Feeding solution
Large catheter tip syringe (30 mL or larger)
Feeding bag with tubing
Water
Measuring cup
Other optional equipment (disposable pad, pH indicator strips, water-soluble lubricant, paper towels)

STEPS

1. Gather equipment and supplies after checking the physician's order for tube feeding.
   RATIONALE: *Checking the order confirms the type of feeding solution, route, and prescribed delivery time. Organization facilitates performance of the skill.*

2. Prepare formula:
   a. Shake can thoroughly. Check expiration date.
   RATIONALE: *Feeding solution may settle and requires mixing before administration. Outdated formula may be contaminated or have lessened nutritional value.*

   b. If formula is in powdered form, mix according to the instructions on the package. Prepare enough for 24 hours only. Use a large-enough container for the mixed amount, and refrigerate any unused formula. Label and date the container. Allow formula to reach room temperature before using.
   RATIONALE: *Formula loses its nutritional value and can harbor microorganisms if kept over 24 hours. Cold formulas can cause abdominal discomfort.*

3. Explain the procedure to the client. *Rationale: Providing information fosters the client's cooperation and understanding.*

4. Wash hands prior to putting on gloves.
   RATIONALE: *Handwashing prevents the spread of microorganisms. Gloves act as a barrier.*

5. Position the client with the head of the bed elevated at least 30 to 40 degrees.
   RATIONALE: *This position discourages aspiration of feeding solution into lungs.*

6. Determine placement of feeding tube by:
   a. Aspirating stomach secretions.
   RATIONALE: *Aspiration of gastric fluid indicates that the tube is correctly placed in the stomach. The*
   (continued)

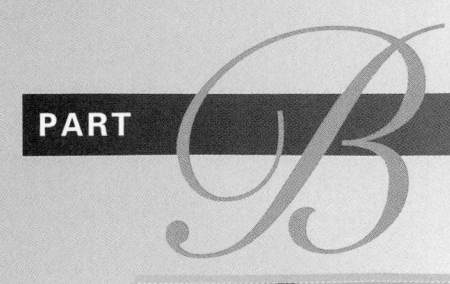
Nursing Care Skills

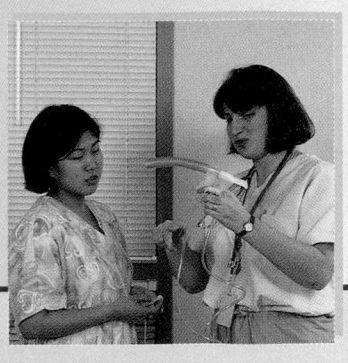

Unit VI

THE NURSING PROCESS

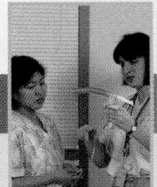

CHAPTER

33

Introduction to the Nursing Process

LEARNING OBJECTIVES

1. Define New Terminology terms.
2. Explain the use of critical thinking to solve problems.
3. Discuss the relationship between critical thinking and problem-solving.
4. Explain the use of the nursing process in nursing practice.
5. Describe the nurse's actions during each step of the nursing process.
6. Compare the seven steps of scientific problem-solving with the correlated steps of the nursing process.

NEW TERMINOLOGY

client-oriented
critical thinking
nursing care plan

nursing process
scientific problem-solving
trial and error

ACRONYM

NCP

A primary goal of nursing is to help individuals meet their basic and higher-level needs (see Chap. 5). Meeting with clients leads to specific interactions, including communication, observation, support, education, and provision of care. Nurses support and encourage individuals in their healthy habits and help clients solve health problems. They provide care to clients by combining scientific problem-solving methods with critical thinking skills to provide care through the nursing process.

PROBLEM-SOLVING

Problem-solving is the basic skill of identifying a problem and taking steps to resolve it. Common sense is helpful in solving many problems. However, when a problem is complex or challenging to define, you may need to use other—more formal—methods of problem-solving.

Trial and Error

Trial and error is an experimental approach to problem-solving that tests ideas to decide which methods work and which do not. Usually the results are completely unknown until tried, because the experimenter simply does not have enough information to anticipate results. Sometimes, you use trial and error to solve problems in your everyday life. Consider your dilemma if you have an allergy to an unknown substance in hand lotion, but also have a problem with dry skin and wish to soften your hands. You try one brand, but develop a rash. You try another brand with the same results. These trials result in errors: the lotions continue to cause an allergic response. Eventually, you find a brand that works without causing a rash, and your trial is successful.

As healthcare evolved throughout history, care providers used trial and error to distinguish between successful and unsuccessful treatments. Errors occurred when people died after treatment with plant berries, leaves, roots, or crude surgery, as care providers tried to find a cure.

A form of trial and error experimentation is used in laboratory studies when testing several solutions to a problem. Solutions that are harmful or ineffective are discarded until helpful solutions are found. In other situations, trial and error is used when unexpected results occur that could possibly have beneficial outcomes for another problem. For example, minoxidil (Rogaine) was first marketed as an antihypertensive drug. However, the unexpected result of hair growth led to experimentation and development of drug forms for the treatment of hair loss.

Many advances in modern healthcare have resulted from this type of experimentation; however, trial and error must be used carefully when working with people because of the possible harmful results. Researchers develop strict guidelines to protect the safety and well-being of individuals and proceed with trial and error experimentation only with the permission and understanding of the individual involved.

Scientific Problem-Solving

Today's society prefers that only safe and proven effective treatments be given to those who are ill. Therefore, healthcare providers rely on previously proven facts to determine which treatments are safe. Scientists and healthcare researchers use a precise method to investigate problems and arrive at solutions. This method, called **scientific problem-solving,** allows researchers to discover the best possible safe and effective treatments for disease or dysfunction. The seven steps of scientific problem-solving are as follows:

1. Identify the problem.
2. Gather information relative to the problem.
3. Formulate tentative solutions (hypotheses); choose preferred solution.
4. Plan action to test suggested solution.
5. Experiment and observe the results.
6. Interpret the results (draw conclusions); understand what the results mean.
7. Evaluate the solution, either concluding or revising the study to test the solution again if results are unsatisfactory. (p. 220[1])

Scientific problem-solving requires both logical thought and imagination. When you use scientific problem-solving, you combine what you have learned from your own experience with facts previously proven through scientific study.

CRITICAL THINKING

Unless you have already been educated as a scientist, you probably confront problems and find solutions without using trial and error or scientific problem-solving. You may use a complicated mix of inquiry, knowledge, intuition, logic, experience, and common sense called **critical thinking.** This kind of thinking enables you to grasp the meaning of multiple clues and to find quick answers when facing difficult problems. Critical thinking is neither trial and error nor a structured scientific problem-solving system.

Critical thinking has some characteristics that are important for solving problems in healthcare. When you think critically, you examine facts and compare these facts with information you already know, thereby being actively curious and critiquing ideas for reasonableness. You form ideas or concepts that are mental pictures of reality. You are reasonable and rational, continuously searching to understand the entire situation. You may think randomly, without a particular method or pattern; however, you do not jump to conclusions. As a critical thinker, you form your own beliefs or ideas rather than automatically accepting the thoughts or ideas of others. You become an open-minded person, flexible to alternatives. You also use your imagination and creativity to systematically gather information and draw conclusions (Figure 33-1).

Consider a simple example of how you use critical thinking when confronted with a problem. Early one morning your car keys are not in their usual location. You have only 30 minutes to get to class for a required exam. What do you do first? You probably search frantically again, but then stop to think about where else you may have left your keys. Perhaps you retrace your steps of the previous day when you last had your keys. You ask yourself, "Where was I? What was I doing? Did I leave them in a pocket? What was I wearing?" By asking yourself logical questions, remembering the facts, creating a mental

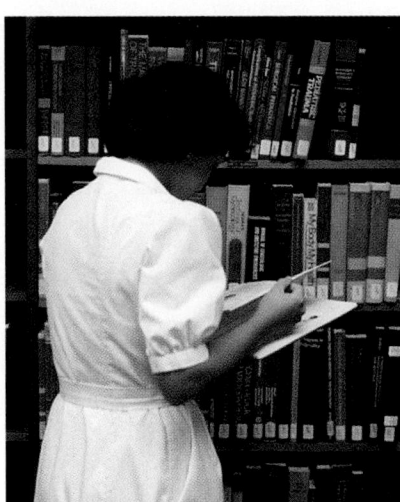

FIGURE 33-1. Critical thinking utilizes previous knowledge, research and analysis, as well as common sense, to solve problems.

image of your activities, and perhaps following a hunch about where the keys are, you may solve your problem quickly and find your keys. If you do not find them within a reasonable time, you begin to think about other ways of handling the problem of getting to the required exam. This process is called critical thinking: remembering facts, using logic, asking key questions, forming a mental image, and analyzing all information.

Most client care problems have many possible causes and many probable solutions. When you think critically, you can grasp the nature and extent of problems more quickly and easily. You can make decisions that are logical, suitable for a particular client, and effective for solving the specific problem. This entire book presents exercises to help you develop your critical thinking skills as you continue to learn about nursing practice.

NURSING PROCESS

Although you will use critical thinking during your nursing career, it alone does not give you a framework for solving problems purposefully and methodically, a necessary safeguard in healthcare. As a nurse, you combine critical thinking skills with a scientific problem-solving method to identify client problems and to provide care in a structured, purposeful, and effective way. This framework for thinking and acting is called the **nursing process.** The nursing process is a special way of thinking about how to care for patients. The nursing process is also described as "a systematic method that directs the nurse and client as they together (1) determine the need for nursing care, (2) plan and implement the care, and (3) evaluate the results." (p. 217[1])

You will use the nursing process framework throughout your nursing practice, but particularly as you learn to become a nurse. The nursing process is the method you use to identify and to treat client care problems. To ensure consistency among all nursing staff, use the nursing process to develop guidelines when caring for each client. These guidelines are the **nursing care plans (NCP).** The nursing process framework enables you to develop plans of care individualized for each client,

identifying what is suitable and desirable for that particular person (see In Practice: Nursing Care Plan 33-1 about an elderly women with pneumonia, and the accompanying photo display depicting the steps of the nursing process in action). The care plan helps you manage your time more effectively as you provide care. Because the nursing care plan is available for other nurses to use as well, it provides consistency in care.

The effective use of the nursing process allows you to identify not only actual problems but also potential problems. The ability to foresee problems may avert painful, as well as costly, complications. The nursing process also enables you to determine if your nursing care helped the client.

You can develop critical thinking and problem-solving skills by working through the nursing process framework repeatedly, as you learn to identify and treat client needs. Often, you will practice the steps of the nursing process as you prepare nursing care plans. Keep in mind that every time you prepare a care plan, you are developing your critical thinking skills and expanding your nursing knowledge. Also, remember that every time you carry through with your plan, you are carrying out the work of nursing. Eventually this process of thinking and doing becomes automatic.

The nursing process framework is used throughout the United States and Canada as a guide for identifying needs and treating clients, though how it is used varies from one area to another. Sometimes, its use varies among types of healthcare facilities and may be related to available staffing. In some areas of practice, registered nurses are more likely to diagnose clients, set overall goals, and plan care. In other areas, licensed practical nurses also diagnose and plan, as well as implement the plan. Determine what your role is expected to be (as a student and as a graduate) in your particular healthcare facility.

Steps in the Nursing Process

The nursing process has specific steps in which you work with the client to plan and to carry out effective nursing care:

Nursing Assessment: the systematic and continuous collection of data (Fig. 33-2)
Nursing Diagnosis: the statement of the client's actual or potential problem
Planning: the development of goals for care and possible activities to meet them
Implementation: the giving of actual nursing care
Evaluation: the measurement of the effectiveness of nursing care

The next three chapters expand on these steps of the nursing process.

Characteristics of the Nursing Process

The steps in the nursing process lead to specific results. The characteristics of the nursing process, as discussed in the following sections, are critical to its effectiveness.

Based on Scientific Problem-Solving
The five steps of the nursing process closely parallel the steps of scientific problem-solving. Table 33-1 shows the relation-

In Practice
Nursing Care Plan 33-1

THE ELDERLY WOMAN HOSPITALIZED WITH PNEUMONIA

Medical History: MT, a 78-year-old female with a history of mild heart failure treated with diuretic therapy and sodium restriction, was brought to the emergency department by her daughter. Oxygen saturation (SaO_2) via pulse oximetry is 93%. Supplemental oxygen is ordered via nasal cannula at 4 L/min. Chest x-ray reveals patchy areas of consolidation in the right middle, and lower lobes. White blood cell count reveals leukocytosis (increased white blood cells). Her daughter states, "I just thought that she had a bad cold but now she's been coughing up some thick yellow mucus and says that it is hard to breathe." A sputum culture obtained was positive for Streptococcus. The client is admitted to the hospital.

Medical Diagnosis: Streptococcal pneumonia.

Data Collection/Nursing Assessment: Client is diaphoretic (sweating profusely) and pale with complaint of shortness of breath. Temperature, 102.6 degrees F (39.2 degrees C) orally; pulse, 126 beats per minute (bpm); respirations, 38 breaths per minute, use of accessory muscles noted; blood pressure (BP), 100/60. Lungs with scattered coarse crackles (moist bubbling sounds as inhaled air comes in contact with secretions) and decreased breath sounds, especially in the right middle and lower lobes. Client describes a productive cough with thick, purulent sputum several times in the last hour. Daughter states, "I've tried to get her to drink some fluids but she just seems so tired, coughing all the time."

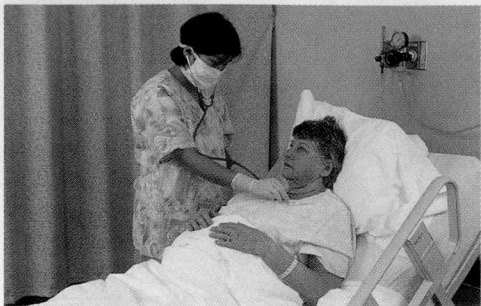

Photo: B. Proud

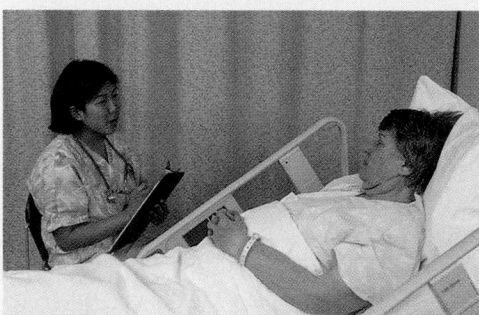

Photo: B. Proud

Nursing Diagnosis: Ineffective airway clearance related to physiologic effects of pneumonia as evidenced by increased sputum, coughing, abnormal breath sounds, tachypnea, and dyspnea.

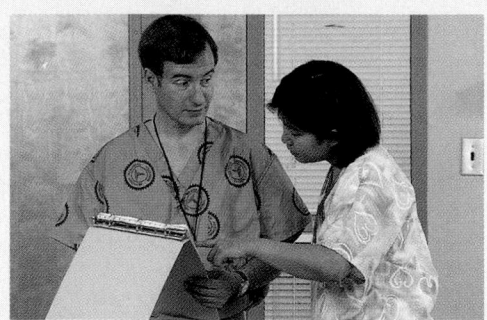

Photo: B. Proud

Planning:

SHORT-TERM GOALS:
#1: Within 4 to 6 hours, oxygen saturation will be maintained at 95% or greater with the use of supplemental oxygen.
#2: Within 24 hours, client will state that breathing is easier.
#3: By day 2 of hospitalization, client's vital signs and arterial blood gas levels will be within expected ranges for age.

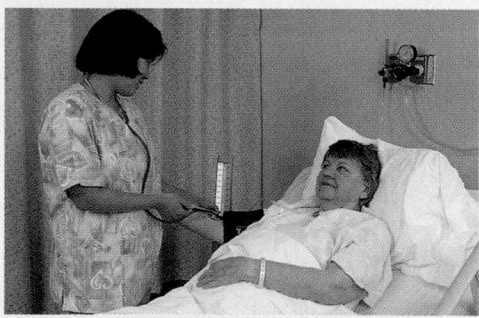

Photo: B. Proud

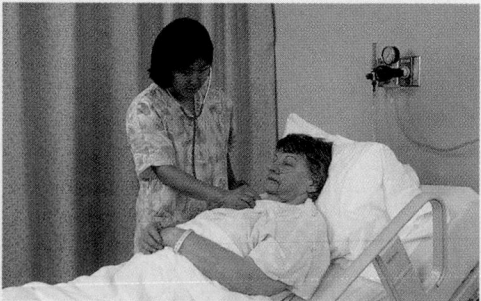

Photo: B. Proud

(continued)

In Practice
Nursing Care Plan 33-1 (*Continued*)

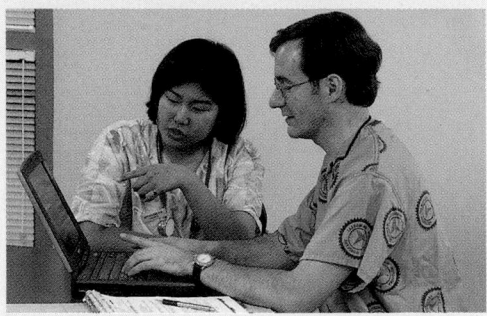

Photo: B. Proud

LONG-TERM GOALS:

#4: By discharge, client's lungs will be clear to auscultation, and oxygen saturation will remain at greater than 95% without the use of supplemental oxygen.

#5: At time of discharge, client and daughter will verbalize measures for continued therapy and followup to prevent a recurrence.

Implementation:

NURSING ACTION: *Administer supplemental humidified oxygen via nasal cannula at the prescribed flow rate.*

RATIONALE: *Supplemental, humidified oxygen aids in improving ventilation, thereby minimizing the risk for hypoxemia without drying the mucous membranes.*

NURSING ACTION: *Monitor oxygen saturation levels via pulse oximetry; assist with obtaining arterial blood gases (ABGs) as ordered.*

RATIONALE: *Oxygen saturation levels and ABGs provide objective evidence of the client's tissue oxygenation.*

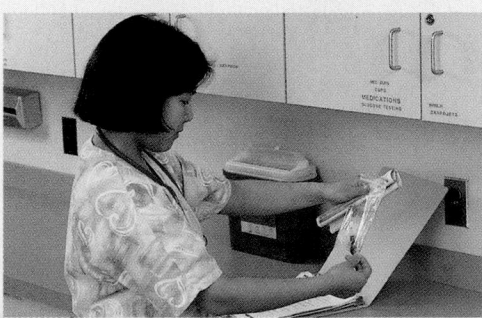

Photo: B. Proud

EVALUATION: SaO$_2$ at 95% via pulse oximetry; ABGs results confirm oxygen saturation at 95% and PaO$_2$ at 92 mm Hg with supplemental oxygen therapy. *Goal #1 met.*

NURSING ACTION: *Assist client to assume semi-Fowler's to high Fowler's position and reposition frequently.*

RATIONALE: *A position in which the client's head is elevated facilitates breathing and promotes optimal lung expansion by relieving pressure on the*

diaphragm. Frequent repositioning prevents pooling and stasis of secretions.

EVALUATION: Decreased use of accessory muscles; client reporting a decrease in shortness of breath and decrease in difficulty breathing. *Goal #2 met.*

NURSING ACTION: *Assess vital signs and respiratory status including auscultation of lung sounds, initially every 1 to 2 hours and then as indicated.*

RATIONALE: *Frequent assessment of the client's status provides evidence of improvement or deterioration in the client's condition.*

EVALUATION: Temperature 100.4 degrees F (38.0 degrees C) orally; pulse, 100 bpm; respirations, 30; BP, 110/64. *Progress to meeting Goal #3.*

NURSING ACTION: *Begin intravenous (IV) fluid therapy as ordered using an infusion pump; prepare antibiotic for IV infusion.*

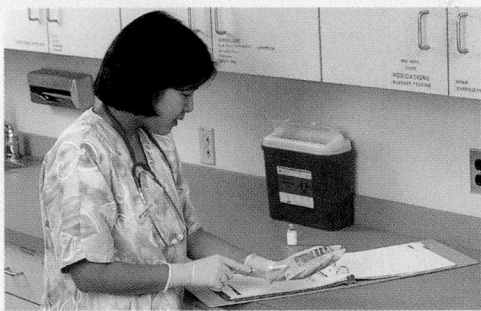

Photo: B. Proud

RATIONALE: *IV fluid therapy aids in replacing increased fluid lost through insensible sources and provides a route for administering IV antibiotic therapy, which is effective against the causative organism. Use of an infusion pump reduces the risk for possible fluid overload.*

EVALUATION: Mucous membranes pale but moist; IV site clean, dry, and intact, running at prescribed rate; IV antibiotic being administered without problems; vital signs within expected ranges. *Goal #3 met.*

NURSING ACTION: *Encourage frequent sips of fluid and administer antipyretics as ordered.*

RATIONALE: *Oral fluid intake is necessary for replacement of fluid, minimizing the risk for possible fluid volume deficit due to increased insensible fluid losses. Antipyretics reduce fever, thus decreasing the amount of insensible fluid lost in this manner.*

EVALUATION: Tolerating approximately 45 mL of fluid every 30 minutes; afebrile.

NURSING ACTION: *Instruct client in coughing and deep breathing and use of incentive spirometer. Assist with prescribed nebulizer therapy as necessary.*

(*continued*)

RATIONALE: *Coughing, deep breathing, and use of incentive spirometer aid in maximizing ventilatory capacity and mobilizing and expectorating secretions. Nebulizer therapy helps to open airways and keep membranes moist, facilitating expectoration.*

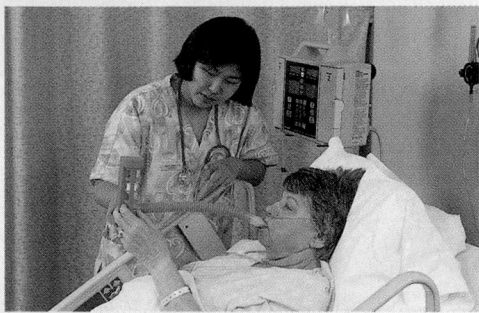

Photo: B. Proud

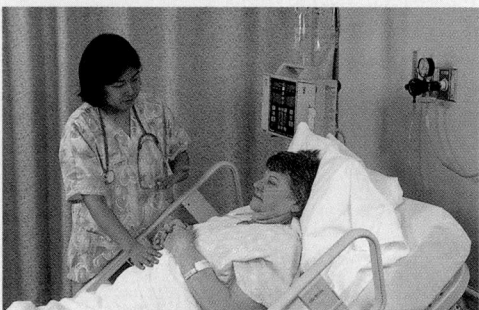

Photo: B. Proud

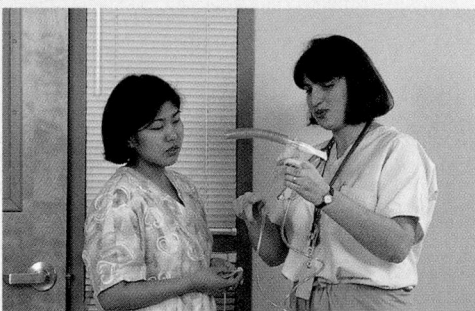

Photo: B. Proud

EVALUATION: Client able to cough and expectorate sputum. Mucus becoming pale yellow and less tenacious; remaining afebrile; lungs clearing; right middle lobe clear to auscultation. *Progress to meeting Goal #4.*
NURSING ACTION: *Gradually increase client's activity level, assisting client out of bed to the chair—using oxygen saturation levels as a guide.*
RATIONALE: *Gradual increase in activity minimizes the risk of exhaustion; increased activity without an accompanying decrease in oxygen saturation levels*

indicates improvement in the client's ability to meet oxygen demands.

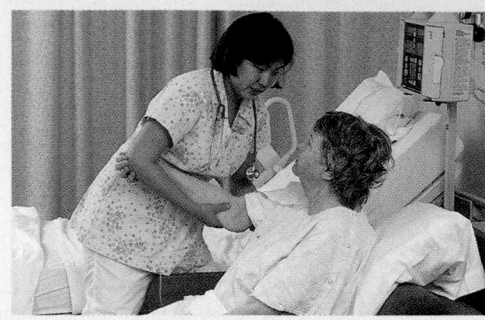

Photo: B. Proud

EVALUATION: Client out of bed to chair for 20 minutes with supplemental oxygen in place; SaO₂ 98%. *Continued progress to meeting Goal #4.*
NURSING ACTION: *Continue monitoring vital signs and respiratory status every 4 hours or as indicated, noting need for oxygen based on oxygen saturation levels.*
RATIONALE: *Continued monitoring provides objective evidence of improvement or deterioration in client's condition.*

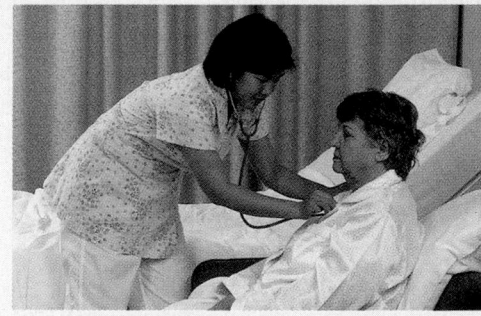

Photo: B. Proud

EVALUATION: Afebrile; pulse, 84; respirations, 22; BP, 116/70; lungs clear to auscultation except for small portion of right lower lobe; client out of bed to chair for 20 minutes without use of oxygen; SaO₂ 98%.
NURSING ACTION: *Administer oral antibiotic as ordered and indicated by improvement in the client's condition.*
RATIONALE: *Continued antibiotic therapy is necessary to ensure complete eradication of the causative organism.*

EVALUATION: Vital signs remaining in expected range for age; afebrile. Lungs clear to auscultation. *Goal #4 met.*
NURSING ACTION: *Instruct client and daughter in measures for continued therapy and followup after discharge.*

(continued)

In Practice
Nursing Care Plan 33-1 (Continued)

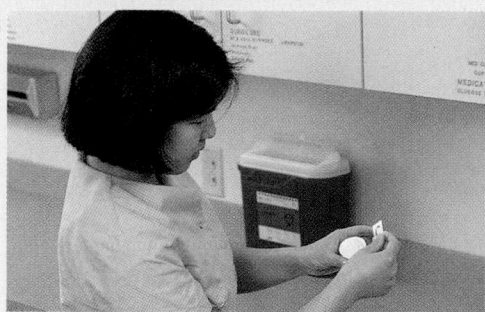

Photo: B. Proud

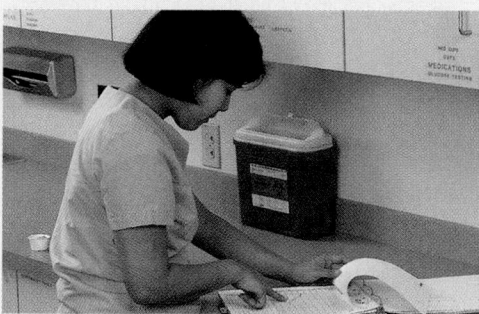

Photo: B. Proud

RATIONALE: *Knowledge about necessary therapy and followup aid in decreasing the risk for recurrence.*

EVALUATION: Daughter reporting return visit to primary care provider scheduled; client and daughter able to state signs and symptoms of recurrence. *Goal #5 met.*

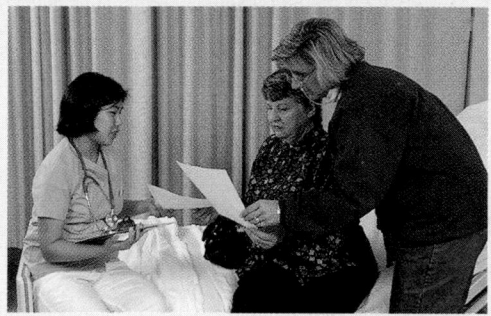

Photo: B. Proud

ship between the steps of the nursing process and those of scientific problem-solving.

Systematic

By following specific steps to identify the client's needs and planning activities to meet them, you will not overlook important information or activities.

Client-Oriented

Through the nursing process, the client (and if appropriate, the family) becomes your partner in determining the goals for care. You focus on meeting individualized client needs rather than on performing specific skills or tasks. Nursing thus becomes **client-oriented,** rather than task-oriented.

▪▪▪ TABLE 33-1 *The* NURSING PROCESS COMPARED WITH SCIENTIFIC PROBLEM-SOLVING

Steps in Scientific Problem Solving	Related Steps in the Nursing Process	Activities to Perform
Gather information relative to the problem	Nursing Assessment	Identify priorities; collect data; update database
Identify the problem	Nursing Diagnosis	Recognize significant data; recognize patterns or clusters; identify strengths and problems; reach conclusions; validate observations; write diagnostic statements
Formulate tentative solutions; describe possible solutions; choose preferred solutions	Planning	Set priorities; establish expected outcomes; select nursing interventions
Plan action to test suggested solutions	Planning	Write a nursing care plan (NCP)
Test solutions	Implementation	Put NCP into action; continue collecting data; communicate care to healthcare team; document care
Evaluate the solution; evaluate the results	Evaluation	Analyze client's responses; identify factors that contributed to success or failure of the NCP
Formulate another tentative solution	Evaluation	Plan for future nursing care; revise plan as needed

Goal-Oriented

With the client and family, you determine what goals should be set and met in nursing care. These goals are ranked according to the client's priority needs and preferences. Some goals are short-term, which means they can be achieved within hours or days. Other goals are long-term, which means they may take weeks or months to achieve.

Continuous

Figure 33-2 shows that the nursing process is continuous or cyclic. Problem-solving goes on throughout your relationship with the client. You continually reassess, reevaluate, and revise the nursing care plan.

Dynamic

The nursing process is dynamic, or ever-changing. Although it contains definite steps, these steps overlap. Sometimes they all occur at once. For example, in an emergency, you may be performing an intervention, while evaluating its effect, while assessing another factor, while planning priorities of what to do next.

Nursing Process and Quality Care

Nursing process is an important tool for providing measurable and observable evidence indicating the effectiveness of nursing care given in any setting. As a licensed nurse, you are responsible, or accountable, for your actions. Chapter 36 discusses accountability in depth.

Although you may work with several clients who have the same medical problem, each person will have special considerations. For example, you have two clients, Mrs. M. and Ms. R., who have just learned they have diabetes. Both clients

must learn to give themselves insulin by injection to control the disease. Mrs. M. has no prior knowledge of diabetes, but Ms. R. cared for her diabetic mother and administered insulin by injection for a number of years. Thus, you can develop care plans for both clients that consider their specific learning needs. Because all the nurses providing care for a client refer to the same care plan, consistency of care is ensured. You can measure how the client is progressing according to the plan. If goals are not being met, a reevaluation will indicate what further needs must be identified.

☞ KEY CONCEPT

The nursing process is scientific, systematic, client-oriented, goal-oriented, continuous, and dynamic. The nursing process consists of the following steps:

- *Nursing Assessment*
- *Nursing Diagnosis*
- *Planning*
- *Implementation*
- *Evaluation*

The steps may overlap, change, repeat themselves, or happen all at once.

✦ STUDENT SYNTHESIS

Key Points

- Scientists have used scientific problem-solving for many years to systematize their research.

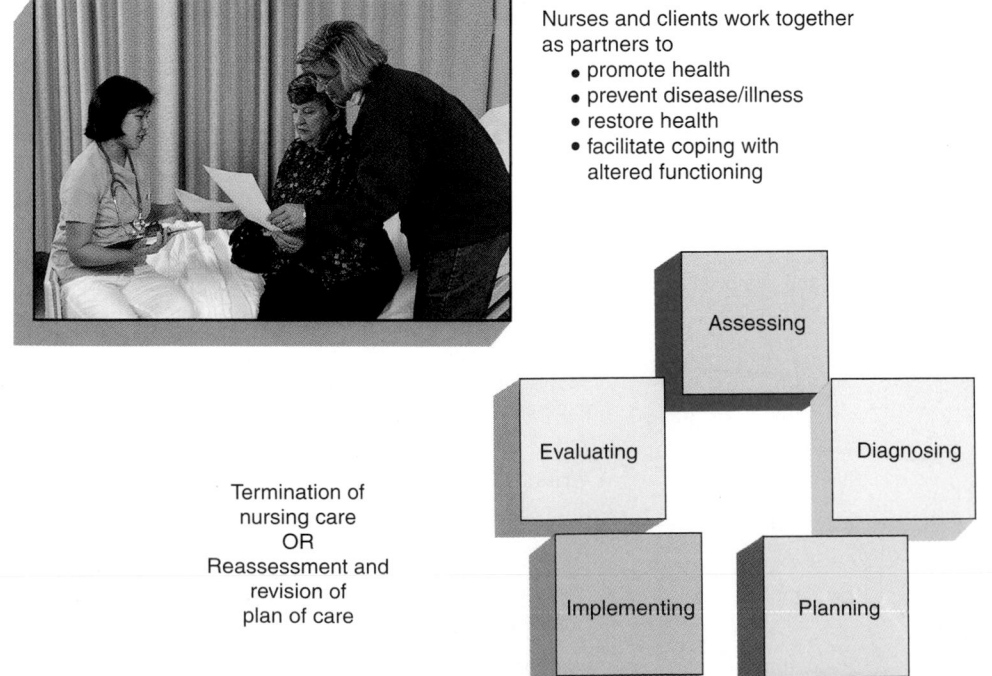

Nurses and clients work together as partners to
- promote health
- prevent disease/illness
- restore health
- facilitate coping with altered functioning

Termination of nursing care OR Reassessment and revision of plan of care

FIGURE 33-2. The nursing process is a continuous, scientific, systematic, client oriented, and goal oriented approach where the nurse and client work together to ensure quality care.

- Critical thinking is an important nursing strategy for problem-solving.
- The nursing process is a framework of scientific problem-solving combined with critical thinking skills.
- The nursing process provides individualized care that is accountable.
- Steps in the nursing process include assessment, nursing diagnosis, planning, implementation, and evaluation.
- The nursing process can be used to identify not only the client's actual problems, but also potential problems.
- The client and the family are involved in developing the nursing care plan.

Critical Thinking Exercises

1. Your client, a 21-year-old woman who delivered a baby girl 3 hours ago, has just told you that she feels nauseated. This is the first time she has reported this symptom. What additional information would you ask her, or seek from other sources, before reporting this information to your team leader? What observations would you make? Explain the rationale for your choice of questions and observations.
2. You are currently working with two clients who have had a stroke. Both clients are paralyzed on the right side. Based on your understanding of holistic nursing and of individualized client care, describe factors that you would expect to consider when working with each client to design a plan of care.

NCLEX-Style Review Questions

1. Which part of the nursing process includes the statement of the client's actual or potential problem?
   a. Assessment
   b. Implementation
   c. Nursing diagnosis
   d. Planning
2. Which of the following is a characteristic of the nursing process?
   a. Instinct forms the basis for the process.
   b. All health professionals use the nursing process.
   c. The process occurs once for each client.
   d. The client is the central focus of the process.
3. Implementation of the nursing process involves:
   a. Collecting data
   b. Giving actual nursing care
   c. Measuring effectiveness of nursing care
   d. Systematically developing goals
4. Which skill does the nurse use to determine the meaning of multiple cues when assessing clients?
   a. Critical thinking
   b. Evaluation
   c. Experimentation
   d. Nursing process
5. The primary reason for nurses to use nursing care plans is to:
   a. Ensure consistency of care among all nursing staff
   b. Identify client problems
   c. Provide justification for nursing care
   d. Utilize critical thinking skills

Reference

1. Taylor, C., Lillis, C., & LeMone, P. (2001). *Fundamentals of nursing: The art and science of nursing care* (4th ed.). Philadelphia: Lippincott Williams & Wilkins.

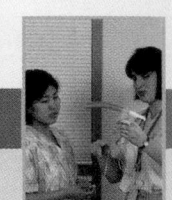

34

Nursing Assessment

LEARNING OBJECTIVES

1. Define New Terminology terms.
2. Discuss the steps in nursing assessment.
3. Differentiate between subjective and objective data.
4. Explain methods of data collection.
5. Identify techniques used in the health interview.
6. Discuss the process of data analysis to determine client problems.

NEW TERMINOLOGY

data analysis

health interview

nursing assessment

nursing history

objective data

observation

subjective data

ACRONYMS

ADL   CC

All steps of the nursing process depend on complete and accurate information about the client. The nurse carefully collects this information, also called *data*, during the first step of the nursing process. This chapter discusses this first step of the nursing process: assessment.

NURSING ASSESSMENT

As you enter the nurse–client relationship, the nursing process begins with assessment (Fig. 34-1). **Nursing assessment** is the systematic and continuous collection and analysis of information about the client. The purpose of assessment is to identify whether the person is well, has risk factors for problems, or has actual problems. If the client has actual problems, assessment further helps to identify whether the client has the necessary strengths to cope with these problems. Throughout assessment, you use critical thinking skills to guide your thoughts and actions. Because clients are partners in their own care, they participate actively in the entire nursing process.

Data Collection

The best sources of information about the client are the client and family. You also consult other members of the healthcare team for their information and analysis of the client. In addition, you learn information from the client's previous and present health record, laboratory reports, and reference books dealing with the client's medical diagnosis or condition.

The physical examination also yields important data (see Chapter 47 for a detailed description of the physical examination). Data to be gathered from the client also are identified in Chapter 45, and throughout this book.

Data collected about a client generally fall into one of two categories: objective or subjective.

Objective Data
Objective data include all the measurable and observable pieces of information about the client and his or her overall state of health. The term *objective* means that only precise, accurate measurements or clear descriptions are used. Therefore, other healthcare providers can verify objective data. Judgments, opinions, or client statements are not considered objective data. As a nurse, you measure the client's vital signs, height, weight, and urine volume. You use specific descriptions about the size and color of a wound. Measurements of body structure and function that involve extent, rate, rhythm, amount, and size are usually made with instruments—such as a stethoscope or sphygmomanometer—or are the results of laboratory tests or radiologic diagnostic tools. Laboratory tests also measure the chemical makeup of the blood and urine.

The critical thinking skills that you use while collecting objective data about the client involve asking key questions. What are the client's vital signs? What can you directly observe? Have you read the physician's history and progress notes? What do the other members of the healthcare team have to say about the client? What do laboratory reports tell you about the client's condition?

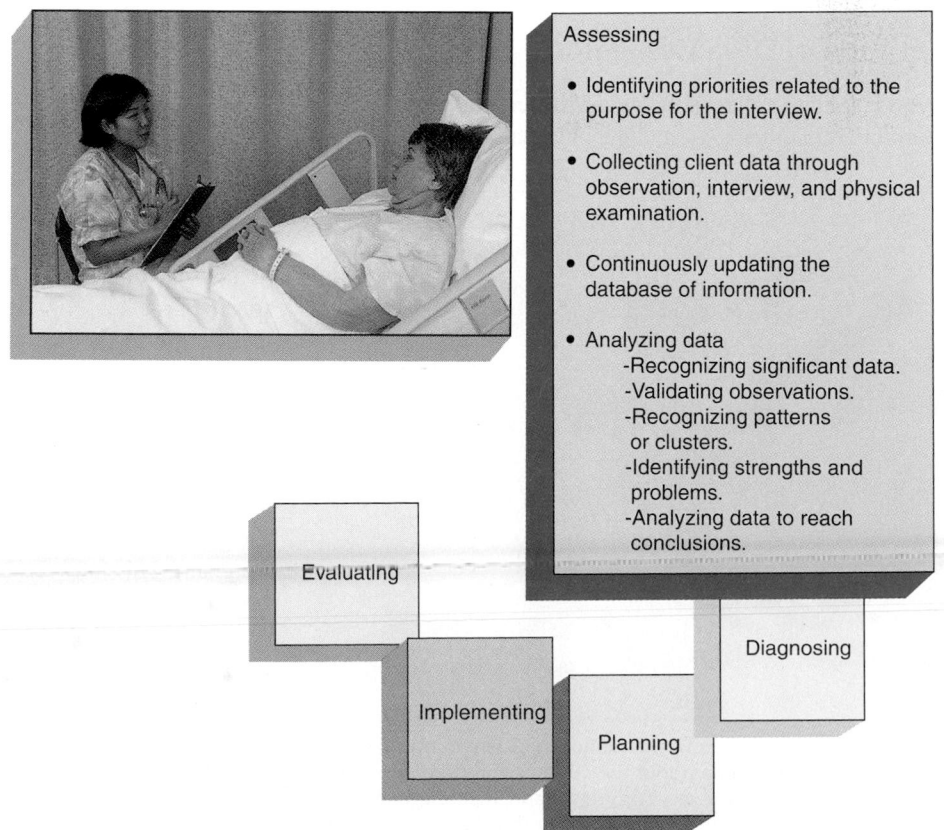

FIGURE 34-1. The nursing process begins with assessment. The nurse collects as much objective and subjective data about the client as possible.

Subjective Data

Subjective data consist of the client's opinions or feelings about what is happening. Only the client can tell you that he or she is afraid or has pain. Sometimes the client communicates through body language: gestures, facial expressions, and body posture. Both spoken and written words and body language tell you the client's opinions and feelings. Often this information cannot be confirmed through any other source (Fig. 34-2). To obtain subjective data, you need sharp interviewing, listening, and observing skills. Always be sure to consider cultural factors, such as specific body postures and use of eye contact, the client's beliefs about health and illness, or the use of special amulets or folk remedies (see Chapter 8 for more information about culture). Chapter 44 discusses therapeutic communication and interviewing in more detail.

The following considerations are critical thinking questions to ask yourself when obtaining subjective data about the client:

- What is the client saying about how he or she is feeling? (*subjective data*)
- Do the client's words and behaviors say the same thing? (*congruence*)
- What does the client say is the reason for coming to the healthcare facility?
- What is working and what is not working?
- How is the client coping with the immediate environment (home, hospital, nursing home)?

☛ KEY CONCEPT

Objective data are things that you directly see *or* measure. *Subjective data are things the client* feels *and* expresses, *either verbally or nonverbally.*

Methods of Data Collection

Methods used to collect data include observation, interview, laboratory and other tests, and the physical examination. By using all of these methods, you can obtain complete and accurate information. When you examine all of this information together, a picture of the total client emerges. Data must be factual, unbiased, and impartial and must be updated continuously.

Observation

Observation is an assessment tool that relies on the use of the five senses (sight, touch, hearing, smell, and taste) to discover information about the client. This information relates to characteristics of the client's appearance, functioning, primary relationships, and environment.

Visual Observation.   Sight provides an abundance of clues that you must continually process when assessing the client. A few examples to consider are body movements, general appearance, mannerisms, facial expressions, mode of dress, nonverbal communication, interaction with others, use of space, skin color and appearance, and cleanliness. You use visual observation to collect subjective data, such as when noting the client's facial expression and body language. You also use visual observation to collect objective data, such as when you inspect the client's skin for rashes or irritation, and note the cleanliness and level of safety of the client's immediate environment.

Tactile Observation.   The sense of touch provides valuable information about the client. For example, touch or *palpation* of the skin assesses factors such as muscle strength, temperature, moisture, edema, rash, or swelling.

Auditory Observation.   Hearing allows you to listen actively to the client and family as they interact with you and other members of the healthcare team. You may also use specialized equipment to listen for information. For example, data collected by auscultation (listening to the heart, lung, or bowel sounds with a stethoscope) depend on your sense of hearing and level of skill in interpreting such sounds. Similarly, you must be able to hear the sounds of the pulse when measuring blood pressure with a sphygmomanometer and stethoscope.

Olfactory or Gustatory Observation.   The sense of smell identifies odors that can be specific to a client's condition or state of health. In turn, the sense of smell can stimulate specific taste sensations. For example, olfactory observation includes noting body and breath odors (which might indicate alcohol intoxication, poor hygiene, or metabolic acidosis). The senses of smell and taste may also help you to detect harmful chemicals in the air.

The Health Interview

The **health interview** is a way of soliciting information from the client. This interview may also be called a **nursing history.** If the interview is conducted when a client is admitted to a healthcare facility, it may be called an *admission interview.* When a physician obtains this information, it is called a *medical history.* In some areas, registered nurses (RNs) take the nursing history, with a nursing student or practical nurse assisting. In other areas, the practical nurse may perform the nursing history. The RN assesses the data and works with the team to formulate a nursing diagnosis and plan of care.

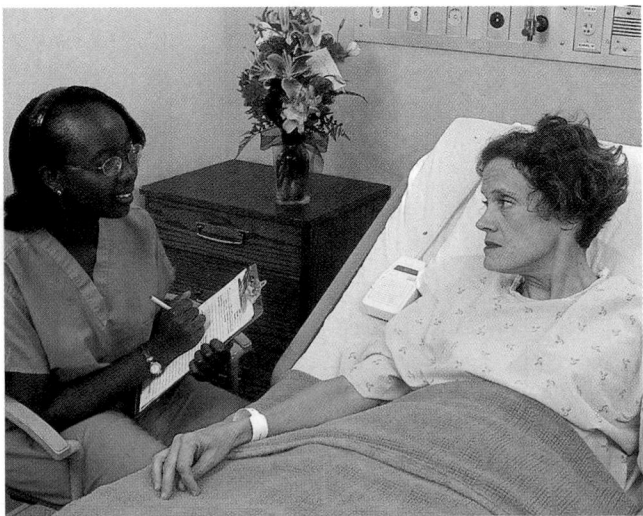

FIGURE 34-2. Effective communication is a key component in obtaining subjective data about the client. The nurse must take into consideration the client's body language, including posture, gestures, and eye contact, as well as what the client says.

Each facility has its own history form for you to complete in partnership with the client. Forms may target the specific needs of the client (eg, if the client wants to lose weight). You may guide the conversation with direct questions, or the client may direct the dialogue by discussing health problems, symptoms, or feelings about the problem (see Chap. 44).

To be most effective and efficient, plan for the interview before meeting the client. Tell the client that the purpose of the interview is to enable the nursing staff to plan effective care. Box 34-1 lists sample questions to ask during an initial interview. Remember that clients have the right to refuse to answer questions that they believe are too personal. In some cases, you may need to talk with family members because some clients are too ill or confused to respond, or too young to speak for themselves. Even when the client can respond, family members may give you additional information. Keep in mind that you must protect the confidentiality of the client, never revealing any information previously unknown to the family without the client's permission.

Components of the Nursing History.   A complete health history helps you develop an effective plan of care for the client. Usually, the following information is essential:

➤➤ BOX 34-1

SAMPLE QUESTIONS TO ASK AT THE INITIAL CLIENT INTERVIEW

Use the following questions as a guide when interviewing the client. Tailor the pace of the interview to what the client can handle; if the client is exhausted or in pain, you may wish to separate the interview into several shorter sessions. Be sure to check to see if the client and family speak English. If not, you may need to seek the help of an interpreter. If family members are providing the answers to any questions, indicate so in your notes (for additional information, see Chap. 45).

By what means did you come to the healthcare facility? Who, if anyone, was with you? Did you come from another facility: hospital? nursing home? another area?

Do you have a living will or other healthcare advance directive? If not, do you need help in preparing one?

Are you under the care of any other physician? If so, what is the physician's name? For what condition are you being treated?

Do you use any types of complementary therapy (for example, chiropractic, homeopathy, acupuncture, therapeutic massage, vibrational therapy, essential oil therapy, meditation, imagery)?

Have you been hospitalized? For what? How long ago? Where? Have you had surgery? For what? How long ago? Have you ever had a broken bone? When? Which bone? What happened?

Are you on a special diet at home? If so, what is the diet and why was it ordered? When did you last eat? Have you had a recent sudden or unexplained weight gain or loss? Do you have any definite food dislikes? Does your religion prohibit you from eating certain foods? If so, what are they?

Do you have any trouble chewing or swallowing? Are your teeth in good condition? Do you wear dentures? If so, do they fit comfortably?

Do you have any allergies to foods? To medications? To other substances? If so, what are they?

Are you taking any prescription medications? Who prescribed the medication(s) you are taking? For what reason? What dosage? For how long have you been taking it (them)? Have you been taking them as ordered? Do you have them with you?

Which nonprescription medications, if any, do you regularly use? Home remedies? Herbal supplements? What do you take for pain? Headaches? Menstrual cramps? Upset stomach? Heartburn? Diarrhea? Constipation? Earache? A cold? To lose weight?

Are you taking an iron preparation? Calcium? Vitamins? Eye drops? Nose drops? Birth control pills? If so, what kind?

What immunizations (vaccines) have you had and when did you receive them?

Do you have difficulty sleeping? If so, what remedy do you take?

Do you smoke? How many packs/day? Use smokeless tobacco? Do you drink alcoholic beverages, coffee, or cola drinks? If so, how often? Do you use marijuana, cocaine, and recreational drugs? Have you had chemical dependency treatment? Did you ever have any serious problems (such as seizures) during withdrawal? When did you last drink or use the substance? What is your longest period of sobriety?

Do you drive regularly? Work around dangerous machinery?

Have you had blood transfusions? When?

Are you regularly exposed to strong solvents or pesticides? Other chemicals? Radiation? Communicable diseases?

Do you have a history of diabetes? If so, do you take any medication (insulin or oral medications) to manage it?

Do you have a history of heart trouble? Unexplained bleeding? High blood pressure? Asthma? Emphysema? Tuberculosis? Urinary problems? Cancer? Mental or emotional disorders? Rheumatic fever? Other diseases? If so, what do you use to manage the condition? What about other members of your family?

Have you ever had a seizure? What were the circumstances? Are you taking anticonvulsive medications?

Do you have any speech problems?

Do you have any cold symptoms? Fever?

(continued)

➤➤ BOX 34-1

SAMPLE QUESTIONS TO ASK AT THE INITIAL CLIENT INTERVIEW (CONTINUED)

Do you have any problems walking by yourself, or do you need assistance?

Do you have a prosthesis (an artificial eye or limb, for example)? If so, please state what it is. Do you have it with you? (This also applies to crutches, canes, walkers, and braces.)

Do you wear glasses? Contact lenses? If so, do you have them with you? Do you have removable partial plates or bridgework, or a retainer? If so, do you have it (them) with you? Do you have a hearing aid? Is it with you? How is your corrected vision or hearing?

Are you sexually active? Do you use condoms? Have you ever had a sexually transmitted disease? Have you ever been tested for human immunodeficiency virus (HIV)? Would you like to be tested? Do you have any sexual concerns?

When was your last bowel movement? Do you have difficulty with bowel movements? Do you regularly take laxatives? Enemas? Do you have any difficulty in voiding (urinating)?

Have you ever passed blood in your stool or urine? Have you ever coughed or vomited blood? Do you have frequent nosebleeds?

Do you have a family? Will they be visiting you here? Do you wish to restrict visitors or phone calls? Whom should we call in case of emergency? Phone number (day and evening)?

Do you have any valuables with you? If so, describe them. Do you plan to lock them in a safe or send them home with your family? (Do not give the client any other choices; send cell phones and pagers home with the family if possible.) What clothing and toilet articles do you have with you?

Are you able to read and write English? How much education have you had?

Do you wish to see a member of the clergy or a chaplain? Do you need assistance in telephoning?

Do you have a place to live? Do you need to apply for medical assistance? Do you need to see someone from the Social Services Department?

For women: When was your last menstrual period? Do you think you may be pregnant? Are you receiving hormone replacement therapy (HRT)? When was your last mammogram? Pap smear? Do you perform regular breast self examination? How many times have you been pregnant? Were there any problems with the pregnancies? Did you breast-feed?

For men: When was your last prostate/testicular examination? Have you had a prostate-specific antigen (PSA) test done? If so, was it normal? Do you perform regular testicular self examination?

Is there any other way in which I can be helpful to you?

Is there anything else I should know?

Biographical data: Includes name, age, birth date, spouse, support person, children, address, phone number, occupation, financial status, insurance, etc.

Reason for coming to the healthcare facility: Addresses the *primary* reason, also described as the client's chief complaint (**CC**) or perception of the illness. What does the client expect to happen in the healthcare facility?

Recent health history: Includes symptoms of recent disease treated with medications and/or surgery, and exposure to communicable diseases.

Important medical history: Includes family history of disease, allergies, immunizations, medications, and use of alternative/complementary therapies and herbal supplements.

Pertinent psychosocial information: Addresses family relationships, employment, living conditions, emotional stability, sexual relationships, substance use or abuse, medications, etc.

Activities of daily living (ADL): Involves how well the client is able to meet basic needs, such as eating, drinking, bathing, dressing, and toileting. Does the client get adequate exercise, food, rest, and sleep?

The Physical Examination

Chapter 47 discusses how to assist with the physical examination. You also will learn some basic skills of the physical

examination so that you may continually monitor the condition of your clients as you care for them.

☛ KEY CONCEPT

You will use the following methods to collect data:

• *Observation (use of the five senses)*
• *Interview (the nursing history)*
• *Physical examination (general survey and specific examinations)*

DATA ANALYSIS

During and after data collection, you must critically examine each piece of information to determine its relevance to the client's health problems and its relationship to other pieces of information. Through systematic **data analysis,** you can draw conclusions about the client's health problems. During data analysis, you also use critical thinking skills to ponder other questions that might be important, or to develop a visual image of what the client is telling you.

Recognizing Significant Data

The information itself may pose difficulty when interpreting data. You may find that you have too much information or not enough information. When preparing to analyze data, ask yourself which items are pertinent to client care and which are not. By doing so, you are thinking critically. As a nursing student, you must discuss your assessments with your team leader or instructor. Once you have gained experience, you will make more decisions on your own.

Validating Observations

One way to validate observations is to "check them out" with the client. Do your observations agree with what the client is experiencing or are they only your interpretations? Sometimes, thinking of clients as "team leaders" who are directing the members of the healthcare team is helpful. You may also consult with your nursing team leader or colleagues to validate your observations.

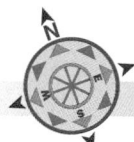 **SPECIAL CONSIDERATIONS:** CULTURE

Observation

When making observations, be sure that you consider cultural and ethnic factors or practices that may influence your findings.

Recognizing Patterns or Clusters

Some data are similar or have a pattern or connection. These data can be grouped together in clusters for further analysis. For example, you will see a relationship among symptoms when a client reports pain and bloating in the abdomen and no bowel movement for 3 days. Recognizing data clusters also helps you determine relevant information.

Identifying Strengths and Problems

While assessing the client, look for strengths the client has that he or she can use in coping with problems. Through careful analysis of data clusters, you may identify actual or potential problems.

Reaching Conclusions

After initiating the preceding steps, you are ready to reach a conclusion. Four conclusions are possible:

1. The client has no problem. No further nursing care is needed; you reinforce the client's current health habits and recommend other health promotion activities.
2. The client may have a problem. You need to gather more information.
3. The client is at risk for a problem. This finding indicates a potential nursing diagnosis. You continue through the nursing process by planning, implementing, and evalu-

ating. The client may deny that a problem exists or may refuse treatment.
4. The client has a clinical problem. The client has a nursing diagnosis or medical diagnosis. The problem is a *nursing diagnosis* if it falls in the domain of nursing and nursing staff may treat it without consulting a physician (see Chapter 35 for further discussion). If the problem requires medical treatment (*medical diagnosis*), you have identified a collaborative problem. When this occurs, you must consult a physician and work together to resolve the problem.

☛ KEY CONCEPT

Nursing assessment is the systematic and continuous collection of data about a client. It includes the following steps:

- *Identifying assessment priorities related to the purpose of the interview*
- *Collecting data about the client from observation, interview, and physical examination*
- *Continuously updating the database of information*
- *Recognizing significant data*
- *Validating observations*
- *Recognizing patterns or clusters*
- *Identifying strengths and problems*
- *Analyzing data to reach conclusions*

➤ STUDENT SYNTHESIS

Key Points

- Nursing assessment is the systematic and continuous gathering and analysis of data about the client.
- Assessment includes observation (the senses), the interview, and the physical examination.
- Data collected include objective data (factual, measurable; what you can directly observe) and subjective (what the client tells you; the client's opinions and feelings).
- Data analysis requires recognizing significant data, validating observations, recognizing patterns or clusters, identifying strengths and problems, and reaching conclusions.

Critical Thinking Exercises

1. Your client has just reported to you that he has the following symptoms: ringing in his ears, swelling of his right ankle, difficulty swallowing, pain in his right knee, a tingling sensation in his right toes, a toothache, and numbness in his right calf. Which symptoms might be related? Do you find more than one cluster? What additional information would help you understand his problem(s)?
2. Identify ways that you can target your assessments to meet the specific needs of clients. What particu-

lar methods would you use for a client who comes from a background different than your own? How would you work with a client who presents with various conditions? How would you handle a situation in which a client appeared non-compliant or did not want to participate in care planning?

NCLEX-Style Review Questions

1. Which of the following is an example of objective data?
   a. Client complains of nausea
   b. Client's respirations are 14/minute
   c. Client states feelings of loneliness
   d. Client reports complaints of pain
2. Which of the following is an example of subjective data?
   a. Client complains of chest pain
   b. Chest radiograph appears normal
   c. Surgical incision 6 centimeters in length
   d. Temperature 98.6° Fahrenheit
3. Which of the following is an example of a client's chief complaint?
   a. "I'm in the hospital for hip surgery."
   b. "I need help with going to the bathroom."
   c. "I prefer potatoes to rice."
   d. "I take medication for my heart."

4. A client is admitted to the hospital with complaints of chest pain during exercise. Which of the following questions would be a priority for the nurse to ask?
   a. "Are you sexually active and do you have any sexual concerns?"
   b. "Do you have any difficulties with bowel movements?"
   c. "Do you need to see someone from social services?"
   d. "What, if anything, helps to relieve your chest pain"?
5. After the nurse completes the nursing history and physical examination, which action is most appropriate?
   a. Assessment
   b. Communication with client's family
   c. Data analysis
   d. Evaluation of nursing plan

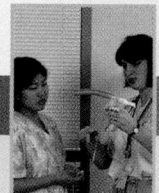

Nursing Diagnosis and Planning

LEARNING OBJECTIVES

1. Define New Terminology terms.
2. Differentiate between nursing diagnosis and medical diagnosis.
3. State the purposes of nursing diagnosis.
4. Explain the components of the nursing diagnostic statement.
5. List the steps in planning client care, and describe how nurses carry out these steps.
6. Describe the purpose and format of the nursing care plan.

NEW TERMINOLOGY

collaborative problem
expected outcome
Kardex
long-term objective
medical diagnosis

nursing diagnosis
planning
prognosis
short-term objective

ACRONYMS

AEB   NANDA   R/T

The first step of the nursing process is data collection, or the *nursing assessment*. Standing alone, the data gathered are useless until you determine what they mean. The second step of the nursing process is identifying the nursing care problem—otherwise called the *nursing diagnosis*—based on your analysis of the data. Only then can you move on to the third step of the nursing process, which is *planning* client care based on the problems or diagnoses you have identified.

NURSING DIAGNOSIS

A **nursing diagnosis** is a statement about the actual or potential health concerns of the client that can be managed through independent nursing interventions (Fig. 35-1). Nursing diagnoses are concise, clear, client-centered, and client-specific statements.

In some areas, practical nurses do not make nursing diagnoses. Keep in mind that a nursing diagnosis identifies the client's care problems. Whether or not you make a nursing diagnosis yourself, you must understand the meaning of a nursing diagnosis and how it is used to plan and to implement nursing care.

Nursing Diagnosis Versus Medical Diagnosis

Nursing diagnosis is not to be confused with medical diagnosis. You are probably more familiar with medical diagnoses. Remember these facts about a **medical diagnosis:**

- It identifies the disease a person has or is believed to have.
- Physicians arrive at a medical diagnosis by studying the physiologic manifestations of the illness and establishing its cause and nature.

- A medical diagnosis provides a basis for **prognosis** (projected client outcome) and medical treatment decisions.

Medicine clearly emphasizes the disease process. Hypertension, pneumonia, diabetes mellitus, and renal failure are examples of medical diagnoses. Nursing, however, focuses on the person: the individual's response to his or her health. Nursing asks how a disease or illness influences an individual's functioning and how his or her needs can be met.

Recall the woman described in the nursing care plan in Chapter 33. Her medical diagnosis is pneumonia. When you look at the data that have been obtained about the client, you are concerned about how she is functioning and what you can do to help her to improve or to adapt. From the assessment data, you determine that the client has abnormal breath sounds, a cough with thick yellow sputum, increased respirations, difficulty breathing, fever, and fatigue. After analyzing the data, problems involving the client's airway (respiratory tract) and activity emerge as the priorities.

Purposes of the Nursing Diagnosis

The nursing diagnosis serves the following purposes:

- Identifies nursing priorities
- Directs nursing interventions to meet the client's high-priority needs
- Provides a common language and forms a basis for communication and understanding between nursing professionals and the healthcare team
- Guides the formulation of expected outcomes for quality assurance requirements of third-party payers

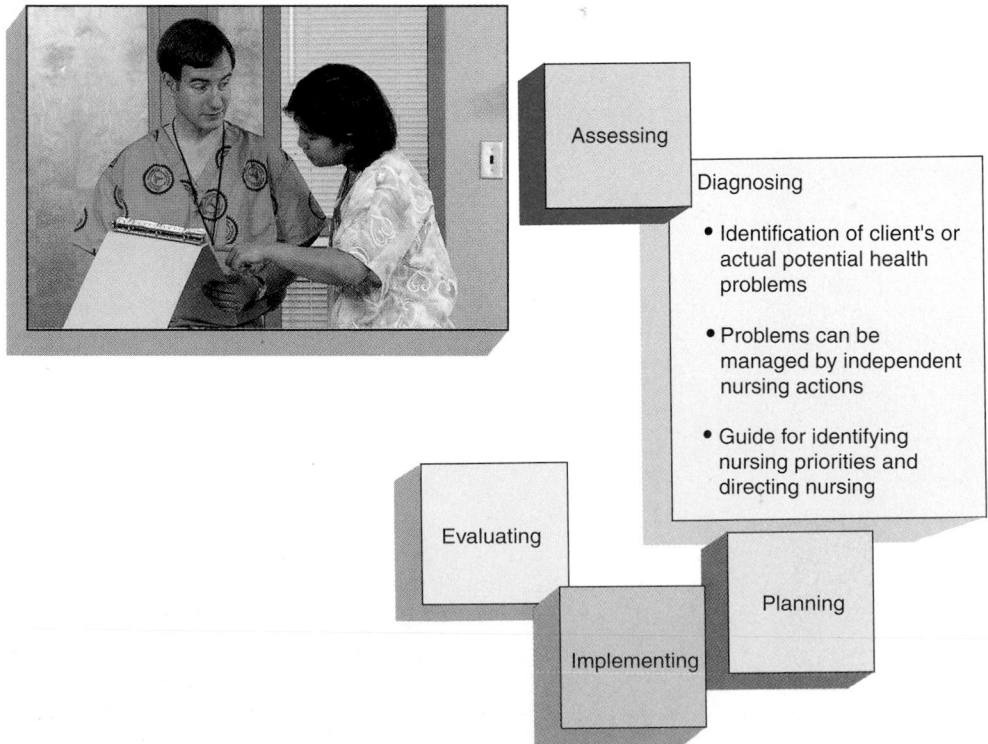

Assessing

Diagnosing

- Identification of client's or actual potential health problems

- Problems can be managed by independent nursing actions

- Guide for identifying nursing priorities and directing nursing

Evaluating

Implementing

Planning

FIGURE 35-1. In the second step of the nursing process, nursing diagnoses are developed based on analysis of the data collected during nursing assessment.

- Provides a basis of evaluation to determine if nursing care was beneficial to the client and cost effective
- Is of help when making staff assignments

NANDA-Approved Nursing Diagnoses

Since 1973, a group of nurse researchers and educators belonging to the North American Nursing Diagnosis Association (**NANDA**) has maintained a list of acceptable nursing diagnoses. These words or terms are actually the diagnostic labels or categories on which the entire client-oriented nursing diagnosis statement is built. Most healthcare facilities have the current NANDA list posted in a central location or in the medical information system for all nurses to use. (See the inside back cover of this text for the current list of NANDA-approved nursing diagnoses.)

The Diagnostic Statement

The client may present with more than one problem. Therefore, the nursing diagnosis may be made up of multiple *diagnostic statements*. Each diagnostic statement has two or three parts, depending on the healthcare facility. The three-part statement consists of the following components:

- Problem
- Etiology
- Signs and symptoms

A two-part diagnostic statement consists of the problem, and signs and symptoms.

Problem

The *problem* portion of a statement describes—clearly and concisely—a health problem a client is having. Use one of the NANDA-approved nursing diagnostic labels to state the problem.

Recall the example from the Nursing Care Plan in Chapter 33 for the woman admitted with pneumonia. After assessing the client and taking the steps leading up to the diagnostic statement, you determine that one of the client's problems is difficulty breathing because her airway is filled with mucus. Following the NANDA guidelines and stating the problem concisely, you state "Ineffective Airway Clearance." This diagnostic label of a problem is the first part of the diagnostic statement.

Etiology

The *etiology* part of the diagnostic statement is the *cause* of the problem. Etiology may be physiologic, psychological, sociologic, spiritual, or environmental. For the woman with pneumonia, the etiology for the problem "Ineffective Airway Clearance" is "the physiologic effects of pneumonia."

Signs and Symptoms

Data collected during the nursing assessment point to the nursing diagnosis. The third part of the diagnostic statement summarizes these data. You may need to include several *signs and symptoms* (remember the clusters). For instance, the client with pneumonia had cough with thick sputum, abnormal breath sounds, increased respirations (tachypnea), and difficulty breathing (dyspnea). For her, the third part of the statement would be "increased sputum, coughing, abnormal breath sounds, tachypnea, and dyspnea."

☛ KEY CONCEPT

A nursing diagnosis has three components:
P—problem (diagnostic label)
E—etiology (cause)
S—signs and symptoms

Writing the Diagnostic Statement

The diagnostic statement connects problem, etiology, and signs and symptoms. The first two parts of the statement are linked by "related to," sometimes abbreviated **R/T**. The last two parts are linked by "as evidenced by," sometimes abbreviated **AEB.** Therefore, the statement for the client with pneumonia described in the Nursing Care Plan in Chapter 33 would read as follows:

> Ineffective Airway Clearance related to physiologic effects of pneumonia as evidenced by increased sputum, coughing, abnormal breath sounds, tachypnea, and dyspnea.

When formulating a nursing diagnosis, make sure that it is something the nursing staff and the client can treat without orders from the physician. Such actions are called *independent nursing actions*. If treatment requires something you cannot do, such as prescribe medication for the cough, the problem is a collaborative problem. A **collaborative problem** means that you will work together with the physician or other healthcare providers. For instance, the physician will prescribe the medication, but the nurse will decide whether or not to administer a PRN (as needed) medication at bedtime.

☛ KEY CONCEPT

The nursing diagnosis is a statement about the client's actual or potential health concerns that can be managed through independent nursing interventions. It contains the following steps:

- *Establishing significant data*
- *Writing a two- or three-part diagnostic statement*

PLANNING CARE

After identifying the nursing diagnoses, you begin planning nursing care. **Planning** is the development of goals to prevent, reduce, or eliminate problems and to identify nursing interventions that will assist clients in meeting these goals. Setting priorities, establishing expected outcomes, and selecting nursing interventions result in a plan of nursing care (Fig. 35-2).

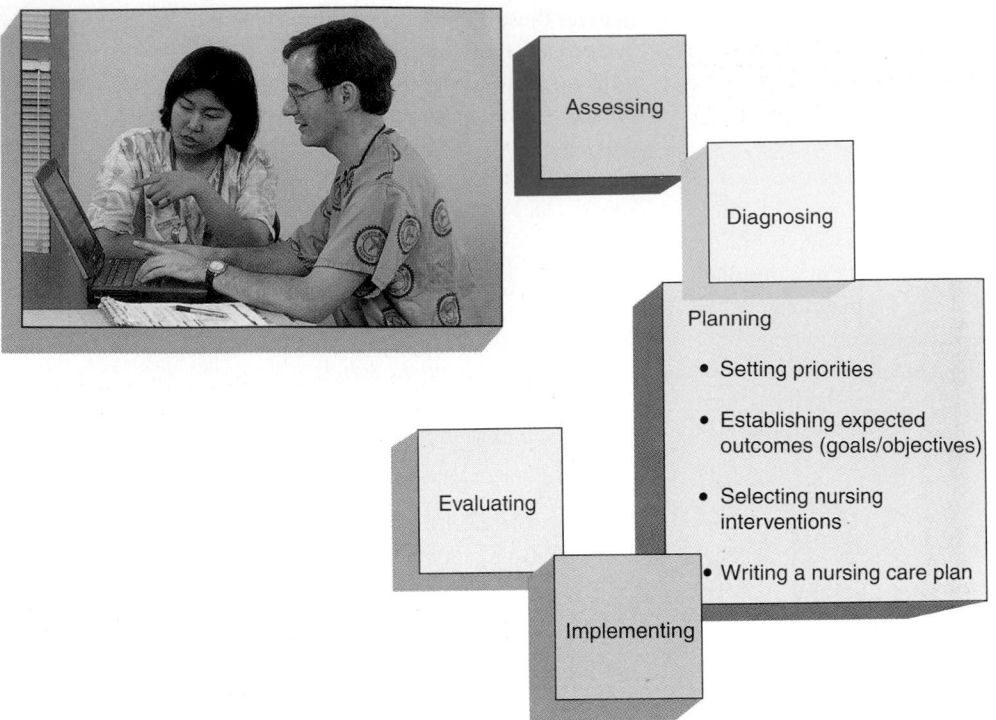

FIGURE 35-2. During planning, the third step of the nursing process, goals are established and interventions are identified to assist the client in meeting the goals.

Setting Priorities

Because some diagnoses have a higher priority than others, they are more important. Nursing diagnoses are ranked in order of importance. Survival needs or imminent life-threatening problems take the highest priority (see Maslow's Hierarchy of Human Needs in Chapter 5). For example, the needs for air, water, and food are survival needs. Nursing diagnostic categories that reflect these high-priority needs include Ineffective Airway Clearance and Deficient Fluid Volume. Safety needs are the next priority, with nursing diagnostic categories such as Risk for Injury or Risk for Suffocation. At a lower level of priority are the social and psychological needs for love, self-esteem, companionship, and fulfillment; some possible nursing diagnostic categories are Ineffective Role Performance, Anxiety, and Social Isolation.

The reason for the client's admission to your facility is the most important concern. The client may have a number of nursing diagnoses that are unrelated to the primary care problem. Attempts to treat them may be unsuccessful because the client has more urgent, immediate needs. These other problems can be deferred until a later time.

In addition, materials and human resources availability, as well as time limitations, affect the order of priority. (Equipment, supplies, and staff must be available.) Keep in mind that you cannot treat every nursing diagnosis that a client may have.

The client also determines the priority of health concerns. For example, a smoker may be fully aware of the health risks of smoking but may choose to continue. In this case, plans to help the client quit smoking will fail, even though the need for oxygen is a requirement for survival, and thus, is a high priority.

Establishing Expected Outcomes

You are familiar with learning objectives or behavioral objectives in your nursing program. A similar type of objective or outcome is established for the client. An **expected outcome** is a measurable client behavior that indicates whether the person has achieved the expected benefit of nursing care. It may also be called a *goal* or *objective.* An expected outcome has the following characteristics:

Client-oriented: The client, not the nurse, is expected to meet this outcome. For instance, "the client will walk around the room at least once per shift."

Specific: Everyone, including the client, knows what is to occur. For instance, "the client will walk up and down the hall for 5 minutes."

Reasonable: The outcome should be within the client's capacity and abilities, considering the confines of his or her condition. For example, if the client is having trouble breathing, walking may be limited to trips to the bathroom.

Measurable: The behavior can be observed and measured. For example, nursing staff can observe a client walking, or the client can state that he or she walked for 5 minutes.

Working together, you and the client should determine outcomes. Box 35-1 gives examples of some verbs commonly used in expected outcome statements.

BOX 35-1

EXAMPLES OF VERBS USED IN EXPECTED OUTCOME STATEMENTS

cough	perform
demonstrate	relate
describe	share
discuss	sit
express	stand
has a decrease in	state
has an absence of	use
has an increase in	verbalize
identify	walk
list	

Expect clients to achieve outcomes in varying lengths of time. A **short-term objective** is an expected outcome or goal that a client can reasonably meet in a matter of hours or a few days. (for example, "The client will walk for 20 minutes longer each day for the first three postoperative days"). A **long-term objective** is an outcome that the client ultimately hopes to achieve, but which requires a longer period of time to accomplish. Sometimes, the longer period means that the client will not still be in the healthcare facility when the objective is achieved. You can help the client put this objective in writing. Then, while working toward self-care, the client can probably identify the desired long-term goal or objective. He or she can learn how to measure the progress toward achieving the objective. For example, the client's long-term goal may be "to return to college" after self-care is achieved.

☞ KEY CONCEPT

Expected outcomes are client oriented, specific, reasonable, and measurable.

Selecting Nursing Interventions

Nursing interventions, also called *nursing orders* or *nursing actions,* are activities that will most likely produce the desired outcomes (short-term or long-term). Sometimes, the client and nursing staff set specific target dates for achieving certain goals, checking them off as they are completed. Nursing orders may include such things as further assessment, client teaching, or referral.

Generally, specific nursing interventions are selected because scientific research has demonstrated that these actions are effective. That is, the interventions are based on the scientific rationale or reason for using them.

Consider again the client with the medical diagnosis of pneumonia described in the Nursing Care Plan in Chapter 33. Follow her nursing care through the next steps of the nursing process. Her nursing diagnosis was "Ineffective Airway Clearance related to the physiologic effects of pneumonia as evi-

denced by increased sputum, cough, abnormal breath sounds, tachypnea, and dyspnea." You want to help the client to experience less difficulty breathing. An expected outcome could be "Within 24 hours, the client will state that breathing is easier." To achieve this outcome, you would select nursing interventions such as the following examples:

- Offering fluids frequently
- Positioning the woman with the head of the bed elevated for optimum breathing
- Teaching the woman deep-breathing exercises
- Monitoring vital signs frequently
- Encouraging correct use of the incentive spirometer
- Administering oxygen as ordered by the physician
- Ensuring that Respiratory Therapy is administering nebulizer treatments as ordered

Writing a Nursing Care Plan

The nursing care plan is the formal guideline for directing the nursing staff to provide client care. The entire nursing team usually formulates the nursing care plan at a meeting called a *nursing care conference* or *team conference* (Fig. 35-3). One or two nurses may create the care plan. Ideally, plans for client care are written to provide instructions and guidelines for the total healthcare team to use for direction and communication.

The nursing care plan usually includes nursing diagnoses or client problems (according to priorities), expected outcomes (short- and long-term objectives or goals), and nursing orders (activities nurses carry out to help the client achieve goals). Nurses develop the care plan shortly after a client is admitted to the facility. However, the plan is an ever-changing guide, which is updated regularly as the client's condition changes. Consequently, some parts of the recorded care plan may be written in pencil. Because each healthcare facility develops its own format according to the particular health needs of its clients, the content and the structure of the written nursing care

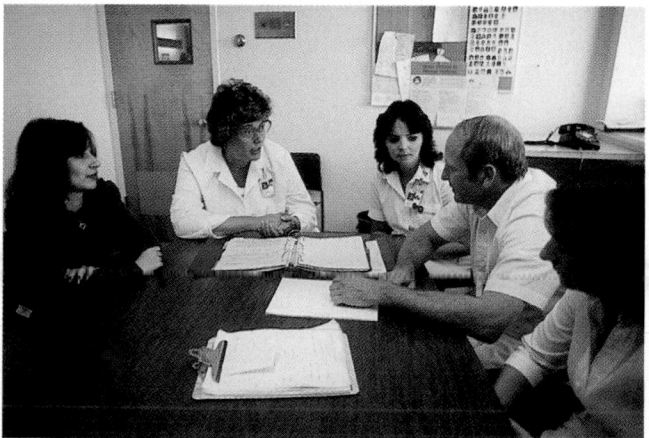

FIGURE 35-3. The nursing team often holds a nursing care conference to develop a Nursing Care Plan for a client with complex healthcare needs.

plan vary. Be sure to familiarize yourself with the format used in your facility.

The written care plan is kept in several ways. Sometimes plans are written on a Kardex for each client. The **Kardex** is a flip-file with card slots, or a notebook, for each client being treated by a unit or nursing care team. The Kardex contains records of background information and care related to the client's medical treatment. You may access your clients' care plans and other information simply by flipping through the cards or the notebook. Healthcare facilities that have computerized medical information systems often keep the nursing care plan as part of a client's computerized health record. Changes to the care plan are entered along with other pertinent client data. For convenience, you may either scroll the computer monitor for the care plan or print out an individualized care plan *each time* you care for the client.

Regardless of the manner in which the care plan is kept, it becomes part of the client's permanent health record. Documentation of a nursing care plan is a requirement of agencies such as the Joint Commission on Accreditation of Healthcare Organizations (JCAHO), nursing home regulators, and Medicare. Personnel from such organizations review health records during site visits to the facility. If a nursing care plan does not exist within 12 to 24 hours of the client's admission, the health care facility will be cited for noncompliance. Penalties can be severe.

The ideal nursing care plan is individualized for each client. Many facilities, however, use a standardized nursing care plan incorporating the usual and expected outcomes for a particular type of nursing care problem or nursing diagnosis. These standardized care plans allow for additions or substitutions so that the care plan can be individualized to the specific client. The standardized care plan is efficient, and a welcome aid when you must work with many clients.

☛ KEY CONCEPT

Planning is the development of goals to prevent, reduce, or eliminate problems and to identify nursing interventions that will assist clients in meeting these goals. Remember the following steps involved in planning:

- *Setting priorities*
- *Establishing expected outcomes*
- *Selecting nursing interventions*
- *Writing a nursing care plan*

✑ STUDENT SYNTHESIS

Key Points

- Nursing diagnosis is a statement about the client's actual or potential health concerns that can be managed through independent nursing interventions.

- Medical diagnosis is concerned with the disease process. Nursing diagnosis is concerned with the person and how the disease affects his or her functioning.
- Nursing diagnosis helps identify nursing priorities and goals to maintain quality and continuity of care.
- Nursing diagnosis is stated in terms of a problem (a statement approved by NANDA), its etiology, and signs and symptoms.
- After establishing the nursing diagnosis, planning nursing care begins. Priorities, expected outcomes, and nursing interventions are selected; a nursing care plan is written.

Critical Thinking Exercises

1. Compare a written nursing care plan for a client in a long-term care facility (eg, nursing home) with that of a client in an acute care facility (eg, hospital). What are the similarities and differences? Because all people have similar needs, why do you think these differences exist?
2. Practice making a nursing diagnosis. From the following data, write a three-part nursing diagnostic statement: A male client, age 69, complains that he has difficulty swallowing because of a severe sore throat. He complains of having a dry tongue and feeling thirsty and lightheaded. He has not urinated in 5 hours and does not feel the urge to urinate now.

NCLEX-Style Review Questions

1. In this nursing diagnosis, "Hyperthermia related to exposure to hot environment as evidenced by temperature 101° Fahrenheit, skin flushed and warm to touch," which part represents the problem?
   a. Exposure to hot environment
   b. Hyperthermia
   c. Skin flushed and warm to touch
   d. Temperature 101° Fahrenheit
2. In this nursing diagnosis, "Chronic pain related to chronic physical disability as evidenced by patient's statement of pain as usually a 6 out of 10 on the pain scale, restlessness, facial grimacing with movement," which part represents the etiology?
   a. Chronic pain
   b. Chronic physical disability
   c. Facial grimacing with movement
   d. Restlessness
3. Which of the following is a correctly written goal?
   a. Client will demonstrate sterile dressing technique by tomorrow (date).
   b. Client will increase ambulation, with assistance.
   c. Client will feel better by end of week.
   d. Client will discuss feelings about illness.

4. Which of the following nursing diagnostic categories has the highest priority?
   a. Ineffective role performance
   b. Anxiety
   c. Functional urinary incontinence
   ✓ d. Ineffective airway clearance

5. When writing nursing care plans, the nurse should develop a plan for the client that is:
   a. Cost effective
   b. Complex
   ✓ c. Individualized
   d. Reasonable

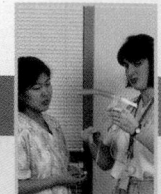

36

Implementing and Evaluating Care

LEARNING OBJECTIVES

1. Define New Terminology terms.
2. List the three action phrases identified with nursing interventions (implementation).
3. Compare and contrast intellectual, interpersonal, and technical skills and describe how they apply to nursing.
4. List the three steps in evaluating nursing care and describe how they might be accomplished.
5. Describe at least three means used for evaluating client care.
6. Define quality assurance.
7. Briefly describe discharge planning.

NEW TERMINOLOGY

accountability
case management
case manager
dependent actions
discharge planning
evaluation
implementation

independent actions
intellectual skills
interdependent actions
interpersonal skills
technical skills
variance

ACRONYMS

CCP   DRG   QA

After collecting data, identifying nursing diagnoses, developing goals, and writing a nursing care plan, your next step is to carry out the plan. This step of the nursing process is called **implementation**, or implementing the plan. Implementation is also called *providing nursing interventions* (Fig. 36-1).

IMPLEMENTING NURSING CARE

"Do it," "share it," and "write it down" are the action phrases of implementation. You "do" nursing care with and for the client. You "share" the results by communicating with the client and other members of the healthcare team, individually or in a planning conference. You "write" information by documenting it so that the next healthcare provider can act with purpose and understanding. Always remember that adequate communication and documentation facilitate the continuity of care (Fig. 36-2).

Nursing Implementation—"Do It"

When implementing care, you perform nursing actions that may be dependent, interdependent, or independent. Actions that carry out a physician's orders regarding medication or treatments are **dependent actions** that you must follow explicitly. Because of regulatory requirements, you may not administer medications or perform certain treatments without physician's orders. **Interdependent actions** are those that you perform collaboratively with other care providers; the physician may write orders for some of these actions. These actions are interventions for collaborative problems. For example, the physician may write an order to give an enema to a client when necessary. You use your nursing judgment to determine when the client needs an enema, although you cannot administer the enema without the physician's order. Together,

you have collaborated to provide client care. **Independent actions** are nursing actions that do not require a physician's orders. Only you—the nursing staff—perform independent nursing actions, which are based on your judgment. Independent actions are those actions that you take to assist the client with activities of daily living (eg, bathing, toileting) or to help reduce stress (eg, backrub).

To understand the different types of nursing actions, consider the example of the woman with pneumonia described in the Nursing Care Plan in Chapter 33. The physician writes an order for supplemental oxygen at a specified flow rate. Administering oxygen, which is considered a medication, is a *dependent action*. So too is administering the client's IV fluid and antibiotic therapy. The physician also writes an order for an antipyretic PRN. Administering the medication is a *dependent action*. You may choose, however, to give the antipyretic medication based on the client's temperature, for example, when the client's temperature is greater than 100.4° Fahrenheit (38.0° Celsius). This action is *interdependent*: you are following the physician's orders, but you are making a decision based on your judgment about timing and effective treatment. Additionally, you may decide, *independently*, to apply cool compresses to aid in reducing the client's fever. Independent actions may be written as nursing orders such as "assist with out of bed to chair at least once daily," "encourage frequent sips of fluid," "assist client to assume semi-Fowler's to high Fowler's position and reposition frequently," "monitor vital signs and respiratory status every 1 to 2 hours." Ask your instructor or team leader if you are unsure about any nursing actions.

You are responsible for all actions you perform, whether they are dependent, interdependent, or independent. This responsibility is also called **accountability,** an important aspect of the legal requirements of nursing practice. Using critical

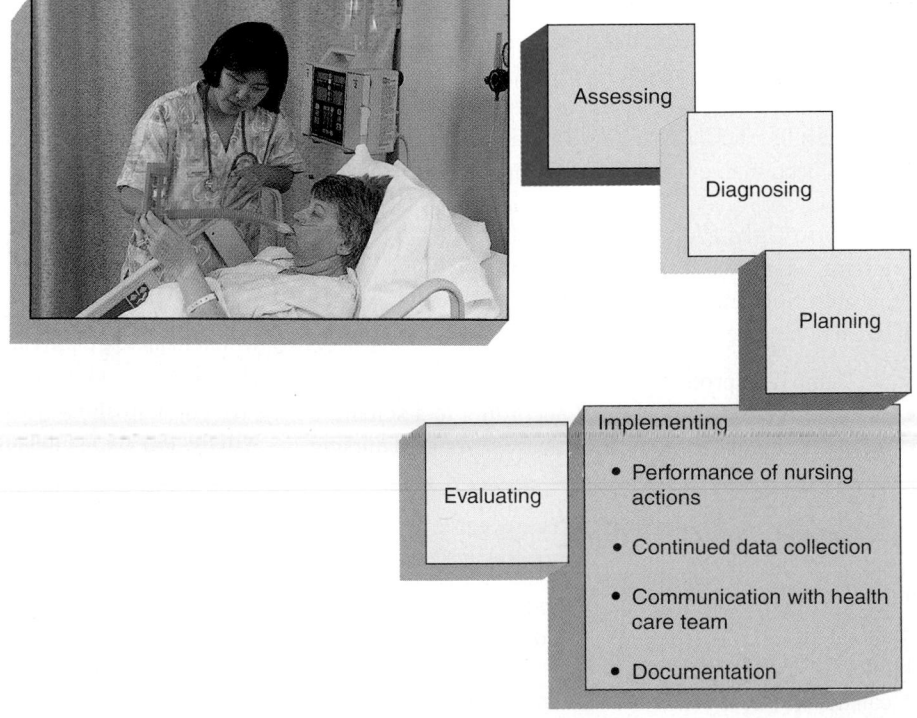

Assessing

Diagnosing

Planning

Implementing
- Performance of nursing actions
- Continued data collection
- Communication with health care team
- Documentation

Evaluating

FIGURE 36-1. During implementation, the fourth step of the nursing process, you put the client's plan of care into action.

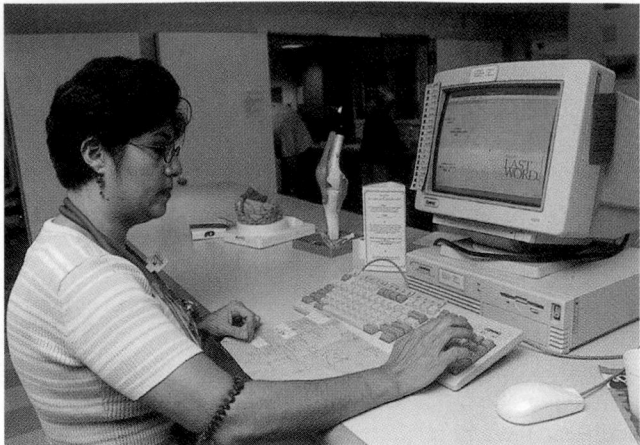

FIGURE 36-2. The nurse may use the computer to document care, print out a nursing care plan, or retrieve data (such as laboratory or x-ray) about the client. The physician may also input orders for a client to be carried out by the nurses. Nursing students and graduates will also find a wealth of healthcare information on the Internet.

thinking skills will greatly assist you to make the safest and most helpful choices for each of your clients.

Skills Used in Implementing Nursing Care

Certain skills influence the implementation of the nursing care plan. These skills include your ability to perform intellectual, interpersonal, and technical skills. **Intellectual skills** involve knowing and understanding essential information (eg, basic sciences, nursing procedures and their underlying rationale) before caring for clients. Critical thinking is one type of intellectual skill essential for making quick decisions and taking swift action. **Interpersonal skills** involve believing, behaving, and relating to others. Solid communication techniques, and client encounters that promote the development of a trusting relationship (rapport), are interpersonal skills (see Chapter 44 for more information about therapeutic communication). Behaving professionally also involves interpersonal skills. **Technical skills,** such as changing a sterile dressing or administering an injection, require safe and competent performance.

The Nursing Care Plan in Action

The nursing team determines if the plan, as written, makes sense. Using critical thinking, ask yourself the following questions when reviewing a care plan:

- Does this plan protect the client's safety?
- Has the plan been developed according to a scientific problem-solving approach? Is it based on sound nursing knowledge?
- Do the nursing orders logically achieve the desired results? Are the orders arranged in an appropriate sequence?
- Do the nursing orders enhance and facilitate the client's care and progress to recovery and goal achievement?
- Did the client have active involvement in this plan and can the client give some ideas about whether it is appro-

priate? (Many facilities encourage the client to read and to sign the nursing care plan after it is written.)

How you manage your time, the client's time, and your activities are important concepts in determining what you and the client accomplish during the day. Prepare a timetable so the client can see the schedule of activities for a full day. Encourage client participation in planning the timetable. Remember to include both the client and the family in this process.

Continuing Collection of Data.   As you care for clients, observe them carefully. Listen to what clients say; watch what they do; check their vital signs. Use critical thinking continually to determine if the nursing orders are effective in moving the client toward meeting his or her specified goals.

Communication With the Healthcare Team—"Share It"

Periodically, a *client planning conference* is held. If the client is to be discharged from healthcare services, this conference serves as a *discharge planning conference.* Interdisciplinary planning conferences offer an excellent way to coordinate your nursing care and to interact with other health disciplines. If you do not personally attend the conference regarding a client for whom you are providing care, you are responsible for giving both verbal and written information to those attending. By doing so, you help ensure that the plan of care is not only coordinated with those of other healthcare providers, but also is evaluated by them.

You also will document ("write it down") all care given to your client. Chapter 37 presents a detailed discussion about documentation and reporting.

☛ KEY CONCEPT

Nursing implementation means the carrying out of the nursing care plan. It includes the following steps:

- *Putting the nursing care plan into action*
- *Continuing the collection of data*
- *Communicating care with the healthcare team*
- *Documenting care*

COST-EFFECTIVE QUALITY CARE

Managed care and case management are two methods by which healthcare providers are attempting to implement cost-effective care while delivering the highest-quality care possible. These methods are a response to third-party payers who will not pay for healthcare that is inefficient or of poor quality. Your understanding of how these systems work will encourage your participation in controlling costs while providing the best care for your clients.

Managed Care

Managed care is a system of healthcare delivery that coordinates the activities of health professionals to address the health needs of clients while ensuring that costs are controlled (see Chap. 3). Usually the managed care system follows plans that determine the treatments and resources most likely to result in the best outcomes (see "Clinical Care Paths" below). Only approved treatments are compensated. Insurance companies, health maintenance organizations (HMOs), and government health plans (Medicare and Medicaid) use this system. Managed care has the following goals:

- Encouraging healthy lifestyles to keep clients well
- Developing and using clinical care standards with well-defined outcomes
- Prioritizing and using efficient resources and services to contain costs
- Monitoring and measuring client outcomes frequently
- Promoting communication, teaching, and continuity of care with client and family
- Identifying and solving client care problems within the managed care system

Clinical Care Paths

A clinical care path (**CCP**) is a planning method in which optimal sequencing and timing of healthcare interventions are identified. The concept of this type of planning is borrowed from the construction industry, where the sequence and timing of a project are critical to successful completion of the whole project. For example, interior finishing of walls cannot be completed until electrical wiring is in place. In healthcare, the client whose leg was amputated below the knee cannot begin walking without crutches until a leg prosthesis (artificial limb) is fitted. This method of planning identifies a maximum length of time to achieve designated client outcomes, while establishing priorities for care and organizing the many activities to be accomplished in a specified period.

The clinical care path differs from the nursing care plan in several ways. One important difference is that the clinical care path designates specific interventions for all members of the healthcare team, not just the nursing team. The nursing care plan may identify many interventions to achieve outcomes, but may not plan a specific time frame or sequence for interventions, which the clinical care path does. The clinical care path designates alternative specific interventions if the ideal interventions do not work or other variations occur. The nursing care plan does not routinely include these variations.

Clinical care paths are developed by a team of healthcare professionals within the facility to meet the particular needs of their clients. Thus, a variety of formats are used in different facilities. Clinical care paths are also called by several other names including *anticipated recovery plans, case management plans, critical pathways, care maps,* and *client care pathways.* The clinical care path is developed for a specific medical diagnosis, treatment problem, or diagnostic-related group (**DRG**). Within the clinical care path, the usual length of admission is determined and a problem list is developed, with an accompanying sequential timeline for treatments and expected outcomes. Related assessments, activities, interventions, and participation by all health team members are noted. Each client is assessed regularly, according to the timeline.

The clinical care path incorporates the goals and principles of managed care to provide efficient, cost-effective, high-quality care. Your agency may use a clinical care path instead of a nursing care plan. When you use a clinical care path, take note of scheduled treatments and procedures on the timeline. Some procedures must be done each hour or more often (such as frequently taking vital signs). Others are designated to be done each shift (such as intake and output) or each day (such as a bed bath). Check off each item that you perform. Your attention to these details will help ensure that your client receives the best care possible and that your employer receives payment for services.

Variances.   If a client does not achieve an expected outcome by the designated time, a variance from the clinical care path has occurred. A report must be written. The written **variance** explains the expected outcome of the clinical care path against the actual outcome. The variance is important—without documentation of a change in the expected pattern of care, a third-party payor may refuse payment. The three types of variances are:

Provider: something the nurse or physician was unable to do (eg, nurse did not have time; physician did not order)
Client: client refused treatment; client developed complications
System: client admitted at night/weekend when ordered services were unavailable; client cannot be discharged from acute mental health unit because no bed is available at state hospital

Case Management

Case management is another method of providing high-quality care while effectively using healthcare resources and controlling costs. In case management, a **case manager** plans and directs all necessary activities to coordinate the client's care. Case management may be most useful when a client is at high risk and care is more complex and costly. Healthcare facilities that employ nurses as case managers select primary care nurses or nurses who are skilled clinicians.

EVALUATING NURSING CARE

Evaluation is measuring the effectiveness of assessing, diagnosing, planning, and implementing. The client is the focus of the evaluation. Steps in the evaluation of nursing care are *analyzing the client's responses, identifying factors contributing to success or failure,* and *planning for future care* (Fig. 36-3).

You can use several means to evaluate the effectiveness of nursing care:

Client: The primary source of evaluation criteria is the client. The family may also be helpful in determining if care given was effective.
Team conference: A conference is helpful not only to plan nursing care, but also is used to evaluate the effectiveness of care and to design a discharge plan.

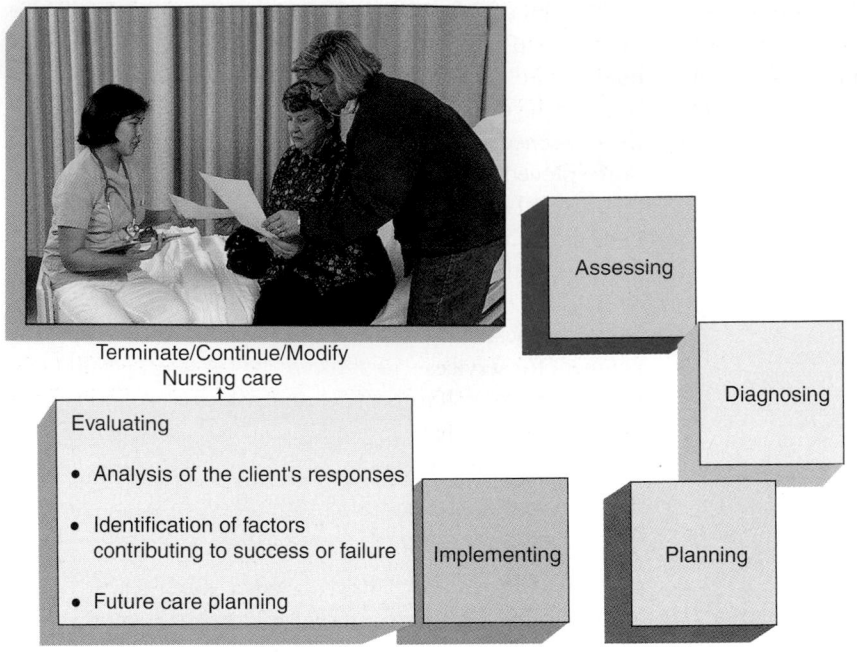

Terminate/Continue/Modify
Nursing care

Evaluating

- Analysis of the client's responses

- Identification of factors
  contributing to success or failure

- Future care planning

Implementing

Planning

Assessing

Diagnosing

FIGURE 36-3. During evaluation, the last step of the nursing process, the nurse and client jointly measure how well the client has achieved the goals that were specified in the plan of care. Any factors that contributed to the client's success or failure are identified and the plan of care is revised as necessary. The client's responses to the plan of care determine whether the plan continues as is, is modified, or is ended.

Community health agencies: Another way of evaluating outcomes of care is to contact healthcare providers in community agencies who are in touch with clients after they leave your facility. Such care providers include public health nurses, school health nurses, social workers, and receptionists and nurses who work in physicians' offices.

Analyzing the Client's Response

The previously established goals and objectives of the nursing care plan become the standards or criteria by which to measure the client's progress. Evaluation of care is based on these criteria. Was each goal met? The evaluation criteria should also consider whether nursing care has helped the client realize self-care goals. For example, for the woman with pneumonia described in the Nursing Care Plan in Chapter 33, resolution of fever, decreased use of accessory muscles, the client's report that her shortness of breath and difficulty breathing were decreasing, changes in the color of sputum, lungs clearing on auscultation, and ability to increase activity level without the use of oxygen provide evidence that the goals identified on the nursing care plan were being met.

Identifying Factors Contributing to Success or Failure

Various factors contribute to the achievement of goals. For example, the client's family may or may not be supportive. The client may be too sick to perform activities. The client may have been uncooperative or may refuse treatments or medications.

Sometimes you, the nurse, may be a factor. For example, you may lack knowledge about how to perform certain actions, or may be thinking about personal problems and therefore perform a procedure incorrectly. *Remember:* You are responsible

for ensuring that your knowledge and skills are always of the highest quality.

Planning Future Nursing Care

The nursing process is dynamic and cyclical. Problems may resolve or change. Resolved problems are noted on the care plan or care path as "resolved." As clients meet their goals, new goals are set. If goals remain unmet, you must consider the reasons why these goals are not being achieved and suggest revisions to the nursing care plan.

For the woman with pneumonia described in Chapter 33, knowledge about the need for followup to prevent a recurrence is a goal. By the time of discharge, both the client and her daughter are able to identify signs and symptoms that would indicate a recurrence. However, if this evidence was lacking, the plan of care would need to be modified to address additional teaching for the client and her daughter.

☛ KEY CONCEPT

Nursing evaluation is the measurement of the effectiveness of assessing, diagnosing, planning, and implementing. Evaluation includes the following steps:

- *Analyzing the client's responses*
- *Identifying factors that contributed to the success or failure of the care plan*
- *Planning for future nursing care*

Quality Assurance

Healthcare evaluation means more than simply measuring individual client outcomes. It also requires careful examination of all aspects of the healthcare organization. A healthcare facility evaluates its overall effectiveness through voluntary surveys from outside accreditation agencies. It also conducts its own performance evaluations to rate the care provided by the facility itself. Together, these evaluative efforts are called quality assurance (**QA**). Chapter 3 describes QA in more detail.

DISCHARGE PLANNING

Discharge planning is the process by which the client is prepared for continued care outside the healthcare facility or for independent living at home. Clients themselves, family, or other healthcare workers may provide continuing care. Planning for discharge begins when a client is admitted to the healthcare system, and is ongoing throughout the client's plan of care. Because clients achieve different levels of care at different times, the discharge plan must be individualized. Some facilities incorporate the discharge plan into the nursing care plan or clinical care path.

➤➤ BOX 36-1

COMPONENTS OF DISCHARGE PLANNING

A discharge plan includes specific components of client teaching, with documentation as to exactly what was taught, who did the teaching and when, who was present (members of the healthcare team, client and/or family), and the client's reaction or expressed level of understanding. Examples of specific components of discharge planning, which must be carefully documented, include the following:

- Equipment needed at home; documentation that the family has obtained it or knows where to get it
- Instruction in the use of any special equipment, including a return demonstration by the client/family caregiver
- Special diet, with documentation by the dietitian as to teaching the client and family and their level of expressed understanding
- Medications to be taken at home; documentation of instructions and special precautions
- Special procedures, such as a dressing change, to be performed at home; instruction must have been given several times and the client allowed to practice under the nurse's supervision.
- Documentation that the family can get needed supplies
- Referral to public health or home care services
- Appointment for next visit to the physician
- Danger signs and when to call the physician
- Instructions regarding activities allowed
- Documentation of verbal teaching and provision of a written instruction sheet for the client
- Describing what was taught

Before the client is ready for discharge from the facility, the healthcare team usually holds a conference with the client (and family, if possible). The purpose of this conference is to identify long-term goals that are still unresolved and to plan for continued assistance to the client.

Working together, the healthcare team and client may set new goals at the discharge conference. The family learns to help the client to meet new—and also former—goals. The primary nurse, or team leader, is responsible for seeing that the client or family has the necessary discharge instructions. All instructions (verbal, and written or printed out) that are given to the client or family must be carefully documented. Discharge plans also include plans for followup. Box 36-1 lists components of discharge planning.

☞ KEY CONCEPT

Discharge teaching begins on admission and continues throughout the client's care. The client and family cannot be expected to remember a large amount of teaching at one time, especially just as the client is leaving the facility.

➤ STUDENT SYNTHESIS

Key Points

- Implementation involves dependent, interdependent, and independent actions.
- Nurses use intellectual, interpersonal, and technical skills to implement care plans.
- During implementation, nurses collect further data and communicate information with other members of the healthcare team.
- Some facilities use a system of managed care to increase cost effectiveness while maintaining quality care.
- During evaluation, client responses are analyzed, factors contributing to the success or failure of the plan are identified, and planning for future care occurs.
- Discharge planning and future planning are based on nursing care plans.

Critical Thinking Exercises

1. Describe various skills a nurse needs to implement care. Give examples of these skills and determine which skills you best perform. Draw up a plan to become more proficient in your weaker skills.
2. Healthcare should be cost effective. Explain how managed care, clinical care paths, and case management help to control costs of healthcare. Give examples.

NCLEX-Style Review Questions

1. Which of the following is an independent nursing action?
   a. Administering medication
   b. Inserting an indwelling urinary catheter
   c. Providing a backrub for a client
   d. Transferring a client to a different unit

2. Which of the following is a dependent nursing action?
   a. Administering a routine medication
   b. Assisting with setting up meal tray
   c. Encouraging a client to attend support group
   d. Placing siderails in up position at night

3. Which type of skill is the nurse using when inserting a nasogastric tube?
   a. Intellectual
   b. Interdependent
   c. Interpersonal
   d. Technical

4. The purpose of a critical care path is to:
   a. Ensure all healthcare members know what nursing care is to be completed
   b. Evaluate nursing activities and client outcomes
   c. Plan for the client's care once the client is discharged
   d. Plan the optimal sequence and timing of healthcare interventions

5. Which of the following is an example that would be used for evaluation of the nursing process?
   a. Client's condition is shared during shift report
   b. Client was too sick to perform activities
   c. Physical assessment is complete.
   d. Wound was irrigated and dressing reapplied

6. Which of the following clients would most likely need a case manager?
   a. Client seen in clinic for the flu
   b. Client with a sprained ankle
   c. Client receiving tube feedings and chemotherapy
   d. Client who has had minor outpatient surgery

CHAPTER

37

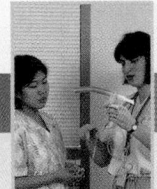

Documenting and Reporting

LEARNING OBJECTIVES

1. State at least three reasons for maintaining a health record.
2. Explain the differences between manual and electronic documentation.
3. List four categories of information included in the health record.
4. Describe various formats for organizing nursing progress notes.
5. State generally accepted guidelines for documentation.
6. Use descriptive terminology for client signs and symptoms when documenting client care.
7. Identify common abbreviations when documenting client care.
8. State the correct way to record a documentation error, and differentiate a documentation error from a client care error.
9. Explain how and when to report to other nursing staff.

NEW TERMINOLOGY

change-of-shift reporting
confidentiality
flow sheet

health record
progress note
walking rounds

ACRONYMS

APIE	MAR	RAP
CBE	MDS	RIE
DAPE	MIS	SOAP
DARE	PIE	SOAPIER

DOCUMENTATION

The *health record* is a manual or electronic (computer) account of a client's relationship with a healthcare facility. Healthcare providers chronologically and systematically record all information regarding the client's health, past and current problems, diagnostic tests, treatments, responses to treatments, and discharge planning through handwritten or keyboard entries. Because you, the nurse, are usually the primary caregiver, the information that you put in the record is very important to inform other caregivers of the client's appearance, behavior, and responses. You must record such information clearly, accurately, and frequently. The commonly used term for documentation is "charting." The client's health record is usually called the "chart."

Purposes of the Health Record

Accurate and complete documentation in the client's health record is essential for *maintaining effective communication among all caregivers,* and for *providing written evidence of accountability* to meet legal, regulatory, and financial requirements. The health record is also used for *research and educational purposes.*

Communication

Because the goal of the healthcare team is to work together to provide the best possible care for the client, the health record is a communication tool that all caregivers use to exchange information with one another. Each caregiver enters information about the client's condition, treatments, responses to treatments, and plans. Instructions for treatment of the client (eg, physician orders, care plans, or care paths) are also included in the health record. Together, these data, notes, and instructions provide a way for healthcare providers to remain in touch about the nature of the client's health problems, possible treatments, treatments given, and client responses.

Think of the health record as a bank where information is deposited, stored, and made available to all who need it. This central resource for information ensures that a client's care is consistent and effective.

Another aspect of communication that is important to the client is the documentation and verification of his or her own health status. A client may require this record of information for specific reasons, such as employment or for a disability application.

Accountability

As you learned in Chapter 36, accountability means responsibility for actions. The health record is *documented evidence* that the healthcare agency and providers have acted responsibly and effectively. Such evidence of accountability is required for legal, regulatory, and financial reasons.

Legal Requirements and Protection.   The healthcare record fulfills a legal requirement mandating all businesses and corporations that provide public services to keep records of their interactions with clients. Thus, the health record is a *legal document.*

The health record is an important piece of evidence when questions of inadequate, incorrect, or poor healthcare arise. If a client, family member, or attorney questions the quality of care given, the well-written and comprehensive health record is the best source of information describing what actually occurred. Accurate, precise, and timely entries into the health record are your protection against accusations of inadequate or poor nursing care.

> ✚👁 **N u r s i n g   A l e r t**
> If your health records are audited or if you go to court, *if it was not documented, it was not done* in the eyes of the law. (This does *not* exempt the nurse who makes an error.)

Regulatory Requirements.   All healthcare agencies must meet certain *standards of care* established by governmental or voluntary regulatory agencies. One standard is record keeping. Another standard is providing safe and effective healthcare and verifying it through quality assurance programs. Complete and accurate healthcare records help agencies prove that they have met both standards.

Financial Accountability.   Just as payment for your groceries requires a receipt listing the items you selected, clients and third-party payers depend on a complete list of services and products provided before paying for healthcare. To facilitate this process, you must record all treatments given, exams administered, and special equipment used (eg, an air mattress). Third-party payers will not reimburse the healthcare facility unless billed-for services and supplies are recorded in the health record. Thus, you must enter every aspect of your care to tell the third-party payer what has been done. Failure to do so may result in a loss of payment to the employing agency, ultimately leading to higher costs for clients and consumers.

Research and Education

Healthcare planners examine health records of individuals and groups to determine patterns of illness, trends, or effective treatment strategies. This research is necessary to select the best treatment for an individual or to search for better treatments for specific health problems. Health records, particularly those kept in computer databases, provide excellent research opportunities in healthcare.

The health record is also an excellent educational tool. Students in healthcare vocations benefit from reading and comparing the data of various clients as they enlarge their knowledge of health, illnesses, treatments, and responses.

Documentation Systems

The **health record** is either a manual (paper) document or an electronic document. Electronic documents are located in a *medical information system* (**MIS**), which is housed in a computer network. Sometimes the health record is a combination of the paper document and the electronic system when a hard copy (printout) of data from the MIS is attached to the manual record. As MISs become more user friendly and cost effective, healthcare facilities are converting from manual to electronic formats because of the advantages of simplified and rapid data management (see Fig. 36-2).

Manual Records

The *manual health record* is a collection of various forms and documents. It tells the story of the client's relationship with the healthcare facility. A notebook or binder kept in a central location (such as the nurses' station or main administrative offices) in the healthcare facility secures these papers. You may keep some of the forms in a client's record at his or her bedside for your convenience—for example, a fluid intake and output sheet or a Daily Nursing Assessment flow sheet.

The manual health record documents assessment data, care plans, medications and treatments, vital signs, treatment outcomes, and the client's daily progress. Care providers enter information by hand in ink at frequent intervals. Table 37-1 lists the purposes of the various forms included in the manual health record.

Electronic Records

The *electronic health record* uses an MIS for storing, processing, and transmitting client data, treatment strategies, and outcomes over a computer network. This network is a series of terminals attached to a central computer that handles the actual storing and processing of information. Usually a terminal consisting of a monitor and keyboard is located in every nursing care unit and in other offices throughout the healthcare facility. Other systems may use laptop computers in the clients' rooms or a hand-held input device that can be carried in a uniform pocket.

For many years, healthcare facilities have used an MIS for diet, laboratory, and pharmacy orders, billing, and statistical data collection. Recent systems also contain mechanisms for recording assessment data, care plans, and nursing information about clients' conditions and responses. You enter information through a keyboard, a light pen, a mouse, or by touching the screen with your finger. Information from a machine to check blood glucose levels may be added to the system via telephone transmission.

All the information included in the MIS is similar to that found in the manual record. Entering and retrieving information, however, is different. Once you have learned to use the computer system, you will understand the advantage of speed and convenience in both the entry and retrieval of information.

Usually the MIS is designed for a healthcare agency's specific needs. Although requirements for documentation are the same for all healthcare facilities, each agency's system is unique. If the healthcare facility where you work uses an MIS, you will need to take orientation classes to learn how to use the system correctly.

Contents of the Health Record

The health record contains four general *categories of information*: assessment documents, plans for care and treatment, progress records, and plans for continuity of care.

Assessment Documents

Assessment documents record all information about the client obtained through interview, examination, diagnostic procedures, or consultation. These documents include the physician's history and physical examination, the nursing admission history, and other records that list or describe related aspects of information about the client. All caregivers contribute to this bank of information. (For specific forms, purposes, and responsible caregivers, see Table 37-1.) The actual formats of the various records and forms vary among agencies. You will acquaint yourself with these forms as part of your orientation with any healthcare employer.

Long-term care and some home care agencies use a standard form called a *minimum data set* (**MDS**) as part of the admitting nursing history. This form is sometimes called a *resident assessment protocol* (**RAP**). This form measures a client's ability to perform the activities of daily living, and identifies functional losses that affect this ability. There are several other assessment forms available to aid the nursing care team in developing an individualized plan of care for each client. Federal and state regulatory agencies require these forms. You must answer all the questions asked on the form to ensure that your employer is complying with regulatory requirements.

The MDS helps to ensure that all clients are assessed in the same way. Because these forms are the same in all agencies, you will find them easy to use if you move from one agency to another.

Plans for Care and Treatment

The purpose of the *plans for care* is to ensure that all caregivers provide the same care and treatments for the client. The physician's plan of care contains goals for treating the client and specific instructions called *orders* to guide the nursing staff. The nursing care plan is usually developed by the registered nurse after a thorough assessment of the client's health status. Sometimes the care plan is not included in the actual chart but is kept in a separate Kardex (see Chapter 35). In this case, the Kardex becomes a part of the permanent record when the client leaves the facility.

The *clinical care path* is a plan that specifies expected outcomes and treatments at specified times for all members of the healthcare team (see Chapter 36). The manual version of this form may have spaces for handwritten entries to respond to the instructions. The electronic version may also require information from the caregiver.

Progress Records

Progress records are periodic entries that describe the treatment and responses of the client at a point in time. The medication administration record, the physicians' and nurses' progress notes, and nursing flow sheets are the usual types of progress records kept.

The *medication administration record* (**MAR**) lists all medications that the physician has ordered for the client, with spaces for the caregiver to mark when medications are given. Sometimes the agency may separate MARs from the rest of the health record for your convenience when you administer med-

■■■ **TABLE 37-1** *C*ONTENTS OF THE HEALTH RECORD

General Category	Specific Form or Screen	Purpose	Responsible Caregiver
Assessment documents: forms/screens	Admission record	Lists client's name, address, sex, age, physician, insurance company, reason for admission	Admitting staff
	Medical history and physical	Records physician's history and physical examination findings	Physician
	Nursing admission history	Records nurse's history	Usually RN but may be LPN in some facilities
	Minimum data set (MDS)	Records information that identifies the client's ability to perform activities of daily living and functional losses that affect this ability	Admitting RN but may be LPN in some facilities
	Laboratory record	Records results of blood, urine, stool, or other body substance analysis	Laboratory personnel: physicians, technicians
	Consultation	Records findings and opinions from consults requested by primary caregivers	Consulting physician or other care provider
Plans for care and treatment	Problem list	Describes physician's goals for treatment	Physician
	Physician's orders	Lists instructions to nurses or technicians to implement client's diagnostic tests, treatments, or medications	Physician
	Nursing care plan	Lists client's expected outcomes of nursing care. Lists nursing actions to achieve outcome	Usually RN but may be LPN in some facilities
	Teaching plan	Identifies client's teaching needs. Lists teaching strategies	Nursing staff
	Clinical care path	Lists diagnostic tests, treatments, and expected client outcomes on a timeline; usually designates responsible caregiver	All caregivers
	Consents for treatment	Explains expected and possible adverse outcomes for treatments; contains client's signature	Admitting personnel; physician; nursing
Progress records: forms/screens	Flow sheets	Documents large amounts of information briefly and concisely by a timeline. Includes intake and output sheets, graphic sheets for vital signs, anesthesia sheets during surgery, routine nursing care sheets, intensive care unit records. Efficient records.	Depending on purpose of flow sheet, all care providers but particularly RN, LPN, perhaps aides
	Medication administration record	Lists ordered medications, amount, route, and ordered time of administration for noting time of actual administration and response to medication	Usually prepared by pharmacy; medication administration documented by RN, LPN
	Progress notes	Describe client's treatment and responses, unusual events, progress toward achieving outcomes	All care providers
Plans for continuity of care form/screen	Teaching record	Lists times and teaching strategies used; client's responses	Usually RN but may be LPN in some facilities
	Transfer form/screen	Summarizes client's condition and responses to treatment to prepare for transfer to another unit, facility, or community health agency	Usually RN but may be LPN in some facilities
	Discharge summary	Summarizes client's condition upon discharge from the healthcare facility	Physician and RN or LPN

ications. (Refer to Unit 9 to learn how to document medication administration.)

The **progress note** is entered at regular intervals to summarize the client's condition or response to treatment. Several systems of data entry are used, often using an acronym to guide your thinking as you organize information. These systems are based on the nursing process as required by regulatory standards for documentation. The **SOAP** system separates **S**ub-jective and **O**bjective data, followed by an **A**nalysis and **P**lan. Variations on the SOAP system include the addition of information about specific **I**nterventions, **E**valuation, and **R**evisions of nursing care (**SOAPIER**). Focus charting systems have several variations (**APIE, PIE, DAPE,** and **DARE**) in which the progress note identifies or focuses on specific problems and incorporates plans, interventions, evaluation, and education related to that specific problem. Charting by exception (**CBE**) is a system that uses a flow sheet to identify expected assessments, and a progress note to identify abnormalities or unexpected findings. Table 37-2 outlines commonly used systems for progress notes.

Nursing progress notes are handwritten in ink in the manual record on pages specified for these notes. The MIS may have screens on which standard or routine types of information are listed. You select the words or phrases about your client by touching with your finger or a light pen or by clicking the mouse. Some systems require you to keyboard a narrative portion of your notes.

A **flow sheet** is a graph or form that records large amounts of information collected at intervals over a specified period in brief, concise entries. Examples of flow sheets include intake and output and vital signs records. Routine nursing care such as bathing, ambulation, and how well the client eats also may be in a flow sheet format.

Both manual and MIS records have flow sheets. The flow sheet in the manual record is a page in the health record or a

separate sheet kept near the client's bedside. The flow sheet in the MIS is a screen that has simple "yes" or "no" responses that can be completed quickly and efficiently, using a light pen or keyboard. The flow sheet may have highlighted blanks for data entry, similar to recording intake and output on paper.

Sometimes the data on the flow sheet are summarized elsewhere in the health record so that not all data are kept. An MIS system is particularly useful for this type of data compilation and storage. If the record is a manual paper chart, the flow sheet itself may be discarded by the primary care nurse or team leader as the summary is recorded in the MIS.

Plans for Continuity of Care

The length of a client's admission to the healthcare agency varies from a few days to a few years, depending on the nature of the illness or disability. During admission, transfer, or discharge from the agency, healthcare personnel use specific forms to ensure that the client's care is continuous, consistent, and effective. Teaching plans, transfer notes, and discharge

▪▪▪ TABLE 37-2 *C*OMMONLY USED NURSING NOTE FORMATS

Format or Acronym	Category	Content
SOAP *or* SOAPE *or* SOAPIE	**S** Subjective	Subjective client data; usually direct quotes from client
	O Objective	Objective client data identified through observation, examination, or interview
	A Assessment or analysis	Conclusions drawn from data; often stated as a nursing diagnosis or client care problem
	P Plan	Expected outcome; if a SOAP note, this states nursing strategies to treat the nursing diagnosis or client care problem
or SOAPIER	**I** Intervention	Nursing strategies to treat the nursing diagnosis or client care problem
	E Evaluation	Outcomes of nursing care; reassessment of client
	R Revision	New plans for treatment of care problem based on client outcomes or responses
APIE	**A** Assessment	Objective and subjective data about the client; may include a conclusion in the form of nursing diagnosis or client care problem. (If system is PIE, A is recorded on a flow sheet at regular intervals.)
or PIE	**P** Plan	Expected outcome listed *or* Planned strategies to treat the nursing diagnosis or client care problem
	I Intervention	Nursing care given
	E Evaluation	Outcomes of nursing care; responses of client; reassessment information
DAPE	**D** Data	Objective and subjective data about client obtained through observation, interview, and examination
	A Assessment	Conclusions drawn from data; may be nursing diagnosis or client care problem
	P Plan	Expected outcomes listed or planned strategies to treat the nursing diagnosis or care problem
	E Evaluation	Outcomes of nursing care; responses of the client; reassessment information
Focus	Focus	Problem stated as nursing diagnosis or client care problem
DARE	**D** Data	Objective and subjective assessment data that support the Focus
	A Action	Nursing interventions to treat the problem
	R Response	Outcomes of interventions; reassessment data
	E Education	Client education
Charting by exception (CBE)	Uses SOAPIER for progress notes Adds: Assessment/intervention flow sheet	See above for content. Routine or client-specific nursing assessments listed at time intervals. Normal or expected data are only checked. Abnormalities or unexpected findings are then listed in progress notes using SOAPIER format.

summaries contain information that enables other caregivers to ensure continuity of care (see Chapters 36 and 45 for more information).

Guidelines for Documentation

The quality of your documentation says much about the kind of care you give. *Accurate* and *complete* documentation is important for effective communication and accountability. Regardless of the particular format your agency uses, always practice the following skills in documentation.

Document What You See

Describe exactly what you observe, and document what you see. Table 37-3 lists descriptive terms to use in documentation. Describe your assessments objectively; do not give your opinions or interpretations. Be specific. For example, when you

observe bleeding, indicate how much blood there is; its color; whether it is gushing, oozing, or running; and its source. When you are describing a client's response, describe the client's activity, not what you think it means. For example, "client crying and rocking back and forth in chair" is an objective and descriptive statement. If you try to interpret the client's actions, however, you may come to several conclusions, with no guarantee that any of them are correct. One interpretation might be "client lonely"; another might be "client out of touch with reality"; and still another might be "client in pain." Such interpretations may be incorrect and serve only to confuse issues and to distract care providers from treating the client's primary problems.

Is the client having trouble moving? Does the client stumble? Can the person stand in a normal fashion? Is speech coherent? Is speech clear and appropriate? Does urine or stool smell foul? Does the client's breath have a foul odor? These are the

(*text continues on page 444*)

■■■ TABLE 37-3 *D*ESCRIPTIVE TERMS COMMONLY USED IN DOCUMENTATION

Points of Observation	Observations to Be Charted	Specific Terms
Abdomen	Bloated; filled with gas Hard; boardlike Large; extends out	Distention, tympanites Rigid Protruding
Amount	Large amount Small amount	Copious, excessive, profuse Scanty, light
Appearance (skin, mucous membranes)	Bluish discoloration Skin appears yellowish	Cyanotic Jaundice
Appetite	Craves certain foods Eats everything served and asks for more food Appears never to get enough food Loss of appetite Eats nonfood items	Parorexia Hearty appetite Insatiable appetite Anorexia Pica
Arm or leg (extremity)	Puffy or swollen	Edematous; edema
Attitude	Afraid; worried Fixed idea (right or wrong) False belief insisted	Anxious; fearful Obsession Delusion
Baths	Given when client arrives Entire body Face, neck, arms, back, and genitals Taken in bed Taken in tub or special tub	Admission bath Complete bath Partial bath Bed bath Tub bath or sitz bath
Belch	To expel gas from stomach through the mouth	Eructation; burp
Bleeding	In large amount and in spurts Very little Nosebleed Blood in vomitus Blood in urine Blood in sputum	Hemorrhage; spurting blood; profuse Oozing; minimal amount Epistaxis Hematemesis Hematuria Hemoptysis
Breast	Large; hard Nipple always depressed	Engorged Inverted nipple

(continued)

■■■ **TABLE 37-3** *D*ESCRIPTIVE TERMS COMMONLY USED IN DOCUMENTATION (CONTINUED)

Points of Observation	Observations to Be Charted	Specific Terms
Breath	Unpleasant odor	Halitosis
Breathing	Difficulty in breathing Short time without breathing Rapid breathing Cannot breathe lying down Snoring sounds made when breathing Increasing dyspnea with periods of nonbreathing	Dyspnea Momentary apnea Hyperpnea Orthopnea Stertorous respiration Cheyne-Stokes respiration
Coma	Does not respond to stimuli	Coma (partially comatose or in profound coma); loss of consciousness
Consciousness (level of)	Aware of surroundings Level of consciousness	Alert; conversant; fully conscious; oriented Evaluated with Glasgow coma scale
Consistency of drainage (exudate)	Watery (from nose) Tears (from eyes) Contains pus Watery and bloody Thick and sticky Mucuslike	Coryza, rhinorrhea Lacrimation Purulent Sanguineous, serosanguineous Concentrated, viscous and tenacious Mucoid
Cough	Coughs all the time Coughs up material Coughs over a long period Coughs without producing material Coughs with a whoop Coughs at certain times Various types of cough	Continuous, spontaneous Productive Persistent Nonproductive Whooping cough Paroxysmal Loose; deep; dry; painful; exhaustive; tight; hacking; hollow
Decay	Tissue	Necrosis; necrotic
Dizziness	Feeling of being unstable; unsteady; dizzy	Vertigo (feeling of rotation); dizziness
Drainage	Fecal (contains stool material)	Fecal
Drainage	Contains mucus and pus Vaginal discharge that occurs for 1 or 2 weeks after childbirth	Mucopurulent Lochia
Dressings	New dressing applied over original one	Reinforced dressing
Ears	Wax in ears Ringing sensation	Cerumen Tinnitus
Edema	Leaves a dent when pressed Exists when body part is hanging down or lowered	Pitting Dependent
Emesis	Vomiting Vomiting forcefully and without warning Descriptive terms	Emesis Projectile Coffee ground, hematemesis (containing frank blood), color (describe), containing solid material (describe), amount
Expectoration	Coughing and spitting up sputum Spitting up blood	Expectorate Hemoptysis
Eyes, vision	Dilation of pupil Small, pinpoint pupils Sees double (two images of a single object)	Enlarged pupil, dilated pupil Contracted pupil; "pinpoint" Diplopia

(continued)

■■■ **TABLE 37-3** 𝒟escriptive Terms Commonly Used in Documentation (CONTINUED)

Points of Observation	Observations to Be Charted	Specific Terms
	Cross-eyes	Strabismus
	Drooping eyelids	Ptosis
	Appear to be staring; eyes appear not to move	Fixed
Face	Scars and pits	Pockmarked
Faint	Losing consciousness; fainting	Syncope
Feces	Resembling clay	Clay-colored BM
	Black (tarlike) color	Tarry BM, charcoal BM
	Inability to control (child)	Encopresis
	Inability to control (adult)	Incontinence (fecal)
	Bowel movement (BM)	Feces; stool; defecation
	Excessive; watery	Diarrhea
	Soft material	Soft, formless, or soft-formed stool: loose
	Constipated	Hard-formed stool expelled with difficulty; pellet like
	Condensed, retains shape	Formed
	Client unable to expel	Impacted
Fever, body temperature	No evidence of fever	Afebrile
	Temperature above normal	Pyrexia
	Temperature greatly above normal	Hyperpyrexia
	Elevated temperature suddenly returns to normal	Crisis
	Elevated temperature gradually returns to normal	Lysis (falling)
Fingers	Appear square across and curved at the end	Clubbed (as in some cardiac conditions)
Gas	Excessive amounts of air and gas in stomach or intestine, causing distention of organs, passing of gas	Flatus, flatulence
Gums	Pulling away from teeth	Receding; shrunken
	Other descriptive terms	Bleeding; spongy; firm; pink; cyanotic
Hair	Absence of hair; baldness	Alopecia
Hallucination	Abnormal sense perceptions not experienced by others	Hallucination
	Hearing	Auditory hallucination (voices, music, or sounds)
	Sight	Visual hallucination (visual images not observed by others)
	Smell	Olfactory hallucination (abnormal odors)
	Taste	Gustatory hallucination
	Touch	Tactile hallucination (feeling something on skin that is not there)
Heartbeat	Irregular beating	Arrhythmia
	Slow	Bradycardia (<60/min)*
	Fast	Tachycardia (>100/min)*
Hives	Hives (raised areas on skin)	Urticaria
	Itching	Pruritus
Lips	Tiny cracks	Fissured; cracked
Memory	Loss of memory	Amnesia
Mental state	Fails to accept reality; overly happy	Euphoric
	Indifferent; showing little or no emotion	Apathetic, flat affect
Muscle	Loss of normal tone or size	Atrophy

(continued)

■■■ **TABLE 37-3** *D*ESCRIPTIVE TERMS COMMONLY USED IN DOCUMENTATION (CONTINUED)

Points of Observation	Observations to Be Charted	Specific Terms
Odor	Spicy Like fruit Unpleasant Belonging to a particular thing	Aromatic Fruity Offensive; foul Characteristic
Perspiration	Excessive perspiration	Diaphoresis
Pain	Descriptive terms	Dull; aching; faint; burning; throbbing; gnawing; grinding; squeezing; acute; chronic; generalized; superficial; excruciating; unyielding; cramping; shooting; darting; colicky; continuous; shifting; agonizing; piercing; intense; cutting; transient; localized; remittent; persistent; unremitting; intractable
Pulse	Number of beats per minute Rhythm Beats missed; not continuous <60/min >100/min Beats indistinct (rapid) Beats hardly perceptible Rapid, distinct beats Cannot be felt	Rate Regular or irregular (may describe arrhythmia) Intermittent Slow, bradycardia* Rapid, tachycardia* Running Thready Bounding, full Imperceptible
Sensation	Feelings that are experienced	Tingling; burning; stinging; prickling; hot; cold
Skin	Descriptive terms Fragile Bruise ("black and blue mark")	Pale; red; moist; dry; clear; warm; coarse; tanned; scaly; thick; loose; rough; tight; discolored; jaundiced; mottled; calloused; edematous; cyanotic; excoriated; abrasion; bruised; oily; painful; scarred; black; brown; white; pink; translucent; clammy; rash; wrinkled; smooth; skin returns quickly (1–2 seconds) when pinched (turgor) Friable Hematoma, ecchymosis
Sleep	Inability to sleep Sleeps more than normal	Insomnia Hypersomnia
Speech	Unable to be understood Meaningless Runs words together Difficulty in speaking Inability to speak Unwillingness Other descriptive terms	Incoherent Rambling; loose; tangential Slurring Dysphasia Aphasia Mute Stammering; stuttering; hoarse; feeble; fluent
Teeth	False teeth Decayed Accumulation of material on teeth Without teeth	Dentures Caries Sordes Edentulous
Thirst	Excessive thirst	Polydipsia
Throat	Difficulty in swallowing Inability to swallow	Dysphagia Aphagia
Tongue	Descriptive terms	Dry; furrowed; cracked; raw; coated; swollen; ulcerated; pink; inflamed; furry
Treatment	Preventive Giving temporary relief but not curing	Prophylactic Palliative

(continued)

■ ■ ■   TABLE 37-3 𝒟ESCRIPTIVE TERMS COMMONLY USED IN DOCUMENTATION (CONTINUED)

Points of Observation	Observations to Be Charted	Specific Terms
Urination	Pass fluid from bladder	Void; micturate; urinate
	Unable to control	Incontinence; involuntary
	Unable to wait to void	Urgency
	Increased excretion of urine	Diuresis
	No urine passes	Anuria
	Frequent urination; large amount of urine	Polyuria
	Unable to start stream	Hesitancy
	Voiding during the night	Nocturia
	Pus in urine	Pyuria
	Blood in urine	Hematuria
	Sugar in urine	Glycosuria
	Albumin in urine	Albuminuria
	Scantiness of urine	Oliguria
	Bed-wetting	Enuresis
	Stones (in urine or elsewhere)	Calculi
	Other descriptive terms	Cloudy; with sediment; straw-colored; coffee-colored; foul-smelling
Weight	Overweight	Obese; morbidly obese
	Very thin; underweight	Emaciated; cachexic
Miscellaneous terms	Came on suddenly, as a symptom	Sudden onset
	Spreading from one part of body to another (eg, cancer)	Metastasis
	How long it (eg, infection) lasts	Duration of (state length of time); prolonged; intermittent; persistent

*Adult average rates (slow pulse is normal in athletes).

types of questions to ask yourself so that your assessments are accurate and your documentation is informative.

Identify the client's reaction to your actions, whether it is to a medication given, client teaching, or nursing interventions. Record the client's response, as well as the time, dosage, description, and any adverse effects. Check the health record for previous adverse reactions to this medication or treatment.

Be Specific

Avoid ambiguous statements and generalizations. For example, "had an uncomfortable night" does not say anything specific, whereas "client was up 10 times with diarrhea during the night" tells *why* the client had an uncomfortable night and *why* sleep was interrupted. Avoid judgmental words such as well, fair, poor, or good.

Use Direct Quotes

Directly quote the client, and differentiate the client's words from your observations. Enclose the client's statements in quotation marks so others will know exactly what the client said. The following statement serves as an example:

Mrs. C. stated, "I have a throbbing pain in my head."

Note that this documented statement is specific, describing how the client interprets the pain.

Do not chart hearsay, such as what someone else has told you about the client, unless you quote it. For example:

Mrs. R.'s husband said, "My wife does not like the food here."

Be Prompt

Document immediately after giving all care, medications, and treatments. The health record does not have memory lapses, although you may. Always document *after* you give a medication or perform a treatment, *never before*. If you forget to document a pertinent fact and add it after you have entered other documentation in the health record, you must identify your entry as a "late entry."

Be Clear and Consistent

Correct spelling, punctuation, and sentence structure are essential. "Bathed in wheelchair in hall" is not a clear statement. "Client had a bed bath given by the nurse and is now sitting in a wheelchair in the hallway" is clear and accurate.

On manual records, write or print neatly in black ink. Make sure the record is continuous and *legible*. Use the format specified by that particular agency. Indicate the date and time of each entry. Be aware that most facilities use the 24-hour clock (Table 37-4).

Use only standard abbreviations (Table 37-5). Do not invent your own. If you are unsure about your institution's acceptance of an abbreviation, refer to the agency's policy and procedure manual. Sign the health record with your first initial or full first name (depending on the agency's policy), last name, and classification (eg, "M. Smith, LPN").

Do not leave vacant lines in the health record. Using every line maintains the chronology of charting. If you continue on the back of a sheet or on a new page, again write the date, time, and "(continued)" before continuing your entry. If a

TABLE 37-4 THE 24-HOUR CLOCK

Time	Conversion to 24-Hour Time
12 AM (midnight)	0000
12:01 AM	0001
6 AM	0600
7:30 AM	0730
12 PM (noon)	1200
1 PM	1300
2 PM	1400
8 PM	2000
11 PM	2300

vacant line is left between entries, draw a line through it, to indicate that the documentation is chronological.

Always replace the health record where it belongs. Do not remove it from the nursing station unless you have consulted the charge nurse or team leader.

Record All Relevant Information

Read the physician's notes. If you have any questions or concerns, bring them to the physician's attention. Document all communications with other members of the healthcare team. Other departments also have policies and procedures that you must follow to protect the client. If, for example, the care plan

TABLE 37-5 COMMON ABBREVIATIONS USED IN DOCUMENTATION

Abbreviation	Meaning	Abbreviation	Meaning
@	at	per	by
aa	of each	PM	afternoon
ac, AC	before meals (Latin: *ante cena*)	po (o)	by mouth; oral (Latin: *per os*)
ad lib	as desired, at liberty	PRN*	when required, as needed (*pro re nata*)
alt hor, QOH	every other hour	pt	pint, patient
AM	morning	pulv, pwd	powder
BID	twice a day (bi-daily; Latin: *bis in die*)	q	every
BRP	bathroom privileges	qd, QD	every day
c̄	with	qh, QH	every hour
cap	capsule	q (2, 3, etc.) h	every (2, 3, etc.) hours
cc	cubic centimeter	q.i.d., QID	four times a day
D/C	discharge, discontinue	QOD	every other day
dr	dram	qs	sufficient amount
dx	diagnosis	R, PR	rectally, per rectum
& (et) ɛ̵	and	℞, Rx	take, prescription, treatment
elix	elixir	s̄	without
fx	fracture	2°	secondary to
Gm, gm, G, g	gram	Sig or S	write on label, instructions
gr	grain	SOS*	if necessary
gt or gtt	drop, or drops	spans	spansule
H, hypo	hypodermic	s̄s̄	one half
h (hr), H	hour	stat, STAT	at once, immediately
hs (HS)	at bedtime (hour of sleep)	subq	subcutaneously
hx	history	supp	suppository
IM	intramuscularly	susp	suspension
IV	intravenously	t.i.d., TID	three times a day (tri-daily; Latin: *ter in die*)
L	liter	tint, tinct	tincture
m, min, or m$_x$	minim, or minims	t, tsp	teaspoon
µg, Mcg	microgram	T, tbsp	tablespoon
mg	milligram	TPN	total parenteral nutrition
mL	milliliter	tx, TX	treatment, traction
NPO	nothing by mouth (Latin: *nil per os*)	ungt, ung	ointment
od	right eye (Latin: *oculo dexter*)	ī	one
oint (ungt)	ointment	īī	two
os	left eye, oculo sinister	v̄	five
ou	both eyes (Latin: *oculi uterque*)	x̄	ten
oz	ounce		
pc, PC	after meals (Latin: *post cena*)		

*Note the difference between these abbreviations: SOS (if necessary) means for one dose only; PRN (when needed, as often as necessary) means the nurse is expected to use judgment about repeating the dose. For instance, the doctor may leave a PRN order for a cathartic, but if the client has an adequate bowel movement, a cathartic is not necessary on that day. Two days later it may be needed. Usually PRN orders specify the frequency (how often) the drug may be given and usually must be rewritten at specific intervals in order to be considered valid.

notes that side rails must be up after 10 pm, document that you have followed this guideline. If you do not carry out this order, you must state the reason in the documentation.

Respect Confidentiality

Confidentiality means that conversations with clients, and nursing observations and assessments, are shared only with the appropriate caregivers in the proper setting. What you record and show to the client and other health professionals is never to be shared with anyone else. Do not discuss clients "over coffee"; your conversation may be overheard. Remember to maintain confidentiality during telephone conversations, taking care that a bystander does not hear confidential information and that you do not violate client confidentiality through telephone conversations with the client's family or friends. Do not allow clients to see the computer screen. Be careful to maintain client confidentiality in the home care setting as well, when family or friends are present and eager to learn about your client. Keep in mind that you may be held liable in court for "breach of confidentiality" (see Chapter 4).

Record Documentation Errors

Erasures and the use of correction fluid on the client's health record are *illegal*. Such measures could be considered as an attempt to hide poor nursing care or an error made in client care. If you make an *error in documenting*, cross out the incorrect statement with a single line, enclose it in parentheses, and write ERROR and your initials above it. (Your original note must be readable.) Some agencies recommend using *recorded in error* (**RIE**) instead. Other agencies use the term "mistaken entry." After filling in the term that your agency uses, record the correct statement. *(An error in client care is an entirely different matter that you must report to your instructor or team leader at once.)*

You may also make an error in the electronic chart. The MIS has a mechanism by which you may review your entries and make an immediate change before final approval of the information. If you later recognize your error and wish to make a change, the MIS has a mechanism for "late entries," in which you may identify your earlier error. Be sure you learn about the methods for making both an immediate change and a late change in the electronic chart during your agency's orientation.

> ### Nursing Alert
> The importance of careful documentation in healthcare cannot be overstated. You must make sure to document all nursing assessments and actions completely and accurately.

REPORTING

Several times during the day the nurse must "report off" to another nurse. The first nurse summarizes the activities and conditions of assigned clients because he or she is leaving the unit for a break or at the end of a shift. The report may be very brief or quite detailed, depending on the purpose of the report and each client's condition. These reports must be efficient and accurate to make effective use of nursing time and to ensure continuity of client care.

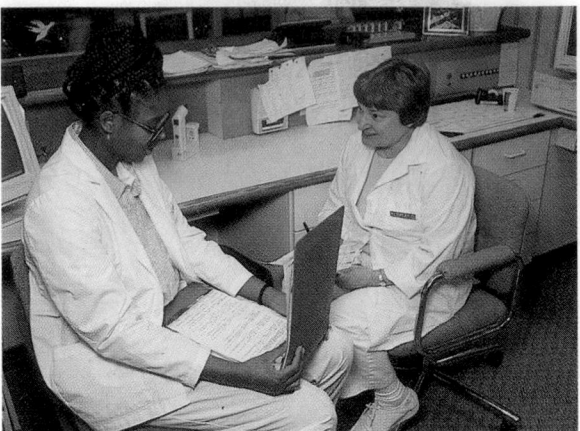

FIGURE 37-1. By reporting to one another, nurses ensure that clients have continuity of care around the clock. This report may be face-to-face, by tape recorder, or in a "walk-around" format.

Change-of-shift reporting is a means of exchanging information between the outgoing and incoming staff on each shift (Fig. 37-1). In Practice: Nursing Care Guidelines 37-1 gives pointers for change-of-shift reporting. The team leader may report to the entire incoming shift, or reports may be given from caregiver to caregiver. The report may be recorded on a tape recorder or may be given in walking rounds. In **walking rounds,** caregivers move from client to client, discussing pertinent information. Walking rounds encourage client participation and enable the new oncoming staff to view equipment, dressings, and other treatments with the previous nurse. The

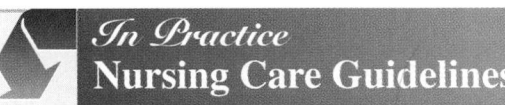

In Practice
Nursing Care Guidelines 37-1

CHANGE-OF-SHIFT REPORTING

- Use the nursing care plan as your guide.
- Identify the client's room number, diagnosis on admission, age (if relevant), physician's name, primary nurse or case manager, significant medical history.
- Report on each nursing diagnosis or listed problem.
- For each nursing diagnosis or problem, identify the following:
  - Significant assessment data
  - Related nursing and medical orders
  - Medications
  - Recent test results
  - Scheduled diagnostic tests or surgery
  - Vital signs
  - Significant events
  - Short- or long-term goals achieved
  - Teaching plans
  - Discharge plans
- Prepare a written summary to give to the oncoming nurse if this is a procedure of your agency.

outgoing nurse introduces the incoming nurse to the client. This technique personalizes client care and helps to establish rapport.

➤ STUDENT SYNTHESIS

Key Points

- The primary purposes of the health record are to facilitate communication among caregivers, to provide evidence of accountability, and to facilitate health research and education. Both manual and electronic records serve these purposes.
- Electronic records are a result of the use of medical information systems (MIS) to enter, store, process, and retrieve client data.
- Assessment documents record all client information.
- Minimum data sets and resident assessment protocols guide nurses to develop individualized care plans, especially in long-term and home care.
- Plans for treatment of the client include the physician's orders and the nursing care plan.
- Progress records describe the treatment and responses of the client.
- Healthcare facilities use various formats to organize nursing progress notes in the health record.
- Plans for the continuity of care include teaching plans, transfer notes, and discharge summaries.
- Accurate and complete documentation ensures effective communication and accountability.
- Confidentiality means a client's right to privacy that healthcare personnel safeguard in both documentation and reporting.
- Reporting is an oral method of communicating that is timely, precise, and accurate.

Critical Thinking Exercises

1. Compare the various progress notes formats found in Table 37-2 with the nursing process. Which phase of the nursing process do each of these formats represent?
2. What do you believe are the advantages and disadvantages of using an electronic chart rather than a manual chart? Would you prefer to use a manual or electronic chart, and why?
3. Confidentiality is an important client right. List ways in which you can ensure confidentiality in both manual and electronic charting.

NCLEX-Style Review Questions

1. The nurse has recorded nursing care in the wrong client's chart. What action should the nurse take?
   a. Cross out the error with a single line and write "error" and his or her initials.
   b. Erase the entry from the chart and write over the space.
   c. Remove the page from the chart and shred the page.
   d. Use correction fluid to cover up the entry.
2. Which of the following is a correct entry that can be made into a client's chart?
   a. Client appears to be worried about something.
   b. Client is such a nice lady.
   c. Client's family is not supportive.
   d. Client's dressing is dry and intact.
3. Which of the following is a correct method for documenting subjective data?
   a. Client states that he has a headache.
   b. Client states that his pain is 8 out of 10 on the pain scale.
   c. Client states, "I feel nauseated."
   d. Client states that her family will arrive at the hospital in 30 minutes.
4. On which form would the nurse document vital signs?
   a. Flow sheet
   b. Medication administration record
   c. Minimum data set
   d. Progress note
5. On which form would the nurse document what a wound looked like during a dressing change procedure?
   a. Flow sheet
   b. Medication administration record
   c. Minimum data set
   d. Progress note
6. A client complains of feeling bloated after surgery. Physical examination reveals the abdomen is filled with gas. The nurse would document the findings as:
   a. Abdomen is rigid
   b. Distended abdomen
   c. Productive abdomen
   d. Thready abdomen

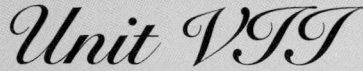

Unit VII

SAFETY IN THE HEALTHCARE FACILITY

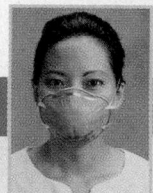

CHAPTER

38

The Healthcare Facility Environment

LEARNING OBJECTIVES

1. List and describe components included in the basic client unit.
2. Compare and contrast the basic client unit in the hospital, long-term care, and home care settings.
3. Discuss the relationship between housekeeping procedures and client safety.
4. Summarize the guidelines for all nursing procedures.
5. Describe at least four direct client care departments in hospitals.
6. Describe the functions of at least four hospital support departments.

NEW TERMINOLOGY

autopsies
client unit
commode
intercom
morgue
neurodiagnostic
nuclear medicine
nursing unit

ophthalmoscope
otoscope
pathologist
protocol
rationale
research laboratory
telecommunications
telehealth

ACRONYMS

ADL	GYN	PICU
ART	HS	PM&R
ASU	ICU	PSYCH
CCU	IV	PT
CDU	MH, MHU	PTA
COTA	MICU	QI
CP	MIS	REHAB
CQI	MRI	RPT
CRU	NEURO	RR
CSR, CSS	NICU	RRA
CT	NMR	RRT
DERM	OB	RT
ECF	OPD	SDSU
ECG/EKG	OR	SICU
ED	ORTHO	TICU
EEG	OT	UAP
EMG	OTR	UROL
GERI	PACU, PARR	US
GU	PEDS	

The needs of clients include the basic needs of all human beings (see Chap. 5) and special needs connected with illness or injury. Essential physiologic needs are oxygen, water, nutrients, waste elimination, sleep and rest, activity and exercise, and shelter. Higher-level needs include safety, emotional and spiritual support, and pleasant surroundings. Additional needs include essential medical and nursing care, encouragement to return to normal or baseline functioning, and diversion. The client's progress toward recovery, comfort, and happiness depends on the extent to which these needs are satisfied. Meeting these needs involves teamwork among all those who come in contact with the client, including the client's family.

Traditionally, most nursing care was provided in a hospital or extended care facility (**ECF**). Changes in the healthcare delivery system have expanded nursing into the community in a variety of settings (Fig. 38-1). Your first experience with clients may be in a hospital or ECF, but it may also be in a community health agency or in homes. Wherever you begin, you need to know the basic equipment used for client care. You also should understand the various departments and support services found in many hospitals and healthcare facilities. This knowledge will enable you to call on appropriate services for clients, and to know and explain the functions of various healthcare personnel.

THE CLIENT UNIT

The **client unit** is the area where most client care is provided. This area may be around the client's bed or in the living room of a person's home. The unit usually includes a bed, other furniture, and equipment used in the client's daily care (Fig. 38-2). In the hospital or ECF, the client may be in a private or semi-private room, or in a ward containing three or more beds. Each bed and the accompanying furniture is considered a client unit. In the home, the client unit is the primary area where the client receives care. It may be the bedroom or the main living area—where the person is most comfortable, and where adequate room is available for essential equipment such as a hospital bed, oxygen, intravenous (**IV**) pole, or commode. In today's healthcare environment, facilities give a great deal of thought to providing clients with surroundings that are homey, pleasant, and also practical. The **nursing unit** is an area containing several client units.

Components of the Basic Client Unit

The following components make up the basic client unit in hospital, ECF, and home care settings:

Furniture: Bed, bedside stand (also called a bedside table or bedside cabinet), chair, lamp, overbed table. Most hospital beds have built-in side rails. The television, telephone, and nurse call signals may also be built into the side rails. Regular beds in the home do not have side rails, and require additional safety considerations. In the home, clients may use a couch or bed or may rent a hospital bed during their illness. Some clients may bring a favorite chair to the long-term care facility.

Linens: Mattress pads, sheets, pillowcases, blankets, bedspread, bath blanket, face towel, washcloth, bedpan cover, gown or pajamas. In the home, personal preferences, living conditions, and limited resources may affect the type and amount of linens available for use.

Toilet equipment: Washbasin, soap dish, toothbrush, toothpaste, denture cup, toothbrush container, emesis basin, comb, bedpan, urinal for male clients. A portable **commode,** or toilet, is lightweight and sturdy and is easily moved in and out of a room. Home care clients may adapt the bathroom with safety equipment to ease toileting and bathing.

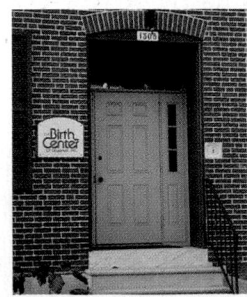
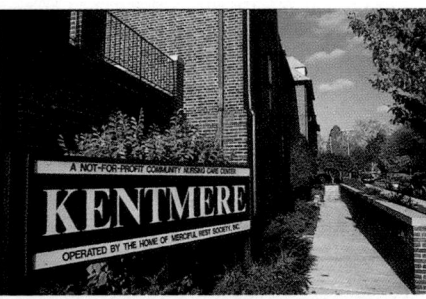
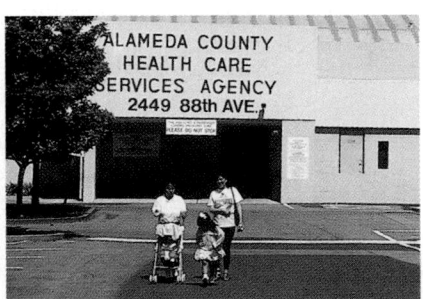
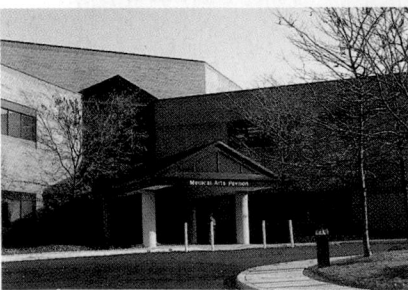
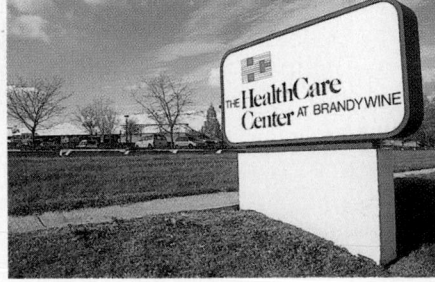
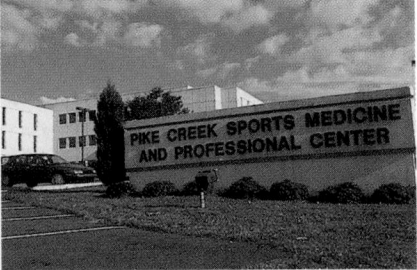

FIGURE 38-1. Traditionally, most nursing care was provided in a hospital or extended care facility. Today, a great deal of our healthcare has moved into the community, including the client's home.

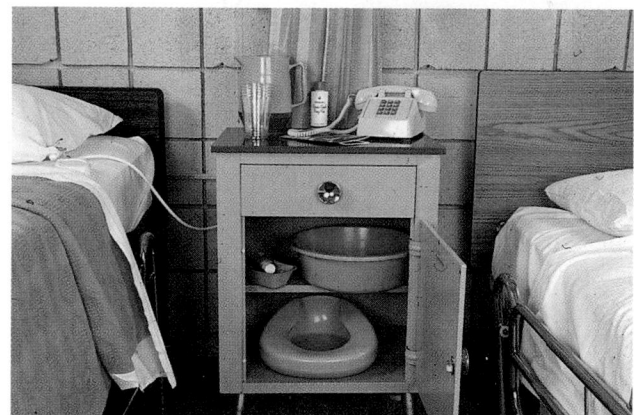

FIGURE 38-2. The basic client unit includes a bed, other furniture, and equipment used in the client's daily care. The curtain behind the bedside table can be used to provide privacy for the client.

Other articles: Water pitcher and drinking glass, thermometer, call bell or button, screen or curtain, TV, VCR, often a telephone. Many hospital units have a built-in blood pressure setup, suction, and oxygen on the wall, as well as an intercommunication, or **intercom,** system. The intercom allows clients to communicate with healthcare providers at the nursing station.

Equipment for nursing treatments may be kept outside the unit or in the treatment room or utility room. The client unit should always be complete and ready for use—to save steps and to prevent delays. Home care nurses may bring blood pressure equipment and other essential items to the home each time they visit. Medical equipment supply companies will deliver beds, oxygen, infusion pumps, and other supplies directly to the client's home.

Furniture
Hospital Bed.   The hospital bed is specially constructed and equipped to provide maximum safety and comfort for clients and their caregivers. Chapter 49 describes the bed, its attachments, and the skills used for bedmaking. Many home care clients rent a hospital bed during their illness because it can be raised and lowered, making care less strenuous for nurses and family caregivers. If the hospital bed is electric, the client or caregivers can raise and lower the head or foot of the bed with little effort.

Overbed Table.   The overbed table fits over the bed. It is useful when the person is eating, reading, or grooming. The table can be opened, revealing a mirror and space for small toiletry articles. The top is adjustable to permit the client to place a book at a comfortable angle to read without having to hold it.

Bedside Stand.   The bedside stand is durable and easy to keep clean. The top is covered with Formica or a similar material that absorbs sound when articles are placed on the surface.

Bedside stands include a drawer and an enclosed storage space containing shelves. The legs are metal or rubber-tipped or have casters that allow the table to be moved easily and quietly. The drawer provides space for personal belongings. Some

facilities have lockers for their clients to store clothing and other personal items in. They usually have a place for clients to lock up valuables or possessions. (However, many facilities encourage clients to leave their valuables at home, particularly for short stays.)

In the home, TV stands, end tables, dressers, or coffee tables may serve as the bedside stand. Often, many personal items and mementos surround the client. Remember the home care setting is not like the more sterile hospital environment. You are providing nursing care in someone's home. Be flexible and work within the client's physical surroundings and cultural practices.

Other Components
The TV and radio controls, buttons to raise and lower the head and foot of the bed, and the intercom button are often built into the bed's side rails.

When you orient the client and family to the room, demonstrate how to operate the equipment. It is frightening to the ill client to be alone in unfamiliar surroundings and not to know how to obtain assistance. First, teach the client how to use the nurse call button. Assure the client that a nurse can respond in person or from the nursing station by using the intercom. Home care clients may use a bell or other device to attract the caregiver's attention. They may also choose to install an alert system that they activate, transmitting a signal to a hospital or other facility in an emergency. Personnel then respond by telephone or through video surveillance.

Safety and Nursing Care Equipment.   Other equipment is available to healthcare personnel. Many units have items such as nasogastric suction equipment, blood pressure apparatus, oxygen, and a hanger for IV infusions built into the wall or ceiling above the bed. Because this equipment may frighten the client, explain that it exists in all units just in case it is needed.

If the client is in a multi-bed room, a curtain will hang around each client's area for privacy. This curtain runs in a track on the ceiling, and can be pushed out of the way when not needed.

Ventilation and Air Quality.   With concern for air quality, most healthcare facilities have taken action to prevent pollution. Hospitals do not allow smoking, although they may designate a special outside smoking area. Usually, the windows do not open, and heating and cooling are controlled centrally. However, you will need to make sure each client is comfortable. Air temperature affects comfort. There must be a balance between heat lost and heat produced. The room temperature that most effectively maintains this balance is between 68° and 72° Fahrenheit (20° and 22.2° Celsius).

Protect your client from chilling. An ill or injured person is often unusually susceptible to feeling cold. Offer extra blankets to the client when in bed. Protect an ambulating client with a warm blanket over the shoulders, a bathrobe, and slippers. Place chairs away from drafts. Cover the client with a bath blanket when giving a bed bath.

Odors.   Illness may make a person extremely sensitive to odors. Remove bedpans, urinals, and soiled dressings from the client's bedside immediately after use. Do not use strong cologne, perfume, or aftershave lotion. The smell of smoke bothers some clients; if you smoke, be sure that your breath is clean and your clothes do not smell of smoke. You may need to explain the facility's smoke-free policy to the client and visitors. (You are also expected to abide by this policy.)

Noise.   Noise can overstimulate or frighten the client and produce fatigue. Therefore, attempt to minimize or eliminate noise as much as possible. Slamming doors or dropping equipment startles clients and may cause restlessness and irritation. Turn radios and TV sets to a low volume. Headphones or under-the-pillow speakers may be available. Clients should use them whenever possible, to prevent annoying other clients. Be especially aware of the noise level at night. Even the sound of two nurses talking can irritate the client who is having difficulty sleeping. Overhead music is often played softly in clinics and other facilities to help make the environment more pleasant and comfortable.

Privacy.   You are obligated to respect and to preserve the privacy of all clients. In consideration of the client's modesty, be sure to use screens, curtains, bath blankets, or other drapes to keep the person covered as much as possible during treatments. Shut the client's door when procedures are being performed. If a client is confused and pulls off covers, pajamas may be more practical to use than a hospital gown.

Respect the client's privacy when visitors call. You may need to help enforce the facility's visiting policy to protect the privacy of other clients. Many facilities permit only one or two visitors at a time. This is sometimes difficult to enforce when a crisis occurs and cultural practices require the presence of many relatives, spiritual leaders, and significant others.

Housekeeping on the Unit

Always keep the unit neat and orderly. Good housekeeping helps prevent accidents and infections and helps you to carry out nursing care efficiently. Arrange equipment and supplies so that all personnel can locate the items easily and quickly. Consistency from room to room helps maintain order. These measures help clients feel secure, and make falls and other accidents less likely.

Restocking the Unit

Replace used supplies promptly. Check equipment and inspect it for breaks, cracks, or rough places that might be harmful. Inspect electrical cords to ensure that they are intact. Replace broken or damaged equipment and report damage to the appropriate person so that equipment can be replaced or repaired. Many facilities keep an inventory of equipment as a basis for ordering new articles or replacing damaged ones. Some facilities have an automated system for tracking supplies and order new supplies as they are used.

Cleaning the Unit After Use

Auxiliary personnel from the housekeeping department are usually responsible for cleaning client units in hospitals and ECFs. However, in an emergency, all nurses should know how to clean a unit according to their facility's policies and the principles of medical asepsis (see Chap. 41). In some situations, you will supervise such procedures.

Always make sure the unit is cleaned after a client has been discharged or transferred to another room, and before another client uses the room. In the hospital or ECF, everything in the unit is considered contaminated and must be discarded or disinfected before it can be used by another client. Such measures prevent the spread of infection and help to allay the client's concerns about the spread of diseases. Cleanliness is just as important in the home, although it is often more difficult to enforce. If you work in home care, you will need to teach clients and their families many important measures for maintaining sanitary and safe conditions. Many of these measures are discussed throughout this unit.

The Clinic Setting

Although equipment in a clinic setting may differ slightly from that found in a hospital or ECF, basic equipment includes the following pieces:

Furniture: Examination table, Mayo stand (holds the equipment used in the examination), chair, examination light, rolling stool. Most examination rooms have a sink and a few cabinets for storing supplies.

Linens: Sheets, disposable paper over the examination table, paper towels, disposable or cloth gown and drapes or small towels for privacy.

Other articles: Many units have a built-in blood pressure setup. An **ophthalmoscope** (an instrument used for examining the eyes) and an **otoscope** (an instrument used to examine inside the ears, nose, and throat) are often mounted on the wall. A scale is available to weigh clients.

PROVISION OF NURSING CARE

The nurse will provide most nursing care directly in the client unit. Healthcare facilities and agencies have specific policies outlining their standards for care. A Procedure, **Protocol,** or Standards book is available to employees and students in that healthcare setting. In Practice: Nursing Care Guidelines 38-1 provides information about general steps to follow for all procedures you conduct, regardless of the setting.

In acute facilities and ECFs, you are likely to perform several specific procedures together for efficiency. These skills may be grouped because they are associated with the same time of day or with a special kind of treatment. Many nurses know these blocks of nursing care by group names. In Practice: Nursing Care Guidelines 38-2 provides some examples of specific types of care according to time of day. Usually, you will have more than one client to care for, and you will need to consider your facility's routines when planning their care. When preparing your work plan, consider meal hours, healthcare provider rounds, and appointments for surgery, x-ray examinations, therapy, and laboratory procedures. You may be asked

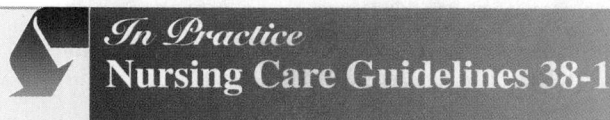

In Practice
Nursing Care Guidelines 38-1

GENERAL GUIDELINES FOR PERFORMING NURSING PROCEDURES

- Check the physician's orders; review the Kardex, nursing care plan, care map, critical pathway, and so forth.
- Identify the client.
- Perform the procedure on time.
- Follow Standard Precautions (Chap. 41).
- Wash your hands before and after every procedure.
- Wear gloves for most procedures (follow your facility's protocol).
- Assemble all necessary equipment so you can carry out the procedure easily, quickly, and efficiently.
- Introduce yourself and explain the procedure to the client to allay fears of pain or discomfort; clients may be apprehensive about machines, sharp instruments, hot or cold applications, or equipment that covers the face.
- Avoid using the words "hurt" or "painful." Say instead, "You may feel some discomfort," or "You will have to lie in one position, but I will help to make you comfortable."
- Emphasize positive aspects: "The procedure won't take long," or "It will make you feel better." A client will usually be more cooperative if he or she knows what to expect. Never tell a client "There's nothing to it," when you know that a procedure has some painful or uncomfortable aspects. Make the client as comfortable as possible before beginning any procedure. Offer prescribed pain medication (as ordered) to the client before carrying out any uncomfortable procedure.
- Ensure the client's privacy by closing the door or using curtains and screens. *Cover the person as much as possible.*
- Stay with the client during examinations and procedures. Explain and answer questions promptly.
- Care for equipment as required, and store it as indicated by the facility's policies (eg, wash, sterilize, store, or return to central supply department).
- Discard all dressings and disposable equipment, following facility protocol.
- Document procedures, the time they are performed, results noted, and unusual client reactions assessed. Report any pertinent symptoms or observations to the appropriate person. Report emergencies immediately.
- *Ask for help when you need it.*

to assist temporarily with emergencies that come up on a busy unit. In all situations, your clients are your first responsibility.

Each nursing procedure is complete in itself. There is a reason, or **rationale,** for each specific step in every nursing procedure. These reasons guide you in making the procedure effective. Although individual steps may vary among health-care facilities, your nursing care will be safe if you do not violate the basic underlying principles. As skills are presented in this book, the rationales for steps are given to guide you in adapting your care to individual situations after graduation. As a student, follow procedures exactly as taught by your instructors until you have a firm grasp on nursing's underlying principles.

☛ KEY CONCEPT

Although some of the steps of a procedure may be carried out differently in your healthcare facility, the underlying principles do not change. (These principles are usually related to safety for the client or for staff and visitors.)

HOSPITAL PERSONNEL AND SERVICES

Hospitals offer a variety of services; therefore, they are staffed with people experienced in many different areas. Many of the following services are also provided in—or linked to—ECFs, clinics, surgery centers, and home care agencies. Even if you do not work in a large hospital, you should have a general understanding of these departments and services because, as a healthcare professional, you will work with people from many of these disciplines. You will also need to explain particular services to clients when providing care. Many abbreviations and acronyms are commonly used in these large facilities. They are listed at the beginning of this chapter and are also included with other abbreviations in Appendix B.

Diagnostic and Treatment Departments

Clinical diagnostic laboratories perform numerous tests to assist providers in diagnosing disorders. **Pathologists** and their associates determine the underlying nature of diseases through their examination and study of tissue specimens. These specimens include blood, sputum, feces, and biopsied tissues. Pathologists also perform **autopsies** (examinations after death [postmortem]). The **morgue** is under a pathologist's direction and is the place where dead bodies are kept until identified and released to a funeral home or family. Autopsies may take place in the hospital or in another outside facility.

Some large teaching hospitals also include a **research laboratory,** where studies and experiments on animals are conducted to understand, cure, or prevent human disease.

The radiology department performs diagnostic x-ray studies to aid healthcare providers in determining the exact location and nature of disorders. Radiation therapy is given to treat certain diseases. Sometimes this entire department is called **nuclear medicine.** Other procedures this department conducts include computed tomography (**CT**) scans, xerography and mammography (breast studies), magnetic resonance imaging (**MRI**) or nuclear magnetic resonance (**NMR**), and ultrasound (**US**) studies. This department also supervises and performs the implantation and injection of radioactive and opaque materials for treatments and examinations.

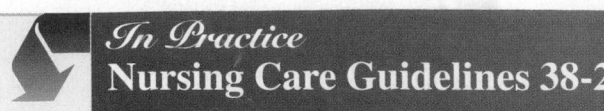

In Practice
Nursing Care Guidelines 38-2

GUIDELINES FOR PERFORMING GROUPED PROCEDURES

You will conduct most of the following procedures when working in acute or some extended care settings, where clients receive a great deal of round-the-clock attention. The times for some of the following procedures may vary, according to each facility's policies. As often as you can, perform these procedures at a time that is most comfortable and therapeutic for the client, not necessarily for your convenience. For example, a client might be accustomed to bathing at night, not in the later morning. It may be possible to accommodate such a preference. Do any painful procedures first, then give a backrub and perform other comfort measures so that the client is better able to rest after the procedure. Also, offer the client a bedpan, urinal, or assist him or her to the toilet before washing his or her hands. Give medications after you have given all other care.

Early Morning (AM) Care

Perform these measures before breakfast for the client's health and comfort.

- Offer a bedpan or urinal, or assist the client to the bathroom.
- Wash, or assist the client to wash, face and hands.
- Brush, or assist the client to brush, his or her teeth.
- Adjust the bed and bedclothes.
- Take the client's temperature, pulse, respiration, and blood pressure.
- Change the client's position for comfort.
- Adjust the table for the breakfast tray.

Later Morning (AM) Care

Perform these measures after the client's breakfast for health and comfort.

- Remove the breakfast tray.
- Offer the client a bedpan or urinal, or assist the client to the bathroom.
- Give the client a bath or assist with bathing (bed bath, tub, or shower depending on the client's condition).

- Make the client's bed. Change linens according to your facility's policies.
- Change the client's position or help him or her to ambulate.
- Comb hair, or assist the client to comb hair.
- Care for the client's nails.
- Perform any AM treatments as ordered.
- Give the client a backrub or massage.
- Tidy the client unit.

Afternoon Care

Perform these measures to relax the client in preparation for visitors.

- Change the client's position or help the client to ambulate.
- Offer the client a bedpan or urinal, or assist him or her to the bathroom.
- Wash, or assist the client to wash, face and hands.
- Perform afternoon treatments, as ordered.
- Give the client a backrub or hand massage.

Evening (HS or "Hour of Sleep" Care)

Perform these measures for health, comfort, and to prepare the client for sleep.
- Complete evening treatments.
- Offer the client a bedpan or urinal, or assist him or her to the bathroom.
- Wash, or assist the client to wash, face and hands.
- Brush, or assist the client to brush, his or her teeth.
- Comb and tidy the client's hair.
- Change the client's position.
- Adjust the bed and bedclothes.
- Give the client a backrub.
- Give HS medications as ordered.
- Tidy up the client unit. Be sure all obstacles are out of the way so that healthcare team members and the client do not fall over them during the night. Turn on the night light.

The electroencephalography (**EEG**) department, also known as the **neurodiagnostic** department, records results of the "brain wave" test, which determines electrical activity within a client's brain. The EEG department also administers evoked-potential examinations, does specialized sleep studies, and monitors clients who have seizures.

The electrocardiogram (**ECG/EKG**), a recording of the heart's electrical activity, may be done by a specialized department or by the intensive care unit (ICU) or EEG department. The electromyogram (**EMG**), a record of the minute electrical impulses within muscles, may be done by the EEG, ECG, phys-

ical therapy, or respiratory care department, or in the clinical laboratory.

Direct Client Care Departments

Therapies

The physical therapy (**PT**) department directs its efforts toward preventing physical disability. PT staff assist clients to regain the best possible function of their affected body parts through individually planned programs of exercise and activity, with emphasis on gross (large) motor muscle activity. PT employees include registered physical therapists (**RPTs**) and physical therapist assistants (**PTAs**).

By using diversional or craft activities, the occupational therapy (**OT**) department helps clients move toward rehabilitation, paying attention to fine motor skills and activities of daily living (**ADL**). OT staff may aid clients in training for a job or in homemaking skills, as well as therapy. Employees include registered occupational therapists (**OTRs:** *occupational therapists, registered*) and certified occupational therapy assistants (**COTAs**).

The respiratory therapy (**RT**) department, also known as the respiratory care department or cardiopulmonary (**CP**) department, is responsible for measures prescribed by healthcare providers to assist clients who have certain cardiac or respiratory disorders. Registered respiratory therapists (**RRT**) and technicians provide treatment and support to clients in other departments. Examples include clients on ventilators in the ICU, or clients with traumatic injuries in the emergency department. Respiratory therapists also provide services to clients on nursing units. They often oversee oxygen administration throughout the hospital. The RT department may draw blood for blood gas analysis and perform special tests, including pulmonary function, vital capacity, and cardiac stress tests. Personnel include respiratory therapists and technicians.

Some facilities also provide music therapy, recreational therapy, and play therapy. These services are most common in facilities that contain rehabilitation, psychiatric, chemical dependency, and children's therapy units, and those that work with people who have some sort of intellectual impairment.

Surgery

The staff in the operating room (**OR**) and the post-anesthesia care unit (**PACU**)—also called the recovery room (**RR**) or the post-anesthesia recovery room (**PARR**)—are concerned with the care of surgical clients immediately before, during, and after surgery. They may also manage a same-day surgery unit (**SDSU**) or ambulatory surgery unit (**ASU**). Many surgery centers outside the hospital provide similar services.

Nursing Care Units

Nurse managers are responsible for the nursing unit (station) or several units. Usually, nurse managers must ensure that the units function well and that quality care is provided in each. *Assistant nurse managers* or *charge nurses* provide direct supervision during their assigned shift. Other nursing personnel include *team leaders, primary nurses,* and *staff nurses* or *clinical nurses,* as well as *nursing assistants* or other *unlicensed assistive personnel* (**UAP**). *Clinical nurse specialists* and *case managers* are often part of the nursing team. Many units have a *secretary.* Various departments or units provide specific care, and may require nursing staff to acquire special in-service education for that particular area of practice.

The pediatric (**PEDS**) unit is responsible for the care of children. In large hospitals, the PEDS department may be divided according to children's ages.

The obstetrics (**OB**) department, sometimes called a "birthing center," provides care to mothers and newborns. Tradi-

tionally, the OB department was divided into a labor room, delivery or birthing room, newborn nursery, and postpartum unit (where women received care after delivery). Many hospitals now provide birthing-center rooms where the woman goes through labor, delivers the newborn, and remains with her baby throughout the postpartum period. In the current healthcare climate, the length of stay in birthing centers is considerably shorter than in the past, and may be less than 24 hours in some facilities (see Unit 10).

The *medical unit* is responsible for caring for adults who have medical conditions or disorders that do not require surgery. The *surgical unit* is involved in the care of clients before and after surgery. In a large hospital, the basic medical-surgical divisions may be subdivided into many divisions. These include orthopedics (**ORTHO**) for musculoskeletal disorders; urology (**UROL**) or genitourinary (**GU**) for disorders of the kidneys, bladder, liver, and male reproductive system; neurology (**NEURO**) for central or peripheral nervous system disorders, including disorders of the brain; geriatrics (**GERI**) for care of older adults; dermatology (**DERM**) for skin disorders; oncology for cancer clients; psychiatry (**PSYCH**) or mental health (**MH**) for mental health and emotional disorders; and gynecology (**GYN**) for female reproductive disorders.

Specialized Client Care Departments

Specialized departments and units are designed to give medical-surgical and nursing care for different degrees of illness:

The emergency department (**ED**) gives care to persons whose conditions require immediate attention. Clients may arrive on their own, by ambulance, or by air transport. Staff is specially certified and prepared to manage traumatic injuries, provide cardiopulmonary resuscitation, and care for clients with a variety of critical and urgent conditions. In some facilities, social workers, chaplains, and crisis teams also provide services in EDs.

The intensive care unit (**ICU**) provides care for critically ill clients. Many hospitals have specialized ICUs, such as neonatal or newborn (**NICU**), pediatric (**PICU**), surgical (**SICU**), medical (**MICU**), and trauma (**TICU**). Many facilities require nurses to obtain critical care certification before they can work in ICUs.

The coronary care unit (**CCU**) cares for clients with serious heart disorders. Nurses who work in CCUs are specially prepared in cardiac care. After their conditions have stabilized, clients may move into a coronary step-down unit or a coronary rehabilitation unit (**CRU**).

The dialysis unit provides care for clients who need chronic renal (kidney) dialysis.

The mental health unit (**MHU**) serves clients with emotional or psychiatric disorders.

The chemical dependency unit (**CDU**) serves persons who abuse chemical substances.

The clinical decision unit (also abbreviated **CDU**) provides care for clients who need additional observation, diagnostic testing, or treatment before hospital admission or discharge. Stays in this unit are usually less than 24 hours.

Many facilities use this area as a chest pain center and treat and observe stable chest pain clients here.

The *intermediate care unit* provides care for clients requiring a moderate amount of skilled nursing care.

The *self-care unit* provides care for clients who are transitioning from the hospital or skilled nursing facility to the home. Clients care for themselves as much as possible; staff provide assistance as needed.

The rehabilitation (**REHAB**) unit, also called physical medicine and rehabilitation (**PM&R**), provides psychosocial support and rehabilitative services to people who have a physical disability and need assistance to regain as much capacity for activity as possible. Many clients in REHAB have experienced trauma, strokes, head injuries, and brain damage from drug overdoses or accidents.

Hospice, also called *palliative care,* gives physical and emotional care to dying individuals. Hospice staff provide clients and families with support and assistance in dealing with terminal illness and death (see Chapter 99).

The outpatient department (**OPD**) provides care for clients after discharge from the facility, or clients who can be treated without being admitted to the hospital.

The *client education department* provides educational services for staff, clients, and the community. Educators teach complex procedures to clients and their family caregivers. In many facilities, this department is also responsible for staff development and community wellness programs.

Support Services

The facility's *administration* oversees the efficiency of all departments. The administrative team may include several executives responsible for different functions, such as nursing, clinical services, human resources, financial services, or physician services. Other support services in the hospital include:

The *dietary* department (*nutritional therapy*) prepares all meals for clients, in accordance with instructions given by healthcare providers. *Dietitians* teach clients and families about special diets. This department also may prepare meals for the staff and visitors.

The *pharmacy* is responsible for dispensing medications ordered by healthcare providers. *Pharmacists* may instruct clients on the use and side effects of prescribed medications.

The central service supply (**CSS**) or central supply room (**CSR**) cleans and sterilizes equipment and instruments for use throughout the facility. In many facilities, most stock supplies are processed through CSS if a central storage area is unavailable.

The *admissions* department and *business office* process clients when they enter and leave the facility. Bills are paid and insurance claims are processed in the business office.

The *medical records* department keeps medical records for all clients who have ever been in the facility. The department is responsible for ensuring that all notations are made on the chart and that the chart is complete. The Accredited Record Technician (**ART**) or Registered Record Administrator (**RRA**) may be called into court with the chart during a legal action.

Volunteer services assists in many ways. *Volunteers* may operate a gift shop; deliver mail, flowers, magazines, toys, and books to clients; operate an information desk in the lobby; or run a coffee shop. They often bring clients to the nursing unit from the admitting department and transport clients for discharge or special tests. Often, volunteers are available to assist families of clients who are having surgery or are in the ICU, or to be with new fathers during delivery.

The *chaplaincy services* provides spiritual support to clients and families during illness, surgery, and death. Many facilities have a chapel. Nondenominational worship services and religious rituals may be provided.

The *social services* department provides counseling and assistance to clients and families in matters of finance, home care, discharge planning, and living arrangements. Social workers may make referrals to outside agencies that can assist families with special needs and often facilitate support groups and family-team meetings. Social services may also assist at discharge, or may help refer clients to a public health nurse or other specialized agency for continuing care after discharge.

The management information services (**MIS**) department provides computer support for the organization. Many hospitals, clinics, and outpatient services are linked through a network and communicate vital information about clients as they use various services in the system. Automated services may include the documenting in client records, billing, reporting lab and x-ray results, ordering tests and services, and collecting data for planning purposes. **Telecommunications** enables healthcare providers to communicate with clients in different locations using a telephone and a computer. Telecommunications allows providers to review images, tests, lab values, and ECGs; to examine skin conditions; and to diagnose conditions without clients needing to come into the facility. This service is tremendously important in rural areas with limited medical and transportation resources.

The *case management* department provides service coordination, health assessment, education, and discharge planning for clients who are at high risk for readmission. Once high-risk clients are identified, case managers follow up with them after discharge into the community to maximize wellness, provide healthcare, and coordinate services.

The quality improvement (**QI**) department, also called continuous quality improvement (**CQI**), promotes the organization's efforts toward ensuring quality care by continually improving systems, services, and processes and enhancing customer service and satisfaction. In the past, this department primarily reviewed records for quality issues. Most organizations are now concerned with meeting and exceeding customer expectations, improving performance throughout the organization, and improving processes to remove barriers to excellent service.

The consulting nurse service (**telehealth**) provides telephone advice to callers who need assistance deciding if and when to seek medical attention. Based on the severity of a caller's symptoms, the service advises callers to seek care immediately, to make an appointment, or to try home care measures. Nurses use approved protocols (which are often computerized) to assess the problem and to provide advice. In many organizations, this service is combined with physician referral services and community health and wellness education services.

➤ STUDENT SYNTHESIS

Key Points

- The needs of clients include the basic needs of all human beings plus special needs connected with illness or injury.
- The client unit is the area in which the nurse delivers most nursing care.
- The client care unit in the hospital, ECF, home, or clinic is designed to meet healthcare needs.
- A clean and orderly unit helps to prevent accidents and infections and to maximize efficiency.
- Certain guidelines are common for all nursing procedures. Some procedures are grouped according to time of day.
- Healthcare facilities offer a wide variety of services and are often staffed with personnel who have special training. Direct client care departments, specialized client care departments, and support services are found within many facilities.
- Many services provided in the hospital are also provided in ECFs, clinics, and the home.

Critical Thinking Exercises

1. Your client is spending the first full day in your care in an acute care facility. Describe the basic activities for that day. Discuss your responsibilities. How will your coordination of activities help your client?
2. Your client is a 35-year-old homemaker and single mother of three small children. She has broken her right arm and is soon to be discharged from acute

care. Describe hospital and community support services that may be used in her care and discharge.
3. How would your role and degree of autonomy change in the following settings: hospital, ECF, clinic, home care, consulting nurse service?
4. Discuss how telecommunications, consulting nurse services (telehealth), and case management can help to provide cost-effective care for the client outside the hospital setting. How does this care reduce healthcare costs?

NCLEX-Style Review Questions

1. Steps of a nursing procedure may vary in different facilities, but the underlying principles do not change and usually are related to:
   a. Maintaining client safety
   b. Providing comfort
   c. Providing privacy
   d. Stabilizing the client
2. When orienting a client to the hospital room, the nurse should first demonstrate how to operate the:
   a. Electronic thermometer
   b. Nurse call signal
   c. Telephone
   d. Television
3. The nurse is going to complete a procedure on a client that is painful. Which statement would be the most appropriate?
   a. "I'm sorry I have to do this painful procedure."
   b. "It will be painful, but only for a short time."
   c. "Most clients say the pain subsides quickly after the procedure."
   d. "You may feel some discomfort with this procedure."
4. A client who is on a special diet is admitted to the nursing unit. Which department would the nurse notify?
   a. Admissions department
   b. Central service supply
   c. Dietary department
   d. Social services department
5. A client needs to have blood drawn for a blood gas analysis. Whom should the nurse notify to complete this procedure?
   a. Ambulatory surgery unit
   b. Respiratory therapy department
   c. Emergency department
   d. Special care unit

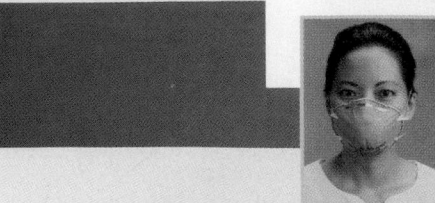

CHAPTER

39

Emergency Preparedness

LEARNING OBJECTIVES

1. List at least 10 nursing measures that help to prevent accidents in the healthcare facility.
2. Identify five potentially hazardous materials.
3. Describe the use of a material safety data sheet (MSDS).
4. Describe at least five safety tips to consider when using and storing hazardous substances.
5. Explain the use of the emergency signal in the client's bathroom.
6. Identify alternate methods of communication when a disruption occurs in telephone service.
7. List at least five things to consider when developing a personal emergency preparedness plan.
8. Discuss the difference between an internal and an external disaster.
9. Describe actions to take when a bomb threat occurs.
10. Define triage.
11. List three things to consider when evacuation from a facility or a client's home is necessary.
12. Explain the acronym RACE and its relationship to the fire plan.
13. List four classes of fire extinguishers and their uses.

NEW TERMINOLOGY

command center
crash cart
employee right-to-know
  laws

external disaster
internal disaster
triage

ACRONYMS

| CPR | MSDS | RACE |
| DMAT | OSHA | START |

Safety promotion and accident prevention are important in the healthcare facility, community, and home. A safe environment is one in which little risk for illness or injury exists. Every person in a healthcare organization is responsible for safety.

The disastrous events of September 11, 2001 have graphically illustrated the need for emergency preparedness at all times by all healthcare facilities. In addition, you must understand the necessity for safety and emergency preparedness, your facility's disaster plan, and your role in emergencies. This knowledge helps you to perform competently and confidently when an emergency occurs.

SAFETY AND PREPAREDNESS

Safety extends to clients, employees, and visitors. The goal is twofold: to prevent accidents and to be prepared for emergencies. Prevention is the key. Nurses are important providers of safety and emergency care. As a nurse, you will be exposed to a number of safety hazards and emergency conditions in healthcare facilities and in the community. Power outages, road closures, and inclement weather can affect the delivery of healthcare. In addition to prevention, you must know where emergency equipment is kept in the facility or in the client's home, and how and whom to call in various emergencies.

The Safety Committee

Every healthcare facility is required to have a designated safety committee, whose goal is to provide a safe environment for clients, employees, and visitors. Some of the committee's responsibilities include establishing principles of worker safety, staff management, and occupational health nursing; analyzing job safety; investigating accidents; and tracking injury and illness rates. This committee usually includes representatives from the departments of administration, infection control, industrial hygiene, fire/safety, engineering, environmental management, human resources, and nursing.

Client Safety

A client has the right to expect that a healthcare facility will protect against injury and disease. Safety measures in healthcare facilities include essential precautions, such as general emergency preparedness, plans for specific emergencies (eg, fire), and plans for evacuation. Other measures include provisions for resuscitation and correct administration of medications and treatments. A more subtle aspect of safety is proper waste disposal to prevent both environmental contamination and exposure to infectious materials. Many clients and healthcare providers are developing a sensitivity to latex. Most healthcare organizations have plans for providing safety for latex-sensitive individuals. (Chapter 42 discusses latex allergies in greater detail.)

Accident Prevention

Most accidents are preventable with proper knowledge and attention to safety hazards. All staff should work together to prevent accidents. Observe and take action in potentially hazardous situations. For example, if you notice a piece of chipped glass on a client's food tray or a spilled substance on the floor, take immediate corrective action. If an accident does occur, follow your facility's procedure for documenting the circumstances in an official accident, incident, or variance report. In Practice: Nursing Care Guidelines 39-1 provides information to help prevent accidents.

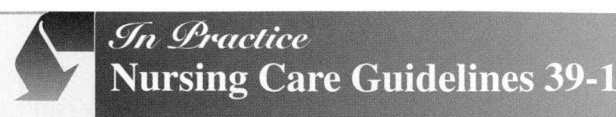

In Practice
Nursing Care Guidelines 39-1

PREVENTING ACCIDENTS

- Keep floors dry and clean to prevent falls. Know the proper and safe method for cleaning up spills of various substances.
- Keep halls free of obstacles, and promote good order at all times.
- Lock medicine carts and do not leave them unattended. Keep the keys on your person at all times. In the home, be sure to have the client and family keep all medicines out of the reach of children.
- Get adequate assistance to move and walk clients. Use a transfer belt when necessary.
- Administer medications properly; ask the nurse manager, team leader, primary nurse, or pharmacist any questions you have. Know how to use drug reference books.
- Provide adequate lighting. In the home, encourage the use of a night light.
- Place the client's necessary items within his or her reach, including the call light or bell.
- Check the temperature of any liquid or solution (including water) before giving it to the client.
- Raise the height of the client's bed to prevent back strain when you work with a client. Keep the bed in a low position at other times.
- Raise side rails as ordered for clients who are very old, very young, disoriented, confused, or sedated. When side rails are down, do not leave these clients unattended.
- Do not perform unfamiliar procedures without proper supervision. You are responsible for learning the procedures specific to your facility.
- Check all equipment routinely to ensure it is working properly. Check electrical cords for tangles, loose plugs, and fraying.
- Make sure sterile packages are dry and unopened and that medications have not expired or are otherwise unfit for use.
- Check on all clients frequently to make sure they are comfortable.
- Always be aware of safety rules. (For example, never leave a client unattended who has a rectal thermometer in place.)
- Do not allow a client to use electrical equipment in the home unless it has been inspected for safety.
- Do not heat blankets, towels, or intravenous solutions in the microwave.

Safety for the Left-Handed Client.   The majority of people are right handed, and thus the typical client environment is arranged to facilitate the movement and action of a right-handed person. However, when the person is left-handed, modifications are necessary to prevent the client from twisting and turning and possibly injuring him- or herself.

Always be sure to ask the client if he or she is right- or left-handed. Then if the client is left-handed, rearrange items appropriately. For example, place the telephone, bedside stand, call signal, and television controls on the client's left side. This way the client can use these items without straining or twisting to reach them. This same principle applies to the client who has the use of only one arm or hand or who has one eye patched. Keep in mind that the client who is left-handed is often "left-footed." Take this into consideration when assisting the client out of bed and when ambulating the client.

Fall-Prone Assessment.   Falls are the most common cause of injury for older adults. Help to prevent falls in the healthcare facility or in the client's home by considering these factors for each client:

- Level of awareness vs. level of confusion or disorientation
- Ability to communicate and understand
- Availability of mobility devices, such as walker or cane
- Potential for unsafely attempting to walk without assistance
- Ability to move about and conduct activities of daily living
- Placement of furniture, use of rugs
- Level of lighting
- Physical condition and medications that might increase the risk of injury
- Presence of small animals/pets in the home
- Availability of caregivers

Assessment of these factors helps to determine if a client is likely to be at risk for falling. This is known as a "fall-prone" or "fall-risk" assessment. Other factors, such as age, substance abuse, or a history of cardiovascular problems, may need to be considered on an individual basis.

Electrical Safety

Electric shocks are preventable. Water conducts electricity. Dry your hands before inserting a plug into or removing it from an electric outlet. Never turn appliances on or off when you are in contact with water. Always disconnect equipment by grasping the plug; do not pull on the cord. Always have frayed or worn cords repaired to prevent fires, short circuits, and blown circuit breakers. Disconnect equipment and turn off motors as soon as you are finished using an electrical apparatus. Teach clients and family members to follow these same measures. If you are working in a hospital or ECF, notify the maintenance department of any malfunction, including excess heat or burning odors from a running motor. Notify your supervisor when you identify safety hazards in the community setting or home. *But first, immediately remove or otherwise address the source of imminent danger.*

Employee Safety

Employee Right-to-Know Laws

Individual states have enacted **employee right-to-know laws,** legislation enforced by the Occupational Safety and Health Administration (**OSHA**). These laws state that employees have the right to be aware of dangers associated with hazardous substances or harmful physical or infectious agents that they might encounter in the workplace (including healthcare facilities) (Table 39-1).

Each facility must have on file a material safety data sheet (**MSDS**) about each substance that is considered hazardous. The MSDS provides information about a substance's potential dangers and describes the product, its ingredients, its physical properties, fire or explosion hazards, and reactivity. The MSDS also gives information on protective equipment required, safe handling information (in case of a spill or leak), and first-aid interventions for accidental exposure. An MSDS is also maintained for potential industrial hazards in the community. This information helps staff provide appropriate treatment and to take necessary protective precautions when exposed to contaminated individuals who arrive in the emergency department. All staff must be instructed in the use of MSDSs and protective gear. MSDSs for toxic substances must be kept for a period of not less than 30 years.

Guidelines for Using Hazardous Substances

Hazardous substances are used daily in healthcare facilities and in the home. Remember the following safety tips when using and storing hazardous substances:

- Have the phone number of the poison control center readily available.
- Read labels carefully and note emergency information.
- Follow instructions for use, storage, and disposal.
- Avoid spills.
- Use protective equipment as recommended.
- Never use any substance that is not labeled.
- Do not store hazardous materials in familiar food or drink containers.
- Keep household chemicals in their original containers.
- Do not use gasoline indoors.
- Do not mix substances.
- Do not use hairspray or other aerosol products around an open flame or contact lenses.
- Avoid breathing mists or vapors; keep areas well ventilated. (Chapter 43 describes first aid for exposure to hazardous materials.)

■■■ **TABLE 39-1** $\mathcal{O}$**CCUPATIONAL HAZARDS**

Hazard	Example
Flammables	Alcohol, oxygen
Poisons	Clorosorb
Skin or eye irritants	Hibiclens
Carcinogens	Formalin
Harmful physical agents	Radiation

- Follow radiation prevention guidelines closely. Radiation is a potential source of accidents.

☛ KEY CONCEPT

Every staff member in a facility should participate in accident prevention and in client and employee safety.

Emergency Preparedness

Nurse's Call Light and Intercom

Place the nurse's call light button within reach of the client at all times and remind the client to use it whenever necessary. Make sure the client can physically reach and operate the call button. Explain to the client how to use the intercom to request assistance. This will help the healthcare staff to respond appropriately in an emergency. Check the client frequently if he or she is sedated, confused, or physically unable to use the call light. A tap bell may be used.

Emergency Signal

In most facilities, using the emergency signal device in the client's bathroom causes an additional light to flash or a buzzer to sound at a central station. This signal may be used by the client when experiencing difficulty while in the bathroom or by the staff to request emergency assistance, for example, when a client goes into cardiac arrest. Staff respond quickly to the emergency signal. If the client is in a multi-bed room, another client can help by pressing the bathroom alarm button and then using the intercom to explain the nature of the emergency.

Many home care clients can activate an alert system when they are having difficulty or feel they have an emergency. The signal is carried by the client and activates an alarm in a designated location, such as an emergency department. The client is then contacted by telephone, a neighbor is alerted to check on the client, or the local emergency medical response providers are contacted and directed to the client's residence.

Emergency Resuscitation

Knowing the location and use of emergency resuscitation equipment is essential. In the hospital and skilled nursing facility (SNF), each nursing unit generally has an emergency cart (**crash cart**) stocked with emergency medications and equipment. Check this cart regularly according to the facility's protocol to make sure all items are there and in good condition.

Know the procedure for calling the cardiopulmonary resuscitation (**CPR**) team in the facility (termed "calling a code") or the emergency response service in the community health setting. "Code Blue" and "Dr. Blue" also are designations commonly used in facilities to designate a cardiopulmonary arrest. Many clinics have some resuscitative equipment or a plan for obtaining help immediately. Most healthcare organizations require CPR certification for all healthcare personnel.

☛ KEY CONCEPT

Each emergency will have its own code name in the facility's public address system. All healthcare providers must learn how to initiate and interpret the code system(s) used in the facility.

Personal Preparedness

Preparing for emergencies is important in the home, workplace, and community. Unexpected emergencies such as an earthquake, wind storm, flood, or inclement weather can disrupt an individual's personal life and ability to care for clients. Nurses who provide care in the home need to be prepared for travel through a weather emergency, disaster area, or other emergency situation. You may be asked to help during an emergency and to provide care in a variety of settings including shelters, clinics, or other hospitals. This may involve working long hours away from your home and family. Taking the time to develop a *personal emergency preparedness plan* will help you to cope with such a situation and its effects on your home, family, and work. Box 39-1 offers a list of pointers for developing your own emergency preparedness plan.

➤➤ BOX 39-1

PERSONAL EMERGENCY PREPAREDNESS

- Plan for prolonged power outages. Store flashlights, battery-powered lamps, and extra batteries.
- Keep a first-aid kit, a portable radio, flashlights, and extra batteries on hand.
- Store 1 gallon of water per person in your household per day, and adequate food supplies to last 4 days. Store additional water and food for pets.
- Maintain sufficient gas in your car, and have cash on hand to last several days. During power outages, gas pumps, cash machines, banks, and most retail stores are closed.
- Store prescriptions, glasses, dentures, hearing aids, and other essential items in a secure and accessible area.
- Develop a family plan. Identify safe areas in the home to hide in during different types of disasters. Establish a meeting place near the home for emergencies such as fire, and away from the home in case you are unable to return to the area due to floods or blocked roadways.
- Select a relative or friend outside your area as a contact point for your family to call and leave messages with. Write down addresses and telephone numbers for family members to keep in their wallets. Knowing your loved ones are safe will help you to focus on your work.
- Carry an emergency kit in your car including walking shoes, flashlight, batteries, maps, water, extra clothing, blankets, flares, jumper cables, wire, duct tape, cellular phone, and gear appropriate for conditions in your area.
- Plan ahead what you would take if you had to evacuate your home. Write it down. Decisions are more difficult to make during a time of crisis.
- Have a plan for child care when school closures occur.
- Identify potential hazards that might block your usual travel route. Identify alternative routes that may not be impeded by water, debris, or other disruption in the roadway.

☞ KEY CONCEPT

Making good decisions and coping with disruptions are easier to do when you are prepared for a disaster or emergency.

THE DISASTER PLAN

A *disaster plan* describes the actions to take in the event of a disaster. The disaster plan is activated when an incident produces casualties of such a number that the routine methods for client care are inadequate. All employees need to know the disaster plan for their organization. Healthcare facilities are required to have regular, periodic fire and disaster drills to allow their staff to practice emergency skills. Each healthcare facility has a plan for natural disasters common to its area of the country. These disasters may include tornadoes, blizzards, hurricanes, earthquakes, avalanches, floods, or mud slides. Facilities also have plans for bomb threats and hazardous materials spills. Find out what the plans are in your organization. If a disaster occurs, you will be prepared and able to protect yourself and your clients calmly. Box 39-2 is an example of a disaster plan for a bomb threat situation.

With any threat, notify the facility's security personnel or the local police immediately. Do not attempt to decide on your own if the threat is real or not. Call and let trained personnel decide what action to take.

Internal Versus External Disasters

Two basic types of disasters exist in healthcare facilities. The first is an **internal disaster,** in which the facility itself is in danger or damaged and function is impaired. An internal disaster may be caused by a fire, an explosion, terrorist activity, radiation, a chemical spill, or a storm. An **external disaster** occurs outside the facility but impairs normal facility operations. It requires the organization to activate the disaster plan to prepare to receive a large number of casualties or to evacuate. It may require the facility to evacuate existing clients to make room to receive incoming disaster casualties. Earthquakes, floods, hurricanes, explosions, airplane crashes, or chemical spills are types of external disasters. Specific plans are executed for each type of disaster. In the event of an earthquake or tornado, the facility may have to prepare for both an internal and an external disaster. A facility that has sustained significant damage may have to evacuate portions of the building while continuing to provide emergency care from another location in the facility.

Staff Notification

Healthcare facilities usually incorporate the use of a cascade call system ("telephone tree") during a disaster. The cascade system is a means of notifying staff by telephone that a disaster has occurred and that their assistance is needed immediately. The system includes both on- and off-duty personnel. Key people are called and they, in turn, call others. The cas-

➤➤ BOX 39-2

SAMPLE BOMB THREAT DISASTER PLAN

If you receive any bomb threat, immediately notify your supervisor. If you receive the threat over the phone, follow these guidelines:

Ask these questions and write down the caller's answers:
- Where is the bomb, exactly?
- What does it look like?
- What will make it explode?
- How can we stop it from exploding?
- When is it going to explode?
- Why was it put there?
- Who are you?

Listen to other cues and note the things you hear:
- Voice characteristics—such as loud, pleasant, intoxicated
- Speech—such as fast, slow, slurred
- Language—such as foul or use of scientific terms
- Accent—such as local, foreign, male or female
- Manner—such as calm, angry, incoherent
- Background noises—such as machines, airplanes, street traffic

General Guidelines
- Stay away from windows or other large glass objects during the search.
- Search the area as directed by your supervisor. Look for something out of place, unusual, or new to the area.
- Look for something that makes a strange or different noise.
- Search the area in sections and from floor to ceiling.
- Notify your supervisor if you find something suspicious. Do not touch or open it. Clear the area.
- Do not use elevators until the situation is cleared.

cade system speeds up the process of notifying staff that they are needed. Personnel are expected to arrive at the facility, if at all possible, within 30 minutes.

When telephone service is disrupted, several other means of communicating with staff and other healthcare providers are available, including:

- Cellular phones
- Amateur radio operators
- Television or radio broadcasts
- Runners (people who transport messages on foot)
- Computers (E-mail)
- Contacts outside the affected area
- Pagers
- Portable or hand-held radios
- Police

Implementation

The healthcare facility's disaster plan describes the duties and responsibilities of individuals within the organization in case of a disaster. Nursing staff are generally instructed to report to their general area of duty or to a centrally designated area for assignment. Persons working at the time of the disaster may be asked to assist in another area or location. Your supervisor will assign you to specific duties.

A disaster plan will identify the location of the **command center,** the purpose of which is to provide overall direction of the facility's activities. Additional responsibilities include communicating with areas receiving those affected, assigning personnel to areas needing assistance, releasing information to the press, and monitoring the extent of the disaster and its potential affect on the facility.

Triage

You may be assigned to assist in **triage,** which is the process of sorting and classifying injured persons to determine priority of needs. All injured people are identified, if possible, along with names of next-of-kin. The triage person also assigns victims to the proper place for treatment. In the event of a major disaster, people with minimal injuries may be asked to assist with those who are in more critical condition.

When a disaster such as a bombing, airplane crash, hurricane, or earthquake strikes, how you triage can mean the difference between life and death. The simple triage and rapid treatment (**START**) system identifies people who are going to die quickly if they do not receive immediate medical care. START is taught to first responders in the community who are trained in advanced first aid. Chapter 43 also discusses triage.

Disaster Medical Assistance Team

Disaster medical assistance team (**DMAT**) provides assistance and support in many environments both inside and outside healthcare facilities. They may set up a temporary hospital or may be called on to relieve facility staff when a large disaster strikes. During a disaster, staff often work long hours and may be stressed physically and emotionally. Healthcare personnel often provide care for those who have been injured when they may have suffered their own personal losses. DMAT can provide relief when there is a shortage of workers and can relieve workers who need to rest. The team includes physicians, nurses, and emergency medical technicians.

Evacuation

Sometimes the threat of fire or disaster is severe enough to require evacuation of the facility. The extent of the emergency will affect the decision to evacuate a portion of the facility or the entire facility. There are a number of ways to evacuate clients. Those who can walk or use wheelchairs are usually evacuated first. Others may require transporting on stretchers, dragging on sheets, or passing the client and sheet along from person to person. Maternity and nursery nurses may wear large aprons that fit several babies at one time. You may be asked to help relocate essential equipment, such as emergency resuscitation carts and intravenous infusion pumps and solutions, for use in another area. Each client should be wearing an ID band. Babies must be identified. Take the client's personal items such as glasses, dentures, and hearing aids as well as medical records, if time permits. Consider taking your own personal belongings as well. Sometimes long delays exist before anyone can re-enter an evacuated area.

During times of disaster, home care agencies usually try to involve family members or friends in evacuating the client. If that resource is not available, local emergency preparedness agencies must be used for transportation. These agencies will need to know the location of the client and the client's specific needs to ensure quick and proper evacuation. If the home care client cannot be moved to the home of family or friends outside the area, he or she may need to be admitted to a hospital or ECF. Most shelters are not equipped to deal with clients with special needs.

Special Situations

Several special situations may arise that are potentially dangerous. Box 39-2 describes the steps to take in the event of a bomb threat. It is vital that you act quickly.

If you suspect that a person is carrying a weapon of any kind and has entered the facility, notify your security personnel or the police immediately. Remember that a weapon is not only a gun; it can be a knife, club, or any other item that can be used to inflict harm.

Kidnapping

The kidnapping of a baby or small child in a healthcare facility involves special procedures. Most hospitals do not allow any baby or small child who is hospitalized to be carried—they must be in a rolling bassinet or crib. If you see a baby or small child in hospital garb being carried, alert your supervisor and call a "code." Many hospitals use the term "Code Pink" to denote a missing baby. In the event of such a code, all entrances to the facility are immediately shut down and guarded, and the facility is thoroughly searched until the child is found.

Work Stoppages

Unfortunately, work stoppages can involve nurses and other healthcare personnel. In the event of a strike in your facility, you must decide whether or not to cross the picket line if you are a part of the involved bargaining unit. If you are not on strike, you will often be expected to work. You may also be asked to work in an area of the facility which is different from your regular assignment.

THE FIRE PLAN

Fire is a major hazard that may be caused by improper management of flammable materials or gases, careless smoking, frayed electrical wiring, or faulty equipment. Most healthcare facilities do not permit smoking. Smoking in the home care environment is more difficult to control; however, you must teach clients and their families about safety hazards. Alert the client and family to the particular dangers of smoking when oxygen is in use (see Chap. 86). In Practice: Educating the Client 39-1 reviews pointers for fire safety in the home.

Fire Prevention

Fire prevention requires a constant state of alertness to possible danger areas or situations. Follow these general preventive measures:

- Enforce "no smoking" regulations.
- Inspect the home care client's home for potential fire hazards.
- Be sure no smoking occurs near oxygen use or storage.
- Make sure all equipment is operating properly.
- Practice electrical safety (eg, no frayed cords, no three-prong adapters, no "cluster plugs," no extension cords).
- Make sure fire alarms, fire doors, and emergency stairs are clearly marked and unobstructed. NEVER prop open a fire door!
- Regularly practice procedures to follow in case of a fire.

General Procedures

If a fire does occur, every staff member must know exactly what to do to protect clients and themselves:
- Know where emergency equipment is located.
- Know the types of extinguishers appropriate for different types of fires.
- Know how to use a fire extinguisher.
- Know the location of fire alarms and the procedure for calling in a fire alarm.
- Know what to do to ensure the safety of clients in the immediate area of the fire.
- Do not panic.

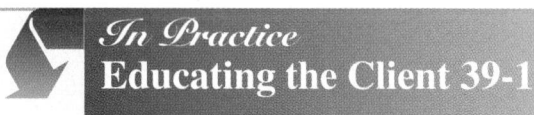

In Practice
Educating the Client 39-1

WAYS TO PROMOTE FIRE SAFETY IN THE HOME

- Check all electrical cords. Place them out of the flow of traffic. Look for frayed or cracked cords. Make sure extension cords are used properly.
- Look for smoke detectors and check that they are working properly. Also check to make sure that the family changes the battery regularly.
- Assist the family with developing an emergency exit plan if they do not have one.
- Check space heaters. Keep them out of the flow of traffic. Keep flammable materials away from heaters.
- Assess the kitchen for adequate ventilation and presence of flammable materials near the stove.
- Make sure potential fire sources are cleared away from the bed.
- Observe storage areas for flammable liquids.

- Keep clients calm.
- Know how to protect clients from injury.
- Use common sense.
- Know the code name for "fire" in your facility's public address system. "Mr. Red," "Dr. Red," and "Code Red" are common names used.

RACE is an acronym that may help you to remember the general order of procedures for a fire:

R = Rescue: Remove clients from the general area
A = Alert/Alarm: Sound alarm
C = Confine: Contain fire (close doors and windows, make sure fire doors close)
E = Extinguish fire

Various facilities may use different acronyms, but the intent is the same.

Rescue
Rescue the client from immediate danger before doing anything else. Lead the client who can walk into the hall. Close the door to the room, then sound the alarm. Assist the client who cannot walk into a chair and remove it from the room, or drag the client out of the room on a sheet. (Do not try to carry a client, unless he or she is a small child.)

Alarm
Use your facility's procedure to get help. Usually you will pull a fire alarm and call the switchboard operator. When you make a telephone call, be sure to tell the person the fire's exact location. Make sure all other clients are in a safe place. Notify other staff.

Confine
After you call in the alarm, close all doors, including fire and room doors. Check to make sure "automatic" doors close. Close open windows on the unit. Do not use elevators during a fire alarm. Do not use the telephone unnecessarily. Turn off or unplug unnecessary electrical appliances. Report to the nurse manager for further instructions.

Extinguish
Attempt to put out a fire only if you are sure you can do it safely. Different types of fire extinguishers are available for different types of fires (Table 39-2). Be sure that you know the type of extinguisher to use, based on the type of fire. Learn the locations of extinguishers in your clinical setting and read the operating instructions. Putting out a fire is the *last* thing to

▪▪▪ TABLE 39-2 *T*ypes of Fire Extinguishers

Type of Fire	Type of Extinguisher
Wood, paper, cloth	Type A
Flammable liquids (grease, anesthetics)	Type B
Electrical	Type C

A type ABC extinguisher can be used on any type of fire.

do after you have protected others and notified the authorities. *Do not* try to put out a fire yourself without first calling for help. Again, use common sense. All fires in a healthcare facility must be reported to the fire department. The fire department is required to respond to all healthcare facility fires, even if the fire has been extinguished to ensure safety.

➤ STUDENT SYNTHESIS

Key Points

- The safety committee functions in evaluating accidents that have occurred and in planning to prevent future occurrences.
- Nurses not only must prevent accidents but also must know what to do if an accident occurs.
- Staff members must be able to identify potentially hazardous substances and describe what to do if exposed to them.
- A personal emergency preparedness plan will help you to cope personally with the disruption caused by a disaster, allowing you to focus on caring for clients.
- A facility's disaster plan is set up to deal with both internal and external emergencies.
- Every staff member in a healthcare facility or community setting must be knowledgeable about fire safety.

Critical Thinking Exercises

1. If a fire occurred in your work area, describe the steps you would take to safely address the situation.
2. You arrive at your client's home to change a dressing and find the client in bed, sleeping, and barely holding onto a burning cigarette. Describe how you might handle this situation. What things are important to consider when assessing the home for safety?
3. A large earthquake occurs in the middle of the night. You are at work in the healthcare facility, which sustains damage. How would you handle this situation? What factors are important to consider? How would you handle communications if the phones were out? How would you check on the safety of your family?
4. How might a disaster or emergency affect your ability to provide care in the community or home?

NCLEX-Style Review Questions

1. What is the purpose of a material safety data sheet (MDSD)?
   a. Ensure all workers are aware of disaster plans.
   b. Explain emergency procedures to healthcare workers.
   c. Provide fire safety information.
   d. Provide information about hazardous materials.
2. The nurse notices that a client's electric bed has a frayed electrical cord. Which nursing action should be completed first?
   a. Apply tape to the frayed area.
   b. Inform the maintenance department.
   c. Remove the bed.
   d. Unplug the bed.
3. A flood in the community area would be classified as:
   a. A simple triage and rapid treatment
   b. A catastrophe
   c. An external disaster
   d. An internal disaster
4. A client is smoking a cigarette in a "no smoking" area. Which action should the nurse take?
   a. Inform the client this is a "no smoking" area and they will need to extinguish the cigarette.
   b. Notify the fire department immediately.
   c. Sound the fire alarm to prevent the spread of the fire.
   d. Take the cigarette from the client and extinguish it.
5. A fire is found in a client's room. A co-worker is removing the client. What action should you take?
   a. Confine the fire by closing all doors.
   b. Run to the nurses' station to notify the other staff.
   c. Sound the fire alarm.
   d. Tell family members to leave immediately.

CHAPTER

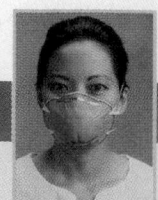

40

Microbiology and Defense Against Disease

LEARNING OBJECTIVES

1. Explain what microorganisms are and why an understanding of them is vital for all healthcare workers.
2. Define the term pathogen.
3. Name and describe the essential factors that influence microbial growth.
4. Describe how culture and sensitivity (C&S) reports and staining aid in the treatment of infectious diseases.
5. Identify the basic characteristics of the five main types of micro-organisms.
6. Describe the way in which bacteria are classified.
7. Discuss ways to prevent the development of drug-resistant bacteria.
8. Explain three basic ways in which infectious diseases are transmitted to people.
9. Name the components of the chain of infection.
10. Suggest ways to stop the spread of infection at each point in the chain.
11. Describe the effect of toxins on the body.
12. Describe factors that help determine if a pathogen will cause disease.

NEW TERMINOLOGY

aerobe	microorganism
anaerobe	mycosis
bacillus	opportunistic
bacteria	parasite
bacteriology	pathogen
coccus	prodromal
communicable	reservoir
contagious	sensitivity
culture	spirillum
endemic	spore
endotoxin	sterile
epidemic	suppurative
etiology	toxin
exotoxin	vector
flagellum	virulence
Gram's stain	virus
incubation period	

ACRONYMS

C&S	pH	TB
DNA	RNA	VRE
MRSA		

Microorganisms (minute living cells not visible to the naked eye) are found almost everywhere in the environment. *Microbiology* is the scientific study of microorganisms. Thousands of species of microorganisms exist in nature. Some are beneficial. For example, sharp, pungent cheeses owe their flavor to molds, and the decomposition of animal and plant wastes (which depends upon microorganisms) accounts for soil's fertile nature. Other microorganisms are harmful. You are likely to have heard and read about many diseases caused by microorganisms. For example, acquired immunodeficiency syndrome (AIDS) is caused by the human immunodeficiency virus (HIV). Lyme disease is caused by bacterium carried by tiny ticks.

Human understanding of methods of disease transmission has enabled the creation of technology that aids in disease prevention. Additionally, today's healthcare industry heavily emphasizes the teaching of sound personal, family, and community health practices to individuals in an effort to prevent the spread of disease. You are likely to care for clients who have infectious or communicable diseases. You will continually take measures to prevent the spread of disease, many of which are discussed throughout this unit and the entire book.

This chapter explains basic facts about microorganisms. It discusses their characteristics, their capacity for harm, their growth, the study of them, and their various forms. It introduces some types of diseases that microorganisms produce. This chapter explains how disease spreads, how to break the chain of infection in healthcare settings, and factors that influence the course of infection.

MICROORGANISMS

Structure and Function

Despite their small size, the cell structures of many microorganisms are similar to the cell structures of larger organisms, such as animals and plants. (However, bacteria lack certain structures, as well as membranes surrounding their genetic material. They do not have nuclei.)

Many large organisms (eg, human beings) take in oxygen, use it to burn food for energy and growth, and then excrete wastes in a process called *metabolism* (see Chaps. 15 and 25). Many microorganisms have this ability as well. They can also increase in size, divide, and produce new members of their species. They react in various ways to environmental changes. Many microorganisms are able to move under their own power. Some microorganisms safeguard themselves by forming protective capsules, or spores. Be aware that *viruses* are one type of microorganism that cannot perform all the essential functions characteristic of living things. These characteristics include: metabolism, growth, reproduction, irritability, motion, and protection.

Nature of Microorganisms

All human beings contain microorganisms in and on their bodies. Most of these microorganisms do not produce disease under normal conditions. These are called **endemic** organisms; those that are present all or most of the time in the environment or in the body. Microorganisms that cause disease are called **pathogens.** Pathogenic microorganisms have the potential to negatively affect a person's health.

Opportunistic microorganisms are those that usually do not cause disease, but can do so if the person is susceptible due to a compromised immune system (such as with AIDS) or other factors. These otherwise benign microorganisms become pathogenic *only to that person.* To more easily understand this idea, consider the following example. Microorganisms are always present in a person's digestive system. Some of them perform important digestive functions. Under usual circumstances, these microorganisms are not harmful and actually contribute to the body's proper functioning. They can cause disease, however, if they somehow gain access to the person's bloodstream or various body tissues.

☞ KEY CONCEPT

A relatively small percentage of microorganisms cause diseases and disorders. Most microorganisms are helpful.

Growth

Microorganisms are said to grow when the number of them at an individual site increases. At the beginning of a bacterial infection, a group of bacterial cells may number only a few hundred. As the bacteria reproduce, they form groups of many millions of individual cells, collectively called *colonies.* Certain environmental factors affect the growth of microorganisms.

Oxygen

Most microorganisms require oxygen for growth; these are called *obligate* **aerobes.** Some, called *obligate* **anaerobes,** cannot survive in the presence of oxygen. Other microorganisms can live in either the presence or absence of oxygen (*facultative anaerobes*).

Nutrients

A key ingredient for microbial growth is the presence of organic (carbon-containing) nutrients. Microorganisms also require other chemical elements, such as nitrogen for the manufacture of protein, and sulfur for protein and vitamin synthesis. Some microorganisms make their own food from raw materials, such as carbon dioxide. Others must find their nutrition ready-made.

Parasites are microorganisms that live on or within another living being (the host). *Saprophytes* live off the organic remains of dead plants and animals.

Temperature

The temperature at which a specific microorganism grows best is its *optimal temperature.* Most pathogenic microorganisms flourish at normal body temperature. Some types of microorganisms prefer either extremely cold or hot environments. Cold temperatures often significantly slow the growth of microorganisms, which is the reason refrigeration is used to control bacterial growth in food. High temperatures usually kill most microorganisms. Steam sterilization and boiling water are two common techniques used to kill pathogenic microorganisms.

Moisture

All microorganisms require water or moisture to grow. The matter in or on which they grow must contain available moisture (such as jellies) or may be a liquid (such as milk or blood).

pH

A substance's **pH** (hydrogen ion concentration; acidity or alkalinity) also affects growth. Generally, microorganisms survive only in environments with a pH that is neither too acidic nor too alkaline (see Chap. 17).

Light

Some microorganisms need light for growth. Other microorganisms, however, flourish in darkness. Many microorganisms die when they are exposed to the sun's ultraviolet rays, although moderately diffused light does not affect them.

Study Methods

Microbiologists can grow most microorganisms under controlled conditions in the laboratory. By studying microbial development, microbiologists learn and devise methods to prevent pathogenic growth.

Cultures

A growth of microorganisms prepared for laboratory study is called a **culture.** Cultures are usually grown in test tubes or on small, flat, covered plastic plates called *Petri dishes.* The material in or on which the microorganisms are placed is the *culture medium.* Various types of culture media serve different purposes. Solid media contain *agar,* which is obtained from a form of seaweed. Liquid media are called *nutrient broths.* All culture media contain specific nutrients designed to promote the growth of one or more types of microorganisms. Culture media must start out **sterile** (free from microbial contamination) for a valid study.

To see and study the individual characteristics of microorganisms grown in cultures, a small amount of the material to be examined is placed on a clean rectangular piece of glass called a *slide.* The slide is prepared especially for observation of the microorganisms. The microorganisms can be viewed in their living, moving state in a drop of liquid culture placed on a slide.

Identifying the microorganism that is causing disease is important to a disease's treatment. A culture and **sensitivity** (**C&S**) test is ordered when infection is suspected or known. The C&S test serves the following purposes:

- Identifies the pathogenic microorganism
- Determines which treatment will eliminate the microorganism
- Monitors the microorganism's response to therapy

The culture and sensitivity report will indicate the name of the test ordered, type of specimen (eg, blood, urine, sputum),

type of report (preliminary [within 24 hours] or final [usually within 48 hours]), colony count, type of microorganism (may be several), and susceptibility testing. The report will indicate the various antibiotics (if any) to which the organism is sensitive. Remember to collect specimens for cultures before administering antibiotic therapy. Antibiotics can temporarily lower the number of pathogens in the person's bloodstream, masking signs of infection. Chapter 52 describes methods of specimen collection.

Stains

Often, microorganisms are stained with a drop of dye so that their features become more clearly visible. One of the most common ways to stain a microorganism is called **Gram's stain,** which uses a series of dyes. Gram's staining is a way to rapidly categorize bacteria into one of two large groups. Gram-positive organisms retain the stain; gram-negative ones do not. Healthcare providers may then use this information to start antibiotic therapy immediately, instead of waiting for the full culture report.

Types

Microorganisms, like all living creatures, are categorized based on a variety of physical and biologic characteristics. Each organism has a name consisting of two parts. The *genus* refers to a general grouping and is listed first; the *species* defines a biologically unique category and is the second name. For example, the common bacterium *Escherichia coli (E. coli)* is found in the colon. Microorganisms fall into a number of large groups: algae, fungi, protozoa, bacteria, and viruses.

Algae

The many types of algae resemble plant cells. Algae are often found on sunlit water, appearing as green scum or green cloudy water. They are an important part of the environmental food chain. Algae rarely cause human disease.

Fungi

Fungi include the single-celled yeasts and the multicellular molds. An infection caused by a fungus is called a **mycosis.** Common *mycoses* (plural) include types of tinea (known as "ringworm" due to ring-shaped lesions). One type of ringworm, tinea capitis, is a lesion of the scalp often found in children. Another form is tinea pedis, also known as athlete's foot.

Yeasts. Yeast cells reproduce by a process called *budding.* Each parent cell produces a "daughter cell" or bud that eventually breaks off and grows in the same manner as the parent cell. Yeasts require sugars in solution as their food. When yeasts metabolize sugars in the absence of oxygen, a chemical change called *fermentation* occurs, producing alcohol and carbon dioxide. Many industries use controlled fermentation to manufacture products such as beer and bread.

An example of a pathogenic yeast is *Candida albicans,* which causes the disease known as *thrush.* Thrush produces a white growth in a person's mouth and on the tongue. *C. albicans* also causes approximately one third of cases of vaginitis (a yeast inflammation of the vagina).

Molds.   Multicellular molds are common in the environment. Some familiar molds appear as fuzzy patches on jelly and fruits, greenish growth on spoiled breads, and blue veins in some cheeses. Many molds grow best at room temperature or with refrigeration and have a characteristic musty smell. They send threads or branches called *hyphae* throughout the material on or in which they grow. Some hyphae extend beyond the surface of the host material and, when mature, produce rounded capsules containing spores at their tips. **Spores** give molds their characteristic colors. The slightest current of air wafts spores about. When spores find a suitable surface, they attach themselves to it and reproduce to form another colony.

Protozoa

Protozoa are single-celled microorganisms visible under an ordinary laboratory microscope. Two common protozoa are the amoeba and the paramecium. Protozoa are able to take in food and excrete wastes. They can reproduce sexually, and generally live in a moisture-rich environment. Some protozoa capture and engulf their food and even feed on bacteria.

Although most protozoa are nonpathogenic, there are some notable exceptions. Amoebic dysentery is caused by *Entamoeba histolytica,* which forms ulcers in the colon and attacks red blood cells. This amoeba produces a capsule (cyst) to protect itself. It then infects people through contact with contaminated food or water. Malaria is caused by a protozoan known as *Plasmodium malariae.* It reproduces in the Anopheles mosquito, and the insect then transmits it to people through bites. *Trichomonas vaginalis* causes vaginal infection in women and urinary tract infection in men. It is often transmitted from an infected individual to an uninfected partner by sexual intercourse.

Bacteria

The study of **bacteria** is called **bacteriology.** Bacteria are part of a group of single-celled organisms that are unique in that they do not have a true nucleus. Their genetic material (**DNA:** deoxyribonucleic acid) is not bounded by a membrane; rather, the DNA float freely within each bacterial cell's cytoplasm.

Classification.   Bacterial groups can be classified according to physical shape, movement, Gram's stain reaction, and relationship to oxygen.

Shape.   Most bacteria fall into one of three categories based on shape (Fig. 40-1). A round or spherical bacterium is called a **coccus** (plural: cocci). A rod-shaped bacterium is known as a **bacillus** (plural: bacilli). A spiral-shaped bacterium has the name **spirillum** (plural: spirilla) or spirochete.

The cells of cocci do not always separate when they reproduce. Sometimes they form pairs (*diplococci*), clusters (*staphylococci*), or chains (*streptococci*). Likewise, *diplobacilli* are paired bacilli and *streptobacilli* are chains of bacilli. Bacilli may have tapered ends (*fusiform* bacilli) or they may be shaped like long threads (*filamentous* bacilli).

Movement.   Some bacteria are capable of locomotion, which is possible because of a cellular organelle called a **flagellum** (plural: flagella). This structure resembles a long whip. Flagella can propel bacteria in different directions, in response to chemical changes in the environment. Some bacteria have a single flagellum at one end; others have a flagellum at each end or a group of flagella at one or both ends. Still other species have flagella distributed over the entire organism (Fig. 40-2).

Gram's Stain.   One of the chief tools a microbiologist uses to identify different species of bacteria is the differential stain, in which dyes react according to the specific type of bacteria tested. Perhaps the most common differential stain is Gram's stain. As a result of Gram's staining, bacteria may be classified as either gram-positive or gram-negative. The first step in Gram's staining involves staining all cells purple. The bacterial sample on a glass slide is next washed with alcohol to selectively decolorize the cells. Gram-positive bacteria have thick cell walls and do not lose their purple color. However, gram-negative bacteria lose their purple color. But they would be difficult to see if another stain were not used. A counterstain turns gram-negative bacteria a color ranging from pink to red. This counterstain does not affect gram-positive bacteria.

Reaction to Oxygen.   Bacteria can be grouped according to the ways in which they use or react to oxygen. For example, some bacilli are obligate aerobes, others are obligate anaerobes, and still others are facultative anaerobes (see "Oxygen" heading). Some bacilli are further divided into those that use oxygen to metabolize sugars (oxidizers) and those that metabolize sugars in the absence of oxygen (fermenters).

☛ Key Concept

Bacteria may be classified according to shape, motility, Gram's stain result, and relationship to oxygen.

Reproduction and Survival.   Bacteria grow or increase in number by duplicating their genetic material and then splitting in two across the middle of the cell. The two new cells share the original DNA equally between them (binary fission).

FIGURE 40-1. Bacteria can be classified according to shape. Cocci are round, and can be found as diplococci, staphylococci, or streptococci. Bacilli are rod shaped. Spirilla are spiral shaped.

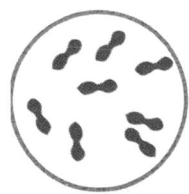
Diplococci

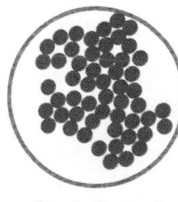
Staphylococci

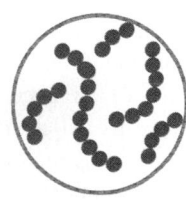
Streptococci

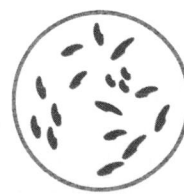
Bacilli

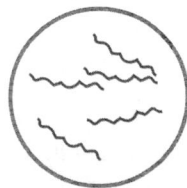
Spirilla (spirochete)

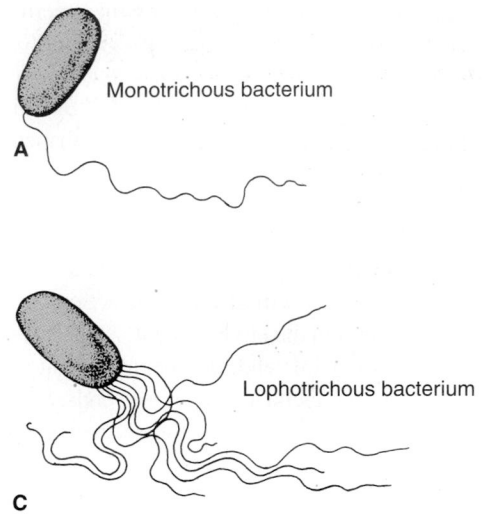

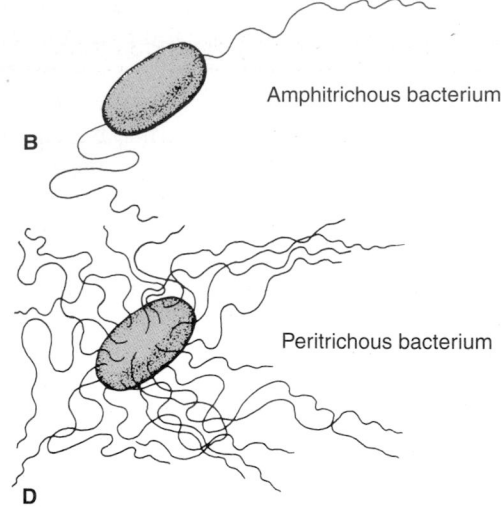

FIGURE 40-2. Four basic types of flagella on bacteria: (**A**) one flagellum at one end; (**B**) one flagellum at each end; (**C**) a tuft of flagella at one end; (**D**) flagella spread over the entire surface. (Adapted from Burton, G. R. W., & Engelkirk, P. G. [1999]. *Microbiology for the health sciences* [6th ed.]. Philadelphia: Lippincott Williams & Wilkins.)

Spores produced by molds in the fungi group are reproductive. Spores related to certain bacteria are for their protection. *Clostridium tetani* and *Bacillus anthracis* are examples of spore formers. When conditions are unfavorable to their growth, these bacilli develop a protective covering (spore) and go into a nonactive (dormant) phase. The spore is resistant to the environment and can survive extreme conditions of light, drying, boiling, and many chemicals. When more favorable conditions return, the spore germinates and the bacteria cell reactivates. Spore-forming bacteria are the most difficult to control and destroy. All pathogenic bacteria die at water's boiling point (100° Celsius or 212° Fahrenheit) *except* the spore formers.

Common Pathogenic Bacteria.   Many bacteria are able to cause disease because of their capsule protection and the makeup of their cell walls. Table 40-1 summarizes some important pathogenic bacteria.

Neisseria are diplococci in shape and cause gonorrhea, upper respiratory infections, and infectious meningitis. The bacillus *Pseudomonas* is responsible for **suppurative** (pus-forming) infections. Bacteria from the genus *Legionella* cause the infamous, pneumonia-like Legionnaires' disease (legionellosis).

Rickettsiae are a special form of bacteria. Some of them are bacilli and others are cocci. They can grow only within the cell of another organism, the host. Rickettsiae are transmitted to people through the bite of an infected insect or tick. Resulting infections range from mild to fatal. One form of rickettsiae causes Rocky Mountain spotted fever. Members of the typhus group cause epidemic and endemic typhus.

Staphylococci are gram-positive bacteria that are always present in the environment and are normal inhabitants of the skin and respiratory tract. *Staphylococcus aureus* is the most dangerous of this group: it produces poisons called *toxins* and frequently resists antibiotics. It can be responsible for serious or fatal infections in newborns and postsurgical clients. An outbreak of "staph" in a healthcare facility is so

serious that all personnel constantly strive to prevent such infections.

Streptococci are also gram-positive; they are common body inhabitants. Members of this group cause "strep throat," pneumococcal pneumonia, and scarlet fever.

Many gram-positive bacilli form spores, such as those from the genus *Clostridium*, one of which causes botulism (a form of food poisoning). These bacilli are particularly difficult to destroy. A respiratory tract infection known as tuberculosis (**TB**) is caused by the tubercle bacillus (a rod) *Mycobacterium tuberculosis.*

Drug-Resistant Bacteria.   Effective antibiotic therapy normally destroys or significantly reduces the number of bacteria causing disease, allowing the body's natural defenses to take over and fight weaker, unwanted microorganisms. Some bacteria, however, are becoming resistant to antibiotic therapy. Methicillin-resistant *Staphylococcus aureus* (**MRSA**), *Clostridium difficile,* and vancomycin-resistant enterococci (**VRE**) are examples of bacteria that are resistant to antibiotic treatment.

The development of antibiotic-resistant strains of bacteria occurs in several ways. The most common way is described here. When antibiotic therapy is incomplete, strong bacteria survive. These bacteria also have the ability to transfer their resistance to other bacteria. Therefore, future antibiotic therapy may be ineffective for other infections. The more these resistant organisms are transmitted into the environment through coughing, sneezing, and direct contact, the greater the chances are that more drug-resistant bacteria will develop. Individuals who do not have a strong immune system to protect their body and to fight these drug-resistant bacteria are at great risk.

To help prevent the development of drug-resistant bacteria and the spread of disease, you can take several measures. It is important to teach these measures to your clients as well:

• Take antibiotics only as prescribed.
• Take antibiotics for the entire period prescribed, even if symptoms of illness disappear.

▪▪▪ TABLE 40-1 ℐome IMPORTANT PATHOGENIC BACTERIA

Bacterium	Diseases	Type	Gram's Stain Reaction*
Bacillus anthracis	Anthrax	Spore-forming rod	+
Bordetella pertussis	Whooping cough	Rod	−
Borrelia burgdorferi	Lyme disease	Spirochete	−
Brucella abortus and B. melitensis	Brucellosis, undulant fever	Rod	−
Chlamydia trachomatis	Lymphogranuloma venereum, trachoma	Coccoid	−
Clostridium botulinum	Botulism (food poisoning)	Spore-forming rod	+
Clostridium perfringens	Gas gangrene, wound infections	Spore-forming rod	+
Clostridium tetani	Tetanus (lockjaw)	Spore-forming rod	+
Corynebacterium diphtheriae	Diphtheria	Rod	+
Escherichia coli	Urinary infections	Rod	−
Francisella tularensis	Tularemia	Rod	−
Haemophilus ducreyi	Chancroid	Rod	−
Haemophilus influenzae	Meningitis, pneumonia	Rod	−
Klebsiella pneumoniae	Pneumonia	Rod	−
Mycobacterium leprae	Leprosy	Rod	+/−
Mycobacterium tuberculosis	Tuberculosis	Rod	+/−
Neisseria gonorrhoeae	Gonorrhea	Diplococcus	−
Neisseria meningitidis	Nasopharyngitis, meningitis	Diplococcus	−
Proleus vulgaris and P. morgani	Gastroenteritis, urinary infections	Rod	−
Pseudomonas aeruginosa	Respiratory and urogenital infections	Rod	−
Rickettsia rickettsii	Rocky Mountain spotted fever	Rod	−
Salmonella typhi	Typhoid fever	Rod	−
Salmonella species	Gastroenteritis	Rod	−
Shigella species	Shigellosis (bacillary dysentery)	Rod	−
Staphylococcus aureus	Boils, carbuncles, pneumonia, septicemia	Cocci in clusters	+
Streptococcus pyogenes	Strep throat, scarlet fever, rheumatic fever, septicemia	Cocci in chains	+
Streptococcus pneumoniae	Pneumonia	Diplococcus	+
Treponema pallidum	Syphilis	Spirochete	−
Vibrio cholerae	Cholera	Curved rod	−
Yersinia pestis	Plague	Rod	−

*+, gram-positive; −, gram-negative; +/−, gram-variable.

From Burton, G. R. W., & Engelkirk, P. G. (1996). *Microbiology for the health sciences* (6th ed.). Philadelphia: Lippincott Williams & Wilkins.

- Do not share antibiotics with others or take their "leftover medications."
- To avoid development of resistant strains, discuss the necessity of antibiotics for mild bacterial infections with your healthcare provider.
- Do not use antibiotics for viral infections.

Viruses

Although scientists long suspected the existence of microorganisms smaller than bacteria, it was not until 1935 that the first **virus** was discovered. Since then, advances in electron and x-ray microscopy and biochemical technology have provided a clearer picture of these elusive structures. Scientists are now able to culture specific viruses, which they can maintain in the laboratory indefinitely.

Viruses are protein-covered sacs containing the genetic material of either DNA or ribonucleic acid (**RNA**) and other organic materials. They lack most characteristics of living organisms. However, when a virus enters the cell of a living organism, the virus's nuclear material is activated. The host cell then becomes a culture medium for viral reproduction. A virus must use the host's ability to make protein and energy, because the virus itself lacks the capacity to carry on metabolism.

Viruses cause a wide range of diseases. Table 40-2 summarizes common viruses. Most pathogenic viruses cannot be easily controlled or destroyed. Immunization is the most effective means of preventing viral infections such as measles and polio. Viruses affect every system and tissue of the body. One of the most well-known and deadly viruses is the human immunodeficiency virus (HIV).

INFECTIOUS DISEASE

An *infection* is a condition in which pathogens invade the body. Diseases caused by pathogenic microorganisms are called *infectious diseases.* The microorganisms increase in number and produce the symptoms of illness. Microbiologists use the term **etiology** to describe the specific cause of a disease. Many diseases caused by microorganisms are **communicable,** meaning they can spread from one person to another. **Contagious** diseases are communicable diseases that are transmitted to many individuals quickly and easily. When a large

■■■ TABLE 40-2 𝒞OMMON PATHOGENIC VIRUSES

Disorder Group	Name	Common Disorders Caused	Comments
Internal disorder producers	Picornavirus (enteric group) Poliovirus	Poliomyelitis	At least three types Vaccine available
	Echovirus	ECHO syndrome (*enteric cytopathogenic human orphan*), aseptic meningitis, diarrhea neonatorum, paralytic disease	At least 30 types No vaccine
	Picornavirus (rhinovirus group)	Common cold, upper respiratory infections	No vaccine
	Coxsackievirus	Aseptic meningitis, myocarditis, pericarditis	At least 30 types No vaccine
Rash producers	Poxvirus	Smallpox	Almost eradicated
	Rubella virus	German measles (rubella)	Vaccine available Can cause birth defects
	Rubeola virus	"Red" measles (rubeola), encephalomyelitis	Vaccine available
	Erythema infectiosum	"Fifth" disease	No vaccine
	Varicella zoster (herpes zoster)	Chickenpox (varicella), shingles (herpes zoster)	No specific vaccine; may use gamma globulin
	Herpesvirus simplex	Cold sores (herpes simplex)	
	Herpesvirus type II	Herpes labialis (genital herpes), encephalitis, vulvovaginitis	No vaccine Two types
	Roseola infantum virus	Roseola infantum ("rose rash," exanthem subitum)	No vaccine
Respiratory disorder producers	Influenza virus (myxovirus types A, B, C)	Influenza ("flu," grippe), croup, pneumonia	Three types Vaccine available (moderate effectiveness)
	Mumps virus (paramyxovirus)	Parotitis (mumps), orchitis (inflammation of testes), meningoencephalitis	Vaccine available
	Infectious mononucleosis virus (Epstein–Barr virus)	Infectious "mono"	No vaccine
	Adenovirus	Conjunctivitis	
Chronic (latent) disorder producers	Hepatitis Type A	Type A hepatitis (formerly called infectious hepatitis)	No vaccine
	Type B ("Dane particle")	Type B hepatitis (formerly called serum hepatitis)	No vaccine
	Type C (non-A, non-B)	Type C hepatitis (parenterally transmitted)	No vaccine
	Type D	Type D hepatitis (can be coinfection with type B)	
	Type E	Type E (transmitted by fecal-oral route)	
	Papovavirus	Warts (verrucae)	
	Arbovirus Group A	Equine encephalitis	Vaccine possible
	Group B	Yellow fever	Vaccine possible
	Diplovirus	Colorado tick fever	No vaccine
	Rabies virus (rhabdovirus)	Rabies (hydrophobia)	Vaccine available
Autoimmune disorder producers	Human immunodeficiency virus (HIV)	Opportunistic infections, such as pneumocystis pneumonia and Kaposi's sarcoma Can develop into full-blown AIDS	Virus has been identified No vaccine available Transmitted via body fluids especially blood and semen

number of people in the same area are infected in a relatively short time, the disease is said to be **epidemic.**

Chain of Infection

Communicable diseases spread easily. Scientists and healthcare workers use knowledge gained in *epidemiology* (the study of ways by which diseases are transmitted to people) to

develop methods for preventing the spread of microbial infections. Disease will spread if the chain of infection (Fig. 40-3) remains unbroken. The chain if infection contains the following elements:

- *Pathogenic microorganism*
- *Reservoir* in which the pathogenic microorganism can live and grow

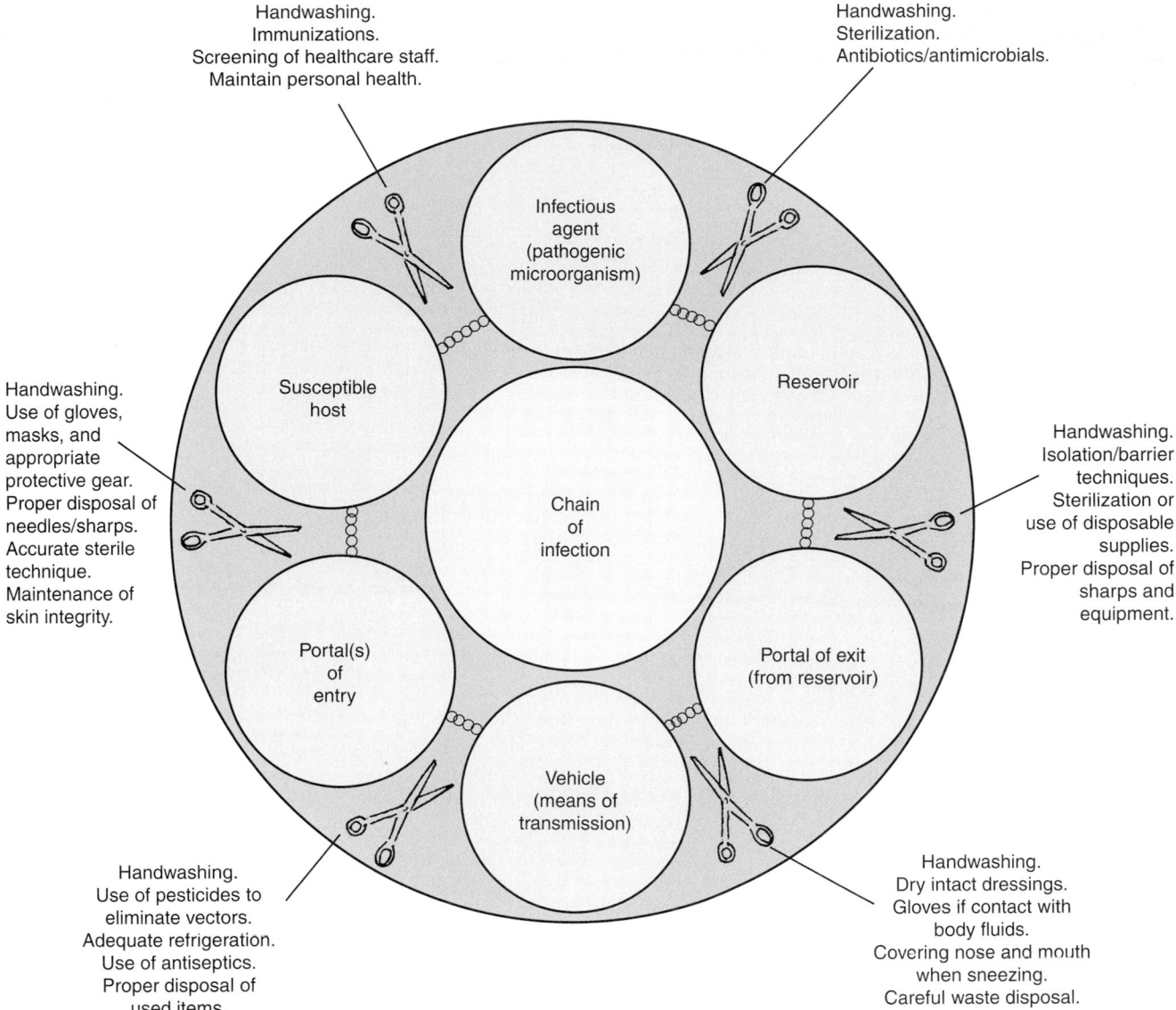

Handwashing.
Immunizations.
Screening of healthcare staff.
Maintain personal health.

Handwashing.
Sterilization.
Antibiotics/antimicrobials.

Infectious
agent
(pathogenic
microorganism)

Susceptible
host

Reservoir

Handwashing.
Use of gloves,
masks, and
appropriate
protective gear.
Proper disposal of
needles/sharps.
Accurate sterile
technique.
Maintenance of
skin integrity.

Chain
of
infection

Handwashing.
Isolation/barrier
techniques.
Sterilization or
use of disposable
supplies.
Proper disposal of
sharps and
equipment.

Portal(s)
of
entry

Portal of exit
(from reservoir)

Vehicle
(means of
transmission)

Handwashing.
Use of pesticides to
eliminate vectors.
Adequate refrigeration.
Use of antiseptics.
Proper disposal of
used items.

Handwashing.
Dry intact dressings.
Gloves if contact with
body fluids.
Covering nose and mouth
when sneezing.
Careful waste disposal.

FIGURE 40-3. The cyclic process through which an infection occurs. To prevent a disease from spreading, the chain of infection must be broken.

- *Portal of exit* from which the microorganism can leave the reservoir
- *Vehicle* to transmit the organism
- *Portal of entry* through which the microorganism can enter the host
- *Susceptible host* in which the microorganism can find a reservoir

Some of these elements are controllable and some are not. The following sections discuss each component of the chain of infection, and measures you can take at each stage to break the chain.

Reservoir

A **reservoir** is any place where a microorganism can survive before moving to a place where it can multiply. Reservoirs may be living beings (eg, people, domesticated or wild animals, and

insects) or inanimate objects (eg, air, soil, food, fluids, bedding, and utensils).

Healthcare personnel can break the chain at this point by destroying the microorganism or retarding its growth through the following measures:

- Sterilizing instruments and dressings used in the operating room and elsewhere.
- Disinfecting floors and equipment.
- Cleaning thermometers and bedpans thoroughly after use.
- Discarding disposable equipment (eg, thermometer probe covers, catheters) in appropriate receptacles after use; discarding other equipment such as bedpans, urinals, and water pitchers when the client is discharged.
- Giving baths using soap and water to remove drainage and dried secretions.
- Changing dressings promptly when they become wet as per physician's order.

- Placing contaminated articles such as dressings, tissues, or linen in moisture-proof bags. Using red, specially labeled biohazard bags when indicated.
- Discarding contaminated needles and syringes and other sharps in the appropriate moisture-resistant, puncture-proof container. Never throwing them in the waste container or putting your fingers inside the sharps container!
- Making sure drainage tubes and collection bags drain properly, and emptying them according to agency policy.
- Never using any sterile package that has become wet or has a broken seal.
- Thoroughly washing hands often.

In addition, healthcare personnel should not work when they might be a source of infection to clients.

Portal of Exit

Microorganisms must have a means of escape from their reservoir. Portals of exit in the human body include all body orifices (openings) and skin discharges. Microorganisms may leave the body in any of its natural discharges: mucus, semen, sputum, saliva, urine, and feces. They may also leave the body in vomitus, drainage, or blood from breaks in the skin.

You can break the chain of infection and prevent microorganisms from escaping with thorough handwashing, appropriate waste disposal, and careful management of secretions and drainage. Avoid talking, sneezing, or coughing directly over open wounds or a sterile field. Always wear gloves when potential contact with body secretions exists. Clients who have airborne infections may need to wear masks or receive ordered medications that prevent coughing. Follow infection control protocols carefully.

Vehicle of Transmission

Microorganisms are transmitted by several means (Table 40-3). *Direct contact* usually involves the spread of pathogens from one person to another through body contact, such as touching, shaking hands, kissing, or sexual intercourse. Many infectious diseases are spread in this fashion. *Indirect contact* implies that an intermediary object harbors the microorganisms and carries them from an infected person to a new victim. Common intermediaries found in healthcare settings include bedding, used tissues, used syringes, drinking cups, and dressings. A *human carrier* does not exhibit the symptoms of a disease, but carries the pathogens and transmits them to others.

Airborne transmission of an infectious disease is accomplished by dust particles carrying microbes or spores that blow from place to place. For instance, infectious diseases can be transmitted by pathogen-containing moisture drops—produced by sneezing or coughing—that are propelled far from the carrier. Common colds and other upper respiratory infections are easily spread by droplet infection.

Public water supplies contaminated with bacteria will produce *water-borne transmission* of diseases. Food poisoning can result from eating foods that have been improperly refrigerated or cooked. The spread of pathogens in this fashion is called *food-borne transmission.*

Living carriers of pathogens are called **vectors.** Mosquitoes, flies, fleas, ticks, and lice are the most common vectors that transmit diseases to human beings. These vectors spread disease by transferring microorganisms from their feet, wings, or bodies to food, which a person eats, unaware that the food is contaminated. Another method of disease spread occurs when vectors become infected themselves and bite a victim, who then also becomes infected.

To break the infection chain at the vehicle of transmission level, burn all trash in nonresidue incinerators. Remove linen without shaking it or allowing it to touch your clothing. Carefully cover all infected wounds. Properly handle and prepare food. Healthcare facility measures include isolation of clients with contagious diseases, sterilization of reusable equipment and supplies, and control of airflow. Be aware of how specific diseases are spread. For example, TB is spread through the air; thus, when treating clients with TB, you should use airborne precautions. If a client has a disease that can spread through body excretions, disinfecting the toilet after use or having the client use a toilet in a separate room may be necessary. Use syringes and needles safely. Do not recap or attempt to break needles. A needle stick from a contaminated needle can spread disease. In all healthcare settings, clients should have their own set of personal care items. Sharing items such as bedpans, urinals, and eating utensils can lead to the transmission of infection. *Handwashing is the single most basic way to prevent the transmission of pathogens.* (Many of the above procedures are further described in Chapters 41 and 42.)

Portal of Entry

Pathogens need a portal of entry to gain access to a person's body. They can enter through the respiratory, gastrointestinal, urinary, and reproductive systems and through breaks in the skin or mucous membranes. Open wounds, incisions, puncture sites from injections, or body orifices into which catheters (tubes) or similar devices are inserted are common portals of

■ ■ ■ TABLE 40-3 𝒯RANSMISSION OF INFECTIOUS DISEASE

Type of Transmission	Examples of Methods
Direct or indirect contact	Touching, kissing, shaking hands, sexual intercourse
Airborne	Dust particles and spores in the air, droplets from sneezing
Food-borne	Spoiled and uncooked food, food contaminated with feces or soil
Water-borne	Feces-contaminated water supply
Vectors	Bites by infected insects, dogs, cats, rodents
Contaminated articles	Dishes, bedding, needles, syringes
Blood-borne	Transfusions, kidney dialysis, injections

entry. To prevent organisms from entering a host, take these measures:

- Keep the client's skin clean and dry. Apply moisturizers to dry skin to prevent cracking.
- Be very careful if clipping a client's nails. Urge clients not to bite their fingernails or cuticles and not to pull on hangnails.
- Avoid positioning clients against tubes or objects that could cause skin breaks.
- Frequently reposition clients who have impaired mobility.
- Provide clean, dry, wrinkle-free linen.
- Make sure urine collection bags are lower than the client.
- Disinfect tubes and ports before collecting specimens from drainage tubes or intravenous lines.
- Keep wounds that are draining and breaks in skin covered.
- Use sterile technique when performing invasive procedures (see Chap. 57).

As a healthcare worker, you are at risk for infection. Wear gloves to protect yourself when handling any blood or body substances or other potential pathogenic reservoirs (ie, contaminated equipment). Wear protective eyewear, masks, gowns, and shoe covers if any danger exists of splashing or spraying body substances. These precautions are particularly important for the prevention of infection with HIV and hepatitis (see Chap. 41). Handwashing and proper wound and catheter care will also break the chain of infection.

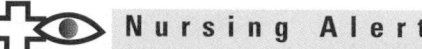

> **Nursing Alert**
> Proper handwashing is the single most useful and effective means of breaking the chain of infection.

Susceptible Host

Normally, healthy people have a variety of defenses against infection, both nonspecific (eg, skin as a barrier, fever, phagocytosis) and specific (eg, immunity). Ill or inactive people or hospitalized clients, however, are more susceptible to infections. Their immune systems may be compromised. Chronic fatigue and poor nutrition weaken the body's ability to respond fully. Infants, young children, and older adults are especially vulnerable. Injury, wounds, shock, and trauma further weaken the body. Side effects of some medications also contribute to a person's susceptibility. Emotional factors, such as anxiety, may play a role in altering the body's defenses.

Help to reduce each client's susceptibility to infection by treating the client's underlying condition. Provide adequate rest and skin care. Give nutritional support. Help to reduce anxiety. Encourage adequate fluid intake. Help with coughing and deep breathing when the client is immobilized. Encourage proper immunization of children and older adults who are at high risk of acquiring communicable diseases. Practice infection control measures. Preventing infection is the daily job of every healthcare worker.

> **Nursing Alert**
> Observe Standard Precautions in all nursing care.

Actions of Pathogens in the Body

Pathogenic microorganisms have two possible damaging effects within the body: local destruction of tissue, or production of poisonous substances that migrate. Although some microorganisms destroy the tissues in which they live, many organisms cause damage to host tissues far from the infection site. These microorganisms produce substances called *toxins,* which are poisonous.

Toxins cause harmful effects by traveling through the circulatory system to damage other body cells. The wide variety of cellular effects include interrupting cellular metabolism, stopping protein synthesis, and destroying cell membranes. Toxins can cause many different symptoms.

Microorganisms produce two types of toxins. **Endotoxins** are part of the cell walls of gram-negative bacteria. When a microorganism dies, the cell wall decays and releases the toxins. **Exotoxins** are toxins manufactured by the microorganism and excreted into the surrounding tissue. They are released into host blood vessels, where they are carried to other body parts.

RESPONSE TO INFECTION

Whether or not a pathogen produces an active infection depends on both the organism and the host. A healthy individual often can muster physical defense mechanisms to ward off disease. Persistent and effective pathogens, however, can overwhelm even the healthiest person.

Normal Course of Infection

When an infection occurs, it usually follows a progressive course. The first stage is the **incubation period,** the time from when the pathogen enters the body to the appearance of the first symptoms of illness. For example, after the varicella organism (which causes chickenpox) enters the body, it takes 2 to 3 weeks before any lesions appear. The second phase is the **prodromal** stage, the period from the onset of initial symptoms (such as fatigue or low-grade fever) to more severe symptoms. Many illnesses are at their most contagious during the prodromal stage. The third phase is the full stage of illness. During this period the symptoms are acute and specific to the type of infection, such as a high fever, lesions covering the body, cough, headache, or congestion. The final stage is the *convalescence* stage. During this period the acute symptoms of the infection subside and the person recovers.

Factors That Influence the Development of Infection

Normally, the body has a variety of defense mechanisms that contribute to its resistance to pathogenic infection. Although the individual is unaware of it, his or her body is almost constantly defending itself against foreign invaders. Chapter 24 discusses nonspecific mechanisms that fight disease, as well as the crucial role the immune system plays in warding off pathogens. Review that chapter for a better understanding of how the human body naturally defends itself against pathogenic microorganisms.

Several factors other than the strength of the body's natural defenses help determine whether or not disease-causing microorganisms will ultimately cause an infection.

Specific Portal of Entry

In general, microorganisms cause disease only if they gain access to the body through a specific portal of entry. For example, *Streptococcus pneumoniae* causes pneumococcal pneumonia only when it enters the respiratory system; use of any other portal of entry does not result in infection. Likewise, the typhoid bacillus must enter the digestive tract. Meningococcus uses the nose as its chief portal of entry.

Number of Microorganisms

Usually, large numbers of microorganisms are needed to cause infection. If the number of pathogens entering the body is small, the body's natural defenses can easily overcome them. The greater the number of pathogens, the greater the opportunity they have to cause disease.

Virulence

A pathogen's strength to cause disease is called its **virulence**. Some bacteria form protective capsules that increase their virulence by making them less likely to be destroyed by the host's white blood cells. Other bacteria produce enzymes that destroy blood cells, stop normal blood clotting, or consume muscle fibers. Each of these enzymes increases the virulence of the particular species that produces them.

Host Resistance

Naturally occurring microorganisms in the body do not cause disease in healthy people. In fact, some of them play a necessary role in disease resistance. The ability of some species of microorganisms to live together is called *symbiosis*. An association in which one species of microorganism prevents the growth or actually destroys members of another species is called *antibiosis*. (The term *antibiotic* is derived from the term *antibiosis*.) Some naturally occurring body flora have this type of antibiotic relationship with pathogens and contribute to an individual's overall health.

If a person is immunocompromised as a result of illness or another factor, he or she will not be able to fight off disease. Examples include people with AIDS, agammaglobulinemia (congenital absence of normal gamma globulin), people undergoing some forms of chemotherapy for cancer, or people recovering from a bone marrow transplant. In these cases, even normally occurring microorganisms can cause disease (*opportunistic infections*).

➔ STUDENT SYNTHESIS

Key Points

- Some microorganisms are beneficial in nature. Others, called pathogens, cause disease in human beings.
- All microorganisms, except viruses, engage in the same life functions as do other plant and animal cells. Their reproduction and infectious spread in human beings depend on the right set of environmental conditions.
- Culture and sensitivity reports and staining identify microorganisms and appropriate treatment for them.
- Microorganisms are classified by their physical and biologic characteristics into basic groups, each with distinguishing means of reproducing and (if they are pathogens) infecting people.
- With the number of drug-resistant and multi-drug–resistant bacteria increasing, prudent use of antibiotics is essential.
- Viruses cause disease by taking over the host cell's metabolism and genetic material and by reproducing in extremely large numbers.
- Most common microbial diseases are communicable and are spread within the population by direct or indirect contact; by contaminated air, water, or food; or through vectors.
- Healthcare professionals who practice antiseptic techniques and Standard Precautions can break the chain of infection.
- Infections follow a progressive course. Many factors contribute to the microorganism's ability to result in disease.

Critical Thinking Exercises

1. Discuss how you would teach the client and family about the spread of disease. What suggestions would you make to control infection and to break the chain of infection in the home, the clinic, and the school setting?
2. What suggestions would you make to the homeless person who comes to the clinic where you work seeking treatment for a severe wound infection on the leg and multiple lesions on the body?

NCLEX-Style Review Questions

1. Which of the following is the single most effective method to break the chain of infection?
   a. Applying gowns
   b. Performing handwashing
   c. Placing clients on isolation
   d. Using protective eyewear

2. Which of the following is the correct sequence for the chain of infection?
   a. Portal of entry, susceptible host, reservoir, portal of exit, vehicle of transmission
   b. Portal of exit, vehicle of transmission, reservoir, portal of entry, susceptible host
   c. Reservoir, portal of exit, vehicle of transmission, portal of entry, susceptible host
   d. Vehicle of transmission, portal of entry, reservoir, portal of exit, susceptible host
3. Why is it vital for nurses to learn about microorganisms?
   a. To assist in diagnosing diseases
   b. To prevent the spread of diseases
   c. To teach clients about illness
   d. To teach the community about diseases

4. Which nursing education measure would be appropriate to help prevent the development of drug-resistant bacteria?
   a. Avoiding contact with persons taking antibiotics
   b. Sharing antibiotics with ill family members
   c. Stopping antibiotics when symptoms disappear
   d. Taking antibiotics as prescribed
5. Which of the following organisms can be classified according to physical shape, movement, Gram's stain reaction, and relationship to oxygen?
   a. Bacteria
   b. Fungi
   c. Protozoa
   d. Viruses

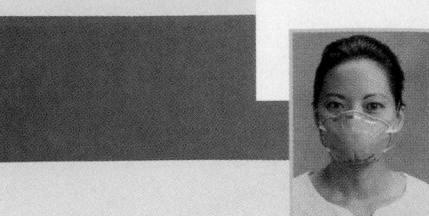

CHAPTER

41

Medical Asepsis

LEARNING OBJECTIVES

1. Define the term nosocomial infection.
2. Differentiate between endogenous and exogenous organisms.
3. Identify at least five factors that predispose clients to nosocomial infections.
4. Define medical asepsis.
5. Describe three elements of medical asepsis.
6. State the single most effective nursing measure in preventing the spread of disease.
7. In the laboratory, demonstrate proper handwashing technique after routine client care, before contact with a severely immunocompromised client, and after performing an invasive procedure.
8. List the most commonly used personal protective equipment.
9. In the skills laboratory, demonstrate the use of barrier techniques.
10. Explain how antimicrobial agents and environmental controls contribute to medical asepsis.
11. In the skills lab, demonstrate the teaching of infection control to a client or family member.
12. Describe the nurse's role in the disposal of biohazardous waste and in cleaning up biohazardous materials.

NEW TERMINOLOGY

antimicrobial agent
asepsis
bacteremia
endogenous

exogenous
invasive
medical asepsis
nosocomial infection

ACRONYM

PPE

In Chapter 40, information was presented about pathogenic microorganisms and how they contribute to the spread of infectious disease. Preventing infections is vital to any healthcare facility's operation and to the provision of healthcare in the community and in the home. Practicing techniques of medical asepsis will help protect you, your clients, and your coworkers from infection. Standard Precautions, which are important to follow in all nursing care, are included in Appendix E.

MEDICAL ASEPSIS

Asepsis refers to practices that *minimize* or *eliminate* organisms that can cause infection and disease. There are two kinds of asepsis: medical and surgical. Medical asepsis (clean technique) is discussed in this chapter; surgical asepsis (sterile technique) is discussed in Chapter 57.

Medical asepsis refers to the practice of *reducing the number* of microorganisms. The goal is to prevent reinfection of the client and to prevent or reduce the transmission of microorganisms from one person (or source) to another. Medical asepsis may also be referred to as *clean technique.* It is used in the care of all clients. Components of medical asepsis include:

* Reducing the number of skin microorganisms through handwashing (the best method of disease prevention), both before and after all client care
* Using barrier techniques (eg, gowns, gloves) to protect staff and clients from microorganisms
* Keeping the environment clean and controlled to reduce disease transmission
* Protecting objects in the client's environment from contamination, or disinfecting them as soon as possible after contamination

Surgical asepsis, on the other hand, aims to *destroy all* organisms.

NOSOCOMIAL INFECTIONS

Nosocomial infections are serious problems for healthcare facilities. They are infections that clients acquire while in the facility. A person's risk of acquiring an infection in a healthcare facility is high for several reasons: A number of disease-causing microorganisms are present in the facility, many of which are resistant to antibiotics. Also, healthcare facilities are environments that house many potential reservoirs for pathogenic growth (eg, infusion fluids, foods, biologic materials, and equipment). A person's risk for developing a nosocomial infection increases when certain conditions exist. Some of these conditions are:

* Antibiotics may be used inappropriately, leading to the development of resistant strains of pathogens, or resistance and allergies in the client.
* Broad-spectrum antibiotics may be used too frequently. This may also promote development of antibiotic-resistant strains of pathogens.

* Healthcare personnel fail to use appropriate prevention techniques and the chain of infection is not interrupted.
* Multiple healthcare personnel provide care for a client, thus increasing the client's possibility of exposure to pathogens.
* A person has lowered resistance to disease because of their current illness, surgery, or injury. People with a chronic illness are more susceptible to illness.
* The very old and very young are also more susceptible.
* People who are ill often have electrolyte imbalances, poor hydration, or poor nutrition, making them more susceptible.
* Clients in the healthcare facility may have ineffective immune systems. due to chemotherapy, radiation, bone marrow transplant, or an immune deficiency disorder such as AIDS.
* The client experiences a prolonged hospitalization, compounding all the risks.

☞ Key Concept

Nosocomial infections can lengthen the person's stay in the healthcare facility, increase the cost of treatment, and even cause death.

According to Miller and Keane, "more than one-third of (nosocomial) infections are easily preventable."[1]

Common Nosocomial Infections

The most common nosocomial infections include:

* Genitourinary infections (the most common nosocomial infections)
* **Bacteremias** (generalized bacterial infection in the blood)
* Respiratory infections (may be secondary to ventilator use or emergency intubation with an oral airway)
* Surgical-site infections
* Gastrointestinal infections

In some cases, **endogenous** (present within the person's body) microorganisms cause the infection (Table 41-1). In other cases, **exogenous** (from outside the body) microorganisms are responsible. *Salmonella, Clostridium tetani,* and *Aspergillus* species are examples of common exogenous microorganisms that cause nosocomial infections. Gram-negative organisms cause most of today's nosocomial infections. However, it is predicted that lesser-known pathogens and new strains will cause more infections in the future.

Clients and Nosocomial Infections

Infections can occur when a *person's resistance is lowered.* Several factors can contribute to a client's lowered resistance:

* *Trauma.* Injury, illness, or emotional shock lowers the body's resistance as it tries to rebuild itself. Trauma can cause breaks in the skin, providing avenues for infection.

TABLE 41-1 *E*XAMPLES OF ENDOGENOUS MICROORGANISMS

Site of Normal Growth	Endogenous Organism	Possible Infection
Skin	*Staphylococcus aureus*	Impetigo, wound infection
	Staphylococcus epidermidis	Acne
Respiratory tract	*Streptococcus pneumoniae*	Bacterial pneumonia
	Neisseria species	Meningitis (inflammation of meninges of nervous system)
Colon	*Escherichia coli*	Urinary tract infection
	Pseudomonas species	Wound infection
Vagina	*Clostridium perfringens*	Diarrhea
	Yeasts	Moniliasis, pneumonia

The central nervous system, bladder, and blood are normally sterile and do not contain endogenous organisms.

Examples include burns, compound fractures (bone exposed), stab wounds, and lacerations (cuts).

- *Pre-existing disease or frequent illness.* Before entering the facility, the client may have an infection or condition that has lowered the body's defenses.
- *Age.* The very young and the very old do not have as many defenses as do people of other age groups. The immunity that breast-fed newborns receive from their mothers does not protect them against all diseases. Older adults may be poorly nourished, have fragile skin, or be inactive, causing impaired resistance.
- *Inactivity.* The person who is ill usually does not get much exercise, which leaves the body weakened against fighting infections.
- *Poor nutrition, inadequate hydration, poor health.* The ill person may be malnourished, dehydrated (not enough fluid in the tissues or in the circulation), or overhydrated (too much fluid). Inadequate circulation may compound the problem.
- *Stress.* Increased stress increases the body's cortisone levels, reducing resistance to disease. Prolonged stress may also result in exhaustion.
- *Fatigue.* The person who is extremely tired cannot effectively fight off disease. Those who are fighting illness or injury or who have had surgery are often fatigued.
- *Invasive therapy.* The term **invasive** means any therapy that enters or *invades* the body (by a means other than normal), either through a skin break or incision or through an instrument that enters an otherwise sterile area. Examples of invasive therapy include any type of surgery, medication injections, intravenous therapy, urinary catheterization, and tracheostomies (a tube inserted into the trachea to open an airway).
- *Frequent use of broad-spectrum antibiotics.* Microorganisms that the person is harboring may develop resistance to antibiotic therapy after repeated exposure to the same antibiotic. In this case, those antibiotics are later ineffective against the resistant pathogen.

- *Inadequate primary and secondary defenses.* The body's primary defenses may be altered due to a break in the skin, low white blood cell count, an autoimmune disorder, or diminished lung function.
- *Immunosuppressive therapy.* This type of therapy deliberately suppresses the body's natural immune system. Types of immunosuppressive therapy include chemotherapy for cancer or bone marrow transplant or administration of high doses of steroids to reduce inflammation.

Nurses and Nosocomial Infections

Nurses play a vital role in preventing nosocomial infections by carefully following all nursing procedures.

Breaking the Chain of Infection

Many nursing procedures are aimed at breaking the chain of infection. Following are the links in the chain of infection. The nurse helps to break this chain (by examples in parentheses):

- *Causative agent.* The nurse helps to reduce the number and/or virulence of pathogens. (Administration of antibiotic medications; following agency protocols for delivery of care; careful handwashing.)
- *Reservoir for growth of pathogens.* The nurse helps to eliminate areas in which pathogens might grow and multiply. (Properly disposing of contaminated dressings or body fluids; disposing of outdated IV solutions; keeping personal immunizations up to date; using disposable equipment and materials; discarding any broken sterile packages; proper handwashing.)
- *Portal of exit.* The nurse gives special attention to the respiratory and gastrointestinal tracts and to body fluids. (Keeping all wounds covered; encouraging safer sex; following correct isolation techniques, proper handwashing.)
- *Vehicle of transmission.* Careful nursing care eliminates the transmission of pathogens between people. (Correctly

using masks and gloves; properly disposing of wound drainage, urine, and feces; carefully disposing of soiled dressings, diapers, or tubing; proper catheterization and injection techniques; keeping urinary drainage equipment sterile; correct handling of all body fluids, using waterproof bags for soiled or wet linens; careful handwashing before and after all nursing procedures.)

- *Portal of entry.* Correct nursing procedures help to prevent pathogens from being allowed to enter a client's system. (Following prescribed protective isolation protocol; cleansing from clean to dirty when giving perineal care; using correct sterile technique for invasive procedures such as medication injections; careful handwashing.)

- *Susceptible host.* Nursing actions are aimed at increasing the client's resistance to disease. (Promoting adequate nutrition, hydration, and rest; following protocol for administration of antibiotics; administering prescribed medications; giving particular attention to the immunocompromised client's care; assisting the client to obtain exercise.)

These are just examples. There are many more ways that nurses help prevent nosocomial infections. The use of Standard Precautions in all nursing care is also an important factor in controlling the spread of infection.

Risks for the Nurse

Just as clients are at risk, nurses too are at risk, because they are in repeated contact with infectious materials and are continually exposed to communicable diseases. Risks for infection in nurses after exposure to diseases such as tuberculosis or hepatitis are of concern. It is important for the nurse to take preventive measures to protect himself or herself.

A major factor in protecting oneself is obtaining appropriate immunizations. Box 41-1 lists immunization recommendations for all healthcare personnel. Careful handwashing and the use of Standard Precautions are also vital in protecting the nurse. In Practice: Nursing Care Guidelines 41-1 lists additional preventive measures to protect healthcare staff from acquiring and spreading nosocomial infections.

➤➤ BOX 41-1

RECOMMENDED IMMUNIZATIONS FOR HEALTHCARE PERSONNEL

Hepatitis B
Measles
Mumps
Rubella
Poliovirus
Tetanus
Diphtheria
Influenza
Pneumococcal disease

The Infection Control Committee

Healthcare facilities are required to monitor nosocomial infections. The Infection Control Committee is charged with this task. The functions of the committee are:

- Watchfulness to locate instances of infection
- Investigation of any infections that occur
- Compiling statistics regarding nosocomial events
- Teaching healthcare staff, clients, and families how to prevent infections
- Serving as a liaison between the healthcare facility and the community

You may be asked to serve as a member of this important committee.

Handwashing

Handwashing is the single most effective measure to prevent the spread of disease. In general, the frequency and products to use in handwashing relate to the duration, type, sequence, and intensity of activities you are performing. For example, touching an item that is not soiled does not require handwashing afterward. However, touching something contaminated with blood or body fluids requires thorough handwashing. *If in doubt, wash your hands!*

The Centers for Disease Control and Prevention (CDC) recommends routine handwashing for a duration of 10 to 15 seconds, and for longer if your hands are visibly soiled. The CDC recommends handwashing in the following situations:[2]

- When hands are visibly soiled
- Before and after contacts with all clients
- After contact with any source of microorganisms (eg, blood or body fluids, mucous membrane, non-intact skin, or objects that might be contaminated)
- Before and after performing invasive procedures
- Before and after removing gloves

Again, if there is any doubt about possible contamination, wash your hands. The type of cleaning agent and handwash depends on several factors. Box 41-2 describes three types of handwashing to use in different healthcare situations. In Practice: Nursing Procedure 41-1 outlines the steps in handwashing for all situations.

☞ Key Concept

Handwashing is the single most important procedure for protecting yourself and your clients against disease transmission.

Barrier Techniques

Barrier techniques include the use of personal protective equipment (**PPE**): gloves, eye protection, gowns, and masks. The principal reasons for wearing PPE are to keep organisms from entering or leaving the respiratory tract (the nurse's or the client's), your eyes, or breaks in the skin. They also help to protect the nurse from the client's body fluids.

(*text continues on page 486*)

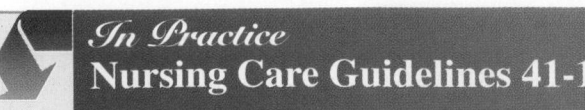

In Practice
Nursing Care Guidelines 41-1

Preventing Infection for Nursing Staff and Clients

- Get plenty of sleep and exercise. Eat nutritious foods.
- Practice good personal hygiene.
- Keep immunizations up to date.
- Consult the clinical facility and physician regarding voluntary immunization for diseases such as hepatitis B and influenza. Have regular PPD tests.
- Attend in-service education classes related to infection control.
- Practice good nursing skills and continually review them.
- Report needle sticks or any breaks in the skin.
- Practice safer sex.
- Do not use nonprescribed medications.
- Stay home from work if ill with an infectious disease.
- Practice good and frequent handwashing.
- Wear gloves when in contact with any body fluids.
- Wear masks, goggles, gowns, shoe protectors, and hair covering when splashing is likely.
- Isolate infected clients and practice good isolation precautions (as discussed in Chap. 42).
- Use sterile techniques for catheterization, injections, dressing changes, etc.
- Do not use a sterile package if the seal is broken, if the wrapper is torn or wet, or if the sterilization monitor is not registered.
- Do not use a sterile package or medication if it has passed the expiration date.
- Keep cupboards closed where sterile materials, linens, or other supplies are stored.
- Store sterile and clean supplies separately.
- Change your clothes immediately if they become soiled with body substances from clients.

- Teach clients hygiene and good techniques of self-care.
- Do not shake linens or place linens on the floor when changing beds. Use covered linen hampers.
- Make sure sitz baths, bathtubs, showers, and other common areas are carefully cleaned and disinfected between clients.
- Do not keep dinner trays for clients; some foods will spoil.
- Ensure that electronic temperature probes are covered and that the covers are disposed of correctly.
- Practice care when working with catheters or IVs.
- Use disposable equipment as much as possible.
- Follow procedures carefully for preoperative and postoperative clients.
- Use waterproof bags to send heavily soiled or moist linens to the laundry.
- Send items to be sterilized to central supply room in plastic bags.
- Ensure that all trash is collected in heavy-duty plastic bags. Most is collected in special containers and incinerated.
- Make sure that any spilled body substances are cleaned up immediately, using the prescribed protocol.
- Report any infection *immediately.*
- Ask questions if you are not sure of a procedure or protocol.
- Monitor the compliance of others regarding infection control practices.
- Encourage other healthcare personnel to practice proper infection control practices.

➤➤ BOX 41-2

HANDWASHING GUIDELINES

Handwash with soap or detergent to remove soil and transient microorganisms in the following situations:

- Routine client care
- Before and after client contact
- When hands are visibly soiled
- After contact with a source of microorganisms
- After removing gloves

Perform *hand antisepsis,* using antimicrobial soap or detergent or alcohol-based handrub, to remove or destroy transient microorganisms in the following situations:

- Before contact with severely immunocompromised clients and all newborns
- After caring for an infected client or one likely to be colonized with microorganisms of epidemiologic concern
- Before and after contact with clients in high-risk units.

Perform a *surgical hand scrub* using antimicrobial soap or detergent or alcohol-based handrub to remove or destroy transient microorganisms and reduce resident flora in the following situation:

- Before and after client contact when performing invasive procedures. (Chapter 56 describes the surgical hand scrub.)

Adapted from APIC guideline for handwashing and hand antisepsis in healthcare settings (Larson, 1996).

In Practice
Nursing Procedure 41-1

HANDWASHING

Supplies and Equipment

Liquid or bar soap
Paper towels

Steps

1. Remove jewelry. A plain wedding band may remain in place.
   RATIONALE: *Rough places in jewelry can harbor microorganisms.*

2. Stand in front of the sink and avoid leaning against it.
   RATIONALE: *This action avoids the transfer of contamination from the sink to the nurse's uniform.*

3. Turn on the water and regulate its flow and temperature. Knee or foot pedals may be available on some sinks. In some facilities, water automatically flows when placing the hands under the faucet.
   RATIONALE: *Controlling the force of flow limits splashing. Warm water is more comfortable and less irritating to the skin. It is much safer not to touch faucet handles.*

4. Wet your hands and forearms with water, keeping the hands lower than the elbows.
   RATIONALE: *This action allows water to flow from the least contaminated area toward the hands, which are the most contaminated area.*

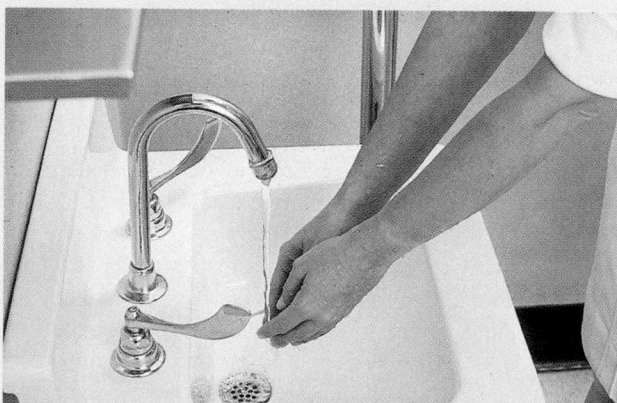

Wetting hands, keeping the most contaminated area lower. (Photo © B. Proud)

5. Apply an antibacterial liquid soap. If you must press a lever to dispense soap, do so with a paper towel. Liquid soap with a foot- or knee-operated dispenser is the most sanitary.

RATIONALE: *The dispenser may be contaminated. Using a paper towel or foot-operated dispenser is important to prevent further contamination.*

6. Wash your hands, wrists, and lower forearms for a minimum of 10–15 seconds (about the length of time it takes to sing "Yankee Doodle"), using a scrubbing motion. Interlace the fingers and rub the hands back and forth.
   RATIONALE: *Friction loosens dirt and bacteria on all surfaces.*

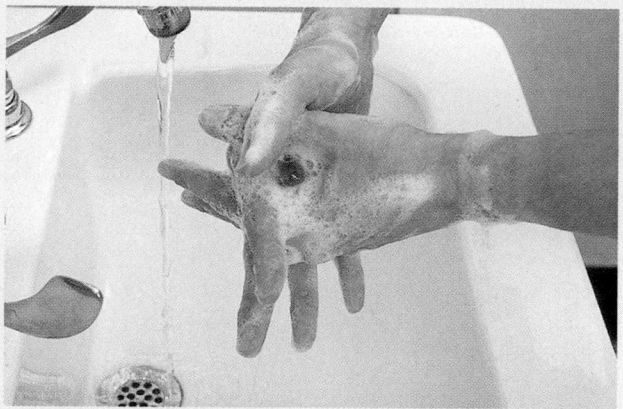

Using scrubbing motion to wash hands. (Photo © B. Proud)

7. Insert the fingernails from one hand under those of the other hand, using a sweeping motion. Repeat with the other hand.
   RATIONALE: *Bacteria tend to accumulate under the fingernails.*

8. Rinse thoroughly, keeping the hands lower than the forearms.
   RATIONALE: *Keeping hands lower than the forearms prevents soap lather from recontaminating clean areas.*

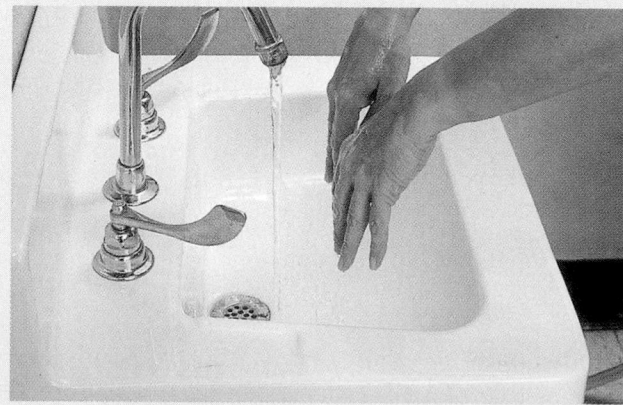

Rinsing thoroughly. (Photo © B. Proud)

(continued)

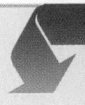

In Practice
Nursing Procedure 41-1 *(Continued)*

9. Repeat the procedure if the hands are very soiled.
   RATIONALE: *This ensures a thorough cleaning.*

10. Dry the hands thoroughly with a paper towel. Discard the towel.
    RATIONALE: *Drying thoroughly prevents chapping. Using paper towels helps prevent spread of microorganisms.*

11. Use a clean paper towel to turn off faucets.
    RATIONALE: *A dry, clean towel prevents recontamination of hands with organisms on faucets. A wet towel would allow the passage of microorganisms back to the hands.*

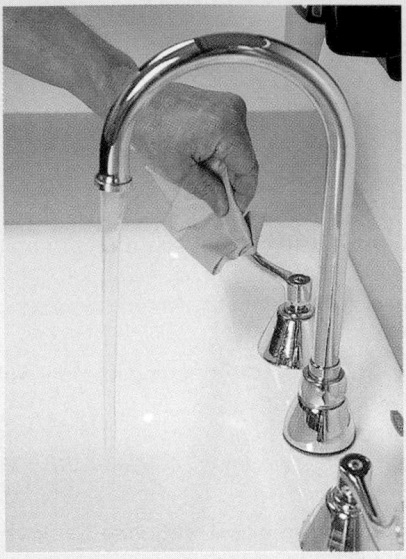

Using a clean paper towel to turn off faucets. (Photo © B. Proud)

Gloves

Gloves provide a protective barrier when touching blood or body fluids. It is vital to use gloves in all client care that involves potential exposure to any body fluids. Gloves provide protection from microorganisms that clients carry. Gloves also help prevent the spread of pathogens from one client to another, from client to healthcare staff, or from healthcare staff to client. Disposable clean gloves are available in all healthcare facilities, including community-based settings. Home care nurses carry gloves with them.

Use gloves when anticipating any contact with a person's blood or body fluids. The nurse must always wear gloves if he or she has any breaks in the skin of the hands. Discard used gloves in the appropriate receptacle in the client's room or examination area. Home care nurses must also carefully dispose of gloves. (Chapter 57 describes the use of sterile gloves.) In Practice: Nursing Procedure 41-2 explains the procedure for putting on and removing gloves.

Nursing Alert

If the integrity of gloves is altered (eg, ripped or punctured), the gloves are no longer effective. They must be discarded.

Latex allergies.   One of the components of all gloves was formerly latex (rubber). It is estimated that 8% to 17% of healthcare workers and 1% to 6% of the general public are sensitive to latex. Be alert for latex sensitivity in clients.

Allergic or *sensitivity reactions* may occur from direct contact and may also occur due to the powder that has been in contact with latex gloves. Latex proteins attach to the powder and cause reactions through contact or breathing. Overall latex sensitivity has increased since 1987 when Universal (General) Precautions were introduced, and healthcare facilities began to enforce stringent recommendations for glove use. Many healthcare organizations are eliminating latex gloves because of the rapid increase in the number of latex-sensitive healthcare workers. Repeated exposure to latex products heightens the reaction for sensitive individuals.

There are three levels of latex sensitivity:

- Skin irritation
- Contact dermatitis
- Generalized anaphylaxis

A simple skin reaction may occur alone. However, sensitivity may progress to the second level, contact dermatitis, which is the most common allergic reaction to latex. Contact dermatitis is a localized reaction. Other localized symptoms of latex sensitivity include hives or a rash (which may become crusty), itching, cracking, scaling, or weeping of the skin. A localized allergic reaction in the lungs may also occur when sensitized individuals are exposed to others who are wearing gloves. When the other healthcare workers remove their gloves, the powder is released and dispersed through the air. The sensitive individual may develop swelling of the face, itchy and red eyes, excessive sneezing, a runny or stuffed nose, an itchy nose or palate, and difficulty breathing.

The third and most serious latex reaction is a systemic reaction. This can quickly progress to general anaphylaxis, which is life-threatening. (Anaphylaxis is discussed in more detail in Chapter 43, in Box 47-1, and elsewhere in the book.)

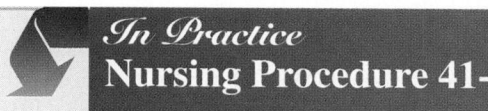
In Practice
Nursing Procedure 41-2

USING CLEAN (NON-STERILE) GLOVES

Supplies and Equipment

Appropriate-size gloves

Donning Gloves

1. Wash the hands and dry thoroughly.
   RATIONALE: *The nurse's hands must be as clean as possible. Gloves may be sticky if the hands are damp.*

2. Choose the correct size glove.
   RATIONALE: *Gloves must fit properly to be effective and comfortable.*

3. Bunch the glove up and then pull it onto the hand; ease the fingers into the glove. Repeat for other hand.
   RATIONALE: *Bunching up allows for ease in pulling gloves on.*

Removing and Disposing of Gloves

1. To remove gloves, grasp the *outside* of one glove, near the cuff, with the thumb and forefinger of the other hand. Pull the glove off, turning it inside out while pulling and holding it in the hand that is still gloved.
   RATIONALE: *Turning the glove inside out during removal confines contamination to the gloves.*

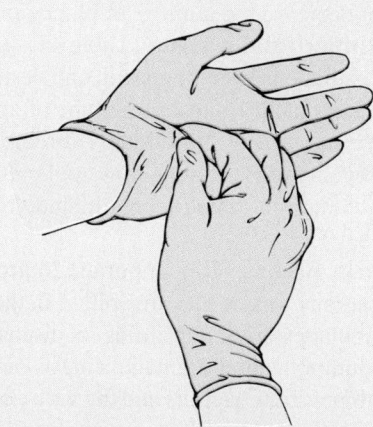
Grasping the outside of the first glove

2. Hook the bare thumb or finger *inside* the other glove and pull it off, turning it inside out and over the already-removed glove.
   RATIONALE: *Hooking the finger on the inside of the other glove prevents contamination of the*

ungloved hand, while confining contamination to the gloves.

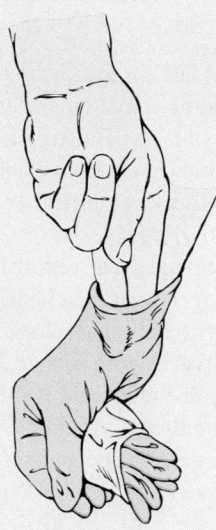
Hooking the bare fingers inside the remaining glove

3. Roll the two gloves together, with the side that was nearest the hands on the outside. The outside of the glove is now considered contaminated to the client. The inside of the glove is considered clean (or contaminated to the nurse).
   RATIONALE: *This action confines contamination.*

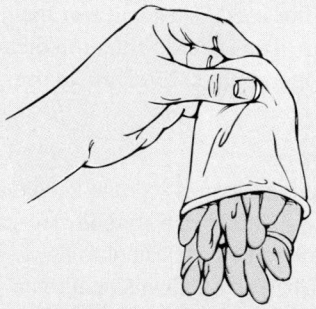
Rolling the two gloves together in preparation for disposal

4. Drop gloves into the appropriate waste receptacle.
   RATIONALE: *Proper disposal assists in preventing the spread of infection.*

5. Wash the hands again.
   RATIONALE: *Handwashing further assists in preventing the spread of infection.*

Some people are more susceptible than others to latex sensitivity. Be particularly watchful of the person who has:

- A history of spina bifida
- A history of genitourinary birth defects
- Daily catheterizations
- Allergies to certain foods (rich fruits such as bananas, kiwi, avocados; and peaches, pears, cherries, chestnuts)
- A history of many surgeries and other invasive procedures
- Frequent use of gloves (such as the nurse)

Although the use of latex-free gloves is becoming common, it is important to remember that other items in the healthcare facility are also made of latex. These include catheters, rubber binders, elastic waistbands, condoms, and many other items. Research continues in the development of substitute, latex-free items.

It is important to include a question about latex allergy during the admission interview of the client. Ask the client if he or she has difficulty with balloons, elastic waistbands, or condoms, or if he or she works with rubber. If the client is latex-sensitive, note this on the chart and Kardex, ask the client to wear an allergy ID band, and obtain latex-free materials for his or her care. Report any suspected personal or client latex sensitivity to your supervisor as soon as possible.

Eye Protection

Wear goggles with side and forehead shields if any danger exists that a client's body fluids may splash or spray onto you. The nurse may wear his or her own glasses with side shields. Goggles are also available that fit over glasses. Use disposable goggles when caring for clients in isolation (see Chap. 42).

In some situations when extra protection is needed, such as in the operating room, emergency department, or morgue, full-face shields are used. These protect the eyes, as well as the nurse's mouth. The specific situation dictates the type of eye and mucous membrane protection to use.

Gowns or Aprons

A gown or protective apron is worn to keep the nurse's clothing clean when a potential exists for body substances to splash. The gown or apron must be resistant to fluids. Follow the following pointers when using gowns or aprons:

- The inside of the gown or apron is clean; the outside is contaminated.
- The gown or apron must be long enough to cover the nurse's uniform or clothing. The apron covers the front and sides, but not the sleeves. The gown or apron opens in the back and must be full enough to overlap at the back. A tie around the waist keeps the gown or apron in place.
- The neck of the gown or apron is considered clean because the nurse does not touch that part with contaminated hands.
- If the nurse is wearing long sleeves, the sleeves are rolled up above the elbows before putting on the gown or apron.
- A supply of clean gowns or aprons is ready outside the client's room to put on before entering.

- After use, remove the gown or apron and dispose of it inside out (contaminated side in). When using a disposable gown or apron, place it in the receptacle for contaminated material. If using a reusable item, place it in the linen hamper for laundering. (Gowns or aprons are not usually hung in the room for reuse.)
- After removing any gown or apron, wash the hands thoroughly before touching anything else.

Masks

Masks protect both clients and healthcare personnel from upper respiratory infections and communicable diseases. Use a mask when giving nursing care to clients with communicable diseases that are transmitted through the respiratory tract. For example, if a client is coughing or sneezing, a mask is worn to cover the nurse's nose and mouth. Each healthcare facility establishes its own policy about the type of mask to use. Everyone who comes into contact with the client, including visitors, should wear a mask. Or, the client may be the only one to wear a mask when outside the room. In the operating room or the newborn nursery, masks protect clients from possible infection by staff members.

Masks are disposable to reduce the risk of cross-contamination. When not using the mask, dispose of it. A mask should never be left to hang around the nurse's neck. This would greatly increase the risk of cross-contamination by providing a reservoir for infectious agents. In Practice: Nursing Procedure 41-3 describes considerations in using a mask.

Clean and Controlled Environment

Using Antimicrobial Agents

Chemicals that decrease the number of pathogens in an area are called **antimicrobial agents** (Table 41-2). They limit and eliminate pathogens by suppressing and destroying their growth. Healthcare facilities use some type of antimicrobial agent to clean equipment. Individuals directly use other antimicrobial agents (eg, through skin application). Examples of common antimicrobial agents include *disinfectants* and *antiseptics*.

Cleaning Up Spills.   It is important to properly clean up any biohazardous wastes that are spilled in the healthcare facility. This includes any body fluids or discharge (blood, urine, feces, sputum, wound drainage, emesis, and so forth). The facility will provide materials and the written protocol for safely cleaning up such spills. It is important to carefully follow the steps in cleaning up and disposing of these wastes, because they are highly contaminated and very likely to spread infection. It is also important to wear gloves when handling any body fluids and to carefully wash the hands after the procedure.

Disposing of Biohazardous Wastes.   After a spill has been cleaned up, the nurse is responsible for properly disposing of the material. In addition to body fluids spilled, other biohazardous wastes include soiled wound dressings, used blood tubes and syringes, and catheters or IVs that have been removed. Each facility has a written protocol to follow. Many

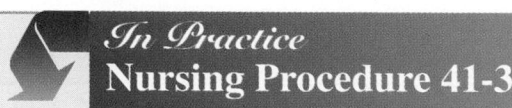

Nursing Procedure 41-3

USING A MASK

Supplies and Equipment

Mask in container

Putting on a Mask

1. Wash the hands.
   RATIONALE: *The nurse's hands must be clean to prevent contaminating the mask.*

2. Remove the mask from the container or package, handling it as little as possible and by the strings only.
   RATIONALE: *Too much handling will reduce the mask's efficiency to screen out microorganisms.*

3. Place the mask so that it completely covers the mouth and nose. Bend the strip at the top of the mask so that it fits tightly around the nose.
   RATIONALE: *The mouth and nose must be completely covered to prevent the transfer of microorganisms. If the nurse wears glasses and if the strip is not tight over the bridge of the nose, the glasses will fog.*

4. To tie the mask, loop the top ties over the ears and tie them under your chin in a bow, not a knot.
   RATIONALE: *Tying is necessary to secure the mask in place; a bow is easiest to untie.*

5. Tie the bottom ties behind the neck in a bow.
   RATIONALE: *By tying the mask in this manner, only one bow needs to be untied to take off the mask. If the top bow is tied behind your head, it may slip down and cause the mask to fall off.*

6. Change the mask when it becomes damp.
   RATIONALE: *A moist mask harbors and transmits organisms.*

Removing a Mask

1. To remove the mask, untie the tie behind the neck. Touch the mask by the strings only. Be careful not to let the mask drop onto the clothes.
   RATIONALE: *The mask is now considered contaminated.*

2. Discard the mask in the proper receptacle.
   RATIONALE: *Proper disposal helps prevent infection spread.*

3. Wash the hands.
   RATIONALE: *Handwashing after mask removal further helps to prevent the spread of infection.*

---

of these items will be placed in a special red "biohazard" bag for disposal. These special bags are handled in a specific manner by the housekeeping staff of the facility. (It is important not to place inappropriate materials in these bags, because there is an additional charge for their disposal.) Remember to put sharps, such as needles, suture removal scissors, or scalpel blades, in the designated "sharps" container. The supervisor is a resource if there are any questions.

The nurse in a community-based setting or in home care is often responsible for disposal of biohazardous wastes and for teaching clients and families. Consult agency protocols for specific procedures.

Leaving a Client's Room

When leaving a client's room, take special care not to spread infection to others. Discard gowns and masks without spreading contamination, and scrub the hands without spreading contamination to the upper arms.

> **Nursing Alert**
>
> All discarded materials used by both nurses and clients are considered contaminated.

Keep in mind the following:

- Use general handwashing techniques. Pay special attention to prevent contamination.
- Always point the hands down when washing them. *Rationale: This reduces the risk of contaminating the upper arms.*
- Do not touch any part of the sink or the faucets. The ideal sink has foot or knee water controls or water that automatically turns on when the nurse's hands are placed under the faucet, as well as a foot-controlled soap dispenser. *Rationale: The sink is contaminated with pathogens. A bar of soap, or soap that requires pushing a button or lever, spreads microorganisms.*
- Use paper towels to dry the hands and discard them in the appropriate waste container. *Rationale: A common towel is contaminated and spreads organisms.*
- Scrub the hands thoroughly at least twice, giving special attention to your nails. Do not wear rings. *Rationale: Rings can harbor microorganisms.*
- Use a dry towel to turn off faucets. *Rationale: A wet towel can allow microorganisms to pass through.*

Terminal Disinfecting

Terminal disinfection refers to the care of a client's unit and belongings after the illness is over. In many facilities, this procedure is carried out by housekeeping personnel, but nurses must understand the underlying principles of the procedure. The nurse may be required to supervise or teach the procedures to other staff or to family members, or to clean a unit in an emergency.

The process is the same whether the client remains in the facility, is discharged, or dies. The facility prescribes the method to use, which should be sufficiently thorough to

TABLE 41-2 Antimicrobial Agents

Type	Mechanism	Example	Use
Soap	Lowers the surface tension of oil on the skin, which holds microorganisms; facilitates removal during rinsing	Dial, Safeguard	Hygiene
Detergent	Same as soap, except detergents do not form a precipitate when mixed with water	Dreft, Tide	Sanitizing eating utensils, laundry
Alcohol	A 70% concentration injures the protein and lipid structures in the inner cellular membrane of some microorganisms	Isopropanol, ethanol	Cleansing skin, instruments
Iodine	Damages the inner cell membrane of microorganisms and disrupts their enzyme functions; not effective against *Pseudomonas,* a common wound pathogen	Betadine	Cleansing skin
Chlorine	Interferes with microbial enzyme systems	Bleach, Clorox	Disinfecting water, utensils, blood spills
Chlorhexidine	Damages the inner cell membrane of microorganisms, but is ineffective against spores and most viruses	Hibiclens	Cleansing skin and equipment
Mercury	Alters microbial cellular proteins	Merthiolate, Mercurochrome	Disinfecting skin
Glutaraldehyde	Inactivates cellular proteins of bacteria, viruses, and microbes that form spores	Cidex	Sterilizing equipment

From Timby, B. K. (1996). *Fundamental skills and concepts in patient care* (6th ed.). Philadelphia: Lippincott-Raven.

destroy the disease-causing organisms. Some organisms are more difficult to destroy than others. Also, some organisms can live up to 6 months on furniture and other surfaces, if these surfaces are not properly cleaned. Terminal disinfection takes into consideration all the links in the chain of infection. It is a vital step in the prevention of nosocomial infections.

Nursing Alert

Anything that touches the client is contaminated and must be decontaminated or sterilized before it can be used for another client. Stop to think before you do anything for the client, or you might become contaminated and spread disease. *One break in technique is all it takes to spread infection!* Remember, good handwashing is vital. *If in doubt, wash your hands!*

CLIENT AND FAMILY TEACHING

Preventing and controlling the spread of infection is part of the daily routine as a nurse. However, families who are caring for clients in the home, and visitors in healthcare facilities, may be unfamiliar with appropriate aseptic techniques. Be sure to teach clients, families, and visitors information about infection, modes of disease transmission, and methods of prevention. Include the following instructions in teaching:

- Handwashing technique
- Hygienic practices that reduce pathogenic growth and spread, including use of disinfectants, proper mouth care, maintenance of skin integrity, and adequate rest
- Proper methods of food handling, preparation, and storage
- Aseptic techniques for self-care activities such as urethral catheterization, medication administration, and wound care
- Proper methods for handling and disposing of contaminated material
- The importance of adequate fluid and food intake and exercise
- The importance of following instructions regarding medications, including taking all of an antibiotic prescription, even if symptoms have improved
- Any special procedures or individual precautions

Be sure to encourage the client and family to ask if they have any questions.

➤ STUDENT SYNTHESIS

Key Points

- Nosocomial infections are those which are acquired by clients in the healthcare facility.

• Clients are more susceptible to infections in healthcare facilities because their resistance to disease is often lowered, and facilities house many pathogens.

• Medical asepsis helps to lower the number of microorganisms in the environment, and reduces their transmission.

• Handwashing is the single most important measure to prevent disease spread.

• Commonly used protective barriers include gloves, eye protection, gowns, and masks.

• Keeping a clean and controlled environment is essential to maintaining medical asepsis.

• Antimicrobial agents limit and destroy pathogens. Commonly used examples include antiseptics and disinfectants.

• Following proper methods of leaving a client's room; use of proper handwashing technique; use of masks, gloves, and gowns; and terminal disinfection help prevent the spread of infections.

• Teaching aseptic practices to clients, families, and visitors is essential for protection against disease, particularly because clients often leave the healthcare facility while they are still ill.

Critical Thinking

1. Discuss possible differences and similarities in practicing medical asepsis in the healthcare facility, the clinic, and the home.

2. From Chapter 40, identify steps in the chain of infection. Describe when and how healthcare personnel could break this chain by using aseptic practices.

3. Discuss why clients in healthcare facilities are more likely to contract infections than other people. Give reasons for your answers.

4. Develop a teaching plan for clients and other nurses regarding asepsis in home care.

NCLEX-Style Review Questions

1. Which method for handwashing should be used after providing care to a client who is infected?
   a. Use soap or detergent to remove soil and transient microorganisms.
   b. Perform a handwashing as usual.
   c. Perform a surgical hand scrub.
   d. Use antimicrobial soap or detergent to perform hand antisepsis.

2. Which of the following infections could be caused by endogenous microorganisms that normally exist in the colon?
   a. Acne
   b. Meningitis
   c. Pneumonia
   d. Wound infection

3. Which is the correct procedure for removing a mask?
   a. Cut the strings and let the mask fall off.
   b. Pull the mask over the head.
   c. Untie the strings behind your neck.
   d. Untie the strings under your chin.

4. The most effective method to prevent the spread of infection is:
   a. Handwashing
   b. Using protective eye gear
   c. Wearing gloves
   d. Wearing a gown

5. If your gloves become ripped during a procedure, the most appropriate action is to:
   a. Apply another pair of gloves over the ripped pair
   b. Discard the gloves, wash hands, and apply a new pair
   c. Finish the procedure and then wash your hands
   d. Remove the gloves and then finish the procedure

References

1. Miller & Keane (1997). *Encyclopedia and dictionary of medicine, nursing and allied health* (6th ed.). Philadelphia: W. B. Saunders.
2. Larson, E. (1996) *APIC infection control and applied epidemiology: Principles and practice*. St. Louis: Mosby.

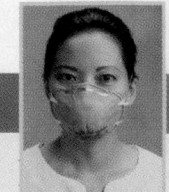

42

Infection Control

LEARNING OBJECTIVES

1. Explain the relationship between standard and transmission-based precautions and infection control.
2. Discuss the purpose, use, and components of Standard Precautions.
3. Explain the purpose, use, and components of transmission-based precautions.
4. Identify how to follow specific airborne, droplet, and contact precautions.
5. Describe how to set up a client's room for isolation, including the appropriate barrier techniques.
6. Demonstrate precautions to take during medication administration, vital sign monitoring, and transport of a client who is potentially infectious.
7. Explain what is meant by protective (neutropenic/reverse) isolation.
8. Identify the role of the infection control committee.

NEW TERMINOLOGY

airborne precautions
colonization
contact precautions
droplet precautions
isolation

neutropenic isolation
protective isolation
Standard Precautions
transmission-based
   precautions

ACRONYMS

BBP
CDC

HICPAC

PPE

Clients in all healthcare settings are at risk for acquiring *nosocomial infections* (infections acquired in the healthcare facility) because of their reduced capacity to resist pathogens; greater exposure to different microorganisms; and invasive procedures that can introduce infectious microorganisms into the body. Nurses are at risk for infection because of frequent exposure to infectious materials and communicable diseases. Although practices of medical asepsis help prevent infections, pathogens are still a danger. Drug-resistant microorganisms are a growing threat, as strains of tuberculosis (TB), gonorrhea, staphylococcus, and other infectious diseases no longer respond to treatment as they did in the past. The threat of contracting human immunodeficiency virus (HIV) and various forms of hepatitis continues to plague society. In an attempt to control the spread of these and other infectious diseases, precautions have been established for infection control in all healthcare facilities. This chapter discusses these precautions and their use. It also discusses isolation practices that are necessary for clients with specific conditions. Infection control precautions help protect healthcare workers, clients, families, and visitors against disease.

INFECTION CONTROL

The best method of infection control is prevention, which is successful when the chain of infection (see Chap. 40) is successfully broken. Healthcare facilities use several types of prevention methods, including the aseptic practices discussed in Chapter 41. The Joint Commission for Accreditation of Healthcare Organizations (JCAHO) requires healthcare facilities to have an effective infection control plan to qualify for accreditation. The plan must include these elements:

- An infection control committee
- Surveillance of nosocomial infections
- Employee health program
- Isolation policies
- Infection control in-service education for employees
- Procedures for environmental sanitation
- Available microbiology laboratory
- Infection control procedures for client care

In 1996, the Centers for Disease Control and Prevention (**CDC**) and the Hospital Infection Control Practices Advisory Committee (**HICPAC**) revised their guidelines for isolation precautions in healthcare facilities, in an attempt to reduce the risk of transmission of microorganisms from both known and unknown sources of infection. The guidelines include two tiers of precautions. The first and most important are Standard Precautions, designed for the care of *all clients, regardless of diagnosis or infection status*. The second tier of precautions, transmission-based precautions, is designed for clients with specific infections or diagnoses.

Standard Precautions

Standard Precautions are a combination of Universal Precautions (designed to reduce the risk of transmission of blood-borne pathogens) and Body Substance Isolation (designed to reduce the transmission of pathogens from moist body substances). These precautions apply to blood; all body fluids, secretions, and excretions (except sweat); nonintact skin; and mucous membranes. They are designed to reduce the risk of transmission of microorganisms from both known and unknown sources of infection.

Standard Precautions state that healthcare facilities must consider all clients as potentially infected with blood-borne pathogens. For that reason, workers must use Standard Precautions in the care of all clients. Appendix E of this book and In Practice: Nursing Care Guidelines 42-1 summarize the basics—you must become familiar with these guidelines. By following Standard Precautions, you protect not only your clients and coworkers, but also yourself.

In 1992, the Occupational Safety and Health Administration (OSHA) implemented "Occupational Exposure to blood borne pathogens (**BBP**)" (Standard 29 CFR 1910.1030). This standard requires and enforces the implementation of policies, procedures, and control measures that will prevent employee exposure to the blood and body fluids of clients. Violations of Standard Precautions carry a severe fine to the healthcare facility. OSHA regulations require the following of healthcare employers:

- Develop an infection control policy that conforms to OSHA guidelines. This policy must identify when personal protective equipment (**PPE**) is required, how to clean up spills of blood or body fluids, how to take specimens to the laboratory, and how to dispose of infectious waste.
- Educate staff about the policies.
- Provide free hepatitis B immunizations to staff who might be exposed to blood/body fluids.
- Provide follow-up care to staff members who are accidentally exposed to splashes of blood/body fluids or needle sticks.
- Supply rapidly accessible PPE.
- Provide proper sharps disposal containers and replace them regularly.

Standard Precautions stress the use of handwashing and PPE to protect against contracting diseases. Table 42-1 lists typical nursing procedures with recommended infection control measures.

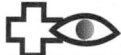 **N u r s i n g   A l e r t**
You must report unusual exposure to potential infection (eg, a needle stick) immediately. OSHA requires initial screening and follow-up care.

Transmission-Based Precautions

Standard Precautions are used when caring for all clients. **Transmission-based precautions** are implemented when caring for clients with a suspected or known infectious disease, based on the disease's route of transmission. Transmission-based precautions are designed to interrupt the transmission of epidemiologically important pathogens in healthcare facilities. These precautions are grouped into three types: airborne precautions, droplet precautions, and contact precautions. When

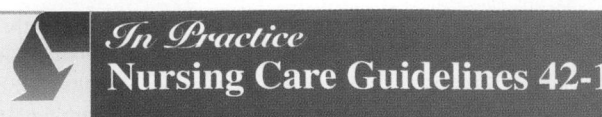

In Practice
Nursing Care Guidelines 42-1

IMPLEMENTING STANDARD PRECAUTIONS

- Wear gloves when in contact with blood, body fluids containing blood, secretions, excretions, nonintact skin, mucous membranes, or contaminated items. *Rationale: These body substances can carry diseases. You may be at risk of contracting a disease or you could spread disease.*
- Change gloves after each contact with a client. *Rationale: The gloves may be contaminated.*
- Wash your hands and skin surfaces immediately and thoroughly if they become contaminated with blood or body fluids; after each client contact; and after removing gloves to prevent transfer of microorganisms between clients or between clients and the environment. *Rationale: Proper handwashing helps stop the spread of infection.*
- Wear a gown or apron when clothing could become soiled. *Rationale: Wearing a gown or apron prevents spreading infection to yourself or others.*
- Wear a mask, eye protection, and face shield if splashing or spraying of blood or body fluids is possible. Healthcare facility protocol will determine the type of eye protection required in each case. *Rationale: Infection could enter your body through the mucous membranes of your mouth or nose or through your eyes.*
- Do not recap or break needles. Place needles and sharp objects in a special, puncture-resistant container after use. Use the needleless system, or safety syringes, if available. *Rationale: Recapping or breaking a needle poses a possibility of accidental finger stick. Protect yourself and housekeeping personnel.*
- Report any exposure to blood or body fluids to your supervisor immediately. *Rationale: OSHA requires initial screening and follow-up of the accident. Reporting protects your safety as well.*
- Clean or process equipment after use for a client. Discard disposable single-use items. *Rationale: Proper cleaning and disposal helps prevent transmission of infectious microorganisms.*
- Place contaminated linen in a leak-proof bag. *Rationale: Using a leak-proof bag prevents skin and mucous membrane exposure.*

Adapted from Centers for Disease Control and Prevention (1996). HICPAC guidelines for isolation procedures in hospitals. *American Journal of Infection Control*, 24, 24.

■■■ **TABLE 42-1** *N*URSING ACTIVITIES AND REQUIRED PPE TO DECREASE BLOOD-BORNE PATHOGEN EXPOSURE

Procedure	Handwashing	Gloves	Gowns	Mask	Eyewear
Talking with client					
Hygienic care	■				
Feeding a client	■	■			
Adjusting IV rate or noninvasive equipment	■				
Examining client without touching blood, body fluids, mucous membranes	■				
Examining client with contact with blood, body fluids, mucous membranes	■	■			
Drawing blood	■	■			
Inserting arterial or venous access devices	■	■	Gown, mask, eyewear are usually required		
Handling soiled waste, linen, other materials	■	■	Use gown, mask, eyewear if splattering is likely		
Operative and other procedures that produce extensive splattering of blood, body fluids	■	■	■	■	■
Handling lab specimens	■	■	Use gown, mask, eyewear if splattering is likely		

Adapted from the CDC and other sources.

treating clients who require any of these precautions, you will use them in addition to Standard Precautions. Table 42-2 presents an overview of transmission-based precautions and the types of diseases for which they are used.

☞ KEY CONCEPT

- *Standard Precautions—Treat blood and all body fluids (except sweat) from all clients as infectious.*
- *Transmission-based precautions—Use barrier precautions for clients with suspected or diagnosed infections.*
- *Special situations—For example, violent client who spits or bites, use PPE as needed.*

Airborne Precautions

Airborne transmission occurs when tiny microorganisms from evaporated droplets remain suspended in the air or are carried on dust particles. Air currents disperse the microorganisms, which a susceptible host can easily inhale. Special air handling and ventilation are required to prevent this type of disease transmission. TB, measles, and chickenpox are examples of airborne-transmitted infections.

Clients requiring **airborne precautions** are placed in a private room that has monitored negative airflow pressure. Six to 12 air changes occur per hour, with the air being discharged to the outdoors or specially filtered before circulating to other

■■■ **TABLE 42-2** 𝒯RANSMISSION-BASED PRECAUTIONS

Client Placement	Protection	Examples of Diseases
Airborne • Private room • Negative air flow pressure* • Discharge of room air to environment or filtered before circulation	• Follow Standard Precautions. • Wear a mask for airborne pathogens, or particulate air filter respirator in the case of TB. • Place a mask on the client if transport is required.	• Tuberculosis • Measles • Chickenpox
Droplet • Private room, or in a room with a similarly infected client(s) or one in which there is at least 3 ft between other client(s) and visitors	• Follow Standard Precautions. • Wear a mask when entering the room, but especially when within 3 ft of the infected client. • Place a mask on the client if transport is required.	• Influenza • Rubella • Meningococcal meningitis
Contact • Private room, or in a room with similarly infected client(s), or • Consult with an infection control professional if the above options are unavailable.	• Follow Standard Precautions. • Don gloves before entering the room. • Remove gloves before leaving the room. • Change gloves after contact with infective material. • Perform handwashing with an antimicrobial agent immediately after removing gloves. • Wear a gown when entering the room if a possibility exists that your clothing will touch the client or items in the room, or if the client is incontinent, has diarrhea, an ileostomy, a colostomy, or wound drainage not contained by a dressing. • Avoid transporting the client, but, if required, use precautions that minimize disease transmission. • Clean bedside equipment and client care items daily. • Use items such as a stethoscope, sphygmomanometer, and other assessment tools exclusively for the infected client and terminally disinfect them when precautions are no longer necessary.	• Gastrointestinal, respiratory, skin, or wound infections that are drug-resistant • Acute diarrhea • Draining abscess • Impetigo

* Negative air pressure pulls air from the hall into the room when the door is opened, as opposed to positive air pressure, which pulls room air into the hall. Adapted from J. S. Garner & Hospital Infection Control Practices Advisory Committee. *Guideline for isolation precautions in hospitals.* Atlanta: Public Health Service, U.S. Department of Health and Human Services, Centers for Disease Control and Prevention. *www.cdc.gov.ncidod/hip/isolat/isolat.htm.* updated 8/28/01

areas of the healthcare facility. Many facilities have special portable air-filtering machines to use when maintaining airborne precautions. Doors to rooms with clients who require airborne precautions are kept closed.

When caring for clients requiring airborne precautions, respiratory protection is necessary. Because of the recent resurgence of TB cases, CDC guidelines recommend the use of a special high-filtration particulate respirator when caring for those with active TB. The air-purifying respirator is a mask that fits the face tighter than the typical surgical mask, and is able to filter out 95% of particulates in the air. Although somewhat controversial, the use of this mask is believed to help protect against exposure to TB (Fig. 42-1).

Droplet Precautions

Droplet transmission occurs when droplets containing microorganisms are propelled through the air from an infected person and deposited on the host's eyes, nose, or mouth. Transmission can occur through sneezing, coughing, talking, or during certain procedures such as suctioning. Examples of illnesses spread by droplets include meningococcal meningitis, streptococcal pharyngitis (in infants and young children), pertussis, influenza, mumps, and rubella.

Clients requiring **droplet precautions** are placed in a private room. However, if a private room is unavailable, he or she can share a room with another client with the same infectious disease. The room's door may remain open. Wear a mask when working within 3 feet of the client. Have the client wear a mask if you must transport him or her to an area outside the room.

Contact Precautions

Contact transmission is the most frequent mode of disease transmission in healthcare facilities. Transmission can occur as a result of *direct contact* between a susceptible host's body

surface and an infected or colonized person. (**Colonization** occurs when a microorganism is present in a client, but he or she shows no clinical signs or symptoms of infection.) *Indirect contact* occurs when a susceptible host comes into contact with an intermediate contaminated object (eg, dirty instrument, needle, or hands). Examples of illnesses spread by contact transmission include drug-resistant gastroenteritis and respiratory, skin, and wound infections. Hepatitis A, herpes simplex virus, impetigo, scabies, and pediculosis are other examples.

A client who requires **contact precautions** can be placed in a room with other clients who are infected with the same microorganism if a private room is unavailable. The door may remain open. Wear gloves when entering the room and remove them before leaving. Change your gloves after contact with a client's infective material (eg, fecal matter or wound drainage). Wash your hands with an antimicrobial agent or waterless antiseptic agent. Wear a gown, gloves, and mask into the room if you anticipate contact with infectious matter, and remove them before leaving the room (Fig. 42-2). When possible, try to restrict the use of noncritical equipment to one client only. Clean and disinfect equipment before using it for other clients.

☛ KEY CONCEPT

Specific procedures for an individual client will often be prescribed, depending on the reason for precautions. Each healthcare organization has its own established local protocols.

ISOLATION

Standard Precautions and transmission-based precautions are the currently followed **isolation** guidelines. Historically, two primary types of isolation systems were used in healthcare: category-specific isolation and disease-specific isolation. Although standard and transmission-based precautions have replaced the common use of these systems, some facilities still follow such systems, in addition to standard and transmission-based precautions.

In *category-specific isolation,* specific categories of isolation (eg, respiratory, contact, enteric, strict, or wound) are identified, using color-coded cards. This form of isolation is based on the client's diagnosis. The cards are posted outside the client's room and state that visitors must check with nurses before entering.

Disease-specific isolation uses a single all-purpose sign. Nurses select the items on the card that are appropriate for the specific disease that is causing isolation.

Nursing Measures in Isolation

Setting Up a Client's Room for Isolation

Clients who require isolation must stay in their own room. All healthcare facilities have policies and procedures for isolation and for the use of specific PPE. Supplies are stored outside the client's room in a cart or bassinet or in a small room adjacent

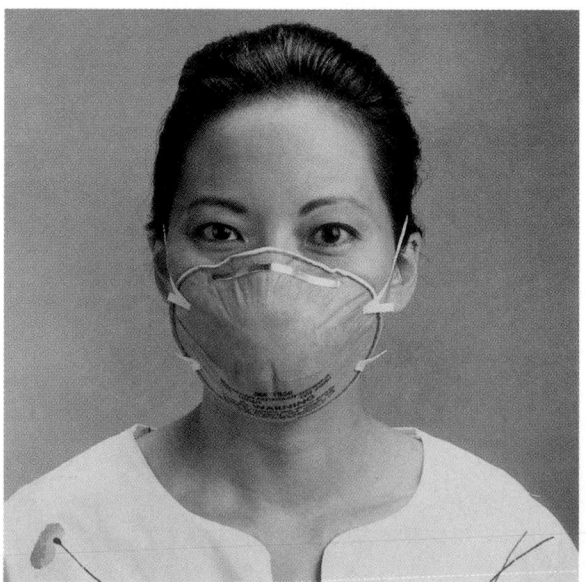

FIGURE 42-1. CDC guidelines recommend the use of a special high-filtration particulate mask when caring for clients with tuberculosis.

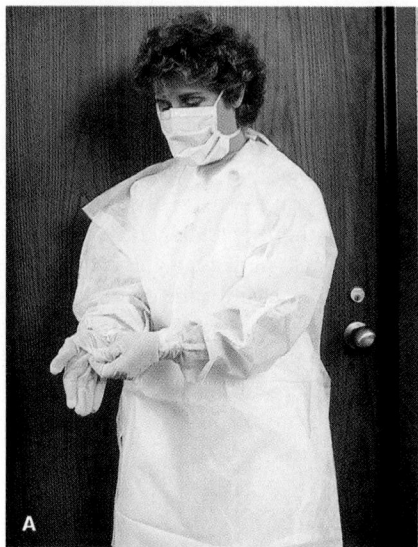
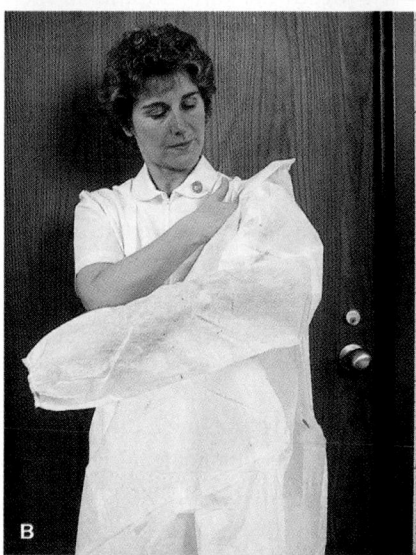

FIGURE 42-2. For the client requiring contact precautions, (**A**) wear a gown, gloves, and mask into the room if you anticipate contact with infectious matter and remove them before leaving the room. (**B**) The nurse uses her ungloved hand to grasp the inside of the gown for removal.

to the client's room. A sink is usually available or nearby for handwashing. Check the healthcare facility's policies and procedures for specific measures to follow if the client needs to be brought out of the room for a treatment or test.

Education and Preparation. When setting up the client's room, explain the reasons for the isolation precautions to the client and family. They will need to understand how easily pathogens spread when specific precautions are not observed. When they understand the reasons for preventive procedures, they are more likely to cooperate. Explain that children are usually not allowed to visit a client with a disease requiring special precautions, because children are so susceptible to infection. Additionally, some children will not be able to follow the special instructions.

Barrier techniques and PPE may frighten clients, who may fear their disease and believe that others are afraid to come

near them. These clients may experience loneliness and miss the companionship of others. Make every effort to visit and communicate with clients in isolation as much as possible. Organize your workload so that you can remain in their room for longer periods. Even when you are not going into their room, stop by and say hello.

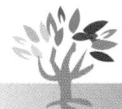

SPECIAL CONSIDERATIONS: THE LIFE SPAN

Nursing Procedures in Pediatric Infection Control

A higher percentage of pediatric admissions involve communicable diseases than do adult admissions. Often, members of the pediatric population are not immune to such diseases. If such diseases are not contained, an outbreak can result. Keep in mind the following:

- Children are at greater risk of acquiring viral infections than are adults.
- Young children may not be able to understand good handwashing and barrier precautions. They require adult supervision.
- Environmental surfaces must be kept as clean as possible because children may have physical and oral contact with them. Children may also put toys and other objects into their mouth. Some toys may be shared in playrooms. Shared toys must have cleanable surfaces. Stuffed animals and dolls cannot be shared.
- Barrier techniques are important to employees who care for children because children require close contact (eg, rocking, cuddling, and feeding).

Supplies. The client's room is usually equipped with a bedpan and urinal; wash basin and soap dish; water pitcher and glass; emesis basin; toilet and facial tissues; toothbrush and dentifrice; and personal items such as shaving equipment, comb or brush, deodorant, shampoo, and cosmetics. (Disposal of these items is necessary on the client's discharge.) Provide the client with a telephone and television, if possible. Additional items may include paper towels; plastic or paper bags to line the wastebasket for trash disposal; washable blankets, pillows, and bedspreads; and impervious laundry bags, as well as the usual linens needed for a client unit. A sink with foot or knee controls and a covered linen bag and stand are ideal. This client should have a private bathroom and shower.

Items to place outside the client's room or in an anteroom include a bedside stand or cabinet stocked with PPE as required for the client's condition. Other items may include clean laundry bags, large trash bags, biohazard bags, and tape or tags for marking contaminated bags. Healthcare facilities require a sign for the door; the sign will vary depending on the specific precautions the client's condition requires.

Administering Medications in Isolation

Follow Standard Precautions when administering medications. Use and dispose of disposable materials in the client's room. The following suggestions review general pointers for medication administration and add specific suggestions for clients in isolation.

- Unwrap medications before going into the client's room. *Rationale: Unwrapping will be difficult to do after you put on gloves.*
- If you will need juice or applesauce in which to mix medications, take it with you into the room. If using a medication tray, be sure it is disposable.
- Do not take medication administration cards or records into the client's room.
- If you are not going to touch the client, you may only need to wear a mask, if required. Do not touch the client or anything in the room, and be sure to scrub carefully.
- If you are giving an injection, wear gloves (per Standard Precautions). Wear a gown and mask as the client's condition indicates. Place needles and syringes into the sharps disposal container in the client's room. To avoid an accidental needle stick, do not break or recap needles, or detach them from syringes. Many facilities use "safety syringes" (see Fig. 63-6).
- Use disposable medication cups.
- Use and discard intravenous (IV) solution bags in the client's room. In the rare case of using an IV bottle, label the bag "glass" and place the bag into the appropriate container in the room.
- Dispose of all materials in the client's room.

Sending a Specimen to the Laboratory

Before collecting a specimen, label the container. If you are sending any specimen to a laboratory, place it on a clean paper towel in the anteroom and carefully scrub the container after you are outside the room. Then, place the specimen into a sealable plastic bag identified with the standard "biohazard" label to inform laboratory personnel of suspected microorganisms. Wash your hands again. Take the specimen to the laboratory as soon as possible. Remember to touch the request cards and the outside of the bag only with your clean hands.

Taking Vital Signs

Usually, necessary equipment to take vital signs is kept in the client's room and is disinfected when the client is discharged from the healthcare facility. Follow these guidelines when taking the vital signs of a client in an isolation room:

- Use the equipment in the room. Do not bring items in with you.

- Wear gloves and whatever other PPE is indicated.
- Remember that there is usually a clock on the wall, so you will not need to use your watch. If you do need to use a watch, however, place it on a paper towel and touch only the bottom of the towel with your contaminated hands, or seal the watch in a plastic bag. Pick up the watch after you have scrubbed outside the room.
- Use disposable thermometers, cuffs, and stethoscopes if available. You also may use a glass clinical thermometer that you will discard after the client's discharge. Many facilities use temperature indicator dots or other disposable systems for measuring the client's temperature. A blood pressure apparatus is usually on the wall. The cuff and stethoscope are disinfected when the client is discharged.

Using Double-Bagging

In some healthcare facilities, refuse and linen are "double bagged" outside the client's room. In other facilities, this procedure is no longer used because refuse and linen from all clients are considered contaminated and treated as such. Two nurses must carry out the double-bagging procedure. The nurse inside the room is considered "contaminated" and the nurse outside is considered "clean." The contaminated nurse places dirty items into a bag and closes the top. This entire bag, inside and out, is considered "contaminated." The clean nurse, outside the room, has a second bag that is considered "clean." He or she folds the top of the clean bag down on the outside to make a collar or cuff. The clean nurse keeps his or her hands protected by this cuff. The contaminated nurse then places the contaminated bag inside the clean bag, while the clean nurse holds the clean bag.

The contaminated nurse touches only the *inside* of the clean bag; the clean nurse touches only the *outside* of the clean bag and does not touch the contaminated bag. The clean nurse folds over the top of the clean bag, seals it carefully, and labels it, touching only the outside of the bag. After this is completed, both nurses wash their hands thoroughly.

Transporting the Client to Other Departments

In rare cases, transporting the client to another part of the healthcare facility for a special procedure or x-ray is necessary. Take the following special precautions when transporting a client in isolation to another area:

- Wear PPE as needed.
- Make sure the client wears appropriate PPE as indicated by his or her condition.
- Control and contain any of the client's drainage.
- Drape the wheelchair or stretcher with a clean sheet or bath blanket. Wrap the client with the clean material.

- Make sure to escort the ambulatory client to any examinations.
- Notify the other department that the client requires special precautions, so that personnel can prepare and perform accordingly.
- Carefully disinfect the wheelchair or stretcher after use.

Caring for the Client's Body After Death

If a client who is in isolation dies, you must take special precautions to prevent the spread of infection. Note that many healthcare facilities follow these precautions for all clients who die. In Practice: Nursing Care Guidelines 42-2 describes care of the body of the person who was in isolation.

Protective (Reverse or Neutropenic) Isolation

Sometimes, the client must be protected from the outside environment. In such a case, isolation procedures are reversed: other people's microorganisms are kept away from the client. This type of isolation is known as **protective isolation** (also called *reverse* or **neutropenic isolation**). Protective isolation attempts to prevent harmful microorganisms from coming into contact with the client. Box 42-1 lists general procedures for protective isolation.

Clients who need protective isolation have a weakened immune response. They may become infected; however, they may not show classic signs and symptoms of infection because they lack the white blood cells necessary to create the normal

---

➤➤ **BOX 42-1**

GENERAL PROCEDURES IN PROTECTIVE/NEUTROPENIC ISOLATION

- The client requires a private room.
- Healthcare workers and visitors may not enter if they have a cold, influenza, or other communicable disease.
- Anyone entering the room must wear a mask and practice strict handwashing before coming into contact with the client.
- The client cannot receive fresh fruit, fresh vegetables, or flowers.
- Rectal temperatures, enemas, suppositories, IV and intramuscular injections, and other invasive procedures are to be avoided if possible.
- The tympanic/ear probe method for monitoring the client's temperature is recommended. Measure the client's temperature at least every 4 hours.
- A blood culture may be necessary if any reason exists to suspect infection.
- In some cases, you will use special linens and wear specially laundered scrub suits and shoe covers. Some facilities require special hair covering. Staff working in these units often wear lab coats when leaving the units.
- Special air purification measures are used.

---

inflammatory response. Individuals who may require placement in protective isolation include those who have experienced burns or bone marrow transplants. Clients with AIDS, who are undergoing chemotherapy for cancer, or who are experiencing low resistance from another cause (eg, agammaglobulinemia) may also require protective isolation.

THE INFECTION CONTROL COMMITTEE

Each accredited healthcare facility has an infection control committee that monitors and evaluates any infection occurring in the facility. When the committee identifies the cause, it can take necessary preventive measures.

Healthcare workers must report any infection that occurs. The infection control committee will investigate to determine the cause. If a break in nursing technique is identified, the committee will propose different procedures to eliminate the problem. In many cases, the educational committee will hold educational sessions to teach new techniques. As a nurse, you may be asked to serve on an infection control committee.

The infection control committee has the following goals:

- Provide a central place for reporting infections.
- Investigate cases of infection.
- Maintain total statistics related to the numbers and types of infections that occur in the facility.
- Determine the cause of infection.

In Practice
Nursing Care Guidelines 42-2

CARING FOR THE BODY OF A DEAD PERSON WHO WAS IN ISOLATION

- Follow the measures for caring for the dead person's body that are listed in Chapter 59.
- Wrap the body while you are in the room. Usually, you will place it in a plastic zippered bag.
- Transfer the body to a cart that has been draped with a clean bath blanket or sheet. A clean person outside the room will wrap the clean blanket around the body.
- Decontaminate the room according to the facility's procedures.
- If you are the person caring for the body inside the room, remember that you are considered contaminated. You must wash your hands when leaving the room. Afterward, you may touch only the outside of the wrapping or shroud.
- Label the body properly. The pathologist treats all bodies as if they have an infectious disease.
- Check your healthcare facility for special procedures.

- Study current literature and identify effective national practices for infection prevention.
- Design local protocol and policies, following national guidelines, to control infection; the committee enforces standard and transmission-based precautions for that particular facility.
- Evaluate the effectiveness of protocols after they have been tried.
- Offer continuing education for healthcare personnel, to prevent infections.
- Serve as consultants in cases of questions or concerns of healthcare personnel.
- Review records of clients to identify organisms that may have become resistant to various drugs.
- Assist in employee health and wellness programs.
- Conduct research related to infection control practice.
- Conduct product evaluations for infection control items.
- Report diseases and infections to local, state, and federal authorities.
- Prevent future recurrences.

✄ STUDENT SYNTHESIS

Key Points

- Infection is best controlled by prevention—breaking the links in the chain of infection.
- JCAHO requires every healthcare facility it accredits to have an infection control plan.
- Standard Precautions consider that every client's blood and body fluids are potentially infectious; thus, Standard Precautions are used in the care of all clients.
- Transmission-based precautions are designed to prevent the spread of specific infections. They include airborne, droplet, and contact precautions. The specific type of transmission-based precautions for a particular client is used in conjunction with Standard Precautions.
- Barrier techniques are designed to prevent microorganisms from leaving a client's room.
- Special filtered respirator masks are often required when caring for a client with known or suspected TB.
- Before entering a client's room, determine the necessity of using PPE and other equipment.
- Isolation is often frightening and misunderstood by clients and families.
- Isolation procedures vary among healthcare facilities. Know your facility's specific procedures.
- Protective isolation helps prevent organisms from coming into contact with clients.
- One duty of an infection control committee is to monitor and evaluate infections in clients and in staff who are exposed.

Critical Thinking Exercises

1. Identify the appropriate PPE you would use in the following situations. Give your rationale for each:

- Discontinuing an IV for a client with no known or suspected infection
- Giving intramuscular medications to a client with no known or suspected infection
- Measuring the vital signs of a client with hepatitis
- Changing a bloody dressing on a client with TB
- Changing bed linen for an incontinent client
- Giving a bath to a client who is HIV positive
- Assisting with wound irrigation for a client with no known or suspected infection

2. Explain how you would expect to use standard and transmission-based precautions in a variety of settings (eg, schools, clinics, industry, and home care). Would your implementation of such measures change in any way from place to place? How would you explain the need for these precautions to clients and their families?

3. You are providing care for a homeless client in a clinic. You find that the client has been diagnosed with TB, but is not taking the medication for it. How would you handle this situation?

NCLEX-Style Review Questions

1. A client is admitted to the nursing unit with an infected wound. The most appropriate nursing action would be to place the client:
   a. In any open room
   b. On airborne precautions
   c. On contact precautions
   d. On droplet precautions

2. For a client on airborne precautions, which of the following is needed?
   a. At least 3 feet of distance to other clients
   b. Negative airflow pressure room
   c. Private room with similarly infected client
   d. Protective isolation

3. Which type of isolation would be appropriate for a client undergoing chemotherapy?
   a. Airborne
   b. Contact
   c. Droplet
   d. Protective

4. Which personal protective equipment would be needed for a client with TB?
   a. Double layer of gloves
   b. Gown
   c. High-filtration particulate respirator
   d. Protective eyewear

5. A client is on contact isolation. Which precaution would be necessary during transportation of this client to another part of the healthcare facility?
   a. Controlling and containing any client drainage
   b. Having the client wear a mask
   c. Notifying family members to transport the client
   d. Refusing to transport an infected client

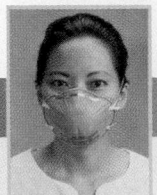

Emergency Care and First Aid

LEARNING OBJECTIVES

1. Discuss the importance of assessing the safety of an emergency scene.
2. Describe the medical identification tag and its purpose.
3. Describe, in order, the steps for assessing an ill or injured person in an emergency.
4. Identify early, common, and progressive signs of shock.
5. Describe at least five common types of shock, including hypovolemic shock, identifying nursing actions in emergency-induced shock.
6. Define sudden death.
7. Differentiate between clinical and biologic death.
8. State and demonstrate the procedure for calling a code in your healthcare facility or agency.
9. Describe general emergency actions for chest, neck, back, and head injuries.
10. Demonstrate in the lab, emergency actions for a puncture wound of the chest.
11. Describe at least three signs of increasing intracranial pressure.
12. Explain symptoms and first aid for injuries caused by exposure to cold, including frostbite and hypothermia.
13. Describe symptoms and immediate first aid for heat-related illnesses and injuries, including heat exhaustion and severe burns.
14. List at least three signs of an inhalation injury following a fire.
15. Discuss first aid for musculoskeletal injuries, including a fracture, demonstrating the ability to safely splint an ulnar or radial fracture using common household materials.
16. Describe the immediate actions of a rescuer in suspected heart attack.
17. Describe emergency care for at least three different types of hemorrhage.
18. Define the term anaphylaxis and describe causes, symptoms, and treatment of anaphylaxis.
19. Identify at least three precautions to take when dealing with hazardous materials.
20. List at least five immediate actions to take when a person is suspected of being poisoned.
21. Define the term triage, and describe how it applies to emergency care.
22. List at least four factors that identify a psychiatric emergency or the potential for suicide.

NEW TERMINOLOGY

ambu bag	hypothermia
anaphylaxis	intrusion injury
antidote	intubation
avulsion injury	mediastinal shift
bandage	near drowning
biologic death	pneumothorax
café coronary	poison
caustic	rabies
clinical death	shock
code	splint
debride	sprain
dislocation	strain
emetic	stridor
epistaxis	sudden death
extrication	syncope
fracture	thrombolytic
frostbite	tourniquet
gastric lavage	toxin
heat cramps	trauma
heat exhaustion	triage
heat stroke	wind chill factor
hemorrhage	

ACRONYMS

ABCDE	DNI	MI
ACLS	DNR	MVA
AED	EMS	PERRLA+C
AVPU	EMT	PTSD
BCLS	HAZMAT	RICE
BLS	ICP	SIRES
CMS	LOC	SIRS
CPR	MAST	

Trauma refers to a wound or injury that is caused by an outside force. Thousands of people die from the effects of trauma and sudden illness every year. Traumatic injuries are caused by events such as motor vehicle accidents (**MVAs**), poisonings, burns, responses to temperature extremes, obstructed airways, and gunshot wounds. Events such as the tragic explosion and collapse of the World Trade Center towers in New York emphasize the need for first-aid training for all healthcare workers, emergency and rescue personnel, law enforcement officers, and the general public.

This chapter describes actions to take when caring for someone who has experienced sudden illness or trauma. Cardiopulmonary resuscitation (**CPR**) and basic life support are not described in detail in this chapter. To learn the detailed methods used in CPR and removal of airway obstruction, the nurse *must* take a specific course. Healthcare facilities and organizations require CPR certification for all employees. It is up to each healthcare provider to take the responsibility for obtaining this training and to keep certification current. This chapter briefly outlines measures in administering basic first aid for selected injuries and accidents.

PRINCIPLES OF EMERGENCY CARE

Simply because you are a nurse, people will expect you to be able to deal with emergencies. Good Samaritan Laws (Box 43-1) require the nurse to assist at the scene of an accident in certain situations. Each nurse must be fully able to meet this expectation. Basic emergency care principles provide the foundation to act appropriately when accidents happen. In an emergency, the first responder must decide *quickly* what to do. A confident, matter-of-fact approach will reassure victims and onlookers. If the first responder appears confident, others will follow instructions and assist.

Without an adequate oxygen supply—due to blood loss or airway obstruction—a person's brain cells begin to die within 4 to 6 minutes. Therefore, you must give care in an emergency quickly. The stress level is usually high during an emergency, so having a predetermined, orderly plan of action and method of assessment is critical.

Assess Safety

Make sure the scene is safe before rushing to assist in an emergency. Check the environment and look for clues. Is there any danger of fire, explosion, or building collapse? Is there danger of being caught in traffic or hit by a car? Are there electrical hazards, live wires, or other hazardous materials? Is the person in danger of drowning? If the scene is unsafe, the first responder may need to call for additional help *before assisting injured persons.* It may also be necessary to move victims away from danger before starting first-aid care. Do not move any injured person, however, if the area is safe. *Rationale: Unnecessary movement can compound or cause additional problems.* If the person is a victim of an automobile accident, remember to assign someone to direct traffic to prevent further injuries.

Identify Problems

Is there anything unusual about the situation? Are containers lying about that suggest attempted suicide, poisoning, or drug abuse? Do medications give a clue to a medical problem (eg, diabetes, epilepsy)? Are there signs of alcohol or drug abuse? Is there any indication of foul play?

☛ KEY CONCEPT
___

If there is any indication of foul play, treat the victim without disturbing what has now become a crime scene.

When reporting an MVA, note the vehicle's condition. Is the vehicle upside down, on its side, or in a ditch? Is the vehicle in the water? Is there a gasoline spill? Note areas of intrusion: the driver's side, passenger's side, roof, front end, or back end. Were victims wearing seatbelts? Were the airbags deployed? Was anyone thrown from the vehicle, and if so, how many feet or yards? If the victim was riding a bicycle or motorcycle, was the victim wearing a helmet and protective clothing? This information can help emergency personnel anticipate certain types of injuries.

Medic Alert Tag

Check accident victims for medical identification or Medic-Alert® tags, which a person may wear as a bracelet or on a chain around the neck (Fig. 43-1). This tag signifies any specific medical problem (eg, diabetes, epilepsy) to be considered when administering first aid. Some emergency medical identification tags provide a 24-hour toll-free telephone number for obtaining additional medical information, as well as the person's identity or next-of-kin, for emergency purposes. If you do not consider such information and treat accordingly, the person may die. It may be necessary to look in an unconscious person's wallet to see if it contains any medical information. Consult the person's family, if possible.

➤ ➤ BOX 43-1

GOOD SAMARITAN LAWS

- Most states have a law that protects emergency care rescuers from legal liability, provided that the rescuers give *reasonable assistance* to the extent possible without danger or peril to the person or themselves.
- Some states consider rescuers guilty of violating the law if they do not give aid to someone who needs it. (In general, if emergency rescue personnel are already on the scene, you are not required to assist, unless you are specifically asked to do so.)
- Nurses are required to assist in an emergency only *to the level of first aid training.* Do only what you are trained to do in an emergency. Become familiar with the laws in the areas in which you work, live, and travel.

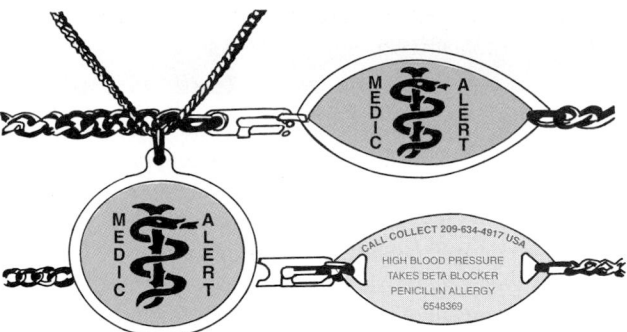

FIGURE 43-1. The First Aid person should always search for medical information on an injured person. Shown here is the *MedicAlert*® tag. This tag may be worn as a bracelet or necklace. Pertinent emergency information is printed on the back, as well as a 24-hour hotline number. By giving the person's ID number (printed on the tag), the person's identity as well as additional medical information and his or her next-of-kin can be determined. If a person has a potentially life-threatening condition, the MedicAlert tag is preferable to information in a wallet or purse. (Reproduced by permission. © 2001 MedicAlert Foundation. All rights reserved. MedicAlert®, a 501(c)(3) nonprofit membership organization, is the nation's leading emergency medical information service. For information, call 800-432-5378 or visit http://www.medicalert.org.)

If a card is found indicating that a person wishes to donate tissues or organs after death, inform emergency personnel at the scene of the accident. In many states, the fact that the victim wishes to be a donor is indicated on his or her driver's license. (Remember that the next-of-kin is required to give permission for organ or tissue donation if a person dies, even if the person has a donor card.)

Perform Triage

Triage is the process of sorting and classifying to determine priority of needs (see Chap. 39). Triage involves determining life-threatening situations and assisting those clients first. If there are a large number of victims, less seriously injured people may be able to assist others. It is also important to *identify* victims and their next-of-kin whenever possible.

The triage nurse and rescue personnel must determine whom to assist first, when and how to call for help, and how untrained bystanders can assist. If there are numerous victims, the local hospital must be notified so that they can activate their disaster plan. Nurses also use triage in emergency departments (EDs) and clinics, whether through telephone screening or on a walk-in basis.

Summon Assistance

Summoning help is an important part of emergency care. A victim's life may depend on rapid response. In most communities in the United States and Canada, the fastest way to summon the emergency medical service (**EMS**) is by telephoning 911. *Be sure to know the local emergency number if it is not 911.* If possible, send someone to call, but make sure the person has all necessary information, including the exact location and the nature of the emergency.

Assess and Treat for Shock

Shock is often the first phase of the body's "alarm reaction" to trauma or severe tissue damage. Many types of shock result when the body loses its ability to circulate an adequate supply of oxygenated blood to all its components, particularly the brain. After an accident, many conditions can lead to shock; however, shock usually results from problems in the cardiovascular system (see Chap. 22).

The body attempts to compensate for any trauma or insult to its integrity. Because the central nervous system (CNS) controls all body functions, it monitors changes and immediately implements *compensatory circulation* to maintain an adequate blood supply to vital organs (eg, the brain and the heart) in an emergency. This compensatory action can quickly adjust the rate and strength of the heart's contractions and the tone of blood vessels in all body parts. It actually shuts down the flow of blood to the skin, digestive system, and kidneys, and *shunts* (transfers) the blood that would normally go to these areas to the heart and brain instead. (The symptoms of shock are largely related to this compensatory mechanism.) Compensatory circulation is a survival mechanism that ensures that the body's most vital organs are adequately perfused with blood until the last possible moment.

However, in some cases (for example, because the injury is so severe), the body cannot compensate. In this case, shock develops. Shock may develop rapidly following trauma (or more slowly in other situations). Consequently, *every injured person* should receive preventive and precautionary treatment for shock. Anything that could cause increased blood loss or otherwise contribute to shock should be avoided. For this reason, never handle or move injured persons roughly or cause them undue anxiety.

Shock may fall into three major categories: *primary*—the nervous system's response immediately after a severe injury; *secondary*—one or more hours after an injury, perhaps up to 24 hours later (*delayed* or *deferred shock*); *hemorrhagic*—due to blood loss, and may be categorized as primary or secondary. The major types of shock, along with less commonly known types, are listed in Box 43-2.

Hypovolemic Shock

Trauma that results in excessive blood loss will decrease the amount of blood volume available for the heart to pump. This will lead to a type of shock called *absolute hypovolemic shock*. It is most commonly referred to as just *hypovolemic shock*. The loss of about one fifth of the body's total blood volume can cause this type of hypovolemic shock.

In addition to hemorrhage, absolute hypovolemic shock may result from: severe dehydration (lowered *intravascular* [within the blood vessels] fluid volume), possibly due to *diaphoresis* (excessive sweating) or diseases such as diabetes insipidus and, in some cases, diabetes mellitus; severe diarrhea; protracted vomiting (over a long period of time); intestinal obstruction; *peritonitis* (inflammation of the peritoneum); acute *pancreatitis* (inflammation of the pancreas); and severe burns.

➤➤ BOX 43-2

TYPES OF SHOCK

Major Types of Shock

- *Anaphylactic (allergic) shock*—a severe, life-threatening reaction to a substance to which the client is sensitive or allergic. (See Box 47-1 in Chapter 47 for a list of symptoms associated with this type of shock.)
- *Cardiogenic (cardiac) shock*—primarily a failure of the heart to accomplish its pumping function. The heart is severely compromised. Possible causes may include: failure or stenosis (narrowing) of heart valves, cardiomyopathy (primary heart disease), or rhythm disturbances. Low cardiac output is often the result of an acute MI (heart attack) or heart failure. (Cardiogenic shock may also occur in high cardiac output. This condition is approximately 80% fatal.)
- *Electric shock*—the immediate effects after the passage of electric current through the body. This type of shock is usually the result of accidental contact with electric circuits or wires, but it may also be caused by lightning. The amount of damage is influenced by the pathway taken by the current, the amount of current, and the skin's resistance. Symptoms include unconsciousness, respiratory paralysis, tetanic muscle contractions (continuous tonic spasm), bone fractures, and cardiac standstill. Immediate defibrillation is often necessary.
- *Hypoglycemic shock (insulin shock, wet shock, "diabetic shock")*—secondary to low blood sugar (less than 40 mg/dL). It may be a result of overdose of insulin, a skipped meal, or strenuous exercise in a person with IDDM (insulin-dependent diabetes mellitus). It may also be caused by an insulin-secreting tumor of the pancreas. (Chapter 78 discusses IDDM in more detail.) Symptoms are often related to a lack of sugar (fuel) in the brain. Treatment includes administration of sugar (glucose) and supporting the blood pressure.
- *Hypovolemic shock (hematogenic shock, hemorrhagic shock, oligemic shock)*—most often a result of hemorrhage. The body has insufficient blood volume to maintain adequate cardiac output, blood pressure, and tissue perfusion (circulation). Oxygen is not delivered to the tissues, and wastes are not removed. Symptoms include physical collapse and prostration. This type of shock is discussed further later in this chapter.
- *Irreversible shock*—the changes produced cannot be corrected by treatment; death is inevitable.
- *Lung shock (shock lung, acute respiratory distress syndrome [ARDS])*—pulmonary damage that occurs early in shock. Symptoms include acute respiratory distress and pulmonary edema. The pulmonary vessels may plug with blood cells and platelets, leading to anoxia, damage to the alveoli and capillaries, and generalized hypoxia of tissues. Decreased surfactant (a lubricating substance that allows lung expansion) may lead to *atelectasis* (collapsed lung).
- *Neurogenic shock*—vasodilation secondary to cerebral trauma, spinal cord injury, very deep general or spinal anesthesia, or CNS (central nervous system) depression caused by toxins. The major mechanism here is that of decreased peripheral vascular resistance.
- *Septic shock (endotoxic shock, endotoxin shock, toxic shock)*—the result of an overwhelming infection throughout the body, secondary to the release of toxins, usually by Gram-negative bacteria (particularly *Escherichia coli*) and by cytokines (see Chapter 24). Other organisms, such as viruses, can also cause septic shock. Endotoxins, stimulated by the infection, act on the vascular system, where a large amount of blood is held in the capillaries and veins and is not available to the general circulation. The blood pressure can fall to a very dangerous low level. Other symptoms include chills, fever, warm and flushed skin, increased cardiac output, and less hypotension than in hypovolemic shock. If therapy is ineffective, the symptoms will be similar to those of hypovolemic shock. Septic or toxic shock is one stage in the systemic inflammatory response syndrome (**SIRS**). Most common in newborns or people over age 50, and in persons with diabetes, cirrhosis of the liver, or compromised immune systems (eg, due to AIDS, cancer chemotherapy, bone marrow transplants).
- *Spinal shock*—loss of spinal reflexes after acute transverse spinal cord injury. Flaccid paralysis (below the level of injury) and loss of reflexes and sensation occur. Arterial hypotension is possible.
- *Toxic shock syndrome*—shock caused by an infection, usually by a staphylococcus organism (associated with tampon use) that can progress to untreatable (irreversible) shock. The bacteria produce a toxin that enters the blood stream, causing a septic condition. Treatment involves removal of the tampon and administration of antibiotics.
- *Traumatic shock*—any shock caused by trauma, injury, or surgery, such as a crushing or cerebral injury; fracture; burn; heart damage following an MI (myocardial infarction); intestinal obstruction; perforation or rupture of viscera (internal organs); strangulated hernia; or torsion of viscera (including ovary or testicle).

Less Commonly Known Types of Shock

- *Anaphylactoid reaction*—pseudoanaphylaxis (not true anaphylactic shock).
- *Anesthesia shock*—due to an overdose of a general anesthetic.
- *Burn shock*—caused by the loss of plasma into a burn wound.
- *Chronic shock*—due to peripheral circulatory insufficiency in older people with debilitating diseases such as cancer, or due to a subnormal blood volume that results from slow bleeding.

(continued)

➤➤ BOX 43-2

TYPES OF SHOCK (CONTINUED)

- *Cultural shock*—distress related to assimilation into a completely new culture or country.
- *Distributive shock*—marked decrease in peripheral vascular resistance, causing hypotension (as in septic, neurogenic, or anaphylactic shock)
- *Epigastric shock*—caused by a blow or extensive surgery to the abdomen.
- *Osmotic shock*—rupture of plasma membrane and loss of cellular contents secondary to exposure to a very hypotonic environment (see Chapter 17), which causes a sudden change in osmotic pressure within the cells.
- *Pleural shock*—a hypotensive condition secondary to *thoracentesis* (withdrawing fluid from the lung cavity), especially if a large amount of fluid is withdrawn at one time. Symptoms include cyanosis (blueness of the skin and mucous membranes), pallor (paleness), dilated pupils, and disturbances of pulse and respiration.
- *Postoperative shock*—shock that occurs after surgery.

- *Protein shock*—secondary to parenteral (central arterial line) administration of proteins.
- *Psychic shock (mental shock)*—secondary to emotional stress, such as an injury or accident, possibly manifested by excessive fear, joy, anger, or grief.
- *Serum shock*—anaphylactic shock secondary to administration of a foreign serum to a sensitized person.
- *Shell shock (battle fatigue)*—a mental disorder in World War I associated with combat. Now known as post-traumatic stress disorder (**PTSD**).
- *Surgical shock*—shock occurring during or after surgery (includes postoperative shock and traumatic shock).
- *Testicular shock*—shock resulting from a sharp blow to the testes.
- *Vasogenic shock*—shock that is secondary to marked vasodilation, usually as a result of severe loss of vascular tone resulting from damage to the vasomotor centers in the brain stem or medulla.

If a person is experiencing absolute hypovolemic shock, look for the following:

- Hypotension (lowered blood pressure, after a slight increase)
- Weak, thready pulse
- Cool, clammy skin
- Tachycardia (increased pulse)
- Tachypnea (increased respiratory rate)
- Hyperpnea (very deep breathing, gasping)
- Restlessness, anxiety (caused by decreased blood flow to the brain)
- Weakness
- Decreased urinary output

Remember, most of these signs and symptoms are related to the compensatory mechanisms of the body.

In the healthcare facility, additional information is obtained by diagnostic procedures such as monitoring of central venous pressure, pulmonary wedge pressure (PWP), and cardiac output; electrocardiogram; serum electrolyte levels; urine volume and specific gravity; arterial blood gases; and complete blood count. Keep in mind that in shock, many of these values are abnormal.

Relative Hypovolemic Shock.   Another type of hypovolemic shock, technically referred to as *relative hypovolemic shock,* is caused by widespread *vasodilation* (enlargement of the blood vessels of the body). This type of shock is caused by a massive infection or severe nervous system injury, rather than by hemorrhage.

In relative hypovolemic shock, blood volume is normal, but it is insufficient to supply the tissues with oxygen because of the increased size of the blood vessels. The symptoms are largely the same as those seen in absolute hypovolemic shock.

Late Signs of Hypovolemic Shock.   Later signs of hypovolemic shock include lowered body temperature, shallow respirations, and a narrowed *pulse pressure* (the difference between the systolic and diastolic blood pressure readings). Late in the process, the stage of *decompensated shock* occurs if the shock is not successfully treated. The client in this stage is extremely hypotensive. This situation is often life threatening.

Sequelae of Hypovolemic Shock.   Hypovolemic shock can lead to serious and life-threatening conditions such as *metabolic acidosis* (due to increased lactic acid), or irreversible cerebral (brain), hepatic (liver), and renal (kidney) damage. A condition known as *disseminated intravascular coagulation* or DIC (widespread blood clots, mostly in the capillaries) can also occur and is very dangerous.

Shock is present in most serious injuries or illnesses, even though the classic signs may not be apparent. Compensatory action may keep a person responsive, and in some cases alert, even when massive blood loss has occurred. Look for signs of a change in the person's level of consciousness (**LOC;** see Chap. 77). Progressive signs indicate that circulation to the brain is inadequate. Falling blood pressure is a *late sign* of shock. In extreme cases, MAST trousers are applied by paramedics. These are described and pictured later in this chapter.

Treatment of Shock.   Treatment of hypovolemic shock is symptomatic (aimed at correcting imbalances and removing the underlying cause—the causative disorder—of the shock). The treatment of most types of shock is approximately the same. In a first-aid situation:

- Efforts are made to increase the blood supply to the brain. (In many cases, this involves elevating the feet or lowering the head.)

- Bleeding sites are identified. If there is bleeding, the bleeding is controlled.
- Fluid loss is replaced.

In addition, the following may be necessary:

- Administering blood and blood components
- Supporting blood pressure with medications such as dopamine or norepinephrine
- Administering IV antibiotics if the cause is an infection (after a culture and sensitivity test)
- Treating an infection: draining abscesses, debriding (removing) necrosed (dead) tissue, removing other possible sources of infection (eg, catheters, IV, drainage tubes, tampons)

In all cases, the underlying causes of the shock are treated. In any emergency situation, *if in doubt, treat for shock.* In Practice: Nursing Care Guidelines 43-1 gives further pointers in the recognition and treatment of shock.

☛ KEY CONCEPT

Look for all signs of shock. *A falling blood pressure is a late sign of shock, and is ominous.*

ASSESSING THE PERSON IN AN EMERGENCY

The *primary assessment* is the assessment performed as soon as rescuers arrive at an emergency scene. During this assessment, life-threatening problems or injuries are identified and handled. If there are no life-threatening problems to correct, the primary assessment usually can be completed within 60 seconds.

The *secondary assessment* involves taking and recording the victim's vital signs (see Chap. 46) and continues with a head-to-toe assessment. This secondary assessment should take from 1 to 2 minutes, unless injuries requiring immediate intervention are identified. If the person has life-threatening

---

In Practice
Nursing Care Guidelines 43-1

TREATING SHOCK IN AN EMERGENCY

- Keep the person lying down and as calm as possible; reassure both the person and bystanders. Have someone call for assistance. Avoid rough handling of the injured person. *Rationale: If the injured person becomes excited, the body's oxygen needs will increase, thus increasing the shock. The person may need advanced life support.*
- Establish, maintain, and monitor the airway, breathing, and circulation. *Rationale: These functions are vital to life.*
- Administer a high concentration of oxygen, if available. Assist breathing as needed. *Rationale: Administration of external oxygen increases the oxygen available in the blood and helps the person to breathe with less effort.*
- Control bleeding. *Rationale: Additional bleeding leads to more blood loss and adds to shock.*
- Maintain body temperature; many people become chilled after an accident. Cover with a blanket or coats, if necessary. Do not overheat the person. *Rationale: The parasympathetic nervous system takes over in an emergency and reroutes blood to the vital organs and away from the skin. Excessively low or high body temperature causes the heart to work harder.*
- Keep the person dry. *Rationale: If a person becomes wet, chilling occurs much more quickly.*
- Give nothing by mouth. *Rationale: The person could aspirate, choke, or vomit.*
- Elevate the lower extremities, unless contraindicated. *Rationale: Elevating the legs helps blood to*

flow toward the brain where it is needed. Some people may need to have the head elevated, to breathe. In head injury, the body is kept level.

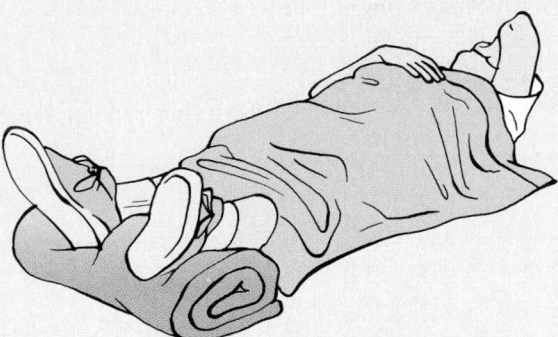

In many emergencies and injuries, the person must be treated for shock. Keep the person lying down. Maintain body temperature with blankets or coats. Elevate the feet and legs unless contraindicated.

- Use the position that is most comfortable for the person and that is within medical limits for that injury. *Rationale: Proper positioning maintains client comfort and prevents further injury.*
- Immobilize fractures. *Rationale: Immobilization prevents further injury.*
- Monitor level of consciousness. Take and record vital signs every 5 minutes. *Rationale: Level of consciousness and vital signs provide important information about the client's status. Emergency and medical personnel must know the person's reactions to the injury.*

problems, the secondary assessment may be delayed until the person is being transported. (Keep in mind that the assessments of the nurse acting as a first-aid person can only be performed to the level of the individual nurse's skills and training.)

Whenever assessing a person in an emergency, use the acronym **ABCDE** to help you remember the order for assessment:

A = Airway and cervical spine
B = Breathing
C = Circulation and bleeding
D = Disability
E = Expose and examine

A: Airway and Cervical Spine

Evaluate the airway's patency to determine whether it is open (*patent*). While doing so, keep in mind the injury's mechanism, location, and scope. For example, the person must be able to breathe before other first-aid measures can be instituted.

If a possibility of spinal injury exists, *stabilize the person's cervical spine* before attempting other activities. If the proper equipment is not available, wait for emergency rescue personnel to arrive. Unless there is an immediate danger, such as of explosion or fire, *do not move the person!*

B: Breathing

Assess breathing by listening for breath sounds, watching for chest movements, and feeling for breath against your cheek and ear.

Maintain the Airway. *Maintain the person's airway* even if breathing is present. Blood, body fluids, and vomitus may accumulate in the person's mouth and should be removed. Be sure the person's tongue is out of the way. (The tongue can occlude the airway in even a minor event, such as fainting.) Position the person on the side if vomiting threatens, while maintaining cervical spine alignment.

Nursing Alert
The most common airway obstruction in an unconscious person is caused by the tongue falling back and occluding the airway.

Observe Respirations. As you assess breathing, note if *respirations* appear to be of a normal rate and depth (see Chap. 46). Examine the person's mouth, gums, lips, and nail beds for color and moisture. Blueness (*cyanosis*) or duskiness in the skin, nail beds, or mucous membranes indicates a lack of oxygen.

Look for Life-Threatening Chest Injuries. If indicated by the injury's mechanism, examine the person's chest for life-threatening injuries. Chest injuries may cause internal bleeding and injury to the heart and lungs. If the body's ability to exchange oxygen and circulate oxygenated blood diminishes, permanent brain damage or death will occur if left uncorrected. Immediately care for injuries such as rib fractures,

punctured lung, stab wounds, gunshot wounds, compression injuries that result in a caved-in or open chest wall, and cardiac contusions. *If the chest wall is not intact, plug the hole at once.*

A serious situation is *flail chest,* which is a loss of stability of the chest wall. Flail chest is caused by several fractured ribs or detachment of the ribs from the sternum, as a result of a crushing injury. The loose portion of the chest moves in a direction opposite from normal when the person breathes (*paradoxical respiration*). In other words, the chest rises on expiration and falls on inspiration. It is important to stabilize the chest wall as much as possible with whatever is available. For example, apply an all cotton elastic (ACE) roller bandage and have the person lie on the affected side, to apply pressure to the chest wall. Transport the person immediately.

Be alert for important signs of chest injuries, which include:

- Pain at the site of injury and on breathing
- Shortness of breath, gasping
- Failure of the chest to expand
- Coughing up blood
- Rapid, weak pulse and low blood pressure
- Cyanotic lips, gums, fingernails, or fingertips
- Panic, agitation, nasal flaring
- Abnormal breathing sounds, such as wheezing or stridor (see Chapters 46 and 47)
- Abnormal chest movements on breathing

C: Circulation and Bleeding

The heart must be pumping effectively for oxygen to be carried to the cells. Also, there must be sufficient blood volume to carry the needed oxygen. Therefore, any disruption in the pumping action of the heart, the blood pressure, or the amount of blood available can compromise the person's condition.

Palpate the Pulse. Palpate the victim's pulse, using the carotid artery in the neck, for 5 to 10 seconds (see Fig. 43-2). If no pulse is present, ask bystanders to call for assistance: This person needs advanced life support as soon as possible. Begin cardiac compressions immediately if qualified. (This technique should be learned in a special CPR course.)

Observe the Pulse. If a pulse is present, note its rate and regularity. Does it seem normal? Do *not* count the pulse at this time; just try to get a sense of its quality. While palpating the pulse, also observe skin color, temperature, and neck veins.

Reassess Breathing. A person may have a heartbeat without having respirations; therefore, reassess breathing. If the person is not breathing, begin rescue breathing immediately. (This technique is also learned in a special CPR course.)

Nursing Alert
Use a one-way filtered breathing mask for CPR whenever possible, to protect the rescuer.

When the EMS personnel arrive, they can "bag" the person with an **Ambu bag.** This is a bag attached to a face mask, which can be used to "breathe for" the person. This method is safer, more effective, and less tiring for the rescuer than rescue breathing. Supplemental oxygen can also be delivered via the ambu bag.

Assess for Progressing Shock.   Always consider the possibility of shock in any injury. Use the *capillary refill test* to evaluate for shock, as follows:

- Press a finger into the middle of the person's forehead until the spot being pressed turns white.
- Remove the finger. Count the seconds it takes for color to return. (Count: one-one thousand; two-one thousand, etc.)
- If it takes more than 2 seconds for color to return, *shock is progressing* (see discussion earlier in this chapter on shock).

Assess and Control Hemorrhage.   The presence of a palpable pulse indicates that the person's heart is beating. However, you must also assess for major bleeding (*hemorrhage*).

Control hemorrhage *immediately* or the person will die from blood loss. With gloved hands, place sterile compresses over wounds and apply pressure. If blood seeps through the compresses, do not remove them but place additional compresses

over the top of those already in place. As necessary, apply additional pressure over the wound.

☞ **KEY CONCEPT**

Follow Standard Precautions whenever possible in administering first aid.

Measures that can be used to stop bleeding include:

- Apply direct pressure (should be done first).
- Elevate a bleeding limb.
- Apply an ice or cold pack, if available; place ice over several layers of dressings to avoid freezing body tissues.
- Apply *indirect pressure:* press the blood vessel at a pressure point against a bone. (See Figure 43-2 for an illustration of pressure points.)
- If severe bleeding continues, reach into the wound and try to grasp the bleeding vessel with your fingers.
- Apply a tourniquet *as a last resort* (see procedure later in this chapter). Mark the tourniquet with the time it was applied. Also mark the client's forehead, so all rescue

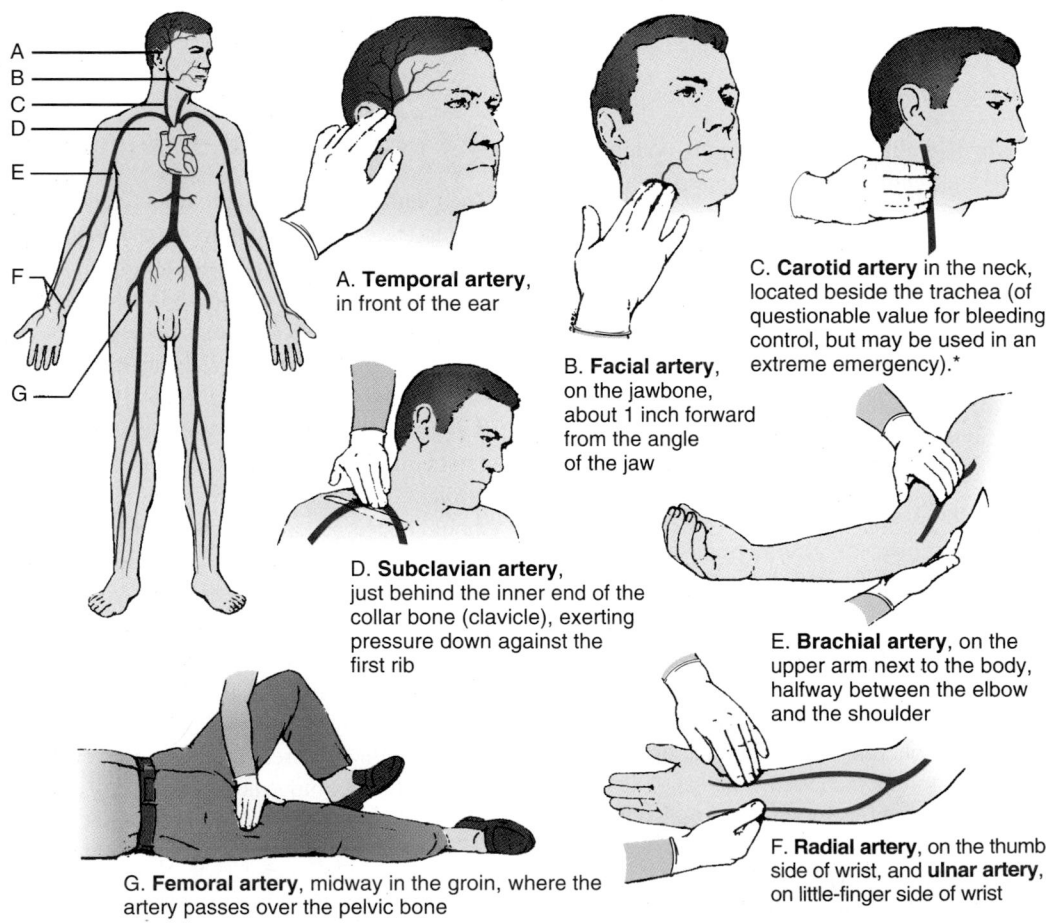

A. **Temporal artery**, in front of the ear

B. **Facial artery**, on the jawbone, about 1 inch forward from the angle of the jaw

C. **Carotid artery** in the neck, located beside the trachea (of questionable value for bleeding control, but may be used in an extreme emergency).*

D. **Subclavian artery**, just behind the inner end of the collar bone (clavicle), exerting pressure down against the first rib

E. **Brachial artery**, on the upper arm next to the body, halfway between the elbow and the shoulder

F. **Radial artery**, on the thumb side of wrist, and **ulnar artery**, on little-finger side of wrist

G. **Femoral artery**, midway in the groin, where the artery passes over the pelvic bone

*****Note**: Do *not* apply pressure to both sides of the neck at the same time. This would cut off the blood supply to the brain.

FIGURE 43-2. Pressure points for hemorrhage control. (Adapted from Smeltzer, S. C., & Bare, B. G. [2000]. *Brunner and Suddarth's textbook of medical-surgical nursing* [9th ed.]. Philadelphia: Lippincott Williams & Wilkins.)

workers know that a tourniquet is in place. *Do not release a tourniquet after it is applied.*

D: Disability

Neurologic Assessment. Conducting a neurologic assessment at an accident scene will help receiving medical personnel in the ER. Identify levels of consciousness. (The acronym **AVPU** will help in remembering these levels.)

  A = Alert: Speaks and moves spontaneously; answers questions about name, place, and date correctly
  V = Responsive to *verbal stimuli* only; answers when directly addressed
  P = Responsive to *painful stimuli* only (eg, rubbing the sternum or pressure on the nail beds)
  U = *Unresponsive*

Eye Signs.   Assess the person's pupillary responses. The pupils of both eyes should be the same (equal). They should be round and should constrict when a bright light quickly shines into them (react to light). The pupils should change size between close and far vision (*accommodation*). Reactions should be the same in both eyes, and they should move together when following a moving object (eyes coordinated). Remember this procedure by following **PERRLA+C**:

  PE = Pupils Equal
  R = Round
  RL = React to Light
  A = Accommodation OK
  C = Coordinated

E: Expose and Examine

Expose and examine any site of possible injury or any area that the person complains about, even if the area was examined previously. After having controlled the immediately life-threatening problems, obtain the person's medical history, including any illnesses or allergies if possible. Sources include the person, the family, or bystanders. Try to find out what happened.

If equipment is available, take vital signs (temperature, pulse, respiration, blood pressure) every 5 minutes after life-threatening problems are under control (see Chap. 46). Count pulse and respirations for at least 30 seconds. This recording establishes a baseline for further treatment. Report the findings to rescue personnel when they arrive.

SUDDEN DEATH AND LIFE SUPPORT

Sudden death occurs any time breathing and the heartbeat stop abruptly or unexpectedly (*cardiopulmonary arrest*). It is important for all nursing students and graduate nurses to maintain current certification in CPR, to be able to assist in a sudden death emergency.
  Causes of sudden death include:

• Electrocution and severe electric shock
• Drowning and near drowning
• Anaphylaxis (severe allergic reaction)
• Drug overdose
• Poisoning
• Shock
• Myocardial infarction (heart attack)
• Stroke (cerebrovascular accident)
• Total airway obstruction or suffocation
• Smoke inhalation, carbon monoxide poisoning, inhalation of other gases
• Severe trauma
• Adverse reaction to general anesthesia

Two definitions for death exist: clinical and biologic. **Clinical death** occurs when a person's breathing and heartbeat stop. This type of sudden death may be reversible, with prompt action by people trained in basic and advanced life support. The term **biologic death** refers to permanent damage of brain cells due to lack of oxygen. Biologic death is irreversible.

Basic Cardiac Life Support

Basic life support (**BLS**), also called basic cardiac life support (**BCLS**), includes rapid entry into the EMS, performance of CPR, and use of techniques to clear an obstructed airway.

The automated external defibrillator (**AED**) is considered the definitive initial treatment of victims in cardiac arrest. The American Heart Association has expanded its standard of care to include the AED in BCLS. The AED is a portable unit, with electrodes that attach to persons who are pulseless, unresponsive, and not breathing. The unit analyzes the heart's rhythm and indicates the appropriate action to take. If it detects a shockable dysrhythmia, the unit will indicate that a shock is necessary and will automatically charge itself, for delivery when the button is pushed. If an AED is available when you are involved in an emergency, defibrillation should be initiated before beginning CPR. (The AED should be used only by trained personnel. This training is often included in CPR classes for healthcare personnel.)

Cardiopulmonary resuscitation is a technique that artificially supports circulation and ventilation for a victim of cardiopulmonary arrest. It helps to provide oxygen to the brain, heart, lungs, and other organs until advanced life support can be given. CPR must be performed immediately after cardiac and respiratory arrest, or it will not reverse clinical death; biologic death will follow. The American Heart Association and the American Red Cross have established guidelines for CPR. They make changes as new medical and emergency techniques are developed. All healthcare workers are expected to keep abreast of the latest techniques. In order to maintain CPR certification, a refresher course is required every two years.

Advanced Cardiac Life Support

Emergency medical technicians (**EMTs**), paramedics, and many nurses are trained in advanced cardiac life support (**ACLS**) techniques. ACLS includes starting intravenous (IV) lines, administering fluids and medications, using defibrillation and cardiac monitoring, administering oxygen, and opening and maintaining the airway (sometimes by inserting a tube into the person's trachea, which is called **intubation**). In certain states, only first responders and EMTs are allowed to use the AED, start IVs, and give certain medications.

In the healthcare facility, nurses usually perform rescue techniques under a physician's supervision, or have standing orders from the physician. At the scene of an accident or in the client's home, however, the nurse does not have such orders and must function as a lay rescuer or first-aid person.

Continued Assistance

As soon as medical or paramedical assistance arrives at the scene of an accident, the nurse's role is to assist.

The Client at Home

When providing care to a client at home, plans for emergencies are included in the client's initial plan of care. Keep in mind the following:

- Know the client's **DNR** (do not resuscitate) and **DNI** (do not intubate) status before beginning care. If the client is DNR/DNI, a copy of the documentation must be in the home care records.
- Review plans for resuscitation with the client and family before administering even routine care. The client's family must be comfortable with the DNR/DNI status, if this is the case.
- Carry a pocket mask and gloves at all times, in case of emergency.
- Teach the family how to perform CPR. This is a helpful skill for all people.

Unless specified as DNR or DNI, the client receiving home care is to be resuscitated. In this case, if the client arrests while you are in the home, do the following:

- Have a family member call 911.
- Begin CPR immediately. (It is important for all home care personnel to have this training.)
- Before the ambulance arrives, have a family member turn on the porch light and watch for the ambulance.
- Ask the family to move furniture to clear a pathway to the client.
- Reassure the family after the event.
- Document the event and its outcome.

Code in a Healthcare Facility

The nurse working in a healthcare facility when an emergency occurs must activate the agency's signal for a **code.** ("Code Blue" or "Dr. Blue" are common signals for a cardiopulmonary emergency.)

Assisting With a Code

Obtain necessary emergency equipment: crash cart, manual breathing bag, emergency medications, heart monitor, stethoscope, blood pressure and oxygen apparatus, IV lines, suctioning equipment, and oral airways. Crash carts are usually standardized throughout the facility so that everyone is familiar with the setup (Fig. 43-3). They may be equipped with Broselow tape for pediatric emergencies; this color-coded system gives equipment sizes, drug doses, and defibrillation settings based on height and body build.

During resuscitation attempts, the nurse assists the code team. Duties include locating emergency medications and administering them as ordered; helping to set up emergency IV, suction, or oxygen equipment; and calling in other personnel as needed.

If resuscitation measures are successful, the person's pulse will resume, pupils will constrict, color will improve, and breathing will begin. The person may cough, move, or vomit. If assisting a code team and suction is available, turn the client's head to the side and suction the mouth. Do not place fingers in the client's mouth. If it is necessary to open the client's mouth, use an instrument such as a tongue depressor or a spoon. *Always wear gloves.*

After the person is resuscitated, a mechanical ventilator, IV therapy, or vasopressor drugs may be needed for maintenance. Until the primary healthcare provider decides that the person is out of danger, the person needs close observation in the ED or intensive care unit in case another emergency resuscitation is required.

The entire procedure is documented, including the time the arrest was discovered and the physician's estimate of when the arrest occurred; emergency measures taken by the first person

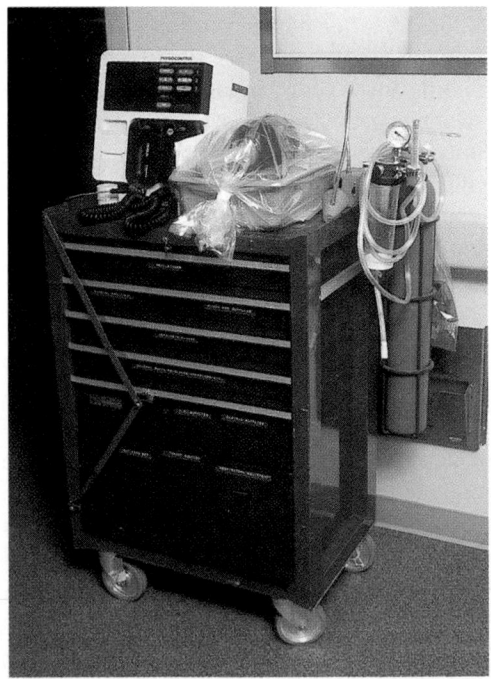

FIGURE 43-3. Crash carts are usually standardized throughout the facility so that everyone is familiar with the set-up.

on the scene; the time the code team arrived; procedures performed from that time on and by whom; medications given, stating dosages and times; the victim's responses to medications and treatment; and laboratory work, electrocardiograms, x-rays, and other tests done. Finally, the outcome of the resuscitation efforts and subsequent nursing care, if appropriate, are noted.

FIRST-AID MEASURES

All nurses are expected to know basic first-aid measures. This knowledge will also prove beneficial to the nurse in his or her role as a parent, sports coach, or neighbor. No one can predict when an injury or sudden illness will occur or when a person may be called upon to assist.

☛ Key Concept

Remember: You are expected to perform first aid only to the level of your training and experience.

Chest, Back, Neck, and Head Injuries

Do not move the person with a chest, back, neck, or head injury until the EMS team arrives, except in unusual situations. For example, you may be on a canoe trip in the wilderness without available EMS assistance, or the person may be in a dangerous situation such as a burning building or a car that may explode. In cases such as these, you will need to supervise the cautious transport of the injured person.

Transporting any injured person requires the utmost care. Careless transport can compound an injury. When moving a person with a neck injury to a stretcher, immobilize his or her neck and back first, then keep the body straight. Sometimes, if the person is lying in an abnormal position, putting the person on the stretcher in this same position may be easier and safer than trying to straighten the body. Enlist as many assistants as needed to move the person effectively and safely. (*Rationale: Doing so protects both the injured person and the rescuer.*) Chapter 48 discusses the transfer and lifting of an immobilized person in more detail.

In some cases, a person must be removed from a badly wrecked vehicle; however, only persons who have special instruction and equipment should do so. The *only time* unqualified people should attempt **extrication** (emergency removal of a victim) is when the person is in great danger if he or she is not moved. For example, in an MVA in which danger of fire or explosion exists, or if the vehicle is under water, the person must be removed from the car, even though moving might aggravate the person's injuries.

Chest Injuries
Blows, stabbings, shootings, and MVAs are the most common causes of chest injuries. CPR may also cause fractured ribs. Fractured ribs may injure soft tissues by puncturing a lung or tearing blood vessels. When such complications are not present, treat fractured ribs by immobilizing the person's chest with an elastic bandage.

Chest compression that results from an explosion or an MVA may rupture a lung and cause death from hemorrhage or suffocation. Wounds that penetrate the chest are serious, and require immediate first aid.

Take emergency action in the case of a puncture wound of the chest. An open chest wound allows air to enter the chest cavity, compressing the lungs. (The normal vacuum within the chest cavity is disrupted.) Normal breathing fails because the lungs cannot adequately expand. This condition is called **pneumothorax.** Signs of pneumothorax include difficult breathing, weak and rapid pulse, restlessness, distended neck veins, hypotension, chest and shoulder pain, and cyanosis.

If it is determined that pneumothorax is present, seal the wound in any way possible—use aluminum foil, petroleum jelly (Vaseline) gauze, plastic wrap, or a rolled-up dressing if necessary. Holding something over an open chest wound for a period of time may be necessary until medical assistance can be obtained. Sealing will help the lungs re-expand. Tape a dressing on three sides so that air can escape when pressure builds in the chest. After the client arrives at a healthcare facility, chest tubes will be inserted for continuous, closed drainage.

When transporting a person with a puncture wound of the chest by a foreign object, make sure that the object remains in place. If the wound is open, cover it at once with an occlusive dressing. Hold the dressing in place with a gloved hand. Oxygen is helpful, and mask-to-mouth or manual breathing bag resuscitation may be needed. If the person's condition seems to worsen, loosen the dressing to let out some air that is building in the chest, to prevent a tension pneumothorax (described below). Then reseal the wound.

A *tension pneumothorax* is particularly dangerous. This situation occurs when air leaks out of the lung or bronchus into the chest cavity and cannot escape. As the leak continues, air collects and pressure builds in the chest. The lung on the same side of the chest as the leak collapses.

In a tension pneumothorax, breath sounds will be greatly diminished or absent on the *affected side*. A tension pneumothorax that remains uncorrected will worsen, resulting in a **mediastinal shift.** The heart, great vessels, and the trachea shift to the side opposite the injury, the *unaffected side,* as a result of the building air pressure. The amount of blood returning to the heart to be pumped to the body will diminish, as will the ability of the heart to pump, resulting in rapid progression toward death. A primary healthcare provider or emergency person may place a large-bore IV needle or chest tube through the chest wall to relieve excess air pressure.

✚👁 Nursing Alert
In an emergency, do not remove an article puncturing the chest if it is still in place. *Rationale: The article will help to seal the hole; its removal may cause added damage. Surgical removal is necessary under controlled conditions.*

Back and Neck Injuries
When a person is a victim of an MVA or a fall, suspect a neck or back injury. A great danger exists for further injury by

moving the person without proper preparation. Always treat the person who has been injured as though he or she has a back or neck injury, until proven otherwise. Immobilizing devices such as the cervical collar, head blocks, or the back board are applied by EMS personnel before the person is moved. It is better to be too careful than to risk causing further injury. (Only specially trained personnel should apply immobilizing devices.)

Head Injuries

Scalp lacerations cause profuse bleeding, making even the smallest wound appear very serious. Determining the extent and cause of the injury is important. A blow to the head that causes a laceration may also cause injury to the skull or brain. Observe for blood or fluid draining from the nose or ears (with no known injury to the nose), bruising behind the ears or under the eyes, persistent bleeding, or a change in behavior since the accident. These are all serious danger signs.

Emergency care for a potential head injury includes having the person lie flat while restricting his or her movements. Do not lower the person's head! Keep the person warm and check for signs of increasing *intracranial pressure* (**ICP**; see below). Apply an ice pack to the swollen area. Instruct family to watch for signs of complications every 2 hours for the first 24 hours. Always advise the client to see a physician after *any* head injury.

> **Nursing Alert**
> Any person who has a head injury, no matter how minor, should be observed carefully for at least 24 hours. Late complications can occur.

Monitoring for signs of increased ICP is crucial. Serious signs of increasing ICP include:

- Confusion, disorientation, or agitation
- Any change in vision, such as blurred vision or double vision
- Decreased LOC or difficulty arousing; extreme lethargy
- Numbness, tingling, or weakness in an arm or leg
- Persistent vomiting
- Severe headache
- Speech problems
- Seizures

If the person with a head injury must be moved, stabilize his or her head in a neutral position and in line with the back. Usually, emergency personnel will bring special immobilizing equipment, such as cervical collars, head blocks, and short and long spine boards, which they will use to prepare the person for transport. Stabilize the person without moving him or her, until proper equipment and assistance arrive.

Cold-Related Injuries

Severe injuries, even death, can result from exposure to cold. Serious injuries can occur even if the temperature is not extreme. Factors influencing cold-related injuries include:

- Temperature of the exposure
- Wind chill factor
- Wetness
- Length of exposure time
- Part of the body exposed
- Person's age and mental status
- Circulatory status
- General physical condition
- Drug or alcohol use

Cold injuries can occur if body parts are exposed, because the body automatically cuts down blood flow to the peripheral structures and redirects it to the vital organs (heart and brain).

Frostbite

Frostbite is the freezing of body tissues that results from exposure to cold temperatures. The body part becomes so cold that ice crystals form in the spaces surrounding the cells; the cells then die. The body is most vulnerable to frostbite when there is a high wind, because blood rushes to the skin to warm it, then cools quickly due to rapid heat loss. The mathematical calculation of temperature and wind speed is called the **wind chill factor.** Skin can freeze when the wind chill factor is below the freezing point, even if the actual air temperature is considerably higher. If the person is wet, this factor also increases the possibility of frostbite.

Frostbite is most likely to affect hands, feet, noses, ears, and cheeks. Noses, ears, and cheeks are vulnerable because they are continually exposed; hands and feet are vulnerable because circulation to these areas is slowest. However, larger body surface areas can be affected as well.

> **Nursing Alert**
> If you work in a public healthcare facility in a cold climate, you will likely see frostbite among homeless people, especially those who are mentally ill, inebriated, elderly, or physically debilitated.

When a body part becomes frostbitten, the area is first painful and then numb. The frostbitten part is pale and cool to the touch, and feels like a block of wood or marble. These symptoms exist initially, regardless of how mild or severe the frostbite. In late stages, hemorrhage may occur; the part may swell and blisters may form. The skin may slough off; gangrene can occur. Box 43-3 presents degrees of frostbite.

A person suffering from frostbite needs immediate assistance. *Do not rub* a frostbitten part to restore circulation. Rubbing, particularly with snow, will only *increase* the damage and can contribute to gangrene. Protect frozen body parts and handle them gently. Loosen tight clothing. Do not allow the person to walk on a frostbitten foot. Separate frozen fingers and toes with cotton wedges; however, do not use bandages, ointments, or salves.

➤➤ BOX 43-3

DEGREES OF FROSTBITE

- **First degree** (*superficial*): Temporary tenderness, reddened skin, some peeling may occur—usually no permanent damage. Sometimes called *frostnip.*
- **Second degree** (*partial-thickness*): Blisters and some tissue and nerve damage—can result in permanent hypersensitivity to cold and increased risk of future frostbite. Subsequent exposure to even mild cold can cause *chilblains* (painful chilling and burning sensations). This condition is sometimes called *pernio* and may persist for years.
- **Third degree** (*full-thickness*): Tissue death—often includes nerve and bone damage. Often leads to *gangrene,* even if treated. Usually requires skin grafting or amputation. Often treated in a Burn Center in the same manner as a burn.

Adapted from "Frostbite—the Big Chill." Burn Center, Hennepin County Medical Center, Minneapolis, Minnesota, 1999.

Place frozen parts in water that is between 98° and 104° Fahrenheit (36.6° and 40° Celsius). If a thermometer is not available, use water temperature that feels *tepid* (lukewarm). Rewarming the affected part in water will take about 20 to 45 minutes. The person may experience some pain as the part warms. The part will turn pink or bright red as circulation resumes. Protect the part against refreezing.

The person with severe frostbite needs immediate medical attention. It sometimes takes providers several days to assess the extent of damage. Treatment is often the same as for a burn, with treatment commonly being provided in a burn unit. If treatment is unsuccessful, amputation may be necessary. In severe frostbite, blisters form quickly. They should not be broken.

Immersion Foot

This condition occurs most often in hikers and canoers, when the feet are kept in moist, cold boots for several days. It can also occur in military personnel who spend several days in the field. In rare cases, this condition can affect the hands. The feet (or hands) should be gently warmed, cleaned, dried, and elevated. Because infection often occurs, antibiotics are often given, as well as a tetanus booster.

Hypothermia

Hypothermia occurs when the body loses heat faster than it can burn food (fuel) to replace it. It is caused when a person is exposed to extreme or fairly extreme cold, or is chilled for a long enough time to lower his or her *core* (internal) *body temperature* to a dangerous level (usually less than 94° F). Profuse sweating over time can also cause this condition. In addition, windy or wet conditions greatly accelerate the onset of hypothermia. Hypothermia caused by such external forces

is known as *accidental hypothermia.* Hypothermia also occurs when the body's temperature regulation malfunctions. In addition, temperature is sometimes intentionally lowered to make surgery safer. This procedure is called *induced* or *surgical hypothermia.* Induced hypothermia confined to one body part is called *local hypothermia.*

Accidentally lowering the body's core temperature even a few degrees can result in serious symptoms and even death. Symptoms of hypothermia include sleepiness, slow and clumsy movements, shaking, cardiac dysrhythmia, loss of reflexes and slowed reaction times, impaired judgment, and respiratory failure. Hallucinations may occur. If the person is in water, drowning is very possible as a result of weakness and confusion. In a first-aid situation, the initial warning signs are confusion, disorientation, slurred speech, and lethargy. Check also to see if the person complains of blurred vision, dizziness, tiredness, or feeling very cold.

☛ KEY CONCEPT

Preventing hypothermia is important, especially for individuals engaged in outdoor activities—for example campers and hikers. Because major heat loss occurs via the uncovered head (which acts like a chimney), wearing a hat is very important. Wool clothing helps, because it is warm even when wet. Wearing layered clothing also is beneficial because the air pockets between layers serve as insulation. Eating enough food and obtaining adequate fluids are also important. Warn campers and hikers to remain dry and to avoid sitting on wet cold ground or cold metal surfaces.

Definitive diagnosis of hypothermia is based on an accurate measurement of core temperature. Special monitoring equipment is necessary because normal clinical thermometers often do not register low enough to measure core temperature accurately.

Treatment of Hypothermia.   Gradual rewarming is necessary. *Rationale: When the body is rewarmed too quickly, cold blood returns to the heart, causing severe dysrhythmia and sometimes cardiac arrest.* Continually monitor the person's cardiac status during rewarming. On a first-aid basis, get the person into warm, dry clothing. Warmed beverages also help, if the person is alert and can swallow.

If the client is unconscious, immediate transfer to a healthcare facility is vital. There, the body is warmed until the core temperature is approximately 94° F (35° C). *Then* the extremities are warmed. Warmed blankets and warming lights are used. Sometimes, the person is placed in warm water. In addition, warmed oxygen and warmed IV infusions may be given. Blood may be circulated through a pump oxygenator and warmed before returning it to the body's core circulation. Warm fluids may be instilled into the gastrointestinal system. Treatment continues until the body's core temperature is near normal (98.6° F; 37° C).

Nursing Considerations.   The person with severe hypothermia must be moved very carefully to prevent cardiac dysrhythmias or arrest. During the rewarming process, nursing care includes careful monitoring of vital signs and IV infusion, close observation of skin condition, special mouth and eye care, and measurement of oral and IV intake and urine output. Monitor the body's core temperature by using a special electronic thermometer. The person who has an IV infusion may suffer from such common complications as bleeding and gastric distention.

During first aid, cover the person's head, hands, and feet. A ground cover provides a barrier against moisture and insulates materials under the person. Keep the person *awake* until medical assistance arrives. Remove wet clothing.

> ### Nursing Alert
>
> Hypothermia that accompanies frostbite is a medical emergency. Give *immediate* emergency care in any case of hypothermia. A person with severe hypothermia is not considered dead until he or she has been rewarmed and still shows no signs of life. Because of the increased risk for cardiac standstill, CPR is not usually recommended for this person until he or she is in the emergency department.

Heat-Related Injuries

Heat-related injuries are most likely to occur on days of high humidity, with temperatures from 95° to 100° F (35° to 37.8° C), and no breeze. *Rationale: The body's major defense against heat accumulation is sweating; evaporation of sweat helps cool the body. When humidity exceeds 75%, particularly when there is no breeze, evaporation decreases.* Heat injuries typically occur in early summer, before people have acclimated themselves to high temperatures. Such injuries can also occur inside enclosed areas, when the outside temperature is low but other heat sources increase a person's internal heat load. For example, on a bright day, a parked car can quickly become a *fatal* enclosed area for children and pets because of the radiant heat produced by the sun. Heat produced in some work areas also can cause illness. Any enclosed area where equipment produces a large amount of heat that accumulates has the potential to cause heat-related illness.

Although sensitivity to heat varies among individuals, certain groups are particularly susceptible. Studies have identified infants, older adults, the very obese, chronic abusers of drugs or alcohol, and persons with underlying illnesses as being at the highest risk for heat-related injuries. Military personnel and athletes are also vulnerable because of the tendency to over-exercise in the heat, sometimes in heavy clothing.

Heat Cramps

Heat cramps are severe muscle spasms that usually occur after hard exertion. They are frequently found in physically fit young people, who usually have been sweating profusely and drinking plain water. These cramps may occur in cool environments as well as hot ones, and are usually located in the legs, arms, or abdomen. Along with heat cramps, the person may show signs of heat exhaustion (see discussion below).

Heat cramps are relieved by drinking very dilute salt solutions. Give the person a mixture of up to ¼ teaspoon of salt per quart of water (or another balanced salt solution). Commercial products such as sports drinks (Gatorade) also contain extra sodium. If symptoms continue longer than an hour, seek medical advice. Salt tablets are not recommended because they are gastric irritants. Moving the person to a cooler environment is helpful, but make sure the person's head is uncovered, and keep him or her calm. Explain what is happening. Tell him or her to avoid exertion for the next 12 hours.

For the future, suggest that the person add some salt (but not too much) to food before exertion. The person should also drink adequate liquids and stop exercising if he or she feels ill. Misting the skin with water also helps.

☞ KEY CONCEPT

Persons in cooler climates, such as mountain climbers, may experience heat cramps because they are dressed too warmly, causing excessive sweating.

Massaging cramped muscles will not cure heat cramps; in fact, it may increase the pain.

Heat Exhaustion

Heat exhaustion often occurs in physically fit people who are exerting themselves in a hot environment over a length of time. Under such conditions, these people do not take in enough water and sodium to replace lost fluids and electrolytes, resulting in a serious blood flow disturbance similar to shock. Pure forms of heat exhaustion are rare. Heat exhaustion that occurs quickly is likely to be related to *water depletion.* (Another type of heat exhaustion, called *salt-depletion heat exhaustion,* develops over time.) True heat exhaustion is rarely life threatening.

As a person loses large amounts of water and salt through sweating, blood flow decreases if water is not replaced. Decreased blood flow affects brain, heart, and lung functioning. When a person loses salt as well as water, heat cramps may occur, along with headache, dizziness, anxiety, nausea, and weakness. Other symptoms of heat exhaustion include excessive sweating, faintness, hypotension, loss of appetite, and unconsciousness (usually brief). Fainting or unconsciousness is most common when the person is standing, because blood pools in the legs, interfering with blood flow to the brain. Skin is pale, cool, and usually sweaty; body temperature may be subnormal and blood pressure is low. The person's eyes are dilated, breathing is rapid and shallow, and pulse is slow and weak. The person may have difficulty walking.

Treatment for heat exhaustion includes cooling the person without chilling him or her. Move the person to a cool place and remove and loosen as much clothing as is practical. Apply cold, wet compresses to the skin. Fanning is helpful. Have the person lie down and elevate his or her feet 8 to 12 inches. *Rationale: Doing so will help increase circulation to the brain.*

Water replacement and rest will usually relieve symptoms of heat exhaustion caused by water depletion. However, the salt-depleted person will usually need sips of a salt solution, given slowly over a period of time. If there are any doubts about the person's condition, transport him or her to a healthcare facility immediately. *Rationale: Telling the difference between heat exhaustion and heat stroke may be difficult. If blood pressure and pulse remain low for more than ½ to 1 hour, suspect heat stroke.*

Heat Stroke

Heat stroke is a potentially *life-threatening condition.* This condition often develops rapidly and requires immediate treatment. *Classic heat stroke* occurs when the body's heat-regulating mechanisms fail and core temperature soars. When a person's core temperature reaches 105° to 110° F, sweating stops, brain cells become damaged or destroyed, and death results. Classic heat stroke usually occurs during a summer heat wave with high temperatures and humidity. Classic heat stroke most often affects the poor, those living in poorly ventilated housing, older individuals who do not take in enough water, and chronically ill persons, who often are taking medications that contribute to heat stress. However, the recent death of a professional football player points out the dangers of extreme heat and humidity for all people, regardless of age or physical conditioning.

Nursing Alert
Certain illnesses, such as cystic fibrosis and scleroderma, restrict the client's ability to sweat. These individuals are more susceptible to heat stroke.

Exertional heat stroke develops from an increased internal heat load due to muscular exertion, along with high external temperature and humidity. It usually occurs rapidly (within a few hours) in young, healthy, athletic individuals, simply because their heat-regulating systems become overwhelmed. In about half the cases of exertional heat stroke, the person is sweating.

Persons with *classic heat stroke* usually are brought to the healthcare facility because of hypotension, fever, and coma. Persons with *exertional heat stroke* are usually brought in because of bizarre behavior or collapse. Both forms of heat stroke can be life threatening and require immediate medical

care. *Rationale: The longer a person goes without treatment, the greater the danger is.*

Persons suffering from either form of heat stroke share many of the symptoms of heat exhaustion. However, some distinct differences exist (Table 43-1). Persons suffering from heat stroke have hot skin, and usually a high body temperature—above 106° F (41.1° C). Persons suffering from heat exhaustion have cool skin, and normal or even slightly below normal body temperature.

After activating the EMS, first-aid treatment for heat stroke includes rapidly cooling the person to at least a temperature of 101° F. Place the person in a cool, shady place and remove his or her clothing. Wrap the person in cold, wet sheets or spray him or her with a cold mist of water. Place ice packs on the person's forehead, under the armpits, and at the neck and groin. If the person is conscious, give sips of cold liquids containing a dilute salt solution. Tell the person not to drink too quickly (to prevent nausea.) Prevent shivering. Monitor the person's airway, breathing, and circulation. If necessary, begin CPR. Watch for seizures. *Immediately transport the person for emergency care.*

Nursing Alert
If the person suffering from any type of heat-related illness vomits, *stop giving fluids.* The person needs IV fluid replacement. (This is usually the only time a person with *heat exhaustion* needs to be hospitalized.) Any person with *heat stroke* needs immediate medical attention.

Burns

Burns occur due to many heat sources. Chapter 74 discusses burns in more detail, including classifications and area calculations. Study Chapter 74 along with this discussion.

The most common emergency cases of burns are caused by thermal, electrical, chemical, and radiation sources. Flames, steam, hot liquids, and hot objects may cause *thermal burns.* Electrical power sources or lightning may cause *electrical burns.* Strong chemicals can cause severe *chemical burns* to

TABLE 43-1 HEAT EXHAUSTION VERSUS HEAT STROKE

Element	Heat Exhaustion	Heat Stroke
Skin	Cool	Hot
Sweat	Person may or may not sweat.	*Classic heat stroke*—person is usually dry. *Exertional heat stroke*—person is usually sweating.
Body temperature	Normal or below normal	High (often > 106°F)
Symptoms	Headache, nausea, dizziness, weakness, faintness, pale skin, weak pulse, tachycardia, anorexia, hypotension, brief periods of unconsciousness, rapid breathing	*Classic heat stroke*—hypotension, fever, coma *Exertional heat stroke*—confusion, bizarre behavior, collapse
Treatment	Cool the person without chilling; elevate his or her feet. *Water depletion*—give water. *Salt depletion*—give salt solution.	Cool person rapidly, monitor airway and circulation, observe seizure precautions.
Medical attention	Seek medical attention if in doubt.	Seek medical attention immediately in all cases.

the skin, respiratory system, or eyes. Radiation sources (eg, power plants) may cause *radiation burns;* sunburns also fall in this category.

First Aid for Sunburn.   Too much exposure to the ultraviolet rays of the sun or a sun lamp causes *sunburn.* Although a person of any skin tone can be sunburned, the effects on an individual vary with the person's skin tone and previous levels of sun exposure. It is important to apply sun block before spending any length of time in the sun, particularly if the person is prone to sunburn. Excessive exposure to the sun is also known to cause certain types of skin cancer.

The person who is sunburned will have reddened skin and may have a fever. Blisters and peeling may develop later. First aid for sunburn involves neutralizing the burning effects. This can be done with vinegar, milk, or certain commercial preparations. The sooner these measures are applied, the less of a chance there is for long-term damage to occur. In cases of severe sunburn, the person may require emergency medical care.

First Aid for Other Types of Burns.   The seriousness of a burn is estimated by its depth, percentage of the body burned, location, age of the victim, and any underlying complications (see Chap. 74). The following are examples of special considerations:

- A burn that involves more than 10% of the body's surface is extremely serious.
- Any second- or third-degree burn is serious.
- Burns to the hands, feet, mouth, throat, and perineum are serious.
- Full-thickness circumferential burns to the limbs or chest are special problems because they can restrict circulation and breathing.
- Diabetic persons of any age have more difficulty recovering from burns because their bodies heal more slowly; they may also have underlying circulatory or other difficulties.
- Any underlying injury can affect a person's recovery after a burn.
- A person with a compromised immune system is at a particularly high risk for infection following a burn.

In Practice: Nursing Care Guidelines 43-2 summarizes immediate first-aid measures for burns.

Associated problems often cause more harm than the burn itself. Be alert for *inhalation injuries and breathing problems,* as well as for broken bones or other injuries. Check for the signs of possible inhalation injury including:

- Burned or singed nasal hairs or burns in or around the mouth
- Flecks of soot in the client's saliva
- Smell of smoke on the client's breath
- Hoarse voice

Remember that a person can experience a burn *internally,* such as from swallowing a caustic substance. These types of inhalation injuries can be life threatening. The trachea and lungs can be burned. The gases in smoke can replace the air in the lungs, rendering the person unable to oxygenate his or her blood. In any case of suspected inhalation injury, immediately transport the person for emergency care.

> **Nursing Alert**
>
> If a burned person was trapped in a confined space and exposed to chemicals or smoke, suspect smoke or heat inhalation injury.

Near Drowning

Drowning is suffocation from submersion in liquid. **Near drowning** implies that recovery has occurred after submersion. Most drownings occur in lakes, rivers, and oceans. However, children can drown in the toilet, bathtub, wading pool, or a bucket. Assess victims of near drowning for associated injuries or illnesses: cardiac arrest, airway obstruction, head injury, spinal injury, and internal injuries. Long-term brain damage may result from extended *anoxia* (absence of oxygen). Submersion in cold water may also cause hypothermia. However, individuals submerged in cold water may survive, because when body temperature is lowered, metabolism slows, which decreases the brain's need for oxygen. Victims of near drowning may appear dead because of the reduction in brain and cardiovascular function. However, rescuers should initiate and continue lifesaving measures, including CPR, until the person can be evaluated with instruments such as an electroencephalogram. People may respond to prolonged resuscitation efforts without sustaining brain damage after near drowning. This is particularly true of children. Treat all near drowning victims for hypothermia and shock. Maintain respirations and blood pressure until the person is cleared medically.

Musculoskeletal Injuries

Musculoskeletal injuries are those involving bones, muscles, or joints.

Fractures, Sprains, and Dislocations

When a person has been involved in an MVA or a fall, look for these possible problems:

- **Fracture:** broken bone
- **Sprain:** twisting of a joint with rupture of ligaments and other possible damage
- **Strain:** twisting or stretching that damages a muscle or tendon
- **Dislocation:** displacement of a bone from a joint

Sometimes, determining whether a sprain or a fracture has occurred is difficult. If in doubt as to an injury's extent, assume that a fracture has occurred and treat the person accordingly until a definite diagnosis is made. Use ice as treatment for a fracture or sprain until medical assistance is available. Usually the person will have pain on movement or weight-bearing after sustaining a fracture. *Do not have the person stand or walk on a suspected fracture to check for pain; doing so is likely to aggravate the injury.*

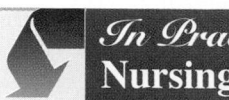

PROVIDING EMERGENCY FIRST AID FOR BURNS

- Stop the burning process by removing the heat source. Make sure burning clothing is *cooled*. Do not remove burning fabric or other materials, unless they fall off. *Rationale: Some materials continue to smolder or melt and must be neutralized; however, removing the clothing could tear the person's skin and damage it further.*
- If rescuers arrive within a few minutes of the incident, flood the area with cool water. Do not apply ice. *Rationale: The goal is to cool the area to stop the burning and to reduce the incidence of scarring. Ice may further irritate the burned area by cooling it too quickly.*
- Continue to flood the area with cool water. *Rationale: Cool water helps to control pain; discontinuation may increase pain temporarily because of damaged nerve endings.*
- Flood most chemical burns with a gentle, continuous flow of plain water until emergency help arrives. *Rationale: Flooding with water will help stop the burning process and cool the area. It will also help to dilute and wash away caustic chemicals.*
- Always check a chemical container for directions on emergency treatment. *Rationale: Some chemicals react adversely when in contact with water.*
- Watch for shivering if you are using water to cool a burn covering more than 10% of the body. Change to dry, sterile dressings if shivering occurs. *Rationale: Exposure to cold may cause hypothermia.*
- Do not put anything other than water or a specifically prescribed substance on a burn. *Rationale:*

Materials such as salves, ointments, or butter occlude the burn so that it becomes difficult to examine. These substances promote infection and pain on removal.
- Remove the injured person's jewelry. *Rationale: It can remain hot and continue the burning process. Swelling usually occurs later, making it impossible to remove rings or other jewelry; if left on, jewelry can cut off circulation.*
- Monitor the person's airway, breathing, and circulation. Be prepared to initiate CPR. *Rationale: Respiratory or cardiac arrest (or both) can occur from the shock.*
- If the burn is extensive, cover it with a dry, non-stick, sterile dressing. Do not use gauze. *Rationale: Gauze will peel off additional tissue and cause more damage. For all large burns, use only a dry, sterile dressing, following removal of the heat source and cooling down period. Rationale: The dressing will help to prevent infection.*
- Keep dressings cool and wet. Be sure to keep person warm and monitor for hypothermia. *Rationale: Wet dressings may promote hypothermia.*
- Prevent contamination of the wound as much as possible. *Rationale: Infection is a major hazard with burns.*
- Treat for shock. *Rationale: Pain, loss of body fluids, and anxiety contribute to shock.*
- Determine what first aid measures others have already given. *Rationale: Some of these measures may be dangerous. Emergency and medical personnel need to be aware of what has been done.*

The cardinal rule of emergency care is *do not move the person*. Get emergency help. Question the person if he or she is conscious. Observe for obviously deformed limbs; cover them with a blanket until you can obtain adequate help. If the person must be moved, the injury should be immobilized.

Never attempt to replace the ends of bones in a fracture, whether or not the skin is broken. (If the fractured ends of the bone protrude through the skin, this is called a *compound fracture*. If the skin is not broken, this is called a *simple fracture*.) Cover any open wounds with a sterile dressing and control excessive bleeding by direct or indirect pressure.

Remember the acronym **RICE** in emergency procedures for sprains and strains:

R = Rest
I = Ice
C = Compression (such as with a roller bandage)
E = Elevation (keep the part above the level of the heart, if possible)

Splinting.　A **splint** is a device applied to *immobilize* a fracture or sprain. You can use any hard, straight item; however, do not attempt to splint a fracture if emergency medical assistance is available. A good emergency splint for an arm is a magazine wrapped around the arm and tied. (Be careful not to tie the splint so tightly as to cut off circulation to the limb.) Numerous commercial splints also are available. Traction splints are best for most major leg fractures and should be applied only by specially trained members of the EMS team. Inflatable splints may also be used.

If a fracture of a knee or elbow is suspected, splint the joint in its existing position. (Rationale: Because of the joint's close proximity to arteries, veins, and nerves, straightening the joint can put pressure on blood vessels, cutting off circulation or sensation to the extremity's distal portion.) An effective splint for a fractured toe is the adjacent toe; tape the digits together ("buddy taping"). The same is true for fingers. An ice cream stick is a handy item to use for a finger splint.

Nursing Alert

When splinting a fracture, check the person's distal pulse *before and after* splinting. An *absent* pulse is a medical emergency. Obtain medical attention *immediately*.

Dressing a Wound. If emergency assistance is unavailable, it may be necessary to apply a dressing to an open wound, such as that which accompanies a fracture. Although many articles can be used as a dressing in an emergency, use a sterile dressing whenever possible. Sterile dressings are available in many sizes and thicknesses. If a sterile dressing is unavailable, use the cleanest material at hand. A clean handkerchief or dish towel is suitable. Fresh newspaper also can be used because it is clean. *Remember to wear gloves, if at all possible.*

Using Bandages. A **bandage** is a piece of material used to hold a dressing or splint in place, to give support, or to apply pressure. When applying a bandage in an emergency, follow these guidelines:

- Apply the bandage firmly but not so tightly that circulation is restricted. Watch for evidence of tightness: blanching of skin, loss of sensation, and absent pulse. Loosen the bandage if necessary.
- Always tie a square knot, because it will not slip and can be easily untied.
- If possible, leave the tips of the person's toes and fingers exposed. *Rationale: Checking for impaired circulation is necessary to ensure adequate tissue perfusion.* Assess for pallor, lack of pulse, pain on passive motion, paresthesia (burning, tingling), or paralysis. (This assessment is known as **CMS**: color, motion, and sensitivity or sensation.) Chapter 76 discusses assessment of musculoskeletal injuries; Chapter 53 discusses the application of bandages in more detail.

Applying Cravat Bandages and Slings. A *triangular* or *handkerchief bandage* can be made from a square of cloth and secured without tape or pins, if necessary. A 36- to 40-inch cloth square is an adequate size. Fold it diagonally through the center to form a triangle. (Fold the cloth several times to make a *strip* or *cravat bandage*.) A triangular bandage also may be used to make a sling for arm support. The steps for applying a sling are described at In Practice: Nursing Procedure 43-1.

Dental Injuries and Missing Teeth

Teeth may be displaced or knocked out accidentally, particularly in children. A tooth that is pushed up into the socket is called an **intrusion injury.** A tooth that is knocked out is called an **avulsion injury.** In either event, *immediate dental care* is necessary.

In an avulsion injury, the dentist may be able to reimplant and reposition the tooth. An avulsed tooth that is reimplanted within 30 minutes has a 90% chance of being saved. It *may* be saved if reimplanted within 2 hours. First aid for avulsed teeth is outlined at In Practice: Nursing Care Guidelines 43-3.

☛ Key Concept

If the person can cooperate, have him or her hold an evulsed tooth under their tongue en route to the dentist. Otherwise, place the evulsed tooth in milk. Rationale: The client's own saliva or the milk will help to preserve the integrity and viability of the tooth's root system.

Foreign Objects

A *foreign object* is any abnormal object or substance lodged in a body orifice or structure.

Foreign Objects in the Eyes

Foreign objects in the eye can be particles of dust or soot or an eyelash resting on the eyelid's lining. Particles also can become embedded in the eyeball. Anything that lodges on the cornea irritates it, especially when the eyelid opens and closes. Foreign objects have a scratchy effect and cause tears to flow. (This is a natural body defense mechanism. Often, the tears will wash out the foreign object and no treatment is needed.)

Caustic substances are those which burn or destroy flesh. A caustic substance in the eye is extremely irritating and very dangerous. Sometimes, in an industrial accident, chemicals enter a person's eye. Quick action must be taken to flush the eye with water. In Practice: Nursing Care Guidelines 43-4 summarizes skills in the emergency care of eye injuries. If any question exists about the injury's severity, seek medical assistance as soon as possible.

Most contact lenses used today can remain in the person's eyes for several hours without incident. If lenses are left in place following an accident, the medical team must be aware of this fact. The person's corneas can become ulcerated if he or she does not blink. Hard or gas permeable contact lenses are more likely to cause corneal ulcers than soft lenses. In some cases, removal of contact lenses at the scene of an accident is necessary. A special suction cup is available for this purpose.

Foreign Objects in the Nose or Ears

Children often insert small objects into their noses or ears. To remove an object from a child's nose, have the child blow the nose gently with *both* nostrils open. Unless the object is clearly visible and at the edge of the nostril, do not attempt to remove it with a finger or instrument. Call for medical assistance. If a foreign object lodges in a person's ear, do not attempt to remove it. Instead, transport the person to a healthcare facility.

Nursing Alert

Be aware that an object such as a bean or a dried pea will swell when moistened. This makes these objects very difficult to remove, especially from the nose.

In Practice
Nursing Procedure 43-1

APPLYING A SLING

1. Put one triangle end over the person's shoulder on the *uninjured* side. The point of the triangle should point toward the elbow of the injured arm and be placed under it.
   RATIONALE: *Placing the sling around the person's neck will support the injured arm.*

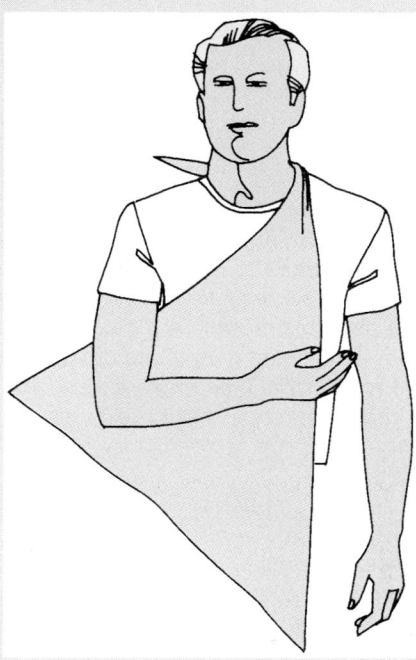

A

2. Bring the other end of the triangle over the person's shoulder on the *injured* side. Tie the two ends of the triangle together at the side of the neck.
   RATIONALE: *Tying the knot on the side of the injury will pull the knot away from the neck, preventing discomfort.*

   If the nature of the injury or another situation makes this impractical, place some sort of padding beneath the knot.
   RATIONALE: *Padding the area minimizes pressure on the neck.*

3. Bring the point of the triangle backward around the person's elbow and pin it to the back of the sling. You can adjust the sling by adjusting the knot or by pinning a tuck in the front of the sling above the person's hand. Elevate the hand 4 to 5 inches above elbow level.
   RATIONALE: *Elevation helps to prevent swelling and pain.*

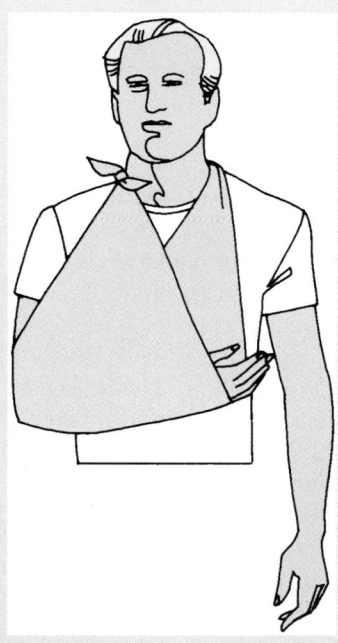

B

Slings. (A) Step 1. (B) Steps 2 and 3.

Airway Obstruction

Foreign objects often become lodged in the throat. If the foreign object is not visible but the victim is able to breathe adequately, call for emergency medical assistance or take the person to an Emergency Department. If the person is not exchanging air and shows signs of respiratory distress, call 911 and use appropriate obstructed-airway techniques if you have been properly trained. (All nursing students should receive CPR training and should renew this certification on a regular basis.) An airway obstructed by a foreign body will quickly cause respiratory arrest. Anytime a person (particularly a child) becomes cyanotic, stops breathing,

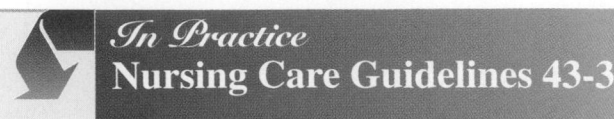

In Practice
Nursing Care Guidelines 43-3

GIVING FIRST AID FOR AN EVULSED TOOTH

- Ask bystanders to look for the missing tooth. Instruct them to pick it up with a sterile piece of gauze by the crown and not to touch the root. *Rationale: Touching the root may damage important structures.*
- Call a dentist immediately. The person must see a dentist or go to an emergency department as soon as possible. *Rationale: The sooner a tooth is repositioned, the more likely it is to be saved.*
- Clean the person's mouth with gauze. Using sterile gauze, have the client gently bite down. *Rationale: Doing so will restrict bleeding and reduce pain.*
- Instruct the person not to put pressure on adjacent teeth. *Rationale: The accident may have loosened adjacent teeth.*
- If possible, have the person bite gently on a dry tea bag. *Rationale: Tannin in tea acts as a natural coagulant and helps to stop bleeding.*
- Do not allow the client to suck on a straw or to smoke. *Rationale: The sucking action may loosen a blood clot and cause more bleeding.*
- Place the tooth on sterile gauze. You may clean it by dipping it in milk, while holding the crown. *Rationale: Using water or any solution other than milk may damage the root.*

and collapses for no apparent reason, suspect an obstructed airway.

Children may put coins or buttons in their mouths. Bits of food or bones can lodge in a child's throat or esophagus. In an adult, foreign body obstruction is usually caused by a large piece of food becoming lodged in the airway. Meat is the most common cause. Poorly fitting dentures and alcohol ingestion also are associated with obstructed airways. Certain medical conditions, including neuromuscular disease, strokes, cleft palate, brain injury, seizure disorders, heavy sedation, decreased saliva production, or a diminished or absent cough or gag reflex, can increase the risk for choking. Older adults who cannot chew food well are also at risk for choking.

Airway obstruction often occurs in restaurants. The person is embarrassed by the incident and suddenly leaves the table. Suspect an obstructed airway when you see a person coughing and gasping, who looks frightened and suddenly leaves the table. Follow the person, and ask if he or she is choking. If this person goes off alone, he or she may die. This common occurrence is called a **café coronary.** The person leaves the table, goes to the restroom, and may be found not breathing and without a heartbeat (an apparent heart attack victim).

The person who has a *partially obstructed airway* with good air exchange will cough forcefully. Wheezing may be

present, but adequate air exchange is obvious. Encourage the person to cough. *Do not interfere* with attempts to expel the obstruction, and do not leave the person. Offer encouragement and continue to monitor him or her. If the person's condition does not rapidly improve, activate the EMS. Poor air exchange may be identified by ineffective coughing and sometimes by high-pitched wheezing sounds called **stridor.** The person often experiences increasing respiratory difficulty and may become cyanotic.

In a *complete airway obstruction,* the person is unable to talk, breathe, or cough. The person may even indicate the condition by using the universal signal for choking, which is clutching the neck between the fingers and thumbs of both hands. In complete airway obstruction, no oxygen enters the lungs. The person will soon become unconscious unless the obstruction is removed. Use the *Heimlich maneuver,* also called *abdominal thrusts,* in the case of complete airway obstruction. The Heimlich maneuver is not described in this chapter. Enroll in a specialized class to learn the basics of this life-saving skill. All nurses should be able to perform this skill.

Cardiovascular Emergencies

Fainting
Fainting (**syncope**) is caused by an insufficient supply of blood and oxygen to the brain. Extreme hunger, tiredness, heat, or being in an oxygen-deprived environment can cause a person to faint. Fainting can also result from an emotional shock. Severe hemorrhage, excruciating pain, and standing in one place for a prolonged period, especially with the knees locked, are other causes.

The symptoms of imminent fainting include dizziness, blackness or spots before the eyes, pallor, and excessive perspiration. The person loses consciousness; the pulse is weak, and breathing is shallow. In Practice: Nursing Procedure 43-2 may be used for the person who has fainted or who feels faint.

Suspected Heart Attack
Chapter 80 discusses the specifics of myocardial infarction (**MI**), commonly known as *heart attack.* In an MI, some of the heart's blood supply is cut off, causing heart muscle tissue to die. This is usually the result of a blockage in a coronary artery (one of the arteries supplying the heart itself). The location and extent of the infarction determines the seriousness of the MI.

The person usually complains of chest pain, which may radiate to the left (or right) arm. Rest usually does not relieve this pain. Other symptoms include pain radiating to the back, neck, jaw, or teeth; the pain may also be mistaken for heartburn or indigestion. Be aware that pain may also occur in other places. The person may have been having symptoms off and on for several days (*unstable angina*). Other common symptoms of MI include: restlessness, panic and a sense of impending doom, difficulty breathing and other signs of respiratory distress, as well as changes in pulse quality and rate. The skin is cold and clammy and the person may be cyanotic

In Practice
Nursing Care Guidelines 43-4

GIVING FIRST AID FOR EYE INJURIES

First Aid for Foreign Objects in the Eye
- Instruct the person not to rub his or her eye. Have the person keep the eye closed and avoid blinking. *Rationale: Rubbing or blinking may drive a foreign object deeper into the eye.*
- Never use an instrument, a toothpick, or a match to remove a foreign object. *Rationale: These items are unsterile and may introduce pathogens into the eye and scratch the cornea.*
- Never attempt to remove a foreign object if the slightest possibility exists that it is embedded in the cornea. *Rationale: You could drive the object deeper into the eye and cause more serious damage.*
- Remove contact lenses. *Rationale: Contact lenses can contribute to further aggravation and injury.*
- Treat both eyes even if only one is injured. *Rationale: A sympathetic injury can occur.*

When the Object is not Embedded
- Pull down the person's lower eyelid to see whether the object is on the eyelid membrane. *Rationale: If the object is on the inside of the eyelid, you may be able to lift it off by touching it gently with the corner of a clean handkerchief or with a cotton-tipped applicator moistened in water.*
- Always moisten the cotton tip of an applicator before touching it to the eye. *Rationale: Small particles of dry cotton can become lodged in the eye.*
- If the object is under the person's upper eyelid, grasp the lashes of the upper eyelid with your forefinger and thumb; ask the person to look upward; gently pull the lid forward and downward over the lower eyelid. *Rationale: Usually this eyelash movement dislodges the foreign body, and tears wash it away.*
- Flush the eye with plain water. *Rationale: Sometimes the pressure of the water will flush an object out of the eye.*

First Aid for Caustic Materials in the Eye
- Flush the eye with large amounts of water or normal saline solution. *Rationale: Eyes are sensitive to chemical or thermal burns. It is vital to use a large amount of water to cleanse the eye.* You can use a sterile medicine dropper or a small sterile bulb syringe. Do not use an unsterile eye cup. *Rationale: Eye cups may introduce pathogens into the eye.*
- Use an eyewash sink or shower if possible. Have the person stand over the sink, with the eyes close

to the jets. Encourage the person to keep the eyes open as much as possible. When the water is turned on, the jets direct a continuous stream of water into the eyes. *Rationale: Large amounts of water are necessary, which are easily provided with an eyewash sink.*

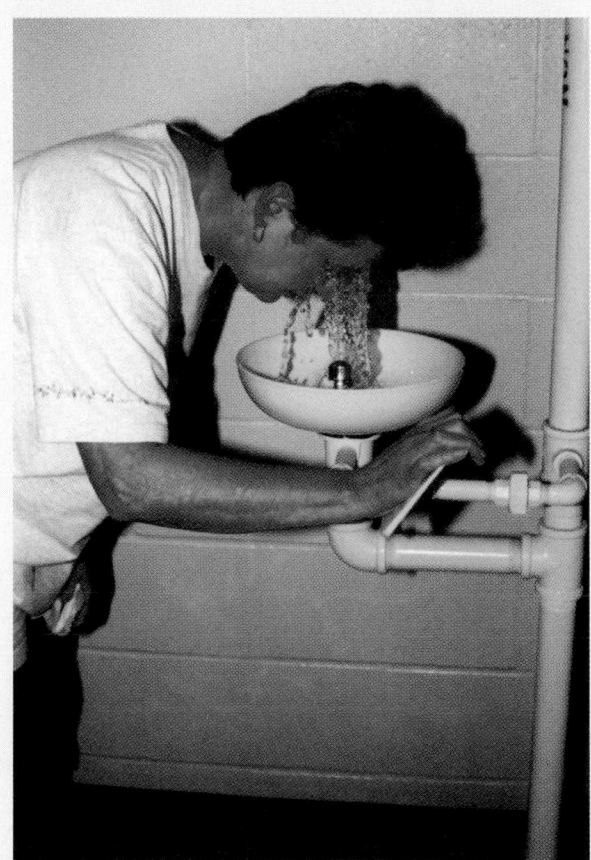

If any caustic material splashes into the eye, *immediately flush the eye* with large amounts of water. (Photo © Kimberly Malcolm Rosdahl)

- Do not instill another substance into the eye in an attempt to neutralize a caustic substance. *Rationale: Putting another substance into the eye could do more damage.*
- Have the person see a physician immediately. *Rationale: Prompt action is necessary to prevent permanent eye damage.*

In Practice
Nursing Procedure 43-2

ASSISTING THE CLIENT WHO IS FAINTING

1. When someone complains of feeling faint, have the person sit or lie down and bend his or her head forward between the knees. Maintain the person in this position.
   RATIONALE: *When the head is lower than the heart, more blood is carried to the brain.*

2. Loosen tight clothing.
   RATIONALE: *Tight clothing can constrict breathing, further reducing the amount of oxygen carried to the brain.*

3. If the person is unconscious, assess for respirations and pulse. Start CPR if necessary.
   RATIONALE: *A life-threatening condition may be the cause of unconsciousness.*

4. When the person regains consciousness, help him or her to rise slowly, first to a sitting and then to a standing position.
   RATIONALE: *The person may feel weak and could fall.*

5. Do not allow the person to move until he or she has fully regained consciousness.
   RATIONALE: *The person's altered LOC may be due to a serious condition, such as a skull fracture, concussion, stroke, cerebral hemorrhage, or shock.*

In Practice
Nursing Care Guidelines 43-5

GIVING FIRST AID IN SUSPECTED HEART ATTACK (MI)

- Have someone call 911. *Rationale: Prompt treatment is vital.*
- Keep the person completely quiet. Do not allow the person to move about, no matter how much better he or she claims to feel. *Rationale: Most people say they feel better. This is part of denial.*
- Loosen any tight clothing. *Rationale: Loosening clothing helps to make breathing easier.*
- Cover the person with a blanket or coat. Put a ground cover under the person, if possible. *Rationale: Keeping the person covered helps to prevent chilling and shock. These complications add exertion to the already stressed heart.*
- Place something under the person's head and upper back. If necessary, assist the person to sit up to breathe. *Rationale: The person usually finds it easier to breathe if the head is elevated.*
- If the person shows signs of shock, keep him or her flat, unless this prohibits breathing. *Rationale: Lying flat helps to control shock. However, the person will become more panicky if he or she can't breathe.*
- Be prepared to initiate CPR. *Rationale: Cardiopulmonary arrest is a relatively common complication of heart attack. If the person can be maintained until arrival at the healthcare facility, the chance for a positive outcome increases.*

(indicating lack of oxygen to the tissues). If a person has any of these symptoms, suspect a heart attack and call for help *immediately.*

Prompt action is the most important factor in whether a person lives or dies following an MI. **Thrombolytic** medications dissolve the clot and clear the blocked blood vessel. These medications have improved the success rate in saving lives when administered within one hour of the attack. In Practice: Nursing Care Guidelines 43-5 presents first aid for the person with a suspected heart attack.

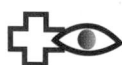

Nursing Alert

The most frequent common denominator in heart attack is *denial.* The person cannot believe that he or she is having a heart attack.

Bleeding

Nosebleed (Epistaxis)

Another name for *nosebleed* is **epistaxis.** In Practice: Nursing Procedure 43-3 gives the basic steps for treating a nosebleed.

Nursing Alert

If the person with a nosebleed has a fractured skull, *do not attempt to stop the bleeding.* Doing so could increase intracranial pressure. In severe hypertension, a nosebleed may be the body's safety valve against a cerebrovascular accident (stroke).

Minor Wounds

Place a sterile pad directly over a minor wound that is bleeding. A prepared commercial adhesive bandage strip (eg, a Band Aid™) is an adequate dressing for a small cut or scratch. Such strips are packaged in various sizes and should be in every home medicine cabinet. Do not touch the part of the sterile dressing that covers the wound; put the dressing exactly where it is to stay. It cannot be moved afterward without contaminating it. Be sure that the bandage or adhesive is firm, yet not so tight as to cut off circulation. Telfa™ (nonstick) pads are much less irritating on removal than conventional gauze bandages.

If a sterile dressing is not readily available, use a clean handkerchief or cloth. Press the dressing firmly on the bleeding

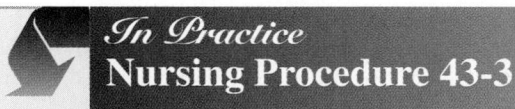

In Practice
Nursing Procedure 43-3

ASSISTING THE CLIENT WHO HAS A NOSEBLEED

Supplies and Equipment

Gloves
Gauze
Cold compresses

Steps

1. Have the person sit down and lean forward slightly. If this position is impossible because of other injuries, have the person lie down, keeping his or her head and shoulders elevated.
   RATIONALE: *The head should be above the heart, to reduce pressure.*

2. Apply pressure to the nostrils or to the bridge of the nose with your thumb and forefinger for 5 to 10 minutes without releasing the pressure.
   RATIONALE: *This location will place pressure on some of the blood vessels supplying the nose. Releasing the pressure too soon will allow a clot to break loose, and bleeding will resume.*

3. Place cold compresses on the person's nose and face.
   RATIONALE: *Cold causes vasoconstriction and slows blood circulation to the area.*

4. If bleeding continues, place small, clean pieces of gauze in one or both nostrils. Do not use cotton. Reapply pressure.
   RATIONALE: *Clean pieces of gauze act to apply pressure locally. Cotton could stick to the bleeding area and cause additional bleeding when removed.*

5. Apply pressure above the person's upper lip if he or she is conscious.
   RATIONALE: *Applying pressure helps to cut off some of the blood supply to the area.*

6. Seek medical assistance if bleeding is uncontrollable.
   RATIONALE: *Continued bleeding may be a symptom of a more serious disorder and may also become life threatening.*

Hemorrhage

When a blood vessel is cut or torn, blood escapes and bleeding occurs. The amount of bleeding depends on the number and size of injured blood vessels. A person can lose a great deal of blood if bleeding is excessive before clotting occurs.

Bleeding that is abundant or uncontrollable is called **hemorrhage.** A severe injury to one large blood vessel can cause a serious hemorrhage; however, an injury to many small vessels or capillaries can cause an equally life-threatening hemorrhage.

In an emergency involving bleeding, the first and most important step is to stop the bleeding. The second step is to treat the shock that accompanies hemorrhage (see discussion earlier in this chapter). Because blood is the chief means of transmission of human immunodeficiency virus and other diseases, be sure to follow Standard Precautions.

When you are faced with a situation involving bleeding, quickly assess for the type of bleeding:

- In *capillary bleeding,* blood oozes slowly out of the wound.
- In *arterial bleeding,* blood comes in spurts with each heartbeat, and is bright-red or pink in color. Arterial bleeding is usually the most severe type of hemorrhage.
- In *venous bleeding,* blood flows steadily and is dark in color. Usually, venous bleeding is minor and stops by itself, unless the person has a bleeding disorder.

In any case of hemorrhage, place the person on a flat surface and slightly elevate his or her feet (unless the person has a head injury).

Applying Direct Pressure.   In external hemorrhage, cut the person's clothes away from the site to reveal the site and amount of bleeding. Apply direct, firm pressure at the site, which will control bleeding in most injuries. Elevate the injured part, unless the possibility of fracture or other trauma to the area exists.

Applying Indirect Pressure.   If direct pressure does not control hemorrhage, you may need to apply *indirect pressure.* This term means that you do not apply pressure directly to the wound, but to an artery at a pressure point between the wound and the heart (see Figure 43-2). You will need a firm surface to press against, to cut off the blood flow from the heart to the wound. Therefore, choose a pressure point in which the supplying artery lies close to a bone.

If bleeding is severe enough to require the use of a pressure point, maintain the pressure until medical assistance arrives. If you release pressure, the clot that formed may dislodge and bleeding will resume. Danger of embolism also exists.

✚👁 Nursing Alert

Never wipe a blood clot from a wound. The clot acts as a plug for ruptured blood vessels. If the clot breaks loose, death may result from *external hemorrhage* or from *embolism.*

Using a Tourniquet.   A **tourniquet** is a tie used on an extremity over a pressure point to stop hemorrhage. Use a

area; then apply a firm bandage to hold the dressing in place. The dressing should stop minor bleeding. If bleeding is more severe, apply an inflated blood pressure cuff or air splint, or insert a firmly rolled sterile pad under the dressing. (A rolled pad allows for more pressure than a flat pad.) Fasten the bandage securely in place. Fasten a dressing on an arm or leg with an ACE-type roller bandage. Be sure not to shut off circulation entirely. (A roller bandage placed over the dressing may also help to control bleeding.)

tourniquet *only as a last resort*. Using a tourniquet may mean that the person will lose the limb as a result. The tourniquet must be tight enough to cut off the blood flow in the artery completely. If it is too loose, it will only prevent the blood from flowing back through the veins, and thus will increase bleeding. In Practice: Nursing Procedure 43-4 outlines the steps for applying a tourniquet.

MAST Trousers. Military antishock trousers (**MAST**) may be used in cases of massive internal hemorrhage or hypovolemia. MAST are pneumatic and serve to provide pressure evenly to the body, support circulation, and lessen shock (Fig. 43-4). MAST trousers are not to be used in pulmonary edema, cardiogenic shock, increased ICP, or evisceration (protrusion of viscera through the skin, most often through an unhealed surgical incision).

You may see paramedics applying MAST, or a person may come into an emergency department with them in place. Only emergency personnel apply MAST. Nurses do not apply or remove them. In some areas, MAST are rarely used because rapid transport of the critically ill person is preferable to taking extra time to apply the trousers.

Indications for the use of MAST trousers include very low or rapidly falling blood pressure; loss of consciousness; decreased or absent leg pulses; pale, mottled, and cold feet; and severe respiratory distress (dyspnea, tachypnea, gasping breaths, cough, pink and frothy sputum).

Internal Bleeding

A person experiencing *internal bleeding* can develop life-threatening shock before the bleeding is discovered. Consider internal bleeding in all cases of trauma, especially in older clients. Possible causes of internal bleeding include blunt trauma, fractures, gastrointestinal bleeding, and vaginal bleeding. A fracture is the most common cause of internal bleeding.

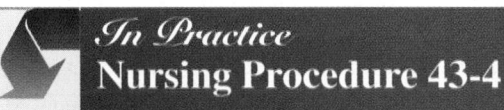

In Practice
Nursing Procedure 43-4

APPLYING A TOURNIQUET

Supplies and Equipment

Gloves
Small object such as a pencil or stick
Piece of cloth
Tightly rolled, firm pad

Steps

1. Try all other methods of controlling hemorrhage (direct and indirect pressure) first. If all other methods fail, prepare to apply the tourniquet.
   RATIONALE: *Use of a tourniquet may necessitate later limb amputation.*

2. Place a compact, rolled piece of material over the artery's pressure point, controlling blood flow to the injury. Wind the tourniquet over this pad.
   RATIONALE: *This measure applies pressure over the blood vessel.*

3. Tie a half knot at the side of the injured limb. Place a stick or similar object over it, and tie a square knot over the stick. Twist the stick tightly enough to control bleeding.
   RATIONALE: *The tourniquet has to be tight enough to inhibit bleeding.*

4. Secure the stick firmly.
   RATIONALE: *The tourniquet may loosen if not secure.*

5. Do not cover the tourniquet; it should be in full view.
   RATIONALE: *Medical personnel have to know it is there. If not, it could remain in place too long, causing severe limb damage.*

6. Do not loosen the tourniquet without a physician's order.
   RATIONALE: *Clots may form, which, if dislodged, could cause embolism.*

7. Tag the client with a note stating the location of the tourniquet and the time of application. It is also a good idea to print a "T" on the person's forehead with a marker or lipstick.
   RATIONALE: *Emergency and medical personnel must know that a tourniquet is in place. Prompt action may help to save the limb.*

8. Keep the bleeding part immobile and elevate it if possible.
   RATIONALE: *This action slows circulation.*

9. Treat the person for shock, and observe for cardiac arrest.
   RATIONALE: *Clients with severe hemorrhage are at high risk for cardiac arrest.*

10. Transport the person to the nearest medical facility immediately.
    RATIONALE: *Medical care is needed to save the extremity and to treat shock or other cardiovascular problems.*

Chapter 43 ➤ Emergency Care and First Aid   525

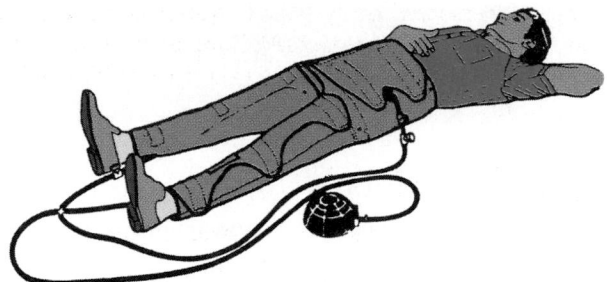

FIGURE 43-4. The military antishock trouser (MAST) is a garment designed to correct internal bleeding and hypovolemia (low blood volume) by the application of counterpressure around the legs and abdomen. This pressure creates an artificial peripheral resistance and helps sustain coronary perfusion. It should be applied as soon as possible after injury, preferably before the client is transferred to the emergency department. (Courtesy of David Clark Co, Inc, Worcester, Massachusetts.)

A fractured pelvis is the most severe fracture related to blood loss. Signs of gastrointestinal bleeding may include vomiting bright red or coffee-ground–like emesis, or passing bloody or black stools. A person with gastrointestinal bleeding can deteriorate very quickly.

Report the following observations to the EMTs or physician immediately if you see them in any person, regardless if the person is in a healthcare facility or not:

- Large or unexplained bruises and contusions
- Bleeding from the mouth, rectum, ears, or other body opening
- Dizziness when rising from a lying to a standing position, without a known cause
- Cold, clammy skin
- Profuse sweating
- Restlessness, anxiety, unexplained combative behavior
- Confusion, without other known causes
- Weak, rapid pulse
- Shallow, rapid breathing
- Extreme thirst
- Unexplained weakness
- Falling blood pressure
- Altered LOC

Treatment is aimed at stopping the bleeding, and replacing blood and fluids lost.

Anaphylaxis

Normally, when the body senses the presence of an antigen, an antigen–antibody reaction occurs (see Chap. 24). This constant neutralizing reaction protects the person from toxins and infections. In the hypersensitive person, the antigen–antibody reaction works to the person's detriment. The release of chemicals in the body, such as histamine, causes reactions affecting several body systems (*systemic*). **Anaphylaxis** (anaphylactic shock) is a type I allergic, life-threatening reaction to a substance. A severe type I reaction occurs within minutes of exposure.

Anaphylaxis is highly individualized; people can be hypersensitive to almost any substance. Common triggers for anaphylaxis include:

- Bee stings
- Certain foods (eg, peanuts and chocolate)
- Food additives or preservatives (eg, sulfite, MSG)
- Medications (eg, antibiotics, aspirin)
- Chemicals
- Inhaled substances

In Practice: Nursing Assessment 43-1 list signs and symptoms of anaphylactic shock. The person's LOC is especially significant. The person will be restless and panicky, and may faint or have a seizure. Loss of consciousness often occurs early in severe anaphylaxis. The time range for an allergic reaction is from a few seconds to several hours. Reactions are often generalized and violent. Each occurrence is more serious than the last. People who have severe allergies should carry medication such as subcutaneous (SQ) epinephrine with them at all times. Family and friends, as well as the person, should learn how to administer the medication. Common medications for anaphylaxis are listed at In Practice: Important Medications 43-1.

Remember the acronym **SIRES** when faced with an allergic or anaphylactic situation:

- **S** = Stabilize
- **I** = Identify the toxin
- **R** = Reverse the effect of the toxin
- **E** = Eliminate the toxin
- **S** = Support (respiration, circulation, and so forth)

First-aid care begins with creating an open airway. Activate the EMS system immediately. Ask the person if appropriate medication is available. If so, the person may need assistance in administering this.

Animal Bites and Scratches

Animal bites and scratches are a common problem, particularly among children. Most often, the child is bitten by a household pet. **Rabies,** a communicable disease transmitted through animal bites, is caused by the rhabdovirus. The virus travels along the person's nerves to the CNS. Untreated rabies is almost always fatal. A specific **antidote** (a substance that neutralizes poisons) for rabies is available, though it is painful and expensive.

Animal bites and scratches can also cause an infection, which may become serious. These infections include *cat-scratch disease (fever),* which is usually mild, resulting only in swelling of regional lymph nodes. *Cat-bite disease* can be more serious. Usually, the cat does not show any signs of dis-

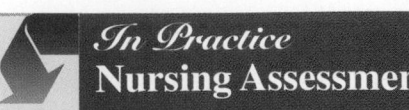

In Practice
Nursing Assessment 43-1

SIGNS AND SYMPTOMS OF ANAPHYLAXIS

Skin
- Raised hive-like patches (*urticaria*)
- Burning of the skin
- Severe itching (*pruritus*)
- Pallor
- Perspiration
- Cold, clammy skin or flushed skin
- Blueness (*cyanosis*) around the lips and nails

Neurologic System
- Dizziness
- Weakness
- Restlessness
- Panic
- Tingling and numbness
- Seizures or stroke
- Coma

Circulatory System
- Dilation of blood vessels
- Blood volume loss
- Decreased cardiac stroke volume
- Decreased cardiac output
- Lowering of blood pressure
- Weak, rapid pulse
- Irregular pulse
- Circulatory collapse

Respiratory System
- Coughing, sneezing, wheezing
- Itching nose
- Swelling of face, tongue, and airway
- Chest tightness
- Dyspnea
- Choking sensation
- Respiratory arrest

Gastrointestinal System
- Nausea and vomiting
- Abdominal cramping
- Diarrhea

Other
- Watery, itching eyes
- Throbbing in the ears
- Incontinence

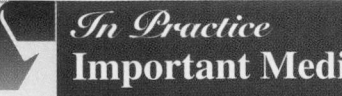

In Practice
Important Medications 43-1

TO TREAT ANAPHYLAXIS

For severe anaphylaxis, the following drugs may be used:

- Epinephrine (Adrenaline)
- Corticosteroids
- Histamine 1 receptor antagonists (antihistamines)

For milder forms of anaphylaxis, medications such as diphenhydramine hydrochloride (Benadryl) or hydroxyzine (Vistaril, Atarax) may be used.

area with sterile normal saline. *Do not delay in obtaining medical care.*

Follow the physician's orders for further care. Usually, the nurse or physician will **debride** (cut away) any loose tissue. A tetanus injection or antibiotics, to prevent or treat infection, may be administered. An antibiotic commonly used in the case of an animal-related injury is dicloxacillin (Dynapen). If a rabies antiserum is required, the manufacturer will include specific instructions for its use. These instructions must be followed exactly.

☞ KEY CONCEPT

In the case of an animal bite, the animal is captured and observed whenever possible. If it cannot be located or captured, obtain an accurate description of the animal and the circumstances. Do not destroy the animal; sometimes a length of time in quarantine is needed to determine if it is diseased or not. In the case of a household pet, a fine may be assessed if the animal has bitten someone previously. The law requires reporting any animal bite to the Public Health Department and the police immediately. (If the animal is not available for observation, the person must undergo painful and expensive anti-rabies treatment.)

Exposure to Hazardous Materials

Hazardous materials (**HAZMATs**) are used in the production of many common products including fuel, medications, plastics, and home cleaning agents. These materials are normally stored, used, and transported safely. However, when they are improperly handled, they may become hazardous to the environment. These powerful chemical products can cause poisoning, burns, exposure to toxic fumes, contamination of groundwater, and explosions. Other environmental emergencies are chemical or oil spills and gas leaks.

Primary exposure is when a person is exposed directly to a hazardous substance, for example by breathing fumes from evaporating liquids. *Secondary exposure* occurs when the rescuer or healthcare provider is exposed to the contaminated person. To prevent exposure, follow these safety measures:

ease in either case. A dog bite can be very serious and disfiguring, especially if it involves the face. Some dog attacks can result in death, particularly in children.

When a person is bitten, cleanse the wound with warm, soapy water and rinse the area thoroughly. Swab the area with Zephiran or alcohol. If a puncture wound is present, flush the

- Do not walk into or touch spilled material.
- Avoid inhalation of gases, fumes, and smoke.
- Do not assume that gases or vapors are harmless because they are odorless.
- Do not go near accident victims if you cannot identify the hazardous material.
- Do not walk into or drive into a gas cloud. If you are accidentally caught in one and are unable to drive out, roll up your car windows, close the vents, turn off the fan, unlock the doors, and wait for assistance.

Emergency personnel specially trained in the management of hazardous materials will respond, to eliminate and prevent contamination. Clients exposed to hazardous materials require specialized care. Take these additional precautions:

- Wear personal protective equipment (PPE) to help prevent secondary exposure.
- Decontaminate the victim. Remove his or her clothing and rinse off the chemical. Most emergency departments have showers available for this purpose.

If a contaminated person presents to the ED or clinic, avoid exposing the entire department to the hazard. After a hazardous chemical enters a building, the area may require evacuation and decontamination. Most EDs have plans for decontaminating victims outside the area using special rooms with an outside entrance, portable self-contained showers, or hoses. Remove the victim's clothes and store them in appropriate bags. Use special decontamination stretchers for clients who are unable to shower. Complete the process as quickly as possible, then treat the victim's injuries. If lifesaving procedures are necessary before decontamination is possible, personnel must wear appropriate protective barriers to avoid contamination.

Poisoning

Any substance that threatens a person's health when it is absorbed or comes into contact with the body is defined as a **poison.** Poisons are in such common substances as household cleaning agents, insecticides, antifreeze, furniture polish, kerosene, and nail polish. Accidental poisoning is a particular danger for children. In Practice: Nursing Care Guidelines 43-6 outlines first-aid care for poisoning. In Practice: Important Medications 43-2 lists common antidotes for poisoning.

In many cases of poisoning, **gastric lavage** ("pumping out the stomach") may be necessary. This procedure is less therapeutic if not performed promptly after ingestion of the poison. In some situations, an **emetic** medication will be ordered, causing the person to vomit. In other situations, vomiting would cause more damage. Follow the instructions from the Poison Control Center.

✚👁 **N u r s i n g   A l e r t**
Never make the person who has ingested poison vomit unless specifically instructed to do so by the Poison Control Center or physician.

Medication Poisoning

All medications are potentially poisonous, but many do not have such effects because they are given in small doses. Accidental drug poisoning may result from misreading a label or taking medicine from an unlabeled bottle or in the dark. Older persons may take extra doses of medications because they may forget that they have already taken them. A drug overdose may be accidental or intentional (eg, a suicide attempt). Care in a suicide attempt is discussed in Chapter 93.

Food Poisoning

Food poisoning is almost always caused by eating contaminated food. Bacteria's normal action on food causes *decomposition,* which forms **toxins** (poisonous substances). Another cause of food poisoning is the accidental eating of poisonous fruits, berries, or vegetables (eg, toadstools or poisonous mushrooms).

Symptoms of food poisoning include abdominal pain, nausea, vomiting, and diarrhea. Onset is acute (within a few hours after eating the contaminated food). The sooner the symptoms occur, the more serious the poisoning is. Symptoms usually disappear in 1 to 2 days, after the person has excreted the toxins.

A severe form of food poisoning, called *botulism,* is caused by the organism *Clostridium botulinum.* About half of the cases of botulism result in death. Home-canned foods that have been improperly sterilized or have lost their seal are a common cause. Symptoms are progressive and include weakness, headache, paralysis of the eye and throat muscles, and finally, respiratory paralysis. Specific antitoxins are effective if given early. Rescue breathing may be required until EMS personnel arrive. They will maintain the person with the ambu bag during transport. The person may need to be maintained via endotracheal tube on a mechanical ventilator until the antitoxin takes effect and spontaneous respirations resume.

✚👁 **N u r s i n g   A l e r t**
Warn clients to never use a home-canned or commercially canned item if the top is bulging, if there is dark leakage around the seams, or if there is any discoloration in the contents of jarred foods. *If there is any doubt, throw it out!*

Psychiatric Emergencies

Psychiatric emergencies affect people of all ages and can occur at any time. A person requires medical attention when severe anxiety results in hallucinations, paranoia, confusion, or suicidal threats or gestures. *Anxiety* or "panic attack" may cause the person's heart to race or his or her respirations to become rapid. Sometimes the person's fingers and hands become numb and tingly. The person may feel incapable of functioning. Assess the person for suicidal tendencies and potential risk for harming self or others. The nurse working in home care or community-based nursing may be the first and only healthcare person to come in contact with the client. Recognizing the symptoms of

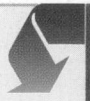

In Practice
Nursing Care Guidelines 43-6

GIVING FIRST AID IN POISONING OR OVERDOSE

- Call for help: 911. *Rationale: Treatment for poisoning depends on the poison ingested. Expert assistance is needed.*
- After calling 911, contact the nearest Poison Control Center. In some EMS areas, 911 dispatchers can connect the call to the Poison Control Center and monitor the call. *Rationale: The Poison Control Center can instruct the caller in proper treatment. In some cases, vomiting is induced; in other cases, vomiting would cause more damage.*

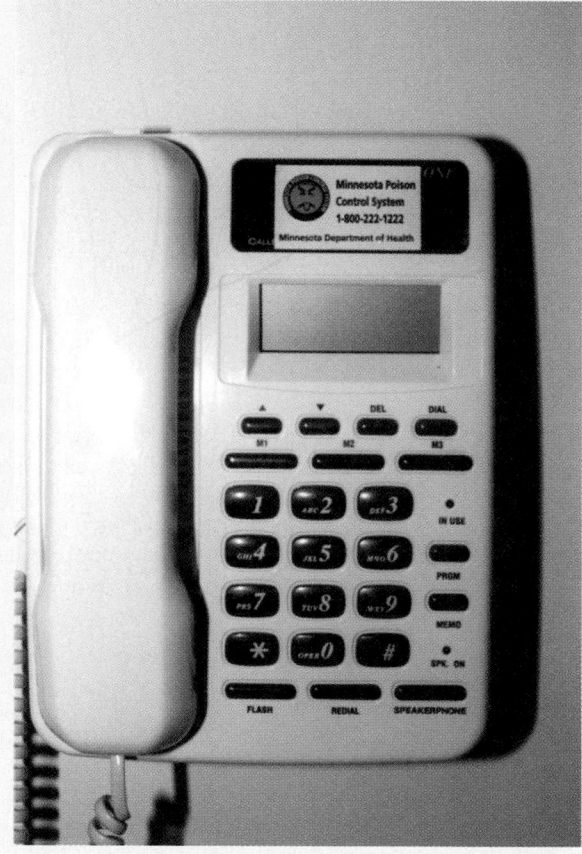

The number of the nearest Poison Control Center should be posted near the phone. (Photo © Kimberly Malcolm Rosdahl).

- Attempt to identify the poison. Question the person, if possible. Save all vomitus, urine, or stools and the remains of food or drugs that may have been responsible. Look for medication bottles or other containers. Bring all these materials to the medical facility with the person. *Rationale: This information is necessary to determine the nature and amount of poison or drug taken.*
- Use the sense of smell to detect the odor of alcohol or other chemicals on the person's breath. *Rationale: Many drugs are more dangerous when combined with alcohol.*
- In cases of suspected overdose, ask questions of the person and the family. Was this a suicide attempt or an accident? Was there a suicide note? Was the person depressed or despondent? How many pills or how much alcohol was taken? *Rationale: This information will be important to the medical team in planning emergency treatment and continuing medical care.*
- Give supportive care. Keep the person warm. Use artificial ventilation if the person is having difficulty breathing. Maintain the heartbeat. If possible, keep the person awake. Follow basic life support procedures if CPR is needed. *Rationale: Poisoning or overdose is a medical emergency. Maintain the person in the most stable condition possible until arrival at the healthcare facility.*
- Follow the instructions of the Poison Control Center. *Rationale: They are the experts in treatment of poisoning or overdose.*
- If syrup of ipecac or activated charcoal are prescribed, follow specific instructions. Do not give either of these unless told to do so by the Poison Control Center. *Rationale: In some cases, the caller will be instructed to make the person vomit; in other cases, vomiting would be very dangerous.*
- Remember the acronym SIRES. *Rationale: This acronym will help to guide your actions.*

---

a psychiatric emergency is important. Call for medical assistance when any of these factors are present in an individual:

- Threat to harm self or others
- Suicidal thoughts, especially if the person has a specific plan (eg, weapons, pills, and so forth) or even if the person does not have a plan
- Refusal to talk further when a psychiatric emergency is suspected

- History of prior suicide attempts
- Severe depression
- Intoxication or drug abuse, combined with suicidal or violent thoughts or actions
- Self-injurious behavior (eg, burning or cutting oneself)
- Out-of-control or bizarre behavior, causing major disturbances in the community
- Evidence of self-harm (eg, empty pill bottles, unresponsiveness, suicide attempt)

In Practice
Important Medications 43-2

FOR POISONING AND DRUG OVERDOSE

The following medications are commonly used for treating poisoning or overdose:

- All-purpose antidote: activated charcoal (Actidose-Aqua, Charcocaps)
- Emetic (causes vomiting): syrup of ipecac
- Acetaminophen overdose: acetylcystine (Mucomyst)

When caring for the person receiving any of these medications, keep in mind the following:

- Never combine these medications.
- Be sure that activated charcoal and syrup of ipecac are available to all first-aid personnel and in every home medicine cabinet.
- Assess the first bowel movement after activated charcoal is given. It will appear black. Watch for constipation; bowel obstruction may occur.
- Do *not* give syrup of ipecac—an emetic that induces vomiting—if the person is unresponsive, inebriated, having seizures, or in severe shock. It should *not* be given after ingestion of caustic substances (which would irritate the throat again when being vomited), or after ingestion of volatile substances such as gasoline (which could be easily aspirated into the lungs).
- Assess for a gag response before giving emetics.
- Follow the instructions on the bottle.
- If you have given syrup of ipecac, do not give activated charcoal until after the person has vomited.

- Evidence of not caring for one's self, such as not eating, not sleeping, living in a trash-strewn house or not taking prescribed medications
- Reports of any of the above by family or neighbors

Assist emotionally disturbed people by remaining calm. Show them respect and make no assumptions or judgments. Ask questions that allow him or her to explain the situation. Avoid questions that elicit yes or no answers; encourage the person to talk. Help generate a positive plan of action. Express a desire to help. Communicate on the client's level. Listen attentively. Obtain medical assistance as soon as possible. The police can assist in taking the person to the hospital if necessary. Chapter 93 describes psychiatric emergencies in more detail.

☛ KEY CONCEPT

When dealing with an emotionally disturbed person, remain calm and speak softly, slowly, and clearly. Maintain a non-threatening posture and tone of voice. Prevent the person from injuring him- or herself or anyone else. Seek assistance as soon as possible.

⮞ STUDENT SYNTHESIS

Key Points

- Nurses are with clients much of the time in the health-care facility. Therefore, the nurse may be in the position to recognize and alert the appropriate staff to deal with cardiopulmonary arrest and other emergencies.
- Nurses must use Standard Precautions when administering first aid (to whatever extent possible).
- In emergencies, nurses and nursing students function *only at their level of first-aid training.* Quick evaluation of the scene and planning for action are crucial.
- Calling 911 will summon the EMS system in almost all areas of the United States and Canada. The nurse must know how to summon assistance in an emergency.
- When assessing an emergency, the most important consideration is to make sure the person is breathing and that his or her heart is beating.
- Be sure to treat the injured person for shock.
- Do not move an injured person, unless the situation is dangerous. Take precautions to prevent further injury.
- All healthcare workers, including nurses, should know how to perform CPR in an emergency. Maintain current CPR certification.
- The nurse may be called on to provide first-aid assistance in a community. Each nurse has the responsibility to be knowledgeable in basic first-aid techniques.
- Chest injuries can result in inadequate air exchange and are immediately life threatening. Ensure that the chest wall is intact. Plug any open wound of the chest. Do not remove any penetrating objects.
- Be aware of the possibility of injury from excessive heat or cold. Take prompt action in life-threatening situations.
- A person who is having a heart attack is often in denial. EMS personnel may need to be very persuasive to get the victim to appropriate medical care.
- The first-aid person must be knowledgeable in methods used to stop bleeding.
- Anaphylaxis is a medical emergency that requires immediate treatment.
- Follow the instructions of the Poison Control Center in the event of poisoning or overdose.
- Remain calm when dealing with an emotionally upset client. Be alert for the possibility of suicide.

Critical Thinking Exercises

1. A motorcyclist has been hit by a car and thrown from the bike. What actions should people on the scene take? What should you do if you are there? Discuss Standard Precautions in relation to the accident scene.

2. You notice a pregnant woman choking and coughing in a restaurant. She runs to the bathroom. What actions would you take and why?

3. You are caring for a client in her home who tells you she wants to die. You believe she has the means and is serious about harming herself. How would you handle this situation?

4. Your neighbor is mowing his lawn when he suddenly falls to the ground. Describe what actions you should take and why.

NCLEX-Style Review Questions

1. Which of the following interventions would be your priority when treating a victim suspected of being in shock?
   a. Establish, maintain, and monitor the airway.
   b. Immobilize fractures.
   c. Maintain body temperature.
   d. Monitor level of consciousness.

2. Most states have laws to protect emergency care rescuers form legal liability. These laws are called:
   a. EMT Protection Laws
   b. Good Samaritan Laws
   c. Rescuer Laws
   d. Safe Care Laws

3. During which condition would heat injuries most likely occur?
   a. High humidity, high temperature, and no breeze
   b. High humidity, high temperature, and strong breeze
   c. High humidity, moderate temperature, and no breeze
   d. Low humidity, high temperature, and no breeze

4. A victim has fallen from a second-story window and complains of pain in the right leg. Which action is most appropriate?
   a. Ask the person to walk on the leg to see if it is broken.
   b. Ask the person why they fell.
   c. Do not move the person.
   d. Remove the victim's pants.

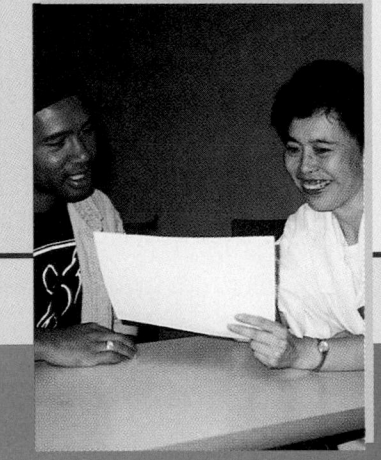

Unit VIII

CLIENT CARE

CHAPTER

44

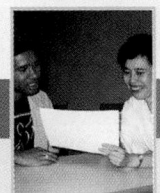

Therapeutic Communication Skills

LEARNING OBJECTIVES

1. Define communication.
2. List the five components of effective communication.
3. Discuss the three parts of the communication process.
4. Explain rapport and its importance in nursing.
5. Differentiate between verbal and nonverbal communication.
6. List at least five nonverbal cues, and discuss each one.
7. Discuss factors that influence the effectiveness of communication.
8. Demonstrate the interviewing and communication skills of questioning, therapeutic silence, and clarifying.
9. In the skills lab, demonstrate a teaching session for the following clients: young children, older adults, visually impaired persons, hearing-impaired persons, unconscious clients, and aphasic individuals.
10. In the skills lab, demonstrate means of communicating with a client who does not speak your language.
11. In the skills lab, demonstrate effective telephone communication skills.

NEW TERMINOLOGY

alias
aphasia
assertiveness
body language
closed-ended question
communication
eye contact

interview
nonverbal communication
open-ended question
personal space
rapport
therapeutic communication
verbal communication

ACRONYMS

AKA   TO   VO
ROI

Communication means the giving, receiving, and interpreting of information through any of the five senses by two or more interacting people. **Therapeutic communication** is helpful and healing for one or more of the participants; the client benefits from knowing that someone cares and understands, and the nurse derives satisfaction from knowing that he or she has been helpful to someone. A nurse must have self-awareness and interpersonal skills to communicate therapeutically. The goal of therapeutic communication is to help clients talk about and resolve their feelings and problems related to health, illness, treatments, and nursing care.[1] Successful therapeutic communication encourages client coping and motivation toward self-care.

Effective use of communication will play an important role in your nursing career and personal life. It is the foundation on which interpersonal relationships are built. The art of therapeutic communication does not come naturally; it must be learned. Pointers for using therapeutic communication are listed in the accompanying feature, In Practice: Nursing Care Guidelines 44-1.

COMMUNICATION

Personal characteristics of genuineness, caring, trust, empathy, and respect spark harmony among individuals. This feeling of harmony is called **rapport.** Conveying these attitudes to another person creates a social climate that communicates goodwill and empathy, even when fears or concerns cannot be fully expressed verbally. To be most helpful, the nurse develops the ability to convey a nonjudgmental attitude, especially if another person's beliefs and values differ from the nurse's own. Accept others as individuals; respect each person's right to his or her own beliefs. Clients must experience this feeling of rapport for them to be willing to share personal, and sometimes embarrassing, information with you.

Components of Communication

Communication requires several components (Fig. 44-1):

> *Sender:* The originator or source of the idea
> *Message:* The idea
> *Medium* or *channel:* A means of transmitting the idea, which can be verbal or nonverbal
> *Receiver:* The person who receives and interprets the message
> *Interaction:* The receiver's response to the message through feedback

Think of communication as a reciprocal process in which both the sender and the receiver of messages participate simultaneously.

All the senses can be involved in communication. We see and hear other people through conversations. Nurses sometimes touch others to express concern or care. The sense of smell or taste can also convey information. Sometimes, various factors affect communication. For example, noise can distort interactions. Conducting therapeutic communication in

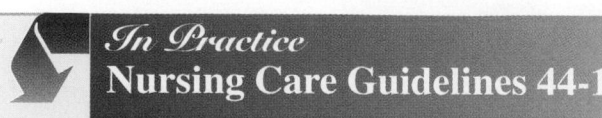

In Practice
Nursing Care Guidelines 44-1

USING THERAPEUTIC COMMUNICATION

The nurse who is using therapeutic communication will:

- Put the client at ease and develop rapport.
- Provide privacy.
- Respect the client's rights.
- Respect the client's personal space.
- Keep information confidential, as appropriate.
- Begin the interview with general information and ask emotionally difficult questions after the client gains confidence.
- Adjust language level as appropriate for the client.
- Not use complex medical terms or "talk down to" the client.
- Ask an interpreter to assist, if the client speaks a language different from that of the staff.
- Be attentive, and concentrate on what the person says.
- Make appropriate and congruent eye contact.
- Try not to write during the interview. Pay close attention. Clarify details with the client later.
- Show sincere interest in the client's responses.
- Ask the client about his or her perceptions. Why did he or she come to the facility?
- Pay attention to the client's choice of words; any repetition; variations in tone of voice; silence; body language; assertiveness; behaviors; and so forth.
- Assess or ask the client's attitudes about touch before using that technique.
- Include the family in conversations, if the client prefers.
- Consider the client's cultural background in all interactions and assessments.

privacy or in a quiet area may avoid distractions that detract from its effectiveness.

Types of Communication

Nurses communicate with clients often and in various ways. Two types of communication are verbal communication (using words) and nonverbal communication (using actions). The most effective communication occurs when words and actions convey the same message; this is essential.

Verbal Communication
Verbal communication is sharing information through the written or spoken word. Nurses use verbal communication extensively. They converse with clients, write care plans, document information and assessments, chart, and give oral or written change-of-shift reports.

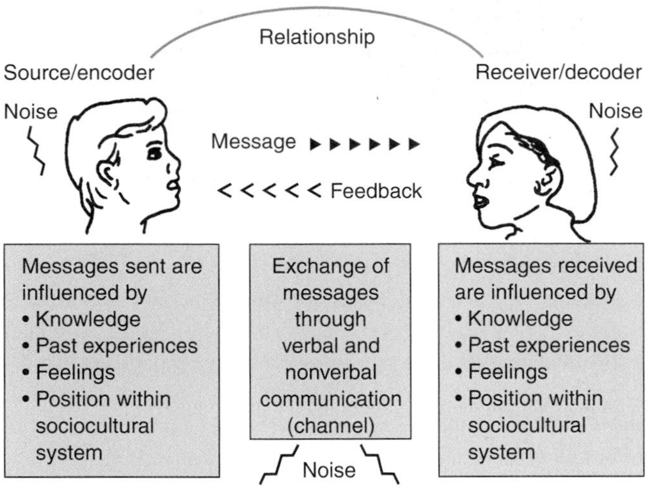

FIGURE 44-1. Various components in the process of communication. (Adapted from Taylor, C., Lillis, C., & LeMone, P. [2001]. *Fundamentals of nursing: The art and science of nursing care* (4th ed.). Philadelphia: Lippincott Williams & Wilkins.)

Much verbal information is related through vocabulary, sentence structure, and pronunciation. People reveal their education, intellectual skills, interests, and ethnic, regional, or national background through verbal communication. Voice inflections and sounds reveal messages. Although a client may say what the nurse wants to hear, his or her tone of voice may imply lack of sincerity. The person may make sounds that indicate true feelings. A snort, for example, may denote disgust.

Be aware that some responses stop the communication process. These blocks are called *verbal barriers*. Table 44-1 lists such barriers and more effective responses that encourage further discussion.

Characteristics of Speech. It is important to note the volume of the client's speech. Speaking loudly may be culturally based. However, it may also indicate conditions such as a hearing impairment or mania. Speaking softly may imply such things as nervousness, paranoia, shyness, or lack of self-confidence. This may also be a reflection of the client's culture.

Consider also the rate and rhythm of the client's speech. Speaking very fast may imply anxiety, mania, flight of ideas, or impatience. Speaking very slowly may be the result of a brain disorder or a mental illness. Hesitation in speaking, thought-blocking, difficulty in finding words, or total aphasia may indicate that the client does not speak English, has a brain disorder, or is hallucinating (seeing or hearing things that others do not perceive). These are just examples; many other factors influence a client's speech patterns.

Aphasia is a defect in or loss of the ability to speak, write, or sign, or of the ability to comprehend speech and communication. Aphasia is usually caused by an injury or disorder of the brain's speech centers. *Expressive aphasia* refers to difficulty in speaking or in finding the correct or desired word. *Receptive aphasia* refers to a disorder of the brain that interferes with the comprehension or understanding of what one is hearing. Chapter 80 describes aphasia, its causes, and related nursing care in more detail.

Nonverbal Communication

Nonverbal communication is sharing information without using words or language. It is also called **body language.** Sometimes body language differs from what the client states verbally. For example, Mr. H., a young diabetic client, begins clenching and unclenching his fists when the nurse asks about his sexual activity. He says, "everything is fine," through gritted teeth. Later, when he trusts the nurse more, he admits that he has been impotent for the past 6 months. Often, body language provides more powerful clues than verbal language, because it points to the person's true feelings.

Messages expressed through body posture, gestures, facial expressions, and other forms of nonverbal behavior provide cues or suggestions to a person's true feelings or beliefs. The nurse must be aware, however, that nonverbal behavior has different meanings for different people and in different situations. The nurse must be cautious when interpreting nonverbal cues. It is important to always check with clients before making assumptions about what their body language means.

■■■ TABLE 44-1 *V*ERBAL BARRIERS

Barrier	More Effective Response
Offering empty reassurances	Reassuring the client with factual responses
Changing the subject	Helping the client express feelings by staying on track
Using trite clichés such as "the doctor knows best"	Involving the client in decision-making
Imposing your ideas or values on clients and giving advice according to your values	Helping the client explore his or her own values when a decision or choice must be made
Disapproving of or judging the client	Accepting each client as unique; considering ethnic and cultural practices in understanding values and behaviors
Voicing personal experiences, especially those that are health-related	Allowing the person to discuss his or her own concerns; answering questions factually; offering client-oriented reference material

☛ KEY CONCEPT

Be sure that verbal and nonverbal communications give the same message to clients. When verbal and nonverbal messages conflict, clients are more likely to believe the nonverbal message.

Personal Space.   Each person has an area around him or her called **personal space;** this area is reserved for only very close friends or intimates. Personal space, a culturally learned behavior, varies greatly across cultures. For example, in traditional Western society, personal space extends outward from the body for 18 and 24 inches, although it may vary slightly from person to person. However, in the Middle East and Far East, the area of personal space is smaller. Consider this concept when working with clients from other cultures. An action that would be considered an invasion of personal space by a client from one culture may be considered acceptable behavior by a client from another culture.

It is important for nurses not to violate the outermost boundary of any person's space. If the nurse comes too close, it is an invasion of the person's space. If the nurse is too far away, the client may feel isolated. When speaking with another person, it is usually possible to sense his or her personal boundaries. Nurses, however, are often forced to invade a client's personal space to provide care. It is important to be sensitive to the discomfort this may cause. The nurse should alert the client before touching him or her. Be careful to touch the client gently on the arm or hand before further intruding into his or her space; this practice offers comfort and reassurance so that the client feels safe in the nurse's presence.

✛👁 **N u r s i n g   A l e r t**

The nurse must be aware that some clients may react in a violent or assaultive manner when touched. This may be particularly true in psychiatry or with a client who has dementia. Do not touch any client without being alert for this possibility.

Sometimes, the client's use of personal space is not cultural, but indicates a mental or physical disorder. For example, the psychiatric client who consistently invades the nurse's personal space may be threatening the nurse. Another client who maintains a very large personal space may be very paranoid and afraid of any contact with others. On the other hand, the client with a hearing or visual disorder may need to be very close to the speaker in order to determine what is being said. It is important to consider the reasons for variations in personal space boundaries when giving nursing care.

Eye Contact.   **Eye contact** means looking directly into the eyes of the other person. Lack of direct eye contact has various meanings among cultures. Sometimes indirect eye contact means that a person is nervous, shy, or lying. However, it may also signify respect, as in Southeast Asian, Hispanic American, and Native American cultures. In these cultures, direct eye contact often signifies defiance or hostility.

Facial Expressions.   **Facial expressions** convey messages of many emotions: joy, sadness, anger, and fear. Some people mask their feelings well, which makes understanding what they are thinking very difficult. Nurses learn to control their facial expressions if they are experiencing emotions that may offend the client or block effective communication. For example, the nurse remains calm, with a neutral expression, when viewing wounds or smelling body secretions.

Body Movements and Posture.   A twitching or bouncing foot may indicate anger, impatience, boredom, nervousness, or side effects of certain medications. A slouched appearance may indicate depression. Wringing hands may indicate fear, pain, or worry. Avoid making assumptions about these body language messages, however. The nurse can ask the client what he or she is feeling if there is concern about these or other visual cues.

Personal Appearance and Grooming.   Personal hygiene and general appearance relate information about clients. These nonverbal messages may convey clients' true feelings about themselves, or they may be misleading, especially in illness. Individuals who are trying to meet their basic physiologic needs, such as oxygenation, may not have the physical or emotional energy to work on higher-order needs, such as cleanliness. Lack of personal care may also be a reflection of emotional factors such as depression. In addition, persons with severe and persistent mental illness or out-of-control chemical dependency often have difficulty managing self-care as well.

Therapeutic Use of Touch.   Touch can say "I care" (Fig. 44-2). A firm touch can discourage a child from doing something dangerous; a light touch can encourage a person to walk down the hall. In some cases, touch makes people anxious. Some people do not like to be touched, feeling that it invades their personal space. Be sensitive to the feelings of all clients. Sometimes, a nurse may need to touch a client to carry out a nursing procedure. In such a case, verbally convey understanding of the client's discomfort.

☛ KEY CONCEPT

Nursing care revolves around communication: giving, receiving, and interpreting information. Communication is both verbal and nonverbal.

Factors Influencing Communication

Many factors influence the effectiveness of communication. Some factors enhance communication. Other seemingly harmless factors create barriers between people.

Attention

A listening or attention barrier can occur because of lack of concentration. Selective listening may also be the culprit. In such a case, a person hears only what he or she wants or expects to hear. The nurse may not be paying attention and may not hear because of emotional responses to what the client is saying. Or, the nurse may be mentally framing the next

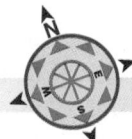

SPECIAL CONSIDERATIONS: CULTURE

Using Unbiased Language When Documenting Client Behaviors

- The nurse objectively describes eye contact, rather than applying judgments. For example, "The client looks at the floor when speaking" is descriptive and nonjudgmental. (A judgmental statement such as "good eye contact" implies that all clients should behave like most Western Europeans or Caucasian Americans.) The nurse might go on to state that (in the nurse's opinion) the client is "insecure and afraid." However, this assessment may be incorrect if, for example, the client is Native American and looking down is considered a sign of respect.

- The nurse objectively describes behavior related to personal space. For example, "client maintains approximately 3 feet of personal space and moves away when approached." In the nurse's opinion, the client might be described as "staff-avoidant." However, this assessment may be incorrect, depending upon the cultural background of the client.

- The nurse describes the tone and volume of the client's verbalizations in objective terms. An objective statement might be, "client speaks very loudly." The judgment that the client is "hostile" may be incorrect, however, when the nurse considers that in some cultures, all people speak very loudly. (On the other hand, the client may be hearing-impaired and may speak loudly as a result of this condition.)

  A male nurse may write about a female client, "client refuses to speak." However, it might be incorrect to say that the client is "paranoid" or "aphasic." It is important for this nurse to remember that in some cultures, women are not permitted to speak to men outside their families.

  Objective documentation may be, "client speaks softly." However, rather than stating that client is "shy" or "afraid," it is important to remember that in some cultures, women are expected to speak softly at all times.

- The use of profanity is common in some cultures and is considered part of everyday language. Documenting what the client says, in quotation marks, rather than making judgments, is objective.

- Many people of the world consider folk medicine or mystical beliefs to be a normal part of life. Therefore, if a client talks about the "evil eye" or a "cold disease," documentation of the actual statement is appropriate and objective. A nurse might wrongly determine that this client is "delusional," for example, when these beliefs are common to most of the members of that client's culture.

- The preceding are examples. The nurse uses the same general guidelines when documenting other nonverbal behaviors, such as reaction to pain, body posture, and general attitudes about health and illness. The nurse will be objective if he or she documents exactly what the client says and does, rather than making judgments based on the interpretation of those statements or actions. (Formal nursing assessments are made using NANDA guidelines. Unit 6 of this book, The Nursing Process, describes these guidelines in more detail.)

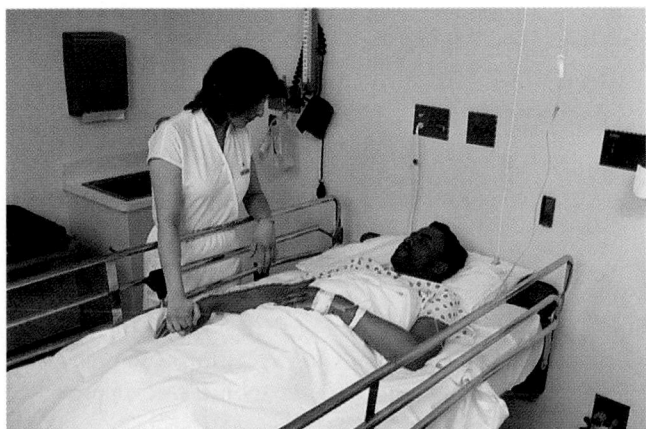

FIGURE 44-2. Therapeutic use of touch is the most potent nonverbal communication technique of all. A gentle and reassuring touch tells the client that the nurse cares and is there to help.

question. Sometimes, a client is experiencing pain or discomfort (physical or emotional) so great that he or she cannot listen or concentrate. The client may also be preoccupied with internal stimuli (such as auditory hallucinations). If both the sender and the receiver do not give, or are not able to give, full attention to the current communication, an effective nurse–client relationship may be stalled.

Age

Age can be an advantage or a disadvantage to effective communication. Very young or very old clients may be unable to communicate fully because of physical or intellectual development. Some clients are uncomfortable with caregivers much younger or older than they are. These clients may prefer to receive care from someone closer to their own age, although this is not always possible.

Gender

Gender roles may influence nurse–client interactions. For example, a man who is accustomed to being in charge may resent being told what to do by a female nurse. A nurse who believes men should be tough may find it difficult to see a male client cry. A female client may be embarrassed by a male nurse performing personal care procedures. Approaching a personal situation matter-of-factly or professionally may eliminate embarrassment.

If a client sexually harasses you, consult with your instructor or team leader to correctly handle this inappropriate behavior. Sexual harassment is defined as any unwanted sexual activity. This includes any inappropriate or unwanted touching, as well as sexual statements, or lewd jokes or comments. The use of profanity and name-calling is also included. If a client continues these inappropriate actions after being warned, the nurse may consider pressing charges.

Culture and Subculture

Cultural norms and traditions influence the behaviors and perceptions of all people, including nurses. Chapters 8 and 31 discuss transcultural aspects of nursing. Each nurse would be well-advised to develop an awareness of his or her own personal beliefs and practices, based on culture and ethnicity. Cultural differences are significant, for example, in relation to concepts such as personal space and eye contact. Understanding and accepting differences is the key to developing therapeutic communication. The effective nurse actively seeks and maintains the client's sense of self-worth by acting in a nonjudgmental manner.

☛ KEY CONCEPT

Remember: A smile is part of the universal human language. It is understood by all.

The Aggressive Client

Some clients are very anxious or angry when admitted to the healthcare facility. They may respond with aggression, which may be directed toward the nurse or the situation in general. It is important for the nurse to remain objective and to practice **assertiveness** (confidence without aggression or passivity). Box 44-1 gives a brief description of aggressive and assertive behaviors and an introduction to assertiveness training for nurses.

Social Factors

Social acceptance of a particular illness plays a role in a person's reaction to the illness. For example, a sexually transmitted disease may be more difficult for the client to cope with

➤➤ BOX 44-1

AGGRESSIVE VS. ASSERTIVE BEHAVIOR

Clients may be upset or afraid upon admission to the healthcare facility, and may react in a manner that is unusual for them. Or, some clients may be aggressive and hostile by nature. Some of these personality traits may make it difficult for the nurse to care for a client objectively. (Nurses may also find these suggestions helpful when working with peers and family members.)

Characteristic	**Suggested Approach**
Passivity: This person does not seem to care what happens, and may be forgetful and/or inefficient. Body language displays indifference.	Involve the client in decisions about his or her care. Explain what is being done. Answer questions thoughtfully.
Aggressiveness: This person seems angry and hostile, disagrees with everything that is said, and displays angry body language. Often stubborn and argumentative.	Remain calm. Do not argue or become angry. Reinforce what is expected of the client in firm, nonjudgmental way.
Passive-Aggressive: This person seems passive but does things to sabotage their care (or the work environment). Includes intentional disregard for physician's orders, intentional inefficiency, telling lies, and engaging in manipulative and obstructive behaviors. May secretly and intentionally sabotage the situation.	Document instructions to the client, along with the client's actions or words in quotes. Remain calm. Practice assertiveness, but not aggressiveness.

Assertive behavior or **assertiveness** is an important skill for nurses to learn. The assertive person is able to make statements without conveying either aggressiveness (dominance) or passivity (submission). The assertive person makes confident statements of fact, without making judgments. *Assertiveness training* is a helpful tool for the nurse to use in all interactions, whether with clients or peers. This training assists the nurse to "express personal feelings freely, speak up for his or her rights, communicate comfortably, persist in expressing a legitimate complaint, and negotiate mutually satisfying solutions to interpersonal situations."*

(*Miller & Keane. (1992). *Encyclopedia and dictionary of medicine, nursing and allied health* (p. 143). Philadelphia: Saunders.)

than a disorder such as glaucoma, because of the attitudes of society. Negative implications are often assigned to sexually transmitted diseases. The client with a sexually transmitted disease may feel embarrassment or shame about this.

Religion
Members of some religious groups do not go to physicians or hospitals (eg, Christian Scientists). Others do not believe in receiving blood transfusions (eg, Jehovah's Witnesses). Some religions believe in faith healing only. Such religious beliefs may directly conflict with the procedures and goals of a healthcare facility. A person may speak out strongly about their religious beliefs in relation to health. It is important for the nurse to be considerate and nonjudgmental.

History of Illness
People who have never been sick may feel threatened or incapacitated by a sense of loss of control. They may react by becoming depressed, hostile, or resistant to those who want to help. Chronic or continuing illness can affect coping skills and motivation toward self-care and independence.

Body Image
How clients feel about themselves and illness affects communication. For example, athletes who value a healthy body may see illness as a threat to self-image and their ability to function productively. The woman who has had a mastectomy may worry about her sexual appeal. The body part affected, its symbolic meaning, and the visibility of bodily changes may influence how the client relates to others.

Physical Disabilities
Clients often have health conditions that impair their ability to communicate. For example, the person with Alzheimer's disease or who has had a stroke may have difficulty communicating. This person may not be able to process what you are saying or may not be able to formulate a response (aphasia). He or she may have difficulty finding the right words to say. Also, the client may not have brought his or her glasses or hearing aid to the healthcare facility, or may have lost them. Thus, a client may not be able to see or hear you. All of these, and other factors, must be taken into consideration in order to administer effective nursing care.

The Healthcare Team
Healthcare team members may influence an individual's attitude toward illness. It is important for nurses to put aside personal needs and anxieties. For example, though the nurse's pain threshold may be higher than a client's, the nurse should not judge the client based on this difference. The nurse learns to set aside personal feelings, understand what the client is experiencing, and offer appropriate pain-relieving measures.

THERAPEUTIC COMMUNICATION TECHNIQUES

Therapeutic communication techniques are strategies to encourage clients to express their thoughts and feelings more effectively. These techniques are the tools for building and maintaining rapport with others. Some techniques are verbal; others are nonverbal (Fig. 44-3).

Interviewing
An **interview** is a goal-directed conversation in which one person seeks information from the other. In nursing, the interview is the communication technique used to evaluate the client's understanding of his or her health concerns.

The effectiveness of the interview depends on the selection of suitable questions for which the client can provide answers. Sometimes, questions require simple responses (eg, "What medications are you taking?" or "Do you have children?"). This type of question is called a **closed-ended question** because only brief and predictable responses are required. An **open-ended question** encourages longer and more thorough answers. Table 44-2 compares these two types of questions.

Nonverbal Therapeutic Techniques
Just as the client's body language provides cues to conversation, the nurse's body language indicates to the client something about the nurse. Nurses learn to use effective nonverbal communication techniques, such as maintaining an openly accepting facial expression or mirroring what the client says or does. It helps to lean toward the client to express acceptance. The nurse who is an effective communicator learns to avoid gestures such as crossing the arms, pointing fingers, or holding the hands on the hips. (The client may interpret these gestures as judgmental or threatening.)

Use of Silence
Silence gives the nurse and the client an opportunity to collect their thoughts and to prepare to continue the conversation. It is very difficult for many nurses to cope with silence; they feel they must say something. However, if the nurse pauses for a few seconds, the client will often answer a question or make a statement that he or she was reluctant to before. Learning to effectively use silence is a valuable communication tool.

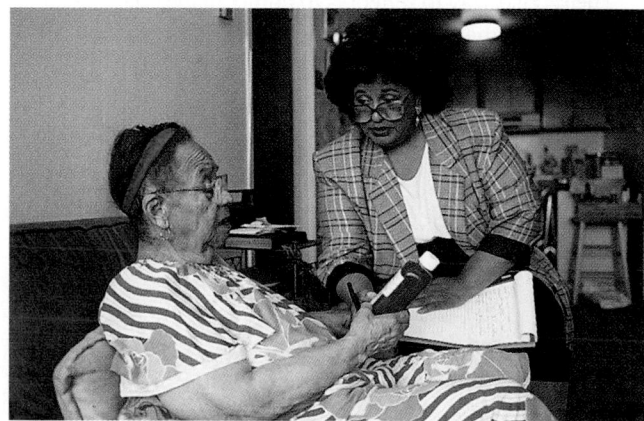

FIGURE 44-3. Therapeutic communication techniques are the tools for building and maintaining rapport with others.

■■■ TABLE 44-2 *E*XAMPLES OF CLOSED- AND OPEN-ENDED QUESTIONS	
Closed-Ended	**Open-Ended**
How well do you sleep?	Tell me about your usual sleep patterns.
Do you like dairy products?	Do you eat foods in the milk and dairy products group? If so, which ones, and how often? Describe any discomfort caused by dairy products.
How many children do you have?	Tell me about your family.
Do you have a normal sex life?	Tell me about your means of sexual expression.
Does your leg hurt often?	Describe the pain in your leg.
Did you have a bowel movement today?	What is your usual pattern of bowel movements?
When was your last period?	Describe your menstrual history.
Are you hearing voices?	Describe your hallucinations.
Do you abuse alcohol? Smoke?	Tell me about your drinking and tobacco use.

☛ KEY CONCEPT

Practice waiting in silence for a client to speak. This is a very effective communication tool, but is difficult for many nurses.

Clarification

Clarification is necessary if the client answers a question and the nurse does not understand the answer. The nurse can ask the client to repeat what was said, or may say, "Tell me more about it," or "Explain that to me."

Reflection

Reflection can be used in two ways. First, the nurse may echo the client's words, allowing the client to hear what he or she just said. In this way, the client can reevaluate the words to determine if they expressed what he or she meant.

> CLIENT: "My life has been one frustration after another."
> NURSE: "Your life has been full of frustrations?"

The second way to reflect is to point out the client's behavior or attitude that seems to be underlying his or her words.

> CLIENT: "I'm just a worthless old man, and no one cares about me!"
> NURSE: "You say that as if you were very angry."
> CLIENT: "I am angry. I raised six children and gave them the best years of my life. If they cared about me, they would come to visit me."

Paraphrasing

Use of paraphrasing helps the nurse to clarify the interpretation of the message by restating it in other words.

> CLIENT: "It was really noisy here last night. It was like Grand Central Station."
> NURSE: "You didn't get a very good night's sleep?"

Summarizing

If the nurse tells the client what he or she heard, it helps the nurse to make sure it was what the client meant. Often the person adds more to the statement or clarifies the nurse's interpretation.

> CLIENT: "I was in the hospital 2 years ago, and I swore I would never come here again. The food was so tasteless I couldn't eat. My roommate died. The noise at night kept me from sleeping. I went home in worse shape than when I came to the hospital."
> NURSE: "You were very uncomfortable and dissatisfied the last time you were here and are apprehensive about being admitted to the hospital again?"

Another example of summarizing is as follows:

> CLIENT: "I don't eat meat. My son says I should, but I don't."
> NURSE: "You don't eat meat?"
> CLIENT: "That's right. I can't chew it any more." *Or,*
> CLIENT: "That's right. I can't afford meat." *Or,*
> CLIENT: "That's right. I have become a vegetarian." *Or,*
> CLIENT: "That's right. I'm afraid of the cholesterol."

By allowing the client to continue talking, the nurse can find the real reason that he or she does not eat meat.

Using Unfinished Statements

Sometimes, if the nurse makes an unfinished statement, the client finishes it. For example:

> NURSE: "You're going to live with your daughter. . .?"
> CLIENT: "Well, I don't know. She really wants to put me in a nursing home, but I don't want to go!"

Communicating in Special Situations

Not all communication can be handled in the same way. Modifications to communication techniques are often necessary when working with children, older adults, mentally ill people, or people with special sensory or behavioral problems.

Communicating at Different Age Levels

The Young Child.   When working with small children, keep normal developmental stages in mind (see Chap. 10), and communicate at an appropriate level for the child's age. Remember that children often regress (revert) to an earlier stage of development when ill. Role playing is often helpful to determine what a child is feeling (Fig. 44-4).

☞ KEY CONCEPT

It is important to remember that play is often the most effective means of communicating with a child.

The Older Adult.   It is important to respect and treat the older adult as you would expect to be treated. The effective nurse tries to communicate with older adults at an appropriate level and to be considerate of personal dignity. It is important to not "talk down to" any of your clients, whether younger or older. Show respect by addressing the person as "Mr." or "Ms." and adding the client's last name. It is disrespectful to refer to an older person by such names as "Grandpa" or "Sweetie." If the client asks to be called by his or her first name, it is acceptable to do so. Think of how you might feel if a younger person did not treat you with respect.

Communicating With the Client Who Has Sensory Problems

The Visually Impaired or Hearing-Impaired Person.   Communication with sensory-impaired people is discussed in more detail in Chapter 79. Remember these important points:

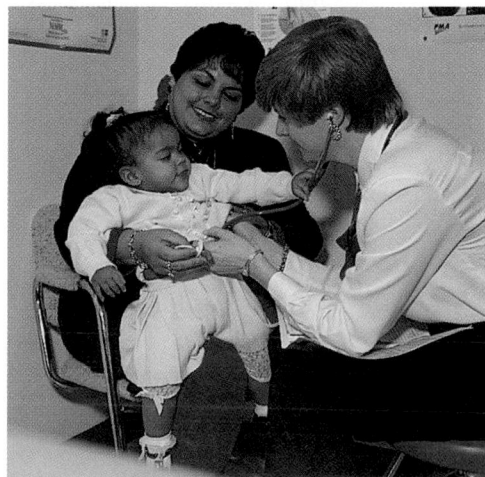

FIGURE 44-4. When working with small children, keep developmental stages in mind and communicate at an appropriate level for the child's age.

Do not frighten the person. The visually impaired person cannot see you coming; the hearing-impaired person cannot hear you. Make sure the person knows you are in the room before you touch him or her.

Remember, the person with a sensory impairment is normal, not abnormal. The visually impaired or hearing-impaired person has strengths, likes, and dislikes, just like any other person. Take a little extra time to stop and communicate with this client.

☞ KEY CONCEPT

Suggestions for communicating with visually impaired or hearing-impaired clients are contained in Chapter 79.

The Unconscious Client.   Use these guidelines for communicating with the unconscious client:

Always assume the client can hear you.
Introduce yourself.
Explain what you are going to do.
Do not talk about the client in his or her presence.

Many people who have been unconscious for some time remember—when they recover—everything that occurred while they were unconscious.

The Aphasic Person.   *Aphasia* is the inability to communicate verbally, usually resulting from a neurologic disorder or injury or a psychiatric disorder. Sometimes, this client cannot write or sign as well, and cannot understand what is said. Clients who have suffered a cerebrovascular accident (stroke) often have some type of aphasia. This state can frustrate clients because their intelligence is often unaffected. Develop some system or method of communication to help prevent withdrawal and social isolation. See Box 44-2 for examples of communication skills to use when working with people who have speech or communication difficulties.

Communicating With a Person Who Speaks a Language Different Than the Nurse's

Speaking different languages may make complete and effective communication difficult, but it need not prevent interaction with others. A smile is understood in all cultures, and people can often use hand signals to communicate their needs. You may use drawings or photographs to explain or ask something. For example, a drawing of a toilet or bedpan may ask the question, "Do you need to use the toilet?" when you cannot ask in the client's native language. A collection of drawings or photos may help the client to tell you when he or she is hungry, thirsty, cold, or in pain.

Learn a few key words in the languages common in your area. Speaking a few words of another language often helps the client to appreciate the nurse's efforts. For more technical communication, find interpreters to speak to the client. Often a family member may assist, but there are risks involved: The family member may add his or her own interpretation to what the client says, or may not be able to translate medical terms correctly. The nurse has no way of knowing the accuracy

➤➤ BOX 44-2

SPECIAL COMMUNICATION TECHNIQUES

The nurse is obligated to establish a means of communication with each client. Suggestions follow:

The Client Who is Not Able to Speak:

• Provide the client with a "magic slate" or pencil and paper. Encourage him or her to write requests and comments.
• Establish hand signals or eye signals that are understood by both client and staff. It is most important to establish signals for "yes" and "no."
• Remember that most clients can hear and can often understand, even if they are unable to speak.
• Treat each person with respect. Do not "talk down to" the client or talk about the client.
• Talk to the client, even if he or she is unable to answer.
• Many clients who cannot speak can use a computer. Assist the person to try this.
• Allow the client time to formulate words. Do not rush.
• Encourage the client to read. This may help the aphasic person to find more words.

The Client Who Speaks a Different Language

• Provide a client's language–to–English language dictionary at the bedside.
• Make sure to schedule a qualified interpreter for physician's visits, team conferences, etc.
• Try to learn a few words of the client's language.
• Ask the client to repeat back what was said. Many people who do not speak the language being spoken will say they understood, even if they did not. It is important to check to make sure that the client understands questions and instructions.
• Computer programs and translation devices are available to assist people to communicate in a language other than their own.

• Try to assign staff who can speak some of the client's language.
• Encourage family members and friends to visit. They can provide encouragement to the client and may be able to give information to the staff.

Both the Client Who is Unable to Speak and the Client Who Speaks a Different Language

• Design a picture board showing commonly requested items. The client can point to items requested. Put the word under each picture.
• If a client is not English-speaking, put the English word and the corresponding word from the client's language under each photo.
• Remember that everyone understands a smile.
• Be conscious of body language. Make sure it is not misunderstood.
• Encourage the person to speak. Reinforce attempts to speak.
• Be patient. Give the person a chance to communicate.
• Remember that hesitation before speaking or avoiding direct eye contact may be a sign of respect.
• Make liberal use of hand gestures.
• Speak slowly and clearly.
• Avoid slang. Keep statements simple.
• Do not yell—the person is not hearing-impaired.
• Do not repeat the same thing over and over. Try to phrase it in a different way.
• Remember that most of these clients can understand more than they can speak.

of the lay person's translations. (See Chapter 8 for more information.)

Other staff may also assist. Appendix A provides a list of Spanish and English words to use to help break down the language barrier.

☞ KEY CONCEPT

The nurse must establish some sort of communication system for all clients.

Dealing With Specific Client Behaviors

Some clients may be anxious. They may be afraid of being hospitalized; fear dying; or feel generally depressed. Some people do not trust anyone and are suspicious. Some clients will question everything the nurse does. Other clients regress and become dependent on the nursing staff. Others become isolated and reject everything the nurse tries to do. Some people may be very fearful or may react with false bravado.

Be patient and open-minded with all clients. Reassure them and make sure that the client is not a danger to self or others. Let all clients know you care, but do not allow them to participate in dangerous or threatening behavior. Encourage independence in all clients.

Chapter 93 further discusses some of these behaviors, along with suggested interventions.

COMMUNICATIONS AMONG THE HEALTHCARE TEAM

The nurse must know how to interact effectively with other members of the healthcare team.

Physician's Orders

One form of communication among members of the healthcare team is the physician's order. Physician's orders may be handwritten in the chart or may be communicated via computer. The physician depends on the nurse to interpret these orders correctly, to make accurate observations concerning the client, and to document those observations. The physician's orders tell nurses what to do, and nursing protocols show how to do it.

The physician may give verbal directions to explain written ones. The team leader or charge nurse must read written orders before the physician leaves, to be sure they are understood. Some orders are absolute and positive; others may require the nurse's judgment. The nurse may need to decide when (or if) to give a PRN (as needed) medication, for example. Judgment is needed to decide which nursing procedures may be safe to perform without an order, and which procedures require clear orders from the physician. Protocol and agency procedures also give guidance to the nursing staff.

Verbal Orders

In some situations, particularly in an emergency, it may be necessary for the physician to give verbal orders. These orders are legal, but must be signed by the physician as soon as possible. If given in person, the verbal order is abbreviated **VO.** If given by telephone, a verbal order is called a telephone order and is abbreviated **TO.**

Verbal orders are not to be taken by nursing students, nursing assistants, or unit secretaries. Only licensed nurses may assume this role. See Chapter 100 for a discussion of the licensed nurse's role in taking verbal orders.

Nursing Alert

The nursing student should never take verbal physician's orders, whether in person or on the telephone. Only a licensed nurse has legal authority to take verbal orders.

Telephone Communication

Whenever a nurse telephones someone, the nurse should give his or her name and the name of the person being called. If the nurse calls a physician, it may be necessary to explain to the physician's office nurse what the call is about and whether or not it is an emergency. (Office nurses usually screen the physician's calls to conserve time.)

The nurse should not chew gum at any time while on duty or when conducting hospital or office business by telephone. It is rude to cover the receiver and continue a conversation with someone else. If the caller must be put on hold, be sure to return every few seconds to inform the caller that the call will be completed as soon as possible. If the wait will be lengthy, it is appropriate to ask if the caller wishes to continue holding, wants to call back, or wants to leave a message.

Answering the Phone

Wherever the nurse works, one of the duties will be to answer the phone. When doing so, be sure to give the name of the department along with your name and position, so callers know to whom they are speaking. For example, you might answer the telephone as follows: "Station Main 2 West, (state your name), nursing student, speaking." The caller then knows if you can help or if someone else is needed.

Answer the telephone as promptly as possible. The call may be an emergency, and the caller may become agitated while waiting for an answer.

Taking Messages

Write down messages carefully. Do not try to remember messages. Repeating the message to the caller helps to clarify and to verify the message. Write the date, time, and your name on all messages you take. Deliver messages promptly, especially in the case of laboratory, pathology, x-ray, or other reports.

Making Emergency Calls

Sometimes a nurse must make an emergency telephone call. If so, give all necessary information. The nurse must be calm and not panic. The prime responsibility of the caller in an emergency is to get assistance, but the caller will be unable to do so effectively unless he or she is calm and gives all the necessary information.

Nursing Alert

Be sure you know the emergency numbers and code names for your agency. For example, "Mr. Red" is a common code name for fire; "Code Blue" or "Dr. Blue" is a common code name for cardiac arrest (see Chap. 39).

Computer Use in the Healthcare Facility

A great deal of information about the client is communicated among departments and among staff members by computer. In addition, client chart information is often computerized. In many facilities, client care is documented on the computer by all staff members. It is often possible to pull up information about a client regarding previous hospitalizations. It is also possible to access the most current laboratory or x-ray tests or surgical reports, even before the hard copy is placed into the permanent record. It is important for you to learn to safely and competently operate your facility's computer system.

Confidentiality about clients is vital. Make sure no unauthorized person can access client information. Remember that the chart (whether computerized or on paper) is a legal document. All information on the chart or client record may be called into court, and nurses may be asked to testify. Think about this whenever you make an entry into the client's record.

Nursing Alert

Remember to protect the client's privacy when using the computer. The nurse must always log off when finished with accessing information or documenting client care. In addition, be careful to keep the screen protected so that unauthorized people or other clients cannot read confidential client information.

Giving Information

Information given to family or friends is limited to protect the client's privacy. No one can legally give out personal information about a client without a signed Release of Information (**ROI**) by the client. If a nurse is unsure about what information is acceptable to give, he or she should consult the team leader or charge nurse for guidance. For example, if someone calls by telephone to ask the client's condition, facility protocol may allow the nurse to state the condition listed on the Kardex. If the caller wants more information, the call is transferred to the team leader or charge nurse. The nurse must avoid revealing any information that destroys the confidentiality of the nurse/client or agency/client relationship.

✚◉ Nursing Alert

Before discussing a client with anyone other than the healthcare team, the nurse must be sure to have a signed "Release of Information" form from the client. Make sure the person who is receiving the information is authorized to receive it.

When giving any information regarding a client, whether in person or by telephone, the nurse must be sure he or she cannot be overheard by other clients or visitors. Protect the client's confidentiality at all times.

"No Information" Status.   Any client can request "no information" status. In this case, the client does not want anyone to even know that he or she is in the healthcare facility. In this case, you cannot acknowledge that the client is there, and he or she does not receive mail, flowers, or visitors. The "no information" status is common in locations such as mental health or chemical dependency units or abortion clinics.

The Alias.   Some clients are admitted into the healthcare facility under an **alias.** This means that they are assigned a name other than their own and all their records, laboratory tests, room tags, diet slips, etc., use this name. Examples of clients admitted under an alias include politicians, movie or rock stars, persons who have committed violent crimes, and other well-known people.

The AKA.   The alias is different from the case of a woman who marries and takes her husband's last name. In this case, the client's records are changed to reflect her new name. This client's previous name is often listed as an **AKA** (also known as) on the chart and Kardex to avoid confusion. (Remember, not all women change their last name when they marry. Some men take their wife's name as well.) In some facilities, all married female clients with different married names have their birth (maiden) names listed on the chart as an AKA, even if they have never been hospitalized before.

In addition, some clients use different names on different admissions. In this case, the records indicate the name currently being used, and list other names the client has used in the past (if any are known). The other names are listed as AKA in the chart, to avoid confusion. For example, some clients are mentally ill or are wanted by the police. They may give a false name on admission to the hospital. If their true name is later learned, it is added to the client's record as an AKA. Sometimes, the client's family is located and family members are asked to make a positive identification.

In some cases, clients from other countries give their name on admission in a format that is different from traditional American names. For example, sometimes it is difficult to determine which is the client's first name and which is the client's last name, or both first and last names may be the same. It can be difficult to determine the English spelling of a foreign name. Therefore, a client's name may be spelled several different ways before it is decided which way is best.

☛ KEY CONCEPT

If a person is registered under an alias, it is important to use the alias when addressing them, even if you know their given name.

☛ KEY CONCEPT

Sometimes, it is possible to help identify a person on the basis of their birth date. However, in some cultures, all people are considered to have been born on January 1. Therefore, it is impossible to differentiate certain clients by using birth date. In this case, it is also not known exactly how old the person is, because his or her age could vary by nearly a year.

John Doe Admissions.   Sometimes an unidentified person is admitted to the healthcare facility, most often as an emergency admission. The common practice in this case is to admit the person as "John Doe" or "Jane Doe." Some facilities admit as "unidentified," including race and gender (eg, "unidentified Asian female"). When the identity of the person is established, the records are changed to indicate the person's name. In some cases, a family member or friend is located who can establish the identity of the person.

Other Types of Communication in the Healthcare Facility

Change-of-Shift Reporting
Nurses are required to give some sort of report or update to oncoming members of the team whenever they go off duty. When the nurse goes to lunch or leaves to take a client to an examination, a brief report is given, including pertinent or life-threatening information. A more complete report is given when the nurse leaves at the end of the shift for the day.

Nursing students will practice reporting-off. Reports may be given to the instructor, team leader, or nurse who is coassigned to the care of clients while students are in the clinical facility.

As a graduate, a nurse reports to the next shift nurse whenever going off duty. This change-of-shift report may be given in person, in writing, or by tape recorder. If the report is verbal, make sure it is given in a location where clients cannot overhear you.

Facilitating Communication in Healthcare
Nurses facilitate communication between clients and members of the nursing team in various ways, including:

- Skillfully interviewing clients to determine their healthcare needs
- Listening attentively to what the client is saying
- Teaching clients and their families certain aspects of care
- Documenting information on the nursing care plan and in the client's chart

- Reporting the condition of the client to other members of the healthcare team, either in person, on tape, by computer, or by writing in the client record
- Participating in team conferences and client care conferences
- Maintaining the confidentiality of all information about clients
- Treating each client as a unique individual; it is important to consider each person's age, sex, ethnic and religious background, state of health, life experiences, body image, feelings about being in the healthcare facility, language preference, and other personal factors
- Using both verbal and nonverbal means of communication and observing clients' verbal and nonverbal reactions
- Using touch as a therapeutic modality, but not invading the client's personal space or threatening the client

All these aspects of communication influence the quality and effectiveness of your client care. How the nurse handles this responsibility will directly influence the client's recovery.

➥ STUDENT SYNTHESIS

Key Points

- Effective communication is the cornerstone to competent nursing care. This is true in any setting.
- Communication involves a sender, a receiver, a channel, a message, and feedback.
- Developing rapport with the client is a basic ingredient of the nurse–client relationship.
- All communication has verbal and nonverbal components. Nonverbal communication is very powerful.
- The nurse considers all personal and cultural factors about each client when communicating.
- Nurses conduct interviews to learn information about clients.
- The nurse can make many important observations, in addition to what the client says when communicating.
- Nurses use techniques other than words to communicate with clients who have special communication difficulties.
- Competent nursing care requires caring, accurate, and ethical communication with clients and the healthcare team.
- A nurse has the challenge to always make a positive impression when answering the telephone.
- It is critical to maintain each client's confidentiality when communicating, whether verbally, by computer, or in writing.
- Continuity of care is enhanced when thorough and accurate reporting occurs between nursing shifts.

Critical Thinking Exercises

1. Your client is Mr. J., 77 years old, who recently had a cerebrovascular accident (stroke) that left him with a receptive aphasia. Although he cannot understand the meaning of language, he does respond to body language. What is an effective method for communicating so that you can meet Mr. J.'s basic needs?
2. Your client is a 5-year-old child, who has a congenital hearing loss. She is hospitalized, recovering from an accident in which she received internal injuries. Before the accident, she had begun to learn sign language, but you do not have this skill. What options do you have to communicate with this child?
3. A 43-year-old client from Somalia has been admitted to your unit. Neither she nor anyone in her family speaks English. You do not speak Somali and an interpreter is not available. Describe ways in which you could establish a communication system with this woman. What orientation would you provide to your coworkers?
4. Review Chapter 8 and discuss therapeutic communication skills as related to specific ethnic and religious beliefs about health and illness.

NCLEX-Style Review Questions

1. Nonverbal communication includes:
   a. Eye contact
   b. Reading
   c. Speaking
   d. Writing
2. Components of communication include:
   a. Assumptions
   b. Conducting
   c. Interaction
   d. Thinking
3. Which of the following is an open-ended question?
   a. Do you like fresh fruits?
   b. Do you want your pain medication?
   c. Have you been coughing today?
   d. Tell me about your family.
4. During an interview, the nurse did not understand an answer to a question. Which therapeutic technique would the nurse use next?
   a. Clarification
   b. Reflection
   c. Silence
   d. Summarizing
5. Which information is communicated when answering a phone in a healthcare facility?
   a. Department and position
   b. Department, your name, and position
   c. Your name and department
   d. Your name, facility name, and date

Reference

1. Craven, R. F., & Hirnle, C. J. (2000). *Fundamentals of nursing: Human health and function* (3rd ed.). Philadelphia: Lippincott Williams & Wilkins.

CHAPTER

45

Admission, Transfer, and Discharge

LEARNING OBJECTIVES

1. Demonstrate in the skills lab how to orient a new client to the health-care facility.
2. Discuss at least three concepts related to caring for the client's clothing and valuable items on admission.
3. List at least five factors related to dehumanization. State how each might be avoided.
4. State at least five nursing considerations related to the admission of a client.
5. Identify information that the nursing student or practical nurse (LPN/LVN) should report to the registered nurse (RN).
6. In the skills lab, demonstrate the ability to transfer a client from one unit to another safely and effectively.
7. Identify at least 10 nursing considerations related to a client's discharge from the healthcare facility.
8. Explain teaching that should occur at the time of a client's discharge.
9. Differentiate among the responsibilities of the healthcare facility, the physician, and the nurse for a client who signs out of the facility against medical advice.

NEW TERMINOLOGY

acuity	litter scale
dehumanization	vital signs

ACRONYMS

AMA	CXR	TPR
AWOL	D/C	VS
BP	ID	W/C

To provide effective nursing care, the nurse must be aware of the client's needs, attitudes, and emotions. Understanding basic human needs guides nurses when planning care. Knowledge of cultural considerations and the stages of human development helps nurses to place different clients in a continuum of life experiences. By maintaining safety and drawing on communication and interviewing skills, nurses help clients to express and work through their feelings about admission. Always keep in mind the feelings of the family of the client as well.

ADMISSION

Admission has more than one meaning in healthcare: Admission to the healthcare facility means the activities surrounding a client's arrival at the facility for the purpose of receiving healthcare. Also, each continuous period of time a client spends in a facility is considered one admission (Box 45-1).

The Admitting Department

The first contact that most clients have on arrival at the healthcare facility is with the admitting department or with the admitting clerk in the outpatient department. (There are specific exceptions. For example, a client might arrive by ambulance for an emergency admission. In addition, some clients are preregistered, including same-day surgery clients or women at the full term of pregnancy. These clients will often go directly to the receiving area.) In any event, the admitting department is responsible for the administrative activities necessary for the client's entry into the facility. During these preliminary procedures, personnel from the admitting department make every effort to put the client at ease. They enter information about the client's age, sex, marital status, next of kin, employer, physician, and health insurance into the health record. They attach an identification band with the client's name (and AKA or alias, if applicable; see Chapter 44) and agency identification number (also called *medical record number* or *history number*) to the client's wrist. Diagnostic tests (eg, x-ray examinations and blood tests) are often performed before the client is escorted to the nursing care unit.

During admission, the client signs documents giving consent for treatments. The client and family also sign documents accepting financial responsibility for costs not covered by insurance and designating insurance payments to be made to the facility.

The client who has an *advance directive* or *living will* submits a copy of the documentation for placement in the chart. (All clients must be advised of their right to create an advance directive while in the healthcare facility. They may need assistance with this process. The fact that the client was offered the opportunity to make an advance directive must be documented in the nursing admission notes. *Remember, if it is not documented, legally it was not done.*)

The Client's Arrival on the Nursing Unit

Before the client's arrival, check to be sure that the unit is completely equipped and that the bed is available. The client may walk in or arrive in a wheelchair or on a gurney. If possible, introduce the client to the charge nurse and staff before taking him or her to the room.

The client forms his or her first impressions of the nursing staff on admission. Routines and procedures that are common for healthcare workers and admitting staff may seem threatening and frightening to the newly admitted person. Explain the purposes for these routines to the client to ease discomfort (Fig. 45-1).

➤➤ **BOX 45-1**

ADMISSION AND DISCHARGE IN VARIOUS FACILITIES

Much of the material in this chapter is geared toward admission and discharge of the client as related to the acute care facility. Some specific procedures apply when the client is to be admitted to or discharged from other areas, such as the long-term care facility, home care, a hospice program, same-day surgery, or an outpatient department. These topics are considered in other chapters of this book:

Chapter 65—the woman in labor and delivery
Chapter 66—the newborn in the nursery
Chapter 70—admission or discharge of a child
Chapter 93—the mental health unit
Chapter 94—the chemical dependency unit
Chapter 96—rehabilitation facilities
Chapter 97—ambulatory care
Chapter 98—home care nursing
Chapter 99—hospice care

In addition, specific admission and discharge procedures are discussed in conjunction with particular disorders in Unit 12.

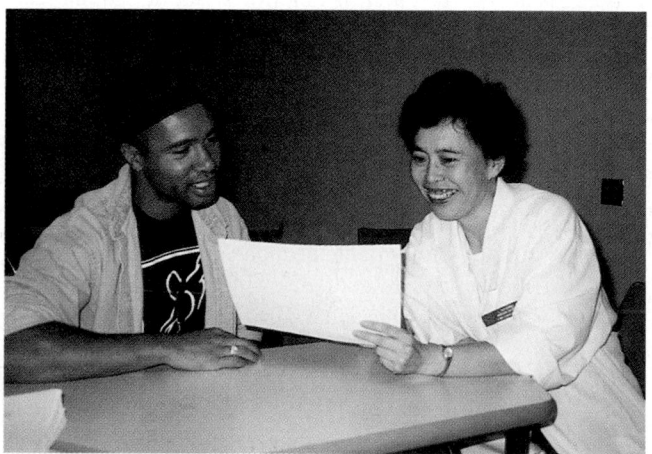

FIGURE 45-1. Explaining the purpose for routines to the client helps ease fear of the unknown in unfamiliar settings.

Upon admission to the hospital, unless reasons exist to the contrary, the client undresses, puts on a healthcare facility gown, and goes to bed in preparation for the admission examination by the nurse and the physician. (In other areas, the client may not be required to undress.)

☛ KEY CONCEPT

Remember that the client's impression of the facility depends in large part upon you. Make the person feel as comfortable and safe as possible.

Removing the Client's Clothes

In the acute care facility or before same-day surgery, give the client whatever assistance is needed to undress. Sometimes a family member will assist, particularly if the client is a child. *Rationale: A child may resist being undressed by a stranger, or may not understand the need for going to bed during the day.* Refer to In Practice: Nursing Procedure 45-1 when undressing an immobile client.

Assisting the Client Into Bed

If a client is weak or tired when admitted, remove his or her shoes and outdoor clothing, and help the person lie down on the bed immediately. Cover him or her with a bath blanket or bedclothes. Lying down helps prevent added fatigue. The client may have already exerted considerable effort in making the trip to the healthcare facility. In the acute care facility, it is usually desirable to have the client put on a hospital gown. *Rationale: Wearing the hospital gown facilitates the physical examination and various treatments. It also prevents soiling of the client's clothes.* As soon as the client is able, assist him or her to put on a hospital gown and explain why this is desirable.

☛ KEY CONCEPT

Nursing data collection and assessment begin immediately upon the nurse's first contact with the client.

Orienting the Client to the Facility

The charge nurse or team leader will tell you what the client's privileges are. If the client is able to be out of bed, indicate the location of the bathroom and closet. Check to see if the client is to give a urine specimen or is on intake and output (a recording of all fluids taken in and urine expelled). If so, give the client a bedpan or urine cup and explain what the client is to do and why. Ask the client not to void directly into the toilet until needed samples are obtained. (Chapter 52 describes the methods for collecting specimens.)

Allow time for the client to unpack, if items have been brought to the facility. (Encourage clients to bring only what is absolutely necessary to the acute care facility. In the long-term care facility, the client will most likely bring a number of personal items.) Help the client if necessary, and tell him or her where you are putting items. Place the bathrobe and slippers in a handy spot. Arrange the client's personal belongings. Place special items, such as eyeglasses, on the bedside table or in the drawer for easy reach. (Make sure all valuables are either sent

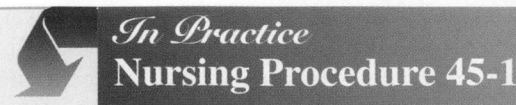

In Practice
Nursing Procedure 45-1

UNDRESSING THE IMMOBILE CLIENT

Supplies and Equipment:

Healthcare facility gown

Steps

1. Push the client's blouse or shirt off one shoulder.
   RATIONALE: *Do one side at a time.*

2. Roll the sleeve on the same side down to the wrist.
   RATIONALE: *This action makes the shirt easier to remove.*

3. Slip off the sleeve.

4. Repeat steps 1 to 3 on the other side.
   RATIONALE: *Avoid straining the client.*

5. Put a gown on the client.
   RATIONALE: *By removing the garments from above the waist first and putting on a gown, you avoid exposing the client while you remove the lower garments.*

6. Unfasten the waistband, and push all lower garments down as far as you can.

7. Ask the client to raise the hips while you pull down the clothes.
   RATIONALE: *Encourage the client to help as much as possible.*

8. If the client cannot raise his or her hips, request assistance from other healthcare personnel.
   RATIONALE: *Avoid overtiring or injuring the client or yourself.*

9. If garments must come off over the head, slip the client's arms from the sleeves, push the clothing up to the hips, and ask the client to raise the hips. Pull the garments up to the shoulders. To get clothing over the shoulders more easily, turn the client's shoulders first to one side and then to the other.
   RATIONALE: *Undress the client as easily and quickly as possible while preventing exposure.*

10. Slip garments over the face by raising the client's head and gathering the clothes together into a roll behind the head. Do not cover the client's face, and avoid dragging clothing over the face.
    RATIONALE: *Many people become frightened if their face is covered. Dragging clothing over the face may cause injury.*

11. When putting the gown on the client, cover him or her with a bath blanket and work under it as much as possible.
    RATIONALE: *Avoid undue exposure or embarrassment and provide warmth.*

home with a family member or locked in the hospital vault for safekeeping.)

Adjust the shades, regulate ventilation, and position the head or foot of the bed for the client's comfort. Put the entire bed in *low position,* regardless of whether the client can get in and out of bed without assistance. Explain how the bed works as you adjust it. Most beds have controls for the client to adjust without assistance.

Tell the client when meals are served and that you will find out what he or she may have to eat and drink and when. Explain that admission routines often take a long time, and encourage the client to be patient and cooperative. Explain the concept of physician's orders to the client; nurses will function under the direction of the physician.

☛ KEY CONCEPT

Make sure a meal is ordered for each new client. Be sure to check the physician's orders to determine if the client is on a special diet.

Introduce the client who is sharing a room to the other client. The nurse does not leave the client until he or she is convinced that the client's questions have been answered and that the person is comfortable. Leave the door or curtains open or closed, as the client wishes.

Intercom System.   Show the client how the communication system works, and place the "nurse call" signal within easy reach. Also show the client where the signal mechanism is located in the bathroom. *Rationale: Taking time to explain things to the client helps alleviate fear and anxiety in unfamiliar surroundings.*

☛ KEY CONCEPT

Explain to the new client that the signal light in the bathroom is for emergencies only. Usually, there is both a button and a pull cord. Using either signal will probably ring an alarm bell, as well as activate the nurse-call light. Ask the client not to use this signal unless it is a true emergency.

Many call systems are equipped with television controls. Clients may become confused when confronted with numerous buttons or controls to push. Turn on the television, and set it on a preferred channel at a comfortable volume.

Toilet Articles.   Every healthcare facility can supply such essential toilet articles as toothbrushes, toothpaste, combs or hair picks, tissues, and soap. Usually these supplies are sold in a pharmacy or gift shop within the facility, or nearby if the facility does not automatically provide them. Many clients have personal preferences and like to choose these articles themselves.

Many facilities provide new clients with a packet of supplies that contains soap, a plastic soap dish, backrub lotion, a plastic water cup, a water carafe, disposable tissues, and mouthwash. Clients may use and discard these articles or take them home on discharge. Sometimes the package also contains an emesis basin, bath basin, bedpan, urinal, comb, toothpaste,

toothbrush, deodorant, shampoo, and mouthwash. Nurses may need to provide other items for individual clients. If a denture cup is needed, be sure to label it, on *both the container and the lid.* If you handle the client's dentures or used tissues, wear gloves (see Chap. 50.) Some facilities also provide disposable blood pressure cuffs, thermometers, and telephones to reduce the risk of cross-contamination.

Gown.   Clients may bring their own pajamas, nightgowns, bathrobes, and slippers with them. The client's family or other caretaker is then responsible for laundering these items. (In extended-care facilities, this laundry service is usually available for a fee.) Acute care facilities have gowns, robes, and slippers available for client use.

☛ KEY CONCEPT

It is advisable for clients who are bleeding, incontinent, or having wound drainage to wear hospital pajamas and robes, rather than their own clothes. (The hospital laundry facility uses special methods to ensure that pathogens are removed from soiled clothing and bedding. The client and family need to be protected from these pathogens. In addition, the hospital gown allows easier access to suture lines, wounds, and equipment such as intravenous lines, and facilitates special tests and procedures.)

For clients confined to bed, using gowns provided by the healthcare facility is customary. The gowns are laundered by the facility's laundry service, using special techniques to prevent cross-contamination. Hospital gowns are easy to put on and to remove. Explain to the client that these gowns are used for convenience, comfort, and safety. They open in the back and fasten with ties, Velcro, or snaps. The sleeves also may open to accommodate intravenous (IV) tubing. Be sure that a client's gown is long and large enough. Be sure the gown's ties are not uncomfortable when secured; tie with bows to the side. Clients should also be provided with a robe and slippers, if they did not bring them.

☛ KEY CONCEPT

Most hospitals provide extra-large gowns and robes. If a client is unusually large, it may be necessary to use two gowns, one opening in the front and one opening in the back. Some facilities, such as mental health units, allow clients to wear extra-large hospital scrub suits.

Individual Equipment.   Inform clients as soon as possible that the equipment in their unit is for their use alone. This equipment includes items such as suction machines, oxygen and inhalation equipment, and so forth. Point out which part of the closet and which drawers are for each client's use. Point out towel rods to be used by each client in a semiprivate room or in a shared bathroom.

Client Identification.   Be sure each client receives and wears an identification (**ID**) band. If the client has allergies, a separate red name band is usually worn. Special precautions, such as seizure precautions, may also be indicated on a special band. Check the information on all ID bands to make sure that it is correct.

Check the tag on or above the bed (if these tags are used in your facility) and make sure the client is correctly identified. In addition to the client's name and the physician's name, the tag or chalkboard usually indicates whether the client is allowed out of bed; the client's diet; and other pertinent information, such as intake and output or seizure precautions. Regularly check this information against the physician's order sheet. A tag indicating the client's first name is often placed near the door of the room as well.

☛ KEY CONCEPT

If name tags are used to identify clients' rooms, only the first name should be used (to protect client confidentiality). In addition, if a master board with all clients' names and room numbers is placed at the nursing station, it should be in such a position that passers-by cannot read the names.

Caring for the Client's Personal Belongings

Clothing.   Each client in the acute care facility has a place for a bathrobe and slippers and a drawer for other articles. Clients are encouraged to keep only essential items in the hospital. (In the long-term care facility, the client has more items and more storage space.)

Fill out a property sheet, including a description of every item of clothing. Follow the system the facility has established; doing so protects the client and the facility. Have the client sign the property sheet after he or she checks the list.

Valuables.   Valuables—such as jewelry, credit cards, and cash—should not be brought to the facility. If they are brought, they should be kept in the facility's safe. When clients learn they cannot keep these belongings with them, they may prefer to send them home with a person they designate. Clients usually keep a small amount of change to buy newspapers and other items from the coffee or gift shop.

☛ KEY CONCEPT

In some situations, such as in an Alzheimer's unit or mental health unit, the hospital does *assume some responsibility for client belongings, because the client is not competent to do so. In this case, your careful listing and description of the client's property becomes even more important. (The hospital may be required to reimburse this client for lost items.) In these units, the client may not be allowed to keep any jewelry (other than a wedding ring) or any money at the bedside.*

The client sometimes keeps a few personal items, such as eyeglasses, dentures, a prosthesis, or a watch or wedding ring, at the bedside. These items are noted and described on the property sheet. Usually the client signs a waiver verifying that these items are to remain at the bedside at his or her own risk. (In the long-term care facility, mental health unit, hospice unit, or chemical dependency unit, the client usually keeps more

personal items. In this case, all items must be labeled with the client's name and room number; this usually includes all the client's clothing in the long-term facility. Cloth name tags are usually recommended for clothing.) When labeling client belongings, be sure to use a label that can be easily removed without damaging the item when the client is discharged.

If the client goes to surgery or has a lengthy examination, items such as a watch or eyeglasses are given to the family for safekeeping or are sent to the hospital vault. The client must sign later to verify that the items have been returned.

☛ KEY CONCEPT

It is very important to carefully list the client's property. Describe items as much as possible. For example, "blue Nike ski jacket" or "3 white t-shirts." When describing jewelry, do not make judgments about values. For example, it is best to say "clear stone" instead of "diamond" or "gold-colored bracelet" instead of "gold bracelet." It the client has valuable jewelry or an amount of money greater than about $20, these items should be sent to the facility's vault or be sent home with the family. If the client chooses to keep a valuable item, such as a wedding ring, this must be noted on the property sheet and the client assumes responsibility for it. (If the client is confused or unable to make decisions, the concept of property becomes a difficult legal question. Consult your instructor or supervisor if you have a question.)

Preventing Dehumanization

Dehumanization is the process of depriving a person of personality, spirit, privacy, and other human qualities. It means neglecting the individuality of clients, ignoring their specific needs, and failing to recognize their need for input about their care. Care must be taken to avoid dehumanization.

The person admitted to the healthcare facility surrenders clothes, belongings, and individuality to follow orders about when to eat, sleep, take a bath, and even when and where to go to the bathroom. A stranger asks when the client last had a menstrual period or a bowel movement. All these factors have the potential to dehumanize the person.

Whether giving care in a hospital, extended-care facility, or in the home, the nurse can take many measures to prevent clients from feeling dehumanized. Handle questions and procedures with the utmost tact and respect for the individual. Always think of each client as a person whose need for physical and emotional support is greater than normal because of illness. Emphasize the client's strengths rather than weaknesses. In this way, the nurse can invaluably assist in the client's recovery. Allow the client to maintain personal dignity.

☛ KEY CONCEPT

Imagine how you would feel if a stranger expected you to answer personal questions about your toileting habits, your menstrual history, and your sex life. Take this into consideration when asking these questions of clients in the healthcare facility.

Anxiety or Apprehension.   A person who is facing illness or surgery often feels anxious or nervous. Individuals may also be worried about the welfare of their family or about finances. What may upset one person, however, may have no effect on another. A person's degree of anxiety may vary with the severity of illness or with the person's previous experience. This anxiety may cause physical and emotional stress that can aggravate the client's health problem.

A state of great anxiety can have varying effects upon the client's coping mechanisms. Remember Maslow's hierarchy of human needs (Chap. 5). If a person's lower-level needs are not being met, he or she will have difficulty concentrating and learning. This person will probably not be able to remember and identify what medications are being given, learn self-care, or participate in the development of his or her care plan.

Levels of anxiety or non-anxiety range from the person who is calm to the person who is in a state of extreme agitation or panic. The client's anxiety level may be estimated as follows:

Calm = Not anxious
+1 anxiety = Increasing uneasiness and apprehension
+2 anxiety = Increasing uneasiness, apprehension, dread
+3 anxiety = Increasing apprehension, dread, paranoia
Panic = Symptoms may include a feeling of choking, difficulty breathing, inability to sit still, chest tightness or pain, trembling, increased pulse rate, headache.

Anxiety may be *rational* (logical or justified) or *irrational* (out of proportion, unrealistic, inappropriate to the situation). Anxiety differs from fear in that the person often cannot identify a specific cause for anxiety. (The source of fear can often be verbalized.) Anxiety and fear can be precipitated by factors such as fear of the unknown, fear of death, fear of body image changes, threat to self-concept, loss of significant other, or financial concerns. Some of these factors may be realistic in the case of a serious illness or accidental trauma. Generalized anxiety or panic is often not realistic, in relationship to the situation.

Nursing interventions aimed at alleviating anxiety and fear include:

* assessment of level of discomfort
* clear explanations and clear answers to questions
* offering the client an opportunity to express feelings
* providing more helpful coping mechanisms

It is important to remember that severe anxiety or panic can interfere with medical care. For example, non-emergency surgery may be canceled if the client is extremely apprehensive.

Fear of the Unknown.   Perhaps the most intense fear is fear of the unknown. The client may be afraid of a serious illness or even of death. Some people may feel that healthcare personnel are not telling the truth about their disease or condition, or that their condition is more serious than it actually is.

Fear of Body Image Changes.   *Body image* refers to the way an individual perceives himself or herself. Different people respond differently to a threat to body image. A person may feel threatened by an illness, especially if treatment involves surgery. This concern exists even when surgery will not cause a visible change in the client's appearance. If surgery involves a procedure such as limb amputation or breast removal, the concern about disfigurement is more real. The client may experience disturbing fears about the family's response to the surgery, the reaction of friends, or the possible loss of a job. Consider the situations of a fashion model, an Olympic-level skier, a mother of a toddler, an 80-year-old, or a construction worker about to have a leg amputated. They may react in different ways to the situation as it relates to their body image and lifestyle.

Financial Concerns.   Another concern of many clients is the fear of financial burden. Insurance coverage varies. Some people do not have insurance to cover the costs of healthcare. Others worry that their insurance will not cover every procedure or treatment they receive. Some clients cannot afford hospitalizations or admittance to extended-care facilities. They may be concerned about how their family will manage while they are away. Such preoccupation with financial problems can affect the client's reaction to illness.

Embarrassment.   Many people are embarrassed when personal services, such as bathing or assistance in toileting, must be performed for them. Providing as much *privacy* as possible and *explaining* what is occurring during treatment are of key importance. Client embarrassment during nursing care may be a result of superstitions, folk medicine beliefs, cultural beliefs about illness, or cultural practices regarding the roles of men and women. Lack of medical knowledge about the body can cause client confusion and misunderstanding.

The Client Who Speaks Another Language.   The client who does not speak or understand English is much more likely to be uncomfortable in a healthcare facility where everyone else speaks only English. This person often does not understand what is happening, and staff are unable to explain things to lessen the client's discomfort. It is vital to obtain interpretive services for this person as soon as possible. Chapter 8 describes, in more detail, some ways to communicate with people of different cultures and Chapter 79 describes ways to communicate with the hearing-impaired person.

Assessment, Reporting, and Documentation

After orienting the client to the nursing unit and the room, the nurse takes the admissions interview and history, unless the client's health needs dictate that this must be done earlier. (In some situations, such as psychiatry, the client may be too agitated to participate in an interview; the interview may need to be postponed.)

Box 34-1, in Chapter 34, lists questions to ask during the admissions interview. In Practice: Nursing Care Guidelines 45-1 gives tips for performing the admission interview.

The nurse takes vital signs (see Chap. 46) and measures height and weight (see In Practice: Nursing Care Guidelines

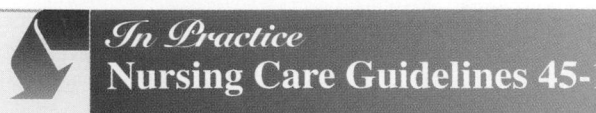

In Practice
Nursing Care Guidelines 45-1

PERFORMING THE ADMISSIONS INTERVIEW

- Gather necessary supplies (eg, health record, physician's orders, charts).
- Become familiar with information from the admitting department before meeting the client.
- Introduce yourself; explain that you will be taking information and discussing routines of the healthcare facility.
- Observe the client's general appearance (eg, posture, ability to ambulate).
- Assess the client's general condition (eg, level of alertness, orientation).
- Observe the client's skin condition (eg, temperature, color, turgor, scars, lesions, abrasions, pressure areas, edema). Briefly describe any abnormalities on the interview form, indicating their location.
- Monitor the client's respiratory status (eg, coughing, wheezing, shortness of breath).
- Assess the client's psychological status, as evidenced by verbal and nonverbal responses.
- Measure weight and height.
- Measure vital signs.

Obtain health history and information regarding current status:

- Reasons for admission
- Past illnesses and dates
- Current medications
- Allergies to medications, foods, and other substances (eg, latex)
- Use of tobacco and alcohol
- Daily eating, sleeping, elimination, and exercise routines
- Use of appliances or prostheses (eg, artificial limbs, hearing aids, contact lenses, dentures)
- Family support (eg, Will people visit regularly or stay in the facility with the client? Is someone available at mealtimes to help feed the client? Who should be contacted in an emergency?)
- Employer or school
- See Box 34-1 for a detailed admissions interview.

In Practice
Nursing Care Guidelines 45-2

WEIGHING THE CLIENT

- Calibrate the scale so it is at zero before weighing the client. (Chairs and litters will automatically deduct the weight of the equipment.) Determine the client's weight by using the weights and indicator on the free-moving balance arm or by using the digital readout. This is done in the same manner for all types of scales.
- The client who is strong enough may stand on a transfer paper or paper towel on the *balance scales* or step-on scale. Assist the client to step onto the scale (to prevent falls).
- Clients who are unable to stand are weighed on *chair scales* or on the bed itself, if it includes a scale. The chair scale resembles the step-on scale, but is equipped with an armchair for the client's comfort. Assist the client to step up onto the platform under the chair and to be seated in the chair.
- An immobile client is weighed lying down on a **litter scale,** a sling-type apparatus that looks like a suspended hammock or a client hydraulic lift. Ask for assistance to place the client on a litter scale (for client safety). The machine raises the client from the bed's surface, then records the weight.

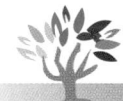 **SPECIAL CONSIDERATIONS:** THE LIFE SPAN

Admission Assessment for Children

- Observe for signs of anxiety and fear of the unknown, as evidenced by crying or temper tantrums.
- Be knowledgeable about developmental stages, to be better able to judge each child's physical and emotional needs.
- Determine if a parent or family member will stay with the child.
- Determine how much self-care the child can perform.
- Be aware that regression often occurs when a child is ill. (The child may move backward to a previous level of functioning.)
- Check with the child to determine how much he or she understands. The nurse may need to find an alternate method for teaching important information to the child. (Pictures, videos, role play, story books, or toys are often used.)

45-2). Urine, stool, or sputum specimens may also be collected at this time (see Chap. 52). A nurse may accompany the client to the radiology department or laboratory for tests. A sample form for admission notes and data base is shown in Figure 45-2.

During time with the client, the nurse must be observant. Report to the team leader if the client complains of severe pain or seems to be very uncomfortable. Look for any physical signs or symptoms. Knowing the client's diagnosis is helpful when observing signs and symptoms (see Chap. 47). Listen to what the client says. Review Chapter 44 for specific interviewing techniques.

FORM 54.41A 9/98

UNIVERSITY OF CHICAGO HOSPITALS

ADMISSION ASSESSMENT

PRIMARY CARE MD:

ARRIVAL	**VITAL SIGNS**	**EMERGENCY CONTACTS**
DATE _____ Time: _____	T _____ P_____ R _____	Name/Rel.: _____
MODE: ☐ amb ☐ cart	BP _____ Ht _____	Home #: _____
☐ wc ☐ other		Work #: _____
VIA: ☐ Clinic ☐ ER	Wt _____ Age _____	Name/Rel: _____
☐ Admitting	Armband on _____	
☐ Other		Work #: _____

VALUABLES / DISPOSITION

	Home	Bedside	Safe	**ORIENTED TO**	**SUBJECTIVE INFORMATION OBTAINED FROM**
☐ Glasses	☐	☐	☐	☐ Room	☐ Patient Other _____
☐ Contact Lenses	☐	☐	☐	☐ Bed	☐ Unable to Obtain:
☐ Dentures	☐	☐	☐	☐ Phone	☐ Language Barrier: _____
☐ Clothes	☐	☐	☐	☐ Call light / TV	☐ Patient Wishes to be Addressed As:
☐ Jewelry	☐	☐	☐	☐ Get well TV	_____
☐ Other:	☐	☐	☐	☐ Visiting hours	_____
				☐ Smoking Policy	

Explained that the hospital is not responsible for valuables or other personal belongings. ☐ YES Initials: _____

Signature _____ Title _____ Date _____

FOR IN-PATIENT PSYCHIATRY (ONLY)

☐ Patient's body/belongings searched. Items taken from patient: _____

Patient's rights reviewed with patient. Initials: _____ ☐ Release(s) of information signed. Initials: _____
List for who/what: _____

CURRENT ADMISSION

Reason for Current Admission: _____

Date of Last Admission _____ (reason) _____

Previous illness, injury or surgery _____

Any other health problems_____
Exposure to communicable disease ☐ Yes ☐ No If yes, state disease _____
Date of last Pap Smear _____ Request during admission ☐ Yes ☐ No Physician notified ☐ Yes ☐ No

ALLERGIES ☐ None ☐ Drug or food _____ ☐ Latex ☐ Iodine ☐ Other

Describe Reactions: _____

Have you ever had or been told you had an allergy or allergic reaction to latex products? ☐ Yes ☐ No

Do you have spinal cord deformities or Congenital Gastrointestinal or Urological anomalies? ☐ Yes ☐ No

When exposed to latex in rubber gloves, balloons, Band-Aids, condoms, rubberbands, rubber toys (like Koosh balls) or other latex items have you ever had:

a) itching or watery eyes, b) itching or swelling of your lips or face, c) sneezing, d) itching on your body, e) hives, f) wheezing, or g) collapse? ☐ Yes ☐ No

*** If one yes answer to these questions then institute Latex Precautions.**

MEDICATIONS: ☐ did not bring ☐ patient has ☐ other (specify) _____

Medications & Strength (over-the-counter meds also)	Freq.	Last Dose	Medications & Strength (over-the-counter meds also)	Freq.	Last Dose

Patient/Caregiver assessed for medication knowledge:	☐ No medication ☐ Independent ☐ Unable to assess ☐ Non-compliant
	☐ Needs teaching: _____

ADVANCE DIRECTIVES Durable Power of Attorney ☐ Yes ☐ No Living Will ☐ Yes ☐ No More information Requested ☐ Yes ☐ No Referral date/initials _____

FIGURE 45-2. Example of one facility's admission assessment.

Weight.   Measure and record the client's weight on admission. (Do not go by what the client says.) This measurement provides a baseline for later comparison. Fluctuating weight may indicate when the client is or is not retaining fluids. The initial weight, compared with the client's height, helps to determine if the client is overweight or underweight. The admission weight also establishes a baseline for further observations or calculations of medication doses or anesthesia. In Practice: Nursing Care Guidelines 45-2 describes the steps in weighing the client. Record weights on the graphic sheet (see Chap. 46) or in the computer as soon as possible, because current weight is necessary for the physician to calculate medication dosages, to determine the effectiveness of special feedings, and assess over- or underweight.

Height.   Measure and record the client's height on admission. When measuring height, ask the client to remove his or her shoes and to stand on the scale with their back against the measuring bar. Ask the person to stand straight. Lower the L-shaped sliding bar so that it lightly touches the top of the client's head. Record the height in inches or centimeters (not feet or meters) on the flow sheet or graphic sheet, according to healthcare facility policy.

If the client cannot stand, the nurse can obtain an approximate height while the client lies in bed. Have the client lie on his or her back and stretch out as much as possible. Place a mark on the sheet under the person's heel and at the top of the head. Then measure between these two marks on the taut bottom sheet. Record as "estimated" height.

Vital Signs.   Measure and record the client's **vital signs** (**VS**) during admission and as ordered while the client is in the healthcare facility. Vital signs include body temperature, pulse (rate of heartbeats), respiration (rate of breathing), and blood pressure (the pressure the blood exerts against the walls of the arteries). These readings are abbreviated as **TPR** (temperature, pulse, respiration) and **BP** (blood pressure). They are called *vital* signs because they must be present for a person's life to continue. Vital signs are important in healthcare. Chapter 46 describes the measurement of vital signs.

Collecting Specimens.   Often, a urine specimen will be ordered. Give the client instructions about the collection. Most often, a midstream or clean-catch urine specimen is to be collected; instruct the client on how it is done. Chapter 52 discusses the procedure in detail.

Other specimens are not usually ordered to be collected by nursing staff immediately upon admission. However, if the physician requests other specimens, collect them per protocol (see Chap. 52).

Radiology and Laboratory Exams.   Some clients are given a chest x-ray (**CXR**) on admission. A chest x-ray provides basic baseline information about heart and lung structure. It can be used to rule out diseases, fractures, or abnormalities in size. Most clients will also require admission blood work to be done by the laboratory. If x-rays or laboratory work are ordered, the nurse may transport the client to the radiology department or laboratory. Be sure to follow the guidelines in Chapter 48 for transporting a client by wheelchair or stretcher.

Reporting the Admission

The Joint Commission on Accreditation of Healthcare Organizations (JCAHO) requires an RN to perform formal admission interviews, nursing diagnoses, and admission charting. When a student or LPN has finished the client orientation and the assigned admission procedures, he or she must notify the team leader or charge nurse. The charge nurse may be busy and may not know the status of the admission process. The charge nurse or team leader is responsible for seeing that the physician is notified of the client's arrival. The charge nurse also checks the physician's orders for the client and confirms that the client's diet order is sent to the food services department. Other orders are also sent to lab, radiology, pharmacy, and other departments as needed.

The LPN/LVN reports preliminary observations and the client's vital signs to the team leader. Head-to-toe observations are important to the admissions interview (see Chap. 47). These observations provide a starting point for the interview. The admitting nurse can then complete the nursing diagnosis, and the entire team can develop the nursing care plan. Box 45-2 lists pointers for admission documentation.

Advance Directives

The law requires all clients to be informed about advance directives upon admission to a healthcare facility. As discussed in Chapter 4, an advance directive is a written document that allows the individual to specify choices of healthcare treatment if he or she becomes terminally ill or has an injury that limits the ability to make or to communicate decisions.[1] As stated previously, ensure and document that the client has received

> ➤ BOX 45-2

ADMISSION DOCUMENTATION

In many facilities, it is the responsibility of the RN to document official interview information, but nursing students and LPNs/LVNs often record the following information:

- Weight and height
- Vital signs
- Whether any laboratory tests were done, blood drawn, or x-ray studies done
- Any other procedures
- Specimens sent to the laboratory: note the amount of urine voided and its appearance, or the client's inability to void
- Any prostheses or appliances the client uses (eg, dentures, contact lenses, glasses); note where these items were placed ("at bedside," "sent home with family," and so forth)
- Listing and location of the client's property. List all items sent to the vault.
- Report any other information or symptoms directly to the charge nurse or team leader.

See also Box 34-1 in Chapter 34.

information regarding advance directives when admitted to the facility. If the client has an advance directive or a living will, be sure to note this on the Kardex and in the client's chart, and in other locations specified by local protocol. A copy of any advance directive must be included in the chart.

TRANSFER TO ANOTHER UNIT

The client may be transferred to another unit for several reasons:

- Assignment to a certain unit is temporary.
- A change in client **acuity** (level of illness) necessitates placing the client in another department.
- The client is becoming agitated by a very busy unit, and requires a quieter environment.
- The client is disturbing others, for example by snoring loudly, and needs a private room.
- The client's condition becomes serious enough to require transfer to an intensive care unit (ICU).
- Another, more acute condition is discovered than that for which the client was first admitted. Another unit specializes in care of clients with that condition.
- The client has delivered a baby and is being moved into a postpartum care room.
- The client has had surgery and is being moved to post-surgical care.

In Practice: Nursing Care Guidelines 45-3 outlines steps to follow when transferring a client.

☞ KEY CONCEPT

The procedures for transfer are carried out in much the same manner if a client is to be transferred to another healthcare facility.

DISCHARGE

Planning for the client's discharge (**D/C**) begins at admission. For example, the client and family are taught about the illness or surgery; they have an opportunity to practice procedures and to learn about medications and special diets; and plans for special care at home can be made. The staff and client work on completing these activities throughout the client's hospitalization. This plan for discharge is very similar in today's rehabilitation centers and in many extended-care facilities, with the goal of returning the client home to self-care as soon as possible.

Chapter 36 introduces discharge planning and client teaching. The total nursing care team, the client, and the family are involved in discharge planning and organizing care at home. Figure 45-3 shows an example of a discharge summary.

Nursing students and LPNs/LVNs assist with teaching the client and family prior to discharge. In Practice: Educating the Client 45-1 lists information to communicate. The facility's protocols will describe staff members' roles in teaching clients and their families. Report any suggestions you have for client teaching. The entire nursing care team needs to know the client's responses to teaching.

To determine that the client and family members understand, it is important that they be able to verbalize information and to perform return demonstrations of procedures. Carefully document all discharge teaching. For example, "client was shown how to change colostomy bag and was able to accurately return demonstration. Plan to have client change bag independently tomorrow."

Before the day arrives for the client to go home, discuss the best time for him or her to leave. Ask when the family will be available to pick up the client. Instruct the family to bring clothing, pillows, or blankets if they will be needed.

The Day the Client is Discharged

On the day of discharge, if the person seems eager to leave and if his or her condition permits, the client can dress in street clothes and rest on the bed until it is time to go. Make sure all the steps in the discharge have been completed before the client leaves the facility. In Practice: Nursing Care Guidelines 45-4 gives pointers on discharging the client.

Documentation

In some healthcare facilities, only RNs perform discharge documentation. A student or LPN/LVN may be asked to assist. The practical nurse's observations are important, whether they are written in the health record directly or reported to another person.

The nurse who discharges the client brings the health record up to date, records the hour of discharge, and documents who accompanied the client and whether the client was in a wheelchair or required an ambulance. A nursing summary that includes the identified nursing problems and their resolution or revision may be required. For example, "42-year-old male diagnosed with coronary artery disease. Placement of two stents successful. Client able to perform wound care independently; verbalize medications with doses, times, and side effects; and describe exercise and diet regimens. Client informed of time/date for post-op examination. Postoperative course has been unremarkable. Client has phone numbers to call if problems."

These measures complete the nursing record of the client's stay in the healthcare facility. The physician is also required to write a discharge summary for the health record within 24 hours of discharge.

LEAVING THE HEALTHCARE FACILITY AGAINST MEDICAL ADVICE

Occasionally a client leaves the healthcare facility without a physician's permission. Such action is called against medical advice (**AMA**). Report to the team leader any client who says he or she is leaving the healthcare facility AMA. A client who leaves AMA is asked to sign a dated release form that absolves the physician and the facility of all responsibility in the event that the client suffers complications. A licensed nurse witnesses the client's signature.

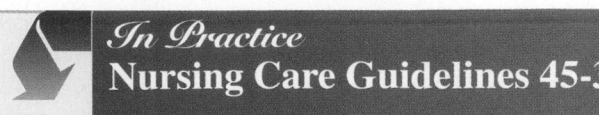

In Practice
Nursing Care Guidelines 45-3

TRANSFERRING THE CLIENT TO ANOTHER UNIT

Preparation for the Transfer

- Explain the transfer to the client and family. Give the reason for the transfer and when the transfer will take place. *Rationale: Clients may become anxious and fearful when moved to an unfamiliar setting.*
- Assemble all the client's personal belongings, charts, x-ray films, and lab reports. Double-check for all clothes and other articles. *Rationale: If items are left behind, the client's care may be compromised because the new unit does not have all pertinent information. In addition, it is more difficult to find items once they have been left behind. It causes more work and frustration for everyone.*
- Determine how the client will be moved. *Rationale: You are responsible for safely moving the client. Type of transportation depends on the client's condition. Seldom is the client allowed to walk.*
- Provide for client safety. Take measures to accommodate IV bottles, drains, and catheters. Protect the client from drafts, and cover the client with a blanket for warmth and privacy. *Rationale: It is important not to worsen the client's condition.*
- Collect all the client's medications, IV bags, tube feedings, and so forth. Check the Kardex or medication administration record for accuracy. *Rationale: All treatments that have been performed and medications given must be documented, to ensure lack of duplication and to prevent omission.*
- Review the client's health record and check for completeness.
- Record the transfer in a transfer note and on the computer (if used). Give the time, the unit to which the transfer occurs, type of transportation (wheelchair or stretcher), and the client's physical and psychosocial condition. The nurse may need to include a brief review of the client's history as well. For example, "1410: Client transferred from Room 312B to Room 110A via **W/C** (wheelchair). Medication,

chart, and belongings given to P. Johnson, RN. Client's V.S. (vital signs) stable, O_2 sat = 97% without oxygen, IV running via pump. C. Bunker, PN student." *Rationale: It is important for the receiving unit to know as much about the client as possible. This will ensure continuity of care from all staff on the new unit, around the clock.*
- Make sure the receiving unit is ready. Usually a short verbal report is given to the receiving nurse. *Rationale: To provide immediate continuity of care on the new unit.*

Transporting the Client

- Keep the client safe during the move. *Rationale: Being moved is traumatic in itself. It is important not to further upset the client.*
- Introduce the client to the staff at the new nurse's station, if his or her condition permits. *Rationale: Make the client feel as much at home as possible.*
- Give a report to the staff on the new unit, if this was not done on the phone before the transfer.
- Leave medications and records.
- Take the client to his or her room.
- Assist the client into bed, and make sure he or she is comfortable.
- When returning to the nursing unit, notify all necessary departments of the transfer. This includes the dietary, business, radiology, and pharmacy departments. Make sure that all scheduled tests and treatments are still scheduled, with the new unit identification. *Rationale: Make sure no important procedures are missed because the client has been moved.*
- Make sure the client's location has been changed on the computer or the admissions office and client information office have been notified. *Rationale: To ensure that the client will continue to receive his or her mail, visitors, flowers.*

If the client refuses to sign, the refusal must be noted on the form. The form is then signed by at least two witnesses. The nursing student should not witness any legal papers, including the AMA form.

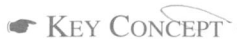

☞ KEY CONCEPT

---

*Sometimes, a client walks off the unit to go home or to leave the facility without being discharged. This client is considered **AWOL** (Absent Without Leave). In many facilities, this client would be officially discharged AMA at*

midnight. If the client who is AWOL returns after midnight, or the next day, he or she usually needs to be readmitted, using the complete admission process. This is considered a new admission for the client. (In some cases, insurance will not cover the client who goes AWOL and returns to the facility.)

Long-term facilities usually identify clients who are likely to leave without permission. These clients wear special transmitters (see Fig. 95-3) that alert personnel if the client tries to leave, so staff can intervene. This is important for safety, particularly if the client is confused.

TO BE COMPLETED BY M.D.   PLEASE PRESS FIRMLY

FORM 44.21 R5/00

THE UNIVERSITY OF CHICAGO HOSPITALS
**MULTIDISCIPLINARY PATIENT
DISCHARGE NOTE**

ADDRESSOGRAPH

ADMISSION DATE:	DISCHARGE DATE:	SERVICE:

PRINCIPAL DIAGNOSIS THIS ADMISSION:

SECONDARY DIAGNOSIS:	1.	3.
ALLERGY:	2.	4.

PRINCIPAL PROCEDURE:	DATE:
SECONDARY PROCEDURE:	DATE:
	DATE:
	DATE:

SIGNIFICANT FINDINGS:

CLINIC PHYSICIANS:	1.
2.	3.

FOLLOW-UP VISITS: **APPROX RETURN:**   **DATE / TIME:**

Dr. _____ in _____ appt _____
CLINIC   LOCATION   PHONE   WEEKS

Dr. _____ in _____ appt _____
CLINIC   LOCATION   PHONE   WEEKS

Dr. _____ in _____ appt _____
CLINIC   LOCATION   PHONE   WEEKS

Dr. _____ in _____ appt _____
CLINIC   LOCATION   PHONE   WEEKS

Pap smear done in hospital _____Yes _____No   Pap smear appt.: _____

MEDICATIONS / TREATMENTS:

MEDICATION / DOSAGE / FREQUENCY

ACTIVITY: _____   **DIET:** _____

Refer problems / questions to _____ Telephone: (_____) _____

DICTATING RESIDENT:	SIGNATURE:	DATE:
DISCHARGING M.D. SIGNATURE:	DATE:	PAGER #:

PLEASE BRING THESE INSTRUCTIONS TO THE NEXT CLINIC APPOINTMENT

FIGURE 45-3. Example of one facility's multidisciplinary patient discharge note.

(*continued*)

TO BE COMPLETED BY NURSE   PLEASE PRESS FIRMLY

ADDRESSOGRAPH

☐ Port-a-cath needle removed.   ☐ Central line Heparinized.

Heplock / IV Removed ☐ Yes ☐ No

If No, reason in place on discharge _____

_____

HOME CARE / EQUIPMENT / SUPPLIES / COMMUNITY SUPPORT SERVICES	AGENCY	PHONE NUMBER

Specific preprinted discharge instructions sent with patient: ☐ Yes ☐ No Titles: _____

_____

(Inpatient Psych) Patient belongings returned to patient: Signed: _____

SPECIAL / ADDITIONAL INSTRUCTIONS:

_____

_____

_____

_____

_____

_____

_____

_____

_____

_____

_____

MEDICATIONS					
MEDICATION	DOSE	FREQ	PURPOSE	NEXT DOSE DUE	PRESCRIPTION GIVEN

ABOVE INSTRUCTIONS REVIEWED WITH: ☐ CHECK IF INSTRUCTIONS CONTINUED ON SUPPLEMENTAL PAGE.

☐ Patient   ☐ Authorized Representative: Print Name and Relationship to Patient _____

I UNDERSTAND THE ABOVE INSTRUCTIONS:

SIGNATURE: _____ DATE: _____ PATIENT PHONE #: _____
Patient / Authorized Representative

Instructions given by: _____ Date / Time: _____ Unit Phone: _____

Patient Accompanied by: _____ Mode: _____

PLEASE BRING THESE INSTRUCTIONS TO THE NEXT CLINIC APPOINTMENT   **PATIENT**

FIGURE 45-3. (*Continued*) Example of one facility's multidisciplinary patient discharge note.

In Practice
Educating the Client 45-1

DISCHARGE PREPARATION

Remember that planning and teaching for discharge begin immediately upon the client's admission to the healthcare facility. Teaching while preparing the client for discharge includes the following:

- Explain the *safe change of dressings*. Give the client a list of needed supplies. Demonstrate the method for removing the old dressings and for safe disposal at home. Demonstrate how to put on the new dressing. Allow the client and family to practice while you watch, to be sure they know how to do the procedure.
- Describe the amount of *rest* the client will need and activities that are allowed and their duration. Describe and demonstrate suggested *exercises,* and detail walking regimens.
- Detail *dietary restrictions,* such as foods the client should eat and their amounts; foods that are required each day; and foods that are not allowed on the client's prescribed diet. A dietitian should consult with the client about special diets and be available to answer questions.
- Show how to *perform personal care;* make the bed, give a bed bath, move and turn the client, give and remove the bedpan, adjust pillows, and maintain body alignment and skin integrity for clients who will be confined to bed at home. Allow family to practice and demonstrate back to you.
- Demonstrate the *operation of equipment* and care of tubes and ask the caregivers to demonstrate back to you.
- Understand and communicate the *client's preferences* for how treatments are performed.
- Emphasize the importance of self-care and building the *client's independence and self-esteem.* Teach the family to encourage self-care by the client as much and as soon as possible.

- Provide information about *public health* and home nursing services. Give the client/family the phone number to call if these services are needed.
- Explain where to buy or rent *equipment,* materials for dressing changes, special beds, and so forth. Give this information to the client in writing.
- Advise the family if substitute pieces of *equipment* can be used. (For example, in some cases a regular bed placed on blocks can replace a special hospital bed.)
- Describe *medication administration,* such as how and when to take medications and undesirable side effects. Give the client/family written guidelines for medication administration and a list of possible side effects. Be sure the client and family understand the need for accuracy.
- Identify situations that require the client to be seen by the *primary care provider.* Write down the name and phone number of this provider and instructions as to how to contact this person for routine and/or emergency needs.
- Write down the phone number of your hospital unit, so the client can call if there are any questions.
- Communicate the date, time, and location of the *next scheduled examination,* if known. This should also be given to the client/family in writing.
- Discuss with the physician the need for a public health nursing referral, if you feel that the client and/or the family will not be able to safely manage the client's care at home.

➤ STUDENT SYNTHESIS

Key Points

- The admission process helps to establish how clients feel about admission and potentially helps to determine the effectiveness of an admission to any healthcare facility.
- Clients may have serious concerns about their physical condition and about the unfamiliar procedures in the healthcare facility.
- Nurses perform an initial nursing assessment.
- No matter what type of healthcare facility or program will be serving the client, some sort of admission procedure is required.

- Clients' belongings must be properly identified and listed; valuables are sent home or to the facility's vaults.
- Careful documentation of admission is important to establish a baseline and to give information to other members of the healthcare team.
- When a client is transferred, explain the procedure to the client; take belongings, records, and medications; and safely transport the client.
- Discharge teaching begins on admission. All teaching is individual and must be documented.
- Make sure the client has all belongings at discharge.
- Escort the client to the door. Usually, clients are required to ride in a wheelchair to their transportation (to reduce the risk of an accident).

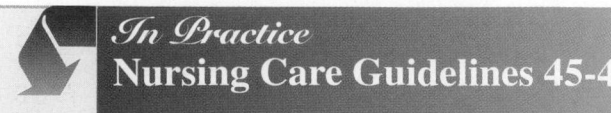

In Practice
Nursing Care Guidelines 45-4

DISCHARGING THE CLIENT

- Verify the discharge order.
- Check for written or telephone orders.
- Check orders for take-home medications, special treatments, or special equipment.
- Check orders for last-minute procedures, laboratory tests, or x-ray examinations.
- Make sure the person has a place to go.
- Coordinate transportation if necessary. You may need to make a telephone call to request an ambulance or taxi service or to contact a neighbor.
- Determine what type of clothing the client is best suited to wear. (If he or she is being discharged to extended care, pajamas or a robe may be appropriate rather than street clothes.)
- Assist the client with packing and dressing for discharge.
- Check the closet and bedside stand for personal items.
- Arrange for a small utility cart or easy conveyance to the exit.
- Secure release of any valuables checked into the vault.
- Check and have the client sign the property record.
- Notify necessary departments of the discharge. Unit clerk reports discharge to admissions, dietary, housekeeping, and business offices.
- Escort the client from the clinical unit.
- Accompany the client to the car or taxi.

- Some clients sign out of the healthcare facility against medical advice (AMA) or leave without permission (AWOL).

Critical Thinking Exercises

1. An 81-year-old woman is admitted to the healthcare facility for tests of the digestive system. She is oriented to time, place, and person. Her verbalizations are logical. Describe what actions or skills you will use when she arrives on the unit, including assessments and reports.
2. Explain the causes, effects, and methods by which you can prevent feelings of dehumanization in your clients.

3. Describe possible effects of illness and surgery on body image. How would you feel if you were suddenly faced with a body-altering disease, condition, or illness? Try to evaluate the reasons for your feelings.
4. Using information from Chapter 36 and this chapter, describe the planning, teaching, discharge procedures, and documentation that must be done when the client leaves the healthcare facility.

NCLEX-Style Review Questions

1. Prior to arriving on the nursing unit, the admissions department usually:
   a. Has the client sign consent for treatment
   b. Itemizes the client's belongings
   c. Obtains the client's height and weight
   d. Reviews the physician's orders
2. When a client arrives on the nursing unit, the student nurse or LPN would be responsible for:
   a. Admission charting
   b. Admission interview
   c. Formulating nursing diagnoses
   d. Obtaining vital signs
3. Which of the following measures will help prevent dehumanization?
   a. Do not tell the client about upcoming diagnostic tests.
   b. Handle procedures with respect and tact.
   c. Share the client's condition and treatment plan with friends and family.
   d. Remind the client of his/her financial obligation for receiving treatment.
4. When a client tells a nursing student that he/she is planning to leave a healthcare facility against medical advice, what action should the student take?
   a. Apply restraints to the client.
   b. Have the client sign a release form.
   c. Inform the team leader of the client's plan.
   d. Notify the hospital security personnel.
5. Nursing documentation at discharge should include a:
   a. Detailed account of the hospital stay
   b. Detailed account of all financial obligations
   c. Nursing summary of client problems and resolution
   d. Summary of personnel who cared for the client

Reference

1. Craven, R. F., & Hirnle, C. J. (2000). *Fundamentals of nursing: Human health and function* (3rd ed.). Philadelphia: Lippincott Williams & Wilkins.

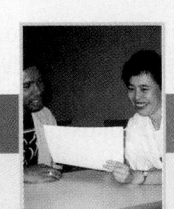

CHAPTER

46

Vital Signs

LEARNING OBJECTIVES

1. Identify the measurements that constitute vital signs. State why they are called vital signs. Describe the relationships among the vital signs.
2. Give examples of reasons for changes in body temperature. Describe the related physiology.
3. State normal adult body temperature as measured in four different body areas.
4. Differentiate among the terms febrile, afebrile, intermittent and remittent fevers, crisis, and lysis.
5. In the skills lab, demonstrate the ability to measure body temperature by the various methods and with the various equipment discussed in this chapter.
6. In the skills lab, demonstrate the ability to measure and to describe radial, apical, and apical-radial pulses.
7. In the skills lab, demonstrate the ability to count and to describe respirations.
8. In the skills lab, demonstrate the ability to accurately measure blood pressure and orthostatic blood pressure using the arm cuff and thigh cuff and using the aneroid manometer and the electronic monitor.
9. State the normal adult pulse rate, respiration rate, and blood pressure ranges.

NEW TERMINOLOGY

apical pulse
apical-radial pulse
apnea
auscultation
axilla
bradycardia
bradypnea
carotid pulse
Cheyne-Stokes respirations
crisis
cyanosis
diastole
dyspnea
eupnea
femoral pulse
fever
hypertension
hypotension
Korotkoff's sounds

Kussmaul's respirations
lysis
oral
orthopnea
palpation
pedal pulse
popliteal pulse
pulse
pulse pressure
radial pulse
rectal
sphygmomanometer
stertorous breathing
stethoscope
systolic
tachycardia
tachypnea
tympanic

ACRONYMS

AP	F	PMI
A-R	HR	PO
Ax	I&O	PR
BPM	MAP	R
C	O	SBP
DBP		

Body temperature, pulse, respiration (TPR), and blood pressure (BP) are basic client assessments. Taken and documented over time, these data demonstrate the course of a client's condition. TPR and BP are called *vital signs* (VS) or *cardinal symptoms* because these measurements are indicators of functions necessary to sustain life.

☛ KEY CONCEPT

The temperature, pulse, respiration, and blood pressure are called vital signs *because they must all be within normal limits to sustain life.*

Temperature, pulse, and respiration are usually observed together. Many acute care facilities routinely require observation of these signs every morning and evening for all clients. For some illnesses, more frequent observation of vital signs is necessary to detect variations indicating a change in the client's condition. Often, variations occur in more than one vital sign. A physician will order more frequent assessments of the client with an unstable condition. The nurse may also use judgment to determine if a client requires more frequent vital signs.

THE GRAPHIC RECORD

The *graphic record* is a type of flowsheet used to easily document large amounts of information for all members of the healthcare team to read. Usually the graphic record documents measurements of vital signs, fluid intake and output (**I&O**), weight, and bowel movements, assessed at regular intervals. Fig. 46-1 shows a sample manual (paper) graphic record. In some facilities, these measurements are entered into electronic health records. When complete, the format of the graphic record results in a picture of the variations that occur throughout the client's illness, whether on paper or a computer monitor.

Recording Vital Signs

Vital signs must be recorded accurately and promptly to provide continuous and current documentation. A record of a client's vital signs helps providers diagnose and respond to the client's changing condition. It also serves as a quick and handy reference for the entire healthcare team.

The nurse needs to know the format for documenting vital signs in his or her agency. Steps for recording vital signs in the manual record include:

- Locate the current date on the graphic record.
- Record temperature by making a dot on the scale parallel to the temperature value under the designated time. Connect the dot to the previous reading with a short line.
- Record pulse rate by making a dot on the scale parallel to the pulse rate under the designated time. Connect the dot to the previous reading with a short line.
- Record respiratory rate at the bottom of the graph with numbers.

- Record BP with written numbers (eg, 120/80) or graph the numbers similarly to the temperature graph.
- Record other information, such as weight, bowel movements, and the totals for I&O, with written numbers in the spaces provided.

On the electronic graphic record, enter TPR, BP, and all other information as designated on the computer screen. Sometimes BP is stated on a graph with dots or check marks. The graph is marked in increments similar to the increments seen in the temperature graph. Many times a BP graph is superimposed on the temperature graph. Sometimes the various readings are charted in different colors.

Frequent Vital Signs Sheet

Sometimes a client's condition is serious enough to require taking vital signs every 5, 10, or 15 minutes. The *frequent vital signs sheet* is the document used in such cases (most often in critical care areas, after surgery, or immediately postpartum). Graph vital signs in the same way on the frequent vital signs sheet as you would on the regular record. In many cases, space is available to record other information, such as intravenous (IV) fluids, I&O, weight, medications, and notes.

ASSESSING BODY TEMPERATURE

Body temperature is the measure of heat inside a person's body (core temperature); it is the balance between heat produced and heat lost. The body generates heat as it burns food and loses heat through the skin and lungs. Normal body temperature using oral (**O;** or per os, **PO**) measurement remains at approximately 37° Celsius or 98.6° Fahrenheit. Temperature measurements that are higher or lower mean that some change in the body's regulatory system is upsetting the balance. The signs of an elevated temperature are easy to recognize: flushed face, hot skin, unusually bright eyes, restlessness, and thirst. A lifeless manner and pale, cold, clammy skin are often signs of a subnormal temperature.

Temperature is measured on the Fahrenheit (**F**) or the Celsius (centigrade) (**C**) scale. Most Americans are more familiar with Fahrenheit values. If a nurse works in an agency that uses Celsius measurements, it is important to learn the Fahrenheit equivalents to easily translate measurements for clients and their family members. Converting measurements from Celsius to Fahrenheit and vice versa is often necessary. Table 46-1 explains conversions and gives equivalents.

Regulation of Body Temperature

The hypothalamus, which is the brain's heat-regulating center, controls body temperature by controlling blood temperature. Heat is a product of metabolism. Muscle and gland activities generate most body heat. When the body is cold, exercising the muscles warms it; if a person is angry or excited, the adrenal glands become very active and he or she feels warm. The digestive process increases body temperature. Cold, shock, and certain drugs depress the nervous system and decrease

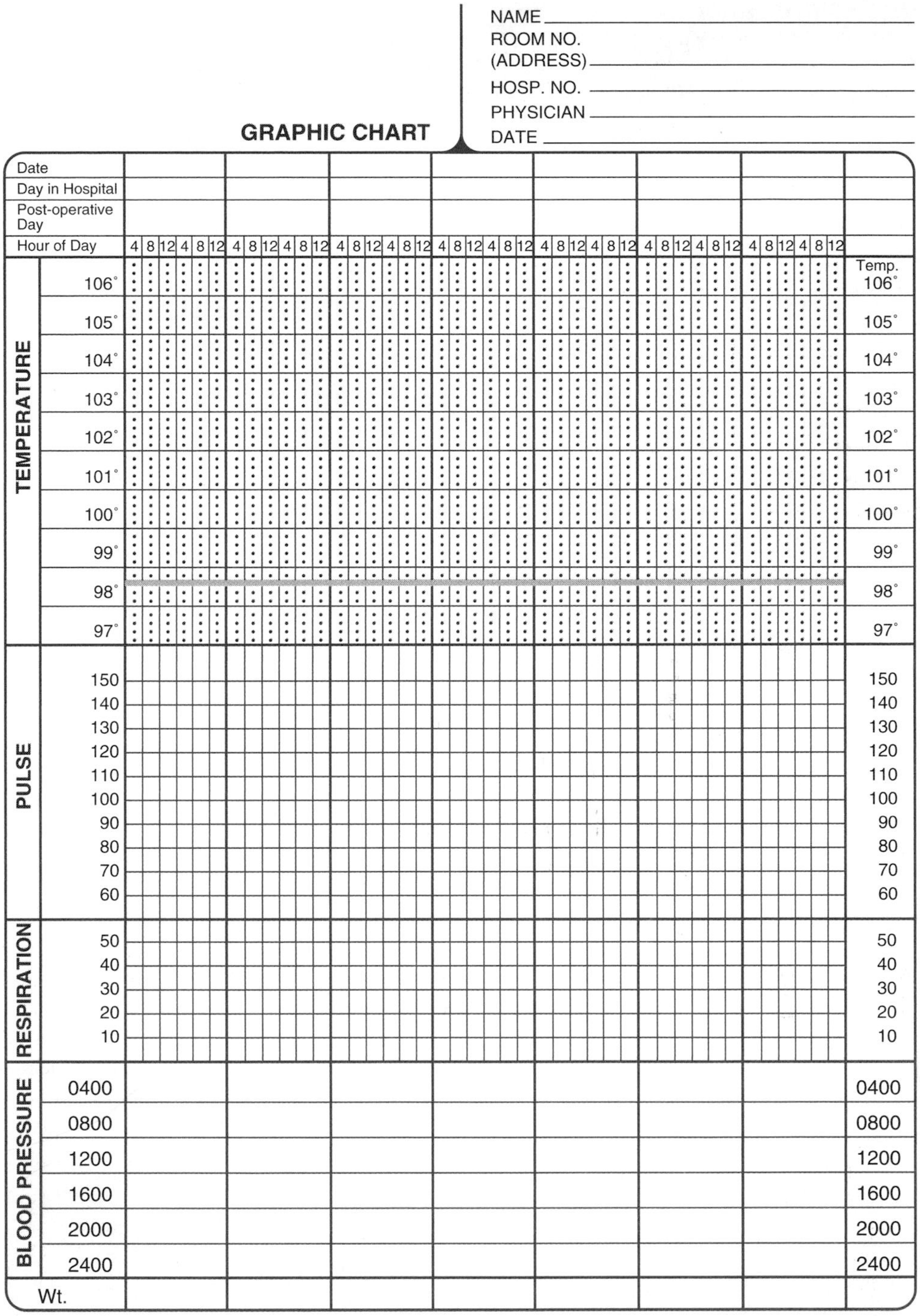

GRAPHIC CHART

NAME _____
ROOM NO. _____
(ADDRESS) _____
HOSP. NO. _____
PHYSICIAN _____
DATE _____

Date								
Day in Hospital								
Post-operative Day								
Hour of Day	4 8 12 4 8 12	4 8 12 4 8 12	4 8 12 4 8 12	4 8 12 4 8 12	4 8 12 4 8 12	4 8 12 4 8 12	4 8 12 4 8 12	4 8 12 4 8 12

TEMPERATURE: 106° 105° 104° 103° 102° 101° 100° 99° 98° 97°

PULSE: 150 140 130 120 110 100 90 80 70 60

RESPIRATION: 50 40 30 20 10

BLOOD PRESSURE: 0400 0800 1200 1600 2000 2400

Wt.

FIGURE 46-1. Vital signs graphic record. (Courtesy of AMI Nacogdoches Medical Center, Nacogdoches, Texas.)

heat production. The hypothalamus senses these changes and makes appropriate adjustments.

Normal Body Temperature. Normal temperature variations are slight. A difference of 0.5° to 1° F either way is usually considered to be within normal limits. Body temperature is usually lowest in the morning and highest in the late afternoon and evening. The oral equivalent of normal temperature for newborns ranges between 98.6° and 99.6° F (37°–37.5° C), although the temperature is measured by axillary or **tympanic** (eardrum) methods. The body temperature gradually lowers to the adult normal temperature as the child matures.

Other influences on normal body temperature include ovulation, childbirth, and individual metabolism. Table 46-2 gives average normal temperatures for adults (who are known as *afebrile*, or without fever). The length of time to keep the thermometer in place for an accurate reading in different body areas is also listed. (Remember that everyone has a *temperature*, but not everyone has a *fever* [elevated temperature].)

Elevated Body Temperature. Temperature rises when the body's heat production increases or heat loss decreases; both may occur simultaneously. If the temperature is elevated, fever (also called *pyrexia*) is present. The person is

TABLE 46-1 Equivalent Celsius and Fahrenheit Temperatures*

Celsius	Fahrenheit	Celsius	Fahrenheit
34.0	93.2	38.5	101.3
35.0	95.0	39.0	102.2
36.0	96.8	40.0	104.0
36.5	97.7	41.0	105.8
37.0	98.6	42.0	107.6
37.5	99.5	43.0	109.4
38.0	100.4	44.0	111.2

*To convert Celsius to Fahrenheit, multiply by ⅘ and add 32. To change Fahrenheit to Celsius, subtract 32 and multiply by ⅚.

slows metabolism and thus decreases the body's need for oxygen. *Clinical hypothermia* is used to perform some surgical procedures; *accidental hypothermia* is life-threatening and requires immediate treatment.

Nursing Alert

An extremely high temperature (*hyperthermia*) or low temperature (*hypothermia*) can be fatal. Survival is rare if the core temperature is above 108° F (42.2° C) or below 93.2° F (34° C).

Hypothermia can also indicate impending death. This is a normal component of the dying process.

said to be *febrile*. **Fever** is a sign of some disorder within the body. It often accompanies illness, or it may signify that the body is fighting an infection. In some cases, a slightly above-normal temperature is useful for fighting microorganisms. For this reason, treating a fever may be delayed until a diagnosis is confirmed.

Oral temperatures in fever range from 100° to 103° F or greater (37.8°–39.4° C). Fig. 46-2 illustrates types of fever.

- A temperature that alternates between a fever and a normal or subnormal reading is an *intermittent fever.*
- A temperature that rises several degrees above normal and returns to normal or near normal is a *remittent fever.*
- A *constant fever* stays elevated.
- A sudden drop from fever to normal temperature is called **crisis.**
- When an elevated temperature gradually returns to normal, it is called **lysis.**
- Fever that returns to normal for at least a day, and then occurs again, is a *relapsing fever.*

Lowered Body Temperature. A temperature significantly below normal is called *hypothermia*. A low body temperatures may precede death or result from overexposure to the elements or cold water—as in near-drowning.

In some instances, body temperature slightly below normal indicates a desirable situation: the lowered body temperature

Equipment

Several types of thermometers measure body temperature. *Glass thermometers* are mostly used outside acute care facilities. Understanding their use is important for teaching, however, because clients and families commonly use glass thermometers in the home. However, clients should be encouraged to use other types of thermometers. Many pharmacies offer a "trade-in" program, whereby a glass thermometer can be exchanged for an electronic model. *Electronic* and *disposable thermometers* are commonly used in healthcare facilities, including hospitals.

Glass Thermometer

Body temperature is sometimes measured by a glass thermometer, which is marked in degrees Fahrenheit, Celsius, or both. The glass thermometer is a hollow glass tube or a stem with a mercury-filled bulb on one end; both ends are sealed.

Heat expands the mercury in the temperature bulb, causing it to rise into the stem; the stem is marked off at full degrees and at two-tenths of each full degree. The markings range from 93° or 94° F (33° or 34.45° C) to about 108° F (42.2° C). These degree ranges encompass possible temperatures in living humans. The reading remains on the thermometer until you briskly shake the mercury down.

Types. The two types of clinical glass thermometers are slender-tipped and bulb-shaped. The *slender-tipped* ther-

TABLE 46-2 Average Normal Temperatures

Route	Normal Reading	Time for Clinical Thermometer	Time for Electronic Thermometer
Oral (mouth)	98.6°F (37°C)	3–5 min	0.5–1.5 min
Rectal (anus)	99.6°F (37.5°C)	3–5 min	0.5–1.5 min
Axillary (armpit)	97.6°–98°F (36.4°–36.7°C)	8–10 min	1–3 min
Tympanic (auditory canal)	Usually charted as tympanic without conversion; possible to convert to oral, rectal, or core equivalents	—	1–2 sec

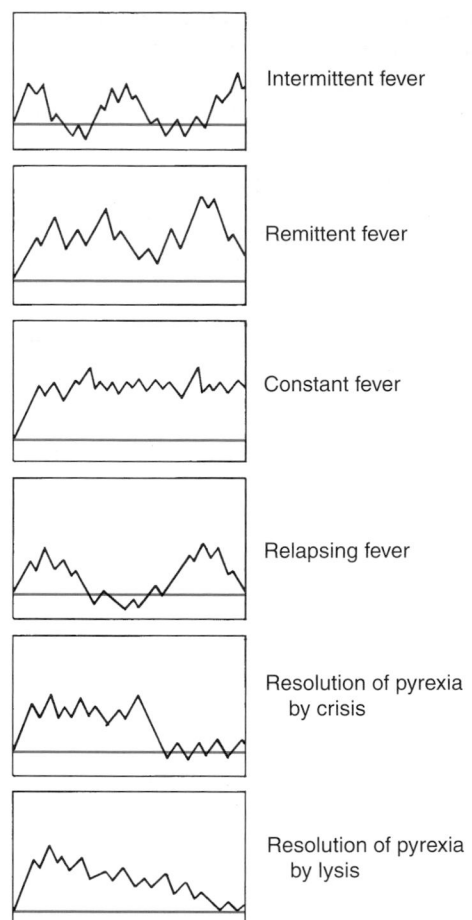

Intermittent fever

Remittent fever

Constant fever

Relapsing fever

Resolution of pyrexia by crisis

Resolution of pyrexia by lysis

FIGURE 46-2. Common courses of fever and its resolution. The colored line represents normal temperature. (Taylor, C., Lillis, C. A., & LeMone, P. [2001]. *Fundamentals of nursing: The art and science of nursing care* [4th ed.]. Philadelphia: Lippincott Williams & Wilkins.)

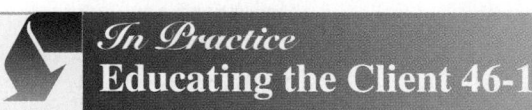

In Practice
Educating the Client 46-1

CLEANING AND DISINFECTING THE GLASS THERMOMETER

- Wash the thermometer in cold water. *Rationale: Heat will break the thermometer.*
- Use detergent to remove lubricant from a rectal thermometer before disinfecting. Rub any thermometer with a soap or detergent solution, and rinse under cold running water. *Rationale: Lubricant interferes with disinfectant. Rubbing and soap loosen debris and organisms. Running water helps to rinse away soap residue, which would interfere with disinfection and taste unpleasant. Water also rinses away many microorganisms.*
- Dry the thermometer, and place in prescribed disinfectant for the designated length of time. In some cases, thermometers are stored in a solution. Be sure to rinse before using. *Rationale: Disinfectants have an unpleasant taste.*
- Encourage clients to use disposable, plastic thermometer covers. This eliminates the need for disinfection in most situations.

---

mometer is used for taking oral (by mouth) temperatures. The *bulb-tipped* thermometer is used for taking rectal (**R;** per rectum, **PR**) temperatures because it allows for safer insertion. Do not use oral and rectal thermometers interchangeably. Thermometers in healthcare facilities may have colored balls attached to the end to avoid confusion about their use. A blue bulb indicates the thermometer is used only for oral temperature measurements; a red bulb designates use for rectal measurements.

Cleaning and Disinfecting.   When glass thermometers are used, each client has an individual thermometer. Follow agency instructions for cleaning, disinfecting, and caring for clinical glass thermometers. If the client uses a glass thermometer at home, instruct him or her in how to clean and disinfect it. In Practice: Educating the Client 46-1 explains general principles for cleaning and disinfecting the glass thermometer.

Electronic Thermometer
Nearly all healthcare facilities use only electronic thermometers. The electronic thermometer is fast, accurate, easy, and safer to use than the glass thermometer. Usually, electronic thermometers can be set to display either Fahrenheit or Celsius temperature readings.

Place the temperature probe in the client's mouth, **axilla** (armpit), or rectum in the same manner as you would the bulb of the glass thermometer. The probe is encased in plastic or in a paper cover that you discard after each use. The electronic probe that registers temperature most quickly is the *tympanic membrane temperature probe* (also called the *otic temperature probe*), which measures the energy given off by the tympanic membrane in the ear (Fig. 46-3).

☛ KEY CONCEPT

All electronic temperature probes are encased in a new cover for each client. One-time use covers are also available for glass thermometers.

Regularly clean and sterilize electronic thermometers following the manufacturer's instructions. Electronic thermometers are rarely used in isolation units because of the difficulty of sterilizing them after use. The disposable single-use thermometer is most often used for the client in isolation.

Disposable Single-Use Thermometer
Temperature indicators made of paper are available for one-time use. These indicators are often used in isolation units and are inexpensive and convenient for use at home. They are also very handy when traveling.

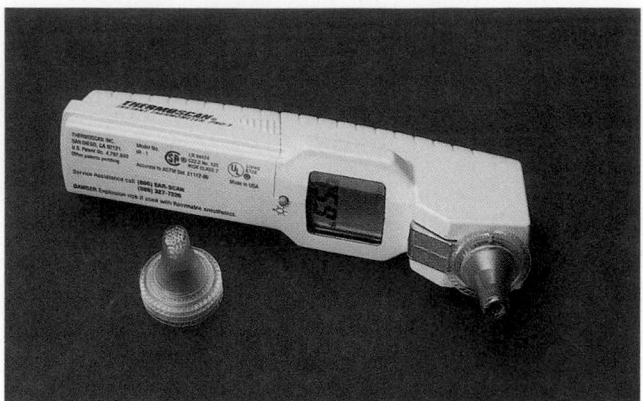

FIGURE 46-3. A tympanic thermometer is inserted into the ear canal to measure body temperature. (Craven, R. F., & Hirnle, C. J. [2000]. *Fundamentals of nursing: Human health and function* [3rd ed.]. Philadelphia: Lippincott Williams & Wilkins.)

To use, remove the wrapper and place the indicator under the client's tongue. Some types of indicators are designed to be held against the client's forehead. Follow the manufacturer's instructions.

Measuring Body Temperature

In Practice: Nursing Procedure 46-1 presents the methods for taking oral, rectal, axillary, and tympanic temperatures. Certain rules apply to using all types of thermometers and body areas:

- Every healthcare agency has an established routine for measuring the client's temperature. Follow guidelines accordingly.
- Place the bulb or probe so that body tissues completely surround it.
- When using the tympanic probe, surround it with the skin of the outer ear, rather than the mucous membrane, to minimize the risk of spreading infection.
- Cover temperature probes and multi-use thermometers during use. Slip the cover tightly over the thermometer, take the temperature, and then remove and discard the cover. Wash your hands between clients.
- Prelubricated covers are available for rectal thermometers.
- Record the temperature to the even two-tenths of a degree on the client's graphic record (unless you use an electronic thermometer, which has a digital readout to one-tenth of a degree). Some special electronic thermometers read the temperature to a more exact measurement.

Oral Temperature

The oral temperature measurement method is often the easiest, least invasive, and most comfortable for the client. If a client has had a hot or a cold drink, wait 15 minutes before taking a mouth temperature; the temporary effects of heat or cold will then disappear from mouth tissues. Use of gum, cigarettes, and smokeless tobacco also can affect oral temperature. Do not use

the oral method for clients who are unconscious, confused, or otherwise not responsible for their actions. Do not use this method with babies or young children because of the danger of injury from a broken thermometer. The oral method is contraindicated in surgery, injuries to the nose or mouth, conditions in which the client must breathe through the mouth, and for the client receiving oxygen.

Rectal Temperature

The rectal temperature is highly accurate because the thermometer or probe is placed in an enclosed cavity. If any question arises about the accuracy of an oral temperature, it should be checked against a rectal temperature. Some healthcare agencies make it a policy to recheck temperature by the rectal method when the oral reading is above a certain level. Take a rectal temperature when caring for unconscious or confused clients, infants and young children, and after mouth surgery, unless contraindicated or tympanic thermometers are available. For easier insertion, use a lubricated probe cover. To prevent injury, hold the thermometer in place in the rectum. This method is contraindicated in conditions such as diarrhea and rectal disease, and following rectal surgery.

Axillary Temperature

The axillary (**Ax**) temperature is the least accurate because the skin surfaces in the axillary space may not come together to form a tightly closed cavity around the thermometer tip. Hold the thermometer tightly in place in the client's armpit when using this method. The axillary method is used routinely for taking the temperature of newborns (see Chap. 66). For all other clients, take axillary temperatures only when conditions make the use of any other method impossible.

Tympanic Temperature

The tympanic temperature thermometer is placed snugly into the client's outer ear canal. It records temperature in 1 to 2 seconds (see Fig. 46-3). Many pediatric and intensive care units use this type of thermometer because it records a temperature so rapidly. Charge and care for this equipment as you would other electronic thermometers.

☛ KEY CONCEPT
___

When assessing body temperature, technique must be correct to get accurate, reliable results. This is especially true of tympanic temperatures.

ASSESSING PULSE

Every heartbeat produces a wave of blood that causes pulsations through the arteries. This vibration is called the **pulse.** The pulse can be felt through the nerves in the fingertips if the fingers are placed over one of the large arteries that lie close to the skin, especially if the artery runs across a bone and has very little soft tissue around it.

(*text continues on page 570*)

In Practice
Nursing Procedure 46-1

MEASURING BODY TEMPERATURES: ORAL TEMPERATURE BY ELECTRONIC THERMOMETER

Supplies and Equipment:

Thermometer with probe
Disposable probe covers
Paper or flow sheet
Pen

Steps:

1. Gather equipment.
   RATIONALE: *Organization facilitates accurate skill performance.*

2. Wash the hands.
   RATIONALE: *Handwashing prevents the spread of infection.*

3. Explain the procedure to the client.
   RATIONALE: *Providing information fosters cooperation and understanding.*

4. Check that the oral probe is attached to the portable thermometer unit. Slide a disposable plastic cover onto the probe until it snaps into place.
   RATIONALE: *The disposable sheath prevents the spread of infection.*

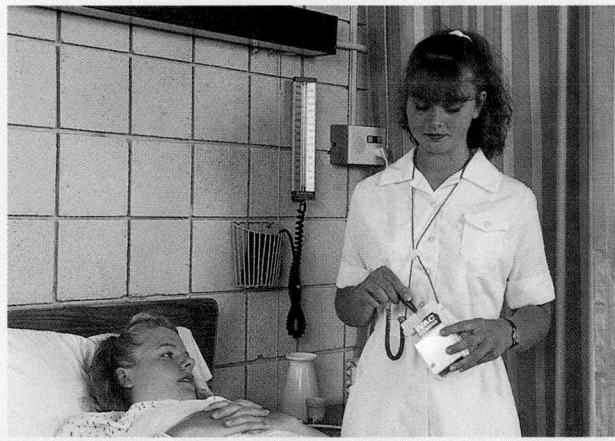

Covering the probe with a plastic sheath.

5. Place the probe under the client's tongue at the base of the sublingual pocket on either side.
   RATIONALE: *Heat from superficial blood vessels in the sublingual pocket produces the temperature reading.*

6. Instruct the client to close the lips (not the teeth) around the probe.
   RATIONALE: *Closing the lips steadies and secures the thermometer. Injury may occur if the client bites the probe.*

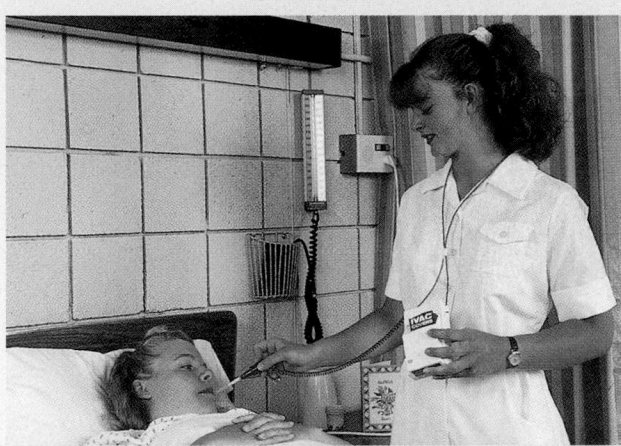

Placing the probe under the client's tongue.

7. Remove the thermometer when a "beep" sounds or the numbers stop flashing and the digital reading of the temperature is displayed.
   RATIONALE: *The signal indicates that temperature has registered and the reading has recorded.*

8. Remove the probe from the client's mouth and read the displayed temperature.
   RATIONALE: *The electronic instrument will display the client's measured temperature.*

9. Push the eject button to discard the plastic probe cover into the wastebasket. Return the oral probe to the portable unit.
   RATIONALE: *The eject button allows you to dispose of the cover without touching it.*

10. Wash the hands.
    RATIONALE: *Handwashing prevents the spread of infection.*

11. Record the client's temperature on paper or the flow sheet. Report an abnormal reading to the appropriate person.
    RATIONALE: *Documentation provides ongoing data collection. Do not try to remember vital signs. Write them down.*

Note: A 15-second timer is usually available on the electronic unit. It can be used to count pulse or respiration. It is activated by pressing the "T" button on the unit.

ORAL TEMPERATURE BY GLASS THERMOMETER
Supplies and Equipment:

Thermometer with plastic wrapper
Soft tissues
Paper or flow sheet
Pen

(continued)

In Practice
Nursing Procedure 46-1 *(Continued)*

Steps:

1. Gather equipment.
   RATIONALE: *Organization facilitates accurate skill performance.*

2. Wash the hands.
   RATIONALE: *Prevent the spread of infection.*

3. Explain the procedure to the client.
   RATIONALE: *Providing information fosters cooperation and understanding.*

4. Wipe the thermometer from the bulb toward your fingers with a tissue.
   RATIONALE: *Wipe from the area where few organisms are present to the area where more organisms are present to limit spread of infection.*

5. Hold the thermometer firmly with the thumb and forefinger; shake it with strong wrist movements until the mercury line falls to at least 35° C (95° F).
   RATIONALE: *Lower the mercury level within the tube so that it is less than the client's potential body temperature.*

6. Place the bulb of the thermometer well under the client's tongue. Instruct the client to close the lips (not the teeth) around the bulb. Ensure that the bulb rests well under the tongue, where it will be in contact with blood vessels close to the surface.
   RATIONALE: *This position helps ensure an accurate temperature reading. Closing the lips steadies and secures the thermometer.*

7. Remove the thermometer after 3 to 5 minutes, according to agency guidelines.
   RATIONALE: *Ensure enough time for accurate measurement.*

8. Remove the thermometer; wipe it once using a firm twisting motion.
   RATIONALE: *Clean the instrument to prevent the spread of infection.*

9. Hold the thermometer at eye level. Read to the nearest tenth.
   RATIONALE: *Ensure accurate and prompt recording.*

10. Dispose the tissue. Wash the thermometer in lukewarm, soapy water. Dry and replace the thermometer in a container at the bedside. Wash your hands.
    RATIONALE: *Cleaning and handwashing prevent the spread of organisms.*

11. Record temperature on paper or flow sheet. Report an abnormal reading to the appropriate person.
    RATIONALE: *Documentation provides ongoing data collection.*

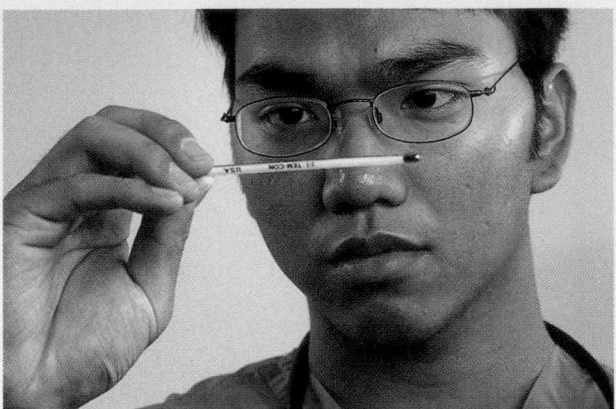

Read the thermometer to the nearest tenth.

RECTAL TEMPERATURE BY GLASS OR ELECTRONIC THERMOMETER

Supplies and Equipment:

Rectal thermometer
Wipes
Tissues
Water-soluble lubricant or lubricated probe cover
Disposable gloves
Graphic record and pen

Steps:

1. Wash the hands and put on gloves.
   RATIONALE: *Washing hands and wearing gloves helps prevent the spread of infection.*

2. Turn the client on one side.
   RATIONALE: *This position exposes the client's rectal area for thermometer placement.*

3. For the glass thermometer, lubricate the bulb and the client's rectal area up to 1 inch above it with lubricant on a wipe. Use a lubricated probe cover with an electronic thermometer.
   RATIONALE: *Lubrication reduces friction and makes it easier to insert the thermometer or probe without injuring body tissues. Applying the lubricant with a wipe prevents contamination of the lubricant supply.*

4. Fold back the bedclothes, and separate the client's buttocks so that the anal opening is clearly visible.
   RATIONALE: *Allow for easy thermometer insertion.*

5. As the client takes a slow, deep breath, insert the thermometer about 1.5 inches. Insertion depth is necessary for blood vessels in the rectum to surround the probe.
   RATIONALE: *Deep, slow breaths allow the client to relax the anal area.*

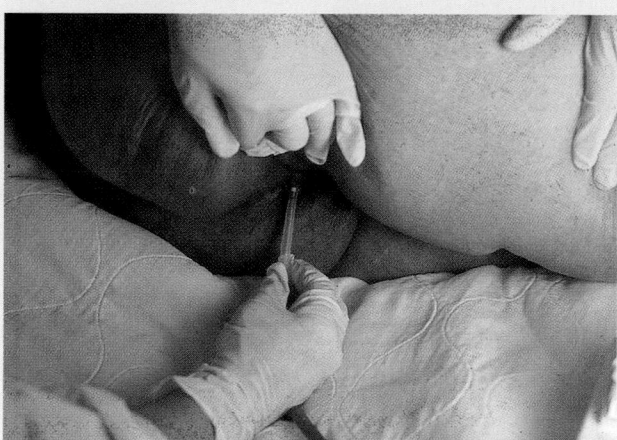
Use a lubricated probe cover with an electronic thermometer.

6. Hold the thermometer in place for 3 to 5 minutes, according to agency protocol.
   RATIONALE: *Hold the thermometer in place for safety and so the client does not expel it. Adequate time is needed for an accurate reading.*

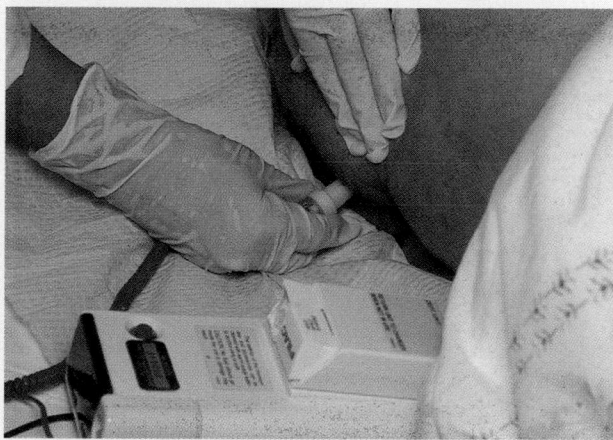
Hold the thermometer in place for 3 to 5 minutes.

7. Remove and wipe the glass thermometer toward the bulb or dispose of the probe cover. Read the temperature.
   RATIONALE: *Fecal matter left on the thermometer would obscure the markings.*

8. Dispose of the equipment properly. Wash the hands.
   RATIONALE: *Prevent the spread of infection.*

9. Document the temperature on the client's graphic record. Indicate that temperature was taken rectally by writing "(R)" next to it.
   RATIONALE: *A difference in normal values exists between oral and rectal temperatures.*

AXILLARY TEMPERATURE BY GLASS OR ELECTRONIC THERMOMETER

Supplies and Equipment:

Appropriate thermometer
Graphic chart
Pen

Steps:

1. Wash the hands.
   RATIONALE: *Prevent the spread of infection.*

2. Be sure the client's axilla is dry. If it is moist, pat it dry gently before inserting the thermometer.
   RATIONALE: *Moisture will alter the reading.*

3. After placing the probe or bulb of the thermometer into the axilla, bring the client's arm down against the body as tightly as possible, with the forearm resting across the chest.
   RATIONALE: *Close contact of the probe or bulb of the thermometer with the superficial blood vessels in the axilla ensures a more accurate temperature registration.*

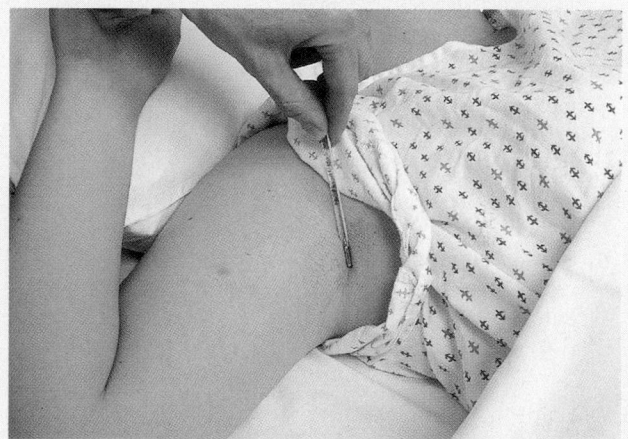
Placing the glass thermometer into the axilla.

4. Hold the glass thermometer in place for 8 to 10 minutes. Hold the electronic thermometer in place until the reading registers directly.
   RATIONALE: *Ensure an accurate reading.*

5. Remove and read the thermometer. Dispose of the equipment properly. Wash the hands.
   RATIONALE: *Prevent the spread of infection.*

6. Record the reading per agency procedures. Indicate that the axillary method was used: "(Ax)."
   RATIONALE: *Axillary temperature readings usually are lower than oral readings. Document to avoid confusion.*

(continued)

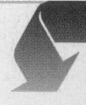

In Practice
Nursing Procedure 46-1 (Continued)

TYMPANIC TEMPERATURE

Supplies and Equipment:

Tympanic thermometer
Disposable probe cover

Steps:

1. Wash the hands.
   RATIONALE: *Prevent the spread of infection.*

2. Explain the procedure to the client. *Rationale: Ensure cooperation and understanding.*

3. Hold the probe in the dominant hand. Use the client's same ear as your hand (eg, use the client's right ear when you use your right hand).
   RATIONALE: *Ensure a firm grasp on the instrument. Promote proper placement of the temperature probe.*

4. Select the desired mode of temperature. Use the rectal equivalent for children under 3 years of age. Wait for a "ready" message to display.
   RATIONALE: *Be sure to use the thermometer correctly.*

5. With your nondominant hand, grasp the adult's external ear at the midpoint. Pull the external ear up and back. For a child of 6 years or younger, use your nondominant hand to pull the ear down and back.
   RATIONALE: *You need to straighten the curved ear canal as much as possible to obtain optimum visualization.*

6. Slowly advance the probe into the client's ear with a back and forth motion until it seals the ear canal.
   RATIONALE: *Sealing the tip of the probe confines radiated heat within the area being measured.*

7. Point the probe's tip in an imaginary line from the client's sideburns to his or her opposite eyebrow.
   RATIONALE: *Be sure to align the probe with the client's tympanic membrane.*

8. As soon as the instrument is in correct position, press the button to activate the thermometer.

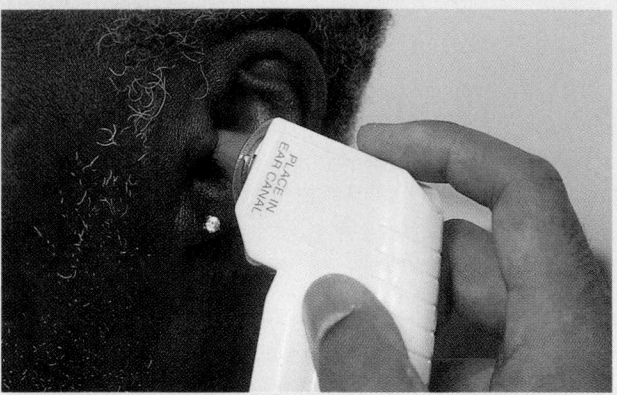

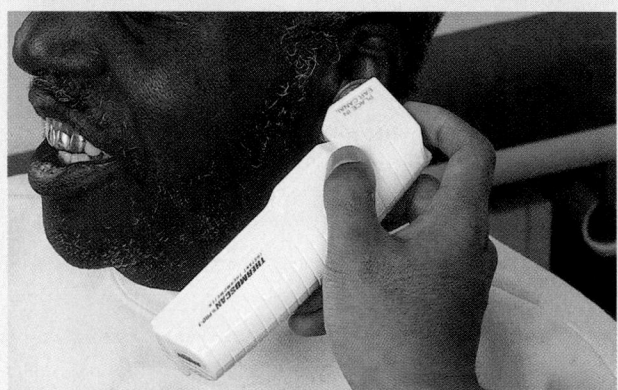

Advance the probe until it seals in the ear canal. Point the probe's tip in an imaginary line from the client's sideburns to his or her opposite eyebrow.

   RATIONALE: *Initiate sensing within 25 seconds to ensure an accurate reading.*

9. Keep the probe in place until the thermometer makes a sound or flashes a light.
   RATIONALE: *Wait for the procedure to be complete.*

10. Read the temperature and discard the probe cover. Replace the thermometer and wash your hands.
    RATIONALE: *Limit the spread of microorganisms.*

11. Record the temperature on the client's record.
    RATIONALE: *Documentation provides ongoing data collection.*

The pulse can be felt most distinctly over the:

- temporal artery just in front of the ear
- mandibular artery on the lower jawbone
- carotid artery on either side of the neck in front
- femoral artery in the groin
- radial artery in the wrist at the base of the thumb

Pulses counted in these areas may be stated as *temporal pulse, mandibular pulse,* **carotid pulse,** or **femoral pulse.**

If nothing is stated, it is assumed that the pulse was a **radial pulse.** (Fig. 43-2 in Chapter 43 illustrates these pulse points, as does Fig. 47-32 in Chapter 47).

Regulation of Pulse

Pulse Rate

The *pulse rate* (or *heart rate,* **HR**) tells how often a person's heart beats per minute. Pulse rate varies with the client's age, size, and weight. The normal adult pulse rate is 60 to 80 beats per minute (**BPM**). Women have a slightly higher average rate than men. The pulse of a newborn ranges from 120 to 140 BPM. Rates for children fall between those for adults and newborns, according to each child's size and age (see Chapter 70).

Activity affects pulse rate. The heart does not work as hard when a person sleeps; thus, pulse rate decreases. After running, vigorous exercise, or strenuous physical work, and during disease, the heart beats faster; thus the pulse rate increases. Excitement, anger, and fear increase the rate, as do some drugs. The pulse rate is faster in persons with a fever or an overactive thyroid gland. It increases in proportion to the body's temperature: pulse rate rises about 10 beats for every 1° F (0.56° C) increase in body temperature.

A condition in which the pulse rate is consistently above normal (>95 BPM) is called **tachycardia.** Many of the previously mentioned conditions cause a temporarily rapid rate. An abnormally rapid rate that persists may signify heart disease, heart failure, hemorrhage, or some other serious disturbance.

Sometimes the pulse rate is continuously slow (< 55 BPM). This condition is called **bradycardia.** Well-conditioned athletes often have a pulse rate that is lower than normal, but often bradycardia suggests an abnormality. Bradycardia may occur during convalescence from a long feverish illness. It is a sign of cerebral hemorrhage, indicating increased pressure on the brain. It also is a sign of complete heart block (nonfunctioning of the heart's electrical conduction system). Certain medications also lower pulse rate.

Pulse Volume

Pulse volume varies with the blood volume in the arteries, the strength of the heart contractions, and the elasticity of blood vessels. When every beat is full and strong, a normal pulse can be felt with moderate finger pressure (stronger finger pressure obliterates the beats). If a pulse is difficult to obliterate, it is strong and is called *full* or *bounding.* In hemorrhage, when a considerable amount of blood has been lost, every pulse beat may be weak or thready and the pulse is easy to obliterate.

Pulse Rhythm

Pulse rhythm is the spacing of the beats. With normal or regular rhythm, intervals between beats are the same. When the pulse occasionally skips a beat, this irregularity is described as an *intermittent* or *irregular pulse.* A pulse may be regular in rhythm but irregular in force; that is, every other beat is weak. These beats may be so weak that they are not felt in the radial pulse at all. This finding is serious because it means the heart is actually beating twice as fast as the pulse rate indicates. This condition can be detected by measurement of the **apical-radial pulse** (simultaneous measurement of the apical and the radial pulse), discussed later in this chapter. Pulse may be irregular in force and rhythm (*dysrhythmia*), a sign of some forms of heart disease or of an overactive thyroid gland (see Chap. 80).

Methods and Equipment

Palpation

Palpation (feeling with the fingers) is used to assess the radial, temporal, mandibular, carotid, and femoral pulse. To locate the area of strongest pulsation, palpate the client's pulse with your first, second, and third fingers of one hand. (Do not use the thumb, which has its own pulse.) Count the initial pulsation as zero. This procedure is detailed in In Practice: Nursing Procedure 46-2.

Auscultation With a Stethoscope

Auscultation (listening to sounds) and counting the **apical pulse,** normally heard at the heart's apex, will usually give the most accurate assessment of pulse rate. This procedure is detailed at In Practice: Nursing Procedure 46-3. For this assessment, use an instrument called a **stethoscope,** which amplifies sounds received in the head of the instrument as they pass through the earpieces. Most stethoscopes have two heads: the diaphragm and the bell. The flat diaphragm is pressed against the skin to test high-frequency sounds: breath, normal heart, and bowel sounds. The cup-shaped bell is pressed lightly on the skin to collect low-frequency sounds, such as abnormal heart sounds. (To change from one head to the other, turn the head until it clicks into place.)

The diaphragm of the stethoscope is placed over the heart's apex to assess apical pulse. (The apex of the heart is about halfway down the center of the left chest.) Each heartbeat consists of two sounds. S_1, the first sound, is caused by closure of the mitral and bicuspid valves, which separate the atria from the ventricles. S_2, the second sound, is caused by the closure of the pulmonic and aortic valves. The result is a muffled "lub-dub" sound, which constitutes one heartbeat (see Chap. 22).

Doppler

An ultrasonic vascular Doppler device is used to detect peripheral pulses. Apply a conductive gel, and place the Doppler transmitter over the artery being assessed. The earpieces or a special speaker attached to the Doppler device amplify the sounds. They may also be recorded on a computer or on a special printout.

Measuring the Pulse

Radial Pulse

The radial artery is most commonly used to count the pulse because of its convenient location. In Practice: Nursing Procedure 46-2 outlines the steps of taking a radial pulse. Use the middle two or three fingers to take the pulse. Do not use the thumb; it has its own pulse that may be stronger than the client's.

Apical Pulse

The apical pulse (**AP**) is more accurate than the radial pulse, and is always the pulse taken for children under 2 years of age. In Practice: Nursing Procedure 46-3 outlines the steps of taking an apical pulse. Always measure the client's apical pulse if

In Practice
Nursing Procedure 46-2

MEASURING RADIAL PULSE

Supplies and Equipment:

Watch with a second hand
Paper or flow sheet
Pen

Steps:

1. Wash your hands.
   RATIONALE: *Handwashing prevents the spread of infection.*

2. Explain the procedure to the client.
   RATIONALE: *Provide information to foster cooperation and understanding.*

3. Position the client's forearm comfortably with the wrist extended and the palm down.
   RATIONALE: *This position allows for easy assessment.*

4. Place the tips of your first, second, and third fingers over the client's radial artery on the inside of the wrist on the thumb side.
   RATIONALE: *The fingertips are sensitive and better able to feel the pulse. Do not use your thumb because it has a strong pulse of its own.*

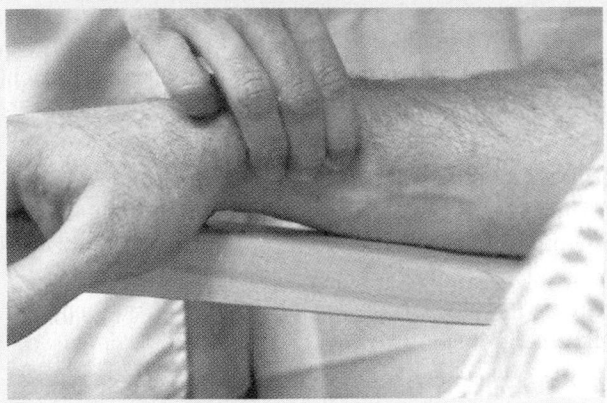

Placing the fingers over the radial pulse.

5. Press gently against the client's radial artery to the point where pulsations can be felt distinctly.
   RATIONALE: *Excessive pressure will obliterate the pulse.*

6. Using a watch, count the pulse beats for 30 seconds and multiply by two to get the rate per minute.
   RATIONALE: *Allow sufficient time to assess the pulse rate when it is regular.*

7. Count the pulse for a full minute if it is abnormal in any way, or take an apical pulse.
   RATIONALE: *Counting a full minute permits a more accurate reading and allows assessment of pulse strength and rhythm.*

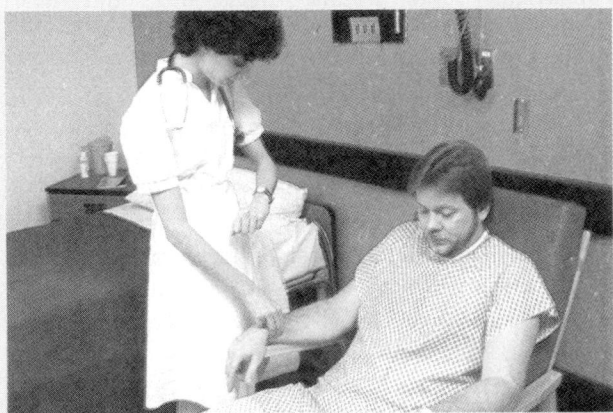

Counting the pulsations.

8. Record the rate (BPM) on paper or the flow sheet. Report any irregular findings to the appropriate person.
   RATIONALE: *Documentation provides ongoing data collection.*

9. Wash your hands.
   RATIONALE: *Handwashing prevents the spread of organisms.*

---

any question arises about the heart's rhythm or rate, or if it appears that the heart has stopped. In some cases, the physician orders apical pulse as a routine order.

Apical-Radial Pulse

An apical-radial pulse (**A-R**) measurement is ordered when it is suspected that the client's heart is not effectively pumping blood. If the apical and radial measurements are not the same, a pulse deficit exists. This must be reported to the physician. In Practice: Nursing Procedure 46-3 gives the steps for taking this measurement.

Pedal Pulse

The **pedal pulse** (foot pulse) is felt over the dorsalis pedis artery or the posterior tibial artery of the foot. The pulse point is located on top of the foot, posterior to the toes (see Fig. 22-4 in Chapter 22). The status of blood circulation to the foot can be determined at these pulse points. A strong pulse indicates that circulation to the lower extremities is unrestricted, whereas a weak and irregular pulse suggests impaired or restricted blood flow. Use caution in palpating the pulse site, so that the pulse is not completely obliterated with excessive pressure. Inspect the feet for color, temperature, and presence of edema.

In Practice
Nursing Procedure 46-3

MEASURING APICAL PULSE

Supplies and Equipment:

Stethoscope
Pen and paper or flow sheet
Watch with second hand

Steps:

1. Wash your hands.
2. Expose the client's chest area.
   RATIONALE: *Noise from clothing and bedclothes will distort pulse sound.* Remember to respect the client's privacy.
3. Locate the point of maximal impulse (**PMI**) over the heart's apex where the apical pulse is best heard or felt. This point is usually at the fifth intercostal space approximately 3 inches left of the chest's midline (just below the left nipple). The apical pulse can be palpated in about half of adults. It is near the pointed bottom of the heart.

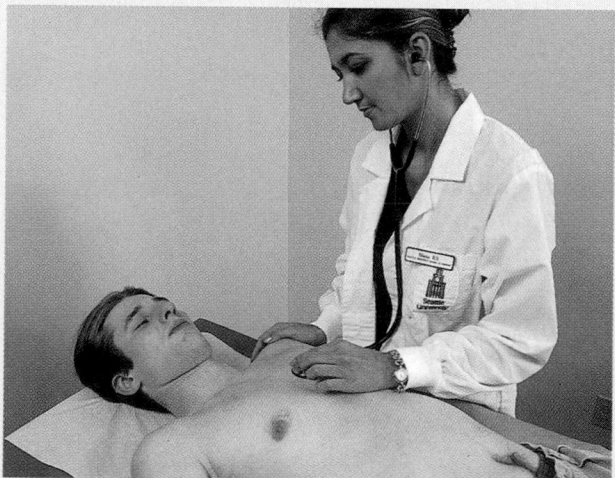

Locate the point of maximal impulse (PMI) over the heart's apex where the pulse is best heard or felt.

4. Warm the stethoscope's diaphragm in the palm of the hand.
   RATIONALE: *A cold metal diaphragm is uncomfortable against the skin. Provide for the client's comfort.*
5. Place the diaphragm firmly over the PMI, and auscultate (listen) for heart sounds.
   RATIONALE: *Lub-dub is the opening and closing of the heart valves to make one beat.*
6. Count for 1 full minute to ensure accuracy.
7. Determine regularity.
   RATIONALE: *Irregularity may indicate a need for further evaluation.*
8. Wash your hands.
9. Record findings on vital sign sheet, and report abnormalities to the charge nurse.

MEASURING APICAL-RADIAL PULSE

Supplies and Equipment:

Stethoscope (one for each nurse)
Pen and paper or flow sheet
Watch with second hand

Steps:

1. Two nurses carry out this procedure.
2. Using the same watch, one nurse counts the client's apical pulse for one minute, while the other nurse counts the radial pulse.
3. Both nurses start counting at the same time. The nurse counting the radial pulse calls for the timing to start and stop and times one minute with the second hand.
4. The nurses then identify and chart the two figures at the end of one minute. For example, "A-R pulse 76/72."
5. Normally, the two readings are the same. If a difference exists between them, it is called the *pulse deficit* and must be promptly reported and recorded. (*Note:* It is impossible for the apical pulse to be lower than the radial. If this finding occurs, you have made a mistake. Take both pulses again.)

Also observe the condition of the client's toenails and cuticles. Always assess pedal pulse bilaterally (in both feet) for comparison.

Popliteal Pulse

The **popliteal pulse** is located posterior to the knee. It is palpated by placing the fingers in the space behind the knee. Use this site to assess the status of circulation to the lower leg or as an alternative means of assessing blood pressure with a large leg cuff.

Carotid Pulse

The carotid pulse, on either side of the neck, can be located directly over the carotid artery. Palpate this pulse along the medial edge of the sternocleidomastoid muscle above the cricoid notch (see Fig. 47-32 in Chapter 47). The carotid artery is easily accessible for checking peripheral pulse. Individuals who must do self-checks often use this method. It is also used in cases of shock when other pulses are not palpable and to determine the need for cardiopulmonary resuscitation (CPR).

The pulse is counted on either side of the neck. The client's head is positioned midline to the body. (Rationale: Such positioning provides easier access to the pulse, which is obliterated when the head is turned to one side or the other.)

Nursing Alert

Never check carotid pulse on both sides of the neck at the same time. *Rationale: Doing so could cut off circulation to the brain, possibly causing cardiac arrest.* Use the fingertips to palpate the carotid pulse. (The thumb has its own pulse.) Do not reach across the person's neck to count carotid pulse. (The client's airway could be occluded by the pressure of the examiner's arm). Measure the carotid pulse in the client's neck on the side facing you.

ASSESSING RESPIRATION

Oxygen keeps body cells alive; accumulated carbon dioxide kills cells. Respiration is the process that brings oxygen into the body and removes carbon dioxide. This exchange takes place in the lungs (see Chap. 25). Observing respiration closely is necessary to detect signs of interference with the breathing process.

Regulation of Respiration

Respiratory Control
The brain's respiratory center, and the proportion of carbon dioxide in the blood, control and regulate respiration. Injury to the respiratory center or to the nerves connecting it with the lungs affects respiration; too little or too much carbon dioxide in the blood also affects breathing.

Respiration is automatic; people breathe without thinking about it. You can control your breathing to some extent by taking deeper or shallower breaths or even by holding your breath for a limited time. When the limit is reached, automatic control takes over, and your chest muscles relax despite your efforts. If this automatic resumption of breathing does not occur, a breathing disorder exists. An example is **apnea** (cessation of breathing), which occurs in sudden infant death syndrome (SIDS), sleep apnea, and other conditions.

The organs that accomplish breathing include the lungs, the chest muscles, and the diaphragm; injuries to these parts of the body affect respiratory functioning.

Rate and Depth
The normal respiration rate for an adult is 12 to 18 breaths per minute. Women have a more rapid rate than men. For newborns, the rate is approximately 40 breaths per minute; for children, the rate varies from 25 to 30 breaths per minute (see Chapter 70).

Nursing Alert

In the adult, a respiration rate below 8 or above 30 breaths per minute is a sign of significant respiratory impairment. Report this situation promptly.

Normal breathing is called **eupnea.** When respirations are abnormally rapid (>20 breaths per minute), **tachypnea** is present. When respirations are abnormally slow and fall below 10 breaths per minute, **bradypnea** occurs. Table 46-3 discusses abnormal breathing patterns.

Excitement, exercise, pain, and fever increase respiratory rate. Rapid respiration is characteristic of lung diseases such as pneumonia and emphysema. Heart disease, hemorrhage, and nephritis also increase the rate, as do some drugs. Rapid respiration indicates that the body is making an increased effort to maintain the correct balance of oxygen and carbon dioxide. The body is also trying to adjust the balance by taking deeper breaths. Note that all people sigh or yawn occasionally, to cleanse the lungs and physiologically expand the small airways and alveoli that are not used during ordinary respiration. (This also helps to equalize the pressure between the outside atmosphere and the middle ear, via the eustachian or auditory tube.) Do not confuse sighing with abnormal or difficult breathing.

Pressure on the brain's respiratory center decreases respiration rate; cerebral hemorrhage also has this effect. Some drugs, such as opium preparations, depress the respiratory center. Poisons that accumulate in the body in uremia and diabetic coma also slow the rate of respiration. In **Kussmaul's respirations,** respirations are abnormally deep, much like gasping. This condition is associated with severe diabetic acidosis and coma. If a client takes in and breathes out small amounts of air, respirations are described as *shallow.*

Respiration Sounds
Snoring occurs when the air passageway is partially blocked. It is common during sleep, when the person's tongue falls back due to relaxation.

Stertorous breathing occurs when air passes through secretions present in the air passages. These bubbling noises or rattles (rales) are characteristic before death, when the air passages fill with mucus. (Sometimes, very loud snoring is referred to as stertorous breathing.) Obstruction near the glottis causes a hissing, crowing sound.

Difficult Breathing (Dyspnea)

When a person is making a distinct effort to obtain oxygen and get rid of carbon dioxide, breathing becomes difficult. The term for difficult or painful breathing is **dyspnea.** This condition may be temporary, such as when a runner breathes in gasps at the end of a race, or when a person runs upstairs and pants to get his or her breath when reaching the top. Obesity also can cause dyspnea, especially on exertion. In some cases, breathing difficulty is more or less constant, as in the acute stages of pneumonia or emphysema, or in some types of heart disease. When the difficulty is so marked that the client can breathe only when in an upright position, it is called **orthopnea.**

Obstructions of the air passages by secretions or foreign objects interfere with breathing. *Asthma* is a condition that causes difficult breathing because of spasms and edema of the bronchi (see Chap. 85).

▪■■ TABLE 46-3 *A*BNORMAL BREATHING PATTERNS

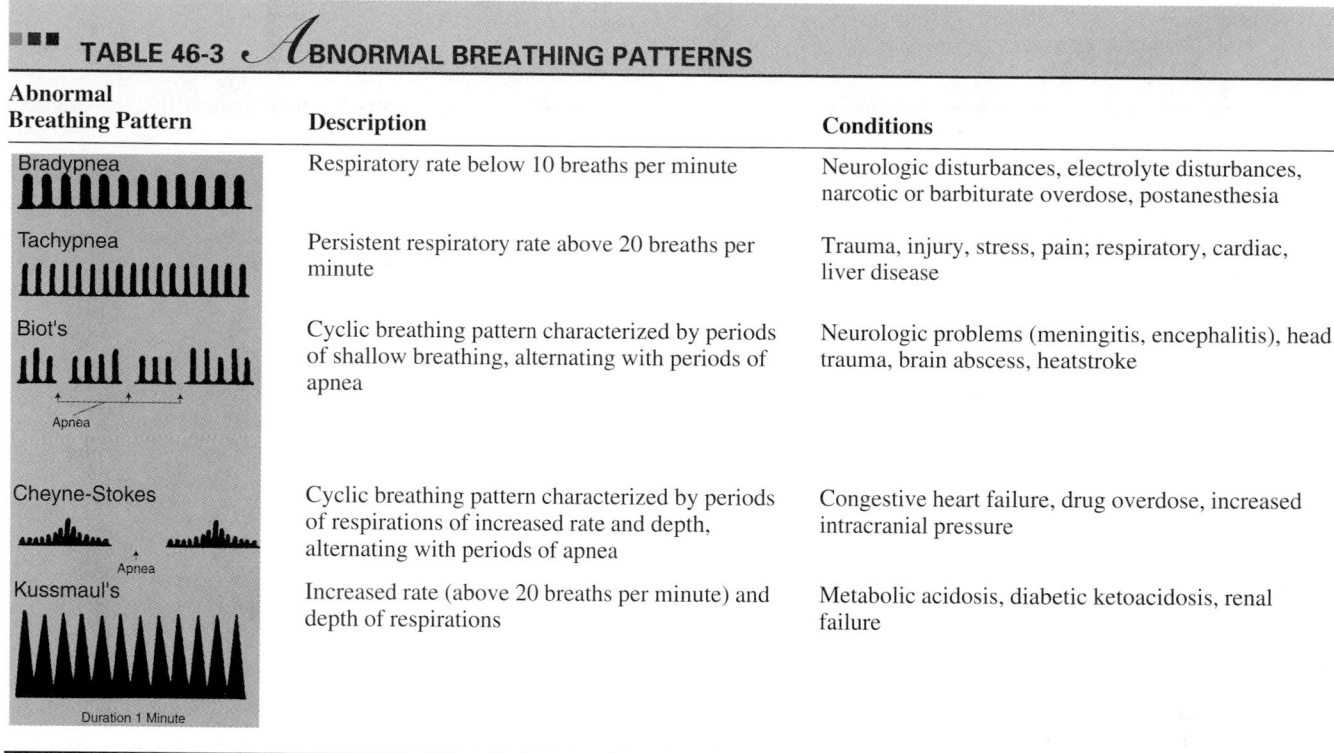

Abnormal Breathing Pattern	Description	Conditions
Bradypnea	Respiratory rate below 10 breaths per minute	Neurologic disturbances, electrolyte disturbances, narcotic or barbiturate overdose, postanesthesia
Tachypnea	Persistent respiratory rate above 20 breaths per minute	Trauma, injury, stress, pain; respiratory, cardiac, liver disease
Biot's	Cyclic breathing pattern characterized by periods of shallow breathing, alternating with periods of apnea	Neurologic problems (meningitis, encephalitis), head trauma, brain abscess, heatstroke
Cheyne-Stokes	Cyclic breathing pattern characterized by periods of respirations of increased rate and depth, alternating with periods of apnea	Congestive heart failure, drug overdose, increased intracranial pressure
Kussmaul's	Increased rate (above 20 breaths per minute) and depth of respirations	Metabolic acidosis, diabetic ketoacidosis, renal failure

Craven, R. F., & Hirnle, C. J. (2000). *Fundamentals of nursing: Human health and function* (3rd ed.). Philadelphia: Lippincott Williams & Wilkins.

Normally, the proportion of respirations to heartbeats is 1:5 in adults. Respirations usually increase if pulse rate increases, but not always in definite proportion. Usually pulse rate increases faster than respiration rate. However, respiration rate increases faster than pulse rate in respiratory diseases.

Characteristic signs of breathing difficulty are heaving of the chest and abdomen, a distressed expression, and **cyanosis** (bluish tinge) in the skin, especially in the lips (*circumoral cyanosis*) and mucous membranes of the mouth. In severe conditions, cyanosis spreads to the nails and extremities and eventually becomes apparent over the client's entire body. An excess of carbon dioxide causes the bluish tinge. Cyanosis also may result from a circulatory or blood disorder. It is much easier to detect in light-skinned people. The condition appears as a dusky gray color in dark-skinned individuals.

Cheyne-Stokes respirations are slow and shallow at first, gradually grow faster and deeper, then taper off until they stop entirely. Periods of apnea may last for several seconds and then the cycle is repeated. When observing this client, document the length of the period of apnea in seconds. Usually the client experiencing Cheyne-Stokes respirations is not cyanotic. Cheyne-Stokes respirations are serious and usually precede death in cerebral hemorrhage, uremia, or heart disease.

Counting Respirations

Respirations are the easiest to assess of all the vital signs. Each time such assessments are made, check them against the baseline information. See In Practice: Nursing Procedure 46-4.

ASSESSING BLOOD PRESSURE

Assessing blood pressure (BP) is especially important for clients with abnormally high or low readings, for postoperative clients, and for clients who have sustained serious injury or shock. The BP reading gives significant information about the client's status and is one of the most important parts of the nursing assessment. In routine client care, BP is assessed at least once or twice daily.

Regulation of Blood Pressure

As the heart forces blood through the arteries, the blood exerts a certain amount of pressure on the arterial walls. Two things determine the degree of pressure: the rate and force of the heartbeat, and the ease with which the blood flows into the arterioles. BP will be within normal limits (about 120/80 for an adult) if the normal elasticity of the arteries and the arterioles has been maintained, blood volume and composition is normal, and the heart's contraction exerts normal force.

If exertion or illness increases heart rate or force, BP also increases. If the quantity of blood within the circulatory system decreases—with other factors remaining the same—BP falls. In contrast, if blood volume is normal but the elasticity or caliber of the arteries is reduced, BP rises. High BP is called **hypertension;** low BP is called **hypotension.**

Systole and Diastole

The BP is at its highest with each heartbeat during heart contraction; this measure is the systolic blood pressure (**SBP**) or

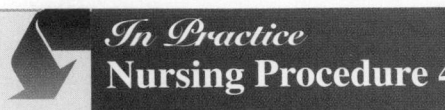

In Practice
Nursing Procedure 46-4

COUNTING RESPIRATIONS
Supplies and Equipment:

Watch with second hand
Paper or flow sheet
Pen

Steps:

1. Prepare to count respirations by keeping the fingertips on the client's pulse.
   RATIONALE: *A client who knows you are counting respirations may not breathe naturally.*

2. Observe the rise and fall of the client's chest (one inspiration and one expiration). Respirations can be counted by placing the hand lightly on the client's chest or abdomen.
   RATIONALE: *One full cycle consists of an inspiration and an expiration.*

3. a. Count respirations for 30 seconds and multiply by 2 to get the rate per minute.
   RATIONALE: *Allow sufficient time to assess respirations when the rate is regular.*

   b. Count respirations for 1 full minute for an infant, a young child, or an adult with an irregular, more rapid rate.
   RATIONALE: *Children normally have an irregular, more rapid rate. Adults with an irregular rate require more careful assessment including depth and rhythm of respirations.*

   c. If the client has an irregular or abnormal breathing pattern, such as Cheyne-Stokes respirations, document the length of apnea as well as the number of breaths.

4. Record the rate on paper or the flow sheet. Report any irregular findings to the appropriate person.
   RATIONALE: *Documentation provides ongoing data collection.*

5. Wash your hands.
   RATIONALE: *Handwashing prevents the spread of microorganisms.*

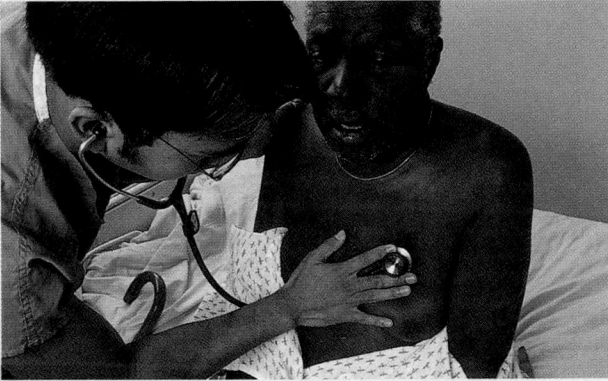

Observe the rise and fall of the client's chest (one inspiration and one expiration), while keeping the stethoscope in place.

systole. Pressure diminishes as the heart relaxes. Pressure is lowest when the heart relaxes before it begins to contract again; this measure is the diastolic blood pressure (**DBP**) or **diastole**. The difference between these two readings is called the **pulse pressure.** A value called the mean arterial pressure (**MAP**) is calculated using a mathematical formula:

$$1 \times \text{systolic} + 2 \times \text{diastolic}/3$$

Or

$$\frac{1 \times \text{systolic} + 2 \times \text{systolic}}{3}$$

MAP is approximately the value of the diastolic pressure plus one-third of the pulse pressure. It denotes the average pressure within the arteries. An electronic device is usually used to determine the accurate average pressure or MAP.

Normal Blood Pressure
Normally, the difference between the systolic pressure and the diastolic pressure (*pulse pressure*) is a number equal to one third to one half of the systolic pressure. Both readings give information; a wide or very narrow difference between the two indicates a problem. Average systolic pressure for an adult aged 20 is approximately 120, and average diastolic pressure is approximately 80. BP increases gradually with age. At age 60, normal systolic pressure can be expected to reach 130 to 140, as a result of the effects of aging on the heart and the arteries. This pressure would be considered alarming in a 20-year-old person. Any pressure that is much higher than normal for the person's age (*hypertension*) is a sign of a circulatory problem. A very low BP (*hypotension*) may indicate hemorrhage or shock. A systolic reading of 80 or less usually indicates shock or another difficulty. A diastolic reading over 90 is usually considered dangerously high. Medications may cause varia-

tions. The normal blood pressure in the child, as with other vital signs, varies with age. Chapter 70 details the normal ranges for children of various ages.

Methods and Equipment

The BP can be measured directly by means of a probe or catheter inserted directly into the client's artery (arterial line). The tip of the catheter has special sensors that measure pressures and transmit this information to an electronic machine that displays the systolic and diastolic pressures in the form of a wave.[1] This is called *direct measurement* of BP. Many critical care units use this type of measurement because constant monitoring is essential.

Sphygmomanometer

In most cases, BP is measured indirectly with a **sphygmomanometer.** This device consists of an inflatable bladder, enclosed in a cuff, that is attached to a bulb or a pump. (The bladder has a deflating mechanism as well.) The cuff is wrapped around the arm. Cuffs come in various sizes, as indicated in Table 46-4. If an incorrect size is used, accurate compression of the artery may not occur and the measurement will be incorrect.

Obtain the *indirect* BP reading with a sphygmomanometer by listening to the heartbeat with a stethoscope, which is placed over the brachial artery on the inside bend of the elbow. The stethoscope magnifies the sound of the heartbeat within the arteries. The sphygmomanometer may be of two types: mercury or aneroid. The placement of the arm wrap and stethoscope is the same.

Mercury Manometer

Healthcare agencies are less likely to use mercury sphygmomanometers, due to the potential hazard of a broken manometer leaking mercury into the environment. However, many are still available. The manometer has a glass tube that contains mercury and has markings to indicate BP level. The mercury manometer is fastened to a stand or a case, or to the wall. The pressure reading is indicated and read on the glass tube (at eye level for an accurate reading).

Aneroid Manometer

With the aneroid (spring-type) manometer, the arm wrap is attached to a dial rather than to a mercury column manometer. Pressure readings are observed on the dial. Estimating the systolic pressure in an emergency is possible with this method because the heartbeats can be seen as the needle bounces. Most facilities mount these manometers near the the client's bedside, although a portable type is frequently used as well.

Electronic Blood Pressure Apparatus

Apply and manipulate the cuff of the electronic BP apparatus in basically the same manner as an aneroid manometer. Place the microphone under the cuff, so the arrow that indicates the artery is in the correct location. Hold the microphone in place while applying the cuff. Systolic and diastolic blood pressures and the client's pulse rate will print out on the screen within a few seconds. The stethoscope may be used to double check. In some cases, the electronic device remains in place to continuously monitor BP. In this case, the cuff inflates and deflates automatically.

Palpation

When a stethoscope is unavailable, blood pressure can be estimated. Palpate pulsations of the artery as pressure is released from the cuff. Estimate the systolic pressure when the pulsation is first felt. Usually, it is only possible to estimate the *systolic* pressure through this technique because pulsations do not diminish as the cuff pressure is released. Palpation may be the only technique for estimating BP if the client is in hypovolemic shock caused by hemorrhage. (In this case, the nurse often cannot hear the sounds.) Electronic BP measurement is more accurate.

Doppler Ultrasound

If sounds are difficult to hear or indistinct, a Doppler ultrasound may be used to amplify sounds instead of the stethoscope. Similar to palpation, only the systolic pressure can be obtained using this method of determining blood pressure values.

Measuring Blood Pressure

In Practice: Nursing Procedure 46-5 presents steps for taking BP using a sphygmomanometer and stethoscope.

☛ KEY CONCEPT

Take BP and pulse initially in both arms, especially if the client has known vascular disease or if the reading is not within normal range. A difference of 5 to 10 mm Hg commonly exists between arms. Readings of greater than 10 mm Hg difference indicate arterial occlusion in the arm with the lower pressure.

■■■ **TABLE 46-4** *R*ECOMMENDED BLADDER DIMENSIONS FOR BLOOD PRESSURE CUFF

Arm Circumference at Midpoint* (cm)	Cuff Name	Bladder Width (cm)	Bladder Length (cm)
5–7.5	Newborn	3	5
7.5–13	Infant	5	8
13–22	Child	8	13
22–32	Adult	13	24
32–42	Wide adult	17	32
42–50+	Thigh	20	42

*Midpoint of arm is defined as half the distance from the acromion to the olecranon.

In patients with very large limbs, the indirect blood pressure should be measured in the leg or forearm.

Reproduced with permission. *Recommendations for human blood pressure determination by sphygmomanometers.* Copyright © American Heart Association.

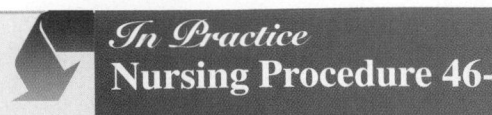

Nursing Procedure 46-5

MEASURING BLOOD PRESSURE

Supplies and Equipment:

Stethoscope
Sphygmomanometer
Blood pressure cuff (appropriate size)
Alcohol wipe
Paper or flow sheet
Pen

Steps:

1. Gather equipment. Select a cuff that is the appropriate size for the client. Cleanse the stethoscope's earpieces and diaphragm with an alcohol wipe.
   RATIONALE: *Organization facilitates performance of the skill. Incorrect cuff size may give an inaccurate reading. Cleansing the stethoscope prevents spread of infection.*

2. Wash your hands.
   RATIONALE: *Handwashing prevents the spread of infection.*

3. Explain the procedure to the client.
   RATIONALE: *Provide information to foster cooperation and understanding.*

4. Assist the client to a comfortable position. Support the selected arm; turn the palm upward. Remove any constrictive clothing.
   RATIONALE: *Ideally, the arm is at heart level for accurate measurement. Rotate it so the brachial pulse is easily accessible and not constricted by clothing. Do not use an arm where circulation is compromised in any way.*

5. Palpate the brachial artery. Center the cuff's bladder approximately 1 inch (2.5 cm) above the site where you palpated the brachial pulse.
   RATIONALE: *Center the bladder to ensure even cuff inflation over the brachial artery.*

6. Wrap the cuff snugly around the client's arm and secure the end appropriately.
   RATIONALE: *The BP reading will be inaccurate if you apply the cuff too loosely.*

7. Check that the mercury manometer is vertical, at eye level, and level with the client's heart.
   RATIONALE: *Improper height can alter perception of reading. (The aneroid manometer does not need to be at eye level.)*

8. Palpate the radial or brachial pulse with one hand. Close the screw clamp on the bulb and inflate the cuff while still checking the pulse with the other hand. Observe the point where pulse is no longer palpable.
   RATIONALE: *Palpation identifies the approximate systolic reading.*

9. Open the screw clamp, deflate the cuff, and wait 30 seconds.
   RATIONALE: *Short interval eases any venous congestion that may have occurred.*

10. Position the stethoscope's earpieces comfortably in your ears (turn tips slightly forward) and place the diaphragm or bell over the client's brachial artery.
    RATIONALE: *BP is easier to hear when you place the stethoscope directly over artery.*

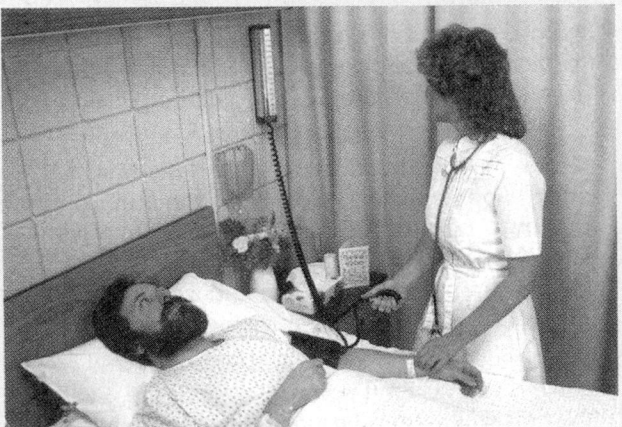

Palpating the radial pulse while inflating the cuff.

11. Close the screw clamp on the bulb and inflate the cuff to a pressure 30 mm Hg above the point where the pulse had disappeared.
    RATIONALE: *Ensure that the systolic reading is not underestimated.*

12. Open the clamp and allow the mercury column or aneroid dial to fall at 2–3 mm Hg per second.
    RATIONALE: *If deflation occurs too rapidly, reading may be inaccurate.*

13. Note the point on the column or dial at which you initially hear a distinct sound.
    RATIONALE: *The first sound heard represents the systolic pressure or the point where the heart is able to force blood into the brachial artery.*

14. Continue deflating the cuff and note the point where the sound disappears.
    RATIONALE: *This is the adult diastolic pressure. It represents the pressure that the artery walls exert on the blood at rest.*

15. Release any remaining air in the cuff and remove it. If the reading must be rechecked for any reason, allow a 1 minute interval before taking BP again.
    RATIONALE: *This interval eases any venous congestion and provides for an accurate reading when you repeat the measurement.*

In Practice
Nursing Procedure 46-5 (*Continued*)

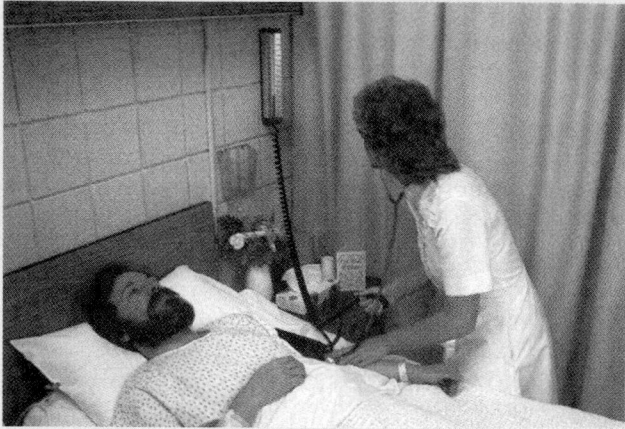

Listening for the systolic and diastolic pressure readings.

16. Assist the client to a comfortable position. Advise the client of the reading.
    RATIONALE: *Indicate your interest in the client's well-being and allow him or her to participate in care.*

17. Wash your hands.
    RATIONALE: *Handwashing prevents the spread of microorganisms.*

18. Record BP on paper or the flow sheet. Write the systolic pressure over the diastolic (using even numbers). For example, record a systolic of 120 and a diastolic of 70 as 120/70. Indicate site where you took the BP, if not brachial. Report any irregular findings.
    RATIONALE: *Documentation provides ongoing data collection.*

MEASURING ORTHOSTATIC BLOOD PRESSURE
Supplies and Equipment:

Stethoscope
Sphygmomanometer

Blood pressure cuff (appropriate size)
Alcohol wipe
Paper or flow sheet
Pen

Steps:

1. The client's blood pressure and pulse are measured with the client lying down.

2. Without removing the BP cuff, the client is asked to stand.
   RATIONALE: *The cuff remains in place to ensure a more accurate measurement.*

3. The BP and P are measured again. A significant drop in blood pressure (25 mm Hg systolic or 10 mm Hg diastolic) must be reported to the physician. This is called *orthostatic hypotension.*

4. A drop in BP may also affect the pulse rate. The pulse rate may decrease, but often it increases. A pulse rate increase of more than 12–15 beats per minute should be reported.

5. The person with orthostatic hypotension may feel dizzy or light-headed on standing and may be prone to falling or fainting. Carry out measures to ensure the client's safety. Instruct the person to rise slowly, to adjust to each new position. A decrease in blood pressure with an accompanying rise in pulse may also indicate low circulating blood volume, as in hemorrhage.

6. Orthostatic blood pressure is recorded as follows:
   ↓ 150/80, P 76   ↑ 120/66, P 92

(*Note:* This particular orthostatic drop in blood pressure, with the accompanying rise in pulse, should be reported to the physician.)

Whenever BP is measured with a manometer, listen to the heartbeat through the stethoscope and watch the manometer at the same time. When the cuff deflates, blood returns through the artery. **Korotkoff's sounds** are heard in the stethoscope. There are five phases of Korotkoff's sounds, as described in Fig. 46-4. The onset of phase I is the recorded systolic pressure. The onset of phase IV indicates diastolic pressure in children, and phase V indicates diastolic pressure in adults.

When using the electronic device, it is not always necessary to listen to heart sounds; the systolic and diastolic pressures are read out. However, it is still more accurate to listen.

Measure BP when the client is resting and quiet. Physical exertion or emotional stress will affect BP. Prepare the client by explaining that the cuff on the arm may feel tight for a second or two; otherwise, the procedure is not bothersome and will only take a few minutes.

Sometimes, it will be impossible to measure BP in the client's arm (eg, in the client with an IV or the client recovering from mastectomy). Use the thigh if a cuff that is wide and long enough (specifically identified as a *thigh cuff*) is available. Wrap the cuff at midthigh with the cuff's bladder in the back. Be careful to use a cuff that is the correct width. Auscultate over the popliteal artery in the back of the knee.

The lower arm also can be used, with auscultation over the radial artery in the wrist. If using an alternate site for taking BP, identify it in the documentation and use the same site continuously throughout the client's care to maintain comparable

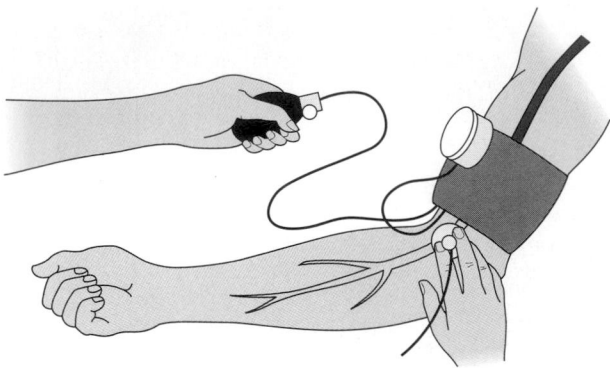

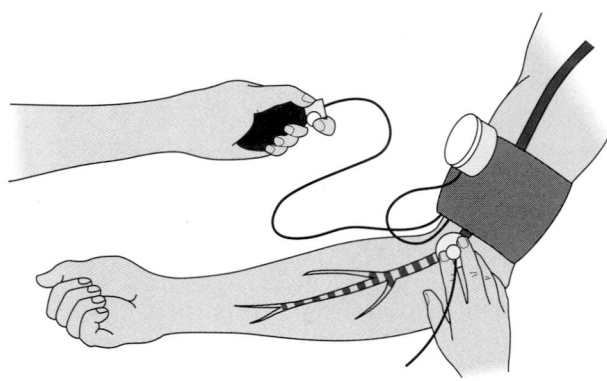

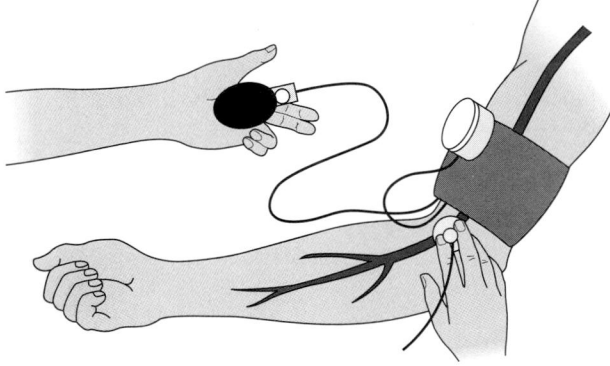

FIGURE 46-4. Five phases of Korotkoff's sounds. PHASE I: Characterized by the first appearance of faint but clear tapping sounds that gradually increase in intensity—the first tapping sound is recorded as the *systolic pressure.* PHASE II: Characterized by muffled or swishing sounds—these sounds may temporarily disappear, especially in hypertensive people. This disappearance of the sound during the latter part of phase I and during phase II is called the *auscultatory gap* and may cover a range of as much as 40 mm Hg. Failing to recognize this gap may cause serious errors—underestimating systolic pressure or overestimating diastolic pressure. PHASE III: Characterized by distinct, loud sounds as the blood flows relatively freely through an increasingly open artery. PHASE IV: Characterized by a distinct, abrupt, muffling sound with a soft, blowing quality—the onset of this phase is recorded as the *diastolic pressure in children.* PHASE V: The last sound heard before a period of continuous silence—the pressure at which the last sound is heard is recorded as the *diastolic pressure in adults.* (Craven, R. F., & Hirnle, C. J. [2000]. *Fundamentals of nursing: Human health and function* [3rd ed.]. Philadelphia: Lippincott Williams & Wilkins.)

data. Be sure to document where BP values were measured if the site is unusual.

Orthostatic Blood Pressure Measurement

Some clients, particularly those who are older or taking certain medications, will experience a drastic drop in BP and/or an increase in pulse when changing from lying to sitting or from sitting to standing. A drop of as much as 25 mm Hg systolic pressure and 10 mm Hg diastolic pressure (or more) can occur. When a severe drop in BP occurs, the condition is known as *orthostatic hypotension.* See In Practice: Nursing Procedure 46-5 for the steps involved in taking an orthostatic blood pressure measurement.

☛ KEY CONCEPT

Certain medications, including many anti-seizure medications and anti-psychotics (used in psychiatry), commonly cause orthostatic hypotension. These clients often have orthostatic blood pressure readings ordered as a routine order.

⮕ STUDENT SYNTHESIS

Key Points

- Temperature, pulse, respiration, and blood pressure are called vital signs (or cardinal symptoms) because they are indicators of functions of the body that are necessary to maintain life.
- Documentation of vital signs is essential to collecting information regarding the client's status and well-being.
- Temperature is the measurement of heat inside the body (core temperature). It is the balance between the heat the body produces and loses.
- Pulse is the vibration of the blood through the arteries as the heart beats. It is measured by rate and rhythm.
- Respiration is the process by which the lungs bring oxygen into the body and remove carbon dioxide.
- Blood pressure measures the pressure the blood exerts on the walls of the arteries. Rate and force of heartbeat, blood vessel condition, and blood volume determine the reading as the ventricles contract and rest.

Critical Thinking Exercises

1. You are measuring a client's temperature by the oral method. You find a variation from normal. What steps do you take next? Why?
2. Using a wall-mounted aneroid sphygmomanometer, you begin wrapping the cuff around the client's upper arm when you realize the cuff is the wrong size. Why is this a problem? What do you do next to ensure an accurate measurement?

3. Your client, Mr. B., is sound asleep when you enter his room to take his vital signs. Should you measure any of his vital signs before waking him? If so, which ones and why? How will you measure them?

4. Mrs. P. has never taken her temperature using an electronic thermometer. She now must monitor her daily temperature because of a recurring infection. Explain what steps she must take to measure and record her body temperature accurately.

NCLEX-Style Review Questions

1. When counting a client's respirations, which action is appropriate?
   a. Count the respirations for 2 minutes
   b. Keep your fingertips on the client's pulse
   c. Record your findings only if they are abnormal
   d. Tell the client to breathe normally

2. For a healthy adult, which vital sign indicates an abnormal finding?
   a. Blood pressure = 120/80
   b. Pulse = 60 BPM
   c. Respirations = 14 per minute
   d. Temperature = 38° C

3. Which type of temperature reading is the easiest, least expensive, and most comfortable for clients?
   a. Axillary
   b. Oral
   c. Rectal
   d. Tympanic

4. Which of the following would have the least effect on an adult's pulse?
   a. Acute pain
   b. Hemorrhage
   c. Time of day
   d. Vigorous exercise

5. When documenting a client's blood pressure, the systolic pressure is recorded as the point at which:
   a. The first Korotkoff's sound appears
   b. The second Korotkoff's sound appears
   c. The fourth Korotkoff's sound disappears
   d. The fifth Korotkoff's sound disappears

Reference

1. Taylor, C., Lillis, C., & LeMone, P. (2001). *Fundamentals of nursing: The art and science of nursing care* (4th ed.). Philadelphia: Lippincott Williams & Wilkins.

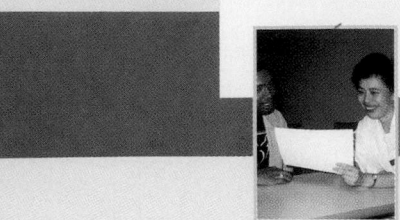

CHAPTER

47

Data Collection in Client Care

LEARNING OBJECTIVES

1. Explain the role of the practical/vocational nurse in assessment and data collection.
2. Identify common risk factors for disease and illness.
3. Define and differentiate between acute and chronic; and primary and secondary illnesses.
4. Describe the effects of inflammation and infection on the body.
5. State the rationale for obtaining a UA, CBC, UTox, or UPT.
6. List four types of tests and procedures that primary healthcare providers use to establish a medical diagnosis. Describe how each is used in this process.
7. Discuss the purpose of the physical examination done by the primary healthcare provider, and the data collected about the client by the registered or practical/vocational nurse.
8. Describe the common examination techniques of observation, inspection, palpation, percussion, and auscultation. In the skills lab, demonstrate each technique.
9. Describe common organizational formats used to perform the physical examination.
10. In the skills lab, perform a daily client data collection on a sample client, distinguishing between normal and abnormal findings.

NEW TERMINOLOGY

abscess	nodule
accommodation	observation
acuity	pallor
acute disease	palpation
auscultation	papule
chronic disease	percussion
cognitive function	primary disease
complication	purulent
conjunctivitis	pustule
crackle	rale
diplopia	rhonchi
dysphasia	risk factor
ecchymosis	scoliosis
emaciation	secondary disease
endoscope	sequela
erythema	serosanguineous
exudate	serous
fistula	sign
granulation tissue	slough
guaiac	strabismus
Hemoccult	striae
hemorrhage	stridor
herniation	suppuration
Homans' sign	symptom
induration	thrombophlebitis
infection	tumor
inflammation	turgor
inspection	ulcer
kyphosis	vesicle
lordosis	wheal
macule	wheeze
malaise	wound sinus
necrosis	

ACRONYMS

ABG	CT	LOC	T&X
CAM	ECG	LP	UA
CBC	EEG	MRI	UPT
C&S	EKG	O&P	UTox

The process of collecting data about the client's condition, combined with the physical examination, identifies and clarifies a client's health status. It identifies any health problems the client may be experiencing. When collecting health data about the client, the nurse asks, "What is the state of the client's health? Does the client have risk factors for health problems? Does the client have variations from usual or normal? Have changes occurred since the last assessment? If so, what are these changes?" To answer these questions, it is important to understand procedures that assist healthcare providers in establishing a medical and nursing diagnosis.

All healthcare providers must be able to distinguish between abnormal and normal physical findings. An organized format of data collection ensures thoroughness. It is also important to use correct language to describe findings, so all members of the team will understand.

Medical Versus Nursing Diagnosis. It is important to understand the roles of all healthcare providers in data collection. Remember the distinction between medical diagnosis and nursing diagnosis, as stated in Chapter 35. *Medical diagnosis* is determined by a primary healthcare provider: a person such as a physician, osteopath, or advance practice nurse. The medical diagnosis emphasizes the disease process and includes the identification of the disease or disorder, as well as the estimation of the course and outcome of the disease (*prognosis*). A diagnosis of pneumonia is a medical diagnosis.

The *nursing diagnosis,* on the other hand, focuses on the person and his or her needs in response to the disease, rather than on the disease itself. Nursing diagnosis is the concise problem-centered description of actual or potential health problems, based on the nursing process and stated in terms of NANDA groupings. Therefore, a nursing diagnosis for the person with pneumonia might be "ineffective airway clearance" because the person is coughing and needs assistance in breathing.

Data Collection to Assist in Diagnosis. The nurse uses two chief methods of data collection: the nursing history or interview (see Chap. 44) and the collection of physical findings about the client. The interview and examination of the client assists the team to make both medical and nursing diagnoses and to develop and implement an effective total plan of care.

☛ KEY CONCEPT

Remember to ask clients if they use complementary and alternative medicine (CAM) treatments such as vitamins, herbs, or homeopathic remedies. Some forms of CAM have been proven to be helpful and safe; others pose serious health risks to the individual when used after self-diagnosis. Care should be taken by the nurse to be nonjudgmental when information is revealed about unconventional treatments.

Assessment of the client occurs in nearly every nursing interaction. For example, as the nurse assists a woman to move from bed to chair, the nurse assesses how she is breathing, whether she is moving more or less stiffly than the day before, or whether she appears to be in pain. After providing nursing care, the nurse documents findings in clear language that every other member of the healthcare team will understand. Learning how to assess breathing, movement, and pain, and knowing accurate terms to describe these observations, can be more readily done if the nurse understands the format and techniques of a systematic physical examination.

FACTORS THAT INFLUENCE ASSESSMENT

Many factors influence disease and the body's response to that disease. Different people react in different ways to physical and emotional disorders. In addition, cultural factors influence how an individual person might respond to a disease process.

Risk Factors for Disease and Illness

Chapter 6 discusses disease and illness in more detail. Some individuals are more susceptible to illness than are others. They may have predisposing physical and emotional conditions, genetic predisposition, or lifestyle practices that increase the likelihood of developing a certain disease or disorder. These are called **risk factors.** Table 47-1 lists common risk factors with examples of diseases that may occur. As part of the nursing history, the nurse asks the client if any of these risk factors are present.

Course of the Disease

An **acute disease** develops suddenly and runs its course in days or weeks. A **chronic disease** may continue for months, years, or even life. **Acuity** means a disorder's level of severity. A **complication** is an unexpected event in the disease's course that often delays the client's recovery. Complications may occur at early, continuing, late, or terminal stages of a disease.

A disease or injury may also be described as independent (primary) or dependent (secondary). A **primary disease** occurs independently (by itself), such as a streptococcal sore throat. A **secondary disease** directly results from or depends on another disorder. An example is rheumatic heart disease, which is secondary to rheumatic fever. Both of these conditions are secondary to a streptococcal infection in the throat or tonsils.

The Body's Response to Disease

When gathering data about a client, the examiner looks for evidence of health or illness. **Signs** are *objective evidence* (data) of disease that can be seen or measured, such as a rash, swelling, or change in vital signs. **Symptoms** are *subjective evidence* (data) of disease, sensations that only the client knows and can report, such as pain, itching, nausea, fear, or lightheadedness. During physical assessment of the client, the examiner looks for evidence of change or abnormalities, and asks the client to describe previous signs and symptoms.

TABLE 47-1 𝓡ISK FACTORS FOR DISEASE

Risk Factor	Example/Explanation	Examples of Possible Disease or Disorder
Diet	Excess intake of fatty foods	Cholecystitis (inflammation of the gallbladder); weight gain
	Excess intake of sodium (salt)	Increased incidence of hypertension; edema and/or water retention
	Lack of vitamin C	Scurvy; slow wound healing
	Low intake of protein	Poor wound healing
	Low intake of calcium	Demineralization of bones, increased incidence of osteoporosis and/or fractures
Immobility, lack of exercise	Leg immobilized in a cast because of fracture of the femur	Atrophy (tissue wasting) of leg muscles
	Refusal of client to exercise or move	Increased incidence of pneumonia, constipation, thrombophlebitis, weight gain
	Individual confided to bed rest	Pressure ulcers on bony prominences
Age	Toddler	Accidental poisoning; other accidents
	Older adult	Chronic constipation; risk of falling, increased risk of fractures; increased incidence of chemical dependency, accidental overdose; enlarged prostate; cataracts; osteoporosis
Obesity	Decreased ability to perform usual physical activities	Shortness of breath; muscle atrophy (wasting); increased incidence of hypertension, diabetes mellitus, accidental injuries, coronary artery disease, certain cancers, gallbladder disease
Smoking	Constant irritation of lung tissue from smoke; systemic effects of nicotine	Cancer of the mouth, larynx, bronchi, or lung; peripheral vascular disease; coronary artery disease, hypertension, COPD (emphysema)
Heredity	Genetically transmitted disorders or pre-disposition	Coronary artery disease; diabetes mellitus; hypertension, hemophilia; sickle cell disease
Race	Disorders specific to certain racial groups	Sickle cell disease, Tay-Sachs

To gather health data accurately, it is important to understand normal characteristics and to use correct examination techniques. While determining objective physical findings in the client, the examiner also needs to ask questions to gather subjective information from the client. Together, objective and subjective information help to clarify the client's health problems. Table 47-2 lists common signs and symptoms of illness and disease, with some possible causes.

Inflammation and Infection

One of the most common health problems is **inflammation** (heat, redness, or swelling in an area). Inflammation is the body's response to some type of injury. Inflammation can affect nearly every body tissue, organ, or system. It results from a rush of white blood cells into an area in an attempt to fight off a foreign body, heal an injury, or prevent an infection from developing. **Infection** is the invasion of cells, tissues, or organs by pathogens. Infection is harmful to the body and may result in tissue destruction, tissue or organ dysfunction, or even cellular, tissue, or organ death. An infection is often the cause of inflammation.

Diagnosis of infection is made when microorganisms are identified as present, through microscopic examination of tissues or drainage from the site of inflammation. The suffix -*itis* is used to designate inflammation in a body part (eg, *appendicitis* is inflammation of the appendix, *cholecystitis* is inflammation of the gallbladder, and *tendonitis* is inflammation of a tendon).

An inflammation or infection may be *local* or *generalized*. A local inflammation is confined to one body part, such as an organ or a limb. A generalized infection affects the entire body. The most common signs of local inflammation are redness, swelling or edema, heat, pain, and loss of function of the area. If an infection becomes generalized, the person may also experience some feelings of general discomfort, such as headache, loss of appetite, and general **malaise** (an overall feeling of illness). A generalized infection is more likely to be life threatening than is a localized infection. Inflammation may also be described as *acute, subacute, or chronic.*

In acute inflammation, an excess of fluid and cells (**exudate**) is usually present in or oozing from tissues. Exudates may be clear drainage from a wound (*serum*) or may be

■■■ **TABLE 47-2** *C*OMMON SIGNS AND SYMPTOMS OF DISEASE AND ILLNESS

Sign	Definition	Selected Causes
Anorexia	Loss of appetite; refusal to eat	Infection; gastrointestinal (GI) disorders; mental illness
Cough	Forceful expiratory effort	Abnormal substances in respiratory tract; noxious irritation to the respiratory mucous membranes; cancer
Cyanosis	Bluish discoloration of skin and mucous membranes	Low oxygen levels in the blood; anemia; lung disorders; circulatory disorders
Diarrhea	Frequent, watery stools	GI inflammation or obstruction; medication side effect; fecal impaction
Dyspnea	Shortness of breath; difficult or painful breathing	Low blood oxygen levels due to respiratory disease or obstruction; chemical imbalances; pneumonia
Edema	Swelling of tissues; fluid retention	Circulatory disease; local inflammation or infection; malnutrition; electrolyte imbalance
Emesis	Vomiting	GI inflammation, infection, or obstruction; irritation of GI lining; electrolyte imbalance
Fatigue	Loss of energy	Sleep loss; poor nutrition; inflammation; infection; depression; circulatory disorders
Hemorrhage	Abnormal or unexpected bleeding	Trauma or injury to tissues; nutritional losses; blood clotting disorders
Jaundice	Yellowish discoloration of skin and mucous membranes	Obstruction of bile pathways due to gallstones, inflammation, tumors; liver disorders
Malaise	Generalized discomfort	Infection; biochemical imbalances; diseased organs; emotional difficulties
Pallor	Paleness; loss of normal skin temperature	Acute or chronic blood loss; nutritional deficiencies (iron); hypothermia; panic
Pyrexia (fever)	Fever; elevated body temperature	Inflammation; infection; brain dysfunction

mucoid, such as the discharge from a nasal cold (*coryza*). Exudates may be fibrinous, which causes *adhesions* (abnormal joining of tissues) to form as tissues are repaired. Bloody exudate is the result of small *hemorrhages* (bleeding) in the area. An exudate described as **purulent** contains pus, because of the presence of bacteria. The formation of pus is called **suppuration.** A collection of pus in a localized area is called an **abscess.**

When bacteria grow within an inflammation site, the disorder has become an *infection,* in which pathogens release *toxins* (poisons) that destroy white blood cells and tissues. Tissue death is called **necrosis.** Destroyed tissue may be cast off (**sloughed,** pronounced "sluffed"), leaving behind an area that fills with new tissue (**granulation tissue**). Sometimes a local unhealed area of epithelial tissue is left, called an **ulcer.** A canal or passage leading to an abscess is called a **wound sinus.** An abnormal tubelike passage that connects two internal organs, or connects an internal organ to the surface of the body, is called a **fistula.** A fistula is often difficult to heal, the most common being an anal fistula in the rectal area.

Chronic inflammation persists over a long period of time, often for the remainder of the individual's life, and does not follow the usual healing process. A *subacute inflammation* is midway in severity between acute and chronic. The person may appear to be clinically well. However, laboratory tests, radiologic (x-ray) examinations, or computed tomography (**CT**) scans may diagnose the condition. For example, a person may be a carrier of a disease, such as hepatitis, but may not show any outward symptoms of the disease him- or herself. An *acute infection* is one that heals and leaves no aftermath or other related disorders (**sequelae**).

MEDICAL DIAGNOSIS

The *medical diagnosis* is formulated by the primary healthcare provider, based on both objective observations and subjective data. In the following procedures, the role of the nurse is to assist in this process by gathering as much information as possible about the client and his or her problems. Data gathered by nurses, in combination with the physical examination and specific diagnostic tests, assists in formulating the medical diagnosis. The nurse needs a basic understanding of all these procedures to effectively collect client data.

Laboratory Tests

Laboratory tests are often done as part of the physical examination. Results of these tests are used in planning the client's care. Some laboratory tests are a routine part of screening; others are specific for certain disorders. Many of these tests will be discussed in relationship to disorders of specific body systems throughout the remainder of this book. Appendix C lists commonly accepted normal values for some of the more frequently performed laboratory tests.

Examples of common laboratory tests include urinalysis (**UA**), complete blood count (**CBC**), stool examinations for blood (**guaiac** or **Hemoccult**) or for ova and parasites (**O&P**), and blood tests for specific antibodies, electrolytes, chemicals, or abnormal blood components. Specimens of body fluids may be cultured to isolate pathogens and to determine

the appropriate medication for treatment: culture and sensitivity (**C&S**). Arterial blood gas analysis (**ABG**) or analysis of a sputum specimen can help determine a client's respiratory status. Specific blood tests can help determine damage to heart (cardiac) muscle and other conditions. The client's blood may be typed and crossmatched (**T&X**) for later blood transfusions. Blood or urine may be tested for levels of various drugs (**UTox**), to evaluate situations such as driving under the influence of alcohol or the amount and identification of a drug used in a suicide attempt. It is common to perform a urine pregnancy test (**UPT**) before prescribing certain medications.

Special Types of Diagnostic Procedures

Many diagnostic procedures are done to determine abnormalities or disorders of various body systems. Preparation of the client and results obtained through many of these examinations are discussed throughout this text. Table 47-3 lists common diagnostic tests for several body systems. Some of these are discussed in more detail below.

▪▪▪ TABLE 47-3 *D*IAGNOSTIC TESTS

Type of Test	Purpose	Procedure
Skin Tests		
Biopsy	Identifies tissue abnormalities (often to determine presence of cancer)	Provider surgically removes a portion of tissue.
Intradermal test	Identifies the client's previous exposure to an allergen; controls may be used to determine if client is anergic (unable to formulate antibodies)	Provider or nurse injects an amount of the allergen intradermally and later examines the area to identify changes in color or temperature, or the presence and size of **induration** (hardened tissue). Frequently used to test for tuberculosis or allergies.
Patch or scratch test	Identifies allergies	*Patch:* Filter paper or gauze impregnated with allergen is applied to skin. *Scratch:* Minute amount of allergen is applied to tiny scratch. These tests read similarly to the intradermal test.
Respiratory Tests		
Chest radiograph (x-ray)	Pictures the structures of the chest cavity, particularly the lungs and heart; identifies tissue changes, fluid collection, narrowed airways, collapsed alveolar tissue, enlarged heart	Client has a flat-plate radiograph taken. Dye may be used.
Pulmonary function tests	Measure lung size and airway patency; identify lung volumes and airflow	Client breathes in and out of a measuring device.
Pulse oximetry	Estimates percentage of oxygenated blood flow through a body part	Sensor is attached to the client's finger or earlobe that uses light to determine the amount of oxygen attached to circulating hemoglobin in the blood.
Bronchoscopy	Allows direct visualization of the airways	Flexible fiberoptic scope with a tiny camera is inserted into airways; an image is projected on a viewing screen.
Arterial blood gases (ABG)	Identifies blood levels of oxygen, carbon dioxide, and alkalinity	A sample of arterial blood is withdrawn through arterial puncture.

(continued)

■■ TABLE 47-3 *D*IAGNOSTIC TESTS (CONTINUED)

Type of Test	Purpose	Procedure
Cardiovascular Tests		
Electrocardiogram (ECG)	Graphically records the electrical impulses of cardiac musculature to identify dysrhythmias or tissue damage	Electrodes are attached to the client's chest wall and limbs to record the electrical impulses of the cardiac muscles.
Stress testing	Identifies changes during cardiovascular stress	Client walks on a treadmill or rides stationary bike with ECG, BP, and pulse recording.
Echocardiogram	Measures heart size and thickness; identifies valve function; measures cardiac output	External probe sounds high-frequency sound waves through the chest wall, creating "echoes" that can determine depth and size of tissue.
Angiography	Outlines blood flow through cardiac vasculature to identify blockages or aneurysms	Small catheter is threaded through a vein or artery into the heart vessels; dye is injected and radiographs are taken.
Cardiac catheterization	Measures pressures within heart chambers to determine muscular strength, valve function, cardiac output, and fluid volume	Catheters are threaded through veins or arteries into heart chambers; catheters have devices to measure pressure. Interior of heart and vessels can be visualized via fiberoptics.
Gastrointestinal Tests		
Oral endoscopy	Allows direct visualization of the esophagus, stomach, duodenum	Flexible fiberoptic scope with a tiny camera is inserted into upper GI system through the mouth and projects an image on a screen.
MRI or CT scan	Allows visualization of body tissues through a series of images recorded in layers	Client is positioned in scanner; images are taken through x-rays (CT scan) or computer imaging system (MRI).
Cholangiogram; cholecystogram	Provides radiologic visualization of the gallbladder and common bile duct	Client ingests a dye that localizes in gallbladder and common bile duct; radiographs are taken.
Proctoscopy or colonoscopy	Allows direct visualization of the colon or rectum to identify abnormalities	Flexible fiberoptic scope with a tiny camera is inserted into lower GI system through the rectum and projects an image on a viewing screen.
Barium enema	Allows x-ray visualization of large intestine	Client is given a retention enema containing barium, a radio-opaque substance.

Endoscopy

An **endoscope** is a long, slender, flexible tube with a fiberoptic scope (similar to a TV camera) on the end. The provider passes this tube through a body orifice to examine internal body areas. The use of endoscopes can help determine a client's digestive or respiratory structure and function. Specially trained providers examine areas such as the esophagus (*esophagoscopy*), stomach (*gastroscopy*), large intestine (*colonoscopy*), or rectum (*sigmoidoscopy*). A *bronchoscope* is used to examine the trachea, bronchi, and lungs (*bronchoscopy*). Minor surgical procedures can also be performed via oral or rectal endoscopy. Procedures such as polyp removal and biopsy are common. These procedures do not require an incision.

Endoscopy is also used for surgery and tests of internal areas of the body, via a tiny incision. Abdominal surgery is done using the *laparoscope;* joint surgery uses the *arthroscope.* These procedures are invasive, but much less invasive than traditional incisional surgery. Chapter 97 describes endoscopic surgery in more detail.

Biopsy

If a growth or body tissue appears questionable, a *biopsy* is performed to determine the presence of cancer or other disorders. The provider obtains a piece of tissue or a small amount of fluid and sends it to a laboratory, where it is examined microscopically. A biopsy specimen may be obtained with an endoscope or needle or by making an incision through the skin. A special syringe may also be used to withdraw a specimen. The examiner may obtain a biopsy specimen of a woman's cervix during pelvic examination.

X-ray, Ultrasound, and Other Examinations

Many tests that do not require surgery can yield valuable diagnostic information about the status of the body's internal organs and structures. They include x-ray and fluoroscopy examinations of all body areas (eg, upper and lower gastro-intestinal series, kidney films, or x-ray examinations of bones to determine fractures and other pathology), ultrasonography (ultrasound), CT scan, magnetic resonance imaging (**MRI**), and electroencephalogram (**EEG**). Spirometry and pulmonary function tests help to determine a client's respiratory status. Tests such as the electrocardiogram (**ECG** or **EKG**) and the treadmill stress test help evaluate a client's cardiovascular status. These procedures are for the most part noninvasive, and require no incisions or injections. Some of these procedures, however, require the injection of dye. Some dyes are radio-active. Box 47-1 describes necessary precautions when dye is used.

Lumbar Puncture

A lumbar puncture (**LP**), also called a *spinal tap*, may be done to determine the status of the client's nervous system. Lumbar

➤ ➤ BOX 47-1

PRECAUTIONS WHEN TESTS ARE PERFORMED USING DYE

In any procedure in which a dye is used, a skin test is often done first to determine if the client is sensitive to that dye. Ask if the client is allergic to shellfish or iodine. (If so, notify the physician immediately. *Many dyes contain iodine or similar chemicals.*)

During and for about one-half hour after the test, be alert for signs of *anaphylaxis* (an exaggerated and life-threatening allergic reaction). Nursing assessment includes noting untoward signs such as:

- Restlessness, apprehension, agitation
- Weakness
- Perspiration; cold, clammy skin
- Tingling sensations; numbness
- Sneezing; nose itching
- Rash; generalized pruritus (itching)
- Watery, itchy eyes
- Throbbing in the ears
- Difficult breathing; wheezing; choking sensation; coughing
- Rapid, thready, or irregular pulse; heart palpitations
- Lowered blood pressure
- Swelling or edema
- Flushed skin
- Incontinence
- Seizure or stroke
- Coma

Usually an anaphylactic reaction involves either respiratory or cardiovascular symptoms, but not both. If you observe any of these symptoms, notify the team leader or the physician immediately. Death can result very quickly (within 1 to 2 minutes) if the allergy is severe and if it is not treated at once.

puncture can determine intracranial pressure (within the head and spinal cord) and the presence of abnormal components such as blood or pus in the cerebrospinal fluid, or it can be done to inject drugs or spinal anesthesia. Chapter 77 discusses this test in more detail.

Preparing the Client for Diagnostic Procedures

Clients must completely understand what is to be done. *Informed consent* is required for most procedures. This means that the client has had a full explanation of the test, the reasons for the test, and what to expect during the procedure. The client must have a full knowledge of possible adverse effects of the test as well. Clients who know what to expect are likely to be less apprehensive and more relaxed during the examination. Chapter 4 discusses informed consent in more detail.

When assisting with all tests and examinations, follow Standard Precautions to protect yourself, clients, and other healthcare staff. In areas of high radiation exposure (eg, radiology department), healthcare workers wear lead shields to protect vital organs from overexposure to radiation. (The staff in these areas can instruct you as to specific precautions.) Many diagnostic tests are discussed throughout this book in connection with specific body disorders.

Nursing Responsibilities in Diagnostic Examinations

The nurse has a number of responsibilities before and during special diagnostic examinations. These include assisting the client to maintain NPO (nothing by mouth) status or to eat a special meal before the examination; giving special medications prior to the examination; and reassuring the client and answering questions. The nurse often transports the client to a designated area of the facility for special tests. It is the nurse's responsibility to make sure that the client's chart is up to date before the test; sometimes a special checklist is used. The nurse assists the client to dress properly (usually in a hospital gown) and assures that the client either voids or does not void before the test, as ordered. The nurse often helps to position and drape the client and may remain during the test. In some cases, frequent vital sign monitoring and other special nursing care is required after the test.

THE PHYSICAL EXAMINATION

The *physical examination* is a tool that healthcare providers use to distinguish between normal and abnormal physical characteristics. Each provider, however, has different goals when performing the examination. A physician will look for abnormalities to establish a medical diagnosis, monitor a disease's progression, or evaluate changes in the client's condition. The physician's examination may be extensive and thorough, or it may focus on a particular body area that the client identifies as symptomatic. A physical therapist will examine the client's functional abilities and ability to move, to develop a treatment plan and monitor the client's responses to treatment. A dentist or dental hygienist will examine only the client's mouth structures to identify problems and monitor treatments.

Nurses have several goals when examining clients. The primary purpose is to determine the client's physical condition, to identify potential or actual problems that can be prevented or treated. Because nurses also carefully assess physical, emotional, psychological, developmental, and spiritual aspects, their examination can help determine how a client's physical condition affects overall health and functioning.[1] This information lays the groundwork for nursing diagnosis and then for developing a plan of nursing care to meet client needs.

If a client complains of physical symptoms, the affected body area is examined for signs that might explain the symptoms. For example, if the client complains of constipation and gas pains, the nurse will inspect, palpate, and perhaps *auscultate* (listen to) the abdomen with a stethoscope to search for physical clues about the pain's cause. Another important purpose of the examination is to evaluate the outcomes of nursing and medical treatments, such as the client's response to medications or physical therapy.

Because all nurses collaborate with other healthcare professionals to provide care, each healthcare worker must report and record continuing assessments promptly so that other providers may act as needed. Carefully documented data about physical findings portrays a picture of the client's condition over time.

The goals of the physical assessment performed by nurses are to:

- Distinguish between normal and abnormal
- Identify potential problems
- Promptly report changes and unusual or abnormal findings to the supervising nurse, the client's physician, or other primary healthcare provider
- Deliver client care within the appropriate scope of practice.

Like the physician, nurses examine the client's entire body regularly to determine changes, or may focus on a particular body part when the client has a complaint. For example, if a nurse has many tasks to perform and other clients who require attention, the nurse may examine only the abdomen when the client complains of constipation and discomfort.

Examination Abilities and Techniques

Nursing students work to develop certain abilities and techniques and, with practice, will be able to perform thorough, accurate, and productive client data collection. Effective oral and written communication skills are essential to successfully interview the client and to accurately document findings. Knowledge of the body's normal structure and function (see Unit 4) is crucial so that the examiner understands the relevance of the findings. Objectivity ensures that all examiners approach the physical examination without any previously set expectations.

The healthcare examiner uses five techniques to find information:

- **Observation** is the technique of looking at the client or watching for *general characteristics,* such as overall appearance, skin color, grooming, body posture, gait, mood, interactions with others, and any other factor that does not require closer scrutiny or the use of measurement aids (eg, a stethoscope).
- **Inspection** is careful, close, and detailed visual examination of a body part.
- **Palpation** is feeling body tissues or parts with your hands or fingers.
- **Auscultation** is listening for sounds from within the body, usually with the aid of a stethoscope or using an ultrasound blood-flow detector (Doppler).
- **Percussion** is tapping or striking the fingers against the body; the resulting sounds indicate the place and density of body tissues or organs. Percussion requires a high level of expertise, developed with experience.

☛ KEY CONCEPT

Appendix D lists and describes many descriptive terms used in the documentation of physical findings. Common abbreviations used in documentation are listed in Table 37-3 in Chapter 37.

Examination Tools

Several tools are used during the physical examination. Although the examiner's own eyes, ears, hands, and nose may be the most important tools, the examiner also uses items such as the thermometer, stethoscope, sphygmomanometer, and tongue blade. The client is also asked to perform a number of activities to test the function of the cranial nerves (see In Practice: Nursing Assessment 47-1).

For more complex examinations, primary care providers use an *ophthalmoscope* (instrument to look at the retinas of the eyes through the pupils), an *otoscope* (instrument to examine the ear canals and eardrum), a *tuning fork* (for checking hearing), and a *reflex hammer* (to test reflexes; see In Practice: Nursing Care Guidelines 47-1). A *vaginal speculum* and a *nasal speculum* are other instruments used for specialized examinations. Primary care providers may also use some type of device to test the tactile senses of sharp, soft, hot, or cold, and use substances to test smell and taste. Figure 47-1 shows several instruments used in physical examinations.

Format of the Examination

A common format for the physical examination is the *head-to-toe method.* It begins with a general appearance examination, then moves to the head, and proceeds to the neck, chest, breasts, abdomen, arms, legs, back, and perineum. As the examiner moves to each area, the focus is not only on the *structures,* but also on the *functions* of these body areas. The head-to-toe method flows smoothly and provides the examiner with a mental road map of directions to follow while conducting the examination.

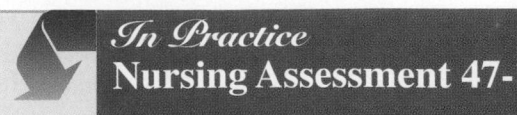

In Practice
Nursing Assessment 47-1

GROSS ASSESSMENT OF CRANIAL NERVE FUNCTION

The gross functioning of most of the cranial nerves can be assessed with simple actions. For example, the examiner asks the client:

Action	Cranial Nerve Involved
To follow a moving finger with the eyes	III Oculomotor
	IV Trochlear
	VI Abducens
To move or clench the jaw	V Mandibular branch of the trigeminal
To smile	VII Facial
To stand with the eyes closed	VIII Vestibular division of the vestibulocochlear
To swallow	IX Glossopharyngeal
To shrug the shoulders and turn the head	XI Accessory
To stick out the tongue and move it from side to side	XII Hypoglossal

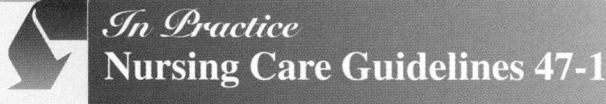

In Practice
Nursing Care Guidelines 47-1

MEASURING REFLEXES

Some reflexes can be observed because they occur spontaneously, such as automatic constriction of the pupil when a light is shined into the eye. Other reflexes must be specifically elicited.

To elicit knee-jerk reflexes:

1. Use a reflex hammer in adults; a finger will work well to elicit most infant reflexes.
2. Hold hammer between thumb and index finger.
3. Position extremity so the tendon is slightly stretched.
4. Have the client relax, or use distraction techniques to assist the client to relax.
5. Strike tendon briskly using a full swinging motion.
6. Repeat this on the other side of the body.
7. Compare results from both sides.
8. Normally, reflexes should be the same on both sides.
9. Reflexes are graded on a 0 to 4+ scale. +2 is considered normal. Above this, reflexes are considered *hyperactive* (very brisk). Below this level, they are considered *hypoactive* (weak) or *absent* (written as "0").
10. Document your findings.
11. Notify the physician or charge nurse with findings that are abnormal or are a change from previous readings.

The other common format used in the physical examination is similar to the head-to-toe, but focuses instead on *body systems:* musculoskeletal, nervous, cardiovascular, respiratory, digestive, and so on. The student will note that this textbook is organized in relationship to body systems.

A variation of this format is the *focused physical examination,* in which one body system is thoroughly examined because the client has a particular complaint or problem in that area. For example, the client admitted to the emergency department complaining of chest pain and severe shortness of breath will have a focused cardiovascular and respiratory examination. The examination of a pregnant woman will focus on her pregnancy and fetus. These several examination formats all have value. Table 47-4 compares the techniques.

Each nurse develops an examination method that is thorough but brief; accurate; and easy to use. This physical examination will include general examination techniques. When the techniques are correct, findings will agree among healthcare providers. The primary healthcare provider is expected to interpret the findings, based on data collected by all members of the team. As the nurse's expertise and knowledge grow, the understanding of the meaning of the findings will grow and develop.

Some healthcare agencies require all nurses to use the same method of data collection and provide documentation data sheets or electronic pages for recording the findings.

The Nursing History

As discussed in Chapter 34, the *nursing history* is the interview in which the nurse asks questions to obtain the client's understanding and perspective on his or her state of health and illness. As the nurse develops his or her examination skills, it will become possible to combine the interview with the examination, to increase efficiency, without sacrificing quality.

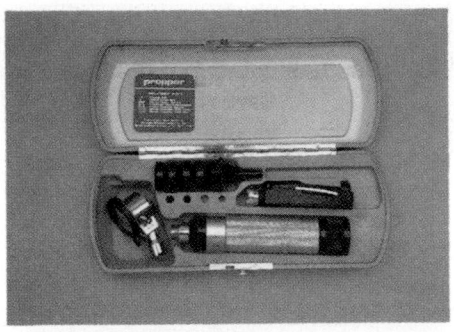

Ophthalmoscope and otoscope set

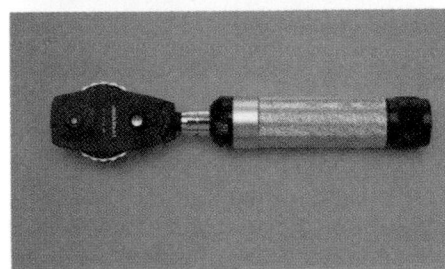

Ophthalmoscope

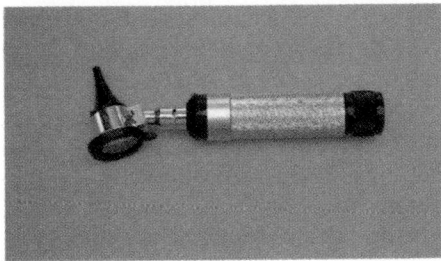

Otoscope

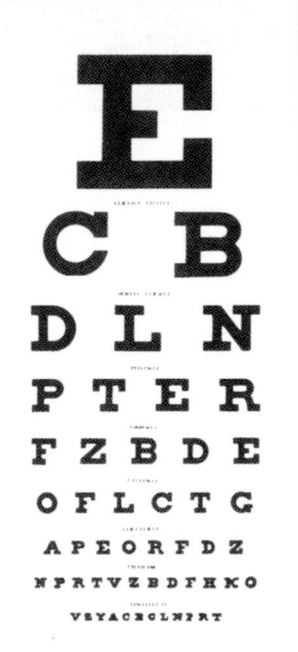

Snellen chart

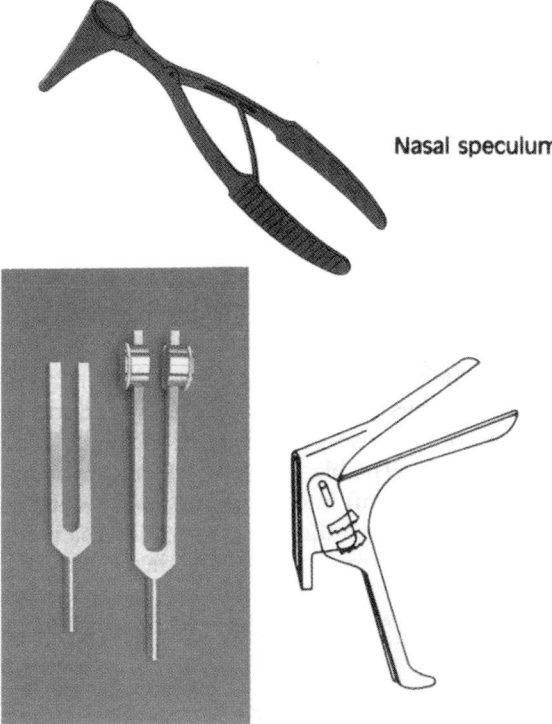

Nasal speculum

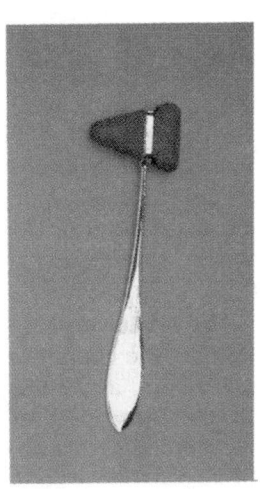

Percussion hammer

Tuning forks

Vaginal speculum

FIGURE 47-1. Instruments healthcare providers commonly use for the physical examination.

■■■ TABLE 47-4 *S*EQUENCE OF MAJOR METHODS OF PHYSICAL EXAMINATION

Adult Head-to-Toe	Infant and Children Head-to-Toe	Systems Approach
General survey	General survey	General survey
Vital signs	Vital signs	Integumentary system
Hair, scalp, cranium, face	Weight	Fluid and electrolyte balance
Eyes and vision	Skin	Musculoskeletal system
Ears and hearing	Heart sounds	Head and neck
Oral cavity	Lung sounds	Extremities
Cranial nerves	Head, scalp, cranium (including measurements)	Nervous system
Thyroid gland	Eyes	Endocrine system
Neck veins and nodes	Oral cavity	Sensory system
Upper extremities	Neck	Cardiovascular system
Nails	Ears	Immune system
Breasts	Musculoskeletal system and reflexes	Respiratory system
Precordium (heart and upper thorax)	Upper extremities	Digestive system
Anterior thorax	Chest and back	Urinary system
Abdomen	Abdomen	Reproductive system
Back	External genitals	
Lower extremities	Lower extremities	
Internal and pelvis		
Anus and rectum		

Preparing for the Physical Examination

Whether a nurse is doing the entire examination or only a portion of it, it is necessary to explain the purpose to the client (Fig. 47-2), answer any questions, and close the door to the room or draw curtains around the bedside to protect the client's privacy. Ask the client to empty the bladder or bowel if necessary. Specific positioning is described in Chapter 48.

Performing the Physical Examination

The following pages contain guidelines and illustrations to help students in performing the head-to-toe assessment of an adult. In addition, special considerations for the physical assessment of the child are presented.

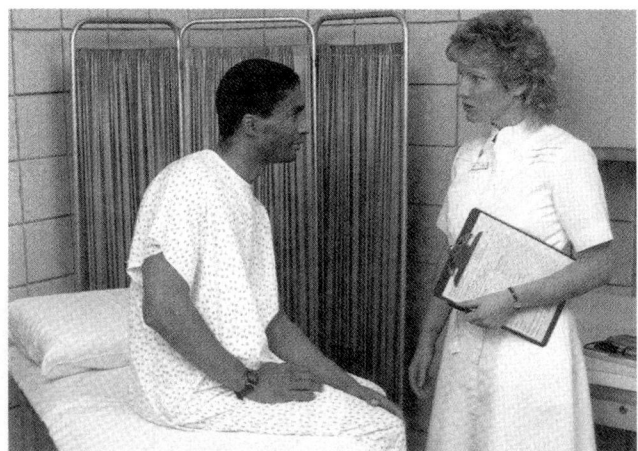

FIGURE 47-2. To begin the examination, introduce yourself and explain your purpose.

➤ STUDENT SYNTHESIS

Key Points

- Healthcare providers perform assessment and physical examination of clients for specific purposes. The primary purposes of nursing assessments are to identify and report abnormal or unusual findings, identify potential problems, and provide needed care measures within the individual nurse's scope of practice.
- Disease is a change in body structure, a definite pathological process. Illness is marked by a pronounced deviation from health: sickness, the individual's response to change in function.
- People who are more likely to develop some diseases may have lifestyle risk factors present such as obesity, smoking, or lack of exercise.
- People may also have a genetic or hereditary predisposition to certain physical disorders or illnesses.
- Diseases are categorized in several ways according to etiology or the effect on the person, such as acute versus chronic illness.
- Inflammation and infection are disease categories that can affect nearly every body system or part.
- Several laboratory and diagnostic tests can help primary healthcare providers to establish medical diagnoses. Nurses need a basic understanding of such procedures, to assist appropriately.
- The healthcare provider performs the physical examination with varying degrees of complexity

and thoroughness, according to the purpose of the examination.

- The most common formats for the physical examination are the head-to-toe examination and the examination done according to body systems.

Critical Thinking Exercises

1. Your client, Mrs. F., is 83 years old and has been residing in a long-term care facility for 2 years because of increasingly disabling arthritis. She requires assistance with her activities of daily living because of weakness, joint stiffness, and pain. She is very alert and interested in many activities around her. On your morning rounds, Mrs. F. tells you that she doesn't feel well, hasn't eaten for 24 hours, and hasn't had a bowel movement for 3 days. Remember that you are to report these concerns to your supervising nurse and document them in the client's health record. What questions can you ask to help clarify the client's problem? What part of the physical assessment examination will help you focus on her problem? What findings will be significant to report and record?

2. Mr. T., 78 years old, has diabetes. His vision has been failing for several years. On your rounds, Mr. T. tells you that he has been having some "tightness" in his chest and is unable to walk to the bathroom without becoming short of breath. What questions can you ask to help clarify his problem? What part of the physical assessment examination will help you focus on his problem? What findings will be significant to report and record?

NCLEX-Style Review Questions

1. The nurse understands the most important use of UTox is to:
   a. Determine if a client is pregnant
   b. Evaluate levels of various drugs in the blood or urine
   c. Study the urine and determine glucose levels
   d. Type and crossmatch for blood transfusion

2. Which of the following assessment data can be indicative of a generalized infection?
   a. Exudate
   b. General malaise
   c. Inflammation
   d. Temperature of 98.6° Fahrenheit

3. Which of the following techniques would be used to detect the presence of edema during the physical examination?
   a. Measure the circumference with a tape measure.
   b. Observe for exudate.
   c. Press finger against suspected edematous area for 10 seconds.
   d. Pull the skin up gently and observe for return to normal position.

4. Which examination technique is most commonly used to examine the lungs?
   a. Auscultation
   b. Inspection
   c. Palpation
   d. Percussion

5. Which of the following formats of examination would be used to evaluate a particular complaint or problem in an area?
   a. Body systems
   b. Function and structure assessment
   c. Head-to-toe method
   d. Focused physical examination

Reference

1. Weber, J., & Kelley, J. (1998). *Health assessment in nursing: Lippincott's learning system* (p. 2). Philadelphia: Lippincott Williams & Wilkins.

◾◾◾ 𝒟ATA COLLECTION IN NURSING

Following are basic guidelines for data collection. These guidelines are not intended to teach the performance of a comprehensive physical examination.

GENERAL EXAMINATION—Assess overall body appearance.

Action/Rationale	Normal Findings	Changes from Normal
The nurse introduces him- or herself and explains what will be done. (*Not all procedures will be performed daily.*)		
Observe the client for signs of distress. (*Alert the primary healthcare provider to immediate concerns. If serious distress is noted, the client may require healthcare interventions before the exam is continued. Chapter 45 describes admission of the client to the healthcare facility.*)		The client shows labored breathing, wheezing, coughing, wincing, sweating, guarding of body part (suggests pain), anxious facial expression, or fidgety movements. (See Chap. 85.)
Observe the client's general appearance: posture, gait, and movement. (*Identify obvious changes.*)	Posture is upright. Gait is smooth and equal for the client's age and development. Limb movements are bilateral.	Posture is stooped or twisted. Limb movements are uneven or unilateral.
Observe the client's facial expression. (*Facial expression suggests mood and mental status and pain.*)	Eyes are alert and in contact with the examiner, as is culturally appropriate. The client smiles or frowns appropriately and has a calm demeanor. The client is able to converse easily. Note if the client needs an interpreter.	Eyes are closed or averted. The client is frowning or grimacing. He or she is unable to answer questions, avoids answering, or is fidgety, and appears anxious. Note if the client does not speak English. (See Chap. 8)
Visually observe the client's height/weight correlation. Height and weight are measured if performing an admission exam (Fig. 47-3). (*Height/weight indicate nutritional status.*) See Chapter 45 for height and weight procedures.	Height and weight are in balance.	Obesity, **emaciation** (physical wasting of tissues), or uneven fat distribution over the client's trunk is observed.
Observe grooming, hygiene, and dress. (*Personal appearance can indicate self-comfort. Identify the client's grooming status, which may suggest his or her ability to perform self-care. The client may have family caregivers who can assist.*)	Clothing reflects gender, age, and climate. Hair, skin, and clothing are clean, groomed, and appropriate for the occasion. Body or mouth odor is absent.	The client wears unusual clothing for gender, age, or climate. Hair is unkempt. Excessive oil or perspiration is on the skin. Body odor is present.
Take vital signs. (*Vital signs provide baseline data.*) See Chap. 46.	Temperature, pulse, respirations, and blood pressure are within normal limits for the client's age.	Abnormal findings include fever, hypothermia, dyspnea, tachypnea, orthopnea, tachycardia, bradycardia, dysrhythmia, hypertension, hypotension, postural hypotension. (See Chap. 46.)

SKIN ASSESSMENT—Assess integumentary structures (skin, hair, nails) and function.

Inspect the backs and palms of the client's hands for skin color (Fig. 47-4). Compare the right and left sides. Make a similar inspection of the feet and toes, comparing the right and left sides. (*Extremities indicate peripheral cardiovascular function.*) See Chap. 80.	Hues range from pale white to deep brown, depending on the client's race and ethnicity. Color variations on dark, pigmented skin may be best seen in the mucous membranes, nail beds, sclera, or lips.	**Erythema,** loss of pigmentation, cyanosis, **pallor,** or jaundice is noted (Table 47-5) (Fig. 47-5).
Palpate the skin over the sternum or forehead for moisture and texture. Pinch and release the skin on the forearm or upper chest (Fig. 47-6). (*Palpation indicates the skin's degree of hydration and* **turgor** *[skin resiliency and plumpness].*)	Plump, firm, elastic skin is slightly moist. Pinched skin that promptly or gently returns to position when released signifies normal turgor. Return to position may be slower in the older person.	The skin is excessively dry or flaking. Moisture, perspiration (*diaphoresis*), or oiliness is noticeable. Pinched skin is very slow to return to normal position. Slow return of skin to normal position often indicates dryness (dehydration).

(continued)

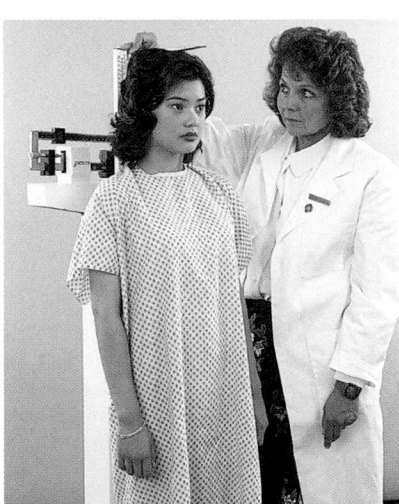

FIGURE 47-3. Use a balance scale for accurate measurement of weight. Height can be measured at the same time.

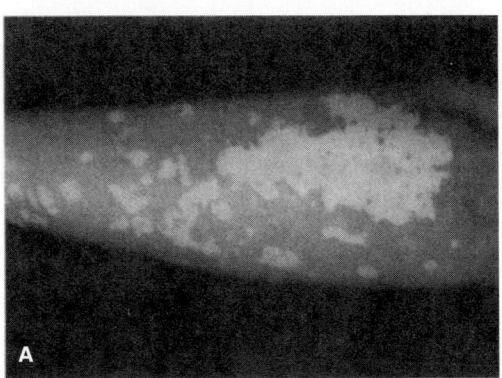

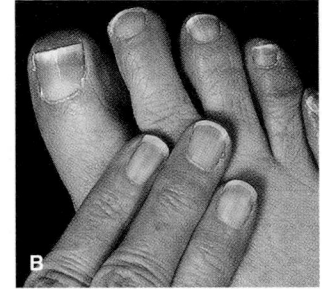

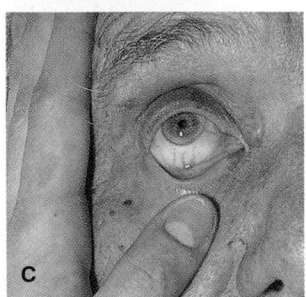

FIGURE 47-5. (**A**) Loss of pigmentation. (**B**) Cyanosis. (**C**) Jaundice.

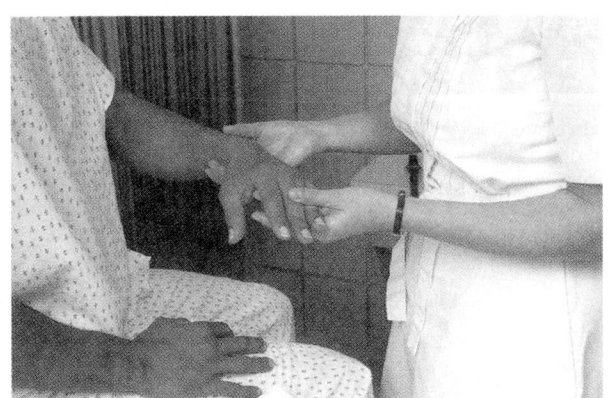

FIGURE 47-4. Inspect the hands and upper arms for skin color and warmth.

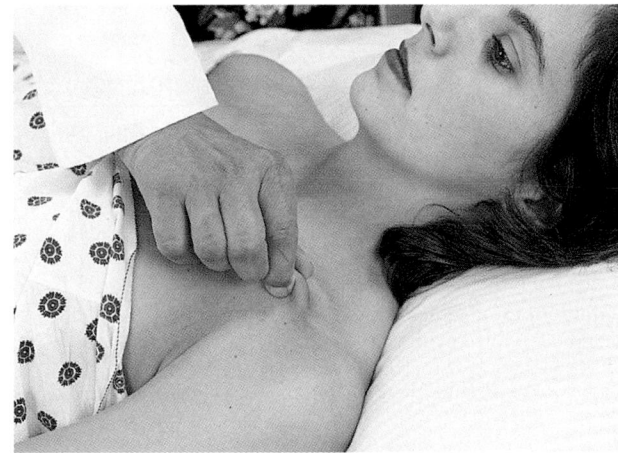

FIGURE 47-6. Check skin **turgor** (tone or fullness) by pinching a fold of skin, releasing it, and watching the skin return to its natural shape. A slow return suggests loss of usual turgor.

𝒟ATA COLLECTION IN NURSING (CONTINUED)

SKIN ASSESSMENT (*Continued*)

Action/Rationale	Normal Findings	Changes from Normal
Palpate the skin's temperature with the back of the hand (Fig. 47-7), particularly noting and examining any reddened areas. Compare the client's left and right hands, arms, and feet (Fig. 47-8). (*Comparison indicates the bilateral status of peripheral circulation.*)	Skin is warm to touch; temperature may vary among body parts. Hands and feet may be cooler than head or trunk. Both hands and arms are the same; both feet are the same.	Skin is very cool or warm to touch; reddened skin areas are warmer than other body parts. Extremities are much cooler, particularly the feet and toes. (Often, cool skin is very pale.) Swelling in the ankles, fingers, or over bony prominences, particularly the sacrum, is noted. (*Edema indicates fluid retention, a sign of circulatory disorders.*) One hand, arm, or foot is noticeably different in temperature from the other.
Inspect and palpate for edema. (See Chap. 75.) Press the fingers against suspected edematous areas for 10 seconds; observe for indentations (Fig. 47-9).	No edema, no abnormal swelling. Skin and tissue return immediately to original shape (no *pitting* [denting] remains.) Skin should resume shape in under 2 seconds.	"Pits" or "dents" remain for more than 2 seconds after pressure is released (*pitting edema*); or edema is obviously present, but skin is shiny and hard and does not dent, even when pressed (*non-pitting edema*).
Press against the nail tip until the flesh under the nail *blanches* (loses color). Release pressure quickly (Fig. 47-10). (*Check capillary refill, an indicator of peripheral vascular function.*) Inspect nails for abnormalities and cleanliness.	Color returns immediately (under 3 seconds) when pressure is released. Nails should have no discoloration, ridges, pitting, thickening, or separation from the base.	Color returns to nail slowly. Client's nails are dirty, broken, or torn. Chewed or torn cuticles. *Clubbing* of fingertips (bulb-type shape on ends of fingers) (Fig. 47-11).

TABLE 47-5 𝒮KIN COLOR VARIATIONS

Color	Possible Cause	Changes in Dark-Skinned Person
Redness called **erythema**	Dilation of superficial blood vessels due to exposure to heat, increased body temperature, local inflammation.	Skin color darkens; may appear purple. Often the skin is also warmer than other body areas; compare temperature with another body area.
Gray-blue around mucous membranes, nail beds, called **cyanosis** (see Fig. 47-5B)	Constriction of superficial blood vessels due to exposure to cold, lowered body temperature; may result from low oxygen levels in blood (**hypoxemia**) due to heart or respiratory disease. Abnormal hemoglobin levels may be due to genetic disorders.	Color loss appears with tinges of blue or deepened color in mucous membranes of mouth and nail beds.
Loss of color or **pallor**	Vasoconstriction due to lower body temperature; shock from loss of blood volume; decreased amount of hemoglobin in blood causing anemia.	Skin appears gray or ashen, particularly in palms or soles or around mouth.
Yellow called **jaundice** (see Fig. 47-5C)	Destruction of red blood cells releasing bilirubin into skin; liver or kidney disease.	Sclera of eyes are yellow; color changes in nail beds or palms.

(continued)

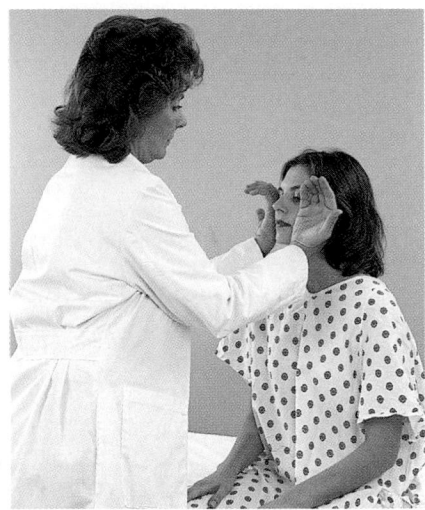

FIGURE 47-7. Palpate the client's skin temperature with the back of your hands.

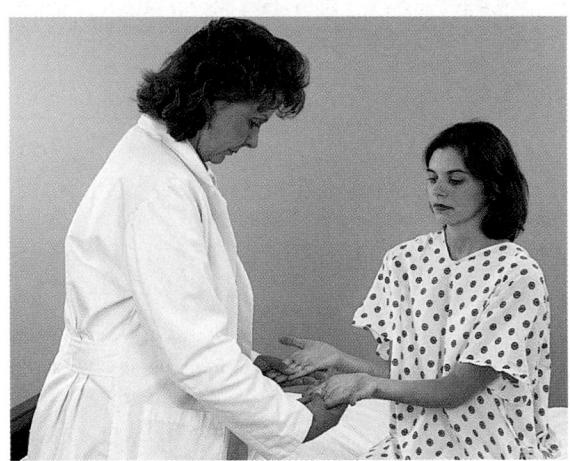

FIGURE 47-8. Compare the client's palms for bilateral status of peripheral circulation.

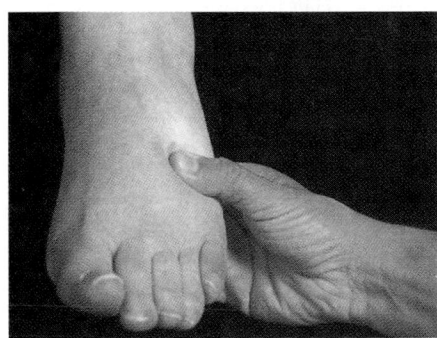

FIGURE 47-9. Gently press against the skin over bony areas of the body, such as the feet and ankles, to determine the presence of edema. In *pitting edema,* a dent will remain after release of pressure.

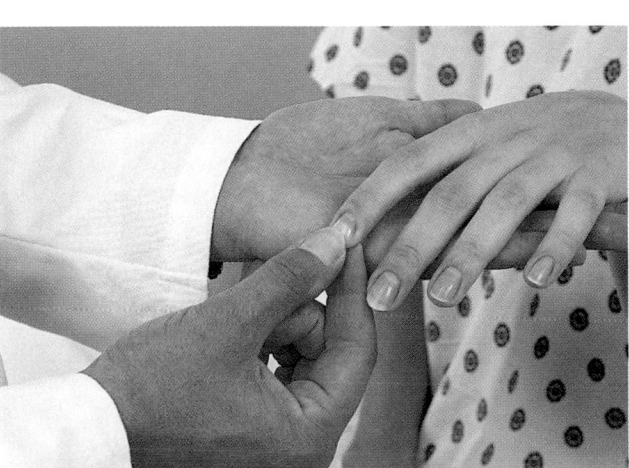

FIGURE 47-10. Check capillary refill by pressing against the nail beds, releasing, and monitoring return of color. (It should return immediately.)

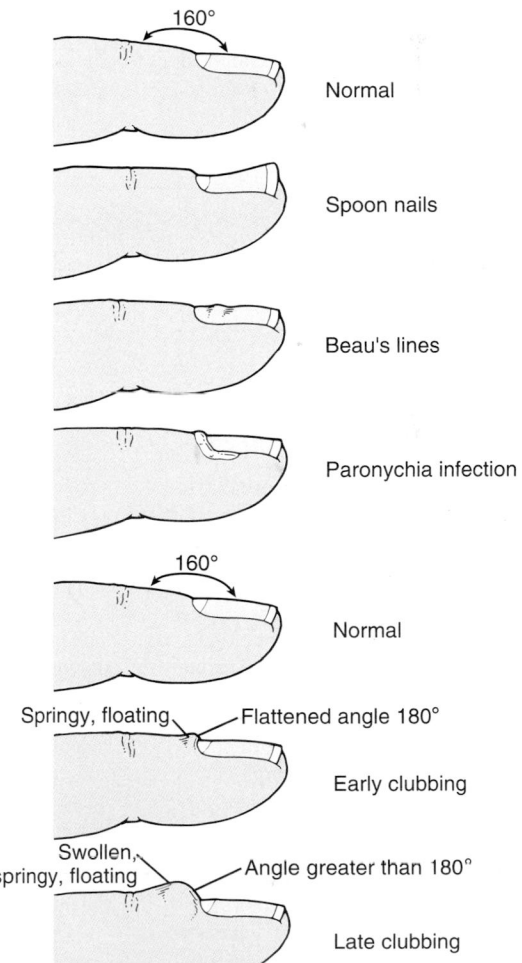

FIGURE 47-11. Normal and abnormal fingernails.

▪▪▪ 𝒟ATA COLLECTION IN NURSING (CONTINUED)

SKIN ASSESSMENT (Continued)

Action/Rationale	Normal Findings	Changes from Normal
Inspect the skin for lesions throughout the remainder of the exam. Note the appearance, size, and location of lesions, and the presence and appearance of any drainage. *(Locate abnormal growths or trauma that suggest abnormal physiologic processes.)* For PPD (TB) skin tests given 48 or 72 hours previously: measure **induration** (swelling) and record. Follow agency protocols.	Skin is intact, without reddened areas but with variations in pigmentation and texture, depending on the area's location and its exposure to light and pressure. (Freckles and moles are normal.)	Abnormal findings include erythema and **ecchymosis** (bruising or discoloration of the skin). Lesions include rashes, **macules, papules, vesicles, wheals, nodules, pustules, tumors,** warts, or **ulcers** (Table 47-6, Fig. 47-12, 13, 14). Wounds include incisions, abrasions, lacerations, pressure ulcers (*decubitus ulcers*) (Fig. 47-15). Exudates from open wounds are present; they may be **serous** (contain clear fluid), **purulent** (contain pus), bloody, or **serosanguineous** (contain bloody and serous fluid). Changes in the size or color of moles and warts may be detected as compared with previous examinations. Malignant melanoma (Fig. 47-16) is a life-threatening skin lesion. Chapter 74 discusses skin disorders.
Inspect the hair for texture, uniform growth and distribution, and scalp lesions (Fig. 47-17). *(Identify abnormalities.)*	Texture varies from fine to coarse; hair should appear glossy with bilateral growth and distribution.	Hair is excessively dry or oily. The client has unilateral or excessive hair loss (Fig. 47-18), dull sheen to the hair, excessive scalp scaliness, or raised lesions. There is evidence of lice (*pediculosis*) or another disorder.

HEAD AND NECK ASSESSMENT—Assess central neurologic function, vision, hearing, and mouth structures.

Observe the face and head for size, shape, and symmetry.	The head is symmetrical, round, and erect in the midline. The eyes, nose, mouth, and ears are symmetrical.	The skull is enlarged or irregularly shaped. Eyes, ears, or mouth are asymmetrical. One side of the face droops or sags abnormally. Unilateral eye drooping (*ptosis*).
Observe the client's ability to respond to verbal commands. *(Responses indicate the client's speech and **cognitive function**—ability to think: the intellectual process by which one becomes aware of, perceives, or comprehends ideas.)*	The client responds appropriately to commands.	The client has confused, disoriented, or inappropriate responses.
Observe the client's level of consciousness **(LOC)**—degree of wakefulness, stages of response to stimuli; and orientation. Ask the client to state his or her own name, current location, and the approximate day, month, or year. Ask who the president of the United States is. (This is orientation to person, place, and surroundings.) *(Responses indicate the client's brain function. LOC is the degree of awareness to environmental stimuli. It varies from full wakefulness and alertness to coma. Orientation is a measure of cognitive function or the ability to think and reason.)* Evaluation of LOC is discussed in further detail in Chapters 43 and 47.	The client is fully awake and alert: eyes are open and follow people or objects. The client is attentive to questions, and responds promptly and accurately to commands; he or she moves willingly. If the client has been sleeping, he or she responds to verbal or physical stimuli, and demonstrates wakefulness and alertness. The client is aware of who he or she is (orientation to person), where he or she is (orientation to place), when it is (orientation to time), and who the president is (orientation to surroundings).	Client has a lowered LOC and shows irritability, short attention span, or dulled perceptions. Client is uncooperative or unable to follow simple commands or answer simple questions. At a lowered LOC, he or she may respond to physical stimuli only (such as deep pain). The lowest extreme is coma, when the eyes are closed and the client fails to respond to verbal or physical stimuli, with no voluntary movements. If LOC is below full awareness but above coma, objectively note the client's eye movements, response to commands, and type of movement: voluntary, withdrawal to stimuli, or withdrawal to noxious stimuli (pain) only.

(continued)

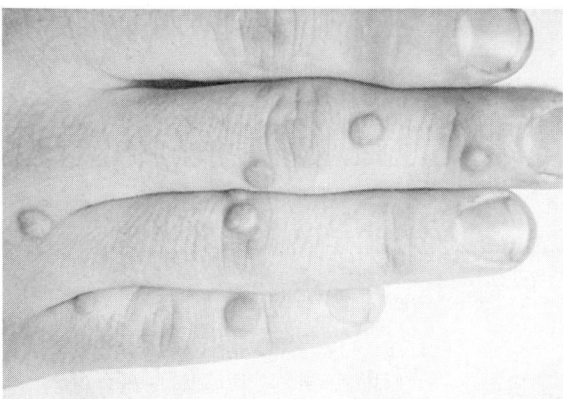

FIGURE 47-12. Warts (a papule).

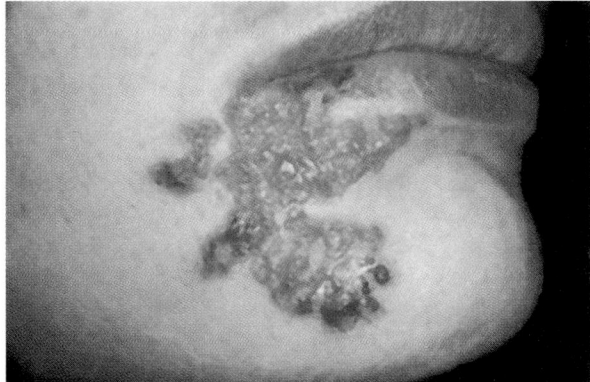

FIGURE 47-13. Herpes simplex (a vesicle).

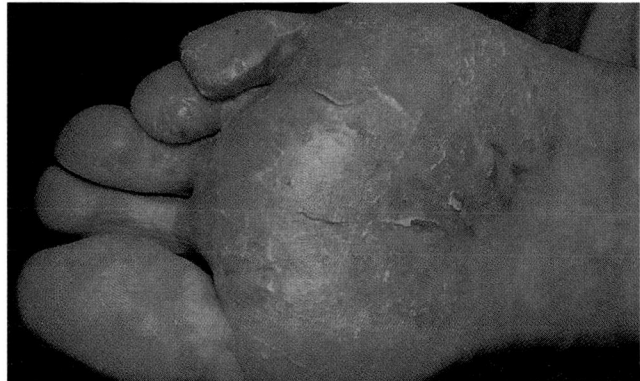

FIGURE 47-14. Athlete's foot (tinea pedis).

Granulation tissue   Epithelial edge

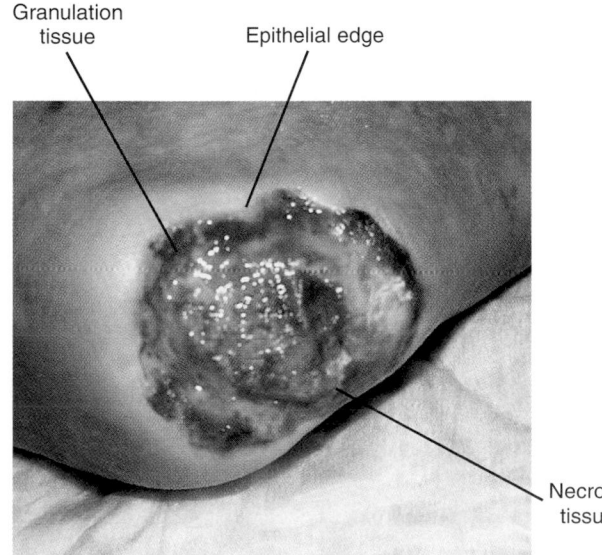

Necrotic tissue

FIGURE 47-15. Pressure ulcer.

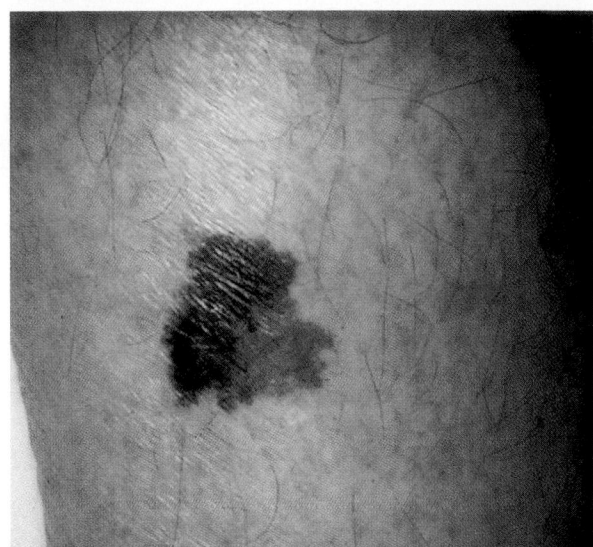

FIGURE 47-16. Malignant melanoma.

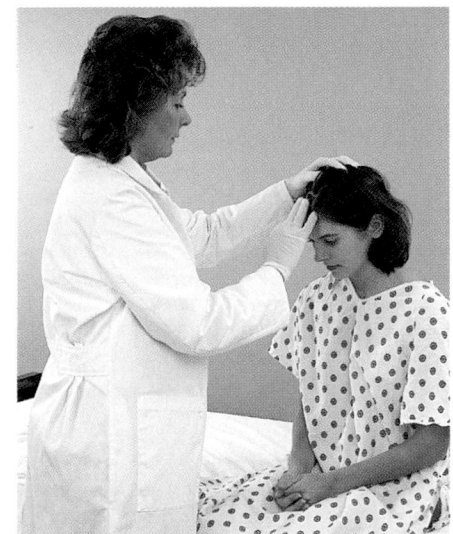

FIGURE 47-17. Inspect the client's hair and scalp.

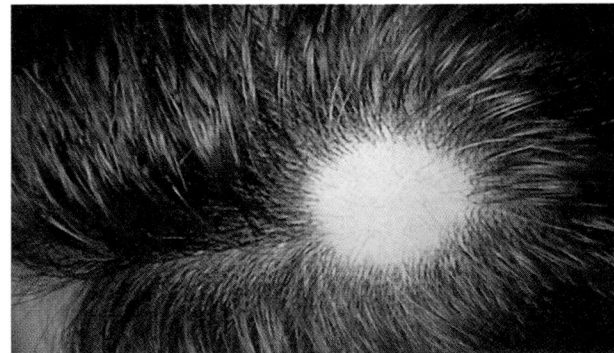

FIGURE 47-18. Excessive hair loss (not the same as male pattern baldness).

■■■ DATA COLLECTION IN NURSING (CONTINUED)

HEAD AND NECK ASSESSMENT (Continued)

Action/Rationale	Normal Findings	Changes from Normal
Observe the client's ability to think, remember, process information, and communicate. (These processes indicate cognitive functioning.)	The client is able to follow commands and repeat and remember information. He or she is able to see and identify objects within the room.	Abnormal findings include **dysphasia** (difficulty in understanding or expressing language), dysarthria (inability to speak), memory loss, disorientation, or hallucinations. The client may also be voluntarily mute (in psychiatry). Dysphasia is discussed further in Chapter 80.
Observe the client's ability to see, hear, smell, and distinguish tactile sensations. Inspect the eyes, ears, and nose. Check for symmetry and intactness of the eyes, ears, and nose. Special hearing and vision tests may be performed by the primary provider. (These tests indicate the functional status of the client's vision, hearing, smell, and tactile sensation.)	The client can hear even though the speaker turns away. He or she identifies objects or reads a clock in the room, and distinguishes between sharp and soft objects. The nose is centered; the ears are symmetrical on the sides of the head. The eyes are moist and symmetrical; the lids open and close on command.	The client cannot hear low tones and must look directly at the speaker to distinguish what is being said. He or she cannot read a clock or distinguish sharp from soft. Eyes, ears, nose, or mouth are asymmetrically placed. Redness or swelling appears around the eyelids or eyes. Excessive tears, **exudate** (abnormal drainage from eyes or ears), or **conjunctivitis** (redness of eyes) is present. Sensory disorders are discussed in Chapter 79.
Inspect and compare the pupils for size, shape, response to light, and ability to focus (accommodation) (Figs. 47-19 and 47-20). Check eye coordination. (Pupillary size, shape, and accommodation are an indicator of the status of brain function and intracranial pressure. Coordination of eye movements indicates brain function and muscular attachments to eyes.)	Pupils are equal, round, and responsive to light, and are able to see objects both near and far away (**accommodation**). Eyes move together to view objects (coordination). This examination is abbreviated as PERRLA + C:	Pupils are unequal and/or unresponsive or sluggishly responsive to light. **Strabismus** ("cross-eyes" or "wall-eyes") present, or eye movements asymmetrical. Client reports **diplopia** (double vision) or blurring of vision. Eyelids are drooping (ptosis) or have asymmetrical movements.
Ask client to open the mouth and say "aah." With gloved hands, insert a tongue blade to open the lips. Inspect inside the mouth. Check the lips, mouth, teeth, gums, and tongue (Fig. 47-21). (Identify abnormalities of these structures.)	Lips are smooth. Oral mucous membranes are pink, moist, and smooth. Teeth are firm, intact, and clean. The tongue is pink, moist, and symmetrical.	Lips are dry and cracked. Mucous membranes show abnormal color changes: pallor, cyanosis, jaundice. Lumps or ulcerations are visible in the mucous membrane. Teeth are loose or absent; gums are receding or bleeding. Halitosis (bad breath) is present. Client shows involuntary tongue or mouth movement.

MUSCULOSKELETAL ASSESSMENT—Assess muscles, joints, body movement, and neuromuscular function.

Action/Rationale	Normal Findings	Changes from Normal
Watch while the client rotates the upper body laterally and back to the midline, leans forward, and then leans backward. (These movements demonstrate the lumbar spine's range of motion.)	Client rotates the upper body approximately 90° and freely moves the body forward and backward.	Client reports pain or exhibits limitation in rotation, flexion, or extension. Abnormal spinal curvatures are evident. Range of motion is discussed in Chapters 18 and 48.

(continued)

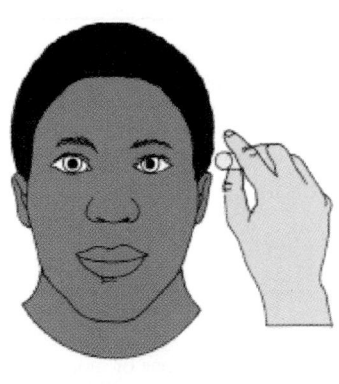

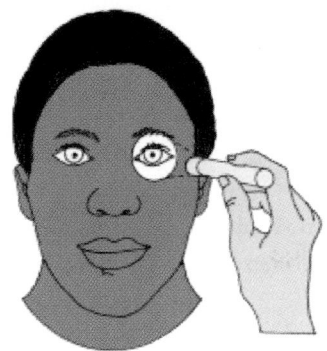

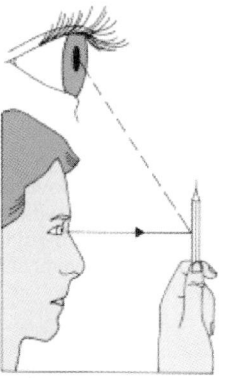

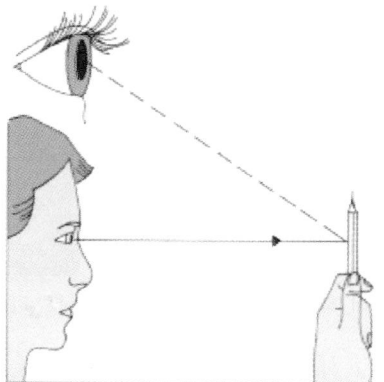

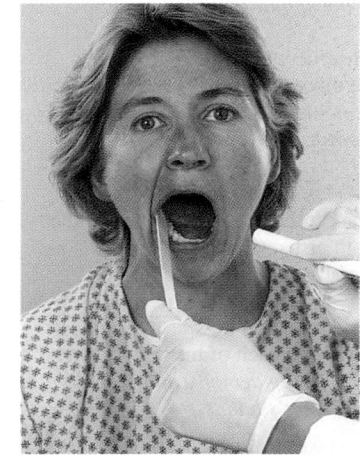

FIGURE 47-19. Monitor the client's pupils for equality of size and reaction to light. To test for reaction to light, a pen light is moved quickly from the side to shine on the client's pupil. The pupil should quickly constrict.

FIGURE 47-20. Check for ability to focus the eyes (**accommodation**).

FIGURE 47-21. Wear clean gloves when inspecting the mouth.

■■■ **TABLE 47-6** 𝒫RIMARY SKIN LESIONS

Lesion	Description	Example
Macule	Small (<1 cm in diameter); well-defined border; flat and nonpalpable on skin surface; no color change	Freckle, some skin rashes
Papule	Small (<0.5 cm diameter); palpable; elevated solid tissue	Mole, wart (see Fig. 47-12)
Wheal	Slightly irregular in shape; transient superficial elevated area of localized edema	Hive, insect bite
Vesicle	Small (<0.5 cm diameter); well-defined border; elevated cavity filled with serous fluid	Blister, chickenpox, herpes simplex (see Fig. 47-13)
Pustule	Well defined border; elevated superficial cavity filled with pus	Acne lesion, impetigo
Fissure	Linear crack in skin	Chapped lips, fungal infection such as athlete's foot (see Fig. 47-14)
Ulcer	Loss of top layers of skin tissue	Pressure ulcer (decubitus ulcer) (see Fig. 47-15)
Nodule	Small (<2 cm diameter); well-defined border; palpable elevated mass	Fatty tumor (**lipoma**), localized scar tissue, cyst
Tumor	Over 1–2 cm in diameter; irregular border; palpable elevated mass	Larger lipoma or malignancy (see Fig. 47-16)

Source: Weber, J., & Kelley, J. (1998). *Health assessment in nursing: Lippincott's learning system* (pp. 140–143). Philadelphia: Lippincott-Raven.

∫PECIAL ASSESSMENT CONSIDERATION FOR CHILDREN (CONTINUED)

MUSCULOSKELETAL ASSESSMENT

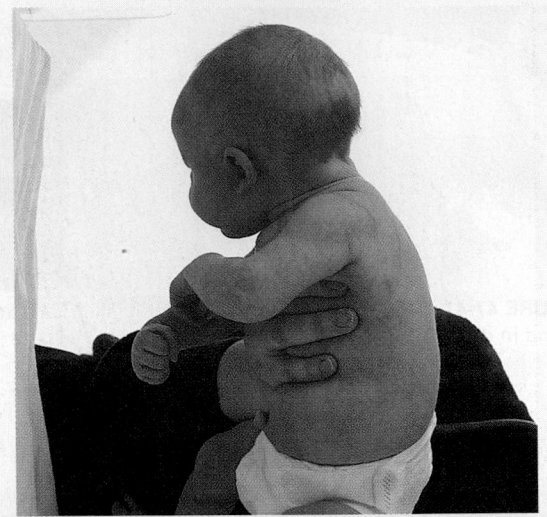

FIGURE 47-45. Infants younger than 3 months of age have rounded spines.

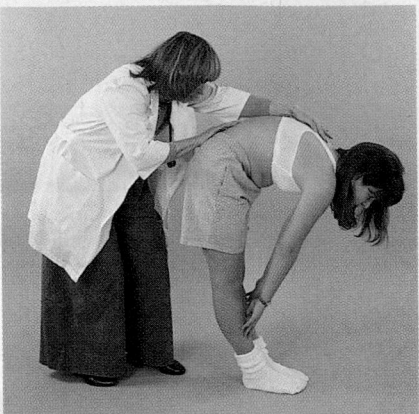

FIGURE 47-46. An important musculoskeletal examination for pre-adolescents and adolescents is checking the spine for **scoliosis** (s-shaped curvature).

ASSESSMENT OF CHEST, ABDOMEN, AND PELVIS

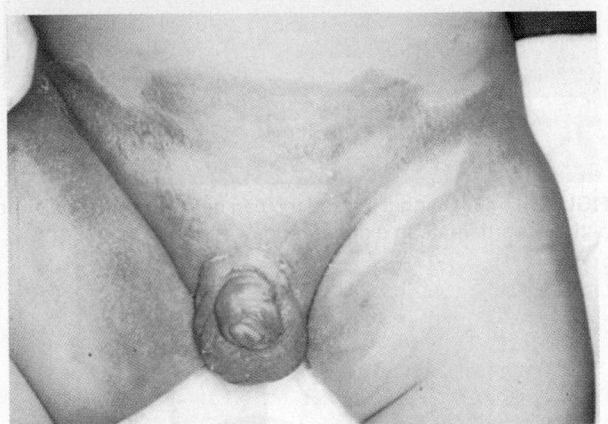

FIGURE 47-47. Diaper rash in infants is common, but must be treated.

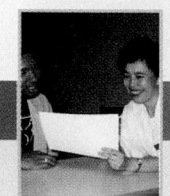

48

Body Mechanics and Positioning

LEARNING OBJECTIVES

1. State the three principles underlying proper body mechanics and relate a nursing consideration for each.
2. In the skills lab, demonstrate safe, comfortable, and appropriate positioning for clients in bed.
3. State the purposes of range of motion exercises.
4. Define and demonstrate the following movements: abduction, adduction, circumduction, flexion, extension, rotation, pronation, and supination.
5. In the skills lab, demonstrate the ability to perform passive range of motion exercises and to supervise active range of motion exercises.
6. Identify at least three principles related to safe movement of clients in and out of bed.
7. In the skills lab, demonstrate the ability to move a partially mobile client safely from bed to chair and back.
8. In the skills lab, demonstrate the ability to use the wheeled stretcher (litter, gurney) safely.
9. In the skills lab, demonstrate the ability to teach each of the crutch-walking gaits to a client. Practice each gait.
10. Demonstrate and practice going up and down stairs with crutches.
11. Describe the types of client reminder devices; state the precautions and nursing care for each; identify the regulations and documentation for each; and state when each is used. Differentiate between client reminder devices and leather safety devices.
12. In the skills lab, demonstrate moving a partially or totally immobile client safely up in bed or to the side of the bed.
13. In the skills lab, demonstrate moving a partially or totally immobile client safely to a chair.
14. State at least six client positions commonly used for examinations and treatments. In the skills lab, demonstrate the ability to position a client safely into each of these positions.

NEW TERMINOLOGY

base of support
body mechanics
center of gravity
circumduction
client reminder device
contracture
contralateral
dangling
dorsal lithotomy
eversion
footdrop
Fowler's position
gait
gait belt
gravital plane
gurney
hemiplegia

inversion
isometric
line of gravity
litter
logroll turn
paralysis
paraplegia
pronation
prone
protective device
recumbent
rotation
transfer belt
transfer board
Sims' position
supination

ACRONYMS

| AROM | OOB | ROM |
| CPM | PROM | |

Nurses often need to teach clients the use of proper body mechanics for safe walking and movement. First, however, the nurse needs to understand and to practice proper body mechanics. People (clients and nurses alike) differ in weight, size, and ability to move. The nurse's physical strength is not as important as how efficiently he or she uses the body. Ultimately, efficient use of one's body will determine how effectively and safely the nurse is able to move clients. It is important to provide safety for both the nurse and the client.

PROPER BODY MECHANICS

Use of the safest and most efficient methods of moving and lifting is called **body mechanics.** This means *applying mechanical principles of movement to the human body.*

Principles of Body Mechanics

The laws of physics govern all movement. From these laws we derive the general principles of body mechanics (Box 48-1). In other words, some ways of moving and carrying objects are more effective than others.

Principles underlying proper body mechanics involve three major factors: center of gravity, base of support, and line of gravity (Fig. 48-1).

Center of Gravity

A person's **center of gravity** is located in the pelvic area. This means that approximately half the body weight is distributed above this area, half below it, when thinking of the body divided horizontally. In addition, half the body weight is to each side, when thinking of the body divided vertically. When lifting an object, bend at the knees and hips, and keep the back straight. By doing so, the center of gravity remains over the feet, giving extra stability. It is thus easier to maintain balance (Fig. 48-2).

> ➤➤ BOX 48-1

BASIC PRINCIPLES OF BODY MECHANICS

1. It is easier to *pull, push,* or *roll* an object than it is to lift it. The movement should be smooth and continuous, rather than jerky.
2. Often less energy or force is required to keep an object moving than it is to start and stop it.
3. It takes less effort to lift an object if the nurse works as close to it as possible. Use the strong leg and arm muscles as much as possible. Use back muscles, which are not as strong, as little as possible. Avoid reaching.
4. The nurse rocks backward or forward on the feet and with his or her body as a force for pulling or pushing.

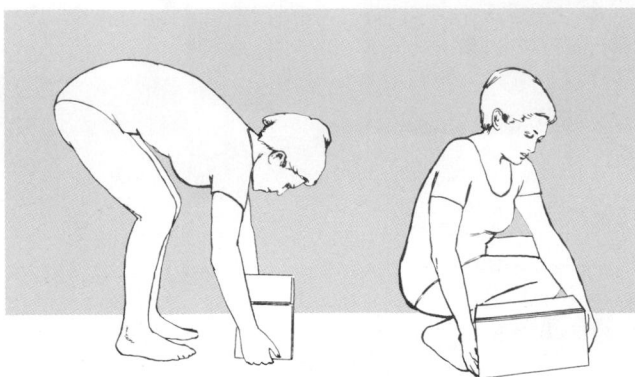

FIGURE 48-1. *Left,* Poor position for lifting. Pull is exerted on the back muscles, and leaning causes the line of gravity to fall outside the base of support. *Right,* Good position for lifting, using the long, strong muscles of the arms and legs and holding the object so that the line of gravity falls within the base of support.

Base of Support

A person's feet provide the **base of support.** The wider the base of support, the more stable the object, within limits. (The nurse's feet must not be too wide apart, as this would cause instability.) The feet are spread sidewise when lifting, to give side-to-side stability. One foot is placed slightly in front of the other for back-to-front stability. The weight is distributed evenly between both feet. The knees are flexed slightly, to absorb jolts. The feet are moved to turn the object being moved. (It is important not to twist the body.)

Line of Gravity

Draw an imaginary vertical (up and down) line through the top of the head, the center of gravity, and the base of support. This becomes the **line of gravity,** or the **gravital plane.** This is the direction of gravitational pull (from the top of the head to the feet). For highest efficiency, this line should be straight from the top of the head to the base of support, with equal weight on each side. Therefore, if a person stands with the back straight and the head erect, the line of gravity will be

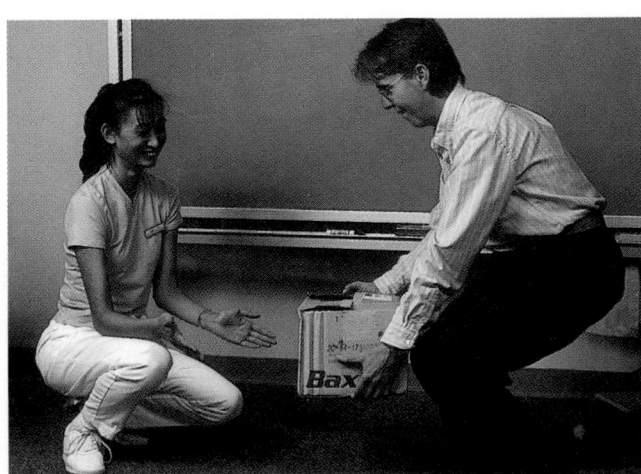

FIGURE 48-2. The nurse instructs a client on proper lifting techniques by using the body's center of gravity, located in the midpelvis, to prevent injury and back strain.

approximately through the center of the body, and proper body mechanics will be in place.

Body Alignment

When lifting, walking, or performing any body activity, proper *body alignment* is essential to maintain balance. When a person's body is in correct alignment, all the muscles work together for the safest and most efficient movement, without muscle strain. Stretching the body as tall as possible produces proper alignment. This can be accomplished through proper posture. When standing, the weight is slightly forward and is supported on the outside part of the feet. Again, the head is erect, the back is straight, and the abdomen is in. (Remember that the client in bed should be in approximately the same position as if he or she were standing.)

POSITIONING THE CLIENT

Encouraging clients to move in bed, get out of bed, or walk serves several positive purposes. Clients may be reluctant to move, or may stay in bed unnecessarily. This immobility can cause a number of disorders, among which are pressure ulcers, constipation, muscle weakness, pneumonia, and joint deformities. By assisting clients to maintain or to regain mobility, you promote self-care practices and help to prevent deformities.

Body Mechanics in Client Positioning

It is important to practice good body mechanics when lifting and moving clients. In this way, the nurse prevents injury to himself or herself and to the client.

Moving and Positioning Clients

As stated before, there are many reasons to change the client's position. These include promoting comfort, restoring body function, preventing deformities, relieving pressure, preventing muscle strain, stimulating proper respiration and circulation, and giving nursing treatments. In Practice: Nursing Care Guidelines 48-1 gives tips on positioning clients for their maximum comfort.

It is important to explain to the client why his or her position is being changed and how it will be done. The client's understanding is important because he or she will be more likely to maintain the new position. If he or she can help, explain how. The client's assistance will save strain on the nurse, and will give the person some exercise; increase independence, self-esteem, and a feeling that he or she is helping; and instill a feeling of control.

Sometimes turning the client is such an important part of treatment that the physician specifies how often to do it. This consideration is especially important for older or immobile clients. Some conditions do not permit turning the client, such as fractures that require traction appliances. In other conditions, such as spinal injuries, turning may be harmful.

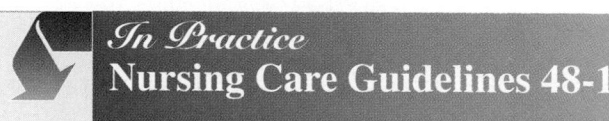

In Practice
Nursing Care Guidelines 48-1

POSITIONING THE CLIENT FOR COMFORT
- Maintain functional client body alignment. (Alignment is similar whether the client is standing or in bed.)
- Maintain client safety.
- Reassure the client to promote comfort and cooperation.
- Properly handle the client's body to prevent pain or injury.
- Follow proper body mechanics.
- Obtain assistance, if needed, to move heavy or immobile clients.
- Follow specific physician's orders.
- An order is needed for a client to be out of bed.
- Do not use special devices (eg, splints, traction) unless ordered.

In some cases, the client is turned only to wash or rub the back or to change the bed. In other cases, the client cannot be turned at all. In this case, the nurse can rub the client's back by asking him or her to pull up slightly on the overhead trapeze. In this way, the client's back is off the bed. The nurse can then gently massage the back with his or her hand held flat. *Rationale: Gentle massage stimulates skin circulation and helps to prevent skin breakdown.*

Most often, clients who cannot turn are placed in a special bed. One of these beds is discussed and pictured in Chapter 49. It operates to relieve pressure and provide back support. In some cases, the client who cannot turn is placed in a *circle bed* (which rotates the client head-to-toe) or a *Stryker frame* (which rotates the client side-to-side). However, with today's methods of immobilization of fractures, these types of beds are not often used.

Turning and Moving Clients

Clients may be able to help move themselves if the nurse explains what will happen and how the client might assist. Be sure to request help from another person if the client is heavy or if you are unsure that you can move a person by yourself.

Turning the Client to a Side-Lying Position
Proper body alignment is always important when turning a client to the side. When a person is to remain in the side-lying position for a long period, he or she is turned in the same manner as if the position were temporary (for example, to receive a backrub). Then, the client is propped into the new position. In Practice: Nursing Procedure 48-1 gives the steps in turning the client to a side-lying position.

In an alternative side-lying position (*modified Sims' position*), the client is asked to bend the knees more (see Box 48-2).

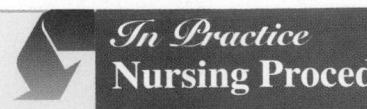

In Practice
Nursing Procedure 48-1

TURNING THE CLIENT TO A SIDE-LYING POSITION
Supplies and Equipment

Pillows
Side rails
Cotton blanket or towels, rolled for support

Steps

1. Wash your hands.
   RATIONALE: *Prevent the spread of infection.*

2. Explain the procedure to the client.
   RATIONALE: *Providing information fosters the client's cooperation and understanding.*

3. Adjust the bed to a comfortable height.
   RATIONALE: *Bed at proper height prevents back strain.*

4. Lower the client's head to as flat a position as he or she can tolerate, and lower the side rail.
   RATIONALE: *A flat bed eliminates the need to pull against gravity.*

5. Move the client to the far side of the bed. Raise the side rail.
   RATIONALE: *Positioning the client near the far side allows adequate room to turn. Raised side rails keep the client safe.*

6. Ask the client to reach for the side rail.

7. Assume a broad stance, tensing your abdominal and gluteal muscles. Roll the client toward you.
   RATIONALE: *This action provides a wide base of support and enables you to use large muscle masses to move the client.*

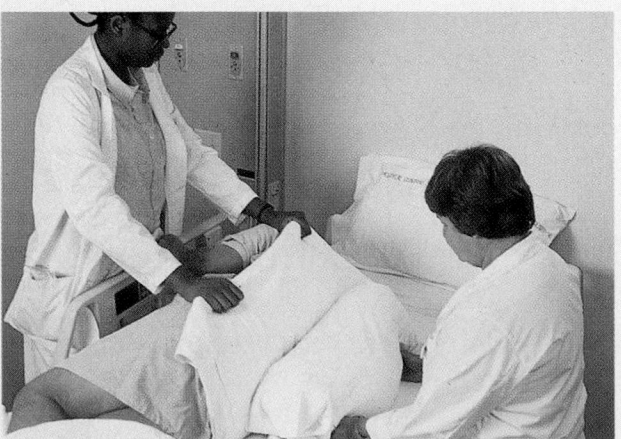

Rolling the client toward you. (Note the client is grasping the siderail).

8. Position the client's legs comfortably.
   RATIONALE: *Prevent strain on the hip joint and minimize pressure on bony prominences.*

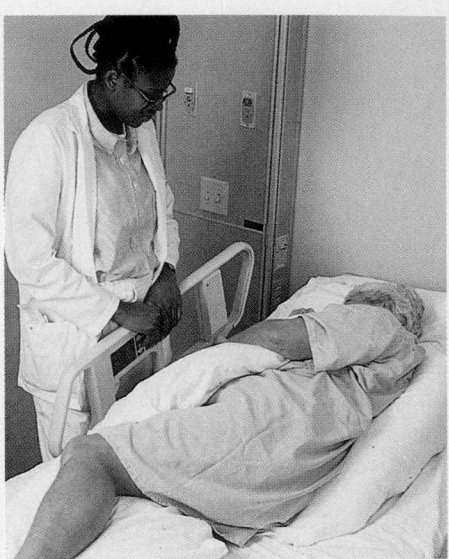

Positioning the client's leg and supporting the client's back.

   a. Flex his or her lower knee and hip slightly.

   b. Bring his or her upper leg forward and place a pillow between the legs.

9. Adjust the client's arms.
   RATIONALE: *Support the client's upper body and prevent pressure on bony prominences:*

   a. Shift his or her lower shoulder toward you slightly.

   b. Support his or her upper arm on a pillow.

10. Wedge a pillow behind the client's back. Use rolled blankets or towels as needed for support.
    RATIONALE: *Pillow helps keep the client on his or her side.*

11. Lower the bed, elevate the head of the bed as the client can tolerate, and raise the side rail.
    RATIONALE: *Repositioning provides for the client's comfort. Side rails ensure safety.*

12. Wash your hands.
    RATIONALE: *Prevent the spread of infection.*

CLIENT POSITIONING FOR EXAMINATIONS AND TREATMENTS

Horizontal Recumbent Position

This position is required for most of the physical examinations. The client lies on the back with the legs extended. The arms are above the head, folded on the chest, or alongside the body. One small pillow may be used. Cover the client with a bath blanket for privacy. *Caution:* This position may be uncomfortable for a person with a back problem.

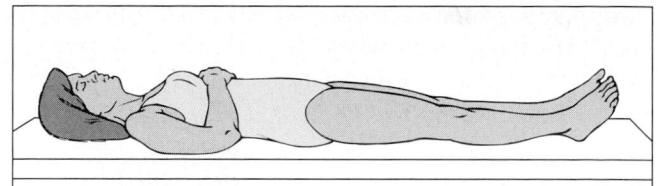

Dorsal Recumbent Position

This position is used for a variety of examinations and procedures. The client lies on the back, with the knees flexed and the soles of the feet flat on the bed. Cover the client with a sheet or a bath blanket folded once across the chest. The second sheet should be crosswise over the client's thighs and legs. Wrap the lower ends of this sheet around the client's legs and feet. Fold the sheet so the genital area is easily exposed. Keep the client covered as much as possible.

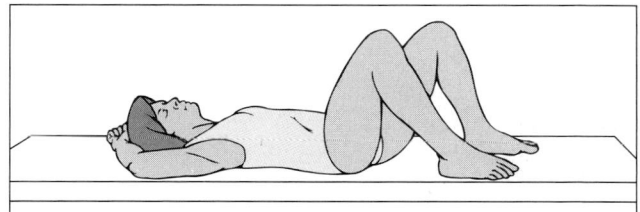

Prone Position

This position is used to examine the spine and back. The client lies on the abdomen with the head turned to the side for comfort. The arms are held above the head or alongside the body. Cover the client with a bath blanket for privacy. *Caution:* Unconscious clients, pregnant women, clients with abdominal incisions, and clients with breathing difficulties cannot lie in this position.

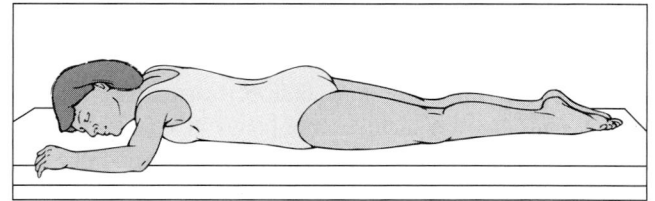

Sims' Position

This position is used for the rectal examination. The client rests on the left side, usually with a small pillow under the head. The right knee is flexed against the abdomen, the left knee is flexed slightly, the left arm is behind the body, and the right arm is in a comfortable position. Cover the client with a bath blanket. *Caution:* The client with leg injuries or arthritis often cannot assume this position.

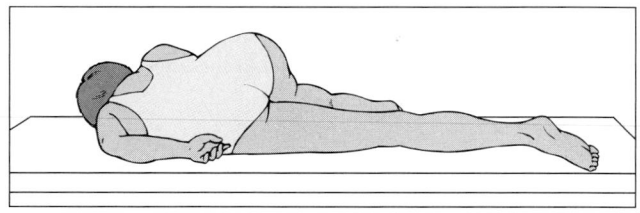

Fowler's Position

This position is used to promote drainage or to make breathing easier. Adjust the head rest to the desired height, and raise the bed section (Gatch bed) under the client's knees. Place a rolled pillow between the client's feet and use the foot of the bed as a brace, if desired. *Caution:* Observe for signs of dizziness or faintness when you raise the head of the bed.

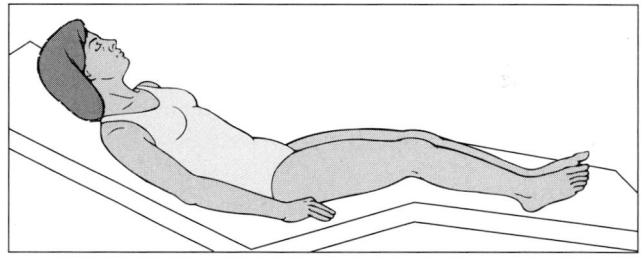

Knee-Chest Position

This position is used for rectal and vaginal examinations and as treatment to bring the uterus into normal position. The client is on the knees with the chest resting on the bed and the elbows rested on the bed, or with the arms above the head. The client's head is turned to one side. The thighs are straight up and down, and the lower legs are flat on the bed. *Caution:* The client may become dizzy or faint and fall. Do not leave the client alone.

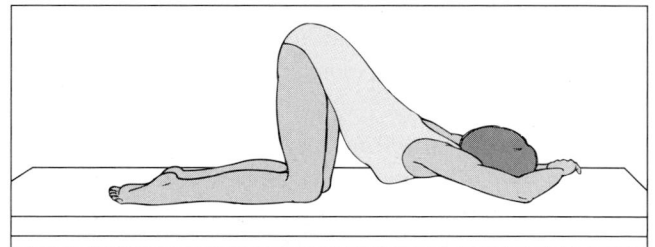

Dorsal Lithotomy Position

This position is used for examinations of the pelvic organs. It is similar to the dorsal recumbent position, except that the client's legs are well separated and the knees are acutely flexed. The nurse will usually place the client's feet in stirrups. Keep the client covered as much as possible for privacy.

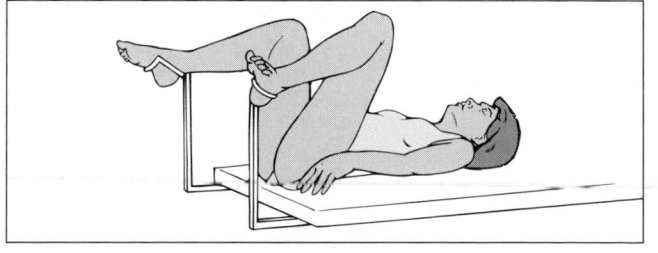

Pillows may be placed as the client wishes, to add to his or her comfort. Use this position for variety, but the client will probably be uncomfortable if lying in the modified Sims' position for very long.

Supporting the Client in a Sitting Position

A client may sit up for a short time to eat meals, work at a table, or change position. Clients with orthopnea need to sit upright continuously to make breathing easier, such as in respiratory or heart conditions. Support may be needed when the body is in a sitting position, if the client is otherwise immobile and unable to adjust support as desired. Pillows support the back, neck, and head to keep the spine in its normal curves. Folded pillows support the arms and keep the shoulders up. Pads in the hands support the wrists and keep the fingers bent slightly and the thumb out, which is the grasping position. The knees are supported in a comfortable position. A slanting footrest (at about the same angle as if the person were standing) is comfortable for the feet and prevents footdrop. (**Footdrop** is a *contracture deformity* in which the foot hangs in a plantarflexed position. This deformity prevents the heel from being placed on the ground, and thus impedes walking.)

The bed mattress may slip to the foot of the bed when the head of the bed is raised. Maintaining proper body alignment becomes difficult. To avoid mattress slippage, place a pillow or a rolled blanket in the space between the edge of the mattress and the lower end of the bed.

Body Alignment With the Client on the Back

Often the client prefers to lie on his or her back most of the time. (This client may turn from a side-lying position to the back, if he or she is not properly supported on the side.) When the client prefers this *supine* or *horizontal recumbent* position, use pillows to support the head, neck, arms, and hands, and a footboard to support the feet (to prevent deformities). This position gives respiratory and digestive organs room to function normally.

If the client's trunk must lie more flatly than the upper part of the body, the person will need only one pillow to support the head and neck. A knee-roll is placed under the knees, and a pad is placed under the ankles to prevent pressure on the heels. The footboard will be more nearly upright in this case.

The Protective Prone Position

The person may be positioned on the stomach (**prone**) for short periods, to provide variety. This position is called the *protective prone* position. This position, however, is uncomfortable for extended lengths of time. Having the head turned sideways can greatly strain the neck and cause headache.

☛ KEY CONCEPT
_____

The client's body alignment when lying down should be approximately the same as if the person were standing. If in doubt about moving any client, ask for assistance.

The Logroll Turn

The **logroll turn** is a method of turning the client that keeps the body in straight alignment (like a tree log). This method is used for clients who have spinal cord injuries or who have had back surgery. Because the goal is to turn the client's body as one intact unit, it is important to prevent further injuries to the back and spine. Two or three nurses are required to turn the client properly in this fashion; however, one nurse may perform this procedure in an emergency, such as if the client is vomiting.

The logroll turn may be used for bed linen changes, change of body position, or to give back care. The client is turned to the side using the logroll turn. This position is helpful in relieving pressure areas over bony prominences and generally adds to the client's comfort. In clients who have a cervical spinal injury, one nurse is required just to maintain the stability of the neck and keep it in alignment. Assess the client's ability to understand instructions and to be cooperative in the turn. In Practice: Nursing Procedure 48-2 explains the detailed steps of the logroll turn.

JOINT MOBILITY AND RANGE OF MOTION

Every body joint has a specific but limited opening and closing motion that is called its range of motion (**ROM**). The limit of the joint's range is between the points of resistance at which the joint will neither open nor close any further. Generally, all people have a similar ROM for their major joints. Factors such as body development, genetic inheritance, presence or absence of disease, and amount of exercise the person usually gets, determine individual differences.

Review the basic musculoskeletal system and its movements as presented in Chapter 18. Box 48-3 (and Figures 47-22 through 47-27 in Chapter 47) will help you review the various motions the body can perform.

Ligaments, muscles, and tendons that connect the bones control joint movement. Clients who have injuries to their tendons, muscles, or ligaments will have limited joint movement.

Every large body joint (ie, neck, shoulder, elbow, wrist, finger, thumb, hip, knee, ankle, and toe) must move regularly several times each day to prevent stiffness and deformities. For healthy and active people, this exercise occurs normally in everyday life. For the ill or immobilized person, however, joint movement may be limited or impaired. To avoid joint abnormalities, the nurse must be sure that clients exercise all joints— several times daily—through ROM exercises.

Nursing and physical therapy share the responsibility of managing ROM exercise programs for clients. Regular exercises prevent joint deformities due to prolonged muscle contractures. A **contracture** is the continuous contraction (shortening of the length) of the muscles that move the bones of the joint. Exercise also helps to prevent conditions such as hypostatic pneumonia, thrombophlebitis, footdrop, circulatory difficulties, skin breakdown, and fecal impactions. Attentive and frequent nursing care can minimize these problems for the immobile client.

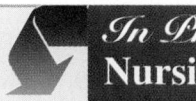

In Practice
Nursing Procedure 48-2

LOGROLL TURN
Steps

1. Determine the number of nurses needed for the move.
   RATIONALE: *Large clients may require the help of three nurses.*

2. Position yourselves together on the same side of the bed, assuming a broad-based stance with one foot slightly ahead of the other.
   RATIONALE: *This position provides easier access to the client and aids in distribution of the client's weight.*

3. Position the client's arms on his or her chest.
   RATIONALE: *Prevent the client's arms from becoming entangled under the body during the turn.*

4. Shift the weight of your trunk and flex the knees, thighs, and ankles.
   RATIONALE: *This position enables nurses to use their large muscle groups.*

5. Slide your arms under the client. If two nurses are turning the client, one nurse should lift the neck region and upper body; the other nurse should lift the hips and thighs. If more than two nurses turn the client, each nurse should take a smaller region of the body.

   RATIONALE: *Allow for even distribution of the client's weight and prevent further injury to the client.*

6. The nurse at the head of the client calls the signals.
   RATIONALE: *Ensure organization and control in the turn.*

7. On the count of three, move the client to the side of the bed.
   RATIONALE: *Maintain body alignment.*

8. On the count of three, roll and position the client on his or her side.
   RATIONALE: *Provide position change.*

9. Place a small pillow under the client's head.
   RATIONALE: *The pillow helps stabilize the neck.*

10. Place one or two pillows under the client's legs.
    RATIONALE: *Pillows help keep the legs aligned.*

11. Place a pillow to the back (optional).
    RATIONALE: *Support the back and provide comfort.*

12. You may use a turning sheet in the logroll turn.
    RATIONALE: *It allows for ease in turning the client, especially if only one nurse is available. Take care to carry out all safety precautions in the turn.*

Passive Range of Motion

If a client is unable to move, the nurse helps by performing passive range of motion (**PROM**) exercises. In Practice: Nursing Procedure 48-3 gives information for providing PROM exercises. The physical therapist may draw up a special PROM plan for a specific client. Figures 47-22 through 47-27 in Chapter 47 illustrate many of the movements.

Continuous Passive Motion

Mechanical devices with which the nurse provides continuous motion to a specific joint, usually the knee or hip, are called continuous passive motion (**CPM**) machines. They are often used after surgery for joint replacement or arthroscopic repair of a joint. The CPM machine moves the client's leg without effort on the part of the nurse or the client. CPM exercises promote joint mobility and speed rehabilitation. It is important for the nurse to carefully explain the purpose of the machine to the client in order to avoid anxiety. Some discomfort may also occur.

The CPM machine is electric, with a padded rack to hold the extremity. The nurse sets the machine for the number of move-

ments per minute it is to move, as ordered by the physician. The client's leg is secured into the rack, with the knee joint far enough away from the end of the rack to allow flexing without rubbing the skin. Be sure the call light is placed within the client's reach. The client is instructed to call if there is severe pain. It is often helpful to give a PRN pain medication approximately 15 minutes before the CPM treatment begins, to relieve pain and allow greater joint movement during the treatment.

☛ KEY CONCEPT

Do not force joint movement when doing PROM exercises. If the client complains of extreme pain, stop and check with your supervisor.

Active Range of Motion

The client doing individual self-directed exercises is performing active range of motion (**AROM**), although supervision may be necessary to ensure that the client moves all joints and muscles to the fullest extent possible.

➤➤ BOX 48-3

RANGE OF MOTION IN BODY MOVEMENTS

Flexion	Decreasing the angle between two bones or bending a part on itself, as in bending the elbow (See Fig. 47-22 [elbow], 47-24 [hand], 47-25 [hip])	**Circumduction**	Moving an extremity in circles; the extremity draws a cone, with the joint as the apex of the cone—as in swinging arms in circles
Extension	Increasing the angle between two bones, as in straightening the arm (See Fig. 47-22)	**Rotation**	Moving a bone on a longitudinal axis (horizontally), as in shaking the head no, or moving in a circle from the waist
Hyperextension	Increasing the angle of an extremity beyond normal (See Fig. 47-24)	**Supination**	Inversion. Turing the palm anteriorly (forward) or the foot inward and upward (so it faces the other foot) (See Fig. 47-23)
Dorsiflexion	Bending a body part toward the dorsum (backwards), as in moving the foot so the toes face toward the back (See Fig. 47-27)	**Pronation**	Turning the hand so the palm faces downward or backward (See Fig. 47-23)
Plantar Flexion	Bending the foot so that the toes are pointed downward (See Fig. 47-27)	**Inversion**	Turning a part so that it faces medially or inside, such as turning the ankle so that the sole of the foot faces the opposite foot
Abduction	Moving a body part away from the midline of the body (See Fig. 47-26)	**Eversion**	Turning the foot so the sole faces away from the other foot
Adduction	Moving a body part toward the midline of the body (See Fig. 47-26)	**Protraction**	Moving forward or anteriorly, as in jutting out the jaw
		Retraction	Moving backward or back into anatomic position

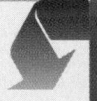

In Practice
Nursing Procedure 48-3

TIPS ON PERFORMING RANGE-OF-MOTION EXERCISES

General Guidelines

- Check the physician's order. A physician's order may be needed for complete ROM exercises (either passive or active). The physician also may order ROM exercises for specific joints only.
- Practice proper personal body mechanics to prevent injury. For example, the nurse puts the bed in high position, and moves the client close so that stretching and bending are not necessary.
- Move slowly and gently, so the client is not injured.
- If the client complains of extreme pain, stop and report it. *Do not force joint movements!*
- Support the dependent part of each extremity while performing passive joint exercises.
- Repeat each movement three times.
- Perform limited ROM movements during treatments such as the bed bath.
- If the client becomes tired, allow reasonable rest periods between exercises.
- Return the bed to low position before leaving the room.

PERFORMING PASSIVE ROM EXERCISES

Steps

1. Wash your hands.
   RATIONALE: *Prevent the spread of infection.*

2. Explain the procedure to the client.
   RATIONALE: *Providing information fosters the client's cooperation and understanding.*

3. Adjust the bed to a comfortable height. Select one side of the bed to begin PROM exercises.
   RATIONALE: *Bed at proper height prevents back strain and eliminates reaching across bed.*

4. Uncover only the limb to be exercised.
   RATIONALE: *Ensure warmth and protect the client's privacy.*

5. Support all joints during exercise activity.
   RATIONALE: *Cradling joints prevents injury and discomfort.*

6. Use slow, gentle movements when performing exercises. Repeat each exercise three times. Stop if the client complains of pain or discomfort.

In Practice
Nursing Procedure 48-3 (Continued)

RATIONALE: *Repetitive motion maintains joint mobility. Discontinuing exercises, if they cause pain, prevents injury to joint.*

7. Begin exercises with the client's neck and work downward.
   RATIONALE: *Performing procedures in a systematic manner ensures that you exercise all joints.*

8. Flex, extend, and rotate the client's neck. Support his or her head with your hands.
   RATIONALE: *Prevent flexion contracture of the neck.*

9. Exercise the client's shoulder and elbow.
   RATIONALE: *Maintain strength in the client's deltoid muscle and prevent contracture.*

   a. Support the client's elbow with one hand and grasp the client's wrist with your other hand.

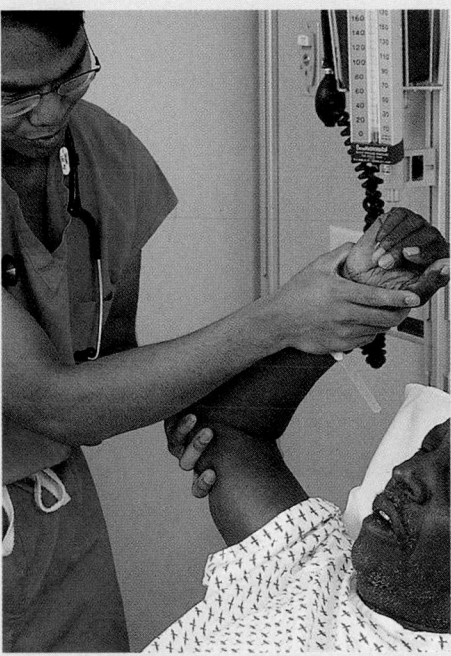

Supporting the joint.

   b. Raise the client's arm from the side to above the head.

   c. Perform internal rotation by moving the client's arm across his or her chest.

   d. Externally rotate the client's shoulder by moving the arm away from the client.

   e. Flex and extend the client's elbow. (See Figure 47-22.)

10. Perform all exercises on the client's wrist and fingers.
    RATIONALE: *Maintain strength and flexibility in the wrist and fingers.*

    a. Flex and extend the wrist.

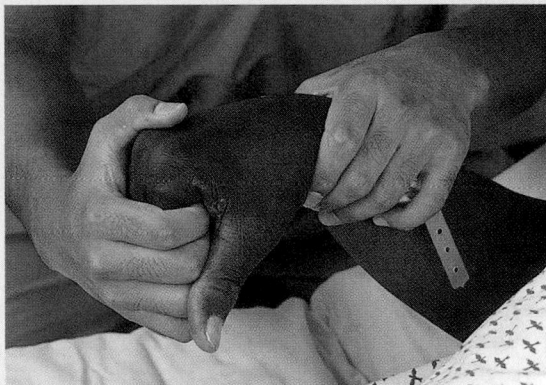

Flexing and extending the wrist.

   b. Abduct and adduct the wrist.

   c. Rotate and pronate the wrist. (See Fig. 47-23.)

   d. Flex and extend the client's fingers.

   e. Abduct and adduct the fingers.

   f. Rotate the thumb.

11. Exercise the client's hip and leg.
    RATIONALE: *A contracted hip or fixed knee severely limits the client's ability to ambulate.*

    a. Flex and extend the hip and knee while supporting the leg. (See Fig. 47-25.)

    b. Abduct and adduct the hip by moving the client's straightened leg toward you and then back to median position. (See Fig. 47-26.)

    c. Perform internal and external rotation of the hip joint by turning the leg inward and then outward.

12. Perform exercises on the ankle and foot.
    RATIONALE: *Protect the feet because they support the body and allow the client to walk.*

    a. Dorsiflex and plantarflex the foot. (See Fig. 47-33.)

    b. Abduct and adduct the toes.

    c. Evert and invert the foot.

13. Move to the other side of the bed and repeat exercises.
    RATIONALE: *Ensure that you exercise all joints.*

14. Reposition and cover the client. Return the bed to low position.
    RATIONALE: *Repositioning allows for the client's comfort. Lowering the bed prevents accidents.*

15. Wash your hands.
    RATIONALE: *Prevent the spread of infection.*

16. Document completion of PROM exercises.
    RATIONALE: *Documentation provides ongoing data collection.*

Isometric (muscle-setting) exercises are those the client performs by tightening and releasing certain muscle groups. These exercises are helpful for strengthening the abdominal, gluteal, and quadriceps muscles, which are necessary for ambulation. Because these exercises only preserve muscle mass, they are not useful in preventing contractures. Therefore, isometrics are useful in preparing the client for crutch-walking; maintaining muscle tone in a casted limb; wheelchair use; or teaching bowel training. The routine that achieves the best results is a repetition of five sets of exercises, each lasting 5 seconds, with a 2-minute rest period between repetitions. (For example, tighten the abdominal muscles; count 1-1,000, 2-1,000, 3-1,000, 4-1,000, and 5-1,000. Rest for 2 minutes. Repeat until five sets have been completed.) The thigh and leg muscles can be strengthened by asking the client to contract the quadriceps femoris, the large muscle on the anterior thigh; the client will feel as though he or she is pushing the popliteal space behind the knee downward into the mattress and pulling the foot forward.

Other exercises are done while sitting up in bed or in a wheelchair. The client lifts the hips by pushing the hands down into the mattress or the chair. For push-ups, the client lies face down with the hands placed flat on the mattress next to the shoulders, with the elbows bent. The client extends the elbows stiffly to raise the head and chest up off the bed.

Some daily activities can be turned into useful exercise (eg, reaching for objects on the bedside table; pulling the overbed table forward and pushing it away; brushing the hair). Most clients confined to bed are given a trapeze, which hangs on a bar above the bed. The client uses it to pull up in bed, thus exercising the arms. Frequent use strengthens muscles, and the client often creates his or her own exercises when the importance of exercise is explained.

The physical therapist may introduce the exercises, but the activities are repeated several times a day, and nurses supervise them. Occupational therapy also provides muscle exercises, often for smaller muscle groups.

ASSISTING THE MOBILE AND PARTIALLY MOBILE CLIENT

Some clients are allowed out of bed (**OOB**) for the entire day; others are up for certain lengths of time each day, as their conditions permit.

Follow these basic principles when assisting clients out of bed:

- Check the physician's order to determine the client's prescribed level of activity.
- Assist the client to put on a bathrobe and slippers. Offer a blanket, to avoid chilling.
- Being up after an illness is tiring. Ask the client to tell you if he or she is becoming tired, faint, or weak.
- Offer PRN (as needed) pain relief medication approximately 30 minutes before the client is to get up. (This will increase client comfort and may increase the length of time he or she is able to be up.)
- Make sure the client's nurse call signal is within reach, if you leave the client while he or she is sitting up.

Dangling ✓

Dangling refers to allowing the client to sit on the edge of the bed, with the legs down and the feet supported on a footstool or on the floor. This helps the client who has been in bed to prepare to sit in a chair and eventually, to walk. *Be careful:* Allow the person to sit for a few minutes before assisting him or her out of bed. The client may experience lightheadedness or weakness due to a temporary fall in blood pressure (*orthostatic hypotension*). It is important for the nurse to be aware of the client's limitations. He or she may be strong enough only to dangle and then lie down again. In Practice: Nursing Procedure 48-4 discusses the steps for dangling.

Helping the Mobile Client out of Bed

Clients who are weak from long periods of bed rest or who are unsteady because of illness require assistance from bed. Care should be taken to ensure that the client has a good sense of balance, before helping him or her out of bed. In Practice: Nursing Procedure 48-5 discusses the steps in helping the mobile client out of bed.

> ### Nursing Alert ✓
> A client may be light-headed or faint when he or she gets out of bed. If this occurs:
> - Help steady the person while he or she sits on the side of the bed. Return to the supine position as soon as possible.
> - If the client is in a chair, have him or her bend over at the waist and lower the head.
> - If walking with a client, help him or her to lean against a wall and bend over. If this does not help and no one else is there, gently ease the client to the floor.
> - Use a transfer belt the next time the client gets up.
>   Remember: the goal is to keep the client safe and free from injury.

Using the Transfer Belt

The nurse can provide secure support to the weak or unsteady person by using a **transfer belt** (also called a **gait belt**). A transfer belt is a sturdy webbed belt with a buckle that easily secures around the client's waist. Figure 48-3 illustrates the use of a transfer belt. Explain to the client that the belt provides safety and protection for both client and nurse. In Practice: Nursing Care Guidelines 48-2 lists considerations in the use of the transfer belt.

> ### Nursing Alert
> Even if a client is falling, the nurse must avoid letting the client grab him or her around the neck. (One's neck cannot withstand the force if the client falls.) If a client grabs for the nurse's neck, the nurse puts the head down so the client cannot get a grip. The nurse must immediately lower the client to safety and explain why he or she reacted in that manner.

In Practice
Nursing Procedure 48-4

DANGLING

Supplies and Equipment

Stethoscope
Blood pressure cuff
Bath blanket
Pillow

Steps

1. Place the bed in low position.
   RATIONALE: *The client can place his or her feet on the floor easily from low position.*
   Explain what will happen.
   RATIONALE: *Prepare the client.*

2. Fan-fold the bed covers to the foot of the bed, and cover the client with a bath blanket.
   RATIONALE: *Protect the client's privacy and prevent chilling.*

3. Measure and record the client's pulse and blood pressure.
   RATIONALE: *This procedure often helps you evaluate how well the client may tolerate being up.*

4. Elevate the head of the bed as high as it will go.
   RATIONALE: *Elevating the head of the bed raises the client without requiring manual lifting.*

5. Place one arm around the client's shoulders and your other arm under his or her knees.
   RATIONALE: *Doing so allows you to turn the client's body as a unit.*

6. Turn the client toward you so that his or her feet touch the floor. For shorter clients, provide a foot-stool.
   RATIONALE: *Supporting the client's feet is crucial.*

7. Roll a pillow and tuck it firmly behind the client's back.
   RATIONALE: *This measure helps support the person in the sitting position.*

8. Dangle the client's legs for as long as ordered, if tolerated. Stay with the person at all times. Help the person to lie down if he or she becomes light-headed or feels faint.

RATIONALE: *When a person sits up for the first time, blood rushes into the legs. The client may feel faint due to orthostatic hypotension.*

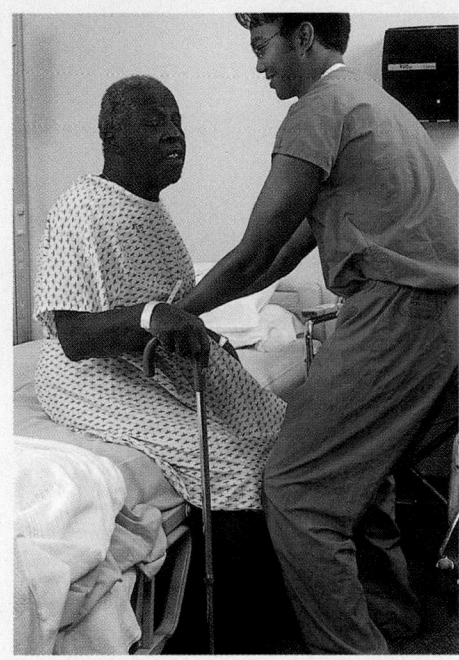

Dangle the client's legs for as long as ordered if tolerated. Stay with the client at all times.

9. After the prescribed time, help the client lie down again by supporting his or her shoulders and knees and turning his or her back around.
   RATIONALE: *Provide support for the client during movement toward the bed.*

10. Measure and record the client's pulse and blood pressure immediately.
    RATIONALE: *These readings, compared against baseline measurements, help the physician determine how well the client tolerated the procedure.*

11. Wash your hands, and document the procedure: how long the client dangled, how he or she tolerated the procedure, and any unusual occurrences.

Helping a Client Move From Bed to Chair

Some clients have difficulty moving (transferring) from bed to chair or back again because of weakness or **paralysis** (inability to move). Generally, the nurse can transfer even the weakest client safely, using effective body mechanics. In Practice: Nursing Procedure 48-6 outlines the steps for assisting a client to move from the bed to a chair. Additional procedures in this chapter describe moving the client who is very weak or paralyzed.

☛ KEY CONCEPT

Always apply body mechanics principles to protect yourself and your clients from unnecessary body fatigue, strain, or injury.

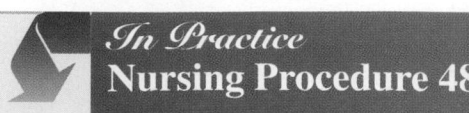

In Practice
Nursing Procedure 48-5

HELPING THE MOBILE CLIENT FROM BED
Supplies and Equipment

Robe

Steps

1. Get assistance if you need it.
   RATIONALE: *Preventing falls is essential.*

2. Position the client as described for dangling.

3. Reassure the client that you will provide necessary protection from falling, and explain how.
   RATIONALE: *The client may worry about falling.*

4. Help the client into clothing or a robe.
   RATIONALE: *Protect the client's modesty; provide warmth.*

5. Choose a chair that will not slide and position it next to the bed.
   RATIONALE: *Most healthcare agency injuries are caused by falls.*

6. Encourage the client to stand. Provide support by holding the client's arm or having the client hold your arm. Get assistance when moving immobile, weak, or unusually heavy clients.
   RATIONALE: *Being in bed, even for a short time, can make a person very weak.*

7. Walk with the client to the chair; gently ease the client down into the chair.
   RATIONALE: *Ensure that the client is safe while walking.*

8. Check your client's pulse rate before and after putting him or her into a chair. Watch for signs of fatigue.

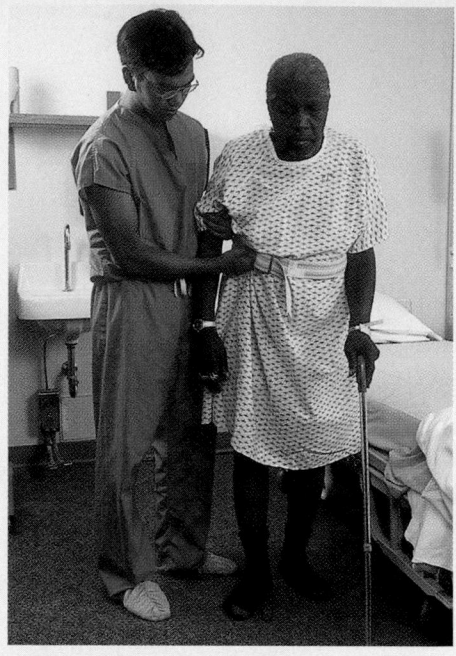
Walk with the client to the chair.

   RATIONALE: *The change in position affects circulation and blood supply to the brain; the client may feel faint.*

9. Place the signal cord within easy reach.
   RATIONALE: *The client must be able to call for assistance if he or she has pain or feels faint.*

10. Check on the client frequently. Provide diversion (eg, television, a book, mail).
    RATIONALE: *Encourage the person to stay up longer.*

Using Mobility Devices

Wheelchairs and Stretchers
Use a wheelchair to move clients who cannot walk or who should be spared fatigue as much as possible. In Practice: Nursing Procedure 48-7 discusses these steps in detail.

After the client is in the wheelchair, check to see that he or she is comfortable. If the client is to stay alone, secure the call signal within easy reach. If the client is unable to remain seated upright or may attempt to stand up, a *client reminder device* or *protective device* may be needed so the person does not fall out of the chair. An order is required for the use of most protective devices (discussed later in this chapter).

Check on the client frequently because he or she may become faint or may have pain. Carefully assist the client back into bed. Be sure to lock the wheels of the wheelchair or stretcher for transfer.

Sometimes, the client will be moved in a wheelchair to another area for examinations or tests. In Practice: Nursing Care Guidelines 48-3 presents skills to use when pushing a wheelchair. These same skills are used when pushing a wheeled stretcher (also called a **litter** or a **gurney**). A *stretcher* is a four-wheeled bed-like cart with a moisture-proof mattress. It is used for moving people who cannot sit or walk.

Canes
A *cane* is a slender, hand-held, curved stick or device meant to provide support while walking. The three basic types of canes are the standard *straight-legged cane,* the *tripod cane* (which has three feet), and the *quad cane* (which has four feet). The cane should have a sturdy handle grip and rubber-tipped feet (Fig. 48-4). The cane supports balance and helps the client to walk. It provides additional support when one side of a per-

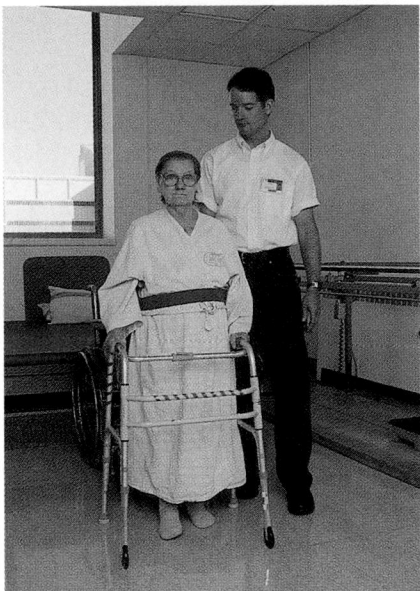

FIGURE 48-3. The transfer belt gives the client more confidence and will help the nurse if the client begins to weaken or fall. The nurse grasps the transfer belt as the client walks with a walker. Always grasp the transfer belt with the fingers inside the belt and pointing upward, with the palm of the hand under the bottom edge of the belt. (Craven, R. F., & Hirnle, C. J. [2001]. *Fundamentals of nursing: Human health and function* [3rd ed.]. Philadelphia: Lippincott Williams & Wilkins.)

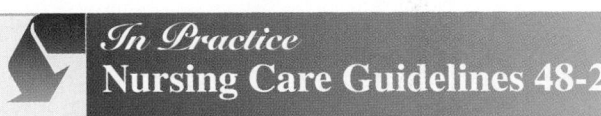

In Practice
Nursing Care Guidelines 48-2

USING THE TRANSFER BELT

- Place the belt securely around the client's waist before he or she gets up. It must be tight enough to support the client's weight, but should not be uncomfortable. The belt also must not be too tight. Fasten the buckle securely, with the loop back through the gripper teeth. *Rationale: The belt must be able to support the client if he or she begins to fall. However, the belt must be loose enough for you to slip your hand into it.*
- Keep one hand inside the back of the belt at all times when transferring or walking with the client. *Rationale: You must be prepared to support the client if he or she begins to fall.*
- Always insert your hand into the belt from the bottom, with your fingers pointing upward and the bottom of the belt in the palm of your hand. *Rationale: If the client slumps or slips, you will be able to support the weight. If you grasp the belt from the top, it will slip out of your hand due to the client's weight.*
- If the client is likely to soil the belt, give him or her a personal belt to keep in the room. *Rationale: Prevent the spread of infection.*
- Store the belt outside the room if the client is depressed, suicidal, or may assault someone else. *Rationale: The buckle could be used as a weapon. The belt could also be used to commit suicide.*
- Assess the client for correct body alignment when the transfer is completed. *Rationale: If the body is twisted or misaligned, and the client is left sitting for long periods, pressure on certain muscle groups and nerves can cause damage.*

son's body is weak. The cane is held on the client's strong side and is adjusted to the appropriate height. In Practice: Nursing Care Guidelines 48-4 describes additional considerations when your client is using a cane. Chapter 96 describes many general principles of rehabilitation.

The Walker

A *walker* is a four-legged tubular device with hand grips. It provides sturdy support for clients who are unable or too unstable to walk with a cane. The standard walker is made of lightweight aluminum. The client grips the device, raises it from the floor, moves it away from the body a few inches, sets it securely on the floor, and walks toward it. A moderate amount of upper body strength is necessary for a client to pick up the walker. Some walkers have rubber-tipped feet; others have wheels in the front or back or both. Some walkers also have a seat. The client must feel secure when walking, and should stand upright (see Fig. 48-5). In Practice: Nursing Care Guidelines 48-5 will give you suggestions for helping the client to use a walker.

Crutches

Crutches are walking aids made of wood or metal in the form of a shaft. They reach from the ground to the client's axillae. For walking ease, crutches must be adjusted correctly for the client. If crutches are too long, they will cause pressure in the axillae. If crutches are too short, the client will be unable to maintain erect posture. To adjust crutches:

- The bottom of each crutch is placed about 6 inches (15 cm) from the outside of the client's feet. The top of the crutch should be two to three finger widths below the client's axillae when his or her elbows are flexed approximately 30° (Fig. 48-6, A & B).
- Placement of the hand bar is just as important. It should be at a height that allows the client to extend the arm almost completely when leaning on the palms. Even if crutches are the correct total length, the position of the hand bar may need to be adjusted. (Some people have long arms in relation to their body height; some people have shorter arms.) If crutches are shortened by more than 1 inch, the position of the hand bar will most likely also need to be changed.
- The crutch tip is made of sturdy rubber that fits snugly. A large vacuum tip is a necessity. *Rationale: This gives confidence to the severely disabled person who must place*

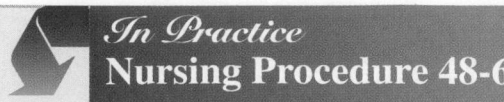

In Practice
Nursing Procedure 48-6

MOVING THE CLIENT FROM BED TO CHAIR

Supplies

Pillow
Blanket
Stockings or shoes

Steps

1. Position the client as described for dangling. (See In Practice: Nursing Procedure 48-4).

2. Place the bed in low position.
   RATIONALE: *Safety is important.*

3. Move a comfortable armchair close to the bed.
   RATIONALE: *The shorter the distance, the safer the move.*

4. Place a pillow on the chair seat, and cover it with a moisture-proof pillowcase if the client is likely to soil.
   RATIONALE: *Provide comfort.*

5. Spread a blanket across the seat, and leave enough of it at the lower end to wrap the blanket around the client's legs and feet as needed.
   RATIONALE: *Keep the client warm.*

6. Get the client's stockings, slippers, or shoes.
   RATIONALE: *Keep the client comfortable.*

7. Transfer the client to the chair or wheelchair in the same manner (see In Practice: Nursing Procedure 48-7).

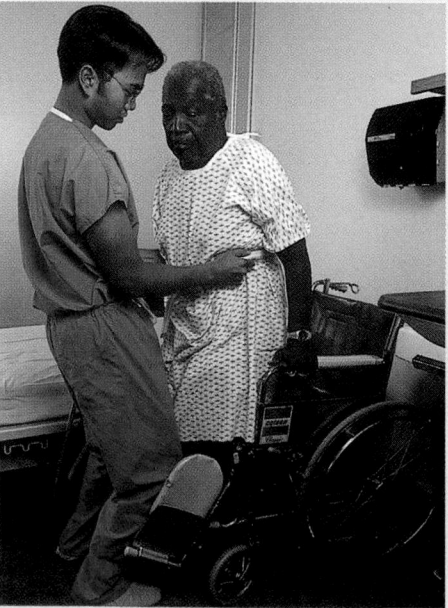

Transfer the client to the chair.

his or her crutches wide to provide a firm base of support. It also prevents slipping.

- Crutches that fit properly and are used correctly do not create pressure under the arms. Make sure that the client places his or her weight on the hands, and does not lean on the tops of the crutches. Properly fitted crutches are comfortable to use. *Rationale: A serious disorder called crutch palsy or brachial palsy can result if the client bears weight in the axilla.*

- Rubber pads may be on the tops of the crutches to protect clothing.

- For safety, the client should wear shoes that fit well, with low, broad heels and straight inner borders. A pair of comfortable shoes is excellent, but the client should not wear bedroom slippers. *Rationale: Slippers provide no support and may seriously damage the foot. They also may have slippery soles.*

➕👁 Nursing Alert ✓

Leaning on crutches can cause a serious disorder called *brachial paralysis* or *crutch palsy*. To prevent this condition, the hands—not the axillae—should bear the weight of the client's body.

The client is assisted to condition and strengthen the upper body. If available, a physical therapist teaches the client to use crutches. Nurses are responsible for helping the client to master this skill. If a physical therapist is unavailable, nurses do the teaching. This teaching includes learning a safe and comfortable crutch-walking gait, as well as learning how to go up and down stairs. Documentation of all teaching is vital.

Conditioning and Strengthening Exercises

Conditioning and strengthening exercises prepare the client's body for action. The client dangles, sits in a chair, and learns to stand by the side of the bed. As the client performs these actions, he or she practices correct posture: head is up, chest is out, back is straight, and abdomen is in. Encourage the client to press the feet down on a footstool to regain the feeling of standing. While the client sits with the arms extended, show him or her how to press the palms down on the bed to exercise the arm muscles, or how to lie on the stomach and do bed push-ups. Short crutches are sometimes used, so the client can practice and build strength while still in bed. Push-ups can also be done in a wheelchair. Some of these exercises were described in more detail earlier in this chapter as range of motion exercises.

Weight-Bearing Restrictions

The physician determines how much weight the client can safely bear on the legs. In some cases, the client cannot put any weight on an injured leg or hip (which is considered *non–weight-bearing*). In other cases, the client may be partially or totally weight-bearing on one or both legs. Crutches are used to support *full–weight-bearing* as a safety measure.

In Practice
Nursing Procedure 48-7

HELPING THE CLIENT INTO A WHEELCHAIR OR CHAIR

Supplies and Equipment

Wheelchair
Slippers or shoes (non-skid soles)
Robe
Transfer belt (optional)

Steps

1. Wash your hands.
   RATIONALE: *Prevent the spread of infection.*

2. Explain the procedure to the client.
   RATIONALE: *Providing information fosters the client's cooperation and understanding.*

3. Position the wheelchair next to the bed or at a 45° angle to the bed. Lock the wheel brakes and remove the footrests or move them to the "up" position.

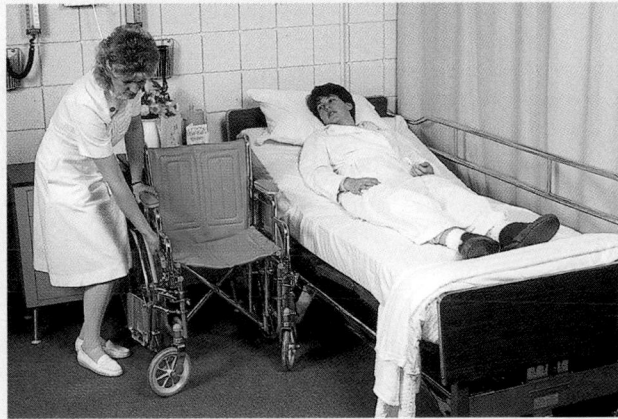

Locking the wheelchair brakes.

4. Prepare to move the client:
   a. Assist the client with putting on robe and slippers.
      RATIONALE: *Slippers with non-skid soles ensure safety and stability.*
   b. Obtain help from another person if the client is immobile, heavy, or connected to multiple pieces of equipment.
      RATIONALE: *Requesting assistance prevents accidents.*

5. Raise the head of the bed so that the client is in the sitting position.
   RATIONALE: *A sitting position facilitates movement out of bed.*

6. Assist the client to sit on the side of the bed.
   RATIONALE: *A gradual change in position lessens the chance of the client developing orthostatic hypotension.*

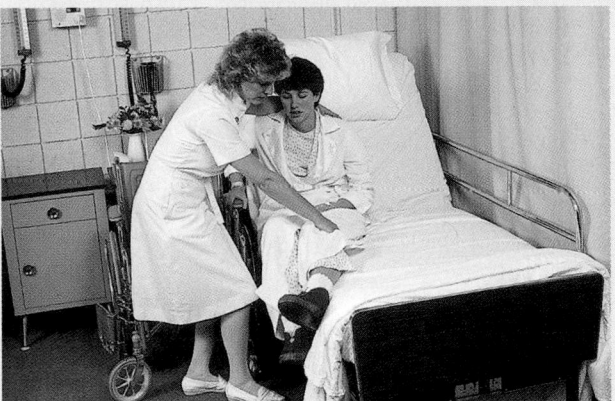

Assisting the client to the side of the bed.

   a. Support the head and neck with one arm.
   b. Use your other arm to move the client's leg over the side of the bed.
   c. Allow the client's feet to rest on the floor.
   d. Maintain the client in this position for a short time.

7. Prepare to raise the client to a standing position.
   RATIONALE: *This position provides stability for the transfer.*
   a. Apply a transfer belt if necessary.
   b. Spread the client's feet and brace your knees against the client's knees.
   c. Place your arms around the client's waist.

8. Use the rocking motion of your legs to assist the client to stand. The client may use his or her hands to help push upward from bed.
   RATIONALE: *Use muscles with large muscle mass to lift the client.*

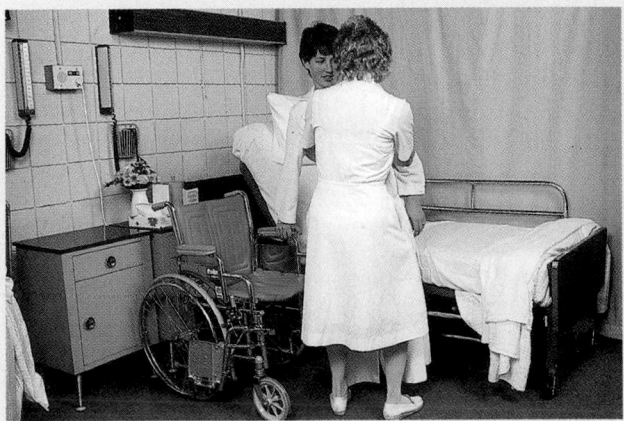

Assisting the client to stand.

(continued)

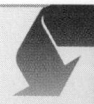
9. Pivot the client into position immediately in front of the wheelchair. Encourage the client to use arm rests for support while you lower him or her into chair.
   RATIONALE: *This position supports and stabilizes the client as he or she moves into the chair.*

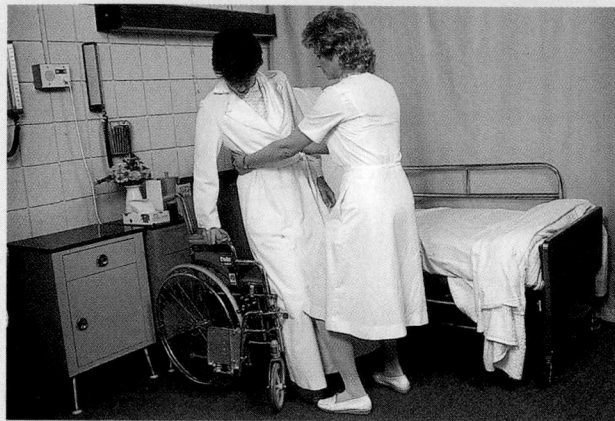

Lowering the client into the wheelchair.

10. Reposition foot rests. Secure the client in a chair with a reminder device if needed. Cover the client with a blanket. Provide the nurse call button.
    RATIONALE: *A client reminder device prevents accidents. The blanket ensures warmth. The client must be able to call for help.*

11. Wash your hands.
    RATIONALE: *Prevent the spread of infection.*

12. Check on the client frequently.
    RATIONALE: *You can then assist if the client feels faint. Provide a feeling of security.*

13. Document the transfer and the client's response.
    RATIONALE: *Documentation provides ongoing data collection.*

In Practice
Nursing Care Guidelines 48-3

PUSHING A WHEELCHAIR OR WHEELED STRETCHER/GURNEY

- Secure restraint straps or safety belts and side rails. *Rationale: Prevent the client from falling.*
- Secure the client's equipment (eg, IV stands, ventilatory machines, and drainage apparatus). *Rationale: Prevent injuries to the client and yourself.*
- Take the client's chart when transporting from one station to another. *Rationale: The chart helps identify the client, and other departments often need the information.*
- Push from the back; do not pull. *Rationale: Prevent back strain.*
- Look for clear traffic path ahead (eg, avoid people approaching, equipment left in hallway, or wet floors). *Rationale: Prevent accidents.*
- Negotiate corners slowly. *Rationale: Prevent the client from falling and prevent hitting someone coming the other way.*
- Use slow to moderate speed in pushing gurney or chair. *Rationale: It is more difficult to stop a faster-moving object.*
- When approaching a downward incline, walk in front of the gurney or chair. Wheel the chair backward. *Rationale: Prevent the gurney or chair from going too fast.*
- When approaching an upward incline, turn the gurney or chair around, so you pull the client head first. *Rationale: It is easier to pull than to push uphill.*
- When approaching a curb or single stair, tip the chair back, and put the small wheels up on the curb or step. Move ahead by lifting or pushing the back wheels over the curb or step. *Rationale: Prevent jarring the client.*
- Do not attempt to go up or down a curb with a gurney. To go down a curb with a wheelchair, turn the chair around and ease the large back wheel off the curb first. *Rationale: This will prevent the possibility of lurching the client forward, possibly out of the chair. The large wheel is easier to roll over the curb and if the wheelchair lurches, the client will just be pushed against the back of the chair and not out of the chair. In addition, the small front wheels often spin sideways and get stuck.*
- When entering or leaving an elevator, use an elevator bridge, if one is available. The bridge is a flat board, with a piece to fit into the slot between the floor of the elevator and the floor to which you are going. The bridge prevents the wheels of the chair from getting stuck in the crack. If no bridge is available, turn the wheelchair around and roll the large back wheel into and out of the elevator first. *Rationale: Provide safety for your client.*

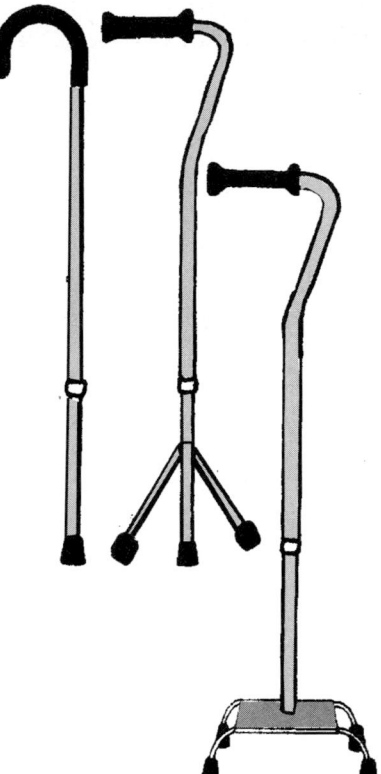

FIGURE 48-4. The three basic types of canes are the standard straight-legged cane, the tripod cane (has three feet), and the quad cane (has four feet). The cane should have a sturdy handle grip and rubber-tipped feet.

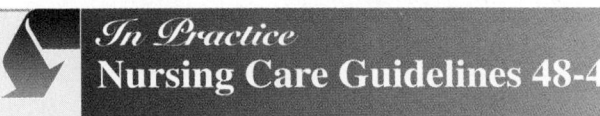

In Practice
Nursing Care Guidelines 48-4

WALKING WITH A CANE

- Adjust the cane's height to allow for a slight bend in the client's elbow. The cane handle should be approximately at hip level. *Rationale: This position is the most comfortable and gives the client the most support.*
- Instruct the client to hold the cane on the strong side, unless specifically contraindicated. *Rationale: This will allow the client to have a normal walking gait, including normal arm swing, while providing maximum support.*
- Check the client's balance. Assist the client by using a transfer belt, if necessary. *Rationale: It is important to prevent falls. Many clients using canes are older or debilitated and need extra practice.*
- Teach the client to move his or her stronger leg forward while carrying his or her weight on the weak side and the cane. The cane and the weaker leg move together as a unit. *Rationale: The cane adds stability and support to the weaker leg. The stronger leg can support the client's weight without assistance.*
- Walk on the client's *affected* side when assisting. *Rationale: It is important for you to be available in case the client slips or stumbles. Be prepared to support the client if this should happen. If the client has weakness or instability, it will be on the affected side.*
- Continue helping the client to walk in this manner. *Rationale: Assist the client to practice correct cane-walking. This will help to promote independence.*

It is important for the nurse to explain these restrictions and the underlying reasons to the client. (Usually, a leg is considered non–weight-bearing if a fracture is not totally immobilized or is not healing well.)

Crutch-Walking Gaits. The client's strength and type of disability are guides to the best possible crutch-walking **gait** or style of walking (Fig. 48-7).

The client should use the muscles and joints as much as possible. Table 48-1 lists the types of crutch-walking gaits. A physician and a physical therapist will determine the gait that is best for each client to use.

- In *two-point gait,* the client is partially weight-bearing on both legs. (A crutch and the opposite leg are considered one "point." The other crutch and leg are the second "point.") The client puts his or her body weight on one leg and on the **contralateral** (opposite side) crutch. The client then brings the other crutch and leg forward together, and shifts the weight to them. This gait is faster and more like walking than the others, and the client can change the gait as muscle power improves. This gait is used following spinal cord injury; when both legs have about the same strength; and when a client is learning to walk again.
- In *three-point gait,* each crutch and only one leg support weight. (Each is considered a "point.") The other leg is non–weight-bearing. The person moves the weak leg

and both crutches forward together, balancing the weight on the unaffected leg, while supporting the weight on the crutches and weak leg. He or she then steps forward with the weight-bearing leg. Steps should be of equal length, and timed so that no pauses occur. This gait is best when one leg is disabled and the other is strong enough to bear all the client's weight. This gait keeps most or all of the weight off the weak leg. However, sometimes the client may place a small amount of weight on the weak leg if partial weight-bearing is allowed. This gait is one means of strengthening the weak leg without endangering the client.

- In *four-point gait,* each crutch and each leg move separately. (Each of the four "points" supports weight.) The client places one crutch forward, and then advances the contralateral foot; he or she then brings the second crutch forward, and the other foot follows. Rhythmic, short, and equal steps are important. Counting helps to develop rhythm: *one,* right crutch forward; *two,* advance left foot;

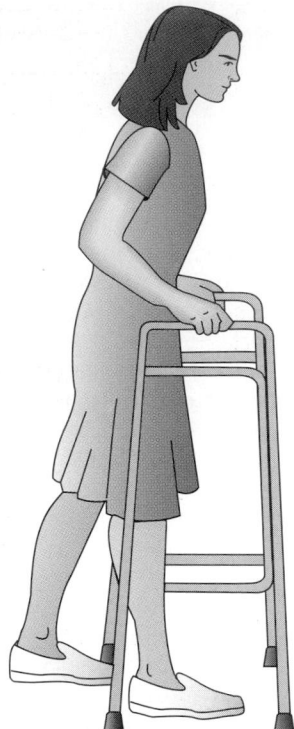

FIGURE 48-5. A walker is a four-legged tubular device with hand grips, that provides sturdy support for clients who are unstable or unable to walk with a cane.

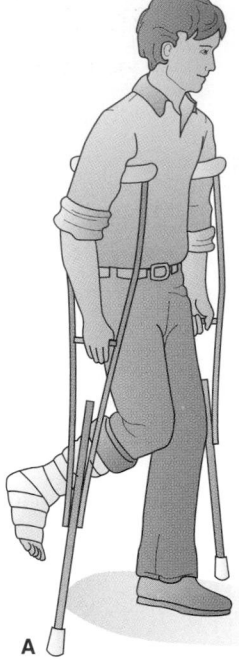
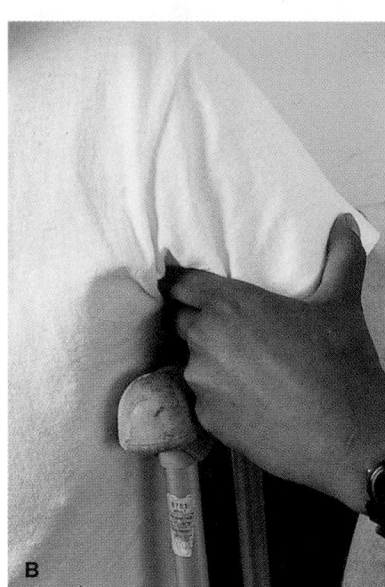

A   B

FIGURE 48-6. Crutches are walking aids that are made of wood or metal in a shaft that reaches from the ground to the client's axillae. Shown here are traditional hand-held crutches. Another type of crutch is pictured in Figure 48-9. (**A**) In the three-point gait, the client is instructed to stand on the unaffected leg while swinging the affected leg and the crutches forward. He then swings the unaffected leg through, while balancing on both crutches. (**B**) Crutches should be adjusted so the weight is borne on the hands. The crutch pads should not touch the axillae and no weight should be borne on the tops of the crutches.

In Practice
Nursing Care Guidelines 48-5

USING A WALKER

- Position the walker in front of the client. Explain the use of the walker. *Rationale: The client must be comfortable with the use of the walker in order to be willing and able to use it.*
- Have the client pick up the walker and move it ahead approximately 6 to 12 inches at a time, with his or her weight equally distributed on both feet. *Rationale: It is important that the client learn to use the walker correctly, to prevent falls and to instill confidence.*
- When both sides are weak, move the client's right foot forward while the client shifts weight to the left side and the arms. *Rationale: Assist the client to maximal use of abilities. The client needs to learn what he or she can and cannot do.*
- Next, move the client's left foot forward while he or she shifts weight to the right side and the arms. Continue helping the client to move forward in this man-

ner. *Rationale: This will help the client to learn how to use the walker most effectively.*
- When only one side of the client's body is weak, first move the walker and the client's weak leg together, while the client carries weight on the strong side. *Rationale: In this case, the walker is used in much the same manner as crutches.*
- Next, move the client's strong or unaffected side while the client carries weight on the weak side and the walker. Continue to assist the person to practice in this manner.
- It is important to note that the wheeled walker is more difficult to use, because it does not stay in one place as easily. The client must be carefully taught to lean on this walker before shifting his or her weight, to prevent the walker from rolling away. This could be a dangerous situation.

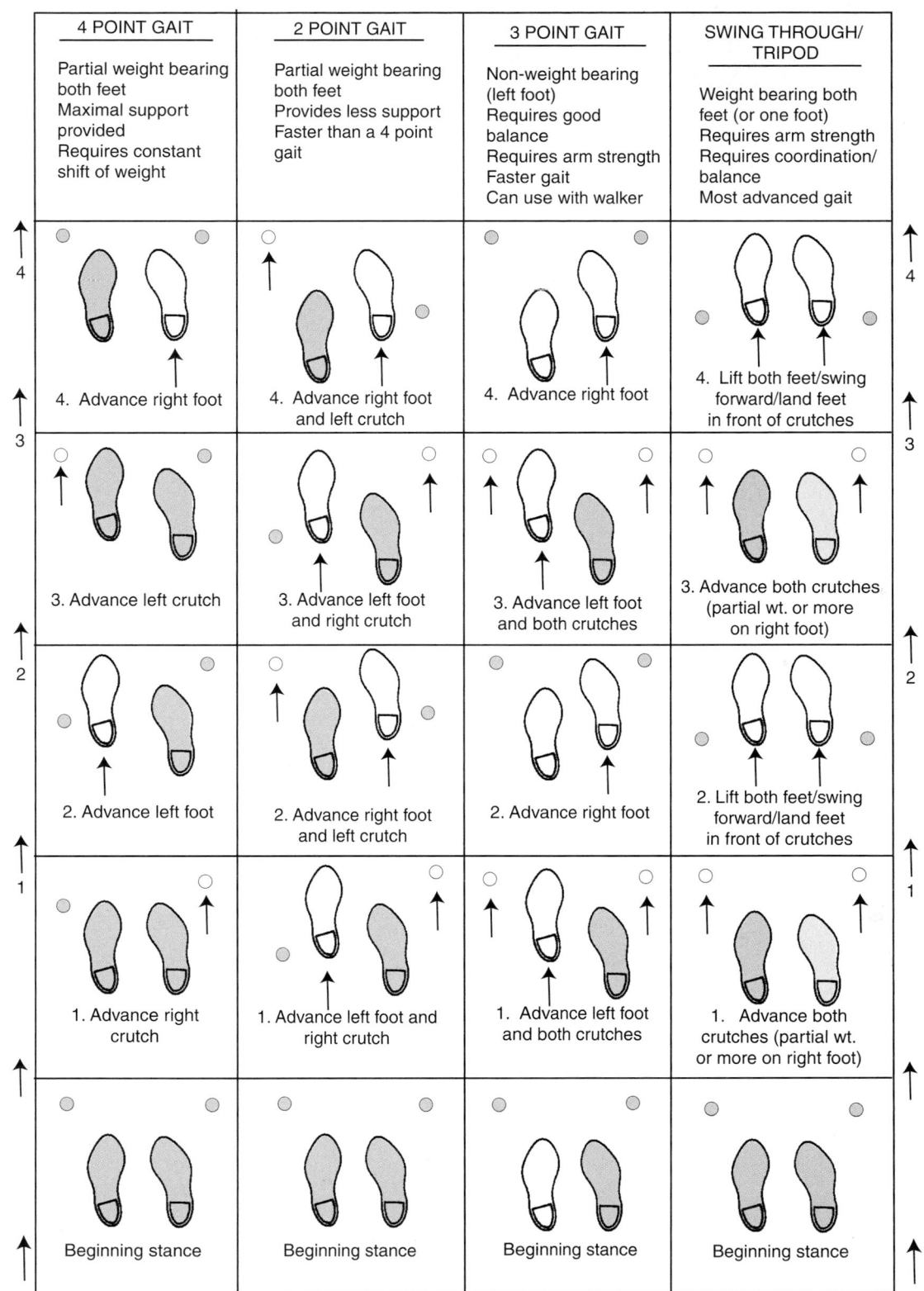

FIGURE 48-7. Crutch-walking gaits. *Shaded* areas indicate weight bearing. *Arrow* indicates advance foot or crutch. (The illustration of each gait begins at the bottom of the picture.)

■■■ TABLE 48-1 *C*RUTCH-WALKING GAITS

Gait	Walking Pattern
Two-point gait	Partial weight-bearing is permitted on both feet. The pattern is a speeded-up version of the four-point gait. *Pattern:* Right crutch and left foot forward at the same time, left crutch and right foot forward at the same time.
Three-point gait	Weight-bearing is permitted only on one foot. The other foot cannot support but may act as a balance. *Pattern:* Both crutches and the non-supportive leg go forward, then the weight-bearing leg comes through; the crutches are brought forward immediately, and the pattern is repeated.
Four-point gait	Weight-bearing is permitted on both feet. *Pattern:* Right crutch forward, left foot forward, left crutch forward, right foot forward.
Swing-through gait	Weight-bearing is permitted on only one foot. *Pattern:* Unaffected foot bears weight while both crutches are brought forward; then both legs swing through between the crutches, and weight-bearing returns to the unaffected leg. (Swing-through gait also can be used by the paraplegic client with weight-bearing on both feet.)

Taylor, C., Lillis, C., & LeMone, P. (2001). *Fundamentals of nursing: The art and science of nursing care.* (4th ed.). Philadelphia: Lippincott Williams & Wilkins.

three, left crutch forward; *four,* advance right foot. This gait is the easiest and the safest to use (the client always has three points of support). The client must be able to bring each leg forward, and clear the floor with each foot. Those who are partially paralyzed or who have fractures of both legs or arthritis can safely use this gait.

- In *swing-through* or *tripod gait,* the client stands on the strong leg, moves both crutches forward the same distance, rests his or her weight on the palms, and swings forward slightly ahead of the crutches. The client then rests the weight again on the good leg and balances for the next step. Because this gait is fast, the client should learn to balance before attempting it. This gait is often used following a fracture, when no weight-bearing is allowed on one leg. It also is used following amputation, when the prosthesis is not in place (particularly for young people). The client who is allowed to put weight on only one leg must hold up the other leg, bending the knee (not bending at the hip). *Rationale: It is important to prevent hip contracture, which can occur rapidly. A contracture is an abnormal shortening of muscles, which can lead to permanent deformity. This technique also improves balance.*

Bending the knee is tiring, and the client should rest frequently with the leg elevated.

Climbing Stairs.   When going up stairs, the client holds the handrail on the unaffected side, if one is available. Both crutches are held on the affected side. The stronger leg advances up the first step, with the client's weight on the crutches and the handrail. Then, the affected leg and the crutches move up to the same step, while the weight is on the stronger leg and the handrail. *Rationale: In this way, the client's weight is borne either by the crutches and the handrail or by the stronger leg. The handrail provides added safety and support.*

When descending stairs, the client reverses this process.

If no handrail is available, climbing stairs is more difficult and dangerous. In this case, as shown in Fig. 48-8, one crutch is held in each hand. The affected leg and the crutches move together as a unit, with the strong leg doing the work of climbing. Excellent balance and a fair amount of strength are necessary to climb stairs using crutches when no handrail is available.

✚👁 N u r s i n g   A l e r t
Adequate teaching is vital. The physical therapist and the nurse bear increased liability if the client does not receive adequate instruction and supervised practice. All instruction *must* be carefully documented.

Using One Crutch.   When the client progresses to using only one crutch, he or she places the crutch on the side of the stronger leg. When the affected leg moves forward, the crutch naturally swings forward with the contralateral hand.

The Lofstrand Crutch.   This type of crutch has a single hand bar for the user to grip, and a cuff that fits around the arm. People with a permanent disability (such as multiple sclerosis or post-polio syndrome) or a long-term disability (such as a spinal cord injury) often prefer this crutch. The person can drop the hand bar and grasp a handrail, or do work without losing the crutch. Although the Lofstrand crutch is more convenient than traditional crutches, it provides less stability (Fig. 48-9).

The Client Lift

A *hydraulic lift* is a mechanical device that elevates and transfers immobile clients from the bed, stretcher, wheelchair, tub, or toilet (Fig. 48-10).

The lift assists the nurse to lift a client who would otherwise be difficult to lift. Several models are available. Usually the device is equipped with a cloth sling that supports the client's body and holds it in alignment while he or she is being moved. The sling is attached to a swivel bar. The lift is pressure driven, and works much like a hydraulic car jack as the lever is pumped up. As you lift the client from one surface to another, the sling holds his or her body securely. When the

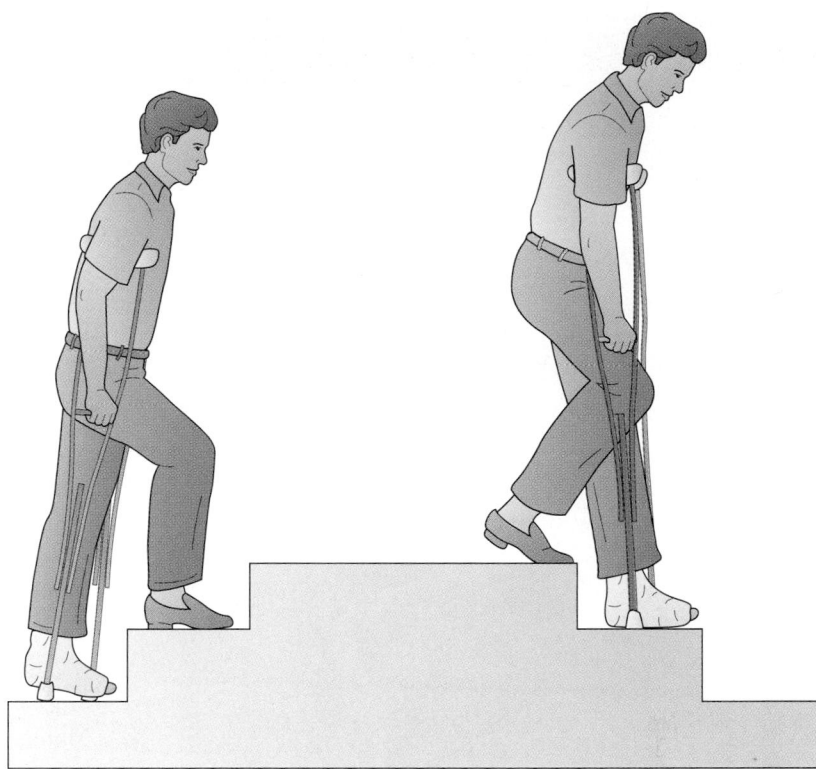

FIGURE 48-8. Stair climbing can be dangerous to the client. Balance must be maintained to prevent falls or injuries. Step "up with the good"; step "down with the bad." Both crutches and the affected foot move as a unit. It is very difficult to climb stairs without a handrail.

next surface is reached, pressure is released and the client is lowered to the new surface. When using these lifts, be familiar with the manufacturer's instructions for use, and maintain safety precautions at all times to prevent falls or injuries. Also secure any client equipment and tubing (eg, catheter drainage tubing) before moving the client.

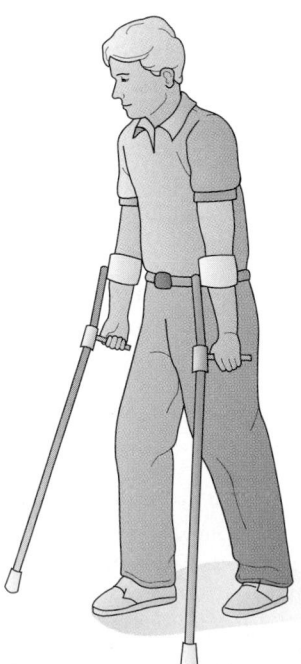

FIGURE 48-9. Lofstrand-style crutches offer forearm support while allowing greater flexibility of activity for the client.

Using Client Reminder Devices

A piece of equipment used to ensure the safety of the client and the healthcare environment is called a **protective device** or a **client reminder device** (In some situations, a device called a *leather restraint* is used. This device is different. Its use is explained in the following section of this chapter.) The client reminder device that is most often used in the general healthcare facility or nursing home is a vest or belt. Often, this device is used to help the client to remain in a chair. In Practice: Nursing Procedure 48-8 explains the uses of some client reminder devices.

Because the use of client reminder devices may be a potential legal violation of the client's freedom and may be dangerous, the nurse must know the agency's policies regarding their use. A client could be injured due to incorrect application or prolonged use without periodic release and reapplication. A client can also injure himself or herself while in such a device. Client reminder devices are applied on the physician's order, or on an emergency order from the charge nurse who has made an independent decision within policy guidelines to apply the reminder device. A physician's written order must be obtained after the emergency application of reminder devices.

Guidelines for nursing care of the client in a reminder device include correct application and frequent release so that the client's condition can be evaluated. Figure 48-11 provides an example of a form that could be utilized when these devices are applied in a non-psychiatric setting.

The client may view reminder devices as a threat, especially when a body part is immobilized. The confused, disoriented, or dangerous client requires careful and empathetic nursing

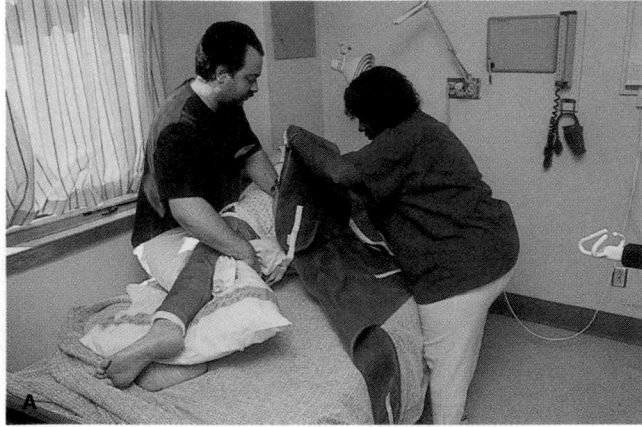

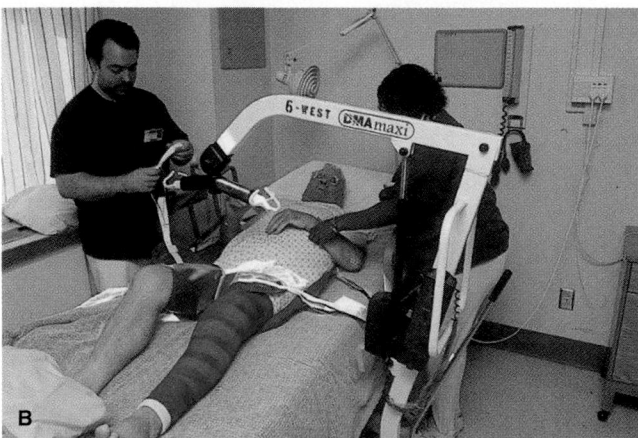

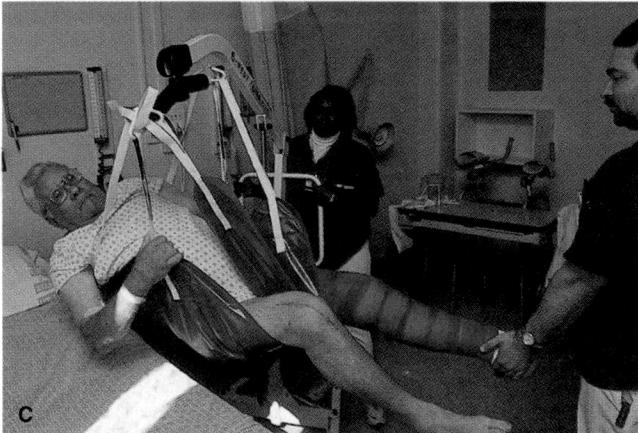

FIGURE 48-10. A hydraulic lift. (**A**) The device is equipped with a cloth sling that supports the client's body and holds it in alignment while he or she is being moved. (**B**) The sling is attached to a swivel bar. (**C**) The lift is pressure driven and works much like a car jack as the lever is pumped up. As you lift the client from one surface to another, the sling holds his or her body securely. When the next surface is reached, pressure is released and the client is lowered to the new surface.

care. Most importantly, the nurse must explain to the client that the device is applied to protect him or her and others from accidental injury. Explain the reason for this measure to family or friends of the client as well, so they understand that the ultimate goal is safety. See Figure 48-11 for information about documenting restraint use.

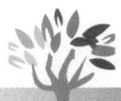

SPECIAL CONSIDERATIONS: THE LIFE SPAN

Client Reminder Devices for Children

In some extreme cases, a child must be controlled or held immobile. There are several means of accomplishing this. However, any type of restraint is used only as a last resort, because the child usually becomes very uncomfortable and frightened. Cases in which a child must be placed in some sort of protective or reminder device include delicate procedures such as circumcision or lumbar puncture. In addition, the child must be prevented from pulling on tubes or IVs, from scratching a rash, or from picking at a suture line. Children often are too young to understand explanations, so some sort of immobilization or reminder device must be employed.

The first choice is for another nurse or the child's mother to hold the child.

If the child must be immobilized or controlled in another way, methods include:

- Mummy restraint—the child is wrapped tightly in a blanket for a short time (to keep still for procedures)
- Mitts—the hands are wrapped in Kerlix, or special mitts are used (to prevent scratching or pulling at tubes or sutures)
- Padded tongue blade reminder device—prevents bending the elbows (to protect suture line or tubes when mitts will not work, such as following cleft lip repair)
- Papoose board—the child is held tightly to a specially-designed board for a very short time (for a surgical procedure such as circumcision)
- Bed net or bubble top—placed on the crib (to prevent child from jumping out)
- Jacket reminder device—similar to that for an adult, but smaller (to keep child in a chair)
- Child can be held or secured in a rocking chair (which allows movement, but prevents scratching or picking at a suture line)

Usually, children are not placed in arm, leg, or waist belts because of the extreme danger of strangulation. Chapter 70 describes child protective devices in more detail.

Nursing Alert

Some people who are restrained in any way become very agitated. They may chew through the device, even if it is leather. It is also possible for clients to strangle or to injure themselves by biting or scratching themselves. Clients may become so hysterical that they become exhausted. Death is possible. These are some of the reasons for very close nursing observation of clients while reminder devices are being used.

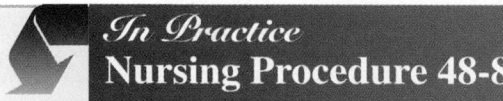

In Practice
Nursing Procedure 48-8

Using Client Reminder or Protective Devices
General Information

1. Use client reminder devices according to physician's order. Be sure you know the protocols for use of specific protective devices.
   RATIONALE: *There are legal implications in client reminder device use.*

2. Explain the procedure to the client and family.
   RATIONALE: *Relieve fear and gain their cooperation.*

3. Document use of protective devices and reasons for use. Be specific as to what device(s) are used. Verbal intervention must be attempted first and documented.

4. Loosen safety devices periodically, exercise the limbs, and check the condition of the skin.
   RATIONALE: *Prevent skin breakdown.*

5. Obtain a physician's order for use of any device, as per agency protocol.
   RATIONALE: *Some protective devices may be left on longer.*

6. Monitor the client on a one-to-one basis while a safety device is being used.
   RATIONALE: *To prevent injury to the client.*

7. Interview the client (usually the next day) to determine concerns and explore alternate means of handling the situation.

Upper Body Devices

There are two types of safety vests, the Criss-Cross Vest and the Posey Jacket Reminder Device.
   Determine which type of client reminder device you are using. If you have any questions, ask your team leader or instructor.
RATIONALE: *Improper application can be dangerous and can cause death from suffocation.*

Criss-Cross Vest

1. Place the vest on the client, with the opening in the front.

2. Pull the long tie on the end of the vest through the slit on the opposite side.

3. Cross over the client's abdomen. Be sure to cross the two sides of the vest in the front.

4. Bring one tie down on each side and tie to chair.

Posey Jacket Reminder Device

1. Put the jacket on with the opening in back. The side seams should be under the arms.

2. Close with zipper, ties, or hooks. Some types have extra ties.
   RATIONALE: *Ensure a snug fit.*

3. Tie shoulder loops around the push handles of a wheelchair.
   RATIONALE: *Prevent the client from falling forward.*

4. Use the loops. Never tie anything around the client's neck. Do not use this jacket on a bed.
   RATIONALE: *It does not allow the client to turn over in the bed. Shoulder loops may choke the client who struggles in bed.*

5. Tie the waist straps to the bars at the bottom back of the wheelchair.
   RATIONALE: *Prevent the client from sliding out of the chair.*

Soft Wrist Protective Devices

1. Apply the padded portion of the device around the wrist.
   RATIONALE: *Prevent skin breakdown.*

2. Protect the wrist with thick gauze or padded dressing under the protective device.
   RATIONALE: *Prevent skin breakdown.*

3. Pull the long tie through the slit in the safety device; apply the Velcro, or close the buckle.

4. Bring both ends of the long tie together, and attach to the *movable portion* of the bed frame or to the chair post.

5. Measure distance of the tie to allow for range of motion (ROM) of the arm, while protecting tubes or equipment from hands.
   RATIONALE: *Total restraint is frightening and can add to a client's confusion, making the client combative.*

Fastening the Straps of Protective Devices

If the client is in a wheelchair, tie the straps on each side to the posts in the bottom at the back. Be sure knots are out of the client's reach.
If the client is in bed, tie the straps to the *movable part* of the bed, and tuck any extra length up under the bedsprings.
   RATIONALE: *If straps are tied to a stationary part of the bed, the client could be injured if the bed is raised. The device must be able to move with the patient.*
Use quick-release knot or a square knot.

Other Types of Client Reminder and Safety Devices

If the client struggles, locked or unlocked leather straps may be necessary.
If the client slides forward, a device with a crotch piece is necessary.

FORM 78.10-A R7/98

THE UNIVERSITY OF CHICAGO HOSPITALS

RESTRAINT DOCUMENTATION
FLOW SHEET
(NON-PSYCHIATRIC UNITS)

		DATE	DATE
M.D. ORDER - NOTE DATE/TIME			

RESTRAINTS MUST BE REORDERED q 24°

TYPE & LOCATION OF RESTRAINT (S):
(CHECK TYPE AND LOCATION)

☐ LEATHER _ _ _ _ _ _ _ _ _ _ _	___ RUE ___ RLE ___ LUE ___ LLE	___ RUE ___ RLE ___ LUE ___	
☐ SOFT _ _ _ _ _ _ _ _ _ _ _ _	___ RUE ___ RLE ___ LUE ___ LLE	___ RUE ___ RLE ___ LUE ___	
☐ MITT _ _ _ _ _ _ _ _ _ _ _ _	___ RIGHT ___ LEFT	___ RIGHT ___ LEFT	
☐ VEST ☐ OTHER			

PATIENT/FAMILY EDUCATION DAILY	11										
Ed. provided to pt/family on	7										
restraint use	3										
Pt/family response to	11										
education	7										
	3										

PATIENT SAFETY CHECK		TIME & INITIAL PT. SAFETY CHECKS AT DESIGNATED TIME INTERVALS									
RESP. STATUS q 1 hr.*	11										
*When posey vest applied	7										
	3										
PROPER APPLICATION/RELEASE q 2 hr.	11										
Check to ensure restraints are applied correctly.	7										
Loosen or remove & assess for reapplication	3										
CIRCULATION q 2 hr.	11										
Check restrained extremity for swelling,	7										
discoloration, abnml. coolness.	3										
JOINT MOBILITY q 2 hr.	11										
Check restrained extrem. for movement of	7										
wrists, fingers, ankles, toes.	3										
SENSATION q 2 hr.	11										
Check to ensure patient perceives touch to	7										
restrained extremities.	3										
SKIN INTEGRITY q 2 hr.	11										
Check skin under restraints for bruising or	7										
abrasions.	3										
POSITION CHANGE q 2 hr.	11										
Note position & time of change	7										
CH = Chair R = Right L = Left B = Back	3										
ROM: ACTIVE/PASSIVE q 8 hr.	11										
Note extremity (RUE, RLE, LUE, LLE)	7										
and time of ROM.	3										
ELIMINATION INTERVENTIONS q 4°	11										
E1 - Incontinent E3 - Defecated	7										
E2 - Urinated E4 - Foley	3										
NUTRITION INTERVENTIONS q 4°	11										
N1 - Ate food N3 - Took Medication	7										
N2 - Took Fluids	3										

PT. RESPONSE q 2°											

R1- Unable to reach   R7- Confused
   therapeutics   R8- Restless
   (foley, IV tubings,   R9- Laughing
   drsg. etc.)   R10- Crying
	11										

R2- Quiet R11- Struggling against R3- Coherent restraints	7										

R4- Eyes closed/   R12- Hallucinating
   respirations regular R13- Physically/verbally
R5- Mute   Threatening
R6- Mumbling/   * = See progress
   incoherent   notes
	3										

INITIAL	FULL SIGNATURE/TITLE	INITIAL	FULL SIGNATURE/TITLE	INITIAL	FULL SIGNATURE/TITLE

FIGURE 48-11. Restraint documentation. (Form courtesy of University of Chicago Hospitals, Chicago, Illinois)

KEY CONCEPT

The Joint Commission on Accreditation of Healthcare Organizations (JCAHO) published new regulations regarding seclusion and restraint in 2001. These regulations have caused local healthcare facilities to write new protocols, to comply with the regulations. Check with your supervisor or instructor if you have questions about the use of client reminder devices or leather restraint safety devices in your particular facility.

The Violent Client

In the case of a violent client, it may be necessary to use a *client safety device* or *leather restraint*. (Different regulations apply to the use of *leather restraints* versus *client reminder devices* [discussed previously].) The leather safety device is most often used in psychiatry, and the regulations that apply are much more stringent. When using a leather safety device, a physician's order must be obtained immediately, and the physician is required to physically see the client within one hour of the emergency application. In addition, one-to-one nursing observation (a member of the nursing team within arm's reach at all times) must be provided for the client in such a device. Nursing staff is required to interview the client after leather safety devices are removed. This interview helps determine the client's feelings about the procedure and to explore alternatives to restraint. In addition, the client's family must be notified immediately upon application of such a device. The use of these devices is discussed in detail in Chapter 93.

MOVING THE CLIENT WHO IS PARALYZED

The person with **paraplegia** is paralyzed from the waist area down. This person has limited or no ability to move the legs, but usually is able to build up adequate arm strength. When assisting this person with a transfer, the nurse will need to move the legs, but the client can help lift with his or her arms. A chair with arms is used. The bed is placed in its lowest position. The nurse moves the client's legs over the side of the bed, and brings the client to a sitting position with the feet on the floor. The client then leans over, with his or her back toward the back of the chair, and grasps the arms of the chair (client's left hand—left arm of chair; client's right hand—right arm of chair). Usually, with minimal assistance, the client can use the arms to swing his or her buttocks into the chair. The nurse moves the legs into position as the client moves the buttocks. If the client is not skilled enough or strong enough to move the upper part of the body, two nurses will be needed to safely complete this transfer (unless the client is very light).

Sliding an Immobile Client From Bed to Chair

The sliding technique is especially useful when an immobile client is too heavy for one person to lift, and no other help is available. It can also be used to transfer a person to a chair or commode. Explain the transfer to the client to lessen anxiety about the process. Safety is important. Correct procedures should be followed, to prevent injury to staff or to the client. In Practice: Nursing Procedure 48-9 discusses these steps in detail.

Moving an Immobile Client From Chair to Elevated Bed

A slightly different technique is used when the surface to which the client will be transferred is higher than the surface the client is transferring from. In Practice: Nursing Procedure 48-10 provides detail for performing this technique correctly.

Using the Transfer Board or Bridge

A **transfer board** (*sliding board* or *bridge*) may be used for the client who is unable to stand. The board is made of hard plastic, and is approximately ½ to ¾ inch thick and long enough to reach from the side of the bed to a chair. It is about 1 to 1½ feet wide. It is lightweight and has handholds on the sides, making it easy to handle. The board's surface is smooth, and allows for ease in sliding the body. Using the board to transfer clients protects them from injury brought about by stretching or pulling on their limbs, and reduces the chance of a client fall. It also conserves the nurse's energy and prevents injury. Explain to the client what will be done and how he or she can help. In Practice: Nursing Procedure 48-11 outlines the steps for using the transfer board or bridge.

Using the Wheeled Stretcher

The wheeled stretcher (also called a gurney or litter) is used to:

Move clients who cannot sit up
Move clients with appliances or casts that do not fit into a wheelchair
Move clients to the operating room, x-ray department, or other rooms for special tests, treatments, or examinations, especially if they are sedated

Safety precautions to follow when using a wheeled stretcher:

Check to ensure that the rubber wheels are intact so the client is not jarred.
The stretcher covering should be clean. Provide enough blankets to keep the client warm.
Protect clients from injury by lifting them correctly and putting them down carefully on the stretcher. Make sure enough people participate to ensure safe lifting of the client.
Never leave a client alone on the stretcher.

Helping a Mobile Client Move From Bed to Wheeled Stretcher or Stretcher to Bed

If the client is able to help, place the stretcher tight against and parallel to the bed. Raise the bed so it is level with the stretcher. Lock the wheels of both the stretcher and the bed.

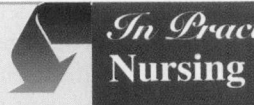

In Practice
Nursing Procedure 48-9

SLIDING THE CLIENT FROM BED TO CHAIR
Steps (for one nurse)

1. Place the bed in low position.
   RATIONALE: *This position is safest for both you and the client.*

2. Lock the wheels on the bed.
   RATIONALE: *A moving bed is a hazard.*

3. Be sure no obstacles are in the area.

4. Place a chair facing the foot and against the bed opposite the client's buttocks.
   RATIONALE: *The bed and chair should be at the same level.*

5. Slide your arms under the client's head and shoulders.
   RATIONALE: *This position supports the client.*

6. Advance one foot.
   RATIONALE: *Give yourself support.*

7. Rock backward, drawing the upper part of the client's body forward for easier sliding.
   RATIONALE: *Momentum will bring the client's body to the edge of the bed.*

8. Standing behind the client at his or her head, reach under the shoulders, and put one arm well under each axillae, resting the head and shoulders against you.
   RATIONALE: *Your body provides support for the client's head.*

9. Move carefully behind the chair, drawing the client into it as you move. Rock back, pulling the

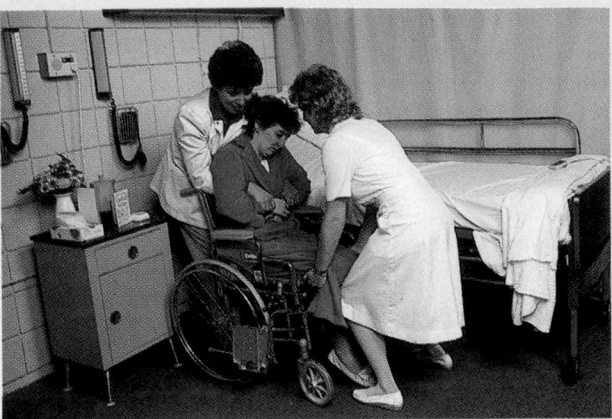

Standing behind the client at his or her head, reach under the shoulders and put one arm well under each axilla, resting the head and shoulders against you. Here, a second nurse moves the client's feet.

client into the chair, and brace yourself by leaning against the chair back. The chair is supported against the bed.
   RATIONALE: *Support the client's body as much as possible, and use proper body mechanics.*

10. Grasp the seat of the chair, and slowly pull the chair back until only the client's feet and ankles are resting on the bed. Be careful not to drop the feet to the floor.
    RATIONALE: *Injury could result.*

11. Flex the client's knees and legs as you lower the feet to the floor, keeping your own knees flexed.
    RATIONALE: *Provide passive exercise for the client's legs, and simulate normal sitting position.*

Cover the client with a blanket, and turn back the bedclothes. *Rationale: Prevent tangling in the bed linens.*

Assist the client to move onto the stretcher. During the move, the nurse braces his or her body tightly against the stretcher, holding the stretcher tightly against the bed. Make sure no space is between the stretcher and the bed. *Rationale: Prevent the client from falling through.* Use a bridge if the client has difficulty moving. (See In Practice: Nursing Procedure 48-11.)

Moving an Immobile Client From Bed to Stretcher

At least three people are needed to move an immobile or non-responsive client to a stretcher (unless the client is very small or a mechanical lift is used). An additional person may also be needed to move a cast or traction apparatus, or the legs of a person who has had spinal anesthesia or with **hemiplegia** (para-

lyzed on one side of the body). If a client is very large, more people are needed. In Practice: Nursing Procedure 48-12 outlines the detailed steps in moving an immobile client from bed to stretcher.

Assisting the Client Confined to Bed

Clients confined to bed need exercise and regular changes in body position to preserve their muscle tone, normal body functions, and morale. A schedule is usually set up to turn such a client at regular intervals. Doing so helps prevent musculoskeletal deformities, respiratory complications, circulatory disorders, constipation, and skin breakdown.

Adjusting the Backrest and Pillows
Raising and lowering the head of the bed is a simple yet easy way to change the client's body position. The nurse lifts the client's head and shoulders to adjust the pillows. In Practice:

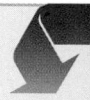

In Practice
Nursing Procedure 48-10

MOVING THE CLIENT FROM CHAIR TO ELEVATED BED
Steps (one nurse)

1. Bring the chair with the client in it to the side of the bed, and keep the client facing the center. If the chair does not roll, slide it to the bed rather than lifting it.

2. Place a transfer belt around the client's waist, if available.

3. Stand in front of the client on one side of the chair and place your arms under the client's axillae, drawing the person close against you. Or grasp the transfer belt on either side of the client's body.
   RATIONALE: *Supporting the upper portion of the client's body on your body reduces the weight to be moved.*

4. Standing with your foot near the chair drawn back, and the other foot forward, rock the client's trunk strongly upward, lifting the entire trunk and buttocks onto the bed.
   RATIONALE: *Using the weight of your body to move the client is an application of body mechanics.*

5. Support the client's thighs by resting against them.
   RATIONALE: *This position prevents falls.*

6. Slide the chair away with your foot.
   RATIONALE: *You need room for the next step.*

7. Pivot the client onto the bed. Brace the client's knees and thighs so they cannot buckle.

8. Lift the client's legs onto the bed, and roll and slide the client onto the bed.
   RATIONALE: *It is easier to lift the client in "sections" rather than all at once.*

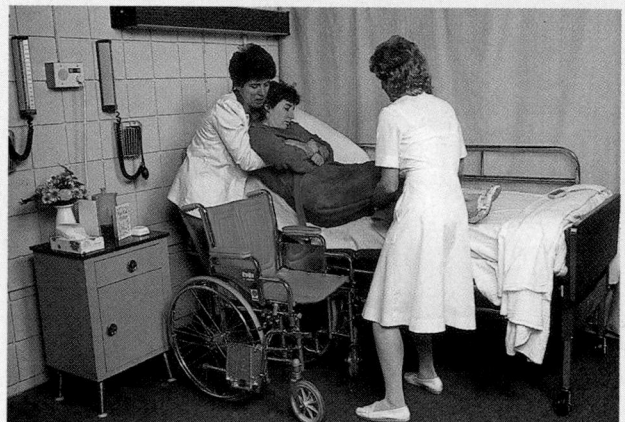

Lift the client's legs onto the bed, and roll and slide the client onto the bed. The procedure is easier with two nurses.

9. Make sure the client is comfortable, and the call light is within reach.

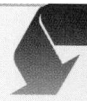

In Practice
Nursing Procedure 48-11

USING A TRANSFER BOARD
Steps

1. Lower bed to chair level. Lock the wheels on the bed.
   RATIONALE: *Prevent bed movement.*

2. Position the chair, commode, or wheelchair close to the head of the bed. Lock the wheelchair brakes.
   RATIONALE: *Prevent chair movement.*

3. Remove the arm rest from the wheelchair or commode.

4. Assist the client to an upright position in bed.
   RATIONALE: *This position prevents orthostatic hypotension.*

5. Insert one end of the board under the client's buttocks.
   RATIONALE: *The board serves as a wedge to accommodate body weight.*

6. Position the other end of the board on the chair.
   RATIONALE: *This establishes the bridge.*

7. Guide the client across the board from the bed to the chair. Make sure the board does not move.
   RATIONALE: *This helps control the transfer.*

8. Assess the client for proper body alignment.
   RATIONALE: *Prevent pressure on bony prominences and allow for adequate circulation.*

9. Apply a seat belt or other restraint if needed.
   RATIONALE: *Provide for client safety.*

In Practice
Nursing Procedure 48-12

MOVING THE CLIENT FROM BED TO WHEELED STRETCHER

Steps

1. Lock the bed wheels, and raise the bed to the same height as the stretcher.

2. Roll the client to one side of the bed and slip a draw sheet under his or her body; roll the client onto his or her back. Cover the client with a bed sheet or bath blanket.

3. Place the stretcher directly next to the bed with side rails down. Lock the stretcher's wheels.
   RATIONALE: *This position allows safe movement of the client.*

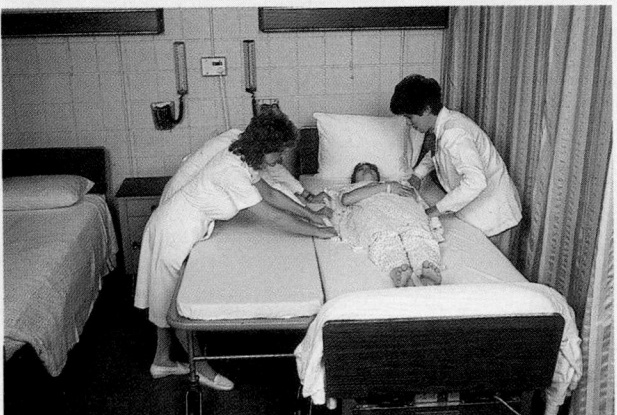

Position two nurses next to the stretcher away from the bed; position one or two nurses on the other side of the client next to the bed.

4. Position two nurses next to the stretcher away from the bed; position one or two nurses on the other side of the client, next to the bed.
   RATIONALE: *Dividing the work of moving the client among all nurses lessens each person's effort and prevents injury.*

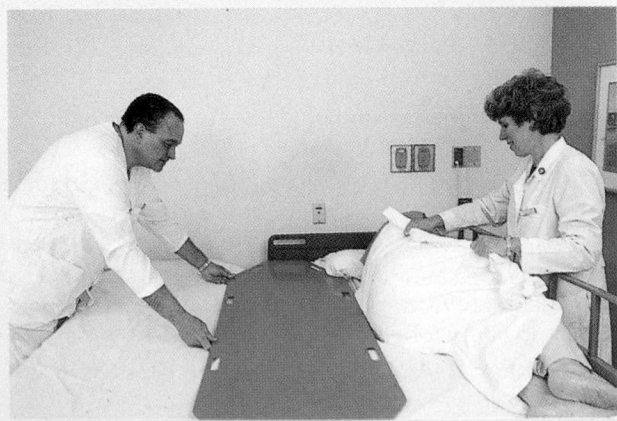

Turn the client on the side with his or her back to the stretcher. Place the transfer board lengthwise between the client and the stretcher.

5. All nurses grasp the edge of the draw sheet (lifting sheet) as close to the client's body as possible.
   RATIONALE: *Create a tight surface to ensure that the client's body is in proper alignment during the transfer.*

6. At an agreed-on signal, all nurses lift the client's body with the lifting sheet and move the client to the bed's edge. Pause, and then lift the client onto the stretcher.

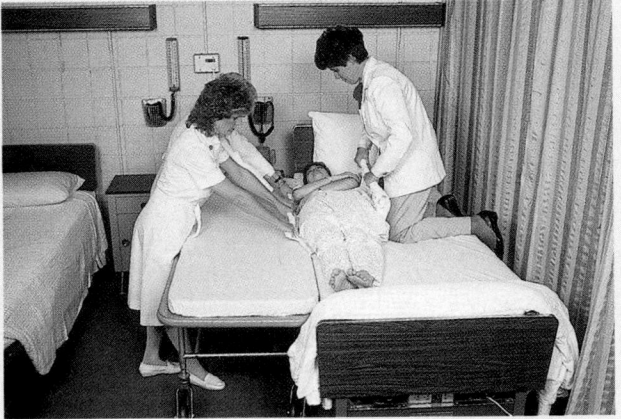

At an agreed-on signal, all nurses lift the client's body with the turning sheet and move the client to the bed's edge. Pause, then lift the client onto the stretcher.

7. Assess the client's body alignment. Cover the client and position reminder devices as needed.
   RATIONALE: *Prevent injury to the client's musculoskeletal system.*

If using a transfer board, after Step 1:

2. Place the stretcher directly next to the bed with the side rails down and lock its wheels.
   RATIONALE: *This position allows safe movement of the client.*

3. Turn the client on the side, with his or her back toward the stretcher. Place the transfer board lengthwise between the client and the stretcher.
   RATIONALE: *This position of the board provides a smooth surface.*

4. Place a draw sheet between the client and the transfer board; turn the client onto his or her back.

5. Grasp the draw sheet and slide the client across the transfer board onto the stretcher.
   RATIONALE: *The smooth surface decreases friction and facilitates easier movement of the client's body.*

6. Remove the transfer board and position the client comfortably; secure protective devices if necessary or raise side rails.[1]

Nursing Procedure 48-13 discusses the steps of adjusting the head of the bed.

Assisting the Immobile Client to Move Up in Bed
In Practice: Nursing Procedure 48-14 applies to moving all bedridden clients. Before beginning, the nurse assesses the client's ability to participate, encourages him or her to help as much as possible, and gives clear instructions on how to help. The nurse must be aware of his or her own limitations and capabilities, and ask for assistance if the client is too heavy to move alone.

The Lifting-Sheet Method.   Another method for moving the totally immobile client is the two-person draw sheet or

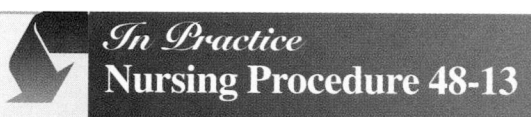

In Practice
Nursing Procedure 48-13

ADJUSTING FOR CLIENT COMFORT
Steps

1. Stand facing the client, with one foot forward and the body bent forward from the hips. RATIONALE: *This position helps you to maintain good body alignment.*

2. Put one arm under the client's shoulders, and put the client's nearer arm over your shoulder and around your neck.

3. Put your other arm under the client's other arm and across the back.

4. Tighten your thigh and hip muscles, and bring your body and the client's body upright together. RATIONALE: *Using proper body mechanics makes moving the client easier.*

5. Continue supporting the client while you adjust the pillows or backrest with your hand under the client's back.

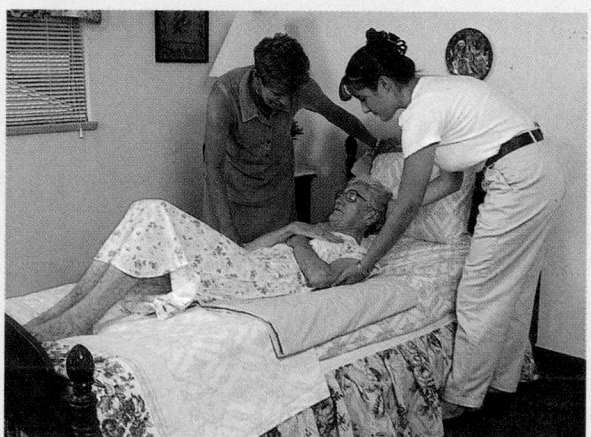

Continue supporting the client while you adjust the pillows or backrest.

lifting-sheet method. First, lock the bed wheels. Slip a wide draw sheet or folded large sheet under the client, from the head to below the buttocks. Roll the sides of the sheet close to the client's body. A piece of plastic under the lifting sheet helps it to slide easier and prevents dragging. *Rationale: The sheet serves as a handle to grasp on each side of the client.*

Two nurses stand across the client's bed from each other and facing each other. Both nurses place the foot closest to the head of the bed slightly behind the other foot (to widen the base of support). Both nurses grasp the rolled lifting sheet, with one hand near the client's neck and the other hand near the client's lumbar region. Together, both nurses lean forward, and then rock backward, away from the bed, lifting the client's body off the bed. Then, moving together, both nurses rock onto the foot that is closer to the head of the bed, also moving the client toward the head of the bed. (The nurses' combined weight lifts the client off the bed and then moves the draw sheet and client up toward the head of the bed.)

The lifting sheet method of moving a client can also be used to move the client to the side of the bed or down in bed. If one nurse is on the far side of a stretcher, this method can also be used to move a client to a stretcher.

This method helps to prevent sheet burns or irritation to the client caused by being pulled across the bed linens. It also helps to prevent client injury, which may be caused by pulling on the client's shoulders or by nurses placing their hands under the client's body. This procedure also saves back strain and injury to nurses. (Special care is necessary, particularly to guard against injuring the older or very ill person.)

Assisting the Immobile Client to Move to the Side of the Bed
Sometimes the nurse needs to move the client to the side of the bed so that he or she is closer for a treatment or injection. Moving the client to the side of the bed also prepares for rolling the client to a side-lying position. One nurse, using proper body mechanics, can move most clients to the side of the bed. Whenever possible, encourage the client to assist in the movement. The client can be encouraged to use the side rail or overhead trapeze to help in moving. The nurse serves as a support to the client. First, the client is assessed to see if he or she is able to understand the instructions. The nurse judges the client's size and weight, as compared with the nurse's capabilities. In Practice: Nursing Care Guideline 48-6 outlines tips for moving this client.

POSITIONING FOR EXAMINATIONS

The client is sometimes helped into a special position as part of a treatment or examination. Many different positions are used for physical examinations, nursing treatments and tests, and to obtain specimens. Because nurses assist clients into some of these positions and will see other positions used, it is important to know how to assist the client and how to place the necessary drapes. Important client positions are *horizontal* **recumbent** (lying on the back), *dorsal recumbent* (lying on the back with the knees flexed), *prone* (lying on the abdomen),

In Practice
Nursing Procedure 48-14

ASSISTING THE IMMOBILE CLIENT TO MOVE UP IN BED

Supplies and Equipment

Pillows
Side rails
Overhead trapeze (optional)
Draw sheet (optional)

Steps

1. Wash your hands.
   RATIONALE: *Prevent the spread of infection.*

2. Explain the procedure to the client.
   RATIONALE: *Providing information fosters the client's cooperation and understanding.*

3. Adjust the bed to a comfortable height.
   RATIONALE: *Bed at proper height prevents back strain.*

4. Lower the bed to as flat a position as the client can tolerate and lower the side rail.
   RATIONALE: *A flat bed eliminates the need to pull against gravity.*

5. Lock the wheels on the bed.
   RATIONALE: *Prevent the bed from rolling.*

6. Remove the pillow from under the client's head and place it against the head of the bed.
   RATIONALE: *Repositioning the pillow prevents injury to the client's head when moved upward.*

7. Assist the client to flex the knees and hips with feet flat on the bed.
   RATIONALE: *Allow the client to assist with the lift using the strength in his or her legs.*

8. Ask the client to assist with the move by:
   a. Folding his or her arms across the chest.
   b. Using an overhead trapeze (if available) to lift and pull the body upward.
   c. Pushing upward with the feet.
   d. Grasping the top of the bed and pulling with both hands.
   RATIONALE: *Encouraging the client to assist with movement fosters independence. Keeping the arms off the bed prevents friction rub of*

sheets when moving upward. Using large muscle groups increases the force of upward movement.*

9. Assume a broad-based stance by flexing your knees and hips with your feet spread and turned toward the head of the bed.
   RATIONALE: *This position lowers your center of gravity and provides a broad base of support before you move the client.*

10. Slide your arms under the client's shoulders and thighs.
    RATIONALE: *Support and evenly distribute the client's weight.*

11. Rock your weight onto your back leg, and shift upward with the client's assistance on the count of three. Repeat steps if necessary to advance the client further up in bed.
    RATIONALE: *Rocking motion assists the client's forward motion.*

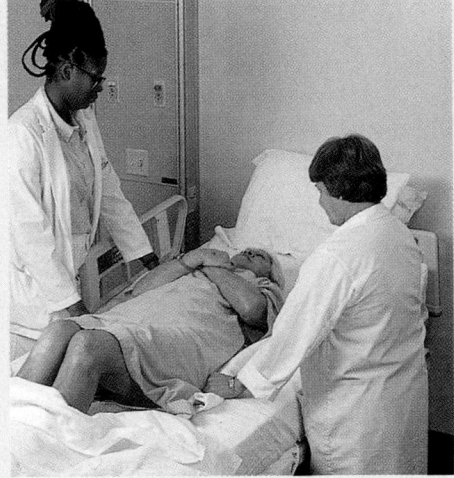

Moving the client in bed.

12. Replace the pillow under the client's head. Lower the bed and elevate the head as the client can tolerate. Raise side rail.
    RATIONALE: *Repositioning provides for the client's comfort. Side rails ensure safety.*

13. Wash your hands.
    RATIONALE: *Prevent the spread of infection.*

In Practice
Nursing Care Guidelines 48-6

MOVING AN IMMOBILE CLIENT TO THE SIDE OF THE BED

- Support the client's head and shoulders with one arm and the middle back with the other arm. *Rationale: By placing your hands in this manner, you move the largest area of the client's body.*
- Do all lifting and moving gently. *Rationale: Prevent injury or irritation to the client's skin.*
- Bend at the knees, move from front foot to back foot, and pull the client toward your body. Do not lift. *Rationale: Use proper body mechanics to avoid injury to yourself.*
- After you have moved the client's shoulders, repeat the same procedure with the hips and legs. *Rationale: Moving the client in two sections reduces the effort needed and makes it easier.*
- When moving a very large client, two nurses are more efficient than one. *Rationale: Although one nurse can move most clients, it is easier and often more comfortable for both the nurse and the client to ask for assistance.*
- Use proper body mechanics at all times, but do not be afraid to ask for help if necessary. *Rationale: It is vital to protect yourself from injury.*

Sims' (lying on the left side with the right knee flexed), **Fowler's** (lying on the back with the head elevated), knee-chest (lying on the knees with the chest resting on the bed), and **dorsal lithotomy** (lying on the back with the feet in stirrups) (see Box 48-2).

Although Chapter 47 describes physical examination in more detail, a few hints are included here. The following measures are carried out before draping the client for examination:

- The client is asked to empty the bladder, unless contraindicated. *Rationale: This helps the person feel more relaxed and helps the examiner to better palpate the area being examined. In some cases, a full bladder aids in the examination.*
- A urine specimen is collected, as ordered.
- The client is encouraged to defecate before a rectal examination.
- The client is provided with an examination gown or bath towel to cover the chest.
- A bath blanket or sheet is provided for warmth and privacy.
- The examination procedure is explained to the client.
- The body is draped appropriately for client privacy and examiner's access.
- The nurse stays with the client during the examination.

➡ STUDENT SYNTHESIS

Key Points

- The nurse can learn to effectively transfer and position clients for maximum safety and comfort for both nurse and client.
- Client reminder devices or protective devices must be used with caution and within agency guidelines.
- Pulling, pushing, or rolling an object is easier than lifting it. Keeping an object moving requires less energy or force than starting and stopping it.
- Rocking backward or forward on the feet uses body weight as a force for pulling or pushing.
- A client may become dizzy or faint when first getting out of bed.
- The nurse should move so that the client cannot grab him or her around the neck during transfers. Such a force can seriously injure the nurse.
- The hospital bed should be in low position, except when giving bedside care.
- The client's body alignment when lying down should be approximately the same as if the person were standing.
- Do not force joint movement when doing PROM.

Critical Thinking Exercises

1. Demonstrate how you would teach principles of body mechanics to a 30-year-old mother of a toddler.
2. Your client is a 25-year-old man who is recovering in traction after a femur fracture. He has been immobilized for several weeks. Now he is ready to begin walking, but will need assistance. He asks you about various kinds of walking aids. Describe your answer.
3. You are caring for an 88-year-old man in a nursing home. His physical therapist has advised him to do isometric exercises. The client is not sure why the exercises are important or what they are. Explain to him the purposes of his exercises and how to do them. How would you lead him through some exercises?

NCLEX-Style Review Questions

1. To prevent injury, the Posey jacket safety device should not be used:
   a. On a bed
   b. On a chair
   c. On a wheelchair
   d. When sitting
2. Prior to moving an immobile client up in bed, how should the bed be positioned?
   a. Fowler's
   b. Head of bed elevated
   c. Head of bed in flat position
   d. Knee elevated with gatch bed

3. Which of the following actions is correct when performing passive range of motion exercises?
   a. Begin exercises with the foot.
   b. Repeat each exercise five times
   c. Support all joints during exercise.
   d. Uncover all limbs to be exercised.
4. A client is having difficulty breathing. Which position should be used to make breathing easier for the client?
   a. Dorsal recumbent
   b. Fowler's
   c. Prone
   d. Sims'

5. Which instruction is most important for the nurse to include in discharge teaching for a client who will be using crutches?
   a. Avoid going up stairs.
   b. Rest underarms on the padded part of the crutch.
   c. Wear shoes that fit and have narrow heels.
   d. Weight bearing should be on the hands.

Reference

1. Taylor, C., Lillis, C., & LeMone, P. (2001). *Fundamentals of nursing: The art and science of nursing care* (4th ed.). Philadelphia: Lippincott Williams & Wilkins.

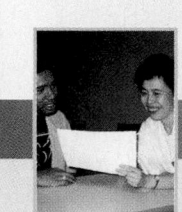

Beds and Bed Making

LEARNING OBJECTIVES

1. State the purposes of bed making in the healthcare facility.
2. Demonstrate the ability to make an unoccupied, occupied, and postoperative bed.
3. Demonstrate the ability to open a bed for a client.
4. Describe the use of a bed cradle.
5. Explain the purpose of side rails.
6. Demonstrate the ability to safely adjust side rails.
7. Describe three devices that may be added to the hospital bed and their uses.
8. Identify the purposes of specialized hospital beds.

NEW TERMINOLOGY

bed cradle
closed bed
egg crate
  mattress

flotation mattress
mitered (corners)
occupied bed
open bed

postoperative bed
traction
trapeze
unoccupied bed

Some clients are so ill that they are totally or partially confined to bed. A bed should provide comfort and correct posture for the client, as well as proper height and accessibility for caregivers. The ideal bed is durable, lightweight, easy to move, and easy to clean.

The most commonly used bed in healthcare facilities adjusts to different positions. (This is called a *Gatch bed.*) This bed is equipped with an electric mechanism that lowers and raises the entire bed so that the client can get in and out easily. The mechanism can lower and raise the head and foot of the bed as well. Often both the client and caregivers can use controls to position the bed as desired.

☛ KEY CONCEPT

The controls on a hospital bed can be locked so the client cannot adjust the bed. This may be necessary in the event of a delicate suture line or unset fracture. In these cases, adjusting the bed could cause client discomfort and could be dangerous to the client.

BED MAKING

The purpose of bed making is to help clients feel comfortable. Necessary supplies include clean linens, a tight bottom sheet to prevent wrinkles that might cause skin irritation, and upper bed clothing that does not weigh on the client's body or restrict movements, but still covers his or her shoulders. Adjustments in basic bed making may be necessary for comfort and to suit individual client conditions.

Schedules for changing beds vary among healthcare agencies. Usually you remake the bed after the client's bath or morning care. Make exceptions if the linen becomes soiled or if changing the bed may prove harmful to the client. For example, a client may be bleeding; receiving a special treatment; or feeling too weak or exhausted to be disturbed. Change stained sheets immediately. In some cases, beds are not changed every day or are partially changed. Even if you do not change the bed, tuck in sheets and blankets to get rid of wrinkles and fluff the pillows.

☛ KEY CONCEPT

Every client needs a smooth, clean bed for comfort. Wrinkles or crumbs can make the client uncomfortable and cause skin breakdown.

Proper body mechanics are an essential part of bed making. Put them into practice by following the guidelines in Chapter 48.

Making an Unoccupied Bed

An **unoccupied bed** is a bed that is empty at the time it is made up and is the easiest bed to make. The unoccupied bed can be made up either as a closed bed or as an open bed. A **closed bed** is a bed that is made up when preparing the unit for a new client. An **open bed** is a bed to which a client is already assigned. After making any bed, step back and survey your work to see if the linens are straight; firmly tucked under the mattress; smooth and without wrinkles; and not hanging onto the floor.

To make a *closed bed,* the top covers are pulled up to the head of the bed over the bottom covers. A pillow is placed on top of the linens, much like you would do in your home. Specific steps in making a closed bed are given in In Practice: Nursing Procedure 49-1. To make the *open bed,* the top covers are fan-folded to the foot of the bed so the client can get into bed easily. Steps in making an open bed are also found at In Practice: Nursing Procedure 49-1.

Making an Occupied Bed

Some clients are unable to get out of bed as a result of their specific condition or generalized weakness. Changing bed linens with the client in the bed is called making an **occupied bed.** Work quickly, and disturb the client as little as possible. This task of bed making may be done alone; however, if the client is large or his or her medical condition is unstable, ask a coworker to assist you. In Practice: Nursing Procedure 49-2 gives the steps in making an occupied bed. If done efficiently, this procedure requires minimum exertion for both you and the client. Some clients need extra blankets for additional warmth, and some may have fractures or injuries that necessitate turning or moving them in a special way.

Opening a Bed for a Client

Open beds allow linens to be turned down, making it easier for the client to get into bed. Open a bed for a new client or leave it open when the client is out of bed for a short time. Follow these steps:

- Turn the bedspread down from the top, and fold it around and over the top edge of the blanket. Then fold the sheet over the top of the blanket and spread. *Rationale: Protect the blanket, keep the rough blanket away from the client's skin, and make it easier for the client to handle the bedclothes.*
- Turn the top bedding down to the foot of the mattress, and fold it back on itself. *Rationale: Show the client that the bed is ready. Helping the person into bed is also easier when the bed is open.*
- Always leave the bed in low position. *Rationale: It is vital to prevent falls.*

Making a Postoperative Bed

When a client is to return from the operating room or from another procedure that requires transfer into bed from a stretcher or wheelchair, a **postoperative bed** is made up. The postoperative bed is made in such a way as to make it easy to transfer the client from a stretcher to the bed. In Practice: Nursing Care Guidelines 49-1 outlines the steps in making this bed.

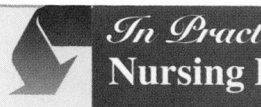

In Practice
Nursing Procedure 49-1

MAKING A CLOSED OR UNOCCUPIED BED
Supplies and Equipment

Gloves (optional)
2 sheets (either 2 flat sheets or 1 flat sheet and
  1 contour bottom sheet)
Draw sheet (optional)
Blanket
Bedspread
Pillowcases
Linen hamper or bag
Mattress pad
Bedside table or chair

Steps

1. Gather linens and supplies.
   RATIONALE: *Organization facilitates accurate skill performance.*

2. Wash your hands.
   RATIONALE: *Handwashing prevents the spread of infection.*

3. Adjust the bed to a comfortable height. Remove the call bell if it is attached.
   RATIONALE: *A bed placed at the proper height prevents back strain.*

4. Wear gloves if the linens are soiled. Loosen all soiled linens. Remove, roll up, and place them in a linen hamper or bag. Never place soiled linens on the floor or hold them against your uniform.
   RATIONALE: *Many microorganisms are on the floor. Soiled linens from the bed or floor can contaminate your uniform, which may come in contact with other clients.*

5. Refold the bedspread or any item that is to be re-used. Place it on the table or on the back of the chair.
   RATIONALE: *Agency policy dictates which linens are to be reused if they are not soiled.*

6. Remove soiled pillowcases and place them in the linen hamper. Move pillows to the chair.
   RATIONALE: *Removing pillows from the bed simplifies bed making.*

7. Slide the mattress toward the head of the bed. Place a mattress pad on the bed.
   RATIONALE: *Moving up the mattress provides more foot room for the client.*

8. Place a bottom sheet on the bed. Open it lengthwise, with the center fold along the bed's center. Unfold the upper layer of the sheet toward the opposite side of the bed. Slide the sheet upward over the top of the bed, leaving the bottom edge of the sheet even with the edge of the mattress. If using a fitted (contour) sheet, tuck it over the mattress at the upper and lower end of that side.

RATIONALE: *Unfolding the sheet in this manner allows you to make the bed on one side.*

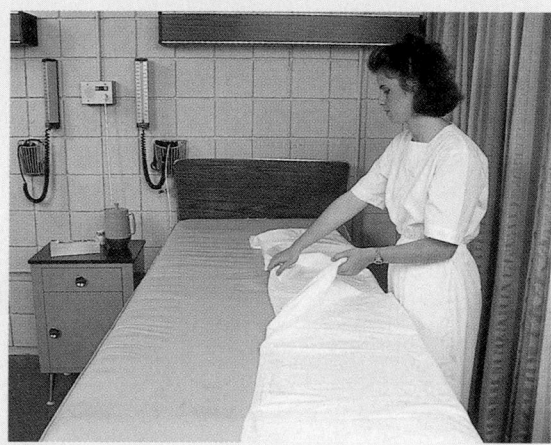

Centering the bottom sheet on the bed.

9. Tuck the sheet securely under the head of the mattress. Make a diagonal or **mitered** (square) corner if the sheet is not fitted. The following figures show you how to make a mitered corner.
   RATIONALE: *A mitered corner has a neat appearance and keeps the sheet securely under the mattress.*

   a. Pick up the selvage edge with your hand nearest the foot of the bed.

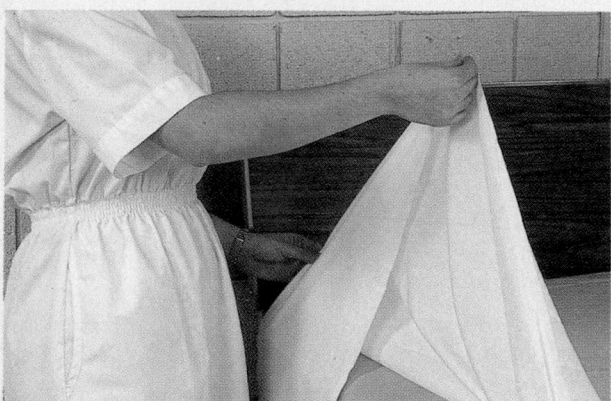

Picking up the selvage edge.

   b. Lay a triangle back on the bed.
   c. Tuck the hanging part of the sheet under the mattress.
   d. Drop the triangle over the side of the bed.
   e. Tuck the hanging edge under the mattress.

10. Tuck the sheet under the entire side of the bed.
    RATIONALE: *Secure the bottom sheet on one side of the bed.*

(continued)

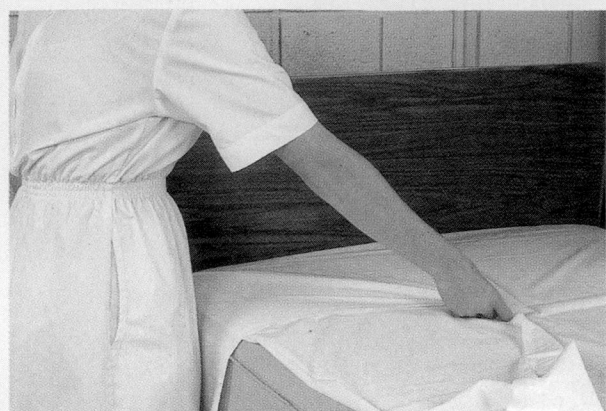

Laying a triangle back on the bed.

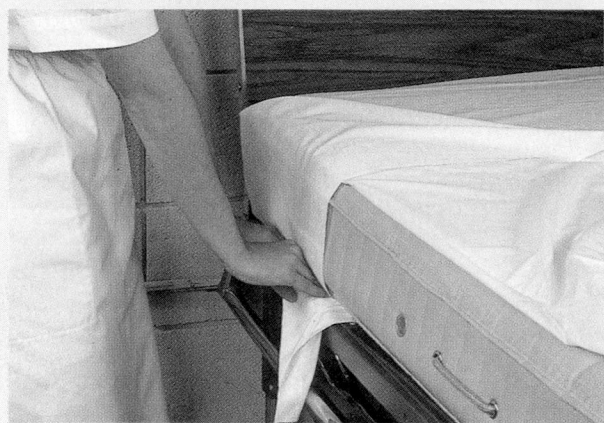

Tucking the hanging part.

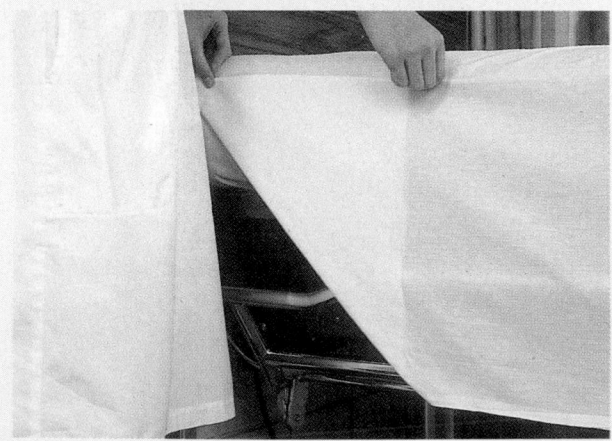

Dropping the triangle over the side of the bed.

11. Place a draw sheet (if used) on the bed, folded in half, with the fold in the center of the bed. Lift the top half toward the other side of the bed. Tuck the draw sheet under the mattress.

RATIONALE: *A draw sheet is an additional protection for the bed and serves as a lifting or turning sheet for an immobile client.*

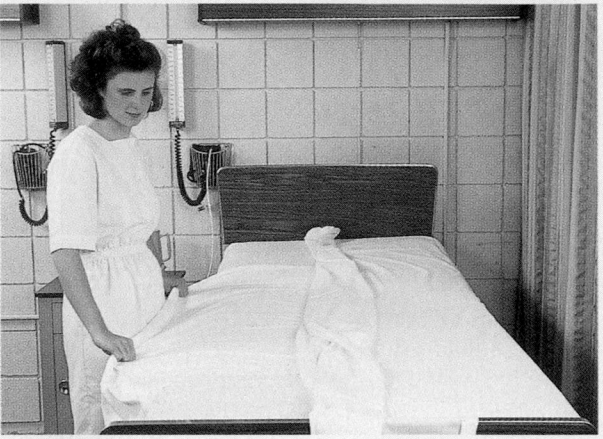

Pulling the draw sheet taut.

12. Place the top sheet on the bed, centering it in the same manner as the bottom sheet. Make sure the upper hem of the top sheet is level with the top of the mattress. Drop the lower end of the sheet over the end of the mattress.
    RATIONALE: *Staying on one side of the bed until it is completely made saves steps and time.*

13. Cover the top sheet with a blanket and/or bedspread. Tuck all these together under the bottom of the mattress. Miter the corner.
    RATIONALE: *Tucking all these pieces together saves time and provides a neat appearance.*

14. Move to the other side of the bed. Tuck in the linens as in step 13. Fold back the cuff at the head of the bed with the sheet and bedspread if the client will be returning to bed.
    RATIONALE: *A blanket provides warmth. A bedspread ensures a neat appearance. The cuff makes it easier to fold back the linens.*

15. Put a clean pillowcase on the pillow.
    RATIONALE: *Using this method minimizes shaking the pillow excessively:*
    a. Rest the pillow on a flat surface.
    b. Grasp the pillowcase in the center on the closed end.
    c. Turn the pillowcase back over your hand.
    d. Grasp the pillow through the pillowcase.
    e. Pull the pillowcase over the pillow.
    f. Adjust the pillowcase smoothly over the pillow. An alternate method is to put one hand inside

In Practice
Nursing Procedure 49-1 (Continued)

the pillowcase and pull the pillow corners into the corners of the pillowcase.

16. Place a pillow at the top of the bed in the center, with the open end away from the door.
    RATIONALE: *A pillow is a comfort measure. The open end may collect dust or microorganisms.*

17. Make a toe pleat at the foot of the bed.
    RATIONALE: *Toe pleats allow freedom of foot movement:*

    a. For a horizontal pleat, gather the linens to make a fold approximately 2–4 inches (5–10 cm) across the foot of the bed.

    b. For a vertical pleat, gather the linens to make a fold approximately 2–4 inches (5–10 cm) perpendicular (up and down) to the foot of the bed.

    The **closed bed:** *If no client is assigned to that client unit, make a* closed bed. *Pull the covers up to the head of the bed. Place the pillow on top. This keeps the bed clean and ready for the next occupant.*

18. *The* **open bed:** If a client is assigned to the bed, you will make an open bed. Fanfold the top of the linens to the bottom third of the bed. This is called an open bed.
    RATIONALE: *This allows the client easier entry into bed.*

19. Replace the call signal on the bed and secure it in place.
    RATIONALE: *Provide safety for the client to call for help.*

20. Move the overbed table next to the bed.
    RATIONALE: *Bedside necessities will be within easy reach for the client.*

21. Return the bed to low position if the client is ambulatory, or high position if the client is returning to the room by stretcher.
    RATIONALE: *Prepare the bed for the client's return.*

22. Discard linens appropriately. Wash your hands.
    RATIONALE: *Handwashing and proper linen disposal prevent the spread of infection.*

In Practice
Nursing Procedure 49-2

MAKING AN OCCUPIED BED

Supplies and Equipment

Gloves (if needed)
2 sheets (either 2 flat sheets or 1 flat sheet and 1 contour bottom sheet)
Draw sheet (optional)
Blanket
Bedspread
Pillowcases
Linen hamper or bag
Mattress pad
Bedside table or chair
Bath blanket (optional)

Steps

1. Gather linens and supplies.
   RATIONALE: *Organization facilitates accurate skill performance.*

2. Explain the procedure to the client.
   RATIONALE: *Providing information fosters cooperation and understanding.*

3. Wash your hands. Put on gloves if the linens are soiled.
   RATIONALE: *Handwashing prevents the spread of infection. Gloves act as a barrier. Wear them to prevent contact with soiled linens, body fluids, or drainage.*

4. Adjust the bed to a comfortable height. Remove the call bell if it is attached to linens. Lower the side rail on the near side, while keeping the other side rail raised.
   RATIONALE: *Proper bed height prevents back strain. The raised side rail prevents the client from falling out of bed.*

5. Lower the head of the bed if the client can tolerate it.
   RATIONALE: *The bed is easier to make when it is in the flat position.*

6. Loosen the top bed linens. Remove the spread, refold it if it will be reused, and place it on the table or back of the chair.
   RATIONALE: *Agency policy indicates which linens to reuse if not soiled.*

(continued)

7. Place a bath blanket over the top sheet and ask the client to hold onto the upper edge if he or she is able to do so. Remove the top sheet, and place it in the linen hamper or bag. If a bath blanket is unavailable, leave the top sheet in place.
   RATIONALE: *The bath blanket and top sheet keep the client warm and protect his or her privacy.*

8. Slide the mattress toward the head of the bed if necessary. Request assistance to do this.
   RATIONALE: *Moving the mattress up provides more foot room for the client.*

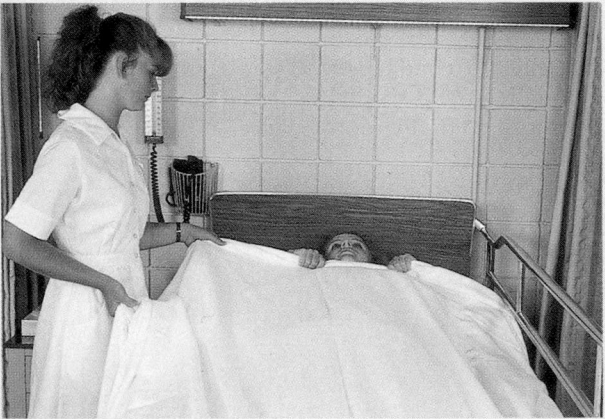

Placing the bath blanket.

9. Assist the client to turn toward the other side of the bed. Adjust the pillow. The client can help by holding onto the side rail, if able.
   RATIONALE: *Moving the client as close to the other side of the bed as possible gives you more room to make the bed.*

10. Loosen bottom bed linens. Fanfold used linens from the side of the bed and wedge them close to the client. Leave the mattress pad in place unless soiled.

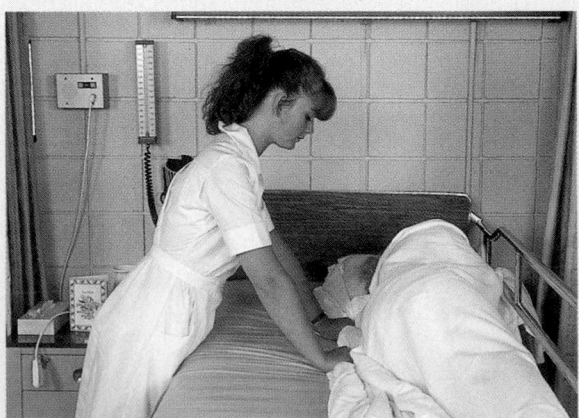

Fan-folding used linen toward the client.

RATIONALE: *Placing folded used linen close to the client allows more space to place the clean bottom sheets.*

11. Place the clean bottom sheet on the bed folded lengthwise, with the center fold as close to the client's back as possible. Adjust the sheet, miter the upper corner, and place the draw sheet (optional) as in Procedure 49-1, Steps 8, 9, and 10. If using a fitted (contour) sheet, tuck it over the mattress at the upper and lower ends. Fold upper half of the sheet and draw it back toward the center. Tuck it under the client and under soiled linens.
    RATIONALE: *Used linens can easily be removed, and clean linens are positioned to make the other side of the bed.*

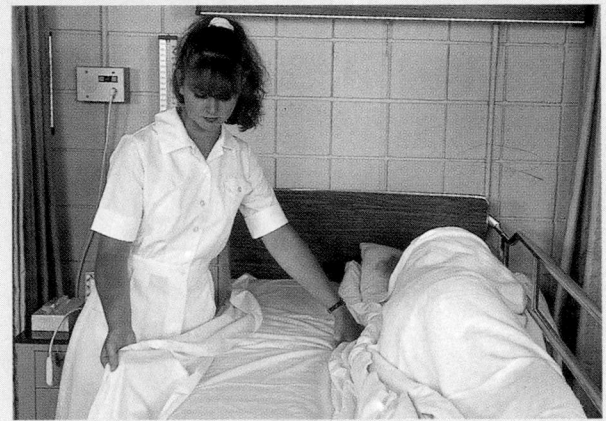

Unfolding the clean linen.

12. Raise the side rail. Move to the bed's other side. Help the client roll over the folded linen to the other side of the bed. Lower the side rail on your side. Readjust the pillow and bath blanket.
    RATIONALE: *Side rails maintain safety. Moving the client to the bed's other side allows you to make the bed on that side.*

13. Remove the used bottom linens. Hold them away from your uniform. Place them in the hamper or bag. Straighten the mattress pad.
    RATIONALE: *Used linens can contaminate your uniform, which may come into contact with other clients.*

14. Grasp clean linens and gently pull them out from under the client. Spread them over the bed's unmade side. Pull the linens taut and tuck in the bottom sheet. Miter the corner. If using a contour sheet, tuck it in both the top and bottom corners. Brace your knee against the bed. Pull the bottom sheet and draw sheet taut, prior to tucking them under the mattress.
    RATIONALE: *Wrinkled linens can cause skin irritation.*

In Practice
Nursing Procedure 49-2 *(Continued)*

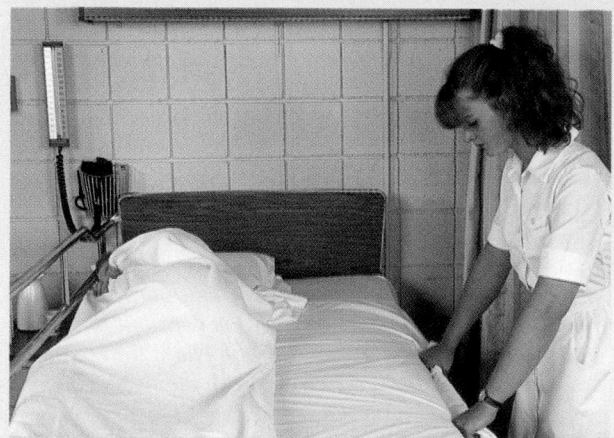
Tucking in the bottom sheets.

15. Assist the client back to the center of the bed. Remove the pillow. Replace the used pillowcase with a clean one and return the pillow to the bed under the client's head.
    RATIONALE: *The pillow is a comfort measure for the client.*

16. Place the top sheet over the bath blanket. Ask the client to hold onto the upper edge. Remove the bath blanket and place it in the linen hamper or bag, or client's closet. Unfold the bedspread over the top sheet. Tuck the lower ends securely under the mattress. Miter corners.
    RATIONALE: *Tucking these pieces together saves time and provides neat, tight corners.*

17. Turn the top edge of the spread back over the sheet.
    RATIONALE: *This technique provides a neat appearance.*

18. Make a toe pleat or loosen the top linens over the client's feet (see Procedure 49-1, step 17).
    RATIONALE: *Toe pleats allow for freedom of foot movement.*

19. Raise side rail. Lower the bed and adjust the head of the bed to a comfortable position. Replace the call signal on the bed.
    RATIONALE: *These measures provide for safety.*

20. Discard linens appropriately. Remove gloves and wash your hands.
    RATIONALE: *These measures prevent the spread of infection.*

ATTACHMENTS AND ACCESSORIES

Bed Cradle

A **bed cradle** is a frame used to prevent the bedclothes from touching all or part of the client's body. It is used for clients with fractures, extensive burns, and open or painful wounds. A wide cradle fits all the way along the bed lengthwise. A narrow one fits along the bed lengthwise; it can be used over one arm or leg. Bed cradles are usually made of metal or plastic. Arrange bed linens over the cradle. In some instances, you will pin the linens to the cradle or frame. Leave the linens long enough at the top to cover the client's shoulders comfortably. Place side rails up for safety. Discourage clients from adjusting the bed controls to avoid displacing the cradle and causing injury to themselves. (You may need to lock the controls so the client does not forget.) In Practice: Nursing Procedure 49-3 shows how to make a bed that includes a bed cradle.

Side Rails

Side rails (safety rails) are bed rails that not only prevent clients from falling out of bed, but also help the client to change position while in bed. They often incorporate TV controls and the nurse call signal as well. Sometimes, however, these bed rails alarm older or confused clients. Most facilities have a standard policy regarding the use of side rails. Make it your practice to be aware of these policies and to follow protocols, always keeping the safety of your clients in mind.

> **Nursing Alert**
> In some cases, having the side rails up can be more dangerous than having them down. For example, an elderly client may continually try to crawl out of bed. In this case, he or she might crawl over the side rails, making a potential fall worse than if it were just from the lower level of the bed.

It is natural for a client to resent side rails. Many people fear being shut in or treated as if they are irresponsible. Explain to the client and family that side rails are for the client's protection. If protecting the client from pressure or possible injury is necessary, cushion the side rails of the bed with a mattress pad, bath blanket, seizure pads, or pillows. Restless or confused clients may press or throw themselves against the hard side rails or may attempt to climb over them.

Other Equipment

A *footboard* may be attached to the foot of the bed to prevent a deformity called *footdrop,* which may occur when a client remains in bed for a prolonged period (see Chapter 48). The

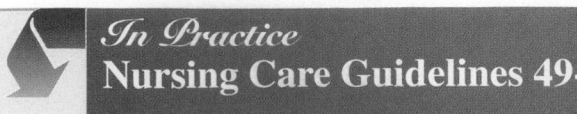

In Practice
Nursing Care Guidelines 49-1

MAKING A POSTOPERATIVE BED

- If the client has had surgery, make the entire bed with clean linen. *Rationale: Reduce the possibility of postoperative infection by removing as much contamination as possible.*
- Wash your hands. *Rationale: Prevent the spread of infection.*
- Make the bottom (or foundation) of the bed as you normally would. The postoperative bed usually requires a draw sheet under the client's hips. You also may wish to place several disposable pads on the bed. Usually another draw sheet is placed under the client's head. *Rationale: By using a draw sheet and pads, changing the entire bed will be unnecessary if the client has emesis or is incontinent. You can then change only the soiled articles. You may also use a drawsheet to lift the client.*
- In some cases, top linens are simply fan-folded to the foot of the bed. In others, a full postoperative bed is made. To do this, put the top linens over the foundation, but do not tuck them in. Fold down the top as you would for an occupied bed. Then fold the bottom of the linens up so that the fold is even with the bottom of the mattress. Do not tuck the linens in. Fanfold the top linens to the side so that they lay opposite from where you will place the client's stretcher. Alternatively, you may fanfold the linens to the foot of the bed. Leave a tab on top for easy grasping. *Rationale: Placing the linens all to one side or folded to the bottom keeps them out of the way for easy transfer of the semiconscious client. The tab on top makes pulling the covers over the client easy after he or she is in bed.*
- Have one or two pillows available, but do not put them on the bed. *Rationale: A pillow may be contraindicated for a client; usually the physician or charge*

nurse will determine when it is safe for the client to have one.
- Be sure all furniture is out of the way. *Rationale: You need to make room so the stretcher can be brought to the bedside easily.*
- Be sure the call light is available, but keep it on the bedside stand until the client is in bed. *Rationale: It is important for the client to be able to summon help immediately if he or she has any postoperative complications. The call light cord is kept out of the way, to facilitate the transfer of the client into bed.*
- Know what surgical procedure your client has had before you determine what special equipment is needed. For the client's convenience and safety, make the following items available: tissues, an emesis basin, a blood pressure cuff and stethoscope, a "frequent vital signs" flow sheet, an intake and output record, and an intravenous (IV) stand. Most clients will require a bedpan; males need a urinal. Often, a bath basin is also required for the first day or so after surgery. You will need to add other items, according to the client's specific requirements. Learn from the Recovery Room nurse's report whether your client needs such items as a suction machine, chest drainage setup, or other special equipment. *Rationale: It is important to have all pieces of equipment available immediately upon the client's arrival. Omission of an important piece of equipment causes inconvenience and could even be life-threatening.*
- Report to your charge nurse when you have completed the postoperative bed and assembled the necessary equipment. *Rationale: The charge nurse will then know when it is safe to authorize the client's transfer from the Recovery Room.*

---

footboard has a slight angle to it and is placed to support the client's feet in a simulated standing position. A *bed board* may be placed under the mattress to support the body in correct alignment. In addition, the headboard and foot end of hospital beds are usually removable, for placement under the client if CPR is needed. In some cases, a separate *CPR board* is attached to the bed; the crash cart contains a CPR board as well. Hospital beds are also equipped with a means for attaching a *standard* that holds bags for intravenous (IV) or blood therapy. (The standard itself is often stored on a rack under the bed, for easy access.) Additional equipment, such as suction bottles, catheter bags, or client reminder devices, may also be clamped onto the bed frame.

A **trapeze,** a horizontal bar hanging on chains, is often attached to a large overhead frame, which itself attaches to the bed. The trapeze is used by the client to pull up to a sitting posi-

tion or to lift the shoulders and hips off the bed. The trapeze is also used to exercise and strengthen the arms, particularly if the client will be using crutches or is a person with paraplegia (paralyzed from the waist down).

The client may be placed in **traction.** Traction consists of a series of ropes, pulleys, and weights that serve to keep a body part, such as a leg, in proper alignment. Chapter 76 describes the care of a client in traction. The ropes and pulleys must be maintained in straight alignment. Do not remove traction weights without your supervisor's instruction.

SPECIAL BEDS AND MATTRESSES

Special types of mattress surfaces are used for clients on prolonged bed rest or for those with poor skin integrity. Examples include the **egg crate mattress,** which is foam rubber

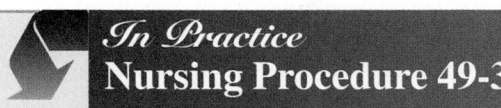

In Practice
Nursing Procedure 49-3

USING A BED CRADLE
Supplies and Equipment

Bed cradle
Linens used for changing a bed
Extra blanket
Bath blanket
Extra top sheet
Extra bedspread

Steps

1. Make the foundation of the bed as you would for any client. A smooth foundation is especially important for the client who spends a great deal of time in bed.

2. Tuck the top sheet under the foot of the bed to hold it in place.

3. Place the cradle. Draw the top sheet over the cradle.
   RATIONALE: *The cradle protects the client's limbs.*

4. Place another top sheet over the first top sheet, overlapping the two as much as is necessary.
   RATIONALE: *Make the linens long enough to cover the client's shoulders when the bed is completed.*

5. Hold the bottom of the second top sheet and the top of the first top sheet, with hems lined up, off the bed. Roll them over each other, making a flat fold crosswise to the bed. Repeat this process as many times as is necessary to obtain the correct length of sheeting.
   RATIONALE: *The goal is to keep the client warm. The double fold will hold the sheets together, and they will seem like one long sheet.*

6. Tuck in the blanket at the bottom of the bed. Pull it up over the bed cradle. Add a second blanket, and fold it the same way as you did for the sheets. Follow the same procedure for the bedspread, folding the covers at the head of the bed as for an open bed.
   RATIONALE: *When all three layers of covers are folded together, they will be long enough to cover the client's shoulders and secure enough to pull up without separating.*

7. Place a bath blanket under the cradle, covering the client as much as he or she desires.
   RATIONALE: *Prevent chilling or overheating the client.*

8. Be sure the signal light is within the client's reach.
   RATIONALE: *The person needs to be able to call you for help. The cradle restricts the client's movements, so he or she will need your assistance with daily needs.*

9. If you are using a cradle that applies heat, you will need specific instructions.
   RATIONALE: *Burns must be prevented.*

---

with a surface shaped like an egg carton, and the **flotation mattress** or pad (for a specific area of the body). The flotation mattress or pad contains a special gel-type material, which supports the body or body part in such a way as to avoid creating pressure points. This mattress provides comfort and helps to prevent skin breakdown by lessening pressure, especially on bony prominences. However, although egg crate mattresses provide client comfort, they do not prevent skin breakdown. Special skin care and measures for prevention of pressure ulcers are described in Chapter 58.

Therapeutic beds are used to treat clients with severe joint contractures, prolonged immobility, or skin wounds such as pressure ulcers or severe burns. These beds reduce or relieve the effects of pressure against the skin through various mechanisms. The surface of such beds often feels like a waterbed. These beds are more comfortable for clients who have severe contractures because their bodies float as if suspended in mid-air. Severe skin wounds are more likely to heal when the effects of pressure are reduced. Examples of these beds are the *air-fluidized bed*, the *airless bed*, and the *micro-computerized bed* (see Fig. 49-1).

Orthopedic beds support clients who must remain immobilized. The *circle bed* has a flat surface attached between two large tubular rings. The bed rotates as the large rings

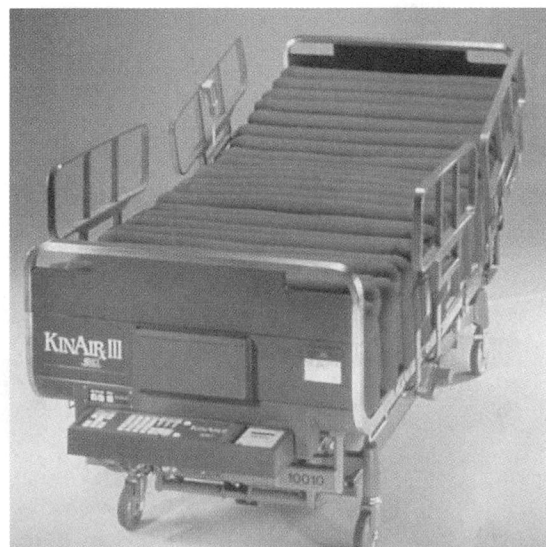

FIGURE 49-1. This micro-computerized bed not only greatly lessens the possibility of pressure area development, but also manages incontinence in the immobile client. It provides drainage for body fluids into the receptacle at the foot of the bed, where it can be measured. It also provides a scale and a heater, and has a quick-release mechanism for CPR. Some beds also have a cleansing and vacuuming system for skin care. (Photo courtesy of KCI Therapeutic Services, San Antonio, Texas.)

rotate; its purpose is to move the client from prone to supine position while keeping the body in straight, flat alignment. Another bed that moves the client from prone to supine is a *rotating frame (Stryker frame)*. The circle bed turns the client from head to toe; the rotating frame turns the client from side to side.

Throughout your nursing career, you will work with clients who need therapeutic beds, many of which are complex to use. Be sure to read carefully the instructions for use, paying particular attention to safety features. You are responsible for the safe and effective use of these therapeutic beds, as well as the safety and well-being of your clients.

➤ STUDENT SYNTHESIS

Key Points

- Organize work. Gather all supplies before making the bed. Strip and make one side of the bed at a time to conserve time and energy.
- To prevent the spread of microorganisms, never shake linen or put it on the floor.
- Hold soiled linen away from your uniform, and never place soiled linen from one client's bed onto another client's bed.
- Place soiled linen in a laundry hamper or on a chair while continuing your work.
- A well-made bed promotes comfort and rest, helps prevent skin breakdown, and provides safety for clients.
- Special attachments and beds are available to meet particular client needs.

Critical Thinking

1. Explain how to use correct body mechanics when you make an occupied bed.
2. A client's son argues with you about side rails being placed in an up position. Describe your explanation of the use of side rails to the son.
3. Do you agree or disagree with the statement that some people are safer with side rails down? Why or why not?
4. A client is returned to his room after surgery and the bed is as it was when he went to the O.R. Describe and justify your concerns. What needs to be done?

NCLEX-Style Review Questions

1. The nurse knows that a properly made bed for a client who is bedridden is important to prevent:
   a. Anxiety
   b. Boredom
   c. Increased confusion
   d. Skin breakdown
2. A closed bed-making technique would be used with a client who has:
   a. Arrived on the unit
   b. Extensive burns
   c. Generalized weakness
   d. Returned from a procedure
3. The nurse will know that a bed cradle is functioning properly if the:
   a. Client remains warm
   b. Client verbalizes less pain
   c. Client's body remains aligned
   d. Linens remain off the client's body
4. A coherent client complains of the side rails being in the up position and has tried to crawl over the rails. The nurse's best action would be:
   a. Instruct the client to use the nurse call light.
   b. Place wrist restraints on the client.
   c. Put the side rails down on one side.
   d. Remove the side rails from the bed.
5. Routine remaking of client's bed is usually done:
   a. After the evening meal prior to bedtime
   b. After the client's bath and morning care
   c. Only when absolutely needed
   d. Prior to giving the client a bath or shower

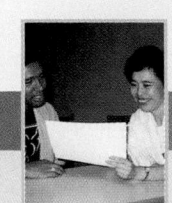

CHAPTER

50

Personal Hygiene and Skin Care

LEARNING OBJECTIVES

1. State at least five reasons for giving mouth care to a client.
2. In the skills laboratory, demonstrate assisting a client with oral care.
3. Demonstrate cleaning and caring for dentures.
4. Identify the steps involved with routine eye and ear care.
5. Demonstrate caring for the client's fingernails and toenails, addressing the reasons for attention to each area.
6. Describe how to assist clients to shave with an electric shaver; with a blade razor.
7. List at least three reasons for performing routine hair care, and describe hair care for damaged or very curly hair.
8. Describe and demonstrate giving a backrub, hand and foot massage, and foot soak.
9. State three types of cleansing baths and when each one is used.
10. Demonstrate how to safely assist a client with each type of cleansing bath.

NEW TERMINOLOGY

cerumen
halitosis
nits
pediculosis

perineal care
pyorrhea
sordes

Feeling clean contributes to people's sense of well-being and comfort, particularly those who are ill. This chapter describes how to assist clients to meet this need when they cannot do it alone.

MOUTH CARE

Frequent *mouth care* benefits everyone, but it is particularly beneficial to the ill person for several reasons:

- Many disease-causing organisms enter the body through the mouth.
- Food particles lodged between the teeth cause decay, breath odor (**halitosis**), and inflammation of the tooth sockets (**pyorrhea**).
- Some illnesses cause irritation, dryness, or brownish deposits (**sordes**) on the tongue and the mouth's mucous membrane.
- Some gum infections are transmitted from one person to another.
- A mouth condition may lessen a person's appetite and lead to nutritional deficiencies.
- Some oral conditions cause infection or pain in other body parts.
- Breath odors or decayed teeth make people self-conscious.

Some people may not have learned good oral health habits. Therefore, teaching the client about good oral hygiene is key. The client who learns to perform good oral hygiene in the healthcare facility may continue to do so at home. Remind the client that practicing good oral hygiene is beneficial because:

- Appearance improves.
- Appetite improves and food tastes better.
- Healthy teeth and gums improve overall health.

Offer the client the opportunity to brush his or her teeth before and after each meal and in the morning and evening. When caring for the client's mouth, observe the condition of the gums, tongue, mucous membranes, and teeth. Record the effects of brushing. Note on the health record any factors such as unusual tenderness, sensitivity to hot or cold, pain, bleeding, unusual redness, swelling, or odor. If the gums or teeth are unusually sensitive to touch or temperature changes, use applicators or a tongue depressor wrapped in gauze, rather than a toothbrush, for oral hygiene. While assisting the client, teach and encourage future self-care.

Routine Daily Mouth Care

Before assisting the client, assemble all supplies and equipment and be sure to wear disposable gloves as protection against contact with body fluids and microorganisms. Then do the following:

- Assist the client to a comfortable upright position with an emesis basin in hand, or assist the client to stand or sit near a sink.
- Protect the client's gown and bedclothing with a towel.

- Instruct the client to brush teeth by placing the bristles at a 45° angle against the teeth. The client should direct the tips of the bristles under the gum line, and rotate the bristles using a vibrating or jiggling motion, following the direction of tooth growth. Continue until all outer and inner surfaces of the teeth and gums are clean. He or she should then brush the tongue and the biting surfaces of the teeth. *Rationale: This cleans all surfaces and stimulates the gums.*
- Encourage the client to rinse with fresh water and to spit into the emesis basin or sink. *Rationale: Rinsing removes any debris that has been loosened with brushing.*
- Assist the client to floss the teeth. Teach the technique of moving the floss on the outer edge of each tooth's surface. Remember to include the teeth located furthest back in the mouth. *Rationale: Using the outer edge of the surface prevents cutting gums with floss.*
- Observe the condition of the client's teeth, gums, and tongue. *Rationale: Observation aids in assessment.*
- Wipe the client's mouth and chin. Rinse the toothbrush and put away supplies.
- Remove gloves and wash your hands.
- Document the procedure.

The Client Who Needs Special Mouth Care

In certain situations, some clients need assistance with mouth care or require special care (for example, clients in whom sordes has collected on the tongue and teeth due to illness). In addition, special mouth care may be needed for clients who:

- Breathe through the mouth
- Are receiving supplemental oxygen or mechanical ventilation
- Are unable to take fluids by mouth, or have fluids restricted
- Need to be encouraged to take food (cleansing the mouth before meals makes food more palatable)
- Are unresponsive or paralyzed
- Are very young, confused, or otherwise unable to perform independent mouth care

Oral cleansing sometimes removes secretions and thus helps to prevent choking. In such cases, mouth care is performed frequently. For the client who is unresponsive and breathing through the mouth, for example, oral hygiene is often ordered every hour. Exact procedures may differ among agencies. A basic procedure is given at In Practice: Nursing Procedure 50-1.

The mouth of a client who is unresponsive may become dry and cracked, creating a portal for harmful microorganisms to enter. Keeping the mouth moist and intact is an important nursing action to prevent infection. Position this client in a side-lying position, with the head of the bed slightly lowered. In this position, gravity causes saliva to run out of the mouth and prevents the client from choking. This position also allows for the client to be suctioned. (Procedures for suctioning are described

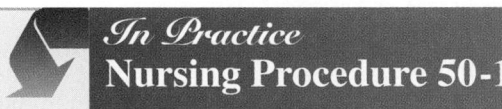

In Practice
Nursing Procedure 50-1

GIVING SPECIAL MOUTH CARE

Supplies and Equipment

Gloves
Toothbrush or sponge toothette
Tongue blade padded with a 4 × 4 gauze sponge
Water, mouthwash, or hydrogen peroxide (H_2O_2)
Towel
Water-soluble lubricant for lips
Suction catheter with suction apparatus (optional)
Emesis basin

Steps

1. Gather supplies.
   RATIONALE: *Organization facilitates accurate skill performance.*

2. Explain the procedure to the client.
   RATIONALE: *Providing information fosters cooperation.*

3. Wash your hands and put on gloves.
   RATIONALE: *Handwashing and use of gloves prevent the spread of infection.*

4. Close the curtain or door to the room.
   RATIONALE: *Closing the curtain or door protects the client's privacy.*

5. Raise the bed to a comfortable height. Lower the near side rail. Turn the client on the side toward you, with the client's head tilted down toward the mattress.
   RATIONALE: *Proper positioning prevents back strain. Tilting the head downward encourages fluid to drain out of the client's mouth.*

6. Place a towel and emesis basin under the client's chin. Have a suction catheter and apparatus available if needed.
   RATIONALE: *The towel protects the client and the bed. The emesis basin and suction equipment facilitate drainage from the client's mouth.*

7. Open the client's mouth and insert the padded tongue blade toward the back molar area. Never insert your fingers into the client's mouth.
   RATIONALE: *The tongue blade assists in keeping the client's mouth open. As a reflex mechanism, the client may bite down if fingers are placed in his or her mouth.*

8. Dip a toothette sponge, soft toothbrush, or another padded tongue blade in water, mouthwash, or diluted H_2O_2. Move it back and forth gently across the client's teeth and chewing areas. Cleanse the roof of the mouth and the inner cheek area.
   RATIONALE: *Friction cleanses the teeth. Cleaning solutions aid in removing residue on the*

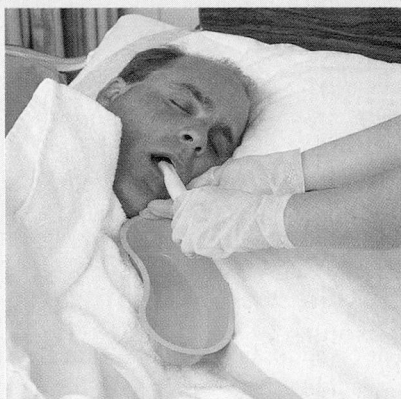

Positioning the mouth open with a padded tongue blade.

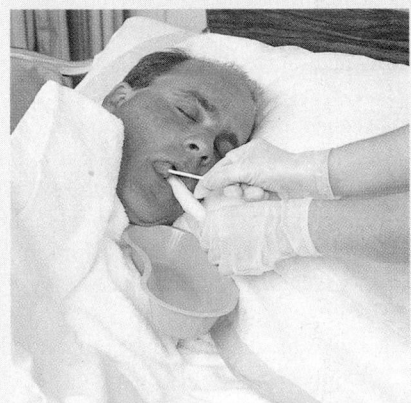

Cleansing the teeth and mouth with a toothette sponge.

client's teeth and in softening encrusted areas.

9. Rinse the areas, using a clean toothette or padded tongue blade moistened in water. Suction any drainage if necessary.
   RATIONALE: *Rinsing or suctioning removes cleaning solution and debris.*

10. Apply water-soluble lubricant to the client's lips.
    RATIONALE: *Applying lubricant prevent lips from drying or cracking.*

11. Reposition the client. Lower the bed and raise the side rail again.
    RATIONALE: *Repositioning with the bed at the proper height and side rails raised provides for the client's comfort and safety.*

12. Remove gloves and wash your hands.
    RATIONALE: *Handwashing prevents the spread of infection.*

13. Document assessments on the health record.
    RATIONALE: *Documentation provides communication and coordination of care.*

in Chapters 85 and 86.) While giving oral hygiene, inspect the gums and the mucosa of the mouth. Also inspect the lips for dryness and cracking. Apply petroleum jelly (Vaseline) or other ointment as ordered.

☛ KEY CONCEPT

Be gentle when giving mouth care; the oral mucosa is fragile and may be injured if mouth care is performed too vigorously. Also be sure to prevent aspiration in clients who are unable to swallow or spit out solutions. Use only a minimum of solution and make sure it is completely suctioned or drained out of the client's mouth.

The Client Who Wears Dentures

Ask the client on admission to the healthcare facility if he or she wears dentures. The presence of dentures should be recorded on the client's chart. The client who wears dentures needs the same mouth care as the client who has natural teeth. Specially designed brushes and preparations for soaking dentures are available to remove deposits. Brush dentures in the same manner as natural teeth. Be sure to rinse them, because the denture cleaner may have a disagreeable taste.

Most dentists encourage their clients to wear their dentures all the time. *Rationale: If clients remove dentures for long periods, their gum lines change and their dentures will no longer fit.* If the client must remove dentures, they should never be stored in cups or glasses that are used for drinking. *Rationale: The client may accidentally swallow the dentures. This would cause choking.*

If the client leaves the dentures out of the mouth, put them in an opaque container, preferably covered, out of sight, and labeled (both the container and the lid) with the client's name and room number. It is best to use a specially marked denture container to avoid confusion. While the dentures are being stored in the container, keep them in water. *Rationale: Dentures must be kept moist to preserve their fit and general quality.* Take extra precautions to ensure that the dentures do not get lost.

Be alert for a client who constantly removes his or her dentures. Question the client about any possible reasons why he or she is removing them. Also, inspect the client's mouth, looking for any irritation or redness that may suggest a problem. For example, the dentures may fit poorly or may cause pain, which is often the reason for bad eating habits and poor nutrition. Sometimes, clients remove dentures during or after mealtime and place them on the food tray. Care should be taken to prevent the dentures from being removed from the room with the meal tray. Be particularly observant of the client who is experiencing confusion.

For the client who wears dentures, respect the client's privacy when cleaning his or her dentures. Wash your hands before and after handling dentures and wear gloves. Handle dentures carefully; they are slippery, fragile, and expensive. To avoid breakage, place a folded washcloth in the bottom of a basin of water or sink, holding the dentures over it. Do not hold them over a hard surface. In Practice: Nursing Procedure 50-2 reviews the general steps associated with denture care.

✚👁 Nursing Alert

Always remove dentures if a client is unresponsive, irrational, having seizures, or going to the operating room. If dentures are removed, document that fact and store them safely.

ROUTINE EYE CARE

Normally, the lacrimal (tear) ducts bathe the eye continuously. However, if lacrimal duct functioning decreases, dried secretions may accumulate on the person's lids and lashes. These secretions can be removed by applying a cotton ball or gauze square moistened with sterile water or normal saline to the eyelids. Some clients also will need supplemental moisture in the form of eye drops, as ordered. In Practice: Nursing Care Guidelines 50-1 describes routine eye care. (Chapter 79 discusses care of the prosthetic eye.)

EAR CARE

A client's external ears are washed routinely during the bed bath. If excessive **cerumen** (ear wax) is present, a special procedure may be necessary to remove it to prevent hearing difficulty. Wax removal is done by irrigating the ear's outer canal with warm water. This procedure must be ordered by the physician or advanced practice nurse. Special training is needed to perform this procedure.

Warn clients never to use bobby pins, cotton swabs (Q-Tips), or toothpicks to clean their ears. *Rationale: These objects can injure the ear canal or puncture the eardrum.*

Care of a Hearing Aid

Clients who have a hearing impairment may use a *hearing aid.* A hearing aid is a battery-operated, sound-amplifying device that consists of an earpiece that fits into the ear and a power source. Hearing aids may be very small and may fit entirely into the outer ear. They may also have a piece which fits behind the outer ear, or may require a separate battery that is carried in a pocket and connected to the device by a cord. The size of the device depends in part on the type of hearing loss that exists. (Some types of hearing aids have a part of the device implanted within the person's body and a part worn externally. One example is a *cochlear implant.*)

When caring for a client with a hearing aid, be sure to include the following:

- Clean the earpiece regularly with saline or the prescribed solution (to prevent cerumen buildup). Do not clean with alcohol. *Rationale: Alcohol may damage the delicate parts of the hearing aid. It may also be irritating to the client's ear canal.*
- Check and replace batteries regularly.
- Adjust the volume to meet the individual's needs.
- Turn off the aid when the client is not using it, to preserve the life of the battery.
- Remove batteries if the client will not use the aid for an extended period.

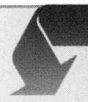

In Practice
Nursing Procedure 50-2

CARING FOR DENTURES

Supplies and Equipment

Gloves
Tissue or gauze square
Denture container
Washcloth
Toothbrush
Denture cleaner
Tap water
Mouthwash
Emesis basin
Towel

Steps

1. Position the client in an upright or side-lying position.
   RATIONALE: *Proper positioning maximizes efficiency.*

2. Wash your hands and put on gloves.
   RATIONALE: *Handwashing and use of gloves prevent the spread of infection.*

3. When possible, encourage the client to remove their own dentures. If the client is unable to do so, use a tissue or a gauze square to grasp the upper plate with your thumb and index finger. Gently move the denture up and down.
   RATIONALE: *Moving the denture up and down breaks the suction that holds the denture in place.*

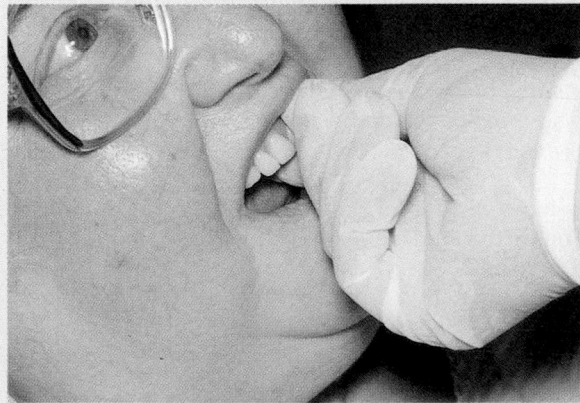

Removing the upper denture.

4. Remove the upper plate from the mouth and place it in the denture container.
   RATIONALE: *Proper placement protects dentures from breakage.*

5. Remove the lower plate from the mouth by turning it to a slight angle.

RATIONALE: *Turning the plate to an angle breaks the suction so that the denture can be removed easily.*

6. Place the lower plate in the denture container.
   RATIONALE: *Proper placement protects dentures from breakage.*

7. Carry the denture container carefully to the sink or to an emesis basin.

8. Place a washcloth in the bottom of the sink or in the emesis basin. Fill the sink or basin with water.
   RATIONALE: *The washcloth provides a cushion and prevents damage if dentures are dropped.*

9. Pick up the dentures one plate at a time and scrub each with denture cleaner that you have applied to the toothbrush.
   RATIONALE: *Using a denture cleaner aids in removal of debris from the denture surface.*

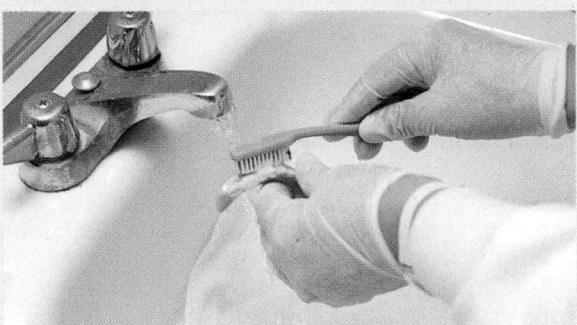

Scrubbing the dentures with a denture cleaner.

10. Rinse the dentures with tap water.
    RATIONALE: *Rinsing removes food particles and denture cleaner. Using very hot water may damage the dentures.*

11. Soak dentures in commercially prepared solution at the client's request.
    RATIONALE: *Soaking aids in further cleaning and in maintaining moisture.*

12. Rinse with tap water.
    RATIONALE: *Rinsing removes the solution and any residual aftertaste due to the solution.*

13. Inspect dentures for breaks, rough edges, missing teeth, and other damage.
    RATIONALE: *Inspection helps to identify any potential problem areas that may cause injury.*

14. Inspect mucosa of the client's mouth for redness or irritation.
    RATIONALE: *Dentures may rub and be uncomfortable. Report irritation immediately.*

(continued)

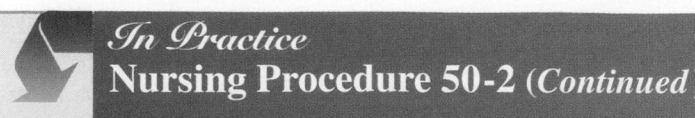
15. Assist the client to rinse the mouth with mouth-wash.
    RATIONALE: *This is refreshing and removes debris.*

16. Apply denture adhesive, if the client requests it. Encourage the client to replace the dentures. If he or she is unable to do so, insert the dentures into the mouth, one plate at a time. Hold plates at a slight angle while inserting.
    RATIONALE: *Proper insertion prevents injury to the lips and surrounding mucosa.*

17. Wipe the client's mouth and chin with a towel.
    RATIONALE: *Keeping the client dry aids in comfort.*

18. If the client chooses not to wear the dentures or is unable to wear them, store the dentures covered with water in the denture container.

RATIONALE: *A covered denture container protects the dentures from possible breakage and maintains the client's privacy. Moisture helps preserve dentures.*

19. Label the container and lid with the client's name and room number.
    RATIONALE: *Identification is important if dentures are misplaced.*

20. Remove and discard gloves and wash your hands.
    RATIONALE: *Handwashing prevents the spread of infection.*

21. Document the procedure on the client's record.
    RATIONALE: *Documentation provides communication and coordination of care.*

In Practice
Nursing Care Guidelines 50-1

CARING FOR THE EYES

- Wash your hands and put on gloves.
  Rationale: Handwashing and gloving prevent the spread of infection.
- Soak cotton balls or gauze squares in sterile water or normal saline solution. *Rationale: Using sterile water or normal saline solution avoids introducing harmful microorganisms to the sensitive eye tissues.*
- Wipe the client's eyelid from the inner (next to nose) to the outer canthus. *Rationale: Proper wiping technique moves debris away from the eye, prevents reinfection or contamination of the eye, and protects the tear ducts.*
- Repeat steps on the other eye, using clean supplies. *Rationale: Using new supplies prevents spreading infection between eyes.*

The Client Who Wears Contact Lenses

- Determine the type of contact lenses the client wears and the client's usual cleaning practices. *Rationale: Different types of lenses require differing cleaning and storage techniques. Some contacts are disposable.*
- Encourage the client or a family member to remove the lenses and place them in cleansing or soaking solution. *Rationale: It is important that permanent lenses do not dry out.*
- Notify the charge nurse or team leader if the client is unable to remove the lenses by him- or herself. *Rationale: A suction cup is available for removal of contact lenses. This must be used by a specially trained person.*
- If lenses cannot be removed, notify the primary healthcare provider. *Rationale: Corneal damage may*

result if the client wears contact lenses for too long a period of time, particularly if the client's eyes are dry or if he or she cannot blink.
- When lenses are removed, store them in the solution specified by the manufacturer or in normal saline. *Rationale: Proper storage maintains the integrity of the lenses. Sterile normal saline can be substituted for contact lens storage solution in an emergency.*
- Be sure to label separate containers for each eye and include the client's name and room number. *Rationale: Contacts have a separate prescription for each eye and can be easily switched. In some cases, a small dot indicates the right eye. The containers also must be labeled with the client's name, to prevent loss.*

Special Eye Care for the Client Who Cannot Blink

- Follow the steps above for routine cleaning of the eyes.
- Instill lubricating drops in the eye, or ointment onto the lower lids, as ordered by the physician. *Rationale: Drops or ointment help to keep eyes moist. See Chap. 63 for procedures.*
- Close the client's eyelids. *Rationale: Closing the eyelids helps to maintain available moisture.* If allowed by the agency, cover the eye with a sterile eye pad and secure with paper tape. (This procedure may vary among clinical agencies; check the standards for care in your agency.)
- Document all procedures on the client's record. *Rationale: Documentation provides communication and coordination of care.*

- Avoid exposing the aid to heat and moisture.
- Turn the volume down completely before inserting the aid into the client's ear.
- Evaluate client complaints about the hearing aid, or repeated removal or refusal to use the aid.

☛ Key Concept

If a hearing aid is working properly and fits properly, the client will be willing to wear it. Refusal to use a hearing aid or repeated removal of the aid usually indicates discomfort or malfunction of the device.

NAIL CARE

A client's general condition and health habits affect the condition of his or her *nails*. Brittle, broken nails may be due to improper diet or fever.

Caring for Fingernails

Emotional tension may cause fingernail or cuticle biting. Some occupations cause nails to be stained or broken. Water, strong soaps, and washing powders make nails and cuticles dry. Nails that are well cared for are pleasing to look at and are a health protection measure.

Conditions such as torn cuticles are an invitation to infection. Therefore, report reddened areas or breaks in the cuticles. Dirty nails can spread infection. If a client's nails are torn or jagged, trim them with nail clippers rather than scissors. Use an emery board or orangewood stick on nails to file the rough edges, to prevent nails from breaking due to snagging on clothing. Do not use a metal nail file because of its sharp point, and because it may be harder on the nails than an emery board. Avoid using scissors to cut nails, to minimize the risk of accidentally nicking the skin.

The best time to complete fingernail care is after the client's hands have been in water. Soap and water loosen dirt and temporarily soften cuticles. Cuticle oil applied to the nails and cuticles softens them as well.

Usual supplies and equipment for nail care include a basin half-full of warm water, soap, lotion, towel, nail brush, nail polish remover (if needed), and an orangewood stick. The client may have other items, such as nail polish, cuticle oil, and an emery board. Clean beneath the client's nails and push back the cuticles daily using an orangewood stick. In Practice: Nursing Care Guidelines 50-2 provides additional information.

Never give equipment that has a sharp point or that is used for cutting to a client who has unsteady hands or who is confused, depressed, or at risk for self-injury. The person who is going to have surgery or who is experiencing respiratory distress usually is asked not to wear nail polish.

Caring for Toenails

Toenails need the same care as fingernails. Long toenails may scratch the client's skin or catch on bedclothes and break. Dirty toenails may cause infection if they scratch the client's skin. However, cutting a client's toenails is an intervention that requires a physician's order. Never cut the toenails of a client with diabetes or hemophilia, or a newborn's toenails. These clients are particularly susceptible to injury. Chapter 78 describes special foot care for the client with diabetes.

Follow the same procedure as for the fingernails, with some exceptions. If toenails are thick and hard, you may have to cut them first (with a physician's order), then smooth them with a file or an emery board. Cut toenails straight across, and do not round off the corners. If the nails tend to grow into the skin at the corners, place a wisp of cotton under the nail to prevent toenail pressure. A notch cut in the center will pull in edges and corners. Sometimes, very thick, hard toenails require the skill of a podiatrist or surgical removal. People who jog or walk a great deal often have thickened toenails, especially on their great toes. Thickened and raised nails can be a sign of a fungal infection.

✚👁 Nursing Alert
Cutting into the corners or rounding the corners of toenails contributes to the development of ingrown toenails. This condition is painful and may become serious enough to require surgical removal.

While caring for toenails, observe whether corns or calluses are present on the client's feet. If so, apply oil to soften them, but nothing else. If the client is distressed by corns, calluses, ingrown toenails, or bunions, report the condition. Corns and calluses may become infected as a result of cutting them with razor blades or using corn removers that contain salicylic acid. Cover an infected area with a sterile dressing. Any additional treatment must be ordered by a physician. Be sure to report and document any such problems. See In Practice: Nursing Care Guidelines 50-2 for further information.

✚👁 Nursing Alert
Special orders are required before cutting the nails of clients with diabetes or hemophilia, or those with very thickened nails, to avoid accidental injury to soft tissues. *Rationale: Wounds heal very slowly in these clients. Very thick nails often need to be cut by a specially trained person, using special equipment and techniques.*

SHAVING

Most adult men shave daily. Clients who are unable to shave every day may feel or look untidy. Many healthcare facilities use electric razors because they are easier and safer to use than blade razors. If the client can shave without assistance, prepare the equipment, provide a mirror, and see that the room is well lighted. Allow as much privacy as possible for clients to carry out this part of their care.

If the client cannot shave without assistance, provide assistance. When using an electric razor, read the instructions carefully. Clean the razor after each use. When shaving a client with a safety razor (blade razor), follow the facility's recommended procedure. Be sure to wear gloves to minimize expo-

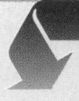

In Practice
Nursing Care Guidelines 50-2

CARING FOR NAILS

Care of Fingernails

- Wear gloves when giving nail care. *Rationale: Wearing gloves prevents the spread of infection.*
- Assist the client to a comfortable upright position. *Rationale: The client often enjoys watching fingernail care. The client may assist as much as possible.*
- Remove nail polish. *Rationale: Removing nail polish enables inspection of the true condition of the client's nails. It also aids in assessing the client's level of oxygenation.*
- Soak the client's fingers in a basin of warm water and mild soap. *Rationale: Soaking helps to cleanse the nails and make it easier to remove dirt and debris. It also softens the nails and cuticle, for easier cleaning.*
- Scrub the client's nails with a soft nail brush. *Rationale: Scrubbing with a soft brush helps to loosen and remove dirt that has collected under the nails.*
- Dry the client's hands thoroughly.
- Trim the client's fingernails straight across with nail clippers. *Rationale: This is the safest way to clip nails.*
- Shape the fingernails with an emery board, rounding the corners and smoothing the edges. *Rationale: The emery board is less dangerous than the metal file. Rounded corners and smooth edges are less likely to catch and tear. Any break in the skin can be a site of infection.*
- Push the cuticle back with the blunt end of an orangewood stick. *Rationale: The stick is blunt and smooth and less likely to injure the nails than a metal nail file.*
- Clean under the client's nails with the more pointed end of an orangewood stick. *Rationale: Using the pointed end of the stick helps to get under the nail to remove any debris.*
- Clip hangnails with manicure scissors or snippers. *Rationale: Clipping hangnails helps to keep them from tearing. This helps to prevent discomfort and infection.*
- Apply lotion to the client's hands and gently massage them. *Rationale: Scrubbing and soaking can dry the hands. Lotion helps prevent chafing and cracking, which can lead to infection. Hand massage helps to relax the client (see discussion later in this chapter).*

Care of Toenails

- Assist the client to a sitting or lying position with the head of the bed elevated. *Rationale: This position enables the client to soak his or her feet and is relaxing.*
- Place the client's feet in a basin of warm water and soak them. *Rationale: The foot soak is soothing and helps to soften nails, so they will be easier to trim.*
- Gently dry the client's feet. *Rationale: Drying prevents areas of moisture, which could lead to irritation and breakdown. Most clients' feet are tender. It is important to be gentle.*
- Scrub the toenails with a soft nail brush. *Rationale: Using a soft nail brush helps to loosen and remove dirt.*
- Trim toenails straight across with clippers. *Rationale: Trimming straight across helps to prevent ingrown toenails.*
- Do not shape corners. *Rationale: Rounded toenail corners are much more likely to become ingrown.*
- Clean under the client's nails with an orangewood stick. *Rationale: The orangewood stick is less irritating than a metal file to remove any debris under the nail.*
- Apply lotion to the client's feet and gently massage them. *Rationale: The lotion helps to restore the natural skin oils and prevents drying. Foot massage is very soothing.*

---

sure to the client's blood if the face or neck should be nicked accidentally during shaving.

If your healthcare facility uses disposable blade razors, take extra precautions. Do not allow a client with unsteady hands or poor eyesight to shave with a blade razor. Also closely supervise clients who are depressed, suicidal, or assaultive. Use the sharps container for disposal. Follow the steps at In Practice: Nursing Procedure 50-3 for shaving both men and women.

☛ KEY CONCEPT

Some women have excessive facial hair (hirsuitism) and may wish to shave. This may be embarrassing for them. Be sensitive to the client's feelings.

HAIR CARE

Brushing and dressing one's hair is part of daily care. It keeps the hair in good condition and makes the person feel better. Encourage clients to comb their own hair; it is good exercise for the shoulder joints and also enhances self-esteem.

Daily Hair Care

Daily *hair care* provides an opportunity for assessing the client's hair and scalp. Brushing stimulates scalp circulation and distributes oil over the hair to give it sheen. Short hair should receive the same care as long hair. In some healthcare agencies, such as long-term care, beauty parlor and barber services are available. Although time typically is not available to

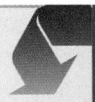

In Practice
Nursing Procedure 50-3

SHAVING A CLIENT

Supplies and Equipment

Razor: safety or electric
Wash basin
Warm water
Disposable gloves
Shaving cream or soap
Aftershave lotion, if desired
Moisturizer
Towels
Some of these supplies may not be needed if an
  electric razor is used.

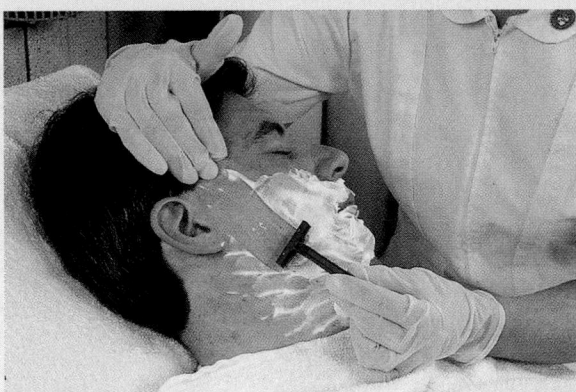

Holding the razor at a 45° angle to the skin.

Steps

1. Explain the procedure to the client.
   RATIONALE: *Explanations gain the client's
   confidence and help to reduce anxiety.*

2. Place the client in a position that is comfortable
   for both the client and nurse.
   RATIONALE: *Proper positioning maximizes efficiency
   and comfort.*

3. Put on gloves.
   RATIONALE: *Use of gloves helps to prevent the
   spread of infection.*

4. Place a warm wet washcloth on the area to be
   shaved for a few seconds.
   RATIONALE: *Moisture softens the beard.*

5. Apply shaving cream or soap to the area, if using
   a blade razor.
   RATIONALE: *Shaving cream or soap makes the hair
   easier to cut.*

6. Hold the skin taut while making strokes.
   RATIONALE: *Keeping the skin taut (especially with
   a blade razor) reduces the risk of cutting
   the skin.*

7. Holding the blade razor at a 45 degree angle to
   the skin, move it across the skin in short strokes in
   the direction the hair grows.
   RATIONALE: *Moving the razor in the direction of
   hair growth helps to reduce skin irritation.*

   a. If using an electric razor, move it across the
      area as needed until all of the beard is cut.

8. Wash the shaven area thoroughly with a clean,
   warm, moistened washcloth.
   RATIONALE: *This will remove any cream, soap, and
   stray hairs.*

9. Pat the area dry.
   RATIONALE: *Patting rather than rubbing prevents
   skin chafing.*

10. For men, apply aftershave lotion if the client
    prefers.
    RATIONALE: *Aftershave stimulates and tones
    capillaries in the epidermis.*

11. If shaving a woman's legs or underarms, apply
    moisturizer if the client prefers.
    RATIONALE: *Shaving may make skin dry.*

12. If a disposable blade razor is used, discard it in
    the sharps container; if using the client's own
    razor, cover the blade and store it in a safe place
    to prevent cuts and loss.
    RATIONALE: *Proper blade razor disposal and care
    prevents injury.*

    a. Clean the client's electric razor thoroughly after
       each use by removing the face plate and
       blades and cleaning the blades and surround-
       ing areas with the small brush provided or a
       disposable toothbrush. Brush out all beard
       stubble and skin debris.
       RATIONALE: *Proper cleaning prevents damage to
       the razor, ensuring that it will be in proper
       working order for the next use.*

    b. Then clean all surfaces around the blades with
       an alcohol wipe and allow to dry before
       reassembling.
       RATIONALE: *Cleaning and wiping ensures
       removal of all debris.*

    c. Plug in the razor for recharging if necessary.
       RATIONALE: *Recharging, if needed, allows the
       razor to be ready for next use.*

13. Properly dispose of gloves and document the
    procedure in the client's record.
    RATIONALE: *Proper glove disposal reduces the
    risk of infection transmission. Documentation
    provides communication and coordination of
    care, noting any unusual skin observations.*

provide elaborate hairstyles for clients, try to style their hair as becomingly as possible in the time allotted. Comb one lock of hair at a time, holding the lock firmly and leaving it slack between your hand and the client's head to avoid pulling.

Braid long hair to prevent tangles. Start braids toward the front so that the client does not have to lie on them. Fasten them at the end with a special rubber band or ribbon. A male client with long hair may wish to have his hair tied in a ponytail. Be sure the braid or ponytail is comfortable when the client lies in bed. Avoid using hairpins or bobby pins; they might be uncomfortable or injure a client's head.

Some clients will wear their hair in fashionable woven braids. Remember to cleanse the scalp regularly to maintain cleanliness and to allow the scalp to be conditioned. In some cases, clients will request that oil be massaged into the scalp (Fig. 50-1).

Wash the client's brush and comb frequently. Doing so helps to keep the hair clean and prevents reinfection of the scalp in infectious conditions. Report and document such conditions as excessive dandruff, falling hair, lice, crusts, or lesions.

Shampoo

A *shampoo* may be needed after lotions or other medications have been applied to the scalp; after an electroencephalogram for which a paste is used; or for cleanliness during a long-term illness. A shampoo may also be part of the treatment for lice (*pediculosis*) or dandruff (*seborrheic dermatitis*).

Giving a Shampoo to a Client Who is Ambulatory
For the client who is ambulatory, the simplest method of shampooing is for the client to shampoo during a shower or bath. If a client cannot shampoo his or her own hair but can ambulate, he or she can have a shampoo in the bathroom, using the lavatory sink. Choose a chair at a level that allows the client's head to rest comfortably on the bowl's edge. Be sure

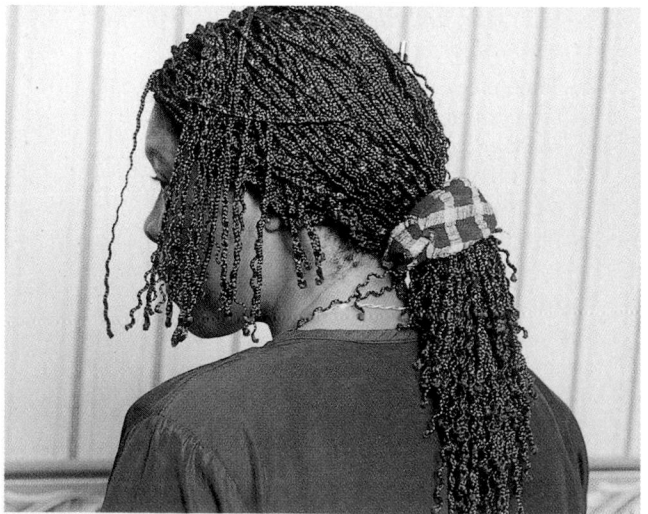

FIGURE 50-1. Hair fashions such as woven braids need daily cleansing and oil preparations to keep the hair and scalp healthy.

to pad the edge of the bowl with towels. The person may prefer to sit facing the sink, resting the forehead on the edge and holding a folded towel over the eyes. If using a spray, adjust the water's temperature before you begin. If the client feels lightheaded or faint, stop the procedure, wrap the client's head in a bath towel, and help him or her back to bed.

The client who can be moved on a stretcher can be wheeled to a convenient sink for a shampoo. The shampoo is done while the client lies on the stretcher with the head near the edge of the sink. Use a trough to funnel the water back into the sink.

Giving a Shampoo to a Client Who is Confined to the Bed
Clients who cannot ambulate must be shampooed while in bed. In Practice: Nursing Procedure 50-4 gives detailed steps for shampooing a client's hair while he or she is in bed.

Hair Care in Special Situations

Some clients require special hair care. In the case of hair that has recently been permed, bleached, or colored, the hair is often damaged. Some clients also have hair that is naturally very curly or kinky. All these types of hair tend to be very dry. Some illnesses also contribute to dry or damaged hair. In these cases, oil may need to be added, to prevent splitting and breaking of the hair. In addition, very dry hair should not be washed often, because washing further dries the hair and removes natural oils.

Some clients prefer to use special hair preparations to replace oils; petroleum jelly (Vaseline) may be used if no specific hair dressing is available. Clients may wish to wear a shower cap, bandana, or hat to keep the natural oil in the hair and to prevent excessive drying.

If the client has very tightly curled hair, use a hair pick instead of a comb. The pick has longer teeth that are further apart than the teeth of a comb. Using a pick helps to prevent pulling and tearing of the hair.

Many clients with very curly hair prefer to wear braids or dreadlocks, especially when they are in the hospital (see Figure 50-1). These styles are fashionable and comfortable. Although they may be time-consuming to create, they are easy to maintain. (The client's family may be willing to assist in doing a special hairstyle.) It is important to comb braids and dreadlocks out on a regular basis, to prevent damage to the hair, and infection or excessive drying of the scalp. When the complex hairstyle is placed into the hair again, an effort should be made to vary the placement of braids or dreadlocks to avoid constant pulling on the same sections of hair.

Some clients prefer to shave their heads, especially when in the hospital. It is important for the person shaving the head to be very careful, to prevent cutting or nicking the scalp. Some clients rub oil on their heads after they have been shaved, to restore the natural oils of the scalp.

Giving Hair Care After an Accident
A client may come to the healthcare agency after an accident with dirt, blood, or glass in the hair. If no scalp wounds are

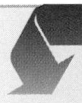

In Practice
Nursing Procedure 50-4

SHAMPOOING A CLIENT'S HAIR IN BED
Supplies and Equipment

Comb or hair pick and brush
1 bath towel, 2 hand towels, 1 washcloth
Plastic for floor and chair
1 large pitcher of water
Cotton balls
1 small pitcher for pouring
Shampoo or mild soap solution
1 pail
Shampoo trough
Moisture-proof pillowcase
Gloves
Conditioner and hair dryer (optional)

Steps

1. Check to ensure that there is a physician's order on the client's health record.
   RATIONALE: *A physician's order is needed for a bed shampoo.*

2. Wash your hands and put on gloves.
   RATIONALE: *Handwashing and using gloves reduces the risk for infection transmission.*

3. Cover the client with a bath blanket and turn back the bedclothing.
   RATIONALE: *Doing so keeps bedclothing dry while also keeping the client covered and warm.*

4. Cover the pillow with a moisture-proof case and place it under the client's head.
   RATIONALE: *A moisture-proof case prevents soiling and wetting the bed linen.*

5. Raise the bed to the highest position and place the head of the bed in the flat position.
   RATIONALE: *Proper positioning enhances efficiency and reduces the nurse's risk for back strain.*

6. Gently move the client's head and shoulders to the edge of the bed nearest the nurse.
   RATIONALE: *Moving the client's head toward the edge of the bed allows for easy access to the hair while providing for client comfort.*

7. Comb and brush the client's hair thoroughly.
   RATIONALE: *Hair is easier to wash when it is combed and brushed.*

8. Place plastic on the floor.
   RATIONALE: *Plastic on the floor maintains safety, keeping the floor dry.*

9. Place the pail on a covered chair.
   RATIONALE: *Placing the pail on a covered chair reduces splashing, because water will splash if it falls a great distance from the shampoo basin.*

10. Place the shampoo basin under the client's head with the trough directed to the side of the bed so that water flows into the pail.
    RATIONALE: *Water will drain continuously.*

11. Cover the client with an extra bath blanket.
    RATIONALE: *Doing so helps prevent chilling.*

12. Secure a folded towel around the client's neck.
    RATIONALE: *The towel absorbs drips, and keeps water from running down the client's neck and back.*

13. Cover the client's eyes with a damp washcloth and place cotton in his or her ears.
    RATIONALE: *Covering the eyes and ears prevents soapy water from entering. These areas cannot drain normally when the client is in a back-lying position.*

14. Place a towel over the client's chest.
    RATIONALE: *A towel on the chest protects the client from getting wet and feeling chilled.*

15. Wet hair thoroughly with warm water (about 105° to 110° F, 40.6° to 42° C).
    RATIONALE: *Warm water prevents burns to the face and scalp.*

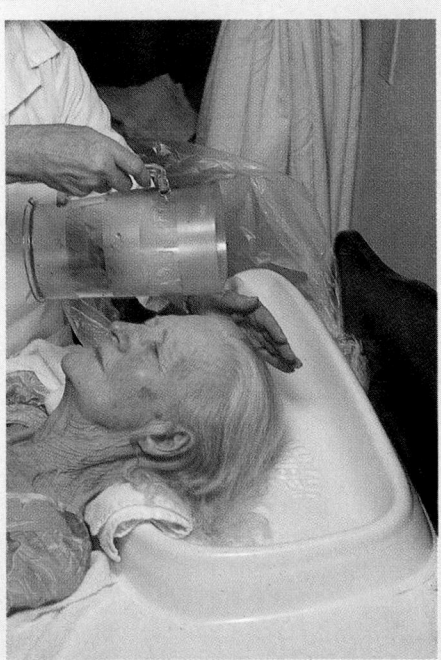
Wetting the hair with warm water.

16. Apply shampoo or mild soap solution—using enough to make a thick lather—and rub it into and massage the scalp as you do so.
    RATIONALE: *Friction loosens dirt particles, and soap and water wash them away.*

(continued)

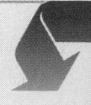

In Practice
Nursing Procedure 50-4 (Continued)

17. Rinse well.
    RATIONALE: *Rinsing removes debris and soap.*

18. Reapply shampoo, massage, and rinse thoroughly.
    RATIONALE: *Oil or other body secretions may collect in the hair of a bedridden client.*

19. Apply conditioner and rinse.
    RATIONALE: *Conditioner prevents drying and makes combing easier.*

20. Squeeze excess water from the hair and wrap a towel around the client's head. Gently pat or rub to dry hair. Wrap a dry towel around the client's damp hair.
    RATIONALE: *Removing extra moisture helps prevent the client and bedclothes from getting wet. Wrapping the client's hair in a towel prevents chilling.*

21. Remove wet towels and equipment.
    RATIONALE: *Removal of wet items prevents chilling the client and makes the client care area comfortable and clean.*

22. Use a hair dryer, comb, or hair pick, and brush as needed.
    RATIONALE: *Individuals have preferences on how their hair is styled.*

23. Dispose of gloves and wash your hands.
    RATIONALE: *Proper glove disposal and handwashing reduce the risk of infection transmission.*

24. Document the procedure and note how the client tolerated it.
    RATIONALE: *Documentation provides communication and coordination of care. Noting any unusual observations or problems alerts caregivers to modifications needed for the future.*

---

apparent, the client's hair may need to be shampooed. (A physician's order is necessary.) The shampoo removes debris and makes the client more comfortable. Shampooing a client's hair also provides an opportunity to examine his or her scalp. Always wear gloves for this procedure. Take care to avoid being cut on glass or debris in the client's hair.

Brush or comb the hair first; combing helps to remove larger pieces of debris. At the same time, check for scalp wounds. If scalp wounds are discovered, report them before continuing with the shampoo. Scalp wounds need attention before a shampoo, because a shampoo would be irritating and might cause further damage. In addition, wounds provide a source for infection.

If the client cannot tolerate a shampoo with water, use dry shampoo instead. Follow the instructions on the package, and be sure to keep the powder out of the client's eyes.

Treatment of Pediculosis

Pediculosis is the term for infestation by lice, tiny insects that suck blood from the person they infect. Pediculosis also causes intense itching. Usually lice are found on hairy body parts. They are tiny, oval, grayish insects. The eggs, called **nits,** look like dandruff, but are solid specks, not flakes. They cling tightly to the hair shafts and are hard to remove or destroy. A special fine-toothed pediculosis comb helps to remove lice and nits.

Head lice (*pediculosis capitis*) are found in the hair and on the scalp. Body lice (*pediculosis corporis*) are found on the body and clothing. "Crab lice" are found on other hairy body parts, especially in the pubic area (*pediculosis pubis*). If scratches are noted in these areas of the client's body, look for nits on the body or in the hair.

Lice spread disease. They cause itching, and the resulting scratches may become infected. They spread via clothing, bedding, and combs and brushes. Look for signs of skin irritation and lice when admitting a client to the healthcare agency.

Both nits and adult lice can be destroyed by a routine treatment, often with a special shampoo or a shower with a specially medicated soap. If you observe lice in a client, report it to your team leader. The physician will order specific treatment. Chapter 74 describes the care of clients with lice and other parasitic skin infestations.

Nursing Alert

If you are shampooing or bathing a client with suspected or confirmed pediculosis, wear a gown to protect your clothing. Dispose of this gown without touching the outside. Always wear gloves. Alert the client's family to the situation and to the necessity of eliminating lice from the home.

SKIN CARE

The skin is the body's primary defense against disease and infection. If this defense system is to be effective, it must remain unbroken and unirritated. The skin also helps regulate body heat; a break in the skin could upset that balance. When giving nursing care, observe for any signs of skin irritation or lack of skin integrity.

Frequent and effective *skin care* is essential to keep the skin intact and to remove dirt, excess oil, and harmful bacteria. If the skin is oily, regular cleansing is needed; if the skin is dry, a daily bath may be harmful. However, everyone's face, underarms, and perineal area need daily cleansing.

Remember that body fluids, such as perspiration, vomitus, urine, and feces are very irritating to the skin. They must be removed immediately. This client often needs special skin care to prevent skin breakdown.

Backrub

Give a *backrub* when bathing the client and as part of evening care. Do it at other times if the client is likely to have skin irritation from bed rest; remember also that the backrub provides relaxation and comfort. The backrub is often the highlight of the day for the client who is confined to bed. It can be relaxing, and it allows direct observation of the client's skin condition. In Practice: Nursing Procedure 50-5 gives the steps in giving a backrub.

Backrub lotion or fine powder is most often used to reduce friction between the nurse's hands and the client's skin. Lotion is preferred, because it soothes and softens the skin. Alcohol is not used, because it is very drying to the skin.

Warm the hands and the lotion to prevent chilling the client. (Immerse a bottle of lotion in warm bath water for a few minutes to heat it.) Be sure that fingernails are short enough to rub the client's back safely. Do not wear jewelry. *Rationale: Long fingernails and jewelry can scratch the client, and both can collect lotion, skin debris, and microorganisms, causing infection.*

Apply appropriate pressure and friction with your hands. Light pressure is soothing; heavy pressure is stimulating. The four movements listed below are the simplest and most effective for the kind of light massage given to stimulate circulation and relax contracted muscles. Perform all four patterns at least three times.

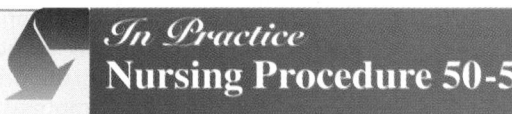

In Practice
Nursing Procedure 50-5

GIVING A BACKRUB

Supplies and Equipment

Backrub lotion or body powder
Gloves, if indicated

Steps

1. Wash your hands. Wear gloves, if indicated.
   RATIONALE: *Handwashing and wearing gloves reduce the risk of infection transmission.*

2. Make sure the room is warm enough.
   RATIONALE: *A large portion of the client's body will be exposed.*

3. Close the door or pull the curtain.
   RATIONALE: *Closing the door or pulling the curtain ensures privacy for the client.*

4. Place the client comfortably on the side, or face downward, with his or her entire back and buttocks exposed.
   RATIONALE: *Proper positioning enhances efficiency and effectiveness.*

5. Apply lotion all over the client's back after warming the lotion in your hands or placing the lotion bottle in warm water.
   RATIONALE: *Warming the lotion prevents chilling the client.*

6. Stand with one foot slightly forward and knees slightly bent.
   RATIONALE: *This position lowers the caregiver's center of gravity and reduces back strain.*

7. Position the client as close to the side of the bed as possible.

   RATIONALE: *Positioning the client near the nurse reduces stretching and straining, and minimizes the risk for back injury to the nurse.*

8. Rock on the feet while rubbing.
   RATIONALE: *Using this position allows the nurse's strong arm and shoulder muscles to do the work and helps prevent back strain.*

9. Using the first three fingers of both hands, rub the neck under the client's hairline with a circular motion.
   RATIONALE: *This motion relaxes the client's neck, a frequent source of tension and headaches.*

10. Using the first three fingers of one hand, rub in the hollow at the back of the neck with a circular motion.
    RATIONALE: *This also helps to relax the client's neck.*

11. Separating the thumb and the fingers of one hand, place the thumb on one side of the client's neck and the fingers on the other. Beginning at the hairline, rub the length of the neck with a circular motion.
    RATIONALE: *Massaging in a circular motion helps to relax the muscles in this area.*

12. Using the first three fingers of both hands, continue the circular motion down each side of the spine to the coccyx, paying special attention to the coccyx.
    RATIONALE: *Tension builds along the spinal column. The coccyx is a bony prominence with very little fatty covering; thus, it is in great danger of skin breakdown. The rubbing motion stimulates circulation.*

In Practice
Nursing Procedure 50-9 *(Continued)*

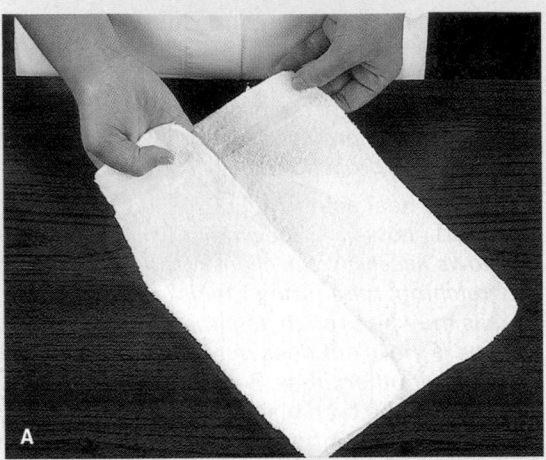

A

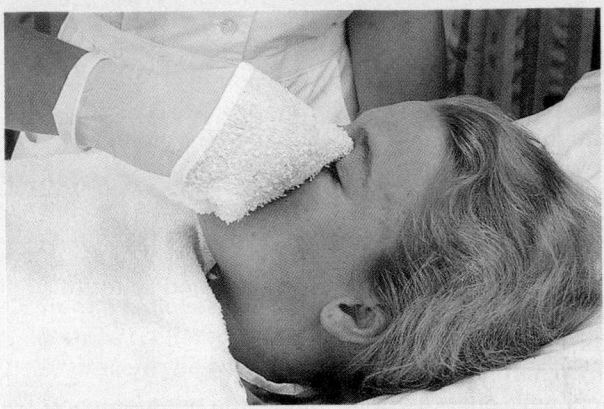

Cleansing the eye, moving from the inner toward the outer corner.

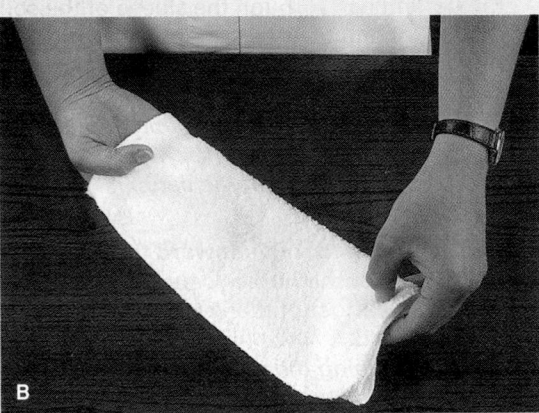

B

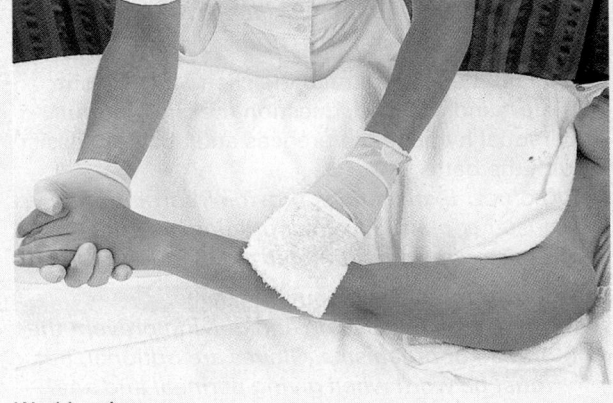

Washing the arm.

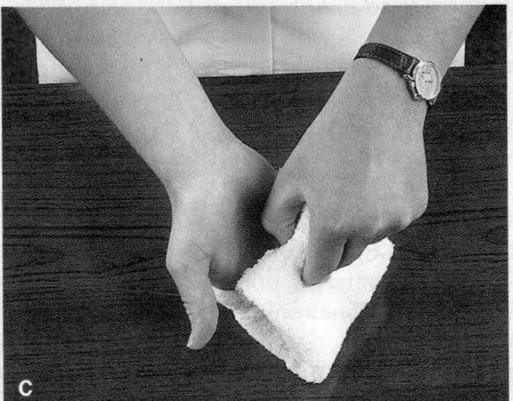

C

Making a mitt.

RATIONALE: *Washing the far side first prevents dripping bath water onto a clean area. Long strokes improve circulation by facilitating venous return. The axilla is a common site of body odor due to perspiration.*

15. Place the basin on a folded towel. Immerse the client's far hand in the water. Wash, rinse, and dry. Cover the client's arm with the bath blanket. Repeat these steps for the client's near arm and hand.
    RATIONALE: *Soaking the hand is comforting and aids in cleansing under the fingernails.*

16. Open a bath towel over the client's chest and fold the bath blanket back. Wash, rinse, and dry the client's chest. Wash, assess, and carefully dry the skin under the female client's breasts. Apply powder if the client desires.

14. Uncover the client's far arm. Place a bath towel under it. Wash with long strokes, rinse, and dry the area. Pay special attention to the axilla.

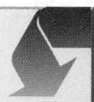

In Practice
Nursing Procedure 50-9 (Continued)

RATIONALE: *Moisture collects in the skin folds under a woman's breasts and may cause irritation or infection. Powder is soothing and helps keep the area dry.*

17. Keeping the towel over the client's chest, lower the bath blanket to just above the pubic area. Wash, rinse, and dry the abdomen, paying special attention to the umbilicus or any skin folds. Then cover the client's chest and abdomen with the bath blanket and remove the towel. The client may put a gown on at this time, leaving it untied at the neck.

    RATIONALE: *The bath blanket continues to provide warmth and privacy. A client who is chilly may feel warmer if he or she wears a gown.*

18. Uncover the client's far leg and place a towel under it. Wash with long strokes, rinse, and dry it.

    RATIONALE: *Washing the far side first prevents dripping bath water on a clean area. Long strokes improve circulation by facilitating venous return.*

19. Place the basin on a folded bath towel and carefully immerse the client's far foot in water. Wash, rinse, and dry the foot, paying particular attention to the area between the toes. Re-cover the leg and foot with the bath blanket. Repeat on the other side.

    RATIONALE: *Soaking the foot is comforting and aids in cleansing between the toes and beneath the toenails.*

20. Raise the side rail and change bath water at this point.

    RATIONALE: *Cool bath water is uncomfortable. The water is probably unclean. Change water earlier if necessary, to maintain the proper temperature or if it becomes dirty.*

21. Lower the near side rail. Assist the client to turn away from you onto his or her side. Uncover the client's back and buttocks. Place an opened towel on the bed, parallel to the client's back. Wash, rinse, and dry the client's back and buttocks. Wash the rectal area. Assess for reddened areas or any skin breakdown.

    RATIONALE: *Skin breakdown usually occurs over bony prominences. Carefully observe the sacral area and back for any indications of skin breakdown or irritation.*

22. Give a backrub at this time. Tie or snap the client's gown at the back or side of the neck.

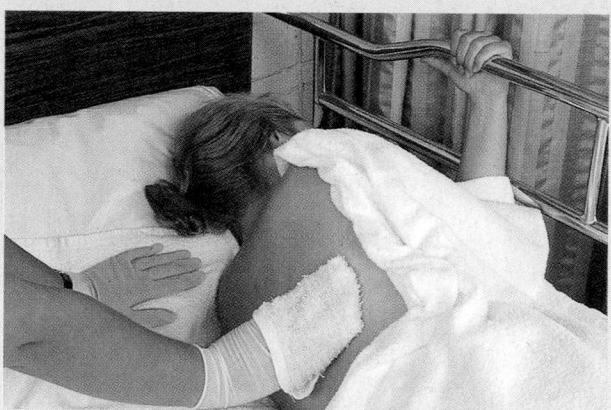

Washing the back.

RATIONALE: *A backrub stimulates circulation and is a comfort measure.*

23. Return the client to his or her back and adjust the bath blanket so that the client is covered. Use side rails for safety, and change bath water again. Use a clean washcloth and towel to wash the client's perineal area (if the client is unable). Otherwise, place necessary equipment within the client's reach and allow him or her to complete this care. Provide privacy. Re-cover the client with the bath blanket. Remove gloves and discard them in the proper receptacle.

    RATIONALE: *Cleaning the perineal area prevents skin irritation and breakdown and decreases the potential for body odor. Self-care may eliminate possible embarrassment for the client.*

24. Help the client put on a gown or pajamas (if this was not done before). Assist the client with personal hygiene, such as deodorant and cologne. Assist with hair care and oral hygiene.

    RATIONALE: *Gown or pajamas provide warmth. Helping with specific hygiene needs personalizes the client's care.*

25. Make the bed with clean linens. Lower the bed and raise the side rails as ordered.

    RATIONALE: *These measures provide for comfort and safety.*

26. Wash your hands.

    RATIONALE: *Handwashing helps to prevent the spread of infection.*

27. Document assessments on flow sheet and chart.

    RATIONALE: *Documentation provides communication and coordination of care.*

Critical Thinking Exercises

1. You are performing personal hygiene on a client. Describe information that can be obtained while giving a sponge or bed bath.
2. Your client is 78 years old and is of the opposite sex. He or she has had a stroke that caused left-sided paralysis. The client responds only occasionally to your questions. He or she does not move independently. Explain how you will assist with this client's bath.

NCLEX-Style Review Questions

1. When teaching the client about oral hygiene, the nurse should include which of the following?
   a. Healthy teeth do not affect overall health.
   b. Oral hygiene diminishes appetite.
   c. Oral hygiene does not affect appearance.
   d. Oral hygiene improves food's taste.
2. Which of the following clients would need hourly oral hygiene?
   a. A child who is teething
   b. A postoperative client
   c. An unresponsive client
   d. A well client
3. When providing eye care, which approach should the nurse take?
   a. Avoid cleaning the eyes.
   b. Cleanse from the inner to the outer canthus.
   c. Cleanse from the outer to the inner canthus.
   d. Moisten a towel and lay over the eyes.
4. The nurse is caring for a client with poor eyesight. Which action is appropriate when shaving this client?
   a. Allow client to shave him- or herself.
   b. Ask a family member to shave the client.
   c. Assist the client with shaving.
   d. Do not shave this client.
5. Which information is most important for the nurse to obtain prior to bathing a client?
   a. Client's condition
   b. Client's normal habits
   c. Client's shampoo preference
   d. Time of client's last bath

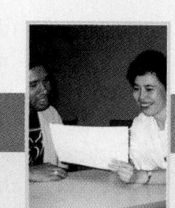

CHAPTER

51

Elimination

LEARNING OBJECTIVES

1. Describe the normal color, clarity, and odor of urine.
2. Describe at least eight abnormal patterns of urination.
3. Identify the normal color and consistency of feces.
4. Explain two deviations from normal as related to feces.
5. Demonstrate the techniques for assisting the client to the bathroom, giving and removing a bedpan or urinal, and transferring the client from bed to commode.
6. Explain the purpose and procedures for competent catheter care.
7. Describe techniques for relieving urinary retention.
8. List the purposes of cleansing, retention, and carminative enemas.
9. Demonstrate the technique for administering a self-contained disposable enema.
10. Describe the procedure for manual disimpaction, including a situation in which this procedure would be used.
11. Discuss nursing care for the client who is vomiting.

NEW TERMINOLOGY

anuria	melena
calculi	micturition
constipation	nocturia
Crede's maneuver	oliguria
cystitis	polyuria
defecation	projectile vomiting
diarrhea	renal colic
dysuria	urgency
enema	urinary catheter
enuresis	urinary frequency
fecal impaction	urinary retention
flatus	voiding
incontinence	vomitus
Kegel exercises	

ACRONYMS

BM	SP	TWE
BRP	SSE	UTI
BS		

The healthy human body smoothly and effectively eats, digests, absorbs, and metabolizes food, to fuel and operate its many functions. Just as smoothly and effectively, the healthy body rids itself of waste products that it does not need, to maintain homeostasis. Elimination of liquid and solid waste products is normally routine and uneventful, unless a change in habits or illness occurs. Changes in bowel or bladder habits may be *signs* of illness, or they may *cause* illness. Assessing the client's products of elimination (urine and feces), observing his or her bladder and bowel function, and assisting the client who is facing a problem with these functions are fundamental nursing responsibilities.

> **N u r s i n g   A l e r t**
>
> Standard Precautions require the use of gloves when coming in contact with any body secretion or drainage from the client. Handwashing before and after all client care is required.

ELIMINATION

Urine is the body's liquid waste product. Passing urine from the body is called *urination,* **micturition,** or **voiding.** Feces, also called a *bowel movement* (**BM**) or *stool,* is the body's solid waste product. **Defecation** refers to the excretion of feces.

Urine and feces are the waste products of the urinary and digestive systems, respectively. Each has typical characteristics when these systems and processes are normal. However, both urine and feces may also contain indicators of dysfunction during illness. Urine and stool specimens are frequently collected as part of nursing assessment and care (see Chap. 52). Becoming familiar with the normal characteristics of these waste products, and understanding the usual functions of elimination, helps to identify variations or abnormalities when they occur.

Urinary Elimination

Urine, formed by the kidneys, is composed of excess water from the body, some carbon dioxide, a small amount of solid wastes, and abnormal substances being filtered from the blood. It is then excreted via the bladder and urethra (see Chap. 27). Normal kidneys produce about 1 milliliter of urine per every kilogram of body weight each hour. This means that an average-sized adult forms and excretes approximately 1,000 to 1,500 milliliters of urine every 24 hours. However, this total output varies, according to a person's fluid intake and the amount he or she excretes through normal respiration, perspiration, and the fluid contained in feces. When the body freely perspires due to hot weather, exercise, or fever, it forms and excretes less urine. If the body retains water because of impaired circulation or kidney function, it forms and excretes less urine.

Fluid output is usually about the same as *fluid intake.* Encourage clients to drink adequate amounts of fluid. To maintain normal fluid balance, each adult needs six to eight 8-ounce glasses of liquid daily. If ordered, the nurse records the client's intake and output (I&O) every shift to assess the fluid balance. This procedure is described in Chapter 52.

Changes in the characteristics of urine or in usual urination patterns may be signs of problems in the urinary system. The nurse is in a unique position to observe the client's elimination patterns. Report any unusual or abnormal signs or symptoms.

Characteristics of Urine

Urine is observed for color, clarity, odor, and volume. The nurse makes these observations as part of routine data collection. Any deviations may indicate an abnormality.

Color.   Freshly voided urine is light yellow or amber in color. The degree of color in urine varies with the body's level of hydration. *Overhydration* (too much fluid) results in dilute urine that is nearly colorless. *Dehydration* (too little fluid) results in concentrated urine that is dark amber or orange-brown.[1] In addition, certain medications and foods can alter the color of urine.

Clarity.   Freshly voided urine is clear or transparent. It appears cloudy if it contains abnormal substances, such as bacteria, blood, mucous shreds, or pus, or if it has been standing for a period of time in a collection container.

Odor.   Freshly voided urine has a characteristic odor that is sometimes called *aromatic.* Dilute urine has fewer odors than concentrated urine. When it has been exposed to the air for some time, urine decomposes and emits a strong, ammonia-like odor. Sometimes foods or medications alter urine's usual odor. Usually a strongly offensive odor from freshly voided urine suggests an abnormality, such as a urinary tract infection.

Volume.   The typical amount of urine that an adult voids at one time ranges between 250 and 400 milliliters. The exact output relates to each person's size, bladder condition, hydration level, and other fluid gains or losses.

Specific Gravity.   Normal urine has a *specific gravity,* when compared with water, of 1.010 to 1.025. Chapter 52 describes how to measure urine specific gravity.

Abnormal Components.   Abnormal components—such as microorganisms—in urine suggest dysfunction or disease somewhere in the body. Sometimes, the urine's appearance is so changed that abnormalities are obvious; other times the urine appears normal to the naked eye. Many urine tests are performed in the laboratory. Specific tests are described throughout this book.

Patterns of Urinary Elimination

Although observation of the appearance of a client's urine can indicate renal (kidney) or urinary problems, a change in the usual pattern of urinary elimination is just as significant a finding. Be familiar with these common signs and symptoms that may occur:

- **Urinary frequency:** Voiding more often than usual without an increase in total urine volume.
- **Urgency:** The desire or sensation of needing to void immediately. Often, the person is unable to delay voiding without some involuntary urine leakage (*incontinence*).

- **Dysuria:** A painful or burning sensation when passing urine (most commonly associated with an infection). The person may also experience cramping or shooting pain in the pelvis.
- **Nocturia:** Frequent or repeated voiding during the night. Sometimes, it occurs when the person drinks a large amount of liquid before bedtime, and may not indicate a structural or organic problem. Usually, frequency accompanies abnormal nocturia.
- **Enuresis:** Involuntary voiding in bed (*bedwetting*). Enuresis is a common problem in children, but may also be a problem for some adults. Enuresis also may be a side effect of certain medications.
- **Polyuria:** An increase in the expected amount of urine a person excretes over a period of time. It may occur when the person drinks a larger than usual amount of liquids, but it may also be a symptom of diabetes mellitus or certain types of kidney disease.
- **Oliguria:** A decrease in the expected amount of urine a person excretes (usually below 30 milliliters in one hour). Kidney disorders or urinary tract obstruction may cause oliguria.
- **Anuria:** The absence of urine excreted by the kidneys (less than 100 mL/d). Anuria is a very serious sign of kidney dysfunction. Other signs of failing kidneys include headache, dizziness, edema, puffiness around the eyes, nausea, and dim vision.
- **Urinary retention:** Inability to empty the bladder of urine. Retention may have several causes. Sometimes, a person is unable to feel the usual urges for voiding or is unable to relax the urethral muscles to allow urination. An obstruction may exist in the urinary tract. Often the person retains urine for 6 to 8 hours. Retention may also mean incomplete emptying of the bladder during usual voiding. Temporary urinary retention following abdominal surgery is common.
- **Incontinence:** The involuntary loss of urine from the bladder. Loss of muscle tone, injury, or paralysis destroys the ability of the urethral muscles to constrict and to keep the urinary outlet closed; thus, urine dribbles, or the muscles relax without the person's control. If the nerve pathways to the brain's control center are injured, the person either does not feel the impulse to urinate, or is unable to control the outlet muscles, and therefore voids involuntarily. If the cause is muscular weakness, bladder retraining often is effective.

Urinary Tract Problems

Urinary Tract Infection (UTI).   Urinary tract infections (**UTI**) are common, often occurring when microorganisms contaminate the usually sterile urinary tract through the urethral opening. UTIs are more common in women than in men because the female urethra is shorter. *Urethritis* technically means inflammation of the urethra; **cystitis** is an inflammation of the bladder; and *nephritis* or *polynephritis* refer to inflammation of the kidneys. Inflammation is most often caused by an infection, and the term *cystitis* is often used to denote any UTI.

The person experiencing a UTI may complain of urgency, frequency, dysuria, chills, abdominal discomfort, and pain. The urine may appear cloudy due to the presence of microorganisms or pus. Encourage the client who complains of these symptoms to drink more liquids than usual. Obtain a clean urine specimen for culture, and report such complaints to the client's healthcare provider. Most UTIs respond quickly to specific antibiotics.

Urinary Calculi.   Urinary calculi are stones. They may occur in the kidney (*renal calculi*) or bladder (*cystic calculi*). Calculi are formed from body waste products when certain conditions—such as infection, urinary retention, or prolonged immobility—are present. In some cases, the specific cause of urinary calculi is unknown. The stones may vary in size from tiny, microscopic pieces of sand to marble-sized accumulations. These stones may obstruct a client's normal urinary flow as they move within the urinary tract. If a stone becomes lodged in a ureter, the person experiences severe, penetrating pain in the lower back called **renal colic.** Calculi often cause UTIs. Chapter 88 describes urinary calculi and their treatment in more detail.

When caring for a client with possible kidney stones, the physician will most likely order the urine to be strained for calculi. In Practice: Nursing Care Guidelines 51-1 describes how to do this.

Bowel Elimination ✳

Similar to urinary elimination, changes in *bowel elimination* may occur because of gastrointestinal illness or illness in another body system. The bowel responds to even the slightest changes in a person's usual eating or exercise habits. Bowel elimination can change quickly when a client is ill or immobilized. Daily assessment includes noting the characteristics of a client's stools and any changes or difficulties that he or she reports.

Characteristics of Feces

Feces (stools), the solid waste products of digestion, consist of the end products of the metabolism and digestion of foods.

Color.   Normally, feces are yellowish-brown (due to the presence of bile). A change in color suggests a change in gastrointestinal functioning or contents of the stool. Gray- or clay-colored stools usually indicate that bile is missing, often a sign of gallbladder disease. Dark, black, or tarry stools usually indicate the presence of digested blood, called **melena,** indicating hemorrhage high in the gastrointestinal tract. Bright-red blood in (or streaked on the outside of) the stool indicates rectal or anal bleeding. Stools that are yellow or greenish in color indicate the abnormal presence of microorganisms, suggesting infection. Some medications or foods may alter stool color as well.

Consistency.   Normal stools are soft and formed. Hard, dry stools result when the rectum has not been emptied as needed and excess liquid has been absorbed. This is called **constipation.** Often, it occurs when a person ignores the impulse to empty the rectum. Constipation may also result if the person has not taken enough fluids or has not had sufficient

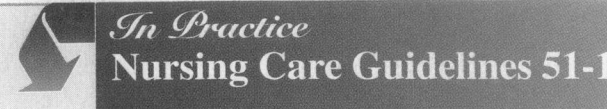

In Practice
Nursing Care Guidelines 51-1

STRAINING URINE FOR CALCULI

Teach the client not to discard any urine until it has been examined. Each time the client voids:

- Wash your hands. Put on clean gloves. *Rationale: Handwashing and using gloves helps to prevent the spread of infection, especially when handling body fluids.*
- Prepare a graduated container with a fine-wire strainer in which clean gauze has been placed. *Rationale: This client is probably under an intake and output [I&O] order, so urine amount needs to be measured. The wire strainer catches any stones [calculi] that might be present. The gauze enables you to see the stones more clearly.*
- Pour urine through the strainer and gauze into the graduated container.
- Look for visible stones. *Rationale: You will need to report size, number, and appearance of any stones that you recover.*
- Inspect any blood clots for the presence of stones by pressing them against the sides of the gauze in the strainer with a tongue blade. *Rationale: A blood clot could hide stones.*
- Report any blood clots or active bleeding. *Rationale: Urinary hemorrhage may occur as a result of calculi. Bleeding may need to be treated, in addition to determining how to deal with the calculi.*
- Retrieve any stones and place them in a specimen container to send to the laboratory for examination. *Rationale: Identification of stone composition is necessary to determine the correct treatment for prevention of future stone formation.*
- Discard gloves and wash your hands. Document findings. *Rationale: Proper glove disposal and handwashing reduce the risk of infection transmission. Documentation provides communication and enhances continuity of care.*

exercise to stimulate peristalsis. Constipation may also result from some types of medications or may occur after surgery.

Diarrhea is the expulsion of loose, watery, unformed stools. Sometimes the person has frequent, watery stools. Continuing diarrhea suggests chronic irritation of the colon, intestinal infection, food poisoning, or a parasitic infection. The person's emotional state may also affect stool consistency, causing either diarrhea or constipation. Diarrhea can also be a sign of **fecal impaction** (accumulation of hardened stool in the rectum), which is discussed later in this section.

Shape. Generally, stools have the same shape as the bowel's interior: round, oval, or cylindrical. Long, thin, pencil-like stools suggest a narrowing of the rectum or anal opening, which could be caused by a mass or tumor. Stool that always assumes the same irregular shape is also suggestive of an abnormal growth in the rectum or anus.

Odor. Stools have a characteristic odor. Note any unusual or very strong odors. Sometimes medications, strong-flavored foods, or the presence of unusual microorganisms change the odor.

Density. *Stool density* is the weight concentration of waste products in relation to water. Normally, stools are heavy enough to sink in water. Stools that float are less dense and suggest undigested fats, especially if they have a fatty or oily appearance. Make a note if stools float; this may be an indication of gallbladder disease.

Abnormal Components. The presence of pus or mucus in stool indicates an inflammation or infection somewhere in the digestive system. The presence of undigested food products may suggest digestive system malfunction. Blood or **melena** suggests hemorrhage from inflammation or irritation.

Fecal Impaction. The term *fecal impaction* denotes stool that is so hard and dry or putty-like that it cannot be expelled by the client. Fecal impaction is usually the result of chronic bowel problems, but can also be the result of immobility or paralysis. Some clients develop a fecal impaction following an x-ray procedure called a *barium enema;* this type of impaction results from retained barium.

Symptoms of fecal impaction include severe abdominal discomfort and a feeling of pressure. The person often feels the urge to defecate, but is unable to do so or is unable to empty the bowel completely. Diarrhea also may be a symptom, with liquid stool leaking out around the impaction. In fecal impaction, a rectal examination reveals a hard or putty-like mass. Digital removal of impacted stool (manual disimpaction) may be required. This procedure is discussed later in this chapter.

☛ KEY CONCEPT

After manual disimpaction, the client may have several bouts of explosive diarrhea before settling into a normal bowel elimination pattern.

Patterns of Bowel Elimination

Defecation usually occurs at regular intervals when the mass of feces moves into the colon through the muscular action of the intestinal wall, called *peristalsis.* The fecal mass causes pressure against the bowel walls, which signals to the person that he or she must empty the bowels. The abdominal muscles help push stool from the rectum.

Patterns of elimination are unique to each individual. Many individuals experience a bowel movement in the morning after breakfast. The feces have accumulated during the night and the food eaten stimulates peristalsis. Nursing assessment determines the *frequency* (how often) and *regularity* (interval between stools) of an individual client's bowel movements. Document if the client reports a change in the frequency, regularity, or characteristics of stools. For example, a change in bowel habits is one of the warning signs of cancer.

☞ KEY CONCEPT

Remember that not everyone has a bowel movement daily. If the person is symptom-free, bowel movements occurring less often are not a cause for concern.

Flatus

Intestinal gas is called **flatus;** the condition of having intestinal gas is called *flatulence.* The normal intestine creates gas as part of the digestive process. Most flatus is reabsorbed through the vasculature of the intestinal wall; some of it is expelled with defecation. Some people are prone to developing and retaining gas in uncomfortable amounts. Different varieties of foods, such as broccoli, beans, and very spicy foods are more gas-forming than others. Flatus may accumulate and cause considerable discomfort and embarrassment.

Abdominal Signs and Symptoms

Data collection and assessment include a specific examination of the abdomen, particularly if the client reports pain or discomfort and changes in bowel habits. The first step is to listen for bowel sounds (**BS**). The action of peristalsis, which causes the products of digestion to move through the intestine, creates distinctive sounds that can be heard with a stethoscope. *Diminished* or *absent* sounds indicate that the bowel is functioning improperly. Report such findings immediately. When listening for bowel sounds, *auscultate* (listen) in each of the four quadrants of the abdomen with a stethoscope. In Practice: Nursing Care Guidelines 51-2 describes the method used to listen for bowel sounds. Table 51-1 tells how to describe and document bowel sounds.

After auscultating for bowel sounds, gently palpate the client's abdomen. Normally, the abdomen is soft and pliable. If the abdomen is hard, swollen, or tender, the client may have flatus, fecal impaction, or an intestinal obstruction. Record and report any changes or unusual discomfort that the client mentions.

☞ KEY CONCEPT

The client may feel uncomfortable or embarrassed when discussing bladder or bowel elimination. Be sure to provide privacy and demonstrate understanding.

ASSISTING WITH TOILETING

Elimination is a function included in the activities of daily living when describing a client's independence level. Helping the client with elimination is a basic nursing responsibility. Various nursing interventions to assist the client with either bowel or bladder elimination are called toileting.

Helping the Client to the Bathroom

The client who is weak, confused, sedated, or extremely tired may require some help getting to and from the bathroom. Be sure that the client has bathroom privileges (**BRPs**), and check to see if I&O are being recorded before the client leaves the

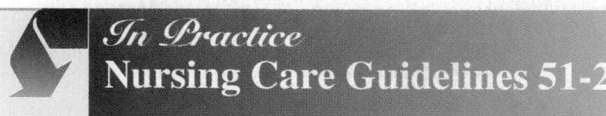

In Practice
Nursing Care Guidelines 51-2

LISTENING FOR BOWEL SOUNDS

- Wash hands and position the client in a dorsal recumbent (supine) position. *Rationale: Positioning the client in this manner allows the major part of the abdomen to be accessible.*
- Expose the abdomen, but keep other areas of the client's body covered. *Rationale: This action maintains the client's privacy while allowing access to the abdomen.*
- Warm the stethoscope in your hands. *Rationale: The shock of a cold stethoscope can temporarily halt bowel sounds.*
- Place the flat side (diaphragm) of the stethoscope against the client's abdomen. *Rationale: The diaphragm offers coverage of a larger area than the bell, and is useful in detecting high-pitched sounds. This improves your chances of hearing all bowel sounds.*
- Imagine the abdomen to be divided into four quadrants or regions (see Fig. 15-5 in Chap. 15). Begin at a particular quadrant and continue in a clockwise fashion around the abdomen. Always use the same pattern. *Rationale: This will help ensure that all areas are auscultated and all occurring bowel sounds are heard.*
- Listen to peristalsis, which makes a gurgling sound that occurs every 5–20 seconds. A sound may last for several seconds. *Rationale: Gas is formed during normal digestion and peristalsis. The sounds are this gas moving within the intestines.*
- If sounds are difficult to hear, listen for 3–5 min before concluding that they are absent. *Rationale: Sometimes, peristaltic movements pause, or there is a minimum of gas for a short time.*
- Wash your hands and document your findings on the client's record. See Table 51-1 for documentation tips. *Rationale: Documentation provides communication about the client's intestinal motility and enhances continuity of care.*

bed. If I&O are being recorded, place a measuring "hat" under the toilet seat so that urine is collected for measurement and recording. (The measuring hat and the procedure for measuring I&O are described in Chapter 52.) Assist the client as needed and check on the client frequently. Explain that he or she can call for assistance by triggering the call signal in the bathroom near the toilet.

Giving and Removing a Bedpan or Urinal

Male clients who are confined to bed will use a *bedpan* for defecation and a *urinal* for voiding. Female clients use the bedpan for both defecating and urinating; a *female urinal* is also

✳ ■■■ **TABLE 51-1** 𝒟ESCRIPTION OF BOWEL SOUNDS

What is Heard	What is Documented
Audible: Heard every 5–20 sec	BS + (normal bowel sounds)
Decreased and soft: Hypoactive, occurs only about once/min	BS ↓ (decreased bowel sounds)
Increased and rapid: Loud and high pitched, occurring at more frequent intervals (every 3–5 sec)	BS ↑ (hyperactive bowel sounds)
Absent: No movement of intestine heard after listening for at least 3 min; may result from surgery, bowel obstruction, inflammation, spinal cord trauma, or other conditions	BS − (bowel sounds absent)

Bowel sounds are usually the same in all four quadrants of the abdomen. If this is not true, record the sound in each quadrant. For example, BS ↓ LUQ (left upper quadrant), and so forth.

available, however. Always wear gloves when working with bedpans or urinals. In Practice: Nursing Procedure 51-1 lists the steps for giving and removing a bedpan.

The Bedpan

Usually the *bedpan* is made of plastic or nylon-resin. *Fracture pans* may be made of metal. Warm the pan with hot water before placing it under the client. A nylon-resin bedpan feels warmer to the touch, is less noisy in handling, and can be cleaned and sterilized by conventional methods. Nylon and plastic bedpans are disposable. A child's bedpan is smaller than the standard size. Use a pediatric bedpan for an adult who requires complete assistance or who is unable to lie on the larger pan. A fracture pan with one flat end is also available. Use this type of bedpan when the client is unable to raise the hips high enough to get on top of the usual bedpan; slip the flat end under the buttocks. However, remember that the fracture bedpan holds less and spills more easily.

Remember that getting onto a bedpan in bed is very difficult; help the client as needed. Raise the head of the bed so that the client is in a more functional sitting position while on the bedpan. Provide as much privacy as possible; otherwise, the client may be unable to relax. If a client is confused or unable to follow directions, protect the bed with a pad and stay with the person.

A full bladder is uncomfortable. Offer a bedpan or urinal to the client before meals and visiting hours, and when he or she settles down for the night. Avoid keeping a client waiting for a bedpan; holding urine or feces weakens sphincter tone in the urethra or rectum and is physically and emotionally distressing. If a client has to wait for assistance, and does not have prompt attention after using the bedpan, he or she may try to walk to the bathroom alone, may upset the bedpan, or may be incontinent in bed.

The Urinal

When the male client asks to use the urinal, encourage him to position it himself. If necessary, help the client to position the urinal. Be sure to wear gloves and provide privacy. Also provide needed articles for handwashing. Sometimes a man can void more easily while standing at the bedside, if this is allowed.

After he urinates, measure the urine, if ordered. Then rinse the urinal, dispose of gloves, and wash the hands.

☛ KEY CONCEPT

Rinse bedpans and urinals in cool-to-warm water. Rationale: Hot water will cause the proteins in waste products to coagulate.

Helping the Client to Use a Commode

The client may find it difficult to urinate and to defecate when using a bedpan. The client who is unable to use the bedpan may be able to use a bedside commode: a straight-backed chair with an open seat and a receptacle beneath.

Wear gloves when helping the client to the commode. Transfer the person from the bed to the commode as you would from the bed to any chair (see Chap. 48). Stay with the client if there is any chance that he or she will become lightheaded or dizzy. Be sure to provide privacy.

The procedure for using a commode is the same as that for using a bedpan. Wash the client's hands, note the contents of the commode container, discard the urine or feces, rinse the commode after use, and wash your hands. Properly dispose of gloves. If the commode cannot be kept out of sight, it may be closed and kept at the bedside.

☛ KEY CONCEPT

Make sure the client has the call signal nearby when using the bedpan or commode. Rationale: Having the call signal nearby will help to protect the client from falling and possibly prevent spills.

ASSISTING WITH URINARY ELIMINATION

The Client Requiring a Urinary Catheter

A **urinary catheter** is a latex or vinyl tube that is inserted to remove urine. It is approximately 24 inches long and is inserted into the bladder through the urethra using sterile

In Practice
Nursing Procedure 51-1

Gɪᴠɪɴɢ ᴀɴᴅ Rᴇᴍᴏᴠɪɴɢ ᴛʜᴇ Bᴇᴅᴘᴀɴ

Supplies and Equipment

Gloves
Cover for bedpan
Hand washing supplies
Bedpan
Toilet tissue
Air freshener (optional)

Steps

1. Obtain a bedpan, if one is not available in the bed-side cabinet.

   Rᴀᴛɪᴏɴᴀʟᴇ: *Organization facilitates accurate skill performance. Each client has a separate bedpan that is disposable and discarded when the client is discharged.*

2. Explain the procedure to the client.

   Rᴀᴛɪᴏɴᴀʟᴇ: *Providing information fosters cooperation.*

3. Wash hands and put on gloves.

   Rᴀᴛɪᴏɴᴀʟᴇ: *Handwashing and using gloves helps to prevent the spread of infection.*

4. Close the curtain or door to the room.

   Rᴀᴛɪᴏɴᴀʟᴇ: *Closing the curtain or door protects the client's privacy.*

5. Raise the bed to a comfortable height. Lower the near side rail.

   Rᴀᴛɪᴏɴᴀʟᴇ: *Proper positioning prevents back strain for the nurse. Lowering the side rail nearest the nurse provides easy access to the client.*

6. Fold the bed linen away from the client, exposing as little of his or her body as possible. Place an incontinence pad on the bed if the client is confused or if using a fracture pan.

   Rᴀᴛɪᴏɴᴀʟᴇ: *This action protects the client's privacy and provides access for placing the bedpan. The incontinence pad protects the bed linens from urine.*

7. Assist the client onto the bedpan. If the client is able to help, encourage him or her to flex the knees and lift the hips:

   a. Place the bedpan under the buttocks, with the rounded curved end toward the client's back, and the narrower open end toward the feet.

      Rᴀᴛɪᴏɴᴀʟᴇ: *Placing a regular bedpan in this position fits the contour of the body, alleviates discomfort, and prevents spilling of waste materials.*

   b. If a client is unable to use a regular bedpan, use a fracture bedpan. Place it under the but-

tocks with the flat end toward the client's back.

Rᴀᴛɪᴏɴᴀʟᴇ: *A fracture pan exerts less pressure on the hips and spine and is easier to place under the client.*

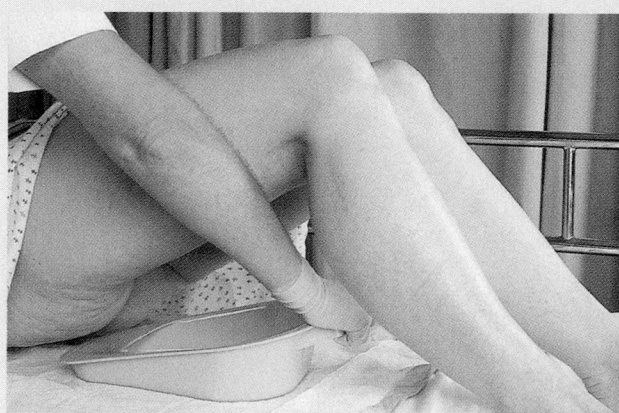

Placing a fracture pan under client.

8. If the client is immobile, roll the client onto his or her side away from you. Position the bedpan against the client's buttocks, hold it firmly in place, and turn the client onto his or her back. Check the pan's location.

   Rᴀᴛɪᴏɴᴀʟᴇ: *Properly positioning the bedpan avoids spillage while ensuring the client's comfort.*

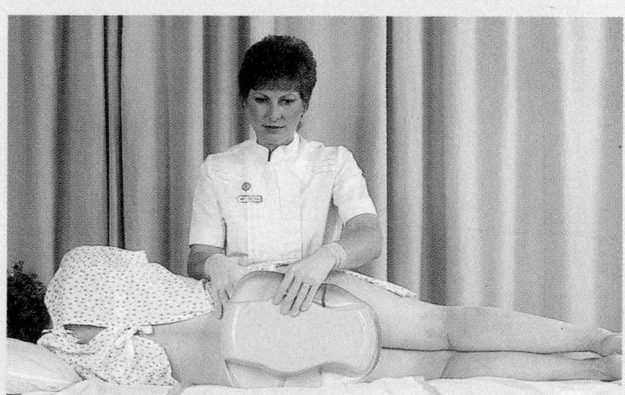

Positioning the bedpan against the buttocks while the client is on his or her side.

9. Replace the bed linen over the client.

   Rᴀᴛɪᴏɴᴀʟᴇ: *Covering the client protects the client's privacy.*

10. Elevate the head of the bed to semi-Fowler's position if the client can tolerate it. Raise the side rail again.

    Rᴀᴛɪᴏɴᴀʟᴇ: *This position most closely resembles the normal position for elimination and uses*

(continued)

In Practice
Nursing Procedure 51-1 (*Continued*)

gravity as an additional force. The raised side rail offers security to the client and provides something for the client to use to help with balance or to move.

11. Place the call light and toilet tissue within the client's reach and leave him or her alone if possible. Tell the client to call if he or she needs help and also when finished. If leaving the bedside, remove gloves and wash hands.
    RATIONALE: *The call bell provides for the client's comfort and security. Leaving the client alone allows for privacy.*

12. To remove the bedpan:
    a. Wash hands and put on gloves.
    b. Lower the side rail and the head of the bed.
    c. Uncover the client.
    d. Fold the toilet tissue and wipe from the front (pubic area) to the back (anus) if the client is unable to do so independently.
    e. Steady the bedpan as the client either lifts the hips or is assisted to turn away from you.
    f. Place the bedpan on the chair and cover it.
    g. Cleanse the area with soap and water if necessary. Shaving-cream lather works well and is soothing. Dry carefully.

RATIONALE: *Holding the bedpan steady and assisting the client off of it prevents spillage of contents. Keeping the client's skin clean and dry helps to prevent skin breakdown.*

13. Offer handwashing supplies to the client.
    RATIONALE: *Handwashing helps to prevent the spread of microorganisms and teaches good hygiene.*

14. Return the client to a comfortable position. Lower the bed and raise the side rail. Use air freshener if necessary.
    RATIONALE: *These steps provide for comfort and safety.*

15. Empty the pan into the toilet and rinse. Measure output or obtain stool sample if ordered. Remove gloves and wash hands.
    RATIONALE: *Proper disposal and cleaning prevent the spread of infection.*

16. Document results according to agency policy on flow sheet, intake and output summary, or chart.
    RATIONALE: *Documentation provides communication and coordination of care.*

---

technique (see Chap. 57). A *straight catheter* is inserted, urine is drained, and the catheter is removed and discarded. A *retention catheter* is inserted, anchored in place, and continuously drains urine from the bladder; sometimes it is called an *indwelling catheter,* which is placed when a client is unable to void naturally or has had surgery. Several types of catheters are available, but the *Foley catheter* is most frequently used. This catheter usually has two tube-like cavities called *lumens* within it. One lumen is connected to a balloon that is inflated inside the bladder to anchor the catheter in place. Another lumen drains the urine. The distal end of the catheter is attached to a drainage bag that collects urine. Some catheters have a third lumen to provide a means for continuous bladder irrigation.

Nursing Alert

Many clients and health care workers are developing *latex sensitivity.* Be sure to ask about latex allergy before inserting a catheter. If the client is allergic to latex, use a vinyl or latex-free catheter.

Never remove a retention catheter without an order. If it should fall out, report this immediately. A new, sterile catheter must be inserted, or the retention catheter may be discontinued if the client is now able to void.

Inserting the Catheter
Chapter 57 describes the technique for inserting a catheter. The insertion of a catheter is a sterile procedure that must be performed with the utmost care to avoid introducing bacteria into the client's bladder. (If bladder or gynecologic surgery is performed, a urologist usually inserts the catheter in the operating room.)

Some retention catheters are packaged with tubing and a drainage bag already connected to avoid contamination. The bag is lightweight and hung on the bed frame, but it can easily be fastened to the client's gown while he or she is out of bed. This closed drainage system collection bag must never be higher than the level of the client's bladder. *Rationale: This would cause urine in the bag to flow back into the bladder, possibly leading to infection.*

Caring for the Catheter
When the client has a retention catheter in place, assess both the equipment and its function frequently. Check that the catheter remains securely in place and that the tubing is not pulling against the urethra or kinked. The tubing should go over the client's leg when the client is in bed. To prevent pulling, tape the catheter to the thigh in the female client and to the abdomen in the male client, allowing for some slack before taping in place. Check that the bag is hung at a proper height below the bed, or below the level of the bladder if the

client is out of bed. Observe for the flow of urine through the transparent plastic tubing leading to the collecting bag. Measure the amount of urine in the bag, and empty the bag regularly. If the catheter is to be changed, change the entire drainage set. In Practice: Nursing Care Guidelines 51-3 gives steps for catheter care.

Emptying the Urinary Drainage Bag

Emptying the drainage bag is done while maintaining the sterility of the closed system. In Practice: Nursing Procedure 51-2 gives steps for emptying the drainage bag.

Irrigating the Catheter

Some catheters are irrigated to ensure patency and to remove clots or debris that may obstruct free urinary flow. Irrigation procedure usually requires a physician's order.

Catheter irrigation is a sterile procedure and is described in Chapter 57.

Using the Suprapubic Catheter

A suprapubic catheter (**SP**) is inserted into the bladder by way of a small surgical incision ("stab wound") through the abdominal and bladder walls (Fig. 51-1). This type of catheter is anchored in place by a balloon or "mushroom" apparatus on the end of the catheter inside the bladder wall (similar to a retention catheter). Often an adhesive seal is applied around the surgical incision to prevent urinary leakage. The catheter is connected to a drainage bag. This catheter is used after some types of gynecologic or urologic surgery, when urine cannot drain normally through the urethra, or to avoid contamination of a surgical wound with urine. However, if the urethra is functioning normally, urine also can be voided naturally while the suprapubic catheter is in place.

In Practice
Nursing Care Guidelines 51-3

PERFORMING CATHETER CARE

- Keep in mind that a catheter is used only when absolutely necessary. Only trained personnel, using strict aseptic technique, should do the catheterization procedure itself. *Rationale: Catheterization is an invasive technique.*
- Ensure that the catheter drainage system is a closed sterile system. *Rationale: Catheterization is performed using sterile technique because the bladder and urinary system are considered sterile.*
- Wash hands and wear gloves when working with catheters. *Rationale: Handwashing and using gloves help to prevent the spread of infection, especially when working with body fluids.*
- Do not disconnect tubing unless there are specific orders. *Rationale: Disconnecting the tubing breaks the integrity of the closed system and places the client at risk for infection.*
- Do not irrigate catheters unless the primary care provider writes specific orders to do so. *Rationale: Irrigation may introduce pathogens into the sterile system.*
- If the client ambulates, make sure that the bag goes along with him or her. *Rationale: Urine is produced continuously and must be collected.*
- Obtain sterile urine specimens from most catheter drainage systems by using a syringe with a small-gauge needle, and aspirating from a designated specimen port area that has been cleansed with an antiseptic agent such as alcohol. Other specimens may be obtained from the bag-emptying plug at the bottom of the bag. However, this specimen is not as accurate, especially for urine cultures.
- Secure the catheter externally. *Rationale: Properly securing the catheter prevents pressure on the

urethra and prevents the catheter from being pulled out.*
- Cleanse the urethral meatus and the catheter near the meatus at least twice a day with an antiseptic agent such as alcohol or pHisoHex soap. *Rationale: Cleansing the meatal area helps to prevent infection.*
- Apply an antimicrobial ointment to the meatal area after the bi-daily cleansing, if recommended by agency policy.
- Check the drainage tubing for the presence of urine, which is secreted constantly and will drip constantly through the drainage tube unless obstructed. Absence of urine draining is a serious sign. *Rationale: Observation of urine flow ensures proper functioning of the drainage system and allows for early identification of problems should any arise.*
- Position the tubing over the client's leg, not under. *Rationale: The weight of the client's leg might slow or stop drainage.*
- Allow some slack in the tubing above bed level. Fasten the tubing to the bed. *Rationale: Slack in the tubing allows the client to turn freely in bed. If the tubing is loose above the level of the bed, drainage will not be impaired. Fastening the tubing to the bed keeps it from falling over the side.*
- Ensure that the tubing falls straight down from the bed to the drainage bag. (This is called *straight drainage.*) It should not hang down or be kinked. *Rationale: If the tubing is kinked or hangs down, drainage will be slowed and infection can occur.*
- Always keep the level of the bag below the level of the bladder. *Rationale: If urine flows back into the bladder, there is danger of infection.*

(continued)

In Practice
Nursing Care Guidelines 51-3 (Continued)

- Remember that drainage systems are closed systems. Do not open the bag except to empty it from the bottom. Follow the instructions for the particular bag being used. *Rationale: Ensuring the integrity of the system is vital to maintaining sterility.*
- Measure and record output in the proper manner. *Rationale: The volume of urine is a valuable piece of information in the care of the catheterized person.*
- Observe the quality and characteristics of the urine. *Rationale: The presence of sediment, dark urine, or cloudy urine often indicates an infection. Very dark*

urine or obvious blood usually indicates bleeding in the urinary system. These are serious findings that must be reported immediately.
- Note the client's body temperature. *Rationale: Fever usually accompanies infection.*
- Dispose of gloves properly and wash hands after catheter care. *Rationale: Proper glove disposal and handwashing are important in reducing the risk for infection transmission.*
- Document all information properly. *Rationale: Documentation ensures communication among health care team members.*

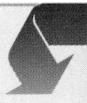

In Practice
Nursing Procedure 51-2

EMPTYING THE DRAINAGE BAG
Supplies and Equipment

Disposable gloves
Measuring container or graduate

Steps

1. Wash hands and put on clean gloves.
   RATIONALE: *Wear gloves when handling any body fluids to reduce the risk of infection transmission.*

2. Carefully pull the drain tube (located on the bottom of the bag) out of the storage pocket, without touching it below the level of the clamp.
   RATIONALE: *Not touching the tube below the level of the clamp helps maintain the sterility of the closed system.*

3. Hold the tube over the container and release the clamp, making sure that the drain tube does not touch anything.
   RATIONALE: *Making sure that the drain tube does not touch anything helps to ensure sterility of the closed system. Touching the lower part or inside of the drain tube is avoided because pathogenic organisms can travel up the system and cause a bladder infection.*

4. When the urine has drained out, clamp the tube and carefully replace it into the storage pocket. Be sure the clamp is far enough up the tube to allow most of the tube to fit into the pocket. Do not move the clamp up on the tube.
   RATIONALE: *These procedures help maintain the sterility of the catheter's closed drainage system.*

5. Collect the urine in a graduated container and measure it.
   RATIONALE: *Measuring urine output provides information about the client's hydration status and kidney function.*

6. Observe the color, odor, and other characteristics of urine.
   RATIONALE: *Observation of urine characteristics helps to identify possible changes from prior assessments, which may be significant.*

7. Discard urine (unless a specimen is required) and rinse the graduated container with cool water.

8. Explain each step of emptying the drainage bag to the client and family if the client will be discharged from the healthcare agency with the catheter.
   RATIONALE: *The client and family need instruction about caring for the drainage system to prevent complications.*

9. Ask the client or a family member to do a return demonstration after you have demonstrated the procedure.
   RATIONALE: *A return demonstration ensures that the client and family understand the procedure, so later they can do it themselves.*

10. Remove and discard gloves and wash hands.
    RATIONALE: *Proper glove disposal and handwashing limit the transfer of microorganisms.*

11. Record output on the appropriate sheet and document and report any special observations about the urine.
    RATIONALE: *Documentation provides communication and continuity of care.*

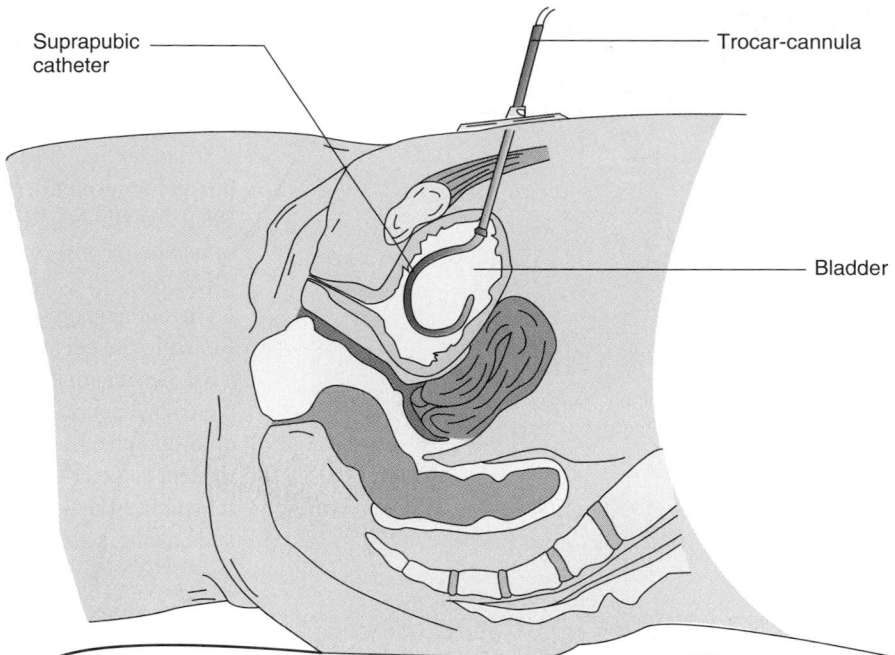

Suprapubic catheter

Trocar-cannula

Bladder

FIGURE 51-1. The *suprapubic catheter* is inserted into the bladder by way of a surgical incision through the abdominal and bladder walls.

➤ **N u r s i n g   A l e r t**
Any catheter placed in the urinary bladder is a potential source of infection. The catheter must be inserted using sterile technique. In addition, care must be taken to maintain the integrity of the sterile system and to prevent contamination.

Using External Catheter Systems

An *external catheter* or *condom catheter* is an elastic rubber sheath that is secured to the male client's penis to collect urine (Fig. 51-2). The open end of the sheath usually has a self-adhesive mechanism that keeps the catheter in place; wrapping surgical tape around the catheter's opening to prevent urine leakage may be necessary. The urethral end of the sheath is attached to the drainage tubing and a bag. The sheath is removed at intervals to expose the penile skin to air, to cleanse and dry the skin, and to avoid prolonged pressure that may cause skin breakdown.

The drainage bag for the external catheter is either a large drainage bag similar to that used with a retention catheter or a small, supple plastic bag that the client wears strapped to the leg. These bags have an outlet at the lower end, which is opened to drain urine. The urine bag is emptied several times daily and rinsed at least once daily with warm water, followed by draining the bag dry. This drainage system is considered clean, not sterilized. When caring for a client with a leg bag, do the following:

- Open the drainage port at the bottom, to allow urine to drain out. Swab with antiseptic to limit transfer of microorganisms. (This is done several times a day.)
- Remove the catheter from the bag connection daily and swab the connections with antiseptic.
- At least once each day, disconnect the leg bag. Wash the leg bag in warm (not hot) soapy water, rinse it thoroughly,

and hang it to dry. When dry, reattach it to the catheter. If the client is incontinent, two bags are often used, so that one can be worn while the other is being cleaned. (Daily washing and rinsing are necessary to remove urine and to avoid odor.)

Urinary Incontinence

Urinary incontinence (inability to hold urine) is a problem that may occur as people age, particularly in women. Several factors can contribute to incontinence. The goal of treatment is to reduce or eliminate incontinent episodes. Most interventions are directed at limiting the effects of incontinence on the client's physical and emotional well-being. The goal is to keep the client as dry and comfortable as possible, while working toward bladder control.

For the male client who is incontinent, the external catheter can be used to collect urine. For the female client who is incontinent, a similar device is not available. However, she can wear a perineal pad or use a disposable incontinent brief. Change the pad or brief frequently to minimize exposure of the skin to urine, gently washing and thoroughly rinsing the perineal area between changes. Assess the skin frequently for signs of breakdown.

➤ **N u r s i n g   A l e r t**
Do not limit fluids for the client who is incontinent.

Bladder Retraining

Some types of incontinence may be controlled by establishing a voiding routine (see Chap. 88). The specific routine usually is determined by the primary care provider or an incontinence specialist.

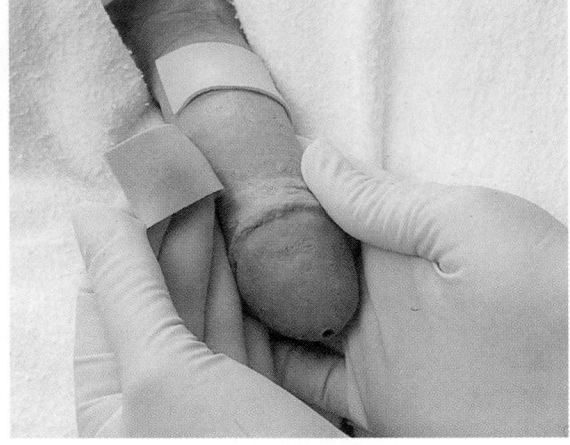

A

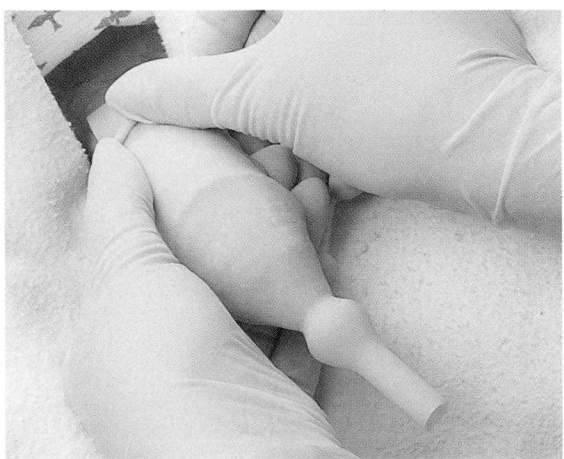

B

FIGURE 51-2. Applying a condom catheter. (**A**) An adhesive strip is applied in a spiral fashion to the penis. (**B**) An *external catheter* or *condom catheter* is secured to the penis.

Begin by documenting when the client's bladder empties to determine if there is a pattern. Either give the client a bedpan or help him or her to the bathroom just before these times to help establish a routine for emptying the client's bladder. Gradually the time between voidings is increased, thus building up the tone of the client's bladder muscles and increasing the bladder's capacity. The bladder eventually becomes trained to empty at regular intervals.

In some cases, the **Crede's maneuver** (pronounced krá-daz) is used. Crede's maneuver is performed by applying firm, gentle pressure to the bladder, with hands held flat, starting at the umbilicus and moving down to the symphysis pubis. This procedure is repeated several times, applying the final pressure directly over the bladder itself.

More often, **Kegel exercises** are recommended. These exercises are designed to increase sphincter tone. The client is taught to tighten the pelvic floor and urethral sphincter and to hold this tightening for up to 10 seconds. The client may wear a disposable pad during the training period. If after 1 year this conservative mode of treatment is not effective, the client may opt for surgery. Medications are also available to help control incontinence.

☛ KEY CONCEPT

The goal of all rehabilitation is to restore the client to a functioning that is as close to normal as possible.

Bladder incontinence is more difficult to control than bowel incontinence, but many clients can establish control. Plenty of fluids and exercise are important. Adequate fluid intake helps prevent urinary stasis and thus helps to prevent infections.

Incontinent episodes may occur during the training period. Reassure the client. Keep a careful record of I&O to maintain a balance and to ensure that urine is not being retained. Complete bladder control is not achieved by every client, but many do accomplish it. Bladder control is important because a permanent catheter in the bladder greatly increases the danger of infection. Additionally, urinary continence adds to self-esteem and enhances self-care.

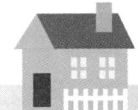

SPECIAL CONSIDERATIONS: HOME CARE

The Incontinent Person

Many clients are released from the healthcare agency without having overcome incontinence. This problem then becomes a family concern. Aggressive client and family teaching is necessary. Demonstrate how to keep the client dry without changing the entire bed. Absorbent pads, covered by a liner, can be placed next to the skin. The pads can be changed easily, and the liner helps to prevent irritation. Disposable pads on the bed or chair are used when possible. If the client has established a routine for voiding, teach the family the importance of maintaining this routine. Explain and demonstrate the use of disposable incontinent briefs. Emphasize the importance of fluids, diet, and cleanliness.

The establishment of continence, or management of incontinence, is a key factor in determining where a client may be able to live. Managing bowel and bladder function can enable an individual to live independently. On the other hand, an individual who is unable to control this function may find it necessary to live in a long-term care facility.

Bladder Retraining With a Closed Drainage System

Bladder retraining may be started while the catheter is connected to the closed drainage system. The goal is to help the client regain the sensation to void by allowing the bladder to refill, which causes the bladder muscles to stretch and signal the brain. Some techniques require temporarily disconnecting the catheter from the drainage tube, but these methods increase the possibility of microorganisms ascending the catheter into the bladder. In Practice: Nursing Procedure 51-3 outlines the steps of bladder retraining by clamping the catheter.

Urinary Retention

Sometimes a client is unable to void in the healthcare facility. Inability to void is a common problem after receiving anesthesia. Sometimes the client who is on bed rest cannot relax the urinary sphincters enough to void when using the bedpan. This temporary retention may be relieved through several simple nursing measures. Hearing the sound of running water, putting the client's hands in warm water, or pouring warm water over a female client's genitalia helps to stimulate the muscles to relax and to release urine. A warm shower or bath may help. If the female client is permitted to sit up in bed or on a commode, she may be able to void. The male client will be more likely to void if he is able to stand.

If urinary retention continues, the bladder is distended, and the client is uncomfortable, this must be reported. Catheterization may be necessary.

ASSISTING WITH BOWEL ELIMINATION

Changes in bowel function may result in fecal retention, either short-term (more commonly called *constipation*) or long-term, resulting in fecal impaction or bowel obstruction. When monitoring bowel function, identify the client who has not had a recent bowel movement and who may require nursing intervention.

Usually ingesting food creates peristaltic waves throughout the intestine that move feces from the colon into the rectum. The fecal mass stimulates nerve endings in the rectum, creating the urge to defecate. If a person ignores this urge, it fades. The feces become dry and hard, and defecation becomes difficult (constipation). The colon and rectum become distended and lose muscle tone as feces accumulate.

Enemas

An **enema** is the introduction of a solution into the rectum and colon to stimulate peristalsis, thereby causing elimina-

---

In Practice
Nursing Procedure 51-3

BLADDER RETRAINING WITH CLOSED URINARY DRAINAGE

Supplies and Equipment

Protective pad for bed
Catheter clamp
Disposable gloves

Steps

1. Explain the procedure to the client.
   RATIONALE: *Explanations help to relieve the client's anxiety and foster the client's cooperation.*

2. Put on disposable gloves.
   RATIONALE: *Gloving helps to prevent the spread of infection.*

3. Position the client in supine position with the head of the bed slightly elevated.
   RATIONALE: *Proper positioning prevents pressure on the bladder.*

4. Place a protective pad under the client.
   RATIONALE: *The pad protects the bed from becoming wet if urine leaks.*

5. Clamp the catheter tubing for 1 to 2 hours.
   RATIONALE: *Clamping allows time for the bladder to fill.*

6. Open the clamp and allow the bladder to drain by gravity into the drainage bag.
   RATIONALE: *This measure empties the bladder and prevents urine stasis. Bladder emptying simulates normal voiding.*

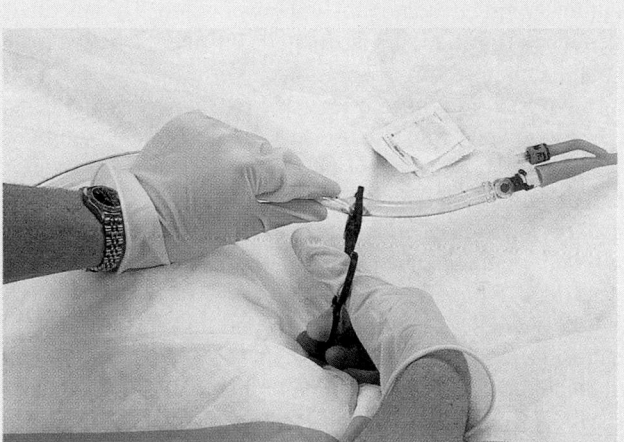

Clamping the catheter tubing for 1 to 2 hours.

7. Repeat the procedure. *Rationale: Repeating the procedure allows for continued training of the bladder.* Increase the time the bladder is clamped off to 3 or 4 hours, as ordered.
   RATIONALE: *Increasing the time for clamping aids in helping to reestablish bladder control.*

8. Dispose of gloves properly and wash hands carefully.
   RATIONALE: *Proper glove disposal and handwashing limit the spread of infectious organisms.*

9. Record the procedure on the client's record, including urinary output.
   RATIONALE: *Documentation provides communication and evidence of the client's progress toward gaining bladder control.*

tion of stool. An enema may also be given to introduce medications or other therapeutic agents. In addition, enemas are sometimes given before a procedure such as a colonoscopy or before bowel surgery, to cleanse the bowel.

Most often, commercially prepared disposable enemas are used. However, a can- or bag- and-tubing type enema is usually used to introduce the contrast solution into the bowel for an x-ray procedure called a *barium enema*. Another type of enema using the can-and-tubing method is called the *Harris flush* or *return flow enema*.

Most commonly, an enema is given because the client is unable to empty the bowel naturally. The enema helps remove feces, but unless normal stimulation and regular defecation are established, the muscles could become weakened and the use of enemas could become a habit. In Practice: Nursing Care Guidelines 51-4 reviews steps in giving any enema.

A primary healthcare provider's order is required for an enema. The order will state the type of enema to be given, as well as how often. The order may be PRN (as needed). Check with the team leader if there is any uncertainty about when to administer the enema.

Types of Enemas

Cleansing Enema.   The *cleansing enema,* also called a *purgative enema,* introduces enough fluid into the colon to soften feces, stimulate peristalsis, and produce a bowel movement that empties the rectum and lower colon. This enema is given when the client is constipated or when the bowel must be emptied before surgery or a special procedure.

The most common solution used for the cleansing enema is plain tap water (tap water enema: **TWE**). Other solutions include normal saline, hypertonic saline, or a soap solution. A small amount of oil (such as cottonseed, mineral, or olive oil) may be given as a *retention enema* to cleanse the bowel. Action may result immediately or it may take longer; usually it occurs in less than 15 minutes.

Adding prepackaged soap concentrate (castile soap) to water is the method of mixing a soap suds enema (**SSE**). Soap irritates the colon's mucous membrane, stimulating peristalsis. Mild soap is used, to avoid excessive irritation. An SSE is usually not used before rectal examinations or for clients known to have rectal disease.

The commercially prepared, disposable enema unit is the most convenient for the nurse or the client to use. The one most commonly used is a brand-name preparation called a *Fleet enema*. It contains a small amount of hypertonic solution, usually 4 ounces (120 mL) for an adult. Smaller units are available for children. Acting through the principle of osmosis, the enema draws fluid from the colon tissues to create fluid bulk. The solution is not irritating and it usually results in effective evacuation in less than 10 minutes. This type of enema is especially useful for clients who are unable to retain larger quantities of fluid or who have anal incontinence. It also helps to prevent fecal impaction in clients who must lie in one position or who are unable to sit up. The Fleet enema is frequently used in preparation for colon examinations or procedures and can be self-administered. Disposable enemas containing other special solutions are also available.

Carminative Enema.   The *carminative enema* is given to stimulate peristalsis so that flatus (gas) is expelled from the intestine.

Anthelminthic Enema.   *Anthelminthic* drugs help destroy intestinal parasites. They usually are given orally, but because they are toxic, they are unsafe for some clients to take orally. In such instances, a solution of an anthelminthic drug may be instilled into the rectum for retention.

Emollient Enema.   An *emollient enema* consists of a small amount of olive or cottonseed oil, given to protect or soothe the mucous membrane of the colon. This enema is to be retained.

Oil Retention Enema.   The *oil retention enema* is given in small amounts because it must be retained to be effective. Large amounts stimulate bowel evacuation. If an oil solution proves ineffective after several hours, following it with a soap suds enema or saline solution enema may be necessary.

Medicated Enema.   The *medicated enema* inserts a drug into the rectum; sometimes, it is the only way to give a drug to a client, possibly because the client is unconscious or has had mouth or throat surgery. It may also be the best way for a specific drug to take effect quickly because some drugs are rapidly absorbed by the colon's mucous membrane. Because this enema must be retained to ensure effective absorption, the drug is combined with a small amount of oil or saline to reduce its irritating effect and to lessen the client's desire to expel it.

Administration

See In Practice: Nursing Care Guidelines 51-4 for the principles for administering any type of enema. In Practice: Nursing Procedure 51-4 explains how to give a cleansing enema by the can (bag)-and-tubing method.

Self-contained disposable enemas, such as Fleet, are frequently used. General principles for administration of all enemas are the same. Specific instructions are on the package. Be sure to use the correct enema solution and size. Fleet enemas are usually stored and administered at room temperature. Warming the solution in a container of warm water or under running warm tap water often makes the enema more comfortable. Figure 51-3 shows how to compress the disposable enema as it is being administered. The client often self-administers this enema before surgery or radiography.

Special Circumstances

The Client Unable to Retain an Enema.   If a client is unable to contract the anal sphincter muscles and hold the solution, place the client on the bedpan, commode, or toilet and administer the enema. If the client is in bed, elevate the head of the bed slightly and place a pillow in the lumbar region to lessen back strain. In some cases, the enema tubing is passed through a ball, and the ball is held against the rectal opening to hold the fluid inside. The advantage of the disposable enema unit for this client is that only a small quantity of solution is required. In addition, the disposable enema

(*text continues on page 693*)

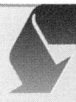

In Practice
Nursing Care Guidelines 51-4

ADMINISTERING AN ENEMA

- Wash hands before and after giving an enema. Always wear gloves. *Rationale: Handwashing and wearing gloves help to prevent the spread of microorganisms. Feces are highly contaminated.*
- Remember that if the can-and-tubing (or bag-and-tubing) method is used, the height of the can (bag) affects the force and speed of its flow. The higher the container is held, the greater the force of the flow. Never hold the container more than 18 in (45 cm) above the mattress. Also, regulate the speed and pressure by which a prepackaged enema is given. *Rationale: Proper positioning of the device and using appropriate pressure help to prevent injury.*
- Give the can-and-tubing (or bag-and-tubing) enema by way of a rectal tube, which is smooth and flexible and not likely to irritate the client's rectum. Rectal tubes come in different sizes. Use a latex-free rectal tube if the client is allergic to latex. *Rationale: The larger the catheter, the faster and the more forcefully the fluid can flow. The faster you instill the fluid, the harder it will be for the client to retain it and the faster he or she will expel it.*
- Know the correct amount of solution to use. The amount of solution to use for a cleansing enema (can-and-tubing method) for an adult ranges from 750 to 1,000 mL. The amount to use for a retention enema ranges from 150 to 200 mL. *Rationale: The larger amount stimulates rapid expulsion; the client will retain the smaller amount longer.*
- For any type of enema, use judgment to decide when to stop instilling fluid, based on the client's statements and reactions. *Rationale: Each person has a different limit to the amount of fluid he or she can retain.*
- Store disposable enema units at room temperature; never store them in a cold place. Warm the solution slightly before insertion. *Rationale: A cold solution is uncomfortable for the client and could cause shock.*
- Ensure that the solution's temperature is at—or slightly higher than—the client's body temperature. Measure the solution's temperature with a thermometer before insertion. It must never exceed 105° F (40.5° C). *Rationale: Using the proper temperature avoids injuring the lining of the client's intestines.*
- Have the client lie on the side (preferably the left) for the cleansing enema. *Rationale: The colon's position within the body makes this position the most effec-*

tive. If the client is in traction or a cast, give the enema with the client lying on his or her back.
- Place the client in a knee-chest position for a retention enema, if the client can tolerate it. *Rationale: This position encourages fluid retention for a longer period. It is very difficult to give an enema effectively with the client sitting up.*
- Drape the client, covering his or her body as much as possible. *Rationale: Proper draping preserves the client's privacy and dignity.*
- For a can-and-tubing enema, lubricate the rectal tube and insert the enema carefully. Insert the tube about 3–4 in (7.5–10 cm). Do not force the tube against resistance. *Rationale: The anus has inside and outside sphincter muscles that together control the opening to the outside of the body. To be effective, the tube must be inserted carefully past both of these sphincters.*
- Instruct the client to take a few short, panting breaths and relax. *Rationale: Relaxation helps with the insertion of the tube and helps the client retain the fluid longer, thus enhancing the effectiveness of the procedure.*
- If using a prepackaged unit with a prelubricated enema tip, check to make sure the lubrication is present. If not, lubricate the tip. *Rationale: Lubrication allows for easier and more comfortable insertion.*
- Give the solution slowly. Instruct the client to retain the enema as long as possible. *Rationale: Both cleansing and retention enemas are held longer if given slowly. Longer retention enhances the enema's effectiveness.*
- Carefully dispose of all materials after the enema is completed. Dispose of gloves and wash your hands. *Rationale: Fecal matter is contaminated. Proper disposal of materials helps to prevent the spread of infection.*
- Check back with the client to make sure that he or she is not having any difficulties. Observe or ask the client about the results. *Rationale: Some clients may become weak or faint or may have difficulty getting to the bathroom. Observing the results helps to determine if the enema was effective.*
- Record administration of the enema, the results, and the client's reactions. Chart the type of solution used and its temperature. *Rationale: Documentation allows communication and continuity of care.*

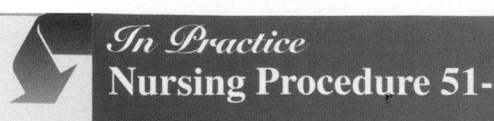

Nursing Procedure 51-4

GIVING A CLEANSING ENEMA: CAN (BUCKET)-AND-TUBING METHOD

Supplies and Equipment

Gloves
Disposable enema setup including container, tubing,
   and clamp (Approximate rectal tube size:
   adult 22-30 Fr, child 12-18 Fr)
Solution as prescribed
Bedpan and cover
Toilet tissue
Waterproof pad
Water-soluble lubricant
Bath blanket
Cleansing supplies
IV pole

Steps

1. Gather supplies. Use a latex-free tube if the client is allergic to latex.
   RATIONALE: *Organization facilitates accurate skill performance.*

2. Explain the procedure to the client.
   RATIONALE: *Providing information fosters cooperation.*

3. Wash your hands and put on gloves.
   RATIONALE: *Handwashing and using gloves help to prevent the spread of infection.*

4. Prepare the enema:
   a. Fill the enema can with prescribed solution at proper temperature (adults, 100° to 110° F; children, 100° F).
   RATIONALE: *Proper temperature prevents thermal injury to the intestinal mucosal tissue.*

   b. Open the clamp and allow fluid to flow through the tubing.
   RATIONALE: *Enema solution clears the tubing of air.*

   c. Reclamp the tubing.

5. Close the curtain or door to the room.
   RATIONALE: *Closing the curtain or door protects the client's privacy.*

6. Raise the bed to a comfortable working height. Lower the near side rail.
   RATIONALE: *Proper positioning prevents back strain. Lowering the near side rail provides for easy access to the client.*

7. Place a waterproof pad under the client's buttocks.
   RATIONALE: *The pad prevents moistening or soiling of bed linens.*

8. Assist the client to turn onto the left side with the right knee flexed. Place a bedpan in the bed, close to the client. If the client is unable to retain the enema solution, place him or her on the bedpan (some clients will be able to go into the bathroom to expel the solution).
   RATIONALE: *Gravity facilitates the flow of the solution when the client is on his or her side. Poor anal sphincter control may make it difficult to retain the enema solution.*

9. Lubricate the tip of the rectal tube for 2–3 in (if it is not pre-lubricated).
   RATIONALE: *Lubricant allows for smooth insertion of the rectal tube without injuring the client's bowel mucosa.*

10. Place the enema can on an IV pole or raise the container approximately 18 in above the client's anus.
    RATIONALE: *Gravity aids in the instillation of the enema solution.*

11. Separate the client's buttocks. Ask the client to take a deep breath. Gently insert the rectal tube 3–4 in toward the umbilicus (2–3 in for a child).
    RATIONALE: *Taking a deep breath helps relax the anal sphincter. Inserting the rectal tube too far can damage or perforate rectal mucosa.*

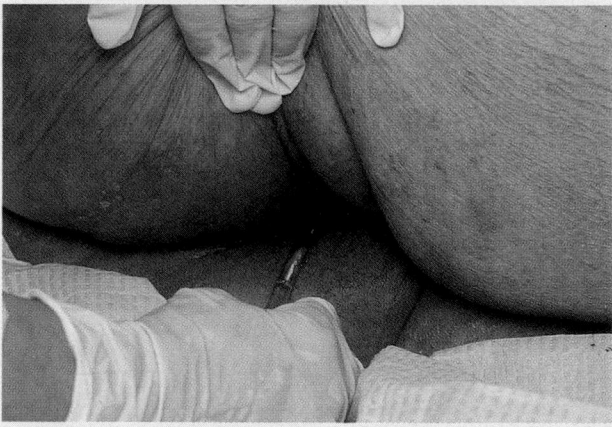

Inserting the tube into the rectum.

12. Hold the tube in place with one hand, while opening the clamp with the other hand. Allow solution to flow slowly into the rectum, while holding the can approximately 18 in above the rectum. Enema should be delivered for 5–10 min. If the client complains of cramping, lower the bag or temporarily clamp the tubing.
    RATIONALE: *The higher the container is positioned, the more rapid the flow of enema solution. Halting the enema for a brief time aids in solution retention.*

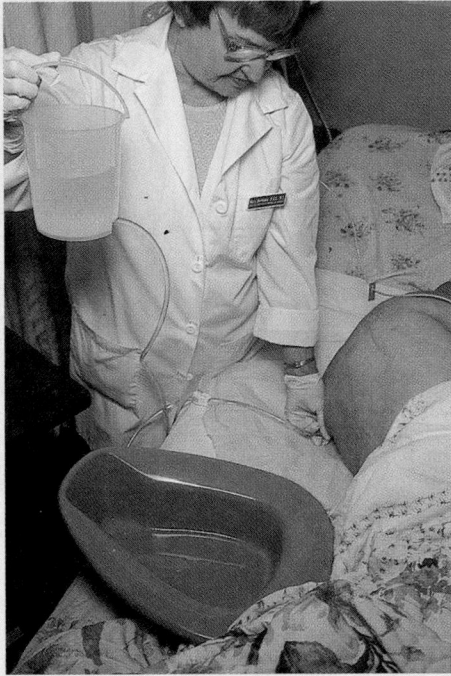

Raising the container 18 inches above the client's anus.

13. Apply the clamp and remove the rectal tube when the enema is completed or when the client is unable to take more solution. Ask the client to retain the solution for as long as possible.

RATIONALE: *Retaining the solution facilitates effective results from the enema.*

14. Assist the client into the bathroom, or onto the bedpan with the head of the bed elevated. Place the call bell within easy reach.
    RATIONALE: *Contracting the abdominal and perineal muscles is easier in a sitting position.*

15. When the client has expelled the enema solution, assist him or her back to bed or off the bedpan. Inspect the enema's results and obtain a specimen, if ordered.
    RATIONALE: *Some diagnostic tests require that enemas be given until the results are clear. Observing results of the enema confirms its effectiveness.*

16. Return the client to a comfortable position. Lower the bed and raise the side rail.
    RATIONALE: *This action provides for comfort and safety.*

17. Remove gloves and wash hands.
    RATIONALE: *Proper glove disposal and handwashing help prevent the spread of infection.*

18. Document enema results and type of enema administered on the flowsheet or chart.
    RATIONALE: *Documentation provides communication and coordination of care.*

---

container can be held against the rectal opening to help in retaining the solution.

The Client Unable to Expel an Enema.   When the sphincters do not respond to stimulation and the client is unable to expel an enema, the nurse must withdraw the solution. Place the bedpan on a chair at the client's bedside, beneath

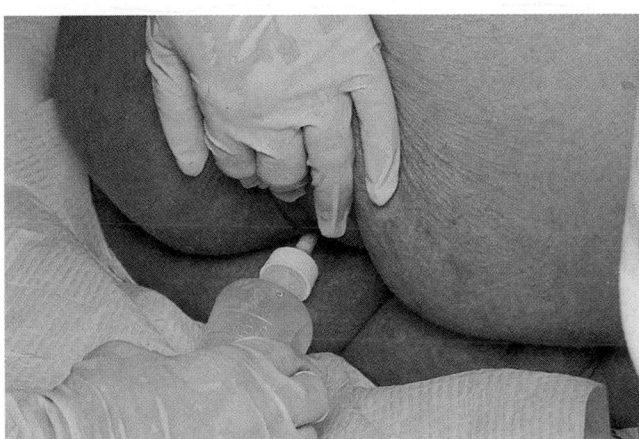

FIGURE 51-3. Compressing the disposable enema as it is being administered.

the level of the rectum. When the rectal tube is directed into the pan, the force of gravity helps to drain off (siphon) the fluid.

Giving an Enema to a Client With Paralysis.   Giving an enema requires a special approach if the person is paralyzed. Often the paralyzed client is unable to retain the enema solution. If the client must have an enema, give it at the same time every day. Later, a suppository at this time may be all that is necessary to stimulate a bowel movement, until finally the client needs neither of these aids. Manual digital pressure to the abdomen or manual disimpaction may also be applied to assist this client with bowel evacuation.

Manual Removal of Impacted Feces

If a fecal impaction does not respond to an enema or if a client has paralysis, a primary care provider may order manual or digital removal of the feces, a procedure known as *manual disimpaction* or *digital evacuation.* Many clients with permanent paralysis perform their own manual disimpaction as part of their activities of daily living. In Practice: Nursing Procedure 51-5 gives the steps for digitally removing impacted feces.

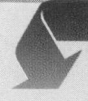

In Practice
Nursing Procedure 51-5

PERFORMING MANUAL DISIMPACTION

Supplies and Equipment

Disposable gloves
Toilet tissue
Bedpan

Steps

1. Wash hands and put on gloves. You may wish to wear two pairs. *Handwashing and wearing gloves help to minimize the risk for infection transmission.*

2. Explain to the client what will be done and why.
   RATIONALE: *Client cooperation and relaxation help to make the procedure more comfortable.*

3. Place a disposable waterproof pad under the buttocks.
   RATIONALE: *A pad helps to prevent soiling of the bed.*

4. Position the client on the left side, with the knees—especially the upper knee—drawn up as far as possible.
   RATIONALE: *This position is comfortable for the client and allows easy view of—and access to—the anal area.*

5. Drape the client.
   RATIONALE: *Proper draping preserves the client's privacy as much as possible.*

6. Instruct the client to take short, panting breaths during the procedure.
   RATIONALE: *Panting helps relax the anal sphincter.*

7. Using clean disposable gloves, lubricate one or two fingers well. Insert one or two fingers *carefully* into the rectum until you feel the stool; then, rotate the finger gently.
   RATIONALE: *This helps break up the stool. Usually this procedure is all that is needed to assist the client to expel impacted feces.*

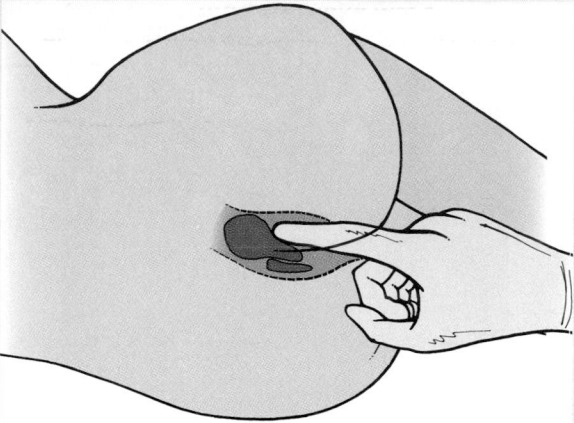
Rotate the finger gently to break up the stool.

8. Before removing your finger, gently stimulate the anal sphincter with a rotating motion.
   RATIONALE: *This stimulation helps cause a natural response to defecate.*

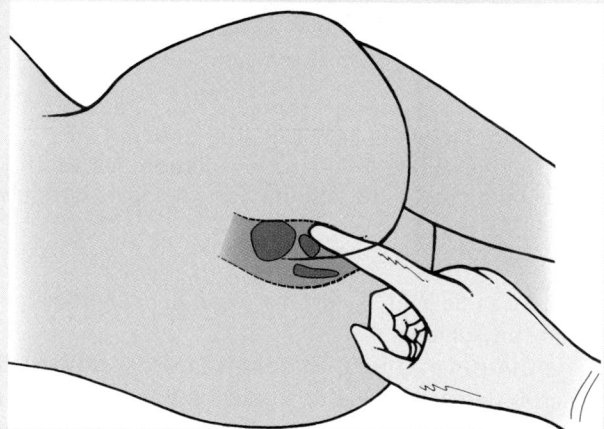
Gently stimulate the anal sphincter with a rotating motion to cause defecation.

9. Dispose of gloves properly and wash hands.
   RATIONALE: *Proper glove disposal and handwashing help to prevent spread of microorganisms from the intestinal tract.*

10. Assist client to bathroom, commode, or bedpan as needed.
    RATIONALE: *Client may be uncomfortable and may need assistance.*

11. Leave the client's signal cord within reach.
    RATIONALE: *The person may need the bedpan again in a short time. Diarrhea often occurs after non-routine manual disimpaction.*

12. Provide a washcloth and soap for the client to use for cleansing the rectal area, or clean the area if the client cannot. Leave the waterproof pad in

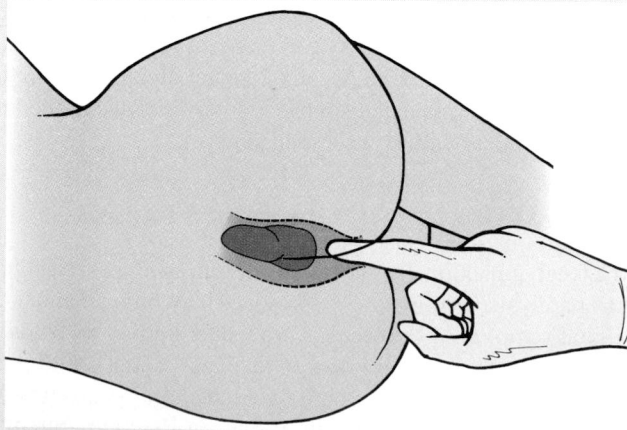
Insert one finger into the rectum until you feel the stool.

place for a few minutes to protect the bed. Dispose of gloves and wash hands. Provide handwashing supplies for the client to wash his or her hands.
RATIONALE: *Keeping the client and the bed area clean helps to prevent spread of micro-organisms.*

13. Document the procedure, noting any special client reactions, as well as the amount, color, consistency, and odor of any stool obtained or expelled. If the client is unable to expel impacted feces, report this immediately.
RATIONALE: *Documentation provides for communication and continuity of care.*

Nursing Alert

Digital removal of feces is contraindicated for most clients with cardiac conditions and after reproductive surgery, abdominoperineal repair, rectal surgery, colostomy, and genitourinary surgery. It is also contraindicated in clients who are receiving radioactive isotope therapy (especially in the abdominopelvic area) or perineal perfusion of anticancer drugs. Clients who have a bleeding tendency, especially in the rectal or vaginal area, should not receive this treatment, nor should pregnant women. *Rationale: The procedure could aggravate the existing condition or could cause damage.*

Stop the procedure immediately if the client complains of pain, faintness, or nausea, or if you note any untoward effect, such as bleeding. Usually, after the stool is broken into pieces, the client is able to expel it. The client may be given an enema for assistance. In some cases, you may remove the particles of feces after breaking up the stool. Remove the stool in as non-invasive a manner as possible.

Bowel Retraining

Bowel retraining may be necessary if the client is unable to have a bowel movement naturally or is incontinent of stool. Because the bowel responds to certain stimuli to function naturally, you may use natural means to stimulate peristalsis. These factors are helpful in bowel training:

Timing: The client is assisted with elimination at the same time each day.
Fluid intake: A high fluid intake is recommended.
Diet: A diet to assist in maintaining a fairly solid fecal consistency without causing constipation or diarrhea is recommended.
Physical activity: The more exercise the client receives, the more likely it is that he or she will be able to achieve bowel control.

A large quantity of liquids and bulk foods (such as fresh fruits and vegetables) in the diet is helpful. Encourage the client to avoid those foods that he or she has found in the past to produce loose stools and excess gas (flatus). If pos-

sible, assist the client to use the bathroom, rather than using a bedpan or commode. *Rationale: Moving about helps to stimulate a bowel movement and enhances the client's self-esteem.*

A successful bowel-retraining program includes the following steps as suggested at In Practice: Nursing Procedure 51-6. Always give the client positive reinforcement for any progress. Bowel retraining is a long process. Some clients are not able to achieve full bowel continence.

Flatus

Sometimes a rectal tube or an Evac-u-sac is used to aid the client in expelling *flatus* from the intestine. Inserted in the rectum, the device provides an outlet for accumulated gas and relieves the discomfort of intestinal distention. In Practice: Nursing Procedure 51-7 gives the steps for removing flatus.

NAUSEA AND VOMITING

Nausea is an unpleasant abdominal sensation, sometimes followed by vomiting. *Vomiting,* also called *emesis,* is an involuntary action that expels stomach contents. Symptoms of nausea leading to vomiting include weakness, frequent swallowing, profuse perspiration, dizziness, pallor (paleness), and shakiness. Pulse and blood pressure may drop during vomiting. In some cases, vomiting is **projectile vomiting** (expelled with great force). This must be reported at once, because projectile vomiting can be a sign of a serious condition such as a brain tumor or brain trauma.

Vomitus means stomach contents. Its appearance and odor may indicate the cause of emesis. Assess for particles, color, odor, and consistency. Vomitus may contain bright-red blood, a sign of gastric bleeding. It may contain coffee-ground material, a sign of bleeding in the lower digestive tract. It may contain mucus or pus. Vomitus that contains bile is yellowish or greenish. Vomitus that has been forced back into the stomach from the intestine has a fecal odor.

Observe vomitus for the presence of medications and specific foods. Measure and document the amount, if possible. Always save any unusual vomitus for inspection and wear gloves when handling specimens. The primary healthcare

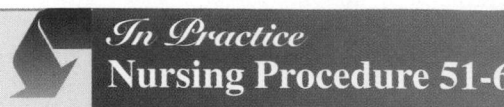

In Practice
Nursing Procedure 51-6

ASSISTING WITH BOWEL RETRAINING
Supplies and Equipment

Oral stool softeners or suppositories
Gloves
Bedpan or bedside commode, if needed

Steps

1. Put on gloves.
   RATIONALE: *Using gloves helps to prevent the spread of infection.*

2. Choose a time that is convenient for the client within his or her daily schedule.
   RATIONALE: *A daily routine will stimulate peristalsis at the same time.*

3. Administer oral stool softeners daily or as ordered, or insert a cleansing suppository at least 30 min before the scheduled time for elimination.
   RATIONALE: *This action initiates retraining of the bowel to react to softeners or a suppository on a regular basis.*

4. Offer a warm cup of liquid or fruit juice.
   RATIONALE: *Warm liquids stimulate peristalsis.*

5. Assist the client to the toilet (or bedpan or bedside commode) at the designated time.
   RATIONALE: *Assisting to the toilet, bedpan, or commode readies the client for defecation.*

6. Provide for privacy.
   RATIONALE: *Elimination is a private matter.*

7. Instruct the client to apply pressure to the lower abdomen, and bear down.
   RATIONALE: *This action stimulates the colon to empty.*

8. Empty and cleanse the elimination receptacle. Discard gloves and wash hands. Assist client to wash his or her hands.
   RATIONALE: *Proper disposal and cleanup reduces the risk of infection transmission.*

9. Document results of bowel movement on the client's record.
   RATIONALE: *Documentation provides for communication and continuity of care, while monitoring the client's progress in bowel retraining.*

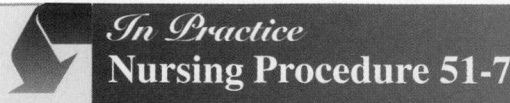

In Practice
Nursing Procedure 51-7

HELPING TO RELIEVE FLATUS
Supplies and Equipment

Rectal tube
Evac-u-sac or cardboard container
Lubricant
Disposable gloves

Steps

1. Wash hands and put on gloves.
   RATIONALE: *Handwashing and using gloves helps to prevent the spread of infection.*

2. Ask the client to lie on his or her side (preferably the left side).
   RATIONALE: *This position promotes client comfort and ease in inserting the tube.*

3. Lubricate the tube. If the client is allergic to latex, be sure to use a latex-free tube.
   RATIONALE: *Adequate lubrication eases the insertion.*

4. Insert the tube 3 to 4 in (7.5–10 cm) into the rectum.
   RATIONALE: *The tube is inserted far enough to bypass any stool in the lower rectum and to reach gas above the stool.*

5. Determine the tube's patency. If the tube is patent (open), gas or feces will return.
   RATIONALE: *The tube can become plugged with stool; it must be kept open.*

6. Place the outer end of the tube in an Evac-u-sac.
   RATIONALE: *An Evac-u-sac or cardboard container helps to absorb odor and sound and helps to minimize the client's embarrassment.*

7. Leave the tube in the rectum for 20–30 min.
   RATIONALE: *After that time, the sphincter muscles become numb and the tube ceases to stimulate peristalsis.*

8. Properly dispose of supplies and wash hands.
   RATIONALE: *Proper disposal of equipment prevents the spread of infection.*

9. Document results on the client's chart: duration of the insertion, amount of gas and feces expelled (if any), and whether the client felt relief.
   RATIONALE: *Documentation provides communication and continuity of care.*

provider may want the entire specimen sent to the laboratory for examination. As with other specimens, place vomitus in a moisture-proof, covered container and properly label it. Take it to the laboratory immediately along with the appropriate laboratory request.

Note the nature of vomiting. Was it violent or projectile? How does the client describe the episode? If you are monitoring the client's I&O, consider vomitus as output. Report the

vomiting episode. Carefully document all observations on the client's chart.

The person who is nauseated or vomiting feels uncomfortable and helpless, and usually does not want to talk. In some cases, vomiting is dangerous and should be prevented. For example, the client who has had recent abdominal surgery or delicate eye surgery may incur an injury as a result of the vio-

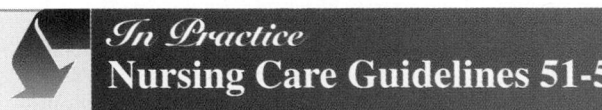

In Practice
Nursing Care Guidelines 51-5

ASSISTING THE CLIENT WHO IS NAUSEOUS OR VOMITING

- Always wear gloves. If vomiting is projectile or any possibility exists that vomitus will splash, also wear eye goggles and gown. *Rationale: Using personal protective equipment helps to prevent the spread of infection, especially when you are in contact with body fluids.*

The Client Who is Nauseated

- Place a cool, damp washcloth on the client's forehead. *Rationale: This is soothing to the client and may help him or her to relax. Relaxation helps prevent vomiting.*
- Tell the client to take slow, deep breaths through the nose. *Rationale: Breathing helps relax the client and distracts from the nauseated feeling. Adding oxygen to the blood, and thus the control center in the medulla of the brain, helps relieve nausea.*
- Have the client lie on the right side. *Rationale: This position moves gastric contents toward the stomach's bottom end and away from the cardiac sphincter, relieving irritation and stimulation of the cardiac sphincter.*
- Give antiemetic (anti-nausea) drugs by injection or rectally, as ordered. *Rationale: Antiemetics cannot be given by mouth because that might cause vomiting.*
- Offer something dry, such as a bite of soda cracker or unbuttered toast. Do not give the food until the worst of the nausea subsides. Use only small amounts of food. *Rationale: Dry food may soak up some excess stomach acid and remove the disagreeable taste from the mouth. Food may cause further upset and irritation; it must be given cautiously.*

The Client Who is Vomiting

- Hold an emesis basin (kidney basin) directly under the client's chin. *Rationale: This basin can catch the emesis.*
- If possible, have the client sit up; if he or she cannot sit up, make sure the client lies on the side. *Rationale: Lying on the back while vomiting is dangerous because vomitus could be aspirated into the lungs.*

- Place a towel under the basin or use a draw sheet at the head of the bed. *Rationale: The sheet or towel protects the client's clothing and the bed linens.*
- Carefully assess the vomitus. Measure it, if possible. *Rationale: The appearance and nature of vomiting can be important to the physician in making a diagnosis. Vomitus is part of the client's daily output and is added to the I&O sheet.*
- Immediately report if there is any blood or unusual material in the vomitus. *Rationale: Particularly with the client who has had recent surgery or who has stomach or esophageal ulcers, the presence of blood may be life threatening.*
- After nausea has subsided, allow the client to rinse the mouth with mouthwash or a weak salt solution. Tell the client not to swallow any solution. *Rationale: Vomiting leaves a disagreeable taste in the mouth. Gastric contents are also irritating to the throat and mouth. Swallowing fluid could cause more nausea.*
- If the client has had recent surgery, carefully inspect the suture line. Report any abnormalities. *Rationale: Vomiting could disrupt new sutures, causing serious complications such as evisceration (protrusion of abdominal contents through the suture line) or disruption of delicate eye sutures.*
- Remove soiled linen and wash the client's face and hands. *Rationale: This action provides for client comfort.*
- Empty the emesis basin and measure vomitus. *Rationale: The sight and smell of vomitus is very disagreeable. Knowing the amount will help the physician make a diagnosis.*
- Wash the emesis basin in cold water. Leave the clean basin close to the client, in case the nausea and vomiting return. *Rationale: Hot water will cause protein material to coagulate.* Check back with the client frequently. *Rationale: Frequent checks with the client help determine if the nausea and vomiting have returned.*
- Dispose of gloves and wash hands. *Rationale: Proper glove disposal and handwashing help to prevent spread of organisms.*
- Carefully document the event and pertinent observations. *Rationale: Documentation provides communication and continuity of care.*

lent action of vomiting. The person who has ingested a caustic substance can experience additional injury by vomiting (the substance burns twice: once going down, and then again as it comes up). Rather than ask questions, assist the person who is nauseated or vomiting with comfort measures. In Practice: Nursing Care Guidelines 51-5 describes the nursing care of this client.

➔ STUDENT SYNTHESIS

Key Points

- Adequate elimination is a basic function critical to health and life.

- Thorough handwashing and wearing gloves are important when coming into contact with any body secretions or drainage from the client.
- Placing the client in as comfortable a position as possible for elimination or when vomiting and allowing for privacy are key.
- In caring for the client with a retention catheter, precautions must be taken to prevent any source of infection from reaching the bladder.
- Diarrhea may be a symptom of impacted stool or a sign of another gastrointestinal disorder.
- Retraining of the bladder and bowel aids the client's health and self-esteem.
- Bladder and bowel continence or management can make the difference between independent living and the need for long-term care.
- Enemas may be used to assist in bowel elimination, to cleanse the bowel, or to instill medications.
- It is important to assist the client who is vomiting, to alleviate discomfort and to prevent complications.

Critical Thinking Exercises

1. You have been assigned to teach a client about the importance of proper elimination and personal hygiene. Describe how you would teach the importance of these self-care activities.
2. Your client, Mrs. R., is 87 years old. She has not had a bowel movement for two days. She has asked for an enema for relief. The physician has ordered SSE PRN or oil retention enema PRN. How would you assess this client to determine whether or not she needs an enema? Describe the reasons for giving each type of enema. How will you determine which type is best for Mrs. R.?

NCLEX-Style Review Questions

1. A client has not had a bowel movement for 3 days, except for a small amount of diarrhea. What nursing action would be most appropriate?
   a. Check the client for fecal impaction.
   b. Continue to monitor the client's status.
   c. Notify the physician immediately.
   d. Start intravenous fluids.

2. A client is complaining of abdominal pain and has had three episodes of diarrhea in the past 6 hours. Which of the following assessment findings would the nurse expect to find?
   a. Absent bowel sounds
   b. Decreased and soft bowel sounds
   c. Increased and rapid bowel sounds
   d. No change in bowel sounds

3. A client is on a bladder retraining program and has just had an episode of incontinence. Which response by the nurse is appropriate?
   a. "I'm really surprised that you haven't had problems sooner."
   b. "It's too bad you had an accident, now we have to start all over."
   c. "Occasional incontinence is expected and is not a sign of failure."
   d. "This is unusual for someone to be incontinent after starting bladder training."

4. Which action by the nurse could help stimulate voiding in a client who has had anesthesia and is having difficulty voiding?
   a. Continue to monitor the client for voiding.
   b. Encourage the client to perform Crede's maneuver.
   c. Encourage the client to listen to stimulating music.
   d. Place the client's hands in warm water.

5. A client is complaining of abdominal pain and starts to vomit. What action should the nurse take?
   a. Administer Mylanta to the client.
   b. Hold the emesis basis directly under the chin.
   c. Place the client in a supine position.
   d. Offer bland foods.

Reference

1. Craven, R. F., & Hirnle, C. J. (2000). *Fundamentals of nursing: Human health and function* (3rd ed.). Philadelphia: Lippincott Williams & Wilkins.

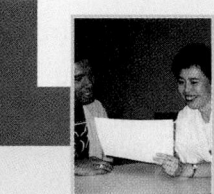

Specimen Collection

LEARNING OBJECTIVES

1. Explain the purpose of monitoring a client's fluid intake and output (I&O).
2. Describe and demonstrate how to keep accurate I&O records.
3. Demonstrate correct measurement of urine volume and urine specific gravity, listing one medical condition associated with high specific gravity and one that is associated with low specific gravity.
4. Identify at least three reasons for laboratory examination of urine.
5. Describe and demonstrate correct collection of the following urine specimens: midstream, 24-hour, fractional, and indwelling urinary catheter.
6. Identify and explain at least one reason for collecting each of the following specimens: stool, sputum, and blood.
7. Demonstrate correct collection of a stool specimen.
8. Demonstrate correct collection of a sputum specimen.

NEW TERMINOLOGY

expectorate
guaiac
Hematest
Hemoccult
hydrometer
occult

specific gravity
urinalysis
urinometer
venipuncture

ACRONYMS

C&S
I&O
mL

NG
O&P

V&S
vol. & spec.

One means by which healthcare providers learn information about the health status of clients is by collecting samples of body fluids for laboratory study. Nurses are often responsible for collecting specimens of urine, stool, sputum, and blood. The nurse may measure or observe such specimens for characteristics or send them to the laboratory for examination. Be aware of the specific agency protocols for specimen collection. Observing these protocols provides quality control and keeps specimens free from contamination, which is essential in ensuring accuracy and consistency in test results. In Practice: Nursing Care Guidelines 52-1 highlights key information when collecting any specimen.

✚👁 Nursing Alert

Always wear clean gloves when collecting specimens of urine, stool, sputum, wound drainage, or blood. Thorough and consistent handwashing before and after any contact with clients and their specimens limits spread of microorganisms that cause disease.

THE URINE SPECIMEN

As the body's liquid waste product, *urine* has typical physical and microscopic characteristics that are excellent indicators of a person's state of health (see Chap. 51). Collecting and examining urine can provide significant information.

In Practice
Nursing Care Guidelines 52-1

COLLECTING SPECIMENS AND SAMPLES

- Label specimen bottles with the client's name and other data before collecting the specimen.
- Always wash your hands before and after collecting the specimen.
- Always observe Standard Precautions when collecting specimens. Expect to wear gloves when collecting most specimens.
- Collect the sample according to the individual facility's policy and procedure.
- Clean the area involved for sample collection.
- Observe sterile technique for sample collection, if needed.
- Place all specimens in biohazard bags to protect staff and other clients.
- Transport the specimen to the laboratory immediately.
- Be sure the specimen is accompanied by the appropriate request or laboratory cards.
- Record the collection and forwarding of the sample to the laboratory on the client's health record.
- Check the client's record later to determine if the results need to brought to the attention of the primary healthcare provider immediately.

Keeping Intake and Output Records

The amount of fluids a client consumes and eliminates during a given period is an excellent indicator of his or her nutritional and fluid balance. Over 24 hours, a person's normal fluid intake and urinary output (**I&O:** intake & output) will be approximately the same, or *balanced*. Fluid I&O that is significantly out of balance because of illness may lead to a life-threatening condition. The client may be retaining fluid, which can lead to edema, or the client may be dehydrated. Records of the client's I&O guide decision-making about increasing or restricting fluids or foods. These records can also be used to assess the effectiveness of certain medications given to the client, as well as to establish his or her elimination patterns. I&O records are usually kept for every shift and then totaled for a 24-hour period at midnight. To measure *total* food and fluid intake, the order is given to "record food and fluid intake" or "I&O+calorie count." In this case, record exactly what the client ate, directly on the client menu. Record fluids on the I&O sheet.

☞ KEY CONCEPT

Some normal situations can cause the fluid intake and output to be quite different. For example, during very hot weather, fluid is lost through perspiration, but it cannot be measured. Or, eating extra salt may cause a temporary retention of water in the tissues.

In most facilities, amounts recorded for I&O are recorded in milliliters (**mL**) or cubic centimeters (cc). The preferred unit of measurement is milliliters. These two measurements are approximately equal (1 cc=1 mL). Fig. 52-1 shows a sample I&O record.

Generally, the I&O sheet is kept near the client's bedside, and each nurse is responsible for recording I&O as it is measured. On the electronic record, an easily accessible screen documents I&O. Sometimes two records are kept. A temporary worksheet records I&O for each shift; this information is transferred to the 24-hour totals in the permanent record.

Measuring Fluid Intake

Fluid *intake* includes all fluids consumed through the gastrointestinal (GI) system (by mouth or a tube feeding) and those fluids taken as part of intravenous (IV) therapy or total parenteral nutrition (TPN).

Generally, when a client is on I&O, measure all fluid intake. Items such as ice, gelatin, ice cream, ice pops, and thin cereal are considered liquid intake. Each healthcare agency has a list describing the quantity of liquid found in various containers and in different foods. Use these standard quantities when recording, unless the client drinks from an unusual vessel. Record all fluids the client takes. Count ice as 50% water (eg, 200 mL of ice would count as 100 mL of fluid intake).

Be sure to find out your facility's policy concerning the recording of water intake from the bedside water pitcher. In some agencies it is recorded when the pitcher is filled and in others, when it is empty. Do not fill a pitcher or empty one unless you are sure of the procedure. Do not empty a bedpan

DAILY INTAKE AND OUTPUT BEDSIDE WORKSHEET

DATE _2/4/02_

John Menendez
#3987624
Dr. Abdul
Green Medicine Service

Record Shift totals on 24 Hr. Nurses Progress Notes

Approximate Measures in mL's	
1 oz.	30 mLs
8 oz. water glass (tea)	240 mLs
8 oz. glass of ice (melted)	135 mLs
Soup bowl	150 mLs
Jello (1 serving)	100 mLs
Small milk carton	240 mLs
8 oz. ice cream cup	90 mLs
Small juice glass	120 mLs
6 oz. hot styrofoam cup	180 mLs
12 oz. tea glass	360 mLs
Coca-cola paper cup	240 mLs
Insulated coffee cup	220 mLs
Canned 12 oz. drinks	360 mLs

FOR ISOLATION PATIENTS

9 oz disposable cups (tea and water)	240 mLs
6 oz. styrofoam cup	180 mLs
5 oz. plastic glass	150 mLs

	INTAKE			OUTPUT			
	ORAL		I.V. FLUIDS	URINE	EMESIS	SUCTION	STOOLS
7-3 0700-1500	*Juice* 120 *Milk* 240 *H₂O* 120 *H₂O* 200 *Jello* 50 *Coffee* 100		*D₅W* 420	0830-200 1045-225 1300-300 1400-125	0930-50	*Paracentesis 350 mL*	
TOTAL	830		420	850	50	350	
3-11 1500-2300	*Juice* 240 *Coffee* 240 *Milk* 140 *Soup* 100 *H₂O* 300 *Ensure* 200		*D₅W* 400 *+50 piggyback 2 meds.*	1530-275 1630-125 1245-200 2100-125 2200-Incont. (lg amts)	1545-50		
TOTAL	1220			725+ incont.	50	0	
11-7 2300-0700	*Water* 100		*D₅W* 395	0030-200 0245-325 0600-350			
	100		395	875			
TOTAL	24 Hr. 2150		1245	2450	100	350	

FIGURE 52-1. Example of an intake and output (I&O) form used at the bedside. (Form courtesy of AMI Nacogdoches Medical Center, Nacogdoches, Texas.)

or urinal without first finding out if the client's I&O is being recorded. Enlist the aid of the client when possible; for example, having the client report when he or she has voided or when the water pitcher is empty.

Measuring Output

Output includes urine and all other fluids leaving the body by any means. Output includes wound drainage, emesis (vomiting), bleeding, watery diarrhea, and nasogastric (**NG**) suction tube returns. When recording output other than urine, be sure to identify what the output was (for example, NG drainage, watery stool). Wound drainage on dressings is measured by weighing the dressing before and after and comparing it to a standardized chart to convert weight to milliliters.

Figure 52-2 shows a device called a toilet hat or "half pan" that can be placed under the toilet seat and used to collect either

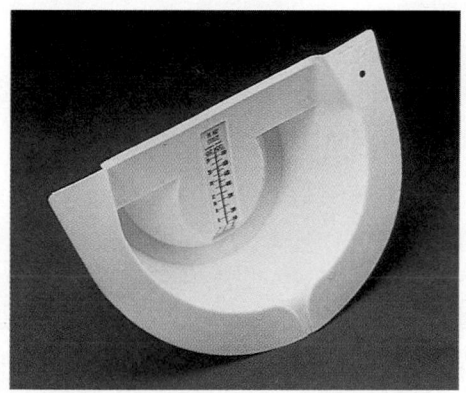

FIGURE 52-2. The urinary "hat" measuring device.

urine or stool without mixing them. The receptacle is positioned to the front to collect urine and to the back to collect stool. It has graduated volume marks on the inside to facilitate measurement of urine. In Practice: Nursing Procedure 52-1 reviews how to measure urine volume.

Often the client's normal bowel movements are also noted as part of the record. Sometimes all stools are weighed so that the physician knows more closely what the total output was.

Maintaining the IV Fluids Record

Many facilities have a separate I&O record for IV fluids. This record notes specific types of IV fluids, additives, amount of IV fluids absorbed, and amount remaining per shift. Make sure

that all IV fluids are included in the 24-hour total. Chapter 63 describes IV administration in more detail.

Measuring Urine Specific Gravity

Often when a urine output recording is ordered, a **specific gravity** (the concentration of urine compared with pure water) measurement to determine the concentration of urine is ordered at the same time. Generally the order calls for urine volume and specific gravity (abbreviated as **vol. & spec.** or **V&S**) to be recorded at specified intervals.

Urine specific gravity is measured with a specialized instrument called a **urinometer** or **hydrometer.** Mea-

---

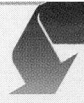

In Practice
Nursing Procedure 52-1

MEASURING URINARY OUTPUT

Supplies and Equipment

Gloves
Measuring graduate
Bedpan, urinal, or toilet hat (half pan)

Steps

1. Wash your hands and put on clean gloves.
   RATIONALE: *Handwashing and using gloves helps to prevent infection transmission.*

2. Ask the client to void in the bedpan, toilet hat, or urinal. Label the hat, urinal, or bedpan with the client's name if he or she is sharing a room or if several clients share the same toilet. Position the toilet hat in the toilet with the collecting receptacle towards the front.
   RATIONALE: *To be accurate, all urine output is measured. Placing the toilet hat in this manner acts as a reminder to the client and allows collection of urine without stool, if the client has a bowel movement. Labeling prevents cross-contamination.*

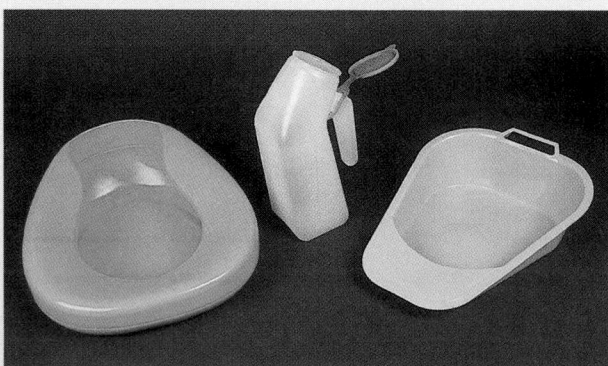

Collection devices for urine. Shown here are (from left to right) the traditional adult bedpan, the male urinal, and the fracture bedpan.

3. Pour the urine into the graduated measuring container, hold it at eye level, and read the urine volume in milliliters.
   RATIONALE: *Using a graduated container ensures accurate measurement.*

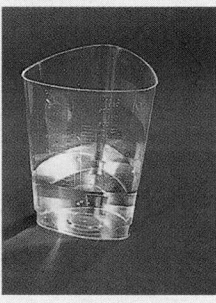

The graduated measuring container (also called a "graduate"). If the graduate is used for I&O, pour the urine into it and read the urine volume in milliliters.

4. Pour the urine into the toilet and flush, unless the urine is to be saved.
   RATIONALE: *Sometimes more than one test is made from one urine sample.*

5. Rinse the bedpan, urinal, or hat and the measuring graduate in cool water.
   RATIONALE: *Hot water will cause any protein substances to coagulate and will break down the urine faster, releasing ammonia.*

6. Encourage the client to wash his or her hands.
   RATIONALE: *Handwashing reinforces proper hygiene and reduces the risk of infection.*

7. Remove and dispose of gloves and wash hands.
   RATIONALE: *Handwashing and proper disposal of gloves limit the transfer of microorganisms.*

8. Record the urine volume on the output sheet.
   RATIONALE: *Immediate documentation ensures greater accuracy, providing communication and continuity of care.*

sure the reading in decimal increments above 1.000, which is the reading for pure water. Because the increments are in thousandths, be very accurate. The normal range of urine specific gravity is from 1.010 (dilute) to 1.025 (highly concentrated). Test urine as soon as possible after obtaining it to avoid inaccurate results. In Practice: Nursing Procedure 52-2 outlines the steps of measuring the specific gravity of urine.

Extremely concentrated urine (high urine specific gravity, approximately 1.025) may indicate either dehydration or fluid retention in the tissues (edema). Low specific gravity (below 1.010) may indicate a disorder such as diabetes insipidus or

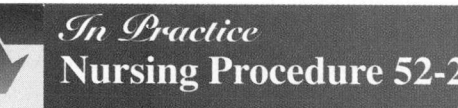

In Practice
Nursing Procedure 52-2

MEASURING URINE-SPECIFIC GRAVITY

Supplies and Equipment

Specific-gravity beaker
Gloves
Hydrometer or urinometer
Bedpan, urinal, or toilet hat

Steps

1. Maintain Standard Precautions.
   RATIONALE: *Standard Precautions reduce the risk of infection transmission.*

2. If ordered, measure urine for volume as described at In Practice: Nursing Procedure 52-1.
   RATIONALE: *Volume measurements are completed before any other testing is done.*

3. Fill the specific-gravity beaker with urine to approximately 1 inch from the top. Gently drop in the measuring instrument, called a *hydrometer* or *urinometer,* while twisting it gently.
   RATIONALE: *A rotating hydrometer is easier to keep away from the side of the beaker. Handling the hydrometer gently avoids breakage.*

4. Be sure the hydrometer is floating freely and not touching the side of the beaker.
   RATIONALE: *If the hydrometer touches anything, the reading will not be accurate.*

5. Hold the beaker at eye level and obtain the reading at the bottom of the meniscus, the slight bulge or curve seen on the liquid's surface.
   RATIONALE: *Liquids are always measured in this way for accuracy and consistency.*

6. Rinse the beaker and hydrometer in cool water.
   RATIONALE: *In addition to coagulating the protein, hot water can break the instrument.*

7. Remove and dispose of gloves and wash your hands.
   RATIONALE: *Handwashing and proper disposal of gloves limit the transfer of microorganisms.*

8. Record the results.
   RATIONALE: *Documentation ensures greater accuracy, providing communication and continuity of care.*

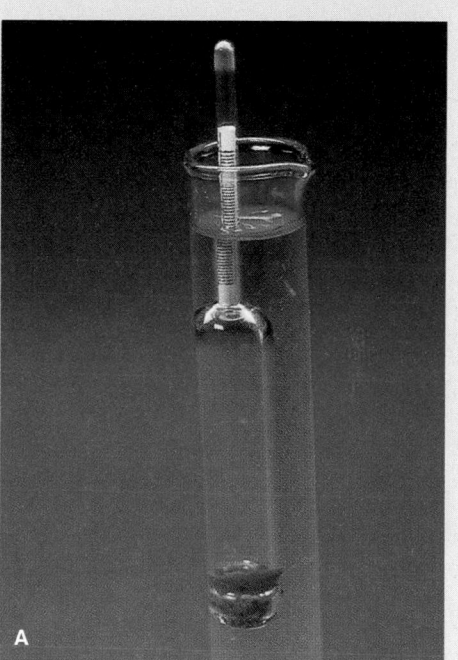

A

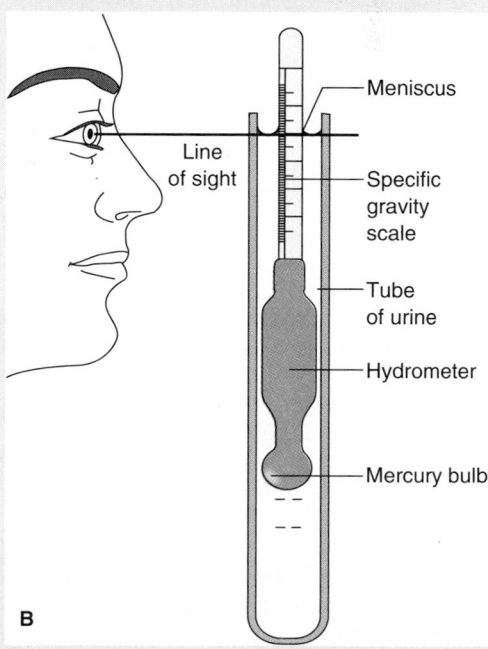

B

Measure specific gravity of urine at eye level for accuracy. Read at the bottom of the meniscus, which is the slight bulge or curve seen on the liquid's surface.

excessive use of diuretic medications. A kidney disorder may cause either a high or low urine specific gravity.

Collecting Urine Specimens for Examination

Urine specimens may be collected and sent to the laboratory for examination. **Urinalysis,** in which the components of urine are identified, is part of every client assessment at the beginning of treatment and during an illness. In addition, urine is commonly collected to determine the presence of legal or illegal drugs, to determine pregnancy, and to assess for the presence of infection. Many other tests can be performed with urine samples, and some urine tests are significant in the diagnosis of physical disorders. In Practice: Nursing Care Guidelines 52-2 highlights important components of collecting urine specimens.

Nursing Alert

Place all specimens in leakproof containers. Keep the outside of these containers clean and dry. Place them into plastic biohazard bags for transport to the laboratory. Label containers before use. In some facilities, you must label the bag as well. Be sure to include requests or lab cards, so the lab staff knows which tests to perform.

Collecting a Single-Voided Urine Specimen

A *single-voided urine specimen* often is ordered. Tests are done to determine the efficiency of the kidneys or to examine the urine for abnormalities. In Practice: Nursing Procedure 52-3 reviews the steps for collecting a single-voided urine specimen.

Collecting a Clean-Catch or Midstream Urine Specimen

By using the *clean-catch* or *midstream* method, a specimen is obtained with minimal contamination from external sources without inserting a sterile catheter. Because the genital area and urethral opening are cleansed before the specimen is obtained, and the sample is taken after some urine has already been passed, any bacteria found in the laboratory tests are most likely from urine in the bladder. In Practice: Nursing Care Guidelines 52-3 describes measures for collecting a clean-catch or midstream urine specimen.

Collecting a 24-Hour Urine Specimen

An accumulated quantity of urine gives more detailed information than a single specimen does because the accumulated specimen better shows the type and quantity of wastes being excreted by the kidneys. The urine is usually collected for 24 hours or for some part of that period, depending on

---

In Practice
Nursing Care Guidelines 52-2

COLLECTING URINE SPECIMENS

- Be aware that the amount and content of a urine specimen vary with the time of day, and with food and fluid intake. The physician may ask for specimens at different times of the day. The urine specimen collected for part of a day is called the *single fractional specimen.*
- Label specimen bottles before the client voids. *Rationale: Doing so reduces handling after the bottle is contaminated and helps the label to adhere to the container better.* Include the client's room or department and the physician's name. *Rationale: Proper labeling prevents errors.*
- Wake a client in the morning to obtain a routine specimen. *Rationale: If all specimens are collected at the same time, the laboratory can establish a baseline. Also, this voided specimen usually represents urine that was collecting in the bladder all night—usually the longest period the client goes without voiding.*
- Note on the specimen label if the female client is menstruating at that time. *Rationale: One of the tests routinely performed is a test for blood in the urine. If a woman is menstruating at the time a urine specimen is taken, a false-positive reading for blood will be obtained.*
- To avoid contamination and the necessity of collecting another specimen, encourage the client to wash the genital area with soap and water immediately

preceding the collection of the specimen. Single, prepackaged wipes are available for this purpose. Teach the female client to use the towelette and clean the urinary meatus from front to back; teach the male client to clean the urinary meatus wiping in a circular pattern from the center outward. *Rationale: Bacteria are normally present on the labia or penis, the perineum, and in the anal area.*
- Use a urinary or toilet hat (half pan) in the toilet if the client is ambulatory. *Rationale: This type of container allows the client to have a bowel movement while collecting only urine.* Use a urinal for a male client.
- If a sterile container is being used to collect the specimen, tell the client not to touch the inside of the container or its cover. *Rationale: Maintaining the sterility of the container helps to ensure accurate results and prevents cross-contamination.*
- Maintain Standard Precautions when collecting all types of urine specimens. *Rationale: Standard Precautions reduce the risk of infection transmission.*
- Wash your hands before and after the procedure and instruct the client to do the same. *Rationale: Handwashing helps to prevent infection transmission.*
- Document the procedure in the designated place and mark it off on the client's flowsheet or Kardex to avoid duplication. *Rationale: Documentation provides communication and continuity of care.*

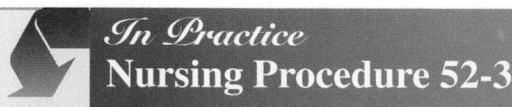

In Practice
Nursing Procedure 52-3

COLLECTING A SINGLE-VOIDED SPECIMEN

Supplies and Equipment

Covered specimen bottle or container
   (wide-mouthed)
Label
Bedpan, toilet hat, or urinal
Gloves
Biohazard bag

Steps

1. Follow previous Nursing Care Guidelines for collecting urine specimens. For most tests, a midstream sample is best if the client can cooperate (see In Practice: Nursing Care Guidelines 52-3).

2. Label the container with the date, client's name and room, department identification, and physician's name. Apply the label to the container before the client voids.
   RATIONALE: *Proper labeling ensures correct identification and avoids mistakes. The label may not stick if the container becomes wet.*

3. Wash hands and put on gloves.
   RATIONALE: *Handwashing and using gloves reduce the risk of infection transmission.*

4. Instruct the client to clean the genital area with soap and water or a specially prepared antiseptic towelette, and then to void into the specimen container or a clean receptacle or bedpan.
   RATIONALE: *Cleansing the genital area helps remove potential sources of contamination. Voiding into a clean receptacle prevents most cross-contamination.*

5. Remove the specimen as soon as possible after the client has voided.
   RATIONALE: *Substances in urine decompose when exposed to air. Decomposition may alter test results.*

6. Pour about 120 mL of urine into the labeled specimen container (unless the client has voided directly into the container). Cover the container.
   RATIONALE: *An adequate amount of urine is needed for the required tests. Covering the bottle retards decomposition and prevents added contamination. Place the bottle in a biohazard bag and send it to the lab immediately.*

7. Remove and discard gloves; wash your hands.
   RATIONALE: *Handwashing and proper glove disposal reduce the risk of infection transmission.*

8. Document in the client's health record that the specimen was obtained.
   RATIONALE: *Documentation provides communication and continuity of care.*

---

the specific information desired. In Practice: Nursing Procedure 52-4 describes the actions for collecting a *24-hour urine specimen.*

Collecting the Fractional Urine Specimen

Twenty-four hour *fractional* specimens are collected to determine amounts and characteristics of urine during various periods ("fractions") of the day. Follow these actions in collecting the 24-hour fractional urine specimen:

- Follow all the steps as when collecting other urine specimens. Be sure to follow Standard Precautions.
- Depending on the order, determine how many bottles you will need. Often fractional specimens are obtained for 6-hour periods of the day: 12 midnight to 6 am; 6 am to 12 noon; 12 noon to 6 pm; and 6 pm to 12 midnight. If this is the case, you need four specimen bottles, covers, and labels. Label all bottles before you begin. Indicate times.
- Begin by asking the client to void. *Rationale: Each new time slot begins with an empty bladder.*
- Collect all urine from the first fraction of the day in bottle #1. Be sure to ask the client to void at the end of that period. *Rationale: Each new time slot begins with an empty bladder.*
- Continue for the other "fractions" of the day. End the total day with an empty bladder.
- Store all specimens on ice or in a specimen refrigerator during the 24-hour collection period.
- Take the specimens to the laboratory immediately at the end of the 24-hour collection period. Document your findings.

Testing Urine for Abnormal Substances

Under normal circumstances, urine is free from sugar, acetone, and protein, but any of these may be present in the urine of the person with diabetes or kidney disease. With the availability of a variety of sophisticated but easy-to-use blood glucose monitors, urine testing for the presence of sugar is done infrequently. However, such testing may be done in the laboratory.

Collecting a Specimen From an Indwelling Catheter

Some clients have catheters (tubes) inserted that drain urine continuously (an *indwelling catheter* or *retention catheter*). Most likely, a catheterized specimen will only be obtained from the person who is unconscious or who already has a retention catheter. Otherwise, the midstream method is most often used to prevent the possibility of contaminating the bladder.

The urinary bladder is a sterile area. Contamination of any part of the retention catheter system can cause an infection because microorganisms can travel up the catheter into the bladder. Therefore, when collecting a catheterized specimen, be particularly careful not to endanger the client by contami-

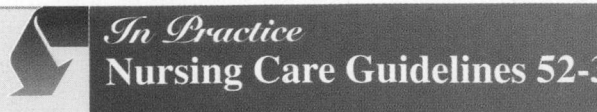

In Practice
Nursing Care Guidelines 52-3

COLLECTING CLEAN-CATCH OR MIDSTREAM URINE SPECIMENS

• Instruct the client to cleanse the urethral area thoroughly. *Rationale: Thorough cleansing limits external bacteria from entering the specimen. It is important to be evaluating only the bacteria that appear in the urine and not the bacteria on the external genitalia.*

• Use prepackaged wipes, if available. *Rationale: These wipes are sterile, which avoids introducing added contamination. They are also convenient.*

• Label the container before giving it to the client. *Rationale: The bottle may become soiled or wet, making it difficult and unsanitary to attach a label. This step also avoids confusion and misidentification.*

• Instruct the female client to cleanse from front to back and to cleanse each side with a separate wipe, saving the last for the urethral area itself. *Rationale: Cleansing in this manner avoids contaminating the vaginal and urethral areas with bacteria from the anal area. This ensures that the urethral area is as clean as possible.*

• Instruct the male client to cleanse the penis using a circular motion and going outward from the urethral meatus. The first wipe is for the urethral meatus. The

next wipe cleanses the end of the penis, and the last wipe again cleanses the urethral opening. *Rationale: The urethral area should be kept the cleanest.*

• Instruct both male and female clients to void only a small amount into the toilet, to rinse out the urethra, and to hold the rest of their urine. *Rationale: The voided urine flushes the urethral meatus of any remaining contaminants.*

• Instruct the client to then void into the sterile container, catching the *midstream urine. Rationale: This is the urine which will yield the most accurate information about the condition of the kidneys and bladder.*

• Finally, instruct the client to void the last of the stream into the toilet. *Rationale: The midstream urine is most characteristic of the urine produced by the kidney and is the best indicator of kidney function. The last part of the voiding does not yield as much information.*

• Take the specimen to the laboratory without delay. *Rationale: Delay could cause a false-positive result, particularly in the case of a urine culture.*

• Be sure to wear gloves when handling all specimens. *Rationale: Using gloves reduces the risk of infection transmission.*

nating the catheter system. Take care not to allow the collecting bag to be elevated above the level of the bladder. This action could result in urine flowing back into the bladder, carrying microorganisms with it. Also do not allow the collecting bag to touch the floor, which is a highly contaminated area. In Practice: Nursing Procedure 52-5 lists instructions for collecting a urine specimen from a urinary catheter.

Obtaining a One-Time Catheterized Urine Specimen

Occasionally, a catheterized urine specimen will be ordered. Generally, catheterization is not performed for urine collection unless the client is to be catheterized for some other reason. One reason for catheterization is to determine the amount of urine that remains in the bladder after voiding (residual urine). Often when catheterization is performed, a urine specimen is sent at the same time. Catheterization places the client at risk for a urinary tract infection. The procedure for performing a urinary catheterization is presented in Chapter 57.

THE STOOL SPECIMEN

The stool specimen provides information about the functioning of the GI system and its accessory organs. The most common test is for the presence of **occult** (hidden) blood in stool, which indicates bleeding somewhere in the GI tract. Another common test is for ova and parasites (**O&P**), which indicates the presence of intestinal parasites or their eggs (ova). In

Practice: Nursing Procedure 52-6 gives details for collecting stool specimens.

In the ambulatory care setting, in the home, or on the nursing unit, stools are tested for occult blood using the **Hemoccult** or **Hematest** brand methods. Sometimes, these tests are referred to as **guaiac** tests, named for the substance used to cause the tested occult blood to change color (Fig. 52-3). In these tests, the nurse places a smear of stool on the testing card and adds a drop of a reagent. After a timed interval, the smear is compared with a color chart to determine the presence of blood. Always check the kits for any special instructions. The test is simple enough to conduct in the client's bathroom or a utility room. As always, be sure to wear clean gloves when handling stool.

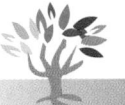

SPECIAL CONSIDERATIONS: THE LIFE SPAN

Collecting a Stool Specimen From a Child

When an infant has diarrhea and the stool specimen is to be examined, place the entire diaper in a biohazard bag, label it, and take or send the diaper to the laboratory immediately. Otherwise, if the stool is formed, remove the stool from the diaper with a tongue blade, as for an adult.

In Practice
Nursing Procedure 52-4

COLLECTING A 24-HOUR URINE SPECIMEN

Supplies and Equipment

2-liter opaque collection bottle
label for container
container of ice or refrigerator for storage
towel
bedpan, urinal, or toilet hat
gloves
biohazard bag

Steps

1. Collect supplies: 2-liter opaque collecting bottle with loose-fitting lid or towel to be used as a cover, label, urinal or toilet hat, urine measuring container, and container of ice (if refrigerator is unavailable for cooling and storing the collecting bottle).
   RATIONALE: *Organization facilitates efficiency, maximizing the accuracy of the results.*

2. Maintain Standard Precautions and follow guidelines for urine collection given earlier in this chapter.
   RATIONALE: *Standard Precautions reduce the risk of infection transmission.*

3. Label the opaque collecting bottle with the client's name and pertinent data before beginning.
   RATIONALE: *Proper labeling ensures correct identification of the urine specimen by the laboratory.*

4. Give the bedpan, toilet hat, or urinal to the client and instruct the client to void. *Discard* this urine and record the time on the client's chart.
   RATIONALE: *Collection begins with an empty bladder. If this collection is made from an indwelling catheter, proceed following the same timetable.*

5. Measure each specimen of urine voided, and pour into the collecting bottle that is placed on ice or being cooled; record each amount.

RATIONALE: *Measuring each voiding ensures that all urine is collected and available for substance analysis.*

6. Keep the collecting bottle opening covered. Label it with the client's name and the time the test started.
   RATIONALE: *Urine decomposes into ammonia when exposed to air; limiting exposure to the air controls odor.*

7. Continue collection for 24 hours from the time the first urine was discarded.
   RATIONALE: *Complete collection of all urine produced in 24 hours ensures accurate test results.*

8. At exactly 24 hours after beginning the collection, instruct the client to void. Pour this voided amount into the bottle.
   RATIONALE: *The last voiding completes the 24-hour total; collection ends with an empty bladder.*

9. State the exact time and amount of the last urine specimen collected, on the bottle label. Cover the bottle tightly, place in a biohazard bag, and label as a 24-hour urine collection with the client's identification information. Maintain cleanliness on the outside of the bag.
   RATIONALE: *Proper labeling and timing ensures accurate results. Keeping the outside clean helps to protect the healthcare worker.*

10. Remove and discard gloves; wash hands.
    RATIONALE: *Proper glove disposal and handwashing reduce the risk of infection transmission.*

11. Take the specimen to the laboratory immediately.
    RATIONALE: *Immediately transporting the specimen to the laboratory avoids any further decomposition of the urine; prompt analysis of the urine ensures accurate results of the test.*

12. Document information about the specimen collection, including time of starting and stopping and total amount collected, and that the specimen has been sent to the laboratory.
    RATIONALE: *Documentation ensures communication and continuity of care.*

Nursing Alert

Be aware that "false-positives" may occur with guaiac tests. False-positives can be caused by eating large amounts of rare red meat or by eating certain foods such as radishes, tomatoes, beets, horseradish, or some melons. In addition, the client should not take more than 250 mg per day of vitamin C and should not take aspirin or nonsteroidal anti-inflammatory drugs (NSAIDs) for 3 days prior to the test. Be sure to let the client know about the possibility of false-positives if you perform a test and it seems to be positive. Usually, three separate specimens are collected on three separate days before a determination of positive or negative is made. If after this time the test is positive, further examinations are necessary.

In Practice
Nursing Procedure 52-5

COLLECTING A URINE SPECIMEN FROM A RETENTION CATHETER (SYRINGE AND NEEDLE SYSTEM)

Supplies and Equipment

Gloves
Clamp or rubber band
Container with label
10–20 mL syringe with 21- to 25-gauge needle
  (for needleless hub)
Biohazard bag
Alcohol prep or disinfectant swab

Steps

1. Gather supplies. Label the container.
   RATIONALE: *Organization facilitates accurate skill performance.*

2. Explain the procedure to the client.
   RATIONALE: *Providing information fosters cooperation.*

3. Wash hands and put on gloves.
   RATIONALE: *Handwashing and using gloves help to prevent the spread of infection.*

4. Clamp the drainage tubing, or fold the tubing over once and secure it with a rubber band below the collection port. Allow adequate time for urine collection, but no longer than 15 min.
   RATIONALE: *Collecting urine from the tubing guarantees a fresh specimen.*

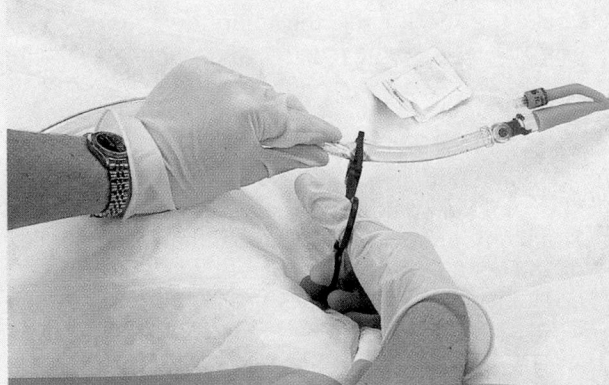
Clamping the drainage tubing.

5. Cleanse the aspiration port with an antiseptic swab, such as an alcohol prep.
   RATIONALE: *Disinfecting the port prevents microorganisms from entering the catheter.*

6. Open the syringe package, maintaining the sterility of the syringe and needle. Insert the needle into the aspiration port and withdraw urine into the syringe. The laboratory test required determines the amount of urine to collect.
   RATIONALE: *This technique provides an uncontaminated urine specimen, while preventing contamination of the client's bladder.*

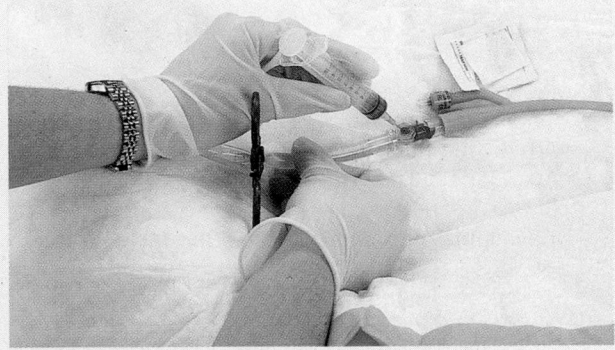
Inserting the needle into the aspiration port.

7. Transfer the urine to the labeled specimen container. The container must be *sterile* for a culture and *clean* for a routine urinalysis.
   RATIONALE: *Careful labeling prevents confusion. Careful transfer of the specimen prevents contamination or confusion of the urine specimen.*

8. Unclamp the catheter.
   RATIONALE: *The catheter must be unclamped to allow free urinary flow and to prevent urinary stasis.*

9. Prepare the container according to the agency's policy for transport to the laboratory.
   RATIONALE: *Proper packaging ensures that the specimen is not an infection risk.*

10. Dispose of used equipment. Remove gloves and wash your hands.
    RATIONALE: *Proper equipment disposal and handwashing help to prevent the spread of infection.*

11. Send the container to the laboratory immediately with the proper documentation.
    RATIONALE: *Microorganisms grow quickly at room temperature.*

12. Document on the flowsheet or the client's record that the specimen was obtained.
    RATIONALE: *Documentation provides communication and coordination of care.*

In Practice
Nursing Procedure 52-6

COLLECTING A STOOL SPECIMEN
Supplies and Equipment

Gloves
Clean bedpan and cover or toilet hat
Closed specimen container and cover
Label
Wooden tongue blades
Biohazard bags

Steps

1. Maintain Standard Precautions. Wash the hands and put on gloves.
   RATIONALE: *Using Standard Precautions and hand-washing reduces the risk of infection transmission.*

2. Explain the procedure to the client. Ask the client to tell you when he or she feels the urge to have a bowel movement.
   RATIONALE: *Most people cannot have a bowel movement on command.*

3. Label the container.
   RATIONALE: *Proper labeling ensures correct identification of the specimen by the laboratory.*

4. Give the bedpan when the client is ready. If the client will be using the toilet, place the toilet hat turned towards the back of the toilet.

RATIONALE: *It is most likely to obtain a usable specimen at this time. The toilet hat allows stool to be collected free of urine.*

5. After the client has moved his or her bowels, use the tongue blade to transfer a portion of the feces to the container. Do not touch the specimen.
   RATIONALE: *It is grossly contaminated.*

6. Take a portion of feces from three different areas of the stool specimen.
   RATIONALE: *Samples from three different areas will enhance the accuracy of the results. Keep in mind that sometimes, examination must be made of the entire stool. In this case, use a larger container.*

7. Cover the container.
   RATIONALE: *Covering the container ensures that no further contamination of the specimen will occur.*

8. Remove and discard gloves; wash your hands.
   RATIONALE: *Proper glove disposal and handwashing reduce the risk of infection transmission.*

9. Take the container immediately to the laboratory with the appropriate request slip.
   RATIONALE: *Stools should be examined when fresh. Examinations for parasites, eggs (ova), and organisms must be made when the stool is warm.*

THE SPUTUM SPECIMEN

For clients with some respiratory disorders, a sputum specimen may be obtained and sent to the laboratory for culture or other examination. This test is most commonly used to determine the presence of the tubercle bacillus, the causative organism for tuberculosis. Often, such specimens are collected for 3 days in a row. The best time to obtain a sputum specimen is soon after the client awakens in the morning. Sputum accumulates in the airways during the night and often is more easily expelled by coughing in the early morning. The first specimen of the morning is considered to be the most accurate. Obtain the specimen before the client eats, uses mouthwash, or brushes the teeth.

Observe Standard Precautions when collecting sputum. Keep the inside of the specimen container sterile. A sterile container ensures that any organisms cultured from the specimen will be due to the specimen and not a contaminated container. Keep the cover on the container as much as possible, to prevent contamination by particles in the air and to prevent the spread of organisms from the sputum speci-

men. When the cover is removed, place the cover with the inside up.

Consuming adequate amounts of fluid and breathing humidified air or aerosolized medications often help to loosen and liquefy secretions, making it easier for the client to **expectorate** (cough them up). If the client has used aerosolized medications, document this fact in the health record, along with the fact that a specimen has been collected. In Practice: Nursing Procedure 52-7 gives tips for collecting a sputum specimen.

The physician may write an order to measure sputum. If so, do this in one of two ways:

(1) If enough sputum is collected in a graduated specimen container, read the amount directly; or (2) pour an equal amount of water into an identical container and measure the water.

In addition, do the following:

• Weigh the specimen, if ordered. Do so on a balance scale, subtracting the initial weight of the container.

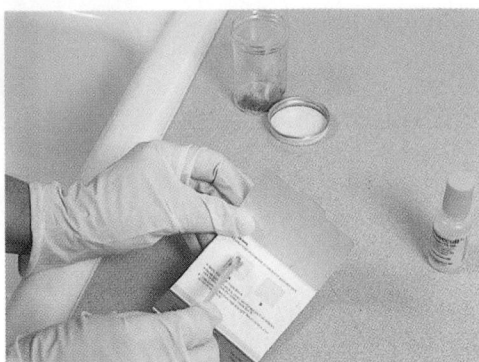

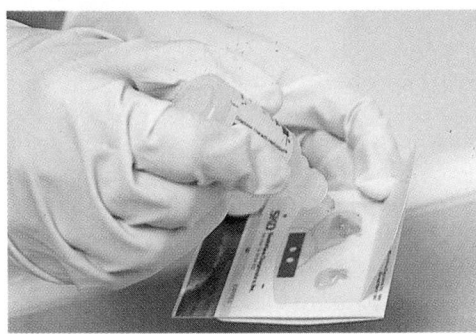

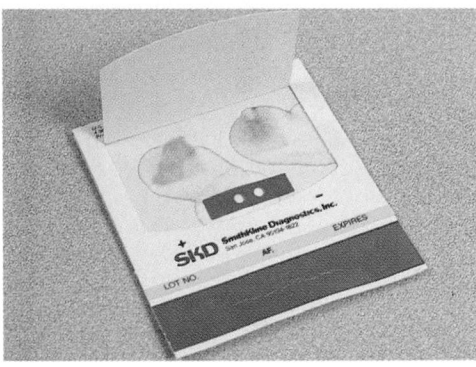

FIGURE 52-3. Hemoccult testing. (**A**) Placing a smear of stool on the testing card. (**B**) Adding a drop of a reagent. (**C**) Observing the smear for a blue discoloration indicating the presence of blood.

- Take the specimen to the laboratory immediately after collection. *Rationale: A delay may alter the result of a culture.*
- Call the attention of the laboratory personnel to the fact that this is a sputum specimen.
- Document the sputum's amount (copious, moderate, small), color, and consistency.

☩👁 Nursing Alert

• The sputum specimen is considered highly contaminated. Treat it with caution.
- Paper tissues used by any client also are considered contaminated. Dispose of them properly.
- Wear gloves when handling tissues and sputum specimens, and when providing nursing care if the client is coughing up sputum.

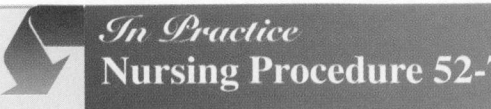

In Practice
Nursing Procedure 52-7

COLLECTING A SPUTUM SPECIMEN
Supplies and Equipment

Sterile, covered sputum container
Tissues
Labels
Gloves
Biohazard bag

Collecting the Specimen

1. Wear gloves when handling a sputum specimen or any used facial tissue.
   RATIONALE: *Sputum, and anything containing it, is considered highly contaminated.*

2. Explain the procedure to the client.
   RATIONALE: *If the person understands the procedure, he or she will cooperate more readily.*

3. Label the container.
   RATIONALE: *Careful labeling ensures accuracy of the report and alerts laboratory personnel to the presence of a contaminated specimen.*

4. Instruct the client to cough up secretions from deep in the respiratory passages.
   RATIONALE: *A sputum specimen should come from the lungs and bronchi. It should be sputum rather than mucus.*

5. Have the client expectorate directly into the sterile container.
   RATIONALE: *Expectorating directly into the container avoids outside contamination of the specimen or contamination of other objects.*

6. Cover the specimen immediately.
   RATIONALE: *Covering the specimen helps prevent contamination.*

7. Remove and discard gloves; wash hands.
   RATIONALE: *Proper glove disposal and handwashing reduce the risk of infection transmission and prevent contamination of other objects, including the label.*

8. Transport specimen to the laboratory immediately.
   RATIONALE: *Immediate transport of the specimen prevents the proliferation of organisms and ensures more accurate results.*

9. Document the collection of the sputum specimen in the client's health record.
   RATIONALE: *Documentation provides communication and continuity of care.*

THE BLOOD SPECIMEN

A blood specimen is usually taken when a person is admitted to a healthcare facility, to assess the blood's normal cells and other components and to determine the presence of abnormalities or disease organisms. In some conditions, different blood cells increase in number or change in shape. For example, the number and the shape of red blood cells give information about the type and severity of anemia; the number and characteristics of white blood cells give information about infection and the body's immune system.

Assisting With Venipuncture

Venipuncture is the procedure of using a needle to withdraw blood from a vein, often from the inside surface of the forearm near the elbow, called the *antecubital space*. Here the veins are near the surface and are easy to see or feel. Other areas where the veins stand out prominently, such as the forearm or dorsum of the hand, may be used. The blood is drawn into a tube or syringe. If only a very small amount of blood is needed, such as for glucose testing, the client's finger is pricked with a lancet, and the blood is placed on a test strip. Laboratory personnel may also draw the blood into a pipette or smear it directly onto a glass slide.

The primary caregiver or the laboratory professional (*phlebotomist*) usually collects the blood specimen by venipuncture. A nurse with specific training also may perform this procedure. Venipuncture is often performed by home care nurses. The skill is explained here because the nursing student or LPN/LVN may be asked to assist with drawing blood or assembling equipment. To assist with obtaining blood samples:

- Collect the proper tubes and labels.
- Have the request or physician's order available to ensure that the proper tests are done.
- Observe Standard Precautions. Always wear gloves.
- Have the client lie on the back with the arm resting comfortably on the bed, or sit in a chair with the arm resting on the overbed table. *Rationale: If the arm is relaxed, the procedure will be easier to perform and will be less uncomfortable for the client.*
- Place a protective sheet under the arm. *Rationale: If there is some bleeding, it will not soil the bed.*

Observe as the person trained in the procedure obtains the sample:

- A tourniquet is placed around the upper arm, tightened, and secured with a slip knot. *Rationale: This procedure helps to distend the veins, which helps to show an appropriate vein.*
- The area over the vein is cleansed with an alcohol swab, wiping from the center out. *Rationale: Cleansing the area helps to prevent the spread of infection; using a circular motion removes organisms away from the intended site of puncture.*
- The vein is palpated to determine the best site and angle for insertion of the needle. *Rationale: Visualizing a vein*

is not as effective as feeling the vein. A vein typically rebounds when it is pressed gently.
- The needle is inserted into the vein, bevel up. A Vacutainer tube is often used. In some cases, a "butterfly" setup, using a scalp vein needle, may be used for specimen collection. *Rationale: The vacuum in this tube draws the blood into the tube without the need for a syringe. The butterfly setup uses a tiny needle and may be more comfortable for the client.*
- When the required amount of blood has been collected, the tourniquet is released, and a sterile gauze square or cotton ball is held over the needle while it is withdrawn. *Rationale: Releasing the tourniquet makes the time of client discomfort as brief as possible. Covering the needle insertion site prevents the introduction of organisms into the needle wound.*
- Assist with encouraging the client to bend the elbow, using the gauze or cotton ball as a compress or taping the gauze in place. *Rationale: This helps to prevent bleeding and bruising.*
- Assist with discarding any used supplies and equipment, for example, gloves and needles. Thoroughly wash the hands. *Rationale: Proper disposal of equipment and careful handwashing help to prevent the spread of organisms and minimize the risk of needlestick injury.*
- Label the specimen and take it to the laboratory immediately with the appropriate request. *Rationale: Some specimens deteriorate with time and when at room temperature.*

Assisting in Obtaining Blood for Culture

Sometimes a blood culture is ordered. The order is often written for the test to be done in case the client spikes a fever (PRN, "as needed") or it may be written as a routine order ("blood for **C&S**" [culture and sensitivity]). The culture identifies the disease-causing organism, and the drug sensitivity test determines what medications will kill or arrest the growth of that organism. If blood is to be drawn PRN, have the equipment located and prepared so that it is ready when needed.

The nurse's role is often that of assistant, with the responsibility of notifying the proper laboratory person when the culture is to be done. Assemble all the materials, and explain the procedure to the client. Use the following actions when assisting with blood cultures:

- Obtain and label the proper tubes or bottles.
- Carefully wash your hands. *Rationale: Handwashing helps to prevent contamination of the culture and infection transmission.*
- Observe Standard Precautions. Put on gloves and provide gloves for the person you are assisting. *Rationale: Standard Precautions reduce the risk of infection transmission.*
- Protect the bed with a pad under the client's arm. *Rationale: In case there is some bleeding, it will not soil*

the bed. Additionally, the materials used to prepare the puncture site may stain the linens or the client's clothing.

• Prepare the skin using the specified protocol. Usually at least two antiseptic wipes are used. *Rationale: The skin must be as close to sterile as possible, to ensure that the culture is that of the blood and not of the skin.*

• Assist the person drawing blood.

• Keep in mind that the blood may be placed into two or more tubes or bottles. Remember that strict sterile technique must be maintained when the blood samples are drawn and placed in the specimen container. *Rationale: Sterile technique is crucial to prevent contamination of the sample. The culture grown must yield organisms present in the blood only.*

• If necessary, help to place a gauze pad, folded into a compress, tightly over the venipuncture site and secure it firmly with tape. Check a few minutes later to make sure all bleeding has stopped. *Rationale: Because a large needle is used, some bleeding may occur. Firm pressure is needed to minimize the risk of bleeding.*

• Assist with properly disposing of supplies, bed pad, and syringes. *Rationale: Proper disposal of equipment helps to prevent the spread of organisms; proper disposal of syringes minimizes the risk of needlestick injury.*

• Carefully wash hands. *Rationale: Handwashing helps to reduce the risk of infection transmission.*

• Document that the procedure was done and by whom. *Rationale: Documentation provides communication and continuity of care.*

• Take the specimen to the laboratory immediately. This is especially important with cultures. *Rationale: The culture medium enhances growth. Culturing must be performed under carefully controlled laboratory conditions.*

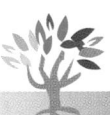 **SPECIAL CONSIDERATIONS:** THE LIFE SPAN

Obtaining a Blood Specimen From a Child

The sites for obtaining a blood specimen in infants and children are the same as those for adults. In some instances, however, the jugular or femoral vein may be used. Having blood drawn is very frightening for a child and it can be painful. Ensure that the specimen is drawn somewhere other than at the child's bedside. Doing so maintains the child's bed as a safe area.

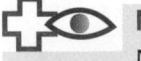 **Nursing Alert**

Nurses who draw blood need specialized instruction and supervised practice in venipuncture.

STUDENT SYNTHESIS

Key Points

• Standard Precautions are used when collecting specimens involving any body fluids.

• Careful handwashing limits the transfer of microorganisms from one person to another and retards the spread of disease.

• Fluid intake includes all fluids consumed through the GI system (by mouth or tube feeding) and fluids taken as part of IV therapy or total parenteral nutrition.

• Output includes urine and all other fluids leaving the body by any means. This includes wound drainage, emesis (vomiting), watery diarrhea, bleeding, and NG suction tube returns.

• Routine specimen collection is usually scheduled for early in the morning.

• Any specimen collected should be transported to the laboratory immediately to ensure the most accurate results.

• Urine specimens collected include single-voided, clean-catch (or midstream), catheterized, 24-hour, and fractional urine specimens.

• Stool specimens are typically evaluated for occult blood and ova and parasites.

• Sputum specimen collection requires the client to expectorate or cough up secretions from lower in the respiratory tract. The early-morning specimen is the most accurate.

• Nurses do not draw blood unless they have specific education and supervised practice.

Critical Thinking Exercises

1. Considering the reasons for keeping accurate I&O records, what are the possible outcomes for the client if the I&O records are inaccurate?

2. If a 24-hour urine collection is not done accurately, how would the results be affected?

NCLEX-Style Review Questions

1. The nurse knows that a false-positive guaiac stool test may occur if the client eats:
   a. Chicken
   b. Beets
   c. Carrots
   d. Pork

2. When teaching a client about obtaining the 24-hour urine specimen, it is most important to instruct the client to:
   a. Avoid fluids during the testing period.
   b. Discard the first and last void of the specimen.
   c. Mix stool with the urine.
   d. Notify the staff with each voiding so the urine may be collected.

3. When obtaining a urine specimen from a retention catheter, which technique should the nurse use to avoid contamination of the system?
   a. Cleanse the aspiration port with a Betadine swab.
   b. Prior to obtaining the sample, clamp tubing for 30 minutes.
   c. Remove urine from the catheter tubing with a sterile needle.
   d. Transfer collected urine to a sterile specimen cup.

4. Which method should the nurse use when collecting a stool specimen?
   a. Obtain specimen from stool with gloved finger and place in sterile cup.
   b. Place collected specimen in a toilet hat and transfer to the laboratory.
   c. Take a portion of feces from three different areas of the stool specimen.
   d. Verify that the client has an infection prior to collecting the specimen.

5. When obtaining a midstream urine specimen from a female client, which instructions would be most important for the nurse to tell the client?
   a. Start voiding directly into the sterile cup.
   b. Void the last of the stream of urine into the sterile cup.
   c. Wash hands after obtaining the specimen.
   d. Wipe from front to back when cleansing the urethral area.

CHAPTER

53

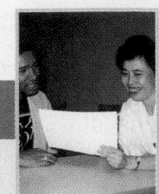

Bandages and Binders

LEARNING OBJECTIVES

1. State at least three purposes for applying binders and bandages.
2. State the most common reasons for applying the roller bandage.
3. Explain how to assess the client's extremity when it is wrapped in a bandage or has an antiembolism stocking applied.
4. Identify the most common use of the T-binder, addressing the differences when used for a male and a female client.
5. State the rationale for using Montgomery straps.
6. In the skills laboratory, demonstrate the ability to perform the following: applying roller bandages and antiembolism stockings, and changing a dressing using Montgomery straps.

NEW TERMINOLOGY

antiembolism stockings   Montgomery straps
Kerlix   T-binder
maceration

ACRONYMS

ACE   ISCD   TED
CMS

When the client's condition requires the application of bandages or binders, understanding the reasons for their use and performing correct, safe application techniques are important.

BANDAGES

A *bandage* is a strip of gauze, cloth, or elasticized material that is wrapped around a body part to give support or to hold dressings in place. Bandages are prepared in various widths and lengths and are usually rolled to simplify application. They may be clean or sterile (see also Chap. 58).

Often elasticized bandages are wrapped around a client's limbs to provide muscle or joint support or to increase circulation. Gentle pressure against the tissues stimulates blood return to the heart and prevents blood from pooling in the extremity. Application that is too tight, however, can squeeze the blood vessels and nerves (*constriction*), resulting in tissue damage. Carefully and frequently assess circulation and nerve function in the client's fingers or toes to make sure that a bandage is not too tight. You can do so by assessing the client's skin color, finger or toe motion, and sensation (color, motion, and sensitivity [**CMS**]). See In Practice: Nursing Assessment 53-1. Note any abnormal signs and alert your team leader to them at once.

Wrapped bandages also can loosen easily, particularly if the client is mobile or restless. Loose bandages are not therapeutic. Just as you will check frequently to see if the bandage is too tight, you must also check to see if it is too loose.

Roller Bandages

The most commonly used bandage is the elastic roller bandage called the *all cotton elastic* (**ACE**) roller bandage (Fig. 53-1). (ACE is a brand name.) Although usually wrapped around a limb to give support, the ACE bandage may also be used to hold a dressing on an extremity or the body's trunk. Sometimes an ACE bandage may be wrapped around a body part to exert pressure over a bleeding point.

Kerlix™

In other cases, a type of gauze with the brand name **Kerlix** is used to hold dressings in place or apply pressure. Kerlix is a stretchy gauze in a long roll. The steps for applying an ACE- or Kerlix-type bandage are described at In Practice: Nursing Care Guidelines 53-1.

Antiembolism Stockings

Many physicians routinely order **antiembolism stockings** (also called thromboembolytic disease [**TED**] stockings) for all postoperative clients. These elastic stockings cover the foot (not the toes) and the leg, up to the knee or mid-thigh. A firmly wrapped ACE bandage may also be applied, but stockings provide firmer and more even pressure against the leg's blood vessels. They help ensure adequate return circulation (*venous circulation*) to the heart and may help prevent blood clots (*emboli* or *thromboemboli*).

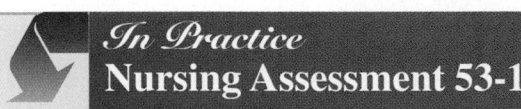

In Practice
Nursing Assessment 53-1

THE CLIENT'S CIRCULATION WHEN USING BANDAGES

Color of Toes or Fingers
- The toes or fingers should be a color appropriate for the client's normal skin tone. They should not be pale, white, cyanotic, or mottled.
- Digits are assessed by pressing them lightly. Skin tone should return to normal immediately after the pressure is removed. If the area that was touched remains lighter, the skin is *blanched* (impaired circulation).

Motion or Mobility
- The client should be able to move the toes or fingers freely without pain.

Sensitivity or Sensation
- The client should be able to feel your touch on his or her toes or fingers.
- The client's subjective feelings—tingling, numbness, or itching; pain (report and follow up); and any tightness (extreme tightness is a significant complication) should be discussed to obtain additional information.
- The client's complaints of severe or excessive pain are significant.

Edema and Swelling
- When you press the client's hand or foot, your indentation should not remain. An imprint indicates edema.

Temperature
- The temperature of the client's toes or fingers should be warm and the same as the rest of his or her body.

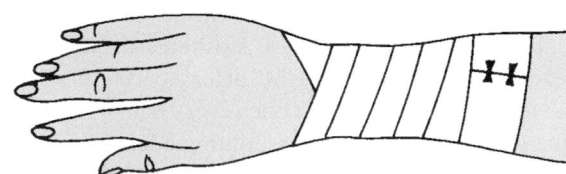

FIGURE 53-1. Roller bandage application. During the wrapping procedure, elevate the client's extremity to the level of his or her body or higher. Place firm, even pressure on the bandage as you apply it. Each successive wrap will cover about half of the previous part of the bandage. (Courtesy of 3M Company, St. Paul, Minnesota, Medical Products Division.)

In Practice
Nursing Care Guidelines 53-1

APPLYING A ROLLER BANDAGE

- Check your agency's policy to see if the physician has ordered dressing changes. If so, the physician's order will indicate the specific part to wrap and how often. *Rationale: The dressings will be changed at the same time as the bandage is rewrapped. It is important to follow the physician's instructions because this is part of the treatment of the wound or the client disorder.*
- Use the correct bandage size. The width of the bandage used is determined by the part to be wrapped. Generally, a bandage wider than 3 in (7.5 cm) is difficult to keep in place on an arm or leg. Wider bandages may be used on the chest or abdomen. More than one roller bandage may be used, if necessary. Simply overlap ends. *Rationale: If a bandage is too narrow, it will pinch and bind. If a bandage is too wide, it will fold over. In either case, the effectiveness of the bandage will be compromised.*
- Explain to the client what you plan to do. *Rationale: Ensure the client's cooperation.*
- Elevate the extremity to be wrapped to the level of the client's recumbent body. *Rationale: Elevation helps to prevent congestion of the blood and lymph in the area to be wrapped.*
- Roll the bandage before beginning to wrap. *Rationale: This will help ensure that even pressure is applied.*
- Begin wrapping the bandage at the client's toes or fingers and move toward the hip or shoulder.

Rationale: Wrapping upward enhances venous circulation.
- Wrap the bandage firmly, but not too tightly. Do not stretch the bandage while wrapping. *Rationale: These precautions will help prevent the bandage from being wrapped too tightly and cutting off circulation.*
- Overlap each layer about half the width of the strip. *Rationale: Overlapping ensures more even pressure.*
- Anchor the top with tape or the attached Velcro strips. *Rationale: Pins or clips may scratch the client.*
- Assess the circulation of the client's toes or fingers after the bandage is in place. *Rationale: A bandage that is too tight can cut off circulation and cause tissue damage. If it is too loose, it will not provide support.*
- Document the procedure, noting the client's reactions. *Rationale: Documentation provides communication and ensures continuity of care.*
- Check the client's color, motion, and sensitivity (**CMS**) in the fingers or toes at least every 2 hours. *Rationale: A bandage that is too tight can cause damage very quickly.*
- Release the bandage at least once every 4 hours, unless ordered otherwise. At this time, help the client exercise the leg or arm and give skin care. *Rationale: Releasing the bandage allows for skin inspection under the area that is bandaged; exercise increases circulation and helps to prevent deformities and discomfort.*

To give proper support, the stockings fit tightly without binding the leg or cutting off circulation. Stockings are available in various sizes. Measure the client's thigh or calf according to the instructions on the package to select the size that ensures proper fit. Apply the stockings before the client gets out of bed or after the client has remained *recumbent* (lying down) for at least 15 minutes. *Rationale: Doing so prevents pooling of fluid or blood in the leg, which increases the pressure from the stockings and alters their effect.* In Practice: Nursing Procedure 53-1 describes application of elastic stockings.

Unlike ACE bandages, these stockings do not become loose; thus, check the client's CMS at least once every 2 hours. Remove the stockings at least once every 8 hours and examine the leg carefully for redness, pitting edema, or skin discoloration. Document your findings. Wash the client's legs gently each day, apply lotion if the skin is dry, and apply clean stockings.

Another type of device, called an *intermittent sequential compression device* (**ISCD**), provides alternating pressure to the legs. This device is used to support circulation and is discussed later in this book.

BINDERS

A *binder* is a wide, flat piece of fabric that is applied to support a specific body part or to hold a dressing in place. Commonly used binders include the *arm sling* and the *T-binder*, a T-shaped strap. Some binders are made of elasticized material. Most use hook-and-loop fasteners (Velcro). In Practice: Nursing Care Guidelines 53-2 highlights information about applying binders.

☛ KEY CONCEPT

Occasionally, a breast binder will be ordered for a woman after childbirth. However, usually the client is instructed to wear a good support bra instead.

T-Binder

A **T-binder** gets its name from its shape. It is made of two strips of material, 3 to 4 inches (7.5 to 10 cm) wide, which are fastened together, forming a T. The T-binder is used to

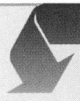

In Practice
Nursing Procedure 53-1

APPLYING ANTIEMBOLISM STOCKINGS (TED STOCKINGS)

Supplies and Equipment

Support stockings
Talcum powder
Tape measure

Steps

1. Explain the procedure to the client.
   RATIONALE: *Providing information fosters cooperation.*

2. Use the tape measure to determine the proper stocking size for the client.
   RATIONALE: *Stockings that are too tight may interfere with circulation. Stockings that are too loose do not encourage venous return.*

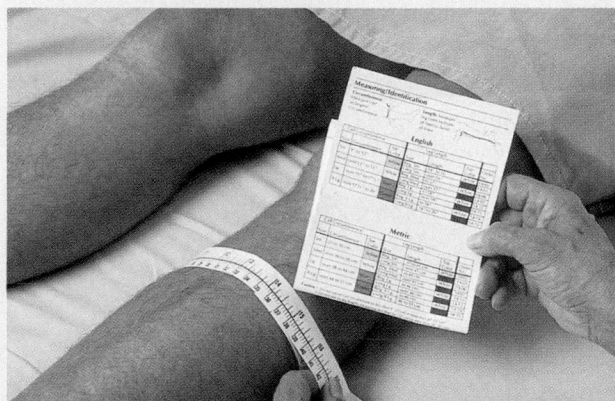

Use a tape measure to determine proper stocking size for the client.

3. Gather supplies.
   RATIONALE: *Organization facilitates accurate skill performance.*

4. Wash the hands. Wear gloves if your skin or the client's skin is not intact.
   RATIONALE: *Handwashing and using gloves help prevent the spread of infection.*

5. Assist the client to the supine position. Allow at least 15 min before applying stockings if the client has had the lower extremities in a dependent position.
   RATIONALE: *Stockings are best applied early in the morning before the client assumes a sitting or standing position; otherwise, the client's veins become distended and edema often occurs.*

6. Apply a small amount of talcum powder to the client's feet and legs, if not contraindicated.
   RATIONALE: *Powder reduces friction and allows easier application of stockings.*

7. Grasp the stocking's heel and turn the stocking inside out.
   RATIONALE: *This action minimizes bunching of the stocking on the client's foot, which constricts circulation.*

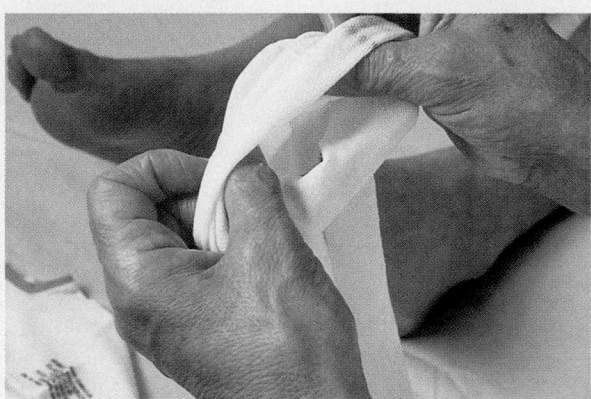

Grasp the stocking's heel and turn it inside out.

8. Slip the client's foot, toes, and heel into the stocking. Center the heel in the stocking's heel pocket. Slip the stocking opening over the toes, so that the toes are mostly exposed. Slide the stocking over the client's foot.
   RATIONALE: *Properly positioning of the stocking on the client's foot prevents injury.*

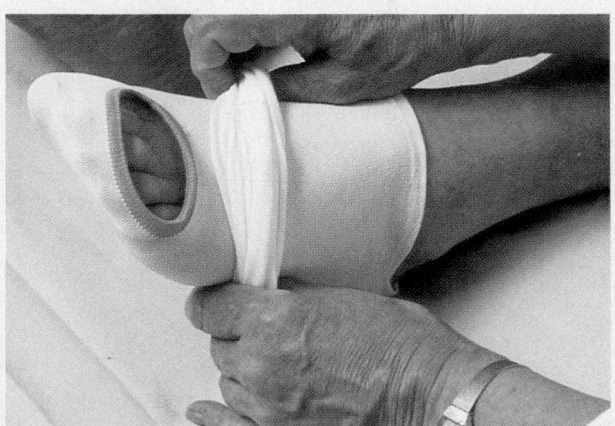

Putting the client's toes, foot, and heel into the stocking.

9. Support the client's ankle and ease the stocking smoothly over the calf and the remainder of the leg.
   RATIONALE: *Smooth application prevents the formation of wrinkles, which can impede circulation.*

(*continued*)

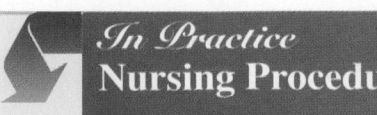

In Practice
Nursing Procedure 53-1 (*Continued*)

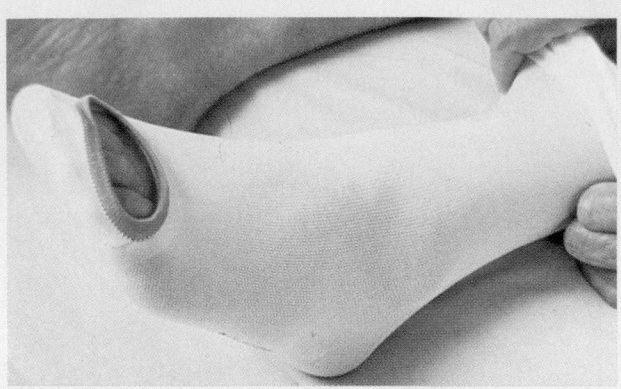

Easing the stocking over the calf.

10. Pull forward slightly on the stocking's toe section.
    RATIONALE: *Pulling forward eases pressure on the client's toes and nails.*

11. Instruct the client to report any extreme discomfort.
    RATIONALE: *Early reporting of complaints aids in preventing complications.*

12. Remove gloves (if worn) and wash the hands.
    RATIONALE: *Handwashing helps prevent the spread of infection.*

13. Document the procedure on the client's record.
    RATIONALE: *Documentation provides communication and ensures continuity of care.*

hold rectal or perineal dressings in place. The perineal strap is split through the middle to make a T-binder for a male client (Fig. 53-2).

When applying a T-binder, wear gloves. Place the band around the client's waist, bring the perineal strap between the legs, and fasten the band and the strip at the midline. Be sure the binder is tight enough to hold the dressings, but not so tight that it is uncomfortable.

Abdominal Binder

An *abdominal binder* is a wide, flat piece of fabric that is secured around the trunk of the client's body to support the abdomen or dressings on the abdomen. It may be used after abdominal surgery or childbirth. To apply the abdominal binder, place the center of the binder at the level of the client's waistline on his or her back. Wrap the ends of the binder snugly over the client's abdomen and secure it with the Velcro straps.

Tape

Instead of bandages and binders, sometimes strips of *hypoallergenic tape* are used to hold a client's dressings in place. Tape also may be used to give support, as for sprained ankles, fractured ribs, or fractured toes. Tape such as 3M Micropore tape allows ventilation and helps to prevent skin **maceration** (skin softening and breakdown due to moisture accumulation and lack of circulation).

Shave the client's skin (particularly on hairy body areas) before applying large tape dressings, because hairs stick to the tape and make removal painful. Always remove tape in the direction of hair growth for less discomfort. If tape is difficult to remove, carefully apply acetone to the skin at the edge of the applied strip to loosen the adhesion. Keep moistening the skin close to the adhesive as you gently peel off the tape.

In Practice
Nursing Care Guidelines 53-2

APPLYING A BINDER

- Wash the hands before and after applying or adjusting a binder. Use Standard Precautions. If the client's skin is intact, gloves are not necessary.
- Apply the binder firmly enough to give support, but not too tightly. *Rationale: If the dressing is not applied firmly in place, bleeding could occur, or the dressing's movement could irritate the area.*
- If using a binder to hold a client's body part in place, be sure it is firm enough to be effective. *Rationale: A binder that is too tight might cause unnecessary discomfort or constrict circulation. A binder that is too loose will not support or hold the body part in place.*
- Fasten the binder from the bottom up to give upward support. *Rationale: Applying it from the top down will exert downward pressure.*
- Be sure the binder is a size appropriate for the client. *Rationale: Using an incorrect size will not be effective.*
- Rewrap the binder every few hours. *Rationale: The client's movements tend to loosen the binder. When rewrapping the binder, assess the client's skin and check the dressing.*

Nursing Alert

Be careful with acetone and other substances used to remove tape adhesive. *Never* use these liquids near an open flame, the client's eyes, or on an open wound! Be alert that some clients may be allergic to acetone. Also, remember that acetone will remove nail polish, paint from surfaces, and may damage other surfaces.

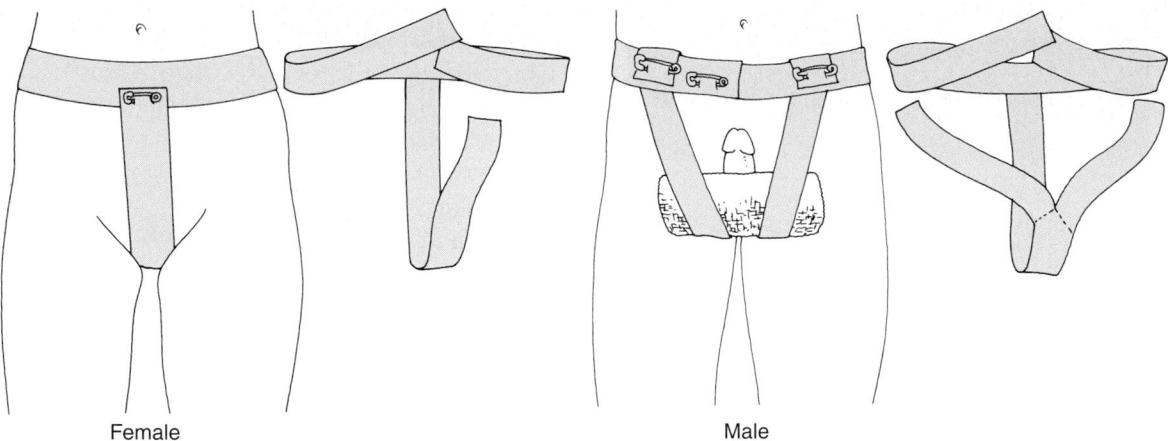

Female   Male

FIGURE 53-2. The T-binder may be adapted to use in the male or female client to hold dressings in place.

Montgomery Straps

Use *tape straps,* also called **Montgomery straps,** if frequent dressing changes are needed. These straps allow the dressing to be changed without having to remove tape from the client's skin with each change (Fig. 53-3). This measure helps prevent skin irritation in two ways: dressings are changed more often and more conveniently, and the tape remains in place, maintaining skin integrity.

The adhesive end of each strap is applied to the client's skin. The dressing is held in place by the nonadhesive end of each strap, which is tied, buckled, or fastened with Velcro to the other straps over the dressing. Change the dressing as often as needed without removing the tape from the skin each time. Use the steps at In Practice: Nursing Procedure 53-2 to apply Montgomery straps.

✚👁 N u r s i n g   A l e r t

If the client complains of pain or itching while any bandage is in place, assess the area immediately for bleeding, exudates, swelling, or changes in skin color. Report abnormalities to your supervisor immediately.

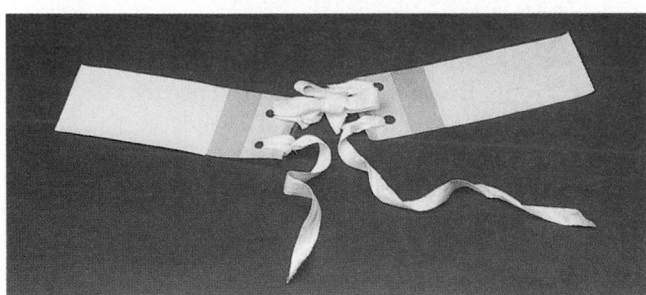

FIGURE 53-3. Commercially prepared Montgomery straps.

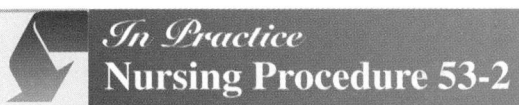

In Practice
Nursing Procedure 53-2

APPLYING MONTGOMERY STRAPS
Supplies and Equipment

Gloves
Dressing
Tape or adhesive-backed material and strings for ties, or commercially available Montgomery straps

Steps

1. Wash the hands. Wear gloves.
   RATIONALE: *Handwashing and using gloves reduce the risk of infection transmission. The soiled dressing is considered to be contaminated.*

2. Use Standard Precautions. Properly dispose of soiled dressings.
   RATIONALE: *Soiled dressings are highly contaminated and a source of many microorganisms.*

3. Cover the incision with the new dressing.
   RATIONALE: *Covering the incision helps keep the incision free of microorganisms.*

4. Use premade products, or make a strap by placing one half of the length of a wide strip of tape or adhesive-backed material to the skin. Fold the other half of the tape onto itself.
   RATIONALE: *Applying straps, either pre-made or nurse-made, allows for dressing changes without removing tape. Folding the tape onto itself creates a flap to secure ties.*

(continued)

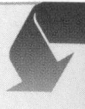

In Practice
Nursing Procedure 53-2
(Continued)

5. Repeat the above steps for the other side of the straps.

6. Cut holes into the ends of the straps if the adhesive-backed strip does not contain them.
   RATIONALE: *This allows strings to be inserted so that the straps can be pulled together to secure the dressing.*

7. Secure the ends of the straps with ties across the dressing or fasten the Velcro.
   RATIONALE: *Tying or fastening secures the dressing.*

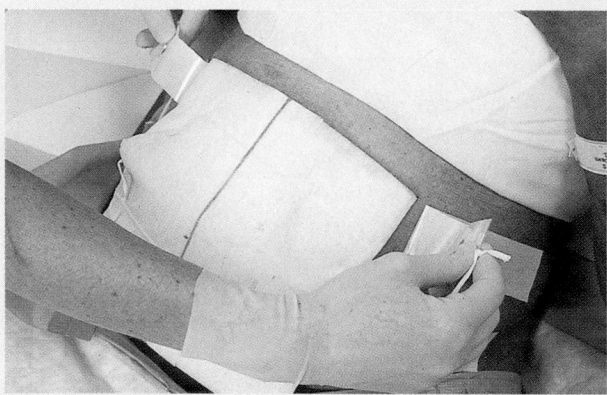

Using two sets of straps to secure a large, bulky dressing.

8. Use two or more sets of straps and ties for a large, bulky dressing.
   RATIONALE: *Two sets provide more support.*

9. Untie straps or unfasten for dressing changes.
   RATIONALE: *Untying the straps provides access to the contaminated dressing.*

10. Leave straps in place until they become soiled or need to be changed or removed.
    RATIONALE: *Leaving the straps in place until soiled or needing to be changed reduces the trauma to the skin from frequent removal.*

11. Dispose of contaminated dressings and carefully wash hands.
    RATIONALE: *Proper disposal of supplies and handwashing reduce the risk for cross-contamination.*

12. Document the procedure and condition of the wound on the client's record.
    RATIONALE: *Documentation provides communication about the presence of straps for future dressing changes and enhances continuity of care.*

➤ STUDENT SYNTHESIS

Key Points

- Elastic roller bandages may be used to encourage and support circulation after surgery. They are often used to support joints.
- Because elastic roller bandages apply direct pressure, they may be used to help control bleeding.
- When used, binders and bandages should be rewrapped every few hours. The client's skin should be assessed at this time.
- Antiembolism stockings should never be allowed to bunch or roll up. This could lead to constricting circulation in the leg.
- When applying antiembolism stockings or an elastic roller bandage to an extremity, even pressure is applied over the extremity.
- The client's CMS is checked frequently when bandages are used.
- Binders are used to supply support for specific body parts. Types of binders include T-binders and abdominal binders.
- When a client requires frequent dressing changes, Montgomery straps can be used to avoid repeated tape removal and subsequent skin irritation with each dressing change.

Critical Thinking Exercises

1. Describe five important elements for checking circulation when using bandages. Describe the significance of each element.
2. A female client has TED stockings in place. She has had a number of complaints during her stay in the facility and is now complaining that the TED stockings are "too tight." Describe your actions and reasoning.

NCLEX-Style Review Questions

1. What instruction is most important for the nurse to include after application of a binder or bandage to a client's extremity?
   a. Do not remove the bandage or binder.
   b. Keep clothing off the bandage or binder.
   c. Keep extremity elevated at all times.
   d. Notify the nurse if extreme pain occurs.
2. When evaluating the effects of a bandage, the nurse should monitor:
   a. Amount of drainage
   b. Circulation and nerve function
   c. Client's orientation level
   d. Temperature and respirations

3. Prior to applying antiembolic stockings, which action by the nurse is most important?
   a. Ensure that the client has been recumbent for at least 15 minutes.
   b. Gather supplies, including Kerlix dressings.
   c. Obtain a set of vital signs.
   d. Offer to medicate for pain because application of stockings is painful.

4. Elastic stockings should be removed every 8 hours to:
   a. Allow for increased venous return in the legs
   b. Ensure the client's comfort
   c. Examine the leg for redness, pitting edema, or skin discoloration
   d. Prevent the leg from becoming macerated

5. A client complains of itching while a bandage is in place. The nurse's first action should be:
   a. Administer anti-itch medication
   b. Apply cool compresses to the area
   c. Assess the area immediately
   d. Continue to monitor the client's condition

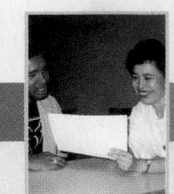

CHAPTER

54

Heat and Cold Applications

LEARNING OBJECTIVES

1. State at least three purposes of applying heat to the body; of applying cold to the body.
2. Explain specific precautions when applying heat; when applying cold.
3. Demonstrate the administration of a leg soak, a sitz bath, and the aquathermia pad.
4. Demonstrate the use of the cooling blanket and the application of an ice collar.

NEW TERMINOLOGY

aquathermia pad   sitz bath
hypothermia blanket   tepid sponge bath
icecap

ACRONYMS

IR   UV   WA
US

Some conditions benefit from the application of either heat or cold. Because complications can occur due to extreme heat or cold, the nurse must be knowledgeable to use these therapies safely and effectively.

HEAT

Heat causes *vasodilation* (enlargement of the blood vessels), which increases the amount of oxygen, nutrients, and white blood cells delivered to body tissues.

Rules for Application

Heat application serves the following purposes:

- Relieves local pain, stiffness, or aching, particularly of muscles and joints
- Assists in wound healing
- Reduces inflammation
- Makes the chilly client more comfortable
- Raises the body's temperature
- Promotes drainage (draws infected material out of wounds)

Because heat must be fairly intense to produce the desired effect, burns may result if heat is applied improperly or for too long. The application must be hot enough to accomplish its purpose, but within a safe temperature range. Remember that heat applied over a large area affords more warmth; however, the potential for injury is greater than that of heat applied over a small area. Protect the client from possible burn injury by observing safety precautions. In Practice: Nursing Care Guidelines 54-1 outlines steps for applying heat therapy.

Both dry heat and moist heat have local effects. Apply *dry heat* with a warm-water bag, waterproof water-filled heating pad (aquathermia pad), heat lamp, electric heat cradle, or electric heating pad.

Moist heat applications warm the skin more quickly and are more penetrating than applications of dry heat, because water is a better heat conductor than air. Apply moist heat with compresses, packs, or soaks, including the sitz bath. Sometimes wet compresses are used in combination with the aquathermia pad to provide longer-lasting moist heat. Skin maceration is a problem that may develop when moisture is applied directly to the skin for long periods. The client's skin may be protected by first applying a thin layer of petroleum jelly, if ordered. Limit application time. (The order typically specifies the length of time for the heat to be on and off. For example, apply moist compresses for 15 minutes every hour while awake.)

Specific Heat Therapies

Dry Heat

Aquathermia Pad. An **aquathermia** (Aqua-K) **pad,** which produces dry heat, is used to treat muscle sprains and mild inflammations, and for pain relief. Temperature-controlled distilled water flows through the waterproof pad. Apply the pad according to the physician's order. Check the pad to make sure it is heating properly and not overheating. Report any malfunctions to the facility's maintenance depart-

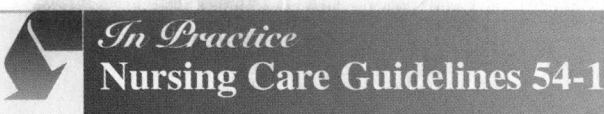

In Practice
Nursing Care Guidelines 54-1

APPLYING HEAT THERAPY

- Heat is only applied when specifically ordered by a physician and with the utmost caution. *Rationale: The nerves in the skin are numbed easily, and the client may not feel the pain of a burn, especially if heat has been applied often.*
- Specific body parts such as the eyelids, neck, and inside the arm are especially sensitive to heat.
- Each person has his or her own sensitivity to heat. Test each person for sensitivity before applying heat. *Rationale: Prior testing helps to determine how much heat is safe and for how long.*
- Infants, older people, and those with fair, thin skin have less heat resistance. Lowered body resistance due to illness also makes body tissues less resistant to heat. *Rationale: It is important to consider each client individually.*
- Clients who are unresponsive or anesthetized and those suffering from neurological disorders or dementia are at increased risk for injury from heat applications. *Rationale: These clients are unable to report that heat is too intense.*
- Impaired circulation and some metabolic diseases make people more susceptible to burns (eg, the client who is in shock or who has diabetes). *Rationale: Changes in body systems interfere with skin integrity and healing, and may impair the client's ability to identify discomfort.*
- Clients receiving radiation therapy or chemotherapy for cancer and those with any degree of paralysis are particularly susceptible to burns. *Rationale: Their immune system or skin integrity is already compromised.*
- Listen to the client. If he or she complains of pain or discomfort, stop the treatment and consult the team leader or primary care provider. *Rationale: Each client is different. Only the client can tell the nurse how the treatment feels.*

ment. In Practice: Nursing Procedure 54-1 reviews the steps in using an aquathermia pad.

Nursing Alert

When disassembling the aquathermia pad for return to the supply or equipment department:
- Unplug the unit before doing anything else to prevent shocks.
- Empty the water out of the pump unit and out of the pad and connecting tubes to prevent any leakage.
- Discard the pad because it is contaminated.
- Return only the heater/pump to the equipment department.
- Carefully wash hands.

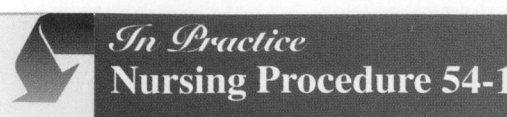

In Practice
Nursing Procedure 54-1

Usɪɴɢ ᴀɴ Aǫᴜᴀᴛʜᴇʀᴍɪᴀ Pᴀᴅ
Supplies and Equipment

Pad
Control unit
Cover for pad
Distilled water

Steps

1. Wash your hands. Make sure that the control unit is connected to the pad. Fill the control unit receptacle two-thirds full with distilled water.
   Rᴀᴛɪᴏɴᴀʟᴇ: *If the control unit is not connected, water will run out. Handwashing helps to prevent infection. Distilled water will not damage the unit as tap water might.*

2. Set the temperature control to 105° F (40.6° C).
   Rᴀᴛɪᴏɴᴀʟᴇ: *This temperature delivers heat to the area without burning it.*

3. Cover the pad with a pad cover, sheet, pillowcase, or towel.
   Rᴀᴛɪᴏɴᴀʟᴇ: *Covering the pad aids in protecting the client's skin.*

4. Plug the control unit into an electrical outlet, and place the control unit on the bedside table.
   Rᴀᴛɪᴏɴᴀʟᴇ: *The aquathermia pad requires electricity to heat the water.*

5. When the pad is heated, apply it to the specific body part, as ordered. The pad should rest on top of the body part in nearly all cases.
   Rᴀᴛɪᴏɴᴀʟᴇ: *Proper application ensures appropriate treatment.*

6. Use tape or a roller bandage to secure the pad in place. Do not use safety pins.

Rᴀᴛɪᴏɴᴀʟᴇ: *Pin-pricks can cause the pad to leak and possibly to short circuit.*

7. Instruct the client avoid lying directly on the pad (the pad should be on top of the body part to be treated). Instruct the client not to change the temperature settings on the control unit.
   Rᴀᴛɪᴏɴᴀʟᴇ: *Lying on top of the pad could lead to burns. Changing the settings could lead to burns if set too high, or to the treatment being ineffective if set too low.*

8. Place the call signal within the client's reach.
   Rationale: *The client must be able to get your attention if he or she is uncomfortable.*

9. Assess the area for redness after 5 min.
   Rᴀᴛɪᴏɴᴀʟᴇ: *Assessment after 5 min allows for followup evaluation and reduces the risk of possible burn injury.*

10. Remove the pad after the specified time for treatment, as ordered.
    Rᴀᴛɪᴏɴᴀʟᴇ: *Maintaining the therapy for the prescribed time enhances its effectiveness. Leaving the pad in place for too long reduces the effectiveness of the treatment and could lead to injury.*

11. Store the pad until the next treatment.
    Rᴀᴛɪᴏɴᴀʟᴇ: *Proper storage ensures ready availability.*

12. Wash the hands.
    Rᴀᴛɪᴏɴᴀʟᴇ: *Handwashing reduces the risk of infection transmission.*

13. Document the procedure on the client's record.
    Rᴀᴛɪᴏɴᴀʟᴇ: *Documentation provides communication and continuity of care.*

Heat Lamp Treatments and Ultrasound. Specially trained personnel give *heat lamp* and *ultrasound* treatments because these personnel must carefully regulate the client's exposure to light rays to prevent injury. The nurse working in a clinic may be trained to administer these treatments.

Infrared rays (**IR**) relax muscles, stimulate circulation, and relieve pain. They have the same effect on the body as other forms of dry heat. Ultraviolet rays (**UV**) are not as penetrating as infrared rays. Sunlight provides mild ultraviolet radiation; prolonged exposure to the sun, however, will burn sensitive skin. Ultraviolet rays are used to treat skin infections and wounds.

Ultrasound (**US**) is a method of applying deep, penetrating heat to muscles and tissues. The timer must be working correctly. A lubricating gel is applied to the client's skin and the ultrasound paddle or wand is kept moving at all times during the treatment to prevent burns.

The Heat Cradle. In rare instances, a *lamp, light bulb,* or special *heater* is mounted on the inside of a bed cradle (see Chap. 49) to provide dry heat. A physician must order this treatment and specify the time limits. (For example, the order may be written, "heat cradle 20 min. Q hr, **WA** [while awake]".) As with any heat application, monitoring the client closely is very important, to prevent burns. It is also important to closely observe the time limits as ordered. Some heat cradles have an automatic timer that shuts the lamp on and off at preset intervals.

Nᴜʀsɪɴɢ Aʟᴇʀᴛ
Do not perform any type of heat lamp treatment without a physician's order and special training in the use of the equipment.

Electric Heating Pad. An *electric heating pad* is a covered network of wires that emits heat when an electric current passes through it. Pads with a waterproof covering are the safest. Never put pins into a heating pad; if a pin touches the electric wires, it can cause shock. If wires are crushed or bent, the pad can overheat and cause burns or a fire. An electric heating pad can easily burn a client, particularly if he or she is older or has neurologic impairment that causes insensitivity to heat changes. Electric heating pads are unsafe to use with children, older adults, irrational and unresponsive persons, clients who are suicidal, or clients who have spinal cord injuries.

Healthcare facilities seldom use the dry electric heating pad because it poses many hazards. Some extended-care facilities occasionally use these pads. However, they are commonly used in the home. In Practice: Educating the Client 54-1 describes the safe use of electric heating pads at home.

Moist Heat

Warm, Moist Compresses and Packs. *Warm, moist compresses* and *packs* apply moist heat to an area to stimulate circulation, ease pain, and promote wound drainage. They may also be used to apply medications.

Warm, moist gauze compresses (such as 4×4 gauze pads) apply heat to a small area. Large warm, moist packs of cotton or terry cloth apply heat over a larger area. Covering the pack with heavy, dry material helps it retain heat longer. Application of an Aqua-K pad over a pack enables the pack to remain heated almost indefinitely. Compresses and packs do not need to be sterile, unless a client's skin is broken.

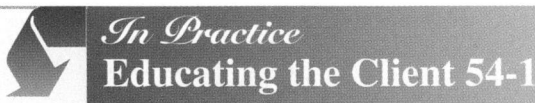

In Practice
Educating the Client 54-1

USING ELECTRIC HEATING PADS AT HOME

- Before applying the pad, connect it to an electric outlet and turn the heating switch to *high* to see whether the pad heats promptly. Then turn it off and disconnect it.
- Check to make sure the cord is intact and there are no frayed wires near the plug. If there is any question, do not use the pad.
- Never use safety pins or water near a heating pad.
- Cover the pad and connect it to an outlet.
- Adjust the pad to *low* temperature and apply it over the body part; do not lie on it.
- Inspect the skin frequently, to prevent burning.
- Leave the setting on *low* at all times.
- Only use the pad for the length of time specified by the primary care provider.
- Make sure there is nobody in the home who might become entangled with the cord. (This includes children, persons who are confused, or those who are suicidal.)

The primary care provider prescribes the type of application, where it is to be applied, and the length of time it is to be left in place. The order also includes the solution to use. Most often, the solution is water, a mild antiseptic solution (such as 2% boric acid), or normal saline.

The pack should be as hot as the client can comfortably tolerate. Apply it slowly so that the client can tell you how the pack feels. The client is the best judge of his or her own comfort. During the procedure, the client may feel chilly, so take precautions to keep the person warm and protected from drafts.

Sometimes, you will need to apply a warm compress to a client's eye. The eyelid and the skin around the eye are thin and delicate structures, easily prone to injury. In this situation, use tepid water, not hot water. Use caution to prevent burning the client's eyelid and skin. Wash your hands carefully and wear clean gloves before applying eye compresses, because the eye is highly susceptible to infection. If the eye is draining, discard each compress when you remove it. Send all reusable equipment for sterilization after the treatment. If applying compresses to both eyes, use separate equipment and wear new gloves for each eye to prevent spreading infection from one eye to the other.

To apply warm, moist compresses and packs to all body parts, follow the general rules as outlined at In Practice: Nursing Procedure 54-2.

Warm Soaks. Another method for applying moist heat consists of immersing the client's affected body part in warm water or a solution for a prescribed time. This procedure is called a *soak*. The following are reasons for giving a *warm soak*:

- Improves circulation
- Increases blood supply to an infected area
- Assists in breaking down infected tissue
- Applies medications
- Cleans draining wounds
- Loosens scabs and crusts from encrusted wounds

Often, a soak may be combined with a whirlpool bath. This is commonly done in the physical therapy department.

Although the tub is usually not sterilized between clients, it must be cleaned thoroughly with soap, disinfectant, and water, per agency protocol. Persons receiving soaks often have open wounds. Therefore, thorough cleaning of the tub helps prevent the spread of infection between clients. Use tap water for soaks unless otherwise specified. A detergent (such as Dreft) or other substance (such as colloidal oatmeal) may be added to the water.

The temperature of the water should be no higher than 105° Fahrenheit (40.5° Celsius). The physician may prescribe a definite temperature. Test the water's temperature frequently, and add hot water slowly, to prevent burning the client. Stir the water to distribute the heat evenly. The usual length of a soak is 15 to 20 minutes. Follow the steps at In Practice: Nursing Procedure 54-3 for giving an arm or leg soak.

Sitz Bath. The purpose of a **sitz bath** (use of a tub or basin filled with warm water) is to provide moist heat to the pelvic or perineal and perianal area. Commercial sitz bath tubs or seats are available. Disposable-type sitz basins are com-

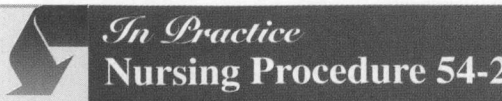

In Practice
Nursing Procedure 54-2

APPLYING WARM, MOIST COMPRESSES AND PACKS
Supplies and Equipment

Compress or pack
Dry pack and moisture-proof cover, if ordered
Hot-pack machine or forceps
Petroleum jelly (petrolatum)
Aquathermia pad
Gloves, if necessary

Steps

1. Wash your hands. Wear gloves if there is a break in your skin or the client's skin.
   RATIONALE: *Handwashing and using gloves help to prevent the spread of infection.*

2. Use a hot-pack machine set at the proper temperature.
   RATIONALE: *Using the hot-pack machine ensures a particular temperature. Because it has an attached wringer, you do not have to wring out the pack by hand. Otherwise, immerse the compress or pack in hot tap water (or heat the pack in a microwave for a one-time application).*

3. Apply petroleum jelly to the client's skin before applying the pack.
   RATIONALE: *The petroleum jelly protects the client's skin from prolonged moisture.*

4. Wring the compress or pack with forceps or wringer, removing as much water as possible.
   RATIONALE: *Hot water dripping on the client's skin could cause a burn. To wring out a pack with forceps, clamp one forcep onto each end of the pack and twist them in opposite directions.*

5. Shake the pack lightly, and apply it to the area gently at first, gradually pressing it against the skin.
   RATIONALE: *Shaking the pack cools it a little. Because air is a poor heat conductor, eliminating air spaces between the compress or pack and skin makes the treatment more effective.*

6. Ask the client if the pack is too hot. If so, remove it and shake it in the air briefly to lower its temperature.
   RATIONALE: *Applying a compress or pack that is too hot will burn the client's skin.*

7. Cover the moist compress or pack with a dry pack and moisture-proof cover.
   RATIONALE: *Covering the pack insulates against heat loss and moisture evaporation. Omit this step if using the aquathermia pad.*

8. Change the pack as often as necessary to keep the area heated.
   RATIONALE: *Keeping the pack warm for the specified time helps to ensure that the therapeutic effect is achieved. Small compresses cool more quickly than large packs. Use an aquathermia pad on top of the large warm, moist pack to keep it warm, if ordered.*

9. Assess the condition of the client's skin at least every 10 min.
   RATIONALE: *Continued exposure to heat and moisture can cause skin breakdown.*

10. Continue treatment for the prescribed time, and then remove the application. Use packs for one client only. Discard them after removal or save them to use again for that same client.
    RATIONALE: *Maintaining the application for the ordered time enhances the effectiveness of the treatment; proper use, disposal, and cleaning of equipment minimizes the risk for infection transmission.*

11. Dry the skin and cover it, as ordered. Be sure to wipe off any excess petrolatum.
    RATIONALE: *Drying the skin and covering the area prevent chilling. Drying also helps to reduce the risk of maceration when the skin is then covered.*

12. Wash the hands. Document the treatment on the client's chart, noting the client's reaction.
    RATIONALE: *Handwashing helps to minimize the risk of infection transmission. Documentation provides communication and continuity of care.*

---

monly used for maternity clients and clients who have undergone rectal or perineal surgery. The basin fits on the inside of the commode and is equipped with a bag, tubing, and nozzle to allow water to flow freely to the perineal area (Fig. 54-1). If no sitz bath is available or if the client is at home, the client can be placed in a regular bathtub containing enough water to cover the client's hips and perineum. In Practice: Nursing Procedure 54-4 describes the use of the portable sitz bath. If a disposable commode basin is used, adapt the procedure to include the following:

- Place the sitz bath on the commode seat and fill the reservoir with warm water at 100° to 105° F (38° to 41° C), as measured with a bath thermometer. Hang the reservoir at a height that will allow the water to flow from it through the tubing and into the basin.

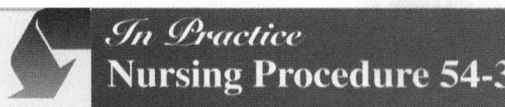

In Practice
Nursing Procedure 54-3

ADMINISTERING AN ARM OR LEG SOAK
Supplies and Equipment

Towel
Gloves
Bath thermometer
Sheet or bath blanket
Sterile dressing
Detergent or other substance as ordered

Steps

1. Cover the tub with a bath towel.
   RATIONALE: *Using a towel pads the tub to prevent bruises.*

2. Cover the client with a protective sheet or bath blanket.
   RATIONALE: *Covering the client protects the client's privacy and prevents chilling.*

3. Prepare the water in the tub (100° to 105° F [37.8° to 40.6° C], unless otherwise specified). Always use a bath thermometer.
   RATIONALE: *Proper temperature prevents burns.*

4. Wear gloves. Remove the dressing from the client's wound, if present. Dispose of the dressing in the prescribed manner.
   RATIONALE: *Wearing gloves and proper disposal help to prevent cross-contamination and spread of infection.*

5. Gradually lower the client's affected body part into the water.

RATIONALE: *Gradually lowering the body part into the water allows the part to adjust to the water temperature and avoids burns and discomfort.*

6. Adjust the padding on the edge of the tub for the knee or elbow to rest on; support the body part with a folded pillow if necessary.
   RATIONALE: *Proper padding and support prevent injury to extremities.*

7. Test the water's temperature frequently with a bath thermometer. Add hot water carefully as needed, and stir the water.
   RATIONALE: *Adding hot water and stirring help to maintain the proper temperature, which promotes vasodilation.*

8. Remove the client's arm or leg from the bath in 15–20 min, or as ordered. Dry the client's skin.
   RATIONALE: *Adhering to the prescribed time limit enhances the treatment's effectiveness and reduces the risk of injury.*

9. Apply a sterile dressing to the wound, if a wound is present. In the case of a draining wound, equipment must be thoroughly sanitized after use. In some cases, disposable tubs are available for use with a single client. Properly dispose of gloves.
   RATIONALE: *Covering the wound and properly caring for equipment after treatment help prevent spread of infection.*

10. Document the treatment and the client's reactions.
    RATIONALE: *Documentation provides communication and continuity of care.*

- Assist the client to sit on the basin. Be sure that the client has a robe or blankets to put over the shoulders to prevent chilling, and that the call signal is within the client's reach.
- Have the client use the clamp on the tubing to regulate the flow of water.
- Assist the client out of the sitz bath and help him or her to dry the buttocks.
- Carefully wash the hands and document the procedure.

COLD

Cold causes *vasoconstriction* (shrinkage of blood vessels), which decreases the amount of blood flow to an area, slowing the body's metabolism and its demand for oxygen. The therapeutic results are controlling hemorrhage, reducing edema, easing inflammation, and blocking pain receptors.

Rules for Application

Cold application prevents escape of heat from the body by slowing circulation, which also relieves congestion and often relieves muscle pain. A cold application commonly serves the following purposes:

- Slows or stops bleeding
- Slows bacterial activity in clients with an infection
- Relieves pain following some types of surgery, tooth extraction, headache, or muscle or joint injury
- Prevents peristalsis in clients with abdominal inflammation
- Relieves pain in engorged breasts
- Reduces swelling in injured tissues, including sprains and fractures
- Controls pain and fluid loss in the initial treatment of burns

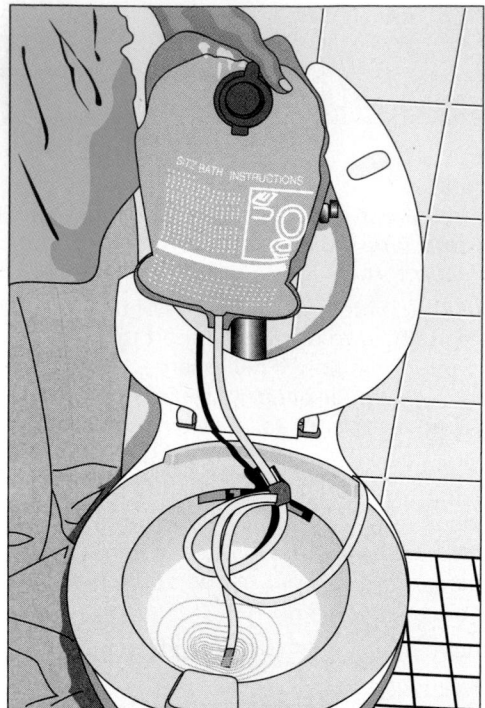

FIGURE 54-1. A disposable sitz bath that fits inside a commode. The warm water from the bag flows through the tubing and into the basin to provide a constant stream of warm water to the area.

Cold application is more effective than heat for sprains or other soft tissue injuries. You may apply cold to prevent swelling (*edema*); however, cold application will not reduce edema that is already present. Methods of *cold application* include the use of a compress, icecap, ice collar, ice pack, sponge bath, and hypothermia (cooling) blanket. In Practice: Nursing Care Guidelines 54-2 lists some important considerations when applying cold therapy.

Specific Cold Therapies

Cold, Moist Compresses

Apply *cold, moist compresses* to reduce swelling and inflammation in soft tissue injuries or after tooth extraction. The size of the compress depends on the area to be treated. Gauze 4×4's are frequently used as cold, moist compresses for tooth pain. Change compresses frequently, because they warm rapidly, thereby losing their effectiveness. In Practice: Nursing Care Guidelines 54-3 highlights important information about applying cold compresses.

Icecap or Ice Collar

An **icecap** is a round, flat rubber bag with a leakproof, screw-in top. The icecap has a wide opening that allows it to be filled easily with ice chunks. An *ice collar* is a narrow rubber or plastic bag, curved to fit the neck. A physician prescribes the

---

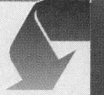

In Practice
Nursing Procedure 54-4

USING A SITZ BATH

Supplies and Equipment

Sitz bath tub
Bath towels
Cotton bath blanket
Bath thermometer

Steps

1. Make sure the sitz tub is clean or is to be used by only one client. Use gloves when cleaning it.
   RATIONALE: *If several clients will use the sitz tub, it must be sanitized between uses. Use the solution and methods as directed by the facility.*

2. Check the order. The physician will prescribe the length of the treatment, which is usually 15–30 min.
   RATIONALE: *Performing the sitz bath for the prescribed length of time promotes effectiveness of treatment.*

3. Fill the sitz tub to the required depth, with water of the specified temperature. The client's body will displace water in proportion to size.
   RATIONALE: *An adequate depth of water is needed to achieve therapeutic effect.*

4. Place a large bath towel in the bottom of the sitz tub. If needed, place the drain adapter in place, so that the sitz tub drains continuously.
   RATIONALE: *The towel makes the sitz tub more comfortable and easier to clean.*

5. Help the client onto the sitz tub, with the client sitting far enough forward to avoid occluding the drain. A short client may need a stool under his or her feet.
   RATIONALE: *The stool prevents pressure on the legs' blood vessels. Place a folded towel in the lumbar area. Rationale: This towel supports the back and keeps the client's body in good alignment.*

6. Cover the upper and lower part of the client's body with a cotton bath blanket.
   RATIONALE: *Covering the client prevents chilling and protects the person from drafts.*

7. Set the water temperature gauge on the faucet to maintain the required temperature. Adjust the water supply and drain to maintain a constant water circulation.
   RATIONALE: *Water of the correct temperature is the most therapeutic and safest.*

(continued)

In Practice
Nursing Procedure 54-4 (Continued)

8. Use a bath thermometer. If the aim of the sitz bath is to apply heat, start the temperature at 95° F (35° C) and gradually increase it to a maximum of 105° F (40.5° C). If giving the sitz bath to cleanse and promote healing, maintain the bath temperature from 94° F to 98° F (34.4° to 36.6° C).
   RATIONALE: *Extremely hot temperatures may damage skin tissues, rather than promote their healing. Sitz tubs in many facilities are set so that the temperature can not exceed 105° F.*

9. Watch the client closely for signs of fainting or weakness.
   RATIONALE: *Heat promotes vasodilation, drawing blood away from the brain.*

10. Help the client out of the sitz bath after the specified time of treatment. Assist the client with drying.
    RATIONALE: *Vasodilation could cause the person to feel faint when standing or walking.*

11. Help the client to bed after the bath.

    RATIONALE: *Heat applied to a large area of the body may make the client feel weak or faint because blood is drawn away from the brain. Resting in bed allows the client's circulation to return to normal.*

12. Cover the client adequately.
    RATIONALE: *Covering the client protects him or her from drafts and chilling.*

13. While wearing gloves, clean the sitz tub, according to the agency's policy for the client's specific condition. If the sitz tub is to be used for only one client, be sure it is labeled with the client's name.
    RATIONALE: *Proper cleaning after client use reduces the risk of cross-contamination.*

14. Wash the hands.
    RATIONALE: *Handwashing helps to prevent transmission of microorganisms.*

15. Document the treatment on the client's chart, noting the client's reactions.
    RATIONALE: *Documentation provides communication and continuity of care.*

application of an icecap or ice collar to a specific part of the body. However, an icecap can be applied for a headache or in an emergency, such as a sprain or nosebleed, without an order. In Practice: Nursing Procedure 54-5 gives steps to follow in applying an icecap or ice collar.

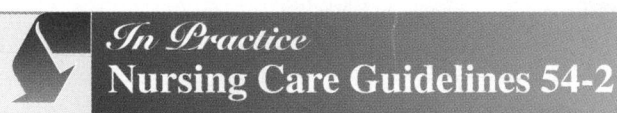

In Practice
Nursing Care Guidelines 54-2

APPLYING COLD THERAPY

- Client complaints of numbness in the area of the cold application—with the skin appearing white or spotty—indicate the need to discontinue the application. *Rationale: Cold numbs nerve endings.*
- As cold decreases the flow of blood in one area of the body, flow increases to other areas. (This explains why cold or chilling drafts striking the body often cause congestion in the nasal passages.)
- Continued application of cold affects deeper tissues. Prolonged exposure to extreme cold may cause actual freezing (*frostbite*).
- Cold often is applied to a sprain, strain, fracture, or burn. *Rationale: This helps to remove blood and lymph congestion in the area and reduces pain.*

Single-Use and Refreezable Ice Packs
Many healthcare agencies and emergency services provide ready-for-use frozen ice packs filled with a solution. These ice packs also are used by sports teams, hikers, and organizations such as the Boy Scouts or Girl Scouts. Generally, these can be reused, but only for one client. Ice packs are also available for one-time emergency use. They have a capsule that, when broken, releases a chemical that causes the bag to become cold. Some gel-filled packs also are available. These packs can be either frozen or heated and used as either a cold or hot pack. These packs are reusable.

Nursing Alert
Many ice bags, particularly ones with the capsule, become *very* cold. They can cause frostbite fairly quickly. Therefore, use extreme caution when applying cold. If the client's skin becomes blanched or extremely red, discontinue treatment immediately and check with the supervisor.

Tepid Sponge Bath
A **tepid sponge bath** is a bath with water below body temperature, usually in the range of 70° to 85° F (21.1° to 29.4° C). This type of bath may be ordered to reduce a client's elevated temperature. The first effect of this water on the skin is blood vessel constriction. Do not use alcohol because it cools too much (it evaporates very quickly).

A tepid sponge bath may be temporarily soothing, but it may not produce a marked temperature drop unless it is used

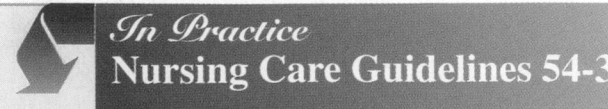

In Practice
Nursing Care Guidelines 54-3

APPLYING COLD COMPRESSES

- Wear gloves if the client has an open wound or has had surgery. *Rationale: Using gloves, if indicated, helps to prevent infection transmission.*
- Put the compresses in a basin containing pieces of ice and a small amount of water. *Rationale: Water soaks and cools the compresses faster than plain ice does.*
- Explain to the client that the treatment will relieve discomfort. *Rationale: A relaxed client will feel relief sooner than a tense client.*
- Wring the compresses thoroughly and apply. *Rationale: If ice water drips, it may startle the client.*
- Change compresses frequently. *Rationale: Compresses warm rapidly as they absorb body heat.*
- Continue the treatment as ordered, usually for 15–20 min. Repeat every 2–4 hours as ordered. Clients who are able can apply the compresses themselves. *Rationale: Applying the cold application for the specified time promotes effectiveness of the treatment.*
- Properly dispose of gloves, if used, and wash the hands. Document treatment on the client's chart, noting duration and the client's reaction. *Rationale: Proper glove disposal and handwashing help to prevent infection transmission. Documentation promotes communication and continuity of care.*

for an extended period. The minimum time is about 30 minutes. If elevated temperature is a threat to the client's life, other treatments are used to bring the temperature within a manageable range more quickly and permanently. In conditions associated with a dangerously high temperature, an *ice mattress* or *hypothermia blanket* (described below) often is used.

Tepid sponge baths are inadvisable for older people with inelastic arteries, clients with arthritis or lowered resistance to disease, and very young children, because of the water's initial effect on depressing body systems. See In Practice: Nursing Care Guidelines 54-4 for further information.

✚👁 **N u r s i n g   A l e r t**

Constantly assess the client's core body temperature with an electronic thermometer during the sponge bath. If the client begins to shiver or if the core temperature falls to within 1.5° F of normal, discontinue the treatment and report the findings to the supervisor.

Hypothermia Blanket

A **hypothermia blanket** (cooling blanket) is a plastic mattress pad through which very cold water flows continuously. Its role is to decrease body temperature. Hypothermia blankets are used primarily in surgery to slow body processes and to prevent complications resulting from unstable temperature regulation. They are also used in cases of extremely high body temperatures that are uncontrollable with medications. These blankets are equipped with electrical control units that can be set to the desired temperature. When using a hypothermia blanket, follow the agency's protocol and the primary care provider's orders. Check frequently to make sure that the client's core temperature is not too low.

In Practice
Nursing Procedure 54-5

APPLYING AN ICECAP OR ICE COLLAR
Supplies and Equipment

Icecap or ice collar
Basin of chipped ice (do not use whole ice cubes)
Paper tape or cloth ties
Bath blanket (if needed)

Steps

1. Wash your hands.
   RATIONALE: *Handwashing reduces the risk of infection transmission.*
2. Inspect the bag's stopper or closure and test the bag for leakage.
   RATIONALE: *Leaks cause the bedclothes to become wet, chilling the client and causing discomfort.*

3. Fill the icecap or collar about three-fourths full, using small pieces of ice.
   RATIONALE: *The bag will fit closely to the body and provide better cooling if the ice pieces are small.*
4. Flatten the bag on a hard surface, and press on it to expel air.
   RATIONALE: *A flat icecap or ice collar is easier to fit to the body.*
5. Screw on the top or fold over the end, making sure that the top is firmly in place and secured. These bags may be closed with hook-and-loop fasteners (Velcro).
   RATIONALE: *Proper closure of the bag or collar prevents leakage as ice melts.*
6. Dry the icecap or collar and cover it with a towel, securing the towel with tape.

(continued)

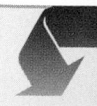
RATIONALE: *Drying prevents moisture from condensing on the outside of the bag, which would make the client uncomfortable.*

7. Adjust the bag on the part of body to be treated.

8. Leave the icecap or collar in place for 15–20 min. Wait 1 hour before reapplying it, unless directed otherwise.
   RATIONALE: *Prolonged application of cold reverses the full beneficial effects and may cause tissue damage. Ice melts in this time as well.*

9. Wash your hands after applying the icecap or ice collar and after removing it.
   RATIONALE: *Handwashing reduces the risk of infection transmission.*

10. Document the treatment on the client's chart, noting "on" and "off" periods and the client's reactions.
    RATIONALE: *Documentation provides communication and continuity of care.*

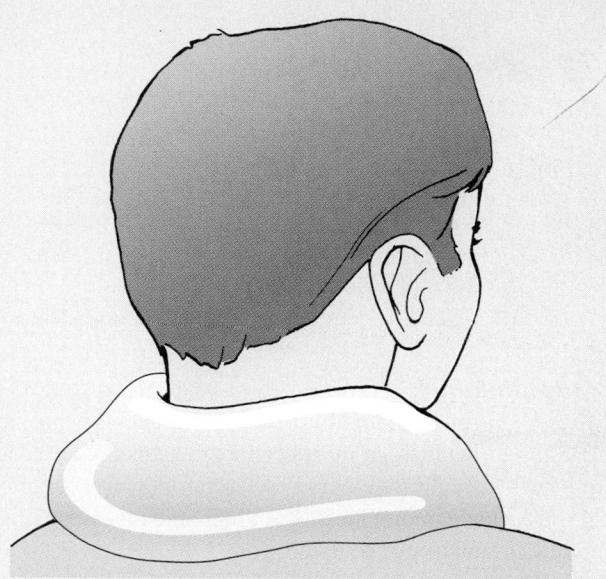

An ice collar applied to the neck.

GIVING A TEPID SPONGE BATH TO REDUCE BODY TEMPERATURE

- Explain the procedure to the client. *Rationale: The bath is less likely to be effective if a client is nervous or fearful.*
- Give the client an opportunity to use a urinal or bedpan before the bath. *Rationale: The client will be more comfortable. You also want to avoid having to stop and restart the bath.*
- Take the client's temperature and record it. *Rationale: The baseline temperature can guide the treatment. Continued monitoring of the client's temperature during the procedure is required, to prevent overcooling.*
- Note whether the client has had an antipyretic to reduce fever. *Rationale: Such medications may influence the sponge bath's effectiveness.*
- Add tepid water to the bath basin (70° to 85° F or 21.1° to 29.4° C). Use a thermometer to test. *Rationale: Temperatures in these ranges are below normal body temperature, so they will be effective in lowering the client's temperature. They are not so cold, however, as to be dangerous.*
- Place moist, cool cloths—wrung out just enough to prevent dripping—in the client's axillae and the groin. *Rationale: The blood vessels in these areas lie close to the skin. Water evaporation there will cool the body efficiently.*

- Be aware that the client's first reaction to a tepid sponge bath is a sensation of chilliness, which disappears as the body adjusts to the water's temperature. Therefore, continue the bath long enough to allow for this adjustment (at least 25–30 min). Monitor the client's body temperature throughout the procedure to determine the treatment's effects. *Rationale: Temperature monitoring provides objective data about the effectiveness of the bath, thus helping to prevent reducing the client's core temperature too much. Remember that temperature will continue to drop after the bath.*
- Sponge each limb for at least 5 min and the back and buttocks for at least 10–15 min. *Rationale: Sponging for this length of time is necessary for fever reduction.*
- Stop the procedure if the client becomes very chilled or begins to shiver. *Rationale: People respond to treatments differently. Stopping the procedure—due to complaints of chilling or evidence of shivering—prevents possible hypothermia.*
- Stop sponging as soon as the client's temperature approaches the normal range (about 100° F or 38.7° C, orally). Give the client a bath blanket.

(*continued*)

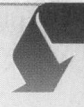

In Practice
Nursing Care Guidelines 54-4 (*Continued*)

Rationale: The client's temperature will continue to drop after the bath is completed. Stopping the bath when the client's temperature is still above normal body temperature prevents it from dropping too low.

- Wash the hands. Document the treatment on the client's chart, noting his or her reactions. Be sure to record the beginning and ending temperatures on the graph sheet. Keep a separate temperature record during the procedure as well. *Rationale: Handwashing helps to prevent infection transmission. Recording the client's responses to treatment is vital, especially if the procedure needs to be repeated.*

- Take the client's temperature 30 min after you complete the bath. *Rationale: The body takes about 25–30 min to fully respond to cold applications.*

Cold Humidity

Cold humidity is commonly ordered for clients who have breathing difficulties. In most healthcare agencies, air conditioning and heating systems provide a constant level of humidity. But if the humidity level is not high enough, an auxiliary humidifier may be placed in the room.

Some clients need constant cold humidity in high concentrations. A child may be placed in a *croupette* or a *humidity (mist) tent*. Oxygen administered to all clients must be humidified to prevent drying of the mucous membranes of the nose and throat. If the client has a tracheostomy, a "trach mask" may be placed over the opening to provide humidity, either with or without auxiliary oxygen. A *face tent* is also available, which may be used to provide a high concentration of moisture in the inhaled air.

⇨ STUDENT SYNTHESIS

Key Points

- Heat dilates surface blood vessels.
- Whenever heat is applied, take measures to protect the client from possible burn injury.
- Warm, moist applications heat the skin more quickly than dry heat applications.
- Water temperature for a soak should be no higher than 105° F (41° C).
- A sitz bath applies heat and water to the pelvic or perineal and perianal area.
- Cold constricts surface blood vessels.
- Cold, moist compresses are applied to small body parts.
- A tepid sponge bath may be used to reduce a client's body temperature.
- Several different pieces of equipment may be used to administer heat or cold treatments.

Critical Thinking Exercises

1. Describe how you would teach a client to use an electric heating pad at home.

2. Using heat or cold, how would you treat localized aching in an extremity? A muscle sprain? A headache? A fever? Why?

NCLEX-Style Review Questions

1. When applying moist heat, which approach should the nurse use?
   a. Always use sterile compresses and equipment.
   b. Apply the treatment for 1 hour.
   c. First, apply a protective layer of petroleum jelly.
   d. Set the heat setting at 110° Fahrenheit.

2. Which technique should be used when performing an ultrasound treatment?
   a. Apply lubricating gel to the client's skin.
   b. Hold the paddle in one place for 30 seconds before moving to another area.
   c. Instruct the client to perform the treatment.
   d. Perform the treatment until the client complains of tingling on the skin.

3. The physician orders a tub soak for a client for 30 minutes at 110° Fahrenheit. Which action should the nurse take?
   a. Administer the bath as ordered.
   b. Question the order with the physician, due to the possibility of burning the client.
   c. Request that someone else provide the bath.
   d. Set the temperature setting at 105° Fahrenheit.

4. Which of the following treatments would be most appropriate for a maternity client who has just delivered a baby and has an episiotomy?
   a. Aqua-K pad to the perineum
   b. Electric pad to the perineum
   c. Sitz bath to the perineum
   d. Warm compress to the perineum

5. To reduce a fever, a tepid sponge bath should be used for approximately:
   a. 5 minutes
   b. 10 minutes
   c. 15 minutes
   d. 30 minutes

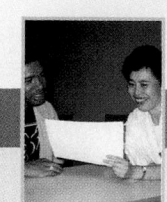

Client Comfort and Pain Management

LEARNING OBJECTIVES

1. Identify at least three causes of pain.
2. Differentiate between the two major types of pain.
3. Discuss the impact of chronic pain on a person's life and family.
4. Describe the function of endorphins in pain management.
5. Identify important nursing considerations for assessing pain.
6. Explain the role of analgesics in pain management.
7. Name three different classes of analgesics, including the specific uses for each.
8. Describe how surgery can provide comfort and pain relief.
9. List and describe at least five physical and cognitive–behavioral measures that can be used to complement pharmacologic pain management.

NEW TERMINOLOGY

acute pain
analgesics
chronic pain
cue
endorphins
guided imagery

intractable pain
neuropathic pain
nociception
nociceptive pain
pain threshold
pain tolerance

ACRONYMS

NSAIDs   PCA   TENS

Pain is the body's signal of distress that cannot be ignored. It is one of the most common reasons that people seek healthcare. People try many remedies to relieve pain, often without success. Relieving pain and providing comfort are common and ongoing nursing challenges.

PAIN

Pain is difficult to define. A noted pain theorist, Margo McCaffery, states in her classic writing that "Pain is whatever the experiencing person says it is, existing whenever he says it does."[1] In its clinical practice guidelines for acute pain management, the Agency for Health Care Policy and Research (AHCPR) states that the client's self-report is the single best indicator of pain.[2] Pain is the body's way of signaling that something is wrong.

Causes of Pain

The person in pain seeks relief from discomfort. Providing relief and comfort through medication administration and various other interventions is an important nursing responsibility.

Determining the pain's cause is key so that effective treatment may begin as soon as possible. The causes of pain vary, and sometimes a definite cause may be difficult to determine. Regardless of the cause, nursing care is directed at relieving pain.

The term used to describe normal pain transmission and interpretation is **nociception.** It has four phases:

* *Transduction:* The nervous system changes painful stimuli in the nerve endings to impulses.
* *Transmission:* The impulses travel from their original site to the brain.
* *Perception:* The brain recognizes, defines, and responds to pain.
* *Modulation:* The body activates needed inhibitory responses to the effects of pain.[3]

Several factors can initiate the pain response. Physical causes include trauma, injury, surgical incision, and tumor growth. Poor nutrition, metabolic factors, and temperature extremes may also influence pain.

Muscle spasms and resulting decreased blood supply to muscles can cause pain. As oxygen supply to muscles decreases, discomfort increases. As discomfort increases, the body's natural response is to tighten muscles further. Fatigue, fear of the unknown, and lack of knowledge about pain management can cause further muscle tightening. A cycle of pain can follow (Fig. 55-1).

Types of Pain

Acute Pain

Acute pain is a sensation that results abruptly. It lasts for only a short period of time, typically 6 months or less. Acute pain results from the nervous system's normal processing of

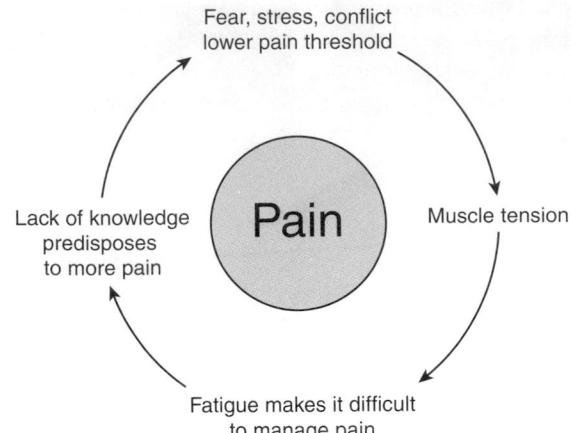

FIGURE 55-1. The pain cycle and some factors affecting it.

trauma to the skin, muscles, and visceral organs. Another term for acute pain is **nociceptive pain.** After the underlying cause is identified and treated, acute pain disappears. Common causes of acute pain are cuts, sore throat, and surgery.

Chronic Pain

Chronic pain (also called **neuropathic pain**) is discomfort that continues for a long period (6 months or longer). Often chronic pain interferes with a person's normal functioning. This type of pain sometimes lasts for life. It results when the nervous system abnormally processes sensory input. Neuropathic pain syndromes are difficult to treat, and the exact mechanisms involved are not yet fully understood. This pain continues beyond what would be expected to be a normal healing period for acute pain. Individuals with neuropathic type of pain report burning, tingling sensations, and shooting pain. Customary interventions for relieving such pain may be ineffective; more aggressive measures are usually necessary. The term used for chronic pain that resists therapeutic interventions is **intractable pain.** This type of pain also can have a known cause, such as an inoperable, invasive tumor.

Chronic pain can be destructive to a person's lifestyle and outlook, especially if the cause is unknown. The person's reaction may be frustration and anger; however, the person may find that expressing these feelings is difficult because family and friends are unresponsive or do not seem to understand. Or the person may fear worrying loved ones, and thus may avoid talking about the pain. The more anger and anxiety the client feels, the more difficult the pain and frustration may become. The client may even begin to feel that no one else believes the pain is real.

When a person fails to express feelings, suppressed anger may turn inward and cause depression. Symptoms of depression include extreme fatigue, inability to sleep, lack of interest in surroundings, lack of or excessive appetite, guilt feelings, sexual impotence, and withdrawal from social activities (see Chap. 93). Persons with depression suffer from lack of self-esteem and may feel worthless or burdensome to others. Severe depression, particularly when combined with chronic pain, can contribute to substance abuse and dependency and possibly suicide.

Continued chronic pain may cause a person to withdraw socially and to become physically inactive. Inactivity aggravates pain because muscles and joints stiffen and begin to deteriorate.

When working with clients, try to recognize those who are experiencing chronic pain as early as possible. Help them and the healthcare team to take aggressive steps toward treatment. Attempt to identify factors that worsen pain because each factor that worsens pain intensifies the pain cycle (Table 55-1).

Aim interventions at breaking the cycle of pain. Treat symptoms surrounding the pain, because it may be difficult to identify the exact cause of the pain. Focus treatment on raising the client's self-esteem and helping him or her to deal with feelings of anger, guilt, and frustration. In Practice: Educating the Client 55-1 lists helpful tips for chronic pain management.

☛ KEY CONCEPT
_____

If a client feels pain, the pain is real.

Factors Affecting Pain Perception

A person's **pain threshold** is the "lowest intensity of a stimulus that causes the subject to recognize pain."[4] **Pain tolerance** denotes the point at which a person can no longer endure pain (see Fig. 55-2).

The body has internal mechanisms that help control pain perception. The central nervous system produces **endorphins,** naturally occurring substances that relieve pain. Endorphins are released with exercise and other forms of physical stimulation. Unfortunately, endorphins dissipate rapidly. Some authorities believe that activities other than exercise, such as laughter, also increase endorphin production. Theorists believe that the intake of certain chemicals and foods, including caffeine, nicotine, alcohol, salt, and sugar, decreases endorphin production.

NURSING ASSESSMENT

Pain is *subjective;* that is, only the client can describe it. Although it cannot be measured objectively, some manifestations of pain can be observed. Keep in mind that the client's culture may affect how the client expresses pain.

■■■ TABLE 55-1 *R*ESULTS OF THE PAIN EXPERIENCE

Characteristics	Suggested Approaches
Loss of control	Regain control over one part of life at a time; set intermediate goals with target dates
Decreased self-esteem	Participate in support groups, affirmations; build on abilities, not disabilities
Decreased communication (family members do not want to hear about pain anymore)	Talk to others with chronic pain; limit talking about pain with family to a specified length each day; attend support group and individual therapy sessions
Inappropriate life goals	Try to control pain while resuming normal activities, trying for a longer period each day; prepare for possible job retraining if necessary
Change in relationships; lack of sexual activity; role changes within family	Attend marriage and family therapy; encourage expressions of love and caring even though sexual activity may be difficult; seek financial counseling; explain to family why life is changed and what activities can continue; encourage family activities; assume leadership again gradually, one step at a time
Anger of family and friends over need to "take care of" client or do client's work	Participate in family therapy; receive vocational counseling; try to find appropriate job within capabilities (start with volunteer work, if necessary)
Decreased activity	Find alternative activities, hobbies, entertainment; attempt to be active in something, such as a club, part-time job, or church
Decreased endurance	Build up strength gradually; find activities that are possible at present, such as walking, stationary bicycle, swimming, low-impact aerobic exercise; participate in activities with other clients who have chronic pain; keep moving, to avoid further deterioration and depression

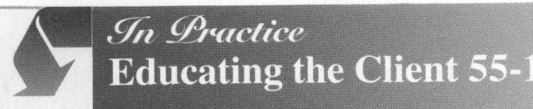

In Practice
Educating the Client 55-1

MANAGING CHRONIC PAIN

- *Medications:* Be sure to follow medication schedules accurately. It is best to take medications on a regular schedule to maintain an adequate blood level, rather than to wait until pain occurs.
- *Exercise:* Stay active. Exercise at a pace and a level that is comfortable. Avoid competing with others. Do your own personal best.
- *Nutrition:* Develop a healthy diet. Enjoy food and pleasant mealtimes. Drink plenty of water and other fluids, including fruit juices.
- *Recreation:* Have fun. Participate in activities that bring pleasure.
- *Relaxation:* Learn to relax both *passively* (self-hypnosis, meditation, deep breathing) and *actively* (knit, sew, read, travel).
- *Support:* Join a support group. Bond with family and friends when pain is intense.
- *Hobbies:* Stay occupied. When possible, do things alone without depending on others. Develop hobbies that are compatible with physical abilities.
- *Rest/sleep:* Investigate stress management techniques. Coping with pain is easier following rest. Be sure to get an adequate amount of sleep. Take naps during the day, if necessary.

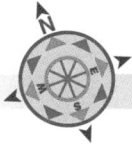

SPECIAL CONSIDERATIONS: CULTURE

Expressions of Pain

The expression of pain is related to cultural and ethnic factors. These factors include, but are not limited to:

- Beliefs about the causes of pain (evil spirits, punishment from God, guilt)
- Manner of expressing the pain in that specific culture (stoicism, crying out, withdrawing, hiding)
- Gender differences in the expression of pain (men versus women)
- Acceptance of traditional versus nontraditional medicine

During the client's admission to the healthcare facility, determine as much as possible about his or her pain. Ask questions about its location, onset, duration, frequency, and quality. Find out what makes the pain better or worse. Identify any factors that seem to precipitate the pain.

Recent changes in Joint Commission on the Accreditation of Healthcare Organizations (JCAHO) regulations state that pain also is to be assessed whenever vital signs are measured. That is, clients are to be asked on a regular basis if they are experiencing pain. Failure to do this may result in a JCAHO citation. See In Practice: Nursing Assessment 55-1 for further information.

The JCAHO also requires healthcare facilities to use pain scales to help clients determine their *level* of pain (Fig. 55-2). For example, one of the pain scales asks a client to rate his or her pain on a numerical scale from 0 (indicating no pain) to 10 (indicating unbearable pain).

Some healthcare facilities use pain questionnaires when assessing pain in the client. The McGill-Melzack Pain Questionnaire is an example (Fig. 55-3).

For clients such as children or adults who may have difficulty expressing themselves, a type of pain scale that has drawings of facial expressions to rate pain can be used. (Fig. 55-4). The client is asked to choose a face that best describes how he or she is feeling because of the hurt or pain being experienced.

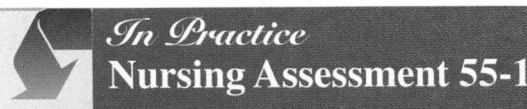

In Practice
Nursing Assessment 55-1

THE PAIN EXPERIENCE

The nurse also notes the client's nonverbal reactions and responses to pain.

Location
- Where is the pain?
- Is it internal or external?
- Does it seem to radiate or spread? Where does it start?

Duration
- How long have you noticed this pain?
- Is the pain constant, occasional, or recurring?
- How long does an episode last?
- How often does it occur?

Quantity/Intensity
- What is the degree of the pain? (Have the client indicate the degree of pain on a distress scale.)

Quality
- How would you describe the pain? Be specific.

Aggravating/Alleviating Factors
- Does anything compound or decrease the pain?

Related Occurrences/Sequelae
- Do you experience any other symptoms before, during, or after the pain?

Adapted from Taylor, C., Lillis, C. & LeMone, P. (2001). *Fundamentals of nursing: The art and science of nursing care.* Philadelphia: Lippincott Williams & Wilkins.

PAIN DISTRESS SCALES

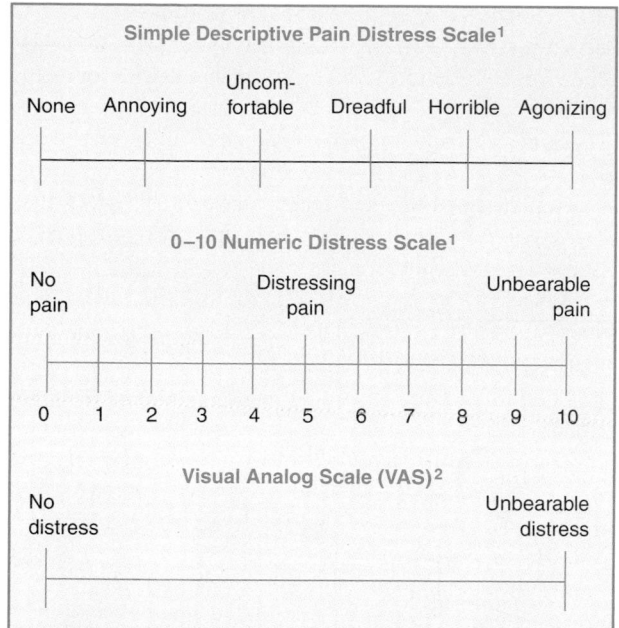

¹ If used as a graphic rating scale, a 10 cm baseline is recommended.
² A 10-cm baseline is recommended for VAS scales.

FIGURE 55-2. Sample pain distress scales. (Adapted from Acute Pain Management Guide Panel, Website: http://www.ahcpr.gov/clinic)

Many terms can be used to describe pain characteristics. Examples may include the following:

- The client may describe the *duration* of pain as *intermittent, spasmodic, or constant.*
- Pain *intensity* may be *mild, slight, moderate,* or *severe.* The client's descriptions of the intensity will help the provider determine appropriate medication or other appropriate intervention.
- The client may describe the *quality* of pain as *boring, burning, constant, cramping, crushing, dull, excruciating, grinding, hammering, intermittent, knifelike, penetrating, piercing, pounding, radiating, sharp, shooting, spasmodic, stabbing, tearing, throbbing,* or *tingling.*
- Associated *sequelae of unrelieved pain* may include *visual disturbance, nausea and vomiting, fatigue and depression, anorexia, muscle spasms, anger and aggression, withdrawal, depression,* and *regression.*

☞ KEY CONCEPT

After pain is identified, focus nursing care and client and family teaching on breaking the cycle of chronic pain as soon as possible.

PAIN MANAGEMENT

Pharmacology is the cornerstone of successful pain management. A physician may order other *complementary interventions* to be given by a specially trained person. *Nursing interventions* include changing the client's position, massaging his or her back, or applying heat or cold. Keep in mind, however, that these methods are used to complement, not replace, pharmacologic interventions. In Practice: The Nursing Process 55-1 applies the nursing process to pain management.

Pharmacologic Techniques

Analgesics are medications that relieve pain. A needed analgesic that is withheld for too long may be ineffective when given. Some clients are allowed to administer their own analgesia through a patient-controlled analgesia (**PCA**) pump (Fig. 55-5).

Analgesics generally provide pain relief by altering the body's sodium and potassium levels, thus slowing or halting pain transmission.[4] Three classes of analgesics are commonly used for pain relief. These include:

- *Nonsteroidal anti-inflammatory drugs* (**NSAIDs**): Examples of NSAIDs include *aspirin, ibuprofen (Motrin),* and *naproxen (Naprosyn, Aleve).* These drugs are usually given to clients who are experiencing mild to moderate pain.
- *Opioids/narcotic analgesics:* The most commonly used example is *morphine* (and its derivative). Opioids are usually used to manage pain in clients with moderate to severe pain.
- *Adjuvant drugs:* Common examples include *anticonvulsants* and *antidepressants.* These medications can help improve the client's mood, thus assisting in muscle relaxation. When muscles are relaxed, pain improves and endorphin production often increases.

Ointments and *liniments* that contain local anesthetics may provide pain relief. Such medications may also draw blood into the painful area to increase temperature and improve circulation. Unit 9 provides a detailed discussion of the many types of medications used in pain management.

The preventive approach is recommended (eg, give analgesics immediately after surgery or before a painful treatment). If medication is given before pain occurs, the pain is often easier to control. Keep in mind that addiction to pain medications does not occur when the client needs relief from acute pain. However, these medications, especially opioids, should not be used on a long-term basis.

Surgical Intervention

Surgery may be necessary to alleviate certain types of chronic pain. For example, when a herniated disk is the cause of lower back pain, the disk may be removed. Physical causes, such as tumors causing pressure or pinched nerves, can be treated with surgical intervention. Nerves transmitting the pain sensation may be cut. However, with the advent of many less invasive techniques, this surgery is rare today. Chapter 56 discusses preoperative and postoperative care for the client who requires surgery.

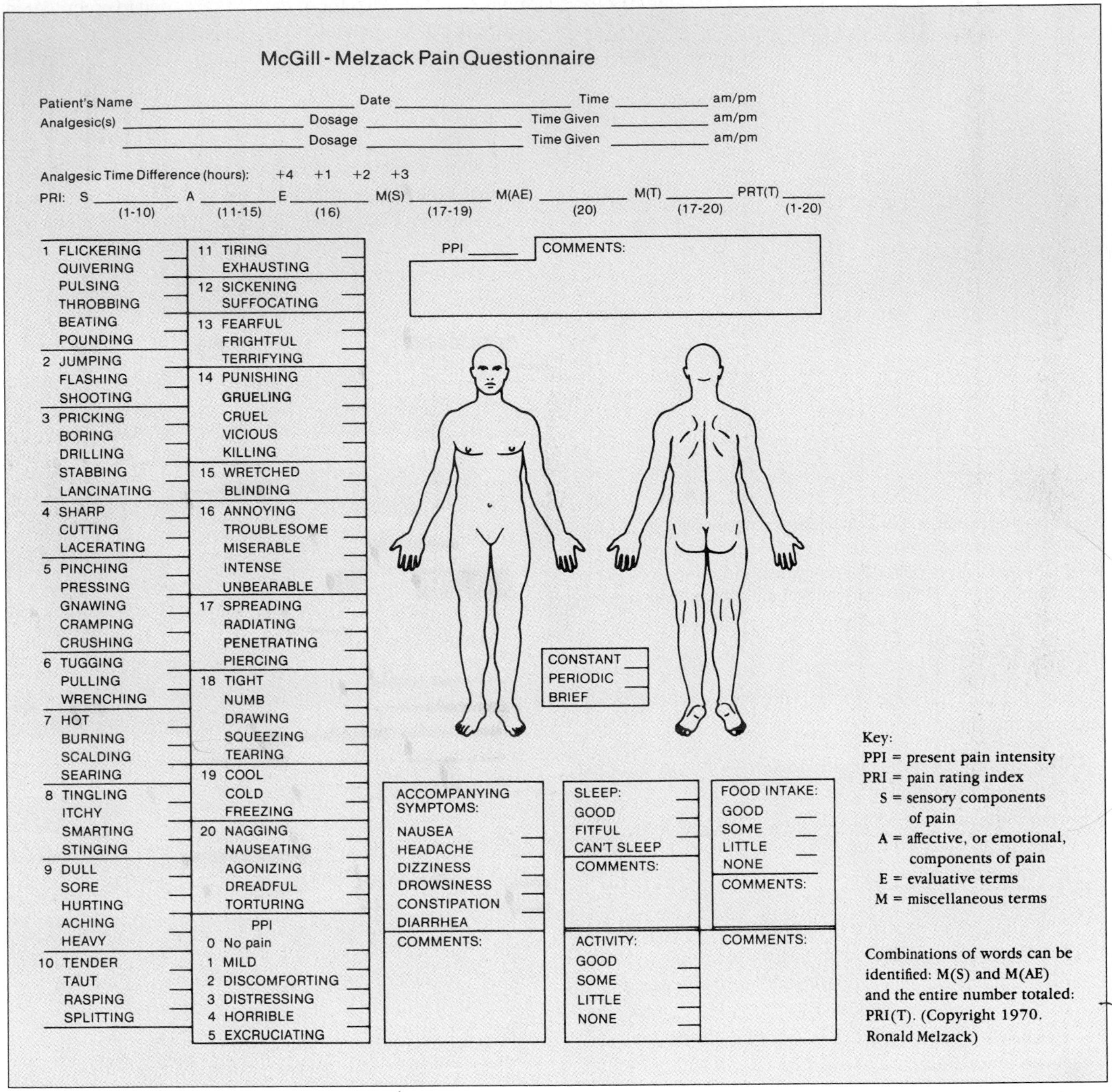

McGill - Melzack Pain Questionnaire

Patient's Name _____ Date _____ Time _____ am/pm
Analgesic(s) _____ Dosage _____ Time Given _____ am/pm
             _____ Dosage _____ Time Given _____ am/pm

Analgesic Time Difference (hours):   +4   +1   +2   +3

PRI: S _____ A _____ E _____ M(S) _____ M(AE) _____ M(T) _____ PRT(T) _____
         (1-10)   (11-15)   (16)   (17-19)   (20)   (17-20)   (1-20)

1 FLICKERING	11 TIRING
QUIVERING	EXHAUSTING
PULSING	12 SICKENING
THROBBING	SUFFOCATING
BEATING	13 FEARFUL
POUNDING	FRIGHTFUL
2 JUMPING	TERRIFYING
FLASHING	14 PUNISHING
SHOOTING	GRUELING
3 PRICKING	CRUEL
BORING	VICIOUS
DRILLING	KILLING
STABBING	15 WRETCHED
LANCINATING	BLINDING
4 SHARP	16 ANNOYING
CUTTING	TROUBLESOME
LACERATING	MISERABLE
5 PINCHING	INTENSE
PRESSING	UNBEARABLE
GNAWING	17 SPREADING
CRAMPING	RADIATING
CRUSHING	PENETRATING
6 TUGGING	PIERCING
PULLING	18 TIGHT
WRENCHING	NUMB
7 HOT	DRAWING
BURNING	SQUEEZING
SCALDING	TEARING
SEARING	19 COOL
8 TINGLING	COLD
ITCHY	FREEZING
SMARTING	20 NAGGING
STINGING	NAUSEATING
9 DULL	AGONIZING
SORE	DREADFUL
HURTING	TORTURING
ACHING	PPI
HEAVY	0 No pain
10 TENDER	1 MILD
TAUT	2 DISCOMFORTING
RASPING	3 DISTRESSING
SPLITTING	4 HORRIBLE
	5 EXCRUCIATING

PPI _____   COMMENTS:

CONSTANT _____
PERIODIC _____
BRIEF _____

ACCOMPANYING SYMPTOMS:
NAUSEA _____
HEADACHE _____
DIZZINESS _____
DROWSINESS _____
CONSTIPATION _____
DIARRHEA _____
COMMENTS:

SLEEP:
GOOD _____
FITFUL _____
CAN'T SLEEP _____
COMMENTS:

FOOD INTAKE:
GOOD _____
SOME _____
LITTLE _____
NONE _____
COMMENTS:

ACTIVITY:
GOOD _____
SOME _____
LITTLE _____
NONE _____
COMMENTS:

Key:
PPI = present pain intensity
PRI = pain rating index
  S = sensory components
      of pain
  A = affective, or emotional,
      components of pain
  E = evaluative terms
  M = miscellaneous terms

Combinations of words can be identified: M(S) and M(AE) and the entire number totaled: PRI(T). (Copyright 1970. Ronald Melzack)

FIGURE 55-3. The McGill-Melzack Pain Questionnaire.

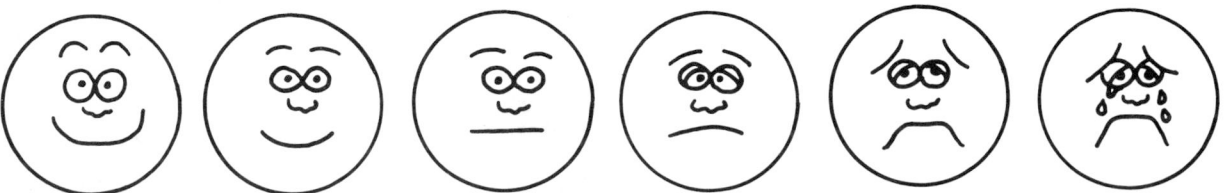

FIGURE 55-4. The Wong/Baker Faces Rating Scale for Pain. (From Wong, D. (1999). *Essentials of pediatric nursing,* 4th ed., St. Louis: Mosby.)

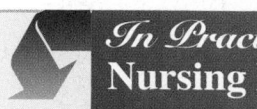

In Practice
Nursing Process 55-1

PAIN MANAGEMENT

Assessment Priorities

- The client's description of the pain, and the pain experience: the pain's location, duration, quantity, quality, and chronology; aggravating factors; and phenomena associated with pain
- What meaning, if any, the pain has for the client
- The client's coping strategies and their success or failure
- Behavioral responses to pain (moving away from the stimuli; grimacing, moaning, crying; restlessness; protecting the painful area; withdrawal)
- Physiologic responses (*sympathetic responses when pain is moderate and superficial:* increased blood pressure, pulse rate, and respirations; pupil dilation; muscle tension and rigidity; pallor; increased adrenaline output and blood glucose level; *parasympathetic responses when pain is severe and deep:* nausea and vomiting; fainting or unconsciousness; decreased blood pressure and pulse rate; rapid and irregular breathing)
- Affective responses (weeping and restlessness, withdrawal, stoicism, anxiety, depression, fear, anger, anorexia, fatigue, hopelessness, powerlessness)

Possible Nursing Diagnoses

- Acute Pain
- Chronic Pain
- Ineffective Coping
- Deficient Knowledge (effective pain-management program)
- Powerlessness
- Compromised family coping

(*Note:* Initially, the nurse must view pain as a symptom and pursue its physical etiology. Interventions for pain that are performed prior to an accurate assessment may mask the true cause of the pain, thus causing further suffering and possibly even death by allowing the progression of signs, symptoms, and the disease process.)

Planning

Design a plan of care with the client and family to achieve the following general goals:

- The client describes a gradual reduction of pain using a scale of 0 (no pain) to 10 (pain as intense as it can get).

- The client demonstrates competent execution of a successful pain-management program.

  For the client with chronic pain, appropriate goals may include the following:

- The client verbalizes (demonstrates) the ability to control pain sufficiently to manage or enjoy everyday living.
- The family relates the feeling of being better able to cope with the client's pain experience.

Implementation

- Establish a supportive and trusting nurse–client relationship.
- Teach about the function of pain, and instill confidence that a successful pain-management program can be developed.
- Remove or alter the cause of pain (whenever possible) and alter factors that decrease pain tolerance.
- Use appropriate noninvasive relief measures: distraction, imagery, relaxation, cutaneous stimulation (massage, application of heat or cold, vibration, pressure).
- Administer the prescribed analgesic; if a patient-controlled analgesia unit (PCA) is being used, instruct the client about its use.
- Learn about the client's use of other pain therapies as appropriate: acupuncture, biofeedback, neurosurgery, electrical nerve stimulation, and others.

Evaluation

Determine the adequacy of the plan of care by evaluating the client's achievement of the preceding goals. If the client is unable to meet key goals, modify the plan. Key evaluative criteria include:

- Client experiences adequate relief.
- Client demonstrates knowledge of pain relief measures.
- Client is satisfied with the pain-management program.
- Client feels sufficiently comfortable to attend to the demands of everyday living.
- Family members are able to recognize and report improvement.

Alternative and Complementary Techniques

Clients may use many *nonpharmacologic measures* to manage pain. Some measures may be considered nontraditional, such as *chiropractic care, acupuncture, hypnosis,* or *biofeed-* back (see Chap. 3). These measures are being integrated into traditional pain control regimens more and more frequently however. Other nontraditional measures include *homeopathy, use of flower essences and aromatic oils,* and *herbal remedies.* These measures are not frequently prescribed by the traditional healthcare system, but have proven to be helpful

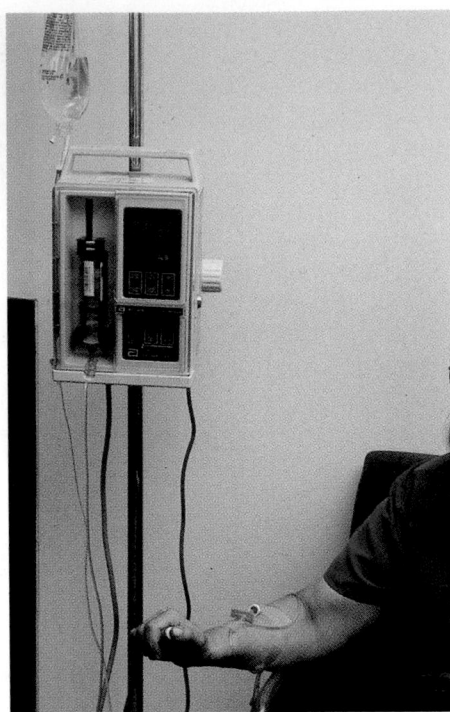

FIGURE 55-5. A patient-controlled analgesia (PCA) pump allows clients to administer their own analgesia.

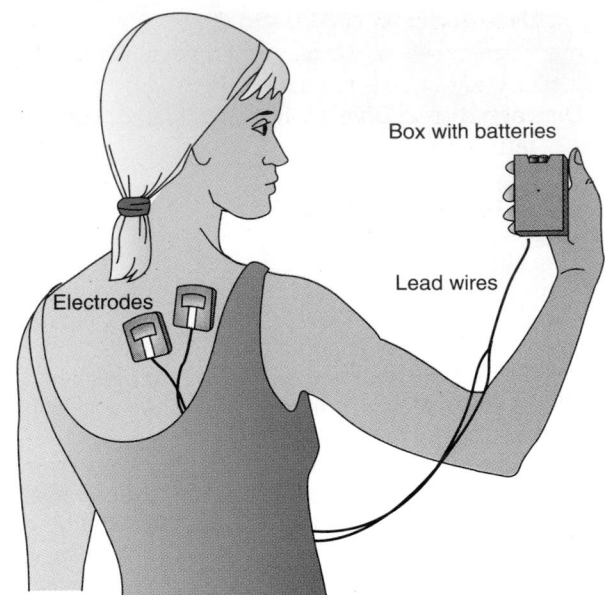

FIGURE 55-6. The transcutaneous electrical nerve stimulation (TENS) unit provides physical stimulation. The client controls electrical stimulation when pain is felt. The gentle electrical shock blocks pain, allowing the relaxation of muscles.

to many clients. Many alternative and complementary techniques allow the client to take ownership for their own pain management. The relief from pain felt by nonpharmacologic measures that results from these techniques seems to be very effective in many cases.

Nurses can provide comfort without an order by positioning the client comfortably, giving back or hand massage, and ensuring proper nutrition. Some clients, especially those with a terminal illness, suffer from long-term intractable pain. Chapter 99 discusses pain management for those special clients.

☞ KEY CONCEPT

The client with chronic pain is vulnerable to unscrupulous practitioners, because the client is desperate and often willing to try anything to relieve the pain. Persons promoting "quack" cure-all schemes may take advantage of these clients.

Physical Measures

Physical measures can be used in addition to pharmacologic pain management interventions.

Physical Stimulus (Cutaneous Stimulation).   Gentle massage or pressure may relieve congestion or promote circulation and oxygenation, and thus help relieve pain. The transcutaneous electrical nerve stimulation (**TENS**) unit provides physical stimulation (Fig. 55-6).

TENS is a noninvasive technique that allows the client to wear an electronic device and trigger an electrical stimulation when he or she feels pain. This gentle electrical shock blocks pain, allowing muscles to relax. The shock

also stimulates the production of endorphins. (Other, more invasive methods may also be used but are beyond the scope of this text.)

Heat and Cold Application.   The application of *heat* or *cold* (see Chap. 54) may help to control localized pain by causing vasodilation or vasoconstriction. Applying heat and cold is one of the few nonpharmacologic techniques proven to relieve pain.

Exercise.   Actively *exercising* specific body parts, with a gradual but steady increase in activity levels, increases joint flexibility and muscle strength. Exercise should be performed only to the body's tolerance. Exercise is required as a part of one's self-care routine to prevent loss of muscle tone and strength. Teach the client what activities are allowed to prevent injury (and thus more pain) from occurring. Be sure activities vary and are enjoyable. Activities performed with other individuals often are more enjoyable than those activities done alone. Encourage participation in group programs.

Exercise and activity programs are designed to increase endurance gradually. The client needs to understand that he or she might feel some pain while exercising the muscles; however, a safe level of pain will help to prevent further injury or deterioration. Increase activity levels a little each day, pushing just beyond each client's discomfort and tolerance level to stimulate endorphin production and increase endurance and strength. Teaching the client to monitor their own body **cues** (feelings that one experiences by listening to body rhythms) places the emphasis on self-care and self-monitoring.

Comfort Measures.   A clean bed, clean face and hands, restful music, a warm room, or a semi-lighted room may promote *relaxation,* which in turn may help lessen pain. Positional changes can also help.

Cognitive–Behavioral Measures

Several *cognitive–behavioral techniques* can also act as complementary pain control measures.

Distraction and Diversion. *Activities* such as visiting, games, television, or craft projects may help divert a client's attention away from focusing on pain.

Deep Relaxation and Guided Imagery. The client can learn deep relaxation techniques that are often helpful. The client is taught to perform specific deep-breathing and relaxation exercises. Next, the client concentrates on a pleasant and relaxing experience. Some clients learn through relaxation therapy to relax taut muscles, thereby relieving pain.

Guided imagery is a process through which the client receives a suggestion to concentrate on an image to control the pain or discomfort. Deep relaxation exercises are performed first, so that the client is totally relaxed. Then the client is guided through specific images. For example, the suggestion may be that pain occurring over a large area of the body is moving down and out of the body. In this way, a smaller area can be involved; the eventual goal is to eliminate the pain entirely. The client can also focus on moving the pain. (This procedure is also used for individuals who have cancer. Clients visualize their defense cells as large and strong and the cancer cells as small and weak.) People in pain learn to visualize themselves as powerful and able to conquer their pain. In addition, they learn to change their pain perceptions so that discomfort is better tolerated.

Support Groups. *Support groups* and *group therapy sessions* can help individuals in pain by giving them an opportunity to express their feelings and talk about pain with others who can relate. Group members often offer suggestions as to how they handled similar situations and concerns (Fig. 55-7). Some support groups provide information about financial assistance to help cope with the costs associated with medications, or vocational counseling to aid in maintaining functional abilities.

Usually, family members of a client in pain can benefit from participation in a support group as well. They learn how to deal with the client's concerns and how to be supportive.

If pain continues for some time, they can learn to deal with their own feelings about the situation. Some support group therapists use a program similar to the 12 steps of Alcoholics Anonymous (see Chap. 94). The first step is accepting that "I am powerless over this pain." If clients can accept feeling powerless, they can work on measures to regain control. Such programs have proven effective in many cases.

Stress Management. A great deal of stress may aggravate pain. The client in pain may find *stress management* techniques helpful. He or she can benefit by developing effective coping mechanisms. Learning to be more assertive may help reduce stress. Other stress-reducing measures include physical activity, recreation, adequate fluids, and a well-balanced diet. Antidepressant medications also may be used (see Chapter 93).

➤ STUDENT SYNTHESIS

Key Points

- Nociception (pain transmission) has four components: transduction, transmission, perception, and modulation.
- Acute pain (nociceptive pain) lasts up to 6 months and is relieved when its cause is identified and treated.
- Chronic pain (neuropathic pain) lasts for more than 6 months. Common treatment measures may fail to relieve such pain.
- Factors that affect pain perception include a person's pain threshold and pain tolerance. Culture also influences the expression of pain. The body's naturally occurring endorphins also influence how a person experiences pain.
- Early intervention in the cycle of pain may help control it.
- Nursing assessment of the client in pain focuses on the client's self-report of the experience and the use of pain scales.
- Pharmacology is the cornerstone of pain management.
- Surgical intervention is sometimes necessary to relieve certain kinds of pain.
- Both physical and cognitive–behavioral techniques are used to complement pharmacologic pain management.

Critical Thinking Exercises

1. You work in an extended care facility where many of your residents have chronic pain. Describe a basic plan and rationale for pain management for a resident with long-standing lower-back pain who refuses to get out of bed.
2. Mrs. T. is taking regular pain medications for intractable pain. She is interested in exploring additional methods. What recommendations would you make? How would you explain different therapies?

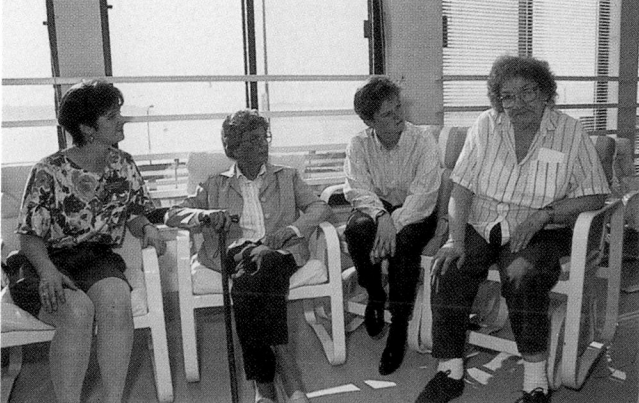

FIGURE 55-7. By sharing common experiences and concerns, members of a support group can enhance their coping skills and find a valuable avenue for understanding and encouragement.

If you were experiencing chronic pain, what alternative and complementary methods would be of most interest to you?

NCLEX-Style Review Questions

1. When evaluating the effects of medication therapy, the nurse should monitor for which of the following?
   a. Decrease in pain tolerance
   b. Increase in pain level
   c. Occurrence of adverse side effects
   d. Participation in activities
2. Which of the following is the best indicator that a client is experiencing pain?
   a. The client has an elevated heart rate.
   b. The client has a grimacing facial expression.
   c. The client has an elevated respiratory rate.
   d. The client states that pain is present.
3. A client who experiences chronic pain is at risk for developing:
   a. Aneurysms
   b. Depression
   c. Hypertension
   d. Pancreatitis
4. Which of the following would be an appropriate nursing intervention for a client experiencing pain?
   a. Administer extra dosage of analgesics.
   b. Apply heat or cold.
   c. Encourage client to lie still in bed.
   d. Encourage client to avoid social interaction.
5. Which of the following medications would the nurse expect to administer to control severe pain?
   a. Aspirin
   b. Ibuprofen
   c. Morphine
   d. Naproxyn

References

1. McCaffery, M. (1968). *Cognition, bodily pain and man–environment interactions.* Los Angeles: University of California.
2. Agency for Health Care Policy and Research. Website: http://www.ahcpr.gov/clinic
3. Craven, R. F., & Hirnle, C. J. (2000). *Fundamentals of nursing: Human health and function* (3rd ed.). Philadelphia: Lippincott Williams & Wilkins.
4. Taylor, C., Lillis, C., & LeMone, P. (2001). *Fundamentals of nursing: The art and science of nursing care* (4th ed.). Philadelphia: Lippincott Williams & Wilkins.

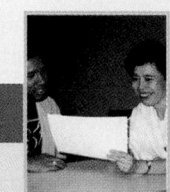

Preoperative and Postoperative Care

LEARNING OBJECTIVES

1. Discuss at least six major classifications that identify a high-risk surgical client.
2. List the two major types of anesthetics.
3. Describe the four stages of general anesthesia.
4. Explain the importance of client teaching, as related to surgery.
5. List at least six important preoperative nursing steps.
6. State the function of the post-anesthesia care unit and describe equipment found there.
7. Describe specific nursing measures when a client returns to the nursing unit from the post-anesthesia recovery area.
8. Identify specific nursing actions used to alleviate postoperative pain, thirst, nausea, distention, and urinary retention, and possible immediate postoperative complications.
9. Outline procedures for turning the postoperative client and promoting respiratory function.

NEW TERMINOLOGY

anesthesia
atelectasis
conscious sedation
dehiscence
elective
embolus
evisceration
hypothermia
hypoxia

intraoperative
perioperative
pneumonia
postoperative
preoperative
splinting
suture
thrombophlebitis
venous access lock

ACRONYMS

MRSA	PACU	TCDB
OR	PAR	

Surgery is performed on a client when the best treatment for his or her disorder is repairing, removing, or replacing body tissues or organs. Surgery is an invasive process because an incision is made into the body or a part is removed. Surgery often is disruptive for clients and families. Careful and attentive nursing care often can make the difference between a negative and a positive surgical experience from which the client recovers quickly.

PERIOPERATIVE CARE

The term **perioperative** refers to the time span that includes preparation for, the process of, and recovery from surgery. Therefore, perioperative nursing consists of the following three phases:

- **Preoperative** nursing care: Before surgery
- **Intraoperative** nursing care: In the operating room (**OR**), post-anesthesia recovery (**PAR**), or post-anesthesia care unit (**PACU**)
- **Postoperative** nursing care: After surgery

Factors in Surgery

Surgery is performed in several different types of healthcare facilities. If surgery is extensive or a person's condition is classified as high risk, the surgery will be conducted in an acute-care facility, such as a hospital. Less complex or less dangerous procedures may be performed in a walk-in or ambulatory center, often called a surgi-center or same-day surgery center. In these facilities, the client enters, has the surgical procedure performed, and goes home the same day. This center may be part of a physician's clinic, a department in a hospital, or a free-standing facility.

The physician will assess each client and weigh the risks of surgery against the need for surgery. The necessity for surgery may outweigh risk factors. Table 56-1 identifies factors that are addressed when assessing the risk status of all clients.

Types of Surgery

Levels of client choice in surgery are:

- *Optional*/**Elective:** The condition is not life threatening. The client may choose whether or not to have the surgery. (Examples include plastic surgery, removal of a non-malignant birthmark, and tubal ligation for sterilization.)
- *Required/Nonelective:* The surgery is necessary at some time. The client has some choice as to when the procedure will be done. (Examples are hernia repair, prolapsed uterus, and hip joint replacement.)
- *Urgent/Nonelective:* The surgery must be performed within a day or two to prevent further damage to the client. (Examples are removal of a malignancy and removal of a severely diseased appendix or tonsils.)
- *Emergency:* The surgery must be performed immediately to save the client's life. (Examples are ectopic pregnancy

rupture, severe internal hemorrhage, ruptured appendix, and angioplasty after a heart attack.)

Nursing Considerations

A variety of nursing diagnoses may be established for the perioperative client and his or her family. Examples may include:

- Fear
- Deficient Knowledge
- Anticipatory Grieving
- Disturbed Body Image
- Risk for Aspiration
- Ineffective Airway Clearance
- Pain
- Hyperthermia
- Hypothermia
- Altered Tissue Perfusion (cerebral, peripheral)
- Deficient Fluid Volume
- Impaired Tissue Integrity
- Impaired Skin Integrity
- Impaired Physical Mobility

The following nursing interventions are common to all surgical procedures, regardless of the type:

- Providing emotional support to the client and family
- Preparing the client physically for the surgery
- Ensuring that all legal matters, such as signing the surgical consent, are carried out
- Ensuring that all required tests, such as ECG, ordered blood tests, and x-rays are done before the date of surgery
- Providing client and family teaching
- Providing routine preoperative and postoperative care

The time available for each of these nursing interventions related to surgery depends in large part on where the surgery is performed and whether or not it is an emergency. For example, if the surgery is an elective procedure and the person is a hospital inpatient, preparation and teaching time will be considerably longer than if the person is brought in by ambulance and must receive emergency surgery.

☛ Key Concept

Clients who are about to undergo surgery almost always experience some level of concern or anxiety, which is made more acute by the fact that nearly all clients go home very soon after surgery. It is a nursing responsibility to teach the client and the family beforehand as much as possible about the procedure and what to expect. When the client is better informed, he or she is likely to be more comfortable about the procedure. If a client is very anxious about surgery, the procedure may need to be postponed.

Anesthesia

Anesthesia is the complete or partial loss of sensation. Medications called *anesthetics* induce anesthesia. The discipline of medicine that administers anesthetics is called *anesthesiology*.

■■■ TABLE 56-1 *F*ACTORS TO ADDRESS WHEN ASSESSING CLIENTS FOR SURGICAL RISK

Category	Risk Factor	Possible Complications
Weight	Obesity	Poor healing (less circulation in fat tissue) Hypostatic pneumonia (less activity) More difficult surgery (more fat tissues to dissect) More underlying disorders likely (eg, diabetes, poor lung function)
	Undernutrition, malnutrition	Poor healing (lack of nutrients) Skin breakdown (less padding over bony prominences, lack of protein)
Hydration status	Dehydration Edema	Reduced circulation (lack of tissue fluid, electrolyte imbalance) Reduced circulation (retention of fluids, pressure within tissues)
Electrolyte balance	Imbalance	Many complications, depending on specific electrolyte
Age	Very young	Respiratory problems (poorly developed lungs) Existence of congenital conditions, possibly causing various complications Inability to understand or follow instructions Dehydration or overhydration, electrolyte imbalances more likely due to small body size
	Very old	Poor healing (reduced circulation) Skin breakdown (friable skin, bony prominences, poor circulation) Confusion (may be caused by anesthesia or change in routine) Hypostatic pneumonia (lack of activity, poor lung-tissue turgor) Dehydration or undernutrition (poor eating habits, confusion) Coexisting disorders more likely
Use of chemicals	Smoking	Lung disorders (inflammation, increased mucous production, diseased lung tissue, chronic bronchitis, and so forth) Circulatory disorders, such as blood clots or poor circulation, hypertension (nicotine constricts blood vessels) Cardiac disorders, such as atherosclerosis in heart vessels Digestive disorders, such as peptic ulcer
	Chemical abuse	Withdrawal symptoms (caused by removal of substance) Addiction (less resistance to dependency because of abuse) High drug tolerance (requiring higher doses of pain medications to achieve comfort) Lung disorders or circulatory disorders (general poor health and poor nutrition)
Use of certain prescription drugs	Risk factors are dependent on specific drug	Bleeding disorders, fluid retention, kidney damage, confusion, and many other complications
Preexisting physical disorders	Risk factors are dependent on disorder	Poor circulation, slowed healing, tendency for blood to clot, pulse disorders, retention of fluids (heart disorders) Hypostatic pneumonia, poor oxygen exchange (lung disorders) Slowed healing, increased incidence of infections, insulin imbalances (diabetes mellitus) Inability to regulate blood sugar levels (diabetes mellitus) Allergic reactions to anesthesia or medications (allergies, asthma) Inability to control seizures (seizure disorders, epilepsy) Slowed healing, high incidence of infections (immune disorders, diabetes, cancer chemotherapy)
Psychological status	Excessive fear	Difficulty in understanding instructions, pulse disorders, cardiac arrest, difficulty in achieving anesthesia
	Intellectual impairment	Inability to understand instructions, lack of follow-through (psychiatric disorders, dementia, mental retardation)
	Depression	Lack of motivation to follow instructions
Physical activity status	Immobility, poor physical condition	Prone to thrombophlebitis, bowel obstruction or impaction, pressure ulcers, orthostatic blood pressure changes, pneumonia, decreased stamina and strength, other postoperative complications
Living situation	Lack of available caregivers	Difficulty in carrying out postoperative instructions, inability to care for oneself, inability to recognize complications

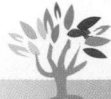

SPECIAL CONSIDERATIONS: THE LIFE SPAN

Perioperative Care in the Older Client

- Height and weight are used to calculate exact dosages of narcotics and anesthetics; older adults are more susceptible to overdose.
- Baseline respiratory assessment is important because older individuals are more susceptible to aspiration and hypostatic pneumonia.
- Early mobility helps prevent complications secondary to immobility, a vital concern for the older client.
- Skin and body fat assessments are made because color, turgor, and temperature assessments are not always reliable.
- Skin tends to be more *friable* (fragile) in the older client. Skin breakdown is a particular danger.
- Blood pressure must be monitored closely because older adults are more susceptible to hypertension or postural hypotension.
- Oxygen saturation must be monitored closely because older clients often have decreased lung function and/or circulation.
- Parenteral fluids may overload circulation because of diminished kidney function.
- Fluid and electrolyte balance changes more quickly in older adults.
- Older adults often have coexisting diseases that increase their surgical risk.
- Older clients often have a slower immune response and may be less able to fight off infection.
- Clients should wear their hearing aids and glasses if possible; be sure the room is well lighted.
- Clients may have poor peripheral vision; be careful not to startle them.
- Clients may react differently to medications than expected (a *paradoxical reaction*); as a result of age-related changes in body systems, they may have difficulty excreting medications.
- Older clients are more susceptible to postoperative urinary retention and constipation.
- Clients may be confused; teach in small doses and remember to include the family (even a minor infection can cause confusion in the otherwise lucid older person).
- Offer to tape wedding rings in place for all clients.

A physician trained in anesthesiology is called an *anesthesiologist,* and a registered nurse trained in anesthesiology is called a *nurse anesthetist.* A visit from the anesthesiologist or nurse anesthetist before surgery enables a client to ask questions that may be troubling him or her. Also, the client may feel more comfortable if he or she can recognize someone in the OR. In Practice: Nursing Care Guidelines 56-1 describes general nursing care for the client receiving anesthetics.

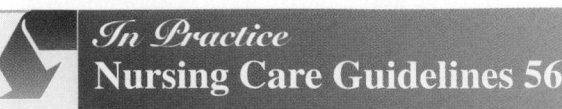

In Practice
Nursing Care Guidelines 56-1

CARING FOR THE CLIENT WHO IS RECEIVING ANESTHESIA

- Check for allergies before any client has surgery and before administering any pre- or postoperative drug.
- Bring any abnormal laboratory results pre- or postoperatively to the physician's attention immediately.
- Notify the surgeon immediately about any extreme apprehension following the administration of preoperative medication.
- When using spinal anesthetics, keep the client flat until the anesthetic has worn off (sometimes up to 12 hours). Observe the client's urine output very carefully. Watch for bladder distention.
- Observe carefully for signs of respiratory distress following the use of neuromuscular blockers or any type of general anesthetic. Be cautious with postoperative narcotics, because of this client's already decreased respiratory drive as a result of anesthesia.
- Watch carefully for signs of circulatory depression following the use of neuromuscular blockers or any general anesthetic.
- Keep in mind that neuromuscular blockers may *potentiate* (increase) effects of anesthesia when used with other central nervous system depressants, including alcohol.
- When epidural or spinal anesthetics or narcotics are used, keep naloxone (Narcan) at an easily accessible location for reversal of untoward effects. Watch for respiratory depression, and safeguard the IV injection site. The same principles apply when the client receives postoperative medications via spinal or epidural routes.
- When using topical anesthetics, watch for skin irritations. The use of eye anesthetics may retard the eye-blink reflex, causing the eyes to become dry.
- Anticipate the need for pain medication early after recovery from anesthesia. The use of many new anesthetics with short durations allow clients to leave surgery more alert than was common in the past. Because the anesthesia may wear off more quickly, clients may require pain medication sooner. Always be alert for adverse effects, even with short-acting medications.

Source: Kathleen McCullough, Hennepin County Medical Center, Minneapolis, Minnesota.

Types

Anesthetics are divided into two main classes: general anesthetics, which suspend all body sensations; and local, regional, or spinal anesthetics, which create insensitivity of specific body parts without causing unconsciousness.

Clients receiving local anesthetic are often given some type of sedation as well.

General anesthetics are administered intravenously (IV), rectally, or by inhalation. Abdominal or chest surgery is usually performed under general anesthesia, as are some orthopedic and many genitourinary procedures. The less anesthetic used, the safer it is for the client; thus, *local anesthesia* is preferred whenever possible. A local anesthetic may be administered topically or by injection. Common procedures performed under local anesthesia include dental work, many types of plastic surgery and skin suturing (stitching), and some types of eye surgery. Much brain surgery is done using local anesthesia.

General Anesthesia. General anesthetics most often given by inhalation are halothane (Fluothane), nitrous oxide, and cyclopropane. The client is usually prepared for inhalation anesthesia with an IV injection of a barbiturate, such as thiopental sodium (Pentothal), or another agent such as etomidate (Amidate), fentanyl citrate with droperidol (Innovar), ketamine hydrochloride (Ketalar), or propofol (Diprivan). The client falls asleep, after which he or she is intubated and maintained on an inhalation anesthetic.

Stages of General Anesthesia. If a slow-acting anesthetic is used, the client passes through recognizable stages of general anesthesia. As the client wakes up from the anesthesia, these stages are reversed.

1. Stage of analgesia/amnesia: Reflexes present, heart rate normal, slower rate and increased depth of respiration, normal blood pressure (BP), some dilation of eyes with reaction to light
2. Stage of dreams and excitement: Active reflexes, increased heart rate, irregular breathing, increased BP, pupils widely dilated and divergent
3. Stage of surgical anesthesia: Four planes with third and fourth plane best for surgery, progressive loss of reflexes, decreased heart rate, progressively depressed respirations until apneic, normal to decreased BP, constricted to slightly dilated and centrally fixed pupils
4. Stage of toxic or extreme depression: No reflexes, weak and thready heart rate, respiration completely flaccid, decreased BP, widely dilated pupils (danger stage)

☞ KEY CONCEPT

The client under general anesthesia is completely dependent on others; he or she cannot control the most basic of body functions, including breathing. This person must be observed and monitored carefully at all times by specially trained anesthesia personnel.

Conscious Sedation. In **conscious sedation,** intravenous sedative medications are used alone or in conjunction with local anesthetics. A client receiving conscious sedation has a depressed level of consciousness but continues to breathe and is able to respond to verbal stimuli. Midazolam HCl (Versed), frequently used to induce sleepiness and relieve anx-

iety, is commonly used for conscious sedation in procedures such as endoscopy. This drug often results in amnesia about the procedure.

PREOPERATIVE NURSING CARE

Before surgery, the surgeon or anesthesiologist writes orders indicating exactly what medications and necessary physical preparations the client needs. Carry out preoperative orders exactly—they affect the surgery's success. While completing preoperative care, remember the feelings of the client and family and their need for reassurance. Many clients are admitted to the healthcare facility the day of surgery and often will not arrive on the nursing unit until after surgery. In emergency surgery, the preoperative period may be short. Within these constraints, remember to provide emotional support to all clients.

✚👁 **N u r s i n g   A l e r t**

In most instances, the client is instructed to stop taking aspirin, ibuprofen (Motrin, Advil) and other NSAIDs or any specific agents affecting blood coagulation for at least 7 days before surgery to reduce the risk of excessive bleeding. Certain herbal supplements are mild anticoagulants and can contribute to the risk of bleeding. These include camomile, cat's claw, feverfew, garlic, ginger, ginkgo, ginseng, goldenseal, grape seed extract, green tea leaf, horse chestnut seed, and turmeric. The preoperative client usually is advised to stop taking herbal supplements also.

Preoperative Checklist

Each healthcare facility has a preoperative checklist to use in the care of all clients requiring surgery. This checklist identifies assessments, medications, and other physical preparations that must be completed before the client is anesthetized. Be sure that all items are checked off before the client is transported to the surgical suite. The list may be shortened if ambulatory surgery is done or if the client is to have a local anesthetic. In Practice: Nursing Care Guidelines 56-2 discusses the organization of preoperative nursing care and lists items regularly included in the checklist. Figure 56-1 shows an example of a preoperative checklist.

✚👁 **N u r s i n g   A l e r t**

Be sure the client has signed the operative permit *before* giving give any pre-sedation medications. Otherwise, the client cannot be held responsible for signing the permit after receiving the medication. His or her next of kin must then be called for permission to operate. In that case, if the next of kin cannot be located, the surgery would need to be postponed.

Surgery may need to be postponed or canceled if preoperative care is performed incorrectly or incompletely or if the checklist items are not documented or documented

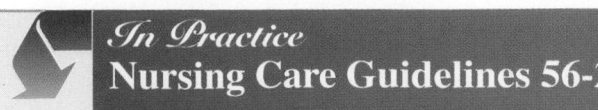

In Practice
Nursing Care Guidelines 56-2

ORGANIZING PREOPERATIVE NURSING CARE

General Measures

- Check the client's record and note the preoperative orders.
- Ensure that the client has signed the surgical permit and that it has been witnessed. (Nursing students should not witness legal papers of any type.)
- Prepare the operative area, as ordered. (Usually the nursing staff is only responsible for supervising a pHisoHex shower, if ordered. The actual surgical preparation and shave is usually done in the operating room.)
- Keep in mind that in the event of brain surgery, the client's head will be shaved. Make sure that the client and family are aware of this beforehand. Let them know that the hair will be saved to make a wig if needed. (In some cases, the eyebrows will be shaved or the eyelashes will be cut. The client needs to know what to expect.)
- Check the client's medical history for any essential respiratory, cardiac, or other drugs he or she takes routinely. Notify the physician of these medications. The client may need to take these drugs despite NPO (nothing by mouth) status.
- See that all specimens and blood samples have been collected and sent to the laboratory.
- Make sure that a history and a physical examination are recorded in the chart.
- Check that results of all testing are on the chart. (Usually an ECG, and sometimes a chest x-ray, are ordered and these results are required as well.)
- Note and attend to any change in diet, as ordered.
- Give a sedative, if ordered.
- Withhold fluids and foods, as directed. Usually, the client is NPO for at least 8 hours before surgery.
- Make sure that any client allergies are noted on the front of the chart and that the client is wearing a special "allergy" identification band.
- Give preoperative instruction and provide emotional support to the client and family.

Immediately Before the Operation

- Check to make sure that the client is wearing his or her identification band.
- Record the client's temperature, pulse, and respiration (TPR); and blood pressure (BP). Report immediately any marked deviation from normal. (The surgeon must be notified.)
- Make sure the client's weight is recorded on the chart. (This helps to determine drug dosages.)
- Help the client with bathing and other hygiene measures. Be sure the client removes all clothes before going to surgery and wears only a clean gown provided by the facility. (In some cases involving local procedures, the client may continue to wear street clothes.)

- Ask the client to remove any prostheses, wigs, contact lenses, hearing aids, false eyelashes, glasses, and false fingernails. (If the client will be expected to participate, as in brain surgery, hearing aids are usually left in place.)
- Remove the client's jewelry and valuables and put them in a safe or give them to the client's family. Be sure to include the client's wedding band. If the client does not want to remove the wedding band, be sure to securely bind or tape the ring to the client's hand. Carefully document what has been done with the valuables.
- Help the client put on elastic stockings, if ordered.
- Help the client to void immediately before going to the operating room (OR). If the client is unable to void, report this and document it on the record.
- Remove any hairpins. For clients with long hair, pull it back and cover it with a surgical cap or a cotton towel. (Hair should be washed the evening before surgery, if possible.)
- Remove any complete or partial dentures and place them in a denture cup with clear water. Label the cup and its cover and put it in a safe place.
- Remove the client's makeup and nail polish. (The anesthetist must be able to observe the client's nail beds and lips. The oximeter sensor may not register properly if nail polish or artificial nails are present.)
- Account for all items on the preparation checklist. Be sure the list is signed and attached to the client's chart. Be sure the chart goes with the client to the OR. (This checklist must be completed by 6:00 AM if the client is first on the OR schedule.) Carry out some procedures the evening before if the client is scheduled for early surgery. In most cases, a nursing student is not allowed to do the final sign-off on the chart. Learn the rules of the healthcare facility.
- Help ensure the client's safety by giving preoperative medications, as ordered, *after* completing all personal care and making sure that the checklist is completed and signed. (The client should not be active after taking a sedative.)
- Be sure the side rails are up and the bed is in low position.
- Be sure that all preoperative charting is up-to-date and signed before the client goes to the OR.
- After the client goes to the OR, begin to prepare the unit for his or her postoperative return.

Note: Some of the above procedures are done in the OR if the client is admitted to the facility the morning of surgery. Also, many of these procedures are carried out by the client at home if the client will not be admitted to the hospital, or if the client will be reporting directly to the surgery department on the day of surgery.

FORM 71.25A R6/98

UNIVERSITY OF CHICAGO HOSPITALS
PRE-OPERATIVE CHECK LIST

CHECK YES, NO OR NA FOR ITEMS 1 THRU 20 AND RECORD INITIALS

	YES	NO	N/A	INITIALS
1. 2 ID bands applied (different extremities)				
2. 2 Blood bands applied #_____ Autologous/donor directed blood avail. (different extremities)				
3. Blood consent signed and witnessed and on chart				
4. If no blood consent, blood refusal form signed and on chart				
5. Advance directives signed and on chart				
6. Consent signed and witnessed and on chart				
7. Laterality identified on the consent form. Surgery will be on the (circle one) Right Left Bilateral Midline				
8. Laterality on the consent form is consistent with the patient's response				
9. Allergies NKA Latex				
_____				
_____				
10. NPO since _____				
11. Pre-op medication Time:_____ Medication _____				
★ 12. Vital Signs BP_____ HR_____ Temp_____ Resp_____				
13. Voided Time _____				
14. Height_____ Wt._____				
★ 15. Patient personal belongings dentures_____ corrective lenses_____ hearing aid_____ jewelry_____ clothing_____ other_____ Disposition ☐ Admission Services ☐ Family Member (_____) ☐ Remains w/Patient name ☐ Other_____				
16. Nail Polish Removed				
17. Isolation *See Isolation Guidelines on opposite side. Type_____				
18. H & P on chart				
19. Previous Medical record with chart				
20. Addressograph plate on chart				

★ Signature_____ Initials:_____

★ If admit assessment form (54.41) is completed in DCAM pre-op or GOR pre-op, mark NA.

ADDRESSOGRAPH

O.R. PRE-OPERATIVE CHECK LIST

CHECK YES, NO OR NA FOR ITEMS 1 THRU 4 AND RECORD INITIALS

	YES	NO	N/A	INITIALS
1. Wearing two I.D. Bands that are legible (one on wrist, one on ankle)				
2. Blood Bank two I.D. Bands in place (one on wrist, one on ankle)				
3. Consent Signed and Witnessed				
4. Laterality on the consent form is consistent with: - the OR schedule - patient response - the pre-op checklist				

5. Allergies

_____

_____

6. Time Arrived in Pre-op Holding _____

7. Chart Checked for Completeness

8. IV Fluids   Amount _____

Signature:_____ Initials:_____

NOTE: _____

_____

_____

STATEMENT OF PATIENT COMPLIANCE

I AM AWARE OF THE DANGER TO ME OF FOOD OR LIQUID (INCLUDING WATER, COFFEE, OR TEA) IN MY STOMACH DURING ANESTHESIA AND I CERTIFY THAT I HAVE HAD NOTHING TO EAT OR DRINK SINCE_____

EXCEPTIONS:_____

I CERTIFY THAT I HAVE AN ESCORT HOME WHOSE NAME IS:

_____

PATIENT:_____

WITNESS:_____ DATE:_____

Isolation Precautions Guidelines		
	May go to Pre-op	May go to PACU
Airborne	No	No
Respiratory (Droplet)	No	No
Strict	No	No
Contact	No	Yes (in isolation room)
Special Handling (CJD)	Yes	Yes
Protective	No	No

FIGURE 56-1. Preoperative checklist. (Courtesy of University of Chicago Hospitals, Chicago, Illinois.)

inaccurately. A preoperative goal is for the client to be in the best possible physical and emotional condition for surgery. A well-prepared client is more likely to have successful surgery and an uneventful course of recovery, leading to optimum rehabilitation. (Remember: Today, nearly all routine preoperative preparation is done at home before surgery.)

☞ KEY CONCEPT

Each step in preoperative preparation has a purpose. If any steps are omitted, the client's safety becomes jeopardized. The client will perform many of these steps at home, when being admitted on the day of surgery. It is the nurse's responsibility to interview the client to make sure all steps in the preoperative preparation have been completed.

Client and Family Support

The client who faces surgery may be apprehensive. Most people fear pain. Some are concerned about losing consciousness; others are afraid they will die. Some are fearful of cancer or of being disabled. The client who has had previous surgery may compare the previous experience to this one. If the previous experience was difficult, the client may be particularly frightened.

The client or family may wish to speak with their spiritual advisor or with a facility chaplain. Help to arrange this meeting. They also often wish to meet with the surgeon before surgery, and the anesthetist or anesthesiologist usually visits with the client before surgery.

To help prepare the family, explain that the client will be taken to surgery 30 to 60 minutes before the scheduled surgical procedure. Inform them that after surgery, the client will be taken to the PACU or PAR area, where specially trained personnel will observe the client until vital signs are stable and full consciousness returns. If the family understands these procedures, they will be less upset by the length of time the client is gone. Inform the family where they may wait for news about the procedure. If the client is to be transferred to another unit after surgery, the family must know where the client will be.

Explaining what will happen during and after surgery is most helpful in preparing the client and family. Those who understand these procedures are usually more relaxed and cooperative. Before surgery, the client practices exercises and uses equipment such as the incentive spirometer (Fig. 56-2). Describe any such postoperative equipment to lessen its frightening effects. (The use of the incentive spirometer is described later in this chapter.)

Teach the client and family what to expect when the client returns from the operating suite. Preoperatively, explain about any equipment such as tubes, IV lines, or suction that might be present after surgery. Explain preparation procedures to the client as they are performed, and tell the client how each step helps both the client and the surgeon.

Preoperative teaching concentrates on several major points, as listed at In Practice: Educating the Client 56-1. When preparing the client:

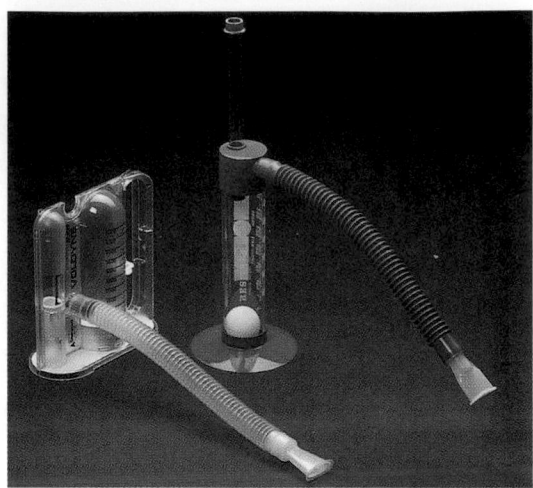

FIGURE 56-2. Two types of incentive spirometers with mouthpieces.

- Organize your teaching.
- Explain what you are going to do.
- Demonstrate the procedure.
- Have the client return the demonstration; make sure that the family caregiver can also accurately perform the procedure, if required.

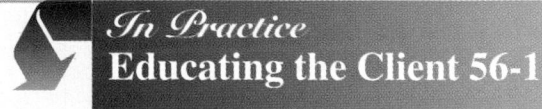

In Practice
Educating the Client 56-1

PREOPERATIVE INSTRUCTION

- Explain the reasons for the special equipment by the bedside.
- Describe what equipment is likely to be present for each individual client in the postoperative period.
- Describe and allow the client to practice how to turn in bed without assistance.
- Allow the client to practice all procedures as needed.
- Describe discomforts to expect and how to alleviate them.
- Show how to splint the incisional area.
- Demonstrate deep-breathing exercises.
- Explain the use of the incentive spirometer.
- Show other exercises to perform postoperatively.
- Describe the amount and kind of ambulation allowed or expected after surgery.
- Provide a description of the operating room and the post-anesthesia care unit. (Sometimes, especially for children, a presurgery tour of these areas is helpful.)
- Describe appropriate wound care.
- Discuss optimum nutrition.
- Explain the importance of communication.

- Supervise the client's practice until the client can perform it independently.
- Reinforce successful behavior.
- Review the procedure.

If a nurse cannot answer a client's questions or does not understand equipment that will be used, be sure to ask someone who is knowledgeable to help.

☛ KEY CONCEPT

If a client will be on a ventilator or otherwise unable to speak after surgery, make arrangements for a communication system. Allow the client to practice this system preoperatively.

Assessments

Prompt, accurate assessments before surgery help to ensure a successful outcome for the client.

Observation. Observe the client carefully during preparation for surgery. Record any unusual reactions or observations in the client's chart and report them at once.

Physical Examination and Laboratory Tests. Before the surgical procedure, the client receives a complete physical examination. Admission vital signs recorded on the client's chart are used as baseline data for comparison during the physician's physical examination, during the surgery itself, and immediately postoperatively. Record the client's weight on the health record in pounds and kilograms because dosages of medications, including anesthetics, are calculated on the basis of the client's weight (usually in kg).

Routine preoperative tests often include the chest x-ray examination, complete blood count (CBC), and urinalysis (UA). Other tests and examinations are performed as needed. An electrocardiogram (ECG) is usually obtained for all clients over age 40. Blood is drawn for a type and crossmatch if any possibility exists that a blood transfusion will be needed during surgery. A bleeding–clotting test, such as the prothrombin time, is often ordered. Notify the physician of routine medications the client takes. Information about allergic reactions is necessary. The accompanying In Practice: The Nursing Process 56-1 applies the nursing process to preoperative care.

Skin Preparation

Because the skin is normally oily and harbors a multitude of bacteria, it is thoroughly cleansed before surgery to help prevent wound contamination. Usually the client is required to shower with antibacterial soap several hours before surgery at home or in the hospital. The operative site is further prepared just before or after the client is anesthetized. The skin is cleaned with an anti-infective agent and possibly shaved because microorganisms adhere to hair. These procedures are known as a surgical preparation or "prep." Most often, this prep and shave are performed in the operating room to reduce the potential risk for infection. If the nurse is expected to perform this procedure, specific instructions will be needed.

Intestinal Preparation

The type of surgery, the anesthetic, and the client's condition determines the type of intestinal preparation needed. In many surgical procedures, the intestinal tract should be as empty of feces as possible. If surgery is in the abdomen or pelvis, and in some other cases, the client will most likely receive an enema to empty his or her bowel (see Chap. 51). Be sure that the client expels the entire enema. (An anesthetized client may expel the remainder on the operating table.) This enema is often done at home. A client also may be required to drink a cathartic solution to cleanse the bowel. Often, the client must take a large amount of solution (as much as several quarts). The client needs encouragement and positive reinforcement to complete this task.

If the client is to have spinal or general anesthesia or conscious sedation, he or she is asked to remain NPO (nothing by mouth) for approximately 8 to 10 hours before surgery to minimize the possibility of nausea and vomiting during anesthesia. In some cases involving extensive local anesthesia, or if there is any chance of an emergency requiring general anesthesia, maintaining NPO status is also needed. If vomiting does occur, aspiration is less likely if the client's stomach is empty.

☛ KEY CONCEPT

The client may be asked to self-administer a small-volume enema or drink a liquid cathartic at home, if the admission to the healthcare facility is on the day of surgery. The client may need instruction in the use of the enema or the cathartic. Encourage the client and reassure him or her that they will be able to do the procedure.

Preoperative Medications

Three types of medications commonly are used preoperatively: sedatives, narcotics, and drying agents.

Because the client should have as much rest as possible before surgery, a *sedative* is usually ordered the evening before surgery so that the client can sleep. This is a one-time only order. Sedation also helps to stabilize BP and pulse.

On the morning of surgery, a preoperative *narcotic* is given to relax the client and to enhance the anesthesia's effects. It may be ordered for a specific time of day or "on call to OR." In the latter case, the medication is taken when the OR calls for the client.

A *drying agent* is given to help inhibit body secretions so that the client produces less mucus, reducing the likelihood of aspiration and *atelectasis* (collapse of the tiny air sacs in the lungs). Production of gastric and intestinal secretions is also reduced, so there is less abdominal distention postoperatively.

☛ KEY CONCEPT

Before giving any preoperative medications, make sure the client does not have any drug allergies and that the surgical permit has been signed and witnessed.

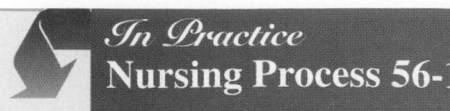

In Practice
Nursing Process 56-1

PREOPERATIVE NURSING CARE

Assessment Priorities
- Nursing history
- Client's understanding of the proposed surgical procedure (clarify any misperceptions)
- Past experiences with surgery
- Fears (fear of the unknown, fear of pain or death, fear of changes in body image or self-concept)
- Factors that increase surgical risk or the potential for postoperative complications:
  Past and present illnesses: Cardiovascular diseases, pulmonary disorders, renal and liver function alterations, metabolic disorders (especially diabetes)
  Medications: Anticoagulants, diuretics, tranquilizers, adrenal steroids, antibiotics
  Lifestyle factors: Nutrition (history of eating disorders, malnutrition, or obesity); use of alcohol, nicotine, or recreational drugs; activity level; use of herbal supplements (many are mild anticoagulants or can adversely interact with medications)
- Adequacy of coping patterns and support systems
- Pertinent sociocultural factors (eg, health beliefs and practices, economic concerns, cultural considerations such as language barrier problems and ethnic beliefs related to surgery and healing)
- Vital signs the morning of surgery (report any significant deviation from normal)
- Accurate height and weight (medications may be calculated on the basis of these data, especially for children)
- General systems review, noting in particular any new cardiopulmonary developments that place the client at high risk during surgery
- Results of all preoperative diagnostic tests recorded in the client's record and if abnormal, reported
- Presence of an escort or driver (for transportation home with same-day surgery)

Possible Nursing Diagnoses
- Anxiety
- Ineffective Coping
- Decisional Conflict
- Fear
- Anticipatory Grieving
- Deficient Knowledge
- Powerlessness

Planning
Design a plan of care with the client and family to achieve the following general client goals. Prior to surgery, the client:

- Demonstrates physical preparedness for surgery (absence of significant deviations from normal in vital signs; no signs of infection)
- Verbalizes any concerns or fears related to the surgery
- Provides *informed consent* for the surgery
- Correctly demonstrates how to turn, deep breathe, use equipment (such as the incentive spirometer), and perform splinting of incision (when appropriate)
- Verbalizes understanding of postoperative pain management program
- Verbalizes understanding of postoperative activity plan
- Demonstrates the presence of adequate caregivers at home after discharge

Implementation
- Establish a supportive and trusting nurse–client relationship.
- Develop and implement a teaching plan that:
  Familiarizes the client and family with what to expect on the day of surgery
  Prepares the client to participate in the pain management program
  Enables the client to state the purpose of deep breathing and to demonstrate it, as well as incentive spirometry, leg exercises, and turning in bed
- Counsel the client and family about helpful coping strategies and available resources. At the client's request, invite a spiritual counselor to see the client.
- Maintain nutrition and hydration; if the client is NPO (nothing by mouth) for 8 to 12 hours prior to surgery, ensure that the client understands the reason for this restriction, and remove all food and fluids from the bedside.
- Evaluate the client's bowel status and determine the need for an order for bowel elimination. If a Foley catheter is ordered prior to surgery, explain its use prior to insertion.
- Carry out preoperative skin and hygiene orders.
- Facilitate sleep and rest in the immediate preoperative period (a sleeping aid may be ordered).
- Remember that many clients are not admitted until the morning of surgery. You must then teach the above preoperative care.

Evaluation
Determine the adequacy of the plan of care by evaluating the client's achievement of the preceding goals. If the client is unable to meet key goals, modify the plan. Key evaluative criteria:

- Client's physical preparedness for surgery
- Client's mental preparedness for surgery
- Client's understanding of and ability to participate in care postoperatively
- An uneventful course of recovery

The client's family is included in all preparation as needed.

Before giving preoperative medications, explain to the client the purpose of the drug and its probable effects. Ask again about any drug allergies. Explain to the client that after the narcotic has been given, the side rails will be raised, that he or she must remain in bed, and that he or she should request assistance to go to the bathroom. Explain to family members that the client has received the medication and that, although they may stay in the room, they should not expect the client to carry on a conversation. In Practice: Important Medications 56-1 provides additional information.

☛ KEY CONCEPT

Be sure to offer a bedpan or urinal to the client immediately before he or she is taken to the operating suite.

Client Transport

If the client is in the hospital preoperatively, prepare the client's room so the OR staff can conveniently move the client. Move furniture so the OR cart can be put next to the bed, and take all items off the bedside stand so they will not be knocked off. Make the client as comfortable as possible. Make sure the preoperative checklist in the client's health record is complete and signed; the record will accompany the client to the OR, where it will be given to the anesthetist or OR nurse. Note on the front of the chart if the client has any drug allergies or is taking cortisone, insulin, an anticonvulsant, or an anticoagulant. In most hospitals, a client with allergies wears a special red name band, along with the regular one. Send a clean bath blanket with the client. Make up a postoperative bed (see Fig. 49-1 in Chap. 49).

Nursing Alert

To prevent errors, always be certain that the client is properly identified before transfer to the OR. *No* client should be allowed to go to the OR without an identification bracelet! Some hospitals require an ID bracelet on both of the client's wrists. The client with an allergy may wear a special ID band as well.

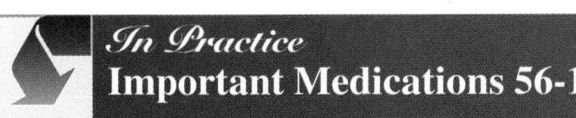

In Practice
Important Medications 56-1

FOR PREOPERATIVE CARE

Sedatives
- Amobarbital sodium (Amytal)
- Chloral hydrate
- Ethchlorvynol (Placidyl)
- Methotrimeprazine HCl (Levoprome, Nozinan)
- Midazolam HCl (Versed) (anesthetic agent)
- Pentobarbital sodium (Nembutal Sodium)
- Secobarbital sodium (Seconal Sodium)

Narcotics
- Fentanyl (Sublimaze)
- Meperidine HCl (Demerol HCl)
- Morphine SO$_4$ (Morphine)
- Sufentanil citrate (Sufenta)

Drying Agents
- Atropine sulfate
- Glycopyrrolate (Robinul; less commonly used)
- Scopolamine hydrobromide (hyoscine hydro-bromide, Scopace; less commonly used)

Nursing Considerations
When sedatives and narcotics are given:
- Observe for respiratory distress or bradypnea. These medications often are contraindicated in clients with severe respiratory disorders.
- Observe for inability to arouse client, extreme lethargy or drowsiness, fatigue, or over-sedation.

- Observe for other central nervous system symptoms, such as dizziness, blurred vision, severe nightmares, ataxia.
- Keep in mind that the medications may potentiate the action of oral anticoagulants and antihypertensive drugs.
- Watch for paradoxical excitement in older adults or children who may have a reaction opposite the desired reaction.

When atropine is given:
- Know that atropine is given cautiously to clients with glaucoma and certain other eye disorders (drug may be contraindicated); it is also contraindicated in clients with certain GI conditions, asthma, COPD, heart conditions, and liver or kidney dysfunction.
- Inform the client about the experience of a dry mouth; relieve with moistened wash cloth, ice chips, sips of water, hard candy, as tolerated and allowed. Report if dry mouth does not gradually resolve.
- Observe for side effects such as dizziness, confusion, constipation or urinary retention, blurred vision, and sensitivity to light.
- Be alert for other more serious side effects including skin rash, eye pain, difficulty breathing, irregular heartbeat, hallucinations, and difficulty swallowing. Report any of these immediately.

INTRAOPERATIVE NURSING CARE

Observing a client undergoing surgery may be a component of a nursing student's experience. Doing so will not only give the student a better idea of surgical procedures, but it will also help in understanding the client's feelings and apprehensions. Many graduate nurses are specially trained to work in the OR or PACU.

☛ Key Concept

Observing surgical procedures aids in understanding why a postoperative client experiences pain and discomfort.

Nurses and surgical technologists assist surgeons in the operating room. The two basic categories of assistant are the sterile assistant and the circulating assistant. The *sterile assistant* (*scrub nurse* or *OR technician*) is scrubbed, gowned, and gloved. He or she functions within the sterile field. Duties include handing instruments to the surgeon, threading needles, cutting sutures, assisting with retraction and suction, and handling specimens (Fig. 56-3).

The *circulating nurse* works outside the sterile field. Duties include opening sterile packs, delivering supplies and instruments to the sterile team, delivering medications to the sterile nurse, labeling specimens, and keeping records during the surgical procedure. This person acts as a client advocate by monitoring the situation and maintaining safety in the operating room. In most cases, the circulating nurse must be a registered nurse.

POSTOPERATIVE NURSING CARE

The Post-anesthesia Care Unit

Nearly all hospitals have a room or suite set aside for the care of clients immediately after surgery. Various names are used to identify this area, including post-anesthesia care unit (PACU) and the post-anesthesia recovery (PAR) area. Here, the client is carefully monitored until he or she is fully recovered from anesthesia. This room is located next to the operating room so surgeons and nurses are readily available. Concentrating postoperative clients in a limited area makes it possible for one nurse to give close attention to two or three clients at the same time.

Articles that may be needed for care are located near the client's unit in the PACU:

- Breathing aids: Oxygen, suction equipment, nasal and oral airways, pulse oximeters, mechanical breathing bag or other resuscitation equipment, emergency equipment such as laryngoscopes, trach sets, endotracheal tubes
- Circulatory aids: BP apparatus, stethoscope, IV solution, tourniquets, syringes and needles, cardiac monitors, cardiac arrest equipment, cardiac drugs and respiratory stimulants, defibrillators
- Drugs: Narcotics, sedatives, and drugs for emergency situations
- Other supplies: Surgical dressings, sandbags, warmed blankets, extra pillows, and various other items

Each client unit has a recovery bed/cart equipped with side rails, poles for IV medications, wheel brakes, and often, a chart rack. The cart can be moved easily and adjusted to elevate or lower the head or feet. The bedside stand holds tissues, an emesis basin, tongue blades, a face cloth, and a towel. Each unit has outlets for piped-in oxygen, suction, and BP and other monitoring equipment. Warmed bath blankets are available to assist

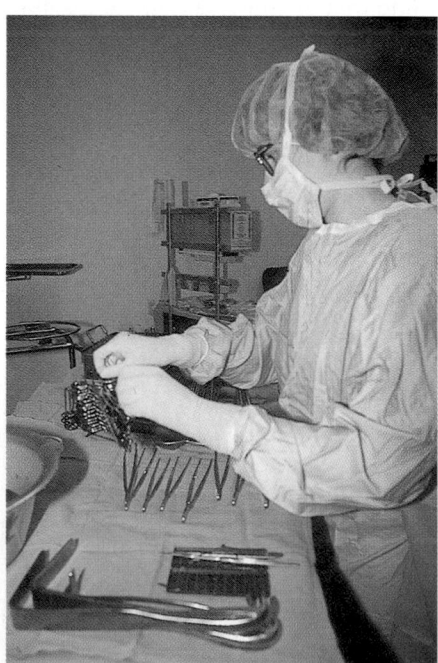

FIGURE 56-3. The scrub nurse prepares sterile instruments for the surgeon's use.

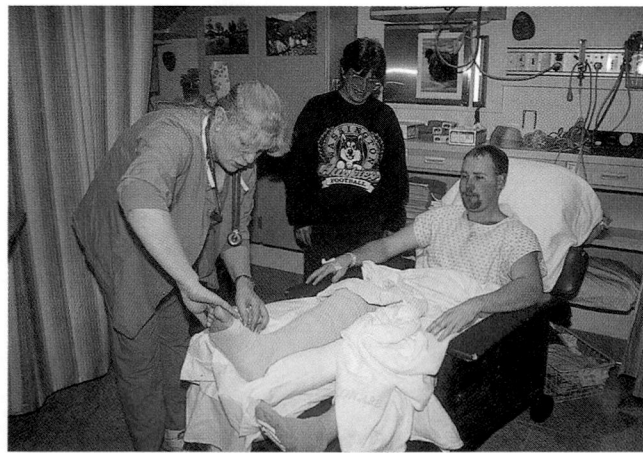

FIGURE 56-4. In ambulatory surgery, the client may be placed in a lounge chair for recovery from anesthesia. The client is assessed to determine if criteria for discharge have been met. Client and family teaching is a vital part of care before discharge from the ambulatory surgery facility.

the client with the normal body chilling that usually follows anesthesia.

☛ KEY CONCEPT

In the case of ambulatory surgery, clients may recover in a special reclining lounge chair. They still require careful nursing observation (see Fig. 56-4).

Moving the Client to the PACU

When a client is moved from the operating room to the PACU, every effort is made to avoid unnecessary strain or injury and to accomplish the transfer as quickly as possible with the least exposure. Enough people must be available to safely transfer the semi-conscious client from the OR table to the PACU cart. The anesthesiologist or nurse anesthetist and circulating nurse go to the PACU with the client to make certain that the client's condition is stable.

The nurse anesthetist or anesthesiologist is responsible for monitoring the client's condition throughout the surgical procedure until that responsibility transfers to PACU nurses. The anesthesia person reports the client's condition to the PACU nurse and leaves the surgeon's postoperative orders and any special instructions required.

Receiving the Client in the Nursing Unit

When the client is nearly awake, PACU staff confers with the anesthesiologist or nurse anesthetist to determine if the client is ready for transfer to the receiving unit, which can be an ambulatory recovery area or a bed in a nursing unit. The PACU staff calls the nursing station before the client's discharge from the PACU to report on the client's condition, indicating what special equipment will be needed for the client when he or she returns to the nursing unit or ambulatory recovery area. The receiving nursing staff will then have time to prepare for the client's arrival. The preparation of a room for a surgical client includes opening the bed by pulling all the top linens to the foot or side of the bed (see Chap. 49). The furniture is arranged so that the client can be easily transferred from the recovery room cart to the bed. All necessary equipment must also be in place before the client arrives.

When the client arrives from the PACU, immediately check his or her vital signs and compare them with those obtained by PACU staff. Any significant variation in vital signs must be reported immediately. The nurse from the PACU will provide a report to the floor staff. In Practice: Nursing Procedure 56-1 reviews information needed for receiving the client from the PACU.

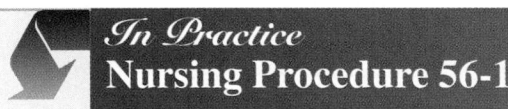

In Practice
Nursing Procedure 56-1

RECEIVING THE CLIENT FROM THE POST-ANESTHESIA CARE UNIT (PACU)

Supplies and Equipment

BP apparatus
emesis basin
frequent vital signs sheet
IV stand
oxygen equipment
stethoscope
suction apparatus
thermometer
tissues
any other supplies or equipment needed for this individual

Steps

1. Carefully identify the client. Check the name band with another nurse. Check the health record with the name band before the PACU nurse gives the report. Wear gloves.
   RATIONALE: *Because the client is not fully conscious, identification depends on the name band. This client has nonintact skin. Wear gloves to protect yourself against exposure to body substances.*

2. Attach any drainage apparatus such as from a wound, catheters, or chest tubes, as ordered, before the PACU nurse leaves. Attach gastric or other tubes to the appropriate suction device. Make sure the IV pump is operating properly and plug it in. Attach any monitors.
   RATIONALE: *These items must be in proper working order. The chest tube suction must operate properly to maintain life.*

3. Keep the client flat (often in Sims' position) until he or she awakens (unless specifically ordered otherwise). If the client is nauseated, position the client on his or her side, unless contraindicated. Keep side rails up.
   RATIONALE: *The semianesthetized client could fall from bed.*

4. Maintain an open airway. Feel for the client's exhaled breath by holding a hand in front of the client's nose. Just because the client's chest or abdomen moves does not necessarily mean that the client is breathing. Watch for any signs of respiratory distress (rapid breathing, cyanosis, panic).
   RATIONALE: *Anesthesia and sedatives can depress respirations.*

(continued)

In Practice
Nursing Procedure 56-1 (*Continued*)

5. Carry out any orders for immediate drug or oxygen administration.
   RATIONALE: *Immediately ordered interventions help stabilize and make the client comfortable as soon as possible.*

6. Assess level of consciousness. If the client received spinal anesthesia, assess sensation in and the ability to move the extremities. Record the advancing level of sensation as it progresses.
   RATIONALE: *This is part of ongoing assessment and documentation.*

7. Take vital signs as ordered. Take BP at least every 15 minutes for the first hour and gradually less often, as ordered, if it is stable. Record vital signs (VS) on the special frequent vital signs sheet. Continuously, watch for signs of shock, such as restlessness or panic (see Box 56-1). Check the client's temperature every 2 to 4 hours.
   RATIONALE: *Complications such as hemorrhage are most likely to occur in the immediate postoperative period. Changing BP values and pulse rate often are the first indicators of hypovolemic shock, which is a consequence of blood loss.*

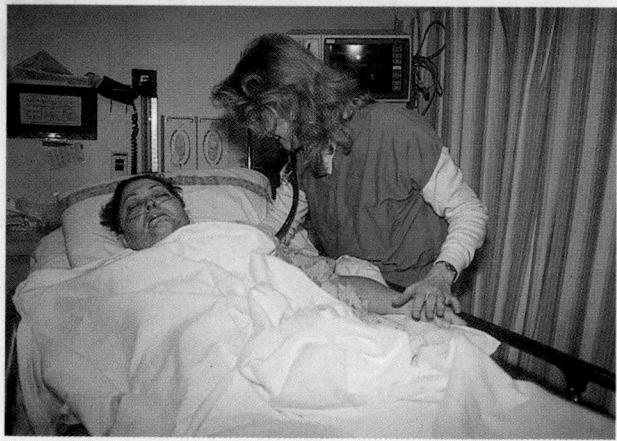

Measure BP every 15 minutes for the first hour, and gradually less often after the client's condition stabilizes.

8. Inspect dressings; note signs of hemorrhage and any unusual amount of drainage. If necessary, reinforce but *do not change* dressings. Report any unusual drainage.
   RATIONALE: *The physician may wish to see the drainage's character; the dressing may be weighed to determine exact blood loss. Removing the dressing might upset the suture line.*

9. If vomiting occurs, turn the client's head to the side. *Rationale: Turning the head to the side helps to empty the mouth, preventing aspiration.* Use the emesis basin to catch the emesis. Check to see if antiemetics can be given.
   RATIONALE: *The emesis basin is specially shaped to fit around the client's neck. Antiemetics help prevent excessive vomiting.*

10. If the client vomits excessively or violently, check to make sure dressings and incisions are intact and that suction equipment operates properly.
    RATIONALE: *The quick and violent movements of vomiting can interfere with the suture line. Stitches or staples can rip out. If vomiting occurs, it may mean the suction is operating improperly.*

11. Measure emesis, noting its time, amount, and nature on the client's health record. Report your findings to the charge nurse. Save the emesis if it appears unusual.
    RATIONALE: *This information is important for monitoring fluid and electrolyte balance; unusual appearance may suggest a possible problem requiring notification of the surgeon.*

12. If the client is receiving IV fluids or blood, check the rate of flow and the time for the next bag (see Chap. 63). Make sure the needle is in the vein. Check the IV site for swelling, warmth, pain, blanching, or redness.
    RATIONALE: *Maintaining a patent (open) IV is necessary for adequate hydration and in case emergency medications must be given. The signs listed may indicate IV infiltration.*

13. Remove and discard gloves and wash the hands.
    RATIONALE: *Proper glove disposal and handwashing help to prevent the risk of infection transmission.*

14. Record intake and output (I&O). Include any oral and IV fluids, as well as drainage, voiding, and emesis.
    RATIONALE: *I&O is monitored to identify normal output and fluid loss.*

15. Document all vital signs, treatments, and the client's reactions. Be sure to include consciousness level and returning sensation in extremities.
    RATIONALE: *Documentation provides communication and continuity of care.*

When the client is settled in bed, and after vital signs have been taken and all immediate orders have been carried out, notify the client's family that the client is back in the room. Although the family should not visit for long, they can help reassure the client by spending a few minutes at the bedside.

Nursing Alert

Leave no client alone until he or she has fully regained consciousness. Check the physician's orders and carry them out immediately.

Immediate Postoperative Complications

Observe the client postoperatively for immediate complications, including hemorrhage, shock, *hypoxia* (inadequate oxygen), and *hypothermia* (below normal body temperature).

Hemorrhage

Hemorrhage during or after surgery can lead to shock, requiring blood transfusions or other fluid replacement. (Usually, the client's blood has been routinely typed and crossmatched before surgery so that compatible blood is available.) Prompt action is necessary in the event of hemorrhage, because excessive bleeding could be fatal.

Secondary hemorrhage sometimes occurs postoperatively; consequently, inspect the client's wound dressings frequently. If bleeding is noted, report it. Also, be sure to look under the client. (Blood may pool there.) However, concealed bleeding, also called *occult* or *internal bleeding,* is revealed mainly through signs of shock.

Shock

The most dangerous type of postoperative shock is known as *circulatory* or *hypovolemic shock,* caused by severe hemorrhage. (See Chapter 43 for a detailed discussion on shock.) Severe blood loss is life threatening: cells cannot live without the oxygen that blood normally carries to them. Be on constant alert for the signs of shock listed in Box 56-1.

If shock occurs, take these steps:

- Call for help.
- Control hemorrhage (use direct pressure, if needed).
- Position the client flat with his or her feet elevated, unless contraindicated. *Rationale: This position drains blood from the feet and legs and increases blood supply to the brain and central organs.*
- Administer oxygen and drugs as ordered by a physician. *Rationale: Administering oxygen helps to prevent hypoxia.*
- Administer blood, plasma, or other parenteral fluids as ordered by the physician. Electrolytes will probably be added to the IV line. *Rationale: These agents help to restore the client's blood volume and fluid balance.*
- Anticipate that the physician may order vasopressor drugs. *Rationale: These drugs increase BP.*

Hypoxia (Hypoxemia)

Anesthetics and preoperative medications sometimes depress respirations and interfere with blood oxygenation, leading to a lack of oxygen in the tissues, a condition known as **hypoxia** or *hypoxemia.* Mucus blocking the trachea or the bronchial passages also lowers the amount of oxygen that enters the lungs, thereby reducing the amount of oxygen available for transport to the tissues. Oxygen and suction equipment should always be readily available for emergency use. Hypoxia is discussed in more detail in Chapters 85 and 86. Symptoms of hypoxia include dyspnea, rapid pulse, initial elevated BP followed by lowered BP, dizziness, and cyanosis. (Some of the symptoms of shock as listed in Box 56-1 are also related to hypoxia.)

Treatment for hypoxia depends on its cause. Usually the client receives oxygen by nasal cannula, or even a mask if higher oxygen concentrations are required. Monitor the client with a *pulse oximeter,* a device that can be attached to the client's nailbed (finger or toe) or earlobe (Fig. 56-5). The physician orders the minimum acceptable oxygen concentration (usually about 95%). If the oxygen saturation falls below the minimum level, the physician is notified and further action

➤➤ BOX 56-1

SIGNS OF SHOCK

- Hypotension
- Narrowed pulse pressure
- Tachycardia; thready pulse
- Restlessness and anxiety
- Difficulty breathing
- Cyanosis or dusky skin color
- Extreme thirst
- Cold, clammy skin
- Hypothermia
- Low oxygen saturation (as measured by pulse oximeter)
- Slowed capillary refill
- Ringing in the ears; difficulty seeing

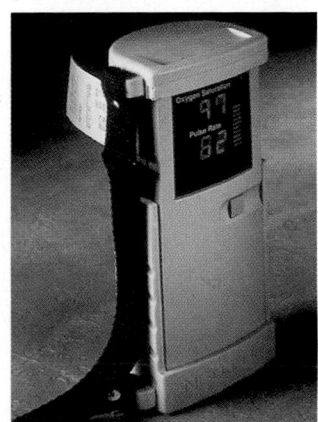

FIGURE 56-5. A portable pulse oximeter. The top reading is the oxygen saturation as a percentage (97%). The bottom reading is the client's pulse rate (62).

is usually taken. In Practice: Nursing Procedure 56-2 lists the steps for using a pulse oximeter.

Hypothermia

Clients often complain of feeling cold after surgery. This is commonly associated with anesthesia. However, severe chilling can cause hypoxia and cardiac stress. The following are significant signs and symptoms of postoperative **hypothermia:**

- Temperature below 97.5° Fahrenheit (36.4° Celsius) rectally

---

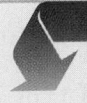

In Practice
Nursing Procedure 56-2

USING A PULSE OXIMETER

Supplies and Equipment

Pulse oximeter machine
Sensor finger clip
Nail polish remover (if needed)

Steps

1. Choose the sensor appropriate for the client's size.
   RATIONALE: *Inappropriate size may cause inaccurate results.*

2. Choose the appropriate location. Place the adhesive sensors and finger clip sensor for adults on their index, middle, or ring finger. Adhesive sensors also can be placed on a client's toe unless the client has decreased circulation in the lower extremities. A small earlobe clip is available for use on small adults, children, and infants. If necessary, place the newborn adhesive sensor on the baby's foot.

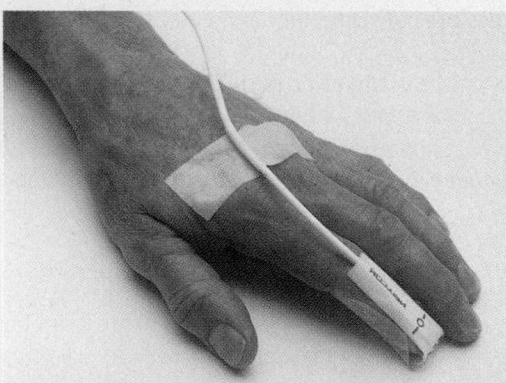

The pulse oximeter sensor is placed on the client's index finger. For a single reading, the sensor need not be taped in place.

3. Before applying the sensor, use an alcohol wipe on the site.
   RATIONALE: *Using alcohol ensures that the site is clean and dry.*

4. Remove any fingernail polish or acrylic nails on the fingers to be used.
   RATIONALE: *The sensor may be unable to provide an accurate reading through nail polish or acrylic nails.*

5. If there are any doubts about the chosen site, check the client's proximal pulse and capillary refill. Check capillary refill by pressing on the client's skin. Normal color should return immediately when pressure is released.
   RATIONALE: *Decreased circulation could skew oxygen saturation readings.*

6. Check the sensor's markings to make sure the light-emitting diode and photo detector are correctly aligned. They should be opposite each other.
   RATIONALE: *If they are not aligned, the sensor will give an inaccurate reading.*

7. Attach the sensor to the client cable and turn it on. The digital read-out or light bar should show readings and alarm settings. The type will depend on the specific monitor being used.
   RATIONALE: *A read-out or light bar indicates that the machine is working.*

8. Obtain a one-time reading or keep the sensor in place and the monitor on continuous monitoring if ordered. If continuous monitoring is ordered, always make sure the alarms are on before leaving the client. The monitors have preset limits that can be changed per physician's order or facility policy. If the monitor is turned off, the alarm limits will default back to the original settings. The continuous pulse oximeter gives audible and visual alarms. The audible alarm can be silenced for 60 seconds at a time by pressing "audio alarm off." Most monitors will reset after 60 seconds.
   RATIONALE: *Setting the alarms ensures notification if the client's values are out of the desired range (indicating a possible problem that requires intervention).*

9. Move an adhesive sensor every 4 hours and a clip type sensor at least every 2 hours. Watch for signs of tissue breakdown or irritation from adhesives or clips.
   RATIONALE: *Moving the sensor helps to prevent tissue irritation and necrosis.*

10. In the client's chart, document each oximeter reading and location of sensor. This is often recorded on the frequent vital sign sheet. Report any downward changes of 3 to 5% in readings.
    RATIONALE: *Documentation provides communication and continuity of care.*

- Shivering and "goose flesh" unrelieved by warm blankets
- Client complaints of being extremely cold

Apply warmed blankets or use an overbed warmer. These measures will raise the client's core temperature. (This is done most often in the PACU.)

Postoperative Discomforts

By the time the client returns from the PACU to the ambulatory receiving area or nursing unit, he or she is usually awake and aware of a number of discomforts. One measure used to relieve these discomforts is the administration of medications. Commonly used medications for postoperative complications are summarized at In Practice: Important Medications 56-2.

Pain.   Pain usually is the first postoperative discomfort the client notices. It is usually most severe immediately after the client's recovery from anesthesia. If the client receives medication early and subsequent doses are spaced properly, he or she will be relatively comfortable. Make sure the client is conscious and that his or her vital signs are stable before you give pain medications. *Rationale: Analgesics are associated with respiratory depression, placing the client at high risk.* Common pain medications are narcotics similar to those given preoperatively, in addition to analgesics such as ibuprofen. Chapter 55 describes ways to assist all clients with pain management.

Thirst.   Thirst is present postoperatively, usually due to a fluid decrease preoperatively, fluid loss during surgery, anesthetic recovery, and dryness caused by drying agents (eg, atropine). Most clients receive IV fluids during surgery and immediately postoperatively. These fluids help prevent thirst, as does rinsing the mouth. In some cases, the client may be allowed to suck on a wet wash cloth, sip water, or suck ice chips in small amounts soon after surgery. Hard candy or chewing gum may also be permitted.

Abdominal Distention.   Temporary paralysis of intestinal peristalsis allows gas to accumulate in the client's intestines, causing abdominal *distention* (bloating). Handling of the intestines, anesthesia, drugs, lack of solid food, and restricted

---

In Practice
Important Medications 56-2

FOR POSTOPERATIVE CARE

Postoperative Nausea
- Cyclizine hydrochloride (Marezine). Given preoperatively to prevent postoperative vomiting.
- Metoclopramide (Reglan). Used for postoperative nausea when nasogastric suction is undesirable. Available in oral, IM, and IV forms. May be given at the end of surgery as a preventive measure.
- Prochlorperazine (Compazine, Stemetil). Given for postoperative nausea. Available in injectable, syrup, rectal suppository, and sustained-release tablet forms.
- Trimethobenzamide HCl (Tebamide, Tigan). Given to prevent emesis. Available in capsules, injectable, and suppositories.
- Ondansetron hydrochloride (Zofran), dolasetron mesylate (Anzemet), and promethazine hydrochloride (Anergan, Phenergan). Used less commonly.

Nursing Considerations
- Allergy to any drug may cause anaphylaxis.
- Side effects include drowsiness, dizziness, lethargy, dry mouth and respiratory passages, orthostatic hypotension, constipation.
- If the client has glaucoma, this condition may be aggravated by drugs. Certain other physical conditions preclude the use of specific medications. The physician will take these factors into consideration when ordering any medications.

Postoperative Constipation
Stool Softener
- Docusate (Colace, Diocto C, Regulax)

Laxatives
- Bisacodyl (Dulcolax)
- Docusate, casanthranol (Peri-Colace)
- Magnesium citrate (Citroma)
- Magnesium hydroxide (Milk of Magnesia, MOM)
- Senna (Senokot)

Bulk-forming Agents
- Bulk-forming psyllium (Metamucil, Hydrocil instant, Genfiber): chewable pieces, effervescent powder, granules, powder, wafers
- Polycarbophil (Fiber-con)

Nursing Considerations
- May stimulate excessive gastrointestinal motility (avoid administering these agents to clients with gastrointestinal bleeding, obstruction, perforation).
- Be alert for possible diarrhea.
- Monitor older clients for possible extrapyramidal side effects (see Chaps. 91 and 93) due to a possible *paradoxical reaction* (opposite reaction).

Postoperative Flatus
- Famotidine (Pepcid)
- Ranitidine (Zantac)
- Simethicone (Gas-X, Mylicon, Flatulex)

Nursing Considerations
- Assess for presence of bowel sounds
- Be alert for possible side effects, including constipation, headache, diarrhea, nausea, and skin lesions.

body movements disturb normal peristalsis during surgery. Accumulated gas (*flatus*) may cause sharp pains that often are more distressing than incisional pain. Moving from side to side, sitting up in bed, or ambulating soon after surgery helps the client to expel flatus. Delay offering solid food until bowel sounds have returned. (See Chapter 51.)

☛ KEY CONCEPT

If a client complains of distention or "gas pains," do not give ice or allow the client to take fluid through a drinking straw. These actions tend to add air to the bowel and increase gas.

If the client's discomfort increases and nursing measures bring no relief, a physician may order insertion of a rectal tube. Medications also may be ordered.

Famotidine (Pepcid) may be given IV and ranitidine (Zantac) may be given intramuscularly (IM) or IV until the client is able to tolerate food. These medications reduce stomach acid and lessen heartburn and gastric distress. When the client is no longer NPO, these medications may be given orally. Simethicone (Mylicon) is also given orally to reduce gas.

During each shift, assess the client for the presence of bowel sounds by listening to his or her abdomen with a stethoscope. In Practice: Nursing Care Guidelines 51-2 in Chapter 51 describes this procedure.

If bowel sounds have not returned within 2 to 3 hours following surgery, report this. If intestinal paralysis persists, a serious complication known as *paralytic ileus* may develop, in which the bowel has no peristaltic activity at all. Any ingested food, fluids, and digestive juices may accumulate and cause considerable discomfort. This may be life threatening, because a bowel obstruction may occur and the bowel may rupture. A nasogastric tube is inserted to decompress or empty the stomach of its contents until peristalsis returns. Emergency surgery may be required to eliminate a bowel obstruction.

Nausea.   If the client complains of nausea, give ordered medications to prevent emesis. Often such medications are given IM or rectally. Some also may be given IV (see In Practice: Important Medications 56-2).

Urinary Retention.   The client may have difficulty voiding because of anesthesia's effects. Help the client sit upright, pour warm water over the vulva or penis, place the client's hands in warm water, and run water so the client can hear it. If the client has not voided within 8 hours after surgery, catheterization may be ordered for relief. Monitor the amount of fluid taken through IV infusion and by mouth to judge the amount of urine likely to be accumulating in the bladder.

☛ KEY CONCEPT

The postoperative client may be permitted to take a sitz bath, a warm shower, or a warm tub bath. This often facilitates voiding and defecation.

Constipation.   Disruption of the normal diet and daily elimination schedule, pain medications, inactivity, and slowed peristalsis because of anesthesia's effects may cause constipation. As soon as the client can eat or drink, encourage fluid intake (specifically fruit juices). Help the client to the commode or bathroom. Encourage ambulation to stimulate peristalsis. Some physicians routinely prescribe a stool softener, such as Colace, both pre-and postoperatively. Usually, routine postoperative orders include a medication to prevent this complication (see In Practice: Important Medications 56-2).

Restlessness and Sleeplessness.   The client may be restless and have difficulty sleeping in the postoperative period. Make every effort to relieve these symptoms through ordinary nursing measures. Medications to promote sleep and relieve pain also play an important part.

Prevention of Later Postoperative Complications

Dangers of prolonged bed rest following surgery include respiratory and circulatory complications including hypostatic pneumonia, development of pressure ulcers, generalized edema, contractures, difficulty in weight bearing and balance, formation of renal calculi, scrotal edema, constipation, urinary retention, loss of appetite, and general mental depression and disorientation. Thus, the sooner the client can move about after surgery, the better it is for the client.

At first, the client may dangle his or her legs over the edge of the bed, then sit in a chair, and finally walk. Early ambulation, preferably on the day of surgery, assists circulation, improves respiration, prevents lung congestion, and aids in voiding and bowel activity. The client who is out of bed and walking around will eat better and sleep more soundly. He or she can become more self-sufficient, promoting a rapid recovery. The nurse helps clients to ambulate as soon as possible after surgical procedures, according to the surgeon's orders. Chapter 48 describes specific procedures for assisting the client to dangle, to move from bed to chair, to walk, and to use crutches or a walker.

Respiratory Complications

The principal respiratory complications following surgery are hypostatic or aspiration **pneumonia** (inflammation of or accumulation of fluid in the lung) and atelectasis.

Pneumonia can result when fluid or mucus is aspirated into the lungs. Inhibition of normal clearance mechanisms (such as coughing) caused by anesthesia can lead to *aspiration pneumonia. Hypostatic pneumonia* is caused by immobility, particularly lying on the back. This condition does not involve invasion by microorganisms. Postoperative pneumonia caused by infectious microorganisms is less common.

Atelectasis is the collapse of air sacs in the lungs, caused by mucous plugs that close the bronchi. Atelectasis may involve all or part of a lung. The postoperative client often is reluctant to cough or breathe deeply because of incisional pain. This can lead to atelectasis. This client may become somewhat cyanotic as respirations and pulse become very rapid and breathing becomes difficult.

An important nursing responsibility is preventing postoperative respiratory complications. Assess lung sounds at least once per shift for evidence of fluid accumulation, dyspnea, atelectasis, or other respiratory symptoms. Other important signs are fever and cyanosis (see Chap. 47).

Prevention of Respiratory Complications.   Respiratory exercises or treatments such as turning, coughing and deep breathing (**TCDB**), chest percussion, and using the incen-

tive spirometer can reduce or eliminate respiratory complications. In Practice: Nursing Care Guidelines 56-3 explains some of these respiratory exercises. Be sure to encourage ambulation as well.

Splinting the incision by supporting the operative area with a pillow, folded bath towel, or blanket helps relieve

---

In Practice
Nursing Care Guidelines 56-3

ASSISTING THE CLIENT WITH POSTOPERATIVE BREATHING EXERCISES

General Guidelines
- Remember that the postoperative client will be better able to perform these exercises if he or she learns them during the preoperative period.
- Wear gloves for these procedures.
- Explain procedures to the client before you assist with them.
- Document all procedures and results.

Splinting an Incision
- Splinting relieves pressure on the abdominal suture line, and thus relieves pain.
- Use a pillow, folded bath blanket, or large towel as a splint to distribute pressure evenly across an incision. Assist the client to use the splint for the first few days after surgery. The client will be able to hold it in place after that.

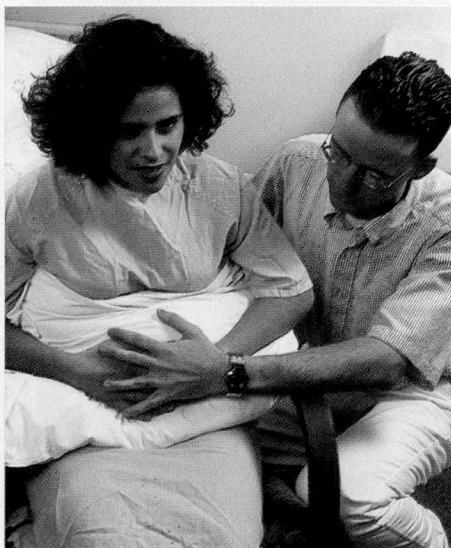

Holding a pillow or a folded bath blanket and pulling it tightly against the incision splints the abdominal or chest incision. This technique helps to make coughing or deep breathing more comfortable and promotes better oxygenation.

- Grasp the pillow or bath blanket at the edges and stretch it across the client's incision. Hold it from behind.
- Apply pressure firmly by pushing down on the splint (for the client who is lying in bed) or by pulling the

splint toward you from behind (when the client is sitting). Do this as the client coughs.
- Anticipate the timing and strength of each client's cough. Count aloud and feel the movement of the client's breathing as he or she prepares to cough.

Turning, Coughing, and Deep Breathing (TCDB)
- Instruct the client to take a deep breath and hold it for 2 to 5 seconds. *Rationale: A deep breath with holding allows air to reach the lung's most severely deflated areas.*
- Instruct the client to do a strong double-cough with the mouth open. *Rationale: The double-cough maneuver helps the client to mobilize and remove secretions.*

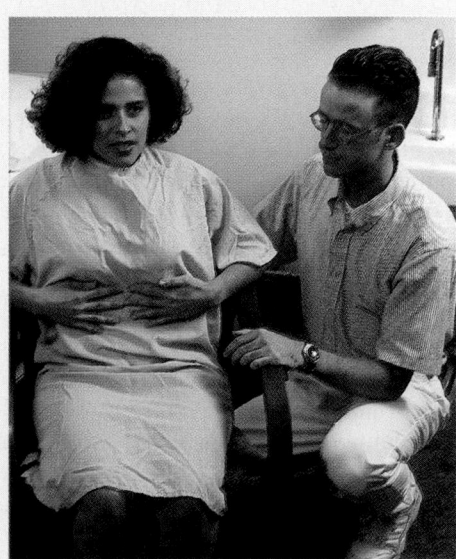

Instruct the client to take a deep breath and hold it for 2 to 5 seconds. Instruct the client to then do a strong double-cough with the mouth open.

- Repeat this process several times each hour, especially for the first few days postoperatively and while the client remains bedridden.

(continued)

In Practice
Nursing Care Guidelines 56-3 (Continued)

Huffing
• Teach the client to take a deep abdominal breath and then force air out in several short, quick breaths. The client should then take a second, deeper breath and force it out in short, panting movements. The client should then take an even deeper third breath and exhale it quickly in a strong huff. *Rationale: This series helps to loosen more secretions than just coughing.*
• Instruct the client to repeat this series of breaths as many times or for as long as is ordered.

Using the Incentive Spirometer
• Position the client as upright as possible without causing discomfort. *Rationale: An upright position allows the client to maximize the use of his or her diaphragm.*
• Explain the operation of the spirometer to the client. (See Fig. 56-2.) Set a goal—number of seconds or specific volume—to be attained. Agree on the number of times and how often the procedure is to be done, within physician's orders.
• Instruct the client to cough to remove as much mucus as possible before the treatment. *Rationale: This action enables the client to achieve the maximum inhalation.*
• Teach the client to take slow, deep breaths and to hold each breath at the end of inspiration for 2 to 5 seconds. *Rationale: Doing so allows air to reach the lung's most severely deflated areas.*
• Repeat the procedure until the client has achieved the established goal or has given his or her best effort at least 8 to 10 times. Ensure that the client does not repeat the process too rapidly. *Rationale: You do not want the client to inadvertently hyperventilate.*
• Instruct the client to repeat coughing or huffing at the procedure's end. *Rationale: The client must clear his or her lungs as much as possible.*
• Dispose of gloves and wash hands thoroughly at the end of the procedure. *Rationale: These procedures reduce the risk of infection transmission.*

Leg Exercises
• Position the client in a semi-Fowler's position.
• Have the client wiggle the toes. *Rationale: This is the first action that the client can do immediately after*

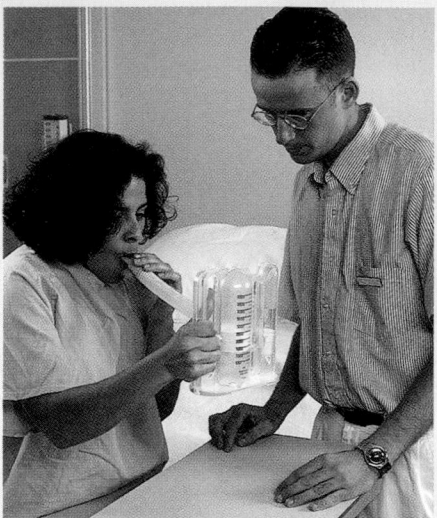

Teach the client to take slow, deep breaths into the spirometer and to hold each breath at the end of inspiration for 2 to 5 seconds.

surgery. This activity helps to promote circulatory function.
• Bend the client's knee and raise his or her foot. Hold this position for a few seconds.
• Extend the client's leg and lower it to the bed.
• Do this five times for each leg. *Rationale: Repetition helps to maintain muscle tone and decrease venous stasis.*
• Have the client trace circles with the feet by bending them down, in toward each other, up, and then out. Repeat this procedure five times with each foot. *Rationale: This motion promotes circulation and contributes to optimal respiratory exchange.*
• Position the client in a side-lying position.
• Flex and extend the client's hip joint by using a bicycling motion. Repeat this five times on each side. *Rationale: This motion promotes contraction of the muscle, which is strengthened with repetition.*
• Encourage the client to exercise his or her legs as much as possible when in bed. *Rationale: These actions promote circulatory function and prevent contractures, foot drop, and other complications.*

some pain and discomfort the client may experience during coughing. Explain why you hold the splint to the client's abdomen or chest, and provide ample analgesia prior to coughing and deep-breathing exercises to maximize pain relief.

The incentive spirometer, which forces the client to concentrate on inspirations while providing immediate feedback, aids deep breathing. Incentive spirometers come in two types:

flow activated and volume activated. The flow-activated incentive spirometer usually consists of one or more balls in a vertical tube. Because deep breaths (volume) are the objective, the length of time the client suspends the ball at the top of the tube determines the depth of the breath. Volume-activated devices come in many shapes, but because they measure volume directly, they make it easier for the client to understand when he or she has accomplished a deep breath.

☞ KEY CONCEPT

Breathing exercises will be more effective if the client learns and practices them preoperatively. The client also takes the incentive spirometer home at discharge, so these exercises can be continued.

Circulatory Complications

Serious circulatory complications can develop postoperatively.

   Thrombophlebitis.   A dangerous circulatory complication is thrombophlebitis, the formation of a blood clot in a vein. It is caused by *venous stasis* (the slowing or stopping of venous blood return) as a result of increased clotting, lack of activity, increased pressure within vessels, and other factors. It most often develops in the calves of the legs.

   To assess for thrombophlebitis, flex the client's foot up toward the knee (dorsiflexion) with the leg straight. If pain occurs behind the knee on dorsiflexion, it is known as a positive Homans' sign, indicating probable thrombophlebitis. Instruct the client to remain in bed, and report this finding immediately.

   If thrombophlebitis occurs, the following supportive measures may be ordered:

* Elevate the affected body part on a soft pillow when in bed.
* Administer anticoagulants as directed.
* Avoid rubbing the body part (may dislodge clot).
* Apply warmth as directed (see Chap. 54).
* In rare cases, the client is maintained on strict bedrest.

   Embolism.   An **embolus** (plural: emboli) is a piece of a clot or thrombus that breaks off and enters the person's circulatory system, usually obstructing the blood flow in a smaller vessel (**embolism**). Symptoms of embolism depend on its location; they include severe pain, nausea and vomiting, and severe shock.

   Probably the most life-threatening embolism is a blood clot that lodges in the small vessels of the lung, a *pulmonary embolism.* Signs of a pulmonary embolism include difficult breathing, sharp chest pain, cough, cyanosis, rapid respirations and heart rate, and severe anxiety.[1] A pulmonary embolism can rapidly be fatal.

   If the embolism is in an arm or leg, circulation distal to the embolus is often cut off with related symptoms, such as numbness, pain, and absence of pulse.

   An embolism often can be treated with the immediate administration of special medications that dissolve existing blood clots (*thrombolytic agents*). Examples include alteplase (Activase), streptokinase (Streptase), and urokinase (Abbokinase).

   One means of avoiding circulatory disorders is to apply elastic stockings, elastic roller bandages, or antiembolytic (TED) stockings as ordered by the physician (see Chap. 53). Other nursing measures used to prevent circulatory disorders include performing leg exercises every 2 hours, complete range of motion exercises every shift, and ambulation as soon as possible after surgery.

Other Complications

Infection.   A temperature elevation occurring 2 or 3 days after surgery, severe pain, and redness or swelling around an incision are usually signs of infection. Be vigilant for signs of infection, to prevent complications. Assess the client's incision at least every 4 hours and document your findings. Sterile technique and careful handwashing are important when changing dressings. Also wear gloves and carefully dispose of all waste materials, according to the agency's protocol. These activities help to prevent infections and the spreading of existing infections to others.

   Treatment of infection includes administration of antibiotics, increased fluids, rest, and an adequate diet to build up resistance. If necessary, the wound is drained. In some cases, the wound is cleaned or flushed with a solution (*wound irrigation*) (see Chap. 58).

   A serious situation today is the development of an infection caused by an antibiotic-resistant organism. Notable is the methicillin-resistant staphylococcus aureus (**MRSA**), which is very difficult to treat.

☞ KEY CONCEPT

An infection acquired in the hospital is known as a nosocomial *infection. Since most postoperative clients return home soon after surgery, it is vital to instruct the client and family about signs and symptoms of an infection. They should be instructed to report any problems immediately.*

   Dehiscence and Evisceration.   **Dehiscence** is the splitting open or separation of the surgical incision; if the incision opens enough so that abdominal organs (viscera) protrude, this is known as **evisceration** (Fig 56-6). Clients at risk for evisceration include those with poor wound healing (eg, diabetic clients), older adults with *friable* (fragile) skin, morbidly obese individuals, and persons with invasive abdominal cancer. Violent coughing or excess movement also can cause dehiscence or evisceration.

   Usually the client describes this sensation by saying "something gave." The condition is uncommon, but be prepared to deal with it. This is an urgent situation. Wear gloves (sterile ones if possible). Cover protruding structures with sterile ABD pads that have been moistened with sterile normal saline. Report the incident immediately. The greatest dangers from dehiscence and evisceration are infection, rupture or intestinal strangulation, and hemorrhage.

Additional Supportive Measures

Providing Adequate Nutrition.   The client should return to oral intake of adequate food and fluids as soon as bowel sounds return. Most people who have had uncomplicated surgery can function on IV therapy for a short time; however, they should resume oral intake as quickly as possible.

   Usually, the client starts with a progressive diet to avoid abdominal distention that may occur if peristalsis is sluggish. Upon the physician's orders, offer the client a clear liquid diet first. Progress to a full liquid diet, and finally a soft or general diet (see Chap. 32). Usually, the sooner the client tolerates

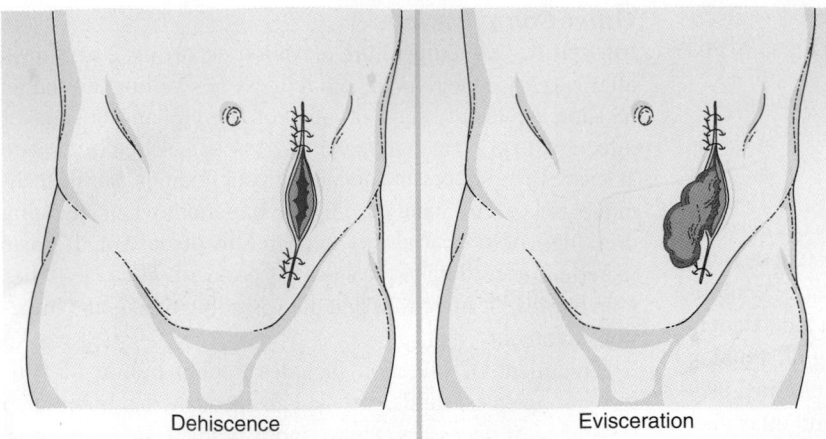

Dehiscence

Evisceration

FIGURE 56-6. Postoperative complications. *Dehiscence* is the splitting open or separation of the surgical incision. *Evisceration* is dehiscence with the protrusion of viscera. Both are emergency situations.

food, the sooner he or she recovers overall. This progression is often ordered as DAT (diet as tolerated).

☛ KEY CONCEPT

In many cases, a nutritional drink, such as Boost or Ensure, is given with meals after surgery, to supplement solid foods. Many clients find that they are able to drink, even if it is difficult to take solids.

Certain clients require more extensive diet therapy and should be evaluated by a dietitian, in cooperation with the physician. Special attention is needed for clients who are:

- Frail and/or older
- Obese
- Severely underweight
- Diabetic
- Suffering from malabsorption disorders, anorexia nervosa, or bulimia
- Diagnosed as having a defect in digestion
- Running a high fever for any length of time
- Experiencing severe trauma or amputation
- Suffering from a large infection
- Severely burned
- Experiencing extensive drainage from any body orifice or wound
- Suffering from severe diarrhea or constipation
- Unable to resume oral intake within 8 to 10 days
- Vomiting for an extended period

To rebuild tissue after the trauma of surgery, the client requires nutrients in excess of normal body needs. Protein is particularly necessary to rebuild wounded or diseased tissue (see also Chap. 32).

Irrigating Wounds.   Many clients have wounds that must be irrigated. A physician will order the type of solution to use, and may suggest a particular irrigation method. Otherwise, check the facility's policies and procedures to determine the method of wound irrigation. In some cases, irrigation follows sterile technique; in others, the procedure is clean. Specific procedures for wound irrigation are described in Chapter 58.

Changing Dressings.   A *dressing reinforcement* is the application of additional dressing materials to an already existing dressing. A *dressing change* is removing the dressing entirely and replacing it with a fresh one. Depending on the institution's policy, nurses can reinforce a dressing without an order, but a physician's order usually is needed to change a dressing. Use aseptic (sterile) technique when changing dressings. Chapter 57 covers the general principles of sterile technique. Always wear gloves and practice careful handwashing when changing dressings.

Removing Sutures and Staples.   Sometimes the nurse removes **sutures** and staples. Check the agency's policies. If assisting with or performing suture removal, use a disposable suture removal kit. A dressing may be applied after the sutures are out. Sutures are readily removed: Use a sterile scissor to cut the suture, and a sterile tweezer to pull out the thread on the side next to the knot.

Staples are used frequently because they are inert, do not cause infection, and are quickly inserted. To remove staples, follow the manufacturer's instructions. A special staple remover is required. Chapter 57 describes sterile technique for suture and staple removal.

Providing IV Therapy.   Most clients leave the operating room with an IV infusion running. Several types of IV solutions are commonly used. These include dextrose 5% and water (D_5W) and dextrose 5% and normal saline (D_5NS). Often, antibiotics and electrolytes are added. In most cases, the IV will be regulated by an electronic pump or controller. Chapter 63 discusses these methods as they relate to medication administration.

Know the techniques necessary when giving daily care, ambulating the client, and positioning the client who has an IV in place. It is important to recognize when the IV line has *infiltrated* (moved out of the vein) and to know how to discontinue it safely. Assess and monitor the infusion site at least once per hour and make sure the infusion is running. Record the amount infused as part of the client's total intake and output (I&O).

The Venous Access Lock.   Almost all clients will have an IV in place during surgery. Some clients will return to the nursing unit with a heparin/saline lock (a **venous access lock**) in place. In this case, fluids and medications can be given via the lock. They may be given with a needle and syringe, needleless system, or by or using an IV bag and tubing. In this case, the tubing is disconnected and the lock remains in place so that it is available to be used again without restarting the IV. The venous access lock is often used postoperatively to administer antibiotics.

Most facilities require venous access locks to be flushed one to three times per day, to keep them patent (open). The solution most often used to flush the venous access lock is sterile normal saline, although heparin may also be ordered.

Removal or discontinuance of the venous access lock is the same as for an IV (see In Practice: Nursing Procedure 63-10 in Chap. 63).

☞ KEY CONCEPT

The client who is having surgery needs not only physical preparation but also kind and gentle emotional support. The nurse is in a unique position to provide that support.

➤ STUDENT SYNTHESIS

Key Points

- Preoperative teaching is the first line of defense against postoperative complications. Teaching also helps to make clients feel more at ease during this stressful time.
- Before giving any pre- or postoperative medication, always check the client for drug allergies.
- Use of narcotics and sedatives can cause serious side effects. Watch carefully for these side effects, especially respiratory depression.
- Early postoperative complications include hemorrhage, shock, hypoxia, and hypothermia. Be alert for early indications of these complications and respond to them quickly.
- Postoperative discomforts may include pain, thirst, abdominal distention, nausea, urinary retention, constipation, restlessness, and sleeplessness. Try to anticipate client needs and take appropriate steps to alleviate these discomforts.
- Pulmonary hygiene is extremely important in the prevention of later postoperative complications.
- Early postoperative mobility helps to decrease the possibility of respiratory or circulatory complications.

Critical Thinking Exercises

1. Discuss the levels of urgency of various types of surgery. Where might each type be performed?

2. Develop a teaching plan for clients who will use the incentive spirometer postoperatively. Practice coaching a classmate in its use.

3. Discuss the importance of teaching the surgical client and the family. What differences exist between the healthcare delivery system of 20 years ago and the current system?

NCLEX-Style Review Questions

1. Clients remain NPO before surgery for approximately 8 to 10 hours to prevent:
   a. Abdominal distention
   b. Nausea and vomiting during anesthesia
   c. Pneumonia and atelectasis after surgery
   d. Weight gain associated with surgery

2. In evaluating the effectiveness of narcotics given preoperatively, the nurse would monitor for:
   a. Aspiration
   b. Pain relief
   c. Normal blood pressure
   d. Relaxation

3. Which of the following statements by a client indicates that the client needs further instructions? "After surgery I will need to":
   a. "ambulate with assistance."
   b. "turn, cough, and deep breathe."
   c. "use the incentive spirometer."
   d. "use pain medication only when my pain is severe."

4. Two days following surgery to remove a client's appendix, the nurse notes that the client has abdominal distention, abdominal pain, and diminished bowel sounds. The most appropriate nursing action would be:
   a. Apply antiembolytic stockings.
   b. Encourage the client to ambulate.
   c. Encourage the client to use the incentive spirometer.
   d. Increase the client's food intake.

5. A client states that "it feels like something gave way." What action would be most appropriate by the nurse?
   a. Assess the surgical site for dehiscence.
   b. Give the client fluids to prevent shock.
   c. Notify the physician immediately.
   d. Notify the surgical team.

Reference

1. Taylor, C., Lillis, C., & LeMone, P. (2001). *Fundamentals of nursing: The art and science of nursing care*. Philadelphia: Lippincott Williams & Wilkins.

CHAPTER

57

Surgical Asepsis

LEARNING OBJECTIVES

1. List at least five examples each of sterile and nonsterile body areas.
2. Differentiate between medical and surgical asepsis.
3. Differentiate between disinfection and sterilization.
4. List guidelines to follow when using sterile technique.
5. Demonstrate the proper technique for opening a sterile tray and sterile package.
6. Demonstrate the correct method for handing sterile supplies to another nurse.
7. Describe the procedures for female and male catheterization, demonstrating each on a lab model.
8. Explain the procedure for removal of a retention catheter.

NEW TERMINOLOGY

autoclave
clean
contaminated
dirty
disinfection

sterile
sterile technique
sterilization
surgical asepsis

Keeping the client and the environment *clean* is necessary to maintain comfort and well-being, as well as to reduce the risk of infection transmission. In addition, in specific circumstances, keeping aspects of the environment *sterile* is critical to ensure that the client does not develop an infection and that he or she is able to recover from illness. This chapter explains the differences between *medical asepsis* (clean technique) and *surgical asepsis* (sterile technique). This chapter discusses steps in surgical asepsis and how to perform selected procedures in which surgical asepsis is necessary.

ASEPSIS

To effectively limit the transfer of microorganisms, the nurse must understand the difference between commonly used terms as they apply to asepsis. **Dirty** is a term for any object that has not been cleaned or sterilized for removal of microorganisms. A dirty object has microorganisms on or in it. Your textbook, pencil, and hands are dirty if you have not washed them. A **contaminated** object was clean or sterile before it touched a dirty object. **Clean** implies that *many* of the most harmful microorganisms have been removed. Mechanical cleansing (scrubbing) and use of disinfectants are sufficient for this purpose. **Sterile** means that the item or area is free of *all* microorganisms and spores. (A *spore* is a resting stage of some microorganisms, and is resistant to environmental changes. See Chap. 40.)

Many body parts are clean but not sterile. Examples include the skin, mouth, gastrointestinal tract, and upper respiratory tract. These areas are open to the outside and are inhabited by microorganisms at all times. Other body parts are sterile. Either they do not normally open to the outside (such as the abdominal cavity or the ovary) or they do not normally contain any microorganisms. Some areas (such as the urinary bladder) are prone to infection, even though they are normally sterile.

Medical Asepsis or Clean Technique

The purpose of maintaining *medical asepsis* is to prevent the spread of disease from one person to another, whether it is from client to nurse, client to client, or nurse to client. Chapter 41 discusses techniques of medical asepsis, also called *clean technique*. Remember that handwashing is the most important medical asepsis technique; skin cannot be sterilized, but it can be cleaned.

Surgical Asepsis or Sterile Technique

To maintain sterility, **surgical asepsis** or **sterile technique** is used. Surgical asepsis differs from medical asepsis in that surgical asepsis uses sterile technique. Use of effective sterile technique means that no organisms are carried to the client. Microorganisms are destroyed before they can enter the body.

Sterile technique is used when changing dressings, administering parenteral (outside the digestive tract) medications, and performing surgical and other procedures, such as urinary catheterization. With surgical asepsis, first articles are sterilized, and then their contact with any unsterile articles is

prevented. When a sterile article touches an unsterile article, it becomes contaminated—it is no longer sterile.

☛ KEY CONCEPT

Sterile to sterile remains sterile. Sterile to clean or dirty becomes contaminated. Always think before you touch anything.

DISINFECTION AND STERILIZATION

Disinfection

Disinfection is a process that results in the destruction of most pathogens, but not necessarily their spores. Common methods of disinfection include the use of alcohol wipes, a hexachlorophene (pHisoHex, Septisol) or chlorhexidine gluconate (Hibiclens) soap scrub, or a povidone-iodine (Betadine) scrub to kill microorganisms on the skin. Stronger disinfectants include phenol and mercury bichloride, which are too strong to be used on living tissue. Boiling also can be used to disinfect inanimate objects. However, it does not destroy all organisms or spores.

Sterilization

Sterilization is the process of exposing articles to steam heat under pressure or to chemical disinfectants long enough to kill all microorganisms and spores. After a client leaves a healthcare facility, equipment he or she used is either sterilized or discarded. For example, at discharge a client usually takes home items such as washbasins, mouth care utensils, and incentive spirometers; if he or she doesn't, then these items are discarded. Occasionally, large or very expensive equipment is sterilized for reuse.

Sterilization is a process that destroys all organisms and spores. Exposure to steam at 18 pounds of pressure at a temperature of 257° Fahrenheit (125° Celsius) for 15 minutes will kill even the toughest organisms. A pressure steam sterilizer is called an **autoclave**.

Some chemicals also can be used to sterilize an object. However, *chemical disinfectants* powerful enough to destroy germs or extreme temperatures cannot be used on certain articles, such as plastic. Thus, most plastic items are disposable. In addition, moist heat such as that found in an autoclave dulls the sharp cutting edges of some instruments; therefore, if the items are not disposable, dry heat or chemicals best sterilize them. Today, however, most sharps—such as scalpels and suture removal scissors—are disposable. Needles used for injections are always discarded.

Other methods of sterilization include *radiation* and *gas sterilization* with ethylene oxide.

STERILE TECHNIQUE

Reasons for Sterile Technique

To prevent the spread of infection, the supplies used for surgical and other sterile procedures must be free of all microorganisms. Anything that touches an open wound or skin break, enters a sterile body cavity, or punctures the skin must be sterile to prevent introducing microorganisms.

Many healthcare facilities prepare sterile supplies in a central supply room (CSR), also called central sterile supply (CSS), or purchase them in a sterile package and dispose of them after use. Some items, such as surgical towels or drapes, are packaged in cloth, paper, or plastic wraps. They are secured with a special type of masking tape, labeled, and sterilized (Fig. 57-1). Items such as syringes and needles are packaged individually and are sterile.

☞ KEY CONCEPT

Disinfection is the destruction of most pathogens but not spores. Sterilization is the destruction of all microorganisms and spores.

Every step in an aseptic procedure is a link in a chain. If one link is broken by contaminating something, the entire chain has been broken and the door is left open for infection.

☞ KEY CONCEPT

Never touch sterile articles with unsterile articles. Discard an article if it becomes contaminated or if you are unsure whether or not it is contaminated. Do not risk using a contaminated instrument or needle.

Learning to perform sterile technique correctly in order to maintain sterility requires understanding the meanings of *dirty, contaminated, clean,* and *sterile.* It also requires a great deal of practice. Equipment or supplies used for many nursing interventions are packaged to maintain sterility. In Practice: Nursing Care Guidelines 57-1 provides general tips for using sterile technique. In Practice: Nursing Procedure 57-1 describes the steps associated with opening a sterile package, which is basic to many sterile procedures.

Healthcare providers entering sterile environments, such as the operating room (OR), must wear sterile protective clothing

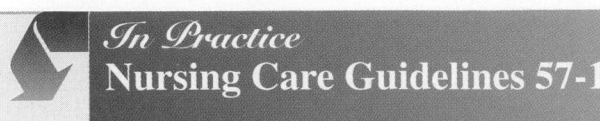

In Practice
Nursing Care Guidelines 57-1

USING STERILE TECHNIQUE

- After sterile gloves or a gown have been put on, the nurse cannot touch anything that is not sterile.
- Reaching over a sterile field contaminates the area, unless sterile clothing is being worn.
- If a sterile wrapper becomes wet, the wrapper and its contents are no longer sterile.
- If a mask becomes wet, it no longer screens out microorganisms; the mask must be changed for a new mask.
- When wearing sterile gloves to perform a sterile procedure, they must be kept in front, between the nipple line and waist. If gloves move above or below these areas, they are considered contaminated.
- A person's back is not sterile, even if a sterile gown is being worn.
- Objects are considered contaminated if there is uncertainty as to whether contamination has occurred. *When in doubt, consider the objects in question to be contaminated.*
- Skin cannot be rendered sterile; it can only be made clean.
- Parts of the body that are not exposed to the outside are considered sterile. These parts include the abdominal cavity, the urinary bladder, and usually the uterus. The GI tract is not sterile, because it is actually a tube within the body that opens to the outside at both ends. In addition, unsterile items (food) enter the GI tract daily.

to prevent contaminating the area with microorganisms that reside on the skin, hair, and clothing. Because many clients today are sent home from the hospital with catheters, IVs, and other tubes in place, it is vital to teach the client and family how to lessen the possibility of infection at home. Typically the client and family are taught how to manage specific equipment at home; this equipment is kept sterile if possible. However, because the client will be exposed to microorganisms within his or her own home, clean technique may be used for some procedures. In these cases, the equipment is considered contaminated specifically to that person. In Practice: Educating the Client 57-1 highlights some examples and tips for teaching.

Hair Covering

In sterile environments (especially the OR) a cap or hood is worn to cover the hair. Remember that no hair can show. If the hair is long, a special type of hood will be worn. If the hair is short, a surgical cap is used. The nurse who has a moustache or beard often wears a surgical hood to cover the entire face, except the eyes.

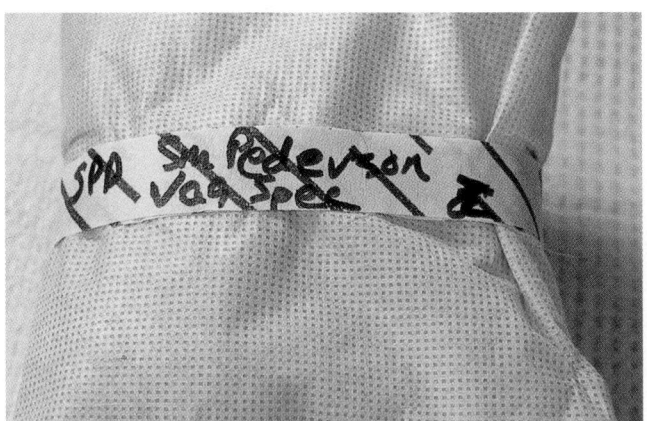

FIGURE 57-1. Some items, such as surgical towels, are packaged in cloth, paper, or plastic wraps. They are secured with a special type of masking tape, labeled, and sterilized. The indicator strip changes color or shows black stripes when sterilized to the correct temperature.

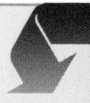

In Practice
Nursing Procedure 57-1

OPENING A STERILE PACKAGE

Supplies and Equipment

Sterile supplies (as needed for procedure)
Waist-high table

Steps

1. Gather supplies. Check the expiration date on sterile supplies.
   RATIONALE: *Organization facilitates accurate skill performance. Outdated packages are considered to be contaminated.*

2. Wash your hands.
   RATIONALE: *Handwashing limits the spread of microorganisms.*

3. Explain the procedure to the client.
   RATIONALE: *Explanation provides information to foster cooperation.*

4. Prepare a waist-high working area.
   RATIONALE: *Sterile objects must be kept above waist level to maintain their sterility.*

5. Place the sterile package on the working area. Remove the outer covering or plastic wrap if present.
   RATIONALE: *The outer covering protects the sterile contents.*

6. Grasp the edge of the outermost flap and open the package away from you, toward the back of the table.
   RATIONALE: *Opening the top flap away from you prevents reaching over a sterile field and contaminating it.*

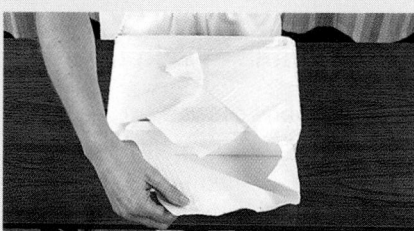

Opening outermost flap away from the body.

7. Fold each side flap down toward the table. While holding the underside of the wrapper, push to bend it up in the middle, pulling the flaps taut so that the flaps will not refold. Lay the package flat on the table.
   RATIONALE: *Folding each side outward allows access to the remaining flap(s); pushing the wrapper up in the middle and pulling the flaps out taut keeps the wrapping from curling back into its original position.*

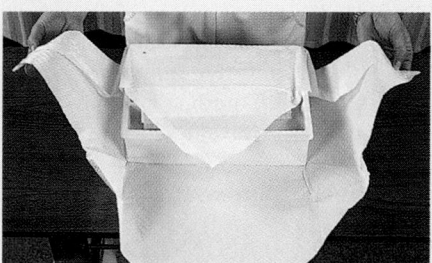

Folding side flaps down.

8. Grasp the tip of the near flap and open it toward you. Pull the flap downward from underneath and pull it taut and into place.
   RATIONALE: *When the flaps are unfolded, the inside is sterile.*

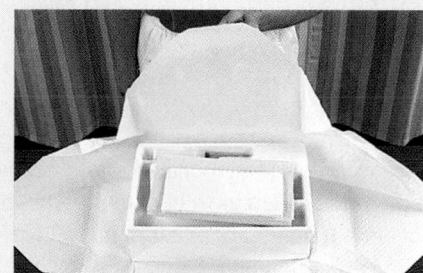

Opening last flap toward the body.

9. Open any additional sterile packages without touching the contents. Drop these items onto the sterile field.
   RATIONALE: *Sterile touching sterile maintains surgical asepsis.*

Surgical Mask

Chapter 41 teaches how to put on a *surgical mask* (see In Practice: Nursing Procedure 41-3.). In strict sterile situations, such as in the OR or with protective isolation, the mask covers the mouth and nose. The purpose of the mask is to form a barrier to stop the transmission of pathogens. In the OR or during other sterile procedures, the mask prevents harmful microorganisms in your respiratory tract from spreading to the client. When the client has an infection, the mask protects you from his or her pathogens.

Sterile Gown

A *sterile gown* is commonly worn in the OR, with protective isolation, and sometimes in the delivery room. The hands

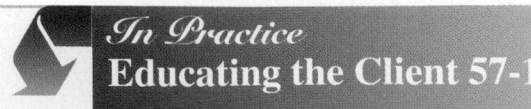

In Practice
Educating the Client 57-1

PREVENTING THE SPREAD OF INFECTION AT HOME

Examples of client and family teaching:

• How to empty the catheter bag
• Methods for safely changing catheter tubing
• Hanging a new IV bag
• How to give injections at home

Additional tips for teaching:

• Demonstrate the skill to be performed.
• Ask the client and family to demonstrate the skill before discharge.
• Explain how to recognize problems or complications, such as postoperative infections.
• Describe when to seek medical care immediately.
• If indicated, make a referral for home care nursing followup.

touch only the parts of the sterile gown that will touch the body after the gown is in place. Thus, touch only the inside of the gown. Someone else must tie the strings. The back of the gown is considered contaminated, even though it was sterile when put on. Any part of the gown below waist level and above nipple level is also considered contaminated. Be careful when wearing a sterile gown not to touch anything that is unsterile.

Sterile Gloves

For some procedures, *sterile gloves* are worn. The instructors will give specific instructions as to how to put on a gown and gloves without contaminating yourself or anything else in the sterile area. Remember that once gloves are put on, touching anything unsterile contaminates them. Therefore, make all preparations before putting on gloves.

☛ KEY CONCEPT

Be sure to keep the hands between the waist and nipple levels whenever sterile gloves are worn. This is true whether or not a sterile gown is worn.

In Practice: Nursing Procedure 57-2 describes a method of gloving called *open gloving*. A procedure called *closed gloving* is often performed when a sterile gown is also used. You will learn that procedure if you work in an OR.

☛ KEY CONCEPT

Whenever the cover on a sterile tray, or a gown, mask, dressing, drape, or other cloth or paper item becomes wet, it is contaminated.

URINARY CATHETERIZATION

The bladder is the reservoir for urine. Normally, when 200 to 250 milliliters collect in the bladder, the urge to void (urinate) occurs. If the bladder cannot empty normally, it becomes distended as urine collects. Urine may dribble from the urethral opening, and chronic kidney disorders can result.

Urinary catheterization is the procedure of inserting a tube (a catheter) through the urethra into the bladder to remove urine. The procedures for urinary catheterization are discussed here because they are performed under sterile conditions to ensure that microorganisms are not introduced into the bladder. Only sterile equipment (usually disposable) is used. A *straight catheter* is used for one sample only and removed. A *retention catheter* (eg, *Foley catheter*) remains in the bladder. The Foley-type catheter is also called an *indwelling catheter*. Other types of indwelling catheters are the *mushroom,* the *Malecot,* and the *Pezzer.*

At one time, catheterization was considered necessary to obtain an uncontaminated urine specimen. Today, however, many providers recommend *midstream* and *clean-catch* methods of urine collection (see Chap. 52). The need for catheterization after surgery has also diminished as early ambulation for surgical clients has increased.

Generally, no more than 750 to 1,000 milliliters of urine are removed from the bladder at any one time, particularly if the client has had retention or distention over a long period. If urine flow seems undiminished after withdrawal of this quantity, clamp or remove the catheter and report it to the primary care provider.

Nursing Alert
A client can go into shock if too much urine is removed from the bladder too fast.

Catheterizing the Female Client

Placement of a retention catheter is often necessary when a woman has had pelvic surgery or bladder tumors. In Practice: Nursing Procedure 57-3 summarizes steps for catheterizing the female client. If a rubber catheter is to be used, be sure to check that the client is not latex sensitive.

The Side-Lying Position
If the client is unable to lie on her back for the procedure, or if she cannot relax her legs because of contractures, use the side-lying position for catheterization. Some nurses prefer to use this position when catheterizing a female client. The side-lying position makes maintaining sterile technique easier, because the nurse needs to hold only one side of labia in position. Contamination of the catheter is less likely because the client maintains this position well, and the nurse does not have to reach over the client's leg.

(*text continues on page 775*)

In Practice
Nursing Procedure 57-2

PUTTING ON STERILE GLOVES
Supplies and Equipment

Sterile gloves of the appropriate size

Steps

1. Wash the hands.
   RATIONALE: *Handwashing limits the spread of microorganisms.*

2. Open the outer glove package, following Nursing Procedure 57-1, on a clean, dry, flat surface at waist level or higher.
   RATIONALE: *Properly opening the sterile package of gloves protects them from becoming contaminated.*

3. If there is an inner package, open it in the same way, keeping the sterile gloves on the inside surface with cuffs toward you.
   RATIONALE: *Ensure that the gloves remain sterile and ready to apply.*

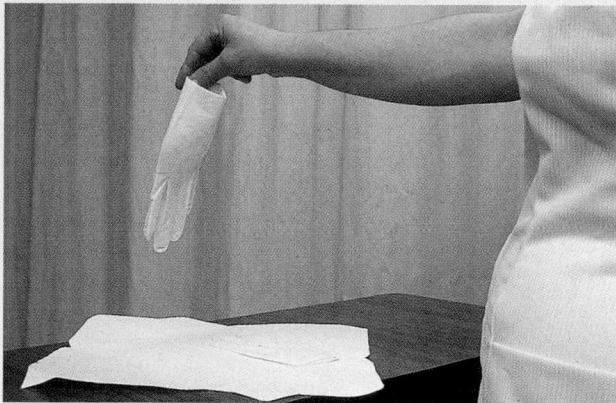

Grasping the cuff and lifting the glove.

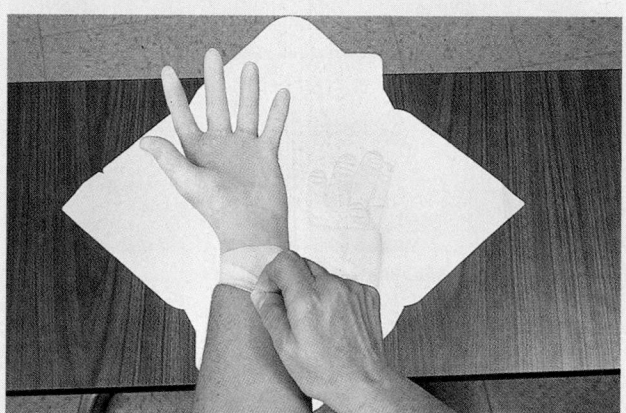

Inserting one hand into the glove.

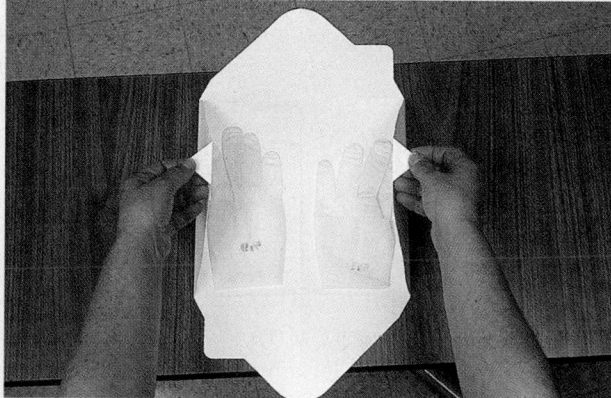

Opening the inner glove package.

4. Use one hand to grasp the *inside* upper surface of the glove's cuff for the opposite hand. Lift the glove up and clear it of the wrapper.
   RATIONALE: *Touching the inner surface of the glove with your clean hand allows the outer surface to remain sterile.*

5. Insert the opposite hand into the glove, placing the thumb and fingers in the proper openings. Pull the glove into place, touching *only* the *inside* of the glove at the cuff. Leave the cuff in place.
   RATIONALE: *Attempts to unfold the glove cuff may result in contamination.*

6. Slip the fingers of the sterile gloved hand under (inside) the cuff of the remaining glove while keeping the thumb pointed outward.
   RATIONALE: *The sterile fingers touch only the out-side of the second sterile glove. This maintains*

sterility. Lift the glove up and clear it of the wrapper.
RATIONALE: *The cuff protects the sterile gloved fingers as the ungloved hand is inserted into the other glove. Holding the thumb outward keeps it out of the way and prevents it from touching the sterile area.*

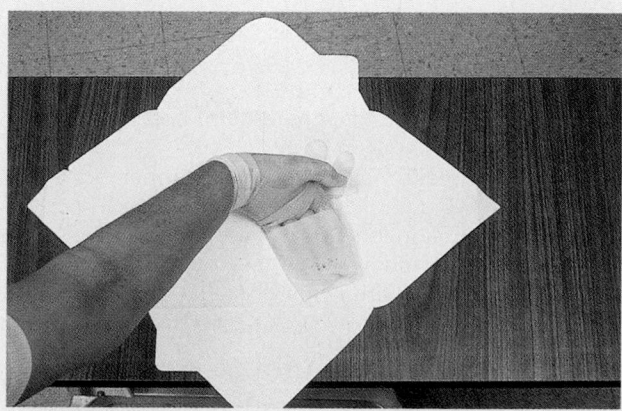

Slipping sterile gloved fingers under sterile cuff.

(*continued*)

In Practice
Nursing Procedure 57-2 (*Continued*)

7. a. Insert the ungloved hand into the glove.

   b. Pull the second glove on, touching *only* the *outside* of the sterile glove with the other sterile gloved hand and keeping the fingers inside the cuff.

   c. Adjust gloves and snap cuffs into place. Avoid touching the inside glove and wrist areas.
      RATIONALE: *Gloves remain sterile when touching other sterile areas.*

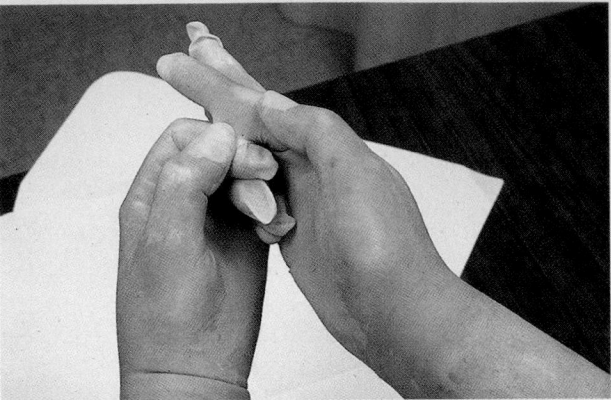

Adjusting gloves, touching only sterile areas.

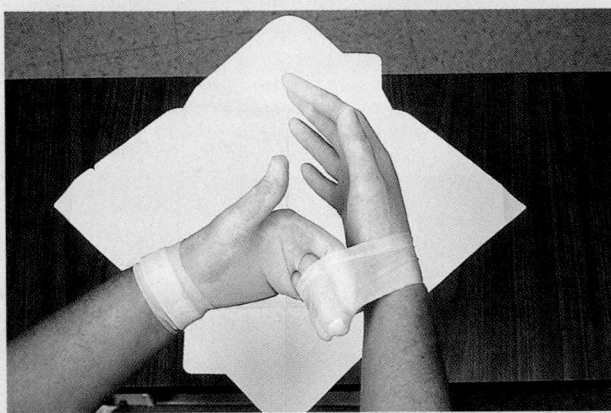

Inserting the opposite hand into glove.

8. Keep the sterile gloved hands above waist level. Make sure not to touch the clothes. Keep hands folded when not performing a procedure.
   RATIONALE: *Holding the hands above waist level keeps them within sight. Keeping the sterile gloved hands folded when not performing a procedure helps to maintain control. Both actions help to prevent accidental contamination.*

In Practice
Nursing Procedure 57-3

CATHETERIZING THE FEMALE CLIENT

Supplies and Equipment

Sterile catheterization tray containing sterile supplies:
   Gloves
   Basin
   Cotton balls
   Antiseptic solution and cup
   Straight or indwelling catheter (size appropriate for client)
   Lubricant (unless the catheter is prelubricated)
   Forceps
   Drapes (plain and fenestrated: containing an opening or window)
   Syringe prefilled with water or saline
   Specimen container
Urine collection bag (may be attached to catheter)
Flashlight or additional lamp
Plastic biohazard bag
Waterproof pad

Velcro leg strap or nonallergenic tape (optional)
Bath blanket
Clean gloves, soap, and water
Washcloth and towel

Steps

1. Explain the procedure to the client.
   RATIONALE: *Providing information fosters cooperation.*

2. Gather supplies after checking the physician's order for catheterization.
   RATIONALE: *Organization facilitates accurate skill performance. Checking the physician's order clarifies insertion of straight or indwelling catheter.*

3. Wash the hands.
   RATIONALE: *Handwashing limits the spread of microorganisms.*

(*continued*)

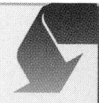

In Practice
Nursing Procedure 57-3 (Continued)

4. Close the door or pull the bed curtain. Adjust the bed to a comfortable working height. If right-handed, stand on the client's right side (if left-handed, stand on the client's left side.)
RATIONALE: *Proper positioning prevents back strain. Closing the curtain or door protects the client's privacy.*

5. Assist the woman into a supine position with her feet spread apart and flat on the mattress and her knees flexed. Use a bath blanket to drape the client.
RATIONALE: *The dorsal recumbent position allows visualization of the urinary meatus. A bath blanket provides warmth and privacy.*

6. Put on the clean gloves. Wash the woman's perineal area with soap and water. Rinse and dry the area. Remove the gloves and wash your hands again.
RATIONALE: *Cleansing the perineal area ensures that the area is as free of microorganisms as possible.*

7. Ensure adequate lighting. Position a lamp at the foot of the bed, or another nurse may hold a flashlight.
RATIONALE: *Good lighting improves visualization of the urinary meatus.*

8. Raise the bedside table to waist height. Open the sterile catheterization tray on the bedside table using appropriate sterile technique (see In Practice: Nursing Procedure 57-1). Put on sterile gloves (see In Practice: Nursing Procedure 57-2). Pick up the sterile drape and gently shake it open. Grasp the upper corners and fold the drape back over the sterile gloves, making a cuff. Keep the hands inside the cuff. Ask the client to lift her buttocks. Place the drape between her thighs with the upper edge under her buttocks.
RATIONALE: *Protecting the gloves with the drape maintains sterility during draping.*

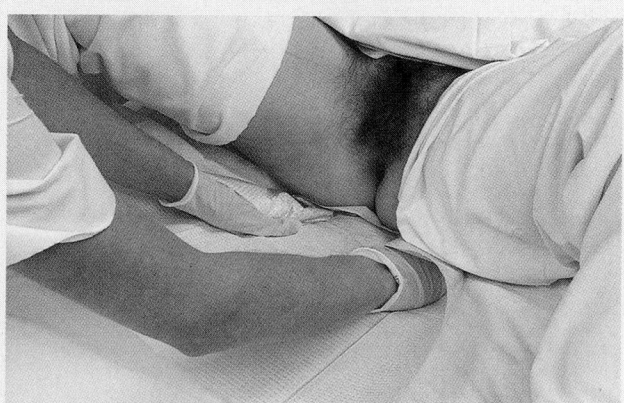

Placing the drape while protecting sterile gloved hands.

9. Set up equipment on the open sterile tray:
   a. Place the cotton balls into the cup. Open the package containing antiseptic and pour it over the cotton balls.
   b. Remove the plastic covering from the catheter. For an indwelling catheter, attach the prefilled syringe to the balloon inflation port and inflate the balloon with the appropriate amount of fluid to test the balloon. After the balloon inflates, aspirate the fluid back into the syringe, leaving the syringe connected to the port and the balloon deflated.

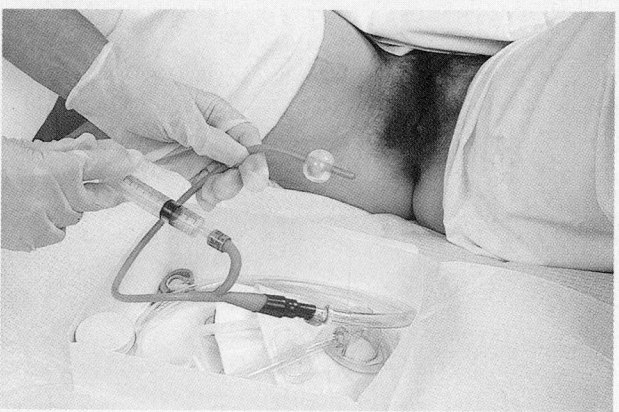

Testing the balloon on an indwelling catheter.

   c. Open the lubricant and lubricate the catheter's tip 1–2 inches. (You may leave the catheter tip inside the sterile lubricant package until you need it.)
   d. Unscrew the cap from the specimen container, if a specimen is ordered.
   e. If a straight catheter is being used, position the drainage end of the catheter in the basin to catch the urine.
   RATIONALE: *Correct preparation ensures that all equipment is present. Inflating the catheter balloon before use checks for leaks or a nonfunctioning balloon. Lubrication of the catheter increases comfort on insertion.*

10. Move the catheterization tray with the equipment onto the sterile drape between the client's thighs.
RATIONALE: *All supplies are easily available, decreasing the likelihood of contaminating equipment.*

11. While using the nondominant hand, separate and gently spread the woman's labia minora to expose her urinary meatus. Keep this hand in this position.
RATIONALE: *The nondominant hand is now considered contaminated. Spreading the labia allows for easier cleansing and visibility.*

(continued)

In Practice
Nursing Procedure 57-3 (Continued)

12. With the dominant hand, use the forceps to pick up cotton balls. Cleanse both labial folds and then the meatus. Use a new cotton ball for each stroke, moving from top to bottom (front to back). Discard each used cotton ball in the plastic biohazard bag. Cleanse the meatus last.
    RATIONALE: *Moving from clean to dirty lessens the chance of introducing microorganisms into the client's bladder. Using a new cotton ball each time helps keep the area as clean as possible.*

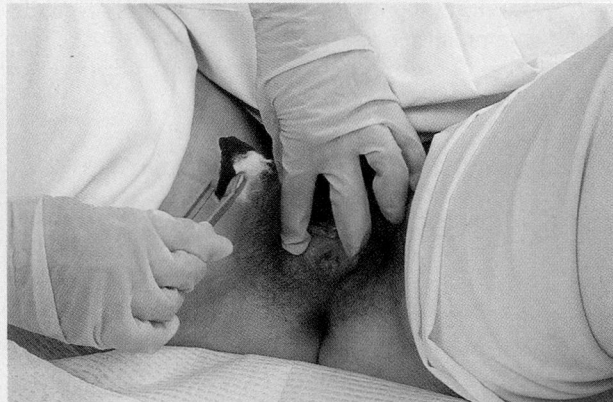

Cleansing from front to back.

13. Pick up the catheter approximately 3 inches from the tip with the dominant hand. Place the drainage end in the basin to catch the urine flow (or if a specimen is to be obtained, place the drainage end into the specimen container). If the catheter is indwelling, it may already be attached to the drainage tubing.
    RATIONALE: *Urine is sterile. Draining urine will not contaminate the sterile setup.*

14. Ask the client to breathe deeply and slowly through her mouth. Insert the catheter gently into the urinary meatus, advancing it 2–3 inches until urine begins to drain. If the catheter is indwelling, advance it another 1–2 inches. Never force insertion of the catheter if resistance is felt. Move the nondominant hand to hold the catheter in place between two fingers, bracing the rest of this hand against the client's perineum. Collect a urine specimen if one is ordered.
    RATIONALE: *Asking the client to focus on breathing relaxes her sphincter and ensures that the catheter meets with less resistance on entering the meatus. Forcing the catheter's advancement may injure the meatus or mucous membranes.*

15. If the catheter is not to be indwelling, allow urine to drain into the basin. Remove the catheter after urine has drained. For an indwelling catheter,

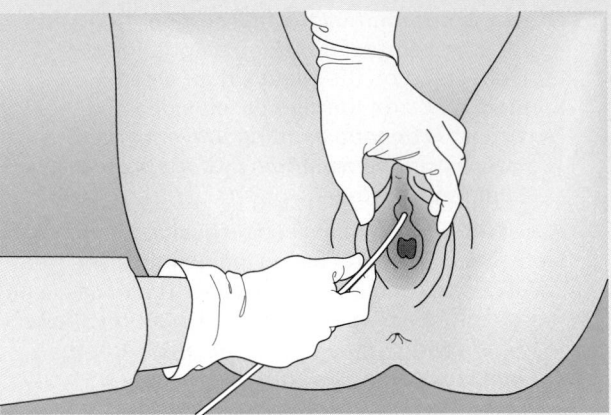

Inserting the catheter gently into the meatus.

inject the fluid to inflate the balloon. Pull gently on the catheter to check that the balloon is inflated and that the catheter is secure.
RATIONALE: *The balloon holds the catheter in place in the bladder.*

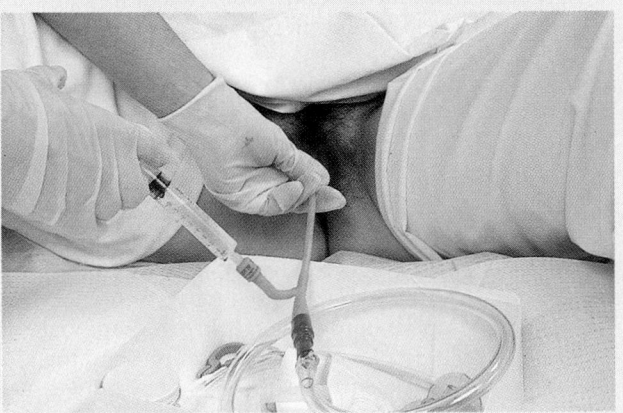

Injecting sterile water to inflate the balloon.

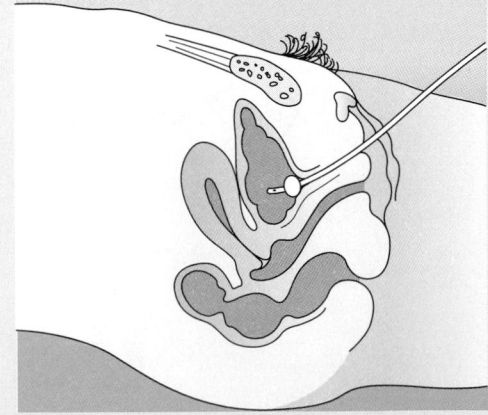

The indwelling catheter in the urinary bladder with the balloon inflated.

(continued)

In Practice
Nursing Procedure 57-3 (Continued)

16. Use a leg strap or tape to anchor the tubing from the indwelling catheter. Position the drainage bag below bladder level. The catheter should pass over the woman's leg.
    RATIONALE: *Properly positioned tubing decreases tension on the catheter. The drainage bag positioned below bladder level uses gravity to*

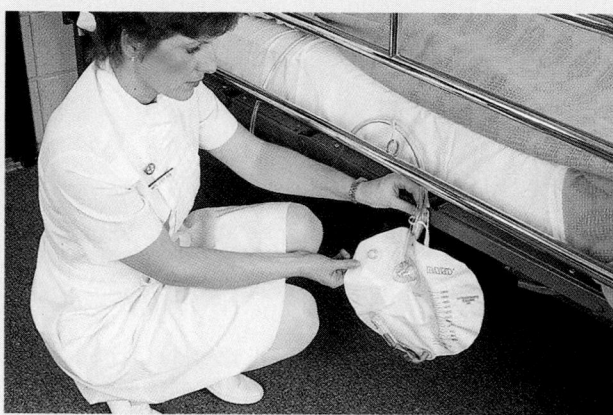

Positioning the drainage bag.

promote urinary flow and decreases the risk of urinary stasis. This also prevents backflow of urine and thus helps to prevent infection.

17. Dry the client's perineal area if necessary. Measure the urine amount. Remove gloves. Reposition and cover the client. Lower the bed. Remove equipment.
    RATIONALE: *These measures ensure comfort and safety.*

18. Dispose of equipment according to agency policy. Dispose of gloves.
    RATIONALE: *Proper disposal prevents transmission of microorganisms.*

19. Wash the hands.
    RATIONALE: *Handwashing limits the spread of microorganisms.*

20. Document the size and type of catheter inserted and the client's response. Record the amount of urine obtained, its appearance, and specimen collection if one was obtained.
    RATIONALE: *Documentation provides communication and coordination of care.*

The client lies on her side with her knees drawn up to her chest. If the nurse is right-handed, the client should lie on her left side, and vice versa. The client's buttocks should be near the side of the bed where the nurse is standing, and the client's shoulders should be near the other side of the bed. Stand behind the client, near her buttocks. Follow the same sterile technique and general steps as those for inserting a catheter for the client lying in the supine position.

Catheterizing the Male Client

Catheterization of the male client is more difficult than catheterization of the female client because the man's urethra is longer and more curved. In addition, sometimes an enlarged prostate gland constricts or obstructs the urethra. Previous urethral infection can also cause strictures. In Practice: Nursing Procedure 57-4 describes the steps for male catheterization.

Caring for the Client After Catheterization

After any client is catheterized, reposition the client to ensure that he or she is comfortable and that the signal cord is within reach. Be sure that the balloon of an indwelling catheter is inflated and that the catheter tubing is secured externally to avoid pulling and discomfort. Use hypoallergenic tape to hold the catheter to the man's abdomen or to the woman's thigh. Explain to the client that he or she may feel the urge to void because of the catheter's presence in the urethra.

The drainage tubing extends straight down from the bed level to the bag (*straight drainage*) with extra tubing placed on the bed with the client, so movement is possible. *Rationale: Loops hanging down can promote urinary stasis and infection.* If a retention catheter is left in place, attach the drainage apparatus to the bed frame (not the side rails), maintaining its sterility. Chapter 51 describes the care of the client with an indwelling catheter in more detail.

Removing the Retention Catheter

Removing a retention catheter is a simple procedure. Take care to prevent urethral trauma. In Practice: Nursing Procedure 57-5 lists actions for removing the retention catheter.

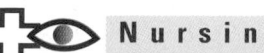 **Nursing Alert**
A catheter is never cut for removal. This could cause the catheter to be pulled back into the urethra or bladder. In that case, surgical removal would probably be necessary. This would also be a source for introducing pathogenic organisms into the urinary bladder.

In Practice
Nursing Procedure 57-4

CATHETERIZING THE MALE CLIENT

Supplies and Equipment

Same as for "Catheterizing the Female Patient" (see In Practice: Nursing Procedure 57-3)

Steps

1. Follow Steps 1 through 4 at In Practice: Nursing Procedure 57-3.

2. Assist the man to lie on his back with his legs slightly apart. Position the drape or bath blanket so that only the penis is uncovered.
   RATIONALE: *Proper positioning and covering prevent chilling and protect the client's privacy.*

3. Put on clean gloves. Wash the penis with soap and water. Rinse and dry. Remove the gloves and wash the hands again.
   RATIONALE: *Cleansing the area ensures that the area is as free of microorganisms as possible.*

4. Open the sterile catheterization tray on the bedside table (see In Practice: Nursing Procedure 57-1). Put on sterile gloves (see In Practice: Nursing Procedure 57-2). Pick up the sterile drape, shake it open, and lay it on the client's thighs. Place the opening of the fenestrated drape over the man's penis.
   RATIONALE: *Using the drape provides a sterile field.*

5. Set up the equipment on the tray, the same as for a female client (see Step 9 at In Practice: Nursing Procedure 57-3). Lubricate the catheter tip for male catheterization 5–7 inches (sometimes lubricant is instilled directly into the urethra).
   RATIONALE: *The man's longer urethra necessitates lubricating a longer portion of the catheter.*

6. Move the catheterization tray onto the sterile drape.
   RATIONALE: *All supplies are easily available, decreasing the likelihood of contaminating equipment.*

7. Use your nondominant hand to grasp the penis. If the client is uncircumcised, retract his foreskin before cleansing. With the forceps, pick up a cotton ball and cleanse from the meatus outward in a circular motion. Repeat three times, using each cotton ball only once.
   RATIONALE: *Moving in a circular motion from the center outward (from clean to dirty) lessens the chance of introducing microorganisms into the man's bladder.*

8. Pick up the catheter approximately 3 inches from the tip with your dominant hand. Place the drainage end in the basin. If the catheter is

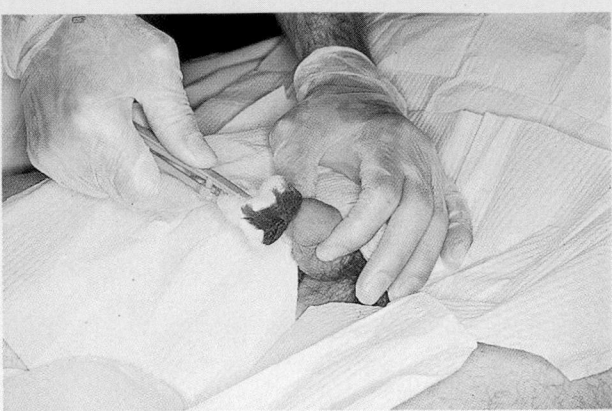
Cleansing the meatus in a circular motion.

indwelling, it may already be attached to drainage tubing.
   RATIONALE: *Draining urine will not contaminate the sterile setup.*

9. Lift the penis to an upright perpendicular position. Gently pressing the end of the penis from two sides may help to open the meatus. Ask the client to bear down as if voiding. Insert the catheter gently into the meatus, advancing it 7–9 inches or until urine begins to drain. If you encounter resistance when passing the catheter, rotate it slightly or withdraw it, rather than forcing it.
   RATIONALE: *Holding the penis upright straightens the urethral canal. Rotating the catheter helps ease it past the client's prostate gland.*

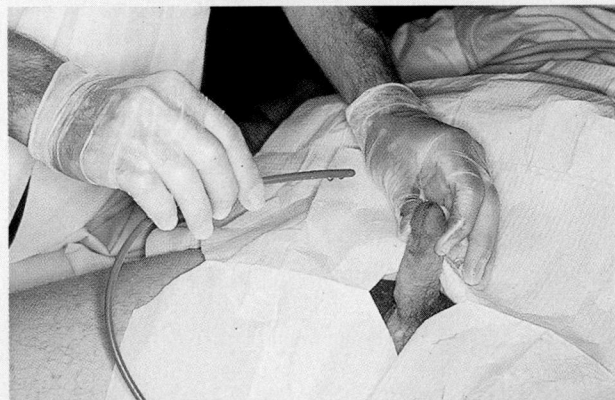
Holding the penis in an upright position for inserting the catheter.

10. For an indwelling catheter, advance it another inch. Collect a urine specimen if one is ordered.
    RATIONALE: *Additional catheter advancement ensures that the balloon inflates in the bladder rather than in the urethral canal.*

(continued)

In Practice
Nursing Procedure 57-4 (Continued)

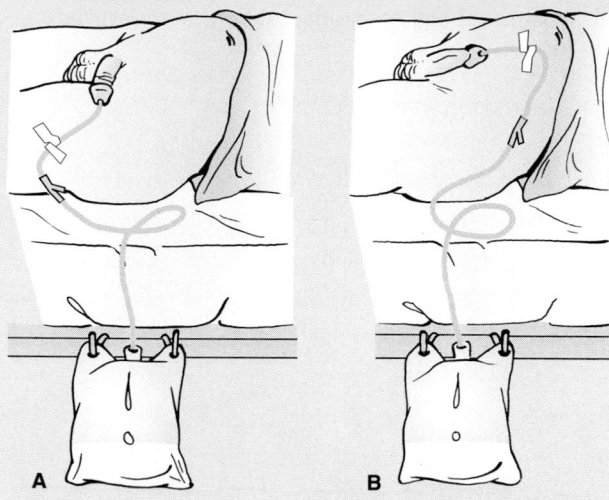

(a) Securing the catheter to the upper thigh. (b) Securing the catheter to the lower abdomen.

11. Follow Steps 15 through 20 at In Practice: Nursing Procedure 57-3. Make the following exceptions for the male client:

a. Tape or secure the catheter to his lower abdomen or upper thigh, allowing some slack in the tubing.

b. Return the foreskin to its original position in the uncircumcised man.

RATIONALE: *Securing the catheter to the lower abdomen may reduce urethral pressure at the angle of the penis and the scrotum. Returning the foreskin to its original position prevents impaired circulation and pressure on the urethra.*

In Practice
Nursing Procedure 57-5

REMOVING THE RETENTION CATHETER

Supplies and Equipment

Gloves
Waterproof pad
Syringe (size is determined by volume of fluid used to inflate balloon)
Soap, water, washcloth, and towel

Steps

1. Explain the procedure to the client.
   RATIONALE: *Providing information fosters cooperation.*

2. Gather supplies after checking the physician's order for catheter removal.
   RATIONALE: *Organization facilitates accurate skill performance.*

3. Wash the hands and put on gloves.
   RATIONALE: *Handwashing limits the spread of infection.*

4. Close the door or pull the bed curtains. Adjust the bed to a comfortable working height. Place a waterproof pad between the client's thighs.

RATIONALE: *Closing the door or curtain protects the client's privacy. Proper positioning prevents back strain. The waterproof pad prevents soiling of the bed linen.*

5. Attach the syringe's hub to the inflation port or insert a needleless hub. Deflate the balloon by completely aspirating all the fluid. *Never* cut a catheter.
   RATIONALE: *The balloon must be completely deflated to prevent urethral trauma on removal. A cut catheter can retract back into the urethra or bladder.*

6. Pull the catheter out gently and slowly.
   RATIONALE: *Easing the catheter through the urethra minimizes the risk of trauma.*

7. Wrap the catheter in a waterproof pad. Remove the catheter, drainage bag, and equipment from the bedside, disposing according to agency policy. Measure urine in the drainage bag and record findings on the intake and output form.
   RATIONALE: *Proper disposal prevents transmission of microorganisms. Urine measurement provides an accurate record of output.*

(continued)

In Practice
Nursing Procedure 57-5 (*Continued*)

8. Assist the client to cleanse and dry the perineal area. Return the client to a position of comfort.
   RATIONALE: *These measures ensure comfort.*

9. Remove gloves and wash the hands.
   RATIONALE: *Handwashing helps to prevent the transmission of microorganisms.*

10. Document catheter removal on the appropriate form.
    RATIONALE: *Documentation provides communication and coordination of care.*

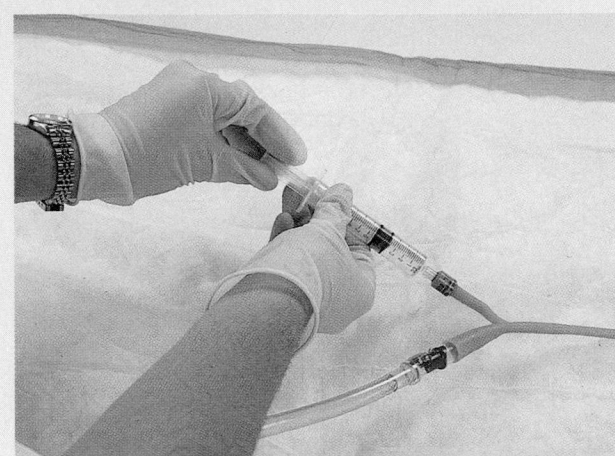

Deflating the balloon. (Photo © B. Proud)

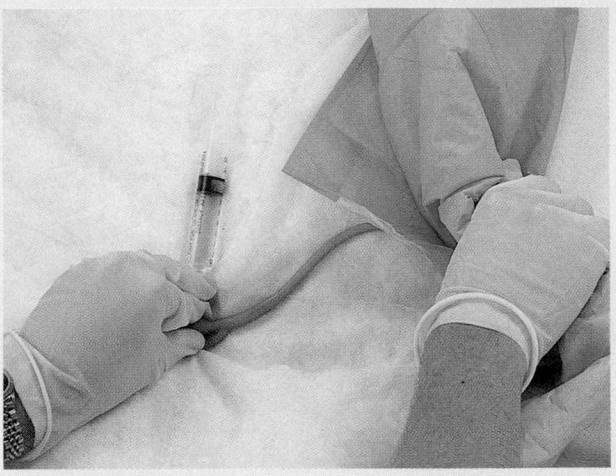

Pulling the catheter out gently and slowly. (Photo © B. Proud)

➤ STUDENT SYNTHESIS

Key Points

- Clean applies to medical asepsis. It means the removal of all gross contamination and many microorganisms.
- Sterile means that the item is free of all micro-organisms and spores.
- When a sterile item touches anything unsterile, it becomes contaminated.
- If a sterile item becomes contaminated or if you are unsure whether or not it is contaminated, the item is considered contaminated and must be discarded.
- Catheterization is the procedure of inserting a flexible tube through the urethra into the bladder to remove urine. This aseptic procedure requires sterile equipment and technique.
- The balloon is deflated when removing a retention catheter. The catheter is never cut for removal.
- Client and family teaching is important, especially if the client or family will need to perform procedures such as IV therapy or catheter care after discharge.

Critical Thinking Exercises

1. Your client is a 48-year-old woman who has been unable to void since having abdominal surgery approximately 6 hours ago. Her bladder is distended (swollen) and she complains of discomfort. The physician has ordered a straight catheterization to relieve her bladder discomfort. How will you explain the procedure to her? Include the purpose, how it will be done, and what she will be required to do.

2. Describe how you would explain to a client of the opposite sex that you are about to perform a catheterization.

NCLEX-Style Review Questions

1. The nurse explains to a client that the most important reason for inserting an indwelling catheter is to:
   a. Allow the client to rest
   b. Ensure adequate blood volume
   c. Prevent bladder infections
   d. Remove urine continuously from the bladder

2. While performing a dressing change, part of the sterile field becomes wet. Which action should the nurse take?
   a. Avoid placing anything on the wet area.
   b. Position all supplies in a dry area on the field.
   c. Set up a new sterile field.
   d. Take the dry supplies and place in a clean area.
3. Prior to inserting a urinary catheter into the male client who is uncircumcised, which action should the nurse take?
   a. Measure the length of the penis.
   b. Retract the foreskin.
   c. Tape the catheter to the leg.
   d. Tilt the penis at a 25° angle.
4. After teaching a client how to change a dressing, it is most important for the nurse to document which information?
   a. Client's ability to perform sterile technique
   b. Family's willingness to assist client
   c. Amount of pain medication used
   d. Type of adhesive tape used
5. When catheterizing a male client, the nurse knows that the catheter is inserted into the bladder when:
   a. 2–3 inches of the catheter are in the client.
   b. 7–9 inches of the catheter are in the client.
   c. The client expresses that the urge to void is gone.
   d. Urine flows into the tubing.

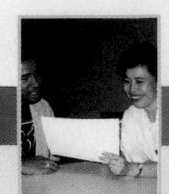

CHAPTER

58

Wound Care

LEARNING OBJECTIVES

1. Identify and describe the following wounds: abrasion, puncture, laceration, and surgical incision.
2. Describe the three types of wound healing.
3. Explain the three purposes of wound dressings.
4. Demonstrate how to change a dry sterile dressing, apply a wet-to-dry dressing, and irrigate a wound.
5. Explain the causes of skin breakdown, including the causes and usual locations of pressure ulcers.
6. Describe nursing measures that help to prevent skin breakdown.
7. Demonstrate assessing, cleaning, and applying medication to a pressure ulcer or other open wound.

NEW TERMINOLOGY

abrasion	pressure ulcer
debridement	puncture
decubitus ulcer	sloughing
eschar	surgical incision
exudate	wet-to-dry dressing
laceration	wound

ACRONYM

ABD

The skin acts as a barrier to protect the body from the potentially harmful external environment. When the skin's *integrity* (intactness) is broken, the body's internal environment is open to microorganisms that cause infection. Any abnormal opening in the skin is a **wound**. As a nurse, inspect the client's skin carefully and frequently for any signs of wounds or breakdown. The primary nursing responsibility is to prevent breakdown; when it occurs, report and treat it as ordered.

WOUNDS

The most common types of wounds nurses encounter are trauma (or accidental) wounds, **surgical incisions**, and **pressure ulcers** (wounds that result from prolonged exposure to pressure). Other types of skin wounds include infections, rashes, lesions, and burns, which are discussed in more detail in Chapter 74.

A **wound** is any disruption in the skin's intactness. It may be *accidental* or *unintentional,* such as an **abrasion** (rubbing off of the skin's surface); a **puncture** wound (stab wound); or a **laceration** (a wound with torn, ragged edges). A wound may also be *intentional,* such as a **surgical incision** (a wound with clean edges). A wound that occurs accidentally is contaminated; intentional wounds are made under sterile conditions.

Healing

Wound healing differs according to how much tissue has been damaged. Wound healing occurs by first, second, and third intention.

- *First intention* healing occurs in wounds with minimal tissue loss, such as surgical incisions or sutured wounds. Edges are *approximated* (close to each other); thus, they seal together rapidly. Scarring and infection rates with first intention healing are low.
- *Second intention* healing occurs with tissue loss, such as in deep lacerations, burns, and pressure ulcers. Because edges do not approximate, openings fill with *granulation tissue* that is soft and pinkish. Later, epithelial cells grow over the granulation tissue. Scarring may occur, and the risk of infection is greater than that for first intention healing.
- *Third intention* healing occurs when there is a delay in the time between the injury and the closure of the wound. For example, a wound may be left open temporarily to allow for drainage or removal of infectious materials. This type of healing sometimes occurs after surgery, when the wound closes later. In the meantime, wound surfaces start to granulate. Scarring is common.

Dressings

Wounds are covered with *dressings* to protect them from contamination, to collect any wound **exudate** (drainage) that may be present, and to protect against further damage during healing. The type of wound and its condition determine the type of dressing to use and the frequency of dressing changes. Sometimes, the primary healthcare provider orders the type and time for dressing changes, but some nurses make these decisions also. Follow the policies of your healthcare agency. Always follow Standard Precautions for any wound care.

Dry, Sterile Dressing

Apply a *dry, sterile dressing* to a wound to protect it from contamination (this is also known as a *dry-to-dry dressing*). This type of dressing is most often used for wounds healing by primary intention. The materials used for this type of dressing include gauze (such as 2×2 or 4×4 gauze), Telfa pads, and sometimes cotton. These materials remove drainage and protect the wound.

Dress a clean, uncontaminated, or uninfected wound (like a surgical incision) with a dry, sterile dressing. Change the dressing to evaluate healing and to apply a new, dry dressing. In Practice: Nursing Procedure 58-1 gives the steps to follow for changing a dry, sterile dressing.

Wet-to-Dry Dressing or Packing
Wet-to-dry dressings are most commonly used for wounds healing by secondary intention. An infected wound has exudate comprising serum, tissue debris, and infectious material or pus. The wound will not heal unless these substances are removed. Removal of infected tissues is called **debridement.** Saturate the sterile dressing with normal saline or other sterile solution, place it on or pack it in the wound, and leave it to dry. When the dried dressing is removed, tissue debris and drainage that sticks to it also will be removed. Using this wet-to-dry dressing is a common technique for debridement. Follow the steps as outlined at In Practice: Nursing Procedure 58-1 to remove the old dressing and complete the sterile dressing change.

In some cases, a packing is placed into a wound. This is done most often in the case of a puncture wound or wounds with sinus tracts. The dressing may be dry or it may be impregnated with petrolatum (Vaseline) or another medication. A special sponge material or gel-foam also may be used for this purpose. In the case of a packing, the entire wound is packed tightly with the material. The material is inserted and removed with a forceps.

Wet-to-Wet Dressing

Wet-to-wet dressings are used on clean, open wounds or on wounds that are granulating. These dressings provide warmth and moisture, which aid the healing process and make the client more comfortable. Thick exudate also can be removed in this manner. Sterile saline or an antibiotic solution is used to saturate the dressing.

Commercially Prepared Gel Dressings
Some wound care products use a specially formulated gel that provides a moist healing environment. These dressings aid in healing while also sealing the wound. An example of the moist dressing is Duo-Derm, which interacts with the moisture on the skin to produce a gel. This type is called a *hydrocolloid dressing.*

In Practice
Nursing Procedure 58-1

CHANGING A DRY, STERILE DRESSING

Supplies and Equipment

Clean gloves
Plastic Biohazard bag
Abdominal (**ABD**) pads
Sterile dressings, as ordered
Sterile saline or water
Bath blanket
Sterile gloves
Tape or Montgomery straps
Waterproof pads
Forceps from sterile suture removal set (optional)

Steps

1. Explain the procedure to the client.
   RATIONALE: *Providing information fosters cooperation.*

2. Gather supplies after checking the physician's order for the dressing change.
   RATIONALE: *Organization facilitates accurate skill performance. Checking the order clarifies the type of dressing ordered, the presence or absence of drainage, and the schedule for the change.*

3. Wash your hands.
   RATIONALE: *Handwashing limits the spread of microorganisms.*

4. Close the door or pull the bed curtains. Assist the client to a comfortable position. Expose only the area to redress, using a bath blanket if necessary. Place a waterproof pad under the client to protect the bed.
   RATIONALE: *Closing the door or pulling the curtain and exposing only the area to be treated protect the client's privacy and comfort.*

5. Prepare a plastic biohazard bag as a receptacle for soiled dressings. Fold back the cuff and place it within reach of your working area.
   RATIONALE: *The plastic bag helps prevent the transmission of microorganisms from the soiled dressing.*

6. Put on clean gloves. Untie the Montgomery straps or gently loosen the tape. Remove the soiled dressing, being careful not to tear the wound or dislodge any drains. Use sterile saline to moisten the dressing if it is sticking to the wound. Lift the soiled side of the dressing away from the client's view.
   RATIONALE: *Gloves act as a barrier. Using caution while removing the dressing maintains the integrity of sutures and prevents discomfort. The sight of drainage or blood may upset the client.*

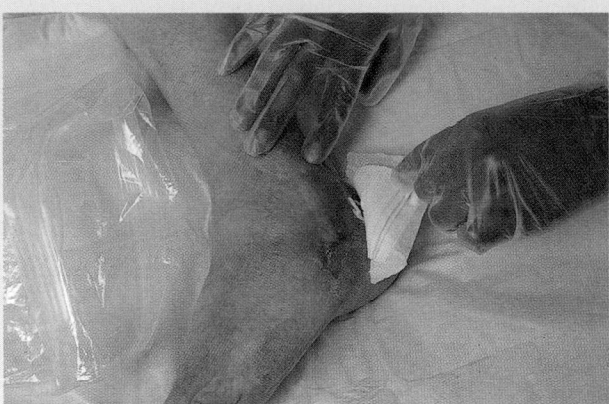
Removing the soiled dressing, being careful not to tear the wound.

7. Assess the drainage's amount, color, odor, and consistency. Observe the wound and surrounding tissues. Measure the wound.
   RATIONALE: *Data collection about the wound provides an indication of the wound's healing and presence or absence of infection.*

8. Remove gloves and place them in the plastic bag.
   RATIONALE: *The gloves are contaminated with wound drainage.*

9. Wash hands. Prepare a sterile field on the bedside table and open sterile dressings onto it. Uncap the sterile saline or other ordered solution to cleanse the wound. Place additional sterile dressings or swabs for cleansing onto the sterile field.
   RATIONALE: *Organization ensures that needed sterile supplies are present and placed in order of use.*

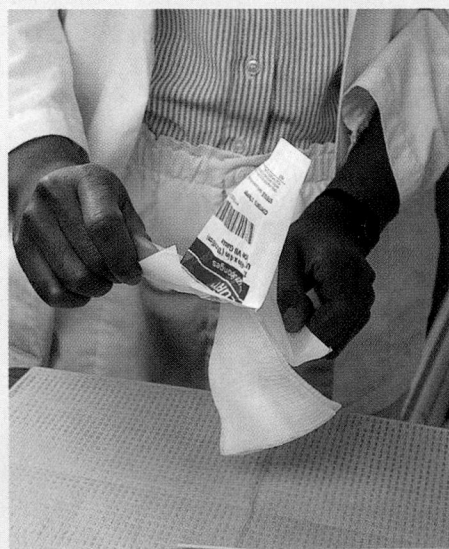
Opening the sterile dressing.

(continued)

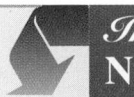

In Practice
Nursing Procedure 58-1 *(Continued)*

10. Put on sterile gloves.
    RATIONALE: *Using sterile gloves maintains surgical asepsis.*

11. Moisten sterile dressings or swabs and cleanse the wound, if ordered, moving from top to bottom or from the center of the wound outward (you may use forceps). Use a new swab or gauze pad for each cleansing motion. If necessary, clean the area around the wound as well. Do not use alcohol or soap.
    RATIONALE: *Cleansing from clean to dirty prevents introducing microorganisms into the wound. Alcohol and soap are drying and may cause further skin breakdown.*

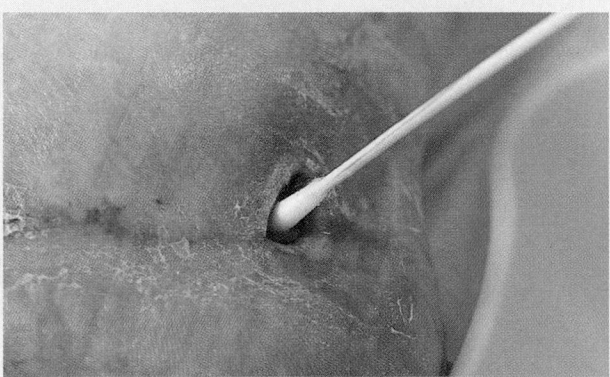

Cleansing the wound.

12. If necessary, use a gauze pad to dry the wound with the same motion as in Step 11. Carefully inspect the wound. Be prepared to accurately describe the wound.
    RATIONALE: *Moisture provides a medium for microorganisms to grow and to multiply. Visual inspection determines if the wound is healing and if there is any evidence of infection.*

13. Apply any ointments or medications to the wound as ordered. Apply a layer of dry sterile dressings over the incision and wound area. Pad with additional dressings and cover with a sterile ABD pad, if required.

RATIONALE: *The inner layer of dressings acts as a wick. Additional dressings and the outer pad absorb drainage and provide further protection for the wound.*

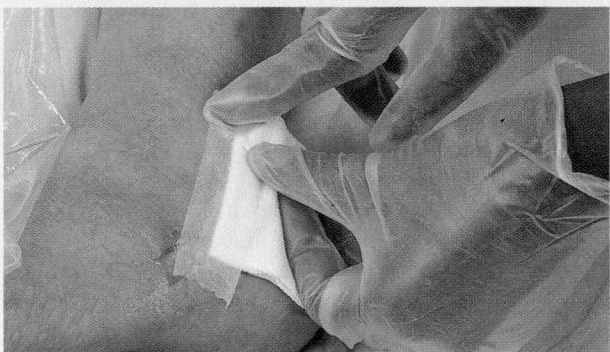

Applying a dry sterile dressing over wound area.

14. Remove gloves and place them in the disposal biohazard bag. Wash the hands. Apply tape or tie the dressing with Montgomery straps.
    RATIONALE: *Tape is easier to apply without gloves, but can also be applied with gloves. Taping or using Montgomery straps secures the dressing in place. Montgomery straps help to prevent skin irritation.*

15. Reposition and cover the client while preventing pressure on the wound. Handle only the outside of the biohazard bag, keeping hands inside (under) the cuff, and carefully closing it. Dispose of the bag with used supplies according to agency policy.
    RATIONALE: *Proper disposal helps prevent transmission of microorganisms. Keeping the pressure off of the wound prevents further damage.*

16. Wash the hands.
    RATIONALE: *Handwashing helps to prevent the spread of microorganisms.*

17. Document wound care and all assessments of the wound and drainage.
    RATIONALE: *Documentation provides communication and coordination of care.*

Sometimes these dressings are covered with a transparent dressing, such as Tegaderm or OpSite. Read the product information for correct application and use.

The Wound Drain

In some cases, a *drain* (a flat or round tube) is placed in a wound to facilitate drainage. A safety pin or other device is attached to the drain near its entrance to the skin, to prevent it from being pulled into the wound. A dressing or receptacle is placed over the end of the drain to catch drainage. The drain may be *advanced* (pulled out) a specified amount each day, until it is totally removed. In this case, careful measurement of the drain length is necessary to make sure that it is being advanced properly. A gentle suction device, such as a HemoVac, which is attached to a drain, may be used to cause more rapid and complete evacuation of the wound materials. The supervising nurse or healthcare provider will decide the specific treatment to provide.

Nursing Alert

Whenever working with any wound drainage, it is vital to wear gloves. If the drainage is excessive or obviously contains blood or pus, double gloving may be desired.

Stitches or Staples

At the time of the dressing change, the nurse may be instructed to remove *sutures* (stitches) or *staples* used to secure the edges of a wound. If so, use a suture removal kit or staple remover, which is discarded after use.

For suture removal, use sterile scissors to cut the suture. Then, with sterile forceps, remove the suture by pulling on it *on the same side as the knot.* Otherwise, if the side opposite the knot is pulled, the knot will be pulled through the incision, possibly causing it to tear the incision.

Remove staples according to the manufacturer's recommendations. Follow the specific procedures of the agency. Figure 58-1 shows an example of a staple remover and one technique used to remove skin staples.

Wound Irrigation

Wounds, even though they may be draining or be infected, are irrigated using sterile technique. A sterile *wound irrigation* is done to remove debris from an open wound following injury or surgery that has been complicated by infection. Sterile technique is used to help prevent introducing additional microorganisms into the wound. Heat or medications also

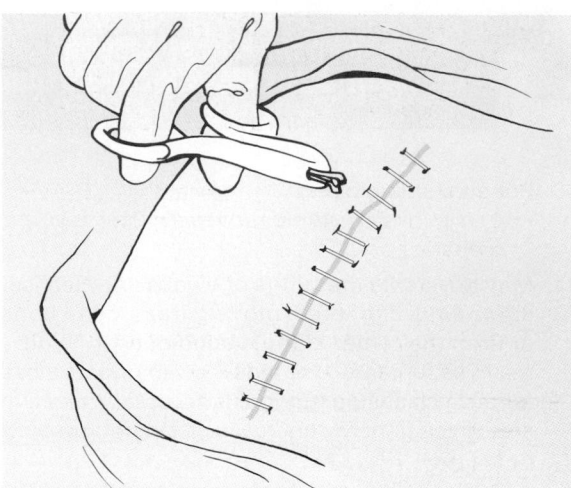

FIGURE 58-1. Skin staples and staple remover.

may be applied using this method. The three major types of wound irrigation are:

- *Manual irrigation* with a hand-held syringe (can be sterile or clean)
- *Continuous wound irrigation* with an infusion-type setup
- *Intermittent irrigation* alone or combined with gentle suction, such as with a HemoVac

In Practice: Nursing Procedure 58-2 describes how to perform a wound irrigation using sterile technique.

In Practice
Nursing Procedure 58-2

PERFORMING A STERILE WOUND IRRIGATION

Supplies and Equipment

Disposable sterile irrigation pack
Irrigation solution, as ordered
Plastic Biohazard bag
Clean gloves
Waterproof bed pad
Eye goggles or face guard
Sterile dressings, as ordered
Clean basin or irrigating pouch

Steps

1. Carefully wash the hands.
   RATIONALE: *Handwashing limits the transfer of microorganisms.*

2. Check the physician's orders.
   RATIONALE: *Orders provide specific information about the solution to use; checking the orders is important because the orders may have changed.*

3. Carefully gather all equipment and supplies.

   RATIONALE: *Organization promotes efficiency. After the wound is exposed, the procedure must be completed as quickly as possible.*

4. Close the door and pull the curtains. Cover the client with a bath blanket.
   RATIONALE: *Closing the door or pulling the curtain and covering the client protect the client's privacy and prevent chilling.*

5. Explain the procedure to the client.
   RATIONALE: *Explanations promote the client's cooperation.*

6. Put on clean gloves and an eye shield or face guard.
   RATIONALE: *Using appropriate barriers minimizes the risk of infection transmission. Gloves protect the hands. If there is any danger of splashing, eye shields or face guards are necessary.*

7. Position the client so that the solution will run from the upper end of the wound downward. Place the waterproof bed pad and clean basin or irrigating pouch under the area to be irrigated.

(continued)

In Practice
Nursing Procedure 58-2 (*Continued*)

RATIONALE: *The bed pad protects the bed linens. The clean basin or pouch will catch the irrigating solution.*

8. Drape the client with a bath blanket to expose only the wound.

   RATIONALE: *Exposing only the area for treatment maintains the client's privacy.*

9. Remove the old dressing and discard it as described at In Practice: Nursing Procedure 58-1. Discard gloves. Wash the hands again.

   RATIONALE: *Handwashing and proper disposal of contaminated equipment help to reduce the risk of infection transmission.*

10. After washing the hands, open the irrigation tray, using sterile technique. Carefully pour the solution, with the label facing the palm, into the irrigation supply bottle. If the bottle has been opened previously, pour off a small amount of the solution.

    RATIONALE: *The outside of the bottle is no longer sterile. You must pour the solution before you put on sterile gloves. Spilled solution will cause contamination and make the label unreadable. Pouring off a small amount of solution washes potential microorganisms from the lip of the container so that solution poured later will not be contaminated.*

11. Place the bottle close to the client on the overbed table. Date and initial the bottle after opening it. Include the client's name.

    RATIONALE: *You will use the solution for one client only. It must be clearly identified and kept handy.*

12. Open the sterile dressing tray if one is to be used, and put on sterile gloves.

    RATIONALE: *Maintaining sterile technique helps prevent the introduction of microorganisms that could cause infection.*

13. Prepare the inside of the irrigation and dressing trays. Place the irrigation syringe into the bottle. Open packs of dressings and prepare other items.

    RATIONALE: *Proper setup of sterile equipment maintains the sterility of the materials.*

14. Carefully assess the amount and character of drainage, and the size and condition of the wound and surrounding tissue.

    RATIONALE: *Data collection about the wound determines the progress of the wound's healing. Be sure to report and to document this information.*

15. While explaining the following steps to the client as you proceed, draw up solution into the syringe.

    RATIONALE: *Explanations foster cooperation and provide the client or family with teaching should irrigation need to be continued at home.*

16. Hold the syringe just above the wound's top edge, and force fluid into the wound, slowly and continuously. Use enough force to flush out debris, but

do not squirt or splash fluid. Irrigate all portions of the wound. Do not force solution into the wound's pockets. Continue irrigating until the solution draining from the wound's bottom end is clear.

RATIONALE: *Flushing the wound until the drainage is clear ensures that debris and infectious products are removed from the wound without damaging the wound.*

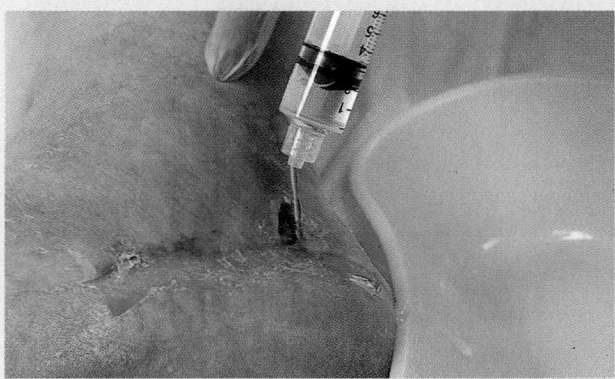

Gently flushing the wound with solution, directing the irrigation from the top of the wound to the bottom.

17. Using sterile 4×4 pads, gently pat dry the wound's edges (unless the wound is to have a wet-to-dry dressing; then dry only the surrounding skin). Work from cleanest to most contaminated.

    RATIONALE: *This measure helps prevent further contamination by removing culture media for microorganisms. The dressings will remain dry longer, and contamination will not spread.*

18. Apply sterile dressings as ordered.

    RATIONALE: *Applying sterile dressings protects the wound from contamination.*

19. Remove gloves and dispose of used supplies according to agency policy. Wash your hands.

    RATIONALE: *Proper disposal helps prevent transmission of microorganisms. Handwashing helps to prevent the spread of microorganisms.*

20. Assist the client to a comfortable position.

    RATIONALE: *Positioning the client comfortably helps minimize any discomfort experienced during the procedure.*

21. Teach the client to observe for excess drainage or severe pain. Teach any other pertinent observations.

    RATIONALE: *The client's observations may alert staff to problems, resulting in quick action. Pertinent observations may assist the team in further care planning.*

22. Document wound care and all assessments.

    RATIONALE: *Documentation provides communication and coordination of care.*

SKIN BREAKDOWN

Disruption of skin integrity, commonly called *skin break-down,* is a constant peril for the hospitalized or bedridden client. Breakdown occurs when skin is torn by friction or when continuous pressure against the skin causes local tissue *ischemia* (lack of blood supply). Ischemic tissues deteriorate and disintegrate, causing skin openings. A skin break is an invitation for infection. Constant safeguards are necessary to prevent skin breakdown.

Pressure Ulcers

Pressure ulcers, also called **decubitus ulcers** or *bedsores,* are the end result of constant skin pressure. Some body areas, including the bony prominences (eg, shoulder blades, elbows, end of the spine, hips, knees, sides of the ankles, and back of the head), as well as areas such as the heels and ears, are more likely to break down than others (Fig. 58-2). These bony areas are not covered by the pads of fat that normally cushion blood vessels. When blood vessels are compressed and blood flow is reduced, oxygen supply diminishes, skin breaks down, and the tissues beneath are destroyed.

Susceptibility to Pressure Ulcers

Because of the generalized lack of fat padding, a thin client is more susceptible to pressure areas than a heavier person. Skin also is more likely to break down if an area is continually moist or is not kept clean. An inadequate diet, especially one low in protein, leaves the skin prone to breakdown. The bedridden client's circulation is affected, and pressure on

bony prominences increases. The danger of developing pressure areas increases if a client must lie in one position or has a cast, splint, or disease that affects circulation.

A wound similar to a pressure ulcer can develop in an obese person, under pendulous breasts, or in abdominal folds. This type of wound is often complicated by a yeast infection. It is important to keep these areas as dry as possible.

Classification of Pressure Ulcers

Pressure ulcers are classified according to their four stages of development (Box 58-1).

In the fourth stage, a leathery black crust of dead tissue, called **eschar,** develops around the edges. Eschar that separates from living tissue is called **sloughing.** Debridement allows healthy tissue to grow, progressing from internal to external tissue.

☞ KEY CONCEPT

Deep open wounds must granulate-in (heal) from the inside outward. If the outside becomes sealed before the area underneath has healed, an abscess will usually form. This abscess may be sterile or infected (containing pathogens). In any event, an abscess is painful and must be treated.

Prevention of Pressure Ulcers

Always remain alert for signs of pressure on the client's body. Be particularly observant when giving a bath or a backrub. The client may talk about painful spots. Report any signs of pressure and be suspicious of reddened areas that stay red after pressure is removed. Preventing breakdown is easier

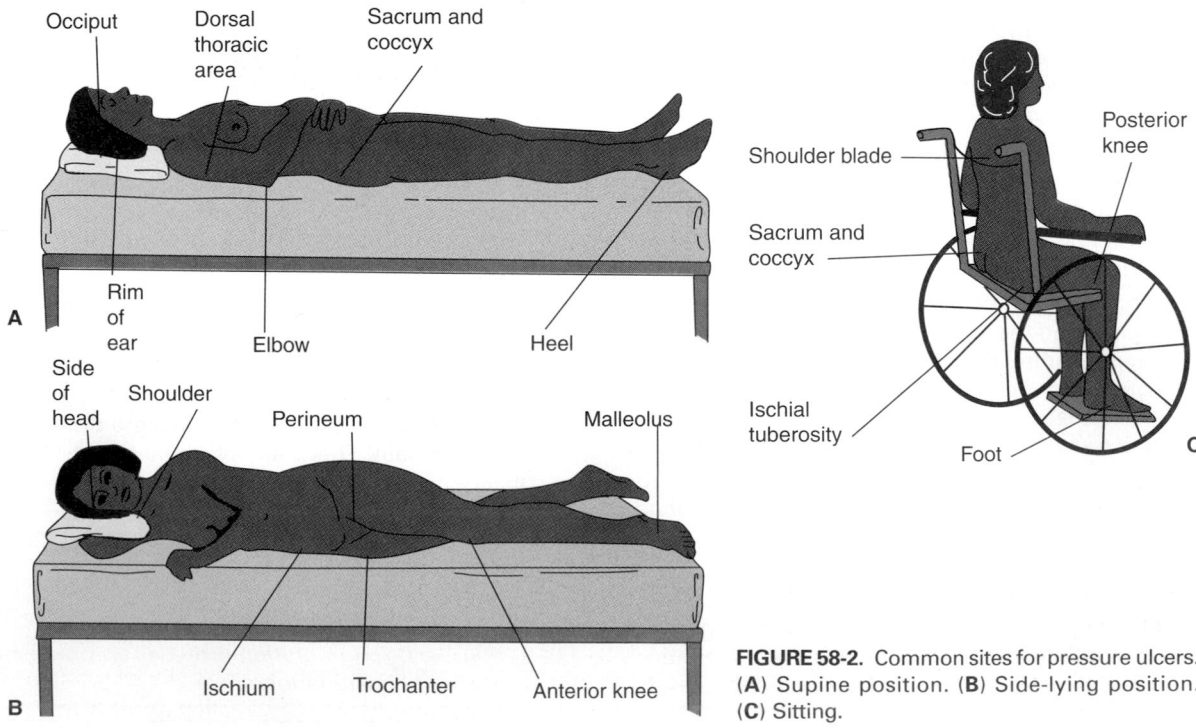

FIGURE 58-2. Common sites for pressure ulcers. **(A)** Supine position. **(B)** Side-lying position. **(C)** Sitting.

➤➤ BOX 58-1

STAGES OF PRESSURE ULCER CLASSIFICATION

Stage 1: Inflammation and redness; no blanching when area is pressed with finger; only epidermis is involved; reversible process, if pressure is relieved

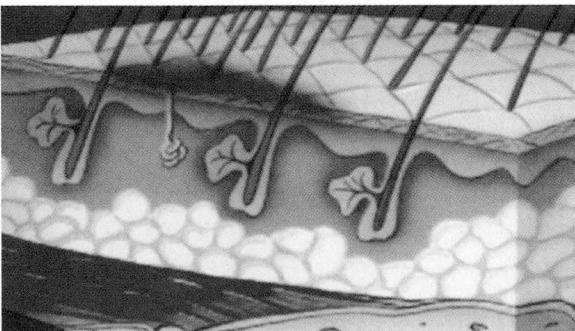

Stage I pressure ulcer.

Stage 2: Loss of epidermis with damage into dermis; appearing as a shallow crater or blister; swollen and painful; several weeks needed to heal after pressure is relieved

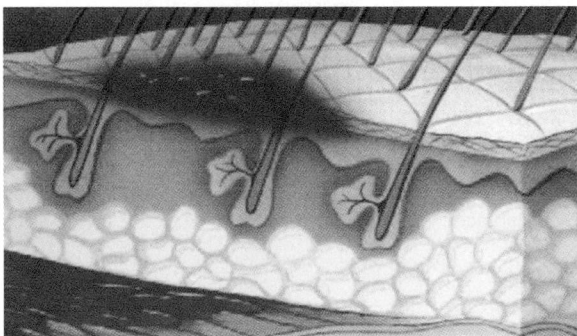

Stage II pressure ulcer.

Stage 3: Subcutaneous tissues involved; not painful; possible foul-smelling drainage; months may be needed to heal after pressure is relieved

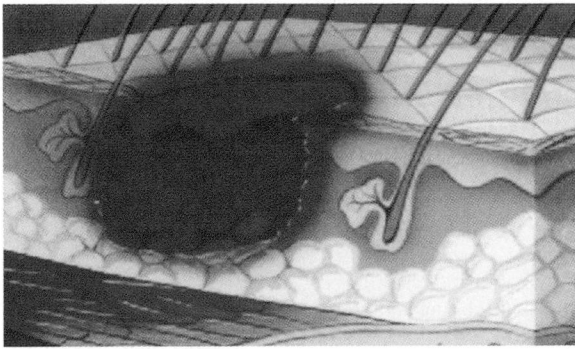

Stage III pressure ulcer.

Stage 4: Extensive damage to underlying structures including tendons, muscles, and bones; wound possibly appearing small on surface, but with extensive tunneling underneath; foul-smelling discharge; months or years may be needed for healing.

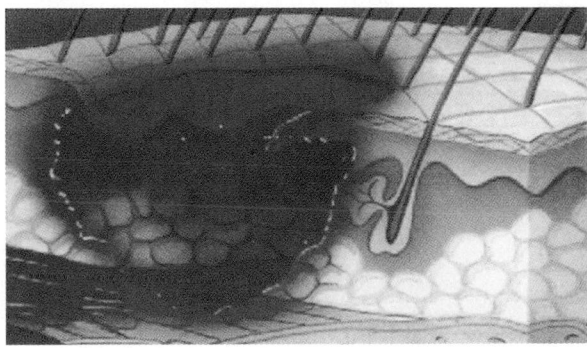

Stage IV pressure ulcer.

than treating it. Table 58-1 lists preventive measures. Remember that as soon as a skin break occurs, the path to infection is open.

The individual client's condition and the probable length of the illness help to determine the most effective prevention efforts. Turn and reposition the client frequently, so that no one body part experiences prolonged pressure. Massage the client's skin frequently to prevent pressure areas from developing. Keep the skin clean, dry, and free of urine, stool, and other secretions. The pelvic area is particularly vulnerable to the development of pressure ulcers in the incontinent client.

Place the client on a bed surface that reduces pressure. A flotation pad, air foam or egg crate mattress, or water- or air-circulating bed helps redistribute pressure evenly across the entire body (see Chap. 49). Occasionally, a lamb skin is prescribed, most likely for use on the seat of a wheelchair. The surface of lamb's wool is effective because it is soft and emits oils (eg, lanolin) that help keep the skin soft. Air spaces in the lamb's wool also help keep skin dry. Lamb skins are expensive; synthetic ones are sometimes used. However, synthetic lamb skins are not as effective as real ones.

Egg crate mattresses provide some comfort but do not really prevent skin breakdown. They do not allow the skin to "breathe" (ie, allow moisture to evaporate) or provide oils like lamb's wool.

Nursing Interventions for Pressure Ulcers

At the first sign of redness, reposition the client to relieve pressure. Keep the area clean and dry. Avoid rubbing or massaging a reddened area, because this added pressure may cause breakdown of small blood vessels, thereby worsening the skin's condition. Avoid skin irritation in all clients, especially

TABLE 58-1 *P*REVENTIVE MEASURES FOR COMMON CAUSES OF WOUNDS

Causes of Wounds	Location	Prevention
Pressure External force great enough to occlude blood in capillaries resulting in tissue anoxia	Bony prominences	Establish a turning schedule at least q2h. Use relieving support. Keep pressure off elbows and heels by elevating them with pillows and by using padding.
Shear Interaction of gravity and friction against the skin's surface	Surfaces exposed to bed or chair, especially if skin turgor is poor; coccyx most common site	Use draw sheet and lifting/turning sheet. Avoid dragging client's body over sheets. Limit elevation of head of bed to 30°. Position feet against footboard before head elevation.
Friction Superficial abrasion resulting from the skin rubbing another surface	Surfaces that rub on bed or chair surfaces	Apply transparent dressings to areas of friction. Move client carefully; avoid dragging across the bed. Use heel or elbow protectors. Keep skin adequately hydrated.
Stripping Unintentional removal of the epidermis by mechanical means such as with adhesive removal	Surfaces where applied	Use only porous tapes and apply without tension. Use saline to help remove dressings that adhere to the skin. Remove tape by slowly pulling tape away with one hand, while supporting surrounding skin with the other. Use alternatives to tape, such as Montgomery straps or Kerlix™ to wrap a limb, or a stockinette.
Urine or Stool Urinary and fecal incontinence	Perianal skin	Use containment equipment: absorptive products, condom catheters, or fecal pouches. Keep perianal skin cleansed, moisturized, and protected with barrier ointments. Investigate cause (eg, urinary infection, need for toileting schedule, impaction, organisms in stool, tube-feeding intolerance).
Perspiration	Areas where moisture can get trapped (eg, skin folds)	Keep areas of skin folds dry. Use barrier ointments. Use antifungal powder (not cream), if yeast is noted.
Arterial Insufficiency Arterial perfusion jeopardized	Feet, toes, and lower leg	Avoid compression. Protect from mechanical, chemical, or thermal injuries. Provide adequate remoisturizing. Take special care with diabetic clients, paralyzed persons, or persons with a bleeding disorder.
Maceration	Under pendulous breasts or folds of abdomen	Wash thoroughly at least once per day. Apply powder or prescribed medicinal cream. Encourage female client to wear a bra, if possible.

those who may be slow to heal, such as older adults, persons with diabetes mellitus, and immunocompromised clients (eg, persons with acquired immunodeficiency syndrome [AIDS] or who are undergoing cancer therapy). Avoid pulling the client across bed linens, which can result in small skin tears or abrasions. Always lift clients who cannot lift themselves.

Assessment and Cleaning.   *Assessment* of all wounds is important. In Practice: Nursing Assessment 58-1 lists items that must be addressed for all wounds.

Be sure to document and report observations. If, despite precautions, a client develops a pressure ulcer, *relieve pressure* on the area as much as possible, and *protect* the broken

A CLIENT'S WOUND

- Exact anatomic location
- Duration of wound (how long has it been there?)
- Size: width, length, and depth (in mm/cm). To measure depth, a cotton-tipped applicator may be inserted and then measured.
- Color of wound bed and surrounding tissue
- Presence of undermining, or tunneling tracts
- Specific appearance of areas of the wound, identified by using the hands of the clock as a reference
- Type of tissue (granulation, subcutaneous, muscle, eschar, leathery, slough, and so forth)
- New tissue formation in margins
- Presence or absence of *exudate* (drainage) and its description (odor, amount, color, general appearance)
- Feeling of warmth, coldness, hardness, and so forth around wound
- Complaints (and description) of pain or other symptoms
- Presence of any foreign bodies (sutures, gauze, dressings, medications)
- Appearance of skin surrounding wound
- Diagram of wound, if irregular in shape
- Other objective assessments (body temperature, blood tests, and so forth)

area from contamination with body substances such as wound drainage, urine, and feces. Keep the ulcerated area *clean and dry*. Moisture, combined with continuous pressure, predisposes the skin to breakdown. Pathogens from an infected wound or feces can be dangerous, particularly where a skin break exists. Always wear gloves when treating a pressure ulcer. Wash hands thoroughly before and after the treatment. See In Practice: Nursing Procedure 58-1 to review the steps for assessing, cleaning, and dressing a wound.

Medications.   Some pressure ulcers and other wounds are treated with *medications*. Usually, the wound is first cleaned and then patted dry with sterile gauze or other dressing. Follow the physician's orders carefully; also read the application instructions packaged with the medication. Apply the medication to the wound itself, but not to the skin's edges, unless ordered otherwise. The medication may be damaging to the surrounding tissues. In many cases, an open wound will be totally filled in with a prescribed cream or ointment medication. In the case of a large wound, this application is most often performed with a tongue blade.

☛ KEY CONCEPT

There are several other types of wounds that may be treated in a manner similar to pressure ulcers:

- *Frostbite (often treated as a burn)*
- *Diabetic ulcers (difficult to treat because of high blood sugar, compromised circulation, poor kidney function, and other complications of diabetes)*
- *Large gunshot wounds (may be left open to heal from the inside outward)*
- *Surgical incisions that have become seriously infected or that have opened (dehiscence)*

Diet.   Encourage the client who is at risk for developing— or who has already developed—a pressure ulcer to eat a healthy and balanced *diet*. To promote wound healing, a high-calorie and high-protein diet with supplemental vitamins (particularly vitamin C) may be ordered. The debilitated client, who is particularly vulnerable to ulcer formation, may require protein supplements between meals as well.

☛ KEY CONCEPT

The major consideration with regard to pressure ulcers is PREVENTION. After an ulcer has developed, it is usually very difficult for it to heal.

➥ STUDENT SYNTHESIS

Key Points

- The skin is a barrier that protects the body's internal environment from invasion by external pathogens.
- A wound is a disruption in the skin's integrity.
- Wounds heal by first, second, or third intention.
- A dressing is applied to a wound to protect it from contamination, to collect any exudate, and to protect against further damage.
- Careful sterile technique is required when dressing any wound.
- A common cause of skin breakdown is pressure against tissues that causes ischemia and tissue death.
- Pressure ulcer prevention focuses on eliminating all causes.
- Standard Precautions are used when changing any dressing, to help prevent the spread of infection to yourself or others and to avoid contaminating the wound. Wear gloves and properly dispose of all used dressings.

Critical Thinking Exercises

1. A 30-year-old man who was injured in an automobile accident is now paralyzed from the neck down. Identify this client's most vulnerable areas for skin breakdown. Explain how you will prevent pressure ulcer formation. What are the special nursing considerations for this particular man?
2. Visit a burn clinic or unit. Carefully describe in writing three wounds you see there. Include measurements, diagrams, and so forth. Ask a burn nurse

to critique your descriptions. Describe the types of dressings used in the burn unit and explain why each is used.

NCLEX-Style Review Questions

1. A client has a painful pressure ulcer that looks like a 1 cm × 2 cm blister. The nurse should document this pressure ulcer and the physician would probably diagnose it as a stage:
   a. One
   b. Two
   c. Three
   d. Four
2. Most surgical wounds heal by:
   a. Primary intention
   b. Removing eschar
   c. Secondary intention
   d. Sloughing
3. The nurse recognizes that which factor in a client's history is most significantly related to his or her formation of a pressure ulcer?
   a. Age 69 years
   b. History of smoking
   c. Restricted to bed
   d. Ten pounds over ideal weight
4. Which of the following foods would the nurse recommend to promote wound healing?
   a. Breads and pasta
   b. Green vegetables and pasta
   c. Fried foods and fruits
   d. Meats and citrus fruits
5. What is the most important goal of care for a client who is receiving sterile wound irrigations?
   a. Cleanse the wound.
   b. Cool the wound.
   c. Increase circulation to the wound bed.
   d. Provide pain relief for the client.

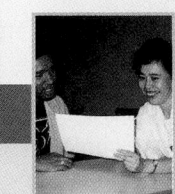

CHAPTER

59

Care of the Dying Person

LEARNING OBJECTIVES

1. Explain the two different types of advance directives.
2. Define and discuss DNR, DNH, and DNI orders that healthcare personnel must understand.
3. Describe and discuss the physical and emotional needs of the dying person.
4. Explain nursing care for the dying person as related to positioning, hygiene, oxygenation, nutrition and hydration, elimination, and pain management.
5. Identify nursing activities that may assist the family to cope with the death of their loved one.
6. Describe the care of the body after death.
7. Discuss how members of the healthcare team can help each other cope with the death of clients.

NEW TERMINOLOGY

autopsy
brain death
Cheyne-Stokes respiration

Kussmaul's breathing
postmortem examination

ACRONYMS

AD	DNI	PSDA
DNH	DNR	TPN

Throughout one's nursing career, facing the death of clients is to be expected. Clients who are dying receive care in hospitals, hospices, long-term care facilities, or their own home. Nursing care also extends to the family of the client. Although death is difficult, a nurse's presence and caring can help the dying client and his or her family to confront pain and loss. Nursing measures can provide needed comfort, respect, empathy, and understanding.

CARE OF THE DYING CLIENT

Before a nurse can help dying individuals and the families that are affected, he or she must effectively examine and begin to address personal feelings about death. Caring for the dying and their loved ones is an opportunity to learn. Although it is a difficult experience, individuals can gain much from it. By drawing on one's own spiritual reserves of strength and by facing the crisis of death, each person can grow emotionally and spiritually. When caring for clients who are dying, assist them with examining their mortality without fear or regret. Offer to secure spiritual counseling for them (Fig. 59-1). Refer to Chapters 14 and 99 for additional discussion of death and dying.

The Client's Wishes

It is important that the client's wishes about his or her care be known to the healthcare staff and be carried out as requested by the client.

Advance Directives

An advance directive (**AD**) is an expression of the client's wishes about the kinds of treatment and care that he or she wants to receive if terminally ill or unable to make decisions about healthcare. In 1990, Congress passed the Patient Self-Determination Act (**PSDA**), a step toward increasing the autonomy of dying persons. Healthcare facilities that receive federal funds must ask the client on admission if he or she has advance directive(s). These facilities must enter the client's response into the health record.

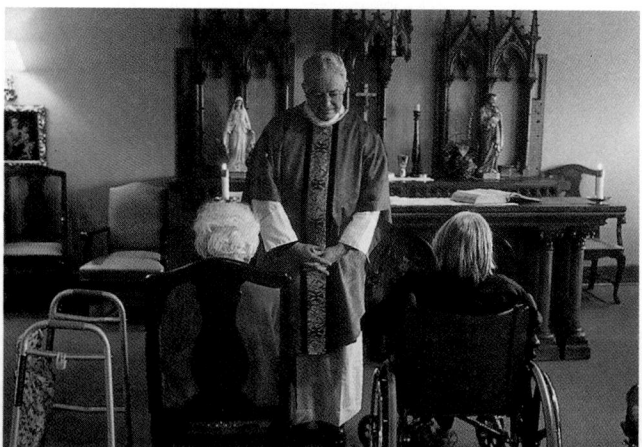

FIGURE 59-1. Direct the client for whom you are caring to examine their mortality without fear or regret. Offer to secure spiritual counseling for them.

An advance directive can take two forms:

- Living will
- Durable power of attorney for healthcare

A *living will* is a document in which clients state the types of treatment they desire to receive or not to receive if a terminal situation arises or if they are unable to make decisions or express their wishes. A *durable power of attorney for healthcare* designates a person of the client's choice to make these healthcare decisions should the client become incompetent (unable to make or express decisions about care) in the future. Chapter 4 discusses advance directives in more detail.

Codes

The advance directive informs healthcare personnel about the measures that should be taken if the client becomes terminally ill. Several healthcare "codes" are involved in these instructions.

An individual may have a do not resuscitate (**DNR**), do not intubate (**DNI**), or both orders in his or her health record. Healthcare personnel are thus informed that if this person experiences cardiopulmonary arrest, a "code blue" (or the code name for arrest in that facility) will not be called. The person will be allowed to die naturally, without mechanical or chemical intervention. He or she will be kept as comfortable as possible and given emotional support.

In the nursing home or in the home, the nurse may see a do not hospitalize (**DNH**) order in addition to a DNR or DNI order. The client needs to inform his or her family and significant other of their wishes regarding hospitalization and resuscitation. A copy of each client's living will should be readily available so it can be taken to the acute care facility in an emergency. The client and family should know the policies of ambulance and emergency transport agencies in their area. Many such service personnel are trained to give cardiopulmonary resuscitation (CPR) to *anyone* under their care. When a client does not wish to be hospitalized or resuscitated, the family needs maximum support in the home if the person's condition becomes serious.

Some individuals with terminal illnesses are on *full code,* meaning that the CPR team is to be called in case of cardiopulmonary arrest, though death is imminent. When working in environments where death occurs frequently, it is vital to know in advance which individuals are DNR and which are full code.

☛ KEY CONCEPT

Healthcare personnel do not determine whether a code should be called or not. Clients, physicians, or family members have already decided in advance, and written instructions are on file. If a client does not have a specific DNR order, a code is always called if the person should experience cardiac arrest.

Organ and Tissue Donation

Many people designate that their organs (eg, liver, kidney, heart, lung) and tissues (eg, cornea, bone, skin) are to be donated after their death. A person's decision is often recorded on his or her driver's license; however, after death most states require the family to give permission as well. Some extraordinary measures may be necessary to preserve organs long enough to be recovered; this problem does not usually arise for tissues.

Nursing Alert

Although a person may designate him- or herself as an organ or tissue donor, the family gains custody of the body at death. Most states have a law (called the Uniform Anatomical Gift Act) that requires healthcare facilities to approach each family regarding donation of their loved one's organs or tissues. Special courses are available to assist nurses in approaching family members at this difficult time. In many cases, being able to help another person by organ or tissue donation assists the family in dealing with the death of their loved one. *Be sure your family knows about your wishes in relationship to organ and tissue donation!*

Nursing Interventions in the Care of the Dying Client

When a client's actual physical process of dying begins, the main task is to assist with supportive and sympathetic care. Allow dying clients to maintain their self-esteem and personal dignity; never do things for clients that they can do themselves (see In Practice: The Nursing Process 59-1).

Care of the Mouth, Nose, and Eyes. Swab the client's mouth with mouthwash as often as necessary to keep it clean. If the client's nose or mouth has excessive secretions (as sometimes happens), turn the client on the side to promote drainage. Free the client's nostrils of crust; moisten and soothe them by applying mineral oil. Keep the eyes clean by wiping them with cotton balls or gauze pads moistened in normal saline. If the client's tongue is dry, moisten it with saline swabs. In extreme cases, a minute amount of a water-soluble lubricant may be applied so that the tongue does not stick to the roof of the mouth. Be sure to keep the client's airway open.

Positioning. Individuals who are dying may be unable to report that they are uncomfortable or that they would like to change position. Therefore, expect to turn them frequently to make them more comfortable. Use pillows for support when clients are lying on their side. Do not leave clients lying on their back because this position may precipitate secretions pooling in the back of the throat, possibly leading to choking or aspiration.

Breathing Difficulties. Various *breathing patterns* may be seen in the client who is dying. **Kussmaul's breathing** often occurs if a person experiences acidosis. This type of breathing is fast (>20 breaths/min), labored, and deep. It can rapidly turn into **Cheyne-Stokes respiration** as heart failure occurs. Alternating periods of *apnea* (absence of breathing) and *hyperpnea* (rapid breathing) characterize Cheyne-Stokes respiration. Gradually, the apneic periods lengthen.

Assist to make respiratory difficulties less distressing by turning the client onto his or her side or propping up the client into a partially sitting position. Always preserve the client's posture and provide enough support. Sometimes, the client slumps when in a sitting position, putting undue pressure on the chest and making it difficult to breathe.

Make certain that the client's tongue does not drop back and obstruct the airway. If it does, pull the tongue forward with gauze, and turn the client onto the side with the head elevated to prevent a recurrence. The collection of mucus and secretions may cause a "death rattle" as the client breathes. Gentle suctioning or a position change may relieve this sound.

In rare cases, the physician may order a very small dose of atropine to dry up secretions. Frequently, oxygen is ordered to increase the client's comfort.

Incontinence, Urinary Retention, and Constipation. Dying clients may be incontinent of stool or urine, or may have a distended bladder or a bowel obstruction. (Urinary incontinence is more common than bowel incontinence in the client who is terminally ill.) Keep clients dry and clean. Notify the primary care provider if a client does not void for 8 hours or as specified in the care plan. (Sometimes, clients produce minimal urine due to kidney failure and electrolyte imbalance.) Also notify the primary care provider if the client's abdomen is severely distended or if the client complains of abdominal pain. In many cases, the very ill client may not have a bowel movement for several days.

Nutrition and Hydration. The dying person usually is not interested in eating or taking fluids. The physician, together with the client and family, determines what course of action is best, using the client's living will or durable power of attorney for healthcare as the guide (if available).

Nausea and *vomiting* are common. Supportive nursing care is given. Medications such as metoclopramide (Reglan) may be used in an attempt to control nausea. In some cases, tube feeding or total parenteral nutrition (**TPN**) is instituted if the client's advance directive permits it.

Self-Esteem. People who are dying need to feel that they are worthwhile and that they are an important member of the family. Many clients want to plan their funeral or write their will. Fixing a client's hair or helping him or her to write a letter can provide comfort. Be sure to help clients perform any self-care that they can manage. Clients may feel inadequate when they are no longer able to perform activities of daily living (ADL) without assistance.

☞ Key Concept

Encourage the family to express their emotions and to let the client see how they feel about the situation. Let them know that it is OK to cry. Some families hide their feelings and refuse to allow the client to talk about death. The danger here is that the client may feel that no one cares that he or she is dying.

Odor Control. There may be foul-smelling drainage or discharge or incontinence. Keep this problem under control for the comfort of both client and family. Keep dressings

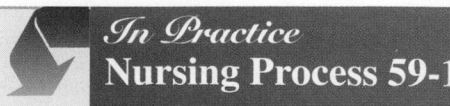

In Practice
Nursing Process 59-1

CARE OF THE DYING PERSON

Assessment Priorities
- Client and family's understanding of medical condition and prognosis
- Client and family's attitude toward death
- Client's preferences concerning death: desire to be at home, in a hospital, or in a hospice setting; decisions concerning resuscitation, aggressive forms of treatment, advanced life support, and organ or tissue donation
- Existence of advance directives, durable power of attorney; all members of the health team must know the authorized decision-maker and the client's wishes
- Religious beliefs
- Cultural influences
- Stage of grief and death reaction (denial and isolation, anger, bargaining, depression, acceptance)
- Adequacy of coping behaviors (client and family)
- Adequacy of resources available to client and family
- Physiologic needs of the client: personal hygiene; pain control; nutritional and fluid needs; movement, elimination, and respiratory needs
- Psychological needs of the client and family: fear of the unknown, pain, separation, leaving loved ones, loss of dignity, unfinished business, financial concerns, powerlessness
- Spiritual needs of the client and family: needs for meaning and purpose, love and relatedness, forgiveness, hope

Possible Nursing Diagnoses
- Anxiety
- Risk for caregiver role strain
- Decisional Conflict
- Ineffective Coping
- Ineffective Denial
- Interrupted Family Processes
- Anticipatory Grieving
- Hopelessness
- Pain
- Powerlessness
- Self-Care Deficit
- Social Isolation
- Spiritual Distress

Other diagnoses will depend on the physiologic responses of the client to the underlying disease process.

Planning
Design a plan of care with the client and family to achieve the following general goals:

- The client and family verbalize that they feel free to express their needs, fears, and emotions.

- The client's preferences concerning death are known and documented.
- The client reports sufficient relief of pain to interact meaningfully with family and to attend to everyday concerns.
- The client participates in self care to the extent possible.
- The client and family demonstrate positive methods of coping.

The long-term goal is death with dignity, which leaves the family unit intact.

Implementation
- Establish a supportive and trusting relationship with the client and family.
- Express warmth, care, and concern in interactions with the client and family; do not be afraid to cry.
- Explain the client's condition and treatment to the client and family.
- Keep the lines of communication open between the medical staff and the client and family, as well as between the client and the family.
- Ensure that the client's physiologic needs are met. Be especially attentive to the client's comfort needs.
- Talk with the client when providing care—even more so if the client is comatose. Provide simple explanations of what is being done and what is to be expected.
- Support the client and family as they work through the stages of grief and dying; refrain from being judgmental.
- Encourage the client and family to take an active role in planning and providing care.
- Arrange for the client's spiritual advisor to visit if the client so requests. Talk with the client about his or her beliefs; pray with the client if asked.
- Encourage family members to be open about their needs and to take necessary time for themselves.
- Help members of the family to understand the emotions and the needs of the dying client.
- Assist the client and family at the time of death, including caring for the body, placing the identification tags, caring for the family, ensuring that the physician has signed the death certificate, answering family questions about autopsy, offering the opportunity for organ and tissue donation, and meeting the needs of other clients.

Evaluation
- The adequacy of the plan of care is determined by evaluating the client's achievement of the above goals. If the client or family is unable to meet key goals, modify the plan. The following are key evaluative criteria:

  - Client's death with dignity
  - Intact family progressing through stages of grief

clean and dry, and drainage bags empty. Subtle deodorizers may be helpful.

Pain Relief.   Medications, including narcotics, are often given to relieve pain. Some authorities recommend that dying clients, even if they are not actually in pain, should have drugs for distress and exhaustion, to make them comfortable and to make dying easier. Large doses of narcotics may be given; physicians usually are no longer worried about the possibility of suppressing respirations and cognitive functions, or of addictions. Patient-controlled analgesia may be used to administer opiates (see Chap. 55). Chapter 99 lists some medications used to assist clients who are dying. Many clients find measures such as self-hypnosis and guided imagery to be helpful. In addition, therapies such as acupuncture and acupressure are often used. Other therapies, such as homeopathy, use of flower essences or essential oils, herbal remedies, or various traditional cultural remedies often prove helpful. Just before death, pain may ease or disappear, often indicating impending death.

Ventilation and Lighting.   Keep the room well ventilated. Allow air to circulate, but prevent it from blowing directly on the client. Oxygen may or may not be helpful at this stage, although it may make breathing slightly easier.

The room should have some lighting, but not so much as to interfere with the client's ability to rest or sleep. At night, keeping a light on in the room is helpful because darkness is frightening to many people. Clients are usually more uncomfortable and afraid if the room is dark.

Signs of Approaching Death

The dying process proceeds from the distal portions of the body inward. Therefore, the legs and then the arms lose sensation and the ability to move before the internal organs cease to function. Peripheral circulation diminishes first and then stops; the client often experiences *diaphoresis* (sweating) or elevated temperature, and then the body cools. The sense of touch is usually diminished, although the person can feel pressure. Box 59-1 lists signs of approaching death.

Failing Circulation.   As circulation fails, the client's body becomes cold and is frequently covered with perspiration. Heavy blankets may make the person restless. Provide light covering, and keep it loose over the client's feet, using a bed cradle if necessary.

Failing Senses.   Research has shown that hearing is the last sense that is lost. Most clients can hear until the final moment. Speak distinctly, and do not whisper or talk about the client to someone else. The dying client is likely to feel a sense of increasing darkness as vision begins to fail, and may turn toward a window or other source of light.

Care of the Client and Family as the Person is Dying

Often a client's family members experience the stress of this period more keenly than the client. They are dealing with a sense of loss, yet they feel they must appear as though everything is normal. Family members should understand that crying and being sad in front of the client are acceptable behaviors and are actually recommended. Showing their feelings tells the client that they care deeply.

If a client is in pain or is very apprehensive, explain to family members that they can make the death easier by taking turns staying with the client. Show the family comfort measures they can take to ease the individual's pain. Encourage family members to continue to communicate with the person, even if he or she does not respond. They can repeatedly tell the individual of their love. They may be reluctant to tell the client that he or she will be missed. However, this will strengthen the person's sense that he or she has made an impression on the world. Family members need to assure

---

➤ ➤ **BOX 59-1**

SIGNS OF APPROACHING DEATH

The following are signs that may be noted in the client who is dying, as death approaches and eventually occurs. Keep in mind that there is no specific order to these changes and each of these changes *may or may not* occur.

- Loss of control over bladder and bowel may occur.
- Intake of food and drink will diminish, and general nutritional requirements are less.
- The extremities will feel colder to the touch, as circulation slows.
- The person experiences increased fatigue and difficulty waking up.
- Recognition of familiar people, places, or objects decreases, and visions of people or things that do not exist may occur.
- Occasionally, restlessness increases.
- Dry mouth and accumulation of thick secretions in the back of the throat often occur.
- Noisy breathing, due to secretions in the mouth or chest, is common.
- The pattern of breathing changes, such as rapid breathing followed by periods where breathing is slow or even absent for as long as 15 sec (Cheyne-Stokes respirations).

At the point of death:

- Breathing, heartbeat, and pulse stop entirely.
- The person is entirely unresponsive to shaking or shouting.
- The person does not respond to painful stimuli.
- The eyelids may be open or closed, and the pupils are dilated and fixed in one direction.
- Loss of urine and bowel control occurs.

NOTE: Not all of these changes occur in each death.

Courtesy of Abbott-Northwestern Home Care, Hospice Unit, St. Louis Park, Minnesota.

the dying person that they can manage after their death. They can reassure their loved one that the love they share will support them in the future. Often, people struggling with death need their closest loved ones to give them permission to move on to the next stage of life's journey, that of death.

Remind the family members, however, of the needs for their personal rest and nourishment. As a sign of caring, offer them a cup of tea or coffee or a snack when a visit with the client has been exhausting. If possible, provide a place for family members to be alone. Sometimes, a place to nap is helpful. If a waiting period is likely to be long, encourage family members to go out for meals and rest, assuring them that they will be called immediately should any change occur. Suggest that they carry a cell phone or beeper for this purpose.

Dying clients can offer comfort to the family by sharing feelings and thoughts. Encourage such communication. Support groups are available for assistance. Families often need help in knowing what to do for their loved ones during the dying process. Explain to them the physical and emotional stages associated with dying.

☛ Key Concept

Clients who have been confused or unconscious may abruptly become lucid and alert when they are about to die. If possible, call family members at this time so that clients have a chance to say a final goodbye.

The Role of Hope

Dying individuals may cling to hope and not give up until the very end, when they finally reach acceptance. Families also may cling to the hope that an unexpected recovery may occur. Individuals and the family may resist entrance into a hospice program (see Chap. 99) because giving up seems impossible or wrong. Do not destroy this hope with logical arguments, but do not give false hope either. The role of the nurse and other healthcare professionals is to be honest with clients and to support them in their own way of coping. Clients and family members may ask, "Is there any hope at all?" An honest answer is that nobody truly knows when a person will die, but that the individual will receive the best care available, and that the healthcare team will do all they can to provide support and comfort (Fig. 59-2).

When Death Occurs

Clinical death occurs when respiration and heartbeat both stop. For the client who is DNR or DNI, note the exact time when respiration stops (usually first), and the exact time when the heart stops beating. Notify the physician or other primary caregivers.

Brain death, *cerebral death,* or *biologic death* is formally defined as the "irreversible cessation of total brain function, determined by clinical examination." Mechanical or chemical means can maintain the client's vital functions even *after* brain death occurs. Therefore, standards for deter-

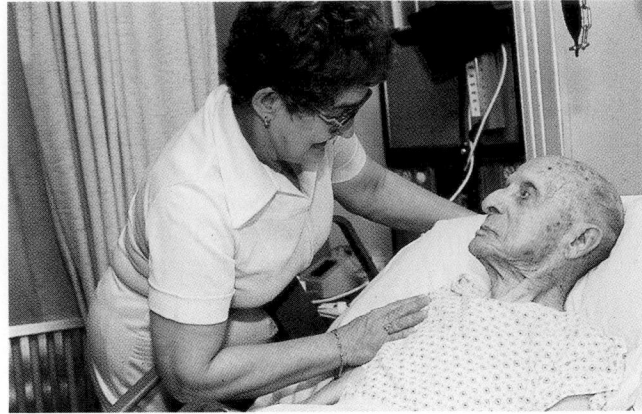

FIGURE 59-2. An honest answer is that no one truly knows if a person will die of an illness, or when; however, the individual will receive the best care available and the healthcare team will do all they can to provide support and comfort.

mining brain death are made under carefully controlled conditions so that in certain situations, a client may be maintained on a ventilator until some of his or her organs may be removed for transplant.

Determination of brain death varies slightly across different states, but generally brain death means that the client's electroencephalogram (EEG) shows no brain wave activity. This EEG determination is often combined with other criteria to pronounce biologic death. Other criteria include:

- Total unresponsiveness to stimuli
- Cessation of all movement, breathing, and heartbeat
- Complete absence of cephalic reflexes
- Fixed, dilated pupils

Cerebral circulation studies also may be done. Two exceptions to the usual criteria for biologic death are a hypothermic condition and central nervous system depression secondary to drug overdose.

☛ Key Concept

The determination of death while the client is being maintained on a ventilator is difficult for the family. They need to fully understand and accept the fact that even though the client appears to be breathing, it is the machine that is actually doing the breathing.

CARE FOLLOWING THE DEATH OF A CLIENT

At the actual time of death, a number of activities must be carried out, either by the nurse or by the family.

Caring for the Family

When a person dies, the family often does not know what to do next. Family members may need time just to sit with the body. Help them to make the transition to bereavement. Give them assistance as they work through their grief.

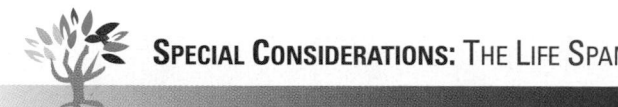

SPECIAL CONSIDERATIONS: THE LIFE SPAN

Family Coping After a Death

Many variables surrounding death may influence how family members will cope. These may include:

- Personalities of the individual family members
- Personality and values of the deceased
- Relationships between the deceased and the other members of the family
- Family stability and unity
- Relationships among the survivors
- Cultural and ethnic practices and customs
- Religious beliefs
- Age of the deceased person (infant, child, adult, or older adult)
- Suddenness of the death (time for preparation and resolution)
- Length and severity of the illness
- Manner of death (natural, accidental, traumatic, homicide, or suicide)

All these factors interact to influence how the family responds to the death. Individual family members most likely will respond in different ways. (Most of these topics have been discussed in some detail elsewhere in this book.)

After a death in a healthcare facility, prepare the body so the family can see it if they wish. Be sure that the body is clean. Place a clean sheet over the client, but do not cover the face. Unless an **autopsy** (examination of the body after death) is likely, remove nasogastric tubes and intravenous (IV) lines, and turn off monitors. Prepare the body so that the client appears comfortable. Allow family members to stay in the room as long as they wish, knowing that help or support is available if needed. Muted lighting is comforting. Offer to call a chaplain, clergyperson, friends, or other family members.

☛ KEY CONCEPT

In the event of a sudden or accidental death, the client's family has had no time to prepare for the event. The nurse working in rescue, or in areas such as the emergency department or the coronary care unit, needs to possess special communication and interpersonal skills. In many cases, special training is available for nurses and other healthcare providers who work in these areas.

The Client Who Chooses to Die at Home

If the client's death has been anticipated, and the client has chosen to die at home, the home care nurse has been discussing the plans with the family beforehand. Usually the nurse is not present at the actual time of death, so the family must be prepared ahead of time. They are told to call the nurse. Most agencies have a nurse on call 24 hours a day to answer questions and to come to the home if necessary.

The Postmortem Examination

In many cases, a **postmortem examination** is desirable or required by law. In the event of a sudden, unexpected death and certainly if there is any suspicion of foul play, a postmortem examination is required. This is known as a "coroner's case." In other situations, such as if the client had been undergoing special therapy or experimental treatment, the physician may feel that an autopsy would be very helpful from a research standpoint. In some cases, an autopsy is requested by the physician or family to establish the exact cause of death, even though the person was known to be ill.

If an autopsy is to be done, the family may have questions about it. Answer their questions as completely and accurately as possible. In nearly all cases, the family may obtain a copy of the autopsy report at a later time.

☛ KEY CONCEPT

When a loved one dies, a family may be required to make three major decisions, involving:

- *Performance of an autopsy*
- *Donation of organs or tissues*
- *Choice of funeral home or crematorium*

Nurses often are involved in assisting the family with these decisions.

Caring for the Dead Person's Body

In the healthcare facility, the primary healthcare provider pronounces that the client is dead, and signs the death certificate. After the family has left the room, nurses prepare the body for transport to the morgue or pickup by the funeral director. In Practice: Nursing Procedure 59-1 reviews caring for the body after death. In the healthcare facility, these procedures are performed by the nursing staff. If the client plans to die at home, the home care nurse is responsible for adapting these procedures and teaching them to the family.

In the home care situation, the family may have been taught and may be willing and able to carry out this preparation. The funeral director is called to come pick up the body directly from the home, unless an autopsy is to be done. In the event of an anticipated death of a hospice client at home, the physician or other healthcare provider usually does not need to travel to the home to pronounce death. In the case of sudden or suspicious death, the coroner is called and pronounces the death and then determines who will manage the scene.

Coping With a Client's Death

One of the greatest challenges facing the nurse is providing care for a dying person. Most nurses cannot just walk away from a situation where a person has died. Colleagues can be an informal help, by allowing time for grieving. Many units in acute care facilities have meetings following the death of

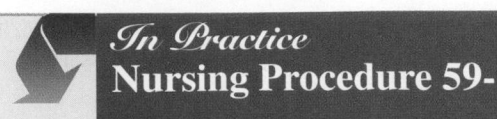

In Practice
Nursing Procedure 59-1

CARING FOR THE BODY AFTER DEATH

Supplies and Equipment

Disposable gloves
Chipped ice (if needed)
Towel
Fresh dressings
Shroud or zippered bag
Identification tags

Steps

1. Wash the hands and wear gloves.
   RATIONALE: *Handwashing and wearing gloves prevent contact with the client's bodily drainage.*

2. Straighten the body, and place a pillow under the head.
   RATIONALE: *Proper positioning immediately after death prevents potential problems later. The body will assume this position in a casket.*

3. If the person's eyes are to be donated, close them, and place a small ice pack on each eye. A glove with a few ice chips works well.
   RATIONALE: *Ice helps prevent swelling and discoloration.*

4. Remove any jewelry. If there is a specific order, tape a wedding ring in place. Carefully document this.
   RATIONALE: *Removing jewelry and documenting its removal make sure that none of the client's property is lost. Some clients never take off their wedding rings.*

5. List all personal belongings, and have the family sign for them and take them. Make sure to check the closet, dresser, and safe of the healthcare facility.
   RATIONALE: *The family will wish to sort through the client's belongings.*

6. Send all flowers and cards home with the family.
   RATIONALE: *These items belong to the client and family; after death, the client's room must be readied for a new client. In addition, the family may wish to write thank you notes.*

7. Close the client's mouth by placing a rolled towel under the chin.
   RATIONALE: *Using a rolled towel closes the mouth and prevents the jaw from falling down.*

8. Remove all IV lines, monitors, and other equipment, unless ordered otherwise.
   RATIONALE: *Equipment is no longer needed.*

9. Remove all extra equipment from the room; remove all top bed linens, except the sheet that covers the client.

RATIONALE: *The equipment is not needed and will be in the way.*

10. Bathe any part of the body that has been soiled with discharges.
    RATIONALE: *Bathing preserves the client's dignity.*

11. Remove soiled dressings, and replace them with clean ones. Pad the wrists and ankles, and tie them loosely together.
    RATIONALE: *This procedure makes handling the body easier and prevents the arms and legs from falling down.*

12. Give the client's dentures and glasses to the funeral director. Most funeral directors prefer to place dentures in the client's mouth themselves. The family may take the client's glasses to the funeral home.
    RATIONALE: *Dentures may be broken when being placed in the mouth. Glasses are important so that the person looks natural; the family can make sure they do not get lost en route.*

13. Attach two tags to the body: one tied to the foot (usually the right great toe) and the other to the hand or wrist. Another may be attached to the covering sheet. These tags are stamped with the address, client's diagnosis, and the date and time of death.
    RATIONALE: *The client must be correctly identified.*

14. Wrap the body before it is taken to the morgue. Check the facility's procedure for wrapping the body. Usually a shroud or zippered bag is provided.
    RATIONALE: *Properly wrapping the body covers the client, demonstrates respect for the client, and maintains his or her dignity.*

15. If the client had a known communicable disease, note this on the shroud or covering.
    RATIONALE: *Special precautions may need to be taken with the body.*

16. Carefully dispose of all dressings, IV lines, and equipment according to the contaminated materials procedures of the facility.
    RATIONALE: *Standard and Transmission-Based Precautions apply.*

17. Remove gloves and properly dispose of them. Wash the hands.
    RATIONALE: *Proper glove disposal and handwashing minimize the risk of infection transmission.*

18. Complete the client's chart, documenting the exact time of death and any pertinent observations.
    RATIONALE: *Documentation provides communication and continuity of care.*

an individual who was receiving care. In such meetings, team members give each other mutual support. Discuss feelings with others who can provide support (eg, supervisor, co-worker, spouse, spiritual advisor). Formal support groups often exist in hospice units where nurses frequently encounter client death. Expressing sadness to the person's family is also appropriate.

✄ STUDENT SYNTHESIS

Key Points

- Advance directives, codes, and organ and tissue donation are three types of client wishes that nurses must be familiar with when caring for dying individuals.
- Changing the dying client's position frequently may promote comfort.
- Positioning the dying person on the side or in a semi-upright position may aid his or her breathing.
- The dying client who is incontinent needs to be kept as clean and dry as possible.
- Tube feeding or total parenteral nutrition may be instituted if the dying client is unable to eat or drink. The client also may choose not to receive nourishment.
- Pain relief may be necessary to ease the dying process.
- Brain death occurs when no brain function can be identified by an EEG and by other means.
- The client's family needs nursing comfort in the form of understanding and support.
- After death, the nurse often gives physical care to the client's body and offers emotional support to the family.
- When a family member chooses to die at home, the family assumes the role of caregiver and usually manages the postmortem care.

Critical Thinking Exercises

1. Review Maslow's hierarchy of human needs (see Chap. 5). Discuss how the needs of the dying person relate to Maslow's basic needs. Make a chart showing the relationships.
2. You are aware of the need for more people to donate organs and tissues for transplant use. The wife of a terminally ill person on a ventilator has been asked to donate his organs for transplant. She is having difficulty deciding what her husband would have wished. She asks you to help her think about her decision. How could you help her?
3. A. M., a 35-year-old Muslim man, is brought to the hospital's emergency room in critical condition fol-

lowing a motor vehicle accident. He is not expected to live. "Donor" is printed on his driver's license. Describe your responsibilities in the nursing care of this man. What issues might the medical and nursing staff discuss with this man's family? What support could you give to the family? What pertinent resources are available in your hospital and in your community? What cultural activities would you expect if this man should die?

NCLEX-Style Review Questions

1. Which of the following would support the client's dignity during the dying process?
   a. Allow the client to complete activities.
   b. Avoid talking about dying.
   c. Encourage the family to only talk about happy memories.
   d. Talk to the client in a soft whisper.
2. When evaluating the effectiveness of atropine administered to a dying person, the nurse would assess for:
   a. Increased alertness
   b. Less secretion
   c. Reduced pain
   d. Stable urine output
3. Which of the following statements reflects the current treatment of dying clients in regard to pain control?
   a. Dosage is closely monitored to prevent addiction.
   b. Large doses may be needed to control pain.
   c. Low doses should be given to prevent cognitive changes.
   d. Medications are discontinued as soon as pain control is achieved.
4. Which of the following indicate that death is approaching?
   a. Client is continent of both bowel and bladder function.
   b. Client states he or she feels rested.
   c. Extremities feel cooler to the touch.
   d. The client recognizes family members and friends.
5. The daughter of a dying client expresses that she feels helpless and does not know what to do. Which of the following would not be an appropriate nursing action?
   a. Assure her that her presence is helpful.
   b. Provide names of local support groups.
   c. Show her how to give her father a backrub.
   d. Tell her that all family members feel this way.

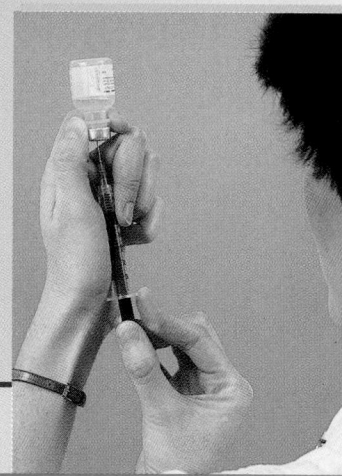

Unit IX

PHARMACOLOGY AND ADMINISTRATION OF MEDICATIONS

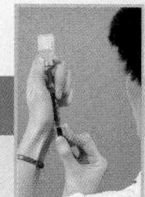

CHAPTER

60

Review of Mathematics

LEARNING OBJECTIVES

1. Explain why an understanding of basic mathematics is essential before learning the basics of pharmacology.
2. Discuss systems of measurement used in the provision of healthcare.
3. Convert among milligrams, grams, and kilograms.
4. Convert among different systems of measurement (household, metric, apothecary).
5. Demonstrate the use of ratio and proportion to calculate medication dosages.

NEW TERMINOLOGY

apothecary
decimal fraction
denominator
gram
liter
meter
metric
minim

numerator
pharmacology
proportion
ratio
significant figure
units

This unit discusses the basics of **pharmacology**, or the study of chemicals and their effects on the body. Pharmacology is closely related to mathematics. A general understanding of mathematics is needed to ensure safety when working with medications and following orders for their administration (Fig. 60-1). This chapter reviews various systems of measurement used in pharmacology, and different methods of dosage calculation.

SYSTEMS OF MEASUREMENT

The *household* (measurement used in the home), *metric* (measurement based on the number 10), and *apothecary* (measurement based on volume and weight) systems of measurement are used in the preparation of medications. Because two or more systems of measurement may be used for the same medication, nurses need to become proficient in converting dosages to and from each system. Table 60-1 gives units of measurement—with their corresponding abbreviations—for these three commonly used systems.

Medications may also be ordered in **units** (a specific measurement used for certain drugs). For example, insulin for the treatment of diabetes mellitus is ordered in units. The term *units* is also used in nutrition.

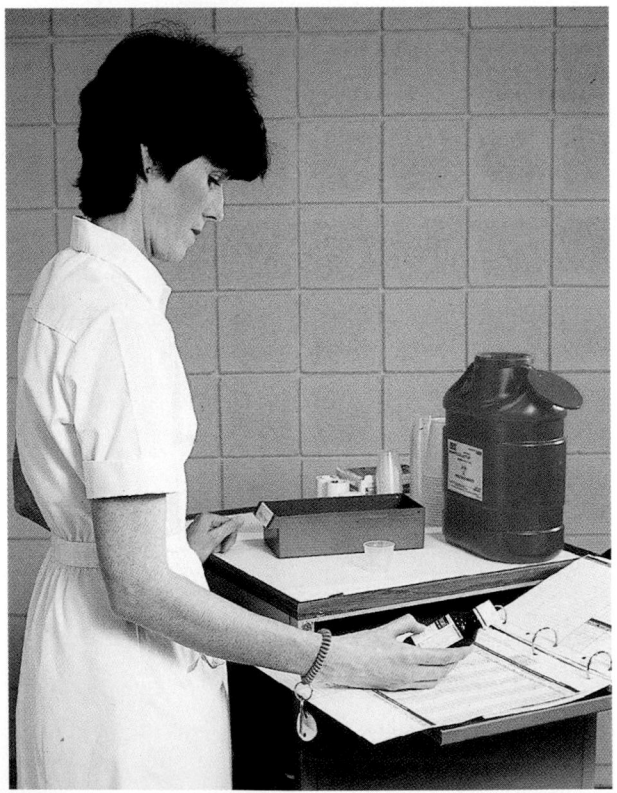

FIGURE 60-1. A basic working knowledge of mathematics is necessary to safely administer the prescribed dose of a medication. Nurses may be required to calculate how many tablets (or portions of tablets) to give or how many milliliters of a liquid medication to draw up into a syringe.

■■■ TABLE 60-1 *S*YSTEMS OF MEASUREMENT

System	Unit	Abbreviation or Symbol
Household	drop	gtt
	teaspoon	t, tsp
	tablespoon	T, tbsp
	cup	c
	pint	pt
	quart	qt
Apothecary	grain	gr
	minim	m, min, ɱ
	dram	dr, ℨ
	ounce	oz, ℥
Metric	milligram	mg
	gram	g, gm, G
	cubic centimeter	cc*
	liter	L
	milliliter	mL
	kilogram	kg
	microgram	mcg, μg

*1 cc equals approximately 1 mL.

🔶👁 **Nursing Alert**

Administering drugs is one of the most important nursing functions. Take this responsibility seriously. A medication error could cause a client's death.

Household Measurement System

Probably the most familiar system, the *household* system of measurement, is that which is used in the home. It includes measurements such as the teaspoon, tablespoon, pint, quart, and gallon. Converting to and from the household system of measurement is done using simple mathematics, following basic guidelines. For example:

    5 mL = 1 teaspoon (approximately)
    Therefore
    15 mL = 3 teaspoons or 1 tablespoon (approximately)

Apothecary System

The **apothecary** system is the oldest system of measurement. It is used in the measurement of weight and volume. Although the apothecary system is used less commonly today than other units of measurement, some physicians still prescribe using this system. Therefore, nurses need to become familiar with it.

The apothecary system uses fractions and Roman numerals. Unlike the metric system, it indicates the units of measurement first, followed by the numeral. For instance, the correct way to write 10 grains would be "gr X"; 3 grains would be written "gr iii." The line and dot above the Roman numerals İ (one), İİ (two), İİİ (three), and so forth are used for clarity of the number. Sometimes, a line is written over 5 and 10 as well, for example, v̄ or x̄. When calculations are made using the apothecary system, however, Arabic numbers are used.

The apothecary system is based on units of volume (using minims, drams, and ounces) and weight (using grains, drams, and ounces). The prefix "fl" is sometimes used to indicate a liquid measurement. A liquid measurement therefore could correctly be referred to as either "fl ounce" or "ounce."

A **minim** is approximately equal to one drop (gtt.). Because differences exist in the size of droppers (and therefore in the size of drops), the dropper must be calibrated if the measurement is to be accurate.

The weight of one *grain* (gr) is based on the average weight of one grain of wheat. A *scruple* is approximately equal to gr $\overline{XX}$ (20 grains). One example of a medication sometimes prescribed in grains is aspirin. A common aspirin dose is "gr x̄," which is equivalent to 650 mg. This system incorporates very old equivalents of measurement. For that reason, it is the least accurate of the three systems of measurement.

Metric System

The **metric** system is the most widely used measurement system in the world today. It is proposed that someday, it will be the only system of measurement used in drug dosages. The metric system is very simple to use. It is a decimal system based on the number 10. The monetary system of the United States is based on the metric system.

For medications, the metric system is based on the meter, gram, and liter. The **meter** (M) is a measurement of length, the **gram** (G, g, or gm) is a measurement of weight, and the **liter** (L) is a measurement of liquid volume. Greek and Latin prefixes are used to describe various increments of these basic units. Refer to Table 60-1 for prefixes most commonly used in computing dosages. For example:

deci—divide by 10; 1/10
centi—divide by 100; 1/100
milli—divide by 1,000; 1/1,000
micro—divide by 1,000,000; 1/1 millionth
deca—multiply by 10; × 10
hecto—multiply by 100; × 100
kilo—multiply by 1,000; × 1,000

In addition to medication administration, nurses use the metric system in other aspects of care. For example, amounts of oral fluid intake and urinary output are measured in milliliters (mL), and newborns are weighed in grams (gm) and measured in centimeters (cm). A client's weight is usually converted to kilograms (kg) to facilitate medication and anesthetic dosage calculations for surgery. When measuring the size of an incision or ulcer, nurses often measure the area in centimeters. Cervical dilation during delivery is always stated in centimeters.

Very often, a prescription for a medication will call for milligrams (mg), but a drug is available only in grams (gm). This requires accurate completion of metric conversions to ensure administration of the proper medication dose. Because the metric system is a decimal system, conversion is very easy by using multiplication or division. For instance, to convert grams (gm) to milligrams (mg), multiply by 1,000. To convert mg to gm, divide by 1,000. Another quick and easy method is to complete the conversion simply by moving the decimal point (see "Decimal Fractions" section for rationale). To convert gm to mg, move the decimal point 3 places to the right; to convert mg to gm, move the decimal point 3 places to the left. Box 60-1 lists some common metric measurements and equivalents.

☞ KEY CONCEPT

To convert from large to small, move the decimal point to the right. Example:

- *g to mg (large to small)*
- *1 g = 1,000 mg*
- *1.5 g = 1,500 mg*

To convert from small to large, move the decimal point to the left. Example:

- *mg to g (small to large)*
- *1,000 mg = 1 g*
- *1,500 mg = 1.5 g*

➤➤ BOX 60-1

COMMON METRIC MEASUREMENTS AND EQUIVALENTS

Some metric equivalents are used more frequently than others. Memorize the following measures and equivalents:

Distance
1 meter (M) = 100 centimeters (cm)
               = 1,000 millimeters (mm)
1 cm = 0.01 M
1 mm = 0.001 M
2.54 cm = 1 inch

Weight
1 kilogram (kg) = 1,000 grams (g) = 2.2 pounds (lb)
1 milligram (mg) = 0.001 g = 1,000 micrograms (mcg)
1 mcg = .001 mg = 0.000001 g
454 g = 1 lb

Volume
1,000 milliliters (mL) = 1 liter (L)
1 mL = 0.001 L
1 mL = 1 cubic centimeter (cc)*

*A milliliter (mL) is equal to a cubic centimeter (cc); the two are often used interchangeably.

Conversion From One System to Another

Converting from one system of measurement to another involves the use of simple mathematics. Table 60-2 identifies systems of measurement and their equivalent relationships. The term *equivalent* does not mean exact or equal. Remember that some discrepancies exist because of the inaccuracies of the apothecary and household systems.

DOSAGE CALCULATION

Ratio and Proportion

Ratio and proportion are frequently used to calculate medication dosages. A **ratio** is the relationship of one quantity to another. A ratio may be written as a fraction or as numbers separated by a colon, for example, $\frac{2}{3}$ or 2:3. When two ratios are set equal to each other, they are said to be *in proportion* to each other. A true **proportion** consists of two equal ratios separated by an equals sign (=) or a double colon (::). For example:

$$\frac{2}{3} = \frac{6}{9}$$

or

2:3 :: 6:9

or

2:3 = 6:9

or

2 is to 3 as 6 is to 9

This is a valuable relationship. When written with the double colon, the first and last numbers are referred to as the *extremes* and the second and third (middle) numbers are the *means*.

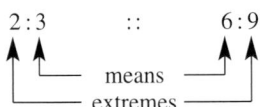

2:3   ::   6:9
means
extremes

TABLE 60-2 *A*PPROXIMATE LIQUID EQUIVALENTS OF HOUSEHOLD, APOTHECARY, AND METRIC MEASUREMENT SYSTEMS

Household	Apothecary	Metric
60 gtt (1 tsp)	1 fl dr	5 mL (cc)
1 tsp	15 min	1 mL (cc)
1 gtt	1 min	0.0616 mL
1 tsp	1 fluid dr	5 mL (cc)
1 tbsp	4 fluid dr	15 mL (cc)
1 c	8 oz	240 mL (cc)
1 pt	16 oz	500 mL (cc)
1 qt	32 oz	1000 mL (cc) (approx.)

There are three rules that apply when using ratios and proportions:

1. The product of the means equals the product of the extremes. The *product* is the answer you get when you multiply. Therefore, $2 \times 9 = 18$ (product of the extremes) and $3 \times 6 = 18$ (product of the means).
2. The product of the means divided by one extreme yields the other extreme. Therefore, $3 \times 6 = 18$ and $18 \div 2 = 9$.
3. The product of the extremes divided by one mean yields the other mean. Therefore, $2 \times 9 = 18$ and $18 \div 6 = 3$.

Therefore, when 3 of the 4 factors of a proportion are known, the missing factor can be found, using simple mathematics.

Dosage Calculations

Ratio and proportion is probably the most commonly used method of calculating dosages. To use the ratio and proportion method, the numbers to be multiplied must be in the same units of measurement. Therefore, it is necessary to convert if this is not true.

#1. EXAMPLE: The prescription is 1 mg Haldol IM (intramuscularly) and the medication is available in an ampule with a strength of 5 mg/1 mL. How many mL should be given?

SOLUTION: Set up a ratio. Known factors:

- Medication available = 5 mg (strength): **Factor 1**
- Volume = 1 mL: **Factor 2**
- Prescribed dosage = 1 mg: **Factor 3**
- Volume (mL) needed to give = X mL: **Unknown factor**

One of the rules of ratios and proportions is that the product of the means, divided by one extreme, equals the other extreme. *Remember:* Units of measure must cancel properly during calculations (see equation below).

Set up units in the same position on each side of the double colon:

5 mg is to 1 mL as 1 mg is to X mL

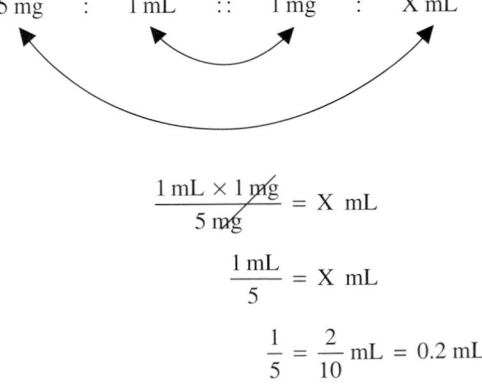

5 mg   :   1 mL   ::   1 mg   :   X mL

$$\frac{1\ mL \times 1\ mg}{5\ mg} = X\ mL$$

$$\frac{1\ mL}{5} = X\ mL$$

$$\frac{1}{5} = \frac{2}{10}\ mL = 0.2\ mL$$

(Above, the fraction $\frac{2}{10}$ mL is converted to the decimal fraction 0.2 mL, because syringe measurements are in decimal tenths of a milliliter.) Measure 0.2 ($\frac{2}{10}$) mL in the syringe.

A nurse can also calculate tenths of a milliliter from a fraction by dividing the numerator (top number) by the denominator (bottom number) (see the section on fractions later in this chapter):

$$\frac{1 \text{ (numerator)}}{5 \text{ (denominator)}} = 5\overline{)1.0}^{\;0.2} = \frac{2}{10} \text{ or } 0.2 \text{ mL}$$
$$\underline{1.0}$$

The nurse would give <u>0.2 mL.</u>

#2. EXAMPLE: The prescription of Penicillin G (oral tablets) is for 375 mg. Tablets are supplied in 250 mg *scored* (able to be divided in half) tablets. How many tablets should be given?

SOLUTION: Set up a ratio:

250 mg is to 1 tablet as 375 mg is to X tablets
250 mg : 1 tablet :: 375 mg : X tablet

Multiply means:
375 mg × 1 tablet = 375 mg tablets
and 375 mg tablet ÷ 250 = X tablets
Therefore, 1.5 tablets = X

$$250\overline{)375.0}^{\;1.5}$$
$$\underline{250.0}$$
$$125.0$$
$$\underline{125.0}$$

The nurse would give <u>1.5 tablets (1 ½ tablets).</u>

One of the scored tablets would need to be split in half. (It is best to divide tablets only where they are scored.) Use a pill splitter whenever dividing tablets if they are scored. (Line up the score line with the blade of the splitter.) Occasionally, tablets are double-scored so they can be divided into halves *or* fourths.

#3. EXAMPLE: The prescription is 75 mg Trazodone. The medication is provided in 150 mg scored tablets. How many tablet(s) are needed?

SOLUTION: Set up a ratio:

150 mg is to 1 tablet as 75 mg is to X tablets
150 mg : 1 tablet :: 75 mg : X tablet

Multiply means:
75 mg × 1 tablet = 75 mg tablets
and 75 mg tablet ÷ 150 = X tablets
Therefore, 0.5 = X tablets

$$150\overline{)75.0}^{\;0.5}$$
$$\underline{75.0}$$

The nurse would give <u>0.5 tablet (½ tablet).</u>

Note: If the dosage for tablets does not come out exactly, the prescribed dosage *cannot* be given.

#4. EXAMPLE: A client is to receive a tube feeding at 75 mL/h. The bag contains 500 mL. How many hours will this feeding bag last?

SOLUTION: Set up a ratio:

75 mL : 1 hour :: 500 mL : X hours

Multiply means:
1 hour × 500 mL = 500 mL/h
and 500 mL/h ÷ 75m/L = Xh
Therefore, 6.66 = X = 6⅔ hours

$$75\overline{)500.00}^{\;6.66...}$$
$$\underline{450}$$
$$500$$
$$\underline{450}$$
$$500$$
$$\underline{450}$$

The bag will last <u>6 hours and 40 minutes (6⅔ hours).</u>

Fractions

A *fraction* is a portion or piece of a whole that indicates division of that whole into equal parts. Fractions can be either common fractions or decimal fractions.

Common Fractions

Common fractions, also called *simple fractions,* have a numerator (the top number) and a denominator (the bottom number). For example:

$$\frac{3 \text{ (numerator)}}{4 \text{ (denominator)}}$$

$\frac{3}{4}$ can be pictured as: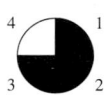

The **numerator** refers to a *part* of the whole, and is the top number (in this example, 3). The **denominator** refers to the *total number of parts,* and is the number on the bottom (in this example, 4). This example is interpreted as *3 parts out of a total of 4 parts.*

Multiplying Fractions.   To multiply fractions:

$$\frac{2}{3} \times \frac{3}{4}$$

1. Multiply the numerators to get the new numerator.

$$\frac{2}{3} \times \frac{3}{4} = \frac{6}{}$$

2. Multiply the denominators to get the new denominator.

$$\frac{2}{3} \times \frac{3}{4} \quad \frac{6}{12}$$

3. Reduce the fraction to its lowest terms. (Here, divide both numbers by their largest common divisor, 6.)

$$\frac{6}{12} = \frac{1}{2}$$

Dividing Fractions.   To divide fractions:

$$\frac{3}{4} \div \frac{2}{3}$$

1. Write the problem.

$$\frac{3}{4} \div \frac{2}{3}$$

2. Invert the divisor.

$$\frac{3}{4} \div \left(\frac{3}{2}\right)$$

3. Multiply the numerators and denominators.

$$\frac{3}{4} \times \frac{3}{2} = \frac{9}{8}$$

4. Reduce the fraction to its lowest terms.

$$\frac{9}{8} = 1\frac{1}{8}$$

Decimal Fractions

Decimal fractions are fractions in which 10 is always the denominator. The 10 is sometimes omitted when fractions are written, and a decimal point is inserted in the numerator, as many places from the right as there are ciphers (zeros) of 10 in the denominator. Therefore, $\frac{1}{10} = 0.1$ and $\frac{1}{100} = 0.01$.

$\frac{3}{4}$ can also be written as a decimal by converting it to tenths, or in this case, hundredths. 4 goes into 100 25 times and 25 times 3 is 75. Therefore, $\frac{3}{4} = \frac{75}{100}$ths or 0.75.

$$\frac{3}{4} = \frac{X}{100} \quad \overset{\text{cross-multiply}}{4X = 300} \quad X = 4\overline{)300} \quad X = 75$$

$$X = \frac{300}{4} \qquad \begin{array}{r} 75 \\ 4\overline{)300} \\ 28 \\ \overline{20} \\ 20 \\ \overline{20} \end{array}$$

In fraction, replace X with 75: $\frac{75}{100} = 0.75$

The Formula Method

When the prescribed or desired dosage is different from what is available or "what is on hand," a dosage calculation is necessary to determine the quantity of drug to give. Use ratio and proportion to solve dosage calculations. Because the calculations are in fractions, follow the rules for working with fractions (see the section on fractions earlier in this chapter).

The formula method can be used when calculating dosages in the *same system* and the *same units of measurement.* The following formula can be used to calculate the amount of medication needed:

$$\frac{\text{Desired amount}}{\text{or prescribed amount (D)}} \times \begin{array}{c} \textbf{Quantity (eg, 1 pill} \\ \text{or 1 tablet} \\ \text{or 5 mL)} = \textbf{X} \end{array}$$

$$\frac{\text{Desired amount}}{\text{Available dosage}} \times \text{Quantity} = \text{amount to give}$$

#1. EXAMPLE: The prescribed dose is $1\frac{1}{4}$ mg clonazepam (Klonopin) and the medication is supplied as $\frac{1}{2}$ mg tablets. Known factors:

- **D**esired amount: $1\frac{1}{4}$ mg (or $\frac{5}{4}$)
- **A**vailable dosage: $\frac{1}{2}$ mg
- In what **Q**uantity: 1 tablet

Set up the problem:

$$\frac{D}{A} \times Q = X \qquad \frac{\frac{5}{4}}{\frac{1}{2}} \times 1 \text{ tablet} = X$$

Use the rules for calculating fractions:

1. Write the problem.

$$\frac{\frac{5}{4}}{\frac{1}{2}} \times 1 \text{ tablet} = X$$

2. Invert the divisor.

$$\frac{5}{4} \div \left(\frac{2}{1}\right) \times 1 \text{ tablet} = X$$

3. Multiply the numerators and denominators.

$$\frac{5}{4} \times \frac{2}{1} \times 1 \text{ tablet} = X$$

$$\frac{10}{4} \times 1 \text{ tablet} = X$$

$$\frac{10}{4} \times 1 = \frac{10}{4}$$

4. Reduce the fraction to its lowest terms.

$$\frac{10}{4} \text{ tablet} = 2\frac{2}{4} = 2\frac{1}{2} \text{ tablets}$$

The nurse would give $2\frac{1}{2}$ tablets.

#2. EXAMPLE: The prescribed dose is $\frac{1}{400}$ gr of a medication. The tablets provided are $\frac{1}{200}$ gr per scored tablet. (Keep in mind that $\frac{1}{400}$ means 1 part out of 400 and $\frac{1}{200}$ means 1 part out of 200.) Known factors:

- **D**esired amount: $\frac{1}{400}$ gr
- **A**vailable dosage: $\frac{1}{200}$ gr
- In what **Q**uantity: 1 tablet

Set up the problem:

$$\frac{D}{A} \times Q = X \quad \frac{\frac{1}{400} \text{ gr}}{\frac{1}{200} \text{ gr}} \times 1 \text{ tablet} = X$$

Use the rules for calculating fractions:

1. Write the problem.

$$\frac{1}{400} \div \frac{1}{200} \times 1 \text{ tablet} = X$$

2. Invert the divisor.

$$\frac{1}{400} \div \left(\frac{200}{1}\right) \times 1 \text{ tablet} = X$$

3. Multiply the numerators and the denominators.

$$\frac{1}{400} \times \frac{200}{1} \times 1 \text{ tablet} = X$$

$$\frac{200}{400} \times 1 \text{ tablet} = X$$

$$\frac{200}{400} \times 1 = \frac{200}{400}$$

4. Reduce the fraction to its lowest terms.

$$\frac{200}{400} \text{ tablet} = \frac{1}{2} \text{ tablet}$$

The nurse would give $\frac{1}{2}$ tablet.

Because the tablets are scored, the nurse can give $\frac{1}{2}$ tablet. (Remember that some tablets cannot be split.)

☛ KEY CONCEPT

In a fraction, a larger denominator denotes that the item is divided into more pieces. Therefore, $\frac{1}{400}$ is half as much as $\frac{1}{200}$.

Significant Figures

The term **significant figure** refers to numbers that have practical meaning or dosages that can be measured. For example, a dosage prescribed is 1.325 mL. When measured with a syringe that has markings of 1.3 mL, 1.4 mL, and 1.5 mL, the last two numbers (the "25") cannot be measured. Therefore, the amount given is 1.3 mL, because this amount is closer to the prescribed dosage than 1.4 mL. (The dosage that can be measured, 1.3 mL, is the *significant figure.*) When rounding, the dosage is rounded to the closest amount. Therefore, using the example, values ranging from 1.301 to 1.349 are rounded down to 1.3, and values from 1.350 to 1.399 are rounded up to 1.4.

☛ KEY CONCEPT

In some cases, a liquid medication is ordered in a dosage that is too small to be measured accurately in a medication cup. In this situation, a syringe can be used to draw up the correct amount of medication, and then the medication can be transferred to a medication cup for administration.

Percentages

The term *percentage* refers to the number per hundred. Therefore, 20% equals 20 per hundred. Percent has no specific units of measure. It is actually a ratio. To convert from percentage to a fraction, the percent number becomes the numerator and 100 is always the denominator. Example:

$20\% = {}^{20}\!/_{100}$

Fraction to Percent. To convert a fraction to a percent, multiply both the numerator and the denominator by the number required for the denominator to equal 100. The numerator becomes the percentage.

#1. EXAMPLE:

${}^{4}\!/_{10} \times {}^{10}\!/_{10} = {}^{40}\!/_{100} = 40\%$ (multiply both sides by 10)

#2. EXAMPLE:

$$\frac{9}{20} = \frac{X}{100} \qquad \begin{array}{c} \text{cross-multiply} \\ 20\,X = 900 \\ X = \dfrac{900}{20} \end{array} \qquad X = 20\overline{)900} $$

Replace X with 45: $\dfrac{9}{20} = \dfrac{45}{100} = 45\%.$

(Alternatively, looking at the original equation, 20 goes into 100 5 times; $9 \times 5 = 45$)

Percent to Fraction. You can also determine the percentage designated by any fraction, by dividing the numerator by the denominator.

$$\frac{9}{20} \qquad 20\overline{)9.00} \qquad 0.45 = \frac{45}{100} = 45\%$$

☛ KEY CONCEPT

Use reference books or tables for any questions about dosage conversions. It is a good idea to have another nurse double-check all calculations of medication dosages.

➥ STUDENT SYNTHESIS

Key Points

- The metric system is the most commonly used measurement system in the world and is used for most measurements and dosages in medicine.
- The nurse must understand how to convert between systems of measurement in the event that a drug order is stated in a different unit of measurement than is available for administration.
- Many symbols and abbreviations are used in medication orders.
- The nurse must be proficient in the use of ratios, proportions, and fractions.
- It is vital to ask if any questions arise about a medication or a dosage.

Critical Thinking Exercises

1. A label on a cephalexin (Keflex) bottle states: "Keflex 250 mg capsules." The physician's order reads "administer 500 mg." How many capsules would be given?
2. A label reads docusate sodium (Colace) 8 oz; 150 mg/15 mL. The physician's order reads 100 mg. How many milliliters would the nurse administer?

NCLEX-Style Review Questions

1. Which system of measurement is the most widely used measurement system and is based on the decimal system?
   a. Apothecary
   b. Household
   c. Metric
   d. Pharmacology
2. The physician has ordered penicillin oral suspension 500 mg. The medication is available 0.25 grams/5mL. How much medication will you administer with each dose?
   a. 0.5 mL
   b. 1 mL
   c. 5 mL
   d. 10 mL
3. The doctor orders nitroglycerin 0.8 mg sublingual now. The medication is available 0.4 mg/tablet. How much medication will you administer with this dose?
   a. 0.5 tablet
   b. 1 tablet
   c. 1.5 tablets
   d. 2 tablets
4. The physician orders 1,000 mL of IV fluid for a client. The first hour, the client is to receive 25% of the fluid. How much should be administered the first hour?
   a. 0.25 mL
   b. 25 mL
   c. 250 mL
   d. 500 mL
5. The physician orders furosemide (Lasix) 20 mg P.O. The medication is available 40 mg/tablet. How much medication should be administered with each dose?
   a. 0.5 tablet
   b. 1 tablet
   c. 1.5 tablet
   d. 2 tablets

CHAPTER

61

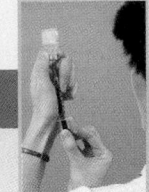

Introduction to Pharmacology

LEARNING OBJECTIVES

1. Define the terms medication and pharmacology.
2. Explain how the Controlled Substances Act regulates specific medications.
3. Describe the proper procedure for monitoring Schedule Drugs in the healthcare facility.
4. Identify the five specific rights of clients as related to prescribed medications.
5. List at least three drug references and one drug-related website that are commonly used by nurses.
6. Define what is meant by chemical, generic, official, and trade names when referring to medications.
7. List at least five different routes of medication administration.
8. Discuss at least six factors that influence the dosage of any specific medication.
9. Differentiate between prescribed and over-the-counter medications.
10. List the seven required components of a prescription.

NEW TERMINOLOGY

agonist	official name
antagonist	paradoxical
brand name	pharmacokinetics
caplet	pharmacology
capsule	potentiating
chemical name	prescription
dosage	synergistic
enteric-coated	tablet
generic name	topical
inhalant	trade name
injectable	transdermal
medication	zydis

ACRONYMS

DEA	OTC	TO
ER	PDR	USD
FDA	RPh	USP
MDI	SR	VO
NF	TD	

A **medication** is a medicinal agent that modifies body functions. *Medications,* also called *drugs,* are used to prevent disease or pregnancy, aid in the diagnosis and treatment of disease, and restore or maintain bodily functions. **Pharmacology** is the science that deals with the origin, nature, chemistry, effects, and uses of medications.

A registered pharmacist (**RPh**) is a healthcare professional who is licensed to prepare and dispense medications on the order of a licensed practitioner of medicine, such as a physician (medical doctor: Doctor of Medicine [MD] or Doctor of Osteopathy [DO]), dentist (Doctor of Dental Surgery [DDS] or Doctor of Medical Dentistry [DMD]), veterinarian (Doctor of Veterinary Medicine [DVM]), and in some states, a physician's assistant (PA) or nurse practitioner (NP) or certified nurse midwife (CNM). This chapter provides an introduction to the basics of pharmacology. It presents general information concerning medications that is important throughout a nurse's career.

The primary nursing obligation is to "do no harm" to clients, especially when administering medications. For this reason, a general knowledge of pharmacology is essential. As the healthcare delivery system continues to evolve, clients are taking more responsibility for their own needs. An important part of nursing practice is teaching clients about medications prescribed for them. Teaching should include the use, administration, actions, and possible adverse reactions or side effects of medications currently prescribed for the client.

☛ KEY CONCEPT

An important part of nursing practice is teaching clients about the effect and possible side effects of medications prescribed for them. Documentation of teaching and the client's response to instruction verifies that teaching did, in fact, take place and that the client understands his or her medication regimen.

LEGAL ASPECTS

Federal Drug Standards

The Federal Food and Drug Administration (**FDA**) operates under the enforcement of the Department of Health and Human Services. The FDA ensures that medications and therapeutic agents are safe and effective for public use. Standards of strength and purity are essential to protect the public against the dangers of impure, inferior, or misused substances. For example, in September 1997, the FDA removed Pondimin and Redux (Phen-Fen) from the market of available prescription medications. Pondimin and Redux were claimed to be "miracle drugs" for the treatment of obesity. These medications were very effective for weight loss; however, federally funded research indicated that one of three clients taking these medications developed life-threatening valvular heart disease, leading to pulmonary complications. Several documented cases of death directly resulted from the use of these drugs.

National publications that define standards for medication approval are the *United States Pharmacopeia* (**USP**) and the *National Formulary* (**NF**). These publications are fully revised every 5 years; however, supplements are published more frequently to provide updated information about medications. These two publications are used most often by pharmacists and primary care providers.

Controlled Substances

The Comprehensive Drug Abuse Prevention and Control Act, passed by Congress in May 1970, is commonly referred to as the "Controlled Substances Act." This federal law, enforced by the Drug Enforcement Agency (**DEA**), regulates the manufacture, prescription, and distribution of psychoactive medications, including narcotics, depressants, stimulants, and hallucinogens. There are five classifications, or "schedules," of controlled substances. The degree of control depends on the medication's classification, which ranges from Schedule I (has a high potential for abuse) to Schedule V (has a relatively low potential for abuse) (Box 61-1).

Protection of Controlled Substances. Controlled substances must be ordered using special forms designed to maintain an accurate inventory and dispersion record of them. In the healthcare facility, controlled substances are kept in a double-locked drawer or cabinet. The keys to the locked cabinet must be in a licensed nurse's possession at all times. Each healthcare facility incorporates the use of specialized forms for documentation of the use of controlled substances. These forms verify the client's name, medication name, dose, time of administration, and the signature of the licensed nurse who administered it. In some cases, the name of the prescribing person also is listed. Some facilities now use computer-operated dispensing units that are easily accessible with the entry of a personal identification number (PIN) assigned to the nurse.

➤➤ BOX 61-1

SCHEDULE OF CONTROLLED SUBSTANCES

Controlled substances (Schedule Drugs) are classified on the following basis:

- *Schedule I (C-I):* High potential for abuse; no accepted medical use (examples: heroin, marijuana, LSD; not kept in healthcare facilities)
- *Schedule II (C-II):* High potential for abuse; severe dependence liability (examples: narcotics, amphetamines, dronabinol, and some barbiturates)
- *Schedule III (C-III):* Lower potential for abuse than Schedule II drugs; moderate dependence liability (examples: nonbarbiturate sedatives, nonamphetamine stimulants, limited amounts of certain narcotics)
- *Schedule IV (C-IV):* Lower potential for abuse than Schedule III drugs; limited dependence liability (examples: some sedatives, antianxiety agents, nonnarcotic analgesics)
- *Schedule V (C-V):* Limited potential for abuse; primarily small amounts of narcotics (codeine) used as antitussives and antidiarrheals (usually not kept locked)

Controlled Drug Count Verification.   To ensure that controlled drugs are properly administered, an "end of the shift count" must correspond with documentation. Two nurses, one going off duty and the other coming on duty, review the documentation and count the number of remaining controlled medications. (The oncoming nurse counts; the outgoing nurse records. This assures the oncoming nurse that all the drugs are there.) The documentation must match the number of remaining medications in the controlled substances cabinet. If the count does not agree, no one is allowed to leave the unit until a search is undertaken and the discrepancy is resolved.

If narcotics are dispensed with a computerized system, a visual count usually is required at least once a day. The daily count is usually done near midnight. Documentation regarding Schedule Drugs is sent to the pharmacy every 24 hours.

The narcotic keys should be in the possession of the nurse to whom they have been assigned. The keys are not to leave the unit at any time. In the event a nurse forgets to give the narcotic keys to the oncoming nurse and takes the keys out of the healthcare facility, he or she must return the keys immediately upon realizing the error. In addition, the locks to the narcotic cabinet containing controlled medications may need to be changed and new keys assigned. As a student, it is good practice to ask the instructor or the nurse to whom the narcotic keys have been assigned to obtain the controlled medications. However, should a student use the keys to obtain medications, they must be returned to the responsible nurse immediately after use. (In most nursing programs, students are not allowed to give controlled medications without direct supervision by their instructors.)

When additional controlled drugs are brought to the nursing unit, only a licensed nurse or pharmacist is allowed to add them to the inventory. In some facilities, two nurses must perform this procedure. A record is signed by the nurse, and verified by the pharmacist, to ensure that all the medications were in fact added to the unit inventory.

Client Rights

Clients have the right to know the name, action, and possible side effects of medications administered to them. They also have the right to refuse to take medications, unless a court order gives a physician the right to administer medications without the client's consent. If clients are endangering themselves or others, medications may be given against their will. Clients also have the right to request the generic form of prescribed medications if available. (Generic forms of medications are often the least expensive.)

Drug References

Many references that provide detailed information about medications are available to healthcare professionals. These references are valuable tools for learning about the classification, use, abuse, desired actions, recommended dosage, and adverse actions of medications.

The *Physician's Desk Reference* (**PDR**) is published annually, with quarterly updates. This recognized source contains extensive information concerning therapeutic dosages,

expected therapeutic effects, possible side effects, contraindications, drug interactions, and FDA pregnancy categories (levels of danger to a fetus). The PDR contains seven color-coded sections that include the manufacturer's index, product name index, product identification section, product information section, and diagnostic product information. This reference also contains a list of poison control centers and a guide to managing overdose. The nursing units of most healthcare facilities contain a copy of the PDR. A companion handbook for nurses is available. A list of drugs removed from the *PDR Nurse's Drug Handbook* is archived on the Internet yearly at http://www.nursespdr.com.

Facts and Comparisons, another drug reference, lists medications under the following classifications: nutritional products, blood modifiers, hormones, diuretics, cardiovascular drugs, autonomic drugs, central nervous system drugs, gastrointestinal drugs, anti-infectives, and biologicals. This resource, which many pharmacies use, is updated monthly and provides the most current medication information available.

The *United States Dispensatory* (**USD**) lists the official and unofficial names of medications. *The United States Pharmacopeia* and the *National Formulary* identify the official names of medications.

Many other publications, such as the *Nursing Drug Reference* and *Handbook of Drugs for Nursing Practice,* are published annually. These publications are designed to meet the needs of nursing students and practicing licensed nurses. They incorporate nursing considerations in addition to mechanisms of action, uses, contraindications, precautions, dosages, preparations, interactions, **pharmacokinetics** (actions of drugs), side effects, and treatments of overdose. These books also emphasize client and family teaching.

In addition to the above sources, much information about medications is available at various Internet websites. Helpful Internet resources include: Rx Med (http://www.rxmed.com), Medscape (http://www.medscape.com), and PharmInfo (http://www.pharminfo.com). Consult such sources when learning about medications. Table 61-1 also lists suggested Internet sites.

Nursing Considerations

When a client is admitted to a healthcare facility, assessment should include a detailed medication history that addresses questions specifically related to allergies or previous adverse reactions to medications. This information will enable the primary care provider to decide which medications are both safe and effective for this client.

Nursing Alert
A client usually does not experience an adverse or allergic reaction on first exposure to a medication. Therefore, stay alert for adverse reactions, even if the client has received the medication previously.

Be knowledgeable about the medications to be administered. Before administering any medication, know its classification, use, recommended dosage, desired effects, possible

■■■ TABLE 61-1 *S*ELECTED INTERNET SITES RELATED TO PHARMACOLOGY AND DRUG THERAPY

Name of Site	Internet Address	Comments
Pharmacology Glossary (Boston University School of Medicine)	http://med-amsa.bu.edu/Pharmacology/Programmed/glossary.html	Information on symbols and terms used in pharmacology
Glaxo Wellcome Pharmacology Guide	http://www.glaxowellcome.co.uk/netscape/science/phguide/index.html	Quick reference guide to most of the important terms and concepts of pharmacology
PharmWeb	http://www.pharmweb.net	Links by subjects to other pharmacology-related information sites for health professionals and patients
PharmInfoNet	http://pharminfo.com	Drug information and links to publications and disease centers
"Virtual" Pharmacy Center (Martindale's Health Science)	http://www.sci.lib.uci.edu:80/-martindale/Pharmacy.html#CPT	Variety of types of information about pharmacology and pharmacy around the world
National Institutes of Health (NIH)	gopher://gopher.nlm.nih.gov:70/11/alerts	Clinical alerts from clinical trials
Drug FAQ: Frequently Asked Questions About Drugs (PharmInfo)	http://pharminfo.com/drugfaq	Information about drugs, links to related articles and resources about the drug, plus questions from patients and health professionals and the answers
U.S. National Library of Medicine	http://text.nlm.nih.gov/ftrs/gateway	Links to AHCPR guidelines; AHCPR Technology Assessments and Reviews; NIH Consensus Development Program; NIH clinical studies
Doctor's Guide to New Drugs or Indications	http://www.pslgroup.com/NEWDRUGS.HTM	Information about new drugs or new indications in United States and worldwide
Drug InfoNet	http://www.druginfonet.com	Information about drugs, diseases; questions to experts; links to other sites; names, addresses, and phone numbers of many pharmaceutical manufacturers
Farmaweb	http://www.farmaweb.com	Information about drugs in Spanish and English
Pharmacokinetics	http://jeffline.tju.edu/CWIS/OAC/pharmacology/pharm-guide/menu.html	Learning module on pharmacokinetics from Thomas Jefferson University
Center Watch	http://www.centerwatch.com	Information about clinical trials in United States and worldwide; also has information about newly approved drugs
Health A to Z—Pharmaceuticals and Drugs	http://www.healthatoz.com/categories/PC.html	Information and links related to drug therapy
Antibiotic Use Guidelines (University of Wisconsin)	http://www.biostat.wisc.edu/clinsci/amcg/amcg.html	Data on antibiotics by drug name, drug class, organism; empiric therapy by site; and antimicrobial treatment of HIV-infected patient
Food and Drug Administration	http://www.fda.gov	Access to information related to drugs and regulation of drugs

Eisenhauer, L., Nichols, L., Spencer, R., & Bergan, F. (1998). *Clinical pharmacology and nursing management* (5th ed.). Philadelphia: Lippincott Williams & Wilkins.

adverse or untoward effects, and route of administration. Confirm that the client has not had a previous adverse or allergic reaction to a medication before administering it. Failure to determine previous untoward effects the client has experienced is not safe nursing practice. This negligence may jeopardize the client's well-being, and possibly, may even be fatal (Fig. 61-1).

☞ KEY CONCEPT

Nurses are obligated to know the classification, use, recommended dosage, desired effects, possible adverse or untoward effects, and route of administration of any medication administered. Should a client experience an adverse reaction

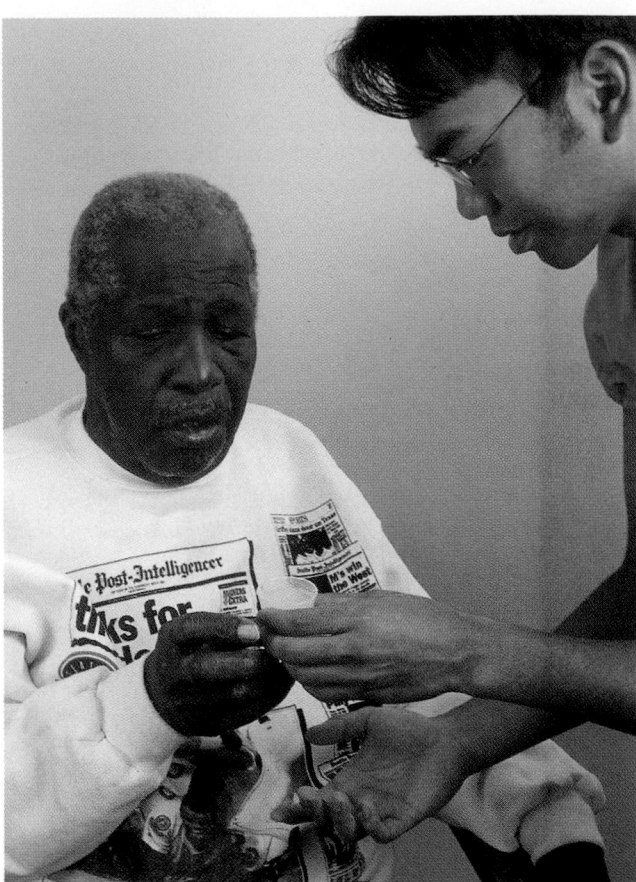

FIGURE 61-1. A nursing student or licensed nurse is responsible for knowing vital information about medications the client is receiving.

that the nurse does not recognize (and thus fails to institute the appropriate action for), a medication error has been committed, just as if the wrong medication had been given.

MEDICATION PREPARATIONS AND ACTIONS

Medications are available in many different forms. The *route of administration* refers to the form of preparation by which the medication is administered. Examples of forms or preparations include *oral* (administered by mouth), **topical** (applied to the skin or mucous membranes), **inhalant** (inhaled or breathed in), **injectable** (given via a needle), and **transdermal** (applied to and absorbed through the skin). Chapter 63 discusses routes of administration in more detail. Some of the different forms are presented later in this chapter.

Medication Names

The number of medications available, as well as the variety of names often given to the same medication, can be confusing. Medications are named in four different categories: chemical, generic, official, and trade or brand name. The **chemical name** describes the medication's chemical composition. The **generic name** is often similar to the chemical name and is

assigned by the medication's first manufacturer. Often, the generic name is simpler than the chemical name and may be used in any country by any manufacturer. The **official name** is the name identified in the *USP* or *NF*. The **trade name** or **brand name** is the copyrighted name assigned by the company making the medication and is followed by the symbol ®. If more than one company makes the same medication, it will have the same generic name, but may have several different trade names. For this reason, many physicians order medications using only the generic name. Box 61-2 gives examples of various names for one medication.

Many medication labels and inserts list both the generic and trade names. Should the physician use one form of the name and the label states another, verify the names to make sure that the correct medication will be given. If unsure of the medication's name, refer to one of the previously listed drug references before administering the medication to the client. These reference books commonly list generic and one or more trade names for most medications.

Medication Actions

A medication that produces a desired response is called an **agonist.** A medication that has an opposing effect, or acts against another medication, is called an **antagonist.** A medication that enhances the effects of another medication has a **synergistic** or **potentiating** effect. (The actions of the synergistic medications taken together are greater than if either medication was taken separately.) The effect of synergistic medications is very important. Smaller doses of each medication should be used, because their combined effects are multiplied.

Adverse Responses to Medications

Be aware not only of the desired actions of various medications, but also of undesired reactions. The nurse must stay alert constantly for adverse reactions and side effects in the client, so that the appropriate actions can be taken.

Side effects are *secondary effects* (other than the desired effect produced by a medication). Side effects are actually considered *adverse reactions.* Sometimes, side effects can be positive or helpful. In discussions with healthcare workers, adverse effects are considered to be those effects that are undesirable, disabling, or life-threatening. However, in drug

➤➤ BOX 61-2

MEDICATION NAMES

The following is an example of the different names used for one medication.

- *Chemical name:* 2-(4-isobutylphenyl) propinoic acid
- *Generic name:* Ibuprofen
- *Official name:* Ibuprofen
- *Brand names:* Motrin, Actiprofen (available in Canada), Advil, Nuprin, Genpril, Haltran, Midol

reference books, all secondary or side effects are listed as adverse effects.

Consider the following example, diphenhydramine (Benadryl):

- *Desired effect:* Antihistamine; relief of itching and allergy symptoms
- *Negative but usually not life-threatening side effects:* Dry mouth, hypotension
- *Positive, helpful side effects:* Cough suppression, relief of motion sickness
- *Mixed side effects:* Sedation that could lead to problems with driving or operating machinery; also helpful as a sleep aid or sedative
- *Life-threatening adverse effects:* Anaphylaxis

Interactions With Herbal Supplements and Homeopathic Remedies

It is important to ask clients if they take supplements of herbs or homeopathic remedies. Record in the clinical record the type and amount of herb or remedy taken and call it to the attention of the primary care provider.

> **Nursing Alert**
>
> If clients take supplements of herbs or homeopathic remedies, the primary care provider may not be aware of this. Herbs and homeopathic remedies may have potential drug interactions with a prescribed medication. The supplement may potentially increase or decrease the desired effect of the medication or treatment. Combinations may also produce life-threatening adverse effects. (See Chapter 56 for a listing of herbal supplements that can contribute to postoperative bleeding.)

Medication Forms

A medication's form, properties, and desired effects determine its method of administration. Medications are available in several forms. These forms include liquids, solids, semisolids, metered-dose inhalants, and transdermal medications. Many medications are available in more than one form for different administration routes. For example, promethazine (Phenergan), an antiemetic, is available in rectal suppository, liquid (syrup), and injectable forms.

Liquids

Liquids are administered orally, *parenterally* (by some means other than the GI tract), or topically. *Oral administration* is used most often for pediatric, psychiatric, and geriatric clients. Oral liquid medications are given to ensure medication compliance, as well as to assist a client who has difficulty swallowing a tablet. Some liquid medications are mixed with juice to mask the taste. A *syrup* is a liquid that contains a sweetener, usually sugar.

Some liquids are designed to be held under the tongue and absorbed through the oral mucosa. (Homeopathic remedies are often given in this way.) Other liquids are designed to be gargled or swished in the mouth and then spit out; for example, "swish and spit" (Magic Mouthwash).

Liquids for topical use include *instillations* (as into the eye) and *irrigations* (as in flushing out a wound). A *tincture* is a form of a liquid medication that contains alcohol.

Solids

Solid medications are often given by mouth. Oral medications may be in the form of pills, tablets, capsules, caplets, or chewing gum. Typically, tablets can be chewed or swallowed. Some solid forms are designed to be placed under the tongue (*sublingual*) and absorbed via the oral mucosa. Nitroglycerin is an example. Capsules may contain medications that are absorbed slowly or rapidly.

Technically, a *pill* is absolutely round. However, tablets, capsules, and caplets are commonly referred to as "pills," even though they are of different compositions and shapes. A **tablet** is a compressed, spherical form of a medication; tablets may be **enteric-coated** (the coating does not dissolve until the tablet reaches the intestine, because the medication can irritate the stomach mucosa), or they may be plain. A **capsule** is a medication in powdered or pellet form enclosed in soluble, cylindrical, gelatin-like material. The capsule may be used to delay the medication's absorption over time, or because the medication has a disagreeable taste. The capsule's covering also makes swallowing easier than using a tablet, which may dissolve in the client's mouth if he or she does not swallow it quickly. A **caplet** is a tablet in the shape of a capsule. The shape makes it easier for the client to swallow. Medications in the forms of tablets, capsules, or caplets may be made to release over time (*slow-release* [**SR**] or extended release [**ER**]) or to release all at one time.

A new form of solid medication is the **zydis** tablet. This tablet is placed on the client's tongue and dissolves instantly, thus ensuring medication compliance. The client touches the tongue to the tablet to remove if from the wrapper. Warn the client not to touch the tablet with the fingers, or it may melt prematurely. Be sure to leave this tablet in its sealed bubble package until it is ready to be administered.

> **Nursing Alert**
>
> Many tablets and pills can be crushed for easier swallowing or to make sure the client takes them. However, not all medications can be crushed safely. Capsules, time-released medications, and enteric-coated tablets should not be crushed or split. Many facilities require a physician's order to crush any medication.

A *powder* is another type of solid. Powders are most often mixed with liquids for oral administration. They may also be applied topically, inhaled, or combined with a sterile diluent for injection.

Chewing gum is used as a medium for delivery of some oral medications. Examples include aspirin (Aspergum) and nicotine (Nicorette gum)—which is used to deliver fixed doses of nicotine for smoking cessation.

Semisolids

Semisolid medications are usually given by the rectal, vaginal, or urethral routes or are administered topically. They are designed to melt at body temperature and are absorbed through mucosa. A suppository is an example of a medication in semisolid form. Suppositories usually are kept refrigerated to maintain their shape. Other semisolid drugs include ointments and pastes.

Inhalers

Oral or nasal *inhalers* deliver medications topically to the area of desired effect (eg, lung or nasal mucosa). Inhalers are metered (metered dose inhaler [**MDI**]) and deliver a measured amount of medication with each inhalation. The advantage of this type of delivery is the reduction of systemic effects on the body, such as rapid heart rate or other uncomfortable side effects. These considerations are especially important when using steroids or sympathomimetics.

Transdermal Medications

Transdermal (**TD**) *medications* are those designed to be absorbed through the skin ("trans" = through; "dermal" = skin) into the body. In this delivery system, the medication is incorporated into a resin and prepared in the form of a patch or paste. The patch is placed on the body, where the skin absorbs the substance in controlled amounts over time. Because transdermal medications bypass the gastrointestinal system, medications that the gastrointestinal system would normally destroy can be given effectively through this route. In most cases, transdermal medications require smaller doses than oral medications to achieve the same desired effects. Examples include fentanyl (Duragesic, Sublimaze), nicotine patches (Habitrol, Nicoderm), nitroglycerin patches (Trans-derm Nitro), and estrogen patches (Estraderm).

Injectable Medications

Injectable medications are given by needle or catheter into a blood vessel. Injectable medications may be given within the layers of the skin (*intradermal*), under the skin into the subcutaneous tissue layer (*subcutaneous*), into the muscle tissue (*intramuscular* [IM]), into the blood vessels (*intravenous* [IV] or *intraarterial* [IA]), or into the area surrounding the spinal cord (*intrathecal*). The latter is a highly invasive method, and is used only when absolutely necessary.

PRESCRIPTION OF MEDICATIONS

A *dose* is a single amount of a medication administered to achieve a therapeutic effect (eg, 250 mg penicillin). A **dosage** contains the dose *and* scheduled times (eg, 750 mg/d in 3 doses, administered at equal intervals). A *therapeutic dose* is the amount of medication required to obtain a desired effect in the majority of clients. (A blood sample may be obtained from a client to determine his or her *blood level* of a drug. This helps to establish the therapeutic dose for a particular client.) The *minimal dose* is the smallest amount of drug necessary to achieve a therapeutic effect. A *loading dose* (larger than the usual continuing dose) may be given as the first dose of a newly prescribed medication to establish a minimum blood level. A *maximal dose* is the largest amount that can be given safely without causing an adverse reaction or toxic effect. A *toxic dose* is the amount of medication that causes symptoms of poisoning or toxicity. A *lethal dose* is the amount of medication that will cause death. These doses may vary from individual to individual.

Factors Affecting Medication Prescription

When healthcare professionals prescribe medications, numerous factors must be considered. These factors are discussed in the following sections.

Age

Children cannot tolerate the same amount of medication as adults because of their smaller size and different metabolism. Older adults also may be unable to tolerate normal adult dosages of medications, because of the effects of the aging process on liver and kidney function, which may lead to incomplete metabolism of some medications. Incomplete medication metabolism can cause the drug to accumulate in the body, or can cause the drug to be excreted without being absorbed. Either situation can result in serious adverse reactions. In addition, older adults, as well as children, may exhibit **paradoxical** responses to medications—the opposite of the desired response.

Gender

Some medications are more soluble in fat; others are more soluble in water. Because women usually have more body fat and tend to be smaller in size, and men have more body fluid, effects of medications differ across genders. (Women usually require smaller doses than men.) Additionally, many medications and herbal supplements cross the placental barrier and can harm the fetus in a pregnant woman. For this reason, pregnant women should avoid all medications without a maternal–child healthcare provider's knowledge and specific consent. Breast milk absorbs some medications in lactating women, which could harm breastfeeding babies. Lactating women should consult their healthcare provider before taking any medications, including over-the-counter and herbal preparations.

Weight

Dosage is often prescribed in relation to a client's weight (this is especially true for children). Heavier clients may require larger dosages than thinner clients to reach therapeutic levels. Body weight is usually expressed in grams or kilograms for dosage calculations.

Client's Condition

A disease's nature and severity may influence the prescribed dosage of a medication. For example, the person in severe pain often will require a higher level of pain-relieving medication than the person experiencing less pain.

Disposition and Psychological State

The client's personality and culture may affect the amount of medication he or she needs. For example, a client with a relatively high pain threshold will require less pain medication than the client with a very low pain threshold. A highly agitated individual may require a larger dose of a sedative than the person who is experiencing less anxiety. A client's cultural values and ethnic background may also affect the client's willingness to take medications. (See Chapter 8 for a more detailed discussion of the cultural aspects of healthcare.)

Method of Administration

Administration route affects the amount of time for the medication to enter the general circulation and become effective. IV and IM injections act more rapidly than oral medications. Rectally administered and transdermally applied medications often are absorbed more slowly than those administered by injection.

Distribution

The body distributes some medications evenly to reach all cells; other medications reach only certain body fluids or tissues. For example: nitroglycerin targets vascular smooth muscles; acetaminophen (Tylenol) reduces fever by acting on the heat-regulating center in the hypothalamus; acyclovir (Zovirax) inhibits the DNA replication of viruses and is used to help manage HIV infections; and simvastatin (Zocor) inhibits a specific enzyme involved in cholesterol synthesis. On the other hand, penicillin kills bacteria throughout the body.

Environmental Factors

Temperature may influence a medication's speed of absorption. For example, heat causes vasodilation and therefore faster absorption, whereas cold causes vasoconstriction and decreases absorption. This might be a factor in administering IM medications.

Some medications are damaged by exposure to light and thus must be stored in dark bottles or opaque containers. Some medications require refrigeration to maintain their effectiveness. Certain liquid medications, when mixed in a syringe or cup, must be given immediately to prevent deterioration due to exposure to room air. Some liquid medications cannot ever be mixed, because they destroy or interact with each other.

Time of Administration

Time is an important factor. For example, the body will absorb a medication taken with meals more slowly than if taken on an empty stomach. A diuretic is best taken in the morning, so frequent voiding does not disrupt the client's sleep. Medications with sedative effects or side effects are usually given in the evening or late afternoon. Certain insulins must be given before meals, while others are administered with meals. (The goal is to provide insulin close to the same time as carbohydrates enter the bloodstream.) A new insulin, Lantus (Glargine), is given in the evening

Elimination

The body eliminates medications through urine, feces, breath, and perspiration. Some medications leave the body in their original forms; others are made inactive by chemical changes in their structure. If these processes are slow, a medication's effects may be prolonged. Medication that leaves the body too quickly may be excreted before it has a therapeutic effect. If the body cannot eliminate the medication because of kidney or liver dysfunction, toxic levels may accumulate in the blood. Chemical changes also may form substances that are harmful to the body if it is unable to dispose of them rapidly enough. Excess fluid intake can flush medications out of the body before they can take effect.

Prescriptions

A **prescription** (medication order) is a written formula for preparing and giving a medication. As stated previously, only certain healthcare providers are licensed to write prescriptions. Federal law requires a prescription for any medication that is considered unsafe for general use without a physician's supervision. (Medications that can be purchased without a prescription are called over-the-counter [**OTC**] drugs.) Many prescriptions cannot be refilled without a physician's written or telephoned authorization. Prescriptions cannot be refilled more than 1 year after the date they were originally written. Some prescriptions, such as those for narcotics, must be rewritten more frequently. Nurses may only give medications on direct orders from one of the healthcare professionals listed at the beginning of this chapter.

A *pharmacist* is the only person qualified and licensed to prepare medications following the directions contained in the prescription. In the healthcare facility, the prescription—written on the physician's order sheet contained in the client's chart, or entered into the computer by the physician—is sent to the hospital pharmacy for preparation. The orders contain a start time and date. The medication is to be given for the specified period stated in the order, or until the order changes or is discontinued. Table 61-2 lists the parts of a prescription. Nurses need to be aware of medical terminology, symbols, and abbreviations used in prescriptions (see Chap. 37 and Appendix B).

Verbal Orders

In emergencies, physicians and other primary care providers may give verbal medication orders, either directly or by telephone. Most acute care facilities allow only registered nurses to accept verbal orders; however, practical/vocational nurses in extended-care facilities usually are allowed to take them as well. Most facilities require that primary care providers sign their verbal orders within 12 to 24 hours.

As a new graduate, if permitted to take a verbal order, be sure to write it in the proper place and note that the order was verbal (**VO**) or by telephone (**TO**). Make sure that the order is co-signed as soon as possible. Documentation provides a permanent record of events for reference and protection of

■■ TABLE 61-2 *𝒫*arts of a Prescription

Part	Purpose
Client's full name	Avoids confusion with another client with the same surname; in some facilities, the client's room number or medical record number may be included.
Date and time of day	Tells when order is to be started; may tell when order is to be discontinued; prescription must be rewritten if medication is to be continued after discharge date.
Name of drug	States the exact name (generic name preferred to trade name); sometimes both are used.
Dosage/amount of drug	States measurement system used by healthcare facility; may also be expressed as number of capsules or tablets or as fluid volume.
Time/frequency of dose	Aids in determining the schedule for administration; nursing service usually determines medication routine schedules, such as the hours for medications ordered 4 times per day or those ordered every 6 hours; the prescribing healthcare provider may give less-definite directions. (However, the nurse needs to know that certain medications must be given before meals, whereas others must be given with or after meals for maximum effect. It is important to differentiate between a medication to be given every 6 hours and one that is to be given 4 times a day.)
Method/route	Determines the route by which the medication is to be given (such as PO, IM). In most situations, giving a medication via the wrong route could be dangerous, possibly even fatal. For example, administration of an IM medication given IV could increase the dose received by the client.
Primary healthcare provider's signature	Identifies the prescribing individual; essential for legal reasons or if some question exists about the order. An unsigned order may mean that the person has not finished writing it, or that it was not written by an authorized person.

healthcare personnel. *Nursing students should not take verbal or telephone orders at any time.*

Clarification of Orders

Nurses are responsible for carrying out orders as given: the nurse cannot make any changes. If there is any reason to question an order, or if it is confusing, clarify it with the healthcare provider who has ordered the medication. (In some cases, the nurse manager, charge nurse, team leader, or supervisor may be able to clarify the order.) If an order is clarified by phone, it is written as a "clarification" under the order in question, dated, and signed by the nurse as a TO. The primary care provider who was consulted is also identified. This clarification is treated as a verbal or telephone order, and must be co-signed by the ordering healthcare provider within 12 to 24 hours.

☛ Key Concept

All medication and other orders must be clear, understandable, and open to only one interpretation before the nurse takes any action. The safe administration of medications is one of the nurse's most important responsibilities.

➢ **STUDENT SYNTHESIS**

Key Points

- Medications are substances that modify body functions. They are used to prevent disease or pregnancy, to aid in diagnosis and treatment of disease, or to restore and maintain bodily functions.
- Many laws, rules, and regulations concern the prescription, storage, and administration of medications.
- Clients have the right to know what medications they are receiving and to request available generic forms of medications. They may refuse to take medications, unless a court order exists to the contrary.
- Medication administration is a nursing task that must be taken very seriously to prevent harm to clients.
- Nurses are required to know how and where to obtain information concerning medications. Several drug references and computer websites are common sources of information.
- Drugs are available in many forms, for example, liquids, solids, semisolids, and transdermal patches.

- Factors that affect medication dosages include the client's age, gender, weight, condition, and psychological state.
- Many medications are considered unsafe for use without a healthcare provider's supervision, and thus require a specific prescription. OTC medications can be purchased by the consumer without a prescription.
- Medication orders must be carried out exactly as written. If any questions arise, the prescribing healthcare provider must be consulted for clarification. No medication can be given legally without a valid and clear order.

Critical Thinking Exercises

1. You are working as a licensed nurse in the healthcare facility. On the way home from work, you realize that you have forgotten to turn over the keys to the medication cabinet. What do you do next? What steps would you take to make sure that you always remember to submit the keys at the end of your shift?
2. An older adult is experiencing what appear to be toxic effects of a medication. Discuss the factors that could be contributing to this finding.

NCLEX-Style Review Questions

1. You are preparing to give a client his medications. He is alert, oriented, and sitting up in bed. The client states that he is allergic to one of the medications you are planning to give. What action should you take?
   a. Ask a family member if the client is allergic to the medication.
   b. Give the client his medication.
   c. Give the medication later in the shift.
   d. Notify the charge nurse and do not give the medication.

2. A controlled substance that is medically accepted and has a high potential for abuse as well as severe dependence is which category of Schedule substances?
   a. I
   b. II
   c. III
   d. IV
3. Which of the following would the client have a right to request as a less expensive alternative to a prescription medication?
   a. Advil
   b. Genpril
   c. Ibuprofen
   d. Motrin
4. Which route of medication would have the most rapid onset?
   a. Intravenous
   b. Oral caplet
   c. Oral tablet
   d. Rectal
5. The nurse is preparing to give medications to a client and is unfamiliar with a medication. The most appropriate action would be:
   a. Administer the medication now, as ordered.
   b. Ask another nurse about the medication before giving the medication.
   c. Ask the client if this medication is taken regularly by him or her.
   d. Hold the medication until you look it up in a reference resource book.

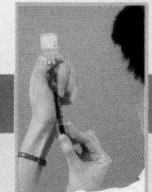

CHAPTER

62

Classification of Medications

LEARNING OBJECTIVES

1. Describe the following classifications of medications including the actions, possible side effects, adverse reactions, nursing considerations, and five examples of each: antibiotics, analgesics and narcotics, hypnotics and sedatives, anticonvulsants, steroids, cardiotonics (give one example), antihypertensives, and diuretics.
2. Describe client and family teaching concerning proper administration of prescribed medications.
3. Discuss the implications associated with drug-resistant bacteria.
4. Discuss the major side effects of prolonged steroid therapy.
5. Describe the most common side effects of narcotics, hypnotics, and sedatives.
6. Demonstrate the ability to accurately research information about medications.

NEW TERMINOLOGY

analgesic	diuretic
antiarrhythmic	emetic
antibiotic	expectorant
anticonvulsant	hypnotic
antihypertensive	insulin
antineoplastic	narrow spectrum
antitussive	nephrotoxicity
bactericidal	opiate
bacteriostatic	ototoxicity
broad spectrum	photosensitivity
bronchodilator	sedative
catecholamine	septicemia
cathartic	steroid
cross-sensitivity	vasoconstrictor
depressant	vasodilator

ACRONYMS

ACE	LASIK	PE
ASA	MOM	PIH
DDAVP	MRSA	PPF
DVT	MS	PT
HCTZ	NSAID	PTT
HRT	NTG	SA
HTN	PCN	TCN
INR		

With the thousands of medications available today, remembering the action and particulars of every available medication would be impossible. Without a system of *classification*, a drug reference would need to be constantly consulted. Quite simply, classification of medications is similar to a filing system, in which medications are filed according to their actions and the body systems affected. Medications are available that specifically affect each body system. Medications with similar actions on a body system can be grouped together. For example, bronchodilators affect the bronchioles, which are part of the respiratory system. Antihypertensive medications lower blood pressure by several different mechanisms.

Accordingly, medications that share common actions may also share common adverse effects (**cross-sensitivity**) (see Chap. 61). Becoming familiar with the classifications of medications helps in recognizing the possible adverse effects that clients may experience, providing a basis for implementing appropriate nursing actions should any undesirable effects occur.

Nursing Alert
Severe, total-body life-threatening adverse reactions are *anaphylactic* reactions and may result from the administration of any drug. Although these reactions are rare, death can result if proper treatment is not instituted immediately.

Classification of medications is also helpful for implementing appropriate nursing actions *before* administering medication to a client. Proper assessment and followup can prevent possible overdose or other adverse reactions that could be life threatening. For example, if an antihypertensive agent is being administered, the nurse would know to check the client's blood pressure before giving the medication. Another example would be to check the current potassium level of a client who is receiving potassium-replacement therapy.

Most drugs are considered to be dangerous to a developing fetus if taken during pregnancy. Drug reference books typically identify a pregnancy category for each medication. Box 62-1 defines these categories.

☛ KEY CONCEPT

A person can be allergic to any medication at any time. Always watch for signs of allergic reaction, including anaphylactic, life-threatening reactions. Also, determine if the client is taking any over-the-counter medications or herbal supplements. Many of these, in combination with prescribed drugs, can cause serious effects.

This chapter is presented as an introduction to the major classifications of medications and their actions. Addressing each and every medication that affects the body systems is impossible in a text of this length; however, some of the most commonly prescribed medications, their classifications, actions, dosages, routes of administration, side effects, adverse effects, and nursing considerations are presented. Tables within

>> BOX 62-1

FOOD AND DRUG ADMINISTRATION (FDA) PREGNANCY CATEGORIES

The FDA has established categories indicating the potential of drugs to cause birth defects. The risks are weighed against the benefits. However, no drugs should be taken during pregnancy unless absolutely necessary, and then only under the direction of the woman's healthcare provider.

The FDA has identified the following pregnancy categories:

- Category A: Adequate studies have not demonstrated a risk to the fetus.
- Category B: Adverse effects in animals have not occurred, and no adequate studies in humans have been done; or adverse effects have occurred in animals, but studies have not shown a risk in humans.
- Category C: Adverse effects have occurred in animals, and no adequate studies in humans have been done; or no animal studies or adequate studies in humans have been done. The benefits to pregnant women may be acceptable despite the risks.
- Category D: There is evidence of human fetal risk; however, potential benefits to the pregnant woman may offset the risks.
- Category X: Studies and reports demonstrate fetal risk; risks outweigh the possible benefits of use by pregnant women.

Adapted from Karch, A. (2002). *Lippincott's nursing drug guide.* (p. 1,351). Philadelphia: Lippincott Williams & Wilkins.

this chapter are available for quick reference and convenience. Some drug reference books also contain photo guides to assist in recognition of pills and capsules (Fig. 62-1).

Nursing Alert
The dosages in this book are based on the current recommendations at the time of publication. The dosages given in all tables in this book are based on the usual adult (ages 20–60) dose. Variations may occur, based on each physician's judgment. Smaller doses are usually prescribed for children and sometimes for older people. *If in doubt about the dose of any medication, look it up!*

Major drug classifications introduced in this chapter include anti-infective agents, and medications that affect the integumentary, nervous, endocrine, sensory, cardiovascular, respiratory, gastrointestinal, and urinary systems. Other books may classify drugs in terms of their specific actions, regardless of the systems affected.

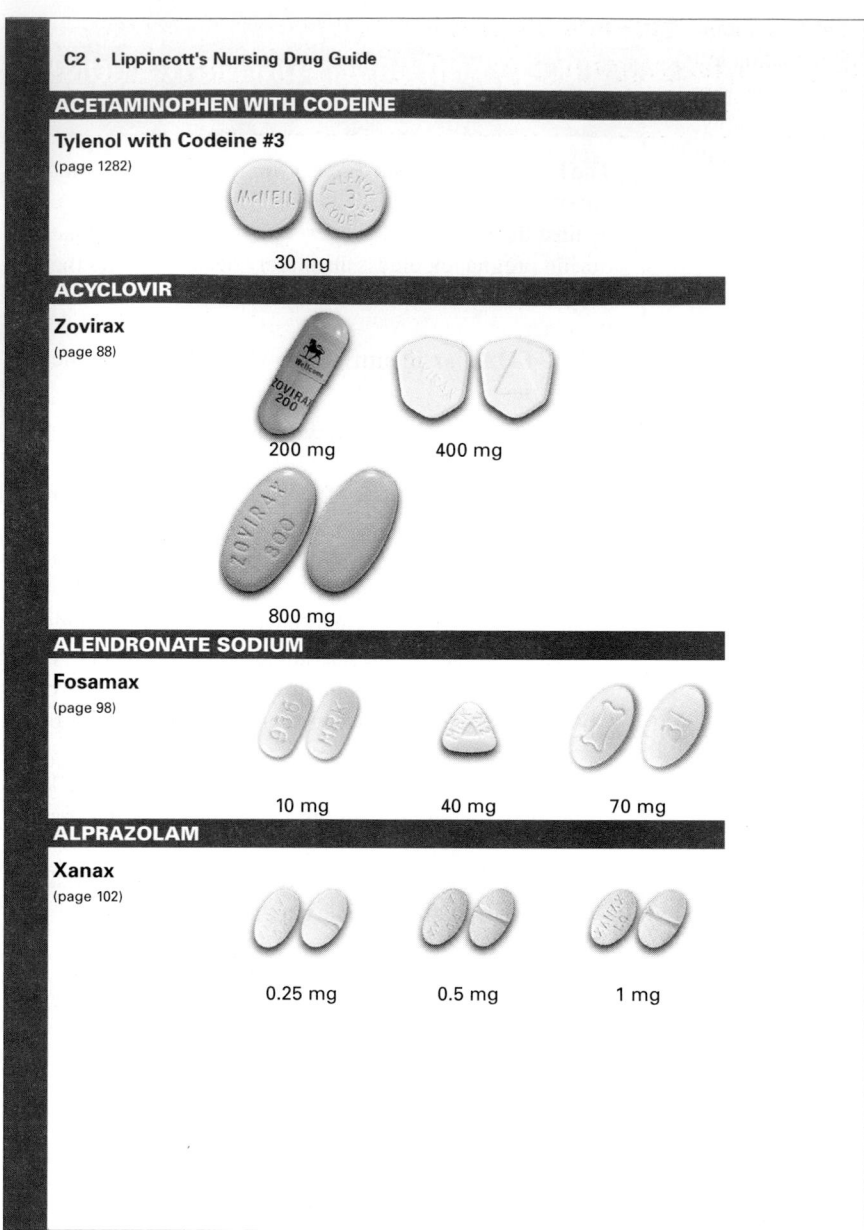

C2 · Lippincott's Nursing Drug Guide

ACETAMINOPHEN WITH CODEINE

Tylenol with Codeine #3
(page 1282)

30 mg

ACYCLOVIR

Zovirax
(page 88)

200 mg   400 mg

800 mg

ALENDRONATE SODIUM

Fosamax
(page 98)

10 mg   40 mg   70 mg

ALPRAZOLAM

Xanax
(page 102)

0.25 mg   0.5 mg   1 mg

FIGURE 62-1. Photo guides are available to assist in recognition of pills and capsules. This portion of a photo guide is found in a reference book. The drugs are labeled with their generic and trade names, as well as strength.

ANTIBIOTICS AND OTHER ANTI-INFECTIVE AGENTS

An anti-infective agent is a medication used to treat an infection. An **antibiotic,** which is one type of anti-infective, is a chemical compound used specifically to treat bacterial infections. It is a product of living cells formed naturally by other living cells (eg, bacteria, yeasts, or molds) or produced semi-synthetically in a laboratory.

Although living cells produce antibiotics, the term "antibiotic" may also be used to mean any medication that acts as an antimicrobial agent. Antibiotics are classified as **broad spectrum** if they are effective against many organisms and **narrow spectrum** or *specific* if they are effective against only a few microorganisms. Antibiotics that retard the growth of bacteria are called **bacteriostatic** agents; those that kill bacteria are referred to as **bactericidal** agents. Table 62-1 lists common anti-infective medications.

☛ Key Concept

Many antibiotics function by reducing the virulence *(strength) of a pathogenic organism* (bacteriostatic). *The body's natural defenses must then take over, to actually kill the pathogen.*

Effectiveness

Several factors must be considered for an antibiotic to be effective. An antibiotic must be soluble in water and diffuse readily into body tissue. It should not cause an adverse or allergic reaction, nor should it affect the normal *flora* (normal and useful bacteria) that usually reside in the human body. Furthermore, if given orally, it should be well absorbed by the gastrointestinal (GI) tract. Finally, it should not be antagonistic to other antibiotics.

(*text continues on page 827*)

■■■ TABLE 62-1 𝒮ELECTED ANTI-INFECTIVE MEDICATIONS

Name of Medication*	Usual Adult Dose	Notes
Penicillins		
amoxicillin (Amoxil, Trimox, Wymox)	Oral only: 250–500 mg q8h	Extended spectrum
ampicillin (Omnipen, Totacillin, Unasyn, Principen)	Oral, IM, IV: 250–500 mg to 1 g q6h	Effective against several strains of bacteria; used as initial therapy for meningitis until results of cultures are completed Polycillin, Principen used for gonorrhea
cloxacillin (Cloxapen, Tegopen)	Oral only: 250–500 mg q6h	Antistaphylococcus activity
dicloxacillin (Dycill, Dynapen, Pathocil)	Oral only: 250–500 mg q6h	Best absorbed of the oral antistaphylococcus drugs
nafcillin (Unipen)	Oral: 250–500 mg q4–6h Oral, IM, IV: 500 mg to 1 g q4–6h	Treatment of penicillin-resistant organisms, especially staphylococcus
oxacillin (Bactocill)	Oral: 500 mg q4–6h By injection: 250 mg q4–6h	Treatment of penicillin-resistant organisms, especially staphylococcus
penicillin G, aqueous	Oral, IM, IV: 5 million to 20 million U/d, in divided doses	Oral form used for mild-to-moderate infections with penicillin-sensitive organisms; parenteral route used for severe infections
penicillin G procaine, aqueous (APPG, Crysticillin, Wycillin)	IM only: 600,000–4,800,000 U/d, in divided doses	Long acting; moderate to severe infections
penicillin V (penicillin V potassium) (Pen-Vee K)	Oral only: 250–500 mg q6h	Mild to moderate bacterial infections; prophylaxis
piperacillin (Pipracil)	IM, IV: 3–4 g q4–6h (max 24 g/d)	Extended spectrum; antipseudomonas activity; mixed infections
ticarcillin (Ticar)	Parenteral only: 2–4 g q4–6h	Antipseudomonas activity; bacterial septicemia
Cephalosporins		
cefadroxil (Duricef, Ultracef)	Oral: 1–2 g q d, in single or divided doses	First-generation cephalosporin used for: skin infections; tonsillitis caused by β-hemolytic streptococcus (can cause renal impairment)
cefazolin (Kefzol, Zolicef)	IM, IV: 250–500 mg to 1 g q6–8h (dose up to 12 g used in life-threatening infection)	First-generation cephalosporin; extended duration of action; used to treat wide range of infection including septicemia
cefdinir (Omnicef)	PO: 300 mg q12h for 10 d	Specific diseases caused by *Haemophilus influenzae* and some staphylococcus organisms
cefepime (Maxipime)	IM, IV: 0.5 to 2 g q12h	Third-generation cephalosporin; possibly nephrotoxic;† may potentiate anticoagulants
cefoperazone (Cefobid)	IM, IV: 1–2 g ql2h	Third-generation cephalosporin; extended duration; antipseudomonas activity (may cause liver or kidney side effects)
cefotaxime (Claforan)	IM, IV: 500 mg–2 g q6–8h	Third-generation cephalosporin; extended spectrum
cefotetan (Cefotan)	IM, IV: 1–4 g/d in divided doses for 5–10 d	Third-generation cephalosporin; bactericidal, wide range; may cause bone marrow depression

(continued)

■■■ **TABLE 62-1** *S*ᴇʟᴇᴄᴛᴇᴅ Aɴᴛɪ-ɪɴғᴇᴄᴛɪᴠᴇ Mᴇᴅɪᴄᴀᴛɪᴏɴs (ᴄᴏɴᴛɪɴᴜᴇᴅ)

Name of Medication*	Usual Adult Dose	Notes
cefoxitin (Mefoxin)	IM, IV: 1–2 g q6–8h	Second-generation cephalosporin; better gram-negative and anaerobic activity
cefprozil (Cefzil)	Oral: 250–500 mg q12h × 10 d (children's dose based on weight)	Second-generation cephalosporin; children's suspension (bubble-gum flavored); used for otitis media, acute sinusitis
cefuroxime axetil (Ceftin); cefuroxime sodium (Kefurox, Zinacef)	Oral: 250–500 mg q12h Uncomplicated UTI: 125–250 mg b.i.d. IM, IV: 750 mg to 1.5 g q8h	Second-generation cephalosporin Used for tonsilitis, uncomplicated UTI, otitis media, sinusitis Preoperative preparation; broad spectrum
cephalexin (Biocef, Keflex)	Oral: 250–500 mg q6h	First-generation cephalosporin Skin infections; otitis media in children
Tetracyclines		
doxycycline (Doryx, Doxy-Caps, Doxychel, Vibramycin, Vibra-Tabs)	Oral: 100–300 mg/d IV: 100–200 mg/d	Oral and IV forms available; long duration of action; can cause photosensitivity Used to treat infections (e.g., some STDs, traveler's diarrhea) and as malaria prophylaxis
minocycline (Minocin)	Oral: 50–100 mg q12h IV: 100–200 mg q12h Loading doses larger	Broad spectrum including acne; carriers of meningococci; gonorrheal infections (oral: may take with food or milk)
tetracycline (Sumycin, Panmycin, Robilet, Tetracap)	Oral: 1–2 g/d in divided doses Loading doses larger	Use in children may cause tooth discoloration Not used in pregnancy May cause photosensitivity Topical form available
Fluoroquinolones		
ciprofloxacin (Cipro)	Oral: 250–750 mg q12h IV: 200–400 mg q12h Eye drops: 0.3%, 1 to 2 drops q4h Ear drops: 0.2%, 3 drops b.i.d. × 5–7 d	Broad spectrum anti-infective Used for UTI, acute sinusitis, bone infections, anthrax exposure Not recommended during pregnancy
gatifloxacin (Tequin)	Oral: 200–400 mg q d IV: 200–400 mg q d	Used for acute sinusitis, UTI, pyelonephritis, community-acquired pneumonia IV form infused over 60 min
levofloxacin (Levaquin)	Oral: 250–500 mg q d IV: 250–500 mg q12h	Used for community acquired pneumonia, UTI IV form infused over 60 to 90 min, not for IM use
Aminoglycosides		
amikacin (Amikin)	IM, IV: 500 mg 2–3 times/d	Treatment of gram-negative infections, including pseudomonas and bacterial septicemia (nephrotoxic, ototoxic)[†]
gentamicin (Garamycin)	Ophthalmic: drops/ointments IM and IV: 3–5 mg/kg/d (in divided doses)	Eye infections Nephrotoxic and ototoxic;[†] reserved for serious gram-negative infections
neomycin (systemic: Neotabs; topical: Myciguent)	Oral: as ordered IM: 15 mg/kg/d in divided doses Topical use as 1% solution or ointment	Toxicity with continued systemic use May be used as bowel prep
streptomycin	IM: 15 mg/kg/d May be given 2–3 × wk	Used to treat *Mycobacterium tuberculosis*, plague, tularemia No longer commonly used

■■■ TABLE 62-1 𝒮ELECTED ANTI-INFECTIVE MEDICATIONS (CONTINUED)

Name of Medication*	Usual Adult Dose	Notes
tobramycin (Nebcin)	IM and IV: 3–5 mg/kg/d in divided doses Ophthalmic solution and ointment, as ordered	Similar to gentamicin in all aspects
Macrolides		
azithromycin (Zithromax)	Oral: 500 mg × 1 d; 250 mg q d × 4 d Oral tablets and suspension Also available as injection	10% cross sensitivity to erythromycin allergies Long acting; client takes for 5 d but medication effect lasts for 10 d Used in children with otitis media Used in adults for community-acquired pneumonia and sexually transmitted diseases
clarithromycin (Biaxin)	Oral: 250–500 mg b.i.d.–t.i.d. 125 mg/5 mL oral suspension	Used for chronic bronchitis, sinusitis, pneumonia; larger doses for duodenal ulcers Used with omperazole and tetracycline to treat *H. pylori*
erythromycin (Erythrocin, E-Mycin, Ilosone)	Oral: 250–500 mg q6h IV: 500 mg to 1 g q6h Topical: as ordered	GI distress with oral forms Ophthalmic ointment available
Sulfonamides and Urinary Antiseptics		
co-trimoxazole (trimethoprim and sulfamethoxazole) (Septra, Bactrim)	Oral: 1 double-strength tablet q12h; may also be given IV	A combination of two sulfa drugs for urinary tract infection and otitis media in children; other infections in adults
nitrofurantoin (Macrodantin, Furadantin)	Oral: 50–100 mg q6h	Oral use only; must be taken with food or milk; urinary antiseptic; urine becomes rust colored
norfloxacin (Noroxin)	Oral: 400 mg b.i.d.	Urinary tract infections; ophthalmic form also available
sulfamethoxazole (Gantanol)	Oral: 2 g initially, then 1 g b.i.d. or t.i.d.	Urinary tract infections
sulfasalazine (Azulfidine)	Oral: 3–4 g/d in divided doses, then 500 mg q.i.d. (around the clock)	Ulcerative colitis; can cause *oligospermia* (lack of sperm cells) and infertility in men (withdrawal of drug reverses effect)
Antifungals		
amphotericin B (Fungizone)	Oral: for thrush; swish and swallow IV: 0.25–1 mg/kg/d	Parenteral antifungal agent; test dose required because of possible anaphylaxis Topical preparations also available
fluconazole (Diflucan)	Oral: 200–400 mg/d initially, then 100–200 mg/d IV: 50–400 mg initially, then as per chart, based on creatinine clearance	Broad-spectrum antifungal 150 mg oral one-time dose for vaginal yeast infections
itraconazole (Sporonox)	Oral: 100 to 200 mg q d to b.i.d.; swish and swallow solution Pulse dose: 200 mg b.i.d. × 7 d; off 21 d, then repeat	Histoplasmosis Pulse dosing for nail infections Used with caution due to numerous drug interactions
ketoconazole (Nizoral)	Topical: 2% cream, once daily Oral: 200–400 mg daily	Antifungal Also available as shampoo
miconazole (Monistat)	IV: 200–3600 mg/d in divided doses Vaginal: OTC	Severe systemic fungal infections For vaginal yeast infection Intrathecal for fungal meningitis Topical preparations available

(continued)

■■■ **TABLE 62-1** *S*ELECTED ANTI-INFECTIVE MEDICATIONS (CONTINUED)

Name of Medication*	Usual Adult Dose	Notes
nystatin (Mycostatin, Nilstat, Nystex)	Oral: 5 mL q.i.d. in suspension (swish and swallow) Oral: 500,000–1,000,000 U t.i.d. Topical: Apply b.i.d. or t.i.d.	Antifungal agent Swish and swallow for thrush; also component in "magic" mouthwash
Antivirals		
acyclovir (Zovirax)	Oral: 200–800 mg 5 times/d IV: 5 mg/kg q8h Topical: Apply q3h × 7 d	Used for herpes simplex virus types I and II and shingles
amantadine (Symadine, Symmetrel)	Oral: 100 mg b.i.d.	Antiviral: influenza type A virus, respiratory tract infections
valacyclovir (Valtrex)	Oral: 1 g t.i.d. × 7 d	Shingles (herpes zoster); most effective if started within 48 hours of onset; also for genital herpes
zidovudine (AZT, Retrovir)	Oral: 200 mg q4h IV: 1–2 mg/kg q4h, infused over 1h	Treatment of HIV infections (AIDS, advanced ARC): adjust dose PRN for hematologic changes
Other Antibiotics and Anti-infectives		
chloramphenicol (Chlormycetin)	Oral: 250 mg–1 g q6h	Very broad spectrum; can be toxic to bone marrow Ophthalmic and ototic preparations also available
chloroquine phosphate (Aralen)	Oral, IV: 300–600 mg/d (base dose); then taper down IM: 200–250 mg/d × 10–12 d	Antimalarial; amebicide; antirheumatoid
clindamycin (Cleocin)	Oral: 150–300 mg q6–8h Vaginal: h.s. × 7d IM, IV: 600–2700 mg/d (in divided doses)	Available in topical, oral, and injectable forms; effective against gram-positive infections
isoniazid (INH)	Oral: Up to 300 mg/d	Treatment of tuberculosis (take with food)
mebendazole (Vermox)	Oral: 100 mg one-time dose (possible dosing b.i.d. × 3d)	Treatment of roundworm, pinworm, whipworm
metronidazole (Flagyl)	IV: 500 mg q6h Oral: 250 mg t.i.d. × 7d, or 2 g as one-time dose	Treatment of anaerobes; treatment of trichomoniasis
polymyxin B (Aerosporin)	IM, IV, intrathecal:‡ 5,000–25,000 U kg/d	Acute infections, especially pseudomonas; urinary tract, meninges, bloodstream (extremely nephrotoxic)
quinine sulfate	Oral: 650 mg q8h Oral: 300–600 mg q d	Antimalarial, low doses for night leg cramps
rifampin (Rifadin)	Oral or IV: 600 mg in single daily dose (used with other TB drugs)	Treatment of tuberculosis (discolors urine); for prophylactic use after *H. influenzae* meningitis exposure
vancomycin (Vancocin)	Oral: 500 mg q6h IV: 500 mg q6h	Used for resistant staph infections in penicillin-allergic patients

*A trade name appears in parentheses following the generic name of the medication.

†Nephrotoxic: damaging to kidney cells; ototoxic: damaging to eighth cranial nerve, causing hearing and balance disorders.

‡Intrathecal: injection through the sheath (theca) of the spinal cord into the subarachnoid space.

Antibiotic-Resistant Organisms

If an antibiotic is used indiscriminately, especially for minor ailments, or is administered improperly, certain pathogens may mutate or build a tolerance to it. Eventually, the antibiotic's action is rendered ineffective against that particular microorganism. Thus, the microorganism is termed *resistant* to the antibiotic. For example, a common pathogenic bacteria that may become penicillin-resistant is *Staphylococcus aureus.* A dangerous organism known as methicillin-resistant staphylococcus aureus (**MRSA**) can cause life-threatening illness, because it does not respond to antibiotics.

☛ KEY CONCEPT

Some clients, who have a particular problem with frequent "strep" infections or a history of rheumatic fever, take a small daily prophylactic (preventive) dose of oral penicillin, sometimes for years. This dosage schedule generally does not build up resistant strains of streptococcus and generally does not have side effects.

Selection of the Appropriate Antibiotic

Physicians often order a *culture and sensitivity* (C&S) test to determine the specific microorganism causing an infection and the medication to which the organism is most sensitive. Cultures may be obtained from blood, sputum, pus, wound drainage (exudate), urine, or drainage from mucous membranes. A culture is grown in the laboratory using special growth media and temperature regulation. The sensitivity of the cultured bacteria is then tested against several antibiotics to determine which antibiotic most successfully inhibits the growth of the bacteria. To ensure the accuracy of test results, antibiotic therapy should not start until after the specimen for C&S is obtained and forwarded to the laboratory for analysis. If antibiotic therapy begins before the specimen is secured, the numbers and types of bacteria present in the specimen could be reduced, which may result in inappropriate, and perhaps ineffective, antibiotic selection. (Methods of collecting specimens are presented in Chapter 52.)

Presently, the most effective and widely used antibiotics include penicillins, cephalosporins, tetracyclines, aminoglycosides, macrolides, and sulfonamides. In some infections, any one of several antibiotics will be effective. In others, only one specific antibiotic will be of value. Sometimes, a combination of antibiotics is required to control an infection. Antibiotics may also be used in conjunction with other medications to improve their effectiveness.

Penicillins

Penicillin (**PCN**), derived from a specific mold, inhibits the growth of susceptible bacteria. It is also *bactericidal* (kills bacteria) in sufficiently high concentrations or blood levels. It is most effective against gram-positive organisms, such as streptococci, staphylococci, and pneumococci. It is also active against some gram-negative organisms, such as gonococci and meningococci, and against the organisms that cause syphilis. It has been proven effective in treating Lyme disease in some cases. PCN is ineffective against the tubercle bacillus, all

viruses, and the organisms causing typhoid fever. Therefore, PCN is a fairly narrow-spectrum antibiotic. It is excreted rapidly in the urine and is remarkably free of toxic effects.

Penicillin, a pregnancy category B drug, is available in liquid, tablet, and parenteral forms. The dosage is measured in units or milligrams and will vary with individual needs and with the type used. It can be given by several routes. The intramuscular (IM) route is most often used with slower-acting PCNs. The intravenous (IV) route is used for severe infections when a high blood level is desired as quickly as possible. The oral route is the easiest and safest way to administer PCN and is usually effective for all but the most severe infections. Gastric secretions destroy some PCN, so the oral dose is often larger than that ordered parenterally. Chapter 63 describes various methods of administering medications in more detail.

Penicillin has few side effects, even in large doses, except for the person who is sensitive or allergic to it. (Penicillin sensitivity occurs in about 5% of North Americans.) In some cases, PCN causes a comparatively mild allergic reaction, such as nausea, sore mouth, or diarrhea. More serious adverse effects, such as hives, a skin rash, fever, dyspnea, or unusual bleeding, should be reported. In milder PCN reactions, symptoms may be delayed and may occur 5 to 14 days after administration.

Nursing Alert
Penicillins share **cross-sensitivity,** or the potential for causing allergic reactions. Some individuals who are allergic to penicillin G, however, may not be allergic to one of the other forms of penicillin. Nevertheless, if a client is allergic to one penicillin, use extreme caution when administering another. Penicillins also share cross-sensitivity to cephalosporins, which are similar in molecular structure.

If the client experiences an anaphylactic reaction (see Chap. 43), treatment includes immediate oxygen administration, epinephrine 1:1000, and intravenous aminophylline or theophylline for respiratory distress. Steroidal anti-inflammatory agents are usually administered after the client's condition stabilizes. A mild allergic reaction is usually treated with an antihistamine, such as diphenhydramine (Benadryl). Clients with a history of previous reaction to a drug should not receive therapy with that drug or related drugs without first being tested for sensitivity.

Cephalosporins

Cephalosporins, like PCN, were originally derived from a mold. Because cephalosporins are structurally similar to PCN, clients receiving cephalosporin therapy should be asked about previous sensitivity to PCN. Monitor these clients very carefully for adverse or allergic reactions. (Approximately 10% of clients with a history of allergy to PCN are also allergic to cephalosporins.)

The cephalosporins are divided into three groups: first, second, and third generations. These divisions are based on the range of the medication's specificity, with third-generation agents being more broad spectrum. Most cephalosporins are bactericidal. They are produced semi-synthetically and are active against gram-positive cocci, including PCN-resistant staphylococci, and gram-negative bacteria including *Escherichia coli, Proteus mirabilis,* and *Klebsiella* species. The cephalosporins are used frequently for mixed infections (those caused by more than one pathogenic organism).

Cephalosporins, pregnancy category B agents, are available in oral and injectable forms. They have become the most popular and widely used antibiotics in the hospital setting. Adverse effects are usually minimal, but may include GI symptoms such as flatulence and diarrhea. If the client uses alcohol while taking a cephalosporin, severe nausea and vomiting are likely. Some cephalosporins can cause more serious adverse effects, such as bone marrow depression. As with any drug, allergic reactions are possible.

Tetracyclines

Tetracyclines (**TCN**) are broad-spectrum antibiotics effective against a wide variety of organisms, including *Rickettsia, Chlamydia,* and *Mycoplasma.* They are well absorbed orally and are also available for IM or IV use. The presence of food and some dairy products (especially milk) in the stomach decreases oral absorption. To promote GI absorption, clients should receive tetracyclines on an empty stomach at least 1 hour after eating. The presence of iron, calcium, magnesium, and aluminum in the stomach also influences tetracycline absorption. Therefore, clients should not take antacids such as Gelusil, Maalox, Mylanta, or Milk of Magnesia.

Tetracyclines, pregnancy category D agents, have relatively few side effects. Side effects usually involve the GI system: nausea, vomiting, or diarrhea. Intestinal infections or digestive difficulties are possible because tetracyclines also may kill the normal flora found in the digestive tract. **Photosensitivity** (sensitivity to light) may develop. Adverse reactions include skin rash, burning eyes, and vaginal or anal itching. Tetracyclines cause a brownish discoloration of the enamel in developing teeth. Thus, they are contraindicated for pregnant women and for children who do not yet have their permanent teeth. Allergic reactions are also possible.

Aminoglycosides

Aminoglycosides are potent bactericidal antibiotics. They are active against many aerobic gram-negative organisms, particularly those causing urinary tract infections, meningitis, and life-threatening **septicemias** (generalized sepsis or infection throughout the body). They are considered the medication of choice for hospital-acquired gram-negative infections. They are also used preoperatively in some clients who are scheduled for surgery of the GI tract, because the action of these medications reduces the number of normal bacterial flora found there. Aminoglycosides are most often administered parenterally.

Aminoglycosides, pregnancy category C agents, can have toxic effects, namely ototoxicity and nephrotoxicity. **Ototoxicity,** caused by damage to the eighth cranial nerve, is manifested by dizziness, tinnitus, and gradual hearing loss that can occur even several days after the medication has been stopped. **Nephrotoxicity** (kidney damage) is manifested by blood and protein in the urine. Monitor clients receiving aminoglycosides carefully for signs and symptoms of any toxicity.

Macrolide Antibiotics

Macrolide antibiotics are narrow-spectrum bacteriostatic agents. Macrolides include azithromycin (Zithromax), clarithromycin (Biaxin), dirithromycin (Dynabac), and erythromycin (Erythrocin). They are effective against most microorganisms that are sensitive to PCN and are used to treat respiratory tract infections in clients who are allergic to PCN. Macrolides, pregnancy category B agents, are usually administered orally; erythromycin also may be administered parenterally. Adverse reactions include skin rashes, abdominal pain, nausea, and cramping. Azithromycin and erythromycin should be given 1 hour before or 2 to 3 hours after a meal. Clarithromycin and dirithromycin should be taken with food.

Sulfonamides and Other Urinary Antiseptics

Sulfonamides (commonly called *sulfa drugs*) are used as antimicrobial agents, chiefly because of their low cost and effectiveness in treating common bacterial infections. They are bacteriostatic agents, requiring normal body processes to eradicate infection. Although the sulfa drugs are very effective, newer and more effective antibiotics with fewer side effects and faster rates of action are replacing them. In addition, the Department of Health and Human Services has voiced concern about increasing bacterial resistance to the sulfonamides. The use of specific sulfonamides is often indicated in the following conditions: chancroid, trachoma, toxoplasmosis, uncomplicated urinary tract infections, specific cases of malaria, meningococcal meningitis, *Haemophilus influenzae* infections of the middle ear, and as an alternative to PCN for PCN-sensitive clients diagnosed with rheumatic fever. Sulfonamides also are prescribed with PCN or erythromycin in conditions such as otitis media. Other sulfonamides are specific for other disorders. In other words, not all sulfonamides are appropriate for all disorders.

Encourage clients taking sulfonamides to drink large amounts of fluids to dilute the urine. Sulfa drugs tend to form crystals in the urine, which causes kidney irritation and possible kidney stone formation. The intake of large of amounts of fluid will minimize the possibility of crystal formation. Observe the client for signs and symptoms of adverse reactions to the sulfonamides, including nausea, vomiting, diarrhea, electrolyte imbalance, cyanosis, or jaundice. Kidney damage or failure is a serious adverse effect that may occur. Sulfonamides are considered pregnancy category C drugs during pregnancy and category D drugs at term.

Sulfamethoxazole/Trimethoprim (Bactrim) is a combination drug often considered the medication of choice for urinary tract infections. As with all other medications, this medication should not be given to infants under the age of 2 months. This medication is *not* the medication of choice for streptococcal infections or infections of the upper respiratory tract.

Other Anti-infectives

The previously discussed antibiotics are the most effective and the most widely used anti-infective agents. Other antibiotics and anti-infectives are also available. Some are used when the causative organism has shown resistance to the more popular antibiotics; others are used in clients allergic to the more popular medications; and some are used to treat nonbacterial infections, such as fungal and viral infections.

The medications in Table 62-1 are not all derived from living organisms, such as mold or algae. Thus, some of those listed are technically not antibiotics. They do have antimicrobial actions and thus are commonly referred to collectively as *antibiotics.*

> ### Nursing Alert
> Symptoms of a serious reaction to clindamycin (Cleocin) include diarrhea with liquid feces and shreds of intestinal lining. Although rare, this reaction can be fatal, especially in children or older adults. Therefore, a client who is receiving clindamycin must report any diarrhea *at once.*

MEDICATIONS THAT AFFECT THE INTEGUMENTARY SYSTEM

The condition of the sweat glands, the state of pores that penetrate the epidermis from the deeper subcutaneous tissue, and the adequacy of blood supply to the area affect absorption of medication through the skin. Absorption increases if the skin is *macerated* (softened), either by water or by perspiration. Chapter 74 describes many skin disorders, related nursing care, and specific methods of administering medications for dermatological conditions.

Medications applied to the skin or into body openings (eg, the ear, eye, or rectum) are called *topical agents. Dermatologic agents* are medications applied to the skin to treat localized skin conditions. Examples include soothing agents, antiseptics, anesthetics, corticosteroids, antifungals, and pediculicides (medications used to kill lice) (Table 62-2). Sterilizing the skin is impossible, but sufficient cleansing will remove most bacteria and loose epithelium. Strong antiseptics can cause skin irritation that may interfere with the skin's protective function as a natural barrier against bacterial invasion. *Transdermal medications* are topical agents designed to be absorbed through the skin for systemic effects. Chapter 63 describes transdermal administration in more detail.

MEDICATIONS THAT AFFECT THE NERVOUS SYSTEM

As presented in Chapter 19, the central nervous system (CNS) regulates the vital control centers of the body, in addition to many other body processes. When CNS functions are disturbed, certain medications may be used to increase or decrease the activity of vital nerve centers in the brain or nerve pathways. *Stimulants* speed up certain mental and physical processes; **depressants** slow them down. Medications used in psychiatry are described and listed in Chapter 93. Abuse and dependency related to stimulants, depressants, and other drugs are described in Chapter 94.

Many medications have a stimulating effect on the CNS, but only a few are medically valuable for this purpose. The most valuable are those used to stimulate the brain's respiratory centers, usually to counteract the toxic effects of depressants, such as barbiturates. Other than to counteract overdose or toxicity, stimulants are rarely prescribed today. In the past, they were prescribed for weight loss; however, such diet medications have a high potential for abuse and for adverse effects, including tachycardia and hypertension.

Medications that depress the activities of the CNS include analgesics; hypnotics and sedatives that bring rest and sleep; and general anesthetics that cause loss of consciousness. In addition to these depressants, some medications are known as *selective depressants,* which are used for the symptomatic treatment of various conditions. Table 62-3 describes many commonly used medications affecting the CNS.

Analgesics

Analgesics are medications that relieve pain. They are divided into two groups: narcotics and nonnarcotics. An example of a narcotic analgesic is morphine. An example of a nonnarcotic analgesic is aspirin (acetylsalicylic acid) or acetaminophen (Tylenol).

Analgesics interfere with a person's perception of pain, but do not cause unconsciousness. Because they relieve pain, they do make a person more comfortable and relaxed, thereby allowing the client to rest and sleep.

Narcotic Agonist Analgesics
Narcotic agonist analgesics are called **opiates** because they are opium derivatives or have opium-like actions. They occur naturally or can be produced synthetically. The most widely prescribed opiates are morphine and codeine, which mainly affect the CNS. These drugs generally are considered pregnancy category C agents.

All medications produced from opium or opium derivatives are very potent. They are highly addictive and subject to narcotic regulation as outlined in the Harrison Narcotic Act of 1914, which was amended by the Controlled Substances Act in 1970 (see Chap. 61).

Opiates have a depressant effect on the brain's cerebral cortex, altering the client's pain conception. Some narcotics are more potent than others.

> ### Nursing Alert
> The first sign of narcotic overdose is often respiratory depression. Therefore, monitoring the client's vital signs, particularly respirations, is extremely important when administering narcotics.

Morphine Sulfate. *Morphine sulfate* (**MS**) is a very potent narcotic analgesic used to relieve severe pain such as that produced by myocardial infarction (MI), passage of renal calculi, or terminal conditions (eg, advanced cancer). Morphine is most effective when given before the client experiences severe pain. Morphine's analgesic effect allows the client to rest more comfortably. Its action also produces a feeling of well-being, reducing fear and anxiety. It may be used preoperatively for this reason. When given preoperatively,

(text continues on page 834)

▪▪▪ TABLE 62-2 ℐSELECTED DERMATOLOGIC AGENTS

Type	Examples*
Soothing Agents Emollient preparations	*glycerin:* In pure form, tendency to dry skin; if mixed with rosewater, moisturizing effect *lanolin:* Used as ointment base; purified fat of sheeps' wool with water *urea:* 2%–40% promotes hydration and removal of excess keratin in dry skin *vitamin A & D ointment* *zinc oxide ointment:* 15% zinc oxide in simple ointment base
Pain Relief Lotions and solution preparations	*capsaicin (Capsin):* apply max. 3–4 × d for temporary arthritis relief *Burow's solution:* Aluminum acetate used for its *astringent* (drying) properties; used for poison ivy, insect bites *Calamine lotion:* Used for *dermatitis* (itching, inflamed skin) caused by poison ivy, insect bites, prickly heat
Anesthetics Benzocaine, lidocaine	Sprays, lotions, or creams used for *pruritus* (itching) and pain due to wounds, minor burns, prickly heat, chickenpox, insect bites, sunburn
Antiseptics	*benzalkonium chloride (Zephiran):* Detergent type of agent; germicidal for a number of pathogens; activity reduced by soap solutions; most effective in 1 : 750 solution *chlorhexidine gluconate (Hibiclens):* Antimicrobial activity against a wide range of microorganisms; used as surgical scrub and cleanser for preoperative bathing and wound cleansing *iodine:* Generally in alcohol solution (*tincture*), in concentration up to 7% *povidone-iodine (Betadine):* Stable compound slowly releases iodine; relatively nonirritating; contains 1% available iodine *thimersol (Merthiolate):* Organic mercury compound; used on abraded skin; concentration of 1 : 1,000; available also as tincture (with alcohol); rarely used today
Antifungals	*butenafine hydrochloride (Mentax):* Used for athlete's foot, ringworm *butoconazole nitrate (Femstat):* Used for vaginal fungal infections; may cause burning *clotrimazole (Lotrimin):* Antifungal used topically for athlete's foot and diaper rash; used vaginally for yeast infection; both forms available OTC *ciclopirox (Luprox; Penla):* Treatment of *onychomycosis* (fungal infection of the nails) in immunocompromised individuals *econazole nitrate (Spectazole):* Antifungal agent; cleanse area before applying *Gentian violet:* External application of solution of 1% of the dye; stains clothing *nystatin (Mycostatin):* Antibiotic; used for fungal infections of skin and mucous membranes; commonly used as vaginal suppository or cream; used in mouthwashes for thrush *naftitine hydrochloride (Naftin):* Antifungal; avoid occlusive dressings; wash hands thoroughly *tolnaftate (Tinactin):* 1% concentration in a cream or solution to treat infections caused by *Trichophyton,* the organism of athlete's foot and other dermatologic infections
Corticosteroids	betamethasone dipropionate (*Diprosone*): Available in varying strengths and emollient bases; used for anti-inflammatory, antipruritic, and antiproliferative actions (avoid contact with eyes; apply sparingly) *desoximetasone (Topicort):* Available as cream, gel, or ointment (use cautiously in viral diseases; may macerate skin if covered with occlusive dressing) *hydrocortisone (Acticort, Bactine HC, Cortef, Hytone, Synacort, Unicort):* Aerosol, cream, gel, lotion, ointment, topical solution, rectal foam (used for dermatitis; may be used on face, groin, axillae, and under breasts; clean area before application; avoid eyes; use as directed)
Pediculosides (Kill lice)	*crotamiton (Eurax):* Thorough massaging into skin needed; bed linens and clothing should be changed the next day *lindane (Kwell):* Available as lotion, ointment, or shampoo (keep away from eyes and mouth; potential for CNS toxicity in infants and children); by prescription only *malathion (Ovide):* Lotion; applied to dry hair and left on for 8 to 12 h; repeated in 7 to 9 d. *permethrin (Nix):* Shampoo (combing of nits [eggs of lice] not required); will prevent reinfection up to 2 wk; available OTC; no CNS toxicity if used as directed

*A trade name appears in parentheses following the generic name of a medication.

▪▪▪ TABLE 62-3 ◢ELECTED CENTRAL NERVOUS SYSTEM MEDICATIONS

Name of Medication*	Usual Adult Dose	Notes
Narcotic Agonist Analgesics		
codeine	Oral or IM: 30–60 mg q4h PRN	Usually given in combination with aspirin (Empirin #3) or acetaminophen (Tylenol #3)
fetanyl (Innovar, Oralet, Sublimaze, Duragesic)	Topical: 25–300 mcg/72 h IV: 1–30 mcg/kg	Dosage depends on use (induction of anesthesia, maintenance of anesthesia vs pain management)
hydromorphone (Dilaudid)	Oral or IM: 2–4 mg q4–6h	Shorter duration of action than morphine
levorphanol (Levo-Dromoran)	IM: 2 mg q4h	For relief of moderate to severe pain
meperidine (Demerol)	IM or oral: 50–100 mg q3–4h	Lacking antitussive (cough suppressant) effect of other narcotics
methadone (Dolophine)	IM and oral: 2.5–10 mg q6–12h	Longer duration of activity; used as narcotic replacement to facilitate withdrawal
morphine	Oral, IV, or IM: 10–15 mg q4h	Used to treat severe pain (eg, MI, cancer)
oxycodone (Percodan, Percocet)	Oral: 5 mg q4h	Often combined with aspirin (Percodan) or acetaminophen (Percocet)
propoxyphene HCl (Darvon†)	Oral: 65 mg q4h	Greater pain relief in combination with aspirin or acetaminophen (Darvon compound); potentiated by alcohol
Narcotic Antagonists		
naloxone (Narcan)	IV: 0.4–2mg q 2–3 min	Used as antidote in narcotic overdose; it prevents or reverses effects of opioids
Nonsteroidal Anti-inflammatory Drugs (NSAIDs)† and Antirheumatics		
acetaminophen (Tylenol)	Oral: 300–650 mg q4–6h	Analgesic and fever reducer; used in aspirin-allergic patients and children
acetylsalicylic acid, ASA, aspirin	Oral or rectal; 81–650 mg (1/4–10 grains) q4–6h	May cause GI distress in high doses; mild anticoagulant Low dose (81 mg) used to prevent stroke and prevent reinfarction following myocardial infarction
auranofin (Ridaura)	Oral: 6 mg/d	Used in arthritis (contains 29% gold)
celcoxib (Celebrex)	Oral: 100–200 mg b.i.d.	Selective COX-2 inhibitor; treatment of osteoarthritis, rheumatoid arthritis Contraindicated if allergic to sulfonamide or NSAID
diclofenac (Voltaren)	25–75 mg b.i.d.	Used in arthritis and ankylosing spondylitis
ibuprofen (Motrin, Advil, Nuprin, Rufen)	Oral: 200–800 mg q6–8h	Given with meals or milk if GI distress occurs. Available OTC in 200-mg strength and sometimes used for fever in children
indomethacin (Indocin)	Oral: 25–50 mg 3 or 4 times/d	Commonly used in arthritis; gastric distress common
naproxen (Naprosyn, Aleve)	Oral: 250–750 mg b.i.d.	Longer-acting drug used for arthritis
piroxicam (Feldene)	Oral: 20 mg q d	Single daily dose in rheumatoid arthritis

(continued)

■■■ TABLE 62-3 *S*ELECTED CENTRAL NERVOUS SYSTEM MEDICATIONS (CONTINUED)

Name of Medication*	Usual Adult Dose	Notes
rofecoxib (Vioxx)	Oral: 12.5, 25, 50 mg qd 12.5 mg/5 mL oral suspension	Selective COX-2 inhibitor; treatment of osteoarthritis, acute pain
sulindac (Clinoril)	Oral: 150–200 mg b.i.d.	For acute and long-term use in arthritis
Nonnarcotic Analgesic		
tramadol (Ultram)	Oral: 50 to 100 mg q4–6h; maximum 400 mg/d	No respiratory depressant effects; used for moderate to severe pain; nonnarcotic
Hypnotic, Sedative, and Antianxiety Medications		
Barbiturates		
amobarbital (Amytal)	Oral: 65–200 mg h.s.	Hypnotic; intermediate duration of action
pentobarbital (Nembutal)	Oral: 100 mg h.s.	Short-acting hypnotic; may be used as preanesthetic
phenobarbital (Solfoton, Luminal)	Oral: 30–120 mg 2–3 times/d	Long-acting sedative; used principally as anticonvulsant
secobarbital (Seconal)	Oral: 100 mg h.s.	Short-acting hypnotic and pre-anesthesia sedative, used occasionally in pregnancy
Benzodiazepines		
alprazolam (Xanax)	Oral: 0.25–2 mg t.i.d.	Intermediate acting; 2-mg dose used to treat panic attacks
chlordiazepoxide (Librium)	Oral: 10–25 mg 3–4 times/d IM: Given deep IM	Long-acting drug to treat anxiety and alcohol withdrawal
diazepam (Valium)	Oral: 2–10 mg up to q.i.d. IV: 5–10 mg PRN	Used to treat seizures, muscle spasm, anxiety; IV form for status epilepticus; used in alcohol detoxification
flurazepam (Dalmane)	Oral: 15–30 mg h.s.	Hypnotic only; use dose of 15 mg in elderly
lorazepam (Ativan)	Oral: 0.5–6 mg/d, in divided doses IM, suspension available	Intermediate acting; sublingual administration absorbed faster than oral
oxazepam (Serax)	IM: Usual dose 1–2 mg Oral: 10–15 mg 3–4 times/d	IM most often used to control dangerous behavior Short-acting drug for anxiety and alcohol withdrawal
temazepam (Restoril)	Oral: 7.5 mg h.s.	Intermediate-acting; prescribed for insomnia
Anticonvulsants and Antiepileptic Agents		
carbemazepine (Tegretol)	Oral: 800–1200 mg/d	Used in mixed seizures, generalized tonic–clonic seizures, and treatment of pain associated with trigeminal neuralgia
clonazepam (Klonopin)	Oral: 1.5 mg/d in 3 divided doses; gradually tapered up to maximum of 20 mg/d	Used in specific seizures not responsive to other drugs; also used for panic attacks
diazepam (Valium)	IV: 1 mg slowly q 2–5 min to maximum of 5 mg	Benzodiazepine; used for treatment of acute seizures, status epilepticus, and alcohol detoxification
magnesium sulfate	Dose variable	Used in emergencies, especially in clients with pregnancy-induced hypertension or magnesium deficiency

■■ TABLE 62-3 𝒮ELECTED CENTRAL NERVOUS SYSTEM MEDICATIONS (CONTINUED)

Name of Medication*	Usual Adult Dose	Notes
phenytoin (Dilantin)	Oral: 300–400 mg/d IV, IM: Variable dosages	Anticonvulsant for generalized tonic–clonic and psychomotor seizures (gingival hyperplasia is frequent side effect)
primidone (Mysoline)	Oral: Taper up to 250 mg t.i.d. to q.i.d. over 10 d	Treatment of generalized tonic–clonic, psychomotor, or focal seizures
Other CNS Medications		
buspirone (BuSpar)	Oral: 5–20 mg t.i.d.	Management of anxiety disorders; not related chemically to benzodiazepines, barbiturates, or other sedative hypnotics; fewer sedative effects than benzodiazepines
carbidopa/levodopa (Sinemet: contains 10 mg carbidopa and 100 mg levodopa)	Oral: 10/100–25/250 t.i.d. Sinemet CR (controlled-release): 50/200	Antiparkinsonism agent May cause hemolytic anemia, cardiac arrhythmias Contraindicated in glaucoma, melanoma; may interact with antihypertensive agents
chloral hydrate (Noctec)	Oral: 500 mg h.s. Rectal: 500 mg–1 g h.s.	Oldest of currently used hypnotics; bitter taste; gel caps and suppositories available
cyclobenzaprine (Flexeril)	Oral: 10 mg t.i.d.	Centrally acting muscle relaxant; structurally related to tricyclics (may cause drowsiness and dry mouth)
dantrolene sodium (Dantrium)	Oral: 25–100 mg 2–4 times/d IV: 2.5 mg/kg 1 1/2 h prior to anesthesia	Skeletal muscle relaxant used for cerebral palsy, multiple sclerosis; also used for malignant hyperthermia
dextroamphetamine (Dexedrine)	Oral: 10 mg/d	Used in adults for narcolepsy (a sleep disorder) Used in children for attention deficit–hyperactivity disorder (ADHD)
meprobamate (Equanil, Miltown)	Oral: 400 mg 3–4 times/d	Antianxiety and sedative with muscle-relaxing properties
methocarbamol (Robaxin)	Oral: 500–700 mg q4h IM, IV: up to 2–3 g/d	Centrally acting muscle relaxant (may cause drowsiness)
methylphenidate (Ritalin)	Oral: 20–30 mg/d in divided doses	Adults: Narcolepsy Children: ADHD
sumatriptan (Imitrex)	SubQ: 6 mg; may repeat in 1 h (limit 12 mg/d)	Treatment of severe migraine headaches; available by prescription (prefilled syringes) for home administration; oral form also available
zolpidem (Ambien)	Oral: 5–10 mg h.s.; maximum 10 mg	Minimal next-day residual effects Dosage decreased in the elderly or in clients with hepatic insufficiency

Antidepressants (See Chap. 93)

*A trade name appears in parentheses following the generic name of the medication.

†NSAIDs are contraindicated when clients are taking any medication that may cause kidney damage, such as lithium.

morphine is usually administered in conjunction with atropine, a drying agent used to reduce secretions of the respiratory tract.

Nausea and vomiting are common morphine side effects that can be relieved by antiemetics. However, antiemetic preparations *potentiate* (increase) the actions of narcotics. Therefore, carefully monitor the client's vital signs, especially if the client is also receiving an antiemetic.

Morphine and other opiates delay stomach emptying and slow peristalsis. They can be used to treat severe diarrhea or used for surgical interventions involving the intestines. This slowed peristalsis, however, can also cause constipation, abdominal pain, and distention. Allergic reactions are common.

Morphine is not recommended for pain that can be relieved by administration of a less-potent analgesic. (Clients receiving morphine may develop a tolerance to it and thus may require increasingly larger doses.)

Morphine poisoning is often the result of attempted suicide. Significant early symptoms of poisoning include decreased respirations (less than 12 per minute), deep sleep, and constricted pupils. Emergency treatment involves the use of narcotic antagonists, such as naloxone (Narcan), that counteract the action of morphine. If respirations are severely depressed, maintain the person's airway, initiate emergency respiratory care measures such as rescue breathing, and be prepared to assist with emergency endotracheal intubation or tracheostomy.

Hydromorphone Hydrochloride. *Hydromorphone hydrochloride* (Dilaudid) is prepared from morphine and has about five times its analgesic effect. Although the effect of Dilaudid is shorter than morphine, it can be prolonged if given by suppository. The medication causes very little drowsiness, nausea, or vomiting, but does depress respiration. Nursing considerations are similar to those for morphine.

Codeine. *Codeine* is a derivative of morphine, but its action is milder. A pregnancy category C agent during pregnancy and a category D agent during labor, this drug is recommended for relief of mild to moderate pain. Codeine has a depressant effect on the cough reflex and is therefore especially effective in relieving cough. It is a common ingredient in cough mixtures. Codeine depresses the CNS to a lesser degree and is less addictive than morphine. However, it may be as constipating as morphine.

Other Narcotic Analgesics. Other narcotic analgesics, such as *meperidine hydrochloride* (Demerol), are effective pain relievers and have fewer adverse reactions than morphine. Demerol, a pregnancy category C agent, is a synthetically produced narcotic analgesic. It is often used instead of morphine to relieve pain whenever possible. Demerol has a quick onset of action, but its effects are not prolonged. It is often used before anesthesia or immediately postoperatively. It also used for postoperative discomfort and may be used during the last stage of labor and delivery. Demerol is less likely to cause nausea and vomiting than is morphine. Demerol also causes less depression of cardiac activity and respirations than morphine. Possible side effects include dizziness, nausea, vomiting, headache, and fainting. A toxic dose may cause dilated pupils, mental confusion, seizures, respiratory depression, and even death.

Methadone hydrochloride (Dolophine), a pregnancy category C agent, is much like morphine in that it is an effective pain reliever and has similarly lasting effects. However, it does not cause euphoria. Methadone is slightly more effective than morphine in relieving chronic pain and is effective in depressing the cough reflex. It may cause nausea and vomiting, itching, constipation, and respiratory depression. The use of methadone in managing withdrawal from morphine or heroin is discussed in Chapter 94.

Oxycodone, typically combined with aspirin (Percodan) or acetaminophen (Percocet), is effective for the treatment of moderate pain. Side effects are similar to those found with other narcotics. Onset of action is approximately 15 minutes. The duration of action is 4 to 5 hours.

Nursing Alert

All opiates and opiate-like medications can be addictive. For that reason, monitor the administration of these medications closely. Evaluate the type and intensity of pain the client experiences. More potent opiate medications, such as morphine, should be used only when the client's pain level is severe. Expect to institute appropriate tapering doses, or substitute less-potent narcotic analgesics, as ordered, as the client's pain level decreases. Be particularly cautious in administering opiates to any person who is otherwise chemically dependent, including alcohol dependent. These clients may become dependent on opiates very quickly.

Nonnarcotic Analgesics and Nonsteroidal Anti-inflammatory Drugs

Nonnarcotic analgesics are less potent than narcotic analgesics and are available over the counter (OTC). Aspirin (**ASA**) and acetaminophen (Tylenol) are the most commonly used examples. *Antipyretic analgesics* are medications that reduce both pain and fever.

Salicylates. The *salicylates* derive from salicylic acid. *Acetylsalicylic acid* (ASA [aspirin]) is available in caplets or tablets (plain or enteric-coated), capsules (regular or time-release), rectal suppositories, oral suspension, and as chewing gum. Flavored chewable tablets are available in dosages appropriate for administration to children, although aspirin often is not recommended for children. (Aspirin is believed to contribute to the development of Reye's syndrome in children.) Aspirin is the most common salicylate used for adults. Aspirin is highly effective for treatment of mild to moderate pain.

Aspirin and other salicylates have three separate actions: analgesic (pain relief), antipyretic (fever reduction), and anti-inflammatory. The *analgesic action* treats headache, arthritis-type pain, neuralgia, and dysmenorrhea. The *antipyretic action* increases heat elimination from the body, thus reducing fever. The *anti-inflammatory action* is particularly effective in the treatment of arthritic conditions and *neuralgia* (pain arising from nerves).

Aspirin also affects the circulatory system by reducing platelet aggregation, thereby reducing the formation of blood clots. Many physicians recommend daily low doses of aspirin to reduce the incidence or severity of stroke and MI. Recent studies indicate that taking aspirin at the onset of an MI may reduce damage to the myocardial tissue supplied by the coronary arteries.[1]

The salicylates have remarkably few side effects. The most common is gastric irritation, which can be eliminated by the use of enteric-coated tablets. Clients with active gastric ulcers or bleeding disorders should not take aspirin, because of its effect on platelet aggregation and blood clot formation. Aspirin also is contraindicated in clients taking warfarin (Coumadin) or other agents that affect blood coagulation, and immediately before and after surgery or obstetrical delivery. It is a pregnancy category D agent.

Overdose or toxicity can occur with the use of aspirin. The most common manifestations include dizziness, tinnitus, and visual disturbances.

☛ KEY CONCEPT

The use of aspirin and other anticoagulants is contraindicated for 7 to 10 days prior to surgery, dental work, or invasive procedures such as biopsy or colonoscopy. In addition, some herbal supplements can contribute to operative and postoperative bleeding. The client should consult a physician for specific instructions.

Non-salicylate Analgesics.   *Acetaminophen* (Tylenol, Panadol, Atasol [in Canada]) has the same analgesic and antipyretic properties as aspirin, but demonstrates fewer side effects. It is classified as a nonnarcotic analgesic. Acetaminophen, a pregnancy category B agent, is often prescribed for people allergic to salicylates, and is usually used for infants and children. It has few GI side effects. Acetaminophen is less effective as an anti-inflammatory agent and therefore, less useful than aspirin for treating arthritis and other inflammatory conditions. The maximum dose is 2,000 milligrams per day.

Tramadol (Ultram) is a centrally acting semi-synthetic analgesic. It does not contain salicylate and is unrelated to the narcotics. Clients who cannot tolerate salicylates or nonsteroidal agents (see next section) often use it. Tramadol, a pregnancy category C agent, does not cause respiratory depression. Side effects include dizziness, constipation, and nausea. Because of the increased risk for seizures, the drug is contraindicated in clients with a seizure disorder.

Nonsteroidal Anti-inflammatory Drugs (NSAIDs).   The **NSAIDs** are used primarily to treat inflammation, but also have analgesic and antipyretic actions. This large class of medications is used to treat mild to moderate pain. Most NSAIDs can cause gastric upset and should be taken with food. They *should not be given* with salicylates or anticoagulants or with certain psychiatric medications (especially lithium) because they reduce renal (kidney) clearance and toxicity may occur. NSAIDs also reduce the effectiveness of some diuretics and antihypertensive agents. Clients receiving cyclosporine (to prevent organ transplant rejection) also should not receive NSAIDs for the same reason. NSAIDs should not be combined with other OTC agents because of the possibility of duplication. These drugs are generally considered pregnancy category B agents, although some variation does exist.

Ibuprofen (Motrin, Advil, Midol-200, Nuprin, Genpril) is a potent NSAID used to relieve mild to moderate pain. Ibuprofen is available without prescription in 200-milligram strength tablets and is indicated for minor aches and pains, fever reduction, and dysmenorrhea. It also is available OTC in children's drops, suspension, and chewable tablets to control pain and fever in children. Monitoring liver and kidney function is necessary for the client receiving ibuprofen.

Indomethacin (Indocin) belongs to the NSAID group, but is chemically unrelated to other medications in this class. It is a pregnancy category B agent during the first two trimesters and a category D agent during the third trimester. Indomethacin is effective in treating arthritis, bursitis, and other joint diseases. Clients should always take it with meals or milk, because it may cause severe gastric distress.

Celecoxib (Celebrex) is a new type of NSAID. It inhibits (blocks) the cyclo-oxygenase–2 (COX-2) enzyme. (COX-2 is an enzyme activated in inflammation.) However, the drug does not inhibit cyclo-oxygenase–1 (COX-1; an enzyme that protects the lining of the GI tract along with playing a role in blood clotting and kidney function). COX-2 inhibitors have excellent anti-inflammatory and analgesic properties, with fewer GI side effects. Celebrex, a pregnancy category C agent, is often the drug of choice for clients with arthritis or peptic ulcer disease. It should not be given to clients who are allergic to sulfonamides, NSAIDs, or aspirin. Side effects include headache, dyspepsia, and diarrhea.

Hypnotics and Sedatives

A **hypnotic** is a medication that produces sleep. It is usually taken at bedtime. A **sedative** is a medication that has a calming or quieting effect. Depending on the dose, medications in this class can have either a hypnotic or sedative effect. To achieve a calming or relaxing effect, small does of sedatives may be administered throughout the day. If given in a large dose at bedtime, a sedative's calming effect may induce sleep.

The ideal hypnotic acts quickly, brings a natural sleep without "hangover," is nonaddictive, and has few or no harmful, adverse effects. The search for this medication has resulted in the manufacture of hundreds of barbiturates, only a few of which approximate these requirements.

Barbiturates

Barbiturates are derived from barbituric acid and have, in the past, been referred to as "sleeping pills." However, the use of barbiturates to produce sleep has greatly decreased since the advent of the benzodiazepines. Nonetheless, some barbiturates are still prescribed. The action of barbiturates is classified as long acting (10 to 16 hours), intermediate acting (6 to 8 hours), or short acting (3 to 4 hours). Long-acting barbiturates, such as phenobarbital (Luminal), are used to control and prevent seizure activity. Intermediate-acting barbiturates, such as amobarbital (Amytal), are used primarily as daytime or day-surgery sedatives and for their sedative effects during labor or before anesthesia. Short-acting barbiturates, such as secobarbital (Seconal), are used primarily at bedtime, or as a pre-anesthetic, because there is less "hangover" due to their short-acting effect (3 to 4 hours). Barbiturates are easily absorbed and can be given orally or parenterally. They are pregnancy category D agents and Schedule II Drugs, subject to the Controlled Substances Act (see Chapter 61).

When barbiturates are used as hypnotics, they interfere with normal sleep patterns, including the dream state identified with rapid eye movement (REM). If barbiturates are used for prolonged periods, REM states return. On discontinuation of the medication, however, the client once again experiences a decrease in REM sleep.

Commonly experienced side effects include "morning hangover" reactions, drowsiness, lethargy, mood change, and depression. Caution clients not to operate machinery. Alcohol potentiates the action of barbiturates.

Clients using barbiturates for extended periods may develop a physical dependency on them. Cessation of barbiturates may cause major withdrawal symptoms that vary with the length of time barbiturates have been administered as well as the dosage used. Stay alert for alterations in vital signs and for hallucinations, delirium, and seizures. Taper doses slowly and never discontinue barbiturate therapy abruptly (see Chapter 94).

☛ KEY CONCEPT

Habituation or addiction to many drugs, especially narcotics and barbiturates, is common. Be alert to this possibility when working with any client. Chapter 94 describes the abuse of many of these drugs and discusses chemical dependency treatment.

Benzodiazepines

In addition to barbiturates, many other medications, including *benzodiazepines,* are used as hypnotics and sedatives. The benzodiazepines were first introduced in the 1960s. They are very safe medications, when compared with barbiturates. A wide margin of safety exists between therapeutic and toxic dosages. In addition to their sedative and hypnotic effects, some benzodiazepines are used as anticonvulsant agents. Others are effective against anxiety. Most of the drugs in this group are pregnancy category D agents. Benzodiazepines are primarily Schedule IV drugs, subject to the Controlled Substances Act.

Common side effects are similar to those of the barbiturates. They include "morning hangover," drowsiness, and lethargy. They also interfere with normal REM sleep.

Because of the risk for addiction, monitor the administration of benzodiazepines closely. If clients discontinue these medications rapidly, severe withdrawal symptoms, similar to those that accompany the abrupt withdrawal of barbiturates, may occur. Withdrawal symptoms may be delayed, possibly appearing several days after discontinuation. For this reason, the dosage of these medications are tapered gradually over 2 to 3 weeks.

Flurazepam (Dalmane), a long-acting benzodiazepine, is useful in the treatment of insomnia. Smokers may metabolize it more quickly. Women taking oral contraceptives may metabolize it more slowly. *Temazepam* (Restoril) is an intermediate-acting hypnotic used to treat insomnia. *Triazolam* (Halcion), a short-acting benzodiazepine, is used primarily as a hypnotic. However, because of the numerous serious side effects, this drug is rarely used today. *Diazepam* (Valium), also a benzodiazepine, is not prescribed often today because of its high potential for abuse.

Midazolam (Versed), a short-acting benzodiazepine, is used mainly as a relaxant and amnesiac preoperatively and during induction of anesthesia. The onset of action with IV administration is 3 to 5 minutes. Afterward, the person usually does not remember the procedure.

Miscellaneous Hypnotics and Sedatives

Many medications can be used for their sedative and hypnotic actions. Several of these medications (including chloral hydrate and paraldehyde) are not classified as either barbiturates or benzodiazepines. These medications affect REM sleep. Clients also may develop a tolerance to them. Prolonged use may lead to addiction.

Side effects are similar to those of the barbiturates and benzodiazepines, including drowsiness, "morning hangover," anxiety, restlessness, generalized weakness, mental depression, hallucinations, delirium, and seizure activity. These medications must be tapered slowly over 2 to 4 weeks to minimize withdrawal symptoms.

Chloral hydrate (Noctec), a pregnancy category C agent, is the oldest of the hypnotics. When mixed with alcohol, this medication has been called "knock-out drops." It is often given to older clients because of its relative safety. It is also used as preoperative sedation because it does not depress respirations or the cough reflex. Its major side effects are gastric irritation and its unpleasant taste; gelcap forms are now available.

Paraldehyde (Paral) is available only in liquid form for oral or rectal administration. It has a very bitter taste and causes a strong, unpleasant breath odor for many hours after ingestion. It is used for its sedative effect, particularly in clients experiencing delirium tremens (DTs) during alcohol withdrawal and detoxification. It may be used to help detoxify pregnant women because it is a category C agent. (Many of the other drugs used for detoxification are category D agents.) *It is important to note that the current goal of therapy is to prevent DTs.*

Paraldehyde may be administered in milk or fruit juice to make it more palatable. Using a straw also may help. It should only be administered in a glass container and should not come into contact with metal, such as a spoon.

Ethchlorvynol (Placidyl), a pregnancy category C agent, is used mainly for its hypnotic effect in the treatment of insomnia. It should be used for short-term treatment only.

Anticonvulsants

Seizures, involuntary and abnormal nervous system activity, are indicative of disorders associated with changes in the brain's electrical activity. The most serious seizure disorders are classified as *epilepsy.* **Anticonvulsants** are CNS depressants that help prevent or control various types of seizure activity, such as tonic-clonic, petit mal, Jacksonian, and complex partial-type seizures. (See Chapter 77 for further discussion of seizure disorders.)

The dosage of anticonvulsant medications is usually adjusted for the individual client, with gradually increasing dosages administered until the desired blood level is achieved or until seizure activity is controlled. Many of these medications require periodic dosage adjustment with prolonged use. Most of these drugs are pregnancy category D agents.

One of the most commonly used anticonvulsants is *phenytoin* (Dilantin). It depresses the brain's sensory areas located in the motor cortex. It is available in tablet, capsule, suspension, and injectable forms. Its most common side effects include muscular incoordination, dizziness, gastric irritation, weight loss, and skin rash.

Clonazepam (Klonopin), a benzodiazepine, is most commonly used for the treatment of petit mal and absence seizures. It is also used in psychiatry, to help calm an anxious client. Common side effects include alterations in behavior, incoordination, and drowsiness. Clients may build up resistance or tolerance to clonazepam.

Carbamazepine (Tegretol) is primarily used to control seizures. However, it has many serious side effects, including heart failure, liver dysfunction, and urinary retention. Lesser side effects include gastric distress, nausea, and vomiting. This medication should not be used if other, less toxic medications are effective to control a client's seizures.

Diazepam (Valium), a benzodiazepine, has been used parenterally for the control of acute seizure activity. A serious adverse reaction that may occur with IV administration is respiratory arrest. Monitor the client's vital signs frequently. Have resuscitation equipment readily available. Diazepam can be used in conjunction with other medications for treatment of seizures. However, used singularly, it is not the medication of choice. Diazepam is also used to manage severe alcohol withdrawal symptoms (see Chap. 94).

Magnesium sulfate is generally used in emergencies to prevent or to treat seizure activity associated with pregnancy-induced hypertension (**PIH**). It is a pregnancy category A agent, making it relatively safe for use in pregnancy. When administered IV, it has an immediate onset of action; however, its duration is approximately 30 minutes. Magnesium sulfate is not generally used to treat seizure activity associated with epilepsy. Toxicity can occur.

Adrenergic Medications

An adrenergic is epinephrine or a substance that acts like epinephrine. Adrenergics mimic the actions of the sympathetic division of the autonomic nervous system (ANS) and, thus, are referred to as sympathomimetics. The major classifications of adrenergics are catecholamines and non-catecholamines.

Catecholamines
Catecholamines are neurotransmitters that play an important part in the body's response to stress. The release of catecholamines at sympathetic nerve endings increases cardiac output (by increasing the strength of contraction of cardiac muscle), constricts peripheral blood vessels, increases blood pressure, and causes bronchodilation. Epinephrine and norepinephrine are catecholamines.

Epinephrine. *Epinephrine's* (Adrenaline) major sympathomimetic action is to constrict peripheral blood vessels. It may be applied locally or administered parenterally. Local application constricts blood vessels and controls capillary bleeding; however, it does not control hemorrhage from larger vessels. Given parenterally, it increases heart rate, raises blood pressure, constricts surface blood vessels, and relaxes smooth muscles in the respiratory tract, causing bronchial dilation. It is the medication of choice for treatment of *anaphylactic* (severe allergic) and hypersensitivity reactions. Epinephrine's bronchodilating effect is also helpful in treating airway obstruction caused by acute asthma attacks, bronchitis, and emphysema. Epinephrine may also be used to reverse cardiac arrest.

Epinephrine is extremely potent, and very small doses are needed to be effective. It is available for subcutaneous (subQ) and IV injection. Its onset of action is almost immediate; however, its duration of action is short, lasting only about 30 minutes. Monitor the client's vital signs. Major side effects include restlessness, nervousness, tachycardia, heart palpitations, dizziness, pallor, tremors, nausea, vomiting, and severe headache. Reassure the client that these reactions are temporary, common side effects. Clients with existing heart disease, hypertension, hyperthyroidism, or diabetes may be more sensitive to epinephrine's adverse effects. Epinephrine crosses the placental barrier and is also secreted in breast milk. A pregnancy category C agent, it is contraindicated during pregnancy and in the woman who is breastfeeding. However, it may be used in an emergency.

Norepinephrine. *Norepinephrine* (Levarterenol, Levophed) is a potent sympathetic neurotransmitter. Its primary action is to increase blood pressure as a result of vasoconstriction of peripheral blood vessels. Increased blood pressure slows the heart rate. Norepinephrine may be used to treat heart failure.

Norepinephrine, a pregnancy category D agent, is available in parenteral form. Side effects include bradycardia and hypotension. Overdose can lead to seizures and severe hypertension. If not administered properly or if IV infiltration occurs, norepinephrine can cause sloughing of tissue. This medication should not be used in the presence of hemorrhage.

Non-catecholamines
Dopamine. *Dopamine hydrochloride* (Dopamine), also a sympathomimetic agent, is not classified as a catecholamine. It is an adrenergic agonist that affects the contractility of the heart muscle and increases blood pressure. It is used to treat severe shock and hypotension. Dopamine is available for IV administration. Side effects include restlessness, nervousness, headache, tachycardia, palpitations, and anginal-type chest pain. The client who is receiving dopamine requires close monitoring.

Other Sympathomimetic Agents. A number of other sympathomimetic amines are available. They often are used to relieve bronchospasm or symptoms of asthma. These agents will be discussed later in this chapter.

MEDICATIONS THAT AFFECT THE ENDOCRINE SYSTEM

The glands of the endocrine system secrete hormones that the bloodstream carries to various target organs, where they have specific regulating effects. Hormone replacement therapy (**HRT**) is given to reduce symptoms caused by various hormonal deficiencies. Endocrine disorders and examples of hormonal agents are discussed in Chapter 78.

Thyroid Replacement Hormones

Thyroid preparations are used to treat primary hypothyroidism and for clients who have had a thyroidectomy. Thyroid replacement hormones consist of one or both thyroid hormones: thyroxine (T_4) and triiodothyronine (T_3).

Steroids

Steroids include the adrenocortical hormones produced by the adrenal glands. The most common adrenocortical hormone is *cortisone,* a very effective anti-inflammatory agent. In addition, steroids have immunosuppressive and salt-retaining effects.

Prolonged cortisone therapy has many serious side effects. The client and family must be aware of these side effects to cope with changes, particularly those related to physical appearance. For example, GI upset may occur. Therefore, administer steroids with food to prevent or to reduce gastric upset. In addition, the client may take antacids with steroid therapy to prevent GI upset or gastric ulcer formation. The client and family also must be able to recognize signs and symptoms of more serious side effects, such as thrombophlebitis. Reassure the client that most of these side effects will disappear on discontinuation of steroid therapy. In Practice: Educating the Client 62-1 lists important side effects associated with long-term steroid therapy.

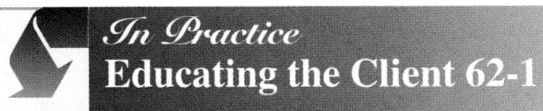

In Practice
Educating the Client 62-1

Side Effects of Long-term Steroid Therapy

- Feelings of euphoria, general well-being
- Increased appetite and subsequent weight gain
- Bruising
- *Hirsutism* (increased facial and body hair)
- Aggravation of adolescent acne
- Generalized weakness
- Hypertension
- Elevated blood glucose levels
- Increased susceptibility to infection
- Cataract formation
- Thrombophlebitis or embolism (or both)
- *Moon facies* (puffy, round face)
- Buffalo hump
- Osteoporosis

Prolonged steroid therapy should be discontinued gradually using a tapered dose system. The effect of negative feedback on the adrenal glands controls the release of naturally occurring cortisone. If cortisone is administered artificially, the adrenal glands are not stimulated to produce this hormone. If cortisone therapy is discontinued abruptly, the adrenal glands are unable to produce sufficient amounts of naturally occurring cortisone until they have, by way of negative feedback, received the message and responded. In the meantime, the client could suffer adrenal crisis, a life-threatening condition requiring immediate intervention.

Prednisone, hydrocortisone (Cortef), and *prednisolone* (Hydrocortone) are examples of other steroidal anti-inflammatory medications. They should be used with caution in individuals with peptic ulcers because of the increased risk for worsening the ulcer. They are contraindicated for individuals with serious infections, such as tuberculosis, because these agents interfere with the immune response.

Insulin

One of the best known replacement hormones is **insulin.** Insulin, produced by the beta cells of the islets of Langerhans in the pancreas, is essential for carbohydrate metabolism. Several types of insulin preparations exist, and new types are being developed constantly. Newer products have fewer allergic properties than older insulins. Insulins are supplied that have various lengths of onset and duration of action. Insulin must be administered subQ (hydrochloric acid in the stomach destroys its action). Only regular insulin can be administered IV. All insulins are now supplied in the U-100 dosage (100 units of insulin per 1 mL).

Clients with type 2 diabetes may control the disease's symptoms by using oral hypoglycemic agents. These agents are not insulin derivatives. They have a number of actions, one of which is the lowering of blood glucose levels by stimulating the pancreas to release available insulin. Chapter 78 discusses diabetes, specific types of insulin and administration, and oral hypoglycemic agents in greater detail.

MEDICATIONS THAT AFFECT THE SENSORY SYSTEM

Medications Affecting the Eye

Ophthalmic medications include agents that dilate or constrict the pupil, antibiotics, and agents that reduce intraocular pressure. Some ophthalmic medications produce their effects by causing the ANS to relax and to contract smooth muscle. Others act directly on eye tissues. *Only those medications clearly marked "for ophthalmic use" should be used in the eyes.*

Mydriatics and Miotics
Mydriatics are ophthalmic preparations used to dilate pupils. They are used primarily during physical examination of the eye. Examples include cyclopentolate (Cyclogel) and homatropine.

Miotics are ophthalmic preparations used to constrict pupils. Examples include dapiprazole (Rev-Eyes) and carbachol (Carbostat). A direct-acting miotic agent that can be used to counteract the drug-induced mydriasis is pilocarpine (Pilocar, Piloptic).

Ophthalmic Antibiotics

Eye infections may be treated with antibiotics or sulfonamides specific to the causative organism and prepared for ophthalmic use in the form of solutions or ointments. Examples include: bacitracin (AK-Tracin), chloramphenicol (Chloromycetin ophthalmic), polymixin B sulfate, natamycin (Natacyn), and gentamicin sulfate (Garamycin).

Agents That Reduce Intraocular Pressure

Elevations in *intraocular* (within the eyeball) pressure can occur, leading to glaucoma or ocular hypertension. *Glaucoma* refers to a group of disorders characterized by an increase in intraocular pressure. The most common type of adult primary glaucoma is open-angle glaucoma. Another type is angle-closure glaucoma, which can be acute or chronic. *Ocular hypertension* is a situation in which intraocular pressure is elevated without any other signs of glaucoma.

A number of medications can be used to treat ocular hypertension and the various types of glaucoma. These may include brimonidine tartrate (Alphagan), brinzolamide (Azopt), demecarium (Humorsol), dipivefrin (Propine, AK Pro), dorzolamide (Trusopt), echothiopate (Phospholine iodide), latanoprost (Xalatan), levobetaxolol (Betaxon), levobunolol (AK Beta, Betagan), metipranolol (OptiPranolol), and unoprostone isopropyl (Resula). Epinephrine (Adrenaline) also may be used to decrease production of aqueous humor.

Other Ophthalmic Medications

Diclofenac (Voltaren ophthalmic) is used in incisional refractive surgery (LASIK), to offset photophobia. Azelastine (Optivar), emedastine (Emadine), fluorometholone (Flarex), ketotifen (Zadito), levocabastine (Livostin), and pemirolast K (Alamast) are used to treat allergic conjunctivitis.

Medications Affecting the Ear

Most medications that affect the ears are applied directly to them to treat localized conditions. Commonly used medications include anti-infectives (to treat ear infections), analgesics (to treat the pain of otitis media, especially for children), and *cerumenolytics* (to loosen and remove impacted earwax). Chapter 79 describes disorders of the sensory system and their treatment in more detail.

MEDICATIONS THAT AFFECT THE CARDIOVASCULAR SYSTEM

Some cardiovascular medications are used for their effects on the heart's action. Others are used for their effects on blood vessels. Medications that stimulate or strengthen the heart's pumping action are called *cardiotonics*. Medications that regulate heart rhythm are called *antiarrhythmics*. Medications

that primarily act on the blood vessels are called *vasoconstrictors* (constrict or narrow the blood vessels) and *vasodilators* (dilate or widen blood vessels). Often, vasodilators are used to control blood pressure. In addition, a number of other medications are used to control blood pressure. Table 62-4 lists common medications used for the cardiovascular system. Cardiovascular disorders and their treatment are discussed in Chapter 80.

Cardiotonics

Cardiotonics are heart stimulants. Commonly used cardiotonics include digoxin (Lanoxin), a derivative of the digitalis leaf. Their main action is to strengthen the force of ventricular contractions, and in doing so, to increase cardiac output. In turn, increased cardiac output results in a slower heart rate and less heart workload. Digoxin is available in oral and parenteral forms. Dosages of digoxin (digitalis) vary according to individual needs. The initial dose, called the *digitalizing dose,* is designed to reduce the heart rate to the desired rate of 60 to 80 beats/min. When a stabilizing dose maintains desired heart rate, the client is placed on a *maintenance dose,* administered daily. Most clients taking digitalis continue the medication for life.

Because heart rate slows in response to digitalis, the *apical pulse* rate is counted for *1 full minute before administration.* If the client's heart rate is below 60 beats per minute, or if irregularities in heart rhythm are present, withhold the medication and report the information. Observe the client receiving digitalis closely for toxicity. Overdose of digitalis can dangerously lower heart rate or cause cardiac arrest. Signs and symptoms of toxicity or overdose include nausea, vomiting, headache, premature ventricular contractions, diarrhea, confusion, drowsiness, blurred vision, or visual disturbances in which lights appear much brighter than they really are, or appear to have halos around them.

> **Nursing Alert**
> Digoxin doses are very small (0.125–0.425 mg/d). Therefore, even a small overdose could be fatal. A similar medication called digitoxin is seldom used today. However, the doses are different. Make sure you know what medication you are giving.

Antiarrhythmics

Antiarrhythmics act on the heart's electrical conduction system to regulate and slow heart rate. *Quinidine sulfate* (Quinidine) is an antiarrhythmic used to treat atrial arrhythmias. Quinidine's action regulates the number of times the atria contract in a given period. It may be administered orally or IM. Side effects include dizziness, headache, ventricular tachycardia, angina, bradycardia, and nausea.

Procainamide hydrochloride (Pronestyl) is used to treat atrial fibrillation; however, it is more commonly used for ventricular arrhythmias, such as ventricular tachycardia or premature ventricular contractions. It can be administered orally, IM,

▪▪▪ TABLE 62-4 𝒮ELECTED CARDIOVASCULAR SYSTEM MEDICATIONS

Name of Medication*	Usual Adult Dose	Notes
Cardiotonic		
digoxin (Lanoxin)	Oral or IV: maintenance dose of 0.125–0.25 mg/d Digitalizing dose: 0.75–1.25 mg/d	Toxicity increased with low potassium levels
Antiarrhythmics		
bretylium (Bretylol)	IV: 5–10 mg/kg, q15–30 min; may use up to 30 mg/kg (may be repeated)	Given slowly in nonemergency situations
disopyramide (Norpace)	Oral: 200–300 mg initially; then 100–150 mg q6h	Depressed contractility of heart
lidocaine (Xylocaine)	IV: 50–100 mg initially, then drip at 1–5 mg/min (may be repeated in emergency)	Action primarily on ventricles; increased toxicity with reduced hepatic function
procainamide (Pronestyl, Procan)	Oral: 250–500 mg q4h (IV for emergency)	Half life of 4h; adverse effects include arthritis-like symptoms
propranolol (Inderal)	Oral: 10–80 mg b.i.d. to q.i.d. Long acting: 80–160 mg/d IV: 1 mg/min up to 10 mg	Decreased conduction, contractility, and automaticity of heart
quinidine sulfate	Oral and IM: 200–400 mg q.i.d.	Similar in action to procainamide; GI distress common
verapamil HCl (Calan, Isoptin)	Oral: 240–320 mg/d in divided doses IV: 0.075–0.15 mg/kg	Calcium-channel blocker; depresses phase 4 of depolarization of heart
Vasoconstrictors and Sympathomimetics†		
dobutamine (Dobutrex)	2.5–10 mcg (μg)/kg/min‡	Less increase in heart rate and cardiac arrhythmias than with other drugs
dopamine (Intropin)	IV: 2–5 mcg (μg)/kg/min (higher doses in emergency)‡	Resultant increased cardiac output and renal blood flow
epinephrine (Adrenalin HCl)	IM or subQ: 0.5 mL of 1:1,000 solution IV: Used in cardiac arrest	Used in *anaphylaxis* (severe allergic reaction) and as *hemostat* (to stop bleeding)
isoproterenol (Isuprel)	IV: 1–10 mcg (μg)/min‡	Cardiac contractility stimulated; increased heart rate and cardiac output
levarterenol, norepinephrine (Levophed)	IV: 2–4 mcg (μg)/min‡	Restored blood pressure in acute hypotensive states
metaraminol (Aramine)	IV: 0.5–5 mg direct IV to restore BP in severe shock Infusion: 15–100 mg in 250–500 mL IV fluid to maintain BP	Increased blood pressure but heart rate usually decreased; may be used as infusion
Vasodilators and Antianginal Agents		
amyl nitrate	Inhalation: Up to 0.3 mL	Relief of acute angina; excessive side effects limit use; may be abused
cyclandelate (Cyclospasmol)	Oral: 200–400 mg b.i.d. to q.i.d.	Direct action on smooth muscle to relax blood vessels
isosorbide dinitrate (Isordil, Sorbitrate)	Oral: 5–30 mg q.i.d. Sublingual: 2.5–10 mg q.i.d.	Prophylactic use in angina pectoris
isosorbide mononitrate (Ismo, Imdur)	Oral: 10–20 mg b.i.d. (regular release); 30–120 mg/d (extended release)	Antianginal agent Regular release form given twice/d, 7 h apart

■■■ **TABLE 62-4** 𝒮ELECTED CARDIOVASCULAR SYSTEM MEDICATIONS (CONTINUED)

Name of Medication*	Usual Adult Dose	Notes
minoxidil§ (Loniten)	Oral: 5–40 mg/d in single dose	Direct-acting vasodilator (major side effect is unusual hair growth)
nitroglycerin (Nitrostat)	Sublingual (most common route): 0.15–0.6 mg PRN for chest pain	Drug of choice in angina; rapid action, short duration
nitroglycerin ointment (Nitro-Bid, Nitrol)	Topical: 1-in spread, usually over chest area; q6h	Prophylactic use; excess dose may cause headache
nitroglycerin transdermal (Nitro-Dur, Transderm Nitro)	Topical: 0.1–0.6 mg/h	Patch applied once daily; alternate application sites; use a location with minimal hair
verapamil (Calan)	Oral: 80–120 mg t.i.d. IV: for acute MI	Used for vasospastic and unstable angina at rest
Antihypertensives atenolol (Tenormin)	Oral: 25–100 mg q d	Used alone or with diuretics; acts mostly on the heart
captopril (Capoten)	Oral: 12.5–50 mg 2–3 times/d (take 1 h before meals)	ACE inhibitor; combined with thiazide diuretics to lower blood pressure. Also used for heart failure.
clonidine (Catapres)	Oral: 0.1–0.4 mg b.i.d. Transdermal patch: Sustained release over 7 d (dose individualized) Continuous epidural infusion for pain management	Sedative effects minimized by bedtime administration
enalapril (Vasotec)	Oral: 2.5–40 mg, single or in two divided doses IV: 0.625–1.25 mg q6h	ACE inhibitor; used for heart failure and hypertension
labetalol (Normodyne)	Oral: 50–300 mg b.i.d. IV: individualized dose based on supine BP	Beta blocker; lowered peripheral resistance with direct action on the heart
lisinopril (Prinivil, Zestril)	Oral: 10 mg/d (max: 20–40 mg/d) IV: 200–400 mg b.i.d.	ACE inhibitor; blockade of angiotensin (a vasoconstrictor), causing vasodilation, increased serum potassium, and sodium and fluid excretion Used in hypertension and as adjunct in CHF
methyldopa (Aldomet) (IV: methyldopate)	Oral and IV: Initial 250 mg b.i.d.; may increase to 500 mg q.i.d. Switch to oral as soon as possible	Drowsiness possible during first days of therapy; with prolonged use, patients can develop positive Coombs' test (indicative of blood disorder)
metoprolol (Lopressor)	Oral: 50–100 mg/d or b.i.d. IV: for acute MI	Action mostly on the heart; beta blocker without side effects of bronchospasm
nadolol (Corgard)	Oral: 40–80 mg q d (may give up to 320 mg/d)	Beta blocker; contraindicated in patients with asthma or bronchospasm
nitroprusside sodium (Nitropress)	IV: 3 mcg/kg/min (may go up to 10 mcg/kg/min)‡	Used in hypertensive crisis—for immediate lowering of blood pressure; and in cyanide toxicity with overdose
prazosin (Minipress)	Oral: Initial 1 mg 2–3 times/d, may increase to 2–5 mg t.i.d.	Reduced peripheral vascular resistance (possible postural hypotension and syncope with first dose; give first dose at bedtime); adrenergic blocker

(continued)

■■■ **TABLE 62-4** 𝒮ELECTED CARDIOVASCULAR SYSTEM MEDICATIONS (CONTINUED)

Name of Medication*	Usual Adult Dose	Notes
propranolol (Inderal)	Oral: 40–240 mg b.i.d. (tablets) (Available ER, SR, and oral concentration liquid) IV form used for life-threatening arrhythmias	Used to treat arrhythmia, angina, migraine, and stage fright; not indicated for asthmatic clients (can cause bronchospasm); beta blocker
verapamil (Calan)	Oral: 80–120 mg t.i.d. (available as SR, ER) IV used in emergency	Calcium-channel blocker (effects observed in first week)

*A trade name appears in parentheses following the generic name of the medication.

†These medications mimic the action of the sympathetic nervous system; they are used to raise blood pressure.

‡This dosage is given in micrograms (μg); a *microgram* is one thousandth of a milligram.

§Minoxidil is also available in 2% topical solution to treat baldness, called Rogaine.

or IV. Side effects include anorexia, nausea, vomiting, skin rash, urticaria (hives), and arthralgia (joint pain).

Verapamil hydrochloride (Isoptin, Verelan, Calan) is the only calcium channel blocker approved for cardiac arrhythmias. It also has antianginal and antihypertensive effects. Verapamil hydrochloride slows the electrical conduction rate of the atrioventricular (AV) node, resulting in a slower heart rate and decreased cardiac workload. Side effects include bradycardia, heart block, and constipation.

Propranolol hydrochloride (Inderal) reduces the irritability of the myocardium and decreases heart rate and the force of ventricular contraction. It results in increased cardiac output and lowered blood pressure. Increased cardiac output improves coronary circulation, which is effective in decreasing vasoconstriction, spasm, and pain associated with angina pectoris. By decreasing the irritability of the myocardium, propranolol is also effective in treating and preventing atrial arrhythmias such as atrial flutter and atrial fibrillation. Propranolol hydrochloride may be administered orally or IV. Side effects include dizziness, fainting, drowsiness, insomnia, weakness, confusion, mental depression, vivid dreams, and loss of libido. Propranolol also is used to prevent migraine headaches and to treat essential tremor, and to help prevent a recurrent MI.

Lidocaine hydrochloride (Xylocaine) is used to treat life-threatening ventricular arrhythmias following MI. It is only available for this use in IV or IM forms and should only be used in intensive care settings.

Other antiarrhythmics include: acebutolol HCL (Sectral), adenosine (Adenocard), disopyramide phosphate (Norpace), dofetilide (Tikosyn), flecainide acetate (Tambocor), ibutilide fumarate (Corvert), and tocainide HCL (Tonocard). The antiarrhythmics are generally pregnancy category C agents.

Medications That Affect the Blood Vessels

Many abnormal conditions can affect the body's arteries and veins. Medications that constrict blood vessels are referred to as *vasoconstrictors;* those that dilate the blood vessels are called *vasodilators.*

Vasoconstrictors

Vasoconstrictors (vasopressors) are used to control superficial hemorrhage, to increase the heart's pumping action, to raise blood pressure, and to relieve nasal congestion.

Norepinephrine bitartrate (Levophed, Levarterenol) is a potent medication used to raise and to sustain blood pressure in acute states of hypotension, such as those caused by hemorrhage or shock. It also is used in cardiac arrest. Given IV in solution, this medication should be administered only in intensive care units.

Metaraminol bitartrate (Aramine), a pregnancy category D agent, indirectly affects the release of norepinephrine, to raise blood pressure. It is used to prevent hypotension or to raise or maintain blood pressure in cases of hemorrhage, hypotension related to spinal anesthesia, trauma, and surgical complications. It may be given IV in a solution of normal saline or it may be given subQ or IM.

Phenylephrine hydrochloride (Neo-Synephrine), a pregnancy category C agent, relieves congestion in mucous membranes. It is also used to treat some types of shock and to raise and stabilize blood pressure. It is available in ophthalmic solution, as chewable tablets, as a decongestant nasal spray, and for injection.

Vasodilators

Medications that dilate blood vessels are used to treat peripheral blood vessel disease, coronary artery disease, and hypertension (**HTN**). **Vasodilators** increase the lumen size of blood vessels and thereby increase blood flow.

Nitrates.   *Nitrates* have been used for many years to treat and to prevent acute episodes of angina pectoris (heart pain). The nitrates dilate blood vessels, particularly in the coronary arteries, by inducing relaxation of peripheral vascular smooth muscle fibers located in the walls of blood vessels. The increased blood flow to myocardial tissue decreases the constriction and spasm of the coronary blood vessels, increases blood flow to the affected tissue, and reduces or relieves the pain associated with angina.

Nitroglycerin (**NTG**), a pregnancy category C agent, is a potent vasodilator and has long been the treatment of choice for acute angina pectoris. Mucous membranes quickly absorb nitroglycerin. Symptom relief usually occurs within 1 to 2 minutes. The duration of action is approximately 30 minutes.

Nitroglycerin is available in several forms, including tablets (for *sublingual* [under the tongue] administration; Nitrostat, Nitroquick) and a spray (for *translingual* administration [sprayed onto the tongue]; Nitrolingual). The tablet form can also be placed in the buccal pouch (cheek), or between the lip and the gum above the incisors. These methods provide immediate symptom relief. Nitroglycerin is also available in long-acting capsules (Nitroglyn, Nitrong), as an ointment for topical administration (Nitrobid), as transdermal patches (Nitro-Dur, Transderm-Nitro), or in IV solution (Nitro-Bid IV, Tridil). Nitroglycerin should be protected from exposure to light. The expiration date is important, because the shelf life of conventional sublingual nitroglycerin tablets is approximately 6 months after initially opening the bottle. The tablet should fizz when placed in the mouth. Tablets should not be crushed or chewed. Sustained-release forms should be given with water. The translingual spray should *not be inhaled*.

> ### Nursing Alert
> Clients who have recently had a myocardial infarction or who have severe asthma, angle closure glaucoma, severe anemia, increased intracranial pressure, or hypotension should not use nitroglycerin.

Amyl nitrate, a pregnancy category C agent, is an antianginal drug used most frequently for the treatment of acute angina. It relaxes the smooth muscles of blood vessel walls, causing vasodilation and increased blood supply to affected myocardial tissue. It is administered by inhalation. It is supplied in liquid form contained in a glass capsule that is wrapped in a protective cloth covering. When administering amyl nitrate, crush the capsule between the thumb and finger and pass the substance back and forth under the client's nose. Amyl nitrate has a very strong, disagreeable odor. Its vasodilating effect is immediate and lasts approximately 3 to 5 minutes. Side effects include nausea, vomiting, headache, dizziness, and flushing. The drug should be protected from light and kept in a cool place. Alcohol use should also be avoided.

Other Vasodilators.   *Hydralazine* (Apresoline), a pregnancy category C agent, relaxes arterial smooth muscle, causing vasodilation. As a result, blood pressure is lowered. It is available in forms appropriate for oral and parenteral administration. Side effects include headache, palpitation, fluid retention, nausea, and vomiting.

Prazosin HCL (Minipress) acts by reducing peripheral vascular resistance, allowing arteries and veins to dilate, thus lowering blood pressure. It is used to treat chronic hypertension. Unlike other agents, such as phentolamine, prazosin does not cause reflex tachycardia. It is available in capsules for oral administration. Side effects include shortness of breath, *orthostatic hypotension* (sudden drop in blood pressure on standing),

pounding heartbeat, fluid retention, dizziness, headache, and drowsiness. Because of the tendency of prazosin to cause fluid retention, it is often prescribed with a diuretic.

Antihypertensives

Medications specifically used to reduce blood pressure on an ongoing basis are called **antihypertensives.** Some antihypertensive agents have been discussed previously. Other medications used for the treatment of chronic hypertension, or in conjunction with other antihypertensives, include diuretics, beta blockers, and calcium channel blockers.

Diuretics
Diuretics are medications that increase the amount of urine excreted by the kidneys. Thus, they decrease the fluid volume circulating in the body, thereby lowering blood pressure. Indications for use of diuretics include edema, hypertension, heart failure, and pregnancy-induced hypertension. One side effect of some diuretics is excessive excretion of potassium (K^+). These diuretics are termed *potassium-wasting diuretics. Hydrochlorothiazide* (HydroDIURIL, **HCTZ**) and *furosemide* (Lasix) are examples of potassium-wasting diuretics. In this case, the client will most likely require supplemental potassium (furnished in several oral forms). Thus, the potassium levels of clients who are taking diuretics are closely monitored. Diuretics also increase sodium excretion, thereby reducing edema. Most diuretics are pregnancy category C agents.

Some diuretics such as *amiloride HCL* (Midamor), *spironolactone* (Aldactone) and *triamterene* (Dyrenium), and the combination *triamterene/hydrochlorothiazide* (Dyazide) are *potassium sparing.* Their action on the kidney tubules promotes potassium reabsorption. Nonetheless, monitor potassium levels.

Beta (β) Blockers
Blood vessels contain adrenergic-blocking receptors, called alpha (α) and beta (β) receptors. Stimulation of alpha receptors causes vasoconstriction, whereas stimulation of beta receptors causes vasodilation. The heart has mainly beta receptors. β adrenergic blockers, pregnancy category C agents, are commonly used as first-line therapy for hypertension. They act directly to decrease heart rate, by depressing atrioventricular node conduction and decreasing the strength of myocardial contraction. Thus, they decrease blood pressure. *Propranolol* (Inderal), *atenolol* (Tenormin), *bisoprolol fumerate* (Zebeta), *carteolol HCl* (Ocupress), *penbutolol* (Levatol) and *metoprolol tartrate* (Lopressor) are examples of β blockers commonly used to treat hypertension.

Calcium Channel Blockers
Calcium channel blockers, pregnancy category C agents, inhibit or block movement of calcium ions across cell membranes, reducing peripheral vascular resistance and resulting in lowered blood pressure. *Diltiazem* (Cardizem) is used to treat chronic hypertension. It is available for oral and IV

administration. Side effects include headache, fatigue, bradycardia, dizziness, and weakness. *Nifedipine* (Procardia) and *verapamil* (Calan) are used to treat hypertension and angina. Verapamil is also used to treat arrhythmias.

Other calcium channel blockers include amlodipine (Norvasc), felodipine (Plendil), isradipine (DynaCirc), and nisoldipine (Sular).

Angiotensin-Converting Enzyme (ACE) Inhibitors

Angiotensin-converting enzyme (**ACE**) inhibitors are medications that reduce peripheral vascular resistance in the hypertensive client by blocking the activation of angiotensin, a powerful vasoconstrictor. ACE inhibitors are often used alone or in combination with thiazide diuretics. They are the most widely prescribed antihypertensive agents. Examples include *captopril* (Capoten), *enalapril* (Vasotec), and *lisinopril* (Prinivil, Zestril). ACE inhibitors are typically pregnancy category C or category D agents.

Miscellaneous Agents

Guanethidine monosulfate (Ismelin) is a potent antihypertensive used to treat chronic and renal hypertension. Side effects include orthostatic hypotension, dizziness, fainting, and bradycardia. Instruct clients to monitor their blood pressure regularly, and caution them to rise slowly from the sitting position. *Methyldopa* (Aldomet) reduces blood pressure by lowering peripheral vascular resistance. These drugs are pregnancy category C agents.

Diazoxide (Hyperstat) relaxes the smooth muscles located in the arterial wall. It is used only in hypertensive emergencies and is administered by IV push. A major side effect is severe hypotension.

MEDICATIONS THAT AFFECT THE BLOOD

Blood is composed of plasma, erythrocytes (red blood cells [RBCs]), leukocytes (white blood cells [WBCs]), and platelets. Erythrocytes carry a substance called *hemoglobin,* the main component of which is iron. When combined with oxygen, *oxyhemoglobin* forms. The circulatory system transports oxyhemoglobin to the body cells, providing them with oxygen. Normally, a balanced diet provides essential iron and other nutrients necessary for blood formation. Blood and lymph disorders are discussed in Chapter 81.

Other medications and products also affect the blood, assisting in blood clotting or preventing clots from forming, and serving to replace blood volume or components lost by events such as hemorrhage.

Iron Replacement Preparations

The adult male only needs small amounts (15 mg) of daily iron intake. Premenopausal and pregnant women need up to four times as much iron as men. Thus, an inadequate intake of iron-rich foods in the diet can contribute to iron deficiency anemia. However, many women need iron supplements, even with a healthy diet.

Prolonged bleeding, such as seen with bleeding ulcers or excessive menstrual bleeding, or injury resulting in hemorrhage, also can lead to iron deficiency anemia. Many women experience iron deficiency anemia during pregnancy because of the increase in demands by the fetus. Iron supplements are commonly given as a routine prophylactic supplement during pregnancy.

Ferrous sulfate (Feosol) is the most commonly used form of iron replacement therapy, available in tablets and liquid. *Ferrous fumarate* (Femiron, Hemocyte) also is available in chewable tablets. Administer the liquid form through a straw to prevent staining the teeth. Remind clients who take the tablet form to swallow the tablet whole. Oral iron preparations can irritate the gastric mucosa; thus, clients should take them with food. Some oral iron preparations are designed for slow absorption and cause less gastric irritation. Iron preparations turn the stool black; alert the client to this normal side effect.

Iron preparations also can be administered parenterally as *iron dextran* (DexFerrum), a pregnancy category B agent. Because injectable iron is irritating to the tissues, it should be administered using the "Z-track" method, deep into the muscle (see Chap. 63). Iron can also discolor the skin if administered superficially.

Iron administration over a prolonged period may cause appetite loss, nausea, vomiting, headache, stomach pain, diarrhea, or constipation. Large doses can cause poisoning, especially in children. Symptoms of iron overdose include headache, fever, and *urticaria* (hives).

Vitamins

Folic acid (folacin, folate, Folvite) is indicated for clients with megaloblastic anemia (a condition characterized by abnormal RBCs). Folic acid stimulates production of RBCs and WBCs and is necessary for normal maturation of RBCs. Folic acid is commonly prescribed in combination with vitamins and minerals before conception and during early pregnancy to reduce the incidence of birth defects in infants. Folic acid therapy has proven particularly effective in preventing neural tube (spinal cord) defects. It also is routinely given to clients who abuse alcohol (see Chap. 94).

Vitamin B_{12} (cyanocobalamin) is necessary for the manufacture of erythrocytes and healthy nervous system functioning. It is absorbed in the small intestine. It cannot be absorbed without the presence of intrinsic factor, which the stomach secretes. Clients who lack intrinsic factor develop pernicious anemia. Injections of vitamin B_{12} (given deep IM) can help to control pernicious anemia. Vitamin B_{12} administration is not usually associated with undesirable side effects.

Coagulants

Medications that promote blood coagulation are called *coagulants. Vitamin K,* a fat-soluble vitamin, is necessary for the formation of prothrombin, which is essential for normal blood clotting. Vitamin K deficiency results in a tendency to hemorrhage. Several preparations of vitamin K are available. *Phytonadione* (Mephyton) is an emulsion of vitamin K that may be administered by the oral or IV route. It is used to control active hemorrhage. *Phytonadione injection* (AquaMEPHYTON) is a colloidal solution of vitamin K that may be administered parenterally, either by the subQ, IM, or IV route. *Absorbable gelatin sponge* (Gelfoam) is used to stop capillary bleeding. It can be left in a surgical wound, where it will be completely absorbed. *Oxidized cellulose* (Oxycel) comes in the form of a treated cotton or gauze pack that is absorbable and can be applied to check hemorrhage.

Anticoagulants

Anticoagulants increase the time it takes blood to coagulate. They are used to treat *thrombophlebitis* (blood clots), to prevent thrombus formation postoperatively, and to treat blood disorders in which blood viscosity is abnormally high. Observe any client receiving anticoagulant therapy for evidence of bleeding, including bleeding gums or unexplained bruising. Check the stool for *occult* (hidden) blood.

Heparin prevents platelets from attaching to the walls of blood vessels, the first step in thrombus formation. Heparin is useful in preventing postoperative thrombosis and embolism. Heparin, a pregnancy category C agent, is administered subQ, most often in the abdominal area, or IV. Apply an ice pack to the area of administration 10 to 15 minutes before injection. This causes vasoconstriction and decreases the possibility of bleeding. *Remember not to aspirate when administering heparin and not to rub the area.*

Laboratory tests, specifically prothrombin time (**PT**), partial thromboplastin time (**PTT**) and/or international normalized ratio (**INR**), are obtained prior to beginning therapy and then used to monitor the effectiveness of anticoagulant therapy.

For the client receiving heparin, check for any use of herbal supplements. Camomile, cat's claw, feverfew, grape seed extract, green tea leaf, gingko, ginseng, horse chestnut seed, garlic, ginger, goldenseal, and turmeric may interfere with heparin, leading to overheparinization. This is also true if the client regularly takes aspirin and, to a lesser degree, NSAIDs (such as ibuprofen). Conversely, psyllium can block the absorption of anticoagulants.

Warfarin (Coumadin), a pregnancy category D agent, is an anticoagulant used to treat venous thrombosis and pulmonary embolism. It prevents thrombophlebitis by inhibiting the synthesis of all types of prothrombin. It is available in tablets for oral administration and also in parenteral form for dilution in sterile water (IV administration is used only when oral administration is not possible). Side effects include skin rash and potential for hemorrhage. Client and family teaching is important because clients are often sent home on warfarin therapy. Monitor PT and PTT values.

Enoxaparin (Lovenox), a pregnancy category B agent, is an injectable anticoagulant that is as effective as heparin. It is indicated for the prevention and treatment of deep venous thrombosis and pulmonary embolism. Enoxaparin specifically targets certain clotting mechanisms and thus is effective in preventing blood clots, with a lesser risk of hemorrhage than is associated with heparin and warfarin. Enoxaparin has been used as postoperative prophylaxis at home after knee and hip replacement surgery. It is administered by deep subQ injection into the abdomen.

Nursing Alert
Clients receiving any anticoagulant therapy should have regular prothrombin time (PT) or partial thromboplastin time (PTT) evaluations to ensure they are not becoming "overheparinized." If the blood clotting time is greater than the prescribed therapeutic range, the anticoagulant dose must be decreased. The "sliding scale" anticoagulant dose is usually based on the outcome of a daily clotting time.

Blood Products

Whole Blood
Whole blood is indicated primarily when there is a rapid loss of both RBCs and plasma, such as in massive hemorrhage. A transfusion of whole blood quickly increases the number of erythrocytes, restoring blood volume and thus raising blood pressure. It may save a client's life when survival depends on quick action. The blood given must be compatible with the client's blood group. For most transfusions, packed red cells are preferred, because they provide only the blood component needed, without extra fluid. (Administration of packed RBCs thus prevents circulatory overload.) Chapter 81 describes the administration of blood and blood products in more detail.

☛ KEY CONCEPT

Careful blood banking and testing techniques ensure a safe, disease-free blood supply. The incidence of disease transmission by blood transfusion is nearly zero today.

Blood Components
Blood components include plasma, plasma proteins, and fractions such as albumin, plasma protein fraction (**PPF**), immune globulin, and antihemophilic factor preparations. (Because of the risk of blood incompatibilities and disease transmission, non-plasma solutions are preferred for rapid fluid replacement.) *Fibrinogen,* a component of blood plasma, can be applied locally to stimulate blood clotting. Another plasma preparation is *antihemophilic factor* (a temporary aid to the person with hemophilia).

Platelets
Platelets also can be removed from a fresh unit of blood. They are administered to clients who have inadequate platelet production, are undergoing intensive cancer chemotherapy, or are receiving large amounts of stored bank blood. Platelets may also be administered to clients with aplastic anemia and leukemia.

ANTINEOPLASTIC MEDICATIONS

Chemotherapy is the administration of **antineoplastic** medications. In some cases, *antineoplastic* ("against cancer") medications are used as a palliative measure for tumors that are no longer curable by surgery, or for cancers such as leukemia that spread throughout the body. Antineoplastic medications can be divided into several large groups based on their probable mode of action. Chapter 82 discusses administration of antineoplastic medications in more detail, as well as side effects and related nursing care.

MEDICATIONS THAT AFFECT THE IMMUNE SYSTEM

Medications Used to Treat Allergies

Antihistamines are most effective in relieving the uncomfortable symptoms of allergic rhinitis and chronic urticaria. These medications are not curative, but do bring temporary relief. Their benefits are short-lived, and they are merely adjuncts to more specific treatment. Many of these specific treatments and related nursing activities are described in Chapter 83. The most common side effects of antihistamines are drowsiness, decreased mental alertness, dry mouth, dizziness, confusion, and constipation. Advise clients to maintain adequate fluid intake, because the action of antihistamines is drying. Clients with asthma should not take antihistamines because of their drying effects on the respiratory tract.

Diphenhydramine (Benadryl) is an antihistamine that is available in oral and injectable forms. It is more sedating than other antihistamines and is sometimes prescribed as a sleep enhancer. *Chlorpheniramine* (Chlor-Trimeton) is slower acting, but has fewer side effects than other antihistamines. Combinations of antihistamines and decongestants (Actifed, Dimetapp) are useful in treating sinusitis, rhinitis, nasal congestion, and postnasal drip. Loratadine (Claritin) and Fexofenadine (Allegra) are newer antihistamines that have few side effects and cause less drowsiness than other antihistamines. However, these newer agents are more expensive.

Corticosteroids, in spray form, have been prescribed when antihistamines are ineffective in controlling the symptoms of allergic rhinitis. They are very effective and the newer forms have few if any side effects. If the inhaled form of corticosteroid is not effective, oral corticosteroids may be needed to bring the situation under control. Oral agents are used only up to a maximum of 10 days. If a person needs to take oral corticosteroids frequently, immunotherapy (allergy shots) should be considered.

Immune Sera and Vaccines

A number of products have been developed to protect children and adults from diseases. The concept of immunity is presented in Chapter 24. Chapter 70 discusses childhood immunizations.

MEDICATIONS THAT AFFECT THE RESPIRATORY SYSTEM

The respiratory system delivers oxygen to the lungs, which in turn help to deliver oxygen to the cells of the body and remove wastes. For these activities to occur, clear airways and a properly functioning respiratory center in the brain's medulla must be present. Chapter 25 describes the anatomy and physiology of the respiratory system; Chapter 85 describes adult respiratory disorders; and Chapter 86 describes the delivery of supplemental oxygen.

Medications that affect the respiratory system include bronchodilators, respiratory stimulants, antitussives, expectorants, antihistamines, and decongestants (Table 62-5). Most of the medications related to the respiratory system are administered by inhalation to reduce systemic effects. If a medication for the respiratory system is given orally, it must reach sufficient blood levels to induce the desired response. Blood samples may be drawn at intervals to measure and determine the appropriateness and effectiveness of the therapy.

Bronchodilators

Bronchodilators act to relax the smooth muscles of the tracheobronchial tree, thereby dilating (increasing) the size of the lumen. Certain diseases, such as asthma and bronchitis, constrict or narrow the size of the lumen, resulting in obstruction of airflow. Bronchodilators remove the obstruction by opening the airways and thus relieving the symptoms.

Epinephrine (Adrenaline) is a potent bronchodilator and is available in several preparations including injection (Ana-Guard), aerosolized mist (Primatene Mist), and solutions for nebulization. (It also is available as a nasal spray and as an ophthalmic solution). Other bronchodilators include albuterol (Proventil, Ventolin), isoproterenol (Isuprel), metaproterenol (Alupent), terbutaline (Brethine), and theophylline (Bronkodyl, Theobid, Theo-Dur). These medications generally are pregnancy category B or D.

Adverse effects of bronchodilators include tremors, nervousness, tachycardia, palpitations, and dizziness. Side effects are dose related and tend to be less severe with inhaled preparations than with those taken orally.

Antiasthmatic Medications

A number of bronchodilators and other medications function specifically to relieve the symptoms of asthma. These include the bronchodilators described previously, as well as other medications including steroids. Steroids are helpful in the treatment of *status asthmaticus* (situation in which the asthma attack does not respond to routine treatment and continues; is life threatening).

Other medications used daily by clients to help prevent asthmatic symptoms include bitolterol mesylate (Tornalate), cromolyn sodium (Intal), isoetharine HCL, levalbuterol (Xopenex), montelukast (Singulair), pirbuterol acetate (Maxair),

TABLE 62-5 ◢ℰℒℰCTED RESPIRATORY SYSTEM MEDICATIONS

Name of Medication*	Usual Adult Dose	Notes
Antitussives (Control Cough)		
benzonatate (Tessalon)	Oral: 100–300 mg t.i.d.	Anesthetizes receptors in respiratory tract to reduce cough reflex
codeine	Oral: 10–20 mg q4–6h	A narcotic, generally combined with other products in cough syrup
dextromethorphan (Delsym, DM Cough, Robidex, Sucrets)	Oral: 10–30 mg q4–8h	Available in many OTC syrups; said to be as effective as codeine for cough
diphenhydramine (Benylin, Benadryl)	Oral: 25–50 mg q4h	An antihistamine with antitussive properties; causes drowsiness
hydrocodone (Hycodan, Hycomine)	Oral: 5–10 mg q4–6h	Schedule III narcotic; depresses cough reflex center in medulla
Expectorants		
guaifenesin (Robitussin)	Oral: 100–400 mg q4–6h	Widely used but some doubt as to clinical efficacy; thins mucus
terpin hydrate	Oral: 85–170 mg t.i.d.–b.i.d.	Antitussive and expectorant
Bronchodilators		
albuterol (Proventil, Ventolin)	By inhalation: 2 puffs q4–6h Also available as tablets, syrup; nebulization	Most selective bronchodilator available
epinephrine (Adrenalin)	SubQ: 0.2–0.5 mg q2h for acute asthma attack (also cardiac arrest)	Short duration; side effects include CNS stimulation and heart palpitations
epinephrine bitartrate (Primatene, Medihaler-Epi)	By inhalation: 1 puff PRN to relieve acute bronchospasm	For temporary use only; available OTC
levalbuterol (Xopenex)	Inhalation: 0.63 mg or 1.25 mg t.i.d. or q6–8h	Used for treatment or prevention of bronchospasm Vials require protection from light
metaproterenol (Alupent)	By inhalation: 2–3 puffs as needed; not to exceed 12/d Oral: 10–20 mg 3–4 times/d	Rapid-acting agent when taken by inhalation route
salmeterol (Serevent)	Aerosol: 25 mcg/puff b.i.d.; 2 puffs; Inhalation powder: 50 mcg b.i.d.	Used for long-term maintenance of asthma and prevention of bronchospasm; not for acute attacks; take before exercise
terbutaline (Brethine, Bricanyl)	Inhalation: 2 puffs q4–6h Oral: 2.5–5 mg q6h, while awake SubQ: 0.25 mg once; repeat in 15–30 min	Not recommended in children under 12; oral form sometimes used to stop contractions in premature labor
theophylline (Theo-Dur, Slo-Phyllin, Bronkodyl, Theon, Theobid)	Oral: Initially 3–5 mg/kg q6h, then 100–200 mg q6h Available as immediate release, timed release, and liquid	GI upset, headache, dizziness, nervousness most common side effects of oral administration; effectiveness decreased by cigarette smoking
Antihistamines		
chlorpheniramine (Chlor-Trimeton)	Oral: 4 mg q4–6h	Available OTC; injectable also available
diphenhydramine (Benadryl)	Oral: 25–50 mg q6–8h	Sedative effects quite pronounced; also indicated for motion sickness and as sleep aid; injectable also available; OTC

(continued)

■■■ TABLE 62-5 *S*ELECTED RESPIRATORY SYSTEM MEDICATIONS (CONTINUED)

Name of Medication*	Usual Adult Dose	Notes
fexofenadine (Allegra)	Oral: 60 mg b.i.d. Children (age 6–11) oral: 30 mg b.i.d.	Used for seasonal allergies Less drowsiness than diphenhydramine
loratidine (Claritin)	Oral (adults and children age 6–11): 10 mg/d Oral syrup: 1 mg/mL	Used for allergic rhinitis and urticaria; rapidly disintegrating tablets available that can be used without water, dissolving in the mouth in seconds; take on empty stomach
promethazine (Phenergan)	Oral: tablets and syrup (25 mg q4–6h) IM: 25–50 mg; repeat in 2–4 h Also available as rectal suppository	Marked sedative action; also used for postoperative nausea and vomiting; may lower seizure threshold
Corticosteroids		
beclomethasone diproprionate (Vanceril, Beclovent)	By oral inhalation: 2 puffs 3–4 times/d	Fewer side effects than systemic steroids Always use 5 min after bronchodilator (not for acute attacks—for preventive use only)
budesonide (Pulmicort)	Oral inhalation powder: 1–2 puffs b.i.d. Inhalation suspension (respules): 0.25–0.5 mg/d to b.i.d.	Used for maintenance treatment of asthma and as prophylactic therapy in children 12 months–8 years Respules administered via nebulizer
flunisolide (Nasalide)	By nasal inhalation: 2 sprays (500 mcg) in each nostril b.i.d.	For treatment of seasonal or perennial rhinitis
fluticasone (Flovent)	Oral inhalation: b.i.d.	Same as beclomethasone
mometasone (Nasonex)	Nasal inhalation: 1 spray in each nostril q d	Long-acting steroid for once-daily dosing Used for seasonal rhinitis
triamcinolone acetonide (Azmacort)	By oral inhalation: 2 puffs 3–4 times/d	Same as beclomethasone
Decongestants		
oxymetazoline (Afrin), in many combination products	Topical: spray or drops in nostrils b.i.d.	Longer duration and less rebound congestion than with other nasal solutions
phenylephrine HCl (Coricidin, Sinex)	Topical: spray or drops in nostrils q3–4h	Oral form also available in many OTC cold preparations
pseudoephedrine (Sudafed, Novafed, Afrinol)	Oral: 30–60 mg 3–4 times/d	Avoid use in patients with hypertension Available OTC
Miscellaneous Products		
cromolyn sodium (Intal)	Capsule for inhalation: 20 mg q.i.d. Solution for nebulization: 20 mg q.i.d. Aerosol spray oral: 2 sprays q.i.d. Aerosol spray nasal: 1 spray each nostril, 3–6 times/d	Drug is antiasthmatic, antiallergic, and mast-cell stabilizer Used for prophylactic management of bronchial asthma (not for acute attacks)
montelukast (Singulair)	Oral: 4–10 mg (tablet or chewable); 10 mg/d	Administered in the evening Used to treat chronic asthma and as prophylaxis in persons 2 y of age and older; not for acute attacks
zafirlukast (Accolate)	Oral: 10–20 mg b.i.d. on empty stomach	Used to decrease daytime asthma symptoms; not for treatment of acute attacks

*The trade name appears in parentheses following the generic name of the medication.

salmeterol (Serevent), and zafirlukast (Accolate). The majority of these medications are pregnancy category C agents.

Respiratory Stimulants

Medications are available that stimulate deeper respirations and an increased rate of respiration, by acting directly on the brain's respiratory center in the medulla. Respiratory depression caused by drug overdose is the most common indication for the use of chemical agents to stimulate respiration.

Naloxone hydrochloride (Narcan), a specific antidote to opiates, is effective in reversing respiratory depression, usually resulting from opiate overdose. It is administered IV. In some cases, Naloxone is also used as a respiratory stimulant after anesthesia administration.

Doxapram HCl (Dopram) is a CNS stimulant used for respiratory depression in the immediate postoperative recovery period. Doxapram is also used to treat acute respiratory failure associated with chronic obstructive pulmonary disease (COPD).

Antitussives

Coughing is a protective reflex to clear the respiratory tract of foreign bodies or secretions. A cough is considered *productive* when it brings up and removes secretions, such as sputum and mucus, as well as exudates from a lung infection. A cough is considered *nonproductive* when it is dry and irritating and no secretions are produced. Treatment of cough is secondary to treatment of the underlying disorder. Medications used to relieve cough include narcotic and nonnarcotic **antitussives.**

Narcotic Antitussives
Narcotics, such as morphine, codeine (most common), and hydrocodone bitartrate (Hycodan), are effective antitussives (cough suppressants). The use of narcotic cough medications usually is limited to a short period of time because of their undesirable side effects (such as constipation) and potential for habituation. (See Chapter 94 for a discussion of substance abuse and dependence.)

Nonnarcotic Antitussives
Nonnarcotic antitussives are widely used, but are less effective than narcotic agents. An example is *dextromethorphan,* which is contained in many OTC cough and cold preparations, such as Benylin, Delsym, Contac, and Robitussin. (Dextromethorphan is often abbreviated as "DM" on cough syrup labels.) Other nonnarcotic antitussives include benzonatate (Tessalon Perles) and terpin hydrate.

Expectorants

Expectorants are medications that liquefy secretions in the bronchi, thus making it easier for the client to cough up and expel mucus. Clients should take expectorants with ample amounts of water or liquid; this will also help to reduce the viscosity of the bronchial secretions.

The most commonly used expectorants include guaifenesin (Breonesin, Genatuss, Liquibid, Tussin) and terpin hydrate (acts as an antitussive and expectorant). These drugs are pregnancy category C agents.

Antihistamines

Antihistamines act by arresting the action of histamine (a body chemical believed to be responsible for causing allergy symptoms). Antihistamines have been used for treatment of various types of allergic reactions (see also previous discussion). Their vasoconstrictive effects have the greatest impact on nasal mucous membranes. They are particularly helpful in controlling the symptoms of allergic rhinitis ("runny nose").

Antihistamines relieve symptoms; however, they do not provide a cure. They should be regarded as accessory agents to more specific treatment. Antihistamines are contraindicated in clients with diabetes mellitus or glaucoma.

Commonly used antihistamines include brompheniramine maleate (Dimetapp), cetirizine (Zyrtec), chlorpheniramine maleate (Chlor-Trimeton), clemastine fumarate (Tavist), diphenhydramine (Benadryl), fexofenadine (Allegra), hydroxyzine (Atarax), loratadine (Claritin), and promethazine (Phenergan). These medications generally are pregnancy category C agents. Many of them are used to treat systemic allergic reactions, not just those limited to the respiratory system.

Decongestants

Decongestants act by reducing the swelling of the nasal membranes and opening up the nasal passages. They may be administered orally as tablets or liquids, or topically in the form of nasal sprays or nose drops. Nasal decongestants should not be used for longer than 3 days' duration, because after this time they cause rebound congestion (the client becomes congested again). Oral decongestants, such as *pseudoephedrine* (Sudafed), are contraindicated in clients who have hypertension.

MEDICATIONS THAT AFFECT THE GASTROINTESTINAL SYSTEM

Medications affect the GI tract in numerous ways (Table 62-6). They cleanse the mouth, stimulate or control peristalsis, and produce or relieve vomiting. Chapter 87 describes many GI disorders and related treatments.

Medications That Affect the Mouth and Teeth

Oral hygiene is the most effective form of mouth care in the prevention of disorders that affect the mucous membranes of the mouth. Mouthwashes are not very potent germ killers, because they cannot be used in strong concentrations without harming the mouth's mucous membrane lining. They are useful in removing mucus from the mouth and throat. They are also helpful in managing *halitosis* (bad breath). A 1% sodium bicarbonate (baking soda) solution (½ teaspoonful in a

■■■ **TABLE 62-6** 𝒮ELECTED GASTROINTESTINAL SYSTEM MEDICATIONS

Name of Medication*	Usual Adult Dose	Notes
Antacids		
aluminum hydroxide (Amphojel, AlternaGEL)	Oral: 600–1500 mg 3–6 times/d, between meals and at bedtime Also available as tablets	May have constipating effect; may impair absorption of certain drugs; OTC
aluminum–magnesium hydroxide (Aludrox, Maalox, Gelusil, Mylanta)	Oral: 15–30 mL 3–6 times/d, between meals and at bedtime	Combination products tend to be less constipating, with equal acid-reducing ability; OTC Some products contain simeth
calcium carbonate (Titralac, Tums)	Oral: 0.5–2 g as needed	High dose may cause hypercalcemia; may reduce absorption of tetracycline antibiotics; OTC May provide calcium
dihydroxy aluminum sodium carbonate (Rolaids)	Oral: 1 or 2 tablets as required	Routine high doses may induce constipation; OTC May provide calcium
Antiemetics		
dimenhydrinate (Dramamine)	Oral: 50–100 mg q4–6h IM: 50 mg q4–6h PRN	An antihistamine; for nausea, vertigo, and motion sickness; OTC
meclizine (Antivert, Bonine)	Oral: 25–100 mg/d in divided doses 25–50 mg 1h before travel	Prevention and treatment of nausea and vomiting associated with motion sickness; treatment of Meniere's Disease
metoclopramide (Reglan)	Oral: 10 mg q.i.d. (1/2 hour a.c. and h.s.) IV: 1–2 mg/kg, repeated q2–3h × 4 then reduce dose	GI stimulant with antiemetic properties; primarily used with cancer chemotherapy
ondansetron (Zofran)	Oral: 4–8 mg q8h, 24 mg tab/day IV: 0.15 mg/kg q4–8h	Used to prevent nausea and vomiting associated with cancer chemotherapy and radiation therapy
prochlorperazine (Compazine)	Oral: 5–10 mg 3–4 times/d IM: 5–10 mg, repeated in 4–6 h PRN Rectal: 25 mg q4–6h	For postoperative nausea and vomiting; also used after cancer chemotherapy or radiation therapy
scopolamine hydrobromide (Transderm-Scop, Scopace)	Transdermal patch (1.5 mg): 1 patch q72h Oral: 0.4 to 0.8 mg q d SubQ or IM: 0.32 to 0.65 mg	Topical patch provides sustained release over 72 hours Used for motion sickness and to relieve spasticity; used preoperatively to reduce secretions.
thiethylperazine (Torecan)	IM, oral: 10–30 mg/d in divided doses	Actions and side effects similar to Compazine; acts directly on vomiting center
trimethobenzamide (Tigan)	Oral: 250 mg 3–4 times/d IM: 200 mg 3–4 times/d Rectal: 200 mg 3–4 times/d	As with most antiemetics, less effective by oral route than by injection
Antispasmodics		
Combination of atropine, scopolamine, hyoscyamine, and phenobarbital (Donnatal)	Oral: 1 tablet 3–4 times/d	Anticholinergic; prevention of nausea, vomiting, or motion sickness
dicyclomine (Bentyl)	Oral: 24–40 mg q.i.d. IM: 20 mg q4–6h (do not give IV)	Slowing of hypermotility of bowel

■■■ **TABLE 62-6** 𝒮ELECTED GASTROINTESTINAL SYSTEM MEDICATIONS (CONTINUED)

Name of Medication*	Usual Adult Dose	Notes
glycopyrrolate (Robinul)	Oral: 1 mg b.i.d. or t.i.d.	Used in peptic ulcer therapy; also used to reduce secretions during anesthesia
propantheline (Pro-Banthine)	Oral: 15 mg q.i.d. (before meals and HS)	Used in peptic ulcer therapy; possesses antisecretory as well as antispasmodic capabilities
Cathartics (Laxatives)		
bisacodyl (Dulcolax)	Oral: 10–15 mg Enema: 2.5 g in water	Must be swallowed whole, not chewed; action occurring in 6–10 h; not to be taken within 1 h of antacids; bowel stimulant; possible urine discoloration
castor oil (Neoloid)	Oral: 15–60 mL	Stimulant laxative generally used as prep prior to bowel x-ray examinations; action occurring in 2–6 h; possible severe abdominal cramping
docusate and casantranol (Peri-Colace)	Oral: 1 capsule up to t.i.d.	Laxative combined with stool softener
glycerin (Fleet Babylax, Sani-supp)	Rectal: 1 suppository; retain for 15 min	Hyperosmolar agent (adds fluid to feces to soften and cause bowel movement); must be inserted high into rectum and retained for 15 min; action occurring in 15–30 min
lactulose (Cephulac, Enulose)	Oral: 15–50 mL	Hyperosmolar agent; mixed with juice or milk to mask taste; action occurring in 24–48 hours
magnesium hydroxide (milk of magnesia, MOM)	Oral: 15–30 mL	Saline laxative with onset of action in ½–3 h; flavored varieties available; also action as antacid
magnesium sulfate (Epsom salts)	Oral: 10–25 g dissolved in water	Saline laxative that attracts and retains fluid in colon and initiates perstalsis; mixed with water; acts in ½–3 h
polycarbophil (Fiber-Con, Konsyl Fiber)	Oral: 1 g 1–4 times PRN; maximum of 6 g/d	Bulk-forming laxative; action occurring in 12–24 hours
polyethylene glycol electrolyte solution (Colyte, Go-LYTELY)	4 L solution (240 mL) q 10 min until all solution is ingested	Bulk-forming laxative; used for bowel cleansing prior to GI examination; action occurring within 1 h; not to be used with bowel obstruction
psyllium (Metamucil, Hydrocil, Konsyl, Genfiber)	Oral: 1 tsp 1–3 times/d	Bulk-forming laxative; considered to be the safest laxative; onset about 12–24 h; mixed with a full glass of juice to mask taste and texture
sodium phosphates (Fleet Phospho-soda)	Oral liquid as laxative: 20–30 mL in glass of water Oral as bowel prep: Amount specified by healthcare provider to be taken in divided doses Enema: 60–135 mL	Used as bowel prep (much less volume to drink than GoLYTELY) and for fecal impaction Not used in abdominal pain or appendicitis; contraindicated in cardiac disorders
senna (Black-Draught, Fletcher's Castoria, Senokot, Ex-lax)	Oral: 1–8 tablets/d h.s. Suppository: 1 @ h.s. Syrup: 10–15 mL q d	Stimulant laxative; possible cramps; action occurring in 6–10 h
Stool Softeners		
mineral oil (MO, Kondremul plain, Milkinol)	Oral: 15–45 mL	Emollient that lubricates intestinal mucosa, softens stool and thus promotes its passage; action occurring in 6–8 h

(continued)

■■■ **TABLE 62-6** *S*ᴇʟᴇᴄᴛᴇᴅ Gᴀsᴛʀᴏɪɴᴛᴇsᴛɪɴᴀʟ Sʏsᴛᴇᴍ Mᴇᴅɪᴄᴀᴛɪᴏɴs (ᴄᴏɴᴛɪɴᴜᴇᴅ)

Name of Medication*	Usual Adult Dose	Notes
docusate (Colace, Surfak, Doxinate)	Oral: 50–250 mg	Fecal softener; take with full glass of water; higher doses required for initial therapy; gentle action, occurring in 24–72 h
Antidiarrheals		
bismuth subsalicylate (Pepto-Bismol)	Oral: 30 mL q½–1h up to 8 doses/d Also available as tablets	Used for "traveler's diarrhea", indigestion, nausea, gas; may cause black, tarry stools
diphenoxylate with atropine (Lomotil)	Oral: 2.5–5 mg q.i.d.; may reduce dosage when controlled (use only liquid for children)	Related to meperidine and therefore subject to drug abuse; used for "traveler's diarrhea"; can be harsh
kaolin-pectin mixture (Kaopectate)	Oral: 60–120 mL after each loose stool	For symptomatic treatment of diarrhea; absorbs excess fluid and reduces intestinal inflammation
loperamide (Imodium)	Oral: Initially 4 mg, then 2 mg after each loose stool, up to 16 mg/d	Clinical improvement should be noted within 48 h; gentle action; possible constipation; OTC for "traveler's diarrhea" Also used in other combination drugs
opium (Paregoric)	Oral: 5–10 mL up to q.i.d. (of 2 mg/5 mL strength)	An opium derivative; sometimes combined with kaolin and pectin CAUTION: Check dosages carefully; some forms contain more morphine
Miscellaneous GI Drugs		
chenodiol (Chenix)	Oral: 250–750 mg b.i.d.; taper dose upward weekly	Used to dissolve gallstones; indicated only in clients at poor surgical risk
cimetidine (Tagamet)	Oral: 200–400 mg b.i.d. to q.i.d.; or 800 mg h.s. IM, IV: 300 mg q6–8h	Inhibits secretion of gastric acid; indicated in treatment of ulcers; sometimes used for gastric reflux or upper GI bleeding
dexpanthenol (Ilopan)	IM, IV: 250–500 mg, repeat at 2 h, then q6h	Indicated in prevention and treatment of adynamic postoperative ileus; used until bowel sounds return
esomeprazole mg (Nexium)	Oral: 40 mg q d for 4–8 wk (acute); 20–40 mg q d (maintenance)	Inhibits gastric secretion; used to treat gastric reflux, esophagitis; may be used with antacids
famotidine (Pepcid)	Oral/IV: Dose dependent on indication for use	Histamine-2 antagonist; OTC
lansoprazole (Prevacid)	Oral: 15 mg q d before eating for 1 wk (acute duodenal ulcer); 10–15 mg q d (maintenance)	Suppresses gastric acid secretion; used to treat duodenal ulcer, gastric reflux
omeprazole (Prilosec)	Oral: 20–40 mg q d	Given q d 4–6 wk; not recommended for more than 2–4 mo of therapy
ranitidine (Zantac)	Oral: 150 mg b.i.d., or 300 mg HS IV and IM solutions also available	Histamine-2 antagonist; similar in almost all respects to cimetidine; longer acting, so is given only twice/d
simethicone (Mylicon)	Oral: 40–80 mg q.i.d., after meals and at bedtime	A defoaming agent used to relieve excess gas in GI tract; may be combined with antacids Also available as tablets, capsules, drops; usually chewable
sucralfate (Carafate)	Oral: 1 q.i.d., before meals and at bedtime	Used in treatment of ulcers; forms a protective barrier at ulcer site to protect against acid

*A trade name appears in parentheses following the generic name of the medication.

glassful of water) also is effective for removing mucus. Additionally, ordinary table salt mixed with water can be used. A solution of warm salt water (saline solution) is also helpful as a gargle for a sore throat. Zinc lozenges also help relieve sore throat pain.

"Swish and swallow" or "swish and spit" mouthwash (Magic Mouthwash), or lozenges, are used to treat oral yeast infections (*thrush*) and other mouth infections in clients with HIV and other immunosuppressive disorders. (Thrush is most often caused by a candida organism.)

Stannous fluoride is recognized as having beneficial effects in preventing tooth decay. It is found in many dentifrices. The American Dental Association has recommended the fluoridation of drinking water as a method for reducing dental decay. A 2% solution of sodium fluoride applied to children's teeth has also been found to be effective in preventing dental caries. Sodium fluoride tablets, drops, solution, and lozenges are available for those who do not have access to fluoridated water. A dentist should be consulted about the specific dose.

Medications That Affect the Stomach

Certain medications are used to control excess production of hydrochloric acid in the stomach and to relieve distention from gas.

Antacids

Antacids are used to treat common "upset stomach." They are also used to reduce and to control stomach acidity, giving peptic ulcers a chance to heal.

Some of the most commonly used antacids include *magnesium-aluminum hydroxide* (Maalox), *magnesium-aluminum hydroxide with simethicone* (Gelusil), and *aluminum hydroxide gel* (Amphojel). Liquid forms are generally more effective than tablet forms.

Histamine (H₂) Antagonists

Histamine (H₂) antagonists are medications that inhibit those gastric secretions that are mediated by histamine. They are used in the treatment of ulcers, gastric reflux, and hypersecretory conditions. Results are usually immediate, but complete healing can take up to 6 weeks or more. Cimetidine (Tagamet), famotidine (Pepcid), nizatidine (Axid), and ranitidine (Zantac) are examples of H₂ antagonists. Most of these medications are pregnancy category B agents.

Proton Pump Inhibitors

Proton pump inhibitors inhibit gastric acid secretion in its final stage. They are used in the treatment of ulcers and in gastroesophageal reflux disease (GERD). Omeprazole (Prilosec), esomeprazole (Nexium), rabeprazole (Aciphex), and pantoprazole (Protonix), and lansoprazole (Prevacid) are proton pump inhibitors. They are also used in the treatment of *H. Pylori* infections.

Antiflatulents

Antiflatulents are used to treat symptoms associated with excess *flatus* (gas) in the digestive tract. Simethicone (Myli-

con) is the most commonly used antiflatulent used alone or in combination.

Antispasmodics

The ideal *antispasmodic* agent reduces gastric secretions and slows GI motility. Although a number of these medications have been developed, they are associated with adverse effects, including blurred vision, dry mouth, and rapid heart rate. Antispasmodics include dicyclomine HCL (Bentyl), glycopyrrolate (Rubinol), methscopolamine (Pamine), and propantheline bromide (Pro-Banthine). One example, tizanidine (Zanaflex) is likely to have the opposite adverse effect of hypotension and bradycardia.

Medications That Produce or Stop Vomiting

Emetics

Emetics are agents given to induce vomiting. Emetics are used as a first-aid measure when prompt stomach evacuation is necessary.

Ipecac syrup is administered orally to produce vomiting in cases of overdose or poisoning. Onset of action is within 30 minutes. Fluids are given after the initial dose of ipecac, to increase the medication's action. Ipecac is available without prescription. The usual dosage is 15 milliliters, with another dose in 30 minutes if no results are seen. Chapter 43 describes emergency care in poisoning in more detail.

> **Nursing Alert**
> In the case of poisoning, contact the local Poison Control Center before inducing vomiting. Vomiting is not induced if a person has ingested a caustic substance. (In this case, charcoal may be used.) Follow the instructions given by the Poison Control Center experts.

Antiemetics

Antiemetics produce symptomatic relief from nausea and vomiting. Numerous preparations are available. Effective long-term treatment, however, usually depends on removal of the cause. Causes of nausea and vomiting include emotional stress, motion sickness, pregnancy, side effects of medications or treatments, chronic illness, or diseases such as influenza.

Dimenhydrinate (Dramamine) inhibits nausea, vomiting, and vertigo, but has a strong sedative effect. It is frequently used to control motion sickness.

Prochlorperazine HCl (Compazine) is an antipsychotic drug that is also used to control nausea and intractable hiccoughs.

Ondansetron (Zofran) is used for the prevention and treatment of nausea and vomiting associated with chemotherapy. It is available for administration IV, or orally in tablets, oral solution, and orally disintegrating tablets. Another drug used to prevent nausea in chemotherapy is *metoclopramide* (Reglan), which is often given 15 to 30 minutes before chemotherapy is administered.

Medications That Affect the Intestine

Cathartics

Cathartics (*laxatives*) are medications used to relieve constipation. A healthy person who eats a normal diet, pays attention to the impulse to defecate, drinks adequate fluids, and exercises sufficiently generally does not need laxatives.

Constipation usually results from a low-residue diet, dehydration, lack of exercise, or stress. Physical activity stimulates peristalsis; thus, clients on bed rest are at risk for constipation. Certain medications, such as opiates and some antipsychotics, also can cause constipation. Institute natural means of relieving constipation before administering laxatives. Prolonged use of cathartics can result in dependency. Do not administer laxatives to clients who are experiencing abdominal pain. (The increased motility of the gut caused by laxatives could result in serious problems. For example, if the abdominal pain was a symptom of *appendicitis* [inflammation of the appendix], increased bowel motility could cause the inflamed or infected appendix to rupture, causing peritonitis, a life threatening infection.)

Many older clients become concerned when they are unable to move their bowels daily. Reassure such clients that many healthy individuals do not have daily bowel movements, and in fact have regular bowel movements only every 3 to 4 days.

Cathartics are classified according to mode of action as follows: bulk-producing agents, irritants, lubricants, saline cathartics, and osmotic agents.

Bulk-Producing Agents. *Bulk-producing agents* stimulate peristalsis by increasing the bulk of feces, thereby modifying stool consistency. The mechanism by which they work is based on a normal stimulus; therefore, these laxatives are among the least harmful substances to the body. However, bulk-producing substances can cause fecal obstruction and impaction. Therefore, give them with adequate fluids and observe the client for any untoward symptoms. An example of a bulk laxative is psyllium hydrophilic mucilloid (Metamucil, Konsyl).

Irritant Cathartics. As the name implies, *irritant cathartics* irritate the large intestine, causing increased peristalsis, which promotes evacuation. Examples of irritant cathartics are cascara sagrada and castor oil.

Lubricant Cathartics. Liquid petrolatum or mineral oil is a *lubricant* used to soften feces. It is given to prevent straining on bowel movements after rectal surgery, or for chronic constipation in less-active persons (such as older adults). Mineral oil taken orally interferes with absorption of the fat-soluble vitamins (A, D, E, and K). Therefore, give it between meals or at bedtime, to avoid interfering with food absorption.

Saline Cathartics. *Saline cathartics* are soluble salts that cause water retention by osmosis. Given with large amounts of water, they increase intestinal bulk and cause distention. The distended colon stimulates smooth muscle contraction, followed by a thorough, quite rapid emptying of the bowel. Examples are milk of magnesia (**MOM**), magnesium citrate, magnesium sulfate, and Fleet's Phospho-Soda. These medications are usually given once a day at bedtime, as needed, or as a bowel prep before surgery or GI examinations.

Osmotic Agents. In some situations, such as preparation for bowel surgery or GI examination, total bowel emptying is required. One common agent for this process is *polyethylene glycol electrolyte solution* (Colyte, GoLYTELY). *Osmotic agents* are not absorbed, and thus do not result in electrolyte imbalance. The client must drink the total amount of solution over 3 hours. Because the total prescribed amount is contained in 4 liters of solution, monitor intake and encourage the client to drink the total amount.

Polyethylene glycol 3350, NF powder (Miralax) is a prescription-only laxative. It softens the stool and increases the frequency of bowel movements. The dose is 17 grams of powder, mixed in 8 ounces of water. It may take 2 to 4 days to produce a bowel movement. It should not be taken for more than 2 weeks.

Fecal Softeners

Fecal softening agents are believed to act like a detergent, by helping to permit water and fatty material to mix with fecal contents. They cause stools to become moist and bulky, thus stimulating the bowel and softening the stool so that it can be expelled more easily. These agents have a wide safety margin and few undesirable side effects. Examples of fecal softening agents include dioctyl potassium sulfosuccinate—docusate potassium (Dialose, Kasof), dioctyl sodium sulfosuccinate—docusate sodium (D-S-S, Colace, Disonate), and dioctyl calcium sulfosuccinate—docusate calcium (Surfak, Pro-Cal-Sof). Mix liquid and powdered forms with fruit juice to mask the taste.

Antidiarrheals

An *antidiarrheal agent* is a medication given to slow GI peristalsis and stop diarrhea, while allowing normal bowel movements. Examples are diphenoxylate hydrochloride in combination with atropine (Lomotil) and loperamide (Imodium).

Lomotil is a Schedule V controlled substance. It reduces intestinal motility and increases intestinal tone. It must not be given to children under the age of 2 years. Side effects include paralytic ileus, toxic megacolon, bloating, constipation, stomach pain, nausea, vomiting, confusion, dizziness, and drowsiness. Encourage clients taking Lomotil to drink at least two liters of fluid daily. Loperamide (Imodium), available without prescription, is as effective as Lomotil, with fewer side effects.

MEDICATIONS THAT AFFECT THE URINARY TRACT

Table 62-7 provides information on common urinary system medications. Chapter 88 discusses urinary disorders and their treatment in more detail.

Diuretics

When urine flow is inadequate, water and salts accumulate in the tissues, causing edema. *Diuretics* rid the body of excess fluids by increasing urine formation. The use of certain diuretics (eg, *furosemide* [Lasix] and *hydrochlorothiazide* [HydroDI-

■■■ **TABLE 62-7** ◟SELECTED DIURETICS AND BLADDER STIMULANTS

Name of Medication*	Usual Adult Dose	Notes
bethanechol (Urecholine)	Oral: 10–50 mg b.i.d. to q.i.d.	Usually used to stimulate bladder contraction
bumetanide (Bumex)	Oral: 0.5–2.0 mg/d IM, IV: 0.5–1 mg given over 2–3 h Do not exceed 10 mg/d	Action similar to furosemide; much smaller doses needed
chlorothiazide (Diuril)	Oral: 500–1000 mg 1–2 times/d	First thiazide diuretic; increases potassium excretion; also used in HTN
chlorthalidone (Hygroton)	Oral: 25–100 mg/d	Long duration of action (up to 72 h); also used in HTN
ethacrynic acid (Edecrin)	Oral: 25–100 mg q d IV: 50 mg; do not give IM or sub Q	More potent than thiazide group; can cause ototoxicity†
furosemide (Lasix)	Oral: 20–80 mg/d; may be repeated IV: 20–40 mg initially; increase in 20-mg increments	*Concomitant* administration (at the same time) with gentamicin may increase ototoxicity; potassium wasting
hydrochlorothiazide (HCTZ, Oretic, HydroDIURIL)	Oral: 25–200 mg/d	Usual initial drug for hypertension treatment
mannitol (Osmitrol)	IV: 50–200 g/24 h	Osmotic diuretic; rapidly excreted
spironolactone (Aldactone)	Oral: 25–200 mg/d	Often combined with hydrochlorothiazide (Aldactazide); potassium-sparing; used in HTN
triamterene (Dyrenium)	Oral: 50–100 mg b.i.d.	Often combined with hydrochlorothiazide (as Dyazide)

*A trade name appears in parentheses following the generic name of the medication.
†Ototoxic: Damaging to eighth cranial nerve, causing hearing and balance disorders.

URIL, HCTZ]) can result in the loss of potassium and sodium. Because these are non–potassium-sparing diuretics (also called potassium-wasting diuretics), clients using them usually require a potassium supplement or must increase sources of potassium in their diet (eg, bananas and orange juice). Diuretics are often prescribed in conjunction with antihypertensive agents to control hypertension.

Xanthine Diuretics. The *xanthine diuretics* include caffeine and theophylline. They are used rarely today because of the availability of newer, more effective diuretics.

Thiazide Diuretics. The *thiazide diuretics* are synthetic medications that are chemically related to sulfonamides. The development of these agents marked a major breakthrough in the search for a potent oral diuretic. All thiazides are equally effective, although dosage and duration of action vary. The thiazides have many advantages over other diuretics: ease of administration (oral), low cost, effectiveness over long periods, low toxicity, and few side effects. Examples include *bendroflumethiazide* (Naturetin), *chlorothiazide* (Diuril), and *hydrochlorothiazide* (HydroDIURIL, Dyazide).

Loop Diuretics. *Furosemide* (Lasix) and *bumetanide* (Bumex) are effective, potent, rapidly acting diuretics. Because of their potency, clients taking them require close supervision of fluid and electrolyte balance. Supplemental potassium is often prescribed when Lasix or Bumex is given. These med-

ications are called *loop diuretics* because they inhibit reabsorption of sodium and chloride in the loop of Henle in the kidney.

Other Diuretics. *Spironolactone* (Aldactone) promotes diuresis and helps counteract potassium loss. It is effective in promoting diuresis in clients who are resistant to more common diuretics.

Triamterene (Dyrenium) is a mild, potassium-sparing diuretic. Its onset of action is slow; for that reason, it should be used in combination with other diuretics when rapid diuresis is required. Dyazide is a combination of *triamterene* and *hydrochlorothiazide*. It is a mild, potassium-sparing diuretic, with a slow onset of action.

Medications That Affect the Muscle Tone of the Urinary Bladder

Bladder dysfunction can result in urinary retention or the sensation of urinary frequency. In either case, the problem is one of poor muscle tone in the bladder. *Neostigmine methylsulfate* (Prostigmin) and *bethanechol chloride* (Urecholine) improve the bladder's muscle tone. *Oxybutynin* (Ditropan) is an antispasmodic used to treat clients who have bladder dysfunction with urinary frequency. *Desmopressin acetate* (**DDAVP**) is a hormone administered as a nasal spray to treat adults with *enuresis* (bed wetting). This condition is often a side effect of certain medications, including psychotropics. DDAVP is also used to treat the excessive voiding of diabetes insipidus.

Urinary Antiseptics and Antispasmodics

Urinary antiseptics are effective agents in the treatment of bacterial infections of the urinary tract. A sulfonamide commonly used to treat urinary tract infections is co-trimoxazole (Bactrim). The tetracyclines, erythromycin, fosfomycin (Monurol), ciprofloxacin (Cipro), and urinary tract anti-infectives such as cinoxacin (Cinobac), methylene blue (Urolene Blue), nalidixic acid (NegGram), and nitrofurantoin (Furadantin) are also used to treat urinary tract infections.

Phenazopyridine (Pyridium) is a urinary antiseptic commonly prescribed for its prompt analgesic effects. The client usually experiences relief of symptoms of urgency and frequency, as well as burning when voiding, within 30 minutes of the initial dose. Advise the client that phenazopyridine will turn the urine reddish orange.

MEDICATIONS THAT AFFECT THE REPRODUCTIVE SYSTEMS

Male Sex Hormones (Androgens)

Androgens are essential for the development and maintenance of male sex characteristics. Both sexes produce male and female hormones, but their effects are antagonistic to each other. Androgen replacement therapy may be administered to men whose circulating hormone levels are insufficient to maintain male sex characteristics. Androgens may also be administered to female clients in an effort to retard the growth of estrogen-dependent tumors. Disorders of the male and female reproductive systems are discussed in Chapters 89 and 90.

Ovarian Hormones

The ovaries secrete two important hormones, *estrogen* and *progesterone* (progestins).

Estrogen. Conjugated estrogens (Premarin) were once prescribed mainly to diminish unpleasant symptoms (such as "hot flashes") associated with menopause. Recent studies, however, have confirmed that estrogen replacement therapy has the additional benefits of helping to prevent osteoporosis and other tissue changes associated with menopause. In addition, estrogen is believed to postpone some of the cardiovascular changes of aging, thus helping to prevent heart disease. For these reasons, estrogen is being prescribed for long-term hormone replacement therapy (HRT) during and after menopause.

Side effects of estrogen replacement therapy include edema, thromboembolism, abdominal cramping, anorexia, bloating, nausea, vomiting, hepatitis, breast tenderness, and breakthrough bleeding. Women with breast cancer or other tumor growth should not receive estrogen replacement therapy.

Estrogen is available in oral, parenteral, and transdermal routes of administration. Other estrogen replacement hormones include Congest (available in Canada), Estrace, and Estraderm. In some cases, men who have cancer of male reproductive

organs receive estrogen as a palliative measure to slow or to retard the growth of male-hormone–dependent tumors.

Progesterone. The corpus luteum secretes progesterone, which influences uterine and ovarian conditions during pregnancy. Progesterone prepares the lining of the uterus for implantation of the ovum. It suppresses ovulation during pregnancy and reduces the irritability of uterine muscle, to prevent premature labor or spontaneous abortion. *Medroxyprogesterone acetate* (Provera) may be used in dysmenorrhea, menorrhagia, metrorrhagia, or threatened spontaneous abortion.

Sometimes, estrogen and progesterone are given in various combinations, such as in Prempro and Premphase.

Medications That Affect the Uterus

The uterus is a highly muscular organ capable of great distention and elasticity. Medications that act on the uterus are used either to increase or to decrease contraction of uterine muscle. Medications used in labor and delivery are discussed further in Chapters 65 and 67.

Medications Used in Family Planning

Oral contraceptives are hormonal preparations that contain estrogen and progesterone and are used to prevent pregnancy. Estrogen suppresses ovulation by affecting the release of follicle-stimulating hormone (FSH). Side effects of oral contraceptives include nausea, vomiting, breast tenderness, headache, nervousness, emotional lability, and *venous thrombosis* (blood clots). Estrogen can promote the growth of existing cancers of the breasts and uterus. Hormonal preparations are also used to enhance fertility in women who have difficulty conceiving (see Chap. 69).

Medications Used in Treating Sexually Transmitted Diseases (STDs)

Antibiotics are used to treat many sexually transmitted diseases (STDs), including syphilis and gonorrhea. Viral STDs, such as herpes, are resistant to antibiotic therapy and must be treated with antiviral agents, such as acyclovir sodium (Zovirax) or zidovudine (Retrovir). Acyclovir and zidovudine are also used to treat HIV/AIDS. Immune disorders and related medications are highlighted in Chapters 83 and 84. Medications used to treat STDs are discussed further in Chapter 69.

➔ STUDENT SYNTHESIS

Key Points

• A wide variety of medications are available to treat or prevent illness or other body dysfunctions. The major groups include antibiotics, analgesics, sedatives, anticonvulsants, and medications specific to disorders affecting each of the body systems.

- Because of the large number of medications available, the nurse must be knowledgeable in the use of drug reference books and related websites. The nurse is legally obligated to know basic information about any medication that he or she is to administer.
- Drugs are classified according to their risk to a developing fetus. However, the pregnant woman should not take any medications without medical supervision.
- In some cases, medications are prescribed even though they have undesirable side effects. Their benefits outweigh the risks and disadvantages.
- It is important to document if a client is taking any herbal supplements or using any homeopathic remedies because these can counteract or potentiate the effects of prescribed medications.
- Medications are often prescribed using their generic name to avoid confusion.

Critical Thinking Exercises

1. The physician writes a medication order which does not seem correct to you. Describe what actions you would take.
2. Choose three commonly used medications from different classifications. Using a drug reference book, write the following information for each: drug class, therapeutic (desired) actions, reasons for use (indications), contraindications and precautions, forms in which the medication is available, average adult dose, pharmacokinetics (including how the drug is distributed to the body or target areas and how it is excreted), adverse effects (identifying those that are life threatening), and nursing considerations and client teaching points.

NCLEX-Style Review Questions

1. When a client is being discharged from the hospital on prolonged steroid therapy, it is most important for the nurse to instruct the client:
   a. Call the physician if questions arise.
   b. Do not stop therapy abruptly.
   c. Return for followup appointment.
   d. Take medication with food.

2. A client is to be started an antibiotic therapy. Which of the following actions is the priority:
   a. Inform client on the type of antibiotic therapy.
   b. Instruct client how to take the medication at home.
   c. Obtain culture before starting antibiotic.
   d. Teach client about potential side effects of the medication.
3. In evaluating the effectiveness of warfarin (Coumadin), the nurse should monitor which laboratory result?
   a. Electrolytes
   b. Glucose
   c. CBC
   d. PTT
4. When evaluating the effectiveness of meperidine hydrochloride (Demerol), the nurse would assess the client's:
   a. Breath sounds
   b. Bowel sounds
   c. Orientation level
   d. Pain level
5. A client is taking digoxin. Which sign exhibited by the client would most clearly indicate that the digoxin could be given safely?
   a. Heart rate of 80 beats per minute
   b. Lung sounds are clear
   c. Oriented to person, place, and time
   d. Tolerating diet well

Reference

1. Karch, A. (2002). *Lippincott's nursing drug guide: Book with mini CD-ROM for Windows and Macintosh.* Philadelphia: Lippincott Williams & Wilkins.

CHAPTER

63

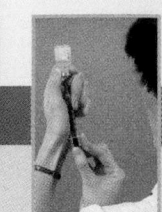

Administration of Medications

LEARNING OBJECTIVES

1. Explain how medications are stored and supplied in healthcare facilities.
2. Discuss the importance of documenting medication administration in the medication administration record, the computerized record, or the client's chart.
3. Differentiate STAT, PRN, and HS medications.
4. Discuss the importance of the "Five Rights" of medication administration, including steps to observe before administering medications.
5. Differentiate between desired and undesired effects, and local and systemic medication effects.
6. Explain what is meant by enteral and parenteral administration.
7. Demonstrate various methods of enteral medication administration.
8. Demonstrate the proper technique for administering subcutaneous, intramuscular, and intradermal injections.
9. Identify nursing considerations for the use of total parenteral nutrition.
10. Discuss the use of infusion pumps, piggyback administration of medications, and intermittent infusion devices such as heparin or saline locks.

NEW TERMINOLOGY

ampule	ophthalmic
anaphylactic effect	otic
anergic	parenteral
diluent	toxicity
enteral	transfusion
hep lock	vial
infiltration	z-track
infusion	

ACRONYMS

D/C	HS	NS
D$_5$½NS	ID	PICC
D$_5$NS	IVPB	SL
D$_5$W	MAR	STAT
DRF	MDI	TPA
G	NaCl	TPN
G-tube	NG	

Administering medications is one of the most important functions for a nurse. It also is one that has an extremely high risk of danger for the client. Administering medications involves much more than just "giving clients pills." The nurse must follow the rules of safe administration faithfully. To ensure each client's safety, each nurse must be familiar with recommended administration routes, dosages, desired actions, possible side effects, and nursing considerations for prescribed medications.

PREPARATION FOR ADMINISTRATION

Before medications can be administered, the nurse needs to interpret the medication orders accurately, including being able to follow administration directions. This involves being familiar with commonly used abbreviations and acronyms. Some commonly used terms are listed as acronyms at the beginning of this chapter and in Appendix B.

In addition, the nurse needs to know how the facility stores and supplies or dispenses the medications and the proper measures for documenting that the client did or did not receive the medications.

Storage

Most healthcare facilities have a "med room" or separate storage area for medications. Many facilities store medications in locked movable carts that allow nurses to prepare medications in close proximity to clients' rooms. Medications are stored in individual drawers contained in the cart. The cart is locked when a licensed nurse is not directly attending it. Some medications require refrigeration to preserve their chemical properties. These medications are kept in a special med room refrigerator. No food or other materials may be stored in this refrigerator. The temperature of this refrigerator must be monitored carefully and documented accurately.

Some facilities have storage areas for medications in special cabinets or drawers, within the client's room or directly outside of it. Like the medication cart, these drawers are locked when not being used for administration by a licensed nurse.

All medications must be properly labeled, with the client's name, medication name, dosage, and expiration date. *If a label is illegible, return the container to the pharmacy for proper identification and labeling. A nurse NEVER relabels a medication.*

All narcotics and other controlled substances are kept double-locked in the medication room or in a "med cart." Nurses must sign out these medications on special sheets as they give them. Such medications must be accounted for at the end of each shift. Nursing students are sometimes allowed to give controlled substances, but only under a clinical instructor's direct supervision. See Chapter 61 for further information.

Dispensing and Supply Systems

Stock Supply
Stock supply refers to medications that may be kept on a nursing unit. Typically, the stock supply includes medications that are frequently ordered for clients on that particular unit. The

medications are stored in locked cabinets and then individual doses are administered from the stock supply when ordered. Sometimes the stock supply is used for a medication that must be given in an emergency. Stock medications often include analgesics such as acetaminophen (Tylenol) and aspirin, comfort medications such as throat lozenges and pseudoephedrine (Sudafed), bowel preparations such as milk of magnesia, and medications specific to a particular nursing unit. Some facilities allow only over-the-counter (OTC) medications to be kept in stock.

Unit-Dose Systems
Many pharmaceutical companies supply tablet, capsule, liquid, and injectable forms of various medications in individual prepackaged containers. Because each dose is packaged separately, this is referred to as a *unit-dose system*. Unit-dose packages are usually marked with the medication's generic and trade name, as well as the dose contained in the package. The unit-dose method provides greater safety in administering medications than does a stock supply, because the medication's name and dose are on each unit dose. Moreover, in acute care facilities, most unit-dose systems provide only a 24-hour supply of the medication for each client. In long-term care facilities, a week's supply of medications is often supplied at one time.

In many facilities, pharmacists label unit doses with each client's name before sending these medications to nursing units. The nurse may take an unopened unit-dose package directly to the client's bedside and open it there. Doing so provides an additional safety check for the nurse and the client, and also prevents waste if for some reason the nurse does not give the medication or the client refuses it (see "Client Refusal" later in this chapter for disposal instructions).

Automated Systems
Some facilities use computerized systems for dispensing medications. Personnel key in coded orders, which a computer relays electronically to a pharmacy. The pharmacy may also be automated for handling of routine medications. Unit-dose medications may be dispensed to the nursing station by means of a conveyor, pneumatic tube system, or courier.

Self-Administered Medications
In some facilities, a responsible client is allowed to keep a medication at his or her bedside and manage its administration. Examples of medications often include creams and ointments, vaginal creams, nicotine chewing gums, throat lozenges, and inhalers. In addition, some clients manage their own pain, using patient controlled analgesia (PCA) pumps. Some clients with diabetes also dispense insulin in this manner.

Medication Records

Healthcare facilities use various systems to document the administration of medications to their clients. Usually, today's medication administration record (**MAR**) is a computer-generated sheet that a pharmacy prepares after receiving its copy of the physician's orders. Nurses keep individual MARs in three-ring binders located on a med cart or in the med room, or directly next to the individual client's medication cabinet or drawer. In some cases, the nurse enters the information into the computer after the medication is given.

An older system seen less often today is the card system, which uses individual medication cards (approximately 2 × 2 inches) that contain the client's name, medication name, and times to administer the medication. The card system is usually color coded, with each particular color representing a different administration route or a different prescribing healthcare provider. The client's medication cards are stored in the Kardex. Another system seen less frequently today is the transcribed (copied) system. Using this system, the charge nurse or nurse manager transcribes the physician's order to a client's MAR.

Whatever system a facility uses, all MARs include the client's name, medication name (usually generic and trade name), dosage, administration route, and scheduled times. The nurse is responsible for checking the MAR's accuracy by comparing it with the original physician's order. An additional precaution to ensure accuracy is a medication and order sheet check performed every 24 hours, usually completed by the charge nurse or nurse manager. (This check is often done during the night shift.)

Setting Up Medications

Although each facility's routine for administering medications varies, the nurse must conscientiously observe universal rules for safe administration. Remember: These safety rules protect not only clients but also healthcare facility personnel from mistakes with very serious consequences. In Practice: Nursing Care Guidelines 63-1 highlights important actions in setting up medications.

In Practice
Nursing Care Guidelines 63-1

SETTING UP MEDICATIONS

- Always pay close attention when setting up medications. *Rationale: A medication error could cause serious injury or death.*
- Check the medication order with the medication administration record (MAR). Make certain that the MAR and physician's orders are identical. If using medication cards, they must match the order *exactly*. *Rationale: This checking mechanism is necessary to prevent an error.*
- Always read the medication label three times: (1) when taking the medication from the shelf or drawer; (2) before removing the medicine from the container; and (3) before putting back or discarding the container. *Rationale: Checking the label three times helps to ensure safe administration.*
- *Never* give a medication from an unlabeled container or if unable to read the label. *Rationale: Doing so increases the risk of a medication error.*
- Make sure the label on the container matches *exactly* with the MAR or the medication card.
- Be familiar with abbreviations, and generic and trade names. Use extreme caution with medications that have similar names. *Rationale: Every effort is necessary to ensure that an error does not occur.*
- Check the medication to make sure it is not spoiled or outdated. *Rationale: The medication may lose its effectiveness or become toxic.*
- If using a unit-dose medication, do not open the package until ready to give the medication. *Rationale: If the client refuses the medication, it will not be wasted. Clients can also be sure they are receiving the correct medication.*
- If not using a unit dose, measure the dose with the appropriate equipment. When measuring liquids, hold the measure at eye level, with the thumbnail on the line of the desired amount, using the meniscus (lower part of the curve at the surface of the liquid) to indicate the level. Pour liquid medications from the unlabeled side of the bottle. *Rationale: Pouring from the unlabeled side helps to avoid soiling the label. A soiled label may be unreadable.*
- If unit-dose medications are unavailable, shake the required number of tablets, capsules, or caplets into the cap of the container. Small paper cups (souffle cups) are usually available for passing medications. Never handle medications with the fingers. *Rationale: If the nurse shakes out too many tablets, he or she can put them back in the container if they have not been touched. If the nurse handles tablets, they are contaminated. They cannot be used or returned to the container.*
- Administer each medication as it is prepared. *Rationale: This action helps to avoid medication errors.*
- *Never* give medications that someone else has prepared. *Rationale: The nurse is personally responsible for all medications he or she gives.*
- Do not leave medications at the client's bedside unless there is a specific physician's order to do so. *Rationale: The nurse is responsible for ensuring that the client receives the ordered medication. Leaving the medication at the bedside makes it difficult for the nurse to ensure that the client actually has taken the medication and when he or she has taken it.*

Nursing Alert

When obtaining a client's history of allergies, inquire as to possible food allergies, as well as allergies to tape and latex (gloves, catheters, and tourniquets all contain latex). Always double-check for allergies *before* giving medications or performing any procedures.

SAFETY

Safe administration of medications is a priority. In Practice Nursing Guideline 63-2 provides tips for the safe administration of medications. It also provides documentation guidelines to follow if clients refuse medications.

The "Five Rights"

The "Five Rights" of medication administration are:

- Right client
- Right medication
- Right dose
- Right time
- Right route

The Right Client

Take special precautions to ensure that the correct medication is given to the *correct client.* Direct total attention to the task at hand, and do not engage in conversation with other people.

Compare the MAR with the client's identification band. Do not administer medications to clients who are not wearing identification armbands or tags. An identification band taped to a bed does not necessarily mean that the person occupying the bed is the client. This case is especially true in long-term or psychiatric facilities, where clients freely move about the

---

In Practice
Nursing Care Guidelines 63-2

ADMINISTERING MEDICATIONS SAFELY

- Always follow the "Five Rights" of medication administration:
  - Right client
  - Right medication
  - Right dose
  - Right time
  - Right route
- Check *very carefully* for medication allergies, including checking the MAR, the client's chart, and the physician's orders. Ask the client if he or she is allergic before giving any medication. Note any allergies on the front of the chart, and apply a special red allergy-identification band to the client. *Rationale: Checking for allergies is essential to prevent client injury.*
- Do not place different types of medications together in a cup unless each is in a separate unit-dose package. *Rationale: The client might miss one medication, and the nurse would be unable to identify for certain which medication was left in the cup.*
- *Never* leave a medicine tray, package, or cup within the reach of clients or visitors. If you must leave the room, take the medication with you. Lock it up if necessary. Lock up the medication cart each time you leave it. *Rationale: The wrong person may take medications.*
- Follow the healthcare facility's policy for established times for medication administration. *Rationale: If medications are not given within the time limits set by the facility, a medication error has occurred.*
- Always chart medications as soon as they are given. *Never* chart a medication before it is given. Record the time, the name of the medication, and the dose.

Rationale: The MAR is a legal document. It is used regularly in planning client care. It must be accurate.
- Add initials and sign full name and status (eg, LPN/LVN, RN, student) at the bottom of the MAR. *Rationale: Doing so ensures that other members of the healthcare team will know who gave the medication. The MAR is a legal document and may be used in court.*
- Record and *report immediately* any unusual client reaction, an unfavorable change in the client's condition, a client's refusal to take medicine, or his or her inability to take all of it. *Rationale: The client may need immediate medical attention.*
- If a medication has been forgotten, report this promptly. *Rationale: This is a medication error.*
- Discard an unused or open dose of a medication: Never return it to a stock container. Dispose of medications according to the facility's policies. Have a witness cosign if a controlled substance is being discarded. *Rationale: Returning medication to a stock container increases the risk of error and possible contamination. The nurse is legally required to maintain an accurate record of all controlled substances used on a unit.*
- If a client refuses a medication, document as usual, then circle the time and write "ref" next to it. Follow the same procedure for any other reason a scheduled medication is not given on time—circle the time, and indicate a reason (eg, "emesis," "on pass," "PT," and so forth). *Rationale: Proper and accurate documentation helps to prevent medication errors. In addition, it provides a means of communication with other healthcare personnel.*

facility. Some clients in these facilities may be easily con-fused, thinking that they are in their own rooms, when in fact they are in someone else's room. Clients may also deliberately mislead the nurse.

After checking the client's identification band, if the client is conscious and oriented, ask the client to state his or her name. Do so in a polite, friendly manner. Do not ask the client "Are you Mr. Brown?" Phrasing a question this way does not help in determining who the client is. Some clients with hear-ing or psychological disorders or who do not speak English well will answer "yes" to any question they are asked.

After determining that the client is indeed the right client, stay with the client until he or she has taken the medication. Make sure the client has swallowed the pill or liquid. Under no circumstances should the medication be left at the bedside for the client to take later. Some clients may dispose of the medication, or the wrong client may take it. In some instances, checking the client's mouth to make sure the medication has been swallowed may be necessary.

The Right Medication

Compare and confirm the *medication's name* and dosage with the client's MAR three times before administering it. The first check is on removing the medication from the storage area; the second is on preparing the medication when placing it in the medication cup; and the third is on opening the medication unit-dose package. These three simple checks will drastically reduce the possibility of a medication error.

NEVER administer a medication that someone else has prepared (unless it is still in its original individual pack-age). A nurse cannot determine what medication he or she is administering if any of the three checks described above are omitted. Any nurse who administers a medication prepared by someone else is committing unsafe nursing practice, and is guilty of a medication error that may place the client's well-being at risk.

The Right Dose

To ensure the *right dose,* double-check that the amount of med-ication supplied matches the amount needed for the ordered dose. In addition, verify that the dose ordered is appropriate for the client. Moreover, always listen to the client. If he or she questions the medication's color, the number of tablets being given, or the administration route, recheck the MAR, order, and medication label *before* giving the medication.

The Right Time

Administer all medications at the *time* for which they are ordered. Most facilities allow 30 minutes on each side of the time for administering scheduled medications. For example, a medication that is ordered for 0900 may be administered any-time between 0830 and 0930 and still be considered "on time." Administering medications as ordered is important to maintain the medication's therapeutic effects. Deviation from the "time window" is a medication error.

Devising a method to ensure delivery of medications at the specified time is advisable. Nurses have devised many differ-

ent systems of "reminders." One method is to draw a chart that contains each client's name and location, with separate boxes for each hour. If a client is to receive a medication at a partic-ular time, enter a check mark or "x" in the appropriate box. This format allows the nurse to check medications for each client each hour, and ensures that the nurse will administer medications on time. Label the last column "Notes" to reserve this area as a reminder for a client's special needs, concerns, or procedures.

The format that the nurse adopts for this task does not mat-ter. However, the nurse needs to use some organizational method that helps in completing medication administration on time. Adopting such a method will also help in planning per-sonal activities. For instance, the schedule must allow time for lunch or for performing special treatments. Consistency with the organizational plan is important.

STAT Doses.   A **STAT** order means that a medication must be administered immediately. First, check the order against the original physician's order. Then transcribe the order to the MAR. Prepare and administer the medication as soon as possible. If the medication is not readily available, inform the supervisor that the medication has been ordered from the phar-macy and it will be administered it as soon as it arrives. As with all medications, *chart STAT medications as soon as they are given.* This measure will prevent duplication of the STAT order. Also write "given," the date, time, and initials next to the original order. This procedure not only informs the physician that the order was carried out and when, but also safeguards against the possibility of duplication. When using the medica-tion card system, tear the card almost in half as soon as the medication is administered, and properly document the proce-dure. Tearing the card indicates that the medication has been administered as ordered. The torn card may be kept for later reference when reporting to the oncoming nurse at the change of shift. *Never chart STAT medications before they are given.*

PRN Doses.   Assessing the client's need for PRN (*as needed* or *on request*) medication is an important nursing responsibility, often learned with experience. If a client asks for a PRN medication, first assess what symptoms have prompted the client's request. For example, if the client is com-plaining of pain, determine the pain's location and discomfort based on a scale of 0 (minimal) to 10 (extreme) (see Chap. 55). Next, consult the MAR to determine when the client last received the medication. If the prescribed period has elapsed, administer the medication as soon as possible. If the pre-scribed period has not elapsed, inform the client when he or she can receive the next dose. PRN medications are usually available for sleep, constipation, and gastric distress, as well as for pain.

Hour of Sleep (HS) Doses.   Physicians often order sedatives and hypnotics, more commonly known as "sleeping pills," on a PRN basis. Technically, the client should request PRN medications. However, he or she may be unaware that the physician has ordered medication to facilitate obtaining a good night's rest. For this reason, tell the client that the doctor has ordered such medication at the hour of sleep (**HS**) and offer to prepare it as requested.

The Right Route

Check the physician's orders and the MAR to verify the *route* by which the medication is to be given (one of the three checks described above). Administering a medication by the wrong route could be fatal.

Medication Errors

Although every nurse hopes never to experience the agony of a medication error, chances are that every nurse will make a medication error sometime during his or her career. Understandably, those chances increase with students, because they are still in the process of learning. Report any medication error to the clinical instructor or charge nurse as soon as it is discovered. (In some cases, immediate emergency action is necessary to prevent undesirable or potentially fatal effects.)

Medication errors include administering to the wrong client, administering the wrong medication or dose, administering at the wrong time, or administering by the wrong route.

For any doubts about a medication, consult a drug reference and ask the supervisor before giving it. If the possibility of a medication error exists, do not hesitate to report it. The greatest error is to avoid reporting. The client's well-being is the major concern. The nurse who discovers an error and does not report it is subject to disciplinary action as well as posing danger to the client.

Client Refusal

A client has the right to refuse a medication (unless there is a court order to the contrary or a medical emergency has been declared). The nurse is obligated to explain to the client the medication's action and the importance of taking the medication as ordered. If the client still refuses, properly dispose of the medication (see below) and document on the MAR as to why the client refused it. In most healthcare facilities, the time for administration is circled and "refused" is written to the side, along with the nurse's initials. Enter additional documentation as to why the client refused the medication into the client's medical record.

Use correct procedure when disposing of medications that a client refuses to take. Disposal methods vary across facilities. If the medication is contained in an unopened unit-dose pack, return it to the client's medication drawer or storage area. If the medication is a controlled substance, another licensed nurse must witness its disposal and also cosign the record. Never sign that you witnessed the disposal of a controlled substance if you did not see the actual disposal.

Nursing Alert

In most healthcare facilities, if a medication is *not* given, the nurse must circle the time it was to be administered on the MAR, initial the entry, and indicate why the medication was held. For example, "⟨0800⟩ NPO CR." or "⟨0800⟩ x-ray CR." Entering this information in the nurse's notes is unnecessary under these circumstances. If the client refuses the medication, however, the nurse must document in the nurse's notes why the client refused.

Documentation

Documentation is an important part of medication administration. Things that are not documented are considered as not having been done. Proper documentation communicates to other members of the healthcare team which medications were administered and when. If a medication is PRN or a first-time administration, documentation will further relay the medication's effects. Chapter 37 presents a comprehensive discussion of documentation in general and that for medication administration. In many facilities, areas for both drug orders and documentation of administration are on the MAR. Nurses in many healthcare facilities record all documentation entries, including medications and treatments, using *military time* (the 24-hour clock). This method eliminates errors in interpreting the exact time the entry was made.

Client Teaching

Client teaching also is an important safety consideration for medication administration. Teach clients the following information concerning medications that they receive:

- What medications they are given
- Why they are taking them
- Dosage and frequency
- How to administer or take them at home
- Expected effects
- Possible undesirable side effects
- How long they will need the medications
- What to do if they miss a dose
- Signs and symptoms that the client should report to the healthcare provider

Clients should be able to verbalize the above information to indicate their understanding of the material. They should also be able to demonstrate specific procedures for their conditions (eg, the injection technique for administering insulin). All teaching *must* be documented, because it is an important component of the nursing care plan and is required by the Joint Commission on Accreditation of Healthcare Organizations. If teaching is not documented, then it is considered to have not been done. Many healthcare facilities provide clients with written information concerning medications, and teaching to reinforce their knowledge and understanding.

GENERAL PRINCIPLES OF MEDICATION ADMINISTRATION

Desired and Undesired Effects

Medications have many effects on the body, both desired and undesired. A *therapeutic effect* is a medication's desired effect, meaning that the medication produces the result for which it was given. An *adverse effect* is a response that is not intended or desired. Some adverse effects are minor (called *side effects*) and, although bothersome, can be ignored or treated easily. Constipation is an example of a side effect. However, others, such as respiratory depression, are potentially fatal.

A medication also may have an anaphylactic effect—the medication causes the client to experience a severe, life-threatening, allergic reaction (**anaphylaxis**) manifested by vasodilation, low blood pressure, and shock. An anaphylactic reaction is a medical emergency that the nurse must recognize and treat promptly. Medication **toxicity** is also an undesired, harmful effect that results from an increased blood level of the medication beyond its therapeutic level. Administering a medication in too large a dose or via the wrong route can lead to drug toxicity. In some cases, the client can also build up a toxicity as a result of a disorder, such as inadequately functioning kidneys.

Local and Systemic Effects

A medication's effects may be local or systemic. *Topical application* (applied directly to the skin or mucous membranes) can cause a *local effect.* Anti-inflammatory medications are examples of medications used for their local effects. These medications may be applied to the mucous membranes of the eye, mouth, nose, throat, vagina, or rectum by instillation, irrigation, swabbing, or spraying. Rectal suppositories are most often used as laxatives; vaginal suppositories are used most often to treat localized vaginal infections. The advantage of local medications is that their effects are limited to the area of application, thus reducing the possibility of undesired systemic reactions.

Drugs that the body absorbs into the general circulation (ie, the blood and lymphatic fluids) and then transports to a specific body area have *systemic effects.* To achieve systemic effects, medications often are administered by mouth or injection (see following discussion). *Transdermal administration* often achieves systemic effects as well. Using this route, a medication patch, for example a nitroglycerin patch, is applied directly to the skin. The medication is absorbed systemically over a prolonged period. Some medications administered rectally also have systemic effects, such as prochlorperazine (Compazine) suppositories to relieve nausea, and aspirin suppositories to reduce fever.

Medication Administration to Children

Children, because of their small size, can tolerate only a fraction of adult dosages. To ensure that correct dosages of medications are administered to children, the nurse needs to calculate pediatric doses. The most common method for calculation of pediatric dosage is milligrams of medication per kilogram of body weight (mg/kg). Body surface area, using the child's height and weight, also can be used for pediatric dosage calculation. Generally, physicians will make these calculations before nurses administer pediatric medications. Review a copy of the healthcare facility's protocol and a drug reference before administering any medications to children.

Enteral Versus Parenteral Administration

Enteral indicates medication administration by way of the digestive tract. This route includes administration orally, buccally (inside the cheek), and via gastrointestinal tubes. Technically, rectal administration also is a form of enteral administration. However, some healthcare personnel consider this route to be *parenteral* because it is not "by mouth."

Parenteral administration means medication administration into any part of the body other than by way of the gastrointestinal tract. This route includes medications administered via the vagina, eye, ear, nose and respiratory tract, skin, and by injection. In common usage, the term has come to refer to medications that are administered by injection. Intramuscular (IM), subcutaneous (subQ or SC), intradermal (**ID**), and intravenous (IV) methods of administration are examples of forms of injections. Table 63-1 shows various routes of administration for medications.

Rate of Absorption and Onset of Action

A medication's rate of absorption depends on its route of administration. Clients usually prefer oral administration, which is used most frequently. A disadvantage of drugs administered orally is the slower absorption rate, which results in a slowed onset of action. Absorption and onset of action with injected medications are more rapid than with orally administered drugs. Of all the injection methods, IV medications are absorbed most rapidly.

> **Nursing Alert**
> Some medications, such as prochlorperazine (Compazine), are available in different forms suitable for oral, injectable, or rectal administration. Other medications are available only in one form.

ENTERAL ADMINISTRATION METHODS

Oral Administration

The oral route of medication administration is used most frequently (see In Practice: Nursing Procedure 63-1). Medications administered orally (by mouth) are referred to as **PO** (Latin: "per os"). A PO medication can be in tablet, capsule, caplet, or liquid form.

Although this method is convenient, economical, and preferred by most clients, there are disadvantages to this method. Some medications have an unpleasant taste or odor; others are harmful to the teeth or mucous membranes of the mouth. Clients experiencing nausea and vomiting should not receive PO medications because they may be unable to retain them. Some clients have difficulty swallowing and therefore risk choking on PO medications, or have just had mouth or throat surgery. Other clients are noncompliant, refusing to swallow medications.

Some liquid medications are given full strength. Other liquid medications are diluted with water, juice, or milk. If a liquid medication has an unpleasant taste, a client may dull the taste buds by sucking on ice chips before taking it. Use a medicine cup to measure liquid medications. However, measure very small amounts in a syringe first and then transfer the amount to the medicine cup.

■■■ TABLE 63-1 *R*OUTES FOR MEDICATION ADMINISTRATION

Route	How Administered	Term Used to Describe Route
Enteral Methods		
By mouth	Client swallows medication	Oral administration (PO)
Applied to mucous membranes	Medication placed under tongue	Sublingual administration (SL)
	Medication placed between cheek and gum (buccal pouch)	Buccal administration
By feeding tube	Medication instilled through feeding tube into stomach or intestine	Types of tubes: Nasogastric (NG) Gastrostomy (GT) Jejunostomy (JT)
Given by suppository	Medication inserted into rectum	Rectal administration (R, PR)
Parenteral Methods		
Suppository or applicator	Medication inserted into vagina	Vaginal administration (V)
Applied to mucous membranes via dropper or tube	Medication instilled into eye	Eye (ophthalmic) administration
	Medication instilled into ear	Ear (otic) administration
Given via respiratory tract	Client inhales the medication	Nasal inhalation
	Client uses nasal spray	Aerosolized administration
	Client receives nasal drops	Nasal gtts (drops)
Given through the skin	Medication patch or ointment placed on the skin	Transdermal administration (TD)
Given by injection	Medication injected into	
	Corium (under epidermis)	Intradermal injection (ID)
	Subcutaneous tissue	Subcutaneous injection (SubQ)
	Muscle tissue	Intramuscular injection (IM)
	Vein	Intravenous injection (IV)
	Large vein (eg, subclavian)	Total parenteral nutrition (TPN)
	Artery	Intra-arterial injection (IA)
	Heart tissue	Intracardiac injection
	Peritoneal cavity	Intraperitoneal injection
	Spinal canal	Intraspinal injection
	Bone	Intraosseous injection
	Subarachnoid space	Intrathecal injection
	Bone marrow cavity	Intramedullary injection

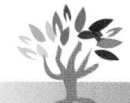

SPECIAL CONSIDERATIONS: THE LIFE SPAN

Liquids and Children

Administer PO liquid medications to small children directly from the syringe or a calibrated pediatric dropper.

Sublingual Administration

Sublingual (**SL**) medications are placed under the tongue, where they are dissolved and absorbed. Clients should not chew or swallow SL medications. Tell clients to keep SL medications under the tongue until the medication dissolves. Nitroglycerin is an example of an SL medication.

Buccal Administration

Buccal administration involves placing the medication between the client's cheek and gum. Clients should not chew or swallow buccal medications, but should leave them between the cheek and gum until such medications dissolve.

Administration Through a Gastric Tube

Clients with nasogastric tubes (**NG**) or other types of gastrointestinal tubes generally receive medications through them. Medications administered by this route should be in liquid form (see In Practice: Nursing Procedure 63-2). If medications are unavailable in liquid form, obtain a physician's order before crushing the medication and mixing it with liquid for administration (see Nursing Procedure 32-1). Do not crush coated or time-release medications.

(*text continues on page 869*)

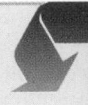

In Practice
Nursing Procedure 63-1

Administering Oral Medications

Supplies and Equipment

MAR or medication card
Disposable medication cups
Mortar and pestle, or pill crusher or tablet cutter (optional)
Water or juice
Medication cart
Straws (optional)

Steps

1. Wash the hands.
   RATIONALE: *Handwashing helps to prevent infection transmission.*

2. Gather equipment. Use the MAR to verify the medication order. Check any inconsistencies with the physician or pharmacist before administration. Check the client's chart for any allergies.
   RATIONALE: *Organization facilitates accurate skill performance and reduces the chance of medication errors. Nurses are responsible for checking the client's allergies to medications.*

3. Prepare one client's medication at a time.
   RATIONALE: *Preparing one client's medication at a time lessens the chances for medication errors.*

4. Unlock the medication cart or drawer.
   RATIONALE: *Keeping the medication setup locked provides security if the area is unattended.*

5. Proceed from top to bottom of the MAR when preparing medications.
   RATIONALE: *Organizing the approach, and being consistent in approach, ensures that any medication orders or specific times are not missed.*

6. Select the correct medication from the drawer or shelf. Compare the label to the medication order on the MAR. Complete any necessary calculations.
   RATIONALE: *Comparing medication to the written order is a check that helps prevent errors.*
   a. Pour a pill from the multidose bottle into the container lid, and transfer the correct amount to a cup.
      RATIONALE: *Pouring medication into the lid eliminates handling it, minimizing the risk of contamination.*
   b. Leave unit-dose medications in wrappers and place them in medication cups.
      RATIONALE: *Unit-dose wrappers keep medications clean and safe, and facilitate identification.*
   c. Measure liquid medications by holding the medicine cup at eye level and reading the level at the bottom of the meniscus. Pour from the

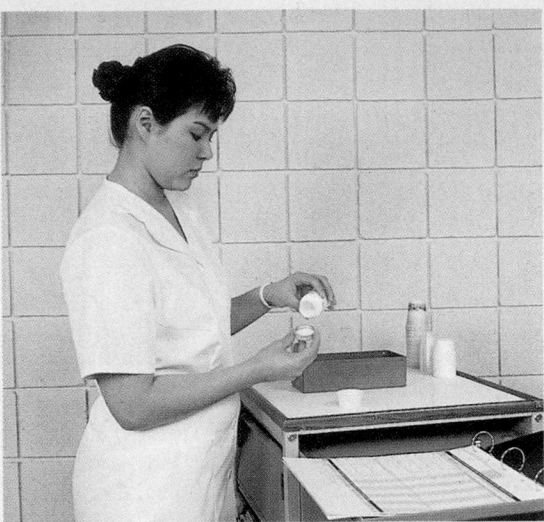

Pouring a pill from a multi-dose vial

bottle with the label uppermost, and wipe the neck with a paper towel if necessary. Sometimes calibrated droppers are provided.
RATIONALE: *Holding a cup at eye level to pour a liquid gives the most accurate measurement. Pouring away from the label and wiping the lip helps keep the label legible.*

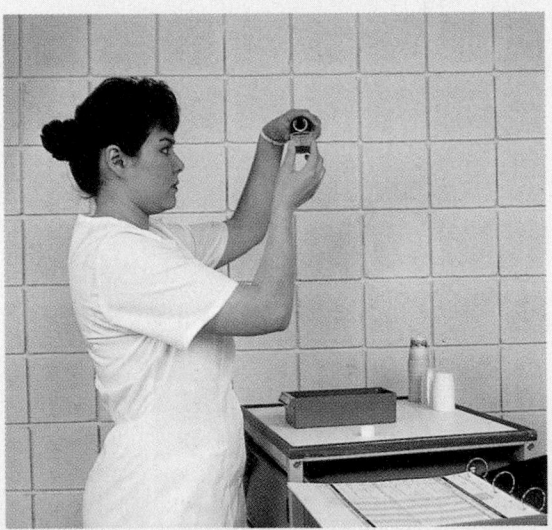

Measuring liquid medication

7. Re-check each medication with the MAR.
   RATIONALE: *Re-checking ensures preparation of the correct dose.*

8. When all medications have been prepared, compare each one again with the medication order.
   RATIONALE: *Checking all medications three times prevents errors.*

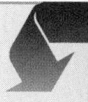

In Practice
Nursing Procedure 63-1 *(Continued)*

9. Crush pills if the client is unable to swallow them.
    RATIONALE: *Crushed medications are often easier to swallow. However, a specific order often is required to crush medications. Some medications cannot be crushed safely.*
    a. Place the pill in a paper souffle cup into a mortar or pill crusher. Cover the pill with another paper souffle cup placed inside the first one. Crush the pill until it is in powder form.
        RATIONALE: *This prevents any medication from getting on the pill crusher.*
    b. Do not crush time-release capsules or enteric-coated tablets.
        RATIONALE: *Enteric-coated tablets that are crushed may irritate the stomach's mucosal lining. Opening and crushing the contents of a time-release capsule may interfere with its absorption.*
    c. Dissolve crushed pills in water or juice, or mix with applesauce or ice cream.
        RATIONALE: *Dissolving helps mask the taste.*
    d. Cut tablets at the score mark only.
        RATIONALE: *Using the score mark ensures accurate dosing.*

10. Take medication to the client after you have prepared it. Give the medication as close to the ordered time as possible.
    RATIONALE: *Agency policy usually considers 30 minutes before or after the ordered time as an acceptable variation.*

11. Identify the client before giving the medication.
    RATIONALE: *Abiding by the "Five Rights" helps prevent medication errors.*
    a. Check the name on the identification bracelet.
        RATIONALE: *Checking the identification bracelet is the most reliable method for client identification.*
    b. Ask the client his or her name.
    c. Ask a staff member to identify the client.

12. Complete necessary assessments before giving medications.
    RATIONALE: *Checking helps reduce the risk of problems after the drug is administered. Checks include asking the client about any allergies and assessing blood pressure, apical pulse rate, or respiratory rate, depending on the medication's action.*

13. Assist the client to a comfortable position.
    RATIONALE: *Sitting as upright as possible makes swallowing the medication easier and less likely to cause aspiration.*

14. Administer the medication.
    a. Offer water or fluids with the medication. Be aware of any fluid restrictions that exist.

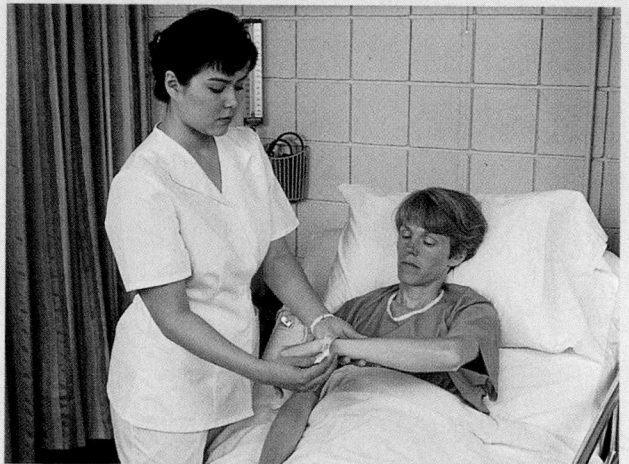

Checking the client's identification bracelet

    b. Ask the client how he or she prefers the medication (eg, one at a time, all at once, from the cup or hand).
        RATIONALE: *Including the client's preferences involves the client in the administration process.*
    c. Open unit-dose medication packages and give the medication to the client.
    d. Review the medication's name and purpose.
    e. Discard any medication that falls on the floor.
        RATIONALE: *Any medication that falls on the floor is considered contaminated.*
    f. Mix powder medications with fluids at the bedside.
        RATIONALE: *Powdered forms of drugs may thicken when mixed with fluid; give them immediately.*
    g. Record fluid intake on the intake and output (I&O) form.
        RATIONALE: *Recording fluid taken with medications maintains accurate documentation.*

15. Remain with the client until he or she has taken all medication. Check the client's mouth, if needed.
    RATIONALE: *Remaining with the client helps to ensure that the client takes the medication. Some clients hide the medication between the gum and cheek [called "cheeking"]. Leaving medication at the bedside is unsafe.*

16. Wash hands.
    RATIONALE: *Handwashing helps to prevent the spread of infection.*

17. Record medication administration on the appropriate form.
    RATIONALE: *Documentation provides coordination of care, and verifies the reason any medica-*
    (continued)

In Practice
Nursing Procedure 63-1 *(Continued)*

tions were omitted as well as the specific nursing assessments needed to safely administer medication.

a. Sign after giving the medication.

b. If a client refused the medication, record according to agency's policy on the record.

c. Document vital signs or particular assessments according to agency's format.

d. Sign in the narcotic book for controlled substances when removing them from the locked area.

    Rᴀᴛɪᴏɴᴀʟᴇ: *Federal law regulates special documentation for controlled substances.*

18. Check the client within 30 minutes after giving medication. This is particularly important following pain medication or any PRN (as needed) medication.

    Rᴀᴛɪᴏɴᴀʟᴇ: *Followup after administration verifies the client's response to the medication—particularly the relief of pain after taking an*

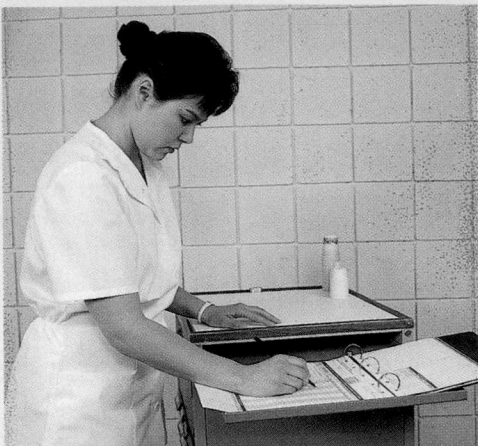

Documenting administration of medication. (Photos © B. Proud)

analgesic. Prompt charting helps prevent duplication in administration.

In Practice
Nursing Procedure 63-2

Aᴅᴍɪɴɪsᴛᴇʀɪɴɢ Mᴇᴅɪᴄᴀᴛɪᴏɴs Tʜʀᴏᴜɢʜ ᴀ Gᴀsᴛʀᴏɪɴᴛᴇsᴛɪɴᴀʟ Tᴜʙᴇ

Supplies and Equipment

MAR
Gloves
Medication
Large syringe
Fluids, as needed
Stethoscope
Mortar and pestle, or pill crusher if an order to crush medications has been obtained

Steps

1. Check the MAR with the original medication order. When giving more than one medication, make sure medications are compatible.

    Rᴀᴛɪᴏɴᴀʟᴇ: *Doing so helps to ensure that the correct medication and correct dosage are administered to the correct client.*

2. Check the MAR and the client's record for allergies to medications.

    Rᴀᴛɪᴏɴᴀʟᴇ: *If the client has previously experienced an allergic reaction to any medication, the medication must not be administered and*

the healthcare provider must be notified immediately.

3. Wash hands.

    Rᴀᴛɪᴏɴᴀʟᴇ: *Handwashing is the single most important method of preventing the spread of infection.*

4. Gather needed equipment.

    Rᴀᴛɪᴏɴᴀʟᴇ: *Organization helps to eliminate the possibility of medication errors.*

5. Set up the medication following the "Five Rights" of administration.

    Rᴀᴛɪᴏɴᴀʟᴇ: *Strictly adhering to safety precautions decreases the possibility of errors.*

6. Proceed to the client's bedside, introducing yourself and explaining what will happen, and identify the client.

    Rᴀᴛɪᴏɴᴀʟᴇ: *Explanation helps to decrease the client's anxiety.*

7. Put on gloves.

    Rᴀᴛɪᴏɴᴀʟᴇ: *Standard Precautions are necessary when a possibility of coming into contact with bodily secretions exists.*

8 a. Using a syringe, check placement of the NG or G-tube.

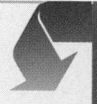

In Practice
Nursing Procedure 63-2 (Continued)

RATIONALE: *Correct placement of the tube ensures that medication will be delivered into the stomach.*

b. Do not aspirate if the client has a button-type G-tube or a jejunal tube.
RATIONALE: *Aspiration can damage the anti-reflux valve.*

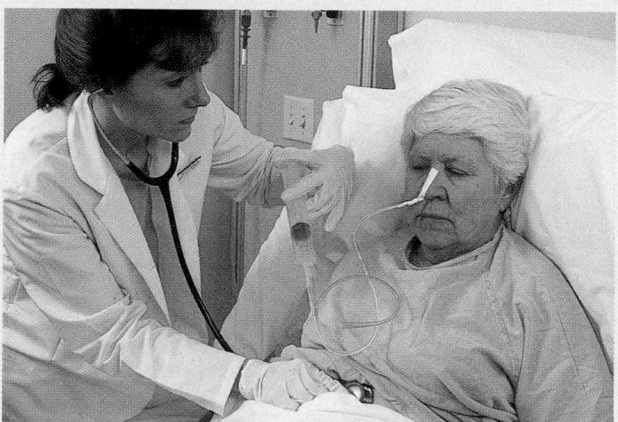

After checking placement of the NG tube, the nurse instills the medication through the tube.

9. After checking the tubing's placement, pinch or clamp the tubing and remove the syringe.
RATIONALE: *Clamping or pinching the tube prevents gastric contents from escaping through the tubing, and ensures that no air enters the stomach and causes discomfort for the client.*

10. Remove the plunger from the syringe and reconnect the syringe to the tube.

RATIONALE: *The syringe will deliver the medication to the tube.*

11. Release the clamp and pour the medication into the syringe. *Note:* If the medication does not flow freely down the tube, insert the plunger and gently apply a *slight* pressure to start the flow. Sometimes this action will start the flow. If medication flow does not start, determine if the NG or G-tube is plugged.
RATIONALE: *If the tube is plugged, the healthcare provider must be notified.*

12. After administering the medication, flush the tube with 15–30 mL of water.
RATIONALE: *Flushing clears the tube and decreases the chance of tube blockage.*

13. Clamp the tubing and remove the syringe.
RATIONALE: *Clamping the tubing and then removing the syringe prevents excessive air from entering the tubing.*

14. Replace the tubing plug; or if a continuous feeding is in effect, reconnect the tubing to the feeding tubing.
RATIONALE: *Replacing the plug prevents air from entering; reconnecting the feeding tube re-establishes the client's nutrition.*

15. Assist the client to a comfortable position.
RATIONALE: *Doing so promotes the client's comfort.*

16. Wash hands and document administration of medication via NG or G-tube.
RATIONALE: *Documentation helps to maintain communication with other members of the healthcare team.*

Crushed medications tend to clog gastrostomy tubes (**G-tubes**). Only those medications specified as *enteral* may be given via G-tubes.

Nursing Alert
To avoid undesired medication effects, consult a drug reference, pharmacist, or charge nurse with any doubts about restrictions or incompatibilities of medications.

Rectal Administration

Typically, medications given rectally are in the form of suppositories. A suppository is a semisolid medication that is designed to melt at body temperature. Suppositories are usually stored in refrigerators. Suppositories should be lubricated with water-soluble lubricants before insertion if not already prelubricated. Additionally, fluid or medication can be instilled

into the rectum as enemas. Chapter 51 discusses the administration of enemas in more detail.

PARENTERAL ADMINISTRATION METHODS

Noninjection Methods

Vaginal Administration
Vaginal medications are supplied in the form of suppositories, foams, creams, and tablets that usually involve the use of an applicator to ensure that the medication is placed correctly. In Practice: Nursing Procedure 63-3 highlights the steps involved when administering a suppository rectally or vaginally.

Eye (Ophthalmic) Administration
Medications that may be instilled or administered directly into the eye (**ophthalmic** medications) include liquid medications, ointments, and medication-impregnated disks that resemble contact lenses (see In Practice: Nursing Procedure 63-4).

In Practice
Nursing Procedure 63-3

Administering a Suppository

Supplies and Equipment

MAR
Gloves
Medication
Lubricant, if needed

Steps

1. Check the MAR against the original physician's order.
   RATIONALE: *Checking ensures adherence to the "Five Rights."*

2. Wash hands.
   RATIONALE: *Handwashing helps prevent the spread of infection.*

3. Put on gloves.
   RATIONALE: *Standard Precautions are necessary when there is the potential for contact with body secretions.*

4. Proceed to the client's bedside and identify the client. Introduce yourself and explain what will happen.
   RATIONALE: *Explanations help to reduce the client's anxiety.*

For Rectal Administration

5. Assist the client to the Sims' position. Generally the left-side lying position is preferable.
   RATIONALE: *This position provides easy visualization of and access to the rectum.*

6. Drape the client properly.
   RATIONALE: *Proper draping ensures privacy.*

7. Insert the suppository into the client's anal canal at least 4 inches for an adult, and 2 inches for a child.
   RATIONALE: *This position ensures placement of the suppository above the client's internal sphincter and maximizes medication absorption.*

8. Ask the client to maintain the Sims' position for 15–20 minutes and not to expel the suppository.
   RATIONALE: *Maintaining the position allows time for the medication to melt.*

9. Dispose of gloves and wash hands.
   RATIONALE: *Proper glove disposal and handwashing help prevent the spread of infection.*

10. Document administration of the suppository.

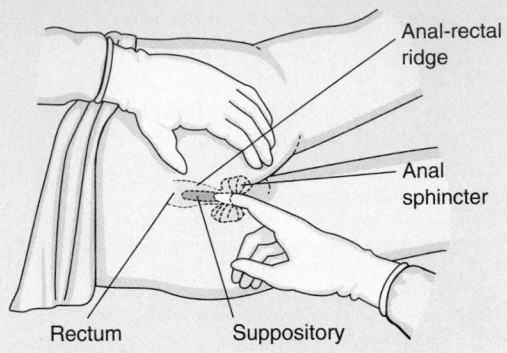

Insert the suppository past the internal anal sphincter against the rectal wall.

RATIONALE: *Documentation maintains communication with other members of the healthcare team and prevents possible medication errors.*

11. Check on the client in 20–30 minutes and document client's response.
    RATIONALE: *Followup determines if the medication was effective, and maintains communication with other members of the healthcare team.*

For Vaginal Administration

5. Position the client in the modified lithotomy position (on her back).
   RATIONALE: *This position enables visualization of the vaginal area and easy access for insertion of the suppository.*

6. Insert the suppository approximately 2 inches into the vagina.
   RATIONALE: *Proper placement will ensure absorption.*

7. Instruct the client to remain on her back for 15–20 minutes.
   RATIONALE: *This position will maximize retention and absorption of the suppository.*

8. Offer the client a sanitary pad.
   RATIONALE: *It will absorb excess drainage and protect the client and bed.*

9. Dispose of gloves and wash hands.
   RATIONALE: *Proper glove disposal and handwashing help prevent the spread of infection.*

10. Document the administration of the suppository and the client's response.
    RATIONALE: *Documentation helps to maintain communication with other members of the healthcare team and prevent possible medication errors.*

In Practice
Nursing Procedure 63-4

ADMINISTERING EYE MEDICATIONS

Supplies and Equipment

MAR
Goggles, if needed
Medication, with dropper if needed
Clean cotton balls
Gloves
Disposable tissues
Separate droppers for each eye, if needed

Steps

1. Check the MAR against the original physician's order.
   RATIONALE: *Checking ensures adherence to the "Five Rights."*

2. Wash hands carefully. If placing drops in both eyes, wash hands before and after treating each eye.
   RATIONALE: *Handwashing is the most effective means of preventing the spread of infection.*

3. Proceed to the client's room and identify the client. Introduce yourself and explain what will happen.
   RATIONALE: *Explanations help reduce the client's anxiety.*

4. Put on gloves (put on goggles if indicated).
   RATIONALE: *Standard Precautions are used if a possibility of coming into contact with bodily fluids or secretions exists.*

5. If administering medication to both eyes, use a clean cotton ball for each eye; cleanse the eyelids by wiping from the inner canthus to the outer canthus.
   RATIONALE: *This action cleans the eyelids and prevents the spread of infection from one eye to the other.*

6. Ask the client to lie down or sit with his or her head tilted backward.
   RATIONALE: *This position will help facilitate the instillation and dispersion of medication.*

7. Provide the client with a tissue.
   RATIONALE: *There may be an overflow of medication or tears.*

For Eye Drops

8. Check the bottle's label; do not instill any medication in the eye unless it is labeled *ophthalmic*.
   RATIONALE: *Other medications could endanger the client's vision.*

9. Gently retract the lower eyelid with your thumb and finger.
   RATIONALE: *Pulling on the lower eyelid exposes the lower conjunctival sac, allowing for proper medication administration.*

10. Brace the thumb on the bone under the eyebrow. Ask the client to look up, and instill the prescribed number of drops into the center of the *everted* (turned outward) lower lid (the *conjunctival surface*).
    RATIONALE: *Instilling the drops into the conjunctival sac will avoid possible corneal injury. The thumb helps give stability.*

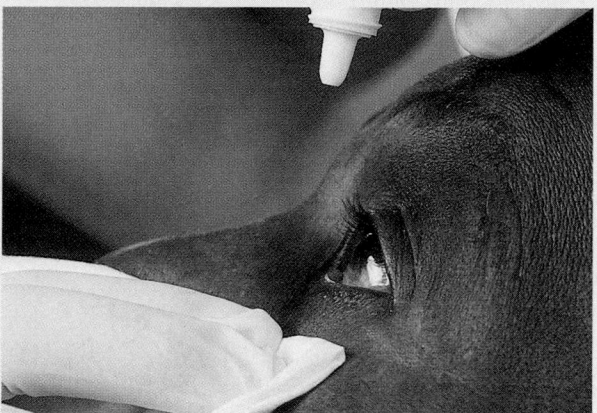

With the client looking up and pressure being applied with two fingers over the cheek's bony prominence, the nurse instills eye drops into the lower conjunctival sac. The thumb can be used to apply pressure downward if it is more convenient.

11. Place gentle pressure on the inner canthus after instilling eye drops.
    RATIONALE: *Applying gentle pressure helps to prevent the solution from draining into the lacrimal duct. It also minimizes the risks of systemic effects or bacteria being washed into the lacrimal duct.*

12. Instruct the client to close the eyelids and apply gentle pressure.
    RATIONALE: *Closing the eyelid while applying gentle pressure allows distribution of the medication.*

13. Wipe off any excess medication with a cotton ball.

14. If ordered, repeat the procedure for the other eye. Use separate droppers, if ordered.

15. Dispose of goggles and gloves. Wash hands.
    RATIONALE: *Proper disposal of items and handwashing helps prevent the spread of infection.*

16. Document the procedure.
    RATIONALE: *Documentation maintains communication with other members of the healthcare team.*

For Eye Ointments

8. Before administration, wipe the tube with a clean cotton ball and discard a small amount of ointment.
   RATIONALE: *Discarding the first portion of ointment maintains the ointment's sterility.*

9. Apply the ointment inside the lower lid, in a thin line, from inner to outer canthus. Do not touch the lower lid or the eye with the applicator tip.

(continued)

In Practice
Nursing Procedure 63-4 *(Continued)*

RATIONALE: *Following this procedure prevents contamination of the applicator tip and subsequent transfer of pathogens to the other eye.*

10. Ask the client to blink a few times.
RATIONALE: *Blinking aids in medication distribution.*

11. Use a cotton ball or tissue to wipe away any excess medication.

12. Dispose of goggles and gloves. Wash your hands.
RATIONALE: *Proper disposal of items and handwashing helps prevent the spread of infection.*

13. Document the procedure on the MAR.
RATIONALE: *Documentation helps to maintain communication with other members of the healthcare team.*

If applying an ointment to both eyes, take great care to avoid spreading the infection from one eye to the other. Do not allow the applicator tip to touch either eye during administration. Give ointments at bedtime because they cause blurred vision.

☛ Kᴇʏ Cᴏɴᴄᴇᴘᴛ

Eye drops are instilled for various reasons: to contract or dilate the pupils, to treat an infection, to provide lubrication, or to produce a local effect (eg, anesthesia). Nurses are often responsible for carrying out the procedure and for instructing clients and their families in the procedure.

Ear (Otic) Administration
Ear (**otic**) medications may be given by instillation from a squeeze bottle or a dropper. To better visualize the ear canal and to help ensure proper medication delivery, position the auditory canal correctly (see In Practice: Nursing Procedure 63-5). Position the squeeze bottle tip or dropper slightly above the ear canal while instilling the drops. Never insert the dropper or applicator tip into the ear canal.

Nasal or Respiratory Administration
Drugs may be given by drops, inhalation, or through aerosol delivery systems for disorders of the respiratory tract.

In Practice
Nursing Procedure 63-5

Aᴅᴍɪɴɪsᴛᴇʀɪɴɢ Eᴀʀ Mᴇᴅɪᴄᴀᴛɪᴏɴs
Supplies and Equipment

MAR
Disposable tissues
Medication
Cotton balls
Gloves

Steps

1. Check the medication order against the original physician's order.
RATIONALE: *Checking helps to ensure adherence to the "Five Rights."*

2. Wash hands carefully.
RATIONALE: *Handwashing helps prevent the spread of infection.*

3. Prepare the medication following the "Five Rights."
RATIONALE: *Adhering to the "Five Rights" helps decrease the possibility of errors.*

4. Proceed to the client's bedside and identify the client. Identify yourself and tell the client what will happen.
RATIONALE: *Explanations help to decrease the client's anxiety.*

5. Put on gloves.
RATIONALE: *Standard Precautions are necessary if a possibility of coming into contact with bodily secretions exists.*

6. Ask the client to lie on the side of the unaffected ear.
RATIONALE: *This position facilitates instillation of medication into the affected ear.*

7. Remove excess drainage with a dry wipe. If the drainage has dried, use a warm wash cloth to clean the area.
RATIONALE: *Dried drainage or crusting may limit the medication's effectiveness.*

8. Expose the external ear canal by properly adjusting the client's ear lobe. For adults, pull the lobe up, back, and outward. For children, pull the lobe down and back.

RATIONALE: *Proper positioning of the ear facilitates delivery of medication into the external auditory canal.*

9 a. Hold the dropper or the tip of the squeeze bottle above the opening of the external auditory canal. Allow the prescribed number of drops to fall on the side of the canal.
   RATIONALE: *Allowing the medication to run into the ear canal toward the tympanic membrane will be more comfortable than the medication falling directly into the canal and on the membrane.*

   b. Do not touch any part of the ear with the dropper or squeeze bottle during administration.
   RATIONALE: *Doing so prevents contamination of the dropper or squeeze-bottle tip.*

10. Instruct the client to remain in the side-lying position for 5–10 minutes with the affected ear upward.
    RATIONALE: *This position allows the medication to run into the ear canal for maximum effectiveness.*

11. If the procedure is ordered for both ears, allow 5–10 minutes between instillations. Repeat the above steps for the other ear.
    RATIONALE: *Waiting allows medication to come into adequate contact with the first ear before treating the second.*

12. Dispose of gloves and wash hands.
    RATIONALE: *Proper disposal and handwashing help prevent the spread of infection.*

13. Document the procedure on the client's MAR.
    RATIONALE: *Documentation maintains communication with other members of the healthcare team.*

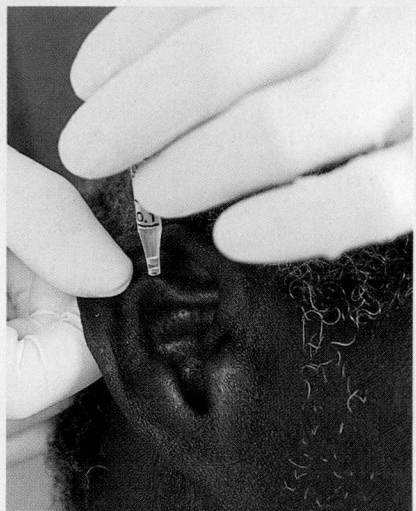

A

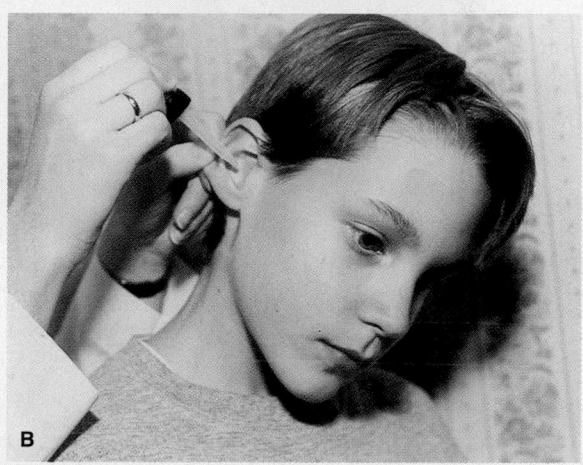

B

(**A**) In an adult, pull the pinna of the ear up and back to straighten the ear canal. (**B**) In a school-aged child, pull the pinna of the ear nearly straight back to straighten the ear canal. (In an infant, the pinna is pulled down and back.) In all cases, ear drops are placed on the side of the canal.

Inhalants and Aerosol Systems.   Medications that are inhaled have a very rapid rate of absorption and onset of action. They may be delivered by an inhaler or aerosol delivery system (Fig. 63-1). *Inhalers* are hand-held devices that deliver a measured dose of medication with each inhalation (metered dose inhaler, **MDI**). Instruct the client to exhale and then to breathe deeply as he or she activates the inhaler by depressing on the canister. The inhaler will deliver a fine mist of medication into the oropharyngeal area, which the client will inhale into the lungs. *Extenders,* also called *spacers* and *chambers,* are available to increase the volume of medication delivered. When using a spacer, the nurse tells the client to close his or her lips around the mouthpiece and then to depress the canister, releasing the medication. The client is then instructed to take and hold a deep breath or to take 2 to 3 short breaths. Each inhalation is referred to as one "puff."

Aerosol or nebulizer administration is based on the use of compressed air or oxygen, which forces a mist of medication through tubing to a mouthpiece or mask. The client then inhales the medication. Most aerosol medications have bronchodilating effects, and are administered by respiratory therapy personnel. However, in smaller healthcare facilities, nurses may regularly administer such treatments. Never leave a client alone during aerosol breathing treatments, due to the effects of the medication. Encourage the client to breathe deeply but not rapidly. Should the client breathe too rapidly, he or she may experience dizziness or possibly tetany. In Practice: Nursing Care Guidelines 63-3 provides more information.

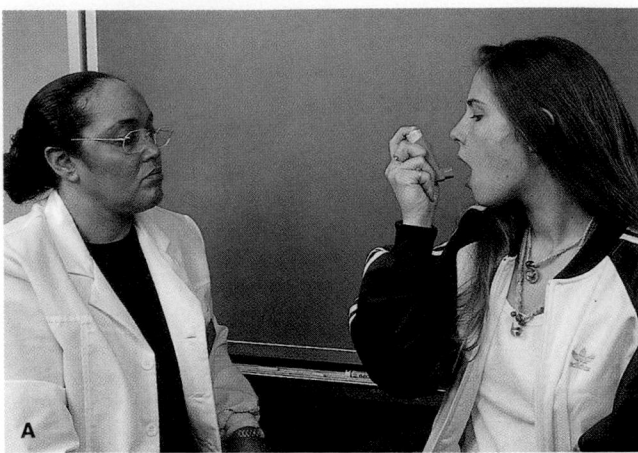

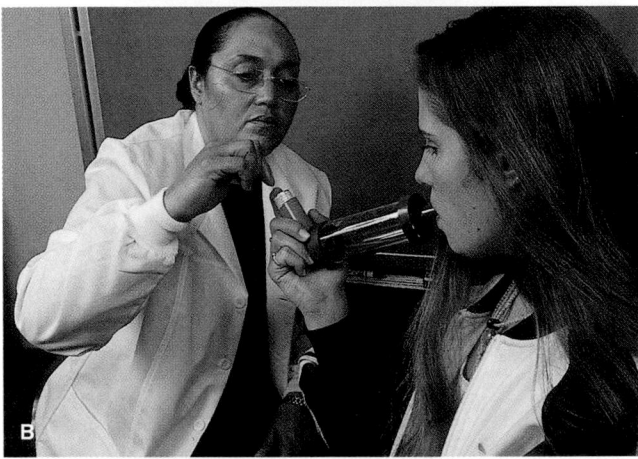

FIGURE 63-1. (A) Using the metered dose inhaler (MDI). **(B)** Using a spacer, which makes administration of aerosolized medications more comfortable and more effective.

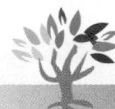

SPECIAL CONSIDERATIONS: THE LIFE SPAN

Aerosol and Inhalation Therapy

To ensure that a young child receives an accurate dose, hold the mouthpiece closely to the nose and mouth or use a mask.

Nasal Sprays or Drops.   Nasal sprays or drops may be ordered for nasal congestion. Follow the steps as for administering any medication, such as checking the MAR, washing hands, preparing the medication, and explaining to the client what will happen. Then use the following as a guide when administering such preparations:

- Assist the client to a high Fowler's or sitting position with the head tilted back. Place the tip of the bottle just inside the nares, aimed toward the nose's midline. Activate the nebulization or squeeze the bottle while the client inhales. *Rationale: This position allows the medication to come into contact with the nasal mucous membranes for maximal therapeutic effect.*
- Instruct the client to maintain this position for approximately 1 to 2 minutes. *Rationale: This position will inhibit drainage of the medication from the nares due to gravity flow.*

When administration is completed, always perform handwashing and document the procedure.

In Practice
Nursing Care Guidelines 63-3

ADMINISTERING AEROSOLIZED MEDICATIONS

General Considerations
- Check the medication order against the physician's original order. *Rationale: This ensures adherence to the five rights.*
- Wash hands and put on gloves if indicated. Set up the medication following safety guidelines. *Rationale: Handwashing and using gloves helps to prevent contamination.*
- Teach the client how to use his or her particular device.
- Avoid treatments immediately before and after meals. *Rationale: Avoiding these times helps to decrease the chance of vomiting or appetite suppression, especially with medications that cause the client to cough or expectorate, or those that are*

taken in conjunction with percussion/bronchial drainage.
- If the client is to continue treatments at home, be sure he or she completely understands the medication and has demonstrated the ability to perform the treatment. *Rationale: At home, the client may not have access to teaching, which could result in incorrect dosing or inability to use or maintain the equipment.*
- Be sure to wash hands before and after the treatment, and document the procedure and the client's response. Document teaching and the client's ability to follow teaching. *Rationale: Documentation provides a means of communication with other healthcare personnel.*

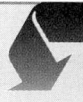

In Practice
Nursing Care Guidelines 63-3 *(Continued)*

For an Inhaler

- Shake the inhaler well immediately prior to use. *Rationale: Shaking aerosolizes the fine particles.*
- Instruct the client to take a deep breath and exhale completely through the nose. Then, have the client position the inhaler to just in front of his or her mouth, push down on the canister, and inhale as slowly and deeply as possible through the mouth; If the client is having difficulty with this, have the client grip the mouthpiece with the lips and then push down on the canister. *Rationale: These steps help to allow the medication to come into contact with the lungs for the maximum amount of time.*
- Instruct the client to hold his or her breath for about 10 seconds and then to slowly exhale with pursed lips.
- Repeat the above steps for each ordered "puff," waiting 5–10 minutes or as prescribed between puffs. *Rationale: This method achieves maximum benefits.*

For a Nebulizer

- Fill the nebulizer cup with the ordered amount of medication. Turn on the oxygen or air at the pre-scribed liter flow. *Rationale: This ensures that the required medication amount is given.*
- Instruct the client to close the lips around the mouthpiece and to breathe through the mouth. (If the client is using a mask, he or she should breathe normally.) *Rationale: Breathing through the mouth or normally with a mask helps the medication travel to the lungs.*
- Instruct the client to continue the treatment until he or she can no longer see a mist on exhalation (from the opposite end of the mouthpiece) or vent holes (in the mask). *Rationale: Lack of mist ensures that the client has inhaled the entire dose.*
- Cleanse the nebulizer cup and mouthpiece with warm, soapy water. Rinse and dry it after each use. Follow facility protocols for the frequency of changing the tubing and cup for each client. *Rationale: Proper cleaning, and following guidelines, decreases the possibility of pathogens entering the client's respiratory tract.*

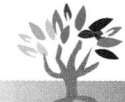

SPECIAL CONSIDERATIONS: THE LIFE SPAN

Administering Nasal Sprays or Drops

A child who must receive nasal medications may be more receptive if a family caregiver administers them. If a family caregiver is unavailable, hold the child with his or her head tilted back while you restrain the arms and legs. Make every effort to administer nasal medications with care. Be gentle and reassuring, especially for a small child.

Transdermal Administration

Many medications are now available in transdermal (**TD**) patches. Many clients use nitroglycerin and hormone replacement patches (eg, estrogen). The skin absorbs these medications systemically. Place transdermal patches on clean, dry, hairless areas (Fig. 63-2). Check with a drug reference, pharmacist, or supervisor if the physician does not include the area of placement in the order. Depending on the medication, the nurse may change the patch daily or weekly. Be sure to follow the steps for any medication administration and then use the following as a guide:

- Note carefully the location of the current patch before removing it. Be sure to cleanse the skin carefully. *Rationale: Patches may sometimes irritate the skin.*
- Locate and remove the old patch. *Rationale: Leaving the previous patch in place may result in increased and undesired dosage of medication.*
- Make sure the application site for the new patch is clean, dry, and hairless. *Rationale: To be effective, the patch must remain in place.*
- Place the new patch in the appropriate area. *Rationale: The body area where the patch is applied may affect its absorption rate.* Be sure to continually rotate the application site. *Rationale: Some medication patches irritate the skin. Changing the site of application will reduce skin irritation.*
- Wash your hands thoroughly. *Rationale: Handwashing helps to prevent any medication from being absorbed through the nurse's skin.* (Wear gloves, as needed)

As with any medication administration, document the administration.

Administration by Injection

Injection is a method of introducing liquid medications into various body tissues. Common methods of injection include ID, subQ, IM, and IV. Other methods include intracardiac,

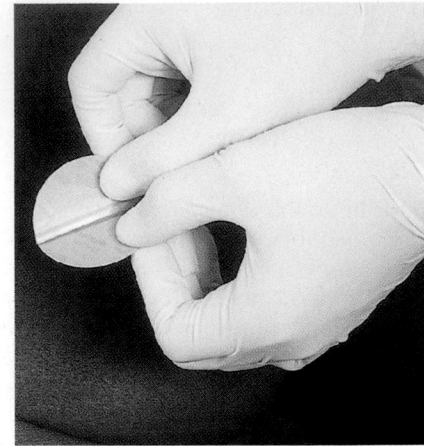

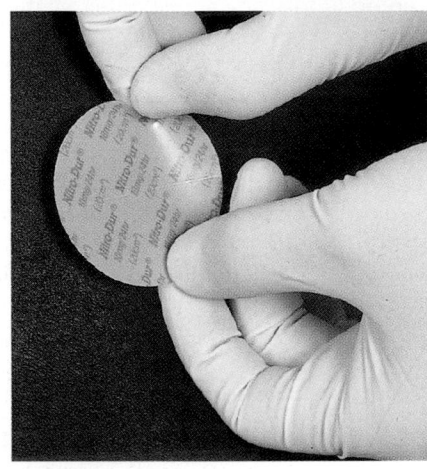

FIGURE 63-2. The transdermal patch. (**A**) First, bend the patch to break the seal. (**B**) Remove protective covering and apply to skin.

intramedullary, intrathecal, intraosseous, and intraperitoneal. Only physicians and specially instructed nurses use these latter routes; for that reason they are not addressed in this text.

Although the nurse may give injections in various ways (ID, subQ, and so forth), general principles apply for every method. Sterile equipment is a must when giving injections to avoid introducing pathogens into the tissues or bloodstream.

A medication may be administered by injection for the following reasons:

- The medication is most effective by injection.
- The medication is unavailable for any other form of administration.
- The client needs the desired action quickly.
- Dosage accuracy is critical.
- The client is nauseated or vomiting and cannot retain oral medications.
- The client's mental or physical condition renders him or her unable or unwilling to swallow oral medications.
- The digestive system cannot absorb the drug.

The body absorbs injected medications much more quickly than it absorbs oral medications. Generally, IV injection achieves the fastest method of systemic absorption.

When administering IM and subQ injections, insert and remove the needle *quickly*. With the wrist, use a quick darting

motion to reduce discomfort that the client may experience when the needle pierces the skin. Gently massage the injection site after withdrawing the needle to speed absorption and to relieve discomfort caused by tissue displacement during the injection. *Do not massage certain areas, such as those sites into which heparin or allergy medications are injected. (The body needs to absorb such medications slowly.)*

The nurse must know the locations of common administration sites and the actions of medications to be injected. An accidental injection into a nerve could result in damage and paralysis. Injection directly into a blood vessel could cause the client's system to absorb the medication too rapidly, with an adverse, perhaps fatal reaction. Failure to inject certain medications, such as injectable steroids, into deep muscular tissue may cause tissue atrophy, with resultant pitting or deformity of the site. Forgetting to rotate the sites of insulin injections, for example, will cause areas of tissue atrophy and indentation (*lipodystrophy*).

Syringes and Needles

Syringes are available in various sizes, ranging from 0.5 to 100 milliliter capacity. All syringes consist of three parts: tip, barrel, and plunger (Fig. 63-3). The *tip* is the portion of the syringe attached to the needle. A syringe may have one of two types of tips: a Luer-Lok or plain tip. The *barrel* is clearly marked with a calibrated measurement scale. When preparing an injection, draw the medication into the barrel section. The *plunger* is the inner portion that fits inside the barrel. Pull out the plunger to create a vacuum and withdraw medication; push in to inject medication.

Milliliters are subdivided into tenths on the syringe. Read the volume of medication drawn into the syringe at the point where the rubber flange of the plunger is even or parallel with the marked measurement scale on the barrel.

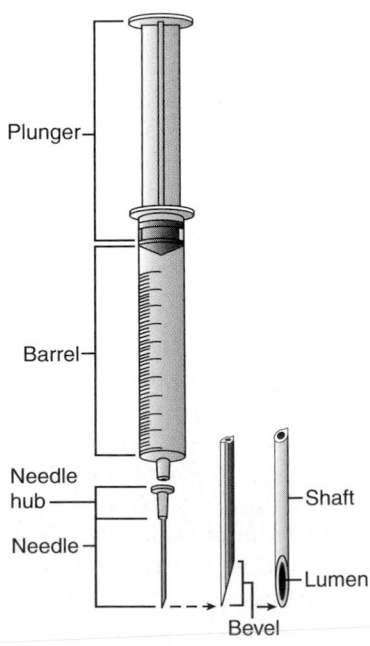

FIGURE 63-3. Parts of a needle and syringe.

Nearly all syringes used today are disposable. Some come equipped with a needle; others do not and the needle must be attached separately. Other syringes, called *cartridges,* contain premeasured amounts of medication (Fig. 63-4). The cartridge-type unit is inserted into a reusable holder that contains a plunger.

Needles also consist of three parts: hub, shaft, and beveled tip. The *hub* or *hilt* is the part that attaches to the tip of the syringe. The *shaft* is the elongated portion. The *bevel* (the area containing the hole or bore) can vary from regular bevel (long, allowing for easy entry through the skin) to intradermal (ID) bevel (blunt, used exclusively for intradermal injections).

Needles are made of stainless steel and come in various sizes. The needle's gauge and length are both important when choosing the correct type for injection. The gauge (**G**) is the needle's inner diameter or bore, through which medication is administered. The gauge is stated using numbers. The larger the number, the smaller the bore. A 25-G needle has a very small opening and would be used for subQ or ID injections; a 23-G needle, which has a larger bore, may be used for IM injections of more viscous liquids; an 18-G needle has a very large bore and may be used for IV injection of large amounts of medication.

Needles range in length from ⅜ to 2 inches. A subQ injection is given with a short needle (⅜ inch in length); an IM injection requires a longer needle with a larger bore, to ensure delivery into the muscular tissue.

Although the physician's order will state the type of injection to give, the size of needle to use depends on the medication's volume (amount) and viscosity. Additionally, some medications, such as steroids, need to be injected into muscles, and therefore will need long needles for accurate delivery.

Needles and syringes are packaged in sterile plastic wrappers. Be sure to maintain their sterility. Check to make sure that wrappers are intact. Also check expiration dates. If in doubt, obtain a different syringe or needle. After use, *always dispose of all syringes and needles in the sharps container provided.*

The Safety Syringe.   A popular syringe-and-needle combination is the *safety syringe,* which has a plastic sheath that is pulled down to protect the needle after drawing up medication (Fig. 63-5). The sheath will click into place, but will not lock if it is pulled straight out. When the nurse is ready to give the injection, he or she pushes the sheath back until it clicks. After giving the injection, the nurse pulls out the sheath again and *twists it until it clicks.* This will lock it into place. The safety syringe prevents needlesticks after it is locked.

Needleless Systems.   Another injection system that prevents needlesticks allows injections into IV tubing without the use of a needle (Fig. 63-6). There are several types of needleless injection systems. They are most commonly used in the hospital setting.

Injection Systems for Various Methods.   *SubQ injections* usually are given using 1- or 2-milliliter syringes with ⅜- to 1-inch needles. When injecting more than 1 milliliter subQ, divide the dose into two syringes and administer two injections.

Depending on the type and amount of medication, *IM injections* usually require 2- to 3-milliliter syringes with 1- to 1½-inch needles. The angle of injection is also different, depending upon the type of injection to be given (Fig. 63-7).

ID (intradermal) injections typically are given using 1-milliliter tuberculin syringes. Needles should be 25 to 26 G with a ⅜-inch intradermal bevel. The intradermal bevel is more blunt than a regular bevel, and allows easier access to the epidermis (see section on "Intradermal (ID) Injections"). Regular-bevel needles are much more difficult to use for ID injections because their added length makes accidental entry into the dermis possible. Because the dermis contains blood vessels, the skin would absorb the medication more quickly than desired, which could cause a systemic reaction.

Preparations

Injectable medications are packaged in many ways. Some are prepared as powders that must be reconstituted with a **diluent.** When mixed with a diluent, these medications deteriorate very rapidly and must be used within the time specified by the manufacturer. Common diluents include sterile water and sterile normal saline. The manufacturer's instructions will specify the diluent. Other medications are premixed. Medications for injection may be supplied in a single-dose ampule, single-dose vial, or multidose vial.

An **ampule** is a glass container that holds a premeasured, single medication dose. Discard any unused portion of an ampule's contents, because no way exists to prevent contamination of an open ampule.

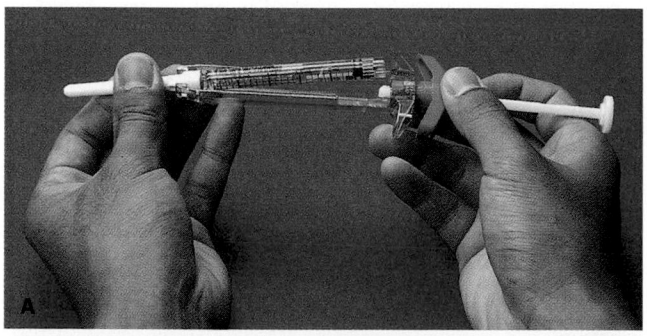

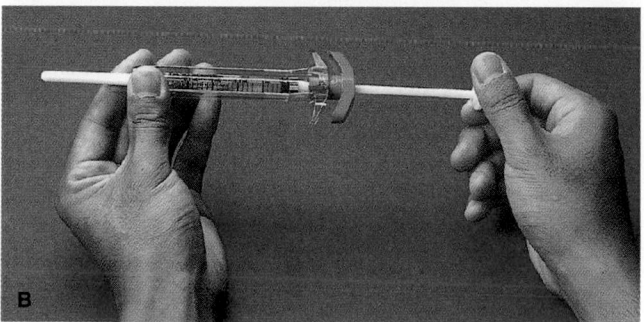

FIGURE 63-4. Using prefilled syringes. (**A**) The prefilled cartridge is inserted into the holder/injection device. (**B**) The device is screwed on to tighten it. This holds the cartridge in place. The cartridge may need to be pushed into place to break its seal prior to injection. The injection is then given as with any syringe.

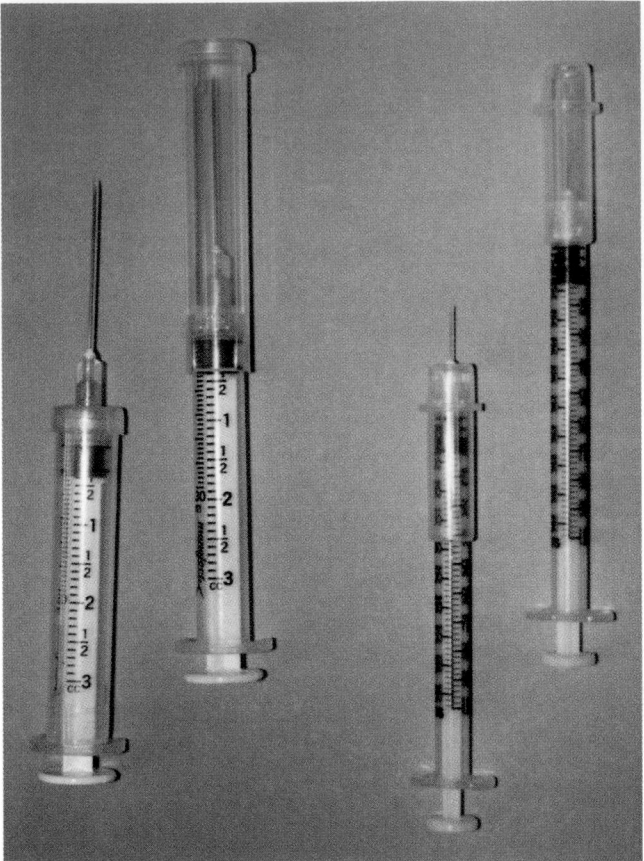

FIGURE 63-5. One type of safety syringe. A sheath covers the needle while it is transported. The sheath is retracted to administer the injection, and is again pulled out and locked when the injection is completed. This technique avoids the dangerous practice of recapping needles and prevents needle stick injuries. Shown are a 3-mL syringe with a 22 gauge, 1½-inch needle (for IM injections); and a 1-mL insulin syringe with a 29 gauge, ½ inch needle. Each needle is shown with the sheath in place and with the sheath retracted. (Photo: Caroline Bunker Rosdahl)

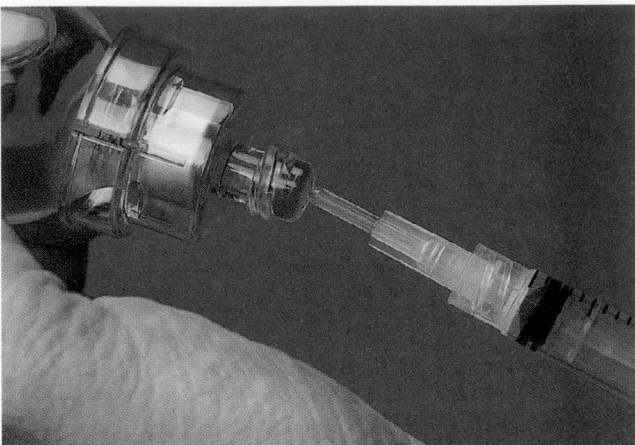

FIGURE 63-6. Some type of needleless system is usually used when administering IV medications or flushing heparin locks. Some needleless systems require the use of a vial adapter, shown here, to draw up medications or saline. The needleless system prevents needle stick injuries.

A **vial** is a glass container equipped with a self-sealing rubber stopper. It may contain a single premeasured medication dose, or it may be a multidose vial. When drawing up any injection, use strict aseptic technique to prevent contamination. Label all multidose vials with the time, date, and initials detailing first use. In Practice: Nursing Procedure 63-6 shows how to draw up medication from an ampule and from a vial.

A *prefilled syringe,* for example Tubex and Carpuject, provides a single medication dose prepared by a manufacturer or pharmacy. If the entire amount of medication is not needed, discard the excess amount into the sink or toilet by pushing the plunger until the correct quantity is obtained. Remember, if the medication is a controlled substance, another licensed nurse must witness this procedure and document it by cosigning the narcotic sheet.

Intradermal (ID) Injections

Intradermal injections, often used for diagnostic testing, are shallow injections given just beneath the epidermis (see Fig. 63-7). The inner aspect of the forearm is the common injec-

tion site. Tuberculin syringes, which identify minims and milliliters and hold a total of 16 minims or 1 milliliter, are commonly used. The *tuberculin syringe* has a very small diameter, graduated in hundredths and tenths for accurate measurement of small amounts of medication (see In Practice: Nursing Procedure 63-7).

If a test is performed to determine sensitivity (such as tuberculin testing; Purified Protein Derivative [PPD] test), check the injection site at 48 hours and 72 hours. Base the evaluation of the injection site on *induration* (hardness). The induration is measured and reported in millimeters. If giving an intradermal injection to determine possible allergies, read the results at approximately 20 minutes. In addition, a control substance (sterile normal saline) may be injected, to determine if the client may be experiencing a false-positive reaction to the injected medication. Some individuals have extremely sensitive skin; any skin manipulation, such as scratching or injection, causes induration to occur. Some clients are **anergic** (absence of ability to generate a sensitivity reaction) due to their immunocompromised status, and show a false-negative reaction.

Subcutaneous (subQ) Injections

Subcutaneous injections are administered into *subcutaneous* or *adipose* tissues located below the dermis. This method is used for small amounts of medication that require slow, systemic absorption. Generally, the duration of subQ medications is longer than that of other parenteral medications. Many medications cannot be given by the subQ route. If the volume of medication is greater than 1 to 2 milliliters, do not use the subQ route.

Subcutaneous medications must be soluble and of sufficient strength to be effective, yet safe for surrounding tissues. Common subQ medications are insulin and heparin. Allergy injections usually are administered subQ.

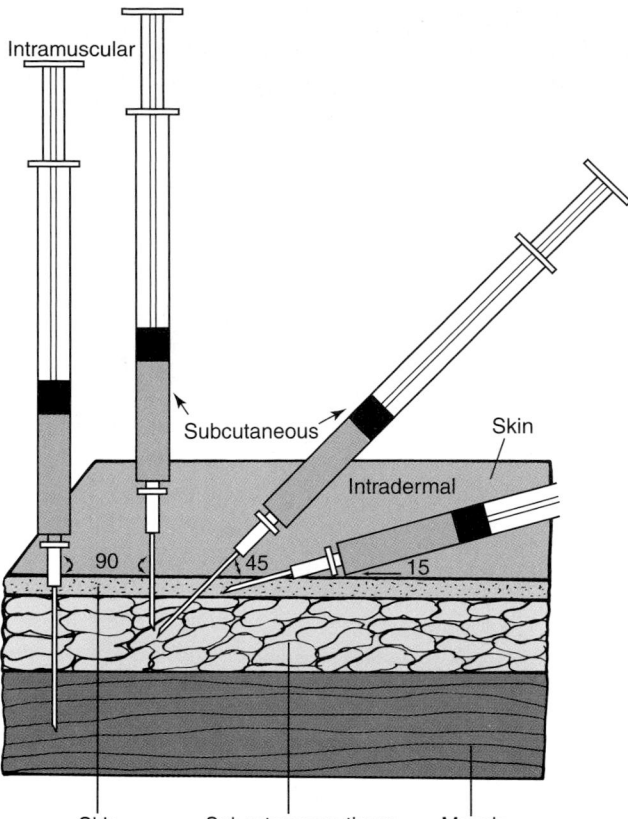

FIGURE 63-7. Comparison of the angles of insertion for IM, SubQ, and intradermal injections. A subcutaneous injection may be given at a 90° angle, if a short needle is used or if the person is heavy.

Give subQ injections in areas where bones and blood vessels are not near the skin's surface. One common site is the outer aspect of the upper arm, slightly above the halfway mark between the elbow and the shoulder. Always rotate injection sites for clients who receive injections on a regular basis.

Assess the client for body mass of subcutaneous tissue and choose the appropriate needle. The angle of injection varies with the amount of available tissue. Most subQ injections are given at a 90° angle. However, a thin client may need to be injected at an angle of a lesser degree. The amount of the client's adipose tissue also determines the length of needle to use (generally between ⅝ and 1 inch). Take care not to inject the medication too closely to the skin's surface. Doing so will allow for faster absorption and onset of action of the medication, and may cause local irritation (see In Practice: Nursing Procedure 63-8).

Intramuscular (IM) Injections

Intramuscular injections are given in muscles situated below the dermal and subcutaneous skin layers. Such medications must be injected deep into muscles. The body absorbs IM injections much more rapidly than subQ injections, because of the greater amount of blood supply to muscle tissue. Thorough familiarity with IM injection sites, and the technique for administering IM injections, is pivotal to nursing practice.

The most common areas for IM administration are the deltoid, vastus lateralis, rectus femoris, ventrogluteal, and

(*text continues on page 883*)

In Practice
Nursing Procedure 63-6

DRAWING UP MEDICATION FROM AN AMPULE OR VIAL

Supplies and Equipment

MAR
Syringe and needle
Ampule or vial of medication
Filter needle (optional)
Alcohol swab
Gloves (optional)

Steps

1. Wash hands and gather equipment. Wear gloves if medication is toxic.
   RATIONALE: *Handwashing helps prevent infection transmission; gathering equipment facilitates organization and efficiency.*

2. Use the MAR to verify the medication order. Check any inconsistency with the physician or pharmacist.
   RATIONALE: *Checking helps to ensure adherence to the "Five Rights."*

For an Ampule

3. Unlock the medication cart or drawer. Check the medication's expiration date.
   RATIONALE: *Keeping the medication setup locked provides security if the area is unattended. Outdated medication may be ineffective or dangerous.*

4. Hold the ampule upright. Use the finger to tap on the ampule's stem, or hold the ampule by the stem and rotate the hand in a circular motion.
   RATIONALE: *All medication in the ampule should be in the lower part prior to snapping off the stem.*

5. Grasp the stem with an alcohol swab.
   RATIONALE: *The swab protects the finger from the glass particles when the stem is removed.*

6. Snap off the ampule's neck away from the hands and face.
   RATIONALE: *Snapping away from the body protects the nurse's face from the small glass particles.*

(*continued*)

In Practice
Nursing Procedure 63-6 (Continued)

18. Change the needle if necessary, recap the needle, or pull the safety sheath over it. Do not twist to lock.
    RATIONALE: *Capping maintains the needle's sterility.*

19. Discard the used single-dose vial, or store the multidose vial according to agency policy.

RATIONALE: *Proper disposal prevents infection transmission; proper storage provides for future use without wasting the medication.*

20. Wash hands.
    RATIONALE: *Handwashing helps prevent infection transmission.*

In Practice
Nursing Procedure 63-7

ADMINISTERING INTRADERMAL INJECTIONS

Supplies and Equipment

MAR
Medication
Alcohol
Swab
Disposable gloves
Sterile tuberculin syringe and 25- to 26-G needle with an intradermal bevel

Steps

1. Check the medication order against the physician's original order.
   RATIONALE: *Checking ensures adherence to the "Five Rights."*

2. Wash hands.
   RATIONALE: *Handwashing helps prevent the spread of infection.*

3. Prepare the medication, observing safety guidelines for administration, including the "Five Rights."
   RATIONALE: *Adhering to the "Five Rights" helps to avoid medication errors.*

4. Proceed to the client's bedside, identify the client, and introduce yourself, explaining what will happen.
   RATIONALE: *Explanations help reduce the client's anxiety.*

5. Put on gloves.
   RATIONALE: *Standard Precautions are used if any chance of coming into contact with body fluids or secretions exists.*

6. a. Choose an injection site on the inner aspect of the forearm that is not heavily pigmented or covered with hair.
   RATIONALE: *Hair or discoloration may interfere with assessment of the site after injection.*

   b. Cleanse the site with an alcohol pad in a circular motion from the center outward. Allow the alcohol to dry.
   RATIONALE: *Cleansing in this manner removes skin microorganisms and prevents contaminating a clean surface with a dirty one.*

7. Use the nondominant hand to pull the skin taut over the injection site.
   RATIONALE: *Firm skin makes injection into the epidermis easier.*

8. a. Hold the syringe as if it were a pencil. Turn the hand slightly so that the syringe and needle are at a right angle to the arm's surface.

   b. Place the needle, bevel down, on the skin surface at approximately a 10° angle.

   c. Rotate the syringe between the index finger and the thumb 180° while exerting slight forward pressure so that the bevel is up when it is inserted. Insert the bevel just under the epidermis.
   RATIONALE: *The rotating action makes insertion into the epidermis much easier and less traumatic to the tissue.*

9. Transfer the thumb to the end of the plunger and slowly inject the medication (usually 0.3 mL). Watch for the formation of a *wheal* (small elevation similar in appearance to a hive).
   RATIONALE: *A wheal indicates correct delivery of the medication into the epidermis.*

10. Withdraw the needle quickly and at the same angle at which it was inserted.
    RATIONALE: *Doing so minimizes skin damage.*

11. Do not massage the site. Instruct the client not to scratch it.
    RATIONALE: *Massage increases absorption. Intradermal medications are to be absorbed slowly.*

sible p
can be
ment o
make t
baby sl
care be
ical in l
before
are diff
mother
hol). T
concep

  1. E
    c
  2. S
    ii
  3. S
    h
    f
  4. F
    a
    is
  5. R
    g
    th
  6. T
    ei
    ci
    H
    al
  7. R
    in
    he

For a
Client 6

Ther
a womai
woman v
may bec
ple woul
before a
United S
of this re
will seek
outcome
care visi
concepti

Stage:

Concep

Human l
(female)
as *fertiliz*
is in the c

15.

16.

Th
for sn
the m
site. /
with t
medic
the vc
quick
Th
upper
63-8C
middl
is 1½ t
and te
in the
Th
rior, l
recom
3 year
group
nerve:

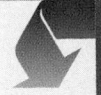
dorsogluteal areas (Fig. 63-8). IM injection is the best technique when medications given less deeply irritate the client's tissues or when large amounts of medication are necessary.

IM injections are given in much the same way as subQ injections. However, a longer needle with a larger bore is used, most often a 1½- to 2-inch, 20- to 22-G needle, depending on the type of medication. Use an angle of 90° for the injection (see In Practice: Nursing Procedure 63-9).

In addition to using a longer and larger-gauge needle, IM injections are more difficult and dangerous than subQ injections. The needle must be injected deeper into the client's body, penetrating the epidermal, dermal, subcutaneous, and muscle tissues. If the medication's viscosity is thick, injecting into the muscle will be more difficult.

Dorsogluteal Site.   The dorsogluteal area is a common IM injection site (see Fig. 63-8A). Never use this site for infants and children under 3 years of age. *Rationale: Their muscles in this area are not yet developed and are not of sufficient mass.*

To use this site, assist the client to a prone position. Instruct him or her to point the toes inward. *Rationale: Pointing the toes inward aids relaxation of the gluteal muscles.* Never administer an IM injection with the client standing, because clear identification of the area is difficult and the muscles will be more tense in this position. In addition, the client may experience a vasovagal reaction and faint, sustaining injury as he or she falls. Remember, the nurse is responsible for keeping the client's well-being in mind at all times. Explain to the client who is reluctant to lie down that doing so is in his or her best interest. Drape the client to maintain privacy while exposing the buttock to determine the proper administration site. Draw an imaginary line from the posterior superior iliac spine to the greater trochanter of the femur (see Fig. 63-8A). Take care not to touch the client's buttocks while drawing this imaginary line (this might cause unnecessary anxiety). Safely give the injection anywhere along the imaginary line below the curve of the iliac crest.

Another method of identifying the correct site is to draw two imaginary lines that cross, separating the buttocks into fourths. The IM injection can be given safely in the upper, outer quadrant, approximately 1 to 2 inches above the intersection of the imaginary lines. Before administering the injection, encourage the client to relax the gluteal muscles. Doing so will ease discomfort due to the medication being injected into the muscular tissue.

Ventrogluteal Site.   The preferred site for injection in the hip area is the ventrogluteal site (see Fig. 63-8B). Use this site if the client is in the side-lying, prone, or supine position. To locate the ventrogluteal site, place the palm on the lateral aspect of the greater trochanter. Move the index, or first, finger to the position of the anterior superior iliac spine. Extend the middle finger to the iliac crest. With the fingers and palm in this position, a "V" is formed between the index and middle fingers. The injection site is in the center of the "V." Ask the client to turn his or her toes inward to relax the muscle used for the injection. Doing so will relieve the discomfort of the medication being injected into the muscle tissue.

The ventrogluteal site is safer and less painful for IM injections than the dorsogluteal site through which the sciatic nerve runs. The fat layer is thinner in this area, and the gluteal muscle is thicker, even in very thin clients. One disadvantage is that the client may never have received an IM injection in this area, which may cause anxiety. Another disadvantage is that the client can see what the nurse is doing, which may also increase anxiety. To avoid this, assist the client to a side-lying position.

Other Sites.   Other sites may be used for IM injections. These sites include the deltoid (upper arm), vastus lateralis (lateral thigh), and rectus femoris. Many clients find the rectus femoris site uncomfortable; it is often used in adults only when other sites are contraindicated.

ception, the embryo is in what is called the *critical phase of human development*. During these weeks, all the organs and structures of the human are formed and are most susceptible to damage.

☛ Key Concept

The first eight weeks of pregnancy are the critical period of human development; *during this time, all major systems of the embryo develop.*

The embryo, and to a lesser degree the fetus, is vulnerable to a number of potentially harmful influences that could result in **congenital** (literally, "born with") defects. Genes determine the basic embryonic structure; therefore, a defective gene may be responsible for certain congenital defects. Environmental factors such as tobacco or alcohol use also can cause *congenital anomalies,* also known as *birth defects* (see Chap. 73).

Period of the Fetus

The period of the **fetus** lasts from the beginning of the ninth week after fertilization through birth, which is usually at about the end of the 40th week of pregnancy. This is a period of increasing growth, differentiation, and functional development

of the tissues that appeared during the embryonic period. At about 20 weeks of gestation, the fetus becomes **viable** (having some chance of life outside the uterus).

Normal fetal growth and development follow a definite and predictable pattern. Growth and development, before and after birth, follows the **cephalocaudal** (head to toe) principle.

Heredity and the mother's nutritional status have some influence on the growth of the fetus. A newborn weighing 10 pounds (4,540 g) or more is often difficult to deliver; however, the smaller the child is at birth, the less likely his or her chances are for survival. A newborn weighing less than 2.2 pounds (1,000 g) is considered immature. With today's newborn intensive care units, however, the chances for survival of very small newborns are improving.

Placenta and Umbilical Cord.   The fetus' chorionic villi eventually meet with an area of uterine tissue to form the **placenta** (see Fig. 64-3), an organ with a rich blood supply that:

- Supplies the developing organism with food and oxygen
- Carries waste away for excretion by the mother
- Slows the maternal immune response so that the mother's body does not reject the fetal tissue
- Produces hormones that help maintain the pregnancy

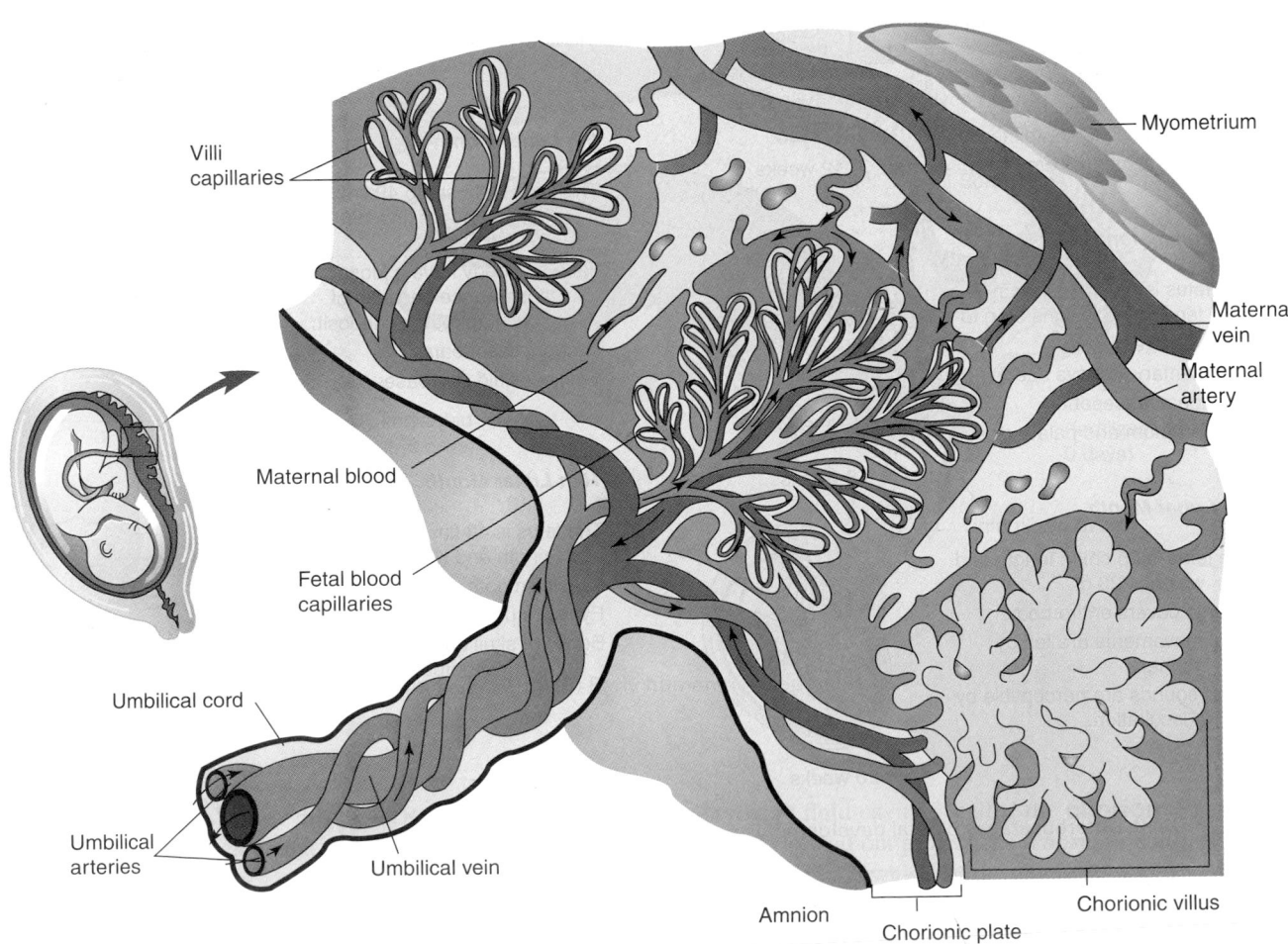

FIGURE 64-3. Placenta.

The fetal blood is entirely within blood vessels. Blood vessels may be found within the fetus' chorionic villi. These villi within the placenta are bathed in a pool of maternal blood, making this area the only place in the body (with the exception of the heart) where blood is not contained within blood vessels. The villi are suspended in this pool of nourishing blood from the mother, much like a cluster of grapes could be dipped in a bowl of water that is continuously circulated by being pumped into the bowl and then drained.

Using its chorionic villi within the placenta, the fetus secures its oxygen and food directly from the mother's blood, instead of using its own lungs and digestive system. The absorption of nutrients, excretion of wastes, and exchange of gases occurs across the walls of the placental villi and the fetal blood vessels they contain. The fetal and the maternal blood are separate.

By term, the placenta is approximately 15 to 20 centimeters in diameter, 2 to 3 centimeters thick, and weighs between 500 and 600 grams. The weight of the placenta is about one-sixth the weight of the infant, if both are healthy.

The *umbilical cord* connects the fetal blood vessels contained in the villi of the placenta with those found within the fetal body. The umbilical cord consists of two arteries and one large vein twisted around each other. The umbilical cord is approximately 20 inches (51 cm) long. A soft, jellylike substance called **Wharton's jelly** protects the cord, which enters the fetus' body approximately in the middle of the abdomen at the **umbilicus,** or *navel.*

Fetal Blood Circulation.   Fetal circulation differs from newborn and adult circulation (Fig. 64-4). The woman's blood supplies food to—and carries wastes away from—the fetus. The uterus expels the placenta, which is also called the *afterbirth,* following the newborn's delivery. While the fetus is *in utero,* the placenta returns *deoxygenated* (low in oxygen) blood from the fetus to the mother through the two *umbilical arteries.* The placenta returns *oxygenated* (oxygen-rich) blood to the fetus via a single vessel, the *umbilical vein.* This process is an exception to the usual pattern, in which all arteries carry oxygenated (bright-red) blood, and all veins carry deoxygenated (dark-red) blood. Some oxygenated blood from the umbilical vein passes through the fetal liver, but most of it enters the fetus' inferior vena cava through the **ductus venosus.** This short duct is found only in the fetus, and atrophies after birth. From the inferior vena cava, the blood flows into the fetus' right atrium.

Because the fetal lungs are not yet functioning, most of the blood is shunted to the heart's left atrium. This shunt occurs through another fetal structure, the **foramen ovale,** which is an opening between the right and left atria. This structure permits most of the blood to bypass the right ventricle. A small amount of blood passes from the right atrium to the right ventricle, and makes its way into the pulmonary artery. This blood is then shunted through the **ductus arteriosus,** a connection between the pulmonary artery and the aorta that allows shunting of blood around the fetal lungs.

Normally, with the newborn's first few respirations, the lungs expand as soon as the pressure within the chest alters. The foramen ovale closes, and the ductus arteriosus and ductus venosus shrivel up and become fibrous ligaments. Congenital heart defects in a child occur when these events do not take place after birth.

Membranes and Amniotic Fluid.   In the earliest human developmental stage, the chorionic plate that gives rise to the villi resembles a fuzzy ball. As the embryo grows, most areas of the villi atrophy, leaving only a disc of villi that develops into the placenta. The rest of the chorion becomes a smooth *outer membrane* for the embryo. Inside it, other cells eventually form a fluid-filled sac, the *amnion,* in which the fetus floats. The **amnion** is the inner membrane surrounding the fetus. These two membranes form a tough, protective bubble for the developing embryo and fetus, protecting it from organisms that might infect the mother's cervix. In addition, the membranes are important to hormone production, and also play a role in the onset of labor. The **amniotic fluid,** kept inside the amnion, performs the following functions:

* It cushions the fetus against injury.
* It regulates temperature.
* It allows the fetus to move freely inside it, which allows normal musculoskeletal development of the fetus.

In late pregnancy, the amniotic fluid is made up primarily of fetal urine and fetal lung fluid. Near term, the fetus swallows almost 400 milliliters of amniotic fluid each day and then excretes it in the urine; therefore, a defect in either the ability of the fetus to swallow or in its kidney function can dramatically change the amount of amniotic fluid. The amount of amniotic fluid increases to about 1,000 milliliters by 37 weeks of gestation, then decreases slowly until 40 weeks, and then decreases much more quickly if the baby is not born by the end of the 40th week. Because of this predictable pattern in the amount of fluid, one measurement of post-term fetal well-being is the volume of amniotic fluid.

Changes in a Woman's Body During Pregnancy

Many of the changes in a woman's body during pregnancy can be seen externally. However, there are also many changes in her internal structure and function. Some of these changes are due to the growing size of the fetus, but even more changes are due to the unique hormonal environment caused by pregnancy. These changes begin to occur soon after fertilization, when the production of hormones changes from that of a normal menstrual cycle.

Signs of Pregnancy

The signs of pregnancy are grouped into three categories:

* Presumptive
* Probable
* Positive

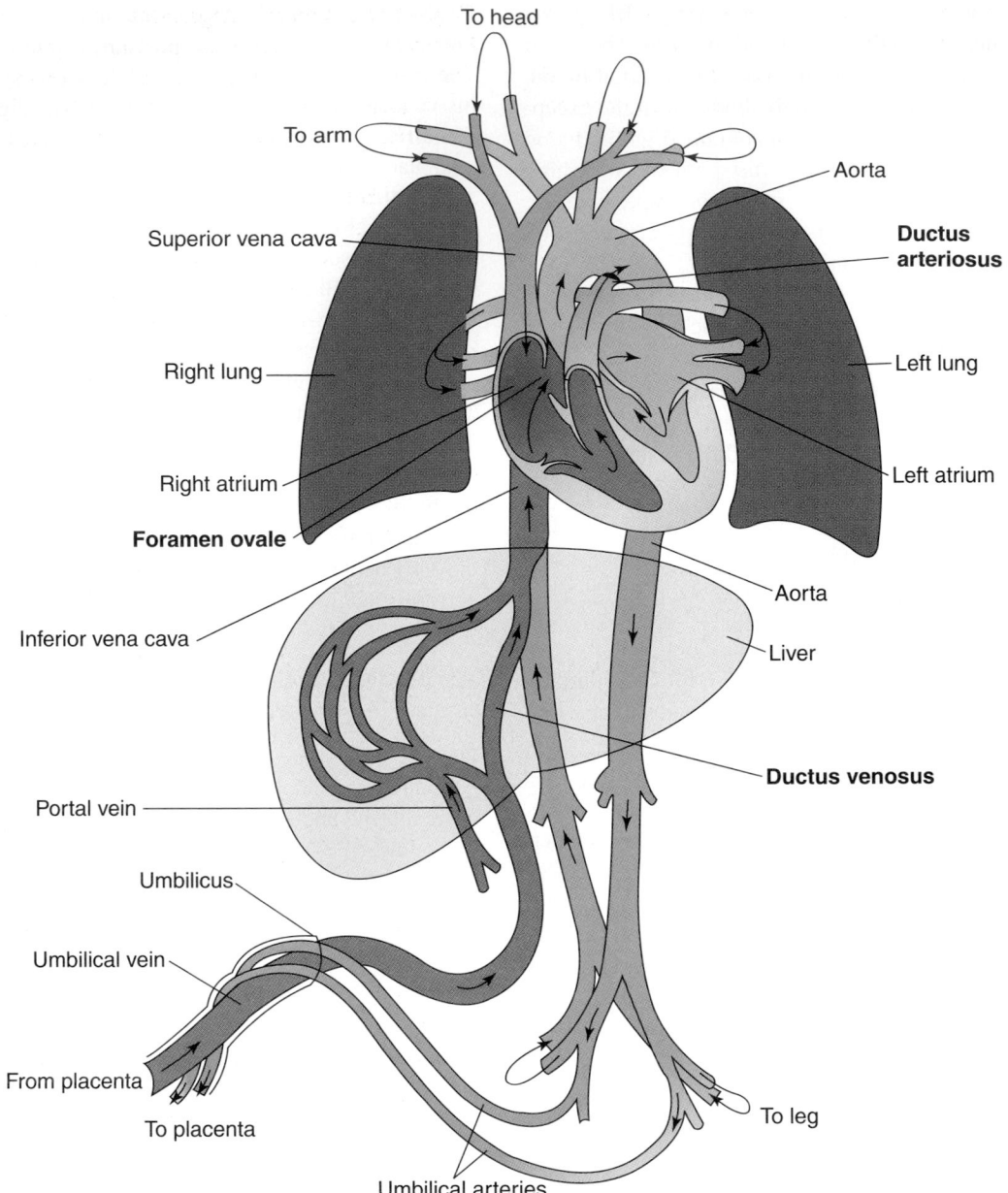

FIGURE 64-4. Fetal circulation. Notice the two arteries, the one vein, the ductus venosus, the ductus arteriosus, and the foramen ovale, which are unique to fetal circulation.

Presumptive and probable signs are primarily due to the hormonal changes that occur during pregnancy. Most *presumptive signs* appear early and are subjective; that is, they may be noted only by the client. When a woman experiences these symptoms, she may assume that she is pregnant. However, these symptoms could indicate a condition other than pregnancy.

Probable signs also appear early in pregnancy but are more objective. Often, both healthcare personnel and the client herself can observe probable signs. Although probable signs are more definite, they still are not absolute.

Only the *positive signs* of pregnancy provide proof that there is a developing fetus.

☛ KEY CONCEPT

Pregnancy is not confirmed until the existence of a fetus can be proved.

Presumptive Signs of Pregnancy

Amenorrhea. *Amenorrhea,* the absence of menstruation, is often one of the first indications of pregnancy. A missed menstrual period, however, does not always signify conception. Pregnancy is dated from the first day of the woman's LNMP. To be considered normal, the period should have come on time, lasted as long as is usual for the woman, and have been the normal flow for her. If any of these three items are not true of that period, ask the client to recall the first day of her previous menstrual period (**PMP**).

Nausea. *Nausea* may begin soon after the first missed menstrual period, and usually disappears after the third month of pregnancy. Approximately half of all pregnant women experience some nausea or vomiting, usually due to hormonal changes. Although it is sometimes called "morning sickness," the nausea or vomiting of pregnancy may happen at any time during the day. If this condition lasts beyond the fourth month, results in a weight loss of 8 pounds or more, or affects the woman's general health, it is considered a complication of pregnancy, **hyperemesis gravidarum.** Chapter 67 further discusses this condition.

Frequent Urination. The enlarging uterus presses against the urinary bladder. This action may cause the woman to feel the need to urinate more frequently than usual. As the uterus grows upward into the abdominal cavity, the pressure eases. Late in the pregnancy, the women again feels the need to empty her bladder frequently. Once again, this is due to pressure, as the fetal head moves downward before birth.

Fatigue. During the early months of pregnancy, the woman may feel drowsy and may tire easily. She may find that she requires more rest and sleep than usual, and that even if she gets the extra rest, she still feels tired. Although the exact causes of this fatigue are unknown, tiredness is probably due to the body's increased use of energy, because it works harder than normal during this time.

Quickening. The first fetal movements that the pregnant woman feels are called **quickening.** The woman usually experiences quickening between 18 and 20 weeks of gestation, but it may occur a week or two earlier in a multigravida. Women describe quickening as a light, "fluttery" sensation. This "feeling of life" is not considered a positive sign of pregnancy, because it cannot be confirmed objectively by anyone other than the woman herself. The movement of gas within the colon can also simulate this feeling.

Breast Changes. The earliest breast changes that occur in pregnancy are similar to those a woman may experience before her menstrual period. However, the sensations during pregnancy are more intense than premenstrual changes. The sensations include enlargement, heaviness, tingling, throbbing, or tenderness. The breasts may be so tender that the discomfort awakens a woman who rolls over onto her stomach during sleep. As the pregnancy progresses, the areolae and the nipples enlarge and darken. By the 14th week, the woman's breasts begin to produce **colostrum.** This clear or slightly milky fluid will be produced in very small amounts throughout the rest of her pregnancy, and in a greater quantity during the first day or two after birth. After that, her true milk will come in.

Pigment Changes. Pregnancy causes some skin changes. A suntanned, bronzed masking may appear across the face of dark-haired women. This is known as **melasma** (or *chloasma gravidarum*), or the "mask of pregnancy." A line of darker pigmentation, known as the **linea nigra,** often appears on the lower abdomen and extends from the umbilicus to the pubic bone. Hormone level changes cause these pigment changes.

Probable Signs of Pregnancy

Probable signs of pregnancy are more objective than the presumptive signs. An obstetrician or midwife may observe them during examination. They are more reliable indicators of pregnancy than the presumptive signs, but still are not proof that a pregnancy exists.

Basal Body Temperature Elevation. The body temperature at rest, or basal body temperature (BBT), rises slightly (usually less than one degree) as one of the earliest signs of pregnancy. For accuracy, however, comparisons require that the temperature also must have been taken and recorded before pregnancy occurred.

Positive Urine Pregnancy Tests. Pregnancy tests check for the presence of the hormone called human chorionic gonadotropin (**HCG,** HCg, or hCG). This hormone is produced by the cells that will become the placenta. It can be found in small amounts in a woman's urine or blood by about the 7th to 10th day of pregnancy.

Home pregnancy testing allows the woman to know she is pregnant at a very early stage, and lets her process the possibility of pregnancy in privacy. She can then make her own decisions about both the pregnancy and her lifestyle. The manufacturers of home pregnancy tests recommend confirmation of the results through professional examination and clinical testing. This advice should be followed because home tests may not have the same accuracy as clinical tests. Errors may occur in as many as 20% to 30% of the home tests performed. The most common error (a false-negative) results from urine testing that is performed too early to obtain an accurate finding. The user must be able to read, follow directions, and perform the test correctly for the results to be accurate.

Cervical Changes. At about the eighth week of gestation, the cervix softens. This is known as **Goodell's sign.** Before pregnancy, the cervix feels firm (like the tip of a nose); during pregnancy, it feels softer (more like the earlobe). The cervix also looks blue or purple when examined; this is **Chadwick's sign,** and may occur as early as the sixth week of pregnancy.

Vulvar and Vaginal Changes. The blueness due to increased blood supply (Chadwick's sign) also occurs on the vulva and vagina.

Uterine Changes. At about 6 weeks, the lower uterine segment (the portion between the body of the uterus and the cervix) softens. This softening is called **Hegar's sign.** A softening of the uterine *fundus,* where the embryo has implanted, also occurs by about the seventh week. The fundus enlarges by the eighth week. The uterus as a whole enlarges steadily throughout the pregnancy. The uterus rises above the symphysis pubis by about the 12th week, and reaches the umbilicus between the 20th and 24th weeks.

Ballottement. After about 16 to 18 weeks of pregnancy, gently tapping one side of the pregnant woman's abdomen will cause the fetus to "bounce" in the amniotic fluid—because the fetus is small compared with the amount of fluid. The examiner can feel this rebound tap, known as **ballottement,** against her hand.

Enlargement of the Abdomen.   As the uterus increases in size, the abdomen is forced outward.

Positive Signs of Pregnancy

The *positive signs* of pregnancy, described below, can only occur in pregnancy.

Visualization of the Fetus.   A fetus can be seen either on an ultrasound or (less commonly) on an X-ray examination. **Ultrasound** is the most common method used to evaluate fetal size, development, and due date. Using ultrasound, it is possible to diagnose pregnancy as early as the fourth week of gestation. The ultrasound examination is safe, painless, and relatively inexpensive.

Fetal Heartbeat.   An examiner can detect the fetal heartbeat (fetal heart tones) by using either a *Doppler* or a special manual stethoscope called a **fetoscope** (Fig. 64-5). The **Doppler** (an electronic stethoscope) converts ultrasonic fre-

quencies (high-frequency sound waves) into audible frequencies or onto a video monitor. An examiner can hear fetal heart tones with the Doppler as early as the 10th week. They can be heard with the fetoscope at about the 18th to 20th week. A normal fetal heart rate ranges from 120 to 160 beats per minute (BPM). When assessing fetal heart rate, the examiner must be aware of two other sounds to avoid confusion. The *funic souffle* is a swishing sound produced by the pulsation of blood as it is propelled through the umbilical cord. Its rate is the same as the fetal heart rate. The *uterine* (or *placental*) *souffle* is a swishing sound produced by the maternal blood as it flows through the large vessels of the uterus. Its rate is the same as the woman's heart rate. The examiner should feel the woman's radial pulse at the same time he or she is assessing the fetal heart rate, to avoid confusing the two. (See In Practice: Nursing Procedure 64-1 for more information on fetal heart tones.)

> **Nursing Alert**
> If you are unable to hear fetal heart tones, you must notify the physician, nurse midwife, or nurse practitioner immediately.

Fetal Movement Felt by an Examiner.   An examiner may be able to feel fetal movement after about week 20. At first, the movements are faint; but as the fetus grows and muscle strength increases, the movements become stronger. These fetal movements must be differentiated from other movements within the woman's body (such as peristalsis).

Important Changes in Maternal Anatomy and Physiology

As you learned at the beginning of this chapter, many of the changes that occur in a woman's body are due to the increasing size of the fetus. Other changes are due to the altered hormonal environment. The placenta produces so many hormones, and in such great quantity, that some people think of it as a "hormone factory." These hormones are needed to help the mother sustain the pregnancy, to nourish the rapidly developing fetus, to prepare for breastfeeding (**lactation**), and for the mother to still have enough energy to support herself.

☛ KEY CONCEPT

Hormones and the size of the growing fetus both result in changes in the woman's body.

External Changes.   After the first trimester of pregnancy, most women look pregnant. Their abdomen changes in contour, becoming increasingly more round as the pregnancy progresses. As the abdomen enlarges and her center of gravity shifts forward, the woman's posture and gait alter as well. She develops an inward curve of the lower back, known as **lordosis.** During late pregnancy, her rib cage flares outward, making more room for the fetus.

Internal Changes.   In addition to the visible changes of pregnancy, a woman's body experiences tremendous internal changes. The hormones of pregnancy cause these changes,

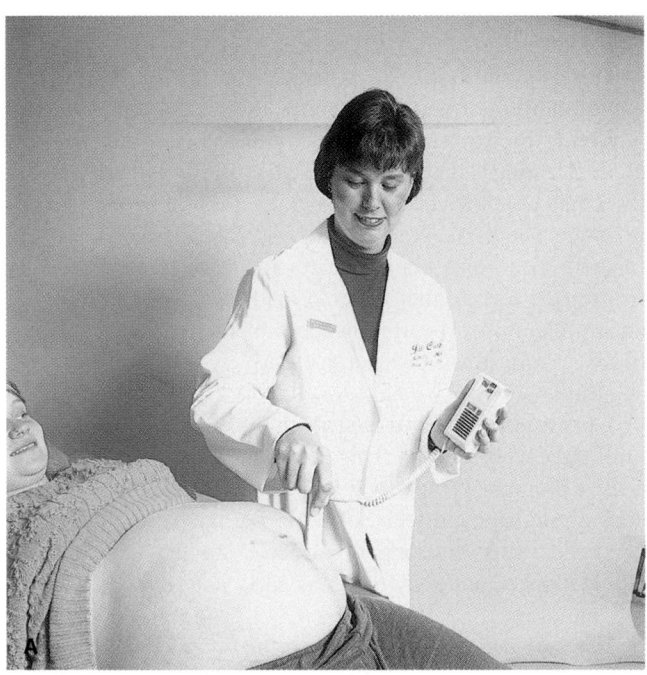

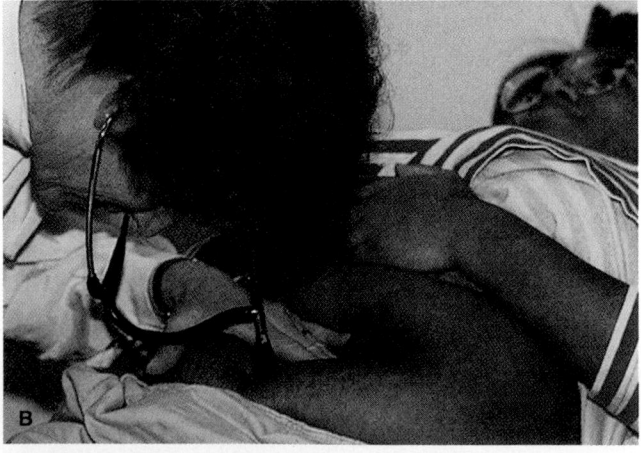

FIGURE 64-5. (A) Checking fetal heart tones (FHTs) using a Doppler. **(B)** Checking FHTs via auscultation, using a fetoscope.

In Practice
Nursing Procedure 64-1

LISTENING TO FETAL HEART TONES (FHTs)

Purpose

To determine the well-being of the fetus

Supplies and Equipment

Fetoscope with tubing <10 inches long or Doppler and water-soluble ultrasound gel

Steps

1. Be sure that the room is quiet.
2. Be sure that the woman has recently emptied her bladder.
3. Wash your hands.
4. Ask the woman to lie down on her back (supine position). If she is more than 28 weeks pregnant, place a small rolled towel under one hip, to tilt her slightly to one side.
5. If you are using a Doppler, apply a small amount of gel to the end of the instrument.
6. If you are using a fetoscope, place the padded cone on the woman's abdomen, just above the pubic bone, and the headpiece solidly against your forehead.
7. Exert a little pressure as you place the instrument immediately above the pubic bone.
8. Slowly rotate it 360° until you hear the baby's heartbeat.
9. If you hear nothing, move the instrument 1 cm at a time up toward the umbilicus, until you are halfway between the pubic bone and the umbilicus. If you have not yet heard the heartbeat, move 1 cm to one side of the midline, and proceed back down toward the pubic bone. If the FHTs are still not heard, do the same on the opposite side.
10. Be sure to rotate the instrument at each new position, as it must be directed at the baby's heart.
11. Count the FHTs for 15 seconds, and multiply by four to get the rate per minute. Chart the FHT rate.
12. In late pregnancy, also chart the location on the woman's abdomen at which you heard the FHTs. This is done by placing an X, or the rate, in a simple diagram of the abdomen:

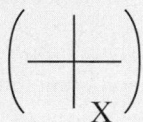

In this diagram, the *curved lines* represent the sides of the abdomen, the *vertical line* is the midline, and the *horizontal line* is an imaginary line drawn through the umbilicus of the woman. The FHTs were heard in the **right lower quadrant** of the abdomen.

13. If no FHTs are heard with a Doppler by 13 weeks, or a fetoscope by 20 weeks, request a sonogram.
    RATIONALE: *Listening to fetal heart tones (FHTs) is an important part of caring for a pregnant woman. FHTs should be evaluated at every prenatal visit, and at very frequent intervals during labor. Chapter 65 discusses labor evaluation in more detail.*

Source: Wheeler, L. (1997). Nurse-midwifery handbook: A practical guide to prenatal and postpartum care. Philadelphia: Lippincott-Raven.

---

which are designed to support the pregnancy and the developing fetus.

Hormone Levels.   A woman's hormone levels change dramatically during pregnancy. Important hormones of pregnancy include progesterone, estrogens, HCG, and **HPL** (human placental lactogen). Levels of estrogens and progesterone rise steadily from early pregnancy until close to term, when they level off (and then may slowly decline). A similar pattern is true of HPL, except that it is not produced until close to the beginning of the second trimester. It then rises rapidly until about 34 weeks, when it decreases. On the other hand, HCG is the primary hormone of early pregnancy; its level drops significantly during the second trimester.

Together, these hormones create an environment that supports the pregnancy. Some of the most important hormonal effects include:

- Maintaining the endometrium so that the embryo can implant
- Causing changes in the mother's metabolism so that nutrients will be available for her own needs as well as the needs of the growing fetus
- Causing an increase in the mother's blood volume and red blood cell mass to provide the extra oxygen needed for the fetus and her own increased demands
- Increasing the blood supply to the gastrointestinal tract, and slowing the peristaltic waves: changes that result in increased absorption of nutrients
- Relaxing the ligaments that connect the pelvic bones, allowing them to spread slightly to increase the space available for the baby to pass through
- Preparing the breasts for lactation, while keeping the milk from coming in until after the baby is born

Anticipatory Guidance About Changes. **Anticipatory guidance** is a term that means education about expected changes prior to their occurrence. By providing anticipatory guidance regarding the unusual and unaccustomed changes the woman is experiencing, you will add to her knowledge of her body, helping her to enjoy (or at least to cope with) these events. Examples of anticipatory guidance about pregnancy changes include:

- A woman should not have bleeding during pregnancy, and she should tell her provider promptly if she does bleed. Note that some women have a spot or two of bleeding when implantation occurs, just about the time they expect a period. However, you should inform the physician, nurse midwife, or nurse practitioner about *any* bleeding that a pregnant woman reports.

- A pregnant woman may wake up feeling very hungry. You might advise her that it could help to eat a starchy food, such as a baked potato, just before bedtime. If she eats sweets, she will probably have a rapid rise in blood sugar, followed by a sharp drop. Either of these changes can cause uncomfortable symptoms. Advise her to try to avoid consuming concentrated sweets to prevent this from occurring.

- As her blood volume rises, the pregnant woman's heart has to work harder (pump more strongly) to deal with the increased workload. She may feel palpitations, or a rapid and pounding heartbeat. This is normal, unless she also feels dizzy or lightheaded.

- The extra blood vessels that form in the gut, combined with the slowed passage of foods, may combine to cause constipation and hemorrhoids. The pregnant woman should consume plenty of fiber and water to prevent this.

- As the ligaments relax and the pregnant woman's center of gravity changes, her balance may be "off." She should avoid wearing high heels, especially during late pregnancy.

- Breast enlargement is normal. The pregnant woman may need to buy a larger-sized bra. Some women need a bra that is larger in both chest size and cup size.

As you study the remainder of this chapter, you will find other information that can form a basis for anticipatory guidance.

Signs of Possible Problems During Pregnancy

Each stage, or trimester, of pregnancy carries its own risks. Any time a woman complains of one or more of the following symptoms, she should be advised to promptly visit her healthcare provider or an emergency department.

Danger Signs During the First Trimester

The primary danger of the first trimester is *spontaneous abortion (miscarriage)* (Box 64-1). Signs of threatened abortion include:

➤➤ **BOX 64-1**

PREGNANCY DANGER SIGNS

First trimester
- Excessive vomiting

At Any Time During Pregnancy
- Vaginal bleeding
- Excessive or irritating vaginal discharge
- Dizziness or fainting
- Decrease in urine output
- Burning with urination
- Persistent vomiting
- Chills or fever
- Chest pain

Late in pregnancy
- Leaking or gushing of amniotic fluid
- Swelling in the woman's extremities or face
- Dyspnea
- Blurred vision or spots before the eyes
- Severe headaches
- Abdominal, epigastric, or severe back pain
- Decreased fetal movement
- Lower abdominal pressure

- *Vaginal bleeding or spotting:* Bleeding does not mean that the woman will miscarry, but it does indicate that she might do so. Bleeding due to a threatened abortion reflects a partial separation of the placenta from the decidua. Blood may appear either bright red, darker red, or brown. The amount of blood loss does not predict the outcome, unless it becomes very heavy (enough to saturate more than one pad per hour).

- *Pelvic/abdominal cramping:* Cramping that increases over time, especially if accompanied by vaginal bleeding, indicates threatened abortion.

- *No longer feeling pregnant:* If the embryo or fetus has died, and the placenta has ceased to function, the hormonal environment changes rapidly. The most common statement about this change is "I just don't feel pregnant any more." Specific symptoms of pregnancy that quickly subside with missed abortions are nausea, breast tenderness, and headaches.

Danger Signs During the Second and Third Trimesters

The complications for which early signs may develop during later pregnancy include incompetent cervix, placenta previa, placental abruption, preterm labor (**PTL**) and/or preterm premature rupture of the membranes (**PPROM** or **PROM**), decreased fetal movement, and pregnancy-induced hypertension (**PIH**). Chapter 67 gives more detail about each of these complications. Danger signs during the second and third trimesters include:

- *Vaginal bleeding, with or without cramping, pressure, or pain:* Painless vaginal bleeding may be a sign of *placenta previa,* a condition in which the placenta lies partly over the cervical opening. The first episode of bleeding often occurs at about 26 to 28 weeks. It may follow sexual activity, or occur spontaneously. The bleeding is generally bright red, and the flow is fairly heavy—at least as heavy as a normal menses.
- *Bleeding with severe abdominal pain:* This symptom is a sign of *placental abruption,* or premature separation of the placenta. The baby can die if not delivered quickly, usually by Cesarean section.
- *Vaginal or lower abdominal pressure:* This may occur when the cervix is *incompetent,* or not strong enough to hold the fetus inside the uterus. This symptom is especially worrisome if the woman also has increased vaginal discharge.
- *PTL:* Early signs include backache, pelvic/abdominal cramping, rhythmic pelvic pressure, diarrhea, change in vaginal discharge, vaginal spotting, leaking fluid, and malaise.
- *PPROM/PROM:* This condition may cause either a gush of fluid or a continuous steady trickle of fluid. The gush is usually easily recognized, but the woman may not realize that a slow, steady leak is a problem.
- *Decreased fetal movement:* Regular fetal movement is a sign of fetal well-being. Each fetus has its own pattern of activity; a marked drop-off in a fetus' activity is a cause for concern about the health of the fetus.

The following symptoms may be signs of PIH:

- *Severe headache,* which does not respond to over-the-counter remedies
- *Visual changes:* double vision, suddenly blurred vision, seeing spots or flashing lights
- *Sudden edema or swelling,* especially of the face, eyes, and hands
- *Epigastric pain,* or pain in the upper abdomen

HEALTHCARE DURING PREGNANCY

The prenatal period refers to the period between conception and the onset of labor. The goals of good prenatal care are to:

- Promote physical and mental wellness of the mother, during the pregnancy and afterwards
- Help the woman give birth safely and without complications
- Ensure a healthy baby

Many women seek prenatal care as soon as they suspect pregnancy. In recent years, the healthcare industry has emphasized health promotion measures, such as preconceptional examination, to encourage positive maternal and child health for the future. Ideally, the woman's health at the end of pregnancy is as good as or better than it was at the beginning. Reg-

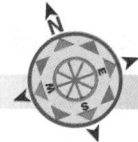

SPECIAL CONSIDERATIONS: CULTURE

Prenatal Care

While Japanese American women are expected to go for prenatal care from early in pregnancy, Gypsy women often avoid prenatal care to avoid having an internal pelvic examination. A different attitude is traditional among Mexican Americans, who may believe that pregnancy is not an illness, so prenatal care is unnecessary; others within that culture seek prenatal care for reassurance of fetal well-being. Some Mexican American women view prenatal care as informal home care received from family members.

ular prenatal care is associated with lower infant mortality and better outcomes on measures of child health, such as weight.

Pregnancy involves all members of the family. Having a baby has a powerful influence on the family system. Each member of the family reacts to pregnancy from his or her own point of view and as related to individual needs, beliefs, and experiences.

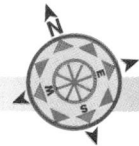

SPECIAL CONSIDERATIONS: CULTURE

Beliefs About Pregnancy

Traditionally, Ethiopians and Eritreans view pregnancy as a dangerous state; the fetus is easy prey for the evil eye and sorcery, which are believed to cause miscarriage, premature delivery, and fetal malformation. For Samoans, pregnancy is considered an illness. Pregnant women cannot eat alone or be left unattended, especially at night. In many Puerto Rican families, pregnancy is a time of indulgence for women, while in Southeast Asian cultures, pregnancy is considered a healthy state.

Pregnancy occurs not only within a family, but also within the environment of a culture. Religious, ethnic, and cultural beliefs influence expectant women. Cultural aspects of prenatal care are extremely important and may affect healthcare practices, pregnancy, childbirth, and family adjustment. Knowledge and understanding of—as well as sensitivity to—cultural differences are invaluable in providing nursing care that addresses the needs of each woman and family in ways that they can understand and accept.

Choosing a Healthcare Provider

Preconceptional and prenatal care, at its best, is a partnership between the woman and the healthcare provider. The woman should choose a provider who will help her make decisions about the best healthcare for herself and her family. Above all else, the provider should be someone who genuinely listens to the woman and her concerns.

A woman may choose a physician, a nurse midwife, or a nurse practitioner for her prenatal care. She may go to a public health clinic, a private office, or a community-based organization. Each of these sites and providers has strengths and limitations. Some examples of questions a woman might ask as she selects a prenatal care provider include:

- Do I want a male or a female provider?
- Should my provider speak the same native language that I do?
- When I have a question or concern about my pregnancy, will my provider talk with me about it?
- Is the location convenient? How will I get to the provider's office? Will I walk, drive, or take the bus?
- Is the staff courteous, friendly, and respectful toward me?
- Do I have a choice of the hospital at which I'll give birth?
- Are there other services (for example, dietician or social worker) available to me through my provider?
- Can my partner come with me for my prenatal visits?

After a woman has chosen a provider, she will have her initial preconceptional or prenatal visit. When possible, the woman's partner should be encouraged to accompany her on the first visit to the practitioner. If the partner is the child's father, he can provide the practitioner with important information about his medical history and any genetic concerns he may have. Any partner who is present to learn important facts about pregnancy will also be in a better position to support and encourage the woman who is expecting. A partner's presence is helpful at subsequent visits, also, to allow the couple to hear and discuss information together.

Components of Prenatal Care

There are three basic components of adequate prenatal care:

1. Early and regular prenatal care
2. Maintenance of maternal health; promotion of good health habits
3. Recognition and treatment of physical, mental, and social/economic problems

Risk Assessments

The goal of risk assessment is to identify women and fetuses who have a chance of having a complication develop during pregnancy, labor, birth, or the neonatal period. After a risk is identified, the healthcare team can provide the appropriate type and level of care, which results in better outcomes. There is no perfect risk-assessment system.

The best health for mother and baby results when the mother has her first visit before the end of the first trimester (before the end of week 13), and then has regular visits until after she has delivered the baby. The usual timing for visits is about once every 4 weeks for the first 28 weeks, then every 2 weeks until 36 weeks, and then weekly until the birth. The

postpartum visit is usually scheduled at 4 or 6 weeks after birth, although many providers also like to see the woman at 2 weeks postpartum.

The Initial Prenatal Visit. The following are key components of the initial prenatal visit.

- *Health history:* The provider takes a complete health history of the woman, and her partner if possible, to learn about past illnesses and any pattern of certain inherited diseases that might affect this pregnancy (such as Tay-Sachs, diabetes, or sickle-cell anemia). The provider is also interested in learning whether a **multifetal** pregnancy (twins or more) has occurred in either family. The physician, nurse midwife, or nurse practitioner needs to know if the woman has had any difficulties during previous pregnancies or births, or if she has had any serious infections, including STDs or HIV. It is also important to assess the woman's lifestyle, including risk due to infections, substance use, or domestic violence. A thorough health history provides an accurate record of the client's past and present health, and gives the provider important data.
- *Physical examination:* A complete physical examination, including a pelvic examination, is part of the initial prenatal visit. This head-to-toe assessment includes examination of the gums, teeth, thyroid gland, heart, lungs, breasts, and all body systems. Also, the woman's height and weight should be measured and recorded at the first prenatal visit. During the pelvic examination, the provider checks the reproductive organs for signs of pregnancy, the bony pelvis for approximate size and shape, and looks for indications of any health problems. Pelvic measurements help in determining whether the bony passageway is large enough for delivery of a normal-sized newborn, an especially important consideration in a primigravida. A Pap test and STD tests (gonorrhea and chlamydia) are also routinely performed as part of the pelvic examination.
- *Laboratory tests:* The woman's blood type and Rh factor are determined. If the woman is Rh negative, she should receive Rh_o(D) immune globulin (**RhoGAM,** Gamulin Rh) at the 28th week of gestation and following any episode of bleeding or any invasive procedure (such as amniocentesis). The purpose of giving RhoGAM is to prevent Rh isoimmunization (see Chap. 67).
- *Other blood tests* that are routinely obtained include a syphilis test (RPR or VDRL), complete blood count (CBC), antibody screen, and rubella titer. A rubella titer is done to determine if the woman is immune to rubella, or German measles. If she is not immune, she is not vaccinated during pregnancy, because the rubella vaccine is live and could possibly have a harmful effect on the fetus. Chapters 67 and 68 discuss this condition further.
- *HIV testing* should be offered to every pregnant woman, according to the Institute of Medicine and the American College of Obstetricians and Gynecologists. If a woman tests positive for the virus and begins treatment for HIV during the pregnancy, the risk of transmitting the virus

to the fetus drops from about 1 in 4 (25%; without treatment) to as low as 1 in 12 (8.3%; with treatment during pregnancy).

- In addition to a pregnancy test (if it is needed to confirm the pregnancy), the woman's *urine* is tested for albumin (protein), glucose, and the presence of harmful bacteria. Each time a urine sample is collected from a pregnant woman, she should be helped to obtain a clean-catch specimen. (See Chapter 51 for the procedure for obtaining a clean-catch specimen.)
- The pregnant woman should be given a *purified protein derivative (PPD) tuberculin skin test,* which must be read between 48 and 72 hours later. In reading the test, only the raised area, not the reddened area, should be measured.
- If the woman or the baby's father has a family history of genetic problems, a referral for *genetic counseling and testing* should be given to the couple.
- *Determining the baby's due date:* A woman who thinks she is pregnant is wise to consult a healthcare provider after she has missed one menstrual period. A full-term pregnancy is approximately 280 days from the first day of the last menstrual period, or 266 days after fertilization. The 280 days equal 40 weeks. Many women do not keep an accurate record of their menstrual periods, or may not have regular periods for many different reasons. In these cases, the practitioner determines the estimated date of delivery (**EDD**), also called the estimated date of confinement (**EDC**), based on the size of the uterus during the physical examination, and/or by an ultrasound estimate of fetal age. See In Practice: Nursing Assessment 64-2 for more information on determining the anticipated birth date. The actual duration of pregnancy varies greatly, and the EDD is an approximate due date. Only about 4% of women actually deliver on their EDD.
- *Initial risk assessment:* The provider determines the degree of risk to the woman and fetus based on information from the history, physical exam, lab results, and due date. Commonly used terms for risk status are *low risk* and *high risk.* Although there is certainly such a thing as moderate risk, it is very hard to define. Based on her risk assessment, an individualized plan of counseling, classes, referrals, and prenatal care appointments is developed with the pregnant woman.

Return Prenatal Visits. At each return appointment, also called a *revisit,* the following measures should be performed and charted by a member of the healthcare team:

- *Weight:* This reading is then compared with her prepregnancy weight and her previous weight measurements.
- *Blood pressure*
- *Urine:* A "dipstick" analysis is performed for protein, glucose, and sometimes nitrites and leukocytes (indicators of bladder infections).
- *Uterus:* Measurement of the size of the uterus, called **fundal height,** and an evaluation of its growth since the last visit are performed.

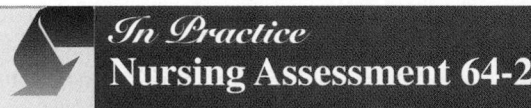

In Practice
Nursing Assessment 64-2

DETERMINING THE ANTICIPATED DATE OF BIRTH OR DUE DATE

Pregnancy is dated from the first day of the woman's last *normal* menstrual period (**LNMP**). To be considered normal, the period should have:

- Come on time
- Lasted as long as is usual for her
- Have been the normal flow for her

If any of these three items are not true of that period, ask her to recall the first day of her previous menstrual period (**PMP**).

When you have an accurate date for her last period, the due date for the baby is determined either by using a gestational wheel or by applying Nägele's rule. The due date is usually called the *estimated date of confinement* (**EDC**), or the *estimated date of delivery* (**EDD**).

Nägele's Rule
- Determine the date of the first day of the woman's LNMP.
- Add 7 days.
- Subtract 3 months.
- The resulting date is the EDD.

- *Fetal heart tones*
- *Edema:* Check the face, hands, legs, and feet for edema.
- *Continuing risk assessments:* At each prenatal visit, the risk profile should be updated. If new information indicates a change in the woman's risk status, the provider will develop a new plan of care with her to address her needs.

The client should be asked about any problems or complications that she has experienced since her last visit; how she is feeling; whether she has any concerns or worries; and how often the fetus is moving (after quickening has occurred).

Additional Tests Performed During Pregnancy. Many women have an ultrasound examination done between 16 and 20 weeks of pregnancy. This is a very accurate time at which to determine gestational age, and also to examine the fetus for normal development. If there is a problem or a concern at a different point during the pregnancy, the ultrasound examination may be repeated.

Between weeks 15 and 19, a blood test called the *maternal serum-alpha fetoprotein* (**MS-AFP**) is done. The primary purpose of this test it to screen for fetal neural tube defects. It may be combined with two other tests (HCG and estriol), which increases the number of neural tube defects that may be identified and also screens for Down syndrome. This test is called a *triple marker screen.*

Between 24 and 28 weeks, all pregnant women should be screened for diabetes. The test used during pregnancy is a 1-hour random glucose tolerance test. The woman eats normally until her prenatal or lab appointment, then drinks a 50-gram glucose beverage. Her blood is drawn 1 hour later to be tested for glucose. Elevated glucose levels may indicate gestational diabetes.

The Rh antibody test is repeated at 26 to 27 weeks, and RhoGAM is given at 28 weeks if the antibody test remains negative (see In Practice: Important Medications 64-1 for more information on RhoGAM).

Many providers repeat STD testing at 36 weeks, and may also do a vaginal culture for group B streptococcus.

Health Promotion

Health promotion through education of the pregnant woman is recognized as an important aspect of prenatal care. Despite the fact that pregnancy is a normal, although unusual, event in a woman's life, the changes from her usual way of being in her own body may come as a shock to her.

In many societies, sexuality and pregnancy are two topics on which caregivers provide very little real information. A great deal of what is learned about these important aspects of life is mythological, or "old wives' tales."

In addition, the scope of knowledge about how to nurture a growing fetus has changed dramatically over the past 30 years.

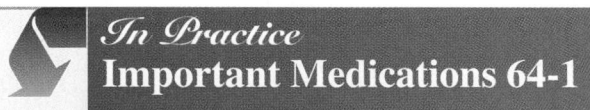

In Practice
Important Medications 64-1

RH IMMUNE GLOBULIN (RHOGAM®)

Microdose: 50 µg (used after spontaneous or elective abortion at <13 weeks gestation)
Full dose: 300 µg at 28 weeks' gestation
Expected effect: In an Rh-negative woman, Rh immune globulin prevents antibodies to Rh-positive fetal blood cells from forming. The 28-week dose provides protection for about 12 weeks; another dose should be given postpartum.
Adverse side effects: Pain, soreness at injection site

Nursing Considerations
• Rh immune globulin should also be given if an Rh-negative woman has any bleeding during the prenatal period, or if she has invasive testing performed, such as chorionic villus sampling or an amniocentesis. Chapter 67 discusses these procedures.
• Rh immune globulin is a blood product, but unlike whole blood or red blood cells, it is a processed immunoglobulin. It is safe for pregnant women to use. The method of its preparation includes viral inactivation. HIV is not a concern with this blood product.
• Because Rh immune globulin is a blood product, women who do not take blood products for religious reasons may refuse to take it.

It was about a generation ago that the first solid recommendations regarding nutrition during pregnancy were published; that fetal alcohol syndrome was recognized as a preventable disorder; and that information about sexuality in pregnancy became available.

Culturally, the feminist movement and the self-care movement worked together to empower women to demand additional knowledge about pregnancy. This includes information about changes within the body, how to improve the chance of having a healthy pregnancy and a healthy baby, and how to deal with the emotional and psychological processes involved in pregnancy.

The combination of these three factors—an inadequate amount of culturally acquired knowledge about pregnancy, an increase in scientifically acquired knowledge, and the pregnant woman's own increased desire to learn about and be an active participant in pregnancy—results in a clear need for health promotion during pregnancy.

Elimination and Hygiene.   A daily bowel movement is preferable for the pregnant woman, although not all women normally have one. A woman who has a tendency toward constipation may face increased difficulties during pregnancy, due to decreased peristalsis. Plenty of water, fruits, vegetables, moderate exercise, and adequate fiber intake encourage regular elimination.

The body's oil and sweat glands are more active than usual during pregnancy, so a daily warm (not hot) bath or shower is important. No proof exists that a tub bath is harmful at any time during pregnancy. Of course, the woman must be careful not to slip or fall in the tub or shower. During the last few weeks of pregnancy, the woman should not take a tub bath if she is home alone because she may have difficulty getting out of the tub and may require assistance. The woman's hair may be oilier than usual and may need frequent shampooing. A woman may safely use hair coloring or permanent waving during pregnancy.

The pregnant woman should practice good oral hygiene. The woman who eats a balanced diet and sees her dentist regularly does not need to worry about tooth damage during pregnancy. Necessary dental work should be performed, and sources of infection treated. Many dentists do not want to perform oral surgery (such as root canal) on pregnant women, unless it is an emergency.

Some women experience an increase in salivation, called **ptyalism,** during pregnancy. Although annoying to the woman, ptyalism does not cause tooth decay or gum irritation.

Some women are advised by non-professional sources, such as mothers or aunts, to douche during pregnancy. This practice is not only unnecessary, but can be harmful. If there is an infection with an odor or itching, the woman should be checked for a vaginal infection. Douching can actually increase her risk of vaginal infection, and sometimes cause an existing infection to be pushed up into the cervix and uterus. Pregnant women should be advised not to douche.

Breast Care.   Except for the use of a supportive bra, elaborate breast care is unnecessary prior to breastfeeding. Studies show that complicated nipple preparation rarely makes a difference in successful breastfeeding. A woman who is considering breastfeeding may decide against it if she is presented with a list of nipple exercises and special creams and ointments she is required to purchase. Women who plan to breastfeed should bathe as usual and use little or no soap on the nipples. They should gently pat their nipples dry. The nipple secretes its own natural moisturizer, which should not be removed with soap or other chemicals. Women should also avoid applying alcohol, tincture of benzoin, and lanolin ointments. These substances may damage the areola and nipple and have not been shown to be effective in preventing sore and cracked nipples. Lanolin is also a common allergen, and may contain insecticide residuals and DDT.

Wearing a nursing bra with the flaps down, and exposing the nipples to air and sunshine, may help to condition them. Harsh treatment may cause sore and cracked nipples and should be avoided. Nipple exercises and stimulation should not be done, especially in the third trimester, when they can cause uterine contractions and premature labor. Flat nipples should be treated with breast shields that are worn during the last trimester and after delivery between feedings. Inverted nipples are rare and can be treated with a nipple shield.

Rest. The pregnant woman tires more easily and should have enough rest to avoid fatigue. Preventing fatigue is better than having to recover from it. The woman should know how much rest she ordinarily requires and plan to get more if needed. Going to bed earlier, getting up later, or taking an afternoon nap may help. Short daytime rest periods are beneficial if the woman really relaxes. Pregnant women are able to carry on normal household activities without harm if they avoid heavy work and get additional rest.

As pregnancy advances, the woman may have a hard time finding a comfortable sleeping posture. Simple measures, such as additional pillows at the back, or a pillow supporting the weight of the abdomen or the top arm while the woman lies on her side, will usually relieve these common problems.

During the pregnancy's last months, the woman should rest on her left side for at least 1 hour in the morning and afternoon (Fig. 64-6A). (This position relieves fetal pressure on the renal veins, helps the kidneys excrete fluid, and increases flow of oxygenated blood to the fetus.)

Advise the pregnant woman not to sleep on her back, or to lie on her back for more than a few minutes. (The weight of the uterus can interfere with the circulation in the aorta and the vena cava, thus depriving the woman and fetus of oxygen; see Fig. 64-6B.)

Exercise and Posture. Exercise improves circulation, appetite, and digestion; it also aids in elimination and helps the woman to sleep better. The woman may safely continue customary exercises.

Swimming in a pool can be beneficial; however, swimming in lake water in later stages of pregnancy is not advised because of the danger of infection. Specific prenatal exercises are a part of childbirth education. Walking in fresh air is excellent exercise. Whatever the exercise, it should not be fatiguing. Exercise should be daily, rather than sporadic. (See In Practice: Educating the Client 64-2 and 64-3 for exercise guidelines and exercise danger signs during pregnancy.)

Activity. Weight gain, stability, or loss involves the balance between energy sources (diet and stored fuel) and energy expenditure. Energy use in this energy equation is the combi-

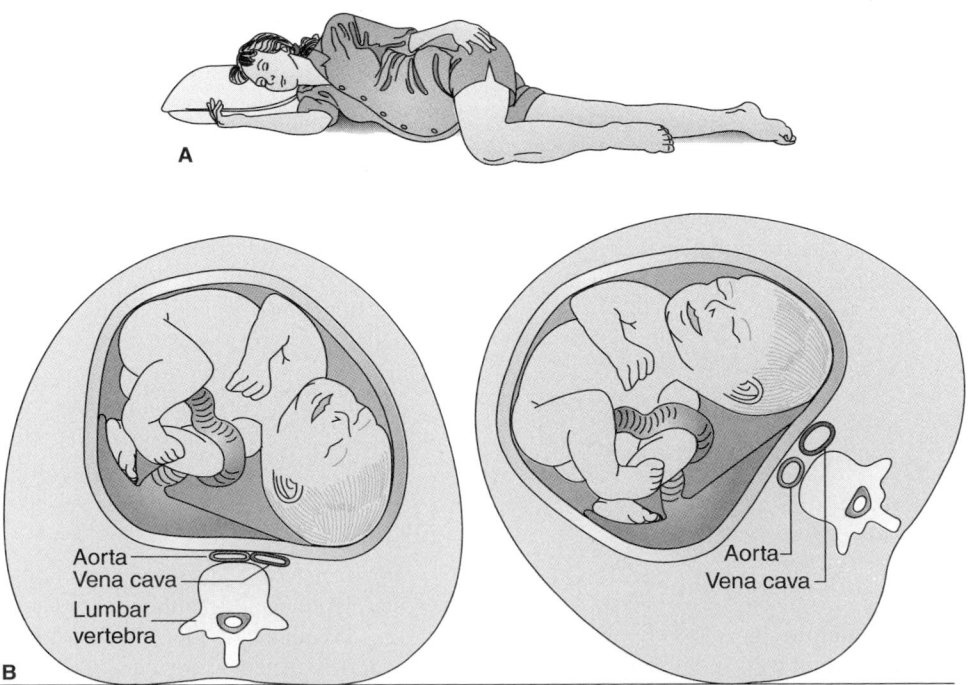

FIGURE 64-6. (A) Rest position during pregnancy. The knees and elbows should be slightly bent, the muscles limp, and the breathing slow and regular. Notice that the weight of the fetus is resting on the bed. **(B)** Supine hypotension can occur if a pregnant woman lies on her back, trapping blood in her lower extremities. If a woman turns on her side, pressure is lifted off of the vena cava.

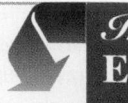

In Practice
Educating the Client 64-2

EXERCISE GUIDELINES DURING PREGNANCY

The goal of prenatal exercise is physical fitness within the limitations of pregnancy. If a woman does not have contraindications to exercising during pregnancy, the following general guidelines should be followed:

- Moderately exercising women with uncomplicated pregnancies can continue to exercise, with these modifications:
  - Reduce the intensity of the exercise by about 25%.
  - Maximum maternal heart rate should not exceed 140 bpm.
  - Periods of strenuous activities should be limited to 15–20 mins, interspersed with low-intensity exercise and rest periods.
- Extremely active women, athletes, and women who perform vigorous aerobic exercise should reduce the level of exertion.
- Sedentary women should begin to exercise very gradually.
- The types of exercise that provide the best cardiovascular and psychological benefits throughout pregnancy are walking, cycling, and swimming.
- Relaxation and stretching exercises (yoga) may be continued throughout pregnancy. Muscle strengthening exercises, such as Kegel exercises to strengthen the pelvic floor, and pelvic tilts or pelvic rocks to strengthen the lower back and relieve back pain, may be done by all pregnant women. These provide no cardiovascular benefits.

- Jogging and weight-bearing aerobic programs should be moderated to avoid injury due to ligament relaxation and increased joint mobility during pregnancy.
- Women who lift weights may continue to lift light weights during pregnancy, with the following modifications:
  - Avoid heavy resistance on machines.
  - Avoid use of heavy free weights.
  - Breathe properly to avoid the Valsalva maneuver.
- Sports which pose a potential risk to the mother or fetus include:
  - Contact sports—football, soccer
  - Sports involving potential joint or ligament damage—basketball, volleyball, gymnastics, downhill skiing, skating
  - Horseback riding
- Sports which are safe to continue during pregnancy include:
  - Racquet sports—tennis, racquetball, squash (avoid heat stress; decrease intensity as pregnancy progresses)
  - Golf (may need to modify golf swing)
  - Slow-pitch softball (avoid sliding into bases, blocking bases)
  - Cross-country skiing
- Avoid any strenuous exercise or sport in adverse conditions—extreme heat, high humidity, air pollution, high altitudes.

---

nation of basal metabolic rate, body heat production, and physical activity. The average total additional energy (calorie) requirement is about 2500 to 3500 calories per day. Changes in daily physical activity are very individual, leading either to an increase or a decrease in energy used throughout the pregnancy.

Sexual Relations.   Pregnancy, although usually a result of sexual activity, is not viewed as a sexual state in our society.

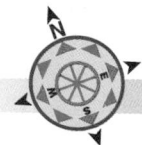

SPECIAL CONSIDERATIONS: CULTURE

Activity and Exercise During Pregnancy

Traditionally, Puerto Rican families view exercise during pregnancy as inappropriate. Contrast that with Haitian women (who are not relieved from their responsibilities, and are expected to fulfill their obligations throughout the pregnancy) and pregnant Cambodian women, who are also active.

Although certain individuals may consider the sight of a pregnant woman beautiful and erotic, she may be seen as misshapen, awkward, and not particularly arousing. In the last decades of the 20th century, pregnancy has commonly been viewed as natural, sensual, and beautiful.

Pregnancy is always a time of challenge to a relationship, both developmentally and sexually. The challenge can result in either crisis or growth.

During pregnancy, a woman continues to have sexual needs. If the pregnant woman has a partner, the partner also continues to have sexual needs. Both partners have needs for intimacy and closeness, which may be different from their sexual needs. Intimacy needs can be categorized into the following three groups:

- *Sexual needs:* The sex drive, or libido, usually changes during pregnancy—although the pattern of the change in libido is quite individual. In addition, the sexual response cycle is affected by pregnancy. These changes, combined with the changes in anatomy and physiology during pregnancy, have varying effects on the relationship of a pregnant couple. Sexual needs may be met through sexual activity with a partner or masturbation. Some women

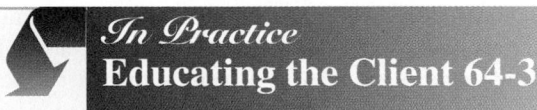

EXERCISE IN PREGNANCY: DANGER SIGNS

A pregnant woman who is exercising should be alert to the following signs and symptoms. If these occur, she should stop exercise, and contact her healthcare provider.

- Pain of any kind
- Uterine contractions (occurring at intervals of fewer than 15 min)
- Vaginal bleeding; leaking amniotic fluid
- Dizziness; faintness
- Shortness of breath
- Palpitations; tachycardia
- Persistent nausea and vomiting
- Back pain
- Pubic or hip pain
- Difficulty in walking
- Generalized edema
- Numbness in any part of the body
- Visual disturbances
- Decreased fetal movement

experience spontaneous orgasm due to the increased pelvic blood supply during pregnancy. Pregnancy diminishes sexual desire in some women and increases it in others. Communication between the pregnant woman and her sexual partner helps to eliminate conflicts.

- *Touch needs:* Pregnancy is a time of a heightened need for touch, which may be met partially by sexual expression, but which can also be met through nonsexual touch, such as massage, caressing, or holding.
- *Comfort and reassurance needs:* The need of the pregnant woman for comfort and reassurance stems both from her changing body image and from the developmental processes of pregnancy. These factors bring fears and concerns for the pregnant woman about safety for herself and the fetus, her desirability, and her need for continued love and support.

Sexual Safety During Pregnancy. In general, expressions of sexuality during pregnancy are quite safe. Sexual intercourse is often physically difficult and awkward late in the pregnancy, and couples may wish to experiment with a variety of positions and sexual practices. Sexual intercourse during pregnancy is not harmful as long as it is not unduly uncomfortable and no high-risk factors are present (such as placenta previa, preterm labor, or ruptured membranes). There are a few exceptions to this rule, and these risks can be categorized by the causative factor. Categories of risk include:

- *Risk due to penetration:* Women who experience bleeding during pregnancy should avoid vaginal penetration until the problem is diagnosed.

- *Risk due to possible infection:* There are two primary areas where infection is a risk with sexual activity: sex with a partner who has a sexually transmissible disease; and sex after the rupture of membranes, which normally protect the fetus and placenta from infection.
- *Risk due to arousal:* For a woman at risk for preterm labor, sexual arousal, and the accompanying increased engorgement of the pelvic organs, might stimulate the initiation of labor. There is no proof that arousal increases the risk of spontaneous abortion. Sexual arousal may be used at term to initiate labor—at this point in the pregnancy, it is no longer a risk.
- *Risk due to orgasm:* The uterine contractions that occur with and follow orgasm may stimulate preterm labor.
- *Risk due to sexual behaviors:* With the exception of STD exposure, the main risky sexual practice during pregnancy is the forceful blowing of air into the vagina, which may result in air embolism.

Clothing. By about the third month, the pregnant woman will discover that her clothing is becoming tight, and she needs to wear looser clothing. Some women wear special maternity clothing; others opt for bigger and looser versions of normal, everyday clothing (eg, oversized sweaters, elasticized pants and skirts). Garters, constrictive knee socks, and knee-high pantyhose should not be used because they restrict blood flow. Women should wear comfortable shoes; flat heels are less awkward and provide a better base of support. The pregnant woman will probably have difficulty tying shoelaces or fastening buckles late in the pregnancy.

The pregnant woman should wear a wide-strapped bra that supports the breasts without causing nipple pressure. An underwire bra is usually more comfortable for the woman with heavy breasts. A good nursing bra is essential after delivery if the woman plans to nurse. She should purchase two or three bras of her normal chest size but with a larger cup size.

Travel and Employment. Most women continue driving during pregnancy, at least until the last months, when it may become uncomfortable (the fetus, woman, and steering wheel cannot occupy the same space at the same time). The woman must be sure to buckle her seat belt under her enlarging abdomen. She should use the shoulder strap, placing it to the side of her abdomen (Fig. 64-7). Seat belts are particularly important during pregnancy to protect the woman and the fetus. A car with air bags provides added protection.

Long trips are exhausting for anyone, but because today's families are often on the move, the pregnant woman may find regular travel necessary. Travel by air or train is recommended for long, tiring trips. If the woman is to travel by car, she should plan to stop at least every 2 hours to go to the bathroom, stretch, relax, and walk around for at least 10 minutes. This movement helps to prevent blood from pooling in the lower extremities. The pregnant woman should never fly in a small plane that is not pressurized because the lower atmospheric pressure decreases the supply of oxygen to the fetus. The expectant woman should consult with her healthcare provider about travel plans, because special conditions and times during pregnancy may rule out traveling. A long trip away from home when the woman is close to term is also unwise.

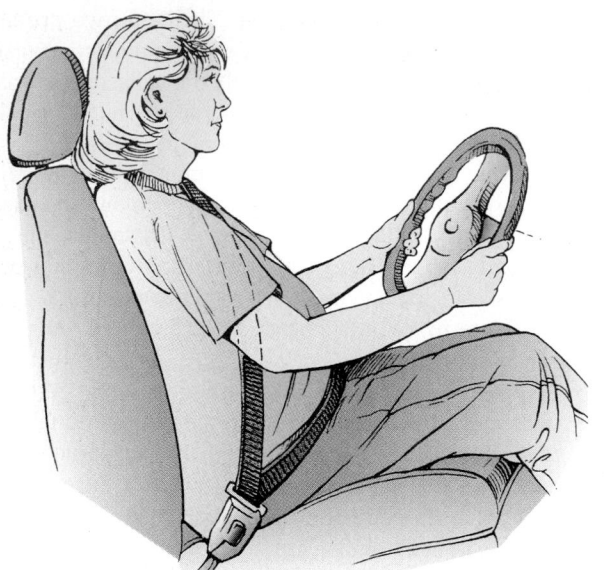

FIGURE 64-7. Pregnant women should wear a seat belt with the shoulder strap above the uterus and below the neck, and a lap belt low and under the abdomen.

Many women continue to work outside the home during pregnancy. The law states that in most situations, a maternity leave of absence, without loss of seniority, must be granted to a woman who requests one. Jobs that involve heavy lifting, operating dangerous machines, continuous standing, or working with toxic substances are contraindicated during pregnancy. Radiation should also be avoided.

Teratogenic Factors.   Some fumes, chemicals, substances, and infections are known to cause fetal defects. These environmental, damaging agents are called *teratogens.* Most teratogenic effects occur in the first trimester of pregnancy, during the critical period of development of the embryo. The woman may not even know yet that she is pregnant.

Teratogenic events occur after fertilization and are not genetic (inherited), although they are congenital (present at birth). Maternal dietary deficiencies and food, air, and water pollutants may play a role. Radiation is particularly dangerous.

In Chapter 67, you will learn about the specific negative effects of many teratogenic factors. The following are some examples of teratogens:

- *Diseases:* Rubella, herpes, toxoplasmosis, syphilis. To avoid the infection of toxoplasmosis, the pregnant woman should not handle cat litter and should cook meat well, especially poultry. She should wash her hands carefully after handling raw meat and wash all raw fruits and vegetables thoroughly before eating them. She should wear gloves while gardening or cleaning.
- *Prescribed medications:* Phenytoin, lithium, valproic acid, isotretinoin, and warfarin have each been associated with teratogenesis.
- *Substances of abuse:* The provider should obtain a complete substance use history at the first preconceptional or antepartum visit. If the mother uses tobacco, alcohol, or recreational drugs, she is strongly advised to stop. Street

or recreational drugs, such as amphetamines and stimulants, can cause fetal difficulties. The danger seems to be greatest early in pregnancy. Alcohol is the most widely used substance, and also the most damaging to the fetus. Heroin can cause congenital addiction. Cocaine may be associated with long-term behavioral and attention problems in the child born to a mother who used it during pregnancy. Other recreational drugs are either known or suspected teratogens. Chapter 94 discusses substance abuse and chemical dependency further. Chapters 67 and 68 present some harmful effects of drugs and alcohol on pregnancy and the fetus in more detail.

- *Ionizing radiation:* This is the type of radiation exposure that is used in treating cancers, or that occurs with a nuclear plant accident.

Nursing Alert

Caution the pregnant woman not to take any herbs, drugs, or medications without asking the healthcare provider. Laxatives, diuretics, stimulants, and depressants are particularly dangerous. Many herbs also are not proven safe for the fetus.

Nursing Alert

If you suspect any type of drug abuse in a pregnant woman, notify the healthcare provider.

Nutrition During Pregnancy.   One of the earliest and most important purposes of prenatal care has been to counsel women and ensure that they receive adequate nutrition to support themselves and their growing fetus during pregnancy. Studies show that a newborn's chances for good health are greater with a reasonably high birth weight. The nutritional requirements of a pregnant woman differ from those of a nonpregnant woman. The woman's caloric needs increase during pregnancy, because she needs to meet energy requirements for fetal, placental, and maternal tissue development. The quality of the diet, not the quantity, matters most, and the pattern of weight gain is more important than the total amount.

Foods for the pregnant woman should be selected from all food groups to obtain the necessary distribution of nutrients. Exclusion of any group may lead to a deficiency of one or more nutrients. The U.S. Department of Agriculture's food pyramid guide (see Fig. 30-1 in Chap. 30) shows the guidelines for daily food choices. The guidelines for pregnant women are basically the same, with a suggested increase in the milk, yogurt, and cheese group to 3 to 4 servings. In addition to the requirements of the basic food guide pyramid, the pregnant woman should make the following dietary adjustments:

- Increase caloric intake by approximately 300 calories daily.
- Increase calcium intake before the last half of the pregnancy. Increase milk intake to 3 to 4 cups daily. Supplemental calcium is sometimes prescribed. (Rationale: Calcium is essential to the development of the fetus' bones and teeth and for blood clotting.)

- Maintain iron intake. Most providers order an iron supplement during pregnancy because of its dietary importance. (Rationale: Iron is essential in the production of hemoglobin. Because breast milk contains little iron, the developing fetus stores iron for use after birth.)
- Maintain folic acid intake. Taking 400 µg daily of folic acid (folate) in a supplement is recommended for all women of childbearing age when not pregnant, in addition to food sources of folate. During pregnancy, the recommendation increases to 600 µg from a supplement, plus food sources. Most prenatal vitamins contain 1 mg of folic acid. (Rationale: Folic acid, a B vitamin, helps to prevent congenital neural tube defects, most notably spina bifida.)
- Increase intake of most vitamins. Many physicians prescribe supplemental vitamins during pregnancy.
- Increase protein intake. (Rationale: Protein is essential to the building and repair of all body tissues, and aids in the production of milk for the nursing mother.)
- Avoid empty calories, including alcohol, sugared soda drinks, other sweets, and salty foods.
- Use iodized salt. (Rationale: It promotes proper functioning of the thyroid gland.)
- Eat a wide variety of foods. (Rationale: Especially during the first few months of pregnancy, if the woman is experiencing nausea, a variety of foods will encourage proper nutrition.)
- Avoid laxatives and enemas unless the physician specifically orders them. Stool softeners, such as docusate sodium (Colace), are ordered more often than laxatives. Fiber is also essential to prevent and to treat constipation.
- Increase fluid intake to 10 glasses daily to assist in kidney and bowel function. Water is the preferred fluid.

When providing prenatal nursing care, keep in mind a woman's general health, age, cultural and religious background, likes and dislikes, food allergies or sensitizations, and socioeconomic status. These factors will affect her diet and pattern of weight gain. Dietary counseling should begin at the first visit and continue throughout all followup visits. Instructing the client to make a sample diet for review is useful in determining needed dietary changes.

Appetite. Changes in the woman's body during the early part of pregnancy may interfere with her appetite, so attention must be given to supplying her with proteins, vitamins, and iron throughout pregnancy.

Many pregnant women find that they are extremely hungry after the first few weeks. They should monitor what they eat and be careful not to fill up on empty calories. Rich, highly spiced, and fried foods are undesirable. In the late months of pregnancy, several small meals daily, rather than three large ones, will probably help her feel better. The pregnant woman will not have as much space in her abdomen for a distended stomach.

Beverages and foods that contain caffeine can be harmful to the pregnant woman. Items containing caffeine include coffee, some teas, most cola drinks, several other soft drinks, and chocolate (in candy or in beverages). Caffeine may contribute to *mastitis,* an inflammation and swelling of breast tissue in the woman that can cause irritability in the fetus, especially if the mother is breastfeeding. Caffeine also crosses the placenta during pregnancy.

Pica is an abnormal craving for nonfood items during pregnancy, such as clay, dirt, and cornstarch. If left untreated, pica can lead to serious nutritional and other physical disorders.

Weight Gain During Pregnancy. The recommended weight gain for each woman depends on her height and what she weighed before she got pregnant. This comparison is known as the body mass index (**BMI**), and provides a starting place to determine how much weight is ideal to gain during this pregnancy. At the initial prenatal visit, the client's height and weight will be measured. She will be asked what she weighed prior to pregnancy. Finally, a BMI chart will be used to determine whether she is underweight, of average weight, overweight, or obese.

The pregnant woman's weight should increase gradually from the sixth week after conception until the end of the full term.

Compare the variables of maternal body size (underweight, normal weight, overweight, obese) and the variables of weight gain during pregnancy (low or high). Recommended weight gain during pregnancy is based on these body size variables. Not only do maternal pre-pregnant body size and weight gain in pregnancy affect birth weight, but they also have an impact on perinatal mortality. For women who are underweight, the risk of perinatal mortality at term is lowest if they gain at least 37 pounds. For women of normal weight prior to pregnancy, the perinatal mortality rate is lowest with a weight gain between 30 and 37 pounds. For obese women with a weight gain of more than 15 pounds, the perinatal mortality begins to increase.

☛ KEY CONCEPT

All pregnant women should gain weight.

In assessing maternal weight gain, other helpful guidelines include the following:

- By the 20th week of gestation, all women except obese women will have gained approximately 10 pounds.
- Any woman who loses more than 8 pounds during the first trimester is at increased risk. Weight loss during pregnancy is never recommended.
- Although weight gain itself is critical, equally important is the quality of food leading to the weight gain. For example: A woman may easily gain weight on a cookie, chips, and soda diet—but may not be well-nourished.

Common Discomforts of Pregnancy. Even in normal pregnancy, it is common for the woman to have some unusual, and sometimes uncomfortable, sensations. These are the so-called "common discomforts of pregnancy." They are considered minor, not in the sense that they do not cause true discomfort, but because they are not serious and do not threaten the life of the fetus or the mother. However, sometimes it is difficult to tell what is truly a common discomfort, or when a symptom may be a warning sign of a more serious problem. Table 64-1 describes the possible causes of many discomforts,

■■■ **TABLE 64-1** 𝒞OMMON DISCOMFORTS OF PREGNANCY

Symptom	Probable Cause or Contributing Factors	Relief Measures	Danger Signs
Integument			
Itching of skin	Stretching of skin over breasts and abdomen	Bathe with baking soda, cornstarch, or colloidal oatmeal in bath water Use little, if any, soap Watch for sensitivity to soaps and detergents Use moisturizers	None
Stretch marks (*striae gravidarum*)	Hormonal changes of pregnancy Heredity	Soothing oils: coconut, olive, vitamin E *Recipe:* ⅓ cup virgin olive oil ¼ cup aloe vera gel 6 capsules vitamin E (cut) 6 capsules vitamin A (cut) Mix; refrigerate. Apply b.i.d. See above if stretch marks itch	None
Melasma	Increased pigmentation	Avoid sun exposure Wear hats; use sunblock Adequate folic acid intake (1.0 mg/day) Advise woman that it may or may not resolve after the birth	None
Nervous			
Sleeplessness	Overexhaustion Dreams Stress Excitement Hard to find a comfortable position	Use pillows to help find comfortable position Herbal teas: chamomile, lemon, marjoram Hot milk with honey No heavy meals before bedtime If can't sleep, get out of bed and read or take a warm bath or shower	Depression
Moodiness	"Superwoman" syndrome Hormonal changes Adaptation to life changes	Emotional self-care Spoil yourself! Nurturing from family and friends	Depression Suicidal thoughts Extremely moody
Musculoskeletal			
Low back pain or backache	Relaxation of joints and ligaments Weight of enlarging uterus Increased lordosis	Good posture Wear flat shoes with good support Pelvic rocking Walking Good body mechanics Apply small amount of salve to back, such as Tiger Balm (camphor, menthol, peppermint, clove, and cajuput)	Kidney infection (one-sided pain) Fever, chills
Braxton-Hicks contractions	Uterus readying itself for labor May occur with breast stimulation or orgasm	Reassurance Warm baths or showers Herbal teas (red raspberry, sarsaparilla)	Preterm labor
Round ligament pain	Enlarging uterus stretches ligaments May be felt on sides of abdomen, in groin, and outside the vagina	Heat, massage, rest Avoid sudden movements Bend slowly toward pain to allow relaxation	Preterm labor Abdominal problem Infection

■■■ **TABLE 64-1** 𝒞OMMON DISCOMFORTS OF PREGNANCY (CONTINUED)

Symptom	Probable Cause or Contributing Factors	Relief Measures	Danger Signs
Reproductive			
Vaginal discharge	Estrogen stimulation of glands of cervix and vagina	Avoid soaps to vulva Wash prn with clear water Do not douche Avoid "anti-itch" creams containing steroids	Severe itching, odor, lesions, pain with intercourse; bleeding after intercourse; pain Partner with complaints of discharge from penis or lesions
Breasts			
Breast enlargement and tenderness	Hormonal changes Preparation for lactation	Supportive bra Good posture Breast care: Wash with water only, to keep the oily secretions from Montgomery's follicles on the nipple and areolae	Breast masses
Nose			
Nasal stuffiness or bleeding	Allergies Common cold Increased number of capillaries	Normal saline nose drops Cold compresses Use cool-mist humidifier Decrease dairy products in diet	Severe nosebleed may indicate high blood pressure
Mouth			
Sore or bleeding gums	Increased blood supply Poor oral hygiene Gingivitis	Vigorous brushing of teeth and gums with soft toothbrush Regular flossing Gum massage Adequate vitamin C	Overgrowth of gums onto teeth (this may require oral surgery)
Excess saliva production (ptyalism)	Cause unknown Ask about pica	Small, balanced, frequent meals Chew gum Suck on oral lozenges or hard candies Increase fluid intake to compensate	None
Gastrointestinal			
Food cravings	May be social custom May indicate lack of certain nutrients in diet	Reassurance Complete diet review Avoid unhealthy foods Limit consumption of non-foods (pica)	Pica may replace nutritious foods Excessive weight gain due to consuming "junk" foods or excessive sweets
Heartburn	Slow stomach emptying Acid reflux into esophagus	Small, frequent meals Avoid caffeine Sip on water, milk, soda water Eat a tablespoon of yogurt Sit up (if happens when lying down) Try to avoid antacids Herbs: Papaya (has digestive enzymes); anise or fennel-seed tea after meals; slippery elm powder (1 tsp. with honey, or in a tea)	Ulcer Gastrointestinal bleeding
Constipation	Slowed GI motility Pressure of uterus on intestines Iron therapy Limited water intake Trying to avoid having BM when it's painful due to hemorrhoids or fissures	Increase fluid intake Increase fiber: bran, fruits, dark breads, vegetables, prunes, raisins If laxative needed, use only bulk laxative, such as Metamucil® Increase activity level	Fecal impaction

(continued)

■■■ **TABLE 64-1** 𝒞OMMON DISCOMFORTS OF PREGNANCY (CONTINUED)

Symptom	Probable Cause or Contributing Factors	Relief Measures	Danger Signs
Nausea and vomiting of pregnancy	Decreased stomach motility Increased hCG level Hereditary, dietary, socio-economic factors	Eat small, frequent meals Eat snacks high in complex carbohydrates at onset of nausea Avoid heavy meals, excessive fats, excessive spices Peppermint tea, soda water, ginger tea Eat sour, salty foods (potato chips and lemonade)	Weight loss >8 pounds Starvation Loss of appetite Eating disorders GI disease (ulcers, gallstones, liver disease)
Hemorrhoids	Varicose veins or hemorrhoidal veins Increased pressure from constipation	Avoid constipation Cold witch-hazel compresses Topical anesthetics Sitz baths Rest on left side with feet slightly raised	Excessive pain Excessive bleeding
Neurologic			
Headaches	Cause usually unknown Possible causes: sinus infection, eye strain	Rest Darkness Acetaminophen prn	One-sided headache Associated sudden visual change Not relieved by acetaminophen
Dizziness Syncope	Pressure of uterus on inferior vena cava when lying down Decreased cardiac return Decreased cardiac output Low blood pressure	Avoid lying on back (supine) after 24–26 weeks' gestation Left lateral position increases blood flow Get up slowly from lying down	Fainting
Urinary			
Frequency, urgency Nocturia	Pressure of enlarging uterus on the bladder	Maintain good fluid intake Void frequently Decrease evening fluid intake	Pain or burning with urination Sweet smell to urine
Cardiovascular			
Varicose veins	Heredity Weight of enlarging uterus Relaxation of smooth muscle in vein walls due to progesterone	Avoid prolonged standing or sitting Rest several times daily with legs elevated Use elastic stockings If varicosities on vulva, apply pressure with a thick sanitary pad inside underwear	Signs of blood clots: heat, swelling, pain Pain with walking
Swollen feet	Increased estrogen and progesterone Decreased venous return to heart	Elevate legs when sitting Elevate legs above heart when lying, or rest on left side Leg exercises while standing and sitting Adequate calcium and potassium	Preeclampsia (high blood pressure, swelling, protein in the urine)

suggestions that may decrease discomfort, and warning signs of more serious problems.

☞ KEY CONCEPT
_____

It is important to differentiate a common discomfort of pregnancy from a warning sign of a complication.

Medical Interventions

Medication Use in Pregnancy.   The pregnant woman should not take any medications, herbs, or nutritional supplements unless they are absolutely necessary and ordered by her healthcare provider. Prescribed medications should be taken in the smallest effective dose and discontinued as soon as possible. The safety of any drug in pregnancy is unpredictable;

even commonly used medications can cause fetal problems. For example, a mother's use of aspirin late in the pregnancy can cause a clotting problem in the fetus. Medications such as nose drops, diet pills, diuretics, and cold remedies can also cause serious difficulties.

Some medications taken during pregnancy cause defects that show up many years later in the child. Diethylstilbestrol (DES), previously taken in pregnancy to prevent miscarriage, has been linked to later cervical cancer in girls and infertility in boys born to women who took DES. Antineoplastic drugs (used to treat cancer) are particularly teratogenic.

The U.S. Food and Drug Administration (FDA) has established five categories of drugs, based on their potential for teratogenic effects in humans. Box 64-2 lists these categories of drug safety in pregnancy as rated by the FDA.

➤➤ BOX 64-2

CATEGORIES OF DRUG SAFETY IN PREGNANCY

The FDA has rated drugs according to their relative safety during pregnancy as follows:

Category A: Controlled studies in women do not demonstrate a risk; possibility of fetal harm appears remote.

Category B: Animal studies fail to demonstrate fetal risks, and there are no controlled studies in women; *or* animal studies show an adverse effect, but the same effect was not confirmed in studies in women.

Category C: Animal studies have demonstrated fetal risks, but no controlled human studies are available; *or* studies in women and animals are not available. Drugs in this category should be given only if the potential benefit to the mother outweighs the possible risk to the fetus.

Category D: Human fetal risks exist, but the benefits of use in pregnant women may be acceptable despite the risk—such as when a life-threatening situation exists, or for a serious disease for which safer drugs cannot be used or are not effective.

Category X: Proven fetal risks exist; drug is contraindicated in women who are or may become pregnant.

Most drug handbooks identify the pregnancy risk for each drug.

Drugs are particularly dangerous to the fetus in the first and third trimesters. In the first trimester, the fetus is being formed and is particularly sensitive to teratogens. Drugs administered in the third trimester are dangerous to the fetus because when the fetus is born, the woman's circulatory system is no longer available to help metabolize or excrete drugs, and the newborn's immature circulatory and excretory systems must take over.

PREPARING TO BE A PARENT

When approaching pregnancy in a holistic manner, there is an obligation to see the woman not just as a container for the fetus, but as an individual in the context of her family and community. It is important to determine how we can best help her and her family members make the necessary transitions. This section examines several aspects of becoming a parent, whether it is for the first or the sixth time.

Adapting to Pregnancy

Pregnancy can be seen as a developmental crisis, a time of both challenge and opportunity. In the earliest stages of pregnancy, it is very common for a woman to feel shock, disbelief, and sometimes denial. To adapt to the pregnancy, there are several stages through which a woman must progress.

Pregnancy Validation: 1st Trimester (Weeks 1 to 13)
The task of this period of the pregnancy is to accept the pregnancy and all that it means as a reality. Common responses include ambivalence, shock, disbelief, self-focus, and fear (particularly if this woman had a prior negative pregnancy experience).

Fetal Embodiment: 2nd Trimester (Weeks 14 to 27)
During this phase, the task of the pregnant woman is to incorporate the fetus into her body image, and to begin to see herself as a mother. Often, the woman becomes more able to identify with her own mother. She may re-live and re-evaluate all aspects of this relationship.

Common responses during the second trimester include increased dependency, excitement when quickening (first sensation of fetal movement) occurs, calmness, increased libido, and buying maternity clothes.

Fetal Distinction: 3rd Trimester (Week 28 to Term)
At this stage, the pregnant woman must learn to see the fetus as separate from herself in preparation for the birth. This is often called a period of "watchful waiting." The woman may exhibit "motherly" behavior, such as reading to the fetus, stroking her abdomen, preparing clothes, choosing a name, and reading books about childbirth and parenting. She also may experience fear related to the birth, her survival, and the survival of the infant. Often these fears lead to dreams of danger. Many women experience a slight depression late in the third trimester.

Separation From the Fetus: Labor and Birth
With the onset of labor, the inevitability of separation becomes clear. Although in many ways this separation is desired, there is usually some ambivalence about the loss of being the center

of attention; the physical separation from the baby; and the fear about the process of labor and birth.

Common manifestations of this fear include frequent visits to the hospital or birth center to assess the onset of labor, and needing constant reassurance that she and the baby are doing well and can complete this step.

Transition to Motherhood: Postpartum

Maternal–infant bonding is a process that begins during the pregnancy and accelerates immediately after the birth. Strong bonding increases the mother's commitment to the infant, and also her ability to be an effective parent. Bonding of the mother and child is helped by immediate maternal–infant touch, visual contact, suckling, and vocalizations by both the mother and the infant. Behaviors that indicate positive attachment include fondling, kissing, cuddling, and gazing.

Preparing for Labor and Birth

As the woman enters the final phase of pregnancy, she becomes more focused on labor and birth, and typically is eager to plan for these events. Planning may include choosing a site for the birth and a birth attendant (if this is not already done), and developing a plan that reflects her desires regarding the conduct of labor and birth, including analgesia and anesthesia alternatives. Safety for herself and the fetus is the overriding concern in planning for labor.

Safety, however, means different things to different people. For some women, safety means immediate access to (and probably use of) the highest level of technology available. For others, the hospital environment may seem inherently unsafe—for these women, safety may lie in attendance by a trusted midwife or physician, maintaining control over any interventions considered, and having family and/or friends whom she chooses stay with her during the labor and birth. For most women, safety lies somewhere in between these two choices.

Only the pregnant woman herself can decide what safety means to her, and how to have the need for safety met during labor and birth. During the prenatal period, she may wish to explore all the alternatives open to her and evaluate them in light of her own values, beliefs, and goals. As a nurse, your task is to support her in the choices she makes.

There are many excellent methods of educating women and their partners or support persons about childbirth. Childbirth education should include:

- Information about the process of birth
- Exploration of individual fears about birth
- Mechanisms for alleviating the pain and working through the fears of childbirth
- Discussion of options in labor and birth, and how to promote having a normal labor. This may include: choosing the site and attendant; discussing positions for labor, activity; hydration during labor; nutrition during labor; analgesia/anesthesia; options surrounding the birth itself (presence of family/friends/siblings, positions for birth,

use of labor/delivery/recovery rooms); episiotomy; immediate contact with the neonate; and immediate breastfeeding.
- Discussion of possible complications, and potential interventions (this should not be the primary focus of the course).
- Postpartum options, such as the amount of contact with and care of her baby; establishing breastfeeding, or breast care if bottle feeding; time of discharge; danger signs; basics of infant care; and postpartum contraception.

Approaches to Childbirth Preparation

Common Methods of Childbirth Preparation. *Natural childbirth* consists of progressive relaxation and abdominal breathing techniques that are taught to the expectant mother and her partner. Hypnosis, when used in childbirth, is a combination of relaxation and conditioned reflexes. It uses a normal breathing pattern. A healthcare provider trained in hypnosis and childbirth works with the mother and her significant other.

The Lamaze Method of Childbirth. The most well-known model for childbirth preparation is the Lamaze method. The two components of this method are education and training, using the theory of conditioned reflex. Expectant women are trained in toning exercises, relaxation exercises, and breathing techniques, which use three levels of chest breathing for different stages of labor.

Current Childbirth Preparation Trends. Currently, the childbirth preparation movement is steering away from specific breathing techniques, and toward assisting the woman to find her natural ways of coping with stress and pain. Many women find the following methods helpful: vocalization, massage, water therapy, visualization, relaxing music, and subdued lighting.

Regardless of the approach to childbirth preparation, it is essential to communicate to the family that the goal of childbirth is to have a healthy mom and baby. Health is more than the physical event of labor and birth; it includes family interactions, bonding with the infant, and the successful transition to a new phase of life.

Responses to Fatherhood

In many pregnancies, the father is the one person whose changing role and developmental tasks do not receive serious consideration. The pregnant woman receives attention, the children in the home receive attention, but the new father's needs are often unrecognized and unmet. Paternal responses to pregnancy include:

- *1st trimester:* Fears losing his wife and the child, and has self-doubt as to his capability as a future father
- *2nd trimester:* Has increased respect and awe as quickening occurs; sees the fetus as a new person; begins to consider names for the fetus
- *3rd trimester:* Fears harming the fetus during sexual intercourse (yet finds that sexual abstinence is difficult); has envy or pride at his wife's creativity; worries

over the birth; and is keenly aware of male and female differences.
- *Throughout the pregnancy:* Has increased romanticism, increased nurturing, increased participation in family life, anxiety about costs, and concern about his lack of skills in infant care

Preparing for the Expanding Family
Family Dynamics. The family unit will evolve with the new changes. Major changes in the family occur, due to the economic cost of pregnancy and a new family member. Healthcare costs escalate during a pregnancy. The pregnant woman may need additional emotional support, as well as additional physical care if a complication develops during the pregnancy. The woman who is at risk of preterm labor, or who is simply 39 weeks' pregnant and ungainly, may not be able to perform her usual household and familial chores.

Siblings often react to a pregnancy by regression in behavior and attitude, because they fear that they will be replaced or unloved. If older children originated in another biologic family (that is, if they are stepchildren, adopted, or living in a blended family), such fears and behaviors may be magnified. It is common for a child to regress in developmental stage, but it is often quite hard for the parents to cope with this occurrence.

The "raging hormones" of pregnancy can keep the woman slightly out of touch with her usual methods of coping. Although she may normally interact and communicate in quite mature ways, during a pregnancy she may become depressed, anxious, withdrawn, or angry as she accomplishes her own developmental tasks. Such behavioral changes can be as hard for a child or spouse to tolerate, as much as the behavioral changes of children are hard for parents to accept.

Preparing for the Newborn
In addition to anticipatory guidance concerning the alterations in family structure and functioning, prenatal preparation for first-time parents involves learning the basics of infant care and preparing for infant feeding, particularly for women who plan to breastfeed. This is a need not only for the woman who will be breastfeeding for the first time, but may be even more important for that woman who had a previous unsuccessful attempt at nursing an infant.

Client Education: Infant Care. Client education regarding general infant care should include:

- The range of normal physical characteristics of newborns
- Neonatal and infant response: adjusting to the needs expressed by the infant (attunement), sleep/wake patterns, vision, hearing, startle reflex, and so forth
- Holding the infant
- Skin care and bathing
- Care of the umbilicus
- Diapering options
- Infant stool patterns

- Newborn and infant safety, including the importance of using a car seat

Client Education: Infant Feedings. There is widespread agreement that breast milk is the best milk for a baby. The only exceptions are women who might transmit a disease (such as HIV) or a medication (such as lithium) through the breast milk.

There is little preparation involved in breastfeeding. In the past, sources recommended a variety of activities to be performed, including nipple toughening, nipple rolling, and nipple pulling. None of these methods has been proven to be of any benefit to lactation, either in establishing suckling or in preventing nipple soreness and cracking, and they are no longer recommended. Some guidelines for lactation teaching are found at In Practice: Educating the Client 64-4.

However, deciding between breastfeeding or formula-feeding a baby is a complicated decision for many women. They may be shy, modest, or have concerns about the reactions of other people if they breastfeed. Throughout the pregnancy, healthcare staff should make the information known that "breast is best," but respect each woman's decision as the best for her.

After a woman has decided which method of feeding her infant she will use, the preparation for that method should be focused on her specific learning needs.

The woman who opts to formula-feed the infant may have educational needs about formula preparation and storage; for example, the frequency and amount of feedings. Each woman should be treated individually, so that education can focus on her particular needs.

For the woman and her family, pregnancy is a time of hope, dreams, anxiety, and fears. Often it is a nurse who makes the difference for a pregnant woman in adjusting to her pregnancy, preparing for her baby, and maintaining a healthy state for herself and her child. By listening, teaching, and caring, you can be the one to make that difference. See In Practice: The Nursing Process 64-1 for an overview of the nursing process during pregnancy.

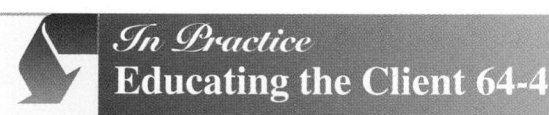

In Practice
Educating the Client 64-4

LACTATION

Generally, new mothers need information regarding the following topics:
- Nutrition and hydration during lactation
- Supply and demand concept
- Nipple care
- Let-down reflex
- Appearance of breast milk
- Positions for breastfeeding
- Expressing/pumping and storing milk

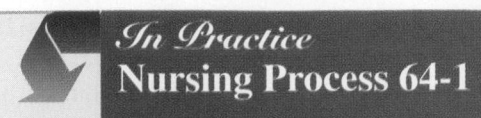

Nursing Process 64-1

OVERVIEW OF THE NURSING PROCESS
DURING A NORMAL PREGNANCY

Assessment Priorities
Possible Nursing Diagnoses
Planning
Implementation
Evaluation
Nursing History
Health history of both parents and their families
Genetic history of both parents
Ethnic background of both parents
Feelings about the pregnancy (reproductive choice)
Obstetric history
Last menstrual period
  First day of period
  Was it normal?
Pertinent lifestyle factors
  Nutrition, balance between activity and rest, sexual
  activity, teratogenic factors (exposure to diseases;
  use of prescription and OTC medications and drugs
  of abuse; use of alcohol, nicotine, and caffeine)
Prepregnant weight
Presence of common discomforts of pregnancy
  Morning sickness, shortness of breath, leg cramps,
  constipation, hemorrhoids, vaginal discharge, gin-
  givitis, edema, varicose veins, stretch marks
Recognition of danger signs in pregnancy and ability
  to state appropriate action
Preparedness for labor and delivery experience
Preparedness for parenting (mother and father)
Effect of pregnancy on self-concept
Adequacy of coping skills and resources
Cultural influences
Concerns, superstitions, and fears
Physical Examination
Initial visit
  Height, weight
  Assist the healthcare provider with the assessment
  and documentation of a complete physical exami-
  nation that includes a pelvic examination
Return visits
  Weight, blood pressure
  Urine dipstick tests for sugar, albumin (protein),
  nitrites, and leukocytes
  Abdominal examination
    Fundal height
    Fetal heart tones
  Presence of edema
Laboratory and Diagnostic Tests
Blood tests as requested
Urine culture if requested
Ultrasound (if indicated)

Possible Nursing Diagnoses
Activity Intolerance
Anxiety
Body Image Disturbance
Ineffective Breathing Pattern
Decisional Conflict

Constipation
Ineffective/Disabling Family Coping
Diversional Activity Deficit
Altered Family Processes
Fatigue
Fear
Fluid Volume Excess
Knowledge Deficit (specify)
Altered Nutrition (less or more than body
  requirements)
High Risk for Altered Parenting
Altered Role Performance
Self-Care Deficit
Self-Esteem Disturbance
Altered Sexuality Patterns
Sleep Pattern Disturbance
Urinary Incontinence, stress

Planning
The nurse designs a plan of care with the woman and
family to achieve the following general goals:

• Throughout the pregnancy, the woman's weight
  gain (overall nutritional status) and general lifestyle
  patterns support fetal growth and development.
• The woman reports she feels able to cope with the
  physical and emotional changes accompanying
  pregnancy.
• The woman and her partner correctly demonstrate
  relaxation techniques for labor.
• The woman describes and uses appropriate
  strategies for dealing with any of the discomforts of
  pregnancy.

The long-term goal is the uncomplicated delivery of a
healthy newborn without maternal harm.

Implementation
• If they request advice and circumstances are appropriate, counsel the woman or couple about reproductive choices.
• Develop and implement a teaching plan that corrects
  any knowledge deficits about conception, fetal
  growth and development, general health practices for
  the woman, and the labor and delivery experience.
• Teach the woman strategies for dealing with any of
  the discomforts of pregnancy that present, such as
  morning sickness or leg cramps.
• Refer the woman to prenatal classes.

Evaluation
Evaluate the adequacy of the plan of care by assessing the woman's and her family's achievement of the
above goals. If they are unable to meet key goals, the
plan must be modified. The basic evaluative criteria
follow:

• Maximum physical and mental health of the woman
  throughout pregnancy
• Uncomplicated delivery
• Healthy mother and newborn after delivery

➤ STUDENT SYNTHESIS

Key Points

- Gravida refers to the number of pregnancies a woman has had; para refers to the outcomes of those pregnancies.
- Preconceptional care includes addressing women's habits, nutrition, and psychosocial needs, as well as risks due to medications, diseases, and genetic defects.
- The fertilized ovum, or zygote, will eventually develop into the fetus and all the supporting structures: placenta, membranes, and umbilical cord.
- The period of the embryo is the critical period of human development, when the organs and systems are formed; the period of the fetus is a period of further growth and development.
- Maternal and fetal blood do not mix under normal circumstances; the placenta provides a place for exchange of gases, nutrients, and fluid between the mother and the fetus.
- In fetal circulation, oxygenated blood travels from the placenta through the umbilical vein, while deoxygenated blood is carried back from the fetus to the placenta through the two umbilical arteries.
- Only the positive signs of pregnancy prove that there is a fetus.
- A woman's body changes in both structure and function due to the size of the growing fetus and the hormones produced during pregnancy.
- Anticipatory guidance about the changes that are coming with pregnancy gives a woman or a couple time to prepare for those changes.
- A healthy lifestyle for a pregnant woman includes maintaining adequate nutrition, avoiding harmful substances, and exercising.
- Good nutrition during pregnancy is dependent upon the mother taking in enough calories to provide energy and enough protein to support herself and the rapidly growing fetus, as well as consuming the recommended amount of vitamins and minerals every day.
- All pregnant women should gain weight; the amount that is ideal for each woman is based on her height and her weight before the pregnancy.
- The common discomforts of pregnancy do not threaten the health of the mother or the fetus, but may be similar to warning signs of more serious problems. It is important to know how to distinguish common discomforts and warning signs and to report them as necessary.
- The psychological changes of pregnancy are just as tremendous as the physical changes; every woman and family deserves support in dealing with these changes.

Critical Thinking Exercises

1. Discuss ways that you would need to individualize a nursing plan of care to address a pregnant woman's cultural beliefs.
2. Plan interventions that you would use to provide supportive care during pregnancy to a woman when the father of the baby is present and involved. How would you adapt the plan to meet the needs of a woman whose partner is not interested or involved? How would you adapt the plan to meet the needs of a woman whose life partner is also a woman?

NCLEX-Style Review Questions

1. Susan is pregnant, and has had two previous pregnancies. She decided to have an elective termination of pregnancy the first time. She also has a 2-year-old son, who was born at 38 weeks of gestation. Her pregnancy history could best be summarized as:
   a. G2 P2
   b. G2 P1011
   c. G3 P2
   d. G3 P1011
2. The period of the embryo ends at what gestational age?
   a. 5 weeks
   b. 8 weeks
   c. 10 weeks
   d. 13 weeks
3. In the umbilical cord, oxygenated blood is carried through the:
   a. Single umbilical artery
   b. Two umbilical arteries
   c. Single umbilical vein
   d. Two umbilical veins
4. The anatomic and physiologic changes in the mother are caused by:
   a. The stress of pregnancy
   b. The growth of the fetus only
   c. The hormones of pregnancy only
   d. The growth of the fetus and the hormones of pregnancy
5. A positive pregnancy test is a:
   a. Possible sign of pregnancy
   b. Probable sign of pregnancy
   c. Positive sign of pregnancy
   d. Presumptive sign of pregnancy

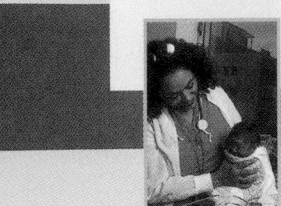

CHAPTER

65

Normal Labor, Delivery, and Postpartum Care

LEARNING OBJECTIVES

1. Identify at least three choices or options for locations for birth. Discuss at least two advantages and disadvantages for each option. Identify at least two nursing considerations for each choice.
2. Define and give at least four differences between true labor and false labor. State at least two nursing considerations related to each type of labor.
3. Explain the significance of lightening, Braxton-Hicks contractions, effacement, dilation, "show," SROM and AROM, engagement, nulliparous, and parous.
4. Differentiate among the following events that occur during contractions: increment, acme, decrement, rest interval, frequency, duration, intensity, and length of relaxation time.
5. Define and discuss at least three nursing considerations for each of the following terms: lie, presentation, station, and position.
6. Discuss the events that indicate the onset of the first stage of labor.
7. Differentiate among the three phases of the first stage of labor. Identify at least three nursing considerations for the latent phase, the active phase, and the transitional phase.
8. Identify the events of the second stage of labor and the significance of bearing down and crowning. Identify at least three nursing considerations related to this stage.
9. Identify the events of the third stage of labor and explain the significance of the expelled placenta. Identify at least three nursing considerations related to this stage.
10. Identify the events of the fourth stage of labor and explain the significance of involution. Identify at least three nursing considerations related to this stage.
11. Compare the advantages and disadvantages of at least four comfort measures related to contractions. State at least four nursing considerations related to epidural and general anesthesia.
12. Discuss at least four nursing considerations related to external fetal monitoring.
13. Differentiate among the following terms: acceleration, decelerations, early deceleration, late deceleration, and decreased variability.
14. Identify at least three nursing responsibilities to the newborn and the mother immediately after birth.

15. Define and differentiate among the following terms: lochia rubra, lochia serosa, and lochia alba. State at least three nursing considerations for each.
16. In the nursing skills lab, demonstrate the techniques of postpartum care, including fundal massage, episiotomy and perineal assessment, peripad changes, Homans' sign, and bladder assessment.
17. In the nursing skills lab, present a client teaching session on the advantages of breastfeeding. Include the following concepts: colostrums, lactation, the "let-down reflex," engorgement, and expression of milk.
18. Discuss the chances of becoming pregnant when a woman is breastfeeding. Differentiate between the return of menstruation and ovulation.

NEW TERMINOLOGY

after-pains	engorgement	lightening
amniohook	epidural	lochia
amniotomy	episiotomy	lochia alba
birth center	fetal monitor	lochia rubra
birth plan	frequency	lochia serosa
birthing room	fundus	nuchal cord
Braxton-Hicks	intensity	postpartum
contractions	interval	presentation
cervical os	intrapartum	show
colostrum	involution	stages of labor
crowning	labor	station
dilation	labor contractions	tocodynamom
duration	lactation	uterine
effacement	lie	contractions
engagement		

ACRONYMS

AROM	FHR	PA	SROM
CNM	LDRP	4 P's	SVE
CRNA	NP		

LABOR AND BIRTH AS NORMAL PROCESSES

In the preceding chapter, you learned about normal pregnancy and how to provide nursing care for the expectant family. In this chapter, you will learn about the process of normal labor and delivery, as well as how to provide nursing care around the time of birth and during the *postpartum* (after delivery) period.

As you recall from the previous chapter, a woman's body is designed for conceiving, carrying, and bearing children. The process of labor is normal, but it is a process that most women experience only a few times in their life. It is an intense process that requires enormous amounts of physical and emotional energy.

In this chapter, you will learn how to promote the normal progression of labor, and how to recognize signs of possible complications. You will also learn to deal with the emotional needs of the laboring woman and her family. Although most families have looked forward to delivery for many months, the individuals involved will have unique concerns. As a nurse, you will be expected to provide encouragement, support, and education to assist family members during this intense event. By using the nursing process, you can provide comprehensive care to the growing family.

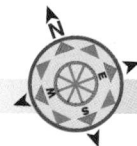

SPECIAL CONSIDERATIONS: CULTURE

Family Involvement in the Birth Process

Most traditional Cuban fathers are not involved in the birth process at all. The level of the father's participation depends on the wife's level of education and assimilation into the American culture. The pregnant woman's mother may be present during the entire labor and delivery. The laboring woman will usually assume a more passive role than her mother, who will try to direct all activity. In Gypsy families, the father stays outside the birth room due to modesty about birth events.

Careful observations of both the mother and newborn are necessary after delivery. You will perform tasks that prevent the development of complications and that promote rapid healing of tissue. You will also function as a teacher to provide knowledge that the family needs for maternal and newborn care. For many women, the most important role of the nurse during the postpartum period is the role of educator. Whether this baby is the client's first child or her fifth, each baby brings changes and challenges to the new parents.

The Four Stages of Labor

Labor is a series of events during which a woman's uterus contracts and expels a fetus by progressing through the four **stages of labor.** In these stages the woman's uterus:

(1) undergoes rhythmic contractions (called **labor contractions** or **uterine contractions**) that cause the **cervical os,** or "mouth" of the uterus, to open and move the fetus downward into the birth canal; (2) continues contracting until the baby is delivered through the vaginal opening; (3) expels the placenta; and (4) contracts again to prevent excessive blood loss.

Although there are many theories, no one is certain what causes labor to begin; but approximately 38 weeks after fertilization (the 40th week after the last menstrual period [LMP]), the fetus is ready to be born. **Intrapartum** is the time period during which labor and delivery take place, and it is followed by the **postpartum** period, which lasts until the end of the 6th week after the birth.

Choices in Labor and Birth

Because each birth is an important life event, many women and their families have a clear sense of what they would like to have occur during the process. There are choices in many areas of intrapartum care. The following are some of the options that should be considered.

Birth Attendant

As discussed in Chapter 64, one of the choices an expectant family makes is its healthcare provider. Many women choose physicians, who may be specialists in either family practice or obstetrics. Other women choose to receive pregnancy and birth care from a Certified Nurse Midwife (**CNM**). Women who have received prenatal care from a nurse practitioner (**NP**) or physician assistant (**PA**) will have a different care provider for the birth; the role of these professionals does not include attending at births.

Birth Setting

Another choice families can make when preparing for birth is the setting for the event. Most women choose to deliver in a hospital setting. In the hospital, they may be assigned to a traditional labor and delivery unit, in which the woman labors in one room and then is taken to a delivery room for the birth. Or, they may be placed in a **birthing room,** in which both the labor and the delivery take place. In some hospitals, these rooms are called **LDRP,** or labor/delivery/recovery/postpartum rooms.

A free-standing (not in a hospital) **birth center** is another option for giving birth. Free-standing birth centers promote the concept of safe, satisfying, and cost-effective childbirth. The National Association of Childbearing Centers has developed standards and criteria for care and safety in childbirth centers.

Finally, women may choose to give birth at home. Home births may be attended by either a CNM or (less frequently) a physician. One reason that some women choose this option is that the home is her territory, which is not the case in either a birth center or a hospital.

Only women in good general health whose pregnancies have progressed normally should be candidates for any type of out-of-hospital birth (birth center or home). At the first signs of complications for the mother or infant, a transfer to a hospital is indicated to ensure the safety of the mother and baby.

Birth Plan

A **birth plan** is a written document in which the expectant mother expresses her desires for labor and birth. Some are brief, while others are long and very detailed. Some items that may be included are:

- The woman's choice of a partner for support during labor
- The type of pain-relief measures the woman desires
- The woman's feelings about having an IV, electronic fetal monitoring, or an episiotomy

It is the nurse's role to inform the mother or couple preparing a birth plan of the policies of the birth setting and birth attendant, and of the need for flexibility if complications develop. The family should discuss the birth plan with their healthcare provider before the onset of labor.

The Process of Labor

Lie, Presentation, Station, Position

In order to understand the process of labor and birth, it is helpful to understand the relationship of the fetal body to the maternal body. There are several terms that are used to describe how the fetus is lying within the mother.

Lie is a term used to compare the position of the fetal spinal cord (the "long part") to that of the woman. The normal lie of the fetus is *longitudinal* (up and down), which means that the fetal spine is parallel to the woman's. In a *transverse lie,* the fetus is lying crosswise in the uterus, and cannot be delivered until the lie is altered.

Presentation refers to the part of the fetus that lies closest to the pelvis, and will first enter the birth canal. The usual presenting part is the head; this is a *cephalic presentation.* Some people call this a *vertex presentation;* however, vertex is only one type of cephalic presentation. Vertex presentation occurs when the fetal head is flexed well against the fetal chest. Other types of cephalic presentations include *face presentation* and *brow presentation* (Fig. 65-1).

When the buttocks, foot, or knee is the presenting (lowest) part, it is called a *breech presentation.* Complicated labor often occurs when body parts other than the fetal head present (see Chap. 67).

Rarely, the shoulder may be the presenting part if the fetus is lying in a transverse (horizontal) position. If the fetus cannot be turned from this shoulder presentation to a cephalic presentation, the baby must be delivered by cesarean birth.

Station refers to the level of descent of the fetal presenting part into the birth canal. Station is measured as the relationship of the fetal presenting part's lowest bony portion to the level of the ischial spines of the woman's pelvic bones (Fig. 65-2).

During pregnancy, the fetus is floating in the amniotic fluid above the level of the symphysis pubis. Near term, the fetal presenting part dips into the pelvis, but can still be dislodged upward. Either before the onset of labor in most *nulliparous* (first time delivery) women, or during labor in most *parous* (have had previous births) women, the head moves downward until it can no longer be pushed up and out of the pelvis. This is called **engagement.**

The station at which the fetus is said to be *fully engaged* is called station 0; that is, the widest part of the presenting part of the fetus has lodged in the pelvic inlet, and the lowest part of the fetal skull is at the level of the mother's ischial spines (see Fig. 65-2). The other stations are measured in centimeters above or below station 0. When the presenting part is higher (above) the level of the ischial spines, the station is expressed with a negative number (−1 station is 1 cm above the spines; −2 station is 2 cm above the spines, and so forth). When the presenting part descends further into the pelvis, the station is expressed as a positive number (eg, +1 station), again using centimeters as the measuring guide. A station of −5 is considered "floating," while a station of +5 means that the fetal head is at the vaginal opening.

Position refers to the relationship between an assigned point on the presenting part of the fetus to one of four quadrants of the woman's pelvis. There are several positions for a fetus in any presentation. The position depends on three things: (1) how much the fetus is flexed (curled) on itself; (2) whether the assigned point of the fetal body is on the mother's right or left side; and (3) whether the designated point is in the anterior or posterior part of the mother's pelvis. The following rules help care providers communicate the part of the fetal body that should be used to determine position.

In *cephalic presentation* positions:

- If the head is well flexed, then the top (*crown*) of the fetal head is presenting, and the *occiput* (back part of the head) is the designated point.
- If the head is fully extended, then the face presents, and the chin (*mentum*) is the assigned point.
- If the head is partially extended, then the brow presents; this assigned point is referred to as the *frontum.*

In *shoulder presentation positions:*

- The fetus is on a *transverse lie.* The shoulder, arm, backside, or abdomen may be the presenting part.

In all types of *breech presentation* positions, the sacrum is the assigned point. Variations of breech position include:

- *Complete breech:* The fetus has both legs drawn up, bent at both the hip and the knee.
- *Frank breech:* The fetus has the hips bent, but the knees are extended.
- *Kneeling breech:* Either one or both legs are extended at the hip, flexed at the knee.
- *Footling breech:* Either one or both legs are extended both at the hip and knee.

After you learn which body part determines position, then you can accurately describe the position of any fetus. For example, the occiput may be on the woman's right or left side, and either in the anterior, posterior, or transverse area of the pelvic opening. These positions are often designated by the obstetric personnel and recorded and initialed in the charts. A fetus with the occiput in the left side of the anterior portion of the mother's pelvis could be described as LOA (left occiput anterior).

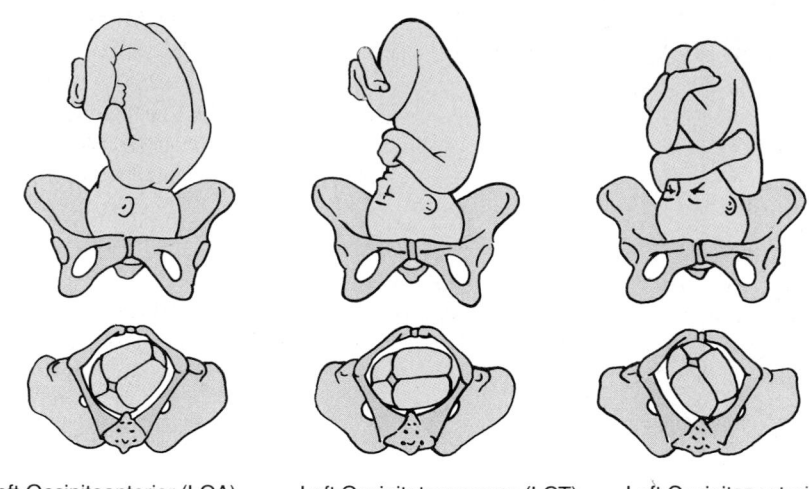

Left Occipitoanterior (LOA)   Left Occipitotransverse (LOT)   Left Occipitoposterior (LOP)

A. Left Vertex (Occiput) Presentations

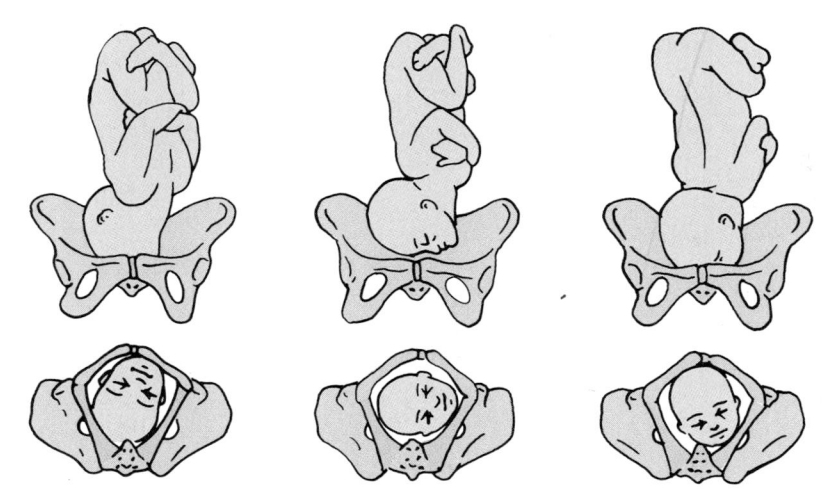

Left Mentoanterior (LMA)   Left Mentotransverse (LMT)   Left Mentoposterior (LMP)

B. Left Face (Mentum) Presentations

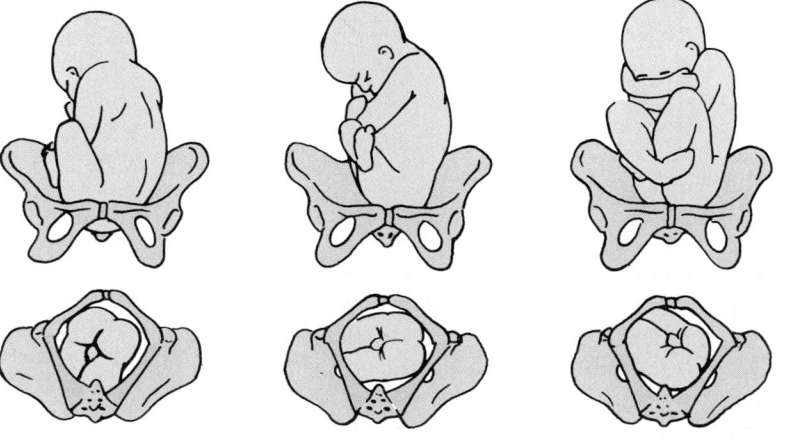

Left Sacroanterior (LSA)   Left Sacrotransverse (LST)   Left Sacroposterior (LSP)

C. Breech (Sacrum) Presentations

FIGURE 65-1. Left fetal presentations. (**A**) Vertex presentations. (**B**) Face presentations. (**C**) Breech presentations. Each position can be left or right, and anterior, posterior, or transverse. Each presentation has a possibility of six positions. For example: LOA—left occiput anterior; LOP—left occiput posterior; LOT—left occiput transverse; ROA—right occiput anterior; ROP—right occiput posterior; ROT—right occiput transverse.

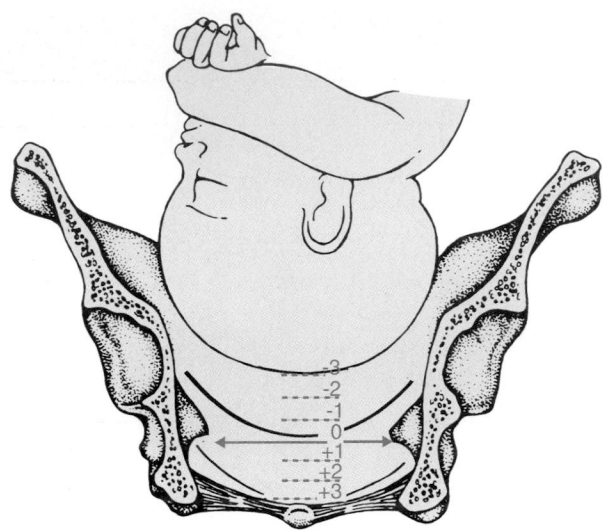

FIGURE 65-2. Stations of the fetal head. This diagram shows the relationship of the fetal head to the pelvic bones, specifically the ischial spines, during the labor and delivery process. Station zero (0) represents the level of the ischial spines.

☛ KEY CONCEPT

Some positions of the fetus make delivery difficult or dangerous. For example, in a footling breech position, there is a chance that the umbilical cord could prolapse because there is so much empty space within the uterus. This could cut off the blood and oxygen supply to the fetus before it is born.

Signs that Labor is Approaching

Commonly known as the **4 P's** of labor, there are four main variables that affect labor: passage, passenger, powers, and psyche. The *passage* includes the diameter of the body pelvis and its soft tissues. The *passenger* includes the fetus, umbilical cord, and placenta. The *powers* are the uterine contractions. The *psyche* includes the process of birthing, the attitude and behaviors of the parents, and the evaluation process of the stages of labor.

Lightening.   **Lightening** is the settling of the fetus into the pelvis. Lay people often say, "the baby has dropped." Lightening usually occurs 2 to 3 weeks before the onset of labor in primigravidas (women having their first child). If the client is a multigravida (has had more than one pregnancy), lightening may not occur until labor begins. Although lightening allows the pregnant woman to breathe more easily, she will notice an increase in pelvic pressure and urinary frequency, and may also have leg cramps and increased edema of the legs.

Braxton-Hicks Contractions.   During pregnancy's late stages, the uterine muscles prepare for labor and delivery by tightening and relaxing at intervals. These contractions, called **Braxton-Hicks contractions,** are usually painless, short, and irregular. They are also known as *false labor.* As labor approaches, these contractions may become stronger and somewhat regular. The woman may sometimes mistake these false labor contractions for true labor. She may experience false labor anytime in the last trimester, but more often during the

final 2 or 3 weeks of pregnancy. A change in activity may provide the woman some relief.

Show.   A mucous plug seals the cervix during pregnancy. Just before labor, the cervix opens slightly and this plug dislodges. At the same time, some capillaries of the cervix rupture, staining the sticky mucus a pinkish color. This process is called the **show,** or *bloody show,* and indicates that labor is about to begin.

True Versus False Labor

A pregnant woman may find that distinguishing between true and false labor contractions is difficult. *False labor* contractions are generally felt low in the abdomen. They occur in an irregular pattern, and their intensity does not grow substantially with time. Although false labor may be annoying, the contractions come and go, and a change of position or activity can relieve the discomfort. In false labor, no change is found in the cervix on internal examination, and there is no bloody show. However, the pelvic exam itself may dislodge the mucous plug and cause some spotting that resembles show.

In *true labor,* on the other hand, the involuntary uterine contractions are rhythmic, grow stronger over time, and begin the true work of labor. These contractions occur at fairly regular intervals, starting at about 20 to 30 minutes apart and increasing until they are about 2 to 3 minutes apart. True labor contractions usually last about 30 seconds initially, and increase in duration as labor progresses. The **interval (frequency)**, or time from the start of one contraction until the start of the next one, in true labor gradually decreases (gets shorter); while the **intensity** (strength) and **duration** (length) of each contraction increases. The bloody show usually appears during this time. Usually, the true labor contraction feels like lower-back pain that moves gradually around to the abdomen. These contractions help create *effacement* (thinning out) and *dilation* (opening) of the softened cervix. The most important difference between true and false labor is whether or not the cervix changes. During labor, the cervix will become 100% effaced, meaning almost paper-thin, and 10 cm dilated, which will permit the fetus to pass through it (Table 65-1).

Onset of Active Labor

Active labor begins when the woman is experiencing regular, rhythmic uterine contractions that are increasing in *duration, frequency,* and *intensity.* When this occurs, the time has come for the woman to notify her practitioner (see In Practice: Educating the Client 65-1).

Contractions.   *Contractions* of the uterine muscles bring about the birth of the fetus. The uterine muscle is a smooth muscle, and the contractions are involuntary; therefore, the woman cannot hurry, slow, lengthen, or shorten them.

During each contraction, the muscle fibers of the uterus tighten. When the contraction ends and the uterus is at rest, the muscles remain slightly shorter than when it started. This is called *retraction* of the muscles. As this process continues over the hours of labor, the shorter muscles pull against the point of least resistance, or the cervix, and cause effacement, and later dilation. The pressure from the taut bag of waters or

■■■ **TABLE 65-1** *False vs. True Labor*

	False Labor	True Labor
Contractions		
Timing	Irregularly spaced	Regular, rhythmic
Duration	Variable	Increases over time
Frequency	Variable	Become closer over time
Intensity	Variable	Become stronger over time
Effect of position or activity change	Contractions lessen	Become stronger with ambulation or activity
Location where felt	Primarily in low abdomen	Start in back, radiate to abdomen
Cervical change	None	Progressive effacement and dilation
Presence of "show"	None	Usually present

the presenting part of the fetus helps maintain the dilation of the cervix. Each labor contraction has three phases:

1. *Increment*—This phase, during which the contraction builds from the resting phase to full strength, is longer than the other two combined.
2. *Acme*—This is the time during which the contraction is at full intensity. This phase becomes longer as labor progresses.
3. *Decrement*—During this phase, the uterine contraction eases, until the resting state is achieved.

The time between contractions is called the *relaxation time* or *rest interval* and is equally as important as the contractions themselves. If the relaxation time is short or absent, the fetus may suffer from lack of oxygen, and the woman may become extremely tired.

 Nursing Alert

Report immediately if contractions come more often than every 2 minutes, or if each contraction lasts 90 seconds or longer. *Rationale: There is not enough relaxation time for the fetus to be well-oxygenated. This event is rare during normal labor, but must be carefully watched for when oxytocin is used for labor augmentation or induction.* (See In Practice: Important Medications 65-1.)

In Practice
Educating the Client 65-1

Contractions

A woman should notify her practitioner when she is having regular, rhythmic contractions that are getting closer together, lasting longer, and becoming stronger. She should also notify her practitioner immediately if the membranes ("bag of waters") break or leak—whether or not she is having any uterine contractions. The practitioner will need to know if the woman is having contractions before, during, or after the membranes rupture.

You will need to estimate the intensity of contractions as *mild, moderate,* or *strong.* The woman may be asked to classify the intensity on a scale from 1 to 10, which helps to quantify a subjective symptom (discomfort). However, remember that a frightened client, who does not understand the labor process and how to work with her body to ease the discomfort, may well cry out in pain or thrash about with very mild contractions. It is important that you independently assess the intensity of contractions by placing your hand on the uterine **fundus,** or upper curve. This is the most muscular portion of the uterus. During a mild contraction, you will be able to press your fingers into the fundus, even at the contraction's peak (*acme*). With moderately strong contractions, you will be able only to dimple the fundus when you press in. With a strong contraction, the uterine fundus feels quite firm, and you cannot press into it when a contraction is at its peak.

Documentation of observations of contractions should include their duration, frequency, intensity, and the length of the relaxation time as well as the client's reactions and statements.

Some people refer to contractions as "labor pains." When giving nursing care, the term *contraction* is preferred to avoid reinforcing the idea of pain. You may inform the client that she may feel some discomfort, and prepare her for the experience. However, if she insists that she is in pain, do not ignore or correct her! Instead, work with her on ways to relieve the pain. Such methods may include relaxation techniques, breathing techniques, vocalizations, and the use of pain medication.

Rupture of the Membranes.   The fetus lies in a two-layered sac filled with amniotic fluid (commonly called the "bag of waters"). By the pregnancy's 40th week, the amni-

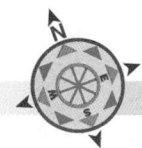 **Special Considerations: Culture**

Expressions of Pain During Labor and Birth

Among most American Indians, stoicism is encouraged and practiced in childbirth. In African American culture, the expression of pain can be quite open and public.

otic fluid volume has reached approximately 1,000 milliliters (about 1 quart). Before the birth of the fetus, the membranes break, and the fluid is released. If left to nature, this usually happens just before delivery and provides additional protection for the fetal head during labor, by serving as a dilating wedge against the opening cervix.

Whenever the membranes break, either a sudden gush or a gentle trickle of fluid results. The breaking of the bag of waters without medical intervention is termed spontaneous rupture of membranes (**SROM**) and occurs in approximately 25% of all births. Even after the rupture of the membranes, more amniotic fluid is produced (the stories of "dry birth" are best categorized as myths).

In the remaining 75% of births, the birth attendant may perform artificial rupture of the membranes (**AROM**), a procedure called **amniotomy.** This procedure is performed using a special hook (**amniohook**) under sterile conditions. This procedure may stimulate true labor to begin, or may speed up the active labor process.

Nursing Alert

Report any yellow, green, or cloudy amniotic fluid. *Rationale: Normal amniotic fluid is clear and colorless, and has a slightly salty odor. Yellow or green fluid may indicate that the fetus has passed meconium, or stool, while still in utero. White or cloudy fluid may indicate the presence of pus in response to an infection.*

A simple test, known as the nitrazine test, will determine if the amniotic sac has ruptured. A strip of nitrazine paper is placed against the client's vaginal wall and is compared with a color standard. The normal pH of the vagina is 5.0 (acidic); the pH of the amniotic fluid is 7.0 to 7.5 (neutral to slightly alkaline). If the paper turns blue, it is probably stained with amniotic fluid, indicating that the amniotic sac has ruptured. If the test or urine strip remains yellow, it is probably in contact with vaginal secretions only. Contact with blood or urine may also turn the paper blue, so it is important to avoid touching these body fluids with the paper.

When providing nursing care to a woman whose membranes have ruptured, record the time, method of rupture (SROM or AROM), color of fluid, and fetal heart rate.

When the membranes are ruptured, microorganisms from the vagina can travel through the cervix and enter the uterus, which poses a risk of infection to both the mother and infant. For this reason, the nurse should obtain a baseline maternal temperature at the time the bag of waters ruptures, and continue to assess the woman's temperature every 2 hours until delivery. If the woman's temperature begins to increase, the practitioner will usually initiate measures to prevent infection of the fetus. These measures may include giving intravenous antibiotics to the mother, and planning the immediate delivery of the infant.

The practitioner will also assess the fetal heart rate for the possibility of a *prolapsed cord* (cord presenting before the fetal head), if the presenting part is not engaged at the time of rupture of the membranes. If there is any question about whether the presenting part is engaged, a woman who was ambulatory should be placed on bed rest. Providers differ in their practices regarding ambulation for a woman with ruptured membranes when the fetus is of normal size, is in cephalic presentation, and is engaged. In this instance, there is little risk of cord prolapse, and ambulation may be permitted or encouraged. The healthcare facility policies and the woman's practitioner provide individual guidelines regarding activity.

Stages of Labor

Labor is divided into four stages:

- The first stage (*dilation*) begins with the onset of true labor contractions and ends with complete cervical effacement and dilation. The first stage has three phases (periods) of recognized achievement.
- The second stage (*expulsion*) begins with complete cervical dilation and effacement and ends with the birth of the newborn.
- The third stage (*placental*) begins with the newborn's delivery and ends with the placenta's delivery.
- The fourth stage (*recovery*) begins after delivery of the placenta and ends when the client's condition is stable (usually about 1 to 4 hours later).

The entire labor process lasts on average between 8 and 18 hours for the primigravida, and between 1 and 14 hours for the multigravida (Table 65-2).

☛ KEY CONCEPT

Effacement of the cervix is expressed in percentages. Full effacement is 100%. Dilation is expressed in centimeters, according to the diameter of the cervical opening. Complete dilation is 10 cm.

The First Stage of Labor (Dilation). In the first stage of labor, the uterine muscles contract to supply the pressure needed for cervical stretching and dilating. The breaking of the bag of waters accompanies this stage, which is divided into three phases: *latent, active,* and *transitional.* Tables 65-2 and 65-3 outline the particulars of each of these phases.

Two distinct cervical changes occur during the first stage of labor: effacement and dilation. **Effacement** refers to the thinning of the cervix. The cervix, normally long and thick

■■ **TABLE 65-2** *Lengths of Phases of Stages of Normal Labor in Hours*

Phase	Nullipara		Multipara	
	Average	Upper Normal	Average	Upper Normal
Latent phase	8.6	20.0	5.3	14.0
Active phase	5.8	12.0	2.5	6.0
Second stage	1	1.5	.25	1

■■■ **TABLE 65-3 $\mathscr{F}$IRST STAGE OF LABOR**

Phase	Frequency of Contractions	Duration of Contractions	Character and Intensity of Contractions	Cervical Dilation	Mother's Behavior
Latent	5–20 min	30–50 sec	Irregular, mild	0–4 cm	Follows directions, excited, talkative
Active	2–4 min	45–60 sec	Regular, moderate to strong	4–8 cm	Serious, apprehensive
Transitional	2–3 min	60–90 sec	Regular, very strong	8–10 cm	Difficulty following directions Frustrated, irritable

(approximately 1–2 cm in length), shortens or thins as a result of contractions. This thinning is measured in percentages. The higher the percentage, the thinner or shorter the cervix. Complete effacement is known as "100% effaced," which describes a cervix that has become almost paper-thin. In **dilation,** the cervical os (opening), normally held closed in a tight circle, begins to open. Dilation is measured in centimeters from 1 to 10. Complete dilation (10 cm or about 3.9 inches) is necessary to allow the uterus to expel the fetus. Cervical dilation is the result of uterine contractions.

Medical personnel are able to estimate the amount of dilation and effacement by feeling the cervix during a rectal or sterile vaginal examination. In a primigravida, effacement usually occurs first, then dilation. In a multigravida, effacement and dilation occur simultaneously.

The Second Stage of Labor (Expulsion). The second stage of labor begins with complete cervical effacement and dilation and ends with the expulsion of the fetus. It lasts about 1 to 2 hours for a primigravida. The second stage of labor for a multigravida usually lasts about 25 minutes, but can take up to 1 hour (about 10 to 15 contractions).

During this stage, the woman's abdominal muscles and diaphragm join the uterine muscles to push the newborn out of the woman's body. The woman may say she feels "pushing pains" or a "bearing down" feeling. The rectum dilates, the perineum bulges, and the top of the fetal head appears. This is known as **crowning.** An expulsive grunt from the woman as she exhales is a classic sign of the second stage.

The birth of the newborn in a normal presentation involves the birth of the head, with the face downward. The head then immediately rotates to one side. The shoulders are born, one at a time, and the rest of the newborn follows quickly. The birth of the body ends the second stage of labor. The cord is clamped in two places and cut between the clamps (Fig. 65-3).

The Third Stage of Labor (Placental). The third stage of labor extends from the time the newborn is delivered until the placenta and membranes are expelled. The placenta is attached to the uterine wall; after the newborn is delivered, the uterine muscles contract. With this contraction, the uterus becomes much smaller in size, and the placenta is sheared away from the wall and then expelled. The third stage of labor can last for up to 30 minutes, but usually takes only 5 to 15 minutes.

The placenta is delivered after the uterus contracts. With the contraction, the uterus rises into the abdomen and becomes round, or globular. As the placenta moves into the vagina, the umbilical cord lengthens, and there may be a sudden trickle or gush of blood. The birth attendant (or the nurse) keeps a hand firmly over the empty uterus until it feels firm and hard, indicating that the muscles and the blood vessels are contracted, and minimal danger of hemorrhage exists. If the placenta is expelled with the shiny (membranous) side out, it is called a Schultze presentation (it helps to remember this as "shiny Schultze"); this is the fetal side of the placenta. Schultze presentation occurs in approximately 80% of births. If it is expelled with the dull side out, it is called a Duncan presentation ("dirty Duncan"). This is the maternal side, which is rough and irregular. Excessive bleeding is more likely with this type of placental presentation.

The birth attendant examines the expelled placenta and membranes to determine if the placenta is intact. Retained placental fragments are a major cause of hemorrhage following delivery. The birth attendant also examines the cervix, vagina, and perineum, and then sutures the episiotomy, if performed, or any lacerations. Blood loss during a normal delivery is usually estimated to be 300 to 350 milliliters.

The Fourth Stage of Labor (Recovery). The fourth stage of labor includes the first 1 to 4 hours following the expulsion of the placenta. During this time, the woman's body begins the process of *involution,* as her reproductive organs begin to return to their normal pre-pregnant size. Total involution takes about 6 weeks. During the fourth stage of labor, the nurse must closely observe for signs of hemorrhage, urinary retention, hypotension, and undesirable side effects from anesthesia.

The other critical event of the fourth stage of labor is *bonding* (attachment) between the parents and infant. The more time that the mother, baby, and other family members spend together during this time, the better the chance of good parental–infant attachment. Bonding is important to the development of a solid relationship between the parents and infant (Fig. 65-4).

NURSING CARE DURING LABOR

Nursing Care During the First Stage of Labor

Maternal Comfort and Care

First-stage nursing care focuses on assessment of the woman's vital signs, contractions, and cervical change, as well as assessment of the fetus' well-being. These findings help the birth attendant to determine the fetus' condition and the woman's

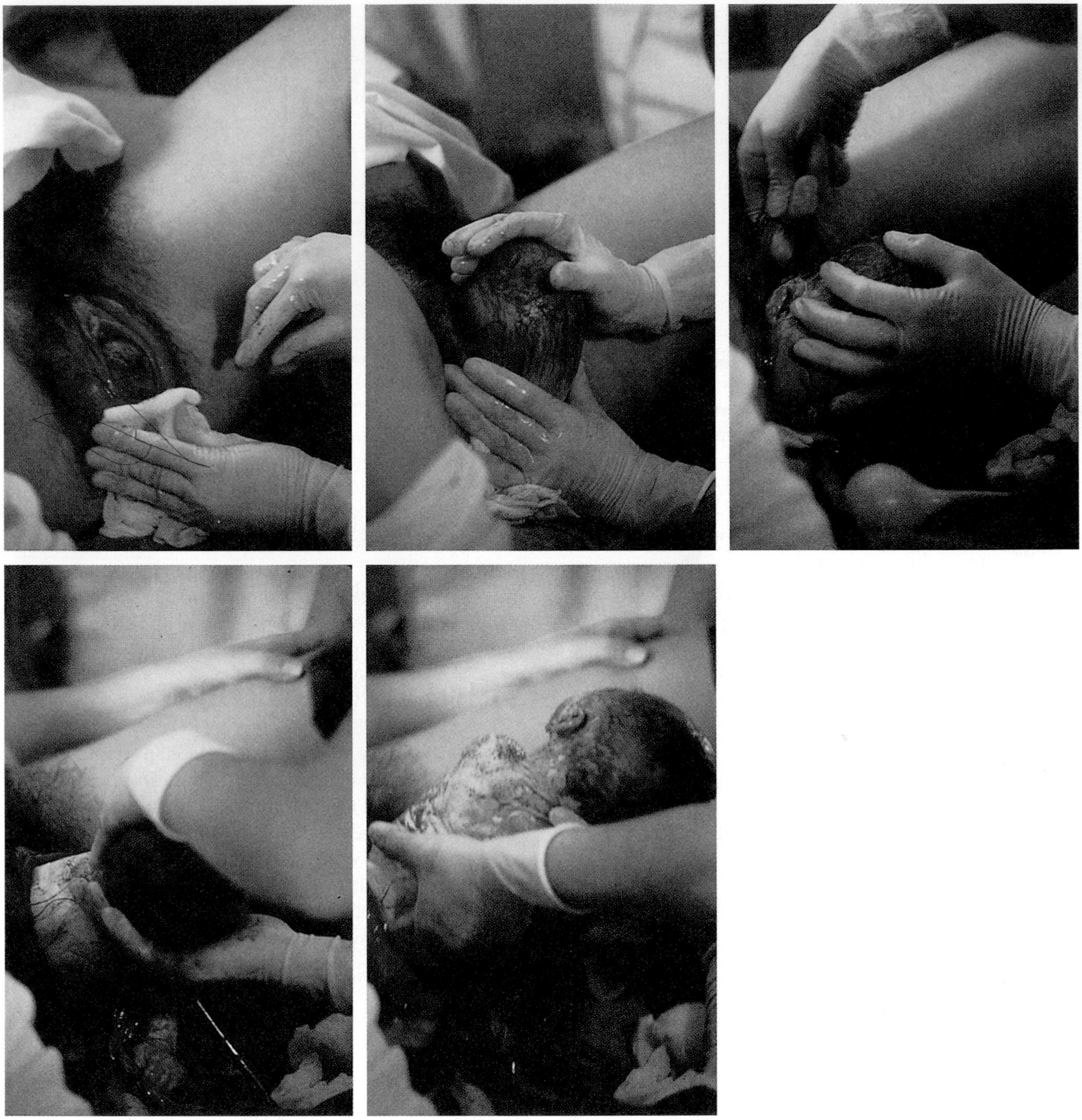

FIGURE 65-3. The normal birth process.

progress. The laboring woman and the fetus she carries need frequent monitoring during this stage to ensure the safety of both. Of equal importance is the role of the nurse in the physical and emotional support of the woman.

Admission.   Admission procedures for women in labor vary among healthcare facilities. The important elements of an admission history, however, are standard in all institutions. The admitting nurse asks about the estimated date of delivery (EDD) and confirms this by comparing the information obtained to the prenatal record, which may already be on file at the hospital or may be brought by the woman. If the

newborn is preterm, special precautions are taken, and special equipment is readied. The nurse also obtains the following information:

- When labor began
- How close the contractions are
- How long each contraction lasts
- Whether the client has noticed any bleeding
- Whether the bag of waters has ruptured

The anesthesiologist or Certified Registered Nurse Anesthetist (**CRNA**) will also want to know when the client last ate.

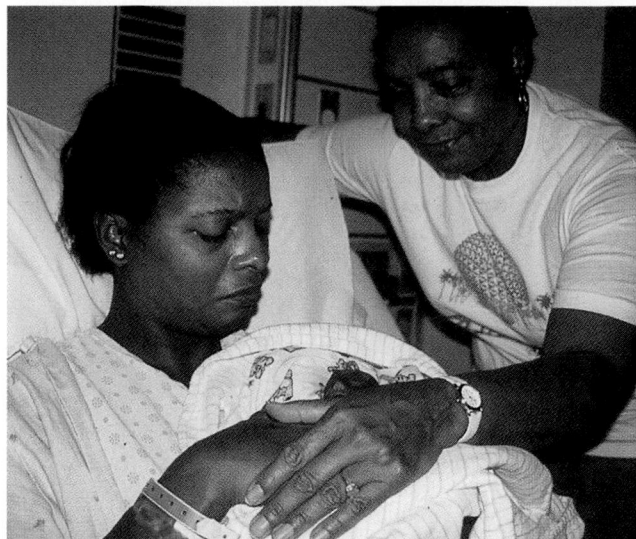

FIGURE 65-4. Bonding during the fourth stage of labor.

✚👁 N u r s i n g   A l e r t

Report any bright-red bleeding at once. *Rationale: A client who is bleeding should never be examined vaginally until ultrasound rules out placenta previa* (see Chap. 67).

Other routine procedures include assessing temperature, pulse, respirations, and blood pressure; urine dipstick testing for sugar and albumin; and blood tests for hemoglobin, hematocrit, and confirmation of the mother's blood type. Assessment of the fetal heart tones should first be done at the time of admission. The birth attendant may examine the woman's heart, lungs, and abdomen; and will also listen to the fetal heartbeat. In most facilities, an external fetal monitor is applied to the woman's abdomen to obtain a baseline fetal heart rate tracing. A sterile vaginal examination often determines how far labor has progressed.

✚👁 N u r s i n g   A l e r t

Be sure to ask the woman upon admission about allergies to povidone-iodine (Betadine), lidocaine (Xylocaine), any other drugs, and latex. *Rationale: Allergic reactions can range from uncomfortable to fatal.*

Remember to keep the woman and her partner informed of progress and to observe closely at all times for any signs of fetal distress. Box 65-1 lists danger signs in labor. You must report any of these signs to the team leader immediately.

Assessment.   Uterine contractions are one means of assessing progress. If the pregnancy is full-term, the uterine fundus (where the strongest muscular contractions can be felt) is located just below the xiphoid process of the sternum. Your hand should rest there lightly to best evaluate uterine contractions. As the uterus contracts, this portion of the abdomen becomes hard and rigid. When the uterus relaxes, you will be able to feel the softening of the uterine muscle beneath your

➤➤ BOX 65-1

DANGER SIGNS IN LABOR

- Sharp, unremitting pain
- Prolonged contractions or failure of the uterus to relax (rigid uterus after a contraction)
- Change in character of the fetal heartbeat; abnormal deceleration pattern on fetal monitor
- Maternal bleeding
- Extreme maternal exhaustion
- Cessation of labor after it has begun
- Hypotension or increased pulse rate of the mother
- Prolapse of the umbilical cord
- Irregular fetal heartbeat
- Passage of meconium-stained amniotic fluid when fetus is in vertex position
- Exaggerated movement of the fetus
- A pH value below 7.2 of fetal blood drawn from scalp veins (indicating fetal acidosis)

hand. You can also assess uterine contractions using external and internal monitors.

A sterile vaginal examination (**SVE**), usually performed by the midwife, obstetrician, or registered nurse, also assesses the labor's progress. In addition to the degree of cervical dilation and effacement, the examiner is able to determine the presenting part, station, size of the pelvic outlet, and status of the membranes.

Nursing students may assist by ensuring that the client is draped properly, and that the examiner has the needed supplies (sterile gloves, lubricant, and, if necessary, an amniohook).

Students should not be asked to perform SVEs. If, as a graduate, you are asked to perform an SVE, you must receive in-service instruction in the procedure from the healthcare facility first.

Emotional and Physical Support.   Nursing support during the first stage of labor is directed toward making the woman as comfortable as possible and encouraging her to do the things (such as breathing) that promote the normal progression of labor. Labor is exactly what it implies, hard work. In the past, women were encouraged to be passive during labor, to lie down and rest. More current thinking is that the woman should be an active participant in the labor process. By laboring in different positions, walking, or even showering during labor, the healthy woman is more likely to have a normal progression of her labor.

Carefully observe the client's physical state during labor and delivery. Measure and record her vital signs at least every 4 hours, and the fetal heart tones at regular intervals (see "Assessing Fetal Well-being" in the following section). Follow healthcare facility routines carefully.

Stay with the client and do everything possible to help her work with the contractions, and relax and rest between them. Encourage the father or support person to be as involved as the couple wishes. Remind the woman to breathe slowly and

SPECIAL CONSIDERATIONS: CULTURE

Activity During Labor

Traditional Puerto Rican women prefer being in bed for labor, while Haitian women may walk, pace, sit, squat, and rub their belly. Samoan women may be either active or passive, as they prefer. Many West Indian women continue with housework during the early stages of labor.

deeply and to use any techniques learned in childbirth preparation classes to relax her muscles and allow the contractions to do the work. Sponge the woman's face and hands occasionally, rub her back, offer her a sip of water or ice chips from time to time, change her gown or bedding if they become damp or soiled, and see that the air in the room is fresh.

Ensure that the client's bladder is empty. A full bladder prevents the fetal head from descending into the woman's pelvis and thereby slows labor's progress. A full bladder during labor may also result in trauma, urinary incontinence during delivery, or urinary retention in the immediate postpartum period, in which case catheterization may become necessary.

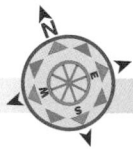

SPECIAL CONSIDERATIONS: CULTURE

Environmental Considerations

Filipino women may want noise and stimulation minimized for fear that too much commotion will increase labor pains.

Early labor is best spent out of the bed. The healthy woman may choose to walk, sit in a rocking chair, shower, and engage in diversionary activities such as card games or conversation. As the labor becomes more intense, she will concentrate more and more on the contractions, and may have little tolerance for suggestions that she earlier would have welcomed.

For those times when the woman is in bed, she might prefer to have the head of the bed elevated. If she does lie flat, however, she should lie on her left side, rather than on her back, to prevent hypotension, which results from compression of the aorta and vena cava by the weight of the uterus falling backward against the spine (see Fig. 64-6B in Chap. 64).

Some hospitals allow the woman to be ambulatory only as long as the bag of waters is intact; other hospitals allow a woman whose membranes have ruptured to be up and about if the fetal presenting part is well applied to the cervix. Be sure to know and follow the policies of your institution and the woman's birth attendant.

Water and clear fluids are usually allowed during the very early stages of labor. Some believe that solid foods may cause the woman to vomit, particularly if she is to have a general

anesthetic; others would prefer that the gastric acid be diluted by oral intake, even if a general anesthetic becomes necessary. It has become common practice in many hospitals to give intravenous (IV) solutions to maintain caloric and fluid intake, and to lessen exhaustion and dehydration. However, be aware that a full liter bag of 5% dextrose contains only about 125 calories, and if given at a slow infusion rate, will not be sufficient to prevent maternal exhaustion.

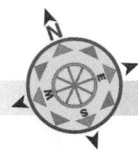

SPECIAL CONSIDERATIONS: CULTURE

Food and Drink During Labor

Offer Korean women lukewarm water only; no ice should be given, in order to maintain the balance between hot and cold. This balance is also seen as precarious during labor in Vietnamese women. Most South Asian women encourage light meals during labor.

Relief of Discomfort.   If the client desires, after labor is well established, she may be given medication to make her more comfortable and relaxed. The type of drug may vary with the locale, the physician, and the woman's condition. Analgesics reduce the discomforts of labor, sedatives promote rest, and tranquilizers relax the client. Sometimes a combination of two drugs is administered. Antiemetics may also be given for women who experience nausea or vomiting during labor.

✚👁 Nursing Alert
After consulting with her provider, a woman often makes a decision about when to use medication during labor. *Rationale: Medications may slow labor if given too early, or may cause the newborn to be lethargic if given too late.*

Many clients receive some form of anesthesia during labor and delivery. One of the most common methods of anesthesia is **epidural** anesthesia, also called the *lumbar epidural block*. A small catheter is inserted into the epidural space within the spinal column. The catheter is taped into place, and a test dose of the anesthetic drug is given. If no undesired side effects arise, the drug can be carefully administered through the catheter during labor and delivery—either intermittently or continuously—using a pump. Most women receive pain relief within 20 minutes. An anesthesiologist should monitor the administration of this type of anesthesia because serious side effects (such as maternal hypotension) can occur.

The woman receiving epidural anesthesia during labor should be positioned on her side, with her head slightly raised. If she lies on her back, a small firm pillow should be placed under her right hip so that the uterus tilts to the left. This measure will help prevent the compression of the woman's aorta and vena cava. Monitor the woman's blood pressure frequently (at least every 15 minutes). The fetal heart rate should be monitored either continuously with an electronic monitor, or frequently with a fetoscope. Disadvantages of delivery using epidural anesthesia include the blocking of the urge to push in the second stage of labor, and an increased chance of forceps delivery.

Other anesthetics can be injected into the spinal canal (*saddle block*), the caudal space (*caudal block*), or the pudendal nerve (*pudendal block*). Sometimes the local anesthetic is injected around the cervix (*cervical block*). Although the client is awake during delivery, she loses sensation in the anesthetized site. The following anesthetic agents are frequently used:

• Tetracaine hydrochloride (Pontocaine)
• Dibucaine hydrochloride (Nupercainal)
• Lidocaine hydrochloride (Dilocaine, Xylocaine)

General anesthesia is rarely used because the client receiving this type of anesthesia is asleep when the newborn arrives. Babies born this way may not breathe spontaneously and may be difficult to awaken. General anesthesia is used in emergencies only (such as an emergency cesarean delivery), due to the possibility of newborn central nervous system depression. In most cesarean deliveries, general anesthesia is not given until after the baby is delivered, with either spinal or epidural anesthesia used prior to that.

Each type of anesthesia has distinct advantages and disadvantages. The client's needs and wishes, and the availability of medications, dictate the form used. Many women view labor as a natural function, and desire to deliver with little or no medication.

Nursing Alert

For the woman receiving anesthesia, report the following findings *immediately:*

• Inability to move the legs
• Numbness in the legs
• Ringing in the ears
• Dizziness
• Metallic taste
• Hypotension or seizures

Rationale: These serious side effects of anesthesia can be fatal to the woman and/or the fetus.

Assessing Fetal Well-being

The well-being of the fetus is of utmost concern during the course of labor. The best indicator of fetal health is the fetal heart rate (**FHR**). The normal FHR is 120 to 160 beats per minute (BPM).

The frequency with which the FHR is evaluated should depend on the absence or presence of risk factors. FHR evaluation may be done using a fetoscope to perform intermittent auscultation, or an electronic monitor may be used for continuous monitoring or periodic test strips. Electronic monitors can be used externally or internally. To permit internal electronic monitoring, the membranes must be ruptured.

Intermittent Auscultation. When there are no risk factors for problems with the mother or the fetus, the stan-

dard practice is to evaluate and record the FHR at least every 30 minutes during the first stage, and at least every 15 minutes during the second stage of labor. When risk factors are present, the FHR should be evaluated at least every 15 minutes during the first stage, and every 5 minutes during the second stage of labor.

☛ Key Concept

The most important factor in fetal monitoring is the relationship *between the fetal heart rate and the contractions of the uterus.*

Electronic Fetal Monitoring. Continuous electronic monitoring of the FHR during labor is routine in many facilities. The purpose of the **fetal monitor** is to record the rate and quality of the fetal heartbeat during contraction and relaxation. It can give an early warning of fetal distress, so that corrective measures can be started immediately. See In Practice: Nursing Procedure 65-1 for information on applying the external monitor. An electronic fetal monitor is usually used in the following situations:

• If the fetus seems to be in distress
• If the delivery is being induced
• If the woman has a chronic health problem
• If a complication of pregnancy exists

External monitoring of the FHT is most commonly used. This approach is based on the Doppler effect, in which high-frequency ultrasound waves directed to the fetal heart bounce back to a transducer strapped onto the woman's abdomen. The receiver amplifies the fetal heart sounds. The signal is converted to sound and is printed on electrocardiograph paper. In addition, a pressure-sensitive device, called a **tocodynamometer,** is used to monitor the frequency of contractions. When placed directly over the woman's fundus, the device transfers an electrical impulse to the monitor, creating a readout. The tocodynamometer does not give information about the strength of uterine contractions. The relationship between the fetal heartbeat and uterine contractions can be studied because the information is printed simultaneously.

Advantages of external monitoring include the fact that it is noninvasive, has no contraindications, and is easy to apply. Disadvantages include the need for frequent adjustments and its sensitivity to fetal and maternal movements.

If the external monitor's printout signals a fetal or maternal problem, an internal or direct monitor is used because it is more accurate. An electrode, such as the *scalp clip* or *spiral,* is passed through the woman's dilated cervix and carefully attached directly to the presenting part of the fetus. The internal monitor can provide precise information, including a fetal electrocardiogram. The external sensor may still be used to measure the frequency and length of uterine contractions, or a catheter (*intrauterine pressure catheter*) may be inserted into the uterus so that the intensity of contractions may also be measured.

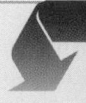

In Practice
Nursing Procedure 65-1

APPLICATION OF EXTERNAL MONITOR

Supplies and Equipment:

Fetal monitor and paper
Ultrasound transducer
Tocodynamometer
Two straps
Conductive jelly

Steps

1. Explain procedure to mother and support person.
   RATIONALE: *Explanation allays fears, gains cooperation, and promotes compliance.*

2. Elevate head of bed 15–30 degrees, or place client in lateral position.
   RATIONALE: *Elevation and uterine displacement decrease aorta and vena caval compression.*

3. Perform Leopold's maneuvers and place two straps under client.
   RATIONALE: *This locates fetal position and best placement of Doppler.*

4. Apply conductive jelly to Doppler, and place on client's abdomen until strong FHR is heard and consistent signal is obtained.
   RATIONALE: *The jelly helps locate the area of maximum FHR signal.*

5. Attach straps to Doppler and secure.
   RATIONALE: *Straps should be snug but not tight.*

6. Push recorder button if not already on.
   RATIONALE: *Machine will not record data if machine is off.*

7. Place tocodynamometer on abdomen between umbilicus and top of fundus.

RATIONALE: *Fundus is the contractile portion of the uterus; care must be taken to avoid placing toco too high on fundus; respirations will record on monitor.*

8. Attach straps to tocodynamometer and secure.
   RATIONALE: *Straps should be snug but not tight; if too tight, pressure-sensitive button will not record data.*

9. Adjust sound and equipment as needed, particularly when a procedure is performed or client's position is changed.
   RATIONALE: *Monitor is sensitive to change or disturbance to equipment.*

10. Review FHR and UA data with client and family. Use thorough descriptions of data.
    RATIONALE: *This review promotes understanding of what client and family will be observing on the monitor.*

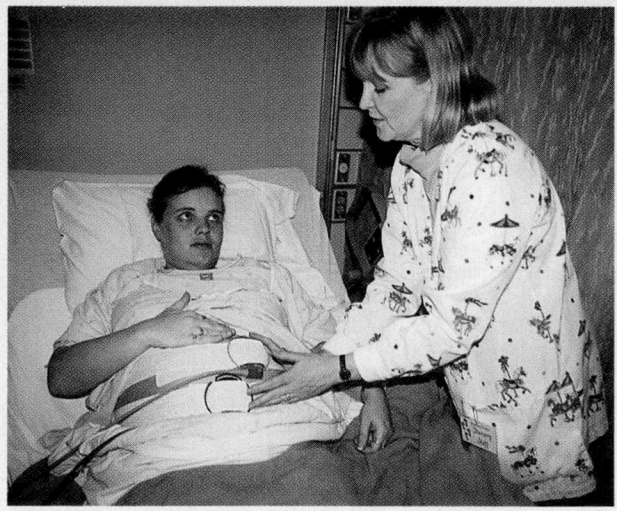

Client being monitored with external transducers secured to her abdomen.

Source: Pillitteri, A. (1999) *Maternal and child health nursing: care of the childbearing & childrearing family.* (3rd ed., p. 1102). Philadelphia: Lippincott Williams & Wilkins.

The advantages of internal monitoring include a high-quality tracing and fewer *artifacts* (interference from other sources) than external monitoring. The disadvantages are that membranes must be ruptured, the cervix must be dilated, and the presenting part must be accessible.

Evaluation of Fetal Monitor Information. As a nursing student or licensed practical/vocational nurse, you most likely will not be responsible for the interpretation of electronic fetal monitoring. However, you should understand basic theory and terminology. Notify the team leader immediately if any signs of fetal distress appear on the fetal monitor, such as:

- *Accelerations:* Accelerations are brief increases of the FHR of 15 BPM or more. It is a sign of a healthy fetus for the FHR to accelerate after movement or stimulation. Any acceleration of 60 BPM or more is considered a complication, and the fetus may be in danger.

- *Decelerations:* Decelerations (slowing) of the FHR are categorized according to when they occur in relation to a contraction. Some decelerations are expected; others are warning signs of possible problems. An *early deceleration* begins early in the contraction, hits its low point at the peak of the contraction, and returns to baseline at the end of the contraction; it mirrors the contraction pattern. Early decelerations are due to vagal nerve stimulation, resulting from pressure on the fetal head, and are considered a normal response of the fetus to labor. A *late deceleration* begins as the contraction eases, and lasts longer than the contraction—into the resting phase of the uterus. This is a sign of a possible problem, and should be reported to your team leader.

- *Decreased variability:* Little to no fluctuation in the FHR on an internal electronic monitor tracing is a danger sign, and may indicate an abnormality in the fetal nervous system. It might also indicate that the mother has taken or been given central nervous system depressants. Report this observation to the team leader for further evaluation.

✚👁 Nursing Alert

Variable decelerations in fetal heart rate occur anytime during or after contractions. They usually indicate umbilical cord compression, and can usually be altered by changing the woman's position or by giving her oxygen. *Late decelerations* begin late in the contraction, and the fetal heart rate recovery occurs after the contraction is over. Decelerations are related to placental insufficiency and indicate fetal distress. The fetal heart rate should not fall below 100 bpm.

Nursing Care During the Second Stage of Labor

Maternal Care

Either an LPN/LVN or RN will assist in delivery. If you are assigned to assist during the birth, you most likely will help with the transfer to the delivery room (that is, in a traditional labor and delivery suite), and then stand at the woman's side, instructing her on how to breathe and when to push, and informing her of what is occurring. If you are assisting the birth attendant, you may be responsible for handing him or her necessary equipment, medications, and other items. If you are caring for the newborn, you will need to make sure that the infant is breathing and is kept warm. You also will perform other routine procedures for the newborn, as described in Chapter 66.

Aseptic conditions must be maintained during delivery. You and any of the woman's support people will wear a clean scrub suit, a cap to cover your hair, and a mask.

If the client is going to deliver in a hospital delivery room, she is transferred on her bed and moved over to the delivery table, with the assistance of the circulating nurse. The table, which is split across the middle, is opened (broken), and the woman's buttocks are positioned at the break in the table. Her feet are placed in stirrups simultaneously to prevent strain on

the pelvic ligaments. Perineal preparation is done to cleanse the skin and to remove secretions from the genitalia. (Shaving is rarely done today.) In some cases, a *birthing chair* or *squat bar* is used.

Coaching the Client.   In the second stage of labor, the woman actively helps the birth process. As each contraction begins, she takes a deep breath and holds it, and then pushes with each contraction. Women often make grunting noises during pushing. If the woman relaxes between contractions, she can work better when the next contraction comes. Encourage the woman to push only with contractions, and to rest between them.

If a woman tells you the baby is coming, you should trust her judgment. Get assistance immediately, and check for crowning. If a delivery occurs suddenly, without advance warning and aseptic preparation, it is called a *precipitous delivery* (this is different from a *precipitous labor,* in which fewer than 3 hours elapse from the onset of labor to birth). A client may "precipitate" in the labor room bed, if her claim that birth is imminent is ignored. Encourage the mother to pant or blow forcefully when told not to push. Remember that only one person should give the woman instructions: during this challenging experience, too many different voices and directions can be overwhelming.

Episiotomy.   Often the birth attendant makes an incision in the perineum, called an **episiotomy,** which enlarges the vaginal opening and allows an easier delivery of the fetus. Some birth attendants believe that episiotomy helps to preserve the structure and strength of the perineal muscles and prevents a jagged laceration or a tear extending to the anus. Other birth attendants believe that a laceration, should one occur, will be less extensive than the episiotomy. Extensive lacerations are difficult to repair and could leave permanent damage.

Note the type of episiotomy (midline, or right or left mediolateral), as well as any lacerations that occurred, on the woman's chart (Fig. 65-5).

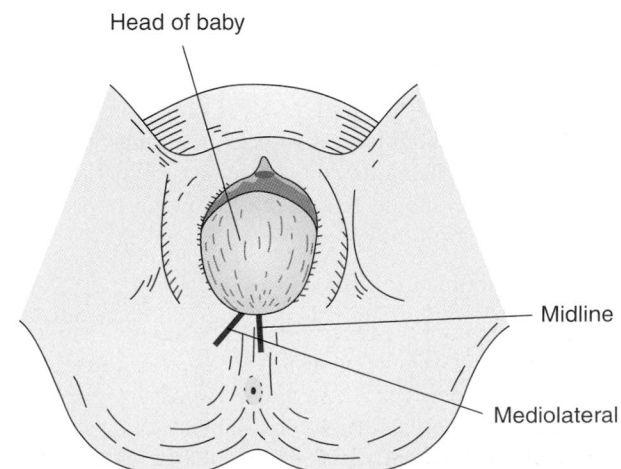

FIGURE 65-5. Position of episiotomy incision in a woman during the second stage of labor. The baby's head is presenting to the vaginal outlet (*crowning*).

Neonatal Care

After the baby's head is delivered, the birth attendant will check for any loops of cord that have become wrapped around the infant's neck (**nuchal cord**) and remove them. Next, he or she will suction the nose and mouth of the newborn with a bulb syringe. The anterior shoulder is delivered, then the posterior shoulder and the remainder of the body. The newborn cries out, and the lungs expand. The time of delivery of the baby should be noted for legal records. This entire portion of the delivery often takes only a few seconds.

The baby may be handed to the mother immediately, before the umbilical cord is clamped. Assist the mother in placing the baby on the bare skin of her chest. Dry the baby, remove any damp towels or sheets, and cover the baby with a clean, dry cloth. Most babies calm quickly after experiencing the warmth of the mother and the security of her embracing arms. You should observe for the infant's breathing pattern and suction the mouth if needed.

When the umbilical cord stops pulsating, two Kelly clamps are applied to it, and the birth attendant or baby's father cuts the cord between them. An umbilical clamp is later applied near the baby's abdomen. Make certain it is attached securely, but does not pinch any folds of skin.

Some hospitals and birth attendants prefer that the infant be stabilized first in a radiant warmer. After the newborn is stable, the parents may hold the infant. However, healthcare personnel are responsible for the newborn's care. Newborns must be kept warm, yet parents should have time to hold and to bond with them. Overhead warmers allow you to observe the newborn.

Observations of the newborn include assessment of the Apgar score at 1 and 5 minutes of life. Details of initial assessment of the newborn are addressed in Chapter 66.

For each delivery, a staff person skilled in neonatal resuscitation should be available to provide resuscitation if needed. If the infant is depressed or not fully responsive to stimulation, the neonatal resuscitation expert should be called immediately. Every minute is critical; never delay summoning help in the hopes that the baby's condition will improve.

Nursing Care During the Third Stage of Labor

The third stage of labor is relatively short, but may be a dangerous period for the mother due to the possibility of hemorrhage. The nurse should record the following information about the delivery of the placenta:

- The exact time the placenta was delivered
- Whether the placenta was delivered spontaneously or removed manually
- Which side of the placenta presented

Following delivery of the placenta, administering an oxytocic medication may be necessary to assist the uterus to contract, and to minimize the risk of bleeding. You may be instructed to administer these oxytocics or to gently massage the fundus to minimize blood loss.

After the birth attendant has examined the cervix and vagina and sutured the episiotomy or lacerations, the vulva and perineum should be cleansed. If stirrups were used, remove the mother's legs from them.

☛ Key Concept

Bring the mother's legs down from the stirrups slowly and together. Rationale: *Doing so helps to avoid further trauma and discomfort.*

Change the woman's gown, apply perineal pads, and cover her with a warm blanket. Some healthcare facilities transfer women to a recovery room; in others, women recover in the room where they deliver.

Before the woman leaves the delivery or birthing room, complete the necessary documentation. Box 65-2 lists information required for the health record.

Nursing Care During the Fourth Stage of Labor

Following delivery, the woman might feel chilled and shake uncontrollably, possibly in response to a cool room, sudden hormonal shifts, or the sudden change in intra-abdominal pressure after the fetus and placenta are expelled. Be sure she has several warm blankets available if needed.

Many healthcare facilities have a recovery room where the mother and newborn are taken after delivery and where the mother and father can fondle and care for their newborn during the first hours. In some facilities, the newborn is first taken to the nursery for an initial admission examination, and then the newborn is returned to the recovery room. Others admit the newborn when the mother arrives in the postpartum area.

Immediately following delivery, the woman may experience extreme fatigue, close to exhaustion, just as she would after any extremely vigorous physical activity or hard work. At

➤➤ BOX 65-2

NECESSARY DOCUMENTATION FOR DELIVERY

- Complete information about the type of delivery and procedures used; who was present
- Sex and condition of the baby (include Apgar score)
- Time of birth
- Time at which the placenta was expelled, and presentation; indicate manual removal or spontaneous delivery
- Condition of the fundus
- Any medication administered
- If an episiotomy was done, and type
- Condition and vital signs of the mother
- Measured maternal blood loss
- Any other events (maternal incontinence, infant resuscitation, perineal tears, etc.)

the same time, she is usually relieved and excited. She is usually interested in seeing and holding her newborn and having a visit with her partner. The bonding between parents and newborn should be encouraged immediately. Allow time for the family to be together as soon as possible. If both mother and infant are stable, you should provide the family with privacy during this time.

Observe the mother closely for several hours after delivery for signs of complications. In addition, document any maternal complaints.

Assessment

Check the mother's blood pressure and pulse at least every 15 minutes for the first 1 or 2 hours or until it is stable, and then every half hour for 1 hour or longer. Usually after the first 12 hours, you will check vital signs every 4 hours for 12 hours and then every 8 hours if no difficulties arise.

When taking vital signs, also check the fundus of the uterus and the perineum. The reason for keeping a close check on the fundus is to ensure that it remains firm and contracted. If it becomes soft and boggy, hemorrhage could occur. Teach the mother to assess her own uterine fundus. If nursing measures are not effective, the physician may order administration of an IV or IM oxytocic drug. Common oxytocic drugs are oxytocin (Pitocin; see In Practice: Important Medications 65-1) and ergonovine maleate (Ergotrate; see In Practice: Important Medications 65-2).

A rising fundus may indicate uterine hemorrhage. If the fundus does not become firm with massage, report this finding immediately. A fundus located to the right of the midline often indicates a full bladder. Voiding will usually return the fundus to its earlier location. If this does not occur, notify the team leader. Check the perineum to make sure the stitches are intact. Be sure no excessive bleeding, edema, or bruising is found.

Lochia is the vaginal discharge that occurs following delivery. It consists of blood and the tissues of the uterine lining as it breaks down. Immediately following delivery, lochia is bloody and should be moderate in amount. While wearing gloves, check lochia during the immediate postpartum period. Assess the amount, character, and color. The next section describes normal lochia changes. The amount is described as scant, light, moderate, or heavy; it should have a fleshy or metallic, never foul, odor (Fig. 65-6).

Observe and record the woman's first voiding after delivery. Failure to void may indicate swelling or injury to the urinary system. Report if the woman feels the urge to void but is unable to do so, or if the fundus shifts to one side. If she is unable to void within 6 to 8 hours after delivery, catheterization may be necessary.

Maternal and Newborn Feeding

The new mother may be thirsty and hungry after delivery. Encourage her to drink fluids to replace those lost during labor and delivery; she can have solid foods as tolerated.

If the mother plans to breastfeed, encourage her to put the newborn to her breast in the delivery or recovery room. The newborn usually is alert at this time, and the stimulation of

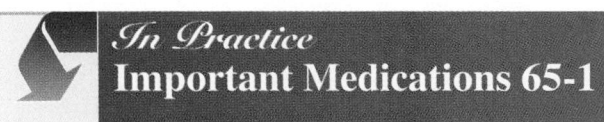

In Practice
Important Medications 65-1

OXYTOCIN (PITOCIN)

Dose
  Labor induction: Initial dose of 1–2 mU; increased 1–2 mU/min until an adequate labor pattern is achieved; maximum recommended dose is 20 mU/min
  Labor augmentation: Initial dose: 0.5–1.0 mU; increased 1–2 mU/min until an adequate labor pattern is achieved; maximum recommended dose is 20 mU/min
  Postpartum: 10–20 mU IM or IV after delivery of the placenta
Expected effect: Used to initiate (induce) labor or augment labor contractions that are weak or ineffective; also used after the delivery of the placenta to contract the uterus
Adverse side effects
  Mother: Unpredictable individual response; hypertonic uterine contractions; tetanic uterine contractions; cervical and vaginal lacerations; amniotic fluid embolism; water intoxication
  Fetus: Fetal distress, birth injury

Nursing Considerations
- *Contraindications to use:* Any obstruction that would interfere with the descent of the fetus; hypertonic or uncoordinated uterine contractions; fetal distress; any contraindication for vaginal birth
- Amount and rate of administration must be carefully controlled; this can be done effectively only by use of the IV route, using an infusion pump.
- Type of solution, amount of oxytocin added, and rate of infusion vary according to agency protocols or physician preference.
- Evaluate fetal heart rate every 15 min when given during labor.
- To prevent water intoxication, give in electrolyte solution, avoid infusing high volumes of fluid, and avoid using high doses of oxytocin for prolonged periods.

the breast encourages the secretion of natural oxytocin to contract the uterus.

Transfer From the Recovery Room

The mother remains in the recovery room, or is closely observed in the birthing room, long enough to ensure that her condition is satisfactory (usually for 1 to 2 hours). When her condition is stable, she is transferred to a postpartum room if she delivered elsewhere.

Record complete information about the delivery and other procedures on the woman's health record before she is moved. Check the charting from the delivery room and the recovery room to make sure that the record is complete. Transfer this documentation with the woman (see Boxes 65-2 and 65-3).

Postpartum Care

Postpartum refers to the first 6 weeks following delivery, the time during which the woman's reproductive organs return to their normal, nonpregnant state. The general care of the postpartum client is similar to that of other clients. Observe the woman's overall state, appetite, activity, patterns of sleep and rest, and interactions with her newborn. Note the client's vital signs. Particular considerations during the postpartum period are described in this section.

Postpartum women are usually discharged from the hospital within a day or two. Client teaching on all aspects of postpartum care, and documentation of this teaching, are vital. The new mother must know what to expect as her body undergoes the rapid changes of the postpartum period, and when to call her practitioner for assistance.

Important Changes in Maternal Anatomy and Physiology

The process by which the reproductive organs return to their nonpregnant state is called **involution.** To provide competent and safe nursing care to the postpartum client, you must understand the physiologic changes that occur following childbirth.

Uterus.   Immediately after delivery, the uterus weighs approximately 2 pounds (900 g) and is about the size of a grapefruit. It can be felt at the level of, or slightly below, the umbilicus. After delivery, it begins to return to its normal position and smaller size. When this process is complete, the uterus will weigh about 2 ounces (50 g) and will be low, at or near the center of the pelvic cavity.

During the postpartum period, the uterus should be positioned midline and feel firm to the touch. The height of the fundus indicates the progress of involution. By palpating the abdomen, the fundus can be located; measure its height in finger widths above or below the umbilicus. Normal involution is occurring when the fundus descends one finger width each day. Record the fundal height as indicated in Box 65-3.

Abnormal findings include:

- If the uterus is deviated to the side, suspect a distended bladder. Increased bladder size will prevent the uterus

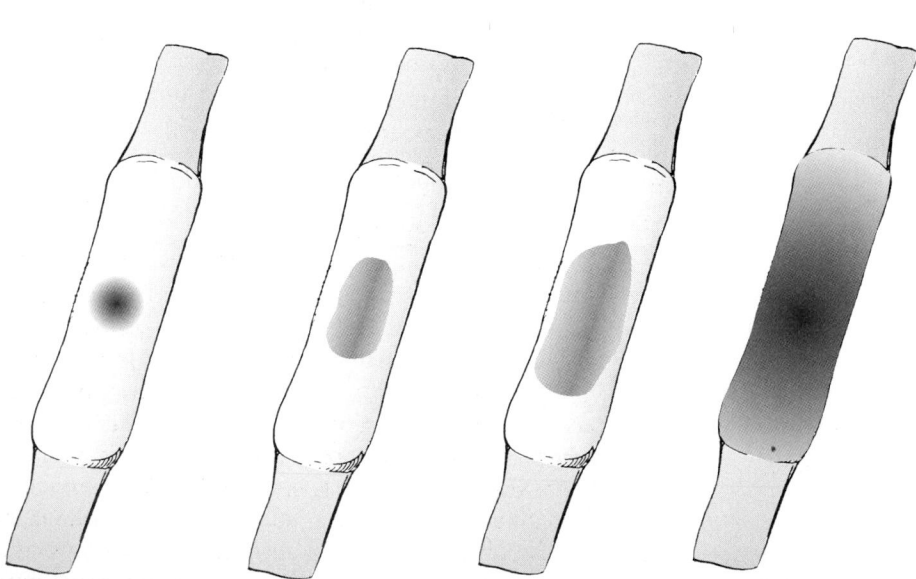

Scant amount
Blood only on tissue when wiped or less than 1-inch stain on peripad.

Light amount
Less than 4-inch stain on peripad.

Moderate amount
Less than 6-inch stain on peripad.

Heavy amount
Saturated peripad within 1 hour.

FIGURE 65-6. Assessing the volume of lochia by peripad saturation.

➤➤ BOX 65-3

NECESSARY DOCUMENTATION REGARDING THE POSTPARTUM WOMAN

Assessment of the fundus:

- Firmness (*consistency*)—firm, boggy (and result of massage)
- At center or deviated (*location*)
- Height (*position*)

Height of the fundus. One possible way of documenting fundal position is shown below:

2/U = 2 finger widths over umbilicus
1/U = 1 finger width over umbilicus
UU = fundus at level of umbilicus
U/1 = 1 finger width below umbilicus
U/2 = 2 finger widths below umbilicus

Lochia:

- Rubra, serosa, alba (*character*)
- Excessive, moderate, scant (*amount*)
- Odor

---

from contracting, and will contribute to excessive bleeding. The uterus should contract after the client voids.

- A soft or boggy uterus indicates relaxation of the uterine muscles, and is also a danger sign.

Lochia. Normally the flow of lochia continues for 3 to 4 weeks, with the following gradual changes:

Lochia rubra is seen for the first 2 days. It is mostly red and bloody. It should smell like blood (slightly metallic); a foul odor indicates infection.

Lochia serosa starts after the bleeding diminishes. The color of the lochia changes to pink or brown-tinged for approximately the next 7 days. Lochia serosa has a slightly earthy odor.

Lochia alba, which is yellow or white, starts on about day 10. At this point, the lochia has decreased greatly in amount. Lochia alba also has an earthy smell.

The amount of lochia after delivery should be about the same as the blood flow during normal menstruation. Abnormal findings include:

- Large clots
- Foul odor
- Lochia that does not change color and characteristics as described

Record the amount, color, and any other characteristics that may be significant. Teach the client to report abnormal lochia.

Cervix and Vagina. The cervix is soft and edematous following delivery. It constricts and firms during the postpartum period. The vagina, too, regains muscle tone, and lacerations and episiotomies heal. The vagina and vulva lose their congested, purplish color and return to their pre-pregnant pinkish hue.

You will not be able to assess cervical and vaginal changes; doing so requires a sterile pelvic examination.

Episiotomy and Perineum. The client should turn on her side to facilitate a better view of the perineal area. If the client has had an episiotomy or lacerations, examine the area carefully to assess the healing process.

Make certain the perineum is intact. You may need a flashlight; the mother will need a mirror. The episiotomy and any lacerations should appear clean, with very slight edema. The sutures should not be pulling against the tissue. Note any hemorrhoids to initiate measures to alleviate them.

Abnormal findings include:

- Inflammation, redness, and discharge from the episiotomy or lacerations
- Hematomas, ecchymosis, and edema

If the client is unable to ambulate, administer perineal care. Apply a fresh perineal pad, usually to the panties, and pull the panties straight up. If using tabbed pads, attach the front first.

Abdominal Wall and Weight Loss. The woman's abdominal wall often remains soft and flabby for several weeks following childbirth, due to extensive stretching of the tissue and loss of muscle tone. By approximately 6 weeks after delivery, the woman should regain muscle tone. The new mother can begin an exercise program gradually as the birth attendant recommends. The length of time it takes for a client to regain her figure depends on the amount of weight she gained during the pregnancy, the amount of weight she lost during the delivery, the amount of exercise she has after delivery, her diet and eating patterns, and whether or not she is breastfeeding. Body weight decreases by approximately 12 to 15 pounds (5,440 to 6,800 g) at delivery and by about 5 pounds (2,270 g) during the next few days due to loss of excess body fluid.

Breasts. Changes in the breasts following childbirth prepare for the newborn's nourishment. During the last half of pregnancy and the first few days postpartum, the breasts produce **colostrum,** a thin yellowish secretion that provides vitamins and immune substances that protect the newborn against infection. On about the second or third day postpartum, the breasts begin to secrete milk.

Each time a newborn is put to breast, milk is secreted. **Lactation,** the production of milk, occurs due to the release of two hormones: prolactin and oxytocin. As the newborn sucks the nipple, a reflex reaction occurs whereby the posterior pituitary gland releases oxytocin, which stimulates cells to produce milk and to move it to the milk ducts. The oxytocic hormone also results in uterine contractions, and mothers often experience abdominal cramping while breastfeeding. This entire process is commonly known as the "let-down reflex"; the milk is said to "let down" or "come in." Because the risks outweigh the benefits, medications to suppress lactation are rarely given to non-breastfeeding mothers.

For the first few days, the breasts should be soft. The nipples should be intact, without drying, cracking, or fissures. When the milk comes in, the breasts will feel full and firm to touch.

Abnormal breast findings are listed below:

- **Engorgement** is the response of the breasts to the presence of an increased volume of milk and a sudden change in hormones. It usually occurs on the third to fifth day postpartum. The breasts become tender, swollen, hot, and hard. The swelling may extend into the axilla. The breasts may look shiny and red. The woman may experience a headache, breast discomfort, and a slight temperature elevation at this time. See In Practice: Educating the Client 65-2 for measures to help relieve engorgement.

Bladder. Pregnancy and labor place added strains on a woman's urinary system. The abdominal muscles may be weakened. In addition, bruising and swelling of the urethra and general loss of muscle tone are common. The involution process places an increased demand on the kidneys and bladder, as the mother's fluid balance is restored. Because of these factors, new mothers may have stress incontinence or difficulty voiding.

Palpate the bladder for a rounded bulge in the suprapubic region, which indicates distention. By questioning the client regarding voiding, you can gain information related to urinary symptoms.

Abnormal urinary system findings include:

- Voiding in small amounts
- Residual urine
- Dysuria
- Bladder infection
- Urinary retention

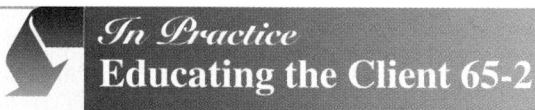

In Practice
Educating the Client 65-2

ENGORGEMENT

The following measures help to relieve the nursing mother's engorgement:

- Wearing a supportive bra
- Frequent breastfeeding
- Applying warm packs to the breast for 15 min prior to nursing. An alternative is to stand in the shower with warm water spraying on the breast for 15 min prior to nursing.

The following measures can help to relieve the non-nursing mother's engorgement:

- Wearing a supportive bra
- Avoiding excessive fluid intake
- Placing cold packs on her breasts three to four times per day
- Avoiding stimulation (eg, hot shower spray)
- Avoiding manual expression or pumping her breasts
- Using medications (usually acetaminophen) as prescribed for discomfort

Gastrointestinal System. The mother may be constipated for 1 to 2 weeks following delivery because the abdominal muscles have been stretched, and the intestines have been inactive.

Whether or not the mother had hemorrhoids during pregnancy, she may have problems with them after the birth.

Extremities. To check for thrombophlebitis, the client's legs should be exposed. Ask the client to straighten her legs on the surface of the bed and to flex her feet toward her face.

Abnormal findings in the legs include:

- Redness, pain, and swelling along the path of a vein may indicate a superficial thrombophlebitis.
- Pain behind the knee on flexion of the feet indicates a positive Homans' sign and suggests thrombophlebitis.

Postpartum Nursing Assessment

To prepare the client for the postpartum assessment, ask her to empty her bladder and then lie flat in bed. Always follow Standard Precautions when contact with body secretions is possible. Teach the woman to check herself frequently.

Measure and record the client's vital signs (see In Practice: Nursing Assessment 65-1). Ask her about any problems she may be having with her breasts, bleeding (lochia), sutures, cramping, constipation, or hemorrhoids.

Begin the postpartum assessment with the fundus. Palpate the fundus. If it is boggy, perform fundal massage. Never massage a contracted fundus. If the boggy uterus does not become firm with massage, notify the team leader. See In Practice: Nursing Procedure 65-2 for instructions on performing a fundal massage.

Observe the amount, color, and odor of the lochia. If large clots are expressed with fundal massage, notify the team leader. For the first few days after delivery, the mother may have painful cramps as the uterine muscles contract. These cramps are called **after-pains** and are more likely to occur in multigravidas. Breastfeeding stimulates uterine contractions, and therefore often brings on the cramping. An analgesic may be ordered as needed for these pains. Heat application is sometimes helpful.

Observe the episiotomy or lacerations for healing. Provide perineal care; change the sanitary pad. While tucking it in at the back, ask the woman to roll onto her left side. Lift the right buttocks and examine the anus for hemorrhoids. Ice packs, witch-hazel pads (Tucks), suppositories, creams, ointments, or sitz baths may be necessary for hemorrhoids.

Wash your hands, and then examine the breasts. Observe the breasts for tightness and redness, and palpate for fullness and temperature. Observe the nipples for drying, cracking, or fissures. Teach the mother to examine the nipples to determine that they are in good condition, and to observe them for cracking, caking, dryness, or bleeding. If the mother is breastfeeding, observe whether her nipples protrude sufficiently for adequate nursing. She can palpate the breasts gently to determine if they are soft, firm, or engorged.

Engorgement in the nursing mother generally subsides within 48 hours if the mother feeds her infant from both breasts every 2 to 3 hours, alternating the breast that she uses

In Practice
Nursing Assessment 65-1

OVERVIEW OF THE NURSING PROCESS DURING THE POSTPARTUM PERIOD

Assessment Priorities
Immediate Postpartum Care
- Check BP and pulse q15 min × 1–2 h or until stable; then q30 min × 1 h; then q4h × 12 h or as ordered.
- Check uterine fundus, lochia, and episiotomy at the same time as BP and pulse.
- Check for any signs of hemorrhage (check the perineal pad, and be alert to the possible pooling of blood under the client).
- First voiding
- Bonding with infant

General Postpartum Care
- After the first 12 h, check vital signs q4 h × 12 h and then q8h.
- Check breasts, fundus of the uterus, lochia, stitches (if present), and legs (for signs of thrombosis) at least once every shift. (Memory aid: BUBBLLEE—breast, uterus, bladder, bowels, legs, lochia, elimination, episiotomy)
- Check voidings and bowel elimination
- Adequacy of self-care behaviors: breast care, perineal care, response to discomforts
- Quality of maternal–newborn bonding and family dynamics
- Adequacy of parenting skills
- Knowledge of what to expect after discharge

Possible Nursing Diagnoses
Impaired Adjustment
Anxiety
Body Image Disturbance
Ineffective Breastfeeding
Decisional Conflict (specify)
Constipation
Ineffective Individual Coping
Altered Family Processes
Anticipatory Grieving
High Risk for Infection
Knowledge Deficit (specify)
Pain
High Risk for Altered Parenting
Personal Identity Disturbance
Altered Role Performance
Self-Care Deficit
Self-Esteem Disturbance
Altered Peripheral Tissue Perfusion
High Risk for Fluid Volume Deficit

Planning
Design a plan of care with the family to achieve the following goals. The mother's body demonstrates the beginning of a return to a normal, nonpregnant state when:

- Fundus remains firm and contracted and moves downward
- Lochia progresses on schedule from lochia rubra to lochia alba
- Breasts
  In the Breastfeeding Mother
  - The breasts begin to produce milk by the third or fourth day
  - The breasts are not engorged
  In the Non-nursing Mother
  - Breast engorgement does not last more than 2 or 3 d.
- Mother demonstrates correct perineal care.
- Incision (episiotomy or cesarean incision, if present) appears to be healing.
- Elimination patterns (urinary and bowel) return to normal, prepregnant state.
- Whenever observed, parent(s) demonstrates adequate bonding with newborn and competence in parent–newborn interactions.
- Parent(s) demonstrate adequate parenting skills: holding newborn, bathing, dressing, feeding.
- Mother repeats discharge instructions.

Implementation
Immediate Postpartum Care
- Facilitate parent—newborn bonding.
- Answer any questions the parent(s) has about the delivery experience, condition of the newborn, or other matters.
- Use warm blankets, if requested, to keep the mother warm.
- If the fundus is soft and spongy, cup a hand around the fundus, and massage it gently until it becomes firm and contracted.
- Use a cold pack or compresses (Tucks) for episiotomy pain if indicated.
- Immediately report any sign of hemorrhage.
- Report delayed voiding (note whether fundus is displaced from midline).
- Give a cleansing bath; use this opportunity to explain breast care, perineal care, care of stitches, and to provide instruction about fluid intake, voiding, ambulation, engorgement, and involution.

General Postpartum Care
- Reinforce teaching about the details of self-care initiated during the initial cleansing bath or bath teaching.
- Allow the mother to talk about her labor and delivery experience.
- Be sensitive to the mother's fluctuating needs to be cared for and to regain her independence.
- Teach both nursing and non-nursing mothers about how to care for the breasts.
- Be sensitive to the client's comfort needs; use positioning, ambulation, massages, compresses, and analgesia as necessary to relieve discomforts and

(continued)

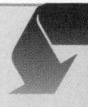

In Practice
Nursing Assessment 65-1 (Continued)

pain. (**Caution:** Never rub or massage a sore calf; evaluate for thrombophlebitis.)
- Observe the mother and newborn during feeding times, and offer suggestions as necessary.
- Teach parenting skills.
- If indicated, role-play healthy interactions with the newborn, and demonstrate care skills.
- Begin discharge teaching as soon as possible; if indicated, refer the family to the public health nurse for followup care.

Evaluation
Determine the adequacy of the plan of care by evaluating the mother or family's achievement of the above goals. If key goals are not met, the plan must be modified. The basic evaluative criteria follow:
- Return of uterus to normal size, incision(s) heals, no infection
- Maximum physical and mental health of mother
- Satisfactory bonding and parenting skills

---

first on each feeding. Engorgement in the non-nursing mother is treated with breast binders and ice packs. Chapter 66 discusses engorgement in more detail.

Constipation is a common problem for new mothers. Diet, adequate fluids, and activity help to regulate this condition. Many birth attendants routinely order stool softeners, such as docusate sodium (Colace; see In Practice: Important Medications 65-3) or mild laxatives, until good bowel function is reestablished. The woman may need a suppository or small enema if a laxative is ineffective.

Nursing Alert

The new mother should never take an enema without a specific physician's order.

Client Teaching

Client teaching begins early (at the time of admission) because mothers are often discharged a short time after delivering. The mother receives instruction in these aspects of self-care:

- Breast care and nursing
- Perineal care and care of the stitches
- Fundus observation
- Fluid intake
- Voiding
- Ambulation
- Engorgement
- Involution

Teach the client how to massage her uterine fundus and document this teaching. The client should use a mirror to check her stitches. Teaching the client the normal sequence of lochia changes is important, as she will probably go home the first or second postpartum day. She must know danger signs so she can spot a problem early and report it to her birth attendant. See In Practice: Educating the Client 65-3 for client information on changing the perineal pad.

Breastfeeding.   Reinforce the benefits of breastfeeding for the client and newborn. Nursing the newborn is beneficial for many reasons. The advantages of breastfeeding are summarized below. Chapter 66 discusses additional aspects of breastfeeding.

- Breast milk is readily available and convenient.
- Breast milk is always the correct temperature.
- Breast milk contains antibodies.
- Nursing helps in the bonding process.
- Nursing speeds involution.
- Breast milk is less likely to cause allergic reactions and other difficulties.
- Breast milk is cheaper than formula.

Most mothers can nurse their babies unless complications such as severely retracted nipples, infections, or breast malformations arise. The first requirement for breastfeeding is a good supply of milk; the woman's emotional status, diet, fluid intake, and amount of rest all influence milk production. Generally, the mother who is happy, who wants to nurse her newborn, and who is not worried or overly tired has an excellent chance to have a good milk supply. An adequate diet based on the food guide pyramid and ample fluids are essential. Intake of dairy products and fluids may be increased. Supplemental vitamins are often prescribed while breastfeeding. Chapter 66 discusses nutrition for a breastfeeding mother.

"Expression of milk" means artificial emptying of the breasts. It may be used when a preterm newborn must be fed in the newborn intensive care unit, or for the convenience of a working mother. An electric breast pump offers the best method for expressing milk because the suction is steady and controlled. Milk also can be expressed by hand. Milk that is to be used later should be collected in a sterile bottle and refrigerated. Refrigerated milk should be used within 48 hours. Breast milk can be kept in a home freezer for 1 month or in a frozen food locker for 6 months.

Bottle Feeding.   Although breast milk is the preferred milk for most infants, there are times when it is not the best milk for a particular baby. For instance, some blood-borne infections such as HIV may be transmitted through breast milk. The client who has chosen to bottle-feed should receive equal support from nursing staff.

The mother who does not choose to nurse her newborn should wear a bra that gives firm support. She may have flu-

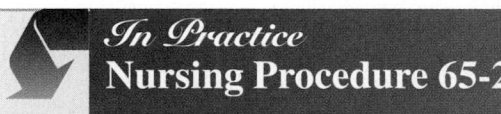

In Practice
Nursing Procedure 65-2

FUNDAL MASSAGE
Purpose

To encourage muscle contraction of the uterus and reduce blood loss.

Supplies and Equipment

Gloves
Perineal wipes or washcloths
Perineal pad

Steps

1. Cup your hand around the uterine fundus (at about the level of the umbilicus).

2. Place your other hand over the symphysis pubis to stabilize the uterus.
3. Rotate your fundal hand *gently.*

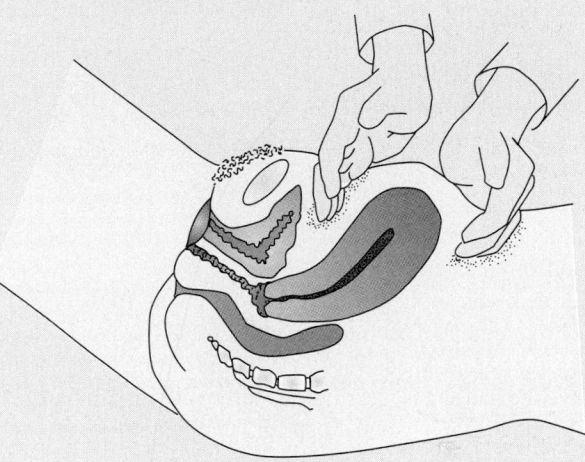

Fundal massage

4. Continue this massage until you feel the uterus become a firm globe.
5. *Do not massage a contracted uterus.*
6. Observe for passage of large clot; notify healthcare practitioner if clots are numerous, frequent, or indicate active hemorrhage.
7. Clean the woman's vulva and perineum.
8. Apply a clean perineal pad.
   RATIONALE: *The uterine muscle responds to stimulation by contracting. When contracted, the figure-8 muscles of the uterus clamp off the blood vessels, reducing bleeding. Massage of an already-contracted uterus may cause it to invert, which can present an emergency situation.*

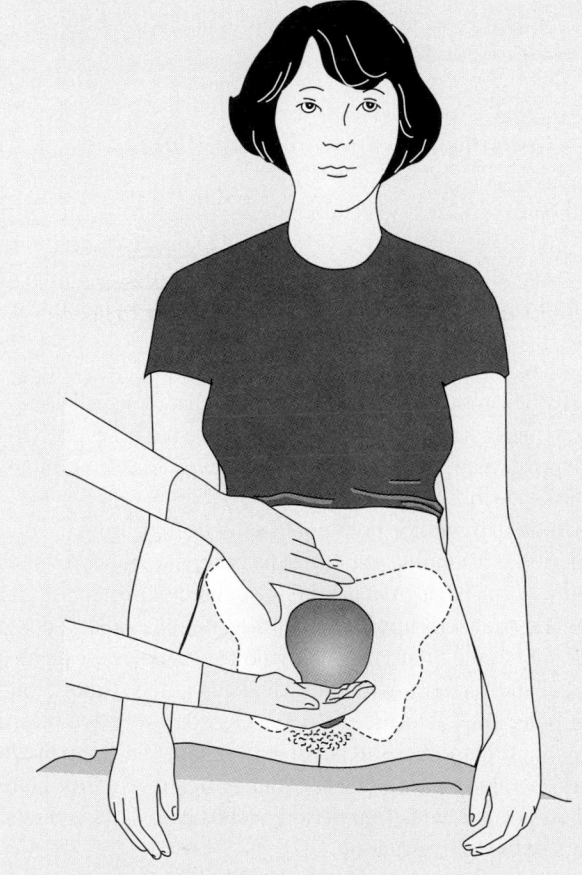

Fundal massage

ids as desired for the first 24 hours after delivery, but after this time, fluids are often restricted. Ice packs and a breast binder can be applied to reduce discomfort.

Perineal Care. Perineal care provides comfort and cleanliness, and prevents odor and infection. Whether or not she has an episiotomy, encourage the client to use a peri-bottle (a flexible plastic bottle containing clear, warm water), a sitz bath, or surgigator (a hand-held sprayer device) after toileting. In addition to promoting healing, these methods help keep the perineum clean and decrease the risk of infection. You may give initial perineal care with the client in bed on a bedpan. When the client is ambulatory, she may attend to it herself.

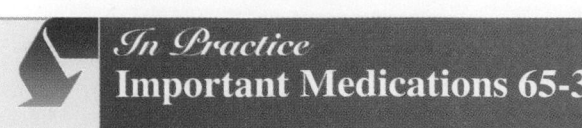

In Practice
Important Medications 65-3

DOCUSATE SODIUM (COLACE)

Dose: 100 mg po tid prn
Expected effect: Stool softener
Adverse side effects: None

Nursing Considerations
• Colace is not a laxative, but simply makes the stool softer to pass.

Methods vary, but the purpose is the same: to avoid contamination from fecal material.

Perineal care is necessary after the client voids or has a bowel movement. Teach the client to wash her hands and to change the perineal pad every 2 to 3 hours during the day. Help remove the pad she is wearing carefully, moving from front to back, and place it in a paper bag for later disposal.

After voiding or a bowel movement, teach the woman to spray tepid water onto the perineum from the peri-bottle, sitz bath, or surgigator. Use fresh toilet tissues to pat dry from front to back, on each side, and then in the middle. Discard the tissues in the toilet. Do not use undue pressure, which can cause discomfort. Without touching the inner surface of the perineal pad, the woman should fasten the tab of the sanitary belt, or attach the adhesive side of the pad to her panties, from front to back so that it will not slip forward.

A soothing analgesic ointment or spray may be applied as ordered. Witch hazel (Tucks) pads may be used. Frequent sitz baths (four times a day) will increase the mother's comfort and promote healing of the episiotomy. Oral analgesics and warm or cold compresses may be ordered to relieve discomfort. Squeezing the buttocks together before sitting down helps provide a cushion.

Bathing.   When the mother is ambulating and stable, she is permitted to take a shower. You will need to assist her the first time, assembling supplies and instructing her on the

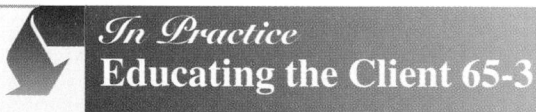

In Practice
Educating the Client 65-3

CHANGING THE PERINEAL PAD

Advise the client to always move the perineal pad from "clean" to "dirty." When removing a soiled pad, the client should pull her panties straight down. If using a sanitary belt, she should unhook the pad from the front first. When applying a clean pad, she should hook it onto the front first, which helps prevent infection.

procedure. Instruct the nursing mother to avoid using soap on the nipples (soap will cause the nipples to dry and crack). The client usually receives a bed bath on the first day after a cesarean delivery.

Activity, Rest, and Diet.   The new mother needs a combination of rest and activity. In most cases, she is up within 4 hours after a normal delivery, which helps to prevent respiratory and circulatory complications. Encourage the client to nap during the day. In some cases, visitors may need to be restricted. Analgesics may facilitate her ability to rest.

Assist the new mother in her initial ambulation. Encourage her to first sit on the edge of the bed and to take deep breaths. If she feels dizzy, she should not get up further until that sensation passes. When she gets up, she should move slowly. Remain with her the first few times until she feels totally stable.

Sometimes the client experiences an increase in lochia while ambulating, which may cause her alarm. Monitor the flow, and assure the client that the increase is likely due to gravity when arising. Explain that the increased lochia helps the uterus to drain and to return to its normal position and size.

The new mother should have a nutritious, balanced diet. If she is nursing, extra quantities of milk and other liquids may be added.

Discharge

Examination by the Birth Attendant.   The birth attendant checks the client before discharging her from the healthcare facility. She is told to return for a followup examination at the end of 6 weeks, and she is usually advised not to have sexual intercourse or use vaginal douches until then.

Discharge Procedures and Teaching.   Routine discharge procedures are followed when mother and her newborn leave the facility, and specific obstetric procedures also are performed. The mother should be informed that menstruation will resume in 6 to 8 weeks if she does not nurse her newborn. If she does nurse, menstruation is usually delayed for 4 to 5 months or until she stops nursing.

Although ovulation does not usually occur during the nursing period, prolonging nursing is no guarantee that pregnancy will not occur. To a great extent, the degree of protection from pregnancy depends upon whether the infant has all its sucking needs met at the breast. A baby who uses a pacifier, sucks on its fists, and so forth, will not provide as much stimulation to the nipple, and therefore provides less contraceptive benefit. Many nursing mothers do become pregnant. The new mother should be made aware that pregnancy is a possibility before the first normal menstrual period because as a rule, ovulation occurs before menstruation.

Discharge teaching should also include normal maternal responses to sex and sexuality, contraception, and when to resume intercourse.

At the time of discharge, rubella vaccine and $Rh_0(D)$ immune globulin (RhoGAM, Gamulin Rh) may be administered to the Rh-negative mother as indicated. The newborn may be given the first hepatitis vaccine. All these medications require informed consent. If the mother receives rubella vaccine, she must be cautioned to avoid pregnancy for 3 months to avoid harm to the next fetus.

The practitioner examines the mother and newborn approximately 6 weeks after delivery. The purpose of this examination includes making sure that the mother's uterus has returned to normal size, that her episiotomy has healed, and that no infection is present. The examiner will advise the mother at that time regarding resumption of regular activities.

➤ STUDENT SYNTHESIS

Key Points

- The role of the labor and delivery nurse is to ensure maternal and fetal well-being.
- The onset of true labor may be difficult to recognize, even for the multigravida.
- Rhythmic uterine contractions causing cervical dilation, and effacement and descent of the fetal presenting part, characterize true labor.
- Normal labor has four distinct stages. In the first stage, cervical dilation and effacement occur, along with fetal descent. The second stage is the birth of the newborn; the third stage is the delivery of the placenta. Family bonding, maternal recovery, and infant stabilization occur in the fourth stage.
- An important nursing responsibility during labor is performing frequent assessments of the woman's progress and any deviations from normal for the woman or fetus.
- FHR can be heard and assessed using a fetoscope, Doppler ultrasound device, or electronic fetal monitor.
- Various patterns of fetal response to uterine activity can be identified with electronic fetal monitors, and appropriate interventions can be started early.
- The fourth stage of labor is a critical time for the mother and her newborn. The major concerns during this time are preventing maternal hemorrhage, maintaining the newborn's respiratory and cardiac function, and initiating family bonding.
- In the postpartum woman, major changes (involution) occur in most body systems, restoring them to their normal pre-pregnant state.
- The uterus decreases in size, the placental site and episiotomy heal, and lochia progresses from rubra to serosa, then to alba, during the 6 weeks following delivery.
- Breasts will begin producing milk within 2 to 4 days postpartum.
- Lactation may be suppressed by mechanical means, such as ice packs and compression binders, and by avoiding breast stimulation. Medications usually are not used because the risks outweigh the benefits.
- Client teaching regarding fundal height and consistency, lochia, perineal care, nursing and breast changes, uterine cramping, backache, and fatigue ensures that these important self-care concepts are learned by the new mother.

Critical Thinking Exercises

1. Discuss expectations of labor with at least three of your female friends. Explore what is common, and what is different in your expectations.
2. Find a source to learn about the labor and birth practices of a different culture. Discuss with colleagues how these practices might be accommodated in our country.

NCLEX-Style Review Questions

1. After lightening occurs, which of the following might be noticed by the mother?
   a. Fewer leg cramps
   b. Less swelling of her legs
   c. Greater difficulty in breathing
   d. Greater pressure on her bladder
2. Which of the following is an accurate statement about true labor?
   a. No cervical change can be detected.
   b. A change in activity causes the contractions to stop.
   c. The contractions are felt primarily in the lower abdomen.
   d. The contractions begin in the back, and move around to the front.
3. During which stage of labor is the placenta delivered?
   a. First stage
   b. Second stage
   c. Third stage
   d. Fourth stage
4. J. H. is a 20-year-old, G1 P0 at 39 weeks' gestation. Which of these statements would you expect to be true about her labor?
   a. Her cervix will efface and dilate simultaneously.
   b. There is no way to predict the pattern of effacement and dilation.
   c. Her cervix will dilate almost completely before much effacement occurs.
   d. Her cervix will efface almost completely before much dilation occurs.
5. R. G. is a 28-year-old G3 P2002 at 38 weeks' gestation who recently immigrated from Cuba. Which of these statements describe how you might help her during labor?
   a. Insist that she remain quiet, and allow no vocalizations.
   b. Be sure to keep her other children away; she will not want them to see her in pain.
   c. Make sure that her husband is actively involved in supporting her during the entire labor.
   d. Find out from her which family members she would like to be with her during labor; help make this possible.

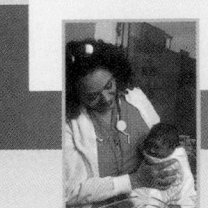

CHAPTER

66

Care of the Normal Newborn

LEARNING OBJECTIVES

1. Describe the respiratory and cardiovascular changes that occur in the newborn during the transition from the fetal to the newborn environment.
2. Identify the four causes of newborn heat loss. State at least one example of each. Identify at least two nursing considerations related to the prevention of cold-stress of the neonate.
3. State the four main goals for immediate care of the newborn.
4. Identify the five components of the APGAR score. Identify at least two nursing considerations related to each component.
5. Discuss the procedure for proper identification of a newborn. State at least three nursing considerations related to each: safety precautions, prevention of nosocomial infections, and completion of birth documentation.
6. State at least two nursing considerations related to each: universal precautions, eye prophylaxis, vitamin K administration, and parental bonding.
7. Discuss the normal ranges of weight and length of the neonate. State at least two nursing considerations related to each: molding, caput succedaneum, cephalhematoma, anterior fontanel, and posterior fontanel.
8. Define and discuss at least two nursing considerations related to the following terms: pseudomenstruation, phimosis, acrocyanosis, milia, Epstein's pearls, erythema toxicum, petechiae, Mongolian spots, lanugo, and vernix caseosa.
9. Define the following reflexes of the newborn: rooting, palmar grasp, Moro's, tonic neck, Babinski's, stepping, and sucking.
10. Identify at least 10 elements of information regarding the process of labor and birth that must be reported to the newborn nursery nurse.
11. Identify the components of the initial assessment of a newborn. Include at least two nursing considerations related to each: the umbilical cord, physical measurements, vital signs, respiratory status, and elimination and meconium.
12. Identify the components of a routine assessment of a newborn. Include at least two nursing considerations related to each: vital signs, weight, urine, and stools.
13. State at least three nursing considerations related to each of the following: holding a newborn, dressing a newborn, cord care, circumcision, and sleep.
14. State the nine main benefits of breastfeeding.

15. Define the following terms: colostrum, foremilk, hindmilk, LATCH. Identify at least two nursing considerations for each ter
16. State at least two nursing considerations related to each of the following common problems of breastfeeding: sore and cracked nipples, engorgement, plugged ducts, and mastitis.
17. Identify at least three teaching considerations regarding nutrition the breastfeeding mother.
18. Identify at least three teaching considerations for the mother who bottle feeding.

NEW TERMINOLOGY

acrocyanosis	inner canthus
alveoli	lanugo
bonding	mastitis
brown fat	meconium
cephalhematoma	milia
caput succedaneum	molding
circumcision	Mongolian spots
desquamate	neonate
en face position	ophthalmia neonatorum
epispadias	outer canthus
Epstein's pearls	phimosis
erythema toxicum	port-wine stain
fontanels	prepuce
foremilk	pseudomenstruation
galactosemia	smegma
hindmilk	stork bite
hypospadias	surfactant
hypothyroidism	vernix caseosa

ACRONYMS

APGAR	LATCH	SIDS
G$_6$PD	PKU	

The care that babies receive, and the bond that they form with their parents in the first several weeks of life, have many effects. These factors influence the growth and development of healthy infants and the closeness of the entire family. As a nurse, you play a special role as a teacher and advocate for family caregivers and their newborns.

A normal baby is born with the reflexes and body systems needed to live outside the woman's body. By no means, however, is the baby ready to live on its own. The infant cannot meet its own basic needs without help. In this chapter, you will learn to assist **neonates** (newborns during the first 28 days of life) and teach their new parents how to care for them. You will learn about immediate care for healthy newborns, their physical and behavioral characteristics, and the typical care of the infant from the time of birth until the time of discharge.

IMPORTANT CONCEPTS IN NEWBORN CARE

At the time of birth, the neonate must quickly make four dramatic changes to adapt to the world outside the shelter of the womb. These changes are temperature regulation, circulation, respiration, and source of nourishment.

The neonate must also complete these transitions quickly; the first 24 hours of life are critical for the newborn. In providing initial care, the focus is on monitoring and assessing the newborn's vital systems and keeping the infant warm. The baby's well-being depends on having a clear airway and effective respiration. Assessing the respiratory and circulatory systems, checking vital signs, and administering cord care are important skills that you will need to master.

Respiration and Circulation

Respiration

The changes in respiration are the greatest challenge for the newborn. The baby must begin breathing immediately after birth. Before birth, all of the fetus' oxygen had been provided through the placenta, where gases and nutrients from the maternal blood diffused into the fetal blood. As soon as the cord is clamped, however, the infant's lungs become the organs of gas exchange.

Excess secretions in the airway can block breathing, and if inhaled can cause aspiration pneumonia. Immediately after delivery of the baby's head, the birth attendant removes secretions from the newborn's mouth and nose with either gloved fingers or with a small, soft-bulb syringe. Sometimes the attendant holds the newborn with the head slightly downward, so that gravity can assist in removing secretions.

The change from being enclosed by the muscular walls of the uterus and the bag of amniotic fluid to an air-filled room with light, noises, and stimulation must be quite a shock. The healthy infant responds to the changes in pressure, temperature, gravity, and stimulation by taking the first breath. When the newborn takes the first breath, he or she usually makes the first sounds.

Although the fetus had some breathing movements *in utero*, the lungs were filled with fluid, and no gas exchange occurred

across the lung sacs (**alveoli**). The first breath expands the air passages and the alveoli. The healthy newborn has enough **surfactant**—a chemical that stabilizes the walls of the alveoli—to allow the sacs to remain open rather than collapsing after each breath. This means that that the next breath will not require as much effort.

The first few breaths set into process events that (1) assist with the conversion from fetal to adult circulation, (2) empty the lungs of liquid, and (3) establish neonatal lung volume and function in the newborn. The baby's respirations may not stabilize for about 2 hours after birth. During that time, some breaths may sound noisy and wet. However, it is abnormal for the respiratory rate to be greater than 60 breaths per minute at 2 hours of life.

> **Nursing Alert**
> By 2 hours of life, the baby's respiratory rate should be less than 60 breaths per minute.

Circulation

Review the information about fetal circulation in Chapter 64 to help you understand the dramatic changes that occur in the circulatory pathway during the first few hours and days of life.

The circulatory pathway changes abruptly when the umbilical cord is clamped and then cut. At birth, the fetal circulatory structures (the foramen ovale, ductus arteriosus, and ductus venosus) must close to allow blood to flow to the heart, lungs, and liver. If these circulatory changes do not occur spontaneously, the newborn will have inadequate oxygenation because of persistent fetal circulation. Correction of this problem requires surgical intervention.

It is important to remember that the changes in the circulatory system happen at the same time as the changes in respiration; the transitions to support life after birth by these two systems are completely interrelated.

Body Temperature

When the fetus was inside the mother's uterus, the temperature was very stable. The fetus had no need to expend energy to maintain its own temperature. After being born, however, the baby must work to keep warm. The baby loses heat by four mechanisms: convection, conduction, radiation, and evaporation (Fig. 66-1).

To counteract the heat loss, the baby has three ways to maintain its temperature: shivering, which is not very efficient; muscle movements, which have only a little benefit; and the production of heat caused by using a stored fat known as **brown fat.** Only infants born at term have much brown fat, and after it is used, the baby cannot create more. This is one reason that it is so important for the nurse to take steps to keep the baby warm. If the baby needs to work hard to keep his or her temperature elevated, the baby may become cold-stressed. A chain of events then occurs that can be harmful to the baby's blood sugar, oxygenation, and acid–base balance.

A newborn's skin has a bluish or dusky tinge at first. As soon as oxygen enters the circulating blood in quantity, the

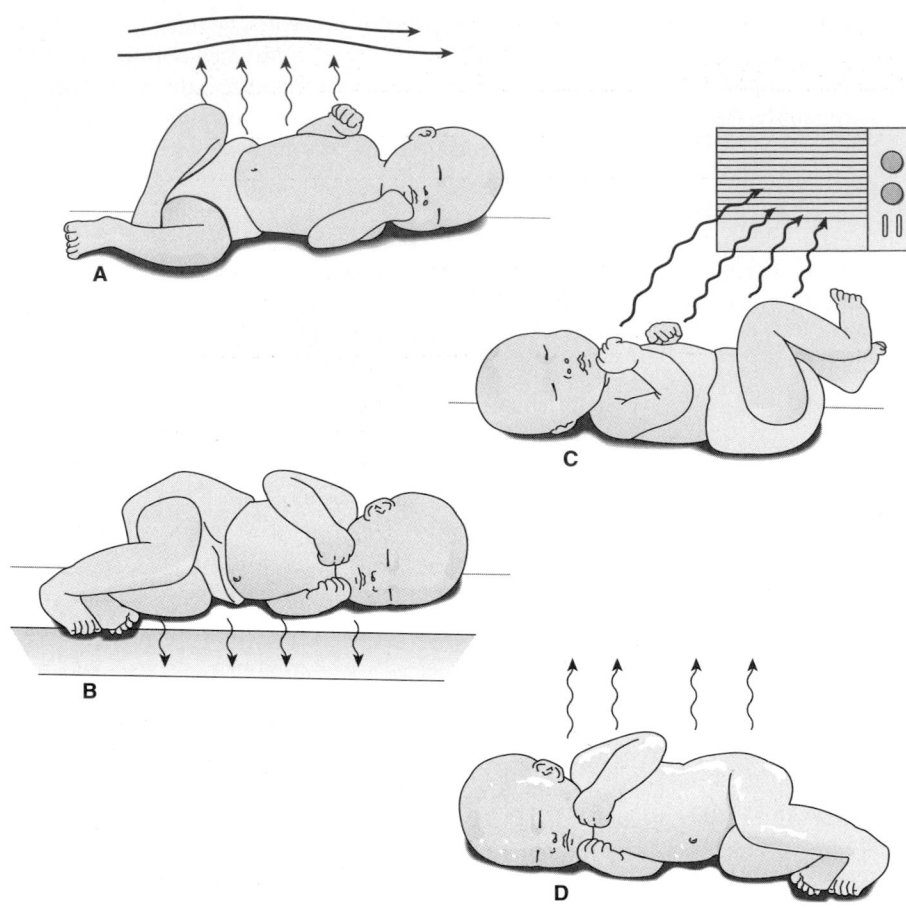

FIGURE 66-1. Heat loss in the newborn can be due to any one, or a combination, of the following factors: (**A**) *Convection:* heat loss due to air movement. (**B**) *Conduction:* heat loss due to direct contact with a colder surface. (**C**) *Radiation:* heat loss via infrared heat rays due to body metabolism. (**D**) *Evaporation:* heat loss due to the cooling effect of water loss on the skin.

white newborn's skin turns lighter and assumes a pink tone. Newborns of other races remain slightly darker. If the mother has been medicated, or has had a long-lasting anesthetic, the newborn may not breathe at once and must be stimulated.

CARE OF THE NEWBORN IMMEDIATELY AFTER BIRTH

It is important to set goals for the immediate care of the newborn. Without goals, actions become merely routines; but if the goals are clear, it is then possible to make a plan to meet them. The importance of each goal and the way that it is addressed will vary from one place to another. Four goals for immediate management of the newborn are to:

1. Establish and maintain an airway and respirations
2. Provide warmth and prevent hypothermia
3. Provide a safe environment and routine preventive measures
4. Promote maternal–infant attachment

Initial Assessment: APGAR Score

The **APGAR** score (Appearance, Pulse, Grimace, Activity, Respiratory effort) was named for the physician who developed it, Dr. Virginia Apgar. It provides a quick and accurate means to assess the newborn's physical condition at the time of birth. The score is used to determine whether the baby needs immediate assistance or resuscitation. It should be determined at 1 minute and again at 5 minutes after birth. The 1-minute score is most accurate in predicting immediate survival, while the 5-minute score may be better in predicting long-term survival and any neurologic damage.

The same five criteria are assessed at 1 and 5 minutes after birth. They include heart rate, respiratory effort, muscle tone, reflexes, irritability, and color. See Table 66-1 for details on scoring each area.

To obtain an Apgar score, give a number from 0 to 2 on each area of the Apgar scoring chart to the infant. Then total all the numbers. Record both the 1- and 5-minute Apgar scores on the newborn's chart. The following list describes the meanings of the Apgar scores:

- If the total score is 10, the newborn is in the best possible condition.
- If the score is 7 to 9, the newborn usually does not need resuscitation.
- If the score is 4 to 6, the newborn is in danger.
- If the score is 0 to 3, the newborn needs emergency resuscitation.

✚👁 N u r s i n g   A l e r t
If the Apgar score is 7 or less, a person who is skilled in neonatal resuscitation should evaluate the infant and provide immediate assistance.

■■ TABLE 66-1 *The* APGAR SCORE

	Score		
	0	**1**	**2**
Heart rate	Absent	<100	>100
Respiratory effort	Absent	Slow, irregular	Good, crying
Muscle tone	Flaccid	Some flexion of extremities	Active motion
Reflexes, Irritability	No response	Weak cry or grimace	Vigorous cry
Color	Blue, pale	Body pink, extremities blue	Completely pink

Neonatal Resuscitation

If breathing does not begin either spontaneously or following tactile stimulation, the newborn's respiratory center is probably depressed. You must take emergency action. The newborn must be resuscitated immediately; permanent brain damage can occur if the newborn is without oxygen for more than approximately 4 minutes.

The purpose of resuscitation is to establish an airway, provide oxygen to the lungs, and stimulate the newborn to breathe. When respiratory difficulties develop in the delivery room, the birth attendant or anesthesiologist assists the newborn. When a baby develops complications in the newborn nursery, however, you may be the person to begin the resuscitation efforts (see In Practice: Nursing Procedure 66-1).

Maintaining Body Temperature

Even with the birthing room temperature set at 75° Fahrenheit, the air is a cold shock to the baby emerging from the warm mother's body, still wet with amniotic fluid. Lifting the newborn onto the mother's bare stomach or chest, perhaps even before the cord is clamped or cut, lets the heat of the mother's body transfer to the newborn. The baby should also be quickly dried, and all wet towels and blankets should be promptly removed and replaced with dry ones. Warm towels or receiving blankets should be placed over mother and newborn. The infant will lose a great deal of heat from its head, so many hospitals and birth centers place a cap on the baby's head to conserve warmth. When it is time for the infant assessment, using a radiant warmer, a pre-warmed mattress, and warm instruments provides a heat-gaining rather than a heat-losing environment (Box 66-1).

Clamping and Cutting the Cord

The birth attendant will decide when to place two Kelly clamps on the umbilical cord. Delaying this procedure allows the infant to receive additional blood from the placenta. Whether or not this is best for the baby depends on the gestational age of the baby, the health of the mother and baby, and other factors. After the cord is clamped, the infant must obtain oxygen through its own respiratory effort. The cord is cut between the two clamps; usually a cord blood sample is obtained from the portion of the cord still attached to the placenta.

After the baby is dried, he or she is handed either to a nurse or to the mother for skin-to-skin contact. This can be done before the Kelly clamp is replaced with a plastic umbilical cord clamp. When replacing the Kelly clamp with a plastic umbilical cord clamp, you must be careful to place the clamp 1 to 2 centimeters above the umbilicus, taking particular care not to clamp any of the baby's skin along with the cord. The Kelly clamp is removed only after the plastic clamp is applied.

➤ **Nursing Alert**
Leave the Kelly clamp on the cord stump until after the plastic umbilical cord clamp has been applied. Otherwise, the infant will lose blood through the cord stump.

Identification

Identification Bands

While the infant is still in the delivery or birth room, it is the nurse's responsibility to prepare and initiate some form of identification. Each hospital differs in what is required; most use flexible plastic bands that come in sets of 3 or 4 with identical numbers on them. The nurse writes the mother's name and admission number; the birth attendant's name; the date and time of birth; and the baby's sex on each band. One band is placed around the mother's wrist, two on the infant (wrist and ankle), and the fourth on the father or significant other. The printed number on the band should be recorded in the baby's and mother's records.

According to the National Center for Missing and Exploited Children,[1] "newborn abductions from hospital facilities dropped 55% between 1991 and 1998. There were no reports of infants abducted from hospitals in 1999," and only one reported abduction in 2000. This decrease is due to improved systems for identifying and monitoring the whereabouts of infants in hospitals.

Properly identifying each newborn following birth is extremely important. Protective measures include identification bands, electronic bracelets, footprinting, and the completion of necessary records.

Electronic Bracelets

Another mechanism of ensuring infant safety is an electronic bracelet that creates an alarm if the baby is taken off the

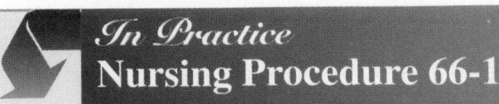

In Practice
Nursing Procedure 66-1

NEONATAL RESUSCITATION
Supplies and Equipment

Gloves
Bulb syringe
Oxygen attached to face mask, or anesthesia bag
and mask

Steps

1. Call for the person most skilled in neonatal resuscitation to come to the area *stat.*

2. Wash your hands thoroughly.

3. Put on gloves.

4. Place the newborn in the supine (back-lying) position, with head slightly lower than the body.
    RATIONALE: *This position facilitates drainage and counteracts shock.*

5. Maintain the neck in a neutral, or "sniffing" position.
    RATIONALE: *Hyperextension can cut off the airway. The purpose of resuscitation is to establish an open airway, provide oxygen to the lungs, and stimulate the newborn to breathe.*

6. Provide gentle suction. If using a bulb syringe, compress the bulb before insertion. Suction the mouth before the nose.
    RATIONALE: *Suctioning the nose first may trigger a reflex gasping motion, which can lead to aspiration of material (meconium or mucus) in the mouth.*

7. Occasionally a newborn needs to be intubated in the delivery room, a procedure that can safely be performed only by anesthesia personnel, the birth attendant, or a specially trained RN.

8. Provide oxygen by mask or anesthesia bag. The mask must be of the proper size to seal over the newborn's mouth and nose.

9. Physical stimulation, such as rubbing the newborn's chest and feet, may help breathing. However, if the baby does not respond to stimulation, do not keep trying it.

10. Medication may be necessary to stimulate the newborn to breathe on his or her own.

11. The newborn usually takes nothing by mouth (NPO) until respiration is stabilized.
    RATIONALE: *This prevents aspiration.*

12. Administration of antibiotics may be necessary if extensive resuscitation has been done.
    RATIONALE: *Because the newborn has been exposed to potentially threatening microorganisms, antibiotics reduce the risk of infection.*

➤➤ BOX 66-1
CONSERVING HEAT FOR A NEWBORN

There are several things you can do to help a newborn baby maintain its temperature.

In the Delivery or Birth Room
- Pre-warm any blankets, towels, hats, or clothing before the birth.
- Dry the baby immediately.
- Replace wet blankets or towels after drying the baby.
- Pre-warm the infant resuscitation area.
- Set birth room temperature at 75° F.
- Do not lay the baby on wet sheets while being suctioned.

In the Nursery
- Transport the newborn in an isolette with the portholes closed.
- Place newborn care areas away from windows, outside walls, doorways, and drafts.
- Keep the newborn's head covered and the body well wrapped for the first 48 hours.
- Postpone the newborn bath until the baby's temperature has been stable for 2 h at about 97.6° to 98.6° F (36.5° to 37° C).
- Bathe the newborn under a radiant heater.
- Do not wash off all vernix (protective material on skin) initially.
- Cover work table and scales so they are not cold.
- Organize work so that the newborn is uncovered only briefly.
- Heat any oxygen or humidified air given.

---

obstetrical unit without the bracelet having been deactivated by hospital personnel.

Footprinting
Some hospitals also use newborn footprints and maternal fingerprints as means of identification. These prints are taken before either the mother or the newborn leaves the delivery room, and they become part of the permanent health record.

Completing Birth Information in the Health Record
The patient record must include information about the newborn's sex, hour of birth, condition, and type of delivery. Document any identifying marks, care of the eyes, vitamin K administration, and the mother's Rh status. You must complete the chart before the newborn leaves the delivery room. Be especially careful if someone in the family has a common name. In all cases, the mother's full name and the date and time of the newborn's birth are of critical importance and should be carefully documented.

The birth attendant who delivered the newborn should complete and sign a certificate of birth as soon as possible. The birth certificate is filed with the State Department of Vital Statistics. To best prevent later confusion, advise parents to choose a name for the newborn before the birth certificate is filed.

Protection Against Disease

Universal Precautions

Infection control is not only very important for the mother and the new infant, but is also important for members of the healthcare team. There are many body fluids and substances involved in the birth process, including amniotic fluid, blood, and sometimes stool. It is essential that all members of the healthcare team practice Universal Precautions, including thorough handwashing and gloving, before handling the baby or providing care to the mother.

Eye Prophylaxis

If the mother has gonorrhea or chlamydia infecting her reproductive organs, the birth process could result in the infant being exposed to those organisms. Even babies born by cesarean section may have been exposed. These organisms can each cause blindness, or **ophthalmia neonatorum,** if left untreated. Therefore, specific protection against them is required in most states.

Erythromycin ointment is effective against both gonorrhea and chlamydia, and is the drug of choice (see In Practice: Important Medications 66-1). Treatment may safely be delayed for 2 to 3 hours while the baby and parents are getting to know each other. See In Practice: Nursing Procedure 66-2 for information on care of the neonate's eyes.

Vitamin K Administration

Newborns are at risk for bleeding problems during the first week of life because their gastrointestinal tract is sterile. The lack of intestinal bacterial flora means that the newborn is

unable to produce an adequate amount of vitamin K, which is important for production of certain clotting factors by the liver. Therefore, an intramuscular injection of 0.5 to 1.0 milligrams of vitamin K is usually administered during the first hour after birth (see In Practice: Important Medications 66-2). The nurse should document and report this injection.

Promoting Parental–Infant Bonding

The best relationship between a parent and infant occurs when they are able to have early and extended contact. The nurse assists in the attachment, or **bonding,** process by encouraging parents to see, touch, and hold their newborn baby. With a healthy baby, practices to promote attachment rarely interfere with its transition to extra-uterine life.

SPECIAL CONSIDERATIONS: CULTURE

In Chinese American families, the new baby is the center of focus and attention. Likewise, Ethiopians and Eritreans consider the mother and baby delicate; every effort is made to protect them from disease and harm. Childbearing is a joyful event; family and neighbors celebrate with food and gift-giving. Korean and Mexican American family members are expected to assist the new mother, so that she can focus on the baby.

Immediately after birth, one of the most important events that occurs is the formation of family relationships. The healthy, unmedicated baby is in a state of "taking in" his or her environment. The mother is in a period called the "maternal sensitive period," which fosters the process of bonding.

Forming a bond with the baby begins during pregnancy. During the first hour after birth, the infant and parents take the next step in bonding, setting the stage for a loving relationship. It may seem obvious, but for bonding to happen, the parents and the baby must be together. Behaviors that indicate this beginning attachment include:

- The mother moves from touching with her fingertips only, to stroking and massaging her baby.
- The mother and baby assume the **en face position,** in which their heads align as they look at each other.
- The parents speak to the infant in high-pitched voices.

The nurse can facilitate bonding by keeping the baby and mother together; placing the naked baby between the mother's breasts (skin-to-skin contact); delaying eye prophylaxis until after this critical time period; and joining in the parents' happy exploration of the miracle of their newborn.

CHARACTERISTICS OF THE NORMAL NEWBORN

Each newborn is different, but there are some characteristics that are common to all newborns.

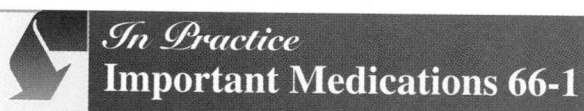

In Practice
Important Medications 66-1

ERYTHROMYCIN 0.5% OPHTHALMIC OINTMENT

Dosage
Apply a thin line, 1–2 cm long, of ointment along the conjunctival sac.
Move from the inner to the outer canthus (See Nursing Procedure 66-2).
Expected effects: Prevention of gonorrheal or chlamydial ophthalmia neonatorum.
Adverse side effects: May cause blurred vision in the neonate.

Nursing Considerations
- Be careful not to touch the newborn's eyelid or eyeball with the tip of the tube.
- Delay administration until after the initial bonding period with the mother and/or father.

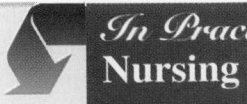

In Practice
Nursing Procedure 66-2

Prophylaxis for the Eyes of the Neonate

Supplies and Equipment

Gloves
Sterile cotton balls
Sterile water
Agent prescribed by physician or by hospital policy:
   Silver nitrate (1%) solution
   Erythromycin (0.5%) ophthalmic ointment or drops
   Tetracycline (1%) ophthalmic ointment or drops

Steps

1. Wash your hands thoroughly.

2. Put on gloves.

3. Clean over the baby's closed eyelids and surrounding area with sterile cotton balls moistened with sterile water.
   RATIONALE: *This action removes blood and body fluids left on the skin following birth, and reduces the risk of transmitting hepatitis B or HIV through the mucous membrane of the eye.*

4. Stabilize the baby's head, and gently separate the lids of one eye.
   RATIONALE: *This allows the medication to reach the conjunctival sac, to prevent blindness due to eye infection with gonorrhea or chlamydia.*

5. If using ophthalmic drops:

   a. Instill 2 drops in the conjunctival sac, and allow to run across the whole sac.
   RATIONALE: *Instillation into the conjunctival sac avoids direct contact with the sensitive cornea.*

   b. Repeat in the other eye. Note: If using silver nitrate, use one ampule for each eye.
   RATIONALE: *This provides the proper amount of medication.*

Ophthalmic ointment:

   a. Place a thin 1- to 2-cm line of ointment along the conjunctival sac, moving from the **inner canthus** (angle of eye nearest the nose) to the **outer canthus**. Be careful not to touch the eyelid or eyeball with the tip of the tube.
   RATIONALE: *The tip of the tube could cause injury to the newborn's eye or eyelid, or carry infection from one eye to the other.*

   b. Repeat in the other eye. Note: If using erythromycin, use one tube for each newborn.
   RATIONALE: *Using a new tube prevents cross-contamination from one baby to another.*

6. Carefully manipulate the eyelids to ensure the proper spread of the drops or ointment.

7. After 1 minute, gently wipe excess solution or ointment from eyelids and surrounding skin with sterile water.
   RATIONALE: *Wiping helps avoid irritation of skin.*

8. Do not irrigate eyes.
   RATIONALE: *Irrigation may decrease the effectiveness of the prophylaxis.*

Source: Reeder, S. J., Martin, L. L., & Koniak-Griffin, D. (1997). *Maternity nursing: Family, newborn, and women's health care* (18th ed., p. 628). Philadelphia: Lippincott-Raven.

Weight and Length

At birth, the weight of a healthy newborn ranges from 5½ to 9½ pounds (2,500 to 4,250 g). The average full-term infant weighs 7½ pounds (3,500 g). Girls usually weigh less than boys. Most newborns lose 5% to 10% of their birth weight during the first few days after birth, and then begin to gain weight. Figure 66-2A depicts a newborn being weighed; see also In Practice: Nursing Procedure 66-3.

Normal newborn length ranges from 18 to 22 inches (46 to 56 cm), with boys usually being approximately one-half inch longer than girls. The easiest way to measure an infant's length is to make a mark on the crib sheet at the top of the baby's head, then stretch the legs downward to their full length. Make another mark on the sheet, and measure between the two marks. In Fig. 66-2B, a newborn is being measured to form a baseline for future growth.

Head and Body

The newborn has a large head, averaging 13 to 14 inches (33 to 35.5 cm) in circumference. A short neck supports it. The chest is somewhat smaller than the head, 10 to 12 inches (25.5 to 30.5 cm) in circumference. The head usually measures 1 to 2 inches (2.5 to 5 cm) more than the chest. Fig. 66-2C depicts the measurement of an infant's head; see In Practice: Nursing Procedure 66-4 regarding measuring head circumference.

Head

The newborn's head may have an irregular shape due to the events of labor and birth. If the newborn was born by cesarean delivery without the mother laboring, the head is usually round. If the newborn was delivered vaginally, the head may show temporary **molding** (elongation) because of the overlap of skull bones during the birth process.

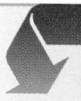

VITAMIN K (PHYTONADIONE, AQUAMEPHYTON)

Dosage: 0.5 to 1.0 mg IM one time within the first hour of life

Expected effects: Vitamin K is used to prevent and treat blood clotting problems in the newborn. It is a necessary component for the production of certain clotting factors by the body. The infant cannot produce vitamin K until the gastrointestinal tract is populated with microorganisms after several days of feedings.

Adverse side effects: Local irritation, such as pain and swelling where injected

Nursing Considerations
• Administer the injection into a large muscle, such as the anterolateral muscle of the newborn's thigh.

Caput succedaneum results from an accumulation of fluid within the newborn's scalp (Fig. 66-3A). This swelling is caused by pressure to the head during delivery. The fluid causes the scalp to be puffy and edematous, and the edema crosses the midline of the baby's scalp. The condition disappears within a few days. **Cephalhematoma** is an accumulation of blood between the bones of the skull and the periosteum, the membrane that covers the skull (Fig. 66-3B). This swelling stops at the midline. The newborn's appearance may upset the parents. It is important to reassure them that the fluids will eventually be absorbed.

Fontanels.   The **fontanels** are the "soft spots" in the newborn's skull, formed at the junction of the individual skull bones. These bones do not fuse completely before birth, so that the head can mold to fit through the mother's birth canal. Two major fontanels can be felt. The *anterior fontanel* is found just above the forehead; it is diamond shaped. The anterior fontanel closes between the ages of 12 and 18 months. The *posterior fontanel*, located on the crown of the head (near the back of the head or *occiput*), is smaller and more triangular. It closes by the third month of life.

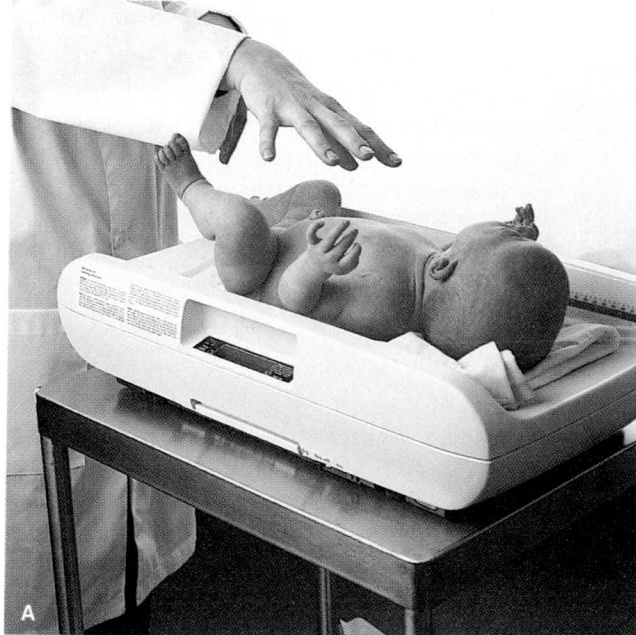

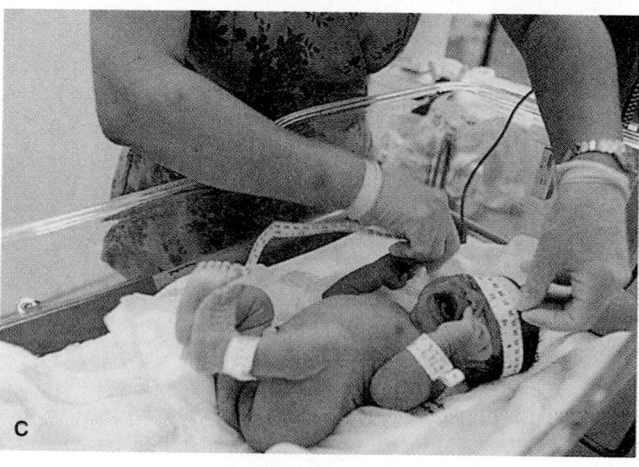

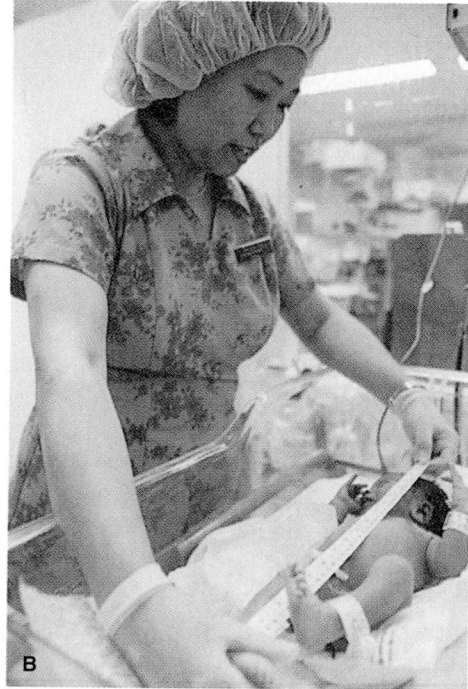

FIGURE 66-2. (A) Weighing a newborn. Notice the protective hand held over the infant. (B) Length should be measured soon after birth, to serve as a baseline from which to judge future growth. (C) The circumference of the head is measured by placing a non-stretchable tape measure just above the eyebrows and over the most prominent part of the occiput.

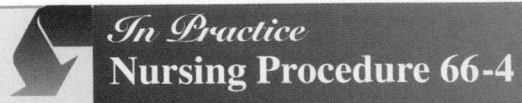

In Practice
Nursing Procedure 66-3

WEIGHING A NEONATE
Supplies and Equipment

Be sure to assemble all needed supplies and equipment before starting to weigh the baby. You may not safely leave the baby unattended, for even a moment, after you begin.

Towel
Transfer paper
Clean diaper
Infant scale

Steps

1. Wash your hands before the procedure. Clean the scale between uses.
   RATIONALE: *Prevent the spread of infection.*

2. Pad the scale with a towel. Deduct the towel's weight to ensure accuracy.
   RATIONALE: *This measure prevents excess heat loss and startling the baby.*

3. Remove all the newborn's clothes. Place a transfer paper on the scale, and weigh the newborn as quickly as possible.
   RATIONALE: *Minimize the newborn's exposure and discomfort.*

4. Keep your hand close above the newborn at all times. Never leave the newborn unattended.
   RATIONALE: *Protect the newborn from falling.*

5. Weigh the baby each day to note the baby's condition and progress.
   RATIONALE: *Expect a weight loss of 5%–10% from the birth weight before the baby begins to gain weight from feedings.*

6. Dress the newborn. Use a clean diaper. Place the newborn back in the crib. Discard the transfer paper. Make sure the baby is safe before cleaning up the area.

7. Wash your hands.
   RATIONALE: *Prevent cross-contamination.*

8. Record the weight in grams on the chart. Convert to pounds for the mother's information.
   RATIONALE: *Use grams for consistency and to promote greater accuracy.*

In Practice
Nursing Procedure 66-4

MEASURING HEAD CIRCUMFERENCE
Supplies and Equipment

Disposable paper tape

Steps

1. Use a disposable paper tape measure.
2. Wash your hands.
3. Gather necessary equipment.
4. Explain to the family caregiver and child (if appropriate) what you are going to do and why.
5. Place the tape measure over the most prominent part of the occiput and around the forehead, just above the supraorbital ridges (eyebrows).
6. Make sure to hold the child's head in a stable position.
7. Tighten the tape so that the reading is accurate.
8. Read the measurement over the forehead. Discard the tape and wash your hands.
9. Record and document the measurement.
10. Compare it with previous measurements. You also may compare it with a growth chart of normal measurements for the child's age.
11. Report and document any significant deviations from normal or previously obtained measurements.

to produce tears because the lacrimal (tear) glands are not yet functioning.

The top of the ear should be at or above an imaginary line drawn from the **inner canthus** of the eye to the **outer canthus.** The ears are functional at birth, but hearing improves over the first 2 or 3 days, as the fluid in the Eustachian tube is replaced with air.

Body

The normal newborn has a round chest and a slightly protruding abdomen. Engorgement of the breasts is common for the first 2 or 3 weeks of life in both boys and girls. This is one result of no longer being under the influence of the hormones of pregnancy from the mother's body. Another effect is that the baby's breasts may produce a small amount of fluid, known by the unusual term "witch's milk." The nurse should assure the parents that this is common, and that trying to express the milk may result in the complication of infection.

The genitals may be swollen, particularly in girls, as well as in any baby who was born in a breech position. The genitals of the female infant may be enlarged and have a mucoid, white, or blood-stained discharge. This is called **pseudomenstrua-**

Face. Newborns typically have small faces, flattened noses and ears, and receding chins. The newborn's eyes appear blue or gray at birth. He or she may look cross-eyed, because the eyes are unable to focus. The newborn usually has eyelashes and eyebrows at birth. He or she keeps the eyes closed most of the time because they are still sensitive to bright lights. During the first several weeks, the newborn is unable

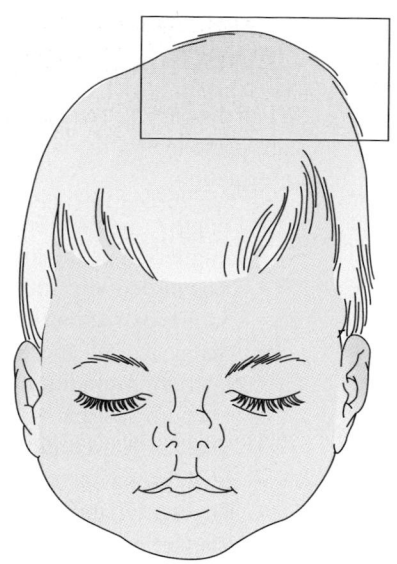

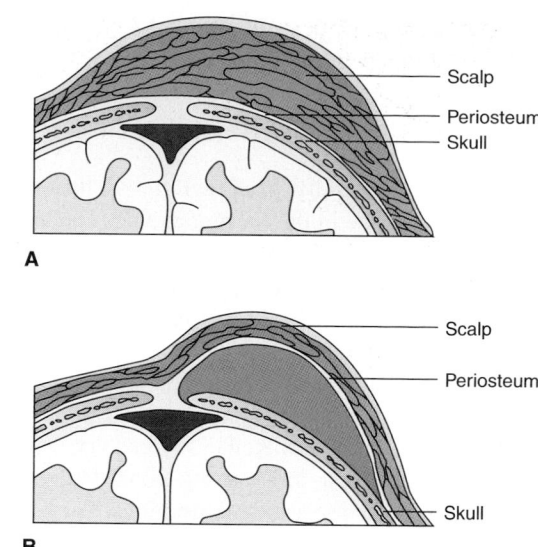

FIGURE 66-3. **(A)** Caput succedaneum: From the pressure of the birth canal, an edematous area is present beneath the scalp. Note how it crosses the midline of the skull. **(B)** Cephalhematoma: A small capillary beneath the periosteum of the skull bone has ruptured, and blood has collected under the periosteum of the bone. Note how the swelling now stops at the midline. Because the blood is contained under the periosteum, it is necessarily stopped by a suture line.

tion. The swelling and discharge will disappear spontaneously within about a week.

In male newborns, the scrotum usually appears relatively large and may have darker pigmentation than the parents expect. This is due to the hormones of the mother, and will fade within a few weeks.

At term, the boy's testes usually can be either felt inside the scrotum, or easily stroked down from the inguinal canal. The foreskin, or **prepuce,** covers the glans of the penis and is often adherent at birth. If the opening of the foreskin is so small that it cannot be pulled back at all, the condition is called **phimosis.** The penis should be inspected to determine the location of the urinary meatus, which should be at the very tip of the penis. If it is located on the underside of the penis (near the scrotum), it is termed **hypospadias.** A less common location is on the upper side of the penis; this is called **epispadias** (see Chap. 68).

Skin

Skin Color and Texture.   A white newborn's skin is pink or red in the first few days after birth. The skin of nonwhite babies may appear pink or tan, with some pigment changes occurring within hours or days of delivery. The newborn's skin should become smooth and of a color typical of its race within 2 weeks.

Because of slowed peripheral circulation, the newborn's arms and legs may appear cyanotic; this condition is called **acrocyanosis.** It is common in the first 24 hours of life, and is more prominent when the newborn is exposed to cold. It is not a serious condition.

Nursing Alert
Report generalized cyanosis or pallor (paleness), which may indicate a heart defect or respiratory disorder. Report at once any jaundice that appears, especially within the first 24 hours.

The newborn's skin may be dry and peeling for a few days, and the skin may even show dry cracks in the folds of the wrists and ankles. The skin also may **desquamate** (peel) in large or small flakes.

Bumps, Rashes, and Other Marks.   The nose and cheeks may have pinhead-sized white spots, caused by unopened oil and sweat glands. These spots are called **milia.** Sometimes white- or grayish-colored bumps known as **Epstein's pearls** are found on the mouth's hard and soft palate.

You may see various types of marks on the skin. Some disappear early in life; others are permanent birthmarks. If forceps or a vacuum extractor have been used for delivery, small bruises or swollen areas may appear on the face or head.

A mark that often appears on the newborn's eyelid or forehead is called a **stork bite.** This type of mark generally fades during infancy, although it sometimes persists into adulthood. A **port-wine stain** is a flat, purple-red area with sharp borders; this is a permanent birthmark.

The skin of some newborns is sensitive; many newborns develop a red, raised rash known as **erythema toxicum.**

Petechiae, small purplish dots on the skin, are due to pressure caused by labor and will fade. Veins may be visible over the entire body. Dark blue areas of discoloration called **Mongolian spots** often appear on the buttocks, lower back, or upper legs of nonwhite babies. These spots usually disappear by early childhood. It is important to know that they have no relationship to "Mongolism," or Down syndrome.

Hair and Vernix.   Fine, downy hair, called **lanugo,** may be seen on the face, shoulders, and back. A white, thick, cheesy material may also cover the skin. It is called the **vernix caseosa** and is composed of epithelial cells and the secretions of glands. It protects the skin from the drying effects of amniotic fluid *in utero,* and is especially noticeable in the hair and skin creases. Both the quantity of lanugo and the amount of vernix decrease with gestational age; a term infant will usually have less than a preterm infant.

Movement and Activities

Maturity.   Generally, each facility will have a gestational age maturity guide in the form of a table. The birth attendant observes the infant's posture, tests flexibility and reflexes, and identifies specific physical characteristics to determine the newborn's physical maturity. The form will allocate scores and identify criteria related to maturity. If the scores are too low, the newborn is treated as premature.

Behavior.   Typical newborns sleep approximately 17 hours a day. They awaken easily and cry when hungry or uncomfortable. Their arms and legs move freely and symmetrically. They often flex their extremities. They are unable to support the weight of the head.

Reflexes.   Certain reflexes are present at birth, even though the newborn's nervous system is immature. These reflexes indicate adequate neurologic functioning; their absence indicates abnormalities.

- *Rooting reflex:* When stroked on the lip or cheek, the newborn reacts by turning the head toward the direction of the stimulus (Fig. 66-4A).
- *Palmar grasp reflex:* The newborn tightly grasps a finger or other object placed into his or her hand. This reflex disappears as the newborn grows older (Fig. 66-4B).
- *Moro's* or *startle reflex:* Sudden noises or jarring movements cause the newborn to throw out the arms and to draw up the legs (Fig. 66-4C).
- *Tonic neck reflex:* When the newborn is lying on the back and turns the head to one side, the leg and arm of that side extend, and those of the opposite side flex (Fig. 66-4D).
- *Babinski's reflex:* When the sole of the foot is scraped from heel to toe, the big toe fans out and hyperextends (Fig. 66-4E).
- *Stepping reflex:* The newborn steps with one foot, and then the other, when held upright with the feet touching a surface (Fig. 66-4F).
- *Sucking reflex:* As the newborn grasps the nipple with the lips, sucking should be automatic.

Other reflexes include gagging, crawling, blinking, sneezing, and coughing.

Senses.   Newborns can see shades of light and darkness following birth. They blink in response to bright lights; however, they are unable to focus their eyes for more than a few seconds at a time. They respond to faces by staring.

Babies can hear at the time of birth. Caregivers should talk to them in soothing tones. It is typical for adults to speak in high-pitched voices to a baby; this is a sign of attachment.

Touch is well developed in newborns. They respond to discomfort, such as pain and wetness. Less is known about the senses of smell and taste. Newborns are known to increase sucking when offered glucose water. Research has shown that newborns at 1 week of age are able to distinguish their mother's milk by smelling their mother's breast pads.

ADMISSION TO THE NEWBORN NURSERY

When the baby is transferred from the delivery room, healthcare personnel in the newborn nursery must receive certain information:

- Length of first and second stages of labor
- Length of time the membranes were ruptured
- Type of delivery and any difficulties; use of forceps or vacuum extraction
- Analgesics and anesthetics that were used in delivery
- Newborn's condition at delivery
- Newborn's Apgar scores
- Whether resuscitation was needed
- Newborn's vital signs
- Whether vitamin K was given
- Whether eye prophylaxis was performed
- Whether or not the baby voided or passed the meconium plug or stool

☞ Key Concept

Report any abnormal signs or symptoms at once. A newborn's condition can change quickly.

Assessment

Initial Assessment

The first hours after birth are a time of continuing transition for the infant as he or she adapts to life outside the mother's uterus. If you work in the newborn nursery, you will assess the newborn on admission. Note physical characteristics, including the newborn's appearance, behavior, and reflexes.

Umbilical Cord.   Observe the cord and make certain that the clamp is securely attached. Count the number of vessels in the umbilical cord. Normally, you will find three vessels: two arteries and one vein. If you observe only two vessels, you must report this, because it indicates a strong possibility of congenital defects in the newborn.

Nursing Alert
Notify the baby's healthcare provider if there are only two umbilical vessels.

Measurements.   Weigh the newborn immediately after his or her arrival in the newborn nursery. Record the weight on the health record in grams, and convert it to pounds for the mother's benefit. Measure the length of the baby along with the head and chest circumference as previously discussed. These measurements are often recorded in centimeters.

Vital Signs.   Take respiration, pulse, and temperature, and record them every hour or two immediately after birth and then every 4 hours for the first 24 hours. In the past, the initial temperature was taken rectally to establish the patency of the rectum. Today, the passage of the *meconium* (stool) is accepted as validation that the anus is patent. Tympanic and axillary

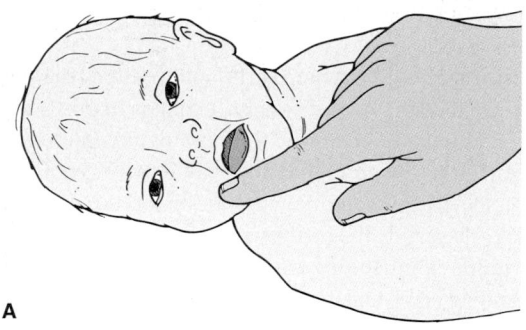

A

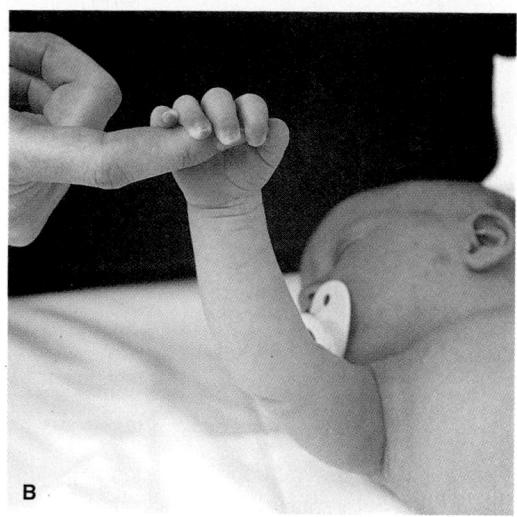

B

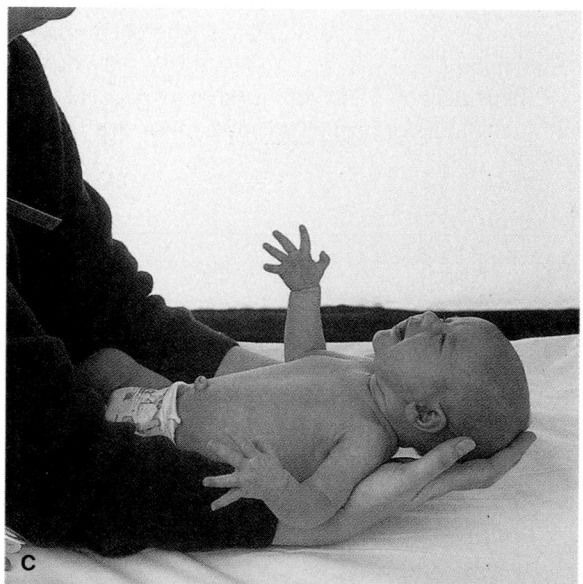

C

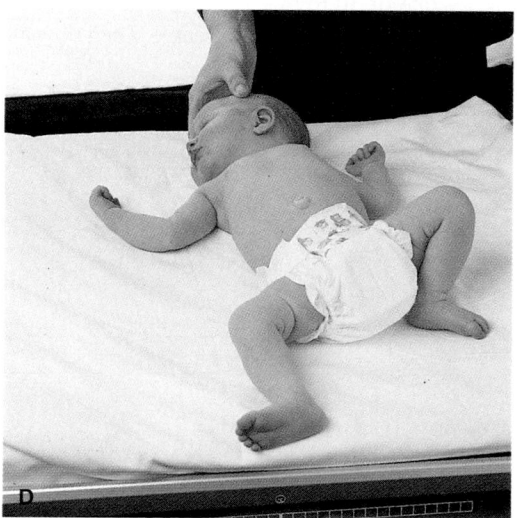

D

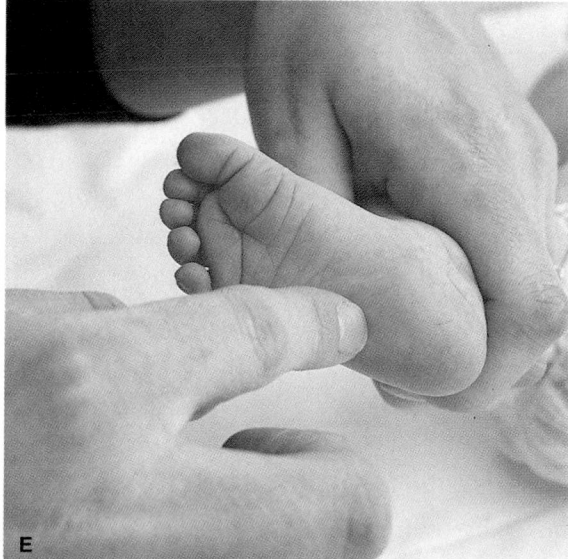

E

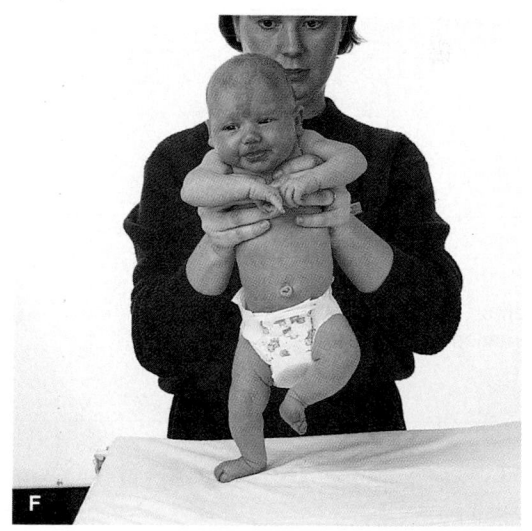

F

FIGURE 66-4. (**A**) When stroked on the lip or cheek, the neonate turns his or her head in the direction of the touch (*rooting reflex*). (**B**) The *palmar grasp reflex* occurs when the infant tightly holds onto an object that is placed in his or her hand. (**C**) The *Moro's reflex* or *startle reflex* occurs as a response to sudden noise. The neonate throws out his or her arms and draws up the legs. (**D**) When an infant is on his or her back, the *tonic neck reflex* occurs when the head turns to one side and the leg and arm of that side extend, while the leg and arm of the opposite side flex. (**E**) To elicit *Babinski's reflex,* hold the newborn's foot and stroke up the lateral edge and across the ball of the foot. Fanning of the toes reflects a positive Babinski's sign. (**F**) A newborn has a *stepping reflex,* which is seen when he or she is held upright so that the feet can touch the ground.

temperatures are considered safe and accurate. Tympanic temperature may be converted to a rectal equivalent.

Ongoing Assessment

Respiratory Status.   For several hours after birth, continue to assess the newborn's respiratory status. Respiratory status is normal if the movements of the newborn's diaphragm and abdominal muscles are synchronized. The newborn's chest should expand as a whole, and the muscles of the chest wall should not show great effort with breathing. The nares should not flare out with the breath, and the baby should not make grunting noises when breathing.

Assess the baby's general condition and evaluate respiratory status by skin color, rate of respiration, and general activity (Fig. 66-5). Newborns are obligatory nose breathers, with a respiratory rate of 30 to 60 breaths per minute. The reflex response of opening the mouth to breathe when the nasal pas-

sage is blocked is absent in most newborns until they are 3 weeks old. Box 66-2 explains the signs of newborn respiratory distress.

Crying.   The newborn cries and tightens the muscles in response to sudden loud sounds, changes in position, the feel of something cold touching the skin, or any interference with movements. Crying is the only way a baby can ask for help. He or she cries when hungry, wet, disturbed, uncomfortable, or sick. The cry of the healthy newborn is lusty. The baby who gets more care usually cries less. Hunger cries are healthy, demanding cries, and the newborn may put fingers in the mouth as an additional sign of hunger. After being fed, the baby is quiet unless he or she has swallowed air from the bottle and needs to bubble. The baby relaxes when held, rocked, and patted lightly.

Elimination.   The infant should pass its first urine within 24 hours of birth. The nurse must record the number

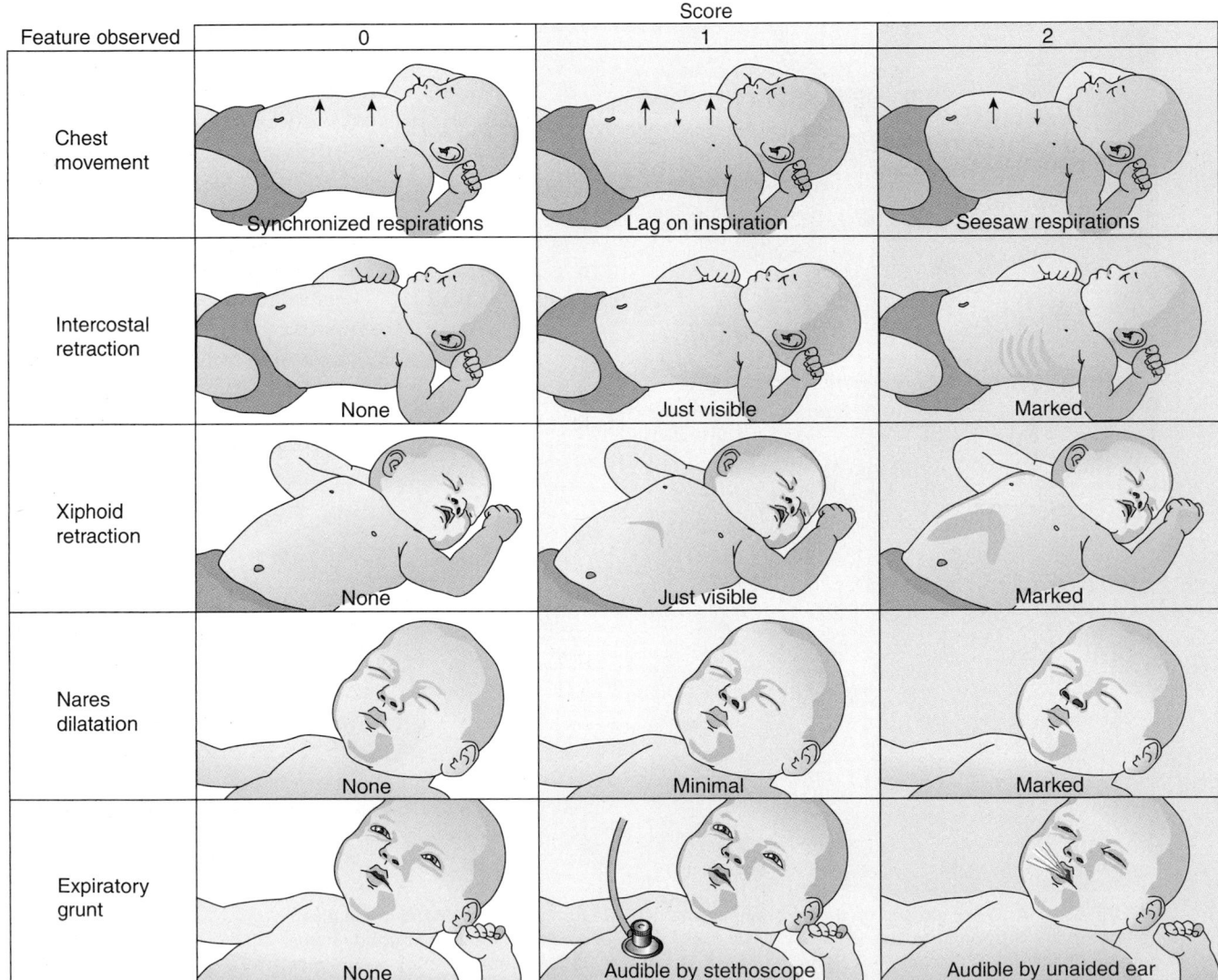

FIGURE 66-5. Grading of neonatal respiratory distress based on the Silverman-Andersen index (Silverman, W. A., & Andersen, D. H. [1956]. A controlled clinical trial of effects of water mist on obstructive respiratory signs, death rate and necroscopy findings among premature infants. *Pediatrics, 17, 1.*)

➤➤ BOX 66-2

SIGNS OF NEWBORN RESPIRATORY DISTRESS

Chest movements	Synchronized movements are normal. A lag on inspiration, or a seesaw movement, is a sign of distress.
Intercostal retractions	The intercostal spaces (spaces between ribs) should not indent. Any indentation is abnormal.
Xiphoid retraction	The xiphoid process (lower tip of the sternum) should not indent. Any degree of indentation is a sign of distress.
Nares dilating (flaring)	With normal breathing, the nares do not flare out. With distress, flaring may range from minimal to marked.
Expiratory grunt	You should not hear a grunting sound with expiration. Grunting, whether heard with a stethoscope or your unaided ear, is abnormal.

Learn additional information about a newborn's respiratory status by observing the color of skin, nailbeds, and oral mucosa; pulse rate; activity level; and character of cry. Gasping and *tachypnea* (rapid breathing) are also abnormal.

You must immediately report any signs of respiratory distress; an infant in distress can worsen very quickly.

See Fig. 66-5 for drawings of these abnormal respiratory movements.

of times the infant urinates daily. Urination is an indication that the kidneys are functioning, and that the baby is getting enough fluid.

The first stool passed by the infant will have a greenish-black, tarry appearance. This stool, called **meconium,** was formed during fetal life, and is composed of shedded skin cells and lanugo hair that the fetus swallowed. The greenish-black color is due to bile pigments. The first stool is usually passed within 12 hours after birth, and should be recorded in the infant's hospital record. If no stool has passed by 24 hours of life, the nurse should report this; it could be due to an anatomic defect of the baby.

Examination by the Healthcare Provider

In addition to the Apgar scoring, the baby's healthcare provider or the birth attendant examines the newborn to determine obvious physical defects. This thorough examination should occur within 24 hours of birth. He or she reviews the chart, including the prenatal as well as the labor and delivery records. The physical examination will include the newborn's circulatory, respiratory, digestive, and neurologic systems. Patency of the nose and esophagus can be determined by passing a number 5 to 8 French suction catheter through the newborn's nares (nose) and into the esophagus. The healthcare provider also carefully observes the reproductive, urinary, musculoskeletal, and endocrine systems. The nurse's assessments and charting during the first few hours are important to this detailed examination.

Maintaining the Infant's Body Temperature

Due to the heat loss described earlier in this chapter and the immaturity of the newborn's temperature control center, he or she is susceptible to cold-stress. When cold-stress occurs, the newborn is at greater risk of respiratory distress syndrome, acidosis, apnea, or increased respiratory rate. Maintaining the newborn's body temperature, therefore, is important (review Box 66-1: Conserving Heat for a Newborn).

If the newborn's temperature is not yet stabilized, an isolette or radiant heat panel should be used. To prevent overheating, the newborn should not wear a diaper or shirt while under the radiant heat panel. The panel responds to the newborn's skin temperature. An automatic sensor is taped to the abdomen, and the other end attaches to the heat panel. The heat panel then provides more or less warmth based on changes in skin temperature. A thermostatic control allows achievement of the exact skin temperature desired.

Cleansing

Procedures for the initial cleansing of the newborn differ. Sometimes, the father is allowed to cleanse the newborn in the delivery room, or a staff member may merely wipe off blood and some vernix. In some facilities, newborns receive a complete body bath and shampoo after they are stable and their body temperature is within normal limits. The nurse should take care to prevent the newborn from being chilled during any bathing procedure. See In Practice: Nursing Procedure 66-5 about bathing a neonate.

Laboratory Screening

When the newborn is a few hours old, hemoglobin and hematocrit tests are often ordered. Because a newborn has increased blood volume for size, the hemoglobin is normally 15 to 18 grams per 100 milliliters of blood. The normal hematocrit for the newborn is 45% to 60%. Hemoglobin

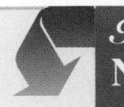

In Practice
Nursing Procedure 66-5

BATHING A NEONATE

Supplies and Equipment

Be sure to assemble all needed supplies and equipment before starting the baby's bath. You may not safely leave the baby unattended, for even a moment, after you begin the bath.

Stethoscope
Pan of warm (98.6° F or 37° C) water
Baby wipes, soft cloth, or other material used in your hospital
Baby soap
Cotton balls
Alcohol or antiseptic for cord stump
Cleanser for buttocks
Clean clothes and diaper
Clean crib linens
Trash bag
Fine comb or brush
Watch or clock with second hand
Temperature probe

Steps

1. Wash your hands thoroughly before beginning the procedure. Use individual equipment and a modified isolation technique.
   RATIONALE: *Preventing the spread of infection among newborns is essential, because their defense mechanisms are immature.*

2. Assemble needed equipment. After you begin, you cannot leave the newborn.

3. Check the baby's respiration, pulse, and temperature first, if ordered. Then undress and weigh the newborn before giving the bath. Be sure to place a cloth or paper barrier between the baby's skin and the cold metal of the scale. If diaper or clothing pins were used, close them on removal, and keep them out of the newborn's reach.

4. Keep the newborn warm and secure. Be sure to support the newborn during the procedure so that he or she does not become frightened.
   RATIONALE: *The first few days of a newborn's life may play a part in shaping his or her attitudes toward the general environment; therefore, promote feelings of safety and security. Bathing the newborn gives the nurse an opportunity to carefully assess the infant's skin, umbilical cord stump, state of alertness, response to touch, and interaction with a caregiver. To be able to assess each of these areas, the bath should be given when the infant is in the quiet alert state.*

5. Assess the newborn as you bathe her. Note any abnormal skin color, blemishes, or rash on the skin; observe muscles for abnormal jerking or twitching; check the genitals of a female baby for bleeding or discharge; observe the baby carefully for any congenital abnormalities.
   RATIONALE: *The girl baby may have some mucous or bloody discharge from the vagina. Both girl and boy babies may have swollen breasts and a few drops of milk production. All of these are a response to no longer receiving the mother's hormones after birth.*

6. Begin the bath by wiping each eye with a cotton ball dampened with clear water only. Stroke from the inner to the outer corner of each eye, using a clean cotton ball for each eye. Wipe the rest of the face with a soft cloth, including the ears, without using any soap.

7. Moisten, wash, and dry the hair. Gently comb or brush it, even if the baby has little hair.

8. Wash the body with clear water, working from the head down. Use soap sparingly, if at all. Give special attention to the folds of the skin, especially those of the legs, groin, and neck.
   RATIONALE: *Soap may dry the skin.*

9. Cleanse the genital area last, assessing for signs of rash or irritation. Use cotton balls or baby wipes to cleanse the vulva and perineum from

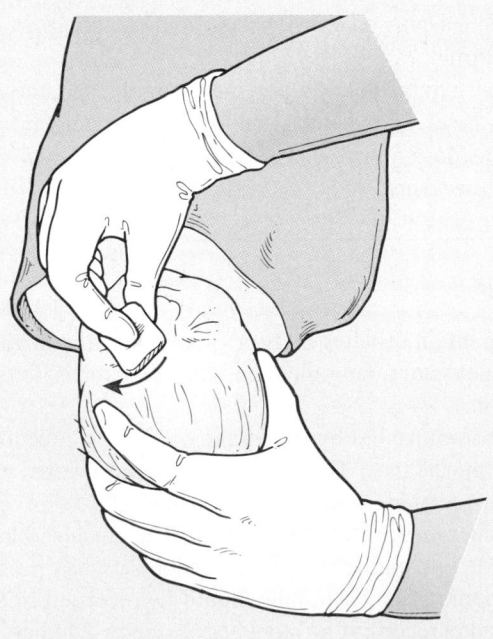

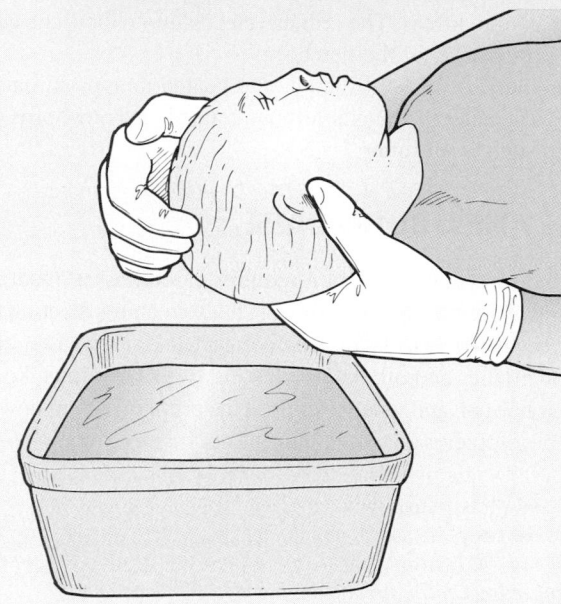

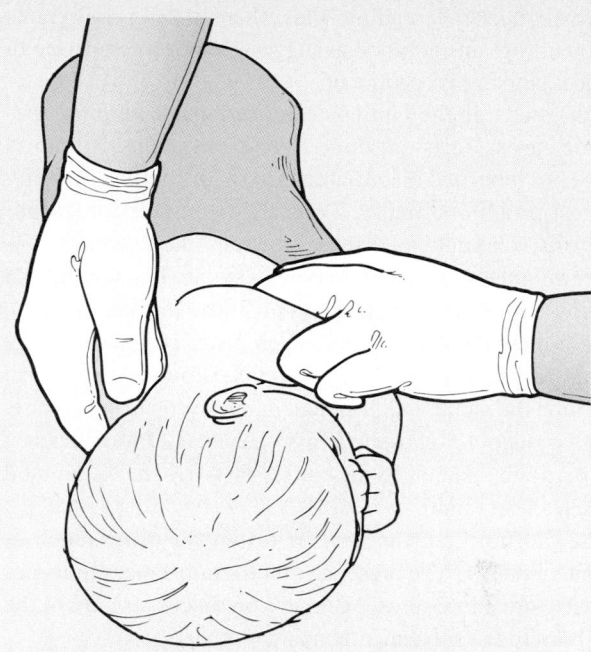

10. If a baby boy has been circumcised, provide care as prescribed at your hospital. Check for any unusual swelling or bleeding. Cleanse the penis carefully; report foreskin adhesions immediately.

11. Do not use lotion or petroleum jelly unless prescribed. Do not use baby powder.
    RATIONALE: *Baby powder tends to cake, and when it is sprinkled on, there is a risk of aspiration.*

12. Do not get the unhealed cord wet. The physician may order alcohol or Triple Dye cleansing, or application of an antibiotic ointment to the cord stump. Be sure to carefully clean the base of the umbilical cord.
    RATIONALE: *These substances help speed healing and prevent infection.*

13. Dress the newborn, folding the diaper below the cord stump, and wrap her in a blanket. Hold the newborn in a football hold with one arm while changing the crib's linen.

14. Wipe all surfaces of the crib with prescribed antiseptic.

15. Discard all trash properly.

16. Place the baby on her back to sleep.

17. Wash your hands before documenting all observations or touching any other baby or nursery surfaces.

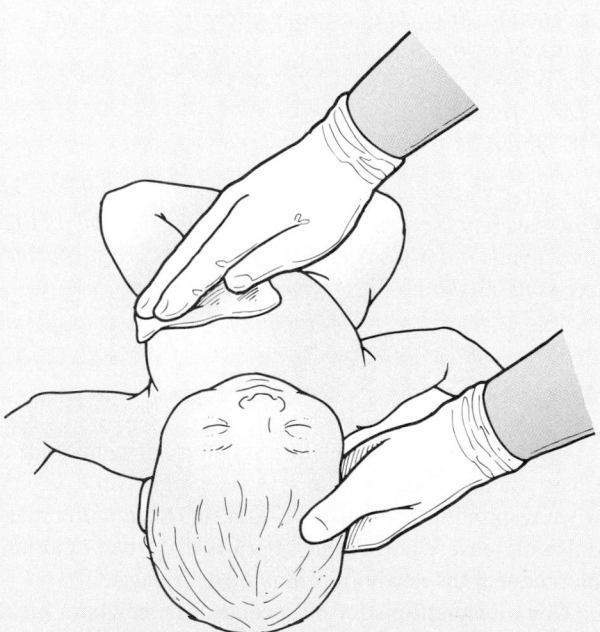

The cleanest areas of the newborn are bathed first: eyes and head, before the chest and back.

front to back for girls, separating the folds of skin and removing all smegma or discharge. For boys, use the soft cloth to clean the penis, scrotum, and perianal area. Be sure to clean carefully between all the folds of skin.

and hematocrit results lower than these normal ranges may indicate anemia.

The physician may also order a test to monitor the newborn's blood glucose level. A small sample of blood is obtained with a heelstick and tested with a blood glucose monitor. If a Dextrostix heelstick reading is less than 40 to 45 milligrams per 100 milligrams of blood, it suggests hypoglycemia (see In Practice: Nursing Procedure 66-6).

Most states in the United States require testing for specific diseases. Tests are done to rule out phenylketonuria (**PKU**), an inherited disorder caused by the body's inability to digest protein normally. Tests are also made for **galactosemia,** a hereditary disease in which the newborn cannot digest galactose, a certain type of sugar. Tests of thyroid function can rule out **hypothyroidism.** Individuals with many of these disorders have a much better prognosis if they are treated before the age of 3 months. Blood tests can also determine the sickle-cell trait and maple syrup urine disease. A test for glucose-6-phosphodehydrogenase (**G₆PD**) deficiency may be done, especially in babies of African, Asian, and Mediterranean origin.

The newborn's urine may be tested for drugs, such as cocaine or heroin. The presence of these substances indicates maternal substance abuse. Chapter 68 discusses care of the baby born to the substance-abusing mother.

In most cases, the heelstick method is used to obtain peripheral blood for examination in the newborn. The heelstick may be a nursing function in your facility.

Protecting the Newborn

Identification. Each time you bring the newborn into the mother's room, double-check the identification bands. Nurses must be diligent in this practice.

Security. Nurses must also be alert to the possibility of infant kidnapping or abduction (Box 66-3). Hospitals should have a written critical incident response plan in case an abduction occurs or a person is observed acting suspiciously.

Sleeping Position. An important measure to teach new parents is that the best sleeping position for newborns is on the back. An alternate position is on the side. This reduces the risk of sudden infant death syndrome (**SIDS**) in infants under 1 year old.

Protection from Nosocomial (Hospital-Acquired) Infection. A newborn nursery can be a dangerous place if an infection is present. Epidemics of skin infections, such as impetigo, and staphylococcus may occur. A fatal type of newborn diarrhea is a particular danger.

Nursery personnel must use techniques that isolate all newborns from direct contact with other babies. Everyone in the nursery, hospital workers and visitors alike, must follow a specific handwashing and scrub technique. Nursery personnel usually wear scrub suits, and visitors wear gowns over their clothes. People with infectious diseases are not allowed in the obstetric area. Each newborn has his or her own equipment and supplies.

☛ KEY CONCEPT

Equipment and supplies are never shared between babies.

When working in the nursery, place each newborn in a separate crib or radiant heat warmer equipped with a firm, waterproof mattress. The crib has clear sides to facilitate constant observation of the newborn.

The nursery is well lighted, and heated to approximately 75° F. The nursery is never left unattended, and newborns are within sight at all times.

DAILY NEWBORN CARE

Routine care of the newborn requires careful assessment for signs of abnormalities or problems. It also requires meeting the basic needs of food, cleanliness, comfort, and safety. Teaching for the mother and other caretakers is vital. They must know what is normal, and when to consult the primary caregiver with possible problems (see In Practice: The Nursing Process 66-1).

☛ KEY CONCEPT

As part of the routine assessment, the nurse should document the following on the newborn's chart:

- *Rate of respirations (note if crying or sleeping)*
- *Type of respirations (note abnormal symptoms, such as retraction, dilation of nares, expiratory grunts, and unusual crying sounds)*
- *Pulse*
- *Temperature*
- *Weight (daily)*

The nurse should make these assessments (with the exception of weight) several times a day for the first day of life and then on a daily basis. If complications are suspected, assessments should be performed more often.

Assessment

Respirations. Count the respirations first, then the pulse. Chart whether the newborn was sleeping, awake, or crying when respiration and pulse were taken. (Respiration rate and pulse increase when the newborn is disturbed. Values are inaccurate if the newborn is moving or crying.)

Count respirations for 60 seconds. The newborn breathes through the nose. Observe the abdomen's rise and fall with each breath. Respirations should be quiet and may be somewhat irregular. The normal respiratory rate ranges from 30 to 60 breaths per minute when the newborn is at rest. Review Box 66-2 for signs of respiratory distress in the newborn that you must report immediately.

Pulse. Take the pulse by listening with a stethoscope over the baby's heart (apical pulse) for 60 seconds. The pulse is rapid and may be slightly irregular; the normal range is 120 to 160 beats per minute (BPM). Warm the stethoscope in your hand before taking the pulse, to avoid chilling the baby.

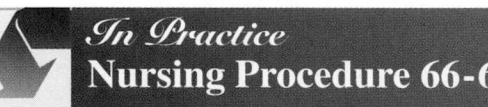

In Practice
Nursing Procedure 66-6

PERFORMING A HEELSTICK PROCEDURE ON A NEWBORN

Supplies and Equipment

Nonsterile latex gloves
Warm, moist compress
Alcohol wipe
Sterile gauze
Disposable lancet
Test strip(s) or capillary tube(s)
Small sterile bandage

Steps

General guidelines:

Surface blood flow can be improved by warming the newborn's foot. Hold it in the palm of your hand or wrap it in a warm (**not hot**) moist compress for 3–5 min.

Do not squeeze the foot too vigorously when obtaining the sample.
  RATIONALE: *This may dilute the blood with tissue fluid, or cause hemolysis or tissue damage.*

If the blood flow slows or stops before the sample is complete, wipe the area with a sterile, dry, gauze square. This may increase the blood flow.
  RATIONALE: *Do not use any liquid on the gauze; that would dilute the blood sample.*

Position the newborn with the foot lower than the body to increase blood flow to the foot.

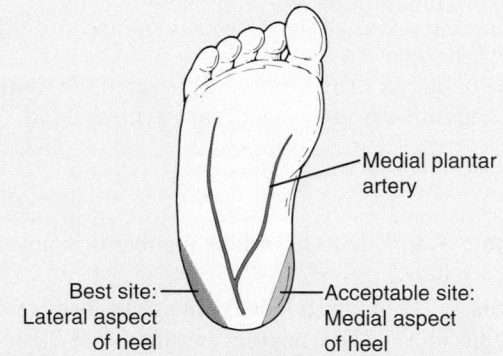

Medial plantar artery

Best site:
Lateral aspect of heel

Acceptable site:
Medial aspect of heel

Approximate sites for the heelstick procedure.

Steps in obtaining the sample:

1. Wash your hands. Put on nonsterile latex gloves.
   RATIONALE: *Observe Universal Precautions.*

2. Hold the foot dorsiflexed (against the shin), with your thumb and forefinger encircling and exposing the heel, and the other fingers stabilizing the ankle.
   RATIONALE: *This will reduce the chance of the infant reflexively withdrawing the foot and jerking it away from the stimulus, resulting in either a laceration or an ineffective puncture.*

3. Clean the heel with alcohol; allow to air dry, or completely dry with a sterile gauze square.
   RATIONALE: *Alcohol should not enter the puncture wound, or dilute the sample.*

4. Use a disposable lancet to make a quick, clean stab in the outer (lateral) surface of the heel. Do not make the puncture wound near the center of the heel or on the sole of the foot.
   RATIONALE: *Minimize tissue trauma. The heel stick is the preferred method for obtaining routine blood samples from a newborn. The sample may be used for glucose, PKU, or other necessary blood tests.*

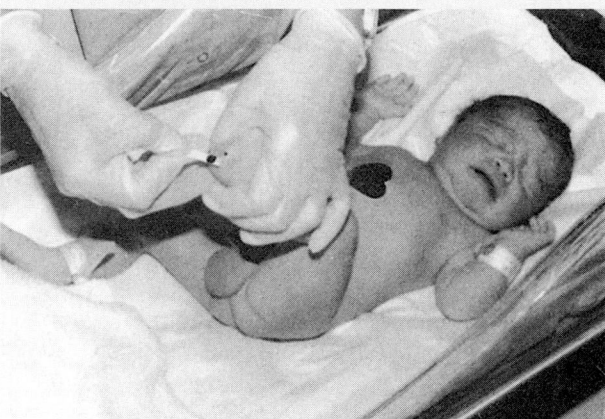

After the site is punctured with a pediatric microlancet, and after elimination of the first drop of blood, the nurse holds the test strip under the heel to collect the second drop of blood.

5. Wipe off the first drop of blood with a sterile gauze square.
   RATIONALE: *Remove blood that could be mixed with skin cells.*

6. When a second large drop forms, without excessive squeezing allow it to fall onto the test strip to completely cover the sensitive area; or lightly touch a capillary tube to the drop of blood.
   RATIONALE: *Squeezing may dilute blood with tissue fluid. Inadequate sampling may give false results.*

7. Follow the manufacturer's directions for the particular test that has been ordered.
   RATIONALE: *Each test has specific timing and sample requirements. Not observing these can result in needing to repeat the test.*

8. Apply a small, sterile bandage to the heel; apply gentle continuous pressure over the wound until bleeding stops.
   RATIONALE: *Any bleeding is controlled.*

9. Remove and discard gloves. Wash your hands.
   RATIONALE: *Observe Universal Precautions.*

➤➤ BOX 66-3

THE "TYPICAL" ABDUCTOR OF A BABY

1. Female, 15 to 44 years old, often overweight
2. Most likely emotionally immature and compulsive
3. Frequently has lost a baby or is incapable of having one
4. Often married or cohabiting; her companion's desire for a child may be the motivation for the abduction
5. Considers the newborn her own after the abduction occurs
6. Usually lives in the community where the abduction takes place
7. In many cases, visits the nursery unit prior to the abduction; asks detailed questions about hospital procedures and the maternity floor layout
8. Plans the abduction but does not necessarily target a specific newborn; when an opportunity presents itself, the abduction is simply a matter of "snatch and run"
9. Frequently impersonates a nurse or other hospital personnel
10. Often acquainted with hospital personnel and even the victim's parents

From *Safeguarding their tomorrows: A resource by NAACOG, National Association of Neonatal Nurses and NCMEC* (1991), as cited by Reeder, S. J., Martin, L. L., & Koniak-Griffin, D. (1997). *Maternity nursing: Family, newborn, and women's health care* (18th ed., p. 628). Philadelphia: Lippincott-Raven.

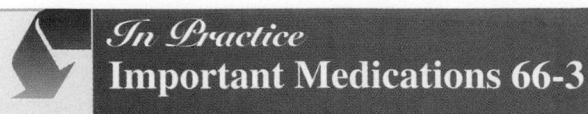

In Practice
Important Medications 66-3

If the mother is *negative* for hepatitis B surface antigen (HbsAg), the infant should receive:

Dosage: Either Recombivax HB® 2.5 µg
or Engerix-B® 10 µg

If the mother is *positive* for HbsAg, the infant should receive:

Dosage: Hepatitis B immune globulin (HBIG)
0.5 ml **AND**
Either Recombivax HB® 5.0 µg
(at a separate injection site)
or Engerix-B® 10 µg (at a separate injection site)

If mother's status for HbsAg is *unknown,* the infant should receive:

Dosage: Either Recombivax HB® 5.0 µg
or Engerix-B® 10 µg

3 doses required:
• First dose within 12 hours after birth
• Second dose at age 1–2 months
• Third dose at 6 months of age

Expected effects: The infant will develop antibodies to hepatitis B, which will protect the child from infection with the virus.
Adverse side effects: Pain with injection

Nursing Considerations
• All newborns receive a first vaccination against hepatitis B shortly after birth.
• Educate the parents about the need for the remaining doses of Hep B to be given according to CDC schedule.
• If the baby has been immunized, even if the mother is a hepatitis carrier, it is still safe to breastfeed.

Temperature.   Most newborn nurseries use the tympanic (ear) method to measure the newborn's temperature. The tympanic temperature probe may be set to convert to the rectal temperature equivalent. Insert the tympanic probe into the newborn's ear, while holding his or her head steady. The probe will record temperature within a few seconds.

If the tympanic method is not used, axillary temperatures may be ordered. The normal newborn's axillary temperature is between 97.6° and 98.6° F (36.5° and 37° Celsius).

In some cases, a rectal temperature may be ordered. To measure rectal temperature, gently insert the temperature probe no more than 0.5 inch (1.3 cm). Hold the newborn's feet with one hand and the probe with the other hand. Place a dry diaper over the newborn's genitals so you will not get wet if he or she voids. Keep the probe in place until the instrument beeps. Hold the probe at all times. Many healthcare facilities no longer perform rectal temperatures because of the potential for injury.

Blood Pressure.   The newborn's blood pressure usually is low, ranging from 50 to 80 mm Hg systolic, and 30 to 50 mm Hg diastolic. Follow protocols for the location to use; the leg is the most commonly used site. Use the smallest size of cuff.

Weight.   Weigh the newborn once a day. Bath time is an excellent time for weighing.

Urine.   Continue to record the number of voidings per day in the hospital record.

Stools.   The stools gradually change in character as the baby begins to eat. These next several stools are called *transitional* stools, and the appearance depends on whether the baby is breast-fed or bottle-fed.

By the fifth day of life, the daily number of stools ranges from four to six. As the baby grows, the number usually drops to one or two per day. During the infant's hospital stay, the number, color, and consistency of stools should be recorded in the hospital record.

Basic Needs

The newborn has the basic human needs for safety, security, and love. Nursing care is designed to provide the newborn with warmth, hygiene, nutrition, rest, and affection, making sure

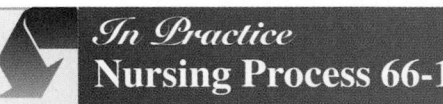

In Practice
Nursing Process 66-1

OVERVIEW OF THE NURSING PROCESS DURING CARE OF THE NORMAL NEWBORN

Assessment Guidelines
Immediate Assessment of the Newborn
- Apgar (heart rate, respiratory effort, muscle tone, reflexes, color)
- Newborn's weight and length (on arrival in the newborn nursery)
- Complete physical examination by healthcare provider on admission to the newborn nursery

Daily Assessment of the Newborn
- Rate and type of respirations (note if the newborn is crying or sleeping while the rate is taken), apical pulse, blood pressure, and temperature
- Vital signs
- Signs of respiratory distress: retractions of the lower chest and xiphoid process, dilation of the nostrils, or expiratory grunts
- Mucus secretions
- Glucose (Dextrostix®) checks (check agency parameters)
- Daily weight (usually in grams)
- Cord condition
- Voiding and stools (describe amount, color, and consistency)
- Skin color, for signs of jaundice or cyanosis
- Sleep–activity patterns, behavior patterns
- Bonding
- Condition of circumcision or perineum
- Adequacy of parenting behaviors
- Any signs of difficulty or abnormalities
- Character of cry (be alert to whining or sharp, high-pitched cries)
- Approximate amount of breast milk taken, measure of bottle feeding taken

Possible Nursing Diagnoses
- Ineffective Airway Clearance
- High Risk for Aspiration
- High Risk for Altered Body Temperature
- Ineffective Breastfeeding
- Ineffective Breathing Pattern
- Impaired Gas Exchange
- Risk for Impaired Skin Integrity related to moist umbilical cord stump
- Impaired Skin Integrity related to peeling and cracking of skin; circumcision
- High Risk for Infection
- Altered Nutrition, Less than Body Requirements
- Altered Growth and Development
- High Risk for Altered Parenting
- Risk for Altered Parent/Infant Attachment
- Family Coping: Potential for Growth related to positive adaptation to parental role
- Ineffective Family Coping

- Altered Family Processes
- Knowledge Deficit related to lack of experience with newborn care; proper newborn care and handling

Planning
The nurse designs a plan of care with the family to achieve the following general client goals:
- The newborn's feeding and daily weight reflect normal growth and development.
- The vital signs fall within the normal newborn range.
- The newborn demonstrates no signs of respiratory distress, infection, or other disease processes.
- The parents demonstrate:
  - Comfort in holding and interacting with the newborn
  - Adequate parenting skills

Implementation
Immediate Care in the Delivery Room
- Suction: Keep the nose and mouth clear of secretions.
- Ensure warmth.
- Administer silver nitrate or antibiotic ointment solution to the newborn's eyes and vitamin K as ordered.
- Place identification bands on the newborn and the mother.
- Take the newborn's footprints and the mother's thumb print.
- Complete the delivery information on the chart before the newborn leaves the delivery room.

Continuing Care
- Follow the facility's procedures for the initial cleansing and daily bathing of the newborn.
- Cleanse the cord three times daily with alcohol or other solution.
- Facilitate the mother's breast or bottle feedings.
- Reposition the newborn on the back or side; sleeping on the stomach is discouraged.
- Role-model healthy parenting behaviors for the parent(s) if indicated.
- Teach parenting skills.
- Refer the mother to appropriate support groups (eg, mothers of twins, breastfeeding group).
- Refer the family to a home health nurse if necessary.
- Instruct the mother about followup care for the newborn after discharge.

Evaluation
Determine the adequacy of the plan of care by evaluating the newborn and family's achievement of the preceding goals. If key goals are unable to be met, the plan must be modified. The basic evaluative criteria are:

- Healthy newborn at discharge
- Parents comfortable with parenting skills and roles
- Siblings prepared to welcome a new family member

that he or she is protected and thriving. You will also teach essential skills to the family to ensure that they will be able to continue to meet the newborns' needs after nursing care ends.

Handling the Newborn.   There is no one right way to hold a baby, but movements should be smooth and firm to help the baby feel secure. Keep in mind that:

- The head, neck, and buttocks need support.
- Newborns wiggle! Be sure you have a firm hold on the baby.
- It is easier to pick up a newborn when he or she is laying on the back (supine) rather than on the stomach (prone). If the infant is on the stomach, turn him or her over before picking up, to make the process more secure.
- Hold the baby close to your body to provide security. The "football" hold is a convenient method because it provides a free hand with which to perform additional tasks.

Dressing and Wrapping the Newborn.   Handle the baby gently but firmly when dressing him or her. Stretch the neck opening of a shirt or gown before bringing it over the head. Reach into the sleeves and pull the baby's hand through, to avoid catching a small finger in the cloth. Fold the diaper beneath the cord stump. Wrap the baby securely in a blanket. This process is known as *swaddling* and helps many babies feel more secure.

Cord Care.   Because the umbilical cord maintained fetal circulation, the newborn faces the danger of rapid hemorrhage through it. Therefore, the clamps or ties must be secure until they can be safely removed. When caring for the newborn, assess the cord for bleeding at frequent intervals during the first few hours of life. The stump of the cord begins to shrivel and darken soon after birth. The clamp is usually removed after 24 hours, as long as no bleeding is evident. (Removal of the clamp prevents tension on the drying stump.)

Triple Dye may be applied to the cut cord and around the umbilicus to prevent infection. One application of Triple Dye is usually sufficient, although some physicians order daily application. The stump is usually swabbed with alcohol with each diaper change. The diaper should not be placed over the stump of the cord, but rather folded beneath it, so that the cord is exposed to the drying effects of room air.

When bathing, do not submerge the baby in tub water until the cord falls off, which is usually 10 to 14 days after birth (see In Practice: Educating the Client 66-1).

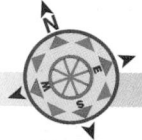

SPECIAL CONSIDERATIONS: CULTURE

Some Native American women stay indoors with their baby for 20 days, or until the cord falls off. The remnant of the umbilical cord may have spiritual value.

Care of the Genitals.   To prevent irritation of the infant's sensitive skin, thoroughly clean his or her buttocks following each voiding and bowel movement. Report any rash or irritation. (Broken skin can be an entry for infection.)

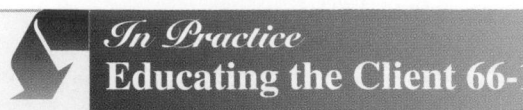

In Practice
Educating the Client 66-1

CORD CARE

- The cord will dry and naturally fall off. This should happen at about 10–14 days after birth.
- Clean the cord stump with isopropyl (rubbing) alcohol at each diaper change. Allow to air dry.
- Fold the diaper below the cord stump.
- Don't give the baby a tub bath until after the cord falls off.
- Call your baby's doctor if the cord shows any of these signs of infection:
  - Red streaks around the cord
  - Foul odor
  - Pus

In male babies, the foreskin (prepuce) covers the glans penis or extends beyond it. The opening may be very small, a condition known as *phimosis*. **Smegma** (excess secretions and dead skin cells) may collect beneath the foreskin, and drops of urine also may remain, causing irritation.

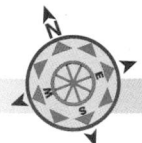

SPECIAL CONSIDERATIONS: CULTURE

Some rural or traditional Puerto Rican families choose not to circumcise the male child for fear of causing pain, bleeding, or harm to the infant. In more urban families, male circumcision is traditionally done soon after birth. Among South Asian cultures, Muslims practice male circumcision as a religious ritual that must be done before 7 years of age. Hindus and Sikhs may perform male circumcision for health reasons.

Some male newborns may be circumcised (part or all of the foreskin is removed). **Circumcision** is most often done for cultural reasons. Ritual circumcision is performed on Jewish male babies, usually on the 8th day of life. If the baby has been circumcised, he must be kept clean and assessed for bleeding, swelling, and voiding. A sterile dressing may be applied after each voiding for 24 to 48 hours, to keep the diaper from sticking. Circumcision is usually performed shortly before the newborn leaves the healthcare facility or after discharge. For this reason, instruct the parents in the care required, and document teaching. Never place the infant on his stomach following circumcision. Assess circumcision every 15 minutes for the first 4 hours. Report any excessive bleeding immediately.

If circumcision is not performed, the physician may order that the foreskin be gently stretched and retracted over the glans penis for cleaning once every day. In some babies, the foreskin will not easily stretch over the glans. Do not force it. Cleaning must be gentle and careful. Replace the foreskin immediately; a tight foreskin causes edema and pain.

In female babies, gently clean between all the folds of the labia, wiping from front to back. You may notice mucus or a blood-tinged discharge from the vagina. This is normal and is caused by the sudden absence of the mother's hormones; it will last only a few days.

Sleep. Except when being fed, the newborn sleeps most of the time, although not deeply. The baby will awaken and cry when hungry or uncomfortable. The baby should be placed on his or her back or side to sleep. Pillows should not be used because of the danger of suffocation.

NUTRITION

Breastfeeding is the best source of nutrition for infants. Differences have been found in the breast milk of mothers of preterm infants and term infants; each mother produces breast milk that is ideally suited for her own baby. However, not all mothers will choose to breastfeed. It is important that the nurse supports each woman in her own choice, and provides client teaching tailored to the needs of each new mother.

Birth attendants differ in their preferences for the first feeding of newborns. It is ideal if mothers who breastfeed are encouraged to do so in the delivery room. A few birth attendants prefer that the newborn remain NPO (nothing by mouth) for 3 to 4 hours after birth. When the first feeding is not from the breast, it usually consists of sterile water and is sometimes given by a nurse. If all is normal, the mother gives the newborn as many other feedings as she wishes.

If the baby eats too much or too fast, or is improperly burped (bubbled), he or she may regurgitate. (Regurgitation is simply an overflow—do not think of it as vomiting.) Food remaining in the esophagus may cause hiccups. Giving the infant sips of water can usually stop the hiccups. However, because of the difference in the method for sucking from a bottle versus the breast, many breastfeeding mothers do not wish the baby to have anything from a bottle. Interestingly enough, many babies can sip from a cup in the early days of life, and this may be a better choice if water is desired.

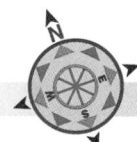

SPECIAL CONSIDERATIONS: CULTURE

Among many Arab Americans, modernization means giving up breastfeeding. In addition, colostrum is believed to be harmful to the baby, so Arab American women may not offer the breast. A similar belief that colostrum is inappropriate for the baby is found among some Cambodian mothers. Russian women are encouraged to breastfeed.

Feeding Schedule

All babies should be fed when they are hungry. Babies are all different, and their nursing patterns will vary. Newborns are usually fed "on demand," or approximately every 2 to 4 hours.

Bringing the Baby to the Mother for Feedings

If the baby and mother are not "rooming-in," an important nursing skill to learn is bringing the newborn to the mother for feeding. The following are recommended guidelines:

- Wash your hands.
- Dress the newborn warmly.
- Some hospitals have a policy that requires that you weigh the breast-fed baby before feeding, and again after feeding. Other authorities believe this is unnecessary, and feel that adequate breastfeeding can be determined by the baby's contentment and number of voids and stools daily.
- Carry the baby carefully; use the football hold.
- Instruct the mother to wash her hands to prevent infection.
- Compare the wristband of the mother with that of the baby, to ensure the right baby is with the right mother.
- Provide privacy.
- Assist the mother into a comfortable position, as she will be in the same position for about 20 minutes.
- Show the mother how to hold and bubble the newborn. Have her do a return demonstration.
- When the feeding is finished, check with the mother about how the baby fed, or determine the amount of formula missing from the bottle. Check if the baby was bubbled.
- Make sure the baby is clean and dry before placing him or her in the crib. Place the baby on the back or side, because sleeping on the back decreases the risk of SIDS.
- Wash your hands and document the feeding on the baby's chart, including how well the baby breast-fed or how much formula was taken, and any other pertinent observations.

Breastfeeding
In summary, breastfeeding provides:

- Better nutrition
- Lower risk of the baby developing allergies
- Reduced risk of infections in the newborn, because maternal antibodies pass through the breast milk
- Enhanced maternal–newborn bonding
- Involution of the uterus promoted by breastfeeding
- Delayed ovulation for women who breastfeed only (no supplements or pacifiers): breastfeeding provides a measure of contraceptive protection for 6 months, or until the woman's first period after the birth (whichever comes first)
- Correct temperature of breast milk
- Availability and convenience of breast milk
- Economical aspects

It is important for the nurse to educate the mother about the advantages of breastfeeding, to enable her to make a decision based on this information and her lifestyle needs. Chapter 65 presents additional details on feeding a newborn.

Assisting a Nursing Mother.   During the first few days, the mother's breasts produce *colostrum,* which is rich in disease-fighting immunities and nutrients. Although the mother's true milk is not in yet, the newborn should nurse often to receive the health benefits of colostrum, to condition the woman's nipples for nursing, and to stimulate milk production. Frequent nursing also prevents engorgement and related complications. The newborn's sucking stimulates milk production.

It is common for newborns to be too sleepy to nurse. Sleepy babies can often be roused by a diaper or clothing change or a sponge bath. Falling asleep while nursing is also normal for newborns.

When the mother's true milk "comes in" by the second, third, or fourth day, a breastfeeding baby typically nurses 8 to 12 times per day. The woman should first offer the breast from which the baby nursed last, because it may not have been emptied completely. Deciding which breast to offer first is often easy, because one feels fuller than the other. The baby should nurse at least 10 minutes on one breast before being offered the other breast. Letting the baby signal when he or she wants to switch is best in order for the newborn to get the right balance of calories. When the baby first begins nursing, he or she gets **foremilk,** which is relatively low in fat. **Hindmilk** appears at the end of the feeding and is higher in fat and calories.

Many women seem concerned about their milk supply after a few weeks because their breasts feel softer and less full. This is normal and due to the body's adjustment to the newborn's needs. Often, a baby who has settled into a nice feeding pattern begins to nurse more often for a day or two. This baby is probably experiencing a growth spurt. Although the mother may not have enough milk the first day, her body will quickly adapt, and her milk supply will increase. Then the baby will once more be satisfied, and will again reduce the frequency of wanting to nurse.

During the early days and months, many babies suck for pleasure, which is called *nonnutritive sucking.* When a baby is actually nursing, the mother will hear a "suck-suck-swallow" pattern. No swallow occurs during nonnutritive sucking.

Signs that the breast-fed newborn is receiving adequate nutrition are at least six to eight wet diapers and at least two stools per day. Once the neonate has finished passing the meconium (within 24 to 48 hours), the breast-fed baby's stool will be loose and unformed, and range in color from pea soup to yellow to tan. The stool may appear seedy and will have little odor. By 6 weeks, most breast-fed babies have only one to two daily soft bowel movements, because breast milk is so well absorbed.

One approach to documenting a mother's progress and success with breastfeeding is the **LATCH** (Latch, Audible swallowing, Type of nipple, Comfort, Hold) breastfeeding charting system, which is described in detail in Table 66-2.

Common Problems of Breastfeeding.   Breast care for the mother who is nursing her newborn varies. The goal is to simplify procedures while avoiding infection. In some facilities, the mother rinses her nipples before each feeding. In other facilities, however, this practice is not followed because it is believed that breast milk contains lactic acid, which acts as a natural cleanser for the nipples. Previous practices of "toughening" the nipples, washing them vigorously, and applying creams are not currently recommended. Nursing mothers are at risk for the following common problems.

Sore and Cracked Nipples. Improper positioning is most often the cause of sore nipples. Prevention of sore nipples is

■■■ TABLE 66-2 ℒATCH BREASTFEEDING CHARTING SYSTEM

		0	1	2
L	Latch	Too sleepy or reluctant. No latch achieved.	Repeated attempts. Hold nipple in mouth. Stimulate to suck.	Grasps breast. Tongue down. Lips flanged. Rhythmic sucking.
A	Audible swallowing	None	A few with stimulation.	Spontaneous and intermittent under 24 h old. Spontaneous and frequent over 24 h old.
T	Type of nipple	Inverted	Flat	Everted (after stimulation)
C	Comfort (breast/nipple)	Engorged. Cracked, bleeding, large blisters or bruises. Severe discomfort.	Filling. Reddened/small blisters or bruises. Mild/moderate discomfort.	Soft, nontender
H	Hold (positioning)	Full assist (staff holds infant at breast)	Minimal assist (ie, place pillows for support, elevate head of bed). Teach one side; mother does other. Staff holds and then mother takes over.	No assist from staff. Mother able to position and hold baby by self.

From Jensen, D., Wallace, S., & Kelsey, P. (1994). LATCH: A breastfeeding charting system and documentation tool. *Journal of Obstetric, Gynecologic, and Neonatal Nursing, 23,* 27.

very important. The suction of the baby at the breast is strongest in the first minutes of feeding, so a longer feeding period may actually reduce the chance of nipple soreness, rather than make it worse. Also, changing the position in which the mother holds the baby at the breast for each feeding session helps to change the area of greatest suction.

In the early days of nursing, a baby with a vigorous suck may cause discomfort. Nipple soreness caused by an enthusiastic baby should ease as the woman's nipples become conditioned. Treatment of sore nipples includes swabbing the affected nipple with breast milk and allowing it to air dry; wearing a nursing bra and leaving the flaps down for a few minutes after feeding to air dry the nipples; changing breast pads when wet; and assisting the infant to "latch on" to the nipple and areola properly.

Other remedies may also be helpful. The tannic acid in brewed tea is believed to help speed healing. The mother can apply it by blotting a steeped, cool tea bag on the sore nipple or areola after feeding. Vitamin E oil may be used sparingly,

but it must be rinsed off with clear water before the next feeding, to prevent the buildup of a toxic level of vitamin E that is ingested from the nipple.

Soap should not be used on the breasts. (It is drying, and promotes nipple cracking.) Flexible nipple shields are available, but may actually contribute to sore nipples by rubbing against the nipple as the baby sucks. In addition, the baby may be unable to effectively grasp the breast for complete emptying at feeding time.

A well-fitting non-waterproof cotton bra is essential. Waterproof bras hold in moisture, which can cause irritation or maceration of the nipples. The breasts should be firmly supported. See In Practice: Educating the Client 66-2 for information about assisting a nursing mother.

Engorgement. Engorgement is extreme fullness of the areola and/or breast. Some degree of engorgement is normal. Two or 3 days after giving birth, a breastfeeding woman may feel the tingling and fullness that indicates her milk is "coming in." It is a good idea to provide anticipatory guidance

---

In Practice
Educating the Client 66-2

ASSISTING A NURSING MOTHER

The mother will often nurse her newborn immediately after birth and again within 4 hours. If the mother does not ask to nurse, the birth attendant may suggest it. You may do so as well. The delivery room staff should cooperate if the mother agrees. Use thermal heat or a radiant warmer to heat the nursing couple if the room is cool, or if the mother is shivering from strenuous labor or medication. Breast-fed newborns usually do not receive supplementary water or bottles in the nursery, to avoid nipple confusion and to encourage nursing at the breast.

Help the breastfeeding mother the first few times so that she learns the best positioning. Proper positioning helps the newborn to receive milk easily. It minimizes nipple soreness, plugged ducts, and mastitis. It also provides comfort for both the mother and the newborn during feedings. The mother can use the cradle or football hold, or she can lie on her side.

Teach the mother the following steps:

- Use the arm to support the newborn. If using the cradle hold, place the back of the newborn's head in the crook of your arm, with your hand holding the newborn's bottom or thigh.
- Support the nursing breast with your opposite hand. Place the hand below the breast on your rib cage. Use as many fingers as necessary to support the breast without covering any of the nipple. Place your thumb above the nipple. This grasp is called the *C-hold* or *palmar grasp*.
- Turn the newborn's body toward yours, so that you are stomach-to-stomach.

- Tickle the newborn's bottom lip or corner of the mouth to trigger the rooting reflex. You will coax the newborn to open his or her mouth. Wait until the newborn's mouth is open wide. *Rationale: If the mouth is not wide open, the newborn will grasp the tip of the nipple, causing soreness.*
- Pull the newborn close. As soon as his or her mouth is wide open, move the baby quickly to the breast so that the nipple passes the gums well into the mouth. The newborn should have the whole areola in the mouth, not just the nipple. Use your arm to support the newborn. His or her chin should touch your breast. If the newborn's nose is covered, press your breast away from the nose, so that the baby can breathe easily.
- To stop nursing, place your finger between the baby's mouth and your areola to break suction.
- If you feel pain while nursing, break suction and begin again. *Rationale: Pain is not a normal part of breastfeeding.*
- Offer both breasts at each feeding, first offering the breast used last at the previous feeding. *Rationale: Each breast needs to be emptied regularly.*

Many women feel a slight tingling sensation when they begin to nurse, called the *let-down reflex*. The newborn's sucking action triggers hormones that cause the woman's brain to release milk from the alveolus. Many "let downs" occur during a single nursing session. The let-down reflex can be impaired when the mother is stressed, cold, or in pain. Alcohol use can also inhibit milk flow.

about this event, and to suggest that she nurse the baby as soon as she feels this sensation. Doing so may help prevent engorgement of the breasts. Frequent nursing also helps in the prevention of engorgement.

If engorgement is already present, have the mother shower or use warm, moist heat before it is time to nurse, and then manually express some milk to soften the breast. This measure allows the newborn to get a proper grasp on the nipple and prevents further pain for the mother. Massaging from the outer breast toward the nipple also helps to soften the engorged breast, to allow for easier hand expression or nursing. The most important treatment is to nurse frequently.

Plugged Ducts. Incomplete emptying of the breasts may cause plugged ducts, or tender lumps in the breasts of an otherwise healthy lactating woman. The treatment is to continue nursing. Massaging the area and applying heat before nursing helps ensure complete emptying. Nursing on the opposite breast first will allow the affected breast to "let down," easing the affected side. Proper positioning also may help. The mother's bra should be checked for proper fit.

Mastitis. **Mastitis** is almost always caused by bacteria from the baby's mouth that enter the mother's breast through a crack in the nipple. Preventive measures are reducing those steps that reduce the chances of soreness and cracking of the nipple: changing positions, nursing more frequently, and nursing at least 10 minutes on each breast.

Signs of mastitis include a sore, red area that feels warm to the touch. Because the bacteria came from the baby's mouth, continued nursing is not harmful to the baby, and is helpful to the mother! The best advice for this client is to continue nursing during treatment for mastitis. Treatment includes heat, antibiotic therapy, rest, and plenty of fluids. There are many antibiotics that are safe for a nursing woman to take; her healthcare provider will select the one that is best for her.

Complications of the postpartum period may also include hematoma, hemorrhage, uterine atony, thrombophlebitis, puerperal infections, cystitis, and depression. These subjects are discussed in Chapter 67.

Nutrition for a Breastfeeding Mother. A well-nourished mother ensures an adequate and nutritious milk supply for her newborn and protects her own health. On the other hand, a poorly nourished mother, or one who is restricting her calories, may not produce enough breast milk. Nursing mothers should receive about 500 calories a day above their nonnursing caloric intake. Adequate fluids are also important for milk production. Usually, following the nutritional guidelines for pregnancy provides the nursing mother with adequate food intake. If she exclusively nurses the infant beyond 4 months of age, her dietary needs will increase as the infant's nutritional needs increase. The nursing mother need not restrict her intake of favorite foods just because she is nursing, although a few foods and beverages cause concern.

Alcohol does appear in breast milk, and large quantities in the maternal diet have been shown to inhibit the let-down reflex. Babies of heavy alcohol drinkers nurse less often and for shorter periods. Alcohol does relax the mother, but there is not sufficient information about a safe level of alcohol intake to assure a mother that drinking any alcohol while nursing is absolutely safe for her baby.

Caffeine also transfers to breast milk. A moderate intake (1 to 2 cups of coffee daily) is fine; however, if the baby appears wakeful, restless, or irritable, the mother should cut down on or eliminate her caffeine intake.

The use of cow's milk by the mother has possibly been linked to colic in newborns. If the baby is colicky, the mother may want to eliminate milk from her diet for 2 weeks to see if it makes a difference. Colic usually worsens if a breast-fed baby is switched to a formula.

Strongly flavored foods may cause temporary colic in some babies. This colic usually lasts approximately 24 hours. Common offenders are onions, garlic, beans, and rhubarb.

Use of Medications While Breastfeeding. Breast milk passes many medications from mother to infant. The nursing mother should consult her baby's pediatrician before taking any drugs (Box 66-4).

Bottle Feeding

Although it is widely accepted that "breast is best," formulas have been developed that are satisfactory breast milk replacements. Breastfeeding may be undesirable when the mother has a chronic disease (such as HIV infection), if the nipples are severely inverted, or if the baby has certain abnormalities.

In the event of a premature delivery and in some other situations, the mother may express her breast milk, which may be bottle fed to the baby. Some women choose to bottle feed for social or personal reasons.

There are many formulas available; each product has its own advantages. The baby's healthcare provider orders the specific formula appropriate for the newborn's needs.

During the first week of feeding, most babies take from 1 to 3 ounces per feeding, with a total intake of 12 to 15 ounces every 24 hours. This amount increases to approximately 20 ounces in 24 hours by the end of the second week. Intake increases rapidly thereafter. By the third week, many babies drop an evening or a night feeding and sleep longer without hunger.

The person feeding the baby must wash his or her hands before receiving the newborn. Use care in keeping the nipple of the bottle clean. Check the rate of flow from the nipple, to make certain that it has a constant drip. Nipple openings are made either with a "cross cut" or with holes. If the opening is not large enough, the hole can be enlarged by putting a red-hot needle through it. If the opening is too large, the baby may tend to choke.

While the baby is eating, the person who is feeding the newborn should tilt the bottle, so that milk is in the neck of the bottle at all times or so the plastic liner folds in on itself, to keep the baby from swallowing air. The baby should be bubbled at intervals during the feeding.

Feeding does not just provide nutrition; it also gives the baby a sense of security and of being loved. The baby should not be left alone with a propped bottle, either in the nursery at the hospital or at home. The mother, father, or other caregiver should always hold the baby and cuddle him or her during the feeding.

➤ ➤ BOX 66-4

MEDICATIONS AND BREASTFEEDING

Many drugs pass into breast milk from the mother. There are many factors that determine whether a medication is safe for a nursing mother to take. Not all drugs pass in the same concentration, or remain in breast milk at a stable concentration. The concentration in the breast milk depends on fat solubility, water solubility, the rate at which the mother's body metabolizes the drug, the time between taking doses of the medication, and other factors. The effect on the nursing baby depends on the drug concentration, as well as on the age and the maturity of the baby.

Just as during pregnancy, a nursing mother should not take any medication or drug without asking her healthcare provider.

Guidelines for Drug Safety in Breastfeeding

Drugs taken by the mother that are *particularly dangerous* to the nursing newborn:

- Anticancer drugs (chemotherapy)
- Radioactive substances (such as those used for diagnostic tests or treatment of cancers)
- Lithium (used to treat psychiatric disorders)
- All drugs of abuse, including

    Amphetamines

    Cocaine

    Heroin

    LSD

    PCP

    Excessive nicotine and alcohol

These drugs are generally considered compatible with breastfeeding:

- Acetaminophen (Tylenol)
- Many antibiotics (penicillins, cephalosporins, erythromycin)
- Codeine
- Phenytoin (Dilantin)
- Pseudoephedrine (Sudafed)

If you are using a bottle to feed a baby, hold him or her exactly as you would the breast-fed baby, and teach family caregivers to do the same. To prevent aspiration of milk and to promote bonding, do not prop the bottle. A propped bottle may also contribute to ear infections because the milk can flow from the throat into the baby's Eustachian tube.

Because bacteria thrive in milk, the parents should be taught to exercise care when preparing the newborn's formula. Many families use either a premixed formula or a formula that is simply mixed with water. If the formula is purchased in small, disposable bottles, the bottles are already sterilized. When using disposable bottles, caregivers must be sure that the plastic bag is securely fastened into the holder and that the baby cannot pull the end of the bag through the side of the holder while

feeding. Also, bottles usually do not need to be disinfected if they are cleaned in an automatic dishwasher.

Formula is usually given at room temperature. A bottle should not be warmed in a microwave; this creates "hot spots" in the formula that may burn the baby's mouth and throat unexpectedly. The person feeding the baby should also check the temperature of the formula. Room or body temperature is appropriate.

Bubbling (Burping) the Baby

☛ KEY CONCEPT

Bubbling must be done whether the baby is breast-fed or bottle-fed.

Newborns must be properly bubbled (burped) during and after each feeding to prevent regurgitation of food and possible aspiration of food into the lungs. The breast-fed baby should be bubbled when switching from one breast to the other; the bottle-fed baby should be bubbled after every ½ to 1 ounce of fluid for the first day or so. All babies should be bubbled after a feeding. The time between bubblings gradually increases, but caregivers must be sure that the baby is not retaining any gas in the stomach at the end of the feeding.

Several methods for holding the baby during bubbling are recommended. Hold the baby so that he or she expels gas in the stomach without regurgitating. You can hold the newborn upright on your knee or against your shoulder. Gently pat or rub the baby's back. Alternatively, you may place the baby prone over your knees, gently rubbing his or her back (Fig. 66-6).

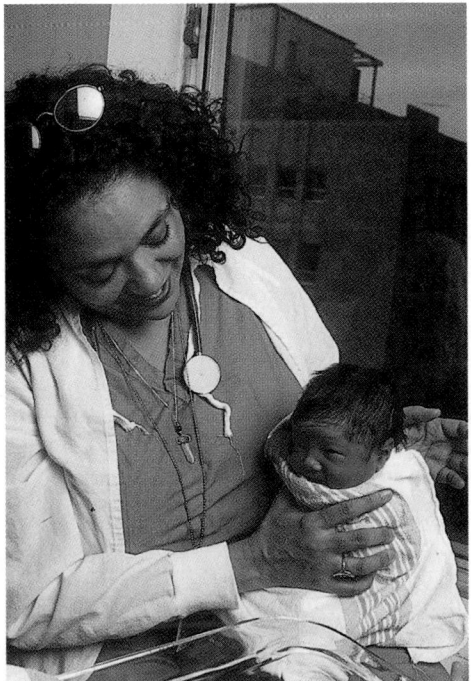

FIGURE 66-6. The nurse demonstrates a sitting position for burping a newborn. The infant's head is supported by the nurse's hand.

Supplements

The physician may suggest that vitamin concentrates be added to feedings when the newborn is 2 to 3 weeks old. Milk contains the other essential nutrients for the first 6 months of life, although iron is often given to prevent iron deficiency anemia.

Breast milk or formula alone is the only source of nutrition that the baby needs for the first 4 to 6 months of life. Parents should be taught that adding other foods, such as cereals, too early can lead to digestive problems and allergies.

DISCHARGE

Prior to discharge, the birth attendant examines the newborn thoroughly. All birth and newborn records are completed. The family is instructed regarding the care of the newborn (see In Practice: Educating the Client 66-3 for newborn tub bath guidelines).

The family also are notified of when the newborn must return to the healthcare provider's office for an examination. Sometimes there is a need for a Public Health Department or home care referral. If so, a visiting nurse will contact the caregivers after they arrive home with their new baby. The home visit is quite common, and is particularly valuable when the mother and baby have been discharged very soon after the birth.

Ensuring Safety

Identification.   At discharge, the nurse should remove one of the newborn's identification bands and place it on the chart, which the mother then signs.

Use of Infant Car Seat.   All babies should be sent home securely restrained in an infant car seat, which is installed as recommended in the back seat of the car. The car seat for the newborn should be rear-facing.

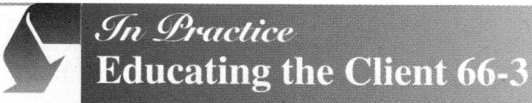

In Practice
Educating the Client 66-3

GIVING THE NEWBORN A TUB BATH

Teach parents and other family caregivers the following steps when bathing their newborn.

- Do not give a tub bath until the baby's cord falls off.
- Be sure that the room is warm enough and that the newborn is protected from drafts.
- Never talk on the telephone or leave the baby unattended—even for a moment!—during the bath, to prevent accidents such as falling or drowning.
- Have all equipment ready and conveniently placed: baby bath tub, bath thermometer, two wash cloths, towels, baby soap, clean clothes and diaper, and lotion. You cannot leave the baby after you start the bath.
- Wash your hands to prevent spreading infection.
- Check the water temperature carefully; it should be warm, not hot (98.6° F or 37° C is the usual maximum temperature).
- Carefully support the newborn's head and body with a moderately firm grip when you put him or her in the tub.
- Use a soft wash cloth, towel, and only a small amount of soap.
- Rinse all soap off.
- Dry the baby, paying particular attention to drying the skinfolds well.
- Look for skin irritation or abnormalities.

STUDENT SYNTHESIS

Key Points

- The Apgar score is used for immediate assessment of the newborn based on heart rate, respiratory effort, muscle tone, reflex irritability, and color. The maximum score is 10. The evaluation is done at 1 minute after birth, and again at 5 minutes. An Apgar score of 7 or less indicates a need for neonatal resuscitation.
- Newborns can lose heat by convection, conduction, radiation, and evaporation.
- To prevent cold-stress, the nurse should keep the baby dry, provide a hat or cap to prevent heat loss from the head, provide a heat source for the baby until his or her temperature stabilizes (skin-to-skin contact with a parent, isolette, or radiant warmer), and maintain the room's temperature at about 75° F.
- At the time of delivery, neonatal assessments include the Apgar score, further evaluation of need for resuscitation, temperature regulation, and neonatal adaptation to life outside the uterus.
- When an infant is admitted to the nursery, ongoing assessments include evaluation of respiratory status, temperature regulation, umbilical cord, body measurements, and elimination.
- Daily newborn assessments include weight, respiration, elimination, and feeding. Each of these items should be reviewed at the time of discharge.
- Newborn identification is essential to ensure that the mother goes home with her own baby.
- Identification measures used in many hospitals include using matching identification bands, taking footprints, using electronic bracelets, and keeping an accurate and complete hospital record. The identification should be confirmed each time the mother and baby are brought together, and again at hospital discharge.
- The normal newborn has a respiratory rate of less than 60 breaths per minute, a heart rate of 110 to

150 beats per minute, and a normal body temperature. The infant may have a variety of temporary or permanent skin markings. Effects of maternal hormones on the baby's breasts and genitals may last for a few weeks.

- When weighing the infant, care should be taken to avoid cold-stress; the baby must never be left alone. In measuring the infant, use the crib sheet to mark where the crown of the head is, then stretch the legs, make another mark, and measure between the marks.
- Daily care of the neonate includes cord care, skin care, assessment of possible problems, and attention to the baby's needs for security, safety, and bonding with the parents.
- A circumcised male infant needs frequent changes of a sterile dressing over the wound and assessment for complications; he should not be laid on his stomach.
- Normal newborn stools progress from meconium to transitional stools as feeding begins. Breast-fed babies have loose, yellow stools; babies drinking formula have more firm stools that may be darker in color.
- The nursing mother needs information regarding helping the baby latch on; taking care of the nipples; alternating breasts; using different positions; and recognizing complications.
- Bottle-fed babies should be held during feedings just as breast-fed babies. The bottle should not be propped, and the infant should not be left unattended.
- All babies should be bubbled during and after feeding. This can be accomplished by sitting the baby on your lap, holding the baby on your shoulder, or laying the baby across your knees and gently patting his or her back until bubbling occurs. Some spitting up is normal.

Critical Thinking Exercises

1. Review the list of newborn reflexes. Why do you think that each of these might exist? Find a book or article that discusses at least one reflex, and write down an explanation that you could give to a new parent as you demonstrate the baby's reflex.
2. Heat loss is a critical factor for newborns. Develop a plan to protect a newborn from the major sources of heat loss in an acute care facility. Compare and contrast that plan with an infant delivered at home.

NCLEX-Style Review Questions

1. A neonate is a child under the age of:
   a. 14 days
   b. 28 days
   c. 6 months
   d. 1 year
2. Baby boy H. B. has a 1-minute Apgar score of 6. What should you do?
   a. Do nothing unless the 5-minute Apgar score has not improved.
   b. Call for someone skilled in neonatal resuscitation to come immediately.
   c. Ask the birth attendant to leave the mother and come take care of the baby.
   d. Stimulate the baby for the next several minutes by briskly rubbing the back.
3. Molding of the newborn's head is:
   a. Swelling of the scalp from pressure during birth
   b. Bruising on the cheeks and temples from the use of forceps
   c. Accumulation of blood between the bones of the skull and the periosteum
   d. Elongation of the head from the bones overlapping as it passed through the birth canal
4. Which of the following statements is true about the characteristics of a preterm baby compared with a term baby:
   a. The preterm baby will have less lanugo and less vernix.
   b. The preterm baby will have less lanugo, but more vernix.
   c. The preterm baby will have more lanugo, but less vernix.
   d. The preterm baby will have more lanugo and more vernix.
5. Medications given in the delivery room to an infant could include:
   a. Erythromycin ointment and vitamin B_{12}
   b. Erythromycin ointment and vitamin K
   c. Triple-antibiotic ointment and vitamin B_{12}
   d. Triple-antibiotic ointment and vitamin K
6. The nurse should report if a newborn does not pass urine by:
   a. 4 hours of age
   b. 8 hours of age
   c. 12 hours of age
   d. 24 hours of age

Reference

1. Simpson, K. R., & Creehan, P. A. (2001). *AWHONN perinatal nursing* (2nd ed., p. 506). Philadelphia: Lippincott Williams & Wilkins.

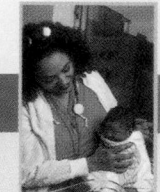

CHAPTER

67

High-Risk Pregnancy and Childbirth

LEARNING OBJECTIVES

1. Explain the term high-risk pregnancy.
2. Define and differentiate between the following tests used to assess fetal status: amniocentesis, ultrasound scanning, OCT, NST, FBP, PUBS, CVS, and MSAFP.
3. Define and differentiate among the following types of abortions: threatened, complete, septic, recurrent spontaneous, inevitable, incomplete, missed, and induced or therapeutic. State at least three nursing considerations for each.
4. State at least three nursing considerations for an ectopic pregnancy.
5. Describe the events leading to gestational trophoblastic disease and state at least three nursing considerations related to the outcome of this condition.
6. Discuss at least five implications to mother and fetus when hyperemesis gravidarum exists.
7. Define PIH, mild and severe preeclampsia, and eclampsia. State at least three nursing considerations for each condition.
8. Discuss at least five nursing implications related to a pregnant woman with existing diabetes mellitus.
9. State at least three nursing implications related to the pregnant woman with an existing cardiac disorder or who has a chemical dependency.
10. Define and discuss the following disorders: maternal infection, Rh sensitization, erythroblastosis fetalis, ABO incompatibility, and polyhydramnios. State at least three nursing concerns for each condition.
11. Define and differentiate among placenta previa, abruptio placentae, and placenta accreta. State at least three nursing considerations for each condition.
12. Discuss at least three nursing implications related to each of the following: prolonged pregnancy, multiple pregnancy, adolescent pregnancy, and pregnancy in the woman over age 40.
13. Develop a nursing care plan for a client with the following complications: maternal hemorrhage, PROM, preterm labor, precipitate labor and delivery, uterine rupture, uterine inertia and fetal dystocia, CPD, and abnormal fetal presentation.
14. Define and differentiate at least three aspects of nursing care related to a prolapsed cord and a nuchal cord.
15. Discuss at least three nursing considerations related to the induction of labor with drugs and amniotomy.
16. Discuss at least three nursing considerations related to version, forceps delivery, and vacuum extraction.
17. Discuss at least three nursing considerations related to preoperative care and postoperative care following a cesarean delivery. Identify at least three special considerations related to care of the newborn.
18. Identify and discuss common complications of the postpartum period, including postpartum hematoma, postpartum hemorrhage, uterine atony, thrombophlebitis, puerperal infection, cystitis, and mastitis.
19. Define and differentiate among postpartum blues, depression, and psychosis.
20. In the skills lab, role-play a scenario in which a newborn has died, using therapeutic communications.

NEW TERMINOLOGY

ABO incompatibility	gestational diabetes	postpartum hemorrhage
abruptio placentae	high-risk pregnancy	preeclampsia
amniocentesis	hydatidiform mole	premature cervical dilatic
amniotomy	hydramnios	products of conception
atony	hyperemesis gravidarum	prolapsed cord
breech		puerperal
cerclage	induction	station
cesarean delivery	macrosomia	stress test
choriocarcinoma	mastitis	thrombophlebiti
cystitis	nuchal cord	uterine inertia
delivery forceps	placenta accreta	transverse lie
dystocia	placenta previa	vacuum extraction
eclampsia	polyhydramnios	version
ectopic	postpartum hematoma	vertex
erythroblastosis fetalis		

ACRONYMS

AB	DIC	MSAFP	PUBS
BOA	FBP	NST	ROP
BPM	FHT	OCT	SVE
CPD	LOP	OP	
CVS	LS	PIH	
D&C	MgSO$_4$	PROM	

Although pregnancy, labor, and delivery are normal physiologic processes, complications can arise at any time, with serious consequences for the woman and fetus. The term **high-risk pregnancy** (or *at-risk pregnancy*) is used when physiologic or psychological factors could significantly increase the chances of mortality or morbidity of the woman or fetus. Early antepartal care helps to identify these problems so that interventions can begin quickly.

Complications related to childbirth have a physical and an emotional impact. The woman faces many hazards to her own well-being, and she has concerns about her baby. For example, prolonged and difficult labor is physically and emotionally draining. This fatigue can interfere with the initial bonding between mother and newborn.

TESTS TO ASSESS FETAL STATUS

Various tests are used to assess fetal status and fetal maturity. The most commonly used tests include amniocentesis, ultrasonic scanning, the oxytocic challenge test, and the nonstress test.

Amniocentesis

Amniocentesis is the insertion of a needle through the maternal abdominal wall into the amniotic sac to withdraw amniotic fluid. This invasive test can be performed in the examiner's office or on an outpatient basis. *An ultrasound scan should always precede amniocentesis,* to determine the location of the placenta and the fetal parts. The examiner confirms the fetal position by palpation, cleanses the area, and anesthetizes the skin site. He or she inserts a long, sterile needle through the woman's abdominal and uterine walls into the amniotic sac. He or she then withdraws approximately 20 milliliters of fluid, removes the needle, and covers the insertion site with a bandage. Amniocentesis involves some risk. Placental and fetal damage, premature labor, or abortion may result, although the use of ultrasound minimizes these risks.

Information Provided. Amniocentesis tests for fetal abnormalities and establishes fetal lung maturity. For example, it can diagnose some disorders causing fetal intellectual impairment, such as *Down syndrome* and *Tay-Sachs disease;* as well as inherited disorders, such as *muscular dystrophy* and *cystic fibrosis;* and some fetal abnormalities, such as *spina bifida.* Amniocentesis is frequently used to determine the status of an Rh-positive fetus in an Rh-negative woman. The birth attendant may order an amniocentesis when he or she suspects intrauterine growth retardation or when exact determination of fetal maturity is essential.

Nursing Considerations. Instruct the client to empty her bladder before the test (to prevent bladder rupture). Monitor the woman's vital signs during the test and for at least 1 hour afterward. Monitor fetal heart tones (**FHTs**) to ensure that the fetus is not in distress; the external fetal monitor is most often used. Instruct the woman to notify the birth attendant if she has any difficulties after returning home, including any bleeding or cramping.

Ultrasonic Scanning

An *ultrasound scan* uses high-frequency sound waves to produce a picture of intrauterine activity. The graphic recording of this picture is called a *sonogram.* From this image, the examiner can learn a great deal about the developing fetus.

A *transducer,* placed on the skin of the abdomen, passes sound waves into the fetus. Because of various densities of body tissues (such as bone and muscle), the waves are echoed back to the transducer at different rates. A computer transforms the echo into an image on the monitor.

Information Provided. An ultrasound scan can determine gestational age, fetal head size, location of the placenta, and some fetal abnormalities. It can identify multiple pregnancies and in some cases, it can also determine the sex of the fetus. Ultrasound is commonly used in conjunction with tests such as amniocentesis. The woman is often allowed to watch the fetus move and listen to the heartbeat. She is usually given a print or videotape of the ultrasound to take home.

Nursing Considerations. Explain to the woman that a full bladder is necessary for the test so that the fetal parts will move up into the abdomen, allowing for better visualization of the fetus. Ask the woman to drink large amounts of liquids. Tell her she will not be allowed to empty her bladder. This test takes 20 minutes, with no known harmful effects. The test is noninvasive.

Oxytocin Challenge Test

Information Provided. The oxytocin challenge test (**OCT**), also known as the **stress test,** is a way to evaluate the response of the fetal heart to contractions. It provides information as to how well the placenta is supplying oxygen to the fetus. Therefore, it is particularly useful in detecting fetuses that are beginning to experience difficulty due to inadequate placental circulation.

Nipple stimulation can initiate uterine contractions, but most often IV oxytocin is used. An IV administration of oxytocin by infusion pump is begun. Its rate of administration increases until three contractions occur within 10 minutes. The reaction of the fetal heart is determined using the fetal monitor. If, toward the end of a contraction, the fetal heart rate decreases (*late deceleration*), uteroplacental insufficiency is indicated, which may lead to fetal death. An OCT is classified as *positive* when there are persistent late decelerations with more than 50% of the contractions. A decision is made about continuing the pregnancy or performing a cesarean delivery.

Nursing Considerations. Although the OCT is not dangerous in itself, it may stimulate labor. Therefore, it is generally performed in the labor and delivery area of the healthcare facility—rather than in the clinic setting—after the fetus is viable; that is, after it is able to survive outside the uterus (20–24 weeks' gestation).

Nonstress Test

The nonstress test (**NST**) provides information on the fetal heart rate in response to fetal activity. The healthy fetus is active in utero, and the fetal heart rate normally increases as the fetus moves in the uterus. To perform the NST, an external fetal monitor is strapped to the woman's abdomen, and she is asked to press a button each time she feels the fetus move. This monitoring process is carried out for approximately 40 minutes.

Information Provided. An NST is classified as *reactive* when at least two episodes of fetal heart rate accelerations of 15 beats per minute (**BPM**) last at least 15 seconds within a continuous 10-minute period. A reactive test shows that the fetal heart rate increases with every fetal movement, and that the fetus is doing well.

A *nonreactive* test shows that the fetal heart rate did not increase with activity, and that the fetus may thus be suffering from lack of oxygen. The fetus may fail to be active during the course of the test. The fetus is then stimulated by other methods, which include palpating or shaking the uterus, making loud noises, or stimulating the woman's nipples.

Fetal Biophysical Profile

The fetal biophysical profile (**FBP**) combines an NST with ultrasonic fetal assessment. Using ultrasound, the examiner evaluates fetal breathing, fetal movement, fetal tone, amniotic fluid volume, and placental grade. These components, including the nonstress test, are scored between 0 (abnormal) to 12 (normal). With a score of 8 to 12, the fetus is considered to be doing well.

Other Tests

Newer tests providing information from direct access to the fetus are percutaneous umbilical blood sampling (**PUBS**) and chorionic villus sampling (**CVS**). These tests diagnose fetal defects early in pregnancy. They are invasive procedures and carry serious risks for both the woman and fetus. Usually these tests are done if the woman is considering an abortion due to a serious genetic defect. PUBS has also become the preferred method of intrauterine blood transfusion for Rh-sensitized fetuses, because it can be done early in the pregnancy.

Maternal serum α-fetoprotein (**MSAFP**) levels are increasingly used as a screening tool to detect the presence of fetal neural tube defects and open abdominal wall defects early in pregnancy.

INTERRUPTED PREGNANCY

Pregnancy may be interrupted due to abortion, premature cervical dilation, ectopic pregnancy, or hydatidiform mole. The loss or termination of a pregnancy has physical, psychological, and emotional consequences for the woman. Nursing care focuses on meeting the woman's immediate needs and providing support.

Abortion

Abortion (**AB**) describes the natural or artificial (through medical intervention) termination of a pregnancy. Abortions occur commonly in nature. Several categories of abortions are discussed in this section.

Medically induced abortion remains a controversial issue. Certain religions oppose most medically initiated abortions for various reasons. Roman Catholic hospitals, for example, may not perform abortions unless specific criteria are met, such as a life-threatening situation for the mother. A healthcare professional may refuse to participate in an induced abortion based on religious or moral grounds.

If the aborting woman is Rh negative, a specific anti-D immune globulin, such as RhoGAM, should be given as a precautionary measure against Rh sensitization. (RhoGAM is discussed in a later section on Rh sensitization.)

There are two major categories of abortion:

Spontaneous: Without medical intervention (that is, by natural causes); often called a *miscarriage* by lay people. Several categories are presented below.
Induced or *therapeutic:* With medical intervention by way of mechanical assistance or medical agents. Therapeutic abortions are discussed below.

Spontaneous Abortion

It is estimated that approximately 10% to 20% of all pregnancies end in *spontaneous abortion*. Fetal abnormalities or defects are the most frequent causes of spontaneous abortion. Maternal alcohol use and cigarette smoking may contribute. Other causes include maternal disorders, trauma (such as a motor vehicle accident), dietary factors, and abnormalities of pregnancy.

Threatened Abortion. This condition exists any time bleeding or cramping occurs in the first 20 weeks of pregnancy without major cervical dilation. Many birth attendants will not take extreme measures to save such a pregnancy because a spontaneous abortion is often nature's way of disposing of a malformed fetus. If bleeding is slight, however, hormones or muscle relaxants may be given. The client is put to bed with her feet elevated for 48 to 72 hours. If bleeding stops, she may resume limited activities. If true uterine contractions occur, the prognosis is more guarded.

Complete Abortion. This occurs when the woman spontaneously expels all the **products of conception** (ie, the placenta and fetus). The uterus then contracts toward normal size, and the cervix closes. The same care that routinely follows a normal delivery is given to the woman. Observe the client closely for signs of hemorrhage. Check her blood pressure to see that it remains stable. Note and report any changes in skin color, especially pallor or cyanosis. Check her pulse (a weak, rapid pulse is a sign of shock). The birth attendant checks to make sure the uterus is contracted. Document the number of perineal pads the client uses and the amount of bleeding.

Septic Abortion. This is the term given when the contents of the uterus become infected before or during an abortion, or when the uterus becomes infected later. *Septic (endotoxic) shock* may occur and may cause maternal death.

Recurrent Spontaneous Abortion. Referred to in the past as *habitual abortion,* this term means that a woman has spontaneously lost three or more successive pregnancies. Recurrent spontaneous abortion is often due to an incompetent cervix that dilates prematurely. In such a case, the birth attendant usually makes every possible effort to save the pregnancy. Attempts are made to determine the cause of the recurrent abortions and to correct the situation if possible. Sometimes surgery may correct a problem causing the loss.

Some habitual and spontaneous abortions are the result of **premature cervical dilation,** during the second or early third trimester of pregnancy. This situation is also called *incompetent cervix*. Premature cervical dilation simply means that the cervix is unable to support a pregnancy. The weight of the fetus is enough to force the cervix to dilate, causing a spontaneous abortion.

Causes of this condition include cervical infections (eg, chlamydia), cervical or vaginal cancer, previous cervical biopsies or conizations, and prior multiple dilatation and curettage procedures. The cervical weakness may be congenital; one such cause is maternal exposure to diethylstilbestrol *in utero*.

Minor surgical procedures are often used for the pregnant woman with an incompetent cervix. A nonabsorbable suture called a cervical **cerclage** (Shirodkar or McDonald technique) or cervical ring is placed around the cervix. This suture holds the cervix closed during the remainder of the pregnancy; when the woman begins labor, the suture or ring is removed. If the cerclage is permanent, the woman requires a cesarean delivery.

Inevitable Abortion. An abortion in which the loss of the products of conception cannot be prevented is known as an *inevitable abortion*. Increased cramping and blood loss, with progressive cervical dilation, characterize this type of abortion.

Incomplete Abortion. This type of abortion occurs when the uterus expels some products of conception, but retains others. Extensive bleeding may occur. In this case, a dilatation and curettage (**D&C**) of the uterus is often performed. In a D&C, the surgeon dilates the cervix and then inserts instruments into the uterus. The uterine walls are scraped to remove any products of conception.

Missed Abortion. A *missed abortion* occurs when the fetus has died, but remains in the uterus. If the fetus is not expelled spontaneously within 1 month, the pregnancy will be terminated and a D&C performed.

For inevitable, incomplete, and missed abortions occurring between 16 and 20 weeks of pregnancy, a drug called dinoprostone (Prostin E2) may be administered to the mother. The drug causes the uterus to expel the fetus.

Induced Abortion

Therapeutic Abortion. A *therapeutic abortion* is the legal termination of pregnancy under a physician's direction. Induced abortion before the 16th to 20th week of gestation is legal in the United States and in many other countries, although an abortion may be difficult to obtain in some areas. It may be done for medical reasons or personal reasons.

A therapeutic abortion may be recommended for a woman whose life is in jeopardy due to the stress of pregnancy. Medical reasons for therapeutic abortion include severe maternal cardiac disease, severe renal or hypertensive disorder, or a fetus with a high probability of congenital anomaly. In some maternal psychiatric disorders or family crises, abortion is performed as an elective procedure.

Certain congenital disorders, which amniocentesis can determine at about the 14th week of gestation, are an indication for abortion to avoid the birth of a severely impaired child. If the woman has rubella (German measles) during pregnancy, especially during the first trimester, the likelihood of fetal defects is strong, and an abortion may be performed (see Chap. 73).

Criminal or Illegal Abortion. An intervention in pregnancy without medical or legal justification is a *criminal* or *illegal abortion*. Abortion is not legal in all situations. Because non-medical people normally carry out illegal abortions in unsterile environments, the risks to the pregnant woman are great. Major risks include hemorrhage and infection.

Complications of Abortion

When the placenta separates from the uterus, large blood vessels are exposed, which can lead to severe infection or hemorrhage. During the time when most abortions were performed illegally and generally under unsanitary conditions, sepsis was a common concern.

Untreated, post-abortion sepsis can be fatal. *Sterility* (the inability to conceive) is another common result. Therefore, maintaining *surgical asepsis* (sterile conditions) and removing all the products of conception from the uterus are vitally important.

Therapeutic abortions involve complex and difficult decisions. Regardless of the decision, depression, guilt, and anger are not uncommon psychological concerns.

> **Nursing Alert**
> A woman's blood pressure that spontaneously and rapidly drops may indicate maternal hemorrhage.

Ectopic Pregnancy

The word **ectopic** means *outside;* therefore, an ectopic pregnancy is one that implants outside the uterus (Fig. 67-1). The most common ectopic pregnancy is a *tubal pregnancy*. In rare cases, *abdominal* and *ovarian pregnancies* are seen.

Factors predisposing to ectopic pregnancy are tubal occlusion, an intrauterine contraceptive device, tumors, pelvic infections, endocrine imbalances, and abnormal tubal development. The symptoms of an ectopic pregnancy begin with spotting or bleeding 2 to 3 weeks after a missed menstrual period. Often pain accompanies the bleeding, which may be quite severe. A tubal pregnancy requires surgical removal of part or all of the affected tube to prevent rupture, a dangerous complication. An untreated ectopic pregnancy can be rapidly fatal due to shock from blood loss after tubal rupture.

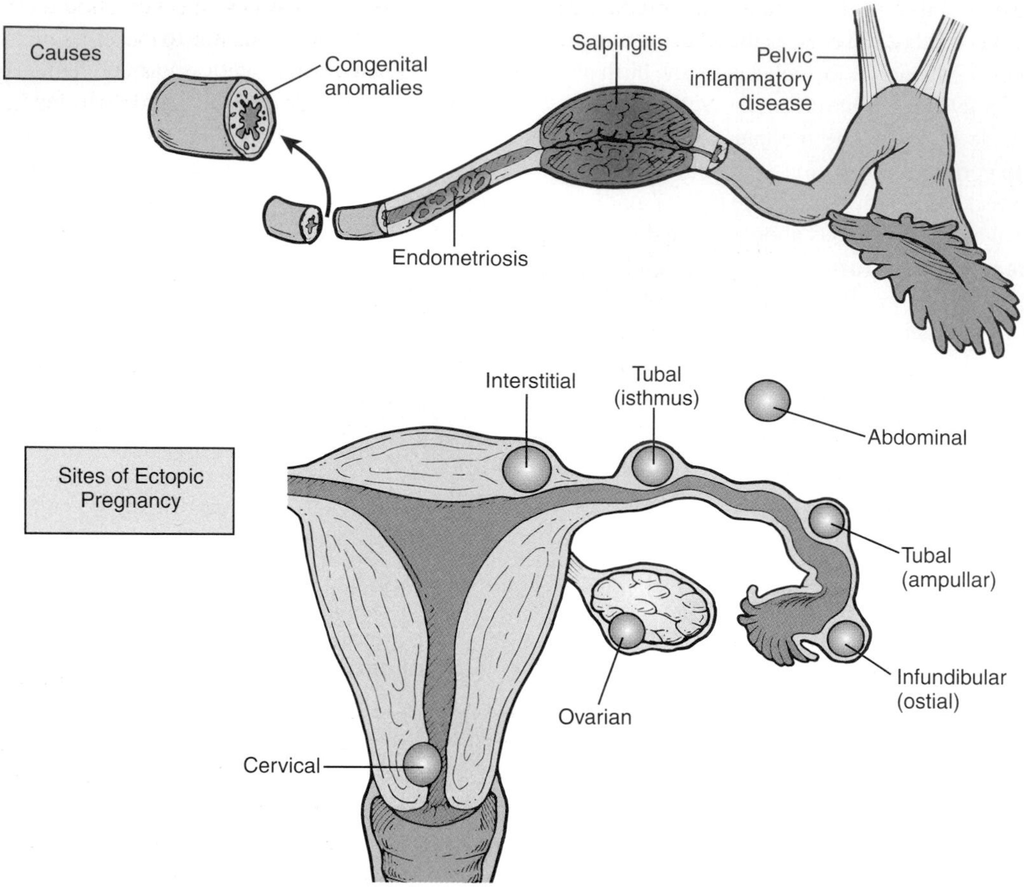

FIGURE 67-1. Causes and sites of ectopic pregnancy. (Reeder, S. J., Martin, L. L., & Koniak-Griffin, D. [1997]. *Maternity nursing: Family, newborn, and women's health care* [18th ed., p. 813]. Philadelphia: Lippincott-Raven.)

Gestational Trophoblastic Disease (Hydatidiform Mole)

In *gestational trophoblastic disease,* also known as **hydatidiform mole,** the embryo dies in utero, and the chorionic villi degenerate, forming grapelike clusters of vesicles. At first, the pregnancy appears normal, but then the uterus enlarges more rapidly than usual. The woman has episodes of spotting and bleeding, with brownish-red discharge of "tapioca-like" vesicles. The mole can become very large.

The signs and symptoms of hydatidiform mole include vaginal bleeding, a uterus that is larger than expected for the weeks of pregnancy, anemia, excessive nausea and vomiting, and signs of pregnancy-induced hypertension occurring before 24 weeks of pregnancy. No fetal heart rate, fetal movement, or palpable fetal parts are detectable. After diagnosis is certain, a physician usually performs a careful D&C.

Documentation following a client's D&C should include the amount and character of the expelled tissue, which should be saved and sent for pathologic examination. Aseptic techniques should be used to avoid infection. Because the experience is frightening, the woman needs a great deal of emotional support.

Followup after delivery of a hydatidiform mole is essential. A *human chorionic gonadotropin titer* must be done; the titer ratio should fall after delivery. Titer that remains high or rises often indicates a situation known as **choriocarcinoma,** which can be fatal and is treated with chemotherapy. The woman should be counseled to avoid pregnancy for at least 1 year, until a series of negative HCG levels are found and chemotherapy treatment is finished. Any contraceptive method, other than an intrauterine device, is acceptable. If the woman is Rh negative, administration of an anti-D gamma globulin (such as RhoGAM) is required to prevent Rh sensitization.

MATERNAL COMPLICATIONS DURING PREGNANCY

Many types of complications can occur during pregnancy that do not necessarily have to result in the loss of the fetus or long-term damage to the mother's health. Many disorders that affect the woman, fetus, placenta, or amniotic fluid require early treatment and careful monitoring. Women with existing medical conditions who become pregnant often have special requirements and need special attention. A woman whose fetus is retained long past her due date faces complications as well.

☛ KEY CONCEPT

Any bleeding in pregnancy or labor is a serious sign and must be reported immediately to the healthcare provider.

The most common disorders related to pregnancy that affect the mother are hyperemesis gravidarum and pregnancy-induced hypertension.

Hyperemesis Gravidarum

Hyperemesis gravidarum, or *pernicious vomiting,* is more severe than regular morning sickness. Its cause is unknown; however, various theories include toxins in the woman's bloodstream, possible hormonal imbalances, and emotional conditions related to digestive disturbances. For example, women whose established reaction to stress involves gastrointestinal disturbances often react the same way to pregnancy.

Morning sickness usually begins between the second and fourth week of gestation and ends at approximately the 12th week, although it may continue throughout the pregnancy. Persistent vomiting to the point of excessive weight loss, dehydration, severe loss of appetite, and acetone in the urine are signs of hyperemesis gravidarum. The woman also may have excessive salivation (*ptyalism*), epigastric and rib discomfort, constipation or diarrhea, nutritional anemia, and electrolyte imbalances. Few drugs are usable without potential harm to the fetus. The woman may receive intravenous (IV) glucose and water with electrolytes, antiemetics, and sedatives. In the more advanced stages, severe headache, mental aberrations, delirium, coma, jaundice, and cyanosis may occur. In severe cases, an abortion may be necessary to save the woman's life.

Pregnancy-Induced Hypertension

Hypertension, edema, and proteinuria are conditions that characterize *pregnancy-induced hypertension* (**PIH**). Not all of these parameters must be present for the diagnosis of PIH. *Edema* is more indicative of advancing disease and multi-organ involvement. PIH may occur antepartally, intrapartally, or postpartally. It is a major contributor to maternal and fetal morbidity and mortality.

The symptoms of PIH result from vasoconstriction and vasospasm of blood vessels throughout the body. The central nervous system, kidneys, and liver may be affected. Decreased blood flow to the placenta and uterus may endanger the fetus.

Prompt treatment of PIH includes controlling symptoms as much as possible, and allowing labor to start normally or initiating it when the safety of the woman and fetus best permits.

Following delivery, the woman with PIH must continue to be monitored. If the elevated blood pressure continues for more than 42 days after delivery, she is diagnosed with *chronic*

hypertension. A 6-week checkup should include extensive evaluation of the woman's blood pressure, complete blood count, blood urea nitrogen, urinalysis, and creatinine. Magnesium sulfate, the drug of choice for PIH, is often continued for 24 hours postpartum.

Pregnancy-induced hypertension is divided into preeclampsia and eclampsia, depending on the symptoms. Table 67-1 describes the signs and symptoms of both stages.

✚👁 **Nursing Alert**
The HELLP syndrome indicates a potentially life-threatening complication of pregnancy-induced hypertension:
• **H**emolysis (destruction of RBCs)
• **E**levated **L**iver enzymes
• **L**ow **P**latelet count

Preeclampsia

The woman who was previously progressing normally, but develops PIH with either edema, proteinuria, or both (usually after the 20th week of gestation) has **preeclampsia.** Preeclampsia develops in approximately 5% of pregnancies, most often in primigravidas and in women with a history of high blood pressure or vascular disorders. Although the symptoms most often allow the obstetrician to intercept it and treat it early, it can occur explosively, perhaps the day after an examination. An expectant woman should report symptoms to her birth attendant immediately.

Predicting preeclampsia is also possible with a test in which the client's blood pressure is measured while she lies on her back, and again while she lies on her left side. This test is referred to as the "roll-over test." It is performed most often in the examiner's office. If the woman's diastolic blood pressure is 20 mm Hg higher (or greater) when she is lying on her back, preeclampsia is likely. She should be advised to rest on her left side as much as possible. The birth attendant usually sees this woman every 2 days during the entire pregnancy.

Mild Preeclampsia.   This condition may be treated at home with sedation or tranquilizers and a regular diet (with salted foods omitted in some cases). Resting in a lateral position (particularly on the left side) aids in placental circulation. The woman is encouraged to rest most of the time and avoid climbing stairs.

Severe Preeclampsia.   The symptoms of severe preeclampsia are identified in Table 67-1. These women must be admitted to a healthcare facility, as the eclampsia that may follow is one of the three leading causes of maternal death in North America.

When treating the woman with preeclampsia, check intake and output and body weight daily. Output must be at least 30 milliliters per hour. The client may have an indwelling catheter. Take vital signs at least every 2 hours; use the fetal monitor to assess fetal status. A low-fat, high-protein diet may be necessary, or the woman may be NPO (nothing by mouth) and have an IV, such as Ringer's solution. Check the urine for albumin at least twice daily. Reduce external stim-

▪▪▪ TABLE 67-1 Signs and Symptoms of Preeclampsia and Eclampsia

Mild Preeclampsia	Severe Preeclampsia	Eclampsia
Weight gain: 1 lb/wk during 2nd and 3rd trimesters; 4½ lb. in a week anytime during pregnancy	Weight gain, as in mild preeclampsia	Symptoms of severe preeclampsia PLUS
1+ or 2+ proteinuria (0.3 g/L in 24h urine)	3+ or 4+ proteinuria (≥5 g in 24h urine) in 2 random urine specimens collected at least 6 h apart	
Urine output ≥30 mL/hr; output = intake	Abnormally small amount of urine secretion (*oliguria*) in relation to fluid intake; with fluid retention and edema. Urine output: ≤30 mL/h or 120 mL/4h	Maximum urine albumin level with scanty urine output
BP ≥ 140/90 mm Hg or elevated by ≥30 mm Hg systolic or ≥15 mm Hg diastolic on two occasions 4–6 h apart	BP ≥ 160 mm Hg systolic or ≥110 mm Hg diastolic or elevation of ≥30 mm Hg diastolic recorded on two occasions, 6 h apart while the client is on bed rest	Very high blood pressure (over 170/110; systolic can be above 200)
Hyperreflexia—no clonus	Hyperreflexia—with clonus	
Edema—fingers, face, legs, feet	Severe, unremitting frontal or occipital headache Nausea and persistent vomiting Abdominal pain, epigastric pain Visual disturbances Localized arterial spasms of retina	Fever Seizures, coma

uli as much as possible. In Practice: Nursing Care Plan 67-1 discusses an adolescent with PIH.

Ensure that the client and her family understand the following precautions:

- Visiting is restricted.
- The room is kept quiet and fairly dark.
- Sedatives are given.
- Padded side rails are up at all times for safety.
- The woman is on bed rest.
- The woman should lie on her left side as much as possible. (Rationale: This helps to facilitate renal circulation in the woman and placental circulation for the fetus.)
- All intake and output are measured.
- Vital signs are taken often; weight is taken daily.
- Level of consciousness and reflexes are checked often.
- Blood will be drawn periodically for testing.
- The fetus will be monitored.

The drug of choice in the treatment of severe preeclampsia (and prevention of eclampsia) is magnesium sulfate (**MgSO₄**) given via IV or intramuscularly (IM). This potent anticonvulsant drug slows neuromuscular conduction and depresses central nervous system irritability, thus reducing muscle excitability and hyperreflexia. Although the vasodilating effects of MgSO₄ will lower the blood pressure slightly, this action is only transient. The main reason for administering MgSO₄ is to prevent seizures, not to lower blood pressure.

Because of the drug's effects on the central nervous system, assess the woman's respirations and deep-tendon reflexes fre-

quently. Observe and report any changes. Also monitor urinary output because oliguria can result from excessively high levels of MgSO₄ in the blood. Calcium gluconate (Kalcinate) is the specific antidote for MgSO₄. It is kept at the bedside at all times while the woman receives MgSO₄ and is used if toxicity occurs.

If MgSO₄ does not control seizures, diazepam (Valium) may be used. Furosemide (Lasix) may be needed to stimulate urine output. Potassium (K⁺) often is given with Lasix.

An IV is usually kept running to administer fluids and to keep the vein open in case emergency drugs must be given. Electrolytes are replaced IV, as blood tests determine needs. If blood pressure remains dangerously elevated, additional medications may be ordered. Hydralazine HCl (Apresoline) is the antihypertensive agent of choice, although labetalol HCl (Normodyne), methyldopa (Aldomet, Dopamet [Canada]), and nifedipine (Adalat, Procardia) are sometimes used. However, the woman's blood pressure should not be reduced too much or too fast, to avoid causing fetal anoxia. Maintain blood pressure in the range of 90 to 100 mm Hg diastolic.

When the client at or near term is stabilized, the fetus will usually be delivered. *Induction*, stimulating labor to begin by using a medication such as oxytocin (Pitocin), will be done if the cervix is ripe. If it is not ripe, cesarean (surgical) delivery is performed. (Induction and cesarean section delivery are discussed in more detail in a later section.) If the fetus is not mature enough to survive, the pregnancy may be sustained for a short time. If the woman's condition worsens, the baby will usually be sacrificed to save the woman's life.

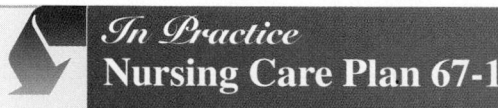

In Practice
Nursing Care Plan 67-1

THE ADOLESCENT CLIENT WITH SEVERE PREECLAMPSIA

MEDICAL HISTORY: *D. L., a 15-year-old, single, prima-para client at 30 weeks of pregnancy, comes to the emergency department complaining of a persistent headache for the past 3 days and blurred vision. Blood pressure is 190/110 with hyperactive deep tendon reflexes and mild clonus. Urine sample is obtained and reveals 3+ for protein. Marked edema is noted in her face and lower extremities. Client states, "I've been to the clinic once since I became pregnant." Client's medical history is negative, except for being underweight for height. Pre-pregnancy weight of 102 lb; height of 5 ft 6 in. Intravenous infusion of magnesium sulfate started. The client is admitted to the hospital for evaluation and treatment.*

MEDICAL DIAGNOSIS: *Pregnancy-induced hypertension, severe preeclampsia*

Data Collection/Nursing Assessment: Client is adolescent female with marked edema of face, ankles, and feet. Edema is +1 pitting. She stated, "I noticed that my feet looked a bit puffy and that my shoes felt tight. And I gained almost 3 pounds since last week." On admission to the unit, client's weight is 124 pounds and vital signs are: Temperature, 98.2° F (36.8° C); pulse, 98 beats per minute and regular; respirations, 22 breaths per minute. Blood pressure is 190/102. Fetal heart rate at 154 beats per minute. Fundal height is 30 cm. Client reports that she has felt the baby move recently. Urine sample obtained reveals 3+ for protein. Client states, "I haven't been going to the bathroom as much over the last couple of days even though I've been drinking a lot of fluids." Urine output for past 2 hours since admission is 50 cc's. Dietary history reveals intake of large amounts of carbohydrates and minimal protein. Hyperactive patellar (knee-jerk) reflex is noted, with mild ankle clonus. (*Although several nursing diagnoses may be appropriate, the priority nursing diagnosis is addressed below.*)

Nursing Diagnosis: Risk for injury (maternal and fetal) related to physiologic effects of severe preeclampsia as evidenced by hypertension, proteinuria, edema, headache, and blurred vision.

Planning:
SHORT-TERM GOALS:
#1. Client's blood pressure gradually is reduced to within acceptable parameters, with diastolic controlled between 90–100 mm Hg.
#2. Fetal heart rate and pattern remain within acceptable parameters.
#3. Client and fetus show no evidence of complications.

LONG-TERM GOALS:
#4. Client is able to maintain pregnancy to term.
#5. Client delivers healthy, term neonate with minimal to no complications.

Implementation:
NURSING ACTION: *Explain condition and necessity for treatment to the client, including measures to help participate in care.*
RATIONALE: *Understanding of events and treatments fosters compliance and helps to alleviate anxiety and stress. Participating in care helps client to regain some control over the situation.*

NURSING ACTION: *Place the client in a private room on bed rest with padded side rails. Dim any lighting and keep the room as quiet as possible. Restrict visitors to only the client's immediate family.*
RATIONALE: *With PIH, the client's central nervous system is irritable. Decreasing external stimuli and stress helps to reduce the risk of seizures. Padding the side rails helps to minimize the risk for injury should a seizure occur.*

Evaluation: Client maintaining bedrest, reporting that headache is lessening. *Progress to meeting Goal #1 and Goal #3.*

NURSING ACTION: *Monitor blood pressure every 5–30 min until stabilized, then every 1–2 h as indicated. Expect to administer antihypertensive agent. Have emergency supplies readily available at the client's bedside.*
RATIONALE: *The client's status can change rapidly. An increase in blood pressure may lead to eclampsia.*

NURSING ACTION: *Monitor intravenous infusion of magnesium sulfate; check level of consciousness, deep-tendon reflexes, and respirations frequently. Have calcium gluconate readily available at the bedside. Assist with obtaining laboratory specimens, including serum magnesium levels, as ordered.*
RATIONALE: *Magnesium sulfate acts to reduce edema and depress central nervous system irritability. Decreases in level of consciousness, respirations, and reflex activity can occur, indicating toxicity. Calcium gluconate is the antidote for magnesium toxicity. Laboratory specimens provide valuable information about the client's condition.*

NURSING ACTION: *Expect to administer antihypertensive agent, such as hydralazine (Apresoline) as ordered. Be prepared to administer other medications, such as sedatives or anticonvulsants, if ordered.*

(continued)

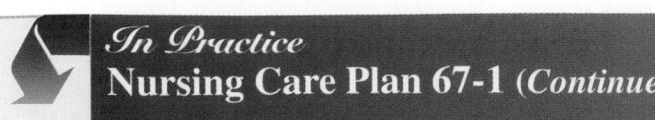

RATIONALE: *An antihypertensive agent is needed to reduce the client's elevated blood pressure. Hydralazine (Apresoline) reduces blood pressure without affecting placental circulation.*

Evaluation: Blood pressure decreasing gradually from initial readings to 140/94. Respirations at 20 breaths per minute; alert and oriented; deep-tendon reflexes brisk but without clonus; serum magnesium level at 7.5 mEq/L; no signs and symptoms of magnesium toxicity or seizures. *Progress to meeting Goal #1 and Goal #3.*

NURSING ACTION: *Assess intake and output frequently. If ordered, insert a retention catheter to monitor urine output hourly. Check urine for protein.*
RATIONALE: *Oliguria is a sign of preeclampsia and also magnesium toxicity. Urine output needs to be at least 30 cc/hr to indicate adequate renal function. Checking urine for protein helps to determine the severity of the preeclampsia.*

Evaluation: Urine output at 48 cc/hr; urine 1+ for protein. *Progress to meeting Goal #1.*

NURSING ACTION: *Encourage client to lie on her side as much as possible.*
RATIONALE: *The side-lying position enhances blood flow to the uterus, the placenta, and the fetus.*

NURSING ACTION: *Monitor fetal status frequently. Obtain fetal heart rate at least every 4 hr. Assess for signs and symptoms of beginning labor.*
RATIONALE: *The mother's hypertension can decrease placental perfusion and subsequently the nutrient and oxygen supply to the fetus. Adolescents have an increased risk for preterm labor.*

Evaluation: Fetal heart rate ranging 144–156 beats per minute; client maintaining side-lying position; client reports no signs and symptoms of labor. Membranes intact. *Progress to meeting Goal #2 and Goal #3.*

NURSING ACTION: *Encourage a moderate-to-high protein, moderate-sodium diet. Monitor daily weights.*
RATIONALE: *Large amounts of protein are being lost in the client's urine and must be replaced. Moderate amounts of sodium are necessary to maintain electrolyte balance. The client's weight is a valuable indicator of fluid balance.*

Evaluation: Weight decreased to 120 lb over past several days. Blood pressure maintained at 132/90. Edema of face, hands, and lower extremities decreased-to-moderate; no pitting noted. *Goal #1 met.*
Fetal heart rate and maternal vital signs within acceptable parameters. *Goal #2 and Goal #3 met; progress to meeting Goal #4 and Goal #5.*

Eclampsia

Because of the availability of successful medical therapies, few women progress to the serious stage called **eclampsia,** which is likely to occur if preeclampsia is left untreated. Eclampsia is one of the most severe complications of pregnancy. Generalized tonic-clonic seizures, very rapid pulse, and very high blood pressure (see Table 67-1) characterize eclampsia, which develops in one out of every 200 women with preeclampsia.

After a seizure, the client may regain consciousness within a few minutes, or she may remain in a coma for several hours or days. Seizures may recur in either instance. Even when a woman awakens after seizures, she may be confused. The treatment for eclampsia is basically the same as that for severe preeclampsia, with delivery performed as soon as possible.

If seizures continue, the coma deepens. The "slushy" respirations characteristic of lung edema are audible, and the woman's prognosis is now poor. The primary causes of maternal death due to hypertension are circulatory collapse, cerebral hemorrhage, and renal failure. A major complication is abruptio placentae (discussed later) with maternal hemorrhage.

EXISTING DISORDERS COMPLICATING PREGNANCY

Some pregnant women have existing conditions that may complicate pregnancy and that require special attention. Such conditions include diabetes mellitus and cardiac disorders. Chemical dependency is another existing condition that requires special considerations to protect both the woman and the fetus. Chapter 68 presents special care considerations for the chemically addicted newborn.

Diabetes Mellitus

Diabetes mellitus is an endocrine disorder in which the pancreas fails to produce sufficient insulin for proper use of glucose. Chapter 78 discusses this condition in more detail. A diabetic woman needs special care and monitoring during pregnancy, because insulin requirements fluctuate. Even when diabetes is monitored carefully, the pregnant woman and her developing fetus are at risk. Women with diabetes ideally should receive optimal care and client education prior to conception, to prevent interrupted pregnancy and congenital malformations in their babies. Tight metabolic control can be achieved with intensive self-management and preparation for pregnancy.

Potential problems during pregnancy include fetal death, **macrosomia** (oversized fetus), a fetus with a respiratory disorder, difficult labor, preeclampsia or eclampsia, polyhydramnios, and congenital malformations. These conditions are discussed elsewhere in this chapter.

Diabetes is usually more difficult to control during pregnancy. The woman may become *hyperglycemic,* with resulting acidosis or diabetic coma. She also may become *hypoglycemic,* with resulting fetal hypoxia. The pregnant woman with insulin-dependent diabetes will need to learn to administer her own insulin injections during the pregnancy. Depending on the condition of the woman and fetus, diabetic women may deliver early (36–38 wk) by induction or cesarean delivery.

➤ **Nursing Alert**

A reaction to too little or too much insulin is a danger to the woman, especially during labor and immediately after delivery. The woman's body reacts to the trauma of birth, and her glucose level is easily upset.

Blood glucose testing, dietary adjustments, and danger signs that must be reported, are necessary teaching for the diabetic woman and her family. Family teaching is important because the woman may be unable to recognize these signs soon enough to be able to take action. Refer to In Practice: Educating the Client 67-1 for additional information.

Diabetic women should be under the care of an internist and an obstetrician during pregnancy. Frequent antepartal visits are essential. Careful fetal monitoring is necessary during labor, and the newborn must be assessed carefully. Generally these newborns are treated as premature babies.

Approximately 4% of pregnant women develop diabetes for the first time during pregnancy, a condition called **gestational diabetes.** Although management of gestational diabetes through diet alone works for some women, others will require insulin. The majority of women will return to pre-pregnancy glucose levels following delivery. Women diagnosed with gestational diabetes mellitus, and women who have delivered a baby weighing more than 9 pounds, are known to develop type 2 diabetes in later years. These women should be advised that they are at possible risk.

Cardiac Disorders

Pregnancy places additional strain on the heart. Due to the increased blood volume, the greatest dangers are during the last trimester, labor, and delivery. During labor, women with a history of cardiac problems should be assessed for dyspnea, chest pain, and pulmonary edema.

During pregnancy, the woman with a cardiac condition should get plenty of rest and avoid activities that result in shortness of breath. She should maintain a diet that will prevent excessive weight gain and water retention. Usually sodium (salt) is restricted. The woman's prognosis depends on her age, and the severity and type of heart disease.

Women with cardiac disorders often successfully deliver their babies. Current belief is that a vaginal delivery is safer for the woman than a cesarean delivery because of the added strain of surgery. Induced labor and early delivery, however, may prevent a difficult labor.

Chemical Dependency

The addicted pregnant woman may be malnourished. Her addiction may result in a failure to seek antepartal care. Drug use may account for a stillbirth, spontaneous abortion, abruptio placentae, and numerous congenital defects. Some of these conditions, as they relate to the newborn, are discussed in more detail in Chapter 68. The chemically dependent mother often lacks parenting skills. Child protection authorities should be involved early in the pregnancy.

DISORDERS AFFECTING THE FETUS

Some disorders present special concerns for fetal health and well-being. Infections including *sexually transmitted diseases* (STDs) not only require careful maternal treatment, but can ultimately compromise fetal health. (Refer to Chapter 69 for more information on STDs.) *Hemolytic conditions,* such as Rh sensitization and ABO incompatibility, also warrant careful evaluation.

Infection

Maternal infections can harm the fetus. For instance, a severe respiratory disease, such as *viral pneumonia,* can cause fetal anoxia. If the woman contracts *rubella* early in pregnancy, fetal malformation is a strong possibility. (Congenital rubella syndrome is discussed in Chapter 68.) A woman whose rubella titer is low (below 1:10) does not have the antibodies to fight rubella. If this woman is exposed to rubella, gamma globulin may be given. An abortion may be an option. After the preg-

---

In Practice
Educating the Client 67-1

THE PREGNANT WOMAN WITH DIABETES

Client and family teaching for the pregnant woman with diabetes includes the following:

- Method for self-testing blood for glucose several times per day
- Insulin and diet adjustments based on glucose level
- Method for insulin injections if the woman has not used insulin previously
- Signs of hyperglycemia and hypoglycemia
- Actions to take if hyperglycemia or hypoglycemia occur
- Signs and symptoms of beginning preeclampsia

nancy, the mother is immunized for rubella. She should be cautioned not to become pregnant for at least 3 months after this immunization, to avoid harm to the next fetus.

Maternal STDs are often transmitted to the fetus. Maternal–fetal circulation transmits syphilis, gonorrhea, herpesvirus 2, and HIV/AIDS. Chapters 69 and 72 discuss these conditions and their effects on newborns and children in more detail.

Rh Sensitization

Rh sensitization is preventable in most cases. In Rh sensitization, the mother is Rh negative, but Rh-positive red blood cells from the fetus cross the placental barrier and enter the maternal circulation. Because the Rh-positive cells become antigens in the Rh-negative woman, they stimulate the formation of antibodies within the woman's circulatory system. These antibodies return to the fetus, destroying the fetal erythrocytes. An Rh-negative woman who has produced these antibodies is said to be *sensitized.* The newborn in this situation is born with a condition known as **erythroblastosis fetalis.**

The sensitization of the woman in erythroblastosis fetalis usually occurs at or near the delivery, so the antibodies do not always affect the fetus being carried at that time. However, in subsequent pregnancies with Rh-positive fetuses, the already sensitized woman usually produces large numbers of antibodies. Some newborns are only mildly affected, whereas others are severely affected. Efforts to save the fetus may include *intrauterine transfusion* (exchange of fetal blood *in utero*) if the pregnancy is less than 32 weeks' duration, or early delivery at 34 to 38 weeks.

Administering *anti-D gamma globulin,* also known as Rh_0(D) immune globulin (RhoGAM, Gamulin Rh), to the Rh-negative woman can prevent erythroblastosis fetalis. This drug should be administered at 28 weeks of gestation and again 72 hours following: the birth of an Rh-positive baby; any abortion; or any invasive procedure, such as an amniocentesis. RhoGAM prevents the woman's body from building up anti–Rh-positive antibodies. Erythroblastosis fetalis is thus prevented, even in Rh-positive fetuses. RhoGAM's availability has made this disorder rare in the United States. RhoGAM is also discussed in Chapter 64.

> ### Nursing Alert
> *Each* time an Rh-negative woman delivers or aborts, RhoGAM must be administered again.

ABO Incompatibility

ABO incompatibility can arise if the woman's blood type is A and the fetus's is B or AB; if the mother is B and the fetus is A or AB; and if the mother is O and the fetus is A, B, or AB (see Chap. 81).

ABO incompatibility is not detectable before birth. It can occur in a first pregnancy and does not increase in severity with subsequent pregnancies. It is usually clinically milder than Rh sensitization. The problem is indicated by jaundice in the newborn within the first 36 hours; *phototherapy* (treatment with an intense fluorescent light) is often useful in treating the jaundice.

PLACENTAL AND AMNIOTIC DISORDERS

Placental disorders include placenta previa and abruptio placentae. *Placenta previa* means that the placenta implants in the wrong place within the woman's uterus. *Abruptio placentae* is a condition in which the placenta tears abruptly and prematurely from the uterus. Both conditions can be life threatening to the woman and fetus. *Polyhydramnios,* or excessive amniotic fluid, presents serious dangers to the fetus.

Placenta Previa

Placenta previa is a serious condition that occurs when the placenta implants in the lower segment of the uterus, rather than in the upper wall (Fig. 67-2). *Low implantation* is placental attachment at the opening or border of the cervical os, but not covering it. If the placenta partially obliterates the cervical os, it is a *partial placenta previa.* Placenta that totally covers the cervical os is called *total placenta previa.*

Predisposing factors are numerous and include closely spaced pregnancies, abnormalities in uterine structure, late fertilization, and old cesarean scars. Painless vaginal bleeding during the later months of pregnancy is the primary symptom, and is due to the separation of the placenta from the uterine wall.

If undetected before labor begins, placenta previa will result in hemorrhage, because the cervical dilation causes increased tearing of the placental tissue. The severity of hemorrhage in relation to the progress of labor determines the method of delivery to be used. In total placenta previa, cesarean delivery is performed. In partial placenta previa, the amount of cervical involvement dictates the method of delivery, although cesarean delivery is usually performed if the previa covers more than 30% of the cervical os when the cervix is fully dilated. A woman may be hospitalized several times before hemorrhaging becomes severe enough to warrant cesarean birth.

Other potential complications of placenta previa are loss of uterine muscle tone (*atony*), uterine rupture, retention of placental tissue, and *air embolism,* a serious complication caused by exposure of uterine sinuses and blood vessels to the air. The fetus is at considerable risk, and fetal shock and maternal or fetal death is possible.

Diagnosis and Management

If vaginal bleeding occurs, the client should be hospitalized *immediately* and placed on bed rest. The need for fetal monitoring, IV and blood administration, possible cesarean delivery, vaginal packing, and emergency infant resuscitation should be anticipated.

Diagnosis is most often obtained by ultrasonography (Doppler ultrasound), which can usually identify the exact placental location. In some situations, x-rays may be used (including *placentography*) to visualize the placenta.

If the fetus is diagnosed as viable, a sterile vaginal examination (**SVE**) may be done (by the physician only) in the operating room. The operating room should be prepared with

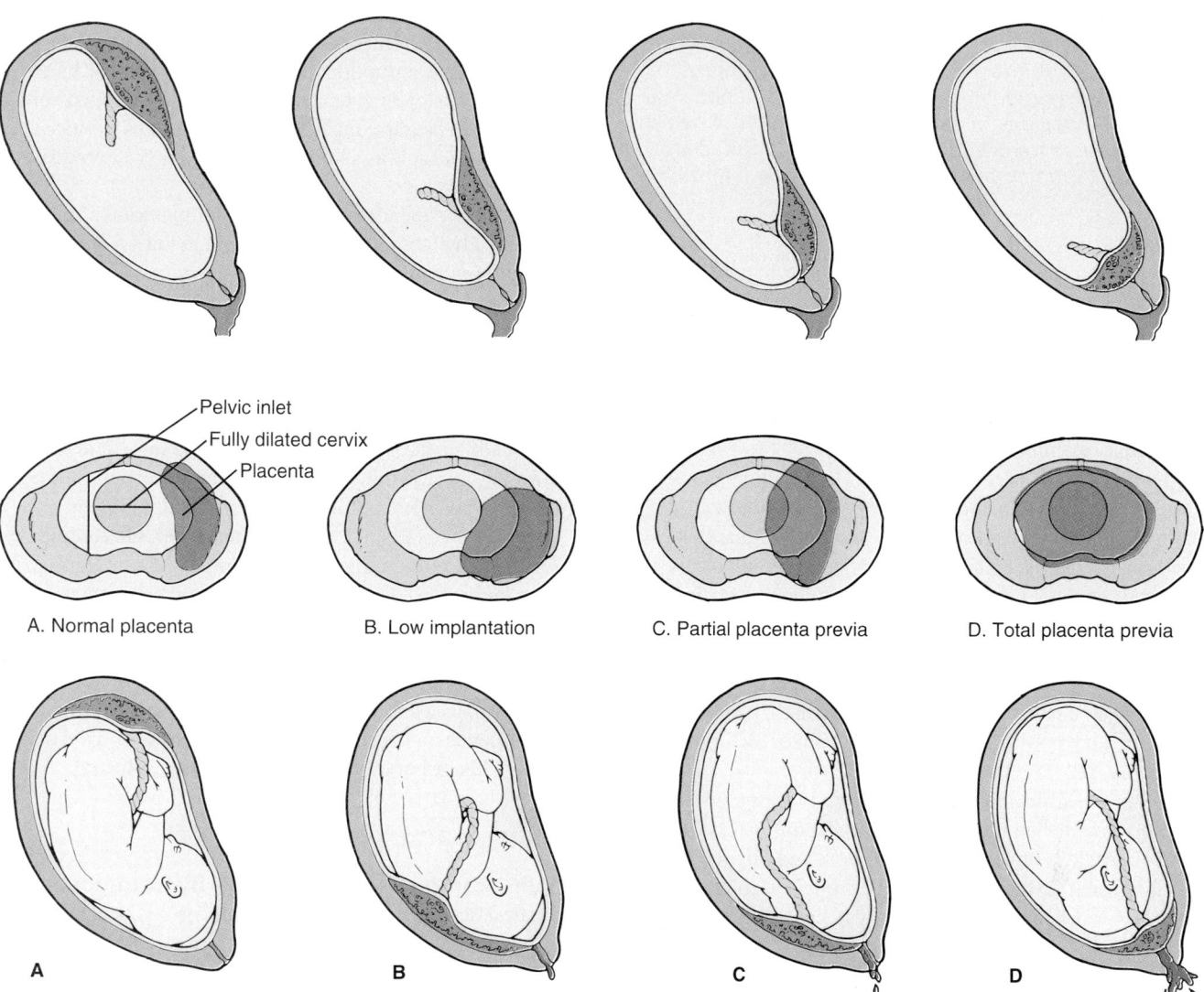

FIGURE 67-2. Placenta previa. (**A**) Normal placenta. (**B**) Low implantation. (**C**) Partial placenta previa. (**D**) Total placenta previa. (Reeder, S. J., Martin, L. L., & Koniak-Griffin, D. [1997]. *Maternity nursing: Family, newborn, and women's health care* [18th ed., p. 822]. Philadelphia: Lippincott-Raven.)

a double setup to allow for an emergency cesarean delivery if necessary.

Vaginal birth is not usually considered unless the previa is minimal. If the fetus is under 36 weeks' gestation, the mother is put on strict bed rest either in the healthcare facility or at home. If no bleeding occurs, ultrasound scanning may be done every 2 to 3 weeks along with nonstress testing and biophysical profile. If bleeding is found, a cesarean delivery is anticipated.

Although placenta previa is still considered serious, modern surgical methods and the use of blood transfusions have greatly reduced maternal mortality. The prognosis for the fetus depends on the effect of maternal hemorrhage on fetal circulation and oxygenation.

Nursing Considerations

Assess the mother carefully for hemorrhage following a placenta previa delivery. If bleeding continues to be severe, and attempts at control are unsuccessful, an emergency hysterectomy may be performed.

Abruptio Placentae

Abruptio placentae, the abrupt premature separation of the normally implanted placenta from the uterine wall, is a grave complication of late pregnancy (Fig. 67-3). It usually develops after the 20th week of gestation, and it often occurs without labor.

Some predisposing factors are hypertension, preeclampsia, poor placental circulation, substance abuse, grand multiparity, and numerous abortions or stillbirths. Physical trauma, such as a motor vehicle accident, also can cause immediate placental separation. The extent of the separation determines the amount of danger to the fetus. Abruptio placentae is a common cause of *stillbirth.*

Diagnosis and Management

Abruptio placentae can occur any time in pregnancy before the birth, giving rise to fetal distress. The bleeding that results from the separation may be apparent or hidden. If bleeding is externally visible, it is often dark. The uterus becomes tender and rigid, and symptoms of maternal shock may occur. Fetal movement may increase or decrease. If the woman experiences extreme pain or the uterine fundus rises, it may indicate bleeding and pooling behind the placenta (*retroplacental hemorrhage*).

Other possible maternal complications include bleeding into the uterine muscle, *precipitous labor* (fast and uncontrolled), loss of uterine tone (*atony*), and oliguria leading to acute renal failure. Disseminated intravascular coagulation (**DIC**) and maternal death may occur. DIC is discussed in Chapter 81. Dangers to the fetus include anemia, anoxia, and death.

Nursing Considerations

The diagnosis of abruptio placentae is based on the client's history, physical examination, and laboratory studies. Sonograms are used to rule out placenta previa, but they are not diagnostic for placental abruption. The amount of vaginal bleeding seen can be misleading, because blood may be trapped behind the placenta. The nurse must be aware of changes in vital signs, and indicators such as sudden extreme pain or aberrations in uterine shape.

Treatment depends on the severity of maternal blood loss, determined by laboratory findings, fetal maturity, and the biophysical condition of both woman and fetus. Continuously monitor the fetus if a fetal heart rate is present. Identify the upper limit of the fundus and mark it on the woman's abdomen with a felt-tip pen. Observe the fundus for changes in shape or movement upward. Measure abdominal *girth* (the distance around) with a flexible tape measure. If the abdomen increases in girth or moves upward, blood may be collecting within the uterus; this dangerous situation usually calls for immediate cesarean delivery.

Before a cesarean birth, lost maternal blood must be replaced and circulating blood volume restored. During this time, monitor maternal vital signs and fetal heart rate (if present) constantly. In a few cases, a hysterectomy may need to be performed to control the bleeding.

With modern treatment, abruptio placentae is rarely fatal to the woman. However, the outlook for the newborn's survival depends on the severity of the separation and the degree to which his or her oxygen supply has been affected.

Polyhydramnios

Polyhydramnios (sometimes called **hydramnios**) means an excessive amount of amniotic fluid (>2 L or 2,000 mL).

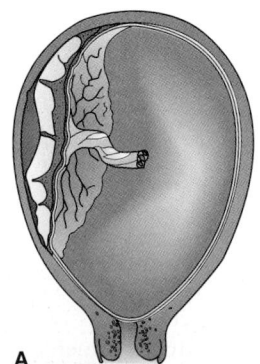 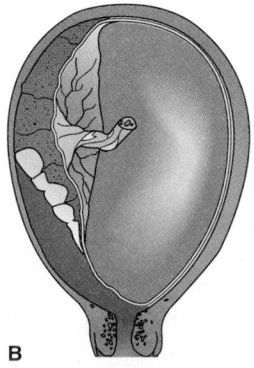 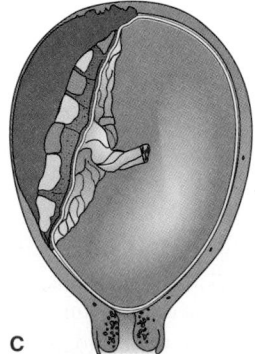

FIGURE 67-3. Premature separation and abruptio placentae. (**A**) Separation is low and incomplete; vaginal hemorrhage is evident. (**B**) Separation is high, causing fundus of uterus to rise. Fetus is in grave danger. External hemorrhage is not present, but amniotic fluid is port-wine color. (**C**) Complete abruption, with fetus in grave danger. External hemorrhage is prevented because fetus's head is in cervical os. (Pillitteri, A. [1998]. *Maternal and child health nursing: Care of the childbearing and childrearing family* [3rd ed., p. 385]. Philadelphia: Lippincott Williams & Wilkins.)

Seen in approximately 10% of pregnant diabetic women, polyhydramnios also accompanies neural tube defects, such as spina bifida and anencephaly. The woman's abdomen is excessively large, producing dyspnea and difficulty with movement. The skin is stretched tightly, and excessive stretch marks (*striae gravidarum*) may be present. Uterine muscles also have been stretched, which may lead to ineffective contractions (*dystocia*) and failure of the uterus to contract following childbirth.

Placenta Accreta

A placenta that fails to separate, fails to be expelled within 20 to 30 minutes after delivery, or leaves remnants in the uterus is a danger to the woman. This condition is called **placenta accreta** or *retained placenta*. The tissue must be removed soon after delivery so that infection or hemorrhage does not develop. Retained placenta may result from partial separation of a normally attached placenta, entrapment of the separated placenta by uterine constriction, mismanagement of labor's third stage, or abnormal adherence to the uterine wall.

The birth attendant may need to remove the placenta manually and may perform a postpartum uterine D&C. Vigorous attempts at removal may lead to hemorrhage, shock, or uterine rupture or inversion. If the uterus ruptures or bleeding is uncontrollable, a hysterectomy may be performed to save the mother's life. Nursing measures include support, and monitoring vital signs.

OTHER HIGH-RISK PREGNANCIES

Prolonged Pregnancy

A pregnancy continuing beyond 42 weeks is known as a *prolonged* (*postdate* or *postterm*) pregnancy. In this case, the obstetrician may induce labor or perform a cesarean delivery. The condition of the fetus is a determining factor. If any indication of fetal distress exists, a cesarean delivery is the most likely option. Risks to be considered include *placental insufficiency,* a condition in which the placenta deteriorates and uteroplacental circulation is compromised. (Preterm delivery is discussed in Chap. 68.)

Multiple Pregnancy

A multiple pregnancy is one in which more than one fetus is developing in the uterus at the same time. If a multiple pregnancy is suspected, ultrasound is diagnostic. Labor is not ordinarily more difficult than in a normal pregnancy, although preterm and *precipitate* (sudden, progressing faster than normal) deliveries are relatively common.

Adolescent Pregnancy

More than 1.2 million adolescent women in the United States become pregnant each year, representing nearly 20% of births. Pregnancy in a girl younger than age 16 places a particular strain on her body; this adolescent is undergoing not only the normal changes of adolescence, but also those needed to sustain a pregnancy. Iron requirements are high for both adolescence and pregnancy, and anemia may result. The young woman may need special dietary instructions or vitamin supplements.

Complications of adolescent pregnancy often involve preeclampsia, eclampsia, and spontaneous abortion. Babies are often preterm and small for their gestational age. Perinatal mortality is increased, and newborns often develop slowly. Pregnant adolescents are at high risk for infections and STDs.

Childbirth preparation classes are offered through local public health departments or healthcare facilities. Pregnant clients, particularly adolescents, should attend these classes to understand their nutritional needs and the process of pregnancy.

The pregnant teen should also receive information about continuing her education. By law, public school education must be made available to pregnant teenagers. Counseling services should be offered, because the girl may be afraid to go to her parents for help. Local church groups or clergy members, Planned Parenthood of America, local social service agencies, and the family physician may provide resources and counseling. Financial assistance also may be available.

Pregnancy in the Woman Over Age 40

The pregnant woman older than 40 years of age encounters more risks than the woman between 16 and 40 years of age. Bodily changes in preparation for menopause may have begun. Primigravidas of this age have an increased incidence of complications in pregnancy (such as ectopic pregnancy, gestational diabetes, and hypertensive disorders) in addition to problems during labor and delivery, such as *hypertonic* or *hypotonic dystocia* (contractions too weak or too strong, respectively) and hemorrhage. They also face greater than normal chances of having cognitively impaired or malformed children. The older grand multipara may be more likely to have a precipitate delivery, placenta previa, hydramnios, hypotonic dystocia, or hemorrhage because of an *atonic uterus* (one that does not contract following delivery).

COMPLICATIONS OF LABOR AND DELIVERY

Approximately 85% of all deliveries are considered *normal;* 15% are considered *complicated.* One nursing duty in the labor and delivery area is to assess for possible complications.

Maternal Hemorrhage

Intrapartum and *postpartum maternal hemorrhage* are life-threatening events that may occur without warning and are often not recognized until the woman experiences profound symptoms. Carefully assess the mother immediately postpartum for signs of hemorrhage or shock. Maternal hemorrhage requires aggressive measures to locate the cause. Begin localized and systemic therapy to avoid maternal mortality. Monitor fundal firmness because *uterine atony* is the number one cause of postpartal hemorrhage.

Premature Rupture of Membranes

Normally, the amniotic sac ruptures with a large gush slightly after the onset of labor. However, in 2% to 18% of all pregnancies, the *amniotic sac,* also referred to as the *bag of waters,* may have a small leak. In this scenario, the client may not go into labor for several days, because the rupture is generally a small leak that may not be detected by the woman. When the amniotic sac loses fluids before the onset of labor, the condition is called premature rupture of membranes (**PROM**). Several complications may arise with PROM:

- Premature labor
- Intrauterine infection (the fetus is particularly susceptible to infections)
- Malpresentations and prolapsed cord

If the bag of waters breaks with a sudden gush, the diagnosis is obvious, but a slow trickling of amniotic fluid is more difficult to diagnose. *Nitrazine* tests may be used to detect amniotic fluid in the vagina.

The woman should be admitted to the healthcare facility when PROM occurs. The woman and fetus are then assessed. Ultrasound and amniocentesis will determine fetal maturity, and labor is induced if the fetus is sufficiently mature.

Preterm Labor

Labor that occurs before the end of the 37th week of gestation is *preterm,* but it often still produces a viable fetus. Because prematurity is a leading cause of infant mortality, the birth attendant often attempts to postpone delivery until the baby is more mature.

The woman is placed on bed rest. *Tocolytic agents* (uterine relaxants) may be given to stop the contractions if there is no fetal distress, the membranes are intact, and the cervix is dilated fewer than 4 centimeters (see In Practice: Important Medications 67-1). Medications are usually administered IV until contractions cease, after which they may be administered orally. The woman and fetus must be followed up closely for the remainder of the pregnancy.

Precipitate Labor and Delivery

A precipitate labor is one that is brief (<3 hours), and in which contractions are unusually severe. It most often occurs in induced labor or multiparity. A precipitate delivery may be so rapid that the woman cannot be taken to the delivery room

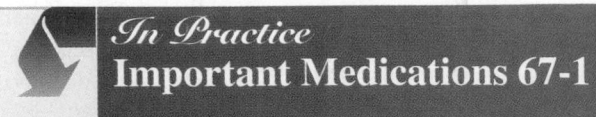

or prepared for delivery; the obstetrician or midwife is not always present.

When providing nursing care for a woman experiencing precipitate labor, stay with her, put the signal light on for help, remain composed, and assist the woman as much as possible until help arrives. Apply the principles of asepsis as the situation allows. Never prevent delivery in any way. Simply assist with the birth and make sure that the newborn is breathing adequately.

Because of the force and speed of labor, possible trauma can occur to the woman and newborn. Dangers to the woman include perineal laceration, hemorrhage, infection, and uterine rupture. Anoxia, subdural hematoma, and fractures may occur in the newborn. Hospitals usually have protocols on determining under what circumstances an infant born out of asepsis (**BOA**) (that is, in an unsterile environment) needs isolation to prevent spread of infection to other infants.

Uterine Rupture

A *ruptured uterus* is one of the most serious complications of labor; fortunately, it is rare. Predisposing factors include a previous cesarean delivery or any uterine scar. Severe tonic contractions with no period of relaxation, dystocia (difficult labor), cephalopelvic disproportion, or injudicious use of drugs, such as oxytocin to stimulate uterine contractions, also may predispose to rupture.

When uterine rupture threatens, the woman complains of continuous and intense pain. A *Bandl's ring* may be noticeable, as a thickened upper segment and a thin distended lower segment of the uterus. The woman appears apprehensive and restless. Contractions are tonic, pulse is rapid, and urination is frequent. If the threat of rupture occurs before delivery, the fetus is usually in great distress, as shown by irregular or absent FHTs.

Constant fetal monitoring is vital. The woman at high risk of, or with, a uterine rupture may need an emergency cesarean delivery to save her life and the life of her fetus. A hysterectomy may be needed to save the mother's life.

Symptoms of rupture are a sharp, tearing pain followed by its sudden cessation. The woman is anxious and shows signs of shock and hypotension; her pulse is rapid and weak. (She is hemorrhaging internally.) Use emergency measures to treat her for shock and hemorrhage. Prepare her at once for an emergency cesarean delivery and possible hysterectomy.

Maternal Dystocia

Dystocia is prolonged, painful labor that does not result in effective cervical dilation or effacement. Therefore, labor is long but does not progress. Dystocia may be related to fetal factors, uterine or passageway abnormalities, or faulty contractions. Dystocia not only exhausts the woman, but also predisposes her and the fetus to possible danger and even death.

Uterine Inertia
Uterine inertia refers to insufficient, uncoordinated contractions that do not produce effective dilation. It is also called *hypotonic dystocia.* Causes include emotional stress, a thick and rigid cervix, and excessive or premature use of analgesic medications. Uterine inertia occurs most often in primigravidas. However, it also is identified in some grand multiparas who have weak uterine muscle tone. Other women may suffer from uterine inertia if they have an overdistended uterus because of an extremely large fetus, a multiple pregnancy, or hydramnios.

Nursing care includes early recognition, prompt notification of the obstetrician, assessment of cervical dilation (if any), accurate evaluation of pain, assessment of the fetal heart rate related to the pattern of contractions by monitor, and positive emotional support and reassurance. Anticipate and be prepared to assist with treatments, such as IV fluids or efforts to stop the ineffective labor with medications such as morphine. Sleep and rest often enable the woman's uterus to achieve a normal pattern when labor resumes. Other treatment may include IV oxytocin infusion or cesarean delivery.

Dystocia Caused by the Fetus

Sometimes the size of the fetus as compared with the size of the woman's pelvis, or the position or presentation of the fetus, causes dystocia.

Cephalopelvic Disproportion
Cephalopelvic disproportion (**CPD**) means that the presenting part, usually the fetal head, is too large to pass through the woman's pelvis. It may be related to maternal diabetes (which often results in large babies), heredity, or maternal nutrition. Cesarean delivery should be anticipated; however,

some birth attendants use cesarean birth as a last resort. An ultrasound or x-ray pelvimetry is performed to determine CPD. Often the woman has dilated and effaced, but the presenting part fails to descend.

Fetal Positions and Presentations
The normal fetal presentation is the **vertex** (head-first) position. If the fetus assumes an abnormal position within the uterus, labor is difficult, and vaginal delivery may be impossible. Depending on the head's position, difficulties may occur. For example, if the face is the presenting part, vaginal delivery is often impossible, because this angle causes a CPD. An abnormal position also may cause a hand or foot or the buttocks to present. Ultrasonography can identify fetal position, as can the location of FHTs. A cesarean delivery may be done for an abnormal position or presentation.

Abnormal Fetal Presentations
Posterior Positions. Normal fetal presentations and positions are discussed in Chapter 65. The most common abnormal fetal presentation is *occiput posterior* where the occiput, or back of the fetal head, is toward the woman's back. Posterior positions are designated right occiput posterior (**ROP**), left occiput posterior (**LOP**), or direct occiput posterior (**OP**). Delivery can be difficult or impossible because the fetal neck is overflexed, the face is uppermost, and the head diameter may be too large to pass through the birth canal. This presentation can occur if the maternal pelvic floor is relaxed. The woman typically complains of a continuous low backache, and FHTs are heard on the woman's *flank* (side).

Medical management may include manual rotation of the fetus (**version**) before engagement, forceps-assisted delivery, or cesarean delivery, which are discussed later in this chapter. Help the woman do pelvic rocking exercises. Pelvic rocking is done while the woman lies flat in bed. She rocks the abdomen from top to bottom, alternating back and forth. First, she presses her backbone against the bed and rocks the hips away from the bed, while tightening the vaginal muscles. She then presses her buttocks into the mattress, while lifting the small of the back. Give emotional support, and massage the woman's lower back.

Transverse Position. The **transverse lie** usually results in a *shoulder presentation.* The fetus lies across the woman's abdomen in the uterus, so a risk of prolapsed cord or descent of a fetal arm exists if the membranes rupture. Management may include version, but a cesarean delivery will most likely be performed.

Face-Brow Presentation. *Face-brow presentation (occipitomental),* occurs when the fetal head is unfavorably positioned for delivery. Predisposing factors include multiparity, polyhydramnios, and a low-lying placenta. The woman may deliver spontaneously if flexion of the fetal neck occurs. Reassure the woman, and anticipate treatment to include an attempted version or cesarean delivery if fetal position cannot be altered.

Breech presentations. **Breech** presentation occurs in 3% of all deliveries. In a *complete breech,* the buttocks present, with the knees bent and the feet next to the buttocks. A *footling breech* is one in which one or both feet present (*single footling* or *double footling*). In a *frank breech,* the buttocks present, with the legs extended straight up (the legs and feet are entwined around the face). Predisposing factors include placenta previa, CPD, multiple pregnancy, small fetus, tumors, and polyhydramnios. If the mother has had a previous breech, a subsequent breech is more likely.

Fetal mortality is higher in breech deliveries than in any other kind of delivery. The risks to the woman include laceration and hemorrhage; to the fetus, the risks include birth injuries and fetal anoxia, which may be caused by early rupture of the bag of waters and by cord prolapse. Also, the head is delivered last, so asphyxia can occur; the fetal head cannot undergo normal molding and may become caught in the birth canal.

Treatment may include diagnostic ultrasound and fetal maturity studies, the use of forceps for the head, or cesarean delivery. Nursing care is the same as for any woman in labor. Anticipate that FHTs will be located at or above the umbilicus, and meconium-stained amniotic fluid may be present. Prepare for newborn resuscitation if a spontaneous delivery occurs.

UMBILICAL CORD COMPLICATIONS

The umbilical cord can be a potential problem during delivery. Possible complications include prolapsed and nuchal cord.

Prolapsed Cord

In a **prolapsed cord,** the umbilical cord precedes the baby. The cord may protrude from the cervix or may drop as low as the vulva. An *occult* (hidden) prolapse is difficult to determine, because the cord is compressed between the fetus and the uterine wall. A prolapsed cord is a serious complication, because as the fetus's head descends, it may press the cord against the hard structures in the woman's pelvis, cutting off fetal circulation. This condition usually requires an emergency cesarean delivery.

A prolapsed cord can result from any factor that interferes with the engagement or adaptation of the presenting part to the pelvis, such as multiple pregnancy, a transverse lie, an abnormal presentation (such as a footling), hydramnios, or a high presenting part when the membranes suddenly rupture.

Sometimes electronic fetal monitoring detects this condition early. The birth attendant or nurse must insert a sterile gloved hand into the vagina to hold the fetal presenting part away from the cord. This measure ensures that fetal circulation is not cut off while the woman is prepared for an emergency cesarean delivery. If the cord has prolapsed outside the vagina, it is covered with sterile towels and moistened with warm, sterile normal saline. This measure prevents drying and caking of the cord and fetal blood. Place the woman in the Trendelenburg or knee–chest position as ordered. Fetal monitoring is essential. Notify the physician at once and prepare for resuscitation of the newborn. A postoperative complication may be maternal puerperal infection.

Nuchal Cord

As the fetus moves within the uterus, the umbilical cord may become wrapped around the neck. This condition is known as **nuchal cord.** If this condition is discovered before labor, cesarean delivery may be done. If it is not discovered until the woman is in labor, the cord may have become so tightly wrapped around the neck that the fetus is unable to receive oxygen. In this case, the birth attendant may use forceps to speed delivery, and the cord is cut immediately. If the nuchal cord is loose, the birth attendant may be able to slip it over the fetus's head.

CONSIDERATIONS RELATED TO DELIVERY

Induction of Labor

The start of labor by medical interventions is called **induction.** Induction of labor may be initiated by a birth attendant for various reasons before labor begins naturally.

Labor is induced only in certain instances, because it is not without risk. Reasons for induction include the possibility of fetal death without labor, worsening signs of PIH, a large or postterm fetus, and maternal diabetes mellitus.

The birth attendant must determine if the woman's birth canal is large enough before inducing labor. If a CPD exists, induction should not be attempted. Fetal maturity also must be evaluated to make sure that the fetus is viable. Amniocentesis can determine maturity by assessing the lecithin–sphingomyelin (**LS**) ratio.

Nursing Considerations

Nursing assessment is important during induction. Carefully monitor the fetus for signs of distress. Take the woman's blood pressure and pulse every 10 to 15 minutes during an IV or suppository induction, and at least every half hour following the rupture of the bag of waters. Any sign of maternal or fetal distress is *an emergency that you must report immediately.* Be sure to provide physical and emotional support to the woman and family during induction.

Induction with Drugs

Drugs may be administered parenterally, orally, or vaginally to induce labor. Nursing considerations can be found at In Practice: Important Medications 67-2. Oxytocin is the most commonly used drug to induce labor. Prostaglandin vaginal suppositories or gel may also be administered prior to oxytocin to ripen the cervix.

Amniotomy

Labor also can be induced by **amniotomy,** which means rupturing the amniotic membranes with a special hook. A physician performs this procedure under sterile conditions, at times with nursing assistance. Labor usually follows quickly. Chart the time of the amniotomy, the color and approximate amount of fluid, and the effects on the woman. If labor does not begin spontaneously after amniotomy, induction with

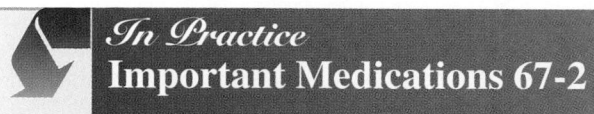

In Practice
Important Medications 67-2

FOR INDUCTION OF LABOR

Oxytocin (Pitocin, Syntocinon)

Nursing Considerations
- Oxytocin is given via IV, using a piggyback setup with a solution of normal saline or D5W (5% dextrose in water) to keep the vein open.
- Adjust the drip rate for optimum rate; character of contractions; and optimum relaxation time between contractions.
- Use the infusion pump to ensure accurate measurement and delivery of the drug.
- Use a fetal monitor to make sure the fetus is not in danger.

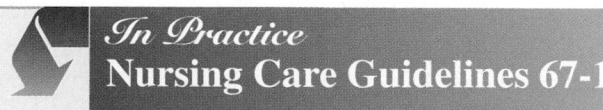

In Practice
Nursing Care Guidelines 67-1

ASSISTING IN AN EMERGENCY DELIVERY

- Provide as much privacy as possible for the woman.
- Wear gloves.
- Do not attempt to prevent delivery.
- Follow aseptic technique as closely as possible.
- Make sure the membranes have ruptured.
- Make sure the newborn's airway is clear before he or she takes the first breath.
- Initiate respiration in the newborn.
- Keep the newborn warm.
- Tie off the umbilical cord in two places.
- Do not cut the umbilical cord.
- Have the mother hold the newborn and put it to breast.
- Get medical assistance as soon as possible.
- Make sure the mother's uterus contracts after delivery of the newborn and placenta.
- Write down the time of birth of the newborn and delivery of the placenta. Write down the mother's name and address.
- Keep the mother warm.
- Reassure the mother.

medications will usually follow. Watch the woman for signs of uterine infection if delivery does not occur within 24 hours.

Emergency Delivery

Sometimes not enough time is available for the woman to get to the healthcare facility for delivery. In this case, police officers, rescue personnel, or nurses may be asked to assist with emergency childbirth. A BOA pack of necessary delivery supplies and equipment is generally kept available at all times in emergency departments and ambulances, and on obstetrical units.

Nursing Considerations

Never delay delivery. Preventing delivery can cause great damage to the woman and fetus. Remain calm and deliver the baby as safely as possible. Follow the best possible aseptic technique. In Practice: Nursing Care Guidelines 67-1 gives additional information on assisting in an emergency delivery.

Usually, few complications arise in a precipitous delivery. Important interventions in the care of the newborn include ensuring respirations and proper body temperature. Cutting the cord is inadvisable, unless the services of the birth attendant are unavailable. However, *tie the cord in two places* when the newborn is breathing or the placenta is delivered. Keep the newborn and placenta together if you anticipate a birth attendant's or hospital's services. Putting the newborn to the mother's breast immediately helps the uterus to contract and prevents maternal hemorrhage. The mother will be examined for retained placental tissue, lacerations, and other complications when she receives medical assistance.

Lacerations

During a precipitous or emergency delivery, a laceration or tear into the perineal tissue and anus may occur. All lacerations are repaired while the woman is still on the delivery table or in the emergency department. Cervical tears are also repaired, to prevent hemorrhage.

Lacerations are classified in several categories.

First degree involves the perineal skin and vaginal mucous membranes.
Second degree involves muscles of the perineal body.
Third degree involves the anal sphincter.
Fourth degree extends to the anal canal.

Operative Obstetrics

Sometimes assisting the woman with the delivery of the baby through operative obstetrics becomes necessary. (Chapter 65 discusses episiotomy.) This section will discuss version, forceps delivery, vacuum extraction, and cesarean birth. The student needs to be familiar with the concepts of normal labor, delivery, and postpartum care presented in Chapter 65.

Version

Version is used to turn the fetus to a more desirable presentation. In *external version,* the woman lies on her back with her knees flexed, and the birth attendant maneuvers the fetus with the hands outside the abdominal wall to a more favorable presentation. In *internal version,* the fetus is turned with the birth attendant's sterile gloved hand inside the uterus. Because the cervix must be dilated to perform the internal version, the fetus is generally delivered at the same time. You must have long, sterile version gloves available for the birth attendant.

Forceps Delivery

Sometimes the birth is assisted with **delivery forceps,** which are double-bladed, curved instruments that fit around the fetal head. Their purpose is to increase traction and to assist in rotating the fetus during delivery. Maternal indications for forceps delivery include exhaustion, heart disease, and prolonged labor. Fetal indications include fetal distress (as indicated by an irregular heartbeat [FHT<100] or a late deceleration pattern on the fetal monitor) and a prolapsed umbilical cord.

Forceps deliveries are classified according to the **station** of the presenting part, that is, the position of the fetal head in relation to the ischial spines (see Fig. 65-2 in Chap 65). *Midforceps* delivery is used when the head is at the ischial spines (*engaged*), and the station is 0. The most commonly used forceps procedure is the *low forceps,* in which the fetal head is on the perineal floor (+3 station).

Before the practitioner applies forceps, the FHTs are checked (preferably with the fetal monitor), an SVE is done to determine whether cervical dilation and effacement are complete, and the membranes are ruptured. The woman is usually catheterized prior to the SVE if forceps delivery is anticipated.

You will be responsible for documenting the time of delivery and the use of forceps and for observing the newborn. If any marks or injuries result from the forceps, document them on the newborn's chart. Document the mother's physical status, vital signs, and emotional reactions.

Vacuum Extraction

An alternative to forceps delivery is **vacuum extraction,** whereby a round, soft plastic cup is placed on the fetal head. Suction is created by a special pump to secure the cup to the presenting part (the fetal head), and traction is exerted to ease the fetus gently out of the birth canal. The woman's cervix must be fully dilated before the vacuum extractor can be used. Document the procedure and observe the newborn and the mother.

Cesarean Delivery

A **cesarean delivery** is a surgical procedure used to deliver the baby through an incision in the abdomen and the uterus. Any complication of labor may be an indication for performing cesarean delivery. In some instances, the woman may have an elective cesarean birth. If the woman has had previous cesarean births, the physician may prefer to do another to avoid the risk of a ruptured uterus. The high number of cesarean births in the United States is controversial.

Preoperative Care.   Cesarean delivery may be scheduled in advance or may be an emergency procedure. A cesarean delivery is not usually done if the fetus is dead.

As a nurse, you will prepare the family for the procedure. Family members are likely to be concerned about the safety of the woman and fetus, as well as the woman's recovery, not only from childbirth, but also from major surgery. A complete explanation of the procedure is given to the partner or coach. Many healthcare facilities allow fathers in the operating room during cesarean delivery, because they can support

the woman during this procedure, just as they can during vaginal delivery.

Chapter 56 discusses preoperative care in abdominal surgery. One difference in cesarean delivery, however, is that the woman does not receive narcotics or strong sedatives, because fetal respiration could easily become depressed. Assess for symptoms of fetal distress or any unusual discomfort the woman might experience.

Generally, the woman is given an *epidural* (spinal anesthetic). In many cases, the woman is not anesthetized further, so the fetus will not be anesthetized. In some cases, local anesthesia is used until the fetus is delivered; the woman then receives general anesthesia for the remainder of the procedure. The woman should be forewarned that she will be awake for at least the first part of the procedure.

Prepare the operating room for abdominal surgery and for care of a newborn. An *isolette* or *radiant heat panel* and resuscitation and suction equipment are required. Surgical nurses and a special nurse to care for the newborn are present at the delivery.

Postoperative Care.   The mother should be given routine postoperative care. Assess vital signs, observe *lochia* (vaginal discharge) and the incision, and check the fundus. Although fundal assessment may be difficult because of the abdominal dressing, it is important to prevent hemorrhage. Record intake and output for 24 to 48 hours. IV fluids are usually continued for 24 hours after surgery. Advance the diet as tolerated. Administer perineal care and oxytocic drugs as ordered. Early ambulation and breathing exercises are important. The client usually goes home on the third or fourth postoperative day.

Care of the Newborn.   Assess the newborn's respiratory status for the first few days of life carefully, because he or she is more likely to experience respiratory distress than a newborn delivered vaginally. During a vaginal delivery, approximately 40% of the fluid in the fetal lungs is squeezed out when the fetal chest compresses while passing through the birth canal. A newborn delivered by cesarean birth does not experience this compression and may suffer respiratory distress due to retained fluids. This newborn also has not had the stimulation of the birth experience.

COMPLICATIONS OF THE POSTPARTUM PERIOD

If undetected and untreated, a postpartal or **puerperal** (occurring following the birth of a baby) complication can become so severe that the mother may require rehospitalization within days of discharge. Therefore, the postpartum assessment provides valuable information in detecting problems. Postpartum complications include circulatory disturbances, infectious processes, and emotional disorders. Common problems of the postpartum period are discussed in Chapter 66.

Postpartum Hematoma

Bleeding into the subcutaneous tissue in the perineal area is called a **postpartum hematoma.** A precipitous delivery, prolonged pressure during labor and delivery, large varicosities in the pelvic area, or a vein that has been cut or pricked during an episiotomy or its repair may cause hematoma. The woman experiences severe pain in the perineal area, especially after a bowel movement or if the bladder becomes overly distended.

Assess the perineal area for discoloration and swelling. You may give the woman cold compresses or a medicated pad, such as Tucks (containing witch hazel); sometimes you will use compresses soaked in a magnesium sulfate solution. Sitz baths may be soothing. You may give analgesics to relieve discomfort. The woman may be returned to the delivery room for incision and ligation of a blood vessel. Small hematomas will be absorbed without treatment.

Postpartum Hemorrhage

Average blood loss during a normal delivery is approximately 300 milliliters; depending on agency guidelines, **postpartum hemorrhage** may be defined as any blood loss from the uterus between 500 and 1,000 milliliters within 24 hours. A postpartal hemorrhage is classified as *early* if it occurs within 24 hours after delivery. A *late* hemorrhage may occur from 2 days to 6 weeks following delivery.

Symptoms of hemorrhage include steady or gushing external vaginal bleeding. The uterus is usually located high in the abdomen and feels boggy. The mother's pulse is often rapid, and the blood pressure drops in relation to the severity of the hemorrhage.

The hemorrhaging woman's life depends on prompt nursing care. Grasp the abdominal area over the uterus, cupping it with both hands. While supporting the lower part of the uterus with one hand, use the other hand to massage gently but firmly. If you cannot locate the uterus because it is boggy, massage the lower abdomen until the uterus contracts. Place the woman into the Trendelenburg position, and monitor her vital signs. Notify the physician, and anticipate IV oxytocin infusion.

If the cause of the bleeding appears to be a laceration or retained placental tissue (see below), the nurse will likely need to prepare the woman for an SVE and treatment, including D&C. If the blood loss is extensive, the client will probably require a blood transfusion.

Uterine Atony and Other Causes

Uterine **atony,** or lack of uterine muscle tone, prevents the uterine muscles from contracting and closing the venous sinuses, which usually causes postpartum hemorrhage. Other causes of hemorrhage are retention of *placental fragments* (which prevents the blood vessels from contracting) and *tears* in the reproductive tract as a result of delivery.

Thrombophlebitis

Thrombophlebitis involves a clot in a blood vessel, with resultant inflammation. In a new mother, thrombophlebitis typically occurs in the femoral vessels in the leg. Early ambulation greatly lessens the occurrence of thrombophlebitis in new mothers.

Symptoms include swelling, slight temperature elevation, pain, and redness or whiteness in the affected area. A positive *Homans' sign* occurs (calf pain on flexion of the foot). The symptoms most often develop in the second postpartal week, and may persist for months.

Treatment consists of bed rest with elevation of the affected part, local application of heat, analgesics, antiembolism stockings, and anticoagulants. After the acute stage has passed, the woman may need to wear a support stocking for some time. Assess lochia, which might become heavier due to anticoagulants.

> **Nursing Alert**
> Carefully assess the woman with thrombophlebitis. *Rationale: If the clot breaks away, it can enter the circulation as an embolism and become fatal.*

Puerperal Infections

Puerperal infection is an infection in any part of the reproductive tract following childbirth. Before the practice of asepsis, it was the major cause of maternal death. Predisposing conditions include the presence of injured tissues or retained pieces of placenta, and lowered maternal resistance. Infection may be mild or severe, local or general; however, like any infection, it is preventable and treatable.

Staphylococcus and *Streptococcus* are common organisms causing puerperal infection. Because healthcare facility personnel can carry these organisms, those who work in the labor room wear caps, clean or sterile suits or gowns, and gloves. In the delivery room, aseptic technique is practiced, and masks are worn. The partner or coach also wears hospital garb in the delivery or birthing room. Handwashing before and after all examinations is absolutely necessary. Practice asepsis when handling the woman's articles, such as peri pads, and teach the woman proper perineal care. Personnel with upper respiratory or gastrointestinal symptoms should not be in contact with the client.

Signs and Symptoms

Fever with a possible chill is the outstanding symptom of puerperal infection. Suspect infection if the woman's temperature elevates to 100.4° Fahrenheit (38° Celsius) orally on any 2 successive days during the first 10 days postpartum. A tender, enlarged uterus, headache, general malaise, and dark-colored, foul-smelling lochia are other symptoms of infection. The episiotomy may appear red, swollen, and tender. The suture line may not be intact. There may be *purulent* (pus-filled) drainage. Assess the characteristics of the lochia, the height of the fundus, and the appearance of the perineum.

The infected mother may be isolated or moved to another floor. The newborn may be isolated and may not be brought to the mother for feeding. Administer antibiotics and encourage fluids. Place the bed in Fowler's position to promote drainage of lochia.

Cystitis

Cystitis, an inflammation of the bladder, is caused by a microorganism. It occurs frequently following childbirth because of urinary retention, residual urine, and trauma to the bladder and urethra during delivery. When urine remains in the bladder, it becomes a breeding place for bacteria.

Signs and Symptoms

The symptoms of cystitis include urination frequency, urgency, pain, burning; hematuria; low abdominal pain; fever; and malaise. After obtaining a urine specimen, administer antibiotics as ordered, and encourage fluids.

Mastitis

Mastitis is a breast infection most commonly caused by *Staphylococcus aureus* (which comes from the baby's mouth), *Escherichia coli,* and rarely *Streptococcus.* These organisms usually enter the body through cracked or injured nipples. The highest incidence occurs in the second or third week postpartum.

Predisposing conditions to mastitis are plugged milk ducts, poor breast drainage, the presence of a pathogenic organism, stress and fatigue, and tight-fitting clothing. Treatment of mastitis includes local massage, moist heat, antibiotic therapy, rest, and frequent nursing. Additional teaching concepts are found at In Practice: Educating the Client 67-2.

Signs and Symptoms

The signs and symptoms of mastitis include localized tenderness, redness, heat, fever, malaise, and sometimes nausea and vomiting. Mastitis should be treated immediately to avoid abscess and chronic mastitis, which may last for up to 4 months and require extensive antibiotic therapy.

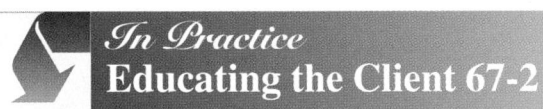

In Practice
Educating the Client 67-2

Prevention of Mastitis Complications

Teach the new mother and family the following measures to prevent mastitis complications:

- Continue to nurse the newborn on both breasts, beginning with the unaffected breast to ease the let-down reflex on the other side.
- Bed rest is mandatory.
- Follow antibiotic therapy regimen as directed by the physician.
- Use hot packs on the breast for comfort.
- Drink plenty of fluids.
- Use mild analgesics (eg, acetaminophen) for pain relief.
- Wear a well-fitting support bra.

Postpartum Blues, Depression, and Psychosis

Women are at risk for "the blues," depression, and psychosis in the months following childbirth. These *mood disorders* are often undiagnosed, and therefore may not be treated. The etiology of the psychological aspect of the postpartum period is most likely due to gonadal hormone imbalances (imbalances in the levels of reproductive hormones). Family and genetic tendencies are also implicated in the development of postpartum mood swings.

Postpartum Blues

Approximately 25% to 85% of all women experience a mild depression, called *postpartum blues,* 3 to 10 days after delivery. Symptoms generally start about 1 week postpartum. The symptoms tend to peak about 5 days post-onset, and generally resolve spontaneously in about 2 weeks.

Typical maternal behaviors may include crying, anxiety, poor appetite, irritability, and insomnia. Many consider these symptoms a normal adjustment phase of the postpartum period. However, these behaviors may also be a warning and indicator of a more serious depression. Treatment generally consists of understanding, reassurance, and support. Members of the family should be made aware of the possible development of "the blues," as well as be told of the importance of follow-up treatment if the symptoms get worse or do not resolve.

Postpartum Depression

Postpartum depression occurs in about 10% to 20% of postpartum women. Depression is more serious than "the blues." Depression begins about 4 weeks after delivery, and women are at increased risk for major depression for several months. The depression may last 6 months or more. A risk factor assessment for depression may be helpful in the early detection of this condition. Risk factors for depression include:

- *Psychological risk factors:* Family history of blues or depression, personal psychiatric history, premenstrual mood swings
- *Social risk factors:* Limited or nonexisting emotional support (from father, parents, or friends), relationship conflict and concerns, stressful living conditions, nominal recreational activities
- *Physical risk factors:* Fatigue, poor general health, thyroid dysfunction, sleep disturbances, use of intramuscular progesterone contraceptive
- *Infant risk factors:* Child health problems, feeding or sleep problems, consensus that the child is a "difficult child"
- *Employment risk factors:* Maternal leave of less than 6 weeks, long work hours with few work rewards

Treatment for depression generally consists of medications such as fluoxetine (Prozac) and/or psychotherapy. The nurse assists by supporting the need for postpartum and well-baby visits. The client's family and other members of her support system should be advised to notify the physician of significant, persistent mood changes between visits.

Postpartum Psychosis

A *postpartum psychosis* can be suspected if the woman exhibits manic-depressive behaviors, generally starting within the first 4 weeks after delivery. Postpartum psychosis occurs in less than 1% of the postpartum population. Initially the symptoms may include irritability, restlessness, sleeplessness, agitation, and avoidance of the infant. The condition may progress to include incoherence, with delusions or hallucinations relating to the child or childbirth. Postpartum psychosis is considered a *medical emergency;* suicide or infanticide is not uncommon.

Treatment consists of hospitalization with suicide precautions and medications such as lithium, antipsychotics, or antidepressants. Child protective services may be necessary. Prognosis, with appropriate medications, is usually good, but the condition may recur following subsequent deliveries. Generally, 95% of these clients improve within 3 months after starting therapy. This condition rarely occurs in women with no previous psychiatric history.

WHEN A NEWBORN DIES

Occasionally, despite excellent antepartal care, a fetus or newborn dies. Obviously, such an event is very difficult for family members. Provide them with as much support as possible and give them a chance to express their feelings. They may appreciate a visit from a chaplain or social worker; ask if the family wishes to have someone special called.

In many healthcare facilities, the woman is moved from the obstetric unit. Intense emotions may be worsened by remaining in a maternity setting. Some facilities prepare a small package of mementos from the baby, such as the tee shirt worn in the nursery, a lock of hair, some photos, an identification bracelet, and the birth certificate. Such articles are given to the mother for her to open or to keep sealed as she chooses. In this way, the baby's existence is acknowledged, along with the loss. Be familiar with policy, and respect the family's wishes. Allow the mother to hold the child and take photos if she wishes. The family also may choose to donate fetal tissues to help other people.

The family should be given the opportunity to have a funeral or cremation. Referral to an organization such as The Compassionate Friends is often helpful.

➜ STUDENT SYNTHESIS

Key Points

- A high-risk pregnancy is one in which complications of the pregnancy or pre-existing health conditions endanger the life or well-being of the woman or fetus.
- Diagnostic techniques for assessing fetal status include amniocentesis, ultrasound, nonstress testing, oxytocin challenge testing, and biophysical profile.
- Some spontaneous abortions occur for unknown reasons; however, fetal maldevelopment and certain maternal factors account for many cases. The type of spontaneous abortion dictates medical and nursing management.
- Ectopic pregnancy is a significant cause of maternal morbidity and mortality.
- Discharge of a woman suffering from hyperemesis gravidarum occurs when she regains fluid and electrolyte balance and begins to gain weight.
- Careful management of the woman with pregnancy-induced hypertension is crucial.
- Existing medical disorders—such as diabetes mellitus, cardiac disorders, and chemical dependency—will complicate pregnancy and require special care.
- Maternal insulin requirements in the woman with insulin-dependent diabetes increase as the pregnancy advances. Control of maternal blood glucose is essential for preventing hydramnios, dystocia, and other complications.
- Placenta previa and premature separation of the placenta are differentiated by the type of bleeding, uterine tone, and the presence or absence of pain.
- Complications of labor and delivery are related to the status of the membranes, the pace of labor, the effectiveness of contractions, the passageway, and the passenger.
- Dystocia is active labor that does not result in effective cervical dilation or effacement.
- Operative obstetrics concerns procedures that involve manipulating the fetus to facilitate birth. Version, forceps, vacuum extraction, and cesarean birth are examples.
- Hemorrhagic (hypovolemic) shock is an emergency in which sufficient blood does not reach vital organs in the mother or newborn; death may ensue.
- The basic purpose of a cesarean delivery is to preserve the life and health of the woman and her fetus.
- Infection control measures are essential to protect the mother and newborn from transmission of infectious organisms.

Critical Thinking Exercises

1. Identify risk factors for noncompliance with the treatment regimen for a woman who is diabetic and pregnant.
2. You are caring for a client who is 32 years old. Three previous pregnancies have been full-term without complications. One previous pregnancy ended in a stillbirth. During this pregnancy, she developed preeclampsia during her third trimester. She is now at 38 weeks' gestation and has been admitted with a large amount of painless, vaginal

bleeding. List nursing interventions according to priority.
3. Compare the effect of amniotomy for induction of labor with various other methods. Consider risks and benefits for the mother and newborn.
4. Place yourself in the position of a woman who has just been told she must have an emergency cesarean birth because of complications. Describe your feelings. Discuss what information you will need and the nursing care you would like to receive.

NCLEX-Style Review Questions

1. Which intervention would be most appropriate for the woman experiencing a complete spontaneous abortion?
   a. Bedrest with feet elevated
   b. Vital signs every hour
   c. Perineal pad count and weight
   d. Administration of Prostin E2
2. Which position is most beneficial for the woman diagnosed with preeclampsia?
   a. Supine
   b. Prone
   c. Left lateral
   d. Right lateral

3. Which statement represents the key to a good maternal–fetal outcome when a pregnancy is complicated by diabetes?
   a. Good control of blood glucose level is of primary importance.
   b. Delivery should occur between 36–38 weeks' gestation to ensure a healthy fetus.
   c. Nonstress tests should be done weekly after 32 weeks' gestation.
   d. Potential problems are avoided with a good, healthy diet.
4. Which statement best reflects the relationship between chemical dependency and pregnancy?
   a. Child protection authorities should be first contacted when the woman is in labor.
   b. The chemically dependent mother often lacks parenting skills.
   c. Drug use is not associated with congenital defects.
   d. The incidence of abruptio placentae is not increased with substance abuse.
5. What is the cause of a firm uterus when abruptio placenta is present?
   a. Uterine contractions
   b. Increased fetal movement
   c. Loss of uterine tone
   d. Blood inside the uterus

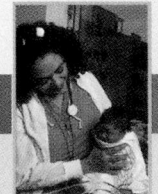

CHAPTER

68

The High-Risk Newborn

LEARNING OBJECTIVES

1. Define the term high-risk newborn.
2. Define and differentiate between the following: AGA, SGA, LGA, LBW, VLBW, RDS, ROP, and macrosomia.
3. Compare and contrast at least three nursing considerations for the care of a preterm infant and a postterm infant.
4. Define and discuss at least three nursing considerations for each of the following: meconium or amniotic fluid aspiration, cyanosis, physiologic jaundice, hyperbilirubinemia, phototherapy, dehydration, NEC, and hypoglycemia.
5. Define and differentiate among Rh sensitization, erythroblastosis fetalis, and ABO incompatibility. State at least three nursing interventions for each of these hemolytic disorders.
6. State the causes of the following types of birth injuries: fractures, intracranial hemorrhage, brachial plexus injury, and facial paralysis. Discuss at least two nursing interventions for each injury.
7. Define and differentiate among congenital disorders, genetic disorders, and teratogenic disorders.
8. Define the following musculoskeletal disorders: talipes, congenital dislocated hip, polydactylism, and syndactylism. State at least two nursing interventions for each disorder.
9. Describe the following nervous system disorders: hydrocephalus, spina bifida, Down syndrome, anencephaly, and microcephaly. State at least two nursing interventions for each disorder.
10. Define the following cardiovascular disorders: patent ductus arteriosus, ASD, VSD, tetralogy of Fallot, and coarctation of the aorta; state at least two nursing interventions for each disorder.
11. Define the respiratory disorder choanal atresia and state two appropriate nursing interventions.
12. Define the following gastrointestinal disorders: cleft lip, cleft palate, esophageal atresia, tracheoesophageal fistula, pyloric stenosis, imperforate anus, PKU, galactosemia, exstrophy of the bladder, hypospadias, and epispadias. List at least two nursing interventions for each disorder.
13. Identify the common infections (TORCH) that can adversely affect the fetus. State at least two nursing interventions for each infection.
14. Define and discuss at least three nursing considerations for FAS.
15. Identify at least three consequences to the fetus if the mother has a chemical dependency on alcohol, cocaine, heroin, or marijuana.

NEW TERMINOLOGY

ABO incompatibility
anencephaly
choanal atresia
cleft lip
cleft palate
congenital
epispadias
erythroblastosis fetalis
esophageal atresia
exstrophy
galactosemia
high-risk newborn
hydrocephalus
hyperbilirubinemia
hypospadias
imperforate anus

macrosomia
microcephaly
pathologic jaundice
phototherapy
physiologic jaundice
polydactylism
postterm
preterm
pyloric stenosis
Rh sensitization
spina bifida
syndactylism
talipes
thrush
toxoplasmosis

ACRONYMS

AGA	LGA	SGA
ASD	NEC	SIDS
CMV	PKU	TORCH
CSF	RDS	VLBW
FAS	ROP	VSD
LBW		

At birth, the newborn assumes the functions of breathing, eating, digesting, eliminating, and stabilizing his or her own body temperature. If problems related to any of these vital functions develop, the newborn is likely to have difficulty surviving. The newborn with a complication is considered a compromised or **high-risk newborn.** Due to advanced technology and improved healthcare measures, high-risk newborns have ever-increasing chances for survival.

Through accurate assessments, the nurse can often detect abnormalities early and report them promptly. Difficulties can often be alleviated or corrected when treatment begins quickly.

The mother, her family, and the high-risk newborn are highly vulnerable. Protecting the newborn by maintaining a warm environment, adequate oxygen, and safety is a priority. The newborn's basic needs for oxygen, nutrition, fluid, and elimination should be constantly monitored and met. The baby's survival and well-being depend on the collaborative efforts of the healthcare team. Remember that the newborn belongs to a family that also has many needs.

Families often are shocked upon learning about a problem in their newborn. At such times, you can provide emotional support. Family members need to express their fears, hopes, and disappointments. Sometimes, they require more knowledge so that they can make decisions related to treatment. Most of all, families appreciate a caring nurse—someone who listens with compassion and understanding.

CLASSIFICATION OF HIGH-RISK NEWBORNS

Newborns may be classified by their size and gestational age (Box 68-1). Neurologic assessments are performed on all newborns to determine their maturity. Newborns whose size falls within standard norms are categorized as appropriate for gestational age (**AGA**). An infant may be at risk even if he or she has reached an acceptable maturation age (after 37 weeks' gestation).

Newborn birth weight is another important classification. Low birth weight (**LBW**) babies can be born as full-term or preterm infants. Very low birth weight (**VLBW**) babies are at a high risk, and are generally born prior to their expected birth date. LBW babies are more likely to be born to adolescent mothers. The incidence of LWB is about 7% in the overall newborn population. In contrast, the adolescent under 15 years of age has nearly double the chance of delivering a LBW baby, at about 13%. The statistics are better for those mothers between 15 and 19 years of age, who have a 9.5% chance of an LBW baby. Box 68-1 gives further information on the classifications of newborns.

Small-for-Gestational-Age Newborn

Causes of newborns born as small for gestational age (**SGA**) include the following:

- Maternal conditions (eg, pregnancy-induced hypertension, cardiac and renal disease, and diabetes mellitus)
- Poor maternal nutrition
- Intrauterine infections
- Maternal substance abuse, including alcohol
- Maternal cigarette smoking
- Congenital malformations
- Multiple births
- Fetal and placental abnormalities

Characteristics of the SGA newborn include an abnormally large head in relation to the body, loose and dry skin, sparse or absent hair, wide skull sutures caused by inadequate bone growth, and diminished muscle and fatty tissue. Specific problems faced by the SGA newborn include hypothermia, hypoglycemia, respiratory distress, prolonged infantile apnea, delayed neurologic development, or sudden infant death syndrome (**SIDS**).

Large-for-Gestational-Age Newborn

In the condition known as **macrosomia,** a newborn is born large for gestational age (**LGA**). These newborns are those with birth weights that exceed the 90th percentile of newborns of the same gestational age. They are born most often to mothers with diabetes.

Although these newborns are large and appear fat, they are not necessarily healthy. Elevated blood glucose levels in the woman increase the glucose available to the fetus, which stimulates additional insulin production by the fetal pancreas. A problem arises when the baby is delivered, and the supply of excess glucose is therefore terminated. This newborn quickly uses all available carbohydrates and may develop *hypoglycemia.*

Other problems facing the LGA newborn include birth injury (eg, fractured clavicle, skull fracture, and brachial nerve palsy), as well as respiratory disorders and brain injuries.

➤➤ **BOX 68-1**

CLASSIFICATION OF NEWBORNS

Based on Size
- *Appropriate for gestational age (AGA):* Growth is within normal limits.
- *Small for gestational age (SGA):* Birth weight is below the 10th percentile expected for that gestational age.
- *Large for gestational age (LGA):* Birth weight is larger than 90% of the babies born at that gestational age.
- *Low birth weight (LBW):* Birth weight is less than 5.5 lb (approximately 2,500 g).
- *Very low birth weight (VLBW):* Birth weight is 1–3.5 lb (500–1,499 g).
- *Immature:* Birth weight is less than 2.2 lb (1,000 g).

Based on Gestational Age
- *Preterm:* Born before the completion of the 37th week of gestation (before 265 days, counting from the first day of the woman's last normal menstrual period)
- *Term:* Born from the 38th week of gestation, but before completion of the 41st week of gestation
- *Post-term:* Born after the completion of the 41st week of gestation

Postterm Newborn

The fetus who remains in the uterus beyond 42 weeks is called **postterm.** Such newborns are not necessarily in better condition than full-term newborns. Postterm newborns often have respiratory or nutritional problems, because the placenta is unable to provide adequately for them after the normal gestation period. As a result, they may be SGA. They often have long fingernails and hair, dry parched skin, and no vernix caseosa. These babies look wrinkled and old at birth. They may have swallowed meconium or aspirated it into their lungs.

Preterm Newborn

Newborns classified as **preterm** are those born prior to the end of the 37th week of gestation. Despite advances in the early identification and treatment of preterm labor, these births account for approximately 7% of all births in the United States. The number of preterm infants born to black women decreased in the last decade of the 20th century. However, the number of preterm births and LBW babies born to African American women is about twice that found in white women.

Causes of preterm delivery include:

- Poor antepartal care
- Maternal age extremes (ie, younger than 19 or older than 35)
- Low socioeconomic status
- Poor maternal nutrition
- Chronic disorders (eg, hypertension, diabetes, renal disorders)
- Antepartum trauma or infection
- Uterine anomalies
- Premature cervical dilation
- Maternal drug or alcohol use
- Maternal smoking

The preterm infant appears thin, with minimal subcutaneous fat. *Lanugo* (fine hair) may appear on the face, back, arms, and legs. Skin is transparent and breast tissue is barely palpable. In male newborns, the testes may be undescended. Breathing is irregular and weak. Body temperature is frequently subnormal, and the baby's cry is weak. Neurologic assessments reflect an immature central nervous system, as demonstrated by diminished or absent reflexes.

Nursing Considerations

To conserve the energy of small newborns, handle them as little as possible. Usually, you will not give them a bath immediately. Controlling their temperature is often difficult; therefore, special care should be taken to keep these babies warm. Dress them in a *stockinette cap,* and take their temperature often. Supply oxygen if necessary. Fig. 68-1 illustrates care provided for a very small newborn in the intensive care unit (ICU). Refer to In Practice: Nursing Care Plan 68-1 for a plan of care for a preterm infant.

Isolette Care. The *isolette* simulates the uterine environment as closely as possible. The isolette is transparent, so

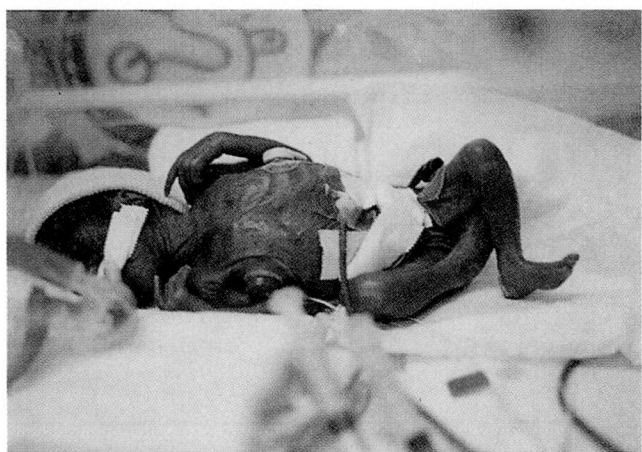

FIGURE 68-1. A newborn in the intensive care unit. Note the electrodes for constant monitoring, and the cap on the head to maintain body heat.

the newborn is visible at all times. The isolette maintains even levels of temperature, humidity, and oxygen. A hood covers it, and nurses can give care through portholes.

Feeding. The *feeding* of small newborns varies. In some instances, small newborns receive no food for 36 hours, because digestion is an additional burden on their bodies. In other instances, they receive formula or expressed breast milk using a nipple or a nasogastric tube (*gavage feeding*). Formula is prescribed in very small amounts on a 2- to 3-hour schedule, to avoid distending their small stomach or adding to respiratory distress.

Elimination. Because their kidneys are not fully developed, small newborns may have difficulty *eliminating* wastes. The nurse should determine accurate output by weighing the diaper before and after the infant urinates. The diaper's weight difference in grams is approximately equal to the amount of milliliters voided.

Protection Against Infection. All who come into contact with the newborn must perform good handwashing, the first defense against infection. Because very small newborns are susceptible to infection, they are isolated, and attended to by nursery personnel with a thorough knowledge of special aseptic techniques. Generally, these newborns are not dressed, so that nurses can observe their breathing. Contact with other people is limited as much as possible. To promote bonding, the parents, wearing gowns and gloves, are encouraged to touch and to hold these newborns (if conditions permit).

Assessments. The very small newborn should be *assessed* carefully. Observations include color (eg, pink, cyanotic, jaundiced), respirations (eg, normal or abnormal, rate, retractions, expiratory grunt, nasal flaring), pulse (eg, rate, strength, regularity), stools and voiding (eg, amount, frequency, description), general appearance, weight, and activity level. Report any abnormal symptoms. If a newborn is having difficulties, attach monitors. Care will be given in the ICU.

Respiratory Status. Respiratory distress syndrome (**RDS**) is a leading cause of death, especially in the preterm newborn. In RDS, the newborn's lungs cannot expand nor-

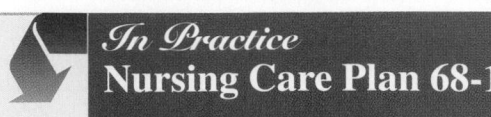

In Practice
Nursing Care Plan 68-1

THE PRETERM NEONATE EXPERIENCING DIFFICULTY REGULATING BODY TEMPERATURE

MEDICAL HISTORY: *Baby boy D., born vaginally at 30 weeks' gestation, has an Apgar score of 4 and 6 (at birth and at 5 minutes, respectively) and weighs 2,250 g. Mother had received betamethasone at 24 and 12 hours prior to birth to enhance lung maturity.*

MEDICAL DIAGNOSIS: *Prematurity*

Data Collection/Nursing Assessment: Neonate born at 30 weeks. Temperature (axillary) fluctuates, ranging between 96.8° F (36° C) and 99.0° F (37.2° C). Client, although preterm, is appropriate for gestational age. Skin appears ruddy with much vernix caseosa and minimal subcutaneous fat. Acrocyanosis is evident. Respirations are slightly irregular at 66 breaths per minute; no bradycardia is noted. (*Although numerous nursing diagnoses may be appropriate, a priority nursing diagnosis is addressed below.*)

Nursing Diagnosis: Ineffective thermoregulation, related to immaturity and large body surface area with minimal fat stores, as evidenced by widely fluctuating axillary temperature readings.

Planning:
SHORT-TERM GOALS:
#1. Client will exhibit no signs of cold stress.
#2. Client will demonstrate gradual stabilization of body temperature within acceptable range for weight.

LONG-TERM GOALS:
#3. Client will maintain body temperature within acceptable parameters out of isolette.

Implementation:
NURSING ACTION: *Dry neonate thoroughly and place in isolette or under a radiant warmer. If using an isolette, minimize the number of times the portholes are opened.*
RATIONALE: *Drying helps to prevent heat loss by evaporation; an isolette or radiant warmer provides a neutral thermal environment. Opening the portholes provides a means for heat to escape from the isolette.*

NURSING ACTION: *Keep handling of the neonate to a minimum. Refrain from bathing the neonate until the temperature is maintained between 97.6° F to 98.6° F (36.5° to 37° C). Consolidate procedures and treatments to avoid tiring the neonate.*

RATIONALE: *Minimizing handling helps the neonate to conserve energy.*

NURSING ACTION: *Cover the neonate's head.*
RATIONALE: *Covering the neonate's head, a large body surface area for heat loss, minimizes the amount of heat lost.*

NURSING ACTION: *Cover any surfaces that the neonate is to lie on and position the neonate away from doors, windows, or other areas that may cause drafts.*
RATIONALE: *Lying on a cold surface increases the loss of body heat via conduction. Keeping the neonate away from areas that may cause drafts minimizes the amount of heat lost via convection and radiation.*

Evaluation: Neonate warm, color pale pink; head covered; axillary temperature at 97.6° F (36.5° C); being maintained in isolette. No evidence of cold stress. *Goal #1 met.*

NURSING ACTION: *Monitor neonate's axillary temperature every 30 min until it begins to stabilize and then every 1– 2 hr.*
RATIONALE: *Frequently monitoring the neonate's temperature provides objective evidence of the neonate's status.*

Evaluation: Neonate's temperature ranging between 97.6° and 98.6° F (36.5° to 37° C) for past 4 hr. *Progress to meeting Goal #2.*

NURSING ACTION: *Continue to monitor neonate's heart rate and respirations for changes indicating possible cold stress. Begin to increase time neonate spends out of isolette, monitoring temperature closely for changes.*
RATIONALE: *Cold stress increases the neonate's consumption of oxygen, increasing the workload of the heart.*

NURSING ACTION: *Weigh the neonate daily and report any significant decreases.*
RATIONALE: *Cold stress can decrease the rate of weight gain in the neonate.*

Evaluation: Neonate's temperature ranging between 97.6° and 98.6° F (36.5° to 37° C); heart rate (120–130 beats/min) and respirations (56–60 breaths/min) within age-acceptable parameters; neonate out of isolette for 10 min 3 times per day with temperature maintained at 97.6° F (36.5° C); weight stabilized. *Goal #2 met; progress to meeting Goal #3.*

mally, and therefore do not receive enough air for proper oxygenation. RDS is caused by a deficiency of a substance called *pulmonary surfactant,* resulting in incomplete lung expansion. *Atelectasis,* partial or complete collapse of a lung, is common. Prevention of preterm birth is a key factor in reducing RDS. Betamethasone, a glucocorticosteroid, is often given to the mother 12 to 24 hours before the preterm birth, to help reduce the severity of RDS.

The newborn with RDS demonstrates *dyspnea* and *cyanosis.* The respiratory rate increases, and the nares (nostrils) flare. (See Fig. 66-5 in Chap. 66.) The chest muscles retract during inspiration, accompanied by *tachycardia* and an *expiratory grunt.* If the condition cannot be corrected, it is usually fatal. If the newborn survives the first few days of life, however, recovery is usually complete.

Administering oxygen in an atmosphere of high humidity, and sometimes using a mechanical ventilator, are treatments for RDS. The newborn is fed by gavage or through a *central line* (large venous catheter providing total parenteral nutrition) to prevent aspiration into the lungs. Antibiotics are usually given.

Retinopathy of prematurity (**ROP**) is a complication of a high concentration of oxygen (especially in the premature newborn), due to vasoconstriction of immature retinal blood vessels. Infants receiving oxygen therapy must have blood oxygen (PO_2) levels monitored to keep oxygen levels as close to normal as possible. In the past, there was no reversing the effects of ROP. Today, *cryosurgery* has proven effective in preserving eyesight.

POTENTIAL COMPLICATIONS IN THE HIGH-RISK NEWBORN

Many of the possible complications in the high-risk newborn are related to respiratory, circulatory, and metabolic functioning.

Meconium or Amniotic Fluid Aspiration

In the *hypoxic* fetus (one who is lacking oxygen), the anal sphincter relaxes, allowing meconium to pass into the amniotic fluid. *Meconium aspiration* can occur *in utero* or at birth. If the first breath is taken prior to suctioning, the newborn may aspirate meconium and amniotic fluid into the lungs.

Any aspirated fluid can lead to atelectasis, pneumonia, and other pulmonary problems. An aspiration bulb is kept at the crib side for the purpose of clearing respiratory passages. Treatment is supportive. Give oxygen, encourage fluids, and regulate temperature. Give antibiotics as ordered.

Cyanosis

If the newborn does not establish initial breathing, he or she turns blue or dusky, a condition known as *cyanosis.* Respiratory difficulty may be due to *prolapsed cord* during delivery, a congenital heart defect, faulty respiratory apparatus, birth injury to the brain, a congenital defect in the brain stem, or

medications (even the analgesic or anesthetic given to the mother during labor).

Prompt initiation of treatment for newborns who do not breathe as soon as they are delivered is crucial. First, determination of whether the air passages are clear of obstructive substances, such as amniotic fluid and mucus, is necessary. Soft catheters, bulb syringes, and mechanical suction are used to remove this material. The newborn's head is lowered, to facilitate postural drainage. The back is rubbed to stimulate respiration. If the baby fails to respond, additional resuscitation measures (eg, mechanical ventilation) are begun.

Physiologic Jaundice

Many newborns have an elevated bilirubin level (**hyperbilirubinemia**), which causes **physiologic jaundice.** *Jaundice* results from the inability of the newborn's immature liver to handle bilirubin, a by-product of red blood cell breakdown. Manifesting about 48 to 72 hours after birth, this type of jaundice is fairly common and generally benign. Excess bilirubin appears in the bloodstream, causing the skin to appear yellow. A heel-stick blood test (see Chap. 66) may be ordered to determine the degree of hyperbilirubinemia. If the level is sufficiently high, phototherapy will be initiated.

Phototherapy is the use of fluorescent lights to alleviate jaundice. The ultraviolet (UV) light of sunshine, or intense fluorescent light, accelerates the elimination of bilirubin in the skin (*photo-oxidation*). To provide maximum skin exposure, keep the newborn naked except for a small diaper. Cover the eyes with dressings to protect the retinas. Then place the newborn under the lights. Nursing considerations during phototherapy include monitoring vital signs, especially temperature. Be aware of *hypothermia* or *hyperthermia.* Generally, the baby is placed on a 3-hour feeding schedule. (Frequent feedings help to speed the excretion of bilirubin.) Supplemental water is necessary, to prevent dehydration. The urine and stool may be green. Remove the newborn from the lights for feeding, obtaining vital signs, and bonding.

> **Nursing Alert**
> Physiologic jaundice usually appears at about the third day of life. Report jaundice that appears immediately after birth. *Rationale: An immediate case of jaundice (pathologic jaundice) is likely to indicate hemolytic disease.*

Dehydration

The greatest concern with newborn vomiting or diarrhea is *dehydration,* which leads to *electrolyte imbalance* if unchecked. Dehydration develops quickly, because the baby has so little reserve fluid. Start treatment immediately, or the newborn may die. Give intravenous fluids, along with humidified oxygen. Lost electrolytes must be replaced.

Newborn *vomiting* may be a symptom of a congenital defect (eg, esophageal atresia), birth injury (eg, intracranial hemorrhage), or infection. A distinct difference exists between vomiting and normal spitting-up in the newborn.

Bacteria most commonly cause *diarrhea,* although an incompatible formula or an allergy may also be the culprit. In newborn diarrhea, the stool is formless, greenish-yellow, and foul-smelling. Dehydration can occur very quickly. Evidence of diarrhea requires isolation of the baby to prevent possible infection of other newborns. Obtain stool cultures.

Necrotizing Enterocolitis

Necrotizing enterocolitis (**NEC**) is a serious disorder that causes varying amounts of the bowel wall to *necrose* (die). It is more common in preterm babies, especially if the woman's membranes ruptured early or if the newborn suffered anoxia; bottle-fed babies are more susceptible. Symptoms include lethargy, abdominal distention, hypothermia, apnea, and irritability. Using a nasogastric tube and suction allows the bowel to rest. Supportive care includes parenteral fluids and total parenteral nutrition, antibiotics, infection control, and surgical resection as needed. X-rays of the bowel are performed frequently to evaluate progress.

Hypoglycemia

All babies have the potential for *hypoglycemia* (decreased blood sugar) soon after birth. The following newborns are at greatest risk:

- LGA newborns
- Newborns of diabetic mothers (see Chap. 67)
- Newborns with erythroblastosis fetalis
- Newborns with heart disease
- Newborns with galactosemia

Additional information regarding these conditions can be found in other sections of this chapter.

Hypoglycemia occurs when the blood glucose level reads below 40 milligrams per deciliter. Signs of hypoglycemia normally relate to the central nervous system and include tremors, irritability, jitteriness, high-pitched or weak cry, and eye rolling. Observable changes in vital signs (such as *apnea* and *tachycardia*) may appear. The newborn may be cyanotic or pale, eat poorly, and have seizures. Treatment consists of a carefully calculated infusion of glucose, decreasing the amount as the newborn is able tolerate oral feedings. Assess the baby carefully for change in status.

HEMOLYTIC CONDITIONS

Hemolytic conditions (destructive to the red blood cells) often result from an Rh or ABO blood incompatibility. In both conditions, the woman builds up antibodies against antigens from her own fetus. **Pathologic jaundice** (hemolytic disease of the newborn) may develop. In contrast to physiologic jaundice, pathologic jaundice can be seen less than 24 hours after birth.

Rh Sensitization

A hemolytic disease of the newborn, **erythroblastosis fetalis,** can occur when an Rh-negative mother is pregnant with an Rh-positive fetus, resulting in **Rh sensitization** (*Rh incompatibility*). The disease does not occur in the first pregnancy, but occurs with increasing severity in future pregnancies. The condition causes the woman's antibodies to destroy fetal red blood cells (see Chap. 67).

This condition is uncommon today because it is preventable. If an Rh-negative women receives *anti-D gamma globulin,* also known as Rh_o(D) immune globulin (RhoGAM, Gamulin Rh) prophylactically at 28 weeks' gestation, following any invasive procedure (eg, amniocentesis) or any abortion, the condition is prevented. It is important to give RhoGAM also following delivery of an Rh-positive baby.

Some cases of erythroblastosis fetalis still occur in women who did not have antepartal care or who did not receive RhoGAM following a previous abortion.

Phototherapy is used to treat milder cases after birth. If such measures do not help, a series of exchange transfusions probably will be performed. In severe cases, the fetus may receive an intrauterine transfusion before birth.

As the newborn grows older, he or she will produce erythrocytes independently and will outgrow the condition.

ABO Incompatibility

ABO incompatibility occurs in the following situations:

- The mother has type O blood and the newborn has type A, B, or AB blood.
- The mother is of the blood group A or B, with a newborn of the opposite blood group or AB.

The disease of ABO incompatibility is usually mild, characterized by jaundice and an enlarged spleen. Treatment usually consists of phototherapy. ABO incompatibility is also discussed in Chapter 67.

BIRTH INJURIES

Various injuries may occur during the birth process. Some are serious but most can be corrected. Chapter 67 provides additional information related to labor, delivery, and possible injuries at birth.

Fractures

Fractures rarely are complicated and usually heal without difficulties. One common birth injury is a *fractured clavicle.* Signs and symptoms of a fractured clavicle include asymmetrical *Moro reflex,* and crying when the affected arm is moved.

Intracranial Hemorrhage

Intracranial hemorrhage can be a dangerous birth injury that is primarily a problem for preterm newborns. Causes other than prematurity include difficult delivery, *precipitate* (sudden, progressing faster than normal) labor and delivery, or prolonged labor. Seizures, respiratory distress, cyanosis, a shrill cry, and muscle weakness are signs. Prognosis varies with the extent of the injury and treatment. To prevent hemorrhage, every newborn receives *vitamin K* intramuscularly soon after delivery, to aid in blood clotting. Treatment is similar to that of an adult.

Position the newborn with intracranial hemorrhage with the head of the bed slightly elevated. Administer oxygen, vitamin K, antibiotics, anticonvulsive medications, and sedatives as ordered. Feeding is by *gavage tube.* Complications that may result include cerebral hemorrhage, cerebral palsy, hydrocephaly, and mental retardation.

Brachial Plexus Injury

Injury to the *brachial plexus* results from trauma during a difficult delivery (eg, shoulder dystocia). One example of brachial plexus injury is *Erb-Duchenne paralysis,* which results from trauma to the fifth and sixth cranial nerves. The baby is unable to elevate the affected arm, which lies limply at the side. Grasp reflex is present. *Lower plexus injury* results in symptoms in the hand and forearm, with the grasp reflex absent. Treatment of both includes range of motion exercises and possible splinting. Prognosis depends on the degree of nerve damage.

Facial Paralysis

Facial paralysis (*Bell's palsy*) occurs when the newborn's facial nerves are injured, usually as a result of forceps delivery. If nerve tissue is damaged, paralysis may be permanent. Usually only one side of the face is affected, and the eyelid and mouth may droop on that side. The baby's sucking mechanism may be impaired, requiring special feeding. The newborn also may need saline irrigation or patching of the eye to retain moisture. Plastic surgery is sometimes effective in improving appearance. Fortunately, most cases of facial and brachial paralysis are temporary.

CONGENITAL DISORDERS

A **congenital** disorder is an abnormality that exists at birth. Congenital disorders may involve any body system. Some disorders involve several systems. Disorders may be classified as the following types:

- *Genetic:* Hereditary in origin, inherited
- *Teratogenic:* Acquired during gestation (eg, due to maternal illness; medications; use of drugs, alcohol, or tobacco; exposure to environmental toxins; vaccinations and inoculations)

Chapters 71, 72, and 73 discuss most of the following disorders in more detail.

Musculoskeletal Disorders

Talipes

Talipes is also known as *clubfoot.* In clubfoot, one or both feet turn out of the normal position. The condition occurs more often in boys. Early diagnosis and treatment usually yield an excellent prognosis. Exercise, corrective shoes, braces, casts, and surgery also may be helpful.

Congenital Dislocated Hip

Congenital dislocated hip occurs more frequently in girls. Faulty embryonic development of the hip joint is the likely cause. The head of the femur fails to situate firmly in the acetabulum. Early treatment is necessary to prevent permanent damage.

The first sign of this condition may be a limitation of abduction on the affected side when the thigh is flexed (*Ortolani's sign*). The affected femur is shorter than the unaffected femur; the skinfolds of the thigh and buttocks are asymmetric, and a slight click may be heard with hip abduction. X-ray studies usually confirm diagnosis.

Treatment usually consists of stabilizing the head of the femur into the acetabulum and holding it there for a period. A "triple" diaper, providing bulk in the groin region to force the leg into abduction, may resolve the problem, as may thick foam pads or splints. In extreme cases, the baby may need a cast (see Chap. 71).

Polydactylism and Syndactylism

The presence of an extra finger or toe is called *polydactylism.* Often the extra digit hangs limp and boneless. In this case, a suture is tied tightly around the appendage, and the digit will fall off. Occasionally surgery is necessary. **Syndactylism** is the fusing together of two or more digits. Separation of the digits may be possible by surgery.

Nervous System Disorders

Hydrocephalus

Hydrocephalus is an excess of cerebrospinal fluid (**CSF**) in the ventricles and subarachnoid spaces of the brain. Untreated, it results in an enlarged head, brain damage, and death. The newborn may also exhibit bulging fontanels and nervous irritability. Hydrocephalus is treated by surgically inserting shunts that drain the ventricles (see Chap. 71).

Spina Bifida

Spina bifida is a congenital neural tube defect in which the vertebral spaces fail to close, allowing a *herniation (bulging)* of the spinal contents into a sac. When the meninges covering the spinal cord herniate through the vertebral space, it is called a *meningocele.* When spinal cord nerve fibers and meninges herniate, it is referred to as a *myelomeningocele.* Surgery may correct these problems; prognosis depends on the deformity's extent. Women who take folic acid (folate) during pregnancy greatly reduce the risk for neural tube defects such as spina bifida in their babies.

Down Syndrome

Down syndrome, also called *trisomy 21,* is a genetic disorder often associated with mothers who give birth after age 40. It is commonly identified in the newborn nursery by typical physical features, although only chromosomal analysis can make a final diagnosis. Physical and mental manifestations may range from mild to severe. One deep crease runs horizontally across the hands. Eyes are slanted, and the tongue is large and protruding. The infant is flaccid. Usually, accompanying mental retardation and heart defects exist, and cataracts and gastrointestinal disorders may be present (see Chap. 73).

Anencephaly and Microcephaly

In children with **anencephaly,** part or all of the brain is missing. The skull is flat, and these newborns live for only a short time, if at all. Children with **microcephaly** have abnormally small heads. They may live or die, depending on the extent of the deformity. Because the brain does not develop as normal, these newborns are almost always mentally retarded.

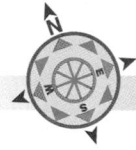

SPECIAL CONSIDERATIONS: CULTURE

Baptism

If a newborn's condition is poor, some Christian families desire baptism to be performed immediately. Anyone can baptize in an emergency; however, if a clergy member or a chaplain is available, this person should baptize the baby. If you are asked to baptize a newborn, pour water over the head or other skin surface and say the following words: "I baptize you in the name of the Father, of the Son, and of the Holy Spirit [Holy Ghost]." Alert the family's priest or minister that baptism has taken place. Insert a record of the procedure on the mother's chart. Two witnesses should be present whenever possible; document their names on the chart.

Cardiovascular Disorders

Several congenital heart and blood vessel defects are seen in newborns. Chapter 71 illustrates some of these conditions. *Cardiovascular defects* include:

- *Patent ductus arteriosus:* The ductus arteriosus fails to close at birth.
- *Atrial septal defect* (**ASD**) and *ventricular septal defect* (**VSD**): Abnormal openings exist between the respective heart chambers.
- *Tetralogy of Fallot:* Four major heart defects occur simultaneously: pulmonary stenosis, ventricular septal defect, overriding aorta, and hypertrophy of the right ventricle.
- *Coarctation of the aorta:* The aorta narrows as it leaves the heart.

One characteristic feature of many congenital heart disorders is cyanosis, which becomes more pronounced when the newborn cries. The birth attendant and nurse must assess carefully for heart murmurs. Other signs may be respiratory difficulty, easy tiring, and abnormal vital signs. The newborn will be treated symptomatically. Medications, such as cardiotonics, may be ordered; surgical repair may be necessary.

Respiratory Disorders

Choanal Atresia

Choanal atresia occurs when the newborn's nostrils are closed at the entrance to the throat, so that air cannot pass through to the lungs. Because newborns are obligatory nose breathers, atresia must be quickly corrected through surgery to open the nostrils.

Gastrointestinal Disorders

Cleft Lip and Palate

Cleft lip, which occurs in approximately 1 in 1,000 births, is a vertical opening in the upper lip. It may appear as a notch in the lip, or extend upward into the nose. When the palate is split, the condition is known as **cleft palate;** this condition occurs less frequently than cleft lip. Cleft palate can be one-sided (*unilateral*) or two-sided (*bilateral*). Clefts also are classified as *complete* or *incomplete.*

Cleft lip and palate cause feeding difficulties if the newborn is unable to suck effectively. In addition, milk that goes into the mouth may be expelled through the nose. Special nipple and feeding devices assist in feedings. The treatment is surgical repair, usually between 6 and 12 weeks of age (see Chap. 71).

Esophageal Atresia

In **esophageal atresia,** the upper end of the newborn's esophagus ends in a blind pouch, making it impossible for the baby to obtain food. Surgery must be performed quickly. The baby sometimes is maintained on total parenteral nutrition until after surgery.

Tracheoesophageal Fistula

When esophageal atresia is accompanied by a tracheal fistula, it is referred to as a *tracheoesophageal fistula.* The situation is life-threatening because the esophagus channels food and mucus directly into the lungs. This condition must be corrected immediately, or the child will suffocate. Emergency surgery is performed immediately, with no feedings prior to surgery.

Pyloric Stenosis

Pyloric stenosis is a congenital anomaly in which an increase in size of the musculature at the junction of the stomach and small intestine occurs, causing the pyloric opening to constrict. Food cannot pass through. The newborn initially vomits a milky substance. Later, the vomiting becomes projectile. The baby is fussy and hungry, loses weight, and becomes dehydrated. Surgical correction is necessary.

Imperforate Anus

In an **imperforate anus,** the baby's rectum ends in a blind pouch, causing an obstruction to the normal passage of feces that must be corrected immediately. Imperforate anus is suspected if the newborn does not pass a stool within 24 hours of delivery.

Phenylketonuria

Phenylketonuria (**PKU**) is a genetic defect that renders the newborn incapable of metabolizing certain amino acids, which spill into the blood and tissues in the form of phenylalanine. No cure exists for this disease, but it can be controlled with a special diet. Treatment is initiated as soon as possible after birth. Untreated, PKU results in mental impairment, behavioral problems, retardation, and other abnormalities. All newborns are tested for PKU prior to discharge from the healthcare facility and at the 6-week checkup (see Chap. 66).

Galactosemia

Galactosemia is a genetic disorder in which the newborn is incapable of metabolizing galactose; thus, galactose builds up in the body and causes vomiting, diarrhea, jaundice, and mental retardation. Early diagnosis and dietary management can help prevent mental retardation.

Genitourinary Disorders

Exstrophy of the Bladder

Bladder **exstrophy** results from abnormal development of the bladder, abdominal wall, and symphysis pubis, causing exposure of the bladder, urethra, and ureteral openings to the abdominal wall. Infection is a common problem, and surgery is necessary. Surgical reconstruction is done in steps and is usually completed by the time the child is of school age.

Hypospadias and Epispadias

The male newborn has **hypospadias** when his urethra opens on the bottom side of the penis. This condition causes problems later during toilet training because the child is unable to direct his urinary stream. Surgical repair involves the use of the foreskin, so circumcision should not be performed on this newborn. Less common is **epispadias,** in which the meatus is located on the upper side of the penis.

INFECTIONS

Infections that are present in the woman during pregnancy or delivery can adversely affect her fetus. Examples of such infections include STDs, rubella, toxoplasmosis, thrush, and cytomegalovirus.

The acronym **TORCH** is used as a nursing reminder of the most serious infections:

T = Toxoplasmosis
O = Other (syphilis, hepatitis, herpes zoster)
R = Rubella
C = Cytomegalovirus
H = Herpes simplex virus

The newborn is at risk for infection following delivery as well. Even with nursery precautions, an infection may spread. One common infection is *bronchopneumonia,* which is dangerous because the newborn is too weak to cough up secretions and may choke. Postural drainage, along with the proper concentrations of oxygen and humidity, aid breathing. Antibiotics and suctioning may be required.

Staphylococcus or *Streptococcus* may cause a skin infection called *impetigo contagiosa.* With the development of antibiotic-resistant strains of staphylococcal organisms, the infection rate with staphylococcal organisms has risen. An outbreak of "staph" in the newborn nursery is dangerous, because it is so difficult to control. Therefore, strict isolation procedures must be followed.

✚◉ N u r s i n g   A l e r t
Infections can be transmitted to nursing personnel. Therefore, follow Standard Precautions in the care of all mothers and newborns.

STDs and the Newborn

Chapter 69 discusses individual sexually transmitted diseases in more detail and discusses the treatment for adults. Particulars for newborns affected by STDs follow.

Gonorrhea

If the organism causing *gonorrhea* gets into the newborn's eyes during delivery, it causes a bilateral *conjunctivitis* (eyelid inflammation). If untreated, this condition can lead to blindness (*ophthalmia neonatorum*). The prophylactic installation of antibiotic ointment into the eyes soon after birth prevents this condition (Fig. 68-2). The law requires this treatment in all states. If a newborn should contract conjunctivitis, he or she receives large doses of antibiotics, and is kept in isolation to prevent spreading the infection to others.

Syphilis

In most states, the law requires testing of pregnant women for *syphilis.* If the test is positive, prompt treatment with penicillin early in pregnancy will prevent harmful effects on the newborn. Untreated syphilis can lead to premature labor and delivery. Complications for the infant include congenital infection, anomalies (defects), and *stillbirth* (born dead).

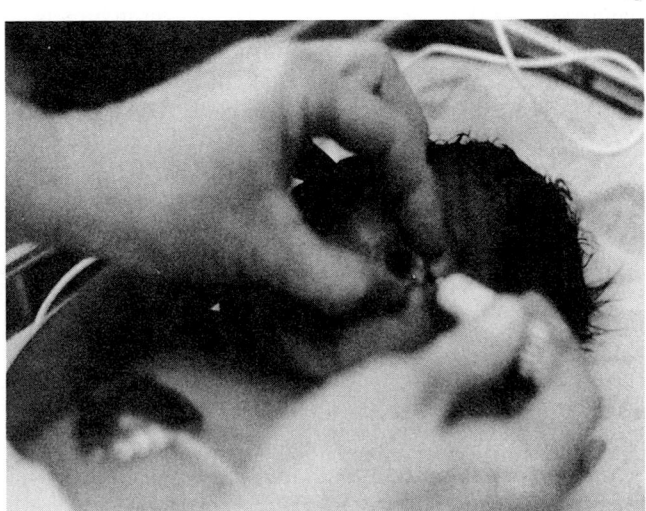

FIGURE 68-2. Ointment is applied to the eyes to prevent infection.

Signs of syphilis in the newborn are general skin eruptions of *rose spots, blebs* (blisters) on the soles and palms, *snuffles* (a catarrhal discharge from the nasal mucous membrane), hoarse cry, cracks and ulcerations around the anus and mouth, and a positive blood test. Isolate the affected newborn and treat him or her with antibiotics as ordered.

Herpes Simplex Virus

Herpes simplex virus (HSV type 1 and type 2) can complicate a pregnancy and can be harmful to the newborn. HSV can be difficult to diagnose, especially if the blisters are not present. It is not possible to differentiate between HSV-1 and HSV-2 without laboratory tests. If the virus becomes active prior to the 20th week of gestation, a spontaneous abortion ("miscarriage") may occur. HSV-2 infection acquired late in pregnancy is very dangerous to the fetus. HSV may cause premature labor or local infection of the eyes, skin, or mucous membranes.

A woman who is known to be infected with herpes and is near term will usually undergo a cesarean delivery, unless the amniotic fluid is considered contaminated. In this case, the fetus probably is already infected. After delivery, the newborn is isolated to prevent transmission of the virus to others in the nursery.

HIV and AIDS

HIV can be transmitted through the placenta or during delivery. The baby with congenital HIV/AIDS may be stillborn; the living newborn may have a guarded prognosis. Although nearly all infants born to HIV-infected mothers test positive for the HIV antibody, research has shown that only about 25% of these infants test positive for the HIV antigen. Current research supports the belief that only the antigen-positive newborns will develop full-blown AIDS. Those who are antigen negative will have a normal life span. Immediate and continued treatment with drugs may be recommended for antigen-positive infants. Chapter 84 discusses HIV/AIDS and its treatment.

Other Infections

Rubella

The virus of *rubella (German measles, 3-day measles)* can be dangerous in pregnancy, but has no permanent ill effects on the woman. It does, however, cause fetal defects, known as *congenital rubella syndrome.* Common defects are cataracts, deafness, congenital heart defects, cardiac disease, and mental retardation.

Toxoplasmosis

The protozoa responsible for **toxoplasmosis** are found in cat feces and in rare or raw meat. Although the pregnant woman may be asymptomatic, possible fetal effects include stillbirth, premature delivery, microcephaly, hydrocephaly, seizures, and mental retardation.

Thrush

Thrush (also known as a *monilial infection*) is a yeast infection, in which milk-like spots form in the newborn's mouth. Thrush is transmitted to the newborn during delivery if the mother has it. Infected healthcare personnel, or family members

who fail to use proper aseptic technique, can also spread thrush. The infected newborn is isolated and treated with nystatin (Mycostatin, Nilstat) by mouth, or less frequently with a 1% to 2% aqueous solution of gentian violet. Clean equipment and good handwashing technique are essential to prevent reinfection. Wiping the newborn's mouth with a gauze sponge after each feeding is important, because lactose (milk sugar) promotes the growth of *Candida albicans,* the causative organism.

Cytomegalovirus

An asymptomatic woman can transmit cytomegalovirus (**CMV**), which belongs to the herpesvirus group, to her fetus through the placenta or through contact during delivery. Possible effects on the newborn include SGA, microcephaly, hydrocephaly, and mental retardation.

CHEMICAL DEPENDENCY AND THE NEWBORN

All drugs, including alcohol and nicotine, can adversely affect a fetus. The newborn of a mother who uses any chemicals is likely to have symptoms, because drugs reach the fetus through the placenta. As a result, this newborn often experiences withdrawal symptoms after birth.

Newborns of mothers who drink, smoke, or use drugs are more likely to be preterm, of low birth weight, and to have intellectual impairments. Spontaneous abortions, abruptio placentae, and stillbirths also are more common in these women.

A large majority of babies born to chemical-using mothers experience withdrawal symptoms serious enough to require treatment. Care of these newborns is based on the type and extent of withdrawal symptoms, and focuses on ensuring adequate respiration, nutrition, and temperature. Keep environmental stimuli to a minimum; sedation may be necessary.

Fetal Alcohol Syndrome

Maternal use of alcohol is a major factor contributing to fetal physical defects. The resulting condition is called fetal alcohol syndrome (**FAS**) (see Fig. 73-1 in Chap. 73). Effects of FAS include growth deficiency, microcephaly, facial abnormalities, cardiac anomalies, and mental retardation. The degree of defect relates to the mother's level of alcohol intake; safe levels of intake are currently unknown. Research has shown that as little as 1 ounce a day of alcohol can adversely affect the fetus.

> ✚👁 **Nursing Alert**
> Advise pregnant women to avoid alcohol completely. *Rationale: Safe levels of alcohol intake during pregnancy have not been established.*

Cocaine and Crack

Cocaine-dependent newborns often experience a significant withdrawal syndrome, which can last 2 to 3 weeks. Newborns experiencing withdrawal from *cocaine* or *crack* may demonstrate the following signs and symptoms:

- Irritability
- Marked jitteriness
- Rapid changes in mood
- Lethargy
- Hypersensitivity to noise and external stimuli
- Poor feeding
- Irregular sleep patterns
- Tachypnea (rapid respirations)
- Tachycardia
- Diarrhea
- Diminished interactive behavior

These newborns may have experienced small strokes *in utero,* due to sudden changes in the mother's blood pressure. Also, fetal exposure to cocaine has been implicated as a cause of SIDS in infancy. Current research indicates that the long-term outlook for these infants, however, is better than in FAS.

☞ KEY CONCEPT

The addicted newborn is hypersensitive. The central nervous system and gastrointestinal system are usually most affected. Suggestions for handling an addicted newborn follow:

- *Provide eye contact.*
- *Touch the newborn gently.*
- *Rock up-and-down (not side-to-side: this makes the newborn more hyperactive).*

Heroin

Signs and symptoms of *heroin* withdrawal include:

- Jitteriness
- Hyperactivity
- Shrill, persistent cry
- Frequent sneezing or yawning
- Increased tendon reflexes
- Decreased *Moro reflex*
- Irregular sleep patterns

See In Practice: Important Medications 68-1 for medications for the heroin-addicted newborn.

Marijuana

Marijuana is one of the most commonly used drugs in the United States, with an estimated 20 million users. It crosses the placenta. If used during pregnancy, marijuana may cause shortened gestation, or a precipitate labor of fewer than 3 hours. Evidence suggests a higher incidence of meconium staining and aspiration. No increased incidence of congenital complications, or effects on growth or physical parameters, are specific to marijuana use alone. When used with alcohol, decreased birth weight and increased risk for FAS are expected. More research is needed for long-term followup studies of these newborns.

➤ STUDENT SYNTHESIS

Key Points

- High-risk newborns have special problems related to maturity, hemolytic conditions, birth injuries, alterations in structure or function, infections, and chemical dependency.
- Classification of newborns according to size and gestational age will direct their plan of care.
- The nurse's main contribution to the newborn's welfare begins with early observations, accurate documentation, and prompt reporting of abnormal signs.
- Interpreting data, making decisions, and providing therapy are crucial nursing skills when caring for the high-risk newborn.
- Nursing care for the preterm infant involves taking into consideration the immaturity of the infant.
- Large-for-gestational-age infants have special problems including hypoglycemia, respiratory disorders, and injuries such as fractures of the clavicle and skull.
- A small number of birth injuries occur, despite competent obstetric care.
- Common disorders occur in the various body systems and carry special nursing care considerations.
- The newborn may acquire an infection while in the uterus, during birth, during resuscitation, or while in the nursery.
- Infections and STDs acquired by the newborn can be life threatening or have long-term sequelae.
- Nurses are often first to observe signs of drug dependency in newborns.
- The onset of signs and symptoms in newborns experiencing withdrawal vary, depending on the drug the mother used.

Critical Thinking Exercises

1. A 2-day-old SGA newborn in your care has developed diarrhea. Describe your actions. Explain why diarrhea is dangerous to this newborn and to other newborns in the ICU.
2. Imagine caring for a newborn with bilateral cleft lip and palate. Describe your reaction to the baby's physical appearance. List your priority nursing

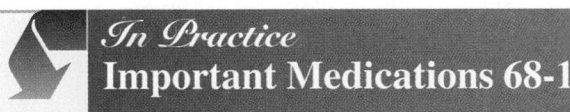

In Practice
Important Medications 68-1

FOR THE HEROIN-ADDICTED NEWBORN

Phenobarbital (Luminal)
Camphorated tincture of opium (paregoric)
Diazepam (Valium)

These drugs may be used singly or in combination.

diagnoses. Explain how you would prepare the family members for caring for their child.

3. A newborn of a cocaine-addicted mother has just arrived in your newborn ICU. Describe what you expect to see in the newborn, and how you will handle each of these problems.

NCLEX-Style Review Questions

1. Which is the best description of a small-for-gestational-age infant?
   a. Weight between 1 and 3.5 pounds
   b. Born before the 37th week of gestation
   c. Weight below the 10th percentile for gestation
   d. Born after the 42nd week of gestation

2. Which is a true statement regarding dehydration in infants?
   a. It rarely occurs.
   b. It can occur due to spitting up after feedings.
   c. It develops quickly.
   d. It results from birth injuries.

3. What action at delivery will decrease the risk of complications when amniotic fluid contains meconium?
   a. Lavage the airway with saline.
   b. Keep the infant in a Trendelenburg position.
   c. Maintain a bulb syringe at the bedside.
   d. Suction the infant prior to taking its first breath.

4. What safety aspect is most important for an infant under phototherapy?
   a. Cover the infant's eyes.
   b. Feed the infant every 3 hours.
   c. Keep the infant's body naked.
   d. Allow maternal–infant bonding time.

5. What statement represents the difference between physiologic and pathologic jaundice?
   a. Pathologic occurs after 24 hours of age.
   b. Pathologic is not treated with phototherapy.
   c. Physiologic occurs at about the third day of life.
   d. Physiologic always requires phototherapy.

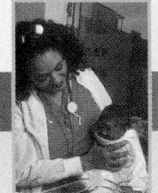

CHAPTER

69

Sexuality, Fertility, and Sexually Transmitted Diseases

LEARNING OBJECTIVES

1. Define and discuss the concepts of sexuality, sexual orientation, heterosexual, homosexual, bisexual, and asexual.
2. Identify at least four nursing considerations for the care of an individual who has been raped.
3. State four causes of sexual dysfunction in both men and women. Describe at least two medical and surgical interventions for each of these disorders.
4. Discuss four nursing interventions for male and female infertility. Identify two diagnostic procedures and two forms of treatment for infertility.
5. Define and discuss the following contraception methods: abstinence, withdrawal, BCPs, emergency contraception, Depo-Provera, Norplant System, Lunelle, IUDs, and mechanical and chemical barrier methods.
6. Discuss at least four aspects of client teaching related to sterilization by vasectomy.
7. Discuss four aspects of client teaching related to sterilization by tubal ligation.
8. Differentiate and discuss at least four aspects of client teaching related to the following types of STDs: HIV/AIDS, chlamydia, gonorrhea, syphilis, HSV, CMV, HPV, chancroid, candidiasis, trichomoniasis, bacterial vaginosis, and pediculosis.
9. Identify the signs and symptoms, diagnostic methods, and treatments for each of the STDs listed above.
10. In the skills lab, prepare a client (mannequin) for the first pelvic exam. Obtain the equipment and assist the healthcare practitioner in obtaining a Pap smear, KOTH slide, and a VDRL.

NEW TERMINOLOGY

artificial insemination	homosexual
asexual	impotence
bacterial vaginosis	infertility
bisexual	lesbian
candidiasis	orgasm
chancre	pediculosis pubis
chancroid	priapism
chlamydia	rape
coitus interruptus	sexual dysfunction
condom	sexual orientation
contraception	sexuality
dyspareunia	sterility
gay	trichomoniasis
genital herpes	tubal ligation
gonorrhea	vaginismus
heterosexual	vasectomy

ACRONYMS

BCP	HPV	LH
CMV	HSV-1	PID
EC	HSV-2	PTSD
ED	IUD	RPR
FAM	IVF	STD
FSH	KOH	VDRL
GnRH		

Sexuality, fertility, and the potential for sexually transmitted diseases (**STDs**) are topics that involve some of the most basic needs and fears that rule the individual. They have affected humans since the beginning of time.

This chapter briefly discusses these topics, which are important for you to understand. When working with clients, you will need to provide them with pertinent information related to sexual concerns. You will also need to communicate effectively and accurately to make clients feel comfortable discussing personal issues and to ensure that they have correct knowledge.

HUMAN SEXUALITY

Sexuality is the way in which individuals physically, mentally, emotionally, and socially experience and express themselves as sexual beings. It involves much more than sexual contact. Sexuality begins at birth and is a vital part of an individual's makeup and personality throughout the life span. It includes anatomy, learned or adopted behaviors, attitudes, feelings, and relationships with all other humans. You must be sensitive to these core human feelings and needs to deliver nursing care in a nonjudgmental manner, in both verbal and nonverbal interactions.

Sexual Orientation

Most individuals have an inherent or acquired tendency to be attracted emotionally and physically to other people. **Sexual orientation** refers to which gender a person finds sexually desirable. An individual's orientation may be heterosexual, homosexual, bisexual, or asexual:

- **Heterosexual:** Individuals who are attracted to the opposite sex
- **Homosexual:** Individuals who are attracted to persons of the same sex
- **Gays:** Men who are sexually attracted to other men, or women who are sexually attracted to other women
- **Lesbians:** Women who are sexually attracted to women
- **Bisexual:** Individuals who are attracted to both sexes
- **Asexual:** Individuals who are not particularly attracted to either sex

☛ KEY CONCEPT

Teach all people, no matter what their sexual orientation, methods of safer sex (eg, sex within a monogamous relationship and the use of condoms and dental dams).

Sexual Assault

Rape is a violent crime in which an individual has been sexually assaulted without her or his consent. Heightened awareness of sexual assault has resulted in more sensitive treatment of its victims. Rape victim support groups are present in nearly every community. Local healthcare facilities are also aware of support groups for victims. Although men are also victims of sexual assault, they are often less likely than women to come forward.

Encourage the victim, whether female or male, to seek physical and psychological treatment immediately following a sexual assault. A person who has been raped should not shower, bathe, or douche before examination. A specific equipment kit, known as a "rape kit," will contain specimen collection containers. The nurse will assist the physician with the pelvic examination and provide emotional support to the rape victim.

The police should be notified; usually a female officer will interview the female victim. Many emergency departments have specially trained healthcare workers that assist during the examination and care of the victim.

It is important to follow hospital and police policies regarding any evidence obtained during the exam. Careful and factual documentation is essential in the client's health record. The nurse should follow protocols regarding the handling of the victim's clothes and other pieces of evidence. Doing so ensures that the victim's rights are protected and that the appropriate information is available for legal purposes. The health record is often used in court as evidence.

Crisis intervention centers, rape centers, and special telephone services are available to provide emergency advice and counseling. In some centers, group therapy sessions are held that aim to help victims regain their emotional health. Chapter 71 addresses the sexual abuse of children.

Often, victims of rape, childhood sexual abuse, or other sexual assault want to put the experience behind them as quickly as possible. They may refuse to seek help or leave treatment early. Many of them later experience flashbacks and other symptoms of post-traumatic stress disorder (**PTSD**). Encourage these individuals to seek help.

Sexual Dysfunction

Sexual dysfunction is the inability to enjoy or to engage in sexual activity. The person may be reluctant to seek help due to difficulty in speaking about a personal problem with a stranger. A variety of physical and psychological factors can cause sexual dysfunction, which may frustrate or incapacitate an individual.

Masters and Johnson in 1966 completed the first and now famous research study on the *sexual response cycle*.[1] The sexual response cycle is divided into four successive phases along a continuum. The phases are the same in both sexes. Masters and Johnson's phases include: *excitement, plateau, orgasm,* and *resolution.* Dysfunctions can occur during any or all of these phases.

Male Sexual Dysfunction

The most common sexual dysfunction in males is **impotence** or *erectile dysfunction* (**ED**). ED is the inability to achieve or to sustain an erection. This condition is also referred to as *sexual arousal disorder.* An occasional episode of impotence is fairly common, and should not alarm the man. The continued inability to perform sexually merits careful investigation.

Medical causes of ED include STDs, chronic health disorders, open-heart surgery, surgery for prostate disorders, hormonal disorders (especially diabetes mellitus), certain medications, chemicals (such as tobacco, alcohol, and cocaine), some types of neurologic damage, and certain degenerative disorders.

Psychological factors are often important concerns in ED. If no physical cause can be found, psychological counseling of both partners is recommended. Extreme tension, feelings of guilt or inadequacy, obesity, and exhaustion can be contributing factors.

In addition to counseling, several treatment options are available. Any medications, including over-the-counter medications, the client uses must be analyzed. After consulting with the client's prescribing provider, it should be determined if the client is affected by any one or a combination of medications. Perhaps the client's medical regimen can be changed. Sometimes it is possible to reduce the dosage of or eliminate drugs that affect sexual function.

Endocrine abnormalities, such as diabetes mellitus or thyroid disorders, should be treated. Occasionally, intramuscular injection of a long-acting testosterone treatment can normalize hormone levels; in some cases, men may use oral testosterone.

ED is often successfully treated by administration of medications designed to induce erection. Sildenafil (Viagra) or yohimbine can chemically stimulate the nerves in the penis to cause an erection. Another method involves the injection of a medication (papaverine) alone or in combination with other drugs (eg, phentolamine) directly into the penile tissue.

These drugs dilate the blood vessels of the penis, allowing them to fill normally with blood, which results in an erection. Hypotension and cardiac complications may result. Another possible complication is **priapism,** continued erection accompanied by pain. The client must be taught that ED drugs have potentially serious side-effects. Chapter 89 has more information on reproductive disorders in men.

Two *surgical options* for treating impotence are available. The first is the placement of a *penile implant*. A variety of implants exist, including the semirigid rod, mechanical devices, the self-contained prosthesis, and the inflatable prosthesis. Each device has its own advantages and disadvantages. The semirigid rod is the easiest device to implant, yet is the least natural. The inflatable prosthesis mimics a natural erection best, but it is the most expensive method.

Another surgical procedure is *penile revascularization*. It involves the reconstruction of the arterial blood supply or the removal of veins that drain blood from the penis too rapidly. Approximately 5% of all impotent men are candidates for penile vascular surgery.

Female Sexual Dysfunction

Sexual function in the woman is a complicated and sometimes misunderstood process. It involves much more than the ability to achieve **orgasm,** which is the culmination of sexual excitement. Up to 30% of normal women do not experience orgasm during intercourse.

Women experiencing sexual dysfunction should be referred for medical and psychological counseling. Medical causes for female sexual dysfunction include:

- **Dyspareunia:** Painful intercourse
- **Vaginismus:** Involuntary contraction of vaginal outlet muscles, which prevents penile penetration
- *Hormonal imbalances* and *chronic illnesses:* For example, diabetes

INFERTILITY

Infertility refers to the inability to conceive and to produce live babies after adequate sexual exposure. Infertility affects approximately 15% of all couples. **Sterility** is the absolute inability to procreate. In other words, the woman does not have or produce eggs; or the man may not have or produce adequate amounts of sperm. Without eggs or sperm in adequate amounts, the woman will not be able to produce a fetus. Approximately 80% of infertility is due to combined male and female factors.

Male Infertility

Approximately 40% of infertility is due to male factors. Several factors must work together, or the ability to reproduce is limited or prevented. The volume of semen ejaculated needs to be about 2 to 5 milliliters, with a density of sperm at about 20 million per milliliter. Also, the *motility, viability,* and *shape (morphology)* of the sperm must be within normal limits.

Undescended testicles, orchitis after mumps, irradiation of the testes, untreated STDs, obesity, internal adhesions, glandular disturbances, infection, impotence, or emotional tension may cause male infertility. Although 1 milliliter of semen contains literally millions of sperm cells, the number of normal active spermatozoa may be comparatively small, which decreases the man's chances of fertilization of the ovum.

Diagnosing Causes

Several tests exist to validate the function of sperm. Cervical mucus penetration tests such as Penetrak, and a sperm penetration assay such as the Hamster Zona Free Ovum test, are examples. Sperm antibody testing and numerical counts of sperm ("sperm counts") may also be required to determine the cause of infertility.

Treatment

Treatment may be *medication* to treat the cause of the problem if it is an infection or hormone disturbance. *Surgery* may be required when the cause (such as an obstruction or a congenital anomaly) is not treatable by medical therapies. An alternative therapy is *artificial insemination,* which is discussed below.

Female Infertility

Approximately 40% of infertility is due to female factors. Many reasons exist for female infertility. Ovulation must occur for pregnancy to take place. To become fertilized by a sperm, the ova must have matured properly.

All the ova that a woman will ever produce are present in her ovaries at her own birth. Damage to the ovaries at any time may cause a permanent inability to produce viable ova. The causes of these situations may be hormonal or anatomic.

Fertilization may be prevented because the ova may not mature or be released properly. The sperm and the egg may fail to unite in the woman's body. The fertilized egg may not implant in the uterus.

The woman may have a displaced uterus, obstructed oviducts, cervical infection or cancer, vaginal infection (such as chlamydia, herpes, or genital warts), ovarian cysts or tumors, scar tissue from pelvic inflammatory disease (**PID**), or a fibroid tumor. Irradiation may have permanently damaged all ova.

PID is a serious complication of infections that invade the female reproductive tract. Sterility, ectopic pregnancies, and chronic pain are common consequences of PID. Figure 69-1 shows a fetus in a fallopian tube that resulted from an ectopic pregnancy. Chapter 90 discusses female reproductive disorders.

Diagnosing Causes

If desired conception does not occur after one year of regular, unprotected intercourse, the concerned parties should consult a physician. Women in their middle to late thirties may wish to consult a specialist earlier if they suspect a problem. A physician will check general health and order tests of semen and of vaginal and cervical secretions.

Inflation of the oviducts with carbon dioxide (*Rubin's test*) may be done to determine *patency* (openness) of the tubes. An x-ray study called a *hysterosalpingogram* looks for problems within the fallopian tubes and uterus. Sometimes, a light *curettage* (scraping) of the uterus is performed, to determine whether the uterine lining is undergoing the normal changes necessary to receive a fertilized ovum.

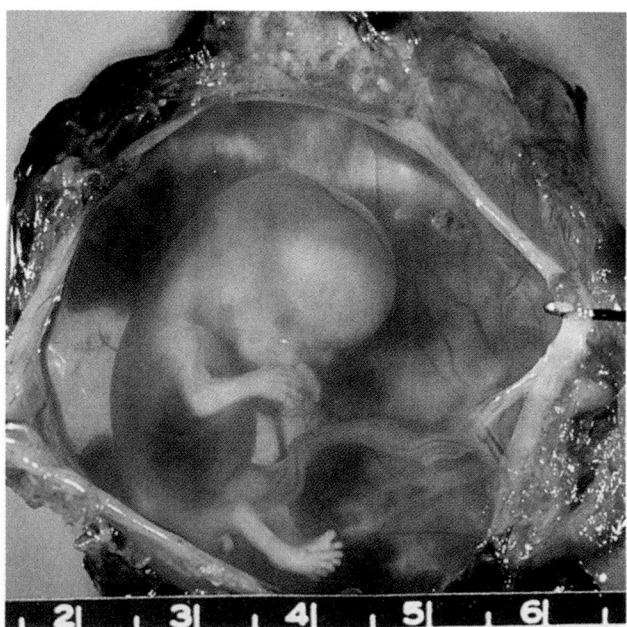

FIGURE 69-1. A fetus in the fallopian tube is an *ectopic pregnancy.* Notice that the fallopian tube is enlarged. It has *been opened here to show the fetus.*

Treatment

In a healthy woman, sexual intercourse at the time of ovulation often results in pregnancy. To determine the dates of ovulation, a woman takes her oral temperature before rising each day and records it on a chart, for 3 to 4 months. A woman can determine when she ovulates by noting an abrupt fall and then a rise in body temperature. At the time of ovulation, temperature should be slightly elevated. Cervical mucus also changes in appearance and consistency during ovulation. The woman correlates a temperature increase and cervical changes as indicators of ovulation. Chapter 29 describes and illustrates the menstrual cycle.

Modern technology now offers a vast number of choices for people experiencing infertility. **Artificial insemination** can be used if the man's sperm count is too low or if the woman's body interferes with sperm motility. A couple or a woman alone may use artificial insemination to enhance the chances of conception. In this process, male sperm (the partner's or a donor's) is artificially implanted through the woman's cervical os. *Fertility drugs* may be ordered. These potent drugs may result in the release of more than one egg, and may consequently cause a multiple pregnancy.

In vitro fertilization (**IVF**) is the fertilization of the woman's or donor's egg outside the woman's body. The resulting fertilized ovum (*zygote*) is then inserted into the woman's uterus. IVF is used if a woman's physical factors interfere with normal sperm motility, if the sperm count is low, or if the woman does not produce viable ova.

These procedures have brought about changes in social mores and medical responsibility. Many legal decisions regarding IVF, sperm banks, surrogate motherhood, and ownership of frozen sperm or frozen fertilized ova have publicly highlighted moral, ethical, and legal dilemmas. Individuals should receive competent counseling before undergoing any of these procedures.

CONTRACEPTION

Many methods of **contraception** (birth control) are available. Any method used should be safe, effective, and inexpensive. It should also have minimal side effects and be easy for individuals to obtain and to use. No single ideal method exists for everyone. The individual using a particular method of contraception must be comfortable with it, and committed to using it correctly to attain optimum effectiveness.

Discussion regarding contraception requires careful communication by the nurse, the client, and the sexual partner(s) to ensure the best method for the individual. The accompanying nursing care plan uses the nursing process as a teaching plan for sharing fertility information. Table 69-1 compares several methods of birth control. Also, see In Practice: Nursing Care Plan 69-1 about a client requesting information about birth control.

Methods of birth control are effective only if the individuals who use them do so correctly. When working with clients to choose a method, consider the following factors:

- Lifestyle
- Age and sexual activity

■■■ TABLE 69-1 *M*ETHODS OF FERTILITY CONTROL AND THE RELATIVE EFFECTIVENESS*

Method	Pregnancy Rate	Drug/Contained/ Brand Name	Action	Comments
No protection	85%–90%	—	—	—
Subcutaneous implant	<1%	Levonorgestrel (Norplant System)	Hormonal	Effective up to 5 years
Injections	<1%	Medroxyprogesterone acetate (Depo-Provera)	Hormonal	Given every 2–3 months
Oral contraceptives	1%–3%	Usually combined— estrogen (such as estradiol, estriol) and progesterone Brand names include the following: *Monophasic* (taken for 20–21 days): Demulen, Levlen, Ovral, Nordette, Ovcon-35, Brevicon, Loestrin *Biphasic* (one color taken for 10 days, next color for 11 days): Nelova 10/11, Ortho-Novum 10/11 *Triphasic* (sequence specified by manufacturer): Tri-Levlen, Triphasil, Tri-Norinyl, Ortho-Novum 7/7/7, Ortho-Tricyclen	Hormonal Simulate pregnancy and depress ovulation	One pill daily (21 days of medication, 7 days without) in various patterns
Emergency contraception ("morning-after" pill)	1%–20%	Estrogen/progestin combined (Ovral)	Hormonal	Emergency only
Intrauterine devices	2%–5%	Progestasert, Copper-T 380A	Prevent implantation in uterus	Replaced yearly Can remain in place for 4 years
Chemical barriers	5%–25%	Spermicidal douches, suppositories, and so forth	Kill or immobilize sperm	Most effective if used with mechanical barrier
Mechanical barriers	10%–15% 5%–20% 2%–10%	Male condoms used alone Condoms (male and female), cervical cap, diaphragm Diaphragm with spermicide Condom with spermicide	Block sperm from fertilizing egg	Most effective when combined with chemical barrier Cervical cap and diaphragm must remain in place in female for several hours after intercourse
Fertility awareness methods (rhythm method)	11%–30%	None	Planned intercourse to coincide with woman's infertile time	Requires mutual cooperation Woman's cycle must be regular
Withdrawal (coitus interruptus)	10%–25% when used with extreme care; usual pregnancy rate higher	None	Withdrawal before ejaculation	Requires mutual cooperation Pre-ejaculation fluid may contain sperm
Male sterilization	<0.15%	Vasectomy	Blocks path of sperm	—
Female sterilization	<0.5%	Tubal ligation	Blocks path of egg (ovum)	—

*Percentages in this table are estimated using a number of sources.

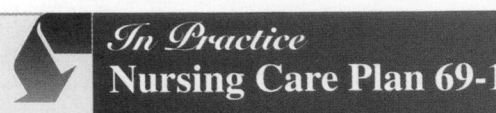

In Practice
Nursing Care Plan 69-1

THE CLIENT REQUESTING INFORMATION ABOUT BIRTH CONTROL

MEDICAL HISTORY: *L. C. is a 21-year-old, Southeast Asian female who just delivered a healthy baby boy at term 2 days ago. Client reports having previously smoked one pack per day prior to becoming pregnant. "I quit as soon as I found out I was pregnant." Otherwise, own medical history is negative for major health problems including sexually transmitted disease. Client's pregnancy progressed without problems or complications. Menarche occurred at age 12 with menstrual cycles averaging approximately every 29 to 30 days with moderate flow lasting approximately 5 to 6 days. Client does report occasional cramping with menses. Family history is positive for kidney stones and heart disease. Client's father died at age 55 from heart attack.*

Data Collection/Nursing Assessment: Client states, "We really didn't plan on having this baby like we did. We've only been married for a little over a year. I'm not sure we can handle more than one child for a while, at least not until we both get ourselves settled. My husband and I talked and we don't know much about the different methods of contraception, and which would be best for us." Client lives with husband, who is enrolled part-time in school. Client is currently on family leave of absence from work as a pharmaceutical sales manager for 6 weeks. *(Although several nursing diagnoses may be appropriate, a priority nursing diagnosis is addressed below.)*

Nursing Diagnosis: Deficient knowledge related to appropriate contraception methods as evidenced by client's questions and statements.

Planning:
SHORT-TERM GOALS:
#1. Client and husband identify possible options available.
#2. Client and husband choose an appropriate method of contraception.

LONG-TERM GOALS:
#3. Client and husband demonstrate correct use of and followup for method chosen.
#4. Client and husband verbalize satisfaction with method chosen.

Implementation:
NURSING ACTION: *Encourage participation of both client and husband.*
RATIONALE: *Joint participation in education enhances sharing of concerns and questions and promotes joint, informed decision making.*

NURSING ACTION: *Determine couple's current knowledge base, correcting any misconceptions or misinformation.*
RATIONALE: *Determining baseline knowledge provides a foundation on which to build an individualized teaching plan.*

Evaluation: Client and husband present at teaching session; couple voicing numerous questions about condoms, oral contraceptives, and diaphragms. *Progress to meeting Goal #1.*

NURSING ACTION: *Review the various methods of contraception available, including action, preparation and use, effectiveness, possible side effects or complications, and risk. Allow the couple time to look over the material and ask questions.*
RATIONALE: *Reviewing the information helps to enhance learning and strengthen understanding. It provides the couple with necessary information from which to make an informed decision. Allowing the couple time to look over the information and ask questions aids in continued decision-making.*

NURSING ACTION: *Provide information using different forms, including diagrams, charts, and pictures.*
RATIONALE: *Individuals learn differently. Providing material in different forms enhances learning.*

Evaluation: Couple focusing discussion on two major methods: oral contraceptives, and condoms and spermicides. Couple choose oral contraceptives. *Goal #1 met; progress to meeting Goal #2.*

NURSING ACTION: *Teach the couple about the method selected, including any specific instructions, such as proper insertion and cleaning techniques, and how to use or take. Have couple return-demonstrate any technique or verbalize specific instructions. Reinforce the need for correct and consistent use of method choice.*
RATIONALE: *Return demonstration or verbalization provides a means for evaluating the couple's understanding. The method is only as effective as it is used consistently and correctly.*

NURSING ACTION: *Review with the couple specific instructions about possible complications and danger signs and necessary followup, such as yearly pelvic examinations and routine screening.*
RATIONALE: *Knowledge of potential complications, danger signs, and necessary followup help to minimize the risks associated with the method chosen.*

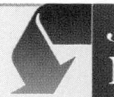

In Practice
Nursing Care Plan 69-1 (Continued)

Evaluation: Couple meeting with healthcare provider for prescription for oral contraceptives; couple verbalizing instructions on how to use oral contraceptives and what to do if pill is missed; client able to verbalize some danger signs and symptoms with assistance from nurse. *Goal #2 met; progress to meeting Goal #3.*

Nursing Action: *Assist with arranging for followup with primary healthcare provider.*

Rationale: *Assisting with followup helps to promote compliance and helps to determine the couple's satisfaction with the method chosen.*

Evaluation: Client followup appointment with healthcare provider; verbalizing danger signs and symptoms independently. Couple stating they are satisfied with their choice. *Goal #3 met; progress to meeting Goal #4.*

- Number of partners
- Need or desire for spontaneity
- Level of maturity
- Understanding of personal health
- Comfort with touching own body
- Religious and cultural beliefs
- Effectiveness
- Reaction to unplanned pregnancy
- Plans for future pregnancy
- Ability to take or to use contraceptives as prescribed
- Risk
- Client's or partner(s)' health history
- History of STDs

☞ Key Concept

There is no "totally safe sex." Use of a condom provides safer sex.

Continual Abstinence

The only 100% effective method of birth control and protection against sexually transmitted diseases is continual *abstinence.* The individual does not have intimate physical contact or intercourse with any partner. The advantages of abstinence include the knowledge that no STDs can be transmitted and no pregnancies will result. However, it may be difficult to abstain from sex for long periods of time.

Periodic Abstinence and Fertility Awareness Methods

Withdrawal

Technically known as **coitus interruptus,** *withdrawal* is an ancient form of birth control. The man must be aware of the approach of his climax (*ejaculation*) and withdraw from the vagina prior to it. This method involves a need for tremendous awareness and disciplined control. It is controversial and risky because most men release small amounts of pre-ejaculatory fluid, which could contain spermatozoa. Unplanned pregnancies are not uncommon with this method. When the best techniques are used, this method has about an 80% to 90%

protection against pregnancy, which is increased to nearly 100% when a condom is used.

Fertility Awareness Method

Fertility awareness methods (**FAMs**) include the *rhythm method,* which involves limiting sexual intercourse to the time during the woman's menstrual cycle when she is most likely to be infertile. This method is reliable only for women who ovulate regularly. Women can determine their cycles through disciplined monitoring of their basal body temperature each morning before rising. (Refer to the earlier section on "Female Infertility.") The woman is generally considered fertile during the 2 days before and the 2 days after ovulation. To avoid pregnancy, she should avoid intercourse during these days. Another option is to use a form of birth control during the time of fertility.

The rhythm method is only about 75% to 99% effective. It does require training and awareness of the days of ovulation. Illness, lack of sleep, and vaginal or other infections may affect temperature patterns. FAMs offer no protection against STDs. FAMs are not expensive and offer alternatives to people who find hormonal or barrier methods of birth control unacceptable.

Over-the-Counter Ovulation Kits. These kits are available in many retail stores. They contain instructions and equipment that assist the woman in determining the specific time of her ovulation.

Hormonal Methods

Hormonal methods of birth control alter a woman's normal hormonal levels to prevent ovulation and thus the chances for conception. Common methods of hormonal birth control are oral contraceptives, Depo-Provera, the Norplant System, and Lunelle.

In the 21st century, oral, injectable, and subdermal implants may be available for men. The World Health Organization and other countries are actively researching potential male hormonal birth control methods.

Oral Contraceptives

Oral contraceptives, also called *birth control pills* (**BCPs**), are widely used in the United States and Canada. They are prescription drugs containing progestin-only or estrogen and progestin. They are available in a variety of doses. The pill prevents ovulation; thus, the effectiveness rate for BCPs is between 95% and 99%. A woman must take birth control pills as prescribed to ensure effectiveness.

Rare but serious health problems can occur with BCPs. Blood clots, *myocardial infarctions* (heart attacks), and cerebrovascular accidents (*strokes*) can occur. Women over 35 who smoke are at the highest risk for these serious conditions.

Non-contraceptive health benefits from oral contraceptives include decreased rates of: PID, cancers of the ovary and endometrium, recurrent ovarian cysts, benign breasts cysts, and fibroadenomas, and discomfort from menstrual cramps. Minor side effects of oral contraceptives are relatively common. These include:

- Weight gain or loss
- Headache or nausea
- Depression
- Breast tenderness
- Loss of or irregular menstrual periods (generally temporary)

Contraindications include:

- High blood pressure
- Heart defects
- Blood disorders (drug promotes clotting)
- Women over age 40
- Heavy smokers
- Obesity
- Diabetes

Emergency Contraception (EC). *Emergency contraception* (**EC**), also incorrectly known as the "morning-after pill," is generally a combination of estrogen and progestin. EC prevents implantation of a fertilized egg by interfering with the hormone balance. It is not considered an "abortion pill" as the zygote has not implanted in the uterus.

To be effective, EC must begin within 72 hours of unprotected sex. Two doses of hormonal pills containing estrogen and progestin are taken 12 hours apart. The effectiveness rate is 75% to 89%; it is most effective when the hormone pills are taken within the first 24 hours after intercourse.

Nausea, vomiting, and cramping are the most common side effects. There is no protection against STDs.

Emergency contraception should not be confused with the prescription oral medication RU-486 or Mifeprex (mifepristone), which can stop pregnancy (cause an abortion) several weeks after it has begun. There are numerous contraindications and precautions for mifepristone. Healthcare providers must be consulted.

Parenteral Contraceptives

Transdermal Patches. *Transdermal patches* with time-released hormones are a new birth control option. They work in the same way as do BCPs. A patch is worn like a Band-Aid and is changed twice per month.

Depo-Provera. *Depo-Provera* (medroxyprogesterone acetate) is a hormone similar to progesterone. It is adminis-

tered by a healthcare provider every 3 months by injection, and is about 99% effective in preventing pregnancy. Medroxyprogesterone works by preventing ovulation. When the drug is discontinued, the return of fertility can take anywhere from 3 to 18 months. Depo-Provera is not effective against STDs.

If a pregnancy does occur, it is more likely to be in a fallopian tube (an *ectopic pregnancy* or *tubal pregnancy*). A ruptured ectopic pregnancy is a medical emergency. Possible side effects of Depo-Provera include:

- Weight gain
- Depression
- Headaches
- Abdominal pain
- Irregular or loss of menstrual cycle
- Nervousness
- Increased or decreased libido
- Breast tenderness or excessive enlargement
- Pulmonary embolism
- May aggravate diabetes mellitus, kidney disease, seizure disorders, cardiac disorders, and mental illness

Contraindications of Depo-Provera include:

- Pregnancy
- Cancer of the breast or reproductive organs
- Previous stroke
- History of liver disease
- History of blood clots in legs

Norplant System. The *Norplant System* and *Norplant System-2* (levonorgestrel) are contraceptive methods that protect against pregnancy for up to 5 years and are relatively easy to use. A healthcare provider implants several rubber-like capsules under the woman's skin, at the undersurface of the upper arm, within the first 7 days after onset of menses. The capsules continually release small amounts of a synthetic hormone that helps prevent ovulation.

Effective within 24 hours of insertion, Norplant can be inserted immediately after childbirth or abortion. If the mother is breastfeeding, she can start Norplant after 6 weeks. The use of Norplant is entirely reversible, with fertility returning in approximately 3 months.

The Norplant System is about 99% effective in preventing ovulation. However, if a pregnancy does occur, it is more likely to be an ectopic pregnancy. Norplant does not provide protection against STDs. A healthcare clinician must remove the capsules.

The following are possible side effects of the Norplant System:

- Irregular menstrual bleeding
- Weight gain or loss
- Nervousness
- Headaches, nausea
- Depression
- Skin changes at site of insertion
- Vertigo
- Aggravated diabetes mellitus or hyperlipidemia
- Visual changes

The following are contraindications of the Norplant System:

- Acute liver disease or jaundice
- Pregnancy
- Thromboembolic disease
- Severe visual impairment

Lunelle. *Lunelle* is an injectable hormone contraceptive containing forms of estrogen and progestin. Injected every month by a healthcare clinician, it prevents ovulation. Lunelle is more than 99% effective. Side effects, mild and severe, are very similar to other combination hormone contraceptives.

Unisex Contraception. Contraception that is effective for *both* men and women is a future goal of reversible contraception. Drugs known as gonadotropin-releasing hormone (**GnRH**) agonists are being researched. GnRH agonists inhibit the release of the gonadotropic hormones follicle-stimulating hormone (**FSH**) and luteinizing hormone (**LH**). Blocking the release of FSH and LH will temporarily inhibit ovulation in females and spermatogenesis in males.

Intrauterine Devices

A physician inserts an *intrauterine device* (**IUD**) into a woman's uterus. The IUD prevents the fertilized ovum from implanting in the uterus. One benefit of the IUD is that it offers continuous protection without the need for the woman's active participation. It is 97% to 99% effective. IUDs give no protection against STDs, and may cause increased incidence of PID, tubal pregnancies, and infertility. STD infection rates increase in women who have many partners. The greatest danger is uterine or cervical perforation, although these situations occur rarely.

Two brands of IUDs are available in the United States: Progestasert and Copper-T 380A. Progestasert is a T-shaped device that releases a small amount of progesterone daily. Yearly removal and replacement are necessary. It is useful if the woman is allergic to copper.

Copper-T 380A also is a T-shaped device, made of copper, that can be left in place for up to 4 years. The nonmedicated IUD avoids the problem of possibly harmful hormonal effects.

Box 69-1 provides considerations for the insertion of an IUD. A physician may decide not to insert an IUD in any of the following situations:

- Recent STD or other pelvic infection. (The IUD also may become a site for infection, which can cause scarring and later infertility.)
- Possible pregnancy. (Insertion of the IUD may cause a spontaneous abortion.) The IUD may be inserted during the menstrual period as a safeguard.
- Abnormally heavy menstrual flow, spotting between periods, or copious vaginal discharge
- Severe menstrual cramps
- Anemia, a bleeding disorder, or fainting spells
- Severely displaced or flexed uterus or another gynecologic problem
- Diabetes, circulatory problems, or atherosclerosis

➤➤ BOX 69-1

IUD INSERTION AND USE

If you are asked to assist with the insertion of an IUD device, keep these points in mind:

- The physician makes sure the client is not pregnant.
- The client should have a Pap test and tests for STDs before having any device inserted.
- Use sterile aseptic technique for insertion.
- The client may feel a sharp pain when the IUD is inserted.
- The client may have cramps for a few days, but these should not continue.
- Menstrual flow may be heavier, or last longer than normal, after IUD insertion.
- The device may be expelled within the first few months. (If the woman does not expel it within 2–3 months, it will probably remain in place.)
- The woman should check monthly to make sure that the IUD is in place. (Slender threads attached to the device can be felt protruding from the cervix.) She should have a yearly Pap test and pelvic examination to assure there is no irritation from the IUD.

N u r s i n g   A l e r t

If a woman becomes pregnant with an IUD in place, the device is usually removed immediately to avoid spontaneous abortion, ectopic pregnancy, septic abortion, or premature labor.

Barrier Methods

Barrier methods interfere with conception by physically preventing sperm from fertilizing ova. Barriers work through mechanical and chemical means. Mechanical devices are more effective when used in combination with chemical barriers.

In order for barrier methods to be effective, the users of them must be consistent and follow appropriate instructions. Some people object to the use of barrier methods, saying they interfere with the spontaneity of sexual arousal.

Mechanical Barriers

Male Barrier Methods. These consist of various types of **condoms,** which are sheaths made of latex, plastic, or animal tissue. A condom is applied to the erect penis before sexual intercourse. Latex condoms help to protect against HIV as well as other STDs. Condom effectiveness ranges from about 85% to 98%. The addition of a spermicide to immobilize sperm increases birth control effectiveness.

Condoms are relatively inexpensive (or free at some clinics), and easily obtainable without a prescription. Some partners may complain of a loss of sensation. Breakage and latex allergies are possible problems.

Female Barrier Methods.   These include the *cervical cap, diaphragm,* and *female condom.* A physician must fit a woman for the cap and the diaphragm, which the woman must insert each time prior to intercourse. The latex female condom attaches to a flexible ring and is inserted into the vagina like a diaphragm. The condom protrudes from the vagina, providing protection for the external genitalia as well. The female condom and new vaginal microbicides will provide better STD prevention as well as act as barrier methods for birth control.

A new vaginal *sponge* is under development and is expected to return to U.S. markets. An earlier version of the sponge had been removed from the United States because of a history of ineffectiveness and associations with toxic shock syndrome. The new sponge is expected to protect against both pregnancy and some STDs. It is made of polyurethane foam and contains spermicidal and microbicidal chemicals.

Chemical Barriers

Chemical barriers include spermicidal creams, vaginal foams, jellies, suppositories, and tablets. They offer added contraceptive protection when used with the mechanical barriers discussed above. The foams are most effective when used with a diaphragm or condom. However, frequent use can irritate vaginal tissues.

Surgical Options

Induced Abortion

Chapter 67 discusses abortion (interruption of an established pregnancy). Abortion is a controversial means of family planning, and is discouraged as a primary means of controlling pregnancy.

Sterilization

Several permanent sterilization procedures are possible. Partners are encouraged to make the decision together concerning which method they will use.

Vasectomy.   A man may have a **vasectomy,** in which the vas deferens (ductus deferens) is *ligated* (tied off) and sometimes partially removed. The vas deferens is part of the long tube that transports the viable sperm in the testes to the outside of the man's body. When it is cut, the sperm cannot reach the ova during intercourse, and pregnancy is prevented.

The man who chooses to have a vasectomy should anticipate that he will remain sterile but will not be impotent. Reversals (reattaching the vas deferens) of vasectomies are not uncommon, but these revision procedures often are unsuccessful.

This procedure is relatively easy and has few complications. It may be performed in the physician's office under local anesthesia. Only two small scrotal incisions are made, and the postoperative course is usually uneventful.

Postoperative complications of vasectomy may be scrotal tenderness, swelling, and impotence for 1 to 2 days. Infection may occur but usually is mild. Sitz baths, ice packs, and analgesics are usually all that are needed to relieve postoperative discomforts.

Regular sperm counts following a vasectomy are important. The client must be told that it may take up to 6 weeks after a vasectomy for the semen to be totally free of sperm, because the body stores semen. A sperm count is usually taken 6 weeks to 2 months postoperatively. If the sperm count is zero, the vasectomy was most likely successful.

Client teaching includes reminding the client to use birth-control measures until his sperm count remains at zero for 6 weeks. However, a sperm count should be taken again after 6 months and then yearly to assess the continuing effectiveness of the surgery. In rare cases, sperm find an alternate pathway, and the man is then no longer sterile.

The man should feel confident in his decision to have a vasectomy. Emotional aspects of vasectomy can be stressful, even more so than physical concerns. Talking with other men who have had a vasectomy may reassure him that he will not lose his sexual potency or drive.

Future goals of vasectomy researchers are to provide a chemical or silicone *inhibitor* (block) within the vas deferens. Chemical vasectomies may be more popular in younger men because they may be reversible.

Tubal Ligation.   **Tubal ligation** is the most common and effective procedure for permanent sterilization in women. A *tubal ligation* involves *ligating* (tying off) the fallopian tubes. The fallopian tubes transport the ova to the uterus. If the ova cannot travel through the fallopian tubes, the woman will not become pregnant.

Tubal ligation is usually done in a same-day surgery center under epidural, spinal, or general anesthesia via endoscope (*laparoscopic* tubal ligation). Each tube is usually ligated in two places, cut, and a portion removed. Only one stitch is necessary in one or two incisions, and it is absorbable, so the woman does not need to return to the surgeon for stitch removal. The woman often needs only a minor dressing; therefore, this operation is referred to as the "Band-Aid tubal."

Often a woman may have a tubal ligation performed after a vaginal delivery. It is easier to perform following childbirth because the *oviducts* (also known as the *fallopian, uterine,* or *ovarian tubes*) are easily accessible. Tubal ligation may be performed at the time of other abdominal surgery through an abdominal incision; all or part of the tube may be removed. It also may be done vaginally.

Mild postoperative cramping may result from manipulation of the ovaries, or referred pain to the shoulder may occur after abdominal distention with carbon dioxide, which is used for better visualization of the tubes.

The client can expect to leave the healthcare facility as soon as she has recovered from the anesthesia. Someone should be available to drive her home after surgery. She may experience a slight vaginal discharge or spotting for a few days postoperatively. Normal menstrual periods and libido should resume after tubal ligation.

Future tubal sterilizations may include methods such as chemical scarring. Phenol (carbolic acid) and quinacrine are introduced into the fallopian tubes. Scar tissue forms, which causes mechanical barriers that prevent conception. This method is in common use in China.

Research anticipates other nonsurgical techniques, such as the introduction of chemicals, or cryosurgery of the tubes. The insertion of liquid silicone that "plugs" the fallopian tubes looks promising as a reversible method of tubal sterilization.

SEXUALLY TRANSMITTED DISEASES

Sexually transmitted diseases are contracted through sexual intercourse or other sexual contact with an infected person. STDs are the most commonly reported infectious diseases in the United States today. Many cases are undiagnosed, and therefore unreported. Adolescents are at a higher risk for infection than are adults. State and national Public Health Departments have requirements for healthcare providers for the reporting of STDs.

Adolescents, particularly females between the ages of 15 and 29, have the highest reported cases of chlamydia and gonorrhea. Risk factors include the likelihood of more sexual partners for shorter durations. These women are more likely to have unprotected sex and to have sex with partners infected with STDs. Younger people often face barriers to receiving STD counseling, protective, and treatment services. Confidentiality, embarrassment, lack of finances or insurance, and lack of transportation also factor into the high rates of adolescent infections.

The increased incidence of STDs cannot be attributed to one cause. Sexual freedom and lifestyle choices have evolved since the 1960s, when the IUD and birth control pills became readily available. One such choice was expanding the number of sexual partners, which increased the risk for and spread of STDs. In the 1980s, when the infection HIV/AIDS was discovered, society was re-energized with the awareness and consequences of STDs.

STDs and birth control must be considered as connected but separate issues. Certain birth control methods—such as withdrawal, IUDs, and oral or implanted contraceptives—factor into the spread of STDs. These birth control methods have no mechanism to prevent the spread of bacteria, viruses, or other microorganisms.

Many barrier methods such as latex condoms provide some protection against both STDs and pregnancy. *Safer sex,* but not *safe sex,* is possible with the use of condoms. Additional precautions such as spermicides provide better protection against STDs. Sexual abstinence is the only guarantee of safe sex.

Treatment of STDs is often difficult. Resistance to antibiotics such as penicillin is problematic. In addition, no specific antibiotic, antiviral, or other treatment has been found that will prevent or cure HIV/AIDS or herpes simplex virus 1 or 2. A person also may have more than one STD simultaneously, which makes treatment difficult. Antibody immunity does not develop in many of the STDs, such as chlamydia, gonorrhea, syphilis, or trichomoniasis, which will be discussed below. Individuals may become infected more than once. Individuals infected with viral STDs are infected for life.

The most widespread bacterial causes of STDs are chlamydia, gonorrhea, and syphilis, with chlamydia and gonorrhea as the two most common infections. Herpes simplex virus 1 and 2 (genital herpes) and *condyloma* (genital warts) are very common. Globally, about 15,000 people a day become infected with HIV.

HIV and AIDS

Chapter 84 discusses HIV/AIDS in more detail. Information regarding women and HIV, general symptoms of HIV, and STDs is reviewed here.

At least half of all cases of HIV/AIDS are spread by heterosexual contact, which is greater than the 40% of HIV/AIDS cases caused by intravenous drug use. Women are the fastest growing population infected with HIV/AIDS in the United States. For young women of color, heterosexual contact is responsible for 62% of HIV/AIDS cases. The vast majority of women infected (84%) are in their childbearing years. The next largest group of women that is becoming infected is women over the age of 50 years.

Women are more easily infected by unprotected sex because the delicate tissues of the female reproductive tract can become scratched or irritated. These little fissures offer direct routes of invasion for the HIV virus.

Women can transfer the virus to their unborn children during pregnancy, birth, or through breastfeeding. Women with HIV can often prevent the transfer of HIV to their unborn children with proper prenatal care.

☛ KEY CONCEPT

Women of childbearing age and women over the age of 50 are the fastest growing population to be infected with HIV. Heterosexual contact with infected males is the primary reason for the trend.

Signs and Symptoms

HIV infection can mimic many other illnesses. Diagnosis by laboratory testing is the only accurate HIV detection method. A person who has had any STD should consider getting tested for HIV. Warning signs of possible HIV infection include:

- Rapid weight loss
- Dry cough
- Fever, night sweats
- Profound fatigue
- Enlarged lymph nodes
- Severe diarrhea lasting more than 1 week
- White spots or unusual blemishes on the tongue or mouth, or in the throat
- Pneumonia
- Red, brown, pink, or purplish blotches on or under the skin
- Memory loss, depression
- Neurologic disorders
- History of STD

Symptoms that women have when they are HIV positive frequently differ than the symptoms men may have. HIV treatment is delayed because the initial symptoms often appear as common female problems. Most women tend to be occasionally annoyed by "female problems" and often self-treat symptoms at home. However, frequent female problems such as yeast infections, abnormal Pap smears, or pelvic pain can be early symptoms of HIV infection.

In keeping with Standard and Universal Precautions, nurses wear gloves when coming in contact with any body fluids, to protect themselves against the possibility that their clients might be HIV positive, or have hepatitis or any other communicable disease.

☛ KEY CONCEPT

A link connecting HIV and other STDs is known. Individuals who are infected with a STD are two to five times more likely to acquire HIV than individuals who do not have a STD. In other words, a person who has a STD and is exposed to HIV, is much more likely to acquire HIV than is a person who does not have a STD. Additionally, an HIV-infected individual who has a STD is more likely to infect a partner with HIV through sexual contact than is an individual with HIV and no STD.

Chlamydia

Chlamydia trachomatis is the bacteria that is the leading cause of preventable infertility in women and the most common STD in the United States. **Chlamydia** is transmitted during vaginal, anal, or oral sex. It can also be passed from an infected mother to her newborn at vaginal childbirth. Box 69-2 looks at the many conditions associated with chlamydia.

Healthcare providers should be aware that teenagers have the highest infection rate of the disease. Often the individual has a history of STDs and does not regularly use condoms. Client teaching should include the awareness that many chlamydia cases are without symptoms and that if left untreated, permanent damage can occur to men, women, and newborns.

Signs and Symptoms

Approximately 50% of affected individuals are asymptomatic; therefore, chlamydia is called the "silent STD." Three out of four women have no symptoms and half of men have no symptoms. Often the infection is not diagnosed until complications develop.

The symptoms of chlamydial infection in men include painful urination, a watery penile discharge, and pain and swelling in the testicles. Untreated chlamydia infection generally causes urethral infections, epididymitis, and potential infertility.

Women may have vulvar itching and burning, grayish-white vaginal discharge, *dysuria* (painful or difficult urination), and spotting between menstrual periods. Symptoms may be mild, absent, or misdiagnosed. PID happens in about 40% of women who do not get treatment for chlamydia. PID often results in chronic pelvic pain, permanent damage to the female reproductive organs, and ectopic pregnancies.

Chlamydia infection can be a cause of preterm birth. In a newborn, chlamydia affects the lungs and eyes, leading to infant pneumonia and *conjunctivitis* ("pink eye") in newborns. Evidence is emerging that suggests an association between chlamydia and infant middle ear infections, nasal passage obstruction, bronchiolitis, and SIDS.

Diagnosis and Treatment

Diagnosis is made with a stained smear test, but this test is less than 50% accurate. Better test results may involve current gene research and gene detection technology. Figure 69-2 shows the nurse assisting the practitioner with smearing a slide for microscopic study.

Medications to treat chlamydia include tetracycline and doxycycline. During pregnancy, or if allergic to tetracycline, erythromycin is used. Because 40% to 60% of clients with gonorrhea also are infected with chlamydia, treatment with ceftriaxone may also be indicated. People with chlamydia must use condoms when engaging in sexual activity, and all sexual partners must be treated simultaneously to avoid reinfection.

Gonorrhea

Gonorrhea is caused by invasion of the bacteria *Neisseria gonorrhoeae*. It is spread through vaginal, oral, or anal sexual

➤➤ BOX 69-2

CHLAMYDIAL INFECTIONS

Chlamydial infections ~~are related to~~ Can Cause many other conditions, including the following:

- Pelvic inflammatory disease, which causes about half of all cases
- Female infertility (due to scars in uterine tubes)
- Male infertility (due to epididymitis)
- Stillbirths
- Premature births
- Newborn infections (such as conjunctivitis)
- Newborn pneumonia, as late as 6 wk after birth
- Ectopic pregnancy
- Urethritis and cystitis in men and women
- Cervical dysplasia and cervicitis (possible precursors to cervical cancer)

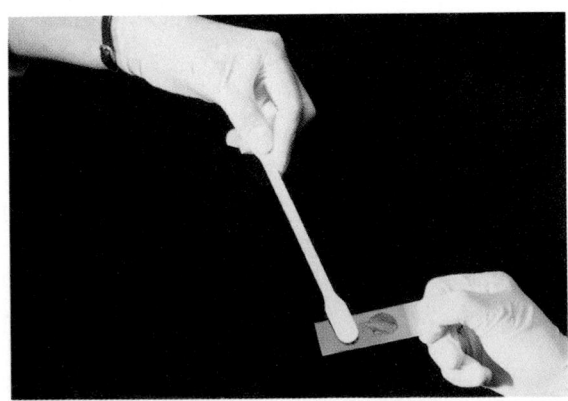

FIGURE 69-2. The nurse is assisting the practitioner during a pelvic exam. Notice that the nurse holds the microscope slide on the frosted portion so that the practitioner can smear the clear portion with vaginal secretions.

contact between partners. Gonorrhea can be spread from one part of the body to another, such as by touching infected genitals and then the eyes.

During delivery, a mother can infect her infant with gonorrhea. Untreated infection in a newborn can lead to blindness, joint infection, or sepsis. Prenatal care and STD screening are important teaching considerations for the nurse. Healthcare facilities have standard criteria, such as administration of antibiotic eye drops to newborns to prevent gonorrheal eye infections.

According to CDC statistics, young adults have the highest incidence of gonorrhea, with 75% of all reported cases found in persons between 15 and 29 years of age. Within this 75%, African Americans had the highest reported number of cases (77%).

Signs and Symptoms

Typical symptoms in men when initially infected are a burning sensation during urination and a yellowish-white discharge from the penis. Painful or swollen testicles are common. Prostatitis, infection of the seminal vesicles, and sterility may develop. Without treatment, the disease progresses to the epididymis.

Approximately 50% of women with gonorrhea are asymptomatic. Clinical findings in women include cervical tenderness, dyspareunia, purulent anal discharge, dysuria, and a yellow-green purulent vaginal discharge. PID and sterility may result. Douching, sexual intercourse, and menstruation may spread the infection to the ovaries and cause abscess.

Gonorrhea can spread to bones, joints, or the bloodstream, resulting in arthritis, heart disease, liver damage, or central nervous system damage. Many individuals who have gonorrhea (40%) also have chlamydia. Treatment consists of antibiotics that treat both infections. Individuals with gonorrhea should also be tested for other STDs, including HIV.

> **Nursing Alert**
> Having gonorrhea once does not confer immunity; the person is particularly susceptible to *reinfection*. Tracing and treating all the person's sexual contacts is important to avoid reinfection ("ping-pong infection"). Reinfection by an asymptomatic carrier is common.

Diagnosis and Treatment

A smear of the discharge is cultured and examined microscopically. Some physicians advocate obtaining urethral, vaginal, and throat cultures.

Treatment of choice for gonorrhea is one intramuscular injection of ceftriaxone (Rocephin) or cefixime (Suprax). Penicillin is no longer used, because many strains of the gonorrhea bacterium have become resistant. All sexual partners also must be treated simultaneously to prevent reinfection.

When the infection is active, teach the client about the use of Standard Precautions; that is, to wear gloves when coming into contact with his or her own body secretions. Frequent and careful handwashing is critical. Eyes are particularly susceptible to gonorrheal infection.

With an advanced infection, the client needs bed rest and may require sitz baths and massive doses of intravenous antibiotics. The individual is not considered disease free until cultures have been negative for at least 7 days without antibiotics.

Syphilis

Syphilis is caused by a destructive bacterial spirochete (*Treponema pallidum*) that can have grave consequences throughout the body. It is known as "the great imitator" because its symptoms resemble those of many other diseases. Annually, the incidence of syphilis is about 100,000 cases, which is much less than the incidence of gonorrhea (about 2 million cases per year). The trend, however, shows a significant explosion of syphilis, particularly in urban minority groups.

Syphilis is spread by direct contact with a syphilitic *lesion* (sore) via vaginal, anal, or oral sex. Lesions generally occur on the external genitals, the vagina, the anus, or in the rectum, on the lips, and in the mouth. The spirochetes can enter through cuts or breaks in the skin. Healthcare workers must use handwashing and gloving precautions.

Pregnant women can pass syphilis to a fetus. Spontaneous abortions (*miscarriages*) are not uncommon in cases of maternal syphilis. An infant born with syphilis may be stillborn (dead at birth) or may die shortly after birth. Some infected newborns do not have symptoms at birth, but develop them within a few weeks. These infants tend to have developmental delays, seizures, or die.

Signs and Symptoms

The spirochetes thrive in moisture, and live for a short time outside the human body. After entering the body, the spirochetes immediately multiply and gain access to the bloodstream. Within 10 days to 3 months, the first syphilitic lesion (**chancre** or *primary lesion*) appears.

Primary Stage. Within 10 to 90 days of infection, the chancre may appear on the penis, on the anus, inside the vagina, on the nipple, or in a crack at the side of the mouth. One or more chancres may appear at the spot where syphilis has entered the body. The chancre lasts 3 to 6 weeks, and heals with or without treatment. The chancre is deep, painless, hard, and oval-shaped, with serous drainage. It contains millions of spirochetes. Sometimes, enlarged lymph nodes also appear. Blood tests (discussed in Table 69-2) are usually positive during the primary stage. Without treatment, the disease progresses to the secondary stage.

> **Nursing Alert**
> A syphilitic chancre is *not* to be confused with the "blisters" of herpes simplex virus type 1 or 2.

Secondary Stage. Approximately 2 to 4 weeks after the initial infection, the *secondary stage* begins; it may last 2 to 6 weeks. A macular copper-colored rash appears on the soles

▪▪▪ TABLE 69-2 *B*LOOD TESTS FOR SYPHILIS

Blood Test	Use
Venereal Disease Research Laboratory (**VDRL**)	70% accurate; can give both false-negative and false-positive results; results are not conclusive until at least 2 weeks after infection. False-positive results may occur in heroin addicts or in people who have recently had measles, infectious hepatitis, infectious mononucleosis, chickenpox, rheumatoid arthritis, or systemic lupus erythematosus.
Rapid Plasma Reagin (**RPR**)	Used for first-line screening
Treponema Pallidum Hemagglutinin Assay (**TPHA**)	Rapid, simple test commonly used for first-line screening; results are not conclusive until at least 2 weeks after infection.
Fluorescent Treponemal Antibody Absorption (**FTA-ABS**)	Detects all stages; very few false-positive results
Treponema Pallidum Immobilization (**TPI**)	Expensive test used for problem diagnoses
Wassermann test	Original test for syphilis (1906); sometimes still used

and palms. Wart-like spots may develop on the mucous membranes or around the anus. These spots are extremely infectious. Patches of the client's hair may come out, and he or she may have a fever, headache, or sore throat. The person may have none of these symptoms and may feel normal and well. This stage also ends spontaneously.

✚👁 N u r s i n g   A l e r t

During the first and second stages of syphilis, the client is highly infectious, even though he or she may show no symptoms. This fact is the main reason for the spread of the disease. The client believes that he or she is cured, or decides that he or she never had syphilis.

Late Syphilis or Latent Stage.   When the symptoms of the secondary stage disappear, the *latent* (hidden) stage begins. This stage may last anywhere from several years to several decades. Serologic lab tests may or may not be positive for the disease. The individual may not be infectious to others during the later stages. *Tertiary syphilis* is the end stage of the disease. Internal organs including the brain, nerves, eyes, heart, blood vessels, liver, bones, and joints begin to show the accumulated damage of the years without treatment. Lack of muscle coordination, paralysis, gradual blindness, dementia, and death occur.

The lack of muscle coordination with syphilis is called *tabes dorsalis (locomotor ataxia),* and involves the nervous system. It is accompanied by a sharp, burning pain in the legs; legs feel numb, and then cold or warm. The person seems not to know where his or her legs are, and cannot walk without watching them closely. The gait is jerky, and the individual cannot find his or her way in the dark. Joint function is lost.

Diagnosis and Treatment

Tests for syphilis and gonorrhea are always done as part of antepartal care. Some states also require premarital blood tests for these disorders.

☛ KEY CONCEPT

The serologic tests for syphilis include the VDRL and the RPR. They should be performed at the same time as the gonococcus smear. The causative organism of syphilis can be transmitted as a "passenger" on the gonorrhea organism.

A smear taken from a syphilitic lesion can provide diagnostic information. More commonly, diagnosis comes from several types of blood tests that are described in Table 69-2.

The best treatment for syphilis at any stage is large doses of intramuscular benzathine penicillin G (Bicillin L-A). Fortunately, resistance to penicillin has not developed. However, although treatment can destroy the syphilis organisms at any stage of the disease, drugs cannot reverse any damage already present. Syphilitic damage is irreversible.

Herpes Simplex Virus

Herpes simplex virus type 1 (**HSV-1**) and herpes simplex virus type 2 (**HSV-2**) are the causes of **genital herpes,** sexually transmitted viral infections. Genital herpes infections have increased 30% since 1970. Genital herpes caused by HSV-1 has increased, and it is often difficult to differentiate primary episodes between HSV-1 and HSV-2. The greatest rate of increase is in young white adolescents. HSV-2 is more common in women and African Americans.

Pregnant women can shed the virus at the time of delivery, causing potentially fatal infections in the newborn. A cesarean delivery is commonly scheduled if a mother has active, or a history of, genital herpes.

The blisters are loaded with the virus, and are the cause for transfer of infections. HSV infection makes individuals more susceptible to HIV infection. Persons with existing HIV infection are more likely to become infected with HSV, as well as other STDs.

HSV-1 is more commonly associated with common *canker sores,* "cold sores," or "fever blisters" of the mouth and lips. HSV-1 is mainly associated with non-genital lesions, but sometimes does involve the genital tract. Direct contact with the saliva of an infected person, such as by kissing, can transmit the infection from one person to another. HSV-1 infection of the genitals is most often caused by oral-genital sexual contact.

HSV-2 is transferred from one partner to another during sexual contact. Assorted considerations for HSV infections are found in Box 69-3. Risk factors for HSV-2 include:

- Multiple sexual partners
- Age over 29 years
- Low socioeconomic status
- Black or Hispanic ethnic origin
- Female gender
- Male homosexual activity
- HIV infection

Signs and Symptoms

Symptoms of HSV range from none to mild to severe. HSV-2 is associated with recurrent episodes of painful genital sores. Persons with a suppressed immune system can have very severe cases of HSV-2.

➤➤ BOX 69-3

CONSIDERATIONS RELATED TO HERPES SIMPLEX VIRUS (HSV)

Predisposing and Precipitating Factors to HSV-1 and HSV-2 Infection
- Existing oral, anal, or vaginal lesions (blisters)
- Multiple sexual partners
- Anxiety or fatigue
- Vaginal or labial irritation
- Sunburn
- Tight clothes, especially synthetics or wet bathing suits
- Fever
- Certain time of menstrual cycle
- Birth control pills
- Hormonal imbalance

Other Considerations
- HSV-2 closely associated with cervical cancer
- HSV-2 closely associated with prostatic cancer
- HSV-2 closely associated with Hodgkin's disease and lymphosarcoma
- Great danger to the newborn if mother has active HSV
- Disease is very contagious at certain times.
- The virus can penetrate a condom.

The initial lesions of HSV-2 resemble fever blisters or the common canker sore. The initial lesions will heal without treatment, although the condition usually recurs. Two thirds of people who have an initial outbreak will have a recurrence. HSV can also be released between episodes of blisters, from skin or mucous membranes that do not have a blister.

In women, the lesions begin on the external genital labia approximately 6 days after exposure. From there, they spread, and usually become painful. They may be painless, however, if they spread into the vagina. The lesions often look like pimples surrounded by a reddened area; they then progresses to papules, vesicles, and finally crusts. This sequence lasts 1 to 3 weeks.

Systemic flu-like symptoms, such as headache, general malaise, fever, and node tenderness, often exist concurrently. Other symptoms of primary infection in women include dysuria, vaginal discharge, perineal discomfort, and dyspareunia. The lesions may be extremely painful. However, approximately 10% of all people infected are unaware of it.

In men, the major symptom is a painful lesion, usually on the penis, which may be mistaken for the chancre of syphilis. The uncircumcised man may carry the herpes simplex virus in the *smegma,* a secretion that collects under the foreskin.

Secondary infections usually are localized, causing painful lesions. Precipitating factors include anxiety, fatigue, excessive sexual activity, excessive vaginal or labial irritation, sunburn, tight clothes (especially synthetics), and fever. Recurrence also seems to be related to hormonal imbalance and to the menstrual cycle. Birth control pills increase the possibility of infection. Oral contraceptives alter vaginal secretions, enabling the virus to grow faster and to be transmitted more easily.

Diagnosis and Treatment

Treatment is generally palliative. Four or five outbreaks per year are common. No cure for genital herpes exists. Antiviral medications can shorten and prevent outbreaks when the client is taking the drugs.

HSV screening should be done at the same time as screening for syphilis and gonorrhea. Cultures should be taken for any suspicious lesion. Diagnosis is possible only when lesions are present. Only viral cultures can differentiate HSV-1 from HSV-2. The virus may bury itself, perhaps in the central nervous system, between outbreaks and become non-observable.

☛ KEY CONCEPT

Diagnosis of herpes simplex virus 2 is possible only *when lesions are present.*

Episodic or *suppressive treatment* exists. Antiviral pills are used. Episodic treatment, that is, antiviral medication taken only during outbreaks, helps to speed healing and shorten the length of the outbreaks. *Suppressive therapy* is used if outbreaks are frequent or severe; antiviral medications are taken every day.

Three main antiviral medications are available and can be taken for either episodic or suppressive treatment. The first antiviral drug, made available in the 1980s, was acyclovir (Zovirax, Avirax). It is related to valacyclovir (Valtrex) and famciclovir (Famvir). Side effects of these antivirals are generally mild, and may include headache, nausea, and diarrhea

HSV is carried in the nerves at the base of the spine, so topical ointments such as dexpanthenol (Panthoderm) may help to ease discomfort, but do not prevent or suppress outbreaks.

Genital herpes is closely associated with cervical and prostate cancer. Any woman who has had HSV should have a Pap test at least every 6 months to rule out cervical cancer. Men who have had HSV should have a rectal examination and a prostatic specific antigen test yearly for prostatic cancer. An association may also exist between genital herpes and Hodgkin's disease and lymphosarcoma. The person with herpes also must have a complete physical examination on a regular basis, to rule out the possibility of these other diseases as well.

Because HSV is not curable, the client needs emotional support. Treatment is mostly symptomatic, and is directed at reducing discomfort and preventing secondary infection. Oral analgesics, such as aspirin, acetaminophen (Tylenol), or other NSAIDs, may reduce systemic discomfort.

Sitz baths may relieve pain but have no effect on the course of the disease. Cleanliness and dryness are essential to promote healing. Cotton underwear is useful. Women may need to be catheterized, although extreme caution must be used to avoid spreading the infection into the bladder.

Individuals with herpes should avoid sexual contact, especially when lesions or any symptoms are present. The virus is small enough to penetrate a condom. Therefore, if herpes is present in the vagina, on the cervix, or on the penis, a condom offers no protection against the spread of the disease.

Client teaching includes instruction on restricting others from using items that come in contact with the lesions, such as a toothbrush. During active outbreaks, an infected person should not share food or engage in kissing. Meticulous handwashing is necessary to prevent spread of the lesions to another part of the body.

☛ KEY CONCEPT

The recurrence of herpes often coincides with the menstrual cycle in the woman or during times of stress.

Cytomegalovirus

Cytomegalovirus (**CMV**), a member of the herpes family, is transmitted by any close contact (eg, intercourse, kissing, breastfeeding). Although individuals with CMV are typically asymptomatic, possible clinical findings include upper respiratory symptoms, fatigue, retinitis, and pneumonia. Treatment includes symptomatic relief, for example through bed rest or acetaminophen; no specific treatment or vaccine for CMV currently exists. Immunocompromised individuals (such as persons with HIV/AIDS or who are undergoing cancer chemotherapy) may be given immunotherapy and an antiviral agent to control symptoms. Pregnant women should avoid contact with CMV if possible.

Genital Human Papillomavirus

Condylomata acuminata are more commonly known as *genital warts* (or *venereal warts*) caused by the human papillomavirus (**HPV**), a large group of viruses. About 30 viruses in this group are sexually transmitted, infecting the genital area, vulva, labia, or anus, and surrounding tissues. HPV infections are very common and have very few signs or symptoms. Any sexually active person is at risk for HPV.

Some of the "high-risk" HPV viruses are linked with abnormal Pap smears and cancer of the cervix, anus, and penis. Precancerous or cancerous changes also may be seen on the cervix. Unexplained, but known to occur, is a link between cigarette smoking and cervical cancer. Therefore, women who have HPV should not smoke. Predisposing factors for genital warts include:

- Oral contraceptive use
- Frequent sexual intercourse
- Multiple sexual partners
- Cigarette smoking
- The presence of other STDs
- Sex without condom use

Signs and Symptoms

Genital warts appear as single or multiple soft, moist, pinkish growths or bumps. Sometimes they form a cauliflower-like shape appearing on and around the genital structures and the anus. Lesions may not appear for several weeks or 2 to 3 months after exposure. Additional clinical signs include *pruritus* (itching), dyspareunia, and chronic vaginal discharge.

➕👁 **N u r s i n g   A l e r t**
The greatest danger with an HPV infection is the *predisposition to cervical cancer.*

Diagnosis and Treatment

HPV infections are diagnosed by inspection and treated by removal of visible genital warts. A Pap smear should be done in all females. The presence of a positive Pap test may be a precancerous warning in a sexually active female. The abnormal Pap test is often the first sign that the HPV is present. There is no cure. HPV infections generally go away without treatment; however, persistent infection is common with the "high-risk" group of HPVs.

A specific test, the ViraPap, can indicate the presence of any human papillomaviruses. The ViraType test can differentiate among strains of HPV. Sophisticated DNA techniques are also available.

Followup is necessary as soon as the Pap test is positive and particularly if the virus is discovered. Lesions must be actively treated as soon as possible to reduce the possibility of cancer. The most common treatment is weekly external application of podophyllin 10% to 25% in benzoin tincture (Pod-Ben-25). The drug is caustic, and the treatment is sometimes painful. This drug cannot be used if the wart or surrounding tissue is irritated or inflamed. It also cannot be used in a diabetic client, if the person has poor circulation, or during pregnancy.

If topical medications are ineffective, carbon dioxide, laser therapy, *cryosurgery* (application of extreme cold), or *cautery* treatments (destruction with an electric current) may be performed. In severe cases, more extensive surgery may be needed.

Treating all sexual partners simultaneously is essential to the prevention of retransmission of the disease. Treatment assists in bringing the virus under control, but does not necessarily cure the person.

The best prevention of genital warts is abstinence from sexual activity. Clients who choose not to abstain should use condoms. Applying spermicidal creams also seems to be helpful in controlling the spread of the virus.

Chancroid

Chancroid is caused by the organism *Haemophilus ducreyi*. The first symptom is a soft sore, different from the hard chancre of syphilis. Chancroid is almost always spread by sexual contact, especially in hot, humid areas. This disease is most common in tropical climates.

Symptoms occur most often in men, but women may be carriers. Lesions appear in the genital area 3 to 5 days after contact and develop into irregular ulcers, surrounded by edema and erythema. They bleed easily when touched. The infection often spreads to the inguinal lymph nodes. Treatment is with antibiotic therapy.

Other STDs

Other common diseases can be spread by sexual contact. *Vaginitis* is a general term that implies inflammation and infection of the vagina. Many causes of vaginitis exist, including personal hygiene products such as soap, laundry detergent, bath oil, commercial douche preparations, spermicidal jellies, tampons, diaphragm, or colored toilet paper.

Although it is not always a *venereal* disease (spread through sexual contact), vaginitis is a very common occurrence in females. Both sexual partners should be treated simultaneously (*concomitant* treatment) to prevent reinfection. (Chapter 90 provides additional information on female reproductive disorders.) The following are the three most common causes of microorganism-produced vaginitis. Figure 69-3 illustrates two of these microorganisms:

- *Candidiasis*, also known as *moniliasis, thrush, fungal infection*, and *yeast infection;* caused primarily by the species *Candida albicans*

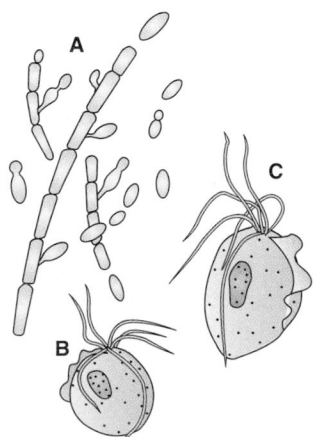

FIGURE 69-3. Organisms that cause vaginal infections include: (**A**) *Candida albicans*. (**B, C**) *Trichomonas vaginalis.*

- *Trichomoniasis,* also known as *trichomonas* or "trich" is caused by the parasitic protozoan *Trichomonas vaginalis*
- *Bacterial vaginosis,* formerly known as *Hemophilus vaginalis* and now referred to as *Gardnerella vaginitis,* is a gram-negative bacteria; it may also be called "nonspecific vaginitis"

Candidiasis

Candidiasis is the most common cause of vaginitis. Organisms of the species *Candida albicans* are commonly found on the skin and in the gastrointestinal tract, and may be found in the woman's vagina. Normally, there is a normal, homeostatic balance among this organism and others in the body. Under certain conditions, such as during a course of antibiotics, the balance is disturbed and there is an overgrowth of candida. Overgrowth of the normal fungal population has been linked to high sugar intake, hormone disturbances, BCPs, corticosteroid therapy, malnutrition, too-frequent douching, immunosuppressed individuals, and diabetes.

Symptoms include intense itching of the vulva, which becomes inflamed and irritated; burning after urination; and a white, cottage cheese–like discharge. Diagnosis is made by putting a sample of the discharge on a microscopic slide. The physician may request a slide prepped with potassium hydroxide (**KOH**).

Treatment is available with prescription and nonprescription medications. Creams or gels inside disposable applicators are used for 1 to 7 days. The 1- and 3-day fungicides are considered to be as effective as the 7-day application, and client compliance with the necessary insertion protocols is more likely to be followed. Diflucan (fluconazole), a single-dose pill, can also be used, especially in cases of reinfection.

Self-reinfection and reinfection from the sexual partner are common. Infection is rare in a circumcised man, but candida can be found commonly under the foreskin in an uncircumcised male. Infection can be transmitted from mother to fetus during pregnancy or during delivery.

Women tend to self-treat this problem due to the availability of over-the-counter medications. Some women state relief from symptoms by swallowing acidophilus capsules, eating yogurt, or instilling yogurt directly into the vagina. Client teaching should include the awareness that a healthcare provider should be seen for persistent problems. Recurrent problems, bad-smelling greenish discharge, or severe pain are not associated with candida.

Trichomoniasis

Trichomoniasis is the second-most common vaginitis. The signs and symptoms of "trich" include itching and burning of the vulva accompanied by a foul-smelling, greenish-yellow or gray, frothy or bubbly discharge. Factors that trigger growth include pregnancy, sexual activity or trauma to the vaginal walls, systemic illness, menstruation, or emotional upsets.

Treatment consists of metronidazole (Flagyl, Metryl, Protostat), which is a highly effective antiprotozoal and antibacterial drug. Side effects include dry mouth, nausea, bitter aftertaste, diarrhea, abdominal cramps, headache, and dizziness. Some individuals cannot take metronidazole orally.

Vaginal gels and suppositories are available, but they are not as effective as oral metronidazole.

Bacterial Vaginosis

Also called "nonspecific vaginitis," **bacterial vaginosis** causes a "stale fish" vaginal odor. The discharge is thin, gray-white leukorrhea that may be mild or very profuse. Generally there is no itching or burning as is associated with candida or trichomonas infection.

Diagnosis is done by obtaining a vaginal smear. The physician may order a KOH prep of the microscope slide.

Treatment is generally successful with metronidazole (Flagyl). Ampicillin and tetracycline may also be used. Sulfonamide creams or suppositories can be used, but are not considered as effective as metronidazole.

Pubic Lice

Pubic lice ("crabs," *Pediculus pubis*) are tiny parasites that attach themselves to pubic hair follicles and cause intense itching. The condition of having lice in the pubic area is known as **pediculosis pubis.** Pediculosis can spread through sexual contact, infested bed linens, and clothing or close physical contact.

Diagnosis is based on viewing the lice or their eggs (*nits*) attached to the hair follicles. Treatment consists of applying a drug such as lindane (Kwell) or pyrethrins (Barc, Pyrinyl, RID) to the affected area, and thoroughly cleaning all clothing and personal articles.

Because Kwell is contraindicated during pregnancy, alternate medications (such as Eurax) must be ordered if the woman is or suspects she is pregnant. The lice die within 24 hours after being separated from the body, but the nits can live for approximately 2 weeks. A repeat treatment is needed at that time. Sexual partners must be treated simultaneously, and household members must be carefully monitored. Other forms of pediculosis are discussed in Chapter 74.

➤ STUDENT SYNTHESIS

Key Points

- Human sexuality involves the whole body, mind, and spirit. It is at the core of each individual's personality.
- Sexual dysfunction is a person's inability to enjoy or engage in sexual activity for any reason.
- Infertility can be caused by male or female factors. Common factors include decreased sperm production, ovulation disorders, tubal obstruction, and endometriosis.
- Infertility carries deep physiologic and psychological effects.
- Contraception is an important consideration for individuals during various stages of their fertile years. Counseling in this area must be nonjudgmental and geared to meet the needs and preferences of the individual.
- STDs have the potential to cause sterility and also, in some cases, death.

Critical Thinking Exercises

1. Consider your own sexuality. How have your sexual orientation, identity, and decisions affected your relationships with others? What sexual choices have shaped the development of your life in terms of family planning?
2. You are working with a couple in their early 30s. They have been trying unsuccessfully for about 6 months to conceive. They are eager to begin fertility testing and have mentioned an interest in discussing fertility drugs and other options with their physician. What is your initial reaction? How would you approach this couple? What advice would you give them?
3. Joey is 15 years old. He comes into the clinic with symptoms indicative of chlamydial infection. Tests confirm this diagnosis. Joey currently has two female sexual partners. What type of information would you discuss with Joey? Explain treatment and other measures for him to avoid reinfection and to prevent infecting others.

NCLEX-Style Review Questions

1. Which is an accurate statement regarding sexuality?
   a. It involves more than sexual contact.
   b. It begins at adolescence.
   c. It is primarily learned through social experiences.
   d. It does not include attitudes and feelings.
2. What is the term used to describe a person attracted to both sexes?
   a. Lesbian
   b. Gay
   c. Homosexual
   d. Bisexual
3. What do you ensure by following protocol during a sexual assault investigation?
   a. The victim's rights
   b. Complete documentation
   c. Emotional closure for the victim
   d. Decreased post-traumatic stress
4. What drug is often used to treat endocrine-based sexual dysfunction?
   a. Viagra
   b. Papaverine
   c. Phentolamine
   d. Testosterone
5. What does the word dyspareunia mean?
   a. Painful intercourse
   b. Involuntary vaginal contraction
   c. Inability to achieve orgasm during intercourse
   d. Difficulty allowing penile penetration

Reference

1. Masters, V. H., & Johnson, V. E., (1966). *Human sexual response.* Boston: Little, Brown.

Unit XI

PEDIATRIC NURSING

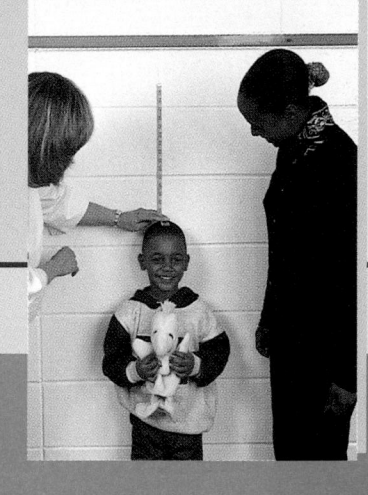

70	FUNDAMENTALS OF PEDIATRIC NURSING
71	CARE OF THE INFANT, TODDLER, OR PRESCHOOLER
72	CARE OF THE SCHOOL-AGE CHILD OR ADOLESCENT
73	THE CHILD OR ADOLESCENT WITH SPECIAL NEEDS

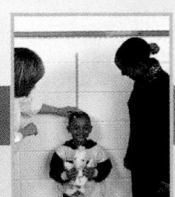

70

Fundamentals of Pediatric Nursing

LEARNING OBJECTIVES

1. Explain the concepts of prevention and health maintenance as they pertain to children.
2. State at least six immunizations provided to children. Identify at least three nursing considerations related to immunizations.
3. Discuss at least five specific nursing observations needed for the care of an infant, toddler, preschooler, school-age child, and adolescent.
4. Provide at least three topics of therapeutic communications with a toddler, preschool-age child, and school-age child.
5. Define and differentiate among the stages of separation anxiety.
6. State the normal limits of pulse, respiration, temperature, blood pressure, height, and weight for infants and children of different ages.
7. Identify at least five concerns related to pediatric safety during a hospital admission.
8. List four types of pediatric restraints. State at least three nursing concerns regarding pediatric restraints.
9. In the skills lab, demonstrate the application of a urine collection device on an infant. State at least three nursing concerns for this procedure.
10. Describe the steps involved in bathing an infant. Identify at least three nursing concerns for this procedure.
11. Define and differentiate among the following: oxygen mask, mist tent, and oxyhood. State at least three nursing concerns for each.
12. Identify at least two reasons for performing each of the following: venipuncture, heelstick, and lumbar puncture. State at least three nursing concerns for each procedure.
13. Differentiate and discuss the treatments for fever lower than 102° F (38.8° C) and higher than 102° F (38.8° C). State at least three nursing concerns for each.
14. State at least three nursing concerns when administering PO and IM medications to an infant, a toddler, a preschool-age child, and a school-age child.
15. State at least eight nursing considerations for a child prior to and following a surgical procedure.
16. Identify at least five concepts that need to be discussed with the caretakers of a child who is scheduled to undergo a surgical procedure.

NEW TERMINOLOGY

circumoral cyanosis	immunization
health maintenance	pediatrician
health supervision	pediatrics

ACRONYMS

AAFP	H flu	OFC
AAP	IPPB	PICC
ACIP	MMR	TPN
DDST	NPO	URI

Pediatrics is the area of care that deals with children and adolescents. Nursing care of children is called *pediatric nursing*. Generally, the provider in this field is a **pediatrician**, although family practitioners, nurse practitioners (NP), and physician assistants (PA) also provide pediatric care. Changes in healthcare delivery have greatly decreased the number of children cared for in hospitals. Many children now have their healthcare needs met in community-based settings and in the home. The primary emphasis in today's pediatric healthcare is on health maintenance and promotion and disease prevention.

As a nurse, you will encounter children in various healthcare settings. You may care for well, ill, physically challenged, and mentally challenged children. Possible settings for healthcare delivery include the home, school, community healthcare facility, day-surgery center, physician's office, summer camp, residential setting, or hospital. The fundamentals of pediatric nursing discussed in this chapter apply regardless of where you provide care. Note that the nursing procedures in this chapter can be used or adapted for children of all ages. Many skills in Unit 8 also are applicable to and adaptable for pediatric nursing. Always consider a child's developmental stage when adapting nursing procedures.

Chapters 66 and 68 present newborn care. Chapter 71 discusses the care of infants, toddlers, and preschoolers who have specific conditions. Chapter 72 examines care of school-age children and adolescents who have specific conditions. Pediatric care for children with special needs is discussed in Chapter 73.

HEALTH MAINTENANCE

Prevention of disease, disorders, and disability is the goal of pediatric nursing. The concept of well-baby and well-child visits for **health maintenance** or **health supervision** has proven to be the most effective method of promoting the growth and development of healthy children. Caregivers must be aware of the importance of routine, scheduled trips to a primary provider or community health facility. Preventive healthcare monitors growth rates and achievement of developmental milestones, and provides opportunities for early detection of health problems.

Well-child visits allow for appointments for immunizations, school and athletic physicals, and screening for eye and ear problems. The child also may visit one of these settings for specific complaints of distress or injury. Well-child visits are also excellent opportunities for the nurse to provide teaching about health, safety, and nutrition issues. The nurse has an opportunity to observe family interactions, and can notify the physician of behaviors that suggest family dysfunction. Counseling of family caregivers can be provided before crises develop. See In Practice: Educating the Client 70-1, which lists some items to discuss with caregivers of children.

Remember that some children are cared for in families headed by persons other than their biologic parents. Gather data that includes information about the relationships within a child's immediate family when you initiate care. Also consider the child's cultural and religious background.

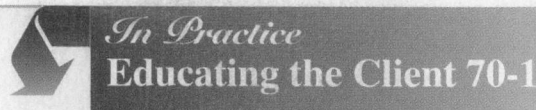

In Practice
Educating the Client 70-1

FAMILY CAREGIVER INSTRUCTION

Infant
- Proper diet and feeding techniques
- Teething
- Feeding routine, colic, and spitting up
- Need to suck; pacifiers
- Positioning and sleep habits
- Diaper rash
- Bathing and bathing safety
- Urinary and bowel habits
- Crib safety
- Use of a car restraint or safety device
- Accident prevention: suffocation, drowning, poisoning, and falling
- Beginning dental care: wipe the infant's gums with a damp cloth to remove excess food

Toddler
- Dental care: dental visits
- Weaning from the bottle
- Diet and solid food
- Behavior patterns: separation anxiety, negativism, and temper tantrums
- Discipline and limit setting
- Poison prevention
- Toilet training

Preschooler
- Eating habits: dawdling over food, "picky" eaters
- Night waking, bedtime fears, and nightmares
- Development of a positive self-concept and body image
- Aggressive behavior and sibling rivalry
- Preparation for school
- Thumb sucking; dental care
- Care for common childhood diseases

☞ KEY CONCEPT

Basic principles of safety and child care apply for both well and ill children.

During each visit, the nurse should obtain specific information related to the child's age. Well-child visit information includes vital signs, height and weight, occipital-frontal circumference (**OFC**) of the head (up to 3 years of age), abdominal girth, and limb measurements. Plot the child's height and weight on a growth chart that allows comparison with other children of the same age. At each visit, the child's growth should be compared with what is considered "normal limits." Early detection of abnormal trends can lead to preventive treatments.

The National Center for Health Statistics, in collaboration with the National Center for Chronic Disease Prevention and

Health Promotion, maintains many growth charts. You can view these charts on their website at http://www.cdc.gov/growthcharts. Separate charts for girls and boys of different ages are included. Some examples of the detailed information that is available include the following graphs:

- Birth to 36 months: Length-for-age and weight-for-age percentiles
- Birth to 36 months: Head circumference for age and weight-for-length percentiles
- 2 to 20 years: Stature-for-age and weight-for-age percentiles
- 2 to 20 years: Body mass index–for–age percentiles

The Denver-II Developmental Screening Test (**DDST**) is a tool used to identify developmental delays in infants, toddlers, and preschoolers. If a delay is identified or suspected, a more detailed evaluation of the child may be performed.

Physical Examination

The primary caregiver will complete a physical examination that will become a reference point for evaluating future illnesses. Many examiners use a head-to-toe checklist. Some assessments utilize a body system approach (eg, cardiovascular, neurological, pulmonary, and so forth). In this way, patterns are established, and nothing is overlooked. When an exception to the established normal trend is noted, it is described in detail on the child's chart.

Immunization

Immunization provides people with temporary or permanent protection against certain diseases. Early immunization is important to protect small children. The immunization program begins shortly after the child's birth and should be continued on a regular schedule. The vast majority of immunizations can be given even when the child has a mild illness.

☞ Key Concept

Families who cannot afford immunizations usually can receive them at no cost (or a reduced rate) from their local health department.

Laws in most states generally follow the recommendations of the American Academy of Pediatrics: five diphtheria, pertussis, tetanus immunizations; four oral polio vaccine immunizations; and two measles, mumps, and rubella (**MMR**) immunizations after the child's first birthday. Immunizations for hepatitis A and hepatitis B, *Haemophilus influenzae* (**H flu**), meningitis, and chickenpox (varicella) are also recommended, and many states are adding these requirements for school entrance.

Family caregivers must present records of immunizations to the child's school; failure to do so may result in the child's exclusion from the school. Table 70-1 presents the recommended immunization schedule of the American Academy of Pediatrics.

Tuberculin testing varies among states. One test is recommended during the child's first 2 years of life or before school admission. Some states require another test during the school years. Additional testing is indicated if tuberculosis exists within a given population.

The requirements of immunization change as the availability of vaccines increases. The Recommended Childhood Immunization Schedule is updated every 6 to 12 months.

Specific Care for Age Groups

Infant Care

Infant health supervision includes family teaching, assessment of developmental milestones, growth assessment, and immunizations. Examinations center around discussion with family caregivers and anticipatory teaching including the topics listed earlier in this chapter.

General observations include the following:

- How family caregivers hold the infant
- If the infant "cuddles" with family caregivers
- General cleanliness of the infant
- The infant's response to painful procedures
- The infant's appearance of health or illness; weight compared to length

Specific observations include the following:

- Equal, active movement of all extremities
- General activity level
- Alertness
- Skin color, warmth, and texture
- Tone and pitch of the infant's cry
- General respiratory status
- Fontanels, reflexes
- Achievement of developmental milestones

Toddler Care

As a toddler's growth progresses, independence and autonomy become important. Well-child assessments include:

- Age of weaning from breast or bottle to cup (usually achieved by age 12 months)
- Ages at which toilet training was started and completed
- Language development
- Play patterns and activities
- Sleep patterns

Discuss with family caregivers their child's behavior patterns and the type of discipline they use at home. Encourage caregivers to begin dental checkups for toddlers as early as 12 months of age.

Assessment and teaching require a strong focus on safety. Toddlers are very mobile but lack the judgment to protect themselves. Observe caregiver–toddler interaction.

Preschooler Care

The physical examination for preschool children focuses on readiness for school. Use a systems checklist to evaluate each child's physical condition. Focus attention also on sleep pat-

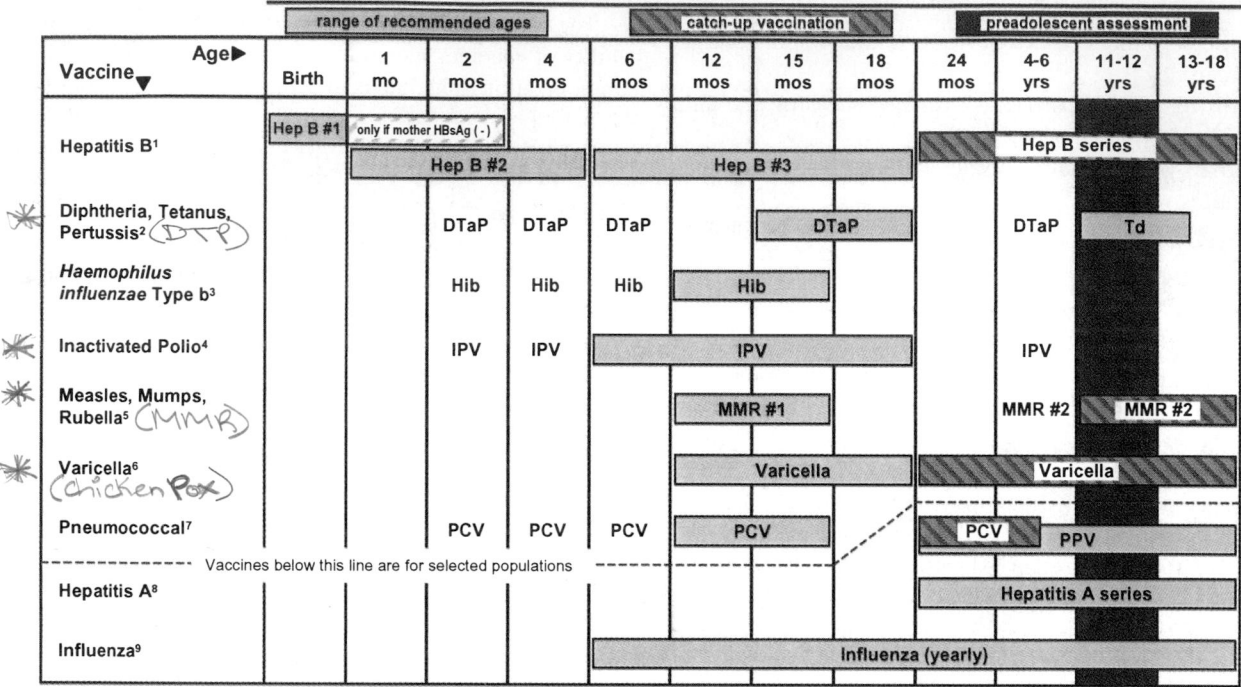

Vaccine ▼ Age ▶	Birth	1 mo	2 mos	4 mos	6 mos	12 mos	15 mos	18 mos	24 mos	4-6 yrs	11-12 yrs	13-18 yrs
										range of recommended ages / catch-up vaccination / preadolescent assessment		
Hepatitis B¹	Hep B #1	only if mother HBsAg (-)	Hep B #2			Hep B #3				Hep B series		
Diphtheria, Tetanus, Pertussis²			DTaP	DTaP	DTaP		DTaP			DTaP	Td	
Haemophilus influenzae Type b³			Hib	Hib	Hib	Hib						
Inactivated Polio⁴			IPV	IPV	IPV					IPV		
Measles, Mumps, Rubella⁵						MMR #1				MMR #2	MMR #2	
Varicella⁶						Varicella				Varicella		
Pneumococcal⁷			PCV	PCV	PCV	PCV				PCV	PPV	
Hepatitis A⁸										Hepatitis A series		
Influenza⁹					Influenza (yearly)							

Vaccines below this line are for selected populations

This schedule indicates the recommended ages for routine administration of currently licensed childhood vaccines, as of December 1, 2001, for children through age 18 years. Any dose not given at the recommended age should be given at any subsequent visit when indicated and feasible. ▨▨▨ Indicates age groups that warrant special effort to administer those vaccines not previously given. Additional vaccines may be licensed and recommended during the year. Licensed combination vaccines may be used whenever any components of the combination are indicated and the vaccine's other components are not contraindicated. Providers should consult the manufacturers' package inserts for detailed recommendations.

1. Hepatitis B vaccine (Hep B). All infants should receive the first dose of hepatitis B vaccine soon after birth and before hospital discharge; the first dose may also be given by age 2 months if the infant's mother is HBsAg-negative. Only monovalent hepatitis B vaccine can be used for the birth dose. Monovalent or combination vaccine containing Hep B may be used to complete the series; four doses of vaccine may be administered if combination vaccine is used. The second dose should be given at least 4 weeks after the first dose, except for Hib-containing vaccine which cannot be administered before age 6 weeks. The third dose should be given at least 16 weeks after the first dose and at least 8 weeks after the second dose. The last dose in the vaccination series (third or fourth dose) should not be administered before age 6 months.

Infants born to HBsAg-positive mothers should receive hepatitis B vaccine and 0.5 mL hepatitis B immune globulin (HBIG) within 12 hours of birth at separate sites. The second dose is recommended at age 1-2 months and the vaccination series should be completed (third or fourth dose) at age 6 months.

Infants born to mothers whose HBsAg status is unknown should receive the first dose of the hepatitis B vaccine series within 12 hours of birth. Maternal blood should be drawn at the time of delivery to determine the mother's HBsAg status; if the HBsAg test is positive, the infant should receive HBIG as soon as possible (no later than age 1 week).

2. Diphtheria and tetanus toxoids and acellular pertussis vaccine (DTaP). The fourth dose of DTaP may be administered as early as age 12 months, provided 6 months have elapsed since the third dose and the child is unlikely to return at age 15-18 months. **Tetanus and diphtheria toxoids (Td)** is recommended at age 11-12 years if at least 5 years have elapsed since the last dose of tetanus and diphtheria toxoid-containing vaccine. Subsequent routine Td boosters are recommended every 10 years.

3. Haemophilus influenzae type b (Hib) conjugate vaccine. Three Hib conjugate vaccines are licensed for infant use. If PRP-OMP (PedvaxHIB® or ComVax® [Merck]) is administered at ages 2 and 4 months, a dose at age 6 months is not required. DTaP/Hib combination products should not be used for primary immunization in infants at age 2, 4 or 6 months, but can be used as boosters following any Hib vaccine.

4. Inactivated poliovirus vaccine (IPV). An all-IPV schedule is recommended for routine childhood poliovirus vaccination in the United States. All children should receive four doses of IPV at age 2 months, 4 months, 6-18 months, and 4-6 years.

5. Measles, mumps, and rubella vaccine (MMR). The second dose of MMR is recommended routinely at age 4-6 years but may be administered during any visit, provided at least 4 weeks have elapsed since the first dose and that both doses are administered beginning at or after age 12 months. Those who have not previously received the second dose should complete the schedule by the visit at 11-12 years.

6. Varicella vaccine. Varicella vaccine is recommended at any visit at or after age 12 months for susceptible children (i.e. those who lack a reliable history of chickenpox). Susceptible persons aged ≥13 years should receive two doses, given at least 4 weeks apart.

7. Pneumococcal vaccine. The heptavalent **pneumococcal conjugate vaccine (PCV)** is recommended for all children aged 2-23 months and for certain children aged 24-59 months. **Pneumococcal polysaccharide vaccine (PPV)** is recommended in addition to PCV for certain high-risk groups. See *MMWR* 2000;49(RR-9);1-37.

8. Hepatitis A vaccine. Hepatitis A vaccine is recommended for use in selected states and regions, and for certain high-risk groups; consult your local public health authority. See *MMWR* 1999;48(RR-12);1-37.

9. Influenza vaccine. Influenza vaccine is recommended annually for children age ≥ 6 months with certain risk factors (including but not limited to asthma, cardiac disease, sickle cell disease, HIV, and diabetes; see *MMWR* 2001;50(RR-4);1-44), and can be administered to all others wishing to obtain immunity. Children aged ≤12 years should receive vaccine in a dosage appropriate for their age (0.25 mL if age 6-35 months or 0.5 mL if aged ≥ 3 years). Children aged ≤ 8 years who are receiving influenza vaccine for the first time should receive two doses separated by at least 4 weeks.

For additional information about vaccines, vaccine supply, and contraindications for immunization, please visit the National Immunization Program Website at www.cdc.gov/nip or call the National Immunization Hotline at 800-232-2522 (English) or 800-232-0233 (Spanish).

Approved by the Advisory Committee on Immunization Practices (www.cdc.gov/nip/acip), the American Academy of Pediatrics (www.aap.org), and the American Academy of Family Physicians (www.aafp.org).

terns, safety, and relationships with peers, siblings, and family caregivers.

Evaluation of speech, hearing, and vision is critical in the preschool years. Each must be within normal limits to facilitate learning. Determine if a child's developmental age is commensurate with his or her chronological age. An adequate attention span is essential, so be sure to assess each child's ability to pay attention, follow directions, and focus on a task. Evaluate gross and fine motor control. These characteristics are evaluated earlier, but they become a special focus in the preschool examination.

School-Age Child Care

Continue to plot the school-age child's heights and weights on the growth grid to establish a comparison with other children of the same age. Emphasize successful completion of schoolwork and relationships with peers, siblings, and family caregivers. Evaluate nutrition, elimination, and sleep patterns. The child needs an MMR booster at age 12 if he or she has not had it between 4 and 6 years of age. In addition, the series of three doses of hepatitis B vaccine should be completed at 12 years of age if it has not been completed earlier. Twelve-year-olds who have not received the varicella vaccine, and do not have a reliable history of chickenpox, should be immunized. Children 13 years of age and older should receive two doses at least 1 month apart.

Adolescent Care

Health supervision issues for adolescents focus on puberty and a smooth transition to young adulthood. Adolescents require an update of the diphtheria-tetanus immunization.

☛ KEY CONCEPT

Adolescents may be too embarrassed to ask questions, particularly about their health. A bulletin board or brochure rack well stocked with informational pamphlets about common concerns can aid communication.

Adolescents are capable of expressing individual concerns; therefore, you will benefit from talking separately with caregivers and with adolescents. A tactful approach to care includes detailed explanations of procedures you are to perform. The transition from childhood to adolescence can be difficult. The adolescent may present with such problems as acne vulgaris, menstrual dysfunction, inadequate nutrition, sexually transmitted diseases, suicidal ideation, or chemical abuse. Many adolescents benefit from professional counseling.

Adolescents need certain accommodations to preserve their self-respect and identity. They do not belong either with young children or only with adults. Adolescents feel more comfortable and are able to relate better with healthcare personnel in a setting customized for them. The healthcare staff should be chosen to work specifically with adolescents. If a specialized setting is unavailable, the adolescent should be placed with others close to his or her age. In any situation, clear rules should be posted so that all adolescents know the setting's guidelines.

Illness or injury can seriously threaten self-image. Many young people worry about damage to their bodies or about death, whether the threat is real or not. In addition they are often acutely aware of their emerging sexuality; therefore, their modesty should be respected. Include adolescents in planning and performing as much care as possible to encourage their emerging independence.

Adolescents need non-biased and accurate information regarding their rapidly changing bodies and the issues they may encounter during this transition to young adulthood. Health education should include information concerning sexually transmitted diseases and prevention, (including HIV/AIDS), homosexuality, pregnancy, and birth control. Teenagers also need clear and nonjudgmental information about substance use and abuse, depression, and suicide.

THE HOSPITAL EXPERIENCE

Short- or long-term hospitalization can be traumatic and disturbing for children and families. Small children usually do not understand what is happening or why they are being taken away from home. Illness threatens body image at any age. You will see nurses in the pediatric department dressed in colorful scrubs rather than the more frightening white uniforms. The units are decorated with pictures of animals or cartoon characters to make the children feel more comfortable.

☛ KEY CONCEPT

Pediatric nurses provide care not just for the sick child, but for the entire family.

Age-Related Concerns

Infants, Toddlers, and Preschoolers

Even before children are 1 year of age, they become frightened of strangers and are aware of their family's absence. From ages 1 to 5 years, children often exhibit severe anxiety when separated from home and family.

Very young children have concrete thought processes and often misinterpret what they hear. The following statements are examples of what to avoid saying when caring for children. (The statements in parentheses give an example of what the child might be thinking):

- "I am going to take your blood pressure." (Where are you taking it?) Instead you might say: "I am going to find out how strong your heart is beating right now."
- "I am going to give you a shot." (Are you going to shoot me with a gun?) Instead you might say: "I am going to give you some medicine."
- "This will only feel like a little bee sting." (Oh, no, I'm afraid of bees!) Instead you might say: "This may hurt a little. Hold your teddy bear tightly to help you."

Keep sentences short, and phrase statements so the child knows what to do, not what to avoid. (For example, if you say: "Don't cross the street alone," the child may only hear: "cross the street alone.") Tell children who are to remain in t pital overnight that nurses work at night also, in case they are worried that they will be alone. See In Practice: Nursing Care Guidelines 70-1 for more suggestions on reducing anxiety in children.

School-Age Children and Adolescents

As a rule, older children are able to understand the need for hospitalization, although they often hide many fears. Younger school-aged children may experience fear of separation when they are ill. Peer relationships are important to children at this age, especially adolescents. Most healthcare facilities allow friends to visit, but activities should be regulated to prevent sick teens from becoming overtired. A telephone should be available for the child client; however; rules for its use should be clearly established.

☞ Key Concept

A smile is a universal language.

Family-Centered Care

Most healthcare facilities make every effort to meet a child's security need to be part of a family unit. Family-centered care may include rooming-in, as illustrated in Figure 70-1. Health-care personnel encourage family caregivers to remain with

---

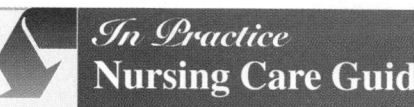

In Practice
Nursing Care Guidelines 70-1

REDUCING ANXIETY AND CALMING CHILDREN FOR ASSESSMENTS AND PROCEDURES

General Guidelines
- Explain the procedure in terms that the child can understand.
- Explain the procedure to family caregivers.
- Never tell the child something will not hurt if it might.
- Avoid performing painful or frightening procedures in the child's bed or the playroom. Use the examination or treatment room. The bed or playroom should be a "safe place."
- Never make a promise to a child that you cannot or will not keep.
- Give an analgesic before a painful procedure, if possible.
- Crying is a normal response to pain and fear. Never tell a child not to cry because it may shame or embarrass him or her.
- After the procedure, explain to the child and family caregivers any undesired effects that they should note, and what to do if they occur.
- Report test results to family caregivers and the child if possible.
- Check the child's condition frequently and reassure the child that you are close by if needed.
- Document any unusual reactions. Also note on the nursing care plan any tips to help make a repeated procedure less disagreeable the next time.

Infants
- Change the infant's diaper before the treatment.
- Feed the infant before the treatment, unless a danger of vomiting exists.
- Offer the baby a pacifier.
- Talk and play with the infant before performing the procedure.
- Position the infant in his or her accustomed sleeping position, if possible.
- Release the thumb for sucking if the infant does not use a pacifier.

- Sing repetitious songs softly to encourage sleep. If singing does not work, try whistling (some babies pause crying long enough to fall asleep).
- Rub the infant's arms and back soothingly.
- Hold the infant in your arms.

Toddlers
- Let the child play with and explore the equipment before the procedure.
- Explain the procedure to the toddler using simple words and short sentences.
- Encourage family caregivers to participate by supporting and comforting the child when possible.
- Allow the child to hold a security object (doll, stuffed animal, or blanket) during the procedure.
- Distract, rather than restrain, whenever possible.
- Praise the child for being "helpful."
- Allow the child to cry without feeling ashamed.
- Allow the child to hold equipment or help whenever possible.
- Allow the child to play with equipment after the procedure.

Preschoolers
- Use simple words to prepare the preschooler for sensations he or she will experience.
- Use dolls or puppets to explain procedures.
- Allow the preschooler to play with the teaching aids.
- Ensure privacy for the preschooler.
- Encourage the preschooler to talk about the procedure; clarify any misunderstandings or questions.
- Encourage the preschooler to help in a reasonable way with the procedure to help him or her achieve a sense of control.
- Verbally praise the preschooler and reward him or her in some way (eg, stickers, stars)

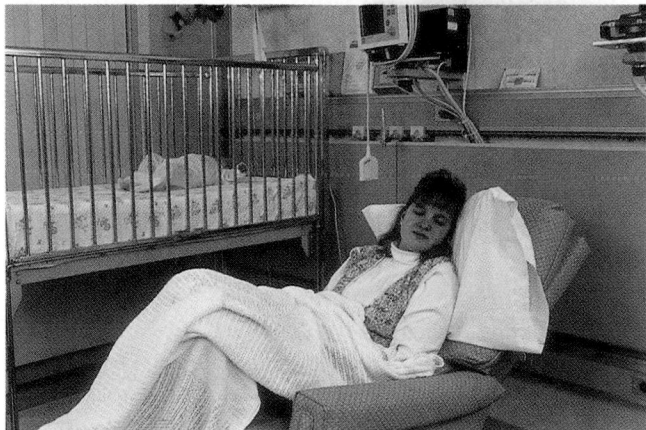

FIGURE 70-1. Rooming-in helps alleviate anxiety for both the child and the caregiver.

children during their hospital experience. Participation in care by family members promotes a less-stressed child and parent.

If family members are unable to remain with their children, caregivers should assure the children that they will return. All caregivers need to state the time of their return in terms that children will understand (eg, "before lunch," "after your nap"). They can also give children a possession to hold until their return. Nurturing measures such as providing a doll, a toy, or a teddy bear can help to relieve anxiety. The object becomes a physical reminder that the family caregiver will return.

Family caregivers react in various ways to hospitalization. Reactions often depend on the following factors:

- The seriousness of the child's illness
- The immediate threat to the child's life
- The situation of the family
- Ego resources of the family caregivers
- The family's former experiences with illness and hospitalization
- The family's style of coping with stress
- The caregivers' beliefs and values

Preparation

Hospitalization often causes apprehension and fear in families. Helping children to successfully adjust is an important nursing goal. One way to ease this adjustment is to prepare children for the experience at their own level of comprehension. Tell children what to expect and help them avoid feeling abandoned or punished. If possible, a tour of the healthcare facility prior to admission provides a foundation for preparing the child. Encourage family caregivers to include the child in packing for the trip to the facility. Remind them to be sure to bring along special items.

Stages of Separation Anxiety

Before accepting the situation of being hospitalized, most children, particularly those aged 3 to 4 years, experience three phrases of separation anxiety: protest, despair, and denial. Each phase extends into the next. The ultimate goal is for the child

to reach a level of acceptance or adjustment to his or her surroundings.

Protest. In the protest phase, the child's need for family caregivers is conscious and sorrowful. The child cries and reacts aggressively, rejecting healthcare personnel. Fear of the unknown and anxiety cause the child to demand his or her own caregivers. Such a reaction is normal and denotes a healthy attachment to the caregivers.

Despair. In the despair stage, the child becomes inactive and sad. Usual comfort measures, such as thumb-sucking and clutching a blanket, become prominent. He or she watches constantly for family caregivers, is quiet and withdrawn, and is uninterested in food or play.

Denial. The denial phase (detachment) may be interpreted as a sign that the child is protecting him- or herself from anxiety by rejecting family caregivers. In truth, the child's need for caregivers is more intense than ever.

Transcultural Considerations

Children and families from a culture that is different from most of the clients or nurses in a healthcare facility may be confused and frightened. Children who do not understand the language may be especially frightened and have a difficult time. Family caregivers should translate for their children if possible. It is helpful for the staff to communicate with children, and make them feel comfortable and relaxed. Allowing them to be with other children as much as possible is also beneficial. Keeping pictures of common items available can help children to communicate their needs, thereby making them feel less isolated.

BASIC PEDIATRIC CARE AND PROCEDURES

Admitting Children to the Healthcare Facility

Although the process of admitting children to a healthcare facility is similar to admitting adults, a special effort should be made to be alert to the needs of both the family caregivers and the child. Make family members as comfortable and secure as possible; it is important to earn their confidence and cooperation. Often if children see that their family caregivers accept and trust you, they become more willing to accept you as well.

Ask family caregivers about their child's special needs, likes and dislikes, allergies, and special vocabulary, especially for items such as the "potty." You can include children in gathering this information by directing the questions to them. You should also introduce them to roommates. The playroom is a non-threatening environment in which the family and nursing staff can get to know each other, thereby helping to put children at ease.

☛ KEY CONCEPT

You can perform much of the admission assessment for a small child while he or she sits on the caregiver's lap.

Assisting With the Physical Examination

The equipment for the physical examination of a child is the same as that for an adult, except that some pieces are smaller. The child's cooperation is of utmost importance. If the child is too young, ill, or frightened to understand how to cooperate, you may need to restrain him or her for parts of the examination. Use restraint only as a last resort, because it only makes children feel more threatened and frightened. A little extra time helping children become comfortable often works wonders. Show the child the equipment and let him or her handle it to promote a sense of control.

Assessing on Admission

Observe the child carefully for any signs of rash, abrasion, discharge, or alteration in consciousness level. Note complaints of pain or other symptoms, as you would for an adult. Carefully document all observations. If you have reason to think a child has been battered or abused in any way, report your beliefs to your supervisor—this is a legal responsibility. Chapter 71 discusses child abuse in more detail.

Vital Signs

Obtain and document vital signs on admission. Table 70-2 lists normal ranges of vital signs for various ages.

Respiration.   Take respirations before taking other vital signs, as you will be unable to obtain an accurate respiratory rate if a child is crying. Count the respiratory rate for 1 full minute. If you cannot obtain a respiratory rate because of crying, observe for signs of respiratory distress by checking skin color, pallor, and the presence of breath sounds. Sites of respiratory distress are seen in Figure 70-2. Signs of respiratory distress include xiphoid retraction, nares dilation, and expiratory grunt. Appropriately document your findings.

Pulse.   For children older than 2 years, you may take the radial pulse; for those younger than 2 years, take the pulse apically. Count the pulse for a full minute. The sizes of the bell and diaphragm of the stethoscope are smaller for children than for adults.

Temperature.   Take an oral or tympanic temperature for children older than 6 years. Take a tympanic, axillary, or rectal temperature for children who are younger than 6 years, disoriented, unconscious, or in severe respiratory distress.

Do not take a rectal temperature if a child has had any immune or hematologic disorder, rectal surgery, or diarrhea. Do not take a tympanic temperature if a child has had ear surgery or has ventilating tubes or infection. Use the axillary method only if other methods are not possible. Regardless of the method you use, remain with the child to ensure safety. Hold the temperature probe in place for the required time. Do not use glass and mercury thermometers.

Blood Pressure.   It is necessary to use a smaller blood pressure cuff for children. When choosing a cuff, measure the width of the cuff against the width of the child's arm. The cuff should cover approximately two thirds of the upper arm. The bladder of the cuff should be long enough to encircle the arm without overlapping. Be sure to use the same size of cuff each time. Cuff size will vary with a child's age and size. The most important aspect is the trend of the blood pressure or temperature: You should determine whether each is going up or down.

> ### ✚👁 Nursing Alert
>
> If taking blood pressure at an infant's thigh, record it as "thigh pressure." In children older than 1 year, thigh pressure is approximately 20 mm Hg *higher* than arm pressure. If you must use the radial artery (wrist), radial blood pressure is 10 mm Hg *lower* than that of the brachial artery. Note use of the radial artery on the record.

Weight and Height.   All children should be weighed upon admission. Weigh small children on an infant or child scale, and measure the weight in kilograms. Often, you will need to convert this weight to pounds for the benefit of family caregivers (2.2 lb = 1 kg). Documenting weight in kilograms allows accurate dosage calculation for medication administration, particularly for intravenous fluids.

To maintain medical asepsis, place a clean paper on the infant scale before weighing a child, and disinfect the scale after the procedure. While weighing children, keep one hand just above them to make sure they do not fall. (See Chapter 66, Fig. 66-2A and In Practice: Nursing Procedure 66-3.) After weighing is finished, discard the paper and document the weight. Wash your hands before and after weighing. Use Standard Precautions throughout the procedure. You should report any deviations in weight immediately. These procedures help

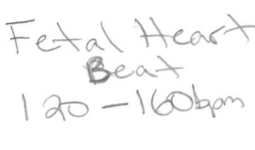

(handwritten) Fetal Heart Beat 120 – 160 bpm

■■■ TABLE 70-2 *A*VERAGE VITAL SIGNS FOR CHILDREN

Age	Average Pulse (beats/min)	Average Respiration (breaths/min)	Systolic Blood Pressure (mm Hg)	Diastolic Blood Pressure (mm Hg)
Infant	80–180	20–40	74–100	50–70
Toddler	80–140	20–30	80–112	50–80
Preschooler	70–115	20–25	82–110	50–78
School-Age	65–110	17–22	84–120	54–80
Adolescent	60–90	15–20	94–140	62–88

Data from Marks, M. G. (1998). *Broadribb's introductory pediatric nursing* (5th ed.). Philadelphia: Lippincott-Raven.

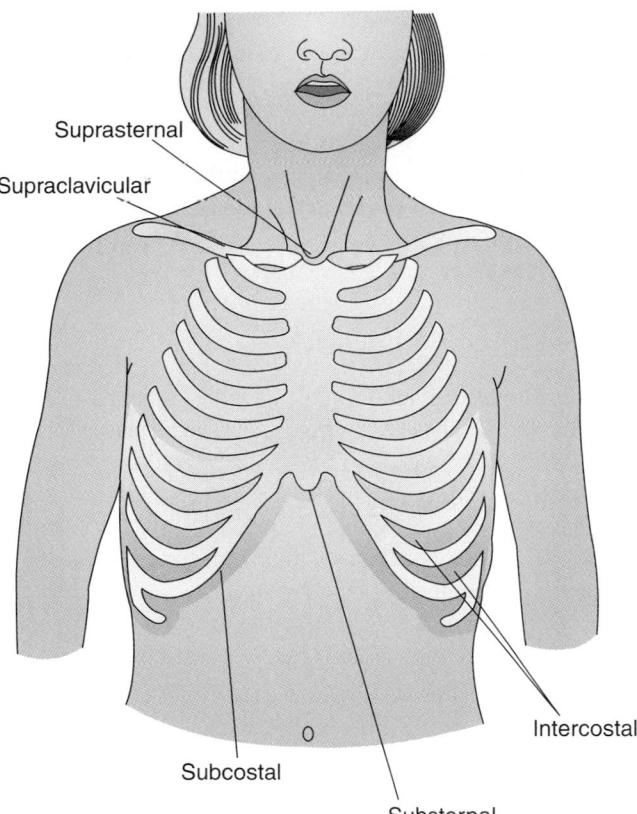

FIGURE 70-2. Sites of respiratory retractions.

(labels: Suprasternal, Supraclavicular, Subcostal, Substernal, Intercostal)

to assess edema, dehydration, and the child's nutritional state. Figure 70-3 demonstrates how to weigh a child.

Figure 66-2B in Chapter 66 shows a nurse measuring an infant's length with a paper tape measure. One way to do so is to mark the child's length from head to toe on the bed and then measure between the marks, rather than trying to mea-

sure a moving baby. Record standing heights for older children as illustrated in Figure 70-4.

Use the following guidelines when weighing an infant:

- Weigh the infant at the same time each day, before feeding.
- Balance the scale carefully before obtaining the infant's weight.
- Weigh the infant without clothes or diaper.
- Note additional equipment being weighed (eg, IV, arm board, brace, cast)

Nursing Alert

Use a disposable paper tape measure when obtaining measurements. *Rationale: A cloth tape measure may stretch and alter measurement findings. Disposable tape measures also prevent cross-contamination.*

Head Circumference

Measure the OFC of the head for children up to 3 years of age and for any child with a questionable head size. (See Chapter 66, Fig. 66-2C and In Practice: Nursing Procedure 66-4.) Plot measurements on a growth chart and compare them against normal sizes for the child's age group to determine any abnormalities.

☞ KEY CONCEPT

The occipital-frontal circumference (OFC) reflects intracranial volume pressure, which is a significant finding. Factors that affect head circumference include brain development, intracranial pressure, hydrocephalus, brain tumor, and some congenital defects, such as microcephaly and hydrocephalus.

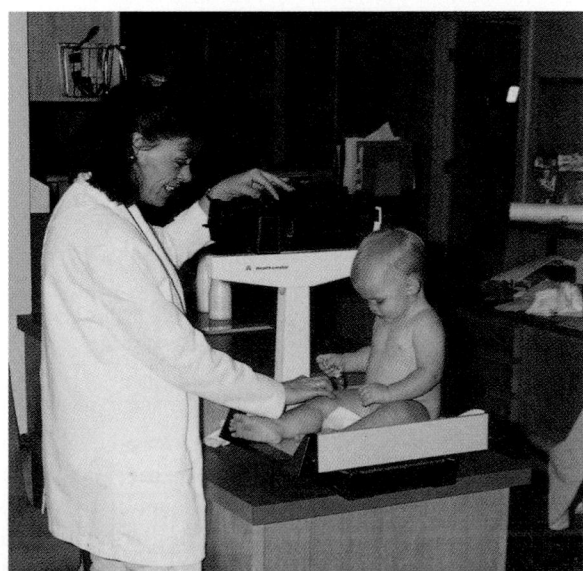

FIGURE 70-3. Children who can sit may be weighed in a sitting position if this is less frightening for them. Infants are weighed lying down.

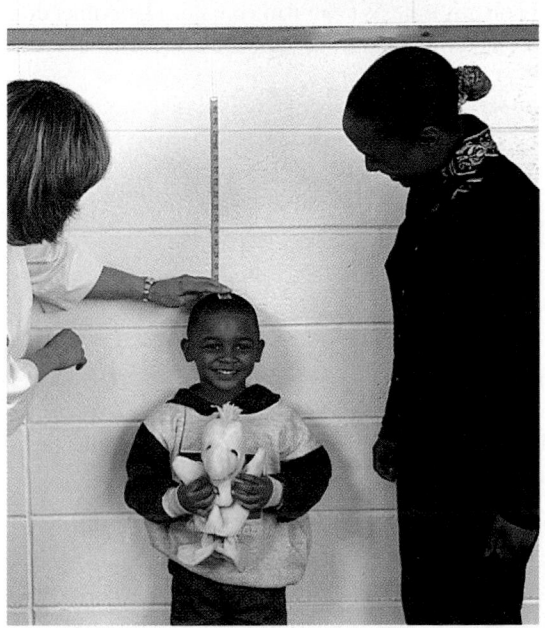

FIGURE 70-4. Measuring the height of an older child.

Chest Circumference

Measure and compare the child's chest circumference with the OFC. Normally the newborn's head is larger than the chest. Chest and head measurements are approximately equal for children aged 1 to 2 years, after which the chest begins to become larger than the head. By age 5, a child's chest is about 2 to 3 inches (5–7.6 cm) larger than the head. Measure the chest at the child's nipple line, using a paper tape.

Other Measurements

Other important measurements include abdominal circumference, extremity length, and extremity circumference. Be sure to note where on the extremity you took a circumference measurement. Measure the abdomen at the child's umbilicus.

Daily Assessing and Documenting

Observe and document all information about the child, including normal behavior and reactions, abnormal symptoms, and unfavorable signs. Check the child's nonverbal signals. A child who is pulling at the ears, for example, may have an ear infection.

Because children often cannot tell how they feel, whether they have voided or had a bowel movement, or how much they have eaten, the nurse is responsible for recording this information.

Diet

Observe how much a child eats and drinks throughout the day. Intake and output (I&O) for children does not mean just fluid I&O; it also means food intake and all types of output. Accuracy is important because it is easy for small children to become dehydrated. Note if an infant spits up formula or if a young child does not want to eat. Many healthcare facilities have special menus that cater to children's appetites. Common menu items include pizza, macaroni, soup, corn dogs, hamburgers, and ice cream. Assess the number, color, and consistency of stools and any emesis (vomiting), voiding, or other drainage. Weigh diapers to obtain an accurate assessment of urine output.

> ### ✚👁 Nursing Alert
> Illness and separation from family and home can greatly change a child's appetite. Be alert for candy and other snacks visitors bring. Eating empty-caloric snack foods can decrease a child's appetite for regular meals. Be sure to include such snacks when documenting intake.

General Appearance

Note the child's activity level, skin color and warmth, comfort level, cry (lusty or weak), response to environment, and general respiratory status.

Family Caregivers' Comments

Note statements that family caregivers make about their child's condition. Family caregivers are more familiar with the child's normal activity and appearance and often notice signs that others miss.

Physical Signs

Be alert for seizures, changes in vital signs, cough, congestion, wheezing, nasal discharge, rash, or any other abnormality.

Visitors

Note whether family caregivers are at the bedside or if they visit frequently. Lack of visits may indicate a family problem. Also observe and report interaction between family caregivers and children.

Discharging Children

Children are discharged from the healthcare facility in much the same way as adults, except that they are taken home by their family caregivers, who are responsible for followup care. Be sure children have been properly discharged by the physician and have appointment slips, prescriptions, and physician's orders. Teach family caregivers followup care, and document this teaching. Family members should carry children to a car or use a wheelchair or wagon to do so. Healthcare personnel must accompany children and family caregivers to the facility's exit. All states require placement of children in a car seat or restraining safety device. Some facilities make car seats available to families who are unable to afford one by the time of discharge. If a car seat or restraining device is not present, one should be made available.

INTERMEDIATE PEDIATRIC CARE AND PROCEDURES

Providing for Pediatric Safety

Nurses are legally responsible for the safety of children in their care. See In Practice: Nursing Care Guidelines 70-2.

Safety Devices

Special measures are necessary to prevent accidents or injuries from falls. Children may also need restraints to remind them not to pull on tubes or pick at suture lines. Sometimes enforcing bed rest by applying a child safety device called a *restraint* is necessary. Small children also should be restrained whenever they are in a high chair, wheelchair, or unattended. Never substitute the safety device, however, for good observation.

A physician's order is usually required for application of any restraint device. Release and reapply restraints every 1 to 2 hours. Check the child's skin and circulation each hour. Document these safety measures. See In Practice: Nursing Care Guidelines 70-3 for more information on pediatric restraints.

Infection Control

Hospitalized children need protection from contagious diseases. Healthcare personnel and family members of children younger than 2 years of age are usually required to wear isolation protection when handling children with contagious diseases, to prevent the spread of infection. Follow standard and transmission-based precautions as appropriate.

Most healthcare facilities use disposable gowns. Change your gown at least once each shift and more often if needed,

In Practice
Nursing Care Guidelines 70-2

PROVIDING PEDIATRIC SAFETY

- Wash your hands before and after giving care. Follow standard and transmission-based precautions as necessary. *Rationale: Pediatric nursing often involves contact with body fluids. Following these guidelines will protect against contamination or exposure to biohazardous substances.*
- Make sure side rails on beds and cribs are up at all times. Beds should always be in the lowest position unless you are performing specific procedures. *Rationale: Prevent injuries from falls.*
- Adequately support children when you carry or transfer them. Always support their heads and necks, and watch the position of their extremities carefully. *Rationale: Correct positioning decreases the possibility of injury and gives children a sense of security.*
- Supervise ambulatory children.
- Be aware of facility procedures for fire, severe weather, external alerts, and so forth. *Rationale: Children will need more attention and assistance than adults in emergencies.*
- Keep children away from electrical equipment, cords, and outlets. Keep them away from heat sources (eg, radiators, lamps, heat vents). If using heat therapy, check the child's temperature and closely monitor the child's skin. *Rationale: A child's skin is more sensitive to heat, and burns more easily than does adult skin.*
- Never leave a child younger than 10 years of age alone in any amount of water. Frequently check on older children. *Rationale: Prevent drowning, which can occur in a very small amount of water for a young child.*
- Use safety restraints when transporting a child. Never leave the child unattended. Always use the provided safety devices when a child is in a high chair.
- Use disposable diapers unless the child is sensitive to them. *Rationale: Disposable diapers do not require pins, and therefore are safer to use.*
- If you must use safety pins, keep them closed whenever you remove them. Do not leave pins exposed, because children can swallow them easily. Put your

fingers between the child's skin and the pin when applying a pin. *Rationale: Prevent choking or injuries to yourself or the child.*
- Check all toys for small, removable, or broken pieces. *Rationale: The child can swallow them and choke.*
- Supervise children who are using pens, pencils, or scissors. *Rationale: Sharp objects can cut children.*
- Use only toys that can be disinfected. Remind family caregivers that toys that cannot be disinfected may need to be thrown away. Disinfect toys regularly (always between use by different children or if dirty or contaminated). *Rationale: Disinfection decreases the possibility of contamination.*
- Do not allow children to use latex balloons; mylar is acceptable. *Rationale: Latex balloons can pop, and the child can aspirate the pieces. Mylar balloons will not pop.*
- Be alert for any broken equipment, furniture, or glass items. *Rationale: Prevent accidents.*
- When taking a child's temperature, assess his or her ability to cooperate. *Rationale: If the child is uncooperative, the thermometer could break, or the reading could be inaccurate.* Check the graphic sheet to see which route to use for temperature taking. Sometimes, the provider orders a specific route. Always stay with a child when you take his or her temperature. Hold the thermometer in place.
- Supervise children when they are out of their room. They should never be in the medication, diet, kitchen, or utility room. *Rationale: Decrease the risk of injury.*
- Never prop bottles. *Rationale: Prevent choking and ear infections.*
- Never leave a young child unattended during eating. Cut food into small bites. Avoid giving foods that are slippery or hard to chew.
- Teach family caregivers good safety practices, and make sure they understand the reasons behind them. *Rationale: Family caregivers will be more receptive to safety practices if they understand the reasons for their use. Teaching helps prevent home accidents.*

---

then discard after use. Scrub before putting on the gown and scrub thoroughly after removing it. Wear gloves if you will come into contact with any body fluids or substances, including stool, emesis, urine, or blood.

Nutrient Intake

At mealtimes, children may sit in high chairs or they may be seated at a small table. Encourage family caregivers to help feed their child, because most children eat better for family

members. Record all food and fluid the child consumes. Always supervise children who are eating.

Fluids

Getting children to take fluids is often difficult because they do not understand the reasons for drinking if they are not thirsty. Ask family caregivers about a child's favorite liquids. Offer small amounts frequently. Aside from actual fluids, acceptable substitutes are ice pops, ice cream, gelatin, soda, and fruit drinks.

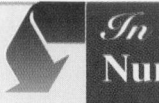

In Practice
Nursing Care Guidelines 70-3

USING PEDIATRIC RESTRAINTS

Explain to family caregivers and the child what you are doing and why. Be sure the child does not view the restraint as punishment. *Rationale: Teaching helps to decrease fears, and prepares family caregivers to see the child in a restraint.*

Commonly Used Restraints

Bubble tops—Made of clear plastic and attached to the top of the crib.

• Be sure it is firmly attached to the crib. *Rationale: Prevent the child from being able to climb out around it or from getting his or her head stuck.*

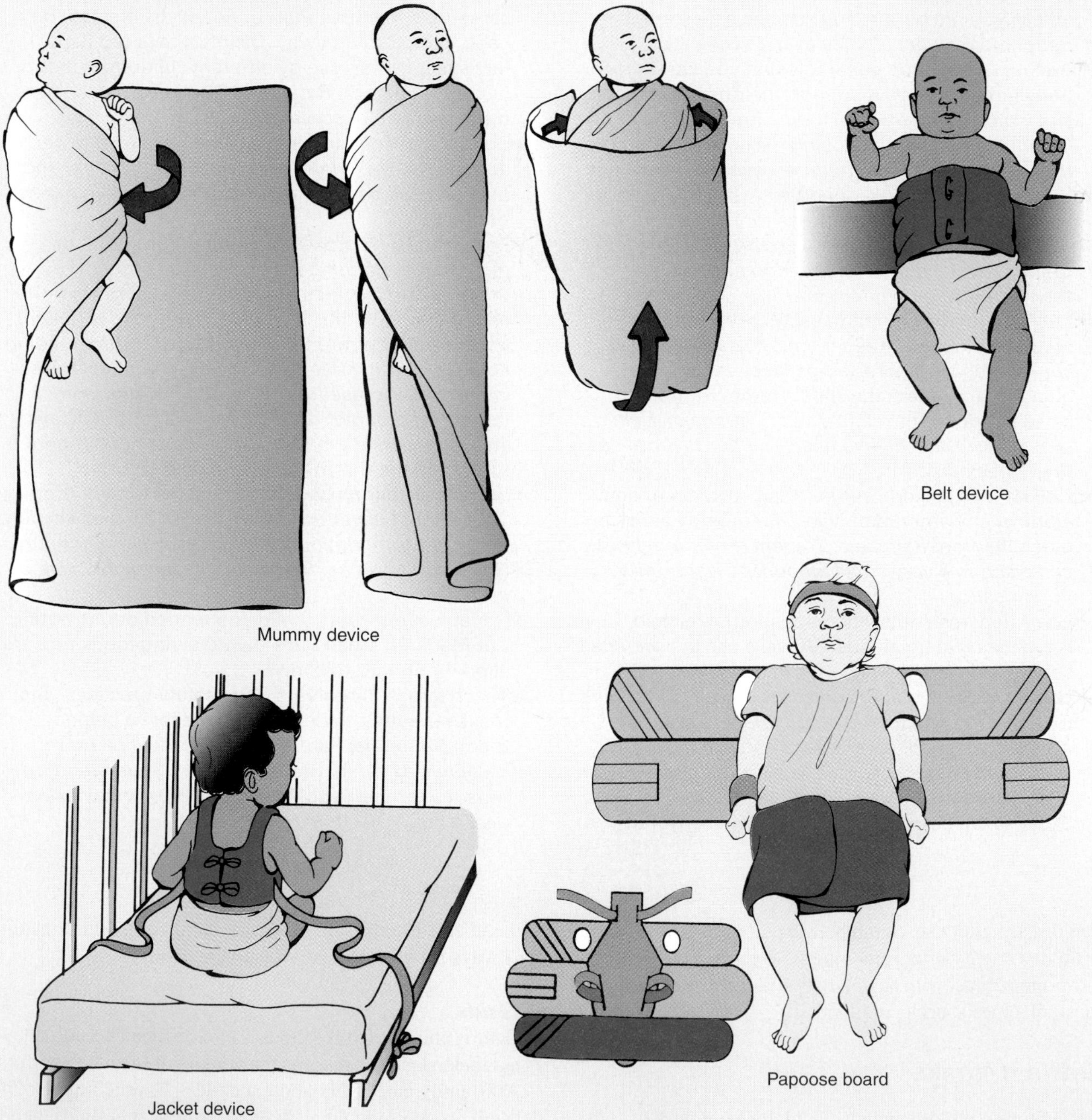

Mummy device

Belt device

Jacket device

Papoose board

Types of pediatric restraints.

- Use for any child who may be able to climb or jump over the sides of the crib.

Jacket—A smaller version of that used for adults; can be used in cribs, highchairs, beds, or wheelchairs.

- Apply over clothing or gowns. *Rationale: Decrease skin irritation.*
- If using a child restraint jacket, the straps come out on each side after applying it. The straps usually cross in front and tie in back. *Rationale: Prevent the child from getting caught in the straps and choking or strangling.*
- Tie the straps to the back of the chair or to the frame of the bed or crib. Tie to a movable part of the bed. Do not tie straps to side rails. *Rationale: Preserve the ability to raise or lower side rails without needing to tighten or loosen restraints. A restraint tied in the wrong place can interfere with the use of equipment or could strangle the child.*
- Check the child's circulation every 1 to 2 hours; allow the child to exercise. *Rationale: These activities prevent skin breakdown, promote circulation, maintain muscle function, and decrease the possibility of respiratory complications.*
- Document and report any evidence of skin irritation.

Clove hitch or commercial wrist device—A Kerlix bandage or stockinette applied in a figure-8 knot, or a manufactured device, can be used to retain one or more extremities (see illustration).

- Remove restraints every 2 hours, and allow the child to exercise the extremity.

Armboards—Used to protect IV sites

- Pad the board with a washcloth or small towel and fasten with tape. *Rationale: The cloth will absorb perspiration and provide comfort. Also, the nurse can change and wash it if it becomes soiled.*
- Secure the armboard to the client's extremity after the IV is in place and secure. *Rationale: Ensure the security of the IV even if the board needs removal.*
- Check the child's circulation to the arm each hour.
- Loosen or reapply tape as needed.
- Document your findings.

Less Commonly Used Restraints
- *Mummy restraint*—Used to restrain the entire body with a small blanket. Only the head is exposed.
- *Crib net*—A net placed over the top of the crib and secured to the bed frame to keep the child from climbing or jumping out of the crib.
- *Papoose board*—A plastic frame onto which the child can be strapped in almost any position. It is commonly used for circumcising infants. It is uncomfortable and should be used only for brief procedures, such as starting an IV.
- *Glove*—Prevents the child from scratching or pulling on tubes.

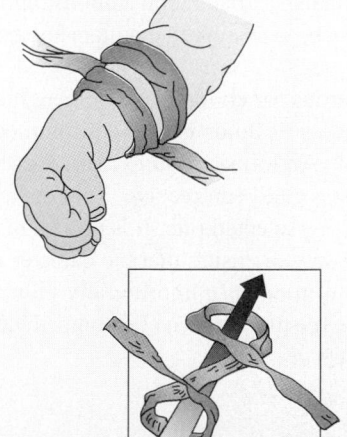 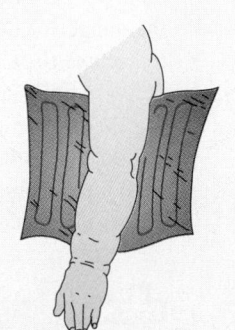 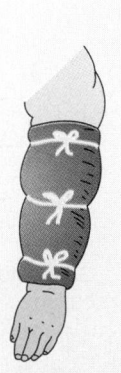 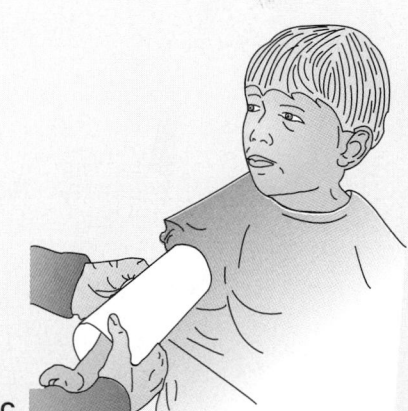

A   **B**   **C**

Types of arm restraints. (**A**) Clove hitch restraint. (**B**) Elbow restraint. (**C**) "No-no" sleeve or commercial elbow restraint.

- Apply padding under the restraint.
- Tie a knot so the device cannot become too tight.
- Check the extremity every hour for circulation and signs of skin breakdown.

- *Sleeve restraint*—Tongue blades are inserted into a sleeve with long pockets and ties. The child's arm is slid into the sleeve and straps are tied under the opposite arm. This device is used to keep a child

(continued)

from bending his or her arm, pulling on tubes or other devices, or disrupting a facial suture line.

Documentation
You may use a checklist to document the use of such devices. This list allows you to state the child's specific reactions and the number of times you applied and removed safety devices.

Knots Used for Restraints
- Make sure straps are not too long. *Rationale: The child might become caught or might strangle.*
- Make sure restraints are not too tight. *Rationale: Prevent impairing the child's circulation.*

Quick-Release Knot
Wind the strap of the restraint twice around the wheelchair post or bed frame. Make a loop by folding the

remainder of the strap in half. Slip the middle of this loop under the part wrapped around the wheelchair post and tighten. You now have "half a bow." If the child pulls on the strap from his or her end, the knot will tighten. However, when you pull on the free end, it will release easily. The free end must be out of the child's reach. This knot is safer than a traditional knot because it can be released quickly in an emergency.

Hold-Fast Bow
To tie a bow that will not come untied spontaneously, wrap the second end all the way around before pulling through the loop to make the second half of the bow. The knot will come untied when you pull on the free end, just like any other bow knot, but will not easily come untied. The knot is handy for shoelaces and for restraints that are tied to each other. It must be kept out of the child's reach.

Gavage Feeding

Sometimes children are fed through a gastrostomy button (Fig. 70-5), which is used because it is less bulky and more comfortable than an external tube. The gavage button is relatively flat on the child's abdominal wall, and connects to a tube that leads into the child's stomach. A syringe or tube-feeding bag is attached to an adapter and is primed with the tube feeding. The adapter is then attached to the button and the tube feeding

is administered. A bolus tube feeding is usually administered over 30 minutes, using only gravity. In some cases, an infusion stomach pump, such as the Kangaroo, is used to give continual feedings.

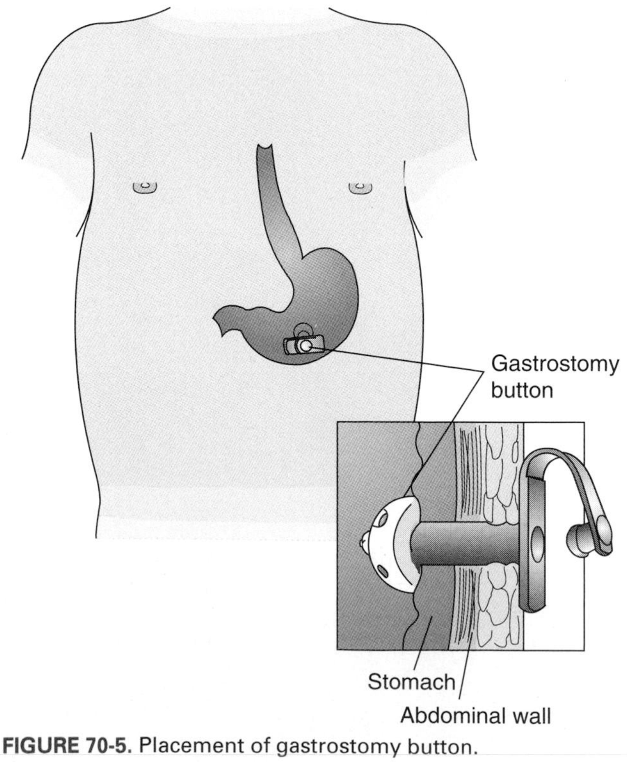

Parenteral Fluid Administration

Because between 65% and 80% of children's weight is water, they become dehydrated more easily than adults. Children who have diarrhea, a high fever, or difficulty excreting wastes may have a fluid or electrolyte imbalance. Parenteral administration of fluids and electrolytes may be necessary to maintain homeostasis.

Too much fluid is dangerous for children. Equipment that controls the rates and amounts of fluids is used to minimize the danger of fluid overload. An infusion pump may be used to control the exact amount a child can receive. This device delivers fluids at a precise, pre-selected rate. It is critical that the IV site is monitored closely to ensure that the catheter is within the vein. Because an infusion pump literally pumps fluid into a person, it is possible that fluid can be pumped into the wrong spaces, causing tissue damage.

Nursing Alert
Do not assume that the alarm on an infusion pump will provide warning of IV infiltration, especially for children.

You may need to restrain the child to prevent him or her from pulling on the tube. The IV may be administered into the scalp or neck veins in infants and toddlers and the arm or neck veins in older children. Protective devices for IV sites are shown in Figure 70-6.

FIGURE 70-5. Placement of gastrostomy button.

Gastrostomy button

Stomach

Abdominal wall

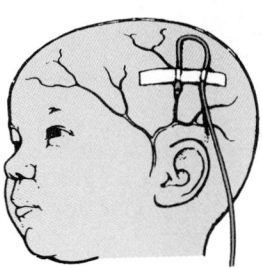

Venipuncture of scalp vein

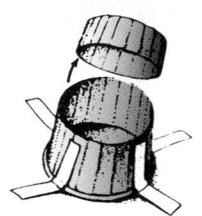

Paper cup taped over venipuncture site for protection. A clear plastic cup may also be used.

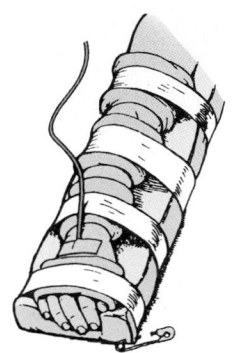

Restraint of arm when hand is site of infusion

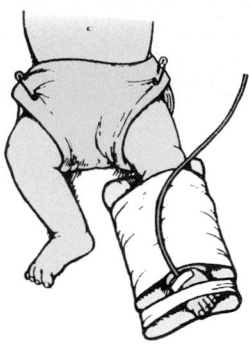

Infant's leg taped to sandbag for immobilization (IV site should be visible)

FIGURE 70-6. IV fluid therapy protective devices.

Children who are receiving long-term cancer chemotherapy or other IV medications may have a central venous line. Examples of these lines include Hickman, Broviac, jugular, and peripherally inserted central catheter (**PICC**) lines. These devices allow for prompt access to blood specimens; the infusion of IV chemotherapy or antibiotics; and total parenteral nutrition (**TPN**) therapy. See In Practice: Nursing Care Guidelines 70-4 for information on assisting a child with long-term IV therapy (see also Chap. 63).

Elimination

For children who are not yet toilet trained, use disposable diapers to promote cleanliness unless they are allergic or have a bad diaper rash. In such cases, use cloth diapers.

Collecting a Urine Specimen

Use the pediatric urine bag to collect a urine specimen. The bag is sterile, disposable, and has an adhesive neck applied to the infant's skin. See In Practice: Nursing Procedure 70-1 about collecting a pediatric urine specimen.

Catheterizing the Child

Children are not catheterized unless it is absolutely necessary, because the procedure can cause distress and damage delicate structures. Catheterization also can introduce bacteria into the bladder, causing urinary tract infections.

If catheterization is necessary, you will need to restrain small children during the procedure. The most common means of restraint is the papoose board. Assistance from another nurse is helpful. Restrain children in this manner for the absolute minimum length of time only.

Administering Enemas

For infants and young children, oral laxatives are usually preferred. If absolutely necessary, an enema is given. Give enemas to children in the same way as you would for adults, but use a smaller quantity of solution. Disposable enemas are most often used. If another type of enema is to be given, follow the protocol of your healthcare facility. Isotonic solutions are nec-

essary. Disposable pediatric enemas are available in measured amounts.

Give disposable enemas at room temperature. For infants, you may use a rubber-tipped bulb syringe. Be careful not to use too much pressure when instilling the fluid; squeeze the container gently.

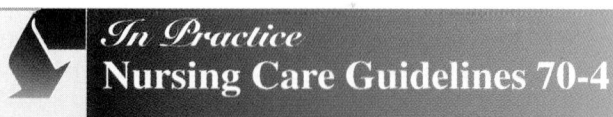

In Practice
Nursing Care Guidelines 70-4

ASSISTING A CHILD WITH LONG-TERM IV THERAPY

- Infection is the most common complication of this type of therapy. Monitor for signs and symptoms of infection at the site: redness, pain, elevated white blood cell count, and temperature. Document observable signs and symptoms with notes made of laboratory findings that may indicate infection.
- Change dressings every 24 hours if using gauze dressing and every 72 hours if using a transparent dressing (such as Tegaderm). Change the dressing any time it becomes wet or loose. Use sterile technique to change dressings (see Chap. 58).
- Carefully monitor the IV catheter and tubing for any tears or leaks.
- Secure connections carefully. Children are more apt to pull on catheters and tubing. Use Luer-Lok or click-lock connectors or tape connections securely.
- Use restraints as necessary to keep children from pulling on IVs.
- Monitor the site for signs of infiltration (eg, hardness, white area, severe pain).
- Teach family caregivers to care for the IV if the child is to be discharged with it in place. Supervise them as they practice with equipment while the child is in the facility.
- After the IV has been removed, monitor the site carefully for hemorrhage.

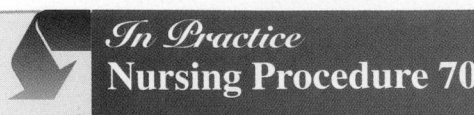

In Practice
Nursing Procedure 70-1

COLLECTING A PEDIATRIC URINE SPECIMEN

Supplies and Equipment

Urine collector of appropriate size and type
Washcloth
Gloves
Water for cleansing
Towel for drying

Steps

1. Offer the child fluids half an hour before applying the collector bag.

2. Gather needed supplies. Check physician's order.

3. Wash your hands and don gloves.

4. Explain to caregivers what you are going to do and why.
   RATIONALE: *Many procedures are unfamiliar and frightening to family caregivers and children. Teaching helps decrease fears and increase cooperation.*

5. Position the child on his or her back with the legs apart and knees bent ("frog-leg" position). You may need another adult's assistance to position the child properly so you can accurately apply the collector. (See illustration.)

6. Gently cleanse and dry the child's perineal area. You may use plain water and a wash cloth to cleanse the labia or penis. Remove any powder or lotion.
   RATIONALE: *Clean, dry skin is necessary for the adhesive to stick.*

7. Peel off the backing of the adhesive surface and apply the bag to the child's perineum. For girls, sealing from the bottom up to the pubis is easiest; do the opposite with boys. Be sure to smooth the skin during application by gently pulling on it as needed.

8. For boys, place the penis in the bag and apply the bag to the pubis and scrotum. In an uncircumcised boy, be sure the foreskin is in its normal position before you apply the bag.
   RATIONALE: *Keep the skin smooth to form a tighter seal and to prevent the specimen from leaking.*

9. Cover the bag with a loose-fitting diaper or underpants.
   RATIONALE: *Doing so discourages the child from pulling on the bag. Tight-fitting diapers or pants may dislodge the bag or cause the seal to burst after the child voids.*

10. Offer fluids after you apply the bag.
    RATIONALE: *Encourage voiding.*

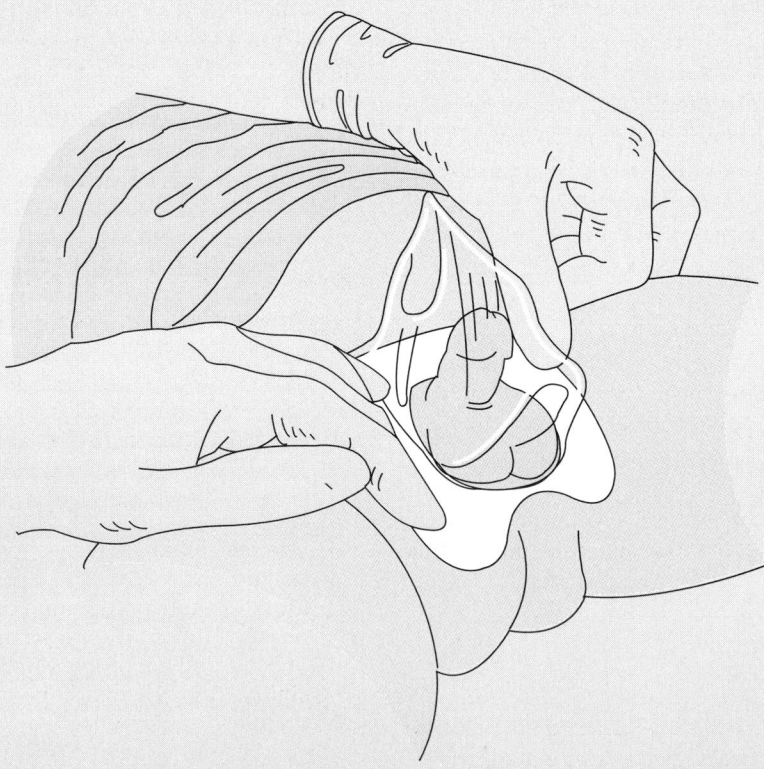

Applying a pediatric urine collection bag. The trick to making the collector adhere is to make sure that the child's skin is dry.

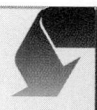

In Practice
Nursing Procedure 70-1 (Continued)

11. Check the bag every 15 to 30 minutes to see if the child has voided.

12. After the child has voided, gently remove the bag as soon as possible.
    RATIONALE: *Prevent loss of the specimen and make the child more comfortable.*

13. Cleanse the child's perineum.

14. Apply a clean diaper or underpants.

15. Place the urine in a specimen cup, through the emptying port provided on the outside of the bag.

16. Discard waste appropriately. Discard gloves.

17. Wash your hands.

18. Send the specimen to the laboratory following your facility's policy.

19. Document that you obtained the specimen. Note the urine's amount and characteristics and how the child tolerated the procedure.

Nursing Alert

A tap-water enema is particularly dangerous for small children because it can cause fluid and electrolyte imbalances and dehydration.

Often, children are unable to retain the solution on their own. Place a child on the bedpan before administering an enema. You may need to restrain a small child or ask for assistance. Remember that this experience is frightening for young children. Praise and reassure them.

Using Suppositories

Drugs commonly administered through suppositories include Tylenol (acetaminophen) and anticonvulsive or anti-nausea drugs. Explain the procedure to the child. Tell the child if the suppository is to be retained or expelled. Insert the suppository and hold it in place by gently pressing on the child's anal sphincter from the outside until the child no longer feels the urge to expel it. Use a clean glove when inserting the suppository. Lubricate the suppository with water-soluble lubricant before insertion if needed. Suppositories may also be used to promote bowel elimination.

Treating Diarrhea

When young children have diarrhea, the main dangers are dehydration and spread of disease. Small children become dehydrated very quickly as a result of diarrhea; therefore, you must take quick preventive measures. Carefully follow Standard Precautions when children have diarrhea. Close observation for signs of dehydration and for skin *excoriation* (breakdown) is essential.

Daily Cleanliness

Infant Bath

Infants are usually given tub baths in small bedside tubs. Be sure to gather all the necessary equipment before you start the bath, because you cannot leave the child alone after you begin the bath. Weigh the child before the bath and cover him or her with a bath blanket or as facility policy requires (see In Practice: Nursing Procedure 70-2).

Oral Hygiene

Give oral hygiene to the infant by wiping the baby's gums with a damp washcloth or gauze pad after each feeding. Pediatric dentists now encourage this type of oral hygiene for all infants. As soon as the child's teeth erupt, begin to use a brush to clean them.

By age 3, children should be able to brush their teeth with adult supervision. By age 8, children should be brushing and flossing independently, with occasional adult supervision. Teach children these procedures if necessary.

Assist children with brushing their teeth. Encourage all children to rinse often with water. If children are mature enough to rinse the mouth and spit out the solution, they may use a well-diluted mouthwash. Do not allow children to swallow toothpaste.

Oxygen

The primary cause of cardiopulmonary arrest in children is respiratory in origin. Small children have respiratory tracts that differ anatomically from adults. These structural differences, in addition to immature immune systems, place infants and young children at high risk for respiratory problems.

If you work as a pediatric nurse, you must be skilled at assessing respiratory status in young children. Babies and small children are unable to tell you that they are having difficulty breathing. A child's status can change quickly, and early signs can be difficult to see.

Nursing Alert

A change in the respiratory rate of an acutely ill child is significant. An infant with a rapid respiratory rate expends a great deal of energy. When the respiratory rate becomes too slow, it may indicate that the infant is becoming too tired. This infant is at high risk for respiratory arrest (see Fig. 66-5 in Chap. 66).

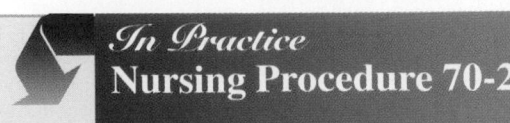

INFANT BATH
Supplies and Equipment

Cotton balls
Baby shampoo
Baby tub (plastic)
Baby soap
Baby lotion
Comb
Washcloth
Towel
Blanket
Baby clothing
Diaper

Steps

1. Cleanse the eyes first with clear water from the inner to outer canthus. (Use a separate cotton ball for each eye.)

2. Wash the rest of the baby's face. Do not probe the outer ear canals.

3. Shampoo the baby's hair daily.

4. Place the infant into the tub. Use this time to talk to the child and make the bath a pleasant experience. Depending on facility guidelines, you may use a mild soap or give the bath with clear water only. Give perineal and genital care.

5. After the bath, dress the infant, and comb and dry the hair.

6. Clean the child's fingernails and toenails. Many healthcare facilities do not allow nails to be trimmed without a specific physician's order.

7. Apply lotion or ointment to irritated areas. Do not use oil because it may lead to clogged pores and possible infection.

8. Assess for signs of diaper rash or any other unusual findings, and report them to your supervisor.

Be alert for restlessness, apprehension, and panic, because these signs may indicate respiratory problems. Darkening of skin color, particularly around the nose, eyes, and mouth (called **circumoral cyanosis**) is a significant sign of poor oxygenation. An infant with an expiratory grunt is at risk for impending respiratory arrest (see Fig. 66-5 and Box 66-2 in Chap. 66).

The following are signs of pediatric respiratory distress:

- Restlessness, apprehension, panic
- Tachycardia
- Tachypnea
- Nasal flaring
- Wheezing
- Stridor
- Change in color (eg, pallor, cyanosis)
- Expiratory grunt
- Retractions: substernal, subcostal, intercostal, suprasternal, supraclavicular (see Fig. 70-2)
- Gasping and shallow, labored breaths
- Head bobbing

> ### Nursing Alert
> Do not use the infant seat for a child with respiratory distress. Because of the lack of head control, the infant's head tends to fall forward, thereby closing off the airway. In addition, the infant tends to "scrunch" down in an infant seat. In this position, the abdominal organs push up on the diaphragm, preventing full lung expansion (*excursion*). The head of the crib is elevated instead.

Administering oxygen to the small child by nasal catheter or face mask is difficult because of the child's limited ability to understand and cooperate. If only humidity is needed, you may use an oxygen mask. Place the mask *near* the child's face, which allows humidity to reach the child without the use of a restricting mask on the face. The child's oxygen saturation should be monitored and recorded at regular intervals during oxygen administration.

> ### Nursing Alert
> Check toys to determine if they are safe and appropriate for the moist, oxygenated atmosphere. Stuffed toys become waterlogged very easily. Electrical or mechanical toys can cause sparks, creating a fire hazard. Toys that are easily wiped clean and do not absorb moisture are best.

Mist Tent

You may place a child with a respiratory condition in a mist tent, which provides oxygen and/or humidity to liquefy secretions and aid breathing. This device may be used to administer humidity, oxygen, or medications.

Place a bath blanket on top of bed linens to absorb moisture so the child stays warm and dry. Flush the tent with oxygen or air before placing the child in it. Tuck the plastic tent securely around the mattress and seal it with a folded bath blanket if the bottom edge does not reach the foot of the bed. Fill the reservoir with distilled water. Document the procedure, its effects, and any signs of dyspnea, cyanosis, or other difficulties. Change linens often. See In Practice: Nursing Procedure 70-3.

Oxyhood

The oxyhood is a clear plastic box that fits over the small child's head. An oxygen–air blender contained in the oxyhood administers oxygen in any concentration. The blender controls the amount of oxygen that mixes with room air and then enters

In Practice
Nursing Procedure 70-3

CARING FOR A CHILD IN A MIST TENT

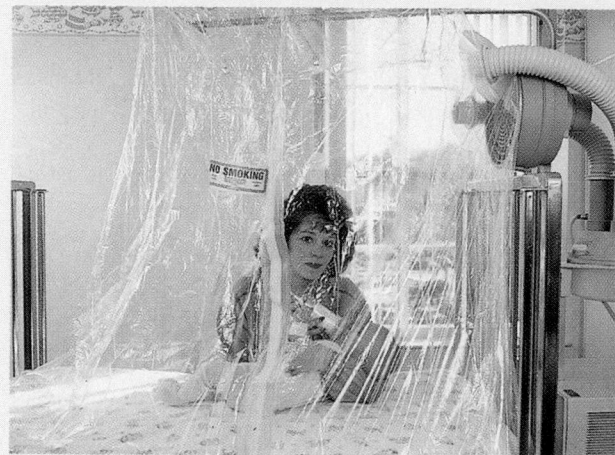

The mist tent supplies humidity and oxygen. The child in a mist tent should be reassured often. (© B. Proud)

Supplies and Equipment

Mist tent
Humidification setup
Oxygen source

Steps

1. Allow the child to explore the tent before placing him or her in it. Explain to family caregivers and the child why and how the tent is used.
   RATIONALE: *Help to reduce fear, which also may reduce the child's need for oxygen.*

2. Wash your hands. Gather necessary equipment. The respiratory therapy department may have the setup responsibility for the tent.

3. Place the child in the tent after it is set up and turned on. Be sure to tuck it in securely.

4. If the child will not stay in the tent, the nurse may need to use a jacket or other type of restraint. If using a restraint, check the child's skin for signs of breakdown at least every 2 hours.

5. Perform a thorough respiratory assessment every 1 to 2 hours or more often if necessary.

6. Observe the child for shivering, lethargy, decreased temperature, or irritability. Change the child's pajamas and bed linens frequently as they become damp. Regularly assess the child's temperature.

7. Monitor the child's I&O. Assess for signs and symptoms of dehydration.

8. Provide diversion; use toys safe for an oxygenated environment that can be cleaned.

9. Teach family caregivers how to interact with the child, and encourage them to spend time with the child.

10. Provide small feedings and frequent rest periods.

11. Document respiratory assessment data and the child's tolerance of the tent. Also document any teaching and the family's response.

12. To provide a clean environment, discard mist tent canopies after use. Use tents for as short a time as possible, because they are difficult to keep germ free and are restrictive.

the oxyhood. The oxygen must be humidified to prevent damage to respiratory mucosa. The flow rate must be high enough so that carbon dioxide flushes out of the hood. The advantage of the oxyhood is that it maintains a constant oxygen concentration, because the child is in a high-flow atmosphere. See In Practice: Nursing Procedure 70-4.

Intermittent Positive Pressure Breathing

Another method of administering oxygen in combination with medication is intermittent positive pressure breathing (**IPPB**). IPPB is used almost exclusively for children with cystic fibrosis and is described in more detail in Chapter 71.

Resuscitation

Resuscitation of children poses a special challenge for all healthcare personnel. The pediatric nurse also must be skilled in emergency medication administration. Pediatric emergency drugs are calculated according to a child's body weight. Pediatric units have a specialized emergency cart, known as a "crash cart" or "code blue cart," which is stocked with med-

ication and equipment of various sizes. Those caring for children in emergencies must be familiar with the sizes and use of this equipment.

Nurses caring for children should receive training each year in pediatric basic life support. Ventilation and chest compressions must be done with the utmost care to prevent further complications.

Diversion and Recreation

Play is an important aspect of growth and development. Play is the work of children. Providing diversional activities in the healthcare facility helps the child physically, socially, and psychologically. Children can express their fears, frustrations, and anxieties through role-playing with dolls and teddy bears. Play activities are more than just ways to entertain children or to pass the time—they are also therapeutic tools that can aid recovery.

Many play activities are suitable for use in the hospital setting. Computers and computer games are appealing to preschool children, school-age children, and adolescents. All

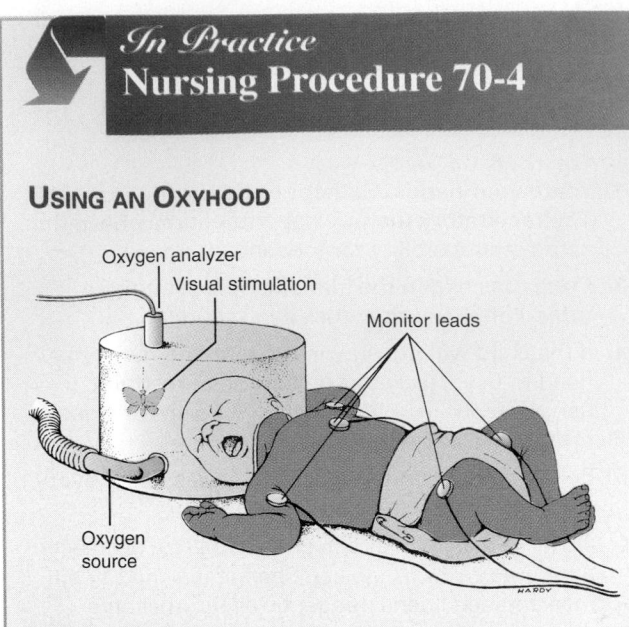

In Practice
Nursing Procedure 70-4

USING AN OXYHOOD

Infant in an oxyhood.

Supplies and Equipment

Oxygen hood (or other device)
Regulator
Oxygen source

Steps

1. Check physician's order. Wash your hands.
2. Collect needed equipment. Be sure you have the correct size of oxyhood.
3. Explain to the caregivers what you are going to do and why.
4. Set up equipment. Most facilities have wall outlets for oxygen.
5. Attach the flow regulator to the oxygen.
6. Connect the tubing to the hood's port and to the flow regulator.
7. Turn the flow meter to the ordered rate to flush the hood.
8. Place the hood over the child's head and neck.
9. Wash your hands.
10. Monitor the child's respiratory status frequently to ensure that the oxygen level is sufficient.
11. Report and document any significant changes or signs of respiratory distress.
12. Document the time you started the oxygen, rate of flow, and assessments of the child.

activities should be selected for their age appropriateness. Children of all ages enjoy reading. Also, they all need to be included in conversations. Children have a great need for someone to listen to them. Therefore, avoid using the television as a "babysitter" for the ill child.

Activities that strengthen the child's muscles and improve coordination should also be planned. Play is important in a child's social development and can be an emotional outlet for the ill child who is experiencing the stress of strange surroundings and painful procedures. Play helps children to learn more about the world. Play can also be used to teach children and to prepare them for certain clinical procedures. For example, you may play-act deep breathing or taking medications. Use dolls or teddy bears to describe planned procedures and to help the child understand what is going to happen.

Many children regress to previous developmental stages when they are frightened, ill, or injured. By observing children at play, you can learn a great deal about their physical, mental, and social states. Healthcare facilities with large pediatric departments have child-life specialists who are specifically trained to address diversional and therapeutic play.

ADVANCED PEDIATRIC CARE AND PROCEDURES

Nurses perform or assist physicians with many procedures. They also assist in comforting children during painful and frightening procedures.

Diagnostic Procedures

Several procedures are used to assist the physician with diagnosis. The role of the nurse is to reassure the child, provide the appropriate equipment, and assist the physician with care. Caregivers of the child may be allowed to stay during the procedure, depending on hospital policy. See In Practice: Nursing Care Guidelines 70-5.

Therapeutic Procedures

Managing a Fever

Fever in a child does not always indicate serious illness; teething or a recent immunization can be the cause. Because fever is one way the body fights pathogens, letting a low-grade fever run its course may be better than giving antipyretic (fever-reducing) medications. See In Practice: Nursing Care Guidelines 70-6 about managing various levels of fever.

> **Nursing Alert**
> Fevers above 104° F (40° C) must be immediately brought under control in children who have neurologic problems, history of febrile illness, or cardiac or respiratory problems (eg, hypoxia).

Medication Administration

More opportunities for errors occur when administering medication to children than to adults. The dosage and routes may differ. There may be specific techniques that need to be adapted to children. Usually the novice must successfully complete a course in medication administration before giving medications to anyone, particularly children. Therefore, nursing students or new graduates sometimes are not allowed to administer med-

DIAGNOSTIC PROCEDURES
Venipuncture

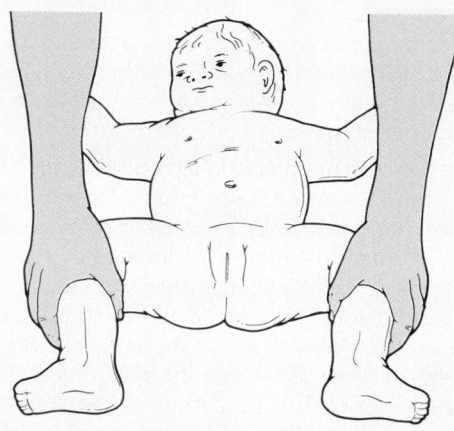

A

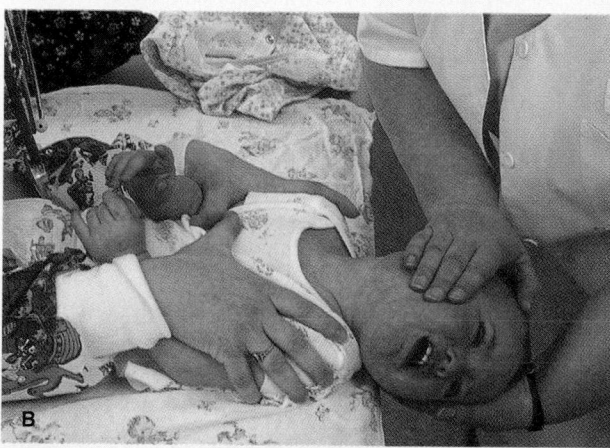

B

(**A**) Position of infant or young child for femoral venipuncture. (**B**) Position for jugular venipuncture. The infant's head is held sideways over the edge of the table by one nurse, while his body is restrained by a second nurse.

• The preferred site for venipuncture in infants is the femoral (thigh) area. When this site is used, stand at the child's head and hold the child on the back with legs spread apart ("frog-leg" position). Hold the child securely while the physician does the procedure. You can easily talk to the child when he or she is in this position. Cover the perineum with a washcloth; apply firm pressure to the puncture site for 5 minutes and check the site every 15 minutes for 1 hour.

• If a blood sample from a very young child is to be taken from the *jugular vein,* assist the physician by holding the child. Restrain the child with the head extended over the edge of the table, and pad the table edge. Hold the child perfectly still. After the procedure, note any signs of swelling or bleeding around the puncture site. Apply firm pressure to the site for the child who is sitting upright.

Heelstick Blood Samples
• Blood may be obtained from an infant by heelstick. Apply a disposable heel warmer first to increase blood supply to the area.
• Use a sterile lancet to obtain the sample after cleansing the area with an alcohol sponge. Chapter 66 details this procedure.

Lumbar Puncture

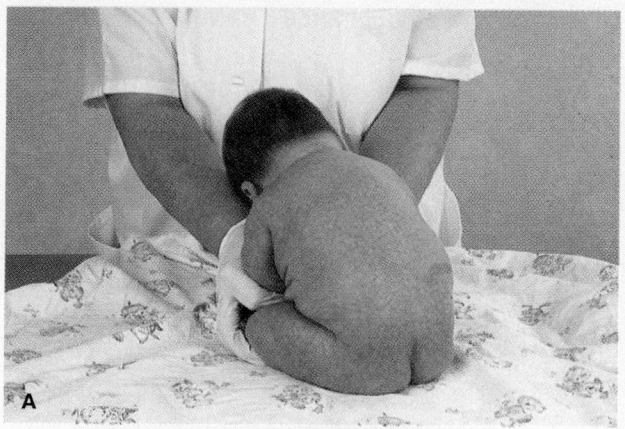

A

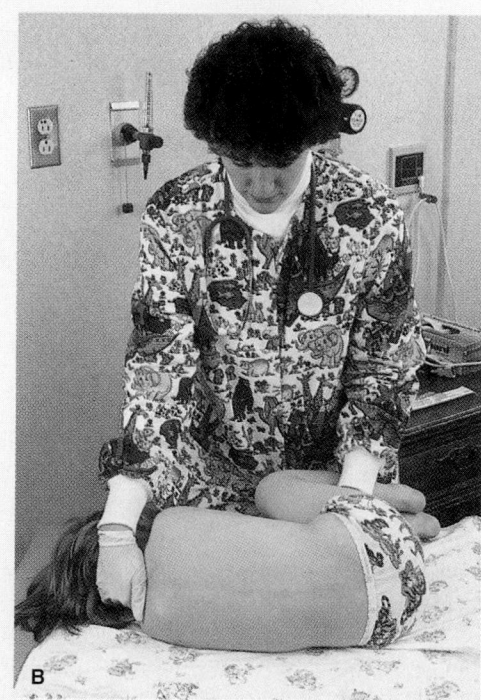

B

(**A**) Positioning an infant for lumbar puncture. (**B**) Positioning a young child for lumbar puncture.

• When lumbar puncture is being performed, hold the infant or child with the back curved while restraining the legs with a sheet. Positioning is illustrated here. The general lumbar puncture procedure is described in Chapter 77.

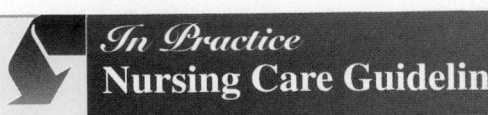

In Practice
Nursing Care Guidelines 70-6

MANAGING A FEVER LOWER THAN 102° F (38.8° C)

- Keep the child quiet. Prevent crying.
- Do not overdress the child; use minimum clothes for comfort.
- Encourage fluids.
- Generally do not use antipyretics unless ordered by the physician or if the child is very uncomfortable.

MANAGING A FEVER HIGHER THAN 102° F (38.8° C)

If the oral temperature is between 102° and 104° F (38.8°–40° C), use the preceding measures and add the following:

- Call the physician; antipyretics may be ordered.
- Put the child to bed.

If the oral temperature is over 104° F (40° C), use all the preceding measures and add the following:

- Give non-aspirin fever-reducing medication. *Do not give aspirin* because of the danger of Reye's syn-

drome (see Chap. 71). Check the child's temperature every 30 min.
- Sponge the child with lukewarm water until you receive further instructions from the physician.
- Check the child's temperature every 10 to 15 minutes during sponging.

Children who do not respond to routine fever treatment may respond to a tepid sponge bath. **Do not use alcohol or ice.** *Rationale: They lead to hypothermia. Alcohol fumes are irritating and may be inhaled or absorbed through the skin.* If the child shows signs of chilling (eg, shivering), discontinue the sponge bath temporarily and wrap the child in a blanket until shivering stops. Generally, the water's temperature should be 85° to 95° F (29.4°–35° C). This procedure is very appropriate for home use. It may be used infrequently in the acute care facility, because a cooling blanket is more efficient. Follow the procedure for giving an adult a tepid sponge bath in Chapter 54, keeping in mind the previous points.

---

ications to young children in a healthcare facility (see In Practice: Nursing Care Guidelines 70-7).

Nursing Alert
Know the side effects of each drug being administered so that your observations of the child will be complete.

THE CHILD HAVING SURGERY

Many pediatric procedures are now completed in a same-day surgery setting. Examples of such procedures include circumcision, insertion of polyethylene tubes, detailed dental work, hernia repairs, and cystoscopy.

Most preparation for surgery is done at home before admission. Because children are discharged from same-day surgery to the home, teaching is of primary importance. Thoroughly instruct family caregivers in the care of the child at home. Documentation of teaching and instructions given to the family is essential. Make certain that the caregivers understand the teaching and instructions.

Although many preoperative and postoperative procedures are similar for adults and children, certain differences exist:

- Children often cannot verbalize discomfort or symptoms they are experiencing. The nurse is responsible for

noting any untoward signs. Make every effort to help children understand what is happening.
- You cannot assess children in the same manner as you would adults. Children's lungs and hearts are smaller, their respirations and heart rates are more rapid, and their urine volumes and blood levels in the body are less. Therefore, small deviations from normal are more significant for children than they are for adults.
- Children will need analgesia appropriate for their body size after surgery to control pain. Children should receive medicine as needed for comfort.
- A characteristically rapid rate of metabolism and growth in children increases the healing ability of their tissues.
- Children become dehydrated very quickly.
- Electrolytes are not as stable in children as they are in adults.
- The high metabolic rate in infants and small children dictates a high caloric intake.

Consider family caregivers and their emotional needs. If you include family members in preoperative and postoperative care, everyone will be more comfortable and cooperative. Teaching care measures are vital.

Family caregivers are usually permitted to be with the child until the child is taken into the operating room. Tell the child exactly where he or she will be and what will happen when he or she awakens. Permit family caregivers to be with the child as soon as possible.

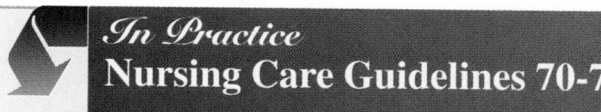

In Practice
Nursing Care Guidelines 70-7

ADMINISTERING MEDICATIONS TO CHILDREN

- Always approach a child in a positive, kind, and firm manner. Never give the child a choice of whether or not to take medicine. Do not say, "Are you ready for your pill now?" Give choices that allow the child some control over the situation, such as the injection site or the number or placement of bandages such as Band-Aids.
- Do not surprise or sneak up on a child or give an injection while the child is sleeping. Doing so will destroy the child's feeling of security, causing psychological trauma.
- Reassure the child that crying is okay.
- After administering an injection, use the term "brave." Do not tell the child he or she has been "good."
- Keep explanations brief and simple. Use words the child will understand.
- Never lie to the child. Do not tell the child an injection will not hurt.
- Avoid prolonging a procedure. Keep the time of administration to a minimum.
- Most medication doses are calculated based on the child's weight in grams or kilograms. Always have another person double-check any calculations before administration.
- Accuracy in administration is vital. Liquids are usually the best method of measurement because you can measure small doses and because you can be sure the child swallows it.
- Children are smaller and have a higher metabolic rate than adults; therefore, they absorb and excrete medications quickly. Watch closely for side effects.
- Catheter-tip syringes are usually used for administering liquids to infants. Use the smallest syringe possible to ensure accuracy. You may give infants liquid medications through a nipple.
- You can crush pills or empty capsules and place their contents in small amounts of applesauce or pudding or dissolve them in ice cream, juice, or formula. Because some medications cannot be mixed with certain types of foods, check a drug reference before using this technique. If adding a medication to any of these foods, use only a small amount of the food. For instance, do not add a medication to an entire bottle of formula or cup of juice. *The child may not finish it and thus may not receive the prescribed medication dose.*
- The anterior thigh (the vastus lateralis muscle) is the preferred site for intramuscular (IM) injections in children younger than 3 years of age. (The child should have been walking for at least 1 year.) *Rationale: Their other muscles are not well enough developed.* You may use the deltoid site if no alternative is available and if there is sufficient muscle mass.
- Never refer to medicine as candy. *Rationale: This could lead to accidental overdose or poisoning.*
- Assess pain through verbal and nonverbal communication. Use pain scales (such as smiling and frowning faces) to assess the child's pain level.
- Be sure to monitor the child's respirations when giving narcotics. *Rationale: Prevent respiratory depression.*
- Always check the child's identification band before giving a medication. *This cardinal rule in giving medications applies to people of all ages.*
- Be sure young children understand that medicine is not a punishment for being "bad" or refusing to cooperate. Use simple terms to explain why they are receiving medication.
- If the child is to receive an IV medication, be sure to explain that after the initial insertion, the child will not get another "poke" with each dose.
- Children may be more likely than adults to experience a *paradoxical* reaction to medication (a reaction *opposite* of what is expected).

A visit from a nurse or anesthesiologist before surgery helps to acquaint the child with those whom he or she will see in surgery, and may help to relieve some anxiety. The child's waiting period should be as short as possible after arriving in the operating room.

Preoperative Care

Prior to elective surgery, children should have an opportunity to tour the facility and touch equipment, as well as to meet the nurses before surgery. If the child is to go directly to the operating room on the morning of surgery, try to alleviate fear of the unknown by giving calm explanations. For additional information see In Practice: Nursing Care Guidelines 70-8.

Postoperative Care

Prepare the room to receive the child. The room should have available an IV stand, emesis basin, tissues, blood pressure apparatus, drainage equipment, and any other necessary supplies.

If the child is being cared for in a same-day surgery unit, he or she will return to the unit in the same bed on which he or she left. However, if the child is returning to a pediatric

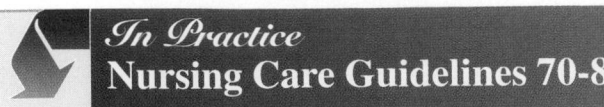

In Practice
Nursing Care Guidelines 70-8

PREOPERATIVE CARE FOR CHILDREN

Many of the same principles prevail for care of children who undergo surgery as for adults. Review general preoperative and postoperative care (see Chap. 56).

Preparation

- Involve family caregivers as much as possible. Most preoperative preparation is done at home by family caregivers, who need careful instructions.
- Send an admission questionnaire home with the family caregivers. They are to complete and return this form to the facility on the child's admission. Provide assistance if the caregivers are unable to read the questionnaire. (Handle such a situation nonjudgmentally to avoid embarrassment.)
- Review the admission questionnaire with family caregivers to ensure it is accurate and understandable.
- The physician, nurse practitioner, or physician's assistant obtains the medical history and performs a physical examination. The licensed practical nurse or nursing student may do part of the nursing history. The family caregivers may come to the facility with the child and stay during the history and physical examination. Be sure to include the family caregivers when obtaining the nursing history.
- General laboratory work is done. Much laboratory testing may be done in a pre-admission appointment. The child may go to the facility a day or so before surgery for pre-admission blood work and x-ray examinations. Blood type and crossmatch are done if necessary. Blood is not given unless absolutely necessary.
- The child returns home and is admitted the morning of surgery to the pediatric or same-day surgery unit.
- The child will probably need to have nothing by mouth (**NPO**) after midnight.
- The family caregivers will have performed preoperative procedures as instructed.
- The family caregiver signs the operative permit because the child is not of legal age. (The nursing student should not be a witness on the operative permit.)

Nursing Assessments

- When the child arrives on the morning of surgery, assess for and document any signs of upper respiratory infection (**URI**), such as fever, cough, or runny nose. URI makes respiratory complications more likely, and will probably cause surgery to be delayed until the infection clears.
- A child is more likely than an adult to have a URI.
- Also be sure to chart the presence of any open wounds, rashes, or other unusual conditions.

Immediate Measures Before Surgery

- Ask the child to void.
- Take and record vital signs. Weight (in grams/kilograms) *must* be recorded.
- Remove any hairpins, barrettes, or jewelry.
- The child should wear an appropriate gown and must wear an identification band.
- Perform ordered surgical preparation, and check to see that all laboratory reports are on the chart and that blood work is complete.
- Take everything, including toys, out of the bed (some facilities permit children to take a special toy or headphones into the surgical suite).
- If the child will be taken to the operating room in a crib, change the sheets.
- Keep the child NPO.
- Preoperative medication is often omitted in children. If you do give medications, an important safety factor is to remind the child and family caregivers to limit activity.
- The child may rest in bed or may be held by a family caregiver, but if he or she has to go to the bathroom, you must provide help if the child has been sedated.
- When everything is ready, sign the chart. Give emotional support to family caregivers and the child. Family members may wish to consult a chaplain or clergy person; facilitate this discussion.
- Tell family members where they can wait during surgery so that the physician will know where to find them. Usually the family caregivers can accompany the child to the door of the operating room.
- Make sure the appropriate parent or guardian has signed the operative permit. Reports of all blood work and preoperative x-ray studies must be on the chart.
- Explain the operative procedure to the family caregiver and child as simply and frankly as possible; explain the general procedures of the post anesthesia care unit (**PACU**), such as what it will be like to wake up after surgery and the likelihood of an IV.
- Explain the need for early ambulation, turning and deep breathing, and encouraging fluids.
- Explain the need for any special equipment, such as nasogastric suction, chest tubes, or catheters.
- Teach family caregivers any care they will provide when they take the child home.
- Carefully document all preoperative procedures and teaching.

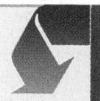

In Practice
Nursing Care Guidelines 70-9

POSTOPERATIVE CARE FOR CHILDREN

- Reorient the child to the room—explain the IV, oxygen, suction and drainage tubes, and dressings to the child and family.
- Notify the family caregivers when the child returns to the unit.
- Assess the child carefully. Check vital signs, according to the facility's policies and the physician's orders. Children's vital signs may change quickly. Most facilities provide a postoperative checklist on which the nurse documents vital signs.
- Inspect the operative site for discharge or bleeding; note equipment in use, such as a retention catheter, suction drainage, bottles, casts, or traction. Be sure everything is connected and operating properly.
- Check color, motion, and sensitivity of toes or fingers if a cast is in place. Reattach weights to traction as ordered.
- Monitor flow of IV, or program the controller or infusion pump; monitor fluid I&O.
- Check the child's positioning; the side or abdominal position is best (to prevent aspiration).
- Turning, coughing, and deep breathing exercises are important, especially for an older child.
- Younger children do not seem to have as much difficulty with postoperative respiratory complications. (Be sure to support the abdominal incisional site with a bath blanket or pillow while encouraging the child to deep breathe.)
- Encourage the older child to move his or her toes, ankles, and legs (if permitted) to prevent thrombophlebitis.
- Check for voiding; take a positive approach, and follow the physician's orders. Many times a child is up

and around the afternoon following surgery. (Remember, the child's oral intake may be diminished, but the child has probably had 500–1,000 mL of IV fluids.) Say that you will "help the child to the bathroom" rather than forcing or coercing the child to void.
- Check for return of peristalsis (eg, flatus, bowel sounds/movement). If bowel sounds are absent, consult your supervisor before you give fluids or ice, to prevent gas pains.
- Give fluids according to physician's orders. Usually about 1 hour after the child returns from the PACU, you can give sips of water or ice chips.
- Refresh the child when permitted; wash the face and hands, and change the gown and bed linens.
- Evaluate pain or discomfort. Use medications as needed. Remember, children experience pain and may have difficulty describing it. Also, children may try to hide pain, so watch them as they move about, to assess their discomfort. Use pain scales (see Fig. 55-4) to help the child express his or her level of discomfort. A simple pain scale for children shows a smiling face on one end and a crying face on the other, with gradations in between. Early ambulation prevents complications.
- Document thoroughly and report accurately.
- Children often recover from surgery quickly. Many children are discharged the afternoon of surgery or the next day. Teach family caregivers specific postoperative procedures and observations for the child's safety and the family's feelings of security. Carefully document all teaching.

---

unit, arrange the room so that the gurney from the recovery room can be easily moved in.

A child usually recovers from anesthesia much more quickly than an adult. However, considerate care and close observation are essential. For more information see In Practice: Nursing Care Guidelines 70-9.

➤ STUDENT SYNTHESIS

Key Points

- Basic care in pediatrics is similar to care for adults, but some procedures need modifications.
- Pediatrics requires knowledge of developmental milestones to help determine developmental delays.
- Children may need assistance to meet basic needs simply because of their age.

- Teaching family caregivers is vital, because most pediatric care is given at home.
- Very young children are especially susceptible to communicable diseases.
- Protecting children from hazards includes monitoring IV infusions, preventing falls, and using safety devices such as restraints.
- Vital signs vary according to a child's size and age.
- Children's respiratory tracts are small and susceptible to infection.
- Play is children's work and their means of communication.
- Administration of medications to children involves precise calculation; it is usually based on body weight in kilograms.
- Special teaching considerations are made for the preoperative and postoperative care of children.

Critical Thinking Exercises

1. Jessie, a 4-year-old girl, is admitted to the acute care facility for abdominal surgery. Using your knowledge of growth and development and client teaching, design a preoperative and postoperative teaching plan for Jessie and her family.
2. Jessie has a teddy bear that she clings to very tightly. When it is time for her to go to surgery, she does not want to let go of the bear. How will you solve this problem to maintain Jessie's confidence without breaking healthcare policy?
3. Matthew, age 2 years, is confined to a mist tent with oxygen because of a respiratory infection. Make a list of appropriate toys he may have. What diversional activities would you plan for him?

NCLEX-Style Review Questions

1. During assessment of a toddler, which of the following data would need further investigation by the nurse?
   a. Diaper in place for a 15-month-old.
   b. Drinks from a cup at age 12 months.
   c. Sleeps through the night.
   d. Two-year-old grunts and points at what he wants.
2. What action should the nurse take when obtaining the pulse from an infant?
   a. If the child is crying, divide the value in half for an accurate rate.
   b. Listen for 30 seconds, and multiply the number by two.
   c. Obtain an apical pulse.
   d. Use a regular adult stethoscope.
3. When administering a bolus feeding, the nurse should:
   a. Administer the feeding with a syringe over 5 minutes.
   b. Administer the feeding over 30 minutes by gravity drainage.
   c. Dilute the feeding with water to half strength.
   d. Warm the feeding prior to administration.
4. Upon admission to the hospital prior to surgery, it is essential that the nurse assess for:
   a. Anxiety in the child
   b. Changes in bladder habits
   c. Crying and agitation
   d. Upper respiratory infection

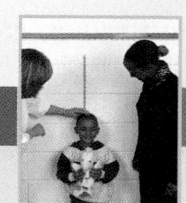

CHAPTER

71

Care of the Infant, Toddler, or Preschooler

LEARNING OBJECTIVES

1. Compare and contrast the symptoms, treatment, and immunizations for the following preventable communicable diseases: diphtheria, tetanus, pertussis, rubeola, mumps, rubella, varicella, and poliomyelitis. State three nursing considerations for each disease.

2. Compare and contrast the symptoms of streptococcal infections and roseola. Identify at least three nursing considerations for each: scarlet fever, "strep throat," and rheumatic fever.

3. Compare and contrast the treatment and control of common parasitic infections in children, including scabies, lice, pinworms, giardiasis, roundworms, and hookworms. Identify at least three family teaching concerns for each.

4. Discuss at least three nursing considerations for each of the following common injuries: fractures, lacerations, cuts and puncture wounds, foreign objects, and animal bites.

5. Identify at least two methods of prevention and treatment for each of the following: burns, poisoning, suffocation, and drowning.

6. In the skills lab, practice a therapeutic communication with the parents of a child who has died of SIDS.

7. Identify at least five potential clues to each: neglect, physical abuse, and sexual abuse. Discuss the nurse's role and responsibility related to these conditions.

8. Describe the physical and/or psychological causes of FTT. State at least three nursing considerations related to FTT.

9. Define and discuss at least three nursing implications of each of the following skin disorders: nevi, rash, and eczema.

10. Define and discuss at least three nursing implications of each of the following musculoskeletal disorders: dysplasia, talipes, and torticollis.

11. Define and discuss at least three nursing implications of each of the following neurologic disorders: Reye's syndrome, meningitis, spina bifida, hydrocephalus, microcephaly, febrile seizures, and breath-holding spells.

12. Define and discuss at least three nursing considerations for each of the following metabolic and nutritional disorders: marasmus, biliary atresia, celiac disease, and PKU.

13. Define and discuss at least three nursing considerations for each of the following eye disorders: strabismus, amblyopia, and cataracts in children.

14. Define and discuss at least three nursing considerations for each of the following ear disorders: otitis media, epistaxis, tonsillitis, cleft lip and cleft palate, and baby bottle syndrome.

15. Differentiate and state at least three nursing considerations for each of the following cardiovascular disorders: ASD/VSD, PDA, TGV, TOF, COA, stenosis, and tricuspid atresia.

16. Differentiate and state at least three nursing considerations for each of the following blood and lymph disorders: Kawasaki disease, iron deficiency anemia, sickle cell anemia, ITP, and hemophilia.

17. Define and differentiate between ALL and AML. State at least three nursing considerations for each type of leukemia.

18. Differentiate and state at least three nursing considerations for each of the following respiratory disorders: URIs, pneumonia, croup, epiglottitis, asthma, bronchiolitis, and cystic fibrosis.

19. Define and state at least three nursing considerations for each of the following gastrointestinal disorders: pyloric stenosis, Meckel's diverticulum, intussusception, and megacolon.

20. Identify the types of hernias commonly seen in children. State three pre- and postoperative nursing considerations for hernias.

21. Discuss at least three nursing considerations for possible electrolyte disturbances and dehydration related to diarrhea in children.

22. Discuss the physical and psychological factors related to encopresis and lactose intolerance.

23. Define and state at least three nursing considerations for each of the following urinary system disorders: enuresis, HUS, urinary obstruction, UTI, pyelonephritis, glomerulonephritis, nephrotic syndrome, Wilms' tumor, hypospadias, and epispadias.

24. Define and state at least three nursing considerations for each of the following reproductive disorders: ambiguous genitalia, cryptorchidism, and hydrocele.

25. Demonstrate a parent–child teaching session related to the nutritional concerns of childhood.

NEW TERMINOLOGY

amblyopia	meningocele
asthma	meningomyelocele
biliary atresia	microcephalic
bronchiolitis	Mongolian spots
celiac disease	mumps
cleft lip	nephrotic syndrome
cleft palate	nevus
colic	otitis media
collagen diseases	pediculosis
cryptorchidism	pertussis
cystic fibrosis	pinworms
diphtheria	plumbism
dysplasia	pneumonia
eczema	poliomyelitis
encephalitis	ptosis
encephalocele	pyelonephritis
encopresis	pyloric stenosis
enuresis	Reye's syndrome
epiglottitis	rheumatic carditis
epispadias	rheumatic fever
epistaxis	rickets
giardiasis	roseola
glomerulonephritis	roundworms
hemangioma	rubella
hemophilia	rubeola
hernia	scabies
herpes zoster	scarlet fever
Hirschsprung's disease	scurvy
Hodgkin's disease	shingles
hookworms	sickle cell crises
hydrocele	sickle cell disease
hydrocephalus	spina bifida
hypospadias	spinal bifida occulta
intussusception	status asthmaticus
Kawasaki disease	strabismus
Koplik's spots	streptococcal "strep"
kwashiorkor	throat
lactose intolerance	talipes
leukemia	tetanus
lymphangiomas	tonsillitis
marasmus	torticollis
Meckel's diverticulum	varicella
megacolon	Wilms' tumor
meningitis	

ACRONYMS

ALL	EEG	PE
AML	ESR	PIA
ASD	FTT	PKU
ASO	GABHS	RSV
BMT	HUS	SGA
BRAT	ITP	SIDS
CLL	LTB	T&A
CML	MDI	TGV
COA	MMR	TOF
CPT	O&P	URI
CRP	ORS	UTI
DTaP	PDA	VSD
DTP		

Chapter 70 introduced general pediatric nursing care. This chapter discusses many conditions that are first seen in infants, toddlers, and preschoolers. A knowledge of normal growth and development patterns and variations is essential (see Chap. 10).

Immunizations protect children from many childhood diseases; however, because of natural curiosity and lack of experience, accidents and traumatic injuries are common for young children. In addition, congenital defects are responsible for a number of health-related disorders requiring nursing support. Many diagnostic, x-ray, and laboratory procedures are similar for children and adults.

COMMUNICABLE DISEASES

The most common diseases in children are *communicable* (transmitted from one person to another). Children with common communicable diseases are cared for at home unless complications develop. When treating children who have highly contagious conditions, use transmission-based precautions.

Preventing exposure to contagious diseases is difficult. One reason for this is that these conditions are often most infectious before symptoms appear. The period between exposure and the development of symptoms is the *incubation period*. With the advent of immunizations (see Table 70-1 in Chap. 70), many children now go through life without experiencing communicable diseases. Children who contract communicable diseases are hospitalized only if they require acute treatment.

Diseases Preventable Through Immunization

The goal of communicable disease management is prevention, which usually occurs through immunization. The ultimate purpose of immunization is to eradicate the disease. Your major responsibility, as a nurse, is to stress to families with children the importance of up-to-date immunizations. Immunizations are frequently administered in clinics for those who are unable to pay.

Diphtheria
Diphtheria, which is transmitted through droplets, begins with a sore throat, fever, and often generalized aching and malaise. Throat inflammation (the disease also may appear in the nose, larynx, or trachea) is followed by the formation of a whitish-gray membrane that is closely adherent and cannot be removed without causing bleeding. The causative bacillus produces a poison that can weaken the child's cardiac muscle. The child is very ill and requires close observation. The mortality rate is between 5% and 10%; the disease is rarely seen today because immunization easily prevents it. People who show no symptoms of diphtheria may be carriers; they are treated prophylactically with antibiotics.

Tetanus
Tetanus is a highly fatal disease characterized by convulsive contractions of all voluntary muscles. Tetanus is preventable through the administration of the tetanus toxoid, which causes

the body to build up antibodies. In the event of an injury, such as a deep cut or puncture wound, tetanus antitoxin is given immediately to provide ready antibodies.

Pertussis

Pertussis or "whooping cough" is a highly contagious respiratory disease occurring most commonly in young children who have not been immunized. It is transmitted through direct contact and through droplets. It can be prevented through the diphtheria, tetanus, acellular pertussis (**DTP, DTaP**) immunization. Incidences of pertussis are rising in the United States. One contributing reason may be that the success of the pertussis immunization has led to complacency among families about ensuring that their children receive it. Others may fear that their children will have a serious reaction to the vaccine. Family caregivers must understand the facts about immunizations. Serious reactions to vaccines are rare.

Whooping cough occurs only rarely in people who are older than 10 years. The incubation period is from 5 to 21 days. Symptoms begin with bronchitis and a slight temperature elevation. The cough steadily worsens, leading to paroxysms of coughing, characterized by a "whooping" sound. The person may cough so hard that he or she vomits or becomes *dyspneic* (labored breathing). The first stage lasts about 1 week. The severe coughing stage lasts from 2 to 3 weeks. It usually takes another 2 to 3 weeks for the cough to disappear, but whooping cough can last for several months. The most serious complication is bronchopneumonia.

When treating children affected with whooping cough, maintain droplet transmission-based precautions throughout the whooping period. Give antibiotics and other medications. These children need close supervision because respiratory difficulties and nutritional problems are likely to occur.

Rubeola

Rubeola (common "measles," "red measles") is caused by a virus found in the nose, mouth, throat, eyes, and their discharges. It is transmitted through direct contact with an affected individual and through airborne droplets. Rubeola is highly communicable, and difficult to recognize in its early stage because the symptoms resemble those of the common cold.

The incubation period is from 10 to 20 days. The disease begins with a slight temperature elevation, a runny nose, and watery eyes. By day 2 or 3, bluish-white pinpoint spots with a red rim, called **Koplik's spots,** appear in the person's mouth. Small dark-red areas appear on the face and spread downward throughout the body. These red areas grow large and group together, giving the skin a blotchy appearance. Respiratory symptoms increase. The child sneezes frequently, the eyes are sore, and the discharge becomes purulent; light hurts the eyes (*photophobia*). The child's throat is also sore, and he or she has a hacking cough. The rash, which may last for up to 10 days, is greatest at about the fourth day. During the second week, the skin begins to flake off in tiny powder-like flakes (*desquamation*) for 5 to 10 days. The child itches all over; therefore, soothing, antipruritic nursing measures are important to manage itching (see Chap. 74).

Measles is rarely fatal, but complications can be serious. The infection may spread to the middle ear (**otitis media**). Pneumonia is a common development, and **encephalitis** (brain inflammation) develops in approximately 1 in 1,000 cases. Permanent brain damage or death can result from measles encephalitis. Measles is most hazardous to the very young child; however, one episode seems to confer immunity.

All children should be immunized because of the seriousness of complications. Measles outbreaks occur periodically in populations in which a large group of individuals have not received necessary immunizations. Two injections of the live, attenuated measles, mumps, and rubella (**MMR**) vaccine are now required for all children.

Mumps

Mumps, also called *epidemic parotitis,* is a viral disease that affects the salivary glands, especially the parotids. It is transmitted through direct and indirect contact and through salivary secretions. Children younger than 2 years and adults seldom contract mumps. However, adults who contract mumps may suffer serious aftereffects, including sterility in men. For this reason, all children should receive the mumps vaccine at about 15 months of age.

Close contact is required for mumps to be transmitted. The incubation period is from 2 to 3 weeks. The first sign is usually a swelling of the parotid gland, on one side or both. Sometimes, the child has a low-grade fever, headache, and general malaise before the swelling appears. The swollen gland is painful, and opening the mouth and eating are uncomfortable. The swelling begins to disappear by the second or third day and is usually gone by day 10. The disease is considered communicable until the swelling disappears. Complications are infrequent; however, if only one side was initially affected, the other side may swell as the first side improves.

Rubella

Rubella or "German measles," a viral infection, is mild and lasts only a short time. The disease is transmitted through direct contact or airborne transmission. Rubella can cause serious fetal malformations if a pregnant woman contracts the disease. All children should be immunized, not only for their own protection, but also for the protection of pregnant women with whom they may come in contact.

The symptoms of rubella are similar to those of rubeola, but are not nearly as severe; spots do not appear on the oral mucous membrane. Sometimes the facial rash is the first noticeable sign of infection. Swelling of the lymph nodes in the occipital region is another symptom often seen. The rash spreads quickly and disappears just as rapidly. Although complications are rare, they can be serious. Immunizations with the MMR vaccine should confer immunity.

Varicella

Varicella or "chickenpox" is the same virus that causes **herpes zoster (shingles),** a condition found in adults. Chickenpox usually begins with a slight, sometimes unnoticeable, fever. The chickenpox virus is found in the nose, throat, blisters, and crusts. The incubation period is from 14 to 21 days.

A rash appears on the face and trunk and then develops into blisters surrounded by a red ring. The eruptions proceed from *papules* (red, elevated skin areas), to *vesicles* (blister-like elevations filled with serous fluid), to *pustules* (filled with lymph or pus), and finally to flat *crusts* that fall off in 1 to 3 weeks. The child is usually maintained on droplet and contact transmission precautions for 10 to 12 days or until dry crusts form. Never give aspirin to the child with chickenpox, to protect against the danger of Reye's syndrome (discussed later in this chapter). A vaccination that can be administered at any time after the child's first birthday provides immunization.

Serious complications are rare. The most common complication is infection due to scratching the blisters, which can leave scars or "pock marks." Antihistamines (Benadryl, Periactin) and antipruritic nursing measures are necessary to relieve intense itching. Ordinarily, the only child for whom chickenpox is very dangerous is the newborn or the immunosuppressed child. The administration of acyclovir (Zovirax) is helpful in reducing symptoms. Family caregivers should keep the child's fingernails short to prevent scratching.

Poliomyelitis

Poliomyelitis ("polio") is a contagious viral disease that attacks the central nervous system (CNS) and can cause temporary or permanent paralysis and weakness in approximately 50% of its sufferers. Vaccines have all but eliminated the disease in the United States. A goal of the World Health Organization is to eliminate polio worldwide in this century. The live oral polio vaccine replicates in the gastrointestinal (GI) tract and can be transmitted to others through fecal material. The only cases of polio in the United States in recent years have been vaccine related. For this reason the administration of the oral live vaccine has been replaced with the inactivated parenteral vaccine.

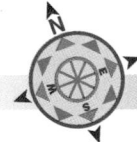

SPECIAL CONSIDERATIONS: CULTURE

Preventive Healthcare

Children of disadvantaged, migrant, transient families often lack preventive healthcare, especially in the area of receiving immunizations. Records are often absent or incomplete. Healthcare is usually only received for severe, acute illnesses.

Some cultures do not value childhood immunizations to prevent childhood disease. The Amish and some religious groups discourage immunizations.

☛ KEY CONCEPT

Teach family caregivers the importance of immunizations.

Vaccines are available to prevent the diseases discussed up to this point. For the remaining contagious diseases, no vaccines are currently available.

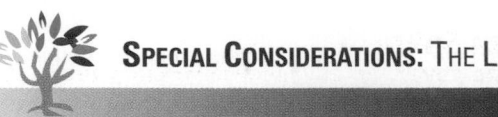

SPECIAL CONSIDERATIONS: THE LIFE SPAN

Immunizations

Infants often receive several parenteral immunizations at the same time. Instead of one nurse administering consecutive injections, several nurses can administer the injections simultaneously to cause the infant less trauma and pain.

Streptococcal Infections

Group A beta-hemolytic streptococcal infections (**GABHS**) are fairly common among children over 2 years of age. GABHS are disease-causing strains of the genus *Streptococcus,* which are gram-positive bacteria normally found in the respiratory, alimentary, and female genital tracts. GABHS is spread by direct contact and large droplets.

Scarlet Fever

Scarlet fever is also known as *scarlatina.* Symptoms develop after an incubation period of 1 to 7 days; they include the appearance of a generalized flush or redness, caused by a sandpaper-like rash of pinpoint-like red spots crowded together (*macular rash*). Desquamation follows. The tongue becomes coated with a white substance that later disappears, leaving prominent papillae ("strawberry tongue"). The most common complications are ear infections, nephritis, arthritis, cardiac problems, and pneumonia. Keep the child on bed rest until symptoms resolve, and administer antibiotics. Prognosis is favorable when scarlet fever is treated promptly.

Streptococcal Sore Throat

Streptococcal "strep throat" is common in young children older than 2 years of age. It is treated with large doses of antibiotics, most often penicillin. To prevent complications, treatment should be started as soon as possible after receiving a positive culture for strep. A rapid diagnostic test ("rapid strep screen") or culture is the only way to differentiate strep throat from a simple viral sore throat. White patches on the tonsils could be due to strep. An elevated temperature that does not fall after giving an antipyretic (acetaminophen, ibuprofen) may also point to strep. If the child complains of a "lump" in the throat rather than a sore throat, and feels "sick all over," strep is the likely cause. A child with a history of strep throat should see a physician, who will take a culture.

The most serious complications of strep throat are rheumatic fever, rheumatic heart disease, and nephritis. The prognosis is good if strep throat is treated promptly. Make certain that family caregivers understand that children who have strep throat must finish their prescribed antibiotic to ensure complete eradication of the bacteria, even if symptoms improve before the medication regimen is completed. A second course of antibiotics may also be necessary.

Rheumatic Fever

Rheumatic fever, an autoimmune reaction to GABHS, belongs to a group of diseases called **collagen diseases** (diseases of connective tissues). It is believed to result from continued streptococcal infections (eg, scarlet fever, **streptococcal sore throat**), in which the child becomes sensitive to streptococci or develops an autoimmune response. Prompt and complete treatment of streptococcal infections greatly reduces the child's risk of contracting rheumatic fever. Rheumatic heart disease is the most common complication of rheumatic fever. The incidences of rheumatic fever and rheumatic heart disease have decreased in countries with access to healthcare resources, although they continue to be a problem in many countries.

Signs and Symptoms.   Symptoms of rheumatic fever vary in degree from mild to severe. Loss of weight and appetite, fatigue, irritability, aches, joint pain, and tenderness in the extremities may be signs. Fever may begin suddenly, especially after a cold or sore throat, and becomes highest in the evening. The most significant symptom of rheumatic fever is *polyarthritis,* in which the child's shoulders, elbows, wrists, or knees swell and become excruciatingly painful. Pain travels from one joint to another (*migrating*) and may affect several joints at the same time. It usually lasts for a few days to a week in each joint, then subsides gradually. Fortunately, the polyarthritis does not cause joint deformities, and the joints usually return to normal after the attack.

Diagnostic tests with the following results may indicate rheumatic fever (not all findings need be present):

- Elevated white blood cell (WBC) count
- Elevated erythrocyte sedimentation rate (**ESR**), commonly known as "sed rate"
- Positive C-reactive protein (**CRP**)
- Elevated antistreptolysin-O (**ASO**) titer

Signs to watch for include jerky, uncontrolled movements of the face, neck, arm, and leg muscles, which are known as *Sydenham's chorea;* small nodules under the skin over the elbows, ankles, legs, knuckles, and at the back of the head; and frequent nosebleeds.

A common and serious complication of rheumatic fever is **rheumatic carditis** (*rheumatic heart disease*), in which valvular lesions (most commonly the mitral valve) impair valve efficiency, thereby increasing the heart's workload. Symptoms range from mild to so severe that cardiac failure occurs.

Medical Treatment.   Most cases of rheumatic fever are treated in the home. When severe instances of carditis or heart failure occur, hospitalization is necessary. The disease's course depends primarily on whether the heart is involved, and if so, to what degree. The degree of carditis directly affects recovery time.

Rheumatic fever's active phase usually lasts from 1 to 4 months, but other outbreaks are likely to follow. The key to treating rheumatic fever is to prevent permanent heart damage. Complete bed rest is maintained until the child is afebrile. Keeping the child inactive is fairly easy during the acute phase

because he or she is very sick; however, aggressive family teaching is important during convalescence, when regulating the child's activity may be difficult.

Drugs such as acetaminophen are given for pain relief and fever reduction. Aspirin may be used for its anti-inflammatory properties. Cortisone reduces inflammation but is prescribed only if absolutely necessary because of associated adverse reactions (see Chap. 62).

An antibiotic (usually penicillin) is administered; if the child is allergic to penicillin, erythromycin is given. Because recurrence is probable, prophylactic medication (penicillin or sulfadiazine) is prescribed for up to 5 years. If the child needs dental work, has an infection, or is having an invasive procedure, penicillin or another antibiotic is given for prophylaxis. Also, if any sign of a strep throat exists, family caregivers should consult a physician immediately. Some people continue on prophylactic penicillin for many years.

The outcome of rheumatic fever depends on the extent of heart damage, with the valves being the most common sites. Neither the chorea nor the arthritis is likely to have serious consequences. The carditis may be fatal, or recovery may be complete. Most children recover from rheumatic fever and lead normal lives.

Children who have had rheumatic fever are susceptible to recurrences, which place them at a greater risk for heart damage. Continuing medical care with antibiotic prophylaxis for dental work and invasive procedures is essential.

Roseola

Roseola is a benign disease of infancy. A very high fever lasting a few days is followed by a rash appearing first on the trunk and then spreading to the neck, face, and extremities when the child's temperature falls. Theorists believe a virus causes roseola, which is not as communicable as many other diseases. The affected child may experience febrile seizures, but other complications are rare. One attack seems to confer lifelong immunity.

PARASITIC INFESTATIONS

Parasites live in or on the body of another living organism. Common parasites that invade humans include bacteria, protozoa, fungi, insects, and worms.

Skin Parasites

Skin parasites spread easily from one person to another. Chapter 74 discusses them in further detail.

Pediculosis

The most common lice infestation (**pediculosis**) in children occurs on the head (*pediculosis capitis*). Children in day care and schools frequently interchange combs, hats, and caps, thereby making them prime targets. Day-care and school nurses should check children periodically. Usually, if more than two cases of lice occur in a school class, the school nurse should check the entire class. Children should be taught not to share combs, brushes, or hats. If a case occurs, the entire family needs to be treated. Teach the family household control measures (see Chap. 74).

Scabies

Scabies is a mite that is easily transmitted among children. The entire family needs to be treated when infestation occurs. Teach the family household-control measures. Chapter 74 discusses scabies infestations in more detail.

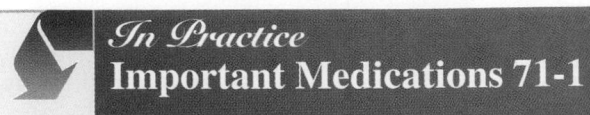

> **Nursing Alert**
> Family caregivers are often embarrassed when they find out that their child has a parasitic infestation. A nonjudgmental and supportive attitude is essential when providing family teaching.

Intestinal Parasites

Intestinal parasites infest the GI tract during their life cycle. Fecal contamination, uncooked animal flesh, and infected plants or water are often the source of infestation. These parasites thrive in environments where human excrement is poorly disposed of, food is inadequately cooked, and poverty and overcrowding exist.

You may collect a stool specimen for ova and parasites (**O&P**) to determine their presence. When handling stool specimens, always wear gloves and take care to avoid self-contamination. See In Practice: Important Medications 71-1 for information on antiparasitic medications.

Pinworms

Pinworms are one of the most common infestations in children, especially those who do not yet have good hygiene habits and often put their dirty fingers into their mouths. Children ingest the eggs, which mature in the cecum. The hatched worms lay ova in anal and perineal folds, causing local itching. Signs that a child may have pinworms include scratching, especially around the anus; teeth grinding during sleep; fatigue; anorexia; and irritability. Worms may appear in the anal region or on stool.

Use a clear cellophane tape test to obtain and identify pinworms. Wind the tape around the end of a tongue blade with the sticky side out. After spreading the child's buttocks, press the tape against the child's anus. Transfer the tape to a clear microscope slide and examine it for eggs. The early morning hours before the child awakens are most favorable for finding ova. Treatment consists of the administration of *anthelmintics* (anti-worm medications), which are given to all family members as well.

Giardiasis

Giardia intestinalis or *Giardia lamblia* is a protozoan that can cause illness. The ingestion of contaminated water caused by the careless disposal of human excrement by campers and backpackers into rivers, lakes, and streams provide the opportunity for infestation.

In Practice
Important Medications 71-1

FOR PARASITES

Some medications are effective against more than one parasite.

Tapeworm—quinacrine HCl (Atabrine), niclosamide (Niclocide)

Roundworms—piperazine (Antepar, Bryel, Entacyl in Canada), mebendazole (Vermox)

Hookworms—tetrachloroethylene

Pinworms—mebendazole (Vermox), pyrantel pamoate (Antiminth)

Lice—Nix, Rid, lindane (Kwell, Scabene)

Scabies—crotamiton (Eurax), lindane (Kwell)

Nursing Considerations

- Teach the child and family caregivers good personal hygiene and careful handwashing. Treat all family members simultaneously, and teach them to avoid food preparation during treatment.
- Discuss careful washing and cleaning of all household items and clothing when teaching about treating for lice.
- Observe carefully the person with a seizure disorder, kidney malfunction, severe malnutrition, or anemia. He or she may be unable to use these medications.
- Observe for side effects of dizziness, drowsiness, headache, seizures, diarrhea, nausea, and vomiting.
- Observe those receiving piperazine for the side effect of hemolytic anemia.
- Observe those taking lindane for skin irritation.
- Avoid applying medications to open lesions, a rash, the face, eyes, mucous membranes, or urethral meatus.
- Avoid inhaling the fumes of lindane. Note that the medication is extremely dangerous if swallowed.
- Apply antipruritic medication if itching continues for a few days after treatment.
- For clients receiving lindane, observe for the potential side effect of CNS toxicity, especially in infants, small children, and older adults.
- Repeat the treatment as needed, especially for lice.

Day-care centers have the greatest prevalence of Giardia. Young children may show signs of the disease, but most often carry the protozoa without symptoms. Their family caregivers often are the ones who become ill. The key to transmission is the survival of the Giardia cysts, even after thorough cleaning and handwashing.

Symptoms of **giardiasis** include diarrhea, *flatulence* (gas), belching, nausea, fatigue, cramps, vomiting, and *anorexia* (refusal to eat). However, people under stress or with immune deficiencies may be sicker, and often have less resistance to the disorder. Metronidazole is the drug of choice for treatment.

Roundworms

Roundworms (*Ascaris* species) are most common in warm climates with unclean living conditions. They primarily affect children aged 1 to 4 years, who contract roundworms through contaminated toys, fingers, and food. Roundworms are transmitted in feces used as fertilizer. The larvae burrow into the person's intestine, enter the bloodstream, and then migrate to the lungs, liver, or heart. Finally, they return to the intestine and mature. The infection may not be suspected until the child passes a worm in stool or vomit. Symptoms may include diarrhea and intestinal obstruction, sometimes with intestinal rupture. Anthelmintic agents kill specific types of worms. Examples include mebendazole and albendazole, which kill roundworms and tapeworms.

Hookworms. **Hookworms** are a type of roundworm. Most often they enter the host through bare feet. They then circulate through the person's bloodstream into the lungs, where they migrate to the mouth and throat. These worms destroy red blood cells (RBCs), thereby causing anemia. The person's abdomen may become distended. Blood or hookworm ova may be found in stool. Iron tablets or blood transfusions may be needed to treat anemia.

TRAUMA

Children are susceptible to injury from accidents, including falling, choking, drowning, poisoning, and burns. Because young children are constantly on the move, watching them every moment is difficult. Children do not have the judgment or experience to protect themselves. As a result, accidents are the number one cause of death in children older than 1 year of age through young adulthood. Family caregivers and others who care for children must constantly be alert to prevent trauma.

Common Injuries

Fractures

Although children's bones are not as brittle as those of adults, children receive more accidental blows and injuries. Consequently, they suffer many fractures. Falls are frequent among children with nervous system disorders, because of their impaired balance and coordination. Some fractures are due to abuse. Treatment of fractures includes casts and traction. When a child is in a cast or traction, check circulation by assessing skin color, sensitivity, temperature, motion, and pulse distal to the injury (see Chap. 76). Fractures most commonly seen in children are those involving the radius, ulna, clavicle, tibia, and femur.

> **Nursing Alert**
> Be aware that children may stuff small objects (toys, coins, marbles, and so forth) into the top of a cast, causing discomfort and a site for possible infection.

Lacerations, Cuts, and Puncture Wounds

Many children come to the emergency department (ED) with cuts and punctures from knives, forks, pencils, or other sharp objects found in the home. The obvious preventive measure is for family caregivers to keep such objects out of children's reach.

Children also may sustain crushing injuries from being caught in car doors or under heavy pieces of furniture, or from being hit by moving vehicles or bicycles. Serious injuries can also occur with electric car windows or garage doors. Bruises and abrasions can result from falls from tricycles, wagons, or playground equipment.

When caring for such injuries, the physician will suture lacerations, apply antiseptics and dressings, and send children for x-ray examinations if necessary to determine the presence of fractures. A tetanus booster will be given depending upon the injury. Advise family caregivers to watch puncture wounds in particular for signs of infection, and to keep such wounds open as much as possible so that they drain and heal from the inside. Instruct caregivers to soak wounds periodically to facilitate drainage.

Foreign Objects

Children learn about the world by exploring. Part of this exploration may include picking up small objects and trying to put them into any convenient body opening, including the mouth, ears, nose, rectum, or vagina. Young children need close observation from family caregivers to avoid injuries resulting from this kind of exploring. See Chapter 43 for details about the removal of foreign objects and appropriate treatment.

Animal Bites and Scratches

Animal bites can be very serious. Children should be warned never to go near a dog that is eating (even their own family dog) or to pet any unfamiliar dog. Sometimes, a dog will bite a child's face, necessitating plastic or reconstructive surgery. When a dog bites a child, determine if the dog has received a rabies immunization. If not, the dog must be isolated and watched for signs of rabies or distemper. If the dog becomes ill or cannot be found, the child must receive prophylactic rabies injections; a tetanus booster also may be necessary. Very few documented cases exist of the survival of humans who were infected with rabies.

A cat scratch often becomes infected more easily than a dog-related injury. As with dogs who bite, cats who scratch must be watched for signs of rabies. Cleanse scratches carefully and apply an antibiotic ointment. Prophylactic antibiotics (amoxicillin plus clavulanate [Augmentin]) may be prescribed. If a scratch becomes infected, the child should see a healthcare provider immediately.

"Cat-scratch fever" (or disease) is a benign, self-limiting illness. The child may have a low-grade fever and malaise. Lymphadenopathy may last 2 to 3 months. Because cats lick their paws frequently, a cat scratch is treated as a bite and requires wound cleaning and antibiotics.

Wild animals also bite people, particularly when trapped or frightened. They are often carriers of rabies or other diseases.

Report such bites, and treat and monitor the victim to avoid serious complications.

Burns

Chapters 43 and 74 discuss burns in more detail. Most information found in these chapters applies to children as well as adults.

The chief nursing concerns in treating burns are combating shock, alleviating pain, and restoring fluid and electrolyte balance. Secondary interventions include the prevention of infection and contractures, and the reconstruction or repair of damage. Children who have been severely burned are best cared for in a specialized burn unit.

Treatment for burns is long term. Pressure garments are frequently used to prevent contractures and scarring. Children may need to wear pressure garments continuously for 12 to 18 months; these garments require replacement to accommodate growth. Family members need understanding and support during a child's rehabilitation period. Children under the age of 5 years have difficulty recovering from burns because their thin skin receives deep burns, they have incomplete immune systems, and they become dehydrated easily.

The extent of burns is determined on a percentage basis. Because a child's body surface differs in proportion from that of an adult, the following method should be used to determine the extent of a burn. Remember that an infant's head is large in proportion to the body.

- *The newborn:* The head is 17% of the entire body surface; each arm, 8%; each leg, 13%; the front or back, 20%; and genitals, 1%.
- *The 3-year-old:* The head is 15%; each arm, 8%; each leg, 14%; the front or back, 20%; and genitals, 1%.
- *The 6-year-old:* The head is 11%; each arm, 8%; each leg, 16%; front or back, 20%; and genitals, 1%.
- *Over age 12:* The "rule of nines" applies (see Chap. 74): the head is 9%; each arm, 9%; each leg, 18%; front or back, 18%; and genitals, 1%.

Burns may be classified as *partial thickness* or *full thickness,* relating to the type of grafting that may be needed.

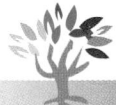 **SPECIAL CONSIDERATIONS:** THE LIFE SPAN

Burns

Even a superficial burn is critical if it covers two thirds or more of an infant's body.

Poisoning

More than 80% of poisonings occur in the home. Inquisitive toddlers, who put anything and everything into the mouth, can easily ingest one or more of these substances. See In Practice: Educating the Client 71-1 for poisoning prevention measures.

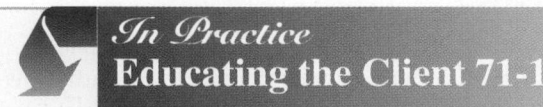 *In Practice*
Educating the Client 71-1

POISON PREVENTION

- Label all poisonous chemicals with warning labels and store them in locked cabinets.
- Keep medications and poisonous materials in their original containers. Never put any poisonous substance in a soda or drink container.
- Use childproof caps whenever possible. Always close them properly.
- Teach children the dangers of poisonous materials and medications. Keep medications in a locked cabinet.
- Keep edibles in separate cabinets from inedibles.
- Never leave children alone when poisonous materials are nearby.
- Never treat medicines and vitamins as though they are candy. Do not purchase medicines resembling candy, animals, people, or cartoon characters.
- Read product labels carefully and follow precautions. Never give medications in the dark.
- Dispose of poisonous materials and medications carefully. Destroy medicines by flushing them down the toilet or washing them down the drain. Do not throw them in the trash.
- Never smoke around children. Keep all fresh or used smoking materials, including ashtrays and butts, away from children.
- Post the local poison control center telephone number on all telephones in the house.
- Keep syrup of ipecac and activated charcoal on hand at all times.
- Watch children when visiting relatives and friends. A new setting is frequently an invitation for children to explore.
- Remain calm in an emergency. Dial the emergency number, give all information, and follow directions.
- Take the container of the medicine or poison to the emergency department with you. If you are uncertain what was ingested, list all possible substances.

Cleaning compounds are a major problem because they are usually kept under the sink or on the floor of the bathroom closet, and are therefore easily accessible. Drug companies attempted to alleviate the problem of medication poisoning by installing safety caps on bottles, and a notable decrease in accidental poisonings has since been seen. However, medications continue to be a culprit in accidental poisonings. Many older adults with arthritic hands ask their pharmacists to dispense prescriptions with a regular cap rather than a safety cap. Unfortunately, grandchildren may find these medications on a bedside table or in some other handy spot and decide to try some.

One difficulty encountered with medications manufactured for children relates to appearance. Most often, these drugs are packaged attractively, taste good, and are in "fun" shapes. As a result, many small children mistake these medications for candy. Children can also be poisoned by consuming an overdose of a medication that had been prescribed for them.

Poisonous house plants and cigarette butts should be kept out of children's reach. Cigarette butts are poisonous if eaten. Lead poisoning (**plumbism**) results from inhaling or eating leaded substances, such as flakes of lead paint (see Chap. 73).

Poison Treatment. In the event of poisoning, family caregivers should call their local poison control center immediately. Special personnel can determine the best treatment for the particular poison. The person calling the center should take the container of the involved item to the telephone so that he or she can give information as quickly as possible. Families should tape the poison control center's number on every telephone in their home. In most areas of the United States and Canada, dialing 911 provides immediate access to emergency assistance.

Physicians recommend that every household keep the emetic, syrup of ipecac. Syrup of ipecac induces vomiting and generally may be purchased over-the-counter. It should be kept with the emergency first-aid supplies, especially when children are present.

Syrup of ipecac is a substance that causes vomiting in 90% of children within 20 minutes. The usual dosage of ipecac is 5 milliliters for children ages 6 to 9 months, 10 milliliters for children 9 to 12 months, 15 milliliters for children 1 to 12 years, and 30 milliliters for children 12 years and older. Always follow the administration of ipecac with water (5 mL/kg to a maximum of 300 mL). Administration can be safely repeated once. If vomiting does not occur within 30 minutes after the second dose, the emetic must be removed by lavage. Unless specifically advised to do so by the poison control center, ipecac should not be given with some poisons, such as caustic substances or petroleum products.

✚👁 Nursing Alert

Do not use ipecac in children under 6 months of age. Vomiting is contraindicated in clients with decreased level of consciousness, those who are convulsing, or those who have ingested hydrocarbons or caustic agents (strong acids or alkalis). *Syrup of ipecac* and *tincture of ipecac* are not the same medication: The tincture is much stronger.

Activated charcoal absorbs poisons, reducing GI absorption. Induced emesis should be done before charcoal is administered orally or by nasogastric tube. Do not mix charcoal with food, or give it with any other drugs, because charcoal absorbs these substances. The dose is approximately 5 to 10 times the amount of poison ingested. The stools will appear black for 2 to 3 days.

When a poisoned child arrives in the ED, specific procedures are performed. Sometimes the stomach is washed out (*gastric lavage*), usually with normal saline, in an effort to remove as much poison as possible. This procedure must be done quickly to prevent as much absorption of the harmful substance into the bloodstream as possible.

Nursing Considerations. The nurse may be asked to assist with gastric lavage. In most EDs the needed equipment is packaged as a "gavage set." A suction machine and ordered drugs and solutions are required. You should assist with procedures, document all pertinent information, and support the child and family.

Also, be ready to assist with suctioning (to prevent aspiration), oxygen administration, resuscitation, catheterization, blood sampling, x-ray studies, and electrocardiograms (ECGs). If several hours have passed since the child ingested the toxin, stomach lavage is usually not performed, because the child has probably already absorbed most of the substance. In this case, the symptoms are treated.

After lavage, the child generally remains in the ED for 1 to 2 hours before discharge, unless his or her bloodstream has absorbed much of the poison. In this case, the child is admitted to the facility for overnight observation. When the child is released from the healthcare facility, instruct family caregivers to watch for unfavorable symptoms. Advise them to return the child to the ED if such symptoms develop.

Nursing care involves assessing the child for any change in level of consciousness (LOC), dizziness, nausea, vomiting, unusual behavior, extreme drowsiness, or excitement. Sometimes irreversible physical or mental changes occur.

Surgery must be performed occasionally to correct physical damage caused by ingested caustic substances. In severe poisonings, the child may have renal failure and may require dialysis or may die. (*Dialysis* is a process whereby wastes are removed from the body when the kidneys are not functioning.)

☞ KEY CONCEPT

Poisonings and accidents sometimes occur during periods of change for the family because adult members are distracted. Typical changes include a move to a new home, the death of a family member, the birth of a new baby, or divorce or separation.

Suffocation

The many causes of suffocation in children include the aspiration of a foreign object or smothering with a pillow or plastic bag. Children should not use pillows until they are able to turn themselves over freely. Mattresses should never be covered with any type of plastic bag.

Infants are obligatory nose breathers who have not yet learned mouth breathing. Suffocation can result if an infant who has an upper respiratory infection (**URI**) cannot cough up mucus plugging the bronchi. Humidity usually helps to loosen secretions. A bulb syringe should be available to assist in keeping the infant's nasal airway clear of mucus accumulation.

See In Practice: Educating the Client 71-2 to learn more about choking prevention.

Children can suffocate if they become trapped in discard refrigerators or other enclosed spaces. Children seeking t

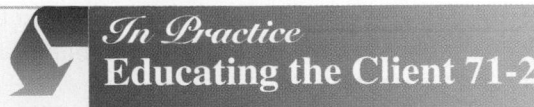

**In Practice
Educating the Client 71-2**

CHOKING PREVENTION

- Cut children's food into small pieces.
- Teach children to eat slowly.
- Teach children not to laugh and talk when they have food in their mouth.
- Serve foods appropriate to a child's age. Avoid serving nuts, popcorn, chewing gum, hard candy, raisins, carrot sticks, and hot dogs to children younger than 4 years of age.
- Keep small objects such as coins, marbles, beads, and small toy pieces away from children younger than 4 years of age.
- Store small household items such as pins, buttons, toothpicks, nails, screws, and thumbtacks away from children's reach. Monitor children when they are in an area where such items are being used.

in large freezers have been known to fall into the freezers and be unable to rescue themselves. Trunks and toy chests can also be fatal traps. State laws generally call for the removal of doors from all discarded refrigerators and upright freezers or for them to be turned tightly against a wall.

Drowning

Danger areas for drowning are age related. Infants are subject to drowning in bathtubs, toilets, or containers of standing water (eg, a dog dish or a pail). According to the Centers for Disease Control and Prevention, between 60% and 90% of drownings of children under 4 years of age occur in residential swimming pools. Adolescents most commonly drown in rivers and lakes. Alcohol use (either by the victim or the supervisor) is linked to between 25% and 50% of deaths. Drownings can occur in any body of water. The outcome depends on the time of submersion and the water's temperature. Vigilance is the key to preventing drowning death and disability. Constantly supervise children. Never allow children to swim alone. Keep small buckets of any fluid away from young children.

☛ KEY CONCEPT

The two most effective ways of preventing drowning are adequate adult supervision at all times and water-safety training.

Sudden Infant Death Syndrome

Sudden infant death syndrome (**SIDS**) is the sudden, unexplained death of a seemingly healthy infant. It occurs while the infant is asleep. SIDS is the number one cause of death in infants 1 month to 1 year of age, and peaks at age 3 months. This

diagnosis can only be made following postmortem examination, when no other cause can be identified.

A condition called prolonged infantile apnea (**PIA**) is defined as cessation of breathing for at least 20 seconds, or for a shorter time with accompanying bradycardia, *cyanosis* (bluish skin), and/or pallor. When this condition is discovered (via a "near miss"), an apnea monitor can be used to prevent SIDS.

Although the etiology of SIDS is unknown, one theory suggests that an abnormality in brain-stem functioning results in faulty respirations. Incomplete bubbling after feeding, secondhand smoke, and sleeping in a prone position have also been connected to SIDS. Small for gestational age (**SGA**) infants are at a greater risk.

In addition to experiencing profound shock and grief, families of SIDS infants often feel overwhelming guilt. When a SIDS tragedy occurs, be particularly sensitive and offer support and compassion. Provide families with information regarding support groups such as The Compassionate Friends and the SIDS Foundation.

Some infants at high risk are placed on an apnea monitor until about 1 year of age. You can teach caregivers how to use the monitor (see In Practice: Nursing Procedure 71-1).

CHILD ABUSE

Abuse of children is a widespread social problem. Many children die or are temporarily or permanently injured each year as a result of abuse.

Child abuse takes several forms, including neglect, physical abuse, and sexual abuse. If you suspect child abuse, you are obligated by law to report it to your supervisor, a physician, or the authorities. See In Practice: Nursing Assessment 71-1 for significant considerations in suspected child abuse.

☛ KEY CONCEPT

A sudden change of behavior in a child of any age is a clue that abuse may be occurring.

Anger is likely to be your first response to any kind of child abuse. Take the time to remain objective. Be aware of possible personal problems of the suspected abuser, such as low self-esteem, rejection, and isolation. Include objective explanations, and be consistent in your approach. Suspected abusers are often in an environment that is out of control, and their way of coping is to abuse their child.

☛ KEY CONCEPT

If you suspect child abuse, you must, by law, report it immediately. Nurses who do not do so are committing a crime. Those reporting suspected abusers are legally protected against recourse.

Parents Anonymous groups throughout the country assist abusers in breaking the cycle. Support groups provide ongoing help to abusers who have completed counseling programs

---

In Practice
Nursing Procedure 71-1

TEACHING USE OF THE APNEA MONITOR

Supplies and Equipment

Apnea monitor with electrodes
Material for cleansing the infant's skin

Steps

1. Wash your hands.
2. Gather equipment.
3. Explain to the infant's caregivers what you are going to do and why.
   RATIONALE: *Teaching helps decrease anxiety and gives caregivers a better understanding of the procedure.*
4. Prepare the infant's skin by making sure it is clean and dry.
   RATIONALE: *When the skin is clean and dry, the electrodes adhere better, with less chance of skin breakdown.*
5. Apply the electrodes (either to the infant or to the electrode belt, depending on the type of monitor being used).
   a. Place the electrode belt at the infant's nipple line. Do not fasten it yet.
   b. Skin electrodes are usually best placed between the infant's nipple and armpit, and may be repositioned somewhat.
      RATIONALE: *Proper electrode placement ensures accurate monitor readings. Moving the electrodes occasionally helps to prevent skin breakdown.*
6. Insert the lead wires into the electrodes. Insert the white lead wire on the infant's right side (mnemonic: white = right). Insert the black wire on the left. Additional color-coded lead wires may appear, depending on the system used.
7. Insert the corresponding lead wires into the cable (the cable is usually color coded to match the lead wires). Insert the cable into the monitor.
8. If using an electrode belt, attach it to the infant. The belt should be snug, but you should be able to insert two fingers under it.

RATIONALE: *Ensure accurate readings without causing respiratory compromise or skin breakdown.*
9. Make sure the monitor is plugged in, the cable is attached, and the alarms are properly set.
10. Turn on the monitor. The indicator lights should be on as well.
11. Settle the infant comfortably, or allow caregivers to hold and comfort their infant.
    RATIONALE: *Comfort helps decrease respiratory distress and makes the infant feel safer.*
12. If the monitor alarms:
    a. Check the infant immediately.
    b. Check the infant's breathing and color. If the infant is pink but not breathing, wait until the 10th beep before starting stimulation. If the infant is not pink, begin stimulation immediately.
       RATIONALE: *The infant may resume breathing without intervention. The alarm may be mechanical in origin, and the infant may not require any stimulation. Believe your observations of the infant before you believe the monitor.*
13. Use this stimulation sequence: Gently touch the infant; flick the infant's heel; slap the infant's foot; rub the infant's back. (Note: Be certain to teach caregivers never to shake the infant.) If the child does not respond, start cardiopulmonary resuscitation (CPR).
    RATIONALE: *Use as little intervention as necessary to help the infant resume breathing. After the problem resolves, the alarm will stop.*
14. Press the reset button to turn off the alarm indicator.
    RATIONALE: *The alarm will stop when the problem resolves, but the alarm needs to be reset.*
15. Document and report any alarms and nursing responses. Document the infant's condition. Always note alarm settings when starting and ending any contact with the infant and at least every hour in between.
    RATIONALE: *Alarms can be altered by other staff or visitors, on purpose or by accident. Check them frequently to ensure they are set correctly.*

---

and need day-to-day assistance in pursuing a non-abusive lifestyle.

Your role in reporting suspected child abuse is important. Reporting abuse is mandated. The following list has guidelines for reporting abuse:

- *Believe the child.* If a child confides in you, always assume that he or she is telling the truth.

- *Observe the child's reactions.* Look not only for marks and bruises, but also for reactions. An abused child may draw away when touched, or avoid contact or interaction with others. The child may attempt to protect the abuser by making excuses for "accidents."

- *Document your observations.* Carefully observe the signs of abuse. Be objective. Identify and document every obser-

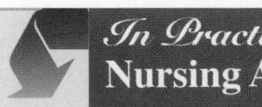

In Practice
Nursing Assessment 71-1

DETECTING CHILD ABUSE

Adults who have risk factors for committing child abuse include:

- Adults who have suffered abuse, neglect, or rejection in their past
- Adults with a history of dependency on others
- Adults with one or more of the following personality traits: hostility, tendency to blame others, punitiveness, low self-esteem, or impulsiveness
- Adults who are caring for out-of-wedlock, unwanted, or foster children
- Young and immature family caregivers
- Individuals in troubled relationships who have unmet needs or who are subject to excessive demands from their partners, rejection, or abuse
- Those who use drugs excessively
- Adults with high expectations of their children, who are overcritical and who do not view the child positively
- Adults who use extreme discipline measures
- Family caregivers who have exhibited a loss of control in disciplining, such as slapping, shaking, and hitting the child
- Those who are overwhelmed by their children's emotional and physical needs and demands
- Individuals who are unable to cope with daily activities, which can lead to irritability and frustration
- Family caregivers who seldom touch or look at their child, react with impatience, or ignore their child's crying

Suspect abuse when you encounter school-age children who exhibit the following behaviors:

- Lying about an injury
- Behavior problems
- Expectation of abusive behavior
- Lawbreaking

- Use and abuse of drugs, especially at an early age
- Truancy
- Self-injurious behavior; suicidal thoughts or attempts
- Promiscuous behavior

Suspect abuse when you encounter infants, toddlers, and preschoolers who exhibit:

- Injuries at various stages of healing (could not have happened at the same time)
- Inappropriate sexual knowledge
- Agreement with family caregivers on illogical causes of injury
- Burns, lacerations, or serious bruises without the appearance of accidents; unexplained fractures; missing chunks of hair
- Attempts to stay away from home
- Attempts to hide scars with clothing
- Frequent injuries
- Extreme fear of adults; fear of being touched
- An appearance of neglect: dirty, unkempt, extremely thin, lethargic
- Stomach problems, colitis, rectal/vaginal bleeding, frequent headaches

Suspect child neglect in the following instances:

- Abandonment of child by caregiver
- Inadequate medical or dental care, hygiene, clothing, supply or quality of food, sleep
- Unmet needs relating to physical or mental problems
- Isolation of family from usual social contacts
- Excessive demands placed upon the child (expected to do all the housework or accept total care of younger siblings)
- Child left without custodial care or supervision

---

vation to the last detail. Measure bruises, abrasions, and other signs of injury. Take photographs.

- *Teach the child.* The child needs to learn what activities are inappropriate, what to do if someone tries to exploit him or her, and that mistreatment is not something he or she "deserves."
- *Call your local child protection agency* if you have any concerns about a child or about appropriate procedure.

For more information, see In Practice: Nursing Care Plan 71-1.

Neglect

Neglect can be divided into emotional and physical realms. An *emotionally neglected* child is deprived of love, affection, and

attention from family caregivers or is continually berated, called derogatory names, and told that he or she is stupid. A *physically neglected* child does not receive adequate food, water, clothing, or medical care (see In Practice: Nursing Assessment 71-1).

Emotionally neglected children may demonstrate self-destructive behaviors or be passive and withdrawn. They may have difficulty sleeping, experience nightmares, and show signs of depression. Physically neglected children may appear disheveled, unclean, and malnourished. They may show evidence of untreated dental problems.

Physical Abuse

Physical abuse has yet to be universally defined. Most often it refers to a situation in which a child has been physically

In Practice
Nursing Care Plan 71-1

THE CHILD WHO MAY BE A VICTIM OF ABUSE

MEDICAL HISTORY: *F. M. is a 4-year-old boy admitted to the pediatric unit from the emergency department following treatment for an asthmatic attack secondary to pneumonia. Client is receiving continuous IV therapy along with nebulized bronchodilators administered every 2 hours. He is receiving oxygen via mask at 4 liters per minute. This is his fifth admission for asthma; his first admission was when he was 30 months old. Past medical history (from previous admission records) reveals visits to the emergency department for spiral fracture of the left forearm and mild concussion.*

MEDICAL DIAGNOSIS: *Asthma, pneumonia; rule out suspected physical abuse*

Data Collection/Nursing Assessment: Four-year-old male sleeping off and on. Client unable to provide any history. On examination, bruises are noted on the back and torso in several stages of healing. Small circular burn-like area approximately ¼ inch in diameter is noted on buttocks (appears to be a cigarette burn). When questioned about the bruises, his family caregivers state, "He's so clumsy and he falls a lot." When questioned about the client's asthma regimen, the caregivers state, "We tried giving them for a while but we stopped." Client demonstrates an extreme fear of adults and an exaggerated eagerness to please his caregivers. Child withdraws when touched. Child abuse is suspected. (*Although other nursing diagnoses may be appropriate, a priority nursing diagnosis is addressed below.*)

Nursing Diagnosis: Impaired Parenting Related to unmet social/emotional/maturational needs of the family caregivers and lack of knowledge about child's needs as evidenced by the bruising and frequent visits to emergency department and hospitalizations.

Planning
SHORT-TERM GOALS:
#1. Child will remain safe and free of further evidence of abuse.
#2. Family caregivers will identify the need for help.

LONG-TERM GOALS:
#3. Family caregivers actively participate in group counseling for parenting.
#4. Family caregivers begin to demonstrate effective parenting skills.

Implementation
NURSING ACTION: *Report the case to Child Protective Services and reassure the child that he is safe in the healthcare facility.*

RATIONALE: *All states have mandatory laws for reporting child maltreatment; reassuring the child helps to foster the development of trust. Maintaining the child's safety is the priority.*

NURSING ACTION: *Provide consistent caregivers to demonstrate acceptance of and affection for the child; implement a program of attention based on play, group interaction with other children, and quiet time with the child. Ensure that someone is in the child's room at all times when caregivers are present.*
RATIONALE: *Meeting the child's anxiety needs is fundamental to care and safety. Acceptance is critical to the child's development. Having someone present when family caregivers are present reduces the risk of trauma to the child.*

Evaluation: Child observed playing quietly in bed with play therapist at bedside. When family caregivers visiting, nurse present at all times. *Progress to meeting to Goal #1.*

NURSING ACTION: *Determine the family caregivers' potential to abuse including any history of abuse as a child, unrealistic expectations of children (role reversal), lack of knowledge of parenting skills, social isolation, and lack of resources to deal with multiple life stresses.*
RATIONALE: *Determining the caregivers' potential for abuse provides a baseline for further investigation and inquiry. Abusive caregivers were often abused as children.*

NURSING ACTION: *Attempt to establish a supportive relationship with caregivers, acknowledging how difficult it can be to raise children (while not condoning abuse), and taking advantage of any opportunities to act as a role model for positive interactions with the child and to teach parenting skills.*
RATIONALE: *Establishing a supportive relationship is essential to building trust with the caregivers and to acceptance of the problem. Role modeling provides an opportunity for teaching.*

NURSING ACTION: *After trust and a supportive relationship are established, assist the caregivers in acknowledging the problem and recommend that the caregivers voluntarily seek professional counseling.*
RATIONALE: *Abusing caregivers have rarely learned to trust others and may feel defensive about their deficiencies. The caregiver needs to acknowledge the problem before being able to seek help.*

(continued)

In Practice
Nursing Care Plan 71-1 (Continued)

Evaluation: Caregivers deny any problem on admission; next evening, caregivers talking about their difficulties as children and being abused by parents. Caregivers requesting to talk to counselor after speaking to child protection worker and learning alternatives. *Goal #2 met.*

NURSING ACTION: *Encourage caregivers in continuing to meet with counselor; continue to role model positive parenting behaviors. Observe caregivers for imitation of these behaviors.*

RATIONALE: *Continuing to meet with a counselor aids in working through the problems. Caregivers demonstrating behaviors indicates learning.*

Evaluation: Caregivers currently attending weekly counseling sessions; caregivers demonstrating beginning awareness of ability to recognize changes in child's behavior. Child without evidence of further injury. *Goal #1 met; progress to meeting Goal #3 and Goal #4.*

---

harmed and injury has occurred. The injury is inflicted intentionally and can vary from minor bruising to death. *Shaken baby syndrome* is an example of physical abuse. In these cases, an adult holds the infant by the shoulders and violently shakes the baby. It usually occurs when the adult becomes frustrated after attempts to quiet the crying infant. The immature development of the infant's neck muscles (leading to lack of head control), along with the violent shaking, results in cerebral trauma or hemorrhage. Death or serious intellectual impairment can result.

Evidence of physical abuse can take a variety of forms. Unexplained bruises in various stages of healing, cigarette burns, scars, and numerous unexplained fractures that have healed are common indicators.

☞ KEY CONCEPT

Accidental brain injury can occur when a child is thrown into the air and caught. Caution caregivers about the dangers of this type of play.

Sexual Abuse

Sexual abuse of children ranges from exposure and fondling to anal, vaginal, or oral intercourse. The typical pattern is one of secrecy. The abuser may be a stranger, someone the child knows well, or a family member (*incest*). He or she can be an adult, adolescent, or an older child. The abused child may be as young as 1 year old.

As the abused child grows older, the abuser tells him or her to keep the abuse a secret and may threaten the child. By the time an abused individual is old enough to realize that what is happening is wrong, he or she is too ashamed and afraid to reveal the truth. His or her reaction is typically guilt and fear. In many cases, the child represses the abuse, only for it to surface in flashbacks, nightmares, and self-injurious or defeating behavior years later. Sexual abuse of children includes child pornography.

Sexual abuse is difficult to identify and harder to prove. The following are signs of sexual abuse:

- Sudden behavioral changes
- Abdominal pain, gastric distress, or headaches
- Emotional disturbances
- Avoidance of touching or physical contact
- Vaginal or rectal bleeding or lesions

Many schools now have programs that teach young children about sexual abuse and incest. These programs demonstrate "good touch and bad touch," and help children learn to say "no" and to seek help. Children learn to avoid strangers and to report any uncomfortable incidents to persons in authority. These programs encourage a strong feeling of self-worth.

Failure to Thrive

Inadequate physical growth is termed failure to thrive (**FTT**). FTT may involve only weight, or it may involve weight and height. Characteristic developmental symptoms include retarded motor development, inadequate social response, and delayed language development. FTT children are withdrawn and apathetic, do not relate to their environment, and do not cry. Psychologically, these children show a *flat affect,* which means that the child has little or no emotional expression in response to external stimulation.

A physiologic problem such as cystic fibrosis, celiac disease, gastroenteritis, parasites, or congenital heart disease may cause FTT. More commonly, FTT has a psychosocial rather than a congenital physical cause. If the cause is related to a difficult social or home situation (most commonly due to a disturbance in the parent–child relationship), the FTT child may appear malnourished and may have spindly arms and legs, a potbelly, and an unnaturally old appearance (Fig. 71-1).

FTT infants may be passive and withdrawn, and may have developmental delays. Family caregivers of FTT children often cannot afford foods, have inadequate nutritional knowledge, or have health beliefs (dietary restrictions) that prevent the child from receiving adequate nutrition. Avoid judgment or blame of family caregivers. Recommend family counseling and education. New or alternative parenting skills can be re-

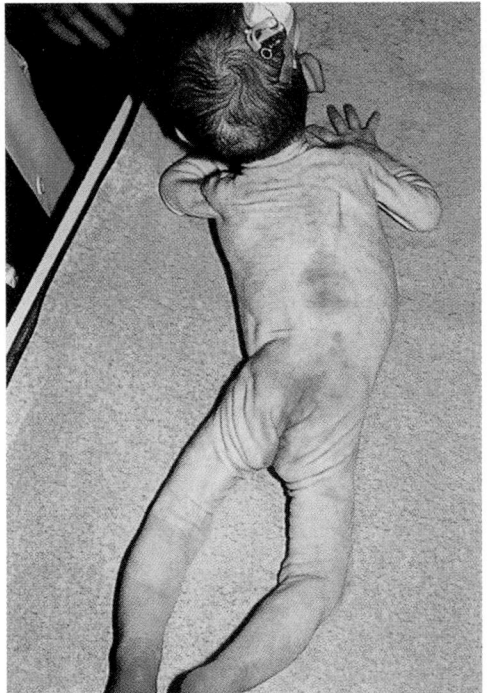

FIGURE 71-1. Failure to thrive. The child with failure to thrive experiences a loss of subcutaneous fat, muscle wasting, and skin breakdown.

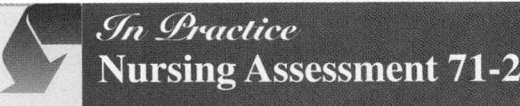

In Practice
Nursing Assessment 71-2

FAILURE TO THRIVE DANGER SIGNALS

Familial Causes
- Early separation of mother from infant, which leads to inappropriate bonding
- Major depression or mental illness of a prominent caregiver early in the child's life
- Major family crisis that disrupts normal family interaction
- Serious illness of the infant, which leads to an inability to form strong familial bonding
- Family caregivers who isolate themselves or who have marital problems
- Very young caregivers or caregivers with minimal parenting skills
- Serious illness or death of caregiver or sibling

Infant-Related Causes
- Prematurity, illness, congenital malformation, malabsorption disorders
- Reduced responsiveness and interaction with others in environment
- Dislike of cuddling, slow social development (eg, does not smile), difficulty in feeding
- Disorders such as severe autism or mental retardation

inforced. Nutritional needs of children of different ages can be another area of focus.

Take a developmental history of FTT children. If the family caregivers are the biologic parents, examine their feelings about pregnancy and having to care for children. See In Practice: Nursing Assessment 71-2 for additional considerations.

The FTT infant is often hospitalized from 10 to 14 days. The child is fed on demand, at least every 2 to 3 hours. If the resulting weight gain is appropriate, FTT is a definite diagnosis. If the child does not gain weight, physiologic reasons must be sought. A physical examination is essential, including a complete blood workup.

Family caregivers should be with their infants to provide care and to spend as much time as possible. Tender loving care and stimulation are essential. Hold such children, and rock and cuddle them. Educate caregivers to look for positive signs (smiles, responsiveness).

Accurate recordings of intake and output (I&O) are essential. Be sure to follow the feeding schedule. In older children, record accurate food and fluid intake.

SKIN DISORDERS

Nevi

A **nevus** (plural: nevi) is an abnormal skin mark that can be either hereditary or acquired as a result of *teratogens* (substances that damage the development of a fetus). A nevus may be pigmented or vascular. Some types are called "birthmarks."

The three major types of nevi are the *intradermal* or common "moles"; the *junctional*, which are flat or raised at the junction of the dermis and epidermis; and the *active junctional*. Active junctional moles are the most likely of the three types to develop into *melanoma* (skin cancer).

Pigmented nevi ("birthmarks" or "moles") are either simple brown spots or dark hairy spots composed of cells containing melanin. Although normally harmless, nevi require close observation because they can develop into malignant melanomas. Pigmented nevi are removed if any chance exists that they are malignant. They are sometimes removed for cosmetic reasons.

A vascular nevus (*angioma*) may be of two types. **Lymphangiomas** are overgrowths of lymph vessels. **Hemangiomas** are overgrowths of blood vessels. A *capillary hemangioma* ("port-wine stain," *nevus flammeus*) is a red or purple lesion that usually does not fade. Port-wine stains, especially on the face, can be treated with a series of pulse-laser treatments under anesthesia. An immature hemangioma ("strawberry mark," *nevus vasculosus*) usually regresses and disappears, making treatment unnecessary. A *cavernous hemangioma* is a raised, red lesion that does not regress.

Mongolian spots are irregular dark, blue-green areas generally found on the lower back. They are almost always present in Asian infants and are frequently found in Mediterranean and African infants. They usually disappear by about the age of 2 to 3 years.

Rash

Many small babies experience rashes of unknown cause. Infant and toddler skin is very delicate and easily irritated. If no cause can be determined, treat the rash symptomatically. Exposure to air generally relieves the rash and symptoms such as itching. The healthcare provider may order an ointment or lotion to ease symptoms as well.

Eczema

Eczema, a severe atopic dermatitis, is characterized by remissions and exacerbations accompanied by vesicle formation, oozing, crusting, excoriations, and itching. Usually beginning on the cheeks, it may move to other parts of the body and usually decreases as the child ages. It appears to worsen in cold weather and tends to run in families. Eczema may occur due to an allergy, although often the cause is unknown.

The baby with severe eczema is miserable; he or she cries and wants to scratch constantly. Scratching can lead to severe excoriation, streptococcal or staphylococcal infection, scarring, or a dangerous complication called *eczema herpeticum* (eczema complicated by herpesvirus). Spending a lot of time with this baby is a good idea, because when the baby is alone he or she will probably need to be restrained to prevent scratching. An effective restraint is the elbow restraint. A child can be restrained in a rocking chair so that he or she can move but cannot scratch.

Dermatitis packs or therapeutic colloidal baths often relieve itching. Sometimes antibiotic or cortisone ointments are applied (see Chap. 74).

Adjust the child's diet to eliminate identified allergy-producing substances. Dietary adjustments often include soybean formulas. Gradually, foods are added to the diet at the rate of one new food per week (known as an *elimination diet*). Instruct family caregivers to use nonallergenic coverings on crib mattresses. Pets may need to find new homes.

"Cradle cap" is seborrheic dermatitis of the scalp. It often occurs when a caregiver is apprehensive about hurting the infant's soft spot. Teach the family caregiver that regular shampooing and brushing of the baby's head is important.

MUSCULOSKELETAL AND ORTHOPEDIC DISORDERS

Chapter 76 discusses orthopedic nursing. Before caring for a child in a cast or in traction, be sure to examine specific related procedures in that chapter.

Developmental Dysplasia

One or both hips may be improperly located in the ball and socket joints; the head of the femur may be displaced, or the acetabulum may develop improperly. These conditions are known as **dysplasia,** causing hip dislocation. If the disorder is unilateral (on one side only), the buttock on the affected side has an additional crease, and the child's two knees are not level when he or she lies on the back with the hips and knees flexed

and the soles flat on the bed (*Allis' sign*). The child's knee on the affected side is lower.

Radiographic studies are diagnostic. In addition, the child shows limited abduction on the affected side when he or she flexes the knees while in the supine position. This condition is more frequent in girls, is uncommon among African Americans, and occurs most often on one side only. It is common in breech intrauterine position, especially frank breech, and in multiple births.

If untreated, the dislocation causes deformity in later life, characterized by a shorter leg and limited abduction on the affected side. Later, the person limps and has *lordosis* (concave curvature of the lumbar spine) and a protruding abdomen.

Medical Treatment.   If dysplasia is diagnosed before complete dislocation occurs, the condition can be treated medically. Most affected infants have dysplasia without dislocation. This disorder is usually discovered when the child is in the newborn nursery or at the 6-week checkup.

To treat dysplasia, the infant is placed in a splint brace or Pavlik harness for 3 to 6 months to maintain the hips in an abducted position (Fig. 71-2). The problem may be corrected in the small infant with the use of multiple diapers, which keep the hips abducted. These measures keep the head of the femur within the acetabulum, promoting bone development.

Early diagnosis and treatment is essential. If the hip has been dislocated, it must be repositioned and maintained in that position. If ligaments or muscles have been torn, the child may wear a spica (body) cast for between 6 weeks and 9 months. Traction may be necessary prior to casting.

When the child has been walking for several years before diagnosis, skeletal traction may be used to try to abduct the

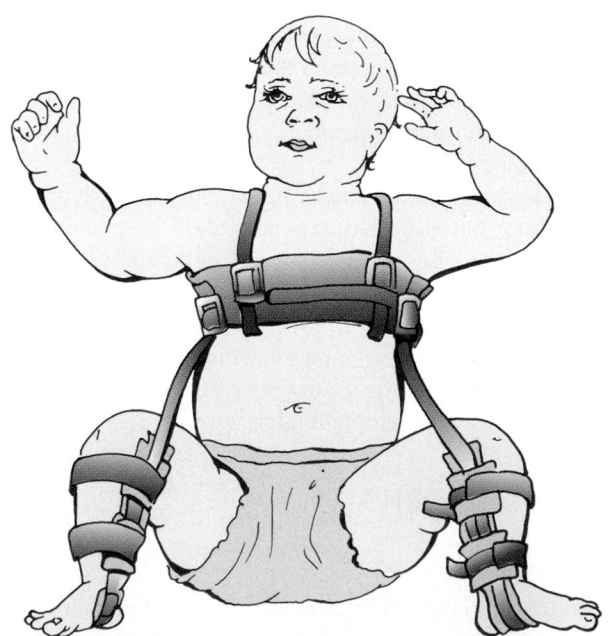

FIGURE 71-2. An infant in a Pavlik harness. The harness consists of shoulder straps, stirrups, and a chest strap. It is placed on both legs even if only one hip is dislocated. (Nettina, S. M. [2000]. *The Lippincott manual of nursing practice* [7th ed.]. Philadelphia: Lippincott Williams & Wilkins.)

hips gradually. If this measure is unsuccessful, surgical repair is necessary. If closed reduction under general anesthesia and casting are unsuccessful, an open reduction (through an incision) is performed. A *tenotomy* (transection of a tendon) may also be necessary. If the child has not been treated and is over 6 years of age, the prognosis for prolonged maintenance of the repair is poor.

Nursing Considerations. Handle the child carefully but pick up him or her to encourage normal social development. Protect the pillow splint or cast from soiling and wetting. Cover the perineal area with moisture-proof protection.

Normal rules for cast care apply (see Chap. 76). Watch for any signs of irritation or pressure. Turn the child often. Help the child to exercise if possible, and take him or her to the play room and to meals.

Instruct family caregivers in the child's care. Obtaining a hospital bed with a Balkan or Bradford frame and overhead trapeze is helpful, so the child can move about in bed.

> **Nursing Alert**
>
> Skin care is especially important for the infant or child in a corrective device. Avoid using powders and lotions because "caking" or "pilling" can occur, causing added skin irritation.

Talipes

The term *clubfoot* or **talipes** describes a foot that is twisted or bent out of shape as a result of hereditary factors or an abnormal fetal position (Fig. 71-3A). It may be flexible (due to intrauterine positioning) or rigid and fixed. The condition occurs more commonly in boys and more often in multiple than in single births. Unilateral clubfoot is slightly more common than bilateral clubfoot.

Medical Treatment. Treatment includes casting or splinting to correct the deformity (Fig. 71-3B); sequential casting at 1- to 2-week intervals is usual. Surgery may be necessary for older children or for those with severe defects. The type of surgery depends on the specific defect. In young children, usually the soft tissues only need to be repositioned because bones are not yet calcified. In older children, the bones may require repositioning and casting.

Nursing Considerations.   Follow the usual procedures and precautions for observing and caring for children in casts. Teach family caregivers what symptoms and complications to look for. Remind them that they need a great deal of patience, because a child may be in a splint or cast for several years.

Torticollis

Torticollis, also called "wryneck," may be congenital or acquired by damage to the nerves or muscles. The congenital type is caused by failure of the sternocleidomastoid muscle to lengthen as the child grows. It must be corrected, or curvature of the upper spine and abnormal elevation of the shoulders will result.

Treatment includes passive or active exercises, surgical correction, or casting. The child must be examined periodically until after puberty to prevent recurrence.

NEUROLOGIC DISORDERS

Reye's Syndrome

Reye's syndrome is an acute and potentially fatal childhood disease. Its etiology is unknown; however, in most cases it follows a viral illness. Reye's syndrome also has been related to aspirin use during a viral illness, although this link is somewhat controversial.

Characteristics of the disease include fever, cerebral edema, impaired liver function, and severely impaired LOC. Elevated blood ammonia levels are also present. Treatment is supportive. Commonly used medications include osmotic diuretics, sedatives, and barbiturates. Assess the child's respiratory status frequently.

Public education regarding the dangers of aspirin use for sick children has been credited for the drastic reduction in incidences of this disease. Early diagnosis and aggressive medical intervention have greatly improved the prognosis for children who contract it. Some children who were once diagnosed with Reye's syndrome are now being diagnosed with other conditions through improved diagnostic techniques.

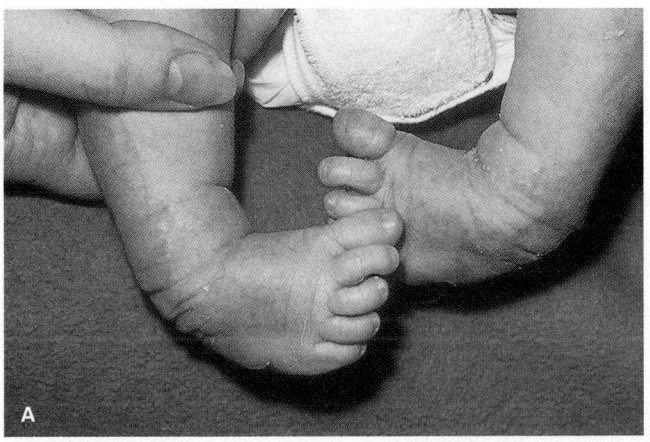
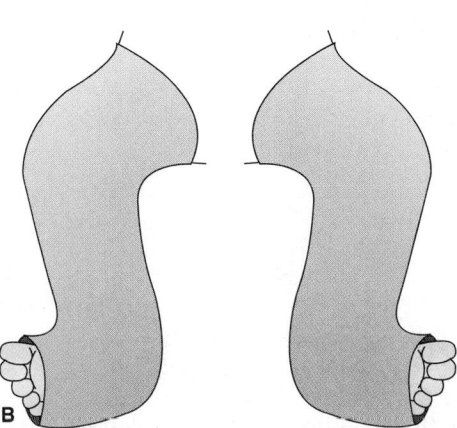

FIGURE 71-3. (A) Talipes equinovarus. **(B)** Casts are applied to treat bilateral clubfoot.

Meningitis

Meningitis is an acute inflammation of the meninges of the brain. It may be caused by bacteria or viruses. In neonates, meningitis is most commonly caused by group B streptococci and *Escherichia coli* organisms. In children older than 2 months, the common organisms are *Haemophilus influenzae* (incidence has decreased since infants have been receiving the Hib immunization), *Streptococcus pneumoniae,* and *Neisseria meningitidis (meningococcal meningitis).*

Symptoms include fever and *nuchal rigidity* (neck stiffness). A lumbar puncture determines the presence of organisms in the spinal fluid. Viral meningitis is treated symptomatically. In bacterial meningitis, intravenous fluids and antibiotics are administered. Isolation is necessary until the child has been on antibiotics for 24 hours. Decreased environmental stimulation and neurologic checks are essential. Elevate the head of the bed to lessen the increased intracranial pressure that is due to edema. Monitor intake and output.

Serious complications may result from meningitis, such as hydrocephalus, learning disabilities, seizure disorders, and deafness. Chemoprophylaxis with rifampin may be necessary for healthcare workers, family members, and daycare workers who come in close contact with meningitis. Provide support to the family and keep them informed of the child's progress. Encourage them to express their feelings of blame and guilt (see Chapter 77 for further discussion of meningitis).

Encephalocele

If the bones in the fetal skull do not close correctly, a portion of the brain may *herniate* (protrude) through the opening. This condition is known as **encephalocele.** The amount of damage to the child's functioning depends on the encephalocele's size and location, and on the presence or absence of strangulation or rupture in the brain. The chief danger in this condition is possible rupture of the meningeal sac, leading almost inevitably to meningitis or encephalitis. The defect can be surgically corrected; surgery is sometimes delayed until the child is 1 year old.

Spina Bifida

Spina bifida is a malformation in which a part of the vertebral or spinal column (usually the lower spine) is open or missing. The condition may be asymptomatic or may cause severe paralysis, depending on how large the opening is and whether the meninges or spinal cord herniate through the opening. Amniocentesis or ultrasound can detect this disorder in a fetus. The examiner checks the amniotic fluid for α-fetoprotein, which, if present, indicates an abnormality. The pregnant woman may have an elective abortion. Genetic counseling may be indicated.

Folic acid (folate) taken during pregnancy helps to prevent spina bifida (and other neural-tube defects). The three forms of this disorder are spina bifida occulta, meningocele, and meningomyelocele:

- **Spinal bifida occulta** is an opening in the child's vertebral column with no apparent symptoms (Fig. 71-4B). It is discovered only if an x-ray examination of the child's spine is done for an unrelated reason, or if an investigation is done because a dimple is present over the backbone. A small tuft of hair or a port-wine stain sometimes appears in the vertebral area. Although this condition may cause the child problems during the pubescent growth spurt, it generally does not cause any difficulty. It may be corrected by surgery if necessary.
- **Meningocele** occurs when one layer of the meninges (the spinal cord covering) herniates through an opening in the vertebral column (Fig. 71-4C). The child with a meningocele will have a visible sac on the back, but may show no disability; conversely, he or she may experience muscle weakness, difficulty with bowel and bladder control, and (rarely) paralysis. Corrective surgery is needed. Generally, the child leads a normal life after surgery.
- **Meningomyelocele** or *myelomeningocele* (see Fig. 71-4D) is the most serious form of spina bifida. The meninges and part of the spinal cord protrude through an opening. The child has a visible sac on the back. He or she is usually paralyzed, and may have bladder and bowel

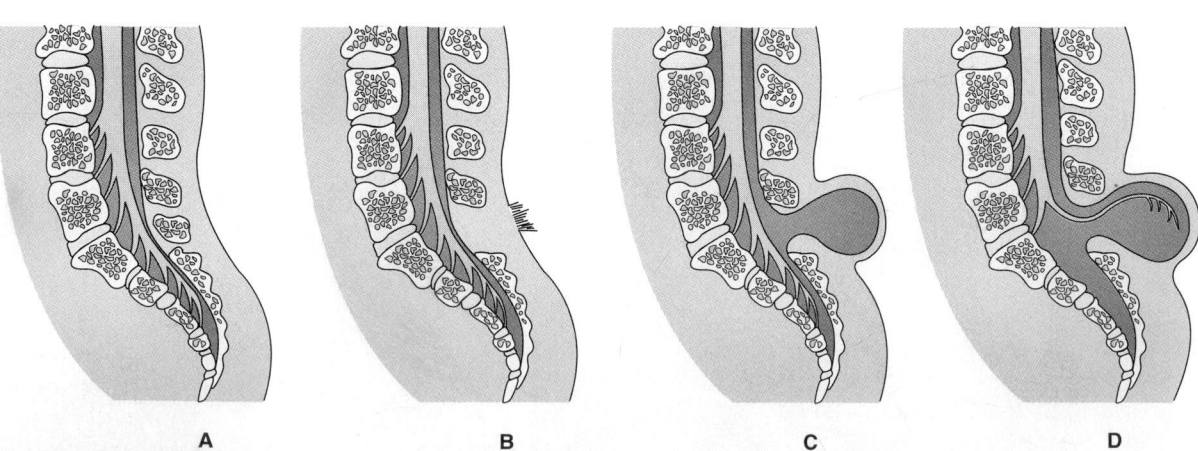

FIGURE 71-4. Spina bifida. (**A**) Normal spine. (**B**) Spina bifida occulta. (**C**) Spina bifida with meningocele. (**D**) Spina bifida with myelomeningocele.

control problems. Serious possible complications include meningitis (inflammation of the meninges covering the spinal cord), encephalitis, and hydrocephalus (see next section). You must handle the defect with great care to avoid injury to the sac or damage to the spinal cord. Surgery is necessary to prevent infection and to preserve as much nerve function as possible. It is often done soon after birth.

Nursing Considerations.

A nursing goal in treating children with spina bifida is to prevent further damage. The most common problem is loss of leg sensation, so be sure to protect the child against possible leg injury. Careful examination also is necessary to assess for pressure areas and tight clothing, which can be irritating and cause skin breakdown or lack of sufficient circulation. Give good skin care, and change diapers immediately and with great care after the child voids or defecates.

Assist in preoperative and postoperative surgical management. Take precautions to protect the child from infection in the area of the defect. Another common site for infection is the bladder, because the child is often catheterized. Teach caregivers to clean the catheter every few hours. The child can be predisposed to infection if the catheter is improperly managed. If kidney damage or other urinary system damage occurs, a urinary tract diversion may be required.

Pay special attention to the child's positioning, because preventing musculoskeletal deformities is important. Also assist the child with range-of-motion exercises (passive or active). A physical therapist usually sees the child regularly. Frequently, orthopedic surgery must be performed to correct accompanying deformities, such as hip dysplasia or clubfoot. Your role as a nurse is to provide psychological support to family caregivers and the child.

Children with spina bifida may need support services involving many specialists throughout their life. Urinary incontinence is one of the most difficult complications that threatens social acceptance.

> ✚👁 **N u r s i n g   A l e r t**
> For some reason, children with spina bifida tend to be extremely sensitive to latex. Make sure such children do not come in contact with items such as tourniquets, catheters, rubber bands, gloves, balloons, or various tubes made of latex.

Hydrocephalus

Spinal fluid, which circulates constantly, encloses the CNS. If this circulation is disrupted, spinal fluid collects, causing head swelling and brain damage. This condition is called **hydrocephalus**. It often results from improper development of the brain or spinal cord or from a spinal cord defect (eg, spina bifida). It can also occur as a complication of meningitis, head injury, or cranial hemorrhage.

Symptoms and Treatment.

The symptoms of hydrocephalus include a progressive increase in the head's circum-ference. The sutures between the cranial bones open, because of increased fluid accumulation. Brain tissue *atrophies* (shrinks) progressively as cranial cavity pressure increases. Be alert to the possibility of seizures. The severely affected or untreated child cannot control voluntary muscle movements and may die from respiratory complications, malnutrition, or infection. Diagnosis of hydrocephalus is made on the basis of lumbar puncture, computed tomography (CT) scan, positron emission tomography (PET) scan, or magnetic resonance imaging (MRI) studies. Sometimes the CT scan is enhanced by the injection of an intravenous dye called iohexol (Omnipaque). An electroencephalogram (**EEG**) may also be done.

Treatment for hydrocephalus is to insert a *shunt* (bypass) surgically, allowing the fluid to circulate around the defect or blockage (Fig. 71-5). Shunts are *ventriculoperitoneal* or *ventriculoatrial* (from the ventricles of the brain to the peritoneal cavity or into the heart). The ventriculoperitoneal shunt is the preferred route. The shunt should be inserted as soon as possible after birth, because brain damage is irreversible.

Nursing Considerations.

Preoperatively, give skin care to prevent skin breakdown, and take precautions to prevent infection. Turn the child frequently from side to side to prevent aspiration and pressure sores. Especially prevent pressure areas on the enlarged, fragile head and the ears.

You may need to give gavage feedings or total parenteral nutrition (TPN) to prevent malnutrition in a child with hydrocephalus, because this child often has difficulty eating. Feed the child carefully and slowly. Place the child's head, neck, and shoulders on a soft pillow, to evenly distribute the pressure that would otherwise be exerted on the infant's head.

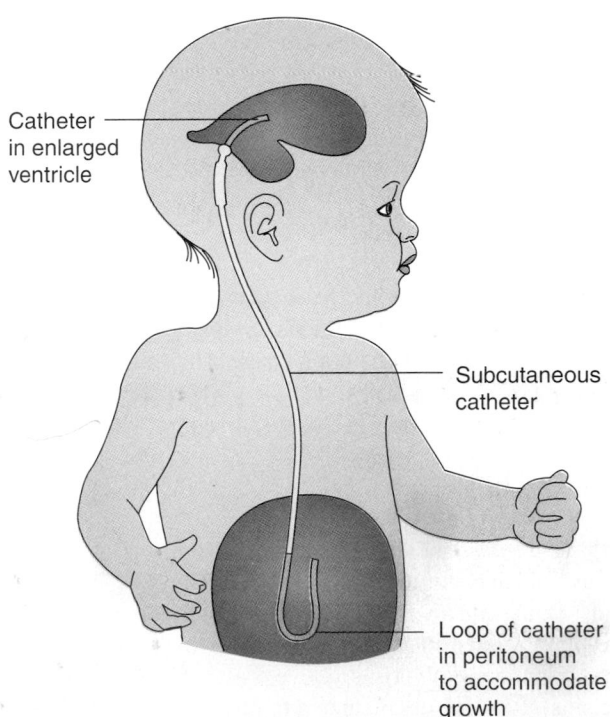

Catheter in enlarged ventricle

Subcutaneous catheter

Loop of catheter in peritoneum to accommodate growth

FIGURE 71-5. A ventriculoperitoneal shunt removes excessive cerebrospinal fluid from the ventricles and shunts it to the peritoneum. A one-way valve is present in the tubing behind the ear.

Assess the child's head carefully. Assess the fontanelles for tension or fullness; measure and record the occipital-frontal circumference (OFC) daily (see Chap. 66). Keep the head clean and dry.

Postoperatively, assess for signs of shock or hemorrhage and check the incisional area for spinal fluid leakage. Take vital signs according to your facility's routines or as directed by the physician.

Position the child away from the operative side to prevent pressure and damage to the shunt valve and the suture line. Record I&O accurately to determine if the child is retaining fluids. Restraints may be needed.

Because shunts are not always effective, observe carefully for any signs of increasing intracranial pressure, such as increasing irritability, bulging fontanelles, and changes in eye signs or LOC. Another frequent complication is infection; report any sign of it immediately. If the shunt is performed before brain damage occurs and is successful, the child can lead a normal life.

Family caregivers need to know major developmental milestones to identify any problems their child has after discharge. Encourage them to prepare goals for their child that are appropriate to his or her ability and potential. Focusing on the child's strengths is important. Referral to special education programs may be necessary.

☞ KEY CONCEPT

Head measurements (OFC and other measurements, as ordered) are an important aspect of nursing care in hydrocephalus. An increase in head size indicates increasing fluid in the brain. For this reason, measure the head's circumference at the same site every time. Mark the head with ink or indicate on a drawing exactly where you are taking measurements. In this way, each nurse will measure in the same location, allowing for accurate comparison. Use a disposable paper tape. Document your measurements carefully, usually in centimeters (cm).

Microcephaly

The **microcephalic** child has a very small brain. The head tends to be small, and the child is intellectually impaired to a degree determined by the brain's size. This condition is congenital. No cure is known, and the child is treated symptomatically. Microcephaly is also discussed in Chapter 68.

Febrile Seizures

Febrile seizures are generalized convulsions of unknown etiology, which occur in children between the ages of 6 months and 3 years, and are more common in males. Febrile seizures are often related to acute illnesses in which a child's body temperature rapidly rises above 101.8° Fahrenheit (38.8° Celsius). Risk factors include a family or personal history of febrile seizures and neurologic disorders.

Treatment of febrile seizures is aimed at controlling fever with antipyretics (acetaminophen, ibuprofen), tepid sponges, or other measures. Medications also may include lorazepam (Ativan) or phenobarbital. Controversy exists over whether or not to institute long-term antiepileptic drug therapy, because febrile seizures are usually benign and related to the high fever only.

Other factors that help determine the appropriateness of long-term drug therapy include EEG findings, the age at which the first seizure occurred, the recurrence of seizures, and the seizure type (generalized versus other types). Chapter 77 contains a discussion of seizure disorders. Reassure the parents of the benign nature of the seizure and of the fact that most children do not develop a seizure disorder. Teach early management of fever and seizures at home.

Breath-Holding Spells

A *breath-holding spell* is an episode during which a child holds his or her breath and becomes unconscious (usually following a period of intense crying). Most authorities counsel parents to ignore these benign episodes because the child will usually outgrow them by 5 years of age.

A typical breath-holding episode may occur following a fall in which the child hits his or her head. The child begins to cry violently and holds his or her breath, resulting in a period of unconsciousness, with some myoclonic (muscle-jerking)-type movements. This activity mimics a seizure, and can be frightening for family caregivers. Assure parents that this is not true seizure activity. The child then begins to breathe spontaneously and recovers. Other injuries and tantrums may result in breath-holding episodes.

METABOLIC AND NUTRITIONAL DISORDERS

Marasmus

Marasmus describes a general failure-to-thrive condition. It seems to be related to such conditions as **kwashiorkor** (protein deficiency), **rickets** (vitamin D deficiency), and **scurvy** (vitamin C deficiency). Marasmus is a separate condition often caused by a general systemic disease, an absorption problem, neglect, or abuse.

Symptoms of marasmus include wasting and atrophy of body tissues. In contrast to kwashiorkor, no edema is present. The child's eyes are sunken, head size is small, and body temperature is low. The child is generally weak and listless. Physical growth lags behind that of other children of the same age. Mental development may or may not be slowed, but severe malnutrition in infancy contributes to slow brain growth and threatens future mental ability. These children are truly starving and will suck on anything available (eg, clothing or fingers).

Nursing care involves restoration of hydration and nutrition, maintenance of body temperature, and general tender loving care. The child usually responds well to treatment.

Many caregivers are not knowledgeable about diets and parenting. An important part of nursing care in such cases is to teach caregivers nutrition and general aspects of child care.

Include the importance of hygiene, affection, and play. Teach caregivers feeding routines (such as giving solids), holding the baby, keeping air out of the neck of the bottle, and bubbling.

Biliary Atresia

One cause of malnutrition may be **biliary atresia,** a defect in the bile ducts that prevents bile from escaping from the liver. The lack of bile causes defective digestion and elimination. In most cases, surgery must be performed to relieve the obstruction. Liver transplantation may also be considered.

Celiac Disease

The most common malabsorption syndrome in children of European descent is **celiac disease,** a chronic intestinal disorder. It involves small bowel inflammation and nutrient malabsorption. Celiac disease is thought to be congenital, although its effects may not appear for several months or years after birth. Usually, however, the condition manifests itself within 6 months after birth.

The basic defect in this disease is an intolerance of the protein *gluten* found in wheat, oats, barley, and rye. When children with celiac disease eat food containing glutens, the small intestine gradually becomes less able to absorb food through the intestinal villi into the bloodstream. These children are specifically unable to absorb fats. Remission usually occurs when family caregivers omit gluten-containing foods from the child's diet. Breastfeeding seems to postpone the appearance of symptoms because breast milk lacks glutens.

Celiac disease is characterized by large, floating, fatty stools; anorexia; undernutrition and FTT; distended abdomen and wasted buttocks; excessive flatus; and arrested growth. A jejunal biopsy and the child's clinical improvement when placed on a gluten-free diet verify the diagnosis. Before treatment, the child may also have a lactose intolerance (see later section), which improves with treatment. More than one child in a family may have the disorder, indicating a familial tendency. The disorder varies in degree from mild to severe. The severe form of the disorder is discussed here.

Medical Treatment.   Treatment of celiac disease includes strict adherence to a gluten-free diet. The person is not allowed any cereal grains, such as wheat, barley, rye, and oats, and is not allowed any malt. The person must follow this difficult diet in some form for life. However, after the growth spurt of adolescence, he or she may introduce a small amount of gluten-containing foods. If any difficulty occurs, the person must remove the foods again.

☛ Key Concept

Celiac disease requires that family caregivers must learn to read labels very carefully to avoid ingredients containing gluten. Gluten is found in prepared soups, processed ice cream, cakes, cookies, other baked goods, pastas, some milk products such as malts, and lunch meat. The school-age child may have an especially difficult time when planning meals away from home.

Phenylketonuria

Phenylketonuria (**PKU**) is a hereditary metabolic disorder. If untreated, PKU causes severe mental retardation that begins during the first months of life. As a result of the absence of the liver enzyme *phenylalanine hydroxylase,* phenylalanine is not converted to tyrosine and phenylketones build up in the blood and tissues, causing permanent brain damage. In addition, melanin is not formed; therefore, persons with PKU are most often blue eyed and blond with sensitive skin. A blood test obtained by a heelstick after the newborn has consumed formula or breast milk for at least 2 days detects PKU (see Chap. 66). The test is required by law in most states. However, because the baby is usually discharged from the birthing facility soon after delivery, the test needs to be repeated when the baby is 2 weeks old. (The blood test is inaccurate until the newborn has had several feedings of formula or breast milk.) If the baby is born at home, caregivers will need to take the baby to a healthcare facility for testing no later than 2 weeks after birth.

Existing damage is irreversible; but treatment, which must begin as soon as possible, prevents further damage. The only treatment is a diet very low in phenylalanine, an essential amino acid necessary for growth and repair of body cells. Family caregivers should use a low-phenylalanine formula such as Lofenalac in place of the usual milk in the diet. The child should avoid phenylalanine-containing foods, including most breads, eggs, meat, milk, cheese, legumes, nuts, and artificial sweeteners containing phenylalanine, such as aspartame (Nutra-Sweet).

The child can eat low-protein natural foods, such as fruits, vegetables, and certain cereals. A dietitian will prescribe a diet that provides a safe amount of phenylalanine, yet will maintain the serum amounts below the toxic level.

These dietary restrictions usually continue until late childhood or adolescence, when the person has achieved most brain growth. The time to discontinue the diet is controversial, with some experts recommending indefinite adherence to the restrictions.

DISORDERS OF THE EYES

Strabismus

Strabismus, commonly known as "squint" or "crossed eyes," is an inability to appropriately move the eyes. Although strabismus is usually congenital, it may result from a childhood disease. The normal newborn appears cross-eyed because he or she has not yet developed control of the eye muscles (*pseudostrabismus*). However, strabismus found in a child older than 6 weeks of age requires evaluation.

The two chief classifications of strabismus are *paralytic strabismus* (the muscles of one eye are underactive) and *concomitant strabismus* (both eyes move, but the deviation of the affected eye is always the same). Other terms associated with strabismus are *convergent* (both eyes looking toward the center), *divergent* (both eyes looking outward), and *vertical* (the affected eye [or eyes] moves only on a vertical plane).

Concomitant strabismus may involve the same eye (*monocular*), both eyes alternately (*alternating*), or both eyes (*binocular*). The person uses the unaffected eye at any particular time. If the child uses one eye all the time, the other eye does not participate in vision, and the resulting double vision (*diplopia*) causes the unused eye to weaken.

In *alternate strabismus,* each eye is dominant at different times and monocular weakness is less likely. In *latent strabismus,* great effort is needed to overcome the muscle imbalance, so the child complains of eye strain, headache, and diplopia.

Medical Treatment.   The unaffected eye is patched to stimulate the unused eye; corrective eyeglasses, which can be prescribed as early as 1 year of age, are ordered. Eye exercises and miotic drugs are prescribed to contract the pupils of the eyes. Treatment begins early to prevent further damage and to improve the child's appearance.

Surgical intervention may be done to the affected muscles to match the unaffected muscles. Sometimes a computer is used to more accurately calculate the correction.

Nursing Considerations.   Prepare the child preoperatively if he or she is to be on bed rest or is to have the eyes covered following surgery. Surgery is done in a same-day or outpatient surgery setting. Often elbow restraints are necessary after surgery to prevent the child from touching the eyes. Speak to, before touching, the child whose eyes are covered, to avoid frightening him or her.

The child is usually up and about soon after surgery. Many children with strabismus have photophobia; sunglasses may help. Teach the child and family caregivers preoperative and postoperative care.

Other Eye Disorders

Infants may have *congenital glaucoma,* an increase in intraocular pressure with symptoms of an enlarged, edematous, and hazy cornea and increased tearing, pain, and photophobia. Surgery may be necessary.

Cataracts may be present at birth or can occur due to eye trauma or disease. The pupil appears to be white and the red reflex cannot be elicited. Surgical removal with insertion of internal contacts is necessary.

Amblyopia ("lazy eye") is subnormal vision in one eye, which may fail to develop due to lack of visual stimulation because the child always uses the good eye for vision. Blindness may develop in the "lazy eye." Strabismus or refractive errors may contribute to amblyopia. Treatment consists of patching the good eye to force the child to use the underdeveloped eye. Correction of strabismus and refractive errors is also essential.

A small child's eye muscles are not developed enough to permit normal pupil accommodation. However, because other factors also may be involved, the child should be examined regularly after 3 years of age (or earlier if symptoms appear). Red, puffy, and watering eyes, or frequent rubbing of the eyes, may indicate difficulty in seeing. The child also may complain of dizziness, headache, or double vision. Determine whether visual difficulties arise from an error of refraction, which can

usually be corrected by eyeglasses, or from another problem, such as a brain tumor.

Ptosis, or drooping eyelids, is usually congenital. In most cases, it is corrected by surgery.

DISORDERS OF THE EARS, NOSE, THROAT, AND MOUTH

Otitis Media

Otitis media, an acute infection of the middle ear, is the most common bacterial infection of early childhood, most often caused by nasopharyngeal reflux or eustachian tube dysfunction. Most children have at least one episode of otitis media. Bacterial organisms can travel through the eustachian tube in an infant or young child much more readily than in an adult. This is due to the fact that the eustachian tube is wider and more horizontal in children, allowing bacteria from the nasopharynx to readily enter the middle ear.

Otitis media is defined as *acute* if its onset is rapid and short, *subacute* if fluid involvement lasts between 3 weeks and 3 months, and *chronic* if it lasts longer than 3 months. Complications include hearing loss, a scarred or ruptured tympanic membrane (eardrum), inner ear infection, mastoiditis (inflammation of the mastoid process), or meningitis.

One primary cause of otitis media is passive smoke inhalation. Infants and young children who live in homes with smokers have a higher incidence of otitis media. Bacterial infections, viral nasopharyngitis, enlargement of nasopharyngeal lymphoid tissue, tumors, foreign bodies, allergies, and other physiologic factors may cause eustachian tube dysfunction. Breast-fed babies have a lower incidence of otitis media, perhaps because they receive immunoglobulin A, which protects against respiratory viruses and allergies. Breast-fed infants are also held in a more upright position than are bottle-fed babies. Propping a baby's bottle may allow fluid to flow through the eustachian tube, causing otitis media.

Pain may be present with otitis media. The infant may express the pain by pulling on or scratching the ear and being irritable. Older children will complain of pain. Signs of infection, a temperature as high as 104° F (40° C), swollen glands, and loss of appetite (sometimes with vomiting) are other symptoms. Occasionally, family caregivers are surprised when a healthcare provider points out a child's red, swollen eardrum, because the child had not indicated any type of ear discomfort.

Definite diagnosis is made when a bulging tympanic membrane is seen on otoscopic examination. Landmarks of the bony prominences are obscured. If the eardrum ruptures, bleeding or purulent drainage may occur.

The most serious complication of otitis media is hearing loss, which may be permanent. Hearing loss occurs from scarring as a result of repeated infections. In many children, hearing loss may go undetected until they enter school. Other complications include mastoiditis and occasionally encephalitis or meningitis. These conditions are rare with the administration of antibiotic therapy.

Medical Treatment.   Antihistamines and decongestants may be administered for otitis media. Warm, moist packs may provide comfort. Some children experience more comfort with an ice pack because it tends to reduce edema. Acetaminophen for fever and (if the child is older than 6 years) codeine for pain may be prescribed. Antibiotics are also prescribed. After 10 days, the healthcare provider inspects the child's ears. If the tympanic membrane remains red or if other symptoms persist, another course of antibiotic therapy may be indicated.

Surgical Treatment. If repeated medical therapies with antibiotics are unsuccessful, surgical options may be considered. Treatment of otitis media involves restoring the normal eustachian tube function and maintaining or improving hearing.

An ear, nose, and throat physician specialist called an *otolaryngologist* may perform an outpatient procedure called a *myringotomy*. This procedure involves making a surgical opening into the eardrum and inserting a polyethylene (**PE**) ventilating tube as a temporary or permanent accessory eustachian tube. The PE tube allows drainage of the accumulated fluid from the middle ear and equalization of pressure on each side of the eardrum (Fig. 71-6). Hearing is usually restored after placement of the PE tube.

The child with a PE tube must avoid getting water into the ears when swimming, taking a shower, or shampooing the hair. Special ear plugs may be prescribed.

Other surgical procedures in otitis media are *tympanoplasty*, which involves reconstruction of the middle ear either with the placement of a homograft transplant of the structure or with a prosthesis, and myringoplasty. A *myringoplasty* is reconstruction of the eardrum, usually with a graft of temporalis fascia.

Epistaxis

Epistaxis (nosebleed) is common in children and usually originates in the anterior portion of the nares. Common causes of epistaxis include foreign objects pushed into the nose, systemic disorders, trauma, allergy, and dry mucous membranes. Dry mucous membranes lead to cracking, crusts, and nose

picking. Treatment consists of applying pressure or cold compresses across the bridge of the nose for 5 to 10 minutes. Usually the bleeding will stop. Have the child sit up and tilt the head forward, to minimize pressure on the nasal blood vessels and to prevent blood from running down the posterior pharynx.

For serious or stubborn nosebleeds, a physician may need to pack the child's nose to stop hemorrhage. A child's blood volume is lower than an adult's, so epistaxis is potentially dangerous. Also the child may swallow blood. Report any symptoms, such as vomiting "coffee-ground" material. Cautery, or application of a substance such as silver nitrate, is used to control epistaxis if it occurs frequently.

> ✚👁 **N u r s i n g   A l e r t**
>
> If a child with a nosebleed also has a head injury, do not stop the bleeding without specific physician's orders. *Rationale: Holding blood inside the nasal cavity can increase intracranial pressure.*

Tonsillitis

Tonsillitis, an inflammation of the tonsils, is caused by a virus or a bacteria. Symptoms include a sore, reddened throat, with swelling and sometimes exudate on the tonsils. Swallowing is difficult, and the child's WBC count and temperature may be elevated. A throat culture can determine the offending organism, and drug sensitivity tests will signify the treatment of choice. Viral infections are treated symptomatically.

☛ Key Concept

Because the tonsils are so close to the eustachian tubes, tonsillitis can easily spread to the middle ear and cause otitis media. Infants and toddlers are most often affected because their eustachian tubes are shorter and straighter than those of adults.

Medical and Surgical Treatment. The child is kept in a high-humidity environment and antibiotics are administered if the cause is bacterial. If the child has difficulty swallowing, a soft diet may be offered. Fluids are encouraged, and antipyretics (acetaminophen, ibuprofen) are given to lower temperature and relieve discomfort.

If the child has had numerous streptococcal infections in a short time, removal of the tonsils (*tonsillectomy*) may be indicated, although this procedure is controversial. Tonsillectomy also may be done in the case of a recurring *peritonsillar* (around the tonsil) abscess. Tonsillectomy is rarely done following a single episode of tonsillitis. Removal of the tonsils and adenoids is called a tonsillectomy and adenoidectomy (**T&A**).

Nursing Considerations. Most T&A surgery is performed in same-day surgery centers. Before surgery, the child must be free of URIs. Accurate assessment is necessary on admission.

Instruct family caregivers in preoperative measures to perform at home. Routine preparation includes giving the child nothing by mouth (NPO) after midnight. When the child arrives

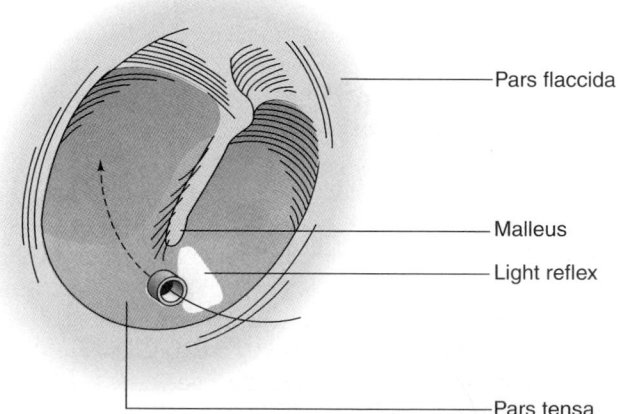

Pars flaccida

Malleus

Light reflex

Pars tensa

FIGURE 71-6. A myringotomy tube provides air to the middle ear to prevent serious otitis media.

at the facility, check to determine if he or she has a URI. Report and document the presence of loose teeth. Preoperative medication may be given to young children.

Direct postoperative nursing care at preventing hemorrhage, the most common complication. Observe the child for spitting up of a great deal of bloody sputum or vomiting of "coffee-ground" material. The child may swallow blood, so some vomiting of dark blood is not unusual. Assess bloody sputum or vomiting. Position the child on the side or abdomen or with the head of the bed elevated to prevent aspiration.

Encourage fluids after the child is awake and fully responding. Clear, bland fluids are best; milk tends to form a film in the throat. Children usually accept ice pops, non-acetic fruit drinks, gelatins, and sherbet very well.

➕👁 **N u r s i n g   A l e r t**
Avoid giving red juices and red frozen pops to the child after T&A surgery. Emesis of red juice may be difficult to differentiate from bloody emesis.

Many physicians write a "diet as tolerated" order. Allow children to help choose the foods and liquids that are most appealing within these limits. Do not permit the child to drink fluids through a straw. Sucking can dislodge clots or stitches and lead to hemorrhage. Normal drinking, chewing, and swallowing promote healing. Supervise gum chewing carefully; chewing gum promotes the flow of saliva, which is soothing and facilitates healing.

Use pain medications as needed so that the child can drink more comfortably and rest more easily. Be alert for an elevated temperature postoperatively, which may indicate dehydration and the need to force fluids. Temperature elevation also may point to infection, although infection is uncommon.

The child is usually discharged the day of or the day after surgery. Sometimes an antibiotic prescription may be given as prevention against infection. Give home care instruction to family caregivers, including signs of hemorrhage and respiratory distress. The child should continue with high fluid intake and soft foods. He or she should play quietly and rest in bed for approximately 1 week before returning to school and other normal activities.

Cleft Lip and Cleft Palate

Cleft lip and **cleft palate** are deformities that commonly occur together at birth. They result from failure of the upper lip and palate to close completely during the second and third gestational months (Fig. 71-7). Each of these defects also may occur separately. Cleft lip is more common in boys; cleft palate is more common in girls. Evidence also indicates a slight tendency for familial occurrence.

Cleft lip may be no more than a notch in the upper lip, or it may extend up into the nostril on one or both sides. The cleft ___e *complete* or *incomplete* and may be complicated by ___ctors, such as a lip muscle separated by the cleft, skin ___nner than normal, missing hair follicles and sweat

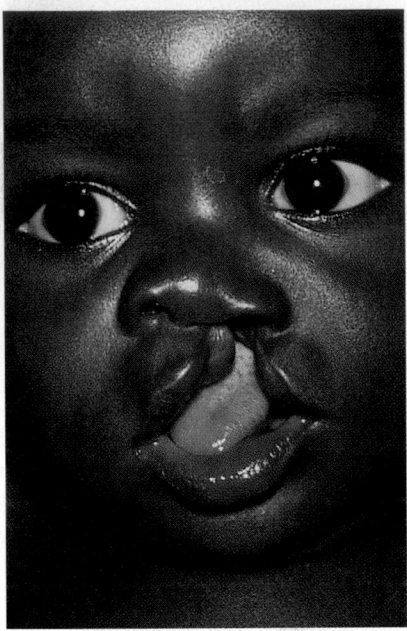

FIGURE 71-7. Unilateral cleft lip. (© 1991 National Medical Slide Bank/CMSP.)

glands, a flattened nostril on the affected side, and a missing part of the jaw and teeth.

Surgical Treatment.   Surgical repair of cleft lip is called a *cheiloplasty.* The cleft is sutured, generally when the child is quite young, to facilitate sucking. Very little preoperative preparation is needed for an infant. The goal of surgery is to restore lip function and to improve the child's appearance.

A skin graft or revision of the scar is often necessary at a later date. The scar is quite prominent immediately after the operation, but usually becomes unnoticeable as the child grows older. A young man may grow a moustache to cover the scar.

Immediate postoperative care is directed toward maintaining the airway, preventing shock or hemorrhage, using proper feeding techniques, and preventing injury to the suture line. Sometimes a Logan bow (curved metal bar) is placed over a repaired cleft lip to decrease tension on the suture line. Often these children need to have PE ventilating tubes inserted in their tympanic membranes to reduce the incidence of ear infections. An elbow restraint may be used to keep children from rubbing the suture lines.

Cleft palate appears as an opening in the roof of the mouth that leads into the nose. Mental retardation is not related to cleft lip or cleft palate. The cleft lip is repaired at a very early age. The cleft palate, however, is repaired later.

Surgical repair of cleft palate is called a *palatoplasty.* It is done when the child is 2 to 6 years old. Repairing the palate before the child develops poor speech habits is desirable. The goals of this surgery are to restore normal speech, to avoid damage to the lip's suture line, and to close the palate as much as possible. The palate may be repaired surgically by placement of a graft, or a dental prosthesis may be used. This prosthesis is either attached to the teeth or used to replace missing teeth and part of the jaw. The prosthesis aids speech by closing the hole between the mouth and nose. Surgical repair of the palate is usually done in one procedure, but it may be carried out in several stages if the cleft is severe.

Dental surgery is often necessary to rebuild missing gums and replace missing teeth. The prosthetic palate may include prosthetic teeth. The mouth must be kept very clean as a protection against tooth decay and infection. Consistent dental care is needed.

Rhinoplasty (repair of the nose) is sometimes necessary to give the nose a balanced appearance; however, it is usually not done until adolescence.

Nursing Considerations. Nursing care begins at birth and involves family teaching. Newborns with these anomalies may upset their families because the defects are so visual. Family members may experience difficult emotions when they first see their child. Also, feelings of guilt may play a great part in the family's adjustment to the child. Be sensitive to the family's feelings. Also be careful not to reveal any personal negative feelings about the infant's appearance.

Feeding. Part of the child's soft palate is missing in cleft palate, and the uvula is almost always absent, as is a part of the hard palate. As a result, the child's mouth and throat are not separated from the nose. Therefore, if the baby is fed by usual methods, he or she regurgitates milk through the nose. If he or she also has a cleft lip, sucking is difficult.

You can feed some of these babies by using a soft nipple with large holes. Hold the baby upright so that he or she does not draw milk into the nose. Occasionally, you may use a special flattened nipple ("duckbill" nipple) or a cleft palate nipple with a flap to cover the hole in the palate. In other cases, you will use a special feeder. Fig. 71-8 illustrates feeders that may be used to facilitate nutrition.

The following are recommendations for feeding infants with cleft lip and/or palate:

- Feed slowly in small amounts, and bubble frequently. Give some clear water last.
- Hold the infant upright, but cuddle and talk to the infant while feeding.
- Clean the mouth and cleft carefully, after each feeding.
- Dilute solids and spoon-feed them.
- In extreme cases, gavage feeding may be necessary until part of the palate is covered.
- Prevent aspiration.

Providing Oral Care. Oral hygiene is essential. Give a small infant sterile water after feeding; encourage the older child to use mouthwash and to brush their teeth often.

Preventing Infection. Because the pathway is open between the mouth and nose, swallowing does not equalize pressure in the eustachian tubes. Infections develop easily and may cause partial hearing loss. Instruct caregivers in ways to prevent ear infections. They should protect these children against colds and URIs.

Addressing Emotional Aspects. How a child adjusts to a cleft lip or palate depends largely on how family caregivers and others react to the deformity. Group discussion with other family caregivers who have faced the same problem provides support. Caregivers can learn to help their child deal with teasing.

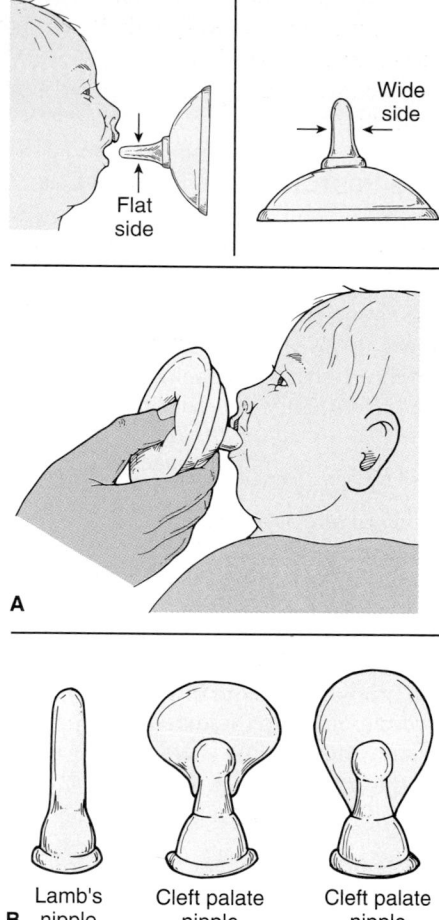

FIGURE 71-8. Nipples used for feeding newborns with cleft lip and palate. **(A)** Beniflex nurser (courtesy of Mead Johnson, Evansville, IN). **(B)** Other types of nipples.

Providing Postoperative Care. Aim nursing care at preventing strain on the suture line and preventing deformities or complications. Do not allow sucking or insert anything into the mouth (see In Practice: Nursing Care Guidelines 71-1).

Baby Bottle Syndrome

If bottle feeding continues after a child has teeth, or if a child uses a bottle as a pacifier, a deformity called *baby bottle syndrome* (nursing bottle mouth) can occur. Baby bottle syndrome is caused by the bottle's contents continually coming into contact with the baby's teeth for prolonged periods, resulting in numerous dental caries. This condition most frequently occurs in children between 18 and 36 months of age. Instruct caregivers how to prevent this condition by following the instructions listed at In Practice: Educating the Client 71-3.

CARDIOVASCULAR DISORDERS

Disorders of the cardiovascular system can result from defects, diseases, hemorrhage, fluid and electrolyte imbalance, neurologic disorders, or poison ingestion. Some

Atresia closing of normal opening

In Practice
Nursing Care Guidelines 71-1

PROVIDING POSTOPERATIVE CARE IN CHEILOPLASTY AND PALATOPLASTY

Cheiloplasty (Cleft Lip Repair)
Use the following care measures:

- Apply a tongue-blade arm restraint or another type of arm restraint. *Rationale: Prevent the child from bending the elbows to touch the suture line.*
- Position the child on the back or side but not the abdomen. *Rationale: Prevent the child from rubbing the surgical site against the bed.*
- Cleanse the suture line after each feeding and as necessary with prescribed solution. *Rationale: Promote healing and prevent undue scarring.*
- Try to ease the child's crying. Provide quiet diversion whenever possible. *Rationale: Keep the child from pulling on the suture line.*
- Give glucose water first, then formula, as per physician's orders. Feed the child with a Brecht nipple, preemie nipple, medicine dropper, syringe, or small spoon, depending on the extent of the repair, the child's age, and the physician's order. *Rationale: Prevent injury to the surgical site, while providing adequate nutrition and medications.*
- Give the child water after the formula. *Rationale: Clear away any mucus that forms, and promote healing of the site.*
- Unless ordered by the physician, do not allow the child to use straws. *Rationale: Straw use may place pressure on the surgical site.*

Palatoplasty (Cleft Palate Repair)
Provide nursing care similar to that for cleft lip repair, except for the following:

- Place the child on the abdomen or side, not on the back. *Rationale: Decrease choking and danger of aspiration.*

- Keep the child's mouth clean and free from irritation. *Rationale: The suture line is inside the mouth. Cleanliness helps promote healing.*
- If the child is old enough to understand, tell him or her not to rub the site with his or her tongue. *Rationale: Help maintain the integrity of the suture line and promote healing.*
- The child may be NPO for the first 24 to 48 hours after surgery. Then advance the diet to liquids (may be necessary for 10 to 14 days postoperatively). After the child tolerates liquids and you receive the physician's order, advance the diet to soft solids. Prevent the child from eating potato chips, popcorn, candy, and other hard or scratchy foods. Teach family caregivers dietary restrictions. *Rationale: Avoid foods that can damage the child's suture line.*
- Discourage the child from sucking and blowing. Do not use a nipple or straw to feed the child; he or she should take fluids from a cup. *Rationale: Sucking can strain the suture line; blowing can force fluids into the eustachian tube.*
- Do not use foods with extremes in temperature. *Rationale: The child may not have sensation in the roof of the mouth, and extremely hot or cold foods could injure the area.*
- Feed the child from the side of a spoon. Do not insert the spoon into the child's mouth. *Rationale: Prevent damage to the suture line.*
- Be sure to teach family caregivers appropriate care and dietary restrictions. *Rationale: Caregivers will provide most care. Teaching provides a chance for practice.*

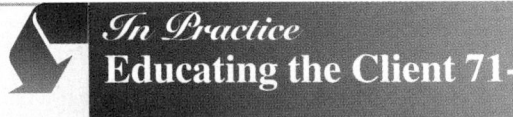

In Practice
Educating the Client 71-3

BABY BOTTLE SYNDROME PREVENTION

- Never prop a bottle.
- Do not give the infant a bottle in bed to fall asleep with.
- Clean the child's mouth and brush his or her teeth after feeding.
- Wean the infant to a cup by 1 year of age.
- Do not allow the child to walk or run around with a bottle.
- Begin regular dental checkups after tooth eruption.
- Give juice in a cup as early as possible.
- Keep pacifiers clean.

children are born with a structural abnormality of the heart, called a *congenital cardiac anomaly* or *defect*. These disorders can quickly result in respiratory distress, shock, and death in the infant or small child. Some cardiac disorders are associated with other conditions, such as Down syndrome, congenital rubella syndrome, or fetal alcohol syndrome (see Chap. 73).

Various types of congenital cardiac anomalies may occur. Major cardiac abnormalities can be divided into cyanotic and acyanotic defects. Refer to Table 71-1 for a comparison of these defects. *Cyanotic defects* may cause a right-to-left shunt, in which venous (deoxygenated) blood is mixed with arterial (oxygenated) blood within the heart and then circulated to the body. The total amount of blood sent to the tissues has a decreased amount of oxygen, because the blood that is sent is only partially saturated with oxygen. *Acyanotic defects* have a left-to-right shunt, which sends oxygenated blood into the venous system.

■■■ TABLE 71-1 *M*AJOR CYANOTIC AND ACYANOTIC HEART DEFECTS

Cyanotic Defects	Right-to-Left Shunt	Acyanotic Defects	Left-to-Right Shunt
Tetraology of Fallot (**TOF**) Transposition of the great vessels (**TGV**)	Deoxygenated (venous) blood on the right side of the heart mixes with oxygenated (arterial) blood on the left side of the heart. The left ventricle sends this blood to the body. The cells of the body do not receive enough oxygenated blood. Signs and symptoms include cyanosis, shortness of breath, and fatigue.	Atrial septal defect (**ASD**) Ventricular septal defect (**VSD**) Coarctation of the aorta (**COA**) Patent ductus arteriosus (**PDA**)	Oxygenated blood on the left side of the heart mixes with deoxygenated blood on the right side of the heart. The heart sends this blood to the lungs, where more oxygen is picked up. Signs and symptoms may not be obvious. Untreated, congestive heart failure (CHF) may develop.

Some congenital heart anomalies cause right-to-left shunting, which permits oxygen-poor blood to circulate in the arterial system. These anomalies are referred to as *cyanotic*. If blood is shunted from the left side to the right side of the heart and oxygen saturation of peripheral arterial blood is greater than 85%, the anomaly is called *acyanotic*.

An infant with a significant heart defect may eventually show evidence of congestive heart failure (CHF) and poor peripheral oxygen tissue perfusion. *Perfusion* refers to the body's ability to send and receive oxygen to the cells. Without adequate oxygen and perfusion of the oxygen, the skin appears *cyanotic* (bluish).

The infant with a heart defect may show signs of cyanosis, depending upon the origin of the condition. Other symptoms include *dyspnea* (difficulty breathing), coughing or choking, persistent tachycardia (greater than 200 beats/minute), heart murmurs, failure to gain weight, difficulty in feeding, listlessness, and a general sickly appearance. Observe the child for symptoms of respiratory distress and changes in pulse rate and rhythm.

The severity of CHF may depend on the severity of the heart defect and the amount of the abnormal mixture of arterial and venous blood within the chambers of the heart. The result of this abnormal mixture is an increase in the work of the cardiac muscle, which *hypertrophies* (enlarges). An enlarged heart is the body's attempt to provide oxygen to tissues throughout the body. This enlarged heart eventually becomes ineffective. Chapter 80 discusses CHF in more detail.

The older, untreated child often has poor physical development, low tolerance for physical activity, clubbing of fingers and toes due to chronic hypoxia, cyanosis in certain cases, elevated blood pressure and pulse rate, and possibly an enlarged heart. Frequently the child may need to squat or sit to facilitate breathing, especially on exertion. With pulse oximetry, providers can measure the child's level of peripheral oxygenation.

SPECIAL CONSIDERATIONS: CULTURE

Cyanosis

Cyanosis is more difficult to determine in dark-skinned children; however, a definite duskiness is present in the skin, lips, and nail beds regardless of the child's skin tone.

Definite diagnosis of congenital heart disease is made by auscultation (listening for heart sounds), x-ray studies, echocardiogram, ECG, careful physical examination, complete blood gases, and a complete history. At times, cardiac catheterization and angiocardiography may be done. However, because these procedures carry some risk, they are done only when necessary.

Children with a congenital heart disease (repaired or unrepaired) need prophylactic antibiotics at times of invasive procedures to prevent subacute bacterial endocarditis.

Several nursing diagnoses are commonly seen in children with congenital heart defects:

- Impaired Gas Exchange related to impaired circulation
- Fluid Volume Excess related to decreased kidney perfusion
- Ineffective Family Coping related to life-threatening diagnosis
- Altered Nutrition: Less than Body Requirements related to fatigue and poor circulation
- Altered Growth and Development related to inadequate nutritional intake and poor circulation

Septal Defects

Ventricular septal defect (**VSD**) is the most frequent congenital anomaly of the circulatory system (Fig. 71-9A). An abnormal opening is found between the left and right ventricles. This defect is usually acyanotic because the greater pressure in the left ventricle causes a shunt from left to right, so the blood pumped to the body is oxygenated. If pulmonary hypertension exists, the shunt may go the other way, and the child will be cyanotic. Open-heart surgery can usually correct such defects; the surgeon places a patch (usually of Teflon) into the opening. If the opening is small and no pulmonary hypertension exists, the child may be asymptomatic and the septum may grow to cover the opening. Surgery may be unnecessary or postponed until the child is older. In some cases, an "umbrella" occluder is placed via catheter, thereby postponing or preventing surgery.

Atrial septal defect (**ASD**) is an abnormal opening between the right and left atria. Most of these defects occur in the area

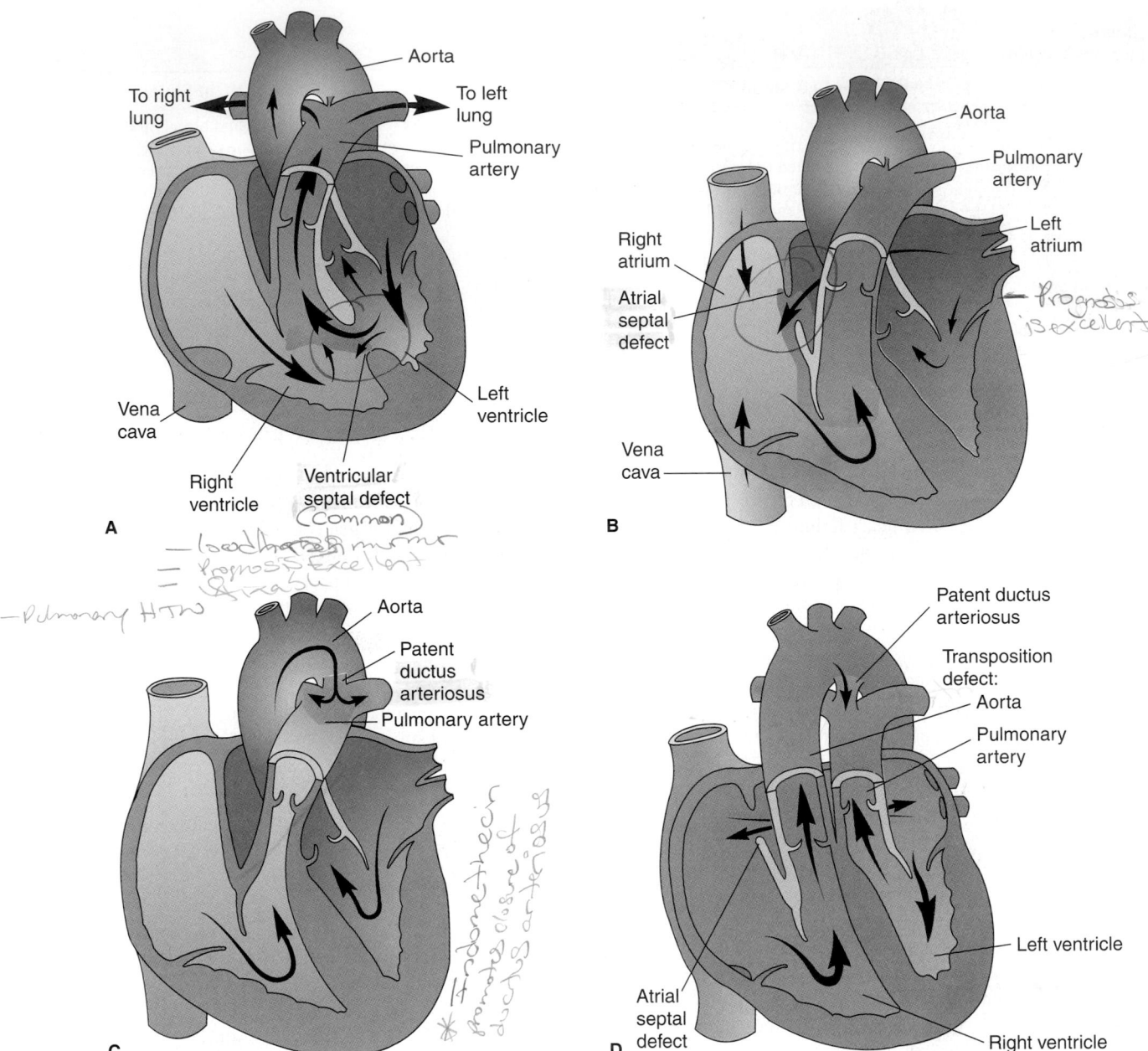

[handwritten annotations: "Prognosis is excellent", "— loud harsh murmur", "— Prognosis Excellent", "fixable", "— Pulmonary HTN", "Indomethacin promotes closure of ductus arteriosus"]

FIGURE 71-9. (A) In a *ventricular septal defect,* a hole is in the wall of the septum that separates the left and right ventricles. Normally, deoxygenated blood flows through the superior vena cava and inferior vena cava into the right atrium, right ventricle, and pulmonary artery. In a ventricular septal defect, some oxygen-rich blood from the left ventricle flows through the defect and recirculates through the lungs. **(B)** In an *atrial septal defect,* an abnormal communication exists between the atria, allowing blood to be shunted from the left atrium to the right atrium through the atrial septum. This hole is usually the area of the foramen ovale, which normally closes at birth. **(C)** A fetal vascular connection called the *ductus arteriosus* directs blood from the pulmonary artery to the aorta. Functional closure of the ductus normally occurs soon after birth. In *patent ductus arteriosus,* the ductus remains patent, and the direction of blood flow in the ductus is reversed due to the higher aortal pressure. **(D)** *Transposition of the great vessels.* The aorta exits the right ventricle; the pulmonary artery exits the left ventricle. The fetal foramen ovale, now an atrial septal defect, allows blood to mix and provide some oxygenation of the blood.

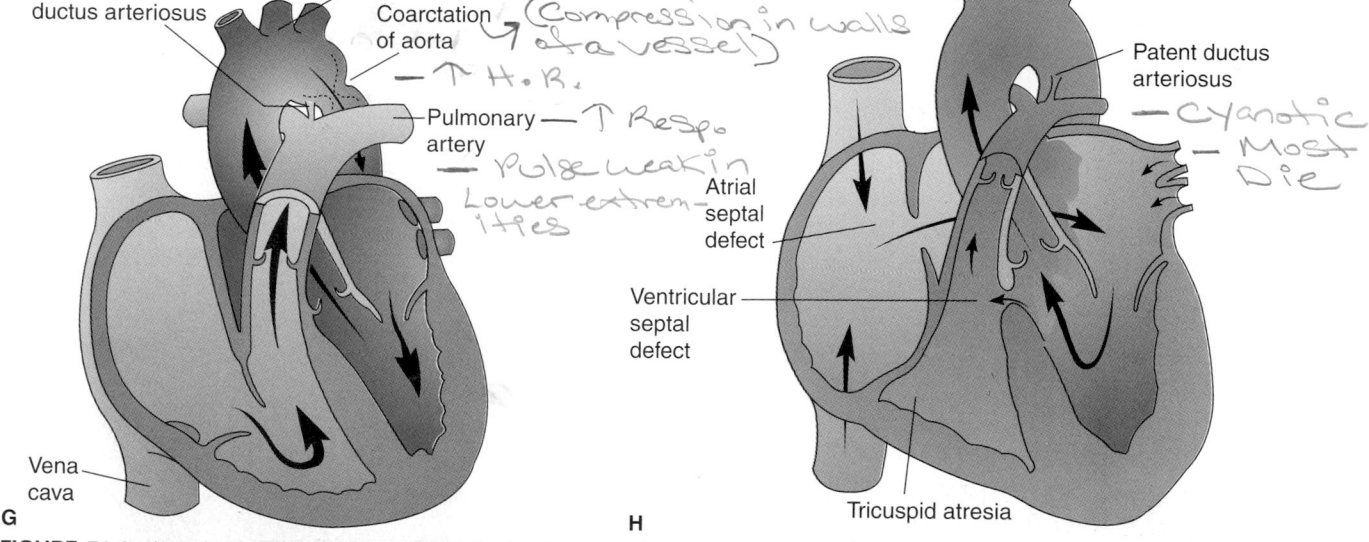

Stenosis of
pulmonary artery

Aorta
overriding
both
ventricles

Hypertrophy
of right ventricle

Ventricular
septal defect

E

Handwritten notes:
✓ cyanotic
✓ Chronically Hypoxic
— Clubbed fingers
— FTT= Failure To Thrive
— Polycythemia
— Prognosis: Excellent d/t heart Surgeries
Tetralogy of Fallot

Aorta
Pulmonary
artery

Pulmonary
stenosis
(Constricted)

Right
atrium

Right ventricle

F

Handwritten notes:
— Hypertrophy (gets bigger) of Rt. side of heart.

Normally closed
ductus arteriosus

Aorta

Coarctation
of aorta

Pulmonary
artery

Vena
cava

G

Handwritten notes:
(Compression in walls of a vessel)
— ↑ H.R.
— ↑ Resp.
— Pulse weak in Lower extremities

Patent ductus
arteriosus

Atrial
septal
defect

Ventricular
septal
defect

Tricuspid atresia

H

Handwritten notes:
— Cyanotic
— Most Die

FIGURE 71-9. *(continued)* **(E)** *Tetralogy of Fallot* is characterized by the combination of four defects: (1) pulmonary stenosis, (2) ventricular septal defect, (3) overriding aorta, and (4) hypertrophy of the right ventricle. It is the most common defect causing cyanosis in children who survive beyond 2 years of age. Severity of symptoms depends on the degree of pulmonary stenosis, the size of the ventricular septal defect, and the degree to which the aorta overrides the septal defect. **(F)** In *pulmonary stenosis,* the right ventricular outflow tract narrows, causing decreased blood flow to the lungs and therefore, decreased oxygenation of the blood. **(G)** In *coarctation of the aorta,* abnormal narrowing of the aorta causes an obstruction of the blood flow from the left side of the heart. Because of this narrowing, pressure in the aorta and left ventricle increases. To help carry blood through the narrowing, blood vessels around it and the left ventricle enlarge. **(H)** *Tricuspid atresia.* The absence of a tricuspid valve prevents blood from entering the right ventricle, causing decreased blood flow to the lungs for oxygenation.

Handwritten notes:
Digoxin — Adult > 60 bpm
— Child > 70 bpm
— Infant > 90 bpm

Tet Position — Squatting; helps breathing.

of the foramen ovale (Fig. 71-9B). Defects found lower in the septum are more likely to involve the mitral and tricuspid valves and the A-V node. Usually, the shunt is from left to right, so the child is acyanotic. Surgery or an occluder can usually close this defect unless severe pulmonary hypertension exists. If the valves are involved, the operation is much more complicated and may include valve replacement.

Patent Ductus Arteriosus

In the fetus, the *ductus arteriosus* is a blood vessel between the aorta and the pulmonary artery that allows the fetal circulation to bypass the lungs. It normally closes before birth or very soon after. If the ductus remains open (*patent*) after birth, the defect is called *patent ductus arteriosus* (**PDA**) (Fig. 71-9C).

In a client with this defect, when the left ventricle pumps blood into the aorta (which should go to the body), some oxygenated blood returns to the pulmonary circulation via the patent ductus, due to the higher pressure in the aorta. Lung pressure thereby increases, as does the volume of oxygenated blood, and may cause pulmonary hypertension. The heart must work harder, and the child's body cells lack oxygen.

Infants may be given indomethacin (Indocin), a prostaglandin inhibitor, to promote closure of a PDA. In some heart anomalies (those with decreased blood flow to the lungs), the patency of the ductus is beneficial to increase blood flow to the lungs for oxygenation. Administration of Prostaglandin E keeps the ductus arteriosus open in conditions where increased blood flow to the lungs is needed (eg, transposition of the great vessels [see below]). A foam plug or an umbrella occluder placed via cardiac catheterization may close the ductus. If these measures do not work, surgical ligation and severing of the ductus is performed. This closed-heart procedure was one of the first surgeries performed. It is usually done even if a child shows no symptoms, because of the danger of lung damage from pulmonary hypertension.

Transposition of the Great Vessels

In *transposition of the great vessels* (**TGV**), the aorta and the pulmonary artery are reversed, so that each connects to the wrong side of the heart. If no shunts or septal defects exist, the child dies early because of lack of sufficient oxygenation to the body cells, because only unoxygenated blood circulates systemically (as shown in Fig. 71-9D).

Immediate intervention includes maintaining patency of the ductus arteriosus to increase pulmonary blood flow, and removal of the atrial septum to facilitate mixing of oxygenated blood into unoxygenated blood. Medication (prostaglandin E) may be given to maintain patency of the ductus arteriosus. Surgical correction involves an arterial switch procedure or construction of an intracardiac baffle to divert the blood to the appropriate vessel.

Tetralogy of Fallot

As shown in Figure 71-9E, *tetralogy of Fallot* (**TOF**) is a combination of four major defects:

- *Pulmonary stenosis:* Narrowing of the pulmonary artery (see following section)
- *VSD:* A hole in the septum separating the ventricles
- *Overriding aorta (dextroposition of the aorta):* The aorta shifts to the right over the septal defect and receives both venous and oxygenated blood
- *Right ventricular hypertrophy:* An enlarged right ventricle due to the heart pumping harder in an attempt to increase blood flow to the lungs for oxygenation

The infant with a severe defect in any of these areas is cyanotic. The repair is done in the first year of life if the infant can withstand surgery. If complete repair is impossible, a temporary repair is performed to increase pulmonary blood flow, usually through a subclavian shunt to the pulmonary vessels.

The infant with this condition may first be seen as an FTT infant. Such infants may go on to have periods of cyanosis and hypoxia, called "blue spells" or "tet spells." If the diagnosis is not made early and the child does not undergo at least palliative surgery, he or she often has increasing pulmonary stenosis. As this child gets older, clubbed fingers and squatting to breathe may become evident.

Improved diagnosis and surgery have greatly decreased the death rate in TOF. Reconstructive surgery is highly successful.

Stenosis

Pulmonary stenosis is the narrowing of the right ventricular outflow tract, including the valve (Fig. 71-9F), which decreases blood flow into the lungs. On rare occasions, pulmonary stenosis also involves a narrowing of the pulmonary artery. If symptoms are present, the valve is surgically corrected (*commissurotomy*). Closed- or open-heart surgery may be indicated, and an artificial valve may replace the valve. If a pulmonary artery is greatly stenosed (*narrowed*), a vessel graft may be done.

In *aortic stenosis*, an aortic valve malfunction causes the heart to work harder to pump blood to the body. The treatment is similar to that for pulmonary stenosis. The aorta itself may also be stenosed.

Coarctation of the Aorta

In *coarctation (constriction) of the aorta* (**COA**), the aorta narrows, obstructing blood flow (Fig. 71-9G). The condition appears similar to aortic stenosis, except that the coarctation is usually further from the heart and therefore causes circulation problems in the arms, head, and lower extremities. Blood pressure is higher in the upper extremities than in the lower extremities. Upper body pulses are usually stronger; lower extremity pulses are weak. In children, conservative medical treatment may be attempted because surgery is difficult. Surgical correction consists of either excising the coarctation and suturing the two ends of the vessel together, or using a blood vessel graft.

Tricuspid Atresia

Tricuspid atresia is the absence of an opening between the right atrium and the right ventricle, allowing no blood to flow from the right atrium to the right ventricle, which greatly decreases pulmonary blood flow (Fig. 71-9H). The only routes by which the blood can get to the lungs are through an atrial or ventricular septal defect or a patent ductus arteriosus. The child dies soon after birth, unless corrective surgery is performed. Because oxygenated blood mixes with unoxygenated blood, the child is cyanotic.

Generally, the older a child is when surgery is performed, the better his or her prognosis will be. However, surgery must be performed earlier for a child who exhibits symptoms of heart failure, pulmonary hypertension, or severe cyanosis.

Sometimes, palliative surgery is performed early, and corrective surgery is attempted when the child is older. In some cases, activity is reduced to lessen strain on the heart, and medications are administered to strengthen the heart's activity and to decrease fluid accumulation, the heart's workload, and the chance of infection.

Medications may include digitalis compounds, diuretics, and antibiotics. Some children regularly receive oxygen. The child should be in the best possible physical and mental condition before surgery.

Open-Heart Surgery

In *open-heart surgery,* bypassing the heart circulation by means of a heart–lung pump (pump oxygenator) is necessary. The heart's action is temporarily stopped. Closed-heart surgery is much safer (although any open-chest surgery is serious). Heart transplant is also possible.

Surgery may be done under hypothermic conditions, which reduces body temperature, thereby slowing all body processes; or hyperbaric conditions, in which the atmospheric pressure is increased to force the blood to carry more oxygen.

BLOOD AND LYMPH DISORDERS

Kawasaki Disease (↑ Platelets)

Kawasaki disease (mucocutaneous lymph node syndrome) is a febrile, multisystem disorder resulting in inflammation of the blood vessels (*vasculitis*). The platelets in the blood tend to be caught in the vessels. It occurs in children younger than 5 years of age. If untreated, as many as 25% of children with Kawasaki disease develop severe cardiac problems. This disease is seen in every racial group, but most commonly in children of Japanese descent. Its cause is unknown.

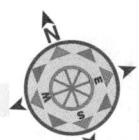

SPECIAL CONSIDERATIONS: CULTURE

Kawasaki Disease

Kawasaki disease was first identified in Japan. The incidence is highest in Asian people.

Symptoms of Kawasaki disease include:

- Prolonged fever of 5 days or more
- Red and infected eyes
- "Strawberry tongue" and cracked, dry lips and oral mucous membranes
- Edema of hands and feet; reddened and peeling soles and palms
- Rash (particularly in the perineal area)
- Swollen lymph nodes
- Pain

Diagnosis of Kawasaki disease is based on assessment of these symptoms. Blood work may reveal increased ESR and anemia; urinalysis may be abnormal.

Medical treatment includes administration of gamma globulin and medications with antipyretic, anti-inflammatory properties (acetaminophen, ibuprofen). Later, an antiplatelet dose is given until the child's platelet count comes down to normal. Nursing care is supportive and should include frequent oral care, skin care, and cardiac monitoring.

Anemia

Anemia results from an abnormally low number of RBCs, low hemoglobin content, or defects in RBC functioning. Some children develop anemia when bottle feeding continues for too long, and they do not eat iron-rich foods. Anemia can also result from hemorrhage, hemolytic disease, malabsorption of vitamin B12, and hereditary factors.

Iron Deficiency Anemia

The most frequent childhood type of anemia is iron deficiency anemia (see Chap. 81). Infants should be kept on breast milk (highly absorbable iron) or an iron-fortified commercial formula until 1 year of age to prevent this condition. Maternal iron stores are exhausted in a term infant by 4 to 6 months of age. Iron-fortified cereal should be the first solid food introduced. Some anemias respond to vitamins and iron. Emphasize to family caregivers the need for the child to follow a nutritious diet, especially with complete proteins, vegetables, and fruits. Caregivers should include foods high in iron: egg yolk, green vegetables (peas, green beans, lettuce, spinach), dried beans, dried peas, peanut butter, organ meats, poultry, fish, and fruits. Orange juice improves the body's iron absorption.

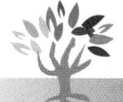

SPECIAL CONSIDERATIONS: THE LIFE SPAN

Anemia

Liquid iron preparations should be well diluted with water or fruit juice and administered through a straw or placed on the back of the tongue with a dropper, to prevent staining of the teeth and to mask the taste. Rinsing of the mouth after ingestion also reduces staining. Iron preparations (FeSol) are best absorbed if taken on an empty stomach. If gastric distress occurs, the medication can be taken with, or immediately after, meals. Orange juice enhances the body's iron absorption if taken at the time of medication administration.

Sickle Cell Disease

Sickle cell disease includes any of the diseases having the presence of hemoglobin S and sickle cells. In the United States, there are several types of sickle cell disease (sickle cell anemia, sickle cell–hemoglobin C disease, sickle cell–hemoglobin D disease, and sickle cell–thalassemia). Sickle cell disease and thalassemia also are discussed in Chapter 81.

Sickle cell disease is a genetic disorder that is primarily seen in descendants of people from Africa, Saudi Arabia, India, and the Mediterranean area. *Sickle cell trait* occurs in the person with one defective gene and one normal gene. *Sickle cell anemia* occurs in the child when both parents carry the recessive gene. The carrier does not show symptoms of the disease. Testing of newborns (*hemoglobin electrophoresis*) can be done to diagnose sickle cell disease or sickle cell trait.

Sickling, or the formation of an abnormal, curved, sickle-shaped RBC, is the key problem of the disorder. These misshapen RBCs are ineffective as oxygen carriers and therefore cause anemia. The sickle shape allows the RBCs to clump together, thereby blocking capillaries. Because blood cannot circulate properly and carry oxygen to the body cells, anemia and circulatory occlusion result.

Clinical symptoms of the disease usually do not appear until the child is about 6 months old because sufficient fetal hemoglobin is still present to prevent sickling. Eventually, the child develops chronic anemia and splenomegaly. Episodes of lethargy, weakness, and fever are sporadic or daily. *Thrombosis* (formation of blood clots) is not uncommon.

Sickle cell crises are severe, painful episodes of sickle cell anemia, which are due to clumping and occlusion of blood vessels. With blood vessel occlusions and without proper oxygenation, tissues become ischemic and can eventually die (*infarction*).

Common sites of pain include the abdomen and the hands and feet; any joint pain may migrate to other joints or be constant. Organs can be damaged, causing cerebrovascular accident (CVA), headaches, convulsions, hearing or visual disturbances, paralysis, pulmonary emboli, and hematuria.

Treatment of sickle cell crisis includes analgesics, transfusions of RBCs, oxygen therapy, and hydration. Constant monitoring of the child during a crisis is necessary because of the possibilities of CVA, shock, or hypoxic episodes. Individuals with a severe active form of the disease usually do not live past middle adulthood.

Nursing considerations include the administration of pain medications, oxygen, and rest. The application of warmth may help diminish pain and promote circulation. (Cold therapy is contraindicated because it can worsen clumping.) Client and family teaching should include suggestions to avoid cold environments and high altitudes, and (when traveling by air) to fly only in a pressurized cabin.

Idiopathic Thrombocytopenic Purpura

Idiopathic thrombocytopenic purpura (**ITP**) is the most common acquired bleeding disorder of childhood. The acute form is seen most often in children between the ages of 3 and 7 years.

Symptoms include easy bruising (often without an obvious cause), *petechiae* (tiny internal hemorrhages) on the mucous membranes, frequent epistaxis, and bleeding into the bladder or GI tract. Symptoms appear suddenly, and the child may look as though he or she has been beaten.

The disease is seldom fatal in children. In most cases, symptoms run an acute course and then clear, with recovery within 6 weeks. The greatest risk is intracranial hemorrhage (5% of cases). Sometimes the cause of the disease cannot be identified, although an affected mother can transmit it to her fetus.

Nursing care involves close observation for hemorrhage, avoidance of injury, and bed rest. Do not give the child intramuscular (IM) injections because of the danger of hematoma formation. Rectal temperatures or enemas are not recommended because of the possibility of trauma to the mucous membranes. Transfusions of platelets are of limited benefit. The child may receive steroids. In extreme cases, a *splenectomy* (surgical removal of the spleen) is performed.

Keep the side rails of the bed raised and pad them to prevent accidental bruising. Use a soft toothbrush for oral care to avoid gum injury. Avoid urinary catheterization because of the danger of hemorrhage and infection. Avoid invasive procedures, such as venipuncture, for the same reason. If venipuncture must be done, exert pressure on the puncture site for at least 20 minutes after inserting the needle to prevent hemorrhage. *Spleen destroying own platelets.*

Hemophilia

Hemophilia is a sex-linked, hereditary bleeding disorder in which a deficiency exists in one or more of the factors necessary for blood clotting. Generally the missing factor is factor VIII or factor IX. Males become symptomatic with hemophilia. Females are carriers of the gene but are very rarely symptomatic.

Internal and external hemorrhage can occur with even a minor injury. Bleeding into soft tissues, the GI tract, and joints (most commonly the hip, knee, ankle, and elbow) results in severe pain. Bleeding into joints may first be noticed when the child begins to walk. Joint contractures can result from scarring and fibrosis of damaged joint synovial membranes. Death can occur as a result of hemorrhage.

In the past, many children with hemophilia died at an early age. Because of improved therapies, most children have good potentials to reach adulthood. In the late 20th century, many hemophiliacs became HIV positive before blood-donor screening and adequate testing of blood products were available.

Nursing considerations include the prevention of injury. Gently touch or move the child. Use measures to try to stop hemorrhage. Take tympanic temperatures to reduce the risk of hemorrhage. Periodic transfusions of blood products may be required. Factor VIII has been genetically produced, and allows for safe replacement of the missing clotting factor.

Teach the family to recognize the symptoms of bleeding, to get medical assistance immediately when needed, and to protect the child from injury without being overprotective.

Additional information about hemophilia is also presented in Chapter 81.

Leukemia

Leukemia is a group of associated disorders characterized by malignancies in the bone marrow and lymphatic system. It is classified into two major types, acute or chronic, and two subtypes, lymphoid or myeloid. Leukemia is also discussed in Chapter 81.

Symptoms. Symptoms of leukemia include fatigue, aches in bones and joints, headaches, fever, swollen lymph nodes, unexplained weight loss, bleeding of gums or nose, frequent bruising, and slow healing. The child is pale and lethargic and bruises easily. Sometimes, the child becomes ill gradually, with increasing weakness and pallor.

Diagnosis. Diagnosis is made on the basis of medical history, which often indicates sudden illness with general malaise, high fever, joint pains, bleeding from body orifices, and enlargement of the liver, spleen, and lymph nodes.

The WBC count is usually elevated, with characteristic abnormal cells. The child is anemic, with a hemoglobin count as low as 4 to 8 g (grams per deciliter [100 mL]). Normal is about 13 to 14 g/dL. Bone marrow and lymph node biopsy can render a positive diagnosis. Further testing may include bone marrow biopsy and genetic studies.

Types of Leukemias

The basic types of leukemias are discussed below along with general information regarding treatments of these cancers. The following are the basic types of leukemia:

- Acute lymphoid leukemia (**ALL**) or Chronic lymphoid leukemia (**CLL**)
- Acute myeloid leukemia (**AML**) or Chronic myeloid leukemia (**CML**)

The most commonly affected group is white males. The elderly are at the highest risk. Adults are 10 times more likely to be diagnosed with leukemia than are children. In children, the highest rates of occurrence occur below the age of 4 years.

Leukemia may also be inherited, especially CLL. Genetic abnormalities, such as those associated with Down syndrome, also carry higher risks for specific forms of leukemia. Risk factors to leukemia include exposure to ionizing radiation and benzene, a chemical found in unleaded gasoline.

A child's survival may depend on the risk factors involved. Factors relating to prognosis include the type of cell involved (ALL has a better prognosis), age at onset (the child aged 2 to 8 years has a better prognosis), initial WBC count (a low WBC count has a better prognosis), and the child's sex (girls have a better prognosis). Rapid remission usually means a better prognosis.

Acute Leukemias

In *acute leukemias,* normal bone marrow is replaced by large numbers of primitive lymphoid or myeloid cells. These primitive cells do not mature normally; therefore, these cells are incapable of functioning as effective WBCs. Over time, the abnormal cells crowd out normal blood cells. Anemia can develop as the primitive cells interfere with the production and maturation of RBCs. In addition, the cancerous cells can collect in lymph nodes and cause swelling. Organ function can be disrupted when these cancerous cells spread.

Acute Lymphoid Leukemia. *Acute lymphoid leukemia* is sometimes called *lymphocytic, lymphatic, lymphoblastic, stem cell,* or *blast cell leukemia.* ALL is the most common kind of cancer (80%) in children under 15 years of age. ALL is rare in adults over age 50.

Children with ALL have a 90% success rate of remission and an 80% 5-year survival rate. Adults have less than 35% survival rates of more than 5 years.

Acute Myeloid Leukemia. *Acute myeloid leukemia* is also called *granulocytic, myelocytic, monocytic, myelogenous, monoblastic,* or *monomyeloblastic leukemia.* AML is the most prevalent form of leukemia in adults (80%), and usually presents in young people—from teenagers to people in their 20s.

Clients with AML can expect about a 70% chance of remission. In many cases, AML returns and the cure rate averages about 50%.

Treatment. Treatment for ALL and AML occurs in phases. A phase is determined by factors such as the client's overall condition and whether the disease is newly diagnosed, in *remission* (controlled but not cured), or in relapse after a remission. Clients will differ in their phases and not all clients have all phases.

Chemotherapy may be given in phase 1 (*induction*) with the goal of putting the disease in remission. The goal of phase 2 (*consolidation*) is to keep the disease in remission. In phase 3 (*prophylaxis*), various chemotherapies may be combined with radiation to prevent metastasis to the brain and CNS. Phase 4 (*maintenance*) consists of scheduled visits to the health provider, who monitors the client's overall condition and reviews laboratory tests.

Recurrent leukemia happens when a client has a relapse or recurrence of the disease. When a relapse occurs, the client is given additional chemotherapies to maintain a remission. Bone marrow transplants may be a treatment of choice for some clients.

Chronic Leukemia

With *chronic leukemias,* the characteristic excessive production of cells occurs in abnormal but apparently mature cells. Chronic leukemia does not attack as swiftly as acute leukemia, and it progresses more slowly. As with acute leukemia cells, the cells of chronic leukemia do not fight infection well. They invade bone marrow and lymph nodes. Clients with CLL and CML have wide ranges of life spans after disease onset. Factors that affect survival rates include early diagnosis, the age of the client, and the individual success of therapies.

Chronic leukemias are categorized by four stages of progressive disease process. *Staging* refers to the criteria related to the spread of the disease.

Chronic Lymphoid Leukemia. *Chronic lymphoid leukemia* accounts for about 30% of all leukemias. It occurs most often in adults between the ages of 60 to 70, but it can also occur in younger adults.

Treatment. Treatment of CLL includes observation, chemotherapy, multiple-drug chemotherapies, and bone marrow transplant, and is gauged by the stage and the general condition of the client. *Stage 0* indicates abnormal numbers of lymphocytes. The criteria for *Stage I* include abnormal lymphocytes and swollen lymph nodes. *Stage II* represents an abnormal number of lymphocytes and swollen lymph nodes, spleen, and liver. In *Stage III,* the RBCs are severely diminished and anemia is prevalent. Anemia may also be present in *Stage IV,* but additionally, there are not enough platelets.

Chronic Myeloid Leukemia. *Chronic myeloid leukemia* accounts for about 25% of adult leukemias. Most often, it affects adults between the ages of 25 to 60 years. CML is often associated with a chromosomal abnormality, which produces a defective gene. The faulty gene may be the cause of CML.

Treatment. Treatment for CML can include chemotherapies, but generally involves bone marrow transplants, which can offer cures.

Medical and Surgical Treatment

Aggressive treatment of leukemia is necessary to inhibit the production of leukemic cells. Treatment includes chemotherapy and radiation, and may include bone marrow transplant or platelet transfusions.

Chemotherapy. *Chemotherapy* consists of potent antineoplastic (*anticancer*) drugs. These drugs must be carefully administered. Many drugs are given intravenously (IV) through a central line in a large vein. Oral drugs are sometimes used, alone or in combination with IV therapy. Medications and protocols vary.

Side effects and adverse reactions of chemotherapy include *alopecia* (hair loss), bleeding, *oliguria* (low urine volume), fluid retention, edema, anorexia, nausea and vomiting, rashes, skin lesions, severe headache, fluctuations in body temperature, and tissue necrosis around the injection site.

Inflammation and ulceration of the GI tract may occur, with ulcerated sores in the mouth often appearing as the first symptom, followed by anal ulcerations. Chapter 82 describes cancer treatment in more detail. Check the child's mouth each day with a flashlight to make sure no ulcerations, reddened areas, or white patches are present. Report any unusual symptoms immediately. See In Practice: Important Medications 71-2 for medications used in leukemia treatment.

Platelet Therapy. *Platelet apheresis* is a process through which the platelets only are removed from a donor's blood. The amount of platelets removed is equivalent to that collected from 6 to 10 units of whole blood. (A well person can safely donate platelets up to twice a week for short periods.) The platelets are then transfused into the leukemic child. Platelet therapy is performed in the hope of forestalling death by hemorrhage until a chemotherapeutic cure is found. This therapy is used primarily in children with AML.

Radiation Therapy. *Radiation therapy* may be a part of the regimen; however, it can cause vomiting, diarrhea, severe electrolyte imbalance, and rapid dehydration. Appropriate nurs-

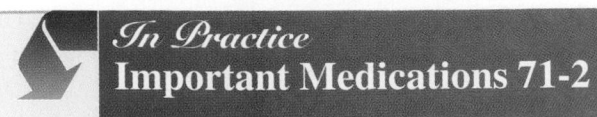

ing considerations are necessary when caring for children receiving radiation therapy (see Chap. 82).

Combination Chemotherapy and Radiation. In some cases, chemotherapeutic agents and radiation are combined for maximum effectiveness. This therapy may be hard on the child, and may reduce antibody levels to the point at which infections occur. The child may be kept in protective isolation during this treatment and during bone marrow transplantation (see Chap. 42).

Bone Marrow Transplantation. If a child does not improve with other treatments, *bone marrow transplantation* (**BMT**) may be done. The donor marrow is usually removed from the pelvic bones. The donor's marrow must match the recipient's; family members are most likely to match. A bone marrow transplantation may be considered a last resort, but up to 70% of children survive more than 2 years after transplantation. Additional information on BMT is found in Chapter 81.

Bone marrow is transplanted through an IV infusion, similar to a blood transfusion. The transplanted marrow naturally grafts itself within the recipient's bones, replacing diseased marrow and making new blood cells.

Nursing Considerations

The child with leukemia can be severely anemic and *thrombocytopenic* (low platelets), which leads to easy bruising and bleeding. Death from hemorrhage is a possibility because of insufficient platelets. Because WBCs are defective, the child is highly susceptible to infection.

The greatest threat to the child during treatment is *bone marrow suppression* (decreased WBCs, RBCs, and platelets), which may lead to life-threatening infection, anemia, or hemorrhage.

Treat symptoms, and make the child as comfortable as possible. Encourage the child to be as active as the disease permits. Prevent infections and injuries. Do not take rectal temperatures because of the danger of injury.

Report a cough or any other symptom of a URI immediately; any infection can result in generalized septicemia and can cause death. Chapters 81 and 82 discuss nursing care for clients receiving chemotherapy, radiation, and blood transfusions.

The child and family need skilled emotional support. Help caregivers accept the course of the disease; always offer hope of remission. The sick child is a part of a family unit; he or she should be involved in family life and friendships as much as possible.

Nursing Alert

The child undergoing treatment for leukemia usually has very low immunity to disease; the greatest danger is infection. Excellent nursing technique is essential for the child's protection.

Other Cancers

Malignant lymphomas, such as **Hodgkin's disease** (discussed in Chapter 81), lymphosarcoma, and other sarcomas (eg, osteogenic sarcoma), are not uncommon in children. Children with such conditions may have a poor prognosis, because malignancies in children often progress quickly and are not detected early. The most common cancers in children are those of the brain, kidney, adrenal glands, bones, and structures of the CNS.

Any brain tumor is serious; the increase in size puts undue pressure on the brain and can cause brain damage. Very young children are less likely to have malignant tumors than are older people. In children, the most common brain tumors are gliomas of the cerebellum, the brain stem, or the optic nerve; *pinealomas* (tumors of the pituitary); and congenital brain tumors. They are most likely to be fast growing and may be inoperable. However, whenever possible, immediate surgery and followup radiation or chemotherapy is required to prevent further complications.

Dealing with the emotional impact of childhood cancer may require the most nursing assistance. Provide emotional support to the child and the family dealing with cancer. See Chapter 81 and 82 for more information about lymphatic system disorders and cancer.

RESPIRATORY TRACT DISORDERS

Sample nursing diagnoses for respiratory illness include:

- Ineffective Airway Clearance related to excessive mucous production, ineffective cough, or swollen airway
- Impaired Gas Exchange related to narrowed airway
- Fear related to breathlessness
- Fatigue related to increased effort of respirations

Upper Respiratory Infection

Upper respiratory infections are common in children and in adults and may be caused by a virus or a bacteria. Symptoms of URI may include a fever; varying degrees of dyspnea with thick, tenacious sputum and mucus; and edema of the throat. If no cough is present, the child may have difficulty getting rid of secretions. Children are usually cared for at home unless complications develop.

General treatment includes antibiotics, humidity, and rest. Oxygen may be necessary. The child may be put in a mist tent, or a bedside cool-air humidifier may be used. If hospitalized, the child with a contagious disease is kept in his or her room, and only adults may visit. At home, caregivers should try to keep ill children separate from well children and encourage the use of separate glasses and utensils. Frequent handwashing is a must.

Pneumonia

Pneumonia, an inflammation of the lungs, usually with consolidation and drainage, is common in children and adults. It may initially be an infectious disease or a disease that is secondary to another disease, or it may result from aspiration. The physician differentiates pneumonia from other URIs by means of a chest x-ray examination. Pneumonia is usually treated with antibiotics, bed rest, and fluids (see Chap. 85).

When caregivers administer antibiotics for any reason, they should understand that the child must take the medication for the prescribed number of days. If the prescribed regimen is not followed, resistant strains of pathogens can develop.

Laryngotracheobronchitis

Laryngotracheobronchitis (**LTB**), a viral infection of the upper airways, usually follows several days of URI. It is also known as *croup*. Croup is a syndrome that results in a harsh, "barky" cough, *inspiratory stridor* (shrill sound on inhalation), hoarseness, and other signs of respiratory distress.

Croup syndromes that affect the larynx, the trachea, and bronchi are serious in children because of the smaller diameter of their airways. Acute spasmodic croup is an inflammation of the subglottic area characterized by the barking cough and varying degrees of respiratory distress occurring primarily at night. Copious tenacious secretions and edema of the airway make breathing difficult. Cyanosis may be present. The child usually has a low fever, rapid pulse, cold and clammy skin, and flushed face. Treatment consists of cool, humidified air and keeping the child calm.

The child is placed in a mist-tent humidifying device (see In Practice: Nursing Procedure 70-3 in Chap. 70). Oxygen may be given to assist respirations. A pulse oximeter may be used to detect hypoxia. A chest x-ray examination may be ordered. Expectorants are often given to loosen secretions and to assist the child in coughing up mucus. A semi-Fowler's position may ease respiratory efforts.

Antipyretics (acetaminophen, ibuprofen) are used to reduce temperature. Oral fluids are encouraged. If the child cannot take fluids orally, IV fluids are given. Offer clear liquids, ice pops, gelatin, and other fluids frequently.

Epiglottitis

Acute **epiglottitis** is an acute, rapidly progressive, life-threatening inflammation of the epiglottis usually caused by a bacteria. Severe respiratory distress, high fever, absence of cough, and drooling of saliva (with refusal to swallow due to an extremely sore throat) are the cardinal symptoms. Intravenous antibiotics result in a rapid recovery. Endotracheal intubation for 1 to 3 days may be necessary to ensure a patent airway.

Influenza B

Nursing Alert

If epiglottitis is suspected, do not attempt to examine the throat, obtain a throat culture, or do anything that might upset the child because this might cause respiratory obstruction.

Asthma

Asthma is a chronic inflammatory disorder of the airways with reactive bronchospasm affecting 15 million people, of which 5 million are children. Airway edema and excessive mucus production may cause airway obstruction. The incidence of asthma has been steadily increasing in both the United States and other parts of the world as a result of increasing air pollution. Asthma has become the most common chronic illness of childhood and is a primary reason for school absences. Asthmatic children are often seen in the ED. Most asthmatic clients have their first symptoms by age 4.

Attacks may occur abruptly or may gradually build over several days. Often the initial attack occurs at night. Wheezing is not always present but is a frequent symptom. *Wheezing* occurs when expired air is pushed through obstructed bronchioles.

Irritants that cause asthmatic attacks include allergens such as trees, shrubs, pollen, molds, dust mites, and foods. Other irritants are animal dander, tobacco smoke, odors, sprays, emotional factors, and some medications. In some children, asthma may result from exercise.

Prevention is the most important aspect of treatment. Children and their families must learn to recognize the symptoms that lead to an attack and begin treatment as soon as possible. The drugs of choice are bronchodilators and steroids administered orally and/or through metered-dose inhalers (**MDI**).

Cromolyn sodium (Intal) may also be used. In an acute attack epinephrine is used. Medications are administered on an as needed basis and are not given over a long period.

The child learns to use the nebulizer or MDI to administer medications. Use of a spacing unit makes the MDI easier to use and aids in delivering the correct dosage of the medication to the lung tissue.

Chest physical therapy (**CPT**) is also a useful addition to treatment; it includes breathing exercises, physical training, postural drainage, and inhalation therapy.

Encourage children with asthma to be active and to take part in managing their own condition. Teach children over 4 years of age to use a *peak expiratory flow meter* (similar to the *incentive spirometer*) to assess the need for preventive measures, indicated by the amount of measured airway exchange as compared with the child's personal best. The child should keep a diary of the peak flow and asthma symptoms. This diary helps the child and family to determine when treatment is needed to prevent a serious attack.

Family caregivers should work toward eliminating any possible allergens in the home. Their children need protection against smoke inhalation. In addition, family caregivers must alert teachers, school nurses, babysitters, and others involved with the child of his or her asthma so that they can provide support as needed.

Nursing Alert

Status asthmaticus, which can be fatal, is a condition that exists when medications do not relieve an acute episode of asthma. Treatment includes administration of IV fluids, bronchodilators (eg, aminophylline), antibiotics, and anti-inflammatory agents.

Bronchiolitis

Bronchiolitis is a viral respiratory infection resulting in inflammation of the bronchioles. It is seen most often in children younger than 2 years and tends to be a seasonal illness, occurring in winter and early spring.

The illness begins with symptoms of a cold, which gradually worsen. Chest x-ray studies reveal air trapping in the lungs. The illness usually resolves within 10 days. A severe case of bronchiolitis may require hospitalization and treatment with IV fluids and oxygen administered by mist tent.

Respiratory syncytial virus (**RSV**) is believed to cause more than half the cases of bronchiolitis. RSV bronchiolitis is particularly prevalent in infants and toddlers and is easily transmissible. Therefore, children with RSV are usually placed on contact isolation. All people caring for these children must observe strict handwashing procedures and wear protective clothing.

Diagnosis of RSV is based on symptoms and a positive nasal culture smear. For high-risk children, treatment may include the use of an antiviral agent called ribavirin, which is administered by mist tent or face mask (see In Practice: Nursing Procedure 71-2).

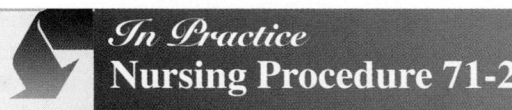

In Practice
Nursing Procedure 71-2

ADMINISTERING RIBAVIRIN THERAPY
Supplies and Equipment

Isolation cart and equipment
Isolation room
Crib or bed to child's needs
Oxygen source and respiratory equipment (oxy-hood, tent, or ventilator for mist humidification)

Steps

1. Wash your hands.
2. Gather equipment and medications. Often the respiratory therapy department sets up the equipment and adds the medication.
3. Explain to family caregivers (and the child, if old enough) what you are going to do and why.
   RATIONALE: *Decrease anxiety and promote cooperation.*
4. Perform a thorough respiratory assessment before beginning and at least every 2 to 4 hours after. Refer to Fig. 66-5 in Chap. 66.
   RATIONALE: *Respiratory infections can cause decreased air exchange. Thorough assessment of the child's respiratory status can determine impending airway obstruction and ensure prompt treatment.*
5. Administer ribavirin using the oxyhood, tent, or ventilator for intubated children. You will usually give it for 3 to 5 days, for 12 to 20 hours per day. The respiratory therapist usually adds 20 mg ribavirin per 1 mL water in a small-particle generator (nebulizer) connected to the oxyhood or tent.
   RATIONALE: *Ribavirin must be administered as a mist to be effective.*
6. If the child is intubated, add antibacterial filters to the circuit of the ventilator tubing; change the filters every 24 hours. Only thoroughly instructed therapists, physicians, and nurses should perform this procedure.
   RATIONALE: *Precipitation of the drug in ventilator tubing around the expiratory valve could obstruct the valve, resulting in high positive-end expiratory pressure and difficulty in exhaling.*
7. Dispose of waste appropriately, and wash your hands.
   RATIONALE: *Prevent the spread of microorganisms.*
8. Document the procedure, medication given, and the child's response. Include respiratory assessment data. Report any signs and symptoms of respiratory distress.

Nursing Alert
Pregnant women should avoid contact with children who are receiving ribavirin. Ribavirin is often teratogenic to the fetus.

Cystic Fibrosis

Cystic fibrosis, a multisystem chronic and incurable condition, is a major dysfunction of the exocrine glands. It is the most common genetic disease in Caucasians, inherited as an autosomal recessive condition. It affects the respiratory system, GI system (pancreas, liver), and in adult men, reproductive organs. It is rare in African Americans and Asian Americans. Many children with cystic fibrosis eventually die from complications; however, with active treatment, children often live past adolescence. In cystic fibrosis, mucous-producing glands secrete abnormal quantities of thick mucus. These secretions collect in the child's lungs, pancreas, and liver, disrupting the normal functions of these organs.

Symptoms and Diagnosis. Symptoms may occur at any age. Some children show symptoms in infancy, including *meconium ileus* (causing bowel obstruction), bile-stained emesis, a distended abdomen, and no stool. The skin of these infants may have a salty taste because of the high sodium chloride content in their sweat. FTT, despite a good appetite, is common. In some children, a hard, nonproductive cough may be the first indication. Frequent respiratory infections follow. A barrel chest, clubbing of the fingers, and signs of malnutrition may be evident.

Diagnosis is based on family history, elevated sodium chloride levels in the sweat (as determined by a sweat test), analysis of duodenal secretions for trypsin content (obtained via a nasogastric tube), and a history of frequent respiratory infections and FTT. If the sweat test is positive for high levels of sodium, only one other criterion must be met for a positive diagnosis.

Medical Treatment. During an acute infection, the client is treated with massive doses of antibiotics to prevent infection. Drugs such as pancreatin and pancrelipase seem to be useful in counteracting pancreatic insufficiency. These pancreatic enzymes are given with meals or snacks to aid in digesting fats and proteins. Pancreatic enzymes have an enteric coating that protects stomach acid from destroying them and delivers them safely to the duodenum. They should be administered at the beginning of the meal with cold, not hot, food because heat decreases the activity of the enzyme.

The high-calorie, high-protein, moderate-fat diet should include supplementary water-soluble forms of fat-soluble vitamins A, D, E, and K, which are necessary because of poor fat digestion. Weight should be frequently monitored. Salt should not be restricted, especially in hot weather. Fluids should be encouraged to prevent dehydration, which causes the mucous to become thicker.

Treatment for maintaining optimum pulmonary function includes chest physical therapy, inhalation therapy, antibacterial drugs for the prophylaxis or treatment of infection as indicated, and immunization against childhood communicable diseases. All immunizations should be maintained and given at appropriate intervals. Encourage physical activity because it improves mucous secretion as well as a positive self-image. Encourage the child to participate in any aerobic activity he or she enjoys. Limit activity, along with physical therapy, only according to the child's endurance.

Inhalation therapy is prescribed as a preventive or therapeutic measure. A bronchodilator drug (albuterol) is usually administered by a hand-held nebulizer. Recombinant human deoxyribonuclease or dornase alfa (DNase, Pulmozyme) are agents that break down DNA molecules in sputum, resulting in a breakup of the thick mucus in the airways. The addition of a mucolytic agent, such as acetylcysteine (Mucomyst), may be prescribed during periods of acute infection. A humidifier can provide a beneficial moist atmosphere. During the summer, a room air conditioner can help provide the child with comfort and controlled humidity.

Chest physical therapy is performed regularly. CPT is a combination of postural drainage and chest *percussion* (clapping and vibrating of the affected areas). Chest percussion that is performed correctly helps to loosen and move secretions out of the lungs. A physical therapist or respiratory therapist can teach family caregivers to perform this routine as an essential part of home care.

The family needs much teaching and support. Caregivers should avoid overprotecting the child. They will need to learn CPT, postural drainage, administration of IV antibiotics, and enzyme regulation, according to the child's needs. In summer the active child may need extra salt. Caring for the child places enormous stress on the family's financial resources. The Cystic Fibrosis Foundation, a national organization, provides education and services for these children and their families. In addition, assistance may be available through local sources. The caregivers must also learn to take time to care for themselves. — Excess mucas plugs openings like glue. Don't live very long.

GASTROINTESTINAL DISORDERS

Review the information on general surgery in Chapter 56 and pediatric surgery in Chapter 70 before caring for children who are undergoing surgery for GI disorders. Sample nursing diagnoses seen in GI disorders include:

- Fluid Volume Deficit related to excessive fluid loss from frequent diarrhea
- Altered Nutrition: Less than Body Requirements related to excessive vomiting
- High Risk for Impaired Skin Integrity related to exposure of skin to frequent loose stools
- Altered Growth and Development related to inadequate intake or absorption of nutrients

Pyloric Stenosis

In **pyloric stenosis,** also called *congenital hypertrophic pyloric stenosis,* the child's pyloric sphincter thickens, narrowing the canal through which food passes from the stomach to the intestine. This condition is more common in boys than in girls. An infant usually does not show signs of pyloric stenosis until he or she is about 2 months old. The stenosis may be so extensive that the obstruction is complete; the pylorus then closes, and food cannot pass into the intestine. As a result, the child regurgitates food into the esophagus, causing severe projectile vomiting. Vomiting is the most common symptom of pyloric stenosis. Other symptoms include loss of weight, hunger, irritability, and dehydration. Often, constipation and oliguria are associated. Diagnosis is made on the basis of an upper GI x-ray examination.

Medical and Surgical Treatment.   The treatment of choice for pyloric stenosis is surgery (*pyloromyotomy*). However, if the child is a poor surgical risk and if the stenosis is not life threatening, medical means of treatment may be used, including sedation, antispasmodic drugs, and thickened feedings. (Medical means of treatment are also used in developing countries, where surgery is not available.)

Nursing Considerations.   Before surgery, IV fluids should be given to correct fluid and electrolyte imbalance due to vomiting. (Electrolyte laboratory studies identify the type of solution to administer.) An accurate record of I&O and the amount and type of vomitus is essential.

Postoperatively, precautions should be taken to prevent aspiration. Position the child on the right side, with his or her head slightly elevated. Schedule care so that you give the child a bath *before* feeding. Glucose water feedings are started 2 to 3 hours after surgery; bubble the child frequently. Increase the amount of feedings when the infant is able to retain more. Progress the diet from glucose water, to half-strength formula, to full-strength formula. Recovery is usually complete and the child experiences no further problems.

Meckel's Diverticulum

Meckel's diverticulum is a congenital disorder in which a small portion of the child's ileum ends in a blind pouch just before its junction with the colon. Symptoms include the passage of bloody or tarry stools. The child experiences no pain unless the diverticulum is inflamed; the condition may exist without ever causing symptoms. When symptoms do occur, surgical removal of the pouch is necessary. Complications are rare. Preoperative and postoperative care is routine.

Hernia

A **hernia** is the protrusion of part of an organ through an abnormal opening. In children, a congenital defect is most often the cause of hernia. Hernias take various forms:

- *Diaphragmatic hernia,* which occurs rarely, is a condition in which a portion of the intestine protrudes through the diaphragm. It is usually diagnosed at birth and repaired through immediate surgery.
- In *umbilical hernia,* a portion of the intestine protrudes through a weak umbilical ring, producing a bulge beneath the person's navel. Because this condition usually disappears by the time the child is 3 to 4 years old, surgery is

usually unnecessary. Strangulation of the protruded part is rare, with surgery necessary only if the protruding part is large or if other congenital defects are present.

- In *indirect inguinal hernia* (most frequent in boys), the intestine protrudes through the round ligament into the inguinal area and may descend into the scrotal sac. Surgery is required if strangulation develops. In girls, an inguinal hernia may involve the ovary or the uterus, and immediate surgery is needed to prevent damage to these structures.

- A *direct inguinal hernia* protrudes through the weakest part of the abdominal wall. Because the peritoneum overlying the protruding abdominal contents is transparent, the contents can be visualized, and all or part of the abdominal contents may be seen. Should the hernia rupture, severe hemorrhage, peritonitis, a generalized septicemia, or strangulation could occur. Surgery is usually performed early in life.

Treatment. The treatment of choice for most hernias is surgery. The specific procedure varies with the condition. Preoperative and postoperative care is routine. Often hernia repair is completed in the same-day surgery suite and may be done by laparoscopy.

Diarrhea

Diarrhea is a sudden increase in frequency of loose and watery stools. It is most often caused by pathogens in the GI tract. Stress, prolonged temperature elevation, and spoiled food are other causes. Certain antibiotics can alter the bacteria normally present in the intestine, resulting in an increased number of stools.

Diarrhea can be very dangerous for young children. Smaller and younger children are at increased risk for fluid and electrolyte imbalance and dehydration. Severe diarrhea can be rapidly fatal in an infant.

Medical Treatment. Mild forms of diarrhea are treated at home. Family caregivers should administer an oral rehydration solution (**ORS**), such as Pedialyte, to children with diarrhea. ORSs are available in different flavors. Clear liquids with sugar and/or caffeine should be avoided. The **BRAT** diet, which consists of ripe banana, rice cereal, applesauce, and toast, once commonly used, has become somewhat controversial because the diet is high in calories, low in energy and proteins, and inadequate in nutrition. An age-appropriate diet should be offered within 24 hours. Family caregivers should avoid giving children with diarrhea salty broth because the salt content may further disturb electrolyte balance.

In severe diarrhea, stools are frequent and forceful, and are green or yellow liquid. The child is lethargic and irritable. Skin turgor is poor, mucous membranes are dry, the eyes and anterior fontanelles are sunken, urination is decreased, and the pulse is weak and rapid, indicating dehydration. Usually IV fluids, based on electrolyte studies, are necessary to replace water loss and to restore fluid and electrolyte balance. A chest x-ray examination determines any complicating respiratory condition, and a stool culture identifies the causative organism. The child is placed on transmission-based precautions to prevent the spread of organisms to others.

Nursing Considerations. Transmission-based precautions should be followed when caring for the child with diarrhea. IV therapy is necessary to replace body fluids; restraints may be necessary during IV infusion. Be sure to comfort the child, and to release the restraints periodically so that the child can change position at will.

Maintain accurate I&O records and carefully describe the amount and character of all stools. Continue food and fluids except in cases of severe vomiting. Teach caregivers to use ORSs and observe the child for any signs of dehydration. Clear fluids and juices are inadequate because they are high in carbohydrates but low in electrolytes. Encourage the early re-introduction of regular nutrients.

Good skin care is essential because the child's buttocks can become sore and irritated. Thorough, gentle cleansing from the front of the perineal area to the back is necessary each time the child defecates. Expose the child's buttocks to air as much as possible. Sitz baths in clear tepid water and protective ointments help ease discomfort.

Encopresis

Encopresis is incontinence of feces without physical cause. It occurs in previously toilet-trained children. Usually, symptoms begin with stool withholding late in infancy.

Treatment should be geared toward improving family relationships and understanding personality patterns. Nursing support and a nonjudgmental, non-punishing approach from family caregivers is fundamental to the therapeutic plan. The child with prolonged encopresis and the caregivers may need counseling. Oil-retention enemas and mineral oil are usually prescribed. Increased dietary fiber and fluids is recommended.

Lactose Intolerance

If a child has frequent attacks of diarrhea, **lactose intolerance,** an inherited disorder characterized by an inability to metabolize lactose in milk and milk products, may be the problem. It is more common in Asian Americans and African Americans than in other groups; about 85% of African Americans have this disorder.

The lactose-intolerant individual cannot drink milk or eat dairy products. Not only does the person's body improperly absorb and metabolize dairy products, but the presence of such substances also interferes with the absorption of other foods. If the problem is not recognized and treated in a child, he or she could die from malnutrition.

Symptoms of lactose intolerance include diarrhea, abdominal pain, vomiting, listlessness, and FTT. These symptoms may appear 1 to 2 weeks after birth. The baby is switched to a lactose-free formula. Yogurt, which has inactive lactase that is activated by the temperature and pH of the duodenum, is an excellent source of calcium. Teach family caregivers to observe for hidden sources of lactose that the child must avoid.

Intussusception

Intussusception is the telescoping of one bowel part into another. It is usually caused by hyperactive peristalsis in one bowel part and hypoactivity in another. Cardinal symptoms include abdominal pain and passage of a currant-jelly stool (clear mucus with blood). One danger of this condition is that the bowel's blood supply may be blocked, causing gangrene and possible bowel rupture.

Intussusception is most common in infants; yet affected babies usually appear to be thriving. A definite diagnosis is based on the findings of a barium enema. The x-ray examination itself may reduce the intussusception; if not, surgery is necessary to prevent complications. Preoperative and postoperative care is routine, and the healthy child seldom has complications.

> ## ✚👁 Nursing Alert
> Passage of a normal stool indicates reduction of the intussusception and should be reported to the physician immediately.

Colic

Colic is paroxysmal abdominal pain, most commonly occurring in the first 3 months of an infant's life. Although colic is not serious, it can be extremely frustrating for family caregivers. Affected babies have frequent crying episodes. These children double up as though they are in great pain. Symptoms seem to worsen in the evenings. Theorists have advanced numerous possible causes of colic: improper feeding or bubbling, an overly emotional family situation, milk or lactose intolerance, secondhand smoke inhalation, and poor responses of caregivers to the infant's crying. None of these theories has been definitely accepted.

Treatment consists of feeding the baby slowly, and reducing the amount of air that the infant swallows. The formula given is usually one with a soy base. In any event, the baby almost always outgrows the condition by the time he or she is 3 to 4 months old. Encourage caregivers to give the infant a pacifier to promote nonnutritive sucking. Soothing the infant through touching, rocking, and gently speaking is also recommended. Family caregivers need a break from the baby's constant crying; encourage them to develop a support system of relatives, friends, and babysitters.

Megacolon

In **megacolon,** also known as **Hirschsprung's disease** or *aganglionic megacolon,* the child's colon lacks parasympathetic nerve supply. Due to a lack of peristalsis, the abdomen becomes abnormally enlarged with stool and flatus. If a large colon segment is affected, palliative treatment may be the only alternative. In 90% of children with megacolon, the aganglionic area is in the rectosigmoid bowel segment. Surgical treatment may be effective, if the damaged or malfunctioning portion can be removed.

✱ Ribbon like stool

Symptoms and Diagnosis. Feces accumulation in the child's bowel causes symptoms that include diarrhea, constipation, nausea, and vomiting. The abdomen becomes distended, and bowel movements are abnormal, resulting in malnutrition. Usually the effects of megacolon appear shortly after birth when the newborn fails to pass meconium within 24 to 48 hours.

Signs of obstruction such as bile-stained or fecal vomiting, abdominal distention, irritability, feeding problems, FTT, or dehydration may occur. The older child exhibits intractable constipation that usually requires laxatives and saline enemas. Surgery is usually required.

Diagnosis is made on the basis of medical history, x-ray studies, barium enema, and palpation of the distended abdomen. A proctoscopy usually reveals an empty rectum and lower colon, and biopsy of the rectal wall usually indicates an absence of nerve fibers.

Medical and Surgical Treatment. If possible, corrective surgery is delayed until the child is about 1 year old and better able to withstand the procedure. During the waiting period, preventing constipation is important. Small saline enemas, stool softeners, and digital removal of fecal impactions are used. Sometimes colonic irrigations are done. These are similar to enemas except that they require a larger tube to be passed into the descending colon.

Drugs that act on the parasympathetic and sympathetic nervous systems may be given to improve peristalsis. Surgery often involves a temporary *colostomy* (opening of the large intestine onto the abdominal wall).

☞ KEY CONCEPT

Watch for abdominal distention, temperature spikes, and irritability after surgery for megacolon. They are signs of possible anastomotic leaks (leakage where the two ends of the bowel are sewn together).

Nursing Considerations. Preoperative preparation includes saline enemas for colon evacuation. Keep accurate records of the quantity of solution you administered. The return solution should be clear of fecal particles. Administer ordered antibiotics as a bowel preparation.

Keep the surgical wound clean and dry postoperatively. Do not take rectal temperatures. The child's first liquid bowel movement will be approximately 3 to 4 days postoperatively. Assess the child's urine for blood because bladder trauma can result from extensive surgical manipulation.

Clear oral feedings usually begin after active bowel sounds are audible. The diet progresses according to the child's tolerance. Instruct family caregivers to watch closely for foods that increase the child's number of stools and to avoid including them in the child's diet at home. Assure caregivers that the child will eventually achieve sphincter control and be able to eat a normal diet. Complete continence may take several years for the child to attain. Encourage caregivers to participate in the child's care as much as possible, to gain confidence in caring for the child at home.

URINARY SYSTEM DISORDERS

Enuresis

Enuresis is the involuntary passage of urine, usually at nighttime, in a child over 5 years of age. More commonly, this condition is known as "bed wetting." Enuresis is more common in boys than in girls. A complete urologic work-up is necessary to discover any physical cause, including severe infection, bladder trauma, diabetes mellitus, small bladder capacity, *meatal stenosis* (narrowing of the urinary opening), or bladder spasm. Any such physical cause is treated directly. Other possible physical factors may be that the child does not empty the bladder completely on voiding, or that he or she is an exceptionally sound sleeper.

If no physical cause is found, providers will investigate a possible underlying emotional problem. Family stress or school problems are associated with enuresis. Family caregivers should not shame or criticize the child for bed wetting. If the condition persists, low dosages of an antidepressant, such as imipramine hydrochloride (Tofranil), have been used to promote continence. Other medications that may be helpful are: flavoxate hydrochloride (Urispas)—used in children under age 12—and oxybutynin chloride (Ditropan), used in children over age 5. Counseling can sometimes assist the child and family.

Hemolytic Uremic Syndrome

✗ Uncommon in adults

Hemolytic uremic syndrome (**HUS**) is a rare, acute condition occurring in children usually between the ages of 1 and 10 years and primarily between the ages of 6 months and 4 years. Three conditions occur in this illness: renal failure, hemolytic anemia, and thrombocytopenia. HUS is the leading cause of acute kidney failure in children.

Two to seven percent of HUS cases are associated with infection by a toxic strain of *E. coli* (0157:H7). E. coli 0157:H7 is an illness caused by numerous sources such as contaminated meat, raw milk, lettuce, and contaminated water. Thorough cooking of meat products is critical in preventing this illness. Person-to-person transmission also occurs because it can be transmitted in diarrheal stools. Proper handwashing is essential.

HUS usually presents as a flu-like illness and gastroenteritis. Nausea, vomiting, abdominal pain, fever, and bloody diarrhea may be present. Pallor, lethargy, and oliguria typically follow the onset of the milder symptoms. The affected child appears pale, bruised, and hypertensive, with diminished or absent urine output.

As the disease progresses, acute renal failure, hemolytic anemia, thrombocytopenia, and microemboli lead to multisystem organ failure. Seizures, disorientation, decreased LOC, and death may follow.

Treatment includes management of hypertension, dialysis, blood transfusions, and nutritional support.

Urinary Obstruction

Urinary obstruction can result from a *neoplasm* (cancer), *calculi* (stones), or severe infection. Relieving the obstruction is necessary to prevent complications such as hydronephrosis. Catheterization or antibiotics can be effective; otherwise, surgery is performed.

Urinary Tract Infection

Infection of the urinary tract (**UTI**) is most commonly caused by perianal microorganisms (*E. coli* in 80% of cases) and is accompanied by frequency, urgency, and dysuria. The short urethra in the female anatomy contributes to a higher incidence in females. Anatomic anomalies may also contribute to the cause of the infection. The occurrence of a UTI in a male warrants urologic evaluation.

Diagnostic evaluation consists of a urine specimen for urinalysis and culture and sensitivity (C&S). Treatment consists of antibiotics, encouraging frequent voiding, and copious fluids. Prevention is the most important goal (see In Practice: Educating the Client 71-4). Children who have chronic UTIs may be maintained on low-dose antibiotics.

Pyelonephritis

Pyelonephritis (*pyelitis*) is a potentially dangerous infection of the upper urinary tract and kidneys (see Chap. 88 for a detailed discussion). The causative bacterial infection can migrate to the kidneys by way of the bloodstream or ascend from the bladder because the urinary tract has a mucous membrane.

Symptoms of pyelonephritis include *dysuria* (painful voiding), urinary frequency and urgency, fever, chills, lower-back pain, and headache. There may be nausea, abdominal tenderness, and pain. C&S tests are done to determine the causative organism so that appropriate antibiotics can be prescribed. Pyelonephritis is curable in most cases if treated promptly.

Glomerulonephritis

Acute **glomerulonephritis,** also called *acute poststreptococcal glomerulonephritis,* is the most common form of nephritis found in young children between the ages of 5 and

✗ Like kidney infection ✗ Smokey urine
✗ 5–10 yos ✗ comes from strep

In Practice
Educating the Client 71-4

PREVENTION OF URINARY TRACT INFECTIONS IN FEMALES

• Wipe the perineal area from front to back.
• Wear white cotton panties because they are not irritating and allow good air circulation.
• Do not use bubble bath because it is irritating.
• Drink plenty of fluids.
• Thoroughly rinse soap off the perineum.
• Use white, unscented toilet paper.

10 years. It results from an immunologic reaction to infection (most often streptococcal) elsewhere in the body. Damage to the glomeruli may cause urinary output to decrease or cease.

The initial and main symptom is smoky urine or hematuria. The child's eyes may be puffy and the blood pressure elevated. A throat culture may reveal GABHS (see "Streptococcal Infections" section). Kidney enlargement may also be present. Blood tests show mildly to moderately elevated blood urea nitrogen (BUN) and creatinine. The urine shows the presence of RBCs (*microscopic* or *gross hematuria*) and elevated WBCs. The urine values, including abnormal protein, indicate impaired renal function. There may be an elevated ASO titer.

The child is kept on bed rest; activity is allowed when the hematuria clears and blood pressure returns to normal. Keep people with URIs away from the child. Provide a diet high in calories and low in sodium, protein, and potassium. Fluids may be restricted. Take daily weights to determine if the child is accumulating fluid in the tissues. Regularly assess vital signs. Antibiotics and corticosteroids may be prescribed, although the use of steroids is controversial.

In most cases, recovery is complete. In a few cases, chronic nephritis may develop, and the client may need to be maintained on dialysis.

Chronic glomerulonephritis may be a complication of acute glomerulonephritis or may occur without preceding illness. Symptoms are unpredictable, and kidney damage usually is progressive. Chronic glomerulonephritis can lead to hypertension, proteinuria, hematuria, and uremia.

The disease tends to progress in three stages. The first stage is the *latent stage,* in which the child shows few outward symptoms. Albumin appears in the urine, and the child may be anemic. No special treatment is needed at this time. In the second stage, called the *edema stage,* the child retains fluid. Treatment includes a high-protein, low-salt diet. Corticosteroid use is controversial; these drugs are sometimes prescribed but are not as widely used as they once were. In the third stage, the stage of *uremia,* the child's kidneys begin to fail. No medical treatment is available for this stage. The child may be maintained on dialysis until a suitable donor for a kidney transplant is located. These children are often excellent candidates for kidney transplantation.

The components of nursing care for chronic glomerulonephritis include:

- Accurate assessment of vital signs, I&O, and daily weight
- Daily assessment of renal function; observation for signs of fluid, electrolyte, and acid–base imbalance
- Low-sodium, high-calorie diet with adequate protein
- Good skin care (because of itching and edema)
- Good oral hygiene (take care not to damage fragile gums)
- Family teaching: the child needs to take medications as ordered and diuretics in the morning so as not to disrupt sleep; report symptoms of urinary tract infections; avoid having the child come into contact with people with URIs
- Explanation to the child and caregivers about side effects of corticosteroids if they are to be given (see Chap. 62)

Nephrotic Syndrome

In *nephrotic syndrome,* changes in the basement membrane of the glomeruli cause the kidneys to excrete massive amounts of protein. It occurs most often in children between 1½ and 5 years of age, and is characterized by generalized edema, proteinuria, and hematuria. Urine output is scanty, and blood pressure is elevated. The abdomen is distended, and the child is uncomfortable. He or she does not eat because fluid in the abdomen and chest causes discomfort. The child is susceptible to other infections.

Palliative measures are symptomatic. Edema is reduced by administering corticosteroids and by limiting fluid and salt intake. Diuretics may be used to reduce edema. Encourage the child to eat. Protect the child against infection. Provide careful skin care and assist the child to move about in bed. If the child is having difficulty breathing, he or she may be more comfortable sitting up.

The child is very ill and needs expert nursing care and emotional support. Corticosteroids may induce a remission, and the prognosis for eventual recovery is good in most cases. Children who respond to steroid therapy have fewer relapses as time progresses. If the disease is diagnosed and treated early, the child can expect to regain normal (or near-normal) renal functioning. Nursing care is similar to that in chronic glomerulonephritis. Check the child's weight at the same time each day, on the same scale, with the child wearing the same amount of clothing. Assess vital signs and I&O regularly. During periods of edema, decrease the child's sodium intake by not adding salt to the diet. A high-protein diet is unnecessary. Do not restrict fluids. Offering frequent small meals (six per day) may help the child's nutritional intake during periods of *exacerbation* (flare-up of symptoms). Protect the child from contact with others who have URIs.

Wilms' Tumor

Wilms' tumor, also called *nephroblastoma,* is a malignant adenosarcoma of the kidney. It is most common in children aged 3 to 4 years. It is one of the most common neoplasms of childhood, and usually only affects one kidney.

In most cases, the child shows no symptoms until the tumor is far advanced. Microscopic hematuria may be present, but usually not until late in the disease's course. Diagnosis is based on palpation of the abdominal mass, x-ray studies, and biopsy during a *laparotomy* (surgical exploration of the abdomen).

Treatment for Wilms' tumor depends on "staging," as shown in Box 71-1. Surgical removal, when done, is followed by irradiation of the tumor site and both sides of the spine. Chemotherapy is often used.

Whenever a child is to have surgery, prepare the family caregivers and child. If the child is old enough to understand, you may use dolls, puppets, and drawings to explain placement of tubes and to play out fears. After surgery, prepare the child and family for the child's hair loss resulting from chemotherapy.

➤ BOX 71-1

Knao ✓

STAGING IN THE PROGRESS OF WILMS' TUMOR

Stage I: The tumor is well encapsulated and is limited to the kidney. It is totally removed by surgery.

Stage II: The tumor extends into the abdominal cavity. Often it can be totally removed.

Stage III: The tumor extends into the abdominal cavity to such an extent that it cannot be removed entirely.

Stage IV: The tumor has metastasized to distant sites (eg, lungs, liver, bone, brain).

Stage V: Bilateral kidney metastasis exists.

Nursing Alert
When treating a child with Wilms' tumor, never unnecessarily palpate the abdomen preoperatively. The tumor could rupture and disseminate. Use extreme caution when handling this child at all times. Post a clear warning sign at the child's bedside.

Hypospadias and Epispadias

In **hypospadias,** the male child's urinary meatus is located on the bottom of the penis; in **epispadias,** the meatus is located on top of the penis. These conditions can usually be surgically corrected and are not life threatening. In severe instances of hypospadias, the newborn's sex may be in doubt because the position of the meatus may appear to be the female urethra, especially when undescended testes are part of the presentation. Chapter 68 also discusses these congenital disorders.

Minor hypospadias is common and usually requires no correction. If surgery is required, it is sometimes done in two stages. Circumcision is contraindicated before surgical correction of this displacement of the urinary meatus, because the foreskin may be used for the procedure. Prepare the caregivers intellectually and emotionally for surgery, which is scheduled between 6 and 18 months of age, before the child develops a strong body image.

REPRODUCTIVE SYSTEM DISORDERS

Ambiguous Genitalia

The newborn who exhibits genitalia that seem to have both male and female characteristics is said to have *ambiguous genitalia.* For instance, in some cases of hypospadias the newborn's sex is unclear. If any doubt exists about a baby's sex, studies are performed immediately. Examiners study the buccal mucosa or skin structure microscopically for a female or male chromosomal pattern. Hormonal and anatomic studies also may be done. Normal social and emotional development demands that a child's sex be established as soon after birth as possible. Depending on the physical problem, surgery may be

necessary to revise or to remove structures. Appropriate hormone administration may also be required.

The term *hermaphrodite* is used when a child has both testes and ovaries, resulting in malformed external genitalia. The term is often interpreted to mean "half-male and half-female," causing confusion and emotional strain for the newborn's family. The importance of correct sexual identification, prompt surgery, and hormonal treatment is foremost in helping the family. Encourage the family to give the child an appropriate, gender-specific name and to identify the child as male or female. Urge the family to openly discuss their concerns with health professionals.

Cryptorchidism

Cryptorchidism is an undescended testicle; Chapter 89 discusses the condition in detail. It is common at birth but usually corrects itself spontaneously. If not, surgical treatment (*orchiopexy*) is performed in early childhood to prevent sterility. Because undescended testes are often associated with hernia and hydrocele (see following section), surgical repairs are usually completed together. If an undescended testicle is found in an older child, surgery must not be postponed. A delay could result in sterility, because sperm cannot tolerate the heat inside the body.

Surgery is usually performed on an outpatient basis. Assess the client to make sure that no symptoms of URI exist; if they are present, surgery will probably be postponed.

Postoperatively, the child is sent home after bowel sounds return and the child takes and retains fluids, voids, and ambulates properly. The child may return from surgery with an abdominal dressing as a result of accompanying hernia repair. Assess the dressing often for drainage. Teach caregivers what to look for if the child goes home soon after surgery.

Hydrocele

A **hydrocele** is an accumulation of serous fluid within the scrotal sac, causing the scrotum to become large and painful. If the fluid is not reabsorbed spontaneously, excision and drainage may be necessary. A hydrocele is often associated with a hernia.

NUTRITIONAL CONSIDERATIONS IN YOUNG CHILDREN

Normal growth implies a state of health and absence of a major chronic disease. Growth parameters of height, weight, head circumference (up to 36 months), and body mass index should be monitored at each well-child visit and graphed on the appropriate chart. (BMI is the ratio of weight in kilograms divided by the height in meters squared.)

The explosive growth during infancy demands adequate nutrition to facilitate proper growth and development. Protein and fat are especially important for CNS development. Infants require 110 to 120 calories per kilogram of body weight per day for the first 6 months, and 95 to 100 for the remainder of the first year.

Human milk has the ideal quality and quantity of nutrients, plus added protection against infections. The American Academy of Pediatrics recommends that breast milk be given to infants exclusively for the first 6 months of life, and then breast milk with added solids be given until the child is at least 1 year old.

Commercial formulas supply 20 calories per ounce and are fortified with vitamins and minerals (especially iron). Formula should be fed at room temperature. Formula should be continued until the child is 1 year old to prevent GI bleeding. Whole cow's milk should not be given until after 1 year of age.

The introduction of solid foods may begin at 4 to 6 months of age when the GI tract has matured and is less sensitive to potentially allergenic foods.

The signs of readiness for the introduction of solid foods include:

- The ingestion of 32 ounces of milk daily without hunger satisfaction
- The disappearance of the extrusion reflex (at about 4 months) *Spoon feed infant; pushes food out w/tongue.*
- The doubling of birth weight
- The ability to sit unsupported and lean forward with an open mouth to receive food or to lean back and turn the head away thereby indicating fullness

The order of solid food introduction is not crucial, but rice cereal is usually introduced first, followed by vegetables and fruit. Highly allergenic foods should be avoided. Parents should introduce one new food at a time in small amounts for a period of 5 to 7 days to determine the infant's response to the food. Solid food should be fed with a spoon and not placed in bottles with formula. As the quantity of solid food increases, the quantity of milk should be decreased to prevent overfeeding. Milk or fruit juice should be introduced in a cup at 6 to 7 months of age, with the goal of weaning completely from the bottle to a cup by 1 year of age to prevent dental caries. Soft, mashed table foods may be introduced gradually.

The toddler's growth slows, requiring decreased energy and caloric requirements (100 kcal/kg/day). Appetite decreases dramatically (*physiologic anorexia*) and the desire for self-feeding increases. Introducing finger foods and allowing food choices facilitates independence. Avoid foods that may induce choking, such as round foods (wieners cut into slices), hard foods (such as raw carrots), or smooth sticky foods (such as peanut butter).

The toddler's diet should consist of a wide range of nutritious foods from all food groups in small-sized servings and should include nutritious snacks. The AAP recommends that children drink whole milk until 2 years of age and avoid excesses of fruit juices and non-nutritive drinks.

The preschool period is not a time of rapid growth and requires only 90 kcal/kg/day. Food fads and strong taste preferences are common. Engaging the child in food preparation, and offering food in small portions in an attractive manner, promotes food acceptance. All snacks should be nutritious and not empty calories. The general consumption of food at this age is about one half of an adult's portion. Children should never be forced to eat. Preschool children tend to be deficient in zinc, calcium, and iron.

➤ STUDENT SYNTHESIS

Key Points

- Many childhood communicable diseases can be prevented through immunization.
- Streptococcal infections can lead to serious cardiac complications.
- Parasitic infections generally involve the entire family and home environment.
- The most common cause of injury to a child is trauma.
- SIDS is the sudden, unexplained death of an apparently healthy child.
- Abuse must be reported.
- Common skin disorders include nevi, rashes, and eczema.
- Neurologic disorders include Reye's syndrome and meningitis.
- Meningomyelocele, the most serious form of spina bifida, may cause paralysis or other disorders.
- Hydrocephalus can be detected by OFC measurements.
- Otitis media may require medical or surgical therapies.
- Children with celiac disease must avoid dietary intake of food containing gluten.
- Structural defects of the heart may result in abnormal shunting of oxygenated and deoxygenated blood.
- Leukemias may be acute or chronic.
- Cystic fibrosis is an autosomal recessive disease of the exocrine glands resulting in serious damage to the lungs, pancreas, and liver.
- Serious respiratory tract illnesses include RSV, LTB, epiglottitis, and asthma.
- Illness of the GI tract places the young child at high risk for fluid and electrolyte imbalance or dehydration.
- Urinary tract problems may be structural, autoimmune, cancerous, or infections.
- The most common reproductive disorder concerns ambiguous genitalia and cryptorchidism.
- Solid foods are generally introduced at 4 to 6 months of age.

Critical Thinking Exercises

1. Describe activities that are appropriate for stimulating a 16-month-old child's growth and development if the child is confined in a hip spica cast for congenital hip dislocation.
2. Jimmie, a 4-year-old boy with nephrotic syndrome, is eating poorly. Although edema gives him a plump appearance, he is actually becoming undernourished. Identify suggestions you will give his caregiver to improve his nutritional intake.

3. You are caring for an infant with a bilateral cleft lip repair. What information will you give the family to help them understand the child's care and how they can assist with protecting their baby from injury?

NCLEX-Style Review Questions

1. When assessing a child suspected of having roseola, which symptom should the nurse expect to find?
   a. Abdominal pain
   b. Tonsillar exudate
   s. High fever
   d. Paroxysmal cough
2. The nurse tells the parent of a child with chicken-pox that administration of which medication could cause a serious neurologic condition?
   a. Phenobarbital
   b. Vermox
   c. Acetaminophen
   d. Aspirin
3. The most serious complication of streptococcal infection of the throat is:
   a. Lymphadenopathy
   b. Scarlet fever
   c. Encephalitis
   d. Rheumatic heart disease
4. The nurse explains to the parents of a child with developmental dysplasia that the special splint serves to keep the child's hips in which position?
   a. Abduction
   b. Adduction
   c. Flexion
   d. Extension
5. When planning care for a child with spina bifida, the nurse should write which statement on the nursing care plan?
   a. Do not palpate abdomen.
   b. Turn every 8 hours.
   c. Avoid exercising extremities.
   d. Do not use latex gloves.

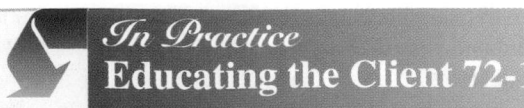

In Practice
Educating the Client 72-1

PREVENTION OF LYME DISEASE

- Wear long sleeves, and long pants with pants tucked into the socks or boots (and tape them). Wear closed shoes or sneakers (no sandals).
- Wear light-colored clothing so ticks can be seen more easily.
- Check skin and clothing frequently.
- Brush clothing off before going indoors.
- Insect repellants such as DEET may be used, but use with caution on infants and children because of toxicity dangers. Permethrin can be sprayed on clothing to prevent tick attachment.
- Apply spray repellants outdoors.
- Walk on paved areas or cleaned paths rather than through brush, if possible.
- Check the entire body after leaving an infected area. Have someone else assist with the inspection.
- Wash clothes after being outdoors.
- To remove a tick, use tweezers; grasp the tick at its head, and slowly pull it straight out without crushing its body. Crushing the body may force some of the infected fluid into the wound.
- Wash the wound with soap and water and apply an antiseptic.
- Use tick and flea collars on pets who are outside in possible infected areas. Inspect them regularly. Common pet ticks do not carry the offending spirochete, but pets can pick up the tick if they are in infested areas outdoors.
- Keep areas where children play free from tall grass, weeds, scrubby areas, and leaf litter.

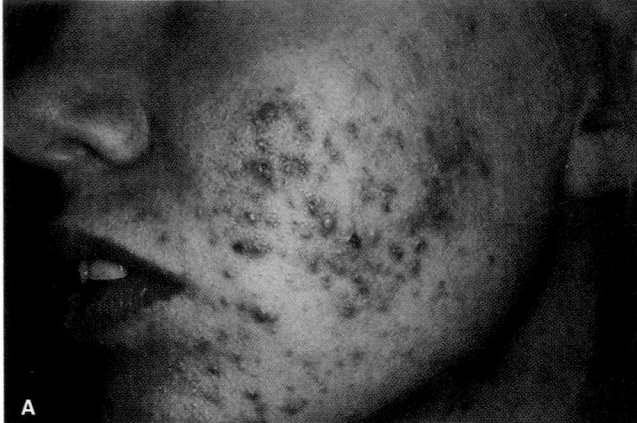

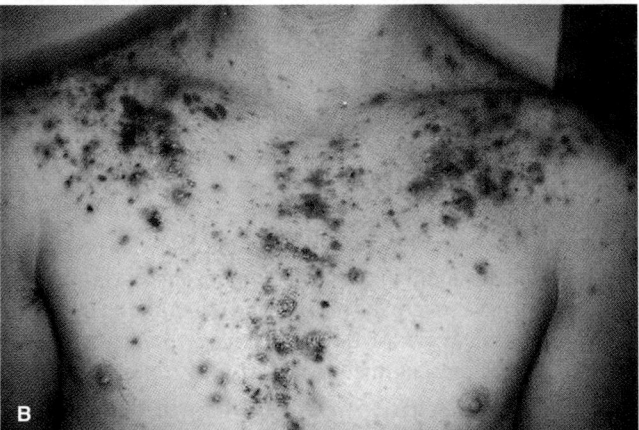

FIGURE 72-2. (**A**) Acne of the face. (**B**) Acne of the chest.

valent in specific geographic areas give rise to more frequent outbreaks. See Chapter 77 for a further discussion on encephalitis.

SKIN DISORDERS

Acne Vulgaris

A skin eruption called **acne vulgaris,** or simply *acne,* affects 85% of the population between 12 and 25 years of age. Blackheads, whiteheads, pimples, cysts, nodules, and scarring characterize acne, which is most commonly seen on the face, back, chest, and upper arms (Fig. 72-2). Acne usually develops first during puberty and is slightly more common in boys than in girls. Research indicates that hormonal changes during puberty accompanied by oversecretion of sebum are acne's underlying causes. Diet plays no significant role in the development or progression of acne; however, a well-balanced, nutritional diet is essential for good overall health. Stress seems to cause acne flare-ups. Severe acne can leave permanent facial scars.

Acne has emotional effects because the condition usually occurs at a time when a young person is agonizingly conscious of personal appearance and peer-group approval. The emotional stress, social withdrawal, and anxiety that accompany acne can greatly affect a young person's development.

Treatment. Treatment includes topical and systemic medications. Key medications for acne are listed at In Practice: Important Medications 72-1. Emotional support is an important aspect of the care for these adolescents. **Dermabrasion,** a surgical means of smoothing the skin, may be considered only after active acne has ceased. This procedure is used to minimize scarring.

Nursing Considerations. Accept and acknowledge that physical appearance is important to the adolescent. Review personal hygiene to help the adolescent prevent infection. Include good general health and diet in the management of acne vulgaris. Be sure to cover instructions regarding medications and skin care regimen. See In Practice: Educating the Client 72-2 for a summary of teaching subjects and In Practice: Nursing Care Plan 72-1.

Impetigo Contagiosa

Impetigo contagiosa is an infection caused by staphylococci, streptococci, or mixed bacteria. Reddened vesicles break open and leave a sticky, honey-colored crust, usually on the

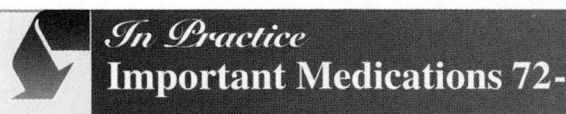

In Practice
Important Medications 72-1

FOR ACNE VULGARIS

Topical Agents
Benzoyl peroxide (Desquam, Fostex, Oxy-10, Clearasil)—antibacterial agent
Retinoic acid, tretinoin (Retin-A)
Tetracycline cream
Erythromycin cream

Systemic Agents
Tetracycline (such as Panmycin, Achromycin)
Isotretinoin (Accutane)—careful monitoring by physician needed because of serious side effects; used only when other agents not effective

Nursing Considerations—Topical Agents
- When combined with other agents, they may cause excessive drying of skin.
- Avoid application to mucous membranes, eyes, inflamed skin, or sunburned skin.
- Use with caution in fair-skinned clients, and in clients with eczema or other skin conditions.
- May cause bleaching of hair or clothing.

Nursing Considerations—Tetracycline
- Take 1 hour before or 2 hours after any food, especially milk, dairy products, or meat.
- May interact negatively with iron, lithium, and oral contraceptives.
- Do not use with renal (kidney) or hepatic (liver) dysfunction; drink plenty of water.

In Practice
Educating the Client 72-2

ACNE CARE
- Follow skin care instructions carefully and patiently. Acne takes a long time to clear up.
- Use gentle cleansing to avoid further skin damage. Avoid scrubbing the face.
- Review side effects and instructions for use of any prescribed medications (especially Accutane).
- Inspect the skin for any adverse reactions following any treatment.
- Avoid pinching or picking at pimples. This results in inflammation and possible scarring, as well as an increased risk of infection.
- Use a clean towel with each washing. Shampoo frequently.
- Maintain good health practices, including regular exercise and balanced nutrition.
- Maintain careful skin care, even after acne lesions have cleared.

face and hands (Fig. 72-3). Impetigo is highly contagious, and transmission-based precautions are necessary to prevent the spread of infection (see Chap. 42).

Aim nursing care at preventing the spread of infection. Remove crusts with soap and water. Good handwashing is essential. Keep the infected person's towels and linens away from others. Discourage the child from scratching or touching infected sites. Antibacterial topical or systemic medications are essential.

Tinea Pedis

Tinea pedis, also known as "athlete's foot," is a common fungal infection that attacks the skin between the toes. Watery blisters that burn and itch, form in moist, weepy spots. The organism responsible for infection (often *Candida albicans*) grows in dark, damp places and is found on the floors of public baths, showers, locker rooms, and pools.

Commercial preparations are available for treating athlete's foot. If the infection does not respond to these preparations, an individual should consult a dermatologist. Medications used in

athlete's foot are Pedi-Dri foot powder, undecylenate acid and zinc undecylenate (Desenex powder, ointment, solution, or cream), tolnaftate (Tinactin), or Lysol solution. Information regarding causes and cures of athlete's foot are helpful to young adults (see In Practice: Educating the Client 72-3).

MUSCULOSKELETAL DISORDERS

Trauma

Because school-age children and adolescents are usually active, they are subject to many kinds of injuries. Fractures, burns, and other forms of trauma are common in this age group. Consult the index for detailed discussions of these conditions.

Postural Defects

Other than trauma, postural defects are the most common musculoskeletal problems affecting school-age children and adolescents. Common defects include lordosis, kyphosis, and scoliosis.

Lordosis is an exaggerated curvature of the lumbar spine in which the pelvis tips forward. It may result from a disease process, or it may be *idiopathic* (of unknown cause). It may be associated with obesity, in which excess abdominal weight distorts the person's center of gravity. It is also associated with hip dislocations or contractures and is accompanied by pain.

Kyphosis is an abnormal curvature of the thoracic spine that results in a "hunchback" appearance. It can result from diseases (such as tuberculosis), compression fractures, or arthritis. Poor posture can also be the cause; in this case, lordosis is

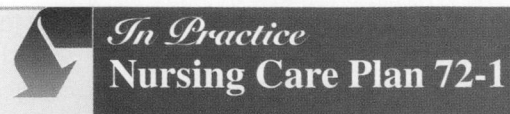

THE ADOLESCENT CLIENT WITH ACNE

MEDICAL HISTORY: *C.H., a 12-year old male, comes to the clinic for a routine health maintenance visit. Growth and development are within range for client, experiencing a 2-inch increase in height in the last year. Small amounts of hair growth noted in axillary and scrotal areas. Based on client's description, pubertal changes have been occurring for the past 9 to 10 months. He states, "Look at my face. It's so ugly with all these pimples." He denies any problems with infections or allergies.*

MEDICAL DIAGNOSIS: *Acne vulgaris*

Data Collection/Nursing Assessment: Client is a well-nourished male reporting that skin eruptions have been occurring for the past 3 to 4 months. "I'm constantly washing my face with a strong soap so that they will go away. And I've been using alcohol to try and dry them up. But nothing seems to work. I've tried to pop them to make them disappear. And I've even stopped eating greasy foods like potato chips." Numerous reddened pustules are scattered on forehead, face, and cheeks. Three small lesions with severely reddened base are noted across the bridge of the client's nose. He complains of tenderness at this site. Client states that he is well otherwise. No other unusual findings are noted. (*Although other nursing diagnoses may be appropriate, a priority nursing diagnosis is addressed below.*)

Nursing Diagnosis: Deficient knowledge related to acne and its causes and treatment as evidenced by client's statements.

Planning
SHORT-TERM GOALS:
#1. Client will identify the causes of acne and preventive measures.
#2. Client will verbalize measures for appropriate skin care and control of acne.

LONG-TERM GOALS:
#3. Client will describe acne, its causes, and treatment accurately.
#4. Client will voice a decrease in lesions by next visit.

Implementation
NURSING ACTION: *Interview client to determine understanding of acne and its causes.*
RATIONALE: *Determining the client's understanding provides a baseline from which to develop teaching plan and appropriate strategies.*

NURSING ACTION: *Review the structure and function of the skin and sebaceous glands, and effects of puberty on their function. Describe how acne develops, clarifying any misconceptions. Engage client in discussion, including having the client describe in his own words what is happening.*
RATIONALE: *Reviewing structure and function and effects of puberty help to clarify what is happening to the client. Clarifying misconceptions provides the client with an accurate knowledge base and better understanding of his condition. Having the client participate in the discussion fosters learning.*

Evaluation: Client able to state how acne develops. *Goal #1 met.*

NURSING ACTION: *Review proper methods of skin care, encouraging client to use a mild soap and water, gently cleansing the areas twice a day. Stress the need to avoid alcohol and too-frequent scrubbing.*
RATIONALE: *Washing too vigorously can rupture the sebaceous glands, worsening the acne. Too-frequent washing or using alcohol is too drying to the skin.*

NURSING ACTION: *Discuss methods of treatment available, emphasizing that improvement does not occur immediately. Notify the primary care provider about the need for a possible referral to a dermatologist.*
RATIONALE: *Discussing available methods provides the client with information about possible options and promotes a feeling of some control over the situation.*

Evaluation: Client states a realistic plan for skin cleansing. He states, "I won't use alcohol on my skin." Client voicing desire to try topical medications. *Progress to meeting Goal #2 and Goal #3.*

NURSING ACTION: *Emphasize the need for a well balanced diet and avoidance of picking or squeezing lesions.*
RATIONALE: *A well-balanced diet is necessary for overall general health; diet plays no significant role in the development or progression of acne. Picking or squeezing the lesions ruptures the gland and spreads the sebum and inflammation, possibly leading to scarring and infection.*

Evaluation: Client states that he will refrain from squeezing or picking the lesions. He verbalizes the lack of significant role that diet has in causing acne. *Goal #2 met. Progress to meeting Goal #3.*

NURSING ACTION: *Arrange for a followup visit in 3 to 4 weeks; have client discuss arranging for visit with dermatologist within the next week to initiate topical medications. Review information presented to client.*
RATIONALE: *Arranging for followup allows time for evaluation, feedback, review of treatment determined by dermatologist, and further teaching. Having client visit with dermatologist within the next week ensures that client will have begun therapy by the next visit, allowing for possible observation of effectiveness of and compliance with treatment chosen.*

Evaluation: Return clinic appointment made for 1 month. Client states he has an appointment with dermatologist on Friday. Client accurately states causes, treatment, and proper measures to prevent and control acne. *Goal #3 met. Progress to meeting Goal #4.*

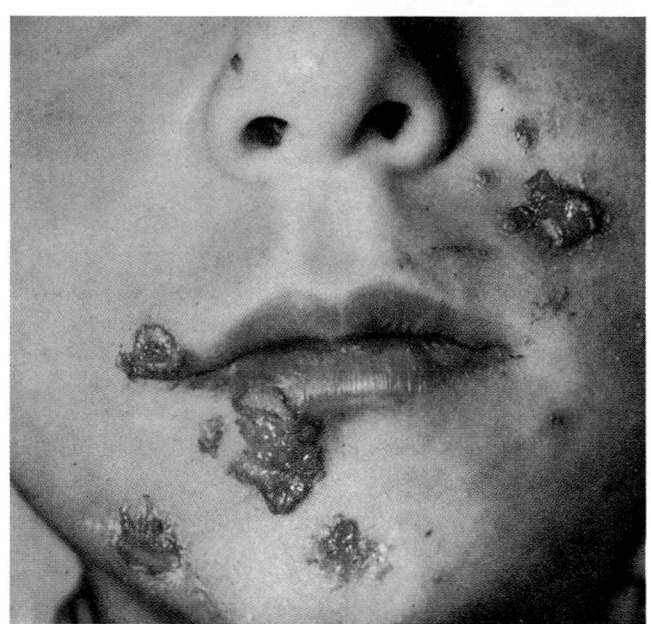

FIGURE 72-3. Impetigo of the face. (Abner Kurten. *Folia Dermatologia.* No. 2. Geigy Pharmaceuticals.)

often present as well, giving the child the appearance of "swayback."

Scoliosis is a lateral curvature, resulting in an S-shaped spinal appearance. Scoliosis is the most common postural defect and is seen more frequently in girls than in boys. There are two types of scoliosis: functional and structural. *Functional scoliosis* results from poor posture. *Structural scoliosis* is rare and is due to defects in spinal muscles or bones.

Diagnosis.   Diagnosis is made by observation and radiography. Postural defects, especially scoliosis, are often dis-

covered by the child's pediatrician or during school screenings (Fig. 72-4). The examination is simple and takes relatively little time. The child faces the screener and stands straight with the feet 2 to 3 inches apart. The examiner looks at the symmetry of the upper torso. He or she then instructs the child to place the chin on the chest and the hands together, and bend over, allowing the hands to hang freely. The screener looks for any asymmetry, such as unequal shoulder height, elbow levels, or hip height. He or she also observes the child for abnormal spinal curvature. If curvature is present, the screener uses a *scoliometer* (leveling device) to detect the curvature's degree. Referral and treatment are based on this degree.

Medical and Surgical Treatment.   Treatment depends on the cause and degree of the postural defect. If the cause is functional, the child may benefit from counseling. Nagging or harassing the child to stand or sit up straight usually does not help.

Many traction devices and braces are used to treat postural defects. Certain exercises also may help in mild cases. The Milwaukee brace is a commonly used device that extends from the chin to the hips and is specially fitted to the child. It is regularly adjusted as the child grows.

A somewhat more controversial method of treatment is the use of electrical stimulation. Electrodes are attached to the muscles of the child's back at night. It is thought that electrical stimulation of the muscles helps correct the curvature by increasing muscle tone.

Surgical intervention may be necessary to correct a postural defect. Surgery includes the application of a device to the spinal column to force realignment. The child usually under-

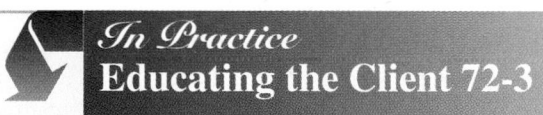

In Practice
Educating the Client 72-3

TINEA PEDIS (ATHLETE'S FOOT)

- Expose the feet to air when possible. Wear sandals and cotton socks.
- Wash the feet daily. Dry thoroughly, particularly between the toes.
- Use a separate towel for each foot; use a clean towel with each bath.
- Apply anti-fungal medication after each bath; continue medication as prescribed.
- Wear shower clogs in public areas, such as swimming pools and locker rooms; step into antiseptic solution at entrance with both feet.
- The fungus may live for a long time in shoes or under toenails.
- Keep shoes ventilated; expose to sunlight and fresh air.
- Alternate wearing at least two pairs of shoes.

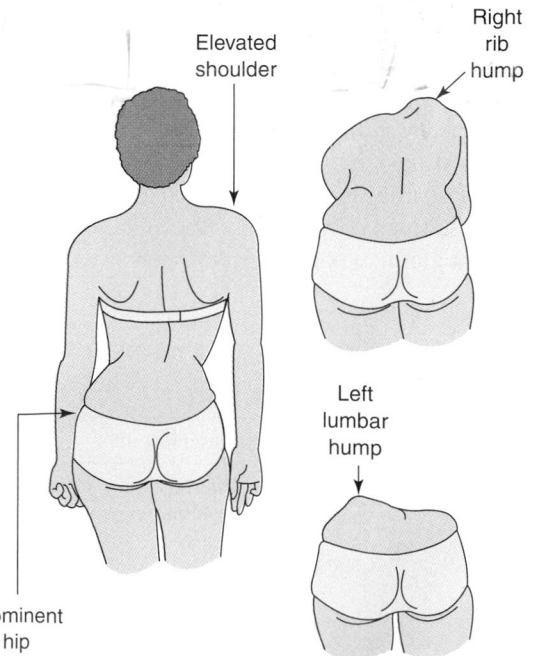

FIGURE 72-4. Scoliosis. Abnormalities to be determined at the initial screening examination. (Gore, D. R., Passhel, R., Sepic, S., & Dalton, A. [1981]. Scoliosis screening: Results of a community project. *Pediatrics, 67*(2). Copyright 1981 by the American Academy of Pediatrics).

goes spinal traction before the surgery. One well-known spinal device is the Harrington rod, which is actually secured to the vertebral bones following spinal fusion. The child's growth is arrested following rod implantation. After surgery, the child may require a cast or brace for immobilization. Surgery is only done after more conservative treatment of the defect is unsuccessful.

Some nursing diagnoses that may be seen on the nursing care plan include:

- Impaired Physical Mobility related to presence of brace, traction, or casts
- Risk for Injury related to restricted movements
- Risk for Impaired Skin Integrity related to presence of brace
- Body Image Disturbance related to chronic skeletal deformity or use of body brace

Clarify the individualized goals of care for the client and family. Make plans to help the client perform activities of daily living as much as possible. Encourage the family to strengthen the affected person's body image and promote as much independence as possible.

☛ KEY CONCEPT

Scoliosis most often affects pre-adolescent girls, who are apt to be concerned with body image. Treatment involves limitations. Provide emotional support.

Juvenile Rheumatoid Arthritis

Juvenile rheumatoid arthritis (**JRA**) is a generalized systemic disease of the entire musculoskeletal system. It can lead to deformities, contractures, and impaired movement. Its cause is unknown. Several research theories have linked JRA to infection or to an abnormal immune response. Girls are more likely to be affected with JRA than are boys.

Symptoms and Treatments. Many characteristic symptoms of arthritis are present, such as painful joint movement and subcutaneous nodules. The child's growth may be arrested; malformation may result from uneven maturation of bones or joints. The primary group of drugs used for treatment are the nonsteroidal anti-inflammatory drugs (**NSAIDs**), which help to relieve fever, pain, and inflammation. Other drugs (eg, injectable gold) are used when NSAIDs are less effective.

Many children experience a spontaneous remission with no recurrence. Only about 20% continue to be affected as adults. Nursing care during the acute phase includes exercising the limbs, helping the child with daily activities, and sometimes applying heat in the form of hot baths, packs, or whirlpool treatments.

Legg-Calve-Perthes Disease

Legg-Calve-Perthes disease results from a lack of blood supply to the hip joint, causing aseptic joint necrosis. The condition has several other names, including *coxa plana, slipped femoral epiphysis, Legg's disease, Legg-Calve disease,* and *Legg-Calve-Waldenstrom disease.* It occurs in children aged 2 to 12 years and is most common in Caucasian boys. It may be caused by an injury or another disease process; it is also associated with low birth weight. Both hips may be affected; however, usually only one hip is affected.

Symptoms include intermittent limp on the affected side and hip pain or soreness, and stiffness. X-rays confirm the diagnosis. The disorder most often clears spontaneously, but treatment is necessary to prevent subsequent hip deformities. Table 72-1 lists stages of the disease.

Medical Treatment. The goal of treatment is to maintain the head of the femur in the acetabulum. Historically, hip immobilization with the child on bed rest was considered necessary. However, keeping a child on bed rest for an extended period of time is very difficult. Treatment now focuses on containing the head of the femur in the acetabulum during the revascularization process to allow the femoral head to form a smoothly functioning joint. A variety of appliances are used that vary with the portion of the femoral head that is affected. Avoidance of weight bearing on the affected limb is essential. The disease is self-limiting, but prognosis depends greatly on how extensively the femoral head had deteriorated before diagnosis and treatment.

■■■ TABLE 72-1 ♪**TAGES OF LEGG-CALVE-PERTHES DISEASE**

Stage	Description	Duration
Stage I	Interruption of circulation to hip joint, resulting in necrosis of femoral head	Approximately 1–3 wk; may last up to 1 y
Stage II	Depositing of new connective tissue because of new blood supply	6 mo to 1 y; child may have definite, constant limp; also may have severe pain, aggravated by activity and relieved by rest
Stage IIIa	Granulation of new bone replaces connective tissue	1–2 y
Stage IIIb	Regeneration and completion of bone growth; shape of joint fixed	2–3 y (depending on whether medical or surgical treatment used)

Surgical Treatment.   Reconstructive surgery that can, within 3 to 4 months, return the child to normal activities is available. Surgery contains the usual risks, but upon evaluation, the child's rapid return to normal may outweigh possible risks.

Dental Malocclusion

Malocclusion refers to faulty tooth positioning, which results in improper alignment of the jaws and teeth. In addition to making teeth difficult to clean, malocclusion may cause facial deformities and difficulty in eating and chewing. The correction of tooth positioning and jaw deformities is called **orthodontia.** Generally, orthodontic care should begin after the child's permanent teeth erupt, between the ages of 8 and 12 years. Sometimes treatment is delayed until the child is older, depending on the problem's severity.

Malignant Bone Tumors

Malignant bone tumors are less common in children than they are in adults. However, tumors tend to grow faster in children than they do in adults. Chapter 82 discusses general nursing care of any person with cancer.

Osteogenic sarcoma is a type of cancerous bone tumor, often seen in young men between the ages of 10 and 30 years. The diaphysis of the long bones is frequently involved, and other bones may be involved as well. The cancer *metastasizes* (spreads) by way of the circulatory system, often to the lungs first. Treatment may involve amputation of the affected extremity, along with radiation and chemotherapy. Aggressive treatment can reduce the person's mortality rate.

Ewing's sarcoma is a bone malignancy that arises from the bone marrow and affects the long and flat bones. It is more commonly seen in young men between the ages of 10 and 20 years. Radiation is used as treatment. The prognosis is guarded.

ENDOCRINE DISORDERS

Of all *endocrine disorders* that can affect school-age children and adolescents, diabetes mellitus is the most significant. Other, relatively uncommon conditions include diabetes insipidus and pituitary disorders that result in changes in growth.

Diabetes Mellitus

Diabetes mellitus type 1 or *insulin-dependent diabetes* (**IDDM**) is the second most chronic illness in childhood and the most common form of diabetes in children, occurring in 1.7 of 1,000 children. The etiologic factors in IDDM include genetics, autoimmune factors, and environmental factors such as viruses and infant nutrition (see Chap. 78 for further discussion). An increasing number of overweight and sedentary children are being diagnosed with *diabetes mellitus type 2* or *non–insulin-dependent diabetes mellitus* (**NIDDM**).

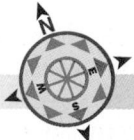

SPECIAL CONSIDERATIONS: CULTURE

Diabetes Mellitus

Different ethnic populations vary in their susceptibility to diabetes mellitus. Scandinavian American and Caucasian American children have a high incidence, while Japanese American, African American, and Hispanic American children have a lower incidence.

Children often have an abrupt onset of the classic symptoms of **polyuria** (dramatic increase in urinary output, probably with enuresis), **polydipsia** (abnormal thirst), and **polyphagia** (increased hunger). These symptoms are usually accompanied by weight loss or failure to gain weight and lack of energy. If the child's symptoms are not noted and the child is not referred for diagnosis, the disorder is likely to rapidly progress to diabetic ketoacidosis and eventually to diabetic coma.

Treatment of diabetes in children includes insulin therapy, meal plans, and exercise. Involve the whole family in the diabetic child's care and treatment.

The child will need close supervision by the healthcare team until he or she adjusts to the insulin dosage and the condition stabilizes. Infections need to receive immediate medical care because they can lead to ketoacidosis. Encourage insulin-dependent diabetic youngsters to test their blood for glucose, self-administer their injections as soon as possible, and lead a normal, independent life (Fig. 72-5).

Diabetic children can learn to regulate insulin intake according to diet and activity. Encourage them to be active, and teach them the importance of exercise in the total program of control. Summer camps are available where diabetic children can learn more about the disease and how to handle it with the least disturbance to everyday life. These children need to understand that other people of their age share their condition. Family caregivers and diabetic children need intensive instruction and support, especially in the early days after diagnosis.

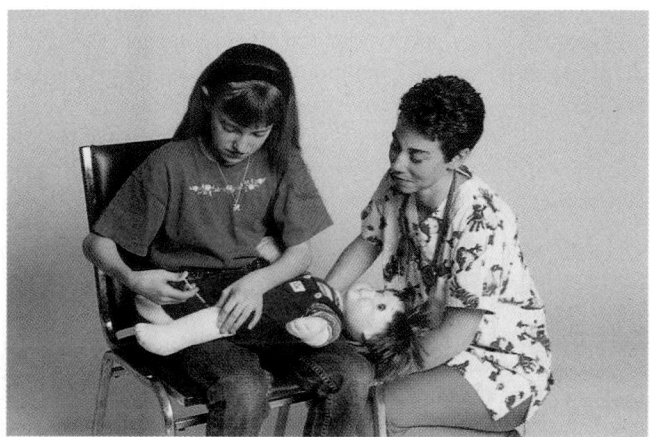

FIGURE 72-5. A school-age child is taught insulin administration using a teaching doll for practice.

Encourage family caregivers to alert all adults who will be responsible for a diabetic child about the child's condition, including teachers, school nurse, camp nurse, scout leader, athletic coach, and so forth. All adults caring for a diabetic child must learn the signs and symptoms of hypoglycemia and hyperglycemia (see Chap. 78) and the proper care for each. Adolescents often go through an adjustment period in which they rebel against treatment. They need understanding and support during this time. Diabetes counseling must emphasize regulation of diet and insulin administration to reflect physical activity.

SENSORY SYSTEM DISORDERS

Retinitis Pigmentosa

Retinitis pigmentosa (**RP**) is characterized by a slowly progressive, bilateral retinal degeneration that often causes blindness. Adolescents are more likely to be affected by RP than are people of other age groups.

Generally, night blindness is the first symptom. The person is often *myopic* (near-sighted) as well. As the disease progresses, the visual field constricts, causing tunnel vision. The physician can often see a characteristic dark retinal pigmentation, which is known as a *bone spicule.* Other ocular defects can occur, including cataracts, glaucoma, or blind spots. Macular degeneration occurs. When the macula is invaded, the person becomes blind. This condition is often associated with hearing disorders.

The person should wear dark glasses in bright sunlight to avoid further eye irritation and to enhance remaining vision. The person may be unable to drive a car at night because of night blindness. The National Retinitis Pigmentosa Foundation provides literature and information about the disorder. RP is a hereditary disease; therefore, genetic counseling is also important.

Juvenile Glaucoma

Glaucoma refers to abnormally high *intraocular* (within the eyeball) pressure, resulting in eye damage and decreased vision. It may be caused by trauma, hemorrhage into the eye, tumor, inflammatory eye disease, or developmental abnormalities during infancy and early childhood. Early symptoms include frequent tearing, *photophobia* (sensitivity to light), and cloudiness of the cornea. Surgery is performed as early as possible to prevent damage to vision. Medications to control intraocular pressure are also used (see Chap. 79).

GASTROINTESTINAL DISORDERS

Inflammatory Bowel Disease

Inflammatory bowel disease (**IBD**) is a chronic gastrointestinal disorder. The two most common types of IBD are Crohn's disease and chronic ulcerative colitis. (Refer to Chapter 87 for more information regarding *Crohn's disease.*)

Chronic ulcerative colitis (CUC) is a relatively common disorder in adolescents and young adults. It results in inflammation of the colon and rectum. One of the most pronounced symptoms of CUC is severe diarrhea (may be bloody), which may be accompanied by weight loss, anorexia, and growth delays. A delay in the appearance of secondary sex characteristics also may be evident if the disease occurs before puberty. The distal colon shows evidence of ulceration, inflammation, and bleeding, which eventually may result in scarring of the gastrointestinal mucosa. An autoimmune component may be associated with this illness.

Medical and Surgical Treatment.   One of the most important methods of treating CUC is through corticosteroid administration. Many side effects, however, are associated with steroid administration, some of which may cause further growth delays (see Chap. 62). A *colectomy,* which removes the diseased portion of the colon, results in the cure of symptoms. Colectomy is done only if conservative treatment fails.

Appendicitis

Appendicitis, an acute infection of the vermiform appendix, is uncommon in children under 2 years of age and is more common in school-age children and adolescents. Abdominal pain begins in the periumbilical area and localizes in the right lower quadrant. Fever, nausea, and vomiting are commonly present. The infection progresses rapidly to perforation and peritonitis due to the gastrointestinal bacteria. *Appendectomy,* a relatively simple surgery, is performed. Generally the young person recovers without difficulty. If the appendix ruptures, the child receives intravenous antibiotics.

REPRODUCTIVE SYSTEM DISORDERS

Many disorders that affect the reproductive systems of older children and adolescents are related to hormonal changes.

Menstrual Difficulties

Menstrual difficulties include delayed onset, discomfort, and altered patterns. Pain occurring with ovulation is referred to as **mittelschmerz. Dysmenorrhea,** painful menstruation, is a common problem for young girls whose bodies are establishing regular cycles. There are two types of dysmenorrhea. *Primary dysmenorrhea* is painful menstruation with no accompanying pelvic disease. Painful menstruation accompanied by organic pelvic disease is called *secondary dysmenorrhea.*

Treatment of primary dysmenorrhea is symptomatic. Administration of NSAIDs (ibuprofen) given 1 to 2 days prior to the beginning of menses prevents the formation of prostaglandins and helps reduce discomfort and inflammation. Warm baths and relaxation techniques also help reduce pain. In severe cases oral contraceptives may be used. When secondary dysmenorrhea occurs, the underlying physical cause is identified and treated as necessary.

Abnormal Sexual Development

With the emphasis on sex appeal in the United States, many adolescents are especially concerned about the development of their secondary sexual characteristics. *Precocious* (early) and delayed sexual development may occur. These conditions are particularly distressing for adolescents because peer pressure is so significant at this developmental stage.

Many adolescents are concerned that they are underdeveloped or overdeveloped compared with their peers. These adolescents deserve sensitive treatment. Consider emotional aspects and each adolescent's perceptions. You may refer especially concerned adolescents to a specialist who can confirm or deny that they have a problem. If a problem does exist, treatment should proceed as needed. Emotional support, including counseling, is essential.

Sexually Transmitted Diseases

As discussed in Chapter 69, most sexually transmitted diseases (STDs) in the United States occur in people younger than age 25. Sexually active young adults with a history of reproductive and/or urinary tract disorders may have STDs that are not obvious or have not been detected. Urge young people to see a physician. Physicians must, by law, treat an adolescent with an STD without reporting the condition to the adolescent's family caregivers. Many free public clinics also provide tests and treatment for STDs.

Certain STDs are most prevalent in adolescents and young adults. They include HIV/AIDS, gonorrhea, chlamydia, genital herpes (herpes simplex virus [HSV]), and genital warts (human papilloma virus [HPV]). The incidence of certain STDs is increasing, even with the massive amount of public education about safer sex and condom use. STDs that are left untreated can cause infertility and sterility. Sexually active school-age children and adolescents should be strongly encouraged to engage in safer sexual practices or abstinence.

SPECIAL CONSIDERATIONS: CULTURE

HIV/AIDS

According to WHO and CDC, HIV/AIDS is the leading cause of death in children worldwide, and the seventh leading cause of childhood mortality in the age group of 1 to 4 years. The number of children diagnosed each year is increasing, primarily cases resulting from transmittal during the perinatal period. Over half of HIV/AIDS infections are transmitted by heterosexual partners. The remaining majority of HIV/AIDS occurs because of contamination related to intravenous drug use.

EMOTIONAL AND PSYCHOLOGICAL DISORDERS

As children get older, they face more challenges and difficult experiences. Adolescents especially encounter many developmental tasks that they must achieve before reaching adulthood. Sometimes, stress becomes overwhelming for adolescents, who develop an emotional disorder in response. In addition to psychological stressors, many of the following conditions may have physical origins or causes. Thorough examination is vital.

Sleep Disorders

Narcolepsy
Narcolepsy is a brief attack of irresistible sleep. An alteration in the young person's emotional status often precipitates this condition; narcolepsy can usually be traced to some type of conflict. Nighttime sleep is basically normal; however, tests usually detect an earlier appearance of rapid eye movement (**REM**) sleep, which under normal circumstances occurs toward morning and is marked by dreams.

Conflict, competition, and unacceptable aggression may be underlying contributing factors. Boys are more likely to be affected than girls. No significant relationship exists between narcolepsy and seizure disorders, although providers must rule out a seizure disorder. Hallucinations may occur just as the person is falling asleep (*hypnagogic hallucinations*). Another symptom is *sleep paralysis*. **Cataplexy,** an attack of muscular weakness and lack of muscle tone, may accompany narcolepsy.

Hypersomnia
Hypersomnia is an uncontrollable urge to sleep, characterized by lengthy sleep periods (12 to 18 hours). Hypersomnia must be differentiated from absence seizures. It may stem from a physiologic cause, such as brain damage, or another physical illness. The disorder may be a manifestation of a psychological problem, in which the person sleeps to "escape the world."

Nightmares and Somnambulism
Nightmares and *somnambulism* are common occurrences that most children outgrow. Nightmares may frighten children, but family caregivers can provide comfort. Children can often recall nightmares in graphic detail the next morning.

Somnambulism (sleep walking) usually occurs during the later stages of non-REM sleep. Children usually do not recall sleep walking episodes the next morning. Sleep-walking episodes can last from several minutes to a half hour or longer. Sleep walking is more common in boys than in girls and is more common when children are fatigued or under stress. Trauma, central nervous system infections, or seizure disorders may be predisposing factors. Most commonly, however, somnambulism is related to anxiety. Often a child sleep walks once or twice and never does it again.

The major concern with sleep walking is physical protection. Do not threaten or abruptly awaken a sleep walker, but observe safety measures to avoid injuries.

Night Terrors or Terror Disorder

Night terrors or *terror disorder (pavor nocturnus)* almost always occurs in children, not in adults. It is not common and is not to be confused with an occasional nightmare. In night terrors, a child awakens screaming and is panicky. Family members cannot console the child, who may be incoherent. After the terror passes, the child usually cannot recall what caused it. The child will usually outgrow this condition. Blood found on a child's pillow after an episode may indicate a psychomotor seizure disorder. A sleep study (*polysomnogram*) can help determine the cause.

Other Sleep Conditions

Somniloquism.   **Somniloquism** (sleep talking) is common in young people. It may or may not be associated with sleep walking. The person can often carry on a logical conversation but will not remember it the next morning.

Insomnia.   **Insomnia** is difficulty falling asleep. It may be caused by *hyperkinesis* (hyperactivity) or may be a symptom of an emotional problem.

Eating Disorders

As children develop, their eating behaviors change. Food can take on new meanings in adolescence as a result of family stress or peer pressure. A few nursing diagnoses that will be on the nursing care plan for a person with an eating disorder follow:

- Altered Nutrition: Less than Body Requirements related to self-induced vomiting, excessive use of laxatives, over-exercise
- Altered Nutrition: More than Body Requirements related to excessive oral intake, lack of exercise
- Risk for Fluid Volume Deficit related to inadequate oral intake, vomiting, laxative abuse
- Body Image Disturbance related to distorted perception of body weight
- Self-esteem Disturbance related to denial of eating disorder
- Constipation related to inadequate diet, laxative abuse
- Ineffective Individual Coping related to altered family dynamics, changes in role expectations

Teaching is of prime importance in the care of a young person with an eating disorder. The adolescent needs to understand normal bodily functions and the need for nourishment to sustain these functions. Developing strong rapport with the adolescent is essential for his or her compliance.

Anorexia Nervosa

Anorexia nervosa is a disorder most commonly seen in Caucasian, upper–middle-class, female adolescents (although some boys are affected). The prevalence is estimated to be 1% to 5% of teenage girls. Anorexia nervosa is characterized by extreme weight loss with no underlying physical cause. Predisposing factors include perfectionist behavior, low self-esteem, and in 40% of the cases, a history of being mildly overweight.

Anorexia nervosa usually begins with moderate efforts to lose weight and progresses to an obsession with any weight gain, causing severe anxiety. Weight loss reduces anxiety. Hunger is extreme and always present. Affected individuals are obsessed with being thin. They have a distorted body image, seeing themselves as overweight, even after they have become dangerously thin. Anorexia nervosa is a long-term psychological problem, involving complex family relationships. Box 72-1 lists symptoms of anorexia nervosa.

Life-threatening complications include lowered blood pressure, bradycardia, *hypokalemia* (low potassium), and congestive heart failure. Death may occur. Severe malnutrition must be treated before long-term counseling can begin. Most severe cases require hospitalization.

Bulimia Nervosa

Bulimia nervosa, known as "gorge-purge syndrome," is an eating disorder characterized by loss of control during overeating followed by purging. Like anorexia nervosa, bulimia is most commonly found in older adolescent and young adult females, although some boys are affected as well.

Typically, affected individuals rapidly eat large amounts of food, usually in secret. Following such binges, they attempt to purge their systems of food through self-induced vomiting or laxative and diuretic use.

Recurrent vomiting can cause dental caries and throat irritation from stomach hydrochloric acid that erodes the enamel from the front teeth. Electrolyte imbalances and even death are possible. Feelings of guilt and depression are common during binges. Long-term counseling is necessary to overcome the disorder. Bulimic individuals are usually of normal weight or overweight; otherwise they fulfill the other criteria for anorexia nervosa.

➤➤ **BOX 72-1**

SIGNS AND SYMPTOMS OF ANOREXIA NERVOSA

Extreme weight loss
Menstrual irregularities
Unexplained amenorrhea
Weakness
Fatigue
Lightheadedness
Constipation
Low blood pressure
Bradycardia (slow pulse)
Hypokalemia (potassium deficiency)
Thinning hair
Distorted body image
Excessive exercising
Low body temperature
Dry skin

Obesity

As assessed by body mass index (**BMI**), the incidence of overweight or near-overweight American children is around 30%. The trend cuts across all sex, age, racial, and ethnic groups. The most obese children are getting heavier, a risk factor for obese adulthood.

Obesity can stem from the regular high consumption of calories, particularly from fats, resulting in excess accumulation of fatty tissue. It is defined as being in excess of 20% of optimum weight. The obese child is most often less active than the leaner child. A hereditary factor is related to obesity. Obesity is rarely caused by slow thyroid function.

Obese children endure many psychological effects. Their socialization skills and self-esteem are greatly affected, which may lead to difficulties making friends and building healthy relationships. Treatment consists of diet and exercise with medical supervision, behavior modification, and counseling. Chapter 30 describes eating patterns and suggestions for healthy diets for children of all ages.

Elimination Disorders

Enuresis (bed wetting) or *encopresis* (involuntary bowel movement) that continues into the school years with no physical cause requires a physician's intervention. The cause is often emotional. Counseling or psychiatric assistance, in combination with medications, usually corrects the problem. Sometimes, a meatal stenosis needs to be surgically corrected. Encopresis most often requires intensive psychotherapy. In any event, family caregivers should not shame or belittle the child—such behavior may cause lasting psychological damage.

Behavioral Problems

Although *behavioral problems* in childhood may have a physical basis, more often the cause is an inability to establish healthy relationships with others. Emotional problems may be manifested by withdrawn or destructive behavior or by bizarre speech. Signs that a child may need professional assistance include an inability to control impulses or behavior, behavior that is very different from others in the same age group, lack of friends, difficulty in learning even though the child tests well, persistent physical symptoms that seem to have no physical basis, and specific deviant behaviors.

The Chronic Lawbreaker. One way a youngster indicates that he or she is having problems is by defying the law. Many police forces employ specialists or counselors to assist young people who are "asking for help" by being in constant trouble with the law. The most effective means of dealing with the problem is through family counseling.

School Phobia. Another problem facing caregivers of school-age children is the development of *school phobia*. The phobia may occur after a summer vacation or a brief illness. A change in school or neighborhood, a new sibling, divorce, or a family member's death may precipitate the child's fear or avoidance of school. School phobia is more common in girls.

Children (usually 5 to 10 years old) who have school phobia suffer from a fear of leaving their caregiver(s). They are often very good students. These children may be so tense that they actually become physically ill; in other instances, they ask to stay home because of minor physical complaints. When family caregivers allow such children to stay home, symptoms and complaints diminish immediately, only to recur the next morning. In a severe case, a child may refuse to leave the house for any reason. School nurses sometimes recognize the symptoms of school phobia in children because these children often spend a great deal of time in their office after they arrive at school. School phobia in adolescents often indicates a more serious problem that requires thorough evaluation.

NUTRITIONAL CONSIDERATIONS

During the school-age period, children are spending more time away from home and assume more control over their daily intake of foods. A minimum of 30% of calories should come from fat, with only 10% coming from saturated fats and a 300-milligram daily maximum of cholesterol to prevent heart disease.

Iron intake is important, especially for girls beginning menses, to prevent iron deficiency anemia. Middle childhood and adolescence is the time to put nutritional practices into effect that will prevent atherosclerosis, obesity, diabetes, and osteoporosis later in life. The Food Guide Pyramid is a useful tool for educating parents of children of all ages about a healthful diet. Nutrition is discussed in Chapters 30, 31, and 32.

School-age children need a nutritious breakfast to prevent hypoglycemia and discomfort due to hunger, which may cause poor concentration and a shorter attention span. The school lunch program is designed to provide nutritious meals that are attractive to children. Advise parents to teach children how to make good food choices and to avoid non-nutritive, high-calorie, high-fat snacks.

When introducing new foods at the table, advise parents to offer them one at a time in small servings. Encourage parents to provide a calm, relaxed atmosphere free of conflict at mealtime.

The rapid growth of adolescents is accompanied by increased nutritional requirements and a ravenous appetite. There is an increased need for protein as body mass increases, and a need for calcium to promote bone density and prevent future osteoporosis. Peer pressure, commitments to activities, and the availability of fast foods often lead to poor food choices and a deficiency of vegetables, fruits, and milk in the diet.

The diabetic child requires the same nutrients as other children, with consistency in quantity of intake and regularity of mealtime. The diet must be individualized to meet the activity pattern of each child. The medical team may recommend the exchange system or the carbohydrate counting system. Whichever method is used to regulate the diet, the regimen of food, insulin, and exercise must be balanced and must meet the requirements for growth and development.

Obesity is estimated to affect 25% to 30% of American children, with less than 5% attributed to underlying disease. This factor translates into poor health outcomes for these children.

Factors that influence childhood obesity include heredity, peer pressure, inactivity, sociocultural influences, and psychological factors. Obsessed with body image and weight, children often engage in fad diets, thereby depriving their bodies of nutrients essential for health. Encourage the family to implement a healthier, moderately low-fat diet and to engage in regular physical activity. To reduce fat and total calories, a 30% decrease in the previous caloric intake is suggested.

Education should focus on ways good nutrition can promote improved appearance. Nonjudgmental involvement of the child in the process of ways to improve their nutrition will have better outcomes.

SPECIAL CONSIDERATIONS IN CHILDREN

Compliance with a therapeutic regimen is a problem for children and families, especially when dietary restrictions, frequent monitoring, or daily pharmacologic interventions are essential. The nurse needs to individualize the treatment plan according to the child's developmental stage, and foster the independence of the child in the management and control of chronic diseases. Client education should focus on the prevention of exacerbations and complications of the disease.

➤ STUDENT SYNTHESIS

Key Points

- Mononucleosis, which is common in young adults, is treated with fluids, rest, and analgesics.
- Lyme disease can be misdiagnosed. Later in life it can cause serious symptoms.
- Acne vulgaris is treatable with topical and systemic medications
- Impetigo is highly contagious
- The most important aspect of treatment of Legg-Calve-Perthes disease is maintaining the affected extremity as non–weight-bearing.
- Scoliosis is more common in girls and must be treated to prevent serious defects related to curvature of the spine.
- Anorexia nervosa and bulimia, although related to nutrition, are psychological disorders requiring long-term treatment.
- JRA can lead to deformities, contractures, and impaired movement.
- Children with IDDM and NIDDM need to closely monitor medications, diet, and exercise.
- RP is characterized by progressive, bilateral retinal degeneration that causes blindness
- IBD in adolescents is seen as Crohn's disease and CUC.
- Dysmenorrhea is the most common menstrual complaint of adolescent girls.

- Over half of HIV/AIDS cases are transmitted by heterosexual partners.

Critical Thinking Exercises

1. Explain developmental characteristics of adolescence that may create adjustment problems for the adolescent diabetic client.
2. While caring for 13-year-old Amy, she confides in you that she is worried about her sexual development. What help and guidance will you give her?
3. Karen, age 13, has recently begun wearing a Milwaukee brace for scoliosis. Previously, she was active in softball, cheerleading, band, and other school activities. Now you find that she has abandoned most of those activities. She claims that she needs more time to study now that she is in the eighth grade. What is your response to her?

NCLEX-Style Review Questions

1. To prevent the spread of mononucleosis among siblings, the nurse should advise the mother to:
   a. Use antibacterial soaps.
   b. Change bed linen daily.
   c. Wash hands after elimination.
   d. Avoid contact with saliva.
2. The nurse teaches a family that the primary cause of Lyme disease is:
   a. Dog saliva
   b. Cat scratches
   c. Tick bites
   d. Deer feces
3. The nurse explains to a pre-adolescent client that acne is primarily caused by:
   a. Hormone changes
   b. Poor nutrition
   c. Inadequate hygiene
   d. Excessive stress
4. A child with multiple honey-colored, crusted lesions on the legs, arms, and face comes to the clinic and is diagnosed with impetigo. The nurse should place priority on teaching the mother to:
   a. Administer analgesics.
   b. Promote oral fluid intake.
   c. Prevent the spread of infection.
   d. Ensure a balanced diet.
5. An adolescent scheduled for dermabrasion asks, "How will this help me?" Which is the best response by the nurse?
   a. "It will remove all the infection."
   b. "It will make your skin smoother."
   c. "All the scars will disappear."
   d. "You will not get acne again."

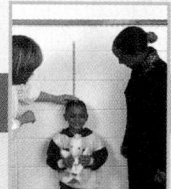

CHAPTER

73

The Child or Adolescent With Special Needs

LEARNING OBJECTIVES

1. Define and differentiate between genetic and acquired congenital disorders.
2. Identify at least five characteristic signs and symptoms of FAS.
3. Identify at least five characteristic signs and symptoms of neonatal abstinence syndrome.
4. Identify at least five characteristic signs and symptoms of pediatric HIV/AIDS.
5. Identify at least four criticisms of standard IQ tests.
6. Define and differentiate among the following levels of mental impairment: borderline, mild, moderate, severe, and profound.
7. Identify at least five characteristics of Down syndrome.
8. Discuss at least four effects that developmental and learning disabilities have on the child and the caregivers and family.
9. Identify at least five characteristics of ADHD.
10. Identify four characteristics of Tourette syndrome and autism.
11. Identify four characteristics and causes of plumbism.
12. Identify the main classifications of cerebral palsy.
13. Differentiate the causes of and treatments for Duchenne muscular dystrophy with Down syndrome and fragile X syndrome.
14. Define and differentiate between the characteristics of childhood depression and childhood schizophrenia.
15. Discuss at least four nursing concerns related to maternal substance abuse and the potential effects on the children involved.
16. Identify at least five nursing considerations related to long-term pediatric rehabilitation.
17. Discuss at least four nursing consideration related to the care and upbringing of special needs children.

NEW TERMINOLOGY

ataxic cerebral palsy	dyslexia
autism	echolalia
BAL in Oil	fragile X syndrome
chelation	genetics
congenital	Gowers' sign
coprolalia	plumbism
developmental disability	schizophrenia
Down syndrome	simian line
Duchenne muscular dystrophy	spastic cerebral palsy
dystrophy	suicidal ideation
dysfluency	teratogen
dyskinetic cerebral palsy	trisomy 21

ACRONYMS

AAP	ARND	FAS
ADDH	ASD	IQ
ADHD	BLL	LSD
AFP	COAS	OCD
ALT	CP	SLD
ARDD	CPK	TS

The process of growth and development can be difficult, even under optimal circumstances. Normal maturation offers opportunities for daily learning experiences for all children. Children with special needs, such as those with a long-term physical or emotional disorder, have additional challenges.

All aspects of the family's daily life are affected when a child has special needs or a chronic illness. The nurse can assist such families by providing support and education. Numerous and varied support groups are available for many conditions and situations. Providing families with accurate information regarding their situation is essential. Families experiencing any difficult process require support and acceptance of their feelings.

☛ KEY CONCEPT

Family caregivers of a physically or mentally challenged child may go through a grieving process, during which they deal with the loss of an anticipated "perfect child." Grieving may occur intermittently, as the child reaches or fails to reach major developmental milestones. Such grieving does not mean that caregivers do not love the child. Your support and understanding can help caregivers cope.

CONGENITAL DISORDERS

Congenital simply means "present at birth"; therefore, a congenital disorder is one that exists at birth. If a congenital defect or disorder results from a defective gene, it is then *hereditary* or *genetic*. A congenital disorder is considered *acquired* if it results from maternal factors or conditions during pregnancy or childbirth.

Genetic Disorders

Genetics is the study of heredity. With the single exceptions of the sperm and ova cells, the nucleus of every human cell contains 23 pairs of chromosomes. Each chromosome contains hundreds of genes, placed in specific locations on the chromosome. Each gene is a unit of heredity and, as such, it is responsible for a specific human characteristics (eg, hair color, nose size, eye color, and so forth). The correct position, shape, and alignment of each gene results in a normal, healthy child. Any abnormality, even of a single gene, can have profound physical and/or mental consequences.

A *genetic disorder* is a physical or mental abnormality resulting from a defect in genetic structure. The defective gene can be *familial*, which means that the biologic parent has the defective gene, and passes it on to the offspring. A defective gene can also occur for no apparent reason. A genetic disorder is inborn and present at birth, but it may not be immediately apparent.

Examples of genetic disorders include:

• *Neurofibromatosis,* which is characterized by "cafe-au-lait" spots and benign skin tumors. The child has neurologic, cognitive, and speech impairments. Attention deficit–hyperactivity disorder and seizures are common symptoms.

• *Tay-Sachs disease* is an inborn error of metabolism, primarily affecting children of Ashkenazi Jewish descent. Symptoms begin at about 1 year of age. The child becomes hypotonic and loses vision. Death due to Tay-Sachs usually occurs before age 4. A blood test is available to determine carriers.

• *Cystic fibrosis, hemophilia, sickle cell disease,* and *phenylketonuria* are among other genetic disorders that are discussed elsewhere in this text. *Duchenne muscular dystrophy* is also a genetic disorder, discussed later in this chapter.

Diagnosis. Some genetic disorders can be diagnosed immediately through identifiable physical characteristics or laboratory studies. Many disorders can be detected prenatally through amniocentesis (see Chap. 67), although the procedure carries a certain risk to the fetus. α-Fetoprotein (**AFP**) testing is performed on amniotic fluid, and increased AFP levels indicate possible neural-tube or ventral-wall defects.

Chromosomal studies are performed when healthcare providers suspect a genetic disorder. A blood sample is taken, and if a chromosomal problem is identified, further studies may be recommended and options discussed.

Counseling. *Genetic counseling* is available for people who are seeking information about the possibility of genetic disorders in their families. A professional counselor specializes in identifying genetic profiles of individuals and families. The counselor takes the individual's or couple's extensive health history, including chronic health problems, miscarriages, birth defects, and causes of death of other family members. The counselor also inquires about employment, ethnic background, and exposure to toxins.

Based on this information, the counselor designs a family tree or genetic profile. Counseling includes education regarding genetics, how disorders are inherited, and individual risks of genetic disorders. The counselor does not make decisions for people about family planning. The counselor provides information and options, and the person or couple makes the necessary decisions. The role of the genetic counselor is one of providing support and information.

Genetic counseling is a form of preventive healthcare that strives to prevent birth defects. Encourage couples or individuals at risk for transmitting genetic disorders to seek counseling before pregnancy. The counselor can help them make educated, informed decisions. Information on genetic counseling can be obtained from the National Foundation of the March of Dimes.

☛ KEY CONCEPT

Genetic counseling is particularly indicated for adults who have known genetic disorders.

Acquired Disorders

Many conditions are congenital but not genetic; they are *acquired.* Examples of acquired disorders are those that are caused by teratogens such as alcohol, drugs, maternal diseases, and toxic substances. **Teratogens** are substances that the pregnant woman uses or comes into contact with, which are known to cause a wide range of fetal abnormalities.

Many substances that may be safe for the mother are unsafe to the unborn child. The Food and Drug Administration has designed pregnancy categories for drugs—an important reference for the nurse. Drugs are listed in five categories: A, B, C, D, and X. These categories are defined in medication reference texts. Essentially, the criteria range from Category A, which has no known effects on the fetus, to Category X, which has known, absolute teratogenic effects.

In addition, trauma or anoxia during the birthing process can cause fetal disorders (see Unit 10). Maternal malnutrition during fetal development and low birth weight are important contributing causes to intellectual impairment. These conditions cause difficulties for the child well beyond infancy.

Fetal Alcohol Syndrome

Fetal alcohol syndrome (**FAS**) results from heavy maternal alcohol consumption. It is estimated that as many as 8,000 cases of FAS occur each year. FAS is one of the leading causes of mental retardation. Many more children are born with associated *alcohol-related neurodevelopmental disorder* (**ARND**) or *alcohol-related developmental disabilities* (**ARDD**). The lifetime consequences of *in utero* alcohol exposure include mental retardation, learning disabilities, and serious behavioral problems. The National Institutes of Health estimate that healthcare costs for treatment of preventable alcohol disorders is nearly two billion dollars per year.

Alcohol in the mother's blood freely crosses the placenta. Birth defects due to alcohol can occur at anytime throughout pregnancy. Abnormal facial features, as well as poor organ and bone development, occur as a result of maternal drinking during the first trimester. Abnormal brain and fetal development occur from drinking at any time during the three trimesters of pregnancy.

The U.S. Public Health Service has indicated that there is no safe level of alcohol intake during pregnancy. Chronic drinking and binge drinking are the most dangerous forms of alcohol intake. Birth defects due to alcohol intake are known to occur in the first 3 to 8 weeks of pregnancy.

Women may not be aware that they are pregnant during the early weeks of pregnancy. The effects of alcohol to a fetus are irreversible. When the woman stops drinking, the health of the fetus improves, but the fetus does not recover from damage that has been done. The U.S. Department of Health and Human Services advises against drinking alcoholic beverages when planning pregnancy and during pregnancy. It is not known why some women who drink heavily during pregnancy do not have children with FAS. Abstinence is the only known prevention of FAS and other alcohol-related disorders.

☛ KEY CONCEPT

Any drink containing alcohol can damage a fetus. The alcohol content is about the same in a four-ounce glass of wine, a standard 12-ounce glass of beer, and a one-ounce shot of straight liquor. Wine coolers, malt beverages, and mixed drinks generally contain more alcohol.

Signs and Symptoms. The majority of infants with FAS experience facial abnormalities, growth retardation, developmental delays, below-normal mental functioning, and dysfunctions of the central nervous system (CNS) (Fig. 73-1). Babies can have some or all of the clinical FAS features. Fetal alcohol effects can be seen to lesser degrees in ARND and ARDD.

These infants tend to be extremely irritable. As they become older, a shortened attention span and hyperactivity are evident. Other features include *microcephaly* (small head); eye, ear, and heart defects, which include septal defects and tetralogy of Fallot; impairment of fine motor movement; and memory deficits.

Diagnosis. Diagnosis is made by obtaining a thorough maternal history and observing characteristic signs and symptoms. Many other conditions may co-exist with alcohol-related disorders. For example, conditions such as growth and developmental delays, hyperactivity, and specific learning disorders may also be diagnosed.

Treatment. Treatment consists of early recognition and referral to support services. Medical management of seizures, surgical repair of physical defects, and special education is commonly necessary. No cure exists for FAS or ARND/ARDD.

Nursing Considerations. Early identification and intervention are necessary to maximize the potential of these children and to prevent further complications. Every pregnant woman should be encouraged to stop drinking any form of alcohol during the entire prenatal period. Peer, significant other, and family support needs to be encouraged. The key to prevention of alcohol-related disorders is public education regarding the dangers of consuming any alcohol during pregnancy.

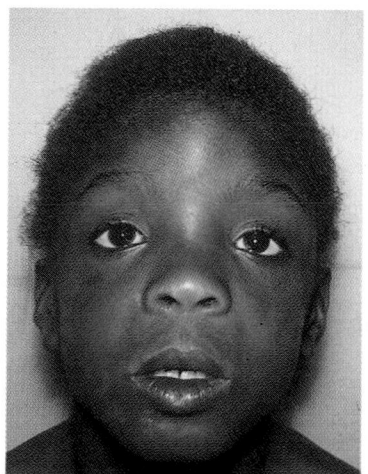

FIGURE 73-1. A child with fetal alcohol syndrome. Babies born to women who are chronic alcoholics are at increased risk for growth deficiency, microcephaly, and mental retardation. Facial characteristics shown here include short palpebral fissures, a wide and flattened philtrum (the vertical groove in the midline of the upper lip), and thin lips.

Neonatal Abstinence Syndrome

The long-term outcome of fetuses exposed to maternal narcotic use is not completely known. After delivery, these newborns show withdrawal symptoms from the narcotic, beginning at 24 to 48 hours after birth and lasting about 2 weeks.

Signs and Symptoms.   Symptom severity depends on the drugs used. Newborn symptoms are more intensified when drugs are used close to birth. Typically the neonates show irritability, tremors, hyperactive Moro reflex, and poor feeding. In addition, these children may have cognitive impairment, behavioral disorders, learning disabilities, and attention deficits.

Diagnosis.   Diagnosis is made by obtaining a maternal history, performing drug screens on the mother and newborn, and documenting the characteristic behaviors of addicted newborns.

Treatment.   Some of the difficulties of addicted newborns may also result from a dysfunctional home environment, in which the mother continues her drug use. In addition, women who use drugs regularly are often malnourished and frequently exposed to infections during pregnancy. Mothers may need help to stop using drugs. Infections need to be treated. Postnatal checkups are very important for both the mother and the baby. Nutritional support and education will promote growth and healthier lifestyles.

Nursing Considerations.   The nurse should provide supportive care of the infant with gentle, but minimal handling. Swaddling, rocking, using pacifiers, and decreasing environmental stimulation should be implemented. Some newborns require medications for withdrawal symptoms (paregoric, phenobarbital).

Narcotic-exposed newborns face long-term social, physical, emotional, and mental challenges. Community resources and family support systems need to be obtained for both mother and infant. Followup phone calls to the mother by the healthcare providers and home health visits are important supportive services.

☛ KEY CONCEPT

Substance abuse is one of the most common causes of cognitive impairment and physical disabilities in children. Behavioral and psychosocial problems may result.

Exposure to Maternal Infections

Many maternal infections critically affect fetuses, with resulting long-term consequences. Fetal exposure to chickenpox or toxoplasmosis can result in mental retardation and microcephaly. Toxoplasmosis also can cause deafness or cognitive impairment. Maternal herpes simplex virus can cause seizures and paralysis in newborns. The outcome of prenatal exposure to rubella (German measles) includes various birth defects, as well as intellectual and visual impairment. (See TORCH infections in Chapter 68.)

HIV/AIDS in Children

About 90% of children who are positive for HIV are infected prenatally or at birth by their HIV-positive mothers. The incidence of pediatric HIV/AIDS has decreased in the last decade since the implementation of prenatal HIV/AIDS counseling and testing. The use of zidovudine (AZT, Retrovir) by HIV-positive pregnant women and their newborns has resulted in fewer cases of pediatric HIV and the reduction of cases of AIDS.

Research has shown that with proper prenatal treatment, newborns may be prevented from being infected by HIV-positive mothers. It is known that HIV-positive mothers may have a high percentage of babies that test positive for the HIV antibody, but only about one in four test positive for the HIV antigen. This means that the infant with only the antibody may not have the actual HIV virus, which is indicated by having the HIV antigen. Therefore, many of these infants have a normal lifespan and most likely will not go on to develop HIV or AIDS. Prenatal and postnatal care for HIV-positive mothers and infants is a critical healthcare factor.

Some children, usually adolescents or older children, became infected with the virus through sexual contact or intravenous (IV) drug use. These children usually develop the multiple symptoms of HIV/AIDS.

Signs and Symptoms.   Before 1 year of age, the human immune system is immature. Therefore, infants who test positive for the HIV antigen are less able to fight off the opportunistic infections associated with HIV/AIDS than are adults. These babies have a more rapid disease progression than do adults who acquire HIV/AIDS. Most children infected perinatally have AIDS diagnosed by the age of 4. Chapter 84 discusses HIV/AIDS in further detail.

Approximately half of these infants develop *Pneumocystis carinii* pneumonia. Diseases such as Kaposi's sarcoma and tuberculosis, although common in adults with HIV/AIDS, are uncommon in children. Infants with HIV/AIDS usually have delayed growth and present as typical failure to thrive (FTT) babies. Most of these infants also have an enlarged liver and many develop lymphoid interstitial pneumonia. These infants and children have a greater incidence of bacterial sepsis and neurologic involvement than do adults.

Diagnosis.   Diagnosis is made by laboratory testing methods: the ELISA (enzyme-linked immunosorbent assay) test for screening and the Western Blot test for confirmation.

Treatment.   Zidovudine (AZT, Retrovir) continues to be the primary treatment for children with HIV/AIDS. Zidovudine is given to HIV-positive pregnant mothers. The drug is continued for up to 1 year in identified infants.

Antibiotics and gamma globulin are used to treat opportunistic infections. Common childhood illnesses such as chickenpox, measles, otitis media, and upper respiratory infections can be deadly to children with HIV/AIDS. Immunizations and isolation from other sick children are critical; a simple case of otitis media can quickly develop into meningitis in children with HIV/AIDS.

Nursing Considerations.   Other factors complicate the care of children with HIV/AIDS. Their mothers may be too ill to care for them. Breastfeeding by HIV-infected mothers is contraindicated. If no other family members are available, foster care may be necessary. Keeping these children separated from sick siblings at home is difficult, as is providing these children with adequate nutrition on limited budgets. Use of universal precautions by healthcare workers and family members is an important teaching concept.

☛ KEY CONCEPT

Some genetic and congenital disorders are not identified until the child fails to achieve certain developmental milestones.

INTELLECTUAL IMPAIRMENT

The individual with **intellectual impairment (cognitive impairment)** demonstrates below-average intellectual abilities, accompanied by difficulty functioning independently. *Mentally retarded, mentally disabled,* and *intellectually challenged* are other terms used to describe those who are impaired.

The severity of a person's handicap or disability is determined in large part by scores the individual achieves on standard intelligence tests. Numerical scores are given that are based on tests using a score of around 100 as a baseline for normal. Tests such as the Wechsler Intelligence Scale for Children-Revised and the Stanford Binet are used to determine degrees of intellectual impairment.

Intelligence quotient (**IQ**) tests are widely used, but are known to have limitations. They are not known to determine success in life. IQ tests are good predictors of academic achievement; however, they are highly criticized for not being able to indicate other types of intelligence. Many indicators of success in life and the working world include factors such as persistence, self-confidence, motivation, interpersonal skills, creativity, intuition, and verbal and nonverbal skills. Standard IQ tests cannot predict work productivity and successful parenting skills.

Cultural, gender, and racial factors are also known to influence scores on standard IQ tests. Minority groups tend to score lower than the predominate culture. Environmental considerations (such as urban, rural, or military) and social resources, the availability of educational resources, and the individual's general health will also affect IQ scores.

Although IQ scores should not be used to determine a child's abilities, the scores usually must be reported so that the child can qualify for special education assistance in public schools. More than one type of testing may be used to determine functional capacity.

Levels of Functioning

Although the use of IQ scores for purposes other than agency placement and funding is discouraged, the following categories of impairment are generally accepted. These IQ categories are modified and adapted from the International Classification of Disease, Ninth Edition, Clinical Modification (ICD-9-CM).

Borderline: IQ Between 70 and 85. The child who has *borderline intellectual impairment* is usually able to function independently with the assistance of special education.

Developmental delays are common among these children, but many of them achieve most developmental milestones.

Mild: IQ Between 50 and 70. The majority of cognitively impaired children fall into the category of *mild impairment.* Most of these children qualify for full-time special education; however, those with higher functioning may develop reading skills at a fifth- or sixth-grade level.

Moderate: IQ Between 35 and 50. The *moderately cognitively impaired* child is unable to function independently and achieves a maximum mental age of 3 to 7 years. Training focuses on activities of daily living (ADL) and the child may eventually require assisted-care living arrangements.

Severe: IQ Between 20 and 35. The child who is *severely impaired* requires a great deal of assistance with ADL but can conform to daily routines and repetitive activities. Language development is minimal.

Profound: IQ Falls Below 20 or Unable to Test. The *profoundly impaired* child requires complete assistance with all aspects of daily life. Some of these children may eventually be toilet-trained; however, many of them are not. Their verbal skills are extremely limited.

The Association for Retarded Citizens in each county assists intellectually impaired people and their families. This association provides support groups, supplies, literature, education, advocacy in housing, employment, and referrals for group homes, respite care, and medical care.

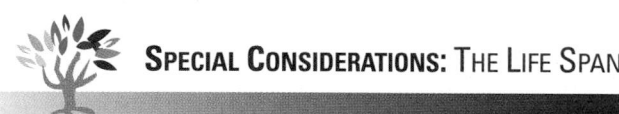

SPECIAL CONSIDERATIONS: THE LIFE SPAN

Intellectually Impaired Older Adults

Aging people who are intellectually impaired face special problems. They are often left alone when their family caregivers die or become disabled. These individuals may have difficulty adjusting to assisted-living situations when they reach middle age or beyond.

Genetic Intellectual Impairment

Causes of cognitive impairment are many and varied. Genetic defects account for some cases, as in Down syndrome and fragile X syndrome.

Down Syndrome

Down syndrome results from a chromosomal abnormality. It is also known as **trisomy 21.** The incidence of Down syndrome is about 1 in 800 births. It is the most common cause of mental retardation. The incidence of Down syndrome increases in children born to women who are older than 35 years of age. A link is also established between mothers younger than 35 years and maternal smoking. The combination of smoking and oral contraceptives increases the risk for Down syndrome.

Signs and Symptoms. Typical physical characteristics of Down syndrome include a small, flat nose and upward, outward, slanting eyes. At birth, the caretakers may notice that the hands of children with Down syndrome have an abnormal crease straight across the palms (**simian line**). Additionally, the hands are usually short and square. These newborns also have short, stubby feet, with a wide space between the big toe and the rest of their toes, and a transverse crease across the soles.

Other characteristic features include white dots on the irises (Brushfield's spots); short, sparse eyelashes; small, low-set ears; and a downward-curved mouth with a protruding tongue (Fig. 73-2). Their muscles are flabby, and their joints can easily be hyperextended without causing pain.

Children with Down syndrome have varying degrees of intellectual impairment.

Diagnosis.   High-risk mothers should be given genetic counseling. Amniocentesis or chorionic villus sampling can determine chromosomal abnormalities prenatally. The mother may elect to proceed with a therapeutic abortion rather than continue the pregnancy. Down syndrome is most often diagnosed at birth through recognizable physical characteristics. Later, chromosomal studies confirm the diagnosis.

Related Disorders.   Multisystem disorders are associated with Down syndrome. Congenital cardiac defects occur in approximately 35% of infants with Down syndrome. These children have an increased incidence of leukemia, severe respiratory illnesses, thyroid disorders, megacolon, and hypotonic abdominal muscles. Developmental delays generally occur in social, sexual, and physical areas.

Treatment.   Treatment is symptomatic. The child may need assistance with feeding because he or she may have difficulty suckling. Surgical repair of cardiac anomalies and other

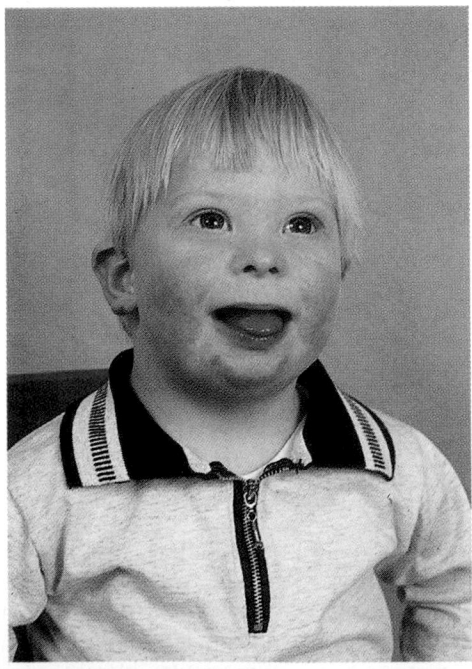

FIGURE 73-2. A child with Down syndrome. Note the physical characteristics. (Marks, M. G. [1998]. *Broadribb's introductory pediatric nursing* [5th ed.]. Philadelphia: Lippincott Williams & Wilkins.)

disorders is common. Children may need chemotherapies for leukemia and antibiotics for infections.

Nursing Considerations.   Nursing interventions for the child with Down syndrome focus on prevention of complications from related disorders, and education and support for the family. Grief counseling is generally necessary. Social, healthcare, and financial resources are needed to provide the care for these children. Special education may also be required. Respite care is often recommended for caregivers.

Education enables children with Down syndrome to live a full life and to feel pride in their accomplishments. Children with Down syndrome, however, need a great deal of repetition to foster learning. Speech development may be slower than motor development. Stammering can occur when these children are under stress. A decrease in relative IQ scores occurs with age, because of the abstract thinking that is required at a higher mental age. Early intervention by professionals is essential for the child to attain optimal health and level of function. In addition to the multisystem disorders associated with this condition, children with Down syndrome experience the same typical childhood problems and disorders, such as pneumonia or appendicitis, that may require hospitalization. In Practice: Nursing Care Plan 73-1 highlights the care of a child with Down syndrome who is hospitalized.

Fragile X Syndrome

Fragile X syndrome is a genetic, sex-linked abnormality of the X chromosome. Women are carriers. The condition manifests most often in boys and to a lesser extent in girls. The condition results in cognitive impairment and distinctive physical features. Intellectual impairment ranges from a specific learning disability to profound mental handicaps. It is the most common form of inherited mental retardation.

Signs and Symptoms.   Male children with fragile X syndrome typically have a large head and chin and a long face. Their eyes may be wide set, and their ears are large and often protruding. They typically have a broad nose, high palate, big hands, and large testicles. There is a noted speech delay; stuttering may be present. Heart murmur, caused by mitral valve prolapse, may be present.

Learning is affected, not only by a lower IQ, but also by a shortened attention span and hyperactivity. These children also may exhibit autistic-type behaviors and temper tantrums.

Diagnosis and Treatment.   Diagnosis is made by chromosomal studies. Treatment is symptomatic. No cure exists for fragile X syndrome.

Nursing Considerations.   Early interventions are essential to maximize the child's potential. Many of the nursing interventions for clients with Down syndrome are appropriate for those with fragile X syndrome. The child will benefit from speech and occupational therapy. Special education assistance is most helpful. Table 73-1 compares the characteristics of Down syndrome and fragile X syndrome.

Acquired Intellectual Impairment

In addition to genetic causes, fetal exposure to infections, drugs, and chemicals, or to maternal malnutrition, play a role

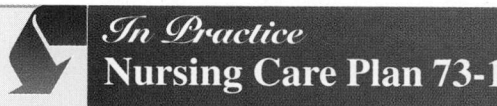

In Practice
Nursing Care Plan 73-1

THE CHILD WITH DOWN SYNDROME WHO IS HOSPITALIZED

MEDICAL HISTORY: *J.B., a 12-year-old boy admitted to the pediatric unit with a diagnosis of appendicitis, is scheduled for an appendectomy later this afternoon. He has had acute abdominal pain with vomiting and loss of appetite for 2 days. Temperature is 100.4° F (41.0° C); child is tachycardic with respirations at 24 breaths per minute. Child is NPO with IV fluids infusing into left hand. Past medical history reveals a diagnosis of Down syndrome. This is the child's first hospitalization.*

MEDICAL DIAGNOSIS: *Appendicitis; Down syndrome*

Data Collection/Nursing Assessment: Child is observed pushing away his father and older sister when they attempt to comfort him. They have stayed with him since admission. Child's eyes are moist and tearing. Child seen lying on left side, staring at the wall, refusing to look at father or sister when they talk to him. His father reports that he is able to function at the level of a 4- or 5-year-old but needs constant supervision and direction. He states, "This is all so new for him. He never had to stay in a hospital before, let alone need surgery." *(Although other nursing diagnoses may apply, a priority nursing diagnosis is addressed below.)*

Nursing Diagnosis: Anxiety related to the new experience of pain and hospitalization, as evidenced by child's withdrawal and parent's statement about the newness of the experience.

Planning
SHORT-TERM GOALS:
#1. Client will demonstrate trust in the nurse.
#2. Client will make needs known to the nurse and staff.

LONG-TERM GOALS:
#3. Client will demonstrate feelings of safety and security by cooperating with care and treatment.

Implementation
NURSING ACTION: *Question father about the child's usual pattern of daily activities, and duplicate this as closely as possible; encourage family members to participate in care if they wish.*
RATIONALE: *Information about the child's usual pattern provides a baseline for individualizing the child's care and modifying the hospital routine to meet the child's needs for consistency.*

NURSING ACTION: *Recommend that the family provide child's personal items, such as own pajamas or favorite toy.*

RATIONALE: *Personal items help to reduce the level of stress, providing a more familiar and comfortable routine, thereby promoting the child's comfort. Changes in routine can be especially threatening to the cognitively challenged child.*

Evaluation: Child lying in bed, tightly clutching the teddy bear that was brought in from home. Father stroking child's head; child looking at nurse when being spoken to. *Progress to meeting goal #1.*

NURSING ACTION: *Assess the child's reaction to illness and hospitalization, noting any verbal or nonverbal expression of common fears of children, such as separation, loss of control, bodily injury and harm based on the child's developmental level, not chronological age.*
RATIONALE: *The child with Down syndrome poses a special challenge, because nursing care is based on the child's unique responses to the stress of illness; entering into the mind and experience of the child offers the best guarantee that the experience of hospitalization will be positive for the child.*

NURSING ACTION: *Explain all procedures simply, in a manner the child can understand and at the child's developmental level. Use dolls or puppets to explain procedures or treatment and allow child to play with them.*
RATIONALE: *Simple explanations at the child's developmental level and help from the family are important to avoid overwhelming the child. Using dolls or puppets aids the child in understanding the information. Allowing the child to play with the teaching materials provides the child with a means to express feelings.*

NURSING ACTION: *Enlist the family's help as necessary. Praise the child for accomplishments and offer assistance as needed.*
RATIONALE: *Providing positive feedback for accomplishments helps to reduce anxiety and to promote a sense of self-esteem. Offering assistance as needed helps to minimize possible feelings of frustration and added stress that this may cause.*

Evaluation: Child observed playing with doll, peeking under abdominal dressing at "scar"; using stethoscope to listen to doll's heart. Father and sister seen playing with child as he plays with doll. Child allows nurse to inspect IV site and listen to abdomen. *Goal #1 met.*

NURSING ACTION: *Be alert to the fact that the cognitively challenged child may revert to the coping*

(continued)

In Practice
Nursing Care Plan 73-1 *(Continued)*

strategies of a younger child: physical resistance, aggression, negativism, and regression; assist the family to understand these behaviors if they present.

RATIONALE: *Most children cope with the stress of illness by regressing to a more dependent and secure level of functioning.*

Evaluation: Child crying loudly and pushing father away when nurse inspects IV infusion site. Child pointing at IV site and yelling, "Go away!" *Progress to meeting Goal #2.*

NURSING ACTION: *Frequently assess the child for evidence of pain. Note verbal and nonverbal behaviors; offer comfort measures as appropriate.*

RATIONALE: *The child may have difficulty understanding events and communicating his comfort need.*

Evaluation: Preoperative preparation completed. Preoperative medication administered IM. Child using doll to show IM injection and what will happen in surgery. Child pointing at abdomen, stating "It hurts bad." Child with tears in eyes, drawing knees up to abdomen. *Progress to meeting Goal #2 and Goal #3.*

---

in intellectual impairment. Preterm and small-for-gestational-age newborns are at risk for cognitive impairment, as are those babies who have cranial defects or trauma. Often, the etiology is unknown.

DEVELOPMENTAL AND LEARNING DISABILITIES

Developmental disabilities are assorted groups of physical, cognitive, psychological, sensory, and speech impairments. According to the National Center on Birth Defects and Developmental Disabilities, about 17% of children under 18 years of age have a developmental disability. Developmental disabilities can begin at any time prior to 18 years of age. The causes for the majority of these disabilities are unknown.

Of the school-age children in the United States, about 2% have serious developmental disabilities, such as mental retar-

dation or cerebral palsy. More than $36 billion dollars each year is spent by federal and state governments for special education programs for children between 3 and 21 years of age.

A **learning disability** is a disorder in one or more of the processes involved in understanding or using language. Learning disabilities can be related to specific aspects of learning, such as memory, attention span, or processing or sequencing of information. A learning disability affects not only school performance, but all aspects of a child's life. Education must be individualized for the child's special needs.

Specific Learning Disability

Specific (special) learning disabilities (**SLD**s) are educational concerns. Most authorities believe that 10% to 20% of school-age children have an SLD. Although an SLD may accompany various other problems (eg, sensory impairment or low IQ), it

---

■■■ TABLE 73-1 *C*HARACTERISTICS OF DOWN SYNDROME AND FRAGILE X SYNDROME

Feature	Down Syndrome	Fragile X Syndrome
Head	Round, small, short	Abnormally large
Face	Flattened profile	Long, large, protruding jaw
Ears	Small, low-set	Large, protruding
Eyes	Upward, outward slant; epicanthal folds; Brushfield's spots	Wide set; epicanthal folds
Nose	Small; depressed nasal bridge	Flattened nasal bridge
Hands	Short, square; simian creases	Simian creases
Mouth	High-arched palate; protruding tongue; mouth curved downward	High-arched palate
Behavioral	Low-normal intelligence to severe intellectual impairment; language delay	Mild to profound intellectual impairment; short attention span, hyperactivity; temper tantrums; autistic-like behaviors; speech delays

does not result from any of these conditions. Children of normal intellectual functioning also have SLDs.

The SLDs include such disorders as the inability to calculate or draw, and *dysphasia* (a speech impairment). SLDs are evidenced by difficulty in speaking, writing, listening, talking, spelling, or calculating. **Dyslexia** is one of the most common disorders in which the person has difficulty with reading, spelling, or writing words. Often the dyslexic child reverses letters or numbers.

When caring for a child with an SLD, learn about the specific disability and set achievable goals. If the child has a problem listening and understanding, give only one or two instructions at a time, and reinforce them periodically. Use visual reminders for the child with a listening deficit. A child with visual processing deficits will benefit from a tape recorder that reinforces information. Provide help and encouragement so the child can achieve progress. Keep in mind that you need to adjust healthcare teaching for the child.

☛ KEY CONCEPT

A child who does not appear to follow directions can cause frustration. The child may continue to play with IV pumps or other equipment even after repeated requests not to do so. Such behavior may indicate a behavioral problem or a learning disorder. In either case, patience and sensitivity are necessary, along with praise and positive reinforcement. The child with an SLD often has low self-esteem. Create a soothing, non-stimulating environment to aid the child to meet expectations.

Attention Deficit-Hyperactivity Disorder

Attention deficit–hyperactivity disorder (**ADHD**) is the most common child behavioral disorder, affecting more than 2 million children in the United States. It may also be called *minimal brain dysfunction* and *attention deficit disorder with hyperactivity* (**ADDH**).

ADHD involves a learning disability and a behavioral disorder. Children with ADHD have difficulties related to attention span, impulsivity, and hyperactivity. The diagnostic criteria for ADHD indicate that the behaviors must persist for at least 6 months to such a degree that they are maladaptive and interfere with developmental milestones.

Signs and Symptoms.   Children with ADHD may manifest inattention by being extremely distractible. They fail to give adequate attention to details (such as in schoolwork or play activities). They seem not to listen to directions, and fail to finish chores or schoolwork. They have difficulty getting started with tasks and sustaining a mental effort with reading or assignments. They often talk excessively. They may lose things necessary for activities such as toys, school assignments, or tools.

Impulsivity can be seen as disruptive and hyperactive behavior. For example, these children may interrupt others by inappropriately intruding on conversations or activities. They have difficulty waiting for their turn in a game.

Hyperactivity can be seen as constant fidgeting with the hands or feet. These children may leave their seat unexpectedly in the classroom, or may run and climb where it is inappropriate. Quiet, leisure activity is often difficult for the ADHD child.

The ADHD child may show poor eye–hand coordination; abnormalities may be seen on their electroencephalograms (**EEG**s). The manifestations of the disorder usually appear both at home and in other settings, such as school.

According to the American Academy of Pediatrics (**AAP**), a 6- to 12-year-old with hyperactivity, inattention, impulsivity, academic underachievement, or behavior problems should be evaluated for ADHD. The onset of the disorder is often before the age of 4 years in approximately half of the cases. ADHD is more common in boys, tends to run in families, and occurs across all socioeconomic strata.

Diagnosis.   The cause of ADHD is controversial; studies are ongoing. A disturbance of the chemical neurotransmitters in the brain has been postulated, but research has not yet identified any specific deficiencies. Understand that although the child with ADHD may develop emotional problems, ADHD is not classified as an emotional disorder.

Diagnosis of ADHD is made only after other medical and psychiatric disorders are ruled out. A child suspected of having ADHD undergoes a multidisciplinary evaluation, which includes speech and language, psychological, medical, and educational testing. A thorough neurologic evaluation is essential, as is feedback from teachers and family caregivers.

Treatment.   Many problems are associated with ADHD, including low self-esteem, poor social interaction, immaturity, and SLDs. Treatment must be addressed with a multidisciplinary approach. A behavioral therapist may set up a behavior-modification program. The school system must address any difficulties with learning and socialization, and the physician is involved with monitoring medication and the child's overall physical health.

Although 80% of children with ADHD will respond to stimulant medications, which have proven to be very effective for some children, they are only part of the total behavioral, educational, and psychological approach to helping the child. The current drug of choice is methylphenidate HCl (Ritalin), a CNS stimulant that affects mental rather than motor activities. Side effects include decreased growth rate, increased heart rate and blood pressure, and sleep disturbances. Pemoline (Cylert) and other cerebral stimulants also may be used. Side effects are similar to those of Ritalin; however, they are not necessarily evident in every child who takes these drugs.

Antidepressants are the second drugs of choice, although some have not proven to be effective. They are less likely to cause sleep disturbances and are not associated with growth retardation.

Nursing Considerations.   Teach family caregivers to minimize environmental stimuli, use consistent discipline, set limits, and focus on positive behaviors. They should give the child just one direction at a time so that the child is not overloaded with directions to remember and organize. Remember, the child wants to be successful just as much as others want him or her to be successful.

Tourette Syndrome

Tourette syndrome (**TS**) is an inherited, neurologic disorder of unknown cause, although a chemical neurotransmitter abnormality is found. *Neurotransmitters* carry signals from one nerve to another. Defects in the body's metabolism of the neurotransmitters dopamine, serotonin, or norepinephrine are suspected. Children with Tourette syndrome exhibit multiple involuntary movements and uncontrollable vocalizations, called *tics.*

Signs and Symptoms.   The tics can be facial such as eye blinking, nose twitching, or grimaces. Tics can also manifest as head jerking, neck stretching, foot stamping, or body twisting. It is not uncommon for a TS client to continuously clear his or her throat, cough, bark, shout, utter obscenities (**coprolalia**), or repeat words of other people (**echolalia**). Actions may be repeated obsessively and unnecessarily. In rare cases, self-harming behaviors are seen (eg, head banging).

The tics may subside for long periods of time and reoccur. They periodically change in number, frequency, type, and location. The individual can control the tic for only a short period of time. During stressful periods, the tic episodes worsen. During sleep, tic activity decreases.

Although children with TS are often of normal intelligence, they may have SLDs and may show ADHD symptoms. Obsessive compulsive disorder (**OCD**), characterized by an intense need to repeat actions such as handwashing, is also found in TS clients. The behavioral symptoms of ADHD or OCD can be more distressing to the individual and family than the tics.

Diagnosis.   Diagnosis is made by physical description of the tics that persist for a period of time. MRI, CT, and EEG studies rule out other causes. There are no laboratory diagnostic studies.

Treatment.   Treatment is symptomatic. Clonidine (Catapres), an anti-hypertensive agent, may be effective in treating some cases of motor tics. Medications such as acetaminophen help ease muscle spasm discomfort. Stimulants such as methylphenidate HCl (Ritalin), combined with haloperidol (Haldol), may help control behavior. A specific medication for TS is pimozide (Orap), which blocks the brain's dopamine receptors.

Nursing Considerations.   Psychiatric counseling does not decrease tics, but may be effective in helping the child and family cope with TS. Many of the tic symptoms decrease as children near adulthood. Occasionally, the condition goes into remission after adolescence. With maturation, other conditions such as depression, mood swings, panic attacks, and antisocial behaviors may increase. There is no cure for TS. Genetic counseling may help the parents understand the risk of TS for other children.

Autism

Autism spectrum disorders (**ASD**) are lifelong, complex developmental disorders characterized by intellectual, social, and communication deficits. Autism is not actually a disease, but a syndrome of specific behaviors that vary widely, thereby making it difficult to diagnose.

The cause of autism is unknown; however, statistics show that more boys are affected than girls. Public interest fostered research into the possible connection of autism with childhood immunizations, particularly measles, mumps, and rubella (MMR). According to the National Immunization Program of the Centers for Disease Control and Prevention (CDC), no association has been found.

The prevalence of autism is estimated to be from two to six children per every 1,000 births. The costs for special education for autistic children range from about $10,000 to $100,000 per year, per child.

Signs and Symptoms.   Autistic children typically demonstrate a profound lack of social interaction. They do not respond to verbal stimuli, and do not like to cuddle or be touched. They may show bizarre attachments to mechanical objects.

Autistic children often display repetitive or ritualistic behaviors such as rocking, head banging, clicking of teeth, or turning the head back and forth. Impaired verbal and nonverbal communication, temper tantrums, and self-destructive behaviors also may be evident. Echolalia is one form of language impairment that may be seen. These children are believed to be preoccupied within themselves, perhaps having fixed delusions and hallucinations. They sometimes become very upset or aggressive when interrupted.

Diagnosis.   There is no specific test or procedure to diagnosis autism. Other physical and emotional disorders need to be ruled out. Autism is often associated with some degree of mental or cognitive impairment. Some autistic children are profoundly impaired. A few children have typical autistic behaviors and additionally may have superior intelligence in one particular area, such as math, art, or music. Others have a photographic memory. These children may be referred to as an autistic "savant."

Treatment.   No known cure exists for autism, and the prognosis varies widely. Psychiatric symptoms occur in approximately half of all autistic children during adolescence. Intervention requires professionals with expertise in speech, language, and behavior control. Education is a lifelong process.

Nursing Considerations.   Emphasize the positive and focus on the child's skills. Teach family caregivers to give the child immediate feedback and to continue interaction with the child using short sentences and simple commands. Remind caregivers to be concerned with the child's safety but to maintain normal daily routines.

Plumbism

Plumbism is *lead poisoning,* which affects approximately 1 million children in the United States. Lead is toxic to the human body. It is a substance that is found almost everywhere: in water, old paint, contaminated dust, and dirt.

Lead poisoning can be acute or chronic. If exposure is sudden, the poisoning is *acute*. If the exposure occurs over a long period of time, lead poisoning is called *chronic*. Symptoms of either acute or chronic poisoning vary widely. Effects of lead on the body depend on the client's age, the amount inhaled or ingested, and how long the client has been exposed to the toxin.

One of the most common causes of lead poisoning in children is the ingestion of leaded paint chips. A 1978 federal law prohibiting the use of lead in paints has reduced the number of lead-poisoning cases.

Water that passes through old pipes that contain lead is also a continual source of plumbism. Additional culprits of poisoning include improperly disposed-of lead in public landfills and industrial sources such as mining, smelting, and recycling processes. Burning batteries releases lead into the environment.

Individuals living in older homes, usually in inner cities, remain at risk. Many times, older homes in deteriorating neighborhoods need repair; they may have chipped paint and plaster. Inquisitive, inadequately nourished, or emotionally deprived children may eat paint chips as well as other inedible things.

☛ KEY CONCEPT

Eating nonfood items is termed pica.

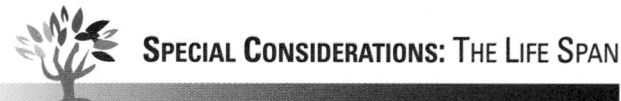

SPECIAL CONSIDERATIONS: THE LIFE SPAN

Lead Poisoning

Low doses of lead can contribute to hypertension in older adults.

✛👁 **N u r s i n g   A l e r t**

Lead is contained in items other than paint, such as: leaded pottery or dishes, home remedies, shoes, old toys, old eating utensils, old pipes and plumbing, soil containing lead from old chipped paint, sand and dirt on playgrounds, air pollution from unleaded gasoline, and family members who bring lead dust home on their clothes. A child who inhales the dust from scraped, leaded paint can suffer the same deleterious effects as the child who eats paint. The buildup of lead can occur gradually.

Signs and Symptoms.   Early symptoms of lead poisoning are so general that they can be easily missed or attributed to other childhood illnesses. Damage can be done to the brain, kidneys, CNS, and red blood cells (RBCs). The most severe complication of lead poisoning is *lead encephalopathy,* which may result in a number of CNS disorders, including seizures, cerebral palsy, cognitive impairment, and ADHD.

Untreated encephalopathy usually results in severe brain damage and death.

Long-term residual effects of plumbism include intellectual impairment, learning disabilities, or seizures. Early recognition of symptoms helps alleviate the long-term consequences of chronic lead poisoning. Damage that is done by lead poisoning cannot be reversed.

The signs and symptoms of plumbism include:

- Blue or blue-black line on the gums near the teeth
- Hyperirritability
- Anorexia, nausea, and vomiting
- Intermittent vomiting (lead colic)
- Abdominal pain
- Joint pain
- Headache
- Fatigue and decreased play
- Anemia, pallor, and decreased RBCs
- Constipation
- Behavior changes (Sudden changes may indicate acute lead poisoning.)
- *Ataxia* (unsteady gait), weakness, or clumsiness
- Decrease in intellectual and mental abilities (eg, memory loss and poor school performance)
- Impaired level of consciousness
- Seizures
- Coma
- *Encephalopathy* (brain degeneration)

Diagnosis.   Blood lead level (**BLL**) should be obtained with children who are at high risk or who demonstrate symptoms. Other disorders need to be eliminated as causes of symptoms.

Treatment.   A multidisciplinary treatment approach involving schools, social services, and the healthcare system is necessary. The individual first must be removed from the lead source. If the case is mild, the child is treated symptomatically. Anemia is treated with diet and iron supplements; seizures are treated with anti-seizure medications.

High-risk children should be screened for elevated BLL. This includes children who live in homes built before 1950, have iron deficiency anemia, are exposed to contaminated dust or soil, or have developmental delays. The CDC and the AAP recommend universal screening in areas where BLLs are elevated, and only target screening of high-risk children in areas where BLLs are low.

Chelation is the administration of medications that bind to lead to remove it from the body. The drug of choice for chelation is edetate acid (EDTA) given IV, and the heavy-metal antagonist, dimercaprol (**BAL in Oil**) given deep intramuscularly. Recently approved by the Food and Drug Administration, 2, 3-dimercaptosuccinic acid (DMSA) has the advantage of oral administration.

Nursing Considerations.   Plumbism may easily be missed as a possible cause of childhood disorders. During well-baby and -child checkups, the nurse should consider plumbism if the child is at risk or demonstrates symptoms. Changes in play activities, new aches and pains, and altered intellectual abilities may be seen by parents but not reported to healthcare providers. The source of lead must be eliminated.

☛ KEY CONCEPT

Public education and prevention are the most effective approaches toward eliminating the problem of lead poisoning.

LONG-TERM NEUROMUSCULAR DISORDERS

Cerebral Palsy

Cerebral palsy (**CP**) is a general term used to describe movement and coordination disorders in children. It may be accompanied by intellectual and learning deficits. Unlike other movement disorders, CP is not progressive. Symptoms may appear at any time before age 2. It is the most common permanent physical disability of childhood. In the United States, about 10,000 babies per year develop CP.

Prenatal causes include maternal infection, excess radiation, fetal anoxia, pregnancy-induced hypertension, maternal diabetes, abnormal placental attachment, and malnutrition. Other causes include birth trauma, brain infections (eg, meningitis or encephalitis), head trauma, prolonged anoxia during childbirth or in very early infancy, brain tumor, and cerebral hemorrhage or clot.

Birth asphyxia and trauma is related to incidences of CP but is not the main cause of this disorder. Research has shown that the fetus has predisposing factors that make the CP infant more susceptible to hypoxia.

According to The National Center on Birth Defects and Developmental Disabilities, a study done in California has identified CP as the most expensive of the childhood disabilities. More than $500,000 per lifetime per child is needed for the care of an individual with CP. Half of these costs are out-of-pocket expenses paid for by families. Families often find it difficult to pay for all the services required by their children. Healthcare professionals must be diligent in the promotion of the recognition of risk factors and the prevention of CP.

Prevention, however, may not be possible in all cases of CP, even using optimal healthcare resources. Studies show that the incidence of CP has not decreased in the later decades of the 20th century in spite of many improvements in obstetric care.

Signs and Symptoms.   Characteristics of CP generally include the following to varying degrees:

- Muscle contractions
- Increased stretch reflexes
- Rapid alteration of muscle contractions and relaxations
- Muscle weakness
- Difficulty sucking or feeding
- *Dysarthria* (speech abnormalities)
- Visual and hearing abnormalities
- Contractures
- Limited range of motion
- Scissors-like gait, such as crossing one foot in front of the other to walk
- Walking on toes
- Seizures
- Delayed motor development, such as with sitting, crawling, or walking
- Learning disabilities
- Mental abilities that range from very intelligent to severe mental retardation
- Hypertension
- Underdevelopment of affected extremities

Classifications.   There are three major classifications of CP. Mixed forms constitute about 20% of CP cases.

Spastic cerebral palsy is the most common type of CP, present in more than 50% of CP clients. Symptoms include increased muscle tone or spasticity, which may affect one or more limbs. Paralysis may be full or partial. Sensory abnormalities such as speech, hearing, and vision deficits may also be present.

Spastic hemiplegia involves one side of the body.
Spastic diplegia involves both legs.
Spastic quadriplegia involves both arms and legs.

Dyskinetic (or *athetoid*) **cerebral palsy** involves about 20% of CP clients. This type of CP is characterized by abnormal involuntary movements, such as twisting, grimacing, and sharp jerks. These movements disappear during sleep and increase with stress. The child has difficulty with speech, due to involuntary facial movements.

Ataxic cerebral palsy involves about 10% of CP clients. It results in tremors, unsteady gait, lack of coordination and balance, *nystagmus* (rapid, repeated movements of the eyeball), muscle weakness, and lack of leg movement during infancy. When the child begins to walk, he or she holds the feet far apart, causing a wide gait. The child with ataxic CP is unable to make fine or sudden movements.

Diagnosis.   Cerebral palsy is diagnosed primarily by symptoms the child demonstrates during infancy. Certain critical observations can direct the healthcare practitioner to look closely for other symptoms. The infant who has difficulty sucking, or has arm or leg tremors with voluntary movement, should be checked for CP.

In children with CP, infantile primitive reflexes persist past the expected age of disappearance. The infant who crosses the legs when lifted from behind, rather than pulling them up, is also of concern. Another sign of CP is difficulty in diapering because the legs are hard to separate. The child tends to use the arms and hands but not the legs.

Other disorders are ruled out by MRI, CT, EEG, and nutritional studies. Hearing and visual screening are necessary to determine the extent of disability.

Treatment.   There is no cure for cerebral palsy. Disabilities associated with CP are permanent; treatment is multidisciplinary and aimed at preventing complications and maximizing the child's potential. Helping the child learn self-care activities is a continuing goal. Improving communication through speech therapy and appropriate educational assistance is important.

Physical and occupational therapy help maintain the child's muscle strength and assist with adaptive measures (Fig. 73-3). Braces, splints, or walkers may aid in ambulation. Orthopedic surgery is sometimes used to correct severe contractures.

Nursing Considerations. Cerebral palsy does not necessarily affect the length of life, but it does profoundly affect the quality of life. Adaptive care devices such as hearing aids, glasses and vision-enhancing equipment, braces, and walkers help with mobility and ADL.

Education needs to be adapted to the needs and capacities of the child. In severe cases, institutionalization may be used instead of home care.

Medications are supportive and used symptomatically. Muscle relaxants can reduce tremors and spasticity. Seizures can be controlled with anticonvulsants.

Surgical interventions require that the nurse provide individualized pre- and postsurgical care, keeping in mind the mental and physical abilities of the client as well as the capacities of the family. Client and family teaching are very important.

Care is necessary for the child as well as the grown adult who has CP. The family and the child will need much emotional support.

☛ KEY CONCEPT

A waterbed is a good idea for many disabled children. The movement of their breathing causes feedback and helps prevent joint pain and skin breakdown. The warmth often adds to comfort.

Duchenne Muscular Dystrophy

Duchenne muscular dystrophy (*Duchenne-Landouzy dystrophy*) is the most common degenerative muscular disorder in children. Almost all cases are inherited, resulting from an X-linked genetic disorder, thereby affecting only boys. A lack of a protein product (dystrophin) in the muscles results in progressive muscle wasting.

Signs and Symptoms. Symptoms begin to appear around the age of 3 years. Prior to this, the child may have noticeable developmental delays. The child's gait appears as a waddle. A positive Gowers' sign occurs (see Fig. 73-4). A positive **Gowers' sign** is exhibited when the child needs to use the upper extremity muscles to compensate for weak hip muscles. The child gets up by pushing to an upright position, using the hands to climb up the legs to a standing position: The child starts at the ankles, alternating hands; he then gradually pushes to an upright position, using the legs as the climbing pole.

The child also may walk on the toes, fall frequently, and have difficulty hopping or running. These children often develop lordosis because of their unusual gait. Delayed intellectual development and borderline IQ may be present. Gradual muscle atrophy occurs, and by age 11 or 12 years, the child is unable to walk and becomes wheelchair bound. Contracture deformities can occur, especially of the hips and knees.

Deterioration of respiratory muscles results in cardiac problems and respiratory failure. In some cases, assisted respiratory ventilation can extend life. However, muscles involved in swallowing are also affected, and tube feeding may be necessary. Boys with Duchenne muscular dystrophy rarely live beyond their twenties.

Diagnosis. Duchenne muscular dystrophy is diagnosed by the presence of symptoms, electromyogram, muscle biopsy, and elevated enzyme levels such as aspartate aminotransferase (**ALT,** formerly SGOT), and creatine phosphokinase (**CPK**).

Treatment. There is no cure for Duchenne muscular dystrophy. Treatment is supportive. Wheelchairs are needed as the child loses the ability to walk. Feeding tubes may be necessary if the child can no longer swallow. As the disease progresses, supportive respiratory therapies such as ventilators may prolong life.

Nursing Considerations. Genetic counseling may be helpful to families who have known or suspected histories of muscular dystrophy. Grief counseling should also be considered. The goal is to maintain physical function as long as possible. This disease is devastating, and emotional support must be provided for the child and family. The mother may experience enormous feelings of guilt because she is the carrier of the defective X gene.

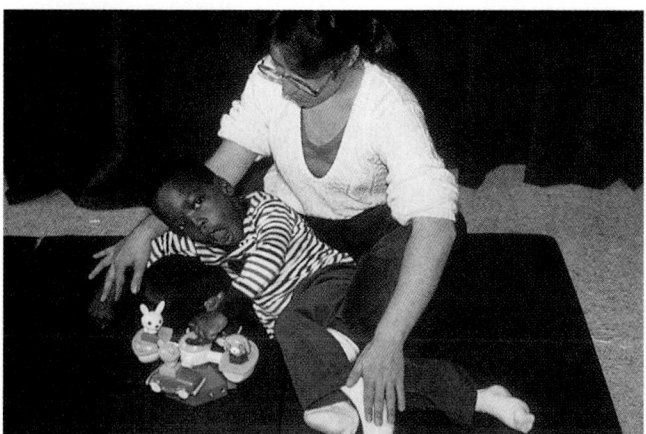

FIGURE 73-3. A physical therapist works with a child with cerebral palsy to maximize mobility.

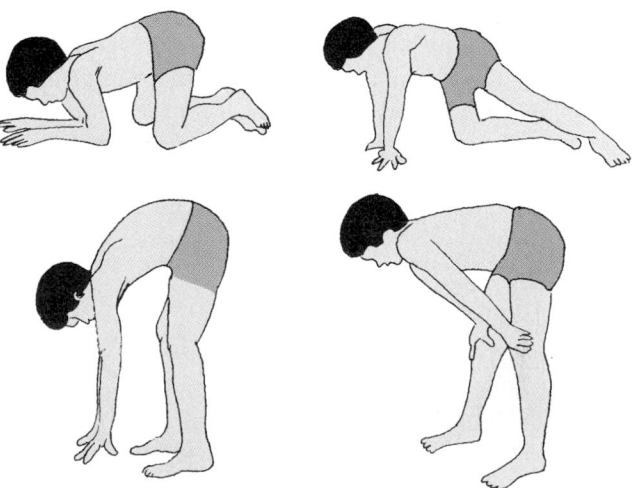

FIGURE 73-4. Positive Gowers' sign.

SENSORY DISORDERS

Children with *sensory disorders* and their families face special challenges. Alterations in the senses greatly affect growth and development, academic performance, development of socialization skills, and communication.

Visual Impairment

The most frequent causes of *visual impairment* include genetic or congenitally acquired cataracts (caused by rubella), optic nerve atrophy, and retrolental fibroplasia resulting from oxygen toxicity. Other causes are amblyopia, retinitis pigmentosa, refractory errors, strabismus, and trauma (see Chaps. 71 and 79).

Severely visually impaired children are dependent on others for learning socialization skills. They lack visual cues, resulting in socialization delays. For older children, special education programs can assist with academics. Audio tapes and instruction in the use of Braille reading are other available learning tools.

Teach family caregivers to remove limitations in the surrounding environment and to promote independent functioning for such children. Clocks with large numbers, calendars with large letters, and books with large print may decrease frustration for children who have partial sight. Encourage nonsighted children to participate in activities with their peers, such as music, guided skiing, swimming, and so forth. Family caregivers should encourage non-sighted infants and toddlers to explore their environment, while at the same time ensuring their safety.

Hearing Impairment

Hearing impairment can result from fetal exposure to cytomegalovirus, herpes, rubella, or syphilis. Meningitis, chronic ear infections, Down syndrome, exposure to loud noises, and certain medications also may cause hearing damage. Manifestations of hearing impairment in a child include avoiding social interaction, playing alone, acting timid, not learning to talk, and displaying poor socialization skills.

Children with impaired hearing face the related problem of poor speech development. Communication and safety are major issues for families with hearing-impaired children. Promoting communication is critical. Speech therapy and sign language are important tools for learning and communication. Assistance with socialization in school is essential; classmates must learn to relate to these children and understand that they are not intellectually impaired.

Speech Impairment

Impairment of speech can result from a hearing deficit, muscular disorders, or cleft lip or palate. Environmental and emotional factors can also influence speech. Disorders in articulation are related to the ability to produce the correct sound. An example of a speech impairment is the child who speaks with a lisp (pronounces "th" instead of "s").

A **dysfluency** is an interruption in the natural flow of speaking. An example is the child who stutters. Stuttering is normal for preschool children because at this age, the ability to understand is more developed than vocabulary and command of the language. Stuttering in school-age children requires evaluation.

Some children benefit from speech therapy. Others require surgical intervention or orthodontics. Evaluation by an otolaryngologist or neurologist also may be appropriate, depending on the specific circumstances. Specialists will test hearing. They will also make necessary referrals to psychologists or counselors for children with emotionally related speech disorders. Computers are especially valuable for these children.

☛ KEY CONCEPT

Hearing disorders are common causes of speech disorders in children. A professional audiologist should test the hearing of a child who is having speech problems. Learning to talk is difficult for one who has never heard anyone speak. If a person loses his or her hearing later, he or she can often maintain speech.

MENTAL ILLNESS

Childhood Depression

Depression in children and adolescents can be difficult to identify. Young children often have difficulties expressing themselves and their feelings, and their depression can go unnoticed. Many adolescents are sometimes moody and withdrawn, and family caregivers may be unable to differentiate such behavior from clinical depression.

Signs and Symptoms. Typical symptoms of depression include isolation and sadness, withdrawal from friends and family, fatigue and decrease in activity level, decrease in appetite, and a change in sleep patterns (such as excessive sleep or an inability to sleep). School grades may decline, and the child may miss school for various reasons. The child may make statements that reflect low self-esteem. The key clue is a marked change in behavior.

Diagnosis. Diagnosis may be difficult. Physicians need to rule out organic causes of diseases. Professional pediatric counselors are generally required to assist in the identification of the proper diagnosis.

Some depression is related to chemical imbalances in the brain. Other cases are situational, occurring in response to a traumatic event such as the death of a family member or pet or the breakup of a relationship. Children with low self-esteem or those overwhelmed with stressful situations are more prone to depression. Depression can also occur in children with a chronic illness or disability.

Treatment. The first step in treating children with depression is identifying the symptoms. Although recognizing depression in children may be difficult, understand that all behavior is meaningful. Investigate characteristics of depression thoroughly to prevent further complications or suicide. Psychotherapy and counseling are necessary, and may be provided on an outpatient basis. More serious cases of depression may require hospitalization. Family counseling is always helpful; antidepressant medications may be necessary.

Nursing Considerations. Depression is a serious disorder in children. Parents, caregivers, and healthcare professionals often miss the symptoms. It is important for the healthcare providers to accept and recognize changes in behaviors. Parents may not identify behavioral changes as abnormal, thinking that all children have adjustment difficulties with some periods of sadness.

Suicide

According to the CDC, suicide is the third leading cause of death in 15- to 24-year-old adolescents. About 15% of all U.S. suicides are committed by individuals under 25 years of age. Though still uncommon, statistics have shown that the percentage of suicides in children 10 to 14 years of age increased over 100% in the 1990s.

Caucasian males account for 72% of all suicides. Combined with the suicides of Caucasian females, this group accounts for 90% of all suicides. Young black men are the group with the most rapidly growing percentage of suicides. Males are four times more likely to die from suicide than females. Females attempt suicide more often than males. Three out of five suicides are committed with a firearm.

Many situations are associated with suicide and suicide attempts. Family problems may be involved, including financial difficulties, divorce, separation, or substance abuse. Adolescents who are experiencing the physical and emotional changes typical of their age group have minimal coping skills to deal with family-related stressors. Depression, personal substance abuse, and low self-esteem are other risk factors. Children with behavioral disorders are also at risk.

Signs and Symptoms. **Suicidal ideation** is the term given to thoughts or ideas of suicide. Suicidal ideation usually precedes a suicide attempt. A *suicide gesture* is an attempt at inflicting personal injury; the injury is not intended to cause death. Suicide ideation and gestures are cries for help. Ignoring these symptoms of despair can result in an adolescent's death. Both are key warning signs that must not be ignored.

Diagnosis. There is no specific test to determine the state of depression or inclination toward suicide. Key warning signals include morbid discussion of and preoccupation with death, giving away important personal belongings, and a sudden cheerfulness following a somber, withdrawn, depressed period. This sudden cheerfulness may indicate that the adolescent has decided to commit suicide and is relieved about the decision. This warning sign can be easily missed. In Practice: Nursing Assessment 73-1 lists danger signals for suicide in adolescents.

Treatment. Warn the family to take suicide ideation, gestures, and attempts seriously. Have the child see a professional therapist immediately. Intensive and long-term psychological counseling is essential. Adolescents with severe depression and suicidal thoughts may require hospitalization and close monitoring until suicide is no longer an immediate threat (see Chap. 93).

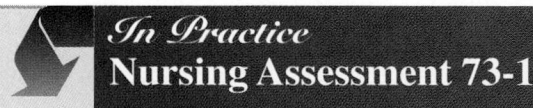

In Practice
Nursing Assessment 73-1

DANGER SIGNALS FOR SUICIDE PREVENTION

Signs that a child or adolescent may be suicidal include:
- Lack of involvement in school activities
- No close friends
- Inability to communicate with family caregivers
- Extreme anxiety, tenseness, abrupt changes in behavior, withdrawal, and sadness
- Change in eating patterns
- Change in sleeping patterns
- Sudden giving away of prized or valuable possessions
- Actual suicide threats, a suicide note, overuse of drugs, constant talk of death, talk of willingness to die or being ready for death, talk of being worthless or no good, talk of death as a release from pressure and pain
- Self-injurious behaviors, such as cutting or scratching oneself, self-inflicted cigarette burns, and so forth
- Very dangerous and life-threatening activities, such as playing "Russian roulette" with a gun or "chicken" with a car
- Deep, lingering depression with loss of energy and desire
- Sudden relief of acute, long-term depression without treatment (may mean that the person has made the actual decision to commit suicide or now has the energy to go through with it)
- Depression, feelings of hopelessness or helplessness, low self-esteem, loneliness and isolation, impulsiveness, ambivalence
- Withdrawal from friends and family
- Unusual neglect of personal appearance
- Radical personality change
- Any suicidal gesture

Nursing Considerations. Be aware of early signs of depression. Listening is more effective than talking to children about sadness, unhappiness, or depression. Consider using a no-suicide contract with the child, wherein the child agrees not to attempt suicide for a specified period, and will contact help immediately if he or she feels suicidal. Children are usually very conscientious about wanting to keep their word, and a no-suicide contract can be effective in some situations.

Childhood Schizophrenia

The schizophrenic person loses contact with reality. **Schizophrenia** sometimes results from a sudden, severe emotional experience, or sometimes from the person's inability to adjust to the environment. Familial tendencies have been noted. Play therapy, behavior modification, and drug therapy may help; however, schizophrenia is often chronic. The person must learn how to manage his or her life with the disorder.

Signs and Symptoms.   The following are characteristics of childhood schizophrenia:

- The onset of schizophrenia can occur as early as 5 or 6 years of age.
- These children share many characteristics with autistic children, such as lack of speech, ritualistic behavior, and intolerance of change.
- Personality and cognitive development are affected.
- Children with schizophrenia often hear voices (*auditory hallucinations*).
- These children have impaired relationships.
- These children are often out of touch with reality, have a distorted sense of what is real, and do not know where they are or what day it is.
- These children have an inappropriate affect (eg, laugh at a sad event).
- Other symptoms include *delusions* (beliefs not based on fact), *paranoia* (unreasonable fear), and aggression toward others.

Diagnosis.   Diagnosis is basically made by the observation of symptoms over a period of time. Other organic and psychological disorders need to be eliminated. Many theories exist as to the cause of childhood schizophrenia. They include biochemical and organic causes, inadequate caregiver relationships, childhood sexual abuse, and ritualistic abuse. Children whose family caregivers suffered from mental health problems may have an increased tendency to develop psychoses.

Treatment.   Treatment emphasizes modifying behavior so schizophrenic children can cope with reality and organize their thoughts. Medications are often helpful in controlling symptoms; however, they sometimes compound symptoms in children. Children require monitoring to ensure medication compliance.

Nursing Considerations.   Because behavior is so difficult for all involved, intensive and long-term therapy is often required. Family and caregivers may need supportive counseling. A program of home care with respite care, medical assistance, and social service assistance is preferred to hospitalization.

The child and the caregivers need to maintain the regimen of medications. When symptoms diminish or disappear, it means that the medications are effective. It is important to differentiate this concept of medical management from the hope that the disease has gone away and the drugs are no longer required.

SUBSTANCE ABUSE IN CHILDREN AND ADOLESCENTS

The transition from childhood to adolescence can be one of confusion and turmoil. Any change in family structure adds additional stress to developmental tasks. Some children view the use of chemicals to alter consciousness as a way of dealing with stress, raising self-esteem, and being accepted by peers. All chemicals have the potential for abuse. In Practice:

Nursing Assessment 73-2 lists signals of substance abuse. Table 73-2 discusses the effects of chronic drug use on body systems.

The most commonly used drugs are alcohol and tobacco. Other common drugs include marijuana, lysergic acid diethylamide (**LSD**), amphetamines, barbiturates, narcotic analgesics, and heroin. Cocaine offers users a euphoric high and can be inhaled as a powder, smoked in free-base form, or smoked in a water pipe ("crack cocaine"). Methamphetamine ("crank," "meth," "crystal") is an inexpensively made drug that produces a longer, more intense high than cocaine.

Huffing is a term given to inhaling chemicals that produce a feeling of delirium or a high. Children may inhale inexpensive household cleaners, hair spray, or paint in aerosol cans. Other common inhalants are fumes from glue, markers, and correction fluid (Box 73-1). Huffing is extremely dangerous because these inhalants are toxic to the CNS. Users may lose

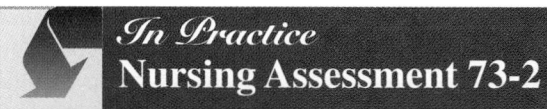

In Practice
Nursing Assessment 73-2

SIGNALS OF CHILDHOOD OR ADOLESCENT SUBSTANCE ABUSE

Signs that a child or adolescent may be abusing substances include:

- Extreme changes in dress
- Sudden loss of interest in personal appearance
- Sudden change in friends
- Extreme changes in eating or sleeping patterns
- Radical changes in normal behavior patterns or interests
- Extreme changes in relationships with family members
- Tardiness or absenteeism
- Unexpected or unusual failure in school
- Seclusion and withdrawal in room for extended periods
- Slurred speech; glazed look; other physical symptoms
- Defense of the right to use alcohol or drugs
- Mood changes that are very prominent
- Sudden refusal to work; not showing up for work or school
- Feelings of being sad or "bummed out"
- Dishonesty; stealing; hiding things
- Wearing dark glasses during the day to hide the eyes
- Wearing long sleeves to hide needle marks
- Sudden need for large amounts of money
- Sudden, unexplained disappearance of items in the home, such as money or jewelry
- Trouble with the law; speeding tickets; driving while intoxicated (DWI) tickets
- Leaving home for several days at a time; unexplained absences

■■■ **TABLE 73-2** ℰFFECTS OF MARIJUANA AND COCAINE ON THE BODY SYSTEMS

System	Marijuana	Cocaine
Nervous	Perceptual difficulties Uncoordinated psychomotor skills Paresthesias Personality/behavioral changes Short-term memory loss	Anxiety, irritability Tactile hallucinations Paranoia, insomnia, aggression
Sensory	Tinnitus Disturbed equilibrium	Visual disturbances
Cardiovascular	Elevated pulse rate Elevated blood pressure	Arrhythmias Acute myocardial infarction Ruptured ascending aorta Cerebrovascular accident
Respiratory	Oropharyngeal irritation Pulmonary damage Precancerous cellular changes	Pulmonary edema Pneumomediastinum Rhinorrhea, rhinitis Ulceration/perforation of nasal septum
Gastrointestinal	Enhanced appetite Xerostomia Vomiting	Weight loss Nausea Intestinal ischemia (gangrene)
Reproductive	Suppressed sexual functioning Possible teratogenicity	Problems maintaining an erection Orgasmic delay Miscarriage/preterm infants

consciousness and have seizures. Unfortunately, quick death can occur with no warning. Permanent damage to the lungs, CNS, or liver may occur. Huffing is often the first form of substance abuse; young children, after experimenting with inhalants, may proceed to other drugs.

➤➤ BOX 73-1

COMMONLY USED INHALANTS

- Aerosol paint cans
- Butane lighter fluid
- Cleaning fluids
- Gasoline vapors
- Kerosene vapors
- Liquid typing-correction fluid
- Model glue
- Nail-polish remover
- Paint sprays
- Paint thinners
- Propellant in whipped-cream spray cans
- Rubber cement
- Shellac
- Solvent
- Upholstery-fabric protection spray
- Varnish

Prevention. One way to prevent substance abuse is through public education. In addition, young people must feel that they are worthwhile. Try to build the self-esteem of all children. Treatment depends on the extent of the abuse, the age at which abuse began, and whether physical dependence exists. Support groups, individual counseling, and family counseling can be beneficial. Chapter 94 describes substance abuse and detoxification.

Children of Alcoholics

Children of alcoholics (**COAS**) are at high risk for developing problems with alcohol and other drugs. These children often experience problems in school and in coping with stress. Children whose family caregivers are alcoholics are more likely to become alcoholics themselves because alcoholism runs in families. These children suffer from school failure, depression, and increased anxiety.

COAS need help to understand that they did not cause a family member's alcoholism and they are not responsible for solving the problem. Encourage COAS to share their thoughts and feelings and help them learn to trust others. Slowly build relationships by doing a regular activity with them and providing some consistent, dependable companionship.

If a child asks for help, follow through by putting him or her in contact with professional counselors. Group therapy sessions help the child realize that others are in the same situation. Asking for help takes an enormous amount of courage;

let the child know that you are aware of this courage and that you respect the child's decision. The younger the child is when help becomes available, the greater the chances for success in breaking unhealthy patterns.

☛ KEY CONCEPT
_____

Probably the most important factor in breaking the cycle of chemical abuse is building a child's positive self-esteem.

NUTRITIONAL CONSIDERATIONS

Many children are affected by a chronic illness or a handicapping condition that affects their nutritional status. Many exhibit feeding problems. An interdisciplinary approach provides the essential assistance and education for parents managing these problems.

Any disorder or disability that reduces energy output places the child at risk for obesity. Children who are obese are at higher risk for diabetes, cardiovascular disease, and psychosocial problems. Focus parental education on slowing the rate of weight gain, not on placing the child on a restricted diet. In other conditions, caloric needs may be elevated due to constant muscle tension or movement (eg, cerebral palsy and muscular dystrophy). Sugar intake has been linked to obesity, hyperactivity, and mood swings.

Nutrition of the child or adolescent with special needs presents many unique nutritional challenges. Because of rapidly advancing medical knowledge, the number of children and adolescents facing life with chronic illness and disability is increasing. Many conditions require therapeutic interventions to prevent malnutrition and promote independent eating ability. Other conditions, such as phenylketonuria or celiac disease, require therapeutic diets to control symptoms or prevent physiologic harm.

Nutritional intervention for the child and family requires patience, flexibility, and sensitivity to individual needs. A multidisciplinary approach is necessary to provide essential education and support for the entire family affected by the condition. While providing for the child's physical needs to maintain growth, consideration must also be given to the psychosocial developmental needs.

Refer the family to a dietitian for explanation of nutritional needs of the specific disability. An occupational therapist can assist the family with specially designed feeding instruments, which will facilitate the child's independence or will assist the family with feeding the child.

SPECIAL CONSIDERATIONS IN CHILDREN

Family-centered care is very important for the family of a child with special needs. The parents' and child's adjustment to the disability will depend on the seriousness of the disability, whether or not the disability is noticeable to others, and the availability of a network of resources and support persons. The family's response may include over-protectiveness, rejection, denial, or acceptance.

The child's response is strongly influenced by the response of the significant others and peers. The child may encounter social exclusion, discrimination, or physical barriers, which make adjustment more difficult. Coping ability is influenced by the child's temperament, self-concept, and developmental stage.

The nurse needs to be knowledgeable about the child's condition and complications that could occur. Recognition and support of the family's ability to care for the child, coupled with healthcare teaching when the need arises, increases their self-esteem. When the child is admitted to the hospital, ask the family their typical way of carrying out a procedure.

Assess the developmental stage, functional level of the child, and parent–child interactions. Assist the family to set realistic short-term goals. Discourage over-protectiveness, which may impede the child's physical and psychosocial development.

Encourage stimulating activities appropriate to the child's developmental stage. Help the family and child to develop better coping strategies. Collaborate with them to develop a manageable plan of care that prevents discouragement and exhaustion. Emphasize the importance of regular followup care with the interdisciplinary team to maintain health and to monitor and manage the disease. Familiarize yourself with resources available for the special needs of the child and family.

Disabled or chronically ill children often miss many school days. Federal laws stipulate that education must be provided for children with special needs. Homebound education may be necessary during acute illness episodes.

Encourage families to allow children with special needs to participate in developmentally appropriate extracurricular activities according to their developmental level and physical limitations. Assign household chores and responsibilities, to develop a sense of accomplishment.

Set firm but reasonable limits on behavior.

SPECIAL CONSIDERATIONS IN PEDIATRIC REHABILITATION

Young people who have permanent disabilities must adjust to them while simultaneously achieving normal developmental tasks. Accomplishing developmental tasks without a physical or emotional disorder is challenging. The individual with specific physical and emotional disorders has different and additional challenges. This individual is, therefore, not considered abnormal. See In Practice: Nursing Care Guidelines 73-1 for more information on caring for children or adolescents with special needs.

Behavior Modification

Behavior modification involves *positive reinforcement,* which encourages a child to repeat desired behavior. The child may

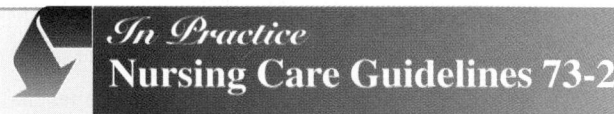

In Practice
Nursing Care Guidelines 73-1

WORKING WITH A CHILD OR ADOLESCENT WITH SPECIAL NEEDS

- Emphasize the positive; stress what the person can do. Reinforce success; praise the person for each accomplishment, no matter how small.
- Encourage the person to be as independent as possible. Encourage self-care. Help the person by showing how to do things. Reinforce by repeating instructions and asking for return demonstrations.
- Encourage development of positive self-esteem. The person may lack role models with similar disabilities, making it more difficult to develop a positive self-image. Encourage participation in support groups.
- Find a balance between the need for assistance and achieving independence in ADL. Encourage family caregivers not to be overprotective.
- Emphasize "normalcy." Encourage the person to do all the "normal" things others do, for instance, music, sports, academic success. Encourage participation in many activities for a well-rounded life. Often the person can do more than he or she may think.
- Encourage normal social contacts. The person should participate in peer activities.
- Encourage regular school attendance when possible. Schools are obligated to provide assistance as needed. Encourage family caregivers to discuss the person's problem and limitations with teachers, the school nurse, counselors, or others in close contact with the child or adolescent.
- Offer emotional support. The person will get discouraged. Listen to his or her problems. Let him or her express him- or herself.
- Observe for depression. A physical or emotional disorder may threaten future plans, resulting in depression.
- Consider the person's family. Involve them in planning and activities. Especially try to involve other siblings who might feel neglected.

need to repeat these skills many times before he or she learns them. If the child is intellectually impaired, make the task as simple as possible. Give praise when the child does a task correctly; do not use punishment.

Usually the intellectually impaired child is unable to generalize from one situation to the next. You must teach each specific skill, task, or behavior. The child needs a routine and needs to do things the same way each time.

There are specific techniques for teaching dressing skills, feeding skills, toilet training, and other ADL. Teaching should occur in a quiet place with few distractions. The site for learning should be neat and kept in the same order at all times. Patience is the most important factor in training the intellectually impaired child.

Feeding Training
Some children with physical, learning, or intellectual impairments have great difficulty eating. Feeding them and teaching them to eat takes patience. See In Practice: Nursing Care Guidelines 73-2 for helpful pointers.

Speech Development
Be patient and encourage children with speech difficulties to say each word slowly and clearly. Do not use baby talk. Encourage children to listen. Even if they cannot answer, be sure to talk to them. Explain to children what you are doing, and try to anticipate their questions. Read to children, and encourage them to look at pictures. Children with speech difficulties may be able to communicate by using computers.

In Practice
Nursing Care Guidelines 73-2

FEEDING THE INTELLECTUALLY IMPAIRED CHILD

- Ensure correct positioning, preferably in a sitting position. *Rationale: This position helps to close the larynx against the epiglottis.* Flex the child's head slightly. You may need to use a pediatric safety device.
- Teach the child to suck by massaging the cheeks or by using a special nipple. A nipple or bottle is appropriate for the infant and young toddler; as the child becomes older, use a cup or glass. A straw may be helpful. Encourage blowing, too. *Rationale: These actions build up muscles used in speech.*
- Assist the person to learn to drink from a cup by using sucking movements.
- Teach or remind the child to chew. If necessary, manipulate the jaw up and down.
- Remind the child to swallow. *Rationale: Prevent aspiration.*
- Place food on the side of the mouth, not in the center. Do not rush. *Rationale: Prevent choking.*
- Encourage the child to use the lips to remove the food from the spoon, to bite off pieces of food, and to move food around in the mouth with the tongue. *Rationale: These exercises also prepare the muscles for speech.*
- Keep the eating atmosphere pleasant. If possible, have several people eat together. Provide role models.
- Allow the person to do as much self-feeding as possible. Keep the table neat and clean.

LONG-TERM CARE

Children with long-term disabilities or degenerative disorders may go to the hospital for extended periods or be readmitted often. These children need special nursing care and attention.

Establish a basic sense of trust with children with long-term disabilities. Ideally, a child who returns frequently to a facility will have the same nurse. These children need to learn self-care as soon as possible; reinforce teaching often. Some facilities give children special responsibilities to increase feelings of self-worth and usefulness. Plan care carefully according to a child's needs and the physician's orders. Consider age, sex, developmental level, family environment, medical problems, and prognosis.

Include the Family. Do not forget that children in long-term care are still members of a family. Be considerate of caregivers, siblings, and other family members. Also, be aware that long-term hospitalization can drain a family's emotional and financial resources.

More children with long-term care problems are being cared for at home. Family caregivers need enormous amounts of support and assistance to successfully provide care. Respite care for the caregivers is important.

Involve the children in their own care. Children must have a sense of security; therefore, their basic needs are important. Allow children to do as much as possible, and assist with other needs without embarrassing them.

Long-term illness usually means treatments and diagnostic tests that can lead to physical discomfort and apprehension. Make an effort to minimize fears by allowing caregivers and children to talk about their concerns. Answer questions simply and truthfully. Focus on what children can do during a painful procedure. Explain treatments just before they are done—discussing them too far in advance can cause a child's imagination to run wild.

Encourage children to maintain social contacts with friends, classmates, and relatives as much as possible. Children with long-term illnesses can become overly dependent, and caregivers may be overprotective. Aim for a careful balance between encouraging independence and expecting too much.

Keep up with school. School-age children and adolescents must have educational needs included in the plan of care. School districts usually provide teachers for children who are in long-term care. Nursing staff should provide sufficient time and a quiet room for teachers and students. When children are receiving home care, family caregivers should plan uninterrupted time for schoolwork.

Use community resources. Use social service agencies in the community to help meet these children's educational, medical, recreational, and financial needs. Public health nursing referrals are helpful. Voluntary associations have special interests in various disorders; often children and caregivers will find talking with other families who have faced similar situations helpful.

Home Care

For the child with special needs to be cared for at home, the medical condition must be stable, the family must be motivated and have the resources, and professionals must be available in the community to provide essential equipment, education, and support.

A family assessment is essential, to identify the family's strengths and potential problem areas. Provide the family with written home care instructions and videotapes of step-by-step procedures for their review as needed. More than one caregiver should receive instructions on all aspects of the child's care. Return demonstrations are the best way to evaluate the caregiver's competency with procedures and use of equipment.

Enormous demands are placed on the family's time, energy, and finances. Assess the family's risk for inability to manage the situational crisis. Support the family's coping mechanisms and promote their optimal functioning.

☛ KEY CONCEPT

- *Encourage the young person with a disability to participate in educational, social, and recreational activities.*
- *Working with people with long-term disorders and their families, offers you the opportunity to use all your technical skills and interpersonal nursing skills.*
- *Keep the lines of communication open by developing active listening skills. Observe verbal and nonverbal cues for potential problems.*

➜ STUDENT SYNTHESIS

Key Points

- A congenital disorder is one that is present at birth. A genetic disorder results from an abnormal gene. A congenitally acquired disorder may result from fetal exposure to teratogens, infections, or trauma.
- Maternal use of alcohol or drugs and other teratogens can result in physical or mental abnormalities in a newborn.
- FAS is prevented by maternal abstinence of alcohol during pregnancy.
- Levels of functioning in the child with intellectual impairment are: borderline, mild, moderate, severe, and profound.
- Children with neuromuscular disabilities often have motor, sensory, and developmental delays, and feeding problems. A multidisciplinary approach is essential.
- Down syndrome and Fragile X syndrome are chromosomal abnormalities with resulting physical and intellectual impairment.
- Developmental and learning disabilities generally require individualized plans for education.

- ADHD children have difficulty with attention span, impulsivity, and hyperactivity.
- Families need support and encouragement when managing the care of a child with special needs.
- Tourette syndrome children may have involuntary movement and uncontrolled vocalizations called ticks.
- Autism is a complex disorder characterized by intellectual, social, and communication deficits.
- Plumbism can be acute, chronic, or fatal. Lead sources in the home and environment are the major causes.
- Cerebral palsy may be a result of birth trauma, brain infections, head trauma, and fetal hypoxia.
- Duchenne muscular dystrophy is an inherited degenerative disorder, which eventually is fatal.
- Visual and hearing impairment in children may be the result of genetic or congenitally acquired problems as a fetus.
- Childhood mental illness may be seen as depression, suicidal ideation, and schizophrenia.
- Substance abuse takes many forms, with permanent damage to the CNS as common.

Critical Thinking Exercises

1. C.J. is a 6-year-old boy who has been diagnosed with ADHD. Using your understanding of ADHD, design a teaching plan to teach him daily health habits.
2. Consider possible concerns for aging family caregivers of an adult child with Down syndrome. Discuss ways to handle such issues.
3. Using your knowledge of growth and development, plan a teaching tool about the hazards of household items that children can inhale as deliriants.
   How many of these items can you find in your own home?

NCLEX-Style Review Questions

1. Upon assessment of a newborn infant, the nurse identifies a small head, facial abnormalities, and limited extremity movement. What should the nurse suspect?
   a. Fetal alcohol syndrome
   b. Hydrocephalus
   c. Acquired immunodeficiency syndrome
   d. Fragile X syndrome
2. Infants infected with the HIV antigen are at high risk for:
   a. Cardiovascular problems
   b. Congenital malformations
   c. Failure to thrive
   d. Fluid and electrolyte problems
3. The physician tells the nursing student that a newborn has a simian line. To assess for this, where should the student look?
   a. Eyes
   b. Hands
   c. Ears
   d. Nose
4. A child with fragile X syndrome will have which characteristics on assessment by the nurse?
   a. Small head
   b. Protruding tongue
   c. Small testicles
   d. Wide-set eyes
5. The nurse counsels a teenager, who is inhaling fumes from aerosol cans, that this abuse practice will cause damage to which body system?
   a. Cardiovascular
   b. Neurologic
   c. Genitourinary
   d. Respiratory

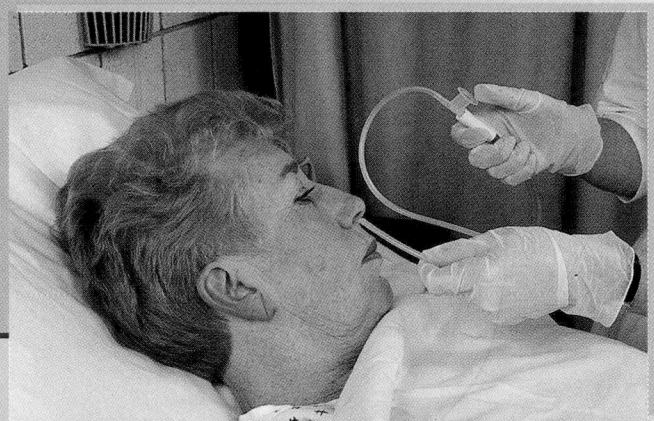

Unit XII

ADULT CARE NURSING

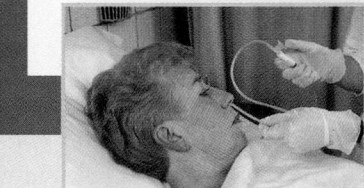

Skin Disorders

LEARNING OBJECTIVES

1. Differentiate among the following diagnostic tests: Wood's light examination, Tzanck's smear, tissue biopsy, and scabies scraping.
2. Discuss the two major types of skin grafts, including at least three nursing considerations for the care of skin grafts.
3. Identify at least eight types of skin lesions, providing an example of each type.
4. State at least four possible nursing diagnoses for a client with a chronic skin disorder.
5. Relate at least three nursing interventions for the care of a client with pruritus.
6. Discuss the following conditions, including at least two nursing considerations for each condition: acute and chronic skin conditions (urticaria, vitiligo, dermatitis, eczema, and psoriasis); infections (warts, condylomata acuminata, impetigo, and folliculitis); parasitic infestations (scabies, lice, bedbugs); and sebaceous gland disorders (sebaceous cysts, seborrhea, seborrheic dermatitis, and dandruff).
7. Identify the four mechanisms that cause burns.
8. Explain how burns are classified according to depth and size.
9. Describe the three phases of recovery in burn therapy, including assessment and treatment of fluid and electrolyte imbalances, respiratory dysfunction, renal changes, infection, and pain.
10. Describe at least four types of dressings, four types of topical medications, and the processes of debridement and skin grafting that may be used when treating burns.
11. Identify at least five complications that occur during burn recovery.
12. Discuss at least four nursing considerations during the rehabilitative stage of burn healing.
13. Identify three common nonmalignant and malignant skin lesions.
14. Discuss at least four interventions that can be used to prevent skin cancer.

NEW TERMINOLOGY

allograft	graft
angioedema	heterograft
angioma	homograft
autograft	impetigo
biopsy	keloid
carbuncle	neoplasm
condylomata acuminata	pruritus
cryosurgery	psoriasis
debridement	scabies
dermatitis	Tzanck's smear
dermatology	urticaria
eczema	vitiligo
electrodessication	warts
eschar	Wood's light
folliculitis	xenograft
furuncle	

ACRONYMS

CEA	UV

The *integumentary system* is composed of the skin (the epidermis and dermis) and its accessory organs, includes epithelial and connective tissue, nerves, and sweat and oil glands (see Chap. 16).

Dermatology is the study of skin diseases; a *dermatologist* is a physician who specializes in this field. Nurses specializing in the care of people with skin disorders are called *dermatologic nurses*. Nurses commonly see skin problems in their clients. For instance, infants sometimes have rashes, and older people may have problems with itching. Common terminology for skin disorders is found in Box 74-1. Some systemic disorders include skin manifestations. These conditions are discussed throughout this unit along with the body system that is primarily involved in the condition.

DIAGNOSTIC TESTS

Direct observation is often the diagnostic tool used first to determine disorders of the integumentary system. However, many skin conditions are manifestations of disorders involving other body systems. Diagnostic tests used to detect such disorders are covered in other chapters of this unit. If a systemic disorder has skin manifestations, the systemic disorder is first diagnosed, and then the symptoms appearing in the skin are treated. Some diagnostic tests used to determine the origin of a skin disorder include allergy skin testing, laboratory tests for blood dyscrasias (eg, leukemia or systemic lupus erythematosus), and blood glucose tests for diabetes mellitus. Other diagnostic tests may include:

- **Wood's light** examination: Use of a special high-pressure mercury lamp that produces long-wave ultraviolet (**UV**) rays to diagnose pigmentary abnormalities and detect superficial fungal and bacterial skin infections.
- **Tzanck's smear:** Examination of cells and fluids—from *vesicles* (blisters), such as those found in herpes zoster and varicella—which are applied to a glass slide, then stained and examined under a microscope.
- **Biopsy:** The procedure of removing of a skin-tissue specimen with scalpel excision, punch instrument, or

shaving technique for microscopic examination to rule out malignancy or to diagnose a skin disorder.
- *Scabies scraping* to diagnose scabies (a parasite that burrows under the skin): Obtained by shaving off the top of a suspected lesion, placing the specimen on a microscope slide that has been covered with immersion oil, and examining the slide under a microscope.

COMMON MEDICAL TREATMENTS

Clients with skin disorders often are uncomfortable. Therefore, treatment is aimed at providing comfort and treating systemic problems. The healthcare provider may order moist dressings, packs, or therapeutic baths. Additional treatments regarding the care of burns is found later in this chapter.

Assisting the Client Who has Pruritus

Pruritus (itching) is often a symptom of a skin disease, but also may arise from other systemic disorders, such as liver disease, iron deficiency, cancer, diabetes mellitus, or thyroid disturbance. Dry skin may cause pruritus, particularly for older adults. The main problem with pruritus is that the client is almost irresistibly compelled to scratch. Scratching may lead to skin breaks, which can become infected and cause scarring.

Telling a client not to scratch probably will be futile. Try to divert his or her attention with other activities. Antianxiety drugs, antihistamines, or topical corticosteroids are sometimes ordered. Educate clients about the proper use of such medications. In Practice: Important Medications 74-1 summarizes the most common medications used to control pruritus.

Hypnosis is often helpful for severe pruritus. Be sure to document the client's reactions, noting which measures are effective. Most clients appreciate advice on how to cope with itching. In Practice: Educating the Client 74-1 highlights some helpful suggestions for preventing and minimizing pruritus.

> **✚👁 Nursing Alert**
> Follow Standard Precautions and appropriate transmission-based precautions when caring for clients with skin problems. Such clients often have open, draining, or weeping wounds. Remember to wear gloves whenever there is possible contact with any body fluids or drainage; wear eye goggles and a gown if any possibility of splashing exists.

Giving Therapeutic Baths

A therapeutic bath is used not only to cleanse the body, but also to soothe the skin. It promotes wound healing, relieves itching, and helps remove **eschar:** the dry crust that results after trauma (eg, decubitus ulcers), infection (eg, skin infections), or injury (eg, burns). Therapeutic baths offer a way of applying medication to the entire body at one time. The therapeutic bath also provides warmth, so that the client can perform physical therapy and range-of-motion exercises more comfortably.

➤➤ BOX 74-1

COMMONLY USED TERMINOLOGY IN SKIN DISORDERS

Abrasion	Scraping of the skin surface
Dermatitis	Skin inflammation
Desquamation	Flaking or shedding of outer layers
Excoriation	Abrasion of the epidermis; scraped area
Laceration	Jagged cut through the skin or tissue
Pruritus	Itching
Purpura	Discoloration of skin due to blood in the tissue outside the blood (eg, ecchymosis, petechiae, or hematoma)

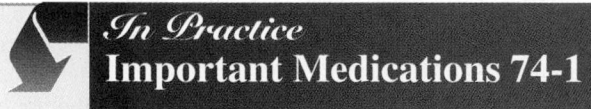

In Practice
Important Medications 74-1

FOR PRURITUS

Antihistamines
- Clemastine fumarate (Tavist)
- Dexchlorpheniramine maleate (Dexchlor, Polargen)
- Diphenhydramine HCl (Benadryl)
- Trimeprazine tartrate (Temaril)

Antianxiety Drugs/Antihistamines
- Hydroxyzine HCl and pamoate (Atarax, Vistaril)

Others
- Menthol (0.25%)
- Camphor (2%)
- Urea (5%–10%)
- Lactic acid (5%–12%)
- Antibiotics (to control infection)

Nursing Considerations
- These medications often cause drowsiness. Warn the client not to drive or work around machinery.
- Alcohol and other sedating drugs potentiate these medications. Urge the client to avoid these.
- Dry mouth is a common side effect. Encourage the client to drink juices and other fluids, not just water. Sucking on hard candy or ice chips, or chewing sugarless gum, is helpful.
- Other side effects include stomach distress, diarrhea, constipation (administer medication with milk or food), and urinary frequency or retention.
- Clemastine fumarate and trimeprazine tartrate may cause a life-threatening blood disorder called *agranulocytosis*.
- Antihistamines are usually contraindicated in people with asthma.
- Before any allergy skin testing, antihistamines should be discontinued for 4 days before the testing, to preserve test accuracy.
- Sunscreen use is recommended to avoid photosensitivity reactions.
- Older adults should use these medications with caution, because the risk for sedative effects is greater in this population.

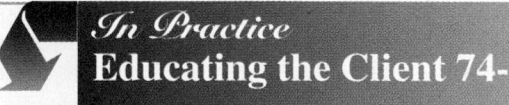

In Practice
Educating the Client 74-1

PRURITUS PREVENTION

- Wear cotton clothing. Keep irritating materials away from the body. Avoid wool or lanolin.
- Wash new clothes before wearing them.
- Rinse clothes in clear water. Avoid using fabric softeners, starch, and antistatic chemicals.
- Take only cool or lukewarm baths.
- Use soothing baths (colloidal oatmeal, starch) or localized skin preparations as ordered.
- Use lotion on dry skin if physician allows.
- Use nonallergenic makeup.
- Perform skin testing to determine allergens. Eliminate allergens if possible.
- Take medications as prescribed.
- Avoid activities that cause the body to become overheated.
- Keep fingernails short. Wear cotton gloves or cotton socks at night.
- Lightly slap, rather than scratch, the itching area. Slapping will provide the same stimulation as scratching but without continued irritation.
- If unable to exercise, sit in a rocking chair to provide some exercise without further skin irritation.
- Use relaxation audiotapes to assist in falling asleep.
- Shower immediately after swimming.

Give a therapeutic bath in a bathtub or whirlpool tank. Disinfect the tub or tank before and after use. Follow the provider's orders regarding the substance to use, the length of time the client is to be in the bath, and other treatments to perform at the same time. (The institution will specify how to clean the tub; colloids and oils used in these baths are often difficult to remove.)

Agents added to bath water often include oatmeal or other cereals, starch, tars, and baking soda. Detergents and antipruritic preparations may be ordered. Do not use soap because of its drying effects. Use medicated bath oil instead. Use tepid water (not hotter than 100° Fahrenheit or 30° Celsius); a very hot bath aggravates pruritus. The tub will be very slippery, particularly if oil is used. Protect the client from falling.

Pat the client's skin dry after the therapeutic bath; rubbing increases irritation or pruritus. Use nonirritating linens, and follow special laundering procedures to avoid leaving potential skin-irritating or allergic chemicals in fresh linens. Place soiled linen in a labeled laundry bag and send it to the laundry. Obtain clean laundry from the central supply in labeled allergy packs.

Applying Moist Dressings

Moist packs are applied to reduce swelling and weeping in acute **dermatitis** (skin inflammation), to soften and remove exudate and crusts, and to relieve pruritus and discomfort. These dressings may be clean or sterile, depending on whether the client's skin is intact. The moist dressing may be closed or open. A *closed dressing* is covered with plastic or a firm material. An *open dressing* is not covered, because the lack of oxygen may cause tissue necrosis. In an open dressing, fluid evaporates rapidly and the dressing requires frequent changing or resoaking. Chapter 54 discusses the basic procedure for applying moist packs.

Many solutions, such as aluminum acetate (Burow's solution), silver nitrate, and potassium permanganate, can be used on moist dressings. The physician or primary care provider will specify which solution to use. In the acute care facility, a pharmacy will mix the solution and send it to the nursing unit.

Explain the procedure to the client. Soak the pack in the solution and apply it, semi-dripping, to the affected area. Keep the pack wet, as ordered. Be sure to change or resaturate the moist pack at least every 2 hours. The bed, the rest of the client's body, and the nurse's body need to be protected from contact with the solution. Use a bed cradle when applying packs to the client's legs or torso. Provide blankets so that the client does not become chilled. Be sure to document the procedure and your observations when removing packs. Used dressings are considered contaminated; dispose of them correctly.

Debriding a Wound

The physician or other care provider will generally remove loose skin, crusts, or *denuded* tissue (protective tissue). This process is called **debridement.** The healthcare provider will also remove eschar. Debridement is a sterile procedure that is often performed when changing moist packs. The nurse may assist with debridement. Receive full instruction in how to carry out the procedure because each client requires different treatment. Debridement and escharotomy are discussed in more detail later in this chapter.

COMMON SURGICAL TREATMENTS

Plastic Surgery

Although skin disorders make clients physically uncomfortable, disfigurement is one of the most damaging psychological effects. Plastic surgery is one way to improve or correct disfigurement. It may be performed for cosmetic effects, to repair congenital defects, or to repair the results of trauma. Plastic surgery is also called *reconstructive surgery.*

Skin and Tissue Grafts

Skin grafts are used to cover areas of skin lost through wounds, burns, or infections. A **graft** is a transplant of skin that is placed on clean, viable tissue. Grafting is a painstaking procedure that may be done in stages. Grafting may take many months, depending on the size and number of areas to be covered, and the success of each step.

There are two major types of grafts. One type is called a *free graft,* which means that skin has been completely removed from its original site and grafted onto the recipient site. The other type is *pedicle graft.* In this type of graft, one end of the graft remains attached to the donor site so that it can continue to receive nourishment until new circulation is established. The other end is attached to the recipient site on the same client's body. In some situations, the client must assume an unnatural position until the graft begins to grow in the new site, at which time the graft can be separated from the donor

site. A pedicle graft is used when a large area of skin is to be replaced, such as on an ear, part of a hand or foot, or a large part of the face.

Other types of grafts are named in relation to the donor, and are described in more detail in the section of this chapter on burns.

Nursing Considerations

Before reconstructive or graft surgery, prepare the client by explaining what he or she can expect. Postoperatively, the surgical site may be swollen and bruised. Pay scrupulous attention to aseptic technique; protect the grafts; keep new grafts immobilized; and prevent infection at donor sites.

Emotional support is an important part of nursing care in reconstructive surgery. The client is often self-conscious about his or her appearance and may avoid others. Encourage family and friends to visit. Provide the client with emotional support and reassurance.

NURSING PROCESS

Data Collection

Carefully observe and assess the skin condition of all clients. Chapter 47 describes nursing assessment of the skin, hair, and nails, which establishes a baseline for future comparison. Report any changes that occur in assessments. Assess skin color (compared with the client's usual color), texture, and turgor. Note whether the skin is intact; examine for any lesions or pressure ulcers. Carefully document the size, color, texture, location, pattern of disruption, or any other distinctive characteristics of the lesion. Table 74-1 highlights several types of common skin lesions. Always use correct terminology to describe variations from normal skin appearance (see Box 74-1). In addition, assess for subjective symptoms, such as itching (pruritis).

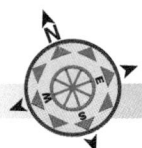

SPECIAL CONSIDERATIONS: CULTURE

Variations in Skin Appearance

Be aware of normal biocultural variations in the skin's appearance. If possible, ask the client or family to describe any variations from normal skin appearance.

Fluid and Electrolyte Balance

Data collection should include an understanding of the client's fluid and electrolyte status. A client's fluid and electrolyte balance and general nutrition may be difficult to maintain, because of developing exudates or serum loss stemming from inflammation or burns. Encourage the client to drink and eat. Provide a high-calorie, high-protein diet. Carefully document the client's intake and output (I&O). Initiate a calorie count for clients who are at risk for poor nutrition. Individuals who

■ ■ ■ **TABLE 74-1** *C*OMMON SKIN LESIONS

Type	Description	Example
Primary Lesions *(originating from previously normal skin)*		
Macule	Flat, discolored spot on skin with sharp borders	Freckle
Papule	Solid elevations without fluid with sharp borders	Mole
Nodule, tumor	Palpable, solid, elevated mass Nodules with distinct borders Tumors extending deep into the dermis	Wart (nodule) Large lipoma (tumor)
Vesicle	Small distinct elevation with fluid	Blister caused by herpes simplex
Bulla	Large distinct elevation with fluid	Large friction or burn blister
Pustule	Vesicle or bulla filled with purulent fluid	Acne, carbuncles

Macule

Papule

Tumor

Vesicle

Bulla

Pustule

(*continued*)

■■■ **TABLE 74-1** *C*OMMON SKIN LESIONS (CONTINUED)

Type	Description	Example
Primary Lesions *(originating from previously normal skin)*		
Wheal	Localized area of edema, often irregular and of variable size and color	Hive, insect bite

Wheal

Plaque	Larger, flat, elevated, solid surface	Psoriasis

Plaque

Secondary Lesions *(originating from a primary lesion)*		
Scale	Thin or thick flake of skin varying in color; usually secondary to desquamated, dead epithelium	Dandruff

Scale

Crust	Dried residue of exudates	Residue of impetigo

Crust

Fissure	Linear crack in the skin	Athlete's foot

Fissure

Ulcer	Opening in the skin caused by sloughing of necrotic tissue, extending past the epidermis	Pressure ulcer, stasis ulcer

Ulcer

have large surface area grafts or deep burn injuries usually require electrolyte replacement.

Allergies

As part of data collection, ask the client if he or she has known food or drug allergies. Food allergies may cause or aggravate skin disorders. Clients may also be sensitive to products such as tape, iodine, latex, or fragrances. Clients may know their allergies, or skin tests may determine them. Use more than one approach with the client when discussing allergies. For example, the client may deny being allergic to all antibiotics. Instead, ask the client specific questions such as, "Have you ever had an unexpected reaction to penicillin, shellfish, peanuts, or other foods or medicines?" Protect the client from exposure to known allergens.

Emotional Support

During data collection, determine your client's support system and coping mechanisms. A relationship may exist between emotional difficulties and skin problems—an underlying psychological problem may manifest itself in some type of skin eruption. Furthermore, the itching that accompanies many skin disorders gives rise to emotional distress: Pruritus is often more irritating and difficult to control than pain.

Observe the client's emotional response to the skin disorder or disease by answering the following questions. Is the client so disabled by pain or itching that he or she needs assistance or encouragement to meet daily needs? Is the disorder so disfiguring that it affects social activities or self-esteem? Is the client anxious or fearful of the outcome? Is the situation life threatening?

Nursing Diagnosis

Based on data collection, a number of nursing diagnoses may be established. The following diagnoses are commonly seen in nursing care plans for clients with skin disorders:

- Risk for Infection related to laceration, rash, skin lesions, skin cancer, burn trauma
- Impaired Tissue Integrity related to trauma or lesions
- Risk for Impaired Tissue Integrity related to chronic disease, impaired circulation
- Excess Fluid Volume related to edema
- Deficient Fluid Volume related to burn trauma
- Ineffective Breathing Pattern related to pain
- Impaired Social Interaction related to disfigurement
- Sexual Dysfunction related to pruritus, pain, skin lesions
- Ineffective Coping related to chronic condition
- Disturbed Body Image related to skin lesions, disfigurement, pruritus, pain
- Pain related to pruritus, burn trauma

Planning and Implementation

Involve the client when planning effective care (based on the nursing diagnoses) to meet his or her needs. Provide pre-

operative and postoperative care for the client undergoing plastic surgery or skin grafting. For the client with severe burns, assist in debridement of dead tissue or in life-sustaining treatments. The client with a skin disorder also may require assistance in meeting daily self-care needs, dealing with itching or pain, or working through the emotional aspects of a disfiguring or chronic disorder. Teach the client about the disorder and its necessary treatments. Develop a nursing care plan to meet each individual's needs.

Planning and implementing care includes relieving pruritus, providing therapeutic baths, and applying dressings, as previously discussed. Basic nursing care such as turning the client, assisting with hygiene, and observing and preventing pressure ulcers also is essential.

Chronic skin problems can present emotional challenges. Often, the same disorder flares up at intervals throughout the client's life. He or she may require assistance to cope. Group therapy may be helpful.

As a result of the skin disorder, the client's outward appearance may be unattractive. Foster an atmosphere of acceptance and support. Allow the client to express his or her feelings, and provide companionship.

The use of touch can be therapeutic. The nurse may touch the client who has a skin condition with clean, ungloved hands, unless the client is contagious or has open or draining lesions. Touch can be equally effective with gloved hands.

Evaluation

Routinely evaluate outcomes of care. Include the client, family, and all members of the healthcare team. Have you met short-term goals? Are long-term goals still realistic? What rehabilitation, home care, or other community services (if any) does the client need, especially if the skin disorder is chronic or requires continued treatment? In planning for further care, consider the client's prognosis, complications, and responses.

ACUTE AND CHRONIC SKIN CONDITIONS

Urticaria

Urticaria, commonly called *hives,* is characterized by the sudden appearance of edematous, raised pink areas called *wheals* that itch and burn. Hives may disappear quickly or they may remain for several days. In most instances, acute urticaria is a manifestation of an allergic reaction to medications, foods, spores, or pollens.

Contact allergens, such as face powder, can cause contact dermatitis. The most common contact allergens are soaps, nickel-based jewelry, perfumes, dyes, and plants such as poison ivy, chemicals, rubber, and insecticides. Stress and anxiety are thought to be important aggravating factors.

Urticaria that lasts more than 6 weeks is called *chronic urticaria.* Its exact cause remains unknown in 80% to 90% of people. Examine the client with an unexplained rash for the possibility of Lyme disease (see Chap. 72).

Edema associated with urticaria is only a temporary annoyance, unless it involves extensive vital areas. However,

angioedema (swelling) can be a life-threatening condition that is similar to urticaria but involves deeper dermal and subcutaneous tissues. Angioedema commonly affects the lips, eyelids, skin, gastrointestinal tract, hands, feet, genitalia, tongue, and larynx. If the larynx becomes edematous, the client may develop severe respiratory distress due to airway obstruction.

The best treatment for urticaria is identification and removal of its cause. Treat mild reactions with cold compresses or tepid colloidal-oatmeal or baking-soda baths. Antipruritic lotions, such as calamine, may help. Nonsedating antihistamines, such as astemizole (Hismanal), are often used for chronic urticaria. In severe cases, epinephrine may be administered. Chapter 83 discusses specific nursing care of the client who has an allergy.

> **Nursing Alert**
> Angioedema associated with urticaria can become life threatening. Assess for the following:
> • Extreme swelling of the lips
> • Swelling around the eyes
> • Dyspnea (difficult breathing)

Vitiligo

Vitiligo occurs when areas of the skin are completely lacking in pigmentation. Pigment cells (*melanocytes*) cannot be detected in the depigmented areas, resulting in patches or areas of very pale, white-looking skin. The condition is more noticeable when the client normally has dark skin. The cause of vitiligo is unknown. No effective remedy is known, although the use of certain drugs, such as methoxsalen (Oxsoralen), followed by exposure to sunlight or UV light, offers temporary darkening of the affected areas. Surgical treatments include mini-grafting and melanocyte transplantation. The treatment is prolonged and time consuming, and must take place under a physician's supervision. Using cosmetics designed to cover birthmarks, and wearing sunscreen, are practical solutions to vitiligo.

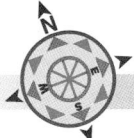

SPECIAL CONSIDERATIONS: CULTURE

Detecting Pigment Changes

Vitiligo is more obvious in darker-skinned individuals.

Eczema

Eczema, also known as *atopic dermatitis,* is a form of dermatitis (Fig. 74-1). This condition causes small vesicles to appear, as well as reddened and pruritic skin. Sometimes the vesicles burst and ooze, forming crusts. Persistent irritation and scratching make the skin appear leathery and thick. Affected individuals may develop viral, bacterial, or fungal skin infections. Eczema may spread to other areas, but is commonly found in the folds of the elbows, the backs of the knees, and on the face, neck, wrists, hands, and feet. It may

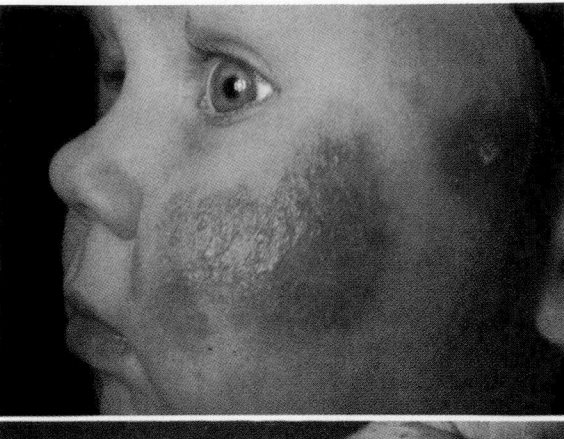
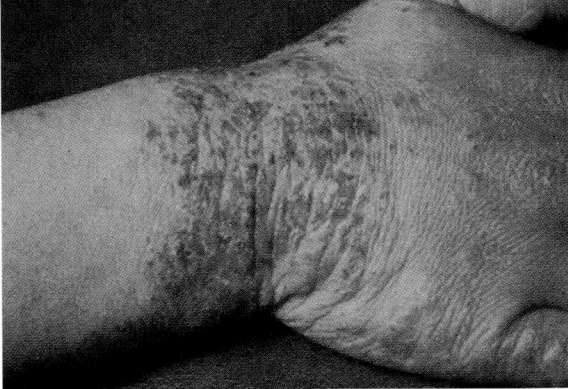

FIGURE 74-1. Examples of atopic dermatitis (eczema).

disappear completely for months or sometimes years, but can recur at any time.

Although the exact cause is unknown, eczema is known to be associated with heredity, allergy, and emotional stress. There may also be an autoimmune component. Sometimes a family history indicates an allergy, such as hay fever or asthma. Children who have eczema often develop these conditions later. As a client grows older, emotional factors can aggravate eczema. Chapter 71 discusses childhood eczema.

The goal of treatment is to prevent skin dryness, cracking, and itching. Treatment consists of applying moisturizing creams, corticosteroid ointments, tar solutions, or wet dressings to inflamed skin, or using starch baths. Antihistamines may relieve the itching, and antianxiety drugs may relieve the tension or anxiety that contributes to the condition. Instruct the client to use soaps that are less alkaline and contain no lanolin. Recommend the use of lanolin-free lotions. Teach clients to avoid contact with wool.

Psoriasis

Psoriasis is a chronic, noncontagious, proliferative skin disorder that most commonly affects young adults and people of early middle age. Epidermal cells rapidly proliferate and form small, scaly patches of skin. The primary cause is unknown, although hereditary, environmental, metabolic, or immune factors contribute to an outbreak of psoriasis. The course of the disorder is unpredictable. In most clients, the disease remains localized. Figure 74-2 shows severe psoriasis of the knees.

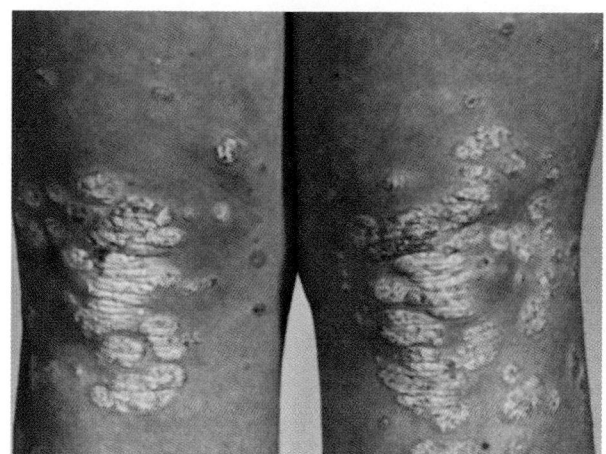

FIGURE 74-2. Severe psoriasis of the knees.

In some individuals, however, the severity is incompatible with a productive life. Spontaneous clearing is rare, but unexplained exacerbations (flare-ups) and improvement are common. Stress and anxiety frequently precede the disease's exacerbations.

Signs and Symptoms
The hallmark of psoriasis is red papules covered with silvery, yellow-white scales that the client constantly sheds. These patches appear mainly on the extensor surfaces of the elbows and knees, on the scalp, and on the lower back. The nails may begin to loosen at the beginning of the fingertips (*onycholysis*).

Medical Treatment
Generally, treatment of psoriasis is never completely successful. The main objective is to reduce scaling and itching. Therapeutic baths, wet dressings, or lubricating ointments may be helpful, followed by application of emollient creams to soften the scaling. Specialized shampoos are used to treat scalp psoriasis. Corticosteroids may be injected into psoriatic lesions. Topical application of a vitamin D preparation called calcipotriene (Dovonex) slows the development of skin cells. UV light treatment or sun exposure may be useful, but requires careful supervision. Methotrexate (Rheumatrex) and oral retinoids (synthetic derivatives of vitamin A) are useful in clients with severe, extensive psoriasis. However, methotrexate may cause hepatic or renal damage, bone marrow suppression, nausea, and fatigue. Photochemotherapy, which combines a photosensitizing agent (psoralen) with UV light, also may be used.

INFECTIONS

Warts

Warts (verrucae) are small, flesh-colored, brown or yellow papules caused by the human papillomavirus (HPV). Most warts are not painful, with the exception of the plantar wart that occurs on the sole of the foot and grows inward due to the pressure of body weight.

Common warts are found most often on the hands, especially of children, or on other sites often subjected to trauma. They may grow anywhere on the skin. *Filiform warts* are slender, soft, thin, finger-like growths seen primarily on the face and neck. *Plantar* or *palmar warts* are firm, elevated, or flat lesions occurring on the soles or palms.

Destruction with **electrodessication** (treatment with short duration high-frequency electrical current) and *curettage* (scraping or suctioning) is the best treatment for common and filiform warts. Warts also are treated by the application of liquid nitrogen (**cryosurgery**); locally applied laser therapy; or keratolytic agents, such as salicylic acid and lactic acid, that are applied in the form of a solution or tape. Some warts resolve without treatment.

Condylomata Acuminata
Condylomata acuminata, or *venereal warts,* are warts that grow in warm, moist body areas. They often develop in areas that rub together, such as skinfolds. They may develop in clusters. These warts are frequently found on the foreskin and penis, particularly in uncircumcised men. They also can develop on vaginal and labial mucosa and in the urethral meatus and perianal (around the anus) area. Condylomata acuminata lesions are becoming more common in young people (see Chap. 69). They are often spread by sexual contact.

Bacterial Skin Infections

Impetigo and folliculitis are the primary bacterial infections of the skin.

Impetigo
Impetigo, most commonly caused by streptococcal or staphylococcal bacteria, is contagious among infants and young children. (Adults are also susceptible to impetigo, but generally have better handwashing techniques than do young children, so adult outbreaks are usually not as severe.) Figure 74-3 illustrates the characteristic vesicles that ooze a clear exudate, which develops a golden-yellow crust that causes local discomfort and pruritis. When the crust is removed, a smooth, red, moist surface remains.

Impetigo is treated with systemic antibiotics (eg, dicloxacillin). Daily bathing with an antibacterial soap or chlorhexidine (Hibiclens) helps remove the crusts. Because the bacteria transfers from the infected client to another person through touch, teach clients to avoid touching the exudates and crusts, to prevent the spread of infection. Wear gloves when bathing the client or treating the lesions.

Folliculitis
Folliculitis is a staphylococcal infection starting around the hair follicle. Prolonged moisture, trauma, and poor hygiene often contribute to this problem. Lesions consist of white pustules or follicular nodules that are superficial or deep. The face is a common site for *deep folliculitis. Superficial folliculitis* may respond to aggressive topical hygiene with antibacterial soaps and the use of topical antibiotics. Folliculitis on the male

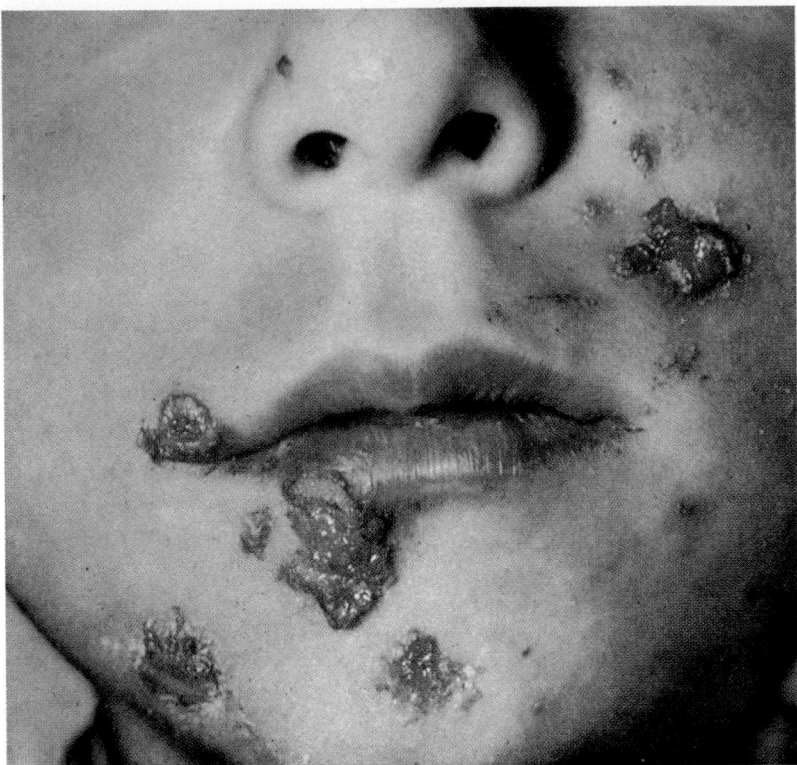

FIGURE 74-3. The lesions of impetigo.

beard can be difficult to treat, and may require the use of systemic antibiotics. Men with curly facial hair often have more difficulty because their hairs easily become ingrown. Teach men to change their razor blade daily and to avoid shaving too closely.

Folliculitis may lead to the production of a **furuncle,** also called a *boil.* A furuncle starts as a firm, red, tender nodule. After a few days, the furuncle may drain pus and finally extrude the core. The core is dead tissue that can drain spontaneously or be reabsorbed into the skin. A boil can also be surgically removed by incision and drainage (I&D). Furuncles are found most frequently in areas of hair-bearing skin that are subject to friction, irritation, and moisture, especially the face, scalp, buttocks, and axillae.

Furunculosis, the term for recurrent boils, develops in individuals who are unable to get rid of the Staphylococcus organism. No evidence has shown that these individuals harbor a particular strain of Staphylococcus or have any deficiency in their host defense mechanisms. A **carbuncle** is composed of several interconnecting boils in a cluster. A carbuncle usually drains at multiple sites; carbuncles are commonly found on the back of the neck, the back, and the thighs.

Wearing clean gloves, apply warm, wet dressings or soaks to localize boil and carbuncle infections to one spot. A physician may carefully incise and drain large boils after they come to a point. After boils are drained, the client will need only topical antibiotics. Furuncles or carbuncles associated with surrounding cellulitis or fever, or that are located on the upper lip, nose, cheek, or forehead, may be treated with oral antibiotics that are active against Staphylococcus organisms. A sensitivity test is obtained before starting treatment, to determine the most effective antibiotic.

> **✚☞👁 Nursing Alert**
> Picking or squeezing a boil is dangerous. Doing so may spread infection to surrounding tissues and possibly to the bloodstream. Advise clients to take special precautions with boils on the face, because the skin area drains directly into the cranial venous sinuses. Microorganisms in that area can cause encephalitis or meningitis.

PARASITIC INFESTATIONS

Parasites live on another organism and take nutrition from it, often damaging the host organism. Scabies, lice, and bedbugs are common parasites found in humans.

Scabies

Scabies is caused by mites (*Sarcoptes scabiei*) that burrow under the outer layer of the host's skin. One month or more after the mites enter the body, the host's skin develops intense itching, especially when heavily covered. Red spots appear, with a row of blackish dots that are one-eighth to one-half inch long with tiny vesicles and depressions. Scabies is found especially between the fingers. Other possible sites include the wrist, front of the elbow, elbow points, axillary folds, nipples, umbilicus, lower abdomen, genitalia, and gluteal cleft (between the buttocks). Adults rarely have scabies above the neck; however, the mites may affect children on any body surface. Mites can live for months or years in persons who are untreated or who have poor hygiene.

Typically, people acquire scabies primarily through close personal contact. However, the infection can be transmitted through clothing, linens, or towels. Because the parasites can live a long time without a host, and usually get into bed clothing and personal garments, use special precautions to keep scabies from spreading. If possible, examine and treat all family members for scabies simultaneously. Begin treatment by having the affected individual bathe and towel dry to remove crusts and open infected spots. Application of the prescribed medication (such as crotamiton [Eurax], 5% permethrin cream [Elimite], or lindane [Kwell] lotion) to the entire body from the neck down is the treatment of choice for children over 2 months of age and non-pregnant adults. Instruct the client to cover all body surfaces, including around the nail beds; between the fingers and toes; the genital area; and the cleft between the buttocks. Inform the client to leave the medication on for 8 to 24 hours, depending on the product used, and then to bathe thoroughly. The client will be instructed to repeat the treatment in 1 week.

Lice

Humans can be infested by three types of lice, called *pediculosis* (head lice; *Pediculus humanus capitis*), *body lice* (*Pediculus humanus corporis*), and *pubic lice* (*Phthirus pubis, Pediculosis pubis*), which inhabit the genital region. Lice may inhabit the hair of the axillae, beard, eyebrows, and eyelashes. Lice survive by sucking blood. They are difficult to eradicate because their eggs, called *nits*, can live for a long time on clothes, bedding, or upholstered furniture. Signs and symptoms include the presence of nits and extreme pruritus (itching). The disease is most common in children. Outbreaks are fairly common in schools and day-care centers.

> ✚👁 **N u r s i n g   A l e r t**
>
> Be alert for the presence of parasites, such as lice or scabies, when caring for a person who has lived on the streets or in shelters. Treat the infected person immediately to prevent transmission to others.

Medical Treatment

Head and pubic lice are best treated by over-the-counter preparations such as permethrin (Elimite, Nix) and pyrethrins (RID). The affected individual applies the agent to the hair for 5 to 10 minutes and then rinses it off with water. Instruct the client to remove nits by combing the hair with a fine-toothed comb. Warn the client not to apply pediculicidal agents near the eyes. Rather, apply petroleum jelly to the eyelashes and eyebrows and remove the nits by hand. For body lice, preparations containing lindane (γ-benzene hexachloride), such as Kwell, Gamma Benzene, or Scabene, are highly effective. These preparations are applied directly to the affected area, allowed to remain for 8 hours, and then completely removed with soap and water. Kwell is also available as a shampoo. The treatment usually is repeated in 1 week. The first treatment should kill most live lice. The second treatment kills lice that hatch after

the first treatment. After each treatment, inspect the client; treated nits are expected to remain. Look for live bugs. (All lice must be killed and nits destroyed to prevent re-infestation.)

Nursing Considerations

Treat everyone in the family and close contacts at the same time. Instruct the client to wear clean clothing. The client should use clean bed linens and should wash and dry clothing, bed linens, and towels using hot laundry water. He or she should have unwashable items dry cleaned and stored in a plastic bag for 30 days.

☞ Key Concept

Be aware of the stigma of uncleanliness that is attached to the presence of lice. Provide emotional support to the person with lice and the family.

Bedbugs

The *bedbug (Cimex lectularius)* measures 4 to 5 millimeters and can survive up to 1 year without food. Bedbugs live in clothing or bedding, and are difficult to eradicate. Bedbug bites appear as red macules that develop into nodules. The bites often appear in groups of three. Bedbugs usually bite the legs and feet, causing itching and burning. Lotions containing menthol, phenol, or 0.5% hydrocortisone are applied to the bitten areas. Spraying all crevices in furniture, mattresses, walls, and floors with an insecticide usually eliminates the insect.

SEBACEOUS GLAND DISORDERS

Sebaceous Cysts

Sebaceous glands secrete oils. When such glands become plugged, small hard nodules form, called *cysts. Sebaceous cysts* are not treated unless they become large and annoying, in which case they are drained or excised surgically.

Seborrhea, Seborrheic Dermatitis, and Dandruff

An excessive sebaceous discharge that forms large scales or cheeselike plugs on the body is known as *seborrhea. Seborrheic dermatitis* is a condition that causes scaling, primarily of the scalp, that is often associated with itching. This inflammatory condition erupts on body areas that have a large concentration of sebaceous glands (eg, scalp, eyebrows, eyelids, ears, axillae, groin, and skin under the ears and the breasts). The dry form of seborrheic dermatitis (also known as *dandruff*) is characterized by scales ranging from small and dry, to thick and powdery, with little to no redness. The oily form of seborrheic dermatitis is characterized by greasy or oily scales and crusts on a red base.

Frequent shampooing is the mainstay of treatment, as advised by a provider. Some shampoos contain selenium sulfide suspension (eg, Selsun Blue); others contain coal tar, salicylic acid and sulfur, or zinc pyrithione. Instruct the client to leave the shampoo on for 5 to 10 minutes. In some cases, lotions or solutions containing corticosteroids are prescribed. The client should use such products sparingly—once or twice daily—according to the provider's directions.

If the seborrheic dermatitis exists in a location other than the scalp, corticosteroid creams or ointments are prescribed. Although no known cure is available, a low-fat diet, exercise, sunlight, stress reduction, and rest can be helpful in management (see In Practice: Educating the Client 74-1).

BURNS

Burns are traumatic injuries that result in tissue loss or damage (see Chap. 43). A burn destroys cells by increasing capillary permeability and damaging cellular proteins. Prevention is key. Warn children and adults about the danger of burns, how to prevent them, and what to do if they occur. In Practice: Educating the Client 74-2 highlights important information about burn prevention.

Burn Classification

Burns may be classified according to the mechanism of injury and according to burn depth and size.

Mechanism of Injury

Thermal burns are the most common type of burn and are caused by steam, hot water scalds, flames, and direct contact with heat sources. *Electrical burns* are potentially life-threatening burns caused by electric shocks due to exposure to electricity or lightning. *Chemical burns* are caused by exposure to acids, alkalis, or other organic substances. *Radiation burns* result from exposure to radioactive sources, such as the ionizing radiation used in industry, or therapeutic radiation. Sunburns are another type of radiation burn.

The severity of injury is related to the burn's depth, extent, location, and length of exposure to the burn agent. Other factors that can affect recovery time include the affected client's age and medical history of concurrent disorders, and amount of respiratory injury from smoke inhalation. Assess the victim during initial care and frequently during the course of burn care.

Suspect inhalation injuries if the burn victim was in a closed area with the fire and smoke. Singed nasal hairs, facial burns, and soot-stained sputum are clear indications of smoke inhalation. Unless the client is suctioned, however, soot-stained sputum may not be apparent. The individual also may be hoarse or have a cough. Inhalation injuries may also be present in chemical exposure.

Burn Depth and Size

Burns are classified as *partial-thickness* and *full-thickness* injuries. Partial-thickness burns are further classified as superficial, moderate, and deep-dermal burns. Table 74-2 summarizes the characteristics of burns of various depths.

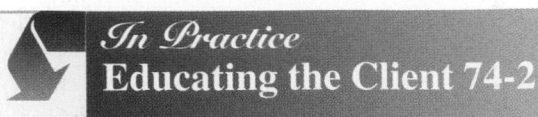

In Practice
Educating the Client 74-2

BURN PREVENTION

The very young and very old are more likely to have accidents. Consider special preventive measures for these people.

- Place portable heaters where no danger of falling over or brushing against them exists. Do not leave portable heaters on when sleeping. Place portable heaters away from curtains, bedspreads, or furniture that can easily catch fire from the heat or flames. Use the type that will shut off automatically if the heater tips over.
- Do not use candles for heat or light. Burn candles only when someone is in the room.
- Place electrical appliances where no one will trip over them. Never use equipment that has a frayed cord. Do not use multiple outlet plugs. Do not run a cord under a rug.
- Use special care around a plugged-in appliance (eg, never use a fork to remove toast from a toaster).
- Hire a qualified electrician to do work in the home.
- Teach children not to touch hot stoves and radiators. Turn handles of pans on the stove inward. Place matches and cigarette lighters in a safe place, out of children's reach. Place hot liquids out of the reach of infants and toddlers.
- Be aware of loose clothing or flowing sleeves that could catch fire when cooking indoors or outdoors. Never add lighter fluid to a fire. Gasoline and kerosene fumes are extremely flammable.
- Carefully follow the manufacturer's instructions for heating pads and other equipment.
- Be aware of overhead wires in the yard or neighborhood. Do not touch wires with metal ladders. Prevent children from climbing poles or flying kites near wires. Have an expert check any wires found disconnected or on the ground, particularly after a storm.
- Place smoke alarms throughout the house; check batteries regularly (one good rule of thumb is to check them in Spring when setting the clocks forward, and in Fall when setting the clocks back).
- Use care when operating electrical appliances around water. Use special lights and equipment for swimming pool areas and for outdoor decorating.
- Avoid overexposure to the sun or to the rays of a tanning bed.
- Wear safety goggles when working with chemicals. Avoid inhaling chemical fumes in enclosed places. Never mix bleach with other cleansers.
- Routinely practice fire drills so family members know what to do in case of a fire. Develop a system in which people will meet after a fire, so the family will know if everyone is out of the house.
- Insist that schools and places of employment have routine fire drills.

■■■ TABLE 74-2 *C*HARACTERISTICS OF BURNS OF VARIOUS DEPTHS

Depth	Tissue Involved	Usual Cause	Characteristics	Extent of Pain
Superficial, partial-thickness (first-degree)	Minimal epithelial damage	Sun	Dry Blisters after 24 hours Pinkish-red color Blanching with pressure	Painful
Superficial, partial-thickness (second-degree)	Epidermis, minimal dermis involvement	Flash burn Hot liquids	Moist Pinkish or mottled-red color Blisters Some blanching	Pain Hyperesthetic (very sensitive)
Deep dermal partial-thickness (second-degree)	Entire epidermis, part of dermis; epidermal-lined hair and sweat glands intact	As above, plus hot solids, flame, and intense radiant injury	Dry, pale, waxy No blanching	Sensitive to pressure
Full-thickness (third-degree)	All of the above and portion of subcutaneous fat; possibly involving connective tissue, muscle, and bone	Sustained flame, electrical, chemical, and steam	Leathery, cracked, avascular, white, cherry red, or black	Little pain

From: Hudak, C. M., Gallow, B. M., & Morton, P. G. (1998). *Critical care nursing: A holistic approach* (7th ed.). Philadelphia: Lippincott Williams & Wilkins.

The extent of burn damage depends on the depth of the burn as well as the extent, location, and size of the injury. Box 74-2 lists criteria for classifying the extent of a burn injury according the American Burn Association. All factors must be considered to assess burn damage and overall recovery time. For example, an individual with a 5% full-thickness burn on the outer forearm can have a quicker recovery than an individual with 3% partial-thickness burns on the hands or face.

Assess and classify burn depth after gently cleansing the burned area. Document your findings on your institution's assessment form.

✚👁 N u r s i n g   A l e r t
Severe burn injuries are often obvious and distressing. Be sure to assess for other concomitant injuries, such as spinal cord injury and fractures.

Most institutions use some modification of the "rule of nines" for estimating percentage of body burned. This method divides the body into multiples of 9%. For instance, one arm equals 9%; the entire back equals 18%. (See comparisons between children and adults described in Chap. 71.)

Phases of Burn Injury Management

The immediate or emergency response to a burn is to stop the burning process and to apply cold packs or cold water to the affected area. As in other emergencies, the care priorities are maintaining the airway, breathing, and circulation (see Chap. 43). When the client is transported to the nearest emergency department, the three phases of burn injury management—resuscitative, acute, and rehabilitative—begin.

✚👁 N u r s i n g   A l e r t
Circumferential burns of the extremities or chest may compromise circulation or breathing. Assess perfusion of distal extremities and respiratory status. An escharotomy may be needed to restore tissue perfusion or ease breathing.

Resuscitative Phase
Usually the burn client is admitted to a specialized nursing unit called the "burn care unit." If this type of unit is unavailable, the client is admitted to an intensive care unit. If the burn injuries meet criteria established by the American Burn Association, the client will be transferred by airlift, if necessary, to the nearest burn center. During the *resuscitative phase,* the client's physiologic condition is unstable; the goal of this phase is to achieve physiologic stability.

When working with a client who has been burned, wash hands thoroughly and frequently, wear sterile gloves, and use aseptic technique when preparing the room and handling supplies. When the client arrives at the healthcare facility, carefully remove his or her clothes, taking care not to further damage burn sites. Place the client on sterile sheets if the burn is severe. Show concern and give encouragement: the client is probably fearful, in pain, and experiencing a sense of loss. The primary provider performs a comprehensive physical examination immediately.

Vital Signs.   Record vital signs, and obtain height and weight measurements. Because the client is subject to shock,

➤➤ BOX 74-2

CRITERIA FOR CLASSIFYING THE EXTENT OF A BURN INJURY (AMERICAN BURN ASSOCIATION)

Minor Burn Injury
- Second-degree burn of <15% total body surface area (TBSA) in adults, or <10% TBSA in children
- Third-degree burn of <2% TBSA, not involving special care areas (eyes, ears, face, hands, feet, perineum, joints)
- Excludes electrical injury, inhalation injury, concurrent trauma, all high-risk clients (ie, extremes of age, concurrent disease)

Moderate, Uncomplicated Burn Injury
- Second-degree burns of 15% to 25% TBSA in adults, or 10% to 20% TBSA in children
- Third-degree burns of <10% TBSA, not involving special care areas
- Excludes electrical injury, inhalation injury, concurrent trauma, all high-risk clients (ie, extremes of age, concurrent disease)

Major Burn Injury
- Second-degree burns of >25% TBSA in adults, or 20% TBSA in children
- All third-degree burns of ≥10% TBSA
- All burns involving eyes, ears, face, hands, feet, perineum, joints
- All inhalation injury, electrical injury, concurrent trauma, high-risk clients

From: Hudak, C. M., Gallow, B. M., & Morton, P. G. (1998). *Critical care nursing: A holistic approach* (7th ed.). Philadelphia: Lippincott Williams & Wilkins.

monitor vital signs frequently. Place a cardiac monitor on him or her. Note any assessment changes, such as tachycardia (which may indicate a worsening condition) or a rise in temperature (which may indicate dehydration or infection).

Nursing Alert
Never apply ointments or salves to an extensive burn; removing them causes further discomfort, and their presence makes determining the extent of the burn difficult. Salves may also introduce pathogens into wounds.

Respiratory Status.   Smoke inhalation is often the cause of death for clients who do not have noticeable external burns. Carefully monitor the client's respiratory status, including the rate and depth of respirations. The client probably inhaled smoke and may have sustained lung burns. Carefully observe individuals who have head and neck area burns because such individuals are more likely to have respiratory damage.

Initiate oxygen therapy. Because of possible respiratory complications, keep an endotracheal tube or tracheostomy set at the bedside. Begin immediate measures to prevent hypostatic pneumonia. Measure pulse oximetry, blood gases, and pH frequently to determine respiratory status and general body status. Monitor serum carbon monoxide level if an inhalation injury is suspected. Administer respiratory therapy as prescribed.

Nursing Alert
Report the presence of a cough immediately. Note the amount and character of any sputum. Black or gray sputum indicates smoke inhalation.

Fluid and Electrolyte Balance.   The client who has experienced burns loses body fluids from capillary leaks and open wounds. Thus, he or she requires large amounts of intravenous fluids. To maintain survival, give such individuals large quantities of sodium-containing fluids. Fluid replacement maintains circulating volume and prevents circulatory collapse that contributes to serious or fatal shock.

Several formulas are available to guide fluid replacement. The *Parkland formula* is commonly used in fluid resuscitation:

4 mL lactated Ringer's solution × kg body weight × % body surface area burned = amount given

Half of this fluid amount is administered over the first 8 hours and the remaining half over the next 16 hours. The client usually has a retention catheter inserted and a nasogastric tube attached to suction. Record I&O accurately. The goal is for a urinary output of 0.5 to 1 milliliters per kilogram per hour, heart rate less than 120 beats per minute, and systolic blood pressure greater than 100 mm Hg.

Carefully assess the client's electrolyte status. Hyperkalemia, hypokalemia, and hyponatremia may occur after a burn injury (see Chap. 75). Monitor serum electrolytes and gastric secretions to determine electrolyte levels. A drug such as cimetidine (Tagamet) may reduce gastric secretions.

Renal Function.   Monitor urine output closely, because renal function commonly slows or stops after the body undergoes severe shock. Measure urinary output at least hourly for the first few days. A very high or a very low urine output is significant. Also monitor the specific gravity of the urine. Note a very high urine specific gravity (very concentrated urine). If the output is too low (less than 30 mL/h), dialysis may be needed. Acidosis also is a frequent complication.

Infection.   Infection is the leading cause of death for people with burns. They are highly susceptible to infection because of their lowered resistance and the many open wounds on the body acting as portals of entry for infectious agents. Clients may be placed in protective isolation to prevent exposure to pathogenic organisms (see Chap. 42). Practice thorough and frequent handwashing and wear sterile gloves. Give IV antibiotics as ordered. Antibacterial body packs or other topical medications may be applied. Expect to administer a tetanus immunization.

● **Key Concept**

Burns disrupt the integumentary system and place the individual at increased risk for infection. Note early signs and symptoms of a developing infection.

Pain Management. Depth of injury, anxiety level, previous experiences with pain, cultural beliefs, and the type of invasive monitoring and wound care procedures needed affect the client's pain level. Individuals with superficial burns experience a great deal of pain. Those with full-thickness burns are not in as much pain, because their nerve endings have been destroyed. Narcotic administration via a patient-controlled analgesia (PCA) device is the standard for pain relief. Morphine is often given to relieve pain; be alert for symptoms of respiratory depression. Imagery, hypnosis, dis-traction, and music therapy may help the client learn to tolerate the pain. See In Practice: Nursing Care Plan 74-1 about a client with burns.

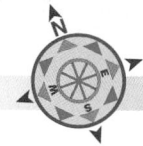

Special Considerations: Culture

Pain Management

Culture influences responses to pain. Recognize cultural differences and avoid stereotyping others. Some cultures commonly practice nonpharmacologic pain relief measures such as biofeedback, yoga breathing techniques, acupuncture, meditation, and hypnosis.

In Practice
Nursing Care Plan 74-1

A Client With Burns

Medical History: *L.D., a 66-year-old man, was admitted to the Regional Burn Center with superficial partial-thickness burns extending over 10% of the right side of his body, involving his upper thigh and lower abdomen. Client reports, "I was making tea and I accidentally spilled a pot of boiling water on myself. Oh, it hurts so much!" Initial IV bolus of morphine sulfate administered with PCA with morphine to be initiated.*

Medical Diagnosis: *Thermal burns*

Data Collection/Nursing Assessment: Client is well-nourished older adult male who is alert and oriented. History reveals no major health problems. Burned areas on upper thigh and lower abdomen appear moist, mottled red, with some blisters and blanching noted. Client moving about in bed and grimacing; rates pain as 9 on a numerical scale of 1 to 10. Vital signs are as follows: Temperature, 98.6° F (40.0° C); pulse, 92 beats per minute and regular; respirations, 26; blood pressure, 146/90. Client reports that pulse rate and blood pressure are elevated from his usual readings. *(Although other nursing diagnoses may be appropriate, a priority nursing diagnosis is addressed below.)*

Nursing Diagnosis: Pain related to thermal burn injury as evidenced by client's rating of 9, grimacing, and elevation in vital signs.

Planning
Short-Term Goals:
#1. Client states that pain has decreased to 5 or less on a numerical pain rating scale.

#2. Client's nonverbal behavior indicates a reduction in pain.

Long-Term Goals:
#3. Client reports pain is controlled at an acceptable level.
#4. Client exhibits no adverse effects of pain management regimen.

Implementation
Nursing Action: *Assist with initiating PCA with morphine. Continue to assess client's vital signs especially respiratory rate and depth, frequently, at least every 2 hours.*
Rationale: *Morphine via PCA is the method of choice for controlling pain associated with burns. Frequently monitoring vital signs, especially respiratory status, is important because morphine is a narcotic analgesic and central nervous system depressant.*

Nursing Action: *Assess client's complaints of pain after initial bolus of morphine and after initiating PCA. Have client rate pain using a numerical pain rating scale. Observe the client for nonverbal indicators of pain.*
Rationale: *Assessment after administration of morphine provides information about the effectiveness of drug therapy. Using the numerical pain rating scale allows for a consistent method of evaluating the client's pain. Nonverbal indicators provide additional evidence for determining effectiveness of pain relief.*

Evaluation: Client reports pain at 7 following bolus injection of morphine, and at 6 following initiation of PCA. Respiratory rate, 20 and regular; pulse rate,

(continued)

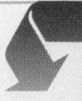

In Practice
Nursing Care Plan 74-1 (*Continued*)

88 beats/minute; blood pressure, 138/88. Client is lying in bed quietly, minimal grimacing is noted. *Progress to meeting Goal #1 and Goal #2.*

NURSING ACTION: *Question client about other non-pharmacologic measures used in the past for pain control. Assist with implementing these measures. Place the client in a position of comfort, using pillows for support as necessary.*
RATIONALE: *Nonpharmacologic measures, including proper positioning, can enhance the effects of analgesia.*

Evaluation: Client lying in bed quietly on his side, listening to music. PCA in use. Client reports decrease in pain, rating it as 4 on numerical rating scale. Vital signs are as follows: pulse, 80 beats/ minute; respira-

tions, 18 and regular; blood pressure, 130/82. *Goal #1 and Goal #2 met; progress to meeting Goal #3.*

NURSING ACTION: *Continue to reinforce use of PCA and music therapy. Assess for possible adverse effects of morphine. Monitor vital signs and level of pain every 3–4 hours.*
RATIONALE: *Continued use of PCA and monitoring is essential to ensure adequate pain relief without complications.*

Evaluation: Client states that pain is controlled and tolerable; continues to listen to music. Vital signs remaining within previous parameters. No evidence of central nervous system depression. *Goal #3 and Goal #4 met.*

Acute Phase

During the *acute phase,* the client remains acutely ill and requires continuing vigilant assessment. After the client's physiologic condition is stabilized, the focus is on managing the burn wound.

Dressings.   Several types of solutions and substances are used as dressings, including gauze impregnated with an antibiotic or drug, and moist packs soaked in a substance such as silver nitrate. Synthetic dressings such as DuoDerm, OpSite, Vigilon, and Biobrane promote wound healing or temporarily cover the wound. Figure 74-4 illustrates the use of Biobrane.

Continue to use aseptic technique and sterile dressings. In Practice: Nursing Care Guidelines 74-1 highlights important considerations.

Open dressings are continuously applied as wet dressings. Because wounds heal better if kept moist, closed dressings are not often used. Often the client wears a tight occlusive

dressing, face mask, or pressure dressing. The pressure may be applied to a specific burn area, such as an arm, or the client may wear a full-body pressure suit. These devices help to prevent the development of **keloid** (scar) tissue.

Topical Agents.   The application of topical agents to the burned area is currently the most widely used therapy. Agents used may include:

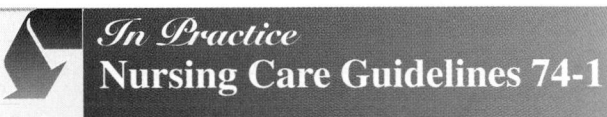

In Practice
Nursing Care Guidelines 74-1

APPLYING BURN DRESSINGS

- Explain the procedure to the client.
- Give as needed (PRN) pain and anxiolytic (antianxiety) medication approximately one-half hour before a dressing change. These medications provide pain relief and relaxation.
- Use aseptic technique throughout the procedure.
- Wear goggles and sterile gloves when changing dressings. Wear gown and mask if splashing is likely.
- Loosen dressings by moistening them with warmed, sterile, normal saline if ordered.
- Assess the burn's condition: extra dry indicates dehydration; wet, soupy, and strong odor indicates infection; redness and swelling at the edge of the wound indicate cellulitis; and clean, pink, and shiny indicates healthy healing.
- Keep in mind that all dressings and packs are contaminated when removed from the body. Dispose of all dressings and packs according to the institution's policies.

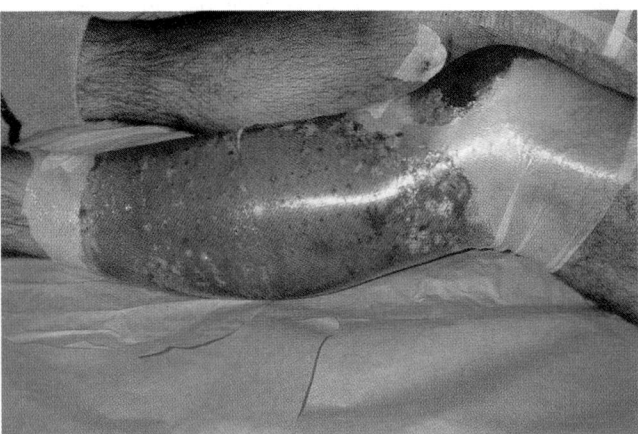

FIGURE 74-4. Biobrane, a type of synthetic, membrane burn dressing, protects the wound from fluid loss and bacterial invasion.

- *Mafenide acetate (Sulfamylon):* An effective bacteriostatic cream used against many gram-negative and gram-positive bacteria; applied in a thick layer to the entire burned area with a sterile, gloved hand; area usually allowed to remain open to the air. Associated with complaints of burning after application, and development of metabolic acidosis.

- *Silver sulfadiazine (Silvadene, Thermazene):* Bacteriocidal cream used against many gram-negative and gram-positive bacteria; applied in a thin layer to the burned area with a sterile, gloved hand; covered with petroleum jelly (Vaseline)-coated Adaptic or sterile dressings, commonly held in place with Kling or Kerlix. Associated with leukopenia; monitor the client's complete blood count. (Some gram-negative bacilli are resistant to the effects of Silvadene. If this condition develops, Silvadene is used in conjunction with other antimicrobial agents.)

- *Bacitracin ointment:* Used for superficial and facial burns applied as a thin layer two or three times per day as ordered.

- *Silver nitrate:* Rarely used today; applied as a 0.5% solution to gauze dressings placed on the burn areas, with dressings kept moist with bulb syringe to apply the solution. Believed that agent's bacteriocidal action on burn areas is so highly effective that cross-contamination does not result; thus, protective isolation technique is usually unnecessary.

✚👁 Nursing Alert

Silver nitrate will blacken anything with which it comes into contact, permanently staining it. Therefore, take measures to prevent staining of clothes, linen, walls, and floors.

Debridement. Eschar is usually thick, dry, and black or dark brown. It must be debrided to expose viable (living) tissue. In this way, grafting can be successfully performed.

Although packs and externally applied medications assist in loosening and softening eschar, the whirlpool is more commonly used for debridement because it is the most comfortable method. Debridement also may be performed in the operating room. Physicians now use laser scalpels for excision (removal) of eschar. This method causes minimal blood loss and less pain than previously used methods. Enzymatic debridement involves the application of proteolytic substances that digest necrotic tissue.

✚👁 Nursing Alert

Offer the client a PRN pain or anxiolytic (antianxiety) medication approximately one-half hour before any painful procedure, such as debridement.

Skin Grafting. Full-thickness burns destroy all skin tissue; therefore, skin grafting is performed to replace tissue that cannot heal by itself. Grafting also is done for cosmetic reasons, to limit the amount of scarring. If the client has enough intact, undamaged skin, an **autograft** (a graft using the client's own skin) is done. When healing begins and the eschar is completely removed, the plastic surgeon cuts paper-thin slices of skin from an unaffected part of the client's body and places these grafts on the affected area.

If the patient's own skin cannot be used, cadaver skin or skin from another person (**homograft** or **allograft**) may be used. Immunosuppressive medications may be given to prevent rejection of the foreign skin. In many cases, the foreign skin is allowed to be rejected, but is in place long enough to allow new tissue growth underneath.

In some severe burns (especially in areas such as the hands, which are prone to contractures) pigskin (a **heterograft** or **xenograft**) is grafted into place. The client's body will reject the pigskin in approximately 1 week, but before this occurs, the pigskin will aid in body fluid retention, protect the open wound from infection, and promote healing.

Clients who are severely burned do not have enough unharmed skin to graft onto injured areas. It is now possible to perform a biopsy on unburned skin and grow new skin. These cultured epithelial autografts (**CEA**) are useful in covering extensive burns.

Skin grafts are delicate; take care not to disturb them so that they can attach to the live tissue underneath and grow. Assess the graft and report if it seems to be detaching. Follow the protocols of the healthcare facility for care of both the graft and the donor sites.

☛ KEY CONCEPT

Wound management in burns is critical. The key to increased survival is early wound closure.

Other Care Management Priorities. Electrolyte imbalances may occur, related to wound leakage and impaired kidney function. Monitor gastric pH, electrolytes, and renal function test results. Administer electrolyte replacement as ordered.

Balanced nutrition with some supplemental nutrients to rebuild injured tissues is vital. The burned client may need as many as 6,000 calories daily. The diet should be high in calories, nitrogen, and protein. Vitamin supplements, extra between-meal protein supplements (such as Resource or Resource Instant Crystals), tube feedings, or total parenteral nutrition (TPN) may be used. If the client is allowed oral intake, urge the client to eat. (Medications ordered earlier to prevent excess acid formation in the stomach may be continued.)

Accurate recording of food intake is often ordered; record exactly what the client eats and any significant observations (such as refusal to eat, choking, difficulty in swallowing, or vomiting). Also monitor daily weights.

Often, stool softeners such as docusate sodium (Colace) are given to avoid straining. Record all bowel movements (time, amount, consistency, and other characteristics).

Rehabilitative Phase

During the *rehabilitative phase,* which can last for months or years, clients require extensive recuperation and healing.

During this phase, the emphasis is on recovery of strength and function.

Services. The client often goes to the physical therapy department for whirlpool treatment and exercises. The whirlpool serves several purposes: it helps clean the body and assists in removing eschar; it can be used to apply external medication; it provides warmth, so that the client can exercise with less pain; and it helps to stimulate viable-tissue growth and wound healing. When the client completes whirlpool treatment, the physical therapist exercises the client's extremities.

The seriously burned client is usually in the healthcare facility for some time and needs diversional activity. He or she also may need counseling or job retraining after discharge, and help in learning how to manage household activities. The occupational therapist provides these services or referrals to vocational counseling.

Due to the long-term nature of the healing of a severe burn, assistance in arranging for care of the client's family during hospitalization and the rehabilitation period may be necessary. Financial assistance may be needed as well. Inform the client and family about available support groups.

Complications. Various complications can occur following a burn, including infection, general gastrointestinal disturbances, hypostatic pneumonia, kidney failure, anemia, skin ulcers, and contractures.

Impaired circulation or difficulty in moving or breathing may occur, as eschar begins to tighten and constrict vital areas. An *escharotomy* (incision into eschar) may be needed to relieve difficulties.

Multiple stomach and duodenal ulcers called *Curling's ulcers* may develop approximately 1 week after the injury, causing significant gastrointestinal bleeding. Curling's ulcers occur when the gastric mucosa becomes ischemic, when there are excess hydrogen ions, or when there is inadequate mucosal cell proliferation. Prevent Curling's ulcers by monitoring gastric pH, providing enteral (tube) feedings, and administering medications such as cimetidine (Tagamet), ranitidine (Zantac), famotidine (Pepcid), sucralfate (Carafate), or antacids. The first symptom of Curling's ulcers often is bleeding, as evidenced by bloody sputum or emesis or by tarry stools.

Contractures, due to abnormal shortening of muscles, tendons, or scar tissue, result in deformity and limited joint movement. Contractures are the most serious long-term complication of burns, but are now usually preventable with passive and active range of motion (ROM) exercises. The client may be reluctant to move because of pain or fear of pain. Therefore, encourage exercise and explain its importance. Splinting the extremities in anti-deformity positions is essential in preventing contractures. If the burn is near a joint, contractures are more likely to form and may need to be released surgically. Give as needed (PRN) medications before exercises to reduce pain.

Emotional Aspects. Many emotional aspects accompany burns. The client may become demanding, expecting much attention in later stages of care because he or she received so much attention immediately after the injury. Allow the client to express his or her feelings. At the same time, be honest, understanding, and firm. Encourage the client and family members to participate in developing a realistic nursing care plan. If the client requires infection control precautions, an added element is loneliness. The client may be realistically concerned about his or her appearance. Help by listening and by encouraging the client to become involved in a support group.

Discharge Planning. Inpatient hospital stays for burn injuries are becoming increasingly shorter. Prepare families for discharge and home care. Teach about wound care, medication use, and signs and symptoms of infection. Make referrals for outpatient care as indicated.

Prognosis. Although the course of treatment is long and arduous, current techniques help the client return to optimum functioning. Most people are able to live productive lives.

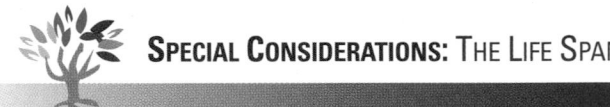

SPECIAL CONSIDERATIONS: THE LIFE SPAN

Burns and the Older Adult

- Older people may not realize they are being burned; they may be paralyzed or confused, or they may be unable to feel the burn.
- People older than 60 years of age may have difficulty recovering from burns because they have very thin skin and usually receive deeper burns. Also, the immune system may be compromised. Older adults are at high risk for hypostatic pneumonia.
- Older adults with cardiovascular disease may be unable to withstand the additional trauma of a burn.

NEOPLASMS

A **neoplasm** is a new growth, often called a *tumor,* which may be *malignant* (invasive) or *benign* (not invasive). Cancer is a malignant neoplasm.

Nonmalignant Tumors

Nonmalignant tumors of the skin include warts, cysts, **angiomas** (birthmarks), keloids, and nevi (see following discussion). A *wart* is a tumor that can be caused by an infection (such as the HPV discussed earlier) or by other nonmalignant neoplasms.

Moles

Moles, or *pigmented nevi,* are usually benign. However, they may become malignant, especially if they are very dark, hairy, and elevated. A biopsy procedure should be performed if a mole has these characteristics.

Angiomas

Angiomas, or *birthmarks,* are vascular skin tumors, involving underlying tissues and blood vessels. Some angiomas, such as the *port-wine angioma*, are difficult to remove. If they are very large, they are inoperable. Other *strawberry angiomas* tend to involute (regress or disappear) spontaneously. Most angiomas are neither very noticeable nor very dangerous.

Keloids

Keloids are painless, benign overgrowths that develop at the site of a scar or trauma. Keloids occur more often in darker-skinned individuals. Plastic surgery, for cosmetic reasons, may be performed to hide these scars.

Skin Cancer

Skin cancer is the most common and most curable form of cancer. Because the lesion is visible, the client usually seeks treatment early. The most common types of skin cancer are basal cell carcinoma, squamous cell carcinoma, and malignant melanoma (Fig. 74-5).

Exposure to the sun is the leading cause of skin cancer. Light-haired, fair-skinned, light-eyed people are at highest risk for skin cancer. Also at high risk are individuals who are prone to sunburn or who do not tan. People over 40 years of age are more susceptible than younger people. A client who as a child had a severe sunburn has an increased chance of developing skin cancer at that site later in life. Smoking also seems to increase susceptibility.

Observation and early investigation of changes in a mole and of new growths is vital; a deeply pigmented mole should be checked. The American Cancer Society has developed a helpful ABCD rule for evaluating a mole:

Asymmetry: One half of the mole does not match the other half.
Border: Edges are irregular, ragged, notched, or blurred.
Color: Color is not uniform, but appears as differing shades of tan, brown, or black, sometimes with patches of red, white, or blue.
Diameter: Size is larger than that of a pencil eraser (about ½ inch) or is increasing.

Teach clients to consult a healthcare provider when any changes in a wart or mole occur, including such factors as size, shape, color, flaking, bleeding, sudden elevation, hair growth, or sudden itching or burning.

Preventive teaching is of utmost importance in controlling skin cancer. Teach all people, especially those at risk, the preventive measures identified at In Practice: Educating the Client 74-3.

Most forms of skin cancer are treated by curettage (scraping), electrodesiccation (removal with intermittent electric sparks), cryosurgery (tissue destruction by freezing), or wide excision (surgery). A pathologist examines the tissue to ensure complete removal. Radiation therapy may supplement surgical removal, or may be used for older adults or for those in whom excision is impractical or impossible. Mohs' micrographic surgery is the treatment of choice for basal cell carcinoma and squamous cell carcinoma. In this process, the tumor is removed layer by layer, until a microscopic examination reveals that all the tumor was removed.

Basal Cell Carcinoma

Basal cell carcinoma appears as a small, fleshy bump or nodule. It usually is found in areas that are repeatedly exposed to the sun or other UV light. It is the most common form of skin cancer in Caucasians. This cancer occurs mostly on the head and neck, is very slow growing, and usually does not metastasize. However, it may extend below the skin to the bone and cause considerable local damage.

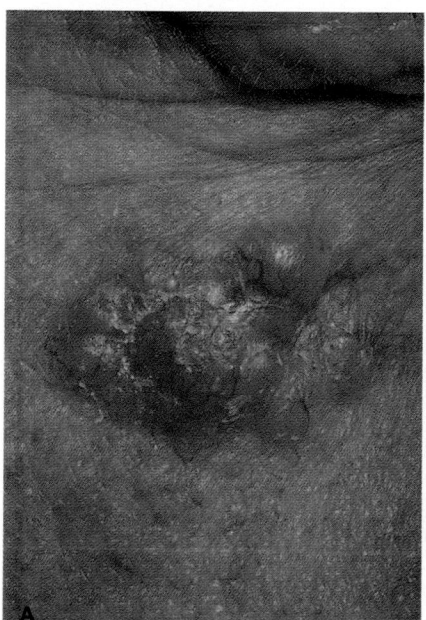
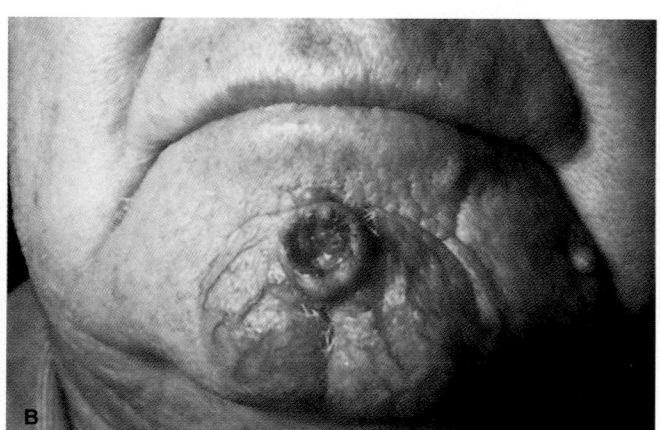
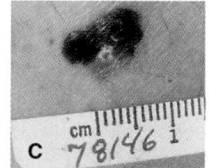

FIGURE 74-5. Skin cancers. (**A**) Basal cell carcinoma. (**B**) Squamous cell carcinoma. (**C**) Malignant melanoma.

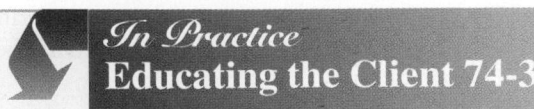

In Practice
Educating the Client 74-3

SKIN CANCER PREVENTION

- Avoid bright sunlight, especially midday or tropical sun, primarily during the hours of 10:00 AM to 3:00 PM.
- Protect your body from sun. Wear sunglasses, a wide-brimmed hat, and long sleeves.
- Use sunscreen with a sun protective factor (SPF) of at least 15.
- Avoid the use of sunlamps and tanning beds.
- Observe the skin for changes in pigmentation; changes in warts or moles; abnormal growths; hair growing in or on a mole; or sudden itching, burning, flaking, or elevation of any skin lesion.
- Observe your childrens' or partner's skin, including the back.
- Have warts or moles removed if they are irritated or exposed to friction from clothing.
- Consult a healthcare provider if any of the above features occur.

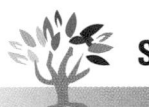

SPECIAL CONSIDERATIONS: THE LIFE SPAN

Skin Cancer

The older adult population has the greatest incidence of precancerous and cancerous skin lesions.

Squamous Cell Carcinoma

Squamous cell carcinoma may appear as a nodule or as a red, scaly patch. Squamous cell carcinoma is the second most common type of skin cancer found in Caucasians. It is typically found on the rim of the ear, face, lips, or mouth. This cancer increases in size and develops into a large mass; the cancer may metastasize. The cure rate for squamous cell carcinoma is 95% with early treatment.

Malignant Melanoma

Malignant melanoma is a darkly pigmented mole or skin tumor—the most virulent of all skin cancers, but almost always curable in its early stages. Melanoma may appear without warning, but it also may begin in or near a mole or other dark spot on the skin. It has a strong tendency to metastasize to the skin, bone, liver, brain, and lung. When colonies of melanoma cells reach vital internal organs, the disease becomes more difficult to treat. The treatment of choice for malignant melanoma is wide excision of the primary lesion. Dacarbazine (DTIC) is the single most effective chemotherapeutic drug

for malignant melanoma. Elective regional node dissection also improves the chances for survival.

STUDENT SYNTHESIS

Key Points

- Dermatology is the study of skin diseases.
- Common diagnostic tests used to determine skin disorders are Wood's light examination, Tzanck's smear, tissue biopsy, and scabies scraping.
- A variety of pharmacologic and nonpharmacologic measures are used to treat pruritus.
- Various allergies may cause urticaria and contact dermatitis.
- Chronic skin disorders include vitiligo, dermatitis, and psoriasis.
- Folliculitis and carbuncles are common bacterial skin infections.
- Parasitic skin infestations include scabies, lice, and bedbugs.
- The four types of burns are thermal, electrical, chemical, and radiation.
- The three major phases of client recovery after a burn are resuscitative, acute, and rehabilitative.
- Extent of burns is determined by a variety of means. Burn depth and percentage of body surface area burned are significant.
- The major types of skin grafts include autografts, allografts, heterografts, and cultured epithelial autografts.
- Moles, angiomas, and keloids are nonmalignant skin tumors.
- Basal cell carcinoma, squamous cell carcinoma, and malignant melanoma are types of skin cancer. Basal cell carcinoma is the most common type of skin cancer and usually does not metastasize.

Critical Thinking Exercises

1. A homeless shelter recently experienced an outbreak of lice. Identify factors that place shelters at risk for lice. How will you instruct the staff at the shelter to manage the problem?
2. You are caring for a client with severe facial burns. His wife desires to visit him; however, she is afraid of his appearance. Discuss how you can support this couple.
3. Your client, who has a circumferential burn to her right forearm, informs you that her fingers are cold and painful. Discuss possible causes and treatments for this finding.
4. You are participating in a health fair at a shopping mall. A teenager asks you if he could develop skin cancer. Describe your assessment of his risk for skin cancer. Discuss specific recommendations for how he could reduce his risk for skin cancer.

NCLEX-Style Review Questions

1. On admission to the hospital, the client has a 10% body surface full-thickness burn. The nurse should give highest priority to:
   a. Applying a dressing
   b. Assessing for stress ulcer
   c. Obtaining vital signs
   d. Preparing for skin grafting
2. The nurse understands that the probable effect of a client's choosing to continue to be exposed to ultraviolet radiation will be:
   a. A healthy tan
   b. Dry flaky scalp
   c. Increased risk of skin cancer
   d. Increased risk of oily skin
3. Which statement by the client who has pruritis indicates that the client has understood teaching regarding the treatment of pruritis?
   a. "I can take a bath with baking soda added to it."
   b. "I should rinse my clothes with a fabric softener."
   c. "I should take hot baths every evening."
   d. "Wearing wool will help control the itching."
4. A client is diagnosed with condylomata acuminata. Which of the following instructions should be included in the teaching plan?
   a. Lesions are not contagious.
   b. Lesions are usually found in the folds of the elbows.
   c. Lesions may be associated with skin cancer.
   d. Lesions may be spread by sexual contact.
5. Which assessment data would the nurse expect with a client who has sustained a full-thickness burn?
   a. Blisters, pinkish-red color
   b. Cherry-red, white, or black color
   c. Dry, blanches with pressure
   d. Mottled-red or pinkish color

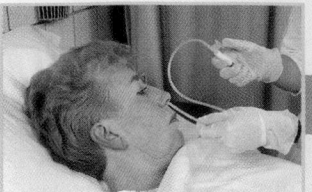

CHAPTER

75

Disorders in Fluid and Electrolyte Balance

LEARNING OBJECTIVES

1. Differentiate among the following fluid compartments: intracellular, extracellular, interstitial, and intravascular.
2. Discuss at least four major nursing responsibilities associated with laboratory tests ordered by a clinician.
3. In the clinical laboratory, demonstrate a client and family teaching session, emphasizing the importance of fluid and electrolyte balance and the types of care that may be needed for the client.
4. Identify at least four possible causes of the two major types of fluid imbalances (fluid volume excess and fluid volume deficit), including at least two nursing considerations for each cause.
5. State at least two nursing considerations for each: dependent edema, sacral edema, pitting and nonpitting edema, and pulmonary edema.
6. State the normal serum levels for the following electrolytes: sodium, potassium, calcium, magnesium, chloride, and phosphorous.
7. Identify at least four causes of each type of electrolyte imbalance.
8. Discuss the major symptoms associated with each type of electrolyte imbalance, stating at least three nursing considerations related to each condition.
9. Differentiate among the four major types of acid–base imbalances: respiratory acidosis, respiratory alkalosis, metabolic acidosis, and metabolic alkalosis.
10. Identify at least four nursing considerations related to the data collection, assessment, monitoring, and care of a client with acidosis and a client with alkalosis.

NEW TERMINOLOGY

acidosis
alkalosis
anascara
ascites
fluid volume deficit
fluid volume excess
metabolic acidosis

metabolic alkalosis
nonpitting edema
overhydration
pitting edema
respiratory acidosis
respiratory alkalosis
turgor

ACRONYMS

ABG
ADH
ATP
Ca^{++}
Cl^-
H^+
HCO_3^-
H_2CO_3
K^+

KCl
LFT
mEq
mEq/L
Mg^{++}
mg/dL
Na^+
P
pH

PO_4^{--}
SI

A normal balance between the body's fluids and electrolytes, and acids and bases, must exist for a person to be healthy. Homeostasis, the dynamic process by which the body constantly adjusts to internal and external stimuli, is disrupted by abnormalities of fluid levels and electrolyte content.

The body constantly uses feedback mechanisms to maintain fluid and electrolyte balance. The nervous and endocrine systems are most intimately involved in feedback. The integumentary, respiratory, digestive, and urinary systems also respond to feedback mechanisms. Feedback mechanisms play a major role in maintaining fluid and electrolyte balance (see Unit 4).

Any disorder, disease, or injury can disrupt homeostasis. The risk of serious disturbances in fluid–electrolyte or acid–base balance increases in clients at the extremes of the age spectrum, in those with burn injuries, and in those with pre-existing conditions or chronic illnesses. Nurses play a major role in monitoring clients for actual or potential threats to homeostasis, with nursing care being directed toward assessing and maintaining this balance.

Chapter 17 introduced the concepts of body fluids, fluid compartments, and electrolyte balance. This chapter continues the discussion of fluids and the major electrolytes. Emphasis is given to data collection and nursing concerns related to excesses or deficiencies of fluids and electrolytes.

DIAGNOSTIC TESTS

Many laboratory tests are aimed at evaluating the body's fluid–electrolyte or acid–base balance. Chemical studies of electrolytes are probably among the most commonly ordered laboratory studies. The healthcare provider may order a determination of levels of a single electrolyte or a combination of electrolytes. Most clinical facilities have standard chemistry panels identified with terms such as "chem. 6," "chem. 8," or "chem. 24." Each facility defines the components of these chemistry panels. Generally, a *chemistry panel* contains a minimum of the basic electrolytes (sodium, potassium, and chloride) plus glucose. Appendix C lists normal chemistry and hematology laboratory values.

Other commonly ordered tests include complete blood counts (CBC) and liver function tests (**LFTs**). In addition, arterial blood gas (**ABG**) evaluations may be performed to determine the **pH** (potential of hydrogen in concentration) of blood, a valuable indicator of acidosis or alkalosis. The components and values of an ABG are listed in Table 17-5 in Chap. 17.

Urine and other body fluids also are studied for composition and abnormal components. In some cases, urine is collected for 24 hours so that an entire day's output can be analyzed.

☛ Key Concept

Fluid and electrolyte disturbances are possible in anyone, but they are particularly common in ill and hospitalized clients (including those undergoing surgical and diagnostic procedures) and in young children and older adults.

COMMON MEDICAL TREATMENTS

When an excess of body water exists in the extracellular fluid (ECF, found in the interstitial and intravascular spaces), or electrolyte excess is detected, medications may be given to facilitate removal of the excessive substance from the body. Oral or rectal medication may be given to draw electrolytes out of the body through the gastrointestinal system. Oral or IV medications may draw fluids or certain electrolytes from the body for elimination through the urinary system.

When a deficit of body water exists in the ECF or electrolyte deficit is determined, fluids, electrolytes, and other substances can be administered to the client to help restore homeostasis. Some substances, such as potassium, can be administered orally. In certain clients, either the body cannot absorb electrolytes taken orally, or the body will not absorb them quickly enough to prevent serious problems. In such cases, IV administration of electrolytes is usually the treatment of choice.

Specific electrolytes may be added to a large-volume infusion (eg, "1,000 mL of D51/2NS with 20 milliequivalents [**mEq**] of potassium chloride [**KCl**]"), or given in a smaller volume via intermittent infusion (eg, "100 mL of NS with 20 mEq KCl via IV piggyback"). In an extreme emergency, a bolus (one-time large dose) of a particular electrolyte may be administered. The person's blood levels are monitored, and the dosage is adjusted accordingly. After critical deficits are corrected, and any oral restrictions are removed, oral fluid or electrolyte replacements may be initiated. Chapter 63 discusses administration of IV fluids.

NURSING PROCESS

Data Collection

Carefully observe and monitor all clients for potential disorders in fluid or electrolyte balance. Obtain ordered laboratory studies and report results to the clinician. Chapter 47 describes nursing assessment and data collection. A baseline is important for future comparison, and to determine the presence of suspected abnormalities. Report any abnormalities or changes in the baseline level.

✚👁 **Nursing Alert**

In the normal flow of information in clinical facilities, the nurse is often the first care provider to see the laboratory results. Although laboratory personnel may have highlighted or noted critical values, generally the nurse is responsible for notifying the primary healthcare provider of significant changes in lab values or of critical lab values. *Critical values* are those laboratory levels that are considered serious or life threatening. The nurse documents that the lab values have been reported, eg, *"0815 Dr. Smith notified by phone of K^+ result of 3.0 mEq. Stat order for K supplement given. 0830 Client received ordered medication."*

When collecting and documenting data about a client's fluid and electrolyte balance, observe factors such as the skin's appearance and **turgor** (elasticity or tonus), the urine's volume and specific gravity, the relative balance between intake and output, and comparisons of daily weights (see In Practice: Nursing Assessment 75-1).

Nursing Diagnosis

Based on data collection, the following nursing diagnoses may be established for the person with a disorder in fluid or electrolyte balance:

- Impaired Oral Mucous Membranes related to dehydration as evidenced by dry tongue and oral lesions with noted poor skin turgor and low urine output
- Impaired Urinary Elimination related to diminished or excessive urinary output
- Excess Fluid Volume related to electrolyte imbalance as evidenced by extremity edema, pulmonary edema, hypertension, **ascites** (fluid in the abdominal cavity), or sodium retention
- Deficient Fluid Volume related to fluid or electrolyte imbalance as evidenced by hypotension, hyperthermia, rapid weight loss, dry skin, poor skin turgor, or concentrated urine
- Impaired Tissue Integrity related to edema or dehydration and poor skin turgor
- Impaired Physical Mobility related to fluid retention or electrolyte disturbances

Planning and Implementation

The healthcare team plans together with the client and family for effective care. The client with a fluid or electrolyte imbalance may require assistance in meeting daily needs, maintaining a balance between input and output (I&O), and understanding more about the disorder, its prognosis, and its treatment. The client needs to follow the prescribed regimen to resolve the imbalance. A nursing plan of care is developed to meet these needs. A critical pathway or care mapping may also be used to help the person meet desired outcomes.

Teaching the Client and Family.   Teach the client and family about fluid and electrolyte problems, especially if the person will be cared for in the home. Include the client and family as much as possible in planning the diet, monitoring dietary restrictions, and following the schedule and amounts of food and fluids to consume. If the client understands the rationale for special diets or limitations, he or she is more likely to comply. This understanding is also important for the individuals who will do the shopping and food preparation in the home. Topics to include in client and family teaching are summarized at In Practice: Educating the Client 75-1.

Treating Edema.   Handle edematous areas carefully. Edematous skin is friable and prone to skin breakdown, sloughing, and ulceration. Change the person's position frequently for maximum comfort. Elevating an edematous body part (usually the feet and ankles) to a position higher than the heart's level helps alleviate the edema.

Assessing Daily Fluid Balance.   Keep accurate I&O records. Normally, fluid I&O amounts are roughly equal. If the amounts differ greatly, evaluate the client's hydration level. Check the urine specific gravity. Evaluate the client's skin turgor by lifting a fold of skin between your thumb and forefinger (Fig. 75-1; see Chap. 47). Assess the extremities or any dependent areas for edema (see "Edema" section). Assess breathing to detect the serious complication of pulmonary edema. Monitor IV fluid administration to prevent circulatory overload. Assess drainage. Note any watery stools and significant *diaphoresis* (sweating). Weigh the client daily to detect rapid unexplained weight loss or gain.

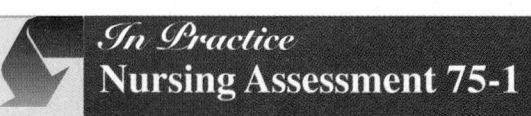

In Practice
Nursing Assessment 75-1

POSSIBLE INDICATORS OF FLUID AND ELECTROLYTE IMBALANCES

- Presence or absence of edema
- Poor skin turgor
- Changes in skin color, moisture level
- Sudden weight gain or loss
- Hypertension or hypotension
- Significant difference between intake and output
- Dyspnea, orthopnea, or rales (fluid in the lungs) on auscultation
- Abnormal electrolyte levels (on laboratory report)
- Elevated temperature
- Decreased or increased urine specific gravity
- Psychological or sensorium abnormalities
- Changes in urine volume
- Thirst

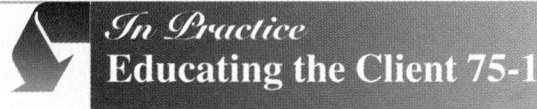

In Practice
Educating the Client 75-1

TEACHING TOPICS ASSOCIATED WITH FLUID OR ELECTROLYTE DISORDERS

- Special procedures to perform
- Special skin care
- Importance of exercise and positioning
- Diet restrictions and diet modifications, with sample diets
- Amount and type of fluids to encourage
- Fluid restrictions
- Changes in lifestyle
- Correct administration of medications, including undesirable side effects
- Precautions to take
- Signs and symptoms of worsening condition and what to report

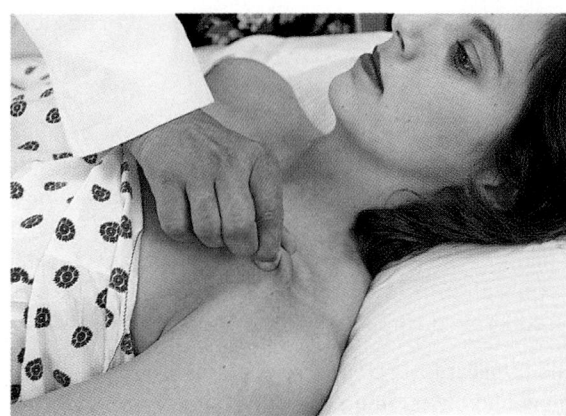

FIGURE 75-1. Testing for skin turgor. The nurse is pinching the skin over the clavicle. Other testing sites include the skin over the sternum and over the forehead. With normal skin turgor, when the skin is released, the skin will return to its normal position immediately. If turgor is diminished, the pinched skin will remain in position briefly. *Tenting* is the term used to describe a finding of poor skin turgor. (© B. Proud.)

Administering Medications. Administer medications as ordered; observe their results and side effects. Correcting an acid–base imbalance may be necessary to correct a fluid–electrolyte imbalance. Give diuretic drugs (to increase urinary output) and electrolytes as ordered. The client's urinary output should increase soon after diuretic therapy is started. Monitor for signs of potassium deficit, dehydration, or acid–base imbalance that may occur with the extended use of diuretics.

Assisting With Mouth and Skin Care. The skin and mucous membranes of the client with a fluid imbalance are prone to breakdown, cracking, and infections. Give the client good mouth and skin care (see Chap. 50). Perform these actions at least every 2 hours.

Evaluation

Periodically, the healthcare team evaluates the outcomes of care. Have short-term goals been met? Are long-term goals still realistic? Planning for further nursing care considers the client's prognosis, any complications, and the client's responses to treatment.

MAINTENANCE OF FLUID BALANCE

A person needs to maintain a homeostatic balance of the amount of water in all body fluid compartments. Fluid is constantly moving among compartments. For example, blood contains *plasma fluids,* which circulate to all body areas. *Tissue fluids* and *lymph fluids* also travel from one fluid compartment to another. *Intracellular fluids* (ICF) are relatively stable. However, if disturbances occur in the ICF balance, the client is critically compromised. If the balance among compartments is upset, several problems can occur, including fluid volume excess and fluid volume deficit (see Chap. 17).

Fluid Volume Excess

Fluid volume excess (FVE) is excessive retention of water and sodium in the ECF. **Overhydration** refers specifically to excess water in the extracellular spaces. The following are possible causes of FVE:

- Increased fluid intake, as in too-rapid administration of IV fluids containing sodium, or too-rapid administration of enteral tube feedings (eg, nasogastric tube feedings)
- Decreased urine output as in kidney or liver disorders
- Physical disorders (eg, heart failure or cardiac insufficiency) that result in a decreased ability of the heart to pump effectively
- Excess ingestion of sodium (eg, from substances that contain large amounts of sodium chloride; overuse of table salt; or medications that contain large amounts of sodium)
- Stress from surgery or other physical trauma that causes aldosterone and antidiuretic hormone (**ADH**) production, resulting in sodium and water retention

Nursing care includes daily assessments as per discussion in earlier chapters; administration and observation of diuretics; and often a sodium-restricted diet.

Edema

The excessive accumulation of interstitial fluid is known as *edema.* As discussed in Chapter 17, edema can be a local or generalized clinical manifestation of many disorders involving FVE, such as:

- *Congestive heart failure, thrombophlebitis, and liver cirrhosis,* all of which increase venous pressure and cause faulty reabsorption of fluids and electrolytes
- *Low protein levels,* due to conditions such as malnutrition or liver disease, which cause fluid to be drawn out of blood vessels and into tissue spaces
- *Poor lymphatic drainage,* which reduces osmotic pressure, causing more fluid to be retained
- *Sodium retention,* due to conditions such as kidney or endocrine disorders, which cause sodium to be reabsorbed rather than excreted; increased sodium levels cause water to be drawn out of the circulation and into the tissues
- *Inflammation,* which dilates the arteries and increases the permeability of the capillary walls
- *Physical stress,* such as surgery, which may cause increased amounts of interstitial fluids (third-spacing) due to tissue trauma and responses by the endocrine system

Dependent edema occurs in an area that hangs down (that is, in a *dependent* position). In an ambulatory person or one who remains in a sitting position, dependent edema is common in the feet and ankles.

Sacral edema, as the name implies, is dependent edema in the sacral area. Typically, sacral edema is noted in the client who remains in bed, and no limb edema is noted.

Pitting edema is the descriptive term used to describe serious observable edema that dents under slight finger pressure. The healthcare provider assesses pitting edema by using a finger to press against the area of swelling. Generally, a scale of +1 to +4 is used to describe the intensity of the edema. For example, the nurse presses against the lower extremity and a slight dent remains after the finger is removed. The dent remains for only a second or so. This example could be described as plus one (+1) pitting edema. When a dent remains for 2, 3, or 4 or more seconds, the observation is charted as +2, +3, or +4 pitting edema, respectively. If the dent in the skin remains for some time in edematous tissue, as in a +4 pitting edema, **anascara** (generalized body edema) may also be noted (Fig. 75-2).

Nonpitting edema, which can also be severe, refers to swelling that does not indent when slight pressure is applied. Be sure to chart that the edema is either pitting or nonpitting on the +1 to +4 scale. Also include the location, and be sure to notify the primary healthcare provider.

Pulmonary edema is an accumulation of interstitial fluid in the lungs. It is a symptom of various heart and blood vessel disorders, nephrosis, cirrhosis of the liver, and IV therapy that is administered too fast.

Fluid Volume Deficit

Fluid volume deficit (FVD) is a deficiency of fluid and electrolytes in the ECF. *Dehydration* refers to a decreased volume

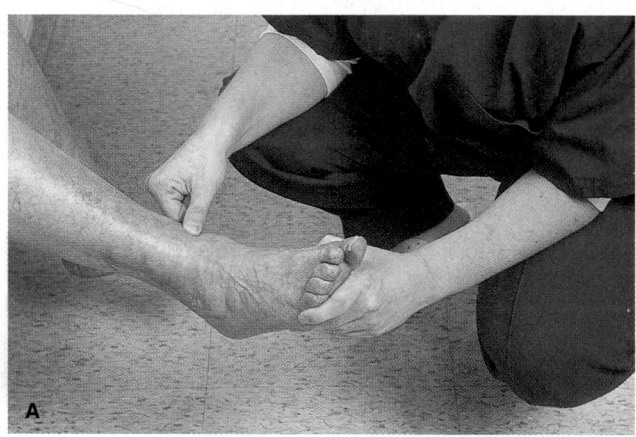

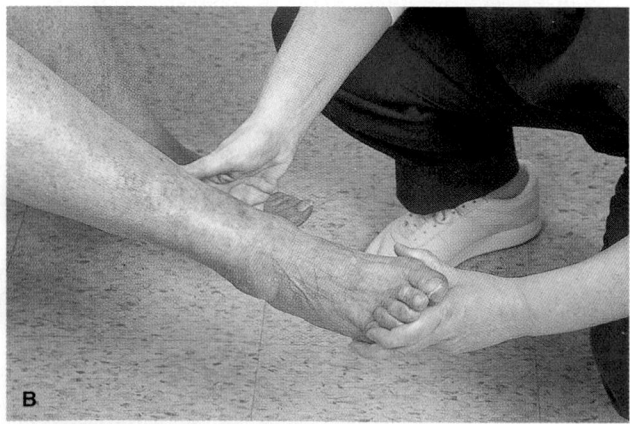

FIGURE 75-2. Testing for pitting edema. **(A)** The nurse is pressing her thumb into the skin on the ankle of the client. **(B)** The impression left by the thumb is called *pitting edema* and indicates significant fluid retention.

of water, but it does not occur without electrolyte changes. The following are possible causes of FVD:

- Inadequate fluid intake and starvation
- Loss of body fluids (eg, from excessive sweating, diarrhea, vomiting, excessive urine output, excessive drainage such as from wounds or burns, or GI suctioning)
- Prolonged fever
- Inability of the body to conserve and reuse water by concentrating the urine (occurs with renal failure or endocrine disorders)

The cause of FVD needs to be identified and treated. Younger and older clients are at the highest risk for dehydration, because of inadequate oral fluid intake. Encourage oral fluid intake unless the person is nauseated or in danger of aspiration. Oral fluids are the easiest and safest way to restore proper hydration. In Practice: Nursing Care Plan 75-1 highlights the care of a client with FVD.

The person with FVD may need fluid replacement therapy or total parenteral nutrition. Chapter 63 discusses IV fluid therapy.

Monitor results from increased fluid intake via observations of skin turgor (see Fig. 75-1) and urine output. When checking skin turgor, if the skin remains elevated, as in a tent, the condition can be described as *tenting*. Skin tenting is an indication of dehydration. A scale of +1 to +4 is commonly used to describe tenting. For example, if the skin does not return to normal position in 4 or so seconds, the nurse would chart, "Poor skin turgor as seen by +4 tenting over sternum."

☛ Kᴇʏ Cᴏɴᴄᴇᴘᴛ

Fluid volume deficit can occur as a result of many disorders. Assess the client's level of hydration and observe for fluid volume deficit in all clients.

MAINTENANCE OF ELECTROLYTE BALANCE

For the body to function properly in all aspects, electrolytes must be properly balanced. Electrolyte imbalances (Table 75-1) can have serious consequences on the body.

Units of measure for electrolytes include milliequivalents per liter (**mEq/L**), which is a calculated concentration of electrolytes in a specific volume of solution. Some laboratories report levels using the International System of Units ("Systeme International," or **SI** units) such as milligrams per deciliter (**mg/dL**). A deciliter is equal to 0.1 liter or 100 milliliters.

Sodium

Sodium (**Na⁺**), as the main extracellular ion, induces water movement between ICF and ECF to help achieve homeostasis of water within those compartments. The severity of symptoms seen with imbalances of sodium concentration is most greatly affected by the cause of the problem, the speed at which the change takes place, and the degree of change in the Na level.

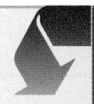

In Practice
Nursing Care Plan 75-1

THE CLIENT WITH FLUID LOSS

MEDICAL HISTORY: *J.J., a 28-year-old female, comes to the emergency department complaining of vomiting for the past 2 days. She states, "I can't keep anything down. I've tried to drink because I'm thirsty, but it's no use. Everybody in my office has been sick with a GI virus." CBC and serum electrolyte levels obtained. Results reveal levels are slightly decreased but within acceptable parameters. Urine specimen obtained for urinalysis. Intravenous fluid therapy initiated at 125 cc's/hour; client is placed on NPO status.*

MEDICAL DIAGNOSIS: *Mild dehydration resulting from gastroenteritis*

Data Collection/Nursing Assessment: Client is alert and oriented. Skin and mucous membranes are pale pink and slightly dry. Skin returns slowly when pinched. Vital signs are as follows: Temperature, 99° F (37.2° C); pulse, 92 beats per minute and regular; respirations, 22; blood pressure, 110/62. Client weighs 132 lbs at present. She states, "I've lost a little over 2 pounds since I've been sick." Client is voiding small amounts of urine, approximately 60 cc's in the past 2 hours. Urine appears concentrated, dark amber in color. Specific gravity is 1.027. (*Although other nursing diagnoses may be appropriate, a priority nursing diagnosis is addressed below.*)

Nursing Diagnosis: Deficient fluid volume related to persistent vomiting from probable gastroenteritis as evidenced by the client's report of vomiting for the past 2 days, minimal to no oral intake, and co-workers being similarly ill.

Planning:

SHORT-TERM GOALS:
#1. Client will report that episodes of vomiting and complaints of thirst are decreasing.
#2. Client will demonstrate ability to tolerate ice chips and sips of clear liquids.
#3. Client will maintain a urine output of at least 30 cc's/hour.

LONG-TERM GOALS:
#4. Client will demonstrate ability to tolerate progressive diet intake.
#5. Client will demonstrate signs and symptoms of adequate fluid balance.

Implementation
NURSING ACTION: *Continue to monitor intake and output, vital signs, mucous membranes, skin turgor, and urine specific gravity at least every 2 hours.*

RATIONALE: *Continued monitoring is necessary to provide a means for evaluating improvement or deterioration in the client's status.*

NURSING ACTION: *Maintain IV fluid therapy as ordered. Maintain NPO status as ordered.*
RATIONALE: *IV fluid replacement therapy is needed to prevent further fluid imbalance that could impact renal function. Maintaining NPO status aids in resting the GI tract.*

Evaluation: Client reports no vomiting for the past 2 hours. Urine output is 80 cc's over the past 2 hours. *Progress to meeting Goal #1 and Goal #3.*

NURSING ACTION: *Begin to offer ice chips and sips of clear fluid, approximately 30 cc's per hour, as ordered. Gradually increase amount according to client's tolerance.*
RATIONALE: *Offering ice chips and small amounts of clear fluids gradually helps to re-establish oral intake without over-stressing the GI tract.*

Evaluation: Client reports ability to tolerate approximately 2 to 3 ounces of fluid over the past hour with decreased complaints of thirst. No episodes of vomiting since admission. Urine output remains at approximately 45 cc's per hour. *Goal #1 met; Goal #2 met; Goal #3 met; progress to meeting Goal #4.*

NURSING ACTION: *Continue to advance oral intake and diet as ordered, offering small amounts of full liquids and then diet as tolerated as ordered. Monitor IV fluid therapy, decreasing rate as ordered.*
RATIONALE: *Advancing oral intake aids in promoting the resumption of pre-illness diet. As oral intake increases, the need for IV fluid replacement decreases.*

Evaluation: Client able to tolerate full-liquid to bland diet. IV fluid therapy discontinued. *Goal #4 met.*

NURSING ACTION: *Obtain weight and compare with baseline. Continue to monitor intake and output and laboratory test results. Assess mucous membranes and skin turgor.*
RATIONALE: *Parameters such as weight, intake and output, mucous membranes, skin turgor, and laboratory test results are reliable indicators of fluid balance.*

Evaluation: Weight is 133 lbs. Urine is clear yellow, with a specific gravity of 1.020; output is approximately 350 cc's in 8 hours. No further episodes of vomiting. Vital signs, CBC, and electrolyte levels are within acceptable parameters. Mucous membranes pink and moist. Skin returns quickly when pinched. *Goal #5 met.*

■■■ TABLE 75-1 *E*LECTROLYTE FUNCTIONS AND IMBALANCES

Electrolyte	Major Functions	Excess	Deficiency
Potassium (K)	Major electrolyte in ICF Controls cellular osmotic pressure Activates enzymes Regulates acid–base balance Maintains nerve and muscle function Influences kidney function Influences sugar uptake	*Hyperkalemia:* Vague muscle weakness (usually the large muscles of the lower extremities) initially, with skeletal muscle weakness possibly progressing to paralysis; paresthesias and dysrhythmias	*Hypokalemia:* Vague fatigue and general malaise initially; muscle weakness, paresthesias, diminished deep tendon reflexes, hypotension, and cardiac dysrhythmias
Sodium (Na)	Major electrolyte in ECF Influences distribution of water Maintains acid–base balance Maintains nerve function	*Hypernatremia:* Thirst, dry mucous membranes, flushed dry skin, and hypotension (if accompanied by FVD); neurologic findings (due to dehydration of the brain cells) such as weakness, lethargy, irritability, twitching, spasticity, seizures, and in extreme cases, coma and death	*Hyponatremia:* Anorexia, nausea, and abdominal muscle cramps; neurologic dysfunction including headache, lethargy, and seizures (due to hyposmolarity and cellular swelling), possibly resulting in coma, respiratory arrest, and death; optic disc possibly swollen (*papilledema*); sternal edema with severe hyponatremia
Calcium (Ca)	Major component of bones and teeth Affects permeability of cell membranes Plays a role in blood coagulation and maintenance of heartbeat Affects nerve function	*Hypercalcemia:* Dysrhythmia, hypertension, muscular weakness, depressed reflexes, and altered states of consciousness progressing to coma	*Hypocalcemia:* Dysrhythmia, hypotension, tetany (muscle spasms), paresthesias, altered mood, and confusion; seizures possibly the primary symptom seen
Magnesium (Mg)	Thought to be needed in activation of enzymes Aids in some neuromuscular functions	*Hypermagnesemia:* Weakness, diminished deep-tendon reflexes, and muscle weakness; hypotension with peripheral vasodilation	*Hypomagnesemia* (symptoms most commonly seen when levels are less than 1 mEq/L; possibly difficult to identify due to hypokalemia and hypocalcemia simultaneously occurring): hyperexcitability with muscle weakness, tremors, and generalized seizures; apathy, confusion, delirium, vertigo, ataxia (defective muscle coordination), and coma; dysrhythmias
Chloride (Cl)	Plays a key role in acid–base balance Helps to maintain water balance	*Hyperchloremia* (usually associated with hypernatremia and metabolic acidosis)	Hypochloremia (usually associated with deficit of sodium and potassium, and metabolic alkalosis)
Phosphorus (P) and phosphate (PO_4)	Component of bone Involved in most metabolic processes	Hyperphosphatemia: few symptoms due to hyperphosphatemia alone; symptoms of hypocalcemia; deposits of calcium phosphate salts around joints and in soft body tissues, causing pain on movement (with long-term hyperphosphatemia)	Hypophosphatemia (common with levels less than 1 mg/dL): Anemia, infections, and bleeding (due to impaired function and survival time of RBCs, WBCs, and platelets); muscle weakness (including the respiratory and cardiac muscles), irritability, and paresthesias progressing to coma; renal symptoms; symptoms related to loss of magnesium and bicarbonate; hypercalciuria (excess Ca^{++} excretion in urine) resulting in osteomalacia (bone softening in adults) and rickets (possible secondary effects)

Hypernatremia, a serum sodium level of 145 mEq/L or greater, is most commonly due to water loss and an excess of sodium. Hypernatremia occurs in endocrine disorders (eg. diabetes insipidus), or in situations involving an increased insensible loss of water (eg, due to hyperventilation or serious burn injuries). Less commonly, it results from sodium gain that cannot be dissolved in body water, such as through excess IV or oral intake.

Hyponatremia, a serum sodium level of less than 135 mEq/L, usually results from excessive water retention. Water retention in excess of salt retention may be caused by an excess production of antidiuretic hormone (ADH), for example due to

SPECIAL CONSIDERATIONS: The Life Span

The Thirst Sensation

Thirst is a major symptom of hypernatremia. However in some individuals, especially the elderly population, the thirst sensation may be diminished or depressed. Individuals with impaired sensations, altered mental status, or communication difficulties may be unable to perceive, communicate, or respond to thirst.

pulmonary disorders such as pneumonia, asthma, oat call carcinoma, or acute respiratory failure; or due to malignancies, such as lymphomas, leukemia, or Hodgkin's disease.

Sodium loss may occur due to diuretic therapy, renal disease, adrenal insufficiency, or loss of gastrointestinal (GI) fluids due to vomiting or GI suction. Sodium deficiencies due to inappropriate intake may be seen with a low-sodium diet, or inappropriate oral or IV fluid (10% dextrose in water [D5W]) intake of water.

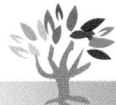

SPECIAL CONSIDERATIONS: The Life Span

Factors Predisposing Older Adults to Fluid and Electrolyte Imbalances

- Older adults have decreased renal and respiratory functioning.
- The thirst mechanisms of older adults are depressed, so encouraging fluids is vital.
- Many medications taken regularly by older adults (eg, blood pressure medications) affect renal and cardiac function and fluid balance.
- Routine procedures, such as administering laxatives before colon x-ray examinations, may induce serious fluid volume deficits in older adults.
- Signs and symptoms of fluid and electrolyte disturbances, such as confusion, may be subtle or atypical.
- Skin turgor is a less valid assessment in older adults because of the decreased elasticity of their skin.
- Older adults may deliberately limit fluid intake to avoid the embarrassment of incontinence. Intervention may be necessary to prevent imbalances.
- Self-medication with enemas, laxatives, or remedies such as baking soda can cause severe electrolyte imbalance.

Potassium

Even though potassium (**K**$^+$) is the major electrolyte in the ICF, the portion of potassium located in the ECF is important for neuromuscular function, especially cardiac function. Excretion of potassium is done primarily by the kidneys (80%). Potas-

sium is also lost through the bowel (15%) and sweat (5%). Potassium cannot be stored; it must be taken in daily. Many different types of drug therapy are associated with potassium imbalances.

Hyperkalemia, a serum potassium level of 5.5 mEq/L or greater, can result from inadequate excretion (eg, renal failure). However, sustained hyperkalemia is not likely for the individual with normal renal function. Shifts of potassium out of body cells that result from *acidosis* (increased hydrogen ion concentration in the blood), tissue damage, or burns, can lead to hyperkalemia. Rapid IV infusion of potassium solutions, excessive intake of salt substitutes, or decreased production of aldosterone are also common causes of hyperkalemia. Because stored blood cells gradually release potassium, transfusion of aged blood can also result in hyperkalemia.

Hypokalemia, a serum potassium level of less than 3.5 mEq/L, can result from decreased potassium intake, possibly associated with starvation and alcoholism. Excessive excretion of potassium can occur in renal disease, vomiting, diarrhea, gastric suctioning, excess sweating, diuretic use, or endocrine disorders. Alkalosis (discussed later in this chapter) can lead to intracellular shifts of potassium, leading to serum potassium deficits. Hypokalemia also contributes to hyperglycemia, due to potassium's effect on both insulin release and organ sensitivity to insulin.

Calcium

Calcium (**Ca**$^{++}$), by exerting a relaxing effect on nerve cells, plays a major role in nerve impulse transmission and muscle contraction. Calcium is also involved in hormone secretion and clotting of blood. Hormonal control of the calcium level is achieved by parathormone (from the parathyroid gland) and calcitonin (from the thyroid gland). Calcitriol, the active form of vitamin D, is a regulator of calcium metabolism.

Hypercalcemia, a total serum calcium level of more than 10.5 mg/dL (5.5 mEq/L), is most commonly due to cancer or primary hyperparathyroidism. However, immobilization, which promotes bone resorption (*decalcification*), other endocrine disorders, medications, and abnormal vitamin D metabolism, could cause hypercalcemia.

Although rare, *hypocalcemia,* a total serum calcium level of less than 9 mg/dL (4.5 mEq/L) or ionized calcium less than 4.6 mg/dL, is most commonly caused by a parathyroid hormone deficit, due to either surgical or primary hypoparathyroidism or abnormal vitamin D metabolism. In many instances, alkalosis causes a decrease in ionized serum calcium. Other conditions—such as hypoalbuminemia, hyperphosphatemia, hypomagnesemia, cancer, acute pancreatitis, malabsorption, chronic alcoholism, and some drugs—cause hypocalcemia.

Magnesium

The balance of magnesium (**Mg**$^{++}$) is dependent upon normal intake, absorption, and renal excretion. Intracellular and extracellular magnesium concentrations are significant for many important cellular processes, including enzyme reactions, neuromuscular transmission, and cardiovascular tone. Mg^{++} is closely related to calcium, phosphorous, and potassium.

Hypermagnesemia, a serum magnesium level of greater than 2.5 mEq/L (3.0 mg/dL), is seen in clients with decreased renal excretion due to diminished renal function. Clients with normal renal function, but who have been aggressively treated with over-the-counter medications (antacids and laxatives) or prescribed doses of magnesium, may develop hypermagnesemia. Calcium gluconate is the specific antidote for magnesium intoxication.

Hypomagnesemia, a total serum magnesium level of less than 1.5 mEq/L or 1.8 mg/dL, is most commonly caused by chronic alcoholism and severe congestive heart failure (CHF) that is being aggressively treated with diuretic therapy. Decreased Mg intake, malabsorption, and GI losses including suctioning, vomiting, diarrhea, and fistulas result in hypomagnesemia. Renal or endocrine diseases, drugs, burns, or shifts of magnesium into cells or bone may also result in hypomagnesemia.

Chloride

Chloride (Cl^-) plays a key role in acid–base balance. An excess is called *hyperchloremia;* a deficit is called *hypochloremia.* Both of these conditions are associated with acid–base imbalance and are discussed later in this chapter.

Phosphorous/Phosphate

Phosphorous (**P**) is a critical component of all tissues. In the human body, phosphorous is often found in the form of phosphate (PO_4^-). More than 70% of P is found in combination with calcium within bones and teeth. To absorb and metabolize phosphorous, vitamin D is needed.

Phosphorous is an important intracellular messenger, and is critical for energy production in the form of adenosine triphosphate (**ATP**). Glycogen needs phosphorus to convert glycogen to glucose. An efficient intestinal tract and normal renal conservation mechanisms are crucial to the normal level of phosphate.

Hyperphosphatemia, an elevation of serum phosphate above 4.5 mg/dL, is commonly caused by decreased renal excretion; redistribution from the ICF to the ECF; or increased intake or intestinal absorption of phosphate. Clients with metabolic acidosis, such as those with renal failure, will often have more ionized calcium present and may exhibit no symptoms of hypocalcemia.

Hypophosphatemia, a serum phosphate of less than 2.5 mg/dL, is unusual but often occurs with respiratory alkalosis (due to prolonged hyperventilation) and extensive burn injury. Decreased oral intake or absorption from the GI tract, a shift of phosphate from ECF to ICF, or a loss of phosphate due to hyperparathyroidism or renal tubule disorder are other causes. Because only 1% of phosphate is in the ECF, decreased serum levels do not necessarily reflect low total-body phosphate.

MAINTENANCE OF ACID–BASE BALANCE

The body must maintain acid–base balance to carry out its functions adequately. The body's cellular activity requires a slightly alkaline medium. ECF is normally maintained at a pH of approximately 7.4, or between 7.35 and 7.45. ICF has a slightly lower pH. Alterations of even a few tenths can be incompatible with cellular activity. An overview of the causes and symptoms of acidosis and alkalosis may be found in Table 75-2. Additional pertinent information is found in Chapter 17.

Acidosis

When the blood is more acidic than normal, a state of **acidosis** exists. A deficit in bicarbonate ions (HCO_3^+) or an excess in hydrogen ions (**H^+**) causes a condition called **metabolic acidosis.** Excess loss of bicarbonate or excessive retention of hydrogen ions due to renal disease is a common cause.

An increase in carbon dioxide in the blood characterizes a condition called **respiratory acidosis.** It may occur in pneu-

■■■ TABLE 75-2 *C*AUSES AND SYMPTOMS OF ACIDOSIS AND ALKALOSIS

Acid–Base Imbalance	Possible Causes	Signs and Symptoms
Metabolic Acidosis	Uncontrolled diabetes mellitus, fasting and starvation (anorexia and bulimia), lactic acidosis, salicylate poisoning (aspirin overdose), alcoholic ketoacidosis, kidney dysfunction and failure, and loss of intestinal secretions (diarrhea, intestinal suctioning, fistulas)	Decreased pH, decreased HCO_3^-, diarrhea, nausea and vomiting, anorexia, weakness, lethargy, malaise, altered mental status, coma, peripheral vasodilation, shock, bradycardia, cardiac dysrhythmias, and warm and flushed skin
Respiratory Acidosis	Respiratory center depression (sedative overdose, head trauma); lung disorders such as pneumonia, emphysema, asthma, pulmonary edema; respiratory distress syndrome; and airway obstruction due to airway or injury to the thorax, extreme obesity, respiratory muscle paralysis, and kyphoscoliosis	Decreased pH, increased PCO_2, hypoventilation, and shallow respirations; headache, weakness, altered mental and behavioral changes (disorientation, confusion, depression, paranoia, hallucinations), tremors, paralysis, stupor, and coma; warm, dry skin; drowsiness; nausea and vomiting; diarrhea; fruity-smelling breath; acidic blood; and acidic urine

▪▪▪ TABLE 75-2 *C*AUSES AND SYMPTOMS OF ACIDOSIS AND ALKALOSIS (CONTINUED)

Acid–Base Imbalance	Possible Causes	Signs and Symptoms
Metabolic Alkalosis	Excess ingestion or administration of sodium bicarbonate, TPN solutions containing acetate, parenteral solutions containing lactate, or blood transfusions containing citrate; GI loss of hydrogen ions via vomiting, gastric suction, bulimia, diuretic therapy, and loss of chloride and body fluids	Increased pH, increased HCO_3^-, confusion, hyperactive reflexes, tetany, convulsions, hypotension, and dysrhythmias
Respiratory Alkalosis	Hysteria, hyperventilation, high fever, salicylate (aspirin) poisoning, elevated blood ammonia levels, encephalitis, and mechanical ventilation	Increased pH, decreased PCO_2, accompanied by deep respirations with rapid breathing; irritability, panic, lightheadedness, dizziness, parasthesia, positive Chvostek's and Trousseau's signs, seizures; nausea, vomiting, and diarrhea; muscle twitching, tetany, and tremors; alkaline urine; and ECG changes

monia, emphysema, and asthma, and after administration of large doses of certain drugs (barbiturates, narcotic analgesics), all of which cause hypoventilation (Fig. 75-3).

The treatment of choice is correction of the underlying condition. Administer IV infusions as ordered. The clinician may order bicarbonate for severe metabolic acidosis; however, it should not be given for respiratory acidosis. Lactated Ringer's solution may be ordered.

Assess the character of respirations. If the respiratory rate or character changes, the person can be compensating for the condition, or the situation may be worsening. Notify the healthcare provider of respiratory changes. The client may need stimulants or narcotic antagonists to reverse respiratory depression caused by medications. Nursing interventions include elevating the head of the bed and administering ordered oxygen. The client may need a mechanical ventilator for severe respiratory acidosis.

Careful assessment is vital; the acidosis may worsen, or the client may become alkalotic as an overreaction to the treatment. Monitor laboratory values carefully. Assess the person's level of consciousness, because the client can lose consciousness if acidosis worsens. Assess the pH of urine. Acidosis can cause electrolytes to shift, leading to electrolyte imbalances. For example, potassium ions may shift out of the cells in response to metabolic acidosis, resulting in hyperkalemia.

Alkalosis

When the blood is more basic than normal, due to a loss of body acids or excessive retention of alkaline substances, a state called **alkalosis** exists. **Metabolic alkalosis** is caused by an excess of bicarbonate, often due to excess bicarbonate antacid administration, or a loss of acids (such as through vomiting or excessive gastric suctioning).

A condition called **respiratory alkalosis** is a deficit of plasma CO_2 (carbonic acid [$\mathbf{H_2CO_3}$]). This situation is usually caused by hyperventilation. Symptoms are similar to those of metabolic alkalosis. Direct treatment at reducing the cause of the hyperventilation. Interventions may involve the client using a re-breathing mask or breathing into a paper bag so that he or she will re-breathe his or her own CO_2, thus replacing the CO_2 needed by the body.

Alkalosis can result in shifts in electrolytes and subsequent electrolyte imbalances. Potassium ions may shift into cells as hydrogen ions shift out of cells in response to metabolic alkalosis. Calcium ions are deionized in states of alkalosis, result-

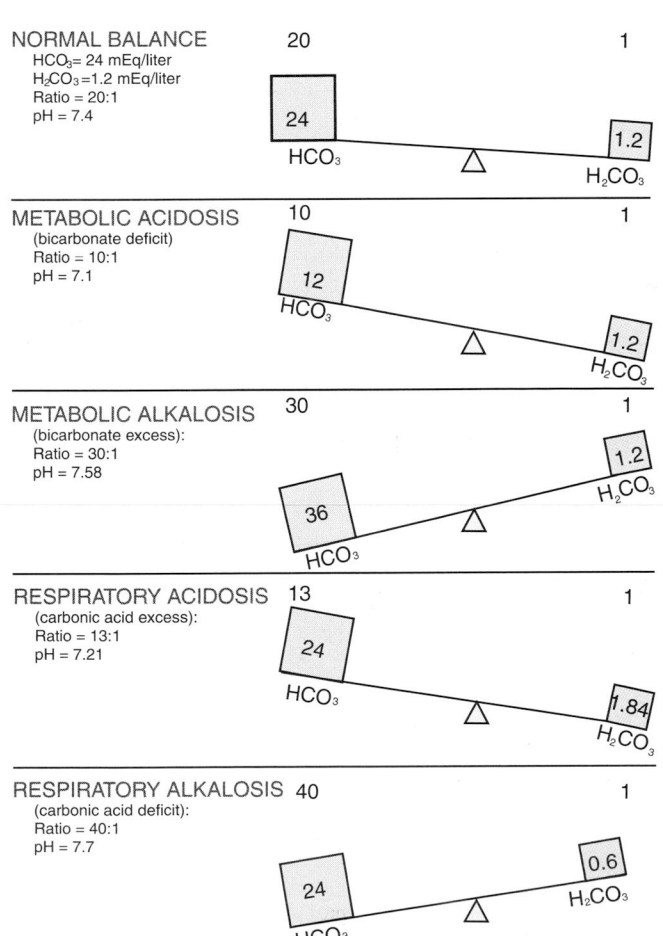

FIGURE 75-3. The pH of fluid is balanced using bicarbonate ion (HCO_3^-), carbonic acid (H_2CO_3), and hydrogen ions (H^+). This figure illustrates pH changes and the balance between HCO_3 and H_2CO_3.

ing in symptoms of hypocalcemia. In cases of respiratory alkalosis, serum phosphate may move into the cells, resulting in hypophosphatemia.

Careful assessment is vital. Monitor laboratory values carefully. Administer IV solutions as ordered to treat any electrolyte imbalances. Treatment of choice for gastrointestinal causes is often sodium chloride or potassium chloride, because these electrolytes are usually lost with hydrochloric acid in vomiting. Make sure the alkalosis does not worsen or result in the opposite imbalance. *Paresthesia* (tingling in the fingers and toes) and muscle twitching are ominous signs of electrolyte loss—particularly the loss of ionized calcium.

➤ STUDENT SYNTHESIS

Key Points

- Fluid and electrolyte disturbances can occur in anyone, but they are commonly seen in ill and hospitalized clients, including those undergoing surgical and diagnostic procedures. The risk of serious disturbances increases in clients who are at the extremes of the age spectrum.
- Measurement of I&O and daily weights is an important component in the assessment of fluid balance.
- Edema is a symptom of many disorders, but most commonly indicates fluid overload. Edematous skin is very friable and prone to breakdown. Good skin care is imperative, as is client positioning.
- Electrolyte imbalances commonly involve either an excess or a deficit of the electrolyte. In certain cases, more than one electrolyte imbalance may be occurring.
- The body's cellular activity requires a slightly alkaline medium. ECF is normally maintained at a pH of approximately 7.4, or between 7.35 and 7.45. ICF has a slightly lower pH. Alterations of even a few tenths can be incompatible with cellular activity.
- Respiratory acidosis, if not corrected, could lead to the need for mechanical ventilation.
- A simple treatment for respiratory alkalosis, usually caused by hyperventilation, is for the client to breathe into a paper bag, thereby retaining needed CO_2 in the body.

Critical Thinking Exercises

1. You have just admitted an older woman from a nursing home. She has poor skin turgor, a dry mouth, and cracked, bleeding lips. She is awake and oriented but refuses oral fluids. What further assessments would you make? What strategies might be effective in restoring her fluid balance?

2. Your client has been diagnosed with respiratory alkalosis due to hyperventilation secondary to head injury. What are the primary symptoms you would monitor for? Which symptoms might be attributed to acid–base imbalance and which might be due to electrolyte imbalance? What might be symptoms of head injury? What major treatments would you expect to administer to this client?

NCLEX-Style Review Questions

1. The client complains of tingling in the fingers and toes. The nurse's best response would be to:
   a. Continue to monitor the client.
   b. Elevate the extremities.
   c. Notify the RN or physician.
   d. Place the extremities in warm water.

2. The laboratory results for a client newly admitted to the hospital reveal a serum sodium level of 140 mEq/L. What action should the nurse take?
   a. Continue to monitor the client.
   b. Notify the RN or physician.
   c. Protect the client from possible seizures.
   d. Start a high-sodium diet.

3. A client is receiving diuretics. Which electrolyte disturbance should the nurse monitor for?
   a. Calcium deficit
   b. Potassium deficit
   c. Potassium excess
   d. Sodium excess

4. Intravenous fluids should be administered at the correct speed and not too fast to prevent:
   a. Acidosis
   b. Alkalosis
   c. Fluid volume deficit
   d. Pulmonary edema

5. A client during active labor is using a fast-panting breathing technique to help her control pain. This client is at risk for developing:
   a. Metabolic acidosis
   b. Metabolic alkalosis
   c. Respiratory acidosis
   d. Respiratory alkalosis

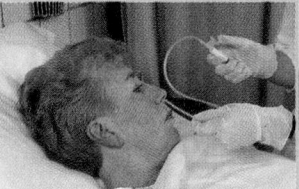

CHAPTER

76

Musculoskeletal Disorders

LEARNING OBJECTIVES

1. In relationship to a client with a musculoskeletal disorder, discuss the diagnostic benefits of the following tests: laboratory tests including ESR, CBC, RF, uric acid, CK, calcium, and phosphorus levels; x-ray; arthrogram; myelogram; CT scan; MRI; bone scan; ultrasound; arthrocentesis; arthroscopy; bone biopsy; and EMG.
2. Describe at least six components of data collection (assessment) for a client with a musculoskeletal disorder.
3. Identify at least four major components of nursing care necessary to protect the client from the hazards of immobilization.
4. Discuss at least six important areas of nursing care for the client who has had an amputation and now has a new limb prosthesis.
5. Explain at least six aspects of nursing care needed for a client who has been surgically treated for IVD or HNP.
6. State at least three nursing considerations for clients with TMJ, muscular dystrophy, and osteoporosis.
7. Differentiate among the following conditions: inflammatory disorders (RA, OA, ankylosing spondylitis, bursitis, and tenosynovitis); repetitive strain injuries (carpal tunnel syndrome and lateral epicondylitis); and systemic disorders with musculoskeletal manifestations (gout, SLE, scleroderma, and rickets or osteomalacia), stating at least four nursing considerations for each disorder.
8. Compare and contrast the following: strain, sprain, and fracture.
9. Identify the four categories and at least five types of common fractures.
10. Describe at least six nursing implications for the care of a client in a cast.
11. Differentiate between skin traction and skeletal traction, including indications and nursing considerations for each type of traction.
12. Discuss at least three nursing measures for care of clients with the following treatments: external fixation, ORIF, and arthroplasty.
13. Identify at least nine complications of fractures or bone surgery.
14. Explain the difference between primary and metastatic bone tumors.

NEW TERMINOLOGY

acrosclerosis	lordosis
amputation	myelogram
ankylosis	orthopedics
arthritis	osteomalacia
arthrocentesis	osteomyelitis
arthrogram	prosthesis
arthroplasty	replantation
arthroscopy	rickets
bursitis	sclerodactyly
cast	scleroderma
dislocation	scoliosis
electromyogram	sequestration
fasciotomy	skeletal traction
fracture	skin traction
gangrene	spinal stenosis
gout	sprain
halo device	strain
kyphosis	synovectomy
laminectomy	tenosynovitis

ACRONYMS

AEA	DJD	ORIF
AKA	ECG	RA
BEA	EEG	RF
BKA	ESR	SLE
CK	HNP	THA
CMS	IVD	TMJ
CPM	OA	TLSO

The specialty of medicine that examines and treats diseases and injuries of the musculoskeletal system is called **orthopedics** (orth/o = straight). Surgeons who specialize in this area of medicine are *orthopedists*. *Orthopedic nursing* involves preventing further complications for clients with musculoskeletal conditions (see Chapter 18 for a review of musculoskeletal anatomy and physiology).

DIAGNOSTIC TESTS

Nursing care for clients with musculoskeletal disorders is likely to involve preparation for physical examinations, radiographic tests, and other diagnostic procedures. Be sure to explain the actual procedures to reduce tension or anxiety that clients may experience. Teach post-procedure activities that ease discomfort and promote wellness. Carry out physical preparation and document all aspects of care.

Laboratory Tests

Several laboratory tests are available to assess the condition of bones and muscles. For example, complete blood cell count (CBC), uric acid levels, and blood levels of calcium and phosphorus help indicate the overall condition of the musculoskeletal system. Erythrocyte sedimentation rate (**ESR**), rheumatoid factor (**RF**), and creatine kinase (**CK**) tests may show inflammation related to an infection or inflammatory condition.

Radiography (X-ray)

Radiography is the most common method of assessing the general state of bones. An x-ray study noninvasively visualizes bones and other internal structures, so that the healthcare provider can diagnose abnormalities and monitor the effectiveness of treatments. Some types of radiographic exams require the use of dye to visualize cavities within bony parts. Before giving a radiopaque dye, assess the client for the presence of any allergies. In addition, before a female client undergoes any x-ray procedure, first determine if she is pregnant. Special precautions must be taken to protect the reproductive organs of all clients from potentially harmful radioactivity.

Arthrogram
An **arthrogram** is an x-ray study of a joint (eg, knee or shoulder). A radiopaque or radiolucent substance is injected, and then a sequence of x-rays films is taken to determine the joint's condition.

Myelogram
The **myelogram** (myel/o = spinal cord; bone marrow) is an x-ray examination of the spinal cord and vertebral canal after injection of a contrast medium or air into the spinal subarachnoid space. This diagnostic procedure is particularly valuable for evaluating spinal cord abnormalities caused by tumors, herniated intervertebral disks, or other lesions.

Computed Tomography
Computed tomography (CT) scanning provides a three-dimensional radiographic view of a body part. CT scanning is painless and can be performed with or without the use of contrast agents. The amount of radiation the client receives is the same as what he or she would receive during a conventional chest x-ray. The scanner takes a series of cross-sectional pictures of the body part in minute slices across the *coronal plane* (vertically, from front to back). A CT scan is useful in diagnosing bone, ligament, and tendon injuries, soft tissue disorders, and tumors.

Other Diagnostic Tests

Magnetic Resonance Imaging
In *magnetic resonance imaging* (MRI), a powerful magnetic field enables a scanning machine to produce detailed images of internal organs without the use of potentially dangerous ionizing radiation or x-rays. The use of a magnetic field and radio frequencies produces measurable signals, which a computer translates into three-dimensional visual images. MRI is safer and less expensive than invasive procedures such as biopsy, surgery, or the use of radioactive isotopes or dyes. For these reasons, many examiners prefer to use MRI whenever possible. MRI units are expensive, however, and not all institutions have MRI capabilities. Portable MRI units are often available for rural facilities.

Nursing Alert
Clients who have metallic implants, such as orthopedic screws, may not be eligible for MRI scanning. Severe damage and death can result if metallic implants are exposed to the intense magnetic fields of a MRI.

Bone Scan
A *bone scan* is used to detect primary bone tumors, metastatic bone disease, osteomyelitis, osteoporosis, inflammation, bone or joint infections, and stress fractures. These conditions are discussed later in this chapter. It requires the intravenous (IV) injection of a radioisotope, such as technetium 99m, which then enhances the visualization of abnormal tissue areas. The client must lie quietly during the entire scan. After the test, instruct the client to drink extra fluids, to increase excretion of the isotope.

Ultrasound
Ultrasound technology—which uses sound waves and their echoes to display images—helps to evaluate soft tissue masses, osteomyelitis, infection, congenital and acquired pediatric disorders, bone mineral density, sports injuries, and fracture healing. This method is noninvasive, inexpensive, readily available, and safe because it does not involve ionizing radiation.

Arthrocentesis
An **arthrocentesis** is aspiration of synovial fluid, blood, or pus from a joint cavity. By examining these fluids, a health-

care provider can diagnose infections, inflammatory conditions, and bleeding. After the test, a compression dressing is applied and the joint is rested for 1 day.

Arthroscopy

Arthroscopy is an invasive procedure using a special endoscope, called an *arthroscope,* which is designed to view joints. The arthroscope has a lens and a light source at its end that transmits a picture to a video monitor in the operating room (OR). Because the flexible scope can bend inside the joint, the surgeon views and operates on the joint's interior, using only a very tiny incision referred to as a "stab wound." The procedure is known as a *closed procedure* because the joint does not need to be laid open.

The procedure is performed in the OR or same-day surgery facility, often under local anesthesia. Surgeons use arthroscopy to diagnose and treat joint disorders. For example, foreign or loose objects (eg, a piece of cartilage, a bone spur) can be removed. A rough and worn joint can be made smoother and more comfortable. Tissue samples can be obtained via biopsy, and a torn meniscus or ligament can be diagnosed and possibly repaired.

Arthroscopic surgery is much safer, more comfortable, and more cost effective than open surgery, and for these reasons it is used whenever possible. Following the procedure, elevate the client's joint and apply ice to control edema and pain. Teach the client how to monitor the site for evidence of infection.

Biopsy

A *biopsy* of bone, tissue, or muscle may be performed using local anesthesia to diagnose tumors, infections, muscle inflammation or atrophy, and various other problems. After the procedure, monitor the biopsy site for bleeding, swelling, infection, or hematoma.

Electromyogram

The **electromyogram** (EMG) is a test of electrical conductivity, similar to the electrocardiogram (**ECG**) or the electroencephalogram (**EEG**). The provider places fine needles into the client's muscles (my/o = muscle), and measures the electrical impulses within the muscles, both at rest and during activity. The provider can then determine whether or not the client's muscles respond appropriately to stimuli.

Nursing Alert
Do not confuse the term *myogram* with the term *myelogram.* The combining form *my/o* refers to muscle, while the combining form *mye/lo* refers to the spinal column.

COMMON MEDICAL TREATMENTS

Joint, bone, and muscle disorders often cause pain and limit movement. Common treatments for these disorders include application of heat or cold through hot baths or soaks, hot or cold compresses or packs, or paraffin baths. Heat causes vasodilation, thereby drawing oxygen, leukocytes, and nutrients to an injured or diseased area to promote healing and prevent infection.

Physical therapy is another common medical treatment for joint, bone, and muscle disorders. The simplest therapies for joints are passive range of motion (PROM) and active range of motion (AROM). *Massage,* if joints are not damaged or inflamed, often helps to soothe aching joints.

Muscle, bone, or joint fractures or diseases accompanied by damage to surrounding soft tissues are treated by external immobilization devices to alleviate pain and discomfort, prevent further injury, and promote healing. External immobilization is achieved through the use of braces, corsets, splints, casts, and traction, which will be discussed later in this chapter.

 **SPECIAL CONSIDERATIONS: THE LIFE SPAN**

Muscles of the Older Adult

With advanced age, a person experiences a decrease in muscle strength. Joints become stiff and slightly more flexed with age.

COMMON SURGICAL TREATMENTS

Common surgical treatments for muscle, bone, and joint disorders are performed to remove or repair damaged or diseased parts. Disorders that may require surgery include fractures, ligament ruptures, arthritic joints, or accidental limb amputation.

Surgery is necessary if a fractured joint or bone cannot heal with external immobilization alone. A bone fracture that results in multiple fragments usually cannot be realigned without surgically opening the body part and reattaching the fragments using surgical hardware such as pins, screws, or plates. *Joint-replacement surgery,* or *arthroplasty,* is a common treatment for the client with either arthritis or severe fractures that may not heal. Various surgical procedures are performed to immobilize or repair the spinal column if trauma or disruption of the spinal space and cord occur. *Amputation* is the surgical choice if a limb is damaged by injury or disease beyond repair. (These procedures are discussed throughout this chapter.)

NURSING PROCESS

Data Collection

Carefully observe and assess the client with a musculoskeletal disorder. Chapter 47 describes physical examination and nursing assessment, which establishes a baseline for future comparison and helps determine the presence of suspected complications. Report any changes from the baseline findings.

Assess for skeletal deformity. Observe posture, coordination, and body build, noting any asymmetry or deformity. Palpate soft tissues, joints, and muscles. Measure muscle mass. Assess skin temperature and document any swelling, crepitation, tenderness, or other abnormality.

Evaluate the client's musculoskeletal function. Assess range of motion (ROM), muscle strength, balance, and gait. A healthcare provider may refer the client to a specialist if limited mobility is suspected. Also evaluate the client's ability to safely use mobility aids, such as a wheelchair, walker, cane, or crutches. Chapter 48 describes the use of these devices in detail.

Observe the client's emotional response to the disorder or disease. Does he or she need assistance to meet daily needs? Does the disorder affect social activities or self-esteem? Is the client anxious or fearful of the outcome?

Assessment With Immobilization Device in Place

Careful assessment of clients who have immobilization devices in place is extremely important to prevent and promptly treat any complications. Areas of concern include pressure, infection (of the wound or bone), and hemorrhage.

A primary concern while observing such clients is to watch for signs of pressure. Undue pressure of any kind can cause serious neurovascular compromise, or damage to nerves and blood vessels. Pressure, and its accompanying lack of blood or nerve supply, can cause tissue *necrosis* (death) and other complications. Other areas of concern include infection (wound or bone) and hemorrhage. In Practice: Nursing Assessment 76-1 provides specific information.

Nursing Alert

Follow Standard Precautions when performing assessments and providing care for clients with compound fractures, wound infections, or the possibility of hemorrhage.

Nursing Diagnosis

Based on data collection, the following nursing diagnoses may be established for clients with musculoskeletal disorders. Some diagnoses may have several causal factors.

- Imbalanced Nutrition: Less Than Body Requirements related to the need for high levels of protein and calcium
- Risk for Infection related to invasive immobilization devices or compound fracture.
- Risk for Trauma related to immobilization device, poor calcification of bones, previous fracture, improper gait, or inability to use crutches, walker, wheelchair properly
- Risk for Ineffective Tissue Perfusion related to compartment syndrome
- Risk for Disuse Syndrome related to immobility, pain
- Impaired Skin Integrity related to fracture, cast
- Self-Care Deficit related to restricted movement, pain, presence of cast
- Ineffective Sexuality Patterns related to immobilization device

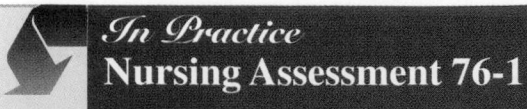
In Practice
Nursing Assessment 76-1

KEY FINDINGS WITH AN IMMOBILIZATION DEVICE IN PLACE

Complications of Pressure
- *Edema:* Swelling under the device, at the edges of the device, or of the entire extremity
- *Skin color:* Blanched, mottled, or cyanotic; inspect the client's fingers and toes frequently and separately for signs of circulatory impairment
- *Numbness, tingling, or the inability to move:* inability to move the fingers or toes and to identify specifically which digit is touched; inability to flex the foot (dorsiflexion and plantar flexion) unless the ankle and foot are in a cast
- *Cool temperature of digits:* Sensation of being colder on affected side if pressure exists
- *Severe pain:* Most likely due to swelling if medication fails to relieve severe pain
- *Lack of distal pulse:* Indicative of inadequate blood flow
- *Slow capillary refill:* Lack of color return in 2 to 4 seconds after nail bed is compressed

Wound Infection
- Elevated temperature, pulse, and respirations; the client may develop hypotension if infection is developing
- Odor of decaying tissue
- Elevated leukocyte count
- Drainage of blood or serous fluid from the fracture area (may be seen at pin insertion sites or in cast window, or may soak through cast)
- Redness and swelling in surrounding tissues
- Pain
- Swelling

Infection of the Bone (Osteomyelitis)
- Fever
- Pain
- Redness and heat
- Elevated leukocyte count
- Nausea, with or without vomiting
- Headache
- Swelling and pressure

Hemorrhage
- Diminished color, motion, and sensitivity of distal limb
- Tachycardia
- Hypotension
- Rapid respirations
- Anxiety, panic, or confusion
- Diaphoresis
- Oliguria (decreased urine output) or anuria (no urine output)

- Impaired Physical Mobility related to pain, immobilization device, inability to use adaptive equipment
- Impaired Home Maintenance Management related to immobility, pain
- Disturbed Body Image related to amputation, or long-term disability resulting from trauma

Planning and Implementation

When planning care, include clients and their families. For clients undergoing surgical procedures (eg, lumbar decompression, joint replacement, insertion of a fixation device or prosthesis), provide preoperative and postoperative care.

Clients with musculoskeletal disorders may also require assistance with mobility, pain control, cast care, nutritional needs, and emotional problems. They need to understand their disorder, prognosis, and treatment. Develop nursing care plans that meet the client's individual needs.

Preventing Disorders of Immobility. Prolonged bed rest is dangerous for clients with musculoskeletal disorders because of the increased risk for complications such as skin breakdown, contractures, constipation, and thromboembolism. Provide teaching to prevent such complications. Work closely with physical therapists to help clients regain mobility.

Providing Comfortable Positioning and Proper Alignment. Some clients must remain in bed. Maintaining proper body alignment is essential. Turn clients frequently to prevent skin breakdown. Pillows, sandbags, splints, and trochanter rolls help prevent footdrop and contractures. PROM and AROM exercises promote and maintain joint mobility and muscle strength. Encourage clients to move independently as much as possible.

Providing Skin Care. Maintain skin integrity and protect against irritation. When bathing clients, minimize the use of soap. Use lotion for cleansing and for soothing dry skin. Reduce friction and shear forces, through proper positioning. Keep sheets smooth and clear of crumbs after meals. If necessary, use special beds, air mattresses, foam pads, and flotation pads to help reduce pressure. However, their use is not a substitute for frequent skin care. Perform a neurovascular assessment and provide skin care during routine repositioning.

If a client has an incision or pins in place, give special care to these skin breaks. Use the protocol prescribed by the healthcare facility. Wear gloves.

Providing Adequate Nutrition. To promote healing, the client with a musculoskeletal disorder should receive a high-protein diet. Increased fiber and fluids help to maintain normal elimination. Record intake and output. Observe for signs of urinary infection or constipation. Give IV fluids as ordered. Many clients receive nutritional supplements, such as Ensure.

Providing Activity and Exercise. Determine how much activity clients are allowed. Both under-exercise and over-exercise can be harmful. Place a trapeze on the bed frame of clients who are confined to bed, so they can help lift their bodies for nursing care. Clients can also use a trapeze for exercise. Encourage clients to exercise unaffected body parts as much as possible.

Remind clients in casts or splints to flex and extend unaffected joints and muscles frequently. Usually, casted extremities are most comfortable when they are elevated. Remind clients to wiggle the fingers or toes of the affected extremities. Instruct clients to do *isometric* (muscle-setting) exercises of immobilized parts as often as possible. A continuous passive motion (**CPM**) machine is sometimes used to exercise extremities. Assist clients to be out of bed as much as possible. Help them use crutches, walkers, or other assistive devices.

Evaluation

Periodically, evaluate outcomes of care with clients, families, and members of the healthcare team. Have short-term goals been met? Are long-term goals still realistic? In planning for further nursing care, such as the need for followup care at home or continued physical therapy, consider prognosis, the presence of any complications, and responses to care.

COMMON MUSCULOSKELETAL DISORDERS

Amputation

Amputation is the absence or removal of all or part of a limb or body organ. An amputation may be congenital or it may result from an injury or surgery. Reasons for surgical amputation include malignancy, trauma, gangrene (which is discussed later in this chapter), infections, and neurovascular compromise related to diabetes mellitus or cardiovascular disease.

A *surgical amputation* is the treatment of choice only when other means cannot control or arrest a disease process. In such cases, amputation is often a lifesaving measure. In malignant disease, surgery may offer improved comfort, increased function, and greater potential longevity. Amputation is not always curative of malignancies.

Level of Amputation

The disease process for which the procedure is necessary determines the level of amputation. Amputation of any extremity is performed at the most distal point possible. When a surgeon is able to preserve joints and maximize limb length, prosthetic fitting is easier and clients retain more functional ability.

Amputations are classified according to the affected limb and the level of the amputation. An amputation of the hand is called a below-the-elbow amputation (**BEA**); an amputation of the forearm and any part of the upper arm is called an above-the-elbow amputation (**AEA**). Amputation of the leg may be below-the-knee amputation (**BKA**) or above-the-knee amputation (**AKA**). Sometimes, only a finger or toe is amputated. An example of this description is "amputation of first finger, right hand, below second knuckle."

Phantom Limb Pain

Phantom limb pain, a frequent aftereffect of amputation, refers to the sensation of pain, pressure, or itching that occurs in the area of the amputation, and the feeling as if the absent body part is still present. If possible, discuss this concept with the client preoperatively, because he or she may be too embarrassed to mention phantom pain when it occurs. Encourage clients who seem to be disturbed and uneasy following amputation to discuss their feelings. If phantom pain or discomfort is causing the distress, explain that the sensation is common and results from damage to the nerves in the stump. Reassure clients that phantom pain will disappear in time. For pain relief, tell clients to move the missing limb. By activating the damaged nerves leading to the amputated limb, clients usually feel great relief. Other interventions include use of analgesics, transcutaneous electrical nerve stimulation (TENS), ultrasound, and visual imaging. Persistent pain can interfere with prosthesis fitting.

Prosthesis

A **prosthesis** is an artificial device that replaces part or all of a missing extremity. Over the years, the design of prostheses has improved, and they have become more lightweight and reliable. The use of computer technology has resulted in better-fitting prosthetic devices that are more functional and natural looking.

Clients are fitted with prostheses as soon as possible after surgery; sometimes surgeons attach temporary prostheses while clients are still anesthetized. Leg prostheses (Fig. 76-1) are most successful. Skirts and trousers can conceal leg prostheses, which can be equipped with shoes that match.

Typically, arm prostheses are more complicated because the hand is an exquisite motor and sensory organ. Functional artificial hands usually do not look real. Above-the-elbow amputees can use either functional or cosmetic prostheses. A practical prosthetic hand is fashioned with a mechanical

hook, consisting of metal prongs placed opposite each other to replace the fingers and thumb. The opposition placement is necessary to allow the amputee to hold articles in a normal manner. Clients can activate their prostheses by body movements or an external electrical power source.

Nursing Considerations

After amputation surgery, a *rigid* or *compression dressing* is applied to the stump to protect the limb, permit healing, control edema, and minimize pain and trauma. Two sets of compression bandages are needed so that bandages can be changed at least twice per day, or more often if a client perspires freely. Teach clients and their family members how to apply bandages. Correct stump wrapping reduces edema and is important to later use of a prosthesis. Wrap the stump so that it forms a cone shape. Obtain instructions for the recommended wrapping of each client's stump.

Preventing Complications. Potential complications following amputation include hemorrhage, infection, failure of the stump incisions to heal, and deformity of proximal structures. Use the following nursing actions to prevent complications:

- Keep a tourniquet within reach at all times to be applied if severe, life-threatening bleeding occurs.
- Observe the dressing for bleeding.
- Change the dressing using aseptic technique.
- If the surgeon has inserted drains, assess drainage for amount, color, consistency, and odor.
- Avoid dislodging drains when turning the client.
- When changing dressings, check the incision closely for signs of healing. Report any signs of dark-red to black tissue, opened areas along the incision line, unusual drainage, or lack of healing. Dark-red or black tissue is a sign of **gangrene,** which is necrosis of tissue due to insufficient or lack of blood supply.
- Encourage the client who has had a leg amputated to lie in a prone position, rather than on the back. To prevent hip contractures, do not place pillows under the stump when the client is on the back. Reduce stump edema by elevating the foot of the bed.
- If ordered, apply skin traction to the stump as soon as the client returns from surgery. A cast of lightweight material is sometimes applied to the stump to maintain its shape.
- If no cast is in place, cleanse, dry, and carefully inspect the stump according to the institution's protocols. Report any redness or irritation because any irritation or skin breakdown will interfere with the use of a prosthesis and may lead to infection.

Client Teaching. Teach and encourage prosthesis self-care as soon as possible. Show clients how to wash, rinse, and dry the stump. Teach clients how to inspect the stump for signs of complications and how to use prostheses. Teach clients who are wearing limb socks to avoid skin problems by keeping the socks free of wrinkles. Instruct clients how to maintain the actual prostheses.

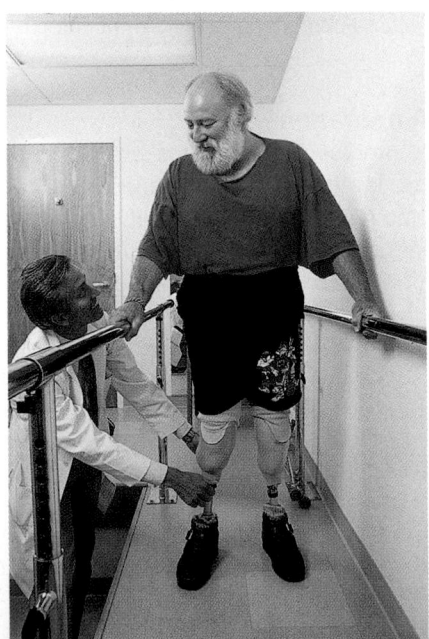

FIGURE 76-1. This double below-knee amputee has received his prostheses, and is learning to walk using parallel bars in physical therapy.

Providing Emotional Support.

Clients who have amputations naturally react with grief because of their limb loss and change in body image. They may exhibit irritability, anger, depression, and other emotions. Allow time for clients to express such feelings. Listen to their concerns and provide support. Refer clients to support or recreation groups. Help family members adjust to the change as well with listening, understanding, and encouragement.

Assisting With Exercise.

When clients undergo foot or leg amputations, they are prepared for walking by increasing strength of upper extremities. Exercises to increase arm strength for crutch walking may start preoperatively. Encourage ROM exercises. Physical therapists may show clients how to maintain muscle tone. Direct your efforts to help clients prevent contractures. Usually, by the first or second postoperative day, most clients can sit up at the edge of the bed and soon progress to a wheelchair. Periodic bed rest is advisable because prolonged sitting may cause contractures and edema. Crutch walking should begin as soon as possible. Amputation changes a person's sense of balance; thus, clients who have experienced amputation require close supervision as they resume movement and ambulation.

Replantation of Severed Limbs

Replantation is the reattachment of a completely severed body part back to the body. With the advent of microvascular surgery, some clients who suffer traumatic amputations may have their limbs successfully replanted. However, this procedure is sometimes impossible. Factors affecting the success of this type of surgery include the availability of a specialist and equipment for the procedure, the client's general condition, and the condition of the severed extremity. Usually, reattachment of lower extremities is less successful than reattachments of upper extremities because of the large and complex sciatic nerve system that innervates the legs.

Postoperative management includes anticoagulation therapy, a caffeine-free diet to prevent vasospasm, wound care, administration of antibiotics, and continuous assessment of the replanted part. Perform a frequent neurovascular assessment of the replanted limb. Monitor for complications such as bleeding, arterial or venous compromise, infection, or decreased ROM.

Chronic Back Pain

Back pain, particularly lower-back pain, is a malady that affects nearly 80% of all individuals. It has many etiologies, but perhaps the most common contributing factor is that the human body stands and walks upright, with most of its weight centering on the lumbar region of the pelvis. The stresses of upright mobility may cause lumbosacral ligament strain and aching muscles. As the body grows older, the combination of prolonged muscular and ligament strain; pressure on the lumbosacral vertebrae; and the aging process itself results in problems such as osteoarthritis, **spinal stenosis** (narrowing of the intervertebral space), and intervertebral disk problems. All of these conditions cause pain due to pressure on the nerves or inflammation of the lower-back muscles.

Back pain may be caused by abnormal or exaggerated curvatures of the vertebral column. **Lordosis** ("swayback") is an abnormal curvature of lumbar vertebra. **Kyphosis** ("humpback" or "hunchback") is an abnormal curvature of the thoracic spine. **Scoliosis** is a lateral (side-to-side) angulation of the spinal column. Abnormal spinal column curvatures may be caused by poor posture, congenital disease, malignancy, compression fractures, osteoarthritis, rheumatoid arthritis, rickets, or aging. Treatment for these conditions will include combinations of therapies, including exercise and electrical muscle stimulation. In more severe cases, braces, casts, or traction may be used. Scoliosis is more common in adolescence and may require insertion of spine-strengthening braces (Milwaukee brace) and support rods (Harrington rod). More information may be found in Chapter 72.

Intervertebral Disk Disease

Intervertebral disk disease (**IVD**) results when a small pad or disk of cartilage (called the *nucleus pulposus*) between two vertebrae presses against the spinal nerves that radiate out from the spinal cord. Generally, disk problems occur in the cervical or lumbar areas. Also known as a herniated nucleus pulposus (**HNP**), the phenomenon is often referred to as a "herniated disk" or "slipped disk." Another term for IVD is *sciatica,* because the sciatic nerve is commonly a site of damage and resulting pain.

Signs and symptoms of IVD include back, shoulder, or neck pain, *paresthesia* (numbness), muscle spasm, depressed deep-tendon reflexes, and neurologic dysfunction. Risk factors include advancing age, smoking, degenerative joint disease, and progressive bone disorders such as osteoporosis. Persons whose occupations require exposure to vibrating equipment; repetitive work movements; or frequent bending, twisting, heavy lifting, pushing, or pulling are at risk for IVD.

Diagnostic Tests.

Diagnosis can be made with a CT scan or MRI, performed in conjunction with the presentation of a positive history and physical examination. The CT scan and MRI can identify spinal stenosis. CT scanning can be combined with myelography using a water-soluble dye to outline nerve root filling. This procedure is particularly useful for clients who have had prior surgery. *Diskography* (x-ray studies) can evaluate the disk's internal structure.

Medical and Surgical Treatment.

Clients are rarely immobilized. Instead, physical therapists recommend a treatment plan that includes regular walking or aquatic exercise. Lumbosacral corsets or braces may be used to improve muscular support of the lower back; however, they do not significantly decrease long-term pain. Additionally, clients wear them only for a short time because prolonged use weakens the supporting abdominal muscles. Antispasmodic and analgesic medications may be helpful. The therapist may also prescribe ultrasound, intermittent traction, or TENS therapies.

If such methods are unsuccessful in relieving symptoms, clients may choose surgery. Spinal disorders caused by pressure on a spinal nerve can often be treated surgically by removing the causes of pressure, if possible.

In an operation called a *lumbar decompression,* the surgeon removes a portion of the vertebra to expose the spinal cord and take out the bone fragment, herniated disk, tumor, or clot pressing on neural elements. A **laminectomy** is a type of lumbar decompression that exposes the spinal canal and allows for relief of compression of the spinal cord and spinal nerve roots. A *diskectomy* removes the herniated disk, which can relieve pressure on the nerves. This procedure can be performed using an endoscope (usually on an outpatient basis), resulting in only a very small incision.

Microdiskectomy may also be used to remove a herniation. The surgeon makes a smaller incision and uses a microscope to help visualize the disk. Because microdiskectomy is quicker and less traumatic, the client experiences a shorter hospital stay and recovers more rapidly.

Sometimes the weakened vertebra can be strengthened by the attachment of a steel rod or by grafting a piece of bone (from the tibia or iliac crest; or donated bone) onto several vertebrae or between a vertebra and the sacrum. This process is called *spinal fusion;* when the graft heals, the spine in that area will be stiff.

Another surgical procedure is the *interbody fusion.* In this procedure, bone grafts or substitutes are placed between the vertebrae, after the disk space is cleaned out. The bone graft is supplemented with a metal fusion cage or other instrument. The surgeon determines the specific type of fusion to be done, after careful testing to determine the cause of spinal instability.

Nursing Considerations.   For the client undergoing surgery, provide routine postoperative care and assist with pain management. Give meticulous wound care to prevent contamination, because infection could lead to meningitis. Watch closely for signs of bleeding and other drainage, leakage of cerebrospinal fluid, or shock caused by trauma. Evaluate the client's neurologic function at frequent intervals. Carefully follow the healthcare provider's orders for the client regarding turning, positioning, and getting out of bed.

When a lumbar decompression has been performed, carefully observe the client's sensation and mobility in the legs. Observe for further complications, such as spinal nerve damage or spinal cord damage that may have occurred during surgery. Immediately report any complaints of tingling, numbness, or difficulty in moving the legs.

Also be alert for the edema that may be an inflammatory response to the trauma of surgery. Edema around the tissues of the surgical site may cause pressure on the spinal cord. Edema may also lead to fluid collection in the legs. In Practice: Nursing Assessment 76-2 provides information on factors to consider following lumbar decompression.

If a cervical laminectomy or decompression was performed, the assessments mentioned above remain important. Additionally, assess the client's upper extremities for evidence of nerve damage or impaired respiratory function.

Although adequate rest is required, encourage clients to move to prevent respiratory complications. Assist the client in participating with the turning procedures prescribed by the healthcare provider. For example, the client can hold the body straight and keep the arms crossed over the chest while being rolled as single entity (*logroll turn*). Use a turning sheet if necessary.

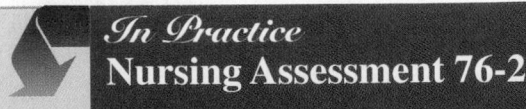

In Practice
Nursing Assessment 76-2

POSTLUMBAR DECOMPRESSION CONCERNS

- *Nerve damage:* Change in sensation or mobility of legs; tingling, numbness of legs, urinary retention
- *Edema:* Collection of fluid in legs; severe pain, which could indicate edema within spinal column
- *Change in level of consciousness:* Possibly indicative of encephalitis or meningitis
- *Muscle spasms:* Leg pain; possibly prevented by exercises
- *Thrombophlebitis:* Leg pain; surgical stockings, exercises, and ambulation can prevent
- *Additional injury:* Prevention by avoiding heavy lifting for a period
- *Infection:* Fever, wound drainage, erythema

Following *cervical* decompression, in addition to the concerns mentioned above (along with other observations appropriate for any postoperative client), also observe for nerve damage suggested by the following:

- Difficulty or change in sensation of arms
- Difficulty in moving arms
- Difficulty in breathing

Manage postoperative pain. Pain medication is often given via a patient-controlled analgesia (PCA) pump or epidural catheter. Offer analgesics before moving, turning, or ambulating the client. Encourage the use of pain medications so that the client is reasonably comfortable at rest and with activity.

The client is usually allowed out of bed on the day of surgery. Assist the client to his or her side, then gradually and smoothly move the legs over the side of the bed as the client pushes up with the arms to a sitting position. Finally, help the client rise to a standing position, while maintaining spinal support and alignment at all times.

Most clients wear a thoracic-lumbar-sacral orthosis (**TLSO**) brace or a corset to support the back and to maintain the effects of surgery. Before applying a brace, put a thin cotton shirt on the client to protect the skin. Be sure to smooth all wrinkles to avoid unnecessary pressure against the skin. Follow the institution's policy and manufacturer's instructions for applying the device. When placing a bedpan, never lift the client, but rather roll the client onto the pan. Always use a fracture bedpan. (Rationale: It is smaller and the client does not arch the back when using it.) Teach the client never to reach or stretch for articles.

During the first few postoperative days, the client may develop muscle spasms, especially in the legs. The physician may order exercises to relieve these spasms. Teach the client isometric exercises for the quadriceps, because he or she can perform these exercises without moving in bed.

Apply antiembolism stockings and pneumatic compression devices. These items help prevent thrombus formation related to immobility.

After lumbar decompression surgery, the client is gradually allowed to do light work but must always avoid heavy lifting. Instruct the client to take caution when lifting anything for at least 1 year after surgery. Also, reinforce proper body mechanics and appropriate lifting techniques. Emphasize that disregarding precautions—even once during convalescence—may result in injury.

If a spinal fusion has been performed, the client may encounter more limitations. He or she usually must wear a brace or corset whenever leaving bed. Occasionally, the physician orders the client to wear the brace at all times. Sometimes, the physician applies a body cast. Tell the client to avoid prolonged sitting because it places extra strain on the back. A client is never moved unless the healthcare provider has ordered it and healthcare personnel have learned how to do it. The client who is paralyzed also needs care appropriate to the degree of paralysis.

After a cervical diskectomy, the client usually wears a cervical collar to limit neck extension, rotation, and flexion. Teach the client to keep his or her neck in a neutral and aligned position. Instruct the client to wear the collar as directed by the physician. Show the client how to open the cervical collar and wash and dry the neck. Assist the client with sitting, by supporting the client's neck and shoulders.

Temporomandibular Joint Disorders

Temporomandibular joint (**TMJ**) disorders are painful, aching disorders involving the facial bones and muscles around the joint between the mandible and the temporal bones. TMJ may affect one side or both sides of the face. Chewing may make the condition worse. The joints may have limited movement and the client may note clicking sounds during chewing. In more severe cases, tinnitus and deafness may be present. Stress, *malocclusion* (malpositioning) of the upper and lower jaw, poorly fitting dentures, rheumatoid arthritis, and neoplasms are the most common causes of TMJ. Successful treatment involves identifying the causative etiology; physical therapy; antiinflammatory agents; and braces or surgery if indicated.

Degenerative Disorders

Muscular Dystrophies

Muscular dystrophies are chronic, degenerative diseases of skeletal muscles that are often inherited. These disorders are characterized by various degrees of progressive weakening and wasting of the muscles.

Although causes of muscular dystrophies are unknown, some researchers believe that they are related to a disruption in enzyme production. Treatment focuses on support. Encourage clients to continue all activities as normally as possible. Exercise programs and splints may help prevent deformities. Often, clients can use special braces to permit ambulation. Inform clients of the need to prevent upper respiratory infec-

tions, to maintain ideal weight, and to strive for general good health. Chapter 73 covers muscular dystrophies in more detail because they usually affect children.

Osteoporosis

Osteoporosis, a condition in which bone mass decreases, is most common in postmenopausal women. Risk factors include advanced age, family history, early menopause, low intake of dietary calcium, excessive alcohol or caffeine intake, sedentary lifestyle, and smoking. Osteoporosis can cause pathologic bone fractures, difficulty in weight bearing, loss of height, and the spinal curvature *kyphosis* (discussed earlier).

Many women take oral calcium in an effort to prevent osteoporosis. Some physicians advise women to take the hormones estrogen and progesterone. A bisphosphonate, alendronate (Fosamax), increases bone density and reduces the risk of fractures and deformities. Osteoporosis is discussed in detail in Chapter 91, which focuses on the care of older adults.

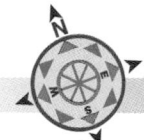

SPECIAL CONSIDERATIONS: CULTURE

Osteoporosis

Women of fair, freckled complexions with blonde or reddish hair, and women from northwest European backgrounds, have a higher incidence of osteoporosis than the general population. Because African Americans have greater bone mass than whites, osteoporosis is rare in African American women.

Repetitive Strain Injuries

Repetitive strain injuries commonly occur in the workplace because of the necessity of performing certain motions (such as keyboarding) repeatedly in some occupations. These injuries may also be identified as *overuse disorders*.

Carpal Tunnel Syndrome

Carpal tunnel syndrome is a compression neuropathy of the median nerve in the wrist. Often, its cause is repetitive movements, such as knitting or keyboarding. Other causes include arthritis, trauma, myxedema, gout, or tumors.

Signs and symptoms include forearm and wrist pain, numbness, and tingling. Symptoms often increase at night. The client's grip is weak. When the provider taps the median nerve, the client experiences paresthesia and pain of the thumb and first three fingers (Tinel's sign).

Treatment includes wrist splinting, rest, NSAIDs, and corticosteroid injections. If these therapies are unsuccessful, surgery may be done to decompress the carpal tunnel.

Lateral Epicondylitis

Repeated forceful wrist and finger movements that stress the origins of muscles cause *lateral epicondylitis*. Lateral epi-

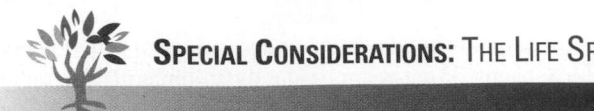

Pregnancy

Pregnant women may experience carpal tunnel syndrome related to fluid retention in that area.

condylitis is often related to activities such as tennis, bowling, pitching, and golf, and thus may be called "tennis elbow."

Clients with lateral epicondylitis often complain of pain along the outer aspect of the elbow, radiating to the forearm. Pain increases on stretching and on resisted wrist and hand flexion.

Common treatments include splinting, analgesics, rest, and corticosteroid injections. Surgery is generally not needed, but is usually successful if performed.

Rotator Cuff Injury

Injury to the rotator muscles in the shoulders may be due to repetitive injury or sudden trauma. The injury can vary in severity. Pain, weakness, and loss of shoulder movement generally result. Less-severe injuries may be treated with extended physical therapy to increase ROM and muscle strength. Often with more severe injuries, surgical intervention is necessary because these injuries tend not to heal by medical intervention alone.

Inflammatory Disorders

Bursitis

The *bursa* is a sac filled with synovial fluid that pads bony prominences in the joints. **Bursitis** is inflammation of a bursa related to mechanical irritation, bacterial infection, trauma, or gout. In response to inflammation, fluid increases, causing distention. With chronic inflammation, calcification may result; pain and tenderness in the joint limit movement.

Usual treatment includes heating and resting the affected part. Anti-inflammatory medications may be indicated. The healthcare provider may inject the bursal sac with corticosteroids or aspirate fluid from it to provide relief. A surgical drainage is performed for infectious bursitis. If these treatments are ineffective, the bursa is excised surgically.

Tenosynovitis

Tenosynovitis, inflammation of the tendon sheath that may result from irritation or an infection, typically affects the wrist or ankle. The infected tendon swells and is painful and disabling. Noninfectious tenosynovitis is caused by strains, blows, or prolonged use of a particular set of tendons (such as in playing the piano over a long period). Symptoms include pain and tenderness, especially on movement. Treatment involves:

- Resting the affected body part; application of a splint
- Application of ice for 1 to 2 days to decrease swelling
- Physical therapy

- Use of nonsteroidal anti-inflammatory drugs (NSAIDs), when indicated
- Surgery (may be needed)
- Antibiotics (may be helpful)
- Elimination of activities that exacerbate symptoms during the inflammatory phase

Arthritis

Arthritis means joint inflammation. More than 100 arthritic disorders are known. The most common types include:

- Rheumatoid arthritis (**RA**)
- Osteoarthritis (**OA**), degenerative joint disease (**DJD**), hypertrophic arthritis
- Ankylosing spondylitis, rheumatoid spondylitis, RA of the spine
- Gouty arthritis
- Systemic lupus erythematosus (**SLE**), lupus
- Scleroderma, progressive systemic sclerosis

Arthritis affects more than 40 million people in the United States. *Monoarticular arthritis* affects one joint; *polyarticular arthritis* affects many joints. Most types of arthritis (except ankylosing spondylitis and gouty arthritis) are more common in women than in men. Table 76-1 compares rheumatoid arthritis with osteoarthritis. Several factors may be associated with causing arthritis:

- Infection of a joint by a virus or microorganism (*infectious arthritis*)
- Direct injury to a joint (*traumatic arthritis*)
- Degeneration or deterioration of a joint (*degenerative arthritis*)
- Metabolic disorder such as gout (*metabolic arthritis*)

Many researchers believe that arthritis has an autoimmune component. In the majority of cases, the cause of the arthritis and its cure are unknown. However, control of the disorder and prevention (or correction) of its crippling effects are possible. Both *acute* and *chronic* forms of arthritis occur. Acute exacerbations may also occur with chronic forms of the disease.

Monocyclic arthritis, accounting for approximately 35% of cases, has a sudden onset, usually responds well to medications, and may never return. *Polycyclic arthritis,* accounting for approximately 50% of cases, is marked by exacerbations and remissions. *Progressive arthritis,* accounting for approximately 15% of cases, continues to worsen, not stopping without treatment.

The clinical features of arthritis include the following:

- Persistent pain and stiffness on arising for 6 weeks or more; stiffness aggravated by damp weather or strenuous activity
- Pain or tenderness in the joints, often symmetrical
- Swelling in the joints
- Recurrence of symptoms, particularly when more than one joint is involved
- Obvious redness and warmth in a joint
- Unexplained weight loss, fever, or weakness combined with joint pain

TABLE 76-1 *Rheumatoid Arthritis Versus Osteoarthritis*

Rheumatoid Arthritis	Osteoarthritis (Degenerative Joint Disease)
Systemic (fatigue, weight loss, anemia)	Not systemic (results from wear and tear)
Fever	No fever
Systemic inflammation	Local inflammation (joint only)
Probably autoimmune origin	Most common type of arthritis
3:1 in women	2:1 in women
Affects young adults (ages 20–30)	Affects middle and older adults (over age 45) Common in women after menopause More common in obese people
Affects small and large joints (symmetrical); most common in fingers, knees, elbows, ankles	Affects primarily large weight-bearing joints and knuckles (knees, hips, knuckles, spine)
May remain the same for life	May progress
Causes inflammatory process in other body parts (lungs, kidneys, eyes)	Sets up local inflammation Can be hereditary
Surgery does not help (condition returns)	May surgically replace or fuse joints (last choice for treatment)
May have lumps (nodules) on joints, which are painful	Often have lumps, but they do not restrict activity and are not painful
Fingers may swell; joints feel cold and moist; bluish color to skin; muscles may become weakened	Joints usually don't swell; muscles remain firm
Joints are distorted and dislocated	Not as likely to be disabling; may remain localized in body
Joints may ankylose (fuse) Abnormal laboratory values (rheumatoid factor, sedimentation rate high; hemoglobin low)	Joints usually do not ankylose

Source: Arthritis Foundation.

- *Bouchard's nodes* (enlargement of proximal interphalangeal joints) or *Heberden's nodes* (growths on the terminal phalangeal joints) with DJD

Box 76-1 describes goals and pain management in the treatment of arthritis.

Rheumatoid Arthritis   *Rheumatoid arthritis* is probably the most painful and crippling form of arthritis. It occurs worldwide and is three times more common in women than in men, until age 65. Theories suggest that a triggering mechanism (possibly a virus) causes the immune system to become overactive. A genetic predisposition to the disorder seems to exist; several members of one family may be affected (see Table 76-1).

Signs and Symptoms.   Chronic inflammatory changes thicken the synovial membrane. The joint capsule swells, the synovial membrane becomes inflamed, and the cartilage is eaten away. An overgrowth of synovial lining occurs. When the cartilage and bone erode, the joint becomes painful because bone rubs against bone.

If the *joint* becomes calcified, movement is impossible. The condition of an immovable joint is called **ankylosis;** however, it does not occur in all persons with RA.

If the opening in the *spinal column* becomes calcified, its diameter becomes smaller, a condition called *spinal stenosis* (discussed earlier). Spinal stenosis can place pressure on the spinal cord.

Rheumatoid arthritis often begins with systemic symptoms such as fatigue, weakness, weight loss, and general body aches. Joints become painful, tender, stiff, swollen, and warm. As tendons and ligaments become shortened and less flexible, joint deformities such as *hyperextension, contractures,* and *subluxation* (**dislocation**) can occur. Figure 76-2 shows subluxation related to RA. These deformities often interfere with the person's ability to perform activities of daily living (ADL).

Medical Treatment.   The goal of treatment is to help the client maintain function and reduce inflammation before joints are permanently damaged. Treatment is multidisciplinary and includes drug therapy (In Practice: Important Med-

› › BOX 76-1

MANAGEMENT OF ARTHRITIS

Goals
- Relieve inflammation (medication)
- Relieve pain (medications, local treatments)
- Maintain optimal functioning (exercise, adaptive devices)
- Educate the client (prevention, treatment)

Pain Management
- Splinting/casting/night splinting/traction
- Positioning
- Heat (paraffin baths, diathermy) and cold (ice packs)
- Physical therapy
- Massage (if joint is not acutely inflamed)
- Medications (most commonly salicylates and NSAIDs)
- Low-impact exercise; isometric exercises (improves muscle strength without overexerting joints)
- Rest (physical and emotional); avoidance of fatigue and overexertion (10 or more hours of rest daily)
- Sleeping on a firm bed
- Placement of bed and chair at same level, to facilitate transfer; chair that helps client to stand is possibly necessary
- Chair 3 to 4 inches higher than regular chair to avoid bending too much at hips (Do not use pillow in chair; promotes slouching, which is tiring.)
- Emotional support
- Adaptive devices to make activities of daily living easier to perform

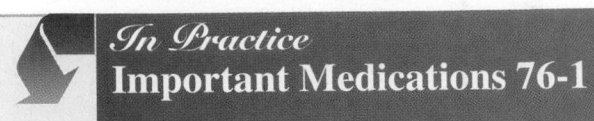

In Practice
Important Medications 76-1

FOR ARTHRITIS

Nonsteroidal Anti-inflammatory Drugs (NSAIDs)
Ibuprofen (Motrin, Advil, Nuprin)
Indomethacin (Indocin)
Piroxicam (Feldene)
Sulindac (Clinoril)
Naproxen (Naprosyn, Aleve)
Ketorolac tromethanine (Toradol)
Fenoprofen (Nalfron)
Diclofenic (Voltaren)
Diflunisal (Dolobid)
Ketoprofen (Orudis)
Nabumetone (Relafen)
Tolmetin (Tolectin)
Rofecoxib (Vioxx)
Celecoxib (Celebrex)

Gold Salts
Auranofin (Ridaura)
Aurothioglucose (Solganal)
Gold sodium thiomalate (Myochrysine)

Antimalarials
Hydroxychloroquine sulfate (Plaquenil sulfate)
Chloroquine (Aralen)

Penicillamine
Penicillamine (Cuprimine, Depen Titratabs)

Corticosteroids
Cortisone (Cortone)
Hydrocortisone
Prednisone

Immunosuppressives
Methotrexate (Amethopterin)
Asathioprine (Imuran)
Cyclophosphamide (Cytoxan)

ications 76-1), client education (In Practice: Educating the Client 76-1), physical therapy, occupational therapy, and psychosocial therapy. Physical therapists design exercise programs that help clients prevent contractures, strengthen muscles, and improve function. Occupational therapists teach clients how to protect their joints and how to use adaptive devices. Measures to increase body resistance to disease, such as rest and a well-balanced diet, are also helpful.

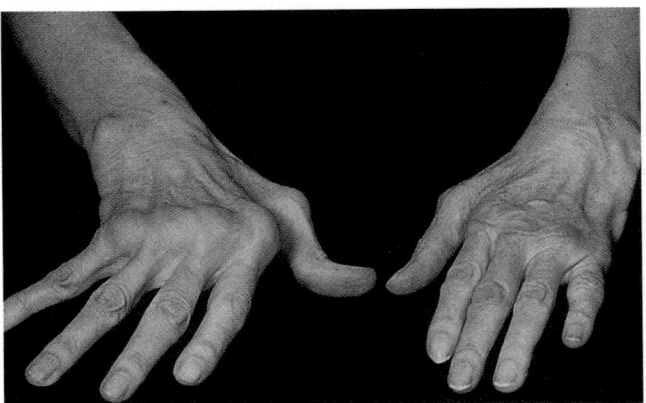

FIGURE 76-2. A severe dislocation called *subluxation of the fingers* in rheumatoid arthritis.

Nursing Alert

Many drugs used to treat arthritis have serious side effects. Be sure to check drug reference sources before administering any drugs. Be alert to possible side effects and report any difficulties immediately.

Osteoarthritis or Degenerative Joint Disease
Osteoarthritis, believed to have a genetic cause or predisposition, is caused by wear and tear on a joint. As illustrated in Figure 76-3, the cartilage wears away and exposes the bone. Next, bony *hypertrophy* (overgrowth) occurs, with the creation of bone spurs. Particles of cartilage break off and float in the joint, making movement painful. **Synovectomy,**

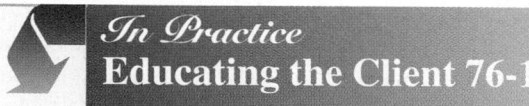

In Practice
Educating the Client 76-1

EXERCISING WITH ARTHRITIS

- Keep your body in the best possible physical condition. Control weight, rest, and exercise.
- Exercise daily even if you have pain. Do specific exercises and not just daily work.
- Apply heat before exercise to lessen pain. Do not overdo exercise because of lessened pain.
- Prepare for exercise with gentle stretching.
- When possible, do active exercise. If not possible, do isometrics or have someone perform passive exercise. You may use a continuous passive motion machine. Stretching and exercise are better when they are done actively (self-movement) rather than passively (by a nurse or therapist).
- Engage in low-impact exercises such as swimming, slow walking, or bicycling.
- Stop exercising if pain becomes too severe.
- Use an adaptive brace or corrective corset or brace as needed.
- Prevent contractures: turn doorknobs to radial (thumb) side when possible. Flatten hand as much as possible.

excision of the synovial membrane, helps to prevent further inflammation in some cases. Arthroscopic surgery may be done to remove loose bodies and bone spurs. Total arthroplasty (joint replacement) is the last resort, and in many cases is effective. In other cases, the joint must be fused to prevent pain. Refer to Table 76-1 for a comparison of OA and RA.

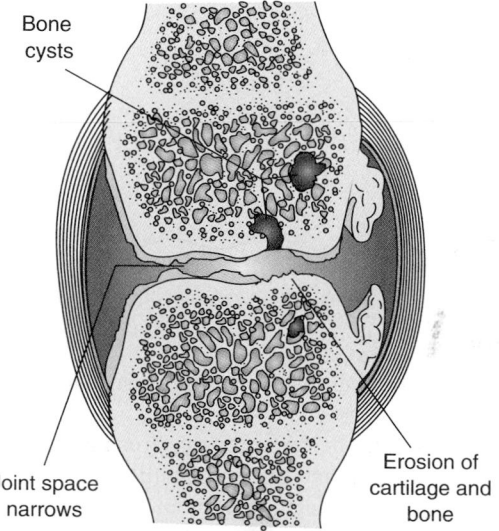

FIGURE 76-3. Joint changes in osteoarthritis. Notice that the *left side* shows early changes, with joint space narrowing and cartilage breakdown. The *right side* shows severe progression, with lost cartilage.

Labels in figure: Bone cysts; Joint space narrows; Erosion of cartilage and bone

Ankylosing Spondylitis   *Ankylosing spondylitis,* also called *rheumatoid arthritis of the spine,* primarily affects the facet joints and the stabilizing ligaments of the spinal column. It mainly affects men and often begins in adolescence or young adulthood. The most common early symptoms are hip and lower-back pain and stiffness. Other symptoms include weight loss, fatigue, fever, and conjunctivitis. Hip contractures and flexion of the neck and back may occur. Breathing may be impaired because chest expansion is impeded. The osteoporotic spine increases the risk of spinal fractures. In severe cases, spinal stiffening also occurs, with resultant humpback and chest curvature. Neck stiffness may make turning the head impossible.

Treatment is similar to that for other types of arthritis. Phenylbutazone (Butazolidin) is sometimes given. Teach the client to refrain from lying on the side, to prevent excess sideways spinal curvature. Light exercise may be more comfortable than prolonged bed rest. The client may wear a back brace.

SYSTEMIC DISORDERS WITH MUSCULOSKELETAL MANIFESTATIONS

Gout

The body produces substances called *purines* during metabolism. If the body is unable to metabolize these substances, uric acid accumulates in the bloodstream and forms crystal deposits in the joints. This arthritic condition, called **gout** or hyperuricemia, usually affects the big toe, instep, ankle, or knee, but it may appear in any joint. Gouty arthritis is more common in men. Alcohol, allergies, surgery, injury, infection, nitrogenous or fatty foods, a fasting diet, emotional stress, or a change in the person's environment can trigger a gout attack.

Signs and Symptoms
Periodic gout attacks are characterized by joint swelling, redness, and severe pain. The slightest touch or weight on the affected area is unbearable during an attack. The person may have fever, *tachycardia* (rapid heartbeat), and anorexia. An attack lasts from 3 to 14 days, after which it disappears suddenly. It may return at any time. However, at other times, the joint is normal. Eventually, repeated attacks permanently damage the joint and limit its ROM. Renal damage and vascular damage (especially atherosclerosis) can follow.

Medical Treatment
Gout cannot be cured, but attacks can be prevented and controlled by adhering to prescribed routines and making regular visits to healthcare providers. Some physicians instruct clients to avoid high-purine foods (such as liver); other physicians prescribe no dietary changes. Gradual weight loss and avoidance of excessive alcohol intake are encouraged.

Colchicine (Colsalide) is usually effective in relieving gout symptoms. If this medication is given early enough, it works within 12 to 24 hours. Side effects include gastrointestinal disturbances (nausea, vomiting, abdominal pain, and diarrhea). The healthcare provider also may order corticosteroids or NSAIDs. Probenecid (Benemid) is used in long-term management because it prevents the kidney's reabsorption of uric acid. Allopurinol (Zyloprim) inhibits uric acid formation. Instruct clients taking any of these medications to drink at least 3 liters of a variety of fluids each day, to promote excretion of a large urine volume. When taking these medications, clients should not take aspirin or any other salicylate because they counteract the effects of gout-relieving drugs.

Nursing Considerations

The affected joint needs protection. If the client is in bed, use a bed cradle to protect it. If necessary, hang a warning sign in a prominent place to prevent jarring or bumping of the bed. Gentle application of warm or cold compresses is sometimes ordered. Elevate the affected joint for comfort. To prevent the joint from stiffening, start ROM exercises as soon as the pain and the redness clear.

Lupus Erythematosus

The two types of *lupus erythematosus* are discoid and systemic. *Discoid lupus erythematosus* is a chronic disease with skin manifestations of disklike patches with raised, reddish edges and depressed centers. *Systemic lupus erythematosus* ("lupus") is an autoimmune systemic disorder that affects many body systems.

Systemic Lupus Erythematosus

People with SLE produce autoantibodies that ultimately contribute to immune-complex formation and tissue damage. SLE primarily affects women. It can be acute or chronic, marked by remissions and exacerbations. It causes widespread damage to the collagen system, affecting any organ system, including the kidneys, heart, and lungs. The characteristic sign of SLE is a butterfly rash on the face. However, a rash may appear over other body parts as well.

Arthritic symptoms include joint pain and muscle aches. Other symptoms include anorexia, nausea, vomiting, swollen glands, and general malaise. In severe cases, the inflammatory process may involve the lining of the lungs and heart with damage to the kidneys, central nervous system, or brain.

Medical Treatment.   Although SLE has no known cure, early intervention can often prevent serious joint damage. Treatment focuses on preventing complications, minimizing disability, and preventing organ dysfunction, and is based on manifestations of symptoms. Commonly used medications include NSAIDs, corticosteroids, and immunosuppressive drugs. Teach clients to avoid sunlight because it can intensify skin manifestations. If clients cannot avoid the sun, instruct them to apply sunscreen lotion with an SPF of at least 22. Adequate rest and prevention of exhaustion are essential. Treatment of the musculoskeletal symptoms of SLE is similar to the treatment of other types of arthritis: medication, exercise, and physical therapy.

Scleroderma

The term **scleroderma** means "hard skin." Scleroderma is considered a collagen disorder that involves chronic hardening and shrinking of connective tissues. Most often, this con-

dition affects women, usually beginning in middle age. Its most severe forms commonly affect men, African Americans, and older people. Scleroderma may have an autoimmune component. The disorder may be localized or generalized.

Localized scleroderma primarily involves the skin, muscles, and bones and is a less-severe form. *Generalized scleroderma* involves the skin, muscles, joints, and internal organs such as the heart, digestive tract, lungs, and kidneys. **Sclerodactyly** is scleroderma of the fingers and toes; **acrosclerosis** is scleroderma of the distal extremities and face.

The disorder begins on the face and hands, where the skin becomes hard and unwrinkled and cannot be raised from the underlying structures. The condition slowly spreads. The person often has joint pain and difficulty moving. *Raynaud's phenomenon,* evidenced by hands or fingers that are cold, numb, tingling, or blanched, is usually an early symptom. Over time, the face appears tight, shiny, and rigid. The fingers may become flexed and atrophied. Death may result from respiratory or renal failure or cardiac dysrhythmias.

Treatment is symptomatic. Joint manifestations are treated in the same manner as in other arthritic conditions. Drug therapy has been ineffective in treating scleroderma.

Nursing Considerations

Because of the client's hardened skin, take measures to prevent skin breakdown. Also consider the condition of the client's hardened skin when giving injections. Teach clients to avoid smoking and exposure to cold. Emotional support is vital.

Rickets and Osteomalacia

Rickets is a disease that results from a deficiency of vitamin D during childhood. The adult form of vitamin D deficiency, which results in softening of the bones, is called **osteomalacia.** The deficiency causes faulty absorption of calcium and phosphorus, both of which the body needs for normal bone hardening.

In rickets, bones remain soft and become distorted as the child grows. When the bones finally do harden, they remain in this deformed state. Severely bowed legs is an example of an effect of rickets. Children with rickets are slow to walk and cut teeth; they are pale, irritable, and inactive. Exposure to sunshine and vitamin D from an early age prevents rickets, making it rare in developed countries. Milk with vitamin D and exposure to sunshine are preventive measures.

TRAUMATIC INJURIES

Sprains

A **sprain** is a traumatic injury to the tissues around a joint. The tissues, such as tendons, muscles, and ligaments, can stretch and tear. Bone fractures may result, as the tearing forces of the tendons and ligaments pull against the bone.

Sprains cause swelling, pain, and interference with movement. At first, a sprain may seem mild with minimal swelling. Rupture of the nearby blood vessels often leaves bruises (*ecchymosis*). If left untreated and the client continues to use the extremity, the tissue damage can become worse. Tissue damage can be mild or quite severe. X-rays examinations may be indicated to rule out fractures.

Treat a sprain by elevating the injured part and using an elastic bandage or splint to immobilize and support the affected area. Relieve pain and swelling by applying ice for 24 to 48 hours. After the first 24 to 48 hours, use warm, moist packs to provide pain relief and prevent muscle spasms. Occasionally, the healthcare provider will apply a cast to keep the area immobile and to facilitate healing. Ligament rupture may require surgical repair.

Strains

A **strain** generally involves damage to the muscle and sometimes to the attached tendon. A strain is a less severe injury than a sprain. Signs and symptoms include pain, swelling, ecchymosis, loss of function, and muscle spasm. Treatment includes application of ice packs for 24 to 48 hours, elevation of the affected part, and rest. Surgical repair may be needed.

Dislocations

When a ligament gives way so completely that a bone displaces from its socket, the resulting injury is called a **dislocation**. Dislocations cause severe pain, abnormal bone position, and inability to manipulate the joint. Following an x-ray examination, the healthcare provider is usually able to put the bone back into position by stretching the ligaments and manipulating the joint. The client may receive sedation or anesthesia for this procedure. Occasionally, the dislocation cannot be reduced. In this case, the area must be surgically opened and realigned. A splint, a brace, or an elastic bandage is applied to immobilize the parts until they heal.

Apply ice to reduce swelling. Assess the affected area's neurovascular status. The joint capsule and surrounding ligaments may take several weeks to return to their normal position.

Fractures

Any break or crack in a bone is called a **fracture** (Fx). Fractures occur when stress placed on a bone is greater than the bone can withstand. *Pathological fractures* are bones that break spontaneously or with nominal trauma, in diseases such as osteomalacia, osteoporosis, bone cancer, and osteomyelitis. An older adult client may experience a pathological fracture to an ankle, hip, or wrist by the ordinary act of getting up out of a chair.

☞ Key Concept

Fractures involving any part of the vertebral column are very serious. Cervical fractures, especially C-1 to C-4, can be immediately life-threatening. Cervical fractures can result in long-term respiratory dependency. All vertebral fractures can result in various levels of paralysis, with motor and nerve impairment. If you suspect any vertebral injury, immobilize the client and call for help immediately.

Most fractures, however, result from significant trauma. Usually surrounding structures such as muscles, blood vessels, ligaments, and tendons are injured as well. Traumatic events that cause fractures include striking a hard surface; a hard fall; or being subject to an indirect force that exerts a strong pulling force on the bone, such as getting a foot caught between rocks and the body falling away from the rocks.

Until age 45, more men than women have fractures; however, after this time, more women are affected because menopausal changes may cause decalcification of bones (osteoporosis). Slippery floors and bathtubs, loose rugs, and dark stairways or corners are hazardous, especially for older adults.

Special Considerations: The Life Span

Child Abuse

Child abuse is a common cause of fractures in children. Suspect abuse in a child who presents with fractures if the child's medical history is inconsistent, the child is less than 1 year old, the fracture is inappropriate for the child's developmental level, fractures have occurred at different times, a sibling is blamed for the injury, other evidence of abuse exists, or family caregivers delay seeking treatment.

Types and Patterns

The following are basic categories of fractures:

- *Complete:* An entire cross-section of the bone is involved; the bone is usually displaced, which means that the bone fragments are out of alignment.
- *Incomplete:* A portion of the cross-section of the bone is involved.
- *Closed:* The overlying skin is intact (this is sometimes called *simple fracture*).
- *Open:* The overlying skin is broken (this is sometimes called *compound fracture*), with various grades of tissue involvement.

The pattern of the break defines some fractures. For instance, there are *transverse, oblique,* and *spiral fractures,* which are defined according to the direction of the fracture in the bone. A fracture may be *depressed,* in which bone splinters are driven into underlying tissue. In a *compression fracture,* the bone collapses in on itself. In a *greenstick fracture,* one side of the bone breaks, while the other side bends. Figure 76-4 illustrates the types and patterns of bone fractures.

Signs and Symptoms

The most pronounced symptom of a fracture is pain that becomes more severe upon movement of the part or when pressure is placed over the affected area. Loss of function and *deformity* (an unnatural position of the part) may accompany

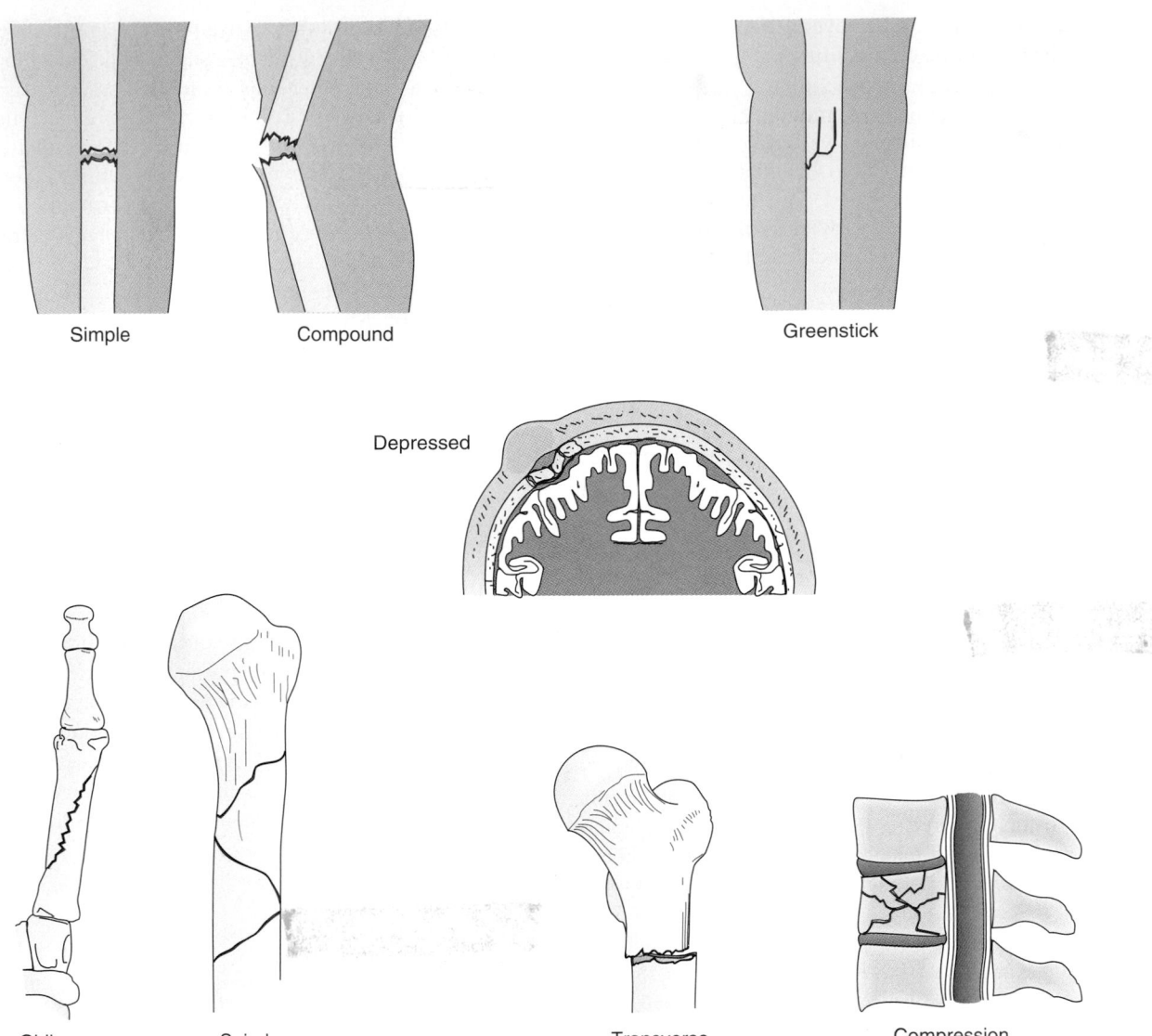

FIGURE 76-4. Fracture types and patterns. Fractures are classified according to type (complete, incomplete, open [compound], or closed [simple]) and the direction of fracture line (transverse, oblique, spiral, depressed or compression, and greenstick).

pain. Other symptoms include swelling over the part and discoloration caused by bleeding within the tissues.

> ### Nursing Alert
> A complicated fracture may result in the loss of the pulse distal to the fracture. Perform frequent neurovascular assessments of the affected extremity.

TRAUMA CARE AND MANAGEMENT

With any traumatic musculoskeletal injury, x-ray films of the injured area are taken to determine the injury and the extent of it, such as a fracture and the resulting positions of bone fragments. A portable high-quality video machine is available to make the first determination of fracture. Such machines help in sports injuries, because they can be carried onto the playing field before the injured person is moved.

The treatment objective is to restore the bone to natural alignment to ensure proper healing. The method chosen depends on the location and extent of the break, and the client's condition and age. The fragments must be brought back into place (*reduction*) and held in that position (*immobilization*) until the broken parts heal. The two types of reduction are closed and open. In *closed reduction*, external manipulation realigns the bone ends; in *open reduction*, surgery accomplishes the realignment.

Different types of immobilization devices may be used, including casts, internal and external fixation, splints, and traction. The use of computers helps determine the exact type of prosthesis or reconstruction needed in some cases.

Many healthcare facilities have a special cast-and-splint room. In large facilities, specialized technicians work in this area. If the nurse is asked to assist, the healthcare provider will specify the desired cast or splint material to use and will direct its application.

Often, clients receive analgesics or anesthetics before cast application; medications are given less frequently for splint application. If a general anesthetic is used, the immobilizing device is applied in the operating room or day-surgery center. Give routine preoperative and postoperative care.

Splints

Immediately after an injury, a temporary splint is necessary to immobilize the affected body part before treatment begins or until swelling subsides. Splints are also used for therapeutic purposes.

A common splint is the *half-cast,* in which a full cast is applied, then sawed in half lengthwise (*bivalved*). The bottom half of the cast may be used alone, or both halves may remain in place. Half-casts are held in place with an elastic roller bandage, which may also be used alone after healing begins, to give support. The half-cast may be taken off at intervals and reapplied, or it may remain in place for the full period of immobilization.

Another type of splint is the *inflatable splint,* consisting of a plastic bag that is inflated inside a second plastic bag with a zipper on one side. Although they are most often used in emergency first aid, acute care facilities also use inflatable splints. These splints are available in different sizes to fit various body parts, including the leg, ankle, and arm.

If an inflatable splint is to remain in place for some time, loosely apply a light stockinette to the affected extremity. Apply the splint, zip it, and inflate it just enough to immobilize the part. This splint is comfortable because it is lightweight. It is also convenient for healthcare personnel to use because it is transparent and does not need to be removed when x-ray films are taken. Be careful not to puncture the bag.

Other splints include *Thomas* or *ring splints* (which may be used in combination with traction), molded aluminum splints, and other metal splints. Nursing care of a client in a splint is similar to that of a client in a cast.

Nursing Alert

Never ignore a complaint of pain or pressure from a person wearing a cast or splint. Check the extremity's circulation, motion, and sensation (**CMS**), elevate the extremity, and report the situation immediately.

Casts

A **cast** is a solid mold that is used to immobilize a fracture, relieve pain through rest, and stabilize an unstable fracture. The cast remains on the affected area until the bones have rejoined, a process called *fusion.* A cast may be applied in a client's room, emergency department, operating room, physician's office, or clinic. Nurses may be asked to assist with cast application. Specific in-service training is usually required. In Practice: Nursing Care Guidelines 76-1 provides more information on casting.

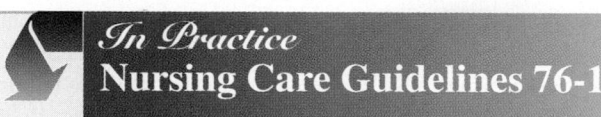

In Practice
Nursing Care Guidelines 76-1

PREPARING FOR CASTING

- Gather all materials beforehand, including a stockinette and padding materials. Be sure a source of water is available.
- Follow the manufacturer's instructions regarding preparation.
- Wear gloves if the fracture involves blood and to protect your hands from the casting materials.
- Prepare the injured area. In many cases, wash the area (without soap), carefully dry it, and shave it. Apply an astringent or alcohol if ordered.
- Lubricate the area, as ordered.
- Have sterile dressings available for an open (broken-skin) compound fracture.
- Position the client as directed.
- Assist or restrain the client as needed.
- Reassure the client during the procedure.
- Be aware that a follow-up x-ray examination is necessary after the cast is applied. Ensure that the client is comfortable.
- Clean up immediately after the procedure, before the cast or splint material hardens and becomes difficult to remove. A special sink with a plaster trap is usually available. *Do not* put plaster or cast material in a regular sink.

Types of Casts

Casts are typically made of plaster or a synthetic material such as fiberglass. Although fiberglass is lighter in weight, longer wearing, and allows better air circulation than plaster, plaster is less expensive than fiberglass and in some cases, can be molded better into the desired shape. Both materials come in strips or rolls that are immersed into water and applied over a layer of cotton or synthetic padding covering the injured area.

Plaster Cast. A plaster cast requires proper care so that it immobilizes the injured part without causing further damage or injury. A large plaster cast remains wet for 24 to 48 hours. Because the cast must dry in its applied shape, support it with pillows to preserve the original contours. Keep the cast uncovered, and turn the client so that all sides of the cast will dry. (Turning also helps prevent other complications.)

Handle the wet cast with palms only, not with fingers. (Rationale: Finger pressure can dent a cast, creating pressure points.) Move the client's extremity by grasping either side of the casted area. Do not grasp the cast unless absolutely necessary.

In some instances, a cast dryer may be used. However, take care not to apply intense heat because it could burn the client, crack the cast, or dry the outside of the cast while the inside stays wet and becomes moldy.

The client may complain of being cold while the cast is drying. Cover the rest of the client's body with a blanket and prevent drafts. If the weather is hot, the client may complain of being too warm. Cool liquids and a cool cloth applied to the forehead may help. If necessary, lower the room temperature slightly. Ice packs can be applied around the cast to offset the heat that the drying plaster emits.

If a cast's edges are rough, cover them with tape, a procedure called *petaling*. If a stockinette is placed inside the cast, cover the rough edges by pulling the edge of the stockinette out, folding it over the cast's edge, and taping it in place. Doing so can help prevent irritation to the extremity caused by plaster crumbs and rough cast edges.

Protect a cast applied near the client's genital area against moisture. Even after a plaster cast dries, it must not become wet or the plaster will dissolve.

Synthetic Cast. Light synthetic casting materials (such as fiberglass) are often more convenient to use than are plaster casts. Today, most casts applied to the extremities are fiberglass. They are sometimes more durable, and they take less time to dry, drying in approximately 15 minutes. Synthetic casts are lighter and stronger than plaster casts. Some synthetic casts can be exposed to some water. X-ray films can be taken through this material. However, there is no give to these casts, and some clients cannot tolerate them.

☞ KEY CONCEPT

If a cast or splint becomes dented, softened, or broken, it will not serve its purpose: immobilization of a body part.

Caring for Clients in Casts

In Practice: Nursing Care Guidelines 76-2 and In Practice: Educating the Client 76-2 provide fundamental information for the nurse, the client, and the family about cast care.

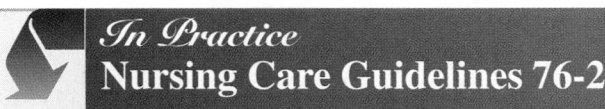

In Practice
Nursing Care Guidelines 76-2

PERFORMING CAST CARE

Synthetic Cast

• Check for rough edges. Petal as necessary. Pull sock or nylon stocking over the cast to prevent it from snagging on clothing.
• Do not immerse the cast totally in water. However, it is not necessary to prevent all contact with water. *Rationale: Although the cast is not likely to dissolve, the padding will become wet and may begin to rot. Also, the underlying skin can itch or necrose.*
• Keep in mind that the fiberglass cast is solid and does not give at all, as does a plaster cast. The fiberglass cast, as a result, may be too tight for comfort.
• Carefully wash, dry, and gently massage the skin around the cast daily.
• Caution the person against being too active. *Rationale: The cast can break, injuring the extremity further.*
• Perform neurovascular assessments frequently. *Rationale: Frequent neurovascular assessments are needed to prevent complications.*

Spica (Body) Cast

• Turn the client frequently. *Rationale: Frequent turning prevents development of pressure points, venostasis, and circulatory complications.*
• Reassure the client when turning him or her. *Rationale: Turning may cause apprehension and fear of falling.*
• Be sure no crumbs or other foreign substances get inside the cast. *Rationale: Foreign material inside the cast can lead to itching and skin breakdown.*
• Provide air conditioning if possible. Hot weather is particularly uncomfortable for the client in a cast.

• Give special attention to bladder and bowel elimination and to the area near the buttocks.
• Use a fracture bedpan for elimination. Remove these bedpans slowly. *Rationale: They overflow easily.*
• Apply powder or lotion to the bedpan before placing it under the client. *Rationale: This helps to slip the pan into place.* Protect the bed with a waterproof pad.
• Report symptoms such as abdominal pain and a bloated feeling. The area of the cast over the stomach should be cut out. *Rationale: Cutting out the area over the stomach helps to prevent superior mesenteric syndrome, also known as body cast syndrome. If the stomach area is not cut out, the stomach has no place for expansion after eating or if the person has gas. This could lead to partial or complete strangulation of the bowel.*
• Encourage the client to exercise as much as possible. *Isometric exercises* should be done inside the cast. *Rationale: Exercises encourage circulation and help prevent complications.*
• Move the client out of the room on a stretcher or in a standing wheelchair.
• Encourage diversional activities.
• Use several people or a hydraulic lift or chair to move the client. *Rationale: Assistance is needed when moving the client to prevent injury to staff and the client.*
• Encourage the client to do as much self-care as possible. *Rationale: Participating in self-care helps to improve self-image and provides meaningful exercise.*

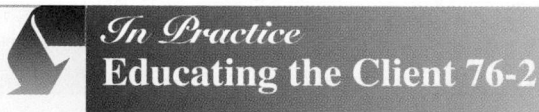

In Practice
Educating the Client 76-2

WEARING A CAST

- Follow the physician's instructions regarding physical activity and limitations.
- Exercise the muscles. Move the fingers or toes frequently to reduce swelling, prevent joint stiffness, and maintain muscle strength. Do muscle-setting exercises (contracting and relaxing without movement) inside the cast to maintain muscle mass, tone, and strength.
- With a foot or leg cast, wear a cast walking shoe at all times, except when sleeping or showering.
- Elevate the cast extremity to prevent swelling.
- Avoid bumping the cast.
- Never stick anything inside the cast. It could result in itching, infection, or decreased circulation. (This consideration is especially important for children.)
- Never trim or cut back the cast.
- Keep a plaster cast dry. If a synthetic cast becomes wet, pat it dry with a towel and dry it with a hair dryer, using the low setting.
- When resting the cast on furniture, protect the furniture with a pad.
- Contact your physician if any of the following problems develop: unrelenting itching; foul odor from cast; drainage present through or around cast; pain unrelieved by medication; cast that feels very tight or too loose; cast that breaks, cracks, or becomes dented; painful rubbing or pressure inside the cast, especially in one particular place; limb that constantly feels cold; fingers or toes that are numb or tingling; fingers or toes that are white, blue, or the color of which does not return when pressed.

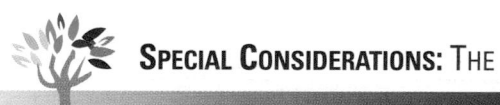

SPECIAL CONSIDERATIONS: THE LIFE SPAN

Casts

Sometimes older clients with casts do not move sufficiently to counteract the dangers of hypostatic pneumonia. Encourage deep breathing exercises and the use of an incentive spirometer as a good preventive measure. Older persons may have difficulty learning to use crutches or other mobility aids safely.

Cast Removal

Casts are removed with a cast saw, which oscillates back and forth although it appears to rotate. The blade moves within only a fraction of an inch and will not cut the client. Because cast removal can be frightening, explain the procedure and show the client the cast saw before removal begins. A client who realizes that cast removal is safe will be better able to tolerate the noise and dust. Wear gloves, protective eyewear, and a mask to avoid irritation and inhalation of small dust particles.

Before a cast is removed, explain to the client that the skin under the cast may be covered with scales or crusts of dead skin. Also inform the client that muscles may appear atrophied and that the limb may be weak or stiff. After cast removal, the client may wear a brace for a week or two to provide additional stability to the injured area. All healthcare team members (eg, physician, nurse, physical therapist) will instruct the client about therapeutic exercises for the affected body part.

Traction

Another means of immobilization is *traction*, which may be used with other types of immobilization, such as surgical internal fixation. Traction exerts a continuous pulling force on broken bones to keep them in the natural position for proper healing. As shown in Figure 76-5, in traction, continuous pulling force is controlled through the use of weights; a physician determines how much weight to apply by using principles of physics. The strength of the *traction forces* (weights) on the bones must be enough to counteract the overall pull of the body's muscles. The location and number of pulleys help determine the direction and degree of the pull. *Countertraction forces* pull against traction forces, and may be produced with weights, bed position, or the client's body weight. An overhead frame attached to the bed holds the traction pulleys and equipment in place. A trapeze may also be attached to the bed so the client can pull his or her head and shoulders off the bed. With any type of traction, never remove or change the weights on *any* traction device without a physician's order. Box 76-2 outlines examples of the two types of traction (skin and skeletal).

Skin Traction

In **skin traction,** the pull is applied to the client's skin, which transmits the pull to the musculoskeletal structures. A belt, head halter, foam rubber wrapped with an elastic bandage, or a foam boot is applied to the client's skin before the appendage is attached to traction. A disadvantage of skin traction is that it can only provide 8 to 10 pounds of pull.

Skeletal Traction

In **skeletal traction** (see Figure 76-5), a physician surgically inserts metal pins or wires into the client's bones so that traction is applied directly to them. Clients with skeletal traction are allowed to move slightly in bed while maintaining the correct position. Skeletal traction can be successful and cost effective in the home setting. To prevent infection, pin insertion sites require the same care as for any incision. Immediately report any signs of infection, and teach clients and family caregivers about these signs. Infection in the incision site can spread to the bone, causing the serious compli-

➤➤ BOX 76-2

TYPES OF TRACTION

Skin Traction

Buck's Traction (Buck's Extension)

The leg is wrapped with an elastic roller bandage or tape. Traction is applied with a weight attached to a spreader bar below the foot. A foam boot may also be used. The traction pull is toward the pulley at the bottom of the bed.

Cervical Head Halter Traction

For neck pain, neck strain, and whiplash, traction can be applied to the cervical spine by means of a head halter. The pull of cervical skin traction should be felt as an upward pull on the back of the neck. A slight change in the level of the head of the bed is often the key to correct application of this type of traction. Because this is a form of skin traction, it cannot be used for prolonged periods. This type of traction is often used by the client at home with the client sitting in a chair.

Russell's Traction (Balanced Traction)

Downward pull, as in Buck's traction, may be applied to the leg, but an additional overhead pulley system is incorporated into the traction apparatus, with the leg supported by a sling. The pull is up (toward the ceiling) and toward the foot of the bed.

Pelvic Traction

Used in pelvic fractures to support separated bones, this traction may be applied by either a belt or a sling. The pelvic belt causes downward pull on the pelvis, while the pelvic sling supports the pelvis off the bed. With a pelvic belt, the upper rim of the belt should rest at the top of the iliac crest and not around the abdomen. This type of traction is used in treating a herniated intervertebral disk or a muscle spasm of the back. It is usually applied intermittently (on 2 hours, off 2 hours) while the client is awake. Weights on the traction are increased gradually.

Skeletal Traction

Skull Traction or Head Traction

This form of skeletal traction is accomplished by inserting the points of a skull tong device (such as Vincke or Crutchfield tongs) into the skull bone. It is used to reduce a fracture of the cervical vertebrae. This type of traction is often used only temporarily until a halo device can be placed.

The Halo Device

This form of skeletal traction allows the client to move about. The combination of the halo, which is attached to the skull, and the vest, which is worn on the body, provides the traction. It is used in vertebral fractures.

The Steinmann Pin or Kirschner Wire

Either of these devices is drilled through the shaft of a bone (commonly in a leg fracture) and attached to the traction apparatus.

---

cation of *osteomyelitis,* a bone infection discussed later in this chapter.

Halo Device.   The **halo device** (Figure 76-6) is a form of skeletal traction used for cervical fractures that is applied to the skull and allows the client to ambulate and perform self-care activities. The four pins holding the halo device in place penetrate the skull only a fraction of an inch. The tightness of the screws influences the amount of traction.

➤ ➤ **N u r s i n g   A l e r t**

The halo device comes with a wrench. Always tape the wrench to the halo device so that the device can be quickly removed in an emergency.

Nurses may assist healthcare providers with applying halo devices. Explain to clients what will be done. Provide the

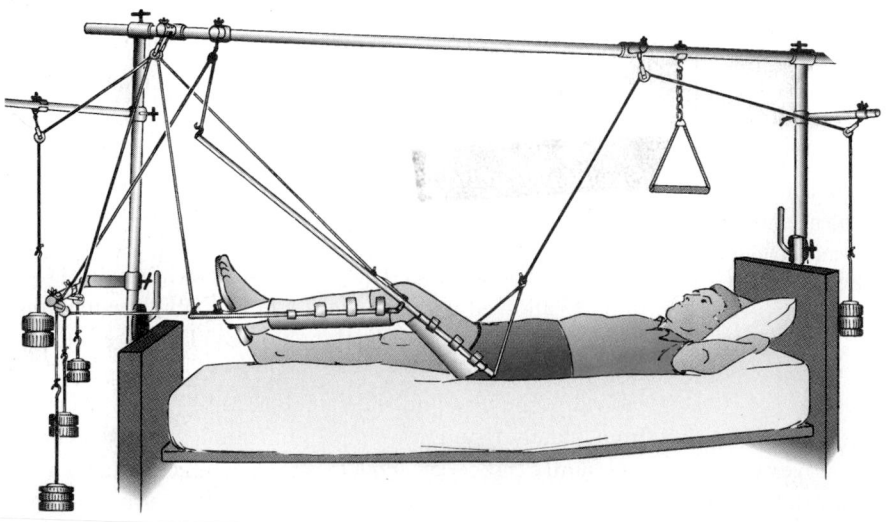

FIGURE 76-5. The client in a balanced suspension traction with a Thomas leg splint. The client uses the trapeze to help move vertically. It is important that the line of pull on the traction is maintained. Note that the weights hang freely at the head and foot of the bed.

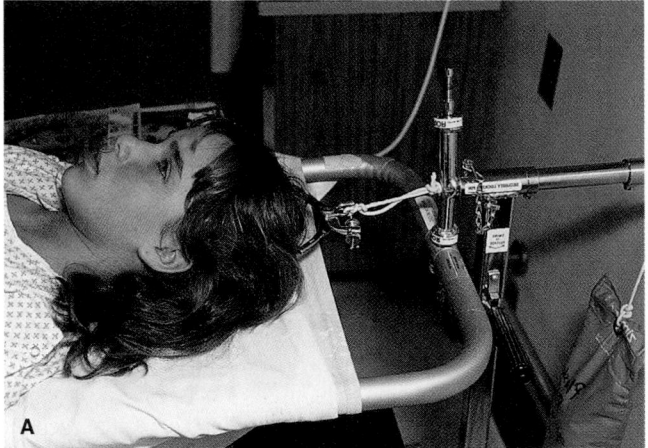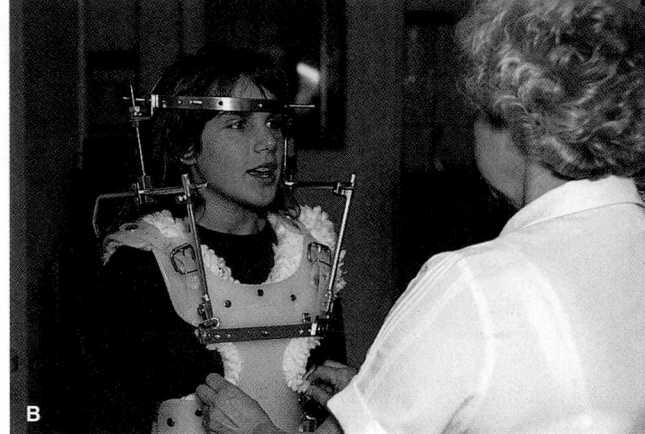

FIGURE 76-6. Methods of cervical skeletal traction. (A) Crutchfield tongs. (B) Halo device.

healthcare provider with the halo, vest, special wrench and positioning plate, regular wrench, and Xylocaine. Use sterile technique and wear gloves.

- Be prepared to place a client in a special bed or chair before the application of the halo device. Use caution not to change the alignment of the head or neck. Support the client's head and neck on movement and during application. After the device is applied, help the client to sit up slowly. (Rationale: The client may become dizzy or faint.) Support the client in a sitting position while the physician adjusts the halo's vertical bars.
- Give good skin care around the device and at the pin sites. Using a sterile cotton-tipped applicator, apply sterile hydrogen peroxide to the pins; rinse with sterile normal saline. Even though the insertion sites are small, watch for evidence of infection. Wear gloves.
- Administer analgesics as ordered. Typically the client may experience some mild discomfort. Immediately report pain that is not relieved by medications.

Nursing Alert

Severe headache is a specific danger sign for the client wearing a halo device.

- Monitor the client for possible complaints of difficulty in swallowing, inability to open the mouth all the way, or persistent neck pain; report such findings immediately because they are signs that the vertical connecting bar is too long.
- Note if the client complains of not being able to see straight ahead, a sign that the apparatus is not straight. If any complications occur, a physician must readjust the apparatus.
- Provide emotional support. Always encourage clients to be as independent as possible. Inform them about community resources and support groups.

Clients will wear the halo device for about 10 to 12 weeks, during which time they or their families will become responsible for care. Teaching is vital. In Practice: Educating the

Client 76-3 summarizes the important concepts. Carefully document all teaching.

Skull Tongs. *Skull tongs* are also used for cervical injuries or fractures. Holes are drilled into the sides of the skull and the tongs are inserted into these holes (see Fig. 76-6). Traction is applied to the tongs to stabilize the cervical spinal cord. The client stays in bed and must remain immobile until the injury heals, surgery is performed, or a halo device is applied. For the client with skull tongs, keep in mind the following:

- Provide client and family teaching and support. (Rationale: If the client has sustained a sudden injury, he or she will be frightened and in addition may be newly paralyzed. Thus, remain with the client during the entire procedure.)
- Explain the procedure to the client. After the client receives local anesthesia, the physician drills shallow holes into the sides of the client's skull. (Be aware that the physician will either shave the area around the tong

In Practice
Educating the Client 76-3

WEARING A HALO DEVICE

- Report the following danger signs immediately: severe headache, difficulty swallowing, inability to open mouth completely, persistent neck pain.
- If the halo device loosens, do not try to tighten it. Report the situation to your healthcare provider.
- Wash the skin under and around the vest. Conduct pin care as directed.
- Report the following signs of infection: fever, drainage, redness, and warmth.
- Report any complaints of not being able to see straight ahead.
- Never use the halo frame for lifting or turning.

insertion sites or instruct the nurse to shave a specific area.) Warn the client that he or she may experience some pain during the drilling (although most clients feel pressure rather than severe pain). The noise from drilling is loud and may be frightening to the client.

- Once the physician inserts the tongs, pay attention to the insertion sites. Check the institution's policies for routine care. Immediately report any signs of infection. (Rationale: The tongs are in close proximity to the brain, and any infection there could be fatal.) Headache is a serious sign that could indicate encephalitis or osteomyelitis. Report a client's headache immediately.
- If possible, place the client in an antidecubitus bed.
- Routinely assess the client's LOC and pupils (eye signs).

Caring for Clients in Traction

The basic principles for care of clients in traction are highlighted at In Practice: Nursing Care Guidelines 76-3.

External Fixation

The *external fixator* is a device used to manage complex fractures that are associated either with soft tissue damage or open wounds in the fracture area. (Rationale: The wounds are easier to treat because casting material is not covering them.) A physician inserts multiple pins that protrude through the client's skin into the bone fragments. The *external fixation device* is a metal frame that, on the outside of the body, holds the pins in place and maintains immobilization (Fig. 76-7). The healthcare provider adjusts the frame to maintain traction and to keep the fracture in proper alignment. This alignment must continue until the bone heals.

Nursing care is consistent with traditional care of a fracture, and also includes care of the pin sites. The physician will order the type and frequency of pin care required. In general, use a sterile cotton-tipped applicator to apply sterile hydrogen peroxide. Rinse with sterile normal saline. If dressings are pres-

---

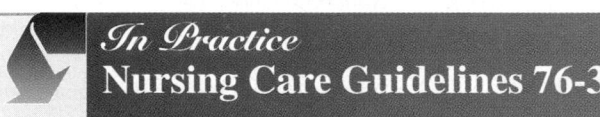

In Practice
Nursing Care Guidelines 76-3

CARING FOR CLIENTS IN TRACTION

- Follow the physician's order for the exact amount of weight to use.
- Be sure the weights hang free; they must never rest on the bed or the floor. Take care not to bump into the weights. *Rationale: Releasing the pull defeats the purpose of traction.*
- When adding weights or attaching traction, release the weights gradually onto the rope. *Rationale: Suddenly adding weights causes an uncomfortable jerk and may disrupt alignment of the fracture.*
- Never remove weights without an order. *Rationale: Traction usually is ordered to be continuous.*
- If the footpiece is touching the pulleys at the bottom of the bed, report it at once. The client should be moved up in bed when this happens. *Rationale: This would negate the effects of traction.*
- Inspect pulleys and ropes regularly. *Rationale: The ropes can slip out of their grooves or become untied.*
- Be certain to understand the physician's orders completely, regarding the client's body positioning; that is, the degree to which the head of the bed may be elevated, and to which side the client with a fracture may turn. *Rationale: Prevent complications and maximize effects of the treatment.*
- Do not use a pillow under an extremity in traction, unless specifically ordered by the physician. *Rationale: Placement of the pillow might counteract the effects of the traction.*
- Encourage the client to exercise the feet periodically and to keep the ankles in neutral position.

Rationale: Make every effort to prevent footdrop, a deformity caused by nerve damage because the foot has been allowed to remain in an abnormal position.
- Maintain the client's body alignment. Be sure to obtain specific guidelines from the physician before allowing the client to change position.
- Reposition frequently as needed. *Rationale: The weight of the traction may tend to pull the client out of alignment.*
- Guide the weights if the client is allowed to use a trapeze to slide up in bed. *Rationale: This ensures that the weights hang freely and are not impeded when the client moves.*
- Follow the physician's orders for ROM exercises. If ROM is not ordered for the client, find out what kind of exercise or positioning is needed.
- Provide diversional activities.
- Use the fracture bedpan. *Rationale: This type of bedpan is easier to slip under the client's hips than the large conventional pan.*
- Maintain skin integrity. Be sure that the rubber strips, elastic roller bandage, or tape does not irritate the client's skin. Clean, dry thoroughly, and gently massage the skin daily.
- Apply lotion to the client's elbows. Frequent skin care is required. *Rationale: These measures prevent skin breakdown.* If the elbows become irritated, apply elbow protectors.
- If the client has skeletal traction, give pin site care as ordered. Wear gloves when caring for the client with skeletal traction.

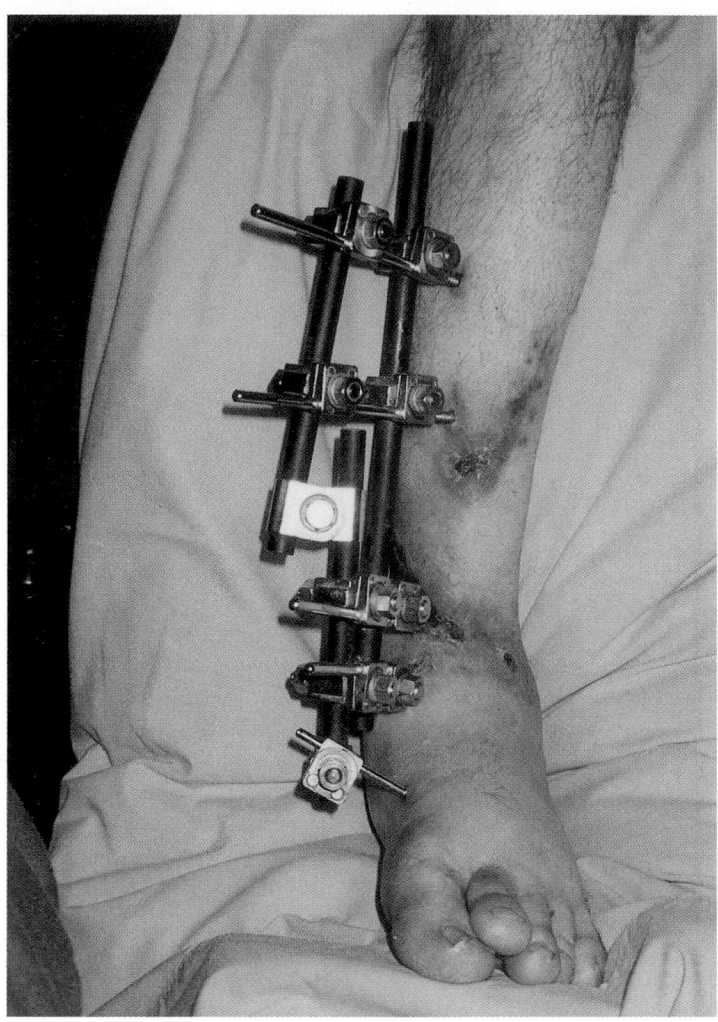

FIGURE 76-7. Pins are inserted directly into the bones in this external fixation device used to realign broken bony parts.

ent, be sure to change them using sterile technique. Avoid the formation of scar tissue around the pin sites; thus, whenever giving pin care, place traction on the skin by slightly and gently pulling the skin away from the pin site. Wear sterile gloves.

Be alert for possible rejection—an adverse reaction to the nails, screws, or plates used. It can occur even though such materials are made of a special metal alloy that is, in most cases, nonirritating.

Nursing Alert

Never move a limb by grasping the frame of the external fixation device.

Open Reduction and Internal Fixation

Surgery, called an open reduction and internal fixation (**ORIF**), is usually necessary if a client has a compound (open) fracture, or if multiple bony fragments are present. With an *open reduction,* the surgeon makes an incision so that the injured or damaged area can be seen. After the wound is *debrided* (dead and damaged tissue removed) and irrigated with antibiotics, peroxide, normal saline, or other solutions, the surgeon visualizes the bone fragments and determines exactly

how to rejoin them. With *internal fixation,* the surgeon places a pin, wire, screw, plate, nail, or rod into or onto the bone to keep it *reduced* (properly aligned), immobilized, or both.

The ORIF is the treatment of choice for certain fractures in which casting is generally impossible (eg, hip fracture), or if multiple fragments are impossible to realign. Internal fixation eliminates the need for traction. Additionally, the client's recovery is usually quicker. Figure 76-8 illustrates types of internal fixation.

Internal fixation can be performed using various devices. It is used most frequently for fractures of the leg's long bones, in which case the spike is called an *intermedullary nail.* Usually internal fixation is done if the client has more than one transverse fracture or if the client's history includes fractures that do not align or heal easily with casting.

The surgeon may apply a metal plate with screws to the outside of the bone; such a device often must remain in place permanently. This procedure is usually performed when a bone is fractured in several places. Screws are sometimes inserted to hold the bone fragments in place without using a plate. Wires may be used to hold fragments of bone together.

Although the client with internal fixation may have no visible form of immobilization, a fracture still exists that requires careful handling. Sometimes, internal fixation is combined

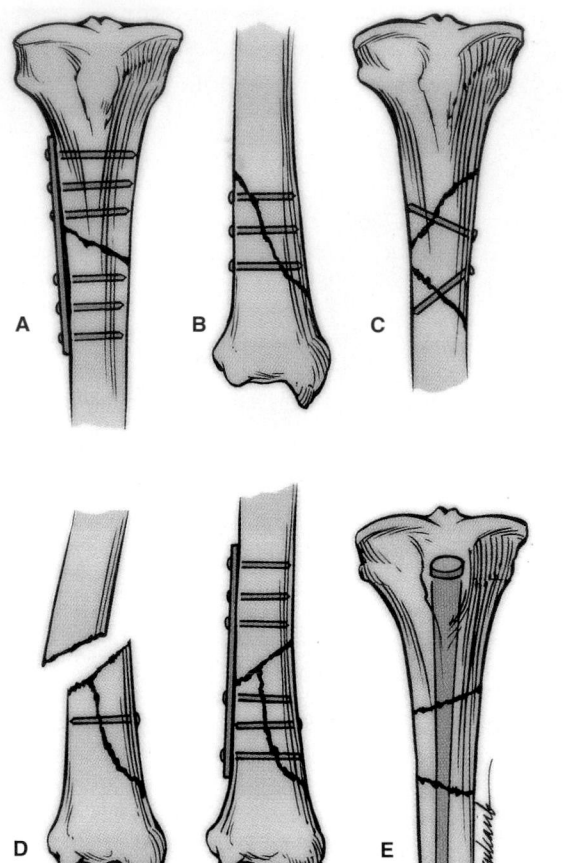

FIGURE 76-8. Types of internal fixation. **(A)** Plate and screws secure a transverse fracture. **(B)** Screws secure a long oblique fracture. **(C)** Screws secure a long butterfly fragment of bone. **(D)** Plates and screws secure a short butterfly fragment. **(E)** A medullary nail secures a segmental fracture of the femur.

with another form of immobilization, such as splinting or casting.

> ### Nursing Alert
> Clients who have internal fixation devices must avoid future MRI studies because of the implanted metal.

Arthroplasty

Repair or replacement of a joint is called **arthroplasty.** For example, in some cases of fractured hip, the femoral head is replaced; in other cases, the hip socket is also replaced with a studded cup, which may be cemented into a deepened hip socket. This procedure is called *total hip replacement* or *total hip arthroplasty* (**THA**). Other joints that can be totally or partially replaced include the ankle, knee, shoulder, elbow, and wrist.

Total joint replacement is done in clients with severe injuries or severe degenerative arthritic disorders, when joints become injured, fused, or too malformed to be functional. Postoperative care is similar to that described for open reduction of the hip or other joint.

Shoulder joint replacement has been less successful than hip joint replacement. Due to minimal bony contact, the shoulder joint is less supported, less stable, and more subject to trauma and disease. For clients with minimal shoulder damage, a *hemiarthroplasty* may be done; in this procedure, only the head of the humerus is replaced.

Hip Fractures

Hip fractures include fractures of the head and neck of the femur or of the trochanter. These fractures often heal poorly, because the healing process in such large bones disrupts nutrition to the bone matrix. In addition, hip fractures are more common in older adults, whose bones heal slowly and who are more likely to have osteoporosis (particularly older women).

Signs and Symptoms

Whenever an older person falls or complains of pain in the hip, groin, or knee, assess for a hip fracture. Although the exact location of the fracture causes symptoms to vary, many hip fractures involve shortening of the leg on the affected side and external foot rotation.

In most cases, if the neck of the femur is fractured, the client complains of severe pain that worsens with movement. If the head of the femur is compacted onto the neck, the client may have less pain and may even be able to bear weight. For this reason, a physician should examine any older person who falls. If the fracture occurs at the trochanter, the client usually has muscle spasms, obvious shortening of the leg, and external rotation of the foot. He or she complains of severe pain, and a large bruise is visible on the hip. Radiographic studies can indicate a specific diagnosis. Bleeding may decrease the person's hemoglobin level; trauma may elevate the person's blood glucose and enzyme levels.

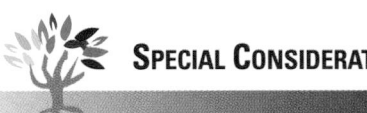

SPECIAL CONSIDERATIONS: THE LIFE SPAN

Hip Fractures

Risk factors for hip fractures include decreased bone mass, advancing age, female gender, difficulty with ambulation, and poor arterial perfusion.

Medical and Surgical Treatment

The fracture will first be immobilized by traction. If a client cannot undergo surgery, traction will continue for about 6 weeks. However, if the client's condition permits an operation, an ORIF of the hip is done as soon as possible. This procedure allows mobility soon after the injury, thus preventing severe complications of immobility, which can be particularly dangerous for older adults.

Sometimes called a "hip pinning," the ORIF involves lining up the bone fragments (reduction), and attaching the bones together (internal fixation) by using pins, nails, screws, metal plates, or by using an intermedullary nail. If these devices fail to provide stabilization, the surgeon removes the head of the femur and replaces it with a prosthesis. Some surgeons implant a hip prosthesis in all cases of fractured hip. Hip prostheses provide stabilization and also prevent complications, such as nonunion of bones and the death of joints, which can result from poor blood supply to joints or bones. Surgeons often perform total hip arthroplasty or replacement, which provides even more comfort and quicker mobility than ORIF.

Nursing Considerations. In addition to routine pre and postoperative care, special teaching is required to prevent hip dislocation after hip replacement surgery. Three major teaching and nursing considerations are necessary for post-operative care of the hip replacement client to maintain alignment of the affected hip:

- Never allow the affected leg to cross the center of the body (eg, do not cross legs when sitting in a chair).
- Never allow the body to bend more than 90 degrees (eg, avoid bending forward to put on shoes).
- Never allow the affected leg to turn inward (eg, avoid bending or flexing the hip when putting on slacks or stockings) (see In Practice: Nursing Care Plan 76-1).

Additional limitations or restrictions concern weight bearing on the affected side. In Practice: Nursing Care Guidelines 76-4 details care for clients with new hip replacements.

In Practice
Nursing Care Plan 76-1

THE OLDER ADULT CLIENT WITH A FRACTURED HIP

MEDICAL HISTORY: *I.M., a 65-year-old widowed female with a history of osteoporosis, was hospitalized after falling at home and fracturing the neck of her left femur. She underwent an open reduction, internal fixation of the left hip 24 hours ago.*

MEDICAL DIAGNOSIS: *Fracture of the left hip with open reduction internal fixation*

Data Collection/Nursing Assessment: Client is alert and oriented, 1 day following open reduction with internal fixation. She reports pain is adequately controlled with analgesic therapy. Surgical site dressing is clean, dry, and intact. Vital signs are within acceptable parameters. Client demonstrating coughing, deep breathing, and incentive spirometry every 2 hours. Client states, "How will I ever be able to walk again? I'm even afraid to move. The doctor said that I have to watch how I move my leg." Prior to client's fall, she was living independently in her own home, frequently babysitting her daughter's children. (*Although other nursing diagnoses may be appropriate, a priority nursing diagnosis is addressed below.*)

Nursing Diagnosis: Impaired Physical Mobility related to repair of fractured hip as evidenced by client's statement about walking and prescribed postoperative restrictions.

Planning
SHORT-TERM GOALS:
#1. Client participates in proper positioning while in bed.
#2. Client demonstrates appropriate exercise techniques.

LONG-TERM GOALS:
#3. Client demonstrates ability to transfer from bed to chair independently.

#4. Client participates in physical therapy program for progressive ambulation.

Implementation
NURSING ACTION: *Carefully check the physician's instructions about position and activity. Maintain hip in neutral position, using trochanter roll.*
RATIONALE: *Specific instructions for activity and positioning are determined by the surgeon. Maintaining the hip in a neutral position prevents stress on the operative site. A trochanter roll reduces the risk of external rotation, which could cause the femoral head to dislocate.*

NURSING ACTION: *When turning client, use an abductor pillow. Enlist the aid of other healthcare personnel to turn the client.*
RATIONALE: *An abductor pillow prevents adduction of the hip joint, which could cause the femoral head to dislocate. Using additional personnel ensures that the client's body is maintained in proper alignment during turning.*

NURSING ACTION: *Before moving the client, explain what will be done and how she can help. Ensure that the bed is equipped with a trapeze bar for client use.*
RATIONALE: *Explanations help to alleviate anxiety and promote client participation in care. Trapeze bar allows the client to participate in moving and repositioning and helps to strengthen upper extremity muscles.*

Evaluation: Trochanter roll used when client lying supine; abductor pillow in place when turning. Client using trapeze bar to help when moving. Client observed crossing ankles; reinforced need to keep legs abducted (apart). *Progress to meeting Goal #1.*

(continued)

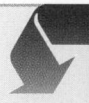

In Practice
Nursing Care Plan 76-1 (Continued)

NURSING ACTION: *Teach exercises the client can do in bed, including isometric, quadriceps-setting, and gluteal-setting exercises. Have client return-demonstrate these exercises. Encourage exercises every 1 to 2 hours; offer support and encouragement.*
RATIONALE: *These exercises help to strengthen the muscles needed for ambulation and aid in venous return.*

Evaluation: Client is maintaining abduction of left lower extremity. Client demonstrates exercises; observed performing exercises at least every 2 hours. Client stated, "I really want to be independent again." *Goal #1 met; progress to meeting Goal #2.*

NURSING ACTION: *As ordered, assist with client transfer from bed to chair, while maintaining proper positioning of the client's extremity and prescribed amount of weight-bearing allowed.*
RATIONALE: *Getting the client out of bed is important to prevent postoperative complications of immobility and to promote a sense of increasing independence.*

Evaluation: Client using trapeze and observed exercising every 1 to 2 hours while in bed; transferred out of

bed to chair with assistance of two persons. *Goal #2 met; progress to meeting Goal #3.*

NURSING ACTION: *As ordered, contact physical therapy for progressive ambulation program. Work with physical therapist and client to promote ambulation.*
RATIONALE: *Physical therapy is indicated to assist the client to achieve the maximum level of independent mobility that is possible. Working with the physical therapist and client is important to foster achievement.*

NURSING ACTION: *Reinforce the ambulation skills the client is learning in physical therapy and use them when assisting the client in transferring, getting out of bed to the bathroom, or for walks. Take proper safety precautions with each interaction. Praise the client's progress.*
RATIONALE: *Ambulation will increase muscle mass, tone, and strength and facilitate mastery.*

Evaluation: Client demonstrates transfer from bed to chair with nurse watching at bedside. Client reports ambulating with walker. *Goal #3 met; progress to meeting Goal #4.*

COMPLICATIONS OF FRACTURES OR BONE SURGERY

Clients who are immobilized with casts or traction, or who undergo surgery to repair joint or bone disease or dysfunction, are susceptible to complications that threaten successful outcomes. Assess the client carefully and frequently for signs and symptoms of these problems.

Neurovascular Pressure

Pressure from an external immobilization device can cause damage to nerves or blood vessels, as well as the skin. Signs and symptoms of neurovascular pressure include complaints of numbness and tingling, loss of sensation, inability to move extremities, pallor, cool skin, or swelling. If the nurse finds pressure from a cast or splint during assessment, measures to provide relief are necessary immediately. A physician may need to remove all or part of a cast or splint. In some cases, the cast will be cut in half lengthwise (bivalved) and held together by an elastic roller bandage, which relieves pressure while maintaining immobilization. Other causes of pressure may be a dent in the cast, swelling of tissue, or crutches that are too long.

Wound Infection

Any compound (open) fracture or open reduction involves a skin break, making infection a possibility. Always use sterile

gloves when caring for clients with any wound. Carefully observe for signs of infection.

Osteomyelitis

Osteomyelitis is a serious bone infection that is curable if it is detected early and treated appropriately. Modern antibiotics have greatly improved the chances for recovery.

Acute Osteomyelitis
Acute osteomyelitis may result from a compound fracture that exposes bone to infection. Because blood supply to the bone is compromised, the bone becomes necrotic. Pus drains through the primary wound. *Acute hematogenous osteomyelitis* is most common in children and occurs when the bloodstream carries organisms (such as staphylococci or streptococci) to the bone from infection elsewhere. Pus forms in the bone's shaft and under its covering (*periosteum*), thereby separating the periosteum from the bone.

Signs and symptoms of osteomyelitis include pain, fever, flushed appearance, elevated white blood cell (WBC) count and ESR, and positive blood cultures. The skin over the affected area may be warm, red, and swollen. Early detection is imperative, to prevent bone necrosis. When osteomyelitis is suspected, blood cultures are obtained and vigorous antibiotic therapy is started. After the offending organism is isolated, specific antibiotics are given IV or directly into the

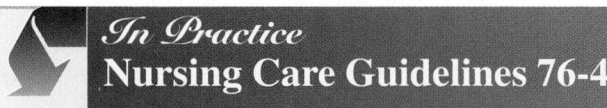

Nursing Care Guidelines 76-4

CARING FOR CLIENTS WITH NEW HIP REPLACEMENTS

- Provide routine postoperative care: deep breathing, high-protein diet, IV and oral fluid administration.
- Perform neurovascular assessments every 15 minutes for 1 hour, every 30 minutes for 1 hour, every hour for 24 hours, every 4 hours for 24 hours, and every 8 hours thereafter.
- Initiate anticoagulation therapy as ordered. Place antiembolism stockings or pneumatic compression devices as ordered.
- Turn clients every 1 to 2 hours (from unaffected side to back). Always check the surgeon's orders before turning a client whose hip fracture was surgically stabilized. Place a special pillow called an *abduction pillow* between the client's legs when turning. *Rationale: The pillow prevents adduction of the legs, which could result in dislocation of the prosthesis.*
  - Have another nurse or technician help turn the client to the *unaffected side* with a pillow between his or her knees to provide good alignment. Position the client comfortably and support him or her with pillows or sandbags and trochanter rolls so that the body is in correct alignment and contractures do not develop. The client usually remains in this position for 2 hours.
  - Turn the client onto the back again. The client usually remains in this position for an hour. Elevate the head of the bed at least 30 degrees when the client is on his or her back, to prevent aspiration.
  - Turn the client to the *unaffected* side again. (*Note:* The client with a hip fracture is usually not placed on the affected side, although some surgeons allow this.)

- Prevent common complications: infection and dislocation of prostheses or pins.
- Frequently evaluate incisions for erythema, intactness, and drainage. If a drainage device is in place, empty it frequently and measure the drainage.
- Change dressings as needed, maintaining sterile technique.
- Provide frequent skin care. Keep skin dry. Relieve pressure areas to prevent skin breakdown.
- Give back care every 2 hours while the client is on bed rest.
- Following insertion of a hip prosthesis (and sometimes following open reduction), maintain the client's leg in an abducted position and in neutral or slight external rotation. Carefully follow the surgeon's orders for positioning and movement.
- Provide active and passive ROM exercises as ordered.
- Place a trapeze on the overhead frame. *Rationale: The trapeze will help the client move and use the bedpan.*
- Encourage early mobility, particularly for older adults. Complications of immobility cause more deaths than surgery itself.
- Assist clients into a chair two to three times per day. Check with the surgeon for any flexion restrictions before helping a client into a chair.
- Begin progressive ambulation as soon as ordered. The physician will determine how much weight a client is allowed to bear on the operative side. Do not ambulate clients before checking this information. Clients often use walkers.
- Instruct clients in routine postoperative procedures and precautions.

---

wound. A surgeon may drain the pus and may place a catheter into the wound for irrigation and drainage. Fragments of dead bone loosen (**sequestration**) and require surgical removal (*sequestrectomy*). Careful attention to rest, nutrition, fluid intake, elimination, and skin care is vital. Instruct clients to move about as ordered to prevent problems associated with prolonged bed rest; however, they must maintain complete immobilization of the affected part. If healing becomes impaired, remaining dead bone tissue (*sequestrum*) must be removed surgically.

Osteomyelitis is so painful that the affected part is sensitive to the slightest touch or motion. Do not move the affected part any more than absolutely necessary. When the part must be moved, support and splint it with a pillow, and lift and move it with the rest of the body. Sandbags, a cast, or a brace help immobilize the limb. Again, take extreme care to avoid jarring the bed.

Promote healing through a diet that is high in proteins, calcium, carbohydrates, and fats. Encourage the client to drink fluids.

Report any swelling, redness, and pain in another body part because these may be signs of spreading infection. Pathologic fractures are possible, although they may not be recognized because the pain is overshadowed by the greater pain of osteomyelitis. Growth of new bone may lengthen the infected bone, or bone destruction may shorten it. A break in aseptic technique when changing dressings could introduce pathogens into the wound. Every attempt must be made to prevent osteomyelitis.

Chronic Osteomyelitis

If antibiotics are ineffective in killing the offending microorganism; the microorganism may be resistant to the antibiotic and the bone infection persists. In these cases, *chronic osteo-*

myelitis occurs. Because of the possibility that a microorganism is drug resistant, a culture and sensitivity test should be done before a course of antibiotic therapy is initiated. Acute osteomyelitis may become chronic in immunosuppressed individuals (eg, those receiving chemotherapy or those with HIV/AIDs.

Signs and symptoms of chronic osteomyelitis include purulent drainage from a sinus tract over the affected bone, pain, swelling, and weakened bone. Changes in the bone's structure are visible on x-ray examination.

The treatment of choice for chronic osteomyelitis is surgical debridement of dead and infected tissue. The physician orders antibiotics and rest of the affected area.

Another type of chronic osteomyelitis is caused by the tubercle bacillus, which settles in the bone or joint (*tuberculosis osteomyelitis*). Signs and symptoms include pain, swelling, localized redness, and warmth. Tuberculosis of the spine, known as *Pott's disease,* is characterized by kyphosis, abscess formation, and possible paralysis. Because skeletal tuberculosis is not spread via the air, it is less contagious than pulmonary tuberculosis. Treatment includes antimicrobial drugs, such as isoniazid, ethambutol, pyrazinamide, and rifampin.

Hypostatic Pneumonia and Atelectasis

Hypostatic pneumonia and *atelectasis* (collapse of all or part of a lung) are preventable complications that result from prolonged immobility. Signs of these conditions include elevated temperature, tachycardia, cough, *dyspnea* (difficulty breathing), decreased oxygen saturation by pulse oximetry, pleural pain, and anxiety. Encourage clients to turn and ambulate as much as possible and to cough and take deep breaths. Show clients how to perform incentive spirometry. Provide respiratory therapies such as suctioning, postural draining, and chest percussion (see Chapter 56 for more discussion).

Embolism

An *embolism* is the sudden blockage of one or more arteries by a piece of foreign material. The foreign material (*embolus*) can be a blood clot, bacteria clump, air bubble, piece of tissue, or piece of an IV catheter. Embolism formation is another possible consequence of immobility, although other factors may be the cause.

The goal is to prevent embolism. Immobilize fractures, minimize fracture manipulation, and support fractured bones when moving clients. If an embolism occurs, be prepared to administer oxygen, steroids, and IV fluids, as ordered.

Fat Embolism

The most common embolism associated with fractures involves a bolus of fat. *Fat embolism* is most common in young people with multiple injuries, particularly fractures of the long bones (such as the femur and humerus), pelvis, and ribs. This type of embolism travels through the circulatory system and causes an obstruction in the brain, the heart, or most commonly, the lungs (see "Pulmonary Embolism" below).

Signs and symptoms of a fat embolism include dyspnea, tachycardia, fever, petechial rash, *hypoxemia* (low blood oxygen), chest pain, and pulmonary edema. Often, *crackles* (abnormal sounds) are heard on lung auscultation. Fat may be present in the blood, urine, or sputum. A change in the client's neurologic status is common. Fat embolism can lead to coma, pneumonia, heart failure, and acute respiratory distress syndrome.

Pulmonary Embolism

An embolism in the lungs is called a *pulmonary embolism.* Risk factors include immobility, prior history of deep-vein thrombophlebitis, or pulmonary embolism, trauma, and orthopedic surgery of the lower extremities or pelvis. Signs and symptoms include dyspnea, *tachypnea* (rapid respiration), hypoxemia, chest pain, tachycardia, cough, and *hemoptysis* (bloody sputum). Pulmonary embolism may cause life-threatening cardiac dysrhythmias.

Prevent pulmonary embolism by encouraging clients to ambulate and to perform active exercises. Administer prophylactic anticoagulant therapy as ordered. Pneumatic compression devices may be used on the legs. Antiembolism stockings or hose, such as TEDS®, must be removed at least every 8 hours and reapplied.

Pulmonary embolism is an emergency that requires immediate reporting and corrective action. Administer oxygen to relieve hypoxemia and dyspnea. Obtain blood gases as ordered. Other common treatments include anticoagulation therapy and thrombolytic therapy. Emergency surgery to remove the embolus may or may not be life saving. Give clients emotional support and calmly explain what is being done.

Deep-Vein Thrombosis

Deep-vein thrombosis (DVT) is a primary complication of prolonged bed rest. *Venostasis* (pooling blood flow) occurs when clients are immobile for long periods, predisposing individuals to clot formation (*thrombosis*). *Venous thrombosis* occurs most often in the legs and pelvis, and can be fatal if the clot moves and obstructs a vital blood vessel (causing an *embolism*). Doppler studies of the lower extremities are used to diagnose DVT.

Signs and symptoms include unequal leg circumference and pain, swelling, and redness of the affected leg. The client may have a positive Homans' sign.

Prevent DVT by applying support stockings or pneumatic compression devices to the legs. The physician may order prophylactic aspirin or low-dose subcutaneous heparin. Teach client's family passive exercises and encourage ambulation as soon as possible.

Hemorrhage

In many fractures, bone fragments damage blood vessels. Be alert for signs of internal hemorrhage such as hypotension, tachycardia, change in mental status, anxiety, increased pain in the affected extremity, and decreased urine output.

Compartment Syndrome

Compartment syndrome and *Volkmann's contracture* (also called *Volkmann's paralysis*) result from inadequate or obstructed blood flow to muscles, nerves, and tissue. These disorders may also result from compression of the muscle compartment, or from an increase in muscle compartment contents related to edema, hemorrhage, fracture, or soft-tissue injury. A tight cast, pneumatic compression stocking, or tissue swelling may cause pressure as well.

Compartment syndrome is a medical emergency. If left uncorrected, permanent muscle and nerve damage will result in 4 to 6 hours. Ischemia leads to muscle necrosis. Contractures develop because fibrous tissue replaces muscle tissue.

The cardinal symptom of compartment syndrome is pain that is unrelieved by medications and aggravated by passive stretching of the ischemic muscle. Other signs and symptoms include swelling, tightness, and *paresthesia* (numbness and tingling) of the affected extremity.

The first treatment for compartment syndrome is to remove the constricting dressing or cast and to elevate the extremity. A **fasciotomy** (excision of the fascia) may be needed to relieve internal pressure.

When caring for any client with a cast, severe sprain, or condition that causes swelling in an extremity, elevate the extremity and apply ice. Be alert for symptoms of nerve compression. Perform routine neurovascular assessments according to the institution's policies. Immediately report any suspicions of compartment syndrome. Teach clients and their families how to monitor for compartment syndrome at home.

Other Complications

Numerous other complications can occur following fractures or musculoskeletal surgery. Confusion is not uncommon, especially in older adults. It often occurs at night, when clients tend to be more confused and restless. Constipation can occur because of age, inactivity, poor eating habits, and insufficient fluids. Kidney stones may form because of poor nutrition, inactivity, changes in mineral composition that may occur during the healing process, or overmedication with salicylates. Skin breakdown may result from poor circulation, immobility, infrequent turning, or poor skin care.

Nonunion (failure of the fracture site to fuse and heal), *malunion* (healing in improper alignment), and *delayed union* (slow healing) are complications of fractures. These complications may result from malnutrition, inadequate mobilization, infection, poor circulation, or older age. Poor positioning or lack of exercise may cause contractures, footdrop, and external rotation.

NEOPLASMS

Common *neoplasms* of the musculoskeletal system are *bone tumors*. Bone tumors are of two types: primary and metastatic. *Primary bone tumors* originate in the bone. They may be benign or malignant. Primary benign bone tumors are usually well circumscribed and slow growing, and seldom spread. They include osteomas, chondromas, giant cell tumors, cysts, and osteoid osteomas. *Primary malignant bone tumors* are rare. They include osteogenic sarcoma, chondrosarcoma, and multiple myelomas (see Chap. 81). These extremely malignant tumors metastasize early, often to the lungs.

Metastatic bone tumors travel to the bone from some other part of the body. They are relatively common. Metastatic bone tumors result from primary lesions in the lung, breast, prostate, kidney, ovary, or thyroid. Metastases occur most commonly in the vertebral bodies, ribs, pelvis, femur, and humerus bones. Carcinomas tend to metastasize to bone more commonly than do sarcomas. The client with metastatic bone disease has a poor prognosis.

Symptoms

Symptoms of bone tumor include pain, swelling, restricted motion, and aching. One of the most significant signs of a malignant bone tumor is pathologic fracture. The bone fractures because it is weakened, even though no external trauma has occurred.

Diagnosis

Diagnosis of bone tumor is made by x-ray, biopsy, frozen section, and laboratory evaluation. Whenever a care provider suspects malignant tumors, chest films are routinely taken to look for *pulmonary metastases* (spread to the lungs). A skeletal radiologic survey (*bone scintigraphy*), MRI, or CT scan is done to locate additional bone lesions.

Treatment

Treatment may consist of surgical removal of a primary tumor, chemotherapy, or radiation therapy. A bone excision or amputation may be necessary to save the person's life. Metastatic bone lesions are usually treated with palliative measures (as opposed to curative). Nursing care focuses on providing comfort, controlling pain, preventing pathologic fractures, and giving emotional support.

➤ STUDENT SYNTHESIS
Key Points

- Tests that are used to diagnose musculoskeletal disorders include blood tests, x-ray, MRI, CT scan, arthrogram, bone scan, ultrasound, arthrocentesis, arthroscopy, biopsy, and electromyogram.
- Careful nursing assessments and knowledge of potential neurovascular complications are essential in orthopedic nursing. Be aware of and try to prevent complications caused by the client's decreased mobility.
- Early treatment of orthopedic complications is necessary to prevent further injury to the area involved.

- Treatment of musculoskeletal disorders and diseases can include drug therapy, exercise, surgery, amputation, physical therapy, diet, or resting the affected part.
- Traumatic musculoskeletal injuries, such as sprains, strains, dislocations, and fractures, require different forms of treatment.
- The many different methods of treating orthopedic injuries include casts, splints, internal fixation, external fixation, traction, and surgeries such as arthroscopy, total joint replacement, and lumbar decompression.
- A cast stabilizes and immobilizes fractures. When clients are wearing casts, carefully assess their neurovascular status, provide pain relief, and protect the casts.
- In skin traction, the pull is applied to the skin; in skeletal traction, the traction is applied directly to the bones.
- Potential orthopedic complications include compartment syndrome, wound infection, osteomyelitis, hypostatic pneumonia, embolism, deep-vein thrombosis, and hemorrhage.
- Primary benign bone tumors grow slowly and rarely spread. Metastatic bone tumors originate elsewhere in the body; the client has a poor prognosis.

Critical Thinking Exercises

1. Your client with arthritis complains that she is having increased difficulty caring for herself. What adjustments could she make? Explain how she can best live with the arthritis and the needed adjustments. Identify other medical professionals or community resources who could assist.
2. You work in an orthopedic unit of a large hospital. An 80-year-old man has a closed leg fracture. Formulate a teaching plan for him. How would your teaching differ if the affected individual is an 8-year-old boy with the same type of fracture?
3. You work in an elementary school. A first-grade girl with an arm cast comes to see you. Her cast is wet and dented. She complains of increased pain; her fingers are cool and white. Discuss possible causes of these findings and how you would intervene.

NCLEX-Style Review Questions

1. A client with a casted left arm complains of increased pain at the site. The client was last medicated 1 hour ago with Demerol 100 milligrams IM. The nurse notes that the fingers are swollen and pressing on the cast. The arm is elevated and the client is unable to separate the fingers on the casted arm. The priority nursing action would be:
   a. Administer Demerol.
   b. Apply ice packs to the fingers.
   c. Call the physician and report findings.
   d. Teach relaxation exercises to relieve the pain.
2. Which of the following statements made by a patient leads the nurse to realize that further teaching is necessary in regard to salicylates?
   a. "I should drink lots of fluids."
   b. "I should expect small amounts of blood in my stools."
   c. "I should take my medication with food."
   d. "The aspirin reduces my fever."
3. Which of the following assessment findings in a client who has had a hip replaced would require immediate nursing intervention?
   a. Legs are crossed.
   b. Legs are in an abducted position.
   c. Patient is lying on the unaffected side.
   d. Toes on the affected side are warm.
4. Which of the following should be included in a preventive teaching plan for osteoporosis?
   a. High-protein, low-carbohydrate diet
   b. Increased calcium and vitamin D in the diet
   c. Low-sodium diet
   d. No change necessary
5. Which of the following statements by a client with gout indicates that the client has understood patient teaching?
   a. "I need to limit drinking alcohol."
   b. "I need to limit the amount of water I drink each day."
   c. "I should avoid exercising my affected joint."
   d. "I should avoid losing any weight."

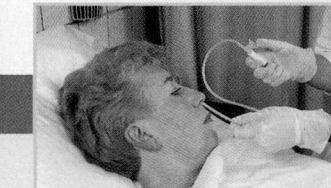

CHAPTER

77

Nervous System Disorders

LEARNING OBJECTIVES

1. Differentiate among the following diagnostic tests: CT, PET, MRI, cerebral angiography, cerebral arteriography, myelography, brain scan, electroencephalography, and videotelemetry.
2. Discuss the nursing care involved for a client before and after an LP.
3. Compare and contrast migraine and cluster headaches, including nursing considerations for each condition.
4. Identify the main characteristics of at least three types of partial seizures and at least six types of general seizures.
5. Identify the key components of nursing care for a client with a seizure disorder, epilepsy, or status epilepticus.
6. Discuss the causes, signs and symptoms, and nursing implications for the following disorders involving nerves: trigeminal neuralgia, Bell's palsy, and herpes zoster.
7. Compare paraplegia with quadriplegia, including a discussion of at least four differences in nursing care for each condition.
8. Describe at least five signs and symptoms of autonomic dysreflexia.
9. Discuss the causes, signs and symptoms, therapies, and at least five nursing considerations for each of the following degenerative disorders: multiple sclerosis, Parkinson's disease, myasthenia gravis, Huntington's disease, and amyotrophic lateral sclerosis.
10. Discuss the causes, signs and symptoms, therapies, and at least five nursing considerations for each of the following inflammatory disorders: brain abscess, meningitis, encephalitis, Guillain-Barré syndrome, post-polio syndrome, and acute transverse myelitis.
11. Explain at least four causes of increased intracranial pressure.
12. Explain the nursing care required for clients with concussion, brain laceration and contusion, skull fractures, and hematoma.
13. State at least three nursing considerations related to care of a client with a brain tumor.
14. Identify at least three pre- and postoperative nursing considerations for a client undergoing craniotomy.

NEW TERMINOLOGY

ataxia
aura
autonomic dysreflexia
bradykinesia
cephalgia
chorea
clonic phase
concussion
contusion
craniotomy
diplopia
dysphagia
dysphasia
epilepsy
flaccidity
focal point
focus
intracranial pressure
laceration

neuralgia
neurology
nuchal rigidity
opisthotonos
otorrhea
paraplegia
parkinsonism
photophobia
ptosis
quadriplegia
rhinorrhea
seizure
shingles
status epilepticus
subdural hematoma
tonic phase
transection
vertigo

ACRONYMS

ALS	HD	LP
CNS	ICP	MG
CSF	↑ICP	MS
EEG	IPV	OPV
GCS	LOC	PPMA

The medical specialty related to the nervous system is **neurology**. Physicians trained in this specialty are called *neurologists*; surgeons are called *neurosurgeons*. Nurses specializing in the care of people with nervous system disorders are called *neuroscience* nurses. The nervous system is a highly specialized major center for communication and control. Chapter 19 reviews the anatomy and physiology of the nervous system.

DIAGNOSTIC TESTS

Many diagnostic tests are used to determine the integrity or functioning of the nervous system.

Visualization Procedures

Numerous tests can be used to visualize nervous system structures. Two commonly used tests are *computerized tomography* (CT) scan, a test that incorporates x-rays and computer technology to produce an image of a transverse body plane; and *magnetic resonance imaging* (MRI), a test that uses a powerful magnetic field to align hydrogen nuclei, which emit signals that are converted into precise images. An MRI can distinguish between normal and abnormal tissues in all parts of the body, even identifying chemical changes within cells. MRI is helpful in identifying cerebrovascular accidents (CVAs) and cancerous lesions before clinical signs and symptoms appear. It is particularly sensitive in identifying multiple sclerosis plaques and other abnormal changes in demyelinating diseases. (See Chapter 47 for more detailed information about these tests.) Other visualization procedures may include positron emission tomography, cerebral angiography and arteriography, myelography, and brain scan.

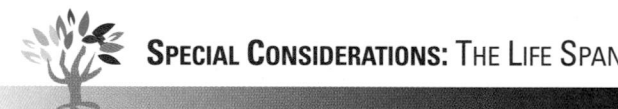

SPECIAL CONSIDERATIONS: THE LIFE SPAN

CT and MRI Scans and Children

A child may be permitted to take a favorite toy or blanket along for the test. For an MRI, make sure the toy contains no metal. Also, because sedation is often required, the child's safety must be maintained.

Positron Emission Tomography

Positron emission tomography (PET) is a type of tomography used to study changes within the brain. Glucose containing a radioisotope is injected into the brain. After the scan, the client remains flat in bed for a few hours and is observed for signs of irritation, such as a stiff neck or pain when bending the head forward. The client is also observed for signs of *anaphylaxis* (severe allergic response).

Cerebral Angiography and Arteriography

In some instances, angiography or arteriography may be performed. An *angiogram* is an x-ray study of any blood vessel,

and an *arteriogram* is an x-ray study of an artery. The procedure involves injecting a radiopaque substance into the carotid or femoral artery. X-rays films are then taken of the brain's blood vessels to detect any abnormalities. Be alert for any signs of allergy to the drug injected for the test. If severe anaphylaxis occurs in a client, it usually occurs immediately.

SPECIAL CONSIDERATIONS: THE LIFE SPAN

Dye Procedures and the Older Adult

Monitor the older adult client's blood urea nitrogen (BUN) and creatinine before and after any procedure that uses dye. The aging population is at increased risk for kidney damage; promptly report any elevations in BUN and creatinine.

Prior to the procedure, obtain a baseline neurologic assessment. A possibility exists that a thrombus can become dislodged, causing an embolus. An embolus could travel to the heart, lung, or brain. During the procedure, also observe for symptoms of muscular weakness, twitching in the face or extremities, and respiratory difficulties. If any of these occur, notify the healthcare provider immediately.

After the procedure, a sandbag or a pressure device (FemoStop) is applied to the insertion site to reduce edema and to prevent bleeding and hematoma formation. Check the area for bleeding every 15 to 30 minutes for several hours. Observe the leg's color, temperature, and pedal pulse if the femoral artery was used as the injection site. Because of the radiopaque dye used, encourage fluids, unless contraindicated.

Nursing Alert

If you cannot find a pulse distal to the injection site, or if active bleeding occurs, notify the healthcare provider immediately.

Myelography

In some cases, a *myelogram* is performed to visualize the spinal cord. However, this test is less commonly used if CT or MRI scanning is available. A lumbar puncture is done and a radiopaque substance is injected into the spinal canal. The client, in the prone position, is tilted so that dye flows around the spinal cord; then x-ray films are taken to detect tumors or a ruptured intervertebral disk. The radiopaque substances used today are water soluble and reabsorbed into the body with little, if any, side effects.

Brain Scan

A *brain scan* involves the injection of a radioactive substance (*radioisotope*), which is then detected by a scanner that generates images as the substance circulates within the brain vasculature. This test is used to evaluate vascular lesions, neoplasms, abscesses, and areas of cerebrovascular ischemia. The rationale for this procedure is that the radioisotope will accumulate in a greater amount at a site of pathology than at normal brain tissue.

Other Diagnostic Tests

Lumbar Puncture

The *lumbar puncture* (**LP**, *spinal tap*) involves the insertion of a hollow needle with a *stylet* (guide) into the subarachnoid space of the lumbar region of the spinal canal, using strict aseptic technique. An LP may be performed to:

* Measure pressure of cerebrospinal fluid (**CSF**)
* Obtain a sample of CSF for culture and sensitivity, blood, pus, or other substance levels (eg, protein, glucose, red blood cells, white blood cells)
* Inject an anesthetic or other drug
* Inject air for special tests

After LP, complications may occur, including the following:

* Severe pounding headache, unrelieved by mild analgesics
* Malaise
* Nausea, with or without vomiting
* Irritation/hematoma at injection site
* Leg or buttock pain (temporary)
* Central nervous system (**CNS**) infection
* Brain herniation (most severe complication, but extremely rare)
* Paralysis (spinal cord injury, which is very rare)

> **✚👁 Nursing Alert**
> Document the client's ability to move all extremities before and after the procedure. If the spinal catheter goes too far, it can damage the spinal cord.

A physician performs the LP under strict sterile conditions. Nurses play a role in assisting with the procedure (see In Practice: Nursing Procedure 77-1).

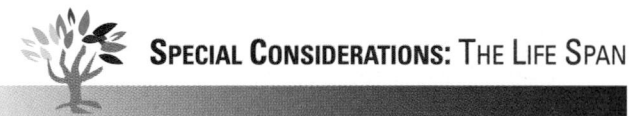

Special Considerations: The Life Span

Lumbar Puncture in Children

Expect the need to hold young children in the proper position for LP, because often they are extremely frightened by someone who is doing something to their back and cannot be seen. They may try to turn over to see what is happening. Sometimes family caregivers are willing to hold the child, which may be less frightening to the child. Because needles are smaller, insertion may be easier in children.

Electroencephalography

Electroencephalography (**EEG**) records the brain's electrical impulses as a graph. This test is used frequently in the diagnosis of seizure disorders, brain tumors, blood clots, infections, and sleep disorders. Another important use of the EEG is to confirm brain death (*electrocerebral silence*).

Electrodes are placed on the client's forehead and scalp by means of a special glue called *collodion;* these electrodes are connected to the machine. In some cases, a cap containing the electrodes is placed on the head; a few clinics use tiny needles. The procedure is painless, has no aftereffects, and requires 1 to 2 hours to conduct.

In preparation for an EEG, the client may be requested not to sleep the night before the test (for a *sleeping EEG*), or he or she may receive sedation (for a *resting EEG*).

Explain to the client that no electric shock will be given and that the EEG procedure cannot determine thoughts or mental ability. Tell the person that he or she will be asked to open and close the eyes and sometimes to perform other movements on command.

In some cases, lights will be flashed, the client will be asked to watch a repeating pattern on a television monitor, or a small electrical stimulus will be given. The brain's responses to these stimuli are recorded. These responses are called *evoked responses* or *evoked potentials.*

If needles are used, there is a slight possibility of infection. After the procedure, the client may need a shampoo to remove collodion.

Videotelemetry Monitoring

Healthcare facilities specializing in neurology and seizure disorders use a diagnostic tool called *videotelemetry monitoring.* It involves video, audio, and EEG monitoring of a person 24 hours a day or all night. When the client experiences a seizure, it can be seen and heard on videotape as well as recorded electrically by EEG.

Seizure precautions are initiated to protect the client from injury. In addition, the client should wear a pajama bottom with a gown for protection of modesty. To allow for visualization of extremities, which may be indicators of the types of seizures, make sure that the client is uncovered, so that these areas can be seen. In addition, make sure the client is within camera range, so the event will be filmed.

NURSING PROCESS

Data Collection

Chapter 47 describes a head-to-toe assessment, including that of the nervous system. This assessment establishes a baseline for future comparison. Report any changes in the baseline level.

Change in behaviors, mentation, level of consciousness (**LOC**), alertness, and orientation could be significant, but subtle. For example, perhaps a client has been alert and cooperative with caregivers. At a later time, however, the nurse notices that this client is irritable and less cooperative. This change of action and behavior could be relevant. The nurse needs to gather further data to determine if the change could be due to a physical dysfunction, such as an embolus in the brain; meta-

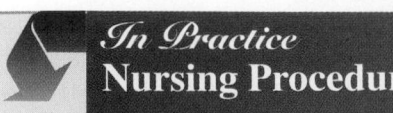

In Practice
Nursing Procedure 77-1

ASSISTING WITH A LUMBAR PUNCTURE

Supplies and Equipment

Sterile gloves
Dressing materials
Local anesthetic solution (sterile), usually lidocaine
   (Xylocaine)
Bath blanket
Prepackaged sterile, disposable LP kit
Clean gloves
Antiseptic solution
Specimen labels
External light source (may be needed)

Steps

1. Be sure the procedure has been thoroughly
   explained to the client and make sure that the client
   has signed the consent form. (Nursing students do
   not witness these permits.)
   RATIONALE: *An LP is an invasive procedure. Informed
   consent is legally required.*

2. Wash hands. Assemble all equipment at the bedside.
   RATIONALE: *Handwashing helps prevent the spread
   of microorganisms; organization of equipment
   maximizes efficiency. Know that the physician
   will wear sterile gloves and may use goggles or
   a face shield, per Standard Precautions.*

3. Identify the client and ask the client to empty the
   bladder.
   RATIONALE: *Proper identification of the client is
   essential to ensure that the procedure is completed for the correct person. Emptying the
   bladder helps the client avoid the discomfort of
   a full bladder.*

4. Assess the client's vital signs before the procedure.
   RATIONALE: *Obtaining vital signs before the procedure provides a baseline assessment for later
   comparison.*

5. Assist the client with removing any clothing and
   putting on a gown that opens in the back. Drape
   the client with a bath blanket or sheet.
   RATIONALE: *The gown provides easy access to the
   proper site. Draping provides privacy and
   warmth, if needed.*

6. Place equipment within the physician's reach.
   Open packs and make sure extra sterile gloves are
   available. Provide extra lighting as necessary.
   RATIONALE: *Organizing supplies and equipment
   enhances efficiency.*

7. Position the client on his or her side with the
   lower part of the back at the edge of the bed. Help
   the client to draw his or her knees up toward the
   chin and to bend his or her head forward.

RATIONALE: *This position increases the space
between the lower vertebrae, making needle
insertion easier.*

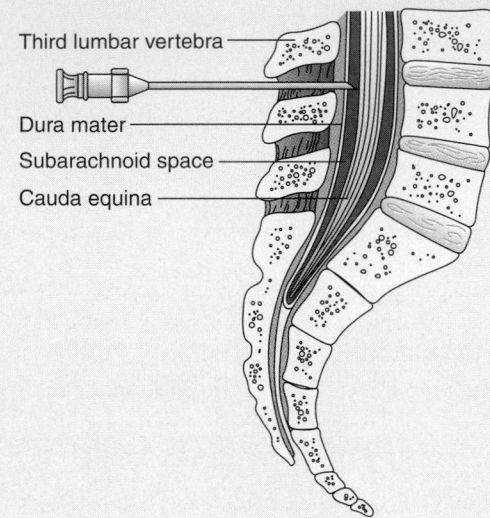

The needle is inserted into the subarachnoid space
above L4.

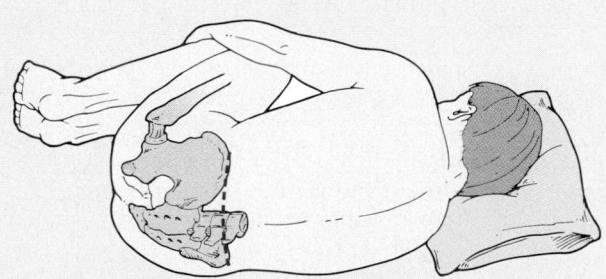

The intervertebral spaces between the spines of L3 and L4 are just
below a line drawn between the anterosuperior iliac spines of the
pelvis.

8. When the procedure begins, move the drape
   to uncover the client's back. Tell the person to
   lie very still, holding the client in place if
   necessary.
   RATIONALE: *Any sudden movement is dangerous
   and could cause spinal cord damage.*

9. Talk to the client during the procedure, offering
   reassurance as necessary.
   RATIONALE: *This procedure can be frightening. The
   client needs to relax and remain still.*

10. Assist as requested, such as with removing caps
    on bottles, labeling specimens, or assisting with
    dressing placement over the LP site.
    RATIONALE: *The procedure must be done using
    strict aseptic technique. Assistance helps to
    minimize the possibility of contamination.*

In Practice
Nursing Procedure 77-1 (*Continued*)

11. Note the beginning CSF pressure, as measured by the physician. Also assess the color and clarity of the CSF, which should be pale and clear.
    RATIONALE: *This information is important in determining the client's disorder.*

12. Monitor the client for any difficulties or problems.
    RATIONALE: *Untoward side effects are rare, but they can occur.*

13. After the procedure, return the client to a comfortable position in bed. Keep the client's head flat (supine) for at least 6 hours, or as otherwise ordered.
    RATIONALE: *Proper positioning promotes comfort while also decreasing the possibility of CSF leakage and postpuncture headache.*

14. Remove and dispose of equipment as indicated. Finish labeling specimens and completing request forms; send specimens to the laboratory immediately in an approved biohazard bag. Properly dispose of gloves. Wash hands. Document the procedure carefully.
    RATIONALE: *Proper disposal of equipment and supplies helps reduce the risk of infection.*

Documentation helps promote communication and continuity of care.

15. Assess the client's vital signs and neurologic signs, comparing them with baseline data. Assess the client's level of consciousness. Report any unusual findings to the physician.
    RATIONALE: *Assessment is necessary to determine any possible side effects the client experiences from the procedure.*

16. Encourage fluids (unless contraindicated) and record I&O. Encourage the client to lie flat.
    RATIONALE: *Rehydrating the client is important, to replace any fluids lost during the procedure; fluids and not elevating the head help minimize headache.*

17. Monitor the insertion site for leakage of CSF, hematoma formation, or edema.
    RATIONALE: *These are possible unwanted results of LP.*

18. Assess severity of headache if it occurs. Report severe headache unrelieved by mild analgesics or lasting more than 24 hours.
    RATIONALE: *Headache may signify potential complications.*

bolic causes, such as low blood sugar; or effects of prescribed medications.

Assess the client's general appearance, mobility level, LOC, muscle tone, strength, balance, coordination, protective reflexes, eye signs, and function of some cranial nerves. In Practice: Nursing Assessment 77-1 lists some of the major components of a neurologic nursing assessment.

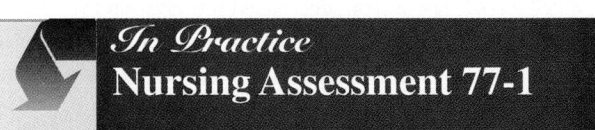

In Practice
Nursing Assessment 77-1

KEY COMPONENTS OF A NEUROLOGIC ASSESSMENT
- Neurologic nursing history, including history as given by family
- Speech patterns
- Level of consciousness (LOC) (particularly changes in LOC)
- Neurologic status, using the Glasgow Coma Scale
- Gross evaluation of muscle tone/strength
- Overview of balance, coordination, and protective reflexes
- Overview of sensory function
- Signs of increased intracranial pressure (↑ICP)
- Function of selected cranial nerves
- Eye signs (sizes in pupillary size and response)

Additionally, observe the client's emotional response to the situation. Does the disorder affect social activities, self-care, and self-esteem? Does the client seem anxious or fearful of outcome?

Nursing Diagnosis

Most nursing diagnoses result from specific neurologic dysfunctions. Some diagnoses may be the same but with different causal factors (see "Imbalanced Nutrition" below). Examples of nursing diagnoses that may appear on nursing care plans of clients with disorders of the nervous system include the following:

- Self-Care Deficit related to sensory and/or motor deficits
- Social Isolation related to unpredictability of seizures
- Ineffective Health Maintenance related to insufficient knowledge of condition and treatment
- Chronic Low Self-Esteem related to changes in body image
- Risk for Disuse Syndrome related to effects of immobility
- Fear related to changes in role responsibilities
- Anxiety related to threat to self-concept
- Imbalanced Nutrition: Less Than Body Requirements related to (1) difficulty in obtaining and preparing food, (2) chewing and swallowing difficulties
- Risk for Infection related to invasive procedures, immobility

- Hopelessness related to deteriorating physiologic condition
- Risk for Injury related to unsteady gait, uncontrolled movements
- Activity Intolerance related to generalized weakness
- Ineffective Cerebral Tissue Perfusion related to stroke, aneurysm, or vasospasm

Planning and Implementation

The healthcare team plans together with the client and family for effective care to meet the client's needs. The client with a neurologic disorder may need help with activities of daily living (ADL), exercises, body alignment and position, elimination, nutrition, and sensory and emotional problems. He or she will need to learn more about the disorder, its prognosis, and its treatment. An individualized nursing care plan is developed to meet these needs.

Assisting With ADL.   The client may need assistance with ADL: skin care, special eye care, mouth care, care of the nails and hair (see Chap. 50), and management of bowel or bladder elimination (see Chap. 51). Be sure to help the client maintain adequate nutritional status to rebuild strength and to prevent further deterioration (see Chap. 32).

Providing Exercise.   The client with impaired mobility needs as much active and passive exercise as possible to prevent contractures, muscle atrophy, and other disuse deformities. Clients who are paralyzed or otherwise physically challenged can use many assistive devices, including lifts, wheelchairs, braces, and splints (see Chaps. 48 and 95).

Providing Comfort With Special Devices.   Clients with neurologic disorders who are immobilized may need to use a special bed, such as Clinitron, the Restcue, or the Kin-Air bed. The most important goals of these specialized beds are to prevent skin breakdown and alleviate pain. For example, the Kin-Air operates on the principle of varying levels of air inflation. It has many configurations for optimum comfort and safety. Follow the manufacturer's specifications when using any of these special beds.

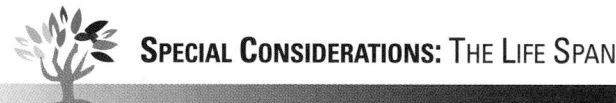

SPECIAL CONSIDERATIONS: THE LIFE SPAN

Skin Care and Special Devices

Often the skin of older adults is very fragile (*friable*), which can increase the client's risk for skin breakdown. Specialized beds or mattresses may be routinely ordered for older clients with fragile skin and neurologic conditions.

Special "neuro chairs" also help to transfer clients in and out of bed and serve as a comfortable place for the client to rest when out of bed. These chairs adjust to various positions and can be placed in high Fowler's or Trendelenburg positions when necessary. Various commercial reclining chairs are also available. When assisting a client to move from the bed to the neuro chair and back, use good body mechanics and place the bed and chair in the flat position and raise both to high position. Maintain the client's safety by locking the wheels of the chair and bed, obtaining additional help to move the client, using safety devices as necessary, and placing the call light within the client's reach.

Evaluation

Periodically the nurse, client, and family evaluate outcomes of care. Have short-term goals been met? For example, is the client able to participate in self-care? Are long-term goals still realistic, especially if the client has a progressive neurologic disorder? Planning for further nursing care must consider prognosis, complications, and the client's response.

CRANIOCEREBRAL DISORDERS

Headaches

Headaches can range in intensity from minor discomfort to extreme pain. Some people suffer from chronic headaches. The most common types are discussed here.

Symptomatic Headache

Cephalgia (headache) is one of the most common symptoms of a neurologic disorder. It is also associated with many other diseases and disorders. Headache is not a disease in itself, but rather it is a symptom of an underlying disorder. Do not confuse the occasional headache that disappears after taking an analgesic with persistent headaches that require further evaluation.

Headaches often appear with conditions such as eye strain, sinusitis, muscle strain, ligament strain, cervical degenerative changes, emotional tension, and stress. It is also associated with brain tumors, hypertension, and *increased intracranial pressure* (↑**ICP**) (see section on "Increased Intracranial Pressure"). Persistent or recurring headaches are frequently associated with true neurologic diseases or disorders, such as brain tumors and aneurysms.

Diagnosis of headaches is made by medical history, family history, and evaluation of the individual patterns of the headaches. Any history of trauma is relevant. Knowledge of changes in behaviors or LOC is particularly important. X-ray examinations of the head and sinuses; food elimination diets (particularly dairy and cheese products); and diagnostic scans such as CT, MRI, or PET can also help to determine the cause of the pain.

Nonjudgmental acknowledgment of the individual's pain is essential, because pain thresholds differ among clients. The nurse may assist by educating the client and family in the various treatment alternatives presented by the healthcare provider. Offer analgesics as needed (PRN) and encourage compliance with the medication regimen. If the headache is triggered by foods, major changes in eating habits may be necessary.

Migraine Headache

The specific cause of *migraine headache* is not known but appears to result from a vascular disturbance in which the brain's blood vessels dilate abnormally. Migraine headaches are also called *vascular headaches.*

The person may have sensory warnings or premonitions (**aura**) that a headache will occur. Various auras include mood changes, anorexia, numbness of a body part, or visual symptoms, such as flashing lights or floating spots. Later, the person will experience unilateral throbbing or steady pain, sometimes accompanied by nausea and vomiting.

Migraine headaches are common in families; they occur more frequently in people who have asthma, hay fever, and food allergies. Stress may bring on migraine headaches. Other triggers include caffeine (or its sudden withdrawal), nicotine, cheese, alcohol, and certain food preservatives (such as monosodium glutamate). Fasting and missing meals may serve as triggers, as may premenstrual fluid retention. Certain drugs, including oral contraceptives and reserpine (Serpasil), an antihypertensive agent, also may be triggers.

In some cases, if treated immediately, the painful experience of the headache can be prevented through various strategies, including relaxation exercises, biofeedback, and some types of medications. Sometimes, an ice pack applied to the back of the neck or at the base of the skull helps to ease pain. Acupuncture also has been helpful to many people. Medications also may be used to treat migraine headaches (see In Practice: Important Medications 77-1).

Cluster Headache

Cluster (histamine) headaches receive their name because they tend to occur in groups or clusters, often at night. Like

migraines, they seem to result from vascular disturbances. These headaches can be severely disabling. They are more common in men than in women.

A cluster headache occurs suddenly and severely, often affecting only one side and involving the eye, neck, and face on that side. The eye may appear to bulge, and other symptoms of vasodilation are seen such as edema, *lacrimation* (tear formation), **rhinorrhea** (runny nose), *diaphoresis* (sweating), and flushing of the affected side. The pupil constricts, and the face and head are sensitive to external touch. The condition may disappear as suddenly as it occurs, although it may continue for several days. Although no specific cure is known, some drugs have been effective in selected cases. These drugs include vasoconstrictor drugs, corticosteroids, and indomethacin (Indocin).

Seizure Disorders

A **seizure,** also known as a *convulsion,* is an episode of abnormal motor, sensory, cognitive, and psychic activity caused by erratic and abnormal electrical discharges of brain cells. Repeated episodes of seizures are called *seizure disorders.* Most seizures are self-limiting and benign, lasting a few seconds to a few minutes. Many individuals may manifest different types of seizures at different times.

Epilepsy is the term used to describe any recurrent pattern of seizures. In most cases, the cause of seizures is unknown. Some known causes include birth trauma, genetic predisposition, head injuries, some types of brain infections and abscesses, toxicity, fever, metabolic and nutritional disorders, tumors, or brain malformations.

Status epilepticus refers to a seizure or a series of seizures, lasting 30 minutes or longer, in which the person does not regain consciousness. Any type of seizure can develop into status epilepticus. The most common types of seizures are discussed below.

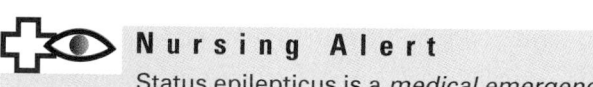

Nursing Alert

Status epilepticus is a *medical emergency.*

Classification

Seizures are classified based on the clinical nature of the seizure's onset: partial, general, or unclassified. Seizures may not be simply of one type: Some seizures begin with one type and progress to another. Partial and general seizures are discussed below. With *unclassified seizures,* the origin of the abnormal electrical activity is not known.

The duration of the seizure is called the *ictal phase.* The period following the seizure is called the *postictal phase.* During the postictal phase, the person may be confused or fall into a deep sleep lasting minutes or hours. Box 77-1 summarizes the classification of seizures.

Partial Seizures.   *Partial seizures* are characterized by abnormal electrical activity involving only one **focus** (point of origin) or lobe of the brain. A partial seizure may also be called a *focal seizure* because of its origination at such a **focal**

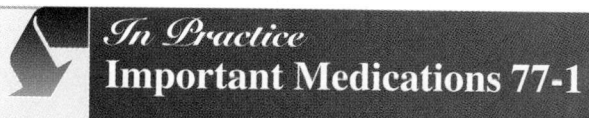

In Practice
Important Medications 77-1

FOR MIGRAINE HEADACHE

- General analgesics: Codeine, ASA (aspirin), ibuprofen (Advil, Motrin), and acetaminophen (Tylenol)
- Combination drugs: Acetaminophen and other drugs (such as Darvon compound)
- Vasoconstrictors or drugs that prevent vasodilation: Ergot alkaloids
- Oxygen
- Other agents: Sumatriptan (Imitrex), self-administered subcutaneously or orally by client at home; propranolol HCl (Inderal); mild diuretics (to control fluid retention associated with menses)

Nursing Considerations
- Some of these drugs, particularly vasoconstrictors, have unpleasant side effects.
- All of these drugs are most effective if given immediately at the first sign of a headache.

➤➤ **BOX 77-1**

CLASSIFICATION OF SEIZURES

Partial or Focal Seizures

A *partial simple* seizure usually results in no loss of consciousness.

- Jacksonian—Rhythmic jerking movements start in one muscle group and spread.
- Adversive—Person may become combative.
- Sensory—Person has unpleasant hallucinations, talks unintelligibly, or experiences vertigo.

A *partial complex* seizure results in impaired consciousness: Person may be motionless or have repetitive movements.

General Seizures

A *general seizure* involves both hemispheres of the brain.

- Tonic-clonic seizures (grand mal)
- Absence seizures (petit mal)
- Tonic seizures
- Atonic seizures
- Infantile spasms
- Myoclonic seizures

Unclassified Epileptic Seizures

Unclassified seizures include all seizures that cannot be classified, due to inadequate or incomplete data.

Adapted from Epilepsy Foundation (2002). Available: *http://www. epa.org* and National Institute of Neurological Disorder and Stroke (2001). Available: *http://www.ninds.nih.gov.*

point. Partial seizures are classified as either simple or complex.

In a *simple partial seizure,* the person usually remains conscious and may have motor, sensory, or autonomic symptoms. During a simple partial seizure, a rhythmic jerking movement begins in one part of the body. The individual is aware that a seizure is occurring, and is unable to stop or control the movement. The seizure is usually brief, lasting less than a minute.

In a *complex partial seizure,* generally consciousness is impaired and cognitive, affective, or behavioral symptoms occur. Complex partial seizures are characterized by motionlessness, or repetitive movements such as lip smacking, chewing or swallowing movements, picking at clothes, or rubbing the nose. After a complex partial seizure, the individual usually experiences a period of confusion and does not remember the incident.

Generalized seizures. *Generalized seizures* are characterized by abnormal electrical activity throughout an entire hemisphere or both hemispheres of the brain. Generalized seizures involve the entire body and brain, with the same motor symptoms on both sides. Generalized seizures can take several forms. Any of these generalized seizure types may occur individually or in clusters.

A *grand mal* or *tonic-clonic seizure* is the most commonly known type of seizure. At the onset of the seizure, the individual may cry out and experience an aura, knowing that a seizure is imminent. The seizure may commence with the person falling down because of brief loss of muscle tone (**flaccidity**). Rigid contraction of body muscles (**tonic phase**), which alternates with rhythmic jerking movements (**clonic phase**), follows. The tonic-clonic or grand mal seizure is perhaps the most life-threatening type of seizure.

Absence seizures, also known as *petit mal seizures,* are characterized by an altered LOC that lasts no longer than about 10 seconds, evidenced as a blank or vacant stare. A warning aura does not typically occur. Loss of muscle tone or minor muscle twitching (*myoclonus*) of the neck and upper extremities occasionally occur. The face may have symmetrical twitching. Return of consciousness is rapid. The individual is unaware that the seizure has occurred, and afterward continues with whatever activity he or she was performing.

Absence seizures may be difficult to spot because the individual appears to be daydreaming. An affected individual can experience as many as 100 absence seizures in a day. They are most commonly seen in children and during the onset of puberty in adolescents.

Other types of generalized seizures include the following:

- A *tonic seizure* is similar to the generalized tonic-clonic seizure but with tonic contractions only. The seizure usually lasts for shorter time periods than tonic-clonic seizures.
- In *atonic seizures,* the muscles become momentarily flaccid and the individual drops to the floor.
- *Infantile spasms* are characterized in infants by clusters of rapid spasm-like movements of the extremities, with neck flexion and arm extension. More than 90% of infants who have infantile spasms have mental deficiencies.
- *Myoclonic seizures* are quick, often repetitive muscle jerks of a single group of muscles, involving the extremities and facial muscles or the entire body. The client may fall but does not lose consciousness.

Diagnostic Tests

Diagnosis of seizure disorders is made based on the client's history, physical examination, laboratory tests, and EEG findings. An accurate description of the seizure itself is essential to identifying the type of seizure and appropriate treatment.

The EEG is a useful diagnostic tool because different seizure types produce specific electrical wave patterns. Just because the EEG looks normal, does not necessarily mean that the person is not experiencing seizures. Videotelemetry monitoring is helpful to the physician in diagnosing the specific seizure type.

☛ KEY CONCEPT

The EEG of a person with a seizure disorder may look normal, especially if no seizure occurs at the time of the EEG.

Other diagnostic procedures may include:

- CT scan and MRI to identify a tumor, bleeding, or a brain lesion
- Angiogram to differentiate between brain tumor and blood-vessel malformation
- Blood work to indicate electrolyte imbalance, drug toxicity, or underlying disorders

Medical and Surgical Treatment

The primary treatment of seizures is pharmacologic therapy with a group of medications referred to as *anticonvulsant drugs*. These drugs work by raising the individual's seizure threshold. Choice of drugs is based on the type of seizure the person experiences. Sometimes several drugs are combined to control the seizures. Routine blood levels of the drug are monitored to ensure a therapeutic dose. If the person is experiencing status epilepticus, anticonvulsant drugs are typically given intravenously (IV) (see In Practice: Important Medications 77-2).

Surgery may be performed in certain circumstances in which the seizure's focal point can be clearly identified in the brain. Electrodes are placed directly on the brain to obtain more specific information as to where the seizure originates. Brain tissue that is thought to initiate the seizure is removed. The neurosurgeon must take great care to protect healthy brain tissue from damage during surgery. A procedure called *brain mapping* is done before surgery to identify the important brain structures to avoid.

Nursing Considerations

When a client with a history of seizures or of taking certain medications is admitted to a healthcare facility, he or she is placed on *seizure precautions,* an expression implying that

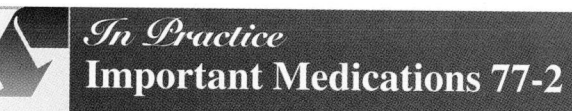

In Practice
Important Medications 77-2

FOR STATUS EPILEPTICUS

- Diazepam (Valium)
- Lorazepam (Ativan)
- Phenobarbital (Luminal)
- Phenytoin (Dilantin)
- Thiopental sodium (Pentothal)

Nursing Considerations

- Keep in mind that when these drugs are given IV for status epilepticus, there is danger of overdose.
- Be alert for CNS signs (such as drowsiness and lethargy), for respiratory depression, and for cardiovascular signs, which may range from hypotension to cardiovascular collapse.
- Monitor kidney function. Some of these drugs may also cause kidney damage.

staff must take special steps to ensure that injury does not result from a seizure. Figure 77-1 illustrates seizure precautions. Necessary equipment should include the following:

- *Oral airway Rationale: It assists in maintaining a patent airway.* Note: Do not insert if seizure activity has already begun.
- *Suction setup Rationale: This is useful if the client has difficulty in handling secretions.*
- Setup of *piggyback port* on an open IV *Rationale: This provides a ready access if the client needs emergency drugs.*
- *Rectal* or *tympanic temperature probe Rationale: Oral thermometers are unsafe to use.*
- *Raised and padded side rails* (all four rails) *Rationale: Raised side rails prevent falls and promote safety.*

The staff must tailor precautions to the type of seizure the client experiences. In Practice: Nursing Care Guidelines 77-1 highlights important measures to ensure the client's safety.

Careful documentation of the seizure helps in identifying the origin of the seizure and developing a treatment plan. Some facilities have an event form on which to document all seizures.

Documentation must include what the person was doing at the seizure's onset, where the seizure began, if and how the person fell, time of day, triggering events, seizure progression and symmetry, eye response, responsiveness, results of commands and memory tests, duration, direction of eye gaze and eye movements, confusion, incontinence, drooling, and diaphoresis. Document what the client says about the seizure and how he or she behaves; check eye signs and LOC. Describe clusters of seizures.

⊁ Nursing Alert

The nurse's role during a seizure is to protect and observe. During a seizure, observe the client for respiratory depression and have emergency airway equipment readily available.

Client and family teaching for seizure disorders is essential. In Practice: Educating the Client 77-1 lists the important topics to address when teaching about seizures. The client needs to know how to adapt his or her lifestyle to the disorder, living as normally as possible. Most people with seizure disorders have seizures that are controlled with medication. Individuals and family members must understand the importance of regular medication administration and periodic medical evaluations.

Cerebrovascular Accident

A sudden or gradual interruption of blood supply to a vital center in the brain is a *cerebrovascular accident* (CVA), also known as a *stroke,* a *brain attack,* or a *central vascular accident.* A CVA may cause complete or partial paralysis or death. CVAs are the third leading cause of death in America. Because the underlying cause of this disorder often involves atherosclerosis of the cerebral blood vessels, this disorder is dis-

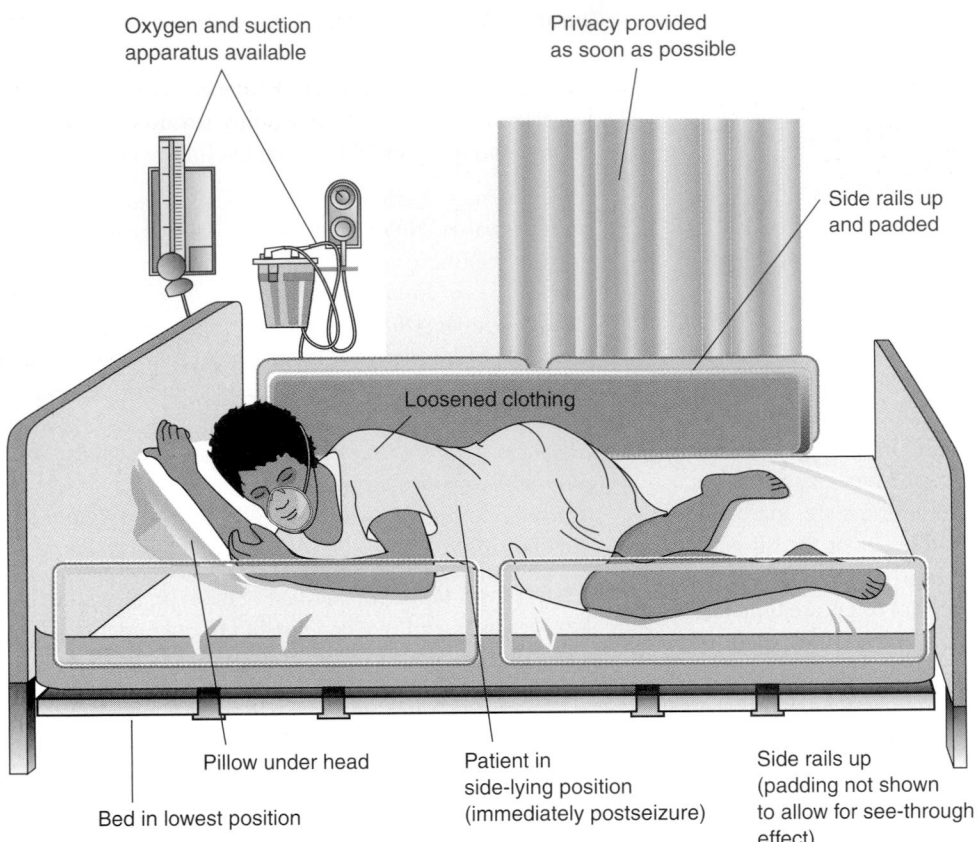

Oxygen and suction apparatus available

Privacy provided as soon as possible

Side rails up and padded

Loosened clothing

Pillow under head

Bed in lowest position

Patient in side-lying position (immediately postseizure)

Side rails up (padding not shown to allow for see-through effect)

FIGURE 77-1. This client unit is set up for seizure precautions. After a seizure, the client is placed in a protective position.

In Practice
Nursing Care Guidelines 77-1

MAINTAINING THE CLIENT'S SAFETY DURING A SEIZURE

- Protect the client from nearby hazards. Move the overbed tray table and other dangerous items away from the client. *Rationale: The client will be unable to control muscle movements or reactions during the seizure.*
- Loosen restrictive clothing, such as a client's tie or shirt collar. *Rationale: Loosening clothing helps to maintain an unobstructed airway.*
- Do not place anything in the person's mouth after a seizure has begun. *Rationale: Doing do could cause the client's teeth to break by forcing an object into the mouth.*
- Do not attempt to restrain the client. *Rationale: Injury may result from forcible restraint against the contraction of the muscles.*
- Place a small soft padding beneath the client's head, such as a folded jacket. *Rationale: Padding the area helps to protect the head from injury.*
- Turn the client's head to the side. *Rationale: Turning the client's head to the side helps to maintain a clear airway and prevent aspiration.*
- Monitor the seizure activity and location carefully. Note the exact time the seizure begins and ends. Test the extremity strength and tone. *Rationale: This information is important to aid in determining the type of seizure that the client experienced.*

- Call the client's name. Give a simple command, such as asking him or her to grab your hand and to let go. *Rationale: Responses to these evaluative techniques assists in evaluating the type and severity of the seizure.*
- Give the client a "memory test" by asking him or her to remember two unrelated words. *Rationale: Whether or not the client is able to remember the words helps provide additional information about the type of seizure.*
- After the seizure, ask the client if there was an *aura* (warning). *Rationale: The client may learn to take protective measures before a seizure occurs.*
- Check the tongue and oral cavity for any bite injuries. *Rationale: The client may have injured him- or herself during the seizure; evidence of injury indicates a need for treatment.*
- Observe and document carefully. *Rationale: Documentation helps to provide communication and assists healthcare personnel in treating the client.*
- Offer reassurance and emotional support. *Rationale: Seizures can be frightening to the client and to those who witnessed the seizure. The client is often embarrassed and may have been incontinent or confused.*

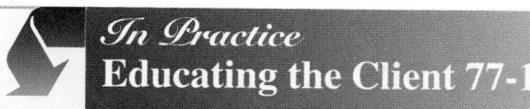

In Practice
Educating the Client 77-1

TEACHING TOPICS TO ADDRESS FOR
SEIZURE DISORDERS

- Explanation of seizure disorder
- Specific information about the particular seizure type the client experienced
- Safety and prevention of injury during a seizure
- Care of the client during and after a seizure
- Importance of taking medications as prescribed
- Medication side effects
- Importance of family observation of seizure, so they can fully describe it to the neurologist
- Importance of adequate sleep, balanced diet, and suitable physical activities
- Avoidance of situations that can precipitate a seizure
- Importance of wearing a Medic-Alert tag and regular followup with physician
- Importance of having blood drawn to determine blood levels of antiepileptic medications

cussed in detail in Chapter 80. In Practice: Nursing Care Plan 77-1 addresses the client experiencing hemiplegia resulting from a CVA.

NERVE DISORDERS

Neuralgia

The term **neuralgia** literally means "pain in a nerve." Neuralgia often applies to fleeting pain in the shoulder and upper arm or pain caused by a herniated intervertebral disk. If application of external heat and administration of analgesics, such as aspirin, do not relieve the pain, medical evaluation is needed.

Trigeminal Neuralgia

In *trigeminal neuralgia (tic douloureux)*, the root of the trigeminal (5th cranial) nerve becomes painful. The cause is unknown and it generally occurs in the older population. The pain is excruciating and comes in spasms that can last for seconds to hours, occurring in the jaw and parts of the face.

The pain may be triggered by the slightest touch to various parts of the face, or even by a breeze, a change in tem-

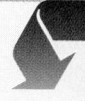

In Practice
Nursing Care Plan 77-1

THE CLIENT WITH A CVA AND HEMIPLEGIA

MEDICAL HISTORY: *I.K., a 55-year-old African American female with a history of hypertension, was admitted to the hospital 3 days ago with a left-sided CVA resulting from cerebral thrombosis. Client has right-sided hemiplegia.*

MEDICAL DIAGNOSIS: *Left CVA, right hemiplegia*

Data Collection/Nursing Assessment: Client is alert and oriented to person, place, time, and situation. Vital signs within acceptable parameters. Slight residual slurring of speech is noted. Gag reflex is intact. Client demonstrates ability to swallow without problems. Client is able to tolerate small amounts of liquids by mouth, approximately 30 to 45 cc's at one time. IV is infusing at a rate of 125 cc's per hour. Right side flaccid and weak. Client is right handed and uses left side to move extremities on the right. Currently, she requires moderate assistance with self-care. Skin inspection reveals quarter-sized reddened areas on right elbow and heel. Urine output is approximately 350 cc's over the past 8 hours. Urine is clear and yellow. Client moved bowels 2 days ago. Scattered crackles auscultated at both bases that clear with coughing. Client lives with 60-year-old husband in a two-story home in the country. Her daughter and son live approximately 20 minutes

away by car. *(Although other nursing diagnoses may be appropriate, a priority nursing diagnosis is addressed below.)*

Nursing Diagnosis: Risk for disuse syndrome related to hemiplegia as evidenced by right-sided flaccidity and weakness and reddened areas on heel and elbow.

Planning
SHORT-TERM GOALS:
#1. Client will exhibit no further evidence of potential skin breakdown.
#2. Client will verbalize measures to reduce or prevent hazards of immobility.

LONG-TERM GOALS:
#3. Client actively participates in measures to reduce or prevent complications.
#4. Client remains free of hazards of immobility.

Implementation
NURSING ACTION: *Change the client's position frequently and provide passive and active range of motion. Encourage the use of a trapeze bar applied to the bed.*
RATIONALE: *Frequent position changes help to prevent disorders caused by immobility–disuse disorders.*

(continued)

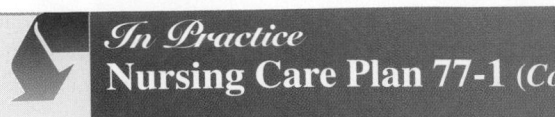

Use of trapeze bar allows the client to assist with position changes and to reduce the shearing forces that can lead to skin breakdown.

NURSING ACTION: *Use special devices, such as pressure relief pads or specialized beds, trochanter rolls, and sandbags as necessary.*
RATIONALE: *These devices help to maintain proper body alignment and positioning, thus helping to prevent orthopedic deformities and minimizing the risk of skin breakdown.*

NURSING ACTION: *Provide special skin care, using lotions and emollients. Make sure the sheets are smooth and the bed is clean.*
RATIONALE: *The skin of the client with hemiplegia is subject to pressure areas and skin breakdown.*

NURSING ACTION: *Protect bony areas from pressure, especially those areas on the left side.*
RATIONALE: *Pressure on bony prominences increases the client's risk for skin breakdown. The client's left-sided hemiplegia contributes to this risk.*

Evaluation: Reddened areas on elbow and heel are pale pink; no change in size is noted. No other reddened areas are noted. *Progress to meeting Goal #1.*

NURSING ACTION: *Teach client about measures to reduce the risk for problems related to immobility. Encourage client to assist with and participate in these measures.*
RATIONALE: *Client participation in the plan of care helps to promote a sense of control over the situation, thereby helping to promote self-esteem.*

NURSING ACTION: *Provide respiratory care as needed; encourage coughing and deep breathing and use of incentive spirometer at least every 2 hours.*
RATIONALE: *Respiratory care measures are necessary to prevent pulmonary complications. Pneumonia is a particularly dangerous complication.*

NURSING ACTION: *Encourage the client to use the trapeze bar and sit up as much as possible, with adequate support. Use a standing wheelchair, tilt table, or "neuro" chair as soon as possible. Use measures to prevent footdrop, such as splints or high-top sneakers.*
RATIONALE: *Mobility will prevent respiratory complications and will help the client to maintain self-esteem. Splints or high-top sneakers aid in maintaining normal anatomical alignment of the joints.*

Evaluation: Client is able to state measures to reduce risk of skin breakdown; asks for assistance with sitting up in bed; actively using trapeze bar to change positions. Client is observed using incentive spirometer every 2 to 3 hours. Lungs clear to auscultation. Areas on left elbow and heel pale pink, approximately the size of a dime. *Goal #1 met; progress to meeting Goal #2 and Goal #3.*

NURSING ACTION: *Encourage fluid intake to approximately 2 to 3 L/day, unless contraindicated; assess urinary output for color and amount; monitor intake and output at least every 4 to 8 hours. Teach the client and family the signs and symptoms of urinary tract infection and kidney stones.*
RATIONALE: *Adequate fluid intake helps to prevent kidney stones and bladder infections. Changes in the color or clarity of the urine may suggest a potential problem. Adequate client understanding of signs and symptoms of potential problems helps to ensure prompt detection and early intervention should any occur.*

NURSING ACTION: *Maintain nutritional status, gradually increasing the client's diet as ordered, including high-fiber foods.*
RATIONALE: *Adequate nutrition is necessary to promote healing and to maintain health. The intake of fiber helps to reduce the risk of constipation.*

NURSING ACTION: *Encourage client to perform active range of motion to left side, and passive range of motion exercises to right side. Contact physical therapy as ordered to assist with muscle strengthening, endurance, and mobility, and occupational therapy to assist with self-care activities.*
RATIONALE: *Continued exercise helps to maintain function of the extremities; contacting physical therapy and occupational therapy professionals promotes development of a beginning rehabilitation plan for the client.*

Evaluation: Client is able to state and actively demonstrates measures to prevent problems of immobility. Client is scheduled to attend physical therapy this afternoon and occupational therapy in the morning. No further evidence of skin breakdown is noted. Lungs are clear to auscultation. Client drank 2.5 L yesterday; voiding clear-yellow urine in adequate amounts. Small amount of soft brown stool passed today. Client states, "I'm looking forward to PT and OT." *Goal #2 and Goal #3 met; progress to meeting Goal #4.*

perature, or a mouthful of food, depending on the trigger zone's location.

Treatment consists of medications or surgery. Some drugs may help temporarily, but surgery is the treatment with the most satisfactory results. Partial removal of the nerve roots eliminates the pain permanently, although it may leave burning, tickling sensations for several weeks or months.

After surgery, various symptoms may occur, depending on which nerve branches were sectioned. The client may have some eye irritation or difficulty eating, in addition to adjusting to a certain amount of numbness. The client learns to avoid situations that previously triggered pain.

Bell's Palsy

Bell's palsy is a temporary, partial, one-sided facial paralysis and weakness caused by ischemia or inflammation of the 7th cranial nerve. A Bell's palsy–type syndrome may result from a brain lesion.

The paralysis may result in a lopsided facial appearance. The eye on the affected side will not close. The client cannot control the mouth on the affected side, which often leads to drooling. In addition, the mouth does not turn up when the client smiles.

These symptoms can be emotionally upsetting for the client. Special eye care may be necessary. Heat and massage may be helpful. In the early stages, prednisone (Meticorten, Orasone) may be used. Usually, symptoms subside gradually, but they may take months to do so.

Herpes Zoster

Herpes zoster, commonly known as **shingles,** is an acute viral inflammation of a nerve caused by the varicella-zoster virus (the same virus that causes chickenpox). The disease results from reactivation of latent virus cells residing in dorsal root or cranial nerve ganglion cells.

Signs and Symptoms. Mild to moderate pruritus (itching), tenderness, or pain frequently precedes the appearance of vesicles. The interval between pain and eruption of vesicles averages 3 to 5 days. Lesions erupt for several days and usually disappear within 3 to 4 weeks. Some clients also experience gastrointestinal upset and general malaise.

Vesicles follow the distribution of sensory nerves, usually on the trunk, causing excruciating pain. Pain can be quite severe, even if vesicles are not visible on the skin. The pain can last for several weeks or months.

Generally, the disorder is self-limiting and localized. Herpes usually heals without complications. The eruption is usually confined to one region of the body. However, the eruption may encircle the trunk—common in clients with HIV/AIDS. Some scarring may occur.

The eruption of herpes zoster vesicles is sometimes associated with other diseases, particularly in clients with suppressed immune systems, such as those with tuberculosis, HIV/AIDS, and lymphoma. Sometimes an injury or an injection of a drug may trigger the inflammation.

In addition, *postherpetic neuralgia* (pain along the nerves after a herpes infection) may cause pain and discomfort for 8 weeks or more. Postherpetic neuralgia is most common in clients older than 60 years of age.

In rare cases, the infection may invade the eyes and cause conjunctivitis. If it is not checked, blindness may result in the affected eye (*ophthalmic zoster*). In clients with serious underlying conditions that suppress the immune system, serious complications may develop.

Treatment. Treatment is symptomatic, focusing on relief of pain and pruritus. Narcotics and/or anti-inflammatory agents may be helpful in obtaining pain and pruritus relief. Wet dressings with Burow's solution may be useful during the vesicular stage of the infection. Calamine lotion and antihistamines may treat pruritus. IV acyclovir (Zovirax) has improved the rate of healing of skin lesions and shortened the period of pain. Oral corticosteroids have been used in clients aged 50 to 60 years and older to decrease postherpetic neuralgia.

Nursing Considerations. All causes of neuralgia need adequate assessment of pain and pain control measures. Environmental conditions may need to be adjusted so that the client can have a quiet environment with minimal stimulus.

With herpes zoster, infection control measures are necessary to prevent cross-contamination. Nurses and visitors who have never had chickenpox or who are pregnant will need to follow transmission-based precautions (see Chap. 42). In addition, all healthcare providers should avoid touching the lesions directly. Be sure to wear gloves whenever there is possible exposure to drainage and secretions.

Instructions on how to avoid pain triggers, and measures for appropriate pain management, are key areas to stress in client and family education. Emotional support also is important because the client may have a disturbed body image related to paralysis, muscle twitching, or outbreaks of vesicles.

SPINAL CORD DISORDERS

An understanding of several basic concepts is necessary when caring for persons with spinal cord disorders. Application of these concepts will help healthcare providers to better understand these disabilities and initiate appropriate care:

- The *spinal cord* is the communication system between the brain and the periphery of the body. It comprises a tight cluster of nerve cell bodies (*gray matter*), surrounded by the ascending (*sensory*) and descending (*motor*) tracts (*white matter*). If the spinal cord is severed or compressed, communication between the brain and the rest of the body is literally cut off.
- The spinal cord lies in an enclosed and confined space called the *vertebral column*. Any invasion into this space can cause devastating effects.
- The spinal cord is responsible for the *reflex arc* (see Chap. 19), which is a built-in protective mechanism. For example, it allows a person to quickly jerk the hand away

from a hot stove, thus bypassing the brain and preventing further injury.

Categories of Spinal Cord Disorders

Spinal cord problems can be divided into three main categories: congenital defects, tumors, and trauma. *Congenital defects of the spinal cord* are malformations that occur in the developing fetus. They most often affect the CNS by disrupting the flow of CSF (see Chap. 71).

A *spinal cord tumor* is located within the vertebral column, taking up space and causing compression of the cord. It interferes with blood supply and CSF circulation. Tumors may be surgically removed. Resulting neurologic deficits will vary, depending on the type of tumor and the length of time compression has occurred. If a tumor involves the cord itself, damage is usually most severe and is often permanent.

Trauma to the spinal cord can be caused by blunt or penetrating forces. Examples of penetrating objects include displaced vertebrae or foreign objects such as bullets. **Transection** (severing) of the cord can be incomplete (partial) or complete. If the transection is *complete,* all sensation and voluntary movement below the site of injury is lost. A *partial* or *incomplete transection* has the best prognosis. In this case, the resulting deficits will depend on whether ascending (sensory) or descending (motor) nerve tracts were severed. Trauma to the spinal cord also includes bruising, in which case the person may regain total function.

Level of Injury

The level of the spinal cord injury determines which body functions are affected. **Paraplegia** means paralysis of the legs and lower body; it usually results from injury to the cord below the first thoracic vertebrae. **Quadriplegia** means paralysis of all four extremities and usually results from an injury above the first thoracic vertebrae.

The extent of all spinal cord injuries depends on the injury's location and severity. Injuries occurring at the second and third cervical vertebrae are usually fatal. Clients who experience any damage at the level of C4 and above require ventilatory assistance because nerve innervation to the respiratory muscles is damaged, and the client cannot breathe independently. Figure 77-2 identifies the structures that are affected by spinal cord injury at various locations.

Sometimes the final outcome of a spinal cord injury is uncertain for a long period. This time can be highly stressful for the person's family and loved ones. When a diagnosis of paralysis is made, the emotional shock to the person and family is usually devastating.

Adjustments, ranging from minor modifications to total alterations in lifestyle, will need to be made. Changes may include adaptations in a home's physical setup, installation of an elevator and ramps, and changes in employment. Assistance with ADL is generally necessary. Adaptations can be made to accommodate the client's needs for transportation, including driving a car. Rehabilitation and occupational therapy can be very helpful.

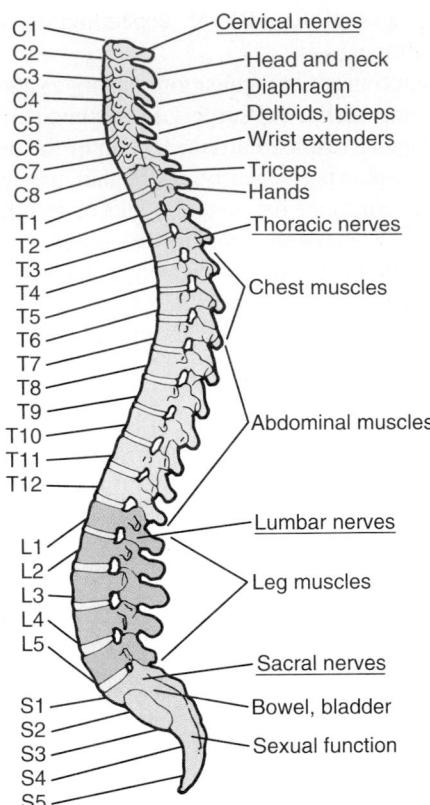

FIGURE 77-2. Structures affected by spinal nerves.

Effects of Injury

Immediately after a spinal injury, the client is at risk for spinal shock and respiratory arrest. Long-term damage to the spinal cord can have various effects. Sensory deficits can range from numbness and tingling in the extremities to total loss of body sensation. Movement disabilities can also range from muscle weakness to partial or complete paralysis.

☛ KEY CONCEPT

Many persons with varying degrees of paralysis have an active sex life. Adaptations and understanding on the partner's part may be necessary. A paralyzed man can father a child and a paralyzed woman can bear a child.

Complications of spinal cord injury include impaired circulation, bowel and bladder incontinence, bone demineralization, skin breakdown, anemia, muscle spasms, contractures, increased body temperature, gastric distention, and respiratory complications. Blood clots may develop in the legs. The lower the location of the cord transection, the fewer the complications will be.

The client may experience severe, shooting pain that results from nerve damage. Many stimuli may trigger the pain: injections, kidney stones, or fecal impactions can aggravate pain. A person may feel *phantom pain* in a paralyzed area of the body because of nerve damage, or it may occur in a ringlike fashion at the level of injury.

Autonomic Dysreflexia. **Autonomic dysreflexia** (also known as *autonomic hyperreflexia*) may be seen in clients with injury to the upper spinal cord. It is characterized by a sudden and dangerous elevation of blood pressure that is a result of an autonomic response to various stimuli (called *noxious stimuli*) that are harmless to people with an intact spinal cord. For example, a distended bladder or fecal impaction can be the trigger. The sudden onset of hypertension can cause seizures, strokes, or hemorrhage. Signs and symptoms of autonomic dysreflexia include:

- Elevated blood pressure (particularly significant)
- Sudden, throbbing headache
- Chills
- Pallor
- Goose flesh (goose bumps)
- Nausea, with a metallic taste

Immediate treatment is required if a client displays these signs and symptoms. Elevate the client's head and notify the healthcare provider. Quickly assess the client for possible causes of pressure, such as a blocked urinary catheter. Monitor the client's blood pressure very closely.

Nurses need to be ever vigilant in assessing the client for possible triggers. Treatment involves elimination of the triggering stimulus. In cases of severe hypertension, antihypertensive medications are used. Teach the client and family preventive measures such as preventing constipation and visually inspecting catheters to ensure that they remain patent.

Emergency Treatment and Diagnostic Tests

After any trauma, extreme care is necessary to prevent further damage when injury to the spine and cord is suspected or known. The head, neck, and spine must be stabilized with the person lying flat on a firm surface. Never lift the person with a known or suspected spinal cord injury by the head, shoulder, or feet. A victim of trauma should never be moved without proper precautions, unless the circumstances are such that the individual's safety is compromised and remaining in place would jeopardize the client's life. Treatment for shock and hemorrhage may also be necessary (see Chap. 43). An x-ray examination to determine the extent of injury is a medical priority.

Nursing Alert
Document the person's ability to move extremities and his or her sense of touch before and after the move.

Medical and Surgical Treatment

If the cause of paralysis is trauma, skeletal traction may be applied to immobilize the damaged cervical vertebrae. Several different devices can be used (see Chap. 76). Surgery may be necessary to remove a portion of vertebral bone pressing on the spinal cord or to stabilize the vertebrae to prevent further damage. If the spinal column is unstable, spinal fusion is done to prevent further damage to the spinal cord and to enable more mobility later.

Rehabilitation must begin immediately on hospitalization to maintain the client's cardiac and pulmonary reserves. The client must be rehabilitated in all spheres—body, mind, and spirit. It is best for the person with a spinal cord injury to enter a rehabilitation center as soon as possible. Usually, most acute-care facilities are not equipped to handle all the lifestyle adjustments that must occur.

Nursing Considerations
The nurse plays a vital part in the care and progress of the client with a spinal cord injury. Observe the client closely when providing care. Check for minute changes in the client's condition that are not yet evident to others.

Rehabilitation focuses on preventing disabilities from becoming worse and on strengthening function. Begin measures immediately to prevent disuse disorders such as skin breakdown and plantarflexion (*footdrop*). Initiate passive and active exercises to develop the client's muscle strength and movement. The degree of success depends on the nature and the extent of nerve damage, as well as the client's own perseverance. Despite paralysis, many clients are able to move about and perform ADL. In Practice: Nursing Care Guidelines 77-2 highlights care for the client with paralysis.

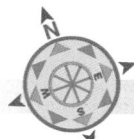

SPECIAL CONSIDERATIONS: CULTURES

Paralysis in Female Clients

For female clients with paralysis from a spinal cord injury:

- Menses usually resume within 3 months following the injury. *Rationale: It takes time for the body to adjust to the injury.*
- The use of tampons is dangerous. *Rationale: The woman may forget that a tampon is in place because she has no sensation.*
- The use of birth control pills is not recommended. *Rationale: They can lead to thrombus formation, particularly if the client is not exercising or is immobile. Effectiveness often decreases because of interactions with other medications.*
- The use of intrauterine devices (IUDs) is not recommended. *Rationale: They can promote thrombus formation or infections. This woman would not be able to tell if the device had fallen out. She also would not be able to feel the pain associated with a perforated uterus.*
- Labor and childbirth may be dangerous. *Rationale: The woman may not be aware of the onset of labor. The likelihood of a cesarean birth is increased, because the woman may not be able to assist with the delivery and the uterus may not have adequate muscle tone. In addition, labor and delivery may serve as a trigger for autonomic dysreflexia.*

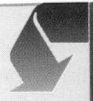

In Practice
Nursing Care Guidelines 77-2

CARING FOR THE CLIENT WITH PARALYSIS

- Use measures to prevent footdrop, such as splints. *Rationale: Splints aid in maintaining normal anatomical alignment of the joints.*
- Change the client's position frequently and provide passive and active range of motion. *Rationale: Prevent disorders caused by immobility– disuse disorders.*
- Give respiratory care as needed. *Rationale: This is necessary to prevent respiratory complications. Pneumonia is a particularly dangerous complication.*
- Encourage the client to sit up as much as possible, with adequate support. Use a standing wheelchair, tilt table, or "neuro" chair as soon as possible. *Rationale: Mobility will prevent respiratory complications and will help the client to maintain self-esteem.*
- Use special devices (beds, chairs, and other mechanical devices) in the early phases of treatment. Trochanter rolls and sandbags may also be used. *Rationale: These devices help to maintain proper body alignment and positioning, thus helping to prevent orthopedic deformities.*
- Give special skin care. Make sure the sheets are smooth and the bed is clean. *Rationale: The skin of the client with paralysis is subject to pressure areas and skin breakdown.*
- If cervical traction, tongs, or a halo device is in place, assess the pin site. Give site care as ordered by the physician. Give incisional care postoperatively. *Rationale: Infection must be prevented, because it can be particularly dangerous to a paralyzed person, whose physical condition is already compromised.*
- Teach the client and family the warning signs of genitourinary infection. *Rationale: Genitourinary infection is a common complication of immobility.*
- Encourage fluid intake. *Rationale: Adequate fluid intake helps to prevent kidney stones and bladder infections.*
- Institute bladder retraining and rehabilitation early, if possible. *Rationale: Bladder retraining and rehabilitation help restore the client's independence and self-esteem.*
- If urinary retention is present, use a urinary appliance, retention catheter, or self-catheterization.

Rationale: The client may not be able to tell when the bladder is filled. Retention of urine can lead to autonomic dysreflexia, infection, or hydronephrosis.
- If a catheter is used, make sure it is draining properly and is handled in as clean a manner as possible. Teach the client and family to care for the indwelling catheter or urinary appliance as early as possible, if bladder retraining is not an option. *Rationale: Proper drainage and care is needed to avoid bladder and urinary tract infections.*
- If disposable pads or incontinence products are used, give special attention to keeping the skin clean and dry. *Rationale: Keeping the skin dry and clean helps to prevent skin irritation, pressure areas, and infection.*
- Teach the client to do manual disimpaction for a fecal impaction. *Rationale: Damage to the bowel can trigger autonomic dysreflexia.* Some clients do a manual disimpaction daily, as their bowel maintenance program.
- Give injections above the level of injury, if possible. *Rationale: Circulation is impaired below the level of injury and the action of the drug is delayed. The skin is more subject to breakdown below the level of injury.*
- Avoid applying external heat to areas of decreased sensation, particularly to the penis or testes. Take care to avoid pressure on the client, and keep sharp objects from touching the client. *Rationale: The client may experience decreased sensation and be unable to detect changes that could result in injury.*
- Monitor temperature of bath water. *Rationale: Burns occur easily because of lack of circulation and sensation: The client would not feel the injury, and skin stimulation can cause autonomic dysreflexia.*
- Maintain nutritional status. *Rationale: Nutrition is necessary to promote healing and to maintain health.*
- Establish some sort of communication system if the client cannot speak. It can involve blinking the eyes, moving a finger, or using a computer. *Rationale: The person's mind is usually active; there must be some way for the person to make needs, wants, and thoughts known to others.*

Encourage the client to make every effort to maximize abilities and perform self-care. Remind the client that at first, even accomplishing the simplest tasks may be overwhelming. The client may become discouraged and angry. Allow the client to express frustration and discouragement and acknowledge these feelings. Provide realistic feedback and encouragement, pointing out the positive gains that the client has made, regardless of how small they may be.

DEGENERATIVE DISORDERS

Degenerative disorders of the nervous system affect people of all ages with loss of neurologic function at various rates. In addition to all the physical problems the person with a degenerative disorder experiences, he or she will often show major emotional and psychological problems. Such problems may include profound mood swings and outbursts of frustration or anger. The person may exhibit inappropriate sexual behavior, signs of regression, and even infantile behavior. Help by allowing clients and their families to express their feelings and anxieties.

Support groups are available for most degenerative disorders. Numerous resources are available. Assist clients and their families to find appropriate support groups. Encourage all family members to talk with other persons who have faced similar situations. Talking can offer reassurance and helpful suggestions for management.

Multiple Sclerosis

Multiple sclerosis (**MS**) is one of the most common nerve disorders in the United States, typically affecting young adults and people living in northern temperate climates. It is slightly more common in females. In MS, the myelin sheath covering the nerves is destroyed. Myelin (see Chap. 19) maintains electrical impulse strength. Loss of myelin (*demyelination*) results in weak electrical impulses and weak muscle contractions.

The cause of MS is unknown. Some experts believe MS is viral in origin. A current theory proposes that MS is an autoimmune disease. Table 77-1 summarizes the four courses of clinical progression of MS. Each course may have mild, moderate, or severe symptoms.

Signs and Symptoms. Initially, MS may be manifested as difficulty walking, tremors, lack of coordination, "pins and needles" numbness, and visual changes including loss of vision. Symptoms may disappear in the early stages, and the person may appear normal and well for years. Each time symptoms reappear, they are more severe and of longer duration. Thus, the disease can be marked by remissions and exacerbations. A person may live 20 years or more after the disease is diagnosed, but disabilities develop over time.

Individuals who have few attacks or who have long intervals between attacks are less likely to develop more severe symptoms. However, clients with early symptoms of difficulty walking, tremors, frequent attacks, and incomplete recoveries have a more rapid progression of the disease.

With recurrent episodes, increasingly severe symptoms such as paralysis, **dysphagia** (difficulty in swallowing), and bladder and bowel dysfunctions develop. Cognitive dysfunction, depression, and emotional upsets are common. The client may complain of fatigue, headaches, and pain. Seizures, tremors, and spasticity, as well as hearing and visual losses, are common. The client experiences dizziness, nausea, or vomiting, or has spastic paraplegia (exaggerated reflexes and muscle tone) and muscle tremors.

The individual may have increasing difficulty thinking, reasoning, and remembering. The person may have sudden emotional upsets, becoming either depressed or exuberant and euphoric. Symptoms are few at first but can increase in number and seriousness over time.

Diagnosis. Diagnosis of MS is difficult until certain symptoms appear together and create widespread disturbances. An MRI best detects changes in the myelin sheath. About 95% of MS clients show plaque changes correlating with the person's symptoms. MRI is said to be conclusive for MS if it identifies two areas of plaque changes.

Other causes of symptoms, such as Lyme disease or collagen–vascular diseases, such as lupus erythematosis, need to be ruled out. Other causes of neurologic lesions may present with similar symptoms but have different etiologies. There are no specific diagnostic blood tests for MS.

Medical Treatment. No cure is known for MS. The client needs to maintain general health with periods of rest, adequate sleep, and a balanced diet. Stress reduction is important. Stressful situations include physical triggers, such as exposure to infection, and emotional triggers, such as employment stress, excitement, and depression.

Preventive interventions may help reduce exacerbation of the symptoms. Physical therapy helps prevent deformities and maintain muscle strength. Occupational therapy may be necessary to provide rehabilitation for lost abilities.

During significant exacerbations, clients may receive IV corticotropin (ACTH) on an outpatient or inpatient basis. ACTH is given for 6 to 7 days and then decreased, with weekly injections for another month.

Nonsteroidal immunosuppressive drugs are effective in treating MS, targeting the disease itself rather than just the symptoms. The interferon drugs beta-1b (Betaseron) and beta-1a (Avonex) are used to reduce the number and severity of acute exacerbations.

■■■ **TABLE 77-1** *The* **CLINICAL PROGRESSION OF MULTIPLE SCLEROSIS**

Course of MS	Characterized by	Comments	Percentage of MS Population
Relapsing-remitting (RRMS)	Partial recovery after attacks (exacerbations with relapses)	Most common form of MS	70%–75% of clients start with RRMS
Secondary-progressive (SPMS)	RRMS course becoming steadily progressive	SPMS develops within 10 years of RRMS	50% of clients
Primary-progressive (PPMS)	Continually progressive disabilities	No periods of remitting (lessening) of symptoms	15% of clients
Progressive-relapsing (PRMS)	Continually progressive, with noticeable periods of acute attacks	Rare	Less than 10% of MS population

Adapted from National Multiple Sclerosis Society website: http://www.nmss.org/Sourcebook_Prognosis.asp.

Nursing Considerations. Nursing care focuses on encouraging the client to schedule periods of rest and adequate sleep. In addition, encourage a well-balanced diet and provide good skin care. As the individual's body manifests more symptoms of muscle wasting and paralysis, the client is less able to prevent the hazards of immobility, such as the complications of contractures, pneumonia, and social isolation.

Elimination problems usually occur. Therefore, monitor diet as well as fluid intake and output. The client may experience urinary incontinence or retention. If the client requires an indwelling urinary catheter, take steps to prevent infection and teach the client and family how to prevent the same. Because constipation often occurs, a bowel training program may be initiated (see Chap. 51).

The client and caregivers need to encourage body repositioning and deep breathing to prevent pneumonia. Give attention to maintaining proper body alignment, because paralysis and weakness can lead to deformities.

Unless physically necessary, do not confine the client to bed. Instead, encourage the person to lead as normal a life as possible. The person with MS can live at home as long as he or she can perform independent physical care or family members are able to assist. Sometimes the client can work at home until the disease's progression makes this impossible.

Provide support to the client with MS and the family. The client and family members may need to alter aspects of their lifestyles and to readjust goals in accordance with the client's condition. Also alert the client and family that stress, temperature changes, fatigue, and illness exacerbate or worsen MS. Frequent rest periods during the day are important.

Parkinson's Disease

Parkinson's disease, also called **parkinsonism,** is second only to Alzheimer's disease as the most common neurologic disease in older adults. It is a chronic progressive disease affecting the dopamine-producing cells of the brain. *Dopamine* is a neurotransmitter (chemical messenger) that sends signals within the brain. Without dopamine, neurons fire out of control, and individuals cannot control muscle movements.

Parkinsonism affects slightly more men than women. Although the disorder usually appears in people in their sixties, it can occur in much younger individuals. It is not considered an inherited disorder. Side effects of some medications, such as tricyclic antidepressants, may present with Parkinson's-like symptoms.

Signs and Symptoms. Early signs and symptoms often go unnoticed because they occur gradually. This progressive brain disease is characterized by **bradykinesia** (slowness of movement) and fine, rhythmic tremors of the hands, arms, legs, jaw, and face. The limbs and trunk become rigid and stiff. The person has difficulty maintaining balance and co-ordination (**ataxia**). A shuffling gait and an unsteady gait are common. Postural instability occurs. The effects of the disorder may lead to a state of immobility.

In the early years, tremors are regular but typically mild so that they are scarcely noticeable. They may affect only one side, then spread to the other side, which may happen immediately or after as long a period as 15 years. Tremors may start in the fingers, extend to the arms, and finally spread to the entire body.

Clients have progressive difficulty with walking, talking, eating, and completing ADL because the disease affects automatic movements. Movement of small muscles that control facial expressions is affected. The person may be unable to blink or smile. As muscles become rigid, the face presents as masklike. The person with parkinsonism often drools. Typical features are seen in Figure 77-3.

Severe tremors are constant—two to five shakes in a second with the thumb beating against the fingers in a sort of pill-rolling movement. Tremors worsen if the person gets excited. However, shaking may cease if he or she moves voluntarily.

Tremors disappear during sleep, except in the disease's final stages. All muscles become rigid, with slightly flexed limbs and slowed movements.

Because the disease can affect the neck muscles, the person sits or stands in a stooped position. The arms no longer swing when the person walks, and he or she is unable to shift position quickly to keep balance. The walking gait is characterized as *shuffling,* a motion that helps to keep the client from falling. If pushed a little, the person loses balance, going faster in the direction of the push.

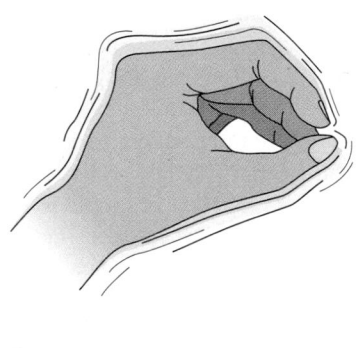

A

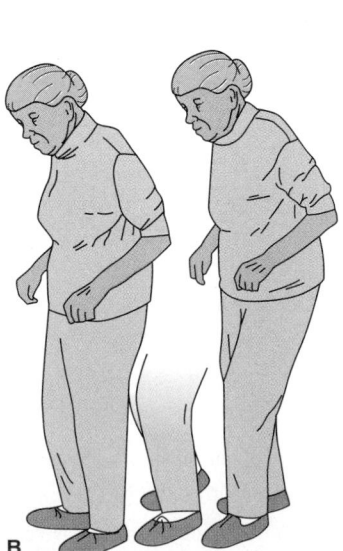

B

FIGURE 77-3. Parkinson's disease signs. (**A**) "Pill-rolling" tremor. (**B**) Forward stoop and shuffling gait.

Although mental changes may accompany this disease, their intensity varies. Common changes include emotional lability (*fluctuations*) and a slowed thinking process. Many people with Parkinson's become clinically depressed.

Medical and Surgical Treatment. Currently there is no test to predict Parkinson's disease. No preventive treatment is known.

Although many medications are used, the most effective antiparkinsonism drug found to date is levodopa (L-dopa) (see In Practice: Important Medications 77-3).

Surgery may be performed in carefully selected cases. It involves the deliberate production of a lesion in the thalamus. The procedure is used less frequently than in the past because of the effectiveness and greater safety of L-dopa.

Nursing Considerations. Physical therapy promotes activity and enables self-feeding, dressing, and transferring from bed to chair. The person can learn range-of-motion (ROM) exercises for the legs and fingers, and ways to maintain balance and to prevent neck muscles from contracting. Exercising does not eliminate tremors but does help prevent rigidity.

Because handling food, chewing, and swallowing are difficult, the person may not eat enough nutritious food. Specific vitamins (except vitamin B) and a high-calorie, high-protein diet are prescribed. Provide teaching for the client and family (see In Practice: Educating the Client 77-2).

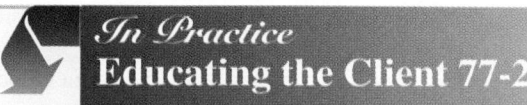

In Practice
Educating the Client 77-2

Parkinson's Disease

- Be as independent as possible.
- Protect against unnecessary stress and fatigue.
- Use adaptive techniques and devices.
- Protect against injuries.
- Take medications on time. Avoid foods and vitamins that negatively interact with medications.
- Be sure to eat a well-balanced diet with plenty of fluids for optimum functioning.
- Have regular eye examinations to check intraocular pressure.
- Follow pertinent exercises as prescribed or recommended.
- Use adaptive feeding utensils as necessary.

While the client is in the healthcare facility, check the consistency of food and teach the client and family about food preparation. They should prepare food that is easy to chew and swallow. Meat should be ground and potatoes mashed; a straw should be provided for liquids. Stress the need to prevent injury, especially burns. The client may be embarrassed by eating difficulties, so encourage him or her to eat. Help the client to make agreeable and safe menu selections.

Constipation may develop due to lack of physical activity, absence of adequate roughage in the diet, or the effects of various medications. Usually a stool softener such as docusate sodium (Colace) is given. Encourage fluid intake (at least 4 to 6 glasses of water and juice each day).

Help the client learn how to use adaptive techniques and devices (see Chaps. 48 and 96). Help the family make adaptations to the home and in homemaking. Families should do a house-safety check and eliminate hazards such as throw rugs and highly waxed floors. (Rationale: The client has poor balance and can easily fall.)

Arrangements for bathroom facilities and a bedroom on the first floor may be necessary. (Rationale: The client should avoid stair climbing, which can be dangerous and may be impossible.) Handrails may need to be installed in bathrooms, stairs, and hallways. Nightlights are also helpful. (Rationale: These measures can help the client to be more self-sufficient.)

Myasthenia Gravis

Myasthenia gravis (**MG**) is a chronic autoimmune disorder characterized by episodes of weakness in the voluntary muscles. One type of *neurotransmitter* (chemical messenger), *acetylcholine,* cannot transmit messages because *antibodies* (immune molecules) block, alter, or destroy its receptors at the neuromuscular junction. The thymus gland, which is abnormal in individuals with MG, develops abnormal clusters of lymphoid tissues, including tumors of the thymus gland

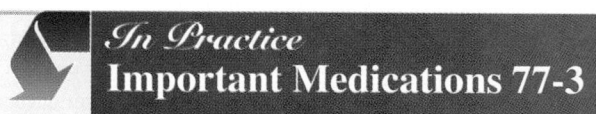

In Practice
Important Medications 77-3

For Parkinson's Disease

Levodopa (L-dopa) (Dopar, Larodopa): Replenishes missing dopamine, a neurotransmitter found in the brain

Nursing Considerations
- L-dopa may cause hemolytic anemia.
- L-dopa must be used carefully in clients with glaucoma. If L-dopa is given, monitor intraocular pressure carefully. *Rationale: One side effect of L-dopa is increased intraocular pressure.*
- L-dopa is contraindicated in undiagnosed skin lesions. *Rationale: The drug may aggravate these conditions.*
- The client taking L-dopa must avoid certain foods, including high-protein foods (which retard absorption of the drug) and foods high in vitamin B_6 (which quickly counteract positive effects of L-dopa). This client must not take certain vitamins.
- The client cannot use drugs classified as monoamine oxidase (MAO) inhibitors. MAO inhibitors often potentiate or counteract L-dopa effects. The client can become hyperactive and hyperexcitable, with increased parkinsonian symptoms and hypertension.

(*thymomas*). Generally these tumors are benign, but malignancies can occur.

Myasthenia gravis most commonly affects women under age 40 and men over age 60. However, it can occur at any age, including in the neonate and during childhood. MG occurs in all ethnic groups. It is not considered an inherited disorder and it is not contagious.

Signs and Symptoms. Most often, the eye muscles are affected first. The client looks sleepy and expressionless. Drooping eyelids (**ptosis**) are common; other facial muscles may be affected, especially those used in chewing, swallowing, coughing, and speaking.

The disease usually evolves gradually. The individual notices that certain muscles feel weak immediately after exercise, but that muscle strength returns with rest. Eventually the person tires with slight exertion.

If respiratory muscles are affected, breathing becomes difficult. If the person is unable to expectorate secretions, pneumonia may develop.

A *myasthenic crisis* occurs rapidly and is considered an emergency situation. Dysphagia, **dysphasia** (difficulty in speaking), ptosis, **diplopia** (double vision), and respiratory distress are the usual manifestations. Maintaining an open (*patent*) airway can be lifesaving. Pulmonary function studies can be used as predictors of respiratory abilities and indicators of potential myasthenic crisis.

Diagnostic Tests. Because the onset of signs and symptoms is slow, diagnosis is often delayed. In addition, similar signs and symptoms also are seen in other disorders.

Antibodies to acetylcholine receptors can be detected by lab testing. Most individuals with MG have abnormally high levels of acetylcholine receptor antibodies.

Typically, an edrophonium test aids in the diagnosis. Edrophonium chloride (Tensilon) is injected IV. The client with MG will experience a temporary relief of symptoms.

Other tests include nerve conduction studies and electromyography. CT and MRI scans can be used to identify thyroid tumors.

Medical Treatment. MG can be controlled with several available therapies used to reduce weakness and improve muscle strength. Muscle strength can be increased by promoting neuromuscular transmission. Anticholinesterase agents, such as neostigmine and pyridostigmine (Mestinon), are commonly used. Potent immunosuppressive drugs such as prednisone, cyclosporine, and azathioprine can suppress the production of the antibody (see In Practice: Important Medications 77-4).

Nursing Alert

For the client with MG, avoid the use of sedatives, tranquilizing drugs, and morphine because these drugs may cause respiratory or cardiac depression.

Plasmapheresis, a procedure in which antibodies are removed from the blood, can be beneficial to the client with MG. Additionally, high doses of intravenous immune globulin may be given, to provide the client with a temporary dose of normal

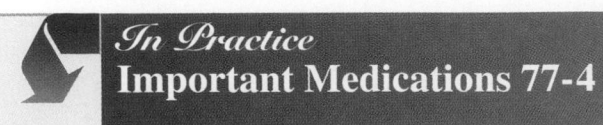

In Practice
Important Medications 77-4

FOR MYASTHENIA GRAVIS
• Neostigmine methylsulfate (Prostigmin)
• Pyridostigmine bromide (Mestinon, Regonol)
• Ambenonium chloride (Mytelase): Used only if client cannot take either of the others

Nursing Considerations
• These medications play a vital role in the client's ability to swallow and to handle respiratory secretions.
• Medications must be given on time and can be given with food (to minimize side effects).
• Side effects must be reported immediately.
• Drugs such as edrophonium chloride (Enlon, Tensilon) can aid in diagnosis and evaluate effectiveness of other drugs.

antibodies. These procedures may be performed during periods of severe weakness.

Surgical Treatment. In more that 50% of clients with MG, signs and symptoms are improved with a *thymectomy* (surgical removal of the thymus gland). A stable, long-term remission is the goal of a thymectomy. Some individuals may be cured by the surgery.

Nursing Considerations. Assure clients that current medications and therapies can greatly improve their muscle strength. Generally, individuals can lead normal or nearly normal lives.

The client should also be aware that emotional upsets and infections can intensify the disease and precipitate a crisis. Teaching is an important aspect of care (see In Practice: Educating the Client 77-3).

During acute episodes, tube feedings or total parenteral nutrition (TPN) may be necessary. Suctioning may be needed to remove secretions. Keep an oral suction machine at the client's bedside; it may be life saving in a case of choking or threatened aspiration.

Warn the client of the signs of myasthenic crisis and instruct him or her to take precautions regarding medical assistance before the crisis develops. Encourage the client to wear a MedicAlert tag, and to have a self-dialing telephone within easy reach. A voice-activated telephone is necessary if the client cannot dial or hold the receiver.

Be prepared to assist with intermittent positive pressure breathing (IPPB) treatments, which are often indicated. In the case of severe respiratory involvement, a tracheostomy may be performed.

Huntington's Disease

Huntington's disease (**HD**), also known as *Huntington's chorea,* is a chronic, progressive, hereditary condition in which

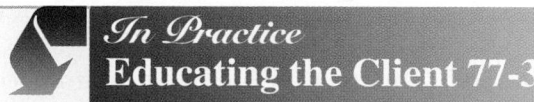

In Practice
Educating the Client 77-3

MYASTHENIA GRAVIS

- Wear a Medic-Alert tag at all times.
- Use a self-dialing telephone or cellular phone. *Rationale: These phones are useful in emergencies.*
- Take medications on time. Use an alarm clock as a reminder. *Rationale: Medications need to be taken on time to maintain a constant blood level.*
- Maintain a regular exercise schedule and conserve energy for essential activities.
- Avoid exposures to temperature extremes. *Rationale: They may trigger myasthenic crisis.*
- Follow a well-balanced diet to maintain optimum health and strength.
- Avoid exposure to infections.
- Be alert for signs of myasthenic crisis: respiratory distress, muscular weakness, dysphagia, fever, and general malaise. Keep a suction device available for emergencies; maintaining an open airway is a priority should crisis occur.

brain cells in the basal ganglia prematurely die. The disorder involves a combination of physical, intellectual, and emotional symptoms.

A child with a parent that has the HD gene has a 50–50 chance of inheriting the gene. Only children that inherit the gene will develop the disease. Only children who inherit the gene can pass on the gene to the next generation. All children who inherit the gene will eventually develop HD. Symptoms generally do not appear until the person is past age 30. The age of onset varies.

Signs and Symptoms. HD usually starts with abnormal involuntary movements, called **chorea,** such as fidgeting, jerking, and spasms. Personality changes include irritability, mood swings, depression, loss of judgment, and carelessness. Early intellectual symptoms include difficulty making decisions and learning new things.

These symptoms progress to constant writhing and uncontrollable movement, changes in speech and ability to swallow, great weakness, severe personality disorders, and psychosis. The disease progresses at different rates.

Eventually the person loses bowel and bladder control and all purposeful movement, and is confined to bedrest. Death usually results from pneumonia or another disorder-related complication associated with immobility.

Diagnostic Tests. A thorough medical and family history is important. A genetic test to search for the HD gene is available. Neurologic tests and laboratory tests can be used to differentiate HD from other nervous-system disorders.

Treatment. There is no cure for HD. Symptoms cannot be reversed. Treatment is aimed at symptomatic relief of phys-

ical symptoms such as fatigue, restlessness, or hyperexcitability. Medications can be given for depression.

Nursing Considerations. Couples at risk may wish to consider genetic counseling before deciding whether to have children.

Initially the client may be able to remain at home, until ADL cannot be managed. Home care adaptations can provide a better quality of life. The person with HD can use lamps with a touch base, and handrails at the proper height that are strong enough to support full body weight. The person can use an electric razor and toothbrush. To steady the hands and arms, he or she can sit down and rest the elbows on a table when shaving or brushing the teeth.

If the person can swallow thin liquids, he or she can use two straws cut to just above the rim of the glass. Sometimes a thickening agent such as Thickit is used to make swallowing easier.

Cutting a spot out of a Styrofoam cup for the person's nose can make drinking easier and safer. (Rationale: The person does not have to tip the head back to drink; this measure prevents choking.)

Amyotrophic Lateral Sclerosis

Amyotrophic lateral sclerosis (**ALS**), also known as *Lou Gehrig's disease,* is a rapidly progressive, fatal neurologic disorder resulting in destruction of motor neurons of the cortex, brain stem, and spinal cord. Voluntary muscle movement gradually degenerates. ALS usually strikes between ages 50 and 70 years and affects more men than women.

Signs and Symptoms. The loss of motor neurons causes muscles to atrophy. Initially the individual may fall frequently and lose motor control of the hands and arms. The individual experiences weakness, fatigue, and spasticity of the arms.

As the disease advances, muscles atrophy, with flaccid quadriplegia. Eventually, the respiratory muscles are involved. The course of the disease is consistent, with no remissions. ALS always progresses to respiratory dysfunction and death, generally within 5 years after onset, although the course of the disease may vary.

Treatment. There is no cure or therapy that will lessen the progress of or reverse the disorder. The first drug shown to prolong survival of ALS clients is riluzole (Rilutek). Additional treatments are palliative only, focusing on support and symptom management.

Nursing Considerations. As with many other neurologic disorders, the nurse can provide physical, emotional, and spiritual support to the client and family. The nurse may provide direction and compassion to the family when discussing subjects such as disease progression and death and dying.

☞ KEY CONCEPT

The individual with ALS retains intellectual and sensory function throughout the course of the disease.

INFLAMMATORY DISORDERS

Brain Abscess

A *brain abscess* is a collection of pus that may result from an infection of the ears, mastoid, sinus, or skull. It can also directly result from brain surgery. If left untreated, the encapsulated pus pocket eventually ruptures and spreads, causing further abscesses and *meningitis*, infection of the meninges.

Findings associated with a brain abscess mimic those of brain tumor (see "Neoplasms" section). The person may also experience a fever if the primary infection site is still infected. Those with brain abscesses are at risk for ↑ICP and seizures, as well as spread of the infection. Surgical treatment is necessary to drain the abscess. Massive doses of IV antibiotics are given preoperatively and postoperatively. The person may be left with some brain damage or may be completely cured.

Meningitis

Meningitis is an inflammation of the meninges, the membranes that cover the brain and the spinal cord. Infection can travel to the meninges from nearby structures, such as the sinuses or the middle ear. The bloodstream also may carry the infection.

Meningitis is a contagious infection. Direct contact with respiratory secretions can transmit the organism from one person to another. People living in close proximity to others, children and caregivers in daycare centers, and individuals who have contact with another person's secretions (as in kissing) are most at risk for meningitis. Specific high-risk groups include refugees, military personnel, college students living in dormitories, and infants and young children. People who are exposed to active or passive tobacco smoke are also at risk.

> ✚👁 **N u r s i n g   A l e r t**
> The best protection against meningitis is
> thorough and frequent handwashing.

Viruses, fungi, or bacteria cause meningitis. Brain damage, hearing loss, disabilities, and death are known to occur more often with bacterial meningitis than with viral meningitis.

The causative organism is related to age. Different organisms infect people of different ages. Meningitis is a serious disease to which children are particularly susceptible.

Three organisms (*Streptococcus pneumoniae, Neisseria meningitides,* and *Haemophilus influenzae,* type b) cause about 70% of bacterial meningitis. Infection with *N. meningitidis* is also known as *meningococcal meningitis,* in which the incubation period is 2 to 10 days and the disease is particularly contagious because the causative organisms are present in the throat as well as in the CSF. A vaccine for some types of *N. meningitidis* is available but is not routinely given in the United States.

Prior to the 1990's, *H. influenzae,* type b (Hib) was a primary cause of meningitis in children. The incidences of Hib have decreased greatly since the development of the vaccine against it. Routine immunization with the Hib vaccine in schoolchildren has prevented the most common cause of meningitis in children.

Infection with *S. pneumoniae,* also known as *pneumonococcal meningitis,* also has a vaccine. However, this vaccine is not effective for children under 2 years of age. It is recommended for some individuals with chronic disorders, and individuals over the age of 65. *Viral meningitis,* also known as *aseptic meningitis,* may resolve without specific treatment. Many types of viruses can be causative agents of meningitis, such as the enteroviruses, herpesviruses, and the mumps virus. Lasting 7 to 10 days, the person generally recovers without disability. No specific medical treatment is currently available. The client needs bed rest, good hydration, and adequate nutrition. Analgesics for headache and fever may provide symptomatic relief.

Signs and Symptoms. Signs and symptoms of meningitis usually appear abruptly. Symptoms of viral and bacterial meningitis are often the same. Many symptoms are due to ↑ICP.

Signs and symptoms include fever, chills, severe headache, nausea and vomiting, **nuchal rigidity** (stiff neck), and irritability. A change in LOC is present. Two neurologic signs are present: positive Kernig's sign and positive Brudzinski's sign (see discussion below).

Photophobia (intolerance to light) and pain when the eyes move from side to side occur. The affected person may have seizures. A petechial purpuric rash is also possible. **Opisthotonos,** an acute spasm in which the body is bowed forward, with the head and heels bent backward, is often present. Children have tense or bulging fontanelles and a high-pitched cry.

Diagnostic Tests. Meningitis is diagnosed based on a general neurologic examination that includes two special neurologic signs:

- *Kernig's sign:* The client lies on the back and brings one leg up so that the hip and knee are both flexed at 90°. He or she then straightens the knee (the sole of the foot toward the ceiling). Pain or resistance indicates meningeal and spinal root inflammation. Kernig's sign is considered a positive indicator of meningitis.
- *Brudzinski's sign:* The client lies on the back and brings the head forward toward the chest. Pain or resistance indicates meningeal irritation, arthritis, or a neck injury. If the person responds by flexing the hips and knees, meningeal inflammation is indicated. Brudzinski's sign is also considered a positive indicator of meningitis. (Fig. 77-4).

Medical Treatment. When a diagnosis of meningitis is suspected, an LP is done. A C&S of CSF may be ordered to determine the causative organism. The client is given antibiotics.

If it is possible to identify the causative organism, the physician prescribes large doses of antibiotics that have been identified as effective in treating the organism. Antibiotics are highly effective in treating bacterial meningitis. If the infection is exceedingly virulent, drugs may prove useless and the

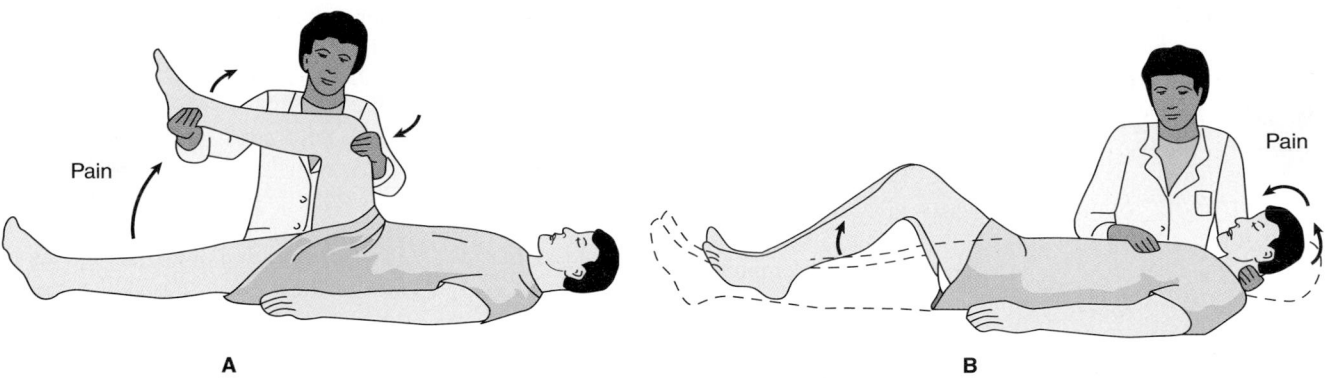

FIGURE 77-4. Signs of meningeal irritation. (**A**) Kernig's sign. (**B**) Brudzinski's sign.

person may die. Sometimes, nerves of sight and hearing are damaged.

Nursing Considerations. Provide nursing care with the awareness that the person is critically ill. The person is generally placed on seizure precautions. Side rails should be raised and padded for the client's protection. Elevate the head of the bed to at least 30°, unless otherwise ordered. Monitor the client's LOC.

A hypothermia blanket and antipyretic medications may be ordered for high fever. Analgesics may be given for pain. Give IV fluids and nourishing liquids as ordered. Tube feedings or TPN may be necessary.

Carefully monitor the person's respiratory status; a tracheostomy may be necessary if the client's respiratory status deteriorates. Keep the client's environment quiet to reduce irritability and to aid relaxation. Minimize traffic in and out of the room.

Caution caregivers and the client not to flex the individual's neck because doing so can obstruct venous flow and increase ICP. The client should also avoid acute hip flexion because it can cause increased intra-abdominal and intrathoracic pressures. These increased pressures interfere with cerebral blood vessel drainage and cause ↑ICP. Caregivers need to be aware that the individual may become confused and disoriented at times. Repeating instructions and closely monitoring the client's status are important.

Because meningitis is communicable, carry out proper infection control precautions (see Chap. 42).

Encephalitis

Encephalitis is an inflammation of the white and gray matter of the brain. It may be associated with meningitis. Encephalitis is caused by a virus, bacteria, or chemicals (such as in lead poisoning). It is characterized by the destruction of nerve cells. It may follow vaccination or a viral infection such as measles. Encephalitis seems to be more prevalent after influenza epidemics. Mosquitoes and ticks are common vectors.

Some types of viral encephalitis are more lethal than others. The death rate varies from 5% to 70%, depending on the infection's cause. Many people who recover from encephalitis are left with mental changes, seizure disorders, or parkinsonian symptoms, all of which become increasingly disabling.

Signs and Symptoms. Encephalitis can attack suddenly, causing violent headache, fever, nausea, vomiting, and drowsiness. The person may show muscular weakness, tremors, or visual disturbances.

Medical Treatment. No drug for the specific treatment of encephalitis has been found. Treatment is similar to the care of a client with meningitis.

Nursing Considerations. Nursing care focuses on reducing fever and maintaining a quiet environment. Warm, moist packs may be ordered to relieve muscle spasms. Tube feedings or TPN is necessary for clients who are unresponsive. If acute respiratory distress occurs, a tracheostomy and mechanical ventilation may be required.

The client with encephalitis is subject to seizures. Side rails should be in place. The family needs instructions for safety to prevent injury. The family also needs to be aware that the client may exhibit mental changes such as irritability and confusion.

Guillain-Barré Syndrome

Guillain-Barré syndrome is an autoimmune disorder of the peripheral nervous system. It may also be called *acute febrile, acute idiopathic,* or *infectious polyneuritis.* In Guillain-Barré syndrome, antibodies start to destroy the myelin sheath of peripheral nerves. When the sheath is damaged, it cannot transmit nerve signals to the muscles. The muscles atrophy and become paralyzed. *Paresthesia* (tingling sensation) develops; the nerves cannot transmit sensory messages such as pain, heat, or texture.

Considered rare, both males and females develop the disorder. It can occur at any age. A viral illness, such as a respiratory or gastrointestinal infection, typically precedes the onset of Guillain-Barré. Surgery or vaccinations also have been identified as triggers of the disorder.

Signs and Symptoms. After the nonspecific febrile illness, onset is often sudden. However, 3 to 4 weeks may pass before the development of signs and symptoms. Symmetrical pain and weakness follow. The syndrome usually begins in the lower extremities, ascends, and may progress to total paralysis. Disability ranges from muscle weakness to total body paralysis. Vital functions such as breathing, heart rate, and blood pressure can be compromised. Eventually the progression of the disease stops and stabilizes. The client generally then begins a gradual recovery.

Diagnosis.   Diagnosis is made after obtaining a careful history and review of systems. No differential diagnostic procedure or laboratory test exists. An LP may be done, possibly revealing increased protein levels in CSF.

Treatment.   Some success has resulted from two types of treatments: plasmapheresis and injection of high-dose immunoglobulins. However, the effects of both are temporary. *Plasmapheresis* may be helpful because it removes the antibodies that are destroying the myelin sheaths. *Immunoglobulin therapy* may be effective because it provides normal support to an immune system that is under abnormal attack.

Steroid therapy is controversial because even though it may reduce symptoms, it may be deleterious to the client's progress.

Nursing Considerations.   The nurse must keep in mind that this client has an excellent chance of total or nearly total recovery. Therefore, excellent nursing care is necessary to prevent permanent damage. Emergency interventions, such as tracheostomy and mechanical ventilation, may be necessary when the respiratory muscles fail.

Maintenance of muscle function is required to prevent atrophy and skeletal deformities. Adequate nutrition may necessitate tube feedings or TPN. Family and other caregivers will need instruction in ROM, skin care, positioning, and ADL.

Recovery is usually slow, lasting weeks, months, or years, depending on the severity of symptoms. Emotional support is essential. This condition is frightening for the client and family. If the acute phase of the disease is correctly managed, however, recovery is often complete.

Poliomyelitis

Poliomyelitis, commonly called "polio," is caused by one of three viruses that attack neurons, affecting the motor nerves between the CNS and the muscles. The virus usually enters the body via the fecal–oral route. The virus then travels along the nerve fibers to nerve cells that are connected with a group of muscles. Cells may be damaged temporarily or they may be destroyed. If enough nerve cells are destroyed, the muscle becomes paralyzed.

Signs and Symptoms.   Signs and symptoms of polio include a general flu-like illness including symptoms such as sore throat and fever, nausea, vomiting, and abdominal pain. Aseptic meningitis follows the early symptoms. The disease can progress to cause paralysis at any level of the spine. Some individuals recover completely, while others have permanent paralysis.

Prevention.   Two types of vaccine are available to prevent polio: inactivated poliovirus vaccine (**IPV**, also referred to as the *Salk vaccine*) and trivalent oral poliovirus vaccine (**OPV,** also referred to as the *Sabin vaccine*). Oral vaccine prevents polio in most cases. The Centers for Disease Control and Prevention and the World Health Organization have aggressive plans for the eradication of polio in the 21st century via a Global Polio Eradication Program. The Pan American Health

Organization was a leader in the eradication of polio in the Western Hemisphere in the early 1990s.

Post-polio Syndrome
Post-polio syndrome or *postpoliomyelitis muscular atrophy* (**PPMA**), affects 25% to 40% of individuals who had paralytic polio in childhood. Thirty or more years after the acute attack of polio, the individuals experience mild to severe muscle pain and weakness as a delayed complication of the first infection. The affected muscles may be the same as those affected earlier, or they may be different.

No treatment is yet known, although the disorder is sometimes treated with the same medications as those used for an autoimmune disorder. The individual is not infectious with the polio virus. Nursing considerations relate to supportive care in ADL and maintenance of muscle tissue. Referral to physical and occupational therapies may be necessary.

Acute Transverse Myelitis

Acute transverse myelitis is an inflammatory condition affecting the spinal cord. It results from inflammation or destruction of the myelin of the spinal cord neurons. The person experiences impaired bowel and bladder function, generalized weakness of the extremities, and loss of sensation.

Acute transverse myelitis has several causes. If the disease is diagnosed as *postinfectious,* it usually begins 5 to 20 days after a viral infection. The cause may also be related to collagen–vascular disease, syphilis, or HIV/AIDS. Prognosis varies; some individuals recover fully, and others do not.

Nursing Considerations.   Nursing care for the client with acute transverse myelitis involves supportive and preventive measures. Be alert for urinary retention, constipation, skin breakdown, thrombus formation, and other complications of immobility.

HEAD TRAUMA

Trauma to the brain is a common cause of motor and sensory symptoms, including brain damage, coma, and paralysis. Normally the skull's thick bones, as well as the tough outer membrane of the meninges (the dura), protect the brain; in addition, CSF acts as a shock absorber.

However, violent blows to the head can cause several kinds of injury to the brain and skull. A major complication of head trauma is increased pressure within the brain caused by swelling, hemorrhage, tumors, or the inflammatory process. Head injuries may be the cause of seizures and epilepsy later in life.

> **Nursing Alert**
> Serious symptoms can appear up to several days after a head injury. Observe the client carefully.

Increased Intracranial Pressure

Intracranial pressure (**ICP**) is the pressure that the brain, blood, and cerebrospinal fluid (CSF) exert inside the cerebrospinal cavity. Normally, ICP is 4 to 13 mm Hg. If one of the normal contents of the cranial or spinal cavity (such as brain tissue, blood, or CSF) increases in size, volume, or shape, pressure increases. This increase in pressure can cause the delicate structures to be moved, damaged, or destroyed.

The increase in pressure is due to the limited space within a rigid bony skull, leaving little or no room for expansion due to edema of the brain, hemorrhage, or increased amounts of CSF. Examples of conditions that may lead to ↑ICP include head injury, brain tumor, CNS infection, brain surgery, stroke, and hydrocephalus.

Normal body functions, such as straining at stool (the *Valsalva maneuver*), may also increase ICP, which may temporarily reach well over 100 mm Hg.

Sustained ICP over 15 to 20 mm Hg is called *increased intracranial pressure* (↑ICP). It is an abnormal and dangerous condition. The first consequence of ↑ICP is venous compression, resulting a decrease in blood flow to the brain. This results in cerebral hypoxia or cellular hypoxia. Brain cells are extremely sensitive to levels of oxygen. Neuron tissue death will begin within 4 to 6 minutes if oxygen is not supplied.

An elevation in ICP can occur suddenly and progress rapidly. Usually, ↑ICP begins on one side of the brain, although both sides quickly become involved. Early detection and treatment are vital before complications occur. The earliest and most important sign of ↑ICP is any change in LOC. In Practice: Nursing Assessment 77-2 presents other signs.

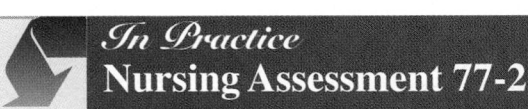

In Practice
Nursing Assessment 77-2

SIGNS OF INCREASED INTRACRANIAL PRESSURE

- Any change in level of consciousness (loss of consciousness, lethargy, confusion, seizures)
- Any change in sensory–motor function (slowed reflexes, slowed response time, restlessness, ataxia, aphasia, slowed speech)
- Headache, which becomes progressively worse or is aggravated by movement
- Change in eye signs or vision (change in pupil size, unequal pupils, slowed or no response to light, inability to follow examiner's finger, difficulty seeing)
- Change in vital signs (pulse <60 or >100, increased blood pressure, widening of pulse pressure, increased or lowered body temperature)
- Change in respirations or evidence of respiratory distress (occurs late—caused by pressure on brain stem)
- ↑ICP, recorded on a monitoring device
- Nausea and vomiting (especially projectile vomiting)
- Urinary incontinence
- Bulging fontanelles (in infant); elevation of bone segments
- Sudden changes in condition
- Leakage of CSF (clear yellow or pinkish) from nose or ear

ICP Monitoring

In special circumstances of ↑ICP, devices that are surgically inserted into the brain can monitor the levels of ICP. The most common monitor is the intraventricular catheter. Other monitors include the subarachnoid (subdural) bolt (or screw), intraparenchymal bolt (fiberoptic), and epidural sensor (least invasive).

The neurosurgeon places such devices using strict sterile technique, using the information that these devices relay via computer to determine the plan of care (Fig. 77-5). These clients are generally in an intensive care unit (ICU), and trained ICU nurses monitor the ICP pressures as part of nursing care. Medications, and possibly surgical interventions, are calculated based on the results of ICP monitoring.

Nursing Alert

Report any break in an ICP monitoring system to the physician immediately. The system must remain sterile. Never move the client's head up or down without specific orders from the physician.

The intraventricular catheter (*ventriculostomy*) may also be used to drain CSF to relieve pressure. The drained CSF can then be sent for laboratory analysis.

Herniation of the Brain

When ↑ICP exerts enough pressure to displace a portion of the brain, *herniation* (an upward, downward, or lateral pushing of a portion of the brain through an opening) can occur. This opening can be a natural intracranial opening, such as the foramen magnum. The brain would herniate (push) through the large foramen (opening) in the occipital bone, which lies between the cranial and spinal cavities.

Herniation can also occur through a previous **craniotomy** (discussed later in text) site, or through an opening caused by trauma. Herniation causes severe injury to the brain because of prolonged hypoxia to parts of the brain that control the vital functions of the body—breathing and blood circulation. The result is brain death, and death of the individual.

When ICP is elevated, an LP is contraindicated because the withdrawal of even a small amount of CSF can cause the brain to shift, or herniate. Therefore, a safer method of determining ICP is ICP monitoring.

Concussion

A **concussion** is the result of any blow to the head. The concussion may not damage any brain structures, but temporary unconsciousness is possible. The length of time that a person remains unconscious varies. Some clients recover from concussions with no apparent ill effects except inability to remember the event; others have blurred vision or severe headaches. A client who has had anything other than a very minor concussion should see a physician immediately for a thorough neurologic examination.

In *coup-contrecoup* injuries, damage occurs both at and opposite to the site of impact. The brain may be hit on one side

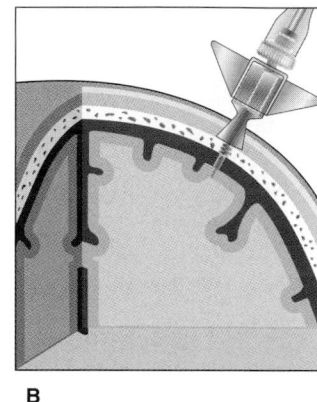

FIGURE 77-5. Intracranial pressure can be monitored by: (**A**) Fiberoptic, transducer-tipped pressure and temperature ventricular monitoring catheter. (**B**) Ventricular bolt that is connected to a pressure transducer and display system.

(*coup*) and then bounce (rebound) off the other side of the skull (*contrecoup*). The brain is partially anchored at the brain stem and floats in CSF within the cranium. With direct and rebound trauma, blood vessels, nerve tracts, brain tissue, and other structures are bruised and torn. Serious injuries may also occur to the brain stem because of the contrecoup action.

After the original injury, a postconcussion syndrome may persist for several weeks to months. Symptoms include headache, anxiety, fatigue, or **vertigo** (a sensation of rotation of self or one's surroundings; not true dizziness).

Laceration and Contusion

A **laceration** is tearing of the brain tissue caused by direct impact or penetrating injury. Lacerations are commonly associated with depressed skull fractures, which are discussed below. In **contusion,** the brain tissue is bruised.

Skull Fractures

A *skull fracture* may be open, closed, simple, depressed, or *comminuted* (fragmented), depending on whether the skull and scalp are intact. Many skull fractures are minor, being no more than cracks in the bone. Usually they heal without difficulty. Any scalp lacerations must be thoroughly examined to determine if the cranium has been opened.

Open skull fractures potentially expose the brain to external microorganisms, which could lead to meningitis or encephalitis. However, open skull fractures are less likely to produce rapid elevations in intracranial pressure. The fracture allows for some brain swelling.

A *depressed skull fracture* is due to a severe blow to the head. The fracture breaks the bone and forces the broken edges to press against the brain, resulting in a significant risk for ↑ICP and meningitis. Effects vary with the injury's severity and location. If, for example, the bone fragment presses on the brain's speech center, the client's speech may be impaired until the pressure is relieved.

A *basilar skull fracture* is a fracture at the base of the skull. It may injure the nerves entering the spinal cord or interfere with CSF circulation. Basilar skull fractures can tear the dura.

In a basilar skull fracture, rhinorrhea, leakage of CSF from the nose (**otorrhea**), or leakage of CSF from the ear may occur. The nurse may be asked to test this fluid for the presence of CSF. A positive test for CSF is known as a *halo sign.* In Practice: Nursing Care Guidelines 77-3 provides two methods of detecting CSF in drainage.

Figure 77-6 illustrates the effects of a basilar fracture with *periorbital ecchymosis* (raccoon's eyes) and *periauricular ecchymosis* (Battle's sign). A basilar skull fracture is an especially dangerous occurrence because of potential damage to the vital centers that control blood pressure and respiration.

Hematoma

A *hematoma* refers to a blood clot within the skull. Hypertension and trauma are the most common causes. With any type of cranial hematoma, ICP may dangerously elevate. The swelling or mass of blood compresses brain tissue, creating further damage. Herniation of brain tissue is possible. There-

In Practice
Nursing Care Guidelines 77-3

DETERMINING CEREBROSPINAL FLUID IN DRAINAGE

- Wet a chemical reagent strip, such as a Dextrostix, with drainage from the nose or ear.
- Observe the color change and whether it indicates the presence of glucose. The presence of glucose in the fluid suggests that the fluid is CSF; test is positive.

However, if the test is positive and there also is blood (which also contains glucose) in the drainage:

- Collect droplets of drainage on a white absorbent pad.
- Inspect the wet area after a few minutes for a *halo sign:* If a yellow ring encircles a central ring that is red, the red ring indicates blood, and the yellow ring suggests CSF.

Adapted from Timby, B. K., Scherer, J. C., & Smith, N. E. (1999). *Introductory medical-surgical nursing* (7th ed., p. 605). Philadelphia: Lippincott Williams & Wilkins.

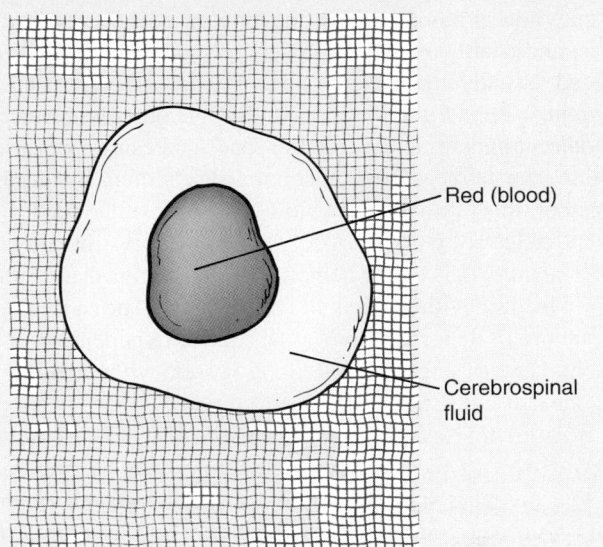

Halo sign. Clear drainage that separates from bloody drainage suggests the presence of CSF

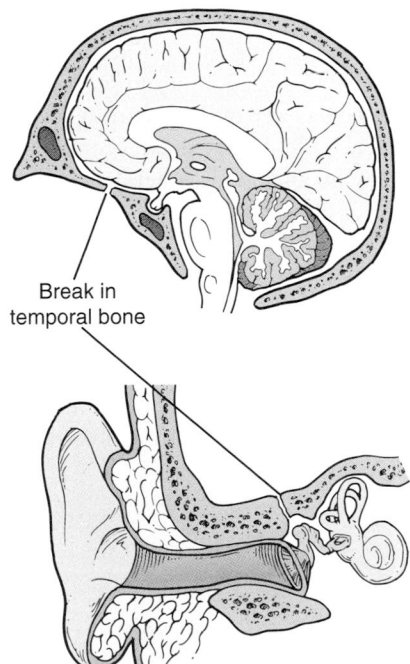

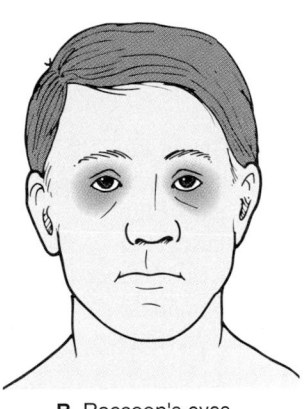

B Raccoon's eyes

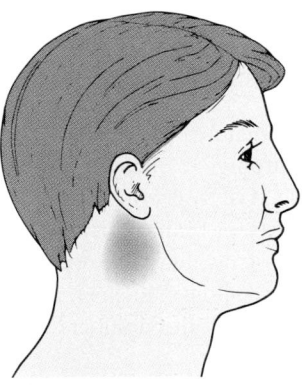

C Battle's sign

FIGURE 77-6. (**A**) Basilar skull fracture in the temporal bone can cause CSF to leak from the nose or ear. (**B**) Periorbital ecchymosis, called *raccoon's eyes*. (**C**) *Battle's sign* over the mastoid process.

fore, carefully observe the client for any signs of ↑ICP. Specific signs and symptoms are determined by the area of the brain affected and the extent of any neurologic damage.

Epidural Hematoma. An *epidural hematoma* is an accumulation of blood, usually from the temporal artery, between the dura and the skull (Figure 77-7A). The pressure of an epidural hematoma can quickly cause seizures, paralysis, and death. One or both of the person's pupils may be dilated. Usually, the person is unconscious immediately after the injury, lucid for a brief period, then unconscious again as blood accumulates in the epidural space and causes pressure. Epidural hematomas are most common in children. The mechanism of injury is typically a blow to the side of the head.

Intracranial Hematoma. An *intracranial (intracerebral) hematoma* is due to hemorrhage and edema that results from bleeding within the skull (Fig. 77-7B). The cause may be rupture of delicate blood vessels due to hypertension or a cerebral aneurysm. Ruptured blood vessels within the brain are one cause of CVAs.

Subdural Hematoma. A **subdural** (below the dura) **hematoma** is typically slow forming (Fig. 77-7C). It is caused by an accumulation of blood, usually from a torn vein on the brain's surface. Symptoms vary with size and location. The person may feel drowsy or lose consciousness, with seizures, paralysis, and muscle weakness. Speech may be affected; confusion is common. Symptoms may not appear for days or even weeks after the accident.

Penetrating Head Injuries

In a *penetrating head injury,* the amount of damage depends on the penetrating object's velocity and location. A high-velocity object, such as a bullet, typically causes more damage than a low-velocity object, such as in a stab wound.

Medical and Surgical Treatment

Immediately after any potential or actual injury to the brain, a neurologic evaluation should be done. The Glasgow coma scale (**GCS**) is commonly used as a broad indicator of the severity of brain injury (Table 77-2). Three areas are given numerical values: eye opening, best verbal response, and best motor response. Each area is evaluated according to standard criteria and the numbers are totaled. The highest possible

number of 15 indicates that the individual has no impairment; the lowest possible number of 3 indicates brain death. The range of 6 to 8 is associated with a coma state.

Medical treatment consists of methods to limit swelling and damage due to ↑ICP. Osmotic diuretics may be given.

Immediate neurosurgery may be necessary to prevent death. Surgery involves tying off the bleeding vessel, and cleaning the area of debris and any accumulated blood or blood clot. Burr holes may be made in the skull or an intraventricular catheter may be inserted, to relieve ↑ICP by draining off CSF or blood.

Nursing Considerations

Head injury will require sensitive nursing care of specific needs as a result of the trauma. Many nursing considerations are listed at In Practice: Educating the Client 77-4.

Loss of consciousness does not always follow a severe head injury. Every client who suffers a blow to the head, no matter how minor it appears, needs careful observation until it is certain that the injury has not damaged the brain. Care providers need to be aware that symptoms of brain damage do not always appear immediately.

The conscious client should remain absolutely quiet, with complete bed rest. Observe for the following signs of ↑ICP: headache, dizziness, visual impairment, hearing loss, dizziness, nausea, or clear or bloody drainage from the ears, nose, or mouth. *Projectile* (forceful) vomiting is indicative of brain injury.

Also observe the client for changes in blood pressure and pupils. If the client is hospitalized, frequently monitor LOC, and note any personality or behavior changes.

Advise a client who is preparing for release after receiving first-aid treatment following a head injury to see a physician immediately if he or she has any of the recurring symptoms mentioned earlier. Teach the family these symptoms also, because the client may be unable to detect deterioration of functioning.

NEOPLASMS

Brain tumors occur in all age groups. Only a small percentage of brain tumors are malignant, and they may result from metastasis from another part of the body. Even a benign brain tumor can be fatal, however, because of the pressure that it

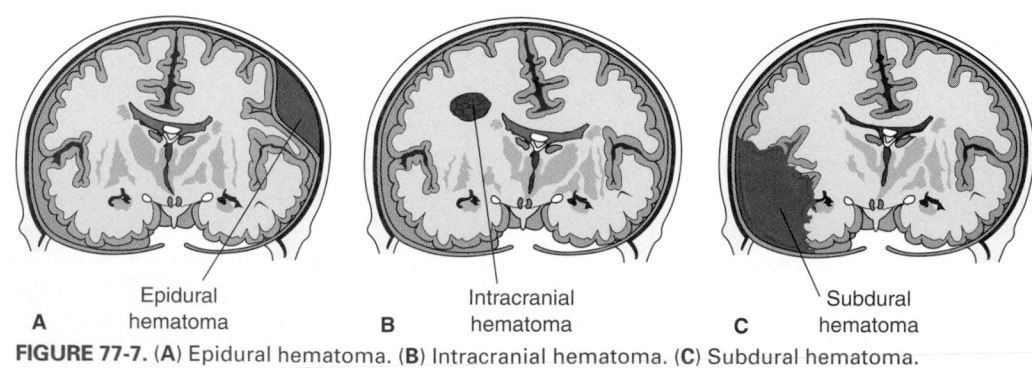

FIGURE 77-7. (A) Epidural hematoma. **(B)** Intracranial hematoma. **(C)** Subdural hematoma.

TABLE 77-2 THE GLASGOW COMA SCALE

Test	Score
Eye Opening (E)	
Spontaneous	4
To call	3
To pain	2
None	1
Motor Response (M)	
Obeys commands	6
Localizes pain	5
Normal flexion (withdrawal)	4
Abnormal flexion (decorticate)	3
Extension (decerebrate)	2
None (flaccid)	1
Verbal Response (V)	
Oriented	5
Confused conversation	4
Inappropriate words	3
Incomprehensible sounds	2
None	1

GSC score = E + M + V. Best possible score = 15; worst possible score = 3.

Source: Smeltzer, S. C. & Bare, B. (2001). *Brunner and Suddarth's textbook of medical-surgical nursing* (9th ed., p. 1682.) Philadelphia: Lippincott Williams & Wilkins.

exerts on the brain. Benign tumors may also later become malignant. Regular followup is essential after treatment for any brain tumor.

Signs and Symptoms

The signs and symptoms of brain tumor include headache, sudden projectile vomiting, and visual abnormalities, all caused by ↑ICP. Additional signs and symptoms may develop, depending on the area of the brain that is affected. For example, if the motor area is affected, numbness or twitching in the arm may occur; a tumor on the brain's frontal lobe may cause personality changes and may affect memory or reasoning abilities.

Often a seizure is the first symptom of a brain tumor. If ↑ICP near the brain stem is unrelieved, severe respiratory difficulties and possibly death due to respiratory failure may occur. As brain tumors grow, signs and symptoms progressively worsen.

Diagnostic Tests

Neurologic assessment and history are necessary to make a diagnosis. By questioning the client and family, the physician can determine the progress of any neurologic deficits. Diagnostic tests, such as the CT scan and EEG, are performed to determine the tumor's location, size, and neurologic effects.

Treatment

Treatment options include surgery, chemotherapy, and radiation therapy, or all three. The specific treatment is determined

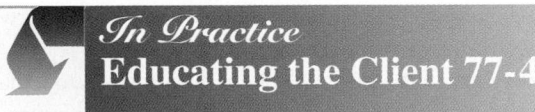

In Practice
Educating the Client 77-4

AFTER A HEAD INJURY

- Know that the client may not be coherent enough to recognize dangerous symptoms.
- Be alert that some symptoms may not appear until several days, weeks, or even months following a head injury.
- Have the client relax for 24 hours so the brain has a chance to recover. Check the client's orientation to time and place every 2 hours for the first 24 hours following any blow to the head.
- Immediately report the following to the physician:
  - Unusual or increased drowsiness
  - Weakness of arms or legs; muscle twitching
  - Nausea and vomiting (especially forceful or projectile vomiting)
  - Headaches—localized or generalized, unrelieved by mild analgesic
  - Dizziness
  - Visual or hearing disturbances, abnormal eye movements
  - Difficulty arousing from sleep, particularly during the first 24 hours
  - Personality changes, such as forgetfulness, irritability, speech difficulties
  - Bleeding or clear drainage from the mouth, nose, or ears
  - Seizures
  - Blood pressure changes

according to the tumor's type and location. One type of surgery is a *craniotomy*, which is discussed next.

Craniotomy. Surgical entry into the skull (cranium) is called a craniotomy. This invasive procedure is performed for many reasons; one of the most common reasons is a brain tumor. Any tumor near the brain is removed, if possible. Its growth would put pressure on the brain. A *craniectomy* is a procedure that removes a portion of skull bone.

Success of surgery for a brain tumor depends on the tumor's location and whether it can be removed without causing brain damage. Some tumors are *inoperable*: impossible to remove without causing severe brain damage or death. Even successful brain surgery can result in neurologic deficits.

Nursing Considerations

Providing Preoperative Care. Before a craniotomy, follow routine preoperative preparation. In addition, the client's head or a portion of it may need to be shaved. If this is the case, inform the client before doing so. Often, hair is not shaved until the client is in the operating room. The client (or legal guardian if the client is a child) must sign an informed consent before hair can be removed or surgery is done. (Shaved hair is put into a paper bag and labeled. This hair can be used later for a wig or hairpiece if the client desires.)

The physician will inform the client if he or she is to remain awake during a craniotomy. Mild sedatives may be given to relax the client, while allowing him or her to respond to various stimuli applied to parts of the brain during surgery. Advise the client beforehand if the surgeon will ask questions or ask for specific movements during surgery. Midazolam (Versed) may be given so the client does not recall the procedure.

The client and family are almost certain to be apprehensive before such surgery. Provide concerned, competent preoperative care. Reassure the client that little pain is involved in brain surgery because the skin is locally anesthetized. Although the procedure can be noisy because the surgeon will drill out a part of the skull bone, the client will feel no pain because the skull and brain have no sensory nerves. However, warn the client about the possibility of a headache after surgery.

Surgery may take from 2 to 6 hours. Anything the nurse can do to make the waiting period easier for family members will be helpful. Take time to say a few words to them at intervals to let them know that they are not forgotten.

Providing Postoperative Care.   During the immediate postoperative period, the client requires expert observation and nursing care, usually provided in the ICU. Monitoring by ICU nurses is done continuously, with comparisons performed between the client's present condition and the initial neurologic examination (the baseline assessment). Any changes, such as signs of ↑ICP, are noted.

Nursing care focuses on the following activities:

- Monitoring the client's vital signs and respiratory status regularly.
- Elevating the head of the bed
- Performing nasogastric suction to help prevent aspiration.
- Positioning the client according to physician's orders
- Checking dressings for blood and CSF, especially at the back and on the side where drainage accumulates by gravity.
- Assessing the client's LOC, orientation to time and place, and ability to speak clearly.
- Checking the client's ability to grasp equally in both hands and to move each foot in any position on command.

These activities are continued even after the client is discharged from the ICU to the nursing unit.

When the client is allowed out of bed, check his or her ability to stand with the eyes closed (*Romberg test*). The client should be able to stand on each foot without holding on to anything. Report any deviation from normal immediately. If in doubt, notify the surgeon. The client's neurologic status can change very rapidly.

During convalescence, the client needs encouragement and understanding. For example, the client may find that it takes time to regain control of bodily movements, or that he or she is spilling food, dropping things, and feeling dizzy when walking. Reassure the client and give assistance as needed.

➤ STUDENT SYNTHESIS

Key Points

- Because the nervous system controls the body's movements, disorders in this system may cause unwanted movement or immobility.

- Seizure disorders have different manifestations, ranging from generalized tonic-clonic movements to uncontrolled movements without loss of consciousness.

- Spinal cord injuries can result in a range of physical and mental deficits, including paralysis.

- Degenerative disorders of the nervous system may cause difficulties in movement, sensory deficits, or varying degrees of alteration in mental status.

- Inflammatory disorders of the nervous system can quickly become life-threatening.

- Increased intracranial pressure has many causes. It is a significant sign of a brain disorder. One of the first and most important signs of increased ICP (and other disorders of the brain) is a change in LOC.

- Most brain tumors are nonmalignant. Benign tumors, however, cause pressure on the brain and can be fatal.

Critical Thinking Exercises

1. Discuss how your nursing care would differ for a client paralyzed from the waist down and a client paralyzed from the neck down. Give explanations for your answers.

2. Mrs. Klein, age 40 years, has recently been diagnosed with MS. She is married with two children, ages 9 and 12. Her husband is very concerned about her condition. When you ask her how she feels about her diagnosis, Mrs. Klein responds, "I don't understand what all the fuss is about. I don't think it's that serious, since I'm feeling fine now." How would you respond to the couple? What types of changes should the family prepare for?

3. You are working with a 70-year-old man who has Parkinson's disease and his family. The client's condition has made it impossible for him to continue to live on his own, and he is planning to move in with his son and daughter-in-law. What types of home care adaptations can be made for the client? What suggestions would you make for the family to successfully adapt to this situation?

NCLEX-Style Review Questions

1. A client has just arrived on your unit with herpes zoster and is complaining of pain. Which nursing intervention should be completed first?
   a. Administer analgesics.
   b. Encourage the client to express his or her feelings.
   c. Order a nutritious meal for the client.
   d. Place the client in a private room on infection control precautions.

2. Following a lumbar puncture, which nursing intervention is appropriate?
   a. Administering antipyretics
   b. Ambulating the client within 2 hours
   c. Instructing the client to remain flat for 6 hours
   d. Keeping the client NPO

3. To prevent further injury in patients with spinal cord injuries, members of the healthcare team should:
   a. Elevate the feet to prevent shock.
   b. Monitor for increased intracranial pressure.
   c. Offer emotional support.
   d. Stabilize the head, neck, and spinal cord.

4. A client was just diagnosed with multiple sclerosis and is bed-bound. The client wants to know if the condition will change. The nurse's best response is:
   a. "You will continue to get progressively worse."
   b. "The disease is marked by remissions and exacerbations."
   c. "You may want to research it on your own."
   d. "The disease usually resolves within 2 years."

5. The nurse teaches clients with seizure disorders to take medications as directed because omitting or stopping medications could result in:
   a. Status epilepticus
   b. Gingival hyperplasia
   c. Focal seizures
   d. A change in the EEG pattern

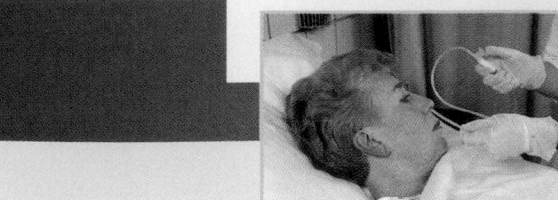

CHAPTER

78

Endocrine Disorders

LEARNING OBJECTIVES

1. Name the common laboratory tests and radiology procedures performed to evaluate functioning of the pituitary, thyroid, parathyroid, and adrenal glands, and pancreas.
2. Differentiate the four major tests used to test blood glucose levels.
3. Describe the difference between gigantism and acromegaly, and SIADH and diabetes insipidus.
4. Compare and contrast Graves' disease, cretinism, and myxedema, including at least three nursing considerations for each.
5. Identify at least five pre- and postoperative nursing considerations for a client who needs a thyroidectomy.
6. Explain the differences between hyperparathyroidism and hypoparathyroidism.
7. Describe the three major adrenal gland disorders: Cushing's syndrome, primary aldosteronism, and Addison's disease.
8. Differentiate among the following: type 1 and type 2 diabetes mellitus, gestational diabetes, and impaired glucose homeostasis.
9. List the three common types of insulins, stating their onset, peak, and duration of action; and the four common groups of oral antidiabetic agents, identifying examples of each group.
10. Compare and contrast hypoglycemia, hyperglycemia, DKA, and nonketotic hyperosmolar state, including causes, signs and symptoms, treatment, and nursing considerations.
11. Identify two examples of macrovascular and microvascular complications of diabetes.
12. Prepare a diabetic client teaching plan that addresses at least ten topics for discussion.
13. Demonstrate the use of a blood glucose monitor in the skills laboratory.

NEW TERMINOLOGY

acromegaly	hypoparathyroidism
Addison's disease	hypothyroidism
cretinism	insulin resistance
Cushing's syndrome	ketoacidosis
diabetes insipidus	myxedema
diabetes mellitus	negative feedback system
endocrinologist	nephropathy
exophthalmos	neuropathy
gigantism	pheochromocytoma
goiter	polydipsia
Graves' disease	polyphagia
Hashimoto's thyroiditis	polyuria
hyperglycemia	retinopathy
hyperparathyroidism	Somogyi phenomenon
hyperthyroidism	thyroidectomy
hypoglycemia	

ACRONYMS

2-h PG	IFG	PTU
ACE	IGH	RAI
ACTH	IGT	RAIU
ADH	IVP	SIADH
BIDS	LH	SMBG
DKA	MMI	STH
FPG	NIDDM	T_3
FSH	NPH	T_4
GDM	OGTT	TFT
GH	PH	TSH
Hb A_{1c}	PTH	VMA
IDDM		

The *endocrine system*, a highly integrated system, is intricately involved in regulating nearly all body processes. The *endocrine glands (ductless glands)* are groups of cells that produce chemical substances called *hormones.* The major sources of the hormones work in concert with other hormones to perform many functions, including the following:

- Helping to control water and electrolyte balance
- Assisting with the regulation of digestion
- Regulating carbohydrate metabolism
- Working as neurotransmitters

- Maintaining stress and inflammation
- Regulating reproductive functions

Endocrine glands and hormones often have more than one name or similar names. (See Chapter 20 for a detailed review of anatomy and physiology.) A physician trained in this specialty is called an **endocrinologist.** Other specialists also treat endocrine disorders.

Most endocrine disorders are caused by overproduction or underproduction of specific hormones. Table 78-1 highlights the major endocrine glands and the functions of the specific hormones each gland produces.

■■■ **TABLE 78-1** *T*HE MAJOR ENDOCRINE GLANDS AND THEIR HORMONES

Gland	Hormone	Principal Functions
Anterior pituitary	GH (growth hormone)	Promotes growth of all body tissues
	TSH (thyroid-stimulating hormone)	Stimulates thyroid gland to produce thyroid hormones
	ACTH (adrenocorticotropic hormone)	Stimulates adrenal cortex to produce cortical hormones; aids in protecting body in stress situations (injury, pain)
	PRL (prolactin)	Stimulates secretion of milk by mammary glands
	FSH (follicle-stimulating hormone)	Stimulates growth and hormone activity of ovarian follicles; stimulates growth of testes; promotes development of sperm cells
	LH (luteinizing hormone); ICSH (interstitial cell-stimulating hormone) in males	Causes development of corpus luteum at site of ruptured ovarian follicle in female; stimulates secretion of testosterone in male
Posterior pituitary	ADH (antidiuretic hormone; vasopressin)	Promotes reabsorption of water in kidney tubules; stimulates smooth muscle tissue of blood vessels to constrict
	Oxytocin	Causes contraction of muscle of uterus; causes ejection of milk from mammary glands
Thyroid	Thyroid hormone (thyroxine and triiodothyronine)	Increases metabolic rate, influencing both physical and mental activities; required for normal growth
	Calcitonin	Decreases calcium level in blood
Parathyroids	Parathyroid hormone (parathormone)	Regulates exchange of calcium between blood and bones; increases calcium level in blood
Adrenal medulla	Epinephrine and norepinephrine	Increases blood pressure and heart rate; activates cells influenced by sympathetic nervous system plus many not affected by sympathetic nerves
Adrenal cortex	Cortisol (95% of glucocorticoids)	Aids in metabolism of carbohydrates, proteins, and fats; active during stress
	Aldosterone (95% of mineralocorticoids)	Aids in regulating electrolytes and water balance
	Sex hormones	May influence secondary sexual characteristics in male
Pancreatic islets	Insulin	Aids transport of glucose into cells; required for cellular metabolism of foods, especially glucose; decreases blood sugar levels
	Glucagon	Stimulates liver to release glucose, thereby increasing blood sugar levels
Testes	Testosterone	Stimulates growth and development of male sexual organs (eg, testes, penis) plus development of secondary sexual characteristics such as hair growth on body and face and deepening of voice; stimulates maturation of sperm cells
Ovaries	Estrogens (eg, estradiol)	Stimulate growth of primary female sexual organs (eg, uterus, fallopian tubes) plus development of secondary sexual organs such as breasts; changes pelvis to ovoid, broader shape
	Progesterone	Stimulates development of secretory parts of mammary glands; prepares uterine lining for implantation of fertilized ovum; aids in maintaining pregnancy

(handwritten annotations: "Females" and "Males" above the LH/ICSH row)

Source: Hosley, J. B., Jones, S. A., & Molle-Matthews, E. A. (1997). *Lippincott's textbook for medical assistants* (p. 643). Philadelphia: Lippincott Williams & Wilkins.

DIAGNOSTIC TESTS

Many blood and urine tests can diagnose endocrine disorders. Other tests, such as computed tomography (CT) and x-ray studies, also may be done. In addition, indirect and direct observation aid in diagnosing endocrine problems because some endocrine disorders lead to defects in growth or appearance.

Pituitary Function Tests

Various tests are used to diagnose disorders of the pituitary gland. Most are specific to the client's suspected condition. Tests include x-ray examinations, CT scans, blood tests, urine tests, and others.

Thyroid Function Tests

Laboratory Tests

The thyroid gland secretes several hormones. Therefore, to assess thyroid function, usually a combination of blood tests is done because no single test gives a complete picture. Multiple tests help determine the cause of the problem, which could be the thyroid gland itself, the pituitary gland that controls it, or both. Table 78-2 presents common thyroid function tests (**TFT**s).

Radiographic Evaluations

Thyroid Scan (Radioscan or Scintiscan). For this test, the client ingests radioactive iodine or receives it intravenously (IV) (see Chap. 47, Box 47-1, for precautions when using dye). Then a scanogram (x-ray study) is obtained to indicate the amount of radioactivity in the entire body. If the thyroid absorbs a great deal of the radioactive iodine, the thyroid is hyperactive, suggesting possible hyperthyroidism. If a decreased amount of iodine appears in the thyroid, the gland is hypoactive, suggesting hypothyroidism or a malignancy. This test may also indicate locations of thyroid malignancy metastases to other parts of the body.

Radioactive Iodine Uptake (RAIU). The *radioactive iodine uptake* (**RAIU**) test measures thyroid gland activity. After a period of fasting, a client drinks a small amount of radioactive iodine dissolved in distilled water, or swallows a capsule of the radioactive substance. At various intervals for up to 24 hours, a scan of the thyroid gland is performed to measure the amount of radioactive material it removes from the bloodstream and absorbs. A normally active thyroid will remove from 15% to 45% within that period; in hyperthyroidism it may remove as much as 90%. Certain drugs can influence the accuracy of a RAIU test, including oral contraceptives, anticoagulants, salicylates, and propylthiouracil (**PTU**) derivatives. Check to make sure that the client is not allergic to iodine or shellfish. Pregnant or lactating women should not take this test.

Before the test, knowing how much iodine the client usually consumes (ocean shellfish, iodized salt, saturated solution of potassium iodide, Lugol's solution) is important. Testers should be aware if clients use iodine-containing antiseptics, or if they have had recent x-ray studies using iodine-based contrast media or other recent studies involving radioactive substances. Question clients about the use of any of the medications mentioned above, plus thyroid-stimulating hormone (**TSH**), estrogen, aspirin, phenothiazines, or barbiturates. Clients must not use any of these substances for a week before the test. In addition, assure clients that the dose of radiation associated with the radioactive iodine is not dangerous. After the substance is given, make sure that the client knows exactly when to return to the laboratory.

Other Tests

Thyroid Ultrasound (Thyroid Echogram). The *thyroid ultrasound* test determines the thyroid gland's size, shape, and position. Abnormal findings may indicate a cyst or a

---

■■■ TABLE 78-2 $\mathcal{T}$**ESTS OF THYROID FUNCTION**

Test	Purpose
FT$_4$I (free thyroxine index)	Measures levels of T$_4$ and T$_3$U
T$_4$ (serum thyroxine)	Measures circulating levels of T$_4$
T$_3$ (serum triiodothyronine)	Measures circulating levels of T$_3$
T$_3$U (T$_3$ resin uptake)	Determines amount of radioactive resin bound to T$_3$
TSH (thyroid-stimulating hormone)	Measures levels of TSH produced by the pituitary gland

Provocative (Response-Inducing) Tests of Thyroid Function

TRH stimulation test	Measures TSH levels repeatedly after thyroid-releasing hormone (normally produced by the hypothalamus to stimulate TSH) is given IV
TSH stimulation test	Measures body's response to TSH by following levels of radioactive iodine uptake and protein-bound iodine uptake
Thyroid suppression test	Measures levels of radioactive iodine uptake and serum T$_4$ after 7 to 10 days of receiving thyroid hormone

solid nodule, which is often cancerous. The test may also be done periodically during treatment to determine the effectiveness of therapy or to evaluate the thyroid during pregnancy (because RAIU examination is dangerous to the fetus).

The ultrasound examination will not hurt, nor will it disturb breathing or swallowing. The test takes approximately 15 minutes. The client will lie on the table, while a liberal amount of water-soluble gel is applied to the neck to ensure transmission of sound waves. The photos and computer printouts will then be evaluated by the healthcare provider. After the test, the client may need assistance to remove the gel from the skin.

Parathyroid Function Tests

Laboratory Tests

Blood tests to evaluate parathyroid function include serum parathormone (also known as parathyroid hormone; **PH, PTH**) levels, serum phosphate and calcium levels, urinary calcium, and serum alkaline phosphatase. Tests of other systems will also be ordered because normal calcium and phosphorus balance involves multiple body systems, including the musculoskeletal, gastrointestinal, and urinary systems.

Other Tests

Ultrasound, magnetic resonance imaging (MRI), thallium scan, and fine-needle biopsy can evaluate the function of the parathyroids and localize parathyroid cysts, tumors, and *hyperplasia* (abnormal increase in size). These tests are described elsewhere in this unit.

Adrenal Function Tests

Laboratory Tests

Blood Tests.   Common blood tests to determine adrenal function include the adrenocorticotropin hormone (**ACTH**) stimulation test, serum ACTH test, and plasma cortisol test. Plasma cortisol and ACTH follow a *diurnal* (daytime) pattern. They can be measured at 8 AM and 4 PM to establish whether or not the normal diurnal pattern is present.

Urine Tests.   Urine tests can also be used to evaluate adrenal function. Measurement of metabolites of catecholamines in the urine is useful in diagnosis. Urinary metanephrine is the most diagnostic urine test of adrenal medulla function. A 24-hour urine specimen may be collected for determining vanillylmandelic acid (**VMA**), a metabolite of catecholamines.

A clonidine suppression test can help determine pheochromocytoma, a catecholamine-secreting adrenal tumor. In this condition, serum and urinary catecholamines are elevated and are not suppressed by clonidine. (Normally, clonidine suppresses catecholamines.) Side effects of the test include hypotension, bradycardia, and *somnolence* (extreme sleepiness).

In addition, a somewhat risky test involves histamine administration, which produces a hypertensive crisis when the client has pheochromocytoma. Similarly, phentolamine (Regitine) can be given to provoke a hypotensive situation. The drop in blood pressure is diagnostic of pheochromocytoma.

A 24-hour urine specimen may be collected for determining metabolites such as 17-hydroxycorticosteroids, 17-ketosteroids, and 17-ketogenic steroids. These 24-hour urine collections require special preservatives. Know the institution's requirements and make sure the appropriate container is available. Proper client education is necessary to ensure the collection of all urine.

Radiographic Evaluations

Radiographic evaluations of adrenal function include the adrenal angiogram and venogram, CT scan of the adrenals, MRI, ultrasonography, and retroperitoneal air sufflation, as well as x-ray study of the sella turcica. These examinations detect benign and malignant tumors of the adrenal glands, as well as *hyperplasia* (excess multiplication of normal cells).

Adrenal Angiogram or Venogram.   These tests involve insertion of a catheter and injection of a contrast medium (dye) so that x-ray contrast studies can be done. The client is usually *NPO* (nothing by mouth) before the test. The major complication is an allergic reaction to the dye. Therefore, be sure to determine the client's allergy to dye before the test, and observe other precautions as listed in Chapter 47. To prevent this complication, propranolol (Inderal), diphenhydramine (Benadryl), or other medications may be administered for several days before and after the test. The test may also cause hemorrhage or dislodging of an atherosclerotic plaque from the wall of the blood vessel used for dye injection. This may cause an infarction. If hemorrhage occurs within the adrenal glands, *Addison's disease* (chronic adrenocortical insufficiency resulting from adrenal gland destruction) may result. If surgery is needed later, it is more difficult when any of these events have occurred.

Angiograms and venograms are also contraindicated in clients who are pregnant, unstable, or uncooperative and in those with hemophilia, a bleeding disorder, or measurable atherosclerosis.

General Pancreatic Function Tests

The pancreas secretes two enzymes: *amylase,* necessary for carbohydrate metabolism; and *lipase,* necessary for fat digestion. Serum levels of both of these enzymes can be obtained. Elevations suggest pancreatitis. Urinary amylase levels also may be obtained. The amylase level in urine remains elevated for a longer time than in serum (see discussion in Chap. 87).

Tests for Diabetes Mellitus

Blood Tests

A number of blood tests indicate the functioning of the endocrine portion of the pancreas. Some of these tests specifically relate to the detection and evaluation of diabetes mellitus.

Fasting Plasma Glucose.   The *fasting plasma glucose* (**FPG**) test, formerly called the *fasting blood sugar,* is used for diabetes screening. In most cases, an elevated *fasting* (without eating) or nonfasting blood glucose level is an indication of *diabetes mellitus* (metabolic condition involving elevated levels of glucose in the blood). The FPG level is defined as the amount of glucose (sugar) present in the blood when the client has been fasting for the prescribed length of time (6–8 hours). The normal range for FPG is 65 to 115 milligrams per deciliter (mg/dL). An FPG greater than or equal to 126 mg/dL and confirmed on a subsequent day indicates diabetes.

Oral Glucose Tolerance Test.   The *oral glucose tolerance test* (**OGTT**) is a timed test used to confirm the diagnosis of diabetes mellitus when the client's FPG is equal to or greater than 126 mg/dL, or when the client's FPG is above normal but below the diagnostic level for diabetes. It is also used in screening for gestational diabetes in both the 1- and 3-hour formats. OGTT also can diagnose functional *hypoglycemia* (abnormally low blood sugar).

- The client should ingest at least 150 grams of carbohydrate daily for 3 days before the test (most individuals following a good general diet easily meet this criterion).
- Tests of both blood and urine are done during the fasting state.
- The client drinks 75 to 100 grams of glucose. He or she must consume this glucose completely and as quickly as possible. (Rationale: The starting point of this timed test must be as precise as possible.)
- Blood and urine specimens are again taken at prescribed intervals: ½ hour, 1 hour, 2 hours, and 3 hours. The collection of specimens is timed from the point of ingestion of glucose.
- The test begins with an empty bladder, although the pretest urine specimen is also saved as one of the fasting specimens to be examined.
- The laboratory technician takes the blood and urine specimens, labels them, and indicates the time when each was collected.
- The client may have water to drink during the test to provide comfort and to make voiding easier. Juice, other fluids, and food are not permitted.
- The client is not allowed to smoke or chew gum.

Normally, plasma glucose levels peak at 160 to 180 milliliters within 30 minutes to 1 hour after administration of an oral glucose solution, and return to fasting levels or lower within 2 to 3 hours. Urine glucose tests should remain negative throughout. Values greater than or equal to 200 mg/dL at 2 hours (2-hour post-load glucose [**2-h PG**]) suggest diabetes. Some factors that may affect the test include thiazide diuretics, oral contraceptives, lithium, caffeine, and nicotinic acid. These substances elevate glucose levels.

Glycosylated Hemoglobin.   The *glycosylated hemoglobin* (**Hb A$_{1c}$**) level reflects the client's average blood glucose level over the previous 6 to 10 weeks. It is measured by determining the amount of glucose attached to a certain portion of hemoglobin in red blood cells. This test is invaluable in monitoring blood glucose control, and allows the client and healthcare team to set measurable goals. Although normal ranges vary depending on the laboratory, most physicians want their clients to be in the range of 5% to 8%, depending on which exact subfactors they are measuring.

Urine Tests

Normal urine is free from sugar (*glucose*), acetone, and protein, but any of these may be present in a diabetic person's urine. Excess glucose in the blood spills over into the urine; acetone appears as a by-product of faulty metabolism. With the availability of a variety of sophisticated (but easy-to-use) blood glucose monitors, urine testing is now done infrequently, both in the healthcare facility and at home. The most common need for urine testing is the test for ketones if a client's blood glucose level is consistently high. Because only clients with type 1 diabetes are prone to diabetic ketoacidosis, these clients learn to test their urine for ketones if their blood glucose readings exceed 240 mg/dL.

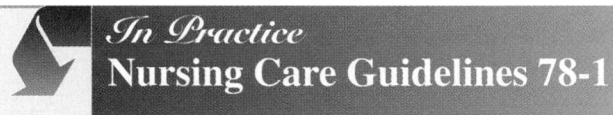

Nursing Alert

The test for urine ketones (acetone) is especially important if the client is vomiting, has a fever, or has a high concentration of glucose in the blood (greater than 240 mg/dL).

Keto-Diastix Test.   *Acetone* is a ketone body that is present when the body cells are starving because of faulty metabolism. Buildup of acetone leads to ketosis, which in turn leads to acidosis. Vomiting or excessive perspiration can alter electrolyte balance. The Keto-Diastix test detects elevated glucose and ketone levels. This simple test as outlined at In Practice: Nursing Care Guidelines 78-1.

In Practice
Nursing Care Guidelines 78-1

USING KETO-DIASTIX

- Wear gloves.
- Ask the client to void and discard the first specimen.
- About half an hour later, ask the client to collect a freshly voided specimen, which is used for testing.
- If withdrawing a specimen from an indwelling catheter, the nurse must obtain the specimen from the port of the catheter tubing and not from the bag. *Rationale: The tubing contains the most recent urine. The bag contains older urine that may have been altered by chemical changes.*
- Dip the test strip quickly into the urine.
- Following instructions regarding time intervals, take the reading for glucose and acetone, using the color chart on the bottle.
- Close the cap of the bottle tightly, because moisture in the air can render the strips ineffective.
- Document your results. Report any abnormal findings to your supervisor.

COMMON MEDICAL AND SURGICAL TREATMENTS

Because such a variety of disorders with an endocrine basis exist, medical treatments are discussed with each condition.

The most common surgical treatment for some pituitary or thyroid disorders is removal of the affected gland. The pituitary gland also may be removed in some cases to slow or stop the spread of certain types of malignancies that are nourished by an endocrine hormone. These surgeries will be discussed later in this chapter.

Diabetes mellitus cannot be treated with surgery, although pancreatic or cellular transplants have had some success in reversing the symptoms. These procedures will be discussed later.

NURSING PROCESS

Data Collection

Using the skills of physical examination and nursing assessment (see Chap. 47), observe and assess clients for possible endocrine disorders. This establishes a baseline for future comparison, and helps determine the presence of suspected endocrine-related complications. Report any changes in baseline levels.

Many assessments of endocrine function are based on laboratory examination of blood. Other testing, such as with x-rays or ultrasound, is also done. Check reports of these evaluations and report any abnormal results immediately. Nurses may perform blood testing for glucose and occasionally urine testing for ketones.

While caring for clients, note any signs and symptoms of endocrine disorders and report them. In addition, observe the client's emotional response to the disorder or disease. Does the client need assistance to meet daily needs? Is the client anxious or fearful of the outcome? Is the person having difficulty accepting a disorder's long-term nature?

Nursing Diagnosis

Based on data collection, numerous nursing diagnoses may be seen in nursing care plans for clients with endocrine disorders. These nursing diagnoses may have more than one causal factor. Some examples of nursing diagnoses include the following:

- Imbalanced Nutrition: Less Than Body Requirements related to endocrine dysfunction
- Imbalanced Nutrition: More Than Body Requirements related to metabolic dysfunction
- Impaired Skin Integrity related to diabetic ulceration, poor tissue healing following surgery or trauma, impaired circulation
- Ineffective Coping related to chronic disorder, lifelong administration of insulin or other hormone
- Ineffective Management of Therapeutic Regimen as evidenced by failure to follow prescribed regimen of diet, exercise, and medication (eg, insulin)
- Impaired Physical Mobility related to foot ulcers, impaired circulation, amputation
- Impaired Home Maintenance Management related to low activity tolerance, impaired mobility, pain
- Deficient Knowledge related to management of hormonal disorder, diet, exercise, medication administration
- Disturbed Body Image related to amputation of limbs, physical manifestations of the disorder, loss of mobility, or chronicity of disorder

Planning and Implementation

Plan together with the healthcare team for effective care to meet the client's needs, based on the nursing diagnoses. Properly prepare clients for diagnostic tests. Provide pre- and postoperative care for clients undergoing surgery.

Because disorders of the endocrine system can affect most body functions, listing all the nursing implications is difficult. An endocrine disorder can be a simple imbalance that is successfully rectified by administration of hormones or other medications. However, in some cases, such as end-stage renal disease caused by diabetes mellitus, a client may require total nursing care and assistance to meet all needs, including those related to death and dying.

Clients may have difficulty accepting an endocrine disorder's chronic nature and the fact that treatments, such as insulin injections or thyroid medications, must continue for life. Most clients need to learn about their disorder, its prognosis, and its treatment.

Evaluation

Periodically, the healthcare team evaluates the outcomes of the client's care. Have short-term goals been met? For example, is the client's blood glucose level being maintained within an acceptable range? Are long-term goals still realistic? Planning for further nursing care considers the client's prognosis, any complications, and the client's response to care given. Client and family teaching is an important component of nursing care. Do the client and family understand the treatment required and the underlying reasons? For example, do they demonstrate an understanding of the need for lifelong thyroid hormonal replacement? Is teaching adequate and documented?

PITUITARY GLAND DISORDERS

Disorders of the Anterior Lobe

The anterior pituitary exerts control by a **negative feedback system**—after it has stimulated a target gland to produce a hormone and the hormone level rises high enough, the anterior pituitary stops stimulating the target gland and stops the hormone release. The anterior lobe alone produces or releases the following hormones: growth hormone (**GH;** somatotropin [**STH**]), ACTH, TSH, prolactin, follicle-stimulating hormone (**FSH**), and luteinizing hormone (**LH**). These hormones are of vital importance in growth, maturation, and reproduction.

Giantism and Acromegaly

Disturbances of the anterior lobe may cause overproduction of the growth hormone STH. If overproduction occurs in childhood, it causes excessive growth of bones, or **gigantism.** In adults, an excess of STH causes overgrowth of tissues, called **acromegaly.** The features of the person with acromegaly coarsen. He or she develops a massive lower jaw, thick lips, a bulbous nose, a bulging forehead, and hands and feet that seem enormous. In women, facial hair also appears (*hirsutism*) and the voice deepens. Headaches are common and partial vision loss may develop. The spleen, heart, and liver enlarge; muscles weaken; and joint pain and stiffness appear. Men may be impotent. Women may not menstruate (*amenorrhea*).

Acromegaly is treated by irradiation of the pituitary gland using proton-beam therapy or surgical intervention. Recently, certain drugs such as bromocriptine mesylate (Parlodel) and somatostatin analogs have shown promise in lowering the levels of STH. Treatment can stop the disease's progression, but therapy cannot alter abnormal growth that has already occurred.

Disorders of the Posterior Lobe

The posterior lobe of the pituitary secretes and releases hormones that affect blood pressure and control water balance in the kidney tubules. It releases *antidiuretic hormone* (**ADH** or *vasopressin*), which regulates the passage of water through the kidneys. It also releases oxytocin in women, which stimulates uterine contractions during labor, and milk release during breastfeeding.

Syndrome of Inappropriate Antidiuretic Hormone (SIADH)

The *syndrome of inappropriate antidiuretic hormone* (**SIADH**) involves the excessive secretion of ADH. Clients with SIADH cannot excrete dilute urine. Fluid retention and ultimately water intoxication occur, along with sodium deficiency. SIADH can result from central nervous system (CNS) disorders, chemotherapy, ADH production by some cancers, and overuse of vasopressin therapy.

Urinary output decreases. The severity of the condition depends on how low the client's serum sodium levels fall (*hyponatremia*), and how much water he or she retains. The client may complain of a headache or experience confusion, lethargy, seizures, and possibly coma if sodium deficiency is severe. Hyponatremia may cause diarrhea. Weight gain also occurs with fluid retention.

Close monitoring of fluid intake and output (I&O), daily weights, and mental status is necessary. Institute safety measures to reduce the risk of possible injury. Fluids usually are restricted to 500 to 1,000 milliliters daily. To correct fluid retention and hyponatremia, medications such as hypertonic saline infusions and diuretics may be ordered. Also, medications such as demeclocycline (Declomycin) and lithium carbonate, which interfere with the antidiuretic action of ADH, may be ordered. Treatment is aimed at correcting the underlying problem.

Diabetes Insipidus

Diabetes insipidus is a disease that results from underproduction of ADH. *Primary nephrogenic insipidus* is rare and is caused by kidney dysfunction, due to a deficiency in ADH or to a lesion in the midbrain. *Secondary central diabetes insipidus* results from a tumor in the gland itself or pressure in the pituitary area from head trauma, infection, or other tumors. It may also occur after pituitary surgery that removes all or a portion of the gland.

In diabetes insipidus, the client voids (copious) amounts of urine, as much as 15 to 20 liters in 24 hours. The urine is dilute, with a specific gravity less than 1.006, and contains no sugar or acetone. The client is constantly thirsty; restricting fluids may have some effect. Keep accurate I&O records to make sure the volume of output is being replaced; closely monitor electrolyte levels. Record daily weights in the early morning before breakfast. Despite an abnormally large appetite, the client is weak and may need assistance with self-care. Treatment consists of giving ADH (vasopressin [Pitressin]) subcutaneously, intramuscularly (IM), or by nasal spray to control urinary output.

> **Nursing Alert**
> Monitor pitressin administration closely, because it can cause coronary artery constriction.

Pituitary Neoplasms

Neoplasms of the pituitary gland can affect various aspects of body function. An overgrowth of eosinophilic cells in the pituitary can result in gigantism. A basophilic tumor in the pituitary can upset production of the hormone that regulates the adrenals, leading to hyperadrenalism (*Cushing's syndrome*). A chromophobic tumor can destroy the pituitary and result in hypopituitarism. A client with this disorder has fine, scanty hair; lowered basal metabolic rate; lowered body temperature; and a tendency toward obesity and slow movements.

Hypophysectomy

Hypophysectomy, surgical removal of the pituitary gland, may be done for a variety of reasons, including malignancy or to decrease diabetic retinopathy. Occasionally the pituitary is removed to control pain associated with metastatic carcinoma of the breast or prostate. Postoperatively, the client usually is admitted to the intensive care unit.

THYROID GLAND DISORDERS

The *thyroid gland* secretes the hormones thyroxine (T_4) and triiodothyronine (T_3), which regulate metabolism by stimulating *catabolism* (the breakdown of cells and foods, with release of energy). Too much of these hormones makes tissues burn oxygen rapidly; too little causes the reverse. The thyroid gland requires iodine to produce these hormones. Thyroid-stimulating hormone from the anterior pituitary gland influences the secretion of T_3 and T_4. In addition, the thyroid gland produces *calcitonin,* which helps to maintain calcium balance in the plasma (see Tables 78-1 and 78-2).

Hyperthyroidism

Hyperthyroidism involves the overproduction of T_4, which leads to an increase in metabolic rate. **Graves' disease** or *exophthalmic* or *toxic diffuse* **goiter** (enlargement of the thyroid gland) is the most common type of hyperthyroidism. The exact cause of this overactivity is unknown, but it may result from infection, physical or emotional strain, or changes related to puberty or pregnancy. Current theories point to an autoimmune origin, in which the person forms antibodies against thyroid cells, specifically the TSH receptor cells. Hyperthyroidism occurs most frequently in women.

Signs and Symptoms

The client is highly excitable and overactive, and may have tremors that make eating impossible without help. The pulse is rapid; the person may have heart palpitations and increased incidence of arrhythmias, which will cause damage if left untreated. The systolic blood pressure is elevated. The person feels hot, and eats voraciously—yet loses weight—because he or she burns calories so rapidly. The skin takes on a characteristic salmon color. In women, menstruation may cease.

Another common symptom is bulging eyes (**exophthalmos**). Figure 78-1 illustrates a woman with Graves' disease. The cause of this symptom is not fully understood. It can lead to blindness caused by stretching of the optic nerve or corneal ulceration. The neck is swollen, and pressure from the thyroid gland may cause hoarseness or difficulty swallowing.

If untreated, this disorder may cause intense nervousness, delirium, and finally death as a result of persistent cardiac overload.

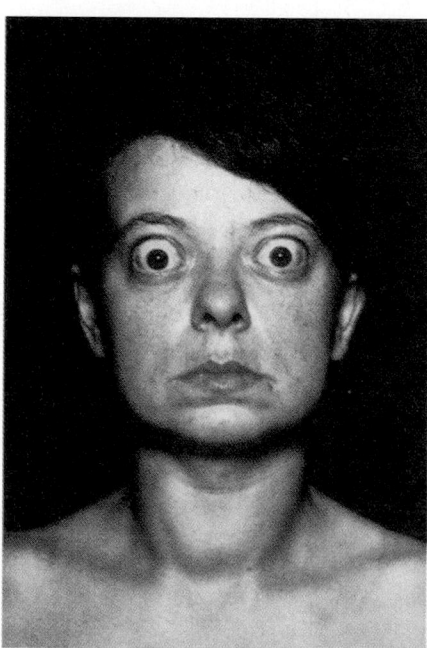

FIGURE 78-1. A woman with Graves' disease. Note the exophthalmos and enlarged thyroid gland.

Treatment

Treatment for hyperthyroidism may be medical or surgical. Medical treatment consists of prescribing antithyroid drugs to block secretion of the thyroid hormone. PTU or methimazole (**MMI;** Tapazole) may be given either as part of a medical treatment or as preparation for surgery. If prescribed as medical therapy, these drugs are given daily, generally over a long time. They may have toxic effects—fever, skin rash, and enlarged lymph nodes, with an increase in white blood cells. Therapeutic doses of radioactive iodine (**RAI**) may also be prescribed. RAI is administered as an oral solution absorbed through the gastrointestinal tract. The radioactive iodine is transported to the thyroid gland, where it destroys the gland's ability to make T_4 and T_3.

Thyroidectomy, removal of the thyroid gland, is no longer the treatment of choice and is done only after anti-thyroid drugs and radioactive iodine have proven unsuccessful, or when the goiter is so large that it constricts structures in the neck region.

Nursing Considerations

Nursing care focuses on minimizing overactivity, improving nutritional status, maintaining a normal body temperature, and improving self-esteem. Assist in providing a calm environment and minimizing the client's expenditure of energy by helping with activities and encouraging alternating periods of rest and activity. Provide increased calories and nutritional support to help improve the client's nutritional status. Diet therapy usually consists of increased caloric and protein needs, vitamins (especially B complex and D), minerals (especially calcium), and fluids. If exophthalmos is present, the client can use eye protection, such as patches, drops, or artificial tears. If body temperature is elevated, give acetaminophen (Tylenol) as ordered and use cooling blankets to reduce body temperature. Because the client is experiencing changes in appearance, appetite, and weight along with overactivity, convey understanding, concern, and willingness to help.

Hypothyroidism

Hypothyroidism occurs when a deficiency of T_4 slows down metabolic processes. It may be due to removal of the thyroid gland or to a decrease in its activity. It is more likely to affect women than men. The congenital form of this deficiency causes a condition called **cretinism.** Advanced hypothyroidism in the adult is called **myxedema.**

Signs and Symptoms

As seen in Figure 78-2, untreated cretinism results in arrested physical and mental development and dystrophy of bones and soft tissues. The person is dwarfed and has a large head, short arms and legs, puffy eyes, and a protruding tongue. The person also has dry skin and movements that are uncoordinated; sterility occurs in almost all cases. Intellectual impairment ranges from moderate to severe (see Chap. 73). If discovered early, this condition can often be successfully treated with administration of T_4 replacement, which must continue for life.

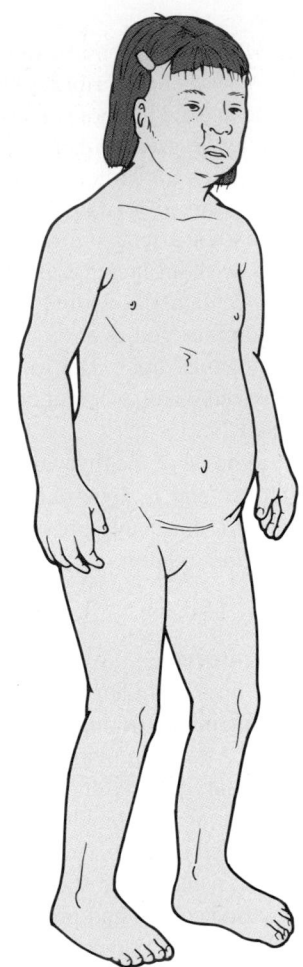

FIGURE 78-2. A client with cretinism.

In adults, myxedema is evidenced by a slowing of physical and mental activity, accompanied by forgetfulness and chronic headache. The client's expression becomes masklike. The skin is dry; the voice is hoarse and low; hair is coarse and tends to fall out; and the client gains weight. The client may become chronically constipated and anemic, and heart rate may be affected. The RAIU uptake rate will almost always be normal; *menorrhagia* (excessive menstrual flow) may occur.

Treatment

Oral thyroid extract such as Armour Thyroid or Proloid (thyroglobulin) may be ordered. More commonly, synthetic thyroid hormones such as levothyroxine sodium (Levothroid) or liothyronine sodium (Cytomel) are given to supply the hormone deficiency. The results are dramatic. The client becomes more alert and the appearance becomes normal. Replacement therapy must be done gradually because a rapid change can be dangerous; for example, the heart rate may increase too rapidly and show signs of strain from increased activity.

Nursing Considerations

Nursing care focuses on the client's improvements in activity tolerance and independence, resuming normal bowel function, improving mental activity, and adhering to the medical

regimen. Anyone with a thyroid deficiency is susceptible to respiratory depression from sedatives or hypnotics. Some people must take thyroid replacement preparations all their lives, but with regulated treatment, they remain well and healthy. Followup visits with healthcare providers for periodic examinations are essential.

> ### ✚👁 Nursing Alert
>
> Do not give sedatives, narcotics, and hypnotic drugs to the person with hypothyroidism, or give them in very small doses. *Rationale: The client's respiratory and heart rates are already slow; additional depressants could cause respiratory or cardiac arrest.*
>
> Be alert for signs of myocardial infarction (MI). *Rationale: MI could result from the long period of slowed circulation to heart muscle.*
>
> Immediately report any complaints of anginal pain, which can occur when thyroid hormone therapy begins. Teach the client signs and symptoms of angina (see Chap. 80). *Rationale: This pain can be the first sign of an MI. A clot may block a portion of the coronary circulation.*

Long-term untreated hypothyroidism can result in *myxedema coma*, a medical emergency necessitating immediate but careful administration of thyroid hormone. Treatment of any depressed respiratory function that occurs and close monitoring of cardiac function are essential.

Hashimoto's Thyroiditis

Hashimoto's thyroiditis is hypothyroidism believed to be autoimmune in origin. It is of the type of autoimmune disorders known as *organ specific* because the body builds up antibodies against thyroid tissue only.

Simple Goiter

Sometimes the thyroid gland, even though enlarged, does not cause toxic symptoms, in which case it is called a *colloid goiter* or a *simple goiter*. The thyroid gland enlarges and the distended spaces are filled with *colloid*, a gelatinous material. No symptoms of T_4 deficiency are noted. (If symptoms of too much T_4 occur [hyperthyroidism], the goiter is referred to as a *toxic goiter*.)

Simple goiter affects women more commonly than men and may appear during pregnancy, adolescence, or infection. Except for its appearance, a simple goiter usually has no harmful effects on health, unless it becomes so large that it interferes with swallowing or breathing.

Usually, a dietary deficiency of iodine causes simple goiter. The thyroid gland must have iodine to produce thyroid hormones. If a sufficient iodine supply is unavailable, the gland enlarges. Sea (salt) water, some soils, and inland drinking water contain iodine. Noncoastal areas—such as mountainous areas, the Pacific Northwest, and the Great Lakes region—are deficient in iodine.

Treatment

Goiter is treated by giving iodine to the client for a period of 2 to 3 weeks and repeating the treatment three or four times during the year, if dietary iodine intake is deficient. Administration of iodine does not cure simple goiter; it prevents it or stops its progression.

The most economical, suitable, and reliable goiter prevention program is the use of iodized table salt. Reinforcing the body's supply of iodine is simple because the thyroid needs a very small amount. Surgery may be necessary if a goiter causes excessive pressure.

Thyroid Neoplasms

A liquid or semisolid cyst sometimes forms in the thyroid. It can be located by ultrasound. A *simple cyst* can be aspirated. A *semisolid cyst* is most often malignant and must be surgically removed. A malignant tumor can occur any time from childhood to late adulthood. If a thyroid tumor is cancerous, it must be removed surgically or treated by irradiation with radioactive isotopes. A biopsy study will tell whether such a growth is malignant. Most common thyroid cancers are slow growing, although a fast-growing adenocarcinoma may metastasize and not respond to radiation therapy.

Thyroidectomy

Thyroidectomy is surgical removal of the thyroid gland. Surgery to remove tissue from the thyroid was once the primary method of treating hyperthyroidism. Today, however, surgery is reserved for special circumstances, such as for pregnant women, those who are allergic to antithyroid medications, and clients with large goiters. Generally, about ⅚ of the gland is removed (*subtotal thyroidectomy*) so that some thyroid hormone production continues postoperatively. Before surgery, PTU or MMI is administered until signs of hyperthyroidism are minimized. In addition, β-adrenergic blocking agents (usually propranolol [Inderal]) may be used to reduce the heart rate. However, if these measures fail to achieve a normal thyroid state, iodine (Lugol's solution or potassium iodide) may be given. Thyroid hormone levels and metabolic rate must be normalized before surgery to reduce the risk of thyroid storm (see discussion below).

A subtotal thyroidectomy usually prevents the recurrence of hyperthyroidism because only enough of the gland is left to maintain normal function. If a *total thyroidectomy* is done (because of injury or malignancy), the client requires thyroid hormone (thyroxine; T_4) for life.

Postoperative Complications

Postoperatively, the client is at risk for complications including hemorrhage, hematoma formation, edema of the glottis, and injury to the recurrent laryngeal nerve. Keep airway equipment near the client's bedside postoperatively in case edema of the laryngeal area causes respiratory distress.

> ✚👁 **N u r s i n g   A l e r t**
>
> Internal hemorrhage, following thyroidectomy, is a threat. Inspect dressings for excessive bleeding. Check for edema in the neck or bleeding at the back of the neck. Keep an endotracheal tube available in the client's room, both preoperatively and postoperatively, because swelling may obstruct the airway, causing respiratory distress. In this event, an endotracheal tube is inserted and the client is taken to the operating room for a tracheostomy.

Another potential and dangerous complication is *tetany*, a generalized continuous muscle spasm of the entire body. It is most often caused by accidental removal of the parathyroid glands during thyroidectomy. *Chvostek's sign* (abnormal spasm of the facial muscles in response to light taps on the facial nerve) and *Trousseau's sign* (an abnormal carpopedal spasm induced by inflating a sphygmomanometer cuff on the upper arm to a pressure exceeding systolic blood pressure for 3 minutes) may be positive (Fig. 78-3). (Trousseau's sign also may be seen in clients with hypocalcemia and hypomagnesemia.) Serum calcium levels also may be low. This condition may be fatal, resulting in seizures and cardiac arrhythmias. Emergency treatment of tetany is the IV administration of calcium gluconate, which must be kept available postoperatively. PTH may be administered, along with calcium gluconate, to treat the condition. If the parathyroid glands have been totally removed, administration of PTH must continue for life.

Thyroid crisis (*thyrotoxicosis* or *thyroid storm*) is another possible complication that can occur in the hospital or possibly after discharge. It is a dangerous condition caused by a sudden increase in T_4. Pre- and postoperatively, be alert for symptoms such as tachycardia, anxiety, and an abrupt increase in vital signs. This extreme form of thyrotoxicosis can cause heart failure. Treatment focuses on maintaining oxygen and glucose levels in the body cells, while reducing fever. Sedatives, tranquilizers, and cardiotonics may be prescribed. Thyroid storm is less prevalent postoperatively with the use of antithyroid

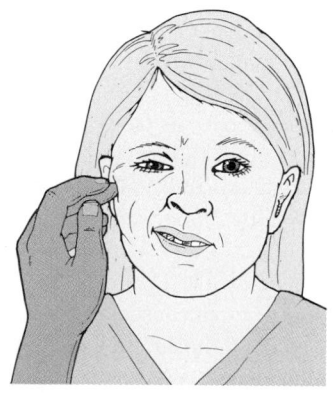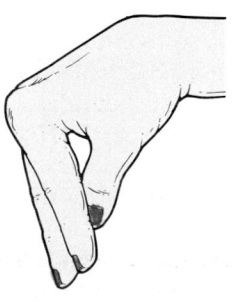

A **B**

FIGURE 78-3. (A) Chvostek's sign. **(B)** Trousseau's sign.

drugs and iodine preparations. In some cases, corticosteroids are given.

Nursing Considerations

Nursing considerations include encouraging the client to rest and avoid excessive physical activity, and to increase nutritional intake to ensure adequate calories, vitamin D, and calcium. Teach the client the importance of continued medication therapy and the signs and symptoms of hypofunction and hyperfunction. Reinforce the need for close followup after surgery. Periodically, the client will need to have thyroid function tests done as part of the followup.

PARATHYROID GLAND DISORDERS

The *parathyroid glands* secrete PTH. Aided by vitamin D, PTH regulates the amount of calcium and phosphorus in the blood, and thus regulates bone formation.

Hyperparathyroidism

Hyperparathyroidism stems from an excess of PTH that causes blood calcium levels to rise, resulting in calcium depletion in bones (*osteomalacia*). Bones become soft and weak, leading to skeletal tenderness. They tend to break easily, even in the absence of pressure or injury (*pathologic fractures*). The skull may enlarge. Muscles weaken, and the client complains of fatigue, nausea, and constipation. Kidney stones, urinary tract infections, and uremia may develop. The person may become disoriented and paranoid and may lose consciousness. This condition may be secondary to chronic nephritis.

Hyperparathyroidism is detected by a consistently high blood level of parathormone and by x-ray indications of skeletal changes or pathologic fractures.

A diuretic agent such as furosemide (Lasix) and large amounts of fluids are often given to prevent renal disorders such as stones, which develop because of the high blood calcium levels. Phosphates may be given cautiously to reduce the serum calcium level. A thyroid lobectomy to remove part of the thyroid gland containing the parathyroid may be done.

Preoperatively, encourage exercise to help prevent the bones from releasing some calcium. Calcium in the diet is limited in some cases. If tetany occurs postoperatively, calcium gluconate is given to restore the blood's calcium–phosphorus balance.

Keep a tracheostomy tray and IV calcium at the bedside for emergency use. The postoperative diet is high in calcium, fat, and carbohydrate. The client needs special care to avoid injury until bones are recalcified.

Hypoparathyroidism

Hypoparathyroidism, the deficiency of PTH, results from lowered production of the hormone, with a consequent reduction in the amount of calcium available to the body and an accumulation of phosphorus in the blood. Accidental removal of the parathyroid glands during a thyroidectomy may cause hypoparathyroidism.

Lack of calcium causes tremors and tetany, the characteristic sign. Cardiac output decreases. A positive Trousseau's sign (carpopedal spasm caused by blocking the blood flow to the arm for 3 minutes using a blood pressure cuff) or a positive Chvostek's sign (twitching of the mouth, nose, and eye after tapping the area over the facial nerve just in front of the parotid gland and anterior to the ear) suggests latent tetany (see Figure 78-3). This extreme muscular irritability may be so pronounced that laryngospasm or seizures occur. Other symptoms include hair loss, skin coarsening, brittle nails, arrhythmias, and possible heart failure.

Treatment is to increase the client's serum calcium level. Calcium salts (calcium gluconate) must be given, usually IV. (Never give calcium preparations IM; they injure tissues.) Large doses of vitamin D are also given because vitamin D helps regulate body calcium levels. Administration of sedatives or anticonvulsants may also be necessary in the acute phase of hypoparathyroidism (to prevent seizures). Client teaching about medications and the need for followup is important.

ADRENAL GLAND DISORDERS

The *adrenal glands* contain two parts: the cortex and the medulla. The *cortex* (outer covering) secretes various types of steroid hormones that control many vital functions. These hormones regulate metabolism to supply quick energy, help maintain fluid and electrolyte balance, and regulate the development of secondary sex characteristics. Disorders involving the hormones of the adrenal cortex are described in this chapter. The *medulla* is stimulated by the sympathetic nervous system and secretes the hormones epinephrine (adrenaline) and norepinephrine. The effects of epinephrine and norepinephrine are discussed in Chapters 19 and 77.

Cushing's Syndrome

Cushing's syndrome (*hyperadrenalism*) results from overproduction of hormones secreted by the adrenal cortex. It can also result from overuse of corticosteroids, or tumors of the adrenal glands or the pituitary.

Fat distribution is abnormal. The face is rounded ("moon face"), the abdomen is heavy and hangs down, and the arms and legs are thin. As the disease progresses, the client becomes weaker, the bones soften, and the client may have a backache. Edema develops and urinary output decreases. *Hypokalemia* (low blood potassium levels) is usually present. *Hypernatremia* (high blood sodium levels) and *hyperglycemia* (abnormally high blood sugar) follow. The client is hypertensive. Wounds do not heal and the client bruises easily. Mood swings are common; the client may be irritable or euphoric. Striae may develop, due to enlarged abdominal girth.

If hyperadrenalism occurs in childhood, puberty starts early for boys. Girls develop masculine traits (such as hirsutism), due to increased secretion of male sex hormones by the adrenal glands.

Nursing Alert

Many young people, especially athletes, use large doses of steroids to enhance muscle development. This dangerous practice often leads to long-term disability and can be fatal. In addition to sexual dysfunction and heart dysrhythmias, the person is at risk for severe behavior problems. In some cases, the person becomes aggressive, loses touch with reality, or shows manic symptoms.

Treatment

Treatment depends on the cause. Surgical removal of the adrenal gland may be indicated. Adrenocortical hormones are given as indicated. After surgery, the client is treated as for Addison's disease. If the cause is pituitary in origin, various controversial methods of treatment are possible.

Nursing Considerations

Nursing care primarily is symptomatic. Institute measures to protect the client from injury and infection, such as assessing skin integrity, promoting good hygiene, and removing or minimizing environmental hazards. Monitor the client's weight daily and assess vital signs frequently. Check electrolyte and glucose levels for changes.

Primary Aldosteronism

This rare condition of the adrenal cortex is characterized by excessive secretion of aldosterone. Symptoms include hypertension and muscle weakness due to low potassium levels. If tumors or excessive growth of the adrenal glands exist, surgery to remove the glands is the treatment of choice.

Addison's Disease

Destruction or degeneration of the adrenal cortex causes a condition called **Addison's disease,** a relatively rare disorder. Tuberculosis, cancer, or a massive infection can be the underlying cause, but in most cases, the gland *atrophies* (wastes away) for unknown reasons. It may be a secondary response to pituitary malfunction. In this case, the pituitary gland fails to produce ACTH in sufficient amounts; thus, adrenal function diminishes.

Signs and Symptoms

With Addison's disease, the production of adrenal hormones decreases, resulting in fluid and electrolyte imbalances and hypoglycemia. In addition, thyroid function is abnormally low, with hyponatremia and hyperkalemia.

The first symptom is usually a darkening of the skin and oral mucous membranes, so that the skin looks bronzed. Dehydration, anemia, and weight loss are seen. Blood pressure drops. The hair thins. Strain or stress of any kind may cause adrenal shock, with abnormally low blood pressure, nausea and vomiting, diarrhea, headache, and restlessness. Tremors and disorientation may arise, progressing to loss of consciousness and seizures.

Addisonian crisis occurs when adrenal function falls to a critically low point. This condition is marked by nausea, vomiting, weight loss, and extreme hypotension, leading to vascular shock, which can be fatal. A stressful situation is usually the precipitating factor.

IV administration of hydrocortisone (Cortef, Hydrocortone) is the treatment of choice. In some cases, vasopressors, such as dopamine hydrochloride (Dopastat, Intropin), are given to raise blood pressure. Salts (sodium and potassium ions) lost by vomiting are replaced in an IV solution of saline with added electrolytes. The exact solution and electrolyte content, to be given several times daily, are determined by the laboratory test results.

Treatment

Treatment consists of supplying needed hormones (fludrocortisone acetate [Florinef]) to restore normal fluid and electrolyte balance. Typically the prescribed diet is high in protein and sodium and low in potassium.

Nursing Considerations

Because this client is dehydrated, fluid replacement is key. Because sodium loss results from previous hormone imbalance, sodium also must be replaced in the diet. Although water intake is restricted, increased sodium will aid in fluid retention without excess fluid intake. (Rationale: Excess water overloads the system.)

Five or six small meals may be prescribed, or the client may receive between-meal snacks of milk and crackers. (Rationale: The person may be too weak to eat a large meal at one time. The diet is planned to combat dehydration.)

Watch the person for dizziness or lowered blood pressure, and protect him or her from falling. Accurately record all food and fluid intake, including the type and amount. Also document the volume and specific gravity of each voiding. Daily weights are important. (Rationale: All these measurements help determine the body's fluid and electrolyte balance. Therapy continues until these values are normal.)

Client teaching is vital. Enlist the client's cooperation and urge the client to maintain regular followup visits with his or her primary healthcare provider and to avoid strain or stress, such as overwork, infection, or exposure to cold. By protecting his or her health, the client with Addison's disease can do very well.

☛ KEY CONCEPT

The client should wear an identification tag with instructions for hormone dosage in case the prescribing physician cannot be contacted.

Adrenal Neoplasms

Pheochromocytoma is a tumor, usually benign, that originates in the adrenal medulla. A tumor of the adrenal medulla increases secretion of the hormones epinephrine and norepinephrine, which in turn causes extreme hypertension, tremor, headache, nausea and vomiting, dizziness, and increased urination. Treatment is surgical removal of the tumor—a dangerous operation because it may cause sudden and extreme changes in blood pressure. Prior to surgery, a 24-hour urine test (VMA test) will be ordered to confirm the diagnosis. In addition, a CT scan of the adrenal glands, along with IV pyelogram (**IVP**) (see Chap. 88), may be used to locate the tumor. After surgery, a repeat 24-hour urine for VMA and catecholamines will be done to evaluate return to normal levels. If the client has a bilateral adrenalectomy, he or she must be treated for Addison's disease postoperatively; adrenal hormones must be supplied artificially for life.

PANCREATIC ENDOCRINE DISORDERS

Hormonal disorders of the pancreas include hypoinsulinism and hyperinsulinism. *Hyperinsulinism* is not common, but it may be a precursor to *hypoinsulinism.* Lowered amounts, lack of, or ineffective use of insulin leads to the disorders of *diabetes mellitus.* Diabetes mellitus has various forms, including type 1 diabetes, type 2 diabetes, gestational diabetes, and impaired glucose tolerance or homeostasis. Understanding the various types, treatments, and implications of diabetes mellitus is critical for any healthcare provider. Table 78-3 looks at the basic concepts of type 1 and type 2 diabetes.

Diabetes Mellitus

Specialized cells of the pancreas produce a hormone called *insulin* to regulate metabolism. Without this hormone, glucose cannot enter body cells and blood glucose levels rise. As a result, the individual may begin to experience symptoms of hyperglycemia. Simply stated, this process is the development of **diabetes mellitus.**

The American Diabetes Association defines diabetes this way:[1]

> Diabetes mellitus is a group of metabolic diseases characterized by hyperglycemia resulting from defects in insulin secretion, insulin action, or both. The chronic hyperglycemia of diabetes is associated with long-term damage, dysfunction, and failure of various organs, especially the eyes, kidneys, nerves, heart, and blood vessels.

At least 16 million people in the United States are believed to have diabetes, half of whom have not yet sought medical attention. Numbers have increased in recent years because so many Americans are overweight. Also, testing accuracy has improved, thus confirming more cases. The number of people with diabetes is expected to double as more people live to middle and old age, when most cases are discovered.

Classification
Diabetes mellitus is classified in the following ways:[1]

- Type 1 (Formerly known as *type I; insulin-dependent diabetes mellitus* [**IDDM**]; or *juvenile diabetes*)
- Type 2 (Formerly known as *type II; non–insulin-dependent diabetes mellitus* [**NIDDM**]; or *adult-onset diabetes*)
- Gestational diabetes mellitus (**GDM**): Occurring during pregnancy and disappearing on delivery
- Impaired fasting glucose (**IFG**) and impaired glucose tolerance (**IGT**): Two categories of *impaired glucose metabolism* (or *impaired glucose homeostasis* [**IGH**]); considered risk factors for future diabetes and cardiovascular diseases

Other specific types of diabetes mellitus include uncommon forms of immune-mediated diabetes and diabetes caused by genetic defects in pancreatic beta-cell function or insulin action, diseases of the exocrine pancreas, endocrinopathies (either drug- or chemical-induced), infections, and other genetic syndromes.

Signs and Symptoms
Diabetes can present a wide variety of signs and symptoms. Often clients have no symptoms; but when present, they may include the three "polys":

Polyuria (excessive urination)
Polydipsia (excessive thirst)
Polyphagia (excessive hunger)

These classic symptoms are found more often in type 1 diabetes and come on rapidly.
Other signs and symptoms may include:

- Fatigue
- Blurred vision
- Mood changes

■■■ **TABLE 78-3** 𝒯YPE 1 AND TYPE 2 DIABETES MELLITUS

Consideration	Type 1	Type 2
Typical age of onset	Under age 30	Over age 30
Classic symptoms	Nearly always present	Usually not present
Hereditary factors	Occasionally present	Usually present
Weight	Normal or underweight	Usually overweight
Prone to ketoacidosis	Yes	No
Usual treatment	Insulin, meal plan, exercise	Meal plan, exercise, possibly oral medications or insulin

- Numbness and tingling in extremities
- Dry skin
- Infections (urinary tract, vaginal yeast infections)
- Weight loss (most often in type 1)

Blood and urine tests for glucose (see discussion at the beginning of this chapter) are used to diagnose diabetes mellitus. Box 78-1 lists diagnostic criteria for diabetes mellitus.

Type 1 Diabetes Mellitus

Type 1 diabetes has two forms: immune-mediated and idiopathic. *Immune-mediated diabetes* results from autoimmune destruction of the pancreatic beta cells. One and usually more of these types of autoantibodies are present in 85% to 95% of individuals when fasting hyperglycemia is initially detected. *Idiopathic diabetes* has developed spontaneously or without an identifiable cause.

Type 1 diabetes accounts for approximately 5% to 10% of cases in the United States. Recent research has shown an inherited tendency for developing the disease, with environmental factors triggering the disease process. These specific factors and how they work are as yet unknown.

Type 1 diabetes also appears to have an autoimmune component, because antibodies to insulin and islet cells are present at the time of diagnosis. In addition, type 1 diabetes is associated with some autoimmune diseases.

When type I diabetes is diagnosed, the goal is to achieve metabolic stabilization, restore body weight, and relieve symptoms of hyperglycemia. Ongoing goals focus on achieving and maintaining normal metabolic functions and minimizing the negative impact of diabetes on the person's life. See In Practice: Nursing Care Plan 78-1 for a nursing care plan for a client with type 1 diabetes.

Type 2 Diabetes Mellitus

Type 2 diabetes can occur at any age, but most cases occur after age 30. More than 80% of clients are overweight and do not always experience classic symptoms. The pancreas is often still functional at diagnosis, which means it still produces insulin. Levels may be normal, low, or elevated. The person may show a decreased tissue sensitivity to insulin, called **insulin resistance.** Clients with type 2 diabetes do not depend on insulin injections to sustain life, but they may require insulin for adequate glucose control.

Approximately 90% to 95% of individuals who have diabetes in the United States have type 2. It is more prevalent in African American, Native American, and Hispanic populations than in Caucasians and is more frequently diagnosed in women than in men. Risk factors for developing diabetes include heredity, obesity, age, stress, and lack of exercise. The individual with type 2 diabetes may have an inherited tendency to develop the disorder, which is triggered by environmental factors. (Type 2 diabetes carries about twice the heredity risk when compared with type 1.) The specific etiology of type 2 diabetes is yet unknown; however, autoimmune destruction of pancreatic beta cells does *not* occur. This type of diabetes develops more frequently in women with prior GDM and in individuals with hypertension or dyslipidemia (abnormal amounts of fat in the blood).

Most clients with this form of diabetes are obese, and obesity itself can cause some degree of insulin resistance: The muscle cells of obese people are less responsive to insulin than are the muscle cells of thinner people, and most glucose breakdown occurs in the muscle cells. Without the normal response to insulin in the muscle cells, the cells cannot take up glucose, leading to increased glucose concentration in the bloodstream (high blood glucose, *hyperglycemia*).

Clients who are not obese may have an increased percentage of body fat in their abdominal regions. Ketoacidosis (see "Hyperglycemia" section) seldom occurs, but may arise in the presence of another illness. This form of diabetes frequently goes undiagnosed for many years. Because hyperglycemia develops gradually, clients may not notice any classic diabetes symptoms. However, they are at increased risk for development of *macrovascular* (large blood vessels) and *microvascular* (small blood vessels) complications, discussed later.

The major goals for treatment are to achieve metabolic control and to prevent vascular complications. Recommended treatment includes meal planning, an exercise program, weight loss, and medication, if needed. Weight management is a primary concern because losing as little as 5 to 10 pounds can significantly improve blood glucose control.

➤➤ BOX 78-1

DIAGNOSTIC CRITERIA FOR DIABETES MELLITUS

In nonpregnant adults, diabetes can be diagnosed in any of the following three ways, confirmed on different days by any of these three tests:

- A fasting plasma glucose (**FPG**) greater than or equal to 126 mg/dL (after no caloric intake for at least 8 hours) (FPG is the preferred test)
- A casual plasma glucose (taken at any time of day without regard to time of last meal) greater than or equal to 200 mg/dL with classic diabetes symptoms (increased urination, thirst, and unexplained weight loss)
- An oral glucose tolerance test (**OGTT**) value greater than or equal to 200 mg/dL in the 2-hour sample

In pregnant women, diagnosis of gestational diabetes is made if two or more blood glucose levels meet or exceed the following during a 100-g oral glucose tolerance test:

Fasting	105 mg/dL
1 h	190 mg/dL
2 h	165 mg/dL
3 h	145 mg/dL

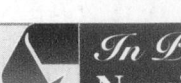

In Practice
Nursing Care Plan 78-1

THE CLIENT WITH TYPE 1 DIABETES

MEDICAL HISTORY: *D.W., a 24-year-old male client, diagnosed with diabetes mellitus type 1 approximately 6 months ago, comes to the clinic for a followup visit. Fasting blood glucose this morning was 210 mg/dL. Vital signs are within acceptable parameters. Currently, he is prescribed insulin twice daily, in the morning and before dinner with self blood glucose monitoring before meals and at bedtime. Client states, "I forgot to check my blood and take my shot last night before dinner."*

MEDICAL DIAGNOSIS: *Diabetes mellitus, type 1, poorly controlled*

Data Collection/Nursing Assessment: Client is an active 24-year-old sales executive. He reports skipping meals several times a week. "When I'm on the road, I stop to get some fast food, like french fries and a milkshake." He reports that he hasn't been keeping a log of his blood glucose results. He stated, "I'm too busy and I don't always have my monitor with me. So, I forget." History reveals that client performs self–blood glucose monitoring on the average of once a day. He states that he has been taking his insulin as prescribed, but does admit to forgetting insulin on the average of 1 to 2 times per week. "I can give myself the injection without a problem, I just can't remember to do all these things." (*Although other nursing diagnoses may be appropriate, a priority nursing diagnosis is addressed below.*)

Nursing Diagnosis: Ineffective therapeutic regimen management related to lack of knowledge about control of blood sugar and difficulty integrating diabetes into daily activities as evidenced by client's statements of skipping meals and insulin and being too busy.

Planning
SHORT-TERM GOALS:
#1. Client will verbalize the importance of adhering to prescribed regimen.
#2. Client will demonstrate understanding of interconnection of diet, activity, insulin administration, and blood glucose monitoring in diabetes control.

LONG-TERM GOALS:
#3. Client will maintain a written log of insulin administration and self blood glucose monitoring, bringing it with him at next visit.
#4. Client will demonstrate ability to integrate diabetes into his lifestyle.

Implementation
NURSING ACTION: *Review underlying physiologic components of the disorder and rationale for specific monitoring activities.*
RATIONALE: *Review of information reinforces the necessity and the reasons for adhering to the regimen.*

NURSING ACTION: *Have client demonstrate techniques for insulin injection and self blood glucose monitoring.*
RATIONALE: *Having the client demonstrate techniques provides an opportunity to evaluate the client's ability to perform them adequately.*

NURSING ACTION: *Question client about usual activities for the day, including time spent in car on the road, at the office, and at home. Work with the client to develop a plan for the day that includes aspects of his diabetic regimen.*
RATIONALE: *Determining the client's usual activities helps to develop an individualized plan for this client. Working with the client provides the client with an opportunity to participate in the plan, providing him with some feelings of control over the situation.*

Evaluation: Client states, "I didn't realize that this disorder could really hurt me and that the insulin was so important." Client able to demonstrate techniques for insulin injection and blood glucose monitoring without difficulty. Client reports that he carries an appointment book with him at all times; appointment book has a planning section with an area for "things to do." *Progress to meeting Goal #1.*

NURSING ACTION: *Discuss the correlation among diet, activity, and insulin. Reinforce the need for a well-balanced diet with periodic snacks.*
RATIONALE: *Discussing the interconnection among diet, activity, and insulin helps to stress the need for adherence to the regimen.*

NURSING ACTION: *Offer suggestions for appropriate food choices when client is on the road. Enlist the aid of a dietician to help with this.*
RATIONALE: *Offering suggestions in conjunction with help from a dietician provides the client with some alternatives and choices, enhancing his feelings of control over the situation.*

Evaluation: Client talking about ways to make sure he eats when out on the road. He stated, "I really need to take better care of myself. It's going to be some work,

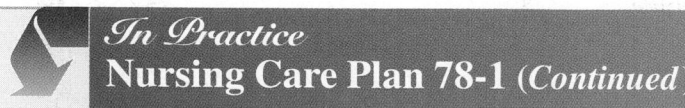

In Practice
Nursing Care Plan 78-1 (Continued)

but it is important to stay healthy." Client will carry blood glucose monitor with him in his briefcase; will record glucose levels in appointment book and bring to next visit. *Goal #1 met; progress to meeting Goal #2 and Goal #3.*

NURSING ACTION: *Question client about ways he will use to monitor his diabetes. Provide feedback and direction as needed.*
RATIONALE: *Having the client propose methods for monitoring promotes client participation in his care and provides a sense of control over the situation, thereby enhancing the chances for success and adherence.*

Evaluation: Client stating that he will take fresh fruit with him to work, and have some snacks readily available in the car when he is on the road; verbalizing

appropriate food choices and times for insulin administration and blood glucose monitoring. *Goal #2 met.*

NURSING ACTION: *Arrange for followup visit for client in 2 weeks, with phone-call followup for review of log and activities in 4 days and at 1 week.*
RATIONALE: *Followup provides a means for determining adherence to instructions and plan, and client's ability to begin implementing the plan.*

Evaluation: Followup phone call on the fourth day: client reported using insulin twice each day and monitoring blood glucose twice the first day, three times the next, and four times the past 2 days; blood glucose values within acceptable ranges. Client reported appropriate food choices. He stated, "I haven't stopped for any fast food since my visit." *Progress to meeting Goal #3 and Goal #4.*

☞ KEY CONCEPT

In type 1 diabetes, insulin deficiency is absolute; insulin injections are necessary for survival. In type 2 diabetes, insulin deficiency ranges from insulin resistance with relative insulin deficiency to a predominantly secretory defect with insulin resistance.

Gestational Diabetes Mellitus

Gestational diabetes mellitus occurs in about 4% of pregnant women, usually in the second or third trimester. Because hormones related to pregnancy stimulate insulin resistance, pregnant women are screened for GDM between 24 and 28 weeks' gestation. GDM usually disappears after delivery. However, women who have had it carry a 25% to 60% risk of developing type 2 diabetes later in life.

Impaired Glucose Homeostasis

In this condition, a client's glucose levels are above normal but not high enough to meet the criteria for a diagnosis of diabetes. As listed previously, IFG and IGT are two categories of IGH. IFG occurs when the client's FPG is greater than 110 but less than 126 mg/dL. IGT means that the results of an OGTT are greater than 140, but less than 200 mg/dL (in the 2-hour sample).

Research has shown that people with IGH are at high risk for developing diabetes and macrovascular complications such as *myocardial infarctions* (heart attack) and cerebrovascular accidents. This condition requires close monitoring. Research (Diabetes Prevention Program) is currently being conducted to

determine whether early treatment can prevent or delay the development of diabetes in people with IGH.

Treatment

All persons with diabetes must maintain a carefully planned and balanced regimen of diet, exercise, and medication as prescribed. The client's understanding of and adherence to a personalized treatment program greatly improves its effectiveness.

The goals of treatment for diabetes include the following:

- Relief of symptoms
- Maintenance of normal weight
- Achievement of normal activity
- Maintenance of blood glucose levels between 70 and 140 mg/dL
- Achievement of acceptable glycosylated hemoglobin (less than 7%)
- Prevention of long-term and short-term complications
- Prevention of hypoglycemic and hyperglycemic reactions

Nutrition Therapy

Nutrition therapy in diabetes is based on an individualized assessment. The dietician generally is responsible for establishing baseline parameters for the client's diet. The nurse reinforces diabetic teachings, encourages diet maintenance, and provides client and family support.

To develop the most individualized dietary plan for the client, the following factors must be assessed:

- Degree of diabetes control
- Presence of complications such as infection, decreased cardiovascular stamina, or neuropathies

- Presence of disabilities such as visual problems, the inability to prepare meals, or financial concerns
- Adequacy of current nutrient intake
- Treatment goals
- Usual eating habits
- Personal schedule and lifestyle
- Client's biochemical indices, such as the glycemic index
- Client's medication regimen

In the early phases of nutritional therapy, clients are often encouraged to obtain blood glucose levels before and after meals. Individuals will vary in their responses to carbohydrates; thus, the glycemic index will vary from person to person. The results of blood glucose monitoring provide the client, the physician, and the dietician with a more individualized picture of the client and his or her response to the diet. Thus, the health-care team has a better understanding of how specific foods affect the individual's glucose level and can adjust foods or medications accordingly.

The current trend in diabetic diet management is to use carbohydrate counting. The rationale for this technique is that blood glucose levels are most affected by the carbohydrates in foods. The total amount of carbohydrate is more important than the source.

Counting carbohydrates can be simpler and less structured than other meal-planning approaches because the client focuses on one nutrient rather than on several food groups. People who follow carbohydrate counting must consult with a registered dietitian. Booklets describing three levels of carbohydrate counting are available from the American Diabetes Association as well as the American Dietetic Association.

Another way to introduce clients to basic diabetes nutritional guidelines is through the Diabetes Food Guide Pyramid. This pyramid is often used to explain the principles of the diabetic diet. Written at a basic level for easy comprehension, this informative pamphlet is ideal for newly diagnosed clients, especially those who are unable to meet with a dietitian immediately.

Not often used, but still available, is the Diabetic Exchange List Diet. A booklet, Exchange Lists for Meal Planning, helps an individual to plan the diet by grouping foods into three categories based on their major nutrient contents. Clients can interchange selections from several lists such as fruit, starch, and milk. The exchange lists include new products on the market, such as reduced-fat or fat-free versions of foods, as well as vegetarian alternatives to meat products.

As with carbohydrate counting, the Exchange Lists emphasize the amount of carbohydrate consumed rather than the type, allowing clients flexibility in choosing their foods at each meal. They can even include carbohydrates, such as cake, into their overall meal plans. Nutrition Tips with each list give clients an overview of the nutrient content of foods. Selection Tips help clients purchase the correct quantities of foods and prepare them in healthy ways.

A very basic approach to diet management is the plate method. Simply stated, the plate is divided into halves or quarters. The dietician or the nurse can demonstrate a typical meal pattern to the client. For example, one half of the plate is a non-starchy vegetable. The other half is divided into two quarters. Proteins make up one quarter and starchy foods make up the remainder.

With any meal planning program, followup appointments with a dietician are important.

Exercise

Although exercise is an important aspect of health promotion for all persons, it is a therapeutic tool for clients with or at risk for diabetes. Exercise increases circulation, helps control weight, decreases blood pressure, and reduces stress. It also helps regulate blood sugar levels. Effects will depend on the individual client and the type of diabetes. Clients must learn which effects may occur, as well as how to reduce the risk of hyperglycemia or hypoglycemia. This understanding is important because their bodies cannot compensate for changes in the same manner as nondiabetic individuals.

Before beginning an exercise program, individuals with diabetes mellitus will undergo a detailed medical evaluation with appropriate diagnostic studies. Medical history and physical examination will focus on signs and symptoms that affect the heart and blood vessels, eyes, kidneys, and nervous system. Clients learn to properly warm up before and cool down after exercise. Precautions involving the feet are essential for people with diabetes. Proper hydration is also important because dehydration can adversely affect blood glucose levels and heart function. Clients must take precautions when exercising in extremely hot or cold environments.

Clients who use medications to control their blood glucose levels must understand the relationship of exercise to food intake and medication use, and learn how and when to exercise. For those with type 1 diabetes, all levels of exercise, including leisure activities, recreational sports, and competitive professional performance, may be appropriate if they have effective glucose control. Exercise does not control this type of diabetes; thus, the purpose of exercise is for its multiple health benefits. These clients must learn to monitor blood glucose before and after exercise, to ingest added carbohydrates if glucose levels are under 100 mg/dL, and to maintain adequate hydration. Making appropriate insulin adjustments based on blood glucose readings is essential.

The possible benefits of exercise for clients with type 2 diabetes are substantial. Long-term studies have shown that regular exercise helps improve carbohydrate metabolism, insulin sensitivity, and blood glucose control. Other possible benefits include weight loss and reduction of hyperlipidemia. The benefits of exercise in the prevention and management of type 2 diabetes are probably greatest when clients start early in the disease's progression.[2]

Insulin

Proper insulin management is essential to ensure the longevity of the diabetic client. Insulin is available in many forms to meet individual needs. All forms are given subcutaneously because digestive enzymes destroy their effectiveness if taken orally. When insulin is present in the blood, it enables glucose to pass through the capillary membranes to the cells for energy. Insulin also helps the liver convert glucose to glycogen, and increases cellular use of oxygen.

Types. Insulin is derived from beef or pork, or can be synthetically manufactured by recombinant DNA technology to resemble human insulin, commonly referred to as *human insulin.* These synthetic preparations tend to work more quickly than those of animal origin. However, clients switching from one type to another can expect different blood sugar responses.

Development of human insulin also has led to decreased *autoimmune* (allergic) reactions in people with diabetes. Antibody levels with human insulin are lower than they are with animal insulin. Therefore, diabetic clients may require lower dosages of human insulin because the body uses it more efficiently. Chances for the breakdown of fat tissue with scarring and malabsorption (called *lipodystrophy*) are also less common with human insulin. Today, most newly diagnosed clients automatically are prescribed human insulin. Many, if not all, clients who previously used beef- or pork-derived insulin are being switched to human insulin as well.

Types of human insulin vary as to their time of onset, peak action, and duration of action. *Regular insulin* is usually referred to as a *short-acting insulin;* Humulin-L and Humulin-N are examples of *intermediate-acting insulins* (**NPH** is also a term used to refer to intermediate-acting insulin); Humulin-U is *long acting.* These differences are shown within Table 78-4.

Lispro (Humalog) is a human insulin analog that is rapid acting. Because it starts working within 15 minutes after administration, clients must take it immediately before a meal. Clients base dosage on the amount of carbohydrates that they will ingest. They must perform blood glucose testing frequently to prevent hypoglycemia.

Lantus is a new long-acting insulin that lasts 24 hours. Unfortunately, it has a low pH. As a result, it cannot be mixed in a syringe with other insulins.

Schedules for insulin vary. During the day, clients usually must repeat doses of rapid or quick-acting insulins, if used alone, because their effects are shorter than are other forms of insulin. Clients must supplement such insulins with a basal dose of intermediate or long-acting insulin once or twice daily. One strength of insulin, U-100 (100 units per milliliter), is widely used in the United States.

Syringes. Syringes for giving insulin are marked in units for measuring the dose. Different types of syringes are available with an attached needle, including 1-milliliter, ½-milliliter, and the ³/₁₀-milliliter disposable syringes. A 1-milliliter syringe can hold up to 100 units of insulin; the ½-milliliter syringe can hold up to 50 units of insulin; the ³/₁₀-milliliter syringe can hold up to 30 units of insulin. Clients use the latter syringes for very small dosages only. Other syringes also are available, including prefilled syringes with short-acting (regular) insulin only, or prefilled syringes with premixed insulin in different ratios. For example, Novolin 70/30 and Humulin 70/30 contain 70% of NPH (intermediate-acting insulin) and 30% regular insulin in one syringe. Other devices such as cartridges and jet injectors also are available for insulin administration. For example, the Novo-pen or Novolin-pen is a cartridge that looks like a pen. The client dials the desired dose of insulin.

Use, Care, and Storage. Insulin deteriorates when it is exposed to excessive heat, cold, light, or agitation. Constant refrigeration is unnecessary as long as the client uses the vial within 30 days. Instruct clients to refrigerate extra bottles until they are needed.

As stated previously, insulin preparations may be mixed to meet an individual's needs. Clients using regular insulin alone at breakfast may have elevated glucose levels by noon. To correct this condition, they may also take a prescribed amount of intermediate-acting insulin. These mixtures can be administered in the same syringe. Syringes may be prepared up to 3 weeks in advance and refrigerated. If 70/30 is the right proportion, Novolin 70/30 or Humulin 70/30 can be used. If lispro is prescribed, clients administer single doses before each meal, and administer intermediate- or long-acting insulin only once

■■■ TABLE 78-4 𝒯YPES OF HUMAN INSULIN

Type of Insulin	Onset (hours)	Peak Effect (hours)	Duration of Effect (hours)	Characteristics
Lispro (Humalog)	Immediate	½–1	3–4	Clear and colorless; can be mixed with Humulin-N and Humulin-U
Regular (Humulin-R)	0.5–1.0	2–4	5–7	Clear and colorless; can be mixed with other human insulins
Lantus	1	5	24	Cloudy; cannot be mixed with any other insulins
Humulin-N	1–2	4–12	24+	Cloudy; can be mixed with regular human insulin and Lispro
Humulin-L	1–3	6–14	24+	Cloudy
Humulin-U	6	16–18	36+	Cloudy; can be mixed with regular human insulin and Lispro

or twice a day as prescribed. Sometimes clients use both regular and lispro insulin before meals. Many combinations can help individuals maintain good glucose control.

When administering insulin in a prefilled syringe to a client, roll and invert the syringe before administration to mix the solution well. Roll and invert insulin between the hands. Do not shake a vial. Shaking causes air bubbles to form, which would alter the dosage.

Vials or prefilled syringes should be crystal clear (regular insulin or lispro) or milky white, depending on the type of insulin. Discard if the liquid is discolored. Also discard vials that do not easily resuspend when you roll them. Other signs of unusable insulin are frosting or coating on the bottle (especially with NPH) and any settling or clumping. Note the expiration date printed on the side of the vial and do not use contents after that date. Make sure insulin is not decomposed. If in doubt, throw it out! Double-checking insulin dosages helps to prevent errors in the healthcare facility; adapt these guidelines for client and family teaching.

☛ KEY CONCEPT

If regular and NPH insulin are to be mixed, the regular insulin must be drawn up first, after injecting air into both vials. Remember: "Clear to partly cloudy."

Insulin Coverage.   Many people who have diabetes experience difficulty regulating insulin when they become ill, particularly from infections. For this reason, clients with diabetes who are hospitalized, regardless of the reason for hospitalization, almost always undergo routine blood testing for glucose and often have insulin coverage to control elevated blood glucose levels. The physician determines a sliding scale of regular insulin, based on the blood glucose levels. Clients receive this coverage three to six times per day, in addition to their usual intermediate-acting dose. Many clients whose conditions are usually well controlled with oral diabetes medications may require insulin during the course of an operation, pregnancy, or systemic disease. A client's insulin requirements are likely to increase during disease and other stressful events.

> ### ✚👁 N u r s i n g   A l e r t
> Many facilities require another nurse to double-check insulin before it is administered. Even if the facility does not have such a policy, it is a good idea. A tiny error in insulin dosage can cause serious adverse reactions.

Insulin Pumps.   As illustrated in Figure 78-4, insulin pumps are mechanical devices that inject insulin automatically. They attempt to mimic pancreatic function by releasing insulin continuously to maintain an acceptable blood glucose level. Clients also may inject a bolus before eating.

Development continues with small implantable devices that automatically monitor blood glucose levels and deliver the appropriate insulin directly into the bloodstream. A type

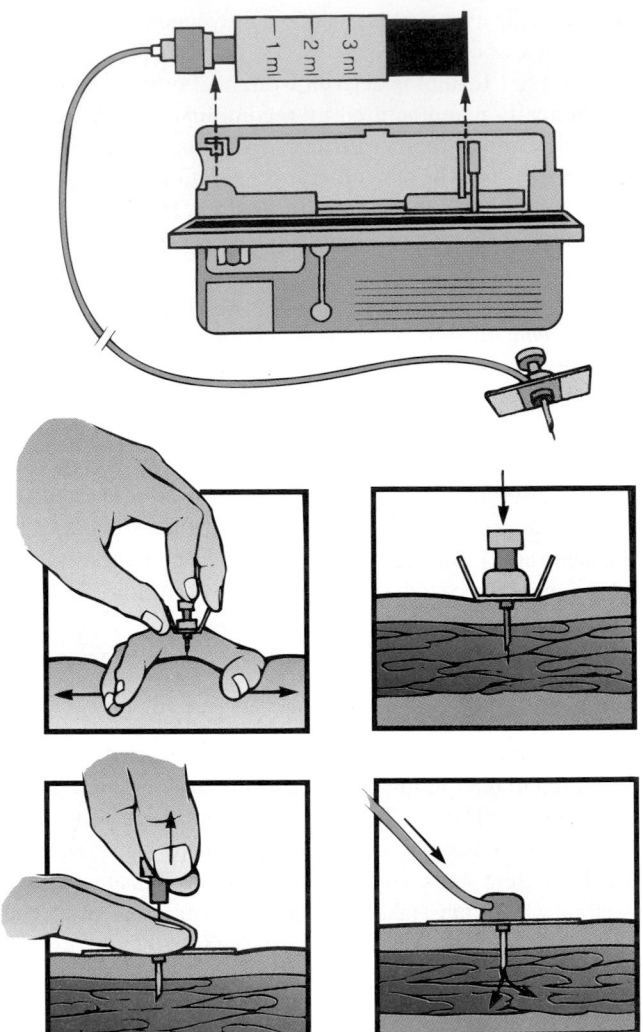

FIGURE 78-4. The insulin pump. Usually attached to the client's clothing, this external insulin pump has an insulin-filled syringe that is attached to a subcutaneous needle via tubing. The pump mimics the physiologic action of the pancreas by injecting small amounts of insulin at intervals.

of insulin called *buffered regular* is often used in the pump. This insulin is not used in any other way.

Oral Diabetes Medications

Unfortunately, insulin itself is ineffective orally, but several groups of medications given orally can lower the blood glucose levels of some clients with type 2 diabetes. These agents are not oral forms of insulin and are not to be regarded as insulin substitutes. Oral agents act within 2 to 6 hours, with effects lasting between 8 and 60 hours. Some oral hypoglycemic agents are given two to three times per day. They can cause hypoglycemia.

Four major mechanisms cause blood glucose levels to elevate in clients with type 2 diabetes. These are:

- Impaired insulin secretion
- Altered carbohydrate absorption
- Increased basal hepatic glucose production
- Decreased insulin-stimulated glucose uptake

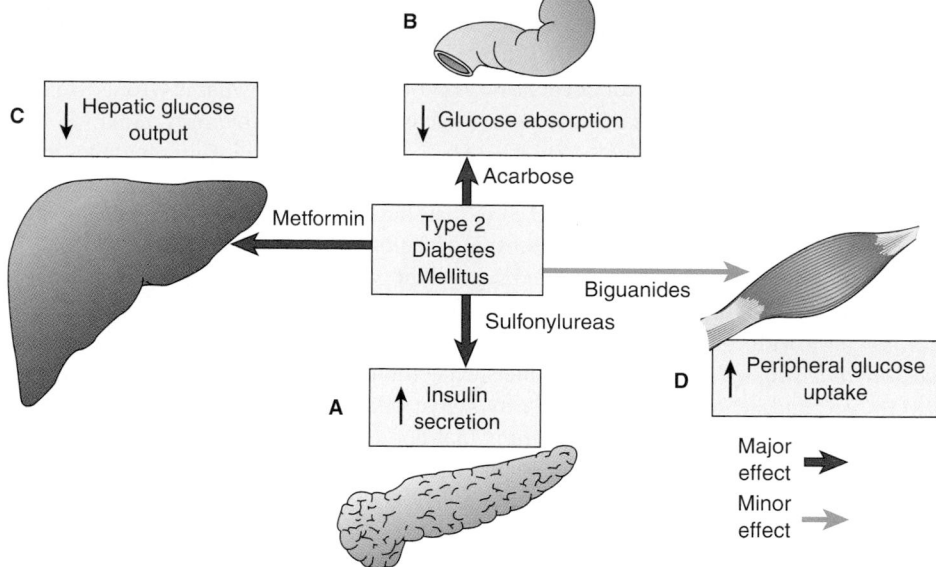

FIGURE 78-5. Oral hypoglycemic drugs use various mechanisms to lower blood glucose levels. There are four main categories of oral hypo-glycemic agents: sulfonylureas, bi-guanides (metformin), α-glucosidase inhibitors (acarbose), and thiazoli-denediones. These drugs have vari-ous effects on the body to lower blood sugar levels. Note how the different categories of drugs have one or more of the following effects: (**A**) increases insulin secretion from the pancreas; (**B**) increases glucose absorption by the cells; (**C**) decreases production of glucose from the liver; and (**D**) in-creases the use of glucose by periph-eral tissues.

The four major categories of oral antidiabetic agents act to interfere with one or more of these mechanisms (Fig. 78-5). These four categories include sulfonylureas (most common), biguanides, α-glucosidase inhibitors, and thiazolidenediones. Table 78-5 looks at the four categories of oral antidiabetic agents.

The actions of the sulfonylureas (Diabinese, Glucotrol, Dia-Beta, Micronase) are not fully understood. These medications are thought to stimulate the pancreas to produce more insulin, to improve the use of insulin at the cell's receptor sites, or to increase the effectiveness of endogenous insulin. Because they

stimulate the pancreas to produce more insulin, they are useful only for people with type 2 diabetes who still produce their own (*endogenous*) insulin.

✚👁 N u r s i n g   A l e r t
Advise clients receiving oral hypoglycemic agents or insulin about the use of alcohol; alcohol can exaggerate the hypoglycemic effect of these drugs. Alert clients that if they drink alcohol, they should do so in moderation and consume it with food (eg, wine at mealtime).

■■■ TABLE 78-5 *C*ATEGORIES OF ORAL ANTIDIABETIC AGENTS

Category	Dosage Range (mg)	Duration of Action (hours)
Sulfonylureas		
First Generation		
Tolbutamide (Orinase)	500–3000	6–12
Tolazamide (Tolinase)	100–1000	12–24
Acetohexamide (Dymelor)	250–2000	12–24
Chlorpropramide (Diabinase)	100–750	60–90
Second Generation		
Glyburide (DiaBeta, Micronase)	1.25–20.0	24
Glipizide (Glucotrol)	2.5–40.0	24
Glimepiride (Amaryl)	1.0–8.0	24
Biguanides		
Metformin (Glucophage)	500–2550	9–17
α-glucosidase inhibitors		
Acarbose (Precose)	75–300	9–15
Miglitol (Glyset)	75–300	9–15
Thiazolidinediones		
Pioglitazone (Actos)	15–30	3–7
Rosiglitazone (Avandia)	2–8	3–5
Troglitazone (Rezulin)	**No longer available**	

Metformin (Glucophage), a biguanide, works by preventing the liver from overproducing glucose. Metformin does not increase insulin secretion and thus does not cause hypoglycemia. This drug is useful for clients who experience early-morning fasting hypoglycemia. It is sometimes given to clients who are also taking sulfonylureas.

Acarbose (Precose), an α-glucosidase inhibitor, blocks enzymes that break down dietary starches so that starches can be absorbed more slowly in the small intestine. It helps clients who experience rapid increases in blood sugar after meals.

Clients can use oral antidiabetic medications alone or in combination with each other or with insulin. *Bedtime insulin and daytime sulfonylureas* (**BIDS**) is one such combination.

Glucophage and Precose do not cause hypoglycemia. However, when they are combined with drugs that do, dramatic lowering of blood glucose levels can occur. The client's participation through *self-monitoring of blood glucose* (**SMBG**) is important in determining which pills or combinations to use, and how effectively the medication regimen controls blood sugar levels.

Pancreas Transplantation

Experimentation with pancreas transplantation in clients with diabetes has been underway for many years. Success has been limited because of the high rate of transplant rejection, but with new anti-rejection medications, results are improving. Research has also shown some success in implanting only the beta cells from the islets of Langerhans.

Complications of Diabetes Mellitus

Hypoglycemic Reaction
Doses of insulin (or oral diabetes medications) are calculated to control blood glucose levels. Too much insulin in relation to the amount of glucose reduces this level below normal. It causes a reaction called **hypoglycemia** (once called *insulin shock*). Hypoglycemia usually means that the person with diabetes has a blood sugar level of under 70 mg/dL. Table 78-6 compares hypoglycemia with hyperglycemia.

Signs and Symptoms. In hypoglycemia, the client experiences symptoms of excess adrenaline, which the body releases in response to low blood sugar. The person feels weak, cold, and suddenly exhausted. This is followed by feelings of hunger and nervousness. The client trembles and perspires. The person may also experience headache, drowsiness, nausea, and vomiting. Without treatment, other symptoms develop, such as dizziness, confusion, and speech loss. The person is unable to control body movements. Vision is double or blurry, and if the condition is still untreated, seizures, loss of consciousness, and permanent brain damage may develop, sometimes causing death.

☛ KEY CONCEPT

All persons with diabetes who use insulin or oral hypoglycemic medications should wear a MedicAlert tag at all times.

Treatment and Nursing Considerations. Hypoglycemia can develop so rapidly that a client may be having seizures or may become unconscious before anyone knows what is wrong. Be quick to recognize the early symptoms of hypoglycemia.

Carbohydrates are needed to counteract the insulin reaction in hypoglycemia. If the client is conscious, give sugar in some form (4 oz orange juice, 4 oz regular soft drink, 6 to 8 Lifesavers, honey, or Karo syrup). Individually packaged glucose tablets are available in pharmacies; give such glucose to individuals who use Precose. (Rationale: The enzymatic action of Precose blocks the absorption of *sucrose,* which is found in table sugar and fruit juice.) Sugar in liquid form is easiest and safest. If the person is unconscious, 50% glucose IV is the initial treatment.

Glucagon administration is another treatment for hypoglycemia. *Glucagon* is not glucose; it is a hormone that causes the liver to release glucose into the bloodstream. It is available as Glucagon for injection (USP) in IV and IM preparations. If the client shows no response within 5 to 10 minutes after the injection, administer 50 milliliters of 50% glucose IV.

✚👁 **N u r s i n g   A l e r t**
Avoid chocolate bars as treatment for a hypoglycemic reaction, because the high fat content prevents quick release of glucose.

Hypoglycemia requires emergency treatment, followed by adjustment of the client's carbohydrate intake and insulin dosage to regulate the disturbed metabolism. Adjusting these factors is difficult in the first 24 hours after the reaction; the client requires close observation for symptom recurrence. Check the client's blood glucose levels frequently.

If medical assistance is unavailable, the client may use a substance called Instant Glucose, which contains 25 grams of pure glucose and is packaged in a tube for squeezing into the client's mouth. If a client is unconscious, place the glucose between the lower lip and front teeth to prevent aspiration. The body will absorb glucose through the oral mucous membranes. Absorption in this manner is much slower than when glucose is given IV.

The **Somogyi phenomenon** occurs when hypoglycemia is followed by a compensatory period of rebound hyperglycemia as the body attempts to correct the initial problem by increasing glucose production. It most commonly develops late at night or early in the morning when the client is asleep. During this time, the body continues to absorb insulin from the injection site, although not enough glucose is available for the insulin to act on it. As a result, the body secretes glucagon, norepinephrine, and corticosteroids to correct the hypoglycemia but exceeds the necessary amounts. Treatment involves reducing insulin dosages until the optimum level is reached.

Hyperglycemia
Diabetic ketoacidosis (**DKA**) results from a lack of effective insulin, causing **hyperglycemia.** Glucose no longer enters

	Hypoglycemic Reaction* (Insulin Reaction)	Hyperglycemia (Acidosis, Diabetic Ketoacidosis, "Diabetic Coma")
Reason	Too much insulin (blood sugar too low); also caused by too little food or too much exercise	Too little insulin (a frequent occurrence during a systemic infection); ketosis results from upset in acid–base balance
Onset	Sudden (may occur in clients who use insulin or who are taking oral hypoglycemics)	Slow—several hours to days (more rapid in active child)
Causes	Skipped meals, overdose of insulin, overexertion, vomiting, excessive dieting	Omitted dose of insulin, spoiled insulin, error in dosage, improperly mixed insulin, increased need for insulin due to stress of illness, exposure, surgery, or improper diet; also, undiagnosed diabetes or not following diet plan (especially in active child or adolescent)
SYMPTOMS†		
Skin	Pale, moist, cool and clammy, sweating	Flushed, dry, hot, no sweating
Behavior	Shaky, nervous, irritable, trembling, confused, disoriented, strange actions, difficulty in problem-solving; later, unconsciousness (rarely, seizures); may first be evidenced by a personality change or drowsiness	Drowsy, lethargic, dizzy, weak; later, delirium and loss of consciousness; anorexia
Breath	Normal odor	Fruity odor (acetone)
Respiration	Normal, rapid, and shallow	Air hunger (Kussmaul's breathing), labored, slow
Blood pressure	Increased	Decreased
Pulse	Increased	Increased
Hunger	Great hunger, often sudden in onset	Anorexia, nausea—may have time of excessive hunger
Thirst	None	Great thirst
Vomiting	Absent	Present, with abdominal pain
Sugar in urine	Absent in second voiding (in unusual circumstances, sugar may be spilled, depending on type and time of insulin administration and kidney function)	Present in high concentrations
Acetone in urine	Absent	Usually present
Urination	Small amount	Frequent, copious, diluted
Blood sugar level	Low, below 60	High, over 140
Chemistry	Electrolytes usually within normal limits	Blood electrolytes and BUN elevated
Other	Blurred or double vision, dizziness, headache, sleepiness	Ringing in ears
Response to treatment	Rapid	Slow
Treatment	Glucose—stop exercising; take simple sugar (regular soft drinks upset the stomach less than orange juice); glucagon for injection is available; 50% glucose; glucose tablets	Force fluids (usually IV), give antiemetics, keep client warm; administer regular insulin in low dosage
Nursing considerations	Prepare to assist with blood samples, urine collection, IV administration of glucose; remain with client until he or she is fully conscious and watch for symptoms of recurrence; client is often nauseated after a reaction; nursing measures should prevent complications of emesis; institute seizure precautions	Prepare to insert catheter, assist with IV, gastric lavage, ECG; prepare to deal with circulatory or respiratory complications and later, with nausea; remain with client and observe

*Note: The symptoms of the hypoglycemic reaction are those of adrenaline overdose, because the body secretes adrenaline when the blood sugar gets too low, in an attempt to raise blood sugar.

†A slow drop in blood sugar is most likely to result in confusion, sleepiness, and headache. A rapid drop in blood sugar (such as caused by exercise) is more likely to result in shakiness, pallor, rapid heart rate, and sweating.

the muscle cells. To make up for the loss of sugar as a source of energy, the body uses more fats and proteins, which it breaks down into ketones and sends to the muscles. If too many ketones accumulate (*ketosis*), body fluids become imbalanced, and a condition called **ketoacidosis** follows. In ketoacidosis, the body produces a volatile substance called *acetone*, which has a characteristic sweetish odor (like nail-polish remover) that can be detected on the client's breath in late stages of ketoacidosis. Any condition that interferes with storage of glycogen in the liver and increases the body's need to burn fat and energy (eg, lack of insulin, vomiting, surgery, or anesthesia) may increase production of ketone bodies.

Signs and Symptoms.   Ketoacidosis develops over time. The client experiences weakness, drowsiness, vomiting, thirst, abdominal pain, and dehydration. He or she has flushed cheeks and dry skin and mouth. The breath may have the sweetish odor mentioned earlier; breathing and pulse may become rapid and deep, and blood pressure low. Unconsciousness may follow. Sometimes the unresponsive client who is admitted to the healthcare facility is unaware that he or she has diabetes. Or a person may have a diabetic condition that is hard to control, even when he or she follows the regimen faithfully.

Treatment and Nursing Considerations.   Intervention must include IV fluids and electrolytes as well as insulin replacement. While laboratory examination of blood and urine specimens is being completed, apply blankets to the unresponsive client to support warmth and combat shock. Check vital signs frequently.

Continuous IV infusion of low-dose regular insulin, with a controlled-flow mechanism, is used. By lowering the body's production of ketones, insulin makes more carbohydrate available to the tissues and builds up the liver's glycogen supply. Regular insulin acts quickly.

Following the initial emergency, test blood specimens for sugar hourly and keep a record of fluid I&O. Monitor blood levels of potassium, chlorides, and bicarbonates hourly and sodium levels every 8 hours. Also check urine or blood ketones every 4 to 8 hours. All these tests are necessary to evaluate the client's progress and to assist the physician in determining how much insulin to prescribe and which electrolytes to replace. When the client's metabolism is in balance again, the physician prescribes a regimen specifically designed for the client.

Nursing Alert

If the nurse is outside the healthcare facility and does not know whether a person is having a hypoglycemic or hyperglycemic reaction, give sugar. *Rationale: If you give sugar, and it is incorrect, an already high blood sugar will only increase slightly. However, if you give insulin and the blood sugar is already too low, the reaction is faster, more severe, and more long lasting. Death is much more likely when insulin, not sugar, is incorrectly given.*

Nonketotic Hyperosmolar State

In this condition, the client has a blood glucose level in the vicinity of 1,000 mg/dL, without typical symptoms of ketosis.

It occurs most often in older adults with no history of diabetes or with a history of type 2 diabetes. The mortality rate is 65%. Underlying causes include advanced age, severe stress, diuretics, undiagnosed diabetes, or response to anticonvulsant or hypnotic sedative drugs.

The client experiences hyperglycemia, hyperosmolarity, severe dehydration, and coma. The body produces some, but not enough, insulin. Hyperglycemia results in severe loss of fluids and electrolytes, resulting in dehydration.

Treatment is a continuous low-dose infusion of insulin and aggressive fluid and electrolyte replacement.

Nursing care focuses on measures to restore the fluid volume and correct the hyperosmolar state. Administer IV fluids and electrolyte replacements as ordered. Monitor fluid and electrolyte balance, I&O, and daily weights. Evaluate blood and urine glucose levels frequently.

Infections

Infections aggravate diabetes. When increased glucose concentration damages blood vessels, clients are more susceptible to infections. Clients with diabetes are particularly susceptible to yeast and fungal infections, carbuncles, and furuncles, as well as common colds and influenza. Because of sugar in the blood and reduced circulation, fighting infection is difficult. Effective diabetes management minimizes blood vessel damage and reduces infections. Injury prevention is important because people with diabetes heal slowly.

Surgical Complications

Persons with diabetes are considered greater surgical risks because of associated circulatory problems and difficulty in regulating insulin balance postoperatively. They are also more prone to infections in any wound, including the surgical incision, and heal less readily because of impaired circulation.

Postoperative nursing care includes frequent blood glucose monitoring, watching for possible complications, encouraging fluids, and following measures to prevent respiratory, circulatory, and wound complications. These individuals are prone to skin breakdowns. Practice meticulous skin care. Clients with type 2 diabetes who do not usually take insulin may require insulin during the perioperative period to control blood glucose elevations.

Macrovascular Complications

High blood glucose levels may increase *arteriosclerosis* (a condition that affects the peripheral blood vessels), especially in the lower extremities and the vessels of the kidneys and heart. These changes are the *macrovascular* (large blood vessels) complications associated with diabetes. When arteriosclerosis narrows the lumen of blood vessels, decreased blood flow causes oxygen deprivation in tissues. Diabetic ulcers can result (Figure 78-6).

Other consequences of arteriosclerosis include hypertension, coronary artery disease, peripheral vascular disease, myocardial infarction, and stroke. Persons with diabetes are two to six times more likely to have a stroke and twice as likely to have a heart attack as the general population. Skin break-

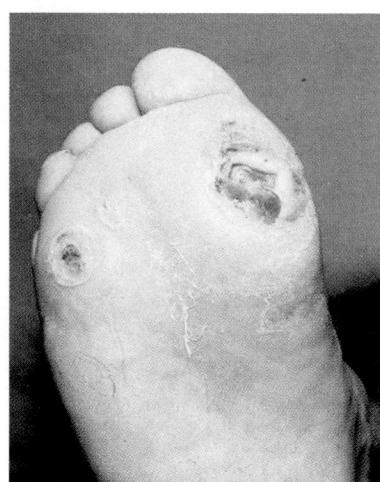

FIGURE 78-6. Diabetic ulcers. Ulcerations, particularly on the legs or feet, are serious for the diabetic client. In many cases, an ulceration heals very slowly or may not heal at all. Gangrene is a serious threat and usually necessitates amputation.

down and a greatly slowed healing process also result from poor circulation and lack of oxygen. Theorists also believe that elevated glycosylated hemoglobin is stickier than normal hemoglobin, so it is more likely to clump, clot, and occlude small blood vessels in the brain, heart, and kidneys.

➤ Nursing Alert

Uncontrolled diabetes mellitus predisposes a person to long-term complications, such as hypertension, stroke, heart and kidney disorders, blindness, and amputation secondary to gangrene. Control of blood glucose levels greatly reduces the possibility of these complications.

Microvascular Complications

Diabetes causes unique microvascular changes in the capillary walls, resulting in diminished blood flow and poor oxygenation of tissues that are highly vascular. The retina of the eye and the kidneys are the primary organs that can be severely damaged by diabetes.

Nephropathy.   Kidney disease (**nephropathy**) caused by microvascular changes can result in death from kidney failure. Kidney infections or albumin or blood in the urine, often the first indications, must be dealt with immediately. Three general approaches to slowing the progress of nephropathy include blood pressure control, blood sugar control, and diet.

Angiotensin-converting enzyme (**ACE**) inhibitors are used to treat high blood pressure and kidney disease in clients with diabetes. Research has shown that people with diabetes who have proteinuria respond better to ACE inhibitors than to other medications used to treat hypertension.

Retinopathy.   One of the leading causes of blindness in this country is diabetic **retinopathy,** which is loss of the functional retinal tissue in the eye due to microvascular damage. Many physicians recommend yearly eye examinations for people with diabetes. Circulatory problems may appear first in the retinal arteries (in the retina of the eye) in the form of hemorrhage or inflammation. Disorders in the retinal blood vessels are usually visible through an ophthalmoscope. The condition of retinal blood vessels reflects the entire circulatory system's general status.

Laser therapy can be used to curtail pathologic eye changes. Damage already done cannot be reversed, but further damage can often be prevented. Cataracts may appear and can be removed surgically if retinal damage is not too great.

Neuropathy

Diabetic **neuropathy** (nerve damage) is another long-term complication of poorly controlled diabetes. It can occur as peripheral or autonomic neuropathy. Various theories exist about what causes the nerve damage. It may result from swelling of nerve cells or axons, caused by the accumulation of sorbitol (a type of sugar), or it may result from accumulation of end products of glucose metabolism.

Peripheral neuropathy usually starts as numbness or tingling in the toes and progresses gradually (over years) to the ankle and then the leg. Symptoms vary from unawareness to extreme pain or numbness. Painful neuropathy can be treated with amitriptyline (Elavil) (50–150 mg/d), carbamazepine (Tegretol), or phenytoin (Dilantin). Lack of sensation in the feet can be dangerous because it can mask injury; ulcers may form that can ultimately lead to amputation.

Autonomic neuropathy can have various effects, including impotence, intestinal involvement (diarrhea with periods of constipation), urinary retention, stomach involvement (*gastroparesis*), *orthostasis* (dizziness on arising), and sweating abnormalities. These neuropathies are treated symptomatically because no cure for autonomic neuropathy exists.

Because neuropathy causes lack of sensation in peripheral tissues of the body, clients are more likely to develop skin infections or injury without being aware of the problem.

Client Teaching

Because clients are ultimately responsible for self-care, the most important aspect of long-term management is educating clients and families to understand diabetes and its management. Much of this teaching is the responsibility of nursing staff and diabetes educators. In Practice: Educating the Client 78-1 provides general guidelines for client and family teaching in diabetes mellitus.

Clients will understand the disease best if it is explained in simple terms. Review this sample explanation when working with diabetic clients:

When you have diabetes, your body can't use the sugar in your blood. That's why your blood sugar level is so high. The sugar stays in your blood instead of going into your body's cells where it can be used for fuel. That's why you have not felt well and have been lacking energy. You will learn the tools to use to control your blood sugar: they consist of healthy food choices, medication, and exercise. There is a lot to learn about diabetes, but there is also a lot of support available to you.

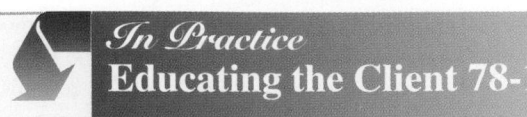

In Practice
Educating the Client 78-1

DIABETES MELLITUS TEACHING PLAN

- Assess the client's and family's knowledge about diabetes.
- Start with the basics. Build on what the person already knows.
- Explain everything in terms the client can understand.
- Give ample opportunity for the client to ask questions, and be willing to repeat information given.
- Ask for return demonstrations. Make sure the person is not "agreeing" just to be cooperative.
- Use booklets and pictures and give materials to the client to keep.
- Recognize each client as an individual with specific needs; structure information to meet these needs. People learn in different ways and at different rates of speed.
- Promote independence to increase self-esteem and safety.
- Stress that seemingly trivial problems can be serious, and that the client must notify the physician immediately.
- Include the following survival skills: basic meal planning, self-monitoring of blood glucose, recognition of hypoglycemia, and insulin preparation and administration (if appropriate).

We can help you take it one step at a time. Eventually you will gain the confidence you will need to self-manage your diabetes. What is it about all of this that you find most difficult?

Clients must understand that diabetes is never cured. It is considered *controlled* or *managed* when the following conditions exist:

- The person feels well.
- The person maintains normal weight on a balanced diet.
- The person's blood glucose level stays within 70 to 140 mg/dL (normal).

Clients must learn that they can reduce long-term complications by controlling their blood glucose levels. Injury prevention is crucial. Special care and regular examinations are necessary for the feet, hands, teeth, and eyes. Illness can quickly upset glucose control.

Clients will be responsible for managing food selection, blood testing, appropriate exercise, and medication administration. Observe performance of these procedures to assess the client's understanding and ability to perform certain tasks. Praise clients when they perform procedures correctly and assist with areas that need reinforcement.

☞ KEY CONCEPT

Persons with diabetes are able to lead normal lives and live longer than in the past. They should maintain tight blood glucose control (70–140 mg/dL) to prevent complications of diabetes.

Physician Contact

The physician will help the client determine the most appropriate schedule for medication dosage, as well as diet and exercise management. Although some clients are able to adjust insulin dosage on their own, clients may need to contact their physician for changes in their blood glucose levels. In addition, clients need to report symptoms such as loss of appetite, hunger, or any gastrointestinal upset persisting for more than 24 hours that is severe enough to prevent eating or to cause diarrhea or vomiting.

Glucose Monitoring

Many nurses in various healthcare facilities monitor blood glucose levels. In Practice: Nursing Procedure 78-1 outlines the skills to use when performing this test.

Adapt these steps to teach clients how to self-monitor blood glucose levels. If they have type 1 diabetes, clients will also learn when and how to test their urine for ketones. These clients must notify their physician if their blood sugar level is consistently above 240 mg/dL for 3 days. Teach clients to perform these tests and document the results in a log or diary. Clients should take these records with them to followup appointments.

SMBG is an important tool in the daily routine for any individual with diabetes. It allows clients to evaluate their diabetes management, aids in problem-solving and insulin adjustments, and provides invaluable information to the diabetes team. Keeping a blood sugar diary helps everyone involved to understand when blood sugar levels fluctuate and why.

Numerous blood glucose meters are available. With recent advances in technology, these meters have become easy to use. Some models are made specifically for the visually impaired. Although they help clients to obtain quick and highly accurate results, these monitoring programs are expensive. However, because monitoring is so useful in preventing chronic hyperglycemia (and long-term complications), the cost is justified and usually covered by third-party payers.

Every meter is different; a healthcare provider who is familiar with the particular technology should teach the client how to select and use a meter. Clients must understand and be able to interpret the data that the meter generates. Blood sugar levels in the normal range can assure clients that self-management techniques are working. Abnormal readings provide opportunities to identify what is not working and can assist clients to make any necessary changes.

Blood glucose testing can be done visually, in which a test strip is compared to a colored chart, or by using a meter in which a test strip is inserted into an electronic device that reads it. Visual testing is rarely used today because blood glucose meters have become easier and quicker to use. Meters are available for clients with visual, hearing, or other problems. SMBG

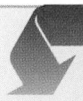

In Practice
Nursing Procedure 78-1

TESTING FOR BLOOD GLUCOSE LEVEL

Supplies and Equipment

Blood glucose testing strips
Glucose testing meter
Sterile lancet
Lancet activating device (optional)
Cotton balls
Alcohol swab
Gloves

Steps

1. Wash your hands.
   RATIONALE: *Handwashing helps prevent the spread of infection.*

2. Gather supplies.
   RATIONALE: *Organization facilitates accurate skill performance.*

3. Explain the procedure to the client.
   RATIONALE: *Explanations help foster the client's cooperation and understanding.*

4. Have the client wash his or her hands with warm water.
   RATIONALE: *Handwashing will cleanse the site for puncture; warm water promotes vasodilation.*

5. Assist the client to a comfortable position.
   RATIONALE: *The puncture site should be easily accessible without causing the client added anxiety.*

6. Remove a test strip from the container. Turn on the glucose testing meter. Check that the code number on the strip matches the code number that appears initially on the monitor screen (or follow the manufacturer's instructions).
   RATIONALE: *Matching code numbers on the strip and the meter ensures that the machine is calibrated correctly.*

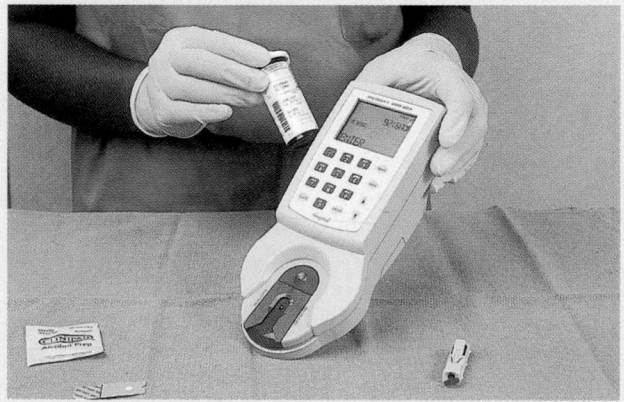

Match the code number on the glucose test strip with the code number on the monitor screen.

7. Prepare the lancet by twisting off the cap. Arm the automatic device by pushing back the plunger until it clicks. Attach the lancet. Remove the cap. Keep the tip sterile.
   RATIONALE: *Maintaining sterility of the lancet reduces the risk of transmission of micro-organisms to the puncture site.*

8. Put on gloves.
   RATIONALE: *Gloves act as a barrier.*

9. Select the site on the client's finger for puncture. Gently massage the finger toward the intended puncture site, keeping the finger in dependent position.
   RATIONALE: *Massage and dependent position encourage blood flow to the area.*

10. Clean the site with alcohol and allow the area to dry thoroughly. (Clients may omit this step at home.)
    RATIONALE: *Alcohol can affect the blood sample and cause destruction of some red blood cells.*

11. Prick the side of the client's finger with a lancet and squeeze gently. Use a cotton ball to wipe away the first drop of blood, if recommended for the particular meter.
    RATIONALE: *Directions for some meters indicate that the first drop of blood should not be used because it may be diluted by serum and give a false reading.*

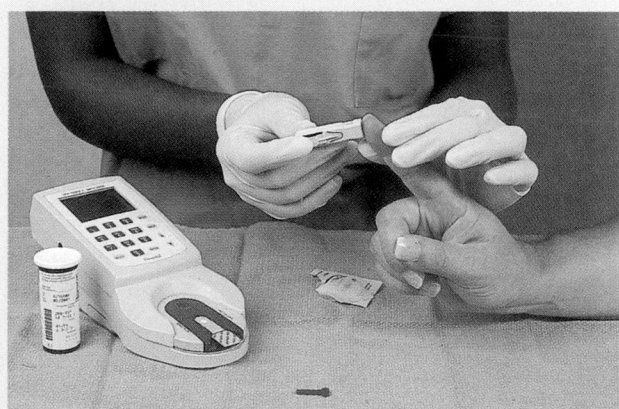

Wearing gloves, prick the side of the client's finger with the lancet.

12. Gently touch the drop of blood to the strip's target area or use a pipette as instructed. Have the client hold a clean cotton ball to the puncture site for a few seconds.
    RATIONALE: *Blood must color the entire target area, but should not be smeared on the strip, or test results will be inaccurate. The person with diabetes often has slowed clotting.*

(continued)

In Practice
Nursing Procedure 78-1 (Continued)

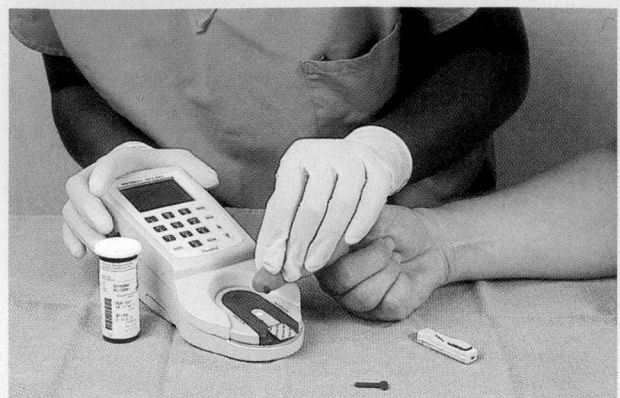
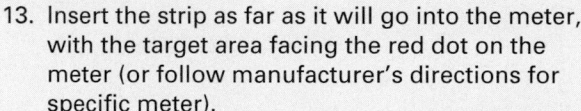

Squeeze the finger gently, and touch the drop of blood on the test strip.

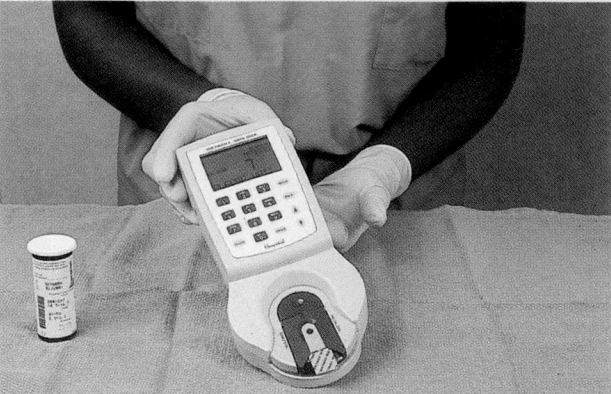

Wait 15 to 60 seconds, depending on manufacturer's instructions, before the monitor screen.

13. Insert the strip as far as it will go into the meter, with the target area facing the red dot on the meter (or follow manufacturer's directions for specific meter).
    RATIONALE: *Inserting the strip correctly enables the machine to determine the client's blood glucose level.*

14. Read test results in 15 to 60 seconds on the meter face. Remove the strip and turn off the meter.
    RATIONALE: *Individual meters read test results within varying time frames.*

15. Dispose of equipment properly. Remove gloves and wash your hands.
    RATIONALE: *Proper disposal of equipment and handwashing prevent the spread of infection.*

16. Record blood glucose reading on proper forms. Check to see if the client is on insulin coverage.
    RATIONALE: *Documentation provides coordination of care. Blood glucose reading may necessitate insulin coverage.*

is recommended for all clients who have diabetes. See Box 78-2 for further details.

Meal Planning
Meal plans for people with diabetes are individualized with help from a registered dietitian. These clients can achieve optimal blood glucose control by making realistic food choices that not only mimic their typical eating patterns, but reflect healthy eating approaches as well. They must be introduced to the concept of carbohydrate awareness. Explain meal plans in terms that clients can easily understand and follow. Foods containing sugar are not forbidden, but clients must count them as part of their total carbohydrate intake. Consider the client's cultural background when planning meals (see Chap. 31). Clients must understand the relationships among diet, medication, and exercise. Alcohol may be allowed, in moderation, provided it is accompanied by food to prevent hypoglycemia.

Lifestyle Factors
Often, clients have many questions about the effect of diabetes on their lifestyles. Assure them that they can participate in activities, as long as they allow for changes in exercise levels

and control their blood sugar level. They should avoid fatigue. Genetic counseling may be advisable before deciding whether to have children.

Smoking
Smoking is definitely contraindicated because the vasoconstrictor effect of nicotine increases the likelihood of circulatory disorders. Strongly urge people with diabetes to stop smoking and provide assistance to do so by giving information about smoking cessation programs.

Insulin Injection
When insulin is prescribed, teach clients about the type of insulin and syringe, along with dosages and self-injection. Usually clients fear the injection itself. Draw up the insulin the first time and immediately let the client inject it to get over the initial fear. After fear and anxiety are relieved, the client is better able to focus on the technique for drawing up the correct amount, site selection, and so forth. Use the type of syringe that the client will use at home. Encourage clients who feel well enough in the healthcare facility to give all their own insulin injections. Doing so will allow the nurse to observe the tech-

> ⮞ BOX 78-2

COMMON GUIDELINES FOR BLOOD GLUCOSE MONITORING

- The calibration number (code or lot number) on the strip bottle must match the meter. The meter calibration can easily be changed if they do not match.
- Make sure the test strips are not outdated.
- Do not expose the meter or strips to extremes of temperature, light, or air more than necessary.
- Check the meter with the procedure and control solution, as indicated by the manufacturer.
- Wash hands with soap and water and dry them well.
- If using alcohol, be sure to let it dry. Repeated use of alcohol will toughen the fingertips and make lancing more difficult.
- Use the lateral aspect of any fingertip for testing. *Rationale: The lateral aspect of the finger has more blood vessels, so blood will be easy to obtain. The lateral aspect also has fewer nerve endings, thus making the procedure more comfortable.*
- Rotate the sites. *Rationale: If sites are not rotated, one site will become irritated and may become infected; the area may also become so hardened that it is impossible to use.*
- Always recap the strip container immediately after removing the strip.
- If the testing procedure calls for removal of blood from the strip, be sure to use the correct material and method (eg, wiping with a cotton ball versus blotting with a tissue).
- Dispose of test strips, lancets, and other materials according to Standard Precautions. Wear gloves.
- Test as often as prescribed by the physician.
- Check the operator's manual for procedure and frequency of cleaning. Certain meters require a high degree of maintenance.

nique and provide reinforcement or correction as appropriate. Children over the age of 7 or 8 are usually able to give their own insulin.

Rotating insulin injection sites will keep skin and tissue healthy and prevent lipodystrophy. Teach clients that standard injection sites include the outside or front of the thighs, the upper-outer part of the buttocks, the outside of the upper arm, and the abdomen. Insulin absorption is fastest from the abdomen. Inform clients to use care when selecting sites. The body will rapidly absorb insulin from sites that are exercised shortly after administration (eg, running after injecting into the thigh can cause too-rapid insulin absorption, resulting in hypoglycemia).

Hypoglycemia and Hyperglycemia
Clients must understand the symptoms of hypoglycemia and hyperglycemia (see Table 78-6). Because these reactions can

be dangerous, clients must know how to identify and manage them. Encourage frequent monitoring of blood glucose levels. Clients who experience frequent reactions should have a sugar supply readily available at all times. Encourage the client to carry a simple carbohydrate snack, such as peanut butter crackers or 5 to 6 pieces of hard candy. A glucagon/glucose emergency kit is recommended for clients receiving insulin; family members and significant others should also learn how to use it.

Also encourage the client to wear a medical alert identification bracelet or tag (eg, MedicAlert). This is very helpful in emergency situations, and the client might not be able to respond.

Sexuality
Many diabetic men experience erectile dysfunction. Approximately 50% of diabetic men are unable to achieve a satisfactory erection; the cause is believed to be neurogenic. Chapter 89 describes treatments for impotence. Encourage male clients to bring this problem to a physician's attention. Some diabetic men use penile implants or prostheses, as well as oral medications such as sildenafil (Viagra).

The literature provides very little discussion about sexual dysfunction in diabetic women, although it occurs. It is not uncommon in women with type 2 diabetes, most likely because many of these clients are postmenopausal with diminished estrogen secretion. Treatments exist for problems in female clients as well.

Exposure to Cold
Clients should be aware that exposure to extreme cold slows blood circulation, especially in the extremities, due to vasoconstriction. Frostbite or hypothermia is a danger, especially because individuals with diabetes do not heal well.

Vision Impairment
Clients with diabetes must understand the importance of annual eye examinations with pupil dilation, which can detect early visual problems. Many assistive devices are available for use by visually impaired clients. Furniture can also be placed where clients are less likely to bump into it—bumps can cause breaks in the skin.

Dental Examination
Persons with diabetes need regular dental examinations. Dental *caries* (decay) can lead to infection, which can upset glucose control. In addition, rough edges can irritate the mouth, exposing the mouth to infections.

Foot Care
Warn people with diabetes against foot injuries. Explain that poor circulation and diminished sensation can result in a wound that isn't detected by the client, and doesn't heal because of poor circulation. Left untreated, a wound can become infected and ultimately result in amputation. Teach preventive foot care to all people with diabetes (see In Practice: Educating the Client 78-2).

In Practice
Educating the Client 78-2

FOOT CARE AND DIABETES MELLITUS

- Inspect feet daily. If necessary, use a mirror to check the undersides of the feet or areas that are difficult to see. *Rationale: Daily inspection allows for prompt intervention should a problem arise.*
- Wash feet daily. Do not soak. *Rationale: Soaking softens the skin too much, making it more easily damaged.*
- Dry feet thoroughly yet gently, especially between the toes. *Rationale: Proper drying prevents cracking and breaks, which could lead to infections.*
- Massage gently with a good quality lotion. Do not use lotion between toes. *Rationale: Lotion keeps the skin soft. Lotion between the toes promotes moisture accumulation, which could lead to skin maceration and breakdown.*
- Cut nails only with a physician's permission. Cut nails straight across with a blunt-tipped scissors. See a podiatrist for treatment of corns, calluses, or ingrown toenails. Self-treatment in any form is dangerous and absolutely forbidden. *Rationale: Proper foot care prevents complications.*
- Never pick at sores or rough spots on the skin.
- Do not walk barefooted. *Rationale: Walking barefoot increases the risk of injury and possible infection.*
- Put lamb's wool between overlapping toes. *Rationale: Lamb's wool prevents rubbing and irritation.*
- Exercise daily. Walking is the best exercise. If you are unable to walk, sit on the edge of the bed and point toes upward, then downward. Do this 10 times. Make a circle with each foot 10 times. *Rationale: Exercise improves circulation.*

- Make sure that shoes fit well, are of high quality, and give good support. Inspect the inside of shoes for any rough areas. *Rationale: Properly fitting shoes prevent the development of any ulcerations or breaks in the skin of the feet. The circulation of the feet may be poor and any ulceration is often difficult to heal.*
- Wear new shoes only for a short period each day for a few days. *Rationale: Minimizing the time in new shoes helps to avoid irritation.*
- Never wear constrictive stockings or socks. Avoid sitting with knees crossed. *Rationale: These actions restrict circulation.*
- Do not use adhesive tape on the skin. *Rationale: Adhesive tape abrades the skin when it is removed.*
- For cold toes, use warm socks and extra blankets at night. Select stockings that allow toe motion.
- Avoid using heating pads and hot water bags because they can be dangerous. *Rationale: Because circulation is poor and neuropathy may be present, the person can be burned more easily.*
- See a physician for a cut or burn, no matter how small it is. If first-aid treatment is necessary, cleanse the area gently with soap and water. Do not use harsh antiseptics. Apply a dry, sterile dressing. It is essential to see a physician as soon as possible. *Rationale: Immediate therapy is necessary to prevent complications. Because of impaired circulation, gangrene is a possibility, which would necessitate amputation.*

Traveling

Persons with diabetes who plan to travel great distances (across several time zones) should consult their physician before such trips. Often, they will need to adjust their daily insulin doses during travel days, until they achieve a regular morning schedule again. Clients must consider diet and exercise in their travel plans. People taking insulin and testing blood glucose levels must keep medications and equipment with them in carry-on luggage and give a spare supply to a companion, in case luggage gets lost. They must also carry a fast-acting carbohydrate and some food with them when traveling. They will probably be asked for a prescription if they try to buy syringes.

Identification

Every person with diabetes should wear a tag, such as a MedicAlert tag, that gives immediate and positive identification of the problem. Many times, a card in the wallet is not easily found. Most paramedics and emergency room personnel are actually forbidden from looking through wallets and purses,

presumably to protect against accusations of stealing and for privacy reasons. A tag worn on the body gives immediate and visible information to healthcare personnel.

➤ STUDENT SYNTHESIS

Key Points

- Endocrine glands secrete hormones that influence metabolism, growth, and development.
- Laboratory diagnostic tests for the endocrine system include serum hormone levels, various glucose tests, several urinalysis tests, radiology procedures, and occasionally iodine uptake tests. Many endocrine disorders affect growth, development, and appearance.
- The majority of endocrine disorders result from overproduction or underproduction of specific hormones.

- Nursing procedures in the care of a postoperative thyroidectomy client include careful monitoring and preparation for emergency care.
- Diabetes mellitus occurs when the pancreas does not make enough insulin or the body becomes resistant to insulin.
- Diabetes mellitus is classified as the following: type 1; type 2; gestational diabetes; and impaired glucose homeostasis (impaired fasting glucose or impaired glucose tolerance). Clients with type 1 diabetes must use insulin as part of their treatment regimen. Clients with type 2 diabetes may use oral antidiabetic agents that affect insulin secretion and/or metabolism. Some type 2 diabetic clients also use insulin.
- Meal planning, exercise, and medications, as needed, are essential components of diabetes management.
- Complications of diabetes affect all aspects of life. Members of the diabetes team work to provide accurate and thorough client teaching and to avoid related complications of the disease.

Critical Thinking Exercises

1. A woman comes to your healthcare facility. She has a rapid pulse and elevated systolic blood pressure. She says that although she has been eating a lot more than usual, she has been losing weight. Her skin is a salmon color, and she has bulging eyes and a swollen neck. Based on these symptoms, what disorder might this client be experiencing? What additional data would you want to collect? What diagnostic test could help confirm the client's condition?
2. Your client is a child with diabetes mellitus. Her parents ask you to explain the differences among the various kinds of diabetes mellitus, particularly the differences between children and adults. Describe what you will tell them.
3. While riding a public bus in your community, you notice a man who is confused, appears sleepy, and is staggering down the aisle. As he bumps next to you, you notice that he is wearing a MedicAlert bracelet that identifies him as diabetic. What do you think may be happening to this man? How will you decide? What can you do to help him?

NCLEX-Style Review Questions

1. A client is admitted to the hospital with a medical diagnosis of hyperthyroidism. When taking a history, which information would be most significant?
   a. Edema, intolerance to cold, lethargy
   b. Peri-orbital edema, lethargy, masklike face
   c. Weight loss, intolerance to cold, muscle wasting
   d. Weight loss, intolerance to heat, exophthalmos
2. Which nursing action is most appropriate for a client in ketoacidosis?
   a. Administering carbohydrates
   b. Administering IV fluids
   c. Applying cold compresses
   d. Giving glucagon IV
3. The nurse assesses a sweet, fruity odor on the breath of a client admitted with diabetes mellitus. This odor may be associated with:
   a. Alcohol intoxication
   b. Insulin shock
   c. Ketoacidosis
   d. Macrovascular complications
4. A client asks what the purpose of the Hb A_{1c} test is. The nurse's best explanation would be that the test measures the average:
   a. Blood sugar levels over a 6–10 week period
   b. Hemoglobin levels over a 6–10 week period
   c. Protein level over a 3-month period
   d. Vanillylmandelic acid levels
5. Which of the following would be the nursing priority for a client just diagnosed with Addison's disease?
   a. Avoiding unnecessary activity
   b. Encouraging client to wear a MedicAlert bracelet
   c. Ensuring that the client is adequately hydrated
   d. Explaining that the client will need lifelong hormone therapy

References

1. American Diabetes Association. (1997). Committee report: Report of the expert committee on the diagnosis and classification of diabetes mellitus. Diabetes Care 20(7) 1183–1197; p. 1183.
2. American Diabetes Association. (1997). Position statement: Diabetes mellitus and exercise. *Diabetes Care 20*(12), 1908–1912.

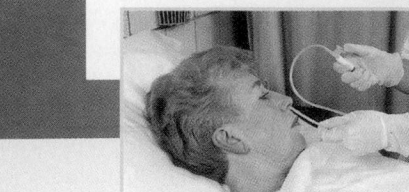

79

Sensory System Disorders

LEARNING OBJECTIVES

1. Identify two nursing considerations for each of the following types of testing: refractive examinations, ophthalmoscope, otoscope, slit lamp, tonometry, ERG, audiometry, caloric test, and ENG.
2. In the skills lab, demonstrate a dry wipe and an ear irrigation, differentiating the techniques used for adults and children.
3. State at least ten nursing considerations for the care of the client with: a visual deficit, including pre- and postoperative nursing considerations; a hearing deficit.
4. Define the following refractive errors: myopia, hyperopia, astigmatism, and presbyopia.
5. Identify the advantages and disadvantages of the following methods of visual correction: eyeglasses, hard contact lenses, soft contact lenses, and extended-wear lenses.
6. Define radial keratotomy, PRK, and LASIK.
7. Describe the following: inflammatory and infectious eye disorders (conjunctivitis, blepharitis, hordeolum, chalazion, trachoma, and keratitis); structural disorders (ectropion, entropion, and ptosis).
8. Differentiate chronic open-angle glaucoma, acute closed-angle glaucoma, and secondary glaucoma, identifying at least three nursing considerations for each disorder.
9. Explain the causes and treatments for cataracts.
10. Identify at least two nursing considerations for each of the following types of eye traumas: hematoma, foreign bodies, hyphema, chemical burns, corneal abrasions, and detached retina.
11. Compare and contrast conductive hearing loss, sensorineural hearing loss, central hearing loss, and functional hearing loss.
12. Discuss the causes and at least two nursing interventions for each of the following: disorders of the external ear (such as impacted earwax, furuncles, foreign objects, external otitis, fungal infections, and punctured tympanic membrane); and disorders of the middle ear (such as otitis media, serous otitis media, acute purulent otitis media, and chronic otitis media).
13. Describe the care for a client who is to undergo a tympanoplasty and myringotomy with insertion of PE tubes.
14. Discuss at least three nursing considerations for a client with Meniere's disease.
15. Identify at least two nursing considerations for clients with a tactile, gustatory, or olfactory disorder.

NEW TERMINOLOGY

astigmatism
cataract
cerumen
diplopia
ectropion
entropion
enucleation
glaucoma
gustation
hyperopia
hyphema
keratoplasty
labyrinthitis
Meniere's disease
myopia
myringotomy

nystagmus
olfaction
otitis externa
otitis media
otosclerosis
ototoxic
phoropter
presbyopia
proprioception
ptosis
tactile sense
tinnitus
tonometer
tympanoplasty
vertigo

ACRONYMS

ENG	IOP	PRK
ERG	LASIK	RGP
IOL	PE	RK

The *sensory system* involves those organs and structures that give individuals information about the surrounding world through the senses of sight, hearing, touch, taste, and smell. The receptors for these senses are located in peripheral parts of the body. The nervous system (see Chap. 19) transmits impulses sent from the sensory system to the brain for interpretation.

Any defect in a sensory organ or the brain itself, or in the transmission of nerve impulses to the brain, can cause a malfunction. Specific disorders of the nervous system and brain are discussed in Chapter 77. This chapter discusses disorders related to the senses of sight and hearing (see Chap. 21), and briefly reviews conditions related to the other special senses.

DIAGNOSTIC TESTS

Eye and Vision Tests

Visual Acuity

The exam for *visual acuity* uses the standard Snellen chart to determine the person's ability to see at specified distances. The chart has a series of progressively smaller rows of letters. The person is usually positioned 20 feet from the chart and is asked to identify letters on a specific line.

The term "20/20" vision means that the person can see an object at 20 feet that the majority of people with normal vision can see at 20 feet. The person with 20/80 vision can see at a distance of 20 feet what a person with 20/20 vision could see at 80 feet. The U.S. definition of blindness is visual acuity equal to or worse than 20/200, or a visual field of 20° or less, in the better eye.

Refractive Examination

The *refractive examination* is used to identify the degree of refractive error and determine the type of lens necessary to correct a visual defect. The pupils may or may not be *dilated* (opened) for examination. Drops such as cyclopentolate HCl (Cyclogyl), phenylephrine HCl (Mydfrin, Neo-Synephrine), scopolamine hydrobromide (Isopto Hyoscine), or tropicamide (Mydriacyl) are used to dilate the pupils.

Dilated pupils provide the examiner with a better view of the interior structures of the eyes and paralyze accommodation (ability to focus at various distances) in younger clients. This allows for more accurate testing for glasses. A **phoropter,** an instrument that simulates different corrective lenses, is placed in front of the client's eyes. Light from the examiner's retinoscope is streaked across the eye, while the lenses from the phoropter are adjusted until the light streak is neutralized. The final corrective lenses are selected by alternating similar lenses and having the client indicate which lens provides the clearest vision.

The Ophthalmoscopic Examination

The *ophthalmoscope* is an instrument used by the examiner to look through the pupil to see the retina and other interior structures (Figure 79-1). The examination provides information about the blood vessels of the inner eye, especially those of the retina, as well as information about the presence of tumors and the condition of the optic nerve.

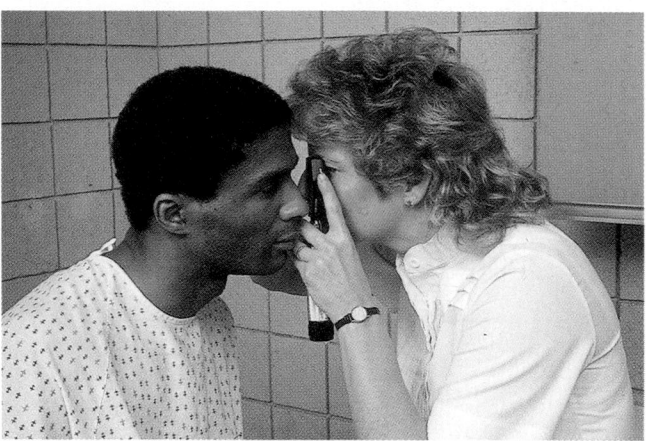

FIGURE 79-1. Technique for the proper use of the ophthalmoscope. The examiner uses the left eye to look into the client's left eye. She uses the index finger to adjust the lens for proper focus.

The blood vessels of the eyes suggest the general condition of blood vessels throughout the rest of the body. Atherosclerotic and hypertensive changes in the blood vessels of the eye are usually a sign that the same conditions exist elsewhere. Complications of diabetes mellitus can often first be seen in the eyes.

Slit Lamp Examination

The *slit lamp* is a special type of microscope that directs a beam of light onto or through the cornea to view the eye's anterior structures. The magnification of the images enables the examiner to identify abnormalities of the conjunctiva, cornea, anterior chamber, iris, lens, and anterior vitreous. The slit lamp also may be used in association with a type of magnifying lens to view the eye's posterior structures.

Tonometry

An instrument called a **tonometer** can indirectly measure intraocular pressure (**IOP**), the pressure within the eye. Two devices, the *Schiotz tonometer* and the more accurate *applanation tonometer,* are used to measure the pressure in the eye and detect glaucoma.

Other Tests

Other tests may be done to evaluate the function of the eyes and vision in specialized situations. The *retinal angiogram* is a visual depiction of the blood vessels in the retina, following the injection of radiopaque dye. *Ocular ultrasound* may also be used.

The *electroretinogram* (**ERG**) records the minute electrical impulses given off by the retina when it is struck by light, in much the same way as an electroencephalogram (EEG) is recorded. The ERG determines whether the retina is functioning. Local anesthesia is used. A contact lens containing the *electrode* (measuring device) is placed on the eye. The patient's head is under a "cone" and much of the test is done while the room is dark. The ERG can confirm a diagnosis of retinitis pigmentosa before the condition can be determined by other means.

Ear and Hearing Tests

The Otoscopic Examination

The *otoscope* is the fundamental piece of equipment used to examine the ear. Using the light and the magnifying lens of the otoscope, the healthcare provider can examine the external ear, the tympanic membrane, and anatomical points beyond the eardrum. Disposable plastic earpieces are used for each client. Several sizes for adults and children are available.

The nurse commonly assists the practitioner with eye and ear exams by providing the appropriate equipment, checking to see that the light is working, and helping the client to remain still during the examination.

Audiometry

Audiometry is a test of hearing. Several types of audiometry may be used. *Pure tone audiometry* tests both conductive and sensorineural hearing deficits (see sections later in chapter about these hearing deficits). *Bone conduction audiometry* tests only conduction loss.

Caloric Test or Caloric Study

This test is designed to determine if an alteration exists in the vestibular origin of the acoustic nerve. Abnormal test results suggest a diseased labyrinth or a tumor of the acoustic nerve. This test can differentiate such disorders from disorders of the brain stem.

Procedure.   The client is either seated or supine, and water is instilled into the external ear canal. Sometimes, warm and cold water are alternated. The affected side is tested first because less of a reaction is expected to occur there.

The normal response to this test is **nystagmus** (rapid, rhythmic eye movements), nausea, vomiting, *vertigo* (a feeling of spinning), and a feeling of falling. Decreased or absence of these responses within 3 minutes indicates an abnormality.

Contraindications.   Water cannot be used for this test if the client's eardrum is punctured. Cold air may be substituted. The client who is having an attack of Meniere's disease (see section later in chapter) should not be tested until the symptoms improve.

Nursing Considerations.   Because nausea and vomiting are likely, keep the client NPO or on clear liquids before the test and provide an emesis basin. The client is usually returned to the room by wheelchair or allowed to lie down until the nausea subsides, which is usually no more than an hour.

Electronystagmography

In *electronystagmography* (**ENG**), electrodes are placed near the client's eyes to assess for alterations in the vestibular system. In ENG, the caloric test is performed while eye movements are recorded on a graph. Other test components are the same as for the caloric test.

Other Tests

Magnetic resonance imaging (MRI) is used to detect tumors of the eighth cranial nerve. An EEG with evoked responses can be used to detect abnormalities of the nerve pathways between the eighth cranial nerve and the brain stem (see Chap. 77).

Another test of the function of the vestibular system and the semicircular canals involves seating the client in a chair that revolves in several planes, and then evaluating the functioning of the client's sense of **proprioception** (location in space) and vestibular system.

COMMON MEDICAL TREATMENTS

Eye Patching

In some cases, a physician orders one or both of a client's eyes to be patched. Several types of patches are available. A *simple single patch* or *double patch* may be used to cover the eye for rest or protection. A *pressure patch* taped in place may be used to keep the eye closed. A metal shield over the patch is also commonly used to protect the eye.

> **Nursing Alert**
>
> If one eye is patched, the client will have a loss of depth perception and peripheral vision. *The client should not drive* or perform duties that could be unsafe to the individual or to others. If both eyes are patched, care for the client in the same way as for a nonsighted person. This client may be apprehensive. Individuals commonly become confused or disoriented when one or both eyes are patched.

Dry Wipe

A *dry wipe* may be ordered to clean drainage out of the external auditory canal and the auricle. The steps for this procedure are described at In Practice: Nursing Procedure 79-1.

Ear Irrigation

An *ear irrigation* may be performed to rinse drainage or medication from the ears and to remove wax or foreign bodies. It is done only with a physician's order. Do not irrigate the ear if the client's eardrum is punctured. As seen in Figure 79-2 irrigating the ear or instilling medications requires different techniques for adults and children. For an adult, straighten the ear canal up and back. For a child, straighten the ear canal down and back. In Practice: Nursing Procedure 79-2 describes the procedure for ear irrigation.

COMMON SURGICAL TREATMENTS

Eye Surgeries

Most surgical procedures on the eye are performed as same-day surgery. In many cases, clients receive local anesthesia and are awake during such procedures. Eye surgeries involve precision. Often they are done with the aid of an operating microscope. The client's cooperation is essential; therefore, preoperative client and family teaching is important, including the following actions:

- Review activities permitted before surgery and restrictions following the procedure.

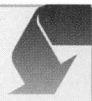

In Practice
Nursing Procedure 79-1

USING A DRY WIPE

Supplies and Equipment

Gloves
Cotton-tipped applicators

Steps

1. Make sure adequate light is available.
   RATIONALE: *The ear is a delicate organ. Ability to see the ear canal is needed to provide gentle and careful care.*

2. Wash hands and put on gloves.
   RATIONALE: *Handwashing and using gloves helps prevent the spread of infection. Drainage may be infectious.*

3. Explain the procedure to the client.
   RATIONALE: *Explanations help to alleviate anxiety and to earn the client's confidence and trust.*

4. Straighten the ear canal, pulling up and back for an adult, or down and back for a child.
   RATIONALE: *Pulling on the pinna helps to straighten the ear canal and provide better visualization.*

5. Insert the sterile, cotton-tipped applicator only as far as can be seen.
   RATIONALE: *Going further than the line of sight could lead to puncturing of the eardrum.*

6. Use each applicator only once, drawing it out and rotating it.
   RATIONALE: *Applicators are not reused because they can spread infection.*

7. Dispose of the soiled applicators and gloves according to Standard Precautions. Wash hands.
   RATIONALE: *Proper disposal of equipment and supplies, and handwashing, help prevent the spread of infection.*

8. Document the procedure. Indicate any observations regarding amount, color, odor, and consistency of drainage.
   RATIONALE: *Documentation provides for communication and continuity of care.*

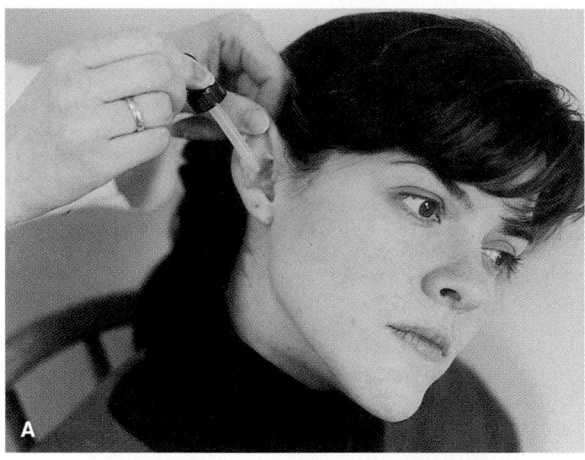

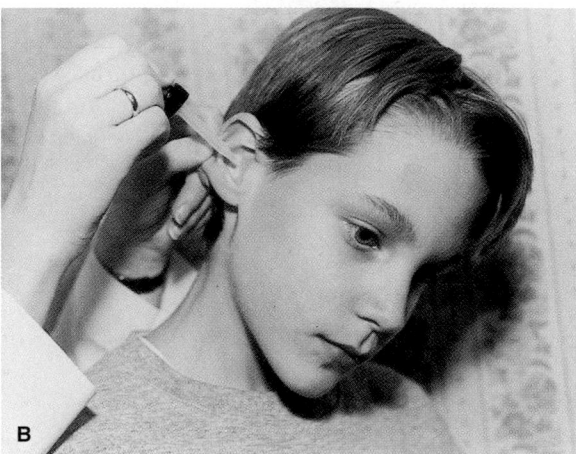

FIGURE 79-2. Technique for irrigation of the external auditory canal or instillation of ear drops. Note the difference in direction of pull on the pinna between **(A)** the adult (up and back) and **(B)** the child (down and back).

- Teach client and family how to administer eye drops or other medication prescribed to dilate the eye or treat infection.
- Review other procedures, such as eye patching.
- Outline the steps of the surgery: what will be done and what is expected of the client.
- Tell the client if he or she will be awake during the procedure.
- Review postoperative care before surgery.

- Remind the family that someone will need to drive the client home after surgery and probably to help him or her for at least a day or two postoperatively.

In Practice: Educating the Client 79-1 highlights additional information regarding client teaching and postoperative care.

Enucleation

Enucleation is removal of the eyeball. This procedure may be done when disease or injury has destroyed the eye or if a malignant tumor develops. After the eye is removed, a metal or plastic implant is buried in the empty eye socket. The eye muscles attached to the capsule move the implant. After healing is complete, a glass or plastic prosthesis shaped like a shell is fitted over the buried implant, for cosmetic purposes. This shell is painted to match the other eye.

Care of the Prosthetic Eye.   The client must learn how to insert and remove the eye and how to care for it. Some types of prostheses are removed at night and placed in a solution. When practicing insertion and removal, the person leans over a soft or padded surface to prevent possible breakage of

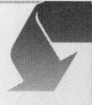

In Practice
Nursing Procedure 79-2

IRRIGATING THE EAR
Supplies and Equipment

Gloves
Plastic cover
Towel
Large emesis basin
Solution
Sterile, rubber-bulb syringe or sterile, large-volume
medication syringe

Steps

1. Warm the solution to body temperature.
   RATIONALE: *Hot or cold solutions can stimulate the inner ear and cause nausea or dizziness.*

2. Wash your hands and put on gloves.
   RATIONALE: *Handwashing and using gloves help prevent the spread of infection.*

3. Explain to the client what will be done.
   RATIONALE: *Explanations help to alleviate the client's anxiety and to earn the client's confidence and trust.*

4. Help the client sit up and provide adequate back support. Have the client turn toward the affected side.
   RATIONALE: *Proper positioning helps to ensure that the client is comfortable. Turning to the affected side allows fluid to drain out.*

5. Drape the client with a plastic cover and towel. Have the client hold a large emesis basin under the ear to be irrigated.
   RATIONALE: *Draping and using an emesis basin help to prevent soiling the client's clothing.*

6. Straighten the ear canal.
   RATIONALE: *This position provides better access to the ear canal.*

7. Expel air from the sterile syringe. Draw up the irrigating solution.
   RATIONALE: *Air is purged from the syringe to avoid introducing air into the client's ear canal. A sterile syringe is used to prevent introducing pathogens into the ear.*

8. Insert the syringe into the meatus for as far as can be seen. Do not plug the canal with the syringe.
   RATIONALE: *Inserting the syringe for as far as can be seen prevents injuring the canal. Not plugging the canal allows the solution to flow out freely and prevents the buildup of too much pressure.*

9. Irrigate gently with the prescribed solution. Note the client's reaction. Stop the procedure if the client finds it very uncomfortable.
   RATIONALE: *This procedure can cause sudden and great discomfort. A person can become dizzy or nauseated. If this happens, let the client rest before continuing.*

10. Allow the client to lie on the affected side.
    RATIONALE: *Lying on the affected side allows the fluid to drain and helps to prevent any great pressure on the eardrum, which could cause it to rupture.*

11. Dry the canal and ear.
    RATIONALE: *Drying promotes client comfort.*

12. Discard waste and gloves per facility's protocol and wash hands.
    RATIONALE: *Proper disposal of wastes and handwashing help prevent the spread of infection.*

13. Document the procedure, including the client's reaction.
    RATIONALE: *Documentation provides for communication and continuity of care.*

---

the prosthesis. The current versions of prostheses are made of plastic and are not easily broken.

If the nurse is required to insert a prosthetic eye, do the following:

- Wear gloves.
- Wet the prosthesis. *Rationale: This action allows it to slip in easily.*
- Lift the upper eyelid. Slip the eye up under the top lid.
- Hold the prosthesis while pulling down gently on the lower lid.
- Slip the lower lid over the edge of the prosthesis.
- Ask the client to blink. Blinking should slip the lid over the prosthesis and seat it in place.

To remove the prosthesis:

- Pull down on the lower lid.
- Press inward on the bottom of the prosthesis, which should cause the prosthesis to slip out.
- Be sure to work over a soft surface, to avoid breaking the prosthesis.

When caring for the eye socket, follow the physician's instructions. Rinsing with tap water or a mild solution available for this purpose is usually recommended.

Providing Care in Eye Surgery
Preoperative Care.   Client and family teaching are essential for all clients who undergo eye surgery, and especially

In Practice
Educating the Client 79-1

AFTER EYE SURGERY

- Do not remove your dressings; leave dressings in place.
- Do not use eye medications until you see the surgeon (usually on the first postoperative day). Bring your eye medications to that appointment.
- If a metal shield is prescribed, wear it while sleeping or napping, for up to 4 weeks to protect the eye from being accidentally bumped or touched.
- If both eyes are patched, be sure to ask your family for assistance; make sure they know how to help you.
- Do not sleep on the operative side for at least a week to prevent fluid and pressure from accumulating on the suture line.
- After the first postoperative day, clean the eye gently to remove mucus. Use cotton balls or tissues moistened with tap water.
- Follow these actions to avoid disrupting the suture line:
  - Avoid sudden movements.
  - Do not press on or rub the operative eye.
  - Avoid bending over with the head below the waist for about 2 weeks.
  - Avoid straining at stool.
  - Avoid vomiting; use antiemetics if prescribed.
  - Avoid activities such as coughing, sneezing, nose blowing, and vomiting.
  - Do not lift more than 10–20 lb for about a week.
  - Try not to bump or shake the head vigorously.
- Shampoo with the head back for at least a week.
- Avoid falls and jolts. Be careful walking on ice or up and down stairs. (Depth perception may be altered postoperatively.)
- Avoid getting soap in the operative eye. Bathing and showering are permitted.
- Read, watch TV, and may ride in or drive a car, as vision permits.
- Follow the surgeon's instructions about your stitches, which may need to be removed or may be absorbable.
- Know that glasses will probably be fitted in about 6 weeks. They may need to be changed during the first year, as the eyes adjust.
- Report any excess drainage, sudden pain, or bleeding to the surgeon immediately.

clients who are older or confused. Make sure to cover and to document all teaching.

When preparing the client for eye surgery, also include the following:

- Make sure to perform all items on the preoperative checklist. The client must sign an informed consent before any preoperative medications are given.

- Check to ensure that the client was NPO after midnight, if an early procedure is scheduled. Also note whether the client has taken a laxative or received an enema the night before surgery, if prescribed.
- Assist the client if he or she is confused or has received a sedative.
- Wash the client's face with surgical soap as ordered. If necessary, ask the male client to shave immediately before surgery.
- Instill eye drops, if ordered.
- If the client's eyelashes are to be clipped, use a blunt scissors coated with petrolatum. *Rationale: The petrolatum catches the eyelashes and prevents them from falling into the eye.*
- Report any signs of a respiratory infection. *Rationale: Infection may necessitate postponing the surgery.*
- If the physician has ordered the client's eyes to be patched preoperatively, find out what type of patch to use. Also check if a metal eye shield may also be ordered.
- Explain the reasons for patching to the client. *Rationale: Explanations reduce apprehension and confusion.*
- Have the client bring a hearing aid (if he or she wears one) to wear during the surgery. *Rationale: The client must be able to hear the surgeon's instructions.* Be sure to document this on the preoperative checklist.
- Perform and to document all preoperative teaching. Answer any questions the client or family may have.

Postoperative Care.   Because the client usually goes home soon after surgery, postoperative care centers around client and family teaching. The client is generally cautioned to avoid coughing, sneezing, lifting objects over 10 to 20 pounds, and sudden head movements. These actions can cause sudden fluctuations in IOP that disrupt suture lines. Focus client teaching on preventing complications, such as hemorrhage, increased IOP, stress on the suture line, and infection (see In Practice: Educating the Client 79-1).

✚👁 Nursing Alert
Report any paralysis of the face or on the operative side or *ptosis* (drooping eyelid) immediately. *Rationale: These findings may indicate damage to the facial nerve or the presence of edema.*

Ear Surgeries

Because many ear surgeries are done on an outpatient basis, nursing care centers around client and family teaching. If the client is in an acute-care facility, the same principles apply.

Cochlear Implant
The *cochlear implant* is a surgically implanted device that emits an auditory signal, bypassing a damaged cochlear system and stimulating the remaining auditory nerve tissue. This procedure is for the profoundly deaf and allows sound perception.

There are several classifications of implants. Location and transmission of the auditory signals and the types of implanted electrodes and stimulation of nerve tissue determine the type and classification of implant.

The potential candidate for cochlear implant must be an otherwise healthy individual with no evidence of mental retardation or psychological disorder. The client must be unable to recognize words spoken away from the line of vision, and be realistic and optimistic about the results.

Encourage clients to talk with others who have had the surgery to learn positive and negative aspects. Postoperatively, treat the client similarly to others who undergo middle ear surgery. Within a few weeks after the surgery, the controls on the implant are adjusted and the rehabilitation process begins. The client must learn to discriminate between sounds and voices. Listening will take patience and training.

Providing Care in Ear Surgery

Preoperative Care.   Preoperative client and family instructions for ear surgery are similar to those for eye surgery. Prepare them for what will occur and what to expect before and after the surgery. The client often is awake for surgery and must be able to follow instructions. Be sure to let the client know this preoperatively. Ear drops may be instilled or the client's ear may require packing with cotton as ordered.

Postoperative Care.   If the client is to go home immediately after surgery, teach the client and family how to perform care. Usually the client is allowed out of bed as soon as he or she leaves the recovery area. Someone must be available to drive the client home. In Practice: Educating the Client 79-2 highlights other items to include.

If the nurse is to change dressings or instill medications, be sure to follow strict aseptic technique and wear gloves. *Rationale: These actions help to prevent infection. Meningitis or encephalitis is possible because of the ear's close proximity to the brain.* Instruct the client not to remove dressings.

NURSING PROCESS

Data Collection

Carefully observe and assess the client with a sensory disorder. The disorder may involve a disruption in vision, hearing, or one of the other senses. Chapter 47 describes assessment, including some aspects of vision and hearing. This assessment establishes a baseline for future comparison and determines the presence of suspected complications. Report any changes in baseline levels. In Practice: Nursing Assessment 79-1 lists some components of nursing assessment for the sensory system.

In addition, observe the client's emotional response to the disorder or disease. Is the client non-sighted? Is the client able to hear? How does the disorder impact the client? If vision or hearing has been lost, is the client able to communicate, and how does he or she communicate? Is he or she able to work? Can the client move from place to place? Does he or she need assistance to meet daily needs? Does the disorder affect social activities or self-esteem? Is the disorder correctable?

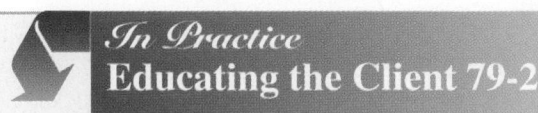

In Practice
Educating the Client 79-2

After Ear Surgery

- Keep any dressings and packs in place for several days or as directed by your surgeon, to avoid disruption of the delicate suture line and to prevent infection.
- Watch for signs of dizziness or prolonged nausea; these are symptoms of inner ear disturbance.
- Avoid vomiting because it can disrupt the delicate suture line. Take antiemetics as ordered.
- Avoid abrupt changes in position. Do not sit up quickly. These actions may overstimulate or upset the semicircular canals of the inner ear.
- Avoid sudden movement, straining, lifting, or acts such as sneezing or coughing. They may disrupt the suture line.
- Do not blow your nose. This can disrupt the suture line and possibly lead to infection.
- Watch for bleeding and any feelings of pressure or pain.
- Follow the surgeon's orders regarding positioning. Some recommend lying on the operative side to facilitate drainage. Some prefer the client to lie on the nonoperative side to prevent fluid and blood accumulation and stretching of the suture line after grafting.
- Watch for any fever, headache, vertigo, or ear pain and notify your surgeon as soon as possible.
- Although you can bathe, do not allow water to enter the operative ear.
- Resume your normal activities in about 2 weeks after being checked by the surgeon.

Nursing Diagnosis

The following are examples of nursing diagnoses for the person with a visual disorder:

- Risk for Imbalanced Nutrition: Less than Body Requirements as evidenced by difficulty in buying, preparing, and eating food, related to vision loss
- Social Isolation related to blindness, visual disorder, inability to drive
- Deficient Diversional Activity related to vision loss, inability to read or sew, inability to drive
- Anxiety/Fear related to plans for future, self-care abilities, rehabilitation, loss of employment, inability to drive
- Risk for Injury related to impairment in vision, eye patching

Based on data collection, the following nursing diagnoses may be established for the person with a hearing disorder:

- Risk for Infection related to ruptured eardrum, chronic respiratory infections

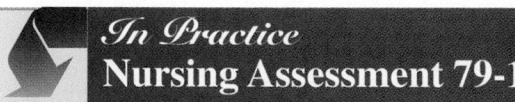

KEY AREAS FOR ASSESSING THE SENSORY SYSTEM

General Areas
- Nursing history, including information from family
- Presence of recent infections
- Medication use and recreational drug use
- General appearance of eyes and ears; examination with ophthalmoscope or otoscope
- Presence of foreign objects
- History of trauma to eyes and ears
- Assessment of cranial nerve function
- Neurologic status
- Signs of cardiovascular disorder (such as stroke)

Vision and Eye Assessment
- Vision assessment with Snellen chart or similar tool (gross determination of visual acuity if person has poor vision)
- Screening for infection or injury
- Screening for color blindness
- Screening for visual field deficits
- Screening for extraocular muscle disorder
- Symptoms and history of vision loss
- Direct observation of disorders such as ptosis

Hearing and Ear Assessment
- Prolonged noise exposure
- Presence of chronic respiratory or ear infections
- Screening with audiometer or similar instrument
- Complaints or symptoms and history of hearing loss

- Risk for Injury related to lack of hearing, hearing deficit, Meniere's disease (risk of falling)
- Impaired Verbal Communication related to congenital deafness, hearing disorder
- Chronic Low Self-Esteem related to loss of hearing
- Pain related to trauma, otitis and other infections, punctured tympanic membrane

Based on data collection, the following nursing diagnoses may be established for the patient with a disorder of one of the special senses of taste, touch, or smell:

- Risk for Imbalanced Nutrition: Less than Body Requirements related to lack of olfactory sense or taste and lessened appeal of food
- Risk for Trauma related to lack of sensory perception and impaired nerve transmission from sensory receptors as manifested by inability to feel or recognize pain, pressure, heat, cold
- Deficient Knowledge related to specific disorder and its treatment

Planning and Implementation

Nursing considerations for clients with sensory deficits include teaching and approaches to effective care for both client and caregivers or family. Whenever possible, make short-term and long-terms goals in conjunction with the client, caregivers, family members, and the healthcare team.

The client with a hearing disorder may require assistance with communication, maintaining balance, and meeting social and recreational needs.

A client with hearing or vision loss may need assistance in dealing with the disorder's emotional aspects. Help all clients to understand more about the disorder, the prognosis, and the treatment. Rehabilitation is designed to promote self-care.

Provide pre- and postoperative care for the client undergoing eye or ear surgery. The suture line is delicate in many of these operations. The client and caregivers at home will need to understand ways to protect these delicate suture lines. because many eye and ear surgeries are done on an outpatient basis.

Nursing Considerations for the Visually Impaired Client

When caring for a client who is visually impaired and is hospitalized, include the following:

- Encourage clients to gradually assume responsibility for their own care.
- Identify yourself when you enter the room.
- Speak before touching clients to prevent frightening them.
- Speak in a normal tone.
- Keep the call light within reach and place the bed in the lowest position.
- Place food on the plate in the same "clock positions" for every meal. Tell the person what is being served and where it is located on the plate.
- When ambulating, walk slowly and allow the person to take your arm. (Do not push.)
- Orient the client to the location of objects in the room such as furniture, the door, grooming articles, and the water pitcher; keep these objects in the same place.
- Let the client know when you are leaving the room.

When a client is visually impaired, simple activities can become difficult or overwhelming. For example, medication administration ordered postoperatively can present problems. The side effects of some eye medications (eg, timolol [Timoptic]) are bradycardia, dizziness, and syncope. Discharge teaching must include the common signs and symptoms of medication side effects. The nurse also can offer suggestions, such as the use of weekly pill reminder dispensers.

A home safety inspection should be performed. Scatter rugs, doors halfway open, and packages left in hallways are common hazards to the person with limited or no sight.

Individuals with a visual disruption often require rehabilitation to resume self-care. The visually impaired individual may need assistance moving around and learning to navigate in familiar surroundings. Meeting daily needs (eg, preparing meals, shopping, hygiene, grooming) brings additional challenges. Moreover, the individual may need assistance in finding new modes of transportation and may experience possible changes in employment.

In addition, other options are available for the visually impaired or non-sighted client. These options include Braille, guide dogs, and white canes.

Braille.   The *Braille alphabet* is a system of raised dots on paper that correspond to the letters of the alphabet and punctuation marks. One of the hardest things that a person who has only recently become visually impaired must do is to become accustomed to the inability to read. Learning to read Braille can be of assistance to many individuals with permanent loss of sight.

The non-sighted person discerns these characters with the fingertips. Learning Braille takes patience. However, many books and other resources are available in Braille and will allow the person to continue to enjoy reading. Direct the person to local agencies for the non-sighted for more information.

Clients can also use books on tape, which are cassette recordings of books and magazines. Special Braille typewriters and computer keyboards are also available. Some magazines and newspapers are available in very large print for partially sighted people. Many are also available in Braille editions.

Guide Dogs.   A *guide dog* (also called a *leader dog* or *seeing eye dog*) is used by many non-sighted individuals. These dogs are trained to recognize danger spots such as curbs, obstacles, or holes. They learn to be careful of traffic. The dog wears a harness fitted with a U-shaped handle that the non-sighted person can grasp; client and dog then communicate through the movements of the harness. A non-sighted person who wishes to use a guide dog must live at a training center for some time to learn how to use and take care of the dog.

The public accords these trained dogs certain privileges. They are allowed to enter restaurants, subways, hotels, and other public places that are usually off-limits to pets. If the client is not moving, the dog will lie quietly nearby. Airlines often reserve space for such dogs in the plane's cabin.

Nursing Alert

Never pet or play with a guide dog. Distracting a dog could place the visually impaired person in danger.

White Canes.   A *white cane* is a signal that the person carrying it is non-sighted. Only a non-sighted person is allowed to use a white cane, and the person has the right-of-way over all traffic. Some non-sighted persons, however, are reluctant to use a white cane unless absolutely necessary.

One type of collapsible white cane that a client can carry in a purse or pocket is longer than a normal walking cane and has a metal or plastic tip that transmits sound, thus providing the person with some guidance about his or her surroundings. As a part of the rehabilitation process, non-sighted people learn to use these canes to locate curbs and other obstructions.

Nursing Considerations for the Hearing-Impaired Client

A person with a marked hearing loss cannot hear sounds that warn of danger. This person loses the thread of a conversation and may ask questions or make comments that have no relation to the discussion. Sometimes, persons with hearing loss lapse into a silence that makes them seem uninterested or inattentive. People who are unable to hear their own voice may talk very loudly or in a monotone. In Practice: Nursing Care Plan 79-1 highlights the care of a client with a hearing impairment.

Many people are generally less tolerant of hearing loss than they are of vision loss, thus they may become impatient when asked to repeat their words.

When caring for a client who is experiencing a hearing impairment, include the following:

- Get the client's attention before beginning to speak.
- Face the client on the same level.
- Place yourself in good light, so the client can see your mouth clearly.
- Do not chew, smoke, put objects in the mouth, or cover it while talking.
- Decrease background noises, such as television and radio.
- Speak slowly and clearly; repeat entire phrases rather than specific words.
- Restate the conversation with different words.
- Use contextual clues such as objects, persons, and hand motions to facilitate the conversation.
- Verify that the person understood the conversation.

Individuals with impaired hearing may stubbornly refuse to admit that they do not hear well. They may deny themselves the help of a hearing aid because of embarrassment. Hearing loss that is due to advancing age (*presbycusis*) cannot be restored, but there are ways of compensating.

Hearing Aids.   *Hearing aids* operate either on the principle of bone conduction or air conduction, depending on the type of hearing loss. The device amplifies sounds. A tiny receiver is inserted in the ear and an earpiece is molded to the wearer's ear. Many hearing aids today are so tiny they are barely noticeable.

The physician will determine whether a hearing aid will help, and which type will be the most beneficial. Unfortunately, a hearing aid usually is less effective in improving hearing than glasses are in improving vision. Adjusting to a hearing aid takes time and patience.

Normally, an individual can adjust to and focus attention on specific sounds, such as human speech. Difficulties that clients encounter when wearing hearing aids include the resultant amplification of all sounds, including background sounds. These sounds can be distracting and annoying.

However, the client can overcome difficulties with perseverance and by wearing the aid at all times, not just occasionally. The earpiece should be washed every day with mild soap and water and dried well. A pipe cleaner will help to clean and dry the cannula. Batteries in hearing aids need to be checked regularly. Getting used to wearing a hearing aid and learning to adjust to it take time and patience.

In Practice
Nursing Care Plan 79-1

THE CLIENT WITH A HEARING IMPAIRMENT

MEDICAL HISTORY: *S.S. is an 85-year-old widowed Native American resident who has just been admitted to a long-term care facility. History reveals hypertension, coronary artery disease, glaucoma, and degenerative joint disease. During her recent stay at the acute care facility, a hearing evaluation was completed and the client received a hearing aid for moderate hearing loss.*

MEDICAL DIAGNOSIS: *Moderate hearing loss; history of hypertension, coronary artery disease, glaucoma, and degenerative joint disease*

Data Collection/Nursing Assessment: Client is alert and oriented. Skin is pale pink, warm, and dry. S.S. has been living alone since the death of her husband 2 years ago. Over the past 2 years, the client's health has declined, necessitating increasing amounts of care. Client has one elderly sister who is in the same facility. Client reports joint stiffness and pain in the morning. "Once I get up and get started moving, they get a little better." Joints demonstrate limited ROM. During interview, client does not always respond to words spoken or responds inappropriately. When questioned about her hearing aid, the client states, "I left it in my bag. Besides, what do I need this thing for? I can hear just fine." Further assessment reveals that client has a hearing deficit that is more severe on the left. When asked, client unable to demonstrate use of hearing aid. (*Although other nursing diagnoses may be appropriate, a priority nursing diagnosis is addressed below.*)

Nursing Diagnosis: Disturbed auditory sensory perception related to diagnosed hearing loss as evidenced by client's difficulty with responses when being spoken to and lack of use of prescribed hearing aid.

Planning

SHORT-TERM GOALS:
#1. Client will acknowledge the need for hearing aid.
#2. Client will respond appropriately to auditory stimuli with the use of the hearing aid.

LONG-TERM GOALS:
#3. Client demonstrates ability to use hearing aid with assistance.
#4. Client uses hearing aid at all times when awake.

Implementation

NURSING ACTION: *Assess the client's feelings and knowledge about hearing loss and using a hearing aid; clarify any misconceptions or misinformation.*

RATIONALE: *Determining the client's feelings and knowledge about the hearing aid provides a baseline from which to plan further actions.*

NURSING ACTION: *Review the reasons for use of hearing aid.*
RATIONALE: *Reviewing the reasons for the hearing aid helps to promote better understanding about the device.*

Evaluation: Client states that she is embarrassed by the use of the hearing aid. Hearing aid applied; client stated, "It does help a bit. Things don't sound so muddled." Client agreed to try using hearing aid for 2 hours per day. *Progress to meeting Goal #1.*

NURSING ACTION: *Get the client's attention before beginning to speak. Face the client on the same level, making sure that lighting is appropriate to allow client to see speaker's mouth.*
RATIONALE: *Getting the client's attention and facing the client when speaking help the client to focus on the nurse and what he or she is saying.*

NURSING ACTION: *Decrease background noises, such as television and radio, and speak slowly and clearly, repeating and restating information as necessary.*
RATIONALE: *Decreasing background noises helps to minimize distractions. Speaking clearly and slowly, repeating and restating, allows the client to focus on what is being said, thereby fostering verbal communication.*

NURSING ACTION: *Use nonverbal behaviors to enhance verbal communication.*
RATIONALE: *Gestures and other nonverbal behaviors can help to clarify the message being communicated.*

Evaluation: Client demonstrates appropriate responses to verbal communication when directly spoken to and with hearing aid in place. Some difficulty with responses is noted when hearing aid not used. Client stated, "I guess I'll try the hearing aid for a while longer." *Goal #1 met; progress to meeting Goal #2.*

NURSING ACTION: *Have client demonstrate the use of the hearing aid, providing feedback and positive reinforcement as indicated.*
RATIONALE: *Feedback and positive reinforcement are necessary to aid in building the client's self-confidence, thereby helping to foster compliance with the use of the hearing aid.*

(continued)

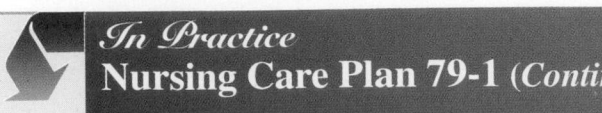

Nursing Care Plan 79-1 (*Continued*)

NURSING ACTION: *Continue to assist and reinforce use of hearing aid. Encourage client to increase time spent using hearing aid.*
RATIONALE: *Continued assistance and reinforcement help to promote learning and to enhance self-confidence.*

NURSING ACTION: *Teach client proper care measures for hearing aid, including cleaning and changing the battery.*

RATIONALE: *Properly caring for hearing aid helps to maintain its function.*

Evaluation: Client needs assistance with inserting aid into ear, stating, "My fingers are so stiff that I can't always get the aid in my ear." Client demonstrates proper technique for cleaning the device. Responses are accurate and appropriate when hearing aid in place. Currently, client wears hearing aid from 8 AM until 12 noon. *Goal #2 and Goal #3 met. Progress to meeting Goal #4.*

Speech Reading. Individuals with a hearing loss may benefit from *lip reading (speech reading)* and facial expressions. To understand lip reading, the hearing-impaired person must directly face the speaking person.

Sign Language. Another means of communication is *sign language (signing).* Certain movements of the fingers and hands form letters of the alphabet and words. People who use sign language constantly are able to speak rapidly with their fingers.

Nursing Alert

Lions International targets vision and hearing improvement as a major goal. If you come into contact with someone who needs eyeglasses, a guide dog, a hearing aid, or surgery, but cannot afford it, put the person in contact with their local Lions Club.

Evaluation

Evaluate outcomes of care with the client, family, and other members of the healthcare team. Have short-term goals been met? For example, has the client's vision or hearing improved after surgery? Are long-term goals still realistic? For example, is the client adjusting to the use of a guide dog? Is the client able to perform self-care? Are family members available to assist? What type of rehabilitation, education, or assistive aids does the client need? Planning for further nursing care considers the client's prognosis, any complications, and the client's responses.

THE EYE AND VISION DISORDERS

Several specialists are involved in treatment of the eye.

- An *ophthalmologist* has received a Doctor of Medicine (MD) degree and has completed at least 3 years of postgraduate training in diseases and surgeries of the eye. This physician is licensed to diagnose and treat eye dis-

orders, prescribe medications, perform surgery, and fit glasses or contact lenses.
- An *optometrist* has received a Doctor of Optometry (OD) degree following undergraduate and graduate studies. He or she is licensed to examine eyes, prescribe eyeglasses or contact lenses, and in many states, treat some eye diseases with medications.
- An *optician* is responsible for grinding lenses and fitting spectacles as specified by either the ophthalmologist or optometrist.
- *Ophthalmic technicians* are certified by the Joint Commission on Allied Health Personnel to assist the ophthalmologist in performing tests on clients.

Visual Changes

Changes in visual acuity are very common, affecting most people sometime during their lifetime. Visual changes may be corrected simply with lenses or surgery, or they may increase in severity until the person is unable to see light at all. The nurse is responsible for identifying early changes, teaching the client how to preserve vision or adapt to changes, and assisting the person when vision is impaired.

Refractive Errors

Vision occurs when light rays of an image pass through the lens and come to a focus point on the retina. From here, neurons send signals about the image to the brain for interpretation.

Refractive errors result when light rays focus in front of or behind the retina due to variations in the shape of the lens. The person experiences blurred vision or other changes in acuity. Holding objects at a distance, squinting, and headaches are some signs of impaired acuity. Common refractive errors are **myopia** (nearsightedness), **hyperopia** (farsightedness), **astigmatism** (abnormal curvature of the cornea or lens), and **presbyopia** (loss of lens elasticity and accommodation due to the aging process). Presbyopia is discussed further in Chapter 91. Table 79-1 summarizes the causes and types of refractive errors.

Correction of Refractive Errors

Refractive errors cause the most common changes in normal vision and are first identified by a Snellen test. The refractive examination pinpoints the degree of the error, which is necessary to determine the treatment. Corrective lenses (eyeglasses) or contact lenses are the most common treatment for refractive errors. The lenses are shaped as either concave or convex, thus *refracting* (bending) the light rays to focus on the retina.

Eyeglasses. *Eyeglasses (spectacles)* are prescribed to correct the refractive errors of myopia, hyperopia, astigmatism, and presbyopia, and for some low-vision ("legally blind") individuals.

Bifocals, two lenses in one, may be prescribed to correct the problem of presbyopia. Each eyeglass lens has two parts: one part corrects the defect in near vision; the other corrects the defect in far vision. *Trifocals* are also available and provide an additional option for vision correction.

Contact Lenses. *Contact lenses* are designed to fit directly on the cornea, where they float on a layer of tears. Contact lenses may provide better vision than eyeglasses by eliminating minification or magnification of objects. Contact lenses may cause corneal ulcerations.

Hard contact lenses are made of rigid gas-permeable plastic (**RGP**) and are paper thin. They are kept in place by capillary attraction and by the upper eyelid. Clients usually wear them daily. The lenses require special cleaning, rinsing, and storage solutions for care.

Soft contact lenses are made of hydrophilic plastic of a larger diameter and greater flexibility than RGP lenses. Soft contact lenses are more likely to be damaged by handling because they can easily tear.

Extended-wear soft contact lenses allow oxygen and carbon dioxide to pass freely through the lens. These lenses may be worn for up to 2 weeks before removal. Extended-wear contact lenses have a 10 to 15 times greater risk of infection than daily-wear contact lenses. Some soft lenses are disposable and are discarded after a period for a new set of lenses.

Many people take contact lenses for granted. Contact lens wearers must realize that prolonged wear or improper care can cause infections and injuries. In some cases, blindness may result from *infectious keratitis* (inflammation of the cornea). Caution clients not to put contact lenses into the mouth to wet or clean them. Doing so can transfer unwanted pathogens to the eye. The greatest danger with the use of any type of contact lens is the possibility of injury to or infection of the cornea, which can permanently affect vision.

In the case of accident or unconsciousness, the wearer could become blind if hard contact lenses are not removed. When the eyes are closed, tears cannot circulate freely, and corneal ulcers can quickly develop. For this reason, clients should not wear contact lenses while sleeping unless they are designed for continuous use.

If the person wearing contact lenses is hit in the eye area, injury to the cornea may result. Contact lenses rarely break while they are in place because the eyeball will give with the blow, and because the surrounding bony structure protects the eye. However, in the event of injury, severe swelling, or infection, a physician may need to remove the lenses.

Surgery. Surgical correction is done by *keratorefractive surgery* (surgical alteration of the corneal curvature), in which a laser or other microsurgical knife reshapes the cornea. Another procedure is *radial keratotomy* (**RK**), in which partial-thickness, radial incisions are made in the cornea to correct the refractive error. *Photorefractive keratotomy* (**PRK**) and *laser-assisted-in-site-keratomileusis* (**LASIK**) are other procedures that correct refractive errors.

Inflammatory and Infectious Disorders

Conjunctivitis

Conjunctivitis, also called *pink eye,* is inflammation of the *conjunctiva,* the membrane lining the eyelids and covering the sclera. Figure 79-3 shows a severe case of conjunctivitis. A bacterial, viral, or rickettsial infection or an allergy may cause conjunctivitis.

Conjunctivitis causes pain, redness, swelling, itching, and sometimes purulent discharge (*pus*). The discharge may be so thick and copious that the eyelids stick together. Following a culture study, antibiotic eye drops or ointments are prescribed for bacterial infections, and antiviral medications for viral infections.

■■■ TABLE 79-1 *Refractive Errors of the Eye*

Refractive Error	Cause	Result
Myopia (nearsightedness)	Elongation of the eyeball	Light rays focus at a point in front of the retina; blurred distant vision.
Hyperopia (farsightedness)	Shorter than normal eyeball	Light rays focus at a point behind the retina; blurred close vision.
Astigmatism	Unequal curvature in shape of lens or cornea	Light rays focus on two different points on the retina; distorted vision.
Presbyopia	Loss of elasticity of lens (poor accommodation)	Light rays focus at a point behind the retina; decreased close vision.

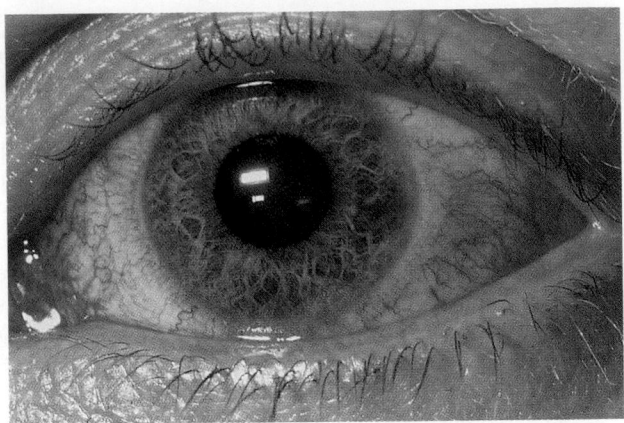

FIGURE 79-3. Conjunctivitis. Note the typical redness of the conjunctiva. (© 1995 Dr. P. Marazzi/Science Photo Library/CMSP.)

Treatment of allergy-related conjunctivitis includes avoiding the offending allergen, taking antihistamines, and undergoing desensitization. Boric acid or saline solution irrigations or warm soaks may remove discharge, reduce swelling, and decrease pain and itching.

Conjunctivitis is contagious. Proper handwashing, use of gloves, and proper cleaning of the client's linen are essential to prevent the spread of infection.

Trachoma.   *Trachoma* is another form of conjunctivitis found in hot, dry climates. Its cause is the organism *Chlamydia trachomatis,* which may also cause the infection *inclusion conjunctivitis.* Trachoma is highly communicable and is one of the world's leading causes of preventable blindness.

Treatment includes topical and systemic antibiotics, which are very effective. Trachoma is rarely seen in the United States.

Blepharitis

Blepharitis is inflammation of the eyelid, and is caused by excessive dryness of the eyes, excessive oiliness of the skin, or infection. This condition is usually characterized by red lid margins and purulent drainage. Treatment consists of applying warm packs to the eye to help loosen crusted drainage. Cleanse the eyelid gently with a mild soap and water once or twice a day. An antibiotic ophthalmic ointment may be prescribed to resolve infection and prevent recurrence.

Hordeolum

A *hordeolum* or *stye* is an acute inflammation of an oil or sweat gland of the eyelid. Styes are red, raised, swollen, and painful. They contain pus. After the area drains, pain is relieved and healing begins.

Treatment includes applying warm, moist compresses and a topical antibiotic ointment to the area to help localize the infection. In severe cases, the abscess is incised and drained. Teach the client not to squeeze a stye, which could spread infection.

Chalazion

A *chalazion (meibomian cyst)* is an accumulation of *lipid* (fatty) material from a chronically obstructed *meibomian* (sebaceous) gland found on the eyelid. If the lesion is small and does not

affect vision, treatment is unnecessary. However, if it becomes infected or interferes with vision or eyelid closure, incising and draining the area may be necessary.

Keratitis

Keratitis is an inflammation of the cornea caused by bacterial, viral, or fungal infections, often after trauma. *Herpes simplex keratitis* is the most common cause of unilateral visual loss from infectious keratitis in the United States.

Symptoms include pain, *photophobia* (sensitivity to light), blurred vision, purulent drainage, and redness of the sclera. Corneal ulceration is a common *sequela* (result). After culture studies are done, treatment consists of eye drops to dilate the pupil. Fortified antibiotic drops may be given hourly for bacterial disease. Antiviral or antifungal therapy as necessary may be given for viral or fungal causes.

Structural Disorders

Structural eye disorders may result from the aging process, injury, or a nervous disorder. They include:

- **Ectropion,** an outward turning of the eyelid due to the aging process. The eye is no longer able to drain effectively and tearing occurs. Surgical intervention is necessary.
- **Entropion,** an inward turning of the lid margin common in older adults. The lower lashes turn inward and are often not visible, but they irritate the conjunctiva and cornea. Corrective surgery may also be necessary.
- **Ptosis,** drooping of the upper eyelid. Ptosis may be due to muscular weakness, damage to the oculomotor nerve, or interference with the sympathetic nerves that maintain the lid's smooth muscle tone. Depending on the cause, corrective surgery and/or correction of the neurologic disorder may be necessary.

Glaucoma

Glaucoma is a condition of increased fluid (aqueous humor) pressure within the eye. It has an insidious onset, usually occurring after age 40 and having familial tendencies. Glaucoma is one of the leading causes of blindness in the United States. A disturbance in the normal balance between production and drainage of eye fluid causes glaucoma, leading to an increase in IOP. This increased pressure permanently damages the retina and the optic nerve. If left untreated, visual changes and blindness can occur. Early diagnosis and treatment are of the utmost importance to prevent vision loss.

Chronic Open-Angle Glaucoma

Chronic (simple) open-angle or *wide-angle glaucoma* is the most common type of glaucoma. In this condition, drainage of the aqueous humor through the *trabecular* (supporting) meshwork (located in the angle of the anterior chamber of the eye) is inadequate. The result is the accumulation of aqueous fluid in the anterior chamber, which causes an increase in IOP. Both eyes are commonly affected.

The onset of chronic open-angle glaucoma is slow, with gradual loss of peripheral vision. Glaucoma is often diagnosed at a routine eye examination when increased IOP is discovered. Often symptoms are absent, mild, or intermittent. Therefore, a serious vision loss may occur before the condition is discovered.

When symptoms occur, they include eye discomfort, temporary blurring of vision, reduced peripheral vision, and headaches. Late signs are the appearance of halos around lights and central blindness.

Treatment. Open-angle glaucoma may be treated by eye drops, to increase aqueous outflow; or oral medication such as acetazolamide (Ak-Zol, Dazamide, Diamox), to decrease production of aqueous humor. Beta-blockers, such as timolol maleate (Timoptic), are used as well. Laser treatment is often used to facilitate the drainage of aqueous humor. In some cases, filtration surgery is required.

Acute Closed-Angle Glaucoma

Acute-angle, acute closed-angle, acute narrow-angle or *angle closure glaucoma* is an emergency requiring immediate recognition and treatment to prevent irreversible visual changes and blindness. Untreated, acute-angle glaucoma can result in blindness in 2 to 5 days. One or both eyes may be affected.

In acute-angle glaucoma, the aqueous humor is blocked by a bulge of the iris at the anterior chamber before it filters through the trabecular meshwork. The result is an accumulation of aqueous humor, with resultant increased IOP.

In some cases, the cause of acute-angle glaucoma may be *iatrogenic* (caused by medical interventions), such as when dilating the pupils with medications for routine eye examinations. Symptoms usually occur suddenly, but may occur gradually and intermittently. They consist of blurred vision, halos around lights, severe eye pain, headaches, and occasionally nausea and vomiting.

Treatment. Treatment of acute-angle glaucoma consists of miotic eye drops (which constrict the pupil). These eye drops are given immediately, to allow drainage of the aqueous humor and decrease IOP. Analgesics are given to relieve pain. The client is kept on bed rest.

Early surgical intervention is indicated and consists of an *iridectomy* (removal of a portion of the iris). This procedure involves making a hole in the iris so that the aqueous humor can flow uninhibited from the posterior chamber to the anterior chamber. Iridectomy is performed with a laser or by traditional surgery.

Secondary Glaucoma

Secondary glaucoma usually results from swelling, infection, hemorrhage, or eye trauma. It usually develops gradually and is painless. Treatment for secondary glaucoma is the same as for open-angle glaucoma.

Nursing Considerations

Client education is important because the prescribed eye medications should be instilled as ordered. Instruct the client to avoid excessive fluid intake and all medications containing atropine. Frequent followup examinations by the ophthalmologist are imperative.

Cataracts

As seen in Figure 79-4, a **cataract** is an opacity or cloudiness of the lens. Because light entering the eye must pass through the lens to reach the retina, vision is impaired when the lens loses its transparency. One of the earliest symptoms of cataract is seeing halos around lights. The person may also notice decreased visual acuity and double vision (**diplopia**).

Cataracts may be congenital; caused by injury to the eye; or occur as part of the aging process. Cataracts have been associated with excessive exposure to ultraviolet rays and radiation; certain drugs, such as steroids; and systemic diseases, including diabetes mellitus. When a cataract occurs due to trauma, it usually develops quickly. A majority of cataracts, however, are associated with changes in the eye related to aging and develop slowly.

Treatment. The only remedy for cataracts is surgery to remove the lens. This procedure is one of the most frequently performed surgeries in the United States. Cataract surgery is usually done as an outpatient procedure using a local anesthetic.

In the person with cataracts, visual acuity that cannot be corrected to be better than 20/60 with eyeglasses is an indication for a cataract extraction. However, the main indication for surgery is when the client complains that vision loss interferes with activities of daily living.

Several types of surgical procedures are used to remove the lens. An *extracapsular cataract extraction* involves removal of the anterior capsule of the lens, followed by intact removal of the lens nucleus through a larger incision. Another alternative is ultrasonic fragmentation (*phacoemulsification*) of the lens nucleus through a smaller incision. An intraocular lens (**IOL**) implant is used with almost every procedure.

TRAUMA TO THE EYE

Contusion and Hematoma

A blunt injury to the eye may cause swelling and bleeding into the soft tissues surrounding the orbit, resulting in a *contusion* or *hematoma,* also known as a "black eye." Apply cold packs for the first 24 to 48 hours to decrease bleeding and edema. When the swelling has stopped, usually after 24 to 48 hours,

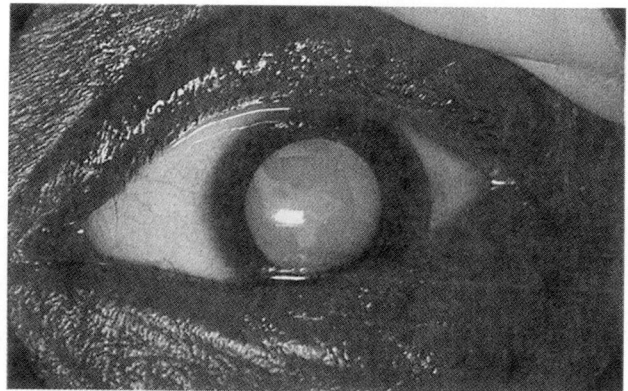

FIGURE 79-4. Cataract. The lens appears cloudy or opaque.

use warm packs on the site to hasten the absorption of the blood from the tissues.

Foreign Bodies

Foreign bodies may be external or internal. External foreign bodies are found on the corneal or conjunctival surface. Internal foreign bodies may penetrate the cornea or sclera and enter the inside of the eye. The latter most often result from pounding metal on metal or trauma such as a gunshot. To prevent damaging internal ocular structures, never attempt to remove a penetrating object from the eye.

Chapter 43 discusses the emergency removal of non-embedded foreign bodies. If the object is imbedded, a topical anesthetic may be ordered for severe ocular pain until the object can be removed. Ultrasound may be used to locate an embedded foreign body, and an electromagnet or surgery may be necessary for removal.

Hyphema

A **hyphema,** a hemorrhage into the anterior chamber of the eye, is usually caused by blunt trauma and can lead to glaucoma and vision loss. Clients should report signs of bleeding in the eye immediately. Treatment consists of mydriatic (dilating) or miotic (constricting) medications. Occasionally, an ophthalmologist may need to evacuate the accumulated blood.

Chemical Burns

Exposure to irritating acidic or alkaline chemicals can severely damage the eyes. Corneal abrasions and ulcerations with subsequent cataract formation may lead to permanent vision loss. The lens and the chambers of the eye can also be affected.

Treatment.   If any accidental substance comes in contact with a person's eye, irrigation with water should be done for a minimum of 5 minutes. During irrigation of the eye, direct the flow of water so the solution does not come in contact with the other eye.

After this initial irrigation, the person should immediately report to an emergency department or an ophthalmologist's office for further treatment. There, the eye is *lavaged* (flushed out) for an extended period. This prolonged irrigation removes acids and alkalis that can continue to melt the eye, even after it seems that thorough irrigation has been performed.

After irrigation is complete, a topical antibiotic ointment is instilled. Continued followup with an ophthalmologist is necessary. *Keratoplasty* (corneal grafting), which is discussed in the next section, may be done.

> ## ✚👁 Nursing Alert
> Extreme caution is necessary when instilling any type of medication into the eye. Containers of eye medications are similar to bottles for other solutions. For example, some non–eye solutions come in small bottles with droppers (eg, guaiac solutions used to test for occult blood). These solutions can be extremely caustic and can cause blindness.

Corneal Abrasions

Corneal abrasions involve the outer (epithelial) layer of the cornea and are often caused by tree branches, fingernails, paper, and contact lens injuries. Symptoms include severe pain, redness, and tearing (*lacrimation*). Corneal abrasions are easily diagnosed using fluorescein dye instillation. Following instillation, the area is viewed with a cobalt blue light. The abrasions appear green.

Treatment.   Treatment of corneal injuries includes instillation of antibiotic drops or ointment and pressure patching. These measures should result in healing within 24 to 48 hours. If healing does not occur, prompt followup is required to prevent complications. A serious complication is *corneal destruction,* which often requires corneal transplantation.

If severe visual impairment results from irreversible changes in the cornea, vision might be restored by corneal transplantation (keratoplasty). **Keratoplasty** involves the replacement of damaged corneal tissue with human donor tissue that is obtained within 6 hours after death. This tissue is rarely rejected because it has minimal blood supply.

Detached Retina

A *detached retina,* shown in Figure 79-5, is a separation of the retina from the choroid, thus depriving the image-receiving layer of its blood supply. Separation of these layers usually follows a hole or tear in the retina, which may result from a blow or injury, myopia, degenerative changes, surgery, tumor, diabetic retinopathy, or extreme hypertension. Because the sensory layer can no longer receive visual stimuli, vision in the affected area is lost.

Signs and Symptoms.   Signs and symptoms may occur suddenly or gradually. If a large part of the central retina is affected, vision loss is greater than if the outer edges are destroyed. The person may see flashes of light (*flashers*) or moving spots (*floaters*). Vision may be blurry, or it may seem

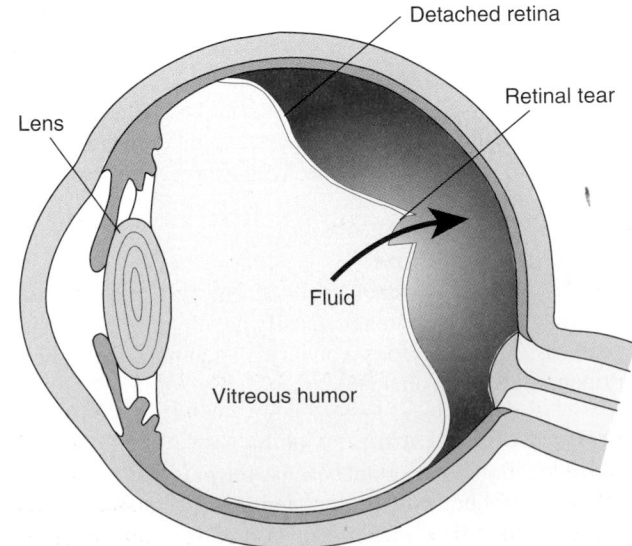

FIGURE 79-5. Retinal detachment. The separation of the retina from the choroid body causes a loss of vision.

as though a shade has been pulled over part of the vision. Usually no pain occurs with a detached retina.

Treatment.   One possible treatment for detached retina is a surgical procedure called *scleral buckling.* This operation shortens the sclera, thus allowing contact between the retina and the choroid. Procedures involving use of a laser beam (*photocoagulation*) and the application of extreme cold (*cryosurgery*) are also used to create an inflammatory reaction and promote healing.

THE EAR AND HEARING DISORDERS

The branch of medicine concerned with ear diseases and disorders is called *otology;* the physician in this specialty is known as an *otologist.* The otologist tests hearing, examines the ear for signs of disease, and determines the treatment. The *audiologist* tests hearing by various means. The *otorhinolaryngologist* or *otolaryngologist* treats disorders of the ear, nose, and throat (ENT). The acronym EENT refers to eye, ear, nose, and throat.

Types of Hearing Loss

Impaired hearing can occur at any age. Undetected hearing defects can be misinterpreted as lack of interest, attention deficit disorders, or mental retardation.

Injuries can affect hearing and cause deafness. Disease, exposure to excessive noise, or congenital factors may also impair hearing. Hearing loss may vary from slight to moderate or may be complete.

Total deafness usually cannot be corrected. A cochlear implant (discussed earlier in this chapter) may be helpful to some deaf clients. Congenital deafness may result in the inability to speak, or in speech that is very difficult to understand.

Conductive Hearing Loss
A *conductive hearing loss* is sometimes referred to as a *transmission hearing loss,* in which the conduction of sound waves to the organs of hearing is disrupted. It may be caused by a disorder in the auditory canal, the eardrum, or the *ossicles* (tiny bones of the middle ear). Fluid in the middle ear is the most common cause. Table 79-2 lists the types and causes of conductive losses. Conductive hearing losses are further classified as follows:

- *Air conduction loss* is due to a defect in the external auditory canal.
- *Bone conduction loss* is due to a defect in the bones of the middle ear.

Sensorineural or Perceptive Hearing Loss
Sensorineural or *perceptive hearing loss* involves a disturbance of the organs of the inner ear or of the transmitting nerve. A sensorineural hearing loss involves the *organ of Corti* (cochlea) or the *auditory nerve* (eighth cranial nerve). See Table 79-2 for a listing of the causes of sensorineural losses. Sensorineural hearing loss is further tested to differentiate between the following types:

TABLE 79-2 *Types and Common Causes of Hearing Loss*	
Type	**Common Causes**
Conductive losses	Otitis media; middle ear disease Perforated eardrum **Otosclerosis** (fixation of the ossicles) Defects of external auditory canal Obstructions of external auditory canal (eg, foreign body or cerumen)
Sensorineural losses	Excessive noise *Presbycusis* (hearing loss related to aging) Ototoxic drugs Tumors (eg, acoustic neuroma) Meniere's disease Congenital factors Trauma, skull fractures, brain damage (eg, cerebrovascular accident) Viral infections (eg, meningitis)

- *Sensory* (cochlear): Factors such as trauma, viral infections, toxic drugs, or Meniere's disease can result in cochlear hearing loss. These sensory conditions are usually not fatal.
- *Neural* (eighth cranial nerve defect): A tumor of the cranial nerve called an *acoustic neuroma* can cause a sensorineural hearing disorder. These tumors are potentially fatal.

Other causes of sensorineural hearing loss include excessive noise and congenital predisposition.

If the organs of hearing are impaired or deteriorating, the person has little chance of escaping deafness, unless the cause of the difficulty is discovered before damage occurs. This process is generally irreversible.

Central Hearing Loss
Central hearing loss refers to the brain's inability to interpret sounds after they have been transmitted. This sometimes occurs in atherosclerosis or after a cerebrovascular accident.

Functional Hearing Loss
In *functional hearing loss,* no organic cause is found and no damage to the auditory nerve is visible. Functional hearing loss is believed to stem from some underlying psychological problem. Professional counseling sometimes helps.

Prevention of Hearing Loss

All individuals should be aware of the dangers of infections and noise in regard to their hearing. The nurse can provide preventive teaching, as outlined at In Practice: Educating the Client 79-3.

Prompt treatment of infectious diseases, such as upper respiratory infections that can spread to the ear, helps to prevent hearing loss. The use of antibiotics early in the course of an ear

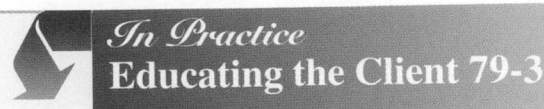

PREVENTION OF HEARING PROBLEMS

- Avoid excessive noise (eg, loud "boom" boxes, televisions, stereos, work environment). Keep volume down and wear protective gear if working in a noisy area.
- Protect ears on cold and windy days. Be aware of dangers of riding in car with windows open, or in motor boats, motorcycles, and so forth.
- Wear ear plugs for swimming if ear problems are present.
- Dry ears thoroughly after bathing or swimming.
- Do not place foreign objects in ears.
- Do not clean ears excessively. Do not pick or pull ears excessively.
- Prevent and treat infection immediately. Ear infection is not to be treated personally; see a professional.
- Have ear piercing be by a physician or trained technician; follow instructions for followup care.
- At symptoms of hearing loss, see a physician immediately.

infection also helps to arrest the disease and to prevent later complications.

Noise pollution is of great concern, particularly for young people and workers in industry. Wearing protective ear devices can prevent many hearing disorders. The Occupational Safety and Health Administration (OSHA) has established standards for industries in general. The loud volume generated from radios and stereo equipment is often harmful to young people's hearing.

Disorders of the External Ear

Most external ear disorders are more annoying than they are serious. If proper treatment is given, the condition tends to heal without difficulty. Unfortunately, many people attempt to treat these disorders by themselves, and consequently complications develop.

Impacted Earwax

Impacted earwax (**cerumen**) in the auditory canal is one example of a minor condition that requires medical attention. Wax can be removed by irrigating the outer ear with a solution warmed to body temperature (98.6° F or 37° C).

Instruct the client not to attempt to remove wax or other objects from the ear. Pushing on a foreign object may damage the eardrum. If the client has a perforated eardrum, irrigation might force the wax and the solution into the middle ear and cause infection. Poking at the wax with a finger, a hairpin, or

an applicator may injure the canal and cause infection. Additionally, the wax can be pushed in further.

Furuncles

Furuncles (boils) are infections in the auditory canal. They often result from picking at the ear to remove wax. They are intensely painful. Heat may be applied, and antibiotics are given.

Foreign Objects

Children or persons who are emotionally or cognitively challenged may put objects into the ear. A healthcare provider must remove any objects. Pushing on the object may cause it to travel further into the canal or cause the eardrum to rupture. If the foreign object is a food substance such as a pea, bean, or piece of corn, moisture will cause swelling and extreme pain, often leading to damage of the eardrum.

Sometimes insects enter the auditory canal. If they remain, they cause extreme distress by their fluttering and buzzing. If a flashlight is held to the ear, the light may draw the insect out. Sometimes a few drops of mineral oil, alcohol, or anesthetic jelly will anesthetize or kill the insect, causing it to float out if the client's head is turned to the affected side. If none of these measures works, the client should see a physician at once. Trying to remove an insect with tweezers is dangerous. Removing an insect from the ear is a delicate process that requires great skill.

External Otitis

External otitis (**otitis externa**), inflammation of the external ear, is most commonly caused by chronic external ear inflammation. Sometimes called "swimmer's ear," prolonged exposure to water often is the cause. The client receives antibiotics and is advised to avoid swimming until the infection clears. The client should then wear ear plugs when swimming.

Application of ear drops, composed of substances such as acetic acid (Domeboro Otic, VoSol Otic), boric acid (Ear-Dry, Swim-Ear), or chloramphenicol (Chloromycetin Otic), can be used for prevention.

Fungal Infections

Fungal infections in the auditory canal tend to occur in warm, damp climates, especially when the auditory canal has not been completely dried. Most of these fungi are opportunistic and feed on cerumen or dead skin cells. Ear drops containing antifungal medications, alcohol, and glycerin can treat such infections, which may resist treatment. Often treatment must continue for a number of weeks.

Punctured Tympanic Membrane

A punctured or perforated *tympanic membrane* (eardrum) is a serious threat to hearing later in life, as well as a possible source of middle ear infection. Although the perforation will often heal spontaneously, surgery is sometimes necessary. Occasionally, a myringotomy (surgical incision into the eardrum and drainage) is done for therapeutic reasons.

Piercing the Earlobes

Ear piercing is commonly done for cosmetic purposes. A physician or a trained technician using the correct sterile equipment and following sterile technique should perform this procedure. Client teaching is important. After the ears are pierced, the client is advised to keep the original earrings in place for at least 2 weeks, to turn them frequently, and to cleanse the earlobes often with an antiseptic solution, such as alcohol. The practice of piercing the external ears above the lobes is often more painful, but not as likely to cause infection, because the earlobes are thicker and not as quick to heal.

Disorders of the Middle Ear

Otitis Media

Otitis media is an inflammation of the middle ear (see Chap. 71). The ear is especially susceptible to upper respiratory infections, which can travel through the eustachian tube from the nose and throat. Children are especially vulnerable to these infections because their auditory tubes are straighter and shorter than those of an adult.

Types of Otitis Media. There are four different types of otitis media: serous, acute purulent, chronic, and chronic purulent. *Serous otitis media* results from fluid that collects in the middle ear, causing an obstruction of the auditory tube. This condition may stem from infection, allergy, tumors, or sudden changes in altitude. Symptoms include crackling sensations and fullness in the ear, with some hearing loss. If this condition is not treated promptly, fluid pressure may rupture the eardrum.

The treatment of choice remains controversial. It consists of antibiotic use or myringotomy. This is followed by analysis and treatment of the original cause of the difficulty, such as removal of a tumor in the nasopharynx.

Acute purulent otitis media is generally caused by an upper respiratory infection spreading through the auditory tube. Pus forms and collects in the middle ear to create pressure on the eardrum. Symptoms include fever, earache, and impaired hearing. The eardrum is inflamed and bulging and may rupture.

Initial treatment is often antibiotics. Myringotomy may also be indicated to prevent rupture of the eardrum. If spontaneous rupture of the eardrum occurs, scarring, which disrupts normal ossicle vibrations, can result. Often this permanently impairs hearing.

Chronic otitis media can develop if acute purulent otitis media is not treated promptly. In the past, mastoiditis was also a complication. However, today this is rarely seen in the United States due to the use of antibiotics. Meningitis is also a possible complication of otitis media because the infection can spread to the brain's meninges.

Other problems include nausea and vomiting, dizziness, injury to the facial nerve causing facial paralysis, or a brain abscess—all of which may start with a simple earache. Fortunately these serious complications are less frequent due to improved treatment for acute infections.

Chronic purulent otitis media is usually associated with a punctured eardrum or may be a complication of acute otitis media, mastoiditis, or a severe upper respiratory infection. Symptoms include ringing in the ears, hearing loss, pain, and purulent drainage. Antibiotics are prescribed, and a mastoidectomy may be necessary in some instances. Steroids may be given to reduce inflammation.

Treatment. Myringotomy is the common procedure used to treat otitis media. It releases pressure and relieves pain. Healing proceeds rapidly. Discharge from the ear is bloody at first, then purulent. To avoid interfering with drainage, do not plug the ear with cotton. Place a small piece of cotton in the outer ear to absorb the drainage and change it frequently. Give ordered antibiotics. Rest, adequate diet, and prevention against chilling are recommended.

Polyethylene (**PE**) tubes are often inserted through the eardrum incision into the middle ear. This procedure is most commonly done in children with recurrent ear infections. PE tubes allow continuous drainage from the middle ear. In this case, the client must use caution to prevent water from entering the ear. Swimming and showering are contraindicated.

Tympanoplasty is the plastic reconstruction of the tiny ossicles of the middle ear. It is done when infection or tumor has destroyed or fused these bones together. The bones reconstructed involve the structures from the oval window to the tympanic membrane. Tympanoplasty is a delicate procedure, performed with the aid of an operating microscope. The goal of the surgery is to preserve and to maximize hearing.

Otosclerosis

Otosclerosis is a bony fixation of the stapes, one of the three ossicles in the middle ear that transmits sound to the inner ear. This condition slows or stops the vibration of the stapes and impairs or destroys hearing.

Otosclerosis usually develops slowly. It appears to have a hereditary basis, because a familial tendency is found in its development. It is the most common cause of conductive deafness.

Signs and Symptoms. One of the first symptoms of otosclerosis is **tinnitus** (ringing in the ears), which is accentuated in quiet surroundings. It may occur for some time before the client notices a hearing loss. The client may not notice that he or she is losing the ability to hear, until ordinary conversation becomes difficult to hear—especially when others speak in low tones or there is background noise. Surgery or use of a hearing aid may help the client with this condition.

Treatment. Surgery to restore vibration of the stapes (*stapes mobilization*) may not be effective. Therefore, usually the client must make a decision about whether to have surgery. The operation is done under local anesthesia with an operating microscope and frees the stapes so it can vibrate. A more common procedure today is the removal of the stapes (*stapedectomy*) and replacement with a prosthesis.

Many clients are able to hear immediately after prosthesis placement. However, the return of hearing is not necessarily permanent; deafness may recur suddenly. Such deafness is due to an infection or to formation of scar tissue. If stapedectomy is unsuccessful, *fenestration* (creation of a new oval window in the ear) may be done.

Disorders of the Inner Ear

Inflammation of the inner ear is called *otitis interna* or **labyrinthitis.** Almost every disorder of the inner ear is difficult to treat. Neither surgery nor hearing aids help inner ear deafness (*perceptive deafness*). Drugs used to treat conditions unrelated to the ear can harm the inner ear (**ototoxic**) and may cause an inner ear disorder. Streptomycin, for instance, may injure the auditory nerve. Some diseases or the aging process may also cause inner ear damage. Treatment often consists of preventing further injury and training in lip reading.

Meniere's Disease

Meniere's disease is a disturbance of the inner ear's semicircular canals, which are responsible for maintaining a sense of stability and balance. Although it is not fatal, Meniere's disease is not curable. No known cause exists, but fluid distention of the labyrinth leads to destruction of the cochlear hair cells.

Signs and Symptoms.   Symptoms are devastating and alarming. The affected individual has sudden attacks of severe and true **vertigo,** a sensation of spinning or rotating, either of oneself or of one's surroundings. (Vertigo is not the same as simple *dizziness,* although sometimes the terms are used interchangeably.)

Other findings include nausea, vomiting, and tinnitus. The person may be unable to walk. He or she definitely should not drive. If the condition is untreated, hearing eventually deteriorates. Bed rest during an acute attack is sometimes necessary.

Sudden attacks of Meniere's syndrome are violent; they may last only a few minutes or several weeks, during which time the quantity of fluid in the space between the semicircular canals increases. During remission, the client's hearing and balance are often normal.

☞ KEY CONCEPT
_____

The person with Meniere's disease is often frightened. Vertigo can occur at any time without warning.

Treatment.   Medical treatment aims at relieving the symptoms. To decrease edema and pressure on the inner ear, the client may require a low-sodium diet. However, the benefits of this diet remain controversial. The person may receive sedatives or tranquilizers to subdue apprehension and accompanying anxiety. Drugs may relieve vertigo and nausea.

The client is advised to omit alcohol, coffee, tea, cola drinks, chocolate, and tobacco from the diet. Sometimes, when only one ear is affected, an operation to cut the auditory nerve is performed. This results in complete deafness in the affected ear.

Nursing Considerations.   When caring for a client with Meniere's disease, avoid jarring the bed, making sudden movements, turning on bright lights, or making loud noises. *Rationale: These actions may precipitate an attack.* Do everything slowly and explain actions to the client ahead of time. Protect the client from falls. *Rationale: If vertigo is severe, the client is in danger of falling.* Side rails should be up; keep the bed in low position at all times to protect against dangerous falls.

Give fluids and foods in small amounts. *Rationale: The nauseated client is better able to tolerate small amounts.* Remember, the attacks are so devastating that the client is understandably apprehensive. Reassure the client that relief is possible.

DISORDERS OF OTHER SPECIAL SENSES

In addition to hearing and vision, the special senses include the senses of touch, taste, and smell.

Tactile Disorders

Tactile sense (sense of touch) includes the ability to feel softness, pressure, pain, heat, and cold. This sense also assists in proprioception, and helps the inner ear to maintain balance. The body's muscles and tendons give information to the ear's labyrinth, which is involved in maintenance of balance.

A tactile sense disorder often results from a neurologic disorder. Persons with spinal cord injuries, nerve transmission deficits, or disorders in the brain's sensory area may be unable to feel or interpret pain. Diabetes mellitus causes peripheral neuropathy with subsequent loss of sensation, especially in the extremities.

Clients with tactile difficulties may be in danger because they cannot react appropriately to external injuries or internal disorders. They may be easily burned, for example, because they do not have the sensation that would warn them of the danger of heat.

In some cases of chronic pain, nerve transmission may be intentionally interrupted by surgery. In other cases, the person is unable to maintain balance, and may easily fall or may be dizzy much of the time.

Gustatory Disorders

Gustatory sense or **gustation,** the sense of taste, involves the sensations of sweet, salty, sour, bitter, and others. Disorders in this sense are usually not life threatening. An absence or alteration in the sense of taste may reduce the person's interest in eating. The loss of the sense of taste is commonly associated with the loss of smell.

Olfactory Disorders

Olfactory sense or **olfaction** (sense of smell) greatly affects the sense of taste. Disorders in olfaction are usually not life threatening, but they may reduce pleasurable sensations in eating or in smelling flowers or perfumes. In certain cases, such as in gas leaks, lack of olfactory sense may be dangerous.

_____
> ⚔ STUDENT SYNTHESIS
Key Points

• The sensory system is important in enabling people to receive information from the surrounding environment.

• Most eye and ear surgeries are done during same-day surgery, using an operating microscope. Careful client and family teaching enables clients to resume daily activities.

• Clients with visual impairments may use eyeglasses, contact lenses, and large-print materials to enhance their sight.

• Visually impaired individuals can learn to read Braille, listen to books on tape, work with seeing eye dogs, and use white canes. Clients with total hearing loss can learn sign language and lip reading. Clients with partial hearing loss may use hearing aids to enhance remaining hearing.

• Refractive disorders result when light rays focus improperly on the retina.

• Most eye infections can be treated with the application of warm compresses and topical antibiotic ointments.

• Early recognition and treatment of glaucoma are essential to prevent visual changes and blindness.

• Surgery is the required treatment for cataracts.

• Hearing deficits may occur at any age. They are caused by diseases and congenital and environmental factors.

• Determination of the cause of a hearing deficit is important because it may point to a more serious problem.

Critical Thinking Exercises

1. You are working in a school. One of your goals is to teach prevention of hearing loss to high school seniors. What would you include in your teaching plan? How will you communicate your teaching to the students?

2. Among the clients on your floor are a hearing-impaired person and a vision-impaired person. Identify ways in which your care would be the same for these two clients. Determine ways in which care would be different. Explain how the care would be different if one person were both hearing and visually impaired.

NCLEX-Style Review Questions

1. What instruction is most important for the nurse to include in discharge teaching for a client who has just had a left cataract extraction?
   a. Glasses will be fitted in about 6 weeks.
   b. Reading is allowed as vision permits.
   c. Do not rub or press on the left eye.
   d. Bathing is permitted.

2. A client has impaired hearing. Which of the following findings has the greatest implication for client care?
   a. Client does not wear ear plugs when swimming.
   b. Client has pierced ears.
   c. Client frequently rides a motorcycle.
   d. Client removes earwax with toothpick.

3. The nurse understands that the probable effect of a client's choosing to continue to be exposed to loud noises is:
   a. Hearing loss
   b. Ear infections
   c. Punctured eardrum
   d. Vertigo

4. Which of the following statements indicates that the patient understands how to care for otitis externa?
   a. "I'm glad I can go swimming today."
   b. "It is a shame I'll never be able to go swimming."
   c. "I'll use a swimming cap when I go swimming."
   d. "I'll be able to go swimming after the infection is gone."

5. The nurse is caring for a patient with blepharitis. Which of the following should the nurse use to safely cleanse the eyelids?
   a. A fatty soap
   b. Hydrogen peroxide
   c. Diluted baby shampoo
   d. An antibacterial soap

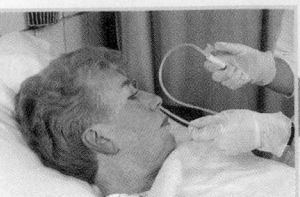

CHAPTER

80

Cardiovascular Disorders

LEARNING OBJECTIVES

1. Explain the rationales for the following laboratory tests: CK, LDH, AST, troponin, and lipid levels.
2. Differentiate an angiocardiogram from an arteriogram, including at least three nursing considerations for each procedure.
3. Describe the role of the nurse during and after the following procedures: echocardiogram, ECG stress test, echocardiogram, and an electrophysiology study.
4. Identify at least four nursing considerations before and after a cardiac catheterization.
5. Identify the rationale for performing a PTCA.
6. Compare and contrast the following surgical procedures: closed-heart surgery, open-heart surgery, heart valve replacement, and heart transplantation, including at least five postoperative nursing interventions for each.
7. Explain the role of each of the following conditions as they contribute to cardiovascular disease: arteriosclerosis, atherosclerosis, hypertension, and hypotension.
8. Differentiate the following cardiac rhythm abnormalities: sinus tachycardia, sinus bradycardia, PVC, heart block, and fibrillation.
9. Discuss the rationale for the use of external and internal defibrillation devices.
10. Describe congestive heart failure, including possible causes, signs and symptoms, diagnostic tests, treatment, and nursing care.
11. Define the following infectious and inflammatory heart disorders: myocarditis, endocarditis, and pericarditis.
12. Identify four major causes of coronary artery disease.
13. Describe three signs and symptoms for angina pectoris and myocardial infarction and four nursing interventions for each condition.
14. Differentiate the following disorders: thrombophlebitis, deep venous thrombosis, phlebitis, and embolism.
15. Identify three nursing considerations for each of the following conditions: intermittent claudication, Buerger's disease, and Raynaud's phenomenon.
16. Identify three main causes and at least four common complications of cerebrovascular accidents.
17. Identify at least six nursing interventions that are important during the various phases of a CVA.

NEW TERMINOLOGY

aneurysm
angina pectoris
angiocardiogram
angioplasty
aphasia
arrhythmia
arteriogram
arteriosclerosis
atherectomy
atherosclerosis
atrial ablation
cardiac catheterization
cardiology
cardioversion
claudication
dysrhythmia
echocardiography
embolus

endocarditis
fibrillation
heart block
hemianopsia
hemiplegia
hemodynamic monitoring
hypertrophy
ischemia
myocarditis
pancarditis
pericarditis
phlebitis
stenosis
stent
stress test
thrombolytic
thrombophlebitis

ACRONYMS

AICD	ECG	PTCA
AST	EPS	PTT
AV	HBD	PVC
CABG	HDL	RIND
CAD	HTN	SBE
CCU	ICD	SGOT
CHF	LDH	SIE
CICU	LDL	TEE
CK, CPK	MI	TIA
CPR	PROM	TMR
CVA	PT	t-PA
DVT		

Cardiovascular disorders include those conditions that interfere with the heart's ability to pump, those that disrupt blood flow within the coronary or cerebral vessels, and those peripheral vascular diseases that disrupt blood flow to a localized area (eg, an extremity). In the United States, collectively these disorders are the leading cause of death among persons over age 25, and the second leading cause of disability among younger persons. The field of medicine that examines the cardiovascular system and its disorders is called **cardiology**; physicians who specialize in this area are cardiologists. Nurses who work in this field are cardiac nurses.

The *coronary care unit* (**CCU**) or *coronary intensive care unit* (**CICU**) is a specialized hospital unit designed for the care of people with heart disorders. The staff is specially trained in emergency measures and coronary care. Training in coronary care includes: normal anatomy and physiology of the heart; normal and abnormal electrocardiogram readings; laboratory tests and their significance; emergency drugs and resuscitation measures; use of special equipment (such as cardiac monitors and defibrillation equipment); hemodynamic monitoring (specialized device to evaluate the pressure in the heart chambers); and the special emotional aspects of coronary care nursing. A detailed discussion of care in a CICU is beyond the scope of this text.

DIAGNOSTIC TESTS

Laboratory Tests

For clients with cardiovascular disorders, measuring the levels of serum enzymes is important. The enzymes include creatinine kinase (**CK;** formerly called creatinine phosphokinase [CPK]), lactic dehydrogenase (**LDH**), aspartate aminotransferase (**AST;** formerly called serum glutamic oxaloacetic transaminase [**SGOT**]), troponin, and myoglobin. These enzymes are released into the bloodstream when muscle damage occurs, as in myocardial infarction (**MI,** "heart attack"). Levels of these enzymes rise and fall at specific times and therefore must be correlated with the client's medical history, as well as with other diagnostic tests. Currently the enzymes relied upon most heavily in conjunction with the medical history are CK and troponin levels.

Blood *lipid* (fat) studies may be ordered to determine *hyperlipidemia* (excess fat in the blood). Cholesterol is a blood lipid often associated with coronary artery disease (**CAD**).

Other important tests measure the serum electrolytes, such as potassium, sodium, and magnesium. An increase or decrease in the level of these electrolytes may cause cardiac *dysrhythmia* (irregular heartbeat).

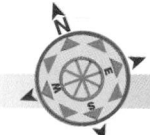

SPECIAL CONSIDERATIONS: CULTURE

False-Positive Results

Women who undergo diagnostic cardiovascular tests experience more false-positive results than men.

X-ray Evaluations

Angiocardiogram and Arteriogram

An **angiocardiogram** (*angiogram*) is an x-ray study of the heart and major vessels performed after injection of a radiopaque dye into a vessel. The angiogram shows the movement of the dye from the heart to the lungs, back to the heart, then out through the aorta. This procedure can provide information about structural abnormalities and calcifications within the vascular system. An **arteriogram** is an x-ray study of any artery.

> **Nursing Alert**
> Ask clients if they are allergic to shellfish or iodine before performing any test using radiopaque dye. This dye could cause a severe anaphylactic reaction.

Because these procedures are uncomfortable and carry some risk, clients must sign an informed consent before these tests can be done.

Nursing Considerations. Usually the client does not eat breakfast before the procedure. He or she may receive a sedative 30 minutes to 1 hour before the test is scheduled. The groin area is often the site for insertion; the area may need to be prepared. Carry out other routine preoperative procedures. Ask the client to void just before the test.

Be alert for a possible allergic reaction to the dye, during or after the procedure. Watch for signs of a delayed reaction after returning to the room, such as rapid pulse, diaphoresis, shakiness, skin rash, or a drop in blood pressure. The client may complain of a swollen throat or difficulty swallowing. The dye is irritating if it comes in contact with the skin, and sometimes the injection site becomes swollen and painful. Ice packs may be prescribed to relieve discomfort. (See Box 47-1 in Chapter 47 for special precautions when dye is used.)

Keep the client on bed rest until he or she is fully awake. Instruct the client not to bend the leg or flex the hip for up to 8 hours if the femoral site was used. Closely observe the insertion site for bleeding, and carefully monitor vital signs to check for internal hemorrhage. Check peripheral pulses distal to the site. Also check the color and warmth of the affected extremity and assess motor and sensory function. Clots or other blockages in blood vessels are possible. If pulses are absent, take emergency measures.

> **Nursing Alert**
> After any study in which the femoral site is used, the client should lie flat for up to 8 hours. Lying flat helps prevent swelling, bruising, and bleeding at the puncture site. Follow physician orders for activity level.

Other Diagnostic Tests

Electrocardiogram

An electrocardiogram (**ECG**) is a graphic record or tracing that represents the heart's electrical action. It provides essential information about the heart, including rate, rhythm, and the presence of certain disorders.

The ECG may be done at the bedside or in a room set aside for this purpose. Tell the client that the test is painless and that he or she must lie very still. *Leads (electrodes)* are placed on the skin (the chest, wrists, and ankles) and connected to a machine called an *electrocardiograph.* Figure 80-1 shows lead placement.

The graph or tracing (ECG) is placed on the chart after the cardiologist has interpreted it and written a statement and summary of the findings. The client does not usually require any special treatment before or after the procedure. The person interpreting the ECG must be informed of any cardiac medications the client is receiving. Data regarding the client's age,

sex, blood pressure, height, weight, and symptoms must be available to the cardiologist. Figure 80-2 illustrates the basic ECG graphic recording, which is read as PQRST waveforms. Deviations from the normal PQRST waveform indicate a variety of cardiac conditions.

Stress Test

The purpose of the **stress test** is to assess the severity of symptomatic and *asymptomatic* (without symptoms) cardiac disease. The client pedals a stationary bicycle or walks on a treadmill while ECG and blood pressure measurements are taken. Various chemicals or medications (thallium, dipyridamole [Persantine], dobutamine HCl [Dobutrex]) may also be injected before or during the test, or used instead of exercise for older adults and those who cannot tolerate activity. The heart's response to physical activity or the medication is determined, and an appropriate exercise program or method of treatment is then prescribed for the individual.

Echocardiogram

Echocardiography uses sound waves to produce a three-dimensional view of the heart and its blood flow. An echocardiogram can assess heart size, detect the presence of excess fluid in the pericardial sac, assess valvular function, and even show the sizes of individual heart chambers. It is especially useful in the diagnosis and differentiation of heart murmurs.

Transesophageal echocardiography (**TEE**) is another means of monitoring of the heart, where the ultrasound probe is inserted directly into the esophagus. This provides for a better visualization of the heart through the esophageal wall. TEE can be performed intraoperatively or in the physician's office.

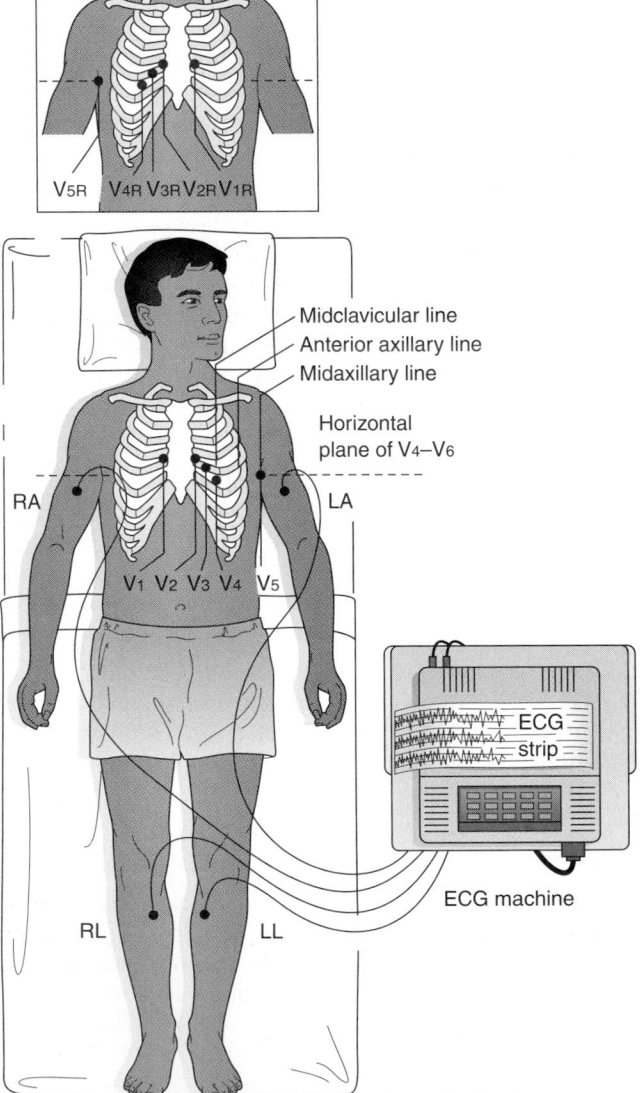

FIGURE 80-1. Twelve-lead ECG electrode placement. (RA—right arm; LA—left arm; LL—left leg; RL—right leg; V₁–V₆—chest leads; aVr—augmented voltage right arm; aVL—augmented voltage left arm; aVF—augmented voltage left foot or leg.)

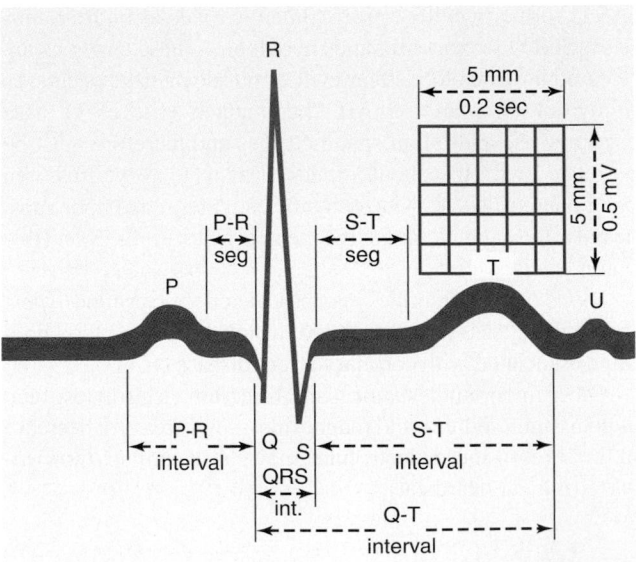

FIGURE 80-2. Diagram of the ECG reading (lead II) and commonly measured components. Each small box on the horizontal axis represents 0.04 seconds; on the vertical axis, each small box represents 1 millimeter or 0.1 millivolt. The P wave represents atrial depolarization, the QRS complex ventricular depolarization, and the T wave ventricular repolarization. Atrial repolarization occurs during ventricular depolarization and is hidden under the QRS complex.

Nuclear Scan

The *nuclear scan* is generally performed to detect *ischemic* patterns (lack of blood supply) and to assess for viable myocardium. During the scan, the client receives a weak radioactive chemical (thallium, technetium, sestamibi, or teboroxime) intravenously (IV) for a better view of the heart's chambers or myocardium.

Electrophysiology Study

The *electrophysiology study* (**EPS**) provides valuable information about the function of the heart by locating the source of a *dysrhythmia* (abnormal heart rhythm) and determining the most effective medication to control it. The EPS is done in the cardiovascular laboratory and takes approximately 2 to 3 hours. The cardiologist will attempt to recreate the abnormal heart rhythm by using a special catheter with multiple electrodes. These electrodes are connected to transducers, to study impulses from conductive tissue and identify abnormalities. After the dysrhythmia occurs, various medications are administered to determine the most effective preventive agent.

Nursing Considerations.   The client must sign an informed consent and will be NPO after midnight. A sedative is sometimes ordered for relaxation before and during the procedure.

After the procedure, the catheter insertion site is covered with a 4 × 4 bandage or Band-Aid. The client will be on bed rest for 1 to 2 hours after the procedure. Check the client's vital signs every 15 minutes initially and less frequently once they have stabilized. This procedure may be done on an outpatient basis.

Cardiac Catheterization

A **cardiac catheterization** is performed to obtain information about congenital or acquired heart defects, to measure oxygen concentration, to determine cardiac output, or to assess the status of the heart's structures and chambers. It may be performed during an angiocardiogram to study the function of the heart or blood supply, or to diagnose congenital anomalies or valvular disease. Therapeutic treatments may be done during the catheterization to repair the heart, open valves, or dilate arteries.

In this procedure, a long, flexible catheter is passed into the heart through a large blood vessel, usually the femoral or brachial artery. However, with the miniaturization of medical devices, a relatively new approach is to use the radial artery (*transradial catheterization*). The pressure is measured as the catheter passes through each location and blood specimens are taken in each area. A dye may also be injected. A team of physicians, nurses, and technicians perform this procedure, which takes from 1 to 3 hours.

Nursing Considerations.   Clients may be apprehensive about the procedure. Explain that it is not painful, although it may be slightly uncomfortable. A local anesthetic is given during the procedure. Warn the client that during the procedure, he or she may feel a sensation of warmth and a "fluttering" in the heart, as the catheter passes through the blood vessels. A signed informed consent is required and the client is NPO for at least 6 hours before the procedure. Exceptions to the NPO order are specific medications ordered by the physician.

Cardiac catheterization usually has no complications, but it is not entirely without danger. Assess the insertion site for bleeding or hematoma. Check the client's peripheral pulses every 15 minutes for an hour after the test and then frequently thereafter for up to 8 hours, depending upon the insertion site used.

> **✚👁 N u r s i n g   A l e r t**
> Report a client's rapid or irregular pulse after cardiac catheterization immediately. It may indicate heart or valve damage, clot formation, or hemorrhage. Also report any complaint of chest or insertion-site pain immediately.

COMMON MEDICAL TREATMENTS

Pharmacologic Therapy

A major aspect of treating cardiovascular disorders is the use of pharmacologic therapy. Numerous drugs are available for the wide range of cardiac conditions. Some of the major drugs are listed at Table 80-1.

Thrombolytic Therapy

Pharmacologic agents called *thrombolytics,* such as streptokinase (Streptase), urokinase (Abbokinase), and alteplase (Activase) (also known as tissue plasminogen activator, **t-PA**), have been shown to dissolve clots in the coronary arteries. (These clots cause *occlusion* [blockage] of the blood flow in situations such as acute MI.) Nurses usually administer the specific drugs through a peripheral vein in the emergency department (ED) or intensive care unit (ICU). Clients for **thrombolytic** therapy are selected by the following criteria:

- History of chest pain within the past 6 hours. *Rationale: Studies have shown that the sooner the pharmacologic agent is administered, the lesser the heart muscle damage that results.*
- **Ischemia** (lack of blood supply) of the heart that persists even after the administration of sublingual nitroglycerin. Ischemia is reflected on the ECG as ST segment depression or T wave inversion, or both.
- No recent history of surgery, organ biopsy, cardiopulmonary resuscitation, cerebrovascular accident (**CVA**), bleeding abnormalities, intracranial neoplasm, recent head injury, pregnancy, or allergy to streptokinase.

General relief of chest pain occurs if the procedure is successful. Assess the client for complications including dysrhythmias, bleeding, allergic reactions, and fever. The client will be in the CCU for 1 to 2 days to facilitate close observation.

COMMON SURGICAL TREATMENTS

Percutaneous Transluminal Coronary Angioplasty

In *percutaneous transluminal coronary angioplasty* (**PTCA**), a surgeon inserts a balloon-tipped catheter into a client's nar-

Type	Uses	Examples
Angiotensin-converting enzyme (ACE) Inhibitors		
Prevent angiotensin activation [vasoconstriction], thus leading to vasodilation	HTN, CHF, CAD, post-MI; persons with weak heart valves	benazepril (Lotensin, Lotrel) captopril (Captopen) enalapril (Vasotec) fosinopril (Monopril) lisinopril (Prinivil, Zestril, Quinapril [Accupril], Ramipril [Altace], Trandolapril [Mavik])
Angiotensin Receptor Blockers		
Prevent angiotensin (hormone that causes blood vessels to constrict) from binding to its receptors on the blood vessel walls	HTN, CHF	Candesartan (Atacand) eprosartan (Teveten) irbesartan (Avapro) losartan (Cozaar) tasosartan (Verdia) telmisartan (Micardis) valsartan (Diovan)
Antiarrhythmics	Control dysrhythmias that are too fast and are life threatening, or those that are not managed by the use of beta blockers, calcium channel blockers, and digoxin (which are now considered first-line treatments of choice)	lidocaine (Xylocaine) amiodarone (Cordorone, Pacerone) bretylium dilsopyramide (Norpace) dofetilide (Tikosyn) flecainide (Tambocor) mexilitine (Mexitil) procainamide (Procan, Pronestyl) quinidine (Cardioquin, Quinatglute) sotolol (Betapace, Tocainamide [Tonocard])
Anticoagulants		
Prevent clot formation and/or dissolve clots	Deep vein thrombosis, embolism	warfarin sodium (Coumadin) dicumarol heparin ardiparin (Normiflo) dalteparin (Fragmin) enoxaparin (Lovenox) nadroparin (Fraxoparine) reviparin (Clivarine)
Antihypertensives		
Include ACE inhibitors, angiotensin blockers, beta blockers, calcium channel blockers, diuretics, and others	HTN	atenolol (Tenormin) captopril (Capoten) alphamethyldopa (Aldomet) clonidine (Catapres) guanfacine (Tenex)
Vasodilators		
Dilate the blood vessels	HTN, peripheral vascular disease	doxazosin (Cardura) guanadrel (Hylorel) guanethedine (Esimil) mecamylamine (Inversine) prazosin (Minipress) hydralazine (Apresoline; acts directly on vessel walls, causing dilation) reserpine (reduces levels of adrenaline-type substance in the body)
Beta Blockers		
Inhibit the binding of adrenaline to the beta receptors on the membranes of heart muscle cells	HTN, control angina, post-MI, CAD, some dysrhythmias, CHF, hypertrophic cardiomyopathy	acebutolol (Sectral) atenolol (Tenormin) betaxolol (Kerlone) bisoprolol (Zebeta) carteolol (Cartrol) carvedilil (Coreg) metoprolol (Lopressor, Toprol) nadolol (Corgard) propranolol (Inderal) timolol (Blocadren)

■■■ **TABLE 80-1** *I*MPORTANT MEDICATIONS FOR THE TREATMENT
OF CARDIOVASCULAR DISEASE (CONTINUED)

Type	Uses	Examples
Calcium Channel Blockers		
Block the influx of calcium into the cells, thereby relaxing muscles in the arterial walls leading to vasodilation, decreased blood pressure, and increased blood supply to the heart	HTN, angina, some dysrhythmias, hypertropic cardiomyopathy; prevent vascular spasm after brain hemorrhage	amlodipine (Norvasc, Lotrel) bepridil (Vascor) diltiazem (Cardizem, Cartia, Dilacor, Diltia, Tiamate) felodipine (Plendil) isradapine (Dynacirc) mibefradil (Posicor) nicardipine (Cardene) nifedipine (Adalat, Procardia) nimodipine (Nimotop, Nisoldipine [Sular]) verapamil (Calan, Covera-HS, Isoptin, Verelan)
Cardiotonics		
Strengthen the heart's contraction by increasing the amount of calcium inside the cells; increase cardiac output; reduce workload and heart rate	Heart failure	digoxin (Crystodigin)
Cholesterol-Reducing Medications		
Fibrates inhibit production of the proteins that contain fat and cholesterol; *resins* bind with the bile that is secreted into the intestines to prevent absorption; *statins* inhibit an enzyme in the liver responsible for the manufacture of cholesterol; *niacin* lowers LDL cholesterol and tryglycerides while raising HDL cholesterol	Hypercholesterolemia/hyperlipidemia	*Fibrates* bezafibrate (Bezalip) clofibrate (Atromid-S) fenofibrate (Tricor) gemfibrozil (Lopid) *Resins* cholestyramine (Cholybar, LoCholest, Questran, Prevalite) colesevelam (Welchol) colestipol (Colestid) *Statins* atorvastatin (Lipitor) cerivastatin (Baycol) fluvastatin (Lescol) itavastatin lovastatin (Mevacor) pravastatin (Pravachol) simvastatin (Zocor) *Niacin*
Diuretics		
Increase excretion of water and some electrolytes	HTN; control of fluid retention	*Loop Diuretics* bumetanide (Bumex) ethacrynic acid (Edecrine) furosemide (Lasix) torsemide (Demadex) *Thiazides* chlorthiazide (Diuril) hydrochlorthiazide (Esidrix, Hydrodiuril, Microzide, Oretec) indapamine (Lozol) metalazone (Zaroxylyn) methyclothiazide (Enduron) *Potassium Sparing* amiloride (Midamor) spironolactone (Aldactone) tramterene (Dyrenium)

(continued)

■■■ **TABLE 80-1** *I*MPORTANT MEDICATIONS FOR THE TREATMENT OF CARDIOVASCULAR DISEASE (CONTINUED)

Type	Uses	Examples
Nitrates and Nitrites		
Resultant vasodilation	Angina	*To Stop an Attack*
		nitrolingual spray
		sublingual nitrostat
		nitrogard
		isosorbide dinitrate (Isordil, Sorbitrate)
		IV nitro-bid
		Tridil
		Prophylaxis
		erythrityl tetranitrate (Cardilate)
		isosorbide dinitrate (Isordil, Sorbitrate)
		isosorbide mononitrate (Imdur, Monoket)
		pentaerythritol tetranitrate (Peritrate)
		nitrobid
		nitrol ointment
		nitrodur
		transderm nitro

Note: Trade names of medications appear in parentheses following generic name. This list may not include all medications in each category. Please refer to Chap. 62 for further information on classification of cardiovascular medications, dosages, and side effects.

rowed coronary artery (Fig. 80-3). Injection of a radiopaque dye allows clear visibility of the coronary arteries by x-ray study so that the surgeon can see the vessels.

Sometimes this procedure is simply called *angioplasty.* **Angioplasty** widens the artery's opening (*lumen*) and improves blood flow to the heart muscles. Another type of angioplasty, called **atherectomy,** involves use of a cutting device (*rotoblator*) with a rotating shaver (*burr*) at the tip of the catheter. This is used to shave away plaque from the coronary artery. *Laser angioplasty* has also been used either alone or in conjunction with the balloon. The laser beam of light vaporizes the plaque in the coronary artery.

In some cases, angioplasty does not maintain arterial patency, and the artery closes. Some surgeons are finding long-term success through angioplasty with placement of a **stent.** The stent is commonly a wire coil similar to the coil of a ballpoint pen, although other types are used. The surgeon leaves the stent in the artery when removing the balloon catheter. Thus the stent keeps the artery open. Researchers have found that the use of a stent reduces arterial closing by 33%.

Cardiac Surgery

Heart surgery may help some people with heart disease. *Closed-heart surgery* refers to surgical procedures that are done without stopping the heart. *Open-heart surgery* involves opening or operating on the heart in such a way that the heart must be stopped and the circulated blood is oxygenated by a device, such as a *pump oxygenator (heart–lung pump).* Use of such a device is called *extracorporeal* (outside the body) *circulation.* As blood circulates through the machine, the machine removes carbon dioxide and adds oxygen through osmosis, filming, or bubbling. The machine also keeps the blood warmed

to body temperature. A trained cardiopulmonary technician maintains the machine and determines if it is properly oxygenating the blood. A person can be maintained for several hours on the heart–lung pump. Various types of heart and blood vessel surgery may be done with the use of the pump oxygenator, or the pump oxygenator may be used as a support device in other types of surgery. In some cases, heart surgery is done after body temperature is lowered (*surgical hypothermia*), or under higher than normal atmospheric pressure with *hyperoxygenation* (in the hyperbaric chamber).

Coronary Artery Bypass Grafting

Coronary artery bypass grafting (**CABG**) is one example of open-heart surgery. Surgeons use a healthy vein, usually the saphenous vein from the leg, and place it around the blockage in the coronary artery. One end of the vein is grafted to the aorta and the other end to the area of the heart that is not receiving blood from the blocked artery. The grafted vein supplies oxygenated blood from the aorta to the heart. This surgery is done when less-invasive measures have failed or are not feasible. Usually, more than one blocked coronary artery requires bypass grafting during the surgery. Figure 80-4 illustrates common grafting sites that revascularize cardiac tissue by rerouting blood flow.

Another relatively new procedure, used only for the treatment of severe CAD in people who are unable to be treated with angioplasty or CABG surgery, is *transmyocardial revascularization* (**TMR**). This procedure uses a high-energy laser to create new channels through the heart muscle from the left ventricle. This allows blood to flow into the heart muscle even though the arteries are blocked. This laser surgery is performed on the beating heart, does not require the use of a heart–lung oxygenator, and usually requires only a small left-chest incision. It is much less invasive than open-heart surgery.

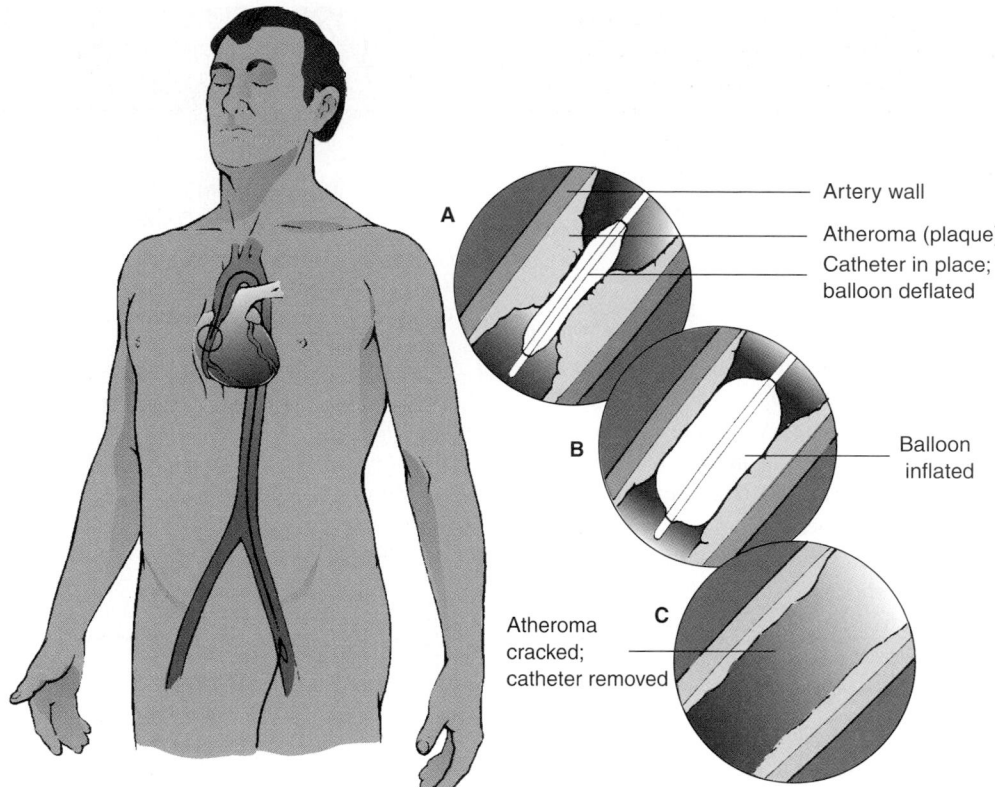

FIGURE 80-3. PTCA is a less invasive procedure than coronary artery bypass surgery in selected individuals. (**A**) A balloon-tipped catheter is passed into the affected coronary artery and placed within the atherosclerotic lesion. (**B**) The balloon is then rapidly inflated and deflated with controlled pressure. (**C**) After the plaque is compressed, the catheter is removed, allowing improved blood flow in the vessel.

Heart Valve Replacement

Congenital defects or diseases can damage the heart valves. In some cases, artificial or mechanical valves are transplanted for *valve replacement.* In other cases, human heart valves are used. Human heart valves have several advantages: 1) they do not need to be replaced as soon (artificial valves last about

10 years); 2) they better control pressures within the heart; 3) they are quiet (some artificial valves click); and 4) they can be preserved until needed. In addition, human heart valves grow with children who receive them. However, because human valves are foreign tissue, recipients must receive more anti-rejection drugs (see discussion of rejection with heart transplantation).

Heart Transplantation

Many problems are associated with heart transplantation, the greatest of which is *rejection* by the body of any foreign object or protein substance. This normal defense mechanism fights infection. However, with transplantation, it works against the person's well-being. Drugs must offset the body's normal antibody response or the new heart will be rejected. *Anti-rejection* or *immunosuppressive* drugs (drugs that suppress the immune response), such as cyclosporine (Sandimmune), azathioprine, and prednisone, are given. The success rate in heart transplantation continually improves. Medical and nursing care in heart transplantation is specialized and beyond the scope of this book.

Providing Care During Cardiac Surgery

Sometimes, people who come into the acute care facility for surgery have been under intensive medical treatment for several weeks. These clients have had time to prepare physically and emotionally for the experience, and many of them wel-

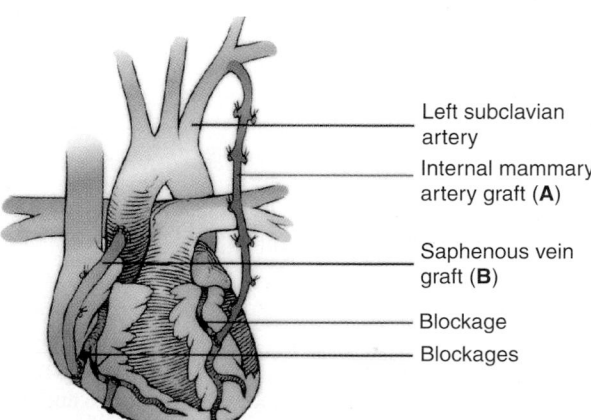

FIGURE 80-4. Coronary artery bypass grafting. (**A**) Mammary artery bypass. The mammary artery is anastomosed to the anterior descending left coronary artery, bypassing the obstructing lesion. (**B**) Saphenous vein bypass graft. The vein segment is sutured to the ascending aorta and the right coronary artery at a point distal to the occluding lesion.

come heart surgery as a new chance at life, realizing that often no other treatment can help them. Other clients have little or no preparation when surgery must be initiated as an emergency measure (eg, following a severe MI). In both cases, new methods of treatment and new surgical techniques allow many people who would not have survived cardiovascular disorders in previous years to live normal lives.

Preoperatively, the following are important considerations: good nutrition; extra oxygen for the body, which has been deprived of an adequate oxygen supply; vitamin therapy; practice in deep breathing; and routine tests and procedures, such as laboratory and x-ray examinations, heart catheterization, and ECGs. In the past, antibiotic therapy was also common, but some healthcare facilities are moving away from this approach because drug-resistant organisms are an ongoing problem. The main objective for all this preparation is to promote the client's best possible physical condition before surgery.

Registered nurses are usually responsible for immediate postoperative nursing care; licensed practical nurses or nursing students may assist. The first 2 days after surgery are the most critical to survival. Postoperatively, nursing care focuses on the following:

- Providing adequate tissue oxygenation
- Assessing cardiac function
- Maintaining fluid and electrolyte balance
- Controlling chest drainage with suction
- Monitoring body temperature
- Relieving pain

NURSING PROCESS

Data Collection

Carefully observe and assess the individual with a cardiac or blood vessel disorder. (See Chapter 47 for physical examination and nursing assessment, including that of the cardiovascular system.) This assessment establishes a baseline for future comparison and determines the presence of suspected cardiovascular complications. Report any changes in baseline assessments.

A complete cardiovascular assessment begins on admission. The nursing assessment includes a complete nursing history, as well as observations. When taking the health history, ask about any potential risk factors, such as smoking, lack of exercise, or poor nutrition. Also include any issues, such as shortness of breath or fatigue, that might interfere with the client's ability to perform activities of daily living.

When doing a cardiovascular assessment, include assessment of heart sounds, blood pressure, and pulse. Note any specific signs and symptoms, such as shortness of breath, while taking the client's vital signs. Difficulty breathing, orthopnea, edema, cyanosis, pain, and fatigue are other possible indications of heart disorders. Observe the client's emotional response to the disorder or disease and the person's understanding of ongoing treatment. In Practice: Nursing Assessment 80-1 highlights important signs and symptoms associated with heart disorders.

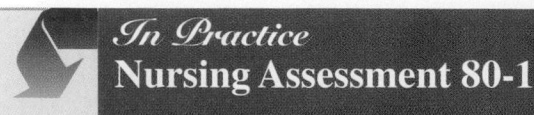

In Practice
Nursing Assessment 80-1

SIGNS AND SYMPTOMS OF CARDIOVASCULAR DISORDERS

- Changes in the rate, quality, and rhythm of the pulse
- Rise or fall in blood pressure or central venous pressure
- Edema, especially in the feet and ankles (faulty heart action causes the collection of fluids in the tissues)
- Weight gain due to excess fluid in the tissues
- Difficulty breathing and the presence of a cough, often due to pulmonary edema
- Cyanosis, due to a lack of oxygen in the blood or a circulatory disorder
- Clubbing of the fingers
- Needing to squat to breathe
- Pain (a significant symptom)
- Fatigue, for no apparent reason
- Intermittent **claudication,** which denotes a decrease in blood supply to the legs and feet (a person with arterial blockage will feel pain within 1 minute after beginning to walk)

Nursing Diagnosis

Based on data collection, the following are examples of nursing diagnoses that may appear on nursing care plans of clients with cardiovascular disorders:

- Excess Fluid Volume related to faulty circulation and inadequate processing of sodium, as evidenced by edema
- Impaired Social Interaction related to limited physical ability, pain
- Fatigue related to inadequate circulation, discomfort
- Disturbed Sleep Pattern related to dyspnea, as evidenced by orthopnea
- Risk for Peripheral Neurovascular Dysfunction related to circulatory disorders, coronary insufficiency

Planning and Implementation

Together, the healthcare team, client, and family plan effective care to meet the client's individualized needs. For the client undergoing diagnostic tests such as cardiac catheterization, and procedures such as angioplasty, provide preoperative and postoperative care. The person with a heart or blood vessel disorder may require assistance in meeting daily needs. The person who has had a CVA (stroke) may need total assistance and nursing care temporarily or on a long-term basis. The person with a chronic disability, such as hemiplegia or a damaged heart, may need assistance in dealing with psychosocial problems. Many clients need to understand more about their disorder, its prognosis, and its treatment. A nursing care plan is developed for each client to meet his or her individual needs.

Teaching About Prevention

To aid in the prevention of cardiovascular disorders, teach about predisposing factors (eg, fat buildup in the arteries, hypertension). Prevention involves a healthy diet to lower weight and cholesterol levels, exercise to strengthen the heart, and cessation of smoking.

The goals of prevention and treatment with many cardiovascular disorders, including hypertension, include: weight reduction, if necessary; reduction or elimination of dietary intake of cholesterol and salt; maintenance of a healthy pattern of sleep, rest, and relaxation; and learning ways to handle emotional upsets. If the client is taking antihypertensive drugs, teaching involves explaining the necessity of taking the prescribed medications even if he or she feels well. Antihypertensives help relieve cardiac stress, relax blood vessels, and reduce tissue fluid and blood volume. Describe possible side effects of these medications (see Chap. 62).

Suggest a consultation with a registered dietitian, or a support group for weight loss and maintenance. Counseling about fat in the diet may be helpful.

Aerobic exercise (in moderation) is good for cardiovascular conditioning and helps in weight loss. Walking, especially at a good pace, is effective and inexpensive. The greatest exercise risk is avoiding it. Teach clients how to warm up before and cool down after exercise. Smoking cessation programs may be necessary for those who wish to stop smoking (see Chaps. 6 and 94 for more information).

Clients can learn how to measure their blood pressure at home. Many authorities believe that when the person is involved in self-care more directly, he or she is more likely to comply with medications and required routines. In Practice: Educating the Client 80-1 lists teaching factors and actions individuals can take to reduce the risk of cardiovascular disease.

Evaluation

Together, the healthcare team, client, and family evaluate outcomes of care. Have short-term goals been met? Is the client stabilized following any initial emergency? For example, have the client's vital signs and heart rate and rhythm stabilized? Are long-term goals realistic? For example, does the client accept the diagnosis of MI and the need for lifestyle changes, or is he or she denying the problem? Will the client need long-term nursing care or short-term rehabilitation placement? Does the client need home health aide/homemaker services or regular in-home medication administration? Has the client been referred to a "stop smoking" program? Do the client and family need a support group? When planning for further nursing care, consider the client's prognosis, as well as any complications, and the client's responses.

ABNORMAL CONDITIONS THAT MAY CAUSE CARDIOVASCULAR DISEASE

Some types of heart disease are curable; others are not, but can be controlled with treatment. A client's attitude toward heart disease affects recovery. Some people are so frightened that they are afraid to move. Others deny the seriousness of

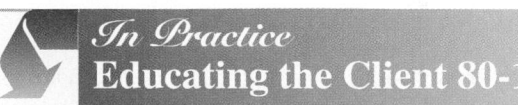

In Practice
Educating the Client 80-1

PREVENTION OF CARDIOVASCULAR DISORDERS

- Stop smoking and avoid smoking's harmful effects. *Rationale: Nicotine is a vasoconstrictor. It also increases heart rate and blood pressure.*
- Reduce sodium (salt) intake. *Rationale: Salt restriction minimizes fluid retention.*
- Maintain weight within standardized guidelines. *Rationale: Obesity increases the workload of the heart.*
- Avoid foods high in animal fats and cholesterol. *Rationale: Excess blood cholesterol can form plaque in blood vessels.* Plan meals following the Food Guide Pyramid (see Chap. 30).
- Avoid foods that contain caffeine: coffee, cola drinks, tea, chocolate. *Rationale: Caffeine is a potent vasoconstrictor.*
- Exercise regularly and moderately (at least three times a week for 30 minutes). Walking is a healthful exercise. *Rationale: Exercise stimulates circulation and builds cardiac strength and endurance.*
- Avoid crossing the legs at the knees when sitting. *Rationale: Crossing the legs at the knees hampers circulation.*
- Have both feet comfortably touch the floor when sitting. *Rationale: This position avoids constriction of blood vessels in the groin area.*
- For a few minutes in the morning and evening, elevate the feet. *Rationale: This position encourages venous return.*
- Avoid constrictive garments, especially around the legs, arms, and waist. Tight-fitting garters or girdles should not be worn. *Rationale: These items restrict circulation.*
- Wear properly fitted shoes. *Rationale: They prevent irritation and skin breakdown. Ulcers on the foot or leg are difficult to heal if peripheral circulation is impaired.*
- Avoid and minimize environmental stress and anxiety-producing factors. Learn ways to handle stress effectively. *Rationale: Stress causes the release of substances called catecholamines, which constrict blood vessels and thus elevate blood pressure.*
- Follow medication regimens for prescribed medications.
- Get plenty of rest and relaxation. Learn relaxation techniques if necessary.

their disease and disregard orders about diet, rest, and smoking. Several types of heart conditions are discussed here that, if left untreated, can lead to more serious cardiovascular conditions. Client teaching can help individuals understand the seriousness of these conditions and the value of diet, exercise, and medication.

Arteriosclerosis and Atherosclerosis

Arteriosclerosis applies to several pathologic conditions in which the walls of the arteries thicken, harden, and lose elasticity. Sometimes it is referred to as "hardening of the arteries." **Atherosclerosis,** the most common type of arteriosclerosis, is characterized by fatty deterioration of the arterial smooth muscle walls. Gradually, over several years, the walls absorb increasing amounts of circulating lipids and the lumen of the arteries narrows (**stenosis**) or may close completely. This buildup of fat and mineral deposits is called *plaque.* Often the terms arteriosclerosis and atherosclerosis are used interchangeably. These diseases may affect the heart valves and may lead to hypertension or CAD.

A diet high in saturated fat is usually associated with an increased blood cholesterol level. Studies have shown that unsaturated fats (eg, olive oil, corn oil) do not raise the blood cholesterol level as much as saturated fats (found in butter, eggs, and meats). Some people seem to metabolize cholesterol differently than others. In treating cardiovascular disorders, the physician periodically measures the client's blood cholesterol level and may attempt to control the amount of cholesterol through diet, medications, and exercise. The balance between high-density lipoprotein (**HDL** or "good" cholesterol) and low-density lipoprotein (**LDL** or "bad" cholesterol) is more important than is the actual total cholesterol value. However, as the total level rises above 150, a person's risk of CAD increases.

Hypertension

Hypertension (**HTN**) or *hypertensive heart disease* means *high blood pressure.* One in five people in America have HTN. Estimates are that two thirds of all Americans over the age of 65, and a growing number of children, have high blood pressure. Under the age of 65, it is more common in men, but over the age of 65, HTN is more common in women. Studies show that African Americans are more likely to have high blood pressure earlier in life, at higher levels, and twice as often as Caucasians.

Hypertension can lead to MI, kidney damage, congestive heart failure, and CVA. Consistent HTN leads to heart damage. With advancing age, blood pressure tends to rise, although the exact reason why is unclear. One thing is certain: the condition of the heart and blood vessels has the greatest effect on blood pressure. Although HTN cannot be cured, treatment can usually bring blood pressure to within the normal range.

High blood pressure is predominantly due to a spasm of the small arterioles. Normal pressure gradients and normal volumes of blood are seen on the graph in Figure 80-5.

An increase in the pressure within the blood vessels can cause significant damage to small arterioles. The spasms increase blood pressure and thus contribute to arteriosclerosis (a vicious circle). Because the heart must pump harder to force blood through the arteries, the result is **hypertrophy** (enlargement) of the heart muscle.

HTN may exist due to a known cause, such as kidney failure, malformations of blood vessels, certain tumors, and some specific endocrine disorders. However, the cause may be unknown (most cases, a condition classified as *essential hypertension*). Symptoms other than elevated blood pressure may not occur for years, and no restrictions are imposed until other symptoms develop. Encourage clients with HTN to exercise, observe moderation in eating, and avoid tension and anxiety. Advise them to avoid smoking, and to limit intake of alcoholic beverages, caffeine, and sodium. Symptoms of HTN may become severe, with headache, fatigue, dyspnea, edema, and nocturia.

Malignant hypertension, which is not cancer, refers to a sudden onset of severely elevated blood pressure that is controllable. It is most often seen in young people. The incidence is highest in African Americans, especially men under age 40. Onset is sudden, and the disease progresses rapidly. In many cases, determining its cause is difficult. Malignant hypertension is known to cause rapid *necrosis* (death) of vital organs,

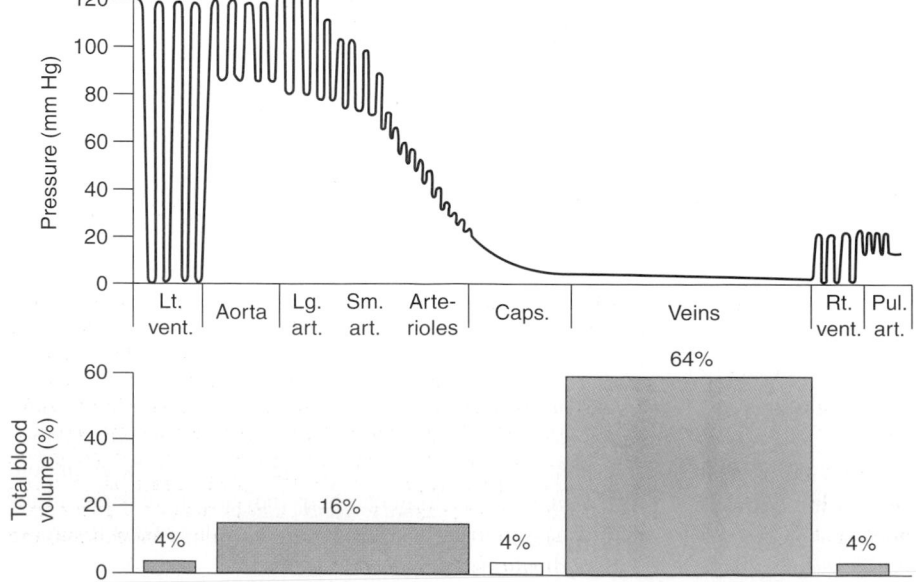

FIGURE 80-5. Pressure and volume distribution in the systemic circulation. The graphs show the inverse relationship between internal pressure and volume in different portions of the circulatory system. Notice that the arterioles and the capillaries have decreased pressure as compared with pressure in the aorta. Arteries are damaged by high pressures, and in turn damage the organs that they service.

such as the heart, brain, and kidney. Clients with malignant hypertension rarely survive more than a few years.

Hypotension

Hypotension is *low blood pressure*. Clinical manifestations differ, depending on the underlying cause. Causes of hypotension can be classified under one of three mechanisms: a heart rate problem, a heart muscle or pump problem, or a volume problem. Treatment will depend on the underlying problem. Variations in blood pressure can also be caused by medications.

Rate problems include a heart rate that is too fast or too slow. *Pump problems* result from MI, *cardiomyopathy* (the heart cavity is enlarged and stretched), acute cardiac or aortic insufficiency, prosthetic valve dysfunction, *cardiac tamponade* (heart compression, due to fluid buildup), pulmonary embolism, and medications that affect or alter the heart's function. Many other clinical problems can also affect how the heart muscle pumps. *Volume problems* include hemorrhage, gastrointestinal fluid loss, renal injury or disease, central nervous system injury, spinal injury, sepsis, medications that affect vascular tone, and any other condition that causes large-volume fluid losses.

HEART DISORDERS

Conditions Affecting the Heart's Rhythm

The heart may be affected by normal physiologic factors (eg, sleep, exercise) and medications (digoxin, calcium channel blockers), which can cause a disturbance in the regularity of the heartbeat. In some cases, the irregularity can be the result of a disturbance in the heart's electrical conduction system.

Cardiac Dysrhythmias

Dysrhythmia, an irregularity in the heartbeat's rhythm, is a complication of numerous disorders, such as MI, electrolyte imbalances (especially potassium), and other heart and circulatory disorders. It may also result from severe trauma or electric shock. (Commonly the term *arrhythmia* is used in place of *dysrhythmia.* Technically, **arrhythmia** means "without heartbeat" (ie, cardiac standstill). *Dysrhythmia* is the correct term meaning "irregularity in heartbeat.") Abnormal electrical impulses occurring in the SA node, AV node, bundle branches, or Purkinje's network can lead to dysrhythmias.

Two common dysrhythmias are:

- *Sinus tachycardia:* Heartbeat is greater than 100 beats per minute. (This rate is normal in children.) It can be present postoperatively and in instances of high fever, extreme emotion, overactive thyroid, or strenuous exercise.
- *Sinus bradycardia:* Heartbeat is less than 60 beats per minute. (This rate may occur in athletes normally.) If it occurs with *digitalization* (administration of digitalis), it is a symptom of *heart block* (an abnormal situation discussed below).

Figure 80-6 depicts a few more common dysrhythmias.

A premature ventricular contraction (**PVC**) is an irregularity in the heart's ventricular rhythm. As the name indicates, a PVC is a contraction that is initiated in the ventricles that is premature. In other words, it occurs prior to the normal SA node–conducted beat. PVCs can be relatively benign; indicators of early cardiac problems; and/or progress to more malignant ventricular dysrhythmias.

Atrioventricular Heart Block

Heart block is not a disease in itself but is associated with many types of heart disease, especially diseases of the coronary arteries and rheumatic heart disease. In atrioventricular (**AV**) heart block, heart contractions are weak and lack sufficient force to send blood from the atria into the ventricles. Pulse rate may be as low as 30 beats per minute.

Electronic Pacemaker. An *electronic pacemaker* may be used to provide external stimulus to the heart. The electronic pacemaker stimulates heart contractions by means of wires connected to electrodes, which are inserted into the heart (Fig. 80-7).

Clients who experience frequent difficulty with heart contractions may have a permanent pacemaker implanted. A portable pacemaker about the size of a small transistor radio is used in the clinical setting. If a permanent pacemaker is indicated, the surgeon implants the pacemaker pack underneath the client's skin, usually in the pectoral or abdominal area.

Premature ventricular contractions (PVC)
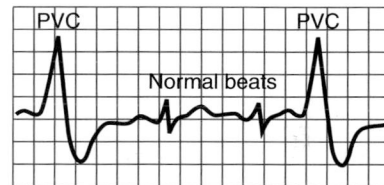

Ventricular tachycardia
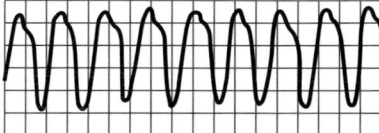

Ventricular fibrillation
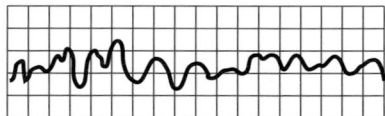

FIGURE 80-6. ECG tracings of ventricular dysrhythmias. With premature ventricular contractions (PVCs) (*top tracing*), the QRS complex is distorted because the impulse is originating from an ectopic focus. Because the ventricle usually cannot repolarize sufficiently to respond to the next impulse that arises in the sino-atrial node, a PVC frequently is followed by a compensatory pause. With ventricular tachycardia (*middle tracing*), the ventricular rate is extremely rapid, ranging from 100 to 250 beats per minute; P waves also are not seen. In ventricular fibrillation (*bottom tracing*), there are no regular or effective ventricular contractions, and the ECG tracing is totally disorganized.

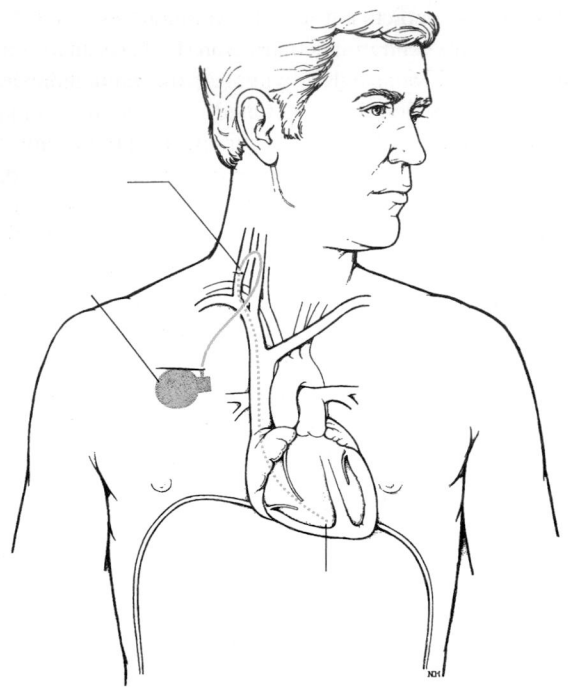

FIGURE 80-7. Pacemaker therapy. The pacemaker delivers an electrical impulse to the heart at specified intervals, causing the heart to beat.

Some clients can discontinue use of the pacemaker gradually, depending on the heart's rhythm. Other clients cannot live without it. A battery replacement is required every 5 to 10 years.

> ### Nursing Alert
> Use of rubber (latex) gloves is recommended when handling pacemaker terminals or generators. *Rationale: Care is necessary to prevent an electrical shock, which could upset the heart rate or stop the pacemaker.* But first, be sure to determine latex allergy in the client.

The critical observation period is 3 days after the pacemaker's insertion. After a client has had a pacemaker implanted, do the following:

- Carry out routine postoperative care.
- Check all electrical equipment in the room for grounding.
- Carefully assess the client's pulse, including cardiac rhythm and rate. The heart rate should correspond to the setting on the pacemaker. Report any deviation at once.
- Assess for neck vein distention or muffled heart sounds, which could indicate cardiac tamponade. These are serious signs that must be reported at once.
- Use sterile technique and keep the incision site clean to prevent infection.
- Provide active or passive range-of-motion exercises and incentive spirometer treatments to prevent complications.
- Reassure the client, who may find adjusting to dependence on the pacemaker difficult.

> ### Nursing Alert
> If the client with a pacemaker notices any symptoms of dizziness or lightheadedness, instruct him or her to move at least 6 feet away from the source of any electrical interference.

A client with a pacemaker should wear a medical alert identification tag or bracelet (MedicAlert). Teach the client how to count the pulse and to report any deviation at once.

Telecommunication or teletransmission of the ECG is used for clients with pacemakers. At a prescribed time and frequency, clients use a special modem to transmit their heart rate, rhythm, and battery life to a central location (usually a hospital or physician's office), where heart rate and rhythm are transformed onto ECG paper for interpretation and followup.

Fibrillation

Fibrillation refers to a quivering of muscle fibers. A disorganized twitching of atrial muscles is known as *atrial fibrillation*. It is sometimes seen in clients with atherosclerosis and rheumatic heart disease. The pulse is irregular, because coordination between the atria and ventricles is interrupted. Treatment depends on the cause, but unless the condition is life threatening, the physician usually prescribes digitalis preparations, beta-blockers, and calcium channel blockers to slow the transmission of electrical impulses from the atria to the ventricles. Anticoagulants may be given to prevent blood clots. Sometimes it is necessary to perform **cardioversion** (changing of the cardiac dysrhythmia, electrically or through medication administration). If all else fails to return the rhythm back to normal, a newly approved treatment, **atrial ablation,** may be used. This procedure uses a catheter to determine the location of the abnormality; then, using radio-frequency energy, it destroys the diseased tissue.

Ventricular fibrillation is a twitching of the ventricular muscles of the heart. The rhythm is totally disorganized and blood does not circulate. It is the most dangerous type of fibrillation and is a medical emergency. It is fatal if untreated because it leads to cardiac arrest.

Defibrillation.   Treatment for ventricular fibrillation is *electrical defibrillation,* which is done by a physician or a specialized critical care nurse. In defibrillation, a high-voltage electrical current is passed through the client's body in an attempt to shock the heart back into a regular beat. The electrical current necessary for cardioversion of atrial fibrillation is much less than that needed for ventricular fibrillation.

> ### Nursing Alert
> During electrical defibrillation, everyone present must be very careful not to touch the client or the bed, or they too will receive the shock and may be injured.

If the client experiences cardiac arrest, external cardiac compression and cardiopulmonary resuscitation (**CPR**) is necessary. In an emergency, perform CPR until the code team arrives to perform electrical defibrillation.

Implantable Cardioverter–Defibrillator. The *implantable cardioverter–defibrillator* (**ICD**) or *automatic implantable cardioverter–defibrillator* (**AICD**) is an effective device in the management of lethal ventricular dysrhythmias for clients whose condition cannot be managed by drug therapy. Use of this device has significantly reduced the mortality rate in these individuals.

The ICD is a lightweight (½ lb) lithium battery–powered pulse generator. It is surgically implanted under the skin, usually in the pectoral or abdominal region (similar to permanent pacemaker placement). Wires (called *leads*) placed in the heart sense the heart's rate and rhythm. Defibrillating heads attached to the heart deliver an electrical shock to the heart muscle when a ventricular dysrhythmia is detected. If the first shock is unsuccessful, the ICD will deliver four to seven more shocks. The latest devices also provide backup pacing of the heart as needed.

After placement of an ICD, the postoperative period allows for close observation of how the device responds to dysrhythmias. Most individuals receive continuous cardiac monitoring during this time. Assist the client with early ambulation, monitor the wound for signs of infection, and provide information and teaching about the device.

Teach the client to lie down when he or she feels a shock from the ICD. If the client is alone when this occurs, he or she should call 911 or the physician; if someone is with him or her, the client should lie down, and the other person should call the physician. When an electrical shock is delivered, it will cause a slight tingling to the individual and to anyone who touches him or her. If the person becomes unconscious, a family member or caretaker should call 911. CPR should not begin unless four to seven shocks have been noted. All family members and caretakers will need to know CPR.

The battery on the ICD needs to be checked every 2 months. Be sure that the client understands the need for wearing a MedicAlert tag.

Conditions Affecting the Heart's Pumping Function

Congestive Heart Failure

Congestive heart failure (**CHF**), also known as *heart failure, cardiac decompensation, cardiac insufficiency,* and *cardiac incompetence,* means that the heart is failing and unable to do its work; it has lost its pumping efficiency. This is called *decompensation.* CHF is a *syndrome* (a group of symptoms) that affects individuals in different ways and to different degrees. The heart will try to keep up with demands made on it; treatment is aimed at helping the heart adjust to the demands placed on it. This is termed *compensation.* Abnormal conditions in the heart may make continued treatment necessary; otherwise, the signs of heart failure will reappear.

Congestive heart failure results from excessive strain on the heart. This may be caused by MI, infection of valves or of heart muscle itself, blood vessel disease, HTN, renal insufficiency,

congenital defects, hyperthyroidism (which speeds up heart action), cardiomyopathy, or rheumatic fever (which damages heart valves). Older people are subject to heart failure because of arteriosclerosis.

Signs and Symptoms. The main cause of right-sided heart failure is left-sided heart failure.

With left-sided heart failure, the left ventricle is not able to pump the blood out to the systemic circulation effectively. Pressure in the left ventricle increases, leading to an increase in pressure in left atrium. As a result, blood flow from the pulmonary vessels into the left atrium decreases, causing increased pressure in the pulmonary vessels and blood congestion in the lungs (*pulmonary edema*). If the body cannot compensate for these changes, pressure increases in the right ventricle.

Failure of the right ventricle to pump results in increased congestion in the systemic circulation, ultimately leading to right-sided heart failure. In short, if a client has failure of one side of the heart, he or she will eventually have failure on the other side, unless treatment is successfully initiated.

The first noticeable signs of a failing heart are excessive fatigue and dyspnea; the person may have to rest after walking halfway up a flight of stairs or may need two pillows at night to breathe comfortably.

The feet or ankles may swell during the day, and although this swelling disappears overnight, it recurs as soon as the person is on the feet again (*dependent edema*). In addition, when a finger presses on the swollen area, an indentation is left that lasts longer than normal (*pitting edema*). An accumulation of fluid in the tissues may cause sudden weight gain. Other symptoms include numbness or tingling in the fingers, albuminuria (the presence of albumin in the urine), cyanosis, engorgement and visible pulsation of neck veins, and engorgement of the liver, with or without jaundice. The heart attempts to compensate for this excess fluid congestion by dilation, hypertrophy, and tachycardia.

Many affected individuals develop a persistent cough, which indicates the start of pulmonary edema—the most serious symptom, which results from left-sided heart failure. When the left heart pumps ineffectively, the pulmonary circuit becomes congested. Symptoms of pulmonary edema include cough, gurgling or crackling lung sounds, dyspnea, and heart palpitations. The person may sound as if he or she has asthma. Sputum may be blood streaked. *Acute pulmonary edema* is a medical emergency and is treated with IV morphine sulfate, supplemental oxygen, and a high Fowler's position.

Diagnostic Tests. The usual tests for detecting heart disease, such as ECG, x-ray examination, echocardiography, and in some cases cardiac catheterization, are performed. Circulation time and arterial and venous blood pressure also are measured. Evaluation of urine reveals a diminished output (*oliguria*), elevated specific gravity, *albuminuria* (the presence of albumin in urine), and the presence of blood (*hemoglobinuria*), and casts (tiny mineral deposits). Blood chemistry shows nitrogen retention by elevated blood urea nitrogen (BUN), uric acid, and creatinine concentrations.

Hemodynamic Monitoring. Heart pressures are increased and a special kind of monitoring, called **hemodynamic monitoring,** is required. In hemodynamic monitoring, an arterial catheter such as a Swan-Ganz catheter is used to measure internal pressures. Placement of the catheter is an invasive procedure and is not without risk. The catheter measures the pressures in the heart and its vessels.

Medical Treatment. Treatment focuses on easing the workload of the heart. Rest, sedation, and proper diet are important. *Cardiotonic glycosides* (such as *digoxin*) are often used to slow the heart's rate, increase the force of systole, and decrease the heart's size. *Digitalis* is a cardiotonic glycoside that is given to slow and regulate the heart rate and to strengthen the heartbeat. ACE inhibitors or other vasodilators should be added as tolerated. These agents expand the blood vessels and decrease vascular resistance. Beta-blockers can be given because they improve left ventricular function. Diuretics help rid the body of excess fluid and salts. Salt (sodium) in the diet is restricted. Fluids also may be restricted, depending on the client's fluid balance status. If these measures are successful, systemic circulation will improve, increasing urinary output and reducing dyspnea and edema.

Nursing Considerations. Key components of nursing care include measuring intake and output (I&O) and weighing the client daily to determine the client's fluid balance status and extent of edema. Give oxygen if the blood is not receiving enough from the lungs. The high Fowler's position usually aids breathing.

Pressure-reducing devices often are used, because the client with CHF is at risk for skin breakdown. Dyspnea and fatigue can interfere with the client's ability to move. Plus, circulation is decreased in areas where edema is present.

Another key aspect of nursing care is administering the prescribed medications to the client and monitoring the client for the effectiveness of therapy. In Practice: Nursing Care Guidelines 80-1 highlights important areas for cardiotonic medication administration.

Nursing Alert

When giving digitalis preparations, be aware of their different names. Be careful not to confuse the *digitalis preparations, digitoxin,* and *digoxin. Digoxin* is fast acting and more rapidly eliminated than *digitoxin.* Dosages of these preparations vary considerably.

• When setting up a digitalis derivative, keep it in its sealed package. Then identify it as the digitalis preparation in a separate medication cup. *Rationale: By setting up in this manner, you will know for certain which medication is digitalis should you need to delay administration.*

Cardiomyopathy

Cardiomyopathy is a very serious disease that interferes with the ability of the heart to pump adequately. The heart muscle usually becomes enlarged, stretched out, and weakened due to a variety of causes. Primary cardiomyopathy cannot be attributed to any specific cause such as HTN, CAD, heart valve diseases, congenital heart defects, or any other specific cause. *Secondary cardiomyopathy* is attributed to a specific cause or disease.

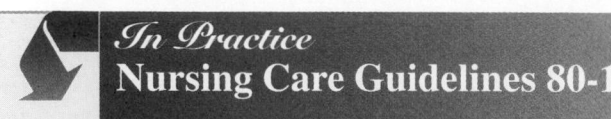

In Practice
Nursing Care Guidelines 80-1

ADMINISTERING CARDIOTONIC DRUGS (DIGITALIS, DIGOXIN, LANOXIN)

• Remember that the first administration of digitalis or its derivative (eg, digoxin) will be larger (*loading dose*) than later doses. The dosage will gradually be decreased, until the amount needed to stabilize the heartbeat (*maintenance dose*) is found. If the dosage is too large, undesirable side effects will occur. When the medication slows the heart rate sufficiently, the client is said to be *digitalized.*

• Before administering any digitalis preparation, take the client's apical pulse for 1 full minute. Do not give the medication if the pulse is below 60 (70 for a child), and report such a finding immediately. *Rationale: Low pulse may indicate overdigitalization.*

• Be alert for possible side effects and adverse reactions of digitalization, including gastrointestinal symptoms, headache, and blurred vision. The client may say that everything has a yellow appearance. Bradycardia also occurs when digitalis slows the heart too much. For this reason, count the client's apical pulse before giving each dose. In some facilities, two nurses check all digitalis preparations before giving such drugs to clients.

• If discharged from the healthcare facility and prescribed a digitalis preparation, teach the client how to count pulse rate; the symptoms of digitalis toxicity; and the significance of notifying the physician of any changes or symptoms. Document all teaching.

The most common form of cardiomyopathy is *dilated* or *congestive cardiomyopathy.* The heart cavity becomes enlarged or dilated and usually progresses to CHF. Dysrhythmias and blood clots may also be problematic because the blood flows more slowly through the enlarged heart. Treatment with anticoagulants and antiarrhythmics can help. Vasodilators may be given to relax the arteries, lower the blood pressure, and decrease the workload of the left ventricle. If the disease progresses despite medical treatment, a heart transplant may be necessary.

Hypertropic cardiomyopathy, another form of the disease, is hereditary in more than half of those diagnosed. The left ventricle hypertrophies, which may decrease the flow of blood from the left ventricle into the aorta. It may also cause mitral valve leakage. Symptoms include dyspnea, dizziness, and angina. Some people have dysrhythmias. Often, a heart murmur can be heard. This form of cardiomyopathy is usually treated with a beta-blocker or calcium channel blocker, antiarrhythmics as needed, or surgical treatment if medication treatment fails.

A less common form of the disease is called *restrictive cardiomyopathy*. The ventricles of the heart become rigid, making it difficult for blood to flow. This form of the disease causes fatigue, dyspnea on exertion, and peripheral edema. Another disease process usually causes this type of cardiomyopathy.

Infectious and Inflammatory Heart Disorders

Chronic Rheumatic Heart Disease

Although adults may develop rheumatic fever, it is usually seen in children between the ages of 5 and 15 years. Fewer than 10% of persons who contract rheumatic fever develop rheumatic heart disease.

Childhood rheumatic fever can result in heart valve malfunction. This chronic condition usually is not evident until about age 40. Symptoms include **myocarditis** (inflammation of the heart's muscular walls), *endocarditis* (inflammation of the heart's inner lining, usually involving the valves; discussed below), or **pancarditis** (inflammation of the entire heart).

The first signs include difficulty breathing, a cough, and sometimes cyanosis and *expectoration* (spitting) of blood. If the condition worsens, the client's feet and ankles swell, the liver enlarges, and the abdominal cavity fills with fluid. Systolic blood pressure may fall. Such signs indicate heart failure.

The most common problem resulting from *chronic rheumatic heart disease* is a narrowing of the mitral valve, a condition called *mitral stenosis.* Because of this, blood collects in the chambers of the left side of the heart, enlarging them and leading to a backup of blood in the pulmonary vessels, which causes pulmonary edema. The left side of the heart is affected first. The condition progresses to the right side and leads to heart failure. Surgical replacement of a valve may be indicated. The physician determines the particular valve design that best fits the client's needs.

To best protect against chronic rheumatic heart disease, a person who has had rheumatic fever should avoid exposure, colds, and streptococcal infections; keep up resistance; get adequate sleep; and eat a balanced diet. Complications may result from tooth extraction, oral surgery, or major surgery. Some clients take a daily maintenance dose of penicillin G as a prophylactic measure. Preventing streptococcal infections or recurrence of rheumatic fever is vital; each time a person has rheumatic fever, cardiac complications become more likely.

Bacterial Endocarditis

The membrane that lines the heart's chambers and valves is called the *endocardium.* Infection of this membrane causes a condition known as **endocarditis** (Fig. 80-8).

Subacute bacterial endocarditis (**SBE**), a serious disease, was once nearly always fatal. Antibiotics have changed this outcome, but bacterial endocarditis is still a health problem. Modern treatment helps control it and prevents it from disabling affected individuals.

People with damaged heart valves, especially those who have had rheumatic fever or who have congenital heart defects, are most susceptible to SBE. Tooth extraction, childbirth,

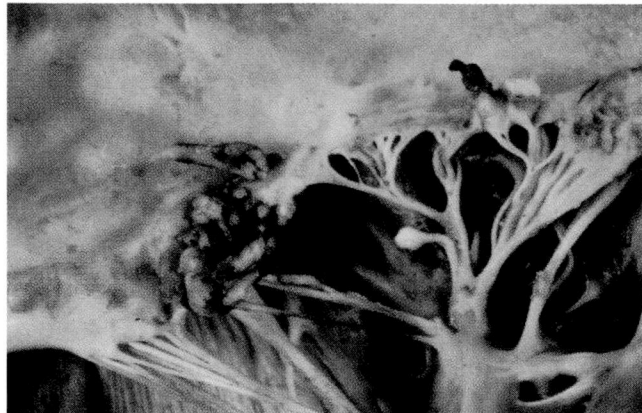

FIGURE 80-8. Bacterial endocarditis. The mitral valve shows destructive vegetations, which have eroded through the free margin of the valve leaflet.

upper respiratory infections, or injecting street drugs directly into veins may release pathogens into the bloodstream that then attack damaged heart valves. Streptococci are frequent offenders.

One of the first signs of bacterial endocarditis is a low-grade fever that gradually increases. The person has chills, perspires, loses his or her appetite, and loses weight. The individual's face may have a brownish tinge, and tiny reddish-purple spots (*petechiae*) appear on the skin and mucous membranes. Usually, the person is *anemic* (not enough oxygen is delivered to body tissues). As the disease progresses, signs of CHF appear.

The course of SBE is rapid and can be fatal if left untreated. However, 90% of cases can be cured without ill effects. Blood culture and sensitivity can usually identify the specific causative organism. Then large doses of antibiotics to which the causative organism is sensitive are given.

Nursing Considerations. Make the person as comfortable as possible and conserve their energy. Note the pulse rate and quality frequently. *Rationale: A change could indicate complications.* Observe closely for fluctuation in body temperature and for any symptoms of complications. *Rationale: Hematuria, pain, or impaired circulation in an extremity might result from a blood clot originating in the diseased valve.*

Pericarditis

Pericarditis, an inflammation of the sac surrounding the heart, may be caused by infection, allergy, malignancy, trauma, or some other nonspecific problem. It is characterized by pain in the *precordial area* (over the heart and lower thorax), which is aggravated by breathing and twisting movements. A *friction rub* is a sign associated with pericarditis, and is audible on auscultation. In most cases, pericardial infections are treated with antibiotics and anti-inflammatory agents.

Coronary Artery Disease

People over age 65 are the most common victims of CAD (also called *ischemic heart disease*), although the risk increases after age 40. During the early middle years, more men than women are affected. However, after menopause, women have an increased risk of two to three times that of men. Although familial tendency toward the disease seems to exist, anyone can be affected. Therefore, all people should take precautions from an early age. In recent years, the healthcare community has given attention to preventing and discovering the disease early, before attacks occur and before atherosclerosis severely damages a person's heart and blood vessels. In addition, health promotion and disease prevention activities have focused on measures to reduce the risk factors for developing CAD, which include:

- Smoking tobacco (each year, one in five coronary heart disease deaths are related to smoking)
- Increased levels of cholesterol and lipids in the bloodstream (10% of adolescents and 15% to 20% of adults have high-risk cholesterol levels)
- Physical inactivity and obesity (rapidly becoming a health threat worldwide)
- Diabetes (this disease affects African Americans almost twice as often as Caucasians)

For additional preventive measures, see In Practice: Educating the Client 80-1.

Angina Pectoris

Literally translated, **angina pectoris** (usually referred to as *angina*) means "pain in the chest." Angina occurs suddenly when extra exertion calls for the arteries to increase blood supply to the heart. Narrowed or obstructed arteries are unable to provide the necessary supply. Consequently, the heart muscle suffers.

In angina, the blood vessels of the heart are unable to supply the heart muscle with adequate amounts of oxygen. If this loss of oxygen supply continues, the result is *ischemia* (prolonged deficiency of oxygenated blood) and necrosis of heart tissue, or MI. For example, a major factor associated with the vessels' inability to supply adequate oxygen to the heart muscle is the development of plaques within the vessels, causing the vessels to narrow or become obstructed. Figure 80-9 illustrates the buildup of plaques that lead to ischemia.

When the underlying disease is coronary atherosclerosis, the client's prognosis may be more encouraging than when other factors are involved. The earlier the age of onset, the poorer the client's prognosis.

There are several types of angina pain. *Intractable angina* does not respond to therapy and often is so persistent that the person cannot work. *Unstable angina* is pain that increases and decreases in frequency, duration, and intensity. *Nocturnal angina* occurs at night; *decubitus angina* occurs when the person is lying down and is relieved when the person sits up.

Signs and Symptoms.   Pain is usually most severe over the chest, although it may spread to the shoulders, arms, neck, jaw, and back. These areas are shown in Figure 80-10.

The person often describes the sensation as tightening, viselike, or choking. Indigestion is often the first complaint. The person is more likely to feel pain in the left arm because this is the direction of aortic branching. However, he or she may feel pain in either arm. The client may be pale, feel faint, or be dyspneic. Pain often stops in less than 5 minutes, but it is intense while it lasts. The pain is a warning signal that the heart is not getting enough blood and oxygen. People who ignore this warning are risking serious illness or sudden death if they do not immediately seek a physician's care. The client may have recurrent angina attacks, but treatment lessens the danger of a fatal attack.

Diagnostic Tests.   Diagnosis is made on the basis of ECG, specific blood tests (especially enzymes), x-ray examinations, the client's medical history, and specific symptoms. If nitroglycerin relieves the attack, it is considered angina. Exercise, exertion, eating, emotions, and exposure often precipitate angina. A person who has diabetes may not feel angina pain because of peripheral neuropathy.

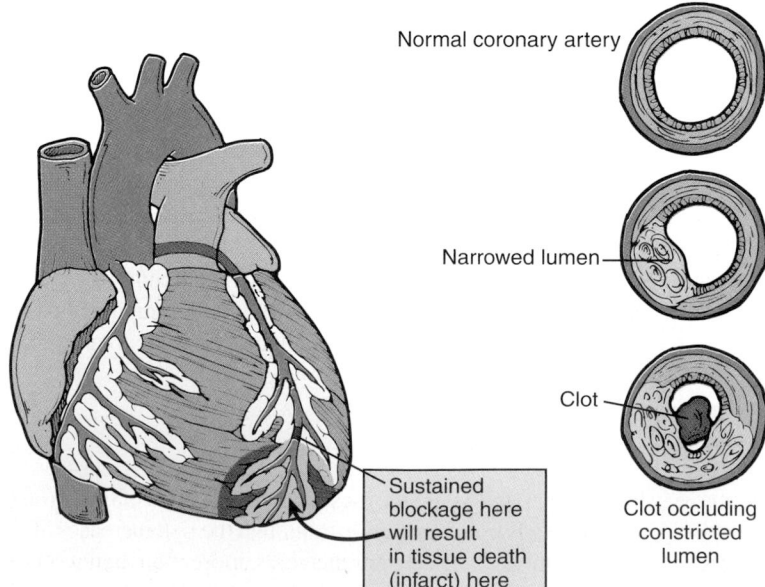

Normal coronary artery

Narrowed lumen

Clot

Clot occluding constricted lumen

Sustained blockage here will result in tissue death (infarct) here

FIGURE 80-9. Progression of atherosclerotic plaque in the blood vessels. Over time, the buildup of fat, cholesterol, fibrin, cellular waste products, and calcium on an artery's endothelial lining may be complicated by hemorrhage, ulceration, calcification, or thrombosis. Infarction, stroke, or gangrene may also occur.

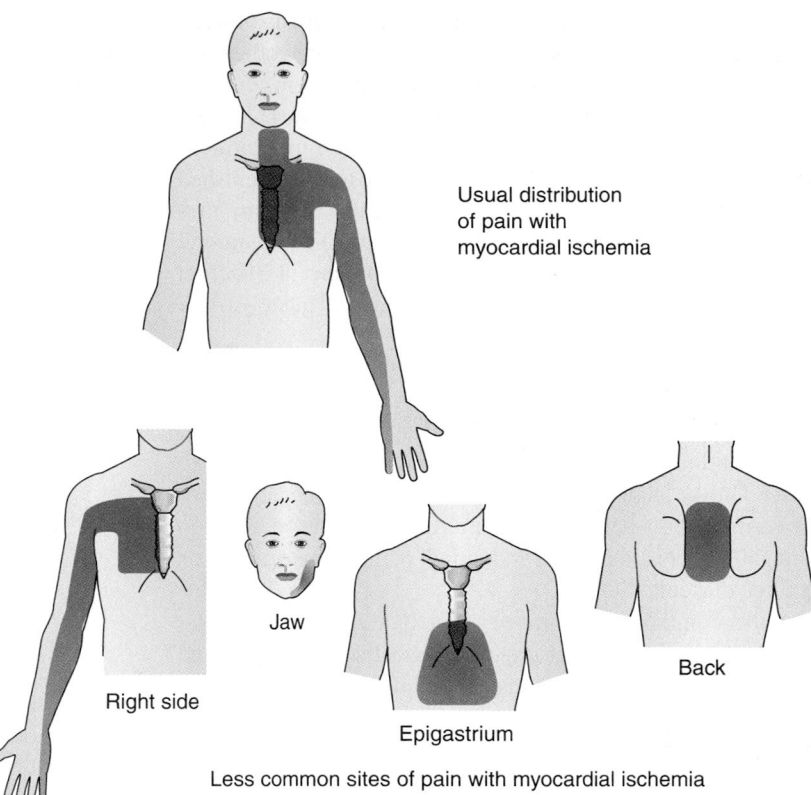

Usual distribution of pain with myocardial ischemia

Jaw

Right side

Epigastrium

Back

Less common sites of pain with myocardial ischemia

FIGURE 80-10. Pain patterns with myocardial ischemia. The usual distribution of pain is referral to all or part of the sternal region, the left side of the chest, the neck, and down the ulnar side of the left forearm and hand. With severe ischemic pain, the right chest and right arm are often involved as well, although isolated involvement of these areas is rare. Other sites sometimes involved, either alone or together with pain in other sites, are the jaw, epigastrium, and back.

Nursing Alert

Angina pain that lasts for more than 15 minutes is considered an MI until proven otherwise. Repeated attacks of angina can be a sign of—or can contribute to—MI.

Medical and Surgical Treatment. Angina can be controlled with nitroglycerin tablets. As soon as an attack begins, the client places a tablet under the tongue, allowing it to dissolve. Nitroglycerin brings quick relief by dilating the coronary arteries; clients can use this drug safely for many years with no ill effects. Topical nitroglycerin ointment or nitroglycerin-impregnated transdermal pads are widely used to protect against anginal pain and promote its relief. (See Table 80-1 and Chap. 62.)

If medication fails to control the person's anginal attacks, PTCA or coronary artery bypass surgery may be necessary.

Nursing Considerations. Help the client by teaching about angina pectoris and how to prevent further attacks. Clients who know that certain stresses bring on angina can learn measures to avoid these stresses or better cope with them. If anginal pain becomes more frequent or more severe, the client may need to curtail certain activities. The best approach is to follow rules for treatment, learn what can and cannot be done, and live accordingly.

Clients with angina need to quit smoking because nicotine constricts the coronary arteries and increases blood pressure and pulse rate. Some teaching points are listed at In Practice: Educating the Client 80-2.

Myocardial Infarction

An MI, also known as *heart attack, coronary thrombosis,* or *coronary occlusion,* is the sudden blockage of one or more coronary arteries. If the blockage involves an extensive area, the

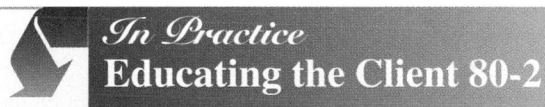

In Practice
Educating the Client 80-2

PREVENTION OF ANGINA PECTORIS

• Use medications properly. Take them at the same time every day. Do not stop or change dosages without a physician's approval.
• Do not expose nitroglycerin to sunlight or moisture. Keep nitroglycerin in its original container. Purchase a fresh supply every 3 months.
• Check with your physician before taking any non-prescription medications. They may cause harmful side effects when combined with the cardiac medications.
• Make necessary lifestyle adjustments. Determine what you can and cannot do. Try to determine things that bring on attacks, so that you can curtail such activities.
• Stop smoking.
• Regular exercise and maintenance of an ideal weight help prevent the disease's progression.
• Keep cholesterol within the 150 to 200 mg/dL range.

person can die. If it involves a smaller area, necrosis of heart tissue and subsequent scarring will occur. However, other vessels can take over for the injured area (*collateral circulation*).

Complications can occur at any time after an acute MI. Complications primarily result from damage to the myocardium and its conduction system that occurred due to the diminished coronary blood flow. The major complications of MI are life-threatening dysrhythmias and cardiac standstill. Abnormal heart rates and rhythms in the person with a recent MI often indicate that the left ventricle is pumping inadequately. As a result, CHF may occur.

Signs and Symptoms.   An MI begins suddenly, with sharp, severe chest pain that sometimes radiates to the left arm, shoulder, and back. Pain is similar to angina pain, but can last longer and is more severe; exertion is not always related to onset. Unlike angina, rest does not relieve the pain, and nitroglycerin does not help. Because an MI may imitate indigestion or a gallbladder attack with abdominal pain, definite diagnosis is often difficult.

Other common symptoms of MI include panic, restlessness, and confusion; a sense of impending death; ashen, cold, and clammy skin; dyspnea; cyanosis; rapid, thready, and irregular pulse; drop in blood pressure; and drop in body temperature. Nausea and vomiting may be present, and the person is often in shock. *Silent coronaries* (ones that show no symptoms) are common, especially among people with diabetes, and may result in greater damage to the heart muscle. Denial occurs in many cases; the person cannot believe that he or she is having an MI. Family members must force individuals experiencing MI symptoms to go to the nearest emergency department for evaluation.

Diagnostic Tests.   Tests help determine the nature of the MI. An ECG and several diagnostic blood tests are done to assess the duration and severity of the MI. The sedimentation rate of the red blood cells is almost always higher after MI, as is the AST level. Troponin levels rise. Cardiac isoenzyme levels will also be elevated after MI. These isoenzymes include fractional CK enzymes (specifically, CK-MB, the cardiac muscle–specific enzyme), LDH, or hydroxybutyric dehydrogenase (**HBD**). Serum myoglobin is tested to estimate the amount of damage to the heart muscle. Within 1 to 2 hours of MI, serum myoglobin starts to rise, reaching a peak within 6 hours after the onset of symptoms. Thrombolytic therapy, to be most effective, must be started as soon as possible after the client develops symptoms. Therefore, the person must seek immediate emergency care.

Medical Treatment.   Individuals complaining of chest pain should be medicated promptly to prevent further damage to the heart muscle. Pain indicates *anoxia* (lack of oxygen). Typically morphine, administered IV, is the drug of choice. Drugs also are given to dilate blood vessels, allowing more oxygen to reach heart muscle.

Oxygen is administered by cannula or mask to assist with breathing and improve oxygenation, thereby relieving pain. A low-cholesterol and restricted-sodium diet is usually ordered. Caffeine-containing beverages are usually not allowed. The client is informed of the hazards of smoking and is encouraged to quit as soon as possible.

Nursing Considerations.   Immediately post-MI, continuous nursing care in the CCU is vital until the person's condition stabilizes. Usually, a cardiac monitor continuously records the client's ECG, blood pressure, pulse, and pulse pressure. Hemodynamic monitoring also is used. Alarms are set to alert the staff if one reading deviates from preset limits. During this acute phase, nursing care typically includes the following elements:

- Frequent vital signs
- Electronic cardiac monitoring
- I&O and daily weight. *Rationale: Lowered urinary output or sudden weight gain often is a sign of fluid retention or kidney disorders secondary to MI.*
- Careful observation for restlessness, dyspnea, or chest pain. *Rationale: These signs indicate that tissue damage is worsening.*
- Assessment for signs of CHF (eg, dyspnea, frequent cough, chest *rales* [abnormal sounds], edema)
- Assessment of skin color. *Rationale: Pallor or cyanosis may indicate anoxia due to impaired circulation.*
- Medications to promote pain relief and improve the heart's functioning
- Emotional support and stress reduction
- Monitoring of diet, IV fluids, or total parenteral nutrition (TPN)

During recovery from MI, rest is a priority (up to approximately 72 hours after an MI). The injured heart must have time to repair itself. The damaged spot in the heart takes from 3 to 6 weeks to heal. Tough scar tissue forms after about 8 weeks. In Practice: Nursing Care Plan 80-1 highlights the nursing care associated with a priority nursing diagnosis.

- Allow clients who are able to use a commode at the bedside for a bowel movement. A commode is preferable to a bedpan. *Rationale: Clients are more likely to strain on the bedpan.* Stool softeners are usually prescribed. *Rationale: Stool softeners prevent straining.*
- Assist the client with *isometric* (muscle-setting) exercises. *Rationale: They provide muscle exercise without causing exhaustion.* Incorporate a planned daily exercise program according to the cardiac rehabilitation program (Box 80-1).
- Use thromboembolic (antiembolism) stockings, as prescribed by the physician. *Rationale: Proper use of stockings prevents thrombophlebitis (inflammation of the vein wall; discussed below).*
- Place all necessary items within the client's reach. Be sure the call light is available. *Rationale: The client must not stretch or strain.*
- Perform physical care (eg, baths, backrubs). *Rationale: Provide rest and comfort.*
- After giving the bath and before making the bed, allow the client to rest for awhile. Positioning in semi-Fowler's position is often preferred. *Rationale: This position assists in breathing and relieves pain.*

Clients who are admitted with a diagnosis of "Rule out MI" are placed on complete bed rest until it is determined whether

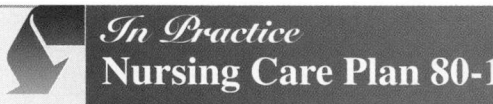

THE PERSON WITH AN ACUTE MI

MEDICAL HISTORY: *C.F., a 37-year-old single white male accountant, presented in the ED with crushing chest pain. Cardiac enzyme levels were obtained revealing a myocardial infarction (anterior wall of the left ventricle). He was admitted to the CCU approximately 18 hours ago. Oxygen at 4L/minute via nasal cannula and intravenous morphine were ordered.*

MEDICAL DIAGNOSIS: *Acute MI of anterior wall of left ventricle*

Data Collection/Nursing Assessment: Client appears pale and slightly diaphoretic. Skin is cool and clammy. Vital signs were as follows: Temperature, 97.2 degrees F (37.2 degrees C); pulse, 120 beats per minute, irregular and thready; respirations, 26 breaths per minute; blood pressure, 90/58. Morphine IV was given with relief; pain currently rated as 2 to 3 on a scale of 1 to 10. Client is currently resting in bed with head of bed elevated 45 degrees; oxygen being administered at 4L/minute. Oxygen saturation via pulse oximeter is at 96%. Continuous cardiac monitoring reveals frequent PVCs (more than 5/minute). Hemodynamic monitoring is in place. Urine output approximately 30 cc/hour. (*Although other nursing diagnoses may be appropriate, a priority nursing diagnosis is addressed below.*)

Nursing Diagnosis: Ineffective cardiopulmonary tissue perfusion related to effects of coronary artery disease and cardiac tissue damage secondary to acute MI as evidenced by low blood pressure, frequent PVCs (abnormal heart rhythm—more than 5/min), irregular, thready pulse, and cool pale skin.

Planning
SHORT-TERM GOALS:
#1. Within 24 hours, client will verbalize a decrease in complaints of pain.
#2. Within 24 hours, client will exhibit pulse rate ranging between 60 to 100 beats per minute, BP within the range of 110–130/64–74, rare to absent premature ventricular contractions (PVCs), hourly urine output greater than 30 mL/h; oxygen saturation of at least 97% with supplemental oxygen.

LONG-TERM GOALS:
#3. By 36 hours of admission, client will maintain vital signs and cardiac status within acceptable parameters.
#4. Within 48 hours of admission, client will be transferred to cardiac nursing unit.

Implementation
NURSING ACTION: *Assess for complaints of chest pain, using a pain rating scale.*
RATIONALE: *Chest pain indicates myocardial ischemia. Using a pain rating scale aids in quantifying the client's pain and provides a means for evaluating relief measures.*

NURSING ACTION: *Assess cardiopulmonary status. Monitor vital signs, especially pulse rate and blood pressure, at least hourly or more frequently if indicated, until stable. Assist with hemodynamic and continuous cardiac monitoring. Monitor respirations and oxygen saturation.*
RATIONALE: *Frequent monitoring is essential to detect changes in the client's condition as soon as possible.*

NURSING ACTION: *Assist with laboratory testing, such as cardiac enzyme levels, as necessary.*
RATIONALE: *Cardiac enzyme levels are important indicators of MI and cardiac tissue damage.*

Evaluation: Client reports pain currently at 2 on a scale of 1 to 10 for the past 2 hours. Pulse rate of 106 with slight irregularity noted; BP at 100/60; respirations 22 and regular; occasional PVCs noted, approximately 1 to 2 per minute. Urine output last hour was 40 cc. Oxygen saturation at 97% with 4 L of oxygen via nasal cannula. Lungs clear to auscultation. *Progress to meeting Goal #1 and Goal #2.*

NURSING ACTION: *Administer morphine as ordered for complaints of pain. Monitor respiratory status closely after administration of morphine. Be prepared to administer other medications, including antianginal agents and vasodilators as ordered.*
RATIONALE: *Morphine is an effective analgesic for chest pain but it is a central nervous system depressant that can cause respiratory depression. Other medications help to improve oxygen delivery to the heart muscle.*

Evaluation: Client states relief of chest pain for the past hour. Pulse rate of 98 beats per minute and regular; BP 106/64; respirations at 22 breaths per minute. Oxygen saturation level at 98% with oxygen at 4L/minute via nasal cannula. One to two PVCs noted in the last 30 minutes. *Goal #1 met; progress to meeting Goal #2.*

NURSING ACTION: *Elevate head of bed to semi- to high-Fowler's position. Encourage client to rest. Plan interactions so client has undisturbed periods of rest (1–2 h intervals); keep environmental stress to a minimum.*

(continued)

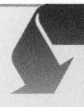

In Practice
Nursing Care Plan 80-1 *(Continued)*

RATIONALE: *Elevating the head of the bed eases the work of breathing. Planning for periods of undisturbed rest and minimizing stress reduces the workload of the heart, decreasing oxygen demand.*

Evaluation: Client reports no further episodes of chest pain. Pulse rate at 72 beats per minute and regular; BP 110/70. Skin is pale pink and warm. Continuous cardiac monitoring reveals no further evidence of PVCs. Urine output of 160 cc's over past 3 hours. Oxygen saturation at 99% with oxygen at 4L/minute. *Goal #2 met.*

NURSING ACTION: *Gradually increase activity as ordered, getting client out of bed to chair or commode. Use cardiac monitoring tracings and oxygen saturation levels as guides.*
RATIONALE: *Gradual increases in activity promote mobility without placing too great a demand on the heart. Cardiac monitoring and oxygen saturation levels provide evidence of client's ability to tolerate increase in activity.*

Evaluation: Client out of bed to chair for 15 minutes; vital signs, oxygen saturation level, and cardiac monitoring tracings within acceptable parameters. *Progress to meeting Goal #3 and Goal #4.*

---

they have had a heart attack. Those who have no pain may feed themselves, even in the acute phase. Plan activities to promote maximum relaxation and to reduce stress.

Clients who have had an MI can live a normal life and can often return to previous employment. The goal is not to change a client's lifestyle completely, but to have the client make necessary modifications to prevent recurrences. Before discharge, instruct clients and their families about patterns of healthy living and how to recognize emotional and physical stress. If the client is taking antihypertensive drugs, emphasize the necessity of taking prescribed medications despite the fact that he or she feels well. Discuss potential side effects when teaching. Also, include teaching about signs and symptoms that require immediate medical help (see In Practice: Educating the Client 80-3). Carefully and completely document this teaching.

➤➤ BOX 80-1

POST-MI REHABILITATION PLAN

- In the healthcare facility, a gradual increase in the client's activity level as ordered by the physician
- Exercise tolerance test and exercise progression
- Graded exercise program with monitoring of tolerance based on blood pressure and pulse
- Emotional support and counseling
- Stress management
- Sexual counseling
- Lifestyle changes, if any
- Risk factor management
- Dietary changes, for example, low-fat diet for hyperlipidemia or weight control
- Smoking cessation
- Hypertension control
- Medication and compliance as ordered

BLOOD VESSEL DISORDERS

Inflammatory Disorders and Complications

Thrombophlebitis
Thrombophlebitis is inflammation of the wall of a vein, in which one or more clots form. *Deep vein thrombosis* (**DVT**) defines the condition wherein a blood clot (*thrombus*) has formed inside a deep blood vessel. The blood clot forms in response to the initial inflammation. **Phlebitis** is the inflammation of a blood vessel without clot formation.

In some situations (eg, following trauma, childbirth, MI, CVA, CHF, or cancer surgery), excessive coagulability of the blood causes thrombophlebitis and thrombosis. Obesity is also a predisposing factor. Women who use birth control pills may have a higher than average risk of developing blood clots.

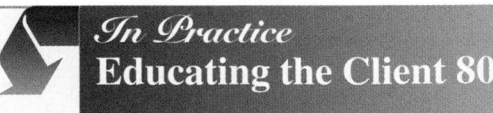 **Nursing Alert**
Never massage or rub a client's leg. *Rationale: Rubbing could dislodge a clot and cause embolism.*

In Practice
Educating the Client 80-3

WHEN TO SEEK MEDICAL HELP POST-MI
- Chest pain unrelieved with sublingual nitroglycerin
- Severe shortness of breath
- Faintness or dizziness
- Unusual fatigue or weakness
- Irregular or rapid heartbeat

Pressure or prolonged inactivity may cause venous thrombosis. It may occur after surgery or any illness in which a person remains in one position for long periods, or when sitting in a car or airplane for an extended length of time. The legs are most likely to be affected because venous blood does not return quickly enough, a condition known as *venous stasis* or *venous standstill*. Prevention of venous stasis is a major reason for early ambulation in illness. Clients with any condition that requires prolonged immobilization often receive low-dose prophylactic anticoagulants. (Some physicians recommend that all adults take aspirin daily, as a preventive measure.)

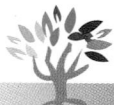 **SPECIAL CONSIDERATIONS: THE LIFE SPAN**

Thrombophlebitis

Older adults and those with heart disease or varicose veins are most susceptible to thrombophlebitis. Prolonged sitting may be a contributing factor. Inform older adults of the importance of frequent position changing. A rocking chair provides some exercise for people who find walking difficult.

Most thrombi form in veins because venous blood moves more slowly than arterial blood. However, a thrombus may form in an artery (*arterial thrombosis*); this condition is usually related to arteriosclerosis, but may be due to infection, injury, or diabetes mellitus.

Signs and Symptoms. Signs and symptoms of thrombophlebitis include pain in the affected leg, redness, swelling, fever, fatigue, and loss of appetite. A positive Homans' sign can indicate thrombophlebitis. (This test is considered positive when calf pain greatly increases with dorsiflexion of the foot.)

Medical Treatment. Imaging studies are performed to differentiate between superficial thrombosis and DVT, because each is treated differently. Clients with DVT only in the calf can be managed with outpatient therapy, receiving low–molecular-weight heparin. Those who must be admitted to the hospital require IV heparinization for 3 to 5 days, in conjunction with overlapping oral anticoagulant therapy, until adequate anticoagulation is achieved. Frequent blood tests to monitor clotting times are used to regulate the dosage of anticoagulants. The client may remain on oral anticoagulants for 3 to 6 months. In addition, clients are usually placed on bed rest for 1 to 5 days, gradually resuming their normal activity.

Nursing Considerations. All clients who are confined to bed should begin an exercise plan as soon as possible. The simplest exercises include periodic contraction and relaxation of the leg muscles and moving of the toes and feet. The bedcovers must be loose enough to permit free movement. Most clients who must remain on bed rest wear antiembolism stockings and may have the foot of the bed elevated to help prevent venous stasis. PROM exercises or the continuous passive motion (CPM) device may be used for clients who are unable to exercise actively. When caring for the client with thrombophlebitis, include the following:

- If exercise is ordered, encourage the client to wiggle the toes, bend the knees, and turn the ankle back and forth.
- In deep thrombophlebitis, immobilize the affected part.
- Prevent vigorous coughing or deep breathing (because of the danger of embolism; see next section). Try to keep the client from straining when defecating; administer stool softeners as ordered.
- Use warm, moist packs (low temperature). *Rationale: Gently stimulate circulation and dissolution of the clot, but avoid overdilation of blood vessels.*
- Enforce bed rest. *Rationale: Moving could cause embolism.* Elevate the affected leg on soft pillows. *Rationale: Promote comfort and enhance venous return from the leg.*

While the client is on anticoagulant therapy, follow the general nursing precautions and procedures to reduce the risks of injury and bleeding. The client usually receives IV heparin during the acute phase and warfarin (Coumadin) as a prophylactic measure later. Routine prothrombin times (**PT**) for monitoring of Coumadin and partial thromboplastin time (**PTT**) clotting tests are done to monitor anticoagulant therapy. The dosage is based on daily blood tests. If clotting time is too high, the medication is temporarily discontinued. Provide education to the client and family about anticoagulants and when to contact the physician at home (eg, in cases of increased bruising, bleeding).

If the client is to wear an antiembolism stocking or an elastic bandage, apply it with even pressure from the toes up to the thigh. *Rationale: Uneven pressure could cause another clot to form.* Remove elastic stockings or bandages at least once per shift for a short time. Gently cleanse the extremity, and apply lotion if necessary. Inspect the extremity carefully for any skin changes.

If the client is required to stay in bed for some time, help him or her to progress gradually from complete bed rest to ambulation, according to physician's orders. Constantly observe for any signs of embolism.

Embolism

Embolism is a severe complication of thrombophlebitis. An **embolus** is a blood clot that is carried through the circulation to some vital organ; it can lodge in a blood vessel and cause death.

Types. A *pulmonary embolism* is the result of a blood clot that travels to the lungs. If the obstruction occurs in a large pulmonary blood vessel (the most common site for the lodging of an embolus originating in the leg), it may cause sudden death. The obstruction of a small vessel may not be so damaging. A pulmonary embolism may cause sudden, sharp chest pain; breathing difficulty; violent cough; and bloody sputum. The client will become cyanotic, and symptoms of shock can develop rapidly. The immediate treatment is to administer oxygen and to provide for complete bed rest in a high semi-Fowler's position. Continuous IV anticoagulation therapy with heparin is a widely used treatment. Pain relief with the use of IV morphine is also indicated.

A *coronary embolus* is a blood clot that travels to a blood vessel in the heart. If the embolus lodges in a blood vessel within the heart, the heart tissue distal to the blockage will necrose. Depending on how large the vessel is, the necrosed area may cause instant death. Symptoms of a lesser blockage are sudden severe chest pain and other characteristic symptoms of MI.

In *cerebral embolism,* the clot blocks one of the brain's blood vessels. The amount of damage depends on the vessel's size and location. This situation is commonly known as a CVA or stroke (covered later in this chapter).

Peripheral embolism and *thrombosis in a limb* involves an embolus that lodges in a blood vessel leading to an extremity. In this case, the first symptom is severe pain at the site of the blockage. The extremity becomes pale and cold to the touch; pulses distal to the blockage are lost. The limb becomes white and cold. Other symptoms of shock are seen if a large blood vessel is obstructed. Amputation below the level of the blockage may be necessary if a clot in a large vessel is not dissolved quickly or surgically removed. Without circulation, gangrene will occur.

Surgical Treatment.   Certain surgical procedures may be performed to combat the danger of embolism. Emboli can be removed from pulmonary arteries, although this procedure is rare. If a thrombus is located in the femoral vein, the blood vessel can be *ligated* (tied off) at the blockage site in a procedure called *femoral ligation.* Sometimes, the vena cava is made smaller (*vena cava ligation*) or a filter is inserted in the vein to prevent clots from traveling to the heart.

Peripheral Vascular Disorders

Most peripheral vascular disorders are evidenced at one time or another by the following symptoms:

- *Intermittent* **claudication:** The person experiences no pain at rest; but exercise, particularly walking, causes excruciating pain in the limb, which disappears when the limb is again at rest. Smoking, vascular spasm, and atherosclerosis aggravate this condition. Intermittent claudication caused by venous stasis is called *venous claudication.*
- *Tingling and numbness:* The extremity or part of the extremity becomes numb, or the person feels a persistent tingling sensation, caused by poor circulation.
- *Coldness and difference in size:* The extremities may feel cold to the touch or the person may sense that the hands and feet are cold. One leg may be markedly different in size, color, and temperature from the other.
- *Lack of new tissue growth:* The skin may become paper thin, shiny, and easily subject to breakdown. Blood vessels are visible.

Simple changes to lifestyle can prevent or arrest peripheral vascular diseases. In Practice: Nursing Care Guidelines 80-2 lists general nursing measures for peripheral vascular disease.

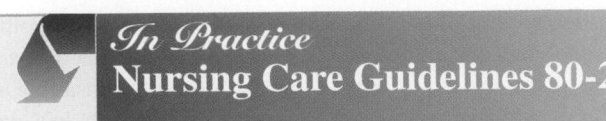

In Practice
Nursing Care Guidelines 80-2

CARING FOR CLIENTS WITH PERIPHERAL VASCULAR DISEASE

- Protect the client's feet and legs from undue pressure of linens. *Rationale: Doing so prevents discomfort and skin breakdown.*
- Take great care in trimming the toenails. *Rationale: Cuts or abrasions on the feet are difficult to heal.*
- Be sure to dry carefully between the toes after washing them. *Rationale: Moisture promotes skin breakdown. Any break in the skin or subsequent infection heals much more slowly when circulation is poor.*
- Be very careful about application of heat. Use extra clothing rather than external heat to warm the extremities. *Rationale: This person is easily burned.*
- Report skin breakdown immediately. *Rationale: Ambitious therapy will be needed.*
- Use warm baths to help increase the circulation; be sure the water is not hot. *Rationale: Heat helps dilate blood vessels. This client is very susceptible to burns. Use a bath thermometer; the maximum temperature is 100° F or 37.8° C.*
- Do not attempt to treat corns or calluses. *Rationale: The client may be accidentally cut or injured, predisposing the client to infection.*

Buerger's Disease

Buerger's disease (thromboangiitis obliterans) results from inflammation that causes obstruction of blood vessels in the extremities, especially the legs. It is more common in men than in women, primarily affecting persons who are heavy smokers. Chilling aggravates the condition. Buerger's disease is less common today than in the past.

Usually the first sign is cramps in the calf muscles, brought on by exercise, which disappear with rest. Other symptoms include tingling, burning, numbness, and edema, which may develop into pitting or *brawny* (hard) edema. Hardened, painful areas develop along the course of blood vessels. When the feet and legs hang down, they take on a mottled purplish-red hue; when raised, they become abnormally pale. Ulcers may develop that, if infected, could result in gangrene, necessitating amputation. As the disease progresses, pain continues even during rest.

Medical and Surgical Treatment.   Affected individuals must avoid anything that worsens this condition, especially chilling of hands and feet. Tobacco in any form is dangerous because nicotine constricts blood vessels. Advise clients to stop smoking or stop using smokeless tobacco immediately.

Mild exercise is recommended if it is not painful. For this purpose, *Buerger-Allen exercises* are prescribed. They consist of alternately raising, lowering, and resting the legs. Sometimes cramps occur with exercise (*intermittent claudication*). Clients may use an electrically operated rocking bed (*oscillating bed*) if they cannot exercise actively. Antibiotics, antiinflammatory agents, and analgesics may be necessary to treat infection and pain. External heat is not used. Rather, clients are encouraged to wear extra clothing. Encourage fluid intake and advise clients to avoid constrictive clothing.

Sometimes a *sympathectomy* is performed, whereby the sympathetic nerves, which innervate the smooth muscles, are cut to relieve vasospasms and increase blood flow to the lower extremities.

Raynaud's Phenomenon

Raynaud's phenomenon is a condition is characterized by spasmodic constriction of arteries supplying the extremities. It especially affects fingers and toes; often it involves only the fingers. It affects women more frequently than men, especially young women. Cold and emotional stress can precipitate the condition. However, the cause is unknown.

Symptoms of Raynaud's phenomenon include blanched and cold extremities. They perspire and feel numb and prickly. Later they become blue—especially the fingernails—and are painful. As heat restores blood flow, the hands become red and warm. In the early stages, these symptoms disappear after an episode, and the hands seem normal again. But as the disease progresses, cyanosis persists between attacks, and ulcers, which are slow to heal, may develop on the fingertips. The skin looks tight and shiny, and the nails become deformed. The fingertips may develop gangrene.

Clients must avoid chilling at all times. They must always wear warm clothing outdoors in winter (eg, wool gloves and socks, and insulated boots). A goosedown or other comforter at night provides steady warmth. Electric blankets may be dangerous because they may be too hot and could burn the client. Clients should avoid emotional upsets and tension of any kind. Smoking is contraindicated. Drugs to relieve spasm of arteries and dilate blood vessels provide considerable relief. A sympathectomy may be necessary.

Varicose Veins

Varicose veins result from weakening of the valves of the veins so that blood pools in the legs or another dependent area. Normal veins fill from below because of valvular action. With varicose veins, the veins fill abnormally. (Hemorrhoids and esophageal varices are also varicose veins.) Predisposing factors include heredity, and weakening of the vein walls resulting from prolonged standing, poor posture, repeated pregnancies, round garters, obesity, tumors, HTN, and chronic diseases of the liver or kidneys. Varicose veins may also result from thrombophlebitis. Women are more commonly affected with varicosities of the legs than men, especially if they have had several pregnancies.

Signs and Symptoms. The main sign of varicose veins in the legs is the appearance of dark, tortuous superficial veins that become more prominent when the person stands and appear as dark protrusions. These superficial veins can some-

times rupture, causing a *varicose ulcer*. Internal or deep varicose veins cause symptoms such as pain, fatigue, a feeling of heaviness, and muscle cramps. Symptoms are much more severe in hot weather and at high altitudes. A diagnostic test involves putting the client into the Trendelenburg position to test blood drainage. Leg veins that do not fill normally on standing signify varicose veins.

Medical and Surgical Treatment. Treatment includes elevating the legs for a few minutes at 2- to 3-hour intervals throughout the day. It also includes avoiding constriction, standing for long periods, or restrictive clothing. The client should wear support hose. All measures aim at promoting venous return from the legs.

In severe cases, surgical ligation and stripping of varicose veins is done. The larger veins are surgically ligated, and smaller ones are stripped out. Occasionally, sclerosing solutions are used for small varicosities: The solution is injected into the vessel that causes irritation and eventually fibrosis.

Nursing Considerations. The client needs teaching about measures that promote venous drainage, to avoid the need for possible surgery. If surgery is necessary, apply antiembolism stockings to the leg postoperatively, and elevate the foot of the bed to encourage venous return. Analgesics may be ordered. Aspirin is often the drug of choice because of its anticoagulant action.

Early ambulation is important after surgical treatment. Often, the client must ambulate as soon as he or she recovers from anesthesia. The client may be alarmed at the idea of walking so soon after the operation, while the legs are stiff and sore, and will most likely need reassurance and an explanation of the need for moving about. The order is often written for the client to walk 5 to 10 minutes each hour during the day and several times at night. Assist and encourage the client to follow this regimen.

Ideas for client teaching after venous stripping appear at In Practice: Educating the Client 80-4. Instruct the client how to apply antiembolism stockings correctly. Teach him or her to avoid knee-high stockings and socks with elastic tops. If weight reduction is suggested, the clinical dietitian will give instructions.

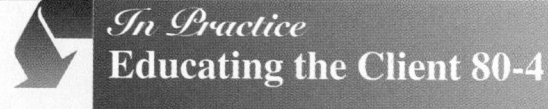

In Practice
Educating the Client 80-4

DISCHARGE TEACHING AFTER VENOUS STRIPPING

- Elevate the legs while sitting.
- Be sure to walk, and to avoid standing still and in one place for any length of time.
- Avoid sitting for a lengthy time.
- Learn how to apply antiembolism stockings correctly.
- If possible, lose weight.
- Do not use tobacco.

Telangiectasia (Spider Veins)

Telangiectasia is a group of small dilated blood vessels. It is treated by *scleropathy,* the injection of a weak sodium chloride solution into nonfunctioning veins. Pressure is applied at specific points and the veins stick together and are gradually absorbed. The lines almost disappear. The treatment is relatively painless.

Aneurysms

An **aneurysm** is an outpouching of a blood vessel. Although it may occur in any vessel, the most common site is the aorta. Figure 80-11 shows several types of aneurysms.

An aneurysm in the aorta or in a cerebral vessel represents an extreme emergency. If it ruptures, surgical intervention may be done if the aneurysm is in an operable site. However, if surgery is not done immediately, the vessel may hemorrhage and the person may die. If the aneurysm is discovered before it ruptures, it is treated by surgical repair, such as clamping or removal. Usually, a synthetic graft is substituted for the portion of the vessel affected.

Aneurysms may be congenital, may occur after trauma, or may develop as a result of the increased pressure of arteriosclerosis. Unknown cerebral aneurysm rupture is often the cause of sudden death in healthy athletes.

Cerebrovascular Accident

A sudden or gradual interruption of blood supply to a vital center in the brain is a *cerebrovascular accident* (CVA), also known as a *stroke, brain attack,* or *central vascular accident.* A CVA may cause complete or partial paralysis or death. CVAs are the third leading cause of death in America.

HTN and smoking are contributing factors to CVAs. Smoking increases the risk of developing a CVA by two to six times. The risk also increases for smokers who use birth control pills over an extended period of time. Postmenopausal women are more likely to have CVAs than younger women. There is a higher incidence of death from CVA in women, although men and women are equally afflicted with the condition.

Causes of CVA

Direct causes of CVA include the following:

- *Cerebral thrombosis:* In this most frequent cause of CVA, a blood clot or piece of plaque blocks an artery that supplies a vital brain center, usually as a result of arteriosclerosis.
- *Cerebral hemorrhage* or *aneurysm:* An artery in the brain bursts because of arteriosclerosis, continuing weakening of the aneurysm wall, or a severe rise in blood pressure, causing hemorrhage and ischemia.

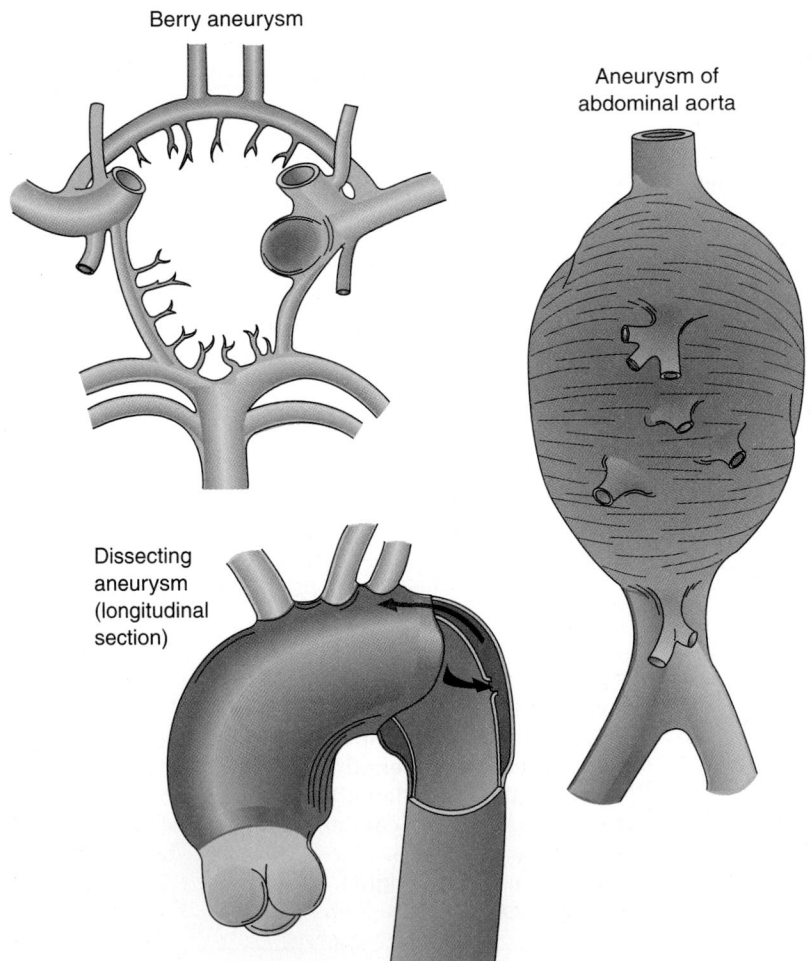

Berry aneurysm

Aneurysm of abdominal aorta

Dissecting aneurysm (longitudinal section)

FIGURE 80-11. Three forms of aneurysms: Berry aneurysm in the circle of Willis, fusiform-type aneurysm of the abdominal aorta, and a dissecting aortic aneurysm.

- *Cerebral embolism:* A blood clot breaks off from a thrombus elsewhere in the body and is carried to the brain, where it lodges in a blood vessel and shuts off blood supply to part of the brain.

Stages of CVA

There are four specific stages of CVA:

- *Transient ischemic attack* (**TIA**) is a sudden, short-lived attack. The person recovers within 24 hours. TIA is often a warning that another, more serious stroke will occur later. The risk of completed stroke (see below) for this person is 25% to 35% greater than in a healthy person.
- *Reversible ischemic neurologic deficit* (**RIND**) is similar to TIA, except that the symptoms last for as long as a week. Recovery is complete or nearly so. RIND is also a warning that a more serious stroke is likely.
- *Stroke in evolution* (**SIE**) is a gradual worsening of symptoms of brain ischemia.
- *Completed stroke* (CS) occurs when symptoms of stroke are present and stabilize over a period. At this point, active rehabilitation can begin.

Signs and Symptoms.   Symptoms of CVA depend on its cause. In some cases of thrombosis, the person has had dizzy spells or sudden memory loss for some time before the actual CVA. No pain accompanies these symptoms, so the client may ignore them. A cerebral hemorrhage may give warning. It causes dizziness and ringing in the ears (*tinnitus*), as well as a violent headache, often with nausea and vomiting. A hemorrhage may follow unusual exertion, such as shoveling snow, heavy eating, or vigorous exercise. Embolism usually occurs without warning, although the person often has a history of cardiovascular disease.

The sudden-onset CVA is usually the most severe. The victim loses consciousness; the face becomes red; breathing is noisy and strained. The pulse is slow, but full and bounding. Blood pressure is elevated, and the person may be in a deep coma. The coma may deepen progressively until death occurs, or the person may gradually regain consciousness and eventually recover. The longer the time period that the person remains unresponsive, the less likely it is that the person will recover. The first few days after onset are critical. The responsive person may show signs of memory loss or inconsistent behavior; he or she may be easily fatigued, lose bowel and bladder control, or have poor balance.

Results of CVA

A CVA can result in numerous effects, depending on the cause and location of the CVA. Some of the major effects are discussed here.

Hemiplegia.   The most common result of a CVA is **hemiplegia,** which is paralysis of one side of the body. Hemiplegia may affect other functions, such as hearing, general sensation, and circulation; the degree of impairment depends on the part of the brain affected.

Generally, hemiplegia progresses through three stages:

1. The *flaccid stage,* in which the affected side exhibits numbness and weakness
2. The *spastic stage,* in which muscles are contracted and tense, and movement is difficult
3. The *recovery stage,* when therapy and rehabilitation methods are most successful

Aphasia and Dysphasia.   Many people with CVA experience **aphasia,** a result of damage to the brain's speech center. Aphasia is a condition in which people are unable to speak. It can be frustrating and frightening because mental functioning usually is unimpaired. In Practice: Nursing Care Guidelines 80-3 highlights key measures for communicating with a client who has aphasia.

Another complication associated with a CVA is *dysphasia,* an inability to say what one wishes to say. Many clients regain some power of speech, but others never do. *Dysphagia* (swallowing difficulty) may also occur.

Brain Damage.   The extent of brain damage resulting from a CVA determines the client's chances for recovery. If the damage is slight, recovery will be more rapid and complete.

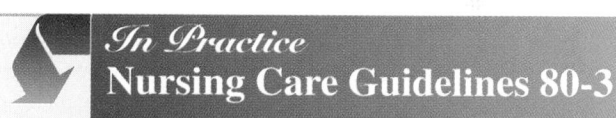

In Practice
Nursing Care Guidelines 80-3

COMMUNICATING WITH THE CLIENT WITH APHASIA

- If the person can write, supply a tablet and pencil or provide a board on which he or she can write.
- If the client cannot write, provide a board or chart on which key words and phrases are printed. The client can point to these words and phrases to make his or her needs known.
- Check to see if the client is able to move a finger or has some way let you know that he or she understands what is being said.
- If the client cannot move at all, ask him or her to blink. The client can blink once for "yes" and twice for "no."
- Talk to the client even if he or she cannot answer. Chat while you perform daily nursing care.
- Do not talk down to the client.
- Never talk about the client to another person—including healthcare personnel—in their presence. Although the client is unable to speak, he or she may be able to hear and understand everything you say.
- Keep in mind that some clients who are unable to speak can use computers. Assistive devices are available for those who cannot use conventional keyboards.
- Expect speech therapy to begin as soon as possible. After the speech therapist has decided what procedures to use, reinforce this with everyone involved in the client's care.

Also, the chances of recovery are better for a younger person who suffers a CVA.

Hemianopsia (Hemianopia). **Hemianopsia** is defined as blindness in half of the visual field of one or both eyes. It is a common occurrence with a CVA. Consider this condition in all aspects of care. For instance, always approach the client from the unaffected side. Teach the client to *scan* (move the head from side to side) to see things.

Pain. Usually very little pain is associated with a CVA. Problems such as infection, kidney or bladder *calculi* (stones), fecal impaction, or emotional disturbances may aggravate any existing pain. Injection of a local anesthetic may provide temporary relief.

Autonomic Disturbances. The person with a CVA may also have autonomic disturbances, such as perspiration or "goose flesh" above the level of the paralysis. He or she may have dilated pupils, high or low blood pressure, or headache. Disturbances of this kind may be treated with atropine-like drugs.

Personality Changes. Personality changes may be functional or organic. The *functional* type results from frustration at being unable to speak or walk, or from the attitudes of other people. In either case, the individual may feel useless or helpless. *Organic changes* may result from blockage of blood supply to part of the brain. In this instance, the person may cry or become easily excited. These conditions cannot be consciously controlled.

Nursing Considerations. The person with a CVA often is admitted to the healthcare facility in an unresponsive state, known as an SIE (described previously). After careful examination and history, this individual may be eligible for thrombolytic therapy to resolve the clot. The quality of nursing care given during the acute phase often considerably affects how much rehabilitation is possible and how quickly it can be accomplished. The following are important nursing activities to implement during this time:

- Note changes in level of consciousness and any changes from the neurologic findings of the initial neurologic examination (see Chap. 77).
- Document every sign of improvement or lack of it.
- Position the unresponsive person on the unaffected side, to keep the airway open and prevent aspiration. *Rationale: Proper positioning prevents contractures and undue pressure on any part.*
- Avoid placing the unresponsive person on the back. *Rationale: The tongue may fall back and occlude the airway; secretions may accumulate in the back of the throat.*
- Provide adequate support for the affected limbs. Extremity splints are now routine. *Rationale: Positioning, support, and splints help prevent contractures.*
- Elevate the head of the bed. *Rationale: Reduce the chance of increased intracranial pressure.*
- Turn the person often, at least once every 2 hours, keeping the body in proper alignment.

- Provide suctioning as necessary. A mechanical airway or tracheostomy may be required. Oxygen will most likely be administered.
- Monitor vital signs carefully. *Rationale: An elevated temperature, and lowered pulse and respiration rates, are signs of increased intracranial pressure—which you must report.*
- Keep the eyes lubricated with soothing eye drops as ordered.
- Talk to the person and explain everything you do as if he or she were responsive. *Rationale: Although the person may not respond, he or she hears. Hearing is the last sense to be lost.*

At the end of the emergency phase, the person is said to have had a CS (*completed stroke,* described previously). When caring for the person who has regained consciousness, do the following:

- Continue to turn the client often, now from the unaffected side to a back-lying position.
- Encourage coughing and deep breathing.
- Encourage movement if possible. *Rationale: Movement prevents hypostatic pneumonia, formation of kidney stones, fecal impaction, urinary retention, and other complications.*
- Provide PROM exercises as ordered.
- Encourage cooperation with the physical therapist.
- Administer ordered drugs (usually heparin, dicumarol, or warfarin) with care. Watch for side effects. *Rationale: These drugs prolong clotting time and prevent further clots from forming. However, danger of hemorrhage accompanies their use. The client usually does not need analgesics.*
- Begin bowel and bladder retraining as the client is ready for it.

Be aware of the various results of CVAs. Treat clients with kindness and understanding. They need support, reassurance, and acceptance most of all (see In Practice: Nursing Care Plan 77-1 in Chap. 77).

Nursing Alert

Hearing and vision on the affected side are usually impaired as a result of a CVA. To avoid having to repeat what is said and perhaps embarrassing the person, approach from the unaffected side.

The Rehabilitation Phase. Immediately on admission, staff should begin planning for rehabilitation. If contractures are prevented, the client can learn to walk again much sooner. If the skin is kept intact, the client will not have to contend with ulcers and infections. If bowel and bladder training have begun, the client will be well on the way to independence. The goal of all rehabilitation is to return the client to the highest level of self-care in ADL. As soon as possible, teach adaptive ADL, such as transferring from bed to chair and to toilet;

dressing; and feeding. Speech therapy also begins as soon as possible. Chapter 95 describes some specific rehabilitation techniques and assistive devices.

Members of the family play a vital role. They need to know what the client can do and how to encourage the person now and after discharge. They should also understand that, because of brain damage, the person may behave differently after a stroke. Whatever the client's disability, members of the family should recognize their own, as well as the client's, emotional needs. They also need to learn how to perform various procedures that help the client, while allowing the person to do as much as possible. The family needs a great deal of emotional support to deal with the client's limitations.

Many resources are available to assist in rehabilitation, including local social service agencies, the American Heart Association, and the state's division of vocational and occupational services. The local public health nursing service can help the family prepare for the client's homecoming, and can assist the client to perform self-care at home.

➤ STUDENT SYNTHESIS

Key Points

• Cardiovascular disorders include conditions that interfere with the heart's rhythm and the heart's pumping ability, and that disrupt the blood flow within the coronary, peripheral, or cerebral arteries.
• Hypertension can lead to such serious problems as myocardial infarction, kidney damage, congestive heart failure, and cerebrovascular accident.
• Some types of heart disease can be cured, whereas others can be controlled by medical or surgical treatment.
• Congestive heart failure means that the heart is failing, has lost its pumping ability, and is unable to do its work. It is a syndrome (group of symptoms) that affects individuals in different ways and to different degrees.
• Coronary artery disease develops over many years, and therefore prevention of controllable risk factors should begin early in life.
• Angina pectoris is a temporary loss of oxygen to the heart muscle. If this loss of oxygen supply continues, the result is ischemia (prolonged deficiency of oxygenated blood), whereas death of heart tissue is called myocardial necrosis.
• Clients who complain of chest pains should be medicated promptly as ordered by the physician, to prevent further damage to heart muscle due to anoxia.
• Hearing and vision are usually impaired on the person's affected side after a CVA; therefore, approach the client from the unaffected side.

Critical Thinking Exercises

1. P. L., aged 25, comes to the healthcare facility for an annual examination. She is concerned because her family has a history of CAD. She asks you her risks and ways that she can prevent CAD. Formulate a plan you could use to teach P. L. preventive measures.
2. I. H. has recently suffered a CVA. He is dysphasic and has recently become very frustrated over his condition. His family members are attentive and concerned; however, I. H. seems unhappy and angry when they are around. What measures could you take to assist I. H. with speech difficulties? How would you address his attitudes toward his family members? How would you help his family cope with his condition?

NCLEX-Style Review Questions

1. Blood screening commonly used to identify heart disorders, especially myocardial infarction, include:
   a. LDH, AST, CBC
   b. CK, troponin, AST
   c. LDH, EPS, PTCA
   d. myoglobin, AST, EPS
2. Three diagnostic tests commonly used in identifying cardiovascular disease include:
   a. Angiocardiogram, thrombolytic therapy, stress test
   b. Electrocardiogram, stress test, CT scan
   c. Echocardiogram, angiogram, electromyogram
   d. Stress test, electrocardiogram, echocardiogram
3. Common surgical methods used to treat cardiovascular disorders include:
   a. Angioplasty, CABG, heart valve replacement
   b. CABG, t-PA, heart valve replacement
   c. PTCA, t-PA, TMR
   d. TMR, t-PA, stent
4. Teaching that is aimed at prevention of cardiovascular disease should include:
   a. Avoiding elevating legs
   b. Increasing moderate exercise
   c. Including high amount of saturated fats in diet
   d. Smoking cessation
5. In what ways are the symptoms of a myocardial infarction different than those of angina?
   a. An MI usually is sudden, sharp, and severe, lasting for a brief period of time.
   b. The pain of an MI is always more severe and lasts longer.
   c. MI pain sometimes radiates to the left arm, shoulder, or back; angina pain radiates to the right arm and shoulder.
   d. Rest and nitroglycerin usually do not relieve the pain of angina.

6. General nursing guidelines for the care of a client with peripheral vascular disease include:
   a. Applying hot packs to improve circulation
   b. Avoiding washing and drying between toes to prevent dryness
   c. Protecting feet and legs from undue pressure of linens
   d. Trimming nails and corns carefully

7. Which of the following would not be associated with causing a CVA?
   a. Cerebral aneurysm
   b. Cerebral claudication
   c. Cerebral embolism
   d. Cerebral thrombosis

8. Which of the following would be unacceptable to use when communicating with the aphasic client?
   a. Enabling the client to feel part of the care by talking about them to other healthcare personnel in the client's presence
   b. Establishing a system for the client to blink "yes" and "no" to questions asked if the client is unable to write
   c. Supplying a tablet and pencil or writing board
   d. Talking to the person while performing daily care, even though they are unable to speak

CHAPTER

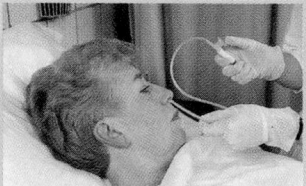

81

Blood and Lymph Disorders

LEARNING OBJECTIVES

1. State the main blood types, including the inherited antibodies and antigens for each blood type.
2. Describe the following diagnostic studies: indirect Coombs' test, direct Coombs' test, type and screen test, and type and crossmatch test.
3. State the functions of each of the following tests: RBC count, Hgb, Hct, WBC count, differential, platelet count, blood smear, PT, PTT, APTT, and bleed time.
4. Identify at least two nursing considerations related to the following: ESR, blood culture, bone marrow biopsy, and lymph node biopsy.
5. Identify at least two advantages and two limitations for colloid solutions.
6. Identify the rationale for the administration of the following blood products: whole blood, packed RBCs, platelet concentrates, FFP, albumin, cryoprecipitates, plasmapheresis, IgG, and IgD.
7. Identify at least three nursing considerations for autologous and allogeneic BMT.
8. Discuss at least three nursing considerations for each of the following RBC disorders: polycythemia, anemia, sickle cell disease, and thalassemia.
9. Compare and contrast the following types of anemia: iron deficiency, hemolytic, hemorrhagic, pernicious, and aplastic.
10. Define the causative factors for the following WBC disorders: neutropenia and leukemia. Identify at least three nursing considerations related to each disorder.
11. Discuss at least three nursing considerations for each of the following platelet disorders: thrombocythemia, ITP, DIC, and hemophilia.
12. Identify the causative factors for the following lymphatic system disorders: Hodgkin's disease, non-Hodgkin's lymphoma, and multiple myeloma.

NEW TERMINOLOGY

agranulocytosis	leukopenia
allogeneic	neutropenia
autologous	oncologist
colloid solutions	pancytopenia
hematology	polycythemia vera
hemophilia	sickle cell disease
Hodgkin's disease	thrombocytopenia
leukemia	thrombocytosis
leukocytosis	

ACRONYMS

ALL	CSF	INR
AML	DIC	ITP
APTT	ESR	NHL
BMT	FFP	PBSC
CLL	GVHD	PT
CML	Ig	PTT

The medical specialty concerned with the hematologic and lymphatic systems is called **hematology**. Physicians educated in this specialty are hematologists. Blood and lymph are closely related to many other body systems and disorders (see Chaps. 22 and 23.) For example, cancer can originate in the blood or lymphatic systems. These transport systems can also be a route by which cancer cells travel and metastasize to other body areas. An **oncologist** (cancer specialist) often treats blood and lymph disorders (see Chap. 82).

Some blood and lymph disorders have systemic consequences and symptoms. Many of these blood and lymph disorders also affect children. To understand these disorders in more detail, also refer to cardiovascular disorders in Chapter 71.

DIAGNOSTIC TESTS

Laboratory Tests

Laboratory examination of blood can reveal the general condition of many body systems and can aid in the diagnosis of many disorders. Medical technologists, other laboratory personnel, and nurses perform many of these tests.

The nurse must be knowledgeable about the types of hematologic studies, the reasons for their use, and the implications of abnormal lab values. In many instances, it is the nurse's responsibility to notify the physician of routine and abnormal lab values. Appendix C has a listing of the most common types of hematologic and chemistry laboratory tests, along with indications for their use.

Blood Typing

Genes are responsible for blood types. Each of the red blood cells (RBCs) has *antigens* that were inherited. It is these antigens or lack of these antigens that determines blood type. Blood is typed according to the antigens of the ABO blood group system. Type A blood has the A antigen and type B blood has the B antigen on an RBC. Type O blood has no antigens on an RBC. Type AB blood has both A and B antigens.

Antibodies in the blood are also inherited. Type A blood has anti-B antibodies. Type B blood has anti-A antibodies. Type O blood has both anti-A and anti-B antibodies. Type AB blood has neither anti-A or anti-B antibodies.

Another aspect of blood types is the D factor or D antigen. This antigen is better known as the Rh factor, named after studies using the rhesus monkey. At birth a person may have the Rh (or D) antigen on the RBC and is therefore Rh-positive; this person does not have the Rh antibody.

At birth an individual may be Rh-negative and have no Rh antigens on the RBC. Under normal circumstances, the individual who is Rh-negative has no antibodies against the Rh factor. However, the individual may become sensitized by receiving Rh-positive blood and develop anti-Rh antibodies. The sensitization of Rh-negative individuals may have occurred during transfusions using Rh-positive blood. In Rh-negative females, this sensitization can occur during pregnancy when the fetus was Rh-positive.

Indirect Coombs' Test.   An *indirect Coombs' test* screens for circulating Rh antibodies. It is ordered on an Rh-negative pregnant woman. If Rh antibodies are detected in the mother, the fetus is in jeopardy of developing *erythroblastosis fetalis* (see Chaps. 64 and 68.) RhoGAM is an anti-Rh antibody preparation that suppresses the mother's production of Rh antibodies.

Direct Coombs' Test.   A *direct Coombs' test* will detect antibodies already attached to the RBC. This test may be ordered prior to blood transfusions and the administration of certain drugs. A positive or abnormal direct Coombs' test may indicate transfusion reactions, erythroblastosis fetalis, hemolytic anemia, infectious mononucleosis, lymphomas, certain cancers and renal disorders, or autoimmune disorders such as rheumatoid arthritis and systemic lupus erythematosus.

Type and Screen Test.   A *type and screen test* of blood determines the ABO blood group, the Rh type, and an indirect Coombs' test. A type and screen is often ordered for clients who have a low to moderate potential of needing a blood transfusion. It is a test that can be completed relatively quickly and reasonably inexpensively.

Type and Crossmatch Test.   A *type and crossmatch test* is a more detailed test usually done for clients who have a greater potential of needing blood transfusions. The type and crossmatch includes testing for ABO groups and Rh factor. An indirect Coombs' test is done on both the donor and the potential recipient. Additional antibody testing may be necessary to identify unusual antibodies. Finally, both the donor's blood and the potential recipient's blood are combined and tested for compatibility. A type and crossmatch may take up to an hour to complete. Therefore, it is necessary to anticipate the need for blood transfusions in advance of their need.

Nursing Considerations.   Nursing considerations related to blood typing include the awareness that blood of different types is often incompatible when mixed. The wrong type of blood could easily be fatal. Even with the safeguards of blood typing, screening, and crossmatching, be sure to observe the client very carefully while he or she receives a blood transfusion because dangerous reactions are still a possibility.

Complete Blood Count

The *complete blood count* (CBC) is the common analysis of blood that provides diagnostic information. A CBC usually includes a numerical estimate of the number of RBCs, white blood cells (WBCs), and platelets found in a blood sample. Deficiencies or excesses of any of the cells may indicate a specific problem. These numbers reflect the functioning of the person's bone marrow, the blood's ability to carry oxygen to the cells, and the client's infection-fighting status and clotting abilities. Normal values of these tests are given in Appendix C. The components of a CBC include:

- RBC count
- Hematocrit
- Hemoglobin
- RBC indices: mean corpuscular volume (MCV), mean corpuscular hemoglobin (MCH), and mean corpuscular hemoglobin concentration (MCHC)
- WBC count

- WBC differential count (granulocytes: neutrophils, basophils, eosinophils; agranulocytes: lymphocytes, monocytes)
- Blood smear

Red Blood Cell Count.

The *RBC count* measures the number of circulating RBCs in a cubic millimeter of peripheral venous blood. Normal values vary according to age and sex.

The test for hemoglobin (Hgb, Hb) identifies the amount of hemoglobin in an RBC. The results of this test indicate the body's ability to carry oxygen to cells. The hematocrit (Hct) test identifies the percentage of RBCs in the blood.

Along with the RBC count, the Hgb and Hct tests can indicate different types of anemias, or an overabundance of RBCs (*polycythemia*). With a client who has adequate overall hydration, the Hct result is about three times the Hgb.

The RBC indices are calculated measurements of the size of an RBC and the amounts of hemoglobin. Using the figures obtained for the MCH, MCHC, and the MCV, the diagnostician can differentiate among different types of anemias including macrocytic, microcytic, thalassemia, aplastic, or pernicious anemias.

White Blood Cell Count and Differential.

A *WBC count* is a valuable diagnostic aid. When an infection is present, the normal count of 5,000 to 10,000/mm^3 may increase to 25,000/mm^3 or higher. WBCs increase in number (*leukocytosis*) or decrease in number (**leukopenia**).

Under a microscope, the technician can estimate the numbers of each of the five types of leukocytes. In some diseases, the proportion of the kinds of WBCs varies. In bacterial infections, the number of neutrophils increases; in viral infections; the numbers of lymphocytes increases. Therefore, a differential count is made, in which the technician compares the number of granular leukocytes with the number of nongranular (agranular) leukocytes. The results are further diagnostic clues for the physician.

The *WBC differential* or "diff" may be ordered specifically to be done by mechanical estimates or to be visualized and counted by a trained laboratory technician.

Leukocytosis (increased total WBC count) is the body's normal response to injury or invading pathogens. The particular type of WBC involved may help to identify the cause of abnormal leukocytosis. For example, an increase in monocytes (*monocytosis*) would indicate mononucleosis. *Lymphocytosis* (increased numbers of lymphocytes), a useful indicator of leukemia, can be used to monitor the client's progress and response to treatment.

Platelet Count.

Platelets or *thrombocytes* are fragments of very large cells (megakaryocytes) formed in the bone marrow. They circulate until needed or are removed every 8 to 12 days, when they are destroyed by the spleen. The platelet count indicates the client's capacity of *hemostasis* (blood clotting).

Low platelet counts are associated with bruising, bleeding disorders, and hemorrhage. *Thrombocytopenia* (low numbers of platelets) can be seen in a number of conditions, including chemotherapy for cancer, radiation therapy, certain types of anemias, and leukemia. **Thrombocytosis** (increased platelets) can be an indication of certain types of anemias, leukemia, pregnancy, and polycythemia vera.

Peripheral Blood Smear.

The *peripheral blood smear* is an informative test performed by a qualified technologist. Under the microscope, the technician views a prepared smear slide for RBCs, WBCs, and platelets. The RBCs are examined for size, shape, color and structure. A differential count of WBCs can be done. The number and appearance of platelets is also monitored.

Coagulation Studies

Prothrombin Time.

The *prothrombin time* (**PT,** Pro Time, PT Ratio/INR) is an actual amount of time that it takes blood to clot, generally given in seconds. This test can indicate the proper functioning of coagulation factors and the coagulation process. The PT will be longer when certain clotting factors are defective or not present in sufficient quantity. The factors that can affect the PT include fibrinogen I and prothrombin II, V, VII, and X. Normally, the PT is less than 12 seconds.

PT is commonly used to monitor the success of oral anticoagulation therapy using warfarin sodium (Coumadin). Adequate amounts of warfarin will prolong clotting time—the desired effect of the therapy. However, too much of the drug can result in bleeding and hemorrhage. Intramuscular (IM) *vitamin K*, which reverses the effects of warfarin in 12 to 24 hours, *is the antidote to warfarin.*

Therapeutic values for anticoagulation therapy of coumadin are 1.5 to 2 times the normal ranges. If the client does not have adequate amounts of the anticoagulation drug, prothrombin times will be normal and *the physician will need to be notified.*

Measuring the PT daily is essential when the client begins anticoagulant drug therapy. When the therapeutic blood level of anticoagulant is stabilized, PT can be determined less often (approximately every 2 weeks). In Practice: Nursing Assessment 81-1 highlights important findings for the client receiving anticoagulant therapy. When a client is receiving anticoagulant therapy, the following are important to reduce the risk of bleeding:

- Avoiding IM injections and needlesticks, if possible
- Not taking temperatures rectally
- Not giving the daily dose of anticoagulant until after blood specimen for the PT is drawn

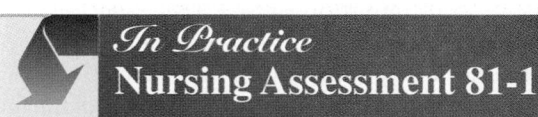

In Practice
Nursing Assessment 81-1

THE CLIENT RECEIVING ANTICOAGULANT THERAPY

- Adverse signs and symptoms
- Bleeding, no matter how slight
- Headache
- Unexplained abdominal pain
- Changes in neurologic signs or level of consciousness

- Reporting results of PT or APTT test (see below) to physician (in case dosage needs to be adjusted)

The *international normalized ratio* (**INR**) is often given along with the PT. The INR is a worldwide standard also used to monitor anticoagulation therapy.

Partial Thromboplastin Time.   Partial thromboplastin time (**PTT**) and activated partial thromboplastin time (**APTT**) are tests used to monitor the pathway of clot formation. The APTT differs from the PTT in that the APTT uses different chemicals in the testing process that accelerate or activate the clotting factors. Defective or deficient clotting factors that may affect the PTT or APTT include factor I, II, V, VIII, IX, X, XI, and XII. The tests can identify deficiencies of the clotting factors, prothrombin, and fibrinogen.

Control or normal values for the PTT range from 60 to 90 seconds. Control or normal values for the APTT range from 25 to 27 seconds.

The PTT and APTT may be used to monitor heparin anticoagulation therapy administered via the IV or subcutaneous route. Therapeutic ranges for both tests would be 1.5 to 2.5 times the normal ranges. Too much heparin may lead to bleeding and hemorrhage. *The antidote for heparin therapy is protamine sulfate.* One milligram of protamine sulfate will reverse the effects of 100 units of heparin.

Nursing Alert

When a client is on anticoagulation therapy, a "normal lab" value may indicate *too little* warfarin (Coumadin) or heparin. Successful anticoagulation therapies require a prolonged time for either the PT (Coumadin) or the PTT/APTT (heparin).

Bleeding Time.   The *bleeding time* is a screening test used to detect platelet disorders, to evaluate for capillary defects, and to assess the client's ability to stop bleeding. It may also be referred to as an *aspirin tolerance test,* a *Duke bleeding time,* an *Ivy bleeding time,* or a *modified Ivy test.*

The bleeding time may be ordered when a family history of bleeding is known or suspected, prior to surgery to assess for hemostasis capability, and during aspirin therapy when used for anticoagulation. Normal bleeding time is 3 to 8 minutes in adults.

Other Hematologic Studies

Erythrocyte Sedimentation Rate.   The *erythrocyte sedimentation rate* (**ESR**) measures the speed (in mm/h) at which RBCs settle to the bottom of a tube of unclotted blood in 1 hour. Normal rate varies with age, sex, and testing method. Inflammation alters blood proteins, resulting in heavier than normal RBCs. The speed with which RBCs fall to the bottom of the tube corresponds to the degree of inflammation present.

Although ESR is a nonspecific test, it is useful in diagnosing infections, inflammatory processes, and autoimmune conditions. When performed in conjunction with a WBC count, the ESR can indicate infection. The ESR is also used to detect inflammatory processes, neoplasms, and necrotic processes. It can help to diagnose diseases and can be used to monitor treatment.

Blood Culture.   A *blood culture* is done to discover the presence of bacteria in the blood or to determine the antibiotics that are most effective against a specific organism.

When obtaining a blood culture, it is important to follow the parameters established by the healthcare facility and the requesting physician for the proper timing. Because this test requires special collection procedures, laboratory technicians often draw the blood.

Hospital policy may indicate that routine blood cultures be taken at certain times of the day, using specific preparations prior to the venous stick. For example, a typical physician's order may read, "Obtain blood cultures times 2 if temperature >101.5° F."

The culture should be obtained before any antibiotic therapy is started, to avoid interference with culture and sensitivity test results. A major nursing responsibility is to notify the laboratory when a client's temperature elevates so that the physician's order is followed promptly.

Bone Marrow Aspiration and Biopsy.   A *bone marrow aspiration and biopsy* is done to evaluate the number, size, and shape of RBCs, WBCs, and *megakaryocytes* (platelet precursors). The aspirate provides a sample of cells that are examined under a microscope for a biopsy determination. This test can be helpful by assisting in the diagnosis and monitoring of many disorders, such as leukemias, hemorrhagic or hemolytic anemias, aplastic anemia, Hodgkin's disease, non-Hodgkin's lymphoma, multiple myeloma, and infections (eg, mononucleosis).

The procedure uses a large-bore needle with an attached syringe. The needle is used to aspirate marrow from the sternum, iliac crest, or anterior or posterior iliac spine (or the proximal tibia in children).

Although physicians generally perform this procedure, nurses assist by ensuring that the client lies still and by providing support to the client. Post-procedure care includes applying pressure to the puncture site and observing carefully for bleeding.

Lymph Node Biopsy.   A biopsy or excision of a lymph node is often performed to diagnose or stage a tumor or to diagnose immunodeficiency disorders. Staging a tumor helps identify its invasiveness.

COMMON TREATMENTS

Transfusions of Colloid Solutions

Colloid solutions, often referred to as *plasma expanders,* are solutions used to replace circulating blood volume. Either a derivative of whole blood or a synthetic product, these solutions work by drawing interstitial fluid into the intravascular compartment. When interstitial fluid enters the intravascular compartment, the plasma fluid (of the intravascular compartment) is increased (expanded). This increase of fluid volume increases blood pressure.

Colloid solutions are given in critical or emergency situations when the client is in jeopardy due to excess loss of fluids (eg, hemorrhage due to trauma, burns, or *anasarca* [total body edema]).

Synthetic colloid products are often used if blood products are not available, if the client refuses blood products, or if the client needs supplementation to the available blood products. Synthetic plasma expanders include hetastarch (Hespan) and dextran (Macrodex, Rheomacrodex). Synthetic colloid products are economical and virus-free alternatives to blood.

Occasionally a client needs more than fluid volume replacement. The client may need hemoglobin and oxygen-carrying capacity, which is not provided by the synthetic colloid products. Recombinant human erythropoietin (EPO, Epogen, Procrit) can be given to stimulate RBC production. At least 10 days prior to surgery, the client receives erythropoietin via IM injection. Additional doses are given on the day of surgery and four days after surgery.

Transfusions of Blood and Blood Products

The intravenous (IV) administration of blood and blood components is called a *blood transfusion*. When blood or blood products from donors is used, the procedure is called an *allogenic transfusion*. A unit of blood can be transfused as whole blood. More commonly, the unit of blood is separated into separate components, which are given for specific purposes.

☛ KEY CONCEPT

In some cultures and religions, clients are not allowed to receive blood products from another person. Respect the client's beliefs.

Administering a blood transfusion involves practicing the essential principles of IV therapy. The added precautions for the administration of transfusions are listed at In Practice: Nursing Care Guidelines 81-1.

Nursing Alert

According to the policies of most healthcare facilities, two licensed personnel must identify both the client who is to receive a blood transfusion and the unit of blood itself. The client should be wearing an identification bracelet before laboratory staff draws the blood sample for type and crossmatch testing (no exceptions should be made). Misidentification of the client, or the wrong test sample or blood unit, can be fatal. Human error is responsible for most fatal transfusion reactions.

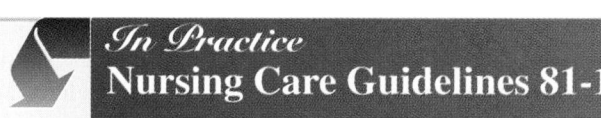

In Practice
Nursing Care Guidelines 81-1

PRECAUTIONS DURING BLOOD TRANSFUSIONS

For each unit to be given, follow all procedures for IV therapy **PLUS**:
- Obtain the unit to be infused just prior to the infusion.
- Double-check the label and the client ID with another nurse.
- Visually inspect the unit for any obvious abnormalities such as gas bubbles, unusual color, or cloudiness (which may indicate contamination or hemolysis).
- Take and record the client's baseline vital signs:
  - Just before starting transfusion
  - After the first 15 minutes of the start of the transfusion
  - Hourly during the transfusion
  - At the end of transfusion
  - 1 hour after completion of the transfusion (or as required by the facility's policy)
- Assess the client's understanding of the procedure and obtain informed consent according to the facility's policy.
- Instruct the client to report unusual symptoms immediately.
- Start the infusion slowly and remain with the client and observe for reactions during the first 15 minutes.
- Monitor the client for reactions throughout the entire transfusion.
- Provide emotional support to the client throughout the transfusion.

- Do not store blood components in nursing unit or other unmonitored refrigerator. Do not keep blood out of a monitored refrigerator for more than 30 minutes before transfusion is started.
- Do not warm blood in an unmonitored water bath, sink, or microwave oven.
- Do not allow any solution other than 0.9% normal saline to come in contact with the blood component or administration set.
- Never add medications, including those intended for IV use, to blood or components. Never infuse through the same administration set as the blood component.
- Immediately stop the infusion and report signs of hemolytic reaction including circulatory overload, sepsis, febrile reaction, allergic reaction, and acute hemolytic reaction.
- Document thoroughly, including the absence of untoward signs and symptoms.
- Return empty blood containers to the transfusion service, if this is facility policy. Many facilities discard blood containers according to a specific protocol.
- Never administer a blood component without the appropriate blood filter; change blood tubing and filter according to hospital policy.
- Do not transfuse a single unit of blood for more than 4 hours.

Adapted from Smeltzer, S., & Bare, B. (2000). *Brunner & Suddarth's textbook of medical-surgical nursing* (9th ed). Philadelphia: Lippincott Williams & Wilkins.

Blood Donation

Blood is obtained typically through blood donations. **Autologous** blood donations are self-donated; it is the safest blood for the client. Several types of autologous transfusion options are available, including preoperative autologous blood donation. Under certain criteria, blood can be collected ahead of time and used for surgery on that client. Autologous blood donations are generally limited to those surgeries that typically require blood transfusions.

Perioperative blood infusions (intraoperative blood salvage and postoperative blood salvage) can use blood that is lost during and immediately after surgical procedures. Special equipment and training is required. *Acute normovolemic hemodilution* is the removal of blood and the simultaneous infusion of other solutions to maintain intravascular volume.

Directed blood donations (designated) are from donors the client selects, such as family members or friends. Directed donations are not as safe as the client's own blood. These blood donations are not equivalent to autologous donations, but are considered as safe as any donation from a general community source.

☛ Key Concept

Even though it is rare, a blood transfusion can transmit blood-borne diseases, such as hepatitis. Tests and procedures for screening blood and selecting blood donors have improved the safety of blood transfusions. When handling tested blood, always follow Standard Precautions.

Blood Products

Whole Blood.   *Whole blood* is rarely used for transfusions today, except to treat massive acute hemorrhage. The normal circulating blood volume in an adult is approximately 6 liters (8–10 pints). Whole blood can be refrigerated for storage up to 35 days.

Packed RBCs.   *Packed RBCs* are produced by *centrifuging* (spinning) whole blood, which forces the RBCs to the bottom of the container. Packed cells can be refrigerated for storage up to 42 days, with the addition of a special preservative. They are given to clients with anemia who do not need increased circulating blood volume.

Platelet Concentrates.   *Platelet concentrates* are used to prevent or to resolve bleeding due to thrombocytopenia, or for active bleeding disorders such as disseminated intravascular coagulation (**DIC**) (discussed later in this chapter).

Fresh Frozen Plasma (FFP).   *Fresh frozen plasma* (FFP) contains unconcentrated plasma with clotting factors. It can be used to produce various derivatives and may be used to supplement infusions of packed RBCs, or for some bleeding disorders such as DIC.

Serum Albumin.   *Serum albumin* is a plasma protein that can be given in concentrated, small amounts to increase colloidal osmotic pressure by pulling interstitial fluids ("third-spaced fluids") into the intravascular compartment. Albumin is used to treat *hypovolemic shock* (low blood volume) or to replace albumin lost because of burns or kidney damage.

Cryoprecipitates.   *Cryoprecipitates* are collected from fresh plasma that has been frozen and thawed. It contains factor VIII and other clotting factors that are used to treat hemophilia and other clotting disorders.

Plasmapheresis.   *Plasmapheresis* or *apheresis* is the separation and removal of specific components of blood. The remainder of the blood is returned to the client at the time of separation. Platelets are often collected by apheresis because a larger amount of the platelets from a single donor can be collected than by separating platelets from a unit of whole blood.

Immune Globulins (Ig).   *Immune globulins* (**Ig**), a family of proteins that act as antibodies, include IgA, IgD, IgE, IgM, and IgG. IgG is the principal immunoglobulin in human serum. IgG is collected from multiple donors and may be given to a person who has been recently exposed to an infectious disease, such as hepatitis. IgD is the major component of RhoGAM, which is used to prevent erythroblastosis fetalis.

Immunoglobulins are a form of passive immunity because their effects are not permanent. Most immune globulins are given IM, except for one form, IV immune globulin.

Blood Administration

The first 10 to 15 minutes of a transfusion are the most critical, and the client must be monitored very carefully during this time. Note that if a major ABO incompatibility exists, the client will usually experience a severe reaction during the first 50 milliliters of transfusion. Therefore, take the client's baseline vital signs before the procedure, begin the transfusion very slowly, and observe the client carefully for the first 15 minutes. In Practice: Nursing Assessment 81-2 highlights the major signs and symptoms of a transfusion reaction. If any of these occur, follow the guidelines of the healthcare facility. In Practice: Nursing Care Guidelines 81-2 provides important information about managing a blood transfusion reaction.

> **Nursing Alert**
>
> Both mild and life-threatening reactions have similar symptoms. Therefore, consider every symptom as potentially serious. Discontinue the transfusion until the cause of the symptom can be determined.

Bone Marrow and Peripheral Stem Cell Transplantations

Bone marrow transplantation (**BMT**) and *peripheral blood stem cell* (**PBSC**) transplantation are treatments that can offer chances for long-term survival to clients with various diseases. The goal of BMT is to provide the client with healthy *stem cells* (immature blood cells). BMT is also discussed in Chapters 71 and 82.

Two major types of BMT are autologous and allogeneic. An *autologous* BMT is one in which the client's own bone marrow is *harvested* (collected). Cancerous cells are treated or destroyed. The BMT is placed in frozen storage and then re-infused into the client when needed.

In an **allogeneic** BMT, the client receives bone marrow from someone else. Three types of allogeneic BMT include:

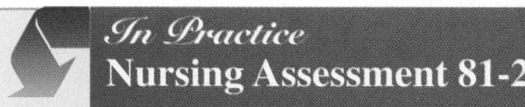

BLOOD TRANSFUSION REACTIONS

Possible signs and symptoms (changes from pre-transfusion data):

General
- Fever (rise of 1° C or 2° F)
- Chills
- Muscle aches, pain
- Back pain, chest pain
- Headache
- Heat at site of infusion or along vein

Integumentary System
- Rashes, *urticaria* (hives), swelling, itching
- *Diaphoresis* (sweating)
- Oozing at surgical site

Nervous System
- Apprehension, impending sense of doom
- Tingling, numbness

Cardiovascular System
- Change in heart rate (slower or faster)
- Change in blood pressure (lower, raised, shock)
- Changes in peripheral circulation (cyanosis, facial flushing, cool/clammy, hot/flushed/dry, edema)
- Bleeding (generalized, oozing at surgical or transfusion site)

Respiratory System
- Increased or decreased respiratory rate
- *Dyspnea* (painful breathing)
- Cough, wheezing, rales

Gastrointestinal System
- Nausea, vomiting
- Pain, abdominal cramping
- Diarrhea (may be bloody)

Urinary System
- Changes in urine volume (less, none)
- Changes in urine color (dark, concentrated, shades of red/brown/amber)

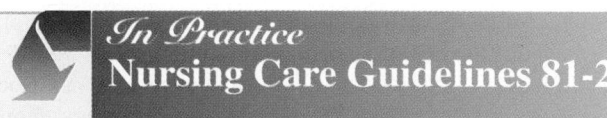

MANAGING A TRANSFUSION REACTION

If a transfusion reaction occurs:
1. STOP THE TRANSFUSION IMMEDIATELY.
2. Keep the IV open with 0.9% normal saline.
3. Report the reaction to both the transfusion service and the attending physician immediately.
4. Do clerical check at the client's bedside: identification band, blood bag, and accompanying materials.
5. Treat symptoms per physician's order and monitor vital signs.
6. Send blood bag with attached administration set and labels to the transfusion service.
7. Collect blood and urine samples and send to laboratory.
8. Document thoroughly on transfusion reaction form and in the client's chart.

---

tion is replacing BMT for most transplant procedures. Only in select cases is it still necessary to use bone marrow for stem cell collection.

Stem cell recipients may experience complications associated with the high-dose chemotherapy which is administered before the actual transplant. The most common complication is infection or sepsis. This is the result of the elimination of the body's neutrophils (which fight infection) along with the destruction of cancer cells. The client is generally placed on protective precautions until the transplanted bone marrow is producing adequate amounts of WBCs.

The use of the client's own stem cells eliminates the complication of graft-versus-host disease (**GVHD**), which can occur in clients who receive bone marrow transplants from a donor. In GVHD, the donated bone marrow attacks tissues such as the liver, skin, and the gastrointestinal (GI) tract. It can occur at any time, up to years, after a transplant. Drugs are given to suppress the risk of GVHD.

☛ KEY CONCEPT

Because matching bone marrow donors to potential recipients is so difficult, donors are always in demand. Contact the local blood bank or donor organization if you are interested in donating.

NURSING PROCESS

Data Collection

Carefully observe and assess the client with a disorder of the blood or lymph. Assess the client's skin for petechiae, bruises, or other evidence of abnormal bleeding. Measure the client's

---

- *Syngeneic*—The donor is the recipient's identical twin.
- *Related*—The donor is related to the recipient (usually a sibling).
- *Unrelated*—The donor is no relation to the recipient.

Traditionally, stem cells were harvested only from bone marrow. Now, however, stem cells can also be found and harvested from peripheral blood. Currently, PBSC transplanta-

blood pressure and pulse. Obtain a thorough nursing history that includes the client's nutritional status, dyspnea, elimination difficulties, difficulty in walking or moving, and pain. Does the person have frequent infections? Are injuries common? Signs and symptoms in these areas may indicate a blood or lymph disorder.

The nursing assessment establishes a baseline for future comparison and determines the presence of suspected blood, lymph, or other disorders. Document and report any changes in this baseline level. Hematologic studies also are important indicators of disease status. Monitor and report abnormal lab values to the physician.

In addition, observe the client's emotional response to the disorder or the disease. Some blood or lymph disorders are chronic, and some are life threatening. What types of assistance does the client require? Does he or she need counseling? Will the client need assistance to meet daily needs? Will he or she need home care? Is the client anxious or fearful about the outcome? Does he or she understand the treatment regimen?

Nursing Diagnosis

Based on data collection, nursing diagnoses are established for the client with a disorder of the blood or lymph. Some diagnoses have more than one causal factor. The following are examples of nursing diagnoses that may appear on nursing care plans of clients with blood or lymph disorders:

- Risk for Infection related to impaired immune system
- Deficient Fluid Volume related to hemorrhage
- Diarrhea related to medication side effects
- Impaired Physical Mobility related to injuries, bruising, bleeding into the tissues, fatigue
- Activity Intolerance related to leukemia, anemia, fatigue
- Disturbed Body Image related to purpura, other visible bleeding disorders
- Chronic Pain related to sickled cells, bone marrow aspiration
- Anticipatory Grieving related to chronic or fatal condition, genetic nature of disorder

Planning and Implementation

Together, plan with the client, family, and other healthcare team members for effective care that will meet the client's needs. Provide pre-test, preoperative, post-test, and postoperative care for the client undergoing procedures such as bone marrow aspiration or BMT. The client with a blood or lymph disorder may require nursing care that ranges from assistance with some daily activities to total nursing care.

In the case of a chronic, genetic, or fatal disorder, help the client and family to deal with the diagnosis, treatment course, and prognosis. Teach about the disorder, prescribed medications, precautions, and treatments to be conducted in the healthcare facility and at home. The nursing plan of care must meet these needs and include both the client and family.

Evaluation

Periodically, the entire team evaluates the outcomes of care. Have short-term goals been met? For example, are the client's laboratory test results returning to within normal parameters? Are long-term goals still realistic? Is the client's prognosis the same or has it changed? Is the client in remission? Is a long-term cure anticipated? Will home care, social services, respite care, or rehabilitation services be necessary? Planning for further nursing care and community services considers the client's prognosis, as well as complications and the response to care given.

HEMATOLOGIC SYSTEM DISORDERS

Red Blood Cell Disorders

Polycythemia

Polycythemia means too many blood cells, particularly red blood cells. Polycythemia may be relative, primary, or secondary.

In *relative polycythemia,* the client has lost *intravascular* (plasma) water but has not lost RBCs. Thus, the numbers of RBCs are higher in relation to the fluid in which the RBCs are found. This condition may occur with dehydration or with excess use of diuretics. Relative polycythemia is treated by increasing total fluid volume by oral or IV fluid intake.

Primary polycythemia is often referred to as **polycythemia vera.** With this disorder, the total numbers of RBCs, WBC, and platelets are increased. It is generally seen in men between 40 and 60 years of age.

Secondary polycythemia is the result of an increase in the hormone *erythropoietin,* which stimulates RBC production. The reason for the stimulus to increase RBC production is hypoxia. Causes of hypoxia and resulting polycythemia include smoking, heart and lung disease, and living at high altitudes.

The client appears dusky red to cyanotic, especially the lips, fingernails, and mucous membranes. Hypertension is common. The client may have headaches, difficulty hearing, and inability to concentrate. Night sweats, itching, and pain in the fingers or toes are common complaints.

Treatment for primary and secondary polycythemia is necessary because the numbers of RBCs and other cells increase the thickness (*viscosity*) of the blood. Headaches, anginal (chest) pain, and difficulty breathing relate to hypoxia and/or occlusions of blood vessels. Hemorrhage, hypertension, and thrombosis (including CVAs, MIs, and deep-vein thrombosis) can occur.

Oxygen therapy is generally initiated to relieve hypoxia. To reduce blood viscosity, the client may have regularly scheduled phlebotomy blood withdrawals on an outpatient basis. The therapeutic phlebotomy will reduce total RBCs and total blood volume. If the disorder is severe, chemotherapy may be given to suppress bone marrow function, thereby reducing the total numbers of RBCs, WBCs, and platelets.

Nursing considerations relate to the effects of hypoxia on the body systems. Client and family teaching should include the awareness of complications of polycythemia, as well as the treatments for the disorder. Encourage fluids, and monitor RBC and WBC counts.

Anemias

Anemia, one of the most common hematologic problems affecting people of all ages, is defined as a condition of a lower than normal level of hemoglobin, and fewer than normal RBCs within the circulation. Anemia is not considered a disease in itself. Rather, it reflects an abnormality in the number, structure, or function of RBCs. Anemia can be a manifestation of many abnormal conditions:

- Dietary deficiencies of iron, vitamin B_{12}, and folic acid
- Bone marrow damage as a result of chemotherapy, radiation, or renal disease
- Malignancies
- Chronic infections
- Overactive spleen
- Bleeding from any organ or tract, or bleeding due to cancer or trauma
- Hereditary disorders (eg, sickle cell disease, thalassemia)

The incidence of anemia is more common in underdeveloped countries because of poor nutrition and the presence of parasites that extract blood from the intestines. Studies suggest that older adults experience a higher incidence of anemia. This finding, however, is not caused by aging alone, but by some other underlying cause.

The seriousness of anemia depends on factors such as its speed of onset, whether it is chronic, and the client's overall health and nutritional status. The more rapidly anemia develops, the more serious it is likely to be.

Signs and Symptoms. Signs and symptoms of anemia relate to the loss of oxygen-carrying capacity, the severity of hypoxia, and the causative factors. Some types of anemia develop slowly so the symptoms are insidious (develops slowly).

Several types of anemia exist, but the signs and symptoms are essentially the same for all. They include any or most of the following:

- Pallor and hypersensitivity to cold
- Fatigue and exercise intolerance
- Dizziness and weakness
- Symptoms of congestive heart failure
- Gastrointestinal complaints (eg, indigestion, loss of appetite)
- Jaundice
- Rapid pulse (heart tries to compensate for lack of oxygen to cells)
- Shortness of breath
- Irritability
- Difficulty sleeping
- Difficulty concentrating
- Menstrual problems; male impotence
- Decreased hemoglobin, hematocrit
- Hypotension
- Bone pain and sternal tenderness (related to increased erythropoietin activity in bone marrow)

Diagnostic Tests. Diagnostic tests include the standard CBC, Hgb and Hct. The simplest method of diagnosing anemia is by determining the blood's Hgb content. Mild anemia is generally diagnosed when the Hgb drops to 10 to 12 g/dL (grams per deciliter). Severe anemia would be indicated by a drop of Hgb to less than 8 g/dL.

Types of Anemia

Iron Deficiency Anemia. Iron deficiency anemia is the most prevalent anemia in all age groups in the world. It results from either an inadequate absorption or an excessive loss of iron. This condition occurs most often in women, young children, and older adults. Primary causes include trauma, excessive menses, bleeding from the gastrointestinal tract, pregnancy, or a diet that lacks iron. Deficiency caused by faulty eating habits is especially prevalent in the adolescent and elderly populations.

Treatment for iron deficiency anemia includes treating the site of blood loss, increasing dietary iron intake, and introducing supplemental iron. In Practice: Nursing Care Guidelines 81-3 and In Practice: Nursing Care Plan 81-1 highlight important considerations when administering iron supplements to any client.

Hemolytic Anemia. Hemolytic anemia is caused by destruction of RBCs prior to their normal lifespan of about 120 days. The client will have an increase of immature RBCs (reticulocytes). Manifestations of hypoxemia symptoms relate to the impaired transport of oxygen and include dyspnea and limited exercise tolerance. The cause of hemolytic anemia is related to defects of the cell membrane of the RBC, inherited enzyme defects, certain drugs and toxins, antibodies, or physical trauma. Treatment of this type of anemia relates to diagnosis and to the causative factors. Corticosteroid hormones and splenectomy may also be of benefit.

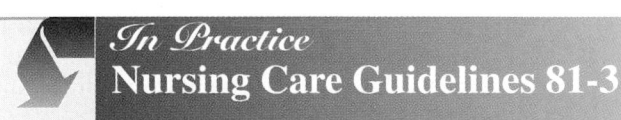

In Practice
Nursing Care Guidelines 81-3

ADMINISTERING IRON SUPPLEMENTS

- Give oral iron preparations with meals.
  Rationale: Iron is irritating to the gastrointestinal tract; it can have an unpleasant metallic taste and is easier to take if given with food.
- Administer Iron dextran (InFeD) deep IM or IV when oral administration is ineffective or impossible.
- Give citrus juices with the iron preparation.
  Rationale: Vitamin C enhances absorption of iron.
- Administer liquid iron through a straw.
  Rationale: Use of a straw avoids discoloring teeth and minimizes unpleasant taste.
- Explain to the client that iron will make stools black, and might cause constipation. Stool softeners may be prescribed.

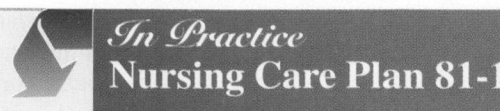

In Practice
Nursing Care Plan 81-1

THE CLIENT WITH IRON DEFICIENCY ANEMIA WHO IS RECEIVING IRON THERAPY

MEDICAL HISTORY: *S.H. is a 32-year-old female who comes to the clinic for a routine visit. During the visit, client reports a history of heavy menstrual bleeding. Complete blood count reveals a hemoglobin level of 10.1 g/dL and RBC count of 3.7 million/mm³. Client is scheduled for a dilation and curettage (D&C) in 3 days. Ferrous sulfate 300 mg is ordered three times a day.*

MEDICAL DIAGNOSIS: *Iron deficiency anemia*

Data Collection/Nursing Assessment: Client's skin is pale, warm, and dry. Mucous membranes and conjunctiva pale. Dietary history reveals adequate intake although client states, "I'm not a big fan of fruits and vegetables." Client asks, "I haven't had to take any medicines except for something for an occasional headache. What is this medication that the doctor has put me on and why?" (*Although other nursing diagnoses may be appropriate, a priority nursing diagnosis is addressed below.*)

Nursing Diagnosis: Deficient knowledge related to iron deficiency anemia and iron therapy as evidenced by client's questions.

Planning
SHORT-TERM GOALS:
#1. Client identifies reason for iron therapy.
#2. Client verbalizes accurate information about iron therapy regimen.

LONG-TERM GOALS:
#3. Client's hemoglobin level rises to within acceptable parameters following initiation of iron therapy and following D&C.

Implementation
NURSING ACTION: *Assess client's current knowledge of iron deficiency anemia and possible causes.*
RATIONALE: *Obtaining a baseline knowledge assessment provides a foundation for further teaching.*

NURSING ACTION: *Explore with client the possible factors contributing to development of iron deficiency anemia.*
RATIONALE: *Chronic blood loss, such as from excessive menses, and inadequate dietary intake of high-iron foods, such as green leafy vegetables, can contribute to iron deficiency anemia.*

NURSING ACTION: *Review rationale for and action of ferrous sulfate.*
RATIONALE: *Ferrous sulfate improves red blood cell formation and replaces iron stores.*

Evaluation: Client reports, "I don't eat as many vegetables as I should and I can see how the loss of blood with my periods would be a problem." *Progress to meeting Goal #1.*

NURSING ACTION: *Assist client with setting up a schedule for taking iron, based on usual activities. Encourage client to take the iron 1 hour before or 2 hours after meals or with meals if stomach upset occurs.*
RATIONALE: *Assisting client with scheduling medication aids in promoting compliance. Taking iron on an empty stomach enhances absorption. However, taking the medication with food can help to reduce irritation to the gastrointestinal tract.*

NURSING ACTION: *Encourage client to take iron with a citrus food or fluid.*
RATIONALE: *The acidity of the citrus food or fluid enhances absorption of the iron.*

Evaluation: Client states, "I'll try before my meals first, but if my stomach gets upset, I'll take the medication with food." Client able to verbalize appropriate choices for citrus foods and fruits. *Goal #1 met; progress to meeting Goal #2.*

NURSING ACTION: *Warn client that the iron can cause constipation, and stools to become black and tarry. Recommend the intake of high-fiber foods to help with constipation.*
RATIONALE: *The client needs to be informed of these common side effects to prevent unnecessary anxiety and possible interruption in therapy. High-fiber foods promote peristalsis.*

NURSING ACTION: *Assist client with scheduling a return followup visit in 2 to 3 weeks.*
RATIONALE: *A return visit helps to determine client's compliance with and effectiveness of therapy.*

Evaluation: Client to return in 2 weeks for followup testing and examination; has clinic phone number to call in case of problems. She states, "I won't worry if my stool looks black. And I'll eat a salad every day for lunch now." *Goal #2 met; progress to meeting Goal #3.*

Acute Hemorrhagic Anemia.   Acute hemorrhagic anemia develops after a rapid and often sudden blood loss. Causes of such blood loss include trauma that leads to blood vessel rupture, aneurysm, or artery erosion caused by a cancerous lesion or ulcer.

Severity and prognosis depend on the total blood volume loss. A total blood volume loss of 20% is considered a marked insufficiency. A loss of 30% will cause failure in the circulatory system, coma, and shock. A loss that reaches 40% can be imminently fatal. In hypovolemic shock, the priority concern is related to the client's needs for fluids to sustain blood pressure. When fluid loss is controlled, the hypoxia due to the loss of RBCs must also be treated.

Immediate treatment is volume replacement, often with administration of IV fluids, such as saline, albumin, or plasma, and transfusions with fresh whole blood.

Chronic Hemorrhagic Anemia.   Chronic hemorrhagic anemia is usually the result of conditions such as peptic ulcers, bleeding hemorrhoids, excessive emesis, or cancerous lesions in the gastrointestinal tract. Chronic blood loss can eventually lead to iron-deficiency anemia because available iron sources are depleted.

Treatment usually includes controlling the site of bleeding and replacing lost iron through diet and supplements.

Pernicious Anemia.   Pernicious anemia is caused by a lack of a gastric substance called intrinsic factor, which is produced in the stomach. The body needs intrinsic factor to absorb vitamin B_{12} from food in the small intestine. Vitamin B_{12} is necessary for the body's proper absorption and use of iron and the protection of nerve fibers.

Pernicious anemia generally affects middle-aged and older adults of northern European descent. Juvenile pernicious anemia, a rare congenital disorder in which the stomach secretes abnormal intrinsic factor, generally affects children under the age of 10 years.

Pernicious anemia develops slowly; therefore, signs and symptoms are usually severe when a diagnosis is finally made. Early signs and symptoms include infection, mood swings, gastrointestinal disorders, and cardiac and renal problems. Late classic signs and symptoms include weakness, fatigue, tingling and numbness of the fingers and feet, sore tongue, difficulty walking, abdominal pain, and loss of appetite and weight.

Dietary modifications alone are ineffective. The client must take vitamin B_{12} (cyanocobalamin, Ener-B) for life by injection. Clients cannot take vitamin B_{12} orally because they lack the intrinsic factor necessary for absorption. Additionally, clients may receive iron supplements, folic acid, and digestants to enhance vitamin metabolism. Sometimes, blood transfusions are also necessary.

Aplastic Anemia.   Aplastic anemia or bone marrow depression, describes a condition in which the bone marrow is underdeveloped or has failed, resulting in a decrease in RBCs, WBCs, and platelets (**pancytopenia**). This condition may occur at any age and develop very slowly or be rapid and very severe.

Causes may include excessive radiation, toxicity to various drugs (eg, chloramphenicol and many anticancer drugs), tumors, insecticides, chemicals, and environmental toxins. It

may develop as a complication of viral illnesses such as hepatitis, HIV/AIDS, and mononucleosis. In many cases the cause is unknown (idiopathic aplastic anemia). Some researchers believe that some cases of aplastic anemia may be autoimmune in origin.

Bone marrow or stem cell transplantation is the most successful therapy. Without transplantation, aplastic anemia has a poor prognosis and a high mortality rate. Prognosis improves dramatically when a stem cell transplant can be done. Antibiotics and transfusions may be given as palliative treatments.

The client with aplastic anemia is extremely susceptible to infection and bleeding. The following measures should be included in nursing care:

- Administering antibiotics per the physician's orders.
- Following sterile technique in all invasive procedures.
- Handling the client carefully.
- Cautioning the client to avoid bruises and cuts. *Rationale: This client has a strong bleeding tendency.*
- Not taking rectal temperatures.
- Using protective isolation during exacerbations of the disease (see Chap. 42).

Sickle Cell Disease
Sickle cell disease is a genetic disease in which the person's RBCs become crescent or sickle shaped when exposed to decreased oxygen (Fig. 81-1). Chapter 71 discusses this disease in more detail.

Sickled cells cannot carry as much oxygen as normal cells. Then, the sickled RBCs become more sickled from a lack of oxygen. Sickle cell anemia develops due to hypoxemia and damaged RBCs. When sickled RBCs can enter the smaller blood vessels, they become caught, obstructing blood flow. Hypoxia ensues, which in turn causes more sickling.

Sickle cell crisis occurs when the deformed RBCs collect (*aggregate*) in small blood vessels. These occlusions are painful due to the hypoxic state of the affected tissues. Permanent damage to organs can develop.

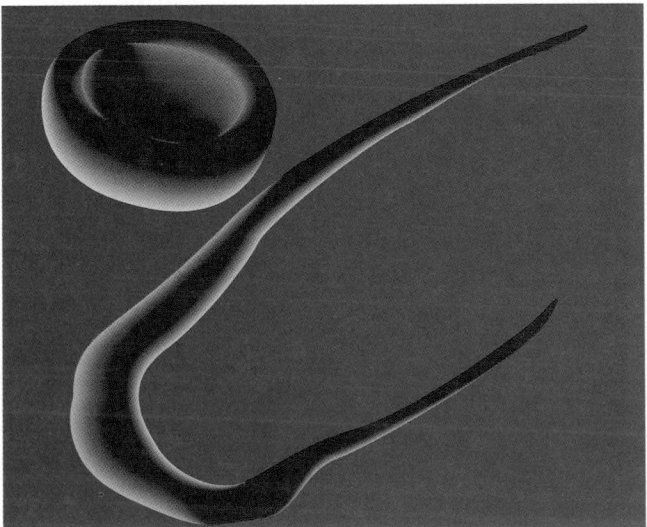

FIGURE 81-1. A sickled and a normal red blood cell.

Symptoms of crisis include severe and unpredictable pain in the extremities and abdomen, jaundice, skin irritation and ulceration, fever, dyspnea, cough, swelling of the hands and feet, and increased infections. Severity of these symptoms relates directly to the percentage of abnormal cells (Hemoglobin S [Hgb S]).

The goal of treatment is to prevent sickle cell crisis. When anemia or crisis does occur, RBC transfusions are the normal therapy. Some clients may be treated with iron-chelating agents to remove excess iron from the blood and to counteract iron overload. Some *cytotoxic* agents (agents that destroy specific cells) are also used in sickle cell disease.

Thalassemia

Thalassemia is an anemia characterized by deficient and damaged chains of Hgb. The thalassemias consist of two main groups of inherited hemolytic anemias caused by autosomal recessive genes. The two categories are alpha-thalassemia and beta-thalassemia. Depending on the number of genes affected, beta-thalassemia may be classified as either minor or major.

Alpha-thalassemia is most common among people of Chinese, Vietnamese, Cambodian, and Laotian descent. Alpha-thalassemia has many varieties, from asymptomatic carriers to infants who are severely hypoxic and are stillborn or die shortly after birth. *Beta-thalassemia* is most common among people of Greek, Italian, and Jewish descent. Both types are common among African Americans.

The signs and symptoms of anemia are related to the severity of the disease. *Thalassemia minor* does not affect a person's life expectancy. Mild anemias may be noted. The client generally has few changes of RBCs.

Thalassemia major, also known as *Cooley's anemia,* is more serious and requires frequent transfusions. Without treatment, signs and symptoms start in infancy, and include fever, failure to thrive, and enlarged spleen. Rapid destruction of RBCs frees large amounts of iron, which can be deposited in the skin, heart, liver, and pancreas. With treatment, the individual's life span is two or three decades.

Growth and sexual development are usually impaired. The heart, liver, and pancreas become fibrotic and lose their capability to function. Congestive heart failure may occur. Signs of thalassemia major also include those of other hemolytic anemias.

Treatment consists of transfusion therapy with packed RBCs. Because these clients receive many transfusions, they are also at risk for iron overload. Bone marrow transplants offer some clients a cure.

☞ KEY CONCEPT

Clients who carry the genetic trait for thalassemia (sickle cell disease) should be referred for genetic counseling.

White Blood Cell Disorders

Neutropenia and Agranulocytosis

Neutropenia, also known as *granulocytopenia,* is a decrease in neutrophils, one of the forms of leukocytes. Severe neutrope-

nia is referred to as *agranulocytosis, granulocytopenia,* or *malignant neutropenia.* Agranulocytosis implies severe reductions of basophils and eosinophils, as well as neutrophils.

Neutropenia can be acquired or congenital. The majority of cases of neutropenia are the result of cytotoxic drugs used in cancer therapy, such as alkylating agents and antimetabolites, which are designed to suppress bone marrow function in clients with types of leukemias and lymphomas. Radiation therapies for cancer can also cause neutropenia.

Drugs other than the antineoplastic drugs can cause toxic idiosyncratic side effects that result in neutropenia. Examples of these drugs include barbiturates, phenothiazine tranquilizers, chloramphenicol (Chloromycetin), certain antipsychotic drugs such as clozapine (Clozaril), and sulfonamides.

Idiopathic cases (of unknown cause) of neutropenia may be related to autoimmune disorders in which antibodies react against the normal human leukocyte antigens (HLA) on WBCs.

Agranulocytosis may also be seen in aplastic anemia. Agranulocytosis can also develop during the course of another disease or from an overwhelming infection.

Signs and symptoms include infection (usually respiratory), chills, fever, headache, malaise, extreme weakness, and fatigue. Bleeding may occur from ulcerations of the mucous membrane on any part of the GI tract, vaginal areas, or skin.

Treatment begins by removing the causative agent. Colony stimulating factor (**CSF**) may be given to stimulate the production, maturation, and differentiation of neutrophils.

Providing protective precautions is an important nursing consideration. Because WBCs are depleted, the person is more susceptible to infection, especially respiratory infections. Extreme care is necessary to protect this person against exposure to pathogens. Antibiotics may be ordered. If the cause is not a neoplastic disorder, bone marrow function may resume in 2 to 3 weeks after the cause is eliminated or resolved.

Leukemia

Leukemia is a malignant hematologic disorder that is characterized by an abundance of abnormal WBCs. Chapter 71 discusses leukemia in more detail.

In leukemia, the factors that normally regulate the process by which cells differentiate and mature are lacking. The type of leukemia depends on which cell line is affected: *lymphoid* or *myeloid.*

Leukemias can also be diagnosed as acute or chronic. In *acute* forms of leukemia, immature cells proliferate and accumulate in the person's bone marrow. In *chronic leukemia,* apparently mature cells become diseased.

With both types of leukemias, abnormal cells take over the normal marrow. The leukemic cells can also be released into the peripheral blood, invading body organs.

Symptom management related to treatment, infection and bleeding precautions, nutritional evaluation and monitoring, and transfusion therapy evaluation and precautions are key elements of nursing care. Clients with leukemia require many treatments, procedures, tests, and frequent hospitalizations. Remember to include the client and family in the plan of care.

In Practice: Educating the Client 81-1 highlights important topic areas to address. Emotional strain is the effect of this disease on the client and family. Provide therapeutic communication techniques to support the client and family. Refer the client and the family to spiritual leaders, social services, and support groups during the course of the disease and treatment.

Acute Leukemias. *Acute leukemias* are generally severe and aggressive. They are characterized by a rapid onset and course. The two types of acute leukemias are *acute lymphoid* (*lymphocytic* or *lymphoblastic*) *leukemia* (**ALL**) and *acute myeloid* (*monoblastic* or *myelogenous*) *leukemia* (**AML**). ALL is most common in children; AML is most common in adults.

Symptoms of ALL result from anemia, neutropenia, and thrombocytopenia. They can include fevers, malaise, fatigue, bone pain, bruising, and bleeding. Clients also may present with enlarged lymph nodes and spleen and liver involvement.

The symptoms of AML also relate to the rapid expansion of leukemic cells. Anemia is generally noted on presentation. Affected individuals usually experience recurrent infections that fail to respond to antibiotics. Clients are nearly always symptomatic when diagnosed with AML, which is not always true for clients with ALL.

Chronic Leukemias. The two forms of *chronic leukemia* are *chronic lymphoid leukemia* (**CLL**) and *chronic myeloid leukemia* (**CML**). Unlike acute leukemias, the WBCs in chronic leukemia appear to be mature but are malignant. The disease progresses slowly; rapid, aggressive onset is rare.

In many cases, CLL is discovered routinely. Clients may present with symptoms such as malaise, anorexia, fatigue, enlarged lymph nodes, and enlarged spleen. Signs and symptoms usually include fatigue, night sweats, anemia, shortness of breath, weight loss, and tenderness over the sternum.

Treatment for CLL and CML are individual or combined therapies of antineoplastic drugs, radiation, and bone marrow transplants. These therapies are discussed in Chapter 71.

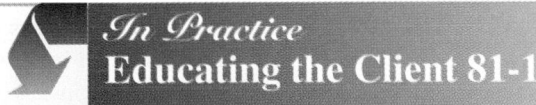

**In Practice
Educating the Client 81-1**

TEACHING TOPIC AREAS FOR LEUKEMIA

- Signs and symptoms of infection and bleeding
- Precautions to avoid infections
- Precautions to prevent tissue damage and bleeding:
  - Good mouth care
  - Use of soft toothbrush only
  - Avoidance of constipation
  - Avoidance of aspirin-containing products
- Good nutrition
- Avoidance of smoking and alcohol
- Possible side effects of chemotherapy and other treatment

Platelets and Clotting Disorders

Platelet disorders can include too many thrombocytes (*thrombocythemia*) and too few thrombocytes (*thrombocytopenia*).

Thrombocythemia

In many cases of *thrombocythemia,* the disease is not detected or may not be treated unless symptoms occur. The platelet counts are greater than 600,000/mm³ and can run as high as one million/mm³. Because the platelets are dysfunctional, hemorrhage and *vasoocclusion* (obstruction of blood vessels) are the primary concerns. Causative risk factors include smoking, peripheral vascular disease, atherosclerosis, and the previous formation of thrombi.

Treatment may be low-dose aspirin therapy or aggressive medications such as hydroxyurea (Hydria) or anagrelide (Agrylin). Both of these medications have significant side effects. Nursing concerns relate to the risks of hemorrhage and the formation of thrombi.

Thrombocytopenia

Thrombocytopenia, a stem cell disorder of the bone marrow, is diagnosed when a client's platelet count falls below 50,000/mm³. It is the most frequent platelet complication of cancer and its treatments. Several types of thrombocytopenia exist.

Idiopathic Thrombocytopenia Purpura (ITP). Idiopathic thrombocytopenic purpura (**ITP**) is one type of thrombocytopenia that can develop at any age, but tends to occur more often in children and young women. The two forms of the disorder are acute and chronic. The acute form usually occurs in children. *Chronic ITP* is usually diagnosed in adults aged 20 to 50 years, with a higher incidence in women.

Acute ITP commonly occurs after a viral illness in children. Thus it may be an autoimmune disorder in which the individual develops antibodies to his or her own platelets. The exact cause remains unknown. ITP may also accompany HIV infection, malignant disease, systemic lupus erythematosus, or pregnancy.

Early signs may include bruises and low platelet counts. *Petechiae* (small hemorrhagic spots in the skin), headache, pain, and swelling, as well as any abnormal bleeding such as from the nose, gums, and gastrointestinal and urinary tracts, may be noted. The severity of ITP depends on the degree of the thrombocytopenia and the extent of the bleeding.

Treatment for ITP is generally corticosteroids. If a drug is the suspected cause (eg, quinine, sulfa-containing medications) the medication is discontinued. A splenectomy may be done. However, the effects of this surgery tend to be limited and transient.

Intravenous gamma globulin is commonly given for ITP. Some clients who are Rh-positive may receive anti-D antibodies against the D antigen. Platelet transfusions may actually result in a further drop in platelet count, but they may be beneficial to a client who is hemorrhaging.

Nursing considerations are similar to those for all blood and bleeding disorders. Obtain a thorough medication history, including over-the-counter medications and sulfa-containing drugs. Because the client may be on corticosteroids, teaching about the tapering regimen may be indicated. Straining with the passage of stool (*Valsalva maneuver*) and constipation should be avoided. Electric razors and soft toothbrushes should be used. Client and family teaching should include information about assessing the client's risk of injury. The client and family need to be aware of the appearance of petechiae, *ecchymosis* (purplish patches), or excessive menses.

✚👁 N u r s i n g   A l e r t

Because blood does not clot correctly in clients with bleeding disorders, even a slight injury can result in a serious hemorrhage. Watch for signs of internal bleeding, such as unusual pallor, rapid pulse, restlessness, and a drop in blood pressure. Protect these clients against injury.

Disseminated Intravascular Coagulation

Disseminated intravascular coagulation (DIC) is a complex and potentially fatal disorder in which clotting occurs in the microvascular system and, at the same time, hemorrhaging develops. It is not a disease, but a result of serious defects in clotting mechanisms related to underlying disorders.

Multiple conditions can cause DIC, including shock, acute bacterial and viral infections, septicemia, hemolytic transfusion reactions, tissue damage from trauma or burns, transplant rejections, various cancers, and complications of obstetrics. The mortality rate for DIC is high.

The disorder usually has a rapid onset, further adding to its severity. Signs of DIC may include petechiae, ecchymosis, or prolonged bleeding from a venipuncture site. Onset may also include severe and uncontrollable hemorrhage.

Treatment of DIC involves the identification of the underlying cause. Symptomatic treatment involves administration of IV fluids, oxygen, and the administration of various clotting factors. Some treatments and agents used to stop the abnormal clotting mechanisms are controversial or investigational.

Heparin, which in most instances is used to prolong bleeding times, may be given. Although somewhat controversial, heparin therapy can inhibit the formation of microthrombi and prevent organ damage. When heparin is initially started, the bleeding may worsen temporarily. Signs of success with heparin are that the abnormal clotting mechanisms of DIC will decrease.

Nursing considerations related to DIC include the awareness of the risk factors. This process may begin suddenly with little or no warning. Clients at risk will need to be closely monitored for signs and symptoms of bleeding, signs of shock, and the formation of thrombi (eg, CVA). Nursing care of the client experiencing DIC will vary depending on severity.

Hemophilia

Hemophilia is a sex-linked genetic disorder in which the person's blood is slow to coagulate due to lack of factor VIII

(*hemophilia A* or *classic hemophilia*) or factor IX (*hemophilia B* or *Christmas disease*) in the plasma. About one third of new hemophilia cases occur without family history of the disease, which suggests new mutations to the gene. Additional information about hemophilia is also presented in Chapter 71.

Almost all affected individuals are males. Children with hemophilia are generally healthy, but are always at risk for bleeding. Severity of bleeding relates to the level of deficiency of the clotting factor.

Unchecked bleeding may be severe. In clients with hemophilia, even a pinprick may cause prolonged oozing of blood. The most minor surgical procedure is risky and is usually preceded by a transfusion of the appropriate blood factor.

Treatment of hemophilia focuses primarily on the prevention of bleeding episodes. When a bleeding episode occurs, treatment involves the replacement of the deficient clotting factor. Recombinant DNA technology has produced safe, virus-free factor VIII. Recombinant DNA is relatively expensive. Clotting factors can be given in the home or at outpatient centers.

Factor VIII gene has been cloned and may eventually be used as part of a cure for hemophilia via gene replacement therapy.

Nursing considerations include awareness of the potential impact of any tiny cut or bruise. Dental work may require special bleeding precautions. Continuously assess the family's needs, and include the family in the plan of care. Key areas of teaching include:

- Maintenance of safety
- Injury prevention
- Lifestyle changes to meet the client's limitations
- Medication teaching
- Methods of administering factor VIII concentrate at home, if appropriate

Lymphatic System Disorders

Malignant lymphomas are a diverse group of diseases that arise from an uncontrolled proliferation of cellular components of the lymphatic system. The lymphomas are divided into two major groups: Hodgkin's disease and non-Hodgkin's lymphoma. Clinical manifestations in both types are similar.

Hodgkin's Disease

Hodgkin's disease **(HD),** the most common cancer occurring in young adults, is slightly more common in men. HD has a high cure rate.

HD studies suggest that it may be related to viral infections and suppressed immune systems. HD may be a result of an autoimmune disorder. Epstein-Barr virus (EBV) is a virus that may be one etiology agent. However, definitive cause or causes are not known.

Painless, enlarged lymph nodes is the common finding in HD. Depending on the age of onset, a particular area seems to be affected first. Then HD travels to other lymphatic sites via the lymphatic network.

Progressive, painless lymph node enlargement continues unless the disease is diagnosed and treated. The client will demonstrate low-grade fever, fatigue, night sweats, itching, anemia, and unexplained weight loss. If the disease is allowed to advance, major organs such as the lungs and liver, the GI tract, and the central nervous system become involved. The individual becomes unable to fight infections.

Diagnosis is made by a biopsy study showing Reed-Sternberg cells in lymph node tissue. (Reed-Sternberg cells may also be found in infectious mononucleosis.) After HD has been diagnosed, *staging* (the extent of disease) must be determined. CT scans, x-ray examinations, lymphangiography, and gallium scans may be done to assist in diagnosis.

Staging will influence the client's treatment decisions. HD spreads in an organized pattern, traveling from one node to another. The criteria for each stage is the number of lymph nodes involved, if the lymph nodes are involved on one or both sides of the diaphragm, and the extent of spread of the disease to the bone marrow or liver (Box 81-1).

Treatment for HD generally includes radiation, chemotherapy, or a combination of both. Stem cell transplantation may also be considered treatment, especially in those who have experienced recurrences. The prognosis for HD depends on the disease's stage at diagnosis. Generally, 60% to 70% of those who achieve complete remission after treatment will be cured.

Research has shown long-term complications for individuals who have had chemotherapies and radiation. This data is developed from the high numbers of cured HD clients. Long-term complications of therapy for Hodgkin's disease include immune dysfunction, herpes infections, acute myeloid leukemia, non-Hodgkin's lymphoma, solid tumors, thyroid cancer, cardiomyopathy, infertility, and impotence. The potential for these serious disorders is weighed against the benefits of cure for HD. Revised treatment protocols in the future may limit the development of complications.

➤➤ **BOX 81-1**

ANN ARBOR STAGING CLASSIFICATION OF HODGKIN'S DISEASE

Modifications of this type of staging are used to classify the severity of the disease as well as to indicate the appropriate mode of therapy.

STAGE I: The disease is limited to a single node or single extralymphatic site.

STAGE II: The disease involves more than a single node, but is confined to one side of the diaphragm.

STAGE III: The disease is present both above and below the diaphragm.

STAGE IV: The disease has extended to one or more extralymphatic organs or tissues.

Nursing considerations are similar to other cancers and are often related to symptomatic relief of the side effects of treatment (eg, nausea, vomiting, hair loss) (see Chap. 82).

Non-Hodgkin's Lymphoma

Non-Hodgkin's lymphoma (**NHL**) is a group of lymphatic neoplasms. Classifications of NHL include low grade, intermediate grade, high grade, T-cell, and Burkitt's.

In contrast to HD, which initially is localized to a single area of nodes, NHL has malignant lymphoid cells that infiltrate in many areas and are unpredictable. Multiple lymph nodes may be infiltrated, as well as tissues outside the lymphoid system, especially the liver, spleen, and bone marrow.

As with HD, the cause of NHL is unknown. The most respected theory is that an immune abnormality causes NHL. In some types of NHL, this abnormality is thought to result from a virus (such as HIV). Exposure to some drugs, such as chemotherapy for previous cancer, has also been associated with a higher risk of NHL.

The most common finding in NHL is a painless, enlarged, single lymph node in the neck. However, other lymph nodes may be affected. Other symptoms include abdominal discomfort, back pain, and gastrointestinal complaints, all of which result from node enlargement. The client with NHL may also experience night sweats, fever, and weight loss.

Diagnosis for NHL is achieved with lymph node biopsy, bone marrow biopsy, and blood studies. CT scans and nuclear medicine studies may be added to determine the stage of the disease.

Treatment for NHL consists of chemotherapy, radiation, or a combination of both. Bone marrow transplantation and peripheral stem cell transplantation may be used.

Nursing considerations for clients with HD or NHL include teaching related to the disease process, treatment options, and possible side effects. Always include the client and family in care. As with leukemia, psychosocial issues and emotional support must be of prime importance.

Multiple Myeloma

Multiple myeloma is a malignant cancer of bone marrow in which the *plasma cells* (the most mature form of B lympho-

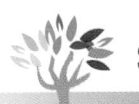

SPECIAL CONSIDERATIONS: THE LIFE SPAN

Hodgkin's Disease and Non-Hodgkin's Lymphoma

The older adult with either of these conditions may experience altered or impaired renal, cardiac, hepatic, or respiratory function caused by the aging process. Remember that many of the treatment options for HD and NHL may also cause impairment of these organs. Monitor these clients carefully. Dose, schedule, or treatment changes and limitations may be indicated.

cytes) proliferate, causing bone pain and anemia. Multiple myeloma is not considered a lymphoma.

It occurs mostly in the middle-aged to older adult population, affecting males more than females. The etiology is unknown and the onset may be *insidious* (slow). The individual may be without symptoms until the disease is advanced. The survival rate is 3 to 5 years after diagnosis. Infection is the usual cause of death.

Signs and Symptoms.   Signs and symptoms of typical multiple myeloma include fractures and hypercalcemia with skeletal deformities. Fatigue and weakness due to anemia occur. The hypercalcemia may lead to excessive thirst, dehydration, constipation, altered LOC, confusion, and coma. Renal failure is possible.

Diagnosis.   Diagnosis is made by detection of monoclonal protein (M-protein) via electrophoresis of serum or urine. The client has an elevated total blood protein. Bone destruction leads to bone pain (especially back pain) that increases with movement; osteoporosis; and fractures. Anemia develops as the bone marrow is destroyed. The individual can become *hypercalcemic* (too much calcium in the blood) due to the excess amounts of calcium lost from bone destruction. X-ray examinations show bone destruction.

Treatment.   Treatment may include combinations of chemotherapy, corticosteroids, and radiation. Radiation is not effective alone in multiple myeloma because the plasma cells proliferate. Tumors can occur in several sites. Bone marrow transplantation can be helpful, even curative, in some clients. Interferon-α can help maintain remissions.

Nursing Considerations.   Nursing considerations focus on pain management, hydration, and prompt detection of fever or other signs of infection. The purpose of plasma cells is to make immunoglobulins, which provide protection against antigens. Without these immunoglobulins, any infection can be life threatening. Client and family teaching will include instructions on activity restrictions (eg, lifting no more than 10 pounds; proper body mechanics). Braces for support are occasionally used. The client generally can control the disease and live a relatively normal lifestyle for many years.

⤚ STUDENT SYNTHESIS

Key Points

- The nurse must be aware of the normal and abnormal laboratory values for common tests of RBCs, WBCs, and platelets.
- Transfusions of blood products require careful identification of recipients, infusion techniques, and followup monitoring.
- Hematologic system disorders frequently manifest by fatigue, bleeding tendencies, infections, and cardiovascular complications.
- Anemias deprive a person of energy and oxygen to carry out the activities of daily living. Treatment of

anemias is designed toward elimination of the causative factor and management of symptoms.
- Sickle cell disease and thalassemia are inherited disorders involving dysfunctional hemoglobin.
- White blood cell disorders affect a person's ability to fight infections.
- Neutropenia is a common side effect of antineoplastic drugs.
- All types of leukemia are generally treated by chemotherapy, radiation, bone marrow transplant, or a combination of these.
- Blood disorders affecting clotting factors can cause serious and life-threatening bleeding problems. Bleeding disorders may result from damage to bone marrow by environmental toxins, autoimmune disorders, or chemotherapy for cancers.
- A major difference in Hodgkin's disease and non-Hodgkin's lymphoma is that Hodgkin's disease initially affects one lymphatic area, while NHL affects many areas.
- An older client with complaints of back pain with movement, hypercalcemia, and fractures should be tested for multiple myeloma.

Critical Thinking Exercises

1. A client who has recently been diagnosed with CML has been referred for a bone marrow transplant. She confides that she is extremely anxious and fearful of the procedure. Describe your response to this client.
2. A child with hemophilia has told you that his mother will not allow him to be involved in any extracurricular school activities. He is angry and asks that you try to convince his mother otherwise. How would you handle this situation? What would you discuss with the mother and the child? Describe how you would include and support the mother in the plan of care.
3. An adolescent client has been diagnosed with iron deficiency anemia. Outline a plan of teaching for this client appropriate for her age and condition.

NCLEX-Style Review Questions

1. A client has Hodgkin's disease, stage I. The nurse knows that this means the disease:
   a. Has extended to extralymphatic organs
   b. Involves more than one node, but is confined to one side of the diaphragm
   c. Is limited to a single node
   d. Is present above and below the diaphragm

2. A client is receiving a blood transfusion and reports to the nurse that she "feels funny." Which action is the priority?
   a. Assess vital signs
   b. Continue the infusion
   c. Notify the RN
   d. Stop the transfusion
3. When administering oral iron preparation, the nurse knows to:
   a. Administer it with orange juice.
   b. Inform the client that stools may become green in color.
   c. Instruct the client to swish the medication in the mouth.
   d. Take the medication on an empty stomach.

4. After a bone marrow biopsy, it is most important for the nurse to record what information?
   a. Absence of bleeding at the puncture site
   b. Amount of marrow removed from the client
   c. Client's level of consciousness
   d. Physician who performed the procedure
5. Following a peripheral stem cell transplantation, the nurse assesses closely for signs of:
   a. Anemia
   b. Infection
   c. Loss of hair
   d. Pain

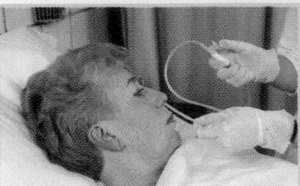

CHAPTER

82

Cancer

LEARNING OBJECTIVES

1. Describe the differences among carcinomas, sarcomas, and mixed-tissue tumors.
2. List the four most common sites of cancer in men and women in the United States.
3. State at least six ways a client can assist with cancer prevention.
4. Define the following tumor markers: enzymes, cancer antigens, oncofetal proteins, hormones, genes, and miscellaneous markers.
5. Identify at least five noninvasive diagnostic procedures used to detect cancer.
6. State the four main modalities for cancer treatment.
7. Identify at least four nursing considerations related to each of the following surgical techniques: incisional biopsy, excisional biopsy, cryosurgery, electrocauterization, fulguration, en bloc resection, exenteration, laser surgery and PDT, prophylactic and palliative surgery, and BMT.
8. State the five main categories of chemotherapeutic agents.
9. Compare and contrast the following biotherapy techniques: MOAB, IFN, CSF, IL, and retinoids. State at least two nursing considerations related to each technique.
10. Differentiate external radiation therapy from brachytherapy, including at least three nursing considerations related to each procedure.
11. Identify at least four concerns related to the safe administration of chemotherapeutic medications, and at least three safety considerations related to exposure to radiation.
12. Discuss at least three nursing considerations related to the following common side effects of cancer therapy: nausea and vomiting, stomatitis, fatigue, alopecia, secondary infections, pain, stress, and hormone therapy.

NEW TERMINOLOGY

adjuvant therapy	cytology
anaplastic	electrocauterization
antineoplastic	fulguration
apoptosis	histology
benign	malignant
biopsy	metastasis
biotherapy	myelosuppression
cancer	neoplasm
carcinogen	oncogene
carcinogenesis	oncology
carcinoma	replication
chemotherapy	sarcoma
cryosurgery	

ACRONYMS

AFP	HCG	MOAB, MoAb
BMT	HGF	PDT
BRM	HLA	PIC
CA	IFN	PICC
CEA	IL	PSA
CSF	LITT	TNM

Oncology is the medical specialty concerned with cancer and its treatment. A nurse who works with cancer clients is an *oncology nurse*. Treatment of cancer also can involve medical and surgical oncology specialists. Closely associated with these specialties is the *radiation oncologist*, who administers radiation therapy.

Clients may be seen and treated in many areas, including specialty care units of large hospitals or cancer specialty hospitals where nurses and physicians focus on the prevention, management, and treatments of cancer. Clients may also be cared for in community hospitals, long-term care facilities, and at home. Hospice care for the terminally ill client may be done at home, in an acute care facility, or in special hospice care facilities.

CANCER DEVELOPMENT

Cancer is characterized by excessive growth (*proliferation*) of cells that lack the capabilities of normal cellular function (see Chapter 15 for a review of basic tissue types and Units 10, 11, and 12 for specific cancer disorders). The development of cancer can occur in any tissue at any age. Although some cancers affect only the young, the adolescent, or the young adult, the overall incidence of cancer increases with age.

Tumors

Tumors or **neoplasms** are growths that arise from normal tissues. (The terms *tumor* and *neoplasm* are interchangeable.) A tumor may be benign or malignant.

Benign tumors, although generally not life threatening, can cause serious problems. In cases where benign tumors push against normal tissues, they can threaten vital structures and functions. The following characterize benign neoplasms:

- Slow growth
- *Encapsulated* (contained within a fibrous cover)
- Composed of *differentiated* cells (resemble the cells of the tissue from which they develop)
- Lack **metastasis** (invasion of other tissues in the body)

Malignant tumors have different characteristics of growth and do invade neighboring tissues. Malignant neoplasms are characterized by the following:

- Rapid growth with uncontrolled, progressive **replication** (reproduction)
- Non-encapsulated, infiltrating and invading other tissues
- Composed of **anaplastic** (*undifferentiated, dedifferentiated*) cells (cells that do not have normal structure or function). The anaplastic cells of malignant tumors lack orderly growth and arrangement, and do not function like the normal tissue cells from which they derive.
- Commonly metastasized, sending the abnormal cells to secondary sites via blood vessels or lymphatic vessels. Secondary sites will also eventually grow into malignant tumors.

Types of Tumors

Based on the study of tissues (**histology**) it is possible to classify cancer into three general categories: carcinomas, sarcomas, and mixed tissue types.

Carcinomas
Carcinomas (CA) are the largest group of cancers. Nearly 90% of all malignancies are carcinomas. These solid tumors develop from epithelial tissues that line skin, glands, gastrointestinal (GI), urinary, and reproductive organs. Examples of carcinomas include gastric adenocarcinoma, hepatomas, adenocarcinomas of the colon, and carcinomas of the glands such as thyroid, adrenals, breast, pancreas, and prostate.

Sarcomas
Sarcomas account for less than 5% of all malignant tumors. These tumors develop from connective tissues such as cartilage, bone, fat, muscle, bone marrow, and the lymphatic system. Connective tissue tumors include the gliomas and neuroblastomas of the brain, as well as osteosarcoma, Ewing's sarcoma, and leiomyosarcoma. Connective tissue sarcomas include the different types of leukemias (bone marrow) and lymphomas (lymph tissue) (see Chaps. 71 and 81).

Mixed-Tissue Tumors
Mixed-tissue tumors are uncommon tumors that develop from both epithelial and connective tissues. Examples of mixed-tissue tumors include Wilms' tumor, a kidney tumor usually found in children, and teratomas, which are common tumors of the ovaries or testes.

Carcinogenesis and Carcinogens

Carcinogenesis, the transformation of a normal cell into a malignant cell, is only partially understood. It is known that a disruption occurs with the normal process of DNA replication occurring during cellular mitosis. The production of new proteins that result from normal DNA mitosis is somehow damaged. Because of this disruption, abnormal, cancerous cells develop and reproduce. The RNA within these abnormal cells sends messages to develop more abnormal proteins.

The malignant cells are not coded correctly by the damaged DNA to continue with normal, needed cellular functions. Instead, the abnormal cells are designed to invade and to spread. The remaining normal cells can become overrun with the damaged cells. The functions that these normal cells would do, such as fight infection, carry nerve transmissions, or make urine, can no longer be accomplished.

Carcinogens are agents that cause damage to cellular DNA that leads to the development of cancer. At least 80% of cancers in the United States are due to smoking, alcohol, diet, and environmental factors. Chronic irritation can predispose an individual to carcinogenesis.

Environmental carcinogens include chemicals, radiation, and viruses. Some cancers are known to be inherited through defects in the DNA or the sperm or egg cells. Different carcinogens are described in Box 82-1.

In addition to carcinogens, oncogenetic and genetic causes are known. DNA can carry a cancer-causing gene called an **oncogene,** a piece of DNA which can cause normal cells to become abnormal, malignant cells when they are activated by a mutation. Certain types of colon cancer and lymphomas are caused by genetically mutated oncogenes. Discovered in 1960 in Philadelphia, the *Philadelphia chromosome* is an oncogene that causes chronic myelogenous leukemia.

Heredity can cause the transfer of defective DNA through the sperm or egg cells. Through genetic screening, individuals can be tested for inherited cancer-causing genes. Inherited genes are implicated in the formation of some breast and ovarian cancers, *retinoblastoma* (retinal tumor), and Wilms' tumor.

Cancer Grading and Staging

To assist in the diagnosis and treatments of cancer, classifications were developed to categorize the extent of cancer. The histologist is looking for differentiation. A normal cell is well differentiated, containing the normal structures of typical, mature cells of a type of tissue.

Grading is a system of looking at abnormal cells under a microscope to determine the cells' degree of dedifferentiation or lack of maturity. Generally, a system of three to five grades is used. *Grade I* tumors closely resemble normal cells. They retain much of their differentiation as specific tissue cells. *Grade IV* or *V* tumors are very anaplastic, often having little or no resemblance to the tissue cells from which they developed. *Grade II* or *III* tumors have intermediate phases of differentiation, ranging from slightly undifferentiated to extremely abnormal cells.

Clients with a grade I tumor have better *prognosis* (probable outcome) than clients with higher grade tumors. Healthcare screening can be done as a detection and early prevention measure, such as with the Papanicolaou (Pap) test of uterine cervical cells. Table 82-1 shows the classifications of a "Pap smear." Other preventive grading can be done to screen tracheal and stomach secretions.

Staging is a method for identifying the spread of a tumor. Typical staging systems look at a tumor's size and local invasiveness, the extent of lymph node involvement, and the evidence of metastasis to distant or secondary sites. The tumor, node, and metastasis system is called the **TNM** system of staging.

Subdivisions of the TNM system are used to designate the size and degree of involvement of each category using a range from 0 to 4 or A to D. For example, a staging of $T_3N_4M_1$ would indicate a fairly large tumor with spread to distant nodes and distant metastasis. A tumor that is staged as $T_1N_0M_0$ is a small tumor without node involvement or metastasis.

The place where cancer starts is called the *primary site. Cancer in situ* refers to tumor cells that have not invaded surrounding sites. Metastatic sites are called *secondary sites* or *secondary lesions.* Cancer may spread through the body by extending directly into nearby tissue or into a body cavity, such as the abdomen or chest. Secondary sites can also occur when cancerous cells travel through blood vessels or the lymphatic system from the primary site to other body parts, especially the lungs, bones, brain, and liver.

Incidence

Cancer is second only to heart disease as the major cause of adult deaths in the United States. About 1,500 people a day die of cancer, and more than half a million Americans die each year of cancer. In the United States, one in four individuals die of cancer. Figure 82-1 represents expected deaths from cancer.

➤➤ **BOX 82-1**

TYPES OF CARCINOGENS

Chemical carcinogens include the hydrocarbons found in cigarettes, cigars, and pipe smoke. More chemical carcinogens are found in automobile exhaust, insecticides, dyes, industrial chemicals, asbestos, and hormones.

Radiation, a form of energy, can be found in sunlight, x-rays, and radioactive materials. When this form of energy interacts with DNA, damage and cellular mutations can occur. Ultraviolet (UV) light radiation can lead to skin cancer. Persons frequently exposed to x-rays can develop leukemias.

Viruses, called *oncogenic viruses,* can cause tumors. Either the DNA or the RNA of viruses can be the causative agent of cancer. RNA viruses are known as *retroviruses.* Examples include:

• Retrovirus of HIV, which causes Kaposi's sarcoma.
• Human T-cell leukemia virus (HTLV) is related to HIV and causes a form of adult leukemia.
• Human papillomavirus (HPV) can cause cervical cancer.
• The Epstein-Barr virus, which is the cause of infectious mononucleosis, can also cause Burkitt's lymphoma, a rare tumor of the lymph node.

■■ **TABLE 82-1** $\mathcal{C}$**LASSIFICATIONS OF PAPANICOLAOU TESTS**

Class	Characteristics
I	Normal test, no atypical cells
II	Atypical cells, but no evidence of malignancy
III	Atypical cells, possible but not conclusive for malignancy
IV	Cells strongly suggestive of malignancy
V	Strong evidence of malignancy

Source: Hosley, J. B., Jones, S. A., & Molle-Matthews, E. A. (1997). *Lippincott's textbook for medical assistants* (p. 789). Philadelphia: Lippincott Williams & Wilkins.

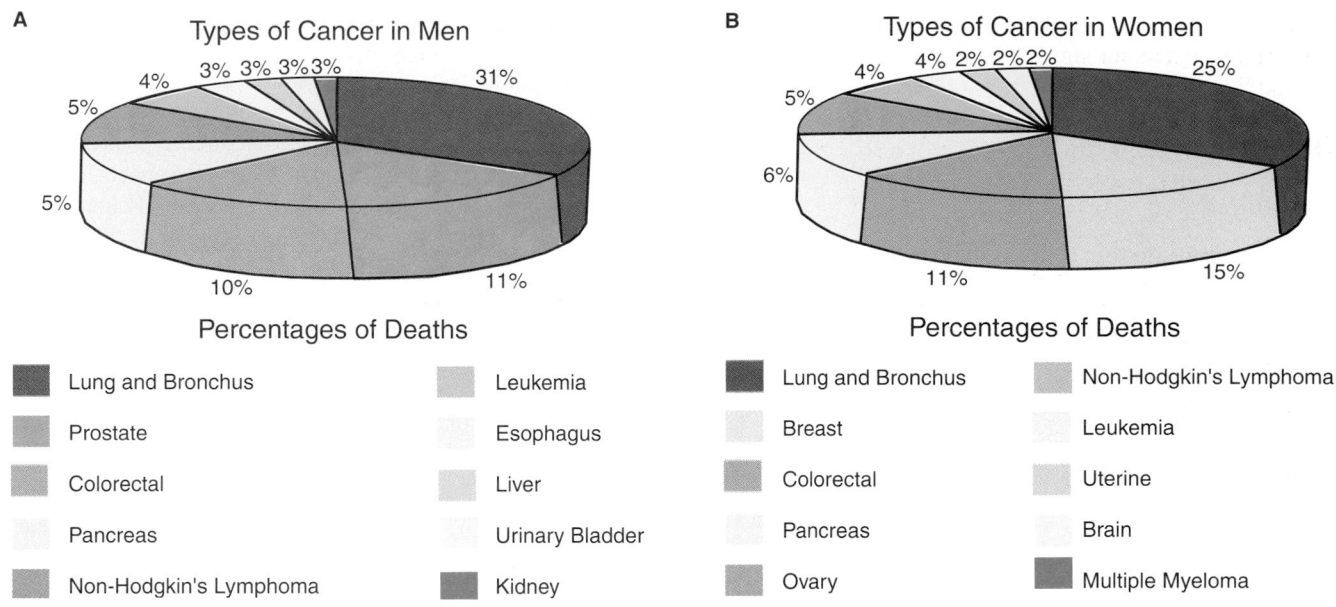

FIGURE 82-1. Leading sites of cancer incidence and death in (**A**) males and (**B**) females. (Adapted from American Cancer Society, Inc. [2002]. *Cancer facts & figures 2002.* Atlanta: Author.)

All people are at risk for developing cancer. About 5% to 10% of cancers are hereditary. All cancers result from a mutation of genes that causes malfunction of cell growth and division. The genes mutate due to either internal factors such as hormones, or external factors such as tobacco, chemicals, and sunlight.

Cancer is also attributed to dietary habits. Of particular concern are diets that are high in fat or calories, or that contain large amounts of any of the following: meats (particularly red meats), salt-cured or nitrate-containing foods, or alcohol.

Occurrence increases as an individual ages. Therefore, most cancers affect adults of middle age or older.

The survival rate for all cancers combined is about 60%, but some cancers have much higher or much lower morbidity rates. Survival rates are based on statistics from clients who live 5 years or more after diagnosis.

The National Institutes of Health estimate that cancer costs nearly $160 billion dollars annually in the United States. About $56 billion is spent directly to pay for medical costs such as hospitalizations, therapies, and healthcare. The remaining estimated 100 billion dollars reflects the indirect costs such as disability, loss of productivity, and premature deaths.

Lung cancer remains the leading cause of cancer death for both men and women. Lung cancer is primarily attributable to cigarette smoking. In fact, smokers are about 10 to 20 times more likely to develop lung cancer than are nonsmokers. In addition, tobacco-related cancers are also associated with cancers of the upper respiratory tract, genitourinary tract, GI tract, and pancreas. A non-smoker who breathes the smoke from tobacco (called *passive smoke* or *secondhand smoke*) has double the risk of cancer.

☛ KEY CONCEPT

The leading cause of cancer deaths in both men and women is lung cancer, which is directly related to cigarette smoking.

The lung cancer rates for men decreased significantly in the last two decades of the 20th century. However, for women, the incidence increased until reaching a plateau in the late 1990s. The incidences of lung cancer reflect the trend of decreased smoking in men, and the increase of smoking in women. Tobacco use by youth increased in the 1990s.

Breast cancer is the second most common cancer in women. *Prostate cancer,* especially in African American men, is the second leading cause of death by cancer in men.

Colorectal cancer is the third most common malignancy and cancer death site for men and women; its incidence is increasing for persons over the age of 50. This malignancy is curable if treated early, indicating a great need for education related to prevention, screening, and detection.

Prevention and Early Detection

Major initiatives by the National Cancer Institute (NCI), the American Cancer Society (ACS), the Oncology Nursing Society (ONS), and the U.S. Department of Health and Human Services (USDHHS) focus on health promotion and cancer prevention and detection. Major activities include emphasizing the following measures to the public:

- *Smoking:* Reduction in the percent of youths who smoke before age 20.
- *Diet:* Reduction in total dietary fats and calories.
- *Sun exposure:* Decrease in total sun exposure and avoidance of artificial sources of ultraviolet light.
- *Self-examinations:* Detection of early signs of breast or prostate cancers.
- *Exercise:* Maintenance of routine and consistent exercise
- *Screening:* Improvement in the screening rates for breast, prostate, and colorectal cancers
- *Education:* Improvement in the educational strategies related to tobacco cessation, diet modification, and screening recommendations.

In Box 82-2, the American Cancer Society shows the CAUTION signals for signs of cancer.

DIAGNOSTIC TESTS

Cytology

Cytology is the study of cells. A cytologic examination is done on sputum, bronchial washings, vaginal and cervical secretions, prostatic secretions, pleural secretions, and gastric washings. Cytology is less accurate than biopsy but has proven diagnostic value, particularly in cervical cancer. The test most frequently used to detect cancer of the cervix and uterus is the Papanicolaou (Pap) test.

☛ KEY CONCEPT

The Pap test is an important part of the physical examination of every woman who is over age 20 or who is sexually active.

➤➤ BOX 82-2

WARNING SIGNALS FOR CANCER

Caution is the byword:[*]

Change in bowel or bladder habits
A sore that does not heal
Unusual bleeding or discharge
Thickening or lump in breast or elsewhere
Indigestion or difficulty swallowing
Obvious change in wart or mole
Nagging cough or hoarseness

Additional concerns that need to be investigated by a healthcare professional:[†]

• Frequent, severe headaches
• Persistent abdominal pain

Signs and symptoms in children that need to be investigated by a healthcare professional:[†]

• Continual, unexplained crying
• Unexplained nausea and vomiting
• Frequent fatigue
• Frequent infections
• General failure to thrive
• Spontaneous bleeding
• Bleeding that does not stop in a normal amount of time
• Bumps, lumps, masses, or swelling anywhere on the body
• Frequent stumbling for no apparent reason

_____
[*] Source: American Cancer Society
[†] Adapted from: Hosley, J. B., Jones, S. A., & Molle-Matthews, E. A. (1997). *Lippincott's textbook for medical assistants* (p. 342). Philadelphia: Lippincott Williams & Wilkins.

Laboratory Tests and Blood Studies

Many laboratory tests and blood studies help to diagnose cancer. Some malignancies can alter the blood's chemical composition, showing specific changes due directly to the cancer. Healthcare providers may begin analysis for cancers by evaluating the results of routine tests such as blood chemistries (eg, enzymes, blood glucose, sodium, potassium, chlorine), a complete blood count with differential (discussed in Chap. 81), and levels of hormones.

Tumor Markers

Tumor markers are specific enzymes, cancer antigens, oncofetal proteins, hormones, or genes that can indicate malignancies. Miscellaneous markers may be types of proteins or chemicals. Tumor markers can be found in the blood and are helpful in monitoring a tumor's response to treatment, assessing the extent of tumor involvement, or detecting cancer recurrences (Table 82-2).

Some tumor markers can lack specificity. Therefore, they are used only as a general screening tool to detect cancer's initial presence. Additional testing is done to verify cancer, such as x-ray, CT, MRI, and ultrasound studies.

Noninvasive Diagnostic Procedures

Radiologic Studies. *Radiologic (x-ray)* studies allow visualization of the body's internal structures. They may be specific to certain areas (eg, chest x-ray examination). These radiographs may visualize the function of an entire system, such as with a barium swallow or barium enema used to detect abnormalities of the GI system.

Mammograms are specific x-ray studies used to detect abnormal cellular growth in the breasts. Generally, if an area of concern is detected, the woman will undergo further testing such as a biopsy.

Computed Tomography (CT). *Computed tomography* (CT) scanning can provide sectional views of various body structures. CT scanning is one of the most useful tools in the staging of malignancies. It is most useful for tumors of the chest, abdominal cavity, and brain.

Ultrasonography. *Ultrasonography* is a noninvasive technique that uses sound waves directed into specific tissues. It is most applicable in detecting tumors within the pelvis, retroperitoneum, and peritoneum. Ultrasound has many clinical diagnostic applications in the detection and diagnosis of disorders of all body systems.

Magnetic Resonance Imaging (MRI). *MRI* can provide detailed sectional images of the body without the use of ionizing radiation. With the use of magnetic fields, it can aid in detecting, localizing, and staging malignant disease in the central nervous system, musculoskeletal system, spine, head, and neck.

Invasive Diagnostic Techniques

Endoscopy. Sometimes, physicians find an abnormality and need to evaluate findings more closely. Instruments such

■■■ TABLE 82-2 *T*UMOR MARKERS

Type of Tumor Marker	Examples
Enzymes	
Higher than normal enzyme levels can indicate specific tumors, or can be nonspecific indicators of a problem	Prostate-specific antigen (**PSA**): Used as a detector for prostate cancer and an indicator of response to therapy
	Lactic dehydrogenase (LDH): Elevated in many types of cancer
	Neuron-specific enolase (NSE): Found in several neuroendocrine tumors and with neuroblastoma
Cancer Antigens	
Type of protein that is associated with a few types of cancerous tumors	CA 125 tumor marker: Ovarian, colorectal, and gastric cancers
	CA 15-3 tumor marker: Metastatic or recurrent breast cancer
	CA 19-9 tumor marker: Helpful for diagnosis of gastrointestinal cancers and treatment of pancreatic cancers
Oncofetal proteins	
Normally found in high levels in the fetus but not normal in the adult	Carcinoembryonic antigen (**CEA**): Breast, colorectal, and lung cancers
	Alpha-fetoprotein (**AFP**): Germ-cell tumors, liver cancer
Hormones	
Elevated levels of some hormones are possibly indicative of benign and malignant tumors	Beta–human chorionic gonadotropin (**HCG**): Testicular and certain types of ovarian cancers
	Thyrocalcitonin: Thyroid and other endocrine disorders and cancers
Genes	
Some genes are linked to specific types of cancer	WT1: Wilms' tumor
	BRCA-1: Breast and ovarian cancers
	Philadelphia chromosome: Chronic myeloid leukemia
Miscellaneous Markers	Beta$_2$-microglobulin: Multiple myeloma and lymphomas
	Paraproteins: Multiple myeloma and lymphomas
	Serum ferritin: Hepatomas
	Thyroglobulin: Thyroid cancer and thyroid disorders

as the *sigmoidoscope, colonoscope, gastroscope, bronchoscope,* and *laryngoscope* may be used for visual observation of internal organs. Examinations with these scopes are discussed in chapters related to specific body systems.

Exploratory Surgery and Biopsy Examination.   In some cases, surgery must be done to visualize, examine, and take a sample (biopsy specimen) of internal lesions or lymph nodes. **Biopsy** examination is the most important means of diagnosing cancer. The pathologist studies a small sample of tissue removed from the organ in question. In almost all cases, biopsy examination can determine whether a lesion is benign or malignant.

Frozen Section.   When a biopsy specimen of a nodule has been removed, or a total specimen has been excised, the tissue is quickly frozen and sliced very thin. The pathologist then studies the specimen under a microscope. This examination can be performed while the client remains anesthetized. The pathologist reports the findings to the surgeon, who then decides on the appropriate surgery.

TREATMENT MODALITIES FOR CANCER

Cancer treatments are individual or combinations of four main modalities:

- Surgery
- Chemotherapy
- Biologic therapy
- Radiation therapy

Surgery

Ideal surgical treatment would be the complete removal of all malignant tissue before it metastasizes. In many types of cancer, *surgery* can prevent the spread of the disease and offer cures. Surgery can involve not only removal of the tumor, but also may include small or large areas of surrounding tissue.

An *incisional tissue biopsy* will help establish diagnosis and staging criteria. The biopsy may be followed by more extensive surgery, radiation, and/or chemotherapy.

An *excisional biopsy* will remove the tumor as well as some of the margin of the tumor, to determine if the cancer has spread and to remove any malignant cells that may have spread to the surrounding area. In cases of small tumors, this procedure can be curative.

To prevent growth and spread, malignant tissues may be frozen (**cryosurgery**), burned (**electrocauterization**), or destroyed by high-frequency current (**fulguration**).

Some tumors may be removed by *en bloc resection,* which involves removal of the tumor and surrounding tissues and lymph nodes. Larger tumors may be treated by *exenteration* (removal of the tumor, the organ involved, and surrounding tissues).

Laser Surgery.   *Laser surgery* can be used to excise precise areas of tumors such as on the glottis. *Laser-induced interstitial thermotherapy* (**LITT**) shrinks or destroys a tumor with heat. Laser surgery can be curative or *palliative.*

In a laser technique known as *photodynamic therapy* (**PDT**), a chemical is introduced to the body. This photosensitizing agent will remain in or around a tumor cell longer than around normal cells. The photosensitized cancer cells are then exposed to the laser, and the laser light is absorbed by the photosensitizing (chemical) agent in or around the tumor. The advantages of this new therapy are that cancer cells can be selectively destroyed, damage to normal cells is minimal, and side effects are fairly mild.

PDT currently can only penetrate tissue that is less than 1 and ⅛ inch (3 cm) thick. Therefore, PDT is used mainly on tumors under the skin or on the lining of internal organs that can be reached by fiberoptic instruments such as a bronchoscope or endoscope. The skin and eyes of clients receiving PDT therapy are very sensitive to direct sunlight and bright indoor lighting for at least 6 weeks after treatment.

Prophylactic Surgery.   *Prophylactic (preventive) surgery* may also be used when certain tumors are known or suspected to be precancerous. Cystic tumors of the ovaries and polypoid tumors from the colon may be removed as preventive measures against progression to cancer.

In addition, some of the endocrine glands known to influence the development of specific cancers can be removed, such as in testicular cancer. In some types of breast cancer, when cancer is discovered in one breast, both breasts are removed as a prophylactic measure.

Palliative Surgery.   *Palliative surgery* may be performed to relieve some of the complications of malignancies that cannot be totally excised. The goal of this type of surgery is not to cure, but to promote comfort for the client. For example, with metastatic lung cancer, a tumor putting pressure on the trachea may be removed to facilitate breathing. Palliative surgery may also be done to promote quality of life as well as to improve longevity.

Bone Marrow Transplant (BMT).   Bone marrow transplant (**BMT**) is a technique used to replace the specialized cells called *stem cells* that develop into blood cells (red blood cells, white blood cells, and platelets). Bone marrow may be obtained surgically from sites on the hip or sternum using very small incisions and a large-bore biopsy needle.

Sources for bone marrow may be the client (*autologous*), a twin (*syngeneic*), or *allogeneic* (any other person). Donated bone marrow is matched to the tissues of the client's human leukocyte-associated (**HLA**) antigen on the surface of the client's white blood cells.

Stem cells are found not only in bone marrow, but also in peripheral blood and in umbilical cord blood. Peripheral blood stem cells (PBSCs) are obtained by *apheresis* (removal through a large vein of blood that is then sent via tubing through special collection filters in a machine). The stem cells are *harvested* (collected) and frozen until needed.

The stem cells that are in the bone marrow of an individual with cancer are commonly damaged by the types of therapies used to treat the abnormal cells, especially chemotherapy and radiation. BMT is commonly used in leukemias and lymphomas (see Chaps. 71 and 81).

The client receives the donated bone marrow after receiving chemotherapy and/or radiation. Preliminary results may be seen in 2 to 4 weeks. However, complete recovery with successful transplants may take 6 months to a year.

Chemotherapy

The term **chemotherapy** implies the use of chemical agents to destroy cancerous cells. The goal of chemotherapy is to damage the DNA within these abnormal cells and cause self-destruction (**apoptosis**).

There are several therapeutic indications for chemotherapy, including:

- To treat widespread or metastatic disease because chemotherapy is a systemic, rather than a local, treatment
- To provide a cure for clients with certain types of cancer, even in advanced stages; for example, acute leukemias, some types of lymphomas, and testicular cancer
- To temporarily control or *palliate* (relieve) tumor-related difficulties—palliative treatment does not cure
- To use as an **adjuvant** (*assistive*) **therapy** after surgery to treat metastases or to attempt to prevent metastases from occurring

Cancer cells have a proportionately higher number of cells dividing at any one time than do normal cells because cancerous cells have unrestrained replication and progressive growth. Another characteristic of tumor cells is that they have limited capacity to repair their own DNA. Thus, they are generally less able to survive DNA damage due to drugs and radiation than are normal cells.

Chemotherapeutic agents are designed to be effective during one or more of the phases of cell division. Because of their abnormal replication process, malignant cells are very susceptible to chemotherapeutic agents.

Chemotherapy can also destroy normal cells. Bone marrow and the cells that line the GI tract also have rapid replication processes. Therefore the normal cells of the bone marrow and GI tract can suffer considerable damage from the potent **antineoplastic** (anticancer) drugs.

Protocols (a written plan) for the administration of chemotherapy have been developed with extensive research and experience. Protocols dictate detailed directions as to specific routes of drug administration, the amount of time between doses, the total dosage of a particular drug, and the types of drugs that should be given in combination. The drugs are continued until the client is in remission. *Remission* is indicated by absence of all signs of the disease. Remission may be partial or complete. Some clients may have a permanent remission and the malignancy never returns (ie, a cure). Unexplained, spontaneous remissions occasionally occur in clients without treatment.

Nursing considerations for clients receiving chemotherapy are discussed later in this chapter.

Chemotherapeutic Agents

Chemotherapeutic agents are classified into five basic categories:

1. Alkylating agents
2. Antibiotics
3. Antimetabolites
4. Antimitotics
5. Hormonal agents

In Practice: Important Medications 82-1 highlights some of the major chemotherapeutic agents in use. The majority of chemotherapeutic agents are associated with **myelosuppression** (bone marrow depression).

In addition to the five major classifications, other drugs such as corticosteroids (eg, prednisone, dexamethasone) may be used. Antiangiogenic drugs (eg, endostatin, angiostatin) interfere with the formation of blood vessels that grow to feed the cancer cells. These drugs may be new additions to the

---

In Practice
Important Medications 82-1

FOR CHEMOTHERAPY*

Antimetabolites (inhibit metabolic functions needed for DNA synthesis or replication)
fluorouracil, 5-fluorouracil, 5-FU (Adrucil, Efudex)
cytarabine (Ara-C)
gencitabine (Genzar)
methotrexate, methotrexate sodium (Folex, Mexate)
fludarabine

Antimitotics: Vinca Alkaloids (interfere with cellular mitosis)
vinblastine sulfate (Velban, Velsar)
vincristine sulfate (Oncovin)
vinorelbine (Navalbine)

Alkylating Agents (interfere with DNA synthesis)
carboplatin (Paraplatin)
dacabarzine (DTIC)
ifosfamide (Ifex)
thiotepa (TESPA, TSPA)
cisplatin (Platinol)
cyclophosphamide (Cytoxan)

Alkylating Agents: Nitrosoureas (interfere with DNA synthesis)
carmustine (BCNU)
lomustine, CCNU (CeeNu)
streptozocin (Zanosar)

Antitumor Antibiotics (prevent DNA replication)
bleomycin (Blenoxane)
idarubicin (Idamycin)
doxorubicin HCl (Adriamycin)
mitomycin-C (Mutamycin)
plicamycin, mithramycin (Mithracin)

Taxanes
paclitaxel (Taxol)
docetaxel (Taxotere)

Miscellaneous Agents
leustatin (Cladribine)
topotecan HCl (Hycamtin)
tretinoin (Vesanoid)

Hormonal Agents (produce temporary regression of metastatic cancers)
tamoxifen (Nolvadex)
flutamide (Eulexin)
leuprolide (Luron)
finasteride (Proscar)

Examples of Combination Chemotherapy Regimens
CHOP: cytoxan, Adriamycin, Oncovin, prednisone
CAF: cytoxan, Adriamycin, fluorouracil
CMF: cytoxan, methotrexate, fluorouracil
CMV: cisplatin, methotrexate, vinblastine

* Note: Most clients receive combinations of agents (regimens).

chemotherapy arsenal in the near future. In Practice: Nursing Care Guidelines 82-1 highlights important aspects of caring for a client receiving chemotherapy.

Biotherapy

Biotherapy (*immunotherapy*) uses the body's own defenses either directly or indirectly against tumor cells. Biologic response modifiers (**BRM**) are produced by normal cells. BRMs repair, stimulate, or enhance substances within the immune system to kill cancer cells. The BRMs, used in biotherapy work, either directly or indirectly to stimulate or enhance the client's immune system.

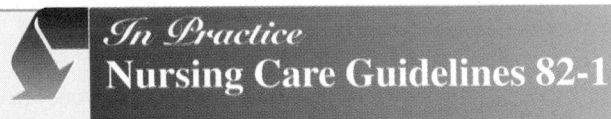

In Practice
Nursing Care Guidelines 82-1

PROVIDING CARE FOR THE PERSON RECEIVING CHEMOTHERAPY

- Provide both emotional and physical support. The client may become discouraged or physically ill and may wish to discontinue treatment. Help by listening to the client and providing encouragement. A support group or a visit from a cancer survivor may be helpful.
- Assist the client with strategies for managing side effects such as constipation, diarrhea, and fatigue.
- Manage nausea and vomiting, the number one side effect of chemotherapy. Strategies include the use of antiemetics and distractors.
- Encourage good oral hygiene. Perform frequent mouth checks to assess for mucositis. (See discussion of special mouth care later in this chapter.)
- Encourage adequate fluid intake, of at least eight glasses per day. Vary the fluids.
- Provide a dietary consultation that includes information on a high-calorie, high-protein diet. Frequent small meals, snacks, and nutritional supplements may provide a solution for a poor nutritional status.
- Provide emotional support when there are changes in body image or sexual dysfunction. For example, when hormonal therapies are used, men's breasts may become enlarged; women may develop a deeper voice and facial hair may appear. There may be a loss of sexual interest; impotence; or vaginal dryness—which may add to decreased self-esteem.
- Plan for a wig, turban, scarf, or hat if hair loss becomes problematic.
- Instruct the client in the implications of low blood counts such as the potential for infection, fatigue, or abnormal bleeding.
- Stress the importance of open and honest communication between the client and family members. Emphasize the overall long-term results of the treatment.

In the future, cancer vaccines may be available as a biologic therapy. The purpose of the vaccines is to encourage the immune system to recognize abnormal, cancerous cells. Cancer vaccines would be given to individuals after detection of small tumors. Clinical trials are evaluating the effectiveness of vaccines in melanoma, lymphomas, and several other areas.

Currently in use are nonspecific biotherapy agents such as bacillus Calmette-Guerin (BCG) and levamisole (Ergamisol), which enhance the immune response. BCG, a vaccine widely used against tuberculosis, seems to work by increasing the inflammatory and immune responses. It may be diluted in a solution and instilled directly into the cancerous tissue, such as is done in bladder cancer. Levamisole may act to restore depressed immune function, and is used along with other chemotherapeutic agents after colon cancer surgery.

Biologic agents that can be produced in a laboratory are referred to as the BRMs. They can be listed in the following categories:

- *Monoclonal antibodies (MOAB)* (eg, rituximab [Rituxan], trastuzumab [Herceptin])
- *Interferons (IFN)* (eg, interferon-α 2a [Roferon, Intron])
- *Colony-stimulating factors (CSF)* (eg, filgrastim [Neupogen], erythropoietin [Epogen])
- *Interleukins (IL)* (eg, aldesleukin [interleukin-2, IL-2])
- *Retinoids* (eg, acitretin [Soriatane], tretinoin [Retin-A])

Monoclonal Antibodies (MOAB, MoAb). *Monoclonal antibodies* (**MOAB, MoAb**) are produced by genetically fusing cancer cells with normal cells. They are highly specific antibodies that seek out and bind to specific targets on cancer cells, causing apoptosis.

MOABs can improve the client's immune response to cancer and interfere with the growth of cancer cells. They can be designed to deliver radioisotopes, other BRMs, or other substances that are toxic to cancerous cells. MOABs may be used as part of the treatment and therapy for BMT.

Currently MOABs are used to combat renal transplant rejection. Additionally, because they can carry radioisotopes to specific areas, they can be used as diagnostic aids for colorectal, prostate, and ovarian cancers.

When MOABs are used, the nurse needs to be aware of the possibility of acute anaphylactic reactions. Anaphylaxis would present initially as generalized flushing, followed by pallor. Respiratory distress may also occur. Other side effects include fever, chills, rigors, diaphoresis, malaise, urticaria, pruritus, nausea, vomiting, dyspnea, and hypotension.

Interferons (IFN). *Interferons* (**IFN**), made by lymphocytes, enhance the effects of the immune system. The three major types of interferon are alpha (α), beta (β), and gamma (γ). They protect normal cells from invasion by intracellular parasites, including viruses. How interferons exert their effects is unknown and unclear; however, all three types appear capable of inducing antitumor activity.

Nursing considerations include client teaching about the usual side effects of flu-like symptoms. However, each client will usually adjust to these symptoms over the course of treatment. These symptoms include chills, fever spikes, fatigue, headaches, myalgia, arthralgia, and malaise. Side effects become more severe as the dose becomes higher.

Colony-Stimulating Factors (CSF). *Colony-stimulating factors* (**CSF**) are part of a group of hematopoietic growth factors (**HGF**), which encourage growth and maturation of blood cell components. Cells that can be influenced by HGFs include granulocytes, macrophages, lymphocytes, monocytes, erythrocytes, and platelets.

When growth factors are successful, myelosuppression is reduced. Accelerated growth of cells, following damage caused by cancer treatment, decreases the resulting *neutropenia* (decreased neutrophils), thereby leading to a decrease in the incidence of infection. With less myelosuppression, the client can receive higher doses of other chemotherapy agents.

Nursing considerations for CSFs generally are influenced by the dose and route of administration. Be alert for low-grade fever, bone pain, fatigue, and anorexia.

Interleukins (IL). *Interleukins* (**IL**) promote the immune response of the T lymphocytes: to stimulate the immune system to destroy neoplasms. High-dose therapy can create severe toxicity. ILs have shown some success in the treatment of metastatic renal cancers and melanoma.

When ILs are administered, be alert for possible hypotension, edema (including pulmonary edema), tachycardia, dyspnea, and tachycardia. Other side effects include chills, fever, headache, malaise, myalgia, arthralgia, fatigue, nasal congestion, and GI upset.

Retinoids. *Retinoids* are a group of compounds derived from retinol or vitamin A. Although not always officially listed as a biotherapy agent, the effects of retinoids include antibody and immune responses. In cancer, retinoids induce cell differentiation and suppress proliferation. Types of cancer that appear to respond to retinoids include promyelocytic leukemia, melanoma, neuroblastoma, and various epithelial cancers.

Retinoic acid syndrome is a serious side effect of this therapy. It can include fevers, respiratory distress, interstitial pulmonary infiltrates, pleural effusions, and weight gain.

Radiation Therapy

Radiation therapy or *radiotherapy* is indicated in many types of cancer and may be used as a primary therapy, as a combined modality with chemotherapy, or as a palliative treatment for symptom relief (eg, pain management). X-ray studies are also used for diagnosis of tumor sites. The purpose of radiotherapy is to direct ionizing radiation to target tissues for damage or destruction of the cells. Radiation damages both normal and abnormal cells. Thus, the therapies must be aimed as directly as possible at the cancerous tissues.

Three types of rays are involved in radiation diagnosis and therapy: alpha, beta, and gamma rays. Alpha and beta rays penetrate only the upper layer of the skin. Gamma rays, on the other hand, penetrate deeply into body tissues.

Safety considerations are a priority for both the client and the healthcare workers when working around any radioactive substance. The critical components to safety when working around any radiation are time, distance, and shielding. Limit

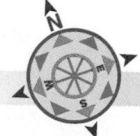

SPECIAL CONSIDERATIONS: CULTURE

Radiation Therapy

Some cultures believe a person's energy is "in sync" with the universe. Therefore, some clients perceive radiation as a threat, or as having the ability to cause disequilibrium of this energy flow.

the time spent near the source of radiation. Increase the distance the individual stands from the source, and use available shielding to block radiation. To monitor exposure to radiation, healthcare workers in radiology units must wear badges such as that shown in Figure 82-2.

> **Nursing Alert**
> If not correctly managed, radiation can be hazardous to the nurse and client. Radiation is particularly dangerous for pregnant women.

There are two main types of radiation therapy: external and internal. *External-beam radiation* uses a treatment machine placed away from the body. *Internal brachytherapy, interstitial irradiation,* or *intracavity irradiation* are radioactive implants that deliver the ionizing radiation directly from within the tumor or a body cavity.

External Radiation

This form of radiation uses both deep and surface x-rays, as well as cobalt, radium, and radioactive isotopes of other elements.

Extreme precautions are taken to protect clients, staff, and healthy cells from the hazards involved in administering radiation therapy. Linear accelerators and betatrons have made delivery of high doses of irradiation to deep-seated malignancies possible, without damaging critical organs or causing severe surface-skin reactions.

Direct nursing care toward ensuring the client's safety and carrying out measures that provide relief of side effects. Side effects depend on the area irradiated and may include decreased appetite, abdominal cramping, diarrhea, and local cutaneous irritation. In Practice: Nursing Care Guidelines 82-2 highlights important aspects of care for the client receiving external radiation therapy.

Internal Radiation

Brachytherapy is the placement of radioactive substances directly into a tumor site. The goal is to deliver large amounts of radiation to a specific site. Internal radiation is an attempt to destroy the cancer cells from within. Radioactive sources are encapsulated so that they do not contaminate body fluids.

Cancers that may be treated with brachytherapy include those of the brain, tongue, lips, esophagus, lung, breast, vagina, cervix, endometrium, rectum, prostate, and bladder.

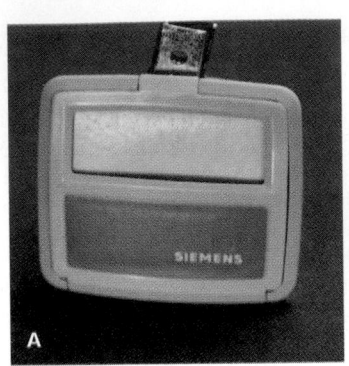
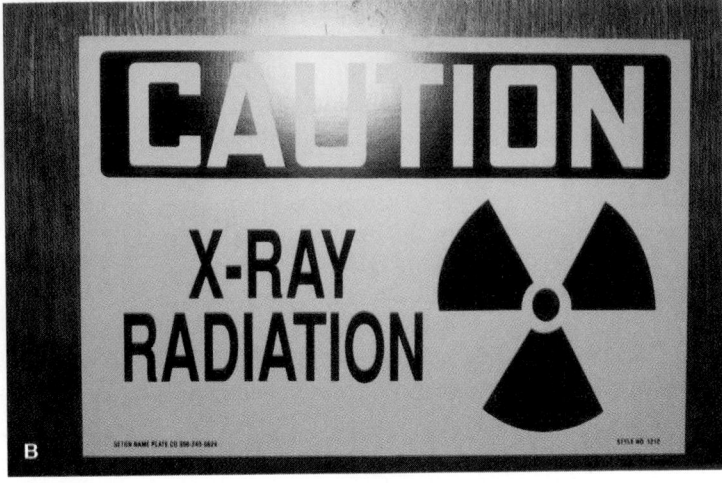

FIGURE 82-2. Radiation from x-ray machines is a health hazard. (**A**) A dosimeter badge is worn by anyone working close to radiation sources. It helps to monitor the amount of exposure by healthcare workers. (**B**) Radiation must be identified by warning signs. Note the universal symbol of radiation. (Source: Hosley, J. B., Jones, S. A., & Molle-Matthews, E. A. [1997]. *Lippincott's textbook for medical assistants* [p. 473]. Philadelphia: Lippincott Williams & Wilkins.

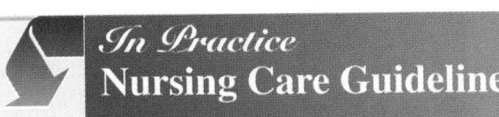

In Practice
Nursing Care Guidelines 82-2

PROVIDING CARE FOR CLIENTS RECEIVING EXTERNAL-BEAM RADIATION THERAPY

• Provide frequent rest periods. *Rationale: The treatment and the disease often cause fatigue.*
• Encourage nutrient intake. *Rationale: A diet high in calories, protein, and vitamins is recommended to increase strength and help offset nausea and diarrhea. Proteins are needed to build new tissue.* Individuals vary in their tolerance to food during radiation therapy. (Guidelines for management of nausea and vomiting are presented elsewhere in this chapter.)
• Provide good oral hygiene. *Rationale: Good oral hygiene helps to prevent breakdown of oral mucosa.*
• Provide special skin care (see In Practice: Educating the Client 82-1; also Chap. 50).
• Keep the radiation site dry and free from irritation. The client's clothing should fit loosely. *Rationale: Friction may cause irritation.*
• Avoid invasive procedures, such as injections and rectal temperatures, if possible. These measures must be particularly avoided within the radiation field. *Rationale: The client's skin is fragile due to radiation. Invasive procedures also introduce a possible route for infection.*
• Follow supportive routine nursing measures for side effects such as gastrointestinal symptoms. If these symptoms are severe, radiation treatment may need to be discontinued or postponed.

NURSING PROCESS

Data Collection

Chapter 47 describes some basic nursing assessment techniques that establish baselines for future comparison and determine the presence of suspected disorders. Report any changes in baseline levels.

With a neoplasm, a client may report unexplained weight loss, a general feeling of discomfort, or a change in elimination habits or other normal functions. In addition, observe the client's emotional and physical response to the disorder or disease. Additional signs and symptoms of cancer are given at In Practice: Nursing Assessment 82-1.

Data collection will generally include questions that provide information about the client's self-care abilities and sup-

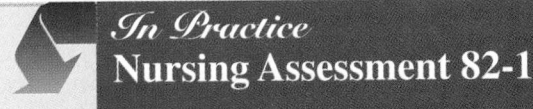

In Practice
Nursing Assessment 82-1

SIGNS AND SYMPTOMS OF CANCER*

In addition to the warning signals, as listed by the American Cancer Society (see Box 82-2):

• General, unexplained feelings of discomfort
• Prickling, tingling, tightness, soreness that does not go away
• Weakness
• Unexplained loss of weight
• Abnormal findings on breast self-examination (BSE) or testicular self-examination (TSE)

* Remember that signs and symptoms in any body system can be a sign of cancer.

port systems. For example, does the client need assistance to meet daily needs? Does the disorder affect social activities or self-esteem? Is the disorder life threatening? Is the client anxious or fearful of the outcome? Is ongoing counseling, rehabilitation, or home care needed? Is a support group available? What are the reactions of family members? Will the client be a candidate for hospice care?

☛ KEY CONCEPT

Early detection promises the highest rate of survival for clients with cancer. Periodic physical examinations and self-examinations are important components of early detection.

Nursing Diagnosis

Based on data collection, nursing diagnoses are formulated for the person with cancer. Nursing diagnoses can relate to any body system, depending on the cancer's location. Some diagnoses have several causal factors. Examples of nursing diagnoses that may be seen on a client's nursing care plan include:

* Pain related to disease, diagnostic procedures, treatment
* Imbalanced Nutrition: Less than Body Requirements related to anorexia, vomiting, nausea, diarrhea
* Impaired Skin Integrity related to radiation therapy, incontinence, tumor invasion
* Risk for Infection related to inadequate secondary defenses, malnutrition, chronic disease process, effects of chemotherapy/radiation
* Spiritual Distress related to challenged belief systems, fear of death
* Anticipatory Grieving related to anticipated loss of life, family, friends, possessions

Planning and Implementation

The client with cancer requires assistance to meet many needs. Education and support are important so that the client and family better understand the disease, treatments, and side effects. The nursing care plan should consider all these needs.

Together with the client, family, and other members of the healthcare team, care is planned to meet the client's needs effectively. Planning for further nursing care should consider prognosis, treatments and their potential complications, as well as the client's functional status.

Evaluation

The healthcare team, client, and family should evaluate outcomes of care. Have short-term goals been met? For example, is the client's pain controlled? Are long-term goals still realistic? For example, will the client be able to return to work? What types of therapy or rehabilitation will the client need?

Cancers related to specific body systems are discussed in each chapter about each body system. Hospice care is discussed in Chapter 99.

NURSING CONSIDERATIONS FOR CLIENTS WITH CANCER

Procedures and Surgery

Diagnostic procedures and treatments for clients with cancer can be mildly uncomfortable to nearly intolerable. Before the procedure or treatment, it is important that the nurse administer medications that may be necessary to suppress nausea, vomiting, and diarrhea.

Supportive care after treatment is important, because the client may feel that the side effects of the therapy are too great to endure. Depression may need to be treated with counseling and medications.

Nursing considerations in cancer surgery include all normal components of preoperative and postoperative teaching (see Chap. 56). In many cases, the client will be very anxious about the results of the surgery. Was the cancer removed, partially removed, or inoperable and not removed? Additionally, the client will be concerned about changes in body image, such as with mastectomy; possible loss of sexual function, such as with prostate surgery; or the presence of ostomies, as is possible with colorectal surgery or kidney surgery.

The importance of education and client teaching cannot be overemphasized. If postoperative exercises are recommended, such as those after mastectomy, teach the client the exercises preoperatively, which will enable the client to perform them more effectively after surgery.

Allow clients to participate in their own treatment plan as much as possible. Individualized adaptations depend on each person's security and self-image. Kindness, understanding, and therapeutic communication techniques can provide an atmosphere in which clients are free to express themselves.

Chemotherapy

Providing care during chemotherapy requires knowledge about the drugs and their side effects. Only nurses who receive special instruction about chemotherapy should administer these potent agents. They must follow safe handling procedures during administration, because chemotherapeutic agents are extremely toxic and can affect the normal cells of a healthcare worker in addition to the cancerous cells of a client. Some facilities have special precautions and limitations for the pregnant nurse who may be on a designated cancer unit or work with chemotherapeutic agents.

Some chemotherapeutic agents can be administered orally. Special handling precautions with oral drugs are generally not considered necessary. However, the nurse must understand the side effects of such agents.

If the nurse is administering parenteral chemotherapy, the following are specific guidelines to follow:

* Wear gloves, gowns, and protective eyewear during preparation and administration. *Rationale: These items protect the nurse against personal injury.*
* Do not allow these agents to come in contact with the eyes or mucous membranes. If such events should occur,

rinse the affected part thoroughly with clear water for at least 5 minutes. Obtain first aid immediately. *Rationale: These agents are extremely toxic and irritating.*

- Be knowledgeable about the medications being administered. *Rationale: Knowledge of the drugs is essential in providing quality client care.*
- Do not administer any chemotherapeutic agent without carefully reviewing administration guidelines and side effects. *Rationale: Administration of chemotherapeutic agents is often based on protocols that must be followed to ensure the maximum effectiveness of the therapy.* (See also In Practice: Nursing Care Guidelines 82-1 earlier in this chapter.)

☛ KEY CONCEPT

The person undergoing chemotherapy will experience both physical and emotional needs. Follow the treatment regimen, protocol, and procedures as established by the healthcare facility and be supportive. A referral to professional counseling or chaplaincy services may be beneficial to the client and family.

Chemotherapy Administration

Chemotherapeutic agents may be given via the following routes: oral, intramuscular, intracavitary, intraperitoneal, topical, intra-arterial, intrapleural, and intravenous (IV).

Devices for Administration.   Vascular access devices are often used if chemotherapy is to be given routinely IV or intra-arterially. Because chemotherapeutic agents can damage tissue, and many cancer clients have poor veins, these devices are ideal. They are more convenient and more comfortable and eliminate the danger inherent in repeated venipunctures.

Selection of a vascular access device should take into consideration the frequency of use, length of treatment, integrity of veins, and the client's preference. Vascular access devices include:

- Peripheral access device, peripheral indwelling catheter (**PIC**) line, peripherally inserted central catheter (**PICC**)
- Central venous access device (subcutaneous port)
- External catheters (Hickman, Groshong)

In some cases, chemotherapeutic agents are administered on a constant basis by means of a chemotherapy infusion pump. A pump may be surgically implanted or worn externally.

Radiation Therapy

Providing care during radiation therapy requires special care for the client and specific precautions for the healthcare providers (see In Practice: Nursing Care Guidelines 82-2 earlier in this chapter).

Adequate explanation of therapy to the client is necessary. The client should understand that the treatment will not hurt, will only take a few minutes, and that the area being treated will not feel hot. The client has a right to understand the goal of therapy, and its possible side effects. In addition, the client needs teaching about properly caring for the skin in the area being irradiated (see In Practice: Educating the Client 82-1).

The client may be afraid to be alone during radiation therapy. Minimize anxiety by explaining that healthcare personnel must avoid radiation exposure for personal protection.

When caring for a client who has a radioactive implant (and in some cases after IV administration of a radioactive isotope), first become familiar with the institution's policies and procedures. Take proper precautions to protect staff, family members, and visitors from excessive radiation. In Practice: Nursing Care Guidelines 82-3 highlights important aspects of care for the nurse providing care to—and the client who is receiving—a radioactive implant.

Management of Side Effects

Nausea and Vomiting

Nausea and vomiting can be extremely unpleasant side effects of chemotherapy and radiation. Some clients are so affected by nausea and vomiting that they decide to postpone or forego treatment.

Many new antiemetics can help to prevent nausea and vomiting. Assess the client's reaction to treatment during each visit or encounter. Become knowledgeable about various medications that are available, and administer antiemetics according to the physician's orders. In Practice: Important Medications 82-2 lists some commonly used antiemetics.

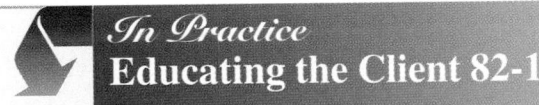

In Practice
Educating the Client 82-1

SKIN CARE DURING RADIATION THERAPY

- Use only plain, tepid water on the skin.
- Use a soft washcloth. Do not scrub.
- Inspect the skin in the treatment area for erythema, pain, and dry or moist peeling.
- If a moisturizing lotion is prescribed, be sure the physician determines the type of lotion to use.
- Do not remove marks placed on the skin by the radiologist. *Rationale: These marks are used as the guide for locating the treatment site.*
- Do not apply deodorant, powder, soap, perfume, cosmetics, scented lotion, or other skin preparations on the treatment area.
- Do not place tight clothing over the treatment area.
- Wear cotton clothing next to the skin. *Rationale: Wool or synthetics may irritate the skin.*
- Do not use any heating or cooling devices on the treatment area. Take steps to prevent burning, such as in the shower.
- Protect the skin from sun (use at least an SPF 15 sunscreen) and from wind and cold. *Rationale: The skin in the treatment area may be permanently hypersensitive and is at risk for burns or frostbite.*

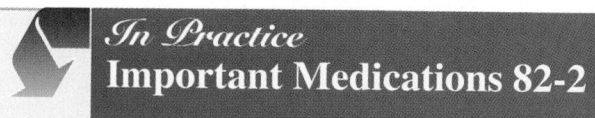

In Practice
Nursing Care Guideline 82-3

PROVIDING CARE FOR CLIENTS WITH IMPLANTED RADIOACTIVE ISOTOPES

- When giving nursing care, do not stay with the client longer than necessary; ask to be reassigned if any possibility of pregnancy exists.
- Plan ahead to make as few trips as possible into the client's room.
- Keep a record of time spent with the client or wear a "radioactive sensor" badge. Usually, a chart is placed on the door of the room, and nurses and physicians sign in and out.
- Do not stand close to the client longer than necessary. Use lead aprons or shields to minimize radiation exposure.
- In addition to Standard Precautions, handle drainage and dressings with extra care. *Rationale: There may be residual radioactivity.*
- Check whether the implant is in place after necessary nursing measures have been completed. Routinely check all equipment such as bedpans, emesis basins, and linens before removing them from the client's room. *Rationale: The implant might become dislodged, in which case it could be lost. If not handled properly, it is dangerous to others. In addition, the client would not be receiving the needed treatment.*
- If an implant does fall out, do not touch it unless absolutely necessary. Notify radiology department staff at once. If an implant must be moved, touch it only with a long forceps. A lead container is kept at the bedside for storage, in the event of an emergency. *Rationale: The implant is highly radioactive.*
- Provide diversionary activity for the client. Encourage friends and family to telephone, if the client's physical condition allows. Provide a television. Encourage friends to write. Offer reading materials or crafts. *Rationale: These actions help to decrease the client's sense of isolation.*
- Teach family members the procedures to follow. Visiting time is limited. *Rationale: Safety must be ensured.*
- Ensure that the radiology department has checked the room and declared it safe before another client is admitted. Sometimes, the room is not cleaned by housekeeping until declared safe by radiology personnel.

In Practice
Important Medications 82-2

FOR CHEMOTHERAPY-INDUCED NAUSEA AND VOMITING

Serotonin Antagonists
ondansetron (Zofran)
granisetron (Kytril)

Dopamine Blocker
metoclopramide (Reglan, Maxeran)

Phenothiazines
prochlorperazine (Compazine)
chlorpromazine (Thorazine)

Corticosteroids
dexamethasone (Decadron)
prednisone (Deltasone)

Butyrophenones
halperidol (Haldol)
droperidol (Inapsine)

mation of the mucous membranes, such as in the mouth and throat) and esophagitis are also common.

Instruct the client to avoid alcohol or foods that may cause irritation. The client should avoid alcohol-containing commercial mouthwashes as well as flossing. He or she should use only a soft brush when cleaning the teeth, and rinse the mouth thoroughly after meal and at bedtime. The following solution can be recommended as an alternative to commercial mouthwash:

- 1 teaspoon salt
- ½ teaspoon baking soda
- 500 milliliters water (1 cup)

If the client develops inflammation, a physician may recommend that the client use a swish and swallow solution that often contains a mixture of diphenhydramine (Benadryl), viscous Xylocaine, and antacid. Another alternative would be to apply vitamin E to affected areas in the mouth.

➤ Nursing Alert
Caution the client to swallow only very small amounts of swish and swallow at a time. *Rationale: The mixture will anesthetize the throat and may cause difficulty in swallowing, talking, or even breathing.*

Fatigue
Fatigue is known to affect almost all people with cancer at one time or another. It may result from the disease, treatment, or psychological distress. After pain, it is the second most distressing symptom reported. About 80% to 99% of all clients

Sometimes clients respond to nonpharmacologic therapies, such as guided imagery, massage, distraction, and relaxation techniques.

Stomatitis
The client receiving radiation or chemotherapy is susceptible to *stomatitis* (inflammation of the mouth). *Mucositis* (inflam-

who receive chemotherapy and 65% to 100% of those who receive radiation experience fatigue.

Assess clients appropriately and make recommendations for interventions, including:

- Optimal nutrition with supplements
- Planned rest and activity periods
- Assistance with prioritization of work
- Support for psychological distress
- Increase in fluids to avoid accumulation of cellular wastes
- Medical management if fatigue is related to anemia

Alopecia

Clients receiving radiation to the upper torso, or chemotherapy, often have *alopecia* (hair loss) because both therapies affect all frequently dividing cells (including cells of the hair follicles in addition to cancerous cells). Hair loss may include eyelashes, eyebrows, pubic hair, and body hair.

One intervention is to encourage clients to purchase attractive wigs before hair is lost so that wigs can be matched to natural hair in color and style. Instruct clients to use only mild shampoos and to avoid all harsh chemicals (such as dyes and permanents) during this time.

Hair loss may be the first visible sign that a client has cancer. It can be an emotional side effect.

Secondary Infections

Radiation or chemotherapy frequently renders the client more susceptible to infections, because the white blood cell count is depressed (*neutropenia*). As dead tissue sloughs, it may leave raw open areas or ulcers. Such open surfaces provide excellent portals of entry for pathogens.

Instruct clients to avoid all activities that could injure cutaneous or mucous tissues. Do not take rectal temperatures or give suppositories. Avoid multiple IV access attempts, and instruct clients to avoid anything that may lead to injury (eg, shave with an electric razor rather than a blade razor).

Inform clients that they should avoid persons and places that present increased risks for infection (eg, daycare centers). Most importantly, be sure to use proper handwashing technique and to instruct clients and all visitors to do the same.

Nursing Alert

Clients receiving radiation or chemotherapy experience lowered platelet and blood cell counts (due to myelosuppression) and therefore have an increased risk of bleeding, anemia and infection. Stress the importance of good handwashing technique. Teach clients precautions to prevent breakdown of skin or mucous membranes.

Pain

Most clients diagnosed with cancer experience pain related to the disease, procedures, or treatments. Studies have proven that nearly all cancer pain is controllable.

Perform a thorough assessment related to pain issues and follow the physician's orders related to the administration of analgesics. Give medications around the clock to consistently control pain.

Try to prevent, rather than treat, pain. Educate the client and family about the myths related to narcotics and addiction; assure them that reporting pain and taking recommended medications are appropriate and safe measures.

Many clients in acute pain manage their own pain using patient-controlled analgesia. The type and dose of pain medication prescribed by the physician are influenced by the pain's origin and severity.

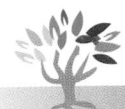

SPECIAL CONSIDERATIONS: THE LIFE SPAN

Pain

Misconceptions related to pain may affect pain management in older adults. Healthcare providers may misperceive pain as deriving from the normal aging process. Believe and evaluate any report of pain a client makes.

Physiologic responses to pain medication with regard to absorption, metabolism, and excretion may be a major concern in the elderly population. Increasing age is associated with a decrease in the hepatic and renal clearance of many medications; therefore, this population may be at higher risk for toxicity.

Stress

A diagnosis of cancer, in combination with its various treatments and lifestyle changes, is stressful. Several techniques are known to be helpful in the reduction of stress.

Therapeutic visualization or guided imagery can provide forms of stress relief as well as pain relief. Clients use audio- or videotapes to guide themselves toward teaching their bodies to respond to cues, and to become more proficient at lessening stress, relieving pain, or combating cancer cells.

Diversional activities are important. The client may enjoy massage therapy, music therapy, art therapy, or exercise as stress relievers.

Hormone-Related Effects

The most common side effects that women receiving tamoxifen therapy for breast cancer experience are those related to menopause. These side effects include amenorrhea, hot flashes, insomnia, and depression. For men on anti-androgen therapy for prostate cancer, the number-one related side effect is hot flashes.

Drug therapy with clonidine HCl (Catapres) or a combination of belladonna, phenobarbital, and ergotamine (Bellergal S) may be effective in eliminating hot flashes for clients receiving hormone therapy. Vitamin E may also be useful.

Many herbal products claim to eliminate hot flashes and may be sold in combination: these include ginseng, cohosh, dong quai, wild yam root, and primrose oil.

Advise the client who is interested in trying a herbal remedy to speak with the physician first and to check for side effects related to these remedies. Many herbal products for menopausal symptoms and hot flashes do contain natural plant estrogen, and are not indicated for women who should not take estrogen-containing products.

Nutritional Needs

Cancer can deplete the body of proteins and affect overall nutritional status. The client may experience oral complications, such as stomatitis, mucositis, and dry mouth. Various taste alterations secondary to chemotherapy and radiation also occur. Thus, nutrition education and side-effect management are important components of the total nursing plan of care. In Practice: Nursing Care Plan 82-1 highlights the care of a client who is experiencing inadequate nutrition due to cancer therapy.

The diet must be high in proteins, carbohydrates, and vitamins. Stress the importance of good nutrition and mainte-

nance of fluid and electrolyte balance to the client and family, particularly with clients who are receiving intensive radiation or chemotherapy. Several small meals are recommended for such clients.

Recognize when clients are experiencing taste changes and recommend alternative food options. You may suggest nutritional supplements, such as Ensure, Sustacal, or Carnation Instant Breakfast, if the need arises. Eating fresh parsley helps build up white blood cells.

Note that many cultures have different food practices, beliefs, and rituals. Therefore, work within the food practices of a client's culture. By doing so, you will improve compliance, communication, and nutritional status.

Client and Family Teaching

As part of routine healthcare, the nurse teaches breast self-examination or testicular self-examination techniques. Pamphlets that reinforce client teaching techniques are readily

---

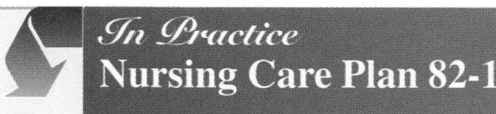

In Practice
Nursing Care Plan 82-1

THE CLIENT WITH CANCER AND INADEQUATE NUTRITION

MEDICAL HISTORY: *H.B., a 72-year-old female who was diagnosed with breast cancer and underwent a modified radical mastectomy, is now receiving chemotherapy. Client has lost approximately 15 pounds since her diagnosis 4 months ago. Weight currently 115 lbs. Client's husband reports that client is having trouble eating.*

MEDICAL DIAGNOSIS: *Breast cancer; chemotherapy-related weight loss due to poor nutrition*

Data Collection/Nursing Assessment: Client is a thin, frail-appearing female. Skin pale pink, returns slowly when pinched. She states, "I'm so tired. It's so hard for me to do anything, especially eat. Nothing tastes good. I've lost so much weight." Client's receiving chemotherapy, currently in her third cycle. She reports occasional nausea but no vomiting. "The medicine that I get before the chemotherapy helps with the vomiting." Dietary history reveals intake of 1 piece of toast with jelly and tea for breakfast, ½ sandwich with 4 oz milk for lunch, and only bites of food at dinner. Husband states, "I don't know how she can survive. She eats like a bird." (*Although other nursing diagnoses may be appropriate, a priority nursing diagnosis is addressed below.*)

Nursing Diagnosis: Imbalanced nutrition, less than body requirements related to effects of chemotherapy as evidenced by client's limited intake on dietary history, weight loss, and client's statements about lack of taste.

Planning
SHORT-TERM GOALS:
#1. Client will state appropriate food choices.
#2. Client and husband will verbalize ways to increase nutritional intake.

LONG-TERM GOALS:
#3. On next visit, client will report an increase in food and fluid intake.
#4. Client will maintain at least current weight through remainder of chemotherapy regimen.

Implementation
NURSING ACTION: *Review with client and husband typical food plan, including food selections, snacks, likes and dislikes. Investigate any cultural or ethnic preferences or practices.*
RATIONALE: *Reviewing client's typical patterns provides a basis for teaching. Culture plays a major role in eating practices.*

NURSING ACTION: *Encourage the use of foods high in protein, carbohydrates, and vitamins. Offer suggestions for ways to enhance nutritional value of foods, such as adding wheat germ to toast or ice cream to milk. Encourage fluid intake to at least 2 liters per day.*
RATIONALE: *Cancer and its therapies can deplete the body of proteins, affecting overall nutritional status.*

Evaluation: Client reports liking milk and milkshakes, peanut butter and fruit; husband will try adding ice cream to milk at lunch; client agrees to trying to eat

(continued)

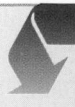

In Practice
Nursing Care Plan 82-1 *(Continued)*

2 to 3 peanut butter crackers as afternoon snack. *Progress to meeting Goal #1 and Goal #2.*

NURSING ACTION: *Encourage rest periods before meals. Suggest small, frequent meals several times per day. Recommend fluids after meals.*
RATIONALE: *Fatigue can interfere with appetite and desire to eat. Smaller, more frequent meals prevent overtiring during eating. Consuming fluids with meals may cause feelings of fullness, interfering with the client's ability to complete the meal.*

NURSING ACTION: *Suggest the use of supplements, such as Ensure or protein bars, as between-meal snacks.*
RATIONALE: *Supplements provide an additional source of necessary nutrients.*

Evaluation: Client identifies appropriate food selections such as fruit and fruit juices from a list of foods; she states, "I'll keep a record of what I eat." Husband states, "I'll get her a supplement and add ice cream to it. It'll be a super milkshake." *Goal #1 and Goal #2 met.*

NURSING ACTION: *Encourage client and husband to keep a record of food intake for next visit. Also suggest that client weigh herself once a week and record this weight, bringing the information with her at the next visit.*
RATIONALE: *Keeping a diary helps in evaluating client's compliance with nutrition, and provides a means for offering additional suggestions and teaching. Weekly weights provide evidence of the client's status.*

Evaluation: Next visit, client and husband report slight increase in intake supported by client's food diary. Weight sustained at 115 lbs. *Goal #3 met; progress to meeting Goal #4.*

---

available from the American Cancer Society. Cancer screening guidelines are also available to encourage the public to participate in decisions regarding screening tests based on age, sex, and risk factors.

Teach all clients to report immediately any of the warning signs identified by the American Cancer Society. Individuals are not always aware of slight changes in the body, which may be perceived as normal changes of aging. Many of these sensations serve as warnings. If signs or symptoms persist, they require investigation.

When diagnosed with any tumor, clients and family members must be involved in decision-making related to cancer, starting with its diagnosis. Begin by asking clients what information they need. Remain cognizant of the extent to which the client and family members are able and willing to learn and to be involved in cancer care. Clients and families can quickly feel overwhelmed, especially during the diagnosis phase.

Provide information and explanations regarding treatment options, various procedures, management of side effects, and other related issues. Also supply written information along with verbal explanations. Repeat information during future meetings. Ensure that clients receive information in a manner they can understand, especially if English is the second language.

Remember also that older adults may have short-term memory loss or vision and hearing problems that could impede learning. Recommending that the client have a family member or friend present during a teaching session is one way to overcome these barriers. Remember to document all teaching for future reference.

A cancer diagnosis is a family crisis. Surviving this crisis means learning how to best manage energy, time, and rela-tionships. Provide information and education that assist the client and family in managing this crisis. Knowledge provides strength. Also provide information related to support systems that they can call on. It would be helpful when assessing these needs to include an oncology social worker and/or chaplain. Learning to manage stress and the pressures of daily life can offer clients and their families insights regarding options and priorities.

☛ KEY CONCEPT

The mere diagnosis of cancer generates fear in most people. Remember to offer reassurance and support. Emphasize that most cancers are curable, especially if treatment begins early. When caring for persons with cancer, interpersonal skills are used in conjunction with nursing skills.

➤ STUDENT SYNTHESIS

Key Points

- Cancer is characterized by excessive growth and proliferation of cells that lack the capabilities of normal cellular function.
- Benign tumors do not metastasize but can interfere with structure and function of tissues. Metastatic tumors are composed of dedifferentiated (undifferentiated) cells that lack orderly growth.
- Carcinomas develop from epithelial tissues and sarcomas develop from connective tissues.

- Carcinogenesis can be caused by chemicals, radiation, and viruses.
- To assist with cancer regimens and protocols, cancers are graded and staged.
- Tumor markers are specific enzymes, antigens, proteins, hormones, or genes that can indicate malignancies.
- Surgical therapies can include biopsy, cryosurgery, electrocauterization, fulguration, exenteration, and laser, preventive, or palliative surgery.
- The main chemotherapeutic agents include alkylating agents, antibiotics, antimetabolites, antimitotics, and hormones.
- Biotherapy uses biologic response modifiers to enhance the immune system and destroy cancerous cells.
- Radiation can be used externally as well as inserted as radioactive devices internally.
- The common side effects of cancer therapies include myelosuppression, nausea, vomiting, fatigue, alopecia, pain, and infections.

Critical Thinking Exercises

1. Your client has been diagnosed with colon cancer. He tells you that his cousin had lung cancer and that the cousin's treatment was different from the treatment he has been undergoing. Your client is very worried about his own diagnosis and prognosis. What would you tell your client regarding the differences between the two cancer types including treatment, prognosis, and expectations?

2. A colleague tells you that an elderly client that she is caring for has become confused and somnolent over the last 24 hours. The client is receiving chemotherapy for ovarian cancer and morphine for pain control. The family has become concerned that the disease is progressing. Your colleague asks your advice. Discuss your assessment and the plan you would present.

3. You have been caring for a client with breast cancer on an outpatient basis. She is currently receiving radiation after lumpectomy. Your client tells you that normal daily activities are becoming difficult, she feels depressed most of the time, and all she wants to do is sleep. Discuss your assessment, plan of care including education, and what supports if any you would suggest.

NCLEX-Style Review Questions

1. The leading cause of new cancer diagnosis in men is for:
   a. Colon cancer
   b. Lung cancer
   c. Prostate cancer
   d. Skin cancer

2. The nurse understands that the probable effect of a client's choosing to continue to smoke cigarettes will be:
   a. Abnormal CA-125 marker
   b. Increased risk for developing lung cancer
   c. Increased risk for neutropenia
   d. Metastasis

3. Which measure, if used by the nurse, would be most effective in preventing the transfer of disease to a client on neutropenic precautions?
   a. Encourage client to eat fresh fruits and vegetables.
   b. Encourage client to use a firm-bristled toothbrush.
   c. Instruct the client to wear a mask at all times.
   d. Instruct visitors to check in with the nurse before entering the client's room.

4. Which method would be most appropriate to control pain for a cancer client?
   a. Administer medication when pain is severe.
   b. Administer medication around the clock.
   c. Administer medication only when the client asks for medication.
   d. Administer medication in small doses.

5. Which diet is appropriate for a client receiving chemotherapy?
   a. High-calorie, high-protein
   b. High-fat, high-carbohydrate
   c. Low-fat, low-calorie
   d. Low-protein, low-calorie

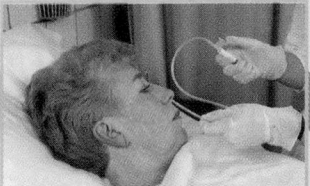

CHAPTER

83

Allergic, Immune, and Autoimmune Disorders

LEARNING OBJECTIVES

1. Differentiate the following: allergy, antigen, immunogens, antibody, and histamine.
2. Demonstrate the procedure for intradermal skin testing.
3. Discuss at least three components of the medical history and the physical exam that relate to the detection of allergies.
4. State three possible skin and three possible respiratory manifestations of the allergic response.
5. Discuss at least five possible gastrointestinal manifestations of the allergic response.
6. Discuss at least three possible manifestations of the allergic response that relate to drugs.
7. State three methods for treating multisystem allergy response.
8. Discuss at least five nursing considerations related to prevention and treatment of anaphylaxis.
9. Compare and contrast organ specific and non–organ-specific auto-immune diseases.

NEW TERMINOLOGY

allergen	induration
allergy	immunogen
anaphylaxis	immunosuppression
autoimmune disorder	immunotherapy
eczema	non–organ-specific
histamine	organ-specific
hives	urticaria

ACRONYMS

AIDS	IgE	SLE
HIV		

As described in Chapters 24 and 40, the complex human immune system protects individuals against "foreign invaders" (*pathogens*). This protection is called the *immune response*. Sometimes, however, the immune system works against a person's best interests, and an allergy, immune, or autoimmune disorder results.

Allergy, defined as hypersensitivity to one or more substances, is a common problem. A person acquires an allergy from exposure to an offending substance. The physician who treats allergies is called an *allergist*, although internal medicine and family practice specialists also treat clients with allergies. In addition, pediatricians see many children with allergies.

Normal immunity is based on the body's ability to recognize foreign proteins and to marshal its defenses to destroy foreign matter. Immune mechanisms are not always positive or beneficial to the body. When an *antigen* (a foreign protein substance) touches or enters the body, the body reacts by producing antibodies for protection against that antigen. The *antigen–antibody* reaction releases chemical mediators, the most common being histamine. These mediators initiate a series of physiologic events in the body's organs. Because antibodies form after initial contact with an antigen, an allergic reaction cannot occur at the first exposure to an antigen. Subsequent contact with the antigen may cause an allergic reaction with a wide variety of symptoms.

One type of immune disorder is an *autoimmune disorder*. Normally the body is able to distinguish "self" from "not self" and takes steps to eliminate substances in the "not self" category. The difficulty in an autoimmune disorder is that the body fails to recognize its own cells as "self" and begins to destroy them.

DIAGNOSTIC TESTS

Determining the cause of an allergy, immune, or autoimmune disorder is often difficult. A person's antigen–antibody response may vary with fatigue, seasons, or hormones. A detailed medical history and physical examination are needed to help establish a diagnosis (Box 83-1). To further establish a diagnosis, laboratory and skin tests are performed.

Laboratory Tests

Laboratory tests include a complete blood count with white blood cell differential and eosinophil count, an eosinophil smear of secretions, and measurement of blood levels of immune response factors such as **IgE** (immunoglobulin E).

Skin Tests

Skin tests are done to confirm suspected disorders or to determine the causes of allergic reactions. Several antigens are tested at one time, with each antigen injected intradermally or applied to a small scratch on the skin (*epicutaneous method*).

➤➤ BOX 83-1

IMPORTANT MEDICAL HISTORY AND PHYSICAL EXAMINATION INFORMATION FOR DIAGNOSING ALLERGIES AND IMMUNE PROBLEMS

Important medical history information includes information about the following:

- Onset, duration, nature, and progression of symptoms
- Factors that aggravate and alleviate symptoms
- Possible environmental or occupational exposures, such as smoking, hobbies, household activities, and animals
- History of family allergies
- Medication usage

Important physical examination information includes the following:

- Skin assessment
  - Color (eg, erythema, cyanosis, pallor)
  - Temperature
  - Rashes
  - Pruritus (itching)
  - Hives ([urticaria] pink edematous elevations)
- Respiratory assessment
  - Nasal edema and congestion
  - Sneezing
  - Rhinorrhea
  - Edema of the oropharynx
  - Hoarseness

- Stridor
- Cough
- Dyspnea
- Wheezing
- Ear assessment
  - Tympanic membrane bulging or retraction
  - Fluid levels
- Gastrointestinal tract assessment
  - Nausea, vomiting
  - Altered peristalsis
  - Cramping
  - Diarrhea
- Cardiovascular assessment
  - Tachycardia
  - Hypotension
  - *Syncope* (fainting)
  - Signs of shock
- Nervous system assessment
  - Anxiety
  - Confusion
  - Seizures
  - Temperature elevation
  - Behavioral changes

These areas are then labeled or otherwise identified. After 20 minutes, the provider reads the skin tests in much the same way as in a tuberculin test. *Erythema* (redness) and most commonly an **induration** (a lump, wheal, or edema) indicate a positive skin test. The degree of edema, measured in millimeters, indicates the severity of the reaction. In this way, the provider can identify which substances are causing the client's reaction and to what extent the client reacts. Despite a positive skin test, a substance may not always cause an allergic reaction. A physician may order antihistamines or "allergy shots" for the client's comfort when tests are done. Figure 83-1 illustrates the technique for intradermal skin testing.

Observe the client closely during a skin test because occasionally a test will cause a severe reaction. Such a reaction is unusual because the amount of the antigen used is very small; however, it may occur if the client is highly sensitive to it. The symptoms of a severe allergic response (*anaphylaxis*) are reviewed later in this chapter and in Chapter 43.

NURSING PROCESS

Data Collection

Carefully observe and assess the client with an allergic or immune disorder. Perform a head-to-toe assessment to establish a baseline for future comparison. Question the client for symptoms such as pruritus, shortness of breath, numbness, and tingling. Examine the client for symptoms such as a rash, urticaria, excessive tearing, rhinorrhea, sneezing, wheezing, or other respiratory signs, and localized edema or erythema. Document and report any abnormal findings or changes in this baseline level.

Report any allergies a client describes or exhibits. For the client's protection, note any medication allergies in large letters on the front of the chart and on the medication record when the client is admitted. A client with allergies usually also wears a special identification band. Keep in mind that a person can

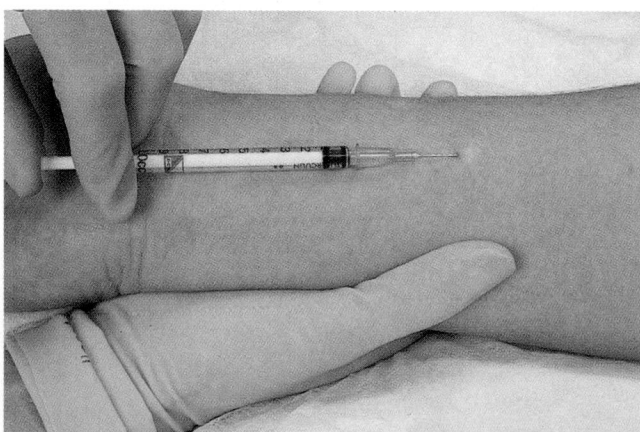

FIGURE 83-1. Skin testing by intradermal injection. With the needle held nearly flat against the skin and the bevel up, the needle is inserted approximately one eighth of an inch under the epidermis. The test agent is injected slowly as a small blister appears. Signs of positive reaction to the agent will appear in 24 to 48 hours.

have an allergic reaction to any medication. The reaction will occur faster and more dramatically if the medication is administered parenterally. Give no medication without first making sure that the client is not allergic to it. If there are any doubts, or if the client has a history of allergies or asthma, the physician may do a skin (*intradermal*) test first. Even then, be prepared to deal with possible anaphylaxis (discussed later).

The client with an immune disorder will generally present with vague symptoms such as fatigue or dyspnea, frequent or recurrent infections, slow wound healing, joint pain, skin rashes, or visual disturbances. Ask the client about any family history of cancer or immune disorders. The physician and other staff can further evaluate any reported abnormalities.

Assessment of the immune system also includes the administration and evaluation of skin tests. These may be administered intradermally or as scratch tests. The client's medical history is particularly important in assessing allergic and immune disorders. In addition, observe the client's emotional response. Does the disorder interfere with the person's daily life? What assistance does the client need?

Nursing Diagnosis

Disorders of the immune system are believed to contribute to or cause many systemic symptoms and problems. For example, allergies are responsible for symptoms that range from rhinorrhea and skin rash to asthma or a total anaphylactic response. Nearly any nursing diagnosis is possible, depending on the specific disorder.

The following are examples of nursing diagnoses that may appear on a nursing care plan for a client with an allergy. Some diagnoses represent more than one causal factor.

- Diarrhea related to food allergy
- Risk for Injury related to severe allergic reaction
- Impaired Skin Integrity related to pruritus, rash
- Risk for Caregiver Role Strain related to a chronicity of an immune or autoimmune disorder
- Disturbed Sleep Pattern related to pruritus, dyspnea
- Fatigue related to asthma, sleep deprivation
- Delayed Growth and Development related to childhood asthma, food allergies
- Disturbed Self-esteem related to rash, itching, difficult breathing

Examples of nursing diagnoses for anaphylaxis include:

- Anxiety/Fear related to inability to breathe
- Ineffective Airway Clearance related to edematous airway
- Impaired Gas Exchange related to severe bronchospasm
- Disturbed Thought Processes related to loss of consciousness

The following nursing diagnoses may be seen on nursing care plans for clients with many autoimmune disorders:

- Chronic Pain related to development of disease
- Imbalanced Nutrition: Less than Body Requirements related to inability to digest nutrients, anorexia

- Impaired Skin Integrity related to diarrhea, reaction to sun, medications
- Impaired Physical Mobility related to decreased strength and endurance, pain

Planning and Implementation

Together the client, nurse, and family plan for effective individualized care to meet the client's needs. Provide supportive care and continuously monitor the client's status. The client may require assistance with activities of daily living and in dealing with the emotional aspects of having a chronic disorder. Teach the client and family about the disorder, its prognosis, and treatment. A sample teaching plan is illustrated in Box 83-2.

Evaluation

Evaluate outcomes of care with the client, family, and other members of the healthcare team. Have you met short-term goals? For example, are the client's acute allergic symptoms controlled? Are long-term goals still realistic? Planning for further nursing care considers the client's prognosis, as well as any complications and the client's response to care given. For example, is the client complying with medications prescribed? The seriousness of the disorder influences the future planning for care and rehabilitation.

ALLERGIES

Antigens that cause an immune response in the body are known as **immunogens.** Sometimes, a tissue reaction may occur, in which case the antigens are called **allergens.** When a person has a tissue reaction to a specific substance, the person is called *sensitive* or *allergic* to the allergen. Allergens can enter the body in various ways, via:

- *Inhalation:* Pollen, dust, mold, grass, various plants, animal dander
- *Ingestion:* Medications (aspirin, penicillin), foods (chocolate, eggs, seafood, strawberries, nuts), preservatives
- *Injection:* Medications (such as antibiotics), insect stings or bites, immunization with animal serum, blood transfusions
- *Direct contact:* Poison ivy, cosmetics, dyes, metals, latex rubber, nylon, wool

➤ ➤ BOX 83-2

SAMPLE TEACHING PLAN FOR A CLIENT WITH AN ALLERGIC OR IMMUNE DISORDER

Key Assessment Areas
- History of allergic or anaphylactic responses
- Knowledge of allergens that trigger allergic or anaphylactic responses
- Understanding of treatment plan

Client and Family Outcomes
- The client and family identify the causes and effects of specific substances that cause allergic responses.
- The client and family make modifications in lifestyle, diet, and environment to avoid allergens.
- The client takes prescribed medications as ordered by the physician.

Implementation Strategies
Teach the client and family to:
- Decrease airborne particles if the allergens are dust or pollen.
- Remove dust-collecting draperies, venetian blinds, upholstered furniture, carpeting.
- Vacuum and wet-mop floors, surfaces daily.
- Place hypoallergenic covers on mattresses, pillows.
- Remove houseplants, pets.
- Avoid contact with grasses, weeds, dry leaves.
- Avoid stuffed animals, pillows, tufted materials.
- Wear a mask when cleaning or when outdoors during seasons of high pollen counts.

- Remain in air-conditioned environment during high pollen counts.
- Heat home with steam or hot water rather than forced air, if possible.
- Replace filters frequently.
- Circulate room air through clean air filters.
- Avoid smoke-filled environments.
- Modify diet if the allergens are found in food substances.
- List all foods or food substances that cause allergic responses.
- Remove all such foods or sources of food substance from diet.
- Select alternative sources of nutrition.
- Identify the purpose and use of medications prescribed to treat the allergy.

Areas for Evaluation
- Ability to identify allergens
- Demonstration or verbalization of changes made in environment and/or diet to eliminate allergen
- Verbalization or demonstration of understanding of medications
- Evidence or report of fewer or no allergic or anaphylactic responses

Source: Adapted from Smeltzer, S., & Bare, B. (2000). *Brunner and Suddarth's textbook of medical-surgical nursing* (9th ed., p. 1397). Philadelphia: Lippincott Williams & Wilkins.

Researchers believe the tendency toward allergic response is inherited, but this does not mean that specific allergies are inherited. The manifestation of allergy relates to many factors, including hormonal responses, type and concentration of allergen, body part involved, exposure to the allergen, and concurrent illness. Allergy symptoms can occur at any age and vary in response from mild to life threatening (as in anaphylaxis).

Allergic reactions may affect the skin and mucous membranes, the respiratory passages, and the gastrointestinal tract. They can result in rash, edema, itching, dyspnea, contractions of the smooth muscles, and in severe cases, total shock and death (as may occur in anaphylaxis; see Chap. 43).

Edema is a symptom that may be related to allergy or to emotional factors. It may occur in one part of the body, such as the lips and eyelids, or it may be generalized. If the swelling presses on a vital organ, such as the larynx, it can severely impair the person's ability to function.

Allergies With a Skin Response

Urticaria (Hives)

Reddened areas (*erythema*), itching (*pruritus*), and burning around swollen patches on the skin may appear. The swellings are called **hives** or **urticaria.** They appear suddenly and may disappear after a few hours or may last for a period of days or weeks. Hives may result from a variety of causes, including foods; additives; medications; viral, bacterial, or parasitic infections; or stress factors (eg, heat, sun, cold, emotional stress). Management includes identification of the causative factor and medications such as antihistamines, epinephrine, or steroids.

Eczema

In **eczema** (atopic dermatitis), tiny blisters that itch and ooze cover the skin, usually in the folds of the neck, elbows, and knees. In *chronic eczema,* the skin becomes scaly and thickened (see Chap. 74).

Contact Dermatitis

A common allergen is poison ivy. In contact with the skin, the plant oils cause itching, swelling, redness, and blisters. Other allergens include soaps, detergents, perfumes, cosmetics, metals in jewelry, leathers, wool, and latex products. In Practice: Nursing Care Plan 83-1 describes the care for a client with contact dermatitis.

Allergies With a Respiratory Response

Allergic Asthma

Spasms of smooth muscles of the bronchi, in addition to edema, create breathing difficulties, which cause cough, mucous accumulation, and wheezing. In a severe attack, the client may become cyanotic; death may follow. Chapter 85 describes asthma in more detail.

Bronchial Asthma

Bronchial asthma is a common condition, characterized by recurring paroxysms of dyspnea of the wheezing type. It is caused by a narrowing of the lumen of the smaller bronchi and bronchioles. It is associated with an allergic reaction in the bronchioles.

Bronchial asthma has several classifications, including *extrinsic asthma* (a reaction to inhaled allergens), *intrinsic asthma* (in which there is no eliciting allergen, but it may be related to infections or environmental stimuli, such as air pollution), and *mixed asthma.* Asthma may also be induced by such factors as exercise, aspirin, stress, or occupational factors (eg, fumes, dust, gases).

Signs and Symptoms.   Signs and symptoms of bronchial asthma include periods of dyspnea, tightness in the chest, wheezing, cough, tenacious sputum, cyanosis, profuse perspiration, and increased pulse rate and respirations. Attacks can be frightening; the person can have a sensation of suffocation. Death can occur in extreme situations.

Treatment.   Treatment includes the use of bronchodilators, corticosteroids, antihistamines, and anticholinergics. Inhalation therapy with adrenergic agonists, cromolyn sodium (Intal, Nalcrom, Opticrom), and steroids is convenient and easy to perform. Narcotics are contraindicated because they cause respiratory depression. Additional treatments include environmental controls such as eliminating dust, fumes, and animal dander. Controlling other precipitating factors is also essential. Dietary control may be necessary for sensitive persons. Exercise is encouraged rather than discouraged. Instruct clients to use their inhalers before exercise (to avoid bronchospasm). Caution clients to wear a face mask in extremely cold weather.

Allergic Rhinitis

Allergic rhinitis (hay fever) is an inflammation of the nasal passages caused by an allergen. Additional responses include sneezing; watery rhinorrhea; edema; burning, itching, and watery eyes; fullness and itching of the ears; and itching of the throat and palate. Potential allergens include all inhalants, pollen, molds, dust, dust mites, perfumes, and animal dander. Symptoms may be seasonal or perennial.

Gastrointestinal Allergy

In this type of allergy, also called *food sensitivity,* the immune system reacts to an otherwise harmless substance. Common food allergens include dairy products, eggs, wheat, soybeans, fish, shellfish, chocolate, nuts, seeds, corn, beer, citrus fruits, and many food additives and preservatives. Common manifestations include nausea and vomiting, diarrhea, abdominal pain and tenderness, swelling of the lips and throat, itching of the palate, rhinoconjunctivitis, sneezing, wheezing, urticaria, and migraine headaches. In many cases, a food that causes burping often also causes allergy.

Drug Allergy

Adverse Reactions

A true drug allergy results from the antigen–antibody response. An *adverse drug reaction* is a noxious or unintended effect of a medication. Drug reactions are linked to about 3% of hospitalizations, and 15% to 30% of hospitalized clients have adverse

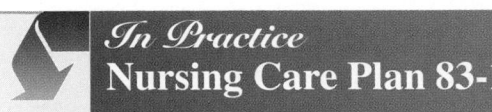

In Practice
Nursing Care Plan 83-1

THE CLIENT WITH CONTACT DERMATITIS

MEDICAL HISTORY: *P.R., a college-aged student, comes to the student health center complaining of severe itching and a rash. Rash is located around neck, axilla, and wrists. Client stated, "It just started this morning after I put on my turtleneck sweater that I just washed yesterday." Client denies any history of other health problems.*

MEDICAL DIAGNOSIS: *Contact dermatitis*

Data Collection/Nursing Assessment: Small, scattered, raised, reddened lesions noted on nape of neck, axilla, and wrist areas. Several small, blister-like areas noted on neck and crease of axilla. Lesions averaging in size from approximately ¼ to ½ cm in diameter. Further investigation reveals client used a new laundry soap to wash his clothes. He states, "The itching is terrible and I've been scratching a lot." Two small areas noted on both wrists as bright red and open, oozing clear fluid. (*Although other nursing diagnoses may be appropriate, a priority nursing diagnosis is addressed below.*)

Nursing Diagnosis: Impaired skin integrity related to contact dermatitis as evidenced by lesions, urticaria, and excoriated areas.

Planning
SHORT-TERM GOALS:
#1. Client will state the reason for rash.
#2. Client will verbalize measures to decrease itching and decrease further development of lesions.

LONG-TERM GOALS:
#3. Client will exhibit no further development of lesions or infection.
#4. Client will demonstrate signs and symptoms of healing.

Implementation
NURSING ACTION: *Explain to client that the cause of the rash is most likely related to use of new laundry detergent.*
RATIONALE: *Explanations aid in helping the client understand suspected cause of the rash.*

NURSING ACTION: *Urge client to refrain from scratching the rash. Offer suggestions to control itching, such as cool compresses or showers, light patting of the area, and distraction. Encourage the client to keep the area clean and dry, but to avoid vigorous rubbing.*
RATIONALE: *Continued scratching promotes continued itching, which could lead to further irritation and skin breakdown. Keeping the area clean helps to reduce the risk of infection. Vigorous rubbing could exacerbate the itching.*

Evaluation: Client states, "I won't ever use that cheap detergent again." Cool compresses applied at clinic with relief. *Goal #1 met; progress to meeting Goal #2.*

NURSING ACTION: *Teach client about topical medications to be prescribed, such as corticosteroids and antihistamine ointments. Stress the need to avoid overuse.*
RATIONALE: *Corticosteroids and antihistamine ointments aid in reducing the inflammation and itching. Overusing the ointments could lead to systemic absorption.*

Evaluation: Client able to state measures to control itching. Hydrocortisone cream prescribed. Client demonstrated how to apply ointment. Client reports continued relief of itching with cool compresses. *Goal #2 met.*

NURSING ACTION: *Arrange for followup visit in 3 days. Teach client signs and symptoms of infection to report immediately.*
RATIONALE: *Followup visits allow for evaluation of effectiveness of therapy and identification of potential complications. Teaching about signs and symptoms of infection allows for prompt identification and notification should any occur.*

Evaluation: Client returns to clinic in 3 days; lesions pale pink, without any drainage. No new lesions are present. Two previously opened areas now closed. Client reports using cool compresses and distraction to control itching. He states, "I rewashed my clothes in my old detergent." *Goal #3 met; progress to meeting Goal #4.*

---

drug reactions. Symptoms vary depending on the drug. Pay close attention if a client claims to be allergic to a substance or drug. Obtain a careful history of the previous reaction and document it in the client's medical record. Encourage persons who are allergic to certain medications or who have had severe reactions to wear a medical alert identification bracelet or tag (eg, MedicAlert).

Serum Sickness or Serum Reaction
Administration of certain drugs may cause a serum reaction. For example, the antiserum used for rabies treatment may cause a severe serum reaction. The client's body mounts a reaction and immunologic attack on the serum or medication administered. Symptoms occur 7 to 14 days after receiving a drug against which the client has no antibodies. Symptoms include

itching and inflammation at the point of injection, skin rash, enlarged lymph nodes, and sometimes swollen joints, as well as a feeling of general weakness and an elevated temperature. Treatment usually includes antihistamines. Corticosteroids are given in more severe cases.

Allergy With Multisystem Response

Some allergies produce symptoms in more than one body system. Initially, the client may experience localized itching and edema, but soon, systemic gastrointestinal or respiratory symptoms may appear. Latex sensitivity is an example of this type of allergic response. Early manifestations include symptoms of contact dermatitis such as pruritus, erythema, and edema, but may progress to vesicles, papules, and crusting of the skin. Respiratory, cardiac, and gastrointestinal symptoms may follow, and in some instances, the life-threatening symptoms of anaphylaxis can occur. The client develops wheezing, dyspnea, laryngeal edema, bronchial spasm, tachycardia, and eventual cardiac arrest.

Treatment

Avoidance of the Substance

Avoiding allergens may be difficult. For instance, a person who is allergic to chocolate can simply stop eating it. But eliminating white flour from the diet or dust from the environment is more complicated. In many cases, when complete avoidance of the allergen is impossible, modifications are helpful. For example, foam rubber or polyester fiber can substitute for feather pillows, and antiallergenic or hypoallergenic cosmetics are available. Encourage the person with allergies, especially to pollens, not to rake leaves or mow the lawn. Some people are able to relocate to pollen-free areas during the pollen season. Other people who are allergic to pet dander may have to give up their pets. When nurses or clients are allergic to latex, they must avoid rubber gloves, catheters, and other latex-based materials. Studies have shown that severe emotional reactions can precipitate or aggravate allergic reactions. See In Practice: Educating the Client 83-1 for more information on understanding allergic conditions.

Immunotherapy

Immunotherapy, also called *desensitization* or *hyposensitization,* consists of giving minute doses of allergens subcutaneously. The doses are gradually increased to enable the client to slowly develop a tolerance to the allergen. Sometimes this treatment eliminates the allergy.

Clients may receive injections weekly or more often. If desensitization is done to treat a seasonal allergy, it must start at least 3 months before the specific allergy season. If the allergy is not seasonal, injections should continue throughout the year. Treatment is fairly expensive but can be helpful to those who have pollen or dust allergies. Treatment may last from 1 to 2 years or longer. Some treatments last for 5 years.

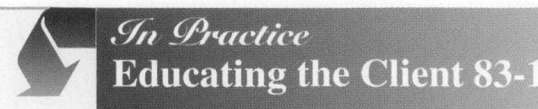

In Practice
Educating the Client 83-1

UNDERSTANDING ALLERGIC CONDITIONS

- Name of allergen and how and where it occurs
- Relationship between symptoms and exposure to causative allergens
- Modifications to environment to reduce exposure to allergens
- Medication and food labels are to be read carefully
- Proper administration of medications, including inhalers and self-injections
- Observations for delayed responses to immunotherapy (allergy shots)
- Compliance and self-responsibility
- Understanding that it may take weeks to months to obtain optimal results

Nursing Alert

Clients should remain in the physician's clinic for 20 minutes following injections for desensitization, due to the possibility of severe reactions.

Medication Therapy

Numerous medications may be given to specifically counteract an allergy or to treat symptoms.

Antihistamines. *Antihistamines* are effective because they inhibit the action of **histamine,** a major chemical mediator involved in the allergic response. These agents provide only temporary relief, however, and clients must use antihistamines frequently if they are to remain free of symptoms. Clients should not use antihistamines for perennial allergies because prolonged use is associated with undesirable effects. These medications may cause drowsiness. In clients who have asthma, antihistamines may dry up the secretions so much that clients cannot swallow or expectorate.

Symptomatic Relief Medications. The type of medication a client uses depends on the symptoms. Decongestants may be used to alleviate symptoms of nasal congestion. In Practice: Important Medications 83-1 highlights some of the more common antihistamines and decongestants.

Clients may receive epinephrine in emergencies to neutralize the adverse effects of histamine. Epinephrine relieves or reduces bronchospasms and reduces congestion of bronchial mucosa by dilating the bronchi. It constricts small blood vessels in the skin and counteracts symptoms of shock. Epinephrine is also used in severe anaphylaxis to treat vasodilation and bronchial constriction. Bronchodilators and expectorants may relieve respiratory symptoms. Cortisone preparations and other anti-inflammatory agents may reduce itching and inflammation in skin lesions. External medications applied to the skin may have cooling and antiseptic effects and reduce itching and other symptoms.

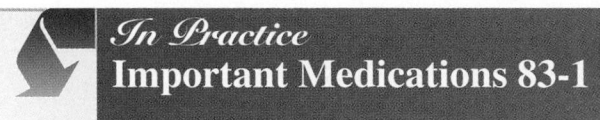

In Practice
Important Medications 83-1

TO TREAT ALLERGY SYMPTOMS

Antihistamines

Sedating Drugs
cetirizime (Zyrtec)
diphenhydramine (Benadryl)
chlorpheniramine (Chlor-Trimeton)
hydroxyzine (Atarax)
promethazine (Phenergen)
Non-Sedating Drugs
fexofenadine (Allegra)
loratadine (Claritin)

Adrenergic Decongestants
oxymetazoline (Afrin, Dristan, Sinex)
phenylephrine (Neo-Synephrine)
pseudoephedrine (Sudafed)

Anaphylaxis

Anaphylaxis refers to a hypersensitivity reaction to an antigen. Severe reactions may lead to vascular collapse, laryngoedema, shock, and death. Any allergen can cause anaphylaxis. Common causes include antibiotics, aspirin, other medications, vaccines, foods, insect venom, and x-ray contrast media containing iodine. In Practice: Nursing Assessment 83-1 lists the signs and symptoms of anaphylaxis.

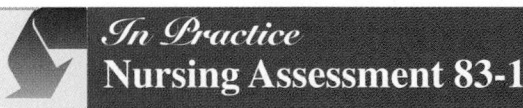

In Practice
Nursing Assessment 83-1

SIGNS AND SYMPTOMS OF ANAPHYLAXIS

- Continuous sneezing
- Edema and itching at the site of injection or sting
- Rash (hives)
- Severe dyspnea; gasping respirations
- Apprehension
- Feeling of choking or suffocation
- Airway obstruction
- Hypotension
- Weak, rapid, thready pulse
- *Diaphoresis* (profuse sweating)
- Pallor or cyanosis
- Pupillary dilation (eyes)
- Seizures
- Loss of consciousness

Treatment

Treatment for anaphylaxis must start immediately because the reaction can become severe very quickly.

The immediate problems are airway obstruction due to laryngeal edema and vasodilation, resulting in hypotension and hypoperfusion of organs. The cardiac output falls and the heart cannot pump enough blood and oxygen to the tissues. The result is anaerobic metabolism and lactic acidosis. The brain is particularly sensitive to alterations in blood perfusion and oxygen content. Severe bronchospasms may also occur.

Treatment of anaphylactic shock involves removal of the causative agent and administration of antihistamines to block the effects of histamine on the blood vessels, bronchioles, and gastrointestinal tract. In severe cases, epinephrine may be used to counteract the vasodilation that occurs. Epinephrine also relaxes the smooth muscle of the airways and inhibits further mediator release.

If the cause is an injection or insect bite, apply a tourniquet above the site to slow the rate of absorption of the antigen into the system. An ice pack to the site will also slow absorption.

> **Nursing Alert**
> During skin testing and allergy shots, clients are at risk for anaphylaxis. Keep epinephrine in 1:1,000 concentration, syringe, tourniquet, and emergency equipment available.

Nursing Considerations

Follow the emergency protocol when dealing with anaphylaxis:

Open the airway—This may require an endotracheal tube, oxygen, or suction. A tracheostomy may be needed.
Support the circulation—Intravenous fluids, placing the client in Trendelenburg position, or initiating cardiopulmonary resuscitation may be necessary
Administer medications—Epinephrine, aminophylline, antihistamines, and corticosteroids are the drugs of choice.

IMMUNE DISORDERS

Immunity is the body's normal adaptive state designed to protect itself from disease. Usually the immune system works on the body's behalf. The point at which a person becomes ill is when, for some reason, the immune system fails to operate as it should. Some immune disorders involve the following:

- *Infectious diseases:* The invading microorganisms are stronger (more *virulent*) or more numerous than the immune system antibodies.
- *Immunosuppression:* The immune system function is depressed, perhaps due to disease, injury, shock, radiation, or drugs. Immunosuppression may also be congenital (*agammaglobulinemia*).
- *Overproduction of gamma globulins:* Malignant blood diseases or chronic infection may be indicated.
- *Severe immune response to an invading antigen (anaphylaxis)*

- *Rejection response:* A beneficial foreign substance placed in the body is rejected, such as graft-versus-host disease after organ or tissue transplant.

Many disorders of immunity are also discussed elsewhere in this book in connection with the study of various body systems. Chapter 84 discusses the human immunodeficiency virus (**HIV**), a virus that cripples a person's immune system and leads to acquired immunodeficiency syndrome (**AIDS**).

AUTOIMMUNE DISORDERS

Sometimes the body does not recognize or tolerate the self as "self." As a result, the body begins to produce antibodies against its own healthy cells or to inhibit normal cell function. This process is called *autoimmunity* or **autoimmune disorder** and it results in damage to the body tissues by the immune system. Resulting diseases can affect almost any body cell or tissue. Although researchers do not yet understand the mechanisms behind autoimmunity, they have suggested the following factors:

- Genetic predisposition and influence of certain antigens in rejection of a person's own tissue.
- Interaction with physical, chemical, and biologic agents that trigger an abnormal immune response.
- Abnormalities in immune cells that lead to an inappropriate immune response.

Examples of autoimmune diseases include diabetes mellitus, rheumatoid arthritis, multiple sclerosis, hemolytic anemia, myasthenia gravis, and systemic lupus erythematosus (**SLE**).

Types

Autoimmune disorders include those that are **organ-specific** (affecting one organ), *systemic* (affecting the entire body), or **non–organ-specific** (affecting one or more organs). Chronic inflammatory changes in a specific organ characterize an organ-specific autoimmune disease. Examples include thyrotoxicosis or Graves' disease (of the thyroid), type 1 diabetes mellitus (pancreas), and autoimmune thyroiditis.

Widespread pathologic changes in many organs and tissues characterize systemic autoimmune disorders. Examples include SLE, rheumatoid arthritis, and myasthenia gravis.

Non–organ-specific autoimmune disorders combine the features of systemic and organ-specific diseases. Examples

include primary biliary cirrhosis and chronic active hepatitis (Table 83-1).

Persons at Risk

Research has indicated that autoimmune diseases (except HIV) show a highly significant familial tendency. Relatives of a client diagnosed with an autoimmune disease are known to be at high risk for developing the same disease (except in HIV and transplant rejection). Also, multiple autoimmune disorders are known to occur in the same client. Women are more likely to develop autoimmune disorders than men, often reaching a 10:1 (female: male) ratio or greater in certain diseases. Scientists believe that thymic hormones, sex hormones, and corticosteroids play a significant role in this ratio.

Examples

Rejection of a Transplanted Organ

To discuss in detail the procedure of organ transplantation is beyond the scope of this book. A transplanted organ, however, is a foreign substance, and the recipient's immune system will reject this foreign substance unless specific measures are taken to prevent it. Before the transplant, tissue typing is done to obtain the most genetically compatible match between donor and recipient. Tissue typing is conducted in much the same manner as blood typing. Another measure taken to suppress the rejection is the use of immunosuppressive drugs for life. Signs of rejection can be similar to other antigen–antibody responses and include fever, chills, diaphoresis, hypertension, hypotension, edema, and signs of organ involvement. If the immunosuppressive drugs are not effective, the organ will be rejected.

Systemic Lupus Erythematosus

Systemic lupus erythematosus is a chronic systemic disorder. Theorists believe it is caused by the development of antibodies that fight the body's own tissues and cells. The result is widespread damage to connective tissues, the hematologic system, skin, kidneys, heart, and brain. Evaluation of SLE includes laboratory tests to document the antibodies and the extent of end-organ involvement. Treatment involves education in rest and stress management, and the use of anti-inflammatory agents and corticosteroids (see Chap. 76 for more information).

▪▪▪ TABLE 83-1 ⱭUTOIMMUNE DISORDERS

Organ Specific	Non–organ Specific	Systemic
Thyrotoxicosis	Primary biliary cirrhosis	Systemic lupus erythematosus
Scleroderma	Chronic active hepatitis	Multiple sclerosis
Inflammatory bowel disease		Pernicious anemia
Type 1 diabetes mellitus		Rheumatoid arthritis
Autoimmune thyroiditis		Myasthenia gravis
Organ transplant rejection syndrome		

Rheumatoid Arthritis

This disorder, characterized by an inflammation of the joints, may also have systemic manifestations. Its origin is generally believed to be autoimmune. It is primarily a disorder of the musculoskeletal system. (see Chapter 76 for more information).

☛ KEY CONCEPT

Autoimmunity is related to many disorders. It is now thought that autoimmunity plays a role in many other previously unexplained disorders.

Treatment

Generally treatment of autoimmune diseases is, for the most part, *symptomatic* (specific symptoms are treated as they occur). It includes the use of mild analgesics to provide pain relief and to reduce inflammation, corticosteroids to treat inflammation (many conditions respond specifically to these drugs), and radiation to suppress the body's abnormal antigen–antibody responses. Systemic autoimmune disorders are difficult to treat successfully because a balance must be sought between suppressing the immune response that is causing the illness and maintaining enough immunity to fight off invasions of actual threatening foreign substances.

➤ STUDENT SYNTHESIS

Key Points

- The immune system leads the "battle" against invading microbes and malignant cells that contact or enter the body.
- Antigens are foreign protein substances that enter the body and stimulate the production of antibodies.
- Individuals can be allergic to almost anything.
- Common manifestations of allergic reactions vary; they may range from mild to life threatening (anaphylaxis).
- Treatment of allergies is directed toward removal of the allergen and counteracting the antibody response.
- The body continually seeks a balance between suppressing the immune response that is causing an illness and maintaining enough immunity to fight the invasion of threatening foreign substances.
- Autoimmune disorders occur when the body fails to recognize its own cells as "self" and begins to destroy those cells.

Critical Thinking Exercises

1. Consider different types of allergies. In addition to their physical impact on clients and family members, what other effects may they have on finances, emotions, long-term plans, hobbies, and so forth?
2. Mrs. G. has just been diagnosed with systemic lupus erythematosus. She comes to you in the healthcare facility and tells you that she does not understand what is meant by an autoimmune disorder. How would you explain the condition? What teaching measures would you use to outline the differences between immunity and autoimmunity?

NCLEX-Style Review Questions

1. Which laboratory test finding would indicate an allergy disorder?
   a. Negative skin testing
   b. Normal chest x-ray
   c. Normal complete blood count
   d. Positive eosinophil smear of nasal secretions
2. During skin testing, which information should the LPN/LVN communicate immediately to the RN or physician?
   a. Complaints of difficulty breathing
   b. Complaints of an itchy nose
   c. Erythema at injection sites
   d. Nausea and runny nose
3. A client complains of burping and mild abdominal pain whenever eating strawberries. What nursing action would be most appropriate?
   a. Instruct client to avoid all fruit.
   b. Instruct client to avoid strawberries.
   c. Instruct client to drink plenty of water.
   d. Instruct client to keep a food journal.
4. A client complains of recurring dyspnea, cough, and thick sputum. This client's symptoms are most clearly an example of which condition?
   a. Anaphylaxis
   b. Bronchial asthma
   c. Food sensitivity
   d. Hives
5. Which of the following is an example of an organ-specific autoimmune disorder?
   a. Chronic active hepatitis
   b. Rheumatoid arthritis
   c. Scleroderma
   d. Systemic lupus erythematosus

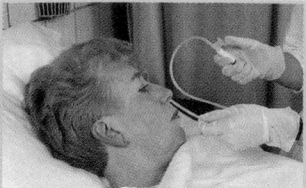

CHAPTER

84

HIV and AIDS

LEARNING OBJECTIVES

1. Define the following: retrovirus, HIV, and AIDS.
2. State at least four routes of transmission for HIV.
3. Discuss the critical nature of T cells and B cells in the immune system.
4. Describe how HIV targets and invades CD4 cells.
5. Differentiate between ELISA testing and Western blot testing for HIV.
6. State at least eight common signs and symptoms of HIV and at least four signs and symptoms of HIV specific to women.
7. Name the three classes of antiretroviral drugs used to treat HIV.
8. Define viral load and differentiate between the technical diagnosis of HIV and AIDS.
9. Discuss at least six opportunistic infections associated with HIV/AIDS.

NEW TERMINOLOGY

antiretroviral therapy	prophylaxis
B cells	retrovirus
HIV-related encephalopathy	T cells
opportunistic infections	viral load
pandemic	

ACRONYMS

ADC	FDA	PCP
AIDS	HIV	PEP
CD4	HIV-RNA	PID
CDC	HPV	STD
CMV	MAC	WHO
ELISA		

As described in Chapters 24, 40, and 83, the immune system protects the body from the adverse effects of invasion by microorganisms and other foreign substances. It also regulates the removal of damaged cells and disposes of abnormal cells that arise within the body. One disorder that affects the work of the immune system is the human immunodeficiency virus (**HIV**) and acquired immunodeficiency syndrome (**AIDS**).

HUMAN IMMUNODEFICIENCY VIRUS

Human immunodeficiency virus first was seen in the early 1980s when several unusual infections were noted in young homosexual men. The virus was identified in 1983, and the Food and Drug Administration (**FDA**) approved an HIV diagnostic test in 1985. Since that time, the disease has reached **pandemic** proportions, meaning that it affects global geographic areas. According to the Centers for Disease Control (**CDC**), in the United States an estimated 650,000 to 900,000 individuals were living with HIV/AIDS in June of 2000, and prior to that, another 435,000 persons had died from AIDS. Although these numbers are large, the number of persons affected by the virus globally is much greater than the number in the U.S. In 1999, the World Health Organization (**WHO**) estimated that 33.6 million persons are living with HIV/AIDS worldwide, and that 2.6 million deaths had occurred. Many of these cases are found in sub-Saharan Africa.

Action of HIV

HIV is an infectious human **retrovirus,** a virus that overtakes the biosynthesis of living cells to duplicate itself. In other words, HIV invades a normal cell and uses that cell's biomechanisms to reproduce new HIV cells. The original purpose or function of the normal cell is destroyed. HIV has a highly sophisticated structure, as seen in Figure 84-1.

This retrovirus commonly invades two types of cells: **T cells** (lymphocytes that mature in the thymus) and **B cells** (lymphocytes that originate in the bone marrow). Normally, T cells and B cells function to fight infection and to produce antibodies for specific immune responses. HIV specifically invades and depletes the helper T4 lymphocytes (T cells are also referred to as **CD4** lymphocytes), thereby compromising the functions of the body's immune system.

Also as a direct consequence of the invasion, the individual is vulnerable to many **opportunistic infections,** infections caused by microorganisms that do not generally cause disease in a person with a normal immune system. However, certain infections can cause serious disease in a person with a weakened immune system. Opportunistic infections and cancers account for a large proportion of deaths related to HIV.

If untreated, HIV depletes an individual's immune system over a number of years, allowing the development of both minor and major opportunistic infections and cancers, eventually leading to death. In an untreated person, the average time from acquisition of HIV until a diagnosis of AIDS is made is about 10 years. However, this time frame varies greatly among individuals.

Since the mid-1990s, strong combinations of medications called **antiretroviral therapy** (medications to specifically combat the retrovirus) have become available, exerting a profound effect on the progression of HIV disease. Individuals who take these medications often see a drop in the amount of circulating virus, and a restoration of immune function as measured by T-cell count. Medication therapies have resulted in a significant decrease in the frequency of opportunistic infections as well as the numbers of deaths in persons infected with HIV.

Transmission

HIV is transmitted through infected body fluids. It can be passed to another through unprotected sexual contact (vaginal, oral, and anal sex are all associated with transmission), sharing of infected needles, accidental exposure of a healthcare worker to infected blood, transmission from an infected pregnant woman to her fetus, and breastfeeding. HIV-infected pregnant women should be treated for HIV because this reduces the risk of infection in the newborn.

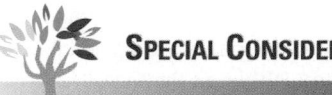

SPECIAL CONSIDERATIONS: THE LIFE SPAN

Prevention of HIV/AIDS in Infants

Early detection and treatment of HIV/AIDS as part of maternal prenatal care can prevent HIV infection in the newborn. Nurses must strongly advocate for HIV testing for all pregnant women.

Prior to 1985, blood transfusion was associated with HIV transmission. Generally, this is not the case now, because blood banks test donors for HIV. Transplant recipients are also poten-

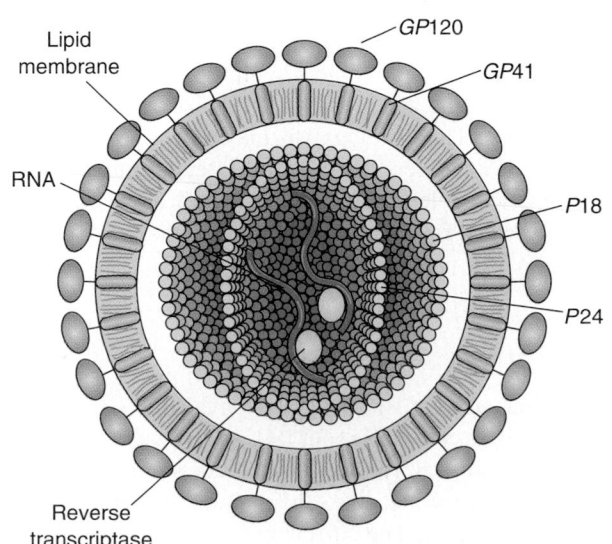

FIGURE 84-1. The human immunodeficiency virus (HIV).

Lipid membrane — GP120
— GP41
RNA
P18
P24
Reverse transcriptase

tially at risk, so transplant donors are tested for HIV infection prior to organ donation.

Women, teenagers, and persons over 50 years of age are currently among the fastest-growing groups of persons becoming infected with HIV. Heterosexual transmission of HIV also is increasing across ethnic groups as well as in assorted age groups.

Diagnostic Tests

HIV Antibody Tests

Antibodies to HIV develop in an infected individual within as little as 3 weeks to as much as 14 months after exposure to the virus. A person can falsely test negative for the virus during this time. HIV antibodies are ineffective agents in the fight against the HIV virus. However, they do allow the identification of infected individuals and blood products.

ELISA and Western Blot

Several blood tests can detect HIV. The enzyme-linked immunosorbent assay (**ELISA**) detects antibodies to HIV proteins. If the ELISA is positive, a second test is done to confirm the presence of antibodies. This confirmatory test is called a Western blot. The Western blot specifically detects HIV. The ELISA is less specific, and can result in false-positive reactions, but because it is easier and less expensive for laboratories to run, it is used for screening before the more specific (and more expensive) Western blot is performed.

Viral Load

After an individual is known to be infected with HIV, two primary lab tests are performed to assess the status of the immune system and the strength (virulence) of the virus. CD4 (T cell) counts are used to measure a person's immune function. Normal values range between 500 and 1,500 cells per cubic millimeter (mm^3). Values under $500/mm^3$ are considered abnormal. The **HIV-RNA** or **viral load** is measured to determine how virulent the virus is. Both the CD4 count and the viral load are performed regularly on infected persons to assess the need for antiretroviral therapy, and the adequacy of response to these medications.

A person who is not infected with HIV has an undetectable viral load. An undetectable reading is also considered to be an excellent response to therapy, although the inability to detect the virus in the blood does not indicate that a person is no longer infected. Clients with HIV that is not controlled with medications may have readings as high as 1,000,000 copies or more of viral cells read as viral load.

Signs and Symptoms of HIV Infection

HIV can be entirely asymptomatic for many years. Box 84-1 summarizes the major clinical manifestations of untreated HIV/AIDS infection.

Generally, the characteristic signs and symptoms associated with infection include:

- Persistent enlargement of lymph nodes (*lymphadenopathy*)
- Fever
- Night sweats
- Diarrhea
- General malaise
- Anorexia
- Weight loss
- Oral thrush
- Herpes zoster infection or shingles

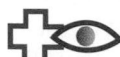 **Nursing Alert**
HIV can be asymptomatic for many years, and persons who have not been tested may not know they are infected. Therefore, learn and rely on Standard Precautions for self-protection from unknown risk.

Women should be aware that HIV infection may be overlooked and attributed to other disorders, such as genital ulcer disease, sexually transmitted diseases (**STD**s), human papillomavirus (**HPV**) infections, and pelvic inflammatory disease (**PID**). Although women may experience the characteristic signs and symptoms, more commonly women experience gynecologic problems as the initial clinical manifestations. In women, other frequent HIV-related signs and symptoms include:

- Recurrent vaginal candidiasis
- Menstrual abnormalities including *amenorrhea* (absence of periods) or bleeding between periods
- Abnormal Pap tests
- Cervical cancer

 **Special Considerations: Culture**

Women's HIV Symptoms

Women often have symptoms of HIV that are more subtle or different from men's symptoms. Women's symptoms may be attributed to other disorders such as PID or STDs. The misdiagnosis may delay early treatment for HIV and lead to inappropriate, incomplete therapies. The delay in treatment may allow the virus to progress and ravage the body, leading to premature death.

Treatment

Medications to treat HIV have been available since the late 1980s, but it was not until about 1995 that new drugs and combinations of drugs were shown to provide significantly better control of the virus and allow the immune system to regenerate to some degree. The current antiretroviral therapy consists of three classes of antiretroviral drugs approved for use

➤ ➤ BOX 84-1

CLINICAL MANIFESTATIONS OF HIV/AIDS

Respiratory Manifestations

Shortness of breath

Dyspnea

Cough

Chest pain

Fever

Associated with:

• *Pneumocystis carinii*
• *Mycobacterium avium* complex
• Cytomegalovirus
• Tuberculosis

Gastrointestinal Manifestations

Anorexia, nausea, vomiting

Malabsorption

Malnutrition

Oral and esophageal candidiasis

Chronic, profound diarrhea resulting in weight loss

Fluid and electrolyte imbalance

Excoriations of mucous membrane

Weakness

Associated with:

• Candidiasis (fungal infections)
• Wasting syndrome

Neurologic Manifestations

Progressive decline in cognition and memory

Headache

Difficulty with concentration

Progressive confusion

Psychomotor slowing

Apathy

Ataxia

Depression, psychosis, hallucinations

Tremors

Incontinence

Seizures

Mutism

Death

Associated with:

• HIV encephalopathy, also known as AIDS dementia complex (**ADC**)

Integumentary Manifestations

Skin lesions and painful vesicles

Associated with:

• Kaposi's sarcoma (lesions brownish-pink to deep-purple, either flat or raised, and surrounded by ecchymoses and edema)
• Herpes zoster and herpes simplex (painful vesicles)

Rash

Associated with:

• Side effect of drug trimethoprim-sulfamethoxazole (TMP-SMZ) that appears as pruritic with pinkish-red macules and papules

Source: Smeltzer, S. C., & Bare, B. G. (2000). *Brunner and Suddarth's textbook of medical-surgical nursing* (9th ed; p. 1354–1357). Philadelphia: Lippincott Williams & Wilkins.

---

by the FDA: nucleoside reverse transcriptase inhibitors, non-nucleoside reverse transcriptase inhibitors, and protease inhibitors. In Practice: Important Medications 84-1 lists information and specific drugs available.

Three or more different drugs are generally administered together to provide powerful control over HIV. This often results in a lowering of the viral load to non-detectable levels. With strong suppression of the virus, the immune system may be able to rebuild. Clients often have an increase in their T cells. As a consequence, they are less susceptible to opportunistic infections. Deaths from HIV and AIDS have been cut drastically since the mid-1990s.

☞ KEY CONCEPT

HIV can be controlled with the use of antiretroviral medications. Some opportunistic infections can be prevented with medications (prophylaxis).

Antiretroviral therapy is not without associated and often significant problems. Many of the drugs produce side effects,

such as severe gastrointestinal upset with nausea, vomiting, and diarrhea; bone marrow suppression; and peripheral neuropathy. These effects can disrupt a client's life. Other illnesses, such as diabetes and increased cholesterol or triglyceride levels, can be attributed to the antiretroviral drugs. Some clients can tolerate medications for only a short period because of toxicity. These medications are also very expensive and may be impossible to obtain without health insurance coverage. The long-term effects and effectiveness of these drugs are still under study.

ACQUIRED IMMUNODEFICIENCY SYNDROME

Acquired immunodeficiency syndrome occurs during the later stages of HIV infection. As the virus progressively destroys the immune system, a variety of infections and cancers can develop. Originally, it was believed that all HIV-infected individuals would ultimately develop AIDS, but with the use of powerful antiretroviral drugs, this may not always be the case. Why the development of AIDS is sometimes delayed is not

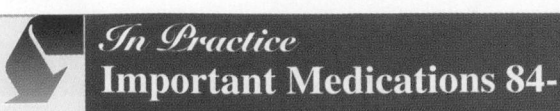

In Practice
Important Medications 84-1

TO TREAT HIV/AIDS

Antiretroviral Medications
Nucleoside Reverse Transcriptase Inhibitors:
abacavir (Ziagen)
didanosine (Videx, ddI)
lamivudine (Epivir, 3TC)
stavudine (Zerit, d4T)
zidovudine (Retrovir, AZT)
zalcitabine (HIVID, ddC)
Non-nucleoside Reverse Transcriptase Inhibitors:
nevirapine (Viramune)
efavirenz (Sustiva)
delavirdine (Rescriptor)
Protease Inhibitors
indinavir (Crixivan)
saquinavir (Fortovase)
nelfinavir (Viracept)
ritonavir (Norvir)
amprenavir (Agenerase)
lopinavir/ritonavir (Kaletra)

Medications to Treat or Prevent Common Opportunistic Infections
Antiviral for Chronic Herpes Simplex Infections and for Shingles:
acyclovir (Zovirax)
Antifungal for Severe Oral Thrush, Candida Esophagitis, Vaginal Candidiasis:
fluconazole (Diflucan)

Antifungal for Mild Oral Thrush, Vaginal Candidiasis, Candida Skin Infections:
clotrimazole (Mycelex) troche, cream, and vaginal suppositories
Antivirals to Treat CMV Retinitis:
cidofovir (Vistide)
foscarnet Na (Foscavir)
ganciclovir Na (Cytovene)
To Treat Tuberculosis or for Prophylaxis:
isoniazid (INH, Nydrazid)
rifampin (Rifadin)
rifabutin (Mycobutin)
pyrazinamide (Tebrazid)
ethambutol
streptomycin
To Treat Diarrhea:
loperamide (Immodium)
To Treat Mycobacterium avium *(MAC) Infections or for* M. avium *Prophylaxis:*
azithromycin (Zithromax)
clarithromycin (Biaxin)
rifabutin (Mycobutin)
ethambutol (Myambutol)
To Prevent or Treat Pneumocystis carinii *Pneumonia:*
trimethoprim/sulfamethoxazole (Septra, Bactrim)
dapsone (Avlosulfan)
aerosolized pentamidine (Nebupent)

well understood. In addition, some individuals seem to maintain a healthy immune system despite HIV infection, without the use of medication. These individuals are called *long-term non-progressors*.

In 1993, the CDC revised its classification system for AIDS. All HIV-positive individuals with a T-cell count below 200/mm³ are now considered to have a diagnosis of AIDS. In addition, persons with HIV and certain opportunistic infections or cancers also meet the case definition for AIDS. Clinical conditions that confer an AIDS diagnosis can be found in Box 84-2.

Opportunistic Infections

When an HIV-positive person's T-cell count falls between 200 and 400/mm³, the first opportunistic infections may appear. Initial infections of the skin and mucous membranes, such as oral thrush, shingles, and severe athlete's foot, may develop. As immunity diminishes further, more life-threatening infections are likely to occur. Some of the more common opportunistic infections include:

- *Candidiasis:* Yeast-like fungus that overgrows, causing infections of the mouth (thrush), respiratory tract, and skin
- *Cryptococcus:* Yeast-like fungus causing infections of the lung, brain, and blood
- *Cytomegalovirus* (**CMV**): One-celled parasitic infection of the gastrointestinal tract causing diarrhea, fever, and weight loss
- *Herpes simplex:* Viral infection causing colitis, pneumonitis, and retinitis
- *Histoplasmosis:* Viral infection causing small, painful blisters on the skin of the lips, nose, or genitalia
- *Mycobacterium avium-intracellulare* (**MAC**): Bacterial disease with fever, malaise, night sweats, anorexia, diarrhea, weight loss, and lung and blood infections
- *Pneumocystis carinii pneumonia* (**PCP**): One-celled organism causing infection of the lungs, with cough, fever, chest pain, and sputum production
- *Toxoplasmosis:* Parasitic infection involving the brain, lungs, and other organs, causing fever, chills, visual disturbances, confusion, hemiparesis, and seizures

➤➤ BOX 84-2

CLINICAL CONDITIONS CONFERRING A DIAGNOSIS OF AIDS

CDC4+ (T-cell count <200–500 cells/mm³)
Candida infection of bronchi, trachea, lungs, or esophagus
Cervical cancer, invasive
Coccidioidomycosis, disseminated or extrapulmonary
Cryptococcosis, extrapulmonary
Cryptosporidiosis, chronic intestinal
Cytomegalovirus (**CMV**) disease (other than liver, spleen, or lymph nodes)
CMV retinitis
Encephalopathy, HIV-related
Herpes simplex: chronic oral ulcers; or bronchitis, pneumonitis, or esophagitis
Histoplasmosis, disseminated or extrapulmonary
HIV-related encephalopathy
Isosporiasis, chronic intestinal
Kaposi's sarcoma
Lymphoma: Burkitt's, immunoblastic, or primary of brain
Mycobacterium avium complex (**MAC**) or *M. kansasii,* disseminated or extrapulmonary
Mycobacterium tuberculosis
Mycobacterium, other species or unidentified species, disseminated or extrapulmonary
Pneumocystic carinii pneumonia
Pneumonia, recurrent
Progressive multifocal leukoencephalopathy
Salmonella septicemia, recurrent
Toxoplasmosis of brain
Wasting syndrome due to HIV

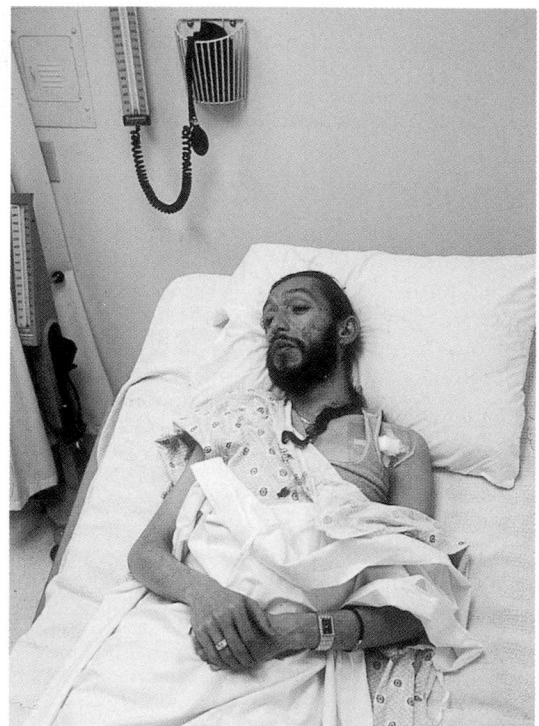

FIGURE 84-2. The wasting syndrome of AIDS. In the later stages of AIDS, the client loses weight and is prone to many opportunistic infections.

ing countries without adequate healthcare, educational programs, or medications, and in impoverished populations in the United States, the mortality rate continues to be high. In Practice: Educating the Client 84-1 highlights how misinformation can cause an increase in the rates of infection. Clients and their families need to have this misinformation corrected.

NURSING PROCESS

Data Collection

Carefully observe and assess the client who has been diagnosed with HIV (see Box 84-1). In addition to a careful nursing assessment, take note of medications. Determine if medication

A variety of other fungal, viral, and bacterial infections may also occur, causing *constitutional disease* (weight loss, diarrhea, fever) and neurologic disorders (dementia, muscle, nerve). For example, in later stages of the disease, a wasting syndrome (Fig. 84-2) and an AIDS-related malignancy (Kaposi's sarcoma [Fig. 84-3]) can occur.

Treatment

The ideal approach to the management of AIDS involves the prevention of opportunistic infections when possible (**prophylaxis**), and the early treatment of such infections when they occur. The use of antiretroviral medications has resulted in the decline (and/or perhaps, delay) in the number of individuals who progress from HIV to AIDS. When T-cell counts are low, prophylaxis is commonly given to prevent PCP and MAC.

Mortality

Since 1995 and the institution of the use of powerful combinations of antiretroviral medications, the mortality rate from HIV has declined in the United States. However, in develop-

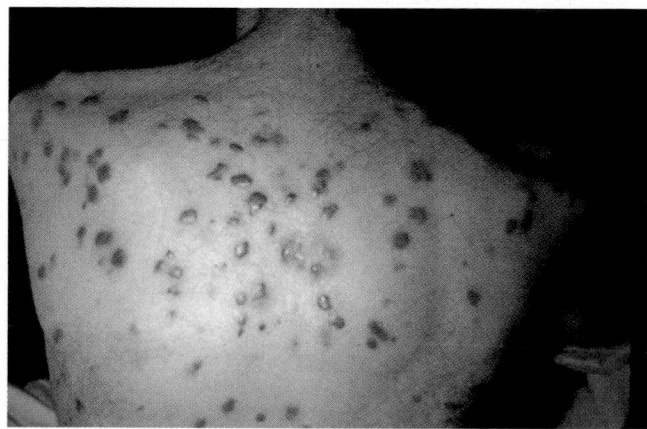

FIGURE 84-3. Lesions called *Kaposi's sarcoma,* an AIDS-related malignancy common in later stages of the disease.

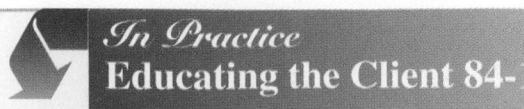

In Practice
Educating the Client 84-1

MISINFORMATION INCREASES RATES OF HIV INFECTION

- The success of the HIV antiretroviral medications has led some individuals to believe that HIV has been controlled or even cured.
- HIV is not curable. It is only treatable.
- Some areas of the United States where rates of HIV had decreased during the 1990s now show an increase in rates of HIV infection. This increase in HIV infections may be related to the lack of adequate knowledge about cure versus treatment.
- Another possible cause of the increase may be that individuals think that medications stop the progression of the disease. The long-term effects of the potent HIV medication combinations are yet to be determined.

➤ BOX 84-3

LEGAL ISSUES AND HIV TESTING

Testing for HIV is associated with many legal implications. Although the laws vary from state to state, they generally hold that:

- An informed consent must be obtained from the client prior to testing.
- Pre- and post-test counseling (usually by a state-approved HIV counselor) is required regardless of the test results.
- Results cannot be given over the telephone. Most laws identify specific standards for whom, when, and how the results can be given.
- Ensuring client confidentiality is essential. Most laboratories use a coding system rather than the client's name.
- The laboratory must be approved by the state for HIV testing.

Source: Adapted from Hosley, J. B., Jones, S. A., & Molle-Matthews E. A. (1997). *Lippincott's textbook for medical assistants.* Philadelphia: Lippincott-Raven.

---

regimens and requirements for taking anti-HIV medications are being followed. Observe for evidence of depression, anxiety, or other symptoms, which may indicate psychological dysfunction or lack of coping mechanisms. When a person has AIDS, specific signs and symptoms may be difficult to identify, because this disorder can affect many body systems. Chapter 47 describes physical examination and nursing assessment, which establish a baseline for future comparison and determine the presence of suspected complications. Document and report any changes in this baseline level. Data collection generally includes specific legal concerns such as consents to obtain HIV infection status. Box 84-3 reviews some legal considerations of HIV/AIDS.

AIDS is a chronic condition and is ultimately fatal. Evaluate the client's physical and emotional response to the disease. What information or help does the client need to cope with the prognosis? Does the client need assistance to meet daily needs? How does the disorder affect social activities or self-esteem? Is the client taking medications as prescribed? What support services do the client and family need? Is professional counseling or a support group available? What rehabilitation or home care services are necessary?

Nursing Diagnosis

Because AIDS destroys the immune system, almost all nursing diagnoses are used at one time or another. The following are examples showing multiple causal factors:

- Imbalanced Nutrition: Less than Body Requirements related to adverse effects of medications, opportunistic infections, anorexia, persistent diarrhea, and general body tissue wasting
- Ineffective Breathing Pattern related to effects of *P. carinii* pneumonia, tuberculosis, or other forms of pneumonia

- Risk for Infection related to impaired immune system function
- Risk for Disuse Syndrome related to immobility, fatigue, decreased level of endurance
- Hopelessness related to deteriorating condition, feeling of abandonment, long-term stress, high costs, poor prognosis
- Impaired Tissue Integrity related to thrush, shingles, athlete's foot, other fungal infections, altered nutritional status, suicide attempts
- Impaired Social Interactions related to fear, fatigue, pain, disability
- Ineffective Coping related to lack of adequate support system, reaction to terminal illness
- Disturbed Thought Processes related to **HIV-related encephalopathy,** suicidal ideation, depression, anxiety

Planning and Implementing

Plan together with the client, family, and other members of the healthcare team for effective individualized care to meet the client's needs. The client may require assistance in meeting all basic and healthcare needs, as well as in dealing with the chronic or terminal nature of the disorder. Teach the client and family about the disorder and prescribed medications and treatment. Counseling, social services, home care, and other community agencies are often involved. A nursing care plan is developed to meet identified needs (see In Practice: Nursing Care Plan 84-1).

In addition to the physical effects of HIV infection, many persons with this diagnosis have experienced stigma, loss of job and insurance, depression, anxiety, and adjustment prob-

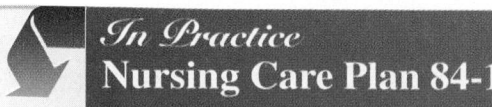
In Practice
Nursing Care Plan 84-1

THE PERSON WITH AIDS-ASSOCIATED WEIGHT LOSS AND WASTING

MEDICAL HISTORY: *C.H., a 39-year-old woman, was admitted to the hospital complaining of anorexia, weight loss, and diarrhea secondary to AIDS. History reveals the use of all possible antiretroviral therapies without success. "Either I had such terrible side effects that I couldn't tolerate or I developed a resistance to them." Client's condition is considered terminal.*

MEDICAL DIAGNOSIS: *AIDS, Anorexia, Wasting syndrome*

Data Collection/Nursing Assessment: Client is thin, frail female, weighing 94 lbs. Client reports episodes of persistent anorexia and diarrhea. Skin thin, pale, and transparent; slow to return when pinched. Skin in perianal area and buttocks reddened and irritated. Client repeatedly talking about the fact that she seems to be getting progressively sicker, and that her weight loss, fatigue, and pain were also increasing in severity. She cried about the fact that her family is becoming exhausted as time goes on. Client lives at home with elderly parents who provide all of the client's care. "My mom is 70 years old and has really bad arthritis. My dad is 73 years old and has a heart condition. I don't know how much more they can take. They're not rich either." When questioned, parents report being tired, stating, "But we want to do everything that we can for her." Client has a younger sister and brother living nearby who come by to help occasionally. "My sister and brother have their families, too." (*Although other nursing diagnoses may be appropriate, a priority nursing diagnosis is addressed below.*)

Nursing Diagnosis: Risk for caregiver role strain related to prolonged disease progression and increasing care responsibilities in conjunction with parental age and physical condition as evidenced by client's statements about current status and parents.

Planning
SHORT-TERM GOALS:
#1. Client will verbalize concerns about her parents to her parents.
#2. Client and family will identify the need for outside assistance.

LONG-TERM GOALS:
#3. Client and family will enlist the aid of home health care and hospice care as appropriate.
#4. Client and family will use resources available to them.

Implementation
NURSING ACTION: *Identify role of client in family and how illness has changed the family roles, noting how she feels about these changes.*
RATIONALE: *Emotional needs are as important as physical needs.*

NURSING ACTION: *Encourage client to talk with parents about the increasing demands on them.*
RATIONALE: *Having the client talk with her parents opens the channels of communication for future action.*

NURSING ACTION: *Note factors, other than illness, that may be affecting family's ability to provide effective care.*
RATIONALE: *Past relationships, time schedules, available space, and finances are some factors that may affect the family's effectiveness.*

Evaluation: Client spoke with parents about increasing demands on them; parents verbalizing desire to help; acknowledge that it is getting more difficult to care for client. *Goal #1 met; progress to meeting Goal #2.*

NURSING ACTION: *Assess information available to and understood by the family regarding outside help.*
RATIONALE: *This basic information will enable the nurse to provide appropriate referral and to encourage the family to seek the help they need.*

NURSING ACTION: *Assist with contacting discharge planner/home health coordinator to discuss with client and family areas in which a home care referral can be beneficial and about the possibility of the need for hospice care.*
RATIONALE: *The discharge planner/home health care coordinator can provide specific information related to the types of services that can be provided for this client in the home.*

NURSING ACTION: *Review information about home health and hospice care. Help family understand that hospice referral is appropriate. Explain the positive role hospice staff can play in late-stage disease.*
RATIONALE: *Hospice personnel are skilled in assisting families and clients to adjust to death and dying as part of the continuum, and to recognize those comfort measures which will contribute to this process.*

Evaluation: Family spoke with discharge planner; plan for home healthcare established; home healthcare

(continued)

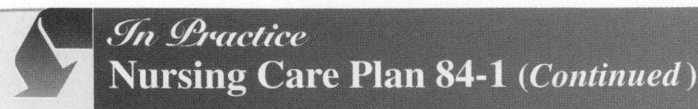

In Practice
Nursing Care Plan 84-1 *(Continued)*

agency contacted, with visit planned for day of client's discharge. *Goal #2 met; Goal #3 met.*

NURSING ACTION: *Request Social Services consult to assist with determining available resources and services for client and family needs (caregivers, housekeeping, support groups/counseling, financial, spiritual).*

RATIONALE: *Social Services has a wide knowledge base to provide assistance in numerous areas.*

Evaluation: Client and family met with Social Services; identified several areas in which it would be beneficial for them to seek help. Client's father to contact community agency for support group. *Progress to meeting Goal #4.*

---

lems. All of these issues must be considered when working with HIV-infected individuals. Legal issues, especially related to confidentiality, are priority considerations.

Nursing Alert

Confidentiality is always a concern for healthcare professionals. For clients with HIV/AIDS, nurses must be diligently alert to the confidential nature of the disease.

Nursing Implications for Clients With HIV

Although many HIV-infected persons can function fully and do not require specialized care beyond that provided by their primary care providers, nursing care can be very helpful in many instances. For example, it is essential to take prescribed antiretrovirals as directed, and persons with HIV often require assistance with medication adherence. The nurse can: help in planning with the client how to take each dose; provide suggestions for pill boxes and calendars; assist in the management of side effects; aid in obtaining refills on time; and teach so that the client and family understand interactions that might occur with food and other drugs. The nurse plays a key role in client and family teaching about all aspects of the disease and care (see In Practice: Educating the Client 84-2).

☞ KEY CONCEPT

HIV/AIDS medication therapy demands strict adherence to a complicated regimen. The client and the nurse must be aware of the requirements of each particular medication.

The psychosocial aspects of being infected with HIV may be significant; persons are stigmatized, may lose the support of friends and family, and may find the restraints on sexual activity difficult. Support from healthcare professionals can assist HIV-positive clients to adjust to their diagnosis. The nurse can make referrals for psychosocial care to counselors and support groups. Some HIV-infected individuals choose to return to school and work, and may benefit from referral to retraining programs or educational counselors. In addition, it is important that those who are infected know how to prevent transmission of HIV to family, friends, and sexual partners.

Nursing Alert

Condoms do not guarantee safe sex. They provide *safer* sex.

Nursing Implications for Clients With AIDS

Individuals in later stages of the disease are more likely to require special nursing care. Because of their weakened condition, many require total nursing care. Some may be able to stay home during their final days. Family members need education about what this entails.

Opportunistic infections require special medications, and clients may need assistance in taking these properly, or in contacting the healthcare provider when problems develop. Intravenous medications may be used, and with such medications comes the associated care of venous access lines. When a person is in the terminal stages of AIDS, the focus is on providing the client with comfort. Emotional support, combined with technical skills, will help clients and families cope with the illness.

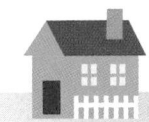

SPECIAL CONSIDERATIONS: HOME CARE

The Person With HIV/AIDS

When a client with HIV/AIDS is being cared for at home, it is important that the client and family know what this entails. A great deal of teaching is needed, including descriptions about how HIV is transmitted and how it is not. Because infection control measures are essential, show the client and family how to care for infectious waste, dispose of sharps, and practice proper hygiene in the kitchen. The nurse may need to schedule regular meetings to provide education, and obtain educational materials to supplement knowledge. Learning about local sources of additional education and community assistance is helpful.

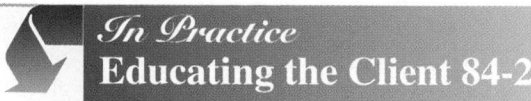

In Practice
Educating the Client 84-2

KEY TEACHING TOPICS FOR UNDERSTANDING HIV AND AIDS

- Disease process, signs and symptoms
- Ways for transmitting and not transmitting HIV
- Infection control measures
- Proper disposal for sharps and contaminated objects
- Maintenance of hygiene in kitchen
- Possible side effects of medication
- Nutritional plans, including the use of dietary supplements
- Psychological support
- Available community resources and services to provide home management
- Sources for hospice care

Evaluation

The entire healthcare team, client, and family will evaluate outcomes of care. Have short-term goals been met? For example, is the client adhering to the prescribed medications? Are the client and family beginning to discuss the disease and its care? Are long-term goals still realistic? What community services are required? Is the client in need of home care services? Does the client need financial assistance? Is a referral for psychiatric care indicated? Planning for further nursing and healthcare considers the client's prognosis and responses to care.

HIV EXPOSURE AND HEALTHCARE WORKERS

Fewer than 1% of HIV infections in healthcare workers result from work-related exposure. Box 84-4 discusses risks to healthcare workers. Most of these exposures are needlestick

➤ ➤ BOX 84-4

PREVENTION OF HIV TRANSMISSION IN HEALTHCARE WORKERS

The risk of HIV infection and AIDS among healthcare workers is small, but it is a definite risk. The nurse is only at risk if he or she is *directly* exposed to blood or other body fluids of HIV-infected persons. *Standard Precautions*, established by the Centers for Disease Control and Prevention (CDC) in Atlanta, must be consistently used for all clients. Practice these precautions with each client, because medical history and examination alone will not reveal all persons infected with HIV. Individuals who sustain needlestick injuries or other potentially hazardous exposures should report to a supervisor or the employee health department immediately.

injuries. Therefore, never recap needles. Postexposure prophylaxis (**PEP**) should begin immediately with thorough washing of the exposed area. All healthcare agencies will have specific protocols to follow if an individual has had possible exposure to HIV. Counseling, lab tests, and followup testing will be included as part of PEP.

➤ STUDENT SYNTHESIS

Key Points

- The terms HIV and AIDS are not synonymous. HIV is the virus responsible for causing AIDS, but the person who is HIV positive does not automatically have AIDS.
- HIV is a retrovirus, a virus that overtakes the biosynthesis of living cells to duplicate itself. HIV invades a normal cell and uses that cell's biomechanisms to reproduce new HIV cells.
- The Centers for Disease Control and Prevention updated the classification of AIDS to include diagnosis based on a T-cell count of fewer than 200 cells/mm³.
- Follow Standard Precautions in caring for all clients, for self-protection and to minimize the risk of contracting HIV and other infections such as hepatitis B and C.
- AIDS is ultimately a terminal condition; the emotional, physical, and financial implications can be enormous.

Critical Thinking Exercises

1. You are working in a clinic. A coworker comes to you and is frantic. He has just accidentally stuck himself with a used needle. What measures would you take? How would you emotionally support the coworker? What should he do?
2. You are working in the home of a client with AIDS. You have provided care to this client for several months. The client is extremely depressed and mentions a few times that he is seriously contemplating suicide. You have worked with the client's family members as well, who are extremely supportive. Last week, the client's daughter mentioned to you that she was worried about her father's emotional state. How would you handle this situation? Give explanations for your response.

NCLEX-Style Review Questions

1. Which test is used as a screening test to detect antibodies to HIV proteins?
   a. Electrolyte screening
   b. ELISA
   c. Prothrombin time
   d. Western blot

2. Which of the following are classes of antiretroviral medications?
   a. Antimetabolites
   b. Hormonal agents
   c. Non-nucleoside reverse transcriptase inhibitors
   d. Vinca alkaloids
3. The nurse explains to a client that the most important reason for obtaining a HIV-RNA (viral load) is to:
   a. Assess the client's immune function
   b. Confirm the results of the ELISA test
   c. Detect the amount of HIV antibodies
   d. Determine how virulent the virus is
4. A client had HIV testing and calls your clinic for the results. The most appropriate response would be:
   a. Explain to the client that results cannot be given over the phone.
   b. Give the client the results and schedule a followup appointment.
   c. Transfer the client to the physician's phone answering service.
   d. Verify the client's identity and give the results.
5. HIV is transmitted by which of the following?
   a. Hugging and kissing
   b. Sharing glasses or eating utensils
   c. Sharing telephones
   d. Unprotected sexual intercourse

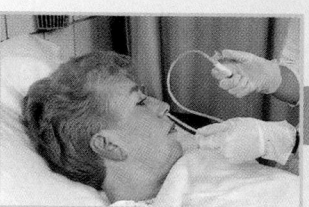

CHAPTER

85

Respiratory Disorders

LEARNING OBJECTIVES

1. State the rationale for the use of each of the following: sputum, lavage, throat culture, and ABG, CXR, lung scan, lung perfusion scan, pulmonary angiography, PFT, and skin testing.
2. Demonstrate the positions of postural drainage.
3. Differentiate the following: thoracentesis, paracentesis, and thoracotomy.
4. Identify at least four nursing considerations related to closed water-seal chest drainage.
5. Identify at least five alterations in normal respiratory status.
6. Identify at least ten interventions that can assist the client who is in respiratory distress.
7. Differentiate the following infectious respiratory disorders: acute rhinitis, streptococcal throat infection, influenza, laryngitis, bronchitis, lung abscesses, pneumonia, pleurisy, histoplasmosis, tuberculosis, and empyema.
8. Compare and contrast the following chronic obstructive pulmonary diseases: asthma, bronchiectasis, chronic bronchitis, and emphysema.
9. Identify three nursing considerations for a client in ARDS.
10. State three common sources of trauma to the lungs, along with three nursing considerations for each.
11. Differentiate benign from malignant lung disorders.
12. Identify three common inflammatory disorders and four structural disorders of the nose.

NEW TERMINOLOGY

anergic	paracentesis
asphyxiation	pleurisy
asthma	pneumonectomy
atelectasis	pneumonia
bronchiectasis	pneumothorax
bronchitis	postural drainage
bronchoscopy	pulmonary emphysema
empyema	rhinitis
epistaxis	rhinoplasty
eupnea	sinusitis
hemothorax	strangulation
histoplasmosis	suffocation
hyperventilation	thoracentesis
incentive spirometer	thoracotomy
laryngectomy	tracheostomy
lobectomy	

ACRONYMS

ABG	CPT	PCP
AIDS	CXR	PFT
ARDS	INH	PPD
BCG	IPPB	SOB
COLD	$PaCO_2$	SOBOE
COPD	PaO_2	TB
CPAP		

The respiratory system is vital to sustaining life. It requires a patent (open) airway for oxygen to reach the lungs. Healthcare professionals may specialize in the field of respiratory care. A physician specializing in respiratory disorders is called a pulmonologist. A related field of respiratory care is *respiratory therapy*, which involves *respiratory therapists* and *respiratory technicians.*

The respiratory system consists of the upper respiratory tract (nose, sinuses, pharynx, and trachea) and the lower respiratory tract (bronchi and lungs) (see Chap. 25). Because blood carries oxygen and carbon dioxide, both the cardiovascular system and the respiratory system must function for life to continue. A person can survive for only a few minutes without oxygen; it is the most vital, basic need of people and animals.

✳DIAGNOSTIC TESTS

Laboratory Tests

Sputum Specimen ✳

Sputum specimens help determine the presence of organisms or blood in a person's sputum. Specimens are best early in the morning when they are most likely to contain sputum, rather than just saliva. Chapter 52 presents the procedure for collecting a sputum specimen.

> ✚👁 **N u r s i n g A l e r t**
> Take precautions in the care and disposal of sputum. Wear gloves when collecting specimens and wash hands after contact with them. Wear a mask and eye shield if splashing is likely. Discard all used facial tissues as contaminated material.

Lavage Specimen

If the client is unable to cough up sputum, the physician may obtain a specimen by bronchoalveolar lavage. In this procedure, sterile saline is instilled into a bronchus. Then, cells and fluid from the bronchioles and alveoli are removed by endoscopy along with the saline. The cells are analyzed in the laboratory, most often to diagnose pulmonary tuberculosis (**TB**).

Throat Culture ✳

A sample of both mucus and secretions from the back of the client's throat can be obtained on a cotton-tipped applicator and applied to a slide or culture medium, which is then incubated in the laboratory to determine the presence of organisms. Drug sensitivity determinations may also be done by placing the specimen on solid media with different concentrations of medications, or in various liquid dilutions of medications to determine which medication is most effective against the organism. This procedure is called a *culture and sensitivity* (C&S) test or *throat culture*. Chapter 52 explains the procedure for collecting a throat culture.

A full culture will determine all organisms present in the specimen. This test takes several days because the organisms must have time to grow. However, a culture may be done within a matter of hours to rule out the presence of streptococci. This

test does not rule out any other organisms. This "quick strep" test is done in cases of suspected strep infection so that appropriate antibiotic therapy can be initiated quickly.

Blood Gas Determinations

The best indicator of oxygen deficiency is the level of arterial blood gases (**ABG**s). The partial pressure of oxygen (PaO_2) value is generally considered normal when it is between 80 and 100 mm Hg (millimeters of mercury). Severe oxygen deficiency exists when the PaO_2 is less than 40 mm Hg. The laboratory can analyze an arterial blood sample and determine the PaO_2, partial pressure of carbon dioxide ($PaCO_2$), and hydrogen ion concentration (pH) of the blood. The physician, nurse, and respiratory therapist then evaluate the blood gas results and plan the most effective treatment for the client.

> ☛ KEY CONCEPT
>
> *Arterial blood gas (ABG) values measure partial pressure of oxygen (PaO_2) and partial pressure of carbon dioxide ($PaCO_2$). These are reported as mm Hg (millimeters of mercury).*
>
> *Values for PaO_2:*
> - *Normal PaO_2 = 80 to 100 mm Hg*
> - *Mild oxygen deficiency = 60 to 80 mm Hg*
> - *Moderate oxygen deficiency = 40 to 60 mm Hg*
> - *Severe oxygen deficiency = less than 40 mm Hg*

X-ray and Fluoroscopy Examinations

Chest X-ray ✳

The *chest x-ray* (**CXR**) examination is no longer done routinely for all clients who are admitted to acute care facilities. It is ordered to determine lung or heart abnormalities. Abnormalities that can be observed on x-ray study include lung tumors or other growths, lung abscesses, pulmonary TB, foreign objects in the lungs, *pneumonia* (inflammation of the lung), or an enlarged heart.

Computed Tomography Scan

The *computed tomography* (**CT**) scan is a series of x-ray films taken to provide a cross-sectional view of the chest or other body part. CT scanning is valuable in the diagnosis of TB, lung abscesses, or tumors.

Lung Scan

After a radioactive medication is introduced into the system by injection or inhalation, a *lung scan (scintiscan)* is done. This test yields a two-dimensional map of various organs and tissues. Disorders are revealed as a difference in density from normal tissue. After the client inhales a special gas, this scan is called a *ventilation scan.*

Lung Perfusion Scan

Albumin tagged with a radioactive material is injected intravenously. These particles pass through the client's venous system and heart, but when they reach the lungs they lodge in the capillaries. The *lung perfusion scan* illustrates different views through which lesions, pneumonia, and other disorders can be located.

Pulmonary Angiography

This test involves injection of radiopaque dye into the pulmonary blood vessels to determine pathology. Chapter 47 describes nursing precautions in the use of radiopaque dye.

Other Diagnostic Tests

Magnetic Resonance Imaging

As with many other body systems, *magnetic resonance imaging* (MRI) can be used to diagnose disorders in the lungs and bronchi. This noninvasive nuclear procedure can produce images of tissues with high fat and water content, which often cannot be seen with conventional x-ray study. Thus, MRI is useful in the diagnosis of lung disorders. It allows the physician to distinguish among cancerous, trauma-induced, and normal tissues because it gives information about their chemical composition.

Pulmonary Function Test

The *pulmonary function test* (**PFT**) measures how much air a client inhales (*inspiration*) and exhales (*expiration*) in one breath, and assesses the client's general respiratory status. Many large hospitals have pulmonary function laboratories for this purpose.

The PFT measures total lung capacity, *vital capacity* (amount of air that is forcibly exhaled after a maximum breath), and *residual volume* (amount of air remaining in the lung after forced exhalation). PFT also measures *tidal volume* (volume of air in an average breath), inspiratory volume, and expiratory volume. The ratios between specific measurements can be determined. The machine used for these tests is the *spirometer*.

☞ KEY CONCEPT

Do not confuse the spirometer *and the* incentive spirometer. *The* spirometer *measures pulmonary function. The* incentive spirometer *also measures pulmonary function, in a sense, but it is used by the client. The incentive spirometer helps the client, such as after surgery, to perform respiratory exercises to maintain lung function.*

PFTs are used to diagnose disorders and to assess effectiveness of therapy. The test helps in assessing pulmonary pathology at an early stage and indicates whether the person has a cardiac or a respiratory disease. The test can evaluate the effectiveness of respiratory therapies and bronchodilator medications and can indicate the surgical risk involved in many cases. When administering this test, encourage the client to breathe as deeply as possible or to follow other instructions.

Bronchoscopy

Bronchoscopy is an invasive procedure in which a *bronchoscope* (a lighted endoscope) is passed through the mouth

and pharynx into the trachea and bronchi. The purpose of this test may be to observe lung tissue, obtain a biopsy or bronchial washings, remove mucous plugs or foreign objects, or determine the location and extent of a mass (tumor). Photographs may be taken. Two types of bronchoscopes are used: the rigid and the fiberoptic. The fiberoptic scope is smaller and more flexible, making it more comfortable for the client and allowing the physician to better visualize the lung within the smaller airways (Fig. 85-1).

Before the test, the person's throat is anesthetized and medications (such as midazolam [Versed]) are administered IV to promote relaxation. These medications may cause a client to experience amnesia about the test. Alert the client to this possibility before the test to prevent concern later.

Food and fluids are withheld for 6 to 8 hours before a bronchoscopy. Give mouth care immediately before the procedure. Explain the procedure to the client, who will most likely remain awake. Be sure that the dentures are removed. Note any loose natural teeth because the bronchoscope may loosen or dislodge a tooth, which could lead to aspiration.

After bronchoscopy, the client remains nothing by mouth (NPO) until the gag reflex returns. The anesthetic numbs the throat, so reflexes are not functional and do not allow the person to cough out secretions. Position the client on his or her side. *Rationale: Doing so keeps the airway open and helps to prevent choking and aspiration.* The side-lying position also helps to facilitate drainage. Note any edema of the throat, bleeding, or dyspnea because if the airway becomes obstructed, an emergency **tracheostomy** (opening into the trachea) may be needed. A sterile endotracheal tube is kept at the bedside until the client is fully awake and reflexes return. In a respiratory emergency, the endotracheal tube can be inserted to assist in keeping the airway open temporarily.

After the client's gag reflex returns, offer clear liquids and monitor the client's ability to tolerate them. Gradually increase the client's diet to soft. Encourage the client to rest and to eat soft foods for 24 hours after this procedure.

Because most bronchoscopy procedures are done on an outpatient basis, be sure to teach the client and family to be alert for possible complications, especially the following:

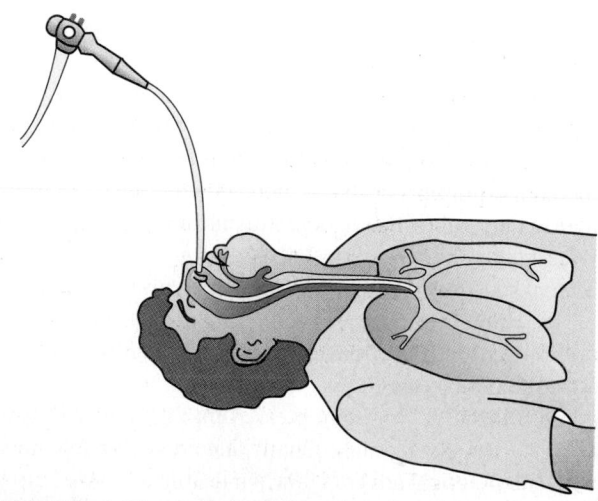

FIGURE 85-1. Fiberoptic bronchoscopy.

- Swelling of the throat
- Difficulty swallowing
- Difficulty breathing
- Bleeding

Be sure to document all teaching completely.

Skin Tests

Skin tests are commonly used to determine if a person has been exposed to tuberculosis or other disorders, such as *histoplasmosis* (a fungal infection discussed later in this chapter). The procedure is the same as that for administering tests to determine allergies to medications or other allergens.

Purified Protein Derivative (PPD) Tuberculin Test.   The *purified protein derivative* (**PPD**) tuberculin test indicates whether a person has ever been exposed to the tubercle bacillus. Approximately 0.1 mL tuberculin serum (PPD) is injected intradermally, with a syringe and needle. The injection site is examined for edema (induration) and redness (erythema) 2 to 3 days (48–72 hours) after the injection. Erythema alone does not indicate a positive reaction; the degrees of positive readings are based on the area of induration, sometimes combined with erythema.

A positive tuberculin test simply means that the person has been exposed to the bacillus at some time, or that he or she has TB antibodies present. A person who is a positive reactor usually remains so for life. Thus, the PPD test is usually not repeated. If a person has a positive reaction to the PPD, a CXR should be done to determine if the lungs are affected. In addition, some individuals may develop a severe allergic reaction to the test.

Use of Controls.   Candida and mumps antigen sera may be injected at the same time as the PPD to determine a person's ability to respond to any foreign agent (antigen). Persons with a healthy immune system should respond to candida or mumps or both. In the immunosuppressed individual, this often does not occur. The term used is *anergy* and the person is considered **anergic** (unable to respond to the foreign agent). In this case, the PPD may have been mistakenly read as negative. In other words, in the anergic individual, the PPD appears to be negative because the person's body cannot appropriately respond to any antigen. This does not mean that the person has not been exposed to TB.

If the person is judged to be anergic, a two-step PPD test may be necessary. The two-step PPD test involves doing two PPD tests, 1 or 2 weeks apart. This method attempts to boost the person's immune system to appropriately respond to the antigen. Many public health departments now do the two-step test routinely.

Tine Test.   Another method of tuberculin testing is the *tine test,* which is simply a different method of injecting the tuberculin serum. It is often used in mass screening. A sterile stainless steel disk with four *tines* (sharp prongs) is impregnated with PPD; the tines are pressed into the person's skin. The disks are packaged individually and are disposable; thus, they offer a practical advantage when testing a large group of people.

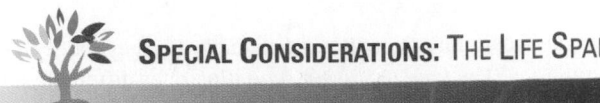

SPECIAL CONSIDERATIONS: THE LIFE SPAN

PPD Tests

A negative result on the PPD test in an elderly person does not necessarily indicate that the person has never been exposed to TB or does not have active TB. Persons over age 65 may be anergic because of immune system failure (not an immunodeficiency disease). If an elderly person tests PPD negative, other tests may be necessary to confirm a diagnosis of TB (sputum culture, chest x-ray examination, or two-step PPD test).

COMMON MEDICAL TREATMENTS

Postural Drainage

Postural drainage uses position and gravity to drain secretions and mucus from the individual's lungs. Figure 85-2 illustrates the basic positions for postural drainage.

The person adopts a head-downward position, which allows the secretions to run far enough into the trachea from the bronchi so that they can be coughed out. The client's exact position will depend on the portion of the lung to be drained. Treatments generally last about 15 to 20 minutes. The procedure is called chest physiotherapy (**CPT**). The nurse must receive specific instructions from a respiratory therapist, physical therapist, or pulmonary physician before performing this procedure. In Practice: Nursing Care Guidelines 85-1 highlights important information about postural drainage.

Often postural bronchial drainage is done in combination with other respiratory treatments, such as inhalations, to loosen and bring up secretions from the lungs and to prevent respiratory complications. Nursing considerations appear in the Nursing Process section later in this chapter.

COMMON SURGICAL TREATMENTS

Thoracentesis

Thoracentesis involves puncturing the chest wall to remove excess fluid or air from the pleural cavity. It is done for diagnostic purposes or to relieve breathing difficulties in clients with TB, cancer of the lung, pleural effusion, pulmonary edema, and chest injuries. Using sterile technique, the physician inserts a *trocar* (large needle with *obturator,* a guide) into the pleural cavity. The obturator is removed and fluid is withdrawn. The specimen is collected in a sterile container and measured. The specimen is then sent to the laboratory for analysis. The fluid is considered contaminated and appropriate infection control measures should be taken.

Throughout the procedure, assist the client and offer support. The procedure is similar to abdominal paracentesis, which is described in Chapter 87. The person will be most comfortable in a sitting position while leaning on a padded overbed table. The physician will need very little assistance, but the client will need considerable emotional support.

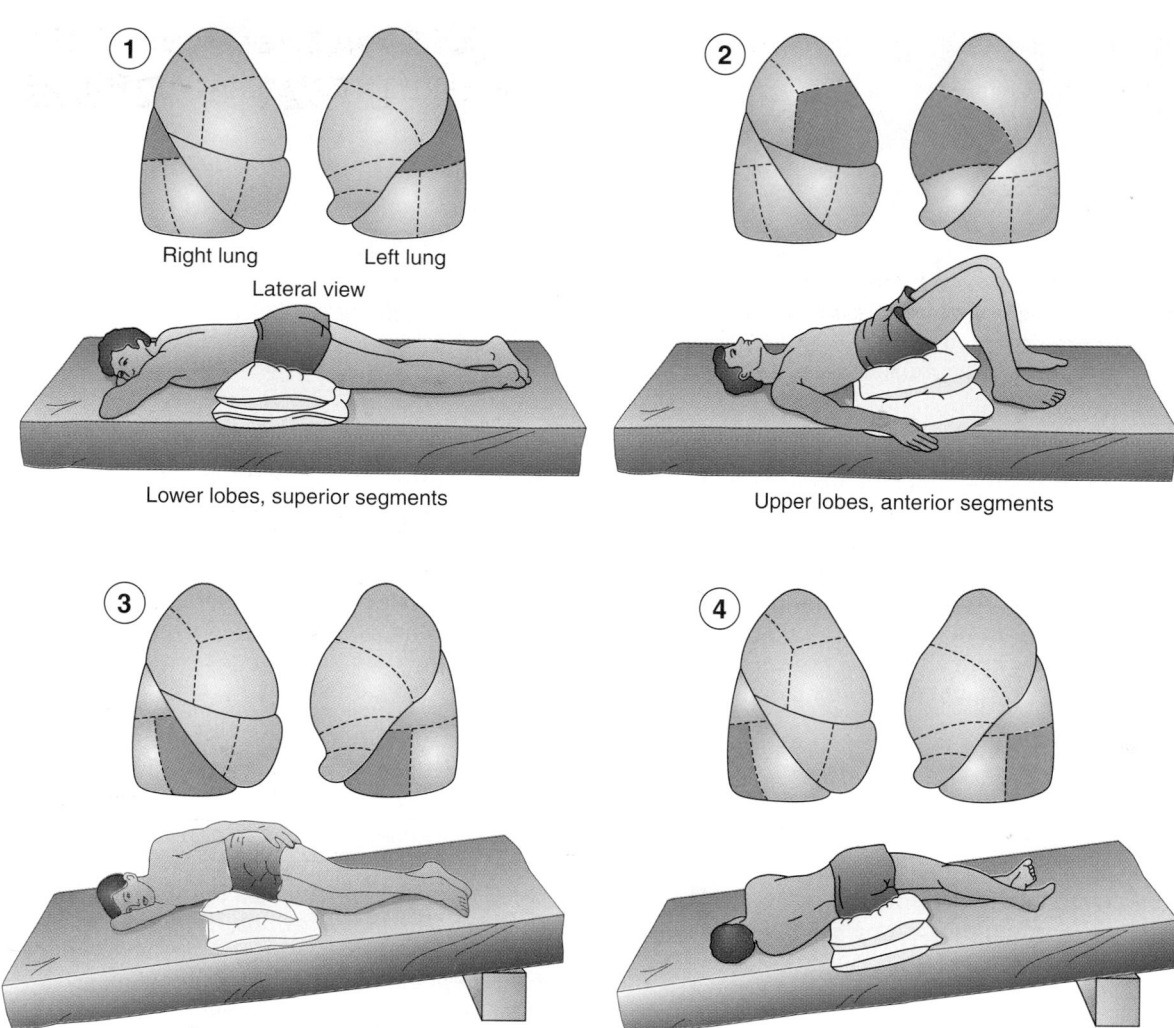

① Right lung   Left lung
Lateral view
Lower lobes, superior segments

② Upper lobes, anterior segments

③ Lower lobes, anterior basal segment

④ Upper lobes, lateral basal segment

FIGURE 85-2. Postural drainage. Usually the bronchi of the lower and middle lobe empty most effectively when the person's head is down. The force of gravity helps drain secretions from the smaller bronchial airways to the main bronchi and the trachea. The individual is then able to cough up secretions. This procedure is most effective early in the morning.

✚👁 Nursing Alert

Because a thoracentesis is an invasive procedure, the client must sign an informed consent before it can begin. Watch the client carefully after the test for signs of fluid leakage or infection. A rare but serious complication is *pneumothorax* (accumulation of air in the pleural space). Clients may have some pain, which analgesics can usually relieve. Be sure to watch for respiratory depression when clients are receiving medications.

Generally, after the procedure, the individual can breathe more easily because the pressure of the fluid, which often causes respiratory distress, has been relieved.

Paracentesis

Paracentesis is defined as the puncturing of a body cavity for aspiration of fluid; however, this process most commonly

refers to puncture of the abdominal cavity. Abdominal distention due to excess fluid immobilizes the diaphragm and interferes with breathing. Therefore, removing fluid from the abdomen can relieve breathing difficulties.

✚👁 Nursing Alert

A large amount of fluid withdrawn (more than 1,000 mL) during paracentesis or thoracentesis can result in vasodilation and *hypovolemia* (decreased circulating fluid volume). These situations can cause *syncope* (temporary loss of consciousness, fainting) and shock. Take the client's blood pressure and pulse immediately after paracentesis or thoracentesis and every 15 minutes until readings are stable and within acceptable levels.

Thoracotomy

Lung surgery is done through a **thoracotomy,** an incision into the thorax or chest cavity.

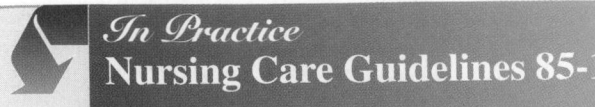

ASSISTING WITH POSTURAL DRAINAGE

- Always wash hands. *Rationale: Handwashing helps prevent the spread of infection.*
- Always wear gloves and handle all soiled tissues as contaminated material. *Rationale: This client may be infectious. Observe Standard Precautions.*
- Explain to the client why the head-downward position is necessary for much of the treatment. *Rationale: This position may be uncomfortable, but if the client understands the reason, he or she will be more likely to cooperate.*
- Improve drainage by striking the client between the shoulder blades with cupped hands (*pummeling*) or by vibrating the client. *Rationale: These techniques help to loosen the secretions.* Be sure to receive instructions in these techniques.
- Have tissues available. *Rationale: The person will probably cough up secretions.*
- Have pillows and pads available. *Rationale: The various positions are easier to assume if a movable bed and pillows are available.*
- Perform this procedure before the person eats. *Rationale: The client may gag, choke, or vomit. Performing postural drainage before eating helps to prevent vomiting and aspiration.*
- Give the client oral hygiene following the procedure. *Rationale: The stagnant or infected mucus may have a foul taste and odor.*
- Dispose of all materials properly and wash hands. *Rationale: Proper disposal of materials and handwashing help reduce the risk of infection transmission.*
- Document the procedure and the client's reactions. *Rationale: Documentation provides for communication and continuity of care.*

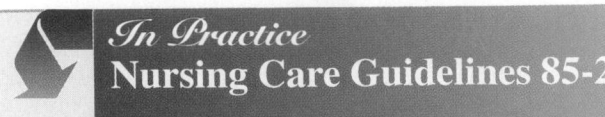

CARING FOR THE PERSON WHO HAS HAD CHEST SURGERY

- Always wash hands and wear gloves. *Rationale: Handwashing and gloves help to prevent infection transmission.*
- Turn the client often. *Rationale: Turning helps to facilitate drainage and prevent hypostatic pneumonia and other complications. The wound will drain the most when the client is lying on the affected side; however, because this can be uncomfortable, coordinate turning to this side with the time when the pain medication effectiveness is optimum.*
- Be sure the client turns and coughs and uses the incentive spirometer, as ordered. *Rationale: Turning, coughing, deep breathing, and using incentive spirometer help to prevent stasis of secretions.*
- Assess for dyspnea, rate of respiration, cyanosis, increased heart rate, chest pain, restlessness, orthopnea, or hemoptysis. *Rationale: These symptoms could indicate that the chest suction is malfunctioning.*
- Help the client to sit comfortably in the chair while the chest suction is operating. *Rationale: Getting the client out of bed helps to minimize the risk for developing complications, in particular, respiratory complications. Sitting in the chair helps to promote lung expansion.*
- If the client is up walking with tubes and drainage bags or bottles, be sure that the hemostatic clamps go along. *Rationale: The client must always be within reach of the clamps in case of accidental dislodgement of tubes.*
- Make sure the client is passing flatus rather than having gas pains or distention difficulties. *Rationale: Abdominal distention can cause difficulty in breathing and extreme discomfort.*
- Encourage ambulation and exercise. *Rationale: Ambulation and exercise help the client recover more quickly and decrease any risks of complications.*
- Maintain a level of comfort acceptable to the client, so that deep breathing and coughing can and will be done. *Rationale: Ease of breathing enhances the client's ability to comply with treatment.*

Caring for the Client With Chest Surgery

Teach the client deep-breathing techniques, as well as range-of-motion (ROM) exercises, before chest surgery. The extent of the client's participation in postoperative care will directly reflect the quality of preoperative instruction given. Postoperative exercises can be vital to recovery and help prevent complications.

Provide routine preoperative and postoperative care. In Practice: Nursing Care Guidelines 85-2 outlines care for a client who has had chest surgery.

The immediate postoperative concern for the person who has had lung surgery is to maintain an adequate airway. Direct care at preventing respiratory complications.

Record vital signs frequently; turn the client often to prevent complications of immobility. Encourage the client to breathe deeply and to cough at least every 2 to 4 hours and to use the incentive spirometer. Coughing is easiest if the person is in an upright position and he or she splints the incision with a pillow (see Chap. 56).

The client must exercise soon after surgery because many muscles are incised during chest surgery and function must be restored; exercise also prevents complications related to immobility. Carry out passive ROM exercises for the client; within a few days he or she should be able to actively participate in ROM. Full ROM exercises, including *isometric* (muscle-setting) exercises, must be provided for the shoulder and arm on the operative side; these exercises may be initiated immediately following surgery. Discontinue any exercises that cause pain or great resistance. Do not overextend or overtire the client's muscles.

> ### Nursing Alert
> If a person with any disorder of the respiratory system is receiving a narcotic, be particularly watchful for respiratory depression. Depressed respirations can be an undesirable side effect in anyone, but the situation is most dangerous for the client whose respiratory function is already compromised.

Chest Suction. Following most types of lung surgery, the client will have large catheters called *chest tubes* inserted into the chest cavity and attached to suction. The breathing mechanism of the lungs works because the pressure of the chest cavity is lower than the pressure of the air outside the lungs. This negative pressure creates a vacuum, which causes air to rush into the lungs and keep them inflated. After the chest cavity has been opened, a vacuum must be created within the chest to reestablish negative pressure. The purpose of suction is to restore the negative pressure within the chest cavity and reinflate the lungs, or to prevent loss of negative pressure and keep the lungs inflated. In addition, secretions and blood that may have accumulated in the chest cavity must be removed.

Closed Water-Seal Drainage. The most common method of reestablishing negative pressure is by *closed water-seal chest drainage.* In this procedure, one or more catheters are inserted into the chest cavity. If more than one catheter is inserted, each may be connected to a separate suction setup, or they may all be joined and attached to one suction setup.

> ### Nursing Alert
> Maintain the integrity of the suction apparatus and water seal at all times. Refill the water chamber if the fluid level gets low. Report at once any client who complains of severe pain or dyspnea. If a bottle or connection breaks, the closed system will be disrupted and this is an emergency! Clamp the chest tubes immediately and summon help.

The water-seal drainage system must remain closed (airtight) so that no air is allowed to enter the chest cavity; otherwise, the lungs collapse. By putting the drainage tubes under water, air is prevented from backing up into the chest. One widely used apparatus of disposable chest drainage systems is called the Pleur-Evac (Fig. 85-3).

This system comes assembled and sterile with instructions for use. It can be connected to suction and provides a water seal. When the chamber is full of blood, it is discarded and replaced with a new one, *only by a trained professional.*

Nursing Implications. Assess for signs of shock, dyspnea, pain in the chest, or a rapid increase in chest tube drainage and report these symptoms immediately. *Rationale: The most serious postoperative complications are hemorrhage into the lung cavity (**hemothorax**) or collection of air in the pleural cavity, causing collapse of all or part of a lung (**pneumothorax**).* In hemothorax, the fluid (blood) collects in the lower part of the pleural cavity. In pneumothorax, the air rises to the top. In Practice: Nursing Assessment 85-1 highlights danger signs for a person with a chest tube. In Practice: Nursing Care Guidelines 85-3 outlines care measures.

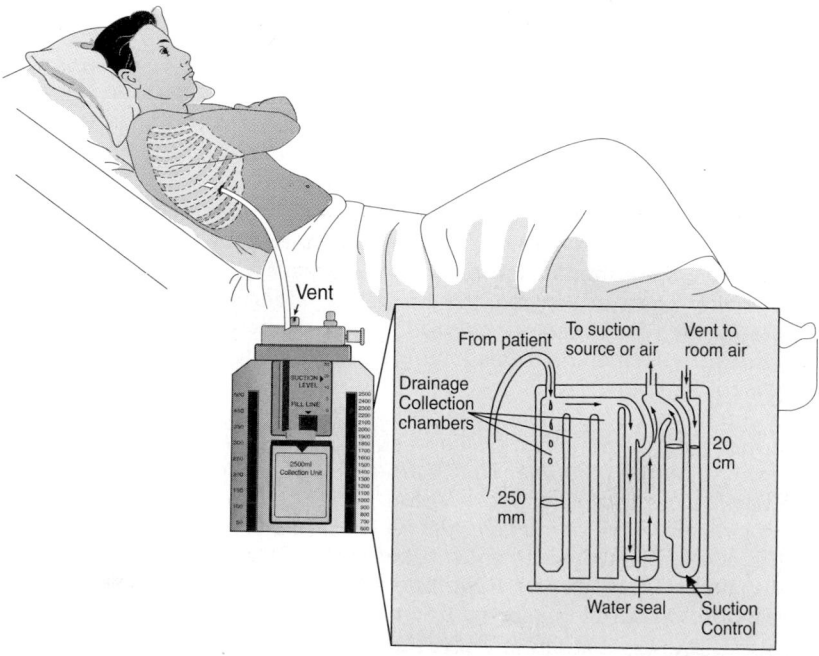

FIGURE 85-3. The Pleur-Evac system of underwater chest drainage. It is prepackaged, sterile, and disposable after use. The *arrows* indicate the flow of air when the lung is inflated properly.

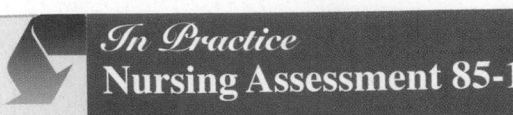

In Practice
Nursing Assessment 85-1

DANGER SIGNS FOR A PERSON WITH A CHEST TUBE

Be alert for the following:

- Leakage of air into the drainage system, whether in a simple water-seal type or a mechanical suction type, is indicated by constant bubbling in the water-seal system or bottle, after the client's lungs have been initially expanded. There will be bubbling in the control bottle—the one connected to suction. If bubbling in the control bottle stops, the suction pressure is too low.
- Air leaks can occur at the insertion site of the chest tube, in connections, in the bottles, or in the stoppers in three-bottle suction; or in the closed drainage system itself.

- To check the location of an air leak, pinch the tubing for a few seconds at intervals between the chest tube and drainage connection. If the bubbling stops, the air leak is due to the system (check all connections). If the bubbling continues, pinch off tubing at intervals between the client and the system; when the pinching is between the source of the air leak and the water chamber, the bubbling will stop.
- Keep all tubes, bags, and other devices below the level of tube insertion. *Rationale: This position prevents reflux.*
- If the client shows signs of cyanosis or dyspnea, or complains of chest pain, investigate the situation immediately. This is an emergency!

In Practice
Nursing Care Guidelines 85-3

CARING FOR THE PERSON WITH CHEST SUCTION

- Always wash your hands and wear gloves. *Rationale: Handwashing and gloves help to reduce the risk for infection.*
- Never attempt to set up any chest suction without assistance. *Rationale: In most facilities, at least two people must check a suction setup before it can be connected to the client. This is a safety precaution.*
- Never disconnect or change chest suction without being absolutely certain about what to do. *Rationale: The person's life depends on the ability to maintain the integrity of the pleural space.*
- Never disconnect chest tubes! *Rationale: These tubes provide the suction that keeps the lungs inflated. If they are disconnected, the lungs will collapse.*
- Keep clamps or hemostats with the client, either clipped to the bedding or to the client's gown (when using the three-bottle system). With the disposable system, a clamp is attached with the tubing. Thus, additional clamps are not necessary. If the client gets out of bed, the clamps go along. *Rationale: The tubes are clamped as an emergency measure in case the tubes become accidentally disconnected.*
- If the tubes become disconnected, double-clamp all tubes close to the chest wall and summon assistance immediately. *Rationale: This is an emergency situation requiring prompt intervention. If air enters the chest cavity, the person's lungs will collapse!*
- Be aware that clamping chest tubes may cause a tension pneumothorax. *Rationale: If any untoward symptoms occur, call for help immediately.*

- Never empty drainage in a closed system. Note the amount as ordered. Discard the entire system when full. *Rationale: The integrity of the closed system must be maintained to prevent lung collapse.*
- Never use pins to fasten the tubes to the bed. *Rationale: A pin might puncture the tube.*
- Never change a chest dressing. *Rationale: The dressing may help maintain the integrity of the chest wall.*
- Never take the plugs out of the bottles without assistance and never pull on chest tubes. *Rationale: These actions may result in air entering the chest cavity.*
- Tape all connections to make sure they are airtight. *Rationale: Taping connections reduces the risk that the tubes may become disconnected.*
- Keep in mind that chest tubes do not need to be *stripped* (cleared) unless there are clots or very thick drainage. In this case, stripping the tubes may be necessary to maintain patency. Hold the tube in place while stripping or milking it, stripping no more than 7 to 9 inches at a time, using short strokes rather than one long stroke. *Rationale: Holding the tube between the hands and the client's chest prevents pulling on the tubes and possibly displacing them. Using short strokes helps to prevent possible tearing of the pleura.*
- If a chest tube becomes kinked, report it immediately. *Rationale: Kinking could disrupt the system and prevent drainage.*
- To set up the drainage after the tube is inserted, wrap a piece of cloth tape around the tube and then

attach the tape to the edge of the bed, so the tube hangs straight down into the bottle. Keep the remainder of the tubing in the bed with the client. *Rationale: Straight drainage provides the best drainage flow. The excess tubing allows the client to turn in bed and move about.*

• Be sure the client does not lie or pull on the tubing. *Rationale: This might obstruct the flow of the drainage.*

• Keep drainage containers lower than the level of the client at all times. *Rationale: This position facilitates drainage and prevents backflow.*

• If possible, use the disposable closed system instead of the bottle system. The bottle system is rarely used today. *Rationale: The plastic container is much less likely to break, and the tubes are more secure in the drainage container.*

• Observe and report accurately. Notify the healthcare provider if there is a marked change. *Rationale: The*

amount, color, and consistency of the drainage is vital information.

• Observe for excessive bleeding or for abrupt absence of drainage. *Rationale: Hemorrhage is a dangerous complication, and abrupt absence of drainage often means that the system is not operating properly.*

• Document any changes in respiratory status, or respiratory distress, and any milking of the tubes. *Rationale: Documentation provides for communication and continuity of care.*

• Put a piece of tape on the drainage bottle to indicate the fluid level, and record the level of the drainage as ordered. *Rationale: The tape identifies the level of drainage, allowing output to be determined.*

• Discard all drainage tubes and other equipment as required by Standard Precautions. *Rationale: Proper disposal of equipment helps prevent the spread of infection.*

NURSING PROCESS

Data Collection

Carefully observe and assess the client with a respiratory disorder. Because adequate oxygenation is vital to life, a disorder in the respiratory system can quickly become life threatening. Chapter 47 describes physical examination and assessment, including that of the respiratory system. This assessment establishes a baseline for future comparison and determines the presence of suspected complications. Report any changes in the baseline level.

When assessing a client's respiratory system, note the client's breathing and oxygenation level. In Practice: Nursing Assessment 85-2 highlights key information.

In addition, observe the individual's emotional response to the disorder or disease. Does the client need assistance to meet daily needs? Does the disorder affect social activities or self-esteem? Is the person anxious or fearful about the outcome?

Noting Alterations in Respiratory Status

Various events, such as illness or injury, can alter a client's respiratory status. Table 85-1 lists possible alterations from **eupnea** (normal breathing).

Aspiration. *Pathologic aspiration* is the inhalation or movement of fluid, mucus, or another unwanted substance into the lungs. It can cause lung disorders or death.

Hyperventilation. In **hyperventilation,** the person breathes abnormally quickly or deeply, resulting in too little carbon dioxide in the blood. The usual cause is anxiety or overexcitement. The hyperventilating person may have muscle spasms, dizziness, or faintness because of excessive oxygen and the depletion of carbon dioxide in the body. The easiest

treatment is asking the client to breathe into a bag. The air the client re-breathes will contain excess carbon dioxide, replacing that which was lost.

Hypoxia

The tissue cells must have a constant oxygen supply to remain alive. Because the body does not store oxygen, the person normally obtains oxygen from the air (air is approximately 21% oxygen). In some types of illness, the body is unable to take in enough oxygen or cannot use it effectively. When the oxygen

In Practice
Nursing Assessment 85-2

THE CLIENT WITH A POSSIBLE RESPIRATORY DISORDER

• Note respiratory rate, depth, and character
• Determine respiratory status
• Observe for signs of respiratory distress, dyspnea, or poor oxygenation
• Be alert for signs or symptoms of *hypoxia* (lack of oxygen)
• Note any symptoms such as cough, hemoptysis, cyanosis
• Listen to lung sounds and breath sounds
• Check results of skin tests related to tuberculosis or other lung conditions
• Observe mouth and throat by visualization and palpation

■■■ **TABLE 85-1** *P*OSSIBLE ALTERATIONS IN RESPIRATORY STATUS

Term	Sign/Symptom of:
Dyspnea: Labored or difficult breathing, painful breathing	Inadequate ventilation, lowered oxygen level in blood
Orthopnea: Difficulty breathing while lying down, relieved by sitting upright (*orthopneic* position)	Cardiac disorders, pulmonary emphysema, congestive heart failure
Tachypnea: Very rapid breathing	High fever, pneumonia, alkalosis, salicylate overdose, brain stem lesions
Hyperpnea: Increase in depth of breaths, maybe increase in rate (no feeling of increased respiratory effort)	Strenuous exercise
Bradypnea: Respiration slower than normal, regular in rhythm	Normal during sleep; sign of drug overdose, disturbance in respiratory center of brain, metabolic disorder
Cheyne-Stokes breathing: Combination of deep and shallow breaths, as well as periods of apnea (may be up to 3 min)	Brain stem lesion, heart failure, brain damage
Apnea: Cessation of breathing 　*Central apnea:* No brain drive to breathe	Undeveloped respiratory center in preterm infants, adult brain stem lesion, high spinal cord injury
Obstructive apnea: No air flow due to upper airway obstruction 　*Mixed apnea:* Central apnea immediately followed by obstruction 　*Adult sleep apnea:* Prolonged and frequent episodes of apnea during sleep	Foreign object in airway, excessive secretions, absent cough reflex *Obstructive* (tongue or throat structures relax), obesity *Central* (brain damage, brain lesion)
Kussmaul's respirations: Dyspnea with rapid (more than 20/min) gasping breaths, air hunger, panting, labored respirations	Metabolic acidosis, renal failure

level in body tissues is inadequate, the client is said to suffer from *hypoxia*. A summary of signs and symptoms of hypoxia is seen in Box 85-1.

One of the most obvious signs of hypoxia is shortness of breath (**SOB**). Earlier signs of hypoxia may be seen with short-

➤ ➤ **BOX 85-1**

SIGNS AND SYMPTOMS OF HYPOXIA

Arterial PaO_2 less than 50 mm Hg
Tachycardia
Mild increase in blood pressure
Cool, moist skin
Confusion
Delirium
Difficulty in problem solving
Loss of judgment
Euphoria
Unruly or combative behavior
Sensory impairment
Mental fatigue
Drowsiness
Stupor and coma (late)
Hypotension (late)
Bradycardia (late)

Source: Porth, C. M. (2002). *Pathophysiology: Concepts of altered health states* (6th ed.). Philadelphia: Lippincott Williams & Wilkins.

ness of breath on exertion (**SOBOE**). When the client expresses this feeling, SOB is called *dyspnea*. The nurse may also assess SOB in the client through clinical observation. Signs include restlessness, apprehension, an anxious facial expression, panic, fatigue, or impaired coordination. As the need for more oxygen continues, the client's rate and depth of respiration may increase.

Severe oxygen deficiency may be manifested by the person's use of accessory breathing muscles of the neck and upper chest. Gasping, wheezing, or retractions of the breastbone or intercostal spaces are also late signs of hypoxia.

Other manifestations include:

- Mental changes, confusion, stupor, and unconsciousness
- Cardiac symptoms such as rapid pulse, dysrhythmias, fibrillation, and cardiac standstill (cardiac arrest) due to the heart's inability to provide blood, and thus oxygen, to the tissues, causing the heart to overwork
- Changes in skin color, such as cyanosis of skin, nail beds, and mucous membranes (resulting from either a marked lack of oxygen or severe blood loss) or pallor

Hypoxemic Hypoxia. *Hypoxemic hypoxia* is a state of decreased blood oxygen level, leading to a decreased amount of oxygen in the tissues. Many situations can result in hypoxemic hypoxia: the client's airway may be blocked, in which case respiration ceases or is ineffective; the lungs may be congested, in which case respiration is difficult and gradually worsens; an injury to the chest or lungs may cause difficulty in breathing; or chronic or acute infections in the lungs may interfere with breathing.

In these instances, oxygen decrease may be sudden or gradual. For example, if a person chokes on a piece of meat, oxygen supply is suddenly cut off and the person will die if the airway is not restored within a matter of minutes. In many infectious or chronic conditions of the lungs, breathing is impaired but not stopped completely. In these instances, most of which are not emergencies, the nurse can assist the person to breathe or to obtain oxygen.

Circulation Hypoxia. *Circulation hypoxia* is due to inadequate blood circulation. If blood cannot get to tissues, the body's oxygen supply is cut off. The two chief circulatory disorders that account for a decrease in oxygen supply are failure of the heart to pump and blockage or rupture of a blood vessel.

Failure of the heart to pump may be caused by a lack of blood to the heart itself, by a weakening of the heart muscle, by stoppage, or by wild, uncontrolled beating of the heart (*fibrillation*). If blood cannot get through a vessel because of a clot or stricture, or because of developing atherosclerosis, the blood supply is reduced or stopped completely. This happens in a cerebrovascular accident (stroke) and in a thrombosis. In a ruptured aneurysm, the vessel explodes and the channel for blood is absent.

Anemic Hypoxia. *Anemic hypoxia* is due to reduction in the blood's oxygen-carrying capacity. Hemoglobin, a constituent of red blood cells (RBCs), carries oxygen to the tissues. Anemia can result from decreased blood volume, decreased hemoglobin within the RBCs, or the inability of hemoglobin to take on oxygen. In sickle cell anemia, the malformed (sickle-shaped) RBCs cannot pass through the capillaries. Carbon monoxide poisoning is a form of anemic hypoxia because the carbon monoxide combines with hemoglobin, leaving no room for oxygen.

Histotoxic Hypoxia. *Histotoxic hypoxia* is due to inability of the tissues to use oxygen. Under the influence of certain chemicals, the cells are unable to use oxygen. The most common example is cyanide poisoning. Persons who have suffered smoke inhalation often have inhaled cyanide gas and may have histotoxic hypoxia.

Nursing Diagnosis

Based on data collection, the following sample nursing diagnoses may be seen on a nursing care plan for the client with a respiratory disorder. Multiple causal factors are listed:

- Excess Fluid Volume related to compromised respiratory mechanism
- Impaired Gas Exchange related to lung disorders, obstruction, trauma, altered oxygen supply
- Ineffective Airway Clearance related to obstruction, trauma, painful/ineffective cough, excess secretions, cerebrovascular accident, infection, spinal cord injury
- Ineffective Breathing Pattern related to neurologic disorder, obstruction, trauma, pain
- Impaired Oral Mucous Membrane related to mouth breathing

- Impaired Verbal Communication related to tracheostomy, obstruction, trauma, physical barriers, brain damage
- Activity Intolerance related to imbalance between oxygen supply and demand, pain, lung disorders, emphysema
- Anxiety related to inability to breathe

Planning and Implementing

Together, the client, family, and healthcare team plan for effective individualized care to meet the client's needs. For the client undergoing lung or chest surgery, provide preoperative and postoperative teaching and care. The client with a respiratory disorder may be anxious. This person may also require assistance in the management of portable oxygen. He or she may need assistance in meeting some or all basic needs, in dealing with emotional problems, and understanding more about the disorder, its prognosis, and its treatment.

Relieving Respiratory Distress

Orthopneic Position. Many people are unable to breathe unless they are in a sitting or semi-sitting position, which is called the *orthopneic position*. Position the client with pillows to support the back. Sometimes it helps if the client leans on a padded overbed table while in this position, or sleeps in a lounge chair. Some people must remain in the sitting position while sleeping. Provide the overbed table and a pillow to lean on.

Turning, Coughing, Deep Breathing. *Turning, coughing, deep breathing* (TCDB) is vital for anyone who is in bed for a long period. Lung complications can occur when a person is immobile, and develop more quickly when a respiratory problem is present. To prevent such complications, be sure that the client continually ventilates and expands the lungs as much as possible.

Administering Respiratory Treatments

Postural Drainage. Because *postural drainage* uses gravity, the person is placed in a head-downward position (see Fig. 85-2 and In Practice: Nursing Care Guidelines 85-1). Request training from the respiratory therapist specific to the individual. *Rationale: Positions vary according to the specific disorder and the lung area being drained.*

Breathing Exercises and Incentive Spirometer. The physician will probably order breathing exercises to help the client build up respiratory capacity. These are usually done with the aid of the **incentive spirometer**. Instructions will depend on the particular type of device the client uses. A major reason for postoperative incentive spirometry is to prevent **atelectasis** (an airless or potentially collapsed lung due to obstruction by mucus or a foreign object).

The client may receive instructions to do other exercises to increase respiratory capacity and function. The nurse may teach the technique of abdominal breathing—pushing the abdominal wall out during inspiration and pulling it in during exhalation.

Breathing Treatments. Several types of breathing treatments may be used. Intermittent positive pressure breathing (**IPPB**) treatment is not often used today, unless aerosolized medications are to be given. The most common uses of IPPB are in cystic fibrosis and neuromuscular disorders. Aerosol nebulizer (mini-nebulizer) treatments provide aerosolized medication via a mask or mouthpiece apparatus attached to oxygen or compressed air. These treatments are further discussed in Chapters 63 and 86.

Oxygen.   Many people with respiratory and other problems receive supplemental oxygen by cannula or mask, which assists them to breathe more easily and provides a higher concentration of oxygen than that of room air. Understand the precautions used when oxygen is administered (see Chap. 86). Provide emotional support because it may be a frightening experience for clients and their families.

Administering Nasal Treatments

People with respiratory disorders often use nasal sprays and nose drops (see Chap. 63). In addition, if the client has a purulent discharge that forms crusts in the nose, a nasal irrigation may be ordered. The irrigation solution flows into one nostril and out through the other. The important point to observe in giving a nasal irrigation is to use the correct amount of pressure. Too much pressure may force the fluid into the sinuses and the eustachian tubes, thus spreading the infection. This procedure is uncommon.

Suctioning to Remove Oral–Nasal Secretions

Many people with respiratory problems require suctioning to remove excess secretions and mucus from the airway. Suctioning may also be indicated in the unconscious person or in clients with ineffective cough. Use a new, sterile, suction kit each time to avoid introducing pathogens into the lungs. The client who cannot swallow may require only oral suctioning. In this case, use a tonsil-suction device and follow clean technique. In Practice: Nursing Procedure 85-1 details the technique. The procedure for suctioning a tracheostomy is similar and is presented in Chapter 86.

 Nursing Alert

Suctioning can cause *dysrhythmia* (irregular heartbeat) and *desaturation* (loss of oxygenation). Continuously assess the person being suctioned.

In Practice
Nursing Procedure 85-1

SUCTIONING TO REMOVE SECRETIONS
Supplies and Equipment

Sterile, disposable suction tube
Gloves
Sterile suction machine in the room

Steps

1. Check the physician's orders.
   RATIONALE: *The orders specifically detail what is to be done.*

2. Assemble equipment and explain the procedure to the client.
   RATIONALE: *Organization enhances efficiency; explanations help to allay the client's fears and anxiety, fostering cooperation.*

3. Place the conscious client in semi-Fowler's position.
   RATIONALE: *This position prevents aspiration.*

4. Wash your hands and set up equipment, opening the sterile suction package.
   RATIONALE: *Handwashing helps to prevent the spread of infection; proper technique is necessary to maintain the sterility of the equipment.*

5. Put on sterile or clean gloves, as ordered.
   RATIONALE: *Using gloves helps prevent introducing pathogens into the client's respiratory tract.*

6. Wear eye protection when performing deep suctioning procedures.
   RATIONALE: *This action adheres to Standard Precautions.*

7. Pick up the sterile catheter and connect it to the suction tubing being held by your nondominant hand, which now becomes unsterile (sterile to clean = contaminated).
   RATIONALE: *The suction tubing is considered contaminated. After this is touched, that hand then is considered contaminated.*

8. Moisten the catheter with sterile saline.
   RATIONALE: *Moistening the catheter lubricates the catheter and helps to minimize trauma to the mucous membranes and increase the client's comfort. Check the suction machine's functioning.*

9. Gently insert the catheter through the client's nostril with the suction off.
   RATIONALE: *Both the catheter and the suctioning can irritate mucous membranes.*

10. Insert the catheter down to the end of the trachea (stimulating the cough reflex); pull the catheter back a few millimeters to reduce irritation to the *carina* (the ridge at the lower end of the trachea which separates the openings of the

In Practice
Nursing Procedure 85-1 (Continued)

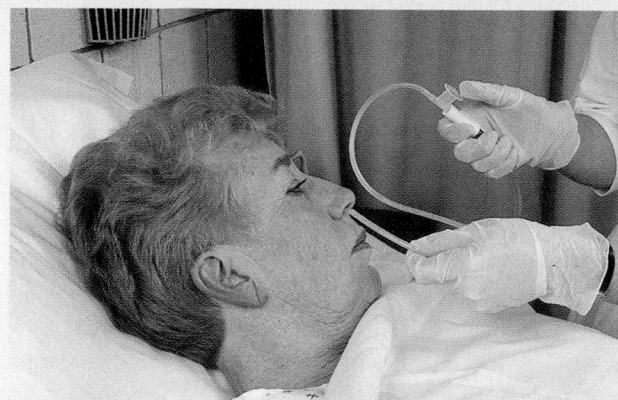

Insert catheter without applying suction. Here a "whistle-tip" catheter is left open to air as the catheter is inserted.

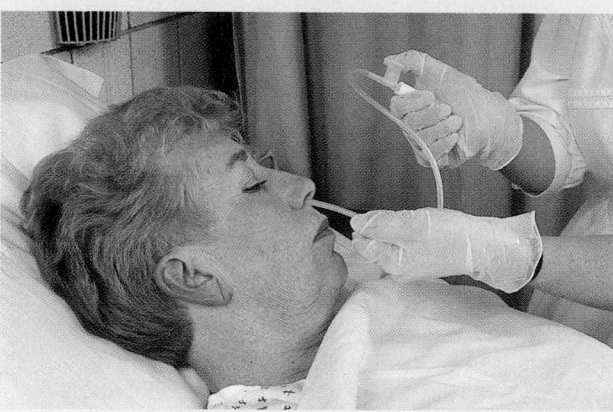

Suction the client by closing the system and creating a vacuum by putting a thumb over the opening as you pull out the catheter.

two bronchi). Begin suctioning, for about 10 to 15 seconds. The entire process of entering, suctioning, and withdrawal should not exceed a total of 20 seconds.
RATIONALE: *Suctioning stops oxygen inhalation, and hypoxia may result. It is also very uncomfortable.*

11. Withdraw the catheter fairly rapidly in a rotating motion while suctioning continues.
RATIONALE: *Rotation helps clean all surfaces of the respiratory passageways.*

12. Repeat suctioning until no mucus returns. Give the client time to rest and breathe normally between suctionings. Give the client oxygen before and after passage of the catheter to relieve panic and reduce the risk of hypoxia.
RATIONALE: *These actions help to prevent hypoxia.*

13. Flush the catheter with sterile normal saline between suctionings. *Rationale: Flushing cleans and clears the catheter and lubricates it for the next suctioning.* Use suctioning pressures of 80 to 100 mm Hg for the adult client.
RATIONALE: *A vacuum pressure in excess of 120 mm Hg causes trauma to the delicate respiratory mucosa; bleeding can result.*

14. Properly dispose of all materials and make sure the client is comfortable. Wash your hands.
RATIONALE: *Proper disposal of equipment and handwashing help prevent the spread of infection.*

15. Document the procedure and the client's reactions.
RATIONALE: *Documentation provides for communication and continuity of care. This procedure can be frightening and uncomfortable.*

Evaluation

Evaluate outcomes of care with the client, family, and other members of the healthcare team. Have short-term goals been met? Has the client shown evidence of improvement in his or her respiratory status? Are long-term goals still realistic? Planning for further nursing care considers the client's prognosis, as well as any complications and the client's response to care given.

INFECTIOUS RESPIRATORY DISORDERS

The Common Cold

The common cold is also known as **acute rhinitis**. *Rhinitis* is a term that means inflammation of the nasal mucous membranes. One or more filterable viruses cause colds; as many as 100 cold viruses have been identified. Colds are easily spread by talking, coughing, or sneezing. Individuals are contagious 48 hours before the appearance of the first symptoms. If fatigue, chilling, or substances that continually irritate the nasal membranes (such as smog) lower the person's resistance, susceptibility to the virus is increased.

The usual symptoms include sneezing, nasal discharge or congestion, headache, sore throat, general malaise, cough, and sometimes a slight fever. The senses of smell and taste are blunted. This unpleasant condition usually lasts from 5 days to 2 weeks.

Treatment.   The most important treatment for a cold is rest. Rest also keeps the person from infecting others. Rest during a cold is especially important for infants, older adults, and debilitated clients because they are more susceptible to serious complications.

Drinking plenty of fluids is essential to help reduce fever, replace lost fluids, and thin secretions. Remind the client to give strict attention to handwashing and using disposable tissues to prevent spreading the infection to others. The client should blow the nose gently to prevent the infection from spreading into the sinuses, ears, or eustachian tubes. Aspirin, acetaminophen, or ibuprofen helps to relieve discomfort and reduce fever. Some authorities believe that vitamin C is helpful in preventing and treating colds. Clients should use nose drops with discretion. Antibiotics are ineffective against cold viruses. They may, however, be prescribed for people who are immunocompromised, to reduce the risk of developing secondary bacterial infections.

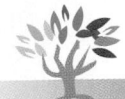

SPECIAL CONSIDERATIONS: THE LIFE SPAN

Use of Salicylates

Never give infants and children aspirin or other salicylates to control fever because of the danger of Reye's syndrome. Use acetaminophen (Tylenol) or ibuprofen.

The person should consult a physician if the fever continues for more than 2 days, if mild analgesics fail to relieve severe headache, and if severe coughing, earache, or chest pain occurs. The client should immediately consult a physician if he or she coughs up dark or bloody sputum. Sometimes, a throat culture is done. Culture can indicate strep throat, but a negative culture for streptococci does not necessarily mean that a strep infection is not present. The person with a chronic respiratory condition, such as asthma, should consult a physician at the first sign of a cold.

If the infection enters the lower respiratory tract, complications such as laryngitis, *bronchitis* (inflammation of the bronchi), and pneumonia can result.

✚👁 Nursing Alert

Usually nurses who have colds may continue working if they feel well. However, it is essential that they follow all principles of infection control, especially handwashing. Some facilities require such nurses to wear masks and to not be assigned to high-risk clients.

Streptococcal Sore Throat

Chapter 71 discusses strep throat in children. In *strep throat,* physical symptoms are more widespread than with ordinary sore throat, with general physical weakness and malaise, high fever, pus on the tonsils, and a headache. Many adults who have recurrent streptococcal throat infections have permanently plugged eustachian tubes; any change in atmospheric pressure is uncomfortable for them. Penicillin is the specific antibiotic prescribed for strep throat unless the person has an allergy or a penicillin-resistant streptococcal infection. The most dangerous complications of strep throat are rheumatic fever and glomerulonephritis (see Chapters 71 and 88).

Influenza

Influenza (commonly called *flu*) is an active contagious respiratory disease caused by one of several strains of filterable viruses: types A, B, C, D, and others. Flu strains may also be described using the name of the place of origin, such as the Hong Kong or Asian flu. Influenza occurs in periodic epidemics, usually due to virus types A and B. Most people recover, but some die from complications such as heart disease, pneumonia, or encephalitis. People may develop parkinsonism many years after having had the flu.

The most dangerous complication of influenza is pneumonia. The person is particularly susceptible to any lung disorder after the flu because of general debility. Other complications are chronic disorders such as bronchitis, *sinusitis* (inflammation of the sinuses; discussed later), and ear infections.

Signs and Symptoms.   The client becomes suddenly very ill, with muscle pains, fever, headache, sensitivity to light, burning eyes, and chills. The person may sneeze, cough, have a nasal discharge, complain of sore throat, feel nauseous, and vomit often. Fever is high (100° to 103° F; 37.8° to 39.4° C) and lasts for 2 to 3 days. Other symptoms, especially the cough, persist longer. A cough may persist for several weeks after the person has had the flu.

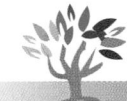

SPECIAL CONSIDERATIONS: THE LIFE SPAN

Complications in Influenza

Infants, older adults, and immunocompromised people are at a much higher risk for developing complications from influenza than other people are.

Treatment and Nursing Considerations.   Give the client large quantities of fluids, including fruit juices and plenty of water. Fluids help the body to flush out wastes created by the virus. (Do not give milk because it tends to form a film in the throat.) Clients may follow a regular diet, although they may be *anorectic* (without appetite). Often, bed rest, as well as mild analgesics to relieve headache, fever, and muscular pains, may be prescribed. Cough syrup may relieve the dry cough; the narcotic contained in some cough preparations (often, codeine) may also assist the client to sleep. Clients should keep warm and avoid exposure to other diseases. Watch for signs of secondary infection, such as chest pains, purulent or rose-colored sputum, a rise in temperature, or an increase in pulse rate.

Prevention.   Encourage individuals at high risk for contracting influenza to be vaccinated yearly in the Fall for protection. Stress the inoculation for older adults, persons with chronic disease, immunosuppressed persons, and healthcare workers. The vaccine is now synthetic, alleviating most side effects seen in the past.

During an outbreak, urge people to stay away from crowds. Sometimes, public gatherings are suspended. People should avoid visiting others in healthcare facilities during this time.

Laryngitis

Laryngitis is an inflammation of the larynx (voice box). It may accompany a respiratory infection or result from overuse of the voice or excessive smoking. The person coughs, is hoarse, and may lose the voice. He or she should avoid talking and smoking, and receive high-humidity inhalations to soothe the throat's mucous membranes. If laryngitis is a complication of another infection, antibiotics may be prescribed. If laryngitis is viral in origin, it is highly contagious; the client should avoid exposing others.

Chronic laryngitis may be a complication of chronic sinusitis or chronic bronchitis or may follow repeated attacks of acute laryngitis. Continued irritation of the throat by public speaking, smoking, or irritating gases may contribute to the problem. People with chronic laryngitis must be carefully examined for signs of cancer, particularly if they smoke cigarettes.

Bronchitis

Bronchitis is an inflammation of the bronchial tubes (bronchi). *Acute bronchitis* often follows a respiratory infection, especially during the Winter months. A dry cough is an early symptom; later, the cough produces mucus and pus. Other symptoms include fever and malaise.

Treatment includes bed rest, a nutritious diet, and plenty of fluids. Humidifiers help by moistening the air, whereas dry air aggravates the cough. Antibiotics are given to treat the infection, and precautions are taken to prevent the infection from spreading. Salicylates are sometimes given.

As in any respiratory disease, instruct the client to cover the mouth when coughing. Dispose of sputum and tissues using Standard Precautions. Acute bronchitis, if untreated, will often develop into *chronic bronchitis*.

Lung Abscess

A *lung abscess* is a localized area of infection in the lung that breaks down and forms pus. It can be caused by a foreign body, or by aspiration of oral fluids or respiratory secretions, and may follow pneumonia. Symptoms include chills and fever, with weight loss and a productive cough with foul, purulent sputum.

Surgery may be required for drainage of the lung abscess. If the cause of the abscess is an aspirated object, bronchoscopy can usually remove the object. Antibiotics usually are an effective treatment, after the cause is eliminated.

Pneumonia

Pneumonia is an inflammation of the lung with consolidation or solidification (Fig. 85-4A). The lung becomes firm as the air sacs are filled with exudate. In past years, one in four persons who had pneumonia died, but modern treatment has greatly reduced the death rate.

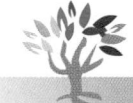

SPECIAL CONSIDERATIONS: THE LIFE SPAN

Pneumonia

Pneumonia accounts for 10% of all hospital admissions in the United States and is often a cause of death in older adults. It often occurs as a complication of another condition.

Pneumonia is classified according to its causative organism. It may be bacterial, viral, fungal, or chemical in origin. It may also be caused by aspiration of fluid or a foreign object into the lungs.

Types

Bacterial Pneumonia.   Persons who are in poor general health or are physically inactive, as well as older people and those with chronic lung disorders, are most susceptible to infectious *bacterial pneumonia*. Persons who abuse substances such as alcohol and cocaine are particularly susceptible.

Pneumococcal pneumonia vaccines are given every 3 to 5 years as a preventive measure, especially for older adults and high-risk populations.

Viral Pneumonia.   A variant of the influenza virus causes *viral pneumonia*. Antibiotics are ineffective; however, they are often used to treat or prevent the secondary infections sometimes seen in viral pneumonia. The person is treated symptomatically. Viral pneumonia is rarely fatal, but it may leave the client in a weakened condition.

Pneumocystis Carinii Pneumonia.   *Pneumocystis carinii* pneumonia (**PCP**) is caused by organisms that are not totally known. Some authorities believe that the causative organism is a protozoan; others blame yeastlike fungi. PCP is most commonly seen as one of the opportunistic diseases in the person with advanced HIV/AIDS infection. PCP is treated with medications such as co-trimoxazole (Bactrim, Septra).

Chemical Pneumonia.   *Chemical pneumonia* is largely associated with aspiration of a chemical substance. Be aware that a person may aspirate into the lungs without any obvious evidence of vomiting. Some people are at an extremely high risk, including the elderly or postoperative clients, clients who abuse substances or are debilitated, and those with swallowing impairments.

Aspiration Pneumonia.   If the person vomits or inhales a foreign object, or substances such as water or large amounts of mucus, the material may be drawn into the lungs. This aspiration not only causes the infectious process, but it can

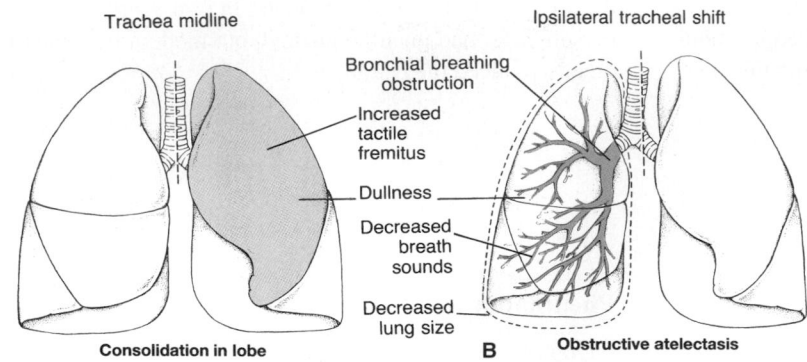

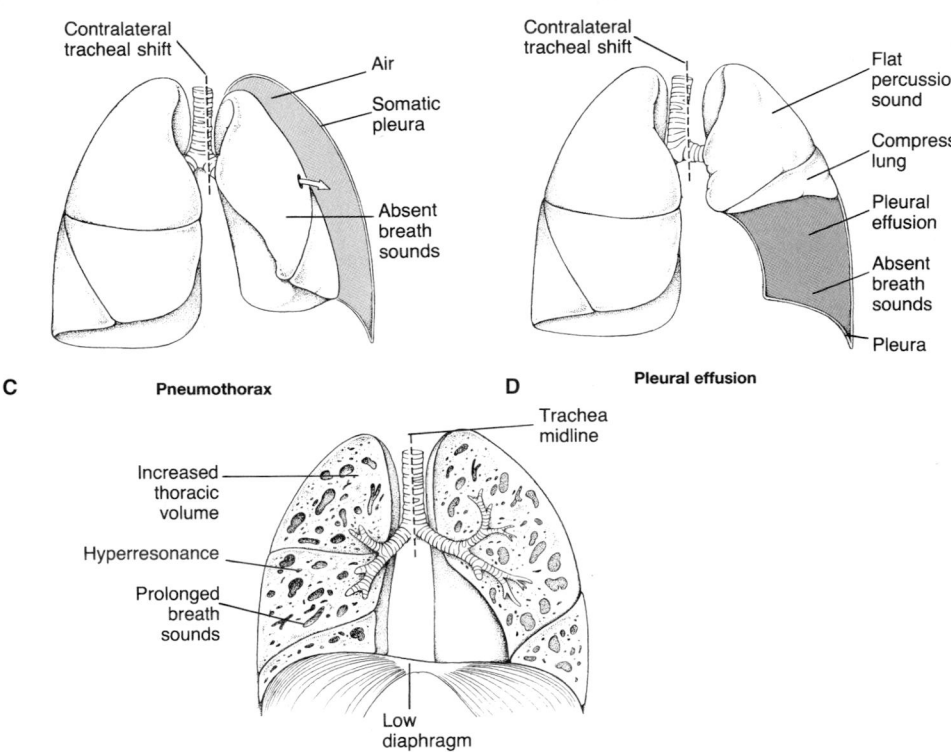

FIGURE 85-4. Respiratory system disorders and their comparative effects on the lungs. (**A**) *Consolidation* within a lobe: trachea in center, dull sound in affected lobe. (**B**) *Obstructive atelectasis:* trachea shifts to affected (ipsilateral) side; decreased lung size, decreased breath sounds. (**C**) *Pneumothorax:* trachea shifts to other (contralateral) side; breath sounds absent on affected side. (**D**) *Pleural effusion or hemothorax* (fluid or blood pooling in pleural cavity): trachea shifts to other side; absent breath sounds in affected lobe; lung compressed. (**E**) *Emphysema:* enlarged (barrel) chest, prolonged breath sounds, *hyperresonance* (echo), trachea in center.

cause additional edema and complications because of the acidity of the gastric contents.

Signs and Symptoms

The onset of pneumonia is characterized by a severe, sharp pain in the chest and chills, followed by fever that may be as high as 105° F or 106° F (40.6° C or 41.1° C). A painful cough, tenacious sputum, and pain on breathing are present. The person's pulse is rapid. Respiration is rapid and expiration is difficult. The individual feels very ill and may be cyanotic. The white blood cell count is high. Mental changes, such as delirium or anxiety, may be present.

Blood cultures and sputum cultures are sent for analysis to determine the causative organism. Sensitivity tests are done to determine which antibiotic is most effective. A CXR will show what part of the lung is affected and to what degree.

Treatment

Treatment focuses on the following:

- Appropriate antibiotic therapy
- Respiratory assessment to measure effectiveness of therapy
- Administration of oxygen
- Adequate fluid intake to ensure hydration
- Small, frequent meals
- Positioning to aid breathing
- Turning, coughing, and deep breathing
- Intake and output records
- Frequent mouth care for comfort

Antibiotics have revolutionized the treatment of pneumonia. They are usually administered IV for rapid action and to maintain a blood level that is effective in eradicating the causative organism. In 24 to 48 hours, the fever usually disappears and the other symptoms improve dramatically.

Nursing Considerations

In Practice: Nursing Care Guidelines 85-4 outlines nursing considerations for the client with pneumonia. Activity is gradually increased as the body convalesces slowly and builds resistance. An CXR is taken to make sure that the infection in the lungs has cleared completely.

Complications

Complications from pneumonia seldom occur today, except in older, debilitated, or immunocompromised clients. If the infection does spread, it also may cause inflammation of the pleura, the middle ear (*otitis media*), sinusitis, or bronchitis.

Pleurisy

Pleurisy, an inflammation of the pleura (the double membrane covering the lungs), can be a complication of pneumonia, caused by a spread of the infection from the lungs. The pleura becomes thickened, and the two membrane surfaces scrape together.

The client feels sharp pain with every breath. Later, as fluid forms, the pain diminishes, and a dry cough replaces it, accompanied by SOB and exhaustion after the slightest effort. (Pleuritic pain may occur with other diseases such as rheumatic fever, systemic lupus erythematosus, and polyarteritis.)

Treatment of pleurisy is similar to that of pneumonia: bed rest and restriction of activity, along with anti-inflammatory agents. Encourage the person to cough, but because coughing may be painful, apply hot or cold packs over the area or have the person lie on the affected side for comfort.

When fluid collection in the pleural space increases, the person is said to have a *pleural effusion* (see Fig. 85-4D). The client may exhibit the same symptoms as pleurisy, but often becomes dyspneic and has a rapid pulse. Pleural effusion can result from congestive heart failure, pulmonary infections (including TB), and malignancies. Treatment relates directly to the underlying cause and may be geared toward specific symptoms.

Histoplasmosis

Histoplasmosis, which mimics "Summer flu" and is often misdiagnosed, is caused by a fungus inhaled in dust from soil rich in the fungus (eg, chicken houses, barns, caves). In the United States, it is most common in the Midwestern states.

Signs and Symptoms. The lungs become inflamed due to invasion by foreign material, which damages the lymph glands and lungs. As a result, scar tissue and calcium deposits may form.

Symptoms are much like those of the flu. Many people are infected with the disease without knowing it because symptoms are so mild. Most people recover after a few weeks. In more severe cases, weight loss and weakness occur, requiring a very long convalescence. In the chronic form, the disease spreads throughout the body, causing weight loss, bleeding, and other severe problems. Occasionally, it is fatal.

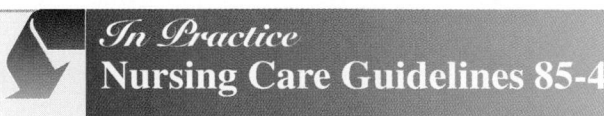

In Practice
Nursing Care Guidelines 85-4

CARING FOR THE PERSON WITH PNEUMONIA

- Always wash your hands and wear gloves, if indicated. *Rationale: Handwashing and gloves help to prevent the spread of infection.*
- Be alert for increasingly labored respirations. *Rationale: If the person has difficulty breathing, he or she is given oxygen, usually by mask or cannula.*
- Adjust the client's position. An orthopneic position may be necessary. *Rationale: Proper positioning helps the person to be more comfortable and to breathe more easily.*
- Place a pillow lengthwise under the back. *Rationale: This action encourages fuller chest expansion.*
- Place a blanket around the shoulders if the person has chills. *Rationale: A blanket provides comfort and warmth, minimizing energy expenditure.*
- Keep the client's bed dry. *Rationale: Wet bed linens can chill the client.*
- Assess the client's vital signs at least every 4 hours. *Rationale: Frequent monitoring is necessary to allow for prompt detection and early intervention if problems arise.*
- Attempt to control fever and discomfort with acetaminophen or ibuprofen, if ordered. Tepid sponges may also be ordered. *Rationale: Fever is often very high and can be dangerous.*
- Maintain the IV site or heparin lock. *Rationale: This client is probably receiving IV antibiotics.*
- Put side rails up if any sign of confusion exists, especially in the older person. *Rationale: The high fever, medications, and disease process may contribute to confusion and lead to injury.*
- Encourage the client to cough and to expectorate secretions while splinting the chest. *Rationale: Keep the lungs as free of secretions as possible. Splinting the chest helps to relieve the discomfort of coughing.*
- Encourage deep breathing. Aerosolized treatments or incentive spirometry may be prescribed. *Rationale: The lungs must be expanded as much as possible.*
- Measure intake and output and daily weights, if ordered. *Rationale: Some clients may have edema. Others will need total parenteral nutrition (TPN) to maintain hydration and nutrition.*
- Give small amounts of fluids frequently. *Rationale: Fluids help to encourage hydration.*
- Provide frequent mouth care; put water-soluble lubricant (not oily) on the client's lips. *Rationale: A fever causes the mucous membranes to be very dry; this person also has probably been breathing through the mouth. Oil might be aspirated and is not used with oxygen.*
- Keep the client's surroundings quiet. *Rationale: Rest promotes healing.*

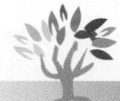

SPECIAL CONSIDERATIONS: THE LIFE SPAN

Histoplasmosis

Very young children and older men are most likely to contract histoplasmosis, and they are especially susceptible to the form that spreads from the lungs to other body parts.

The fungus may be identified by isolation in culture, and occasionally, both sputum and urine must be cultured. A skin test, administered intradermally, can indicate the presence of the fungus.

Treatment.   In the disease's mild form, treatment is similar to that for the flu. Usually, symptoms clear by themselves. In more severe cases, amphotericin B (Fungizone) or another antifungal medication is given IV for several weeks.

Tuberculosis

Tuberculosis (TB), an infectious disease, is caused by the tubercle bacillus, *Mycobacterium tuberculosis*. This organism encases itself in a waxy coating (*spore*) that makes its destruction difficult. Many people have tubercle bacilli in their bodies but do not actually have active TB. TB develops when poor nutrition, stress, or lack of rest lowers the person's resistance. The organisms multiply and become active. Arresting the disease to the point where it is not infectious and remains inactive is possible.

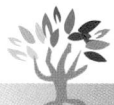

SPECIAL CONSIDERATIONS: THE LIFE SPAN

Tuberculosis

The initial treatment of tuberculosis in children and pregnant women will be with INH alone for 6 to 9 months. Sputum cultures must be followed up closely.

Tuberculosis spreads by inhalation of infected droplets that a person with an active infection releases into the air. Physical contact with an infected person and contact with contaminated utensils or equipment can spread TB. Unpasteurized milk from an infected cow can spread the disease (called *bovine TB*).

The tubercle bacilli most frequently attack the lungs, but the blood can carry the organisms to other body parts, including the kidneys and the bones.

Cases of TB are increasing. Worldwide, more people die of TB than any other single infectious disease. The following conditions increase the risk for TB infection:

- HIV positive
- Chronic renal failure
- Advanced age
- Immunosuppression from steroids or cancers
- Diabetes

- Unclean living conditions, or crowded living conditions with one or more occupants having TB
- Homelessness
- Poor diet
- Immigrants from certain parts of the world

☞ KEY CONCEPT

The number of cases of TB has increased dramatically over the last several years because of the large number of persons with HIV infection who are susceptible to and infected with TB. Another factor is the continued immigration of infected persons, especially from Southeast Asia, Africa, and Latin America.

Types

Pulmonary Tuberculosis.   When the bacillus enters the lungs, it precipitates an infection called *pulmonary TB*. It may be so mild that it produces no symptoms, in which case the infection clears and the person is unaware that he or she was infected. However, the tuberculin test is positive and a CXR will reveal a small scar, a sign that at some time the bacillus was active. The scar is the result of efforts of the white blood cells to surround and destroy the bacilli. The bacilli are then encased in a lump called a *tubercle*. The tubercle (known as the *primary lesion* or *primary TB*) may remain inactive for life. However, if the person's resistance is lowered, the capsule enclosing the tubercle breaks down, and the bacilli spread and cause active illness.

Pott's Disease and Miliary Tuberculosis.   Tuberculosis of bones and joints is another form. Should the bloodstream carry bacilli to the spine, the resulting disease is called *Pott's disease*. The vertebrae collapse and there is pronounced spinal curvature (*kyphosis* or *humpback*). This disease rarely occurs in the United States today. Seeding by the bloodstream may carry the bacilli to other bones and joints, especially the hips and the knees. If disease spreads throughout the body, it is called *miliary TB*.

Infection may spread to the oviducts, ovaries, and uterus; surgical removal of the diseased organ may be required. The gastrointestinal tract, the kidneys, and the meninges are other possible sites.

Atypical Tuberculosis.   *Atypical TB* is often spread to individuals who are immunosuppressed. It is a classification of TB that is becoming more common because of the increased numbers of persons infected with HIV and their increased susceptibility to TB. It may also occur in the person undergoing chemotherapy or radiation treatment for cancer. Atypical TB is highly resistant to treatment.

Drug-Resistant Tuberculosis.   *Drug-resistant TB* is on the rise. In a small percentage of cases, the treatment regimen does not successfully eliminate the TB. This may be due to the client's non-compliance with the medication program, the medication may not be absorbed properly, or the individual may have contracted TB from a person with drug-resistant TB. This type is very difficult to treat. The individual will remain on different medications for a much longer period of time.

Signs and Symptoms and Diagnosis

Tuberculosis usually develops slowly. Signs and symptoms of pulmonary TB include:

- Cough
- Lack of pain (presence of pain may indicate extension to the pleura)
- Thick sputum (possibly blood streaked)
- Expectoration of blood (indicating pleural hemorrhage)
- Positive or negative sputum culture
- Fatigue
- Gradual weight loss (may lead to emaciation, if not treated)
- Low-grade fever, especially in the afternoon
- *Nocturnal diaphoresis* (profuse sweating at night)
- Severe chest pains, persistent cough, and dyspnea as disease progresses

The tuberculin skin test may indicate the presence of the tubercle bacillus in the body, but not necessarily that the person has active TB. In conjunction with preliminary tuberculin tests, CXR and positive sputum cultures for the tubercle bacillus are the most reliable means of detecting pulmonary TB. Only 10% of those who have been infected will actually develop TB.

Treatment

Medication therapy is the specific treatment for active TB, regardless of the organ involved. The goal of medication therapy is to arrest the growth of the bacillus so that natural body defenses (leukocytes and antibodies) can take over and eliminate the disease. In Practice: Important Medications highlights the medications that are used to treat TB.

TB infection is usually treated with isoniazid (**INH**) alone because it is quite effective. INH has few toxic effects, although in rare instances it has been known to cause anemia, neutropenia, gastrointestinal distress, and hepatitis. In combination with other medications, INH is prescribed in almost all cases of TB disease. Rifampin is highly effective in the treatment of TB as well; however, it is more toxic than INH and much more expensive. Ethambutol is usually given with INH and has low toxicity. Vitamin B6 is commonly given with INH in the treatment of TB to prevent peripheral neuropathy.

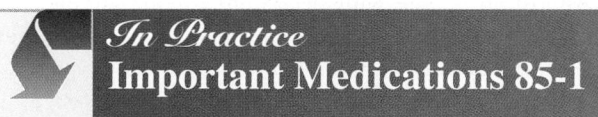

In Practice
Important Medications 85-1

DRUGS OF CHOICE FOR TUBERCULOSIS

isoniazid/INH (Nydrazid, Laniazid)
ethambutol (Myambutol)
pyrazinamide/PZA (PMS Pyrazinamide, Tebrazid, Zinamide)
rifampin (Rimactane, Rifadin)
streptomycin

The regimen for medication administration is important and must be followed faithfully. It may be necessary to treat the client with two to four medications for a period of 6 to 12 months. Treatment time may be longer for immunosuppressed individuals, possibly taking up to 2 years for those with drug-resistant TB.

Surgical procedures include *total* **pneumonectomy** (removal of an entire lung), *partial pneumonectomy* (removal of the affected part of a lung), **lobectomy** (removal of a lobe of a lung), and *wedge resection* or *segmental resection* (removal of one or more bronchopulmonary segments). Because effective medications are now available, surgery is rarely necessary.

Nursing Considerations

Tuberculosis is a long-term illness. Nursing care consists of several elements:

- Careful administration of medications. Following a time schedule is important to maintain a constant blood level of the medications. Give medications at the same time each day, if a daily dose, or spread doses throughout the day. (If b.i.d., instruct the person to take every 12 hours; if t.i.d., take every 8 hours; if q.i.d., take every 6 hours, rather than four times during waking hours, for example.)
- Teaching the client about the importance of continuing medications, even if symptoms seem to have subsided
- A well-balanced diet, high in protein and vitamins A and C
- Prevention of spread of the disease, with careful handwashing, and use of personal protective equipment
- Transmission-based precautions, if disease is active
- Plenty of rest
- Smoke-free environment
- Diversionary activities

Prevention

Nurses can take an active part in community health by seeking ways to prevent TB. The following are some suggestions:

- Educate the public in good, general health practices.
- In home care, burn all used tissues (the TB bacillus can survive for months in dried sputum). If unable to burn tissues, follow community guidelines for the disposal of biohazardous waste.
- Trace active cases and start early treatment of contacts to stop further spread of the disease.
- Follow up with all persons who have had active TB. Regular examination is necessary for life to determine if there is a recurrence and to treat it immediately.
- Screen members of high-risk groups such as immigrants from Southeast Asia, Africa, or Latin America and medically underserved persons of low-income populations.
- Give long-term residents of nursing homes, mental institutions, and correctional facilities the PPD tuberculin test on admission and at intervals thereafter.
- Screen healthcare workers yearly.

The American Society of Thoracic Physicians believes that prophylactic medication treatment (long-term administration of antituberculosis medications) should be recommended for the following individuals:

- Household members and other close contacts of the person with recently diagnosed TB
- Persons with positive tuberculin tests who have CXR findings indicative of TB
- Newly infected persons
- Persons with positive TB tests who have been on steroids, have received immunosuppressant medications, and have hematologic diseases, silicosis, or diabetes mellitus
- Others who have positive reactions, such as infants, teens, and elderly people
- Persons who are immunosuppressed as a result of HIV or AIDS

Vaccine.   A live TB vaccine, known as bacille Calmette-Guerin (**BCG**), is available. It is a weakened strain of the bacterium. This should be used prophylactically on TB-negative persons who are repeatedly exposed to people with untreated or ineffectively treated TB. It can also be given to those in groups with repeatedly high rates of new TB infections.

Empyema

Empyema, sometimes called *pyothorax,* is a collection of *purulent* (pus-containing) exudate in the pleural cavity. It can be acute or chronic.

Acute Empyema

Acute empyema is a secondary infection that may follow TB, lung abscess, or pneumonia. It may also result from an infection of the chest wall or other surrounding tissue or may be introduced directly by a chest wound or surgery. Because it is almost always a secondary infection, empyema is difficult to diagnose. The primary problem usually masks symptoms.

Symptoms of empyema include chest pain (usually on one side), cough, fever, dyspnea, and general malaise. If empyema is suspected, more decisive information can be obtained by CXR and thoracentesis. The offending organism can also be determined by a C&S test on fluid aspirated by thoracentesis.

Antibiotics to combat the infection and measures to drain the empyema cavity are started. The latter may be done by closed drainage or by thoracentesis, in which case an antibiotic may be injected directly into the pleural cavity. Bed rest and sedative cough preparations are also given. If this is not successful, open drainage is done.

Chronic Empyema

Chronic empyema may be a complication of acute empyema or may be caused by bronchopleural fistula, osteomyelitis of the rib cage, or an aspirated foreign body. It may also be a complication of TB or a fungal infection of the lungs.

Soft rubber drainage tubes are inserted in the wound, and large, absorbent dressings and pads are applied. Usually the drainage is profuse at first, so the dressings must be changed frequently. In open drainage, usually a rib is removed, causing some pain.

CHRONIC RESPIRATORY DISORDERS

Snoring

Snoring (or *stertorous breathing*) is a respiratory disorder that is common in some people when they sleep. Not usually a serious problem, snoring is considered a pathologic condition if the person cannot stop snoring, no matter what sleeping position he or she uses; if others can hear the snoring two or three rooms away; or if another person has to leave the room to be able to sleep. In extreme cases, surgery may be done. A procedure called *palatopharyngoplasty,* which removes extra material from the upper throat, has been successful in some cases. A relatively new, inexpensive external device (a tape strip) can be applied to the nasal bridge to help open the nasal passages. Other remedies include: elevating the head of the bed; using a special pillow; sewing an object such as a ball on the back of the pajamas (so the person does not sleep on the back); avoiding heavy evening meals, smoking, sleeping pills, or alcohol; losing weight; and using decongestants.

Sleep Apnea Syndrome

Sleep apnea syndrome causes the person to wake up many times during the night. It is most common in middle-aged, overweight men. The formal definition of sleep apnea is more than five cessations of airflow for at least 10 seconds each per hour of sleep. It is believed to occur because soft tissues at the back of the throat fall back and occlude the airway. This airway occlusion can last as long as 90 seconds. The person suddenly awakens due to lack of oxygen. Hundreds of episodes can occur during a single night.

Diagnosis is based on symptoms and history including:

- Extreme tiredness all day
- Difficulty in concentration
- Memory loss
- Inability to perform one's job
- Falling asleep during the day
- Episodes witnessed by sleeping partner

Almost all people with sleep apnea snore, although the reverse is not necessarily true. The person is at risk for auto or industrial accidents; high blood pressure with related disorder; or social and employment problems.

Treatment.   Recommended treatment includes:

- Weight reduction
- Smoking cessation
- Avoidance of alcohol, especially before bedtime
- Elevation of the head of the bed
- Use of continuous positive airway pressure (**CPAP**) oxygenation (Box 85-2)

Possible surgery (*uvulopalatopharyngoplasty*) can now be done with lasers. Only about half of the people who have this

BOX 85-2

CONTINUOUS POSITIVE AIRWAY PRESSURE (CPAP) OXYGENATION

The continuous positive airway pressure (**CPAP**) apparatus is commonly used to assist persons with sleep apnea. This machine looks like an oxygen-delivery system and is used at night, so the person can sleep. It delivers air, and sometimes oxygen, to the person at a continuous positive pressure that holds the alveoli open. (They usually close at the end of expiration.) This positive pressure prevents respiratory obstruction, increases oxygenation, and reduces breathing effort.

procedure done find significant improvement, however. Respiratory stimulant medications have not proven helpful. In severe cases, tracheostomy (which is plugged during the day) may be required to bypass upper airway obstruction.

Allergic Rhinitis

Rhinitis is an inflammation of the nasal mucous passages. **Allergic rhinitis** ("hay fever") is a condition that occurs when inflammation results from an allergic reaction to a protein substance. It may be due to pollen from weeds, flowers, or grasses at certain seasons, or it may be a reaction to dust, feathers, or animal dander. People with a family history of allergy are more susceptible to hay fever, as are those who have asthma or eczema. At least 10% of the U.S. population has a hereditary tendency. Persons of all ages are affected; hay fever may appear suddenly at any age and may just as suddenly disappear.

Signs and Symptoms.   Allergic rhinitis is disagreeable and inconvenient. Symptoms include edema, an itchy nose, excessive sneezing, and profuse, watery discharge from the nose and eyes. The condition worsens on windy days and in the mornings and evenings. Determining the cause is difficult, and detailed questioning and many skin tests may be needed to identify the offending substance. Sometimes several substances are the offenders. Chapter 83 discusses allergies and describes and illustrates allergy tests in more detail.

Treatment.   The first step in treatment is to avoid the offending substance. It may mean eliminating a food from the diet, avoiding contact with animals, or avoiding dusty places. Air conditioning or filtering or purifying air can also help. Antihistamines relieve symptoms, and desensitization injections may eliminate them entirely. Corticosteroids may be given for severe attacks. An untreated allergy of this kind may lead to asthma, sinusitis, or nasal polyps.

Pneumoconioses

Pneumoconioses are "dust diseases" caused by habitual inhalation and retention in the lungs of certain heavy, harmful dusts. The most common disease is *silicosis,* common in miners, which is caused by breathing silica, or quartz dust. *Asbestosis*

is another common form. As the person inhales dangerous dusts, the dusts eventually slow down or stop the ciliary action in the nose and lungs, and the dusts accumulate there. The dusts can cause irritation or allergic and chemical reactions.

Usually the first symptom of dust diseases is dyspnea. Later, the person develops a chronic cough and expectorates the offending particles in thick mucus. Chest pains are often a later result. Serious complications include TB, pneumonia, chronic bronchitis, and emphysema. Vast evidence now indicates that the presence of asbestos directly relates to a specific lung cancer (*mesothelioma*).

Treatment focuses on prevention because these diseases are difficult to treat after extensive areas of the lungs are involved. The only treatment at present is to reduce exposure to the dust. Damage previously done cannot be reversed.

Chronic Obstructive Pulmonary Disease

Chronic obstructive pulmonary disease (**COPD**), also called *chronic obstructive lung disease* (**COLD**), is a broad classification of disorders that includes bronchial asthma, bronchiectasis (discussed later), chronic bronchitis, and pulmonary emphysema (discussed later). COPD is irreversible and is associated with persistent dyspnea on exertion and reduced airflow of less than one half of normal. It affects 25% of the adult population and is the fifth most common cause of death in the United States.

Care of the client with COPD involves physical, psychological, and environmental measures. The goals of treatment are to improve ventilation and to overcome hypoxic states through the following measures:

- Avoidance of irritants: smoking, allergens, industrial chemicals
- Use of medications: bronchodilators, expectorants, liquefying agents
- Postural drainage
- Increased fluid intake (1000–2000 mL/d)
- Cautious use of oxygen
- Breathing exercises
- Activity as tolerated
- Avoidance of extremes of heat and cold
- Positioning to facilitate breathing (Fowler's or orthopneic)
- Small, frequent meals

Fluid intake is important. Encourage the client to drink at least 2 to 3 quarts daily to thin mucus and make it easier to expectorate.

Oxygen must be administered with caution. The amount should not exceed 3 liters per minute, because many people with COPD retain carbon dioxide. Too high a level of oxygen could suppress their respiratory drive.

Breathing exercises, combined with other respiratory treatments, increase the volume of air that the person is able to exhale. Inhaling and holding the breath also improves breathing. Practicing pursed-lip breathing, especially during periods of dyspnea, is effective. *Rationale: This technique forces air into the lungs.* Avoid rapid or forceful exhalation because it may cause the terminal bronchioles to collapse. The person must be faithful in consistently carrying out breathing exercises.

Advise the person to keep active, but to pace activity with rest before and after. *Rationale: Give the client support and direction to enable him or her to accept the fact that therapy is a lifelong commitment.* Teach the client to limit activities to whatever the heart and breathing capacities can tolerate. The individual has the potential to lead a fairly active life if he or she chooses.

Persons with COPD have special needs because of the chronic nature of the disease. Help these individuals to live optimally through the following measures:

- Assist with developing energy-conserving measures in daily living.
- Teach relaxation techniques to use in situations of respiratory distress.
- Teach management of acute exacerbations of the disease and when to call for help.
- Help to identify situations or other factors that "trigger" symptoms, and assist to find ways to modify or remove these triggers.

If the client is having difficulty with one or more aspects of managing COPD, a pulmonary rehabilitation program may be helpful. This is a program that includes medical management, breathing retraining, emotional support, exercise, nutritional information, and education about living with this disease. A multidisciplinary team of pulmonary experts works with the client to optimize quality of life.

Bronchial Asthma

Asthma is a chronic condition characterized by inflammation of the lining of the bronchial airways. Cells that line the bronchi release chemicals that cause inflammation when they are stimulated by irritants and allergens. When the airway is inflamed, swollen, and narrowed, it becomes more sensitive to things that may trigger an asthma attack. Obstruction of the airway is further complicated by tightening and narrowing of the surrounding muscles (*bronchospasms*). In some cases, mucous glands in the airways secrete thick mucus, which further obstructs the airways.

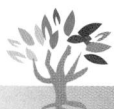 SPECIAL CONSIDERATIONS: THE LIFE SPAN

Asthma

The pregnant women must take her medications faithfully and follow her asthma action plan. If her asthma is not under control, she is not getting enough oxygen to her lungs, or to the baby's lungs.

The cause of asthma is unknown, but it does appear to be familial. Seventeen million people in the United States have asthma; 10% of those are children. As with any chronic dis-

ease, there is an emotional component. An asthma attack is a frightening experience for the person struggling to get air into the lungs. Chapter 71 briefly describes asthma in children. It is the most common chronic disease in childhood.

Signs and Symptoms. Onset of an asthma attack is sudden. The person experiences coughing, wheezing, SOB, and chest tightness. The individual may be very pale and dyspneic, especially on expiration. As the attack subsides, the person may cough up thick, white mucus.

Asthma attacks may be occasional or frequent, but the individual is often symptom free between episodes. Poorly managed asthma with frequent attacks may lead to emphysema. Those who have hay fever or chronic bronchitis are especially susceptible. Asthma can occur at any age and at any time. Chronic, severe respiratory conditions may lead to the clubbing of fingers (Figure 85-5).

Children with asthma usually have fewer symptoms as they grow older, but symptoms for asthmatic adults grow worse with age. Sudden change in temperature, extreme physical exertion, contact with animal dander, overeating, emotional stress, and exposure to antigens may trigger attacks.

An attack that persists for more than 24 hours and that does not respond to treatment is called *status asthmaticus,* a medical emergency that can lead to death. Worldwide, there are about 100,000 deaths from asthma each year.

Treatment. The main treatment objective in an acute attack is to relieve breathing difficulties. In the long term, it is important to assist the client in proper medical management of asthma to improve overall quality of life. This strategy will include the use of several classifications of medications (see In Practice: Important Medications 85-2). All people with moderate to severe asthma should be taking anti-inflammatory inhalers as front-line therapy. The inhaled steroids improve lung function, decrease inflammation, and decrease asthma symptoms and flare-ups (attacks).

Goals include decreasing symptoms and complications, improving physical conditioning and emotional well-being, and encouraging self-management (which will reduce hospitalizations). These goals can be accomplished by the introduction of an action plan (or crisis intervention plan) that assists the client in the determination of how to best manage his or her

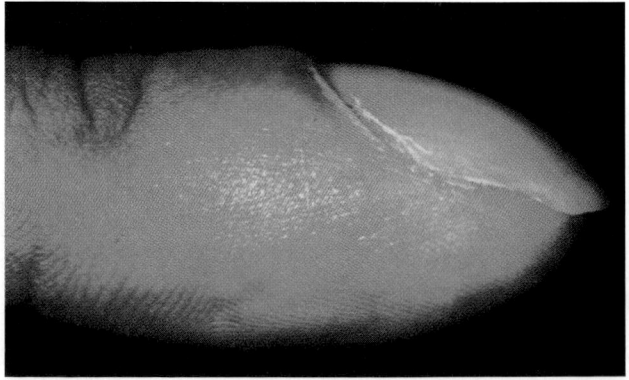

FIGURE 85-5. Clubbing of the finger. Normally, there is an obtuse angle of about 160° between the base of the nail and the adjacent dorsal surface of the finger; with clubbing, this angle exceeds 180°.

➤ *In Practice*
Important Medications 85-2

MEDICATIONS USED FOR TREATING ASTHMA

Anticholinergics
These bronchodilators work on the nervous system to control airway size:

atropine methylnitrate
ipratropium bromide (Atrovent)

Beta-Agonists
These medications dilate bronchial airways by working on the nervous system that controls the muscle tissue around the airway:

albuterol (Asmavent, Proventil, Ventolin, Volmax)
bitolterol mesylate (Tornalate)
epinephrine (Adrenalin, AsthmaNefrin, Epifrin, microNefrin, Sus-Phrine)
levalbuterol HCL (Xopenex)
metaproterenol sulfate (Alupent)
pirbuterol acetate (Maxair Inhaler)
salmeterol xinaforte (Serevent)
terbutaline sulfate (Brethine, Bricanyl)

Corticosteroids
These act as anti-inflammatory agents:

beclomethasone (Vanceril, Beclovent, Beconase)
budesonide (Pulmicort, Rhinocort)
flunisolide (AeroBid, Nasalide)
fluticasone propionate (Flovent, Flonase)
methylprednisone (Medrol)

nedocromil (Tilade)
prednisone (Meticorten, Orasone, Deltasone)
triamcinolone (Azmacort)

Leukotriene Antagonists
These medications block the inflammatory biochemical pathway, making the airway less sensitive to asthma triggers:

montelukast sodium (Singulair)
zafirlukast (Accolate)
zileuton (Zyflo)

Methylxanthines
These bronchodilators relax the smooth muscle of the bronchials:

aminophylline/theophylline ethylenediamine (Truphylline)
theophylline (Theo-Dur, Theovent, Slo-Phyllin, Uni-Dur, Uniphyl)

Mast Cell Stabilizers
These agents inhibit the allergen-triggered release of histamine and slow-releasing substance of anaphylaxis (leukotriene) from the mast cells:

cromolyn sodium (Intal, Nasalcrom)

---

asthma. Education, with full understanding noted by the client and family, is essential. Teaching must include:

- Use of routine (maintenance) medications and emergency (rescue) medications
- Use of a peak flow meter, a small piece of equipment used to determine lung function by showing how fast a person can exhale after deep inhalation
- When to call the physician
- When to go to the hospital for emergency care.

Many people with asthma have the condition well controlled.

Nursing Considerations.   Asthma can be frustrating and frightening. Be calm and supportive and promptly administer the prescribed medications during an attack. Chapter 63 gives guidelines for the use of inhalers. Subjects for client and family teaching are highlighted at In Practice: Educating the Client 85-1.

Bronchiectasis
Bronchiectasis is a chronic dilation of the bronchi in which the walls become permanently distended. The main cause is infection following TB, influenza, pneumonia, chronic sinusitis, upper respiratory infection, measles, or aspiration of a foreign body. Often bronchiectasis begins in early adulthood and progresses slowly over a long period. In a child, it may be a complication of cystic fibrosis and immunodeficiency diseases. It is rarely fatal but may have serious complications. It is usually chronic; the client must modify his or her lifestyle.

Signs and Symptoms.   The characteristic symptom is a chronic cough, most often occurring when the client arises in the morning. The cough produces greenish-yellow sputum with a foul odor. As the disease progresses, the amount of sputum increases. Sometimes the person coughs up blood. In fact, bronchiectasis is the most common cause of *hemoptysis* (bloody sputum). The person loses weight because of poor appetite and may experience chronic fatigue.

Treatment.   Drainage of the purulent material is part of the treatment. Drainage is accomplished by postural drainage, in which the head is lower than the chest (see Fig. 85-2). Encourage the person to cough and breathe deeply. Humidification of air is recommended to help thin secretions and make expectoration easier. Expectorant cough medicines may be prescribed. Give ordered antibiotics to control the infection.

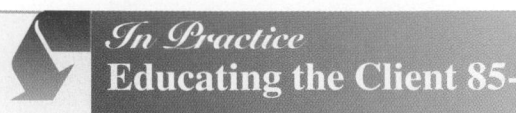

In Practice
Educating the Client 85-1

ASTHMA

- Have an action plan for asthma management.
- Know what medications you are using.
- Use the peak flow meter to determine how your lungs are functioning.
- Know your values for your personal best lung function and when you are at 50% to 80% of your personal best.
- Check with your primary healthcare provider about situations in which you should start adding or changing medications, notify the provider, or seek emergency care.
- Know what triggers your asthma, and take steps to identify and avoid things that may trigger an asthma attack.
- Rinse your mouth with water after using a steroid inhaler to help prevent fungal infections of the mouth.
- Rinse your inhaler mouthpiece daily.
- Use your inhaler properly as shown. Inhalers are not helpful if used incorrectly.
- Take your medications on time. Using medications regularly helps to prevent difficulties and complications.

Good nutrition, fresh air, and rest are also important. The person should not smoke. Give special mouth care to overcome the offensive taste and breath odor and to make food more palatable.

Prompt attention to such conditions as bronchial asthma and bronchitis helps to prevent bronchiectasis. Surgical intervention may be necessary for individuals who continue to have bouts of pneumonia after treatment. Because bronchiectasis can be prevented, it is seen less frequently than in the past. Teaching is summarized at In Practice: Educating the Client 85-2.

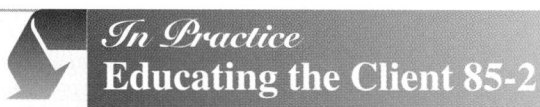

In Practice
Educating the Client 85-2

PREVENTION OF BRONCHIECTASIS

- Have children vaccinated against whooping cough (pertussis) and measles.
- Be sure any adults are vaccinated against influenza.
- Maintain general health at optimum level.
- Seek prompt attention if a foreign object or fluid is aspirated into the lungs, or if a respiratory infection develops.

Chronic Bronchitis

Chronic bronchitis is more serious than acute bronchitis. It often develops so gradually that the person disregards its most significant symptom, a chronic cough. Consequently, the disease is firmly established before the person decides that treatment is needed. Chronic bronchitis is a form of COPD. It usually leads to pulmonary emphysema. Repeated attacks of acute bronchitis may lead to a chronic condition, or it may develop after an acute respiratory infection such as influenza or pneumonia.

Cigarette smoking is one of the most common causes of bronchial irritation; air pollution may also be responsible. People exposed to irritating dusts or chemicals seem to be more likely to develop bronchitis. It affects people of all ages but is most common in persons over age 40 (tendency to postpone treatment over many years could be one reason for this).

Signs and Symptoms.   Chronic bronchitis begins with a dry cough (also known as "smoker's cough") that is most severe when the person rises in the morning. As time goes on, the person coughs up mucus and pus, sometimes with streaks of blood. SOB becomes apparent with exertion. As the disease progresses, it persists even when the individual is quiet. The client's history of a cough, as well as his or her living habits, helps the physician in making a diagnosis. CXR, fluoroscopic examinations, and sputum tests also aid in diagnosis. Table 85-2 lists characteristics of chronic bronchitis and emphysema.

Treatment.   Treatment is slow and continuous; no medication will work a miracle cure. However, treatment reduces symptoms and helps prevent complications. Untreated, the disease may progress until the bronchioles of the lungs are permanently damaged, or it may lead to asthma, emphysema, or heart failure.

Aerosolized treatments, postural drainage, and chest percussion are done. These treatments help to facilitate secretion removal. Build up the person's general health and remind the client to use precautions to avoid exposure to infections. The individual should have plenty of rest and be free from emotional stress. Assist the client with measures to help avoid situations of excessive dust or other factors that aggravate the bronchitis. The client must avoid cigarette smoking. Antibiotics will help to clear coexisting respiratory infections that complicate the condition.

Pulmonary Emphysema

Pulmonary emphysema is abnormal, permanent enlargement of the alveoli and alveolar ducts with destruction of the alveolar walls, which results in lack of elasticity (see Fig. 85-4E and Table 85-2). It is a form of COPD.

In emphysema, air that is normally exchanged becomes trapped in the alveoli. The client is unable to exhale, the lungs become distended, and the muscles suffer from lack of oxygen, becoming less elastic. The condition worsens as more and more air becomes trapped in the alveoli. As a result, the heart must work harder to pump blood through the body and get oxygen to the muscles and other body tissues. The end result of emphysema is often congestive heart failure or right heart failure.

■■■ **TABLE 85-2** $\mathcal{C}$HARACTERISTICS OF CHRONIC BRONCHITIS AND EMPHYSEMATOUS TYPES OF CHRONIC OBSTRUCTIVE LUNG DISEASE

Characteristic	Type A Pulmonary Emphysema ("Pink Puffers")	Type B Chronic Bronchitis ("Blue Bloaters")
Smoking history	Usually	Usually
Age of onset	40 to 50 years of age	30 to 40 years of age; disability in middle age
Clinical features		
Barrel chest (hyperinflation of the lungs)	Often dramatic	May be present
Weight loss	May be severe in advanced disease	Infrequent
Shortness of breath	May be absent early in disease	Predominant early symptoms, insidious in onset, exertional
Decreased breath sounds	Characteristic	Variable
Wheezing	Usually absent	Variable
Rhonchi	Usually absent or minimal	Often prominent
Sputum	May be absent or may develop late in the course	Frequent early manifestation, frequent infections, abundant purulent sputum
Cyanosis	Often absent, event late in the disease when there is slow PaO_2	Often dramatic
Blood gases	Relatively normal until late in the disease process	Hypercapnia may be present Hypoxemia may be present
Cor pulmonale	Only in advanced cases	Frequent Peripheral edema
Polycythemia	Only in advanced cases	Frequent
Prognosis	Slowly debilitating disease	Numerous life-threatening episodes due to acute exacerbations

Authorities believe that chronic bronchitis is the direct cause of chronic pulmonary emphysema, although it may also follow chronic bronchial asthma, TB, and bronchiectasis. The number of cases of emphysema relates directly to cigarette smoking. Evidence also indicates that some families carry a deficiency of a substance (α_1-antitrypsin) that protects the lung tissue during respiratory tract infections. Members of these families are prone to emphysema.

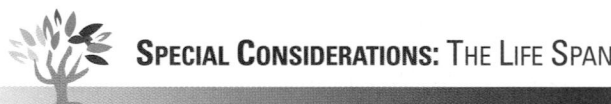 **SPECIAL CONSIDERATIONS:** THE LIFE SPAN

Emphysema

Emphysema may occur in older people simply because lungs lose their elasticity during the aging process.

Some less common types of emphysema include *hypoplastic emphysema* (a developmental defect in which the person has fewer, abnormally large alveoli), *interlobular emphysema* (accumulation of air between the lobules of the lungs), and *interstitial emphysema* (escape of air from the alveoli, caused by chest trauma or bronchiolar obstruction).

Congenital or infantile *lobar emphysema* causes respiratory distress in infants and is characterized by lung overinflation. Another type of emphysema that occurs in young adulthood is caused by the congenital deficiency of α_1-antitrypsin, a plasma protein.

Signs and Symptoms. The first symptom of emphysema is difficulty in breathing after exertion. As the condition progresses, the person has persistent difficulty in breathing. Other symptoms include wheezing and a chronic cough. The person is pale and drawn and is afraid of choking. Many individuals use abdominal muscles as well as other accessory muscles to aid in breathing. The person is afraid to lie down, so he or she sits up, leaning forward and contracting the neck muscles with every breath. The person also raises the shoulder girdle and shows retraction above the clavicles when breathing. The chest becomes barrel shaped, and the individual looks anxious. In the advanced stages, as carbon dioxide accumulates in the blood, the person becomes listless and drowsy. The disease runs its course over a period of many years.

Prevention. Preventive treatment is most important to correct the conditions that cause emphysema, because changes in lung tissue or the blood vessels of the lungs are irreversible. This means, for one thing, alerting the public to the danger signs, such as "morning cough" or "smoker's cough."

☛ KEY CONCEPT

Cigarette smoking causes or predisposes individuals to many diseases of the respiratory system and other systems. It is the single most common cause of disease in the United States today.

Adult Respiratory Distress Syndrome

Adult respiratory distress syndrome (**ARDS**) is also called *noncardiogenic pulmonary edema.* ARDS is a state of progressive oxygen deprivation following a serious illness or injury. Causes include aspiration, medication overdose, cardiac surgery (especially bypass), pancreatitis, end-stage renal disease, embolism, major surgery, and trauma. The person is in acute respiratory failure and usually requires mechanical ventilation and blood pressure medications. If the cause can be determined, it can be treated. However, the mortality rate is greater than 50%.

TRAUMA

An accident may cause respiratory problems or death. If there is no air exchange in the lungs, the person will die within a matter of minutes.

Absence of Air Exchange

Asphyxiation is the condition in which the blood lacks oxygen and the blood and tissues contain excess carbon dioxide. Any form of **suffocation,** or stoppage of breathing, can cause asphyxiation. Suffocation may result from externally applied pressure to the throat (*strangulation*), drowning (*aspiration*), electric shock, or gases (such as carbon monoxide or gases in smoke from a house fire) that enter the lungs and prevent the exchange of oxygen and carbon dioxide. Choking on a foreign object that plugs the airway, or covering the nose and mouth with an object (such as a pillow or plastic bag) can also cause suffocation.

Strangulation refers to respiratory arrest due to an obstruction of the air passage. Most commonly, this term applies to trauma caused by another person, hanging, or an accident.

Chest Trauma

Asphyxiation can result from a sudden blow to the chest. It may cause pneumothorax or airway blockage. Accumulation of blood in the lungs can cause asphyxiation by drowning.

A puncture wound to the chest from a knife or a bullet is an emergency. If a foreign object is in place, do not remove it. Get emergency assistance immediately. *Rationale: The object may plug the hole and maintain the negative pressure within the lungs until help arrives.*

If an object, such as a bullet, has caused an open hole in the chest wall, plug the hole immediately. *Rationale: If the hole is left open, the lungs will collapse because the negative pressure will have been lost.* Keep the hole plugged until emergency assistance arrives.

✚👁 **N u r s i n g A l e r t**

Cardiopulmonary resuscitation (CPR) is ineffective if the person's airway is blocked or if there is an open chest wound. Clear the airway and/or apply pressure to occlude an open chest wound before initiating CPR.

Respiratory Complications in Drug Poisoning

In many cases of drug overdose, the person's respirations are depressed. In some cases, depression of the respiratory system to the point of apnea causes death. This development is called *respiratory arrest.* Drugs most likely to cause respiratory arrest include narcotics (eg, codeine, morphine, and heroin) and depressants (eg, barbiturates).

✚👁 **N u r s i n g A l e r t**

If a person is not breathing, CPR is necessary. It is done with an airway and a manual breathing bag if available. *Rationale: This is less strenuous for the rescuer and prevents the spread of infection from the client to the healthcare worker.* If an airway and manual breathing bag are unavailable, mouth-to-mouth breathing is required.

In the case of an overdose of stimulants (eg, cocaine or amphetamines), respirations may increase. In this type of overdose, overstimulation may lead to seizures, hypertension, stroke, and death.

Drowning/Near Drowning

The medical term for fluid in the lungs is *aspiration.* Fluid or foreign bodies aspirated into the nose, throat, or the lungs during inspiration can prevent adequate air exchange in the lungs. This leads to *aspiration pneumonia,* a serious complication.

Near drowning occurs when an individual has been submerged under water without ventilation. The person will be hypoxic. Begin rescue ventilation and perfusion as quickly as possible. Do not attempt to clear the airway of water because the body can only aspirate a small amount into the lungs and quickly absorbs it into the bloodstream. A small percentage of victims will not aspirate at all, due to breath holding or laryngospasm. In such cases, individuals die because of the lack of oxygen and inability to breathe, but no water is actually in the lungs.

✚👁 **N u r s i n g A l e r t**

Be careful in giving fluids to a person who has difficulty swallowing or who is confused. Never give an unconscious person fluids by mouth. Aspiration can cause pneumonia or death. If aspiration occurs, notify the physician immediately and take measures to prevent complications.

Pneumothorax

Pneumothorax is the presence of air in the pleural cavity or between the pleura and the chest wall. It may result from trauma or be a complication of chest surgery or chest-tube drainage. It usually causes the collapse of a lung, which is a serious complication because less air is exchanged. Pneumothorax is an emergency. Check for the following signs of pneumothorax:

- SOB or severe dyspnea
- Asymmetrical chest
- Mediastinal shift toward the affected side
- Sudden, sharp chest pain
- Drop in blood pressure
- Weak, rapid pulse
- Cessation of breathing (chest) movement on affected side
- Cyanosis
- Change in level of consciousness

Immediately report if any of these signs occur. If the client has chest tubes, clamp them and get help as soon as possible. Additional information regarding closed water-seal drainage for pneumothorax and hemothorax is found in the earlier section on chest surgery (see In Practice: Nursing Care Guidelines 85-3).

NEOPLASMS

Benign Neoplasms

A *benign lung tumor,* or *cyst,* is characterized on the x-ray film by smooth edges and sharply defined margins. Peripheral tumors usually have no symptoms. If the tumor is in the bronchi, there may be obstruction, causing infection or atelectasis distal to the obstruction (see Fig. 85-4B). Bronchoscopy and biopsy are usually done to determine the reason for an abnormal shadow in the lung. Treatment is symptomatic.

Lung Cancer

Lung cancer affects men and women equally. It is now the leading cause of cancer death in both men and women in America (see Chap. 82). Lung cancer is most common in people between the ages of 45 and 70, and is on the rise in women, probably due to the increased number of women who smoke. As the number of teenage girls who smoke continues to rise, so will the increasing incidence of lung cancer in women.

In 80% to 90% of lung cancer deaths, the victims were cigarette smokers. From available research, stopping or not smoking is the best preventive measure. Other causes of lung cancer include environmental exposure to secondhand (passive) cigarette smoke, air pollution, asbestos and other talc dusts, and radon gas in the home or workplace.

Detecting lung cancer in the early stage is difficult because symptoms do not appear until the disease is well advanced. A routine CXR will often reveal the cancer. Lung cancer usually arises in the bronchi and produces no symptoms until

it enlarges. The disease is fatal within 5 years in over 85% of cases.

The first indication of trouble generally occurs when the person begins to cough up mucus and blood-streaked sputum. The client may experience dyspnea, chills, and fever. Even then, the person may think he or she is merely smoking too much and may resolve to cut down. Later, fatigue, unexplained weight loss, and chest pains occur. By the time the client consults a physician, the disease is likely to be in an advanced stage. Bronchoscopy, CXR, sputum examination, and lung scan confirm the diagnosis.

Treatment. If the tumor is localized, immediate surgery, with removal of part or all of the lung, may be curative. Removal of a lobe of the lung is called a *lobectomy;* removal of one entire lung is called a *pneumonectomy.* If the tumor is extensive and involves lymph nodes, radiation or chemotherapy (or both) may be used. These treatments will not usually cure the disease, but they often improve the individual's quality of life. There have been advances in the treatment modalities over the past decade, but the individual must be referred to a cancer specialist or oncologist as soon as diagnosis is made.

If the person has widespread lung cancer, with metastasis to other organs, a combination of chemotherapeutic medications may be instituted. Responses to this treatment vary. At this time, chemotherapeutic agents cannot cure lung cancer, but they are useful in controlling pain and in reducing the pleural effusions caused by the cancer.

DISORDERS OF THE NOSE

Inflammatory Disorders

Sinusitis

Sinusitis is inflammation of one or more of the sinuses located in the head. The maxillary sinus (*antrum*) is most frequently affected by infection spreading from the nasal passages. If the individual's resistance is low, the person is more susceptible to sinus infection. A sinus infection is uncomfortable. Allergy, frequent colds, and nasal obstruction of any kind increase susceptibility to repeated attacks. If neglected, sinusitis becomes chronic and damages the mucous membranes; treatment is then less effective. Of all possible complications of sinusitis, infections of the middle ear and the brain are most serious. Sinusitis may also lead to bronchiectasis or osteomyelitis in the adjacent bone. Early treatment is important to prevent these complications.

Acute Sinusitis

Acute sinusitis begins with pain and pressure. The person feels pain in the cheek or the upper teeth if the maxillary sinuses are affected. Frontal sinus pain occurs over the eyes. The person may have a low-grade fever, fatigue, and a poor appetite. A purulent nasal discharge accompanies postnasal drip, causing throat irritation. Sinus congestion shows on x-ray examination.

Treatment includes increased fluids, antibiotics to control infection, analgesics to relieve pain, and, in severe cases, bed rest. Nose drops containing phenylephrine (Neo-Synephrine) may be prescribed to shrink the swollen turbinates and to encourage drainage; antihistamines are also used. Steam inhalation or hot, moist packs to the forehead can be effective.

If drainage is obstructed in an acute sinus infection, the sinus may be irrigated with warm saline solution, a comparatively painless procedure. However, it may be necessary to puncture the bony wall between the nose and the sinus cavity (Caldwell-Luc procedure) or to enter the frontal sinus through the inner aspect of the eyebrow. These surgical procedures are painful for the client, who may become frightened and feel dizzy or faint.

Chronic Sinusitis

Many people mistakenly think that nothing can be done for sinusitis, and unfortunately allow it to become chronic. *Chronic sinusitis* is characterized by repeated flare-ups of the infection, despite treatment. Symptoms include:

- Cough, due to postnasal drip
- Chronic headaches in the affected area
- Facial pain
- Nasal stuffiness
- Fatigue

Sometimes a relatively simple operation to create a new sinus opening may be ordered. Because many cases of chronic sinusitis are allergic in nature, allergy tests may be done and desensitization injections given.

Structural Disorders

Deviated Septum

The nasal septum is a partition made of bone and cartilage that divides the nose into right and left cavities. The septum is rarely absolutely straight, but unless the deviation is marked, it usually causes no trouble. An unusually crooked septum can interfere with drainage in one nostril or with insertion of a nasogastric tube. An injury that causes a deformity in the septum should have a physician's attention; if left uncorrected, the deformity can cause sinusitis. The operation to correct such a deformity is called a *submucous resection* or *septoplasty*.

Nasal Polyps

Polyps are tumors that look like small bunches of tiny grapes. Nasal polyps obstruct breathing and sinus drainage. They are easily removed through surgery under local anesthesia, but tend to return, in which case the operation must be repeated. A biopsy of the tissue should be done to determine if the growth is malignant.

Plastic Surgery

Plastic surgery of the nose (**rhinoplasty**) may be done for cosmetic reasons or to correct deformities resulting from injury.

Care of the Client Undergoing Nasal Surgery

Most surgery on the nose is performed on an outpatient basis. Therefore, client and family teaching is essential. Be sure to carefully and completely document all teaching.

The nose is highly vascular; hemorrhage is always a possibility. Therefore, teach the client and family important signs and symptoms for which to observe. The procedure can also be painful. In addition, nasal procedures can interfere with normal respiration and can cause anxiety. In Practice: Nursing Care Guidelines 85-5 discusses nursing care in nasal surgery.

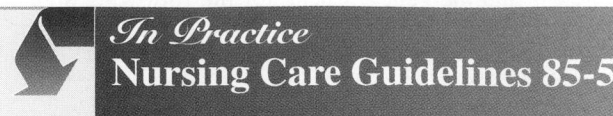

In Practice
Nursing Care Guidelines 85-5

CARING FOR THE PERSON WHO HAS HAD NASAL SURGERY

- Always wash your hands.
- Wear gloves.
- Teach precautions to the client or family and carefully document teaching. *Rationale: Most nasal surgery is done on an outpatient basis. The person will be going home immediately after surgery.*

Promoting Respiration

- Keep in mind that the client is often very uncomfortable. *Rationale: The initial postoperative period can be very painful. The person will probably have to breathe through the mouth.*
- Give frequent oral hygiene. *Rationale: Breathing through the mouth is very drying to the mucous membranes.*
- Elevate the head of the bed. *Rationale: Head elevation facilitates breathing.*
- Observe carefully for choking. Suctioning may be needed. *Rationale: Considerable mucous drainage is usual, because the nasal mucosa has been irritated.*
- Observe for signs of respiratory distress. *Rationale: Swelling or bleeding may cause respiratory difficulties. Aspiration into the lungs is always a threat.*

Assessment for Hemorrhage

- Observe for nausea, coffee-ground emesis, dark-colored emesis, frequent spitting of blood, blood on the dressing, and any signs of shock. *Rationale: The nose is very vascular and may bleed profusely.*
- At regular intervals, examine the back of the throat for draining of blood by using a flashlight and tongue depressor. *Rationale: In surgery of the nose or nosebleed (epistaxis), blood may run down the back of the throat and be swallowed.*
- Remember that the nostrils are usually packed with gauze, which is removed 24 to 48 hours following surgery. Observe carefully for hemorrhage after removal of a pack. *Rationale: The nose is very vascular and may bleed profusely.*
- Apply a *mustache dressing* (a gauze pad impregnated with petrolatum and held in place with strips of adhesive), beneath the nostrils, if necessary. *Rationale: This dressing is applied to absorb drainage.*

Nasal Trauma

Fractures

A fractured nose is a relatively common occurrence. It should be set (moved back into place) promptly to avoid later deformity. Usually, no other treatment is needed.

Epistaxis

Irritation or injury to a small mass of capillaries on the nasal septum may cause nosebleed or epistaxis. Hypertension can give rise to bleeding, in which case the bleeding is more likely to be severe and not easily controlled. Certain blood disorders, cancer, and rheumatic fever are other possible causes. Nosebleeds are fairly common, but when severe, they can be serious.

First aid for nosebleed (**epistaxis**) is simple and described in Chapter 43. If initial treatment is ineffective, pack the nasal cavity with gauze to create pressure on the bleeding area. This can usually be accomplished by passing a string through the nose and bringing it out through the mouth. The pack on the string is pulled back through the nose until the packing is in the back of the nasal cavity. The other end of the string extends out through the nostril.

Bleeding points may also be painted with silver nitrate or other solutions that tend to stop bleeding, or they may be cauterized to cause coagulation.

DISORDERS OF THE THROAT

The throat (*pharynx*) is the muscular tube communicating with the nasal cavity (*nasopharynx*), the oral cavity (*oropharynx*), and the laryngeal cavity (*laryngopharynx*). Two throat disorders, common in children but occurring occasionally in adults, are tonsillitis and streptococcal sore throat (see Chap. 71).

Trauma

Aspiration of Foreign Bodies

A foreign body lodged in the trachea that obstructs breathing is an emergency. In most cases, a sharp blow between the shoulder blades while the person's head is lowered, or the abdominal thrust (see Chap. 43), will dislodge the object. If these measures fail and the person cannot breathe, an emergency tracheostomy or intubation with an airway must be done (if someone available is able to perform the procedure). Artificial ventilation will probably be required after the airway is opened. Tracheostomy is described in Chapter 86.

A client may aspirate a small object into the lung without causing asphyxiation; it will result in infection and atelectasis of all or part of the lung (see Fig. 85-4B) and must be removed. For this, bronchoscopy usually is effective. Open-lung surgery may be performed if the object has lodged deep in a bronchus.

Cancer of the Larynx

Cancer of the larynx most often afflicts men over the age of 45, although cases are increasing among women who smoke. Those who have chronic laryngitis, strain their voices, or are heavy drinkers or smokers are the most likely to develop laryn-

geal cancer. Theorists believe that heredity may also play a role. Symptoms are chronic hoarseness, and, in some instances, inability to speak above a whisper.

Treatment

If the condition is detected early, radiation may be effective. Surgery is often successful in inducing a complete cure. The operation consists of removing either the tumorous part or the entire larynx. The surgery is called **laryngectomy.** A person who has a total laryngectomy is referred to as a *laryngectomee.* If the cancer has spread beyond the vocal cords, a simple or radical neck dissection is done.

After the larynx is removed, air enters and leaves through the trachea. Provision for this is made by inserting a tube into the trachea through an opening in the lower part of the neck. This procedure is called a *tracheostomy;* it is permanent, even after the airway tube is removed. Teaching is summarized at In Practice: Educating the Client 85-3.

Nursing Considerations

Client teaching and support are greatly important. The person faces not only the knowledge that he or she must permanently breathe through a hole in the neck, but also must deal with the diagnosis of cancer. Reduce the client's fears about loss of speech by assuring the individual that, although he or she will lose the natural voice, voice training (esophageal or pharyngeal speech) or a mechanical device will make conversation possible. If only a partial laryngectomy was performed, reassure the client that speech usually returns quickly. A visit

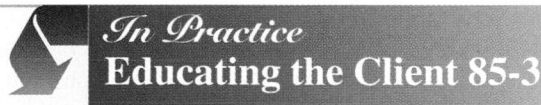

In Practice
Educating the Client 85-3

POST-LARYNGECTOMY

While the client recovers from laryngectomy, the client and family are able to:

- Describe care of the tube such as cleaning, suctioning (if necessary), and how to handle emergencies.
- Explain or demonstrate various communication techniques.
- Identify support groups available for persons and families after laryngectomy or a diagnosis of cancer.
- Show how the permanent laryngectomy opening may be covered by a necktie, a crew or turtleneck shirt, a scarf, or jewelry.
- Demonstrate how to prevent aspiration of fluids or foreign objects into the laryngectomy tube.
- Explain why showering must be done with care and swimming is often prohibited.
- Identify the need to wear a scarf over the opening in extremely cold weather and to avoid thin, filmy scarves because they may be sucked into the tracheostomy and obstruct breathing.

from another person who has made a good recovery after a laryngectomy may help.

Because esophageal reconstruction is likely, inform the client that, for a time, feeding may be done through a nasal or gastrostomy tube (until the esophagus heals) and that the tracheostomy opening will be permanent. The client needs good oral hygiene, which provides comfort and helps keep the surgical site as clean as possible.

When respiratory passages become irritated, mucous secretions increase; they must be removed frequently by suction through the tracheostomy tube. Keep a suction machine at the bedside, and never leave the client alone without a call light. A family member may stay with the client for the first few postoperative days. Chapter 86 presents the procedure for suctioning and care of the tracheostomy tube.

Because the client cannot cry out for help, he or she may fear choking and being unable to breathe. If oxygen is to be administered, apply it by mask or by T-piece (blow-by) over the tracheostomy tube. There is also the danger of hemorrhage, as evidenced by *hemoptysis* (coughing or spitting up of blood) or by symptoms of shock. Give the client a signal bell or call light.

Drainage from the wound following a neck dissection, or other procedure in this area, is usually handled with a portable wound-suction device, such as Hem-O-Vac. This device stays with the individual at all times. Empty and measure the drainage. Follow the facility's protocol.

The client probably will be allowed out of bed the first postoperative day, and soon will learn how to suction the tube and take care of it. Everyone involved in the client's care should know how to perform this procedure. When the airway becomes obstructed, the individual quickly becomes cyanotic and could die within a few minutes if the obstruction is not removed. In this emergency, call for help and suction the tracheostomy opening. Unless the physician has previously instructed the nurses as to what emergency procedures to use, nursing staff should consult the physician to see if the tracheostomy tube can be removed as an emergency measure.

The person usually loses the sense of smell temporarily after surgery. However, it will begin to return as he or she learns to breathe through the tracheostomy tube. The sense of smell will be best recovered in the individual who learns esophageal speech.

☛ KEY CONCEPT

Sometimes, the person must write notes to communicate. In this case, make sure the person's dominant hand is not encumbered with an IV. A child's "Magic Slate" often works well temporarily. Alphabet and picture cards may also be useful. Be sure to answer this person's signal light immediately; he or she will be unable to tell the nurse what is wrong on the intercom. (A tap bell may be used for emergencies.)

Communication and Speech.   Before the surgery, discuss the method of postoperative communication with the client. Clients who know that some type of communication will be available after surgery will be less anxious. Immedi-

ately postoperatively, set up a workable communication system. Provide the client with writing materials. If they try to tell you something, make every attempt to find out what it is.

Speech therapy should begin as soon as possible. The technique of *esophageal speech* consists of swallowing air and using it to make speech sounds while regurgitating the air. It takes patience and constant practice to learn how to do this; some individuals learn the technique in 2 to 3 weeks. Esophageal speech is not smooth, although it is the easiest to learn.

Most people progress to *pharyngeal speech*. The air they use in this case is that which enters the nose and mouth; it is blocked by quick tongue action. The pharynx becomes the sounding board. Pharyngeal speech takes much more practice, but it is smoother and has a more natural sound than esophageal speech.

The third speech technique devised for the person who is unable to learn esophageal or pharyngeal speech is the *artificial larynx*. This is an electronic device that the person holds against the throat. Currently, many physicians during surgery are implanting an electronic device that aids in making speech sound more normal.

Tracheoesophageal puncture is another speech alternative after a total laryngectomy. Movement of air from the lungs through a puncture in the posterior wall of the trachea, into the esophagus, and out of the mouth makes sounds. A prosthesis is placed over the puncture site after it has healed. In some individuals, speech is possible by placing a finger over the tracheostomy opening after taking a breath.

Identification as a Laryngectomee.   Identification as a laryngectomee is important. The individual must wear an identifying tag, such as a MedicAlert tag, so others will know that he or she breathes through a neck opening. This consideration is especially important if the client has not yet begun speech training. Remember, if the opening is plugged, the laryngectomee will die of asphyxiation.

Supportive Resources.   Supportive resources, such as clubs and organizations for laryngectomees, sponsored by the International Association of Laryngectomees, are available in some communities. Members give each other encouragement and emotional support. They are often willing to visit new laryngectomees in hospitals, encouraging them to begin rehabilitation.

Water Dangers.   Anyone who has a tracheostomy or a permanent laryngectomy tube must always be careful to prevent water from getting into the opening. This person must use great caution when showering. A snorkel device is available to fit over the laryngectomee's stoma to allow for swimming. Strenuous water sports are contraindicated.

➤ **STUDENT SYNTHESIS**

Key Points

- The respiratory and cardiovascular systems are vital to the entire body's functioning because they provide and transport oxygen to cells, and wastes away from cells.

- Nursing assessment of a client with a respiratory disorder is critical in determining the severity of respiratory distress, the immediacy of the situation, and necessary care.
- Disorders of the respiratory system may be caused by infections (bacteria, virus, fungi), irritants (smoking, allergens, environmental chemicals), masses (cancerous tumors), or trauma.
- Respiratory disorders may be characterized by multiple clinical manifestations such as cough, changes in respiratory pattern, and abnormal breath sounds.
- When hypoxia (lack of oxygen) occurs, subsequent changes in the neurologic and cardiovascular systems may develop.
- Key elements in the treatment of respiratory disorders include medications specific to the disease; oxygen administration; postural drainage; positioning; turning, coughing, and deep breathing; and breathing exercises.
- The goals of nursing management for persons with respiratory disorders are a patent (open) airway, effective breathing pattern, and improved gas exchange.

Critical Thinking Exercises

1. Your client and his wife are discussing general health concerns with you during the client's checkup. The client mentions that his snoring has worsened and is causing problems between the couple. What factors may contribute to snoring? What measures might help the client and his wife?
2. You are asked to design a prevention program for junior high school students about the dangers of cigarette smoking. What strategies would you use? How would you encourage these students not to smoke? What measures would you use to encourage their families to support these children?

NCLEX-Style Review Questions

1. For a client who is experiencing shortness of breath, which nursing intervention would be most appropriate to do first?
   a. Apply IPPB.
   b. Instruct on turning, coughing, and deep breathing.
   c. Place in orthopneic position.
   d. Perform postural drainage.
2. What is the priority intervention for a client whose Pleur-Evac system has become disconnected from the client's chest tube?
   a. Double-clamp the chest tube.
   b. Notify the MD.
   c. Place client in orthopneic position.
   d. Sound the alarm for a cardiac arrest.
3. The nurse determines that a client is experiencing severe hypoxemia when the client displays:
   a. Confusion
   b. Hypotension
   c. PO_2 of 80 mm Hg
   d. Unruly behavior
4. Which assessment data relate most directly to a diagnosis of pulmonary emphysema?
   a. Cyanosis, hypercapnia, peripheral edema
   b. Decreased breath sounds, barrel chest, SOB
   c. Polycythemia, peripheral edema, weight gain
   d. Symmetrical chest, wheezing, SOB
5. A client is admitted to the hospital with pneumonia. Which assessment finding would indicate that the infection has spread?
   a. Client feels ill
   b. Fever
   c. Painful cough
   d. Presence of pleural friction rub
6. Which of the following is the primary risk factor for developing lung cancer?
   a. Decreased alveolar function
   b. Exposure to coal dust
   c. Exposure to radiation
   d. Smoking cigarettes

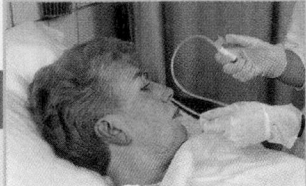

CHAPTER

86

Oxygen Therapy and Respiratory Care

LEARNING OBJECTIVES

1. State the three major goals of oxygen therapy.
2. Discuss at least four key safety factors and hazards in oxygen administration.
3. Describe the use of the pulse oximeter.
4. Identify at least five sources of oxygen and describe how they differ.
5. List at least eight key points in nursing assessment of the client who is receiving oxygen.
6. Differentiate the following types of oxygen delivery systems: simple mask, partial-rebreathing mask, non-rebreathing mask, Venturi mask, IPPB, aerosol mist treatments, and manual breathing bag.
7. State at least three key safety factors or nursing considerations with the use of each of the oxygen delivery systems.
8. Demonstrate how to set up basic oxygen equipment.
9. Discuss at least five nursing considerations for the client receiving oxygen on mechanical ventilation and/or with a tracheostomy.

NEW TERMINOLOGY

Ambu bag
hyperbaric
manual breathing bag
mechanical ventilator
nasal cannula
pulse oximeter

respirator
simple mask
tracheostomy
ventilatory failure
Venturi mask

ACRONYMS

ABG	IPPB	PRM
ARDS	L/min	psi
COPD	LPM	PSV
CPAP	NRM	SIMV
HBO	O_2 sat	

Oxygen is a gaseous element that is essential to life. If a person is deprived of oxygen, death will occur in a matter of minutes. Normally, all people extract sufficient oxygen from the air they breathe. *Therapeutic* (supplemental) oxygen is necessary only when a client is unable to obtain sufficient oxygen for the body's needs, due to a breathing or blood deficiency.

Excess oxygen is not helpful; in fact, it can be harmful. Therefore, oxygen is prescribed as a medication and is administered under controlled conditions. Oxygen is necessary for anything to burn, and increasing oxygen allows common flammable materials to burn faster and hotter. Thus, the more oxygen that is in the air, the greater the danger is for fire. Therefore, safety is of the utmost importance. This chapter discusses the client who is receiving supplemental oxygen, as well as the person whose breathing is supported by a *mechanical ventilator* (machine that forces air into the lungs) or who has a *tracheostomy* (artificial opening in the trachea through which a tube is inserted to aid a person in breathing).

OXYGEN PROVISION

By increasing the concentration of oxygen the person inhales, more oxygen becomes available for the body's consumption. Oxygen may be administered to clients with pneumonia, carbon monoxide poisoning, severe asthma, heart failure, or myocardial infarction, or after chest or abdominal surgery. It provides comfort for the client and allows him or her to breathe more easily.

Goals of Oxygen Therapy

Increasing the concentration (or percentage) of oxygen the client inhales accomplishes three goals:

- Reverses *hypoxemia* (low oxygen concentration in the blood)
- Decreases the work of the respiratory system: If the client receives supplemental oxygen, the respiratory muscles do not work as hard to pump air in and out of the lungs and to maintain a sufficient blood oxygen supply.
- Decreases the heart's work in pumping blood: The heart tries to compensate for hypoxemia by increasing output; supplemental oxygen can ease the heart's load.

Hazards of Oxygen Therapy

Like the safe administration of medications, oxygen must be administered safely. Oxygen given in high concentration over many days can result in oxygen toxicity, manifested as changes in lung tissue. (Recall that excess oxygen in newborns can cause vision difficulties.) In some people, increased oxygen concentrations also affect their ventilatory drive control mechanisms, which actually weakens the stimulus to breathe. Therefore, treat oxygen like a medication and administer it with the same care as in administering any medication.

A physician evaluates the client's need for oxygen and writes a specific order for oxygen therapy with the appropriate dosage. Administration of oxygen by mask or cannula is expressed in liters per minute (**LPM** or **L/min**); some devices control the specific oxygen concentration to administer. When using mechanical ventilators, oxygen concentration can be more easily controlled.

Everyone, including the client, visitors, and others in the unit, must know and follow the necessary precautions when oxygen is administered. If oxygen comes in contact with any combustible material, even a small spark can ignite an explosive (flash) fire. A list of precautionary measures when providing oxygen are presented at In Practice: Nursing Care Guidelines 86-1.

Assessment of Respiratory Status

Whenever a client is receiving oxygen, the client's respiratory status must be continually monitored to ensure that treatment has the desired effects. In Practice: Nursing Assessment 86-1 lists important considerations when assessing respiratory status (see Chap. 47 for adults and Chaps. 70 and 71 for infants). If any signs of respiratory difficulty or distress occur, notify a physician immediately.

Use of the Pulse Oximeter

The **pulse oximeter** is a convenient monitor that measures the amount (percentage) of oxygen saturation in the blood. Through a finger clip or an ear probe, the oximeter shines a light beam through soft tissue. Its measurement is noninvasive (unlike drawing blood for arterial blood gas [**ABG**] analysis) and it can be used continuously or intermittently. The oximeter is read as percent oxygen saturation (O_2 **sat**). The pulse oximeter has limited accuracy. Readings must be interpreted with an awareness of the client's blood components and other variables. Still, it is a useful adjunct to other evaluations of respiratory status. Chapter 56 describes and illustrates the use of the pulse oximeter.

Sources of Oxygen

Large healthcare facilities most frequently use the large bulk storage tank, with its convenient in-room piping system. They normally also have smaller oxygen tanks (cylinders) and oxygen strollers available to provide portable or emergency oxygen supplies. Some smaller facilities that use oxygen supplies less frequently have cylinders.

Wall Outlets

With bulk storage and in-room piping systems, a wall outlet is installed next to each bed. Wall outlets and adapters vary, not only by the type of gas they supply, but in terms of shape, color, and connection method. Be familiar with the wall outlet system used in the facility. Practice inserting the adapter into the outlet so that it can be done quickly and easily during an emergency. Use the following steps:

- Obtain a flowmeter and firmly and quickly push the adapter into the outlet.

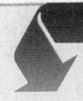

In Practice
Nursing Care Guidelines 86-1

PROVIDING OXYGEN

- Explain about the dangers of lighting matches or smoking cigarettes, cigars, or pipes. Be sure the client has no matches, cigarettes, or smoking materials in the bedside table. *Rationale: Oxygen is highly combustible.*
- Make sure that warning signs are posted on the client's door and above the client's bed (even if the entire facility is nonsmoking). *Rationale: All persons coming in contact with the client need to be aware that oxygen is in use.*
- Use caution with all electrical devices, such as heating pads, electric blankets, or the ordinary call light. *Rationale: Oxygen is highly combustible.* Many healthcare facilities provide call lights with grounding devices or give such clients tap bells instead.
- Do not use oil on oxygen equipment. *Rationale: Oil can ignite if exposed to oxygen.* Be sure no traces of oil are on hands before adjusting an oxygen apparatus.
- Be aware of all potential sources of sparks, especially when administering oxygen by means of a containment device (such as a tent or isolette). *Note:* Items that appear innocuous (such as friction toys, electric razors) have caused explosive fires. *Rationale: Oxygen is highly combustible.*
- With all oxygen delivery systems, turn the oxygen on before applying the mask.
- Gain the client's cooperation. Inform the client of the therapeutic uses of oxygen before bringing equipment into the room. Reassure the client and family. *Rationale: They may be afraid that the use of oxygen is a sign of deteriorating condition. The client's need for oxygen will be reduced if he or she relaxes.*
- Instruct the client not to change the position of the mask, cannula, or any of the equipment after it is in place. *Rationale: Changing position could alter the amount of oxygen being delivered.*
- Maintain a constant oxygen concentration for the client to breathe; monitor equipment at regular intervals. *Rationale: Maintaining the appropriate flow rate enhances effectiveness of oxygen therapy.*

- Give pain medications as needed, prevent chilling, and try to ensure that the client gets needed rest. Be alert to cues about hunger and elimination. *Rationale: The client's physical comfort is important and decreases the demand for oxygen by the tissues.*
- Watch for respiratory depression or distress. *Rationale: Oxygen can depress the respiratory drive in some clients.*
- Encourage or assist the client to move about in bed. *Rationale: Movement helps to prevent hypostatic pneumonia or circulatory difficulties.* Many clients are reluctant to move because they are afraid of the oxygen apparatus.
- Make sure the tubing is patent at all times and that the equipment is working properly. *Rationale: To be effective, the client needs to receive the proper concentration of oxygen.*
- Assess, document, and report the client's condition regularly. *Rationale: Regular assessment of the client's condition is necessary to determine the effectiveness of oxygen therapy.*
- Provide frequent mouth care. Make sure the oxygen contains proper humidification. *Rationale: Oxygen can be drying to mucous membranes.*
- Keep in mind that oxygen does not control every breathing difficulty, but where it is indicated, it can dramatically improve a client's condition. The person breathes more easily, the pulse rate drops, and an anxious attitude may change to a relaxed one.
- Discontinue oxygen only after a physician has evaluated the client. Generally, you should not abruptly discontinue oxygen given in medium-to-high concentrations (above 30%). Gradually decrease it in stages, and monitor the client's arterial blood gases or oxygen saturation level. *Rationale: These steps determine whether the client needs continued support.*
- Wear gloves any time there is a possibility of coming into contact with the client's respiratory secretions. *Rationale: Proper use of gloves helps prevent the spread of infection.*

- Give a gentle pull outward. *Rationale: This action ensures that the adapter is locked in place.*
- After the adapter is inserted, check to see that no oxygen leaks around the edges. If oxygen is escaping, remove and reinsert the adapter.
- To remove the adapter, push it in slightly, then firmly pull it out. Do not be startled by the loud popping sound—it is the release of pressure of the contained oxygen behind the wall source.

Oxygen Cylinders

Oxygen cylinders are available in many sizes, but are grouped into two main categories: large and small. A large cylinder is identifiable not only by its size, but also by the presence of a metal cap screwed onto its top to protect the valve from damage. Also, the valve itself has an attached handle and threaded connection site. Large cylinders are generally used when high flow rates are essential or when a client requires oxygen for an extended period.

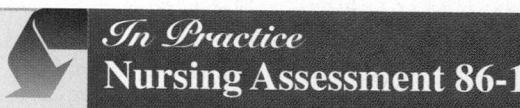

In Practice
Nursing Assessment 86-1

RESPIRATORY STATUS OF A CLIENT WHO IS RECEIVING OXYGEN

- Observe the client's respirations. Assess their rate, depth, and character.
- Document difficulty in breathing: abnormal movements, retractions, irregular breathing patterns, abnormal breathing sounds.
- Assess lung sounds. (Document abnormal lung sounds.)
- Assess the client's level of comfort. Determine if the client is anxious, very restless, or not getting enough oxygen.
- Measure the client's pulse rate often. (In respiratory distress, pulse rate often rises.)
- Monitor results of arterial blood gases (**ABGs**), which are often drawn and analyzed regularly. This involves an arterial stick (as opposed to a venipuncture) and drawing blood from an artery.
- Check pulse oximeter readings, which are often used to determine the client's oxygen saturation. This procedure is noninvasive.
- If indicated, monitor the client electronically (pulse, respiration, blood pressure, oxygen saturation).
- Assess for evidence of cyanosis.
- Monitor the oxygen delivery device for proper fit and usage. Check for signs of leakage.
- Closely observe the client whose oxygen has been discontinued. If the client becomes short of breath, shows signs of cyanosis, or has a markedly increased pulse rate, call the physician at once and resume oxygen.

A small cylinder is identifiable by its rectangular valve with no handle and three holes on one side. Small cylinders are used when transporting clients or for short-term emergencies. Many clients also use small cylinders at home.

Careful handling and use of cylinders provides for safety. Because the gas contained within a cylinder is under extremely high pressure, the pressure must be reduced to a safe level before the cylinder is connected to a person. A regulator is a device that can reduce this pressure. A flowmeter and pressure gauge are attached to most regulators. The flowmeter is either round or similar to the flowmeter used with wall outlets. It indicates the oxygen flow to the client in LPM. The pressure gauge is round, but usually smaller than the (round) flowmeter. It indicates the pressure in the cylinder in pounds per square inch (**psi**) of pressure.

Safety in using oxygen cylinders is vital. They are under high pressure. If a cylinder must be moved, make sure to secure it in a cylinder cart. If the top breaks off, the cylinder becomes "jet-propelled." Be sure to turn off the valve when the cylinder

is not in use. Keep all cylinders away from heat. If asked to administer oxygen or another gas using a cylinder, request instruction in oxygen administration, including the use and management of regulators.

Oxygen Strollers

Portable oxygen can also be provided by a liquid-oxygen stroller, also nicknamed a "walker" or "companion" by manufacturers. The liquid-oxygen portable unit consists of a Thermos-type vessel in a shoulder bag or small carrying case. Liquid oxygen is more dense than gaseous oxygen, so a portable stroller can carry more oxygen and yet be lighter and more compact than a steel gas cylinder. Liquid oxygen is allowed to evaporate within a warming coil into its gaseous state. It is then metered to the person through tubing connected to an oxygen delivery device. Liquid oxygen strollers are generally quite safe.

Remember the following guidelines when operating a portable liquid-oxygen stroller:

- The tank must be kept upright at all times. *Rationale: If tipped, the tank will vent the oxygen contents quickly.*
- Strollers can be refilled from a larger stationary reservoir unit.
- A stroller is considered full or empty depending on its relative weight.
- As liquid oxygen warms, it evaporates. Thus, strollers gradually empty by themselves. For this reason, strollers cannot totally replace cylinders as sources of emergency portable oxygen.

Oxygen Concentrator

Oxygen concentrators are widely used in home and extended care settings. They compress room air and extract oxygen, providing concentrated oxygen flows in the range of 1 to 5 LPM. An oxygen concentrator is much safer and more convenient to use than an oxygen tank. It also does not need to be refilled. However, it does require periodic maintenance by a technician, needs electricity to operate, and is not portable.

Hyperbaric Chamber

Some large facilities have a **hyperbaric** chamber, which simulates deep-sea diving by increasing atmospheric pressure. This method is called *hyperbaric oxygenation* (**HBO**) or *high-pressure oxygenation*. In the chamber, the person can take oxygen into the body in concentrations higher than is possible at normal atmospheric pressure. With the increased pressure, the client's hemoglobin and other blood components can carry more oxygen. HBO is used to treat air or gas embolism, carbon monoxide poisoning, and anaerobic infections (such as gas gangrene); to administer some types of radiation therapy for cancer; and to perform some surgeries (especially heart surgery). It is also used to treat crush injuries or traumatic ischemias and to enhance wound healing in necrotizing soft tissue infections, compromised skin grafts and flaps, thermal burns, and chronic osteomyelitis.

THE CLIENT WHO IS HAVING DIFFICULTY BREATHING

When administering oxygen to an individual who is having difficulty breathing, the type of device that is used is critically important. The primary concern is delivery of the desired concentration (percentage) of oxygen. Monitoring the client's blood gases and assessing for comfort, compliance, and safety are essential.

Oxygen delivery devices can be classified into two types: low-flow and high-flow devices. Low-flow devices do not provide exact oxygen concentrations; the client's breathing pattern influences the concentration of oxygen obtained. With high-flow oxygen devices, the oxygen percentage is constant (as long as the device is set up properly).

With most oxygen devices, humidification is provided. *Rationale: Oxygen from a tank or bulk system is absolutely dry and can be irritating to the respiratory mucosa.* A humidifier sends oxygen through small holes into water that creates bubbles and adds water molecules to the gas. The humidifier is connected to the threaded outlet at the bottom of the flowmeter or regulator. A small universal connector extends from the front or top of the humidifier for connection to the oxygen device.

Nasal Cannula

The **nasal cannula** (nasal prongs) is a device used to deliver small to moderate increases in oxygen concentration. The cannula has two short tubes that fit into the nostrils. This low-flow device can deliver 24% to 44% oxygen at flow rates of 1 to 6 LPM. Most people prefer cannulas because they are less confining and do not interfere with eating or talking.

Use cannulas with caution for clients who have irregular breathing patterns. *Rationale: The percentage of oxygen that reaches the lungs depends on the rate and depth of respirations.* In Practice: Nursing Procedure 86-1 describes nursing actions in the use of nasal cannulas.

Simple Mask

The **simple mask** is a transparent mask with a simple nipple adapter. It fits over the client's nose, mouth, and chin. It is a low-flow device that provides an oxygen concentration in the

---

In Practice
Nursing Procedure 86-1

SUPPLYING OXYGEN WITH THE NASAL CANNULA

Supplies and Equipment

Flowmeter
Oxygen source
Nasal cannula and tubing
Humidifier and sterile water (optional)
"Oxygen in Use" sign
Gloves

Steps

1. Check the physician's orders and gather supplies.
   RATIONALE: *Oxygen is considered a medication. Checking the orders ensures that the proper flow rate and device are used. Organization facilitates accurate skill performance.*

2. Wash hands and put on gloves, if contact with client's respiratory secretions is possible.
   RATIONALE: *Proper handwashing and use of gloves helps prevent the spread of infection.*

3. Explain the procedure to the client.
   RATIONALE: *Providing information fosters the client's cooperation.*

4. Prepare the oxygen equipment:
   a. Plug the flowmeter into the wall outlet or oxygen tank.
   b. Attach the humidifier to the flowmeter.
   c. Fill the humidifier with sterile water.
   d. Attach the cannula with the connecting tubing to the adapter on the humidifier.
   RATIONALE: *Humidification prevents drying of the nasal mucosa. The agency's policy will dictate whether low flow of oxygen (3 liters or less) requires humidification.*

5. Adjust the flowmeter's setting to the ordered flow rate. Check that oxygen is flowing out of the prongs. The flow rate via the cannula should not exceed 6 LPM.
   RATIONALE: *Higher rates may cause excess drying of nasal mucosa.*

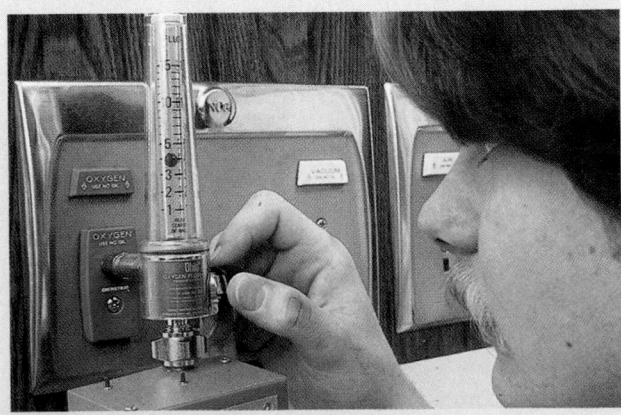

Regulating oxygen flow rate.

In Practice
Nursing Procedure 86-1 (Continued)

6. Insert the prongs into the client's nostrils. Adjust the tubing behind the client's ears, and slide the plastic adapter under the client's chin until he or she is comfortable.
   RATIONALE: *Proper positioning allows unobstructed oxygen flow and eases the client's respirations.*

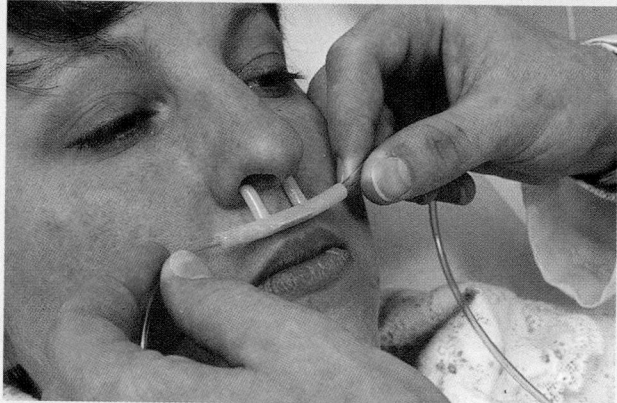

Applying the nasal cannula.

7. Encourage the client to breathe through the nose rather than the mouth.
   RATIONALE: *Breathing through the nose allows the client to inhale more oxygen that will move into*

the trachea and thus is less likely to be exhaled through the mouth.

8. Assess the client's comfort level. Leave the call signal within reach.
   RATIONALE: *Anxiety increases the demand for oxygen.*

9. Dispose of gloves (if used) and wash hands.
   RATIONALE: *Proper glove disposal and handwashing help prevent the spread of infection.*

10. Place "Oxygen in Use" sign at entry into the room.
    RATIONALE: *This sign reminds the client and visitors to use care.*

11. Document the procedure and record the client's reaction.
    RATIONALE: *Documentation provides for coordination of care.*

12. Check the oxygen setup, including the water level in the humidifier, frequently. Clean the cannula and assess the client's nares at least every 8 hours. (*Sterile water must be added when the level falls below the line on the humidification container. Nares may become dry and irritated and require the use of water-soluble lubricant.*)

40% to 60% range, with a liter flow from 6 to 10 LPM. In Practice: Nursing Procedure 86-2 highlights the steps for using the simple mask.

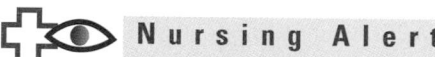

Nursing Alert
The simple mask requires a minimum oxygen flow rate of 6 LPM to prevent carbon dioxide buildup.

Partial-Rebreathing Mask

The *partial-rebreathing mask* (**PRM**) is a low-flow device that can be identified by the presence of a bag and by the absence of valves (Fig. 86-1A). This device can achieve oxygen concentrations between 60% and 90%. In Practice: Nursing Procedure 86-3 highlights the steps involved in providing oxygen with the PRM.

☛ KEY CONCEPT

The PRM is never run at a specific oxygen flow rate; rather, it is run at whatever flow rate is necessary to keep the bag at least one-third inflated. Rationale: The correct flow rate prevents the client from rebreathing his or her own carbon dioxide. *A minimum flow rate of 6 LPM is required with this mask, however.*

Non-Rebreathing Mask

The *non-rebreathing mask* (**NRM**) can be distinguished from the PRM by the presence of valves on the outside of the mask, as well as valves between the mask and bag (see Fig. 86-1B). The NRM can provide oxygen in the 90% to 100% range. Like the PRM, the NRM is never run at a specified liter flow. The bag of the NRM must also remain at least one-third inflated.

To use the NRM, follow the same procedures as for the PRM. Continuous observation of the client's respirations and proper bag deflation is essential. Cardiac monitoring with alarms is strongly recommended.

Because the NRM produces extremely high oxygen concentrations, oxygen toxicity may occur in as little as 72 hours. Never leave the person who is wearing an NRM alone.

Nursing Alert
The NRM is used only in intensive care units or in one-to-one client care situations. *Rationale: Insufficient or interrupted oxygen flow will seal the mask against the person's face, potentially suffocating him or her. The client needs constant monitoring.*

USING THE SIMPLE MASK

Supplies and Equipment

Oxygen mask
Source of oxygen
Gloves, if needed

Steps

1. Check physician's orders.
   RATIONALE: *Oxygen is considered a medication. Checking the orders ensures that the proper flow rate and device are used.*

2. Wash hands and put on gloves, if indicated.
   RATIONALE: *These actions help prevent transmission of microorganisms.*

3. Explain the procedure and the need for oxygen to the client.
   RATIONALE: *The client has a right to know what is happening and why; explanations help decrease anxiety, thereby decreasing oxygen demand.*

4. Attach the humidifier to the threaded outlet of the flowmeter or regulator, and connect the tubing from the simple mask to the nipple outlet on the humidifier.
   RATIONALE: *Proper setup is necessary for proper functioning.*

5. Set the oxygen at the prescribed flow rate.
   RATIONALE: *The oxygen must be flowing before the mask is applied to the client.*

6. To apply the mask, guide the elastic strap over the top of the client's head. Bring the strap down to just below the client's ears.

RATIONALE: *This position will hold the mask most firmly.*

7. Gently, but firmly, pull the strap extensions to center the mask on the client's face with a tight seal.
   RATIONALE: *The seal prevents leaks as much as possible.*

8. Make sure that the client is comfortable.
   RATIONALE: *Comfort helps relieve apprehension, and lowers oxygen need.*

9. Place the call signal within the client's reach before leaving the room.
   RATIONALE: *The client may be unable to call for help with the mask in place.*

10. Remove and properly dispose of gloves; wash hands.
    RATIONALE: *Proper disposal of gloves and handwashing help prevent the spread of infection.*

11. Document the procedure and record the client's reactions.
    RATIONALE: *Documentation provides for communication and continuity of care.*

12. Check periodically for depressed respirations or increased pulse.
    RATIONALE: *These are signs that the oxygen may not be effective or that the client is experiencing further respiratory problems.*

13. Periodically, check for reddened pressure areas under the straps.
    RATIONALE: *The straps, when snug, place pressure on the underlying skin areas.*

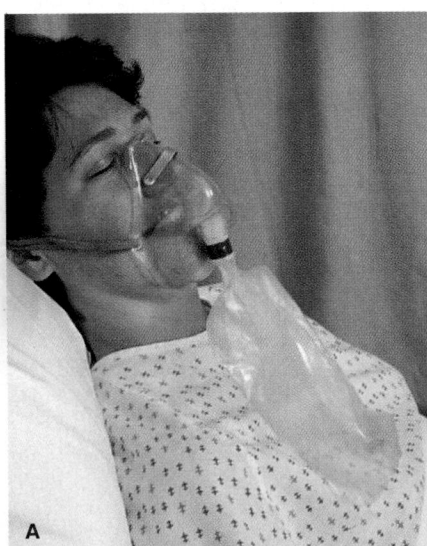 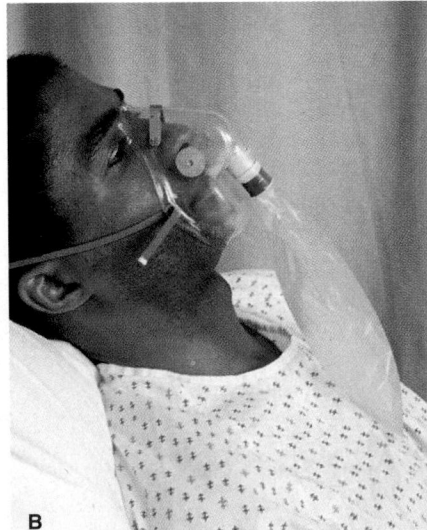 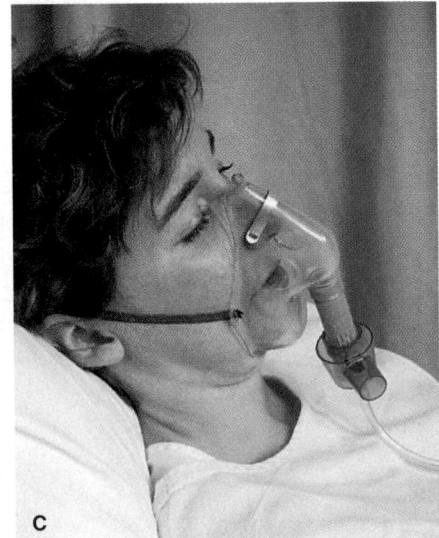

FIGURE 86-1. Types of oxygen masks. (**A**) Partial-rebreathing mask. (**B**) Non-rebreathing mask. (**C**) Venturi mask. (© Ken Kasper)

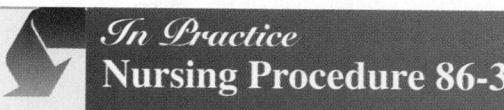

In Practice
Nursing Procedure 86-3

APPLYING THE PARTIAL-REBREATHING MASK

Supplies and Equipment

Mask
Oxygen source
Gloves, if needed

Steps

1. Check the physician's orders.
   RATIONALE: *Oxygen is considered a medication. Checking the orders ensures that the proper flow rate and device are used.*

2. Wash hands and put on gloves, if indicated.
   RATIONALE: *These actions help prevent transmission of microorganisms.*

3. Explain the procedure and need for oxygen to the client.
   RATIONALE: *The client has a right to know what is happening and why; explanations help decrease anxiety.*

4. Do not connect a humidifier, which is unnecessary and often is not recommended.
   RATIONALE: *The humidifier can restrict airflow so much that the device cannot keep up with the client's demand.*

5. Attach the mask to the oxygen source and the set the oxygen flow rate at 12 to 15 LPM. (*Attaching the mask and setting the flow rate must be done before applying the mask to the client to ensure that the equipment is functioning properly.*)

6. Place a finger inside the mask over the hole that leads out of the bag.
   RATIONALE: *Doing so will cause the bag to inflate with oxygen.*

7. Place the mask over the bridge of the client's nose. Bring the mask down over the client's chin. Guide the elastic strap over the client's head and secure it as for the simple mask.
   RATIONALE: *This position will hold the mask most firmly.*

8. Ask the client to take a few breaths, and observe to make sure that the bag deflates with each inspiration, but not to less than one-third full.
   RATIONALE: *If the bag does not inflate and deflate, it is either malfunctioning or incorrectly sealed.*

9. Reduce or raise the flow rate to the minimum possible level at which proper deflation occurs (but not less than 6 LPM).
   RATIONALE: *Regulation of the flow rate is based on the person's breathing, as related to the bag's deflation and inflation.*

10. Make sure that the client is comfortable. Place the call signal within reach before leaving the room.
    RATIONALE: *Comfort decreases the demand for oxygen. Having the call signal within reach enables the client to notify the staff if a problem or need arises.*

11. Remove and dispose of gloves (if used) and wash hands.
    RATIONALE: *Proper glove disposal and hand-washing help prevent the transmission of microorganisms.*

12. Document the procedure, recording the client's reactions.
    RATIONALE: *Documentation provides for communication and continuity of care.*

13. Check the client periodically.
    RATIONALE: *Frequent monitoring helps determine the effectiveness of oxygen therapy.*

Venturi Mask

Of all the facial devices, the high-flow **Venturi mask** provides the most reliable and consistent oxygen enrichment. This mask can be identified by the presence of a hard plastic adapter, with large windows on the adapter's sides (see Fig. 86-1C).

Venturi masks offer specific oxygen concentrations ranging from 24% to 50%. Exact concentrations vary with manufacturers. By drawing room air in through its windows, the Venturi mask mixes a low flow of gas (oxygen) with a high flow of room air. The resulting effect is a high flow of gas to the client with a specific oxygen concentration. Oxygen concentrations can be changed by changing adapters, window openings, or both. Always refer to the specific manufacturer's directions. The directions should specify the oxygen flowmeter setting to use for each desired oxygen percentage. Consult respiratory care personnel with any questions and concerns. In Practice: Nursing Procedure 86-4 highlights the steps for using a Venturi mask.

Nursing Alert

• Do NOT use a humidifier with a Venturi mask. *Rationale: Significant back-pressure may activate the safety pressure valve on the humidifier, causing it to burst. The large amount of room air that a Venturi mask uses will humidify the gas adequately.*

• Ensure that the windows of the Venturi mask remain exposed to room air. Sheets or blankets must not cover the windows or the end of the adapter. *Rationale: Prevent occlusion of the oxygen flow, which would alter the desired oxygen concentration.*

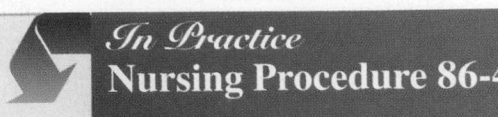

In Practice
Nursing Procedure 86-4

APPLYING THE VENTURI MASK
Supplies and Equipment

Mask
Oxygen source
Gloves, if indicated

Steps

1. Check the physician's orders.
   RATIONALE: *Oxygen is considered a medication. Checking the orders ensures that the proper flow rate and device are used.*

2. Wash hands and put on gloves, if indicated.
   RATIONALE: *These actions help prevent transmission of microorganisms.*

3. Explain the procedure and the need for oxygen to the client.
   RATIONALE: *The client has a right to know what is happening and why; explanations help to decrease anxiety.*

4. Attach the wing nut and tailpiece to the flowmeter's threaded outlet. Then connect the tubing from the Venturi mask to the tailpiece. Attach the mask to the oxygen source.
   RATIONALE: *Properly setting up the device ensures proper function.*

5. Attach the appropriate adapter or set the window openings, in accordance with the manufacturer's directions for the prescribed oxygen percentage.
   RATIONALE: *Using the proper adapter or window opening ensures that the client will receive the prescribed amount of oxygen.*

6. Set the flowmeter to the manufacturer's recommended flow rate for the prescribed oxygen percentage.

RATIONALE: *Using the manufacturer's recommended flow rate is important to make sure that the client receives the appropriate oxygen concentration.*

7. Place the mask over the bridge of the client's nose and then down onto the chin. Guide the elastic strap over the client's head and secure it as you would the simple mask.
   RATIONALE: *This action ensures a snug fit without leaks.*

8. Make sure the client is comfortable. Place the call signal within reach.
   RATIONALE: *Comfort decreases the demand for oxygen. Having the call signal within reach enables the client to notify the staff if a problem or need arises.*

9. Place the bed linen so as not to cover the Venturi adapter.
   RATIONALE: *The linens could plug the windows and disrupt the desired oxygen concentration.*

10. Remove and dispose of gloves, if used; wash hands.
    RATIONALE: *These measures help to prevent transmission of microorganisms.*

11. Document the procedure, recording the client's reactions.
    RATIONALE: *Documentation provides for communication and continuity of care.*

12. Check periodically for depressed respirations and increased pulse.
    RATIONALE: *These are signs that the oxygen may not be effective or that the client is experiencing further respiratory problems.*

13. Check for reddened pressure areas under the straps.
    RATIONALE: *The straps, when snug, place pressure on underlying skin areas.*

Intermittent Positive Pressure Breathing

Intermittent positive pressure breathing (**IPPB**) treatments may be ordered for children or adults who have chronic lung conditions. They are most often ordered for people who have cystic fibrosis. Nurses often administer these treatments, after instruction from respiratory care personnel (eg, respiratory therapists).

The goal of IPPB is to assist the client to breathe more easily by liquefying mucus. The IPPB mechanical device forces room air or oxygen-rich air, combined with medications, deep into the client's airway. The client's lungs expand more completely, making secretions easier to remove. In this way, respiratory disorders are treated and complications are prevented.

In Practice: Nursing Care Guidelines 86-2 provides additional information.

Aerosol Mist Treatment

Aerosol mist treatment refers to suspension of microscopic liquid particles in the air. It serves the following purposes:

- Adds humidity to certain oxygen-delivery devices
- Hydrates thick sputum
- Administers bronchodilator medications to relax bronchioles narrowed by bronchospasm
- Administers anti-inflammatory or anti-asthma medications
- Delivers antibiotics to the lungs to fight infection

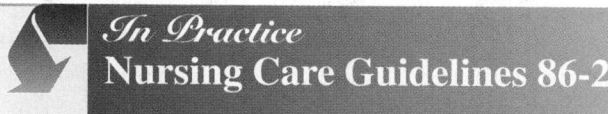

In Practice
Nursing Care Guidelines 86-2

USING INTERMITTENT POSITIVE PRESSURE BREATHING

- Obtain specific instructions for operation of the machine being used.
- Use IPPB only with aerosolized medications.
- Check physician's orders. The pressure may be ordered by the physician.
- Instruct the client to take slow, deep breaths 7 to 10 times per minute. *Rationale: Diaphragmatic breathing causes more air to enter the lungs.*
- Advise the client that each inspiration and expiration should last 2 to 4 seconds. Forceful exhalation is unnecessary and may be harmful. *Rationale: Forcing exhalation may cause lung damage. The client should not hyperventilate.*
- Encourage the client to cough up mucus. Suctioning may be necessary, to ensure that mucus is removed. *Rationale: The client could aspirate mucus, which could cause further obstruction; mucus also provides a culture medium for pathogens.*
- Combine IPPB with postural drainage when instructed, for additional removal of secretions.
- Continue IPPB treatment for 10 to 20 minutes. Consider the treatment finished when the prescribed amount of medications is used up, or if the client cannot tolerate further therapy. *Rationale: The therapy must be continued to be effective.*
- Assess the client carefully for signs of difficulty. *Rationale: Bronchodilators, as well as the treatment itself, can cause tachycardia and dysrhythmias and may lead to dizziness, headache, nausea, or palpitations.*

The *mini-nebulizer* is a hand-held apparatus commonly used for aerosol therapy. People with chronic obstructive pulmonary disease (**COPD**) and asthma commonly use mini-nebulizers to deliver inhaled medications. A mask or mouthpiece apparatus is attached to a chamber containing the prescribed solution (Fig. 86-2). The chamber is attached via tubing to oxygen or a compressed air source. When used, a visible mist appears. The person inhales the medication in the form of mist.

THE CLIENT WHO IS UNABLE TO BREATHE

Manual Breathing Bag

The **manual breathing bag** (sometimes called the *manual resuscitator* or the **Ambu bag** after a popular brand) affords high oxygen concentrations and more effective and sanitary resuscitation than the mouth-to-mouth method (see Chap. 43).

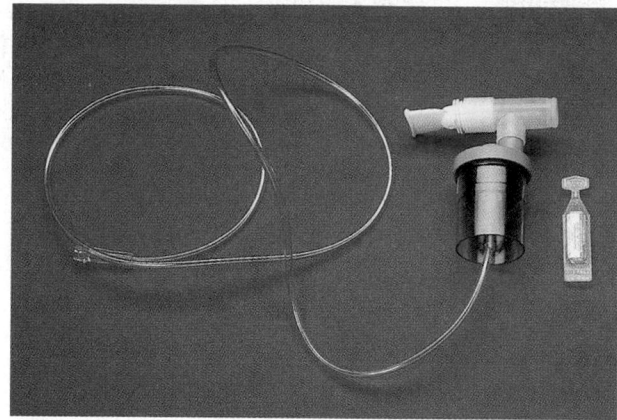

FIGURE 86-2. A mini-nebulizer device with mouthpiece.

The face mask of the manual breathing bag is first placed over the client's nose, then over his or her mouth. Room air may be used. For more oxygenation, the bag can be connected to an oxygen source. The most important considerations are to ensure that the client's airway is *patent* (open) and to start treatment immediately.

Sudden death may occur in acute respiratory failure. Resuscitation must be initiated at once or brain death will result within 4 to 6 minutes. When the nurse first notices that a client is not breathing, immediately initiate respirations and compressions. Call a code for immediate assistance.

Nursing Alert
Do not hyperextend the neck of a person who has experienced a spinal cord injury. *Rationale: Doing so may cause further injury.*

Ventilatory Support

An individual in a state of **ventilatory failure** (unable to breathe adequately alone) needs support from a **mechanical ventilator.** A mechanical ventilator (sometimes called a **respirator**) is a machine that forces air into the lungs.

Negative Pressure Ventilator

The *negative pressure ventilator* encloses all or part of the body. By lowering pressure around the chest, it causes the chest to expand and air to flow into the lungs. Because negative pressure ventilators (such as the iron lung) are cumbersome and restrict access to the client, they are seldom used today. A small device of this type may be used in the home, however.

Positive Pressure Ventilator

The *positive pressure ventilator* pushes air into the lungs through a circuit that joins the machine and the client. Positive pressure ventilators are classified as *volume* or *pressure* ventilators. They are further classified as to whether they assist in or control breathing.

- *Volume ventilator:* Delivers a consistent, preset volume of air with each breath, ensuring adequate breathing.

- *Pressure ventilator:* Pushes air into the lungs until a preset pressure is achieved. (The pressure ventilator is not always as effective as the volume ventilator.)
- *Assisted-breath ventilator:* Helps support clients who are breathing on their own but inadequately; this support may be necessary to avoid ventilatory failure or hypoxia.
- *Controlled-breath ventilator:* Breathes for the client, forcing a breath at set time intervals. (Controlled-breath ventilators prevent the person from controlling his or her own breathing.)

Care for the Client Receiving Mechanical Ventilation

A client is placed on a mechanical ventilator when he or she is unable to move enough air into and out of the lungs. Clients may require mechanical ventilation in acute situations, such as surgery, trauma, or drug overdose. Some clients require chronic mechanical ventilation due to neuromuscular disease (eg, spinal cord injury) or lung disease (eg, emphysema). Most clients need ventilatory support for short periods and are withdrawn from it as their condition improves. The respiratory care department usually provides technical and respiratory care to persons on mechanical ventilators. Consult respiratory care staff for any questions about care or operation of a ventilator.

Assisting the Client on a Mechanical Ventilator. Assist the client who is on a ventilator to turn from side to side at least every 2 hours. *Rationale: Turning helps to improve lung function and to prevent immobility disorders, such as pressure ulcers or thrombophlebitis.* Many of these clients are on special airflow beds. They may require suctioning of lung secretions that they are unable to mobilize. Carefully observe any secretions that the client expectorates or that are suctioned.

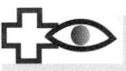 **N u r s i n g   A l e r t**
Report any blood in a client's mucus immediately.

Weaning the Client From the Ventilator. As the client's condition improves and he or she begins to breathe without assistance, the number of positive pressure breaths is gradually reduced. The person who has been on a ventilator for some time may need gradual removal (*weaning*) from it. Weaning can be done in several ways, depending on the situation. Some people have a difficult time breathing after having been on a ventilator. The problem may result from a true physical inability to breathe. However, it also may have an emotional basis (ventilator dependency and fear). These clients need emotional support and encouragement. If a client has required a high degree of ventilatory and oxygen support, he or she may show signs of adult respiratory distress syndrome (**ARDS**), which may make weaning more difficult. (Chapter 85 describes this frequently fatal condition.)

One strategy to facilitate weaning from the ventilator is *synchronized intermittent mandatory ventilation* (**SIMV**). SIMV gives the client a preset number of mechanical breaths at a certain volume. In addition, the client can take as many breaths at his or her own volume as desired. With progress, machine-controlled breaths are decreased in volume or rate. Thus, the client takes on more work of breathing gradually, and progresses to breathing without mechanical assistance.

Another ventilatory mode is called *pressure support ventilation* (**PSV**). In PSV, constant pressure is applied as the person inspires, which lessens the inspiratory effort or work needed. *Continuous positive airway pressure* (**CPAP**) allows inspiratory and expiratory airway pressures to be maintained above atmospheric pressure. CPAP helps keep the client's lungs inflated and tends to improve lung function, even though breathing is spontaneous.

☞ Key Concept

Clients on ventilators are usually sedated, which will decrease their responsiveness and ability to communicate. Sedation may also depress respiratory effort. In addition, artificial airways prevent clients from speaking. Be sensitive to the needs of these clients. For clients on long-term ventilation, use various communication aids (eg, chalk board, letter-pointing board, Magic Slate) and continue to talk to the clients, explaining everything that is being done.

Tracheostomy

Insertion of the Tracheostomy Tube

A **tracheostomy** tube may be inserted directly into a person's trachea as a lifesaving measure when there is sudden blockage of the mouth or throat. A tracheostomy tube may also be a permanent breathing orifice (opening) for the person who has had throat surgery, or for anyone who requires long-term mechanical ventilation. Nurses in intensive care units or emergency departments may be asked to assist physicians with the tracheostomy ("trach") procedure. Most often, an endotracheal airway is inserted first and the person is transported to the operating room for this sterile procedure.

The tracheostomy tube has three parts: an outer tube (*outer cannula*), sometimes with a cuff (an inflatable attachment designed to occlude the space between the trachea walls and the tube for mechanical ventilation), an inner tube (*inner cannula*), and a solid round-ended obturator (*guide*). The physician inserts the obturator into the outer cannula. He or she then inserts the outer cannula and obturator, as one unit, into the client's tracheal opening. When the outer cannula is in place, the physician withdraws the obturator and replaces it with the inner cannula (tube), which is locked into position. Cloth tape attached to each side of the outer tube and tied behind the neck holds the apparatus firmly in position. A cuff is inflated with air. In Practice: Nursing Procedure 86-5 outlines steps to take when assisting at a tracheostomy procedure.

Care of the Tracheostomy Tube

If a client accidentally coughs out the cannula (which rarely happens), a physician or nurse trained in the procedure must replace the cannula immediately. An extra tracheostomy set should remain in the client's room at all times, in case of emergency.

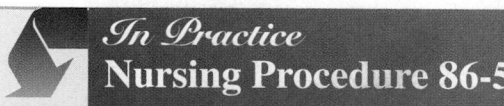

In Practice
Nursing Procedure 86-5

ASSISTING AT A TRACHEOSTOMY
Supplies and Equipment

Sterile, disposable tracheostomy tray
Local anesthetic, such as procaine hydrochloride (Novocain) or lidocaine (Xylocaine)
Syringes and small-gauge needles
Sterile and clean gloves for physician and nurse
Strong light
Emergency breathing apparatus (such as manual breathing bag)
Source of oxygen
Source of suction

Steps

1. Set up the equipment, which usually comes as a disposable trach tray.
   RATIONALE: *Knowing what is supposed to be on the tray allows the nurse to anticipate other needs for the procedure.*

2. Explain the procedure to the client.
   RATIONALE: *Explanations can help the client cooperate and relax.*

3. Put on clean gloves. The physician will don a gown and sterile gloves.
   RATIONALE: *Gloving helps prevent transmission of microorganisms and cross-contamination.*

4. Hold the client's head during the procedure, if requested by the physician. If necessary, place a folded towel behind the client's neck to hyperextend it and to expose the surgical site.

RATIONALE: *The site must be immobilized during the procedure.*

5. Provide strong emotional support.
   RATIONALE: *The client must lie very still throughout this frightening procedure. A lack of oxygen may cause extreme apprehension.*

6. Provide oxygen through an endotracheal tube while the tracheostomy is being done. This is most often done using a manual-breathing bag.
   RATIONALE: *The client needs to maintain an adequate supply of oxygen to his or her tissues.*

7. Dispose of equipment following Standard Precautions. Dispose of gloves. Wash your hands.
   RATIONALE: *Proper disposal of equipment and adherence to Standard Precautions help prevent the spread of infection.*

8. Record pertinent information about what was done and by whom.
   RATIONALE: *Documentation provides for communication and continuity of care.*

9. After the procedure, assess the site for swelling. Check to see if the client has difficulty swallowing or is bleeding.
   RATIONALE: *Any of these situations could impede respiration.*

10. Make sure the individual is now able to breathe freely.
    RATIONALE: *A patent airway is the purpose of a tracheostomy.*

Keep all equipment for cleaning and caring for the tube at the client's bedside. Each facility has a specific routine for tracheostomy care. For the person with a temporary tracheostomy tube, a humidifier must artificially warm and moisten the air to be breathed. *Rationale: In normal breathing, the action of the nose and throat warms and cleans air. Humidification helps to prevent secretions from becoming dry and tenacious.* If a person has a permanent tracheostomy, the body becomes adjusted to room air.

Suctioning should be done using a new catheter each time with strict sterile technique. Typically, sterile gloves and a sterile container for the solution are found in the suctioning kit.

The client needs continued reassurance. *Rationale: Until he or she is accustomed to breathing through the tube, the client may be very apprehensive, easily upset by coughing, and concerned about being unable to communicate verbally.* Keep a call light within the client's reach at all times. *Rationale: This person cannot talk or call out for help.* Provide the client with

some means of communicating (eg, Magic Slate, talking board, or pad and pencil). Sometimes, a client can whisper into a stethoscope for the nurse to hear and understand him or her.

Assess for signs of respiratory difficulty, and take immediate action if respiratory distress occurs. Suctioning may be needed. In Practice: Nursing Procedure 86-6 discusses tracheostomy suctioning and care. Follow the facility's protocols appropriately.

Home Care of the Mechanically Ventilated Client

Clients today are able to receive mechanical ventilation at home. Mechanical ventilation and the care of the client on a ventilator must be ordered by a physician. Continuous monitoring and daily care in the home, however, may be provided by the person themselves, family members, or other caregivers. This care is provided in conjunction with the physician, registered nurse, licensed practical/vocational nurse,

In Practice
Nursing Procedure 86-6

SUCTIONING AND PROVIDING TRACHEOSTOMY CARE

Supplies and Equipment

Tracheostomy suctioning kit containing the following
 sterile supplies:
 Gloves
 Suction catheter
 Basins or containers
 Sterile normal saline
 Portable or wall suction apparatus
 Sterile tracheostomy dressing
 Twill tape or Velcro trach ties
 Hydrogen peroxide
 Sterile gauze pads
 Disposable inner cannula (optional)
Goggles and gown (optional)
Clean towel or plastic drape (optional)

Steps

1. Check the physician's order.
   RATIONALE: *An order is needed for suctioning.
   The order also may indicate special considerations that need to be implemented for
   this client.*

2. Gather supplies.
   RATIONALE: *Organization facilitates accurate skill
   performance.*

3. Explain the procedure to the client.
   RATIONALE: *Providing information fosters the
   client's cooperation.*

4. Wash your hands.
   RATIONALE: *Handwashing helps prevent the spread
   of infection.*

5. Adjust bed to a comfortable working height.
   RATIONALE: *Bed at proper height prevents back
   strain.*

6. Assist the conscious client to a semi- or high-
   Fowler's position. Place the unconscious client
   on his or her side, facing the nurse.
   RATIONALE: *Upright positions promote drainage
   and prevent airway obstruction.*

7. Place a towel or drape across the client's chest.
   Put on a gown or goggles (optional). Turn on
   suction to the appropriate level. Put on gloves.
   RATIONALE: *Gown, goggles, and gloves act as
   barriers and protect the nurse from the client's
   secretions; the towel or drape protects the client.*

8. Prepare the suction equipment:
   a. Open the sterile tracheostomy suctioning kit and
      cleaning supplies on the bedside tray or table.
   b. Pick up the sterile container, open it, and pour
      sterile saline into it.
   c. Put on sterile gloves.

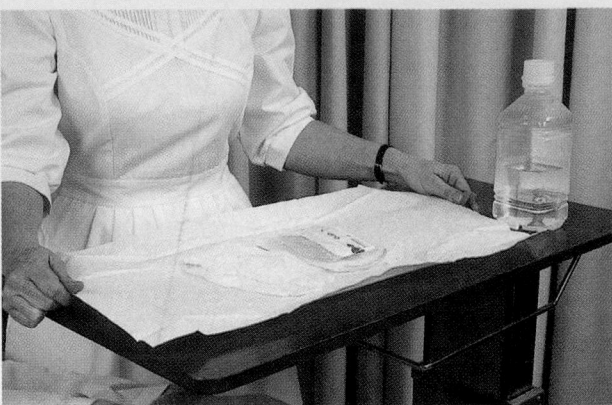

Opening the sterile suctioning kit.

   d. Pick up the sterile suction catheter with your
      dominant hand.
   e. Use your nondominant hand to connect the
      wall or portable suction catheter tubing to the
      sterile suction catheter.
   RATIONALE: *Surgical asepsis decreases the potential for introducing organisms into the client's
   respiratory tract. The nondominant hand is
   unclean after it touches the nonsterile tubing.*

9. Dip the suction catheter into the basin with sterile
   saline. Use the thumb on your nondominant hand
   to occlude the suction port.
   RATIONALE: *Occluding the port applies suction and
   ensures that equipment is functioning.*

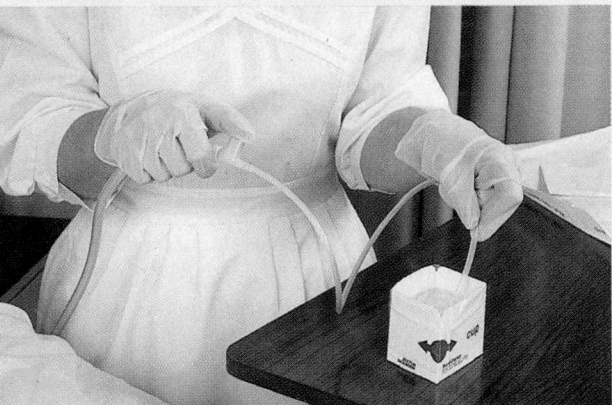

Dipping the suction catheter into the saline solution.

10. Remove the oxygen delivery system with the non-
    dominant hand.
    RATIONALE: *Doing so facilitates tracheostomy tube
    suctioning while maintaining the sterility of the
    dominant hand.*

11. Use the dominant hand to insert the catheter
    into the trachea 4 to 5 inches or until the client
    coughs. Do not apply suction while inserting the
    catheter.

RATIONALE: *Applying suction while inserting the catheter may damage mucosa in the trachea and promote hypoxia.*

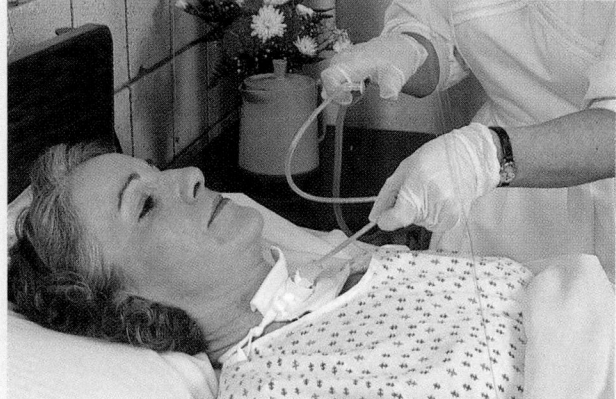

Inserting the suction catheter into the tracheostomy.

12. Occlude the suction port with the nondominant thumb while rotating and removing the catheter. Suctioning should not continue for longer than 10-second intervals.
    RATIONALE: *Rotating the catheter provides effective removal of secretions from the trachea. Limiting suctioning to 10-second intervals reduces the development of hypoxia.*

13. Dip the catheter into saline solution while applying the suction. Repeat the suctioning procedure if necessary. Allow 1 minute between suctioning. Reapply the oxygen delivery system while waiting to continue the procedure.
    RATIONALE: *Saline clears the catheter. Intervals between suctioning reduce development of hypoxia. Reapplying the oxygen system maintains the oxygen supply.*

14. Before removing gloves, cleanse the cannula. If the inner cannula is disposable, remove it and replace it with a clean cannula. For the replaceable cannula:
    a. Unlock the cannula and carefully remove it.
    b. Hold it over the sterile basin.
    c. Rinse it with sterile saline.
    d. Gently replace the inner cannula and lock it in place.
    RATIONALE: *Rinsing with saline or replacing the cannula prevents accumulation of tracheal secretions.*

15. Cleanse around the tracheostomy stoma and under the tracheostomy tube faceplate with sterile cotton-tipped swabs dipped in hydrogen peroxide.
    RATIONALE: *Hydrogen peroxide aids in the removal of accumulated and encrusted secretions.*

16. Rinse the area using cotton-tipped swabs moistened in normal saline.
    RATIONALE: *Normal saline removes hydrogen peroxide and additional secretions.*

17. Dry the area with a dry, sterile, gauze pad.
    RATIONALE: *Moisture provides a medium for growth of bacteria.*

18. Change the tracheostomy tube tape if necessary:
    a. Have an assistant hold the tracheostomy tube in place with a sterile hand. If unassisted, leave the soiled tapes in place until new ones are inserted and secured.
    RATIONALE: *Keeping the tracheostomy tube secure while changing the tape prevents the client from accidentally coughing up the tube.*
    b. Pass the ends of the tape through the opening on the faceplate and bring them behind the client's neck to the other opening on the opposite side of the faceplate.
    c. Insert tape through the opening, pull securely, and tie or Velcro into place.
    d. If necessary, remove the soiled tape.

19. Place a sterile tracheostomy dressing under the faceplate. Tegaderm also may be applied under the gauze.
    RATIONALE: *Sterile dressing absorbs drainage.*

20. Reattach the oxygen delivery system over the tracheostomy tube.
    RATIONALE: *Reattaching the oxygen delivery system provides for adequate oxygenation.*

21. Remove gloves by pulling the glove over the suction catheter; also remove goggles and gown (if worn). Reposition the client. Lower the bed.
    RATIONALE: *These measures ensure the client's safety and comfort.*

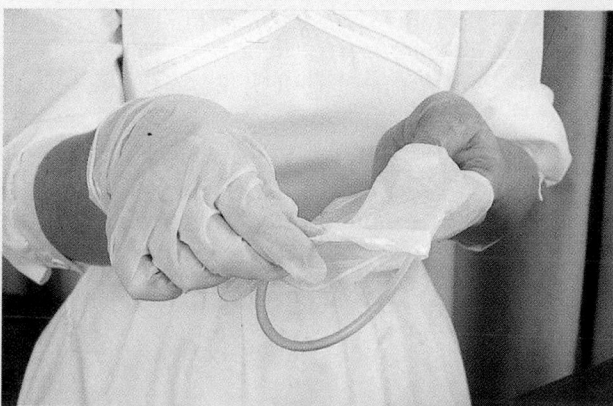

Removing gloves.

22. Wash hands.
    RATIONALE: *Handwashing helps prevent the spread of microorganisms.* (*continued*)

In Practice
Nursing Procedure 86-6 (Continued)

23. Dispose of equipment according to your agency's policy.
    RATIONALE: *Proper disposal helps prevent transmission of microorganisms.*

24. Document the suctioning procedure, nature and amount of secretions, and the client's response. Record respiratory assessments following suctioning procedure.

RATIONALE: *Documentation provides for communication and coordination of care.*

25. Replace bed to its lowest level. Ensure that side rails are up and that the call light is within the client's easy reach.
    RATIONALE: *These measures ensure the client's safety.*

---

respiratory therapist, and other home healthcare team members as necessary. The client and caregivers must be able to recognize abnormalities or problems so that prompt attention and intervention can be initiated. All healthcare team members involved with the client's care must be able to do the same, within the level of the individual's training. Be sure to

include all aspects of care that are pertinent to this client in the nursing care plan.

Regardless of whether the client is in a facility or at home, the nursing process (see Chaps. 33–37, Chap. 85) is used while caring for the client who is receiving mechanical ventilation. See In Practice: The Nursing Process 86-1.

In Practice
Nursing Process 86-1

THE CLIENT RECEIVING MECHANICAL VENTILATION

Assessment Priorities
- Observe client's ventilator settings and verify with physician's orders
- Assess stability of tracheostomy tube
- Assess level of secretions
- Observe chest motion and auscultate lung sounds
- Check pulse oximeter reading (if available)
- Assess level of consciousness
- Assess skin color, pallor, capillary refill
- Assess client's level of comfort
- Ensure that an emergency manual breathing bag, extra tracheostomy tubes, 10-cc syringe, tracheostomy tape, dressing supplies, and normal saline are at the bedside.
- Ensure that there is a list of emergency phone numbers for the physician, local hospital emergency department, mechanical ventilation equipment dealers, and family/other caregivers for the client.

Possible Nursing Diagnoses
- Ineffective breathing pattern related to mechanical ventilation
- Impaired gas exchange related to changes in the alveolar capillary membrane
- Risk for Disuse Syndrome related to effects of immobility

Planning
Design a plan of care with the client and family to achieve the following general goals:

- Client will demonstrate adequate levels of oxygenation
- Client will remain free of complications associated with immobility
- Family will demonstrate measures to care for ventilator and tracheostomy
- Client and family will demonstrate measures to prevent complications associated with mechanical ventilation and immobility

Implementation
- Observe respiratory rate and depth regularly because increased work of breathing adds to fatigue. Client may be fighting the ventilator.
- Observe for tube misplacement. Tape tube securely in place.
- Inspect chest wall for symmetry of movement. Asymmetry may indicate pneumothorax or hemothorax.
- Maintain ventilator settings as ordered.
- Measure client's tidal volume and vital capacity, which indicate the volume of air moving into and out of the lungs.
  Elevate the head of the bed or help client into a chair. This position facilitates diaphragm contraction and helps prevent aspiration.
- Assess the client for pain because it may prevent him or her from coughing and deep breathing. Medicate for pain as needed.
- Monitor ABG test results and pulse oximeter readings.
- Assess level of consciousness, listlessness, or irritability because these signs may indicate hypoxia.

In Practice
Nursing Process 86-1 *(Continued)*

- Assess skin color and capillary refill to determine that there is adequate flow of oxygen to tissues.
- Observe for obstruction. Suction as needed because there may be a mucous plug and inadequate ventilation.
- Turn and reposition client every 1–2 hours, which helps to adequately perfuse and ventilate all lung lobes.
- Assess for psychosocial alterations. Assess for anxiety, depression, inability to communicate, isolation, and change in family dynamics.
- Observe skin integrity for pressure ulcers and use pressure-relief mattress.
- Maintain muscle strength with range-of-motion exercises—this client as at high risk for developing contractures.

Evaluation
Determine the adequacy of the plan of care by evaluating the client's achievement of the preceding goals.

If the client is unable to meet key goals, modify the plan. Key evaluative criteria include:

- Client demonstrates effective breathing pattern techniques with ventilator.
- Client exhibits signs of adequate gas exchange, including oxygen saturation levels within normal limits for client.
- Client is free of ventilatory obstructions.
- Tracheostomy tube remains secure.
- The client will remain comfortable.
- Level of consciousness will remain stable.
- Skin color and capillary refill will remain within normal limits.
- Client will make feelings known.
- Skin will remain intact with no ulcers or sores; muscle strength will be maintained with no contractures noted.

Nursing Alert
Making and implementing ventilator changes in the home care setting may take longer than in the hospital or acute care setting.

➤ STUDENT SYNTHESIS

Key Points

- Oxygen is essential to life. Without oxygen, a person will die in a matter of minutes. Oxygen administration can assist a person to breathe or can totally support life.
- Therapeutic oxygen is like a medication. It requires a physician's prescription and has associated safety considerations that must be understood and followed.
- Oxygen supports combustion: take great care when using oxygen because a fire can start and be explosive.
- Oxygen is administered to support breathing using several devices or methods: nasal cannula, simple mask, partial-rebreathing mask, non-rebreathing mask, Venturi mask, intermittent positive pressure breathing, and aerosol mist.
- Manual breathing bags, ventilators, and tracheostomy tubes are methods of assisting the person to breathe who cannot do so on his or her own.
- The nurse works with the respiratory care professionals in oxygen administration.

Critical Thinking Exercises

1. One of your clients needs assistance in breathing. He is receiving oxygen by nasal cannula. Describe teaching for this client. What teaching measures would you address with visitors? With the client's family?
2. Your client needs a tracheostomy. She is unclear as to what this procedure means and entails. How would you describe the tracheostomy procedure to the client? What are your nursing responsibilities during the procedure?

NCLEX-Style Review Questions

1. Oxygen sources for people who use oxygen in the home differ from sources used in healthcare facilities. Examples of oxygen sources available for home use are:
   a. Wall outlets and oxygen cylinders
   b. Oxygen cylinders, strollers, and concentrators
   c. Wall outlets and oxygen strollers
   d. Hyperbaric chambers
2. The hyperbaric chamber provides high-pressure oxygenation. It is used in the treatment of all of the following EXCEPT:
   a. Air or gas embolism, carbon monoxide poisoning, gas gangrene
   b. Crush injuries or traumatic ischemias, skin grafts and flaps
   c. To deliver chemotherapy in certain types of cancer
   d. Thermal burns and chronic osteomyelitis

3. Ventilators are classified as either positive pressure or negative pressure ventilators. Which of the following statements are true:
   a. Positive pressure ventilators enclose all or part of the body.
   b. Positive pressure ventilators pull air into the lungs.
   c. Negative pressure ventilators increase the pressure around the chest, causing the chest to expand and air to flow into the lungs.
   d. Positive pressure ventilators can deliver a consistent volume of air with each breath, a preset pressure of air, or total breathing for the client at set intervals.

4. Synchronized intermittent mandatory ventilation is often used to wean the client from a ventilator. Which of the following is true of SIMV:
   a. The number of positive pressure breaths at a certain volume are gradually increased as the client's condition improves.
   b. The client has fewer opportunities to control his or her own breathing.
   c. With progress, the machine-controlled breaths are increased in volume or rate.
   d. The client takes on more work of breathing and gradually progresses to breathing without mechanical assistance.

5. All of the following are true for the client who is on a mechanical ventilator EXCEPT:
   a. Once the client goes home, anyone can independently care for the person in the home if the client so wishes.
   b. Mechanical ventilation, and the care of the client on a ventilator, must be ordered by a physician.
   c. The recognition of abnormal status must be acted upon in a consistent manner, within the level of training.
   d. The nursing process is used while caring for the client who is receiving mechanical ventilation.

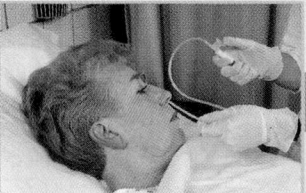

CHAPTER

87

Digestive Disorders

LEARNING OBJECTIVES

1. Identify eight common LFT.
2. Describe preparation that the client needs to complete for an upper and lower GI series using barium contrast medium.
3. Discuss nursing considerations for endoscopic procedures.
4. Describe nursing considerations for care of the client with a GI tube.
5. Define and differentiate between enteral tube feedings and TPN.
6. Differentiate between an ostomy fecal diversion and a continent fecal diversion.
7. Identify at least five major nursing considerations related to care of an ostomy.
8. Describe the nurse's role in caring for the client with stomatitis.
9. Discuss three nursing considerations related to the care of GERD.
10. Discuss three nursing considerations related to the care of peptic ulcers.
11. Define and differentiate at least three nursing considerations related to the care of IBS and IBD.
12. Describe risk factors for colorectal cancer.
13. Identify the types and causes of the major types of hepatitis.
14. Identify at least three nursing concerns related to a client who is obese, anorexic, or bulimic.

NEW TERMINOLOGY

anastomosis	hernia
ascites	ileostomy
cachexia	insufflation
caries	intussusception
colostomy	melena
dumping syndrome	paralytic ileus
dyspepsia	peritonitis
eructation	polypectomy
evisceration	steatorrhea
fistula	stoma
gastrectomy	tenesmus
gastroscopy	volvulus

ACRONYMS

EGD	HDV	LES
ERCP	HEV	LFT
ET	HGV	NG
GERD	IBD	PICC
HAV	IBS	PPI
HBV	LEP	TPN
HCV		

The major organs of digestion are those within the gastro-intestinal (GI) tract, which begins with the mouth and ends with the anus. The accessory organs of digestion include the liver, gallbladder, and pancreas. The digestive system is responsible for digestion (mechanical and chemical) of food, absorption of nutrients and vitamins, and elimination of waste materials. Chapter 26 presents a detailed review of anatomy and physiology of the GI system.

Digestive disorders can be due to structural malfunction, infection, inflammation, or disease. The physician who specializes in treating digestive disorders is called a *gastroenterologist*, although specialists in internal medicine also treat clients with GI conditions. GI tests and procedures may be done in an outpatient setting or a clinic called a GI lab. The *enterostomal therapist* (ET) is a nurse who assists people with learning to care for surgically adapted openings, called ostomies, into the stomach (*gastrostomy*), intestine (*ileostomy*), or colon (*colostomy*).

DIAGNOSTIC TESTS

Laboratory Studies

Laboratory studies used to diagnose digestive disorders include blood tests, urine studies, and stool tests. Urine tests, such as urine bilirubin and urobilinogen, can assess liver function. Urine amylase and lipase levels also may increase in pancreatitis. In Practice: Nursing Assessment 87-1 lists important considerations when assessing digestive status.

Blood Tests
Blood studies are performed to assess, diagnose, and monitor the digestive system. The healthcare provider will start with generalized tests such as a CBC, UA, and routine chemistries to obtain basic data; more specialized tests including carcinoembryonic antigen (CEA), serum cholesterol, and triglycerides may then be ordered.

Liver function tests (**LFT**) are valuable as indicators of liver function and for assessing trends of abnormal liver processes. When the physician orders LFT, check your facility's laboratory manual to determine exactly which tests will be included. Some of the most commonly ordered LFT include:

- Albumin
- Total protein
- Alkaline phosphatase
- Serum γ-glutamyl transpeptidase (GGT)
- Serum aminotransferase (AST); formerly serum glutamic oxaloacetic transaminase (SGOT)
- Serum alanine aminotransferase (ALT); formerly serum glutamate pyruvate transaminase (SGPT)
- Lactate dehydrogenase
- Cholesterol
- Triglyceride levels
- Prothrombin

Appendix C contains normal reference values.

Hepatitis profiles are done to identify the presence of antibodies or antigens for the hepatitis A, B, or C virus. Pancreatic enzyme tests such as serum amylase and lipase may be ordered to detect inflammation or disease of the pancreas, or obstruction of surrounding ducts.

Stool Tests
Stool tests are performed to detect the presence of pathogens, parasites, eggs (ova), blood, and fat. A culture and sensitivity study may be ordered for suspected pathogenic causes of severe diarrhea such as *Salmonella, Shigella dysenteriae, Staphylococcus aureus,* or *Clostridium difficile.*

Fecal occult blood testing is used to test for *occult* (not visible) blood. The Hematest is the most inexpensive and simplest test used to detect occult blood in the stool; the client can perform the test at home or the nurse or physician can perform the test in the office, clinic, or hospital. HemoQuant stool testing not only determines the presence of blood, but also quantifies the amount (*fecal hemoglobin*). The HemoQuant can be done only in the laboratory. Thus, it is slower and less convenient than the Hematest. Each method of testing has its own manufacturer's instructions that must be followed to obtain accurate results. The procedure for collecting a stool specimen is discussed at Chapter 52.

Radiographic Evaluations

Radiography (x-ray) is commonly ordered in addition to laboratory tests to diagnose and assess digestive disorders, including suspected abscesses, bowel obstructions and perforations, or intestinal paralysis (**paralytic ileus**).

Angiography and arteriography may be done to evaluate vascular structures, and computed tomography (CT) scans are used to identify various abnormalities or tumors. Nuclear uptake scans using a radionuclide such as technetium 99 (Tc-99m sulfide) will show size, structure, and abnormalities of the stomach, liver, and hepatobiliary system. Abdominal ultrasounds may be performed to visualize the liver, gallbladder and biliary system, pancreas, and abdomen. Ultrasound can identify gallstones or abdominal tumors. This test is becoming the preferred diagnostic tool, especially to rule out gallstones, pancreatic cysts, and cancerous tumors. No preparation, other than nothing by mouth (NPO) after midnight, is required for ultrasound.

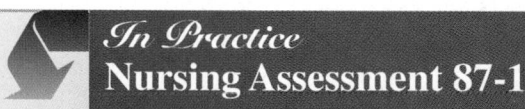

In Practice
Nursing Assessment 87-1

DIGESTIVE DISORDERS
Nutritional history
Recent weight gain or loss
Ability to purchase, prepare, and store food
Ability to chew and swallow
Any symptoms of digestive disorders
Pattern of bowel elimination

Barium Studies

Two barium studies used to visualize the GI tract are the upper GI series and the lower GI series. Before the start of any procedure using barium, chest and/or abdominal ultrasounds and CT scans must be completed; barium may interfere with the visualization of the GI structures.

Upper GI series. An *upper GI series,* often called a *barium swallow,* is conducted for examination of the esophagus, stomach, and duodenum. A radiopaque or contrast material such as barium or dye is used to view the contours of the GI tract. Prior to the start of the procedure, the client will be given a drink containing barium, which is thick and chalky. Several flavored commercial preparations are available such as Gastrografin.

To examine structures under study, fluoroscopy, a type of x-ray examination, is used to visualize the contrast material. The outline of the esophagus, stomach, sphincters, and intestinal tract may be observed as the barium progresses. After 1 to 2 hours, x-ray films are taken of the small bowel. The rate at which the barium travels through the small intestine is significant in some diseases of the GI tract.

Lower GI Series. A *lower GI series,* or *barium enema,* is given to examine the contours of the lower bowel. The barium preparation is given rectally by enema. The client may worry about being able to retain the solution. Tell the client that he or she will have a chance to go to the bathroom immediately after the procedure. One more x-ray film will be taken after the client expels the solution.

Nursing Considerations. Client teaching is important before and after barium studies. The client must understand the appropriate dietary and bowel preparations and should know what the procedure entails. Generally, the entire GI tract is prepared, emptying it as thoroughly as possible, using liquid diets for several days before the procedure, and using enemas or cathartic drinks the day before and/or the morning of the procedure. After the procedure, check with the x-ray department to make sure that the GI series has been completed before giving the client anything to eat or drink. In Practice: Nursing Care Guidelines 87-1 contains additional information about nursing care in barium studies.

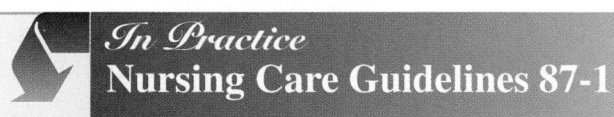

In Practice
Nursing Care Guidelines 87-1

PROVIDING CARE FOR BARIUM STUDIES

- An informed consent is required for any invasive procedure.
- Observe the client's stools following the procedure.
- Note if the client passes the barium (will be white and chalky).
- Observe for constipation.
- Watch for signs of bowel obstruction.
- Give laxatives or stool softeners as ordered.

A substance commonly used to cleanse the bowel for many procedures is called GoLYTELY. It contains electrolytes that cause complete bowel evacuation. The client is required to drink several quarts of this mixture in divided doses the evening before the procedure. This is commonly called the "bowel prep." Tell the client to mix the solution beforehand, carefully following the package instructions. The solution is usually easiest to drink if it is chilled first. Caution the client to be close to a bathroom during the preparation process. With GoLYTELY, the nurse should instruct the client to eat a light supper (some physicians require clear liquids) in the evening and then to be NPO, except for the bowel prep, after supper. The client may brush the teeth, but tell him or her not to drink any water.

If the client is unable to drink the large amount of fluid required for GoLYTELY, an alternative is Fleet Phospho Soda or magnesium citrate. This procedure involves drinking about two thirds of a glass of fluid in the evening and again in the morning. This preparation is considered a purgative because it forces evacuation of the bowel. It is contraindicated in clients with abdominal pain, heart disorders, impaired renal function, rectal or anal lesions, or who are pregnant. This preparation removes electrolytes and can cause dehydration.

Cholecystogram

A *cholecystogram* (gallbladder series) may be ordered to show the outline of the gallbladder and any existing gallstones. Prior to a cholecystogram, it is important that the client completes pre-procedure preparations, which include:

- Eating a fat-free supper the night before the x-ray study.
- Taking a radiopaque dye by mouth. The liver excretes the dye into the bile, which then goes to the gallbladder. The physician will specify the time it is to be taken.
- Eating nothing for the next 12 hours (after taking the radiopaque dye), which allows time for the dye to concentrate in the gallbladder. The client may have water until bedtime, after which he or she is NPO.
- Stopping smoking and chewing gum, which cause premature emptying of the dye from the gallbladder.
- Administering an enema in the morning, if ordered.

If the client vomits before the test, postponement may be necessary because he or she may have lost some of the dye, rendering the test inaccurate. Provide a high-fat meal sometime after the initial x-ray study, if ordered. Another x-ray film may be obtained as indicated to show how well the gallbladder is emptying.

Endoscopic Procedures

Endoscopy is direct visualization of the body's interior through the intestinal tract using specialized instruments called *endoscopes.* Endoscopes are soft, flexible tubes containing specially designed fiberoptic strands connected to a light source. The fiberoptic scope (*fiberscope*) transmits light rays so that a clear image of the internal tissue is directed back up the scope to the lens and eyepiece, which the physician (*endoscopist*) manipulates. This technology is known as fiberoptic illumination (Fig. 87-1). The examination is usually performed in an endoscopy department by a trained endoscopist. He or she may be a gastroenterologist, surgeon, or internist. No incisions are made for routine endoscopy procedures.

The introduction of video imaging allows viewing of internal tissue on a monitor or television-like screen. The physician, nurse, assistant, and even the client can see inside the intestinal tract. Excellent colored photography is possible. It can document a client's condition and healing process. Rapid advancement of endoscopic technology and its related equipment makes endoscopy a safe and effective diagnostic and treatment tool.

These procedures allow identification of growths, strictures, ulcers, or inflammatory disease. In addition to identification of abnormal conditions, endoscopy may be used to *biopsy* or *excise* (cut out) polyps or tumors; *dilate* (stretch) strictured areas; localize and stop active hemorrhaging or bleeding; and remove or crush biliary stones. In addition, palliative measures, such as stent and feeding tube placement, can ease the symptoms caused by a tumor obstructing the biliary tract and allow nutritional support to a debilitated client.

The endoscope will pass through the client's mouth or rectum. However, different types of fiberoptic scopes are used, depending on the part of the digestive tract to be examined. The most common types of endoscopy include:

- *Esophagoscopy* for direct visualization of the esophagus
- *Esophagogastroduodenoscopy* (**EGD**) for direct visualization of the esophagus, stomach, and duodenum
- *Endoscopic retrograde cholangiopancreatography* (**ERCP**), an extended version of the EGD plus direct visualization of the ducts of the pancreas and biliary tract structures
- **Gastroscopy** for direct visualization of the stomach and duodenum

- *Colonoscopy* for direct visualization of the large intestine (colon)
- *Sigmoidoscopy* or *proctosigmoidoscopy* for the direct visualization of the anus, rectum, and sigmoid colon

ERCP and colonoscopy are discussed below. Nursing interventions for other endoscopic procedures are similar.

ERCP

ERCP uses side-viewing flexible scopes to view the bile duct, pancreatic duct, and hepatic ducts to assess for pancreatitis, tumors of the pancreas, stones of the common bile duct, and biliary tract disease. If the physician notices the presence of stones that block ducts, it is possible to enlarge the opening (*sphincterotomy*) to facilitate the passage of the stone. Stones in the area of the common bile duct can be removed mechanically with the endoscope or crushed using a lithotriptor. Surgical intervention is indicated if passage of the stone is not accomplished by ERCP with sphincterotomy.

Before the test, the client may be instructed to avoid aspirin, ibuprofen, or anticoagulants for 5 to 7 days because these medications prolong bleeding times and may cause excessive bleeding if tissue is removed during the procedure. A technique called *conscious sedation* is used for these procedures. The adult client is usually sedated with a short-acting intravenous (IV) analgesic such as fentanyl (Sublimaze) or a sedative such as midazolam (Versed). The medication allows introduction and manipulation of the endoscope, yet relaxes the client, who can respond and maintain vital functions.

A mouthpiece protects the client's mouth and the endoscope tube. Inform the client that the endoscope tube will not hinder normal breathing. The procedure takes 15 minutes to 1 hour. During the procedure air is instilled into the stomach. The client will feel fullness and pressure, which is necessary to expand the stomach fully so that the entire interior surface can be visualized.

Nursing Considerations.   As part of pre-procedure teaching, tell the client that another driver must be available

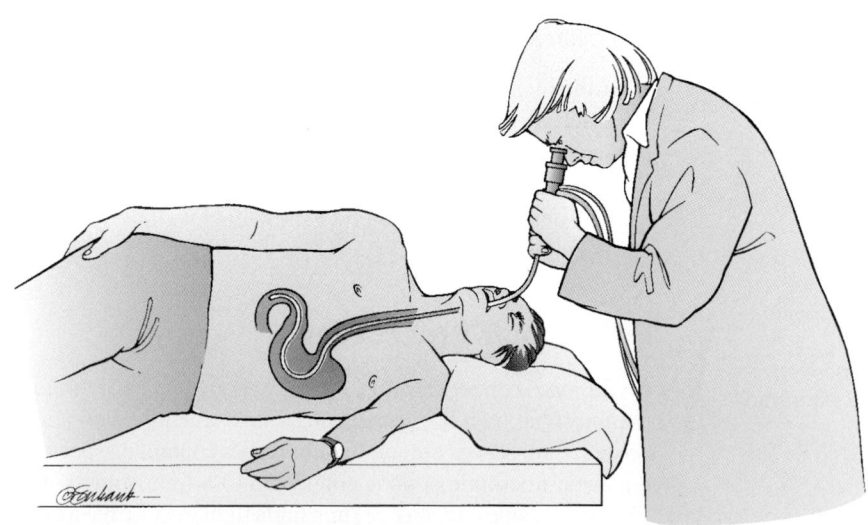

FIGURE 87-1. The flexible endoscope has been inserted through the mouth, down the esophagus, and into the stomach and duodenum for visualization of these organs.

to take him or her home after the procedure because of possible sustained effects of conscious sedation. Carry out any prescribed preparations for the client. Do not give any food or fluids until the client's gag reflex returns and he or she is fully aware.

☛ KEY CONCEPT

Client teaching before any endoscopy is important. Clients need to know what to expect before, during, and after the procedure and what complications are possible. Be sure to document all teaching.

After oral endoscopy, observe the client closely for *dyspnea* (difficult breathing) because the passage of the tube may have irritated the throat or caused swelling. If the client has undergone a *dilatation* (stretching) procedure, observe for bleeding, pain, *dysphagia* (difficulty in swallowing), dyspnea, or a change in vital signs.

Because the dye is sequestered in the GI tract, diarrhea is a common side effect. Pancreatitis and hemorrhage are the most common complications. After an ERCP with sphincterotomy monitor the client's pain intensity and effective response to analgesics closely. Routine vital signs, IV hydration, antibiotics, and followup laboratory work are important for the next 12 to 24 hours.

Colonoscopy

Colonoscopy can be used to follow up on abnormal x-ray examinations. It can help identify growths and inflammatory disease of the lower GI tract. Small polyps and lesions may be *excised* (cut out) or *cauterized* (sealed off by heat or electric current). Growths also may be biopsied. These excising and cauterizing techniques are possible due to the availability of various specialized tools for use with endoscopes. These tools are built so that they can be passed down the lumen of the fiberoptic scope.

Conscious sedation may be used in fiberoptic examinations of the lower GI tract. A colonoscopy is performed with the client lying on the back or left side (Fig. 87-2). The procedure takes 30 minutes to 1 hour. The colonoscopy procedure is most uncomfortable when the scope "goes around the turns" in the colon. Most clients feel the air being instilled into the bowel (**insufflation**) and the endoscope tube being passed. Clients usually describe a mild cramping sensation or pressure. This sensation is mainly caused by the passage of the tube through the anal sphincter and the colon.

Nursing Considerations.   Assist by encouraging the client to take a few deep breaths and to relax each time the scope passes through the colon, particularly around the curves in the large bowel. After the procedure, take and document vital signs.

Teach the client that lying on the right side after the test, with the knees bent and relaxed, will promote the passage of residual air in the colon. Measures to increase peristalsis and comfort include rolling from side to side to stimulate passage of air out of the colon, walking, and a warm bath. Be sensitive to the client's privacy at this time.

The first meal after the procedure should be light; the client should avoid highly concentrated fats. To avoid the feeling of being gaseous, the client should eliminate foods that cause gas production. Accumulated air in the lower GI tract may cause cramps. Instruct the client to observe stools for gross bleeding for 2 to 3 days after the procedure, particularly if polyps were removed or if biopsy was performed.

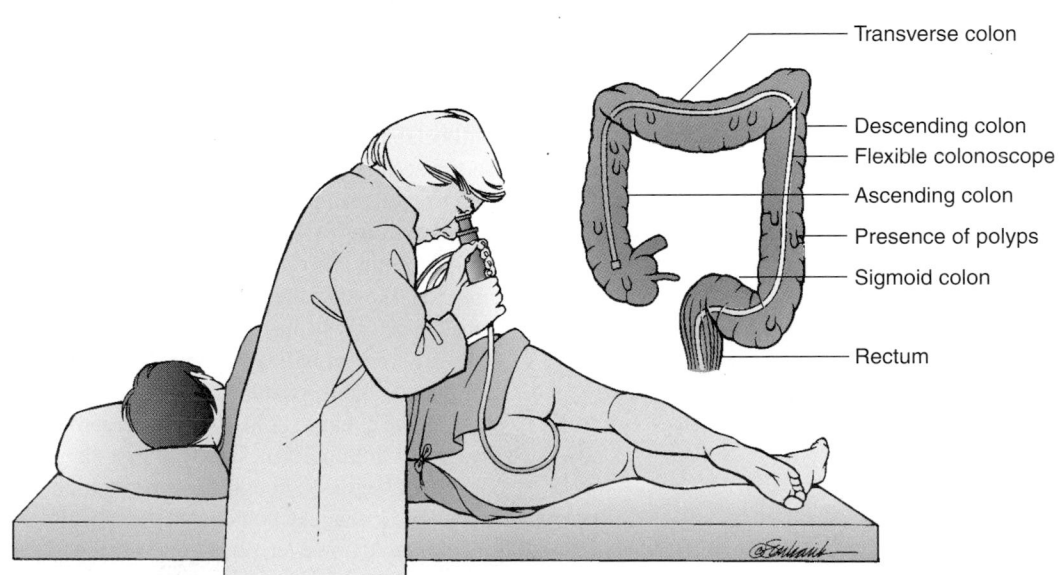

FIGURE 87-2. In colonoscopy, a flexible scope is passed through the rectum and sigmoid colon into the descending, transverse, and ascending colon.

COMMON MEDICAL AND SURGICAL TREATMENTS

Gastrointestinal Intubation

Gastrointestinal intubation involves the insertion of a tube through the nostrils, mouth, or abdominal wall (*gastrostomy* or *jejunostomy*) into the stomach, duodenum, or intestines. Gastrostomy and jejunostomy are used for long-term tube feedings and are discussed briefly at "Enteral Nutrition." Tubes inserted through the nose into the stomach are called nasogastric (**NG**) tubes. NG tubes are short, and are used predominately for suctioning stomach secretions; they may be used for short-term feedings and medication administration. The Levin tube, a single-lumen multipurpose plastic tube, is the most common NG tube (Fig. 87-3). A Salem sump tube is a double-lumen tube with a "pigtail"; this tube is often used for intermittent or continuous suction. Table 87-1 describes several NG tubes commonly used for NG suctioning.

Tubes passed from the nostrils into the duodenum or jejunum are called *nasoenteric*. These tubes can be either

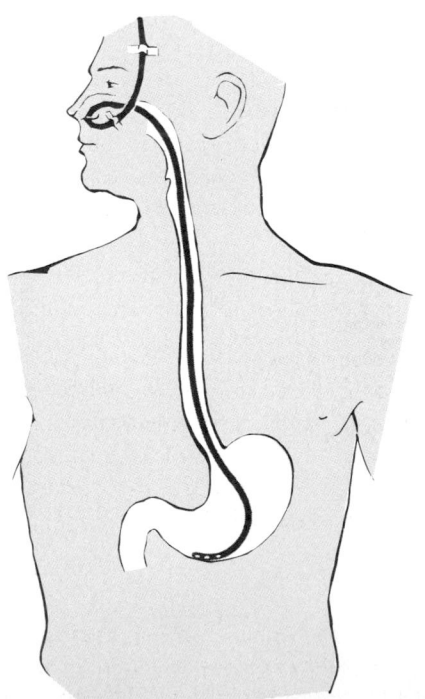

FIGURE 87-3. One type of NG tube: Levin. It remains in place in the stomach. The tube is taped to the face and attached to suction. It is used to keep the stomach emptied or to obtain a specimen of stomach contents.

medium or long in length. Medium-length nasoenteric tubes (eg, Dobbhoff) are generally used for feeding. Long, rubber nasoenteric tubes (eg, Miller-Abbott and Cantor) are used for decompression, aspiration, and to help unblock intestinal obstructions.

Nursing Considerations

Never insert an NG tube without previous careful instruction in the procedure. The nursing student generally is not asked to insert the tubes but may be asked to assist. Be sure to explain the procedure to the client before beginning. The physician will insert nasoenteric tubes, but the nurse may need to assist with advancing these tubes into the intestines.

Providing Oral and Skin Care.   Give soothing mouth rinses, and apply a lubricant to the client's lips and nostril. Apply a water-soluble jelly (eg, K-Y jelly) to the catheter where it touches the nostril because the client's nose and throat may become irritated and dry.

Do not use a humidifier because of bacteria in the air. If possible, the client should brush his or her own teeth; instruct the client to rinse the mouth well with mouthwash but not to swallow. Be sure to reposition the tape and give good skin care to prevent skin breakdown on the nose or cheek.

Assessing the Tube.   Verify the NG tube placement in the stomach by aspiration of a small amount of stomach contents or by auscultation. Inject a small amount of air (15–20 mL) while you listen with a stethoscope approximately 3 inches (8 cm) below the sternum. If the tube is in the stomach, you will be able to hear the air enter (a "whooshing" sound). If inserted at the bedside, nasoenteric tube placement can be verified by x-ray study.

Removing the Tube.   Temporarily clamp the tube before removal to make sure that the client can tolerate its absence. Usually, the physician removes the long nasoenteric tubes. You may be instructed to remove shorter tubes. If a tube with any type of balloon is being used, be sure to remove any substance that keeps the balloons inflated.

Ask the client to hold his or her breath and remove the tube by simply pulling it out, slowly at first, then more rapidly when the client begins to cough. Crimp or pinch the tube as it exits to prevent leakage of contents of the tube. Resistance is seldom encountered; however, do not remove the tube if you encounter any resistance. Generally, another attempt in an hour or so will be successful.

Place the tube in a towel after you have removed it and discard it in the appropriate receptacle. Be sure to remove any tape

■■■ **TABLE 87-1** 𝒞OMMON GI SUCTION TUBES*

Tube Type	Description	Purpose	Nursing Considerations
Levin or Wangensteen	Single lumen Short tube (20–24 in) Multiple holes at distal tip (see Fig. 87-3)	Provides intermittent suction of gastric contents	Irrigate frequently with small amounts of saline or air to keep patent.
Salem Sump	Double lumen (two ports) Short tube (20–24 in) Multiple holes at distal tip	One port provides airflow. Second port allows suction of gastric contents with continuous suction.	Clear the air port with air to keep open and prevent distal tip from sucking against the wall of the stomach, which causes irritation.
Sengstaken-Blakemore	Triple lumens, consisting of one channel and two balloons	The channel provides irrigation and intermittent suction of gastric contents. One balloon provides pressure on the cardiac sphincter area when inflated just inside the stomach. Second balloon provides pressure along the wall of the esophagus to stop bleeding varices.	Rarely utilized due to client discomfort, dangers of tube movement within the esophagus that may cause respiratory distress, and newer more effective treatments to eliminate esophageal hemorrhage Nasotracheal suction is often needed, because swallowing is impossible.

*Mercury-weighted tubes are no longer used for any internal body placement (because of the risk of mercury poisoning). Tungsten-weighted tubes may be used.

marks from the client's face. Provide mouth care and be alert for complaints of discomfort, distention, or nausea after tube removal. Do not give liquids or food without a physician's order.

Gastric Suction

Suction is used for periodic or continuous drainage in many GI conditions, such as the following:

- To obtain a specimen of stomach or intestinal contents for examination
- To treat intestinal obstruction
- To prevent and treat postoperative distention by removing gas and toxic fluid materials from the stomach or intestines
- To empty the stomach before emergency surgery or after poisoning
- To protect the suture line after GI surgery

The *proximal* (outer) end might have a clamp attached to keep it closed. To connect the NG tube to suction, a plastic connector might link it to a longer tube attached to an electric suction machine. Suction may be continuous or intermittent, depending on the type of tube or the needs of the client. NG suction is usually intermittent and low pressure unless the physician specifically orders otherwise.

Nursing Considerations

Note the amount of drainage of gastric fluid and consider it as part of output when calculating fluid intake and output (I&O). The plastic containers of gastric fluid are discarded generally

every 24 hours or according to facility policy. Report vomiting at once; it often indicates a malfunction of the suction apparatus. If the apparatus appears to be functioning improperly, report it at once, and note the situation on the client's chart.

The NG tube will be connected to a mechanical intermittent suction machine, such as the Gomco suction. Be alert to the mechanical functioning of the machine. Document the amount of suction pressure used and what was suctioned (eg, "NG tube attached to low intermittent suction at 30 mm Hg via Gomco; light green watery fluid noted in suction container"). The nurse must be aware of the continual output of fluid as well as its color, consistency, and amount (see In Practice: Nursing Assessment 87-2).

NG Tube Irrigation

A physician's order is needed for irrigating the NG tube. This order should include the type and amount of solution to use and the frequency of irrigation (sometimes it is "as needed or PRN"). The client's condition and different surgical procedures dictate the specific methods to use. In Practice: Nursing Procedure 87-1 details this skill.

Gastric Lavage

If a client has ingested a caustic poison, placing a large single- or double-lumen tube into the stomach may be necessary to dilute or neutralize (using charcoal) the poison, remove the stomach contents, and wash out the stomach. This procedure is called *lavage*.

The steps are basically the same as for inserting the NG tube, except that the lavage tube is larger and is often in-

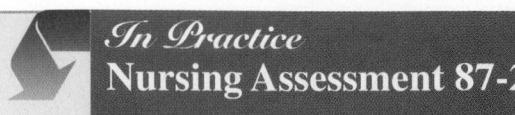

In Practice
Nursing Assessment 87-2

CHECKING DRAINAGE IN GASTRIC SUCTION

- Check the hookup of the bottle and its fluid level.
- Check the drainage for the following characteristics:
  - *Color:* Normal (greenish-yellow); more yellow after injury or surgery and becoming darker and brownish as bile secretion returns; maroon or red (with smell like blood) if blood is present
  - *Odor:* Normal (acidic or sour); foul (indicates presence of infection); bloodlike (indicates gastric bleeding)
  - *Consistency:* Thin, thick, tenacious, presence of chunks or particles, strands of mucus
- Monitor fluid I&O, including drainage:
  - Amount (if tube is irrigated or client has oral fluids, deduct these amounts from gastric output)
  - Presence of vomitus (amount and character)—add to output
- Check for symptoms of electrolyte imbalance. Monitor daily blood level results.
- Check daily weights, if ordered.
- Assess time, amount, and characteristics of stools, if any.
- Assess for any other symptoms (including pain, cramping, nausea, edema, or jaundice).

serted through the mouth instead of the nose. The stomach is then irrigated or "washed" of its contents ("pumping the stomach").

For acute bleeding stomach ulcers and less commonly for bleeding esophageal varices (outpouching blood vessels; discussed later), the stomach is lavaged with saline or tap water to clear blood and stomach contents before performing endoscopic procedures to arrest and treat GI bleeding. Iced lavage is not often used today because it is believed to inhibit platelet function, thus prolonging bleeding.

Enteral Nutrition

Enteral nutrition, also known as *tube feedings,* assists the client to obtain nutritional intake when he or she is unable to obtain adequate calories, appropriate nutrients, solid foods, or liquids by mouth. For enteral tube feedings it is essential that the client have a normally functioning GI tract. Good nutritional status greatly assists the client by providing shorter healing and recovery times. In some cases, enteral nutrition is life-sustaining or lifesaving.

Long-term tube feeding is accomplished either via the nose by utilizing a small-bore, tungsten-weighted nasoenteric catheter (eg, Dobbhoff) or by endoscope-guided tube placement through a "stab wound" in the stomach (*gastrostomy*). Direct insertion of tubes into the stomach can be done via gastric tubes; a PEG tube or even the basic Foley catheter may be used. Figure 87-4 shows a typical dressing for a gastric tube. Chapter 32

In Practice
Nursing Procedure 87-1

IRRIGATING THE NG TUBE
Supplies and Equipment

Irrigation set
Room-temperature tap water or saline
Stethoscope
Disposable pad or bath towel
Clamp
Disposable gloves

Steps

1. Wash your hands, following clean technique. (When supplies are set up for the first time, they are sterile.) In many facilities a new setup is used each time. Precautions are needed to prevent the spread of infection from person to person, but sterile technique is not necessary.
   RATIONALE: *The digestive tract is not sterile.*

2. Assemble the appropriate equipment and solutions at the client's bedside. Explain to the client what you are going to do.

3. Put on gloves.
   RATIONALE: *Prevent spread of infection.*

4. Pour the ordered solution into the irrigation bottle. The most commonly used solution is tap water at room temperature. Measure the amount of solution used.
   RATIONALE: *Subtract the amount of any solution not aspirated from the total amount of drainage for the day so that the I&O record will be accurate.*

5. Disconnect the NG tube from the suction, and check to make sure it is in the stomach. Place your stethoscope over the stomach and listen for a gurgling sound when 10 to 15 cc's of air are injected rapidly into the NG tube.
   RATIONALE: *If the tube is in the lungs, death can result.*

6. Slowly introduce the solution, using the specified irrigating syringe. Do not use excessive force.
   RATIONALE: *Avoid damage to the stomach mucosa or a suture line.*

In Practice
Nursing Procedure 87-1 (*Continued*)

7. Reconnect the tube to low or intermediate continuous or intermittent suction as ordered. The tube should remain *patent* (open) without putting undue stress, due to suction, on the gastric mucosa. The gastric contents should return freely when the tube is reconnected to suction.

8. Note the amount, color, and consistency of any drainage. Fluids that do not return freely may signify a plugged NG tube. Report such a finding immediately.

RATIONALE: *Distention can cause discomfort and respiratory compromise, and pull sutures apart.*

9. Dispose of gloves, wash your hands, and properly dispose of equipment.

10. Document the procedure, noting the time, description of the drainage, and relevant client reactions. Note the amount of fluid instilled or aspirated on the I&O sheet.

---

discusses the specific procedures for administering a tube feeding and related nursing care. Give site care to maintain the skin surrounding a through-the-skin feeding tube.

Parenteral Nutrition

Parenteral nutrition involves direct IV administration of fluids and nutrients into the circulatory system. This method is referred to as parenteral nutrition because it does not access the digestive system (the enteral route). *Total parenteral nutrition* (**TPN**) is sometimes called *total parenteral alimentation. Hyperalimentation* is incorrect terminology because the amounts given are not excessive. If the stomach is functioning normally, it is safer and more appropriate to use enteral nutrition. However, parenteral nutrition may be necessary for many clients. TPN may provide total nutritional support, or it may be supplemental. TPN provides large quantities of fluids and nutrients, including proteins, fats, water, electrolytes, vitamins, and minerals. Each client will have a specifically prescribed TPN solution designed for his or her use.

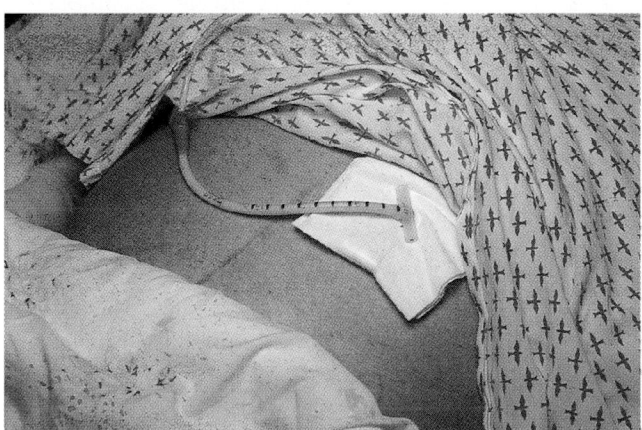

FIGURE 87-4. Protection at the gastrostomy site. A PEG tube may be protected by a dressing that allows access to the tube but covers the exit site. Typically the tube is stabilized with tape over the dressing.

☞ **KEY CONCEPT**

TPN can provide all nutrients needed to sustain life, which is not true for traditional IV therapy. Never use the TPN line to administer medications or blood.

Various access devices are used as infusion devices for TPN. A *central line* involves surgical placement of a small catheter directly into a large blood vessel, often the superior vena cava; the catheter is then sutured in place. This central line allows long-term accessibility and unrestricted movement of the client when the line is not being used. Central lines may be temporary or semi-permanent. The *Hickman catheter* is an example of a central line (Fig. 87-5A). It leaves a small-caliber tube exiting 10 to 14 inches from the upper chest. The *Port-A-Cath* system is accessible by a special needle and is just under the skin's surface, again on the upper chest. Both systems require periodic heparinization (injection of a dilute solution of IV heparin) to keep the blood from coagulating inside the lumen of the catheter.

Another central line is the *peripherally inserted central catheter* (**PICC**) line. A long catheter is inserted into a blood vessel, usually the subclavian vein (Fig. 87-5B). The catheter can be made of several substances, including plastic and Teflon. A physician inserts the catheter under strict sterile techniques and advances it into the superior vena cava.

Nursing Considerations

Several precautions are essential when caring for the client receiving TPN (see In Practice: Nursing Assessment 87-3). First, be sure to check your agency's procedure manual regarding TPN. Most healthcare facilities have specific protocols for administration of nutrients by TPN. In addition, facility policies often require specialized training to work with central lines and TPN solutions.

Follow strict sterile technique when changing bottles, tubing, filters, and dressings. Contamination can quickly disseminate throughout the client's body, leading to sepsis, because the catheter is placed directly into a large blood vessel. Dressings at the insertion site must be sterile. To prevent external

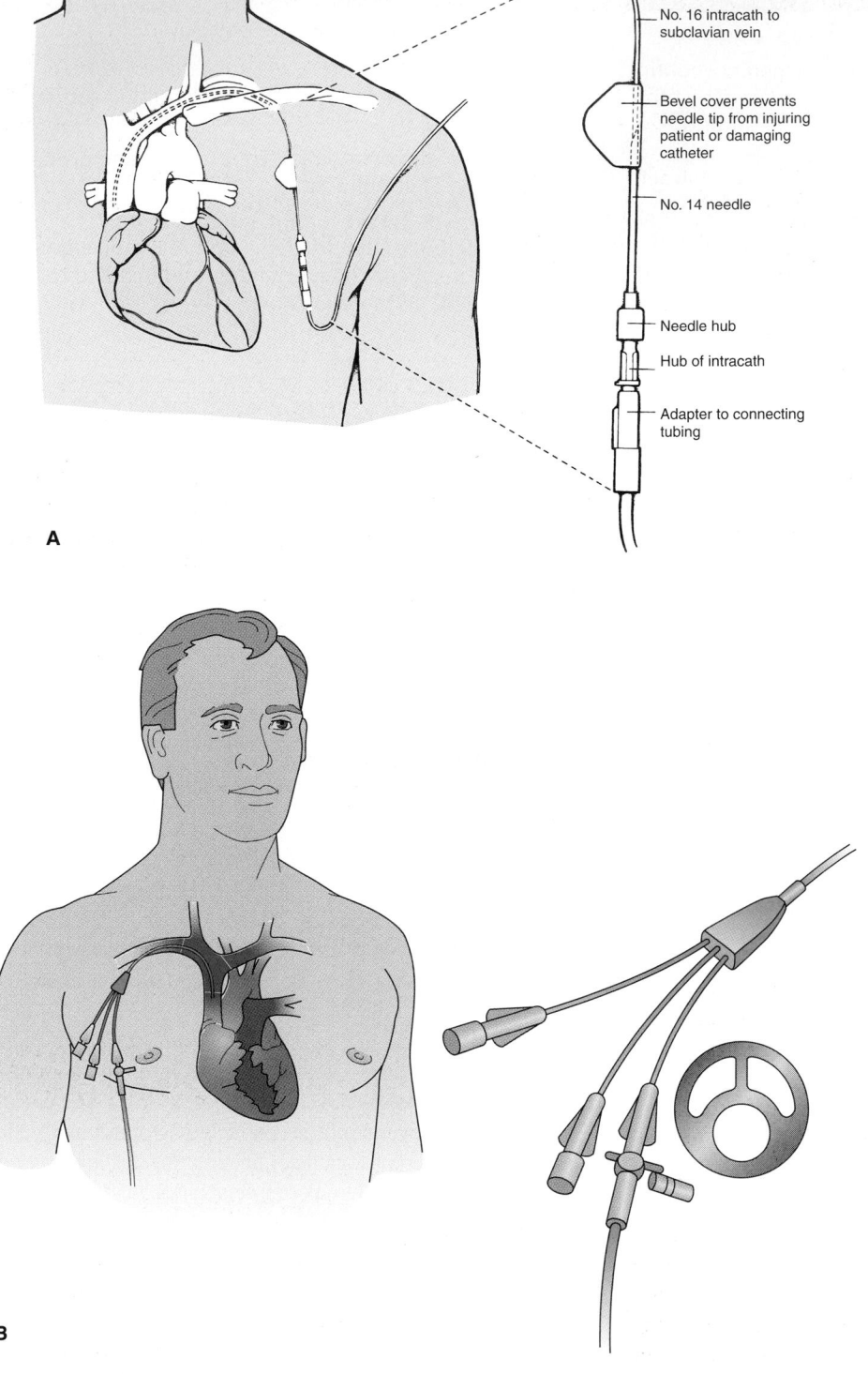

Black silk suture to
secure catheter to skin
and prevent movement
or inadvertent removal

No. 16 intracath to
subclavian vein

Bevel cover prevents
needle tip from injuring
patient or damaging
catheter

No. 14 needle

Needle hub

Hub of intracath

Adapter to connecting
tubing

A

B

FIGURE 87-5. TPN catheters. (**A**) Hickman catheter central line for TPN. The central line enters a large blood vessel such as the subclavian vein, which has access to the superior vena cava. Monitor for bleeding at the site. Always use sterile dressing changes according to hospital policy. (**B**) Subclavian triple-lumen catheter used for TPN and other adjunctive therapy. The subclavian triple-lumen is threaded through the subclavian vein and placed in the vena cava (*left*). Each lumen is an avenue for solution administration; these are secured with Luer-Lok caps when not in use. Hemorrhage and contamination of the catheter or insertion site are major complications (*right*).

hemorrhage from a disconnected central line, tape the catheter securely at the insertion site. To prevent dislodgment internally, use extreme care when working with the catheter or around the site. All connections must be secure. The client's hands may need to be restrained if pulling on the tube is a problem. Assess and document the skin's integrity and the tube at least once each shift.

The rate of infusion for TPN must be constant to prevent episodes of circulatory overload, hypoglycemia, or hyperglycemia. The rate of flow is carefully controlled using a volumetric infusion pump. Discard any unused nutrient solution after 24 hours to reduce the chance of infection. Blood glucose monitoring may be ordered routinely because the solutions contain glucose as well as insulin. Clients may go home on

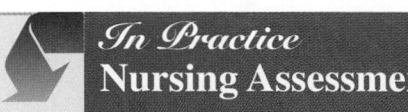

In Practice
Nursing Assessment 87-3

THE CLIENT RECEIVING TPN

- Monitor vital signs frequently, especially temperature, for signs of infection.
- Assess carefully for signs of pneumothorax, hemothorax, internal bleeding, or cardiovascular difficulties (especially during the first 24 hours).
- Monitor rate of infusion at least every hour. *Rationale: Ensure a constant rate of flow and prevent circulatory overload.*
- Monitor I&O. *Rationale: Prevent edema or circulatory overload.*
- Check daily weights.
- Check for dislocation of the catheter.
- Change site dressing and inspect site according to agency protocols.
- Assess for bleeding.
- Check for patency of the centrally inserted intravenous catheter.
- Monitor electrolyte levels as well as blood and urine glucose levels.

TPN and manage lines there. Teach the client and family how to manage and become confident in the care of the lines. Document all teaching.

Biopsy

Many endoscopic procedures of the lower bowel allow biopsy samples to be taken concurrently. The removed tissue is examined for the presence of cancer cells and other abnormalities. **Polypectomy** allows polyps to be removed and examined. In many cases, polyps are considered precancerous.

Liver biopsies are most often performed to verify suspected liver cancer or to detect other liver disorders. However, a biopsy is not done if the client has a bleeding tendency because of the possibility of hemorrhage; the liver is a highly vascular organ.

A small sample of liver tissue is obtained using a long needle with an inner, cutting cannula. The skin is anesthetized before the large needle is inserted. Instruct the client not to breathe during insertion of the needle to avoid inserting the needle into adjacent structures. The needle is inserted with the aid of a stylet inside the needle. The stylet is then withdrawn, and the inner cannula is inserted beyond the end of the needle, and rotated to obtain a specimen. The specimen is then withdrawn. A sample also may be obtained by suction. The sample is examined microscopically. Locating a specific liver site or suspected tumor can require radiologic or ultrasound assistance to aid the physician in performing the liver biopsy.

Nursing Considerations

Explain the procedure and assist the client to maintain the proper position while the procedure is in progress. Wear gloves. This procedure is often uncomfortable. Stay with the client, and offer encouragement and support during the procedure.

Following a liver biopsy, position the client on the right side. Apply pressure to the biopsied site (usually the right side) for 4 to 6 hours, using a sandbag or folded bath blanket to help prevent bleeding.

Take vital signs every 15 minutes for 1 hour; every 30 minutes for 4 hours; and then hourly for 8 hours. Observe the client closely for signs of bleeding. Hemorrhage may be into the abdomen (watch for signs of shock) or from the puncture site.

Gastric Surgery

A *total* **gastrectomy** is a surgical procedure to remove the entire stomach. It may be used in advanced cancer of the stomach when other treatments fail. A *subtotal gastrectomy* is removal of two thirds to three fourths of the stomach, the pylorus, and the first part of the duodenum. A *gastrojejunostomy* joins the stomach to the jejunum. A *vagotomy* is surgery to divide the vagus nerve, reducing the stimulus to create hydrochloric acid. A vagotomy is usually done at the same time as gastric surgery because it limits the stomach's ability to produce secretions. Box 87-1 reviews common gastric surgeries.

Postoperative Complications

Be aware of the possible development of anemia, such as pernicious anemia or iron deficiency anemia (see Chap. 81). Electrolyte disturbances also may result from NG suction, malabsorption, anemia, diarrhea, and vitamin deficiencies.

The suture line is delicate and may rupture and hemorrhage. Signs of shock will appear with massive hemorrhage. Assess

➤ ➤ BOX 87-1

TYPES OF GASTRIC SURGERIES

Common gastric surgeries include the following:

- *Gastroduodenostomy (Billroth I):* A subtotal gastrectomy with removal of distal stomach; anastomosis to duodenum
- *Gastrojejunostomy (Billroth II):* A subtotal gastrectomy with removal of distal stomach and antrum; anastomosis to jejunum
- *Total gastrectomy:* Removal of entire stomach
- *Vagotomy:* Resection of vagus nerves; may be done to reduce gastric acid secretion in selected segments of the stomach
- *Pyloroplasty:* Incision made into the pylorus to enlarge the outlet and relax the muscle; may be done with vagotomy to produce less gastric acid and promote gastric emptying

the gastric drainage carefully for signs of bright-red or partially digested blood. The NG tube must operate properly to avoid distention.

Overeating or eating foods that are not recommended will usually cause immediate discomfort. This condition is called **dumping syndrome.** Foods most likely to cause dumping are those high in carbohydrates and electrolytes, especially salt. Food containing monosodium glutamate is often particularly irritating. Symptoms include palpitation, sweating, faintness, excessive weakness, and diarrhea or vomiting. Signs of shock also may develop. Small, frequent, dry meals (without liquids) usually prevent this problem. Antispasmodic medications also help.

Dehiscence is separation of a surgical incision. **Evisceration** is protrusion of abdominal contents out of the body through the suture line. Both of these conditions are possible, although rare, complications, especially with abdominal surgery. Should either occur, contact a physician immediately. First aid consists of applying a large, sterile compress soaked in saline. Observe sterile technique. Never attempt to push the abdominal contents back into the abdomen.

Some clients, especially those who have had a vagotomy, are susceptible to diarrhea, which may become chronic. Treatment is symptomatic. Other complications specific to gastrectomy include a leaking **anastomosis** (the place where the two ends of the digestive system are joined together). Fever and abdominal distention may be the initial signs of problems. Also, obstruction may cause regurgitation.

Nursing Considerations

Preoperative nursing considerations for the client undergoing gastrectomy include the administration of antibiotics or sulfonamides as ordered. They eliminate bacteria from the bowel and lessen the likelihood of postoperative infection.

Encourage the client to maintain adequate nutrition. The client may need additional vitamin and mineral supplements. TPN may be ordered to provide necessary nutrients. An NG tube may be ordered preoperatively for several days to suction drainage. The NG tube and TPN help to rest the stomach.

The stomach and colon must be empty when the client arrives in the operating room. Therefore, enemas may be ordered preoperatively. Explain to the client that after surgery he or she may need to follow a new dietary regimen that may require changes in meal schedules, nutrient consistency, and types of foods eaten. Allow time for therapeutic conversations to help the client to verbalize feelings and to relax as much as possible. A social worker or chaplain might help the client solve personal, financial, and family problems.

Postoperative nursing considerations include the following:

- Keep the client NPO as ordered.
- Use NG suctioning for 2 to 3 days as ordered. *Rationale: Keeps the operative area clean and eliminates pressure from accumulated fluids.*
- Keep the NG tube patent at all times. Irrigate the NG tube as ordered (usually with approximately 20 mL normal saline). *Rationale: Irrigating the NG tube incorrectly could disrupt the suture line.*

- Assess NG drainage carefully. It may be tinged with bright-red blood at first. Report if the amount of red blood increases or remains bright red. *Rationale: It is a sign of hemorrhage.* The NG fluid should progress toward a normal greenish-yellow color.
- Keep the client in semi-Fowler's position to facilitate drainage.
- Monitor chest tube drainage and chest tube suction. *Rationale: The chest may be opened during the surgery, necessitating the use of chest tubes and suction postoperatively.*
- Provide routine postoperative care, including attention to mouth care and to early ambulation.
- Include deep breathing and incentive spirometer exercises. Encourage the client to cough gently. Support the incision with a small pillow.
- Monitor and control postsurgical pain. Give pain medications as prescribed. The client may be reluctant to breathe deeply or cough because of incisional pain. Medications facilitate exercise, which decreases postoperative complications.
- Assess dressings for excess drainage. Reinforce dressings as needed. Usually the surgeon observes the incision and does the first dressing change. Excess drainage indicates infection or a rupture of the suture line.
- When bowel sounds return to normal, an order will be given to clamp the NG tube for 6 to 8 hours. Monitor for potential complications, such as nausea, vomiting, abdominal pain, and decreased bowel sounds. If no complications occur, then the order may be given to remove the NG tube.
- Give clear liquids when bowel sounds are present. The diet progresses as tolerated.
- Decrease feedings if the client complains of nausea or abdominal distention. *Rationale: These are signs of complications. The NG tube may need to be reinserted.*
- Malnutrition may cause anemia or deficiency disorders. Vitamins and minerals are usually supplemented; the client must receive vitamin B_{12} for life. *Rationale: The stomach is no longer present to secrete the intrinsic factor necessary to metabolize vitamin B_{12} from foods.*
- Instruct the client to increase gradually the amount of food he or she eats at one time until he or she can tolerate three meals a day.
- Teach the client to plan regular rest periods. *Rationale: Prevent overexertion.*
- Regular medical followup is essential.

Fecal Diversions

When a portion or all of the ileum or bowel is removed, an artificial opening for bowel elimination must be created. An incision is made in the abdomen, and a loop of intestine is brought through the incision and opened to allow for drainage of feces. The opening is called a **stoma** or *ostomy.* The person with an ostomy of any type is referred to as an *ostomate.* Ostomy surgeries may be performed to remove all or part of the small or large intestine.

A **colostomy** is an opening into the colon, whereas an **ileostomy** is an opening into the ileum. A stoma may be an end (one stoma), double-barreled (two stomas—both cut ends of the intestine are brought to the outside), or loop (the bowel is not completely severed, so the one stoma has two openings).

The new stoma, which is mucous membrane, should be moist. It ranges from dark red to rich pink, looks like pursed lips, and immediately after surgery, is swollen and may bleed occasionally. External placement of the stoma depends on how much bowel is removed. In Practice: Nursing Assessment 87-4 provides more detail on assessment of a new stoma.

A colostomy or an ileostomy may be temporary if treatment to eliminate or relieve the underlying condition is successful. A colostomy in the transverse colon is usually temporary and is located on the abdomen's right, left, or midline. A temporary stoma may be in place for several weeks to several months, depending on the underlying disease or disorder. Sometimes an anastomosis is possible, which allows the diseased segment to be removed and the normal tissue ends to be reconnected. A *wedge resection* is the removal of only a small amount of bowel. A *bowel resection* is the removal of a larger portion of the bowel. A temporary stoma often consists of a double-barrel stoma. With the double-barrel stoma, the proximal end drains fecal material into the stoma appliance. The distal does not receive nutrients so it does not contain feces. When the underlying condition is healed, a takedown procedure is performed to reconnect (*anastomose*) the cut ends of the double-barrel intestine and close the abdominal wall. The goal is to have the individual resume excretion through the normal rectal outlet.

The colostomy or ileostomy will be permanent if surgery necessitates removal of the colon or the rectum. A permanent colostomy is usually made at the level of the descending or sigmoid colon and is usually located on the abdomen's left side. An ileostomy indicates that the entire large intestine has been removed. The stoma is usually located on the abdomen's lower right side.

Colostomy Irrigation

Colostomy irrigation is a type of bowel management. It enables the person to regulate the colostomy so that he or she may not need to wear a pouch. Prior to the widespread use of disposable, odor-proof ostomy equipment, nearly all clients with colostomies used irrigation for bowel management.

Colostomy irrigation is similar to an enema (see Chap. 51). It is usually done with a cone tip and bag; the fluid drains into the toilet through an irrigating sleeve. The ET nurse often teaches the client the procedure. You may be asked to perform this procedure if you are working in home care.

Most clients irrigate with approximately 1,000 milliliters of tap water every other day. Clients who wish to regulate their bowel by irrigating usually do not learn to do so until at least 6 weeks after surgery, to allow healing. Colostomy irrigation can be time consuming because it usually takes 1 to 1½ hours to irrigate all stool from the bowel. Now that ostomy equipment is odor proof, most clients elect the easier and less time-consuming option of wearing a pouch.

Ostomy Appliances

Types of Appliances.   When the client returns from the operating room, a plastic disposable bag, called a *pouch*, covers the stoma. A faceplate on one end of the pouch has a hole that is the size of the stoma cut into it; the faceplate is then secured to the area around the stoma with a skin barrier that creates a seal. Typical appliances are shown in Figure 87-6.

The opposite end of the pouch, which is not sealed, must be closed with either a special ostomy clamp or binder clip. Stool drains through the stoma and collects in the pouch. Ideally, a snug fit of the faceplate and effective application of a skin barrier prevent stool from contact with the skin. Leaking of fecal material onto the skin causes *peristomal* (around the stoma) skin irritation and can result in skin breakdown.

When the pouch is one-third to one-half full with stool or flatus, it is emptied into a bedpan or other receptacle. If ambulatory and able, the client sits on the toilet, removes the closure clamp, and empties the pouch contents between his or her legs into the toilet.

As it heals, the stoma decreases in size. After approximately 6 weeks, the stoma can be measured for a permanent appliance if one is indicated. A permanent appliance is a faceplate combined with pouch that is secured to the skin with a

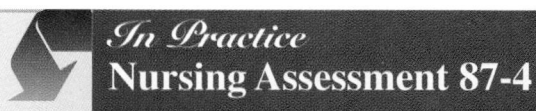

In Practice
Nursing Assessment 87-4

STOMA CONDITION IN THE NEW COLOSTOMY OR ILEOSTOMY

Abnormal and Danger Signs
- Abnormal sounds
- Excessive bleeding (more likely to occur in ileostomy)
- Darkening in color (indicating stenosis around the stoma, which cuts off the blood supply)
- Blanching or extreme lightening in color (indicating lack of circulation to the stoma)
- Drying of the stoma
- Edema of the stoma
- *Prolapse* (stoma pulls back into abdomen)
- Skin irritation around stoma (see In Practice: Nursing Care Guidelines 87-3)
- Signs of infection
- Herniation around stoma

Routine Assessments
- Size of the appliance (It must be large enough so that it does not cut off circulation but small enough so that it does not leak.)
- I&O records
- Daily weights
- Electrolyte balance or imbalance; results of bloodwork
- Amount, character of stool
- Vital signs

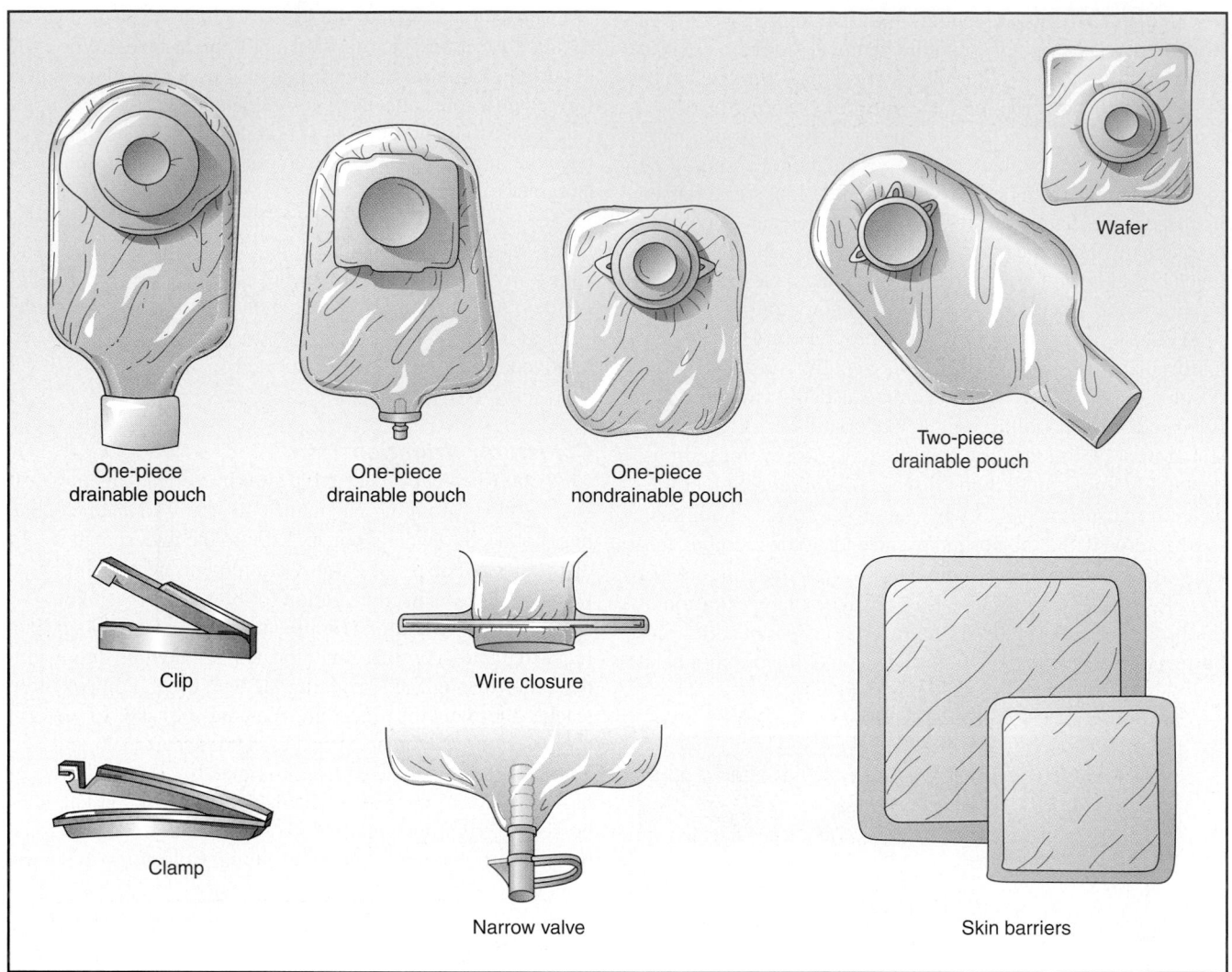

One-piece
drainable pouch

One-piece
drainable pouch

One-piece
nondrainable pouch

Two-piece
drainable pouch

Wafer

Clip

Wire closure

Clamp

Narrow valve

Skin barriers

FIGURE 87-6. Selected ostomy pouches and accessories.

barrier for extended periods of time. A disposable appliance is a pouch that can be secured to a faceplate or wafer and removed as needed. This avoids repeated irritation of the peristomal skin, which can happen with frequent changing of the pouch-faceplate combination.

Ostomy appliances with a faceplate and pouch come in different styles and sizes. The ET nurse and the staff nurse will assist the client in choosing the appropriate appliance, depending on the person's abdominal contours and amount and type of drainage. The client will be fitted with a cut-to-fit pouch while in the healthcare facility (so the size of the stoma opening can be adjusted as stoma edema decreases).

Other permanent appliances have both faceplate and pouch; both must be removed regularly, emptied, rinsed, and replaced over the stoma. For most ostomies, the client can use disposable pouches if a secure seal can be achieved. After a prescribed number of days, the entire appliance is removed and discarded.

Changing the Appliance.   Skin barriers on appliance and pouching systems eventually deteriorate. Depending on the brand used, the person should change the appliance one to

two times per week. Following the recommended time guidelines will prevent deterioration of the skin adhesive and prevent skin breakdown around the stoma.

After approximately 4 to 6 weeks, the nurse can fit the client into a precut appliance, which will eliminate the need for cutting out each pouch before changing it. See In Practice: Nursing Procedure 87-2 for skills in ostomy management. In Practice: Nursing Assessment 87-4 lists considerations when assessing the stoma. Ostomy equipment is stocked at medical suppliers, although some pharmacies also carry it. Most insurance companies cover at least part of the cost.

Nursing Considerations

Nursing considerations for ostomy care are summarized at In Practice: Nursing Care Guidelines 87-2. The most commonly discussed topics follow:

Clothing.   If possible, it is highly beneficial for the ET nurse and the surgeon to discuss the placement of the stoma preoperatively so that long-term care can be anticipated. Immediately after surgery, many clients choose to wear loose-fitting clothing. However, clients will discover that even when wear-

In Practice
Nursing Procedure 87-2

CHANGING THE OSTOMY APPLIANCE

Supplies and Equipment

Pouch or pattern
Pouch adhesive wafer
Closure clip
Stomahesive paste (optional)
Cotton balls or gauze
Scissors
Pen or pencil
Tissues
Water
Soft towel
Liquid deodorant
Plastic waste bag
Gloves

Steps

1. Wash your hands, and apply gloves.

2. Arrange all needed equipment within the client's reach.
   RATIONALE: *The client must become accustomed to self-care as soon as possible.*

3. Teach the client to cuff (turn back) the tail of the pouch before emptying.
   RATIONALE: *Keep the opening free of stool.*
   Empty the old appliance into the toilet and flush.
   RATIONALE: *Remove odor.*

4. Locate the stoma size pattern drawn by the ET nurse. With a pen, trace this size hole on the paper backing of the pouch adhesive. Cut out the opening.
   RATIONALE: *The pouch opening should be only 1/16 inch larger than stoma size to prevent skin irritation from chronic exposure to stool.*

5. Remove the paper backing from the pouch adhesive (wafer). Apply a thin bead of Stomahesive paste to the edge of the adhesive you have just cut.
   RATIONALE: *The paste is a kind of caulking to help seal the pouch around the stoma and prevent leakage.*

6. Gently remove the old appliance, and wipe around the stoma with tissue.
   RATIONALE: *You want to remove mucus or fecal drainage.*

7. Dispose of the old appliance in a plastic bag. Save the closure clip.
   RATIONALE: *Control odor and contamination.*

8. Inspect the skin. Wash the area with warm water, but do not use soap.
   RATIONALE: *Soap can leave a residue on the skin that interferes with pouch adhesion.*

9. Carefully dry the skin. Apply the new appliance. Hold your hand on the appliance for 2 minutes.
   RATIONALE: *The warmth of your hand helps warm the skin barrier and paste so the adhesives seal well to the client's abdominal wall.*

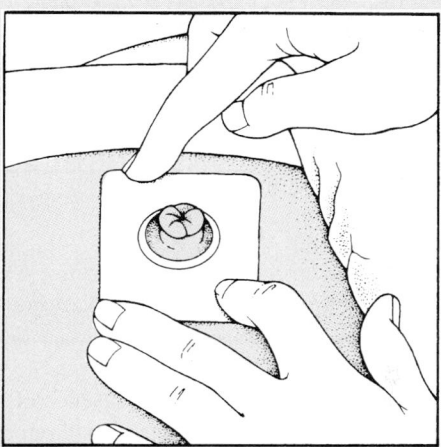

Stomahesive wafer with flange (1½, 1¾, 2¼, 2¾ inch openings) can be applied directly to the periostomal area after it has been thoroughly cleaned and dried.

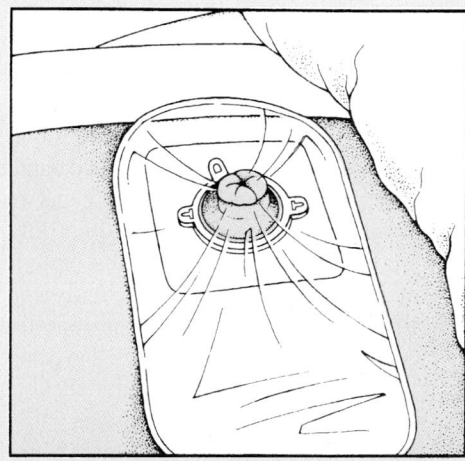

An opaque or transparent drainable pouch is positioned at the desired angle over stoma.

10. Add a few drops of the deodorant to the pouch, and clamp it closed.
    RATIONALE: *The deodorant neutralizes odors.*

11. Properly dispose of waste material and gloves.

12. Wash your hands, and document the procedure, noting the client's reactions.

13. Remove or drain the pouch if it is ½ to ⅔ full.

(continued)

In Practice
Nursing Procedure 87-2 *(Continued)*

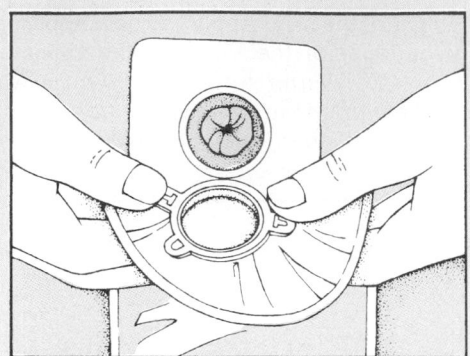

Pouch may be removed without removing wafer.

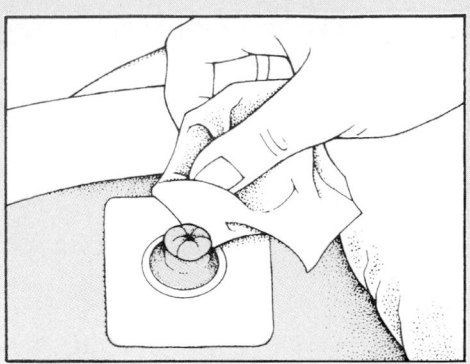

Stoma may be assessed without removing wafer.

14. Assess the stoma every 6 to 12 hours. A new stoma may need more frequent observations.

ing tight-fitting clothing or jeans, the presence of the pouch underneath is not noticeable. Most clients will return to wearing the same clothes as before surgery. The client should not wear a leather belt over the stoma, to prevent irritation. Men who have their stoma site at the beltline may need to use suspenders. Clients can wear the ostomy pouch tucked into their underwear, or they can wear bikini underwear beneath the pouch.

Bathing. All pouching systems are waterproof, so clients can bathe, shower, or swim while wearing them. Clients may choose to remove soiled pouches and shower without them; this is not advisable for the person with an ileostomy. Bowel function with an ileostomy is fairly frequent and unpredictable.

Activity. Heavy lifting is prohibited for 6 to 8 weeks after any abdominal surgery. The person should not lift anything heavier than 5 pounds during this important period of tissue healing. Following this restriction is particularly important in order for the ostomate to avoid a **hernia** (an abnormal protrusion of intestine through the muscle), which can develop in the incision or around the stoma. After the initial postoperative period, the ostomate has no activity limitations.

Diet. After any bowel surgery, the client should follow a low-fiber diet for approximately 1 month. The bowel is generally edematous after surgery, and high-fiber foods may have difficulty passing through it. After 1 month, the person with a colostomy can follow a regular diet.

The person with an ileostomy needs to monitor the diet more closely. The most common complication following an ileostomy is food blockage. Foods that tend to cause blockage include dried fruits, popcorn, many vegetables, nuts, and meats in casings, such as frankfurters. Undigested food obstructs the bowel just prior to the stoma, preventing stool passage. A person with an ileostomy must chew food very well. This person may also have difficulty with odor from flatus; eliminating common gas-forming foods usually helps.

The person with an ileostomy needs plenty of fluids. This person has less formed stools and therefore loses more fluids during elimination. In addition to losing increased water, this person tends to lose sodium and potassium in the stool. Therefore, the person should drink not just plain water, but also fluids that contain electrolytes, such as Gatorade and broth.

Skin Care. Ileal drainage is much more irritating than colostomy drainage, so give special attention to skin care and protection. Cleanse the skin carefully to prevent irritation and dry it thoroughly. If the skin is not completely dry, the appliance will not stick. Remove the pouch gently and carefully to avoid pulling or tearing the skin. For more information on skin care see In Practice: Nursing Care Guidelines 87-3.

Client and Family Teaching. The client who is to have a colostomy or ileostomy may need assistance with adjustment. Naturally, the client wonders how life will be disrupted and may be particularly concerned about the effect on sexual relationships, care of the colostomy or ileostomy, and acceptance of family and friends.

Every nurse must be trained to care for an ostomy. Many healthcare facilities have certified ET nurses who are specially trained to teach clients with ostomies and to provide supportive counsel. The ET nurse is a resource and support person who is commonly called to assist with new, difficult, or unusual conditions that may need special training. However, the ET nurse will not be available at all times. Therefore, the staff nurse must be able to work with an ostomy.

The staff nurse should contact the ET nurse before the client's surgery. The physician, the staff nurse, and the ET nurse assist the client and family with the various aspects of ostomy care. As the stoma changes after surgery, the type of care may change. Several teaching sessions will be necessary to prepare the client and family for life with an ostomy. Assist and teach the client as needed. The goal is to promote self-care.

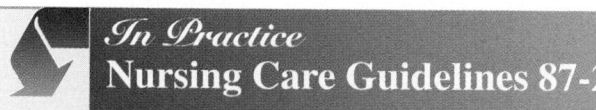

PROVIDING CARE IN COLOSTOMY, ILEOSTOMY, OR OTHER STOMAS

- Be gentle, yet professional, about everything you do for the client.
- Carefully assess the condition of the new stoma.
- If the client has had an abdominal-perineal resection, change the rectal dressing as often as necessary.
- Rectal dressings can be held in place by mesh panties (or a T-binder for a man).
- Give special skin care around the stoma. (See In Practice: Nursing Care Guidelines 87-3.)
- Sitz baths are often recommended. *Rationale: Provide cleanliness and comfort.*
- Cleanliness is important. Change everything that becomes soiled. *Rationale: The client needs to feel clean. Prevent infection.*
- Make every attempt to have the client meticulously clean before mealtime. *Rationale: Minimize the effect of the surgery on the client's appetite.*
- When changing an ileostomy appliance, check for undissolved tablets or capsules. *Rationale: The digestive tract may be functioning incorrectly. If medication is excreted unchanged, the client is not getting the benefit of the drug.*
- Spend time with the client. *Rationale: Allow the client to express feelings. It might be a long time before the client can truly accept the stoma, although the client may be able to care for it physically within 4 to 5 days. Grief reaction to loss of body function is common.* Encourage questions and correct any misconceptions the client might have.
- Encourage and teach the client to be independent as soon as possible: how to remove and apply a new appliance, how to perform skin care around the stoma, and how and what to report about bowel changes.

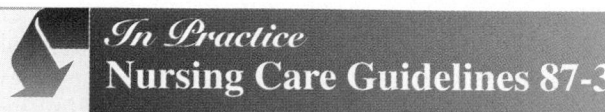

GIVING SPECIAL SKIN CARE IN GASTROSTOMY, COLOSTOMY, AND ILEOSTOMY

- Wipe the new gastrostomy or stoma, as ordered with water or saline.
- Carefully assess the condition of the stoma and surrounding skin daily.
- Do not use alcohol. *Rationale: It is too drying.*
- After the gastrostomy or stoma has healed, clean it with soap and water. (Do not use soap if it irritates the client's skin.)
- Expose the area to air. *Rationale: To keep it dry.*
- If redness or a yeast-appearing growth appears, treat with an antifungal, such as nystatin (Mycostatin) powder.
- A wafer of Stomahesive to *peritube* (around the tube) skin will protect it from drainage. Stomahesive paste also may be used.
- A drain tube attachment device (DTAD) can help to secure the tube.

Parks S pouch is shaped like an S; or the Parks J pouch is shaped like a J. The Parks procedures are usually done in two stages. In stage 1, the entire colon and lining of the rectum are removed, and the reservoir is fashioned. The anal sphincter is retained, and the reservoir (pouch) is sewn to it. A temporary ileostomy is done. The client then eliminates stool through the ileostomy stoma for 6 weeks to 3 months, while resting the bowel. Stage 2 is surgical take-down of the ileostomy. The Parks pouch acts as the sigmoid colon, and the client usually achieves sphincter control.

The ileoanal reservoir procedure requires a longer recuperation time than the standard ileostomy, but greatly improves the quality of life for clients in whom it can be used. The person will pass stool four to eight times in 24 hours and does not have a permanent stoma.

Kock Pouch

Another procedure, called the *Kock pouch* or the *continent ileostomy,* is often more acceptable than the standard ileostomy. The Kock procedure removes the colon, rectum, and anus. A permanent ileostomy is created, and an internal abdominal reservoir is fashioned from about 45 centimeters of the small intestine.

This reservoir is attached to the ileostomy and collects the stool. A one-way nipple valve is created with the ileal tissue and a flush (flat) stoma is present on the abdominal wall. Postoperatively, the pouch is catheterized and irrigated with 20 to 50 milliliters of normal saline every 2 hours. The return flows out by gravity. Check the skin around the stoma and the tube several times daily and change dressings. Be sure that the catheter is securely anchored.

Continent Fecal Diversions

In some cases, the use of surgical techniques results in the removal and rerouting of intestinal tissues internally, thus avoiding external ostomies. In these instances, the client's own tissues may be formed into internal receptacles for stool. Many of these cases result in fecal control without the use of external pouches. Each of these surgeries is highly individualized to the client, the disease, condition of available tissues, and surgical capabilities.

Ileoanal Reservoir

The *ileoanal reservoir* is the surgical creation of a pouch fashioned from the small intestine that collects ileal drainage. The

This procedure is usually impossible if the client is obese or at high risk, or has Crohn's disease, toxic megacolon, diabetes mellitus, or active colitis. The client is usually able to achieve the same continence as with a colostomy by periodic catheterization and use of a small absorbent patch. Complications of either internal pouch procedure include stool seepage and *pouchitis* (inflammation of the pouch).

Other Procedures

In *total colectomy with ileorectal anastomosis,* the colon is removed and the ileum is sewn to the rectum. The client eliminates stool through the anus. A risk of cancer exists, however, in the retained rectum. Stools usually number three to eight daily. In other cases, the ileum is sewn directly to the anus. In this case, continence may not be as good, but still there is no stoma.

Abdominal Paracentesis

Abdominal paracentesis (abdominal tap) is a procedure that may be necessary for diagnostic purposes or to relieve **ascites** (fluid accumulation in the peritoneal cavity). It is considered diagnostic when fluid is withdrawn for microscopic study or for culturing when bleeding or infection is suspected. Therapeutic abdominal tap is done when the client is distended with ascitic fluid. The abdominal cavity is punctured to obtain a specimen for analysis or to drain excess fluid. Because the client also may have difficulty breathing, removal of this fluid will frequently relieve the condition. Ultrasound may be utilized to guide the aspiration of fluid from the abdomen with a large syringe and needle. Sometimes a catheter is inserted into the abdominal cavity for continuous drainage.

Nursing Considerations

Nursing considerations for an abdominal paracentesis include the following measures:

- Ask the client to void immediately before the procedure. *Rationale: Helps to avoid rupture of the urinary bladder by the needle.*
- Assist the client into a comfortable position for the procedure.
- Sterile scrub the abdomen in preparation for insertion of the needle.
- Monitor vital signs during and after the procedure. Watch for fainting or dizziness.
- Measure the amount of fluid obtained.
- Send the appropriate specimens to the laboratory.
- After the procedure, observe the client for bleeding or any signs of shock.
- Check the dressing to make sure it is tightly applied and dry. *Rationale: Prevent and check for bleeding.*
- Keep the client in Fowler's position, unless ordered otherwise. *Rationale: Facilitate drainage and assist breathing.*
- Observe urine output. Check the male client's scrotum for edema. *Rationale: Evaluate the effectiveness of the procedure and determine if complications exist.*

- Tell the client to observe for any signs of infection.
- Carefully document the procedure and all teaching.

NURSING PROCESS

Data Collection

Using the skills of physical examination and nursing assessment (see Chap. 47), observe and assess the client who has a digestive disorder. This establishes a baseline for future comparison and determines the presence of suspected digestive-related complications. Report any changes in baseline levels.

Assess the client's height compared with weight and ask about eating habits and recent weight gain or loss. Determine whether the person is able to chew and swallow and whether food preparation is a problem. In addition, observe the client's emotional response to the disorder or disease. Does the client need assistance to meet daily needs? Does the disorder affect social activities or self-esteem (eg, does the client have a colostomy)? Is the disorder life-threatening? Is the client anxious or fearful about the outcome? Are a support group, home care nursing, Meals on Wheels, and other community programs appropriate?

Nursing Diagnosis

Based on data collection, many nursing diagnoses may be seen on the nursing care plan established for the client with a digestive disorder. Some diagnoses may have more than one causal factor. Examples of nursing diagnoses for digestive disorders include the following:

- Activity Intolerance related to abdominal surgery, diarrhea, or generalized weakness
- Bowel Incontinence related to inability to digest food
- Imbalanced Nutrition: Less than Body Requirements related to inability to digest food, inability to absorb nutrients, or refusal to eat
- Disturbed Body Image related to weight loss or gain, colostomy, or persistent diarrhea
- Deficient Knowledge related to lack of exposure to concepts of diagnostic tests, tube feeding, or ostomy care
- Pain related to abdominal surgery
- Risk for Deficient Fluid Volume related to diarrhea, intestinal obstruction, indwelling tubes, and medications
- Risk for Impaired Skin Integrity related to ileostomy or colostomy, TPN feeding, physical immobilization, and cancer treatment

Planning and Implementing

Plan with the client, family, and other members of the healthcare team for effective care to meet the client's needs based on the nursing diagnoses. Provide preoperative and postoperative care for the client undergoing endoscopy, liver biopsy, or surgery on the stomach or related organs.

The client with a digestive disorder also may require assistance in meeting nutritional or self-care needs. Many digestive disorders have strong emotional components that may aggravate the disorder or be related to the disease's course. Clients often need assistance to understand more about the disorder, including its prognosis and treatment. The client may need to perform special procedures at home; thus, client teaching is vital. Develop a nursing care plan to meet each client's needs.

Evaluation

Evaluate outcomes of care by answering the following questions: Have short-term goals been met? Are additional teaching or rehabilitative measures needed? Is additional treatment or surgery necessary? Are long-term goals still realistic? Are community services required? Is a support group available? Planning for further nursing care considers the client's prognosis, complications, and responses to care given.

DISORDERS OF THE MOUTH

Mouth disorders are uncomfortable, often painful, and at times disfiguring or cosmetically unattractive. They can also disrupt nutritional intake or lead to other undesirable or more serious conditions and lifestyle changes.

Dental Problems

Dental **caries** (tooth decay) result from an erosive process that breaks down tooth enamel and later invades the dental pulp; this causes discomfort and sometimes necessitates tooth removal. The major cause of decay is bacteria nourished by food particles left on the teeth as a result of faulty brushing and lack of flossing. Acids in the mouth and their effectiveness in destroying bacteria; presence of plaque on the teeth and sugar in the mouth promoting bacterial growth; susceptibility of the teeth to decay; and the length of time between brushings play a part in the decay process.

Good brushing is essential to preserve a healthy mouth and prevent tooth decay. Many dentists recommend using fluoridated water or having the dentist apply fluoride. Flossing helps to clean between teeth and to prevent gum disease. Professional dental care also is important. Adults should have their teeth checked and cleaned professionally twice a year.

Dentures are better known as "false teeth." The term for "without teeth" is *edentulous.* Many people delay or ignore dental care. People often mistakenly believe that dentures are a normal part of aging. They may not have access to appropriate gum and dental care, which leads to infected teeth and tooth loss that could have been avoided. Additionally, the individual is being exposed to infection that can become systemic.

In some cases, dentures are the best solution for dental problems. At other times, reconstructive partial inserts can be used. Dentures may be slightly uncomfortable when they are first fitted, but the dentist can remove sources of irritation. The only way to become accustomed to dentures is to wear them all the time, especially when awake. Dentures also help preserve the face's normal shape.

Periodontal Disease

Periodontal disease affects the bones and tissues around the teeth. It can result from poor oral hygiene, inadequate dental care, or poor nutrition.

Gingivitis

Gingivitis, a form of periodontal disease, is inflammation of the gums. General symptoms include bleeding, erythematous, edematous, and tender gums. Gingivitis has many causes, but is most frequently associated with accumulation of bacterial plaque on the teeth as a result of ineffective oral hygiene. Gingivitis also may be a sign of vitamin deficiencies, diabetes mellitus, anemia, and leukemia. It can lead to more serious disorders, such as inflammation of tissues that directly surround a tooth. Proper care of the teeth and gums, including daily flossing and an adequate diet, are the best preventive measures.

Pyorrhea Alveolaris

Pyorrhea alveolaris is an inflammation of the gums and teeth, sometimes with a purulent discharge. It usually begins with *periodontitis* (inflammation of the tissues around and supporting the teeth). Pyorrhea is caused by the collection of food, bacteria, and tartar deposits between the gum line and the tooth root. Untreated periodontitis spreads to the underlying bony structure. The teeth loosen because their support structure breaks down, making chewing impossible.

Treatment includes impeccable tooth, gum, and mouth care: regular flossing, surgical scraping and drainage of the infected area, antibiotics, or extraction of the affected teeth. Surgical scraping is painful, so other measures are tried first. Left untreated, pyorrhea can result in an abscess or a systemic infection.

Stomatitis

Causes of *stomatitis* (inflammation of the mouth) include primary lesions of the mouth; secondary lesions of the mouth (as a result of chemotherapy or radiation); mechanical trauma (mouth breathing, cheek biting); and chemical trauma (sensitivities/allergies of the oral mucosa to ingested substances).

Stomatitis may be a clinical manifestation of a systemic condition or the result of an infection in the oral cavity. Nutritional disorders and bone marrow disorders are some of the systemic causes of inflammation of the oral mucosa. Treatment of this problem depends on the cause and usually involves avoiding oral irritants and providing comfort with frequent oral hygiene. Topical antibiotic ointments may be prescribed to treat bacterial infections.

Canker sores (*aphthous stomatitis*) are recurrent, small, white, painful ulcers that appear on the inner cheeks, lips, gums, tongue, palate, and pharynx. No one knows their exact cause; however, many local and systemic factors, such as food and drug allergies (immune reaction) and physical and emotional stress, have been suggested. Canker sores have been linked to highly salted foods and some forms of nuts. Dental trauma is the most common factor in recurrent canker sores. Premenstrual flare-ups are common. Canker sores may be associated with chronic ulcerative colitis, Crohn's disease, and malabsorption syndromes.

No effective treatment has been found. The sores usually heal without intervention in a few days. The use of topical anesthetics (eg, benzocaine or lidocaine) may help to relieve pain. Silver nitrate stick application destroys nerve endings and may provide pain relief. Application of a solution of tetracycline may improve healing in some clients. Oral lysine also is believed to be helpful.

Candidiasis

Candidiasis, known as *thrush* or *moniliasis,* is a fungal infection caused by the organism *Candida albicans,* which is part of the normal flora of the oral cavity. It is common in newborns, immunosuppressed clients, and clients with chronic debilitating diseases such as HIV/AIDS, diabetes, or alcoholism. Antibiotic therapies also can lead to candidiasis. The infection appears as small, white patches on the mucous membranes of the mouth or tongue. It may extend into the entire GI tract.

Oral pharyngeal cultures are recommended when this infection is suspected. Prophylactic treatment of high-risk clients is indicated. Treatment consists of nystatin (Mycostatin), saline, and hydrogen peroxide mouth rinses, or vaginal suppositories.

Precancerous Lesions

Leukoplakia buccalis (smoker's patch) is the most common precancerous lesion. It is a creamy white, nonsloughing patch on the mucous membranes of the mouth or tongue. This lesion is common in middle-aged people who smoke or who have extensive dental caries. It often disappears if the client stops smoking. A biopsy or oral cytology study is usually recommended.

Herpes Simplex Infections

Cold sores or *fever blisters* are painful vesicles that occur on the face, lips, perioral (around the mouth) area, cheeks, and nose. They are usually caused by herpes simplex virus type I, and can be precipitated by stress. Cold sores usually disappear after a few days, and treatment is not usually required.

Medication may be prescribed for comfort, but is not curative. Five percent acyclovir (Zovirax) ointment may be applied to the lesions. The lesions are infectious, so wear gloves when treating them. Although the ointment may not speed healing, it may decrease the shedding of the virus. Drying agents, such as benzoin or alum, also may be applied to the lesions to speed healing. Bacteria may infect cold sores secondarily.

Trauma

Various types of injuries, such as fracture of the jaw, laceration of the lips, and traumatic loss of teeth, can cause mouth injury. Chapter 43 describes first aid for traumatic tooth loss (*avulsion*).

With simple suturing, lacerations of the lips heal without complications because of a good blood supply. If the entire lip is severed, however, the person may experience problems with lip movement. For lip and other types of facial surgery, a plastic surgeon may perform the suturing.

For a jaw fracture, usually the upper and lower jaws are wired or fastened together so that they heal without displacement. This is called *intermaxillary fixation.* This client cannot open his or her mouth. Consequently you must be ready to assist as necessary. The client needs help with meals because he or she sips foods through a straw or from a spoon. NG tube feedings or TPN may be necessary.

If the client has his or her jaws wired or fastened together, keep a wire cutter with the client at all times for emergency use. If the client is choking or vomiting, the wires must be cut, or the client could die from lack of oxygen. The client's head is kept slightly elevated, and oral suctioning equipment is nearby. Antiemetic drugs are usually administered for the first few days after injury. A tracheostomy or an airway might be a required emergency measure.

If an *extraoral* (outside the mouth) device is in place, give special attention to the position of the client's head for maximum comfort. The device often goes around the client's head. Teach the client not to roll onto the device, which might result in bending or dislodging the wires.

Cancer of the Mouth

Many cancers of the mouth are asymptomatic until they have spread. Mouth cancer can be treated successfully if discovered early. Those who ingest large amounts of alcohol, or engage in risky behaviors such as smoking or using forms of smokeless tobacco (leaf, plug, or snuff), have an increased risk for developing oral cancer. Many people tend to ignore sores or irritations in the mouth because they think such symptoms are insignificant.

Treatment

Cancer of the mouth may be treated with surgery, radium implants, or deep x-ray therapy. Combination therapies with chemotherapy are also common. If possible, the malignancy is removed with as wide an excision as necessary to remove all affected structures and lymph nodes. NG or gastrostomy feedings might be indicated. The operation is often followed by reconstructive surgery to correct facial defects.

Nursing Considerations

Nursing considerations revolve around caring for the client preoperatively and postoperatively. Before surgery, design communication techniques, because the client may be unable to speak as he or she did before surgery. Postoperatively, observe for hemorrhage and airway obstruction caused by facial edema or aspiration. Suction secretions and elevate the head of the bed to make breathing easier. As you support the client's head by placing your hands on either side, instruct the client to breathe deeply and to use the incentive spirometer. Do not encourage coughing unless congestion is present. These measures are needed to prevent hypostatic pneumonia. An emergency airway should be available at the client's bedside.

Give mouth care carefully to improve the client's comfort and prevent odor. Take great care to prevent disruption of the suture line. Give liquids through an NG tube until the client is able to swallow. Self-care is the goal.

DISORDERS OF THE ESOPHAGUS
Esophageal Varices

Esophageal varices are abnormal dilations of the blood vessels of the esophagus. They are most often associated with cirrhosis of the liver, which is a serious and chronic condition. Treatment is imperative; untreated varices can hemorrhage profusely, and the client may die. An EGD may be used in the diagnosis and treatment of esophageal varices. *Sclerotherapy* is an endoscopic procedure whereby caustic agents are injected into the tissue near the varices. This procedure, done in a series of treatments, causes scar tissue to form and stops hemorrhaging. Assess the client for hemorrhage after each treatment and before and after surgery. *Band ligation* is another endoscopic procedure in which small rubber bands are placed on and around bleeding varices on the esophageal wall. These bands stop the bleeding; when the tissue is healed they slough off, leaving scar tissue, which is less likely to bleed. Varices are further discussed at "Cirrhosis" later in this chapter.

Esophageal Diverticulum

Esophageal diverticulum or *Zenker's diverticulum* is an outpouching of the esophagus, usually where the esophagus passes through the neck area. The client first complains of bad breath, which is caused by bits of food that have accumulated in the diverticulum. X-ray studies determine the nature and location of the outpouchings.

In most cases, the diverticulum is small, causes no dysfunction, and requires no treatment. In more serious cases, the client's dietary status is evaluated. The client can be treated medically with a bland diet, antacids, and other measures to prevent *reflux* (return flow) of food and fluid. Surgery may be necessary if symptoms do not diminish with conscientious medical management, or if the client is debilitated and aspiration of the food or fluid trapped in the diverticulum is considered a danger.

Nursing considerations include placing the client in a semi-Fowler's position, serving small meals, and fitting the client with loose clothing. Encourage the client to maintain an appropriate weight to prevent an enlarged stomach or excess fatty tissue from pushing up on the esophagus.

Hiatal Hernia

Hiatal hernia is a condition in which part of the stomach protrudes through the diaphragm's esophageal hiatus (gap or cleft through which the esophagus passes). Weakening of the diaphragmatic muscles at the gastroesophageal junction,

trauma, or congenital causes may contribute to development of a hernia.

Factors that increase intra-abdominal pressure, such as coughing, straining at stool, bending, or lifting heavy objects, may exacerbate the condition. Many people older than 50 years of age have asymptomatic hiatal hernias. A large hiatal hernia is likely to cause symptoms, such as a feeling of fullness, abnormal stomach sounds, ulceration, bleeding, and pain. Hiatal hernia does not cause heartburn, although a person with a hiatal hernia may have heartburn from another cause.

Treatment
Management is directed at keeping the stomach's acid contents from maintaining long contact with the esophageal lining. If a hernia is small and causes little distress, treatment is unnecessary. When surgical treatment is indicated, postoperative edema of the stomach and esophagus may make eating a problem for the first few days. Therefore, the client may receive IV fluids or TPN for several days.

Nursing Considerations
After surgery assess the NG tube drainage carefully, looking particularly for blood. A small amount of blood may be evident immediately after the operation, but after this disappears, the drainage should have the yellowish-green color of normal gastric secretions. Frank bleeding signals a hemorrhage.

If the client has had chest surgery, give special attention to chest tube management and deep breathing. The client should use the incentive spirometer. Administer oxygen and give care to the chest's drainage site. Observe carefully for vomiting or aspiration, particularly when the client begins to take solid or semisolid foods. *Rationale: Regurgitated food may irritate the suture line, and aspiration can cause postoperative pneumonia.* Other postoperative care is routine.

Achalasia

Achalasia is a motility disorder of the lower portion of the esophagus in which food cannot pass into the stomach. Causes include absence of effective or coordinated esophageal peristalsis or failure of the cardiac sphincter to relax.

The most prominent symptom of achalasia is difficulty swallowing. Achalasia is chronic and progressive. Clients often use large volumes of fluids or bulk in an attempt to force open the cardiac sphincter and allow food to move into the stomach. Thus, they may develop malnutrition and vitamin deficiencies. These clients also are susceptible to respiratory problems caused by aspiration of regurgitated esophageal contents.

A special test called *esophageal manometry* is used to measure and record the motility patterns of the esophagus. A barium swallow with esophagoscopy may be done to assist in diagnosis. These procedures also can be used to monitor the disorder's progression.

Treatment
Surgical treatment often involves dilation of the cardiac sphincter to the point of weakening or disrupting its ability to

close. Dilation is done by endoscopy with a variety of balloons and dilators. Medical treatment is directed toward educating the client.

Nursing Considerations

Teaching involves improving dietary and eating habits. Teach the client to eat slowly and in a peaceful setting. Chewing food thoroughly and drinking plenty of liquids during the meal help food move into the stomach. For more information see In Practice: Educating the Client 87-1.

Heartburn

Heartburn (also called *indigestion,* **dyspepsia,** and *pyrosis*) is a common clinical manifestation of esophageal disease. Heartburn is an uncomfortable burning sensation in the lower chest, which often radiates upwards toward the neck. It is exacerbated by postural changes, ingestion of alcohol, and gulping of food or fluids. Clients often state that the pain is cramping and wavelike. Other symptoms include nausea, indigestion, belching, a bloated feeling, and a sore throat due to acid reflux.

As a healthcare provider, determine exactly what "heartburn" means to the client who uses it to describe a symptom, because "heartburn" may be used to describe many different sensations. Treatment of heartburn is directed at alleviating or minimizing the causes.

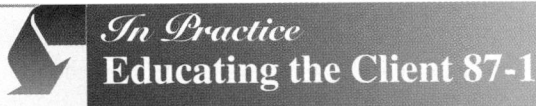

Nursing Alert
Differentiating between heartburn and heart attack pain is difficult. If a person has any question, he or she should seek medical attention immediately. Symptoms of heart attack that differ from heartburn include intense chest pain that radiates to the neck, jaw, back, or arms; difficulty breathing or breathlessness; fainting; limb numbness; sudden nausea and vomiting; and cold, clammy skin accompanied by sweating.

Gastroesophageal Reflux Disease (GERD)

Esophageal reflux or **GERD** occurs when the lower esophageal sphincter (**LES**) leading into the stomach is weak or relaxes inappropriately. With a sphincter that does not close firmly, acidic stomach contents can move back up into the esophagus. Aspiration of stomach acid may cause asthma, pneumonia, and chronic lung disease. Obesity and "desk jobs" are considered to be important contributing factors to the development of GERD.

Esophagitis is the acute or chronic inflammation and irritation of the lining of the esophagus, which may be caused by LES weakness. The presence of a hiatal hernia may aggravate the condition. Many medications and foods aggravate GERD or esophagitis, including aspirin, chocolate, peppermint, spicy foods, coffee, tomato products, citrus fruits, and fried foods. Cigarette smoking greatly decreases LES pressure and aggravates heartburn. Drinking alcohol and overeating exacerbate the condition. Hot or cold liquids may intensify the sensation. Bacterial or yeast infections also may be causes.

Treatment

Treatment of GERD is directed at alleviating or minimizing the causes, and preventing complications. If the client's diet is aggravating the condition, nutritional counseling is in order. Medications that may help include H_2 blockers, proton pump inhibitors (PPIs), GI stimulants, cholinergics, and antacids such as Mylanta, Rolaids, or Tums.

Surgical management is reserved for those clients who do not respond to medical management. Three surgical procedures, the Nissan fundoplication, the Hill operation, and the Belsey operation, may be completed by either laparoscopic or an open surgical approach.

Nursing Considerations

Nursing considerations center around client teaching and postoperative care. The client should stop smoking, elevate the head of the bed, avoid gastric irritants, eat small meals, and maintain proper weight. Explain that drinking adequate fluids and chewing food thoroughly assist in food passage. Instruct the client not to lie down for at least 2 hours after meals and not to wear tight belts or waistbands. Encourage those with GERD to move

---

In Practice
Educating the Client 87-1

HEARTBURN, HIATAL HERNIA, OR ACHALASIA

- Avoid gastric irritants (eg, caffeine, alcohol, spicy foods, nicotine).
- Avoid aspirin and nonsteroidal anti-inflammatory drugs (NSAIDs), unless specifically ordered by a physician.
- Avoid large, bulky meals, especially as the last meal of the day.
- Chew foods slowly and thoroughly.
- Do not eat food 2 hours before retiring or lying down.
- Do not wear tight belts, girdles, or clothing that constricts the waist.
- Avoid sitting for long periods of time. Intermittently stand and stretch to relieve increased abdominal pressure caused by the sitting position.
- Avoid foods that aggravate symptoms. Common culprits are gas formers such as cucumber, onion, cabbage, beans, and pepper.
- Avoid juices high in acidity (citrus types) when symptoms are present.
- Elevate the head of the bed 6 to 8 inches to allow gravity to keep the stomach's contents in the lower portion when lying down. Use books, bricks, or blocks of wood. A wedge pillow or extra pillows cause bending at the midsection, which increases internal abdominal pressure and is undesirable.

away from their desks and stretch intermittently to discourage reflux.

When an open surgical approach is used, postoperative nursing considerations are similar to those for hiatal hernia repair (described previously). Clients who undergo a surgical procedure for GERD are still encouraged to follow an anti-reflux regimen of lifestyle changes, medications, and diet changes due to a significant recurrence rate.

Barrett's Esophagus

Barrett's esophagus is a condition of extreme and chronic irritation of the lower esophagus. It changes the esophageal lining's cell formation from the normal squamous-cell type to the columnar-cell type, which is found in the stomach's wall. Barrett's esophagus is thought to be a precancerous condition that requires careful medical management and annual endoscopic surveillance for development of malignancy.

Esophageal Cancer

Esophageal malignancies usually consist of squamous cell carcinoma or adenocarcinoma of the esophageal mucosa. The incidence of adenocarcinoma of the esophagus and upper stomach has increased significantly in the past few decades. Cancer of the esophagus is most common in men and in smokers. It is also associated with alcoholism. Esophageal cancer often is diagnosed late in its development and the client's prognosis is usually poor.

Signs and Symptoms

One early clinical manifestation is dysphagia, which progresses from mild and intermittent in the first stages of the disease to constant and accompanied by an increase in salivation and mucus in the throat. As obstruction becomes more evident, the client may even be unable to swallow liquids. Any attempt at swallowing causes the person to regurgitate the food, creating discomfort and a disagreeable taste and odor in the client's mouth.

Diagnosis is made on the basis of an esophagogram, upper GI series, and laboratory cytology. Fiberoptic esophagoscopy may be done to visualize the tumor and to take a biopsy sample. CT scans can be used to define the size of the primary lesion and reveal nodal involvement.

Treatment

Surgery is the only effective treatment for esophageal cancer that allows the client to eat normally. Innovative developments in chest surgery have resulted in rapid advances in treatment. Surgery may be performed for cure or palliation, depending on the extent of the disease. Even if removing all the cancerous tissue is impossible because the disease has spread, surgery may help the client eat normally.

Often the malignancy is incurable because it is in an inoperable area or is discovered after the cancer has metastasized. Metastasis is fairly common because the esophagus is close to other vital structures. All malignant tissue that can be isolated is removed. Three common surgical treatments include eso-

phagectomy with graft replacement, esophagogastrostomy, and esophagoenterostomy (colon interposition). Often the client requires parenteral fluids and TPN after surgery. Radiation therapy is a palliative treatment usually included before or after surgery or both. Chemotherapy and photodynamic therapy may be used to inhibit growth of the malignant lesion (see Chap. 82).

Nursing Considerations

Nursing considerations relate to management of symptoms, providing sources of nutrition, and routine postoperative care. Special considerations for clients with cancer are discussed in Chapter 82.

DISORDERS OF THE STOMACH

Gastritis

Gastritis (stomach inflammation), commonly called *indigestion,* occurs in acute, chronic, and toxic forms. Overeating, ingesting irritating medications (eg, aspirin or steroids) or poisonous food, abusing alcohol, or microbial infection are causes of acute gastritis. *Acute gastritis* is characterized by abdominal pain, often with *anorexia* (refusal to eat), nausea, and *enteritis* (intestinal inflammation). Treatment involves removing offending foods or medications and giving a bland diet of liquids or soft foods, along with antacids.

Chronic gastritis continues over time. Pain may occur after eating, but often the person has no pain. Causes include excessive alcohol use, vitamin deficiencies, hiatal hernia, ulcers, and abnormalities in gastric secretions. Treatment is similar to that for peptic ulcer (see below).

Toxic gastritis follows ingestion of poison. It is characterized by burning stomach pain, cramps, nausea, vomiting, and diarrhea. Emesis or diarrhea may be bloody. Toxic gastritis is an emergency. Poison-control specialists in the emergency department treat the client by either flushing out the poison by gavage or neutralizing the poison, if possible, with a substance such as activated charcoal.

Ulcers

An *ulcer* is an open sore in the skin or mucous membrane that is accompanied by sloughing of inflamed and necrotic tissue. A *peptic ulcer* is a break in the integrity of the mucosa of the esophagus, stomach, or duodenum. Peptic ulcers include gastric ulcers and duodenal ulcers.

Gastric ulcers (stomach ulcers) are thought to result from a break in the mucous barrier mechanisms that normally protect the stomach's lining. *Duodenal ulcers* (ulcers in the duodenum) are characterized by increased gastric secretion of hydrochloric acid. The presence of the gram-negative bacteria *Helicobacter pylori* is strongly associated with antral gastritis, duodenal ulcers, and to a lesser degree, gastric ulcers and cancer. *H. Pylori* is not linked to esophageal ulcers.

Signs and Symptoms

Table 87-2 compares gastric and duodenal ulcers. The stool should be tested for occult blood. **Melena** (black, tarry stool

■■■ TABLE 87-2 *Comparing Gastric and Duodenal Ulcers*

	Gastric Ulcer	Duodenal Ulcer
Etiology	Most common in people over age 65 Most common in older women High mortality rate; higher incidence of malignancy than duodenal ulcer	Most common in people under age 65 Three times more common in men than women Four times more common than gastric ulcer
Risk Factors	Stress Alcohol abuse Smoking Nonsteroidal anti-inflammatory drugs and aspirin use (commonly prescribed for arthritis), which contributes to gastric ulcer formation Infection with *Helicobacter pylori*	Stress Alcohol abuse Smoking Pulmonary disease Cirrhosis of the liver Chronic pancreatitis Chronic renal failure Infection with *H. pylori*
Symptoms	High-epigastrium pain 1 to 2 hours after meals; eating may not relieve Weight loss	Mid-epigastrium pain 2 to 4 hours after meals and during night; often relieved by eating Weight gain More likely to perforate than gastric ulcer

containing blood) from bleeding in the stomach may occur and is a significant finding. Gastroscopy and x-ray examination help diagnose peptic ulcer and differentiate it from a cancerous lesion. Diagnosis of *H. pylori* infection can be accomplished by a gastric mucosal biopsy procedure, a serum blood test for antibodies to the *H. pylori* antigen, or a breath test.

Complications

In the event of complications, an NG tube attached to suction will be inserted. The client will be kept NPO for at least 24 hours, and IV fluids will be administered.

Abdominal Infection.   Massive doses of antibiotics will be given to counteract *abdominal infection.* Continued distention without passage of flatus or feces is a sign of serious disruption of peristalsis, causing paralytic ileus.

Hemorrhage.   *Hemorrhage* is another serious and frequent complication of ulcers, occurring when an ulcer penetrates a blood vessel. If the blood vessel is small, bleeding may be so slight that the client does not notice it. Vomiting blood or passing melena is evidence of more extensive hemorrhage. If bleeding is massive, signs of shock appear and include pallor, weak and rapid pulse, low blood pressure, faintness, and collapse. A significant sign of hemorrhage is *coffee-ground emesis* (emesis of partially digested blood). If blood loss is great and sudden, the client is most likely to vomit; if it is small and gradual, the client will most likely pass blood in the stool.

Endoscopic procedures can be performed to seal off bleeding vessels with a small heat probe or bipolar cautery probe passed down an inner channel of an endoscope. Injection of epinephrine by sclerotherapy technique also will stop acute bleeding. Treatment of a bleeding ulcer includes rest, enforced by sedatives. Blood transfusion and IV fluids are often necessary. Surgery will probably be necessary if bleeding continues.

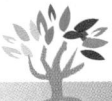 **SPECIAL CONSIDERATIONS: THE LIFE SPAN**

Bleeding With Ulcers

The risk of bleeding is greater in older people, especially if they are taking NSAIDs, such as ibuprofen.

Perforation.   *Perforation* occurs when an ulcer penetrates the wall of the stomach or intestine, allowing the contents to escape into the abdomen, causing *peritonitis* (inflammation of the serous membrane lining the walls of the pelvis and abdomen).

Symptoms of perforation begin with sudden, viciously sharp abdominal pains. Physical signs include pallor and diaphoresis. The abdomen hardens and is tender and painful. The client breathes rapidly and draws up the knees in an attempt to relieve the pain. The client's face later becomes flushed and feverish. This condition can be fatal. It requires immediate surgery to close the perforation. A perforation can occur without warning and may not be preceded by marked signs of digestive disturbance.

Obstruction.   Obstruction may occur when scar tissue builds to the point where it obstructs food passage through the pyloric sphincter. Symptoms include vomiting undigested food and stomach pain. Only vomiting relieves the pain. Peritonitis is a major threat.

Treatment

A variety of treatment modalities are available depending on the severity of symptoms. Diet and medications are effective treatment in most cases. Rest and stress management are also generally indicated. More invasive treatments are indicated in the event of complications as described above.

Medications.   Regimens using bismuth compounds (such as Pepto-Bismol) and antibiotics to eradicate *H. pylori* are proving effective in healing and preventing recurrence of ulcers and gastritis. Other medications used include antacid preparations, histamine (H_2) receptor antagonists, proton pump inhibitors (**PPIs**), and cytoprotective agents, including misoprostol (Cytotec) and sucralfate (Carafate).

Antacid preparations *buffer* (neutralize) gastric hyperacidity. Antacids that contain aluminum hydroxide (such as Amphojel) may cause constipation, and those that contain magnesium hydroxide (such as Mylanta) may cause diarrhea. Maalox and Gelusil combine magnesium and aluminum salts and are less likely to cause electrolyte depletion.

Because antacids can disrupt a person's electrolyte balance, they are often rotated to maintain acid–base balance. Inform the client not to use bicarbonate of soda (baking soda) regularly because it upsets the body's acid–base balance more so than do commercial antacids. The client must chew antacid tablets slowly before swallowing them to obtain their maximum benefits. See In Practice: Important Medications 87-1 for more information.

Histamine (H_2) receptor antagonists inhibit acid secretion in response to all stimuli. Therefore, they reduce gastric acid secretions. The H_2 blockers are well absorbed from the GI tract and begin working within 30 to 60 minutes. IV administration is possible for faster effects. The H_2 blockers usually provide healing for acute gastric and duodenal ulcers in 6 to 8 weeks. They also have been proven safe and effective in long-term management of chronic gastric ulcers and related conditions such as esophagitis and gastritis.

Proton pump inhibitors (PPIs) inhibit the secretion of gastric acid by binding to the proton pump of the stomach's parietal cells. PPIs are potent and widely used due to their effectiveness and the lack of side effects associated with their use. PPIs may be safely administered via NG tube by dissolving them in an alkaline solution.

Misoprostol (Cytotec) is a synthetic prostaglandin (hormone-like medication) that is prescribed in conjunction with nonsteroidal anti-inflammatory drug (NSAID) therapy for arthritic conditions. It enhances gastric mucosal defenses and inhibits gastric secretion to prevent gastric ulcers. Clients with arthritis are at the greatest risk for gastric ulcers, especially if they are female and over 65 years of age. Diarrhea and loose stools are the most commonly reported side effects of misoprostol. Sucralfate (Carafate) provides an additional protective mucous coating to the lining of the stomach and duodenum. It allows healing of ulcers or gastritis. Its most common side effect is constipation.

Diet.   Recent research in diet therapies has shown that the frequency of meals is as important as their content. The client may follow a bland diet while pain is present. For the first few weeks, the client should eliminate gas-forming and highly seasoned foods, and foods high in roughage (eg, fresh fruits, popcorn, and nuts).

The client should also omit coffee, tea, cola beverages, chocolate, alcohol, and cigarette smoking because they stimulate secretion of hydrochloric acid. The patient can include milk and cream, although not in large quantities. The current dietary trend in ulcer management is three normal meals and a bedtime snack.

☛ KEY CONCEPT

Cigarette smokers are twice as likely to have ulcers as nonsmokers. Alcohol use also predisposes a client to ulcer formation.

Rest and Stress Management.   Rest is important, but it does not necessarily have to be bedrest. Relaxation is even more important; many clients are hospitalized at the onset of treatment to force relaxation. Tranquilizers also may be prescribed. After the course of treatment is established, the client maintains the routine at home.

Nursing Considerations

The goals in ulcer treatment are to prevent irritating the lesion, lessen acidic secretions, reduce activity of the stomach and intestine, and manage emotional stress. Client teaching is an important component. Encourage the client to verbalize his or

---

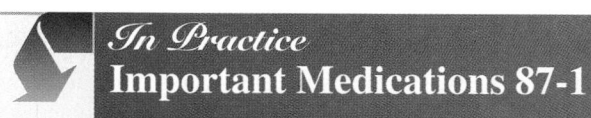

MEDICATIONS FOR TREATING ULCERS

Antibiotics: A 7- to 14-day course of clarithromycin (Biaxin) and metronidazole (Flagyl) in combination with an H_2 blocker or PPI is utilized for the treatment of *Helicobacter pylori*.

Antacids: Amphogel, Mylanta, Maalox, Gelusil, Di-Gel, Riopan

Histamine (H_2) receptor antagonists (H_2 blockers): cimetidine (Tagamet), ranitidine (Zantac), famotidine (Pepcid), nizatidine (Axid)

Proton-pump inhibitors: omeprazole (Prilosec), lansoprazole (Prevacid), pantoprozole (Protonix), rabeprozole (Aciphex), esomeprozole (Nexium)

Mucous enhancer or gastric-secretion inhibitor (protects against drug-induced ulcer formation): misoprostol (Cytotec)

Antipeptic: sucralfate (Carafate)

Nursing Considerations

• Remind the client to allow at least 1 hour between eating or taking doses of antacid, and taking H_2 blocker medication. *Rationale: Antacids and food delay absorption of the H_2 blockers, although the therapeutic effect will eventually be the same.*

• Some drugs, such as Zantac and Tagamet, can cause leukopenia. Other side effects include constipation, diarrhea, headache, and dizziness.

her concerns, rather than to internalize them. Physical activity also may help to alleviate frustrations. Stress management workshops and support groups often are beneficial. See In Practice: Educating the Client 87-2.

Stomach Cancer

Stomach cancer is known as the "silent neoplasm" because it is usually not detected until after metastasis to adjacent structures. Thus the client's prognosis is often poor. Signs and symptoms include sudden *dyspepsia* (indigestion) unrelieved by eating, which is the most important symptom. In addition, the person experiences unexplained weight loss and generalized weakness. Coffee-ground emesis and the absence of free hydrochloric acid in the stomach are other significant findings (Box 87-2). Diagnosis is generally made after microscopic examination of gastric contents show cancer cells. Other routine laboratory and x-ray studies confirm the presence of a neoplasm and its exact location.

Treatment generally involves surgery to completely remove the tumor. A total or subtotal gastrectomy may be performed, depending on the tumor's size and location. The spleen and many structures surrounding the stomach may be removed as well. Metastasis to the spleen, lymph nodes, liver, pancreas, and esophagus is common. Nursing considerations will include pre- and postoperative teaching as previously discussed for gastric surgeries. Client and family grief counseling may be necessary.

DISORDERS OF THE SMALL OR LARGE BOWEL

Diverticulosis and Diverticulitis

Diverticulosis refers to a condition in which outpouches (ruptures) occur along the intestinal wall. Diverticula can occur anywhere in the GI tract. Symptoms that accompany diverticular disease are vague or absent. Diverticula often are found during diagnostic procedures performed for other problems. A barium enema can confirm the presence of diverticula, but the barium may become trapped in the diverticula and form hard masses. Endoscopy can confirm the diagnosis by permitting direct visualization of the lesions.

Diverticulitis occurs when the diverticula become inflamed, usually due to obstruction of the diverticula and bacterial invasion. Signs and symptoms of diverticulitis include nagging, cramping pain and tenderness in the left lower abdomen, abdominal distention, flatulence, and elevated temperature. Increased pressure within the lumen of the bowel can cause rupture of the diverticulum and result in abscess formation and peritonitis.

Treatment

Treatment of diverticulosis and diverticulitis consists of dietary management of symptoms, medications, and possible surgery. Consumption of high-residue foods is recommended to prevent the formation of diverticula and to prevent acute onsets of diverticulitis. When diverticula are present and inflamed, stool softeners and bulk-forming agents, such as psyllium (Metamucil), help to produce soft, nonirritating, and unforced bowel movements.

When fever and abdominal pain are present, indicating infection along with inflammation, antibiotics are prescribed. A low-residue diet, including avoidance of milk products, is recommended. During an acute episode of diverticulitis, the client may be assigned NPO status and have an NG tube in place for suctioning to allow the bowel to rest. When acute

---

> ➤ **BOX 87-2**

SYMPTOMS OF ULCERS AND STOMACH CANCER

Ulcers
- Frequent dyspepsia
- Burning sensation in stomach (may be seasonal)
- Pain that always begins in same place
- Pain relieved by eating or, possibly, vomiting
- Black, tarry stools (*melena*)
- Free hydrochloric acid in stomach
- Tenseness, irritability
- Difficulty sleeping
- Weight often maintained

Stomach Cancer
- Sudden dyspepsia
- Absence of pain until cancer is advanced ("silent neoplasm")
- Pain unrelieved by eating or vomiting
- Coffee-ground emesis
- Absence of free hydrochloric acid in stomach
- Weakness, lethargy, tiredness much of the time
- Unexplained weight loss
- Cancer cells possibly visible in slides of gastric contents

---

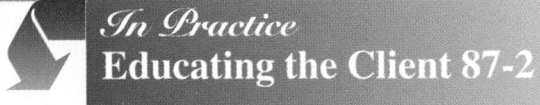

In Practice
Educating the Client 87-2

ULCER MANAGEMENT
- Three meals and a bedtime snack should be routine.
- Meal size and portions should be at a comfortable and tolerated level. Avoid overdistention.
- Determine and eliminate foods that aggravate symptoms.
- Eat foods slowly and chew them well.
- Contact a physician if diarrhea or increased discomfort occur or if the condition is not improving.
- Use methods of relaxation.
- Verbalize concerns.
- Establish a personal balance between exercise and physical and emotional rest, especially during stressful periods.

diverticulitis resolves, the client should begin to add high-fiber foods to the diet and continue to use bulking agents.

Nursing Considerations

Client and family dietary teaching are important aspects of prevention of attacks, management of symptoms, and treatment during attacks. Adequate water intake of 6 to 8 glasses each day is important. Regular bowel habits, regular exercise, and plenty of fruit, vegetables, and fiber are key factors in preventing future problems. Teach the client when to use high-fiber and low-fiber foods.

Hernias

Hernias develop when abdominal muscle weakness causes a portion of the GI tract to protrude through muscle. Herniation often occurs when intra-abdominal pressure increases due to obesity, heavy lifting, coughing, blunt trauma to the abdomen, or pregnancy. A hernia may be reducible, irreducible, incarcerated, or strangulated. A *reducible hernia* is one that may be pushed back into the intestine by lying down and pressing on the abdomen. An *irreducible hernia* cannot be manipulated back into the body cavity. An *incarcerated hernia* occurs when the intestine's peristaltic flow is obstructed. A *strangulated hernia* requires immediate surgical intervention because it interrupts blood flow to the tissue, resulting in tissue necrosis (infarction).

Types of Hernias

Types of hernias include hiatal, inguinal, femoral, umbilical, abdominal, and incisional. Congenital defects are responsible for a large number of hernias; these are often detected soon after birth. An acquired hernia may result from heavy lifting, pregnancy, coughing, or sneezing. Later in life, obesity and muscle weakness may cause hernias.

Hiatal hernias are discussed earlier in this chapter in the section on the esophagus. *Inguinal hernias* are the most common type of hernia. They protrude through the inguinal area in the groin, especially in males. *Femoral hernias* are weaknesses of the femoral canal that carries blood vessels and nerves into the thigh. *Umbilical hernias* protrude through the umbilicus. An *abdominal hernia* is a protrusion of the intestine through the abdominal wall. The abdominal wall is weak in spots, and it is at these points that a hernia can develop. An *incisional hernia* may develop in an incisional area following surgery.

Signs and Symptoms

Signs and symptoms of hernia vary, depending on the location. Some hernias are asymptomatic, although if they are left untreated they often enlarge and cause pain. If the condition is allowed to progress, the intestine may become constricted and the blood supply is cut off (a *strangulated hernia*). This development is an obvious emergency.

Treatment

The person may wear a truss or abdominal support over the herniated area to minimize or reduce the hernia. *Herniorrhaphy* is performed to surgically repair a hernia. It can be done using a laparoscopic extraperitoneal approach (**LEP**) after abdominal insufflation with carbon dioxide. The client will only have two or three small "stab wounds" instead of an incision, resulting in less pain and a shorter postoperative recovery period. This method also results in higher success rates than with traditional herniorrhaphy and less recurrence.

If the hernia has gone untreated for many years, herniorrhaphy may not hold because the tissues are weakened and do not heal easily. In this case, a *hernioplasty* may be done. This reconstructive repair includes reinforcement with mesh to prevent future weakness and herniation.

Nursing Considerations

Nursing care after herniorrhaphy typically is not complicated; the client is allowed out of bed the day of the operation and can have food and fluids. In many cases, this procedure is done on an outpatient basis. Make sure that the client has voided postoperatively; urinary retention is a common problem. Encourage the client to move around but to avoid straining and lifting for several weeks or months. Returning to routine activities after laparoscopic surgery, especially if mesh reinforcement was used, occurs quickly. The male client's scrotum may become swollen and painful after inguinal hernia repair. An ice pack and a scrotal support may be ordered for relief.

The client's return to work depends on the hernia's nature and extent and the client's age, weight, and type of employment. If the work is heavy or strenuous, vocational counseling and retraining may be necessary. If a repair with mesh has been done, the person will most likely not have any long-term lifting restrictions. A referral to local vocational rehabilitation services and public health nursing services may be helpful.

Intestinal Obstruction

Ileus is obstruction of the intestine. It may be due to a mechanical or functional difficulty and occurs when gas or fluid cannot move normally through the bowel. *Mechanical obstructions* occur when there is a blockage in the lumen or pressure exerted from outside the intestine. Examples include:

- Stenosis, strictures, and adhesion scars from previous surgery
- **Volvulus** (twisting of the bowel)
- Foreign bodies, such as a fruit pit
- **Intussusception** (telescoping of the bowel)
- Polyps and tumors (eg, diverticulosis)
- Abscesses

Functional obstructions occur when the intestinal motility (*peristalsis*) is defective. Examples include:

- Paralytic ileus
- Muscle spasms (*spastic ileus*)
- Disorders (eg, muscular dystrophy, diabetes mellitus, and Parkinson's disease)

A vascular obstruction, such as atherosclerosis or thrombus formation, also can cause gradual cessation of peristalsis due to decreased blood supply. Pneumonia, pancreatitis, and peritonitis can produce obstruction of infectious origin. A decrease or interruption of the nerve stimulus—which may result from post-anesthesia paralysis, trauma to the autonomic nervous system, complications from peritonitis, inactivity, large doses of narcotics, or other nerve damage—causes paralytic obstruction (*paralytic ileus*) of the intestine.

Signs and Symptoms

Clinical manifestations of intestinal obstruction depend on the type of lesion causing the obstruction, the level and length of bowel involved, the extent to which the obstruction interferes with the blood supply to the intestine, and the completeness of the obstruction.

Abdominal distention, severe cramps, nausea, and vomiting are typical. If the obstruction is high in the GI tract, the client will vomit to empty the stomach of accumulated digestive fluids. As these materials continue to accumulate, the vomitus becomes thick, dark, and foul smelling because the number of bacteria normally present in the digestive tract increases. If the obstruction is further down, vomiting may be absent. The client is listless, generally weak, thirsty, and has a feeling of fullness and constipation. Symptoms of small bowel obstruction develop and progress rapidly; symptoms of large bowel obstruction progress more slowly. If left untreated, the client will become very ill, with symptoms of dehydration and shock.

> **Nursing Alert**
> An intestinal obstruction can be an emergency; it must be treated immediately.

As a tumor in the intestine becomes larger, it may block the lumen of the intestine. An abdominal series will indicate large quantities of fluid or gas in the bowel. Laboratory studies may show infection, electrolyte disruptions, and dehydration.

Treatment

Treatment of the obstruction depends on its cause. Complete obstruction in the small intestine usually necessitates surgery; obstruction in the lower part of the large intestine may be treated medically.

Medical treatment of large bowel obstruction includes intestinal decompression, involving intubation with a nasoenteric tube. Constant suction via a rectal tube is used to keep the intestine empty. The bowel is allowed to rest. A colonoscopy may be done to attempt to untwist or unblock the bowel.

Nursing Considerations

Assist with fluid and electrolyte replacement. It is important to note the quality of bowel sounds. If the client's condition deteriorates, emergency surgery becomes necessary. Postoperative nursing care follows the protocol for abdominal surgery.

Irritable Bowel Syndrome

Irritable bowel syndrome (**IBS**) is also known as *spastic colon, spastic colitis, mucous colitis,* and *irritable colon.* This condition is the most common functional disorder of the GI tract causing increased motility of the small or large intestine. It affects the intestine's structure, but its specific cause is unknown. IBS does not lead to, or cause, ulcerative colitis or cancer.

Signs and Symptoms

IBS causes alternately tense and flaccid bowel segments. Resulting symptoms can include nausea, abdominal pain, cramps, *flatulence* (gas), altered bowel function (constipation or diarrhea), and hypersecretion of colonic mucus. Symptoms vary in intensity and pattern, and may be aggravated by foods, alcohol ingestion, stress, and fatigue.

Diagnosis is accomplished by tests such as the upper GI series and barium enema. Colonoscopy is appropriate for older adults, because these tests also eliminate other pathologies with similar symptoms.

> **Nursing Alert**
> Rectal bleeding and fever are not associated symptoms of IBS. The person with these symptoms should report to a physician for evaluation.

Treatment

An integrated, individualized approach is recommended for treatment of IBS. Clients must be willing to explore their lifestyle patterns and emotional stressors. They may require lifestyle changes to manage this chronic and frustrating condition. Counseling may be needed, along with biofeedback and relaxation training, which has proven helpful for people with IBS.

A high-fiber diet and agents that add bulk (eg, Metamucil, Effersyllium) help to promote an even and consistent stool to pass through the bowel. The diet also should include adequate oral fluids and regular meal patterns. If the client is subject to lactose intolerance, limitation of dairy products is helpful.

Medications may be prescribed to provide symptomatic relief. For example, sedatives or tranquilizers such as alprazolam (Xanax) help to quiet the bowel's activity and provide relaxation. Dicyclomine hydrochloride (Bentyl) and hyoscyamine (Donnatal) are antispasmodic agents that can relieve pain and cramping symptoms if used routinely during periods of increased bowel irritability. Common side effects are dry mouth, blurred vision, and dizziness. Some clients require occasional antidiarrheal agents, such as loperamide (Imodium), to help them maintain normal activity.

Nursing Considerations

Remind the client to be consistent and follow the prescribed treatment plan closely. Many times clients with IBS get discouraged by seemingly slow improvement or small setbacks, which may keep them from allowing the bowel to establish a more normal pattern. Keeping a log or diary can help the client track progress or identify needed changes.

Constipation

Constipation is a condition in which the client has infrequent, hard bowel movements accompanied by mucus. Constipation may be an acute or chronic condition. The client may have a fecal impaction with loose, watery stool and mucus traveling around the constipated stool. Dehydration, cancer, chemical dependency, or mechanical obstruction may cause this condition. It also may be a psychosomatic disorder. Because prolonged constipation can be a sign of serious difficulty, such as intestinal obstruction or paralytic ileus, immediate action is needed to determine the cause.

Warn the client not to strain while having a stool. Encourage the client to avoid worrying about constipation because undue concern can compound the problem. Teach the client to drink a great deal of fluids, drink prune juice or eat bran, increase dietary bulk, exercise, and follow a regular schedule for defecation. Explain the importance of evacuating the bowel whenever the client feels the urge; postponing the act desensitizes the bowel to the presence of feces.

Removal of feces and flatus can be accomplished by enemas. The client with a disorder of the digestive system may need an enema to prepare for a diagnostic test or surgery, to alleviate symptoms of constipation or distention, or to administer specific medications and fluids.

Digital removal of fecal impaction may be necessary for severely constipated or paralyzed clients. The procedure is done only after stool softeners and enemas have failed to remove the mass.

Fecal impaction can develop after a barium enema or barium swallow and should be considered a possible complication of these procedures. Chapter 51 explains the symptoms of fecal impaction and the procedure for its removal.

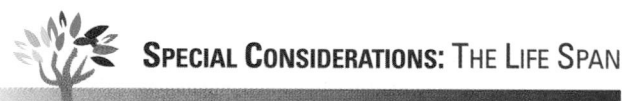

SPECIAL CONSIDERATIONS: THE LIFE SPAN

Constipation

Older adults are especially prone to constipation and its complications. They commonly take multiple medications, which may decrease peristalsis, cause water loss, or interfere with intestinal absorption. In addition, they may have limited mobility or exercise, limited access to proper dietary fiber, and difficulty with chewing, swallowing, or digesting. Daily stool softeners are often suggested; however, regular laxative use should be avoided. Assess an older client complaining of abdominal pain for constipation. Constipation may lead to the serious complications of impaction and infarction.

Caution: Loose, watery stools may not be diarrhea; they may signify severe constipation with leakage of water around the blockage. Assess the client for fecal impaction.

Diarrhea

Diarrhea consists of stools that are liquid or semiliquid, and often very light colored. They may be foul smelling, and con-

tain mucus, pus, blood, or fats. Diarrhea often is accompanied by flatus and severe, painful abdominal cramps or spasms (**tenesmus**), which defecation relieves. Complications of severe or chronic diarrhea include dehydration, electrolyte disturbances, cardiac dysrhythmias, and hypovolemic shock.

Diarrhea is generally a symptom of some underlying condition, such as bacterial invasion by *S. dysenteriae* or *Salmonella. Clostridium botulinum* is an anaerobic bacterium that is often the cause of nosocomial diarrhea. This infection occurs most frequently in acutely ill clients who have received numerous courses of antibiotics. IBS or *inflammatory bowel disease* (**IBD;** discussed later) often is the cause of diarrhea. Medications, such as certain antibiotics, can cause diarrhea that stops when treatment stops.

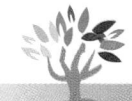

SPECIAL CONSIDERATIONS: THE LIFE SPAN

Giardiasis

Giardiasis, caused by the protozoan *Giardia lamblia,* is commonly associated with contaminated water or food. Daycare centers have experienced outbreaks of diarrhea associated with poor handwashing between diaper changes and children sharing toys that have been in their mouths. Symptoms may be mild or severe with non-bloody diarrhea, abdominal pain, and distention. Metronidazole (Flagyl) for adults and furazolidone (furozone) for children are the usual antibiotic treatments. The entire family or daycare may need stool testing to completely eradicate giardia infection.

Diagnosis

If chronic and not self-limiting, diarrhea symptoms must be evaluated for possible causes (particularly before the client self-medicates). Diarrhea that continually awakens a client from normal sleep often indicates intestinal pathology. A bacterial infection and IBS or IBD should be ruled out.

Stool tests, including cultures, occult blood tests, and O&P smears, are performed. Hematology studies indicate infection or inflammatory processes. Lower GI barium examinations are done to rule out pathologic causes.

Treatment

Treatment is geared toward eliminating the cause of the diarrhea. IV fluids and electrolytes may be needed, especially in the young and in older clients. See In Practice: Important Medications 87-2 for more information.

Nursing Considerations

Assess the client's fluid I&O and weight. Monitor for signs and symptoms of electrolyte disturbances and electrolyte levels, because diarrhea can severely disrupt electrolyte balance. Record the exact time, amount, and character (TAC) of each stool. You may need to restrict the client's diet to clear liquids

In Practice
Important Medications 87-2

MEDICATIONS FOR TREATING DIARRHEA

Motility reduction: loperamide (Imodium), diphe-
noxylate (Lomotil)
Bile salt-binding agent: cholestyramine (Questran)
Antibiotics: to treat bacterial/microbial diarrhea

Nursing Considerations

• These medications are contraindicated in poisoning until the poison is removed from the digestive
  tract.
• Loperamide and diphenoxylate have the potential
  for drug dependence. They may cause sedation,
  dizziness, constipation, and drying of mucous
  membranes.
• Diphenoxylate is not recommended for use in
  pregnancy.
• Cholestyramine may cause constipation, nausea,
  bloating, abdominal pain, and rash. To administer,
  sprinkle powder on surface of liquid or wet food;
  carbonated beverages may foam excessively. Do
  not administer with other medications because it
  blocks their absorption.

and then reintroduce fluids and foods slowly to observe for
improvement or worsening. Client and family teaching include
criteria to prevent food contamination with *S. aureus* and *Salmonella,* which are often sources of diarrhea.

Inflammatory Bowel Disease (IBD)

Inflammatory bowel disease is a general term for ulcerative
colitis and Crohn's disease. Research suggests that environmental, immunologic, hereditary, age, and cultural factors
influence this disease. The cause and cure of IBD, however, are
unknown.

Ulcerative colitis involves inflammation and ulceration of
mucosa and submucosa (the colon's lining). This disease can
span the entire length of the colon, but most frequently begins
in the rectum and distal colon. *Chronic ulcerative colitis* (CUC)
implies long-standing disease. A client's risk of colon cancer
increases if CUC lasts longer than 8 to 10 years.

Crohn's disease can occur in any part of the intestinal tract,
the most common location being the terminal ileum. Unlike
colitis, it involves inflammatory processes of the entire thickness of the bowel wall. It is usually patchy and often skips segments of healthy bowel. The risk of cancer for the client with
Crohn's disease is the same as that for the general population.
Table 87-3 compares ulcerative colitis with Crohn's disease.

Signs and Symptoms

Typical symptoms of ulcerative colitis and Crohn's disease
are diarrhea, blood and mucus in the stool, abdominal pain,

cramps, urgency, bowel incontinence, appetite loss, weight
loss, fever, nausea, and vomiting. Electrolyte imbalance may
result from loss of body fluids. Symptoms may develop gradually or suddenly. Most clients experience patterns of *exacerbation* (attacks) and remission.

Complications

In IBD, bowel obstruction and perforation are threats. They
may result from scar tissue or a **fistula** (abnormal channeling
between loops of bowel) and are the most serious complications of these diseases. Perforation is an emergency. Hemorrhage and peritonitis may develop; removal of the colon and
permanent ileostomy are often necessary. Symptoms of perforation include rapid, thready pulse; extreme anxiety; severe
abdominal pain; fever; abdominal rigidity (boardlike); and
cold, clammy skin. Symptoms of peritonitis are discussed later
in this chapter at "Appendicitis."

Treatment

Advances in medical treatment allow most clients to manage
and cope with IBD. Antidiarrheal medications can allow the
client to maintain normal work and daily activity patterns.

Steroids such as cortisone, which reduce inflammation and
generate healing, are given IV, orally, or rectally (foam, suppositories, or enema). Aminosalicylates (Sulfasalazine, Mesal-
amine, and Olsalazine) are the most commonly used drugs
to treat IBD, especially ulcerative colitis. Mercaptopurine,
methotrexate, and azathioprine are potent immunosuppressants
that are useful in treating IBD, especially Crohn's disease.
Infliximab blocks tumor necrosis factor, which acts to suppress
intestinal inflammation. Close monitoring of blood counts and
the client's clinical condition is necessary with these medications. IV antibiotics may be indicated during severe flare-ups.

Nursing Alert

Clients are weaned off steroid medications
slowly and systematically. They must not stop these
medications suddenly. Steroids suppress normal secretions of the adrenal gland, and abrupt discontinuation
can trigger life-threatening adrenal insufficiency problems. Milder withdrawal symptoms include yawning,
gooseflesh, and muscle aches and pains. See Chapter 62
for side effects of steroids.

Ulcerative colitis is eliminated by removal of the entire
colon, which is the treatment of choice when surgery is necessary. The standard ileostomy allows fecal waste to collect in
an appliance attached to the abdomen. Approximately 66% of
clients with Crohn's disease require surgery, and 40% of these
require a second surgery. These high percentages are due to
the typical recurrence of Crohn's disease in another bowel
segment. The continent fecal diversion procedure of ileoanal
reservoir has been effective for those with Crohn's disease.

Nursing Considerations

The client who presents with severe symptoms is weak, miserable, and often frightened. Nursing care and medical manage-

■■■ **TABLE 87-3** *C*OMPARISON OF INFLAMMATORY BOWEL DISEASES

	Ulcerative Colitis	Crohn's Disease
Also Known As	Ulcerative proctitis	Transmural colitis Regional enteritis Granulomatous colitis
Cause	Unknown, possibly *Escherichia coli*	Unknown, possibly altered immune system
Influences	Environment, heredity, allergies, age, culture, women more than men	Same as for ulcerative colitis
Location	Mucosa and submucosa of colon and rectum; may be localized but ultimately spreads throughout colon, commonly in left colon and rectum	Entire thickness of wall of small or large intestine in segmented areas; commonly in right colon and ileum
Pathology	Recurrent inflammation and ulceration of colon with formation of abscesses, purulent drainage, and sloughing of mucosa; capillaries become weak and bleed	Acute and chronic inflammation that erodes wall of intestine; fistulas, fissures, and abscesses form.
Signs & Symptoms	Nausea, vomiting, anorexia, weight loss, fever, abdominal pain and cramping, diarrhea with pus and blood, bowel incontinence Stools: 10–20 liquid stools per day with blood and pus (no fat)	Nausea, vomiting, anorexia, weight loss, abdominal pain and cramping, diarrhea mostly without blood, **steatorrhea** (fat in stool) Stools: Three or more times per day; diarrhea not as severe, occasional blood, steatorrhea
Complications	*Toxic megacolon* (severe dilation of colon), electrolyte disturbances, abscesses, fistulas, perforation of colon, increased risk of colorectal cancer	Malabsorption of nutrients, electrolyte disturbances, abscesses, fistulas, bowel obstruction, perforation of colon, increased risk of cancer with age
Medical Interventions	Bowel rest, low-residue and increased protein diet, decreased lactose intake, vitamin supplements, IV therapy with electrolyte replacement, TPN, sedation, antidiarrheal medications, sulfonamides, antibiotics, corticosteroids	Same as for ulcerative colitis
Surgical Interventions	Colostomy (curative if entire colon is removed)	Segmental or total colectomy, removal of diseased areas with anastomosis of bowel (not curative)
Nursing Implications	Avoid laxatives and enemas; monitor I&O, nutrient status, lab values; encourage client to express feelings; offer support and encouragement	Same as for ulcerative colitis

ment, including the use of anticholinergic, antidiarrheal, and antispasmodic agents, are used to promote optimal bowel rest.

The client is NPO or limited to clear liquids. TPN is often used when a client has not responded to medical intervention, and is being prepared for, or has undergone, intestinal resection. The client may receive oral supplements only if tolerated.

Nutritional deficiencies are very common in IBD. The prescribed diet for the person with IBD will probably be high in protein and calories, low residue, and lactose restricted. Anemia and vitamin deficiencies can be treated nutritionally or with supplements.

Even though recent studies have indicated that emotional stress does not contribute to the development of the disease, emotional stress can aggravate and stimulate physical symptoms. Be sensitive and supportive to help the client cope with disease-related stressors, which include symptoms, diagnostic

tests, bowel preparation, dietary restrictions, activity limitations, and medication side effects.

Appendicitis

Appendicitis is an inflammation of the approximately 4 inches (10 cm) of slender blind tube that open off the tip of the cecum. The appendix may become obstructed by a hard mass of feces, with subsequent inflammation, infection, gangrene, and possible perforation. A ruptured appendix is serious because intestinal contents can escape into the abdomen and cause peritonitis or an abscess.

Signs and Symptoms

An acute attack of appendicitis usually begins with progressively severe generalized abdominal pain, which later localizes as pain and tenderness in the lower right quadrant midway between the umbilicus and the crest of the ilium (*McBurney's point*). An attack of appendicitis may subside and recur.

Ultrasound can often diagnose an enlarged appendix. Rebound tenderness usually is present: when the examiner quickly releases pressure during a palpation assessment, the pain becomes greater than when the pressure was directly on the site.

The quality of the tenderness relates to the exact location of the appendix. Usually nausea, vomiting, a mild to moderate fever, and an increase in leukocytes accompany the pain. A ruptured appendix will result in more severe symptoms associated with peritonitis.

Treatment

Prompt surgical treatment is necessary to remove an acute appendix before it ruptures. Trends toward minimally invasive surgery techniques, such as laparoscopic appendectomy, have lessened the chances of wound infection. Incisions are smaller and recovery periods are shorter.

In most instances, the client recovers rapidly, is permitted fluids and food, and is allowed out of bed soon after the operation. The client may return to work in 10 to 15 days, with cautions to avoid heavy lifting.

If the appendix ruptures, treatment for peritonitis is necessary. Treatment includes an incisional drainage tube and large doses of IV antibiotics. Rupture is a serious and possibly fatal complication. However, modern treatment with suction devices, irrigation of the peritoneum, IV fluids, and antibiotics has greatly reduced this danger.

Nursing Considerations

Many people mistake abdominal pain, nausea, and vomiting as a temporary intestinal upset. Teach all clients what to do, and especially what not to do, for severe abdominal pain as presented at In Practice: Educating the Client 87-3.

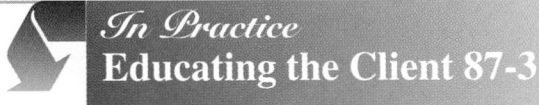

In Practice
Educating the Client 87-3

ACTIONS TO TAKE IN SEVERE ABDOMINAL PAIN

- Do not take an enema or a cathartic. *Rationale: They increase peristalsis, and the result may be a perforated appendix and peritonitis.* If an enema is ordered as a preoperative measure, it must be given low and very slowly.
- Do not take anything by mouth, not even water.
- Call a physician for any attack of severe pain or for pain that persists.
- Do not apply heat to the abdomen. *Rationale: Heat could spread infection.*
- Do not take aspirin or any other analgesic. *Rationale: They tend to mask symptoms. Aspirin and ibuprofen are anticoagulants.*

Peritonitis

Peritonitis is inflammation of the peritoneum, the membrane that lines the abdominal cavity and covers the abdominal organs. Peritonitis usually results from perforation of the intestine or appendix, through which intestinal contents escape into the abdomen. Because the intestinal tract is normally filled with bacteria, the resulting perforation may cause inflammation and peritoneal infection. The most common causes of perforation are appendicitis, ulcer, IBD, abscessed diverticula, and cancer. An infected uterine tube, a ruptured tubal pregnancy, or a ruptured uterus may cause pelvic peritonitis. Peritonitis may be generalized, extending throughout the peritoneum, or it may be localized as an abscess.

Signs and Symptoms

Peritonitis often develops suddenly, with severe abdominal pain, nausea, and vomiting, a gradual temperature increase, a weak and rapid pulse, and low blood pressure. The client's respirations are shallow because breathing hurts the abdomen; the client tries to avoid moving the abdomen and draws up the knees to prevent pressure from the bedclothes and to relieve pain. The abdomen is tense and boardlike and becomes very distended.

Flatus and intestinal contents are stationary in the intestinal tract, and paralytic ileus may develop. If the infection does not respond to treatment, the client grows weaker. The pulse is thready, breathing becomes shallow, temperature falls, and death follows. Diagnosis of peritonitis is made by evaluation of symptoms, laboratory studies, abdominal x-ray examination, ultrasounds, or CT scans. White blood cell counts can be quite high and the client presents as acutely ill.

Treatment

Surgery is sometimes necessary to close the perforation and promote drainage, although the perforation may close by itself. During surgery, the peritoneum is irrigated, usually with a saline and antibiotic solution. Peritonitis is less common today, and recovery is more likely, largely due to improvements in surgery and the use of antibiotics.

Nursing Considerations

Nursing considerations focus on postoperative care of the client. Administer antibiotics to fight infection and analgesics to relieve pain and provide rest. Elevate the head of the bed to the semi-Fowler's position, and closely observe the abdominal wound, pulse, and temperature. Monitor incisional or drainage-tube output (amount and type), vomiting, drainage through the GI tube, and fluid I&O; replace fluids and electrolytes.

Document bowel sounds, and gas and feces passing through the rectum; these signs indicate return of normal GI function. Prevent abdominal distention by using a rectal or NG tube; excess distention is uncomfortable and can disrupt the suture line or cause other difficulties due to pressure. Give special attention to mouth care because the client has no fluids by mouth; fever and the GI tube make the mouth dry and parched. Encourage early, progressive activity to promote peristaltic movement and normal GI function.

Cancer of the Small Intestine

Cancer occurs rarely in the small intestine. However, an increased risk of cancer accompanies ulcerative colitis. If cancer does occur in the small intestine, the person's prognosis is usually poor because the disease is difficult to discover in its early stage. Usually it is asymptomatic. As the cancer advances, pain may be present. The client may have diarrhea (with or without blood), anorexia, nausea, and vomiting. Perforation or obstruction may occur.

The portion of the bowel containing the tumor may be removed and the ends of the bowel joined. Such anastomosis is impossible if malignancy is extensive. Suction relieves distention, IV fluids are given, and antibiotics may be prescribed. Postoperative nursing care is routine.

Colon Cancer

Colon cancer is believed to arise from a single polypoid lesion. Early detection requires surveillance for polyps. The American Cancer Society recommends screening procedures in an effort to locate polyps. Monitoring for occult blood also may be done as part of screening.

☛ KEY CONCEPT

Screening tests, such as rectal examination, proctoscopy (sigmoidoscopy), and colonoscopy, can discover colorectal cancer early. These tests are often recommended for clients older than 40 years of age who are at risk. Risk factors include:

- *Family history of cancer, especially of the rectum, bowel, or female reproductive organs*
- *Family history of ulcerative colitis or Crohn's disease*
- *Presence of precancerous or bleeding polyps*
- *Change in bowel habits (constipation and diarrhea)*
- *Rectal bleeding or blood in the stool*
- *High-fat diet*
- *Low-residue diet*
- *Over 40 years of age*

Signs and symptoms include nausea, vomiting, weight loss, abdominal cramping or fullness, change in bowel habits (diarrhea or constipation or both), excessive flatus, anemia, rectal bleeding, anorexia, and **cachexia** (general ill health and malnutrition). Diagnosis is made by colonoscopy with biopsy of polyps. Treatment generally consists of various regimens of chemotherapy, radiation, and surgery (as discussed in Chap. 82). Nursing considerations relate to the stage of the disease and the course of treatment. Ostomy care is discussed earlier in this chapter.

DISORDERS OF THE SIGMOID COLON AND RECTUM

Hemorrhoids

Hemorrhoids are swollen (*varicose*) veins of the anus or rectum. *External hemorrhoids* protrude as lumps around the anus. They are painful, especially if the client is constipated and strains to have a bowel movement. They may alternately appear and disappear.

Signs and Symptoms

Usually, external hemorrhoids do not bleed, but they may become large, painful, and itchy. Uterine pressure on the rectum during pregnancy, intra-abdominal tumors, constipation, diarrhea, obesity, congestive heart failure, and portal hypertension are major causes. *Internal hemorrhoids* develop inside the anal sphincter; they may bleed but are unlikely to be painful if they do not protrude. Signs of bleeding may be no more than a drop of blood on the toilet paper, or bleeding may be so extensive and continuous that it causes anemia. Internal hemorrhoids almost always protrude on defecation, but at first the client can push them back with the finger. As hemorrhoids grow larger, pushing them back is no longer possible, and they discharge blood and mucus. The proctoscope allows the provider to inspect inside the rectum, to visualize hemorrhoids, and to take a biopsy sample.

Treatment

Sometimes hemorrhoids disappear without treatment. Often warm sitz baths, anesthetic ointments, or witch hazel compresses (Tucks) will relieve them. Keeping stools soft through proper diet and stool softeners may help. Correcting constipation can prevent and eliminate hemorrhoids.

If surgery is necessary, the veins are tied off and excised (*hemorrhoidectomy*) or cauterized. Sometimes a solution is injected to shrink (*sclerose*) the tissues. Occasionally, hemorrhoidectomy must be done if the hemorrhoid is thrombosed, causing vascular obstruction. This situation is not life threatening; surgery is done to relieve pain.

Nursing Considerations

The client receives a cleansing enema at home the night before surgery. Enemas are given "until returns run clear" the morning of the operation. Cleanse the rectal area and shave it, in addition to other prescribed routines.

When the client returns from the operating room, position him or her on the side or abdomen to relieve pressure on the operative area. Give analgesics as ordered. A liquid diet is permitted for the first meal after the operation; thereafter, a full diet is allowed.

Allow the client to sit up. A rubber ring or flotation pad under the buttocks helps relieve pressure on the operative area. The client needs to move as soon as possible to prevent postoperative complications. On the operative day or the next day, the physician will want the client to ambulate.

Several daily sitz baths may be ordered. Assist the client with getting in and out of the tub. The heat of the bath may make the person feel faint. Many facilities have eliminated the sitz bath structures and replaced them with personal, portable sitz units that fit on top of the commode. The client should continue therapy for about 20 minutes, with the water's temperature at 110° F (43.3° C). The water is best if it circulates.

Because removal of hemorrhoids involves excision of portions of blood vessels, bleeding may occur. Assess for signs of bleeding, either on the dressings or as indicated by symptoms of faintness, weakness, lowered blood pressure, or other signs of shock.

The client will need assistance with the first bowel movement following any rectal surgery. The client is naturally apprehensive. Explain that stool softeners are given to make the bowel movement easier. The client may feel some pain but probably much less than he or she imagines beforehand.

Encourage the client to heed the urge to defecate; otherwise, constipation may develop. He or she should not use toilet paper because it may damage the suture line. Tucks are often used to cleanse and soothe the anal area and to relieve itching.

Petrolatum applied around the rectal area when moist compresses are being used helps maintain the skin's elasticity and integrity. If the client is unable to defecate by the second postoperative day, report this finding to the physician. If defecation has not occurred by the third day, an enema will probably be ordered.

Because the surgery was performed in close proximity to the urinary structures, anesthesia or manipulation may make voiding difficult. If the client does not void, distention could cause complications and discomfort, and catheterization will be needed.

Anal Fissure

An *anal fissure* is an ulcer in the skin of the anal wall. It causes severe pain on defecation and sometimes slight bleeding. The client may dread the pain so much that he or she delays defecation and becomes constipated. Sitz baths and local anesthetic ointments are commonly used to treat anal fissure; a stool softener also helps. The only cure for this condition is surgical removal of the ulcer.

Anal Abscess and Anal Fistula

An *anal abscess* is caused by infected tissue around the rectal area. This condition is painful and may be accompanied by fever and chills. The abscess is usually incised and drained, or it may rupture spontaneously. An *anal fistula* usually develops as a result of an anal abscess. A small tunnel forms in the tissues that discharges pus and feces through one or more openings onto the skin.

Treatment

Surgery is necessary to open the fistulous tract; medication-impregnated packing is inserted to keep the wound's edges apart. These measures allow the tissues to heal by granulation, thus eliminating the fistula. The fistula must heal from the inside out, or another abscess will form.

Nursing Considerations

Generally, nursing care is similar to that for any client after rectal surgery, with the following differences. Pack the fistula wound with petroleum gauze and change the dressing every day. Drainage from the abscess is profuse, purulent, and foul smelling. You need to change the dressing on the wound frequently. Dispose of dressings properly and wear gloves to prevent the spread of disease. Keep the fistula draining. If it stops draining before the entire area is filled in with granulation tissue, another abscess will form.

Cancer of the Rectum

The exact cause of rectal cancer is not known; risk factors include a family history of colon or rectal cancer, history of rectal polyps, history of IBD, and a diet high in fat and protein and low in fiber. Symptoms of rectal cancer include rectal pain, alternating constipation and diarrhea, feeling of incomplete evacuation after a bowel movement, bloody stool, and tenesmus (ineffective, painful straining at stool). Rectal cancer is not as common as colon cancer. Diagnosis is made by sigmoidoscopy with biopsy of polyps.

Treatment

If a cancerous growth is in the upper part of the rectum, it can be removed without removal of the rectal sphincter; ultimately, the bowel will function normally. If the tumor involves the rectal opening, a dual operation is necessary through the abdomen from above (including a colostomy) and through the perineum from below. This second type of surgery is called an *abdominal-perineal resection*. With surgical staplers and other newer instruments, some surgeons have successfully retained the rectal sphincter, performing a low resection and anastomosis to eliminate the need for a permanent colostomy.

Nursing Considerations

Nursing care for the client who has had surgery for rectal cancer is extensive. Carefully assess vital signs. Check dressings for bleeding at regular intervals. The danger of shock after this surgery is great. Nursing measures often include caring for a colostomy, administering parenteral fluids (including blood transfusion), NG suctioning, caring for bladder drainage (a Foley catheter is usually inserted in the bladder), and irrigating and caring for drainage from the perineal wound. Turn the client frequently to prevent respiratory complications and thrombophlebitis; finding a comfortable position may be difficult. If the client's condition permits, encourage him or her to ambulate as soon as possible postoperatively, usually within 2 days. Recovery is much faster if the client ambulates soon; however, he or she will require your assistance.

DISORDERS OF THE LIVER

Liver Failure

Liver failure (hepatic coma) is a failure of the liver cells to clear toxins. The waste products build up in the body, resulting in diminished cerebral function. Liver failure can be an acute or chronic condition. Causes include extensive damage to liver cells, such as may occur after massive GI hemorrhage, as a complication of some surgical procedures, after massive infections, and following an overdose of certain drugs. It also occurs in the client with alcoholic liver disease such as cirrhosis.

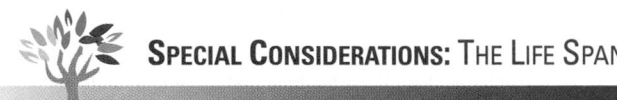

SPECIAL CONSIDERATIONS: THE LIFE SPAN

Overdose on Acetaminophen

Clients who overdose on acetaminophen (Tylenol) are at risk for fulminant hepatic failure. Small children who accidentally ingest even a few tablets could have significant problems. Appropriate therapy should begin within 24 hours of ingestion.

Signs and Symptoms

Liver failure is characterized by tremors and mental changes, including seizures, stupor, and coma. Fulminant hepatic failure involves progressive multisystem failure resulting from massive liver cell death. Acute hepatitis B infections may be the initial causative agent. Clients are confused, *somnolent* (very sleepy), or comatose and usually have ascites, edema, *coagulopathy* (clotting disorder), and a shrinking liver. The mortality rate from this condition is high, and care is supportive. Diagnosis is made by liver function tests. Blood ammonia levels are high because the liver cells cannot convert ammonia to urea. Ammonia, a by-product of protein metabolism, is toxic to the brain.

Treatment

Treatment of liver failure is symptomatic, including control of bleeding, a low-protein diet, and careful management of fluid and electrolyte balance. Antibiotics may be given, and in some cases, corticosteroids. The client's prognosis is guarded, and the possibility of successful treatment decreases with each episode. See In Practice: Nursing Care Guidelines 87-4 for nursing care of the client with a liver disorder.

Cirrhosis

Cirrhosis is a chronic, degenerative disease of the parenchymal cells (the normal architecture and functioning cells) of the liver. Ultimately the liver can no longer do its work. The hepatocytes become infiltrated with fatty and fibrous tissue that cannot detoxify body waste. *Intrahepatic obstructive jaundice* results when hepatocytes are no longer able to function. All body functions eventually deteriorate.

Uncontrolled cirrhosis may result in *hepatorenal syndrome* and *hepatic coma*. Toxins absorbed by the GI tract are not metabolized properly and are allowed to circulate freely in the brain, producing *hepatic encephalopathy*.

In an effort to repair itself, the liver may become so enlarged (*hepatomegaly*) that the blood vessels serving it become ob-

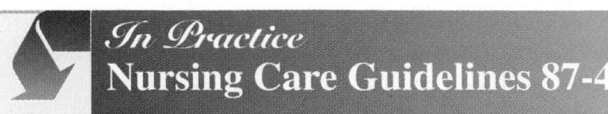

In Practice
Nursing Care Guidelines 87-4

CARING FOR THE CLIENT WITH A LIVER DISORDER

- Use starch baths, calamine lotion, and tepid sponging for relief from itching.
- Place calamine lotion and cotton at the bedside, so the client can apply lotion to spots that itch. Make sure that nails are trimmed. *Rationale: Pruritus is a common symptom in liver disorders.*
- If ascites is present, place the client in a high- or semi-Fowler's position. *Rationale: Facilitate respiration and gas exchange.*
- Assess for signs of blood in the stool and urine, or on the toothbrush when the client brushes the teeth. Look for black-and-blue marks. *Rationale: These are signs of a bleeding disorder, a common complication of liver disease.*
- Exert pressure on the puncture site for a longer time than usual after the needle is withdrawn during any procedure. *Rationale: Prevent a hematoma that would ooze blood and make it impossible to use the vein again. This is important, because people with liver conditions need frequent blood tests. A central line or heparin lock is often in place. (Apply pressure to the site of an intramuscular injection as well.)*
- Provide support and explain jaundice. *Rationale: The sense of self-worth can be impaired because of the client's yellow appearance.*

structed (*portal hypertension*). Deranged liver metabolism also permits the accumulation of hormones that regulate sodium and water, which can lead to a further increase in portal hypertension and ascites.

Increased pressure in the hepatic portal system, combined with decreased production of albumin by hepatocytes and the development of ascites, leads to the formation of esophageal varices. Esophageal varices often rupture, causing massive *hematemesis* (bloody emesis) and hypovolemic shock. If the person survives the hemorrhage, the body's defenses are reduced, and he or she is more susceptible to infection.

Cirrhosis is more prevalent among men than women and occurs most often in people between the ages of 45 and 65. Chronic, long-term alcohol abuse is the most common cause of liver failure, cirrhosis, ascites, and esophageal varices. Drugs, toxins, and certain general anesthetics as well as several types of viral hepatitis also can lead to liver dysfunction, cirrhosis, and ascites.

Signs and Symptoms

Cirrhosis may develop so gradually that the client may not realize that anything is wrong and may only experience indigestion and anorexia. The client may be unaware of a low-grade fever or of weight loss because an increase in abdominal girth (due to ascites) offsets the weight loss. As cirrhosis advances, the client has abdominal pain and a rapid pulse, and breathing becomes difficult because of the enlarged abdomen.

The client tends to bleed easily; blood appears in vomitus or as a nosebleed, and veins are dilated because of portal hypertension. The client is jaundiced, and the skin is dry. He or she feels weak and confused. Hemorrhaging and infection may develop. Diagnosis is made on the basis of symptoms, medical history, x-ray studies, and biopsy. Serial liver function tests are usually done to monitor the extent of the condition.

Treatment

Treatment for liver cirrhosis aims at helping the liver repair itself to maximize liver function. It extends over a long period. In the client with liver failure, at least 2 months are needed before improvements can be noted. The treatment goal is to stop or delay the progression of symptoms.

Alcohol avoidance is a must. Client teaching and referrals to proper agencies that may assist the client to abstain from drinking alcoholic products are important initial steps. Dietary management may require the restriction of dietary protein. Maintaining electrolyte balance will also help lower the ammonia levels. The medication lactulose (Cephulac) will promote ammonia retention and excretion through the GI tract. To relieve pressure from the fluid of ascites, an abdominal paracentesis may be performed.

Providing a safe and controlled environment will prolong life and stabilize the condition. Care must be taken to prevent complications associated with the client's activity intolerance, such as pneumonia and thrombophlebitis.

Nursing Considerations

Teach the client that compliance with dietary and fluid restrictions is necessary to promote health. The diet is high in vitamins, moderate in carbohydrates and fats, and low in sodium; the amount of protein depends on the liver's functional level. If these essential nutrients are not supplied, the body burns up its store of protein, thus increasing accumulation of ammonia (a waste product) in the blood. Teach the client to omit alcohol, tobacco, and fatty foods (pork, bacon, gravies, pastries). Give small liquid or semisolid meals frequently because they are usually more appealing to the person with a poor appetite.

Frequent oral hygiene may promote an increase in appetite. The diet is often supplemented with multivitamins and vitamin B_{12}. Vitamin K is given (usually subcutaneously) to reduce the risk of hemorrhage. Watch for bruising on the skin (*petechiae*) and bleeding following an injection.

Diuretics and reduced sodium intake are ordered. Monitor daily weights and accurate I&O, which will indicate if the liver is functioning. Take abdominal girth measurements as often as ordered. Position the client in a semi-Fowler's position to aid breathing. Good skin care is important. Emollient baths may be ordered to reduce *pruritus* (itching) and to soothe the skin. Care for the client with a liver disorder is summarized at In Practice: Nursing Care Guidelines 87-4. Clients who show signs and symptoms of hepatic encephalopathy need much attention and monitoring because of their altered level of consciousness.

Hepatitis

Hepatitis is an acute or chronic condition of liver inflammation that also may be accompanied by liver tissue damage. Viruses are the most prevalent causes of hepatitis, affecting several hundred million people throughout the world. Alcohol, some drugs, and some autoimmune conditions also cause forms of hepatitis. Table 87-4 compares causes of various types of hepatitis.

Signs and Symptoms

Signs and symptoms of hepatitis are varied and often subtle, making diagnosis and prevention difficult. Box 87-3 lists common presenting signs and symptoms. Diagnosis is made by general liver function tests and specific antibody testing for viruses. Medical knowledge about hepatitis has grown significantly in the past two decades. Blood tests can distinguish among many of the viruses that cause most cases of hepatitis.

Types of Hepatitis

Hepatitis A (HAV).   **HAV,** formerly called *infectious hepatitis,* is the most common form of viral hepatitis. It is spread by the oral–fecal route and is transmitted through contaminated food, water, or infected food handlers. Oral–anal sexual practices also can transmit the virus. HAV primarily affects

■ ■ ■ TABLE 87-4 *Comparing Causes of Hepatitis*

	Hepatitis A	Hepatitis B	Hepatitis C	Hepatitis D	Hepatitis E	Toxic Hepatitis
Routes of Transmission	Enteric (oral–fecal)	Blood and body fluids	Blood and body fluids	Blood and body fluids	Enteric (oral–fecal)	Inhalation, ingestion, injection of anesthetic gases, chemicals
Notes	Self-limiting; may be asymptomatic Frequently found in daycare centers	Linked to chronic hepatitis Increased risk of liver cancer	Linked to chronic hepatitis Increased risk of liver cancer and cirrhosis	Linked to chronic hepatitis Coinfection with hepatitis B	Self-limiting Rare in the United States	Chemicals damage liver tissue or cannot be excreted

➤ **BOX 87-3**

COMMON PRESENTING SIGNS AND SYMPTOMS OF HEPATITIS

- Fatigue and lethargy
- Nausea (sometimes vomiting and diarrhea)
- Loss of appetite
- Abdominal pain
- Joint and muscle aches
- Mild fever (more common in hepatitis A)
- Malaise (generalized feeling and complaint of illness)
- Jaundice
- Liver enlargement (*hepatomegaly*)
- Dark urine

children and young adults. This disease is attributed to poor sanitation, crowded conditions, and difficulty in recognizing disease carriers. It is preventable by immunization. In HAV, the greatest excretion of the virus occurs before jaundice appears. As the disease runs its course, the person becomes less infectious. Thus, the client may unknowingly spread the disease to others. A person who has been exposed may be given immune serum globulin as a prophylactic measure, which is effective against HAV.

Generally the client is noninfectious approximately 1 month after becoming ill. A person may harbor the virus without actually having the clinical disease. No adequate protection against carriers is known. Clients generally recover fully in 4 to 6 weeks with rest and supportive care. They acquire a lifelong immunity to HAV infection and do not develop chronic hepatitis.

Hepatitis B (HBV).   **HBV,** formerly called *serum hepatitis,* is transmitted by three mechanisms:

1. Percutaneous transmission through infected blood, blood products, or instruments
2. Sexual transmission in semen or saliva
3. Perinatal transmission from an infected mother to her child at birth

Those at risk of exposure include IV drug users who share needles, sexually active homosexual individuals, clients receiving hemodialysis, individuals in mental institutions, and infants of women who are HBV carriers. Healthcare workers are at significant risk, and should follow precautions rigorously to protect themselves. The Centers for Disease Control and Prevention recommends pre-exposure HBV vaccination for people working in medical, dental, laboratory, and associated groups.

The synthetic vaccinations, Recombivax-B or Engerix-B, are given in three intramuscular injections at 0, 1, and 6 months. A titer blood test confirms the presence of antibodies. If the vaccine recipient does not produce antibodies, he or she may receive a booster. If the person still does not form antibodies, he or she is classified as a "nonreactor." A significant percentage of healthy people are nonreactors; the reason is unknown. Many institutions are providing these vaccinations for their at-risk healthcare workers free of charge.

Tracing the exact source of the disease is often difficult because the incubation period of HBV is from 60 to 110 days. The acute symptoms of HBV are more clinically severe and longer lasting than those of HAV, although they may include any of those listed in the previous section.

Recovery and resolution of HBV infection occurs in all but approximately 17% of infected people. Overwhelming acute HBV infection and liver tissue damage can progress to fulminant hepatic failure and death within weeks of clinical onset. Also, a small percentage (5% to 10%) of people do not clear the virus from their blood within 6 months and become chronic carriers of HBV. Persistent HBV infection also increases one's risk of liver cancer.

Hepatitis C (HCV).   Hepatitis C (**HCV**) was formerly called *parenteral non-A, non-B hepatitis.* Individuals with the greatest risk of contracting HCV are IV drug users and individuals who received blood products before changes in laboratory testing for HCV. There are at least four different subtypes of HCV active within the United States.

The incubation of the virus ranges from 35 to 70 days. The clinical manifestations of HCV are typical of the other viral hepatitis infections. Often symptoms are mild enough for the affected individual to overlook and not seek medical intervention. However, 50% of these clients later present with chronic disease, and of those, 20% develop liver cirrhosis. Half of all people newly infected with HCV will become lifetime carriers of the virus. Liver cancer also is associated with HCV. Interferons such as Interferon alfa-2b (Intron), and Robiviran, an antiviral medication, are used to ease symptoms and slow the progression of chronic hepatitis. These clients are often good candidates for liver transplant.

Hepatitis D (HDV).   Only individuals infected with HBV can contract **HDV** as a *coinfection* or a *suprainfection* (at the same time). The severity seems to be related to the severity and virulence of the HBV infection. Interferon is helping those who have developed the chronic form of HDV. Transmission, expected recovery outcomes, and prevention are the same as for HBV.

Hepatitis E (HEV).   Although **HEV** is rare in the United States, it is sporadically epidemic in countries with poor water and sanitation systems, such as India, Pakistan, Mexico, and Peru. Individuals who are traveling to foreign countries need a clear understanding of prevailing conditions and necessary precautions for safe and healthy visits. A client should alert a physician if he or she contracts symptoms in a suspect country. The mode of transmission is oral–fecal. HEV resembles HAV in symptom presentation and clinical course. Recovery is usually complete and lifetime immunity to HEV occurs. A high mortality rate exists in infected pregnant women, however.

Hepatitis G (HGV).   A newly discovered form of hepatitis, **HGV** is transmitted primarily by contact with blood and is seen in IV drug abusers, infants born to infected mothers, and clients who have had drug transfusions or hemodialysis. The disease may manifest with no symptoms or mild disease.

Drug-Induced or Toxic Hepatitis.   Liver injury can result from ingestion or exposure to known or unknown drugs, chemicals, or fumes. These chemicals damage liver tissue or collect in the body and the liver cannot excrete them. These events may cause no symptoms other than elevated liver function tests; a person may, however, exhibit fully developing fulminant hepatic failure. The liver has great regenerating ability, and treatment focuses on clearing the offending agent.

Nursing Considerations

Supportive rest and care while monitoring liver function and electrolyte balance are necessary. Treatment and nursing care are similar for all forms of viral and nonviral hepatitis.

Reduce fatigue by emphasizing bed rest and avoidance of any strenuous physical activity during the acute phase of infection and when presenting symptoms are present, especially jaundice, abdominal discomfort, and abnormal liver tests.

Too much activity too soon is likely to bring on a symptom recurrence. This period may be boring for the client, especially if he or she was active before the illness. Helping the client to gain knowledge of liver disease and understanding of the particular viral infection will help the person consider possible consequences and lifestyle changes. This time can be frightening or enlightening. Supportive listening is an effective tool to help clients recover.

Older adults or those who develop ascites or encephalopathy may require in-hospital management. This treatment includes maintenance of a nutritionally balanced diet, which includes IV hydration and electrolyte management. Injections of vitamin K and fresh frozen plasma may be beneficial. These individuals should use medications sparingly, and avoid alcohol completely.

Closely observe standard precautions when caring for clients with hepatitis. Warn clients never to donate blood if they have ever had an HBV or HCV infection. *Rationale: The virus can be present in the blood and body fluids for an entire lifetime.*

Liver Abscess

Liver abscesses are caused by the spread of infection from some part of the intestinal tract, perhaps the appendix or gallbladder, or by obstruction of the bile tracts. Symptoms are chills, fluctuating temperature (intermittent fever), extreme weight loss, nausea and vomiting, abdominal distention, and right-sided pain in the abdomen and shoulder. Jaundice occurs frequently. Pain over the liver is a later symptom.

If the abscess bursts, it scatters infection through the abdominal or chest cavity. Antibiotics are given, and the outcome depends on how successful the person is at combating the infection. Sometimes an attempt is made to establish drainage by surgery. Standard Precautions help prevent the spread of infection.

Trauma

Frequently, the liver is injured in an accident. Extensive damage is likely to be fatal, and the client may die from hemorrhage before reaching an emergency department. Signs and symptoms may include orthostatic hypotension, low blood pressure,

tachycardia, and shock. Diagnosis may be made using these symptoms and a history of recent trauma. Many clients with a ruptured liver die.

Generally, surgery is necessary to control bleeding or to remove a portion of the damaged liver. One great danger accompanying liver surgery is hemovolemic shock, because the liver is such a vascular organ. Nursing considerations include careful monitoring of vital signs, abdominal assessment, and assisting in treating shock. Use careful sterile technique to prevent infection. Observe the color of wound drainage for indications of bile or blood; either could indicate a rupture of the suture line.

Liver Transplantation

Life-threatening end-stage liver diseases have been treated with transplants. The success of the transplant relates closely to the body's acceptance of the foreign organ, technical difficulties, the hazards of immunosuppression, and the availability of a functioning liver for transplant. The transplanted liver may be a total replacement or a liver segment. During the surgical procedure, hemorrhage is likely and many units of blood are needed.

Liver Cancer

The liver is rarely the site of a primary cancer; more often cancer of the liver is metastatic. A cancer that does begin in the liver can be removed surgically by removing the affected part of the liver. If cancer is due to metastasis, surgery usually is not indicated; the client is treated palliatively with radiation or chemotherapy. Antineoplastic drugs may be infused directly into the liver (*intrahepatic*).

GALLBLADDER DISORDERS

Cholecystitis and Cholelithiasis

Cholecystitis and cholelithiasis are common forms of gallbladder disease. *Cholecystitis* is inflammation of the gallbladder and *cholelithiasis* indicates gallstones. These often occur together and each aggravates the other. The stones may block the duct that leads from the gallbladder. They may injure the wall, leading to infection. Bacterial contamination of bile often develops, causing serious complications.

The most likely victims of gallbladder disease are obese women over 45 years of age. Changes in the form of diet (eg, the use of processed cheese versus natural cheese) are suspected causes of the significant increase in gallbladder diseases in first-generation American Hispanics. Frequent pregnancies also seem to make women more susceptible. Asian Americans seldom have cholecystitis or cholelithiasis.

The cause of gallstones (*calculi*) is unknown. Formation of most gallstones is believed to be due to abnormally thick bile, which is high in cholesterol and low in bile acids. The gallbladder absorbs water, causing the bile to change into crystals, then sludge, and then form gallstones. Some gallstones also have a calcium base; these are harder than cholesterol-based stones.

Nursing Alert

Strenuous dieting and rapid weight loss can precipitate a gallbladder attack or the formation of stones. Lack of fat in the diet causes bile to pool in the gallbladder because it is not needed for fat digestion.

Sometimes the infected gallbladder fills with pus (*empyema of the gallbladder*) and may rupture, causing peritonitis. Chronic gallbladder disease also may permanently damage the liver.

Signs and Symptoms
The symptoms of cholecystitis or cholelithiasis include:

* Sudden onset of acute pain, called *gallstone colic,* in the upper right abdominal quadrant that may radiate to the back or right shoulder; pain usually begins a few hours after eating, although some individuals have no pain
* Indigestion and complaints of feeling "full" after eating; fatty foods make this condition worse
* Light-colored stools, **steatorrhea** (fatty stools that float), excessive flatus, and foul-smelling stools.
* Nausea, vomiting, **eructation** (belching), fever, jaundice, and malaise

Diagnosis is usually made by evaluation of symptoms, and laboratory, ultrasound, or x-ray study. A cholecystogram will be done if time permits. EGD or ERCP of the duodenum or biliary ducts may be performed.

☛ KEY CONCEPT
_____

Some clients describe the pain of gallstone colic as the feeling of a "huge bubble" in the upper abdomen or chest area. It is important to differentiate between gallstone colic and the chest pain related to heart attack.

Treatment
The diet is restricted to non-fat foods. Such foods as cheese, cream, greasy fried foods, fatty meats, and gas-forming vegetables are not given. The client may have lean meat (never fried), plain mashed or baked potato, or rice. Alcoholic beverages are contraindicated. Immediately after an attack, the client receives liquids only. If the attack is severe, meperidine (Demerol) may be given. Morphine should not be used because it is believed to increase the spasms.

In some cases, drugs may be effective in dissolving cholesterol-based gallstones. Chenodiol (Chenix) has been used for several years. A new drug, ursodiol (Actigall), is a naturally occurring bile acid that is taken orally and dissolves non-calcium stones by diluting the thick bile that is present.

Surgical procedures include *cholecystostomy* (opening and draining the gallbladder), *cholecystectomy* (removal of the gallbladder), *choledochostomy* (incision into the common bile duct), and *choledocholithotomy* (incision into the duct and removal of calculi). Cholecystectomy is often done through a laparoscope as an outpatient procedure. The gallbladder is excised by laser and removed through the scope. Recovery is usually fast following this procedure.

Nursing Considerations
Assist with various diagnostic tests. Preoperative preparations are similar to those for other abdominal procedures. Tell the client about the tubes and drains that will be in place postoperatively.

Postoperative nursing care for the client after a cholecystectomy depends on what surgical approach is used. If abdominal laparotomy is done, nursing care is essentially the same as for any major surgery, with the additional responsibilities of assessing and monitoring the amount of bile drainage, protecting the skin around the tube, and providing client teaching regarding bile drainage and tube care. The client is expected to turn, deep breathe, and use the incentive spirometer to prevent pneumonia.

An NG tube is often in place to empty the stomach immediately postoperatively. Many surgeons place a tube into the wound for drainage following surgery. Others allow the ducts to readjust and take over bile drainage spontaneously.

If the client has a drainage tube (most often a T-tube), the physician may order the drainage bag to remain at floor level for a short time to allow the release of excess bile. Later, the bag is raised. Note the level of the container on the nursing care plan, and gradually wean the client from the drainage tube. Measure and record the amount and character of the bile every 24 hours. If the amount does not diminish in a few days, it may indicate that the bile is not entering the intestine properly.

Protect the skin surrounding the tube with zinc oxide or petrolatum. Observe the client's stools and urine for the presence or absence of bile. The bile should disappear, and the stools and urine should become normal in color and consistency as function returns. Document accurate fluid I&O.

Teach the client to maintain low Fowler's position to facilitate drainage. Monitor the tube closely to prevent blockage or dislodgment of the T-tube. After the T-tube has drained for 24 hours, you may be asked to clamp it for 1 to 2 days before removal.

The client may go home with the T-tube in place. Teach the client clamping procedures and what to watch for before discharge. Document all teaching. The client must watch for signs of jaundice or discomfort when the tube is clamped or removed.

Most physicians order a regular diet, as tolerated, after surgery. Most clients have no trouble digesting a small amount of fat. Generally, the client who has had gallbladder surgery should avoid foods that caused preoperative discomfort, such as gas-forming foods and alcohol. The client may be referred to a dietitian for counseling.

Common Bile Duct Obstruction

A client may retain or develop biliary stones that block bile flow within the common bile duct. Flow blockage may even follow a cholecystectomy. The client with a common bile duct obstruction is very ill. He or she complains of severe abdominal pain, nausea, and vomiting. On examination, other symptoms include fever, jaundice, elevated white blood cell count, or elevated liver and pancreatic enzymes.

Cancer of the Gallbladder

Early cancer of the gallbladder is not detected easily. Symptoms are similar to those of cholecystitis. Surgery might be attempted, but because the liver is often invaded as well, prognosis is usually poor. More women than men develop cancer of the gallbladder.

DISORDERS OF THE PANCREAS

Pancreatitis

Pancreatitis is inflammation of the pancreas. It may develop from infectious or traumatic damage, alcohol, or drugs. Cysts may occasionally occur. Pancreatitis can be acute or chronic.

Normally, bile does not enter the pancreas; if it does, the pancreas may become acutely inflamed. This process destroys pancreatic tissue and leads to hemorrhage, edema, steatorrhea, and severe pain. Pancreatic enzymes being secreted directly into the pancreas, rather than into the duodenum, also cause pancreatitis. Another cause is a gallstone that traveled backward in the duct.

Signs and Symptoms
Signs and symptoms include intractable pain in the epigastric area that may radiate to the back or upper left side. Fever, anorexia, nausea, and vomiting are common. Jaundice may exist if the common bile duct is obstructed.

Diagnosis is made by ultrasound, CT scans, and/or endoscopic examinations in combination with physical examination and results of laboratory pancreatic enzyme tests. ERCP can diagnose the presence and specific location of a tumor in the head or tail of the pancreas, which is helpful preoperative information for the surgeon.

Treatment
Treatment includes analgesics to relieve pain and spasm. The prescribed diet is low in fat and high in protein and carbohydrates. If the islets of Langerhans are affected, treatment for diabetes mellitus is also necessary. If distress is severe, an NG tube may be inserted to remove gastric secretions, and the client may be given IV fluids or TPN. Rest and freedom from emotional strain and upsets are important. Because the pain is so intense, non–morphine-type narcotics are usually necessary. Surgery may be necessary to remove an inflamed gallbladder, neighboring ducts, or *cystadenomas* (nonmalignant tumors) that could be the cause of the pancreatitis.

Pancreatic Cancer

Tumors of the pancreas are usually malignant. Cancer of the body or tail of the pancreas is usually not detected until metastasis has occurred. The client's prognosis is poor. In addition to other symptoms of biliary obstruction and pancreatitis, jaundice is sometimes the first symptom of pancreatic cancer. Diagnosis and treatment are the same as for pancreatitis. Surgery (*pancreatectomy*) is necessary to remove any cancerous growth. Before the operation, attention is given to building the client's nutritional status.

Nursing considerations focus on postoperative care. Pain management is important because postoperative pain can be excruciating. The client may need to gain weight; however, his or her appetite is usually poor. TPN is often used to restore nutritional deficits. After surgery, the client must be maintained with insulin and digestive enzymes.

CONDITIONS OF OVERNUTRITION AND UNDERNUTRITION

Obesity

Obesity is the condition of being over fat, not necessarily overweight. Obesity is defined as being more than 45% over ideal body weight (IBW). Body Mass Index (BMI) is another method of quantifying obesity. A BMI of above 27 kg/m^2 is characteristic of obesity. Charts of "desirable weight" are available, usually from insurance companies, listing desirable weights in relation to height, bone structure, sex, and age. The ideal percentage of body fat in an adult man is 20%; in an adult woman, the percentage is 25%. A person exceeding this amount is over fat. Some people, such as athletes, may be overweight (exceeding the figures on the chart), but the weight may be from muscle tissue and not excess fat. The percentage of fat is estimated by using calipers to measure skinfold thickness or is measured directly by weighing the person underwater on a special scale.

Complications
Obesity contributes to many physical disorders. The person runs a greater than normal risk for circulatory disorders (eg, arteriosclerosis, atherosclerosis, hypertension, heart attack, or stroke), diabetes mellitus (four times the rate of people of normal weight), and general respiratory difficulties, ranging from shortness of breath and dyspnea to actual lung pathology.

The obese person often suffers from musculoskeletal disorders and is more susceptible to contagious diseases. *Hyperlipidemia* (excess fat in the blood) develops and fat is deposited in the liver, causing liver damage. Dermatitis in moist skinfolds, chafing, excessive perspiration, and heat intolerance are associated problems.

Treatment
If a physical cause for obesity is found, it is treated. A nutritionally sound diet and exercise program are planned. The client must see a provider at regular intervals to ensure that he or she is maintaining weight loss and new eating patterns and that no other physical problems develop. Any person wishing to lose a large amount of weight should do so under a physician's supervision.

Nursing Alert

Weight-loss programs requiring ingestion of large amounts of water may be dangerous to the person with glaucoma (it may increase intraocular pressure) or certain kidney or liver disorders. The nursing mother should not be on a drastic weight-loss program because toxins and pollutants, which are stored in fat tissue, enter the mother's blood and can pass to the baby.

Various diets and group counseling systems (eg, Weight Watchers) are available. They may help a person reach and maintain a sensible body weight. If such a program is unsuccessful, the client may seek medical assistance. Many physicians prescribe diets. Morbidly obese clients need much emotional support as well.

Surgery may be performed for extremely obese individuals in whom all other forms of treatment have failed. The most common procedure is gastric partitioning or stapling, which reduces stomach volume by 90%. Surgery for morbid obesity (100 lb overweight) is normally considered high risk. One type of surgery for morbid obesity includes the intestinal bypass (Roux en Y procedure), in which a large portion of the intestine is removed, eliminating the body's ability to absorb calories. In-depth teaching and pre- and postoperative counseling are required. The person must understand the added surgical risk and must alter eating patterns or he or she will regain the weight. Complications of gastric stapling or intestinal bypass include fluid and electrolyte imbalance and dumping syndrome.

Nursing Considerations

In Practice: Nursing Care Guidelines 87-5 lists measures for obese clients receiving care in the hospital. Client and family teaching concepts include the knowledge that obesity occurs when the number of calories a person takes into the body exceeds the number of calories he or she expends. Exercise can be highly beneficial for the obese person. Explain that the types of exercise do not have to be high intensity but should be routine, at least 3 to 4 times per week. Also, teach the client that eating the wrong types of foods (especially fats) and emotional stress contribute to obesity. Reinforce the concept that obesity usually occurs with time, and successful weight loss also takes time.

☛ KEY CONCEPT

Most diet recommendations include reduction of fat in the diet. Controlling fat-gram intake is important. Many obese people try "crash diets," but many of them fail because the person never learns how to change long-term eating habits. After the person stops the diet, he or she usually regains the weight. This "yo-yo" effect of fast weight loss and immediate weight regain can be as dangerous as the original obesity. Education is vital in the long-term maintenance of weight loss.

Anorexia Nervosa and Bulimia

Anorexia nervosa is characterized by self-imposed starvation. No physiologic cause has been found. Anorexia often begins

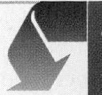

In Practice
Nursing Care Guidelines 87-5

CARING FOR THE HOSPITALIZED OBESE CLIENT

- Two gowns may be needed, one forward and one backward. Help tie the gown.
- One hospital bed may not be large enough; securely tie two beds together and place the mattresses crosswise. Keep the beds in low position and the side rails up at the foot of the bed.
- An overbed trapeze helps the client to move in bed. The person may need to sit up to breathe. You may place blocks under the head of the bed because the gatch mechanism is not appropriate. If the person is in one bed, he or she may be too heavy to lift if using a crank-style bed, or the electric gatch may not work.
- When assisting the client to get up, get help if needed. *Rationale: You will not be able to support the client alone. Always use a transfer belt; you can join two together if needed.*
- Put the bed in a position so the client's feet just touch the floor. *Rationale: If it is too high, the client may fall; if it is too low, the client may not be able to stand up.*
- Have the client wear rubber-soled shoes (not slippers); assist the person to tie the shoes.
- Use a heavy-duty walker, wheelchair, or stretcher. A commode or wheelchair with removable arms may be needed if a large device is unavailable. *Rationale: This strategy will allow the client to fit.*
- Assist the person with personal care; dressing alone may be impossible. The client may not be able to comb the hair.
- Skin care is particularly important in skinfolds and the perineum. *Rationale: The client often cannot reach to do self-care, and chafing or dermatitis is common.*
- A shower is usually safer than a bath in the tub; help the client to sit in the shower.
- Use a large-enough blood pressure cuff, and keep the cuff at the bedside to ensure consistency.
- Use longer needles for intramuscular injections.
- Assist the client in collection of urine specimens. *Rationale: The person may not be able to position the bottle or bedpan properly.*
- If the apical pulse is difficult to hear, use the bell side of the stethoscope, and mark the chest at the optimum location.
- Consider the self-esteem needs of the person. Accentuate the person's achievements and skills.

during the adolescent years and 95% of clients are women. Clients believe that they are fat, when actually they are very thin, often to the point of emaciation. This eating disorder usually results in being severely underweight, with significant functional malnutrition along with electrolyte imbalances. Other conditions include dental caries, muscle wasting, slow pulse and hypotension, blotchy skin, loss of hair (*alopecia*) or abnormal hair growth (*hirsutism*), and susceptibility to infections. Anorectic women almost always experience amenorrhea (absence of menses). They may be hyperactive, even though they are undernourished. The mortality rate is 5% to 15%, with death usually caused by circulatory collapse or cardiac failure secondary to the electrolyte imbalances.

Bulimia is known as the "binge" syndrome. As in anorexia nervosa, a high percentage of bulimics are young women. The bulimic client may either *binge* (gorge with food) or binge-purge. In the *binge-purge* form of the disorder, the bulimic eats thousands of calories at one sitting and, in an effort to avoid weight gain, purges the body of food, either by self-induced vomiting or by excessive doses of laxatives. The non-purging bulimic often is obese. The person who binges and purges is usually thin, sometimes to the point of starvation.

✚👁 Nursing Alert

Obesity, anorexia nervosa, and bulimia can be life threatening.

Signs and Symptoms

Symptoms and conditions common to anorexia nervosa and bulimia are:

- Higher incidence of depression, obesity, and chemical dependency in the family than in the general population
- Overprotective parents with rigid rules and high expectations
- Usually very good students and school leaders
- Feeling of helplessness or being out of control, yet with manipulative behavior
- Intense fear of becoming "fat"
- Inaccurate self-image
- Low self-esteem, but unrealistically high goals
- Often great weight loss in a short time with no physical disorder
- Electrolyte imbalances
- Hiding or hoarding of food
- Preoccupation with food or gourmet cooking
- "Playing" with food; moving it around on the plate without eating it
- Shyness about eating with others
- Secretive behavior
- Going to the bathroom immediately after each meal
- Spending a great deal of time locked in the bathroom
- Going to various physicians, requesting prescriptions for vague physical complaints
- Hiding medications

There is no specific laboratory test to diagnose anorexia nervosa or bulimia. Diagnosis is made by evaluation of the client, nutritional status, and risk factors as listed above.

Treatment

Treatment can be difficult and consists of behavioral counseling, inpatient treatments, and diet therapy.

Nursing Considerations

During a crisis, treatment is symptomatic with enforced feeding, tube feeding, or TPN, or oral replacement of missing electrolytes. The nurse may give oxygen to assist with respirations. Daily nursing assessments include regular vital signs, weight, total calorie count, and I&O. Be sure to explain all procedures and the reasons for them to gain the client's cooperation. Explain the abnormal laboratory findings and their relationship to diet and to physical well-being.

The person needs to understand the functions of electrolytes in the body and the consequences of starvation. Offer small amounts of high-protein food or fluids often. High-protein, high-calorie liquids may be more tolerable than solids. Monitor fluid intake, so the person takes a variety of fluids, including fruit juices; make sure the person does not drink excessive amounts of plain water. *Rationale: Avoid electrolyte imbalance.* After the crisis, extensive psychotherapy and family counseling are needed. Group therapy often is helpful.

➤ STUDENT SYNTHESIS

Key Points

- Diagnostic tests for disorders of the GI tract include liver function tests, blood urea nitrogen, creatinine, and a CBC. Invasive testing of the GI tract includes endoscopies, EGD, and ERCP.
- Nursing care of the client with a digestive disorder includes management of NG tubes (eg, lavage, suction, irrigation), stoma care (eg, colostomies and ileostomies), and the ability to obtain data concerning nutritional history and disorders.
- Ulcers can be found in both the stomach and the duodenum. Surgical intervention may be necessary to prevent or treat hemorrhage; however, medications are also effective in ulcer management.
- IBS is annoying and usually treated symptomatically. IBD (ie, ulcerative colitis and Crohn's disease) is long-term, progressive, and often life threatening.
- The liver is subject to several forms of debilitating illness. Toxins, drugs, and many viruses can result in acute forms of hepatitis. Alcohol is related to cirrhosis and esophageal varices.
- Diseases of the accessory organs of the GI tract include cholecystitis, cholelithiasis, pancreatitis, and appendicitis.
- Cancer of many areas of the GI tract is often not found until metastasis has occurred. Common signs of GI cancer include alterations in eating habits and bowel elimination, weight loss, and rectal bleeding.

Critical Thinking Exercises

1. State the role endoscopy has in diagnosing and treating GI disorders. Contrast its use with x-ray studies and incisional surgery.

2. List factors that are known to aggravate digestive conditions. Explain how you can use these factors in instructing a client to prevent problems with hiatal hernia.
3. Alcohol is a known toxin of the liver. Develop a teaching project for high school students discussing the health hazards of alcohol.

NCLEX-Style Review Questions

1. Prior to removing a nasogastric tube, the nurse should:
   a. Clamp it temporarily to determine if client can tolerate its absence.
   b. Inject 50 cc of sterile water through the tube to clear secretions.
   c. Place suction on high to clear the tube of secretions.
   d. Push air through the tube while gently pulling on it.
2. When a client has his or her jaws wired together, which nursing measure is essential to his or her care?
   a. Elevate the head of bed.
   b. Instruct the client to use saline mouth rinses.
   c. Keep a wire cutter with the client at all times.
   d. Provide pain medications as needed.
3. Antacid preparations that contain magnesium hydroxide, such as Mylanta, may cause:
   a. Acid reflux
   b. Constipation
   c. Diarrhea
   d. Vomiting
4. To promote passage of residual air following a colonoscopy, the nurse should instruct the client to:
   a. Drink plenty of fluids.
   b. Lie on the right side with knees bent and flexed.
   c. Place a pillow under the right hip.
   d. Turn side to side every 4 hours.
5. Clients who have had hepatitis are instructed to:
   a. Avoid large crowds.
   b. Follow up every 3 months.
   c. Make out a will.
   d. Never donate blood.

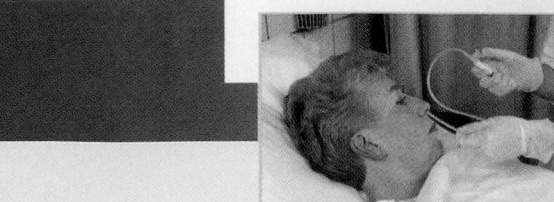

Urinary Disorders

LEARNING OBJECTIVES

1. Identify the components of a normal urinalysis.
2. Discuss the rationale for using the following tests of renal function: BUN, serum creatinine, creatinine clearance, and uric acid.
3. Describe the role imaging studies play in diagnosis of urinary disorders.
4. Identify at least four nursing considerations related to pre- and post-procedure cystoscopy care.
5. Describe the role of urodynamic tests in diagnosing urinary disorders.
6. Discuss medical and surgical approaches to treat incontinence.
7. Discuss client teaching necessary for the client with recurrent cystitis.
8. Define and discuss hydronephrosis and calculi.
9. Identify at least six nursing considerations for the client with calculi.
10. Prepare a nursing care plan for a client who has been recently diagnosed with a metastatic kidney tumor.
11. State at least four nursing considerations for a client with a urinary diversion.
12. Define and differentiate between acute renal failure and ESRD.
13. Identify nursing considerations for a client receiving dialysis.

NEW TERMINOLOGY

anasarca	incontinence
anuria	lithiasis
bacteriuria	lithotripsy
calculi	micturition
casts	nephroma
crystalluria	oliguria
cystectomy	pessary
cystoscope	pyuria
dysuria	reflux
fistula	shunt
hematuria	stent
hypotonic	suprapubic

ACRONYMS

BUN	ESRD	UA
CAPD	ESWL	UPP
CMG	IC	UTI
C&S	IVP	VCUG
EMG	TURBT	

The urinary tract can be divided into the *upper tract* (kidneys and ureters) and the *lower tract* (bladder and urethra). The upper urinary tract filters the by-products of metabolism and adjusts the body's fluid and electrolyte balance. It also delivers urine to the lower tract. The lower urinary tract acts as a storage area until **micturition** (voiding, urination) occurs. Urine then flows through the structures of the lower urinary tract and out of the body. See Chapter 27 for anatomy and physiology of the urinary system.

Common problems affecting the lower urinary tract include infection and incontinence. Damage to the lower tract, while rarely life threatening, can greatly affect a client's quality of life. Damage to the upper urinary tract usually stems from obstruction, which causes **reflux** (backflow) of urine into the kidneys. In addition, infection and inflammation can damage the sensitive tissues of the nephrons, resulting in decreased kidney function. Damage to the upper urinary tract is life threatening. Any systemic condition that affects blood flow will affect kidney functioning. Examples of such conditions include hypertension, heart failure, trauma, and changes in small blood vessels related to diabetes mellitus or collagen/vascular diseases.

☛ KEY CONCEPT

Many kidney disorders result from circulatory disorders that cause renal vascular insufficiency.

The *urologist* is a physician who treats diseases and disorders of the urinary tract system. A *nephrologist*, who specializes in medical aspects of kidney disease, may treat some disorders of the urinary tract. A *dialysis nurse* assists client in a dialysis clinic or may bring dialysis equipment to the bedside of a hospitalized client. Because many terms in urology are similar, they can be confusing. Common combining forms that appear in this chapter are listed in Table 88-1.

■■■ TABLE 88-1 *C*OMBINING FORMS IN UROLOGY

Prefixes/Suffix	Meaning
cyst(o)-	Pertaining to any bladder
lith(o)-	Stone
nephr(o)-	Pertaining to the kidney
pyel(o)-	Pertaining to the renal pelvis
ureter(o)-	Pertaining to the ureter (tubes from kidneys to bladder)
urethr(o)-	Pertaining to the urethra (from bladder to outside of body)
vesic(o)-	Pertaining to a bladder, usually the urinary bladder
-tripsy	Crushing

DIAGNOSTIC TESTS

Laboratory Tests

Blood and urine tests are commonly ordered as screening tools for many urinary tract disorders. Chemistry levels may indicate normal ranges of electrolytes (eg, potassium, calcium, and sodium). Serum and urine glucose and protein levels are also often obtained. These levels help indicate the body's overall fluid and electrolyte balance. Blood and urine levels can help evaluate the nature of renal diseases such as renal failure.

Urinalysis

A *urinalysis* (**UA**) provides much information about the condition of the bladder and kidneys. It tells whether disease is interfering with the function of different kidney parts (renal tubules, nephrons, and glomeruli). It shows whether pathogens are at work in the kidney or bladder, or whether food materials, such as glucose or protein, that should go to body cells are escaping into urine.

Routine or Random UA. A *routine UA* includes tests for pH, specific gravity, glucose (sugar), ketones, albumin (protein), blood (**hematuria**), and bilirubin. An abnormal reading in any of these tests may indicate a kidney dysfunction. This information is generally provided on a diagnostic test strip inserted briefly into the urine and then read.

Urine normally has a specific gravity of 1.010 to 1.025, and a pH of 4.6 to 8. No glucose, ketones, bacteria, albumin, or bilirubin should appear in normal urine. When examined microscopically, urine should contain no (or very few) red blood cells (RBCs) or white blood cells (WBCs). If RBCs are seen under the microscope, hemorrhage could be indicated. The bleeding could be seen as trace amounts with numerous RBC seen or as frank hemorrhage. Frank hemorrhage usually can be noted by gross inspection (visual inspection) of the urine. The presence of WBCs indicates infection.

A routine UA also will check for urine color, appearance, odor, and foam content. Table 88-2 lists conditions that are indicated by abnormalities found in urine. The laboratory also will test the urine for *casts (cylindruria)*. **Casts** are epithelial, fatty, or waxy tissue abnormally forced out of the renal tubules. Additional abnormal findings include the presence of crystals (**crystalluria**) or pus (**pyuria**). Urine calcium may be measured to help detect bone disease; high amounts of calcium indicate degeneration of bone tissue. The urine also may be tested for the presence of other minerals, various drugs, and abnormal components.

☛ KEY CONCEPT

An accurately timed and correctly performed urine sample collection is fundamental in the diagnosis of urinary dysfunction.

Urine Culture. The laboratory performs a *urine culture* by placing small amounts of a urine sample on a culture medium and allowing it to *incubate* (grow). The culture will reveal any organisms present in the urine. If a culture reveals the presence of an organism in the urine, the organism is tested with various medications (usually an antibiotic) to see which

▪▪▪ TABLE 88-2 Conditions Indicated by Abnormalities in the Urine

Abnormality or Abnormal Substance in Urine	Possible Conditions
Abnormal pH	Gout, calculi, infections
Abnormal specific gravity	Kidney disease, electrolyte imbalances, liver disorders, burns
Proteinuria or albuminuria (protein)	Nephritis, kidney stones, renal circulatory difficulties, infection, trauma, preeclampsia (of pregnancy)
Glycosuria (sugar)	Diabetes mellitus, shock, head injury
Ketonuria (ketones)	Diabetes, starvation, bulimia, other digestive disturbances (such as faulty fat metabolism)
Bilirubin	Liver dysfunction, biliary obstruction, hepatitis
Hemoglobinuria or hematuria	Infection, calculi, cancer, trauma, overdose of an anticoagulant, bleeding disorder

one is most effective in eradicating it (*sensitivity test*). The client then receives that medication. Culture and sensitivity (**C&S**) tests for urine are usually ordered together.

Nursing Considerations.   Collected urine may consist of a single random specimen or an accumulated fractional specimen, such as a 24-hour collection. Obtain a clean-catch midstream urine sample from the client for a C&S. Instruct the client to clean the perineal area. In a woman, teach her to separate and clean the area with the openings to the urethra and vagina. For a man, teach him to clean the tip of the penis. Teach the client to start voiding and then to insert the collection container under the urine stream to obtain the sample.

Wear gloves while packaging the urine, and be careful not to contaminate the specimen with any outside organisms so that a true culture of only the client's urine is performed. Contamination commonly occurs when replacing the cap on the specimen container. After the urine is collected for culture, send it to the laboratory immediately. If urine is allowed to stand, microorganisms can grow in it, thereby altering the test's accuracy. If a sterile specimen is required and there is a question as to the client's ability to collect it, the specimen may be obtained by urinary catheter.

Renal Function Tests

The most common diagnostic studies for evaluation of kidney function are blood urea nitrogen (BUN), serum creatinine, urine creatinine, creatinine clearance, and a serum BUN:creatinine ratio. Serum and urine uric acid levels also may be ordered.

The *blood urea nitrogen* (**BUN**) test determines how efficiently the glomeruli remove the nitrogenous wastes (*urea*) that result from protein metabolism. The most common cause of an elevated BUN is kidney disease, although BUN also may be elevated in clients with high dietary protein intake, diabetes, some malignancies, or improper protein metabolism.

Serum creatinine, a product of protein metabolism, is related to muscle mass and excreted by the kidneys. *Creatinine* is the chief nitrogenous waste of protein (muscle) metabolism. The glomerular filtration rate must be reduced by at least 50% for significant elevation of serum creatinine to occur. Therefore, serum creatinine is a much more accurate indicator of renal function than serum BUN. An elevated serum creatinine level usually indicates a serious kidney disorder, such as impaired kidney function or obstruction. Additional information can be obtained by a BUN:creatinine ratio.

The *creatinine clearance test* uses a collected urine specimen to indicate glomerular filtration rate and renal insufficiency. Commonly, a creatinine clearance test is ordered in addition to a *morning serum creatinine*. *Serum creatinine* is found at a basically constant level. Serum and urine creatinine levels are compared, and a creatinine clearance ratio is calculated. Creatinine clearance is one of the most valuable tests to identify early kidney disease and is useful in monitoring the renal function of clients with known kidney disease. To obtain a creatinine clearance test, a 12- or 24-hour urine collection is made, noting the exact time the collection started and ended. *Rationale: Exactness is vital to obtain the full 24-hour specimen.*

Uric acid studies may be obtained from urine or serum. The main diagnostic purpose of obtaining a uric acid level is to evaluate the client for gouty arthritis or kidney disease. A urine uric acid study is generally performed with a 24-hour collected specimen.

Imaging Studies

General imaging studies include x-ray and ultrasound examinations, computed tomography (CT) scans, and magnetic resonance imaging (MRI); more specialized imaging studies used to study the urinary tract include intravenous pyelogram, radioactive renogram, bone scan, nephrotomogram, renal arteriogram, cystogram and voiding cystourethrogram (**VCUG**), and retrograde pyelogram. In addition, a bone scan (*scintiscan*) is indicated when bony metastases are suspected in cases of renal, bladder, or prostatic cancer.

The kidney-ureter-bladder x-ray examination, commonly referred to as a "KUB flat plate of the abdomen," is a good screening test for kidney or bladder stones. Ultrasound may be used to view the kidneys and other urinary structures. CT scans will reveal any kidney abnormalities, such as cysts, tumors, or *calculi* (stones). Spiral CT is used to image the kidneys to evaluate tumors and stones. In addition, MRI may be used to distinguish normal from abnormal tissue.

Intravenous Pyelogram

Intravenous pyelogram (**IVP**) is composed of a series of x-ray films taken after a radiopaque dye has been injected intravenously. These films reveal the outline of the client's kidneys, ureters, and bladder. Before the IVP is done, the healthcare providers must determine whether the client is allergic to iodine or shellfish, because the dye is iodine based. The client is NPO for 8 to 10 hours before the test. He or she usually receives a laxative the night before to rid the bowel of any feces or gas that could obstruct the view of urinary structures. The client may brush the teeth in the morning but should not swallow any water.

The radiology technician takes and develops one x-ray film, commonly a KUB. A radiopaque dye is then administered via the IV route into the client. The technician takes several more x-ray films at intervals to visualize the dye concentration in the kidneys.

A *nephrotomogram* may be performed along with IVP; it allows x-ray films to be taken of kidney layers and the structures within the layers, using a rotating x-ray tube after IV injection of a contrast medium. Preparation and care of the client are the same as for IVP.

Nursing Considerations. Notify the radiology department of known allergies, and if the client is diabetic. Diabetic clients often have decreased renal function and cannot clear the dye quickly through the kidneys. Monitor and observe the client for untoward reactions to the dye. Instruct the client and family to provide at least 2 to 4 liters of fluids for 24 hours after the test to help remove the dye and relieve any dehydration that may have resulted from the client's NPO status before the test. Contrast dye can damage the kidneys if not flushed out quickly.

Radioactive Renogram

A *radioactive renogram (renal scan)* tests the kidneys by means of radioactive substances. The scan will show blood vessels, obstructions, and each kidney. Tumors may be detected, because they "pick up" more of the radioactive substance than normal tissue does.

Cystogram and Voiding Cystourethrogram

A *cystogram* is an x-ray study of the bladder and urethra, made possible by instillation of dye directly into the bladder through a catheter. Using fluoroscopy, the x-ray cystogram will show the bladder's outline and the ureters (if reflux is present). It is used to evaluate the degree of *vesicoureteral reflux* (backflow of urine into the ureters) and the presence of bladder injury.

A *voiding cystourethrogram* (**VCUG**) is a fluoroscopic test done to diagnose vesicoureteral reflux. The first part of the test is very similar to the cystogram, in that a contrast agent is instilled into the bladder via a urethral catheter. When the client feels the urge to void, the catheter is removed and the client voids while x-ray films are taken (reflux often occurs when the client voids).

Retrograde Pyelogram

A *retrograde pyelogram* is used to show the kidneys and ureters. After the bladder is outlined on x-ray film by instillation of dye by catheter, smaller catheters are introduced into the ureters and then passed into the kidney pelvis, where dye is injected into them. X-ray films are then taken that show the kidneys and ureters.

This procedure is combined with cystoscopy (described below). Preparation includes giving the client a low-residue diet the day before, and a laxative or enema in the evening and immediately before the test. Observation following the test is the same as that required for any other test using dye.

Renal Arteriogram

Renal arteriogram is obtained by injecting a contrast dye through a catheter into the aorta at the level of the renal blood vessels. The kidneys are thereby visualized to determine the presence of a pathologic condition (such as a tumor). Care of the client after this examination is the same as for any arteriogram.

Endoscopic Procedure: Cystoscopy

A *cystoscopy* examination allows the physician to view the inside of the bladder through a tubular instrument, the **cystoscope**, which has a mirror and an electric lamp or fiberoptic lens on its end (Fig. 88-1). The physician passes the cystoscope into the client's bladder through the urethra. This examination can detect inflammation or a tumor that may be causing blood to appear in the urine.

Cystoscopy also enables visualization of the openings of the ureters into the bladder; fine, opaque, wax catheters can be threaded into these openings for collection of separate urine specimens from each kidney to determine which kidney is diseased. Dye also may be instilled through these catheters. Because the fluid medium is infused into the bladder at high pressures, infected urine can be forced up into the kidney, causing an infection of the kidney. Therefore, it is important to obtain a urinalysis and urine culture prior to this procedure to determine if a client has a kidney infection.

The physician may use a cystoscope to view the ureters while inserting ureteral catheters. Cystoscopy also may be used to remove a polyp or a tumor, perform a biopsy, or remove kidney stones. The surgeon may conduct electrosurgery (*fulguration*) through a cystoscope to remove small tumors or to coagulate (*cauterize*) small, bleeding blood vessels.

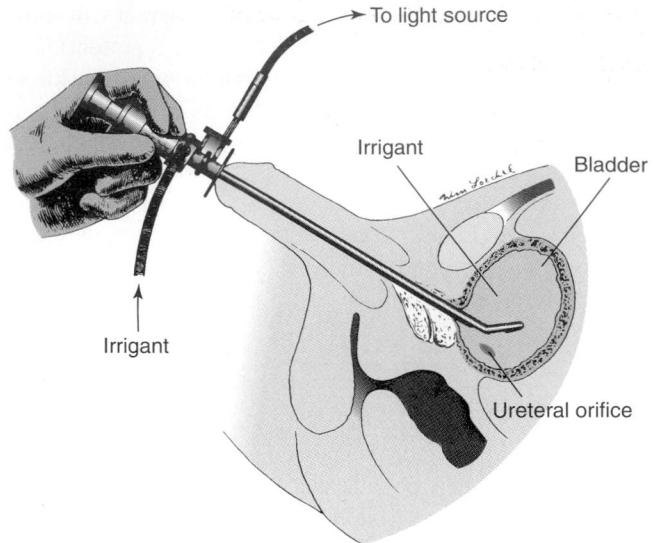

FIGURE 88-1. Examination of the inside of the bladder using a cystoscope.

Because a cystoscopy is usually done in an operating room, the client requires routine preoperative preparation. A cystoscopy may be performed with general anesthesia. Local anesthesia involves administering a tranquilizer or sedative before the examination to relax the client, and instilling Xylocaine jelly into the urethra. Make sure the client is not allergic to lidocaine, Xylocaine, Novocain, or Marcaine before using these agents.

Urine specimens obtained are examined in the laboratory. A mild analgesic may be prescribed after the procedure because voiding may be uncomfortable for 1 to 2 days. The urine occasionally has a reddish tinge immediately after cystoscopy.

Nursing Considerations

Nursing considerations will include reporting a blood-tinged urine for more than 24 hours or darkening urine. Encourage the client to drink fluids to prevent urinary stasis and flush any remaining dye from the body. Help the client with sitz baths to ease voiding and to soothe the affected area. Remind the client to report signs or symptoms of a urinary tract infection or increasing blood in the urine.

Biopsy

Following identification of a mass by imaging studies, a needle biopsy of the kidney may be done for a specific diagnosis. The kidney is located by x-ray or ultrasound and the client's back is marked so that the needle can be inserted at the correct place.

Give the client a sedative as ordered. Place the client in a prone position, with a sandbag under the abdomen. *Rationale: The sandbag helps bring the kidney into a more accessible position.* A local anesthetic is injected into the skin, and the biopsy needle is inserted.

After the procedure, apply pressure to the site to minimize bleeding. Keep the client lying flat for 24 hours and watch him

or her very carefully for any signs of hemorrhage. *Rationale: Hemorrhage is a complication of needle biopsy because the kidney is very vascular.* Take blood pressure, pulse, and respirations and document them at frequent intervals.

Urodynamic Tests

Urodynamic testing is a series of tests that best determines the actual function of the *detrusor muscle* of the bladder (which pushes the urine out), the external sphincter muscle, and the pelvic (pubococcygeal) muscles. Urodynamic tests also evaluate the ability of these muscles to work in sequence.

☛ KEY CONCEPT

Because urodynamic tests are safer than x-ray procedures that require an IV dye, they are the tests of choice in many cases.

A urodynamic evaluation is usually done in two phases—phase one is the filling phase of the study; phase two is the emptying phase of the study. The *filling phase* tests sensation of the bladder, capacity, the muscle activity, and the stretch of the bladder wall (*accommodation* or *compliance*) as well as the ability of the bladder and pelvic muscles to hold the urine in without leaking. The *emptying phase* (*voiding* or *micturition* studies) tests how well the bladder empties and what strategies the client uses to empty completely.

Uroflowmetry

Uroflowmetry is a noninvasive assessment of the status of micturition and generally the first test done in an urodynamic evaluation. The client voids into a funneled commode connected to an electronic measuring device. This device calculates the volume of the urine flow, and the time it takes the client to void, in order to determine a flow rate. This information is recorded on a graph.

Before the test, instruct the client to void in the same fashion as usual. Leave the client alone (if possible) to prevent "bashful bladder syndrome" (the client is too tense to urinate). Further testing will be needed to differentiate between bladder outlet obstruction and **hypotonic** bladder (poor muscle tone).

Residual Urine Volume

A *residual urine volume* test is done to determine if the client emptied the bladder completely. Before obtaining a residual volume, the client voids as much as possible using whatever techniques he or she usually uses to empty as well as possible. Some healthcare facilities require the client to void, followed by a second voiding 5 minutes later. This procedure is referred to as *double voiding technique*. The client is then immediately catheterized with a straight catheter (one that is inserted to obtain a specimen and then removed) to collect whatever urine remains in the bladder.

A noninvasive technique called *bladder scanning* may also be used to assess residual volume. The client voids as discussed above; then the nurse moves the ultrasound scanning device over the bladder area to determine the urine volume in the bladder.

If residual volume is greater than 150 to 200 milliliters, a disorder of the bladder or urethra is probably causing urinary retention. The physician may order a catheter to remain in place if the residual volume is over a certain amount, or the nurse may be ordered to teach the client how to intermittently catheterize himself or herself at home.

Cystometrogram

A *cystometrogram* (**CMG**) is a measurement of bladder pressure during filling. A urethral catheter is inserted, and the bladder is filled either with a liquid, such as normal saline, or with x-ray contrast media. Instruct the client to notify the physician when he or she begins to feel a sense of fullness, again when the bladder actually feels full, and again when the client can hold no more fluid because of discomfort or a feeling that he or she will leak. Normally, bladder pressure remains the same during bladder filling until the volume is approximately 500 milliliters.

If the urodynamic evaluation is being done to assess the continence status of the client, the filling phase may be interrupted several times during the test to have the client cough or bear down. If the client leaks urine during these maneuvers, a leak-point pressure is obtained. The leak-point pressure assists the surgeon in determining if the client is suitable for anti-incontinence surgery.

Urethral Pressure Profile

A *urethral pressure profile* (**UPP**) is another way to evaluate the smooth muscle activity along the urethra. This procedure is often done following a CMG. For the UPP, the bladder is filled either with a fluid, such as normal saline or water, or with contrast media using a catheter. A puller mechanism provides a slow, even rate of catheter withdrawal, while resistance exerted by the urethral wall is registered as a pressure rise on a graph. If the client is found to have a low-pressure urethra, a procedure that improves urethral closure is appropriate.

Perineal Electromyogram

The *perineal electromyogram* (**EMG**) is a test of pelvic muscle (pubococcygeal or levator muscle) function. Several methods are used to record perineal EMG. Patch electrodes are used more commonly today than needle electrodes and are more comfortable for the client.

The perineal EMG is usually combined with the CMG because the major function of the EMG is to evaluate the relationship of perineal muscle activity and detrusor muscle contraction. If the pelvic muscles are inappropriately relaxed during the filling phase of the urodynamic evaluation, then the client may leak urine. If the pelvic muscles cannot relax during the emptying phase of the study, the client may not be able to empty the bladder at all or may have a residual volume remaining after micturition. A *voiding study* also may be done. The CMG sensor is usually left in place along with the abdominal sensor and the EMG patches. The client is then asked to void. Measurements are taken during the procedure.

NURSING PROCESS

Data Collection

Carefully observe and assess the client with a urinary disorder. Chapter 47 describes physical examination and nursing assessment, including that of the urinary system. This assessment establishes a baseline for future comparison and determines the presence of suspected complications. Report any changes in the baseline level, and try to recognize and treat kidney malfunctions early. In Practice: Nursing Assessment 88-1 lists some components of the urologic nursing assessment.

In addition, observe the client's emotional response to the disorder or disease, asking the following questions. Would a support group be helpful? Does the client need assistance to meet daily needs? Do family caregivers understand needed medications and treatments? Is home care or public health nursing necessary? Does the disorder affect social activities or self-esteem? Is the condition chronic or life threatening? Is it reversible or treatable? Does the client need periodic dialysis or other regular treatment? Is the client anxious or fearful of the outcome? Does the client need financial assistance?

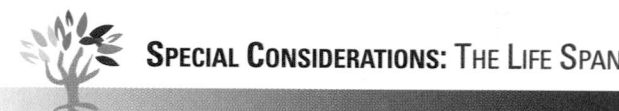 **Special Considerations: The Life Span**

Taking a Complete History in Pediatric Clients

Obtain an accurate history when admitting pediatric clients. Voiding patterns and behaviors may be your only clue to detecting abnormalities. Encourage the child to describe his or her toileting habits for you. *Rationale: Frequently children do not recognize that something is abnormal, so they do not know to tell family members about their symptoms. However, family members can also give valuable information.*

Nursing Diagnosis

Based on data collection, the following nursing diagnoses may be established for the client with a urologic disorder:

- Risk for Infection related to dehydration, excess wastes in the body, tissue breakdown and damage
- Risk for Deficient or Excess Fluid Volume related to the kidney's inability to effectively concentrate urine, fluid restrictions, electrolyte imbalance
- Stress Urinary Incontinence/Reflex Urinary Incontinence/ Functional Urinary Incontinence related to sphincter incompetence, neurologic disorders, impaired mental status, medications, fistula, cancer, surgery, trauma, obstruction
- Urinary Retention related to obstruction, sphincter incompetence, cancer, trauma
- Impaired Tissue Integrity related to dehydration, mucous membrane friability and breakdown, general malaise
- Social Isolation related to incontinence, presence of ureterostomy or urinary diversion appliance

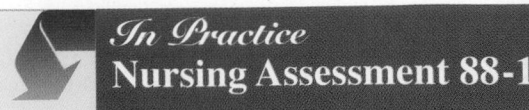

In Practice
Nursing Assessment 88-1

URINARY SYSTEM

Urinary history, including previous providers and
   treatments
General health history
Family health history
Exposure to toxins
Presence of related disorders (eg, type 1 diabetes
   mellitus, heart or blood vessel disorders,
   infections, cancer)
Character of urine, abnormal components
Intake and output amounts
Urinary residual
Difficulty or pain in voiding
Any incontinence and type
Sudden weight gain or loss
Diet and fluids
Presence of symptoms, such as edema or poor
   skin turgor

- Ineffective Sexuality Patterns related to indwelling catheter, dialysis, urinary diversion
- Pain related to surgery, invasive diagnostic tests, urinary tract infections, pyelonephritis, calculi

Planning and Implementing

Plan with the client, family, and other members of the healthcare team for effective care based on the nursing diagnoses (a sample nursing care plan for a client with a urinary tract disorder is provided later in the chapter). Provide preoperative and postoperative care for the client undergoing lithotripsy, renal surgery, dialysis, or invasive diagnostic tests (postoperative care is discussed below). The client with a urinary disorder also may require total assistance in meeting daily needs, dealing with emotional problems, and understanding more about the disorder, its prognosis, and treatment.

Renal disease may require regular dialysis or a kidney transplant, or it may be life threatening with minimal available treatment. A nursing care plan is developed to meet the individual's needs. Damage to the kidneys can be life threatening if not recognized and treated promptly. The goal of nursing care is to prevent further damage or decline in function.

General Nursing Considerations

General nursing considerations when caring for clients with urinary tract disorders include monitoring vital signs and results from diagnostic tests, and assessing the effects and side effects of medications. Assistance with ADL may be necessary in some clients. However, encourage clients to provide self-care whenever possible. The following list summarizes the major nursing considerations:

- Obtaining frequent vital signs, especially blood pressure
- Managing related symptoms, such as diarrhea, nausea, vomiting, headache, anemia, and pain
- Administering prescribed diuretics, mineral supplements, and antibiotics
- Providing skin and mouth care (because of dehydration, edema, and general tissue friability)
- Managing pruritus
- Assessing skin condition, tissue turgor, and presence of edema or dehydration
- Measuring and recording intake and output (I&O), color and clarity, and urine specific gravity
- Taking daily weights to assess for edema and urinary retention
- Monitoring fluid intake with maintenance of fluid restrictions (to help control edema and electrolyte imbalances)
- Encouraging fluid intake, when indicated, to dilute urine and lessen **dysuria** (painful urination)
- Assisting with voiding and with continence training
- Providing medications and emotional support for dysuria and painful intercourse
- Inserting urinary catheters using appropriately ordered catheters; urologists may order specific types of indwelling catheters and may insert these catheters themselves
- Managing and caring for an indwelling catheter or **suprapubic** Cystocath
- Managing incontinence, frequency, urgency, and other urinary symptoms
- Giving sitz baths and warm moist packs to offset pain
- Movement and activity to prevent disorders of immobility, such as deep-vein thrombosis, pneumonia, and urinary tract infections

☛ KEY CONCEPT

Infection of the urinary tract can result in life-threatening damage to the kidney if not treated promptly; therefore, prevention or early treatment is vital.

Postoperative Care

Provide postoperative care for the client after lithotripsy, renal surgery, dialysis, or invasive diagnostic tests. Whether surgery is done for stone removal, cancer, or kidney transplantation, deep breathing and turning can be painful postoperatively. *Rationale: A flank incision is usually made for a ureterolithotomy or a nephrotomy and is done through a number of major muscle groups.* Care of the client who has undergone urologic surgery follows usual postoperative nursing care.

✚👁 N u r s i n g   A l e r t

Instruct the client and family members to report chills and fever. *Rationale: They are signs of infection.* Other symptoms of complications include sharp abdominal pain, hematuria, *anuria* (absence of urine formation), *dysuria* (painful urination), or urine retention.

Additional measures include:

- Clients need prescribed pain medications before turning and deep breathing. Encourage the use of the incentive spirometer.
- The client may have multiple tubes for urinary drainage postoperatively. Be aware of the location, size, and kind of tubes and expected drainage from each. Assess each tube and its drainage regularly.
- Assessment also includes careful observation for any indication of excessive bleeding. Hemorrhage can easily occur after surgery for renal calculi because the kidneys are so vascular.
- Large amounts of urinary drainage may be present on dressings after urologic surgery, but drainage should not be bright red; bright-red drainage indicates frank bleeding. The color most often used to describe normal bloody discharge following nephrolithotomy is "rose."
- The client will often have a urinary catheter or suprapubic Cystocath postoperatively.

☞ KEY CONCEPT

Because many diagnostic and minor urologic surgical procedures are performed on an outpatient basis, aggressive client and family teaching is required. Clients and families must know how to perform preoperative preparation, and untoward signs to look for after the procedure. Carefully document this teaching.

Evaluation

Evaluate outcomes of care with the client, family, and other members of the healthcare team. Have you met short-term goals? Are long-term goals still realistic? Will the client receive care at home? Are additional home care services required? Is a support group indicated? Do the client and family understand the treatment plan? Does the client have a way to get to dialysis, or will it be done at home? Planning for further nursing care considers the client's prognosis, any complications, and the client's and family's responses to care given.

URINARY INCONTINENCE

Urinary **incontinence** refers to involuntary voiding or urine loss. In men, two well-defined sphincter muscles control voiding. The *internal sphincter* controls the bladder's opening into the urethra, and the *external sphincter* (the pelvic muscles) controls the opening of the urethra below the prostate. In women, there is little definition between the internal and external sphincters. Normally, sufficient urine collects in the bladder and stimulates the involved nerve endings, causing the urge to urinate. When a person loses control of this function, incontinence results.

Types of Incontinence

Transient (Temporary) Incontinence

Transient (temporary) incontinence refers to incontinence that can be reversed with diagnosis and treatment. Factors causing transient incontinence include reversible contributing factors such as changes in mental status, infections, medications, fluid intake, mobility problems, or stool impaction. After the precipitating cause is discovered and treated, the incontinence usually resolves without further intervention. A type of transient incontinence, *iatrogenic incontinence,* is similar to transient incontinence in that the cause of the incontinence is usually the result of outside factors. However, iatrogenic incontinence is specifically caused by medical interventions or treatments. A new medication, restraints, or postsurgical mobility problems are the most common reasons for this type of incontinence. Sometimes iatrogenic incontinence can be reversed and other times it may be permanent (eg, when medications cannot be changed).

True or Total Incontinence

True or *total incontinence* is defined as urinary leakage that is nearly continuous.

The most common cause of true incontinence in men is surgical removal of the prostate (*prostatectomy*) (see Chap. 89). Other causes of true incontinence include:

- Injury to the male's external (voluntary) urethral sphincter
- Injury to the female's perineal musculature (muscles)
- Congenital or acquired neurogenic disease (eg, spina bifida or spinal cord injury)
- Congenital anomaly in which the urinary bladder is exposed on the lower abdomen (*extrophy*)
- Abnormally placed ureteral orifices in the female (opening distal to the neck of the bladder or into the vagina)
- *Vesicovaginal fistula* secondary to situations such as injuries during delivery or surgery (may include defects caused by an infection after surgery)
- Invasive cancer of the cervix or prostate
- Radiation injury after treatment of cervical cancer
- Abdominal perineal resection for rectal cancer in men and women

Stress Incontinence

Stress incontinence is urinary leakage following a sudden increase in intra-abdominal pressure (eg, coughing, sneezing, or other physical strain). Urine leakage may be a few drops or a stream of urine; however, clients can almost always tell the healthcare provider when it occurs and what they do to prevent the leakage. Stress incontinence primarily affects women with pelvic relaxation caused by childbirth, trauma, loss of tissue tone, or aging. Males frequently have stress incontinence after surgery to the prostate. Urodynamic tests are often used to confirm or rule out stress incontinence.

Reflex Incontinence and Urge Incontinence

Reflex incontinence and urge incontinence are similar in that in both types clients experience urgency before voiding caused by bladder spasm. *Reflex incontinence* is due to bladder instability as a result of upper motor lesions or neuropathies. *Urge incontinence* is due to irritation of the bladder wall, possibly due to urine components. In both conditions, involuntary loss of urine follows a sudden, strong desire to urinate. Clients usually cannot stop their urinary stream once it starts, and often cannot get to a bathroom in time.

The client often reduces his or her fluid intake to decrease incontinent episodes. However, this concentrates the urine further and increases spasms. Clients with urge incontinence also use the toilet frequently and void small amounts to prevent incontinent episodes. Again, however, this frequency ultimately decreases the bladder's functional capacity. If the client continues this practice for a long time, the detrusor muscle weakens. Distention of the bladder then causes it to spasm at lower volumes of urine.

Overflow Incontinence

Overflow incontinence happens when the bladder overfills with urine and is not able to release it because either the detrusor muscle no longer contracts (usually due to local nerve injury as in diabetes, or central spinal cord injury) or there is a blockage preventing the urine from emptying. Examples of obstruction include benign prostatic hyperplasia (BPH), cancer of the prostate that presses on the urethra, and postoperative urinary retention (see Chap. 89).

The client typically has a large, distended bladder but dribbles urine either continuously or with stress maneuvers like coughing or bearing down. If the incontinence is caused by a blockage, it is very important to either remove the blockage or bypass the blockage by using a catheter, before reflux of the urine into the kidneys causes kidney damage. In addition, clients who have this type of incontinence are generally more prone to urinary tract infections because the stagnant urine provides an ideal place for bacteria to grow.

Treatment

Treatment will depend on the underlying cause of the urinary incontinence. Conservative (medical) treatment is effective in milder cases of incontinence, especially for young people, in clients who are poor surgical risks, or in clients who do not wish to undergo surgery. Conservative treatment includes use of a bladder-retraining program, Kegel exercises, electrical stimulation, pessaries, medication therapy (eg, tricyclic antidepressants), Credé's maneuver, and a catheter to empty the bladder completely (in cases of incontinence caused by neurogenic bladder). Treatment for overflow incontinence caused by obstruction is relief of the obstruction; surgical intervention may be necessary.

Credé's Maneuver

This technique is used to manage overflow incontinence. In *Credé's maneuver,* the healthcare provider applies firm, gentle pressure above the bladder. The technique involves placing hands on the abdomen to press down with flat hands, starting at the umbilicus and moving down to the symphysis pubis. The procedure is repeated several times, applying the final pressure directly over the client's bladder.

Kegel Exercises

These exercises often are used as a treatment for stress and urge incontinence. They are probably the most useful tool the

nurse can teach the client to manage incontinence (see In Practice: Educating the Client 88-1). *Kegel exercises* are designed to increase sphincter tone and to help the client prevent leaking on the way to the bathroom. The client will need to wear a disposable pad during the training period to catch any urine. If after 3 to 6 months of working on an exercise program there is no noticeable improvement in the level of incontinence, the client may opt for surgery or medications for better manage-

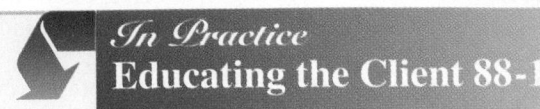

In Practice
Educating the Client 88-1

TEACHING KEGEL EXERCISES

- Instruct the client to be patient. Improved continence takes 3 to 6 months of *faithfully* doing the exercises daily.
- When examining the client's perineum, observe if when they contract the muscles, the anus pulls up and in (an anal wink). If the anal wink is absent, send the client on to urology for assessment and special treatment.
- In the supine position, with knees up, have the client visualize not letting *flatus* (gas) out. Observe the pulling up of the anus. If the client uses the bigger muscles of the buttocks, legs, or abdomen, they are doing the exercise poorly and must be taught to isolate just the pelvic floor muscles. Assist the client to identify the muscles by inserting a finger into the vagina or rectum and asking them to squeeze around the finger.
- Count how long the client can hold the squeeze before it begins to weaken. This is how long the client should hold the squeeze at home.
- It usually is easier for clients to identify the pelvic muscles when in a supine position because gravity is not working to pull the muscles down.
- If the client experiences use of the bigger muscles when doing the squeezes, they are either doing too many squeezes or attempting to hold them too long. The client should do fewer squeezes until the muscle is strong enough to sustain the hold and the desired number of contractions.
- In general, it is best to start the client out doing only four to five squeezes for 5 to 10 seconds, having them rest for 20 seconds between squeezes. A series of squeezes should be done 3 to 4 times a day. Generally before rising in the morning, at noon, at supper, and before falling asleep at night works best.
- The goal is to work up to three to four sets of 10 squeezes held for 10 seconds each.
- Do not tell the client to do their exercises by trying to stop the flow of urine. This trains the client to have an interrupted urine stream that could lead to retention.

ment of incontinence. *Biofeedback* may be used if Kegel exercises are ineffective in controlling urine flow. Biofeedback uses a computer or other electronic device to help monitor how well the client can do Kegel exercises.

Electrical Stimulation

Electrical stimulation (pelvic muscle stimulation) is another method of helping the client to strengthen the pelvic muscles and decrease the bladder activity that causes urge incontinence. A small electrode connected to a generator is placed in the vagina or rectum. When an electrical impulse occurs, the pelvic muscles contract; when no impulse is sent, the muscles relax. This treatment is very comfortable and easy to do at home. It is very useful in clients with neurologic problems or in those who have difficulty figuring out which muscles to use in Kegel exercises.

Pessary

Pessary placement is a nonsurgical option for females with stress urinary incontinence. A **pessary** is a device that is inserted into the vagina to support the organs of the pelvis. These devices vary in size and shape and can be left in the vagina for long periods of time (4 to 8 weeks) without the need for removal for cleaning or maintenance.

If used to help support a prolapsed bladder, the client may improve her ability to empty the bladder completely. A pessary can also be used to help push the neck of the bladder closed, thereby lessening incontinence. Pessaries are useful devices for both the short- and long-term management of incontinence when clients either do not wish to have surgery or are not considered good surgical risks.

Medications

Medications often are used in conjunction with bladder retraining techniques, Kegel exercises, and biofeedback. Medications available to treat urge incontinence include anticholinergics (eg, oxybutynin) and tricyclic antidepressants (eg, imipramine); both of these drug classes work to inhibit bladder spasms.

Tricyclic antidepressants also are used to treat stress incontinence because another effect of these drugs is increased bladder neck resistance. Other drugs used to treat stress incontinence include pseudoephedrine and phenylpropanolamine. Another medication treatment choice is estrogen therapy for women with vaginal atrophy.

Surgery

When a **fistula** (connection) between the bladder and another organ is the cause of incontinence, surgery is almost always needed to repair the opening. Electrocautery may be used to seal the hole. *Electrocautery* refers to both the procedure and the instrument that is used. In this procedure, the urologist *cauterizes* (destroys) defective tissue with an electrode that emits either alternating or direct electrical current. Larger holes may require a more major surgery to patch the hole or correct the defect.

If a fistula is large or is caused by radiation therapy or invasive cancer, the client may require *ileal diversion* (urinary diversion) to correct the incontinence. Urinary diversions are described later in this chapter. *Surgical ureteral reimplantation* can correct abnormally placed ureteral orifices. In this procedure, the urologist attaches the ureters to the urinary bladder.

Many operative procedures are used to correct stress incontinence. The underlying principles of these procedures are the same—elevating the neck of the bladder and suturing it into place to restore the bladder's normal curvature. With the curvature of the bladder neck restored, the person usually regains continence. If the client has an open bladder neck because of nerve damage or scarring from previous surgeries, the goal is to close the bladder neck rather than to elevate it to a more functional position.

Another option for the client with a nonfunctioning urethra is the placement of an artificial sphincter. This artificial device consists of a cuff, which is placed around the bladder neck and is connected to a reservoir bulb. The bulb is implanted in the pelvis. The operating button is implanted in the scrotum or labia. The cuff is inflated with fluid from one of the reservoirs to maintain continence and then deflated when the client wants to empty the bladder.

If the above measures do not work, surgery for increasing the bladder size, *augmentation cystoplasty*, may be considered to increase the bladder's functional capacity. This is a measure of last resort in a population without neurologic problems, and is rarely done unless the problem of urgency is extreme in nature.

An implantable electrical stimulation (Interstim) device was approved for cases of severe urgency and frequency. The device uses a fine electrode attached to the sacral spinal cord to deliver an electrical current that is believed to both relax the bladder and block the sensation of urgency from the bladder.

Nursing Considerations

Nursing considerations for urge and reflex incontinence include encouraging fluids to dilute the urine and to flush irritating substances from the bladder. The nurse also can teach the client measures to empty the bladder completely (see In Practice: Educating the Client 88-2). Bladder retraining can increase the time between voiding episodes and increase the bladder's functional capacity (see In Practice: Nursing Care Guidelines 88-1). Biofeedback and Kegel exercises are recommended to assist with bladder retraining, so that the client learns to contract the pubococcygeal muscles until he or she reaches toileting facilities.

Bladder incontinence is more difficult to control than bowel incontinence, but with perseverance, many clients can establish control. For the client's physical and emotional well-being, achieving continence is important. The client may choose to continue to wear a Peri-Pad or incontinence briefs for urinary containment. See In Practice: Educating the Client 88-3 for management of chronic incontinence.

Chapter 51 discusses nursing care of the client with urinary incontinence and bladder rehabilitation techniques. The

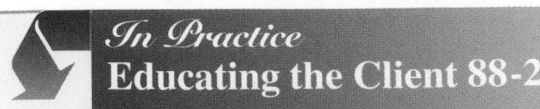

In Practice
Educating the Client 88-2

EMPTYING THE BLADDER COMPLETELY

- Teach the client to take ample time to toilet. If they try to rush through toileting, the pelvic muscle will tighten before their bladder is empty.
- Encourage the client who has "shy bladder syndrome" to find a private, quiet bathroom to toilet.
- The sound of running water will help the bladder that has difficulty starting to urinate.
- Tapping above the pubic bone, tapping the clitoris, or tickling the base of the bladder are all techniques that can be used to initiate a stream.
- It is better to avoid bearing down to empty, but rather push on the belly above the pubic bone during the stream (Credé's maneuver) to empty the bladder completely.
- The client can use a double-void technique to empty the bladder completely.
- In female clients who have prolapse, the client can lift the base of the bladder using a finger in the vagina to tip it into a position that will help emptying.

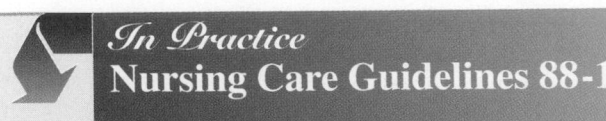

In Practice
Nursing Care Guidelines 88-1

BLADDER RETRAINING

Alternative One

1. The client must be able to follow one-step commands.
2. Use a voiding diary (to determine frequency and continence status).
3. Establish a baseline pattern of voiding with the voiding diary.
4. Set the interval goal at slightly under the average interval between incontinent or voiding episodes, as shown in the voiding diary.
5. After the client consistently empties the bladder when toileting, begin to increase the interval between toileting times.
6. Encourage the client to resist the urge to toilet for 5 to 10 minutes (by using distraction or relaxation techniques).
7. Gradually increase the length of time the client is to resist the urge to toilet until a target goal is reached (usually 20 minutes).
   - Gradually increase the length of time between voiding to the target goal of 3 to 4 hours.

Alternative Two

1. When the client can do a strong Kegel exercise, have them use the contraction to help them increase the length of time between toileting.
2. When the client feels the urge to toilet, they should stop their activity and do two to three quick, strong Kegel contractions that are not held more than 1 to 3 seconds with a 3 second rest between squeezes.
3. They should then count to 30 and see if the urge to toilet is still there. If it is, they should *walk, not run,* to the bathroom and urinate.
4. If the urge is gone they should continue their activity.
5. This sequence should be repeated as needed. This will quickly lengthen the time between voiding episodes.
6. Remind the client that as the muscles get stronger, the better the likelihood that there will be no leaking on the way to the toilet. It is best to practice these techniques when the client is at home initially, until the client begins to develop some control.

nurse is responsible for assisting the person to manage a urethral or suprapubic catheter (see Chap. 51). Chapter 57 describes the sterile insertion, removal, and irrigation of urethral catheters. The physician inserts suprapubic and other types of catheters. In some cases, the client learns to perform regular self-catheterization.

URINARY TRACT INFECTIONS

Acute Cystitis

Cystitis means inflammation of the urinary bladder. It is probably more commonly called a *urinary tract infection* (**UTI**). A UTI is an infection along any part of the urinary tract. Women are more susceptible to cystitis than are men because their urethra is shorter.

Normally the inside of the bladder is sterile, but microorganisms can enter from the urethra (the most common route), through the bloodstream, or directly through a fistula. The UTI may then ascend from the bladder into the ureters and into the kidney structures causing serious, often lifelong renal complications. The most common causative agent is *Escherichia coli,* followed by occasional cases caused by *Staphylococcus saprophyticus, Klebsiella, Proteus mirabilis,* or *Chlamydia trachomatis.*

Factors that may make a person more susceptible to UTI include catheterization, which can advance bacteria into the bladder (sterile technique during catheterization is a must), systemic disease (eg, diabetes), and changes in the vaginal pH in women.

Signs and Symptoms

The cardinal signs of urinary tract infection are frequency, dysuria, hematuria, or other abnormal components of urine, such as WBCs or pus, and a positive urine culture. Many times the symptoms of UTI are missed, especially in an elderly client or during pregnancy.

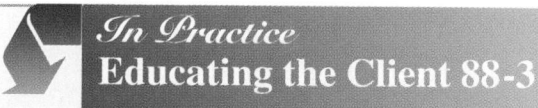

Educating the Client 88-3

MANAGEMENT OF CHRONIC INCONTINENCE

- Incontinence is often correctable and usually can be reduced.
- Use an incontinent pad on the bed and wheelchair to prevent soiling.
- Teach principles of bladder retraining, including Credé's maneuver, if necessary.
- Self-catheterization may be required for long-term management.
- The client may wear an appliance, condom catheter, or incontinent briefs or pads.
- Wash appliances regularly.
- Skin care is important to maintain good skin integrity.
- Female clients should wipe from front to back to help prevent urinary tract infections.
- Wash hands after toileting.

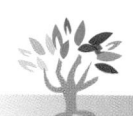

SPECIAL CONSIDERATIONS: THE LIFE SPAN

Urinary Tract Infections in Older Adults

- The only presenting symptom of urinary tract infections in older adults may be a change in mental status. Suspect this type of infection in all older clients who present with sudden, acute changes in mental status.
- Older adults metabolize medications more slowly than do younger clients. Consider this fact when choosing doses and times for PRN medications.
- Older adults often have several chronic disorders. Always be aware of how these disorders and their treatments influence kidney function. Be alert to subtle changes in behavior, personality, or daily functioning. Report these changes to the physician. Document your assessments carefully.

The client with cystitis has a desire to urinate frequently even though the bladder does not need emptying. The client voids very small amounts each time. A painful, burning sensation accompanies urination; sometimes blood is in the urine, and the client complains of a "heavy feeling" in the abdomen or perineum. Diagnosis of UTI is made by urinalysis and C&S.

Treatment

Antibiotics or sulfonamides are ordered as a result of sensitivity testing. Mild analgesics may be necessary for a few days. Drugs given for UTI may cause urinary discoloration; for example, phenazopyridine hydrochloride (Pyridium) causes the urine to appear orange-red.

Nursing Considerations

Teach preventative measures such as the importance of fluids, avoiding tight-fitting nonabsorbent underwear, and avoiding irritants such as soaps and bubble baths. Also explain that diets high in sugar promote bacterial growth and cystitis. Explain to women that sexual activity increases the risk of acquiring a UTI; voiding immediately after sexual intercourse reduces the risk. Teach women and girls to wipe the perineal area from front to back, which minimizes contamination of the urinary meatus with microorganisms from the rectum or vaginal areas.

Tell the client that warm packs can help alleviate the pain associated with infection. Explain the importance of taking antibiotics as ordered to eliminate the causative agents. Inform clients of the possibility of a change in color of urine when taking Pyridium. This discoloration may stain fabric and toilet fixtures. During antibiotic treatment, fluid intake of 3 to 4 liters daily is recommended, unless contraindicated. *Rationale: Additional fluid helps dilute the urine, thus lessening burning on urination.* Fluid intake also encourages elimination, thus preventing urinary stasis, in which bacteria can multiply. Flushing out the urinary system prevents the formation of crystals that may develop from sulfonamide therapy. In addition, the client may take vitamin C tablets (2 g per day) to acidify the urine and prevent growth of bacteria.

Chronic Cystitis

Clients will occasionally develop *recurrent UTI* or *chronic cystitis*. Signs and symptoms include urinary frequency, *nocturia* (nighttime voiding), and incontinence; dysuria will probably not be present. High bacterial counts often are obtained in a culture, yet the client may not be aware of a problem. Infections must be treated before damage is done to the kidneys. Clients with chronic cystitis often will be placed on long-term antibiotic therapy lasting 3 to 6 months.

Nursing Considerations

Nursing care of the client with chronic cystitis is the same as for clients with acute cystitis, but additional client teaching is necessary. The client prone to chronic cystitis should shower instead of bathe to avoid pushing bacteria up the urinary tract. In addition, remind women clients to empty their bladder before and after intercourse and to use a lubricant with intercourse if the vagina is dry. *Rationale: Friction irritates the urethra, increasing the risk of infection.*

Teach women to wipe from front to back to prevent sweeping bacteria into the urethra. Monitor the client on long-term antibiotics for yeast infection. Signs and symptoms of yeast infection need to be explained (see Chap. 90). Sometimes clients on long-term antibiotic therapy have breakthrough infections. Provide the client with a sterile container to bring in a specimen if the individual experiences increased urinary symptoms. For best urine culture results, obtain a clean-catch midstream specimen or obtain the specimen with intermittent straight catheterization.

Acute Pyelonephritis

Acute pyelonephritis, inflammation of the renal pelvis and medulla, is the most common form of kidney disease. Pyuria is noted in a urinalysis. It usually stems from infection with microorganisms that have migrated from another body part; *E. coli* contamination is common. Pyelonephritis may result from an ascending infection from the lower urinary tract or from an indwelling urinary catheter. Microorganisms also may reach the kidney through the bloodstream, causing inflammation, edema, and sometimes many small abscesses.

Signs and Symptoms

Signs and symptoms of acute pyelonephritis are rapid onset of fever and chills, with flank pain, pyuria, nausea, vomiting, and headache. The client with this condition is very ill. If the bladder also is infected, the client will have a desire to urinate frequently and burning will accompany voiding. A urine test reveals bacteria in the urine (**bacteriuria**) as well as WBCs and casts.

Nursing Alert

Because many diagnostic and minor urologic surgical procedures are performed on an outpatient basis, aggressive client and family teaching is required. Clients and families must know how to perform preoperative preparation, and untoward signs to look for after the procedure. Carefully document this teaching.

Treatment

Treatment is antimicrobial therapy for at least 10 to 14 days. Antibiotics, sulfonamides, or urinary antiseptics are ordered to combat the specific causative microorganisms. If the client has nausea or vomiting, an IV line to prevent dehydration may be ordered.

Nursing Considerations

The client with flank pain, fever, and nausea requires immediate medical attention. Bed rest, plenty of fluids, attention to mouth and skin care, proper nourishment, pain management, and change of position are needed to provide comfort and prevent deformities or further infection. See In Practice: Educating the Client 88-4.

Chronic Pyelonephritis

Chronic pyelonephritis may develop if an acute infection recurs or if an obstruction prevents the passage of urine. The kidney becomes permanently damaged, and because kidney tissue is not replaced, renal function is lost. Chronic pyelonephritis develops more slowly after the initial acute infection. Relapses of pyelonephritis are common. Causes may be related to obstructions. Treatment consists of long-term antimicrobial therapy and continued efforts to prevent more damage. Chronic pyelonephritis may advance to renal failure and death.

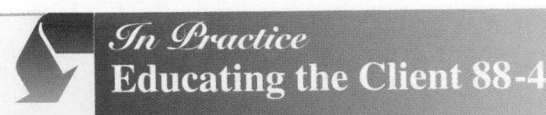

In Practice
Educating the Client 88-4

SIGNS OF INFECTION

- Dysuria
- Frequency
- Nocturia
- Cloudy urine
- Hematuria
- Fever, chills, flank pain in acute pyelonephritis

INFLAMMATORY DISORDERS

Interstitial Cystitis

Interstitial cystitis (**IC**) is a disease of the bladder that may be both autoimmune and inflammatory in nature. The lining of the bladder becomes "leaky" and allows irritants from the urine to contact the muscular wall of the bladder, causing irritability. This disease is more common in women, usually occurring between the ages of 20 and 50. Researchers have indicated that men who have abacterial prostatitis may actually have IC.

Signs and Symptoms

The client experiences a strong urge to void extremely frequently (every 5 to 30 minutes), often for many days without relief. The client may also experience pelvic pain and have painful intercourse. Unlike cystitis, voiding is usually not painful, but instead provides relief from the bladder pain and spasms. Men with this problem have may have penile-tip pain and perineal pain. The major characteristic of IC is that the urine is free of bacteria although the client experiences urgency, frequency, and pain. Clients usually can recall the exact time that their symptoms began, and the onset usually is associated with either a UTI or instrumentation of the bladder.

Diagnosis

In a small percentage of clients undergoing hydrodistention of the bladder, when the bladder is distended with fluid, lesions called *Hunner's ulcers* appear. More typically, petechial hemorrhages occur. Either of these findings is diagnostic of IC. Bladder biopsy examination shows changes typical of IC.

Treatment

Treatment of this chronic disease is difficult and consists of symptom management; there is no cure. Hydrodistention may improve symptoms several weeks after it is initially done, although the client may experience increased symptoms the first few weeks after the procedure.

A number of medications are helpful in symptom management; however, only one medication (Elmiron) is approved to specifically treat this disease. This medication rebuilds the protective layer of the bladder lining. Clients should be cautioned that they might need to take this medication for 3 to 6 months before their symptoms begin to improve. Some physicians administer bladder instillations of a cocktail of medications that includes DMSO, hydrocortisone, heparin, and sometimes lidocaine, weekly for 6 weeks for symptom flare-ups.

Bladder irritants should be removed from the diet and reintroduced gradually one at a time to see if symptoms improve. Fluids should be encouraged to help dilute the urine and remove toxic wastes from the bladder. Physical therapy and stress reduction techniques are helpful in the long-term management of the disease.

Nursing Considerations

Clients with IC should see the same provider at each visit while a urology specialist coordinates the long-term care and management of their disease. Instrumentation frequently causes flare-ups of symptoms, so it is important to do as little manipulation of the pelvic area as possible.

Intercourse is usually painful (*dyspareunia*) and clients are often severely depressed, causing long-term relationships to suffer. The disease worsens when the client is under stress, so it is important to work with employers and family members to help them understand how stress affects the client's symptoms. Social support is very important for these clients.

The pain caused by this disease in advanced cases can be extreme. These clients should be under the care of a urologist and may need counseling and support groups to help them cope with the disease.

Glomerulonephritis

Glomerulonephritis (Bright disease) is a group of diseases in which the kidneys are damaged and partly destroyed by inflammation of the glomeruli. Glomerulonephritis may be a result of an acute infection, as with *poststreptococcal glomerulonephritis*. This type of inflammation may result in an antigen and antibody reaction (an *autoimmune response*). *Nephritic syndrome (nephrosis)* may result from glomerulonephritis and is characterized by marked protein in the urine and edema.

Acute Glomerulonephritis

Acute glomerulonephritis often appears approximately 2 to 3 weeks after an upper respiratory infection or scarlet fever. The organism is usually the same streptococcus that causes "strep" throat. This form of glomerulonephritis is most common in children.

Signs and Symptoms.   The client may not notice the initial symptoms of glomerulonephritis. Family members may be the first to sense that something is wrong when they become aware of the client's pale, puffy face and swollen tissues (*edema*). The client gets up many times at night to void.

Diagnosis.   The urine is diluted due to lack of proper filtering in the glomeruli. Hematuria or smoky urine may be present. The client experiences headaches and irritability. Albumin, RBCs, and casts are present in the urine. Blood pressure often rises, and the client may have seizures. In the absence of treatment, serious complications, and possibly death, may follow.

Treatment.   The treatment goal is to restore the kidney to its best possible function. Antibiotics, such as penicillin, are given to counteract any existing infection. The client must remain in bed, sometimes for several weeks, to rest the body and to put as little strain on the urinary system as possible. Dietary management is determined by laboratory test results.

With treatment, almost all clients recover from acute glomerulonephritis. They are not considered well, however, until their urine has been continuously free of albumin and RBCs for several months.

Nursing Considerations.   Document the client's daily I&O and weight. Give fluids to balance output. Provide skin care and oral hygiene to prevent skin breakdown and infection; remember that this client's skin is fragile. Passive or active exercises help prevent respiratory and circulatory complications.

Chronic Glomerulonephritis

Chronic glomerulonephritis may develop immediately after an acute episode or after the client has been free of symptoms for an extended time. It also is possible for a person to contract chronic nephritis without having been aware that he or she had acute nephritis. *End-stage renal disease* (**ESRD**), also known as *chronic renal failure,* may develop. Chronic glomerulonephritis is much more serious than acute glomerulonephritis because it permanently damages the kidney by destroying nephrons and thereby disrupting function.

> ### Nursing Alert
> Chronic glomerulonephritis can have serious complications, including pulmonary edema, increased blood pressure, anemia, cerebral hemorrhage, congestive heart failure, and ultimately, renal failure.

Signs and Symptoms.   Signs and symptoms are similar to those of the acute stage. In the beginning, few physical symptoms occur other than mild general malaise, albumin in the urine, pale and dilute urine, slight anemia, hypertension, and marked edema or **anasarca** (generalized body edema).

The disease flares up at intervals, but the client usually feels well between attacks. During the course of the disease, which may be 10 to 30 years (with symptoms under control), signs of renal insufficiency develop. In advanced stages, complications include blurred vision followed by blindness. Nosebleed (*epistaxis*) and gastrointestinal bleeding are common in terminally ill clients.

Treatment.   Treatment includes treating edema with antihypertensive medications and restricting salt and water intake. If ESRD occurs, as evidenced by previous symptoms and elevated BUN and serum creatinine, the client receives the same treatment as for chronic renal failure.

Nursing Considerations.   When signs of a flare-up of chronic glomerulonephritis appear, place the client on bed rest to reduce metabolic waste and preserve strength. Lower the client's salt and fluid intake. A low-protein diet may be necessary to reduce the amount of protein breakdown products such as ammonia.

Avoid exposing the client to infection of any kind. Transfusions may be given for anemia. Place the client in the orthopneic position to facilitate breathing. With this treatment, symptoms usually subside in approximately 3 weeks, and the client gradually returns to normal. In the absence of dialysis or a kidney transplant, however, prognosis is poor.

☛ KEY CONCEPT

The person with chronic glomerulonephritis is very ill and needs close observation and skilled nursing care to monitor for and treat related renal failure.

OBSTRUCTIVE DISORDERS

Calculi, growths, spasms of the ureter, kinks in the ureter, or infectious scarring can obstruct the urinary system. An enlarged prostate gland (benign or malignant) can interfere with passage of urine. Other causes of obstruction may be meatal stenosis, blood clots, tumor, fibrosis, urethral stricture, neurogenic bladder, precipitates (materials precipitated out of urine), adhesions, or scar tissue.

☛ KEY CONCEPT

Complete obstruction anywhere in the urinary tract system is a medical emergency and must be treated quickly before renal damage occurs.

Hydronephrosis

Hydronephrosis develops when urinary obstructions block the outflow of the kidneys. Hydronephrosis may be gradual, partial, or intermittent.

Signs and Symptoms

In this condition, urine forms, but the flow of urine from the kidney is obstructed. Depending on where the obstruction occurs, waste products accumulate in the kidney and back up into the blood, leading to ESRD. If the obstruction is in the ureter, only one kidney is involved; if it is in the urethra, the bladder abnormally retains urine and both kidneys usually are affected. A bladder infection also is likely because the urine is allowed to stagnate. In addition, stagnant urine is the ideal environment for stone formation.

Treatment

Generally, *acute hydronephrosis* is reversible. The cause of obstruction must be removed as soon as possible to prevent the development of *chronic hydronephrosis*.

Calculi

Calculi form primarily in the kidneys and descend through the urinary passages. This condition, called **lithiasis,** affects about 3% of the population (Fig. 88-2). Urinary calculi are more common in men and occur most often in people between the ages of 20 and 40. The reason for stone formation is unknown; however, theorists believe that infection, dehydration, and urinary stasis are contributing factors.

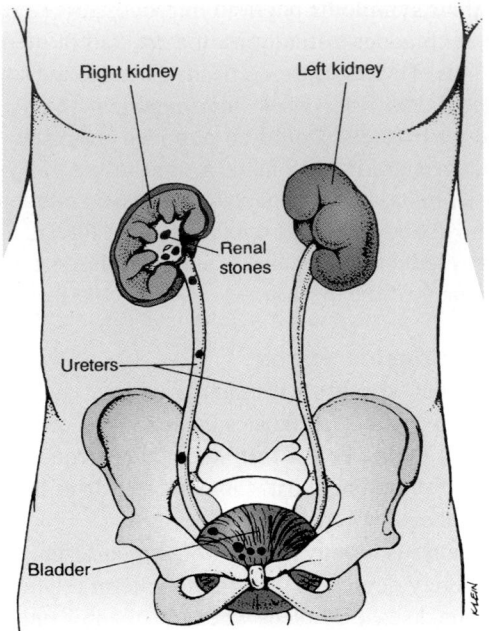

FIGURE 88-2. Locations of calculi formation in the urinary tract.

Urine contains various salts, including uric acid, calcium, and oxalate, which, if they do not dissolve, form stones. Uric acid can elevate and lead to gouty arthritis. Calcium stones are the most common. People susceptible to calcium stones usually must restrict intake of dairy products because foods with high calcium content contribute to stone formation. Often the stones are analyzed for mineral content so that certain minerals can be restricted in the diet.

Clients with a long-term illness who are immobilized for extended periods also are vulnerable. The most important preventative measure in stone formation is adequate hydration (3 to 4 liters of fluid per day).

Signs and Symptoms

With kidney stones, pain in the region of the obstruction is the primary symptom. Often this pain is called *colic,* an excruciating pain that comes in waves as the ureter tries to force the obstructing stone onward. This pain is violent and unbearable. Gross hematuria may occur if the stone traumatizes the ureter. Signs of UTI may be present. If the stone is very small, the spasm may move it along, allowing the client to pass it spontaneously.

✚👁 **Nursing Alert**

Investigate hematuria because it is a sign of infections, stones, and cancers. The usual investigation starts with a specimen for urinalysis and culture (obtain by catheter in women). An IVP is used to image the kidneys for stones and masses and a cystoscopy is used to investigate the bladder for lesions, stones, and inflammation.

Bladder stones are generally less troublesome than kidney or ureteral stones. Stones in the bladder may be asymptomatic or may cause mild hematuria or urgency and urge incontinence. If they do not obstruct the urethra, the client is generally unaware of them until they are found incidentally in diagnostic testing. Removal of bladder stones often relieves symptoms such as urgency, frequency, and repeat UTI.

Clients with multiple sclerosis or diabetes are at risk for formation of bladder stones. Individuals who have an indwelling catheter are at high risk for bladder stone formation. Clients who have repeat UTI may actually have stones, which act as an instigator of infections; until the stones are removed, the infections will be difficult to eliminate. Diagnosis of lithiasis occurs with a KUB x-ray examination or a CT scan of the abdomen or pelvic area.

Treatment

If colicky attacks recur, surgery is usually necessary to remove the obstruction. In some cases, stones are dissolved with medications, although this procedure is not used often. Only a strong analgesic will relieve the pain associated with kidney stones; antispasmodics also may be ordered. After a stone passes through the ureter into the bladder, the client usually has no difficulty passing it out of the body in the urine. If the stone does not pass through the ureteral channel spontaneously, it must be removed.

Unless bladder stones are symptomatic or cause obstruction, they are not treated. However, bladder stones can grow quite large and may need to be removed surgically. If this is the case, the client will need a suprapubic tube to drain the bladder until the suture line is healed. Smaller stones can be removed using a cystoscope (described later in this chapter).

ESWL. *Extracorporeal* (outside the body) *shock wave lithotripsy* (**ESWL**) is used in cases of calculi in the kidney or upper ureter (Fig. 88-3). In this treatment, the stones are "blasted" by shock waves that are so intense that they break

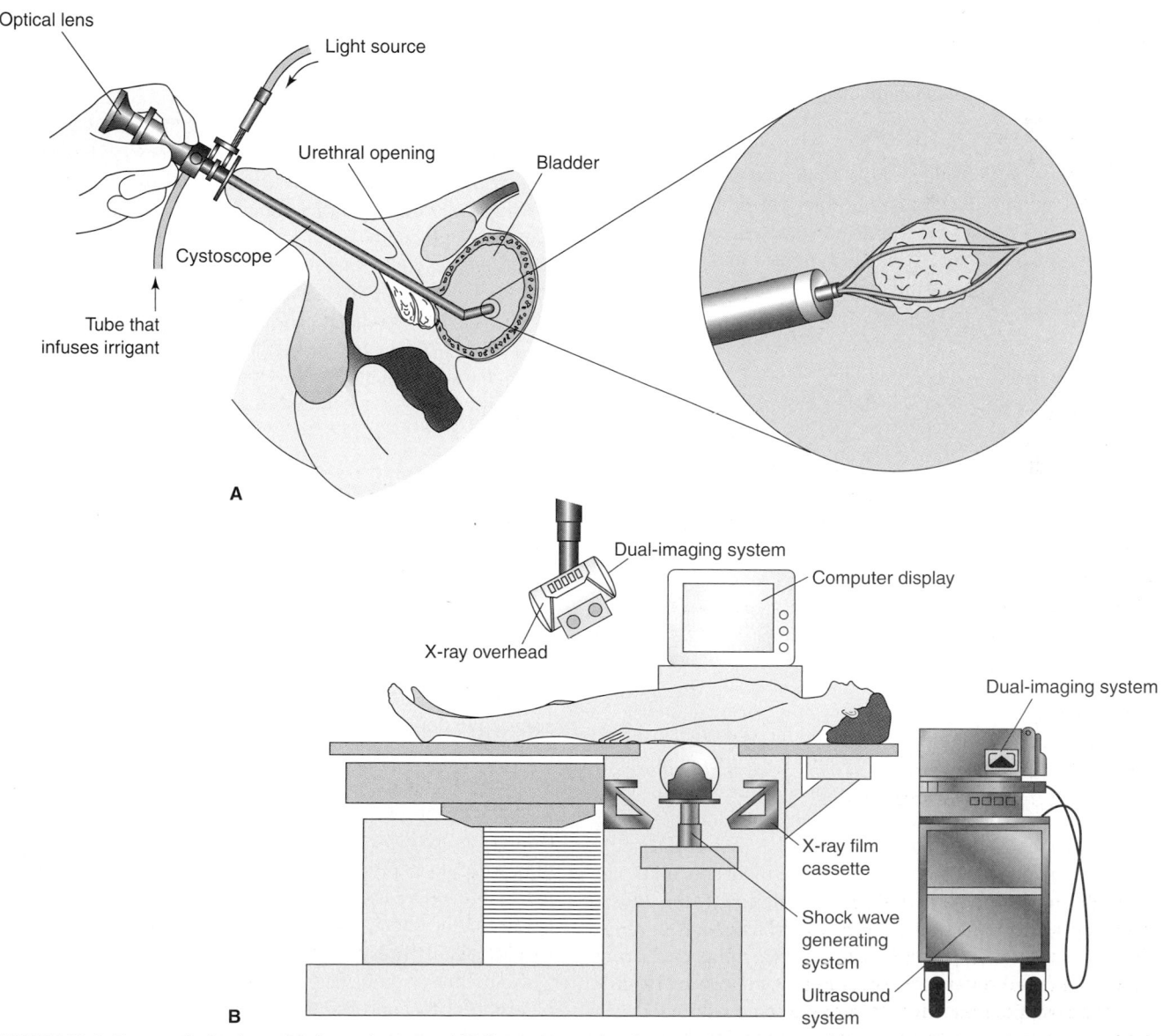

FIGURE 88-3. Removal of urinary and renal stones. (**A**) Stone is removed using a ureteroscope, which captures the stone. (**B**) Extracorporeal shock wave lithotripsy (ESWL).

the stones into small, gravel-like fragments. If a stone is in the lower ureter, it can be pushed up into the upper ureter or kidney and treated with ESWL.

ESWL is not used in the lower ureter or bladder because it can be traumatic, and these tissues are more delicate. ESWL is a specialized and potentially hazardous procedure that must be performed by carefully trained physicians and technicians.

Percutaneous Nephrolithotomy. In this procedure to remove stones from the kidney, a small "stab wound" is made in the flank and a catheter is inserted. An ultrasonic probe is inserted through the catheter. Then ultrasound waves are directed at the stone. These waves break the stone into pieces that are small enough to be withdrawn through the catheter. After the procedure, the catheter is left in place for 1 or 2 days, until edema subsides. At this time, normal passage of urine into the ureter and bladder can resume. A newer but similar method uses a homium laser to break up the stones.

Urethroscopic Calculi Removal. In some cases, stone removal without crushing is possible through an ureteroscopy procedure. The surgeon grabs the stone and pulls it out of the client's ureter, using a special tong-like instrument called a *stone basket.* Some bleeding is common after this procedure because of the trauma caused by the passing of the scope and/or stone.

Lithotripsy. **Lithotripsy** refers to the crushing of stones. It can be done in the bladder or the urethra by passing a crushing instrument into the urethra or urinary bladder through the urethroscope. The purpose of crushing the stone is to make the fragments small enough for the client to pass in the urine.

After urethroscopic calculi removal and lithotripsy, a **stent** (a hollow tube used to support structures) is placed so that it bridges the area where the stone was. The tube supports the structures and allows urine to drain easily. It is important that remaining fragments are washed out. The area will be swollen and traumatized after stone manipulation. It is important that the client returns for followup treatments for stent removal or changing of the stent.

Surgical Removal. An *ureterolithotomy,* surgical removal of calculi in the ureter, may be done in a few cases in which a stone blocking a ureter requires an incision for removal. Surgical *nephrolithotomy* is the method of kidney stone removal least likely to be used today. This major surgery includes an incision into the kidney and removal of the stone.

Nursing Considerations

Straining Urine for Calculi. If kidney or other urinary tract stones are suspected, the physician will order all urine to be strained. You can do this by pouring the urine through gauze, cheesecloth, or a strainer. Save any calculi. Calculi that are passed spontaneously may be as small as grains of sand or as large as pebbles. Measure and discard the urine, and save any material strained out of it for examination by the physician or laboratory personnel. See In Practice: Nursing Care Plan 88-1 for care of the client with renal calculi.

Caring for the Client Undergoing Stone Removal. Pre- and postoperative care for surgical removal of stones is basically the same as for other abdominal procedures, with careful observation and straining of the urine and care of drainage tubes postoperatively (see "Postoperative Care" within the "Nursing Process" section of this chapter).

For the client undergoing ESWL, explain the procedure. Depending on the method of ESWL used, the client will either be placed on a treatment table that has a built-in water cushion or the client will be immersed in a tub of water. If using the submersion tank, place small water wings on the client's arms to keep the arms afloat and out of the way. A mild sedative is usually ordered before the procedure and general anesthesia may be administered. The procedure is not totally without discomfort. Document all teaching.

Nursing assessment after ESWL includes observation of urine, which will be slightly bloody for 24 to 48 hours. The color is most often described as "rose." The bleeding results from ureteral trauma caused by the gravel-like stone fragments passing through in the urine. Strain the urine and encourage fluids. The client may be bruised in the area of the lateral pelvic bones.

The client must follow certain precautions after discharge from the healthcare facility. Urge the client to force fluids and strain all urine. Teach the client how to monitor for signs of infection and hematuria, and to report these findings to the physician. Explain that medications must be taken as prescribed, and that the client may find comfort by applying warm packs.

Client Teaching. The client who has had one kidney stone has an increased chance of forming another one. A key factor in preventing kidney stone formation is intake of water. Encourage the client to drink at least eight 8-ounce glasses of water every day to dilute the urine. Teach the client to increase fluid intake in hot weather to avoid dehydration. Also, depending on the analysis of the stone, teach the client to limit intake of certain foods.

Ureteral or Urethral Strictures

Fibrous bands can form anywhere along the ureters or the urethra, narrowing it and interfering with urine passage. This condition is more common in men than in women because the male urethra is longer. *Strictures* cause difficulty in voiding. The client feels the need to void frequently, but an intense burning sensation accompanies voiding. A thorough medical history, urodynamic flow testing, and other diagnostic studies are used to diagnose strictures.

Treatment

A stricture can be stretched by inserting metal instruments (*sounds, bougies*) of graduated sizes into the urethra, beginning with the size that goes past the strictures and gradually increasing to larger ones. Because strictures have a tendency to reform, the client will need to return to the healthcare facility periodically to have this dilatation process repeated.

Sometimes surgery is necessary to cut the constricting bands; this procedure is referred to as an *urethrotomy.* Recurrence of the stricture is rare after urethrotomy.

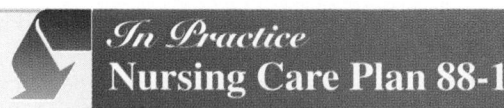

**In Practice
Nursing Care Plan 88-1**

THE CLIENT WITH RENAL CALCULI

MEDICAL HISTORY: *R.M., a 61-year old male, comes to the emergency department complaining of severe colic-like pain in the left flank area that radiates to the thigh. Client states, "I feel like I have to urinate, but then when I try, only a little urine comes out and it hurts." Urinalysis shows hematuria. Diagnostic tests reveal presence of several stones in the kidney and ureter. Client's family history is positive for renal calculi.*

MEDICAL DIAGNOSIS: *Renal calculi, recurrent episode*

Data Collection/Nursing Assessment: Client is a well-nourished male, visibly in pain, holding side and lower back area, rubbing left thigh. He states, "The pain is terrible." He rates pain as 10 on a scale of 1 to 10. Client reports one previous episode of renal calculi treated with analgesics. "Last time I was able to pass the stone." Urine appears cloudy and concentrated; voicing complaints of dysuria and frequency with small amounts of urine passed with each voiding. Voiding amounts ranging from 50 to 75 cc's each time. Temperature slightly elevated at 100.8° F (38.2° C); other vital signs within acceptable parameters. (*Although other nursing diagnoses may be appropriate, a priority nursing diagnosis is addressed below.*)

Nursing Diagnosis: Impaired urinary elimination related to obstruction from renal calculi as evidenced by client's complaints of dysuria, frequency, and voiding in small amounts.

Planning

SHORT-TERM GOALS:

#1. Client will demonstrate an increase in amount of urine voided each time.

#2. Client will verbalize that pain (both flank pain and pain on voiding) has decreased to tolerable level.

LONG-TERM GOALS:

#3. Client demonstrates evidence of passage of stone.

#4. Client voids without difficulty or pain.

Implementation

NURSING ACTION: *Administer analgesics as prescribed; assist client to assume a position of comfort; apply warmth as ordered.*

RATIONALE: *The pain associated with renal calculi can be severe; pain relief is essential for the client's comfort and cooperation.*

NURSING ACTION: *Monitor client's vital signs and urine output closely. Check amount of urine voided each time.*
RATIONALE: *Vital sign monitoring allows for early detection of possible infection. Monitoring urine output, including checking the amount voided each time, provides an objective measure of the client's condition.*

NURSING ACTION: *Encourage fluid intake, to at least 3L/d.*
RATIONALE: *Increased fluid intake is necessary to help move the stones (if possible) through the urinary tract.*

Evaluation: Client rates pain as 7 on a scale of 1 to 10 after administration of analgesic. He reports continued dysuria; 100 cc's of urine passed with each of last 2 voidings; fluid intake of 600 cc's over past 3 hours. *Progress to meeting Goal #1 and Goal #2.*

NURSING ACTION: *Strain all urine for stones; teach client how to do the same.*
RATIONALE: *Straining helps to identify passage of stones.*

NURSING ACTION: *Continue to monitor vital signs, pain, and urine output; obtain urine samples as ordered for testing.*
RATIONALE: *Continued monitoring is essential to determine progress or deterioration in client's condition.*

NURSING ACTION: *Encourage the client to ambulate if possible.*
RATIONALE: *Ambulation aids in moving the stone(s) through the urinary tract.*

Evaluation: Client reports pain after continued analgesic administration now controlled at 2 on a scale of 1 to 10; ambulated twice in hall. He states, "I think I passed some stones." Urine checked; small granules noted and sent to laboratory. Currently voiding approximately 150 cc's at each voiding; states, "It doesn't hurt that bad anymore and I feel like I can urinate more easily." *Goal #1 and Goal #2 met; progress to meeting Goal #3 and Goal #4.*

Nursing Considerations

Monitor clients for bleeding after treatment with bougies or urethrotomy. Other postoperative care is routine, including monitoring urinary output for symptoms of UTI.

URINARY TRACT TUMORS

Benign Renal Cysts

Cysts of the kidney may be single (*monocystic*) or multiple (*polycystic*). *Monocystic kidney disease* or a single cyst is usually benign and asymptomatic. However, depending on the size of the cyst, it can cause pain or decrease kidney function. *Polycystic kidney disease,* also consisting of benign tumors, has been found to be a familial problem. The extent of the disease is much greater than with a single cyst. Generally diagnosed shortly after birth, the cysts become so enlarged within the kidney that a mass is often palpable. This disorder may progress to ESRD. Emotional support for the family is crucial.

Cancer of the Kidney

Nephroma is cancer of the kidney. A primary cancer of the kidney is called a *hypernephroma.* Kidney tumors are almost always malignant. They occur more frequently in men and are rare in people under 30 years of age. Renal cancer is aggressive, often invading the aorta or vena cava. Clients often have distant metastases and local invasion of nearby organs. Renal cancer accounts for about 2% of all cancers.

Signs and Symptoms

Cancer of the kidney is usually advanced before signs appear. The first sign may be blood in the urine (painless hematuria). Other symptoms are fever, loss of weight, and malaise; a palpable flank mass and pain may appear later. X-ray, CT scan, renal arteriography, or ultrasound study confirm the diagnosis.

Treatment

If the kidney is a primary site, the cancer is discovered early enough, and the other kidney is healthy, then removal of the kidney using nephrectomy may be curative. Before surgery, the kidney function is brought to as normal a level as possible. Radiation, chemotherapy, or both are used when the cancer has spread to the lymph nodes.

☛ KEY CONCEPT

Neoplasms may present with problems to renal function by obstructing urinary flow. Chemotherapy may damage renal function.

Bladder Tumors

The bladder is the most common site of urinary system cancer. Bladder cancer occurs most often in men between the ages of 50 and 70. Tumors may be embedded in the bladder wall or may appear as small warts on the inside surface. Most bladder tumors are malignant.

Occupational exposure to chemicals increases the risk of this cancer. Cigarette smoking and lung cancer also are associated with increased incidence of bladder cancer. A correlation also seems to exist between caffeine intake and use of certain artificial sweeteners with the occurrence of bladder cancer.

Signs and Symptoms

Most often, the presenting sign of bladder cancer is painless hematuria. Bladder cancer is diagnosed with a combination of CT scan, x-ray, cystoscopy with biopsy, or urine cytology studies.

Treatment

Treatment for bladder cancer varies, depending on the tumor's extent. Carcinoma *in situ* may be treated using chemotherapy instilled into the bladder through a catheter and then allowed to remain in the bladder for an hour. Treatments take place weekly for 6 weeks and then are repeated at 3-month intervals for a year.

A transurethral resection of a bladder tumor (**TURBT**) is removal of a superficial tumor by endoscopic *resection* (cutting out) or *fulguration* (destruction by electricity). The surgeon uses a special cystoscope called a *resectoscope,* which is inserted into the bladder through the urethra. Laser therapy also may be used. Clients with this type of tumor return at 6-month intervals for cystoscopic examination to determine recurrence or further tumor development.

Cystotomy, an incision made into the bladder, can remove larger or more extensive tumors. If the bladder is not totally removed, a catheter may be placed in the bladder and brought out through the skin as a cutaneous cystostomy or suprapubic Cystocath.

If the tumor is large and invasive, the entire bladder may be removed (**cystectomy**), necessitating urinary diversion (discussed below). Anytime the bladder is removed, a *stent* (tube- or spring-shaped support) is placed in the ureters where they are connected to the ileum to keep them open and prevent edema or excess drainage from causing urinary obstruction during the postoperative period. The stents are usually removed about 2 weeks postoperatively.

Bladder tumors often metastasize to the lymph nodes, then to the bones of the pelvis, ribs, and vertebrae, and sometimes to the kidneys, liver, or lungs. Radiation therapy and chemotherapy are usually combined with tumor removal to prevent or minimize metastases. If the client receives radiation therapy, changes in the bladder wall (if the bladder was not totally removed) make it appear roughened and reddened. In addition, the bladder will lose its compliance and will not hold as much urine. These typically permanent changes are called *radiation cystitis* and can make the client miserable. Treatments used for urge incontinence can be used to help these clients.

Urinary Diversions

If the bladder is removed, urinary diversion is required. There are basically two types of urinary diversion—cutaneous urinary diversion and continent urinary diversion. Box 88-1 summarizes types of urinary diversions. Many factors influence the type of urinary diversion that is used.

Cutaneous Diversions.   *Cutaneous diversions* involve the drainage of urine through a surgical opening (*stoma*) created in the abdominal wall (Fig. 88-4). The client must wear an appliance at all times over the surgically designed stoma, which continuously collects urine drainage. The client often has no voluntary control of urinary flow. Chapter 87 provides information on ostomy appliances and nursing care. Cutaneous diversions include:

- *Ileal conduit:* A loop of ileum is connected to the ureters and brought out through the skin. This is the most commonly used method for excretion of urine. It requires that the client wear an appliance over the stoma to contain urine. See In Practice: Educating the Client 88-5.
- *Cutaneous ureterostomy:* The ureter is brought out to the skin of the abdomen. This procedure is rarely done, due to the high incidence of stricture, which necessitates re-operation.
- *Vesicotomy:* An opening is made into the abdominal and bladder walls to allow for bladder drainage.
- *Cutaneous nephrostomy:* A tube is placed into the kidney and is brought out through the skin.

Continent Diversions.   *Continent diversions* involve surgical creation of a new reservoir for urine from a portion of the intestine. This type of diversion is done depending on the client's preference and anatomy. These methods of urinary diversions may provide the client with voluntary bladder control (Fig. 88-5).

➤➤ BOX 88-1

TYPES OF URINARY DIVERSION

Ileal conduit: Segment of ileum close to the ileocecal valve resected; ureters reanastamosed to it. Proximal end of ileal segment closed; distal end brought to abdominal wall as stoma.

Cutaneous ureterostomy: Ureters brought to abdominal wall as stoma.

Continent diversion (Kock pouch): Two ileal limbs present; each is intussuscepted to create nipple valve. Efferent limb brought to skin as stoma. Ureters stitched to afferent limb, which prevents reflux.

Continent diversion (Indiana pouch): Segment of cecum and ileum resected from the bowel. Ureters tunnelled into colon to prevent reflux. Continence maintained by ileocecal valve. Ileum brought to skin as stoma (pleated to be smaller).

Ureterosigmoidostomy: Transplantation of ureters into intact sigmoid colon; urine and stool elimination controlled by anal sphincter.

Neobladder: Internal urinary reservoir that empties through urethra.

A *Kock pouch* is a type of continent diversion in which the middle portion of the ileum is folded and opened onto itself to create a pouch, with a nipple-valve stoma. A small gauze pad covers the stoma, which is catheterized on a regular schedule. The high re-operation rate to repair leaking nipple valves tends to discourage many clients from this option.

Ureterosigmoidostomy involves connecting the ureters to a loop of bowel so that urine can drain out through the rectum. Ureterosigmoidostomy is rarely done. Postoperative followup has shown an increased risk of colon cancer and sepsis, due to reflux of *E. coli* organisms into the kidneys. In addition, the stool is liquid, causing frequent toileting, if not incontinence.

The *neobladder* is a relatively new procedure that is used for the client who has no tumor in the base of the bladder, so that the urethra can be salvaged (rather than removed). After the cystectomy, a new bladder is constructed using small bowel tissue, which is connected to the existing bladder neck. This allows the client to void naturally through the urethra.

Nursing Considerations.   Urinary diversion may strongly affect the person's body image. Bladder removal for men is often associated with permanent sexual dysfunction. Adapting to cancer, loss of the bladder, and loss of body image can be devastating. Be supportive. Client teaching is an important aspect of nursing care.

☛ Key Concept

Urinary diversions are provided to promote the elimination of urine from the body. Unobstructed intact stomas or other urinary structures are crucial, along with good skin care, emotional support, and client teaching.

URINARY TRACT TRAUMA

Trauma to the kidney can be dangerous because the kidney receives a large amount of blood from the abdominal aorta. Because a small kidney laceration can cause massive hemorrhage, the client will need immediate surgery to repair the tear. Occasionally, a damaged kidney must be removed to prevent further hemorrhage. Bruising of the kidney can result in edema and blocked urine flow.

A fairly common injury sustained in motor vehicle and other accidents is *bladder rupture,* which results in shock, sepsis, and hemorrhage. The client must have emergency surgery, after which a urinary drainage system and other drains will be in place. Postoperative care is routine, with special attention to urinary drainage. Complications may include impotence or incontinence.

General health teaching includes attention to frequent voiding, and the necessity of keeping the bladder empty when the client is traveling or participating in sports or other activities.

RENAL FAILURE

Changes in renal function often are graded on a continuum. *Renal impairment* is identified by specific urine concentration and dilution tests. *Renal insufficiency* becomes apparent when the kidneys cannot meet the demands of dietary or metabolic

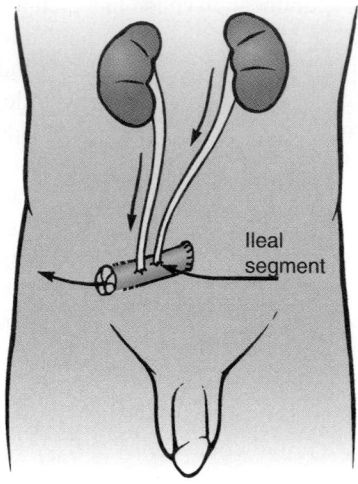

Conventional ileal conduit. The surgeon transplants the ureters to an isolated section of the terminal ileum (ileal conduit), bringing one end to the abdominal wall. The ureter may also be transplanted into the transverse sigmoid colon (colon conduit) or proximal jejunum (jejunal conduit).

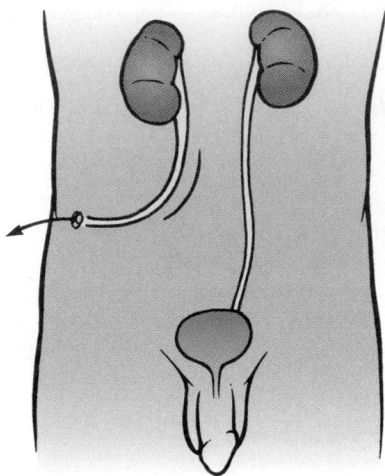

Cutaneous ureterostomy. The surgeon brings the detached ureter through the abdominal wall and attaches it to an opening in the skin.

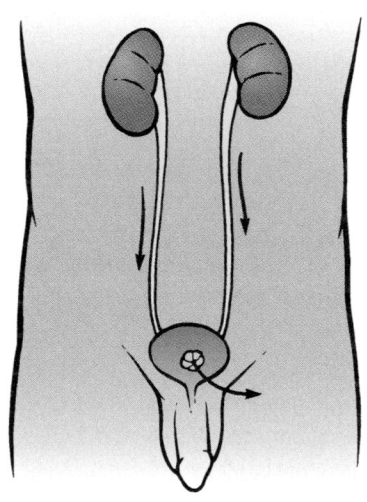

Vesicostomy. The surgeon sutures the bladder to the abdominal wall and creates an opening (stoma) through the abdominal and bladder walls for urinary drainage.

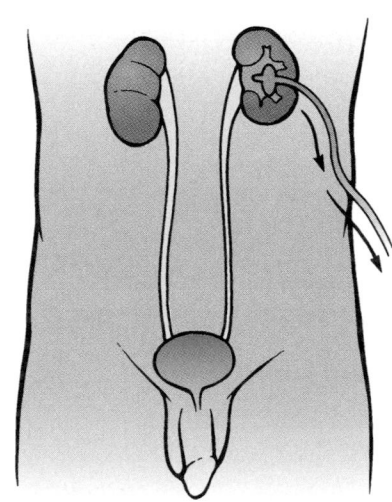

Nephrostomy. The surgeon inserts a catheter into the renal pelvis via an incision into the flank or, by percutaneous catheter placement, into the kidney.

FIGURE 88-4. Examples of cutaneous urinary diversion procedures, after which the client must wear a urinary collecting device.

stress. *Renal failure* exists when the kidneys no longer meet everyday demands. As renal function diminishes, the kidneys lose their ability to adapt to varying intakes of foods and fluids.

Early in renal failure, the creatinine clearance test evaluates effectiveness of treatment. In chronic renal failure, the serum creatinine level reflects the level of renal function; as the disease progresses, the serum creatinine level increases. The phases of renal failure may be characterized by oliguria (lack of urine) or diuresis (increased urine), or they may fluctuate depending on the cause.

In renal failure, the kidneys become unable to remove waste products from the blood and body cells and excrete them in the urine. This toxic condition is associated with renal insufficiency and retention of nitrogenous substances in the blood. Renal failure may result from injury, kidney disease, urinary tract disturbances, or conditions that decrease blood supply to the kidneys. It may follow acute glomerulonephritis, drug overdose or poisoning, excessive inhalation of a highly toxic substance (such as sulfur or carbon tetrachloride), severe transfusion reactions, and other severe shocks to the system. The

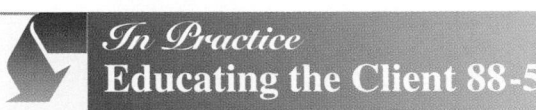

In Practice
Educating the Client 88-5

CARE OF THE ILEAL CONDUIT

- Change appliance every 5 to 7 days.
- Use solvent to loosen appliance; do not "tear" the appliance off.
- Clean the skin with water and mild soap.
- To remove encrustations, use gauze soaked with a 1:3 part solution of vinegar and water.
- Examine the stoma; healthy stoma tissue is deep pink to dark red, and shiny. If the stoma is macerated, dusky, or wet looking, notify the physician.
- Dry the skin area gently, but thoroughly, before applying the new appliance.
- If the tissue is excoriated, apply medication as ordered by the enterostomal therapist.
- Use a synthetic barrier cream that contains little or no karaya (urine destroys karaya).
- Strands of mucus may appear in the urine (from the mucus-producing cells of the ileum).
- Increase fluid intake to 3 L/d (to flush out sediment and mucus and to prevent clogging of the stoma).

vascular changes of Type 1 diabetes mellitus often lead to chronic renal failure. Renal failure also may occur more slowly as a result of nephrotoxic drugs given for unrelated disorders. Box 88-2 lists common nephrotoxic drugs.

☞ **KEY CONCEPT**

The nephrotoxicity of a drug must be determined before the agent is given to a client. Whenever administering medications, watch for signs of kidney dysfunction, and report them to the physician at once.

Acute Renal Failure

Acute renal failure occurs suddenly. Its cause may be factors outside the kidney (prerenal failure), as when the cardiovascular system fails to perfuse the kidneys adequately with blood.

Obstructions in urinary flow that damage the proximal structures or damage the kidney tissue itself are other possible causes. Tubular damage, referred to as *acute tubular necrosis,* is the most common form of intrinsic renal dysfunction.

Signs and Symptoms

Oliguria is common in the early phases of renal failure (*prerenal failure*) and occurs when the urinary output is less than 400 milliliters in a 24-hour period (in newborns, less than 1 mL/kg per hour). **Anuria,** output of less than 100 milliliters per day, may also occur. Laboratory values for serum sodium are

decreased, and the serum creatinine and BUN are elevated. This phase may last from 8 to 14 days.

In obstructive failure, the client may experience an initial diuresis when production of urine increases. The client may be *polyuric* with urine output greater than 6 liters per day.

Although urine volume eventually increases in most anuric or oliguric clients, the quality of this urine is inadequate and the client's body is retaining waste products. This is evidenced in the remaining elevation of BUN and serum creatinine levels. The recovery phase begins when the client's BUN stabilizes or is in the normal range. In this case, urine volume is normal, and the client returns to normal activity. This process may take several months. Some clients do not improve and develop ESRD.

☞ **KEY CONCEPT**

Recognize signs of acute renal failure and treat them promptly to prevent progression to permanent renal failure. Symptoms vary, but close monitoring of intake and output as well as creatinine, BUN, and electrolytes can provide valuable data to try to arrest the disorder.

Treatment

During acute renal failure, laboratory studies are performed frequently to monitor BUN, creatinine, and sodium and potassium levels. Early dialysis is often effective for clients with this disorder.

Nursing Considerations

Institute appropriate dietary measures to help control the complications of the condition. You may need to control sodium, potassium, protein, or fluids, based on the type of renal failure. Very accurate measurements of I&O are essential. To help the client conserve energy, assist with ADL.

End-Stage Renal Disease (ESRD)

ESRD, also known as *chronic renal failure,* is irreversible. By definition, this condition includes chronic abnormalities in the internal environment of the kidneys. ESRD requires maintenance with dialysis or kidney transplantation if the client is to survive. See In Practice: Nursing Assessment 88-2 for symptoms of ESRD.

If the underlying condition cannot be corrected, the client may die. Ideally, when a client is known to have ESRD, he or she should be referred to a dialysis center with family members.

Nursing Considerations

Nursing and medical care plans are designed to treat the primary cause of ESRD and to treat symptoms as they occur. Keep the client in as normal a state as possible, and make every attempt to prevent further kidney damage. Nursing considerations in ESRD include:

- Give sedatives for restlessness, transfusions for anemia, and cardiac medications for tachycardia or dysrhythmias as ordered.

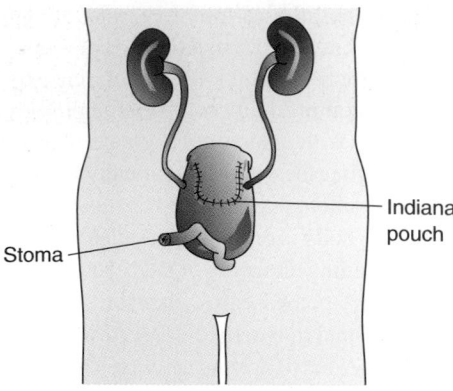

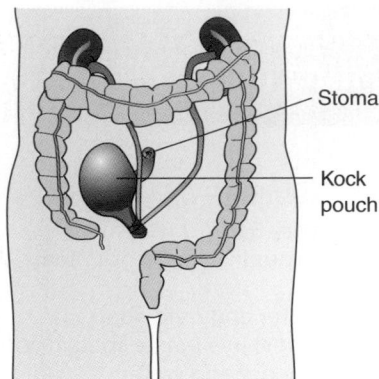

Indiana pouch. The surgeon introduces the ureters into a segment of ileum and cecum. Urine is drained periodically by inserting a catheter into the stoma.

Continent ileal urinary diversions (Kock pouch). The surgeon transplants the ureters to an isolated segment of small bowel, ascending colon, or ileocolonic segment and develops an effective continence mechanism or valve. Urine is drained by inserting a catheter into the stoma.

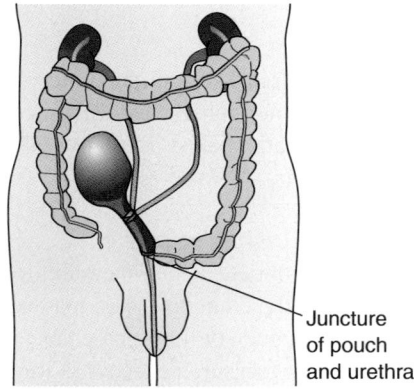

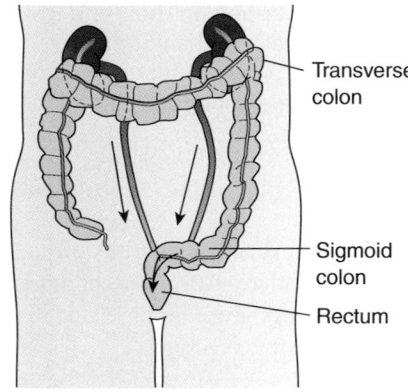

In male patients, the *Kock pouch* can be modified by attaching one end of the pouch to the urethra, allowing more normal voiding. The female urethra is too short for this modification.

Ureterosigmoidostomy. The surgeon introduces the ureters into the sigmoid, thereby allowing urine to flow through the colon and out of the rectum.

FIGURE 88-5. Various types of continent urinary diversions performed when the bladder is removed.

- Restrict fluids because the kidneys are not excreting urine. Vary fluids. Urge the client to spread fluid allowance throughout the day.
- Alkaline solutions are necessary for acidosis. A diet high in fat and carbohydrates and low in protein, sodium, and potassium is helpful, although restrictions may vary for each client.
- Maintain fluid and electrolyte balance as much as possible. Frequent blood chemistry studies will be done, and the physician needs reports as soon as possible. Make adjustments as needed for electrolytes given IV.
- Accurately document I&O: Determining exactly how much urine the kidneys are secreting helps to determine the extent of the disease.
- Take daily weights to detect fluid retention or edema.

- Good skin care and special mouth care are important. To relieve the itching and crusting brought on by pruritus and uremic frost, the client should bathe with tepid water, use no soap, and place a small amount of vinegar or baking soda in the bath water.
- Prevent chilling and exposure to infections because the client has few natural defenses to fight off infection. Also, many antibodies are excreted through the kidneys. Be alert for respiratory or cardiac complications.

Dialysis

Dialysis is a process that assumes the work of a damaged, nonfunctioning kidney. It can be a long-term procedure for chronic disorders such as kidney disease secondary to shock, diabetes mellitus, or chronic hypertension. Clients with severe

➤➤ BOX 88-2

COMMON DRUGS AND SUBSTANCES THAT CAN BECOME NEPHROTOXIC

Common Drugs and Possible Renal Damage

Penicillins: Allergic reactions

Sulfonamides: Allergic reactions

Cephalosporins (eg, cefaclor, cefazolin Na [Ancef], cefoxitin Na [Mefoxin], cephalothin Na [Keflin], cephradine [Velosef]): Damaged kidney cells

Allopurinol (Zyloprim, Lopurin): Allergies; also altered liver function

Aminoglycosides (eg, gentamicin, neomycin, streptomycin): Damaged kidney cells

Amphotericin B (Fungizone): Used to treat fungal infections; can cause permanent renal damage

Lithium (psychiatric drug): Renal toxicity

Cimetidine (Tagamet): Used to treat peptic ulcer; can cause creatinine elevation

Phenytoin (Dilantin): Used to control seizures; can cause toxic hepatitis

Nonsteroidal anti-inflammatory, analgesic drugs (eg, ibuprofen, indomethacin [Indocin], ketoprofen [Orudis]): Used to control pain; can cause acute renal failure or nephrotic syndrome

Antineoplastics: Used to treat cancers; can damage renal cells

Other Substances Toxic to the Kidneys

Heavy metals
Aniline dyes
Iodine-based contrast media
Carbon tetrachloride
Ethylene glycol
Benzene

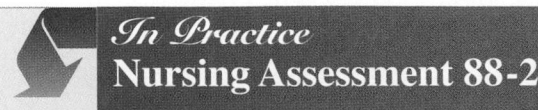

In Practice
Nursing Assessment 88-2

SYMPTOMS OF END-STAGE RENAL DISEASE

ESRD includes any or all of the following symptoms:

Anemia
Itching (*pruritus*)
Uremic frost (waste products crystallizing on the skin)
Loss of appetite (anorexia)
Hiccups (*singultus*)
Nausea
Vomiting
Fatigue
Fluid accumulation (*edema*)
Generalized body edema (*anasarca*)
Potassium retention
Sodium retention
Hypertension (high blood pressure)
Gastrointestinal bleeding
Bleeding disorders
Bone disease
Nerve-conduction defects
Congestive heart failure
Inflammation of the pericardial sac
Decreased immune response
Decreased platelet function
Retardation of growth (in children)
Dementia
Sexual dysfunction
Malnutrition
Decreased vitamin metabolism
Metabolic acidosis

drug overdose or poisoning may be treated with acute dialysis. The purposes of dialysis are to:

- Remove waste products of protein metabolism from the blood
- Remove poisons or toxins from the blood
- Remove excess water
- Establish or maintain proper levels of electrolytes
- Maintain acid–base balance
- Instill medications (such as antibiotics), electrolytes, or other substances

Some people are maintained for many years on intermittent dialysis. People who are awaiting kidney transplants are maintained on dialysis until a suitable kidney is available.

Two types of dialysis, peritoneal dialysis and hemodialysis, that are performed in a hospital or dialysis center, remove body wastes through a semipermeable membrane by osmosis, diffusion, and ultrafiltration.

Peritoneal Dialysis. In *peritoneal dialysis,* the connective tissue of the intestine (*peritoneum*) serves as the semi-

permeable membrane. Peritoneal dialysis is not used if the client has a known peritonitis or has had recent abdominal surgery. It is most often used on a short-term basis (eg, in the case of poisoning).

A catheter is inserted into the visceral cavity through which the dialysis solution (*dialysate*) is instilled into the abdominal cavity. The solution remains in the peritoneum for the time specified by the physician. It then flows freely out of the catheter into the container, which is lowered to facilitate gravity flow. This process may be continuous or repeated intermittently (Fig. 88-6).

Possible complications of peritoneal dialysis include:

- Bacterial or chemical *peritonitis* (inflammation of the peritoneum)—cloudy, odoriferous outflow
- Pain—abdomen, back, or shoulder (referred)
- Shortness of breath
- Protein loss
- Fluid overload or loss
- Electrolyte imbalance
- Constipation
- Infection
- Bleeding—bloody returns

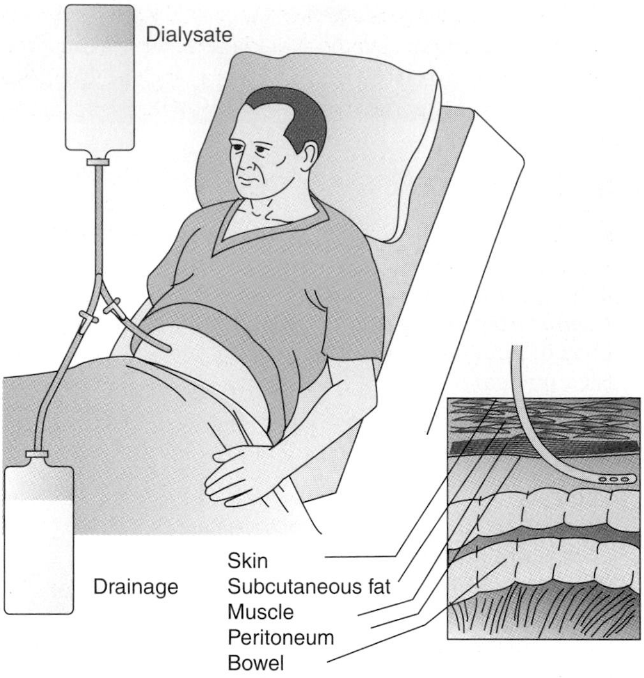

FIGURE 88-6. Peritoneal dialysis, in which the dialysate is infused into the peritoneal cavity by gravity. After remaining in the peritoneum for a period of time, the drainage tube is unclamped and the peritoneal cavity is drained by gravity.

✠👁 **N u r s i n g A l e r t**
Nursing assessment in peritoneal dialysis includes observation for signs of drug reactions, abdominal distention or pain, bleeding or shock, respiratory problems, infection, and leakage around the catheter leading into the peritoneum.

Continuous Ambulatory Peritoneal Dialysis (CAPD). **CAPD** is used in the home. The dialysate remains intraperitoneally. The client exchanges the dialysate four to five times per day. This procedure offers the client freedom from the constriction of machines. Other advantages are that steady blood chemistry levels are easily obtained, the process is shorter and less expensive, and training is less complicated than that for home hemodialysis.

Hemodialysis. Hemodialysis is performed by circulating the client's blood through a machine outside the body. This procedure is also known as *extracorporeal hemodialysis.* An external shunt or an arteriovenous (AV) fistula usually is inserted into one of the client's blood vessels to facilitate repeated hemodialysis. The client's nondominant arm is used for this process. Joining a large vein to an artery creates a *fistula.* A *bruit* (whooshing sound) and a *thrill* (fine vibration) can be detected at the site of an AV shunt. The **shunt** consists of an implanted U-shaped tube, which is usually placed between the radial artery and the arm's cephalic vein. This shunt allows the circulation to bypass the capillary network in that area and provides access to the arterial system. At the time of dialysis, two venipunctures are made into the shunt, one for the arterial blood source and the other for the venous return.

☞ **Key Concept**

Whether the client has a cannula or a fistula, he or she should be taught to check its patency daily by feeling the thrill *(vibration) and hearing the* bruit *(whooshing sound of high-volume blood flow). Clients should also be taught to avoid blood pressures and venipuncture in the affected arm.*

Hemodialysis is conducted within the machine by means of blood flow from the client. This shunt remains in place because the client needs dialysis treatment two to three times per week for 3 to 8 hours per treatment to maintain life.

Other access sites for hemodialysis include a cannula or a subclavian catheter. A *cannula* is an external device composed of two small plastic tubes. This cannula is placed in the client's arm or leg. One tube is placed in an artery and the other in a vein. Each tube comes through the skin at an exit site and rests outside the body. When the client is not on dialysis, the two parts of the cannula are connected together with plastic and usually covered with an occlusive dressing. The blood can then flow from the artery to the vein through this shunt.

✠👁 **N u r s i n g A l e r t**
Cannula separation is a life-threatening emergency. The client can *exsangiuinate* (lose all their blood) in a matter of minutes. Whenever a client has a cannula placement, he should be taught to always have two clamps attached to the dressing, to quickly clamp the ends of the separated cannula until they can be reattached.

A *subclavian catheter,* an IV device, is fairly large and is placed into subclavian blood vessels in the neck region. It has two ports, one for the arterial blood source and one for venous return.

Possible complications of hemodialysis are provided in Box 88-3 and below:

- Septicemia
- Air emboli
- Hemolytic anemia
- Disequilibrium syndrome
- Hepatitis
- Hypotension
- Pain, cramps
- Nausea and vomiting
- *Exsanguination* (severe, immediately life-threatening hemorrhage)

Nursing Considerations. The nurse may be asked to prepare a client for dialysis or to care for the client after a dialysis treatment. Some clients have a dialysis machine at home and do their dialysis during the day or at night. In this case, a family member must learn to assist and to recognize complications. In some cases, specially trained dialysis nurses assist in the home.

➤➤ BOX 88-3

COMPLICATIONS OF CONTINUED DIALYSIS

- The cannula can fall out and the client might bleed to death. More severe bleeding can also occur because the cannula is heparinized.
- The membrane within the dialysis machine can rupture, causing hemorrhage.
- If the chemical agents used are the wrong ones, or if the chemistry workup is incorrect, the client's electrolyte balance will be disrupted even further.
- Because most clients on dialysis have high blood pressure (caused by renal damage), they may go into shock when connected to the machine.
- The blood in the machine must be warm, or the client can suffer cardiac arrest from the shock of cold blood.
- Infection or septicemia is always a possibility. Because this client has especially low resistance, infection can be dangerous.
- Blood can clot in the cannula and cause phlebitis.
- Male clients often become impotent, although this problem may correct itself as the condition is stabilized.
- Excesses in alcohol or food intake will not be excreted between dialysis runs.

Many smaller facilities are served by regional dialysis centers that send personnel to assist on a rotating basis. In this way, clients can be treated in their own town.

Before the dialysis "run" (treatment), be sure the client is wearing a name band. Measure and record the client's vital signs and weight. The client is often NPO after midnight for a morning dialysis run. Blood may be drawn just prior to dialysis.

During the peritoneal dialysis run, keep the puncture site and dialysate sterile. Document the process, including the client's I&O through normal body orifices and a complete record of the dialysate (type, and amounts in and out). The dialysate is warmed prior to the treatment, often using a warm-water bath. Do not use the microwave to warm dialysate. Carefully record the amount and type of solution used, medications or electrolytes added, and times the solution was instilled and drained.

Specially trained personnel will monitor the hemodialysis run. If you are the client's primary nurse, you can provide vital information regarding the client's baseline status, particularly if you suspect changes in neurologic status, an early sign of deteriorating hemodynamic status. Provide any routine IV medications the client requires during the dialysis period that will not be removed from the blood.

In all types of dialysis, monitor and document the client's vital signs, daily weight, and level of consciousness. Never constrict blood flow in an arm with a shunt or fistula (eg, taking blood pressure). Constriction of blood flow can lead to clotting of the device.

Following the dialysis treatment, take vital signs frequently. The nursing care plan should include frequent turning, deep breathing, good skin care, and careful oral hygiene. The client generally feels better the day after dialysis than immediately following dialysis.

When a client is on dialysis, enforce strict dietary restrictions. For example, the client cannot excrete alcohol; therefore he or she should not consume it. Intake of sodium and potassium varies depending on the client's status, type of renal failure, and type of dialysis.

Use meticulous sterile technique when caring for the hemodialysis shunt. *Rationale: Because the shunt is inserted within the circulatory system, any infection would quickly spread throughout the body.* Keep the shunt clean and dry and observe it frequently for clotting and signs of infection. See In Practice: Nursing Care Guidelines 88-2 for more information.

Kidney Transplant

Surgeons can take a kidney from a well human being or a recent cadaver and transplant it into the body of another person to replace a diseased kidney. The kidney is "typed" before transplant for as good a match between donor and recipient as possible. This process is similar to blood typing for a transfusion. Tissue typing of this sort allows the most suitable match for the client. Often, the client's living relatives have compatible tissue matches and are considered as kidney donors. The donor must have two well-functioning kidneys and no underlying disease.

Medical authorities have agreed that a kidney transplant should be attempted only when it has a reasonable chance to succeed and when all other options have been attempted and failed. Transplant surgeons have special training. Kidney transplant is less complex than most other types of transplant.

More kidney transplants are done than any other type, and a high percentage of them are successful. A major advantage is that a live donor can sacrifice one kidney and continue to live without difficulty. Also, cadaver donors can supply two kidneys for two potential clients. Moreover, the client can be carefully prepared for a long time because he or she can be maintained by renal dialysis.

☛ KEY CONCEPT

Kidney transplantation represents a potential cure for the client with renal failure. Proper matching of recipient and donor is crucial.

Rejection of Transplanted Organs. The chief difficulty with all transplants is the body's natural reaction: to reject the foreign substance. Certain factors cause rejection. For example, if the person has been exposed to foreign proteins in the process of previous transplant attempts or multiple blood transfusions, rejection is more likely.

Many medications are available today to suppress rejection, and clients with transplanted organs have a much greater prospect for success. The rejection syndrome in kidney transplantation is usually easier to manage than that in other organ transplants.

In Practice
Nursing Care Guidelines 88-2

CARING FOR THE CLIENT RECEIVING DIALYSIS

- Always wear gloves. *Rationale: You will be exposed directly to the client's blood. Many people double-glove.*
- Check the shunt every 2 to 4 hours for vibration (*thrill*), which you can feel. Listen with a stethoscope for the whooshing sound of blood moving through the shunt (*bruit*).
- Notify the physician immediately if you detect a change in the intensity of these sounds or sensations or if they are absent. *Rationale: This could be life threatening.*
- Keep two clamps on the dressing over the external cannula at all times. *Rationale: In case of cannula separation.*
- Do not draw blood on the arm with a cannula or fistula. *Rationale: To avoid disturbing the shunt.*
- Do not measure blood pressure on the arm with a cannula or fistula. *Rationale: To prevent cannula separation.*
- You may need to take the client's blood pressure with an electronic device. *Rationale: You may be unable to hear it with a stethoscope.*
- If an arteriovenous fistula bleeds, apply pressure until the bleeding stops. *Rationale: Bleeding can be a life-threatening emergency.*
- Usually, you will not flush the port. *Rationale: It is not likely to clot and you want to avoid further possibility of injection.*
- Many clients on dialysis are diabetic and require insulin.

- These clients usually will not void. *Rationale: They do not produce urine because of lack of kidney functioning.*
- Do not give these clients orange juice. Give apple or grape juice instead. *Rationale: Orange juice is high in potassium. Elevated potassium is common in these clients and is dangerous. Hyperkalemia (elevated potassium) can cause fluid overload, shortness of breath, and irregular heartbeat, which can lead to cardiac arrest.*
- Blood for potassium and other electrolyte-level tests is usually drawn daily. *Rationale: To determine what should be included in the next run.*
- Follow medication times exactly. *Rationale: To maintain therapeutic blood levels and to avoid overload.*
- Measure the client's daily weight. *Rationale: To evaluate fluid retention.*
- The client's blood pressure may be elevated. *Rationale: Monitor blood pressure carefully.*
- "Guaiac all stools" is often ordered. *Rationale: To check for internal bleeding from the vascular kidney.*
- Teach the client and family about care of the cannula or fistula and other aspects. *Rationale: They must understand that disconnection of these devices is an emergency, requiring immediate attention.*
- Carefully and completely document all teaching.

Complications of Antirejection Medications.   Side effects of medications that suppress tissue rejection are common because these drugs also suppress the client's immune response.

Assessment includes observation for:

- Development of malignancies
- Susceptibility to viruses
- Susceptibility to infections of all types
- Gastric ulcers
- Gastrointestinal bleeding
- Psychiatric disorders
- Bone disorders

If a client rejects the first kidney transplant, a second transplant may be performed. A concern in all transplants today is that of transmission of diseases, such as HIV/AIDS, to the recipient. Specific tests are becoming more accurate in detecting human HIV and hepatitis B and thus preventing the transplantation of an infected organ.

➔ STUDENT SYNTHESIS

Key Points

- Blood tests to detect renal function include BUN, creatinine clearance, and uric acid.
- Incontinence can be temporary, iatrogenic, total, stress, reflux, or paradoxical.
- Kidney disease can start as an acute infection and reoccur as chronic conditions.
- Nursing care of the client with a urinary disorder focuses on maintaining and preserving renal function, decreasing discomfort, preventing infection, promoting skin integrity, maintaining fluid balance, and restoring and maintaining the client's self-esteem.
- Early symptoms of renal disease are subtle. The nurse's ability to detect small changes in the client is crucial to early treatment.

- Nephrolithiasis can be treated by ESWL and percutaneous nephrolithotomy.
- Common urinary diversions include the ileal conduit and the Kock pouch.
- Kidney and bladder tumors are often metastatic before they are discovered.
- Dialysis is a life-saving treatment.

Critical Thinking Exercises

1. Identify the critical elements you would include in an assessment tool to determine urinary function. Explain why each is important.
2. A client has renal calculi. Explain how nutritional intake could contribute to the development of different renal calculi.
3. Discuss when dialysis might be used for clients who are not in chronic renal failure.

NCLEX-Style Review Questions

1. The nurse should encourage fluids after an IVP to:
   a. Ensure that the kidneys are functioning
   b. Flush blood from the urinary system
   c. Prevent the client from becoming dehydrated
   d. Remove the dye from the client's system

2. Your client complains of dribbling small amounts of urine when laughing or coughing. She asks you why this happens. You explain:
   a. Bladder spasms are causing her to leak urine.
   b. The sudden increase in intra-abdominal pressure causes leakage.
   c. This is a transient condition and it will pass.
   d. You do not know why she is leaking urine.

3. The client is being discharged from the hospital with chronic glomerulonephritis. It is most important for the nurse to include a referral to:
   a. Chaplain or spiritual advisor
   b. Dietitian
   c. Hospice nurse
   d. Physical therapy

4. The client with urinary lithiasis should be instructed to:
   a. Avoid foods high in protein.
   b. Assess urine for pus.
   c. Drink 1 liter of fluid per day.
   d. Pour urine through gauze.

5. A life-threatening complication of hemodialysis is:
   a. Anemia
   b. Cramps
   c. Exsanguinations
   d. Hypotension

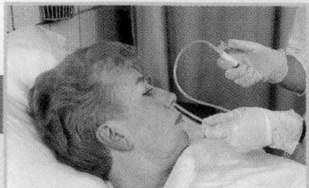

CHAPTER

89

Male Reproductive Disorders

LEARNING OBJECTIVES

1. Differentiate the following laboratory tests: testosterone level, PSA level, and free PSA level.
2. Describe the circumstances that would be necessary for the physician to order an NPT test, a duplex Doppler ultrasonography, and a prostatic biopsy.
3. Differentiate the medical and surgical treatments for erectile disorders.
4. Discuss at least five causes of erectile dysfunction.
5. Define and discuss at least four causes of priapism.
6. Compare and contrast the signs and symptoms of the following: Peyronie's disease, hypospadias, epispadias, cryptorchidism, phimosis, torsion of the spermatic cord, varicocele, and hydrocele.
7. Identify the signs and symptoms of the following: epididymitis, orchitis, prostatitis (acute and chronic), and nonbacterial prostatitis.
8. Describe the differences in signs and symptoms for BPH and cancer of the prostate.
9. In the skills lab, demonstrate how to care for a three-way bladder irrigation.
10. Discuss at least four postoperative nursing considerations when caring for a client who has had TURP.
11. Discuss the etiologies, signs, and symptoms of prostate cancer as compared with testicular cancer and penile cancer.
12. Prepare a teaching plan for TSE.

NEW TERMINOLOGY

cryptorchidism
epididymitis
epispadias
erectile dysfunction
hydrocele
hypospadias
orchiopexy

orchitis
phimosis
plication
priapism
prostatectomy
prostatitis
varicocele

ACRONYMS

ABP	NPT	TSE
BPH	PSA	TURP
CBP		

The male reproductive system is closely linked to the urinary system. For this reason, *urologists* (see Chap. 88) often treat male reproductive disorders.

DIAGNOSTIC TESTS

Laboratory Tests

Testosterone Level

A *testosterone level* or levels of other hormones may be checked in cases of erectile dysfunction (sometimes called *impotence*) or sexual dysfunction. Testosterone is partly responsible for sperm production and *libido* (sexual desire).

Prostate-Specific Antigen

The *prostate-specific antigen* (**PSA**) is a blood test that detects a glycoprotein found only in the tissue of the prostate gland. PSA can be elevated in *prostatitis* (inflammation of the prostate gland), benign prostatic hyperplasia (**BPH**), and adenocarcinoma. PSA is best used in combination with a rectal examination for early detection of prostate cancer. The American Urologic Association recommends annual digital rectal examination and PSA testing beginning at age 50 when there is no preexisting risk factor for prostate cancer.

The *free PSA* is a simple blood test that determines the percentage of free PSA in the overall PSA. Free PSA is commonly used to help determine whether elevated PSA is due to BPH or prostate cancer.

Tests to Diagnose Penile Disorders

Nocturnal Penile Tumescence Tests

Nocturnal penile tumescence (**NPT**) tests help determine if a client is having nighttime erections. Some NPT systems can often show the degree of the erection and duration, and provide definitive clues as to the cause of the condition.

Duplex Doppler Ultrasonography

Duplex Doppler ultrasonography relies on imaging the cavernous arteries at the base of the penis before and after injection of a vasodilator into the corpora cavernosa of the penis. An ultrasound study of the penile arteries may detect an arterial problem of the penis. This test can also suggest a venous problem by ruling out the arterial problem.

Nursing Considerations.   The client may experience some discomfort when the medication is injected. Tell him that these injections usually induce an erection that may not go away. He will need to be monitored until the erection has resolved or has been medically reversed by the physician.

Other Diagnostic Tests

Prostatic Biopsy

A *transrectal biopsy* may be performed to diagnose prostate cancer after a suspicious rectal examination. The urologist uses an ultrasound probe combined with a special biopsy needle that is activated by a rapidly firing spring. The biopsy needle obtains a tissue sample in a fraction of a second. The client feels pressure and mild discomfort during the ultrasound and biopsy procedures. The urologist inserts the probe through the rectum for a clear picture of the prostate on a television screen. The urologist can then guide the biopsy needle to the location of the suspected cancer.

Another type of prostatic biopsy is performed through endoscopy. The endoscope is inserted through the urethra to the prostate, where a small tissue sample is removed. Usually this is done as part of a *transurethral resection of the prostate* (**TURP**).

COMMON MEDICAL TREATMENTS

Bladder Irrigation

Because the urethra passes through the prostate gland as it empties urine from the bladder, *bladder irrigation* is performed to maintain patency of the urethra after prostate surgery. Nursing care for bladder irrigation is discussed later in this chapter at "Prostatectomy."

Radiation Therapy

Radiation therapy may be used following removal of a cancerous prostate to destroy any remaining malignant cells. Refer to the "Prostatectomy" section later in this chapter for nursing considerations.

NURSING PROCESS

Data Collection

Carefully observe and assess the male client who has a reproductive system disorder. Chapter 47 includes assessment of the male reproductive system, which establishes a baseline for future comparison and determines the presence of suspected complications. Report any changes in the baseline level. In Practice: Nursing Assessment 89-1 provides additional information about key assessment areas. Because of the close relationship between the urinary and reproductive systems in the

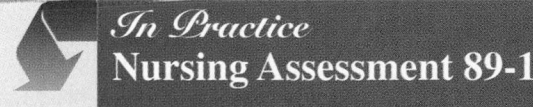
In Practice
Nursing Assessment 89-1

MALE REPRODUCTIVE SYSTEM
- Urinary and reproductive history
- General health history
- History of sexually transmitted diseases or exposure
- Erectile dysfunction
- Urinary dysfunction
- Inspection of external reproductive structures
- Prostate examination
- Testicular examination

male, many of the questions are asked to assess both areas. Remember that some clients are uncomfortable discussing their sexual or urinary systems, which they consider personal and private concerns.

☛ Key Concept

The client may be embarrassed and concerned about any disorder related to the reproductive system. He may see the disorder as a threat to his manhood. Female nurses should be especially conscious of such concerns and be sensitive to the client's feelings.

Observe the client's emotional response to the disorder or disease. Does the client need assistance to meet daily needs? Is the disorder correctable? Does it affect social activities or self-esteem? Is it life threatening? Is the client anxious or fearful of the outcome? What additional services does he need?

Nursing Diagnosis

Based on data collection, nursing diagnoses are established. Some diagnoses may have different causal factors. The following are examples of nursing diagnoses that may appear on nursing care plans for men with reproductive disorders:

- Impaired Urinary Elimination related to bladder outlet obstruction, surgical trauma, postoperative incontinence
- Urinary Retention related to bladder outlet obstruction
- Impaired Tissue Integrity related to prostatic disorders, radiation therapy
- Sexual Dysfunction related to erectile dysfunction, medications, altered body image, effects of therapy (radiation, chemotherapy, hormonal, surgical)
- Ineffective Sexuality Patterns related to erectile dysfunction, structural defects, infections, surgical trauma
- Situational Low Self-Esteem related to erectile dysfunction, incontinence
- Fear related to poor prognosis
- Deficient Knowledge related to testicular self-examination

Planning and Implementing

Together, the members of the healthcare team plan with the client and family for effective individualized care to meet the client's needs. Be sure to provide preoperative and postoperative care and teaching for clients undergoing surgical procedures. The male client with a reproductive system disorder may also require assistance in meeting daily needs, dealing with emotional problems, and understanding more about the disorder, its prognosis, and treatment.

Evaluation

Periodically evaluate outcomes of care with the client, family, and other members of the healthcare team. Have short-term goals been met? Are long-term goals still realistic? Planning for further nursing care takes into consideration the client's

prognosis, as well as any complications and the client's response to care given. Be sure to deal with the emotional aspects that accompany reproductive disorders; refer the client or family member to an appropriate support group or counselor.

ERECTILE DISORDERS

Erectile Dysfunction

Erectile dysfunction (ED) (sometimes called *impotence*) refers to the inability to achieve or maintain an erection sufficient to complete sexual intercourse. As summarized in Box 89-1, ED can be *organic* in origin, meaning it is caused by disease, medication, or environmental factors. It also can be psychogenic in origin, although most specialists believe that organic causes are more likely. All men with ED, except those who have a specific known cause for their erectile dysfunction (such as diabetes or prostate surgery), need an evaluation of hormone levels; nocturnal rigidity measurement; or duplex Doppler ultrasonography to determine causes and identify treatment options.

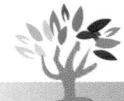 **Special Considerations:** The Life Span

Sexual Problems

Many men remain sexually active throughout life. However, erectile dysfunction and loss of libido are common in older men, particularly when illness is present. The incidence of erectile dysfunction increases with age. The erection can take longer to achieve and ejaculation can be less intense with aging—this mainly stems from medication side effects, neuropathy, or vascular problems. Although sperm viability decreases with age, sperm production continues at the same level throughout life. As the prostate enlarges, the amount of seminal fluid decreases.

➤➤ BOX 89-1

FACTORS CONTRIBUTING TO ERECTILE DYSFUNCTION

- Drug use: Hormones, immunosuppressive agents, diuretics, anti-Parkinson's agents, antihypertensives; antidepressants, psychotropics, tobacco, alcohol, amphetamines, barbiturates, marijuana, cocaine
- Chronic diseases: Renal failure, heart failure, atherosclerosis, multiple sclerosis
- Endocrine disorders: Diabetes mellitus, thyroid disorders, adrenal disorders, pituitary disorders
- Trauma: Spinal cord injury
- Cardiovascular disorders: Stroke, heart disorders, inadequate vascularization
- Surgery: Prostatectomy, ileostomy, colostomy

Medical and Surgical Treatment

An *erection* is caused by spinal reflex arcs activated by tactile stimuli and *psychogenic* factors (auditory, visual, and psychological stimulation). If the client's ED is determined to be truly psychogenic in nature, counseling in conjunction with treatment options may help the client regain function. In cases of organic impotence, counseling also may be valuable along with treatment.

A variety of different treatment options are available. Give a nonjudgmental overview of the pros and cons of each option and let the client select what is best for him and his partner.

Oral Medications.   Oral medications include sildenafil citrate (Viagra). Viagra is a vasodilator taken in pill form that helps the penis to fill with blood. It must be taken with caution due to possible systemic side effects such as hypotension.

> ### Nursing Alert
> Viagra is contraindicated for clients who use nitroglycerin products. Life-threatening hypotension may result.

Other medications also may be used. In Practice: Important Medications 89-1 highlights some selected medications used.

Intraurethral Suppositories.   Medications such as prostaglandin E_1 (MUSE) are urethral suppositories, smaller than a grain of rice, which the client self-injects into the urethra. The pellet melts and the medication is absorbed into the corpora cavernosa. The medication causes the tissue to vasodilate, pulling blood into the area, which causes an erection. This drug has a more localized arteriole-dilating effect than Viagra.

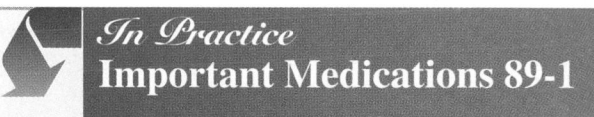

In Practice
Important Medications 89-1

TO TREAT ERECTILE DYSFUNCTIONS

Oral Medications
sildenafil citrate (Viagra)
yohimbine alkaloid
ephedrine (Vaponefrin)
imipramine (Tofranil)

Intraurethral Suppositories
prostaglandin E1 (MUSE)

Vasoactive Intracorporeal Pharmacotherapy
papaverine (Pavabid, Cerespan)
alprostadil
prostaglandin E1 (Caverject, Edex)
phentolamine HCl (Regitine)

Transdermal Agents
nitroglycerin paste

Vasoactive Intracorporeal Pharmacotherapy.   Medications such as papaverine, alprostadil, or prostaglandin E_1 (Caverject, Edex) can be used to induce an erection. The client self-injects a vasodilating medication into the penis.

> ### Nursing Alert
> The client who receives vasodilating medications such as Viagra, MUSE, Caverject, or Edex may have a side effect known as *priapism* (a prolonged, uncomfortable erection for 2–3 hours or longer). Medical intervention may be necessary.

Mechanical Devices.   Mechanical devices, such as *vacuum erection devices* or *vacuum constriction devices,* are noninvasive. They create an erection by mechanically pulling blood into the penis.

Penile Implants.   Several types of devices can be implanted in the penis to help the client achieve and maintain an erection. The device may be malleable, or a two- or three-piece inflatable prosthesis. With the malleable device, the penis looks erect all the time. The inflatable prosthesis can be inflated and deflated, thus simulating a natural erection.

Each device has advantages and disadvantages. These, along with the risk of the implant procedure, need to be clearly explained to the client by his physician. Counsel the client who has a penile implant to avoid sexual activity until his physician gives medical clearance for intercourse. *Rationale: The site needs time to heal completely.*

Penile Revascularization.   Only about 5% of all men with ED are candidates for *penile vascular surgery,* which involves reconstruction of the arterial blood supply or removal of veins that drain blood from the penis too rapidly. However, because this procedure rarely produces a successful outcome, it is rarely performed.

Priapism

Priapism refers to abnormal and persistent penile erection without sexual stimulation. It is extremely painful and may last several hours, or even days. The client must seek immediate medical attention.

Priapism can have many causes, including penile or spinal cord injury, tumor, and cerebrospinal syphilis. Pelvic vascular thrombosis is most often identified as the cause. However, priapism may also result from prolonged sexual activity, leukemia, sickle cell anemia, or other blood disorders. Priapism is common in infections such as prostatitis, urethritis, and cystitis, particularly if renal calculi are also present. It may be a side effect of medications, including trazodone (Desyrel), chlorpromazine (Thorazine), prazosin (Minipress), tolbutamide (Orinase), certain antihypertensives, anticoagulants, and corticosteroids. This condition may also be an undesirable result of therapy for ED, particularly with Viagra, MUSE, and injection therapy.

Signs and Symptoms

The client has an erection that will not go away, along with penile pain and tenderness. The condition is emotionally upsetting. The corpora cavernosa contain thick, dark, venous blood; the corpus spongiosum and glans penis are not involved.

Medical and Surgical Treatment

Priapism can be difficult to treat and sometimes treatment may be unsuccessful. The goal is to improve the venous drainage of the corpora cavernosa while preventing ischemia that may result in impotence. Injection of a solution of phenylephrine into the corpora cavernosa may reverse priapism. *Cavernostomy* with a butterfly needle (to allow drainage) and irrigation may be used, or surgery may be required. Caudal or spinal anesthesia may relieve priapism. Certain medications, such as anticoagulants, may be effective if used immediately. Surgical approaches include creation of a *fistula* (connection) between the glans penis and corpus spongiosum, and semi-permanent diversion with a saphenous vein shunt.

Premature Ejaculation

Premature ejaculation is a consistent problem in which the client ejaculates before, during, or immediately after penetration. Evaluation and treatment is recommended if the client believes the problem affects his ability to have intercourse. Treatment may include wearing condoms, performing a special squeeze technique, application of lidocaine gel, and medications such as serotonin reuptake inhibitors.

Peyronie's Disease

Peyronie's disease is an accumulation of plaques or scar tissue along the corpora cavernosa, causing a painful curvature of the penis when erect. This plaque or scar tissue formation is idiopathic and benign. The erect penis curves in varying degrees and directions, resulting in painful and sometimes impossible penetration. Treatment includes oral medications: aminobenzoate potassium (Potaba), vitamin E, and nonsteroidal anti-inflammatory drugs (NSAIDs). The plaque or scar tissue may be removed by surgery.

STRUCTURAL DISORDERS

Undescended Testicle (Cryptorchidism)

Normally the testes of the male fetus descend into the scrotal sac during the third trimester of pregnancy. A small percentage of male babies, however, are born with a testicle or testicles that have not descended to their normal position in the scrotum, a condition called *undescended testicle* or **cryptorchidism.** This may be a unilateral or bilateral condition, although it is unusual for both testes to be undescended. Sometimes the testicles descend without treatment. If this does not occur, they should be correctly positioned early in life to allow for successful sperm production, because internal body temperature is too warm for the development of viable sperm. If one testis is normally descended, the man will most likely be able to reproduce.

If both testes remain in the client's abdomen past puberty, they may be malformed or progressively atrophy. The boy may not develop secondary sex characteristics because the testes cannot secrete the appropriate hormones. The client may need to receive hormones throughout life. Testes that lodge in the inguinal canal may secrete adequate hormones, but most likely will not produce spermatozoa.

Hormonal therapy is appropriate medical treatment for this condition. If hormonal therapy is ineffective, corrective surgery (*orchiopexy*) is usually done between the ages of 5 and 7 years. **Orchiopexy** involves suturing the testes to the scrotal sac to secure them. Because these clients have an increased risk of testicular cancer, they are encouraged to perform routine testicular self-examination (TSE).

Abnormal Urethral Placement

A urethral meatus located on the underside of the penis is called **hypospadias.** A meatus located on the upper surface is called **epispadias** (Fig. 89-1). These congenital conditions are usually repaired surgically at a young age if they are severe.

Phimosis

Men who have not been circumcised at birth can develop a condition known as **phimosis.** The foreskin becomes so tight that it will not retract over the glans penis. Injury may also cause phimosis. Circumcision can relieve the condition.

Torsion of the Spermatic Cord

Torsion (twisting) of the testicle is caused by a twisting of the spermatic cord, resulting in an interruption in blood flow to the testicle. Torsion is uncommon and occurs most often in adolescents and young men. It may be caused by bilateral and congenital absence of the lateral attachments of the testes and epididymis to the scrotum. Torsion can follow an activity that puts a sudden pull on the cremasteric muscle, which elevates the testis. Extreme cold, such as with jumping into very cold water, may also cause torsion. Occasionally, torsion is spontaneous or occurs during sleep.

Signs and Symptoms

Symptoms include an acute onset of sudden severe scrotal pain, vomiting, abdominal pain, and nausea. This condition can cause testicular infarction and necrosis if left untreated for more than a few hours. Thus, it is considered a surgical emergency.

Surgical Treatment

Surgical *detorsion* (untwisting) and bilateral *orchiopexy* (surgical fixation of the testes) are treatments to fixate each testis and prevent recurrence. If torsion has caused testicle necrosis, the testicle must be removed (*orchiectomy*). An orchiopexy is then performed on the unaffected side to prevent torsion of that testis.

Varicocele

A **varicocele** is an abnormal dilatation of the testicular veins in the scrotum, causing a reflux of blood down to the scrotum

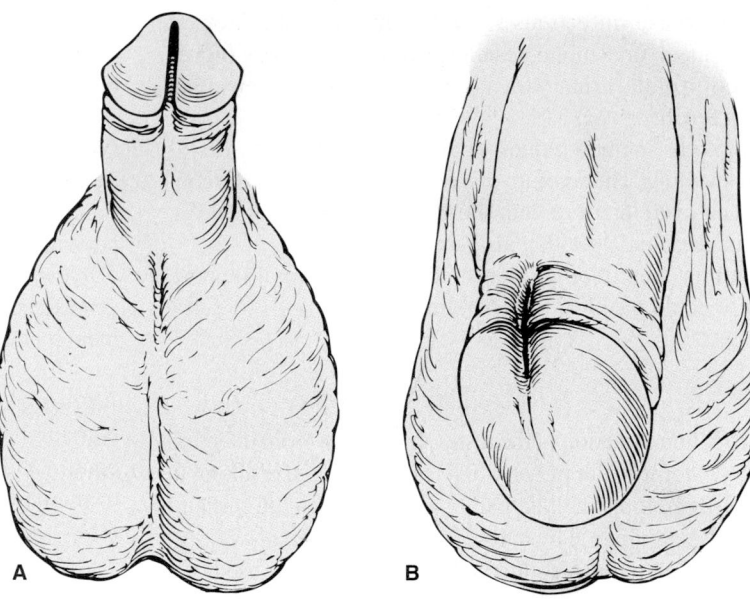

FIGURE 89-1. (**A**) Hypospadias. (**B**) Epispadias.

when standing or straining. The scrotal temperature is higher than normal because of the blood pooling in the area. Heat impairs spermatogenesis and sperm storage, resulting in a low sperm count and infertility. Infertility clinics report an incidence of varicoceles in 30% to 40% of men with male factor infertility.

Signs and Symptoms

Varicocele can cause pain in the testicle or pain radiating to the other side. Symptoms of varicocele include swelling and a nagging dull pain in the scrotum. A varicocele may not be clinically evident until puberty. The veins become dilated and tortuous, and on palpation are often described as similar to a "bag of worms." Varicocele may be unilateral or bilateral. However, this condition is more commonly seen on the left side. This is probably because the left spermatic vein is longer than the right. Presence of a right-sided varicocele may suggest obstruction of the intra-abdominal venous drainage, which could be caused by a tumor.

Surgical Treatment

Correction is done surgically through a number of different types of incisions, laparoscopically, and radiographically. Surgical repair of varicocele may be necessary to eliminate or control pain. Repair can improve the semen count in 60% of men with infertility. However, if semen analysis is normal, infertile men with varicoceles do not require treatment.

Hydrocele

A **hydrocele** is an accumulation of fluid in the space between the membrane covering the testicle and the testicle itself (Fig. 89-2). It may be due to infection (*orchitis*) or an injury. The scrotum enlarges; pain and swelling may be present. However, the client with a hydrocele is often asymptomatic.

Hydrocele may be treated by aspirating the fluid, although this treatment is rarely satisfactory in the adult. Sometimes the sac requires surgical removal. **Plication,** the stitching of folds

or tucks in the hydrocele wall to reduce its size, will usually prevent redevelopment of the hydrocele.

Symptomatic treatment includes applying cold packs, providing support for the scrotum, and providing emotional reassurance that the condition will resolve and will not affect future fertility. A drain is often used if a plication is not performed.

INFLAMMATORY DISORDERS

Epididymitis

Epididymitis is inflammation of the epididymis. In adults under 40 years of age, *Chlamydia trachomatis* is often the causative organism. In older men, gram-negative bacteria are

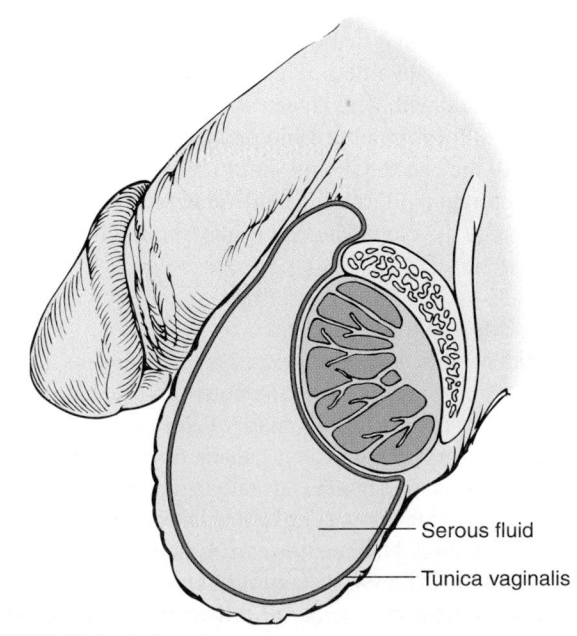

Serous fluid

Tunica vaginalis

FIGURE 89-2. Hydrocele.

the likely cause. Infections spread from the urine, urethra, prostate gland, or seminal vesicles. Epididymitis may follow an infection of the urinary tract or prostate gland. It can affect a man's fertility.

Symptoms include redness, pain, and various degrees of scrotal swelling. The scrotum can enlarge greatly, and the condition can even interfere with the client's ambulation. Chills, fever, nausea, and vomiting also are possible.

Administer antibiotics as ordered, provide scrotal support, and apply cold packs to the scrotum.

Orchitis

Orchitis, inflammation of the testes, may result from infection or injury. Mumps after puberty may cause orchitis, resulting in sterility. Symptoms include pain and swelling in the scrotum and sometimes urethral irritation. A scrotal support is used. An ice bag applied to the scrotum is helpful. Heat is not used.

Prostatitis

Prostatitis, inflammation of the prostate gland, is classified as *acute bacterial, chronic bacterial,* and *nonbacterial.* Urinalysis is often helpful in determining the cause of acute and chronic prostatitis. Bacteria and white blood cells (more than 2,000/L) are present with a bacterial infection. A urine culture and sensitivity test is positive in acute bacterial prostatitis and negative in nonbacterial prostatitis.

Acute Bacterial Prostatitis
Acute bacterial prostatitis (**ABP**) usually results from an ascending urinary tract infection, such as with *Escherichia coli.* The client with acute prostatitis has a very tender, enlarged, and asymmetrical prostate on digital rectal examination. He may also complain of chills, fever, *myalgia* (muscle pain), general malaise, scrotal and low back pain, perineal pain, and pain after ejaculation. Urinary symptoms include *hematuria* (blood in the urine) and urgency on urination or obstructive symptoms such as *nocturia* (frequent voiding at night), hesitancy, or dribbling.

ABP is treated with wide-spectrum antibiotics, analgesics, and sitz baths. A urine culture and/or ultrasound may be done to determine the cause. Clients should receive a long course of an appropriate antibiotic. If inadequately treated, chronic prostatitis may develop. The client may require hospitalization until afebrile.

Chronic Bacterial Prostatitis
Clients with *chronic bacterial prostatitis* (**CBP**) are not acutely ill. The condition results from an acute episode that did not resolve with treatment. The hallmark of chronic bacterial prostatitis is a history of relapsing urinary tract infection. The client with chronic prostatitis is usually asymptomatic, but he may complain of back or perineal pain. The prostate is usually normal on palpation. Diagnosis is established with isolation of bacteria from the expressed secretions obtained from prostatic massage. The client's white blood cell count also is elevated. The urine culture is usually negative. However, if bacteriuria

is present, the initial treatment is a short course of antibiotics. If not successful, additional antibiotic therapy may last 3 to 6 months.

Nonbacterial Prostatitis
Nonbacterial prostatitis is a common form of symptomatic prostatic inflammation. Inflammatory cells are present in expressed prostatic secretions but cultures are negative. *Chlamydia* and *Trichomonas* have been implicated as possible causative pathogens. Results of rectal examination are normal. Empirical treatment includes long periods of antibiotics.

Nursing Considerations
Nursing measures for the client with prostatitis include pain control and warm compresses or sitz baths. Remind the client to increase fluid intake to flush bacteria out of the bladder. Stool softeners help prevent constipation.

NEOPLASMS
Benign Prostatic Hyperplasia

Benign prostatic hyperplasia (BPH) is a common condition in which the prostate gland enlarges. The gland begins to grow at adolescence, continuing to enlarge with advancing age. Because of increasing longevity among men, the incidence of BPH is rising. Most men by the age of 50 have some nonmalignant prostatic enlargement, which is termed BPH. Because the prostate is a donut-like structure surrounding the urethra, BPH often impinges on the urinary stream.

Signs and Symptoms
Growth of the prostate is not harmful, but the symptoms it produces may have many consequences. Initial symptoms may be urinary difficulties. The client does not empty his bladder completely when he voids and finds that he must void frequently, often during the night. He may also find starting to void increasingly difficult or painful and may notice traces of blood in his urine. Cystitis may result.

Diagnostic Tests
The condition is diagnosed by digital rectal examination, urodynamic testing, endoscopy, PSA to rule out prostate cancer, and ultrasound of the prostate. Severe cases will show changes in urinalysis, urine culture, serum creatinine, and blood urea nitrogen.

Medical and Surgical Treatment
Treatment includes watchful waiting until the client is symptomatic. Medications that can be beneficial for these symptoms include doxazosin (Cardura), terazosin (Hytrin), tamsulosin (Flomax), and finasteride (Proscar). Prostate size can be reduced by a number of different methods, such as *simple prostatectomy* (removal of the prostate), transurethral incision, transurethral microwave thermotherapy, and transurethral needle ablation. TURP remains the standard surgical treatment for obstructive BPH. The method selected is dependent upon the client and the preference of the physician.

Complications

The two primary complications of BPH are urinary tract infection and acute urinary retention. Urinary tract infection results from residual urine, which causes decreased resistance to bacterial invasion. Acute urinary retention is a surprisingly common complication, due to the obstructive nature of the enlarged prostate.

> ### Nursing Alert
> If a client experiences an episode of acute urinary retention at home, he can try a warm shower or bath to relax the sphincter muscles. Advise him to allow the urine to flow in the shower or tub. If a shower or bath does not work, he should go to the emergency department for immediate treatment.

Cancer of the Prostate

Excluding skin cancer, cancer of the prostate is the most common cancer in men. It is also the second leading cause of cancer deaths in men. The incidence increases with age. It primarily occurs in men over 50 years of age, with a peak incidence at around age 75. The American Cancer Society recommends that all men over 50 who have at least a 10-year life expectancy have an annual digital rectal examination and a PSA blood test. Men who have risk factors for prostate cancer should start screening at age 45.

Risk factors for prostate cancer include:

- Age over 50 years
- African American heritage
- Excessive alcohol use
- Diet high in animal fats
- Family history of prostate cancer
- Environmental exposure
- PSA elevation

Signs and Symptoms

Early cancer of the prostate does not usually produce symptoms. The first signs of prostatic cancer, if any, typically involve difficulty in voiding, which occurs due to the position of the prostate gland surrounding the urethra and subsequent obstruction of urethral patency. Signs of difficulty in voiding include:

- Decrease in force and size of urinary stream
- Urgency
- Frequency
- Nocturia
- *Hesitancy* (difficulty in starting the stream)
- *Dysuria* (painful voiding) in some cases
- Hematuria

If the client does not seek medical followup for these symptoms, complete urinary retention may result, which is an emergency.

Prostate cancer commonly metastasizes to the bones, lymph nodes, brain, and lungs. The bones involved are usually in the region of the prostate and include the lower spine and hips, leading to symptoms such as backache, hip pain, perineal discomfort, and weakness.

Diagnostic Tests

The prostate gland is palpated rectally for nodular growths. Because most tumors arise in the posterior lobe, the examiner can readily palpate these growths through the wall of the rectum. On examination, a cancerous prostate feels irregular and may have hard nodules. A PSA blood test is performed to look for an elevation. Cancer of the prostate is distinguished from prostatitis with biopsy and PSA.

Treatment Options

Treatment depends on the disease's stage and the client's age and symptoms. Thirty to forty percent of men with prostate cancer have some type of metastatic cancer. Treatment options include radical prostatectomy, radioactive seed implantation, cryosurgery, radiation therapy, or hormone ablation therapy. Erectile dysfunction occurs in 70% to 80% of clients; incontinence is less common (20%).

Prostate Surgery

Preoperative Nursing Considerations. As part of the preoperative preparation for a radical prostatectomy, alert the client to the strong possibility of postoperative erectile dysfunction. About 90% of men are impotent after surgery, except those who have the nerve-sparing procedure. Depending on the client's age, the impotence rate with nerve sparing is only about 30%; younger men are less likely to become impotent. Because 80% of prostate cancers are androgen dependent, a treatment goal will also be to decrease circulating androgens, which further affect the man's ability to achieve an erection.

Encourage the client who wishes to have children to consider sperm banking before the surgery. Review the types of available treatment options for erectile dysfunction and how they work.

Discuss the possibility that the client will have a suprapubic cystoscopy catheter and some sort of continuous bladder irrigation for approximately 2 to 3 days postoperatively.

Before the prostatectomy, the client may have a catheter inserted for continuous urinary drainage, to prevent accumulation of stagnant urine in the bladder. Give him plenty of fluids, with proper diet and rest. Antibiotics are often given prophylactically.

Transurethral Resection of the Prostate (TURP). This is the most common procedure, particularly for older men or those are a poor surgical risk. Figure 89-3 illustrates common techniques. In TURP, the surgeon removes prostate tissue through the urethra by means of a *resectoscope*, which has a cutting edge or electric wire that slices the prostate away bit by bit (Fig. 89-3A). Because the surgeon does the operation through the urethra, no incision is necessary. Recovery after TURP is shorter than after other approaches. Complications of TURP include hemorrhage, urinary retention, stress incontinence, and erectile dysfunction.

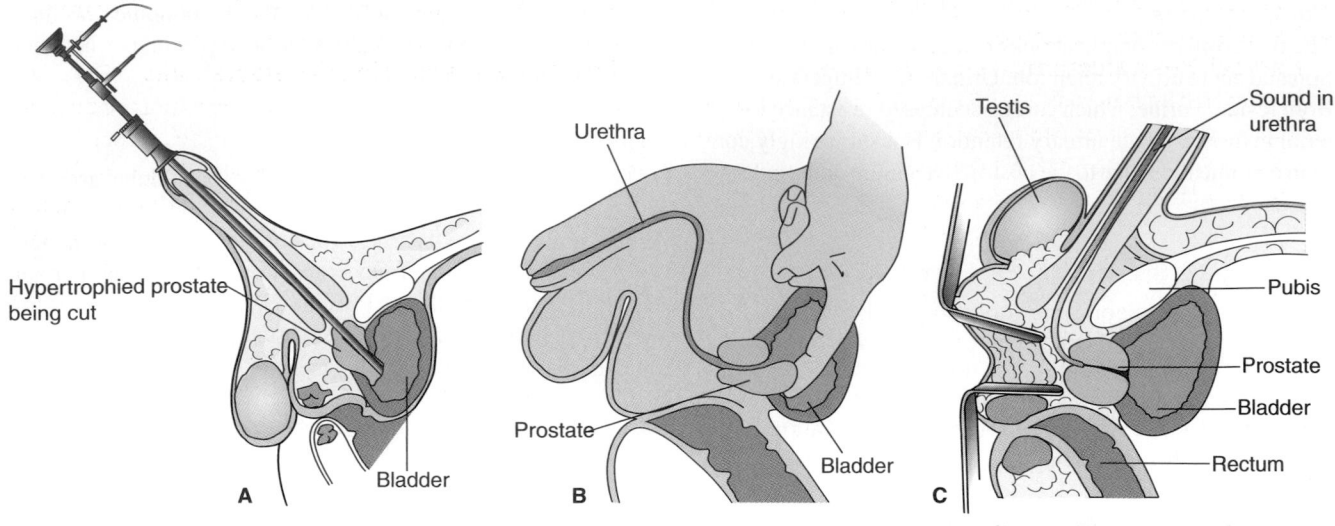

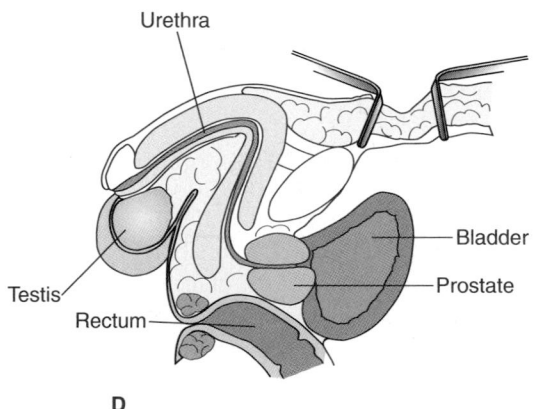

FIGURE 89-3. Types of prostatectomy. (**A**) In TURP, the surgeon connects a wire to a loop of current that is rotated in a cytoscope to remove shavings of the prostate. (**B**) In suprapubic prostatectomy, the surgeon enters through the client's abdomen, and uses his or her fingers to shell out the prostate. (**C**) In perineal prostatectomy, the surgeon uses retractors to view the prostate. (**D**) In retropubic prostatectomy, the surgeon makes a low abdominal incision, and working behind the pubic bone, removes the prostate.

Prostatectomy.   Another surgical treatment for prostatic cancer (and also BPH) is removal of the excess or abnormal prostate tissue (**prostatectomy**) through various approaches. The surgeon can dissect the prostate through an incision through the bladder (*suprapubic prostatectomy* or *suprapubic resection*), a perineal incision (*perineal prostatectomy* or *perineal resection*), or an incision below the bladder (*retropubic prostatectomy*). Dissection is also possible using a *cystoscope* (resectoscope) through the urethra.

Suprapubic Prostatectomy.   The surgeon usually performs the suprapubic procedure if the client's gland is greatly enlarged (greater than 100 g). Surgery may be done in two stages. First, the surgeon performs a *cystostomy* (incision into the bladder) to relieve urinary retention; second, he or she removes the prostate tissue (see Fig. 89-3B). After the two-stage suprapubic operation, the client returns with two indwell-ing catheters in place, one in the urethra and the other in the suprapubic wound (a *suprapubic Cystocath*). These catheters are attached to separate drainage containers, allowing for more accurate output measurement. The urethral catheter is attached to a closed drainage system and the wound catheter is attached to an irrigation apparatus. (The physician may prefer that any bladder irrigation be done through the urethral catheter.)

Perineal Prostatectomy.   If the surgeon removes gland tissue through an incision in the perineum, catheter drainage is through the perineal incision only (see Fig. 89-3C). In this case, the client will find sitting up to be difficult. Fecal contamination of the incision may occur due to its location.

Nerve-Sparing Radical Prostatectomy (Retro-pubic Prostatectomy).   Nerve-sparing radical prostatectomy removes the prostate through an incision below the umbilicus and above the symphysis pubis (see Fig. 89-3D).

This procedure causes less erectile dysfunction, incontinence, and bleeding than other methods.

Radical Prostatectomy. A *radical prostatectomy* (removal of the prostate gland, seminal vesicles, and part of the urethra) sometimes cures prostatic cancer that has not metastasized. A radical prostatectomy is an open procedure because an abdominal incision is necessary. Complications of radical prostatectomy include stress incontinence, epididymitis, urethral stricture, fistula, and erectile dysfunction.

Cryosurgery. A less-invasive procedure used to remove prostatic cancer is *cryosurgery*. An incision is made in the perineum and a special tool is inserted to the area of the prostate cancer to freeze the tissue. This procedure is believed to kill the cancer. The risks involved in cryosurgery are similar to those for other prostate-removal procedures. The success of the procedure is still under investigation.

Postoperative Nursing Considerations. The client will require routine postoperative care such as antiembolism stockings, early ambulation, and incentive spirometry (see In Practice: Nursing Care Plan 89-1). Encourage fluid intake and monitor intake and output. Give stool softeners as ordered. Help the client and his partner deal with any psychological and emotional problems. In Practice: The Nursing Process 89-1 applies the nursing process to preparing the client to go home after a prostatectomy.

A urethral catheter is left in place for about 2 weeks after a radical prostatectomy. The catheter helps put pressure on the *vesicoureteral* (bladder and ureter) incision to control bleeding.

In Practice
Nursing Care Plan 89-1

THE CLIENT WITH ERECTILE DYSFUNCTION FOLLOWING A RADICAL PROSTATECTOMY

MEDICAL HISTORY: *F.O., a 63-year-old married man who presented with urinary hesitancy and straining, decrease in size and force of stream and frequency, and nocturia was diagnosed with prostate cancer. A radical prostatectomy was performed about 8 to 9 months ago. The client comes to the physician's office for an evaluation. During the history, the client reports that he is having difficulty experiencing erections.*

MEDICAL DIAGNOSIS: *Erectile dysfunction; post–radical prostatectomy for prostate cancer*

Data Collection/Nursing Assessment: Client is well-nourished male accompanied by his wife. Client expressing concerns regarding his sexual inability in relation to his marriage and fears of the cancer recurring. Upset with eyes visibly tearing, the client stated, "My wife and I have always been very close, both physically and emotionally. It's so frustrating for me; I'm not a man anymore. I feel like such a failure." (*Although other nursing diagnoses may be appropriate, a priority nursing diagnosis is addressed below.*).

Nursing Diagnosis: Situational low self-esteem related to effects of surgery as evidenced by client's statements of being a failure and not being a man.

Planning
SHORT-TERM GOALS:
#1. Client will verbalize positive statements about himself.
#2. Couple will identify impact of erectile dysfunction on their relationship.

#3. Couple will identify measures to cope with erectile dysfunction.

LONG-TERM GOALS:
#4. Couple will participate in plan to manage erectile dysfunction, ultimately achieving satisfaction with method chosen.

Implementation
NURSING ACTION: *Encourage the client to verbalize his concerns and sexual needs—listen to his comments about the situation and what it means for him. Have him describe himself, noting how he sees and how he believes others see options. Be aware of the client's self-concept in relation to cultural or social values.*
RATIONALE: *Verbalization allows client to openly express his feelings, helping to provide a clear indication of the client's perception of himself and his problem.*

NURSING ACTION: *If client is agreeable, engage client's wife in the discussion, allowing her to verbalize her concerns, feelings, and beliefs about the situation. Correct or clarify any misconceptions or inaccuracies.*
RATIONALE: *Allowing the wife to participate fosters a sense of cooperation between the husband and wife. Clarifying aids in learning and strengthening understanding.*

Evaluation: Client able to state that he is a good provider and supportive person. Wife reinforced these statements. Client and wife beginning to discuss effect of erectile dysfunction on their life and relationship. *Goal #1 met; progress to meeting Goal #2.*

(continued)

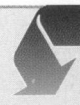

In Practice
Nursing Care Plan 89-1 (*Continued*)

NURSING ACTION: *Allow the client to go through the grieving process; be open and receptive to behavior changes during this time. Expect some expression of negative feelings.*
RATIONALE: *Each client grieves in his own way and time.*

NURSING ACTION: *Recognize behaviors indicating over-concern with the body and its processes. Assist with setting appropriate limits and in helping the client learn how to deal with his feelings and release his emotions in a positive manner.*
RATIONALE: *Limits provide structure and direction.*

NURSING ACTION: *Assess the interaction of the client and his wife. Encourage continuation of open communication of their feelings with each other.*
RATIONALE: *Open, effective communication is necessary for a good relationship.*

Evaluation: Client and wife openly discussing feelings. Wife offering positive support to client. Client verbalizing desire to learn about options for treating dysfunction. *Goal #2 met; progress to meeting Goal #3.*

NURSING ACTION: *Assess the client and wife's knowledge regarding options for erectile dysfunction.*

Help them obtain information regarding coping strategies. Provide information at their level of acceptance.
RATIONALE: *Assessing the couple's knowledge level is important in developing appropriate teaching strategies. Adequate knowledge and understanding is necessary for the couple to make informed decisions about what alternatives are best for them. Providing information at their level helps to prevent them from becoming overwhelmed.*

NURSING ACTION: *Provide client and wife with educational material on various options for erectile dysfunction; contact surgeon for possible referral to a physician specializing in treatment of erectile dysfunction.*
RATIONALE: *Providing the couple with material about available options enhances their understanding and promotes informed decision-making. Contacting the physician for a referral helps the couple to follow through with decision-making.*

Evaluation: Client and wife are observed reading pamphlets on options available; client has an appointment in 2 weeks with a physician who specializes in the treatment of erectile dysfunction. *Goal #3 met; progress to meeting Goal #4.*

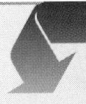

In Practice
Nursing Process 89-1

AT HOME AFTER PROSTATECTOMY

Assessment Priorities
- Ability to monitor for potential voiding complications
- Ability to monitor and manage an indwelling Foley catheter
- Ability to provide wound care
- Ability to manage returning bowel function
- Need for psychological counseling due to potential for depression due to diagnosis of cancer, loss of sterility, loss of sexual function, and/or incontinence.
- Ability to follow recommended treatment plan.

Possible Nursing Diagnoses
Impaired Urinary Elimination related to bladder outlet obstruction, surgical trauma, postoperative incontinence
Urinary Retention related to the surgical procedure and complications of the procedure

Impaired Tissue Integrity related to incision and potential for fecal contamination
Sexual Dysfunction related to erectile dysfunction, altered body image, and effects of the procedure
Ineffective Sexuality Patterns related to erectile dysfunction, surgery, Foley catheter
Situational Low Self-Esteem related to erectile dysfunction, incontinence
Fear related to poor prognosis, diagnosis

Planning
Design a plan of care with the client and family to achieve the following general goals:

- Client voids without difficulty.
- Client is able to demonstrate catheter maintenance, as appropriate.
- Client is able to demonstrate dressing changes and wound maintenance.

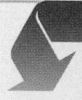

In Practice
Nursing Process 89-1 *(Continued)*

- Client's wound will heal without complications.
- Client's bowel function returns to normal.
- Client is able to verbalize treatment plan and follow up after surgery.
- Client expresses feelings regarding loss of sexual function, incontinence, and sterility.
- Client discusses potential treatment options for erectile dysfunction.
- Client expresses optimistic expectations for the future.

Implementation
- Review discharge instructions with the client.
- Have client demonstrate measures for catheter maintenance, including cleaning and changing of equipment per instructions.
- Explain bowel maintenance program, including use of stool softeners.
- Encourage ambulation.
- Encourage fluids.

- Demonstrate wound cleaning and dressing changes and have client return-demonstrate procedure using clean technique and sterile dressing as appropriate.
- Teach client about bladder retraining and Kegel exercises.
- Assist client with setting up necessary followup appointments, including post-surgical appointments, appointments for evaluation and treatment of ED when necessary, and appointments for counseling when necessary.

Evaluation
- Client has normal bowel function.
- Client reports that he is continent.
- Client's wound demonstrates healing without complications.
- Client reports success with his ED medication.
- Client has followup appointments for his prostate disease.

Keep the catheter straight to avoid obstruction of urine flow. Accidental catheter removal may require the client to return to surgery for its reinsertion.

After TURP, the client will return from the operating room with a bladder irrigation in place. (This procedure may also be used after other genitourinary procedures.) The surgeon inserts a *triple-lumen catheter* (with three separate tubes or openings) immediately after the prostate is removed in the operating room. One lumen inflates the balloon that holds the catheter in place, while a second lumen drains the bladder into a drainage bag (similar to a Foley catheter). The third lumen is used to instill a bladder solution that irrigates the bladder.

Irrigation may be continuous to intermittent after surgery. Continuous irrigation washes out blood before it can form clots; intermittent irrigation washes out clots that plug the catheter. When the catheter becomes clogged, overdistention of the bladder may cause the client great discomfort. In many cases, a pump or controller regulates the flow of irrigant. Figure 89-4 illustrates TURP irrigation, or three-way bladder irrigation, which is used after the procedure. In Practice: Nursing Care Guidelines 89-1 provides information related to TURP irrigation.

✚👁 Nursing Alert
When caring for a client with a continuous TURP bladder irrigation, shut off the irrigation if:

- The client complains of bladder fullness, urinary urgency, or bladder or flank pain.
- Drainage from the TURP tube stops.
- Check to see if an order exists for a manual irrigation.

Carefully monitor intake and output in the immediate postoperative period. Pay particular attention to the color of the draining urine. The postoperative client will have bloody drainage, which should steadily decrease. Because hemorrhage is a major postoperative complication, report and document

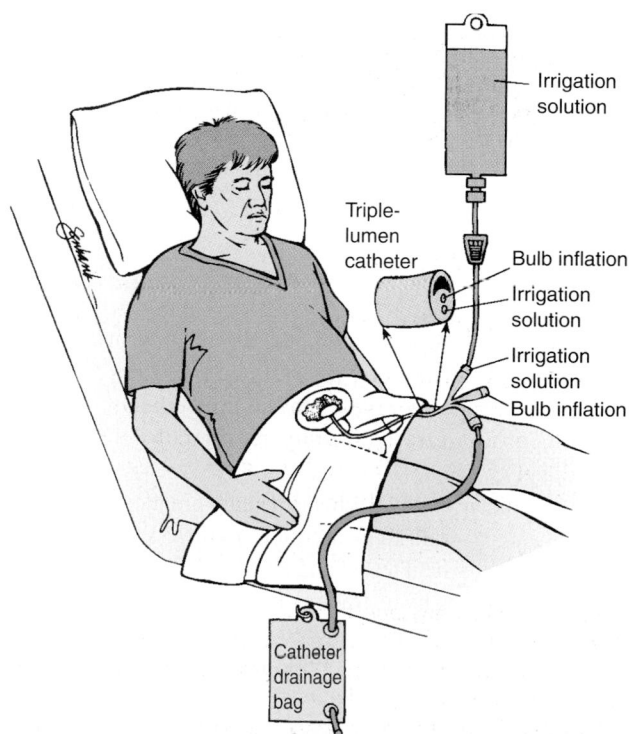

FIGURE 89-4. Three-way bladder irrigation used after prostate or bladder surgery.

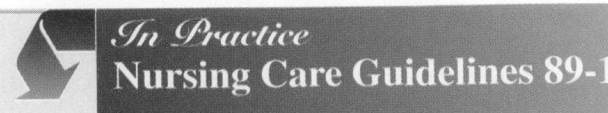

In Practice
Nursing Care Guidelines 89-1

MANAGING CONTINUOUS TURP OR BLADDER IRRIGATION

- Record the amount of irrigating solution instilled into the bladder and the total output. *Rationale: An accurate record of the client's actual urinary output is needed. Subtract the amount of irrigation solution from the total output to determine urine volume.*
- Carefully monitor the TURP setup to make sure all the tubes are open and that they are not twisted or kinked. *Rationale: The tubing needs to remain patent and drain freely to prevent overdistention of the bladder.*
- Because many men who have TURPs are older and may become confused, make sure clients do not pull on the catheters or change rates of flow of the solutions. Catheters must remain taped in place. *Rationale: Damage may occur to the operative site.*
- Often the physician orders that traction be placed on the penis, which is kept taped securely in place on the hip or abdomen and is not allowed to hang down. *Rationale: Traction facilitates drainage and prevents clotting, but may be uncomfortable.*
- It may be necessary to irrigate the catheter manually. Be sure the physician has written an order. There is often a standing order to irrigate the catheter as needed. *Rationale: Manual irrigation helps to dislodge any clots that may be obstructing the catheter.*
- Take special note if the client complains of a feeling of fullness, urgency, or bladder or flank pain, or if the drainage stops flowing from the tube. In any of these situations, shut off the continuous irrigation and notify the team leader or physician immediately. *Rationale: The client is at risk for hemorrhage.*

any sudden increase of blood in the drainage. If urinary flow slows or stops, the catheter may require irrigation to remove obstructing tissue or clots. If the drainage becomes bright red with gushes of fresh bleeding, report to the charge nurse immediately.

After catheter removal, clients usually are incontinent until they are able to train their external urethral sphincter to do the work of both the internal and external sphincters. Assist in sphincter retraining by instructing the client in Kegel exercises.

Sitz baths are usually ordered after a perineal prostatectomy. After a bowel movement, take care to avoid contaminating the wound. Use meticulous aseptic technique to cleanse the perineum.

A wound catheter may be in place following radial prostatectomy. Some urine will dribble onto dressings after removal of the wound catheter. Keep the skin clean and dry by frequent dressing changes. The wound may take a month or more to heal.

Painful bladder spasms are common postoperatively when a client has had prostate surgery. Antispasmodics are administered to control this pain. Pain relief for incisional pain is also needed, but aspirin is avoided because of its anticoagulation effects.

Medical Treatments

Radiation Therapy.   Radiation may be used for cancer of the prostate to reduce tumor size or actually to cure some stages of cancer. It may also be considered a palliative measure for the client with bony metastases, thus alleviating some pain.

Radioactive seed implantation is a common method of treating prostate cancer. Small radioactive seeds (about the size of a grain of rice) are implanted directly into the prostate. This procedure puts radiation in the exact location of the cancer, thereby reducing side effects and risks associated with other types of radiation therapy.

Radiation cystitis is a common problem following radiation therapy after prostatectomy. Antispasmodics, analgesics, and increased fluid intake are forms of treatment. Monitor the client's skin condition during radiation therapy. Clients are prone to excoriation and yeast infections.

The client may experience *proctitis,* an inflammation of the rectum and anus, with preoperative chemotherapy. Use of a low-residue diet and antidiarrheal medications may help alleviate symptoms. The client may experience urethral stricture, due to scarring. Teach the client signs of urinary retention and monitor urine output closely.

Hormone Ablation Therapy.   Prostate cancer needs testosterone to grow. Therefore, removing testosterone will destroy the prostate cancer's chance of survival and growth. An orchiectomy will simply solve this problem, and clients do, in some cases, choose this option. A *partial orchiectomy* can also be performed to remove the portion of the testicle that produces testosterone. There are also medications clients can take to decrease or stop testosterone production; these are gonadotropin-releasing hormone (GnRH) analogs (Lupron, Zoladex) and antiandrogens (Eulexin, Casodex, Nilandron).

Pain Management in Advanced Disease

If the client has distant metastases, the goal of management usually focuses on providing comfort for the client and support for family members. Narcotics are given on a routine schedule (not as needed). Oral administration is preferred because it allows the client more control in his pain management. In later stages of the disease, continuous morphine may be given intravenously for pain control. Chapters 59 and 99 describe care of terminally ill clients.

Cancer of the Testes

Testicular cancer is the most common form of cancer in men between 20 and 34 years of age, with the exception of leukemia and lymphoma. These cancers can often metastasize before diagnosis. The incidence of testicular cancer is higher in men with cryptorchidism. The cause is unknown but may be related to infections and genetic and endocrine factors.

Risk factors for testicular cancer include:

- Age 20 to 34
- History of undescended testicle at birth (regardless of surgical correction)
- Caucasian race
- History of testicular swelling with mumps
- History of maternal use of oral contraceptives and diethylstilbestrol (DES) during pregnancy
- Higher social class
- Unmarried or married late
- Not sexually active

Symptoms appear very gradually. A painless mass develops as the testis enlarges. A feeling of scrotal heaviness occurs. Advanced symptoms of metastatic disease include backache, pain in the abdomen, weakness, and weight loss.

There are two categories of testicular tumors, each of which is treated differently. The first type of testicular tumor is the *seminoma,* which is more common and often remains localized until late in the course of disease. After a *unilateral*

orchiectomy (removal of the testis), any residual tumor will be irradiated.

The second type of testicular tumor is the *nonseminoma.* After a unilateral orchiectomy is performed, the client will undergo a *retroperitoneal* (behind the peritoneum) lymph node dissection. This procedure involves removal of the lymph nodes along the aorta, iliac vessels, and inguinal area on the affected side. Further treatment for possible residual tumor involves the administration of chemotherapy or radiation therapy.

Orchiectomy has little effect on libido and ability to have an orgasm. However, it may impair fertility. Offer clients who must undergo orchiectomy the opportunity to preserve sperm before treatment. Infertility centers have services available for the cryopreservation and storage of sperm.

Testicular Self-Examination

Every male, from the age of 13 or 14 years, is encouraged to perform monthly **TSE** (see In Practice: Educating the Client 89-1). Although the overall incidence of testicular cancer is rare, it is the most common cancer in young men. Caucasians are four times more likely to have testicular cancer than are non-Caucasian men. With early detection, the cure rate is almost 100%, which reinforces the importance of the monthly TSE.

In Practice
Educating the Client 89-1

TESTICULAR SELF-EXAM

Instruct the client to perform the following procedure once each month.

1. Use both hands to palpate the testis; the normal testicle is smooth and uniform in consistency.
2. With the index and middle fingers under the testis and the thumb on top, roll the testis gently in a horizontal plane between the thumb and fingers.
3. Feel for any evidence of a small lump or abnormality.
4. Follow the same procedure and palpate upward along the testis.

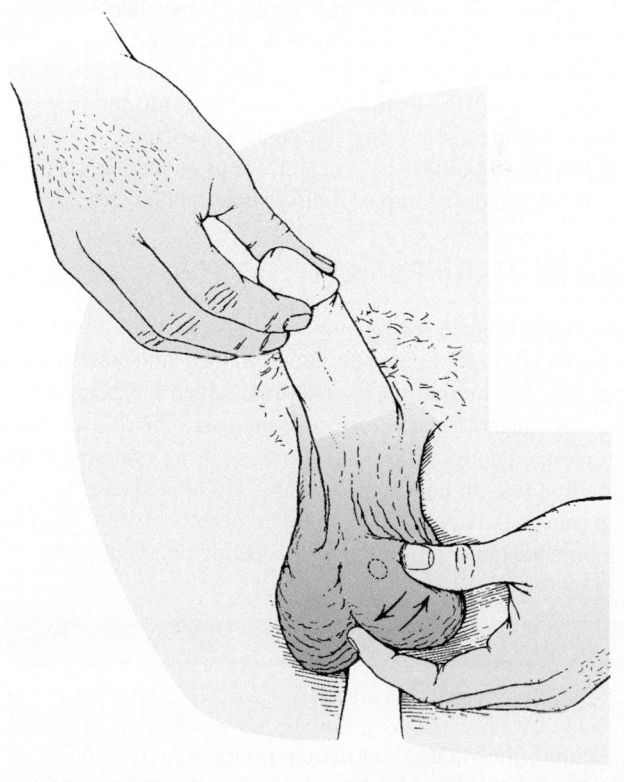

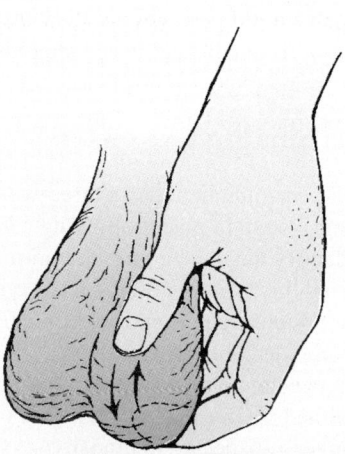

Testicular self-exam.

(continued)

In Practice
Educating the Client 89-1 (Continued)

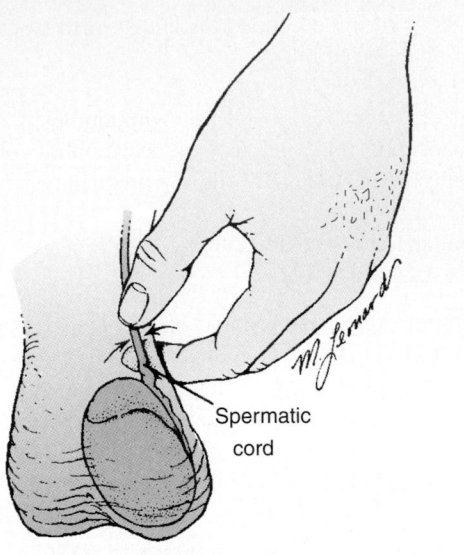

5. Locate the epididymis, a cordlike structure on the top and back of the testicle that stores and transports sperm.
6. Repeat the examination for the other testis. (It is normal to find that one testis is larger than the other.)
7. If you find any evidence of a small, pealike lump, consult your physician. It may be due to an infection or a tumor growth.

Spermatic cord

The TSE is best performed after a bath or shower because warm water relaxes the scrotal sac. The client should avoid touching the scrotum with cold hands; it may stimulate the cremasteric reflex, which causes the scrotum to contract close to the body.

The procedure is simple and painless if the client uses gentle pressure. Normally, the testicle is rubbery and smooth. The epididymis is on top of and behind the testicle. Instruct the client to palpate the testicle between his thumb and first two fingers, progressing along the posterior surface to the epididymis. He should notify a healthcare provider if he palpates any small, painless lump or if his testicle is enlarged.

Cancer of the Penis

Cancer of the penis is relatively rare, especially in circumcised men. It tends to occur in uncircumcised men who practice poor hygiene. The human papillomavirus, which has been implicated in cancer of the cervix, also increases the risk of penile carcinoma. Penile carcinoma often appears as a painless ulceration that fails to heal. Small lesions are treated locally, as in skin cancer. Advanced lesions that involve the shaft or inguinal lymph nodes may require penile resection or amputation.

➪ STUDENT SYNTHESIS

Key Points

• Conditions that affect male reproductive function potentially affect body image and self-esteem.
• Erectile dysfunction is generally organic in nature.

• Torsion of the spermatic cord is an emergency; if unrelieved, it may cause necrosis of the affected testicle.
• Recurrent or chronic infection of the genitourinary tract may affect fertility.
• There are three types of prostatitis, each with different management strategies.
• Inform clients contemplating surgical treatment of benign prostatic hyperplasia that they may experience some incontinence and/or erectile dysfunction after surgery.
• All men over 50 with a 10-year life expectancy should have a yearly rectal digital examination and PSA; those with increased risk of prostate cancer should start screening at 45.
• Most testicular cancers occur between ages 20 and 34. All men should perform monthly testicular self-examination from early adolescence onward.

Critical Thinking Exercises

1. Your 75-year-old client has a three-way bladder irrigation system in place following a TURP procedure. Identify the most common complication of TURP and this type of drainage. Describe when to stop continuous irrigation. Develop a teaching plan for the client and his family.
2. A client presents with a complaint of scrotal edema. Review the possible causes. Design a treatment plan for each suspected diagnosis.

NCLEX-Style Review Questions

1. Testosterone level or other hormone levels are evaluated in clients with:
   a. Cancer of the penis
   b. Erectile dysfunction
   c. History of urinary surgery
   d. Sexual diseases

2. A 30-year-old client is seen at the clinic with a medical diagnosis of epididymitis. When taking his history, which information would be most significant?
   a. Fertility
   b. Pelvic surgery
   c. Sexual activity
   d. Urgency

3. Health teaching for the uncircumcised male should include proper personal hygiene to prevent:
   a. Cryptorchidism
   b. Phimosis
   c. Priapism
   d. Penile cancer

4. A client is admitted with a diagnosis of benign prostatic hypertrophy. This condition is most often manifested by:
   a. A feeling of incomplete bladder emptying after voiding
   b. A feeling of scrotal fullness
   c. Difficulty maintaining an erection
   d. Urethral discharge

5. A client who has had TURP asks why his catheter is taped tightly to his leg, because it is uncomfortable. The nurse explains:
   a. "This facilitates administration of antibiotics."
   b. "This facilitates drainage and prevents clotting."
   c. "This prevents the catheter from falling out."
   d. "This prevents blood clots from forming."

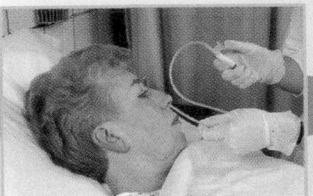

Female Reproductive Disorders

LEARNING OBJECTIVES

1. Describe the rationale, procedure, and nursing implications for the following diagnostic tests: pelvic examination, Pap test, breast examination, mammography, breast ultrasound, and ultrasonography.
2. Define the following: laparoscopy, culdoscopy, colposcopy, cervical biopsy, and conization.
3. Describe at least five nursing implications for a client who needs a D&C.
4. List at least eight factors involved in the nursing assessment of a breast or reproductive disorder.
5. Relate at least eight teaching components related to each of the following: feminine hygiene and breast self-examination.
6. Demonstrate in the skills lab the following procedures: providing perineal care, providing sitz baths, inserting a vaginal suppository, and performing a vaginal irrigation.
7. Differentiate the following menstrual disorders: amenorrhea, menorrhagia, metrorrhagia, dysmenorrhea, and extreme irregularity.
8. Describe the causes, signs and symptoms, and at least three teaching components of nursing care for PMS and TSS.
9. Identify at least four common client concerns related to menopause and HRT.
10. Define the following structural disorders: vaginal fistula, cystocele, rectocele, prolapsed uterus, and abnormal flexion of the uterus.
11. Differentiate the following disorders: vulvitis, vaginitis, trichomoniasis, candidiasis, bacterial vaginosis, atrophic vaginitis, cervicitis, endometriosis, PID, vulvodynia, and STDs.
12. Compare and contrast ovarian cancer, uterine cancer, and cervical cancer.
13. Identify the pre- and postoperative nursing care of a client undergoing a hysterectomy.
14. Explain the steps of breast self-examination.
15. Explain the pre- and postoperative nursing care of a client undergoing breast biopsy, mastectomy, or reconstructive breast surgery.

NEW TERMINOLOGY

amenorrhea	mammography
cervicitis	mammoplasty
colposcopy	mastalgia
conization	mastectomy
culdoscopy	menorrhagia
cystocele	metrorrhagia
dysmenorrhea	Pap (Papanicolaou) test
dyspareunia	pelvic exenteration
endometriosis	prolapse
gynecology	rectocele
hysterectomy	sentinel lymph node
laparoscopy	vaginitis
leukorrhea	vulvitis

ACRONYMS

ACS	IUD	PID
AP	JP	PMS
CA125	LEEP	STD
D&C	NIH	TSS
HRT	OB/GYN	

The medical specialty that focuses on the female reproductive system is called **gynecology**. Physicians who work in this area are called *gynecologists*. Gynecologists who also perform childbirth management are called *obstetrician-gynecologists* (**OB/GYN**) (see Unit 10).

General nursing interventions involving the female reproductive system include teaching about anatomy, self-care related to hygiene, and breast self-examination. Nurses who are specially trained in sexual counseling may provide more detailed care measures.

The female reproductive system comprises a complex and specialized set of organs. See Chapter 29 for more information.

DIAGNOSTIC TESTS

Pelvic Examination

Every woman past the age of puberty should have a complete pelvic examination, including a Pap test, every 1 to 3 years. When any pathology is present or the woman has a family history of pathology, she should have the examination more than once a year. The pelvic examination offers the physician an opportunity to visualize the woman's cervix, vagina, and perineum. A cervical biopsy also can be done during a pelvic examination. Additionally, cauterization, removal, or coagulation of a portion of the cervix using electricity or laser can be performed during a pelvic examination.

In preparation for the examination, ask the client to empty her bladder. Encourage the woman to breathe deeply and relax to minimize the discomfort associated with the examination. Provide the healthcare provider with the necessary equipment, including a water-soluble lubricant, vaginal speculum, and gloves.

After the client is placed in the lithotomy position (Fig. 90-1), the healthcare provider examines the client's external genitalia. Next, the uterus and ovaries are palpated after the healthcare provider inserts a gloved finger into the vagina and places the other hand on the abdomen. The examination also may include rectovaginal examination, in which the healthcare provider places one finger in the client's vagina and another finger into the client's rectum. By palpating in this manner, abnormalities in the rectal area and problems of the posterior genital organs can be detected.

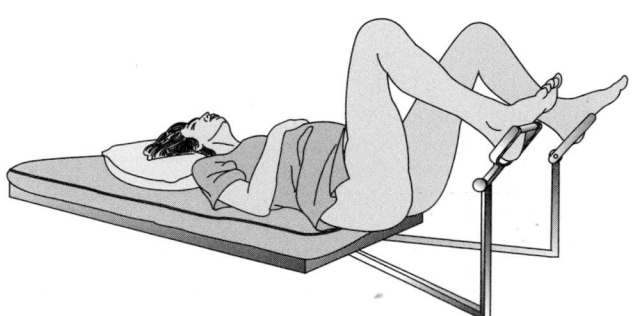

FIGURE 90-1. The client is placed in the lithotomy position for a pelvic examination. The nurse places drapes around the client to preserve privacy.

Laboratory Tests

Pap Test

A malignant growth in the uterus or cervix sometimes sheds cancerous cells into uterine and vaginal secretions. Microscopic examination of a smear from these secretions may help detect cancer before symptoms appear. This examination is known as the **Pap (Papanicolaou) test** or *Pap smear*. Theorists believe this test to be more than 90% accurate in detecting cervical cancer. It is less accurate in detecting cancer of the endometrium or of the uterus.

Cervical cancer is one of the most common cancers in women. If a Pap test is positive or the cervix looks suspicious, further testing is necessary. One half of women with newly diagnosed invasive cervical cancer have never had a Pap test. Unscreened populations include older women and the uninsured. In many cultures, the examination of such a private body part, particularly by a man, is a strong taboo. With early detection, successful treatment of cervical cancer is common.

The National Institutes of Health (**NIH**) recommend that a Pap test be done every 1 to 3 years if the two previous test results were negative. The NIH guidelines state that regular testing should begin at puberty, especially if the person is sexually active, and should continue to at least age 65. The American Cancer Society (**ACS**) and the American College of Obstetricians and Gynecologists (**ACOG**) continue to recommend yearly Pap tests for sexually active women, at least to age 75.

The nurse may be asked to assist the healthcare provider in performing the Pap test, which is most commonly performed during the pelvic examination. The procedure for positioning the client is the same as for any routine pelvic examination. In addition to equipment needed for the pelvic examination, necessary Pap test equipment includes glass slides and the applicator or Y-shaped wooden stick that is inserted through the speculum to obtain a smear of cervical mucosa. This material is smeared onto the glass slide; a spray fixative is sprayed over the slide so that the specimen adheres to the glass.

✚👁 Nursing Alert

Pap tests should be done between a woman's menstrual periods. Tests are less accurate when a woman is menstruating. Some women have a higher than normal chance of contracting cervical cancer. These women require regular screening, sometimes more often than once a year.

Abnormal test results do not necessarily mean that a woman has cancer; however, they do necessitate further testing and evaluation.

☛ KEY CONCEPT

All women must understand the importance of regular Pap tests. Early treatment of cervical cancer is effective in a high percentage of cases. Teach clients that abnormal Pap tests do not necessarily indicate cancer.

Tests for Endometrial Cancer

A positive Pap test may indicate endometrial cancer. However, in 30% to 40% of cases, the Pap test shows a false negative for this type of cancer. Aspiration of the *endocervix* (the internal portion of the cervix) provides more accurate information (approximately 70% accurate). A biopsy of the endometrium itself has proven more than 90% accurate.

Blood Tests

Several blood tests are used in conjunction with biopsy (of the cervix or breast) to determine specific types of cancer. These tests include estrogen and progesterone receptor analysis. Blood tests also determine the effectiveness of cancer treatment. They are not reliable for initial screening to determine whether or not a client has cancer.

Breast Examination

A woman should have a *clinical breast exam* performed by her healthcare provider at least once a year (more often if she has a cystic disorder). However, if any unusual symptoms appear, the woman should have her breasts examined immediately. Palpation by the healthcare provider is essentially the same as that done by the woman during breast self-examination. (Breast self-examination is discussed later in this chapter.)

Mammography

Mammography is an x-ray examination of the breasts that is capable of detecting some cancers 1 to 2 years before they reach palpable size. Up to 40% of all early breast cancers are discovered in this manner.

A baseline mammogram is recommended for women between the ages of 35 and 40 years. Women over 40 are encouraged to have a mammogram every year. Routine mammography is strongly recommended for women who have any of the following characteristics:

- Previous cancer
- Cystic breast disorders
- No children or birth of first child after age 30
- No breast-fed children
- Family history of breast cancer
- Strong family history of any type of cancer
- Female hormone (estrogen) therapy
- Extreme fear of cancer (need mammography for reassurance)

Procedure.   The procedure is simple and does not require the injection of dye. However, a specially trained radiologist must interpret the mammary x-rays.

Some laboratories request that the woman refrain from using deodorant or powder before the test because they may contain zinc or other metals that will interfere with x-rays. The client wears a gown that opens in front and is asked to remove neck jewelry and clothing above the waist. Help by explaining that she will be asked to assume several positions and that her breasts will be flat on the x-ray plate. A compressor is pressed from above or the side to flatten each breast as much as possible. The procedure may be uncomfortable but should not be painful.

A more definitive diagnosis can be obtained by xerography (xeroradiography). However, this test exposes the client to higher radiation levels.

Interpretation.   Tumors may show up on mammography as denser than normal breast tissue. However, not all breast abnormalities are identified on a mammogram. Mammography only identifies abnormal breast architecture or tumors with calcium deposits (approximately 70% of the breast tumors that can be diagnosed). The radiologist can speculate whether a tumor is malignant or benign due to its shape, location, and size. If a lesion is present, a biopsy is usually done.

Breast Ultrasound

The ultrasound examination can distinguish a breast cyst from a solid mass, which usually requires a biopsy examination to determine malignancy. Breast ultrasound is not used for routine screening. Ultrasound is being used more frequently with young women with dense breast tissue who present with breast lumps.

Breast Biopsy

Breast biopsy definitively determines the presence of cancer. The pathologist examines breast tissue or fluid to determine the presence and type of cancer cells. In the case of tissue, a *frozen section* is usually done and is examined microscopically. Breast biopsy can be performed in several ways:

- *Aspiration (fine-needle aspiration):* Cells from a lump are drawn into a syringe. (In the case of some cysts, fluid is aspirated, collapsing the cyst. Often, this cyst requires no further treatment.)
- *Needle biopsy:* A needle with a cutting edge is inserted into a lump and rotated to remove a core sample.
- *Excisional biopsy:* An entire lump is removed and analyzed. If cancer is localized in this lump, no further treatment may be required.
- *Incisional biopsy:* Part of a lump is removed as a sample.

Other Diagnostic Tests

Abdominal or Pelvic Ultrasonography

Ultrasonography uses high-frequency sound waves directed back at a transducer placed over the client's abdominal or pelvic region. The sound waves are converted into electrical impulses, which can be viewed on a special monitor. By scanning the abdomen and viewing the results on the screen, the healthcare provider can evaluate reproductive conditions, such as tumors, cysts, and other pelvic diseases. A secondary approach using ultrasound is with a special probe through the vagina (*vaginal ultrasound*) to view pelvic organs that cannot be seen any other way.

X-ray Examinations

Several x-ray procedures determine patency of the oviducts or the presence of abnormalities in the uterus and oviducts. The most common is the *hysterosalpingogram,* in which the uterus and oviducts can be visualized following an injection of contrast dye. The ovaries also may be visualized. These procedures are most often necessary to locate the cause of infertility or to determine the presence of a tumor.

Laparoscopy

Laparoscopy is a diagnostic technique that provides direct visualization of the uterus and accessory organs, including the ovaries and oviducts. Figure 90-2 illustrates the equipment and the procedure.

For this procedure, a small incision is made in the area of the umbilicus, and the abdomen is then distended (*insufflated*) with approximately 2 liters of carbon dioxide or oxygen. Gas is used because it allows for a clear view of the organs, separate from the intestines. The laparoscope is inserted into the peritoneal cavity, and the internal organs are viewed.

Laparoscopy is usually performed using general or spinal anesthesia. Two or three small incisions may be made in more extensive procedures; an absorbable suture is placed in the incisions.

The client usually ambulates on the operative day. Document client and family teaching. Usually, the woman will be discharged from the day-surgery center to home.

> ### ✚👁 Nursing Alert
> Severe pain following laparoscopy can indicate internal hemorrhage. This needs to be reported to the healthcare provider. Shoulder strap pain may occur as a result of gas instilled in the abdomen during the procedure. It may be trapped under the diaphragm but is referred to the shoulder. It is a temporary pain but is quite uncomfortable. It is not a heart attack.

Culdoscopy

Culdoscopy furnishes direct visualization of the uterus, oviducts, broad ligaments, colon, and small intestine. An endoscope is passed through the vaginal wall behind the cervix after a small incision is made in the posterior vaginal cul-de-sac. The procedure is usually done in the operating room with the client in a knee-chest position. The client may have local, regional, or general anesthesia. Usually, no sutures are involved, and routine postoperative care is given.

During the culdoscopy, photographs may be taken of the cervix and the vaginal vault; cold *conization* (removal of a cone-shaped portion of the cervix; discussed below) also may be done. This procedure also is used to diagnose pelvic pain, tubal pregnancy, and pelvic masses.

Colposcopy

High-risk women often are screened routinely with **colposcopy,** which allows better visualization of the vagina and cervix than with the regular speculum. The colposcope is a lighted, magnifying speculum that is inserted into the vaginal vault. Many believe that the results are more reliable than those from the Pap test. Accurate diagnosis often requires biopsy, however.

Cervical Biopsy

A *cervical biopsy* involves the microscopic examination of a small piece of cervical tissue. It is performed when the physician observes cervical irregularities or when a Pap test is questionable. One means of obtaining this tissue is through a punch procedure (punching out a button of tissue for examination).

The loop electrosurgical excision procedure (**LEEP**) is a common office procedure in which tissue is removed for diagnosis and treatment of cervical abnormalities. A wire loop and

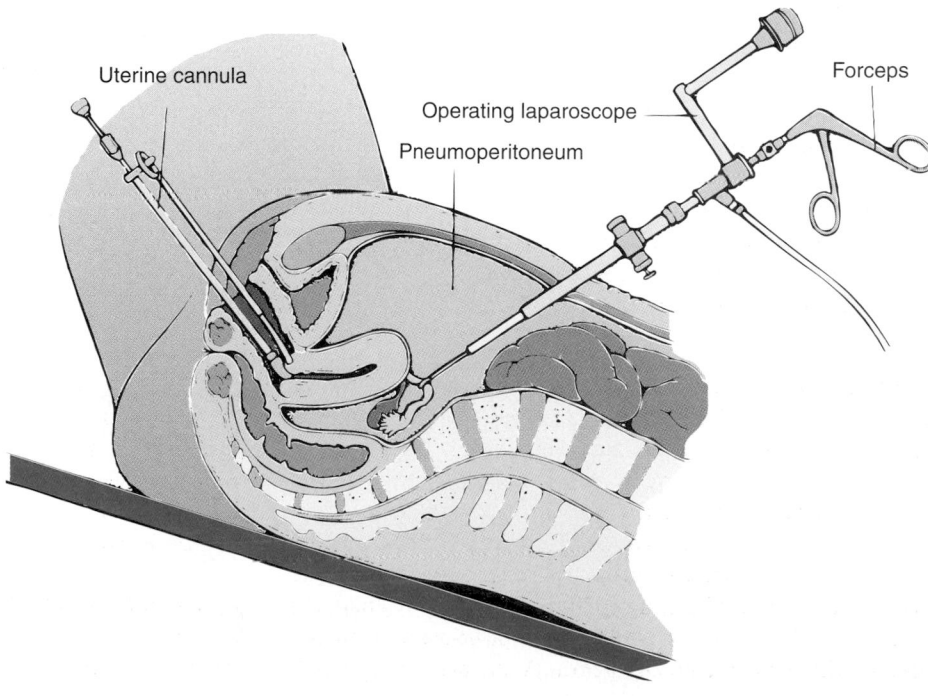

Uterine cannula

Operating laparoscope

Pneumoperitoneum

Forceps

FIGURE 90-2. Laparoscopy. The laparoscope is inserted through a tiny incision near the umbilicus. Gas is inserted to create an air pocket within the peritoneum, which enables the examiner to view the operative area.

a low level of electricity are used to remove a lesion. Minimal bleeding and cramping are the only side effects.

Conization (Cone Biopsy)

Conization is usually done in the operating room with the client under general or spinal anesthesia. The surgeon removes a cone-shaped piece of the cervix for examination. *Cold conization* is done with a specially cooled knife and sometimes preserves the cells better. A small percentage of women (3% to 12%) may have some bleeding after cervical conization. Watch for symptoms. The client also should check for delayed bleeding after the procedure.

☛ KEY CONCEPT
───────────────────────────────────────

Some women who have had cervical conizations or other biopsies have difficulty in later pregnancies. They may need a special procedure, called cerclage, *to prevent premature dilation of the cervix, leading to miscarriage (see Chap. 67).*

COMMON SURGICAL TREATMENTS

Some diagnostic surgical procedures mentioned previously also may be used for treatment. These procedures include laparoscopy, culdoscopy, colposcopy, and biopsy of the cervix, uterine lining, or breasts.

Dilation and Curettage

Dilation and curettage (**D&C**) is the most frequently performed gynecologic surgery. It can be used to diagnose disorders and to treat some disorders. In D&C, the cervix is *dilated* (widened) using calibrated rods. A spoon-shaped instrument (*curette*) is then passed into the uterus, and the endometrial lining is scraped out (*curettage*). D&C takes approximately 15 minutes; it is often done in the day-surgery department on an outpatient basis.

Purposes.   A D&C is used as a diagnostic procedure in women with abnormal vaginal bleeding or to obtain tissue for examination after a positive Pap test. The uterine scrapings are examined for evidence of malignant or nonmalignant growths or other abnormalities. Sometimes a D&C is done just before the menstrual period in an effort to find the cause of female infertility. D&C is frequently used to evaluate *endometrial hypoplasia* (incomplete development of the uterine lining), *menorrhagia* (excessive menstrual flow; discussed later), and *metrorrhagia* (bleeding between menses; discussed later). In some cases, the D&C is all that is needed to eliminate the problem.

A D&C is used as treatment in other instances. It may be used after an abortion, whether spontaneous or therapeutic, to remove the retained products of conception. A D&C is always performed after an incomplete abortion.

Nursing Considerations.   Preoperative preparation is similar to that for any person about to receive anesthesia. In many cases, general anesthesia is used.

The client usually makes an uneventful postoperative recovery. She will need to wear a perineal pad and receive perineal care. A mild analgesic, such as acetaminophen (Tylenol) or ibuprofen (Advil), usually relieves minor discomforts.

In rare instances, the vagina is packed with gauze at the time of the surgery, which may make voiding difficult. The pack is usually removed the next day. Carefully assess the client to make sure that she can void and that she does not experience urinary retention.

Because the D&C is often done on an outpatient basis, teaching is vital. Vaginal discharge will be bloody at first but should quickly become serosanguineous. This drainage typically does not last more than a few days. Teach the client signs of abdominal distention and how to perform perineal care. Instruct the client to call the physician if any problems occur. Carefully document all teaching.

Hysterectomy and Pelvic Exenteration

A **hysterectomy** is the surgical removal of the uterus. It may be performed for a variety of reasons: cancer of the cervix, ovaries, or uterus or to treat uterine fibroids, severe endometriosis, or a *prolapsed* ("fallen") uterus. In some cases, such as a ruptured uterus during labor, an emergency hysterectomy must be performed. The uterus may be removed by means of a *vaginal hysterectomy* (through the vagina) or an *abdominal hysterectomy* (through an abdominal incision). Nursing care for women undergoing hysterectomy is discussed at "Caring for the Woman Undergoing a Hysterectomy."

In some cases of advanced malignancy, especially if the client is young, a **pelvic exenteration** is performed, in which the entire contents of the pelvis are removed. This complex procedure has a high mortality rate. The client will have urine and feces draining through openings (*ostomies*) on the abdominal wall postoperatively.

Cosmetic Breast Surgery

Corrective surgery may be performed on healthy breasts. A plastic surgery revision of the breast is referred to as a **mammoplasty.** If the breast is to be made larger, the term *augmentation mammoplasty* is used; if the breast is to be made smaller, the appropriate term is *reduction mammoplasty.*

Following breast surgery, reconstructive mammoplasty is often done. Usually, these operations are not serious and cause no adverse effects. Occasionally, however, the woman's body rejects materials implanted during the augmentation mammoplasty and the materials must be removed. Because of concerns for safety, implants must be used cautiously with follow-up monitoring.

Mastectomy

Mastectomy is surgical removal of a breast. It is discussed in the section on breast cancer later in this chapter.

NURSING PROCESS

Data Collection

Carefully observe and assess the woman with a reproductive disorder. Chapter 47 describes physical examination and assessment, including that of the female reproductive system.

This assessment establishes a baseline for future comparison and determines the presence of suspected disorders and complications. Report any changes in the baseline level.

When performing a nursing assessment of the female client, obtain a reproductive and sexual history, which assists the physician in making a diagnosis. In Practice: Nursing Assessment 90-1 lists some components of the nursing assessment.

Many clients are reluctant to discuss sexual or reproductive concerns. One nursing objective is to express concern and to put the client at ease when discussing sexuality or sexually related concerns. In addition, observe the client's emotional response to the disorder or disease. Does the client need assistance to meet daily needs? Is the disorder life threatening? Does the disorder affect social activities, sexual identity, or self-esteem? Is the client anxious or fearful of the outcome?

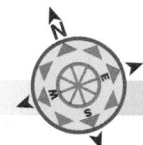

SPECIAL CONSIDERATIONS: CULTURE

When the client is from a culture that the nurse is unfamiliar with, attempt to gather sufficient data about how cultural differences may affect care. For example, in some cultures the woman must pass information through her husband, who will then convey it to the nurse. In some cultures, all decisions are made by family consensus or by the assigned matriarch (eg, grandmother, elder aunt, or mother). The woman may need to consult the patriarch or male decision-maker for the family. In some cases, decisions are made with the good of the society or the family as the highest goal, and the desires of the individual are less important. Any intervention that does not consider such cultural norms will be ineffective.

Nursing Diagnosis

Based on data collection, the following sample nursing diagnoses may be seen on nursing care plans for the female client

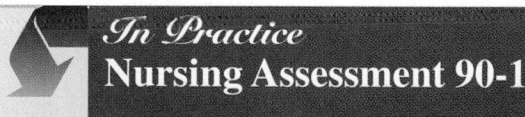

In Practice
Nursing Assessment 90-1

FEMALE REPRODUCTIVE SYSTEM

- Sexual history
- Reproductive history (pregnancies, abortions)
- Method of birth control used
- Menstrual history; date of last menstrual period
- History of STDs and other gynecological infections
- Visual observation of external genitalia
- Breast examination; teaching of breast self-examination

with a reproductive disorder. Some diagnoses may have more than one causative factor.

- Risk for Imbalanced Body Temperature related to infection
- Impaired Urinary Elimination related to female structural abnormalities, pregnancy, multiple pregnancies, pelvic inflammatory disease (**PID**), surgical trauma, abdominopelvic malignancy
- Impaired Tissue Integrity related to PID, injury, radiation therapy
- Ineffective Tissue Perfusion: Peripheral (right or left arm) related to mastectomy
- Ineffective Sexuality Patterns or Sexual Dysfunction related to genital infection, genital deformities, injury, altered self-esteem, sexually transmitted disease (**STD**)
- Disturbed Body Image Disturbance or Low Self-Esteem related to mastectomy, hysterectomy, sexual dysfunction, inability to conceive, STD
- Diarrhea, Bowel Incontinence, or Constipation related to structural abnormalities, infection, multiple childbirth injuries
- Anxiety related to body changes, uncertain or threatening diagnoses

Planning and Implementing

Together with the client, family, and other members of the healthcare team, plan for effective individualized care to meet the client's needs. Provide preoperative and postoperative care for the client undergoing procedures such as hysterectomy and mastectomy. The client with a reproductive disorder also may require teaching about preventive measures, such as breast self-examination. The client may need assistance in meeting needs, dealing with emotional problems, and understanding more about the disorder, its prognosis, and treatment.

Teaching Feminine Hygiene

Nurses are in an excellent position to teach clients about personal hygiene. Many women do not realize that after urinating or defecating they should wipe from front to back to prevent urinary tract and vaginal infections. Caution the woman who is susceptible to infections against using bubble baths, bath oils, and nylon panties or pantyhose. Also stress the importance of thorough handwashing and perineal care, especially during menses. Menstrual discharge is an excellent culture medium for microorganisms. Techniques to prevent vaginal infections are presented at In Practice: Educating the Client 90-1.

Teach the client the procedure for breast self-examination and reaffirm the necessity of a yearly Pap test, breast examination, and serology tests for STDs. Stress the need for adequate nutrition, including vitamin D and calcium intake as well as fruits and vegetables. Teach the client about the dangers of smoking.

Teaching Breast Self-Examination

The ACS recommends that each woman examine her breasts monthly, approximately 1 week following menses, to check

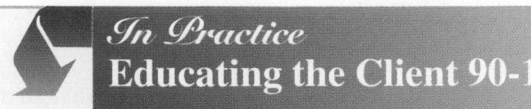

In Practice
Educating the Client 90-1

PREVENTION OF VAGINAL INFECTIONS

- Wipe from front to back after going to the bathroom.
- Wash hands thoroughly after using the bathroom or changing perineal pads.
- Change tampons or sanitary pads frequently. Dispose of them safely. Place them in sealed plastic bags in the trash or burn them, if possible.
- Pull panties, with perineal pad attached, straight down to avoid spreading infection during menses.
- Remove a tampon immediately and call a physician if fever, nausea, vomiting, diarrhea, weakness (signs of toxic shock syndrome) appear. Do not use deodorant tampons.
- Do not use vaginal deodorant sprays or scented powders.
- Douche only when absolutely necessary. Use the cleanest technique possible. Dispose of all equipment each time in a safe way.
- Clean the bathtub carefully before use, or take showers.
- Do not use bubble bath or bath oil, especially if prone to infection.
- Do not use colored or scented toilet tissue.
- Wear only cotton panties, ventilated pantyhose, or hose with garters; avoid nylon panties.
- Avoid tight pants or jeans, nonventilated clothes, or tight exercise clothing.
- Change out of a wet bathing suit immediately after swimming. Stay out of swimming pools or hot tubs if you are prone to infection. (The chlorine in the pool may predispose to infection. An infected person also can spread the infection to others.)
- Cut down on intake of sugar.
- Have the male partner wear a condom when having sexual intercourse. A water-soluble lubricant, such as K-Y jelly, may be needed to increase comfort and prevent irritation.
- Check with a physician at the earliest sign of an infection. (Sexual partner should be checked also.)
- Consult physician regarding use of oral contraceptives or other hormones.

---

examination techniques are discussed and demonstrated at In Practice: Educating the Client 90-2.

☛ KEY CONCEPT

Women discover approximately 40% of all breast cancers by self-examination. A woman who has had a mastectomy should check her chest wall and the scar area because these sites are common areas for recurrence.

Providing Perineal Care
Give perineal care to women after any perineal surgery. Many women need instruction in this procedure (see Chap. 65).

Providing Sitz Baths
Sitz baths are frequently ordered for a female client following a vaginal hysterectomy or delivery. The procedures involved have been described previously (see Chap. 54). Remember to clean equipment after each use and to inform the client why the procedure is necessary (whether it is done to cleanse the area, to aid in the healing process, or to make the client more comfortable).

Performing a Douche or Vaginal Irrigation
The *douche* or *vaginal irrigation* is prescribed less frequently than in the past. Frequent douching is believed to irritate the vaginal mucosa and predispose the client to infection. The secretions from the mucous membrane protect the area from infection. Therefore, it is not desirable to wash away these secretions unless necessary.

If a vaginal irrigation is ordered, explain the procedure and purpose to the client. Vaginal irrigation cleanses the vaginal canal of excess discharge, supplies heat or medication, and relieves pain and inflammation.

The healthcare provider orders the solution to use. Common solutions include povidone-iodine (Betadine), saline solution, sterile water, or a solution of acetic acid (vinegar in water). Disposable douches also are available. In Practice: Nursing Procedure 90-1 outlines the procedure and rationale for vaginal irrigations.

Inserting a Vaginal Suppository
Medication is applied to the vaginal canal by means of vaginal suppositories. Most suppositories must be kept refrigerated until ready for use.

Evaluation

Evaluate outcomes of care with the client, family, and other members of the healthcare team. Have short-term goals been met? For example, is the client ready for discharge following a hysterectomy? Are long-term goals still realistic? Does the woman need followup care or education? Is long-term therapy required, for example, radiation therapy or chemotherapy for cancer? Planning for further nursing care takes into consideration the client's prognosis, any complications, and the client's response to care given.

---

for any lumps, nodules, or thickening. If the woman is postmenopausal, she should examine her breasts on the same date each month. The key is to note any change from the previous month.

Self-examination of the breasts is done in several steps. Using the flat of the fingers, rather than the fingertips, the woman palpates her breast, checking her nipples for lumps, tenderness, discharge, or any changes. The ACS publishes a booklet entitled "How to Examine Your Breasts," which describes and illustrates the entire procedure. Breast self-

In Practice
Educating the Client 90-2

BREAST SELF-EXAMINATION

Instruct the client to perform the following self-examination monthly.

Before a Mirror
1. Inspect the breasts with your arms at the sides.
2. Raise your hands above the head. Breast movement should be free and equal on both sides. Look for changes in the contour of each breast (discharge, puckering, dimpling, or scaling of the skin).

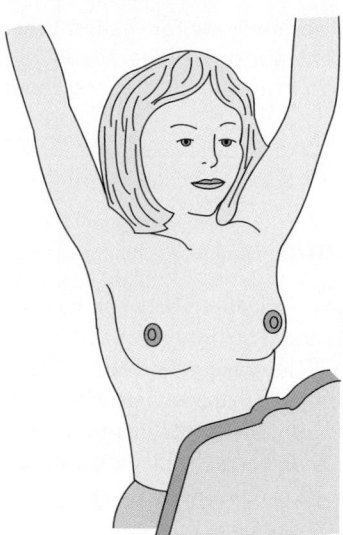

3. Press your hands firmly on the hips and bow slightly toward the mirror, pulling your shoulders and elbows forward. Note any changes in breast contours.

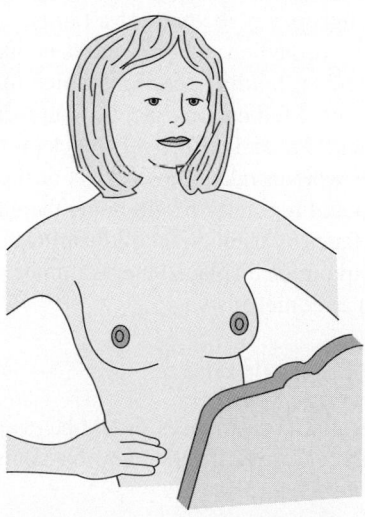

4. Squeeze the nipple of each breast gently between the thumb and index finger. Report any discharge (clear or bloody) to the physician immediately.

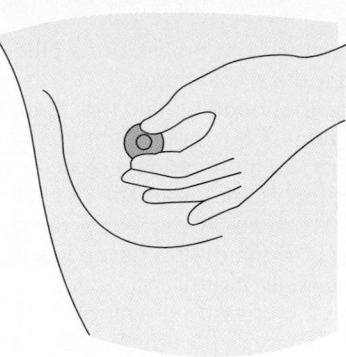

In the Shower
1. Keeping your fingers flat, move them gently over each part of the breast. Use the right hand to examine the left breast, and the left hand to examine the right breast. Check for any lump, hard knot, or thickening.

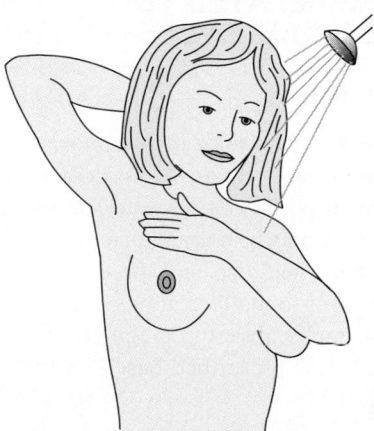

2. Check the axillae for any unusual signs (rash, lesions, lumps, absence of hair, unusual pigmentation).

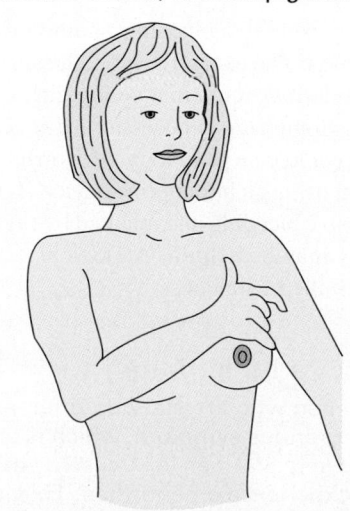

(continued)

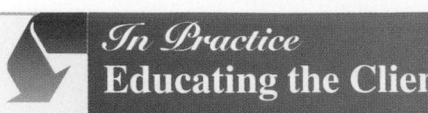
In Practice
Educating the Client 90-2 (Continued)

Lying Down
1. To examine the right breast, put a pillow or folded towel under the right shoulder.
2. Place your right hand behind the head. With your left hand, fingers flat, press gently in small circular motions around an imaginary clock face. Begin at outermost top of left breast for 12 o'clock. Move to 1 o'clock and so on, all the way around, back to 12 o'clock. (A ridge of firm tissue in the lower curve of each breast is normal.)
3. Move in an inch toward the nipple and keep circling to examine every part of the breast, including the collar bone and breast bone. Vary your pattern of checking between the circular pattern and a vertical pattern.

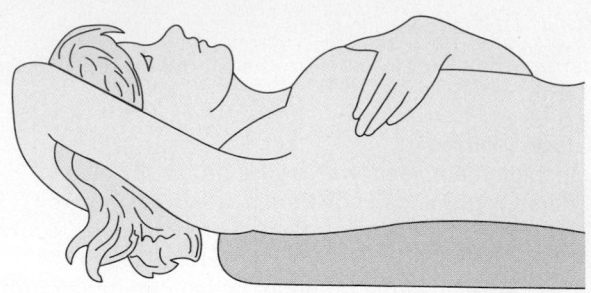

4. Repeat the above steps for the left breast.
5. If you find any abnormalities, measure the distance and direction from the nipple, and report to the physician.

DISORDERS RELATED TO THE MENSTRUAL CYCLE

Amenorrhea

Amenorrhea is the absence of or abnormal stoppage of menses (*menstruation*). If an adolescent female has not begun to menstruate by her 15th year, she should be examined. The difficulty may be hormonal, requiring a specialist's attention. Amenorrhea also may be due to nutritional or emotional causes or to malformations of the female organs. (Menses are normally absent in pregnancy and after menopause.) Treatment is prescribed based on the cause of the client's amenorrhea.

Menorrhagia

Menorrhagia is excessive bleeding in amount or duration during menstruation. The excessive blood loss results in anemia. If this irregularity occurs in a young girl, it may adjust itself. However, monitoring is necessary. If it occurs during menopause, it may indicate pathology. Menorrhagia also may occur in the client using an intrauterine device (**IUD**) for birth control. In excessive bleeding unexplained by organic causes, hormone therapy may be helpful. A D&C also may be performed as therapeutic treatment.

Nursing Alert

Women who are starving often experience amenorrhea, a serious symptom, which is one sign of anorexia or bulimia. Women in intensive athletic training also may experience amenorrhea. They should be under the supervision of an experienced sports medicine specialist.

Metrorrhagia

Metrorrhagia is bleeding between menstrual periods. It is abnormal and should be brought to a physician's attention because it may indicate cancer, or retained placental tissue in the postpartum woman or in the woman who has had a spontaneous or induced abortion. Metrorrhagia may indicate fibroid tumors and is frequently associated with the use of oral contraceptives; in this instance, it is referred to as *breakthrough bleeding*.

Dysmenorrhea

Dysmenorrhea is painful menstruation. Normal menstruation is not painful. Functional causes of menstrual pain may stem from constipation, insufficient exercise, poor posture, fatigue, or improper placement of a tampon. These conditions are easily remedied. Very severe pain may be due to an increase in prostaglandin secretion, which intensifies uterine contractions. Medications such as ibuprofen (Motrin) or mefenamic acid (Ponstel) effectively block prostaglandin production. The woman takes these drugs at the beginning of menstruation and regularly for 48 hours thereafter. Dysmenorrhea often fades by itself after childbearing but occasionally can be a symptom of displaced uterus, tumor, endocrine disturbances, or endometriosis.

Extreme Irregularity

Extreme irregularity of menses should be evaluated because it may indicate a hormonal deficiency that could result in later sterility.

Premenstrual Syndrome (PMS)

Premenstrual syndrome (**PMS**), also called *premenstrual tension*, is associated with symptoms that are common in as many

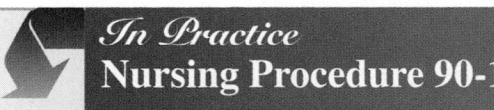

In Practice
Nursing Procedure 90-1

PERFORMING A VAGINAL IRRIGATION

Supplies and Equipment

Gloves
Irrigating bag, tubing, and clamp, or disposable
  douche
Disposable douche tip
Bedpan
Solution, as prescribed
Standard (short intravenous stand)
Bath thermometer
Protective waterproof pad for the bed
Perineal pad (sanitary napkin), if needed
Tissues
Bath blanket
Mineral oil, if needed

Steps

1. Wash hands, and put on gloves. Wear goggles if
   necessary.
   RATIONALE: *These actions prevent the spread of
   infection.*

2. Ask the client to void.
   RATIONALE: *A full bladder will interfere with the
   insertion of the douche nozzle and may cause
   discomfort. The douche may stimulate voiding
   if the bladder is full.*

3. Protect the bed with a waterproof pad. Have the
   bedpan ready before preparing the solution.
   RATIONALE: *Some fluid might spill; using a waterproof pad protects the bed from becoming wet
   and avoids having to change the linens.*

4. Prepare approximately 1,500 mL of the prescribed
   solution at the required temperature, 100° to
   110° F (37.8° to 43.3° C), according to the treatment's purpose.
   RATIONALE: *The fluid will cool; be sure to administer it at the correct temperature. Heat relieves
   inflammation, but a solution that is too warm
   will burn the mucous membranes and the skin
   around the meatus when flowing back.*

5. If the solution is ordered at a temperature above
   105° F (40.6° C), apply mineral oil or petrolatum to
   the vulva and perineum. Maximum temperature
   is 115° F (46.8° C).
   RATIONALE: *The vulva and perineum are more
   sensitive than the vagina.*

6. Carefully inspect the douche tip to make sure it is
   not cracked or rough.
   RATIONALE: *This action prevents injury to delicate
   vaginal tissue.*

7. Have the client lie back with a rolled bath blanket
   under her head, and place her on the bedpan or
   ask the client on the toilet to lean back.
   RATIONALE: *In this position, gravity will help direct
   the solution over the entire vagina.*

8. Place the irrigating bag slightly above the level
   of the client's hips, never more than 18 inches
   (48 cm).
   RATIONALE: *This placement ensures a continuous,
   but gentle, flow of solution. If the bag is higher,
   it can drive infection into the uterus.*

9. Release the clamp to let air out to the tubing
   before inserting the nozzle.
   RATIONALE: *Air might distend the uterus or vagina.*

10. Separate the labia, and gently insert the nozzle,
    directing it downward and backward. If necessary,
    lubricate the tip of the nozzle with water-soluble
    lubricant.
    RATIONALE: *This direction is the same as the slant
    of the vaginal canal; a small amount of water-
    soluble lubricant, such as K-Y jelly, aids
    insertion.*

11. Gently release the clamp, and allow the fluid
    to flow slowly. Rotate the nozzle gently during
    treatment.
    RATIONALE: *A natural pocket forms between the
    cervix and the vagina's rear wall. Rotating the
    douche tip rinses material out of this pocket
    and directs fluid over all parts of the vagina.*

12. Clamp the tubing, and gently withdraw the tip
    from the vagina.
    RATIONALE: *Clamping the tubing prevents the
    solution from spilling as the tip is removed.*

13. Discard the entire douche system in the
    prescribed manner.
    RATIONALE: *Proper disposal helps prevent the
    spread of infection.*

14. If the client is able, have her sit up on the bedpan
    or toilet for a few minutes.
    RATIONALE: *This position will help the fluid drain
    from the vagina.*

15. Place a sanitary pad over the vulva.
    RATIONALE: *The sanitary pad helps protect the bed
    and client from additional drainage.*

16. Dispose of gloves. Wash hands, and document
    the treatment on the client's chart.
    RATIONALE: *Proper glove disposal and hand-
    washing help prevent the spread of infection.
    Documentation provides for communication
    and continuity of care.*

as 40% to 50% of women, with more severe symptoms occurring in women over 35 years of age. In some cases, symptoms increase with age.

Signs and Symptoms.   Signs and symptoms of PMS are cyclic in nature, generally developing 7 to 14 days before the onset of menses and disappearing with its onset. More than 100 symptoms of PMS have been identified; they fall into general categories of mood alterations, symptoms related to fluid retention, and neurologic, vascular, gastrointestinal, and respiratory symptoms. Common symptoms include abdominal distention, backache, headache, generalized edema, abnormal sleep patterns, acne, visual disturbances, food cravings, occasional vomiting, irritability, and moodiness. **Mastalgia** (breast pain) is a common symptom. A diminished chemical in the brain, serotonin, has been linked to many PMS symptoms. PMS also seems to be an allergic reaction in some women.

In many women, dysmenorrhea replaces PMS at the onset of menses. Menstrual headache in some instances is severe and may need to be treated with medications.

Treatment and Nursing Considerations.   The use of a low-salt diet for 1 to 2 weeks during the premenstrual cycle and medications that increase the excretion of sodium ions may be useful (see In Practice: Important Medications 90-1). Increasing protein and decreasing sugar intake also may be helpful. If allergens can be identified, their elimination can greatly reduce symptoms. Positive stress management is helpful, especially when combined with an active exercise program and omission of caffeine. If the condition becomes severe, antianxiety agents may be prescribed. A support group may be helpful in extreme cases.

Toxic Shock Syndrome

The use of tampons, particularly those with plastic inserters, has been associated with a serious condition known as *toxic shock syndrome* (**TSS**). A bacterial toxin (*Staphylococcus aureus*) is believed to be the cause. TSS is characterized by fever of 102° F (38.8° C) or greater, with vomiting or diarrhea. The woman may experience a sudden drop in blood pressure and accompanying weakness and dizziness. A red rash may occur, which later may result in peeling of the skin. Hemoglobin levels may drop. Urine output is diminished. (Wound infections also may be caused by the same staphylococcal organism that causes TSS.)

If any of these symptoms occur, instruct the client to remove any tampon and to call her physician immediately. This disease can be life threatening.

The chance of developing TSS is negligible if a woman does not use tampons. Instruct clients who use tampons about the need to change them frequently and use them intermittently during menstruation. Tampons require careful insertion to avoid abrasions of the vaginal tract. Urge thorough handwashing before insertion.

Instances of TSS have dropped dramatically since 1980, when efforts were made to decrease the absorbency of tampons and to make them from materials less likely to support bacterial growth. However, the risk is still present.

✚👁 N u r s i n g   A l e r t
Toxic shock syndrome or another serious infection may develop if a woman forgets that a tampon is in place or if she moves it so high that she cannot remove it. If the string breaks or a tampon cannot be removed for another reason, the woman should see her physician immediately.

Discomforts of Menopause

Menopause (climacteric), the cessation of menstruation, usually occurs between the ages of 45 and 50, although it may occur earlier or later. Menopause signifies that the woman's production of estrogen and progesterone has stopped and that ovulation has ceased. Menopause is a normal body change that should not be viewed as an illness. However, some women experience difficulties as a result of changes in hormonal balance, particularly the decrease in estrogen and progesterone.

One of the first signs of approaching menopause is a change in the menses. The amount of flow lessens, and the cycle becomes irregular. Finally, the menses stop altogether. In a few women, bleeding becomes heavier for a time. Because the ovaries produce less estrogen, levels may be inadequate, resulting in symptoms.

The most common symptom is the *hot flash,* with accompanying perspiration, palpitation, and fatigue. Although hot flashes are not serious, they are annoying and may embarrass the client. Another possible symptom of menopause is vaginal dryness and atrophy. The vagina loses its normal lubrication and elasticity. Some women also experience weight gain, skin dryness, sagging breasts, and signs of calcium deficiency (*osteoporosis*).

Sometimes women experience symptoms during menopause that affect their sense of psychological well-being or

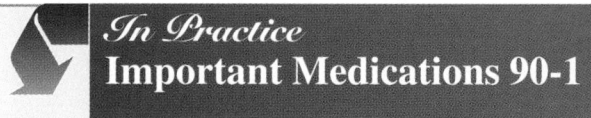

In Practice
Important Medications 90-1

FOR PMS
Diuretic Medications
hydrochlorothiazide (HCTZ) (HydroDIURIL, Esidrix)

Hormones
oral contraceptives
progesterone

Antianxiety Agents
alprazolam (Xanax)
diazepam (Valium)

Supplements
vitamin B supplements, especially pyridoxine
magnesium supplements

quality of life. These include insomnia, anxiety, crying spells, fatigue, mood swings, and depression.

Treatment.   Hormone replacement therapy (**HRT**) may be prescribed to treat severe symptoms and discomforts. This therapy delays menopausal symptoms and can help the woman's body adjust more gradually. Some researchers have theorized that hormone use increases a woman's tendency toward uterine cancer. Other research shows that conjugated estrogens, in combination with medroxyprogesterone acetate (Provera, Amen), help reduce the risk of later cervical cancer. Estrogen replacement therapy lasting longer than 8 years has been associated with a higher risk of breast cancer.

Vaginal dryness is a particularly distressing symptom accompanying menopause. It is so extreme in some women that they have difficulty walking. Over-the-counter products are available for treatment, including Replens, Gyne-Motrin, and Lubrin. Their effectiveness lasts approximately 3 days. The woman may use other products to make sexual intercourse easier, such as water-based lubricants (eg, Astroglide, K-Y jelly). For women with vaginal atrophy, a vaginal dilator may be helpful before intercourse.

To ease menopausal symptoms, many women are interested in herbal therapies, some of which contain plant estrogens. Women are generally encouraged to begin treatment with 400 International Units (IU) of vitamin E twice daily. If this is ineffective, the woman may try ginseng root, evening primrose oil, soy, or other herbals. The safety and effectiveness of these treatments has not been completely established.

Nursing Considerations.   A woman often needs emotional support during menopause. Teach her to realize that menopause is a normal physiologic function. Instruct about helpful health measures: a balanced diet, stress-relieving exercise, adequate rest, leisure activities, and relaxation techniques.

Induced Menopause.   After hysterectomy and *bilateral oophorectomy* (removal of both ovaries) or radiation therapy for cancer, artificial or surgical menopause occurs. If only the uterus is removed, the woman will have no menstrual flow; however, normal hormonal cycles will continue. A young woman who has had both ovaries and the uterus removed will often be maintained on estrogen therapy.

☛ KEY CONCEPT

The premenopausal woman who experiences surgical menopause may have more difficulties than the older woman who undergoes a normal menopause. The younger the woman is, the more likely she is to have difficulties with surgical menopause without estrogen-replacement therapy.

STRUCTURAL DISORDERS

Vaginal Fistula

A *fistula* is an opening between two organs that normally do not open into each other. It results from an ulcerating process, such as cancer or irritation, or from a childbirth injury. A fistula may develop between the ureter and vagina (*ureterovaginal*), bladder and vagina (*vesicovaginal*), or vagina and rectum (*rectovaginal*).

Any fistula is troublesome. If it is ureterovaginal or vesicovaginal, urine will leak into the vagina. If it is rectovaginal, it will cause fecal incontinence. A long-standing fistula is difficult to repair successfully because the tissues are eroded. Infection can become an additional problem.

In many cases, particularly in young women, an attempt is made to surgically repair the fistula. A successful repair is difficult because of the associated problems. The incision must granulate from the inside out to prevent an abscess. The closeness of the urinary tract to the bowel makes infection a common postoperative complication. Repaired fistulas tend to recur because of continued irritation.

Make efforts to assist the healing process by building up the woman's resistance and by keeping her as clean as possible, without perineal irritation. The woman with an unrepairable fistula is distressed by the odor and constant drainage. Sitz baths and deodorizing douches help maintain cleanliness.

Cystocele

Cystocele is the downward displacement of the bladder toward the vaginal orifice. It is most often seen in women who have experienced frequent deliveries or deliveries close together. Sometimes it results from injuries during childbirth.

Cystocele can cause nagging discomforts: pelvic pain, backache, fatigue, and a sagging pelvic weight. The client may experience stress incontinence, or dribbling of urine on coughing, straining, sneezing, or laughing. She also may have urinary urgency and frequency, and residual urine.

If the condition is not advanced, perineal exercises (*Kegel exercises*) may be prescribed to strengthen the muscles (see In Practice: Educating the Client 90-3). Surgery may be necessary, whereby the anterior vaginal wall is repaired (*anterior colporrhaphy* or *anterior repair*) and the bladder is returned to and secured in its normal position.

Rectocele

Rectocele is the upward displacement of the rectum toward the vaginal orifice. Rectocele is most often the result of injuries during childbirth. The woman with rectocele will experience backache, fatigue, heaviness in the pelvic region, and bowel difficulties. She will have incontinence, flatus, and alternating constipation and diarrhea. Surgical repair of the posterior vaginal wall, with a return of the rectum to its normal position, is known as *posterior colporrhaphy* or *posterior repair* and is often very painful. The woman who has had repair of a cystocele *and* a rectocele is said to have had an anteroposterior (**AP**) repair.

Another procedure sometimes performed is called the *Marshall-Marchetti*. In this surgery, the urethra is supported by sutures through the anterior wall of the vagina on either side of the urethra. The sutures are then passed through the outer covering layer (*periosteum*) of the pubic bone and secured.

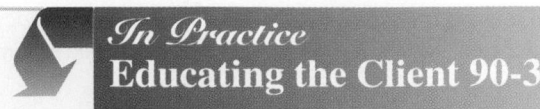

KEGEL EXERCISES

- Locate the muscles surrounding the vagina by sitting on the toilet and starting and stopping the flow of urine.
- Test the baseline strength of the muscles by inserting a finger in the opening of the vagina and contracting the muscles.
- Exercise A: Squeeze the muscles together and hold the squeeze for 3 seconds. Relax the muscles. Repeat.
- Exercise B: Contract and relax the muscles as rapidly as possible 10 to 25 times. Repeat.
- Exercise C: Imagine sitting in a pan of water and sucking water into the vagina. Hold for 3 seconds.
- Exercise D: Push out as during a bowel movement, only with the vagina. Hold for 3 seconds.
- Repeat exercises A, C, and D 10 times each and exercise B once. Repeat the entire series three times a day.

Regular practice of Kegel exercises can restore muscle tone. Benefits include control of stress incontinence, increased vaginal lubrication during sexual arousal, relief of constipation, increased flexibility of episiotomy scars, and stronger gripping of the base of the penis during intercourse.

Nursing Considerations. Prior to an AP repair or other gynecologic procedure, the client may receive an enema and have a catheter inserted, unless a suprapubic Cystocath will be used. For the anterior colporrhaphy, the catheter is left in place for several days, and a residual urine volume test or culture may be ordered when the catheter is removed. Showers and sitz baths promote comfort and healing. Instruct the client to avoid lifting, sexual intercourse, and prolonged sitting and standing until full healing has occurred (usually 6 to 8 weeks).

Prolapsed Uterus

A **prolapsed** uterus is one that sags or herniates into the vagina or in severe cases, even falls outside the vagina. The most common cause is damage during childbirth. A prolapsed uterus is most frequently seen in menopausal women or women nearing menopause. The woman is examined while standing or bearing down. The prolapse is classified as: *first degree* (the cervix can be seen when labia are spread, without straining or traction); *second degree* (the cervix protrudes out to the level of the perineum); or *third degree* (also called *procidentia*) (the entire uterus or most of it protrudes out the vagina onto the perineum).

The client with a prolapsed uterus complains of nagging backache, constipation, and stress incontinence. She may feel pain with intercourse (**dyspareunia**). Rubbing on the

underwear may irritate the cervix. A hysterectomy may be performed to eliminate a severe prolapse. Some physicians prefer to re-suspend the uterus back into its normal position, particularly for younger women.

If surgery is contraindicated because the woman is elderly or in poor physical condition, one of several types of pessaries (*pessary*—a ring-shaped device) may be needed. It is inserted snugly, similarly to a diaphragm, against the cervix and prevents the uterus from moving downward. The woman may feel some discomfort when the pessary presses on the vaginal muscles because it is larger and firmer than a diaphragm. Teach the woman how to insert and remove the pessary, and to clean it with warm, soapy water at least once a week. Most pessaries also must be removed for comfortable sexual intercourse and sometimes for bowel movements.

Abnormal Flexion of the Uterus

A displaced uterus is usually congenital, but it may result from childbearing. Figure 90-3 shows diagrams of abnormal flexion positions. Forward displacement can be termed *anteversion* or *anteflexion*. Backward displacement can be termed *retroversion* or *retroflexion*.

A displaced uterus may cause backache, dysmenorrhea, or sterility. Surgery can correct uterine displacement. With surgery, the uterus is sutured in its proper position.

INFLAMMATORY DISORDERS

Vulvitis

Vulvitis, inflammation of the vulva, may result from trauma due to scratching, improper cleansing, birth control pills, or irritating vaginal discharge. Most often, its cause is some type of infection. Common signs and symptoms include severe itching and burning; pain during urination, defecation, or intercourse; and swelling and redness. The goal of treatment is to determine and eliminate the cause.

Vaginitis

Vaginitis is inflammation of the vagina. Normally, vaginal secretions protect against infection. However, two organisms often cause vaginal infection: *Trichomonas vaginalis* and *Candida albicans* (formerly known as *monilia;* commonly known as *yeast infection*). Trichomoniasis is likely to be transmitted sexually, whereas candidiasis is more easily spread in other ways. However, both are considered STDs.

The most prominent symptom of vaginitis is a whitish vaginal discharge called **leukorrhea.** The discharge is odorous and profuse (more so in trichomoniasis), causing burning and itching in the perineum, vagina, and urethral area. The discharge may be frothy or thick and whitish.

In trichomoniasis and candidiasis, the sexual partner must be treated at the same time so that the infection will not be spread back and forth (see In Practice: Important Medications 90-2). Circumcision of the male may be necessary to help control a recurring infection.

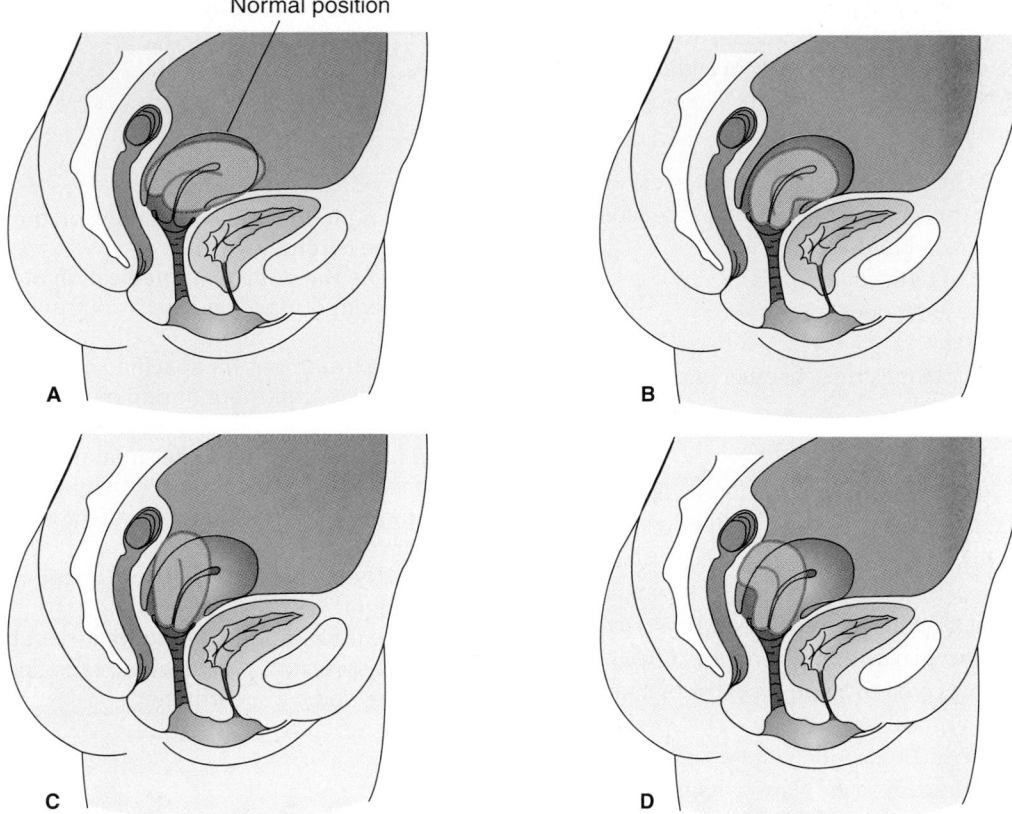

FIGURE 90-3. Variations in uterine position. (**A**) Anteversion. (**B**) Anteflexion. (**C**) Retroversion. (**D**) Retroflexion.

Vaginitis can be difficult to cure. It can be extremely irritating and persist for a long time. Recurrence is fairly common. Early and persistent treatment is the only way to prevent this disorder from becoming chronic. The client may find that wearing sanitary napkins is necessary to absorb the profuse drainage. Frequent napkin replacement, perineal care, and sitz baths will help prevent odor and irritation. Sometimes, mild antianxiety agents or analgesics lessen the effects of *pruritus* (itching).

Trichomonas Vaginalis (Trichomoniasis)

Trichomoniasis is an infection caused by a one-celled parasite. Its prominent feature is a very foul-smelling discharge that is foamy white or greenish-yellow in the woman; the man usually has no symptoms. The condition may be persistent and difficult to cure. Trichomoniasis is considered an STD (see Chap. 69).

Trichomoniasis is most often treated with oral tablets of metronidazole (Flagyl), taken by both sexual partners simultaneously. Clients should abstain from alcohol during treatment because severe gastrointestinal distress almost always results. Sometimes, if the infection is stubborn, metronidazole or antibiotics are inserted vaginally.

Nursing Alert

If a pregnant woman contracts trichomoniasis, treatment is necessary, although it is usually postponed until the second or third trimester because of the unknown effects of the drug on the developing fetus. Untreated trichomoniasis can lead to a fragile cervix that will be unable to maintain pregnancy or withstand delivery.

Candidiasis

Candidiasis is a stubborn fungal infection that is difficult to cure. It is often referred to as a vaginal *yeast infection*. It is common; three fourths of all women will have at least one such infection. Candidiasis may be transmitted sexually or in other ways.

The causative organism, *Candida albicans,* is often present in the vagina under normal circumstances, but certain factors

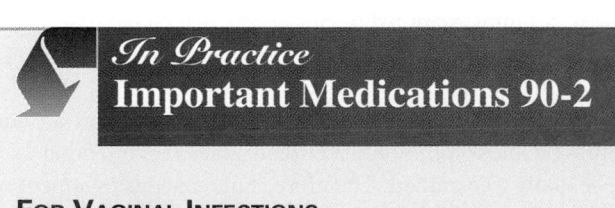

In Practice
Important Medications 90-2

FOR VAGINAL INFECTIONS

Treats Trichomonas and Bacterial Vaginosis
metronidazole (Flagyl)

Treats Candidiasis
nystatin (Mycostatin, Nilstat)
miconazole nitrate (Monistat, Micatin)

or changes can activate the infection. The two major factors that lead to infection are the presence of glucose or glycogen in the urine and a change in vaginal pH. In addition to these two factors, other factors can influence the development of a vaginal yeast infection. These include:

- Hormonal changes during the menstrual cycle or pregnancy or for any other reason (eg, taking exogenous hormones, estrogens, steroids)
- Long-term use of birth control pills
- Use of systemic antibiotics
- Diabetes mellitus
- Spilling of sugar in the urine, whether client is diabetic or not
- Compromised immunity

Signs and Symptoms. Women with candidiasis complain of vaginal itching, ranging from mild to intense. The itching is inside the vagina and on the outer structures in approximately 80% of cases. The woman often complains of soreness, irritation, and burning, especially during sexual intercourse. Vaginal discharge may be profuse and is often clumpy and white, resembling cottage cheese. Redness or a rash may be noted around the vagina.

The male partner often has no symptoms. However, he may have a red, blotchy rash on the penis, which may itch. An abnormal discharge also may be present. He should be sure to tell the physician that his partner has a yeast infection.

Primary care providers should be consulted at the first sign of a vaginal infection by women with:

- First vaginal infection
- Uncertainty that it is a yeast infection
- Risk for human immunodeficiency virus (HIV) or acquired immunodeficiency syndrome (AIDS)
- Diabetes
- Fever over 100° F (40.8° C) orally
- Age under 12 years
- Pregnancy
- New pain, including that of the lower abdomen, back, or either shoulder
- Malodorous vaginal discharge
- Thick, cottage cheese–like vaginal discharge

Nursing Considerations. Frequent bathing provides temporary relief from irritation and itching. Over-the-counter medications, such as nystatin (Mycostatin, Nilstat) and miconazole nitrate (Monistat, Micatin), are available. These medications are supplied in various systems of delivery including creams with several different types of applicators, tablets that dissolve inside the body, and suppositories. A combination pack containing suppositories and cream is available to treat internal and external symptoms.

Teaching is particularly important, because many women will treat their own infections at home and may not see a physician. Instructions are basically the same in all treatment systems. Self-care in vaginitis is discussed at In Practice: Educating the Client 90-4.

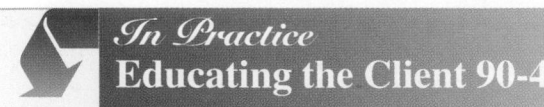

In Practice
Educating the Client 90-4

SELF-CARE WITH A YEAST INFECTION

- Read and follow the instructions on the medication package carefully.
- Insert the full dosage of medication at bedtime.
- Use cream during the day to control external itching.
- Use the treatment for specified consecutive days.
- Do not skip treatment during menses.
- Refrain from sexual intercourse during treatment and for at least 3 days after treatment is completed.
- Remember that a condom or diaphragm used during treatment will not be effective because the medication weakens latex.
- Use only unscented sanitary napkins during treatment.
- Do not use tampons during treatment because they absorb some medication, reducing the dosage, and can be irritating.

Women who are treating a vaginal infection should consult their primary care provider when there is:

- No sign of improvement after 3 days of treatment
- Worsening of symptoms within 3 days
- No relief of symptoms after 7 days of treatment
- Return of symptoms within 2 months

The latter cases indicate the presence of an infection or condition other than candidiasis.

Bacterial Vaginosis
Bacterial vaginosis (formerly called *nonspecific vaginitis*), a relatively common disorder, is believed to be caused by a combination of organisms. However, this complex condition is not completely understood. The client complains of increased white, gray, or yellowish vaginal discharge with or without irritation. An unpleasant fishy odor occurs, which increases after intercourse or washing with soap. Redness and edema are not usually significant.

The usual treatment consists of a 7-day course of an oral antibiotic, most commonly metronidazole. This infection may be sexually transmitted. Therefore, simultaneous treatment of the sexual partner is recommended.

Atrophic (Senile) Vaginitis
Atrophic vaginitis often occurs in postmenopausal women. It is caused by atrophy of the vaginal mucous membranes and decreased mucus and other vaginal secretions, resulting from lowered estrogen production.

Atrophic vaginitis is treated by using a water-soluble lubricant (such as K-Y jelly) during intercourse. An estrogen-based cream also may be helpful.

Cervicitis

Several organisms cause **cervicitis** (inflammation of the cervix), notably *Staphylococcus, Streptococcus,* and *Gonococcus.* Cervicitis occurs often during childbirth because of trauma to and sometimes tearing of the cervix. It also can be related to frequent douching, STDs, or a forgotten tampon. Cervicitis also may result from continued use of contraceptive foams or jellies. The main symptoms are leukorrhea and bleeding. Pain on sexual intercourse also may be occur.

Unless cervicitis is treated promptly, it may be difficult to cure. Periodic vaginal examinations help in diagnosis. Antibiotics are the mainstay of treatment. Sometimes the cervix must be cauterized. After cauterization, a watery discharge appears, which may become foul smelling. It takes about 6 to 8 weeks for the area to heal after cauterization. Some precautions taken to prevent vaginal infection also help prevent cervical infection.

Endometriosis

Normally endometrial tissue is confined to the inside of the uterus. In **endometriosis,** tissue resembling endometrial tissue appears in various places in the pelvic cavity, such as on the ovaries, oviducts, bladder, intestine, rectum, or pelvic wall. The cause of endometriosis is unknown, but it usually affects women between the ages of 25 and 45. There is an especially high incidence in women who have never experienced childbirth.

The client experiences pelvic pain, abnormal uterine or rectal bleeding, symptoms of pelvic pressure, and dysmenorrhea. She also experiences dyspareunia and may possibly be infertile.

Treatment is directed toward symptom relief. Healthcare providers often recommend pregnancy for two reasons. First, endometriosis may eventually result in sterility; and second, because endometriosis is influenced by hormonal changes, symptoms often improve after pregnancy.

If pregnancy is undesirable, medications may shrink the endometrial tissue, thereby decreasing the symptoms. In Practice: Important Medications 90-3 outlines some of these medications. Sometimes, endometriosis recurs when medication is stopped. Extensive and chronic endometriosis may require drastic surgical treatment, such as hysterectomy, *salpingectomy* (removal of oviducts), and oophorectomy. A woman experiencing endometriosis will require a great deal of emotional support.

Pelvic Inflammatory Disease (PID)

Pelvic inflammatory disease, an infection of the ovaries (*oophoritis*), oviducts (*salpingitis*), uterus, or pelvic cavity, enters the body through the vagina, peritoneum, lymphatic system, or bloodstream. *Gonococcus* is often the cause of pel-

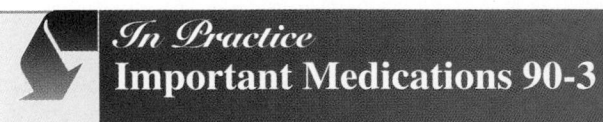

In Practice
Important Medications 90-3

FOR ENDOMETRIOSIS

Combination (estrogen–progestin) oral contraceptives
Progestins
Synthetic estrogen, danazol (Danocrine, Cyclomen)
Gonadotropin-releasing hormone agonists (cause lowered estrogen levels):
 leuprolide (Lupron)
 nafarelin acetate (Synarel)

Note: Medications used to treat endometriosis can cause any or all of the following side effects: abdominal swelling, breast tenderness, breakthrough bleeding, atrophic vaginitis, weight gain, edema, hot flashes, emotional lability.

vic infection, although *Streptococcus,* chlamydial infections (accounting for approximately half of all PID), and other diseases may also cause PID. The microorganisms most often pass up through the vagina and uterus. These microorganisms are more common in women who have had an abortion or those with an IUD in place. Figure 90-4 illustrates routes of PID invasion.

A foul-smelling vaginal discharge is a common symptom of PID. The client also complains of backache, pelvic pain, fever, chills, malaise, nausea, and vomiting.

Treatment. Antibiotics are usually effective in destroying the causative bacteria, unless the PID is caused by herpes virus II, which is not affected by antibiotics. Antibiotics used to treat PID are often administered intravenously. The sexual partner is also treated if necessary. Sexual intercourse is discouraged as long as the woman has any trace of infection. If PID is not treated, it may become chronic and cause sterility, due to the formation of scar tissue that blocks the oviducts.

Nursing Alert

A woman who has had PID is more likely to have an ectopic pregnancy than a woman with normal health.

Nursing Considerations. The client hospitalized with PID is placed in the Fowler's position. *Rationale: This position helps encourage pelvic drainage.* Sitz baths may be ordered. *Rationale: They help relieve pain.*

Take precautions to dispose of soiled pads and dressings as contaminated material. Always wear gloves when caring for this client, and follow Standard Precautions. Give perineal care to the client after removing the pad and after the client uses the bedpan. Sometimes an abscess forms, and the surgeon institutes drainage through an abdominal incision.

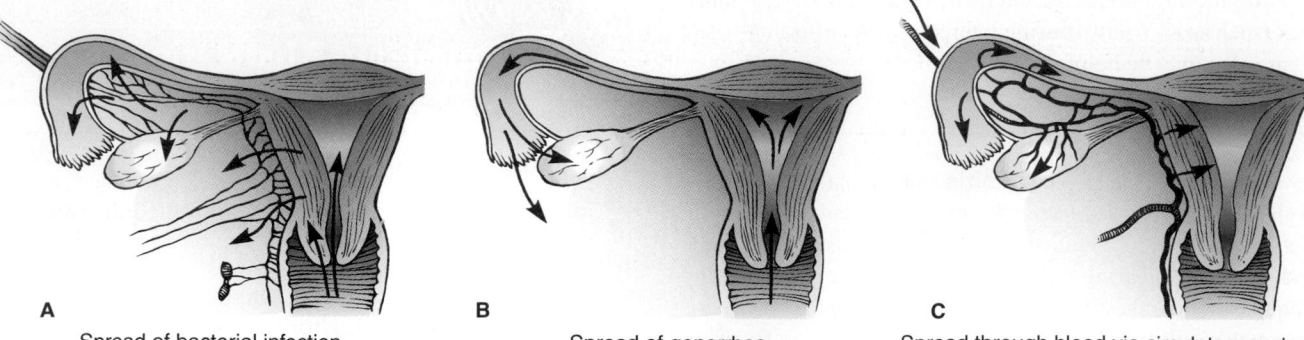

A Spread of bacterial infection   **B** Spread of gonorrhea   **C** Spread through blood via circulatory system

FIGURE 90-4. Pathways by which microorganisms enter the pelvis. (**A**) Bacteria enters through the vagina into the uterus and through the lymph system. (**B**) Gonorrhea spreads from the vagina into the uterus and into the tubes and ovaries. (**C**) Bacterial infection may enter the reproductive organs through the bloodstream.

During the active disease process, the client should avoid douches and sexual intercourse. Teaching, and the cooperation of the sexual partner, are vital in the treatment of PID.

Vulvodynia

Although not actually an infection, *vulvodynia* can cause great discomfort and extreme and disabling pain in the vulvar area. Most women with vulvodynia are aged 20 to 40, and most are Caucasian. This disorder has not been seen in African American women.

The pain is believed to be caused by excess calcium oxalate crystals in the urine. Only recently has treatment been known for this disorder. Calcium citrate is given orally to block formation of oxalate. Calcium citrate also prevents formation of calcium oxalate kidney stones. In addition, following a low-oxalate diet helps some clients. This diet eliminates spinach, green beans, celery, sweet potatoes, tomato sauce, peanuts, chocolate, tea, and coffee. A healthcare provider must manage the client's treatment.

Sexually Transmitted Diseases

Many STDs cause inflammation or other disorders of the female reproductive tract. Review the causes and treatments of STDs, discussed in detail in Chapter 69.

TRAUMA

Many women are victims of trauma, including battering, automobile accidents, and falls. Many times, this trauma involves the reproductive organs.

Most rape victims are women. Rape may cause physical disorders, including vaginal, cervical, or anal bruising or tearing; tampon impaction; or STDs.

Other trauma can cause various types of injury to the reproductive organs. These injuries are diagnosed and treated symptomatically, depending on the nature of the injury.

NEOPLASMS

Tumors of the Ovary

Benign Ovarian Tumors

Also known as *cysts,* these benign growths may form from fluid retained in the ovary or from other causes. Although they usually do not cause any trouble, cysts may enlarge and press on other abdominal organs and cause pain if they rupture or twist.

Malignant Ovarian Tumors

Women who have a personal or family history of cancer have a higher than average chance of developing ovarian cancer. Cancers that seem the most predictive of ovarian cancer include those of the breast, uterus, colon, and ovary. If a woman has had a tubal ligation, her chances of ovarian cancer seem to decrease to one third the risk of other women. Some researchers believe this is because carcinogens travel up the oviducts to the ovaries.

Vaginal ultrasound and the **CA125** blood test can make the diagnosis. Cancer of the ovary often displays no early symptoms and usually is detected only after metastasis has occurred. Ovarian cancer is a fairly frequent cause of death in young women because it is often not discovered in time to provide a long-term cure.

Cancer of the ovary is treated surgically. The procedure involves a total abdominal hysterectomy and removal of both tubes and both ovaries. Hormones are not given because they seem to nourish this particular type of cancer cell. Radiation therapy and chemotherapy are usually prescribed after the surgery.

Table 90-1 reviews warning signs, risk factors, detection, and treatment modalities of ovarian cancer and the other major cancers of the female reproductive system.

Tumors of the Uterus

Benign Uterine Tumors

The *fibroid tumor* is the most common type of benign uterine tumor. Fibroid tumors range in size, usually growing slowly and arising from muscle cells. They are believed to result from

TABLE 90-1 *C*ANCERS OF THE FEMALE REPRODUCTIVE SYSTEM

	Warning Signs	Risk Factors	Early Detection	Treatment (Dependent on Involvement)
Breast Cancer	Breast changes: Lump, pain, thickening, swelling, tenderness, distortion, retraction, dimpling, scaliness	Over age 40 (risk increases with age), history of breast cancer, early menarche, nulliparity, first birth at late age	Monthly self-examination; mammogram by age 40, every 2 years between ages 40 and 49, and every year after age 50 in asymptomatic women	Lumpectomy, mastectomy, radiation therapy, chemotherapy, hormone manipulation therapy
Cervical Cancer	Often asymptomatic; symptoms, if present, can include irregular bleeding or abnormal vaginal discharge	Intercourse at an early age, multiple sex partners, cigarette smoking, history of certain sexually transmitted diseases such as human papillomavirus	Annual Pap test for women over age 18 or who are sexually active; after three consecutive normal tests, Pap tests may be done less often at the physician's discretion	Carcinoma in situ: Cryotherapy, electro-coagulation, local excision Metastatic cancer: Surgery or radiation therapy or both
Endometrial Cancer	Irregular bleeding outside of menses, unusual vaginal discharge, excessive bleeding during menstruation, post-menopausal bleeding	Obesity, early menarche, multiple sex partners, late menopause, history of infertility, anovulation (not ovulating), unopposed estrogen or tamoxifen therapy, family history of endometrial cancer	Endometrial biopsy at menopause (for high-risk women)	Precancerous changes: Progesterone therapy Diagnosed cancer: Surgery or radiation therapy or both
Ovarian Cancer	Often asymptomatic; symptoms, if present, can include abdominal enlargement, vague digestive disorders, discomfort, gas distention	Risk increases with age (especially after age 60), nulliparity, history of breast cancer	Periodic, complete pelvic examination; cancer-related checkup every year after age 40	Surgery, including oophorectomy (excision of an ovary), hystero-salpingo-oophorectomy, salpingo-oophorectomy, excision of all intra-abdominal disease; radiation therapy; chemotherapy

Source: Hosley, J. B., Jones, S. A., & Molle-Matthews, E. A. (1997). *Lippincott's textbook for medical assistants* (p. 789). Philadelphia: Lippincott-Raven.

hormonal influences. The first symptom is abnormal vaginal bleeding, associated with a feeling of heaviness and pressure in the pelvic region. A fibroid tumor, or *myoma,* may become so large that it presses on the urethra or bowel, causing urinary retention or constipation.

Treatment. Treatment for fibroids depends somewhat on the client's age. Often it is possible to remove a nonmalignant tumor from the uterus without removing the uterus itself, an especially important consideration for a woman of childbearing years. Other treatments include medroxyprogesterone (Depo-Provera) injections or oral contraceptives to suppress the uterine lining, thus shrinking the tumors. Leuprolide (Lupron) injection therapy is showing promise in shrinking fibroids as well.

☛ KEY CONCEPT

Most nonmalignant tumors shrink after menopause; hence, postmenopausal bleeding is seldom caused by a myoma.

Cancer of the Fundus or Endometrium

The *fundus,* which is the body of uterus, is not attacked as frequently by cancer as is the cervix. However, malignant growths do occur in the endometrium and fundus. Cancers of the fundus and the endometrium are most likely to occur in postmenopausal women. Women who have previously taken estrogens also are at an increased risk. Therefore, hormone therapy is prescribed with caution.

Vaginal bleeding is the first sign of uterine cancer, possibly beginning as a watery, blood-tinged discharge. If it occurs before menopause, it may be mistaken for menstrual irregularity. A diagnostic curettage to obtain uterine scrapings is performed if the Pap test suggests cancer. If the results of the tests of the scrapings are positive, a hysterectomy is performed, followed by radium implantation, x-ray therapy, or both, to the pelvic cavity. This client may have postoperative chemotherapy but usually not hormone therapy.

Cancer of the Cervix

Of the cancers affecting the female reproductive system, cancer of the cervix is common, being surpassed only by breast cancer. Cervical cancer occurs most commonly in women between the ages of 40 and 55. Box 90-1 lists factors that place women at a higher risk of developing cervical cancer.

In the past, theorists believed that cervical cancer was linked to uncircumcised sexual partners, but this has not been proven. In addition, some researchers believe that a causative relationship exists between long-term use of female hormones, including many oral contraceptives, and development of cervical cancer. This also is unproven. Gynecologists should follow up carefully with women at risk. These women should have frequent Pap tests.

Signs and Symptoms.   Bleeding is the first sign of cervical cancer, but it does not occur in the early stages, when a positive Pap test would indicate the presence of cancer cells. The bleeding usually appears first as spotting between periods or after intercourse. The condition also can occur after menopause.

Staging of Cervical Cancer.   Cervical cancer has been staged similarly to many other types of cancer to standardize treatment depending on location and extent of spread:

- Stage 0: Carcinoma *in situ* (cancer limited to the epithelial layer with no signs of invasion of deeper tissue or of surrounding area)
- Stage I: Cancer is confined to cervix
- Stage II: Cancer extends beyond the cervix but not into the pelvic wall, or involves vagina but not the lower one-third
- Stage III: Cancer extends to the pelvic wall and involves lower one-third of vagina
- Stage IV: Cancer is widely spread throughout the pelvic region or throughout the body.

Treatment.   Early cervical cancer (*in situ* and some types of stage I) is susceptible to radiation therapy (usually radon implantation). In addition, early cervical cancer is more easily localized and therefore more easily excised. In these

➤➤ BOX 90-1

RISK FACTORS FOR DEVELOPING CERVICAL CANCER

- Infection with human papillomavirus (HPV)
- Sexual activity at a young age
- Frequent sexual activity
- Multiple sex partners
- Presence of genital warts (condyloma)
- Presence of herpes virus II
- Maternal history of cancer, especially cervical cancer
- Maternal use of diethylstilbestrol (DES) during pregnancy with this daughter (especially if mother had toxicity to DES)

early states, conization with cryosurgery or laser surgery is frequently used. If conization is performed, Pap tests should be done every 3 months for the first year and every 6 months after that time. These procedures may be done on an outpatient basis in selected cases. Hysterectomy also may be done for early cervical cancer if the woman does not wish to remain able to reproduce.

In the early and middle stages, conization or hysterectomy may be done. In the middle stages, hysterectomy is the treatment of choice. Many of these surgical procedures are combined with radiation or chemotherapy, particularly in stages other than cancer *in situ*.

Cervical Cancer in the Pregnant Woman

If a woman is pregnant and cervical cancer *in situ* is discovered, treatment is delayed until after delivery, which may be allowed to occur vaginally. If invasive cancer is discovered early in the pregnancy, the pregnancy is terminated, and the cancer is treated as in the nonpregnant woman. If invasive cancer is discovered late in pregnancy (third trimester), treatment is delayed until the fetus is viable, and cesarean delivery is done.

✚👁 N u r s i n g   A l e r t
The importance of the Pap test for women past puberty, particularly sexually active women, cannot be overstated. Cervical cancer is almost 100% curable if it is discovered early and treated before it spreads.

Caring for the Woman Undergoing a Hysterectomy

Hysterectomy is a term that describes the removal of portions or all of the female reproductive system. The type of hysterectomy depends on which organs are affected and the goal of surgery. If the entire uterus, including the cervix, is removed, it is called a *total hysterectomy (panhysterectomy)*. Today, the cervix is rarely left in place. However, if it is, and the body and fundus of the uterus are removed, it is called a *subtotal hysterectomy*. Removal of the attached oviducts as well is called a *salpingectomy;* the total procedure is called a *panhysterosalpingectomy*. Removal of both ovaries combined with total removal of the uterus and both oviducts is known as a *panhysterosalpingo-oophorectomy*. If one ovary is removed, the operation is a *unilateral oophorectomy;* if both are removed, it is *bilateral*.

If cancer has metastasized to the entire abdomen, radiation therapy with or without chemotherapy may be used palliatively, and surgery may be unnecessary. In some cases, however, radical surgery is performed.

Preoperative Considerations.   In addition to the usual preparation for abdominal or perineal surgery, the client may have a vaginal irrigation or douche. She will most likely have at least one enema to cleanse the colon of feces.

The client must receive instruction in the administration of the enema and other procedures to be done the evening before surgery. She will be allowed nothing by mouth (NPO) after midnight. This client will probably come into the healthcare facility on the morning of the surgery.

A Foley catheter is often inserted in the client surgical preparation room to lessen the danger of bladder perforation during removal of the uterus. The Foley catheter is usually removed on the first postoperative day and is not replaced unless the client is unable to void. If the bladder also is repaired, the surgeon may insert a suprapubic Cystocath during surgery to drain urine and rest the bladder. Antiembolism stockings usually are applied to the legs to prevent thrombophlebitis.

Be sure to answer all the client's questions fully. Include the woman's husband or partner in teaching. A hospital chaplain or the client's spiritual leader can be a source of needed support and reassurance. Be sure to document all teaching.

Postoperative Nursing Considerations. Plan nursing care according to the type of hysterectomy performed. Provide the same postoperative care for the woman who has had an abdominal hysterectomy as for any person who has had an abdominal incision. The client recovers more quickly from the vaginal procedure than from the abdominal procedure.

Give routine postoperative care to prevent complications. Early ambulation is important. The client often has a urethral catheter in place. After it is removed, make sure the woman is able to void.

Perineal pads are worn postoperatively. Teach the client to pull the underwear and pad straight down to avoid fecal contamination of the operative area. Assess the amount, color, and odor of vaginal drainage. Give frequent perineal care. The use of the peri bottle will keep the perineum clean and the client more comfortable. Teach the client how to perform perineal self-care. Frequent sitz baths may be helpful to increase the client's comfort.

Vaginal packing may be inserted during surgery. This is usually removed on the first or second postoperative day. The client may complain of severe back pain while the pack is in place. Reassure her that removal of the packing will relieve much of the pain.

Before discharge from the healthcare facility, inform the client of complications that might occur and when to notify the physician. Carefully document all teaching. (See In Practice: Nursing Care Plan 90-1.)

In Practice
Nursing Care Plan 90-1

THE CLIENT WHO IS AT RISK FOR COMPLICATIONS FOLLOWING A HYSTERECTOMY

MEDICAL HISTORY: *J.W.B., a 41-year-old Native American, was admitted with severe vaginal bleeding due to uterine fibroids. Her hemoglobin and hematocrit were 8.7 g/dL and 36.6%, respectively. An abdominal hysterectomy was performed. Indwelling urinary catheter was inserted during surgery. IV infusing at 125 cc/hour. Vital signs within acceptable parameters following surgery. Client has a history of varicose veins and of deep-vein thrombosis after the delivery of both of her children. Antiembolism stockings in place.*

MEDICAL DIAGNOSIS: *Abdominal hysterectomy, postoperative day 1*

Data Collection/Nursing Assessment: Client alert and oriented to person, place, and time. Client is complaining of moderate abdominal pain, rating it a 6 on a scale of 1 to 10. Meperidine 75 mg IM is given as ordered, with relief. Vital signs are within acceptable parameters. Abdominal incision with dressing is clean, dry, and intact. Mucous membranes are pale pink. IV infusing at ordered rate into left wrist. IV site is clean, dry, and intact. Catheter draining clear yellow urine, 420 cc's in the past 8 hours. Antiembolism stockings in place. Pedal pulses present and equal bilaterally. Toes are pink and warm; capillary refill 2 seconds. (*Although other nursing diagnoses may be appropriate, a priority nursing diagnosis is addressed below.*)

Nursing Diagnosis: Risk for Ineffective Peripheral Tissue Perfusion related to presence of risk factors as noted by history and client positioning during surgery.

Planning
SHORT-TERM GOALS:
#1. Client will demonstrate methods to enhance venous return while in bed.
#2. By the end of the day, client will ambulate 5 feet in the hallway.
#3. Client will exhibit no signs and symptoms of deep-vein thrombosis.

LONG-TERM GOALS:
#4. By discharge, the client will demonstrate measures to prevent deep-vein thrombosis while in and out of bed.

Implementation
NURSING ACTION: *Assess lower extremities for changes; note color, temperature, pulses, sensations, and capillary refill. Assess for positive Homans' sign. Document and report any suspicious findings.*
RATIONALE: *Changes in the status of the lower extremities may indicate early development of thrombosis, allowing for prompt initiation of treatment.*

(continued)

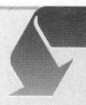

In Practice
Nursing Care Plan 90-1 (*Continued*)

NURSING ACTION: *Inspect lower extremities for swelling; if noted, measure calf circumference and compare measurements bilaterally.*
RATIONALE: *Swelling is an early sign of deep-vein thrombosis. Comparing measurements bilaterally quantifies the swelling, if present, and aids in determining its severity.*

NURSING ACTION: *Remove and then reapply anti-embolism stockings during bathing.*
RATIONALE: *Removing the stockings during bathing allows for close inspection of the skin.*

NURSING ACTION: *Encourage the client to change position while in bed at least every 2 hours. Teach and encourage client to do leg exercises while in bed.*
RATIONALE: *Changing positions in bed frequently and performing leg exercises help to promote venous return from the lower extremities.*

Evaluation: Lower extremities pale pink; no redness, swelling, or warmth noted; pedal pulses present bilaterally; quick capillary refill. Negative Homans' sign. Antiembolism stockings reapplied after bath. Client observed doing range-of-motion to feet after bath. *Progress to meeting Goal #1 and Goal #3.*

NURSING ACTION: *Gradually increase client's activity beginning with sitting at the edge of the bed, sitting in a chair, and then ambulating as ordered. Administer analgesic as ordered, before getting the client out of bed.*
RATIONALE: *These activities help promote venous return from lower extremities. Premedicating the client helps to minimize the amount of pain that the client may experience when getting out of bed.*

NURSING ACTION: *Elevate the client's lower extremities on a stool when out of bed in the chair.*
RATIONALE: *Elevating the extremities helps to prevent venous pooling due to gravity.*

Evaluation: Client assisted out of bed to chair for 15 minutes with legs on stool; antiembolism stock-

ings in place; complained of becoming lightheaded; assisted back to bed. *Progress to meeting Goal #1.*

NURSING ACTION: *Reinforce the need for client to avoid placing any pressure under knees, and to not rub the calves of her legs.*
RATIONALE: *Putting pressure under the knees increases the risk for thrombus formation; rubbing the calves could lead to an embolus if a thrombus is present.*

NURSING ACTION: *Teach client measures to prevent venous pooling, such as avoiding constricting clothing, elevating legs when sitting, and avoiding crossing the legs and standing for long periods of time.*
RATIONALE: *These activities lead to venous pooling, increasing the client's risk for thrombus formation.*

Evaluation: Client assisted out of bed; ambulated from bed to doorway, approximately 10 feet. Assisted back to bed; observed exercising lower extremities. No signs and symptoms of deep-vein thrombus evident. *Goal #1 met; Goal #2 met; progress to meeting Goal #3.*

NURSING ACTION: *Review measures to increase activity level as tolerated, with emphasis on measures to promote venous return. Encourage the use of antiembolism stockings even after discharge.*
RATIONALE: *Adequate venous return, including activity and use of antiembolism stockings, helps to prevent deep-vein thrombosis.*

NURSING ACTION: *Teach client the signs and symptoms of deep-vein thrombosis to report immediately.*
RATIONALE: *Client teaching is important to reduce the client's risk of potential complications postoperatively, including after discharge.*

Evaluation: Client wearing antiembolism stockings, doing leg exercises while in bed, and up and ambulating in hallway with assistance from husband. Assessment of lower extremities reveals no signs of deep-vein thrombosis. Client able to verbalize signs of possible complications. *Goal #3 met; progress to meeting Goal #4.*

Breast Neoplasms

Most breast lesions are benign. Benign lesions tend to be round or oval with a smooth border and usually show no secondary signs. Furthermore, benign lesions are likely to be movable. Malignant lesions are more likely to be irregularly shaped and hard, and often show secondary signs such as enlarged lymph nodes in the axillary area, asymmetry of the breast, retraction of the nipple, bloody discharge, dimpling, or elevation of one

breast. Additionally, malignant lesions are often attached to the surrounding skin, underlying structures, or breast tissue. Diagnosis, however, requires a laboratory analysis of tissue or biopsy study.

Benign Neoplasms

Chronic Cystic Mastitis. *Cystic disease* is the most common breast disorder in women between the ages of 30 and 50. It is believed to result from a hormonal imbalance and is related to the activity of the ovaries. Cyst formation decreases after menopause.

Breast tissue cells collect together and form a mass. This cell mass shuts off the ducts and forms cysts. These masses may form fibrous tumors (*fibromas*) or breast lumps. A biopsy may be performed to rule out cancer. Most lumps removed from the breast are benign. A cyst may be excised or drained without removal of any of the surrounding tissue. On rare occasions, particularly if the woman is extremely anxious, the physician may perform a simple mastectomy, in which only the breast is removed as a preventive measure. Cysts are not precancerous, but they may sometimes mask a cancerous lesion. Caffeine aggravates cyst formation. Women with a cystic condition are therefore advised to avoid coffee, tea, chocolate, and cola drinks. Researchers suggest that these women have a yearly mammogram or ultrasound or both.

Breast Cancer

Cancer of the breast is the most common type of cancer in women and the second most common cause of cancer death in women. (Lung cancer is the most common cause.) Approximately 1 in 9 women will develop breast cancer. More than 180,000 American women develop breast cancer every year. More than half are cured, but the number would be higher if more cases were discovered and treated earlier. Research shows that if breast cancer is treated within 3 months of its discovery, 5-year survival rates are much higher. Breast cancer in men occurs but is rare. Factors predisposing to breast cancer are presented in Box 90-2.

☞ KEY CONCEPT

According to research, some breast cancers may exist for as long as 6 years before they are detected by palpation. Thus, regular mammography, in conjunction with breast self-examination and annual clinical breast examination by a healthcare provider, are recommended for every woman over age 40.

Screening mammography is able to detect some breast cancers up to 2 years before they can be identified through palpation or other signs and symptoms. A radiologist often works up such abnormalities in a diagnostic breast center. The workup might include specialized mammography (compression views, magnification views, cone down views), ultrasound, and stereotactic core needle biopsies. The goal of these diagnostic breast centers is to decrease the period of anxiety for a woman with an abnormality by carrying out the entire workup within 24 to 48 hours.

Signs and Symptoms.   Signs of breast cancer usually become evident as cancer advances. Women are urged to consult a physician if they notice a lump, thickening, or any other change in the breast. Possible noticeable changes include nipple discharge (particularly bloody discharge), history of pain or tingling without a palpable mass, breast enlargement or thickening, nipple retraction, redness with swelling and heat, or puckering in any area of the breast.

> ➤ BOX 90-2

RISK FACTORS FOR DEVELOPING BREAST CANCER

The following categories of women have an increased risk for developing breast cancer; however, breast cancer can occur in women with no known risk factors.

- Menarche prior to age 12 (1st period)
- Late menopause (over age 50)
- Long or irregular menstrual cycles
- Women over age 40 (approximately 25% are between the ages of 40 and 49; approximately 70% are over age 50)
- Family history of breast cancer, especially in mother, maternal grandmother, maternal aunt, sister, or daughter
- History of fibrocystic breast disease
- History of cancer of the other breast
- History of endometrial or ovarian cancer
- Women who have never had a baby
- Women who had their first baby after age 30
- Women who have not breast-fed
- Women on antihypertensive therapy
- Radiation exposure before age 30
- Diet high in fat
- Obesity
- Alcohol and tobacco use
- Previous breast surgery (biopsies, implants, cosmetic mammoplasty)
- Estrogen replacement therapy longer than 8 years

Prompt action may mean the difference between life and death. The ACS states that more than two thirds of women who consult a physician immediately after finding a lump in the breast are alive 5 years later.

Diagnostic Tests.   A mammogram will often (but not always) show a mass and may help to indicate the type of lesion. Breast ultrasonography also may help differentiate between malignant and nonmalignant lesions. Breast biopsy is the only diagnostic test for breast cancer. At the time of biopsy, tests are done on the tissue to help determine the appropriate type of treatment.

Treatment.   The physician's first concern in treating breast cancer is to remove the cancer from the breast. Local treatment includes surgery and radiation therapy. Most women have a choice in selecting local treatment. *Partial mastectomy* (sometimes called *breast-sparing surgery* or *lumpectomy*) with radiation to the remaining breast tissue is as effective as *total mastectomy* (removal of the entire breast) in treating many breast cancers. A mastectomy may be necessary if more than one tumor is in a breast, if the tumor is extremely large or fast growing, or if a cosmetic consideration precludes radiation. Before surgery for a malignant lesion, the surgeon discusses the safety of the surgery or surgery/radiation option with the client and her partner. The recommended treatment mode includes consideration of the client's preferences (eg, accessibility to a radiation center), cultural and personal beliefs about radiation, and the client's feelings about keeping her breast. Oncology clinical nurse specialists often assist clients in making surgical decisions by discussing options and helping clients clarify their preferences and values. Referral of clients to sources that assist in decision-making is a nursing responsibility.

The second consideration in the care of the person with breast cancer is the identification, prevention, and treatment of systemic or metastatic disease. If the cancer has spread from the breast to another part of the body, the client is said to have *metastatic disease*. Metastatic disease requires systemic treatment such as chemotherapy or hormonal therapy. Clients at high risk for metastatic disease are also treated systemically. Determining which clients should receive systemic treatment requires diagnostic skill and a knowledge of prognostic factors. The tumor's size and the presence of cancer cells in the lymph nodes under the arm are the two best predictors of metastatic disease. For this reason, many surgeons remove some lymph nodes at the time of surgery.

Removal of the lymph nodes is a diagnostic procedure, but it does have long-term complications. An estimated 30% to 50% of women who have had the lymph nodes removed develop a condition called *lymphedema*, in which lymphatic fluid accumulates in the tissues, leading to arm discomfort and disability. For this reason, removal of the lymph nodes is becoming a controversial practice in the oncology field. Many physicians believe that lymph node dissection should be done only when the information gained from testing the nodes will influence treatment.

Most premenopausal women with invasive breast cancer are treated with chemotherapy regardless of evidence of positive lymph nodes or metastases. Some would say no value exists in taking the lymph nodes from such women. Others would say that knowing the number of lymph nodes involved might influence the oncologist to recommend more aggressive chemotherapy, and so there may be value in knowing lymph node status in these women. In other cases, such as in older women with large tumors that are estrogen-receptor positive, treatment almost always includes prescribing a hormone-blocking drug. In such a case knowing lymph node status may not influence treatment. Some centers are doing a newer procedure called *sentinel node biopsy,* in which the node that drains the area of the breast involved by tumor (**sentinel lymph node**) is identified and removed. If this node is cancer free, then it is assumed no cancer cells would be in the other nodes either; thus they are not removed.

Chemotherapy regimens for breast cancer include the use of *combination therapy* (the simultaneous use of multiple drugs). Preparing the woman for chemotherapy is important and is often done by the oncologist, clinical nurse specialist, or chemotherapy nurse. Ensuring that the woman has access to expert preparation falls within the role of the nurse who is responsible for the client.

Hormone therapy usually refers to the use of a drug that blocks estrogen's action on the cancer cells (see In Practice: Important Medications 90-4). This therapy is used only when the cells have been tested and are determined to be responsive

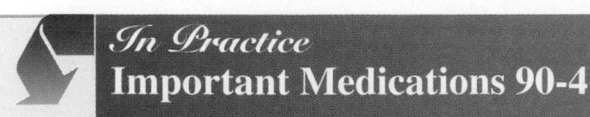

In Practice
Important Medications 90-4

FOR BREAST CANCER CHEMOTHERAPY

AC Regimen
doxorubicin (Adriamycin)
cyclophosphamide (Cytoxan)

CMF Regimen (Combination Chemotherapy)
cyclophosphamide (Cytoxan)
methotrexate (MTX)
5-fluorouracil (5-FU)

Taxanes
paclitaxel (Taxol)
docetaxel (Taxotere)
trastuzumab (Heceptin)

Prevention of Spread and Recurrence
tamoxifen (Nolvadex)
letrozole (Femara)
anastrazole (Arimidex)

to estrogen (*estrogen-receptor positive*). When deprived of an estrogen-rich environment, the cancer cells die off. Estrogen-blocking drugs act like estrogen in that they help reduce cardiovascular disease and osteoporosis; however, they increase the presence of postmenopausal symptoms. One side effect is that they increase proliferation of cells in the uterine lining, sometimes causing uterine cancer. Women taking these medications must have periodic biopsy or ultrasound of the uterine lining performed. Hormonal treatments have been shown to effectively manage breast cancer when used alone and in combination with chemotherapy. Hormone therapies are generally given for 5 years.

The client must discuss all therapy choices thoroughly with the oncologist. Decisions about therapy are made on the basis of the type and extent of the tumor and the client's wishes.

Reconstructive Surgery.   Women who have had a mastectomy have the option of breast reconstruction. National laws require insurance companies to cover the costs of reconstruction in women who lose a breast to cancer. There are two major types of reconstructive breast surgery. The plastic surgeon may implant a saline-, silicone-, or soy-filled envelope under one of the chest muscles to form a breast. Or the surgeon may move skin, muscle, and fat from another part of the body to the breast area and shape it to form a realistic-looking breast. Later the surgeon can form a nipple by bunching up tissue, and create an areola by tattooing the tissue to create color.

Breast reconstruction can be done at the time of surgery, or it can be delayed to a later time. The client will make this decision in discussion with the physicians involved in her care. It is often viewed as better to wait, if the woman will be receiving chemotherapy or radiation therapy. Because a reconstructed breast never looks completely like the original breast, many women decide to have a bilateral mastectomy and reconstruction for symmetry.

Prosthesis. A *prosthesis* is an artificial breast form that is inserted in a bra. It must be fitted to match the remaining breast. A prosthesis creates a natural appearance in clothing. For large-breasted women, prostheses are problematic because they may be made of silicone, which can be heavy. Many women purchase a prosthesis but later decide not to wear it due to resulting shoulder pain. For these women, lighter-weight prostheses are available, but many elect to use cotton forms.

The woman generally does not purchase a prosthesis until all swelling is gone from the surgical area and healing is complete. The physician or a Reach to Recovery volunteer often recommends a particular store or medical supply house where the prosthesis can be fitted. The cost of the prosthesis and the special bras that hold it are usually partially covered by insurance if the physician writes a prescription.

Nursing Considerations. Preparation begins as soon as the woman learns that she will need a breast biopsy or surgery. She must understand the procedure for the biopsy and that most breast lesions are benign. If she is to have a frozen section performed at the time of biopsy, she will want to know when she will receive the test's results. Most surgeons will see the client as soon as they get the result (usually 15 to 20 minutes after surgery) and tell her the result and what the next steps are, if any.

In the presurgical suite, physical preoperative preparations are done, such as shaving and preparing the client for the type of anesthesia to be used. The client should understand that if the frozen section is positive, the surgeon may need to do more extensive surgery later. Discuss the safety of the alternatives presented to her by the surgeon and the implications of the various surgical alternatives (lumpectomy with radiation, mastectomy, and mastectomy with reconstruction). If the client will need future surgery, she will need assistance with decision-making prior to scheduling it.

Many cancer centers have found that women are happiest with their decision if they have adequate time to make an informed decision, followed by a brief time to change their mind if they so desire. In most cases, women need from 1 to 2 weeks. If the woman decides to have immediate reconstruction, she may need a slightly longer period to provide for coordination between the surgeon and the plastic surgeon.

Preoperative teaching includes information about the care of any drains, such as a Jackson-Pratt (**JP**) drain if they are to be inserted during surgery. In many facilities, lumpectomy is a same-day procedure, so teaching must be done preoperatively. If lymph node surgery is to be done, teach postoperative exercises of the arm and allow the client to practice. Include the client's partner and other family members in discussions if possible.

The woman who is going to have a breast biopsy is understandably apprehensive about the possibility of breast cancer. Listen with understanding and support the client and family. Extreme emotional reactions are possible. Breast cancer affects the entire family, and each family member may need assistance with coping. Almost all women who are diagnosed

with breast cancer, no matter how good the prognosis, respond with thoughts and fears of dying. Women who are to have a mastectomy are fearful about how they will adjust. They may be concerned about their sexual appeal to their partners. Those who are about to have the lymph nodes removed are anxious about possible metastases.

If the biopsy sample reveals the presence of breast cancer, assist the client to verbalize her fears and allow her to express emotion. The client is often in such shock that she hears nothing other than the word cancer. Assist by providing anticipatory guidance and focusing on the next steps. Taking action is one of the best ways of coping, and there will be many actions to take and decisions to make in the next few days. After the biopsy procedure, apply an ice bag to the area to reduce bleeding and swelling. At home the client may want to continue the cold application.

Following definitive surgery, give routine postoperative care. Encourage the client to walk and move around. Monitor drains that are placed in the surgical wound to drain excess fluid and prevent edema. Note the amount of drainage and determine its character. One complication of mastectomy may be excessive bleeding. If this occurs, the client may need to return to surgery to stop the bleeding. Check dressings frequently for drainage around the drain insertion site.

Elevate the affected arm for several days to minimize development of edema. Expect some edema if surgery involves the lymphatic system. Surgeons differ in their beliefs about the value of postoperative arm exercises for the woman who has had lymph node surgery. Some encourage exercise to prevent the loss of arm function. Others prohibit exercise because it can lead to formation of a *seroma* (serum-filled mass) in the axillary area. Mild shoulder shrugging and movement of the elbow and hand are usually permitted. Occasionally a snug elastic sleeve will be used to decrease or prevent swelling. A low-sodium diet and diuretics also may be ordered.

> ## ✚👁 Nursing Alert
>
> The most common cause of lymphedema in the woman who has had her lymph nodes removed is infection. Many precautions are necessary to prevent damage to the skin and tissues. Avoid taking blood pressure, giving injections, or drawing blood on the operative side. Protect the arm against future infection. Report signs of infection in the arm or the hand immediately. In many facilities, a pink arm band is applied to the affected arm to alert staff to these precautions.

The post-mastectomy client will need emotional support. She is likely to experience grief over the loss of her breast. She may direct anger at the surgeon, nursing staff, or family members. Many clients are relieved that the surgery is over and do not exhibit negative emotions in the immediate postoperative period. Because of preoperative tension and anxiety, many clients are exhausted postoperatively.

The ACS publishes a booklet called "Reach to Recovery: Exercises after Mastectomy." This booklet describes post-mastectomy exercises that the woman can do at home. Figure 90-5 illustrates several post-mastectomy exercises.

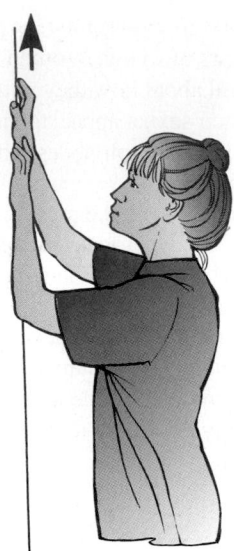

1. *Wall handclimbing.* Stand facing the wall with feet apart and toes as close to the wall as possible. With elbows slightly bent, place the palms of the hand on the wall at shoulder level. By flexing the fingers, work the hands up the wall until arms are fully extended. Then reverse the process, working the hands down to the starting point.

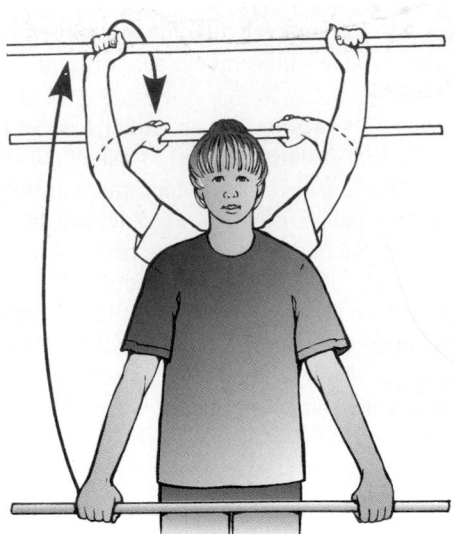

3. *Rod or broomstick lifting.* Grasp a rod with both hands, held about 2 feet apart. Keeping the arms straight, raise the rod over the head. Bend elbows to lower the rod behind the head. Reverse maneuver, raising the rod above the head, then return to the starting position.

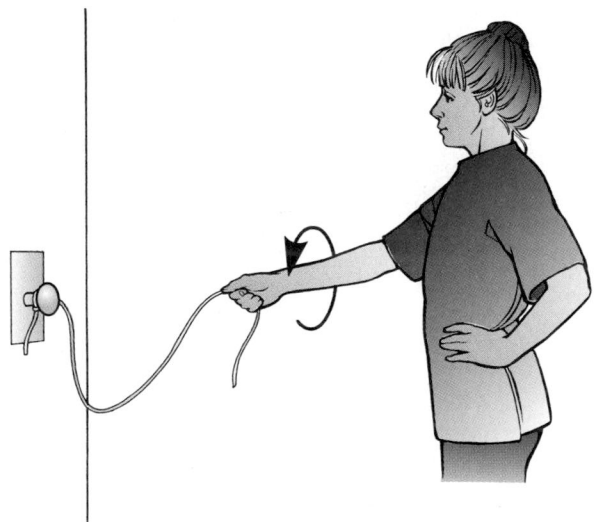

2. *Rope turning.* Tie a light rope to a doorknob. Stand facing the door. Take the free end of the rope in the hand on the side of surgery. Place the other hand on the hip. With the rope-holding arm extended and held away from the body (nearly parallel with the floor), turn the rope, making as wide swings as possible. Begin slowly at first; speed up later.

FIGURE 90-5. Postoperative exercises for the mastectomy client.

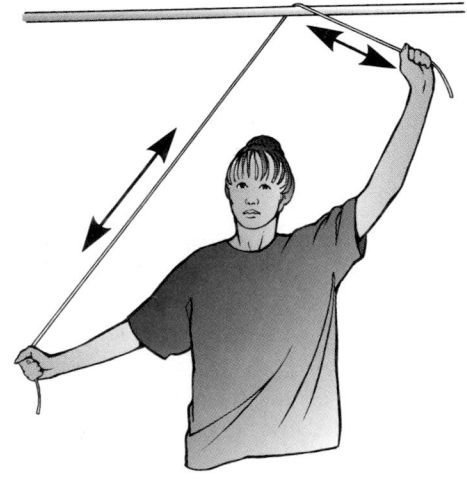

4. *Pulley tugging.* Toss a light rope over a shower curtain rod or doorway curtain rod. Stand as nearly under the rope as possible. Grasp an end in each hand. Extend the arms straight and away from the body. Pull the left arm up by tugging down with the right arm, then the right arm up and the left down in a see-sawing motion.

The client can combine some exercises with ordinary daily activities, such as sliding a towel back and forth to wipe the back, brushing the hair, and reaching with the arms when making a bed. The client should know how to exercise the muscles before she goes home. Some facilities offer post-mastectomy classes so that clients can exercise together.

☛ KEY CONCEPT

A visit from a representative of the American Cancer Society's Reach to Recovery program may help while the client is still in the hospital or shortly after she goes home. Reach to Recovery volunteers are cancer survivors who have had the same surgery as clients. They learn to assist clients with postoperative exercises and to answer common questions about the breast cancer experience. Volunteers can recommend places that sell prostheses for women who have had a mastectomy. They often try to bring temporary prostheses for clients to wear home from the hospital. They also can offer much-needed emotional support and answer questions.

STUDENT SYNTHESIS

Key Points

- A sexual history is important in defining areas of concern.
- Breast self-examination and observation of one's own menstrual cycle patterns are helpful in the early diagnosis of female reproductive disorders.
- Diagnostic studies are necessary (although sometimes uncomfortable) processes. Nurses are invaluable in preparing the client and relieving her concerns.
- Nursing skills performed to assist the female client include perineal care, vaginal irrigation, and insertion of vaginal suppositories.
- Explanation and followup with a client who must undergo surgical treatment is important. The client may not have heard or understood all that was explained to her.
- High cure rates exist in certain cancers if discovered early (especially breast and cervical cancer).

Critical Thinking Exercises

1. Suggest how you would approach and reassure an adolescent who is having her first gynecologic examination. Discuss, in addition to your approach, specific actions you would take.
2. While teaching a woman to do breast self-examination, the nurse must emphasize the importance of doing these examinations regularly. Determine important points the woman should know. State how the teaching would differ between a 28-year-old woman and a 60-year-old woman.
3. Your client has frequent vaginal infections. State important points to use in teaching prevention.
4. Your client is a 38-year-old Hmong woman who sits passively while you explain that she must go to a surgeon for evaluation of a breast lump. How would you proceed?

NCLEX-Style Review Questions

1. When discussing an abnormal Pap test with a client, the nurse tells her that:
   a. Abnormal Pap tests may not necessarily indicate cancer.
   b. Reducing her sexual activity for a few months will allow the cells to return to normal.
   c. She has cervical cancer, which can be removed surgically.
   d. She should have another Pap test in 1 year to confirm the findings.
2. Mammograms are recommended:
   a. Annually for all women over age 40
   b. Annually only for women having risk factors for breast cancer
   c. Because they detect 100% of breast cancer at an early age
   d. Primarily for women under age 70
3. When teaching a client breast self-examination, the nurse:
   a. Describes various causes of breast lumps and what cancer usually feels like
   b. Discusses the American Cancer Society's guidelines on how to perform breast self-examination
   c. Palpates the entire breast for the client, looking for lumps and thickening
   d. Shows the client how to use the tips of her fingers to feel for lumps and thickening in the breast
4. In a woman who has had a hysterectomy, antiembolism stockings are applied postoperatively to:
   a. Assist with leg exercise
   b. Decrease the risk of thrombus and embolism
   c. Place pressure under the knees during ambulation
   d. Promote venous stasis in the lower extremities
5. Toxic shock syndrome is:
   a. An allergy associated with tampon use
   b. Best treated with a low-sodium diet
   c. An infection associated with tampon use
   d. The irritability that occurs 1 to 2 weeks before menses
6. Advantages of hormone replacement therapy for menopause include:
   a. Decreasing bone mineral density
   b. Extension of time in which the woman is fertile
   c. Improvement in vaginal tone and lubrication
   d. Prevention of breast cancer
7. Following a mastectomy, the best option for the woman's appearance is:
   a. Total breast reconstruction
   b. A removable breast prosthesis
   c. Saline breast implant
   d. The option she prefers

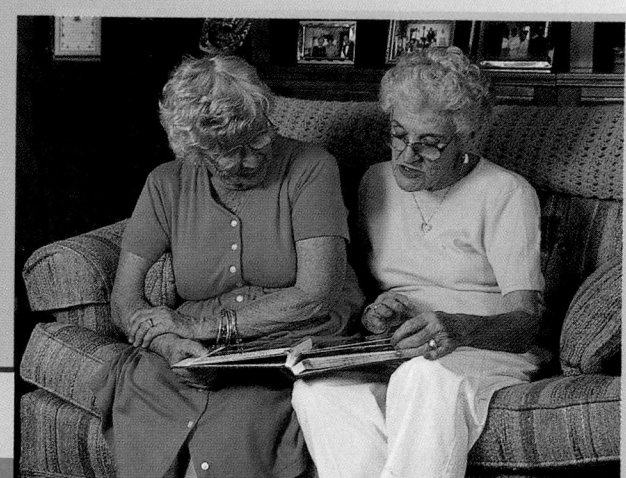

Unit XIII

GERONTOLOGICAL NURSING

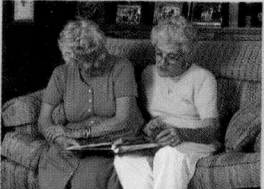

CHAPTER

91

Gerontology: The Aging Adult

LEARNING OBJECTIVES

1. List at least five care settings for older adults. Note the advantages and disadvantages of each.
2. Describe the characteristics of a high-quality long-term care facility.
3. Identify at least three nursing measures to assist an older adult to meet nutritional, elimination, and personal hygiene needs.
4. List at least four common mental health problems in older adults. Identify at least three nursing considerations for each concern.
5. Explain why depression and chemical dependency are important concerns for the older person. Identify at least three nursing considerations for each.
6. Discuss two emotional and psychological therapies and how they help the older person.
7. Explain the importance of relationships and stimulation for older adults.
8. Define presbyopia and presbycusis. List at least four nursing measures to assist an older person to meet communication needs.
9. State at least three nursing measures to assist an older person to compensate for impaired proprioception.
10. State at least five warning signs of elder abuse. Identify at least three nursing interventions that are necessary for suspected elder abuse.
11. Discuss the concept of cumulative loss in aging adults.

NEW TERMINOLOGY

aphasia
aspiration
caregiver stress
chemical restraint
edentulous
elder abuse
friable
geriatrics
gerontology
halitosis

hirsutism
kyphosis
presbycusis
presbyopia
proprioception
pseudodementia
respite
Sjögren's syndrome
vulnerable adult

ACRONYM

LTC

Many important concerns and considerations for the care of older adults have been presented throughout the chapters of this book, including the normal physical changes associated with aging (in Unit 4) and ways to adapt client care measures for older adults (in Unit 8). The changes of aging affect all people to some extent, although each individual's experience is unique. This chapter discusses health-related needs that result from the normal aging process. Chapter 92 discusses assistance for the older adult who is facing the additional challenges of dementia and related conditions. These conditions are abnormal disorders that sometimes develop in older adults.

Gerontology is the study of the effects of normal aging and age-related diseases. **Geriatrics** is the branch of medicine concerned with the problems and illnesses of aging and their treatment. The branch of nursing that assists people to age in a healthy manner and to promote and maintain wellness in late life is called *gerontologic nursing*. Care of ill older adults is called *geriatric nursing*.

Normal aging does not cause specific illnesses. The vast majority of older adults are active and healthy. Although chronic illnesses are more common in older adults than in the rest of the population, acute illnesses are less common (although higher rates of complications and death are associated with acute illnesses in the elderly). When caring for older adults, the nurse will need to understand the process of normal aging versus pathologies associated with disease. Normal aging changes related to body systems are listed in tables at the end of each chapter in Unit 4. Many problems commonly associated with aging are disease processes that result from a combination of heart disease, poor dietary habits, and lack of exercise.

The changes related to the normal aging processes include:

Decreased functioning of organs
Changes in visual and auditory acuity
Decreased reaction time
Unsteady gait; decreased sense of balance
Decreased tactile sensations
Stiff joints
Increased emotional, socioeconomic, and physical losses
Decreased capacity for recovery from injury or illness

Table 91-1 summarizes the common effects of aging on the systems of the body. Being aware of normal aging processes enables the nurse to better assist older clients to continue to meet their basic needs. Normally, seniors retain the ability to learn, adapt, and change, even when the aging process requires modifications.

CARE SETTINGS FOR OLDER ADULTS

The development of a plan of care for an older adult requires observation and an assessment of the person's current lifestyle. Remember that a very high percentage of seniors live in their own homes; however, some need assistance or special care. Care settings for seniors vary, and each has advantages and disadvantages. Cultural considerations, finances, and personal preferences often dictate available choices. The person's ability for self-care and potential for rehabilitation also are issues that require assessment. Care settings for older adults include home care, adult daycare centers, retirement communities, assisted living facilities, acute care hospitals, long-term facilities, and hospice care.

Factors determining the choice of residence for an aging adult include:

The person's ability to provide for physical, financial, and emotional self-care needs
Physical, financial, and emotional support from family and friends
Access to healthcare and rehabilitation services, including availability and transportation
Need for protection and supervision

Home Care

The majority of aging adults live in their own homes and are able to care for their own needs independently. For aging adults with manageable conditions, the current trend in healthcare is to provide needed care in the client's home. To some degree, measures such as financial aid, Medicaid, food stamps, and rental and fuel assistance help aging adults to remain in their homes.

When complicated physical needs require ongoing assistance, home care agencies have a substantial variety of services available 24 hours a day. Other services, such as home health aides, homemakers, or occupational, physical, speech, or respiratory therapists, also are available. These services, plus homebound meals and transportation, also help older adults remain in their homes (Fig. 91-1).

Circumstances may require older adults to move into the home of one of their children. In this situation, roles can reverse, as the child becomes the caregiver and the parent is the care receiver.

Senior Centers

Senior centers provide social interaction and opportunities for peer group relationships. Many centers provide travel, educational discussions, games, meals, and other services. Some centers also provide senior daycare. Caretakers of seniors can obtain temporary relief and rest (**respite**) from the responsibilities of caring for frail adults.

Retirement Complexes

An increasing number of independent-living complexes are being designed and built exclusively for older adults. They are called *retirement* or *life care communities*. They offer older adults the freedom and privacy of their own apartment while providing conveniences, security, and services to lighten their responsibilities. Such complexes are not nursing homes, although many have assisted-living options, units reserved for clients with dementia, and nursing care units available for the resident whose health declines, requiring various levels of skilled nursing care. Ambulatory and independent residents can eat meals in a common dining room, although a small kitchen

■■■ TABLE 91-1 𝓔FFECTS OF AGING ON BODY SYSTEMS

	Systemic Changes	Manifestations	Client Teaching
Integumentary System	Loss of subcutaneous fat	Wrinkling, sagging, decreased ability to maintain hydration, less protection against temperature changes	Encourage the client to drink plenty of fluids and dress appropriately for climate changes.
	Loss of pigment	Paler skin, graying hair, less protection against sun damage	Encourage the use of sunscreens with appropriate UV protection. Suggest using good lubricating lotions and bathing less often. Caution the client to guard against injuries.
	Loss of elasticity	Increased incidence of trauma	
	Receding capillaries	Sallow skin, thicker nails	
	Slower reproduction of hair and skin cells	Balding; thin, fine hair; slower healing	Suggest ways to guard against injuries.
	Diminished oil and sweat production	Dry, fragile skin; intolerance to heat	Encourage the client to use good lubricating lotions and bathe less often. Suggest ways to avoid becoming overheated.
	Erratic pigment and cell production	Senile lentigines (liver spots) and keratoses (skin thickening)	Show the client how to conduct skin checks and consult a dermatologist with any concerns.
Musculoskeletal System	Loss of muscle strength and size	Loss of strength, flexibility, and endurance	Suggest frequent exercise appropriate to the patient's age and ability.
	Loss of bone density	Vertebral compression with diminished height and a dowager's hump (abnormal spinal curvature); osteoporosis (abnormal bone porosity) with frequent fractures	Educate the client regarding weight-bearing exercises. Encourage the client to conduct a home safety check to avoid falls. The physician may recommend calcium supplements, dietary consultations, or estrogen replacement.
	Degenerative joint cartilage	Less clear margins with spurs of bone that restrict movement, degenerative joint disease (DJD), arthritis	The physician may limit phosphorus intake.
Nervous System	Slower nerve conduction	Slower reaction time, slower learning, slower perception of pain with resulting increase in injuries	Allow extra time as needed and educate the client about possible hazards of delayed reaction times. Aim teaching at comprehension level. Encourage the client to conduct home safety checks.
	Reduced cerebral circulation	Loss of balance and vertigo (whirling sensation), frequent falls	Have the client install bath rails, remove throw rugs, conduct a home safety check. Encourage the client to use ambulatory aids.
	Referred circulatory problems	Increase in cardiovascular diseases (atherosclerosis, arteriosclerosis) reflected as cerebrovascular accidents (CVA) (brain ischemia due to vessel occlusion), cerebral hypoxia, and transient ischemic attacks	Educate the client and family about the danger signs for cerebrovascular accidents and transient ischemic attacks.
Eyes	Less time spent in deep sleep	Less restful sleep, more frequent naps	Allow the client rest periods as needed.
	Diminished adjustment of lens to accommodation	**Presbyopia** (farsightedness)	Obtain a referral to an ophthalmologist. Provide adequate lighting and use large-print books.
	Lens cloud	Cataracts (lens opacity) that dim vision as less light reaches the retina	Obtain a referral to an ophthalmologist. Provide adequate lighting.

(*continued*)

■■■ **TABLE 91-1** 𝓔FFECTS OF AGING ON BODY SYSTEMS (CONTINUED)

	Systemic Changes	Manifestations	Client Teaching
	Loss of ciliary function	Glaucoma (increased intraocular pressure as the pupils press on the canal of Schlemm), intolerance to light or glare, poor night vision	Obtain a referral to an ophthalmologist. Provide adequate lighting and have the client avoid night driving.
Ears	Loss of auditory hair cells (organ of Corti)	Hearing loss in upper frequencies, problems distinguishing Ch, S, Sh, and Z	Obtain a referral to an otologist. Speak clearly, facing the client, in an area with few distractions.
	Ossicle becomes fixed	**Presbycusis** (hearing loss), strains to hear, misses cues, inappropriate responses	Obtain a referral to an otologist. Speak clearly, facing the client, in an area with few distractions.
Other Senses	Diminished sense of smell	Loss of appetite, poor nutrition	Suggest dietary consultation.
	Diminished sense of taste	Loss of appetite, poor nutrition, may increase use of salt or spices	Suggest dietary consultation. Encourage the use of spices rather than salt.
Cardiovascular System	Atherosclerosis and arteriosclerosis, narrowing of vessels	Loss of peripheral circulation, fatty plaques with resulting myocardial infarctions and CVAs, cold extremities, slower healing time, hypertension	Encourage the client to exercise and to eat a balanced, low-fat, low-salt diet. Have the client dress appropriately for temperature changes and conduct a home safety check.
	Slower response time to demands for increased output	Complaints of fatigue on exertion	Help the client pace exercise and exertion.
	Diminished function	Pulmonary involvement with edema, dyspnea	Educate the client regarding low-salt diets and orthopneic position.
Respiratory System	Stiffening costal cartilage	Decreased expansion and contraction, barrel chest, decreased lung capacity	Educate the client about smoking hazards and emphysema. Encourage moderate exercise.
	Decreased gas exchange	Fatigue and breathlessness on exertion, impaired healing due to insufficient oxygen, syncope (sudden drop in blood pressure)	Encourage the client to exercise, as appropriate, and to use ambulatory aids. Caution the client to guard against upper respiratory infections and to conduct a home safety check.
	General loss of muscle mass	Difficulty coughing deeply (may lead to pneumonia)	Encourage the client to drink adequate fluids to liquefy respiratory secretions.
Gastrointestinal System	Drying of secretions, including saliva	Dry mouth, dysphagia (difficulty swallowing)	Educate the client regarding oral hygiene and adequate fluid intake.
	Decreased enzyme activity	Incomplete digestion, poor conversion of nutrients with malnourishment	Encourage the client to eat small, frequent, well-balanced meals.
	Slower peristalsis	Constipation, flatulence, indigestion	Suggest the client increase fluid and fiber intake. Have the client avoid laxative dependency.
	Loss of teeth	Poor chewing function, choking on large pieces, loss of appetite, poor nutrition	Refer the client to dentist and provide instruction regarding good oral hygiene. Suggest dietary counseling.
Urinary System	Decreased bladder capacity	Urinary frequency	Encourage the client to respond to the initial urge to void.
	Decreased bladder muscle tone	Urinary retention with resulting urinary tract infections or incontinence	Suggest exercises for strengthening the pelvic floor. Urge the client to completely empty the bladder with each voiding.

■■■ TABLE 91-1 *E*FFECTS OF AGING ON BODY SYSTEMS (CONTINUED)

	Systemic Changes	Manifestations	Client Teaching
	Fewer functioning nephrons	Less blood flowing through the kidneys to be cleaned of wastes, creating possible lethal levels of medications or normal body wastes	Have the client increase fluid intake to maintain hydration.
Endocrine System	Decreased enzyme activity	Menopause, glucose intolerance with non–insulin-dependent diabetes mellitus, slower metabolism	The physician will supplement as needed.
Immune System	Diminished production and function of T cells and B cells	Less resistance to illness	Encourage the client to obtain immunizations as age appropriate.
	Diminished ability to distinguish self from other	Increase in autoimmune diseases	Educate the client regarding symptoms of autoimmunity.
	Diminished defenses elsewhere (eg, gastrointestinal enzymes)	Overload on compromised immune system and more frequent serious illnesses	Encourage the client to obtain immunizations as age appropriate and to guard against communicable diseases.
Female Reproductive System	Decreased egg production	Menopause or climacteric	The physician may prescribe supplemental estrogen.
	Decreased estrogen production	"Hot flashes"; thinner, drier vaginal walls with vaginal itching and painful intercourse; osteoporosis	The physician may prescribe supplemental estrogen.
	Poor perineal muscle tone	Rectocele, cystocele, stress incontinence	Suggest exercises for strengthening the pelvic floor.
Male Reproductive System	Decreased penile and testicle size	Loss of libido	The physician may refer the client for counseling.
	Atherosclerosis and arteriosclerosis	Impotence	The physician may refer the client for counseling. Educate the client regarding good nutrition to avoid atherosclerosis.
	Benign prostatic hyperplasia (BPH)	Urgency, frequency, nocturia, retention	Encourage the client to have yearly checks for BPH, and provide instruction regarding testicular self-examination.

Source: Hosley, J. B., Jones, S. A., & Molle-Matthews E. A. (1997). *Lippincott's textbook for medical assistants* (p. 1024–1026). Philadelphia: Lippincott Williams & Wilkins.

is available in the living quarters as well. Laundry services are often available. Some of these complexes require a deposit or "buy in" fee in addition to a monthly charge. Some use a "sliding scale" rent. Older adults who live in a retirement complex have the advantage of living in close proximity to others of their age group, while having access to assistance and protective services when needed.

Long-Term Care Options

Long-term facilities have developed into specialized areas for care of older adults as well as for chronically ill younger people. Choosing a facility depends on availability of services, finances, and client needs. Some facilities have separate units in one building that serve the different needs of the clients. All

facilities should provide the best possible nursing care, in as homelike an atmosphere as possible (Box 91-1).

Long-term facilities offer four general options or levels of care:

1. *Assisted-living facility* provides room and board, laundry, and some personal nursing services; standards and regulations vary.
2. *Rehabilitative care facility* is often a unit within another facility; a client may transfer from an acute care facility and receive physical, occupational, or speech therapy. The facility provides 24-hour care for a few weeks or months, but the client eventually returns home after recovery from a disabling (eg, cerebrovascular accident) or traumatic (eg, hip fracture) experience.

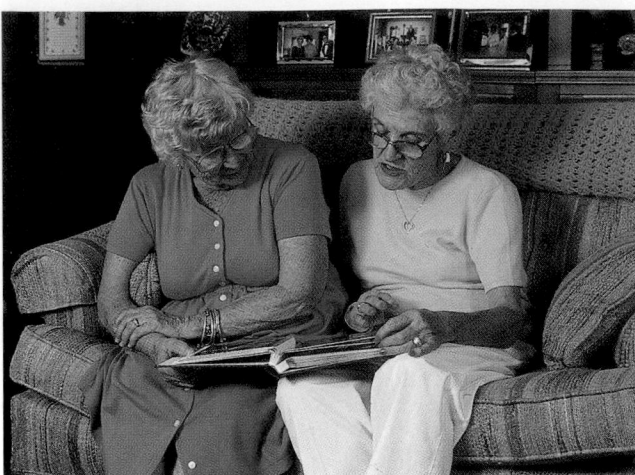

FIGURE 91-1. These older women, living at home, are using reminiscence to fulfill needs for friendship and stimulation.

➤➤ BOX 91-1

CHARACTERISTICS OF A HIGH-QUALITY SKILLED LONG-TERM CARE FACILITY

- Is licensed and regularly inspected by state or local government and is free of serious deficiencies
- Meets Medicare or Medicaid requirements
- Has a medical director (physician) who makes regular visits and is actively involved
- Has a staff of licensed nurses available 24 hours a day, 7 days a week
- Provides other healthcare and therapeutic care
- Provides special services for residents, such as a beautician or barber
- Provides rehabilitation services by trained personnel and encourages all residents to work toward rehabilitation
- Has an in-service program for all staff members
- Conducts routine staff member evaluations
- Maintains high standards of safety for residents and staff
- Provides nutritionally adequate food and special diets if needed
- Provides for social needs of the residents in a home-like atmosphere
- Has a well-planned and purposeful activities program
- Provides a recreational program
- Maintains a medical record, Kardex, and nursing assessment and care plan for each resident
- Makes provisions for obtaining necessary diagnostic laboratory and radiology services for the residents
- Encourages family and friends to visit often
- Encourages visits by young children (and many times by pets)
- Recognizes and provides for spiritual needs of residents

3. *Long-term care facility* (**LTC**) is often referred to as a *nursing home.* Clients are generally referred to as *residents* because the facility is their home or residence. The facility offers care from nurses, nurses' aides, and other healthcare workers who function as an interdisciplinary team. Each facility has a medical director and functions similarly to an acute care facility. However, LTC facilities generally do not have some of the on-site services that can be found in an acute care facility (eg, radiology). Services such as occupational therapy, physical therapy, rehabilitation, and hospice may be available and used according the each resident's individual needs. Other services are brought into the facility as needed (eg, portable x-ray equipment), or the resident may be transported to the location of the service (eg, CAT scan).

   Residents of LTC facilities have an attending physician who provides monitored care. In recent years, extensive governmental regulations have been instituted for LTC facilities, and the care given in such facilities has improved greatly. Nurses who work in LTC facilities have a significant amount of responsibility. These nurses, often LVN/LPNs, require special knowledge of the normal and abnormal progressions of aging, the nursing process, physical and mental dysfunctions, nutrition, and pharmacology.

   LTC facilities encourage family members to visit and provide care whenever appropriate. Healthcare professionals need to be aware of the importance of family and friends.

4. *Subacute care facility* is a recent addition to the range of long-term care facilities available. Typically, residents require more complex care and higher staffing levels than the usual long-term care resident, but not the intensity of care provided by an acute hospital. A subacute care unit can be a separate section within a hospital or long-term care facility, or a separate facility that exists solely for this purpose.

HELPING THE OLDER PERSON MEET BASIC NEEDS

Because of cumulative losses due to aging, older adults may need assistance from nurses or other healthcare workers to meet their basic needs. Clients have a tremendous diversity of needs. For example, some individuals need assistance with daily physical requirements; priorities for others may include financial, emotional, or social needs. The nurse must be aware of specific variations in a client's needs. Each environment in which a senior lives has advantages and resources, as well as disadvantages and limitations. Living at home helps the client retain independence. However, the home environment may limit social interaction or it may not provide adequate physical resources to maintain basic hygiene, nutritional, and healthcare needs.

Nutritional Needs

Individuals must maintain lifelong satisfactory nutritional status to prevent the premature deterioration of body systems.

Estimates are that one third to one half of all health problems of older adults relate directly or indirectly to inadequate nutrition and fluid intake. Balanced nutrition results in increased energy and a healthy mental outlook. In addition, medical or surgical conditions heal more rapidly with fewer complications when clients meet their nutrient needs. Chapter 30 discusses the basic nutritional needs of all people, and considers nutritional concerns for clients when planning care.

Proper nutrients must be available to build the thousands of compounds needed to maintain the body. The body must absorb, store, reorganize, or otherwise convert consumed nutrients into useful substances. To do so, the gastrointestinal system, pancreas, and liver must be healthy.

Older adults absorb nutrients more slowly, and their caloric needs are reduced due to the slowing of metabolism. In general, older adults need to consume fewer calories while meeting their specific nutrient requirements, which vary only slightly from younger people. Protein requirements do not change: a minimum of 1 gram of protein per kilogram of body weight is necessary for maintenance. An older adult whose body needs to build and repair tissues after injury (eg, pressure ulcer) or illness (eg, cancer) has greatly increased daily protein requirements. The older adult's fat intake should not exceed approximately 35% of total caloric intake. Fats with essential fatty acids are more nutrient dense than empty-calorie fats, such as in fried foods, alcohol, or chocolate. Vitamins and minerals are important; most can and should be obtained through a healthy diet, rather than supplements.

Factors such as the inconvenience and effort of food shopping, storage, and preparation also affect a person's nutritional status. The older person may have a reduced appetite because taste perception declines and he or she may be less physically active, or unable to shop or cook food as often. Poorly fitting dentures often limit a client's ability to eat. In care settings other than the home, a client may feel rushed during meals or may not like to eat at the times meals are served.

Weight control is harder as the person ages. The body's overall metabolic rate declines, making fat more difficult to eliminate than in younger years. Excess weight can seriously affect self-esteem and health. Disorders such as diabetes mellitus, hypertension, myocardial infarction, stroke, back and joint pains, and falling are related to obesity. To help control weight, a low-fat, low-calorie, nutrient-dense diet may be recommended. The quality versus the quantity of food intake becomes important. Increasing caloric expenditure through regular exercise can greatly assist in weight control.

Assessing Nutritional Status

Assessing nutritional status includes not only observing the person's food and fluid intake, but also understanding other factors that affect specific nutrients needed and consumed. Such factors include availability of food; the client's ability to purchase, shop for, and prepare food; health conditions that change nutritional needs; oral health; elimination patterns; independence in eating; mood and mental status; energy level; activity; cultural preferences; food likes and dislikes; effects of medications; and presence of symptoms (eg, pain, shortness of breath, nausea). You should assess the client's current weight and compare it with his or her usual weight. Weight loss within the past month that is greater than 5% of the total body weight, or a loss of 10% or more of body weight within the past 6 months, is significant. Report and discuss such findings with the client's physician. Encourage the client to eat. For clients with eating problems, try to determine why they do not want to eat, rather than forcing nutrition.

Special Considerations

Teeth and Chewing. Although tooth loss is not a normal event of aging, many older people wear dentures or have few teeth. These individuals must adapt food so that they can chew it and eat it. Oral care and denture care can facilitate the eating success of **edentulous** (without teeth) clients. Food that is adapted (eg, chopped, pureed, liquid) must be nutritionally balanced and attractively served.

Swallowing Difficulties. Older adults may have conditions that impair their swallowing mechanisms. Make certain that provided food is of a consistency that the client can swallow. The client may better tolerate semisolid foods and thickened liquids; they may prefer small, frequent meals to large, less frequent meals.

For meals, elevate the head of the bed, or if possible, have the client sit in a chair. Cutting food into edible bites will enable the client to chew it easily, and helps prevent choking. Suggesting that the client bend the chin toward the chest while swallowing can help in preventing **aspiration** (choking). Having a suction apparatus available at meals may be helpful. The client who has great difficulty swallowing or who refuses to eat can use special adaptive techniques; a speech therapist can provide suggestions for the client's specific condition.

Medications and Supplements. Table 91-2 describes implications of medication administration as related to the changes of aging. The nurse must be aware of the unique risks associated with medications for older clients. Because older adults have a high risk of complications associated with medications, be certain to educate clients about their purpose, proper administration, expected side effects, adverse effects, and special precautions.

The nurse may assist older clients to take oral medications by crushing tablets or by putting them into custard, cereal, applesauce, or ice cream. Do not crush enteric-coated tablets because they are not meant to be digested in the stomach. Be aware of medication–food interactions, including contraindications and side effects. "Tricking" a person into taking a medication by hiding it in food is illegal. Every person has the right to refuse medications unless a specific court order exists stating otherwise.

In a home setting, establishing a routine for medication administration is important. Additionally, the client is more likely to be compliant with a complicated medication regimen if a system is established. As seen in Figure 91-2, inexpensive organizers can be set up for the client for a day, a week, or longer. A list of current medications, times, and doses should be placed on the refrigerator (where emergency personnel can see it) as well as put into the client's wallet or purse (near the insurance card).

■■■ **TABLE 91-2** *C*HANGES IN AGING AS RELATED TO MEDICATION ADMINISTRATION

Factor	Nursing Implications
Decreased sense of thirst, dry oral mucosa	Difficulty swallowing meds; decreased absorption
Decreased total body fluid volume or percentage	Higher concentration of water-soluble drugs in blood
Decreased muscle tissue	Slower or decreased absorption of intramuscular medications, shorter needle may be needed
Increased percentage of fatty tissue	Accumulation of fat-soluble drugs; more difficulty locating site for intramuscular injection
Decreased general circulation	Slowed absorption; slowed transport of drugs to cells; slowed removal of drugs or wastes from cells
Decreased circulation to colon, vagina	Slower melting of suppositories
Decreased blood flow to liver and kidneys; decreased liver enzymes	Slowed metabolism and absorption; slowed excretion
Fewer functioning (kidney) nephrons; decreased tubular reabsorption	Slowed or faulty excretion; retention of drugs in body for longer time
Decreased stomach acids and other digestive fluids; lower stomach pH	Slowed absorption
Confusion, forgetfulness	Noncompliance with medication program

✚👁 **N u r s i n g A l e r t**

Observe for side effects when giving medications to older adults. The usual adult dose of an antidepressant is often toxic to the elderly person. In addition, any drug given to the older person may cause an effect opposite to that in a younger person (*paradoxical effect*).

Supplementation with vitamins and minerals is an area of continuing research. Vitamin deficiencies can greatly affect nutritional status in older adults. Excessive quantities of vitamins and minerals, however, are harmful and expensive. Calcium supplementation is often combined with exercise and estrogen as part of postmenopausal therapy for women. Self-administration of supplements is common in older adults. More research is needed to determine the benefits or dangers of vitamin and mineral supplements. Teaching is an important nursing consideration in the use of medications and supplements.

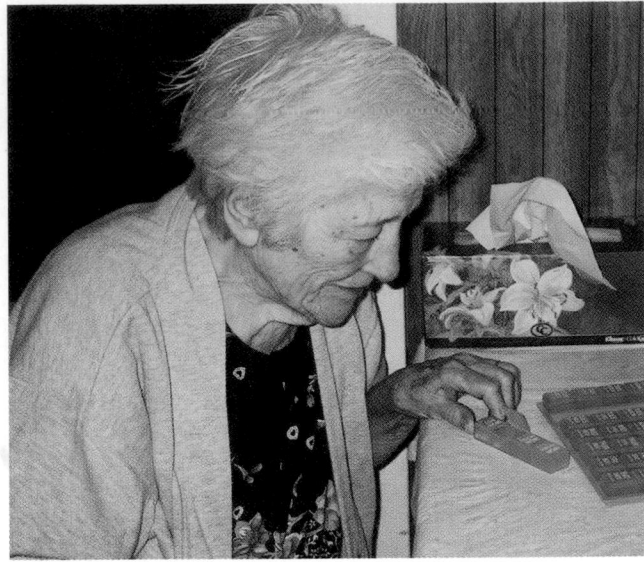

FIGURE 91-2. This older woman uses a multiple-dose, multiple-day medication dispenser to ensure that she takes her prescribed medications on time and in safe doses.

Water. Older adults need encouragement to drink adequate amounts of water. Generally, seniors have lower fluid reserves to protect them during periods of excess fluid loss or reduced fluid intake. Many older adults do not experience thirst as strongly as younger people. Immobile adults often do not drink adequate fluids. Sometimes the older adult avoids drinking fluids due to problems with urinary incontinence, urinary retention, or frequency. Dehydration is a serious and frequently overlooked problem in this age group. The nurse should offer a variety of fluids and provide assistance to clients who are unable to consume fluids independently.

☞ KEY CONCEPT

Older adults have proportionately less body fluid than younger persons and dehydrate very easily.

Supplementing Oral Intake

In many cases, the older person, particularly one who is ill, cannot eat and drink enough to maintain adequate nutritional status. In this event, an alternate means of supplying nutrients is needed to supplement or replace oral intake. The first choice involves oral supplements, such as Ensure or Resource. If these are not possible, other means must be used. Three major types of mechanical nutrient supplementation are intravenous therapy, total parenteral nutrition (TPN), and tube feedings.

Personal Hygiene Needs

Skin Care

Changes in the skin and circulatory system may cause older clients to be more susceptible to the development of pressure areas and skin breakdown. Because aging skin has few oils and is fragile, daily bathing is not always necessary and, in fact, can be harmful. However, daily hygiene measures remain important throughout the life span. Bed baths or sponge baths at the sink can be alternative hygiene measures. To promote circulation and a sense of independence, encourage older clients to do as much of their own hygiene as possible. Care can progress through the stages of dependent bed bath, sitting in a chair at the sink, assisted shower or bath, and finally self-care. This progression is a therapeutic measure to increase activity and promote self-esteem.

If a client is incontinent, keep the skin clean and dry to prevent irritation and breakdown. An older person's skin can become very dry, thin, and **friable** (easily broken). The nurse may apply lotion to keep the client's skin soft and to promote peripheral circulation. Special bath oils are available to keep the skin supple; the client should avoid harsh soaps.

☞ KEY CONCEPT

When bath oil is used, the tub may become slippery. Be careful to prevent falls.

Oral Hygiene

Encourage the client to care for the mouth to prevent dental difficulties and **halitosis** (bad breath). Clients with natural teeth need to brush and floss regularly; the use of mouthwash or swabs alone is not sufficient. Clients who have arthritis, cerebrovascular accidents, altered mental status, or other difficulties often require assistance with oral care. They may be embarrassed or unable to ask for assistance; therefore, you must actively provide the opportunity for oral hygiene. Make sure that the confused person does not lose his or her dentures.

> **Nursing Alert**
> Encourage older people with dentures to check the condition of their gums regularly. Irritation can result from poorly fitting dentures. Cancer of the mouth sometimes occurs and may go undetected.

Hair Care

Clients should shampoo their hair as needed to promote comfort and cleanliness. Because the older person's hair is often dry and brittle, he or she should not shampoo too often. A fresh hairdo or haircut may give the client a more positive self-image and improve self-esteem. Massaging the scalp during a shampoo can be relaxing. Most long-term care facilities and retirement communities have a hair salon with hairdressers available for the residents.

☞ KEY CONCEPT

Self-care of the hair is an excellent opportunity for active range-of-motion exercise.

Nail and Foot Care

The fingernails of older adults grow more slowly and are more brittle than those of younger persons. Toenails often become hard and thick, requiring a podiatrist to trim and care for them. Nails should be cut straight across. Corns and calluses can be soaked in warm water but are never cut; they also require a podiatrist's care and treatment. Encourage clients to wear proper-fitting flat or low-heeled shoes and comfortable hosiery. Clients should wash, thoroughly dry, and inspect their feet daily. When caring for a client's feet, document any injuries or discolored areas and report them to the client's physician. Even in healthy seniors, infection is possible, and wound healing is often slow in the extremities.

> **Nursing Alert**
> Most healthcare facilities do not allow nurses to cut the toenails or fingernails of diabetic clients.

Shaving

The self-esteem of older male clients may benefit from regular shaving. Allow the client to do as much for himself as possible. Be sure he is safe and responsible. Assist when needed, remembering that the skin may be more sensitive than that of a younger man. Be careful to prevent cuts. Postmenopausal women may occasionally have facial hair (**hirsutism**) that the client may want removed for cosmetic purposes.

Clothing

Choice of clothing depends on physical limitations and environment. Because aging adults often need more clothing to maintain internal warmth, layering of clothing is common. Allow residents of nursing homes to wear their own clothes, and encourage clients to dress in street clothes each day. Compliment their efforts to appear clean and well groomed. Sometimes a new shirt or dress can greatly enhance a client's morale. Encourage and assist women to apply cosmetics, if this has been part of their daily routine.

Elimination Needs

Difficulties with elimination stem from many causes. Peristalsis slows with age. Many people exercise less, and lack a good diet that promotes normal elimination. Foods such as whole grains, fruits, and vegetables provide needed fiber, complex carbohydrates, vitamins, and minerals. Generally, older clients do not take in enough fluids. They may deliberately reduce fluid intake as problems with voiding and defecation develop. Foods that they once tolerated now may be irritating.

Constipation

Older people may be misinformed about or preoccupied with bowel function. A daily bowel movement is not necessary for all individuals; if the client is eliminating regularly without discomfort and straining, he or she is not constipated. Discourage excessive use of laxatives or enemas because they can disturb or even eliminate the normal urge to defecate. Encourage clients to respond to the urge to defecate as soon as possible. Changes in fluid and food intake can often eliminate constipation. Prune juice, bran flakes, oatmeal, or apple-sauce are good alternatives to laxatives. Sometimes a laxative or mild stool softener (such as docusate sodium [Colace]) is required. Three or more days without a stool may indicate constipation, impaction, or infarction of the bowel. Nursing care in acute and long-term facilities requires daily monitoring of gastrointestinal function.

Bladder or Bowel Incontinence

Older clients may have difficulty controlling bladder and bowel functions. To overcome this problem, retraining is possible by following a regular schedule. Most clients eagerly accept a bladder or bowel retraining program because it can alleviate embarrassment.

Incontinence may embarrass clients. Be sensitive to treating this situation with dignity and discretion. Do not chide or scold clients for episodes. Provide assistance in cleaning the skin and changing clothes, as needed. Evaluate incontinence to identify its cause; some forms can be eliminated with correction of the underlying problem. Clients may be able to purchase and wear protective garments. Catheters are not the treatment of choice for urinary incontinence because they can introduce infection-causing microorganisms into the urinary tract.

Difficulty in Voiding

Anatomic changes in aging adults may cause difficulties with normal voiding. Weaker bladder muscles can contribute to the bladder retaining some urine after voiding. Fecal impaction is a common cause of urinary retention. Accurate intake and output records may be required to monitor excretory status.

Many older men have difficulty voiding because the prostate gland enlarges and obstructs urinary flow. This problem can be painful and embarrassing. Older men with an enlarged prostate must be examined on a regular basis. Surgery may be necessary in some cases.

☛ KEY CONCEPT

Even if the urine has dried, the skin of the incontinent client needs thorough cleansing to prevent skin breakdown from the irritating substances contained in urine.

HELPING THE OLDER ADULT MEET EMOTIONAL NEEDS

Psychological health is just as important as physical health. Because older adults often face *cumulative losses* (physical, financial, social), mental health problems are common. Health-care providers may overlook depression, anxiety, chemical dependency, and the possibility of suicide in older clients. Box 91-2 identifies possible signs of stress.

Encourage clients to remain self-sufficient and mentally active. Keeping mentally active helps prevent feelings of boredom and depression. Older adults should maintain as much independence as possible. Include clients in care planning and

➤➤ **BOX 91-2**

PHYSICAL, EMOTIONAL, AND MENTAL SIGNS OF STRESS IN THE AGING ADULT

- Elevated blood pressure
- Urinary frequency, loss of continence
- Diarrhea, loss of bowel continence
- Increased heart rate
- Dyspnea
- Insomnia or hypersomnia
- Fatigue
- Lack of attention to details
- Lack of concentration
- Lack of interest
- Lack of awareness to external stimuli
- Living in the past
- Forgetfulness
- Tearfulness
- Withdrawal
- Paranoia
- Depression
- Irritability
- Feelings of worthlessness

other activities. Provide maximum opportunities for them to participate in decision-making.

Mental Health Concerns in Older Clients

Chapter 93 discusses mental health and psychiatric issues in detail. Common mental health concerns for older adults follow.

Anxiety

Anxiety is a feeling of uneasiness or apprehension in response to some threat. The threat can be real (eg, disease pathology) or perceived (eg, fear of the unknown). Some limited anxiety is normal and can stimulate an individual to purposeful actions. Excessive or chronic (long-standing) anxiety can interfere with rational thinking and independent functioning. For aging clients, threats to self-image and self-esteem are common. These individuals may face loss of health, independence, the familial home, family contacts, and life itself. Anxiety can result in withdrawal, isolation, confusion, or combative or maladaptive behaviors. Anxiety is especially evident in older persons who are physically ill.

Treatment.   The nurse should first assess the level of the client's anxiety (mild, moderate, or panic-like). Available physical and emotional defense mechanisms should then be identified. Many times, increased knowledge reduces stress; the fear disappears because the stressor is identified and understood. Remain calm, provide outlets for excess energy, answer questions honestly, and give reassurance to the client. In some instances, referral of the client to a psychiatrist or other mental healthcare professional is necessary for evaluation and treatment.

Depression

Although depression is extremely common in older adults, it is not a normal part of aging. An estimated 10% to 50% of the elderly population exhibit some symptoms of depression. Cumulative losses and numerous changes, most of which are beyond a person's control, can lead to depression. Many older clients are reluctant to admit they are depressed. The stigma attached to psychiatric diagnoses is of much concern. Older clients may assume that they should be able to solve their own problems. They may believe that depression, fear, and loneliness are normal aspects of aging, or they may not even realize that they are depressed.

Clinical depression is often not diagnosed in older adults. Disease processes, side effects of medications, or adjustment to life cycle changes are possible causes of depression. Do not confuse clinical depression with *dementias,* which often contain an element of depression (see Chap. 92). Depression also can be a symptom of long-standing chemical dependency. Symptoms of depression include lack of interest in surroundings and in self-care, lack of energy and appetite, and altered sleep patterns. Suicidal ideation is a possibility. Depression in the elderly may also manifest itself in physical complaints (eg, constipation, anorexia, insomnia). (See In Practice: Educating the Client 91-1.)

Pseudodementia is a term used to describe a condition in depressed clients in which they give the impression of being demented when their behaviors actually are related to depression. Depression may be precipitated by a specific event but usually results from a combination of factors, including:

- Chemical imbalance
- Poor nutrition
- Financial difficulties
- Poverty-level subsistence
- Loss of spouse, friends, pets, roles
- Serious, chronic illness
- Debilitating disease
- Lack of mental or physical exercise
- Medication side effects; oversedation
- Drug or alcohol abuse

Treatment.   Reluctance to seek assistance, or failure of caregivers or healthcare providers to recognize symptoms, can hinder treatment for geriatric depression. The lack of medical professionals who specialize in geriatric psychiatry also limits therapy. The goal of therapy aims at increasing the client's self-esteem. Involvement in social, recreational, and cultural events is remotivating. Participating in volunteer services and caring for pets may be helpful. Many general suggestions for stress relief also relate to the treatment of depression. Encourage the older adult to get adequate exercise and to eat a balanced diet. Be sure that any general physical problems are being treated. Sometimes referral to a psychiatrist or other mental health provider is necessary. Various antidepressant medica-

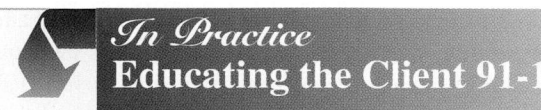

**In Practice
Educating the Client 91-1**

PREVENTION OF DEPRESSION AND ISOLATION IN THE OLDER PERSON

- Pursue an active social life with people of all ages. The place of worship usually has social gatherings. Senior citizen centers offer appropriate activities and encourage people to meet other people.
- Go back to school. The Elderhostel (Elder College) program offers educational programs throughout the United States and other countries. These programs stimulate the mind and offer opportunities for socializing.
- Join a support group. Share concerns, and gain insight from others in the group.
- Volunteer at the local hospital or civic organization. Some communities have babysitting services or daycare centers run by older people.
- Provide consulting service by joining a group such as SCORE (Service Corps of Retired Executives).
- Acquire a pet. This builds a sense of being needed and provides companionship.
- Go back to work. Many companies are encouraging retired people to come back to work. The older worker is reliable and dependable. It is also therapeutic for the person to have a place to go and to have responsibility and pride in having a job.
- Maintain good health practices (balanced diet, exercise, adequate rest).

tions also may be helpful. Remind clients and their caregivers that clients will need to use most antidepressants for 1 month (or more) before effects are noticeable. See In Practice: Educating the Client 91-1 for further suggestions on treating depression.

Suicide.   Suicide is a serious potential consequence of depression. The elderly population is the number one high-risk group for suicide, particularly older white men. The nurse should always take threats or gestures of suicide seriously.

Substance Abuse

Substance abuse is a special problem in the older population. Many factors contribute to geriatric chemical dependency. Loneliness and depression are especially significant.

The older substance abuser is often a widow or widower who no longer has a regular job. He or she may feel there is "nothing to do." The person's self-esteem suffers from a feeling of worthlessness and lack of purpose. Some people try to deal with these feelings by overusing chemicals, most often alcohol or prescription drugs. They may also abuse substances to deal with anxiety. Some older adults believe that substance abuse is a problem of the young. They may deny the possibility that they or others of their age group could have a chemical dependency problem.

Alcoholism in older persons may be difficult to detect. Family and friends may not be aware of their loved one's situation. For older adults who do not have frequent visitors, covering up chemical dependency during occasional visits is easy.

Relatives may think the person is "just confused," when in fact he or she is under the influence of alcohol. If the person is widowed, the former spouse may have covered up and enabled the alcoholism for a long time. The lack of a known alcohol problem can cause family members to disbelieve that their elder relative is an alcoholic. The situation often does not get out of control until the person is alone or retired.

Approximately 40% of all adverse drug reactions occur in people over 65 years of age, a rate that is approximately five times that of younger people. One sixth of all hospital admissions of people over age 70 relate to medication complications. There are several contributing factors. Medications react differently in older persons. Many individuals have little knowledge of medication interactions. Some older adults see no harm in sharing medications with friends or a spouse, or in using medications after the expiration date. They may mix several different medications in the same container or misuse over-the-counter medications. They may forget how much medication they took, or even if they took medications at all. They may be using chemicals as self-medication and taking doses larger than those prescribed. Some individuals may deliberately search out several physicians to obtain added prescriptions.

Even conscientious elders can experience difficulties by taking duplicate prescriptions, because some are labeled in generic names, whereas others use brand names. Some seniors have several physicians who prescribe separate, and often conflicting, medications. (The use of a single pharmacy that can maintain a drug profile for the client can prove useful and spare the older adult unnecessary expense and complications.)

Treatment of substance abuse in older adults is difficult. Older clients may be more resistant than younger chemically dependent people. They may resent younger people, especially their own children, telling them what to do. Denial of the problem is common. Before treatment can begin, the individual must accept help and be prepared to change lifestyle patterns.

Measures for Emotional and Psychological Support

☛ KEY CONCEPT

Evaluate confusion in older adults for organic pathologies and substance abuse.

Remotivation Techniques.   *Remotivation* is an important adjunct to therapy. This reality orientation attempts to focus attention on the present, calling on memories from the client's past (*reminiscence*). Sharing memories encourages participation. Reminiscence and reality orientation are useful strategies to promote mental stimulation and validation of life's past events (see Fig. 91-1).

Recreation.   Recreation is important at any age. In a long-term care facility, an activity or recreation director plans and directs events designed to promote creativity. The goal is to motivate seniors to use their physical and mental capabilities.

Cognitive Function.   Age alone does not result in a loss of cognitive function; older adults normally comprehend and appropriately use and understand language, perform basic calculations, and retain and recall information. Intelligence does not decline with age, but rather reflects lifelong intellectual capacity. Although short-term memory loss is common, exercise of memory function helps to maintain and improve it. Older adults are able to learn, although they require adjustments for slower responses, sensory deficits, and physical limitations. Motivation and readiness to learn are important. Lack of direction and decreased stimulation contribute to decreased mental alertness and comprehension. Changes in cognitive function can accompany a wide range of physical and mental health problems. When cognitive changes are noted, evaluation is warranted.

Social Life and Activities.   Encourage the client to carry on a normal social life and to engage in as many previous activities as possible. Include family members in the plan of care. Encourage them to visit and to take the older person with them on trips and outings.

Older people naturally love to see grandchildren and other children. They usually are interested in young people and will enjoy sharing their own youthful recollections with them. Often, nursing students are favorites among residents of long-term care centers.

Pet Therapy.   Many older clients welcome pets. Pets can provide companionship, stimulate the sense of touch, facilitate interactions, and encourage a sense of responsibility. Many confused clients respond to animals, even when they fail to respond to other people. Pet therapy has proven beneficial in geriatrics and is an accepted activity in many nursing homes.

Religious Support.   Religious practices can be extremely therapeutic. Studies have shown that older adults who engage in religious practices have higher levels of health and function than those who do not. Support clients in their religious practices. Provide privacy when a member of the clergy comes to visit. Many hospitals and long-term care facilities have visiting clergy who conduct religious services; encourage residents to attend if they so desire. If attending services is impossible due to limitations, you may be able to arrange tape recordings of services, or arrange for visitors to read scripture or pray with the client.

Use of Volunteers.   Most community organizations for older adults have volunteers who assist in the agency's activity programs. These volunteers are essential; always encourage their participation when you work with them. Volunteers provide many important services to clients, such as visiting those who have no other visitors, taking residents of long-term care facilities on outings, helping with craft activities, providing parties and entertainment, and assisting with reading or writing letters.

Church groups or service clubs often work with nursing-home residents as a special service. Because nursing-home residents especially enjoy the company of younger people, teens and young adults should be encouraged to assist in the activities of local nursing homes. Not only is this practice meaningful to the residents, but it is also rewarding for young people.

A staff member should coordinate the duties of volunteers to make certain they are helping residents. Encourage all volunteers to keep confidences and to treat clients with respect. If a volunteer makes a commitment to be at the facility on a certain day, he or she needs to meet this obligation. Residents rely on and look forward to visits and may become upset when volunteers miss their appointments. Volunteers should develop empathy. They need patience to help residents perform independently, because it is not helpful just to do things for them.

Many older adults make good volunteers as well. They often have the time and patience required to make valuable contributions. Their involvement as volunteers can add meaningful activities and a sense of purpose to their own lives, while at the same time helping others.

SPECIAL CONCERNS OF THE AGING ADULT

Communication

The senses of older adults are less acute than those of younger people due to the physiologic changes of aging. Hearing and visual deficits can cause many older people to have difficulties in communication. Conditions such as stroke and dementia can alter language comprehension and use.

Age barriers may add to the difficulties of engaging in social interaction. Older adults can avoid feelings of isolation and rejection if they regularly talk with others. In a hospital or nursing-home setting, placing older clients in double rooms is usually best, to help prevent isolation and provide more environmental stimulation. Encourage older clients with whom you work to participate in social events.

Communication is a two-way process. Therapeutic and social communication have different approaches. Be aware of the meanings of touch and body language. Make appropriate eye contact and show genuine interest when visiting. Listen attentively and sit down when speaking to demonstrate interest and respect. Encourage visits from family, friends, and family pets.

Visual Impairment

Although many older people have difficulty seeing because of cataracts or other eye disorders, encourage their participation in activities as much as they are able. Provide aids for the visually impaired, such as large numbers on the telephone and calendar, or magnifying glasses for reading. Remove obstacles that could cause falls. Protect these clients from falling because they may be unaware of safety risks in their environment. Teach them what hazards exist and how to avoid them.

Presbyopia. **Presbyopia** is the specific name for impaired vision that results from normal aging. Presbyopia is caused by a loss of elasticity in the lens of the eye. As the person ages, the lens becomes more inflexible and therefore does not become convex enough to focus on nearby objects. The first symptom often is an inability to read small print, such as the telephone book. Eyeglasses can usually correct this condition. The client will probably need bifocals to allow for far and near vision.

The older person will find that he or she needs more light for reading because the pupils cannot adapt as well. As a rule, illumination (footcandle level) must double for each added 13 years of age beyond 40. Night blindness also increases with age. A night light in the client's room helps prevent injury.

☛ KEY CONCEPT

Clients should clean eyeglasses daily with a soft, dry cloth. Teach them to avoid using paper products to clean because they may scratch the lenses.

Dry eyes can be uncomfortable and irritating, thereby affecting vision. Although dry eyes are a common outcome of normal aging, for some individuals they result from an autoimmune disease called Sjögren's syndrome. This disease causes a drying of the mucous membranes, including the eyes. Persons with Sjögren's syndrome often feel that something is in their eyes and may rub them, causing irritation. Eye drops, such as artificial tears (HypoTears, Isopto Alkaline, Liquifilm Forte, Refresh), are often prescribed.

Hearing Loss

A specific hearing disorder of aging is called *presbycusis*. It begins at approximately age 40 and progresses with age. **Presbycusis** is a sensorineural hearing problem that first affects the client's ability to hear high-frequency sounds (eg, f, ph, s, and sh sounds). As presbycusis progresses, other sounds are affected as well.

Evaluate the client who has a hearing loss to determine if a hearing aid can assist. If so, encourage the client to wear the hearing aid, even if the client is reluctant to do so. Special devices are available for telephones and televisions to enable hearing-impaired persons to hear them better.

Encourage the client to let people know if speech is not heard. Sometimes, using different words to communicate the same message can be helpful. Eliminate distracting background noises. If a client totally loses hearing, communication can be written or signed with the hands. Newspapers and magazines will help keep the hearing-impaired client aware of current events.

Speech Impairment

Aphasia is the inability to use or understand speech. It is often a mixture of deficits, such as slow speech, incorrect speech, or the use of incorrect words and sounds. Aphasia often occurs after a cerebrovascular accident. The client may be unaware of the communication problem. He or she may not be able to understand speech or writing, or may have trouble naming objects. Remember to converse with the client, even if the client is unable to speak. Encourage the client to communicate in other ways (gestures, picture boards, diagrams, writing). Speech therapy is often helpful. Patience is necessary when communicating with aphasic people; they are probably frustrated, and hurrying makes the situation worse.

☛ KEY CONCEPT

Talk to the person, not about the person. Often, the person with aphasia has clear thinking processes.

Safety

Accidents, particularly falls, increase significantly with age and are a leading cause of disability and death after age 65. In addition to falls, the greatest dangers are fire, suffocation, and poisoning. The most common locations for accidents are the bedroom, bathroom, and kitchen. Most accidents are preventable.

Older people may be unsteady on their feet or may misjudge their physical capabilities. Medications or age-related changes can contribute to *orthostatic (postural) hypotension.* The client may become lightheaded and fall when getting out of a bed or chair. Changes in visual acuity and depth perception disturb the person's ability to judge distance. An assessment of the presence of risk factors for falls can be useful in identifying risks and planning measures to reduce them.

Educate the older adult and family about home hazards. Safety teaching is important (see In Practice: Educating the Client 91-2). Be sure all people on the staff of the healthcare facility know about these safety measures.

Loss of Proprioception

Proprioception is the awareness of posture, movement, and changes in equilibrium in relation to other objects. As people age, they may lose or experience alterations in their sense of proprioception. Many older people are unsure of where they are stepping, especially if they are walking on dark floors, bare ground, or dark paved areas. They have more difficulty staying erect without looking. Older adults who have a loss of proprioception may lose their balance when hyperextending the neck to look up at a clock or a high shelf. Lost balance is hard to regain. Teach clients to be aware of obstacles and uneven ground. When walking with older persons, allow them to take your arm, and do not push or pull. Also, avoid quick turns to prevent loss of balance.

✚👁 Nursing Alert

Many older people are afraid of falling and may grab you or furniture when they are lifted or moved. Never rush or frighten clients when assisting them.

Safety Devices

Numerous safety devices for the home and healthcare facility are available. Bathtubs and showers can be equipped with anti-slip surfaces, hand bars, and rails. Night lights are essential for bathrooms and bedrooms. Adaptive devices that make getting on and off the toilet more safely are available. To assist with balance, the older person may use a cane, walker, or other assistive device.

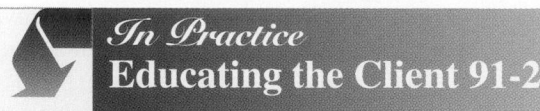

In Practice
Educating the Client 91-2

SAFETY PRECAUTIONS FOR THE AGING ADULT IN THE HOME

• Move with caution, especially on stairs and at curbs.
• Stand up slowly to avoid postural hypotension or dizziness.
• Safe-proof the house. Cover cords that might cause falls. Place furniture where it will not be tripped over. Grab bars should be placed on tubs, showers, toilets, and stairways.
• Ensure adequate lighting in all living areas. Night lights must be used at night in bedroom, bathroom, and stairs.
• Use ambulatory devices (canes, walkers, wheelchairs) as needed.
• Follow good housekeeping practices. Clean clutter and spills.
• Establish an emergency calling system with family and friends, neighbors, and local emergency medical services.
• Place a telephone near the bed for night emergencies.
• Place a fire extinguisher in the kitchen, and know how to use it. Know how to use smoke detectors, and check batteries regularly. Do not smoke in bed.
• Carry a list of medications. Understand use of medications and side effects. Review use of medications periodically. Do not drive while taking medications that cause drowsiness or dizziness.
• Wear suitable and safe clothing: Avoid flowing robes and nightgowns, flowing sleeves, floppy slippers, long shoelaces.
• Understand problems with loss in proprioception.
• Obtain help with banking, especially with Social Security check. Ensure safety on the street when coming from the bank, going to the mailbox, and so forth.
• Prevent scams. Caution the client about financial "deals," especially from strangers. Banks can establish an "alert" if a great amount of money is withdrawn or if more than a certain amount is withdrawn.

In the Hospital
• Use call lights and ask for assistance, especially if getting out of bed at night to go to the bathroom.
• Keep beds in low position.
• Use a transfer belt when assisting an unsteady person to walk.

N u r s i n g   A l e r t
Whenever you use a mechanical lift to assist a client into or out of a tub or bed, you must have thorough familiarity with the equipment's operation and safety factors.

Restraints (Client Safety Devices)

All healthcare providers and families need to learn about the use and abuse of restraints. In addition to devices placed on the wrists and waist to restrict movement, anything that limits the client's free movement is considered a *restraint.* For example, a tray attached to wheelchair that prevents the client from freely moving is a restraint. Another restraint is the **chemical restraint,** in which medications are given to control behavior.

If restraints are necessary, use them only after alternatives have failed to help. Generally a physician's order is required to apply restraints. Consult with the physician when you and other healthcare providers have exhausted other options. Explain to both the client and family or visitors that the purpose of the restraint is to keep the client safe. Never use restraints for your own convenience. A call light must always be within the client's reach if restraints are used. Proper application and frequent monitoring are necessary to prevent injury and ensure safety. Some clinical facilities have special forms for documentation of the use of the restraint, the times that the restraint is checked, and the documentation of the behaviors that necessitate a restraint.

Although intended to reduce accidents, restraints can result in serious injury, such as strangulation, which may be a risk if a client attempts to escape from the physical restraint. The client often feels powerless and without any control of his or her situation. He or she will often exert much energy in an attempt to get out, and will fight against the restraint, causing self-injury. A chemically restrained client often becomes confused and suffers impaired mental function; this client can fall and become injured. Because of these potential hazards, federal and state agencies that monitor and regulate healthcare facilities have placed restrictions on the use of restraints of any nature. Nurses should be aware of the policies that affect them and their employers.

Alternatives to physical or chemical restraints should be considered whenever possible. Frequently remind the client to ask for assistance, and provide reassurance that someone is available and willing to assist if needed. This information may help the client feel more powerful and make him or her less likely to attempt escape. If the client is awake, aware, and cooperative but is at risk of falling due to physical weakness or impairment, consider using a "soft restraint," which is usually a fabric belt or jacket-type device that is secured with Velcro rather than a buckle or tie. The client can undo the restraint if desired. If you place this type of restraint on the client, explain that the device is used to keep him or her safe, and that the restraint will remind him or her to call for help if he or she wishes to move.

Side rails are another form of restraint. Both side rails should not be up on all beds unless proper justification exists. However, keep in mind that having one side rail up may assist the client when moving in or out of bed. To prevent falls, beds should remain in the lowest possible position. Instruct the client to ask for assistance when getting out of bed. Hospital beds are available for home use.

N u r s i n g   A l e r t
In some situations, the client is in more danger with the side rails of the bed up. A bed left in low position is safer than the client climbing over the side rails and falling.

Physical Activity and Exercise

Physical activity is an important part of a total health program for all people. Exercise is vital to maintain circulation, muscle tone, and general health, and to prevent disuse deformities. The client should participate in exercise that complements his or her lifestyle. The benefits of exercise are reviewed in Table 91-3. The ambulatory person can walk, stretch, swim, do t'ai chi and yoga, or participate in competitive activities. Exercises may be modified to suit individual needs. Encourage clients of all ages to participate in active range-of-motion exercises; if this not possible, provide passive range of motion.

☛ KEY CONCEPT

Almost everyone can walk. Walking is the single most highly recommended exercise for older adults.

Immobility is a significant threat to older adults. The dangers of bed rest, even of short duration, and lengthy sitting include contractures, pressure ulcers, constipation, renal and

■■■ **TABLE 91-3** 𝓑ENEFITS OF EXERCISE

System Targeted	Benefits
Cardiovascular	Increases endurance Lowers cholesterol to avoid atherosclerosis Maintains vascular elasticity to delay arteriosclerosis
Musculoskeletal	Increases bone mass to reduce osteoporosis Decreases fat:muscle ratio to maintain metabolism Retains strength and flexibility to ensure mobility and improve posture
Nervous	Improves mental health by reducing stress, fatigue, tension, and boredom Maintains or restores balance to reduce falls

Source: Hosley, J. B., Jones, S. A., & Molle-Matthews E. A. (1997). *Lippincott's textbook for medical assistants* (p. 1029). Philadelphia: Lippincott Williams & Wilkins.

pulmonary complications (especially pneumonia), cardio-vascular disorders, depression, and social isolation.

Osteoporosis is common. Radiologic examination may detect loss of bone density, fractures, or loss of vertebral height (Fig. 91-3). Bone tissue loses density and strength without exercise; thus, fractures may occur very easily. Exercise can assist in reducing mineral loss from the bones. **Kyphosis** (curvature of the spine) can be associated with osteoporosis; this typically causes a humpbacked appearance ("dowager's hump" or "widow's hump"). Appropriate diet, increased calcium intake, supplementary vitamin D, and fluoride may be helpful. Post-menopausal women may be treated with calcium and cyclic estrogen administration. Physical activities promote physical and mental stimulation and help prevent such problems from developing.

Sexuality

The older adult generally maintains the ability and desire to engage in sexual activity. Physical changes due to aging may require some modifications. Menopause has no effect on sexual desire. Physical acts of affection, with or without intercourse, are important for an individual's physical and emotional well-being. The closeness of hugging and holding hands can alleviate feelings of loneliness. Touch can be therapeutic and beneficial at any age. Recognize the value of physical contact for older clients and assure them that the desire to be sexually attractive and active is normal. Encourage clients to discuss with their healthcare provider the impact of health conditions on sexual activity.

ELDER ABUSE

Elder abuse includes emotional, physical, and sexual abuse, financial exploitation, or neglect of older persons. Abuse or neglect may relate to health status and care, personal freedom, property, or income. Abuse takes many forms: any action that places a person in jeopardy may be considered abusive or neglectful. For example, sales gimmicks, medical quackery, fear tactics, and "con games" are considered exploitation of the older person. Organizations such as insurance companies, mail-order sales companies, or religious groups may defraud older adults intentionally or accidentally. Many older people are considered **vulnerable adults.** Abuse of vulnerable adults is a crime, and all people, including family members and healthcare workers, are subject to laws protecting vulnerable adults. The most common elder abusers are, in descending order, adult children, other relatives, spouses, service providers, friends or neighbors, grandchildren, and siblings.

The exhaustion and frustration of daily obligations related to the care of an older person can be overwhelming and is called **caregiver stress.** Be alert to signs of caregiver stress in a family because it may lead to mistreatment. Older adults often fail to report abuse; witnesses are difficult to obtain, and many older victims often fear retaliation. Box 91-3 lists warning signs of elder abuse.

Prevention of elder abuse begins with the recognition of high-risk families, including those families with a recent disruption in lifestyle or living arrangements, financial problems, substance abuse, a history of violence, or mental illness. The greater the number of risk factors, the greater the tendency toward abuse. When working with older clients, remember to address the needs of caregivers as well as those of the client. Caregivers need to know what resources are available; a respite from daily care can offer them relief. Accessible community resources include social service agencies, home healthcare and homemaker services, and Meals on Wheels.

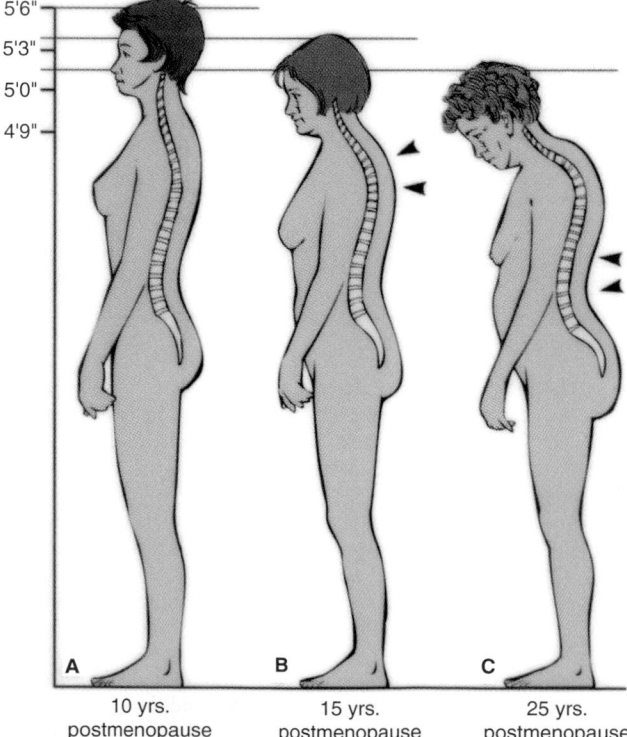

FIGURE 91-3. Typical loss of height associated with osteoporosis and aging. **(A)** Loss at 10 years postmenopause. **(B)** Loss at 15 years postmenopause: 1.5 inches. **(C)** Loss at 25 years postmenopause: 3.5 inches.

➤➤ BOX 91-3

WARNING SIGNS OF ELDER ABUSE

- Frequent trips to healthcare facility
- History of unexplained injuries
- Untreated conditions or wounds
- Malnutrition or weight loss
- Poor grooming
- Inability to perform activities of daily living
- Inappropriate medication administration
- Depression, withdrawal, substance abuse
- Excessive fear
- Spending or donating large sums of money

☛ KEY CONCEPT

Be observant and aware of the possibility of elder abuse. In most states, it is illegal for a healthcare professional not to report abuse.

➤ STUDENT SYNTHESIS

Key Points

- The normal aging process does not cause specific illnesses. Lifestyle adjustments are necessary, however, to compensate for physical changes.
- Most seniors live at home. Some older adults live in specially adapted living situations.
- Many health problems in older adults relate directly or indirectly to nutrition.
- Older adults may need adjustments to basic personal hygiene measures. Skin care, nail and foot care, and adapted clothing are special areas of concern.
- Appropriate preventive care for constipation includes adequate fiber and fluids. Clients should avoid dependence on laxatives.
- Medications are a primary cause of problems for elderly clients. Responses to medications include confusion, dizziness, potentiation of drugs, increased sensitivity to drug dosages, and an increased number of side effects.
- Anatomic changes may lead to problems with continence.
- Presbyopia, presbycusis, and aphasia are three conditions that may hinder an older person's ability to communicate.
- Safety is an important consideration for older adults, due to the loss of the sense of proprioception.
- Older clients must remain physically and mentally active to prevent anxiety, depression, and disorders related to immobility.
- The nurse must report cases of suspected elder abuse.

Critical Thinking Exercises

1. A client for whom you provide care lives with his daughter, her husband, and their children. He spends 2 days a week in adult daycare. What are the advantages for the client, for adult caregivers, and for grandchildren in the home? What are possible disadvantages?
2. Discuss the ways future generations of older adults could differ from today's elderly population. Give reasons for your responses.
3. An older adult you meet in a community screening program is malnourished. Develop a plan to assist in improving the client's nutritional status. What might be causative factors?

NCLEX-Style Review Questions

1. An older adult client has difficulty swallowing. What nursing action would be appropriate?
   a. Break enteric-coated tables into smaller pieces.
   b. Crush tablets and put in applesauce.
   c. Hide the medication in the client's food.
   d. Offer vitamin and mineral replacements.
2. A nurse is caring for an older adult client who has serious health problems and whose spouse has just died. The nurse knows that the client is at risk of developing:
   a. Anxiety
   b. Constipation
   c. Depression
   d. Heart failure
3. A older adult client complains of not being able to read because the print is too small. The nurse will document this as:
   a. Aphasia
   b. Loss of proprioception
   c. Presbycusis
   d. Presbyopia

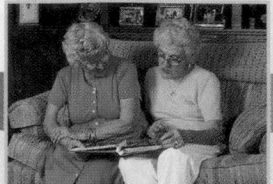

CHAPTER

92

Dementias and Related Disorders

LEARNING OBJECTIVES

1. Differentiate among confusion, delirium, and dementia.
2. List the components of dementia as defined by the American Psychiatric Association.
3. Describe Alzheimer's disease, its physiologic changes, and theories about its cause.
4. Identify the stages of Alzheimer's disease, with accompanying common behaviors. State at least four nursing concerns for each stage.
5. Name at least two common medications used to treat Alzheimer's disease and two common adverse reactions to the medications.
6. Explain why all medication must be used with caution in older adults.
7. Identify how multi-infarct dementia differs from Alzheimer's disease.
8. Describe common methods used to diagnose dementias.
9. Discuss functional assessment of the person with dementia.
10. Apply the nursing process as it relates to clients with dementia.

NEW TERMINOLOGY

ambiguous loss
apraxia
balking
catastrophic reaction
confabulation
confusion
delirium

dementia
organic brain syndrome
paranoia
pseudodementia
respite care
senility

ACRONYMS

AD	MID	SDAT
ALT	MRI	SGPT
CJD	PET	SPECT
HD		

The previous chapter discussed normal changes associated with aging, as well as common problems in late life. This chapter examines some forms of dementia that may occur in the later years, and discusses nursing implications associated with these dementias.

☛ KEY CONCEPT

The American Psychiatric Association states that classification of dementia is based on the irreversible, progressive nature of the problem and its underlying pathology.

CONFUSION, DELIRIUM, AND DEMENTIA

reversible

Confusion, an impairment of mental function, means poor judgment, impaired memory, and disorientation to time, place, situation, or person. The confused individual may lack orderly thought processes or be unable to make decisions. Confusion may be a symptom of an acute problem, such as dehydration or severe emotional stress, or it may be associated with a chronic, organic mental disorder, such as Alzheimer's disease. Confusion always indicates an abnormality because loss of cognitive function is not an expected component of the aging process.

Delirium begins with confusion, sleep disturbances, and restlessness. It progresses to anxiety, delusions, hallucinations, or fear. Delirium has a sudden onset (often hours or days) and usually is reversible. In the past, delirium was referred to as *acute brain syndrome.* Causes of delirium include physical illness, diabetic reaction, drug or alcohol toxicity, dehydration, malnutrition, head trauma, sensory deprivation or overload, systemic infection, electrolyte disturbance, stress, severe sleep deprivation, and reaction to being in an unfamiliar environment (eg, hospitalization or admission to a nursing home).

Although delirium can occur at any age, older adults are more vulnerable to occasional episodes. Delirium does not result from the normal aging process. Older clients simply have more physical and metabolic difficulties due to deterioration of physical systems, and can easily experience conditions that disrupt the body's balance and cause altered mental status. In addition, older persons are more likely to take multiple medications, which can produce delirium as an adverse effect.

In addition to changes in cognition, delirium typically causes an altered level of consciousness. The client's level of consciousness can vary from extreme drowsiness to hyperactivity. Early recognition of the signs of delirium will ensure timely treatment and reverse the problem.

Dementia literally means "mind away." *Progressive dementia* is a chronic, irreversible condition that affects cognitive function, which is the ability to think, understand, and interact with the surrounding world. Eventually dementia interferes with a person's ability to function normally and provide self-care. Although rare, some forms of dementia are caused by nutritional deficiencies or infections and may be reversed. Progressive dementias are characterized by deterioration of intellect, memory, judgment, basic arithmetic abilities, language, and independence. Dementia does not affect level of consciousness.

Formerly, dementia was referred to as **senility** or **organic brain syndrome.** More than 60 causes of dementia exist, with Alzheimer's disease being the most common.

Pseudodementia is a term used to describe a condition in which a client has the appearance of dementia, but whose confusion results from depression. Usually, the confusion clears when the depression is treated.

☛ KEY CONCEPT

When first meeting an individual who has a cognitive dysfunction, the nurse may find it difficult to determine if the disruption is due to confusion, delirium, or dementia. Learning about the history of onset and assessing the client's level of consciousness can help differentiate the condition.

TYPES OF DEMENTIAS

In early stages, individuals and their families may not notice the signs and symptoms of dementia (eg, difficulty with simple calculations, poor memory, and impaired abstract thinking). Changes are usually *insidious* (gradual and cumulative). As the condition progresses, the person has increasing difficulty with social interactions and functional skills. Personality changes occur; exaggerated emotions are common. The prevalence of dementia increases with age. Alzheimer's disease accounts for more than half the cases of dementia. Multi-infarct dementia accounts for approximately 10% to 20% of the cases. Other causes include:

- Parkinson's disease
- Wernicke-Korsakoff syndrome (related to chronic alcohol abuse)
- Pick's disease
- Creutzfeldt-Jakob disease (infectious)
- Huntington's disease (HD, hereditary)
- Dementia caused by acquired immunodeficiency syndrome (AIDS)
- Crack-related dementia; dementias caused by other illegal drugs
- Normal-pressure hydrocephalus
- Brain trauma
- Metabolic disorders (such as diabetes mellitus or end-stage renal disease)
- Drug overdose (toxic dementia)
- Dementia of tertiary syphilis (Bayle's disease)

Before a person can be diagnosed as having an irreversible condition causing dementia, other possible causes of the symptoms must be eliminated. Box 92-1 lists some factors to consider in the identification of dementia.

Alzheimer's Disease (AD)

Alzheimer's disease (**AD**), sometimes called *senile dementia of the Alzheimer's type* (**SDAT**), is a progressive, irreversible, fatal neurologic disorder that affects an estimated 4 million American adults. Estimates are that by the year 2040,

IDENTIFICATION OF DEMENTIA

- Short-term and long-term memory impairment
- At least one of the following: impairment of executive functioning (such as abstract thinking, judgment, or planning); disturbances of higher cortical functioning (such as aphasia or apraxia); inability to identify or recognize common objects (with sensory function intact); or personality change
- Above disturbances significantly interfere with work, social activities, or relationships with others
- Absence of delirium or intoxication (which could cause the same symptoms); absence of known organic cause
- Insidious onset with progressive deterioration

Exclusion of other causes of the symptoms:

- Rule out possible causes, such as stroke or brain tumors.
- Determine if the patient has abnormal blood tests, including serum folate and serum B_{12}.
- Computed tomographic scan shows cerebral atrophy only (no other disorders).
- Electroencephalogram shows slow-wave activity only (no other disorders).

_____
Adapted from American Psychiatric Association (2000). *Diagnostic and statistical manual of mental disorders* (4th ed., text rev.). Washington, DC: Author.

approximately 14 million Americans will be diagnosed with AD. Researchers believe that the number of people with AD will triple in the next 50 years. The disease's duration averages 2 to 10 years, but can last for up to 20 years. This epidemic is not confined to sex (although it is more common in women), race, or social or economic class. The public sometimes refers to this disorder as "senility," although the term "Alzheimer's" is becoming more common. (Allow clients and their families to use terminology with which they are comfortable.)

☛ KEY CONCEPT

Although the incidence of AD increases with each decade of life, this condition is not a normal outcome of aging.

Theories of Causes

Scientists have not identified a single cause of AD, although various hypotheses are continually being tested. Some theories are supported by results of research; others are controversial. Several causes have been hypothesized:

Genetic: A familial tendency may exist, possibly related to a defective chromosome. (Approximately 85% of people with Down syndrome develop AD in midlife.)
Viral: Viruses cause other dementias (kuru, Creutzfeldt-Jakob). A slow virus (one that remains inactive in the body for a long time) hypothesis is being tested.

Toxic: Aluminum has received publicity as a possible cause; however, aluminum deposits in the brain may be a result of AD rather than a cause. Other *toxins* (poisons) are possible causes.
Immunologic: Autoimmune processes ("antibrain antibodies") have been identified.
Trauma: Tissue injury due to serious head injury has been studied.
Biochemical: Neurotransmitter deficiency caused by degeneration is under investigation.
Nutritional: Malnutrition may play a role in predisposing a person to AD.

Box 92-2 lists risk factors for AD.

Physiologic Changes

The microscopic changes seen in the brain (cerebral cortex) of a person with AD have a distinct appearance. The pathophysiology of AD is based on biochemical, morphologic studies of brain tissue obtained by biopsy or autopsy. Three major changes occur in the brain:

- Cerebral cortex atrophy
- Loss of neurons
- Changes in brain cells

Brain cell changes include:

Abnormal neurons, arranged in filaments called *neurofibrillary tangles*—delicate abnormal fibers or threads of proteins
Senile (neuritic) plaques—round or ovoid clusters of destroyed synapses, embedded in a central amyloid core

RISK FACTORS FOR ALZHEIMER'S DISEASE

- *Age*—Prevalence:
  - 2% to 4% in ages 65–85
  - More than 20% in age 85+
  - Greatest incidence over age 85
- *Sex*—Incidence equal when adjusted for age (women live longer)
- *Serious head injuries*—15% to 20% of patients have had serious head injury (up to 35 years before onset)
- *History of thyroid disorders*—Some increase in incidence noted, rationale uncertain
- *Genetics*—Evidence suggests autosomal dominant inheritance; not proven
- *Age of onset*—Varies (even in identical twins)
- *Metabolic or environmental factors*—Suspected, not proven
- *Chromosomal abnormalities*—Alzheimer's seen in approximately 85% of adults with Down syndrome over age 40; other chromosomal abnormalities reported

Granulovacuolar degeneration—the inside of the cell is crowded with fluid-filled vacuoles and granular material

A significant decrease in the brain's ability to make acetylcholine, a vital neurotransmitter, also occurs.

☞ KEY CONCEPT

The pattern and progression of symptoms can vary greatly among clients with AD.

Description

Behavioral, intellectual, and emotional changes develop in fairly regular patterns. Symptoms are always progressive, but each affected individual's rate of change varies greatly. The disease is characterized by the random manner in which the process affects brain tissue. Rapid decline occurs in a few cases, but more commonly several months pass with gradual changes. For our purposes, general patterns are grouped in four stages, which are further illustrated in Box 92-3. Figure 92-1 shows a nurse working at the bedside of a client with AD.

Early Stage. In the early stage, intermittent symptoms develop that clients and family members may disregard or fail to recognize. Clients in this stage may have trouble with num-

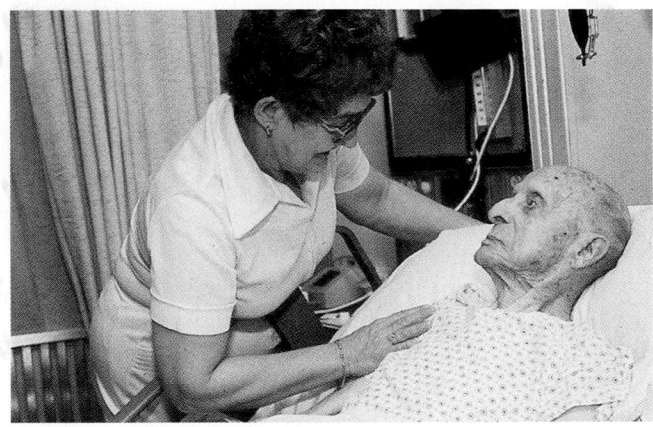

FIGURE 92-1. The nurse speaks calmly and distinctly to the client with Alzheimer's disease.

bers, language patterns, or handwriting. Examples of typical behaviors include forgetting to turn off the oven, misplacing things, taking longer than normal to complete routine chores, repeating questions, and mismanaging money. The client may use **confabulation** (fabricating details of events) to cover up lack of memory.

➤➤ BOX 92-3

STAGES OF PROGRESSIVE DEGENERATIVE DEMENTIA OF THE ALZHEIMER'S TYPE

Early
Forgetfulness
Short-term memory loss
Gradual lack of interest in life
Cannot remember facts, faces, names
Indifferent to social courtesies
Isolative
Indecisive; vague
Decreased reaction time
Difficulty in learning
Uncomfortable in new situations
Recognizes that a problem exists and becomes increasingly frustrated and angry

Advanced
Significant decline in memory
Difficulty with familiar tasks
Confuses day and night; insomnia
Responds slowly
May complain of neglect
May deny problems
Loses things
Has trouble with directions
Inability to care for self; poor activities of daily living (ADL)
Apraxia
Increasing aphasia
Outbursts of anger; aggressiveness (in some people)

More withdrawn and passive (in some people)
Changes in personal relationships
Loss of balance; gait changes
Inability to make decisions

Later or Severe
Loss of sense of time
Severe lapses in memory
Disoriented to place, person; unable to recognize family (sometimes)
Insomnia
Rambling speech; incoherent
Motor ability deteriorates
Paranoid; great frustration, anger
Confused; memory deteriorates more, remembers only distant past
Wanders; gets lost
Unable to perform most ADL; needs custodial care

Final/Terminal
Incapable of self-care
Total memory loss
Periods of anger, hostility, and combativeness
Unable to recognize family, friends
Ataxia (unable to walk)
Incontinent of stool and urine
Mute, or speech unrecognizable
Extreme physical decline
Death

Advanced Stage.   As the disease progresses, **apraxia** (problems carrying out purposeful movements) and *aphasia* (problems with language) worsen. Concentration, orientation, judgment, and planning abilities are affected. Clients in this stage may neglect personal hygiene and health. During this stage, family members become increasingly aware that a problem exists.

Later or Severe Stage.   During this period, clients with AD may have sudden mood shifts (*emotional lability*) or become depressed, suspicious (*paranoid*), fearful, or violent. They may not recognize their family and friends. Major communication problems develop. Behavior may become abusive, causing difficulties for caregivers.

Final or Terminal Stage.   In the last stages of the disease, clients become incontinent and unable to walk. Other people must provide all basic care. Many clients become semi-comatose before death. Some remain in the fetal position.

☛ KEY CONCEPT

The following are the specific and most common symptoms of AD:

- *Memory loss*
- *Inability to learn and retain new information*
- *Loss of judgment and planning skills*
- *Personality and mood changes*
- *Decreased reasoning and abstract thinking skills*
- *Loss of language skills*
- *Inability to care for self*

More than 50% of all nursing home residents are diagnosed as having AD or another dementia. The cost of institutional care for people with dementia has been estimated to exceed $25 billion per year in the United States.

Pharmacologic Treatment

Several medications that affect the transmission of chemicals across synapses are under study. No known medication will stop the progression of AD. Tacrine HCl (Cognex), approved by the Food and Drug Administration in 1993, seems to slow the progression of memory impairment. It has the ability to increase neurotransmissions in the brain by acting on specific enzymes. Although it does not cure AD, this medication seems to help the client and family by enhancing the client's memory capabilities; however, improvement is temporary. Side effects of this drug, which can be troublesome and dangerous, include bradycardia, nausea, vomiting, diarrhea, ulcers, jaundice, and rash. The stool may change color and become light or very dark. Abrupt changes in dosage, either up or down, can cause serious side effects.

Tacrine requires regular monitoring of enzymes such as alanine aminotransferase (**ALT**), also known as serum glutamate pyruvate transaminase (**SGPT**), to prevent liver damage. It must be used cautiously when clients have surgery, because it potentiates the action of muscle relaxants. Clients with pre-existing heart or liver disorders require careful management and frequent assessment.

Donepezil (Aricept) is another drug in this classification that is less toxic than tacrine. Other medications are available to help manage difficult symptoms and behaviors; see In Practice: Important Medications 92-1. Female hormones have seemed to help in some clients. Medication therapy is generally palliative rather than curative. All medications must be used with caution in older people, who metabolize medications less rapidly than younger people. Medications may have opposite effects than those desired (*paradoxical effects*). Some medications increase confusion.

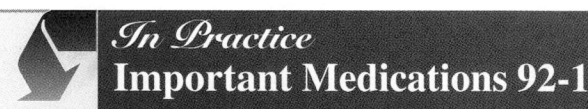

Nursing Alert

Be aware that medications should be a *last resort* in managing behavior problems in AD because of their numerous side effects. Attempt nursing management approaches to these problems *before* the use of chemicals. The Nursing Process section of this chapter presents specific nursing care measures in detail.

Multi-infarct Dementia (MID)

Multi-infarct dementia (**MID**), also called *vascular dementia,* is caused by several brain *infarcts* (loss of blood supply resulting in necrosis) that stem from vascular problems. Cerebrovascular disease and hypertension are the most common causes of MID. Older people who have had a series of small strokes can lose mental abilities as nerve cells die due to lack of oxygen and nutrients.

MID can be distinguished from AD in the following ways:

- It has a faster onset.
- It progresses in a stepwise fashion (not gradually and continuously).
- It usually coexists with other conditions (eg, diabetes, high blood pressure, cardiac disease, previous strokes).

Magnetic resonance imaging (**MRI**) can usually detect small strokes. If detected early, treatment is available to prevent future strokes and MID.

In Practice
Important Medications 92-1

FOR ALZHEIMER'S DISEASE

Slows memory impairment: tacrine hydrochloride (Cognex); donepezil hydrochloride (Aricept)
Antipsychotics: haloperidol (Haldol); thiothixene (Navane); thioridazine hydrochloride (Mellaril); and chlorpromazine hydrochloride (Thorazine)
Antidepressants: trazodone hydrochloride (Desyrel) and fluoxetine HCl (Prozac)
Hypnotics/sedatives: estazolam (ProSom); quazepam (Doral); temazepam (Restoril); flurazepam hydrochloride (Dalmane); and chloral hydrate

Parkinson's Disease

More than 25% of clients with Parkinson's disease have dementia. Often, dementia related to Parkinson's disease is difficult to distinguish from AD, because many clients with AD have motor symptoms similar to those associated with parkinsonism. The client with Parkinson's disease has a history of tremors before the onset of dementia. Figure 92-2 illustrates the symptoms of parkinsonism.

Wernicke-Korsakoff Syndrome

Wernicke-Korsakoff syndrome is the most common type of alcohol-related dementia. It is thought to result from direct damage to the brain by alcohol. It may be caused by nutritional factors, or it may result indirectly from liver damage. Short-term memory is most impaired, although people with this syndrome also may demonstrate poor judgment, lack of insight, diminished attention, and slowed thinking. They may not have the language or perceptual problems common in AD. The characteristic belligerent behavior patterns of some clients with Wernicke-Korsakoff syndrome make them difficult to care for.

Pick's Disease

Pick's disease, which is rare, may be mistaken for AD. These two diseases can only be differentiated through autopsy. AD brain tissue shows plaques and tangles, but in Pick's disease the nerve cells are pale and swollen and contain globules of protein (*Pick's bodies*). The brain looks spongy, due to the increase of non-nerve supporting cells. Symptoms are similar to those of AD. Pick's disease involves primarily the brain's frontal and temporal lobes. Symptoms, therefore, are present as behavioral or language problems. Pick's disease has an earlier onset than AD, most commonly between ages 40 and 50. The average survival time is approximately 7 years.

Creutzfeldt-Jakob Disease

Creutzfeldt-Jacob disease (**CJD**) is a rare dementia is caused by a slow virus, meaning that the incubation period for harboring the organism and developing the disease is measured in years, rather than days, weeks, or months. CJD is an infectious dementia that is considered transmissible. Despite its long incubation period, its course is rapid; death almost always occurs within 2 years of onset.

AIDS Dementia

The client in the late stages of AIDS may become demented. The pathology and exact mechanisms of *AIDS dementia* are subjects of research. Dementia does not occur in all clients with AIDS, and in some people with AIDS dementia, periods of lucidity remain until late in the disease. AIDS dementia is now the most common dementia known to be caused by infection.

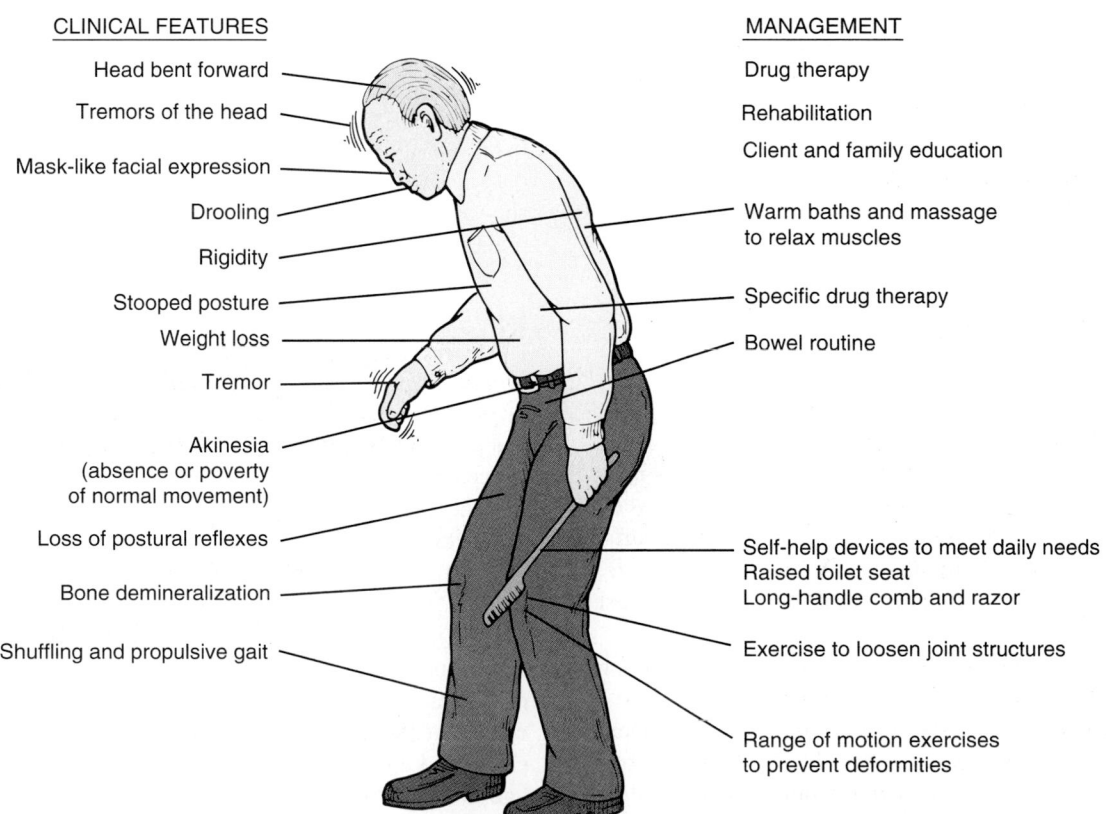

CLINICAL FEATURES

Head bent forward
Tremors of the head
Mask-like facial expression
Drooling
Rigidity
Stooped posture
Weight loss
Tremor
Akinesia (absence or poverty of normal movement)
Loss of postural reflexes
Bone demineralization
Shuffling and propulsive gait

MANAGEMENT

Drug therapy
Rehabilitation
Client and family education
Warm baths and massage to relax muscles
Specific drug therapy
Bowel routine
Self-help devices to meet daily needs
Raised toilet seat
Long-handle comb and razor
Exercise to loosen joint structures
Range of motion exercises to prevent deformities

FIGURE 92-2. The Parkinson's client. Physical tremors appear before cognitive dysfunctions.

Crack-Related Dementia

A form of dementia that is becoming more common is related to the abuse of cocaine, particularly crack cocaine. Relatively little is known about *crack-related dementia*. It is believed to be irreversible. In addition to confusion, memory loss, and speech disorders, people with crack-related dementia often become violent.

Other Causes of Dementia

Numerous physical disorders can cause brain injury that results in dementia. *Toxic dementias* are related to drug overdoses. *Metabolic dementias* can occur after untreated end-stage renal disease (*uremia*), hypoglycemia, hyperglycemia, hypothyroidism, hyperthyroidism, or hepatic failure. Structural problems caused by closed-head trauma, brain tumors, HD, and irradiation to the frontal lobes may also cause dementia.

☛ KEY CONCEPT

The physician must perform a comprehensive physical and mental status evaluation to determine the cause of dementia. Definite diagnosis of AD can only be made by biopsy or autopsy, but a thorough examination can rule out other, more treatable, disorders.

DIAGNOSIS OF DEMENTIA

History

The specific mental and physical changes reported by the client and the family are crucial when searching for possible causes of cognitive decline. The physician establishes the age when changes began, how symptoms progressed, exact functions lost, whether changes were associated with medical or emotional events, and what medications the client was and is taking. This history helps to determine the tests to perform to rule out specific diseases. It alerts the physician to look for specific signs on examination.

Physical and Neurologic Examination

A *physical examination* examines the client's basic general health. The *neurologic examination* is a crucial component in which the physician asks the client to perform maneuvers or answer questions to aid in determining how specific parts of the brain are functioning. This examination includes tests of vision, eye movement, muscle tone and strength, reflexes, coordination, and mental status.

Psychiatric assessment is an important part of the overall examination. A psychiatric assessment may determine the presence of underlying factors that may exacerbate memory loss, including some forms of depression. The findings of the physician's history and physical examination help to differentiate among types of dementia.

☛ KEY CONCEPT

There is no way to predict which skills a client with dementia will lose. One part of the brain may be affected but not another. Some clients retain specific skills until late in the disease. A thorough evaluation is necessary to determine the disease's extent and progression.

Laboratory Tests

Laboratory tests (Table 92-1) are performed to rule out and treat reversible causes of cognitive impairment. They are helpful in identifying risk factors associated with some forms of dementia. Clients with AD usually have normal laboratory test results.

CT Scan, MRI, PET Scan, and EEG

Computed tomography (CT) scanning and MRI provide visualization of the brain's anatomy. This visualization will sometimes show progressive atrophy beyond that of normal aging. These tests are helpful in eliminating conditions such as cerebrovascular accidents, closed-head trauma, hydrocephalus, vascular disease, tumors, and hematomas. They are not reliable in confirming any diagnosis of dementia. Atrophy of the brain's hippocampus is one of the first signs seen in AD. (The *hippocampus* is the area of the brain associated with short-term memory and consolidation of short- and long-term memory.) Positron emission tomography (**PET**) may show decreased metabolism in some areas. A newer scan called the single photon emission computed tomography (**SPECT**) is helpful in evaluating blood *perfusion* (flow) to the brain and the brain's metabolic activity.

The electroencephalograph (EEG) records the brain's electrical activity. This test is not always performed, but may rule out seizure disorders or other brain pathology. In AD, the EEG shows a generalized slowing of brain-wave activity. Distinctive EEG changes are also seen in CJD.

Psychometric Testing

Usually the physician will perform a brief mental status examination as a screening tool to test the client's orientation to time and place; ability to register and recall information; attention, concentration, and calculation ability; and language skills. In AD, the first functions clients lose are memory of recent events, abstract reasoning, mathematic calculations, and the ability to concentrate and complete complex tasks. If a client fails the mental status examination, a psychologist can then perform more comprehensive *psychometric* (neuropsychological) testing. Tests could include standardized intelligence scales, memory scales, testing for judgment and planning abilities, and more comprehensive language testing. (Results of these tests are compared against those of unimpaired people in the same age group.) Psychiatric testing also may be done to rule out psychoses.

▪▪▪ TABLE 92-1 *L*ABORATORY STUDIES AND CAUSES OF DEMENTIA

Test	Possible Cause of Problem	Rationale
Complete blood count	Anemia	Lack of oxygen (ischemia) in brain causes confusion.
Chemistry screening	Toxicity	Metabolic disturbances, kidney disease, and liver disease cause toxic, confused states.
Fasting blood sugar and other tests for insulin-dependent diabetes mellitus	Diabetes mellitus	Excessively high or low blood sugar levels can cause mental disturbances; nutritional disorders also can contribute to delirium and dementia.
VDRL, RPR, MHA-TP, or FTA-ABS	Syphilis	Tertiary syphilis causes dementia.
Erythrocyte sedimentation rate	Infection, immune disorders	Infectious agents can lead to toxicity; chronic inflammation can lead to ischemia.
Urinalysis	Urinary tract disorders	Uremia, infections, and toxicity can lead to dementia.
Thyroid panel	Hyperthyroidism, hypothyroidism	Confusion and depression can occur with abnormal thyroid levels.
Vitamin B_{12} and folate	Anemias	Inability to make or use red blood cells can cause ischemia to brain; also folate and B_{12} are low in chronic alcoholism.
Cerebrospinal fluid assay	Infection/hydrocephalus	Some organic causes other than Alzheimer's disease can be identified.
Autoimmune testing	Vasculitis	Elevated in some cases of multi-infarct dementias.

Tests for HIV
  HIV-1 antigen (P24)
  HIV-1 antibody
	AIDS	Later stages of AIDS can cause dementia.

Alcohol (ETOH); other chemical screening	Drug or alcohol-related dementia	Rule out Wernicke-Korsakoff syndrome, crack-related dementias, other chemical toxicities.
Electrolyte levels	Electrolyte imbalance	Excess or deficiency of some electrolytes can cause dementia.

AIDS, acquired immunodeficiency syndrome; FTA-ABS, fluorescent treponemal antibody absorption; HIV, human immunodeficiency virus; MHA-TP, microhemagglutination assay-*Treponema pallidum;* RPR, rapid plasma reagin; VDRL, Venereal Disease Research Laboratory

Functional Assessment

A *functional assessment* is part of the diagnostic workup for dementias. The client is evaluated for the ability to perform basic skills required for daily functioning—the activities of daily living (ADL). Included in this assessment is the ability to perform instrumental ADL: meal preparation, shopping, telephone use, and transportation.

☛ KEY CONCEPT

The person with dementia who resides in a long-term care facility may state, "I want to go home." Do not try to convince the resident that this is his or her home. It is not the "home" he or she knows. The nurse can make statements, such as "You are staying here. You are safe here." Distracting the person by initiating an activity may also help.

NURSING PROCESS

Data Collection

The healthcare team initially establishes baseline data for the client with AD or any other dementia for later comparison with deterioration trends. An assessment of the client's support systems (family, friends, finances) also is essential when determining short- and long-term treatment options.

Physical Assessment

After the physician performs a thorough history and physical, the nurse will complete the assessment. Include basic information, such as the client's immunizations, particularly flu shots and Pneumovax 23 (protection against pneumococcal pneumonia), on the client's chart. Assess a variety of other areas, particularly sensory deficits. Be sure to obtain substantial information about the client. The following information from the client or family aids in the overall picture.

Visual Acuity Examination. Determine the date of the client's last vision examination. Determine if the client has been checked recently for glaucoma or cataracts, and whether he or she wears glasses. People with dementias often neglect personal healthcare measures. Perceptual problems are common. (They often believe something is wrong with their glasses and refuse to wear them.) They may lose or break their glasses. They may find it difficult to position themselves in relation to objects, and may misperceive the edges of chairs or stairs, resulting in frequent falls.

Audiometric Testing. Find out if the client's hearing has been evaluated. Determine whether the client has had a hearing aid prescribed and whether he or she wears it. Also ask if it works; be sure that batteries are functional. (Limited or misinterpreted stimuli may contribute to confusion.)

Nutritional Status. Discuss the history of weight gain or loss and the time frame in which it occurred. Clients may forget to eat or forget that they just ate. Ask about ability to chew and swallow. Ask if the client wears dentures.

Sleep Pattern Disturbances. Ask about the total number of hours of rest the client gets at night and during the day. Ask if the person gets up during the night, and if so, how many times and for what reasons. Determine if a client's sleep problems are disruptive for family members.

Skin Care. Evaluate the client's skin condition. Check for dryness, bruises, sores, pressure areas, and cracked heels. Check fingernails and toenails.

Oral Care. Assess whether the client is able to brush the teeth or care for dentures. Ask if dentures fit properly, if the client wears them regularly, and if he or she has checked the gums recently for sores or irritated areas.

Psychological Assessment

Psychological assessment includes identification of past and present behaviors. Identifying behavior problems allows the healthcare team to develop a realistic nursing care plan, which includes family education. Behaviors are often responses to environmental cues; clients with dementia may be confused by these cues or may easily misinterpret them. Also, the nurse should be aware of overstimulation or understimulation of clients with AD. Some common behaviors seen in AD and some other dementias are listed below.

Aggression or Agitation. Some clients undergo personality changes. A previously mild-mannered person may become loud, begin to curse and swear, and lash out at people. *Verbal abuse* (using hostile language, cursing, or making verbal threats) is the most common aggressive behavior found in clients living in community-based care settings. Clients also can be *physically aggressive,* especially with strangers (eg, healthcare workers) who invade their personal space. Many hostile behaviors are responses to situations that confused clients perceive as threatening. Using a calm approach and keeping the environment and activities as stable and consistent as possible can assist in relieving anxiety.

☛ **KEY CONCEPT**

Be sure to monitor the bowel elimination patterns of clients who have altered cognition. They often are unable to identify and communicate the absence of regular bowel movements. Fecal impactions may result.

Anxiety or Paranoia. As clients lose short-term memory and time orientation, they cannot understand what has recently happened or what will happen next. They may show *anxiety* by rummaging through drawers, wringing their hands, pacing, or displaying worried looks. As they misplace things or cannot recall their location, clients may believe that items have been stolen. *Paranoia* may lead to accusations. Some clients may cover windows and move furniture in front of doors because they are afraid. In nursing facilities, simple tasks, such as bathing or showering, may frighten clients because they do not understand what is happening. Breaking activities into simple steps and providing short comments may help (eg, "I'm going to wash your face now.").

Hallucinations and Delusions. *Hallucinations* are false sensory perceptions that may be auditory (eg, hearing voices) or visual (eg, seeing a person). Hallucinations may also involve the senses of taste, touch, and smell. Sometimes, clients believe that people on television are in the room with them or that their own reflection is another person. *Delusions* may cause confused ideas, such as believing that a bank has confiscated all the client's money or that a spouse is going to kill the client. These symptoms usually are related to organic changes in the brain; trying to reason with the client will not work.

Withdrawal and Depression. Clients who retain insight into their cognitive and physical losses may become depressed. Report a client's feelings of worthlessness to a physician. *Suicide* (accidental or intentional) is a risk during the early stages of AD. Some clients respond to antidepressants. In many clients, symptoms of depression seem to decrease as the dementia progresses.

Assessment of Functional ADL

An important part of assessment is determining a client's ability to carry out basic daily tasks.

Dressing, Bathing, and Grooming. Determine if the client is able to dress appropriately. Danger signs include soiled clothes worn repeatedly, and clothes put on in an incorrect sequence (eg, clients may wear two dresses, or underwear on the outside). Determine whether the client bathes. Danger signs include an inability to set water temperature or a lack of grooming. Assessment includes asking about the client's ability to shave, comb hair, brush teeth, or use makeup. Determine if these abilities have changed recently. (Solutions for meeting basic ADL are discussed later in this chapter.)

✚👁 **N u r s i n g   A l e r t**
The most common cause of burns in older people is hot water. Take steps to control the water temperature available to clients with dementia. These clients also may be afraid of water and may be particularly confused in the shower.

Toileting: Bowel and Bladder Control. Evaluate whether the client is able to remain continent, locate and use the bathroom independently, perform the tasks in the right order, and accomplish basic hygiene practices. If incontinence exists, determine if it can be managed by scheduled toileting.

Drugs such as haloperidol (Haldol) can cause urinary retention. Reducing the Haldol dose may help prevent overflow incontinence. Regular toileting maintains usual urinary function.

Ambulation and Transfer. Determine if the client can walk without assistance. If the client uses a cane or walker, evaluate the ability to use it safely. Danger signs include a history of falls or unsteady gait, wandering off and getting lost, unexplained cuts and bruises, or several falls within the past year.

The family (or the long-term care facility, if the client resides there) also should have a recent photo of the person, in case he or she becomes lost and police need to assist in the search. (A photo will help with identification.) The Alzheimer's Association sponsors a program called "Safe Return." For a nominal fee, it provides clients with ID bracelets and clothing labels.

> **✚👁 N u r s i n g   A l e r t**
>
> Clients with dementia must wear some sort of identification in case they wander and become lost. They can wear ID bracelets or sewn-on name tags. Hospital identification bands may work well because they cannot be removed easily. Placing bands around ankles rather than wrists might be better because the bands are then out of a client's sight. At least two telephone numbers should be on the identification. Identify the client as memory impaired.

Eating. Determine whether the client can use utensils and cut food. If the client needs to be fed, assess whether he or she is cooperative, can chew, and remembers to swallow. Danger signs include a history of choking, confusion with utensils, and refusal to eat. Be sure to monitor food and fluid intake and weight.

Communication Skills. Although variable for each client, language skills gradually deteriorate as dementia progresses. To assess communication skills, ask if the client repeats questions or stories, has difficulty finding words or naming objects, or makes up nonsense words or phrases. Skills deteriorate in different ways and at different times. For example, some people lose the ability to speak, but still understand written language; others lose the ability to understand all forms of language. Music and social skills tend to remain intact until late in the process.

Assessment of Complex or Instrumental ADL

Management of Finances. Determine if the person is able to handle a checkbook, pay bills, and make change. Clients with dementia may pay bills more than once or forget to pay them at all. They may make large contributions to charity because requests look like bills. They also may become victims of con artists. Clients may hide or lose checks. Danger signs include many unpaid bills, disconnected utilities, or misplacing or donating large amounts of money. Solutions include having Social Security checks deposited directly, bills sent to a family member or guardian, and a cosigner required for all checks.

Driving. Determine if the client is able to drive safely. Is he or she having accidents, getting lost, or trying to get out of moving cars? Danger signs include near misses, accidents, or signs of poor judgment. It may be necessary to request that the state remove the person's driver's license or retest him or her. The family may need to remove any car keys from the client so that driving is not possible. In some cases, the person's car must be sold. Vocational rehabilitation, the American Automobile Association, and the Veteran's Administration will give driving evaluations if the client's judgment and ability are questioned.

Public Transportation. Evaluate whether the person can take a bus or train without getting lost, can make correct change, and can get transfers.

Food Preparation. Determine whether the client is able to follow recipes and instructions. Check if he or she leaves on burners, burns pots or pans, or stores food unsafely. Danger signs include spoiled foods, evidence of fires or burned pans, or hoarding large amounts of food. The solution is to contact Meals on Wheels for assistance, and disconnect the stove.

Shopping, Housekeeping, and Laundry. Determine the client's ability to shop. Note if he or she has changed from previous patterns of cleaning, and if he or she can figure out how to set the washing machine, measure detergent, and load clothes. Danger signs include large amounts of the same items in the house, items stored in the wrong places (such as frozen foods in the cupboard), messy home environment (in a previously neat home), presence of insects and rodents, washing everything by hand, and soiled clothing in closets or drawers. The solution is for family members to perform or to supervise these tasks, or to arrange for help through homemaker services.

Telephone Use. Determine the client's ability to dial and recall phone numbers for emergencies. Danger signs include inability to dial telephones, repeated calls, or calls in the middle of the night to others. The solution is to keep a list of numbers near the telephone. Install a computer dialing device and have family members or friends call often to check on the client and caregiver.

Safety in the Community. Determine if the client can take measures to ensure his or her own safety. Danger signs include opening doors to strangers, giving strangers or neighbors money, and becoming victims of scams. Persons with AD also may have problems in neighborhoods, such as walking into other people's houses, hitchhiking, or requesting money from neighbors.

Assessment of Support Systems

The Family. Alzheimer's disease and other dementias are overwhelming for family members. In many ways, the disease strikes not only the client but the family as well. An important part of assessing the person with dementia includes understanding the needs of family members and other primary caregivers. Sometimes, complex networks of friends and neighbors provide necessary supervision or care for clients affected with dementia. Family or caregiver teaching is vital.

Alzheimer's disease has been called the "dementia from which the client dies twice": first in mind and then in body. Caring for a person with AD in the early stages interferes with the family's recreational time. In later stages, caregivers spend most of their time supervising confused and emotional clients. They need to balance their caregiving with personal activities that bring pleasure.

Female and Aging Caregivers.   Most caregivers are women. Conflicts can arise among the demanding roles of caregiver, wife, mother, employee, and homemaker. Spouses of people with dementias are often older adults themselves. Caregivers may be unable to handle the physical and psychological demands necessary to manage the constantly increasing level of care. Support groups and respite care (discussed later) can prove beneficial to the health and well-being of caregivers.

Nursing Diagnosis

A number of nursing diagnoses for clients, family members, or caregivers are identifiable from information the nurse gathers. Examples of some nursing diagnoses that may be seen on nursing care plans for the client with dementia include:

    Bowel Incontinence; Constipation; or Diarrhea
    Impaired Verbal Communication
    Ineffective Family Coping
    Hopelessness
    Risk for Injury (falls, wandering away)
    Knowledge Deficit regarding disease and its treatment
    Self-Care Deficit (ADL)—specify
    Urinary Elimination, Altered; Urinary Retention

Planning and Implementing

Management of the person with dementia includes caring for basic personal needs; but it also requires a basic understanding of communication and behavior management techniques. Teach caregivers and serve as a role model. Assisting clients to perform ADL is an essential function. The nurse can use special skills in communication and teach these skills to families and other caregivers. Daily routines may help clients. The entire family needs a great deal of support. Listen to their concerns and be aware of problems that are arising. In Practice: Nursing Care Plan 92-1 highlights a priority nursing diagnosis for the client with AD who is hospitalized. See also In Practice: Educating the Client 92-1.

Assisting With Daily Care
Bathing.   Bathing is frightening for clients with dementia. When assisting with baths, be calm. Give baths at preferred times for clients. (Rested clients are more cooperative than those who are overtired.) Use low water levels, and have everything prepared before the client enters the bathtub. Avoid the noise and confusion of a whirlpool or shower. Pad the walls to reduce echoing (overstimulation). Use positive reinforcement ("You look so handsome."). Use gestures; do not shout to be heard.

Dressing.   For clients with dementia, dressing becomes complicated. Lay out clean clothes, and remove dirty clothes (to prevent confusion). Offer clothing in sequence, one piece at a time.

Do not give several verbal commands at once because they can overwhelm clients. Use simple clothing (Velcro, elastic waistbands). Suggest that clients wear cardigan or button-down shirts or blouses instead of those put on over the head (covering the head is frightening). Clients may be unable to manage buttons without help.

Pain Control.   Pain control is important because clients with dementia may experience pain but be unable to express it. Older clients often have arthritis or other physical disorders. Give pain medications before performing care measures, such as bathing or dressing.

> ### Nursing Alert
> Monitor the person's weight. If weight loss is evident, the person is probably forgetting to eat. Agitation and pacing also take a great deal of energy. Remind the person to chew and swallow. Observe for choking.

Nutrition and Hydration.   Maintaining nutrition and hydration is important. As people age, their sense of thirst becomes less acute. Many older people tend to forget to drink or eat. Offer small amounts of fluid each time you interact with clients. Vary choices by providing gelatins, ices, juices, herbal teas, and soups; do not give plain water all the time. Avoid very hot liquids (people with poor judgment are likely to spill liquids and be burned). Limit the variety of foods to prevent confusion. Cut meats to appropriate sizes to prevent choking. Place clients near people they should mimic. If a client is able to feed himself or herself, place the spoon (forks may be dangerous) in his or her hand. Give finger foods if the person cannot manage the utensil.

The person living at home is in danger due to the stove. Gas is particularly dangerous. Remove the knobs or install a master shut-off for either electric or gas stoves.

> ### Nursing Alert
> Increase fluids for clients who have dementia to prevent urinary tract infections and to allow the bladder (which is a muscle) to contract properly. Some medications promote urinary retention; therefore, closely monitor clients who are taking such medications. Check for edema; assess skin turgor.

Bladder and Bowel Management.   Bladder and bowel management often becomes necessary for clients with dementia because incontinence is common in later stages. Clients can avoid daytime episodes by regular toileting. Label the bathroom; give one-step instructions and make each step simple, identifying one activity with each step. ("Come with me. Pull down your pants. Sit down.") Families need education in the use of continence products at home. Document

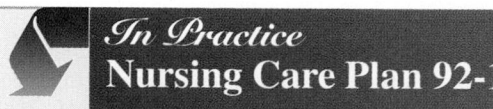

In Practice
Nursing Care Plan 92-1

THE CLIENT WITH ALZHEIMER'S DISEASE WHO IS HOSPITALIZED

MEDICAL HISTORY: *J.S. is a 66-year-old married African American male with a history of AD who is admitted to the hospital for surgical repair of benign prostatic hypertrophy. An intravenous pyelogram and cystography are scheduled. He is to undergo a transurethral resection of the prostate (TURP).*

MEDICAL DIAGNOSIS: *BPH; AD*

Data Collection/Nursing Assessment: Client is alert at present, able to state his name and where he is, but unable to state day of week, month, or year. Currently, client lives at home with wife. She states, "The doctor has said that he is in the advanced stages of his disease." She reports increasing problems with memory, reasoning, judgment, and social interaction. "At times, he gets lost, gets clumsy, and frequently roams and paces around the house." She reports that client awakens frequently at night. Client's speech is somewhat slow. Wife reports that she has to coach him along to do things, especially be washed and dressed. "Sometimes he gets so irritable when I do this, but if I don't, he won't do it. It took everything I had to have him get dressed this morning."

Nursing Diagnosis: Self-care deficit (bathing/hygiene, dressing/grooming) related to altered thought processes secondary to AD as evidenced by wife's statements about difficulty with washing and dressing.

Planning

SHORT-TERM GOALS:

#1. Client will participate in one aspect of self-care activity each time.

#2. Client will demonstrate episodes of minimal frustration with self-care.

LONG-TERM GOALS:

#3. Client will participate in self-care activities within the limits of his disease.

Implementation

NURSING ACTION: *Discuss with client's wife the client's usual routine of care.*

RATIONALE: *Adapting care to meet the client's routine helps in promoting a sense of well-being and comfort, thereby minimizing anxiety.*

NURSING ACTION: *Attempt to maintain an atmosphere and routine of care similar to that experienced by the client at home. Encourage wife to bring in personal care items from home.*

RATIONALE: *Familiarity helps to allay anxiety and reduce the number of new situations to be faced that could cause the client to feel threatened.*

NURSING ACTION: *Label articles for the client's use, such as urinal, call signal, toothbrush, and wash basin.*

RATIONALE: *Labeling articles can help the client's memory.*

NURSING ACTION: *Have one nurse assigned consistently to care for client.*

RATIONALE: *Maintaining consistency with staffing helps to prevent unfamiliar situations for the client.*

NURSING ACTION: *Provide slow, step-by-step instructions for the client when providing hygiene. Provide positive comments.*

RATIONALE: *Slow, step-by-step instructions help the client to focus on the task and complete it with minimal frustration.*

Evaluation: Hygiene activities scheduled in evening as per client's usual routine at home. Client's toothbrush and hairbrush brought in from home and labeled. Client participated in washing face and hands with verbal guidance. *Progress to meeting Goal #1.*

NURSING ACTION: *Explain each intervention, test, or treatment and what is expected of client in simple terms. Speak clearly and calmly to the client.*

RATIONALE: *Explanations with expectations help to alleviate possible anxiety and fear associated with the newness of the situation.*

Evaluation: Client continuing to participate in washing face and hands with verbal guidance; able to provide urine specimen as requested and instructed. No episodes of frustration noted. *Goal #1 met; progress to meeting Goal #2 and Goal #3.*

NURSING ACTION: *Enlist the aid of the client's wife with new situations.*

RATIONALE: *Having the client's wife present can help to allay the client's anxiety and fears.*

NURSING ACTION: *Encourage the client to verbalize feelings of fear, frustration, and anger when they occur.*

RATIONALE: *Verbalization helps to reduce these feelings.*

Evaluation: *Client participating in washing hands, face, and perineal area. Threw hairbrush when asked to brush hair. Progress to meeting goal #3. Continued work needed for Goal #2.*

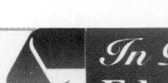

In Practice
Educating the Client 92-1

PROVISION OF A SAFE ENVIRONMENT FOR PEOPLE WITH COGNITIVE DYSFUNCTION

- Do not allow the client to drive (remove keys, disable car, revoke license).
- Remove guns and ammunition from the house.
- Supervise smoking; lock up supplies; use only ashtrays that will not tip or melt. Encourage smoking cessation.
- Disable stove or supervise cooking.
- Supervise use of knives and forks; lock up utensils.
- Turn down temperature of water heater.
- Remove dangerous power tools; supervise use of small power tools.
- Supervise use of razors (allow *only* an electric razor) and supervise use of electrical appliances; do not allow appliance use around water; do not allow use of dangerous appliances (food processor, garbage disposal).
- Supervise use of electric fans or air conditioners.
- Lock up all medications, over-the-counter remedies, poisons, paints, cleaning solutions. Make sure the primary caregiver knows how and when to administer medications; do not leave with client to take unsupervised.
- Supervise use of china and glass dishes to prevent injury from breakage.
- Put a control on thermostat or disable it to prevent the person from constantly adjusting temperature.
- Reduce potential for falls by keeping floors clear of debris (but not highly polished), wiping up spills, and not using throw rugs. Have good railings on stairways. See that the person's shoes fit well. Have halls and stairs well-lighted.
- Install safety locks and buzzers on doors (in case person wanders). Make sure person has identification at all times. Many persons can get through locks and dismantle doors. Fence yard; control access to dangerous areas (swimming pool, beach, highway).
- Keep emergency numbers next to each phone; a preprogrammed phone is a good idea.
- Find a good home for pets, if this person is no longer able to safely care for a pet.

bowel movements; be alert for constipation or impaction. If a client develops diarrhea, check for lactose intolerance, constipation, or drug reactions. Blood electrolyte levels may be ordered if diarrhea continues.

Assisting With Communication
Use all the communication skills you have learned. Your verbal and nonverbal communication skills greatly influence how others respond. If you remain calm, you will have a calming effect on clients. If you are quiet and gentle, clients are more likely to cooperate with you. If you are agitated and in a hurry, clients will respond to your behavior and become upset and belligerent. See In Practice: Nursing Care Guidelines 92-1 for communication guidelines.

Assisting With Behavior Management
Anxiety. *Anxiety* is common in persons who have dementias. Often, these clients display frustrating behaviors, such as pacing or rummaging through closets or drawers, which help them to feel more in control. Reassure anxious clients. Keep commands simple, and reward successes. Work in small groups, and encourage family members to visit one or two at a time. Keep the client's environment and daily routines consistent; assign the same caregivers daily if possible. Allow clients to move around. Eliminate caffeine and limit sugar in the diet. Avoid overstimulation.

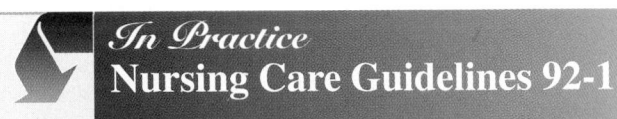

In Practice
Nursing Care Guidelines 92-1

COMMUNICATING WITH THE PERSON WHO HAS DEMENTIA

The following are measures to take when communicating with a person who has dementia:

- Identify yourself—do not make the client guess; he or she may not remember you or be able to read your name tag.
- Tell the person what you are going to do in simple language.
- Maintain direct eye contact. (The person can often respond to nonverbal cues after speech is lost.)
- Stay at the client's eye level. If the person is in a wheelchair, kneel or sit.
- Use a low-pitched voice; speak slowly. (The client will mirror an angry or tense tone of voice.)
- Eliminate background noise. (Avoid overstimulating the confused client; make sure he or she can hear you.)
- Use short, simple sentences; give one-step commands.
- Avoid using questions, such as "Why did you . . .?" or "What do you want?" (These require complex reasoning and memory.)
- Label the environment if the client can read ("John's closet," "bathroom").
- Give the person "reassurance cards" ("Your wife is coming at 3 PM"). The client can refer to these cards if anxious.
- Post a simple daily schedule to structure the day. Post the day and date. Have a clock visible.
- Be aware of nonverbal language; smile, nod your head, approach the client from the front, avoid restraining the person, gently touch the person (unless this is frightening to him or her).
- Use gestures, such as waving goodbye.

Balking. **Balking,** which means refusing to do things, often occurs when clients do not understand what is expected. If a client balks, go away briefly, and come back later with a pleasant tone of voice. Model expected behavior, or have clients mimic others (eg, eating at a table with others).

Persons with dementias commonly display **catastrophic reactions** in which they become overly agitated when confronted with situations that are too overwhelming or difficult for them. The best approach when this occurs is to cease the activity and allow quiet time or time out.

Paranoia. **Paranoia** or fearfulness is common. Keep the environment calm and predictable; remove excess stimulation or items that can contribute to misperceptions (eg, mirrors, intercoms, lamps that cast shadows). Do not try to reason with paranoid clients, but reassure them that they are safe.

Aggressiveness. *Aggressiveness* can be physical (striking out), verbal (name calling, cursing), or sexual. Use a calm approach. Do not confront or try to reason with clients; scolding aggravates aggressive responses. If necessary, remove clients from the group (to avoid upsetting others). Validate their feelings ("You seem angry or frightened."). Give reassurance ("You are safe."). If a client strikes out when you try to perform nursing care, leave temporarily. Allow the client time to calm down, and then return. Remember that your tone of voice can either soothe or upset clients. Try to identify factors (triggers) that cause these outbursts so that you can plan to avoid or minimize them.

Assisting Caregivers

Social scientist Pauline Boss has coined the term **ambiguous loss** to describe the "debilitating confusion" created when the client is "physically present, but psychologically absent." Boss feels that ambiguous loss is the main source of stress for caregivers of AD clients, because "the client is unable to emotionally interact with—or later even to recognize—the caregiver."[1] Dealing with Alzheimer's has also been described as "the long goodbye."[2]

✚👁 Nursing Alert

Someone should be enlisted to check on the primary caregiver of the demented person, particularly if the caregiver also is an older person. A neighbor or relative should call at least twice a day to make sure everything is under control. If something should happen to the primary caregiver, help may be delayed because the demented person may not know what to do.

Support Groups. Support groups for families of clients with AD and other dementias are available. The most prominent is the Alzheimer's Disease and Related Disorders Association, Inc.

Clients and family members can obtain support from many areas. Help them to identify their needs and be open to adaptations. Some needs are educational; for example, learning what the family needs to know to care for the client. Practical solutions, such as transportation assistance, legal assistance, answers for insurance and Medicare questions, medical equipment, and meal services at home are available in most locations. The family as a unit may need counseling because the situation is overwhelming.

Respite Care. **Respite care** allows caregivers some time to themselves by having others care for clients on a short-term basis. Respite is crucial for caregivers—they need relief from the constant responsibility of caring for their loved one, to maintain their own physical and mental health. A resource for families entitled "Homes of Help" is sponsored by the Alzheimer's Association. Many long-term care facilities arrange short-term stays to provide respite. Community alternatives exist, including senior volunteers, home health services, and adult daycare. Adult daycare programs afford caregivers a break from their caregiving responsibilities for a portion of the day, so that they can work or fulfill other responsibilities. Sometimes caregivers feel guilty about not providing care or assistance or cannot afford to provide it. A referral to social service may be needed. Caregivers may be willing to try a supplemental service on a temporary basis. When they find how helpful it is, they may be less reluctant to seek help in the future.

Education. The healthcare team helps with a plan for the family. Document all teaching. The Alzheimer's Association has a newsletter for caregivers and professionals, and support groups throughout the United States. These resources provide education and group support.

Advance Directives. Normally, individuals make their own decisions and grant consent for healthcare, diagnostic, and treatment options. Persons with dementias are unable to give informed consent for procedures, and responsibility for decision-making often falls on the family. The family may feel uneasy making decisions or may be unsure of the client's preferences. A means to ease their burden is to recommend that the client complete an advance directive while still mentally competent to understand and make health decisions. An *advance directive* states the client's preferences for caregiving procedures, treatments, and life-sustaining measures. At a later time, if the client is unable to competently make decisions, the family can make decisions on behalf of the client, using the client's expressed preferences. All individuals should be encouraged to complete advance directives.

Family Dynamics. Boss states that the family must be assisted to go through a "premature grieving process."[1] The person they knew is really gone, and a childlike person has replaced their loved one. The family needs assistance in some areas:

Identify problems: Realize the ambiguity of the situation. The adult is now like a child; the former decision-maker is no longer able to make decisions.

Validate their perceptions: Verify their feelings and perceptions to make sure they correctly understand the situation.

Clarify: Restate and clarify their perceptions and feelings to make sure you understand how they are feeling.

Devise solutions: Assist the family to create solutions for the problems presented.

Test: Test the solutions.
Evaluate: Evaluate, reassess, and revise the care plan.

This procedure parallels the nursing process.

Evaluation

The healthcare team, along with the client and family, evaluate outcomes of care. Have short-term goals been met? Are long-term goals still realistic?

When planning for further nursing care, consider the client's prognosis, as well as any complications and the client's response to care given. Evaluate the caregiver to see how he or she is coping.

➤ STUDENT SYNTHESIS

Key Points

- Many reversible causes of confusion and delirium exist, including physical illness, metabolic disturbances, drug or alcohol toxicity, malnutrition, and sensory deprivation.
- Although confusion can occur at any age, the older adult is more vulnerable because of decreased physiologic reserve and the number of medications taken.
- Dementias affect the brain and nerve cells. They include AD, MID, Parkinson's disease, Wernicke-Korsakoff syndrome, Pick's disease, CJD, AIDS dementia, HD, and crack-related dementia.
- Diagnosis of dementia is often difficult; usually only brain tissue biopsy or autopsy can confirm the diagnosis. Other tests are helpful in ruling out treatable causes of dementia.
- Alzheimer's disease develops in stages, beginning with memory difficulty and progressing to increasing difficulties with memory, language, and movement. In the final stage, the client is no longer able to perform daily activities.
- Treatment for Alzheimer's is palliative; there is no known cure.
- Nursing assessment of physical and mental abilities, needs, and resources is integral in the treatment of dementia.
- One nursing goal is assessment of the client's abilities in performing basic and complex ADL.
- Nursing actions when caring for the demented client include assisting with ADL, using communication skills, and managing difficult behaviors.
- The family or caregivers of the demented client require assessment of their needs, assistance with education and respite care, and referrals to support groups.

Critical Thinking Exercises

1. Some long-term care facilities have special units for residents with dementias, whereas others mix these residents with residents who have normal cognitive function. Discuss the pros and cons of these approaches.
2. The wife of a man with AD confides in you that she feels guilty because she promised her husband that she would never put him in a nursing home, but is now considering it. She says that she is feeling exhausted and gets so overwhelmed with the situation that she has slapped her husband several times when he has resisted care. Discuss your response to her and the options you could recommend.
3. Review the causes of some dementias and describe lifestyle changes people can make early in life to decrease their risk for developing these dementias.

NCLEX-Style Review Questions

1. An older adult is admitted to the hospital. The client exhibits anxiety, severe sleep deprivation, and hallucinations. These data correlate most directly to:
   a. Delirium
   b. Dementia
   c. Organic brain syndrome
   d. Senility
2. Which data findings are associated with the early stage of Alzheimer's disease?
   a. Apraxia
   b. Misplacing items
   c. Neglecting personal hygiene
   d. Sudden mood shifts
3. Which of the following would the nurse assess when completing a functional assessment of a client with dementia?
   a. Ability to complete activities of daily living
   b. Mental status assessment
   c. Support system
   d. Range of motion

References

1. Boss, P. (1988). Alzheimer's and the family: Scientist studies how people cope with "loss" of living loved-one (p. 1–3). *News.* Minneapolis: University of Minnesota, College of Home Economics.
2. Combs, L. (1998). *A long goodbye and beyond: Coping with Alzheimer's.* Wilsonville, OR: Book Partners, Inc.

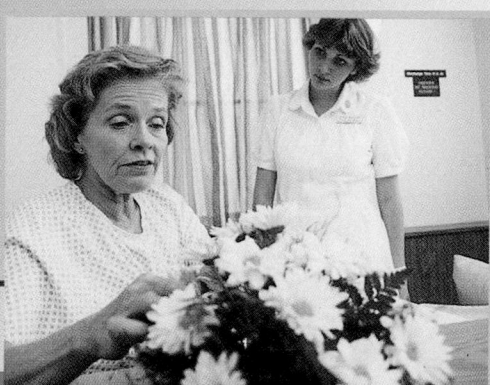

Unit XIV

MENTAL HEALTH NURSING

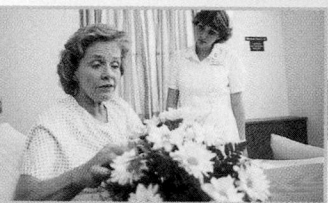

Psychiatric Nursing

LEARNING OBJECTIVES

1. Define the most important terms and acronyms relating to mental health and its deviations.
2. Explain the normal role of defense mechanisms. Describe the results when defense mechanisms are overused.
3. Differentiate between functional and organic mental illnesses.
4. List at least five organic causes of mental illness.
5. Describe the role of neuropsychological and neurodiagnostic testing in diagnosing mental illness.
6. List at least five general symptoms of a mental disorder.
7. Describe the diagnostic criteria for a mood disorder.
8. Explain the differences between a major depressive episode and dysthymia.
9. Describe the behavioral characteristics of the person with bipolar disorder.
10. List and describe at least four personality disorders. Describe in detail common behaviors of people with borderline personality disorder.
11. Define psychosis and list its most common symptoms.
12. Describe the relationships between substance abuse and mental illness.
13. Identify key members of the mental healthcare team and describe their roles.
14. Describe outpatient services commonly available for people with mental illnesses.
15. Identify at least three types of structured living available to clients with mental disorders.
16. Discuss the legal categories of admission to the acute mental health-care setting.
17. Discuss therapies available to clients with mental illness.
18. Describe electroconvulsive therapy, indications for its use, and associated nursing implications.
19. Identify the most commonly used classifications of medications in psychiatry. Give at least three examples of each classification. Describe the undesirable side effects of neuroleptic therapy.
20. Discuss the legal rights of clients with mental illnesses.
21. Target approaches for dealing with aggressive or assaultive persons.
22. State the people most likely to attempt suicide and describe suicide precautions in the acute mental healthcare setting.
23. Discuss nursing responsibilities when working with each of the following: overactive, withdrawn, depressed, hypomanic, regressive, or self-injuring clients.

NEW TERMINOLOGY

affect
agoraphobia
akathisia
anhedonia
anxiety
assaultive
athetoid
benzodiazepine
bipolar disorder
catalepsy
catatonia
cogwheeling movement
commitment
compulsion
cyclothymic
decanoate
defense mechanism
delusion
dual diagnosis
dyskinesia
dysthymia
dystonia
echolalia
echopraxia
entitlement
euthymia
extrapyramidal side effects
forensic
functional disorder
grandiosity
hallucination
hypersomnia
hypervigilance

hypomania
intrusive
lability
malingering
mania
milieu therapy
mood
mutism
neologism
neuroleptic
neuroleptic malignant
 syndrome
obsession
oculogyric crisis
opisthotonos
organic disorder
orthostatic hypotension
paranoia
perseverate
phobia
polydipsic
psychiatrist
psychometric
psychosis
psychotropic
rapport
regression
sally port
schizophrenia
self-esteem
tardive dyskinesia
vulnerable adult
Zydis

ACRONYMS

ABR	EP	PD
AER	EPR	Ψ
AH	EPSE	PTSD
AIMS	ETOH, EtOH	REBT
ALC	FAI	RT
AMSIT	FOI	72 hr./72°
ANAD	GP	SA
A&O ×3	HDRS	SI
AOB	HI	SIB
AP	HID	SIRS
APA	KELS	SIW
APE	LQR	SP
AWOL	LSR	SSRI
B-52	MAOI	TA
BDI	MDD	TAT
BPRS	MI/CD	TCA
CHI	MI&D	TCD
CHT	MI/MR	TD
CIC	MMPI	TDK
CMHC	MMSE	T-Hold
CPMI	NOS	TR
DCH	NSAID	U-Tox
DISCUS	OCD	VH
DSM-IV	OD	vol
ECR	PADS	W/D
ECT	PCA	

The vast majority of clients with alterations in mental health are treated in the community. The trend toward community-based mental healthcare is expected to continue in the 21st century. Some clients, however, who have severe problems or sudden exacerbations of mental illness, receive inpatient care in acute or long-term facilities.

Basic principles of mental health apply to the care of all clients, no matter what the setting. Remember that some people with physical illnesses also develop emotional or psychiatric problems that interfere with or influence their recovery. If a person displays unpredictable, dangerous behavior, his or her mental health and safety (and possibly the safety of others) is threatened.

MENTAL HEALTH

In order to help people with mental health concerns, it is important to understand the meaning of mental health. The World Health Organization (WHO) defines health as "a state of physical and mental well-being." The following are possible definitions of a mentally healthy person:

- One who is responsible for his or her own behavior
- One who is able to manage his or her own activities of daily living, such as eating, grooming, managing money, and finding a safe place to live
- One who is able to adjust to new situations and to handle personal problems without severe discomfort, yet who

still has enough energy to be a constructive member of society
- One who has intellectual insight into personal strengths and weaknesses, and is able to accept weaknesses and to use strengths positively
- One who is able to accept frustration without resorting to harmful, self-defeating, or dangerous behavior (against themselves or others)

In the early 1900s, Sigmund Freud, a pioneer in the psychiatric field, called certain reactions to stress *defense mechanisms*. **Defense mechanisms** help individuals to resolve mental conflicts, reduce **anxiety** (fear of impending danger), protect **self-esteem** (self-value), and maintain a sense of security. All people use various defense mechanisms at times. When a person uses them to excess, however, they threaten that individual's mental health.

Examples of common defense mechanisms include:

Suppression: Consciously inhibiting an unacceptable impulse or emotion
Repression: Unconsciously inhibiting an unacceptable impulse or emotion
Reaction-formation: Displaying a behavior, attitude, or feeling opposite to that which one would normally exhibit in the situation
Rationalization: Trying logically to justify irrational or unacceptable behaviors or feelings
Displacement: Unconsciously transferring feelings onto another person or object
Denial: Disavowing the existence of unpleasant realities
Projection: Attributing to another person one's unacceptable thoughts and feelings
Sublimation: Diverting unacceptable urges into personally and socially acceptable channels
Intellectualization: Unconsciously transferring emotions into the realm of intellect; using reasoning as a means of avoiding confrontation with objectionable impulses

Remember: It is when these defense mechanisms are used to excess that a deviation from mental health exists.

☞ KEY CONCEPT

Be aware of your own feelings, reactions, and use of defense mechanisms. At the same time, recognize the use of defense mechanisms in your clients, so you can plan nursing care to be most effective.

Table 93-1 gives examples of how persons may use the defense mechanisms listed above in everyday life.

MENTAL ILLNESS

Everyone has feelings and behaviors that they must control. *Mental illness* often means a difference in degree of behavior, rather than completely different behavior. Many people who are mentally ill cannot control their socially unaccept-

■■■ **TABLE 93-1** *E*XAMPLES OF DEFENSE MECHANISMS

Defense Mechanism	Example
Suppression	Joe does not want to discuss his mother's recent death and continually tells his wife, "We'll talk about it tomorrow."
Repression	Lauren, who was in an automobile accident in which she did not lose consciousness or suffer any brain damage, cannot recall anything that happened directly before, during, or after the event.
Reaction-formation	Peter does not like his stepfather but is overly polite and kind to him.
Rationalization	Twelve-year-old Jill fails to be elected to student council. She says that "The elections were probably fixed, and student council is for nerds, anyway."
Displacement	Michelle is upset with her husband, but yells at her preschool-age daughter, who in turn yells at the family dog.
Denial	Gordon, recently diagnosed with terminal cancer, tells his family that he feels fine and the doctors do not know what they're talking about.
Projection	Chuck accidentally erases files from his computer. He yells at his son, "See what you made me do with all that noise," and calls the computer names.
Sublimation	Madeline, who has always been very shy and nervous, forces herself to join the college drama team.
Intellectualization	Lincoln, going through a messy divorce, refuses to become emotional about the situation. He continually philosophizes about the meaning of relationships and love, saying things like "Nothing lasts forever."

able behavior. Recent research indicates that nearly half of all people in the United States will experience a deviation from mental health at some point. Psychiatric disorders can arise from external conditions, life stressors, or brain disorders. Some mental disorders arise from unknown causes. The Greek letter psi (Ψ) often is used to denote psychiatry.

Mental illness affects all spheres of a person's life including physical health, employment, housing, finances, and relationships. It may be influenced by or may be a cause of substance abuse and other addictions.

Diagnosis

A psychiatrist, psychologist, advance practice nurse, and other team members work together to determine if a client has a mental disorder and its cause and type. Nursing observations are important input for this evaluation. A complete physical examination is done to rule out a physical disease or injury that may have caused the illness. Specific diagnoses are identified, based on the taxonomy presented in the American Psychiatric Association's (**APA,** 1994) *Diagnostic and Statistical Manual of Mental Disorders* (**DSM-IV**). This taxonomy is a system consisting of five axes, each of which addresses a specific category and includes criteria that, when combined, allow the examiner to develop a complete psychiatric diagnosis (Box 93-1).

Organic Versus Functional

In some cases, the healthcare team identifies a physical (*organic*) cause for the client's mental disorder (**organic disorder**). An endocrine disorder (especially of the thyroid), infection, hypoglycemia, drug overdose (**OD**), psychoactive drug or alcohol abuse, cerebrovascular disease, brain lesion, and conditions such as Huntington's disease or acquired immunodeficiency disorder (AIDS) may cause an organic disorder. Closed head trauma (**CHT**), also known as a closed head injury (**CHI**), may also cause temporary or permanent *psychosis* (discussed later). This development often follows a motor vehicle accident (MVA) or an assault. If an organic cause is identified, treatment of it may alleviate the mental

> ➤ BOX 93-1

THE MULTIAXIAL SYSTEM OF PSYCHIATRIC DIAGNOSES

Axis I: Clinical psychiatric syndromes
Axis II: Personality disorders and mental retardation
Axis III: General medical conditions
Axis IV: Psychosocial and environmental problems
Axis V: Global assessment of functioning

illness. In many cases, however, no specific causative agent is located. This type of mental illness is called a **functional disorder.**

Psychometric Tests

A psychologist and psychometrist aid the psychiatrist to make a differential diagnosis of mental illness. *Neuropsychiatric* (**psychometric**) testing includes an in-depth interview and various tests. Commonly used tests include the Brief Psychiatric Rating Scale (**BPRS**) and Mini Mental Status Exam (**MMSE**). Sometimes, the results of a mental status exam are stated in terms of appearance, mood, sensorium, intelligence, and thought process (**AMSIT**) in the chart. These tests evaluate the client's orientation to time and place and require the person to perform simple tasks. A common abbreviation to describe orientation is **A&O ×3** (alert and oriented to person, place, and time). Other projective and memory tests include the Rorschach inkblot, "Draw-a-Person," sentence-completion, Bender-Gestalt, word-association, and thematic apperception tests (**TAT**). Personality inventories, such as the Minnesota Multiphasic Personality Inventory (**MMPI**), are used extensively. Intelligence tests may also be given. The client's living situation is evaluated; for example, it is determined whether a client needs assistance with activities of daily living (ADL). One such test is the **KELS,** the Kohlman Evaluation of Living Skills.

In addition, a special test may be performed to rule out the client who is **malingering:** feigning or faking symptoms so that he or she can stay in the hospital, receive medications, or get attention. This is called the Structured Interview of Reported Symptoms (**SIRS**).

Neurologic Tests

Neurodiagnostic tests can rule out an organic cause of the disorder. These tests include the computed tomography (CT) scan, magnetic resonance imaging (MRI), positron emission tomography (PET), single photon emission computed tomography (SPECT), and the transcranial Doppler (**TCD**). In addition, a cerebral angiogram (brain x-ray study using contrast media), digital subtraction angiogram, or electroencephalography (EEG) may be needed. Measurement of the evoked potentials of the cerebral cortex (auditory brain response [**ABR**] or auditory evoked response [**AER**]) is also made in the EEG department, as are sleep studies. These tests can often rule out such conditions as brain tumor, abscess, cerebral vascular disease, cerebral atrophy, some forms of dementia, and sometimes, the organic changes associated with schizophrenia. The tests can diagnose some cases of Parkinson's syndrome or seizure disorders and they can locate the origination site of some seizures. They can also diagnose sleep disorders and some metabolic disorders.

A lumbar puncture (LP) may be done. In this invasive procedure, a needle is introduced into the subarachnoid space around the spinal cord (see Chap. 77). The lumbar puncture can determine intracranial pressure (ICP) or the presence of microorganisms, blood, or abnormal proteins in the cerebrospinal fluid.

Symptoms

In most instances, the following behavior patterns signify a mental disorder. All these symptoms affect a person's identity and often lead to poor self-esteem:

- Noticeable behavioral changes—exaggerated feelings, inappropriate responses, unexplained depression, inappropriate elation
- Sudden lack of concern about physical appearance, inability to perform basic ADL
- Not eating, binge eating, excess fluid intake
- Not sleeping or sleeping all the time
- Physical symptoms without apparent medical cause
- Overuse of defense mechanisms
- Loss of contact with reality—altered perceptions and sensory changes such as increased watchfulness (**hypervigilance**), **hallucinations** (hearing, seeing, feeling things that are not there), misperceptions, distorted thinking, difficulty in filtering out irrelevant stimuli, **paranoia** (unreasonable fears), delusional thinking
- Cognitive confusion—disorientation, thought blocking, loose associations, poor abstract thinking, illogical thinking, inability to problem-solve, inability to cope with stress, preoccupation, poor concentration, poor memory, speech latency
- Morbid fascination with death—talk of wanting to die or of committing suicide; thoughts of hurting oneself or others
- Total immobility; suddenly becoming mute

Types

Mental illness varies considerably in degree and type. Clinical diagnosis is often stated as:

- Acute or chronic
- In remission
- Prior history

The following text describes general psychiatric categories.

Mood Disorders

Mood disorders are a group of clinical conditions characterized by disturbance of **mood** (internal, subjective emotional state), along with a loss of control and a subjective feeling of distress. (**Euthymia** is the term that means normal mood.)

Major Depressive Episode.   *Depression* is the most common mood disorder, with over 15 million people in the United States experiencing it in a given year. At least 50% of all suicides can be attributed to a depressive disorder.

Diagnosis of a Major Depressive Episode includes five or more of the following signs and symptoms, which must be present frequently during the same 2-week period and must represent a change from previous functional levels. (Many of these signs and symptoms are observable by other people.)

At least one symptom must be (A) depressed mood most of the day, or (B) markedly diminished/loss of interest or pleasure in all, or most, activities (**anhedonia**).

Four or more additional signs and symptoms must be present from the following list:

- Weight or appetite changes—significant weight loss when not dieting; significant weight gain (>5% in 1 month); marked appetite decrease or increase; inability to eat/drink without physical cause
- Sleep disturbances—*insomnia* (difficulty falling or staying asleep) or **hypersomnia** (sleeping too much); severe nightmares; sleeping only in the daytime
- *Psychomotor retardation* (very slow movements or responses) or psychomotor agitation
- Fatigue; loss of energy
- Feelings of worthlessness (low self-esteem) or excessive or inappropriate guilt—may be **delusional** (fixed false belief not shared by others)
- Diminished ability to think/concentrate; indecisiveness; thought blocking (difficulty finishing sentences or thoughts); preoccupation
- Recurrent thoughts of death or suicidal ideation, with or without a specific plan

The nurse may observe other signs of depression in clients, including crying spells, poor grooming, anxiety, self-blame, isolation, loneliness, irritability, and vague physical complaints. Symptoms of depression cause significant distress or impairment in social, occupational, and other areas of functioning.

Physical (organic) causes of depression may be found. For example, some medications cause depression (eg, corticosteroids). Disorders such as hypothyroidism, stroke, and multiple sclerosis often lead to depression, as does the use of drugs (eg, cocaine, alcohol).

Situational depression is caused by a specific event or factors in one's life. Examples include depression that follows the death of a loved one or loss of a job. Sometimes, several stressors occur simultaneously, and a person feels overwhelmed. Resolution of stressors or therapy to help deal with them can often relieve situational depression. The person who experiences situational depression often never has another episode.

Depression in senior citizens is becoming more significant. Older people often have situational stressors such as loss of a spouse, loneliness, financial problems, physical disorders, chronic illness, pain, and fear of death.

Dysthymia. **Dysthymia** is defined as a depressed mood for most of the day, most days. The client subjectively describes this state, which may be observed by others. To be classified as dysthymia, the situation must be present for at least 2 years. Additional symptoms include sleep disturbances, appetite changes, decreased energy, low self-esteem, poor concentration, and feelings of hopelessness. Dysthymia tends to be less severe, but longer lasting, than major depressive disorder (**MDD**).

Bipolar Disorder (BPD). Broad mood variations from mania to major depression are symptoms of **bipolar disorder** (BPD). Agitation, elation, hyperactivity, and hyperexcitability characterize **mania.** The person shows accelerated thinking and speaking, **grandiosity** (feelings of invincibility and self-importance), distractibility (inability to concentrate), and excessive involvement in pleasurable activities that have a high potential for painful or undesirable consequences. (To meet the definition of mania, symptoms must be present for at least 1 week.)

Mania and depression alternate in BPD. Some people are "rapid cyclers," having short periods of mania that alternate with short periods of depression. Others have much longer cycles or stay mostly in the manic or the depressed end of the scale. Some people have periods of normal behavior between cycles, particularly if medications control the condition.

A *mixed episode* of BPD results when symptoms of both a manic and a major depressive episode occur simultaneously for at least one week.

Personality Disorders

All people have traits that define and mold their personalities. When a personality trait becomes dysfunctional, it is described as a personality (Axis II) disorder. Personality disorders must follow a pattern of inner experience and outward behavior that deviates markedly from the expectations of the person's culture. This pattern of deviation manifests itself in two or more of the following ways:

- Cognition (how a person thinks)
- Affectivity (**affect** is the outward manifestation of subjective emotions)
- Interpersonal functioning (relationships with others)
- Poor impulse control; **intrusive** (interfering) behavior; bizarre behaviors

Personality disorders may be of several types. An individual may also show characteristics of more than one type at any given time. Personality disorders are on a continuum, ranging from slight deviations from normal to highly unacceptable behaviors.

Paranoid personality disorder: Pervasive distrust and suspiciousness of others; marked hypervigilance

Schizoid personality disorder: Pattern of detachment from social relationships and restricted range of emotions in interpersonal settings

Schizotypal personality disorder: Pattern of social and interpersonal deficits, marked by acute discomfort with and reduced capacity for close relationships; also includes cognitive or perceptual distortions and behavioral eccentricities

Antisocial personality disorder: Pattern of disregard for and violation of the rights of others, with no remorse for actions

Borderline personality disorder: Pervasive pattern of instability in interpersonal relationships and affect; low self-image; includes marked impulsivity, with displays of self-destructive or self-injurious behavior (**SIB**), self-inflicted wounds (**SIW**), and suicide gestures. (These people often have a history of sexual abuse, are most often female, and are frequently lesbian. They may have frequent hospitalizations and complain of many physical symptoms. Obesity is often present in severely ill people.)

Histrionic personality disorder: Pattern of excessive emotionality and attention-seeking behavior

Narcissistic personality disorder: Pattern of grandiosity, need for admiration, lack of *empathy* (understanding for others' state of mind) and sense of **entitlement** ("the world owes me everything")

Avoidant personality disorder: Pattern of social inhibition, feelings of inadequacy, and hypersensitivity to negative evaluation; inability to be with other people

Dependent personality disorder: A pervasive and excessive need to be taken care of, leading to submissive, clingy behavior and fear of separation

People with personality disorders are often difficult and frustrating to work with. One reason is that many of them are blind to their behaviors and tend to create more distress for others than for themselves. Diagnosis of pathology on Axis II usually depends more on the clinician's observation of signs than on the client's responses, which may be defensive.

Anxiety Disorders

Some clients exhibit *anxiety disorders.* Components of anxiety disorders can be present in other disorders as well.

Panic Attacks.   The *panic attack* is characterized by intense fear, with no known cause. Symptoms include shaking, diaphoresis, a smothering or choking feeling, nausea, chest pain, and dizziness. This person may falsely believe that he or she is dying.

Phobias.   A specific **phobia** is an excessive, unreasonable, and severe fear of a particular thing or event. The object of fear may be anything, from snakes to flying. A person's exposure to the phobic stimulus causes severe panic. The person realizes intellectually that the fear is illogical, but is powerless to control it without therapy.

One common phobia is called **agoraphobia,** the fear of being in a place from which escape may be difficult or embarrassing. The agoraphobic individual is often afraid to be in a crowd or other tightly enclosed space. Some people are so disabled by this disorder that they are unable to leave the home.

Obsessive-Compulsive Disorder (OCD).   *Obsessive-compulsive disorder* (**OCD**) is marked by obsessions and compulsions. An **obsession** is a recurrent, persistent, intrusive thought or belief that the person cannot ignore. A **compulsion** is a repetitive behavior (eg, handwashing, cleaning) or a mental act (eg, counting, praying) that the person feels driven to perform, sometimes constantly. The person usually imposes rigid rules onto the act. OCD can cause great distress; its ritualistic behaviors can interfere partially or totally with the person's life. In some cases, the person spends the entire day performing these rituals and cannot do anything else. The person realizes that these obsessions and compulsions are products of his or her own mind, but cannot change actions without therapy.

Post-Traumatic Stress Disorder (PTSD).   The DSM-IV describes *post-traumatic stress disorder* (**PTSD**) in terms of several diagnostic criteria. The person has been exposed to a traumatic event or series of events (eg, sexual abuse, torture) in which the response was intense fear or helplessness. Symptoms of PTSD include recurrent and intrusive flashbacks to or dreams of the event, insomnia, inability to concentrate, persistent avoidance of stimuli associated with the event, and inability to recall all or part of it. The person often exhibits symptoms—such as hypervigilance, paranoia, exaggerated startle response, and irritability—that were not present before the trauma. Many clients with PTSD isolate themselves, but they feel lonely and as though they have no future. They are sometimes suicidal or self-injurious.

Psychosis

Marked deviation from normal behavior and seriously inappropriate conduct may indicate **psychosis,** a thought disorder that interferes with one's ability to recognize and to deal with reality. A psychosis also interferes with the person's ability to communicate. Symptoms include delusions, *hallucinations* (false sensory perceptions, without relevant external stimulation), and *impaired reality testing* (impaired fundamental functions, including the ability to differentiate between the external and internal world and between self and the environment). Behavior is unusual and noticeable in most cases. Psychosis can be organic or functional. The person who is severely disturbed is said to be having an acute psychotic episode (**APE**).

☛ KEY CONCEPT

Types of hallucinations *(sensory impressions without objective external stimulus):*

- *Auditory—hearing voices, music, or other sounds (the most common)*
- *Visual—seeing things that others do not see*
- *Tactile (haptic)—hallucination of touch*
- *Gustatory—hallucination of taste*
- *Olfactory—hallucination of smell*

"Command hallucinations" are those that instruct clients to do something, often to hurt themselves or others.

Schizophrenia.   **Schizophrenia** is a group of psychotic disorders that have two or more of the following *positive symptoms:* delusions, hallucinations, disorganized speech, grossly disorganized behavior, and **catatonia** (stupor, muscle rigidity). *Negative symptoms* include withdrawal, isolation, and a flat affect. Symptoms interfere with social, occupational, and self-care abilities. They must be present for at least 6 months for a diagnosis of schizophrenia.

Types of schizophrenia include:

Paranoid: The person is preoccupied either with delusions or frequent auditory hallucinations or both. Paranoid people are fearful and suspicious, thinking someone or something will hurt or kill them. They often feel they are being followed or observed from a distance.

Disorganized: The person exhibits disorganized speech or behavior (or both), flat or inappropriate affect, and inability to perform self-care.

Undifferentiated: The person meets the criteria for schizophrenia, but not for a specific paranoid, disorganized, or catatonic type.

Residual: The person has a history of one schizophrenic episode, but prominent delusions, hallucinations, disorganized speech, and grossly disorganized or catatonic behavior are absent.

Catatonic: The person shows two or more of the following:

- **catalepsy** (the person maintains the body position in which he or she is placed)
- stupor
- excessive, purposeless motor activity
- motiveless resistance to all instructions
- maintenance of rigid posture against attempts to be moved
- **mutism** (refusal to speak)
- voluntary assumption of inappropriate or bizarre postures (*posturing*)
- stereotyped and repetitive movements
- prominent mannerisms or grimacing
- **echolalia** (repetition of another person's words or phrases)
- **echopraxia** (repetition of another person's movements)

Acute lethal catatonia (**ALC**) exists when the person does not move and is unable to eat or care for himself or herself. In this case, prompt medical intervention is required, to save the person's life.

Other Psychoses. *Substance-induced psychosis* is characterized by prominent hallucinations, delusions, or other symptoms of schizophrenia described above that develop during or within a month of substance intoxication or withdrawal. Commonly offending substances include alcohol, MDMA, and cocaine and related drugs, such as crack.

Schizoaffective disorder is a psychotic disorder with symptoms of both a mood disorder (eg, major depression or mania or both) and schizophrenia.

A *delusional disorder* is characterized by persistent, nonbizarre delusions involving situations that may occur in real life. The person may believe that they are being followed, poisoned, infected, diseased (*somatic delusion*), loved by a distant admirer (*erotomania*), or deceived by one's lover (*jealous-type delusion*). Delusions may also be *grandiose* (eg, believing that one has a special relationship with God or is royalty, "delusions of grandeur"). The person may also feel that he or she is being treated in an evil way (*delusions of persecution*). To meet the criteria of this diagnosis, delusions must be present for at least 1 month. Apart from the impact of delusions, everyday functioning is not markedly impaired and behavior is not obviously odd. Delusions are often fixed and of long standing; they may be very difficult to treat. A person may have a fixed delusion for life and may expand and elaborate on it as time goes on.

Brief Psychotic Disorder. A person may have a *brief psychotic disorder*. This disorder is characterized by the presence of one or more of the following symptoms, for at least one day, but for less than 1 month: delusions, hallucinations, disorganized speech (incoherent), or grossly disorganized or

catatonic behavior. The individual has eventual full return to usual functional levels. A brief psychotic disorder may occur with a marked stressor (*brief reactive psychosis*), without a marked stressor, or with postpartum onset.

Psychotic disorder, **NOS** (not otherwise specified) includes psychotic symptoms, but a specific diagnosis cannot be made.

Psychotic Disorder Caused by a Medical Condition. A medical condition can cause a psychotic disorder, often with hallucinations or delusions. Evidence from the person's history, physical examination, or laboratory findings indicate that the disturbance is a direct consequence of a general medical condition. Possible causative conditions are infection, high fever, brain neoplasm (cancer), head trauma, AIDS dementia, tertiary syphilis, or other preexisting dementia.

☛ KEY CONCEPT

A person can have symptoms of several mental disorders simultaneously. For example, a person with depression may also have hallucinations. An individual's diagnosis may change over time. Therefore, the nurse must learn how to deal with various behaviors and not to classify people in terms of their original diagnosis.

Dual Diagnoses

The term **dual diagnosis** literally means that the person has two separate chronic conditions at the same time. It can be a combination of any two factors, such as mental illness and sexual addiction, or anorexia and chemical dependency. Some people with mental illness also exhibit some level of intellectual impairment (mental retardation) (**MI/MR**). However, the term *dual diagnosis* has commonly come to mean mental illness combined with chemical dependency (**MI/CD**). People with serious mental illness are at high risk (approximately 50%) for substance abuse or dependency (see Chap. 94).

Identifying whether substance abuse or mental illness occurred first is difficult in many clients with MI/CD. Some clients drink or use drugs to mask voices or other psychotic symptoms. Others became psychotic after using chemicals. People with no previous psychosis may experience symptoms during withdrawal from alcohol or drugs. Long-standing chemical abuse can also cause *organic psychosis,* secondary to brain damage.

Chemical abuse often aggravates mental illness. For example, alcohol is a depressant; when combined with underlying depression, symptoms worsen. People with normal moods may become depressed when drinking. When working with clients carrying a dual diagnosis, consider the following factors:

- Many clients are *polysubstance abusers* (abuse more than one substance).
- In many cases, chemical abuse *exacerbates* (worsens) mental illness.
- Alcohol (**ETOH, EtOH**) and other mood-altering chemicals have adverse reactions with *neuroleptic* (antipsychotic) and other prescribed medications. These chemicals may negate the desired effects of these

medications or may dangerously increase their effects. These combinations seriously interfere with treatment and can be life threatening.

- Many psychiatric clients are particularly susceptible to the effects of drugs because of their underlying mental instability.
- The presence of mental illness may make it difficult for the client to understand or follow a chemical dependency treatment program.
- Clients are often vulnerable and are easy prey for those who distribute drugs.
- Some after-care and chemical dependency treatment programs and support groups wrongly advise clients not to take their *psychotropic* (mood-modifying) medications.

☞ KEY CONCEPT

Whenever a client is admitted to the mental health unit, consider the possibility of withdrawal from alcohol or drugs. The use of these substances is very common in this population and withdrawal can be life threatening (see Chap. 94).

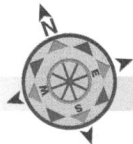

SPECIAL CONSIDERATIONS: CULTURE

Reactions to and Treatment of Mental Illness

Clients come from many cultures with differing beliefs and behaviors. Normal and abnormal behaviors often depend on one's cultural perspective. Conditions such as schizophrenia, bipolar disorder, and major depression are believed to occur worldwide. However, cultural reactions to them differ. For example, in some cultures, guilt and suicidal ideation do not accompany depression. North America has incidences of many culture-bound illnesses (eg, "nervous breakdown" and anorexia nervosa) that are not common in other cultures. Misdiagnosis is a common problem for groups who differ from the typical behaviors of North American culture.

Different cultures also have varying customs and beliefs related to such concepts as eye contact, personal space, or causation of illness. In some cultures, the person who experiences hallucinations is believed to be directly communicating with God and this is considered to be a special "gift." Many of the world's peoples believe in the effect of the "evil eye" or in "possession by demons." Others believe in "hot and cold" effects of foods in causation and treatment of disease. It is important to consider these and other cultural beliefs in your care of clients in the mental health unit. The fact that a client holds the belief of most people in his or her culture should not be considered a mental deviation just because these beliefs differ from traditional Western cultural beliefs.

THE MENTAL HEALTHCARE TEAM

Mental illness affects the client's entire life and that of the family. The team approach is vital to provide the best assistance.

Psychiatrist

A **psychiatrist** is a physician (MD or DO) who has received advanced education in the treatment of mental disorders. Psychiatrists use a holistic approach that considers each client's mental, physical, and emotional characteristics. The mental healthcare team addresses the client's physical disorders as either causative, coexisting, or secondary disorders. The psychiatrist directs the team.

Nurse

The *nurse* is an important member of the mental health team. By creating a therapeutic environment (milieu), nurses assist people to return to as near normal functioning as possible in the shortest possible time. Baccalaureate-prepared RNs can receive national clinical certification in Psychiatric and Mental Health Nursing or Advanced Practice Certification in Psychiatry. The Clinical Nurse Specialist is a Master's degree-prepared nurse with a specialty in psychiatry. This person is often licensed to provide psychiatric therapy and to prescribe medications.

As nurses work with psychiatric clients, it is important to consider the whole person and maintain an awareness of his or her rights (discussed later in this chapter).

Other Team Members

Psychiatric technicians, mental health workers, and *human service workers* also deal directly with clients on the mental health unit. These workers, often unlicensed, may provide a large proportion of the daily physical care required by clients.

Psychologists have either a Master's degree or a doctorate in psychology and provide testing, counseling, and therapy. *Psychometrists* administer psychological tests.

Recreation therapists and *music therapists* provide diversional and personal growth activities and often take clients on outings off the unit. *Occupational therapists* evaluate and instruct clients in ADL, homemaking, crafts, and some job-retraining or employment skills. *Vocational rehabilitation* and *veteran's services* sometimes make school attendance or employment possible. *Chaplains* offer spiritual counseling and support.

Social workers prepare clients for and assist with discharge. They often act as the liaison among clients, family members and friends, and the community. Social workers may help clients find a safe place to live, obtain financial assistance, or access other community resources.

Other specialists may assist with individual cases. These specialists include *medical/surgical specialists, interpreters, diabetic* or *stoma specialists, dietitians, pharmacists,* and *respiratory therapists. EEG, electrocardiographic (ECG), laboratory,* and *radiologic technicians* perform specialized examinations. *Volunteers* may provide pet therapy, gifts for holidays, and other services.

Treatment Centers and Resources

Many resources are available today to assist people with mental health concerns and illnesses. They include a variety of community agencies, as well as acute and semi-acute inpatient units. The range of care varies from independent living to total care and constant supervision.

Community-Based Programs

The trend is toward the least restrictive treatment possible. Therefore, most people with mental illnesses are currently treated, and managed, in the community.

Outpatient Mental Health Clinics or Centers.   The *outpatient mental health clinic* or *community mental health center* provides ongoing therapy and counseling for people who do not require hospitalization. Clients visit daily or weekly; home visits by staff may be included. Medications are prescribed, and compliance and effectiveness are evaluated regularly. In some cases, blood work is done (eg, Clozaril maintenance); or long-acting neuroleptic injections (**decanoates**) are given.

Psychiatric Home Care/Community Outreach.   The trend toward community living for chronically and persistently mentally ill (**CPMI**) clients has necessitated the initiation of home care services for them. Usually, a public health nurse, home care nurse, and other workers visit a client regularly to manage his or her disorder. If a client experiences symptoms or problems, a nurse makes additional visits to evaluate the situation. In some cases, an outreach worker refers the client to the mental health center or inpatient psychiatric unit. If necessary, police may assist in transfer to a hospital for clients who are combative or suicidal, or who refuse voluntary admission and are considered dangerous to themselves or others.

Many challenges are involved in delivering home care to mentally ill clients. Care must focus largely on rehabilitation and teaching. Because home care is provided directly in the client's home, staff are better able to appreciate the client's and family's daily problems. Nurses address issues such as medication compliance, symptom recurrence, sleep disorders, homemaking and home safety, and poor eating habits. They help clients to keep appointments, structure their time, and attend treatment or support group meetings. These nurses also assist with interpersonal skills, helping clients to live comfortably with others. They teach family members about medications and other treatments.

Nursing Alert

The nurse working in home care must be alert to his or her own personal safety. Often nurses making home visits, particularly to mentally ill clients, travel in pairs or carry a cell phone. If a situation feels unsafe to you, leave and consult your supervisor. Do not enter a potentially unsafe situation without backup. (See Chap. 98.)

Some clients need physical care or assistance with homemaking skills. The personal care attendant/aide (**PCA**), also known as a health care attendant/aide (HCA) or home health aide (HHA), makes home visits to assist these clients. PCAs remind clients to take medications and make sure they eat properly. Some homemaking assistance may also be available (eg, homemaker services).

Telephone Services.   Telephone services are often available so people can call and talk to knowledgeable persons about their problems. Such services have proven particularly effective in crisis intervention, such as suicide, drug, and rape counseling. Advantages include anonymity and immediate accessibility.

Other Community Services.   There are federally-mandated Community Mental Health Centers (**CMHC**) around the country. These drop-in centers provide clients with structured recreation and opportunities to meet others with similar disorders. These centers often assist clients with employment, volunteer opportunities, money management, and housing arrangements. They may sponsor dances, holiday parties, and outings for their clients. Community programs assist clients with training in independent living, so that they can live alone or in a minimally supervised situation safely.

Individual communities have organizations that offer support to clients and families. One such example is the Minnesota Bio-Brain Association, which offers speakers and support groups to clients and their families. National organizations also have local affiliates.

Community-Based Living Facilities.   Clients who do not need care in a hospital or extended-care facility are discharged into the community. Some live alone in regular apartments or subsidized housing (such as "Section 8" housing). Others live in shelters or boarding houses. Additional supervision is sometimes necessary for those with chronic and persistent mental illnesses. The following are some of the facilities providing extra care:

Board-and-Care, Licensed Group Homes, and Nursing Homes. Some clients need increasing levels of structure and supervision to remain in the community. They may live in a *board-and-care* (B&C) home that provides meals and other services, with minimal supervision. *Licensed group homes* provide more structure by supervising medications and offering group activities. To qualify for a group home, the client usually must attend a day program, have a volunteer position, or be employed for a minimum number of hours per week. If a client needs more supervision and physical care, a *nursing home* may be necessary. In some cases, the client requires a locked nursing-home unit.

The Halfway House. Many communities offer "halfway houses" for mentally ill clients. This provides a buffer between the hospital and the community. The client lives there for a short time after discharge from the hospital, until he or she can find other housing. This way, readjustment into the community is less traumatic.

Sheltered Workshops and Vocational Rehabilitation. A client may need assistance with employment. *Sheltered workshops* provide an entry into the working world. In many cases, they provide skill training, often paying clients a small wage during training. Some clients continue to work in sheltered workshops; others are able to seek competitive employment in the community. *Vocational rehabilitation services* may also be available to assist clients to enter competitive employment. Vocational rehabilitation counselors may also work with employers, to assist them to better understand mental illness.

Respite Care. Family members often find the supervision of a chronically mentally ill loved one exhausting. They may place clients in inpatient settings for a few days to allow themselves some rest and a chance to regroup. This measure is called *respite care* because it gives families a *respite,* or break. Sometimes, insurance or public assistance pays for respite care for family caregivers.

☞ Kᴇʏ Cᴏɴᴄᴇᴘᴛ

Some mentally ill people are unable to find or maintain an adequate living situation; they may be homeless. Communities have outreach workers who attempt to locate homeless mentally ill people and assist them to find safer places to live. In addition, free medical and dental care, examinations, immunizations, and medication therapy are often provided. Organizations such as the Salvation Army sometimes deliver meals to shelters and camps and provide basic health screening.

Partial Hospitalization Programs

Some psychiatric hospitals have established a service whereby clients spend nights at the facility and hold regular jobs in the daytime (*night hospital*). This plan provides some supervision for these clients, while removing them from potentially dangerous or stressful homes.

In other cases, clients live at home and attend *day-treatment centers* or *partial hospitalization programs.* Activities include group, occupational, and recreational therapies. Clients learn about their medications and illnesses. For chemically dependent individuals, group therapy after discharge from the acute treatment center is vital and often continues indefinitely.

Emergency Services

Many healthcare facilities offer emergency services to people with disruptions in mental health. A *crisis intervention center* (**CIC**) or *emergency mental health clinic* is often part of a hospital's emergency department (ED). Here, clients receive emergency evaluation and assistance. Crisis centers offer many services. They conduct interventions that include prescribing medications and referring clients to mental health centers for therapy and case management. These centers also facilitate admission to inpatient psychiatric units for people who are seriously disturbed and present a danger to themselves or others.

The Inpatient Psychiatry Unit

If mental illness is severe or if a person is dangerous to the self or others, he or she is admitted to a hospital's *acute-care* or *inpatient psychiatry unit.* Hospitalization helps prevent the illness from escalating by reducing emotional stress and offering medication and other therapies. The hospital provides a safer environment for the client in danger. In this instance, the hospital also provides a therapeutic environment. The goal is to help the person learn to function effectively and to be able to function safely in the community upon discharge from the hospital.

Admission Status.   The terms of admission to a mental health facility vary among states and provinces and even within an area. Several general types of admission exist:

Voluntary admission ("vol"): Person comes to the hospital voluntarily
Emergency hold: Placed by a physician, usually for 72 hours, for evaluation of clients who are judged to be dangerous to themselves or others ("**72 hr.** hold, **72°** hold"). The client needs to be told that the 72-hour time frame usually does not include weekends and holidays (because the courts are closed).
Transportation hold: Placed by the police, to bring the person to the hospital in an emergency ("**T-Hold**")
*District court hold (**DCH**):* Placed by a judge before a preliminary commitment hearing
Assessment hold: Placed by the court to assess a person to determine if he or she is mentally competent to stand trial for a crime
Court commitment: Usually to a state, veteran's administration, county hospital, chemical dependency treatment center, or other care facility for treatment
*Mentally ill/chemically dependent (**MI/CD**):* Dual diagnosis, both of which need treatment
*Mentally ill and dangerous (**MI&D**):* Commitment to a security hospital

✚🏥👁 **N u r s i n g   A l e r t**
       Some clients refuse to talk when being admitted to a mental health unit. However, it is *vital* to obtain the following data. Try to get the client just to answer the five questions below. If the client will not answer, try looking at old charts or talking with relatives.

• Do you have allergies?
• Are you feeling like hurting yourself (*suicidal ideation*)?
• Are you feeling like hurting someone else (*homicidal ideation*)?
• Are you hearing voices (*auditory hallucinations*)?
• Why did you come to the hospital?

Commitment.   Long-term hospitalization is often conducted at a state facility (state hospital or treatment center). Although many state hospitals admit people voluntarily, sometimes for special treatment (such as chemical dependency), more people are admitted involuntarily (**commitment**). Commitment is imposed by the court and often follows a stay in a private or county facility. Most clients in state hospitals are supported by public funds. Funding availability varies between states.

Special Circumstances. A client may be admitted to a mental health unit under "no information status." In this case, the client does not want anyone to know he or she is there, and no information can be given out regarding the person. The hospital and nursing station will not even acknowledge that the person is there. In other cases, a high-profile client may be admitted under an *alias* (not their true name). This person is "also known as" (AKA) and all the records are filed under the alias. In other cases, an unknown person is admitted and is registered as "John Doe" or "Jane Doe" until their true identity can be discovered.

Discharge Planning. Planning for discharge as soon as possible is in the best interests of both the client and the family. However, the hospital has a responsibility to both the client and the community. Clients cannot be discharged from a hospital unless the treatment team feels that they are not dangerous to themselves or to others. Everything possible is done to facilitate readjustment into the community after discharge. Management of symptoms and client safety is of primary concern; efforts are made to place people in safe and comfortable living situations.

Provisional Discharge. The person may be discharged on a provisional basis. The terms of the provisional discharge (**PD**) are spelled out. If the client does not meet these terms, he or she is returned to the hospital. Common terms of a PD are: complying with the prescribed medication regimen, keeping followup appointments, maintaining sobriety, attending a day-treatment program or support group, and staying out of legal trouble.

Payment for Mental Healthcare. *Third-party payers* may cover the cost of mental healthcare, including chemical dependency treatment. Requirements for inpatient care, however, have become more stringent in recent years. Inpatient hospital stays are usually short, covering the crisis period only.

Persons with CPMI usually receive governmental financial assistance. It may be from Social Security Disability Income (SSDI), Medicaid, general assistance, or another funding program.

METHODS OF PSYCHIATRIC THERAPY

The goal of therapy is to alleviate symptoms and to modify the client's behavior so that he or she can meet life's demands and return to an optimum level of wellness. Therapy is based on specific behavioral problems and individual needs. Because therapists and nurses work together, nurses are aware of therapeutic goals and incorporate them into nursing care.

☛ Key Concept

The major overriding goal of all psychiatric care is safety of the client, his or her family, and others in the community.

Psychotherapy

Many different methods and theories of *psychotherapy* have been developed. General concepts are presented here.

Individual Psychotherapy

Individual psychotherapy is based on a personal relationship between the client and therapist. The aim is to relieve symptoms and eventually to resolve the disabling conflicts that caused them. Treatment encourages people to tell their stories, discuss problems, and devise socially acceptable and healthy ways of dealing with issues. Hypnosis, psychoanalysis, and counseling are among methods that may be used.

Group Psychotherapy

Group psychotherapy involves several clients and provides an opportunity for everyone to participate by discussing their individual problems (Fig. 93-1). Thereby, each individual learns to focus on others by becoming concerned about them. The client is drawn out of his or her private world to become part of the larger world. Clients often have keen insight into the behavior of others and can express feelings and offer constructive ideas. Group members usually have a special empathy and learn that they are not alone in certain feelings and behaviors. They are often very accepting of suggestions and constructive criticism from peers, perhaps more so than from staff. Group therapy is especially effective for the treatment of addictive behaviors and for grief and loss counseling.

Verbal and Other Therapies

Behavior Modification

Also known as *behavior shaping*, this method is used to deal with emotionally disturbed, mentally ill, and intellectually challenged people. *Behavior modification* is based on the theory that people respond well when rewarded for positive behavior. This positive reinforcement encourages the person to perform the same activity again to win another reward. To be effective, the expected task or behavior must be geared to the client's abilities; success must be possible. The client must clearly know what behavior is being rewarded. An effective form of positive reinforcement is a special food or

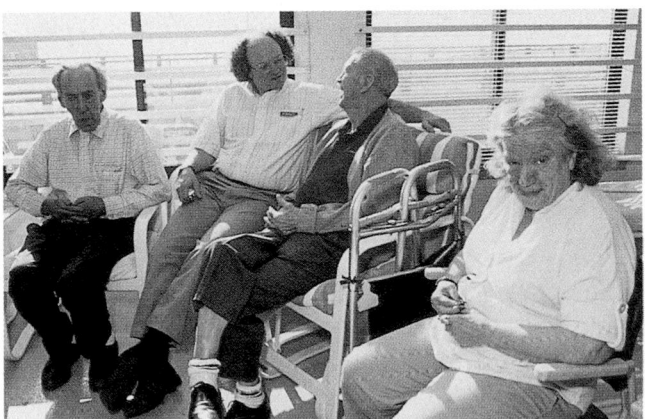

FIGURE 93-1. Group therapy is often used in mental health, rehabilitation, and chemical dependency units. Peers have special empathy and frequently offer helpful insights to others. Often, clients are very receptive to what peers say. It is helpful for clients to realize they are not alone in their feelings about the challenges of life.

another form of physical gratification, although almost any other reward, including attention from staff, can be reinforcing when used correctly. What is rewarding for one client may not necessarily be rewarding for another. *Negative reinforcement* (punishment) is usually ineffective because it does not promote and teach positive behavior. Rewarding appropriate behavior and ignoring inappropriate behavior is most effective.

When using behavior modification, show the person what you want, help them accomplish it, then reward the person for a job well done. The reward is most effective if given immediately. Gradually let the person assume more responsibility for doing tasks alone. Consistency is important. "A classic use of behavior modification techniques is in the treatment of phobias by relaxation and desensitization."[1]

☛ KEY CONCEPT

Giving attention to any person is a powerful modifier of his or her behavior. It is important to give attention for positive behaviors, as much as is possible. Giving attention for negative behaviors reinforces the unwanted behavior.

Remotivation

Many mental health and geriatric units use *remotivation technique* or *reality orientation*. Groups are structured so that participating clients discuss things that are meaningful to them. To stimulate conversation, poems or scrapbooks filled with pictures of familiar items can be helpful. Photo albums, newspapers, or pictures of recent events can also spur discussion.

Everyone is included in the discussion; all members are encouraged to participate. The method and direction of the discussion are based on the group's abilities. For example, in a group of severely regressed or demented people, the discussion would be simple, and the leader would ask many questions to maintain the discussion.

☛ KEY CONCEPT

All individuals need to know who they are, where they are, who other people are, and what day it is, to be comfortable.

Reality Therapy

All people have a need to love and be loved, and to feel worthwhile as human beings to themselves (*self-esteem*) and others (*acceptance*). If a person is unable to meet these needs in a socially acceptable way, he or she may act inappropriately. The goal of *reality therapy* is to help people face reality, reject irresponsible behavior, and learn new and more socially acceptable ways of behaving.

Reality therapy does not necessarily take a traditional approach to mental illness. It differs from conventional psychotherapy by concentrating on the present, rather than the past. In reality therapy, understanding the reasons why clients think or act is less important than solving immediate problems and dealing with behaviors. The reality therapist approaches behaviors as they occur, rather than examining feelings or underlying causes.

☛ KEY CONCEPT

The nurse using reality therapy *indicates to the client that what has happened in the past cannot be changed. The client is encouraged to look toward the future and to live accordingly. Behaviors can be taught, which will be helpful in meeting future goals and in learning to live comfortably outside the hospital.*

Rational Emotive Therapy

Albert Ellis developed this approach, which is also called *rational emotive behavior therapy* (**REBT**), *rational recovery,* and *cognitive behavior therapy*. It is used in psychiatry, chemical dependency treatment, and rehabilitation. It is most "effective with groups whose members have similar problems."[2] This theory disputes irrational beliefs and accentuates rational and positive behaviors. Confrontation is used "as a means of helping (clients) restructure irrational beliefs and behavior . . . Thus, by changing thoughts, a person can change feelings and behavior."[2] The principles of REBT are:

- People are accepted unconditionally because they are alive and human, whether or not they perform well.
- Nothing is awful or terrible, even though it may be frustrating and difficult.

"Mental health rehabilitation is defined as therapeutic counseling, designed to facilitate the emotional development of individuals with mental and physical disabilities, that enables them to lead more productive lives."[3] This approach is less effective if the client is out of contact with reality, highly manic, brain injured, or mentally retarded. Chapter 94 discusses the REBT approach in more detail. If a facility uses this approach, the staff will need to receive specific training.

Transactional Analysis

All interactions between people have meaning and are based on the way people feel at the moment. The goal of *transactional analysis* (**TA**) is to teach people to react in ways that produce positive responses from others, rather than hostile responses.

TA is based on the concept that all people react, at different times, as either the child, parent, or adult. At any particular time, one of these roles predominates. Two roles, those of parent and child, are actually from a person's past. When a person assumes the parent role, he or she will often react as their own parents did. When a person assumes the child role, he or she will often react as they did when they were a child. The goal is to react as a *reasonable adult* in as many situations as possible.

One-to-One Therapy

The *one-to-one* setting provides a therapeutic, non-threatening environment. Clients are encouraged to express concerns and feelings and to indicate how staff can be most helpful. Many people are willing to reveal thoughts and feelings to one person that they would be less willing to share in a group setting. It is most helpful for a client to have the same staff person for several days, in order to build trust. Guidelines for therapeutic communication are listed in Chapter 44.

Psychodrama

The use of *role-playing* (acting out one's feelings) offers many people, especially children and adolescents, the opportunity to release emotions. Many people are able to act out situations in their lives that they are unable to verbalize, such as relationships with a spouse or parents. Close observation of this *psychodrama* by staff is an aid in planning the most effective measures for treatment and nursing care.

Occupational Therapy

Not only is *occupational therapy* (OT) highly therapeutic, it also acts as a source of enjoyment and satisfaction for many people. Clients are able to become active in creative projects, such as arts and crafts, while socializing with staff and other clients. Through the creative process, people gain a sense of success and increased self-esteem. The overactive person is able to release some energy while working on a project; the underactive person is encouraged to participate. Projects can be designed to be appropriate for any skill level. Fine motor skills can be developed, as well as coordination. The OT staff also evaluates the client's concentration, ability to plan, ability to follow instructions, and ability to relate to others. The non–English-speaking person also can comfortably participate in OT.

Occupational therapists also evaluate an individual's ability to function independently. One evaluation is done using the KELS; another is called the Functional Assessment Inventory (**FAI**). These tests help determine the safest living situation for each client after discharge. In many facilities, OT staff assist in career planning, occupational skill training, or training in daily living skills such as cooking, laundry, managing money, or grocery shopping. Occupational therapists may also work in a sheltered workshop, group home, or halfway house, assisting clients who have been discharged from inpatient psychiatric settings.

Recreational Therapy/Therapeutic Recreation

Therapeutic recreation (**TR**), also called *recreational therapy* (**RT**), is an important component of the treatment program. Through planned recreational activities, on and off the mental health unit, the person is helped to reenter the world. A group may go bowling, to a sports event, to a movie, or out to eat. They may also engage in games, activities, and music on the inpatient unit, or they may assist in cooking a meal or dessert. Going to the gym or swimming pool or participating in an active game such as bowling or shuffleboard can help to work off excess energy in the person who is hyperactive. Games such as "Life Stories" help clients to share their feelings. Games requiring scorekeeping help the person to regain math skills. Reading the newspaper together or celebrating holidays and birthdays helps clients keep up with current events. A grooming group encourages clients to look their best (Fig. 93-2). By using these and other activities, the TR staff assist clients to adapt to life outside the hospital as clients

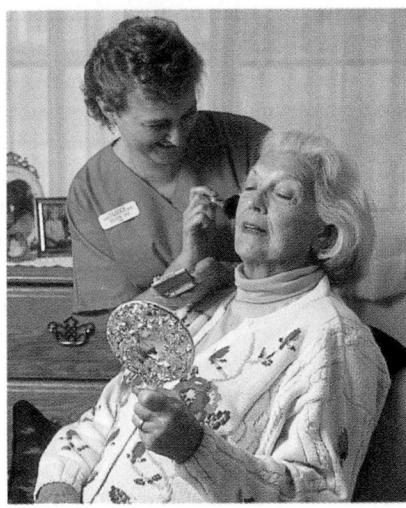

FIGURE 93-2. Clients in mental health units are assisted to build self-esteem, particularly if they are depressed. A new hairdo and makeup encourage this woman to feel better about herself and to make her more able to safely return to independent living.

gradually become re-accustomed to interacting with others. The person who does not speak English can comfortably participate in many TR activities.

Music Therapy

Music is a universal language. Because many nonverbal or non–English-speaking people enjoy music, they often enthusiastically join in by singing or playing rhythm instruments. These individuals are able to communicate and develop social skills without being forced to speak. Music also is a source of gratification and fun. (Sometimes, clients use music to help drown out "voices"; often, they have tape players with headphones. This is less disruptive to others.)

Pet Therapy

Many facilities have great success with visiting animals. Even the most regressed person usually responds positively to a kitten or puppy. Many mentally ill people relate better to animals at first than they do to other people, because animals pose less of a threat than do other people. *Pet therapy* can help prepare individuals for future human interactions and responsibilities. Many mental health units have a resident pet and the clients assist in its care. It is important for staff to closely supervise interactions with pets, to prevent injury to the clients or to the animals.

Play Therapy

There are two types of *play therapy*. The first is used to assist children (and occasionally adults) with disruptions in mental health. The play therapist guides their behavior, slowly helping them to socialize with others and to adjust to the outside world. The therapist can also learn about children and some of the origins of their mental disorders by observing their play.

The second type of play therapy is used with adults. One example is the "New Games" approach. These games are designed for various activity and attention levels and different numbers of participants. Many of these games are incorporated into activity plans for clients in mental health, rehabilitation, geriatric, and chemical dependency units. Clients play games using rules that they can apply to the real world. The games teach people to take psychological and physical risks, to develop trust and a sense of community, to realize that winning is not as important as effort, and to emphasize challenge, rather than competition. Imagery and ritual promote a sense of freedom and decrease inhibition. Staff members must be flexible and feel free to change to another game if the one chosen is not therapeutic. Games can also be changed and adapted to suit the group. "Play hard, play fair, nobody hurt" is the slogan of the New Games Foundation.[4]

Hydrotherapy

Most large mental health units have *hydrotherapy* facilities or swimming pools. Most people enjoy swimming or relaxing in a whirlpool and can work off frustrations or relax. Always closely supervise anyone who is swimming or in a tub.

Electroconvulsive Therapy

Electroconvulsive therapy (**ECT**), formerly referred to as *electroshock therapy,* causes a seizure by sending an electric current through the brain. Theorists believe that the seizure affects the brain's levels of neurotransmitters, which can radically improve the person's mood. Current practice restricts the use of ECT to a limited group of clients. It is most commonly used to treat depression in middle-aged and older adults who do not respond to antidepressant medications. Occasionally, it is used in other situations. Disadvantages of ECT are the person's anxiety before treatment and short-term memory loss in some clients. See In Practice: Nursing Care Guidelines 93-1 for information on caring for the client who is to have ECT.

Medication Therapy

Introduced in the 1950s, *antipsychotic medications* revolutionized the treatment of mental disorders. Certain medications arrest or greatly alleviate the adverse symptoms of many psychiatric disorders, enabling affected persons to function in the community. As a result of antipsychotic medications, the number of long-term clients in mental hospitals has greatly decreased. See In Practice: Nursing Care Guidelines 93-2 for information on administering medication therapy. Table 93-2 identifies commonly used medications, their actions, and nursing considerations. Box 93-2 lists the forms of medications used in psychiatry.

Psychotropic Drugs

Psychotropic drugs (mood modifiers) include antipsychotics, antianxiety sedative-hypnotics, mood stabilizers, and antidepressants. These drugs are used primarily in mental health units and by mental health clients after discharge. However, clients may also use them in other healthcare settings. Pregnant women should not take these medications without medical supervision.

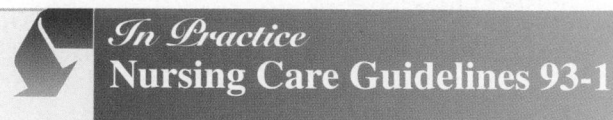

In Practice
Nursing Care Guidelines 93-1

CARING FOR THE CLIENT WHO IS TO HAVE ELECTROCONVULSIVE THERAPY

- ECT is usually carried out in the recovery room or a special treatment room. Routine preoperative preparations are carried out.
- Make sure the person voids before the treatment. (Incontinence may occur.)
- A mental status exam is performed before and after ECT (to assess any change in cognitive skills).
- Explain to the client and family what will happen during the procedure. (A videotape may be available to aid in teaching.)
- An IV is usually started (to administer routine medications and in case of an emergency).
- Paralysis is achieved by use of short-acting anesthetic agents (to prevent injury).
- A tourniquet is applied to one limb (so that the seizure occurs). The tourniquet obstructs the entry of the anesthetic into the limb, restricting the seizure to one limb.
- A common fear relates to suffocation. Make sure the person understands that respiration will be supported during the procedure.
- The person may complain of a sore throat after ECT (as a result of endotracheal tube placement).
- Prevent injury during and after ECT. Monitor vital signs during ECT and report deviations. (ECT is an invasive procedure, in terms of its effects.)
- After ECT, continue to monitor vital signs until the client is stable.
- Allow the person to sleep.
- Headache and *myalgia* (muscle pain) are frequent side effects that can be effectively treated with ibuprofen.

Antipsychotic (Neuroleptic) Drugs

Antipsychotics are also known as **neuroleptics** ("major tranquilizers"). The classic antipsychotic medications (eg, haloperidol [Haldol], chlorpromazine [Thorazine], fluphenazine [Prolixin], perphenazine [Trilafon]) are most effective in treating "positive" symptoms of psychosis. These positive symptoms include: hallucinations, delusions, paranoia, severe agitation, hyperactivity, combativeness, and feelings of unreality. These medications work in the brain's postsynaptic dopamine receptors.

New classes of antipsychotics were introduced in the past 20 years, including clozapine (Clozaril), loxapine (Loxitane), risperidone (Risperdal), and olanzapine (Zyprexa). These medications also work selectively on the dopamine receptors in the brain. Generally, they have fewer side effects and are less likely to cause *tardive dyskinesia* (discussed later). They treat "negative" symptoms of psychosis (apathy, social and emotional withdrawal, poor hygiene, lack of insight, poor

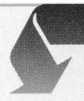

In Practice
Nursing Care Guidelines 93-2

ADMINISTERING MEDICATION THERAPY IN THE MENTAL HEALTH UNIT

- Follow the "five rights" for correct medication administration (see Chap. 63).
- Leave medications in their packages if using a unit-dose system. *Rationale: Allow the paranoid person to see the package being opened or to open it himself or herself; medication need not be wasted if it is refused, and the nurse can more easily identify and teach about medications. If a client loses control and hits the med tray, the medications will not be lost.*
- Use clear medication cups. *Rationale: The nurse will be able to see if there are any pills remaining. Plastic cups are harder to crush in an effort to hide pills.*
- If a liquid medication is to be given, it should be poured up shortly before administration. If it is supplied in a brown bottle, it must be covered while on the med tray. (*These medications are not always stable when exposed to air.*)
- Some liquid medications cannot safely be combined. If there is any doubt, use separate medicine cups for each.
- Identify the person before giving any medication. Always check the person's name band. *Rationale: The person may be confused or may deliberately try to mislead you.* If the person does not have a name band, ask him or her to tell you his or her name; confirm with another nurse if there is any question. Do not ask, "Are you Mr. Jones?" Many clients will answer "yes," even if this is incorrect.
- Ask the client to drink an entire cup of water. It may be necessary to look in the client's mouth, under the tongue, and in the cheeks. *Rationale: Many psychiatric clients attempt to "cheek" [hide] medications and not take them.*
- Assess and document the effectiveness of medications. Desired effects include the following:
  Lessening episodes of *hallucinations* (perceiving something that is not there). These hallucinations are usually *auditory* (hearing voices) or *visual* (seeing things). Less common are *gustatory* (taste), *olfactory* (smell), or *tactile* (touch) hallucinations.
  Decreasing *delusional* thinking (false beliefs that cannot be changed by reasoning).
  Diminishing *distortions* in the thought process.
  Lessening of *destructive behavior* to self or others.
  Improvement in self-care, sleep, or eating habits.
- Observe and document the client's willingness to take medications. Some clients argue about taking medications, but do take them. If the person refuses, document this and the reasons the person gives for refusing. The person has a right to refuse medications and many do. (*Exception: If the client has been court-ordered to take medications or is out of control, drugs can be forced. The client's reasons for refusal or reluctance to take medications are important because they are often related to side effects.*)
- The client with a history of medication noncompliance may be given the liquid or Zydis (instantly dissolving) form of a medication, may have medications crushed, or may receive decanoate (long-lasting) injections, which are given every 2 to 3 weeks. In some cases, clients are not allowed to enter their room for a period of time after receiving medications. *Rationale: Prevent clients from spitting out medications or forcing themselves to vomit.*
- If the Zydis form of a medication is to be given, it cannot be touched or exposed to the air. *Rationale: It will disintegrate, especially if it is damp.*
- Assess and document side effects. Note exactly what the side effect was and how it progressed. Part of the documentation includes steps taken to alleviate side effects. Common side effects of antipsychotic medications are excessive weight gain, dry mouth, constipation, hypotension or hypertension, blurred vision, drowsiness, muscle cramping, drooling, the urge to pace, and sexual dysfunction. However, some side effects are disabling and some can be fatal. *Rationale: A major reason for refusal to take medications is the fear of undesirable side effects, especially tardive dyskinesia, a potentially disabling side effect.*
- Teach the client and family about medications, the importance of following administration times and dosages, possible side effects, and what to do if these occur. *Rationale: Side effects can occur at any time, even after the client has been taking a medication for some time.*
- Assess for more severe side effects. These often are *extrapyramidal* (response of the autonomic nervous system to the medications), such as the following:
  Dystonia: Involuntary and irregular movements of the muscles of the trunk and extremities
  Akathisia: Extreme inability to sit still, motor restlessness, or muscle-quivering tremors
  Parkinsonian syndrome: Symptoms similar to Parkinson's disease (resting tremor, rigidity, slowness in motor activity, and postural abnormalities)
  Tardive dyskinesia syndrome: Involuntary movements, especially of lips and tongue, associated with long-term use of some antipsychotics
  Neuroleptic malignant syndrome: A potentially fatal disorder caused by antipsychotic drugs
- If there is a court order forcing the client to take medications, if a medical emergency has been declared, or if a client is out of control, medications can be forced by IM injection and occasionally are given IV or by nasogastric (NG) tube. *Rationale: In these situations, the client does not have the right to refuse treatment. In some cases, the forcing of medications is lifesaving.*

■■■ TABLE 93-2 *K*EY MEDICATIONS USED IN PSYCHIATRY

Name of Drug*	Usual Adult Dose	Notes
Benzodiazepines		
alprazolam (Xanax)	Oral: 0.25–2 mg t.i.d.; max. 10 mg/d	Intermediate acting; 2-mg dose used to treat panic attacks
chlordiazepoxide (Librium)	Oral: 10–25 mg 3–4 times daily IM: given deep IM	Long-acting drug to treat anxiety and alcohol withdrawal
diazepam (Valium)	Oral: 2–10 mg up to q.i.d. IV: 5–10 mg PRN	Used to treat status epilepticus, muscle spasm, anxiety; IV form for status epilepticus; used in alcohol detoxification
flurazepam (Dalmane)	Oral: 15–30 mg h.s.	Hypnotic only; use dose of 15 mg in elderly
lorazepam (Ativan)	Oral: 0.5–6 mg/d, in divided doses; max. 10 mg/d IM: Usual dose is 1–2 mg	Intermediate acting; sublingual administration absorbed faster than oral; used for anxiety and insomnia secondary to anxiety IM most often used to control dangerous behavior
oxazepam (Serax)	Oral: 15–30 mg 3–4 times daily	Short-acting drug for anxiety and alcohol withdrawal
triazolam (Halcion)	Oral: 0.125–0.5 mg h.s.	Shortest-acting hypnotic in this class; may have dangerous side effects, including amnesia
Miscellaneous		
buspirone (BuSpar)	Oral: 5–20 mg t.i.d.	Management of anxiety disorders; not related chemically to benzodiazepines, barbiturates, or other sedative hypnotics; less sedative effect than benzodiazepines
chloral hydrate (Noctec)	Oral: 500 mg h.s. Rectal: 500 mg–1 g h.s.	Oldest of currently used hypnotics; bitter taste; gel caps and suppositories available
meprobamate (Equanil, Miltown)	Oral: 400 mg 3–4 times daily; max. 2,400 mg/d	Antianxiety agent and sedative with muscle-relaxing properties. Abrupt withdrawal after prolonged use may lead to severe tonic–clonic seizures.
Psychotherapeutic Drugs		
Antipsychotic Drugs		
chlorpromazine (Thorazine)	Oral: 25–200 mg q.i.d. IM: 25–50 mg q1–4h	Higher doses may be used initially and then tapered down.
clozapine (Clozaril)	Oral: 25 mg b.i.d.; gradually titrated upward; max. 900 mg/d	Used to treat schizophrenia and schizoaffective disorders which do not respond to other drugs. Can cause severe blood dyscrasia; client must have weekly WBC. Client must be carefully monitored.
fluphenazine HCl (Prolixin)	Oral: 2.5–10 mg t.i.d.–q.i.d.; IM: 1/2 oral dose IM decanoate (long-acting): 12.5–25 mg q 1–3 wk	Used to treat psychotic disorders. Can cause blood dyscrasias.
haloperidol (Haldol)	Oral: 0.5–10 mg 2–3 times daily IM: 2–5 mg q4–8h IM decanoate: 10–15 g times the oral daily dose q 4 wk	Low sedative properties, high extrapyramidal effects (tics, muscle spasms); higher doses may be used. Higher risk of tardive dyskinesia than with newer drugs.
loxapine (Loxitane)	Oral: 10 mg b.i.d.–q.i.d.; titrate up to maintenance dose: 60–100 mg/d	Use cautiously in respiratory disorders, glaucoma, epilepsy, or ulcers.
olanzapine (Zyprexa)	Oral: 5–10 mg/d; titrate up PRN; max. 20 mg/d	Side effects include increased appetite and weight gain; sedation (give at h.s.)
perphenazine (Trilafon)	Oral: 4–16 mg q.i.d. IM: 5 mg q6h	IM form used as an antiemetic; side effects similar to Haldol

■■■ TABLE 93-2 $\mathcal{K}$EY MEDICATIONS USED IN PSYCHIATRY (CONTINUED)

Name of Drug*	Usual Adult Dose	Notes
risperidone (Risperdal)	Oral: 1 mg b.i.d.; titrate up to 3 mg b.i.d.	Dose titrated over several days; low risk of extrapyramidal side effects (EPSE)
thioridazine (Mellaril)	Oral: 50–100 mg t.i.d.; max. 800 mg/d	Higher doses may be used; side effects similar to Haldol
thiothixene (Navane)	Oral: 5 mg b.i.d.–q.i.d.; max. 30 mg/d	Side effects similar to Haldol
trifluoperazine (Stelazine)	Oral: 2–5 mg b.i.d.; usual dose: 15–20 mg/d	IM injection available to control acute symptoms
ziprasidone (Geodon)	Oral: 20–40 mg b.i.d. with food; taper up over several weeks; max. 80 mg b.i.d. IM form now available.	Atypical antipsychotic; used to treat schizophrenia; lower risk of EPSE; may cause weight gain, GI symptoms, sedation
Antidepressants†		
amitriptyline (Elavil, Endep)	Oral: 50–100 mg/d IM use also	Total daily dose may be given at bedtime to reduce day-time sedative side effects (tricyclic).
bupropion HCl (Wellbutrin)	Oral: 100 mg b.i.d.; slow titration up to 150 mg t.i.d.	Contraindicated in clients with seizure disorders and eating disorders. (Same medication as in Zyban, used for smoking cessation) Unrelated to other antidepressants.
citalopram (Celexa)	Oral: 20 mg/d; max. 60 mg/d	Increases prothrombin time; avoid use with St. John's wort
desipramine (Norpramin, Pertofrane)	Oral: 75–150 mg/d	Fewer anticholinergic and sedative effects than other tricyclics; rarely used
doxepin (Sinequan, Adapin)	Oral: 25–75 mg/d; max. 300 mg/d	Tricyclic; once daily dose at bedtime; can cause hypotension
fluoxetine (Prozac)	Oral: 20 mg q/d; max. 80 mg/d	Usually stimulating; avoid h.s. use; may cause anxiety; SSRI
fluvoxamine (Luvox)	Oral: 100–300 mg b.i.d.; give in divided doses; max. 300 mg/d	SSRI; effective in obsessive-compulsive disorder (OCD); avoid with cisapride, diazepam, primozide, and MAOIs
imipramine (Tofranil)	Oral: 75–100 mg/d; max. 300 mg/d	Mild anticholinergic and sedative effects (tricyclic)
mirtazapine (Remeron)	Oral: 15–45 mg/d	May cause agranulocytosis (0.1%); contraindicated in myocardial infarction (MI); tricyclic
nefazodone (Serzone)	Oral: 150–300 mg b.i.d.; max. 600 mg/d	Avoid with cisapride, triazolam, and MAOIs
paroxetine (Paxil)	Oral: 20–50 mg/d; max. 50 mg/d	Effective in OCD, panic disorder, social phobias; potentiates effects of serotonin
sertraline (Zoloft)	Oral: 50–150 mg/d; max. 200 mg/d	Effective in panic disorder and post-traumatic stress disorder (PTSD), as well as major depressive disorder (MDD); SSRI
tranylcypromine sulfate (Parnate)	Oral: 10 mg b.i.d.; max. 60 mg/d	Monoamine oxidase inhibitor (MAOI) (avoid certain foods) (see Nursing Alert on p. 1589); do NOT use with tricyclics
trazodone (Desyrel)	Oral: 150–400 mg/d; max. 600 mg/d	Effects noted earlier than those of other drugs in this class May be used also to aid sleep in depressed client. Priapism is serious side effect; SSRI Effective as sleep aid in older clients (dose is reduced to 25–75 mg).

(continued)

■■■ TABLE 93-2 𝒦EY MEDICATIONS USED IN PSYCHIATRY (CONTINUED)

Name of Drug*	Usual Adult Dose	Notes
Mood Stabilizers		
carbemazepine (Tegretol)	Oral: 800–1200 mg/d in divided doses Dose based on blood level (Optimum: 8.0–12.0 μ/mL)	Treatment of bipolar disorder, as well as generalized tonic–clonic seizures and pain associated with trigeminal neuralgia
Lithium lithium carbonate (Lithobid, Eskalith) lithium citrate (liquid form)	Oral: 300–600 mg b.i.d.–t.i.d. Dose based on blood level. (Optimum: 0.8–1.4 mEq/L)	Treatment of bipolar disorder Maintain salt and fluid intake. Avoid alcohol. Toxicity by symptoms are diarrhea, vomiting, muscle weakness. Avoid NSAIDs.
valproic acid (Depakote)	250–500 mg b.i.d.–t.i.d.	Treatment of bipolar disorder, as well as generalized seizures
sodium valproate (Depakene —liquid form)	Dose based on blood level (Optimum: 50–100 μ/mL)	Reduce dose in liver disease
Other Drugs		
carbidopa/levodopa (Sinemet: contains 10 mg carbidopa and 100 mg levodopa)	Oral: 10/100 to 25/250 t.i.d. Titrated to 8 tabs/d Sinemet CR (controlled release): 50/200	Antiparkinsonism agent. May cause hemolytic anemia, cardiac arrhythmias. Contraindicated in narrow-angle glaucoma, melanoma; may interact adversely with antihypertension drugs.
cyclobenzaprine (Flexeril)	Oral: 10 mg t.i.d.; max. 60 mg/d; max. duration: 2–3 wk	Centrally acting muscle relaxant; structurally related to tricyclics (may cause drowsiness and dry mouth) Contraindicated in acute MI, heart block, congestive heart failure (CHF). Do not use within 14 days of taking an MAOI.
dantrolene sodium (Dantrium)	Oral: 25–100 mg 2–4 times daily; max. 400 mg/d (evaluate response in 1 wk) IV: 1 mg/kg; max. cumulative dose: 10 mg/kg D/C in 45 d if no response	Skeletal muscle relaxant used for cerebral palsy, multiple sclerosis; used to manage malignant hyperthermia Contraindicated in active liver disease.
droperidol (Inapsine)	2.5–10 mg IM/IV	Anesthetic used to control very assaultive or dangerous clients. Fast acting. Monitor for hypotension or respiratory depression.
methocarbamol (Robaxin)	Oral: 1.5 g q.i.d. × 2–3 d IM: 500 mg q8h IV: up to 2–3 g daily	Centrally acting muscle relaxant (may cause drowsiness); also used in supportive therapy for tetanus management
methylphenidate (Ritalin)	Adult: Oral: 10 mg b.i.d.–t.i.d. Children: 5–10 mg b.i.d.; max. 60 mg/d	Adults: Narcolepsy, attention deficit hyperactivity disorder (ADHD) Children: ADHD Potential for abuse
phenytoin (Dilantin)	Oral: 300–400 mg/d IV, IM: Variable dosages based on serum level	Anticonvulsant for generalized tonic–clonic and psychomotor seizures (gingival hyperplasia is side effect in long-term use)
primidone (Mysoline)	Oral: 250 mg 3–4 times daily	Treatment of generalized tonic–clonic and complex–partial psychomotor seizures.
sumatriptan (Imitrex)	Oral: 25 mg (may repeat in 2 h); max: 100 mg/d Sub Q: 6 mg (may repeat in 1 h); max. 12 mg/d Nasal: 5–20 mg (may repeat in 2 h) max. 40 mg/24 h	Treatment of severe migraine headaches; available by prescription (prefilled syringes, oral tablets, nasal spray) for home administration

*A trade name appears in parentheses following the generic name of the drug.

†Tricyclics, such as amitriptyline, imipramine, and doxepin, can cause annoying and severe side effects (i.e., ECG changes, tachycardia, hypertension).

SSRI, selective serotonin reuptake inhibitor

➤➤ BOX 93-2

FORMS OF MEDICATIONS USED IN PSYCHIATRY

Medication noncompliance is a major concern in psychiatry. Therefore, several forms of medications are used to ensure better compliance.

Oral Medications
- Tablet, capsule: For the person who takes his or her medications
- Crushed tablets: May be in juice, ice cream, or applesauce
- Liquid form of medications (difficult not to swallow, also liquids act faster than tablets—put in juice to disguise the taste)
- **Zydis** form (dissolves instantly on contact with the tongue—do not touch with your fingers or expose to air for any length of time)
- NG tube administration

Injections
- IM injections
- Decanoate injections (last several weeks)
- IV injections (in emergency to control extremely dangerous behavior or to reverse life-threatening side effects)

The person who is noncompliant is placed on "cheeking precautions" in the hospital. The nurse observes the client after giving medications, to make sure the client does not hold them in his or her cheek and then spit them out. In some cases, the client must stay in the lounge for a specified length of time after taking medications, to make sure they are swallowed or dissolved. The client's bathroom also may be locked for a specified length of time.

judgment, and lack of spontaneity and pleasure) more effectively than do classic antipsychotics.

Side Effects.   Multiple side effects are associated with the use of neuroleptics. For example, clozapine can potentially cause agranulocytosis. Therefore, weekly complete and differential blood counts are required, which significantly increases treatment costs. Because of these costs, clients must have at least two failures with other classes of neuroleptics before beginning clozapine. Because of the potential for bone marrow suppression, clozapine must not be given with any other medications that also have this effect.

Extrapyramidal side effects (EPSE) (adverse neurologic effects) are common. These include involuntary movements and symptoms, such as:

- *Parkinsonism:* Muscle stiffness or spasm, shuffling gait, drooling, masklike face, tremors
- *Restlessness and* **akathisia:** Inability to sit still, agitation, tapping, rocking, pacing, and marching in place

- *General* **dyskinesia:** Involuntary, coordinated rhythmic movements; jerking; tremors; twisting; abnormal tongue movements; tonic tongue; toe movements; tics
- *Other muscular side effects:* Jaw spasms, impaired breathing or swallowing, grimaces
- **Opisthotonos:** Severe head and neck extension
- **Oculogyric crisis:** Involuntary upward rolling of eyes
- *Nonmovement side effects:* Dry mouth, blurred vision, constipation, thick tongue, weight gain, sleepiness, tachycardia, impotence, and decreased libido
- **Orthostatic hypotension:** Fall in blood pressure on standing, often including dizziness
- **Dystonia:** Impaired muscle tone and movement
- **Cogwheeling movements** of the arms, a specific side effect of neuroleptic medications. (When the client relaxes the arm and the examiner moves it, the movement is jerky and seems to catch, as would a cogwheel while rotating.)
- *Tardive dyskinesia:* Described below

Another serious and sometimes life-threatening side effect of neuroleptics is *neuroleptic malignant syndrome,* also described below.

Anticholinergic Medications.   These medications are used to prevent or treat many side effects of neuroleptics. The most commonly used anticholinergic medications are amantadine (Symmetrel); benztropine mesylate (Cogentin); orphenadrine citrate (Norflex); trihexyphenidyl (Artane); and the antihistamine, diphenhydramine (Benadryl), and biperiden (Akineton), an antiparkinson drug.

Tardive Dyskinesia.   **Tardive dyskinesia (TD** or **TDK)** is a syndrome of involuntary movements. It is a serious and permanent side effect that results from long-term use of neuroleptics. "At least 20% of persons treated with neuroleptics in the long term develop TD."[5] TD rarely results within the first year of neuroleptic use. Any neuroleptic, except clozapine (Clozaril), can cause TD. TD may also occur as a result of taking amoxapine (Asendin), an antidepressant; the gastric drug metoclopramide (Reglan); or the anti-nausea drug prochlorperazine (Compazine). Early identification of TD is essential to prevent worsening of movements. TD usually cannot be reversed and may continue, even after the causative drug is discontinued. TD can be very upsetting and, in some cases, the involuntary muscle movements are disfiguring and disabling.

The person with TD often has obvious mouth movements; in rare cases, breathing and walking are affected. TD usually starts with abnormal tongue movements; the first sign is a small, wriggling movement under the surface. It can progress to grimacing or rhythmic movements of the tongue, lips, eyes, or face, including facial tics. Sometimes it appears as a chewing movement. Tongue movements include intermittent darting in and out of the mouth; "tongue in cheek"; tongue tremors; or a stationary, protruding tongue. The syndrome may extend to include involuntary **athetoid** (writhing) movements of the fingers, toes, and extremities; pill-rolling movements of the fingers; back and sideways head jerks, usually to one side; and shrugging of the shoulders. Movements stop during sleep; they may be aggravated when the person tries to perform a purposeful movement or speak.

☛ KEY CONCEPT

A person may have early tardive dyskinesia, but mild symptoms may be masked by the neuroleptic medications that he or she is taking. Only when the symptoms become worse do they 'break through' and become obvious. At that point, it is not possible to reverse the symptoms that are already present.

If no other effective psychotropic drug can be found, the client with TD may opt to continue with a lower dose, to control psychotic symptoms. Because clozapine (Clozaril) has not been found to cause TD, this drug may be used. No effective treatment exists for TD, but its progression can be arrested by decreasing or discontinuing the offending medication. Fear of TD is a common reason for clients to refuse or stop taking medication.

Several evaluation scales, such as **DISCUS** (Dyskinesia Identification System–Condensed User Scale) and **AIMS** (Abnormal Involuntary Movement Scale), are used to assess the presence or absence of and severity of TD. Special training in administration of these tests is required. Tests for TD determine if specific abnormal movements are present most of the time, including:

- Facial tics, grimaces
- Chewing or sucking; lip smacking
- Excessive blinking or bursts of blinking
- Abnormal tongue movements (including tremors)—thrusting, tonic tongue
- Abnormal twisting or jerking of the fingers or arms (not including tremor), or writhing or pill-rolling
- Athetoid movements of fingers
- Abnormal toe or foot movements, writhing toes, or overlapped toes due to cramping
- Abnormal head or neck movements or jerking
- Abnormal, rigid body posturing

☛ KEY CONCEPT

Certain common extrapyramidal side effects (EPSE) are not considered to be indicative of TD. These include, but are not limited to:

- *Arm or hand tremors*
- *Cogwheeling*
- *Akathisia, pacing, leg jerks*
- *Rocking*
- *Opisthotonos*
- *Oculogyric crisis*
- *Stiff neck*
- *Difficulty swallowing*
- *Difficulty breathing*
- *Abnormal verbalizations*

The person with milder manifestations of these symptoms, such as tremor, usually does not need to have the medication discontinued or changed. More severe symptoms indicate a need to change the dosage of the medication or to change to a related medication.

The most frightening of these symptoms, particularly opisthotonos, oculogyric crisis, or difficulty breathing, can usually be quickly reversed by administration of diphenhydramine (Benadryl) either orally (in liquid form) or by IM injection.

Neuroleptic Malignant Syndrome (NMS). **Neuroleptic malignant syndrome** (**NMS**) is a rare, life-threatening complication of neuroleptic medications. It is a medical emergency, with a mortality rate of 20% to 25%. (Respiratory or renal failure and pulmonary embolism are the most frequent causes of death.) NMS can occur soon after first administration of a neuroleptic medication. If you suspect NMS, stop the medication and provide emergency care. If NMS is detected and treated early, symptoms will resolve in several days with no permanent damage. Symptoms of NMS include:

- Altered level of consciousness (LOC); mental status changes
- Rapid onset of rigidity
- Autonomic nervous system disturbances (eg, sudden hyperthermia, diaphoresis, tachypnea, tachycardia, fluctuating blood pressure)
- *Dystonia* (sustained contractions of axial or appendicular muscles) and posturing
- Difficulty swallowing
- *Akathisia* (motor restlessness)
- Poor response to anticholinergic medications
- Sleep disturbances
- Abnormal laboratory values: elevated white blood cell count; elevated creatine phosphokinase (CPK), indicating muscle damage due to rigidity; and myoglobin in the urine, also indicating muscle damage
- Respiratory distress is frequent and may be life threatening.

Treatment involves immediately discontinuing neuroleptic medications, maintaining the person's airway, and monitoring vital signs and LOC. Ongoing treatment includes monitoring the client's intake and output, nutritional status, and daily weight. This client will need to be maintained on an unrelated neuroleptic medication in the future.

Antianxiety Agents

Antianxiety agents are central nervous system (CNS) depressants. The most common group of antianxiety medications are the **benzodiazepines.** They are all equally effective in their sedative–hypnotic actions but differ in rate of absorption, speed of onset, and half-life.

Barbiturates have been used for many years; they were once used for anyone who needed behavioral control. They have several disadvantages when compared with benzodiazepines, including rapid development of tolerance and physical dependence (except phenobarbital). Barbiturates have a narrow safety margin, cause sedation and hangovers, interfere with metabolism of other medications (including anticoagulants and other psychotropics), and suppress rapid eye movement (REM) sleep.

Buspirone (BuSpar) is an antianxiety medication that is not a CNS depressant and does not cause euphoria or sedation. Its mechanism of action is unclear. It has a lag period of several weeks before effects begin, so is not useful as a PRN medication. Side effects are usually mild but can be troublesome. They include hypotension, headache, nausea, dry mouth, constipation, decreased libido, and impotence.

Disadvantages of Antianxiety Medications.   Alcohol potentiates the effects of antianxiety agents, often causing severe depression. In addition, individuals become dependent, both emotionally and physically, on benzodiazepines and barbiturates. Severe withdrawal symptoms follow abrupt discontinuation. (Withdrawal symptoms are often worse when the client uses these medications for a long time.)

Mood Stabilizers

Mood stabilizers are used to treat both elevated mood (*mania*) and depressed mood (*major depression*). These medications help to prevent instability when the client is in an *euthymic* (normal) mood. They work by chemically stabilizing the brain's membranes.

Lithium.   *Lithium* is the most commonly used mood stabilizer in the treatment of bipolar and schizoaffective disorders, major depression, and intermittent explosive disorder. It is also used to reduce impulsivity and mood **lability** (sudden changes) when treating personality disorders. Lithium is effective for about 70% of individuals with mood disorders. It is available in an oral liquid form, as well as tablets and capsules.

The client taking lithium must maintain a consistent intake of fluids daily (about 8 glasses). Clients may have polyuria and may tend to drink less fluid in an effort to control this. Salt should not be restricted without medical supervision. Clients should not use nonsteroidal anti-inflammatory drugs (**NSAIDs**) because they can lead to lithium toxicity. Lithium can cause renal insufficiency and hypothyroidism; clients should be monitored for changes in renal and thyroid function annually.

Side effects of lithium use include lethargy, polyuria, polydipsia, coarse hand tremor, nausea, vomiting, diarrhea, muscle weakness, edema of the extremities and face, hypothyroidism, excessive weight gain, increased leukocyte counts, and mild hypoglycemia.

Anticonvulsants as Mood Stabilizers.   Another group of medications, the *anticonvulsants,* have proven effective in treating mood disorders. Carbamazepine (Tegretol) and valproate (Depakote) are both used, alone or in conjunction with lithium. It is unclear why they work, but theorists believe that the same mechanism used to control seizures is used in another part of the brain to stabilize mood.

Side effects of carbamazepine include nausea, vomiting, sedation, dizziness, lightheadedness, ataxia, rash, blurred vision, dry mouth, urinary retention or hesitancy, impotence, and bone marrow suppression.

Side effects of valproate include liver toxicity, bone marrow depression, nausea, vomiting, *amenorrhea* (cessation of menstruation), *alopecia* (excessive hair loss), and sedation.

☞ KEY CONCEPT

Several classifications of medications used in psychiatry have sexual side effects, such as impotence and decreased libido, in both men and women. These side effects are noted to be a major reason why clients refuse medications or stop taking them after discharge from the hospital.

Antidepressants

Antidepressants are commonly used to treat major depression. They are effective in alleviating symptoms in about 70% of those treated. They work by increasing activity of norepinephrine or serotonin (or both) at the brain's postsynaptic membrane receptors. There are four classifications of antidepressants: tricyclics, selective serotonin reuptake inhibitors (**SSRI**), monamine oxidase inhibitors (**MAOI**), and other non-MAOI antidepressants.

The SSRI and non-MAOI antidepressants are most frequently used. Tricyclic antidepressants (**TCA**) are very effective, but have more side effects and can be lethal in overdose. MAOI antidepressants are very effective, but require the client to adhere strictly to dietary restrictions. All antidepressants take 1 to 6 weeks from initiation of administration for symptom relief to occur. The client is at great risk of being overwhelmed by depressive symptoms while waiting for relief.

✚👁 Nursing Alert

Warn clients taking MAOIs against eating foods with high tyramine content (eg, caffeinated beverages, ripened cheeses, beef or chicken liver, meats prepared with tenderizer, beer, and raisins). Other prohibited foods include wine, chocolate, bananas, and herring. These clients should also avoid OTC medications that contain sympathomimetic amines (mimic the sympathetic nervous system), which could produce hypertensive crises when mixed with MAOIs. (Such medications include many cold and hay fever products.) Some herbal preparations can cause serious side effects if combined with MAOIs.

Side effects of all antidepressants include dry mouth, which can be very annoying. Many of these medications also cause sexual dysfunction. Other side effects of tricyclics include urinary hesitancy or retention, constipation, weight gain, tachycardia, sedation, and orthostatic hypotension. Side effects of SSRIs include nausea, vomiting, headache, sedation, nervousness, and insomnia. Side effects of MAOIs are orthostatic hypotension, weight gain, edema, and insomnia. Other non-MAOI antidepressants can cause sweating, seizures, and nausea. Side effects are a major reason for client noncompliance with these medications.

All of the above classifications of medications are listed in Table 93-2.

THE CLIENT IN AN INPATIENT SETTING

Although this chapter is geared primarily to the care of the person diagnosed with a mental health problem, many of these skills apply to clients in other areas as well. The nurse will encounter people experiencing threats to mental health in all areas of the healthcare facility, as well as in daily life.

☛ Kᴇʏ Cᴏɴᴄᴇᴘᴛ

People who are ill or injured often respond in ways that differ from their usual behavior. You may find symptoms of a mental health disorder in many general medical-surgical clients. Often, their undesirable behavior disappears after their medical problem is under control.

The Therapeutic Environment

A therapeutic environment (**milieu therapy**) is one in which all aspects of the surroundings (physical and social) are designed to promote health and to enable clients to cope with life's demands. The eventual goal is safety and comfort in the community after discharge from the facility. The *therapeutic environment* is a community within the facility that encourages people to interact with one another and to improve their interpersonal relationships. The goal is to gain insight into actions and to change undesirable behaviors. Clients form a "government" and, with supervision, set up rules and regulations. In this way, they are able to test ways of coping. The therapeutic environment can fulfill its function only if people learn to live in such a way as to prepare them for eventual discharge.

Rights of the Client

Chapter 4 described the Bill of Rights that applies for all healthcare clients. Some differences exist in mental health units. Because safety must be maintained, limitations to a client's freedom of movement—by seclusion or giving medications against the client's will—are sometimes necessary. Clients may also be held against their will if they pose a danger to themselves or others. Treatment, such as with ECT, can also be imposed against a client's will if there is a court order to do so.

Civil Rights Legislation.   Civil rights laws provide for the equal treatment of all clients, regardless of ethnic or religious background. Clients can refuse treatment, unless a medical emergency has been declared, there is a court order, or a client is out of control or dangerous. A healthcare facility cannot violate a client's civil rights, even though the person is committed by law to the facility. For example, the facility must allow the client to receive mail and telephone calls without censoring them. Clients have the right to see visitors. The only time these rights change is if preserving them would compromise the safety of the client or of other persons.

Vulnerable Adult Legislation.   Legislation is in place to protect those who cannot protect themselves. This law is called the **vulnerable adult** law; it protects intellectually impaired and mentally ill people who are unable to protect themselves. Physical, sexual, or verbal abuse or neglect of any person is illegal. Clients must also be protected from abuse by other clients (peers).

Advocacy.   Most healthcare institutions employ counselors or advocates (*ombudspersons*) who advise people about their civil rights. These advocates act as effective "watchdogs" and pursue any complaints. Any suspected abuse must be reported, or the person who observed the abuse, in addition to the abusive person, may be prosecuted.

Prevention of Dehumanization

A mental health unit is a controlled environment. To maintain safety for everyone in the group, all members must follow the rules. As in all healthcare facilities, measures must be taken to prevent a dehumanizing atmosphere. Clients must be able to maintain their individuality; each person should be treated with dignity. In Practice: Nursing Care Guidelines 93-3 discusses ways to prevent dehumanization. Also see Fig. 93-3.

Visitors

Nurses should gain the good will and cooperation of visitors. They can help by offering observations of a client's behavior and background. They may be upset by the client's condition and will need support and understanding. They may have been dealing with the person's unpredictable or difficult behavior for many years and may be very frustrated.

To avoid surprises, tell clients about any known anticipated visits. Help them to bathe and dress, if needed. Refer all requests from visitors about a client's condition to the client, the client's nurse, or the charge nurse. Remember, it is illegal to give any information about a client without the client's (or guardian's) permission and a signed release of information. See In Practice: Nursing Care Guidelines 93-4.

Outings

Make sure clients understand the expectations that apply to outings before they leave the mental health unit. Usually, clients must sign out and indicate where they are going and with whom. Clients may be allowed to leave only with staff or may be given independent passes or passes with family. Inform clients of the curfew and the consequences if they are late. A physician's order is required before clients can leave; make sure orders are written and signed. Clients must also sign a "pass waiver" in which they promise to return and release the facility from liability while they are gone. The staff is responsible if any client is allowed to leave without an order, without signing a pass waiver, or without signing out against medical advice (AMA).

When clients return from outings, note whether or not they return on time. Identify who accompanied them. Ask what they did and how the outing went. Ask clients if they brought anything back, and if they did, check it in. Chart comments, nonverbal behaviors, physical appearance, and any unusual reactions. Be sure to note, for example, if the person seems unusually agitated or depressed or if you can detect alcohol on their breath (**AOB**). In some cases, the physician orders a routine urine toxicology screen (**U-Tox**) for drugs or a Breathalyzer test for alcohol on return from passes.

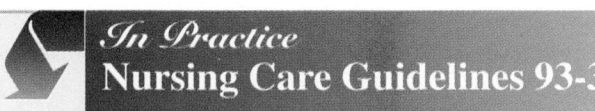

In Practice
Nursing Care Guidelines 93-3

MAINTAINING THE CLIENT'S DIGNITY IN MENTAL HEALTH UNITS

- Allow clients as much choice as possible in such matters as clothes, hairstyle, food, and hours for performing certain activities.
- Encourage the client to participate in ward activities and to help plan these activities.
- Make sure the client has as much privacy as is safe when going to the bathroom, bathing, and performing other personal-care tasks.
- Allow the person to keep as many personal possessions as possible. Make sure the client has hearing aids, false teeth, or glasses, if needed.
- Allow as much freedom as possible; for example, let the client make his or her own purchases in a hospital gift shop or cafeteria.
- Allow freedom in sending and receiving mail and gifts, and in receiving visitors.
- Call the client by the name he or she prefers. Do not use nicknames, unless requested. Use only appropriate nicknames.
- Help the person achieve the best possible appearance. Help with personal cleanliness, makeup, and hairstyles, if necessary.
- Encourage the client not to just "play the game" to be discharged from the hospital; strive for recovery.
- Praise the person as much as possible; encourage a positive self-image. Listen attentively to what the client has to say.
- Explain treatments to the client before they are given; make him or her an active participant in treatment.
- Do not confuse the person. Be consistent.
- Give the person consideration—keep promises; be on time.
- Treat the person with respect.
- Do not set inappropriate limits, but do maintain safety.

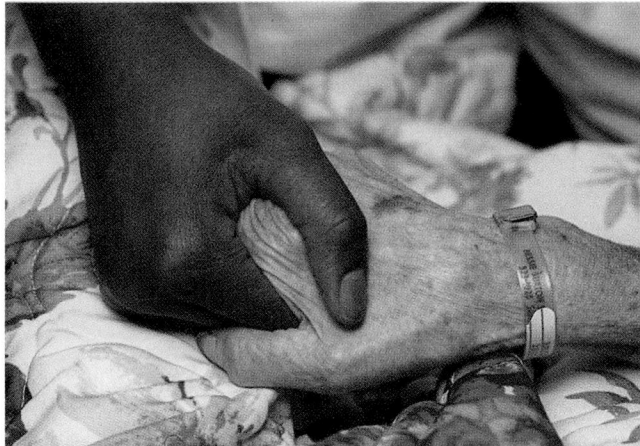

FIGURE 93-3. Often a gentle touch can be soothing. However, it is important to gain the permission of the client in the mental health unit before touching him or her. If this person is surprised, it could be perceived as invasive or threatening, and the client may strike out.

mon assistance. Letting clients know this device is being used will help prevent violence. Most units also have a "panic button" for use in an emergency only. The staff needs to intervene and set firm limits on inappropriate behavior as quickly as possible, in an attempt to prevent acting out.

☛ KEY CONCEPT

Personnel working on a mental health unit must maintain safety at all times. Be alert to what is going on in the unit and be ready to assist if there is any danger to a client, a coworker, or a visitor. Most hospitals have security personnel available to assist in an emergency. Remember, however, that it may take a few minutes for them to get to the unit; you must maintain safety until help arrives.

Restraints and Client Safety Devices

Restraints (*client safety devices* and *reminder devices*) may be necessary to keep clients from hurting themselves or others. They are also used to prevent clients from destroying property, interfering with necessary treatments, or removing dressings or intravenous (IV) lines. Civil rights laws are intended to prevent the use of inappropriate client safety devices. Restraints should only be used in the most extreme circumstances. Always use the least restrictive controls. (Hospital funding agencies are now moving toward abolishing the use of all physical restraints.)

There are two categories of restraints or safety mechanisms used in psychiatry:

- Certain medications are considered *emergency chemical restraints* (**ECR**) or *pharmacological restraints*. An example of a very potent ECR is injectable droperidol (Inapsine). A combination frequently used is known as a "**B-52**" (Benadryl 50 mg, Haldol 5 mg, and Ativan 2 mg). A B-52 can be given orally as pills or liquid, or may be injected IM.
- The *emergency physical restraint* (**EPR**) or *client safety device* is used only if absolutely necessary. If a client

Security

Mentally ill persons need a secure environment and protection against harm for self and others. The healthcare facility is responsible for providing this protection. Rarely are mentally ill people dangerous to others; nevertheless, all facilities treat some clients who could be physically **assaultive** (threatening to hurt others or actually striking someone). The nurse's duties include preventing injuries to self, other personnel, and other clients. In addition, some clients attempt actions of self-mutilation, such as scratching, cutting, biting, burning, or beating themselves or attempting suicide. In a unit where people may become violent or self-injurious, it is helpful to carry an electronic signal (if one is available) that can be used to sum-

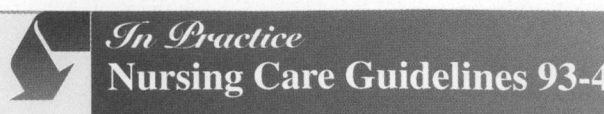

In Practice
Nursing Care Guidelines 93-4

SUPERVISED VISITS

For observation of supervised visits follow these guidelines:

• Check with the client to see if he or she is willing to see the visitor.
• Prevent a vulnerable client from signing papers.
• See that clients open packages or suitcases in the nurse's presence; keep all dangerous items in a safe place away from clients. Record items brought by visitors on the client's property sheet. Take cash, checks, credit cards, and other valuables to the hospital vault.
• Check flowers and plants to make sure they are not in ceramic or glass pots. Balloons should not be latex. Strings or cords may also be dangerous.
• Permit no smoking, except in designated areas.
• Watch for suicide attempts or efforts of clients to leave without permission.
• If the client is on a special diet, monitor food brought by visitors.
• Terminate a visit if the client becomes unduly disturbed.
• Document the client's reaction to the visit. Document interaction with visitors, noting who the visitors were, if possible.
• Observe to make sure visitors are not taking advantage of vulnerable clients. (Examples include pressure for the client to give them money or cigarettes, let them use a car or apartment, or buy drugs.)
• Observe to make sure visitors are not bringing drugs or other contraband onto the unit.
• If a visitor has been drinking, is under the influence of drugs, is abusive, or is otherwise inappropriate to visit, request that the visitor leave. In some cases, this person may need to be escorted out by security staff. (Many clients are too vulnerable or fearful to ask their visitor to leave; the staff will usually need to do this.)
• If a visitor brings small children onto the unit, make sure there is a safe place for the visit to take place.
• Thank the visitors for coming and encourage them to come again, if the visit seemed to go well.
• Document the visit in the client's chart, noting the client's reaction and comments before, during, and after the visit.

must be physically restrained, a device such as the leather Posey belt may be used in psychiatry. Sometimes leg and arm cuffs are required as well.

If any restraint becomes necessary, take specific precautions, as noted at In Practice: Nursing Care Guidelines 93-5. Substitutes for physical restraint are therapeutic treatments

(such as verbal intervention and de-escalation), routine drug therapy, diversion, and seclusion. Use EPR as a last resort only.

Seclusion

Sometimes a person can bring undesirable behavior under control if he or she is placed in a room alone. Try a voluntary time-out first. If the person does not cooperate, it may be necessary to place him or her in a locked seclusion room (**LSR**), also called the locked quiet room (**LQR**), with or without restraints. This process is called *seclusion;* it should be used with care. A written order is required for locked seclusion. Safety within the milieu is the primary goal of all treatment.

Observe the person in seclusion carefully. (If the room is locked, one-to-one observation is required.) As soon as possible, release the client. The room temperature should be comfortable, with plenty of fresh air. Give water or juice. Serve meals on non-fragile dishes. The person should have exercise and frequent opportunities for toileting; however, the bathroom is usually kept locked when not in use, for safety.

The person who is physically restrained is vulnerable. Locked seclusion is required in this case, to protect the client. One-to-one nursing supervision is also required if a client is physically restrained. A call to the client's family is usually also required.

Carefully document any forced seclusion. Note the times, the client's reactions, food and fluids given, and exercise and bathroom breaks. If possible, after release from seclusion, encourage the client to discuss the situation and alternative ways in which it might have been handled, both by the client and the staff.

In some facilities, a room with exercise equipment and a punching bag is provided, as an alternative to seclusion. This allows the client to work out aggressions in a socially acceptable manner. The client must be supervised at all times in this area to provide safety.

Nursing Care of the Severely Disturbed Client

The program of nursing care for the severely disturbed client is threefold: physical care, teaching safe life skills, and building occupational or recreational skills.

Physical Care

Encourage clients to bathe regularly and provide them with suitable clothing. Even the most deteriorated people often respond positively to having their hair fixed, getting new clothes, or having their clothes laundered. Disregard for personal appearance hastens disorganization; therefore, pay attention to helping people keep themselves presentable. Assist as needed in caring for a client's nails, hair, and teeth. Encourage clients to perform as much self-care as possible. The nurse is responsible for seeing that clients carry out such self-care; these activities should be performed only for clients who cannot do so themselves. In rare cases, a bed bath or forced shower may be necessary. Sometimes, a forced haircut is also necessary.

USING CLIENT SAFETY DEVICES FOR THE MENTALLY ILL

- Leather restraints may be required in psychiatry to control extremely assaultive or dangerous behaviors.
- Wear gloves while doing any restraint. Wear eye goggles if the client is likely to spit. Be careful not to be bitten.
- Residents in restraints or safety devices are vulnerable to abuse. The client must have one-to-one nursing care. Usually the person is in a locked seclusion room for their own protection. He or she is often under constant camera surveillance as well.
- A specific written order to use restraints must be in place. (In an emergency, this may be obtained *immediately after* the incident.) This order can only be written for 4 hours at a time. Carefully document the application of restraints, the reason for the restraints, and observation of the person.
- A physician must physically see the client within 1 hour after restraints are applied.
- When restraining the arms and legs (*4-point restraints*), be careful not to make the device too tight.
- Use a stockinette or a soft bandage under the safety device (to prevent injury).
- Some facilities require the use of a waist restraint if the limbs are to be restrained. (The person is then in *5-point restraints.*)
- Patient safety devices are usually locked. Every nurse must have a key available, so that the client can be immediately released in an emergency.
- One type of locked leather restraint has a tiny knob or catch, which must be depressed before the lock can be pushed in, to lock the buckle. Be sure all staff members know how to manipulate the restraints used in the facility.
- When applying restraints, check the buckle to make sure it is locked.
- If the person is out of control, medications may be forced (by IM injection), unless the person agrees to take them orally (liquid oral medications are usually used in this case).
- Offer the client an opportunity to use the urinal or bedpan or to go to the bathroom at least every 1 to 2 hours.
- Offer fluids and food frequently. Use styrofoam trays and dishes to prevent injury to staff or the client. Some clients cannot be given plastic eating utensils because they can be used as weapons.
- Do not fasten the arms and legs in an uncomfortable position. If a person must be placed in such a position to prevent injury to others, change the position as soon as possible. Remove the safety device every hour, and allow the person to exercise the limb. Release one limb at a time. Keep the other limbs secure, to prevent injury to staff.
- Most of the time, the client is placed on the stomach when first restrained. (This helps to facilitate IM injections and provides better control of the client. The client may also be carried into the room in a face-down position, to prevent injury to staff and to maintain better control of the client.)
- If it can be avoided, do not apply a safety device over the chest. This can cause the person to panic. A waist restraint may be needed.
- Never restrain only one side of the body. Even if it seems unnecessary to restrain both hands or both feet, restrain the hand and foot on the opposite side, too. In some facilities, limbs on "opposite corners" can be restrained. When releasing the person from restraints, release one extremity at a time, and alternate "corners." Do not release both extremities on the same side at the same time. (Some facilities never allow only two limbs to be restrained.)
- Frequently feel the pulse of the person who is struggling against a safety device, and watch his or her general condition carefully. Death can result from exhaustion. The person also can work down in the bed and strangle on a restraint.
- Be aware that the person may try to do destructive things while restrained, such as tearing the bed linens or biting holes in the mattress. It is also possible for a severely agitated client to chew through a leather restraint.
- The person also may try to harm himself or herself. He or she must be kept safe. For example, if the person in full restraints bites their shoulder, a cervical collar ("whiplash" collar) can be used.
- Whenever a client is placed in seclusion or restraints, he or she must be *thoroughly searched* for any dangerous objects. This includes matches, plastic tableware, plastic bags, pens, pencils, paper clips, staples, any sharps, liquids such as shampoo or hand lotion, and any other potentially dangerous items.
- If a client is out of control, do not attempt to carry out a restraint without assistance. Sometimes, a "show of force" is sufficient. However, the team must be prepared for violence on the part of the person. The team must be ready to apply involuntary restraints if needed for safety and to maintain the safety of others on the unit.
- If a staff member or client is injured during a restraint, report it immediately and file an incident report. Tests for infectious diseases may be required.
- If a client is extremely dangerous, but has been in restraints for some time, he or she may be allowed to be on the unit wearing a type of shackles called **PADS** (preventive aggression device system). PADS are a form of self-contained personal assault prevention device. The arms are restrained by wrist cuffs to a waist belt. The amount of freedom of the arms can be controlled by the staff. If the client is likely to kick, ankle cuffs are also worn. The distance between the ankle cuffs can also be adjusted. These restraints have locking devices like Posey waist belts. PADS are sometimes required when a dangerous client is taken to court, or to another area of the hospital, such as radiology.

Because some people are unable to care for their own physical needs, incontinence can be a problem. At regular intervals, take disorganized clients to the bathroom. Prevent dehumanization as much as possible. Persons who refuse or who cannot get out of bed may need skin care to prevent breakdown. Incontinence briefs and bed pads can help manage incontinence. Assist women to maintain feminine hygiene, especially during menses.

Teaching Life Skills

The goal of hospitalization is to prepare clients to return to the community. In some cases, clients need to learn acceptable social behaviors and how to care for personal needs.

Eating may be a problem. Many people eat too much and too rapidly; others eat insufficient amounts of food. Some clients drink too much or too little water. Clients often must learn how to buy and prepare food for themselves before going home. Hospitalized clients are given tableware, usually plastic, unless even this is a safety consideration. If necessary, monitor a client's intake.

Behavior modification techniques are often used with severely disturbed clients; usually retraining in many ADL is successful. Long-term clients often benefit from remotivation therapy and from contact with others.

Recreation and activity at an appropriate level are important for all clients, who often enjoy simple activities, such as walks, games, and crafts. Such activities also tend to lessen combative and destructive behavior, as clients work off tensions in a healthy manner. Recreational activities also help to teach social skills. Remember that everyone needs some social contacts, no matter how ill they are. Many people with mental illnesses are very lonely, making them very vulnerable.

Building Employment or Occupational Skills

Persons, particularly those in long-term care facilities, benefit from exposure to the world of work. A job or duty in the unit itself, such as maintaining one's own living quarters, may be the first attempt. As the client masters this task, he or she may progress to helping in the laundry, kitchen, coffee shop, garden, or gift shop. Many clients receive a small amount of pay for such work.

As a person is rehabilitated, he or she may be able to work in a sheltered workshop setting. Employment and earning money can add to any person's self-esteem. Before discharge, most people need vocational rehabilitation to train them for work, if they are well enough to be employed. Many people also benefit from volunteer work.

Some clients are too ill to be employed, even as volunteers. However, they can learn ways to spend leisure time in safe, low-cost, and beneficial ways. They can usually learn to care for their own sleeping or living quarters.

MENTAL HEALTH NURSING SKILLS

Mental health skills and skills in dealing with undesired behavior are needed in all nursing fields. Care of clients with deviations in mental health, however, provides a challenging opportunity; the nurse will need to use these abilities fully.

By working closely with clients in such settings, the nurse becomes a source of stability and consistency. He or she must be emotionally available, able to listen, non-punitive, supportive, understanding, and encouraging. Nurses must also carry out many technical psychiatry nursing skills. Some of these skills are common to all areas of nursing. Other skills are specific to mental health nursing.

☛ KEY CONCEPT

Common orders for precautions on the mental health unit include:

- *AP: assault precautions*
- *EP: escape (elopement) precautions*
- *GP/SP: general (suicide) precautions*
- *Sx: sexual precautions*
- *Sz: seizure precautions*
- *W/D (ETOH W/D): withdrawal or alcohol withdrawal*

Physical Care

The nurse may need to assist clients with severe mental disorders to perform routine physical care. Aspects or this care include:

Assisting with ADL that the person cannot perform without encouragement or assistance; teaching, supervising, and evaluating ADL. Urge the client to do as much as possible for himself or herself.

Ensuring adequate nutritional and hydration status. Some clients are **polydipsic** (drink excess amounts) and their fluids are restricted. Some clients are on calorie-controlled diets. Other clients must be encouraged to take food and fluids; some need nutritional supplements or tube feedings. Clients may be on special diets, as in the case of the diabetic client. Clients on certain medications, such as MAOIs, must follow a strict diet.

Handling inappropriate or dangerous behaviors. Staff must protect themselves from injury, while also preventing injury to the client who is acting out, as well as to other clients and visitors. A behavioral control class is usually provided for psychiatry staff.

Administering prescribed medications, observing for side effects, and teaching clients about medications. Offer as-needed (PRN) medications for side effects or behavior control.

Assisting the sleep-deprived client to get some sleep. Administer PRN medications as ordered. Offer the client measures designed to assist in sleep: relaxation tapes, a snack before bedtime, or a place to sleep in which he or she feels the most safe (Fig. 93-4).

Administering physical treatments as ordered. (Many clients have a physical disorder as well as a mental disorder.)

Emotional Support

The client and family need emotional support. The nurse can give such support in many ways:

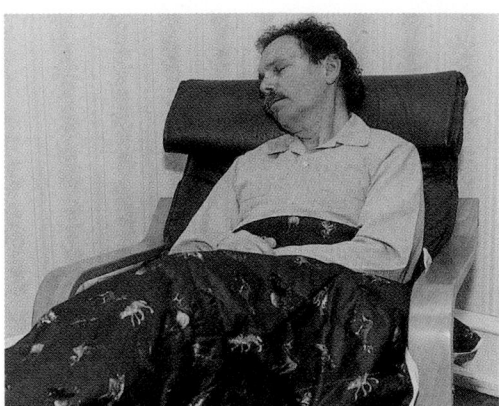

FIGURE 93-4. This paranoid client is afraid to sleep in his own room because of hallucinations and paranoid delusions. He is allowed to sleep in the lounge or commons area near the desk, where he feels more secure, until he becomes less fearful.

- Establish **rapport** (harmonious relationship). Box 93-3 lists some aspects of positive nurse–client relationships.
- Create a therapeutic and safe environment within the mental health setting.
- Provide emotional support to the client and family.
- Provide leadership in socialization activities with a person or group.
- Aid in group therapy sessions.
- Conduct remotivation sessions.
- Assist the client and family to access other resources, such as Alcoholics Anonymous, a community drop-in center, or a community social worker.

Other Skills

In psychiatry, nurses function not only as nurses, but also as counselors, teachers, and support persons (see Chap. 2).

- As a *socializing agent,* the nurse helps clients to participate in group activities and interact normally with others.
- As a *counselor,* the nurse listens to others and encourages them to work through problems.
- As a *teacher,* the nurse helps guide people into socially acceptable activities and teaches them about medications and treatments.
- As a *support person,* the nurse provides physical and emotional care, while encouraging people to face reality independently.

Observation

Observations that are documented carefully, objectively, and accurately can greatly assist the therapist, physician, or social worker. The purpose of ward observations and notes is to observe the client's ongoing behavior and condition (Fig. 93-5). Documentation consists mostly of descriptions of behavior; observation may be done without the client's knowledge. Clients have the right to review their medical records. (In some facilities, a physician's order is required. The client may not be allowed to read the record until the

➤➤ BOX 93-3

THE NURSE–CLIENT RELATIONSHIP

To establish a good relationship with any person, the nurse may do the following:

- Introduce himself or herself and offer to shake hands.
- Be polite, tactful, and friendly to everyone.
- Be truthful, but not brutally so. Avoid answering questions evasively.
- Be even-tempered and uncritical; remember that the person is ill.
- Have poise—it gives the nurse confidence and the client is more likely to have confidence in the nurse.
- Be an *interested* listener.
- Sit down to visit with clients. Do not stand over them. Sometimes it may be necessary to pace with a client.
- Have empathy, an essential characteristic of effective interpersonal relationships. It is not enough to imagine how *you* would feel in the person's situation; it is important to try to understand how *he* or *she* feels.
- Concentrate on the person's strengths and not on weaknesses.
- Appreciate individual differences. Not everyone has the same goals and values as the nurse.
- Be consistent. Tell the truth.
- Do not talk down to the clients or belittle them. Treat adults as adults, no matter how childish their behavior is. Do not argue with them.
- Set appropriate limits.
- Reward positive behaviors and steps toward wellness, however small they may be.
- Remember "The Patient's Bill of Rights."
- Do not force a client to have a long interview if it is uncomfortable for him or her. Instead, initiate a number of short interactions.
- Respect the client's living quarters as a private space. Allow appropriate personal space; avoid being intrusive.
- Never have any outside social contact with current or discharged clients.
- Maintain confidentiality. For example, if a nurse meets a former client on the street, the nurse should allow the person to acknowledge him or her first. The nurse learns to respect the client's privacy by not saying anything unless the client speaks first.
- Be cordial to the client's visitors.
- Maintain safety at all times.
- Do not talk loudly or yell in response to a client who yells. Keep the voice volume calm and low and the tone modulated.

physician determines that it would not be detrimental to the plan of care.) A staff member should be present whenever a client is reading his or her chart to interpret data, answer client questions, and prevent the client from defacing or destroying any part of the record.

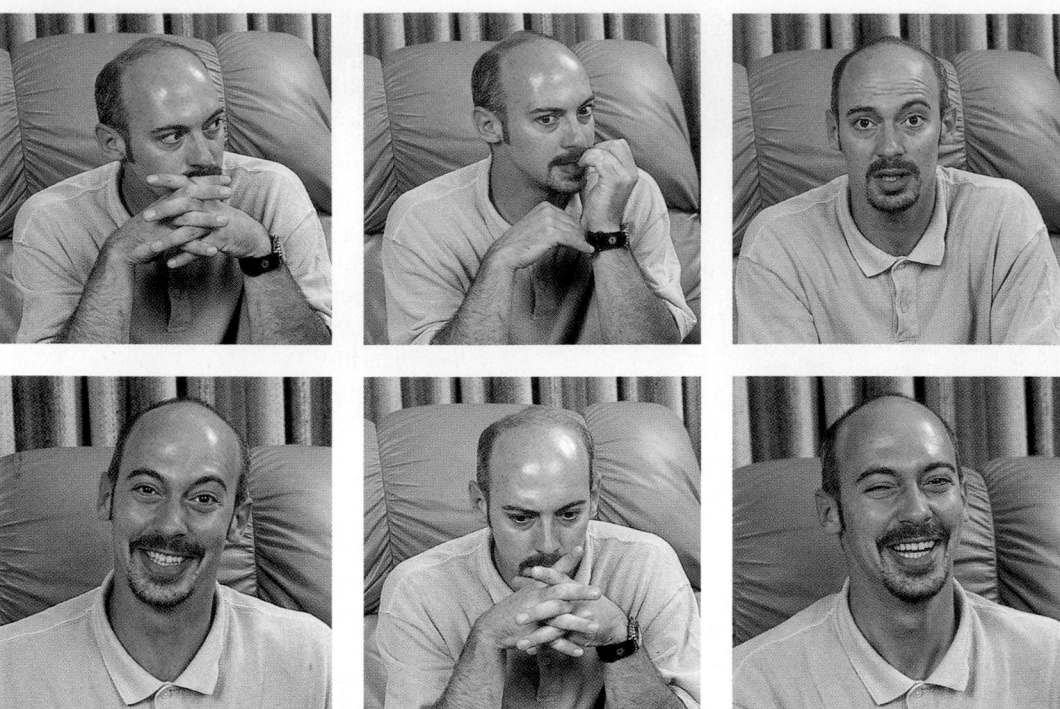

FIGURE 93-5. Nonverbal cues, such as body language and eye contact, are observed and documented. They can give clues as to how the client is feeling. The client's affect may be described using terms such as "bright," "blunted," "flat," or "angry." Document if the client has a wide range of or constricted affect, and if the affect is appropriate to the situation. Document if the client laughs inappropriately or is tearful.

☛ KEY CONCEPT

Some behaviors and speech patterns strongly indicate that individuals are responding to internal stimuli (auditory or visual hallucinations). Examples include talking to themselves, thought blocking, speech latency, and preoccupation. Some clients use a radio and headphones, earmuffs, or cotton in the ears to try to block out voices. Some clients experiencing hallucinations are very uncomfortable. Psychotropic medications may help.

In many settings, clients document their own feelings, thoughts, and activities in their chart, for the benefit of the healthcare team. The individual often has more insight into his or her own behaviors than does the staff. Many clients find it easier to write thoughts than to express them to the psychiatrist or healthcare team. Place all such documents in the client's chart, after dating and initialing them. Consider the factors listed at In Practice: Nursing Assessment 93-1 when assessing, planning, and documenting behavior.

☛ KEY CONCEPT

A meaningful nursing assessment is an art for the nurse to cultivate. Excellent observation and assessment skills are necessary for mental health nursing.

The nurse should observe the client in the following ways:

- Carefully and accurately document behaviors while in the mental health unit and on outings outside the facility.

- Pay attention to personal appearance and grooming, as well as other ADL.
- Record any physical symptoms.
- Carefully observe and document the client's interactions with others. Note if differences exist in interactions with other clients, staff, or family members. Observe also the client's interactions on the phone. Put direct statements in quotes in the client's chart.
- Assess vital signs at least daily and weight at least weekly.
- Document attempts to escape, to leave the unit without permission, or clients who return late from passes.
- In many cases, the client who is absent without leave (**AWOL**) and not under a court order is discharged at midnight. If this client returns after that time, he or she must be totally readmitted. (Third-party payers may not pay for the subsequent hospitalization after a client goes AWOL.)

If a Client Escapes

Even though a nursing unit is locked and a client is on escape/elopement precautions (**EP**), it is still possible to escape (*elope*). A client may walk away from a recreation group or may leave when another person leaves the unit. A client may also take staff keys. This client is said to be AWOL and certain measures are taken. If the client was on a court hold or legally committed to a facility, the physician and (in most cases) the police are notified. It is important to maintain the client's safety. The nurse should be able to describe the client and to give the police an idea where he or she might have gone. Some

In Practice
Nursing Assessment 93-1

THE PERSON IN THE MENTAL HEALTH UNIT

Appearance
- Assess whether the person is neat and clean, or dirty and untidy.
- Check the clothes to be sure they are appropriate for the situation and activity.
- Check makeup and hair.
- Record lack of adequate grooming.
- Describe bizarre or inappropriate clothing or makeup.
- Describe the client's room order; is his or her room messy and dirty, or neat and tidy?
- Is the client's bathroom clean? Does the client void or defecate on the floor?
- Does the client leave the sheets and mattress on the bed, use a pillowcase, and use towels appropriately?
- Does the person remain in hospital clothing all day?

Sociability
- Determine whether the person associates freely with others or prefers to be alone.
- Document if the person associates only with staff, with peers, or with visitors.
- Document if the person stays in bed all day, and if he or she is asleep or awake in bed.

Behavior
- Assess behavior to determine if the person is orderly or disorderly, still or restless, quiet or noisy, friendly or indifferent, interested or uninterested, cooperative or destructive.
- Document irritability, intrusiveness, and threatening behavior.
- Determine how the client spends time, if his or her conduct is always the same, and if the person complies with treatments and medications.
- Document group attendance or refusal.

Emotional Reactions
- Notice if and how clients express emotions (eg, crying, anxiety, depression, fear, suspicion, happiness, sadness, loneliness, or anger).
- Observe if the person is irritable, hostile, or excited; acts impulsively; or has unprovoked bursts of excitement, temper tantrums, or assaultive tendencies.
- Assess the client's overall emotional state and determine if his or her emotions are relatively consistent.
- Be specific in your assessment and documentation. Give examples whenever possible.

Speech
Assessment of speech involves determining answers to the following questions:
- Does the client's speech seem natural? Is it rapid, loose, disorganized and disconnected, or slow and retarded? Does the client speak English? Does the client speak with a "faked" accent or in several accents?
- Does speech indicate that the person understands what is said or requested? Does the person repeat or rhyme words or phrases? Does he or she repeat someone else's words (echolalia)? Does he or she coin new words that are not really words (**neologisms**)?
- Does the person pause before speaking when asked a question (*speech latency*)? Document the length of any latent periods. Does the person stop talking halfway through a sentence and seem unable to continue (*thought blocking*)?
- Does the person talk to himself or herself? How loudly? Is he or she argumentative? Does he or she seem frightened?
- Does the person have any particular speech defect, (eg, stuttering, lisping, stammering)?
- Is the person's hearing adequate?
- How much does the person talk? Does he or she talk voluntarily or only when questioned? Does the person initiate conversation with staff or peers? Does he or she talk constantly? Is the speech pressured?
- Is the client noisy (with words, singing, or just sounds)? Does he or she not speak (mutism)? If the client is mute with staff, does this continue with peers, with visitors, and on the phone?
- Does conversation make sense? Does the client dwell on one subject (**perseverate**) or always return to the same subject? Is the person able to concentrate on a topic? Is speech tangential and loose?
- What does the person talk about? Do meaningless *word salad* sentences occur? Does the person use unusual profanity? Are responses relevant and coherent? Does the client's conversation jump from one subject to another without order or apparent connection—*flight of ideas* (FOI)? Is the client religiously preoccupied?
- Does the person remember things? Is memory loss for recent events or events in the past? Is he or she oriented to time and place?

Document pertinent statements as direct quotes in quotation marks, as much as possible.

Nonverbal Behavior
- How clients behave is often more important than what they say. Posture, facial expression, and personal hygiene can indicate a great deal about self-image and worldview. Sometimes clients react differently when staff is not there, as opposed to when they know staff is watching. Do they act out when being observed or when they think no one is looking?
- Document a client's inappropriate behavior, such as smearing of feces or food, eating garbage, masturbating in public, undressing in public, or writing on walls.

(continued)

- Document any characteristic, ritualistic, and repeated gestures or mannerisms.
- Determine if the client looks at a person when talking and makes *eye contact*. (Consider culture in regard to eye contact and personal space, as discussed in Chap. 8.) (See Fig. 93-5.)
- Describe the client's *affect* (external expression of emotions). Is it flat, blunted, bright, anxious, or fearful (Fig. 93-5)? Does the person cry often?
- How does the client respond to children? To animals?

Physical Complaints
- Carefully document any complaints of pain or discomfort, including voiding difficulties, drooling, GI complaints, dizziness, or blurred vision, which can signify adverse side effects of medications.
- Document specific signs of extrapyramidal side effects (**EPSE**), such as difficulty in moving or swallowing, stiffness, tremor, inability to sit still (*akathisia*), marching in place, cogwheeling, or oculogyric crisis.
- Document vital signs and report abnormalities at once.

Physical Condition
- Note the person's general physical condition. Many clients have not been able to care for themselves, or have not had access to adequate medical care.
- Many clients are homeless and suffer from problems such as malnutrition, frostbite, or parasitic infestation. They may have a number of other physical disorders. Physically ill clients will have orders for medications and treatments in addition to psychiatric orders.
- Manage physical disorders such as diabetes: perform blood sugar testing, observe ADA diet, and so forth.

Movements
- Document whether the person is coordinated.
- Document and describe tremors.
- Does the person move quickly or slowly?
- Does he or she pace continuously or march in place; is the gait even and controlled?
- Does the client remain in one position for long periods?
- Does the person seem to get "stuck" in one position (*catatonia*)?
- If the person's arm is moved, will he or she maintain that position (*waxy flexibility*)?
- Is there unusual posturing (eg, ritualistic movement, karate stances)?

Sleep
- Determine the person's sleep pattern, including length and frequency.
- Is it normal? Disturbed?

- Does the client talk or cry out at night?
- Are nightmares reported?
- Does the person sleepwalk/talk?
- Is it difficult for the person to get out of bed in the morning? Is the person unusually sedated?
- Is he or she afraid at night? Sleep deprived?
- Does the client snore?
- Document the number of hours the person sleeps during the day, as well as at night.

Appetite
- Document the person's attitude toward food.
- Does he or she eat willingly, or must the staff urge and coax the client to eat?
- Is the person losing or gaining weight?
- Does evidence exist of an eating disorder such as anorexia nervosa and associated disorders (**ANAD**) or bulimia?
- Is the person obese or extremely thin?
- Note any peculiar behaviors or rituals in relation to food or eating.
- Assess the person's table manners (or lack thereof).
- Does the person eat or drink constantly? Drink plain water constantly?
- Does he or she have a fluid restriction on intake and output?
- Does he or she follow dietary orders?
- Does the person tell you that food is poisoned or unclean?
- Does he or she refuse to eat? If so, will the person eat food brought in by family members?

Elimination and Menstruation
- Observe elimination habits.
- Does the person maintain cleanliness?
- Document menstruation in women of reproductive age.
- Assist with maintaining hygiene if the person is unable to do so.

Other Observations
- Document any unusual occurrences, such as injuries or altercations between clients, along with the names of witnesses.
- Document attempts to escape.
- Document any overnight visits and passes outside the facility. What was the client's response to the pass?
- Document the condition of the client's living space:
  - Is it neat or messy?
  - Does the person need guidance in putting things away?
  - Does the client display any rituals in dealing with personal items?
  - Does the person lose things?

hospitals have a photo of each client for use by the police. Often, clients escape and then return in a short time on their own or are brought back by a family member.

If a nursing unit is a forensic unit, additional security is usually needed. **Forensic** clients are often those who are brought to the hospital from a jail or prison. In many cases, forensic clients have been accused of a serious crime, such as murder. They are often in the hospital to be evaluated to see if they are competent to stand trial. Forensic units often have sally-port doors, similar to those in a jail. In order to get in and out, people must pass through a **sally port,** an area with a locked door on each end. One door must be closed and locked before the other can be opened. This way, if a client is able to escape through the first door, he or she is held in the sally port and cannot escape. Some clients also have around-the-clock guards.

Nursing Actions in Specific Behaviors

Although broad psychiatric diagnoses are presented earlier in this chapter, not all people can be easily categorized. Therefore, nursing care involves dealing with behaviors. The following behaviors and approaches are specific to mental health nursing, but can be adapted to other areas. These are only guidelines: the nurse must adapt for each person and situation.

The Suicidal Person

Suicidal ideation (**SI**) and suicide attempts (**SA**) are the most common reasons clients are admitted to inpatient mental health units. These clients present a great nursing challenge. They are placed on suicide precautions (**SP**) or general precautions (**GP**) until the physician determines that they are no longer a danger to themselves. Any mental health resident presents a potential risk, but certain types of clients are more likely to attempt suicide than others. Refer to the accompanying In Practice: Nursing Care Guidelines 93-6.

Risk Factors.   Certain factors place clients at higher risk for suicide than normal. These risk factors include:

- Depression, dysthymia
- Sense of failure, guilt, low self-esteem, low motivation
- Previous SAs—A person who has previously attempted suicide is at least 25% more likely to attempt again.
- Well thought-out plan (consider how lethal the plan is)
- Sex—Women attempt more often; men complete more often.
- Age—Teenagers and senior citizens are at highest risk.
- Coexisting substance abuse
- Other mental illness (in addition to depression), especially schizophrenia and other psychoses, and bipolar disorder
- Poor support systems—Lack of religious beliefs, no family/friends (single people without children are at higher risk), no job, homeless
- Physical illnesses, especially progressive illnesses such as multiple sclerosis, HIV/AIDS, Huntington's disease, or cancer

- Personality disorders (such as borderline personality disorder) often contribute to suicide attempts; sometimes these clients are *accidentally* successful.

Certain groups of symptoms are considered significant. For example, the cluster of headache, insomnia, and depression (**HID**) may point to suicidal ideation. Psychological tests are available to assess depression. These include the Beck Depression Inventory (**BDI**) and the Hamilton Depression Rating Scale (**HDRS**).

Reporting and Documentation.   Consider any attempt at suicide serious: report any suicide threat or attempt, however minor it seems. Document and report any conversation in which a client expresses hopelessness or a desire to die. Suicide prevention involves constant and effective supervision and continuous, undemanding emotional support.

Carefully document a client's SI. Document, in quotes, any statement the client makes about feeling suicidal, wanting to die, or "not wanting to be around any more." Ask if the client has a suicide plan and document the responses. (If the client has a suicide plan, consider its lethality.) Document any statements made by friends and family about the client. They may detect subtle changes in the client's behavior. If the client expresses any form of SI, take immediate precautions to maintain safety and notify the physician or primary care provider. Document safety measures taken and who was notified.

☛ KEY CONCEPT

Nurses in all areas of a healthcare facility should be aware of the possibility of depression and suicidal ideation in their clients. Clients at greatest risk include those who have been diagnosed with a chronic illness or who are terminally ill, and women who have had a spontaneous abortion or an ill or dying child. Many hospice clients and chemically dependent people consider suicide during their treatment. If symptoms of depression are observed in any client, report it immediately and carefully observe the person.

Suicide Attempts.   People who injure themselves or others may have been given increased privileges too soon. Sometimes, self-injurious behavior is aimed at getting attention, or it may be in response to *command hallucinations.* People may attempt suicide in the healthcare facility using readily available articles or materials.

Watch people closely while they are working in OT shops to prevent them from securing tools, bits of metal and glass, or similar objects (see In Practice: Nursing Care Guidelines 93-6). Any type of plastic bag, cord, or rope can be dangerous (eg, electric cords, bathrobe ties, shoelaces, belts). Keep all medications under lock and key. People also attempt suicide or deliberate self-injury in other ways, such as diving to the floor from a window ledge, attempting to jump out the window, or ramming their head into a wall.

The early morning hours are a crucial time for depressed people because they often dread facing another day. Deeply depressed people are usually too exhausted to attempt suicide.

In Practice
Nursing Care Guidelines 93-6

SUICIDE PREVENTION

Types of People Who Need Particularly Close Observation
- New clients on the mental health unit
- Depressed people, especially those in early and late stages
- People suffering from insomnia or sleep deprivation
- Persons who abuse alcohol, especially during withdrawal
- Persons who abuse other drugs, especially depressants (including cocaine and related drugs)
- People responding to "command hallucinations"
- People with paranoia and certain types of delusions (eg, persecution, incurable illness)
- People with terminal or very serious illnesses (eg, cancer, AIDS)
- Confused people
- People with extreme mood swings
- People who have chronic, progressive illnesses (eg, Huntington's, Parkinson's, ALS)
- People who have made previous suicide attempts
- People who talk about suicide and express the wish to die
- People with self-injurious behaviors (may accidentally commit suicide)

Examples of Suicide Methods Attempted in the Hospital
- Cutting arteries with plastic, glass, or sharp instruments (including scissors)
- Hanging by sheets, blankets, belts, electrical cords, ties, shoelaces, or other items
- Standing in high places and falling
- Banging the head on such things as the floor, wall, or furniture
- Tipping over backward in a chair while sitting, attempting to break the neck
- Drinking poison from dressing trays, cleaning solutions, or sterilizing solutions; saving up medications and taking them all at once
- Biting and swallowing glass, needles, nails, and other items
- Bribing privileged clients or visitors to obtain destructive articles
- Drowning in the toilet, bathtub, or swimming pool
- Setting fires
- Suffocation (*Be extremely careful with plastic bags.*)
- Attempting to jump out windows or from another high place
- Attempting self-injury while on an outing

Preventive Measures
- Know whereabouts and condition of each resident at all times; 15-minute checks are a minimum.
- Make sure the client is breathing. If a client is in the bathroom, make sure they answer you—or go in.

- Provide a sense of security that encourages confidence.
- All clients should have a regularly scheduled one-to-one conference with the primary nurse at least daily, and should be given a conference whenever they request one.
- If a client is in bed with the covers pulled up over his or her head, make sure he or she is breathing.
- Most clients must be supervised when smoking. The staff usually keeps matches and lighters, and dispenses client cigarettes. If the institution is smoke free, provide supervision if the client is permitted to smoke outdoors. Make sure the person understands the limits of the area. If the facility allows smoking, there is usually a designated smoking area and limited smoking times. A lighter is often built-in or chained to the wall.
- Keep all medications under lock and key, not just narcotics.
- Because suicidal people are often integrated into the general psychiatric population, sharp and dangerous objects are often removed from *all* people on the mental health unit. Cans and any glass items are not allowed. In some units, shoelaces and belts are not allowed.
- Keep elevator doors and dumbwaiters locked.
- Question clients about suicidal or self-injurious ideation and have clients contract for safety. (This includes promising not to hurt themselves and promising to let staff know if they feel like hurting themselves at a later time.) If a client cannot contract for safety, he or she will probably require one-to-one observation.

Care of "Specialed" Residents (One-to-One Observation)
- Watch carefully every movement of the client. The nurse must stay at arm's length *at all times.*
- Permit no strings, belts, shoelaces, or ties on the person's clothing.
- Supervise the person *very* closely while he or she is using sharp objects, electrical appliances, and other dangerous items. In some cases, the client is not allowed to use these items.
- The person should get out of bed and get dressed each day. Encourage him or her to be independent.
- Do not leave the person alone when reporting off duty or going on a break; wait until relief arrives.
- Supervise bathroom use. Leave the door ajar. Listen carefully. Usually tub baths are not allowed, but showers are required. If there is any question, a staff person must go into the bathroom with the client.

- Occupy the person with suitable games when possible. Encourage reading, but do not read to him or her. Inspire the person to accomplish things.
- Anticipate behavior by being aware of mood changes. Occasionally, people will pretend improvement to gain an opportunity for suicide.
- Be sure the person is given any prescribed medication intended to help his or her condition.

- Find out if remotivation techniques have been recommended; they often benefit suicidal people.
- This person usually is not allowed to leave the unit except for ECT or a special test. He or she must be accompanied at all times.

However, as they begin to recover and regain their energy, they become more likely to attempt suicide. Depressed persons who are recovering appear more optimistic than they were before; nurses may fail to watch them as closely. Such persons may seem optimistic because they have devised a suicide plan. Routinely observe clients for signs of suicidal plans or attempts during the early stages of illness and convalescence. Be especially alert at changes of nursing shifts and at night, when fewer staff may actually be on the unit.

Actively suicidal people should be "specialed" (given a single staff person who works with one person exclusively) 24 hours a day. A person specialed in a mental health unit is never left alone. A nurse stays within the client's arm reach, even if the client is in the bathroom. Refer to In Practice: Nursing Care Guidelines 93-6 for care of "specialed" clients.

Suicide Prevention Centers. Some cities have established suicide prevention centers and telephone hotlines to help people who are contemplating suicide. The caller can speak with a knowledgeable person who will listen and discuss the situation; the counselor tries to persuade the person to delay acting. Some centers will rush help—often the police—to the person to prevent him or her from carrying out the suicide threat. Statistics of how many suicides are prevented through crisis prevention centers are unavailable; many callers remain anonymous. However, theorists believe that just talking with another person when the crisis is most severe stops many people from taking their own life. (The suicide crisis counselor also attempts to refer the caller for continuing assistance after the crisis call.)

The Overactive Person

Activity is a normal characteristic of life. Certain people are more animated and forceful than others by nature. Other factors, such as medications, can influence a person's activity level. Just as the degree of activity varies among all people, so does the overactive behavior of mentally disturbed people. Activity levels range from slightly agitated, to agitated and excitable, to extreme states of frenzy. Nursing care for overactive people differs. Also, marked changes may occur in the same person at different times; nursing care is adjusted accordingly. A quiet atmosphere is important. Use a calm,

soft voice; do not talk loudly; and avoid long discussions. Do not force issues; but set limits, be consistent, and prevent harm and injury. The person may need to take a time-out to prevent injury to self or others. The person may benefit from large-muscle activities (eg, basketball, dancing, a workout in the gym, or swimming). Medications may need to be forced to control unsafe behavior, or PRN medications may be requested by the client.

The Hypomanic or Manic Person

Types of Mania. The two degrees of mania are *hypomania* and *mania,* disorders characterized by elation, agitation, hyperactivity, hyperexcitability, and accelerated thinking and speaking (*flight of ideas* [**FOI**]). These people may be grandiose, believing, for example, that they are God, royalty, or millionaires. They may have spent thousands of dollars more than they could afford or may have spent the maximum on a number of credit cards. These people are sometimes "airport admissions," having flown thousands of miles with no specific destination in mind. When confronted by airport security officers, they may become hostile and aggressive, and therefore are brought to the hospital.

Hypomania (below mania) has less-intense characteristics and usually does not require hospitalization when it occurs alone. However, hypomania can cause the person to lose a job or to be evicted from an apartment, and can be very difficult for the family.

Characteristics of Mania. Manic people can be very challenging. Often they are witty, breezy, and enterprising; because of their keen memory and quick conversation, others may not recognize them as truly disturbed. These individuals are apt to be intrusive, domineering, and irritable. They often have rapid mood swings and lability. They rarely accept hospitalization willingly. They may be very entitled, believing that everyone should wait on them. They often make many unreasonable demands. These people are always busy; the chief problem in nursing care is channeling their activity. These individuals are oriented to time and place, but may have delusions. They are often unable or unwilling to sleep; as they become more sleep deprived, they often become more irritable, intrusive, and may become assaultive (see In Practice: Nursing Care Guidelines 93-7).

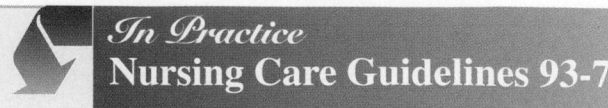

In Practice
Nursing Care Guidelines 93-7

CARE OF THE PERSON WHO IS MANIC/HYPOMANIC

- A small unit is usually best for the manic person (to limit stimulation and restrict activity).
- Be firm, but kind, and avoid familiarity.
- Do not argue with these people.
- Try to keep the person from irritating others and try to keep him or her safely occupied.
- If the manic person does not yet have privileges to participate in outings, use crafts, writing, or reading material for activity.
- Manic persons often benefit from competitive games, such as badminton, but such games require careful supervision. Avoid contact sports (because these clients are likely to play too rough and hurt others). They may enjoy using a punching bag or stationary bike.
- Encourage quiet, non–physically stimulating activities, such as cards and board games.
- Frequently, these people are unable to limit their own activity and must be carefully controlled.
- Their attention span may be quite short (they are easily distractable).
- Treatment usually involves mood stabilizer medications.
- Manic people may be resistant to taking medications (feeling that they are not ill and not wanting to be sedated). Many people enjoy being hypomanic; they become uncontrolled when they progress to mania.
- The client may need a great deal of encouragement to take medications early in treatment.
- Medications may need to be forced (to maintain safety for the client and others).
- Take care to supply extra nourishment and fluids to a hyperactive person (he or she expends much energy and requires additional calories).

The medications most commonly used to assist the person who is manic are:

Lithium carbonate (Eskalith, Lithonate) in oral tablets/capsules or lithium citrate in liquid form (to ensure compliance)

Valproate (Depakote), available in tablets, including extended release tablets and in liquid form (Depakene syrup)

Benzodiazepines and neuroleptic medications may be used during the acute phase, to control behavior and maintain safety.

See Table 93-2 for additional details.

The Highly Disturbed Person

Management and nursing care of the highly disturbed person includes physical protection. Allow active people a wide scope of activity for their surplus energy. In many cases these clients need direct physical care or supervision of ADL. Encourage the client to bathe and to remain clothed. Offer adequate food and fluids and make sure this client gets adequate nourishment. Encourage good mouth and skin care and pay attention to cuts or bruises. Direct nursing care toward limiting overstimulation. Do not force groups. (The person would probably be very disruptive to the group.)

The Hostile or Combative Person

Hostile persons may threaten to injure others and may become physically violent. These individuals usually require assault precautions (**AP**). Document if a client has homicidal ideation (**HI**), threatening to injure or kill others. The person with homicidal ideation may be threatening to everyone or may have a specific person who is the target of his or her hostility (see In Practice: Nursing Care Guidelines 93-8 and Box 93-4).

☛ KEY CONCEPT

When giving any treatment to a highly disturbed client, be sure there is adequate assistance. All staff must work together to maintain each person's safety. (Sometimes a show of force *is needed.) Set firm limits on undesirable and dangerous behavior. Use time-outs in the client's room (5–30 minutes) to assist the person to calm down; doing so provides stability for the entire unit. In an emergency, medications may be forced to control dangerous behavior.* Immediate de-escalation of dangerous behavior is vital!

Always use the least restrictive methods of behavior control:

- *Talk to the client*
- *Encourage a voluntary time-out*
- *Force a time-out*
- *Place the client in seclusion*
- *Use physical or chemical restraints*

Release the client from any seclusion or restraint as soon as possible.

The Person With Delusions or Hallucinations

People may have false beliefs (*delusions*) or perceive false sensory stimuli (*hallucinations*).

Delusions.   A *delusional* belief may be anything, from the status of the individual client to the situation in the world around them. If a person has a fixed delusion about another person, a psychiatrist may need to warn that individual. Delusional clients may harass or stalk love objects. They may seek to hurt the person in their delusion, or may believe that the other person is in love with them and welcomes their advances.

✚👁 Nursing Alert
Any threats against government officials require healthcare professionals to notify the U.S. Secret Service.

Hallucinations.   The nurse working in mental health will meet many people who experience *hallucinations*. Hallucinations are sensory perceptions not based in reality. They

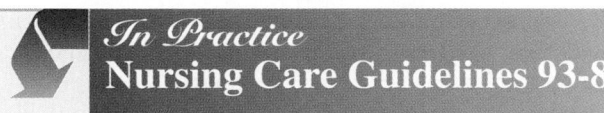

In Practice
Nursing Care Guidelines 93-8

CARE OF THE COMBATIVE OR ASSAULTIVE PERSON

If a Client is Argumentative

• In a verbal confrontation, the nurse's first impulse may be self-defense, but responding defensively is ineffective. *It is also dangerous.* (A defensive response will further escalate the combative person's behavior.)

• An effective response recognizes the person's feelings without judgment. Do not belittle the person.

• Allow the person to talk and express feelings. Do not argue.

• A firm but understanding approach may prevent a hostile person from acting aggressively.

• Speak to such clients calmly and quietly (see Box 93-4).

• Clients who are confused, out of touch with reality, hearing unwelcome voices, or experiencing delusions are often reacting to their situations in the only way they know. They may be very upset by being locked in and may feel "trapped" and afraid.

• Try to look beyond a client's anger and determine what is causing it. Ask the client to work with you to solve the problem.

• Emphasize the positive, and reward appropriate behavior. (Punishing negative behavior is much less effective.)

• Choose appropriate and safe outlets for physical energy. Activities such as outdoor walks, a punching bag, or time in the gym require staff supervision, but are often helpful.

If a Client Strikes Out

• If a person becomes assaultive, threatening to hurt others or actually striking someone, use seclusion (to protect the client and others). Seclusion requires written physician's orders and one-to-one nursing supervision.

• Neuroleptic medications can usually control the manic person, although the person may refuse to take them orally. Medications may be forced (by injection) in an emergency.

• In an extreme case, a powerful antipsychotic medication or an anesthetic, such as droperidol (Inapsine), may be used. (Neuroleptics help to clear thinking and diminish hallucinations. They also promote sleep, which the client often needs; many of these clients are sleep deprived.)

➤➤ BOX 93-4

GUIDELINES FOR DEALING WITH A COMBATIVE CLIENT

• Understand the client. Anticipate and try to prevent the client from acting out.

• Anticipate what the staff is going to do.

• Be careful with eye contact; the client may interpret it as a challenge.

• Avoid becoming excited; speak in a calm and level manner. Speak softly, but firmly.

• Do not make statements or use body language that can be interpreted as a challenge.

• Do not allow the person to move behind a staff person. Do not allow the person to move between staff and the door.

• Protect yourself physically, but do not injure the client.

• If the facility has an electronic alarm system, carry the electronic signaling device at all times, and let the clients know that you have it.

• Call for assistance; have someone clear the area of other clients.

• Be careful not to injure or insult a client in any way.

• Do not retaliate. Remember, the client may not be responsible for his or her actions.

• Seclusion and patient safety devices may be needed to prevent injury to staff or peers.

• If a person attacks a staff person or peer, use non-painful methods to protect everyone. Call for assistance.

• Generally, this client will be placed in a locked seclusion room until his or her behavior is under control. Have PRN medications available. If the client is out of control, medications may need to be forced (by injection).

---

crawling on or inside the body (*tactile*). Delusions and hallucinations often occur simultaneously. See In Practice: Nursing Care Guidelines 93-9.

The Confused or Demented Person

Many people with mental illnesses are confused as a result of their illness. In addition, some medications can contribute to disorientation. A person can also show dementia as a result of Alzheimer's disease, or as a result of brain damage caused by an accident, drug abuse, or as a result of an infection such as encephalitis or AIDS (see In Practice: Nursing Care Guidelines 93-10 and Chap. 92).

The Withdrawn Person

People who are withdrawn choose to be left alone. Matters of major concern to other people, such as food, grooming, and elimination, are often unimportant to them. Conversations with other people are difficult; therefore, withdrawn individuals do not interact with peers. This person may choose to spend the entire day in bed, often with the covers over his or

---

may take the form of sounds, music, or voices (*auditory hallucinations* [**AH**]), the most common type; or images, sights, shadows, or visions (*visual hallucinations* [**VH**]), the second most common type (AH are most common in schizophrenia). Other types of hallucinations are odors (*olfactory*); tastes (*gustatory*); or sensations of being touched or of something

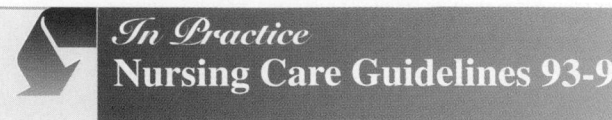

In Practice
Nursing Care Guidelines 93-9

ASSISTING THE CLIENT WHO HAS DELUSIONS OR HALLUCINATIONS

- Try not to reinforce the presence of the false perceptions. Ask the person to describe their delusion or hallucination, but state calmly that you do not see or hear what they are perceiving. It is often helpful to say, "That seems to be part of your illness."
- Remember that these hallucinations and delusions are very real to the client, but it is often therapeutic for the client to realize that others do not hear, see, or believe the same things he or she does.
- Do not argue about the delusion or hallucination.
- Build the person's trust by being consistent.
- Use a soothing voice.
- Document exactly what the person says, in quotes.

her head. Documentation often describes such persons as isolating themselves. (*Autism,* an extreme form of withdrawal, is discussed in Chapter 73.) The withdrawn person may be depressed and suicidal and should be monitored carefully, to maintain safety.

The Depressed Person

In major depressive disorder, the person is usually inactive and shares many characteristics with the withdrawn person. A major treatment objective is suicide prevention; therefore, this person requires particularly close observation. The person is most at risk when he or she begins outwardly to improve, but still is depressed. Other nursing care is the same as for other withdrawn and inactive people. See In Practice: Nursing Care Guidelines 93-6 and 93-11 and In Practice: The Nursing Process 93-1.

☞ KEY CONCEPT

Remind the client that it takes several weeks for antidepressant medications to take effect. This will be a difficult time for the client and he or she will need a great deal of encouragement.

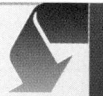

In Practice
Nursing Care Guidelines 93-10

ASSISTING THE PERSON WHO IS CONFUSED OR DEMENTED

- This person needs a calm, quiet environment, regulated by routine and free from danger and anxiety.
- The major treatment goal is to reorient such persons to reality.
- Try to involve the person in activities. Although it is a good idea to encourage these clients to participate and to converse with others, do not force socialization.
- This person may be able to talk to one other person, but is unlikely to be comfortable in a group.
- Nursing care includes helping to maintain grooming, bowel and bladder continence, and menstrual hygiene.
- Check for constipation, a frequent side effect of medications. This client is unlikely to volunteer this information.
- Observe clients for symptoms of physical disease (they may not complain of pain).
- Monitor vital signs.
- It may be necessary to document intake and offer nutritional supplements, such as Resource or Ensure. An IV line or feeding tube may be needed in extreme cases.
- Encourage the person to eat by sitting with him or her or by allowing the client to eat in his or her own room.
- Notify the physician if the person does not have adequate food or fluid intake.
- Weigh the client regularly.

- Encourage participation in remotivation sessions, small group activities, and occupational therapy.
- This person often relates very well to a pet on the unit or to children who come to visit.
- Because disorientation to time and place is common, provide a calendar and clock. To further reinforce time and place, mark off each day on the calendar.
- Remind the person about holidays or birthdays.
- A large sign on the client's door ("Judy's room") can remind him or her not to enter other rooms.
- To avoid further confusion, speak in short, clear, simple sentences and have the person repeat them if necessary.
- Question the client's statements for clarity and try to understand what they are saying.
- Give instructions one at a time and assist the person to perform tasks as needed.
- The nursing staff may need to manage assaultive behavior in this person.
- Medications may or may not be helpful in managing behavior, particularly in the older person. (Some older people have a *paradoxical* [opposite] reaction to medications. In other cases, medications *disinhibit* the person, causing even more antisocial behavior.)

Chapter 92 describes the nursing care of the confused person or the person with dementia in more detail.

In Practice
Nursing Care Guidelines 93-11

ASSISTING THE PERSON WHO IS WITHDRAWN OR DEPRESSED

- Speak softly and calmly.
- Encourage this person to eat. It may be necessary to monitor intake and output.
- Provide a cheerful, well-lighted living area.
- Encourage the person to spend time out of bed or out of his or her room.
- Try not to place depressed or withdrawn people in groups of exuberant people in efforts to cheer them up (this attempt usually has the opposite effect, and tends to make them more conscious of their own unhappiness).
- Encourage participation in activities, but do not force.
- Although occupational therapy is of great value, it should be simple and brief (these people often tire quickly and have short attention spans).
- Introduce the person to *one other person* at a time, not to large groups.
- As convalescence progresses, reading, games, puzzles, and small parties are helpful.
- Indecision is typical, so give the person only one or two choices.
- Many withdrawn people are preoccupied, often as a result of auditory hallucinations. (Be patient. If the person is suicidal, follow the guidelines presented at In Practice: Nursing Care Guidelines 93-6.)
- Antidepressant drugs are often helpful to persons with depression. Remember that it takes a number of weeks for these drugs to begin to take effect.

Chapter 55 discusses depression as it relates to chronic pain.

In Practice
Nursing Process 93-1

CARING FOR DEPRESSED CLIENTS

Assessment Priorities
Nursing History
- Expressions of feeling sad, unhappy, blue, "down in the dumps"
- Loss of interest or pleasure in usual activities (*anhedonia*)
- Anxiety
- Feelings of inadequacy, helplessness, inability to make decisions
- Feelings of fatigue, lassitude, wanting to stay in bed or sleep all day
- Pessimism, hopelessness
- Feelings of worthlessness, self-reproach, or excessive or inappropriate guilt
- Complaints of sleep disturbances, gastrointestinal disturbances, decreased *libido* (sexual drive), extreme weight changes (10%), unusual aches and pains

Data Collection
- Psychomotor agitation or retardation
- Stooped posture
- Poor personal hygiene
- Excessive tearfulness
- Intensity of anger, guilt, and feelings of worthlessness may precipitate suicidal thoughts, feelings, and gestures.
- Verbalizes suicidal ideation with or without plan or intent
- Sudden change in activity level—becomes hyperactive or if highly agitated, suddenly becomes calm

Possible Nursing Diagnoses
Impaired Adjustment
Anxiety
Ineffective Individual Coping
Dysfunctional Grieving
Altered Health Maintenance
Hopelessness
Altered Nutrition: Less than Body Requirements
Altered Nutrition: More than Body Requirements
Powerlessness
Self-Care Deficit
Self-Esteem Disturbance
Sexual Dysfunction
Sleep Pattern Disturbance
Social Isolation
Spiritual Distress
Altered Thought Processes
High Risk for Self-Directed Violence

Planning
Design a plan of care with the client (and family) to achieve the following goals:
- The person's physiologic needs are met, as evidenced by the fact that he or she (1) maintains weight (specify range); and (2) maintains muscle tone and strength.
- The person's safety needs are met, as evidenced by absence of any self-inflicted harm.

(continued)

- The person verbalizes emotions appropriate to the situation.
- The person begins to show interest in everyday concerns, beginning with personal hygiene.
- The person resumes independent self-care activities.
- The person describes (demonstrates the use of) adequate coping strategies.
- The person expresses a new sense of control over his or her goals and future (decreased expression of negative thoughts, helplessness, and pessimism).
- The person expresses increased self-esteem (decreased expression of worthlessness or guilt).

Implementation
- The first priority is to maintain a safe environment for the person: (1) observe closely (specify); (2) remove all potentially harmful objects from the room of any client with self-destructive behaviors; (3) make a contract with the suicidal person that he or she agrees *not* to act on suicidal thoughts unless first contacting the nurse.
- Ensure that the client's physiologic needs are met; encourage the client's maximum participation in self-care.
- Allow the person to express his or her feelings.
- Redirect the client's self-preoccupation to interests in the outside world: (1) involve the person in meaningful, productive tasks and activities; (2) increase the person's level of socialization.

- Promote the client's increased self-esteem: (1) identify significant others that he or she trusts, and facilitate healthy interpersonal relationships; (2) identify and reinforce the person's strengths; (3) encourage good hygiene and grooming and maintenance of sleeping areas.
- Assist the person to replace maladaptive coping mechanisms with healthy coping mechanisms; mobilize social support systems he or she can tap (family and community); and initiate referrals if appropriate.
- Administer prescribed antidepressants, and teach the person about the pharmacologic management of depression.
- Assist with other treatment modalities, such as electroconvulsive therapy (ECT).
- Support the family during the person's treatment and help them to get answers to their questions.
- Ask for a consultation with a Clinical Nurse Specialist or a psychiatric liaison consultation.

Evaluation
The adequacy of the plan of care is determined by evaluating the client's achievement of the above goals. If he or she is unable to meet key goals, the plan must be modified. Key evaluative criteria include:
- Healthy resolution of depression with a return to independent, meaningful living
- Absence of self-inflicted harm
- Verbalization of goals and plans for the future

In Practice
Nursing Care Guidelines 93-12

ASSISTING THE PERSON WHO IS REGRESSED
- Remotivation and behavior modification are useful. Assist the person to learn how to live comfortably in the world.
- Direct nursing care toward helping regressed persons focus on reality. Stimulate their interest in current events and keep them in contact with the present.
- Encourage self-respect by allowing the person to do as much for himself or herself as possible.
- Work to gain the person's confidence by being truthful and by keeping promises.
- Do not reprimand these people for inappropriate behavior; instead reward for appropriate behavior.
- Often regressed people are extremely sensitive and become embarrassed, despite seeming oblivious to everything.
- Set up an appropriate bathroom schedule; reward and praise success. Adult diapers may be

helpful at first, but try to eliminate them as soon as possible.
- Try to design interesting and simple activities.
- Encourage contact with peers, one or two at a time.
- Initiate games, and participate in them with clients.
- Be alert for violent outbursts and suicide attempts.
- Encourage verbalization of feelings and accept any verbalization, no matter how minimal.
- If these clients use profanity, gently guide them to more acceptable forms of verbalization.
- Discourage inappropriate behaviors by distracting the client.
- Today, clients are rarely bedridden. All clients *should* be up and out of bed and should be dressed for the day, unless physically ill. Being dressed in street clothes, rather than hospital garb, helps to reinforce appropriate adult behaviors.

The Person With Both Overactive and Underactive Behavior

In some disorders, the client's behavior alternates between overactivity (hypomania or mania) and underactivity (withdrawal or depression). A **cyclothymic** disorder is a mild form of this condition. (The more severe form is known as bipolar disorder.) Both extremes require symptomatic treatment. Medications are often helpful in controlling this condition, although the person may independently discontinue them after leaving the facility, causing a relapse.

The Regressed Person

Regression is a return to infantile or childish behavior. Examples include eating with the hands, urinating on the floor, soiling instead of using the toilet, openly masturbating, and being naked in public. Re-teaching basic social skills to regressive adults takes patience, and many people are usually involved in their care (see In Practice: Nursing Care Guidelines 93-12).

Nursing Alert

It is *inappropriate, unethical,* and *illegal* to have any social contact with a hospitalized or discharged psychiatric client; this person is usually considered a *vulnerable adult.* Always set limits and maintain high professional standards.

➥ STUDENT SYNTHESIS

Key Points

- Today, most mentally ill people are treated in the community.
- Everyone uses defense mechanisms. When they are used to an extreme, a deviation from mental health exists.
- Several organic causes of mental illness exist. If healthcare professionals can locate such a cause, they can more successfully treat the illness.
- Neurologic and neuropsychological tests help to establish the diagnosis of mental illness and help to determine the plan for treatment.
- One of the most common mood disorders is major depressive disorder, which is a major contributor to the act of suicide.
- The person with bipolar disorder has mood swings, from mania to depression.
- Clients with personality disorders may be very difficult to work with.
- A psychosis is a thought disorder, with major deviations from normal behavior and lack of contact with reality. Hallucinations, delusions, and paranoia are common symptoms.

- Many mentally ill people are also chemically dependent. The two conditions complicate and contribute to one another.
- Outpatient and emergency services are available to serve clients with mental illness. They include a variety of structured and less-structured living situations.
- Clients may come into the healthcare facility voluntarily or may be brought in under one of several legal categories.
- Electroconvulsive therapy is used in some cases of intractable depression or when medication is contraindicated. Nurses are responsible for monitoring the client before and after the treatment and for evaluating any loss of short-term memory or cognitive changes.
- People receiving treatment for mental illness have the same rights as all other clients. Sometimes, a court order may be required to force treatment.
- Many medications that treat mental illness have unpleasant side effects. Some side effects are life threatening.
- Many psychiatric clients who use their medication are able to live productively in the community.
- Nurses must be careful with the use of patient safety devices, to avoid injuring clients.
- Most clients on the mental health unit are legally considered vulnerable adults.
- It is illegal and unethical for the nurse to have social contact with vulnerable clients outside of the healthcare facility.

Critical Thinking Exercises

1. J., 43 years old, comes to your community mental health center for the first time. He says he "feels like killing himself" and recently bought a gun. He states, "My mother talked me into coming here." J.'s wife recently left him, taking their two children with her. Since then, J. has been depressed and drinking heavily. He says he also "used a little crack yesterday." He denies long-term substance abuse. He says, "I don't know what to do. I feel hopeless. I can't even work. I'm afraid my boss is going to fire me. Nothing like this has ever happened to me before."
   a. Describe your initial nursing actions on meeting J. Make a list of pertinent factors to consider when developing a nursing care plan for him.
   b. How does J.'s case differ from a case of chronic, severe depression, lasting about 10 years or more?
2. The police bring an unidentified older woman into the crisis center where you work. She is wearing handcuffs and leg shackles. The woman has reportedly lived in the city park for several years. She has two shopping bags of dirty clothes and other belongings.

Recently, she has been extremely agitated, talking to herself and yelling at passersby. Today, she entered a nearby church and began throwing statues on the floor. "Jane Doe" is wearing two dirty dresses, a sweater, a jacket, a knitted cap, unmatched socks, and dirty tennis shoes. (The temperature today is 92° F.) Her gray hair is snarled and she scratches her head often. She is malodorous; her breath is stale. She is thin and is missing her front teeth. She appears to have a partially healed wound on her left lower leg. When she is asked her name, she replies, "God." She is uncommunicative, except to demand cigarettes. When placed in a holding room, she moves into a far corner and strikes out when anyone approaches. She refuses to sit on the bed. She seems very fearful. Jane Doe did not allow all her vital signs to be taken, but her weight is 97 pounds, her pulse is 120 and her respirations 22. She has a productive cough.

a. Describe ways to approach Jane Doe. What immediate nursing actions are likely? List important factors to consider when developing a nursing care plan for this client. Consider short and long-term goals. What possible (medical and psychiatric) diagnoses might be made?

b. Describe types of patient safety devices and other safety measures that might be used in the client's care.

c. What medications might be prescribed to control the client's behavior and to help make her more comfortable?

d. Identify possible community resources to contact that can help her function better on discharge.

NCLEX-Style Review Questions

1. A client is admitted to the hospital with a diagnosis of major depression. When taking his or her history, which information would be most significant?
   a. Feelings of distress
   b. Lack of energy
   c. Thoughts of self-harm
   d. Weight loss

2. When evaluating the effectiveness of neuroleptic medications, the nurse would monitor for:
   a. Apathy
   b. Decreased hallucinations
   c. Severe agitation
   d. Tardive dyskinesia

3. Prior to electroconvulsive therapy, the nurse would instruct the client that common side effects of the therapy include:
   a. Myalgia and headache
   b. Nausea and vomiting
   c. Pain and seizures
   d. Vomiting and disorientation

References

1. Barry, P. (1998). *Mental health and mental illness* (6th ed., p. 367). Philadelphia: Lippincott Williams & Wilkins.
2. Shives, L. (1998). *Basic concepts of psychiatric-mental health nursing* (4th ed., p. 134). Philadelphia: Lippincott Williams & Wilkins.
3. Gandy, G. (1995). *Mental health rehabilitation: Disputing irrational beliefs* (p. 14). Springfield, IL: Charles Thomas Publishers.
4. New Games Foundation. P.O. Box 1641. Mendocino, CA 95460. 707-962-6514.
5. Videbeck, S. (2001). *Psychiatric mental health nursing* (p. 29). Philadelphia: Lippincott Williams & Wilkins.

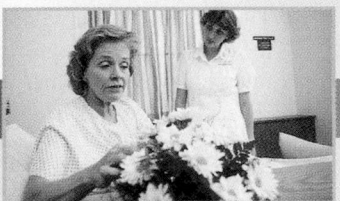

CHAPTER

94

Substance Abuse

LEARNING OBJECTIVES

1. List at least three criteria for a diagnosis of substance abuse and at least four additional criteria for a diagnosis of chemical dependency.
2. Discuss three theories put forth as possible contributing factors to development of chemical dependency. Identify the most common characteristics of the chemically dependent person.
3. List four specific steps in managing chemical dependency.
4. Describe signs that you might see in a client that indicate substance abuse, including characteristic behavior changes and physical signs. Describe the steps of progression to chemical dependency.
5. Identify at least 10 pertinent questions to ask in a nursing assessment for chemical dependency.
6. Describe nursing measures in detoxification. State the chemical from which withdrawal is life threatening.
7. Explain the meaning of refeeding syndrome.
8. Identify and describe at least three programs or theories for the long-term treatment of chemical dependency.
9. List and describe the three stages of unmanaged alcohol withdrawal. Define delirium tremors, and alcohol hallucinosis.
10. Describe specific nursing care in alcohol withdrawal.
11. Describe the role of the codependent in alcoholism. Identify how the cycle of dependence is interrupted.
12. List the signs of abuse and withdrawal symptoms for sedatives, cannabis, narcotics, amphetamines, cocaine, hallucinogens, anabolic steroids, nicotine, and caffeine.
13. Explain how opiate-blocker drugs (opiate agonists) are used in maintenance programs for narcotic substance abuse.
14. Discuss the dangers of abuse of hallucinogens and volatile substances.
15. Describe problems related to abuse of over-the-counter drugs.
16. Identify and discuss special problems associated with drug abuse in pregnant women, adolescents, and older adults.
17. Discuss legal obligations of nurses who believe coworkers are abusing drugs or alcohol.

NEW TERMINOLOGY

after-care
agonist therapy
alcohol hallucinosis
aversion therapy
blackout
cirrhosis
codependent
detoxification
dual disorder
enabler
macropsia

micropsia
polysubstance dependent
refeeding syndrome
remission
substance abuse
substance dependence
tolerance
Wernicke-Korsakoff
   syndrome
withdrawal

ACRONYMS

AA	ETOH, EtOH	MJ
ACOA	FAS	NA
ARLD	GBA	OBS
ASI	GHB	PCP
CD	HPPD	REBT
DARE	LSD	RET
DIS	MADD	STP
DOM	MDA/MDMA	THC
DTs	$MgSO_4$	WKS
DUI/DWI		

Individuals respond to stress in numerous ways. One way is through using harmful, mood-altering chemicals. In addition to stress, another factor very often related to the use of such substances is low self-esteem.

Although addictions can be to chemicals, such as alcohol and other drugs, they may also include obsessions with substances and activities such as work, sex, food, or gambling. Many people use addictions to avoid relationships and painful problems. Addictions know no racial, religious, gender, age, or socioeconomic barriers. Recognizing and caring for those with addictions requires high-level nursing assessment, nursing skills, patience, and compassion.

CHEMICAL ABUSE AND CHEMICAL DEPENDENCY

Chemical Abuse

The American Psychiatric Association (APA) has defined the abuse of chemicals (**substance abuse**) as "a maladaptive pattern of substance use leading to clinically significant impairment or distress" with one or more of the following in a 12-month period:[1]

- Failure to fulfill role obligations (work, school, home)
- Use that presents a danger (eg, while driving or using other heavy machinery)
- Recurrent use-related legal problems (eg, driving under the influence, disorderly conduct)
- Continued use, despite related interpersonal problems

Any drug can be abused, including alcohol, marijuana, or drugs prescribed by a physician.

Chemical Dependency

The APA defines **substance dependence** or *chemical dependency* (**CD**) as including the signs listed above, plus adding at least three or more of the following criteria, at any time, within a 12-month period:

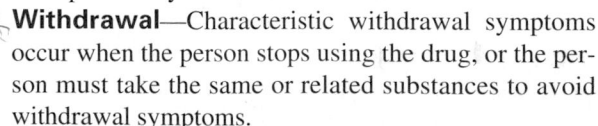

- **Tolerance**—The person needs more of the drug to cause intoxication, or the person experiences decreased effects from previously sufficient amounts.
- **Withdrawal**—Characteristic withdrawal symptoms occur when the person stops using the drug, or the person must take the same or related substances to avoid withdrawal symptoms.
- The person uses the drug in larger amounts or for a longer time than planned (eg, person goes on a "binge" and cannot stop).
- The person wishes to stop using or cut down, but is unable to do so.
- The person spends much time and energy planning to obtain the drug (eg, multiple physicians, traveling out of town, robbing stores to get money, hiding bottles).
- The person gives up formerly important activities (eg, organizations, entertainment, family) secondary to drug use.

- The person continues to use even though he or she knows the drug is causing significant physical, psychological, or interpersonal problems.

In addition, the person who is chemically dependent spends increasing amounts of money on the drugs, even though doing so jeopardizes his or her personal and family finances. Chemical dependencies also are often combined with other compulsive behaviors, such as gambling, adding extra financial burdens. Chemical dependency can exist with or without physiologic dependence. Note that use can be daily or episodic and still be considered abuse or dependence.

There are many evaluation tools used to identify chemical dependency. These include the Diagnostic Interview Schedule (**DIS**), which is specific for alcoholism, and the Addiction Severity Index (**ASI**), which determines degrees of addiction to any drug.

The medical community first recognized CD as a disease in the 1950s. Untreated CD is potentially fatal and will worsen without intervention. Chemical dependency is classified as:

- Active
- In **remission** (not currently active, but still existing)
- On agonist/blocking therapy
- In a controlled environment

These categories are explained later in this chapter. The healthcare industry is continually learning better ways to manage clients with CD.

Chemical dependency can lead to various mental disorders, including delirium, dementia, psychosis, sexual dysfunction, and sleep disorders. In addition, various physical disorders can result from abuse of chemical substances. Examples of physical disorders caused by abuse of drugs include cirrhosis of the liver, organic brain damage, and pancreatitis.

Causes

Despite all that has been written about the causes of CD, no one has yet identified a sole causative factor. The following are possible theories about causation.

Physical Factors Theory

According to this theory, excessive consumption of substances is the most immediate cause of addiction. For example, some investigators believe alcoholics have a nutritional deficiency that they remedy by drinking alcohol. Research is being conducted to learn whether an endocrine factor (similar to diabetes) exists in alcoholism.

Another theory is that ingestion of alcohol and certain other drugs causes an *allergic response,* or an altered reaction of body tissues to a specific substance (alcohol), that would not produce the same effect in non-sensitive people.

Many people use substances "just to feel better" or to "escape from life and its problems."

Genetic Theory

Considerable research has been conducted to target genetic causes. It has yet to be determined whether addiction to alcohol and other drugs is based on direct biologic transmission, or is a learned behavior in children who constantly interact with alcoholic or substance-abusing family members.

Emotional and Psychological Theories

Psychological explanations of substance abuse vary in detail but generally agree that the person abuses the substance to escape stress. Low self-esteem is often considered the most potent precipitating factor in substance abuse. The dependent person needs the drug to feel good about life and self. The stress theory is compatible with this idea, because stress can be caused by low self-worth, as the person continuously tries to be good enough to satisfy his or her own personal ideals.

Some generalizations about the substance abuser's personality have been formulated:

- Low self-esteem
- Difficulties in interpersonal relations
- General uneasiness and dissatisfaction with life
- Low tolerance for frustration
- Tendency toward excessive and self-destructive acts
- Co-existing mental illness (in many cases)

As with most exclusively psychological theories, it is unclear whether these characteristics are typical of the potential substance abuser or result from the abuse.

Dual Disorders

As discussed in Chapter 93, many chemically dependent people also have a coexisting mental illness that complicates both conditions. This **dual disorder** is called mental illness combined with chemical dependency (MI/CD). Many mentally ill people are depressed and use chemicals in an attempt to ease depression or to commit suicide. Many mentally ill people suffer from "voices" (auditory hallucinations) and use chemicals in an effort to "make the voices go away." In addition, these people may have difficulty locating appropriate therapists or support groups. (Some Alcoholics Anonymous [**AA**] groups, for example, do not understand that the MI/CD client needs to take psych medications, even though they should not use other chemicals.) A substance abuser's depression may deepen after use and may also be accompanied by guilt. In addition, many commonly abused drugs, including alcohol, sedatives, and narcotics, are depressants and compound the person's original depression. Figure 94-1 illustrates the complexity of interrelated social factors that contribute to and result from MI/CD.

Nature

Progressive Nature

The progressive nature of CD corresponds to its psychological cause. The typical progression is summarized as follows:

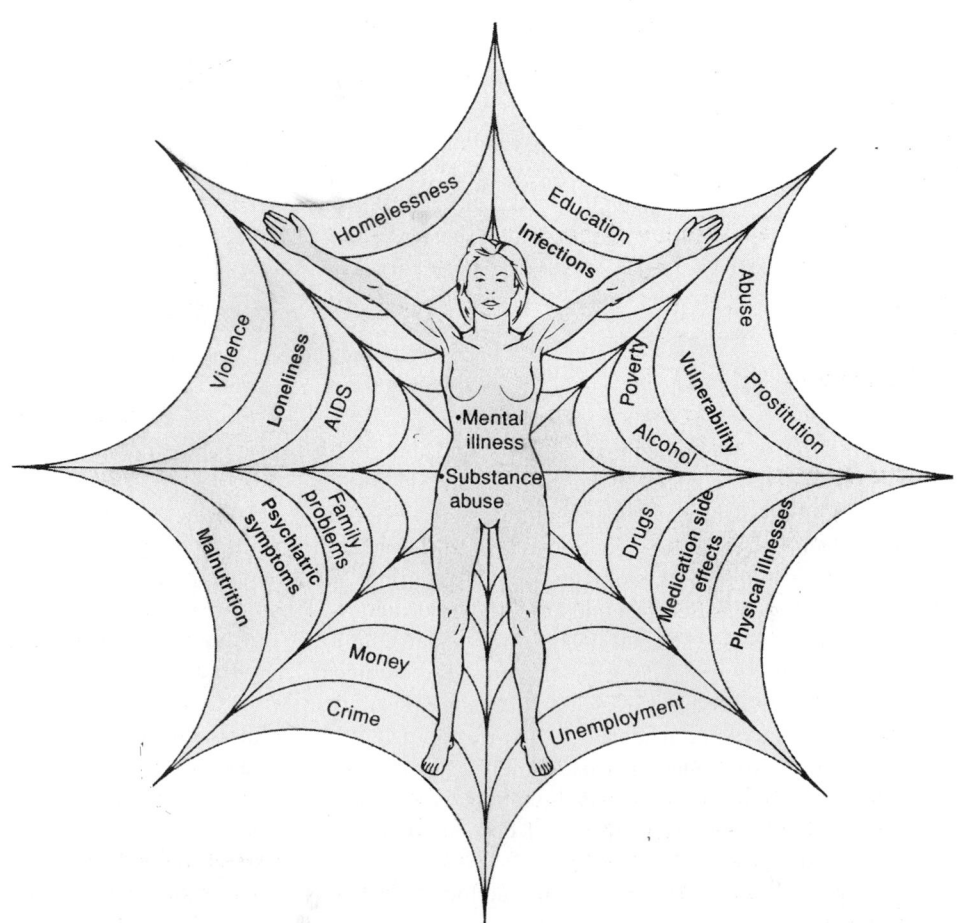

FIGURE 94-1. Clients with a dual diagnosis of mental illness and chemical dependency are often confronted with a myriad of social, financial, physical, and relationship problems. (Source: Substance Abuse and Mental Health Services Administration [Ed]. *Treatment for alcohol and other drug abuse: Opportunities for coordination.* DHHS Publications No. [SMA] 94-2075. Rockville, MD.)

1. "I use it to feel better." In early stages of CD, the chemical temporarily alleviates the person's feelings of low self-worth and stress. Therefore, the person uses it to escape and to feel better.
2. "I use it to keep from feeling bad." As CD progresses, the person must use increased amounts of the substance to stop feeling sick or depressed. The person begins to need the substance to keep from feeling bad, but he or she never really feels good.
3. "I'm losing control." The person now finds that even a small amount of the chemical causes illness or severe intoxication. **Blackouts** (periods of total amnesia) often occur with excessive use. At this point, immediate intervention is vital, often to save the person's life.

Defense Mechanisms

Of the many defense mechanisms people use (see Chap. 93), denial, rationalization, and projection are most important in substance abuse.

Denial: The user usually denies any difficulty in controlling intake or denies that drug use is causing problems, long after those around him or her realize that the person is out of control.
Rationalization: Many users argue that they could not possibly have a problem and they offer rationalizations. Examples of these rationalizations include "I do not use during the day," "I get to work each day," "I only use on weekends," "I don't hide bottles or drink at home," "I never drink before 5 o'clock," "I only drink beer," or "I can quit whenever I want."
Projection: When the person admits to having a problem, he or she often blames others. A typical complaint is related to family problems: "If you were a better parent or spouse, I would not have to drink," or "If my kids were better behaved, I would not need drugs."

Management

The following concepts are basic to the management of all dependencies:

1. *Recognition:* Someone must recognize the condition. The first person to do so is very often someone other than the chemically dependent person.
2. *Intervention:* Active intervention must occur. If no one intervenes in the process of CD, it usually continues.
3. *Treatment:* CD often responds to structured therapy. The person may need a particular milieu to gain control over the habit. In rare cases, the person sees the impact of the destructive behavior and stops using. Usually, however, the client needs assistance to stop using. In addition to abstinence, treatment should address such issues as malnutrition, heart dysfunction, liver disease, brain damage, general health, social changes, and interpersonal relationships.
4. *Recovery:* Many therapies assist chemically dependent people to lead a successful and productive life.

Many such programs use the 12-step approach of AA. They also apply principles of behavior modification. Some programs are briefly described later in this chapter.

NURSING CARE MEASURES

Caring for clients who are dealing with addictions occurs in various settings, including outpatient treatment, extended-care facilities, specific treatment centers and clinics, and hospitals. It is important to note that up to 45% of clients who are receiving care for general medical-surgical conditions have underlying substance abuse problems; the great majority of these clients are alcoholics. More than 33% of emergency department admissions and 20% of acute hospital admissions of older adults can be traced to complications related to substance abuse. Because many insurance plans no longer cover inpatient treatment for addictions, many people with CD are admitted under another diagnosis. Many diagnoses are either associated with or directly result from alcoholism or other substance abuse. Common related diagnoses include motor vehicle accidents (MVA), depression, pancreatitis, cirrhosis and other liver problems, gastrointestinal (GI) disorders, headaches, and cardiovascular disorders such as suspected heart attack and hypertension. See In Practice: The Nursing Process 94-1 for more information in dealing with clients who are substance abusers or chemically dependent.

Identification of the Chemically Dependent Person

Substance abusers use defense mechanisms regularly. They often convince healthcare professionals that their medical disorder is not related to any form of substance abuse; therefore, the chemical problem goes undetected. Beware of stereotypes; it is not possible to identify a substance abuser by appearance (Fig. 94-2).

Nursing Alert

Be alert for signs and symptoms of CD or withdrawal in all clients. Clients in the healthcare facility who are deprived of their drug of choice may suddenly begin having serious or life-threatening withdrawal symptoms. *Remember:* Clients in the emergency department, day surgery, labor and delivery, or any other area may experience withdrawal symptoms. Also, be alert to cross-dependence: abusers of one drug often have built up tolerance to related drugs as well.

Nursing Assessment

Although the practical/vocational nurse or nursing student does not obtain a formal admission history or make a nursing diagnosis in the hospital, all nurses should know the items to include. Often, a practical/vocational nurse assists with the admission and talks with the client and family. Report pertinent observations to the person doing the written admission and writing the nursing care plan.

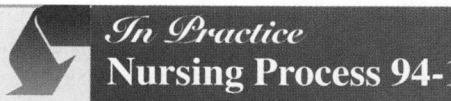

In Practice
Nursing Process 94-1

SUBSTANCE ABUSE

Assessment Priorities
Behavior Changes
- Erratic or inappropriate behavior
- Sudden changes in mood
- Poor school or job attendance or performance
- Antisocial acts, such as stealing, embezzling, prostitution, or selling drugs
- Declining social status or an incongruent economic situation
- Avoidance of previously enjoyed activities
- Frequent visits to an emergency department for depression or suicide threats; anhedonia

Physical Signs
- Withdrawal symptoms (Table 94-1)
- Needle tracks, often covered by long sleeves
- Chronic nasal congestion and cold symptoms with drug snorting; after heavy use, the septum may perforate
- Dilated pupils, often masked by sunglasses
- Unkempt appearance, not usual for client
- Unexplained weight loss
- Abnormal electrolyte levels, anemia

Complications With Overdose
- Cerebrovascular spasm as shown by hemorrhage, seizures, hypertensive or hypotensive crisis; angina; myocardial infarction; dysrhythmias; abnormal respirations (Cheyne-Stokes); hyperthermia; tachycardia or bradycardia
- (Note: If you suspect substance abuse in a person who presents in the emergency department, ask the physician to order a toxicology screen.)

Possible Nursing Diagnoses
Impaired Adjustment
Anxiety
Ineffective Individual Coping
Fear
Altered Growth and Development (fetal)
Altered Health Maintenance
High Risk for Infection
High Risk for Injury
Knowledge Deficit (specify)
Noncompliance (specify)
Altered Nutrition: Less than Body Requirements
Altered Parenting
Personal Identity Disturbance
Powerlessness
Altered Role Performance
Self-Care Deficit
Self-Esteem Disturbance
Sensory/Perceptual Alterations
Impaired Social Interaction

Altered Thought Processes
High Risk for Violence: Self-Directed or Directed at Others

Planning
Design a plan of care with the client to achieve the following general goals:

- The person safely detoxifies
- The person admits that substance abuse has hurt him or her.
- The person admits that he or she needs help to stop using the drug.
- The person agrees to participate in a substance abuse program.
- The person's behavior and physical signs demonstrate decreased or discontinued substance abuse.
- The person tests drug free (urine tests, toxicology screening).
- The person agrees to continue with after-care.

Implementation
- Refer the client to a psychiatric liaison nurse or a drug abuse counselor.
- If a known substance abuser denies abuse, do not withdraw from the case or become angry; continue to break down the denial by pointing out how the addiction has contributed to the person's medical, social, or legal problems.
- If all else fails, provide the person with information about getting help; write down a hotline number or other community resource.
- Support the family of the substance abuser if they are present, and respond honestly to their questions; the family may be enlisted to encourage the client to seek help (*intervention*).
- For emergency department nursing care of the drug-dependent person, see In Practice: Nursing Care Guidelines 94-1.
- In some cases, forced treatment may be required.

Evaluation
Determine the adequacy of the plan of care by evaluating the client's achievement of the above goals. If the person is unable to meet key goals, modify the plan. Key evaluative criteria include the following:

- The client is drug free.
- The client returns to pre–substance-abuse role performance.
- The client seeks and continues treatment and participates in continued followup (such as attendance at AA).

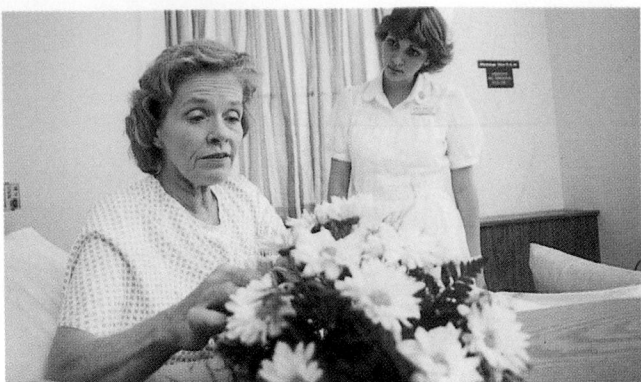

FIGURE 94-2. The nurse must be alert to signs of alcohol or drug withdrawal in all areas of the healthcare facility. Many chemically dependent people do not fit the usual stereotype and are admitted for non–chemical-related problems.

An initial assessment of the client's use of mood-altering chemicals can be incorporated naturally into every nursing history. Ask the person, "How much alcohol do you use? What other drugs do you use? How often? How much?" If the person responds negatively to these questions, ask him or her, "When was the last time you used alcohol or drugs?" When you ask nonjudgmental questions, clients are less likely to deny use. If a client acknowledges any use, ever, obtain additional information. Ask open-ended questions such as, "Tell me about your drinking or drug use." (It is usually not as effective to ask a question such as, "Do you drink alcohol?" It is too easy for the client to just say, "No".)

If this approach does not yield enough information, probe further by asking specific questions:

What do you take to relieve stress? Pain?
Do you drink or use chemicals alone or with others? Are you usually at home or in a bar?
What type of beverages do you drink?
Do you combine alcohol and other drugs?
Do you drink at work?
Do you drink and drive?
Have you ever had a **DUI/DWI** (driving while under the influence, driving while intoxicated)?
Have you had any legal problems because of drug use? Have you been in jail/prison?
How often do you miss work?
On what day of the week do you usually call in sick? (Routinely calling in sick on Mondays [or Fridays] is a danger signal for chemical dependency.)
Are you unemployed?
How much of each chemical (alcohol, marijuana, cocaine, or other chemicals) do you use in a day? How much do you use in a week?
How much does it cost? Where do you get the money?
In what form do you use the drug (such as cocaine, crack, crank)?
Do you inhale, smoke, or inject the drug?
When was your last drink? Drug use?
Have you ever had problems with withdrawal? Seizures?

The last two questions are very important in terms of predicting withdrawal. (For example, the person who has been drinking in the past few days must be closely observed for life-threatening withdrawal symptoms for at least 72 hours.)

☛ KEY CONCEPT

The questions listed above are very significant for clients who are being prepared for surgery or to deliver babies. They can suddenly go into unexpected withdrawal.

Remember that how often and how much a person drinks or uses drugs are not always the best criteria for determining whether someone is alcoholic or chemically dependent. Rather, explore the role that drugs play in the individual's life. *Loss of control and an inability to stop drinking or using are the cardinal signs of CD. If a person's use affects his or her job, interpersonal relationships, or family, he or she has an abuse problem.*

Dealing With an Intoxicated Person in the Healthcare Facility

The admission of an intoxicated person, either in the CD unit, emergency department, mental health unit, general hospital, nursing home, or outpatient clinic is a challenge for any nurse. In Practice: Nursing Care Guidelines 94-1 identifies nursing skills used in an emergency department. Many of these skills apply to other settings as well. Remember the following general points:

- The healthcare staff has no way of knowing definitely what drugs a client has used without specific laboratory tests. Anticipate all possible behaviors.
- A thorough history is required for safety during detoxification and in the event of complications related to chemical abuse, detoxification, or withdrawal. (Not all clients will be willing or able to give an accurate drug/alcohol use history.)
- It is particularly important to determine when the last alcohol or drug use was and if the person has ever had serious withdrawal symptoms.
- Carefully document all information.

The physician or other healthcare provider often orders blood alcohol testing and urine toxicology (U-Tox). This client is usually screened for many drugs, both illegal and legal, over-the-counter (OTC) and prescribed.

The physician writes orders for the client based on the physical examination, the client's history, the history given by the family, the admission nursing history and diagnosis, and laboratory tests.

☛ KEY CONCEPT

Visitors may enter a healthcare facility in an intoxicated state. Allowing them to enter a client's room is unwise. Call the nursing supervisor, charge nurse, or security personnel if such a situation arises. The intoxicated person may be excitable and dangerous. Do not attempt to force an intoxicated person to leave without assistance.

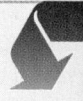

In Practice
Nursing Care Guidelines 94-1

CARING FOR THE ALCOHOL OR DRUG-USING PERSON IN THE EMERGENCY DEPARTMENT

If a client comes into the department and seems intoxicated or seems to have used street drugs:

- Monitor the client's respiratory status; artificial respiratory support or ventilation may be necessary. *Rationale: Respirations may be dangerously depressed in overdose.*
- Maintain an open airway. *Rationale: The person may have depressed reflexes, or secretions that block his or her airway.*
- Monitor the client's cardiac status. *Rationale: Arrhythmias are common.*
- Monitor level of consciousness. Check neurologic eye signs and other responses. *Rationale: Lowering of level of consciousness (LOC) is a dangerous sign.*
- Watch for tremors, involuntary movements, or seizures. *Rationale: Withdrawal symptoms may occur without warning and may be life threatening.*
- Monitor vital signs. *Rationale: Elevated vital signs are often the first indicator of withdrawal, especially from alcohol.*
- Remain with the person at all times during emergency treatment. *Rationale: The person may be very frightened, disoriented, or combative.*
- Provide a quiet, calm environment. Speak softly and calmly. Remove as much stimulation as possible. *Rationale: This client may be hyperirritable and overly sensitive to environmental stimuli.*

If you are afraid, the client will probably sense your fear.
- Tell the client frequently where he or she is. *Rationale: These clients are often disoriented.*
- Assure the person of your concern. *Rationale: Offer support and calm the client.*
- Try not to use waist or limb restraints, unless absolutely necessary. *Rationale: The person may become more frightened and may be injured while fighting the restraints.*
- Remove harmful objects from the immediate environment. *Rationale: In a confused or agitated state, the client might not recognize familiar objects. Maintain safety for the client and others.*
- Do not touch the client unless he or she understands what you are going to do. *Rationale: This person may misperceive and react violently to physical contact.*
- If a client begins to lose control, get assistance. Bring the situation under immediate control. *Rationale: A person on certain types of drugs can become violent very quickly. Prevent the client from hurting self or others.*
- Report any unusual signs or symptoms immediately. *Rationale: Many people abuse several drugs. Therefore, almost any unusual reaction can be a sign of withdrawal.*
- Remember that an injury or accident can precipitate withdrawal symptoms.

DETOXIFICATION AND RECOVERY

Detoxification is the process of removing a drug and its physiologic effects from the person's body. Total detoxification may take many days, depending on the drug(s) used, amounts, level of dependence, liver and kidney function, and the client's size and general health.

The most important goals in detoxification management are comfort and safety during withdrawal. Use sedation and emotional support to allow the client to rest and recover and to prevent injury or exhaustion. Treatment depends in part on the specifically abused substance(s). Remember that detoxification must occur before long-term CD treatment can be effective.

Motivation for CD Treatment

Several reasons exist for the substance abuser to seek treatment. The person may really want to stop and may realize that employment, loved ones, health, and freedom of action are in jeopardy if the habit continues.

The user may want to phase out reliance on the drug. Although some clients express the desire to "cut down," avoid-

ing relapse is almost impossible while the person continues to use any amount of the drug. Abstinence is the only sure method for detoxification and recovery.

A person might enter treatment in response to a court order. In many states, people who are arrested or involved in an MVA while intoxicated are ordered into treatment for several weeks. (Usually, jail is the only other option.) When the person enters treatment, he or she is often very angry and the motivation and desire to succeed may be weak. An underlying rationale for the court order is the hope that exposure to a good treatment program will encourage the person to participate in recovery. Peer pressure is very strong; in many cases, this person begins to take the program seriously.

Nursing Alert

When a person reduces intake of drugs, such as barbiturates or cocaine, the future danger of overdose exists. After the person stops the drug, tolerance is reduced. If the user then takes the dose customarily used before detoxification, this constitutes an *overdose* and can cause death.

The Detoxification Center

A substance abuser may begin recovery in a *detoxification center*. Often, the person is transported to the "detox center" by the police. Here, the person detoxifies under medical supervision. The emphasis is on supportive care and referral to continuing therapy after detoxification, so the person can deal with the underlying motivations that led to the chemical abuse.

The Therapeutic Community

In a *therapeutic community,* clients are isolated from the substance-oriented environment. Their lifestyle changes in basic ways as they learn drug-free coping skills. Recovering drug abusers and alcoholics organize and administer many such programs. Clients are assigned to work or study groups and are given assigned readings that help them to learn more about the disease and assume responsibility. Group therapy is a common component of treatment programs. Sometimes the groups are gender-specific and focus on particular concerns of either men or women. The goals of treatment are to assist clients to address physical and emotional problems associated with abuse and to understand the cycle of dependence. When clients have accomplished these goals, they are ready to begin true recovery.

> ### Nursing Alert
>
> Clients in the early stages of withdrawal often show common signs and symptoms, including anxiety, uncontrollable fear, tremors (internal and external), irritability, agitation, hyperactive reflexes, GI disturbances (especially nausea and vomiting), diaphoresis, and insomnia. In alcohol withdrawal, all vital signs are usually elevated; in withdrawal from some other drugs, vital signs fluctuate.
>
> Detoxification requires careful and correct management, especially for those who abuse alcohol. *Rationale: If managed improperly, the client may progress to a dangerous withdrawal that includes terrifying hallucinations. Seizures may occur. Coma and death may follow.*

Immediate Treatment in Detoxification

A complete medical workup is important when a client is admitted for detoxification. Blood work determines liver, kidney, and thyroid function. Blood chemistry levels indicate vitamin deficiencies, lipid (fat) levels, uric acid levels, and enzyme levels that might indicate physical damage. Urine toxicology reveals which drugs the client has used. In some cases, blood tests are also done to determine more exact drug levels.

Before administering medications (eg, benzodiazepines), the provider evaluates the client for the severity of withdrawal symptoms. (Many chemically dependent people are medication-seeking and ask for medications, even if they are not having true symptoms.)

Assessment and the decision to administer or withhold medications is based on the presence or absence of factors such as nausea and vomiting, internal or external tremors, *diaphoresis* (excessive sweating), anxiety, agitation, hallucinations, headache, or confusion. Usually, several factors must be present, or one must be severe, for medications to be initiated. Several formal rating scales are available to assist the nurse to determine the true severity of withdrawal symptoms. (Clients with liver failure, esophageal varices (enlarged blood vessels in esophagus; varicosities), brain damage, congestive heart failure, or dyspnea, or who are elderly, may need different considerations in their evaluations.)

Reassess the client every hour or more often during the intensive detoxification period. See In Practice: Important Medications 94-1 for a list of medications often used in detoxification.

Withdrawal Symptoms

To begin detoxification, the client's body is denied access to the drug. When the drug of choice is removed, many chemically dependent people experience withdrawal (W/D) symptoms of varying severity. Some clients withdraw with minimal discomfort; others experience very difficult and dangerous withdrawals. Intensity depends on several factors, including the drug used, amount, previous withdrawals, and general health and nutritional status. Liver function and the client's history of previous withdrawal episodes are especially important. Predicting the progression of any withdrawal episode, however, is impossible.

Those experiencing withdrawal are in psychological and medical jeopardy. They immediately present many potential nursing problems. Detoxification from alcohol and certain other drugs is a serious medical problem; the process can be fatal. (Alcohol withdrawal is one of the most dangerous.) Table 94-1 lists common withdrawal signs and symptoms and related nursing considerations for selected drugs. In Practice: Nursing Care Guidelines 94-2 describes general nursing measures used to assist clients during the withdrawal period.

Nutrition and General Health.   In addition to treatment for CD, healthcare must address issues of nutrition and general health. Many clients are seriously malnourished as a direct result of drug abuse and also because of client indifference to health. Assess the client's general physical condition. Usually liver function tests (to rule out cirrhosis and other disorders) and evaluation of GI function (to rule out conditions such as ulcers, diverticulitis, esophageal varices, or colon cancer) are necessary. Evaluate general nutritional status. If the client is severely malnourished, carefully supervise his or her weight gain. Give supplemental vitamins as ordered.

Treat any coexisting conditions, such as injuries, skin rashes, and diabetes mellitus, as ordered. Many times, physical disorders, such as liver or GI damage, require medical attention. Some clients require long-term treatment for generalized infections, including tuberculosis and acquired immunodeficiency syndrome (AIDS), which often relate directly to the drug-abusing lifestyle.

Refeeding Syndrome.   If a drug abuser is severely malnourished or starving, careful dietary management is vital. Rehydrate such clients slowly, with small and carefully planned

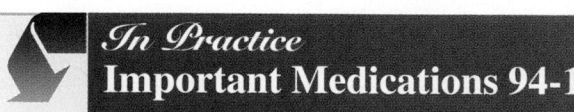

In Practice
Important Medications 94-1

MEDICATIONS USED IN CHEMICAL DEPENDENCY TREATMENT

The client must be assessed for severity of withdrawal symptoms before benzodiazepines are given because of their *abuse potential*. Most chemically dependent people will have a cross-tolerance to many of the drugs used in detoxification. (*See explanation in text.*)

To Control or Prevent Seizures; to Provide Sedation (Benzodiazepines)
Long-Acting

chlordiazepoxide (Librium) 50–100 mg, repeat q1–4h Max. 600 mg/d; taper down over 3–5 d	Work for cumulative effects Oral, IV preferred Given until client mildly sedated, then divided into 4 daily doses
diazepam (Valium) 10–40 mg, repeat q1–4h; taper down over 3–5 d	If symptoms return, give previous day's dose Give IV if withdrawal severe

Short-Acting

lorazepam (Ativan) 2–4 mg, repeat q1–2h during acute symptoms; taper down over 5–7 d	Short-acting preferred in elderly or if liver is damaged IM preferred route; may be given IV Avoid sudden dis- continuation.
oxazepam (Serax) 30–60 mg, repeat q1–2h; taper down over 7 d	

Nursing Considerations
• The goal is safe, comfortable withdrawal.
• Monitor vital signs—*do not overmedicate*—these medications depress the CNS. Death may occur due to respiratory depression or cardiovascular collapse.
• Give Ativan or Valium until the client is mildly sedated. When the client is stable, divide the dose into 4 doses per day.
• When medications are discontinued, they must be tapered down. The general rule is to taper 25% per day.
• Give supplements to reduce nutritional deficiencies and electrolyte imbalances and to arrest brain damage (vitamin C, thiamine, folate, multivitamins, added iron).
• For long-term seizure prevention, phenytoin (Dilantin) or divalproex sodium (Depakote) may be used.
• In emergency, magnesium sulfate (**MgSO₄**) can be given IV to prevent or treat seizures.
• Medications used to prevent seizures also help promote sleep.
• Benzodiazepines have abuse/dependency potential. Taper down as soon as possible, usually within 2 to 4 days.

Adjunct Medications
β-Blockers—to help reduce autonomic nervous system hyperactivity (eg, tachycardia, diaphoresis, hypertension)
  atenolol (Tenormin)
  propranolol HCl (Inderal)

Nursing Considerations
Benzodiazepines are often contraindicated in congestive heart failure, asthma, diabetes mellitus.

Other Drugs

clonidine HCl (Catapres)	May relieve withdrawal symptoms with or without benzodiazepines
nifedipine (Procardia)	Enhances heart action
haloperidol (Haldol, folacin)	May be used in small dose (0.5–2 mg) to control agitated behavior

Vitamins

multivitamins	To treat malnutrition
supplemental iron	To treat anemia
vitamin B₉ (folate, folacin)	To prevent neurologic disorders; not well absorbed in alcoholism
vitamin B₁ (thiamine)	Most clients with chronic alcohol abuse have thiamine deficiency.
vitamin C (ascorbic acid)	To treat nutritional deficiency

Nursing Considerations
• Many chemically dependent people are malnourished. The vitamins listed above are given to the alcohol-dependent person and often to other chemical abusers as well.
• In the chronic alcohol abuser, undiluted IV glucose can worsen thiamine depletion. The IV fluid of choice is usually D₅½ NS. Thiamine is often added, and MgSO₄ may be added to prevent seizures.

Specific Drugs Used to Counteract Overdose

Drug Overdosed	*Antidote*
drugs causing CNS depression	doxapram HCl (Dopram)
benzodiazepines (such as Valium or Ativan)	flumazenil (Romazicon) (contraindicated in mixed drug overdose or chronic benzodiazepine use)
narcotics (such as codeine, morphine, Talwin, Darvon)	naloxone HCl (Narcan) nalmefene (Revex)

▪▪▪ TABLE 94-1 *W*ITHDRAWAL POINTERS FOR SELECTED DRUGS

Signs and Symptoms During Unmanaged Withdrawal	Nursing Considerations
Alcohol	
Alcohol is often used in combination with mood-altering drugs—withdrawal may be a mixed picture of various and unexpected symptoms Acute detoxification begins within 72 hours of last ingestion Risk of suicide increases during detox period Tremors (internal first, then hands, then entire body) Agitation, irritability, depressed mood Anxiety Diaphoresis Delusions, hallucinations (auditory and visual—delirium tremens) Dementia may be exacerbated Hypertension, tachycardia, hyperthermia Nausea, vomiting, anorexia Sleep disorders, especially insomnia Tonic–clonic seizures Vitamin deficiency (especially thiamine and folate) Hypoglycemia, electrolyte imbalance Dilated pupils Confusion, disorientation, coma, delirium, amnesia Blackouts, memory loss Cardiac arrest	Carefully observe vital signs and level of consciousness. Follow detoxification protocol of agency. Client evaluated for other health problems, such as malnutrition, liver damage, cardiac malfunction, infections, tuberculosis, vitamin deficiencies. Follow seizure precautions. Monitor blood sugar levels. Encourage food and fluids; monitor intake and output. Follow suicide precautions. Manage nausea and vomiting. Reorient client, as needed. Give PRN medications to manage symptoms and control blood pressure. (Alcohol causes fetal alcohol syndrome when used by pregnant woman.)
Sedatives, Hypnotics, Anxiolytics	
May range from delirium to loss of consciousness Tonic–clonic seizures Sleep disorders, particularly insomnia Confusion, delirium, amnesia Psychotic disorders, mood disorders Tremor Severe anxiety EEG changes Slowed or absent reflexes Respiratory changes, apnea Abnormal lung sounds Dementia may persist after withdrawal	Follow specific protocol of facility. Follow seizure precautions. Reorient client as needed. Assess vital signs and level of consciousness often. Keep client from hurting self or others. Maintain patent airway. Monitor respiratory status.
Heroin (and other Narcotics)	
Nausea, vomiting Diarrhea Tearing, runny nose, sore throat Dilated pupils Tremors, weakness Diaphoresis, chills Gooseflesh (hair on extremities stands on end) Depression to loss of consciousness or irritability and hyperactivity Confusion, disorientation Delusions, hallucinations Muscle and joint pain Constant yawning Insomnia, sleep disturbances Mild hypertension Lowered temperature (in some cases, temperature rises) Fast, weak, irregular pulse Slowed respirations	Follow protocol of facility. Frequently assess vital signs and level of consciousness. Withdrawal is more dangerous if client has concurrent medical disorder, such as heart disease, lung disease, or diabetes. Client often is malnourished. Assess for infections, abscesses, and other complications of injections. Perform blood test for HIV, hepatitis. Sexual dysfunction is common. Follow seizure precautions.
Amphetamines	
Irritability, agitation Depressed mood Insomnia Anxiety Other general withdrawal symptoms	Follow agency protocol. Provide safety for client and others. Maintain calm, quiet atmosphere.

■■■ TABLE 94-1 *W*ITHDRAWAL POINTERS FOR SELECTED DRUGS (CONTINUED)

Signs and Symptoms During Withdrawal	Nursing Considerations
Cocaine	
Acute detoxification is 4–5 wk	Follow protocol of specific facility.
Depression, irritability	Treat specific symptoms.
Extreme mood swings (lability)	Maintain quiet environment with minimum stimulation.
Lack of enjoyment (anhedonia)	Seizure precautions often used.
Pressured speech, grandiosity, hyperactivity, intrusiveness	Assess level of consciousness and vital signs frequently.
Anxiety, paranoia, crying jags	Control hypertension.
Confusion, poor memory	Assess mental status and orientation.
Tactile hallucinations ("cocaine bugs")	Keep from hurting self or others.
Sleep disturbances, nightmares	Encourage adequate nutrition and fluid intake.
Gastrointestinal symptoms, nausea, vomiting, difficulties with digestion	Assess sleeping habits.
Low urine output (oliguria)	Reorient as needed.
Headache, bone pain, muscle cramps	Monitor intake and output; report oliguria (a serious sign).
Runny nose, nasal congestion, eyes tearing	Manage nausea and vomiting.
Dilated pupils	Monitor respiratory status (respiratory depression can be dangerous). Respiratory stimulants may be needed.
Respiratory depression	(Cocaine is particularly dangerous to mother and fetus when used by a pregnant woman.)
Sudden increase in temperature	
Extreme hypertension	
Tachycardia	
Approximately fourth week—intense craving (high risk for relapse)	
Possible organic brain syndrome (brain damage)	
Caffeine	
Anxiety	Caffeine is contained in coffee, tea, cola drinks, other sodas such as Mountain Dew and Jolt, chocolate, some over-the-counter medications.
Sleep disorders	Caffeine-free beverages are available.
GI disturbance	
Cardiac arrhythmia	
Headache	
Irritability	
Nicotine	
Dysphoria, depression	Many programs are available to assist in smoking cessation.
Insomnia	Nicotine transdermal patches, nicotine gum, special inhalers, and so forth are used.
Irritability, frustration	High incidence of relapse.
Anxiety, restlessness	"Cutting down" usually not effective
Poor concentration	
Bradycardia	
Hunger, weight gain	

In Practice Nursing Care Guidelines 94-2

NURSING CARE IN WITHDRAWAL

The following nursing measures are followed in the care of the client withdrawing from alcohol. Most of these procedures apply to withdrawal from other drugs as well:

- An individual nursing care plan should be developed. Close observation is needed to make a comprehensive plan. *Rationale: If withdrawal symptoms are going to occur, they usually begin within 72 hours.*
- Follow a detoxification protocol/checklist that includes careful observation and assessment according to the specific facility's protocol.

Rationale: Each client withdraws differently. Follow a general protocol to avoid missing any symptoms.
- Make observations, including checking vital signs, *every 15 minutes* for the first few hours or until the client's condition is stable, then every 30 minutes for 12 hours, and then every 1 to 4 hours for 12 more hours. Observations are made at least every 4 hours until 72 hours (3 days) after the person's last drink or use. *Rationale: The client's condition can deteriorate rapidly.*

(continued)

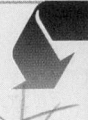

In Practice
Nursing Care Guidelines 94-2 (Continued)

- Closely monitor vital signs and take swift action if they rise. Measure the pulse apically.
- Elevation of all vital signs usually occurs in alcohol withdrawal; in abuse of other drugs, levels may fluctuate. Monitor neurologic eye signs, especially if the client is confused or unconscious. (Dilated pupils are common in withdrawal from many drugs.) Hypertension often occurs. Make attempts to control blood pressure as much as possible, but not to lower blood pressure too quickly. *Rationale: PRN drug dosage is based, in part, on vital signs. The client's condition can change rapidly. Hypertension is caused by hyperactivity of the autonomic nervous system. Peripheral circulatory collapse may occur if blood pressure drops too rapidly.*
- Provide a quiet atmosphere. Remove or turn off the television or radio during intense periods. Provide subdued lighting. *Rationale: Reduce stress and stimuli.*
- Stay with the client as much as possible. In some cases, family or a friend may be available to assist. Carefully observe the client. *Rationale: The client's condition can change rapidly. In addition, this client is at risk for suicide.*
- Nursing assessment is important. *Rationale: Medications, such as diazepam (Valium), are given PRN, based on nursing judgment. Refer to In Practice: Important Medications 94-1 for guidelines.*
- Record intake and output, calorie count, and daily weight. Encourage a variety of fluids. Assess skin turgor and look for other signs of dehydration. *Rationale: Restoring fluid and electrolyte balance improves nutritional status. Drinking only plain water contributes to electrolyte imbalance.*
- Give frequent, small feedings. Manage malnourished clients carefully. *Rationale: Small meals place less stress on the body; the client usually has a decreased appetite and may be nauseated. A life-threatening condition called refeeding syndrome is discussed in this chapter.*
- Monitor the client's blood sugar levels. The person may receive carefully planned supplements. *Rationale: Hypoglycemia may occur during withdrawal because alcohol depletes the glycogen stored in the liver. Alcoholism also impairs glycogenesis because it damages the liver, as in cirrhosis. However, excess sugar can cause refeeding syndrome and worsen thiamine depletion, so sugar intake is carefully balanced.*

- Give intravenous (IV) fluids as ordered. Carefully monitor electrolytes, which may be given IV. The IV fluid of choice in alcoholism withdrawal is usually $D_5\frac{1}{2}$ NS, rather than D_5W. *Rationale: Dehydration and electrolyte imbalances often result from intestinal malabsorption, starvation, diaphoresis, vomiting, and client hyperactivity.*
- Carefully monitor body temperature. *Rationale: Life-threatening hyperthermia is possible.*
- Administer supplemental vitamins as ordered. Routinely used supplements, particularly in chronic alcohol abuse, include thiamine (B_1), folic acid (B_9, folate), and a multivitamin with iron. Vitamin C may be given. A high-protein diet is often ordered. *Rationale: Many chemically dependent people are malnourished. Specific vitamin deficiencies are caused by the inability of the proximal small intestine to absorb certain vitamins, such as thiamine and folate. A chronic deficiency of thiamine can lead to Wernicke-Korsakoff syndrome.*
- Monitor the client's respiratory, hepatic, and cardiovascular systems carefully. Report any distress immediately. Monitor the results of blood tests. An electrocardiogram is often done. *Rationale: Complications of detoxification include respiratory distress, pneumonia, liver damage and disease, and cardiac failure. This client is also at risk for infections.*
- The client usually is not restrained. Side rails should be up when the person is in bed. *Rationale: Restraints could agitate the person further. The absence of restraints is another reason for close observation. This person is at risk for falls.*
- Turn and reposition the client every 2 hours. *Rationale: Prevent disorders related to inactivity. The person may be confused or unconscious.*
- If the person is nauseated or vomiting, position him or her on the side. *Rationale: Prevent aspiration.*
- Follow seizure precautions. Anticonvulsant drugs are prescribed. *Rationale: Seizures are a common complication if detoxification is not managed successfully.*
- Treat other common symptoms (eg, diaphoresis and dry mouth) symptomatically. *Rationale: They are not life threatening.*
- If the client becomes agitated or threatening, request assistance. *(It may be dangerous to attempt to restrain this person. The person may injure him or herself or the staff. Experts may need to advise the staff as to the best treatment for an individual client, depending on the drug(s) used.)*

fluids and feedings. Do not give excess sugar or other carbohydrates. **Refeeding syndrome** is life threatening and can occur when a starving person receives carbohydrates too quickly. Carbohydrates include dextrose IV solutions, tube-feeding mixtures, and liquid dietary supplements. The sudden influx of carbohydrates stimulates insulin production and other events that seriously upset electrolyte balance. Refeeding syndrome can also cause cardiac failure, hypertension, peripheral edema, neurologic complications (including seizures or coma), respiratory failure, and death.

☛ KEY CONCEPT

Nursing care in detoxification is the same in general aspects, no matter what drug the client has abused.

Long-Term Followup and Treatment

The period after detoxification is very important. Usually the client remembers vividly the extreme discomfort experienced and may now be willing to enter CD treatment. The role of the nurse includes discussing the possibility of a CD evaluation with a physician. A person may be diagnosed as a *substance abuser, alcoholic dependent, chemically dependent,* **polysubstance dependent** (dependent on several drugs), or some combination of these diagnoses. Many chemically dependent people are also codependents, living with another person who is an abuser of alcohol or other drugs.

Inpatient or Outpatient Treatment

Treatment for chemical dependency can be on an inpatient basis in a treatment center or on an outpatient basis. The client's attitude, family support, insurance coverage, and the client's work and personal situation often determine what type of treatment is possible. Treatment centers usually base their treatment on one or more of the following programs:

The 12-step program, based on AA
Albert Ellis's rational emotive behavior therapy
Milton Cudney's self-defeating behavior theory
Personal and group counseling
Client and family education about the disease
Family counseling
Improving nutritional and general health

Programs often include general group therapy, gender-related issues, goal setting, grief management, anger management, esteem building, and referrals to sexual assault or violence anonymous groups. Groups may teach relaxation skills, financial management, stress management, and safer sex practices. Many treatment facilities have developed special groups. For example, a writing group teaches the therapeutic benefits of creative expression and keeping a journal. Special programs are available for young children, adolescents, seniors, and chemically dependent mentally ill people. Family groups are common. Programs are offered at various times of day.

An adjunct may be administration of agonist or adverse conditioning medications, discussed later in this chapter.

12-Step Programs. The 12-step groups, such as AA and Narcotics Anonymous (**NA**), teach that untreated CD is a progressive, incurable disease. The disease is considered to be *arrested* or *in remission* when the person is not using. *The person is never cured of the disease.* The 12-step programs do not actually sponsor or endorse any particular treatment program; rather, they are based on helping the individual admit his or her powerlessness over the chemical and that his or her life has become unmanageable because of it. The person then accepts the existence of a "higher power," determines whom he or she has harmed and makes amends, turns his or her life over to the individual higher power, and assists others to do the same. The premise of 12-step programs is, "I have a disease. It's not my fault. I need assistance to stop using."

Rational Recovery. Rational emotive therapy (**RET**) (rational emotive behavior therapy [REBT], rational recovery) was introduced in Chapter 93. **REBT** is built on the premise that an individual's values and beliefs control behavior. Therefore, a person's illogical beliefs in turn influence irrational behaviors. For example, the substance abuser might say, "I am weak; I am worthless; I do not deserve to be happy."[2] Therefore, he or she continues the addiction even though he or she knows it is harmful, because of his or her derogatory self-perceptions. Rational recovery asks the question, "Why do I keep doing the same thing over and over when I know what the result is going to be, and I know I won't like it?"[2]

Rational recovery is based on Milton Cudney's theory of self-defeating behavior and Albert Ellis's REBT. Its treatment premise is helping the person to recognize that "Only I have control over my own behavior . . . I abuse chemicals because I choose to do so, and I quit because I no longer choose to abuse chemicals."[2] Rational recovery assists clients to believe that they are valuable and rational human beings and to understand that abuse of chemicals is irrational. Clients then learn to reject irrational behaviors and replace them with healthy actions for productive and comfortable lives.

Family Counseling. Treating the substance abuser alone is not enough; the family also needs intensive counseling. Treatment centers include treatment programs for families, conducted simultaneously with the client's treatment. The person and family must realize that they all need followup care, which is vital in order for the client to maintain sobriety. The client and family need encouragement and support to deal with normal familial stressors, plus the added challenges of recovering from CD.

☛ KEY CONCEPT

A person's recovery is less likely to be successful if the family is not also in the recovery mode. The family and client may also require social service referrals to assist in obtaining support groups, education/retraining, employment, financial assistance, or housing.

After-Care

The chemically dependent person needs a followup plan for support after detoxification or intensive CD treatment; this **after-care** is often the most important factor in maintaining sobriety. Ongoing support and understanding from a counselor or group, such as AA, must continue for at least 2 years to give the person a good start in the recovery process.

☛ KEY CONCEPT

The substance abuser needs followup care, such as with Alcoholics Anonymous or Rational Recovery, for at least 2 years after completing the intensive treatment stage. Some people need this support for life.

ALCOHOL ABUSE AND DEPENDENCE

Alcohol (**ETOH, EtOH**) abuse is a major public health problem. It causes or contributes to more than 100,000 deaths (5% of all deaths) each year in the United States alone, many of which stem from alcohol-related MVA. Groups such as **MADD** (Mothers Against Drunk Driving) have initiated programs to strongly encourage people not to drive while drinking or using drugs. They have lobbied for stricter laws; stiff penalties for DUI are in place in most states. Groups such as MADD also sponsor programs such as selecting a designated driver and offering free taxi rides on New Year's Eve.

A program sponsored by local police departments, called **DARE** (Drug Abuse Resistance Education), is in place in schools to encourage young people not to begin using alcohol or drugs.

However, it is estimated that at least 15 million people in the United States have problems with alcohol. Unfortunately, an increasing number of young people are abusing alcohol. Another concern is alcohol abuse by pregnant women, which causes fetal alcohol syndrome (**FAS**; see Chap. 68).

Signs and Symptoms

Alcohol is a central nervous system (CNS) depressant. Signs and symptoms that a person is under its influence include slurred speech, unsteady gait, confusion, and behavioral changes. The chronic alcohol abuser may have a swollen nose, prominent or spidery veins (*spider angiomas*), and thickened and reddened palms (*palmar erythema*). Chronic alcoholism can also lead to dementia, amnesia, sleep disorders, and psychotic symptoms, including delusions and hallucinations. Chronic alcoholics are at major risk for suicide.

Blood alcohol levels are important in detoxification. The maximum legal level for driving varies among states, but generally is 0.08 to 0.10 grams per deciliter (g/dL). A person with a level of 0.3 g/dL will usually be vomiting and incoherent, aggressive, or in a stupor. Coma usually occurs at about 0.4 g/dL, and severe respiratory depression and death can occur at 0.5 g/dL. The nurse may be asked to perform a breathalyzer test to determine a person's blood alcohol level. (Follow the instructions on the breathalyzer machine.)

> ### ✚👁 Nursing Alert
>
> **Suspect alcohol dependence** if the Breathalyzer level is 0.1 to 0.15 g/dL and the person does not appear drunk. *Grams/Deciliter*

Routine blood work to determine the physical status of a person who abuses alcohol usually includes evaluation of liver function, measuring levels of enzymes such as aspartate transaminase (AST), alanine transaminase (ALT), lactic dehydrogenase (LDH), alkaline phosphatase (ALP), and γ-glutamyl-transpeptidase/serum γ-glutamyl-transferase (GGTP/SGGT). Elevated enzyme levels indicate liver damage. GGTP/SGGT is elevated in about 75% of chronic alcoholics.

Thiamine and folate (folic acid) levels are usually low. The red blood cell count is often low as well (*anemia*). The blood sugar level is usually low (*hypoglycemia*), and malnutrition may be evident. Lipid and uric acid levels are often increased (*hyperlipidemia* and *hyperuricemia*).

Specific Disorders Caused by Alcohol Abuse

Dietary Deficiencies. Because alcohol is primarily absorbed in the proximal small intestine, absorption of other nutrients may be impaired, causing dietary deficiencies. The most common deficiencies in alcoholism are vitamin B_1 (thiamine) and vitamin B_9 (folic acid, folate). Routine administration of these vitamins, in addition to iron and a multivitamin, is part of the treatment protocol.

Untreated thiamine deficiency in chronic alcoholism causes a severe neurologic disorder, **Wernicke-Korsakoff syndrome** (**WKS**). Many untreated chronic alcohol abusers exhibit symptoms of this disorder including dementia, *diplopia* (double vision), ataxia, *somnolence* (extreme sleepiness), stupor, and *horizontal nystagmus* (rapid eyeball movement, in this case, from side to side). Ocular symptoms are treatable, but ataxia and dementia are generally irreversible. The mortality rate in the acute phase of Wernicke-Korsakoff's is as high as 15%. Prophylactic administration of oral thiamine can prevent WKS, if started early enough.

Cirrhosis of the Liver and Hepatitis. Liver **cirrhosis** (chronic interstitial inflammation) is commonly associated with chronic alcoholism (*Laennec's cirrhosis*). The person may also have acute alcoholic hepatitis, with fever and dehydration. These disorders are sometimes referred to as *alcohol-related liver disease* (**ARLD**). Because the liver has many vital functions, restoring it to maximum health is particularly crucial. (Liver disorders are discussed more fully in Chap. 87.)

Other Disorders. Other disorders directly related to alcohol abuse are esophageal varices and bleeding; cancer of the mouth and esophagus; gastritis, gastric ulcers, and other GI disturbances; kidney disorders; and heart disorders, including coronary artery disease. Sexual impotence is common. Newborns of alcohol-abusing mothers often have FAS (see Chap. 68).

🔑 KEY CONCEPT

A person who has built up alcohol tolerance is likely to be cross-tolerant to other CNS depressants, such as benzodiazepines, which are commonly used to treat mental illnesses. Analgesics, such as morphine, will also have less potent effects for such an individual.

Alcohol absorption varies and is influenced by many factors. For example, carbonation increases absorption; therefore, faster intoxication occurs from drinking champagne. Medications such as aspirin, cimetidine (Tagamet), and ranitidine (Zantac) enhance absorption of alcohol.

Women become intoxicated faster than men because their GI absorption rate is faster, their body fluid composition is different, the ratio of muscle to fat is different, and they are usually smaller in size.

Treatment

Treatment of alcohol abuse is complex. After the person completes detoxification and general medical conditions are treated, ongoing followup begins. The client and family are referred to an ongoing support program. In addition to vitamin replacement and other therapy, specific medications are available to assist intractable alcoholics to maintain sobriety.

Stages of Withdrawal

Alcohol withdrawal (ETOH W/D), unlike withdrawal from most other drugs, progresses through three distinct stages, if medical management is ineffective. The goal of managed alcohol detoxification is to keep the client as comfortable and safe as possible and to prevent progression into the second and third stages of withdrawal, which are life threatening. The following are the stages of *unmanaged alcohol withdrawal:*

1. *Autonomic hyperactivity:* Symptoms include elevated vital signs (pulse >100), nervousness, restlessness, and psychomotor agitation. This stage includes anxiety, sleep disturbances (including insomnia and vivid nightmares), irritability, diaphoresis, flushed face, anorexia, and nausea (with copious vomiting and later, "dry heaves"). A significant sign is the presence of tremors ("shakes"). Subjective, internal tremors occur first. The client can describe these tremors, but they are not observable to the nurse. Hand tremors are the first objective sign others will observe. Stage 1 often occurs within 12 to 18 hours after the person's last drink.

2. *Neuronal excitation:* Symptoms include severe tremors (internal and external), panic, insomnia, and increased agitation. The person may experience transient hallucinations of frightening events (eg, drowning while drunk) or frightening auditory hallucinations. The person may become paranoid, believing that he or she is being persecuted. This person is at high risk for suicide. Stage 2 often occurs within 24 to 36 hours after the last drink.

3. *Sensory-perceptual disturbances:* Symptoms include vivid visual hallucinations (eg, "pink elephants," flashing lights), generalized tonic–clonic seizures, and severe agitation and panic, leading to profound confusion and coma. Death may occur during a seizure or due to exhaustion. This stage is a medical emergency. Untreated, the mortality rate is 25% in this stage. Stage 3 often occurs within 3 to 4 days after the person's last drink.

☛ KEY CONCEPT

The client withdrawing from alcohol often may have abused other drugs as well. Be alert for mixed withdrawal signs and symptoms.

An indicator of a severe toxic state in stage 3 is the presence of *delirium tremens* (**DTs**). Symptoms include delusions and vivid and terrifying auditory, visual, and tactile hallucinations

called **alcohol hallucinosis** (eg, "bugs crawling on the skin"), which may last from a few days to several weeks. The person often retains consciousness during DTs, so the experience is extremely frightening. This person is critically ill. Vomiting may be present; severe diarrhea is common. Vital signs are very high; fever may be 100° to 103° Fahrenheit or even higher. Tachycardia is present, with pulse in the range of 130 to 150 beats per minute. Seizures may be present. A situation called "rum fits" exists when the person has two to eight tonic–clonic seizures close together. Death may occur in this stage due to exhaustion, circulatory collapse (resulting from blood volume depletion), or *hyperthermia* (very high fever).

✚👁 **Nursing Alert**
Surgery, delivery of a newborn, or an acute injury or infection may precipitate DTs in an alcohol-dependent person. *Delirium Tremens*

Many factors determine the severity of withdrawal, including the individual's physical makeup, how much he or she drinks and how often, what other drugs the person combines with alcohol, history of previous severe withdrawal symptoms, and other underlying disorders such as liver damage or diabetes mellitus. Uncomplicated withdrawal is usually completed within 3 to 7 days.

✚👁 **Nursing Alert**
The nurse working in a healthcare facility's medical-surgical unit must be aware of the possibility of serious withdrawal symptoms in a client who is admitted for an acute infection or severe injury. Evaluate all people who have been involved in serious motor vehicle accidents, fights, and street crime for possible alcohol or drug use. *Any other client* could also experience withdrawal. AVOID STEREOTYPES.

Family Considerations

Alcoholism is a family disease. In addition to the abuser, the people most affected by alcoholism are the spouse or significant other and children.

The following are characteristics of the alcoholic family:

- Control—The alcoholic person needs to control the rest of the family.
- Rigidity or perfectionism (or both)—Everyone tries too hard.
- Mistrust of others
- Tension, or overly cheerful and social behavior that seems forced—Constant coverup of real feelings
- Communication deficits; forced interactions
- Overuse of certain defense mechanisms, such as projection, rationalization, and denial

Young people raised in alcoholic families have special problems, including low self-esteem, feelings of failure, and a sense of responsibility to take care of everyone else. Many of these children falsely believe that they somehow caused their loved one's alcoholism. Adult children of alcoholics (**ACOA**) are often clinically depressed or suicidal; they frequently become alcoholic or chemically dependent themselves.

The Codependent or Enabler.   Most alcoholics have one or more *codependents*. Hazelden defines a **codependent,** also called an **enabler,** as "one who has let someone else's behavior affect him or her. The codependent is obsessed with controlling (the user's) behavior."[3] The codependent (often the alcoholic's spouse or partner) is the person who tries to keep the family together, fends off the creditors, drives the drunk person home after a party, and helps while he or she vomits the next morning. The codependent calls in sick for the alcoholic, tells the children that "mother can't cook tonight because she has a headache" or "Daddy doesn't feel well, so don't bother him." The codependent, however, is often the person the alcoholic blames for the entire problem; in turn, the codependent accepts that blame. He or she says, "Maybe if I took better care of myself and looked better, he/she wouldn't have this problem." (In the abuse of many other mood-altering chemicals, the codependent does not always play as important a role as he or she does in alcoholism.)

To break the cycle of dependence, codependents must realize that monitoring another person's behavior and being honest about their own feelings are impossible to reconcile. Preventing crises and shielding the alcoholic will not solve the problem. Many alcoholics and other substance abusers become motivated to seek help only when their well-being or the "status quo" is threatened. To begin recovery, codependents must stop covering up and protecting the alcoholic. They must come to understand that alcoholics have a bad disease but are not bad people. Codependents must also realize that some abusers will not stop; they then must decide to "let go" in whatever way is comfortable. Often, when codependents get help for themselves and stop enabling, alcoholics no longer continue the cycle of abuse because no one is available to blame for their problems but themselves.

☛ KEY CONCEPT
_____

Allow clients to verbalize and take control of their own lives, but do not fall into the enabling trap. Remember: "Enabling isn't kindness . . . it's like letting a life-threatening situation progress unhindered . . . Don't let a substance abuser exploit your (professional concern and) kindness."[4]

Family Programs.   Al-Anon, Al-A-Tot, and Al-A-Teen, sponsored by AA, offer support and encouragement to families of alcoholics. Al-Anon is usually for the alcoholic's spouse or significant other. Al-A-Tot and Al-A-Teen are designed for children of alcoholics (COA) (see Chap. 72). A program in Minnesota, "Children are People," encourages active intervention and therapy for very young children, as young as 3 to 4 years. There are also special programs for ACOA and codependents.

Medication Therapy
Antabuse.   A medication called *disulfiram* (Antabuse, Cronetal) is sometimes used as **aversion therapy** or *adverse*

conditioning in the chronic alcoholic who is unable to maintain sobriety. It is used only if the client is preoccupied with alcohol or is craving alcohol and has had multiple failed treatments in the past. The relapse history often includes impulsive, unpremeditated use. Antabuse may also be court ordered. The oral loading dose is 500 milligrams per day for 2 weeks, followed by a daily maintenance dose of about 250 milligrams.

If the person taking Antabuse drinks, even a very small amount, he or she becomes violently ill. (Antabuse blocks oxidation of ethanol [alcohol], causing buildup of acetaldehyde.) Resulting symptoms include flushing, throbbing headache, dyspnea, hypotension or fluctuating blood pressure, nausea with violent and copious vomiting, tremors, diaphoresis, thirst, anxiety, weakness, dizziness, and confusion. In a severe reaction, respiratory depression, cardiovascular collapse, heart attack, seizures, coma, and death can result.

Obviously, this dangerous drug is used only when everything else has failed. It is implemented only under close medical and nursing supervision. The person with ARLD is not eligible to use it. Antabuse is contraindicated in heart disease, after a stroke, and in diabetes. The client must be motivated to stop drinking and agree to fully cooperate with the treatment program. Therapy continues until the client can independently maintain sobriety—sometimes as long as several years. For more information see In Practice: Nursing Care Guidelines 94-3.

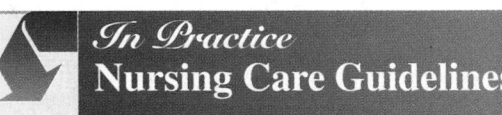

In Practice
Nursing Care Guidelines 94-3

NURSING CONSIDERATIONS IN ANTABUSE THERAPY

It is important to teach the client and the family about these concepts when using Antabuse therapy:

• Do not give Antabuse within 12 hours of alcohol ingestion.
• Adverse interactions occur with several other drugs, in addition to alcohol.
• The drug is contraindicated during pregnancy and in the nursing mother.
• The client must be in acceptable physical condition; a complete physical and psychological workup is required before administration.
• The client must avoid all sources of alcohol, including cough syrup, some mouthwashes, and possible transdermal sources, such as shaving lotion and rubbing alcohol.
• Some adverse side effects may occur, including impotence, decreased libido, fatigue, and an unpleasant taste in the mouth. These usually disappear within a few weeks.

✳Naltrexone. Naltrexone (Trexan, ReVia) was approved for treatment of alcoholism in 1995. It is a blocking agent used to treat opioid abuse, but it is now used as an adjunct treatment for alcoholism. It reduces subjective effects of alcohol, making the person enjoy drinking less. This drug is not used in those with hepatitis or liver failure. The client must be completely detoxified from coexisting opioids before beginning treatment.

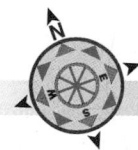

SPECIAL CONSIDERATIONS: CULTURE

Culture and Chemical Dependency Treatment

A major goal in caring for all individuals is to be respectful of clients' diverse cultures and beliefs. In many cultures, chemical dependency is hidden, denied, and is a source of embarrassment or shame. In other cultures, alcohol consumption, for example, is an expected and regular daily practice.

In some cases, there seems to be an ethnic predisposition to chemical dependency and/or alcoholism. The nurse must also take this factor into consideration when working with clients of various ethnic groups.

It is important for the nurse working in chemical dependency to be knowledgeable about cultural beliefs as they apply to this nursing specialty. Often the best source of that information is the client or the family. Being aware of specific beliefs and practices helps the nurse to be respectful of each individual and to incorporate that information into practice. However, it is also important to avoid stereotypes about an entire cultural or ethnic group.

In making referrals to treatment programs, be aware of programs targeting specific ethnic groups, age groups (including adolescents), and gender-specific groups. There are also specific programs for gay clients, for religious personnel, as well as for couples, families, and young children. Offering these options helps clients to better assimilate into and accept the treatment process.

ABUSE OF SUBSTANCES OTHER THAN ALCOHOL

Drug abuse of substances other than alcohol ranges from common drugs found in the home medicine cabinet to marijuana and other illegal drugs, such as crack or heroin. Many people also abuse nicotine and caffeine.

☛ KEY CONCEPT

A large percentage of substance abusers use more than one substance (polysubstance abuse). *Many abusers combine alcohol with other mood-altering chemicals, especially cocaine and marijuana. Many characteristics of the alcoholic also apply to the polysubstance abuser.*

Ethnicity and peer pressure can affect chemical use, sometimes influencing a particular person's drug of choice. Drugs are widely available, but finances may influence what drugs a person uses and in what amounts. Advertising may also influence a person's drug use.

Marijuana, and cocaine and related drugs (eg, "crack," "rock," and "crank"), are more commonly used in the general population than are substances like heroin. However, heroin use is again increasing. Sometimes, people try drugs like marijuana or cocaine for excitement. Unfortunately, dependence can occur very quickly, and the person becomes unable to stop using.

Much of the counseling and psychological treatment for the drug-dependent person is the same as, or similar to, treatment for the alcohol-dependent person. Physical care during detoxification is also similar. Check the agency's protocol when treating each specific drug-related case.

☛ KEY CONCEPT

With alcohol or any other drug, detoxification must precede counseling and long-term recovery.

Sedatives, Hypnotics, and Anxiolytic Drugs

This group of drugs is large and includes barbiturates and antianxiety agents, such as benzodiazepines. The illegal street use of these drugs is increasing. Frequently abused drugs in these groups include:

Barbiturates: amobarbital (Amytal), butabarbital (Butalan, Butisol, Butibel), mephobarbital (Mebaral), pentobarbital (Nembutal), phenobarbital (Luminal), secobarbital (Seconal, "reds"), amobarbital combined with secobarbital (Tuinal)

Benzodiazepines: alprazolam (Xanax), chlordiazepoxide (Librium), diazepam (Valium), lorazepam (Ativan), oxazepam (Serax)

Other abused drugs: chloral hydrate (Noctec), ethchlorvynol (Placidyl), glutethimide (Doriden), meprobamate (Equanil, Miltown), zolpidem tartrate (Ambien), hydroxyzine (Atarax, Vistaril), gamma hydroxybutyrate (GHB; many nicknames)

Symptoms of Abuse. Drugs in these groups are processed by the liver, as is alcohol. Concurrent use of such drugs and alcohol can intensify liver damage. Sedatives, hypnotics, and anxiolytics cause symptoms of generalized body depression, including slurred speech, unsteady gait, nystagmus, decreased memory and attention span, stupor, or coma. Psychological effects can be extreme, including delirium, amnesia, hallucinations, mood or anxiety disorders, and irreversible dementia. A particular danger of overdose with these depressants is life-threatening respiratory depression. (Chap. 93 lists a number of mood-altering drugs, their uses, desired effects, and side effects.) All such drugs have a potential for physical and psychological dependence.

Many abusers have severely damaged livers that cannot properly process these drugs, causing toxic waste products to build up in the body. Therefore, combining any drugs with alcohol is particularly dangerous. In some cases, the combination of drugs and alcohol *potentiates* the effects of both. (The combined effect is greater that the sum of the individual drugs.) Potentiation can cause overdose and can be fatal.

Withdrawal. In acute ("cold turkey") withdrawal from sedative, hypnotic, and anxiolytic drugs, seizures are possible. Withdrawal must be gradual (although this withdrawal is not as life threatening as that from alcohol). Overdose and acute withdrawal are medical emergencies requiring hospitalization. A specific antidote for overdose of benzodiazepines is flumazenil (Romazicon).

GHB (Gamma Hydroxybutyrate)[5]

A newer and very dangerous street drug showing increasing abuse is **GHB**. GHB is also known as "the date-rape drug," "G," and "liquid ecstasy" (it is not the same as "ecstasy"). GHB is colorless, odorless, and tasteless. It is available alone and is also contained in a number of dietary supplements, many of which are marketed on the Internet. (The active ingredient may be listed as furanone or lactone.) GHB causes a decrease in inhibitions and often causes amnesia. However, death may occur, even with first-time use.

Precursors of GHB, such as GBL and 1,4 BD, are marketed on the Internet as "cleaning products," but are intended for abuse and ingestion. The sale, manufacture, or possession of GHB is illegal, but Internet sales cannot be monitored.

Symptoms of Abuse. Acute toxicity symptoms are highly variable and unpredictable. The person may be extremely labile, alternating abruptly between combativeness and somnolence (characteristic presentation). Other signs and symptoms include: facial tics, fist-clenching, self-injurious behavior (such as head-banging), nystagmus, "chain-saw" snoring, hypothermia, urinary/fecal incontinence, nausea/vomiting, bradycardia, amnesia, respiratory depression/arrest, coma, seizure-like activity, and death. Many GHB abusers come into the Emergency Room following an MVA or rape. Other trauma, such as a fracture, can occur as a result of the sudden loss of muscle control ("head-snap") or collapse ("carpeting-out"). A number of fatalities have been documented, particularly when GHB is combined with alcohol or other depressants.

Withdrawal. Symptoms may be similar to the DTs of alcohol withdrawal, but vital signs are often normal or only slightly elevated. Because addiction requires around-the-clock dosing, withdrawal may begin within 2 to 5 hours.

Early withdrawal symptoms include anxiety, diaphoresis, hypervigilance, tachycardia, hypertension, paranoia, and severe insomnia. These symptoms may quickly progress to severe withdrawal, with extreme agitation and combativeness,

hallucinations, paranoia, and delirium. These symptoms may alternate with somnolence and coma. (Arousal from coma may be dangerous, resulting in *emergence delirium*.) Withdrawal symptoms may last 7 to 12 days and may be fatal.

Nursing and medical care are supportive. High doses of sedatives, including benzodiazepines such as diazepam (Valium) or lorazepam (Ativan), or a specialized drug called propofol (Diprivan), may be needed. The anesthetic, droperidol (Inapsine), may also be used. Intubation may be required to support respiration.

Nursing Alert

Motor vehicle accidents, DUI, and sexual assault are common with GHB use. If GHB use is suspected, collect 100 mL of the first voiding, as well as a blood sample (usually in a gray-top tube). *Refrigerate both and report immediately.* (GHB is not detected in most routine U-tox screening tests and requires a special test.)

Cannabis-Related Drugs

The active ingredient in these drugs is tetrahydrocannabinol (**THC**), sometimes referred to as *cannabis*. These drugs are made from the hemp plant and are classified as hallucinogens. Preparations include bhang, ganja, marijuana ("Mary Jane" [**MJ**], "pot," or "weed"), and hashish ("hash"). Marijuana is usually dried and smoked. Hashish is more potent than marijuana and is usually smoked or chewed. Marijuana cigarettes dipped in formaldehyde ("wets"), often cause permanent brain damage.

Nursing Alert

If a person obtains hashish, believing it is marijuana, a fatal overdose is likely.

Symptoms of Abuse. The most common effect of THC is a dreamy state, characterized by euphoria; the person's perception of space and time may be distorted. The user often shows poor motor coordination, restlessness, impaired judgment, tachycardia, dyspnea, palpitations, hunger, nausea, and dry mouth. Signs of intoxication include delirium, delusions, hallucinations, anxiety or panic, and a feeling of choking or suffocation. Cannabis can induce psychological and physical dependence; negative effects can result from continued use. No evidence has shown that smoking marijuana directly leads to the use of opiates or other drugs. However, most people who use "harder" drugs smoked marijuana first.

THC is used medically as dronabinol (Marinol). It is prescribed to treat the nausea and vomiting associated with cancer chemotherapy and to treat anorexia in clients with AIDS. It may exacerbate bipolar illness, schizophrenia, hypertension, and heart disease. Dronabinol usually is locked with narcotics and should be refrigerated.

Withdrawal. Withdrawal symptoms related to THC abuse usually do not appear until about 1 week after use (but may begin within 12 hours). Symptoms often are not recognized as being related to the use of marijuana. Symptoms include diarrhea, "wet dog" shakes, excessive salivation and yawning, *ptosis* (drooping eyelids), restlessness, irritability, insomnia, diaphoresis, runny nose (*rhinorrhea*), hiccups, anorexia, hot flashes, and mild flu-like symptoms. Withdrawal is not usually life threatening.

Narcotics

The narcotics group includes opiates and opiate agonists, such as opium, heroin, morphine, meperidine HCl (Demerol), codeine, methadone (Dolophine), butorphanol (Stadol), hydromorphone (Dilaudid), pentazocine (Talwin), and other drugs. With the exception of codeine, all these drugs are highly addictive and rapidly induce tolerance and physical and psychological dependence.

Symptoms of Abuse.   Symptoms of narcotic intoxication include drowsiness or coma, slurred speech, decreased memory and attention span, *bradypnea* (respiratory depression), dysphoria, and depression. Suicide is a great risk.

Withdrawal.   Narcotic withdrawal, although uncomfortable, is less dangerous than barbiturate or alcohol withdrawal. Symptoms resemble those of a cold or allergic response, with sore throat, rhinorrhea, *lacrimation* (tearing of eyes), diaphoresis, and insomnia. Yawning and dilated pupils are specific signs. In more severe cases, the person appears very ill, with joint and muscle pains, GI discomfort (nausea, vomiting, diarrhea), and fever. A specific antidote for narcotic overdose is naloxone HCl (Narcan). *antidote for*
※ *narcotics*

Nursing Alert

A narcotic or benzodiazepine overdose may occur accidentally or intentionally (as a *suicide attempt*). This life-threatening emergency requires immediate medical attention.

Agonist and Drug Replacement Therapy

Opiates, such as heroin, are very addictive; withdrawal is difficult. Outpatient therapy alone is often ineffective. Inpatient therapy accomplishes detoxification, but clients often relapse when released from the controlled environment.

Several drugs, some without pharmacologic effects of their own, are used as adjunct therapy in selected cases. They act in differing ways. Some "take over" or occupy opioid receptors, blocking the opioid's effects (**agonist therapy**); some displace previously administered opioids (*opioid blockers*).

Naltrexone (Trexan).   The client usually takes this long-acting opioid blocker three times weekly. Opiate blockers occupy the brain's specific opiate receptors, so that clients do not experience the addicting subjective effects (euphoria, psychological dependence) of opiate use. Before the person can use Trexan, he or she must be completely detoxified, to prevent severe withdrawal symptoms. Persons addicted to short-acting opioids (eg, heroin, meperidine) must wait at least 7 days before administration; those addicted to longer-acting drugs, such as methadone, must wait 10 days. This client must be motivated to continue treatment on a long-term basis. Trexan may cause liver damage and other adverse effects.

If a person taking Trexan has pain, he or she should not use opioid analgesics, except in an emergency. In this case, opioid doses must be large, and severe respiratory depression may occur. Pain is best managed using non-opioid analgesics, such as nonsteroidal anti-inflammatory drugs (NSAIDs). If this client is scheduled for surgery, Trexan can be discontinued 3 days preoperatively. When administering postoperative opioids, carefully titrate the opioid upward, and closely monitor the client. (Decreased level of consciousness and impaired respiratory function are danger signs.) Re-addiction is a strong possibility.

Methadone.   Methadone HCl (Dolophine, Methadose), an opiate analgesic, was released in 1972 for the treatment of heroin-dependent individuals. It binds with opiate receptors at several sites in the CNS. Methadone is substituted for heroin (or IV morphine) because it does not produce heroin's "high" or sedation. It suppresses opiate withdrawal symptoms for 24 to 48 hours. Side effects include sedation, nausea, diaphoresis, hypotension, constipation, and urine retention. Life-threatening side effects include seizures (with large doses) and respiratory depression. Some physicians are reluctant to use methadone because it is addictive; withdrawal can be dangerous (although it is usually milder than withdrawal from other narcotics).

After the client reaches a maintenance dose of methadone, he or she can be discharged from a treatment facility and receive the drug daily as a clinic outpatient. Doses are highly individualized, but an average daily dose is 20 to 120 milligrams. (Any higher dose requires state/federal approval.) Oral administration is required by law. Powder is mixed in at least 120 milliliters of orange juice or citrus drink to mask the taste and amount of drug. In most cases, the client must come into a Methadone Clinic daily to obtain his or her dose of methadone.

Regular, supervised urine specimens are required. The client's urine is analyzed for the presence of opiates, barbiturates, or other drugs while using methadone. Repeated evidence of other drug abuse usually results in dismissal from the program. Many methadone maintenance programs also require the client to participate in some form of group therapy to help the person find new ways of problem-solving in a drug-free environment. Some programs build educational programs around health and occupational issues as well.

ORLAAM.   Levomethadyl acetate HCl (ORLAAM, LAAM) is a long-acting synthetic opioid agonist that permits dosing three times a week. Its schedule is more convenient for clients and encourages compliance. ORLAAM is used only for clients who are serious about long-term therapy. Pregnant or lactating women and persons under age 18 cannot use ORLAAM. It is only available as oral liquid (10 mg/mL) and may not be used at home; clients must come to a federal- or state-approved clinic for dosing. Although individual doses vary, the average dose of ORLAAM is 60 to 90 milligrams, three times a week. This drug is never given daily. ORLAAM is diluted before administration and is mixed in a different color juice than orange to prevent confusing it with methadone. In some cases, persons on methadone switch to ORLAAM because fewer trips to the clinic are necessary. If weekend withdrawal frequently occurs, the third dose of the week can be increased.

Side effects include palpitations, syncope (fainting), abdominal pain, diaphoresis, nervousness, cough, and sexual dysfunction. Warn clients that effects of ORLAAM build over time. Thus, use of any other mood-altering drug (including alcohol or psychoactive drugs) can result in a fatal overdose. This situation is most dangerous during initiation of treatment or if the person has relapsed during treatment.

> **Nursing Alert**
>
> Clients in any of the agonist or opiate-blocker programs must meet certain criteria. Generally, they must have been opiate dependent for at least a year and have failed in other treatment programs. Many of these people abuse multiple drugs. They may also have co-existing psychiatric disorders and medical problems.

Central Nervous System (Cerebral) Stimulants

The CNS stimulants include cocaine-related drugs and amphetamines. These drugs induce tolerance and psychological dependence. Caffeine is considered a milder cerebral stimulant.

Amphetamines

Amphetamines are mood elevators and appetite depressants, and they combat drowsiness and simple fatigue. Many amphetamines are sold illegally in the United States. Caffeine potentiates the action of amphetamines. Some drugs in this class are amphetamine sulfate (SO_4), dextroamphetamine SO_4 (Dexedrine), benzphetamine HCl (Didrex, "benzedrine," "bennies"), and methamphetamine HCl (Desoxyn, "Methedrine," "meth"). Street names for amphetamine-like drugs include "ecstasy" (gamma butyric acid, **GBA**) and "ice." "Crystal meth" is a particularly potent and dangerous amphetamine.

Symptoms of Abuse.   Behavioral symptoms of amphetamine intoxication include euphoria, blunted affect, confusion, anger and irritability, and poor judgment. Psychiatric symptoms include hypervigilance, paranoia, and delirium, as well as depression and other mood disorders. Physical symptoms include dilated pupils, pulse and blood pressure disturbances, GI symptoms (eg, nausea, vomiting, and weight loss), chest pain, muscle weakness, anxiety, sexual dysfunction, and sleep disorders. Life-threatening symptoms include respiratory depression, cardiac arrhythmias, seizures, and coma.

Withdrawal.   Withdrawal usually causes depression and in some cases, paranoid psychoses that require hospitalization. Clients may have vivid nightmares, insomnia or hypersomnia, increased appetite, and psychomotor changes. The behavior of people addicted to amphetamine is highly unpredictable; they require careful, consistent, calm, and non-threatening care.

Amphetamine abusers often alternate amphetamines with sedatives, such as barbiturates or alcohol. They may take sedatives to "even out" the high and avoid the "crash" of stimulant withdrawal. Some abusers take sedatives to help them sleep and amphetamines to wake up in the morning. Therefore, they may need to withdraw from several drugs at the same time. The alternating "highs" and "lows" are life threatening if continued.

☛ KEY CONCEPT

Persons withdrawing from amphetamines must be prevented from injuring themselves or others.

Cocaine and Related Drugs

Cocaine is an alkaloid derived from the coca plant or manufactured synthetically. It is one of the most widely used drugs across all socioeconomic groups in the United States. Dependence on cocaine occurs quickly; it may occur with the first use. The cocaine derivative known as "crack," or "freebase" cocaine, is even more dangerous and addictive. Derivatives such as "crank" and "rock" continue to emerge. Cocaine can be absorbed by all mucous surfaces, injected IV, or smoked. Because cocaine is often snorted, the user may have chronic inflammation of the nasal mucous membranes; perforation of the nasal septum may occur.

The use of cocaine and related drugs is particularly dangerous in pregnancy and leads to fetal damage and illness (see Chap. 68). A child protection agency usually becomes involved when a pregnant woman is identified as a cocaine user. Many mothers who use cocaine are not allowed access to their babies until they have detoxified and entered a long-term treatment and management program.

A cocaine habit is very expensive. The cocaine-dependent person may obtain money to support the habit through illegal means, such as burglary or prostitution. Many violent crimes are related to cocaine, crack, and crank activity.

Symptoms of Abuse.   Many symptoms of cocaine intoxication are similar to those of amphetamines, including sexual dysfunction and sleep disorders. Cocaine frequently causes delirium and mood and anxiety disorders. Permanent brain damage, causing psychosis, is possible. Many clients experience vivid hallucinations and grandiose delusions. Cardiac arrest, severe hypertension, and very high fever can result from cocaine overdose, which can be rapidly fatal and which is becoming more common.

☛ KEY CONCEPT

Even small amounts of cocaine can cause permanent brain damage. This organic brain syndrome *(**OBS**) cannot be reversed.*

Withdrawal.   The client in severe withdrawal usually needs intensive care or a special duty nurse. A high potential exists for users to return to cocaine because it is so addicting. If the cocaine abuser also uses heroin, the general procedure is to give naloxone as a prophylactic measure.

Hallucinogens

Hallucinogenic drugs are not believed to cause actual physical dependence, but they do produce psychological dependence and mild tolerance. The three types of hallucinogens are:

- Traditional psychedelics (eg, lysergic acid diethylamide [**LSD**]; the anesthetic, sodium thiopental or sodium pentothal; phencyclidine hydrochloride [PCP]; mescaline)
- Amphetamine-like drugs (including **DOM**, **MDA/MDMA**, GBA ["ecstasy", XTC], and Khat)
- Anticholinergics (eg, belladonna, methantheline bromide [Banthine], scopolamine [Hyoscine])

LSD, Mescaline, and "Mushrooms." Hallucinogens include LSD, mescaline, and psilocybin ("mushrooms"). LSD is, by far, the most potent of these drugs. Tolerance to such drugs is highly variable. Their most characteristic effects are auditory hallucinations and intense visual hallucinations (eg, vivid colors, light flashes, or geometric shapes). The person may see "trails of light" or "halos" around objects. Objects may appear larger (**macropsia**) or smaller (**micropsia**) than normal. Medications are not usually used in detoxification.

Major problems associated with hallucinogens are "flashbacks" (*hallucinogen persisting perception disorder* [HPPD]), sometimes years later, causing severe panic attacks. The abuser also may injure himself or herself by thinking that he or she can fly, walk on water, or stop traffic on a busy freeway. Providing a safe, controlled environment is essential. If a person has a "bad trip," speak calmly and quietly; give reassurance. This person can also have permanent brain damage, especially if he or she combined several drugs.

Phencyclidine Hydrochloride. Phencyclidine hydrochloride (**PCP**, "angel dust") is a hallucinogen that was originally developed as an animal anesthetic. It has been abused since the late 1970s because of its low cost and easy availability. Because it has a simple chemical structure, it is believed that most PCP on the streets is illegally manufactured. Its effects are similar to those of hallucinogens and CNS stimulants. Some theorists believe that PCP prevents the individual from filtering out irrelevant sensory input, so the person becomes overwhelmed by environmental stimuli. The drug's most characteristic effect is an alteration in body image, frequently accompanied by uncomfortable feelings of unreality. Some individuals experience intense feelings of loneliness and isolation.

The most effective way to assist a person on a "bad trip" due to PCP is to provide a quiet environment with reduced stimuli. Verbal reassurance will not benefit this person. Do not talk at all (an approach that differs from treatment of withdrawal from other hallucinogens). PCP use can result in permanent brain damage.

> **✚👁 Nursing Alert**
> Do not touch any detoxifying person without warning him or her. The person may misperceive the actions and strike back, resulting in serious injury to the staff.

Volatile Substances. *Volatile substances* are CNS depressants that, when inhaled, produce altered states of consciousness and varied degrees of intoxication. Most commonly, younger teens and children participate in glue sniffing, gasoline sniffing, or inhaling vapor from aerosol cans or helium balloons. Such inhalant abuse causes hazy euphoria, slurred speech, loss of coordination, lessening of inhibitions, lethargy, dizziness, nystagmus, and blurred vision or diplopia. Serious effects include hallucinations, marked behavioral and personality changes, and impaired perception and judgment. Stupor, coma, or even death may result, even in first-time users. Inhaling these substances often causes serious lung, brain, liver, and kidney damage.

Anabolic Steroids

These substances derive from the male hormone, testosterone. They promote growth of skeletal muscles and increase lean muscle mass in the body. They are abused primarily by athletes in an effort to increase strength and performance in athletic events and to improve physical appearance. Users usually take steroids intermittently (*cycling*), often combining several types.

Undesired side effects include liver damage and cancer, endocrine and sexual dysfunction, electrolyte imbalance, acne, edema, headache, fatigue, and insomnia. The user can become very irritable, aggressive, and violent, and can be very dangerous. The person may also develop psychiatric symptoms, such as mood *lability* (rapid changes) and *paranoia* (unreasonable fear or panic). Some of these symptoms are considered to be withdrawal symptoms. Death can occur due to endocrine imbalances, myocardial infarct, or stroke. Withdrawal can be very difficult and uncomfortable. Relapse is common.

Nicotine

Nicotine is a substance in cigarettes and in chewing and other tobaccos. It is considered one of the most addicting drugs available. Nicotine contributes to or causes cancer, heart and blood vessel disorders, and congenital disorders, as well as many other physical disorders. In response to the Surgeon General's Report in 1964, the U.S. Federal Trade Commission requires each cigarette pack to carry a warning. Two such warnings are, "SURGEON GENERAL'S WARNING: Smoking causes lung cancer, heart disease, emphysema, and may complicate pregnancy" and "Smoking by pregnant women may result in fetal injury, premature birth, and low birth weight."

Nicotine stimulates constriction of blood vessels in the skin, causing a decrease in skin temperature and an increase in blood pressure. Cigarette smoke contains approximately 1% carbon monoxide, which binds with hemoglobin to diminish the blood's oxygen-carrying capacity. In addition, tobacco contains many other dangerous and addicting additives, especially in cigarettes. Over time, tobacco use causes direct damage to many body tissues, especially the lungs and cardiovascular system. Smokeless tobacco ('snuff') is not harmless, as some people think. It can cause many of the same physical reactions and disorders as smoked tobacco.

> **✚👁 Nursing Alert**
> It is important to note that the use of smokeless tobacco can cause cancers of the mouth, throat, esophagus, or stomach, as well as other system orders.

Nicotine withdrawal causes dysphoria and depression, as well as insomnia, irritability, restlessness, and anxiety. Heart rate decreases (*bradycardia*) and the person often feels hungry and gains weight.

There are many free or low-cost local and national self-help programs to help smokers and smokeless tobacco users quit. The nurse can help clients find a program best suited to their personal requirements—often individuals must try several programs before finding one that works. The American Cancer Society, American Lung Association, and local health maintenance organizations are sources for information on smoking cessation. A nicotine patch or nicotine-containing gum is frequently used as an adjunct to a smoking cessation program. A quick test ("COT") can determine if a person has been smoking.

Caffeine

Caffeine is found not only in coffee, but also in tea, some alcoholic beverages, soft drinks (eg, colas and diet colas, root beer, and drinks such as Surge, Mello Yellow, and Mountain Dew), and chocolate. Caffeine is also a component of many OTC and prescription analgesic preparations such as Excedrin, Fiorinal, Anacin, Norgesic, Vanquish, and Cope. Ergotamine and caffeine are combined as Ercaf or Cafergot for migraines. Caffeine is sold OTC as NoDoz and Vivarin ("stay awake pills"). It is sometimes used medically as a CNS stimulant and to treat newborn apnea. Table 94-2 lists approximate caffeine levels in beverages (per 355 mL [12 oz], the size of a regular soda can).

∎∎∎ TABLE 94-2 𝒞AFFEINE LEVELS OF COMMON SUBSTANCES*

Beverage, 355 mL (12 oz)	Caffeine Levels
Cola beverages	30–100 mg
Root beer beverages	23–40 mg
"Mello Yellow"-type beverages	53–70 mg
Brewed coffee	100–200 mg
Instant coffee	100–300 mg
Decaffeinated coffee	2–12 mg
Regular tea	80–200 mg
Medications	**Caffeine Levels**
NoDoz, Vivarin, Ultra Pep Back (maximum strength) (Caffeine is also available in injectable forms for medical use.)	200 mg tablets
Regular Anacin	32 mg
Excedrin (extra strength, Migraine)	65 mg
Excedrin PM	0 mg

*Some soda manufacturers refused to divulge the amounts of caffeine in their products.

Caffeine acts directly on blood vessels, causing them to dilate. It is effective as a mild stimulant and diuretic. Evidence shows that 200 to 300 milligrams of caffeine will partially offset fatigue; caffeine appears to enhance a person's capacity to function beyond his or her normal limit. Caffeine also seems to assuage boredom and increase attention span. Symptoms of overuse include restlessness, nervousness, agitation, insomnia, flushed face, and GI discomfort. Caffeine does not reverse alcohol's intoxicating or depressant effects, and may actually add to depression.

Caffeine is not without dangerous side effects. At levels of 500 milligrams or higher, heart rate increases; with high blood levels of caffeine, the heartbeat may become irregular. In a person with limited tolerance, even a small amount of caffeine makes falling asleep difficult and interferes with normal sleep patterns. Aggravation of cystic breast disease is related to caffeine use. Other conditions may also be related to caffeine intake. Research is ongoing to evaluate potential adverse effects of caffeine use. Dependence on caffeine is a physical reality. Notable withdrawal symptoms are tiredness, severe headache, and irritability.

Over-the-Counter Drugs and Herbals

The OTC drugs are those available without a prescription. Medications and herbal preparations can be purchased OTC at local drugstores and health food stores. Americans spend billions of dollars every year for these medications and herbal supplements. In some cases, self-medication is dangerous; overdose and adverse drug interactions are possible. Adequate nutrition (with vitamin, calcium, and iron supplements, if needed) and attention to proper rest, sleep, and activity are usually enough to maintain health and prevent discomfort. Nurses have many opportunities to teach people about dangers related to self-medication.

☞ KEY CONCEPT

Any substance has the potential for abuse, including mouthwash (especially those containing alcohol) and caustic substances (eg, rubbing alcohol and cleaning solutions). Various non-tobacco items can be smoked. Anything, in excess, can be harmful. *Some practices may cause serious health problems and death. Addictions, other than those to chemicals and drugs, include sex, gambling, and constant overuse of exercise. Herbals can inhibit clotting, add to hypertension, and adversely interact with medications.*

SPECIAL ABUSERS

Pregnant Women

Drug, alcohol, or nicotine use greatly complicates pregnancy, labor, and delivery, with profound effects on both mother and baby. Babies born to drug- or alcohol-abusing mothers are often of low birth weight, with many related problems. Preterm labor is common. Heroin withdrawal symptoms in a newborn may occur within hours after delivery; most affected babies demonstrate symptoms within 24 hours. The number of cocaine- and crack-addicted babies continues to increase.

Many babies born to chemically dependent mothers have permanent physical and/or mental disorders, including birth defects. Long-term adverse effects on the child are particularly evident in the case of the mother who abuses alcohol during pregnancy. In addition, many of these mothers lack adequate parenting skills due to their drug or alcohol addiction. Chapters 67 and 68 describe disorders in newborns related to maternal drug use.

☛ KEY CONCEPT

In many cases of maternal drug or alcohol addiction, the child or children are managed in foster homes and supervised by a Child Protection Agency until the mother can properly care for them.

Adolescents

Substance abuse is a serious problem among adolescents and school-age children. Peer pressure and low self-esteem are common problems in these age groups. Potent forces contribute to chemical abuse. Cigarette smoking alcohol use are also on the increase among adolescents. Chapter 72 discusses adolescent CD in more detail.

Older Adults

Many older adults take large amounts of prescribed and OTC medications. The senior client may be confused and accidentally take a double dose of medications. The person may also intentionally take extra sleeping pills or tranquilizers to counteract loneliness, depression, worries about health problems or financial status, or feelings of loss and hopelessness. Suicide attempts with medications and/or alcohol are possible. Many seniors also overuse medications such as cathartics and antacids. In addition, it is not unusual for older people to change their own medication dosages without consulting a healthcare practitioner.

> **✚👁 Nursing Alert**
>
> The nurse must remember that older people often have a paradoxical reaction to drugs or alcohol. For example, they may become very agitated, confused, or assaultive instead of becoming sedated.

Alcohol abuse is very common among seniors and is a rapidly growing national health problem (Fig. 94-3). Alcohol is particularly dangerous when combined with sleeping pills or tranquilizers.

In interactions with older clients, teach them about medications. Remember that an accurate drug history is an important part of data collection in nursing (see Chap. 91).

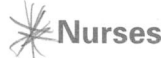
Nurses

Drugs are readily available in healthcare facilities; nurses are at risk for substance abuse (Box 94-1). Research indicates

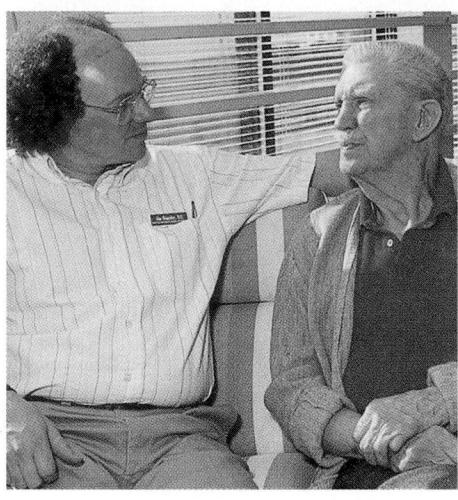

FIGURE 94-3. Chemical dependency and alcoholism among older people are increasing public health problems. Many seniors overuse prescription medications, over-the-counter drugs, or alcohol as a result of loneliness, depression, or confusion. Seniors often live alone and the problem is not recognized until it has become very serious. Shame, embarrassment, sense of loss, and low self-esteem are major components of the illness in this age group. In this photo, an understanding counselor allows a client to express his specific concerns on a one-to-one basis.

> ➤ **BOX 94-1**
>
> ### ✳ SIGNS OF SUBSTANCE ABUSE IN A NURSE
>
> - Consistently signs out more controlled drugs than other staff members
> - Consistently wants to be the medication nurse
> - Opens medication cabinet only when alone
> - Frequently breaks or spills drugs and has to dispose of ("waste") them
> - Makes many medication errors
> - Spends a great deal of time in the bathroom
> - Always wears long sleeves
> - Spends a great deal of time on the unit when not on duty; "hangs around"
> - Noticeable discrepancies regarding relief gained by medications occur between reports of clients assigned to this nurse and reports of clients assigned to other staff members
> - Incorrect narcotic medication count when this nurse gives medications
> - Medication vials appear altered; medication appears different from normal
> - Behavior that might indicate substance use, illogical or unreadable charting, often arriving late to work, extreme mood swings, defensiveness, frequent absences, overuse of sick leave

that nurses are 50% more likely to become chemically dependent than the general population.

The nurse is bound by law, the nursing code of ethics, and the pledge taken on entering nursing to report any staff person suspected of abusing drugs or alcohol. Reporting is necessary to assist others to get help and to protect clients with whom abusers might come in contact. The safe care of all clients rests in each nurse's hands.

☛ KEY CONCEPT

Remember that addiction can occur despite knowledge.

➤ STUDENT SYNTHESIS

Key Points

- Substance abuse and chemical dependency are serious public health problems that cost millions of dollars and take many lives yearly.
- Major precipitating factors of chemical abuse include stress and low self-esteem.
- The person with a dual disorder, such as mental illness and chemical dependency, may experience more difficulty in achieving a successful recovery.
- Management of substance abuse involves recognition, intervention, treatment, and ongoing recovery.
- Clients admitted to any healthcare facility may be substance abusers. Watch for withdrawal symptoms in all clients. Do not assume that any client is exempt from the possibility of chemical abuse.
- Care of a client during detoxification requires excellent assessment and nursing skills.
- Detoxification differs, depending on the abused drug and other physical and emotional factors.
- Certain blocker or agonist medications may be used as adjunct treatment for long-term management of chronic, intractable chemical dependency.
- Most clients require long-term followup and aftercare following detoxification and intensive chemical dependency treatment.
- The codependent or enabler is a key figure in alcoholism.
- Substance abuse is an especially serious problem for selected groups, including pregnant women, adolescents, and older adults.
- Nurses are more likely to abuse substances than the general population.

Critical Thinking Exercises

1. M., 15 years old, is 6 months pregnant. She comes to your clinic for her first prenatal visit. She says that she never uses condoms and has had two previous abortions. She acknowledges that she drinks alcohol ("a few beers each day") and "smokes weed once in a while." Her weight is well below that expected for her height. She has a constant, hacking, and productive cough. She smokes 2 packs of cigarettes and drinks 4 to 5 cups of coffee each day. She has recently been living at the Salvation Army shelter in their "special needs" area. She has no contact with her family and does not know what immunizations she had as a child. She wants to have "a healthy baby" and plans to keep her child. She refuses to discuss chemical dependency treatment.

What implications do alcohol and tobacco use have for M.'s general health and for that of her fetus?

What are the social implications of her lifestyle?

Describe your approach to this client. What nursing measures should you perform? What medical, laboratory, and other examinations or tests would you expect to be ordered to evaluate M. and her fetus? What disorders could she have?

What services could you offer to assist M. to learn parenting skills? What community resources might be available to assist with housing, medical care, education, financial support, and other needs for M. and her baby in your community? What is your personal reaction to this situation?

2. Father O. was admitted to your facility's surgical unit following a major gastric resection for ulcers. He performed his preoperative preparation at home and, reportedly, was in good spirits while on the way to the operating room. His vital signs on admission were 122/82, 98.0° F, 70, and 12. Father O. received IV morphine in the operating room to prevent immediate pain. Since then, he has received Demerol injections; he consistently asks for them more frequently than they are ordered. He is becoming restless and irritable and says he feels "shaky." He has slept about 3 hours in the past 24 hours, once waking up after a nightmare.

You are assigned to care for Father O. When you enter his room, he is irritable and demanding. His face is flushed, and he complains of severe pain, although it has only been 2 hours since his last Demerol injection. He begins crying when talking about the pain. Father O's vital signs are now 152/92, 99.9° F, 104, and 20. When you took his blood pressure, you noticed that his arm was shaking. He complained that the "cuff was too tight." He also says his "insides feel shaky all over" and his "chest hurts." He says he feels nauseated and has a "terrible headache."

Describe your interpersonal approach to Father O. What questions might you ask him to gather helpful data? What specific nursing actions do you think you should take and why? Would you call a physician or would you write your observations in the chart's nursing notes at the end of the shift? If you call the physician, what would you report? Would you expect any additional or different orders to be written? Why or why not?

Describe potential implications of Father O.'s condition since surgery. What important points should be included in the nursing care plan? What is your personal reaction to this situation?

NCLEX-Style Review Questions

1. A client presents in the emergency department with a suspected drug overdose. It is most important for the nurse to:
   a. Admit the client to the hospital
   b. Encourage fluids
   c. Monitor respirations
   d. Notify family members
2. A client is admitted to the hospital with alcohol withdrawal. Which of the following medications will the nurse expect to administer during the acute phase to prevent seizures and provide sedation?
   a. clonidine (Catapres)
   b. lorazepam (Ativan)
   c. nifedipine (Procardia)
   d. vitamin B₉ (folate)
3. Which of the following statements by a client indicates the use of rationalization as a defense mechanism?
   a. "I can quit whenever I want."
   b. "I do not have a problem."
   c. "I wouldn't need drugs if I had a better spouse."
   d. "My kids have driven me to use drugs."

4. Which percentage of general medical-surgical patients has underlying substance abuse problems?
   a. 10%
   b. 25%
   c. 30%
   d. 45%
5. Which of the following indicate that a client is experiencing delirium tremens?
   a. Anxiety
   b. Hallucinations
   c. Internal tremors
   d. Restlessness

References

1. American Psychiatric Association. (1994). *Diagnostic and statistical manual of mental disorders* (4th ed.). Washington, DC: Author.
2. Johnson, B. (1997). *Psychiatric-mental health nursing: Adaptation and growth* (4th ed.). Philadelphia: Lippincott-Raven.
3. Hazelden Staff. (1996). *Alcoholism.* Center City, MN: Hazelden Foundation.
4. Navarra, T. (1995). Enabling behavior: The tender trap. *American Journal of Nursing 95*(1), 50–52.
5. Adapted from presentation by Deborah L. Zvosek, PhD (2002). Minneapolis: Hennepin County Medical Center.

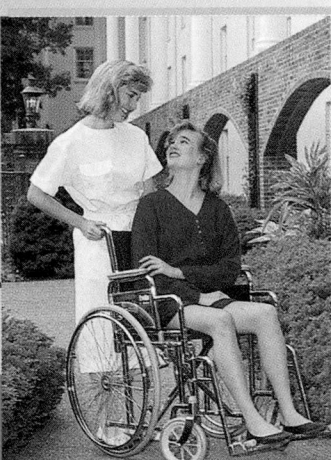

Unit XV

NURSING IN A VARIETY OF SETTINGS

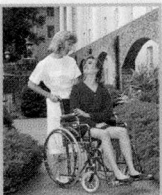

Extended Care

LEARNING OBJECTIVES

1. Describe the continuum of healthcare from acute care to independent living.
2. Differentiate among the major types of long-term facilities.
3. Describe and discuss the concept of transitional facilities.
4. List community resources available to persons living in their own homes.
5. Identify optional services or amenities that may be available at an extended-care facility.

NEW TERMINOLOGY

assisted living
congregate housing
medically complex
  nursing unit

ombudsperson
payee
subacute care
vulnerable adult

ACRONYMS

AARP	COE	NAHC
ADL	ECF	SNF
CLTC	ICF	UAP
CM	LTC	

Until now, much of your clinical experience has been in the acute-care setting. This chapter describes some lifestyle options and housing alternatives available to clients outside hospitals: extended-care facilities and independent living options. An individual may choose different lifestyle options on this continuum at various times, depending on his or her particular circumstances.

☛ KEY CONCEPT

A continuum of lifestyle options is found outside the acute healthcare facility. It includes independent living in a senior citizens' apartment building, independent living with community-based services, assisted living in one's own home or in an assisted-living apartment complex, home care, subacute placement, skilled nursing care, and short- or long-term care or rehabilitation in a healthcare facility. In some cases, the same corporation owns or manages the different services and facilities, and residents can move from one to another with a minimum of "red tape." Sometimes, all of these types of living situations exist under one roof or on one campus. A client may move back and forth between these options, depending upon the client's current state of health and level of independence.

Extended-care facilities and **assisted living** services provide many job opportunities for graduate nurses. With today's nursing shortage, these job opportunities are increasing. Several groups, including the American Nurses' Association, have joined together to address the problem of nurse staffing, particularly in nursing homes.

From the nurse's standpoint, a position in extended care enables the nurse to integrate many nursing skills. Working in extended care also provides the nurse with an opportunity to work with clients over a longer period of time. Unlike in the acute-care facility, the client stays in these areas longer, sometimes for years. You will also be able to work more closely with the client's family and to get to know them and observe their interaction with the client. This situation will provide you with a much broader picture of total nursing care for the total client. National certification in long-term care is available for LPNs (see Chap. 102).

Throughout your nursing program, you have studied procedures and learned the underlying rationales for what you do. In some healthcare facilities, you may need to make minor modifications to adapt to specific situations. Basic principles of asepsis, Standard Precautions, nursing care planning, interpersonal communication, and safety always apply in every setting. Wherever you are employed, your facility will expect you to follow their specific nursing protocols, while keeping the underlying rationales in mind.

EXTENDED CARE OPTIONS

Hospitals are rapidly becoming healthcare facilities that deal almost exclusively with cases of acute injury or illness. Clients often receive care from other facilities for chronic conditions or after the end of the initial crisis period. A broad continuum of care and assistance is available after the acute phase of illness or injury is resolved (Fig. 95-1). Some facilities are referred to as *extended-care facilities* (**ECF**s) because they "extend" or continue care started in the hospital. Facilities that are considered ECFs may include:

- Subacute-care or transitional facilities
- Medically complex care facilities
- Short-term rehabilitation units
- Long-term care (**LTC**) facilities (nursing homes)

☛ KEY CONCEPT

Remember that the hospital is often the first step in the continuum of care for the injured or disabled person. The hospital stabilizes the person during the acute phase of the illness or immediately after the injury. The person then enters a rehabilitation facility or accesses other services in the community to continue on the road to the maximum possible level of functioning.

Many clients also live at home and receive home-based community services (see Chap. 98), or take advantage of independent living options (see later in chapter).

The Continuum of Extended Care

Even within a particular type of facility, there are usually levels of care. For example, a previous LTC facility now may have the broader designation of ECF. This ECF often includes wings or areas that are designated as *skilled nursing care, subacute care,* and *custodial* or *nursing home* beds. Many facilities also include an area specifically designated for clients with dementia, particularly Alzheimer's. Other specialized units may also be included.

Continuum of Lifestyle Options

Intensive Care Unit (ICU)	Acute Nursing (Hospital)	Subacute Care (Transitional Facility)	Medically Complex Care	Skilled Nursing Facility (SNF)	Intermediate Care Facility (ICF)	Assisted Living	Board and Care (B&C)	Congregate Housing	Independent Living

FIGURE 95-1. Many lifestyle options are available for older adults and those with physical or mental challenges. Options range from total care to total independence.

Subacute-Care or Transitional Facilities

Subacute-care facilities provide an "in-between" level of care. They are also called *transitional care* or *continual care facilities*. Although they provide highly sophisticated care, subacute-care facilities are less expensive than hospitals. Many free-standing skilled nursing facilities (SNFs; described later in text) have sections that provide subacute care. *Subacute care* has become primarily a reimbursement designation. The person designated as occupying a *subacute bed* may just need one treatment that is classified as a *skilled nursing care* procedure. The rest of that client's care does not require skilled nursing interventions. (A person may be classified as "subacute" for 20 days under Medicare and then their status must be reevaluated.)

Generally, clients remain in subacute-care facilities for 2 to 4 weeks. Nurses who work in such settings often have previous experience in an intensive care unit, emergency department, or acute medical-surgical unit. Nursing functions include intravenous (IV) therapy, cardiac monitoring, ventilator care, tube feeding (enteral) administration of peritoneal dialysis, and management of severe wounds. Examples of clients in subacute-care facilities include people recovering from extensive surgery, strokes, or hip fractures. These facilities release many clients to independent living when their conditions improve. Other clients enter long-term care facilities or rehabilitation units from the subacute-care unit.

Medically Complex Care Units

A specialized step in the continuum of care is the **medically complex nursing unit.** This unit cares for clients who require more specialized, high-tech care than is provided in traditional SNFs, but who do not require hospitalization or care in subacute units. Nursing procedures include IV therapy, specialized wound care, and some daily nursing care. The medically complex unit is often a section in an SNF.

Short-Term Rehabilitation Units

Facilities may have *short-term rehabilitation units* specially designed to serve residents who are recovering from accidents or acute illnesses. These units usually provide physical, occupational, and speech therapy, as well as other services. Chapter 96 describes rehabilitation in more detail.

Long-Term Care (LTC) Facilities

There are two major types of LTC facilities, which are sometimes called *nursing homes* or *nursing care centers*. These two types are the *skilled nursing facility* and the *intermediate care facility*. Both types of facilities are licensed by the state and must follow prescribed regulations. Nursing assistants must be trained and, in some states, certified. Facilities are expected to provide clean, safe, and homelike environments. They provide room, board, and nursing care; emergency medical care must also be available. Chapter 91 discusses the choice of facilities and other aspects related to geriatric nursing.

The Skilled Nursing Facility (SNF)

One type of LTC facility is the *skilled nursing facility* (**SNF**). The SNF provides 24-hour care and must always have a licensed nurse on duty. This facility provides rehabilitation services, special diets, and access to pharmacy and laboratory services. Occupational, physical, recreational, and speech therapists are usually on staff or serve as consultants. Podiatry and dental services are often provided, as well as the services of counselors and psychologists. Social services may also be available. Other services such as therapeutic recreation, reminiscence therapy, pet therapy, and music therapy may be provided.

The primary care or "medical oversight" is often provided by an advanced practice nurse (nurse practitioner). Physicians are on call and are required to make regular visits to residents, as well as to provide supervision for the advanced practice nurse. Often, facilities provide for consultations with specialized physicians, the more common specialties being internal medicine, endocrinology, urology, and orthopedics.

The situations of the residents of the SNF may vary. In some cases, clients plan to live there indefinitely. In other cases, clients come to the SNF to recuperate following injury or severe debilitating illness, but plan to return to independent living. (A stay in an intermediate care facility may occur between the SNF and the client's home.) Nursing care in the SNF may include such procedures as IV therapy, enteral feeding, ostomy care, wound care, pain management, diabetes management, or bowel and bladder retraining programs, as well as physical rehabilitation.

The Intermediate Care Facility (ICF)

The second type of LTC facility is the intermediate care facility (**ICF**). The ICF provides fewer services and less extensive care than the SNF. ICFs provide room, board, and some nursing care. Generally, a licensed nurse is not required to be on duty 24 hours a day, although a nurse is usually on call.

Components of LTC Facilities

Meal Programs.   Meal programs in LTC facilities vary. Often, residents can elect the meal program they prefer. One choice is three full meals a day, with snacks. However, the person may also be able to select a program that includes a certain number of meals per week, or they may choose to have one full meal each day. Another program issues a meal ticket that has a dollar amount. This ticket is punched with whatever amount of food the person chooses until the dollar amount is used up.

☞ KEY CONCEPT

One of the problems with elective meal programs in extended-care facilities is that of finances. The client may feel that he or she cannot afford to pay for the full meal program, or may skip meals with the "punch card" system. The client's health may suffer as a result. The case manager must oversee the client's dietary intake, to make sure that the client is receiving sufficient nutrition.

Activities and Services. A good facility has many activities and services available to its residents (Fig. 95-2). Support groups, pastoral care and weekly worship services, libraries, van transportation for shopping or recreation, and resident councils are common. Many facilities also have lounges, fireplaces, gardens, and TV/video rooms on site for residents and their families. Facilities may also provide special services such as snack bars, gift shops, small convenience stores, banks, and ATMs.

Other services provided in some facilities include beauty/barber shops, therapeutic massage services, exercise rooms, computer rooms (sometimes staffed), and Internet and fax access. The person may also be allowed to install a special phone line in their living unit so that they can use their own personal computer to access the Internet.

A recreation program of some sort is a requirement in LTC facilities. These programs vary in complexity and extent. In some measure, the programs depend upon the level of functioning of the residents of the facility. Common recreational activities include making crafts, playing cards and other games, and having supervised outings within the community. Sports activities such as golf, fishing, or boating may also be pro-

vided. The residents may organize musical programs or plays, as well as a dance band, orchestra, or choir to perform for their peers. Dance and concert events may be scheduled. A special activities room may be available where these activities and other social events may be held.

In some facilities, particularly those sponsored by a church, temple, or mosque, a formal chapel is available for services and individual prayer. A chaplain is often on hand as well.

In many cases, a swimming pool or a sauna may be available. Therapeutic swimming programs play a part in rehabilitation by providing safer exercises. Sometimes, a person who is otherwise unable to walk is able to "walk" in the pool, which provides exercise and entertainment as well as therapy for the client. By moving in the water, the client is helping to prevent the disabilities associated with inactivity. In addition, the person benefits from the encouragement of the staff and an increase in his or her self-esteem. Other common therapies supplied in LTC facilities are occupational therapy, physical therapy, and recreational therapy.

A wellness clinic in an LTC facility is a plus. In some cases, specialists from various disciplines are available in the clinic on certain days. Some facilities also have a full health-

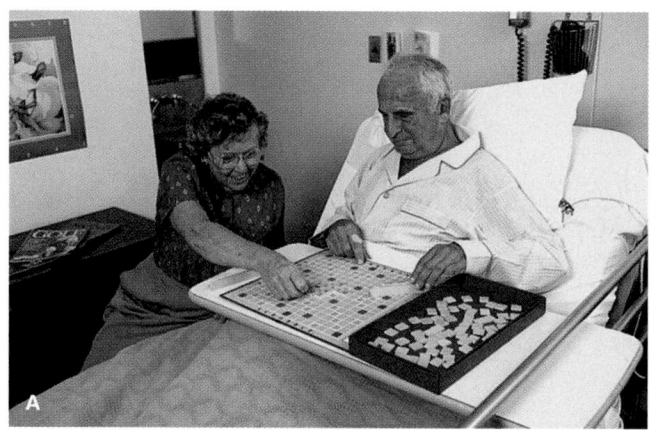

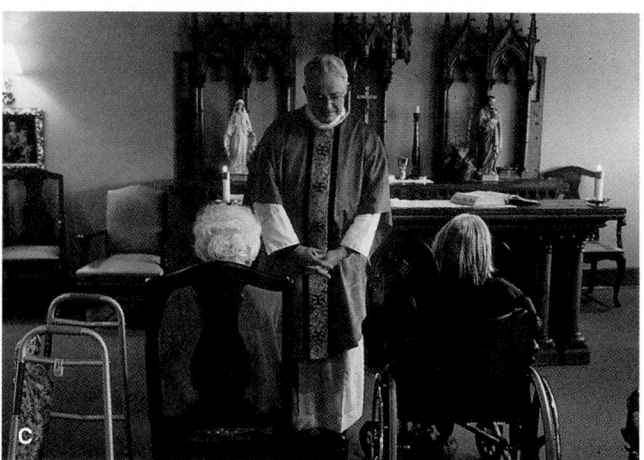

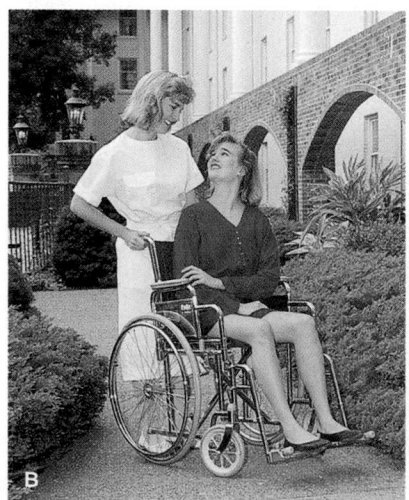

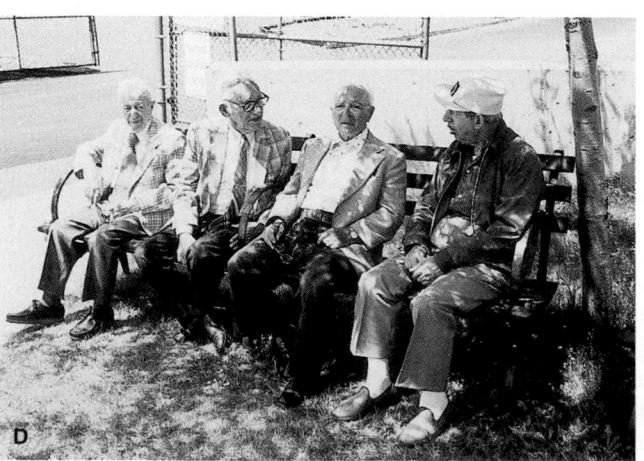

FIGURE 95-2. A good long-term care facility offers many programs for its residents. Opportunities are provided for (**A**) games and visiting with friends and relatives, (**B**) walks out of doors and other outings, (**C**) expression of one's religious faith, and (**D**) socializing with one's peers.

care center on site: This consists of a complete medical office and pharmacy, with physicians, advanced practice nurses, podiatrists, dentists, mental health professionals, pharmacists, and other healthcare professionals in attendance. Clients can receive their primary healthcare here. In some cases, these clinics are designated as official community health centers.

Many facilities have guest rooms available for a small fee so that the client's family members can visit overnight. Often they can share a meal together in the dining room at a reasonable price.

The Ombudsperson. Federal law requires each state to have an LTC **ombudsperson** who provides assistance and information to residents and families. Most clients in LTC facilities are designated as **vulnerable adults.** Therefore, they are protected by law from abuse or neglect. The ombudsperson is responsible for seeing that the client's rights are not violated. Any client complaints are referred to the facility's local administration. If they cannot be resolved at that level, the state ombudsperson may be called in to assist.

Payment for Long-Term Care. Private insurance and other third-party payers, such as Medicare, may cover all or part of the cost of LTC facilities. However, Medicare was designed to pay for acute illnesses or incidents and not to manage chronic conditions (see Chapter 98). Medicaid was designed to meet the needs of the most needy people and is not consistent among the states. Therefore, many people are left with no way to pay for LTC. In addition, clients must usually use all of their private insurance and often, most of their financial resources, before government funding can apply. For this reason, many people are purchasing individual LTC insurance.

In 1999, a coalition of organizations, including the American Association of Retired Persons (**AARP**), the Alzheimer's Association, and the National Association for Home Care (**NAHC**), formed a group called the Citizens for Long Term Care (**CLTC**). The CLTC's goal was to review LTC financing in the United States and make recommendations for improvement. A February, 2001 report released by the CLTC, entitled *Defining Common Ground: Long-term Care Financing Reform,* discusses the devastating financial burdens of LTC upon individuals and families. This report acknowledges that Medicare and Medicaid are unable to adequately cover the costs of LTC. It also sets out "8 Pillars of Financing Reform" to assure that every American will have access to needed LTC services. The goal is to "help maximize personal independence, self-determination, dignity, and fulfillment."

The Case Manager or Care Manager. Each client should have a *case manager* or *care manager* (**CM**), who oversees the client's care. The case manager is the local advocate for the client and is responsible for making sure that the client is receiving appropriate care. The case manager is often responsible for seeing that the client can manage his or her money. If the client is unable to do this, the case manager may be designated as the client's **payee,** receiving the client's monthly check and disbursing the funds appropriately.

Specialized Communities. Some corporations are developing communities for clients who have special needs. Examples of these communities may include young clients,

clients with specific disorders (eg, multiple sclerosis, head injury, Huntington's disease, Parkinson's disease, or clients on permanent ventilators), or clients of particular cultural or ethnic groups. The Centers of Excellence (**COE**) Programs have developed several centers to accommodate groups with special needs. These multidisciplinary programs include assessment, treatment, and rehabilitation therapy. One such COE is the Shepherd Program in Atlanta for clients with multiple sclerosis.

The impact of new "restraint-free" policies has caused changes in the treatment of clients with memory loss. Often, there is a separate unit for clients with dementia disorders such as Alzheimer's disease. These units are locked and alarmed and the elevators are kept locked. In many cases, these units are specially designed by an architect to provide a safe and secure space for the person to wander and to pace without feeling "hemmed in." The client who may wander away may wear a special Wanderguard or Ambularm device (Fig. 95-3). This device warns nursing staff if the person tries to leave the unit without permission. A buzzer located under the mattress warns staff of the unsteady client who attempts to get out of bed. The ultimate goal is to provide safety for the clients.

Respite Care and Daycare Programs. *Medical daycare programs* are often private or government non-profit organizations that provide respite care. This means that the client spends part of their time in a healthcare facility, giving the family some time to themselves (a *respite*). However, caregivers must be available to care for the client before and after the respite care. These respite programs often provide support groups for the family as well.

Services Provided to the Community by Long-term Care Facilities. Long-term care facilities may provide home care or assisted living services in the wider community. Meals, respite care, parish nursing, or hospital visitations are often provided. Some facilities belong to a consortium of healthcare providers in the community. The consortium allows community

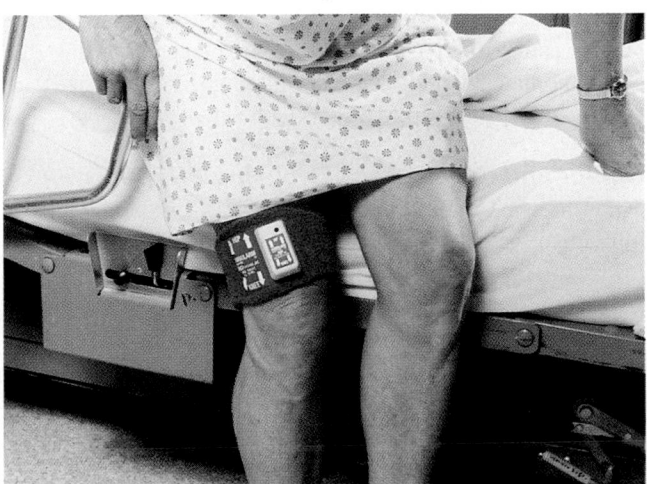

FIGURE 95-3. Changes in regulations have greatly limited the use of client safety devices (restraints) to prevent clients with dementia from wandering away. To provide safety, this client is wearing an Ambularm device, which will alert the staff if the client tries to leave the immediate area. (Photo courtesy of AlertCare, Inc.)

residents to receive dental, hearing, and vision care; podiatry and pharmacy services; as well as acute hospital care, without being residents of an LTC facility. Some facilities provide on-site medical clinics where persons from the community can visit their primary caregiver.

Services Provided by Volunteers. Long-term care facilities, and sometimes subacute-care facilities, have a cadre of volunteers who provide many services to residents. They may help run the gift shop, help with craft activities, provide beauty and barber shop services, take residents on outings, or visit with residents who do not have family nearby. Volunteers often read to residents or help them write letters. The volunteers may organize a bake sale or other fund-raising program to help raise money for special programs and activities. They often provide special items for the residents, such as craft materials, quilts, sweaters, toiletries, or stationery and stamps. They may give parties on special holidays and birthdays and may organize special programs and entertainment throughout the year. Some facilities have volunteers who help with the daily care of residents, serving as bed-makers or helping to feed residents who cannot feed themselves. Many of these services help provide more time for the nursing staff to provide skilled nursing care.

☛ Key Concept

The goal of all care is to provide the least restrictive living arrangement possible, while providing maximum safety and quality of life.

Independent Living Options

Many older adults and people with physical or mental disabilities are too healthy to be in an ECF, but still need help to live independently.

Community Programs

Programs in the community help clients to remain independent longer. Many community services are available, including subsidized and congregate housing, assisted living, home nursing care, and homemaker services. Chapters 97 and 98 discuss ambulatory and home care nursing. Many services are also available for hospice clients (see Chap. 99).

Senior and Other Special Housing Programs

Many housing variations are available for older adults and individuals with disabilities. A special high-rise or other building (**congregate housing**) may be designated for a specific group. These buildings may contain free-standing apartments and may have no supervision or minimal supervision. A person must qualify to live there and, in most cases, receives subsidized rent on a sliding scale based on income. Community services such as assisted living (see below) are available to residents of these apartment complexes. (This is known as "Section 8" housing in some states.)

A person may live in a *board-and-care home,* which provides room, board, and minimal supervision. Many people with mental illnesses and/or physical disabilities live in board-and-care homes.

The next level of housing is the *supervised group home* (known as a "Rule 36" facility in some states). In this facility, clients are supervised while taking their medications and they may be required to participate in some sort of treatment program or to work or volunteer some of their time. Meals and activities are provided. Many people with mental illnesses live in these homes, as do persons with physical disabilities. Chapter 93 describes facilities for persons with mental illnesses in more detail.

Other types of congregate living facilities provide more services for older clients or for those with disabilities. These facilities may serve one or more meals a day in a common dining room; they often provide planned recreational activities. Personnel from the facility usually check on each resident at least daily. Each apartment or room has a signal bell, so the resident can easily call for help in an emergency.

Hospice care, for persons who are terminally ill, may be provided to individuals in congregate living facilities. However, most hospice care is provided in the client's own home. Chapter 99 describes hospice care in more detail.

Assisted Living

Assisted living is the largest area of growth in long-term care and is one way to facilitate independent living. Assisted living programs are administered by both not-for-profit and proprietary organizations. Assisted living programs give older adults the opportunity to age in place in their own homes, while maintaining their independence, individuality, privacy, and dignity. Some people with mental and physical disabilities also need assisted living. Clients, together with their case managers, can choose necessary and helpful services. Available services include Meals on Wheels, laundry services, transportation to appointments, visiting pet programs, grocery delivery, or assistance with finances or housekeeping. Home care nurses may visit at regular intervals to evaluate clients, set up medications, or perform treatments, such as drawing blood for tests (see Chap. 98). They may set up a daily medication reminder box for clients. In these boxes, each day's medications are placed into compartments marked for that day and divided into administration times during the day.

Assistants may also help clients with activities of daily living (**ADL**), run errands, or provide companionship. Some clients require instruction in basic homemaking skills before they can live independently.

Some states have formal statewide assisted living facilities. These facilities require a certificate of need. The manager of each site must be certified. Certification of the site manager requires education, including classroom instruction and community clinical experience, as well as passing a state-administered test. Controversy surrounds this position because unlicensed assistants are allowed to administer certain medications. Visiting nurse associations may be asked to monitor these unlicensed assistive personnel (**UAP**). People who regularly receive services from UAP usually live alone or have inadequate support from family or friends. In other cases, family members learn to administer medications and to provide certain treatments to their loved ones.

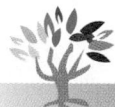

SPECIAL CONSIDERATIONS: THE LIFE SPAN

Today, people are living much longer than in previous generations: This presents unique challenges for healthcare. For example, the very old person may no longer have a satisfactory caregiver, because this person's spouse and children are now becoming old as well. What happens when the 75-year-old daughter can no longer care for her 98-year-old mother? What happens when the 80-year-old mother can no longer care for a son who is 58 and mentally retarded? These are situations brought on by the aging of America that must be addressed by today's healthcare and social services systems.

☛ KEY CONCEPT

Older adults and people with disabilities are spending less time in nursing-care facilities. The average stay is expected to continue to drop in the years to come. A great majority of these people now live independently.

There are many lifestyle choices for people, especially as they age. These options range from totally independent living to total care. The options between these two extremes include care facilities with varying levels of nursing care, assisted living in one's own home, short- and long-term rehabilitation units, and nursing home care. The goal of this care is to provide a safe and comfortable living environment, while allowing each person to be as independent as possible.

➔ STUDENT SYNTHESIS

Key Points

- Many lifestyle options are available for people who need varying levels of assistance.
- Clients may move from one type of lifestyle option to another, as their needs change.
- The least restrictive type of care should be given, to promote the client's independent functioning.
- The vast majority of older adults and people with physical and mental challenges live independently.
- Today's long-term care facilities offer safe and comfortable living. Many offer a wide variety of amenities.

Critical Thinking Exercises

1. Imagine that your aunt is 79, and her memory is failing. Her physical health is generally good, except that she is overweight and has type II diabetes mellitus. She smokes 1 to 2 packs of cigarettes a day and has a chronic cough. Your uncle (her husband) is living with her and is in good health. He stopped smoking more than 20 years ago. Knowing that you are a nurse, your uncle calls you in despair and says, "I can't take care of her any more!" The couple's only child (your cousin) is widowed and lives 75 miles away. He has one teenage child at home and one in college.
   a. What additional information do you need from your uncle in order to help him? What agencies or people would you suggest he call for advice and information?
   b. Identify community resources that are most likely to be available in your uncle's home town (or in the nearest large city).
   c. What questions should your uncle ask his family physician?
   d. If nursing home placement is needed, how can your relatives choose the best one?
   e. What level of long-term care would you recommend for your aunt?
   f. What role could your cousin play in the care of his mother?
   g. What are your personal feelings about this situation?
2. Interview a person in an assisted living program and one in a nursing home. What services do they receive? Compare and contrast the two in terms of the following:
   a. Client self-esteem
   b. Relationships with family
   c. Cost
   d. Services provided and desired
   e. Social interactions with peers
   f. Independence
   g. Role of the nurse

NCLEX-Style Review Questions

1. Which of the following clients would the nurse expect to care for in a subacute-care facility?
   a. Client with end-stage Alzheimer's disease
   b. Client recovering from hip fracture
   c. Client with permanent disabilities
   d. Mentally ill client
2. Which of the following describes a skilled nursing facility?
   a. Provides 24-hour care with a licensed nurse on duty
   b. Provides basic care with a licensed nurse on call
   c. Provides basic nursing care and families are required to bring in meals
   d. Provides housing and very little support care such as physical therapy
3. A client is living at home but complains of difficulty preparing meals. Which services would you recommend to assist the client?
   a. Arrange for grocery delivery
   b. Consult with a dietitian
   c. Recommend eating at a restaurant
   d. Recommend Meals on Wheels

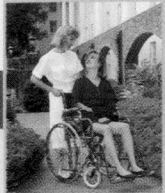

CHAPTER

96

Rehabilitation Nursing

LEARNING OBJECTIVES

1. Explain the goals of rehabilitation.
2. Describe the stages of adjustment to a disabling illness or injury.
3. Identify members of the rehabilitation team and their roles.
4. Relate rehabilitation to Maslow's hierarchy of needs.
5. Differentiate between functional and instrumental activities of daily living (ADL).
6. Explain adaptive equipment and home modifications that assist clients to independently perform ADL.
7. Describe rehabilitation in terms of mobility.
8. Discuss the major elements of a continence program.
9. Describe general rehabilitation for people with disabling musculoskeletal, cardiovascular, or neurologic disorders.
10. Give examples of community resources for people with physical and mental challenges.
11. Define the term architectural barrier and identify several in your community.
12. Identify barriers to rehabilitation for individuals and communities.

NEW TERMINOLOGY

architectural barriers
exoskeleton
hemiplegia
mainstreaming
neurogenic
orthotics

paraplegia
physiatrist
prosthetics
quadriplegia
rehabilitation

ACRONYMS

ALS	FES	MS
CF	HD	PM&R
CVA	IADL	PPS
FADL	MD	TBI

Many times rehabilitation is needed when a person is physically or mentally challenged, often as a result of injury or severe illness. Many people, in addition to the client, are involved in rehabilitation, including nurses, therapists, and family members. As a graduate nurse, you will find many opportunities for employment in rehabilitation nursing. Rehabilitation can occur in the healthcare facility, in the community health center, or in the client's home.

REHABILITATION SERVICES

Definitions of Rehabilitation

Many definitions of *rehabilitation* exist. In general, **rehabilitation** means restoring a person who becomes physically or mentally challenged to his or her former abilities as much as possible. If complete restoration is impossible, rehabilitation assists the client to adjust. Rehabilitation emphasizes coping with physical or mental challenges and learning to adapt one's environment to facilitate independence and safety.

Another definition states that the goal of rehabilitation is to restore the person to a quality of life that is highly satisfactory. Rehabilitation should offer clients optimal happiness and the ability to use all available assets. It should offer clients the most independence possible, not just survival or pain relief.

The outcome of rehabilitation is measured in terms of change in function resulting from the medical intervention. Each individual is assisted to become a participating member of society as much as is possible.

It is important to differentiate between treatment for an acute illness or injury and long-term rehabilitation services. An acute illness or injury is treated and the person often recovers and returns to normal activities, having encountered only a brief interruption. In long-term illness or disabling injury, the person must be assisted over time (in rehabilitation) and may never recover fully to the level that was enjoyed before the event.

The person requiring long-term rehabilitation often has many additional physical and emotional problems. For example, the person who has had a major *stroke (cerebrovascular accident* [**CVA**]) must overcome paralysis. Rehabilitation also addresses problems such as spasticity, skin integrity, *aphasia* (difficulty in speaking), *dyspraxia* (difficulty in performing coordinated movements), *dysphagia* (difficulty swallowing), vocational concerns, sexuality, incontinence, emotional lability, and the prevention of complications such as pneumonia or contractures.

☛ KEY CONCEPT

Remember that most long-term rehabilitation occurs in the community. Only the initial phase of the process occurs in rehabilitation facilities.

Rehabilitation and Maslow's Hierarchy of Needs

The principles of rehabilitation are based upon early recognition and individualized planning for each client. When Maslow's hierarchy of needs is applied to rehabilitation, the person in the acute stage of illness or injury first requires assistance with basic survival needs, such as maintaining an open airway and maintaining an adequate oxygenation level, obtaining food and water, and eliminating wastes. Next, activities of daily living (ADL) are addressed, such as being able to feed, dress, and bathe oneself; moving independently; and being able to communicate. Later, the person learns to work toward self-actualization and to be a creative and contributing member of society. (See Chap. 5 for a complete discussion of Maslow's hierarchy of needs.)

Rehabilitation presents many challenges and opportunities for members of the healthcare team. An extensive discussion of rehabilitation nursing is beyond the scope of this book, but this introduction illustrates that the principles and purposes of rehabilitation remain the same, regardless of the person's specific situation. The particular nursing skills and procedures needed in rehabilitation have been presented throughout this book and throughout your nursing program.

The goal of all rehabilitation nursing is to assist clients to approach normal functioning as much as possible; that is, to minimize the person's limitations and maximize his or her capabilities. Emphasis should be placed on the quality of life (Box 96-1).

Stages of Adjustment to a Disability

During adjustment to a physical or mental challenge, a person usually experiences grief reactions similar to those experienced when dealing with any loss (see Chap. 14).

➤➤ **BOX 96-1**

GOALS SET FORTH BY THE UNITED NATIONS PROCLAMATION OF 1981 AS THE "INTERNATIONAL YEAR OF THE DISABLED"*

1. Help people with disabilities in their physical and psychological adjustment to society.
2. Promote all national and international efforts to provide them with proper assistance, training, care, and guidance to make available opportunities for suitable work and to ensure full integration into society.
3. Encourage study and research projects designed to facilitate practical participation in daily life, such as improving access to public buildings and transportation.
4. Educate and inform the public of the rights of all people to participate in and contribute to various aspects of economic, social, and political life.
5. Promote effective measures for the prevention of disabilities and the rehabilitation of people who are disabled.

---
* These are appropriate goals for any rehabilitation program.

- Early reactions may be defense, shock, and denial. ("This can't be happening to me! I must be dreaming.") The person often is confident of recovery, assuming that the problem is not really happening. Conversely, the person may experience fear and anxiety.
- The client often experiences anger and wants to retaliate, asking, "Why me? I'll get even with someone for this!"
- Many people try to bargain with God or make deals. "I will be a better person if I can just recover from this."
- Eventually, the client with any disability must face reality and may experience depression or mourning for lost abilities.
- Hopefully, the client will come to accept limitations and actively participate in developing realistic long-range goals. Some people have great difficulty in attaining acceptance. Sometimes, psychiatric assistance or counseling is an essential part of rehabilitation. Children and adolescents who have been injured or who have degenerative diseases face additional challenges because they are dealing with disability or disease along with the usual challenges of maturation.

The Rehabilitation Team

The rehabilitation team includes the physician, nurse, advanced practice nurse or certified rehabilitation nurse, and therapists (physical, occupational, speech, music, recreation), as well as the vocational counselor, social worker, and psychologist. The client's case manager (care manager) is becoming an increasingly important member of the team. Physicians who specialize in rehabilitation are sometimes called **physiatrists** or physical medicine and rehabilitation (**PM&R**) specialists. Team conferences are held regularly during the rehabilitation process so that all members can establish common goals.

Preparation for Rehabilitation

The Home Assessment.   Clients and their families are vital members of the healthcare team. A home assessment evaluates the home environment and helps determine the appropriateness and possibility of considering home-based rehabilitation. Questions such as the following must be answered: Is it possible for the client to live at home safely? Are there stairs to negotiate? Are vital areas of the home accessible to the client? Are the floors too slippery to be safe? Do adaptations need to be made in the home?

In many cases, the family must make adaptations to prepare the home for the care of the client. Ramps up to the doors may be needed; railings in hallways, stairs, and bathrooms may need to be installed; doors may require expansion to accommodate a wheelchair or walker; and an open shower may need to be constructed. If the client is required to go up stairs, an elevator or lift may need to be installed (Fig. 96-1).

Availability of Primary Caregivers.   In addition to the physical layout of the home, the home assessment includes an assessment of available caregivers. Taken into considera-

tion are the caregivers' availability, skill level, and willingness and commitment to assist in the rehabilitation process. In many cases, the lack of an appropriate caregiver precludes allowing a client to live independently. The family or significant other must become primary caregivers in most cases (see Chaps. 98 and 99). They must understand the care involved and be willing to make a commitment to providing it. The client's motivation is also an important determining factor in the decision for the client to live at home.

Evaluation of the Disability.   Before rehabilitation can begin, the client is evaluated to determine the level of disability. Common tests include electromyography (EMG) (to determine electrical activity and potential of muscles), and a motor nerve conduction study (at rest, or stimulated [*elicited*]). Gait analysis evaluates how well the person can walk. Vision, hearing, speech, and language production are assessed. Psychological and neurologic testing determine the person's motivation, attitudes, and neurologic deficits. A functional evaluation determines the client's ability to perform ADL. Vocational assessment identifies skills, potential for homemaking or employment, and retraining needs. The team gathers all information and makes a plan for care.

☛ KEY CONCEPT

It is important for the nurse to assess the client for the use of complementary therapies and herbal supplements. Many clients do not consider these treatments as "therapy" and will not mention their use unless they are specifically asked. However, these therapies can significantly impact other therapies that the client may be receiving.

Nursing Considerations in Rehabilitation

Rehabilitation begins with treatment to halt destructive processes and repair body damage. It continues with preventing further injury and then restoring normal functions whenever possible. Increasing strength is often a goal of rehabilitation—this is important to regain or maintain independence, to allow mobility, and to reduce the possibility of falls. Because insurance may not cover the cost of a physical therapist, the nurse may be called upon to perform muscle-strengthening exercises.

In addition to physical support, rehabilitation nursing provides clients with emotional support. The rehabilitation nurse's most important quality is empathy. Rehabilitation nurses must be sensitive and offer encouragement and assistance. If you work in rehabilitation, you will help clients meet unique, complex and multidimensional needs, build interventions based on the client's strengths and resources, and envision rehabilitation as a logical and essential component in the health process across the life span. The scope of rehabilitation nursing practice extends from primary prevention, through acute and subacute levels, and beyond tertiary intervention into community and lifelong care.

Activities of Daily Living

It is important to encourage clients to become as independent as possible. Assist clients by giving them physical care and

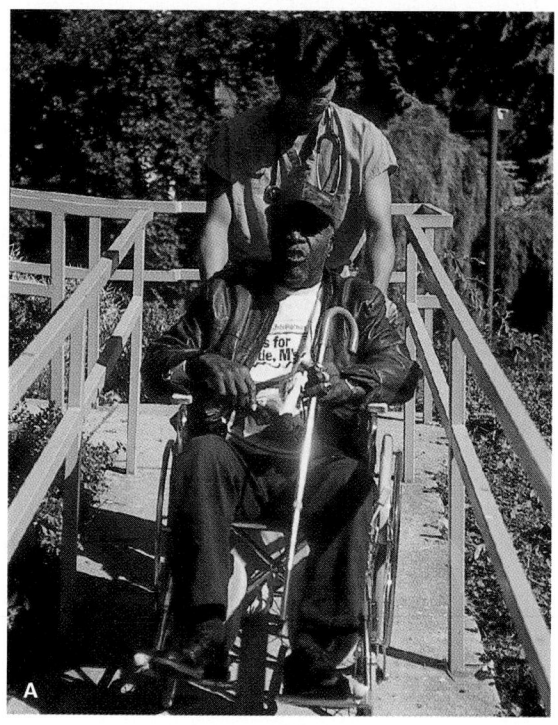
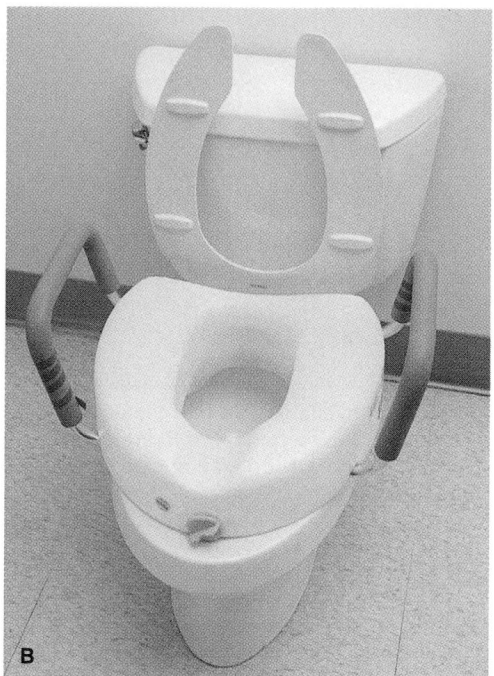
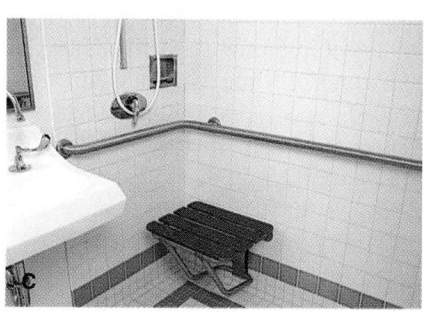
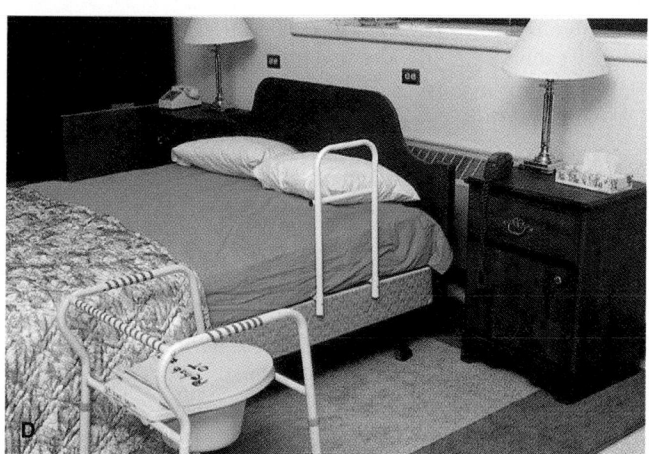

FIGURE 96-1. Simple adaptations allow a client to return home after an illness or injury. (A) A ramp to the door replaces stairs, to allow entrance by a wheelchair. (B) A raised toilet seat and grab bars make it easier and safer for the client to sit and stand. (C) This remodeled bathroom includes an open shower, shown with a built-in seat and sturdy handrails. Free-standing shower chairs and stools are also available. (D) Bed rails provide safety and give the person something to grab, to facilitate getting in and out of bed. A bedside commode is available so that the client does not need to walk to the bathroom. (This commode can also be placed over the toilet seat, to provide privacy and safety in the bathroom.)

encouragement, and helping them with self-care. It is vital for all clients to perform as much self-care as possible. Help them to move as quickly as possible through the stages of adjustment, so that they maximize their self-care abilities. Patience and perseverance are necessary. Clients and their families also must understand the extent of the disability and how it is possible to regain some—perhaps all—normal functions. Even in progressive or degenerative disorders, clients should be encouraged in self-care for as long as possible.

Certain specialized nursing care is important in the care of any person with a disability. Most procedures and condition-related protocols are described with individual physical con-

ditions in Unit 12. The index in the back of this book will help you find particular procedures or conditions. A paramount goal of rehabilitation is aimed at assisting the client to regain the ability to perform as many ADL as possible. Not only does this goal reduce the workload of the primary caregivers; it enhances the client's self-esteem.

When the rehabilitation team has thoroughly evaluated the client and determined what functional capacity is realistic, a program of retraining in ADL is initiated.

Functional ADL.   The basic functional ADL (FADL) include aspects of self-care such as dressing, bathing, toileting and continence, transfer, mobility, and eating (Fig. 96-2).

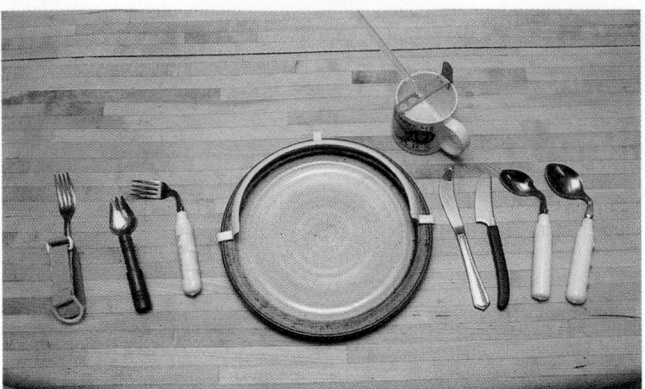

FIGURE 96-2. Many devices are available to allow clients with disabilities to feed themselves. Shown here (*L to R*) are: a fork with a hand strap, a combination fork/spoon, an angled fork, a plate guard to prevent food from being pushed off the plate, a partially covered cup with easy-to-grab handle and drinking straw, a small easy-to-handle knife, a partially rocking knife, and angled spoons with enlarged handles.

Sensory and communication levels (hearing, vision, and speech) should be evaluated. Because of disability, adaptations may be necessary so that clients can perform self-care activities. Teach and guide clients while remaining flexible. Box 96-2 contains examples of FADL.

Instrumental ADL. Instrumental ADL (**IADL**) are more complex living skills, such as food preparation, laundry, and money management. These IADL may or may not be achievable by individual clients. An important IADL is being able to purchase groceries and prepare meals.

The healthcare staff maintains an ADL record that informs all members of the healthcare team of the activities the client is able to do and those that he or she is attempting. Nursing care plans are continually updated with improvements or regressions in progress. See Box 96-2 for examples of IADL.

Modified Equipment and Adaptive Devices

There is a great deal of adaptive equipment available to people with disabilities. Much of this equipment has been invented and developed by people with disabilities to help themselves and others.

The Homemaker With a Disability. Devices have been designed to assist homemakers in caring for themselves, their homes, and their families (Fig. 96-3). Box 96-3 describes some of these adaptations.

☛ KEY CONCEPT

It is important to protect the disabled homemaker from burns or fires while cooking. For example, the person is taught to use a walker for support, rather than trying to stand alone. A fire extinguisher is kept within easy reach and the client is taught how to use it. The level of the stovetop may need to be lowered, in order to accommodate the homemaker in a wheelchair.

Adaptive Equipment. Clients with disabilities often need equipment modifications. Occupational therapists can

➤➤ BOX 96-2

EXAMPLES OF ADL

Functional ADL (FADL)
- Dressing skills (assistance needed)
- Cleanliness and self-care (bathing, grooming, care of teeth, nails, hair; assistance needed)
- Elimination (toileting skills, continence level)
- Taking of food and fluids (self-feeding, ability to chew and swallow, assessment of dysphagia)
- Communication (ability to talk or communicate in other ways)
- Activity and mobility level (walking and transfers, use of walker or wheelchair, skin condition)
- Ability to obtain rest and sleep

Instrumental ADL (IADL)
- ADL skills needed at home or at work (homemaking, laundry, vocational rehabilitation/retraining)
- Ability to use the telephone or computer
- Ability to shop for groceries and essentials
- Ability to prepare meals
- Management of money (paying bills, writing checks, using an ATM)
- Ability to drive or use public transportation safely
- Ability to read and write
- Ability to make appropriate choices of clothing for weather conditions, safety, and activities
- Ability to monitor medications (taking medications daily and on time), order medication refills when needed, report adverse side effects
- Ability to manage special sleep problems (PRN sleep medications, equipment to manage sleep apnea)
- Ability to manage special medical problems (eg, diabetes, emphysema, need for oxygen)
- Ability to manage special elimination devices (eg, incontinence pads, catheters, ostomy bags)
- Ability to make and keep appointments with physicians and therapists
- Ability to maintain safety (eg, making wise decisions about traveling, investments, and so forth)
- Ability to recognize physical and emotional difficulties and seek assistance when needed
- Participation in recreational and diversional activities, visiting with friends and relatives, being comfortable with going out in public

assist in improvising equipment. It is important to provide as much independence as possible, to increase the client's self-esteem. If there is adapted equipment available, it should be provided to the client (see Fig. 96-3 and Box 96-3).

Home Modifications. Adaptations to the home may be necessary to make it more comfortable and convenient for the client. For example, bathrooms and kitchens may be modified to allow access by a wheelchair. This may involve enlarging

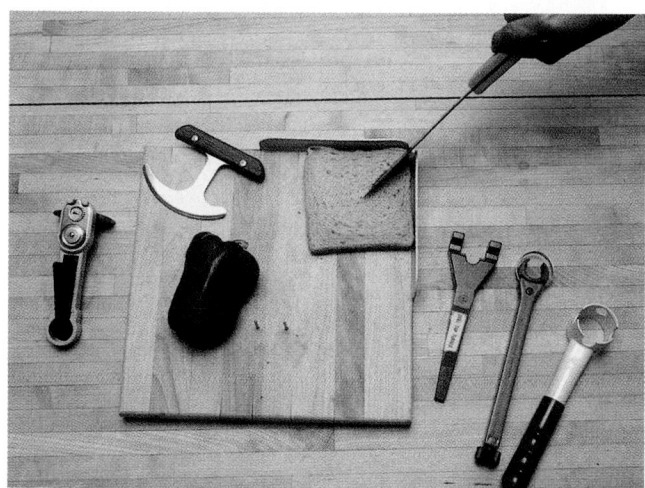

FIGURE 96-3. Adapted equipment can assist the homemaker with a disability to be independent in meal preparation. Shown here (*L to R*) are: a one-handed can opener, a rocking knife, and a food preparation board. This board has spikes to hold food for peeling or chopping and a guard in the corner, to allow bread to be buttered or cut. Items shown to the right assist in opening bottles and other containers.

the room or lowering sinks and counters. It is important for the person to be able to easily bathe, cook, and wash the hands. In some cases, funds are available to help the family with the expense of these remodeling projects.

Adaptive Clothing. A few changes or adjustments to regular clothing can often allow clients to dress alone or to be more comfortable (see Box 96-3 for some common clothing modifications). Many of these modified garments are used by the general public as well, so the person with a disability does not need to feel "different."

☛ Key Concept

Companies selling specialized clothing for persons with disabilities will often meet with groups of clients in a healthcare facility. Many clients are not aware of the attractive and easy-to-use clothing that is available.

Clients with disabilities can also learn how to dress more easily. For instance, clients with **hemiplegia** (paralyzed on one side of the body) can learn to place clothing on the affected arm or leg first and to undress the unaffected arm or leg first. The strong side is thereby free to help the weak side. Much of this teaching is just common sense. For example, clients can learn to put on socks before pants, so toenails will not catch on the pants. Toenails should be kept cut short, to avoid catching on socks. Most adaptive clothing is geared toward independence in dressing oneself.

Mobility

The nurse can teach clients basic bed movements and transfers from bed to chair, onto the toilet, and into the bathtub or shower. Independence is further enhanced when the client can leave home. Teaching transfer from the wheelchair to the car

is an important component of this independence (Fig. 96-4). Not only does mobility enhance independence and self-esteem, it also helps to prevent complications such as hypostatic pneumonia, pressure areas, thrombophlebitis, and constipation.

Wheelchairs and Scooters. Some clients are confined to wheelchairs or motorized scooters. Motorized wheelchairs are also available for those with limited hand or arm strength. Some clients can move about their homes using a walker, but need a wheelchair or scooter to move around outside the home.

Special wheelchairs are available for racing and sports. Some wheelchairs are equipped with various adaptive devices. A "rescue" wheelchair is available to assist in evacuation of wheelchair-bound individuals in an emergency. A standing wheelchair, although expensive, allows the client to meet people at eye level, providing additional mobility and self-esteem. Wheelchair lifts and hand controls are available for cars, enabling many clients to maintain independence in transportation. Various types of slings and pulleys exist, which allow the person with upper extremity weakness to write, eat, or perform other ADL.

☛ Key Concept

When talking to clients confined to wheelchairs or scooters, sit or kneel, so you are at their eye level.

Canes and Walkers. Many clients can achieve mobility just by using a cane or walker for support.

Several types of canes are available. The most common type is the half-circle cane, which is used by the person requiring minimal support. Another type of cane has a straight handle to assist the person who has hand weakness. The cane with four feet (quad cane) gives more support and aids in balance. The Lofstrand crutch or forearm-support crutch has a strap that fastens around the arm, freeing up the hand when needed (Figure 96-5). All canes must have good rubber feet, to grip and to prevent falls. Spikes are also available for canes, to provide better traction in slippery conditions. All canes and crutches are adjustable to the client's height. Many people paint or otherwise decorate their canes or use fancy canes, to express their individuality.

Several varieties of walkers are also available. Walkers are generally used for support and are moved along while the client walks. One type of walker has four rubber-tipped feet. Another type has two rubber-tipped feet and two small wheels. Still another type has four small wheels. Some walkers have a built-in seat, so the client can rest. Other walkers have a basket or shelf, to facilitate carrying things. Each client is evaluated to determine which type of walker will be the most comfortable and safe to use. The walker can be adjusted to the client's height.

It is important to encourage the client to move independently as much as possible. Chapter 48 describes and illustrates various types of crutches, walkers, and crutch-walking gaits.

Braces and Splints. Clients may need special braces or splints to support affected limbs or to maintain correct

➤➤ BOX 96-3

ADAPTIVE OR ASSISTIVE DEVICES USED IN REHABILITATION

Many items have been developed or modified for use by people with disabilities. Some of the general types of equipment are:

Personal Care and ADL Adaptations
- Long-handled comb or brush—allows the person with limited or painful arm mobility to comb the hair
- Long-handled shoe horn—allows the person to put on shoes without assistance
- Velcro closures instead of buttons—Velcro on shoes, pants, blouses, and so forth simplifies dressing for the person with limited manual dexterity
- Elastic waistbands—make dressing easier
- Elastic shoelaces—convert tie shoes to slip-ons, for easier access
- Large rings on zippers—for easier grasping
- Garter clips on long ribbon—to aid in putting on stockings
- Front-hooking bra or bra without hooks—to make putting it on easier
- Gowns or slips with front zippers—for ease in putting them on
- Gowns or dresses that fasten at the shoulder, instead of in the back
- Electric toothbrush—allows the person to brush the teeth with minimal physical effort
- Padded or enlarged handles on silverware or toothbrush, rubber handles, and handles with a loop for the entire hand—allow the person with difficulty grasping to feed himself or herself or brush the teeth
- Rocking knife—allows cutting by rocking the knife, instead of using a sawing motion. The food does not have to be secured with the other hand (see Fig. 96-3)
- Plate holder—to keep plate in place so a person can eat with one hand, or so a person with spasticity will not move the plate
- Food guard—acts as edge on the plate, so food will not be pushed off (see Fig. 96-2)
- Child's "sippy" cup—to prevent spills
- Smaller spoon, fork—for a person with arm or hand weakness
- Angled spoon, fork—for easier picking up of food and easier access to mouth (see Fig. 96-2)
- Divided plate—for a person with spasticity
- Shower stool or chair—to provide safety and independence for a person with weakness or instability. Some chairs have suction-cup feet, to further prevent falls.
- Bedside commode—for use at night, to prevent falls (see Fig. 96-1D)
- Flame-resistant, flame-retardant materials in clothing and bedding—for added safety
- Various slings, braces, etc.—to facilitate movement

Home Adaptations
- Ramp instead of stairs—facilitates entry into home by wheelchair, walker, scooter, or crutches (see Fig. 96-1A)
- Lever-style doorknobs—allows the person who cannot grasp a conventional doorknob to open doors
- Raised electrical plug-ins—allow the person to reach them from a wheelchair or without bending over
- Closets and cupboards with automatic lights—the light goes on when the door is opened, to avoid searching and reaching for the light switch
- Wider doors—to facilitate wheelchairs, walkers, or scooters
- Low pile on carpet—allows easier movement of wheelchairs, walkers, or scooters
- Removal of scatter rugs and low coffee tables—for easier wheelchair access and to prevent falls or stumbling
- Electric lift—allows people who cannot climb stairs to go up and down
- Raised toilet seat—allows people to sit down and stand up easier (see Fig. 96-1B)
- Location of toilet paper holder—may need to be moved to client's stronger side
- L-shaped toilet-paper holders—facilitate changing rolls
- Curtain instead of bathroom door—gives more room for wheelchair or walker
- Flush mechanism on toilet—must be easy to maneuver and to reach. Foot pedal may be used for those with limited hand mobility.
- Large shower—to facilitate bathing on a shower stool or chair, or in a wheelchair. Many people cannot get in and out of a bathtub safely (see Fig. 96-1C).
- Special-color and fluorescent tape on first and last stair—to warn the person of the stairs and prevent falls
- Small lights in darker areas—to prevent falls. Tap lights may be used for small corners and areas without lights.
- Tile instead of carpet, especially in bathroom and kitchen—to facilitate cleaning (and make movement easier)
- Flotation pads, egg crate mattresses, etc.—to prevent skin breakdown
- Seizure pads and side rails on beds—to prevent falls (see Fig. 96-1D)

Homemaking Adaptations
- Peeling board—the board has protruding spikes or nails to hold vegetables for peeling and slicing (see Fig. 95-3)
- Stationary scrub brush—the brush(es) mount inside the sink, to facilitate scrubbing hands, dishes, or vegetables
- One-handed equipment—various items are adapted for use with one hand. These include rolling pins, can openers, egg beaters.
- Bowl holder—a board with a hole in it can be used to hold a bowl while mixing foods
- Adjusted height—stoves, countertops, sinks can be lowered to benefit the homemaker in a wheelchair
- Removal of cupboard doors—for easier visibility and access
- Burner knobs placed on front of stove—for easier wheelchair access

(continued)

➤➤ BOX 96-3

ADAPTIVE OR ASSISTIVE DEVICES USED IN REHABILITATION (CONTINUED)

• Lift-type faucet controls—for those who cannot grasp knob
• Wheels on garbage cans—to facilitate moving out for disposal

Mobility Adaptations
• Canes and crutches—to give support and provide safety
• Wheelchairs and walkers
• Motorized scooters
• Wheelchair and walker baskets or tables—attached tables allow the person to work while in the wheelchair or walker. Attached bags or baskets allow the person to carry items.
• Backpack—allows the person to carry items and have both hands free
• Railings and grab bars—should be installed in bathrooms, hallways, stairs, and wherever needed. The person must be able to maneuver and must feel safe in the home. It is important to prevent falls.
• Telescoping cane—can be used when needed and then collapsed for easy storage. This cane also allows adjustment for the client's height.
• Cane spikes—to place on the tip of the cane for walking in snowy or icy conditions
• Chair lift or elevator chairs—lift the person up, so he or she can stand up easier
• Spikes for shoes or boots—for safety in slippery outdoor conditions
• Automobile lift for wheelchair—to allow access
• Hand controls to operate automobile—for a person with limited leg movement
• Special "handicapped" permit for automobile—to allow safer and more convenient parking
• "Geri chair"—to provide safe movement and a work or eating surface; helps to prevent falls that might occur if a wheelchair is used
• Braces, splints, prostheses—to provide support and facilitate movement

Adapted Equipment for People with Limited Vision or Hearing
• Large remote control for TV—allows the person with limited vision to see the numbers
• Large numbers on phone and alarm clock—for a person with limited vision
• Cards with large numbers or with Braille numbers—allow people with limited vision to see the numbers
• Appliance knobs in large print or Braille—for the vision impaired
• Appliance instructions and recipes on tape—for the vision impaired
• Volume control on telephone—allows people to hear better
• High-wattage light bulbs in lamps, with dimmer switches—allow clients with vision impairments to obtain more light; others can turn down the lights

• Talking thermometer—allows the non-sighted person to take a temperature
• Talking/chiming watch—for a person with limited vision or who is non-sighted
• Service animals—to assist and provide safety

Recreational Items
• TV remote control—allows people who have difficulty moving to change the channels and volume
• Magnetic game boards, boards with pegs, or boards with holes to hold the game pieces—allow people with spasticity or severe tremors to play games without losing the pieces
• Games with larger pieces—for easier handling
• Prism eyeglasses—allow people to read while lying down, without having to hold the book up
• Checkers or chess pieces with loops—for easier grasping
• Hand-held computer games—easy to manipulate and popular

Miscellaneous Items
• Long-handled tongs or specially designed grasping device ("grabbers")—allow people to reach and pick up items easier
• Computer—multiple uses. Helps people with aphasia to communicate. Enables visually impaired people to read because print can be enlarged. Allows homebound people to communicate or to work via e-mail.
• Electronic voice synthesizer—to facilitate speech for people with mechanical speech disorders
• Pill splitter—allows accurate dividing of pills for those who do not have the strength to break a pill in half
• Daily medication box—allows the client's medications to be sorted out by day and time of day. This technique helps the client to remember to take the medications and helps prevent duplication of doses.
• Electronic medication carousel and dispenser—sounds an alarm when medications are due to remind the client; dispenses correct dosage
• Panic alarms and automatic telephone dialers—allow the client to call for help in an emergency
• Hip, knee, or elbow pads—to prevent injury in the event of a fall
• Helmets—to prevent head injury
• "Handicap-accessible" buses—to increase mobility
• Self-adjusting blood pressure cuff—to make blood pressure measurement easier
• Easy-to-use blood glucose testing equipment
• Ambularm—for use by persons who are confused, to provide safety and to alert caregivers if the person leaves a particular area. Provides more freedom for the client (see Fig. 95-3)
• Large ashtray—for easier access and more safety

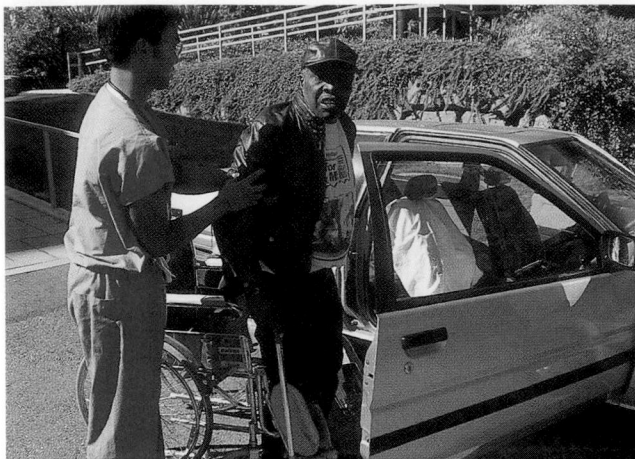

FIGURE 96-4. To regain mobility in the community, the client must be taught to safely transfer from wheelchair to car.

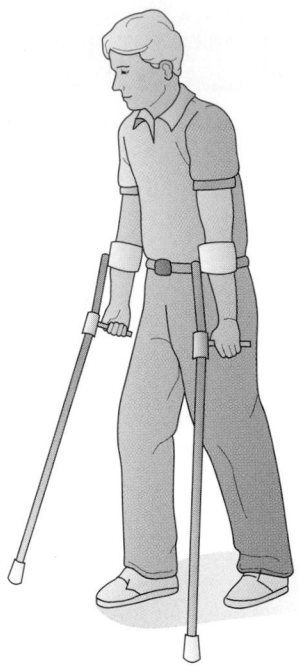

FIGURE 96-5. Lofstrand or forearm-support crutches are often used by the person with a permanent disability. These crutches allow use of the hands while still providing support.

positioning. The medical specialty involved in the fabrication of braces and splints is called **orthotics.**

Splints are available in two forms: *resting splints*, which hold the body part stationary and prevent the hand or limb from becoming contracted; and *dynamic* (moving) *hand splints*, which enable clients to function more easily than would be possible without them. Another type of splint is combined with a hook device for grasping objects (Fig. 96-6).

Braces are often applied to the legs for support, especially for clients with **paraplegia** (lower limb paralysis) or hemiplegia. Physical therapists teach clients to apply and remove braces, and nursing personnel reinforce this teaching. If a client has **quadriplegia** (all four extremities and possibly the trunk paralyzed), he or she may need a neck or back brace. This client may also use a type of inflatable trousers (**exoskeleton**) to maintain an upright position and prevent vascular collapse. Many clients also require special shoes or shoe inserts.

Artificial Limbs.   People who have had all or part of a leg or arm amputated are often fitted with artificial limbs. This specialty is called **prosthetics,** the fabrication and adjustment of prostheses. You may be familiar with the arm

prosthesis that resembles a "hook." This prosthesis provides movement and control similar to normal thumb–finger opposition (see Fig. 96-6). A leg prosthesis is fitted over the amputation stump and allows the person to walk and participate in sports (Fig. 96-7).

Today's technology has advanced the science of prosthetics. Artificial hands are available that look much like a natural hand, but still have the flexibility of the hook prosthesis. Some prostheses are electronic and/or computer-driven.

☛ KEY CONCEPT

Children may be fitted with prostheses or braces. It is important to change the size of prostheses or orthotics as the child grows.

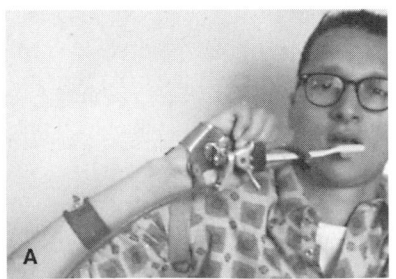
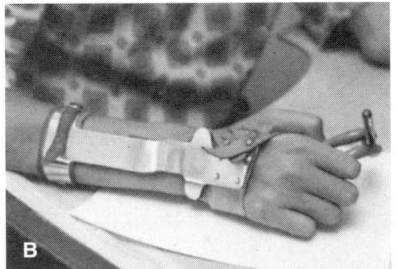
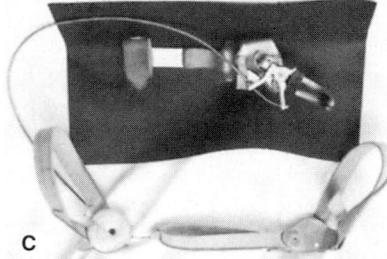

FIGURE 96-6. Many types of splints and slings are available. (**A** and **B**) Handihook, with an adaptive splint, aids in holding a toothbrush or pencil. The splint also helps prevent additional contractures of the fingers. (**C**) Handihook, showing shoulder harness and cable-activated clamp (hook). Movements of the shoulder and upper arm control operations of the hook. This type of device replaces the hand for a person who has had an amputation, or provides function for a person with impaired hand mobility. It offers grasping ability similar to the thumb–finger opposition of the normal hand.

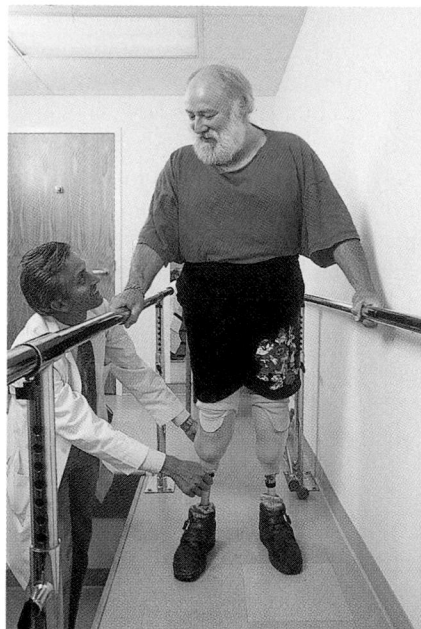

FIGURE 96-7. Persons with amputated lower limbs often receive prostheses soon after surgery. Therapists and nurses assist the person in learning to walk with the new prostheses.

Range of Motion and Flexibility.   Clients must perform range-of-motion (ROM) exercises to move all naturally moving joints. Physical and occupational therapists, as well as nursing staff, assist clients with ROM exercises. These exercises prevent joint stiffness and muscle shortening. ROM exercises are passive (PROM; done by the staff) or active (AROM; done by the client), depending upon the client's disability. Clients also may use the continuous passive motion (CPM) machine. Clients should be informed that exercise is important to build muscle strength, maintain joint mobility, and build endurance (see Chap. 48). Clients who spend long periods lying in bed or sitting in wheelchairs may become *hypotensive* (low blood pressure) when they stand. They should gradually adjust to being upright by using a tilt table.

Skin Care

Clients with impaired sensation or mobility are at high risk for skin breakdown. Measures for preventing pressure areas have been emphasized throughout this book. The following are nursing measures that do not require a physician's order:

- Keeping the client's skin dry and clean
- Using lotion instead of alcohol (which is drying) on the skin
- Keeping bedding free of wrinkles
- Changing bedding or clothing immediately if wet or soiled
- Using diapers or bed pads as needed
- Encouraging frequent toileting
- Encouraging adequate and varied fluids, including cranberry juice
- Repositioning the client at least every 2 hours
- Encouraging the client to be out of bed as much as possible

- Keeping crumbs out of the client's bed
- Giving backrubs; massaging bony prominences
- Using special devices for assistance (such as the hydraulic lift or turning sheet)
- Promptly reporting and treating any redness, skin irritation, or skin breakdown

The primary care provider may order the following devices or measures:

- Special padding or a flotation pad
- A special bed
- A high-protein diet
- Light or heat treatments
- Dietary supplements
- Vitamin or mineral supplements
- Antibiotics
- Special creams or ointments
- Special dressings, such as Duo-Derm or Tegaderm

Chapter 50 describes skin care in detail.

☛ KEY CONCEPT

Clients may visit an enterostomal therapist to assist in skin and wound care, as well as in the care of a colostomy or ileostomy. Clients are often referred to wound care or burn centers for evaluation, treatment, and teaching, in order to maintain skin integrity. Excellent skin care is vital in clients who lack sensation in a portion of the body, who are unable to move independently, or whose skin is particularly friable (fragile).

Elimination

A rapidly growing area of rehabilitation services involves caring for and treating clients with incontinence. Management of incontinence is a major factor in a person's quality of life. A person's independence and ability to live at home, versus being required to live in a healthcare facility, is directly related to continence vs. incontinence. Fortunately, treatment is available for most types of incontinence and nursing is actively involved (see Chap. 88). Increasing the care and treatment provided has led many clients, male and female, out of isolation. As they gain control of the bowel and/or bladder, they are often able to be out of the home, or some clients are able to get into single-room housing facilities or off the streets. At the very least, nurses need to realize that there are options for most people with incontinence.

A client who is paralyzed may have a **neurogenic** (lacking nerve stimulation) bladder or bowel. The lower the level of spinal cord injury, the less likely the client is to have difficulty with elimination. If the injury is high in the spinal cord, the client will often need bowel or bladder retraining to reestablish independent elimination patterns (see Chaps. 51 and 88). In some cases, bladder continence is not possible. This client may wear a leg bag for urine collection (Fig. 96-8).

Bowel Elimination.   If a person is paralyzed or lacks sensation below the waist, fecal impaction can become a problem. Some people manually disimpact themselves daily

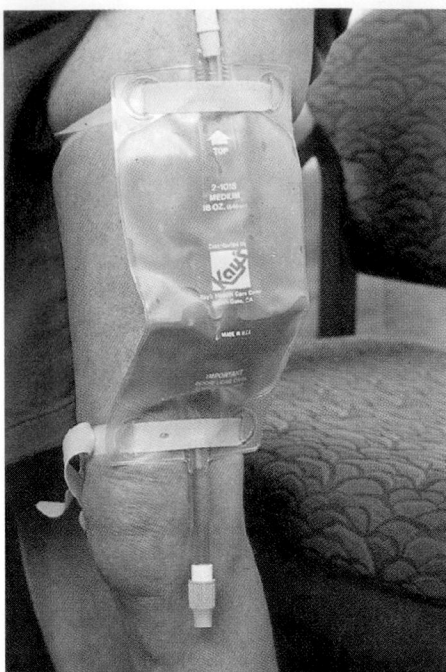

FIGURE 96-8. The person with untreatable urinary incontinence may wear a permanent leg bag, to facilitate cleanliness and independence.

as part of their bowel program. A well-balanced diet, adequate fluids, exercise, and regular times for bowel elimination are helpful preventive measures.

Bladder Elimination. Care of the client who has a neurogenic bladder is complex. Encourage fluid intake to approximately 3,000 milliliters per day. Help clients to establish regular patterns of voiding, beginning with voiding approximately every 2 hours and gradually increasing the interval. Teach clients to apply manual pressure over the suprapubic area (Credé's maneuver). Many people manage their bladder elimination by self-catheterization. As the bladder-training program is being established, clients may need to be awakened during the night to void.

Encourage the client who is incontinent to take fluids. Some people avoid fluids and do not have adequate fluid intake because getting to the bathroom is difficult or because they are afraid of incontinence. It is important to prevent dehydration in these clients.

☛ Key Concept

Some nurses specialize in continence care and set up programs for continence rehabilitation. *They assist clients who have bowel or bladder incontinence to achieve control and to manage their own elimination programs.*

Diversional Activities

All people who are hospitalized for extended periods or who have disabilities must find activities to occupy their free time and to increase their self-esteem. Occupational and physical therapists not only assist clients to find activities of interest, but also initiate exercises for specific muscles, to prevent deformi-

ties. Counselors help clients find appropriate job retraining and employment. Computers can assist many clients who have aphasia and other speech problems, as well as those with impaired vision, to communicate more easily.

Recreation and Sports. Many games have been adapted for use by people with various disabilities. Occupational or recreational therapists will have suggestions for diversional activities. Some activities have specific goals in mind. Examples include improving fine motor skills and eye–hand coordination by tying fishing flies or crocheting, or improving large-muscle strength by weaving on a large loom with weights attached.

National and local athletic events for people with physical and mental challenges are increasing (Fig. 96-9). Marathons have wheeled divisions for persons confined to wheelchairs. Many wheelchair-bound individuals also enjoy bowling, playing golf or tennis, or going fishing or sailing. Skiing, horseback riding, and many other activities are available to persons with disabilities. There are a growing number of wheelchair sports teams in basketball, table tennis, softball, and other sports. Adaptations of golf carts are available to allow golfers who cannot walk to enjoy the game. Some people also play golf or softball one-handed.

The National and International Special Olympics offer fun and competition and allow large numbers of people with physical or mental challenges to participate. Most of these people would otherwise be unable to compete in athletic events. The emphasis here is not so much upon winning as it is on "doing your best" and "fair competition."

Various programs and camps provide outdoor experiences for people with disabilities. With the availability of cell

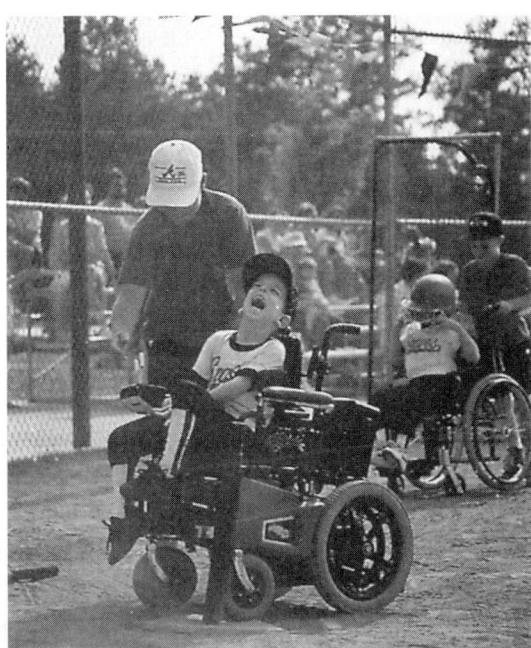

FIGURE 96-9. People of all ages who have physical disabilities are participating in and enjoying sports and other physical activities. Here, a boy plays in the Little League Challenger Handicapped Division.

phones, camping and wilderness experience has become much safer. Wilderness Inquiry is one such program that provides an opportunity to camp and canoe in the wilderness. Camp Courage is a camp in Minnesota designed specifically for clients with disabilities. Medical specialists are on hand during each session to provide therapy and to handle emergencies. Programs and camps such as these exist in all parts of the country, and many have volunteer opportunities for nurses and nursing students. For information, contact your local YMCA, Red Cross, Easter Seal Society, Huntington's Disease Society, or County Social Services department.

Pet Therapy.   Many clients benefit from having pets. Pets provide diversion and companionship and encourage responsibility. In addition, some facilities have resident pets or pets who visit on a regular basis. It is important to make sure that these pets have received their immunizations. The pet must be gentle and not afraid of strangers. Cats are usually declawed and are not allowed to go outside. Training is required on the part of the pet and the owner before they are allowed to make therapeutic visits to healthcare facilities. In addition to search and rescue dogs, therapy dogs were used during the World Trade Center crisis, to provide needed diversion for overworked firefighters and police officers.

Service Animals.   Service animals are useful as aids to persons with special challenges. Leader or guide dogs assist non-sighted persons to move safely about the community.

Hearing dogs assist deaf persons by alerting them to the telephone, doorbell, or intruders. Dogs and Simian monkeys assist clients with limited mobility. These animals can perform tasks such as delivering items to clients, turning on lights, and opening doors. Service animals are exempt from restrictions against pets entering public buildings and restaurants or flying on commercial airlines.

The Importance of Family and Friends.   All people need to feel worthwhile and part of a social group. Encourage the client's family and friends to visit in the facility and to take the client on outings. Special relationships often develop between generations. Both the client and the family can benefit from a special story or a game (Fig. 96-10). Some long-term care facilities operate child daycare centers where the residents serve as volunteers or paid employees. This arrangement provides mutual enjoyment and benefits to the children and to the facility and its residents.

The Scope of Rehabilitative Services

Many clients receive care from inpatient rehabilitation services at one time or another. Clients in rehabilitation facilities may have chronic conditions such as cystic fibrosis (**CF**), progressive multiple sclerosis (**MS**), Huntington's disease (**HD**), muscular dystrophy (**MD**), or acquired immune-deficiency syndrome (**AIDS**). These clients may remain in

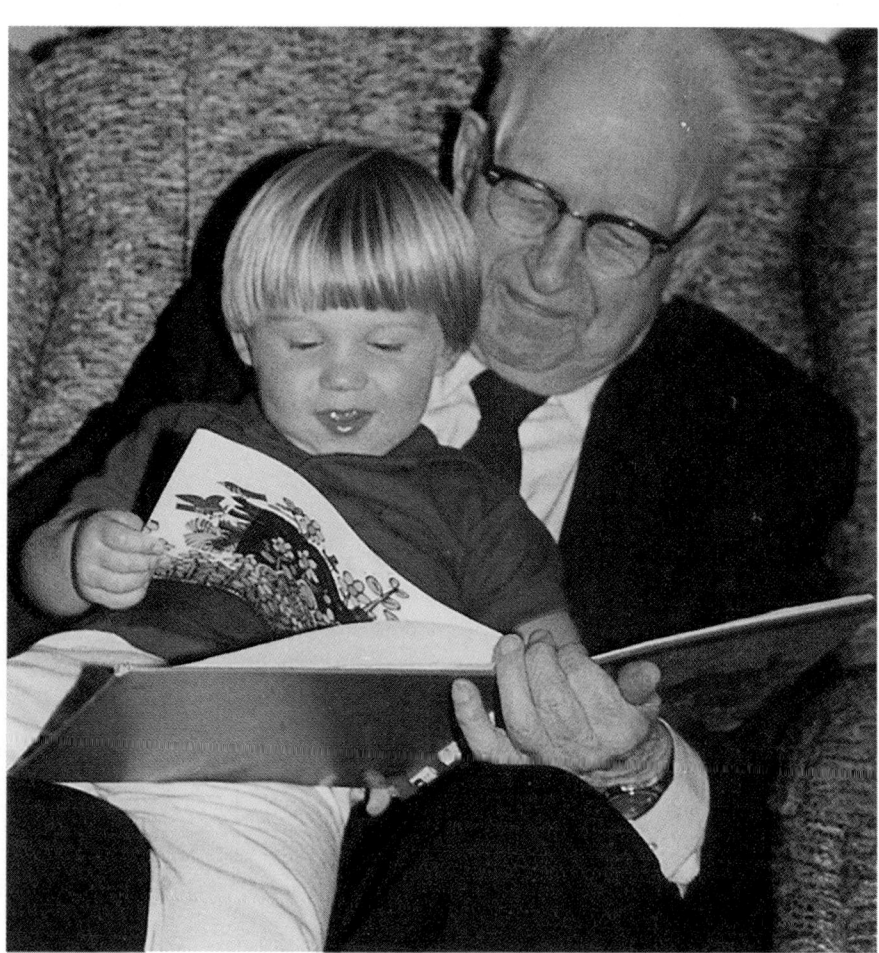

FIGURE 96-10. The importance of family and friends to the rehabilitation process cannot be overestimated. Both the grandfather and grandson benefit from a cozy story time together.

extended care for a long period of time. Other clients may be recovering from acute situations such as a gunshot wound, a traumatic head injury, a severe burn, a CVA, or a hip-joint replacement, and may leave the facility fairly quickly. Therefore, nurses who work in such settings must be able to perform a myriad of skills.

Burn Rehabilitation

The person who has been severely burned faces many challenges. After the initial crisis period, maintaining mobility, preventing deformities, and managing pain and itching are primary concerns. Restoring skin integrity is particularly important. Assist clients with passive and, later, active ROM and strengthening exercises to prevent contractures and hypertrophy of muscles. Clients may use braces and other orthotic appliances. Rehabilitation centers use various means to prevent scarring and contractures. Face masks and special tight gloves or body wraps provide tissue compression and vascular support. Skin and other grafting may be done. Special medicinal substances are often applied. Whirlpool treatments and hydrotherapy are common. Surgery and therapeutic exercise may be required to release contractures. Special face masks can enhance the appearance of clients with disfiguring burns. Clients often must deal with many emotional concerns. They often benefit from counseling and group therapy. They may also need teaching to learn to perform ADL or employment. Chapter 74 discusses burns and their treatment in more detail.

☛ Key Concept

The return to work or school following a severe burn, especially to the face, can be very emotionally challenging. This person needs a great deal of support from the healthcare system. The person's supervisor or teacher should also receive counseling and support, so that they can be most supportive to the recovering person.

Rehabilitation for Musculoskeletal Disorders

Many types of therapy are used to assist in movement and to relieve pain. Chronic conditions such as arthritis and low back pain often require ongoing nonpharmacologic pain management, as well as strengthening and stretching exercises. Clients who have fractured their hip or who have had a CVA will often need gait training and may need assistive devices to walk. Clients with spinal column disorders (eg, scoliosis or spina bifida) require varying levels of therapy, depending on the severity of the disorder.

Therapeutic heat and cold are used extensively (see Chap. 54). Varied equipment is used to provide heat, including diathermy and ultraviolet light (eg, sun lamps, black light). Ultrasound and lasers may be used as well.

Electrical therapy in the form of transdermal electrical nerve stimulation (TENS) assists in pain management. Functional electrical stimulation (**FES**) sends a stimulus to the nerves to move muscles. FES assists clients to move or walk, to improve gait, to reduce spasticity, or to better use hands and fingers.

Acupuncture can manage pain and other symptoms (see Chap. 55). Hypnosis and guided imagery are other possibili-

ties for pain management. Therapeutic exercise and physical therapy are essential treatments. They help clients maintain mobility of joints and muscles, develop coordination, and build strength and endurance.

In many cases, corrective or reconstructive surgery is performed. Joints, such as the hip, knee, and shoulder, are routinely replaced. Clients with amputations are fitted with prostheses and learn how to use and care for them. Chapter 76 discusses musculoskeletal disorders in more detail.

Rehabilitation for Neurologic Disorders

Clients with spinal cord injuries or severe head trauma usually require extensive rehabilitation. Many cities have special centers for rehabilitation of persons with traumatic brain injuries (**TBI**). Special home care programs are also available for these clients. When a client faces permanent *paralysis* (inability to move a part of the body), serious physical complications can occur. Major complications include contractures, pressure areas, and bladder and bowel disturbances. Many people with progressive disorders such as Alzheimer's disease (AD), HD, or amyotrophic lateral sclerosis (**ALS**) can also benefit from rehabilitation. See Chapter 77 for a more detailed discussion of neurologic disorders.

Sexuality.   Sexuality may be a concern for persons who are paralyzed or otherwise disabled. Many people with varying degrees of paralysis are able to participate in sexual activity.

Paralyzed men may need a penile implant (see Chap. 89). Proper positioning may facilitate intercourse. Women who are paralyzed can have sexual intercourse, become pregnant, and deliver normal children. Delivery may be by the vaginal route or cesarean method. Women with limited mobility and sensation may be concerned about vaginal or bladder infections. Frequent examinations by the healthcare provider will usually detect the presence of infection before it becomes a serious problem. Teach clients to maintain an adequate fluid intake. Dietary prevention of bladder infections also includes drinking cranberry juice and acidophilus.

Some counselors are skilled in dealing with human sexuality. They conduct workshops and seminars to discuss specific sexual problems of paralyzed individuals. Family members should also be encouraged to speak freely, express their feelings, and ask questions. Chapter 69 discusses sexuality and sexual disorders in more detail.

☛ Key Concept

Clients require individual counseling regarding sexuality because each case is different. The client and the partner should be carefully interviewed. In some cases, specific training is required. In other cases, all that is needed for satisfactory sexual intercourse is a position change. Other special adaptations to improve sexual expression are also possible. Love and understanding are necessary on the part of both partners.

Rehabilitation for Sensory Disorders

Clients with limited vision or who are non-sighted can learn to perform ADL. They may receive instruction in the use of

Braille for reading or use "talking books" (books on tape or CD). They may learn to use guide or leader dogs. In selected cases, surgery and/or the implantation of a special electronic device enables non-sighted people to have some very limited vision.

Clients with hearing disorders may use hearing aids. Changing technology in the development of hearing aids has provided hearing to many people who were not able to hear in the past. In the case of deafness, surgical procedures such as placing a cochlear implant may be effective. Specialized rehabilitation teams help clients to adjust to the world of sound and teach them how to care for and use the equipment involved. Chapter 79 discusses sensory disorders in more detail.

Computers are helpful both to the person with limited sight and the person with limited hearing, as well as to those who have difficulty in speaking.

Cardiovascular Rehabilitation

Following myocardial infarction (MI, heart attack), clients often need rehabilitation to return to normal activities. They must build endurance, without overtaxing the damaged heart. These clients need a great deal of encouragement and reassurance to overcome fear of another MI. Sexual issues may also be a major concern.

Following a CVA, clients often need extensive rehabilitation. Hemiplegia and aphasia are frequent problems following a CVA. These clients often need assistance with transfers, walking, speaking, eating, and visual impairments. They may be confused or emotionally labile. They may require vocational rehabilitation to function independently in the home or at work. See Chapter 80 for more discussion of cardiovascular disorders.

☛ KEY CONCEPT

Prevention is important in cardiac rehabilitation. The client is counseled about specific high-risk behaviors, in an effort to change behavior and prevent another heart attack or further cardiac damage.

Cancer Rehabilitation

Although cancer is quickly becoming a chronic rather than an acute illness, many people each year are diagnosed with the disease. These clients require various rehabilitative services. For example, men may require a penile implant after prostatectomy. After radical mastectomy, women may require special exercises and compression appliances to reduce *lymphedema* (swelling of lymph nodes). Breast reconstruction or breast prostheses are often used following a mastectomy. The person with either a malignant or a benign brain tumor may have symptoms similar to those of a client who has had a CVA. The person with lung cancer may need pulmonary rehabilitation. The person with cancer of an extremity may need assistance in learning to use a prosthesis. The possibilities for rehabilitation are endless, because cancer can be located in any part of the body. See Chapter 82 for a more detailed discussion of cancer and its treatment.

Rehabilitation in Respiratory Disorders

The rehabilitation team has intense involvement with clients who have chronic respiratory disorders, such as CF, or a chronic obstructive pulmonary disease (COPD) such as emphysema. These clients need chest physiotherapy, postural drainage, breathing exercises, inhalation treatments, and spirometry exercises. Chapter 85 describes respiratory disorders in more detail.

Psychiatric Rehabilitation

Most people with psychiatric disabilities are now living as members of the greater community, rather than in institutions. Some clients require a payee (see Chap. 95) to manage their money. Others only require instruction in IADL, such as grocery shopping, meal preparation, laundry, money management, and managing public transportation. They are then able to live on their own, without further services. Other clients require ongoing community services and support. Programs such as assisted living, homemaking, meal delivery, and ombudsperson/social service contacts may be all that are needed for the client to stay out of the hospital. A case manager helps to determine the services that are needed.

A major nursing role in the management and rehabilitation of the psychiatric client often involves assistance with medications or supervision of medication compliance. The nurse may make a weekly visit to set up the client's medications for the next week and to determine if the client has been taking prescribed medications. Injections of *decanoate* (long-acting) psychotropic medications may be given every few weeks. Clients who are taking the medication clozapine (Clozaril) require a weekly blood draw to continue receiving the medication. The nurse also observes the client for adverse medication side effects. The home nurse evaluates all clients to determine if they are managing adequately in the community or if hospitalization is needed at this time. Some clients need assistance in managing physical problems such as diabetes, asthma, urinary incontinence, or electrolyte imbalance.

If the client with a psychiatric disability cannot live independently, he or she may live in an extended-care facility such as a nursing home, a group home, or a board-and-care home. The client may live in a healthcare facility for a long period of time or the facility may serve as a transitional step between the hospital and independent living. See Chapter 93 for additional discussion of psychiatric nursing.

☛ KEY CONCEPT

Be respectful to any person who is physically or mentally challenged. Maintain the dignity of all people. Offer to assist clients if needed, but do not force your help. Do not touch the person's equipment, because many clients consider equipment as an extension of themselves. It is recommended to refer to such clients as "a person with a disability," rather than as a "disabled person." Each person has many abilities and only a few disabilities.

Community Resources

Members of the rehabilitation team must explore community resources with the client and family to plan for care and discharge. Public health nurses can be involved in preparing clients for home care, for which clients and their family need complete instructions (see Chap. 98). Family members should have actively participated in care while clients were in the rehabilitation center. By doing so, family members will have a clear understanding of the client's limitations and capabilities and of how to perform needed treatments after discharge. Public health nursing and home care services can assist these clients and their caregivers. Available home care services include home nursing, home health aide or homemaker services, social work, and physical, occupational, and speech therapy.

Each client should have a case manager, a requirement for reimbursement by Medicare and Medicaid. However, agencies appoint case managers for other clients as well. The case manager oversees the care and treatment of the client and acts as the client's advocate.

☛ KEY CONCEPT

Facilities to assist people with disabilities are available at no cost or for a low fee. For example, the Shriners' hospitals throughout the country provide free hospitalization, surgery, and rehabilitation for children with physical disabilities. Rehabilitation facilities, such as the Sister Kenny Institute in Minneapolis, often operate on a sliding-fee scale, based on the client's ability to pay.

Various health agencies and private companies have equipment such as hospital beds or wheelchairs available for loan, rent, or purchase. Almost every person can regain a certain amount of function by using special devices and aids. An occupational therapy assessment of the home is particularly helpful in recommending adaptations for the homemaker. The government provides vocational rehabilitation testing and counseling services and financial aid for retraining.

Most young people who are physically or mentally challenged attend regular classes in schools. This process is called **mainstreaming.** These young people participate in school activities and have the opportunity to mingle with others their own age.

Legislation

In recent years, laws have been passed to aid people with disabilities to live more independently. Not only does this reduce tax burdens, but it also enhances the self-esteem of clients.

Architectural Barriers. Government policies emphasize the need to make public buildings accessible and safe for all people. All new construction must include ramps for wheelchairs, elevators, and pneumatic doors. This reduction of **architectural barriers** has enabled many people with disabilities to become employed and to lead more satisfying and productive lives. Removal of architectural barriers also allows people to do everyday things such as shopping, going to school and church, or attending athletic events and concerts.

Parking for People With Disabilities. Clients with mobility limitations usually receive special parking permits. Areas near public buildings must be designated as parking for those with disabilities. These areas must have ramps over curbs and extra space for wheelchairs and scooters to maneuver. It is illegal for anyone else to park in these designated spots.

✚👁 N u r s i n g   A l e r t

Work with your legislators to remove *architectural barriers* that limit the mobility of people in wheelchairs. It is illegal for any non-disabled person to park in a designated "disabled" parking spot, even for a minute. Most states issue substantial fines for violations. Report anyone who illegally uses designated "wheelchair" parking spaces.

Preferential Seating. Airlines reserve special seats for people with disabilities. For example, bulkhead seats may be more comfortable for persons with leg braces or artificial limbs. Sports arenas and theaters have spaces for people using wheelchairs, with adjacent seats for the persons accompanying them.

Barriers to Rehabilitation

Some clients encounter obstacles that interfere with their access to rehabilitation services. Some of these barriers to rehabilitation are described below.

Legislative Barriers. The laws relating to delivery of and reimbursement for rehabilitation and long-term care services are continually changing. At the time of this writing, additional changes in the prospective payment system (**PPS**) were being proposed and written into law and into the rules and regulations of agencies such as Medicare. For example, since October of 2000, home care services have been paid on a PPS basis by Medicare. This system will be implemented in extended-care facilities in the near future. As eligibility requirements change, the pool of clients who are served will change as well. Clients may find this very confusing and cumbersome, as well as frightening.

Agencies delivering these services often find that the amount of paperwork required is overwhelming. Nurses may feel that they must spend too much time filing reimbursement requests and filling out forms, instead of delivering client care.

Financial Barriers. The cost of long-term care and rehabilitation services is staggering. Many families do not have adequate—or in some cases *any*—insurance coverage. They may not be able to afford needed care. In many cases, a person's entire life savings is used to pay for one illness or rehabilitation after an injury. Many people now have long-term care insurance to guard against this possibility. Additional discussion of payment for long-term care and home care is contained in Chapter 98.

☛ KEY CONCEPT

In addition to the entire range of long-term care and rehabilitation facilities, there is a broad range of financial reimbursement programs.

- *Private insurance*
- *Medicare or Medicaid reimbursement*
- *Organizational support, such as homes that are sponsored by an organization, a church, or an employer. If the resident's funds are depleted, the client will continue to be cared for by the organization.*
- *Subsidized coverage*
- *Care paid for totally by personal finances*

Attitudinal Barriers. Some clients and families are embarrassed about requiring rehabilitation services. They may feel that they should be able to take care of the family member without assistance, and may feel guilty when this is not possible. Many people feel that they should be able to keep "Grandma" at home even though she requires full-time nursing care.

The client may also feel guilty about the amount of family time and money being spent on his or her care; this impacts the dynamics of the entire family. Some clients become very depressed and may "give up." This makes rehabilitation very difficult. These clients may be so devastated by the illness or injury that they do not have the energy to begin or to continue the slow process of rehabilitation.

✚👁 **N u r s i n g   A l e r t**
Be aware that suicide is a possibility for the client who must undergo a long rehabilitation or who has a progressively worsening condition.

Body image is greatly affected, especially if a young person has been seriously injured or paralyzed. This constitutes a barrier to rehabilitation if the person is not able to accept the situation and the limitations it imposes.

In some cases, family members are not supportive or are unable to assist with care. In the case of many older peopl_ a suitable primary caregiver is not available. The sp__able any children the couple have may also be older__er rela_ to care for their family member. The person__orking full-tives are often living in another area and __ay not realize the time, making them unable to provid__o difficult for some

Educational Barriers. So_ rehabilitation begins, benefits of rehabilitation serv_. An important component people to understand th__ts and their families about the the more likely it is __tation. of nursing care is t_ goals and ben__

___sider the client's ethnic and religi__lita-
☛ K_ _planning, carrying out, or evaluating__o the
_-term care. Reactions to illness or in___sonal.
tion process may be cultural, rather t

It is the job of the rehabilitation team to work with clients and families in an effort to eliminate the barriers to rehabilitation and to encourage the client to live a happy and productive life.

➤ **STUDENT SYNTHESIS**

Key Points

- Rehabilitation aims to restore a person to full functioning or to maximize the client's remaining abilities.
- Professionals from many different disciplines function as part of the rehabilitation team.
- The client and the primary caregivers are vital members of the rehabilitation team.
- Clients and families often work through predictable stages of grief in dealing with serious illness or a disabling injury.
- Rehabilitation team members assist clients in performing strengthening exercises to prevent falls or other injuries and to provide mobility.
- Adaptive materials are available to assist the person with a disability to perform ADL.
- Many pieces of equipment, including wheelchairs, scooters, walkers, splints, and braces, help provide mobility to people with disabilities.
- Continence management is a major component of rehabilitation.
- Many community esources and agencies are available to assist peope who have disabilities or chronic conditions and th_r families.

Critical Thinking Exercises

1. A young marred woman who has paraplegia comes to you with qestions about her sexuality. Anticipate what qrestions she might a_. Formulate possible answers

2. Mr. Y. Abdul, a 34-y__-old man from Ethiopia, has been in the U__ States for 7 months. His wife an_ family are __ Ethiopia. He was planning to _eturn to Ethi__ next week, when his visa expired. Three week__o, Mr. Y. sustained a severe spinal cord inju__d a fractured right femur in a motor vehicle __sh. He was transferred to your rehabilita-on __ after the acute period of stabilization. H_ has __n classified as paraplegic, although he h_ so__ sensation in his legs. The physicians h_ hewill eventually be able to achieve b_ bladder control. He has no difficult__ eating. His skin is intact. He spe__ __at you English. He is unemployed an__an to

   a. Describe major aspects __ need to address in h_

   b. How would you __ evolve in you_

c. Discuss the following aspects of Mr. Y's care: mobility, bowel and bladder continence, sexuality, skin integrity, nutrition, communication, diversion, emotional and financial support, and spirituality.

d. What type of living arrangements might be available for Mr. Y after discharge from the rehabilitation unit?

NCLEX-Style Review Questions

1. A client is leaving the acute-care facility and asks what is meant by rehabilitation. Which of the following statements would be appropriate for the nurse? "Rehabilitation means:
   a. actively seeking the cause of the client's current condition."
   b. motivating the client to change past behavior patterns."
   c. preventing the client from having similar problems in the future."
   d. restoring a person to his or her former abilities as much as possible."

2. Which of the following is an example of instrumental activities of daily living?
   a. Ambulating to the bathroom
   b. Food preparation for a meal
   c. Getting dressed in the morning
   d. Showering without assistance

3. A client is incontinent of urine and has decreased oral intake to prevent incontinent episodes. Which action is a priority for the nurse?
   a. Instruct client to increase fluids to prevent dehydration.
   b. Manually remove impacted feces.
   c. Offer to assist the client to the bathroom at least every 6 hours.
   d. Teach client how to perform the Créde's maneuver.

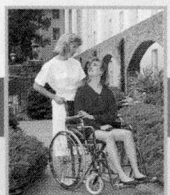

CHAPTER

97

Ambulatory Nursing

LEARNING OBJECTIVES

1. Explain what is meant by the "trend toward community-based healthcare delivery."
2. Describe the functions of the nurse who works in a physician's office, in an emergency room or urgent-care center, and in the same-day surgery center.
3. Discuss the benefits of same-day surgery.
4. Describe scientific developments that have made same-day surgery possible.
5. List and describe the classifications of potential clients for same-day surgery.
6. Describe the importance of client and family teaching in ambulatory healthcare.

NEW TERMINOLOGY

cardioversion	port
emergi-center	stabilization (stāb) room
endoscopy	telehealth
managed care protocol	vertical clients

ACRONYMS

ACS	EHS	PCP
CHC	FHC	SRO
CIC	HMO	

The early chapters of this text introduced you to the concept of community-based healthcare. Chapters 95 and 96 discussed nursing in extended-care and rehabilitation settings. In this chapter, nursing in other community-based settings is discussed.

Community-based healthcare is, by far, the fastest-growing segment of the healthcare industry. In these settings, you will encounter many exciting challenges and learning opportunities. Graduates of all nursing programs are finding increased employment in community-based healthcare.

AMBULATORY HEALTHCARE

Chapter 7 discussed the concept of the community health center as a major provider of primary healthcare. It also briefly referred to public health departments and visiting nurse organizations. This chapter continues that discussion by focusing on ambulatory healthcare. The term *ambulatory healthcare* refers to the care of those clients who do not need to be in an acute-care hospital setting. Many clients receive all of their basic healthcare in community-based facilities and are never hospitalized.

☛ Key Concept

Ambulatory healthcare and home care are, by far, the fastest-growing segments of the healthcare industry.

It is understood that primary client care may be delivered by either a physician or by another primary care provider (**PCP**). Persons such as the clinical nurse specialist, the advance practice nurse, or the trained physician's assistant may deliver primary healthcare. This person is considered to be the client's PCP. PCPs work in coordination with a physician.

The Role of the Nurse

In ambulatory clinics or community healthcare centers, nurses have the opportunity to use many of the skills learned in basic nursing programs. In addition to routine client care skills, nurses in ambulatory settings perform other duties not usually performed by nurses in acute-care settings.

Nursing Alert

Remember: The underlying principles of nursing care, such as safety, asepsis, and confidentiality, apply in all healthcare settings.

Some functions of the nurse in ambulatory care are unique. As this type of nurse, you might:

- Make appointments and set up schedules for physicians and PCPs. Call to remind clients of their appointments.
- Initially triage all clients, to determine clinical acuity and the need to be seen immediately. (In some states, initial triage must be performed by an RN.)
- Make sure the client's charts are all pulled and complete before the client sees the PCP.
- Perform a baseline intake assessment, including height, weight, and vital signs.
- Interview the client to determine the client's "chief complaint": the reason for today's visit to the clinic or care center. Document any special concerns or symptoms.
- Ensure that clients are seen quickly, efficiently, and with a minimum of paperwork and "red tape."
- Assign clients to examining rooms and keep the schedule moving on time. Notify waiting clients if their wait will be excessively long.
- Instruct clients as to what will be required. For example, "Take off all your clothes above the waist and put on this gown, with the opening in the front."
- Assist with examinations, including gynecologic, general physical, and neurologic examinations.
- Assist with sterile procedures, including placement of sutures and some ambulatory surgery.
- Perform special procedures, as ordered by the PCP. These procedures might include suture removal, cast removal, vision and hearing screening, or flushing the client's ears. The nurse may draw blood for special tests or may do a fingerstick to determine the client's blood glucose level.
- Prepare and collect specimens and slides.
- Administer special treatments, such as ultrasound, heat treatments, or application of medicinal creams and ointments.
- Take basic x-ray films in some settings.
- Perform special, non-nursing procedures, such as laboratory procedures, electrocardiograms (ECGs), and inhalation/nebulizer treatments.
- Assist with teaching clients and families. Answer their questions.
- Call in prescriptions to pharmacies, following specific orders from a physician, osteopath, dentist, or advanced practice nurse. (In some states, only RNs can make such telephone calls.)
- Schedule clients for additional tests or surgery.
- Assist with referrals to other physicians and specialists.
- Arrange for hospital admission when necessary.
- Qualify clients for third-party payer reimbursement, and process insurance claims.
- Wrap and sterilize supplies by autoclave or other methods.
- Keep records, including billing, appointments, and laboratory reports.
- Track preventive and health-promotion procedures, such as immunizations and periodic health screenings.
- Administer injections such as antibiotics, tetanus toxoid, and immunizations.
- Administer skin-scratch tests and intradermal screening tests such as the PPD (for tuberculosis [TB]) and appropriate controls.
- Clean and restock rooms and order supplies.
- Follow up with clients by telephone to see how they are doing.

Types of Ambulatory Facilities

There are several general types of ambulatory healthcare facilities. These include private clinics, specialized clinics, community health centers, and emergency care centers.

Private Clinics

Private physicians or groups of physicians often practice in clinics, which may be associated with hospitals or may be free-standing. Other professionals who work in these clinics include advance practice nurses, general staff nurses (RNs and LPNs), and various specialists and office personnel. Some of these clinics make walk-in services available, although many require appointments. Services are usually provided on a fee-for-service basis and clients may be required to have insurance coverage for nonemergency care.

Because community health centers are rapidly becoming the healthcare provider for many special populations, private clinics tend to see only those clients with insurance. Special populations, such as the homeless and the elderly, are more likely to receive primary care at the community health center, as are many of the local neighborhood's residents.

Specialized Clinics and Services

Target Populations and Mobile Clinics. Specialized clinics serve target populations. For example, they may be open a few days a week in a shelter or downtown area to specifically serve homeless or elderly individuals. In other situations, a mobile outreach clinic is housed in a van and comes into the community to provide healthcare to its residents. The van visits sites including retirement centers, soup kitchens, homeless shelters, boarding houses, and single-room occupancy (**SRO**) hotels (Fig. 97-1). They may also set up in a shopping mall or busy downtown district on certain days of the week.

Clients can receive basic healthcare and screening at these clinics without appointments. If the client has a primary

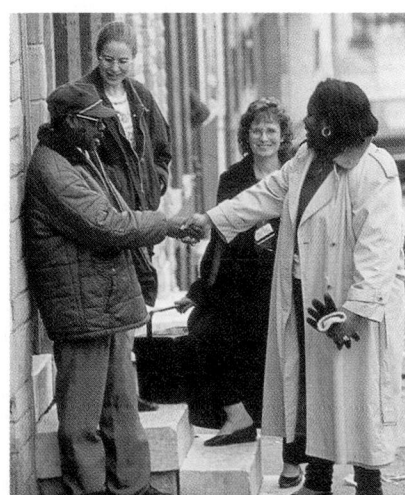

FIGURE 97-1. Community healthcare can be delivered wherever people are located. This may include a shopping center, a retirement center, a homeless shelter, or a single-room occupancy hotel.

healthcare provider elsewhere, these clinics report their findings, so that necessary followup measures can be taken. However, the mobile clinic or community clinic is the only source of healthcare for many clients.

Staff members in the mobile clinic take vital signs, measure blood sugar levels, perform gross vision or hearing screenings, and may hold special events such as health fairs, immunization clinics, or screening for scoliosis, diabetes, or high blood pressure. Screening for other conditions, such as human immunodeficiency virus (HIV), TB, or hepatitis, may also be done. Staff members also perform a great deal of health promotion and teaching.

Rural Services. In some rural counties, vans visit different towns each day to provide needed services that cannot be provided by the local small hospital. Examples include computed tomography (CT) scan, magnetic resonance imaging (MRI), mammography, or dialysis.

Another type of specialized mobile clinic is one that is provided for a particular ethnic group, such as Native Americans or Alaska Natives. In Alaska, for example, a healthcare team flies to a different village each day to provide primary healthcare (including vision and dental care) to the residents.

Clinics for Particular Conditions. Some clinics or resource centers specialize in particular disorders or diseases. Examples include HIV/acquired immunodeficiency syndrome (AIDS), including confidential testing for the virus. Other clinics specialize in conditions such as closed head trauma, cystic fibrosis, scoliosis, or Huntington's disease.

The School-Based Health Service. The school-based health service is becoming increasingly important in the delivery of primary healthcare to children and young people. This health service may be located at the elementary school, middle school, high school, or college. In addition to school nurses, many of these programs also employ an advance practice nurse. In this manner, primary healthcare can be provided. Many school sites are designated as community health centers. The comprehensive school health service has proven to be significant in reducing lost days of school.

Services provided by the school-based health service often include:

- Diagnosis of common illnesses
- Treatment of common childhood diseases
- Basic hearing and vision screening and referral
- Administration of immunizations and skin tests for TB
- Administration of medications
- Treatments such as dressing changes, care of a colostomy or ileostomy, management of a urinary catheter, aerosolized nebulizer treatments, or assistance with special orthopedic exercises
- Screening for conditions such as scoliosis, diabetes, or asthma
- Assistance with splints, casts, crutches, and management of skin breakdown or related problems
- Analysis and correction of architectural barriers within the facility
- Accident reduction
- Diagnosis of complex medical conditions

- Referral to specialists for complex medical care
- Services to adolescent parents and their babies
- Services for children with severe disabilities. In some cases, an attendant is provided for a child, to assist him or her during the entire day.
- Followup of students with excessive absences
- Health counseling for students regarding concerns such as eating disorders, prevention of pregnancy and sexually transmitted diseases (STDs), smoking cessation, drug abuse, anger management, rape prevention, and so forth
- Support groups for recovering alcoholics and students with addictions
- Reporting of suspected child abuse
- Teaching in all areas of health and wellness

The Employee Health Service.   Many large employers have an employee health service (**EHS**) that provides some primary healthcare to the company's employees. Immunizations, health screening, health counseling, and referrals to specialists are usually available. In some companies, the EHS must assess the employee who has been ill and grant permission before the employee can return to work. The EHS also works with Workers' Compensation and the Occupational Safety and Health Administration (OSHA) in many companies.

Telehealth.   Many hospitals, health maintenance organizations (**HMO**s), and visiting nurse services offer call-in services, which may be in the form of crisis lines or "nurse lines" (**telehealth**). These services provide general health information, counseling, and referrals. The nurse uses a computer to triage each call, to determine its disposition. The caller may be referred immediately to emergency services, may be instructed to see his or her PCP the next day, or may be given suggestions for managing current healthcare concerns independently.

Support Groups.   Some community agencies facilitate support groups. Common group designations include coping with cancer, grief and loss (bereavement groups), and mutual support groups for primary caregivers and families of mentally ill people or people with Alzheimer's disease. Hospice nursing and related support groups are addressed in Chapter 99.

The Community/Family Health Center

The government publication *Healthy People 2010* continues to promote the idea of the community/family health center (**CHC** or **FHC**) as a provider of primary care for a large segment of the population (Fig. 97-2). In the year 2000, the National Association of Community Health Centers stated that nearly 47,800,000 people in the United States had no other source of primary healthcare. Therefore, community health centers are major providers of ambulatory and primary care in the United States.

In the year 2000, there were 867 separate CHC/FHCs in the United States. The vast majority of these centers (687) were non-profit and federally designated and funded. Another 180 centers were classified as "look-alikes" and were funded by other sources. In 2000, these 867 centers provided primary healthcare at 3,301 sites, serving nearly 10.5 million people. (This is an increase of several hundred sites since 1996.)

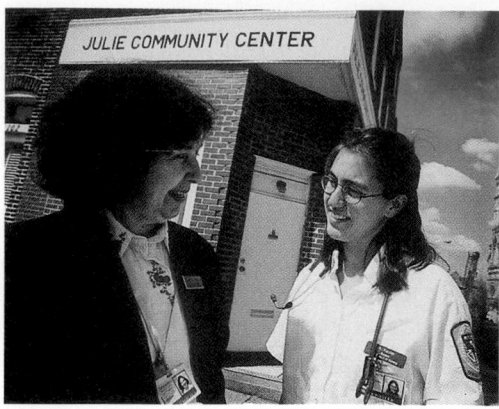

FIGURE 97-2. Community health centers are the only providers of primary healthcare for nearly 48 million people in the United States.

☛ KEY CONCEPT

Many people consider the community health center to be their "family doctor."

Reimbursement for healthcare in these community centers is a mix, with clients having insurance (usually Medicaid), a managed care contract with the local community, or receiving state-financed "uncompensated" care. In the latter case, the state covers some of the cost of care for the uninsured. Local communities sometimes pay for some care for clients who receive general assistance. Many centers offer clients a sliding fee scale.

The target population of CHC/FHCs consists of low-income and medically underserved communities, especially those with few other health resources. These people frequently are homeless and, in many cases, are very old or very young. However, many of the centers appeal to the local community, and the majority of the residents in that neighborhood may receive their primary care at the center.

CHC/FHCs are staffed by physicians, nurses, dentists, therapists, and other health professionals. The centers employ more than 50,000 people nationwide, many of whom live in the neighborhoods they serve. Many centers employ LPNs. In some cases, the staff members volunteer some of their time.

The CHC/FHCs offer a wide range of services, including primary and preventive healthcare and education, social services, and various therapies (eg, physical therapy, occupational therapy and job retraining, dietetic counseling, diabetic teaching, and speech therapy). These centers are also involved with community outreach, transportation, and educational programs, including literacy programs. They cooperate with other community agencies such as schools, homeless shelters, and Head Start programs. The centers serve more than 4.5 million children per year. In 1995, 10% of all births in the United States were under the auspices of these centers.

The Role of the Advance Practice Nurse.   Advanced practice nurses (nurse practitioners) provide most of the primary care in the CHC/FHC. They provide primary healthcare to people of all ages. In other words, they act as "family doctors." Some conditions are considered ambulatory care sensitive (**ACS**) and clients with these conditions are often seen in these settings. Examples include asthma, diabetes mellitus, seizure disorders, and hypertension. For many of these chronic disorders, providers are required to follow specific **managed care protocols.** These formally established guidelines are based on national criteria and detail the required management of specific disorders.

The Emergency Department and Emergi-Center

Most hospitals have emergency departments (emergency rooms [ER]) that care for clients with traumatic or life-threatening conditions. Some hospitals also have urgent-care departments (*urgi-centers*) as well; they care for less critically ill clients. Free-standing **emergi-centers** (urgi-centers, urgent-care centers) and walk-in clinics are also available, but are not attached to hospitals. Many such centers are found in shopping malls or CHC/FHCs.

Hospitals may also have an area of the ER specifically reserved for pediatric clients. They may have a specific area that handles the triage and treatment of clients. Most large hospitals have separate areas set aside to handle psychiatric emergencies, called *mental health crisis centers* or *crisis intervention centers* (**CIC**).

Many emergi-centers are open longer hours than are physician's offices; sometimes they are open 24 hours a day. Free-standing clinics may treat **vertical clients** (clients with non-critical conditions) only; they refer more critically ill or injured clients to hospital ERs.

☞ KEY CONCEPT

A client's primary care provider (PCP) usually must give permission for the client to receive care from an emergency department or other clinic if the client belongs to an HMO. Followup information for the PCP is becoming increasingly important. In many cases, clinics and PCP offices transfer information to one another by computers. If a PCP has questions, he or she can call the clinic for more information.

HMOs evaluate primary care providers based on how many of that provider's clients are seen in emergency rooms or how many times an individual client goes to the ER.

Nursing Care. Nursing care in emergency departments differs from nursing in inpatient settings. Many times, the person working there is a RN, although many rural and small hospitals and urgent-care centers employ LPN/LVNs as well. Advance practice nurses and emergency medical technicians (EMTs) treat clients with less emergent problems. Life-threatening illnesses and injuries are treated by physicians.

✚👁 **N u r s i n g   A l e r t**
It is important to remember that special training and experience is necessary before any nurse can be employed in the Emergency Room.

In addition to performing many routine procedures, staff members in emergency care departments perform the following:

- Providing crisis support and counseling to families
- Using specialized emergency equipment, such as endotracheal airways and hand-held ventilating bags (Ambu bag)
- Communicating with ambulance and rescue personnel who are en route
- Opening and utilizing supplies and equipment contained in the crash cart or storage areas. The nurse must know where all supplies and equipment are kept, so that they can be accessed quickly.
- Setting up examination and treatment areas appropriately to receive clients when ambulances or helicopters arrive, and assembling necessary equipment and supplies
- Notifying appropriate personnel to prepare for the arrival of incoming clients
- Assisting in the **stabilization (stāb) room** while clients are being triaged and stabilized for transfer to operating rooms or other areas
- Assisting with **cardioversion** (defibrillation) or other emergency procedures
- Taking primary responsibility for monitoring intravenous (IV) lines (after specialized training)
- Calling all family members and appropriate clergy members
- Continuously monitoring critically ill clients while they are being examined
- Notifying appropriate individuals if difficulties arise
- Obtaining necessary permits for treatments or surgery from the client or next-of-kin
- Performing triage in the event of multiple admissions at one time, to determine which clients require immediate attention
- Keeping accurate records of emergency procedures performed and medications given, by whom, and at what time—documentation is so essential that one nurse may be assigned only to document, without any other duties
- Arranging for special tests, such as MRI, CT scan, ultrasound, or x-ray examination
- Taking clients to x-ray or other diagnostic areas—many nurses assist with x-ray, ultrasound, or other examinations in emergencies
- Assisting with drawing blood or obtaining other specimens for laboratory analysis—in some situations, nurses draw blood and perform some laboratory tests
- Obtaining ECGs for evaluation by physicians
- Coordinating transcription of physician's orders (see Chap. 100), filling out requests, or entering information into computers for laboratory tests, x-ray examinations, and other procedures
- Arranging for emergency transfer to the operating room
- Making arrangements for hospital admission
- Assisting with non-sterile procedures, such as cast, splint, or traction application
- Assisting with emergency sterile procedures, such as suturing, removal of foreign objects from body orifices, or catheterization
- Applying cold or warm packs and performing other noninvasive procedures

- Administering medications, as ordered—this may include emergency medications during triage, as well as more routine injections, such as tetanus toxoid or antibiotics
- Assisting with selecting crutches or canes and with teaching the client to use these devices
- Obtaining necessary permissions from HMOs or other third-party payers for emergency care to be given, if possible
- Approaching family members regarding organ/tissue donation (following specialized training)
- Notifying other family members or clergy, as requested by the family or client

Nursing Alert

Remember that, even though a person has designated himself or herself as a donor on their driver's license or on a donor card, the next-of-kin must give permission for donation after a person's death.

The steadily increasing volume of cases coming into ERs and urgent-care centers has increased the load on each staff person. The length of time a non-critical client spends in the ER has increased as well. A client may be required to spend several hours in the ER during triage and stabilization before being treated and discharged. The triage process enables the staff to see those clients with life-threatening problems first. Therefore, the person with a severe asthma attack or diabetic reaction will be seen before the person requiring a tetanus injection and several sutures in a non-hemorrhaging wound.

The Same-Day-Surgery or Ambulatory Surgery Center

These centers are called same-day surgery, day-surgery, or ambulatory surgery centers. Clients visit here for many procedures that once required inpatient hospitalization. In addition to pressure from third party payers, the development of specialized equipment and innovative procedures has contributed to this trend.

Some of the specialized equipment and procedures found in these centers are:

The laparoscope and arthroscope: Allow visualization and manipulation of internal structures through a small "stab wound"

The laser: Provides cutting and vessel cauterization at a distance

Fiberoptics: Provide light and magnification at a distance

Ultrasound, MRI, and CT scans: Allow accurate visualization and location of internal structures and lesions

Procedures such as extracorporeal lithotripsy: To pulverize kidney and bladder stones

Stent placement: To eliminate the need for blood vessel bypass

Increased sophistication of local, spinal, and block anesthesia: Eliminates the need for general anesthesia

Availability of client-managed pain-control pump systems (patient-controlled analgesia [PCA]): Allows the client to self-manage pain

The operating microscope: Allows accurate visualization of tiny structures

Use of today's equipment and procedures eliminates, in many cases, the need for a large incision, or any incision. Local anesthesia greatly reduces the risk of postoperative complications. The PCA pump allows the client to effectively manage pain. All these factors speed the recovery process, add to client comfort, and eliminate the need for inpatient hospitalization. In addition, clients often find visiting a day-surgery center just for the surgery and then recovering at home to be more comfortable and conducive to relaxation than recuperating in a hospital.

Same-day-surgery clinics are often located in the operative area of a hospital or are managed by an operating room staff. Free-standing day-surgery centers have also been established by groups of surgeons who have formed a comprehensive group surgery practice. All such centers must be licensed and are inspected and regulated carefully.

Endoscopy.   As stated above, the concept of **endoscopy,** the use of small scopes to visualize and manipulate internal structures, has changed the way in which surgery is performed. The *laparoscope* is used to visualize internal structures in the abdomen. The *arthroscope* is used similarly inside joints.

Complex surgery can be done using several entry points (**ports**), via small "stab wounds." Surgeons can use various angles and several instruments simultaneously. For example, one port accommodates suction, another the scalpel, another cautery, and so on. Other ports accommodate fiberoptics, lasers, crushing instruments, various equipment for obtaining biopsy samples, clamps, pickup forceps, and retractors. Surgeons can insert materials, such as reinforcement meshes for hernia repair, through the ports. They can also remove tissue, such as the gallbladder or uterus, and biopsy samples through the ports.

Procedures Performed.   Criteria have been established to assist in determining appropriate clients for outpatient surgery. Box 97-1 describes these categories and gives examples. It is important to remember that the appropriateness of a client for same-day ambulatory surgery is determined not only by the complexity of the surgery, but also by the underlying physical and mental condition of the client, and the availability of appropriate after-care.

The number of procedures performed in day surgery is expanding continuously. Many procedures performed in day surgery today were inpatient procedures just a few years ago. Examples of procedures currently performed in day surgery include such varied procedures as tonsillectomy, carpal-tunnel release, debridement, open reduction of some fractures, *arthroscopic* procedures (joint surgery) and many other orthopedic procedures (eg, release of hammer toe, and bunion repair). Most eye surgery, such as cataract removal, glaucoma release, or ptosis correction, are performed in day surgery. Most biopsies, and procedures such as vasectomy and colon or bladder polyp removal, are also performed here. Obstetric and gynecologic procedures performed in same-day surgery include dilation and curettage (D&C), tubal ligation, ectopic preg-

➤➤ BOX 97-1

CLIENT CRITERIA FOR OUTPATIENT (SAME-DAY) SURGERY*

Class I
- No underlying organic, physiologic, or biochemical condition (examples include: brittle insulin-dependent diabetes, emphysema, multiple sclerosis, bleeding disorders, immune disorders such as AIDS, seizure disorders, serious eating disorders, or previous adverse reactions to anesthesia)
- No underlying adverse factor such as severe obesity, chronic chemical abuse and dependency, or extreme age (very old or very young)
- No serious psychiatric disturbance or uncontrollable fear
- Absence of severe dementia or intellectual impairment
- Conditions requiring surgery are localized (non-systemic)
- Client has primary caregivers available

Examples of appropriate Class I procedures include: tonsillectomy, tubal ligation, biopsy, cervical conization, cryosurgery removal of nonmalignant lesions, arthroscopy and joint repair, kidney-stone removal, polyp removal, cataract removal, breast lumpectomy, cranial burr holes, D&C, and toe amputation

Class II
- Increasing levels of systemic disturbance, with Class I-type procedures

- More complex surgery, without complicating physiological or psychological factors

Examples of appropriate Class II procedures include: removal of tubal pregnancy, hysterectomy, stent placement (in blood vessel), cholecystectomy, coronary artery arthroplasty (balloon or "Roto-rooter" procedures), lobectomy (lung), hernia repair, simple nephrectomy (kidney), biopsy of brain tumor, patent ductus repair, and partial foot amputation

Class III
- Serious underlying organic disorder that is life threatening
- Severe psychosis or intellectual impairment, rendering the client unable to cooperate or to care for himself or herself following surgery
- Systemic condition requiring extensive surgery

Examples of Class III procedures include: total colon resection, radical mastectomy, coronary artery bypass, hysterectomy with anterior and posterior repair, total gastric resection, total pneumonectomy (lung removal), craniotomy and removal of brain tumor, limb amputation, bone marrow transplant, repair of coronary septal defects, and heart, liver, or lung transplant

---

*Nearly all clients in Class I and some clients in Class II are candidates for outpatient (same-day) surgery. Clients in Class III are too ill, or the surgery is too complex or life threatening, for them to be candidates. In some cases, the lack of an available caregiver may move the client to a higher classification and rule out same-day surgery.

---

nancy removal, hysterectomy, and removal of some uterine tumors. Digestive system procedures such as herniorrhaphy (inguinal is most common), hemorrhoidectomy, partial bowel resection, and cholecystectomy are common same-day surgical procedures. Even more complex procedures, such as placement of a stent in a blood vessel, simple *nephrectomy* (kidney removal), and removal of a lobe of a lung or a lung wedge resection, can be done on an ambulatory basis. Additional examples are contained in Box 97-1.

The client must have a caregiver at home, to assist in followup postoperative care. Ambulatory surgery centers may refer clients to home care services for a few visits, to ensure safe followup. However, if the client cannot pay, available home care services often are very limited.

Nursing Care.   Nursing responsibilities in same-day surgery are more inclusive that in the inpatient setting (see Chap. 56). In addition to routine nursing functions, the nurse in same-day surgery is expected to perform the functions listed below.

Teaching the Client and Family.   One of the most important functions of the nurse in the day-surgery center is that of teaching the client and the family. This nurse is responsible for the following:

- Teach clients about preoperative preparation. Clients or family members will need to perform many preoperative measures at home, including following special diets, maintaining nothing by mouth (NPO) status for a specified number of hours preoperatively, giving pHisoHex scrubs or showers, and administering enemas or other types of bowel prep. (Home care nurses may help clients perform some of these procedures. They may also help to provide preoperative teaching.)
- Refer the client and family to appropriate sources for equipment and supplies that will be needed postoperatively.
- Give instructions verbally by telephone and in writing, and again at the last preoperative office visit, which may be several days before the scheduled procedure. The nurse reinforces these verbal instructions with written followup. (Many commercially and locally prepared booklets can assist clients with learning.) Obtain an interpreter, if necessary.
- Document all teaching. (If teaching has not been accurately documented, it would be considered, in a court of law, not to have been done.) Quiz the client and family, to make sure they understand fully.

- Instruct clients to call if any change occurs in their physical status. For example, canceling surgery or conducting it in an acute-care facility may be necessary if a client has a cold or influenza.
- Be sure the client knows whether or not he or she will be awake during the procedure. Explain that many clients are given conscious sedation, such as Versed, to help them relax and to provide some amnesia about the procedure.
- Let the client know that, in many cases, he or she will be allowed to play tapes or a radio with headphones during the procedure. This helps many clients to relax.
- Teach clients what to expect after surgery and help them to practice postoperative exercises.
- Take the client on a tour of the operating suite before surgery, if this is permitted.
- Make sure arrangements have been made for the person to get home after surgery. Clients are not allowed to drive after day surgery or other outpatient procedures involving sedation.
- Make sure the client has someone to stay with him or her at home for at least 24 hours postoperatively.
- Provide postoperative client and family teaching on the day of the procedure. Explain appropriate care for clients, and describe untoward symptoms and medication side effects for the primary caregiver to monitor.

☛ KEY CONCEPT

It is very important to provide instructions that the client can follow. Find out the client's language of choice. Provide an interpreter, if necessary. Written instructions should be provided in the person's first language or in Braille, if the client is vision impaired. If the client cannot read, taped instructions should be provided. Verbal instructions must be given by signing for the hearing impaired.

Be sure to have the client and/or family repeat instructions back to you, to make sure they understand. Just asking if they understand is not sufficient, because many people will say "yes" to avoid embarrassment or to be polite, even if they do not understand.

☛ KEY CONCEPT

The physician usually instructs that no aspirin or ibuprofen be taken for 7 days prior to a surgical procedure. In addition, the nurse should ask the client if he or she is taking herbal supplements. In particular, St. John's wort reduces the effectiveness of some medications, such as Versed. Other herbals can contribute to bleeding postoperatively.

Functions of the Nurse on the Operative Day. The nurse in same-day surgery is actively involved on the day of surgery (see Chap. 56). This nurse will:

- Perform specific preparations, such as the preoperative scrub and shave or drawing of blood, as ordered.

- Follow the preoperative checklist. Check to see that laboratory and ECG results are on the client's chart. Remove the client's dentures, contact lenses, prostheses, or other such devices. Measure the client's weight and vital signs. Assist the client to change into hospital garb.
- Make sure clients sign the operative permit before they receive any medications. Double-check about possible allergies.
- Make sure the client voids immediately before surgery.
- Introduce the client to anesthesia personnel and operating room personnel. Make sure they are comfortable in the pre-induction room.
- Scrub in and assist surgeons during procedures in the day-surgery center, as needed.
- Support and remain with clients during induction of anesthesia (if the procedure is done under general anesthesia). Anesthesia personnel will maintain the client who is receiving general anesthesia during the procedure. Remain with the client for the entire procedure if it is done under local anesthetic.

☛ KEY CONCEPT

Most clients are admitted on the morning of surgery, even if they are to be admitted to the hospital postoperatively. These clients will be required to do their preoperative preparation at home.

Postoperative Nursing Functions. The nurse in day surgery also functions as the recovery room nurse after surgery. This nurse will:

- Stay with clients postoperatively until they are fully awake. Observe for any complications. Monitor vital signs and perform other routine postoperative procedures.
- Check dressings to make sure there is no excessive bleeding.
- Check to make sure drains, IVs, and equipment are working properly.
- Verify again that the family understands the postoperative care and when to call for assistance. Tell them that you will call tomorrow to see how the client is doing.
- Assist the client to dress and help him or her into the car for the trip home. Be sure to furnish an emesis basin or box of tissues, as needed.
- Telephone clients on the first postoperative day. Determine if they are having any complications. Know what questions to ask.
- Make recommendations for necessary referrals to public health or home care services.

Because most third-party payers do not give clients choices about whether or not to have ambulatory surgery, the nurse plays a vital role in assisting clients and their family members to feel comfortable. Assure clients that ambulatory surgery poses less risk for infection than inpatient surgery.

A relaxed, friendly atmosphere in the day-surgery center is conducive to confidence and recovery. Clients may not need preoperative medications because of the more relaxed atmosphere; they can walk into the operating room feeling more in control. Many clients recover faster and have fewer complications after same-day surgery because they have local anesthesia, they have only small incisions or no incision at all, because they do not receive heavy sedation, and because they are more comfortable at home. Clients are also able to ambulate sooner after surgery, helping to prevent the complications of immobilization. Most people are strongly motivated to recover and to cooperate. Ambulatory surgery will be more and more common as we move through the 21st Century.

➤ STUDENT SYNTHESIS

Key Points

- Ambulatory nursing care may be delivered in a physician's office or clinic, urgent-care center, community health center, day-surgery center, or in the client's home.
- Nurses function as direct assistants to physicians in many ambulatory care settings.
- Nurses who work in ambulatory settings need multiple skills. They may require additional training to perform some skills.
- The family/community health center provides primary care and secondary services for many people. These centers employ large numbers of nurses.
- Clients coming in for same-day surgery or in the morning for inpatient surgery need a great deal of instruction because most preoperative preparation is done at home.
- Same-day surgery clients and many clients discharged soon after surgery (as well as their caregivers) need followup care after discharge to ensure proper recovery.
- Documentation is vital in all phases of ambulatory care, as it is in inpatient settings.

Critical Thinking Exercises

1. Visit an ambulatory clinic in a neighborhood. Talk to a nurse about his or her duties and responsibilities. What are the types and ages of the clients who visit? What disorders are most commonly seen?
2. Observe in an ambulatory surgery center and interview several clients. What were their feelings about same-day surgery? What are the feelings of the nurses who work there? How well prepared do you feel you would be to function as a nurse in these settings?

NCLEX-Style Review Questions

1. Which of the following developments have made same-day surgery possible?
   a. Advanced directives and living wills
   b. HMOs and PPOs
   c. Managed care and decreased insurance coverage
   d. New equipment and procedures
2. Which of the following clients would be a strong candidate for outpatient surgery? Client undergoing a:
   a. Amputation of a limb
   b. Hernia repair
   c. Radical mastectomy
   d. Total colon resection
3. Prior to discharge from an outpatient setting, which of the following would be most important for the client who has a hearing deficit?
   a. Provide written instructions in the client's first language.
   b. Speak very slowly and loudly.
   c. Repeat instructions several times.
   d. Utilize sign language during your teaching.

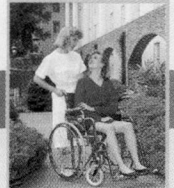

CHAPTER

98

Home Care Nursing

LEARNING OBJECTIVES

1. Identify the reasons for and benefits of home care.
2. Describe situations in which home care might be most appropriate.
3. Identify several nursing functions in home care.
4. Discuss important safety practices for home care nurses.
5. Describe and discuss the influences of regulatory agencies upon delivery of home healthcare.
6. Describe recent changes in reimbursement for home care.

ACRONYMS

CHHA	HHA	OASIS
CNO	HHRG	PPS
HCA	NAHC	

Home care is a major component in the trend to offer most healthcare within an individual's own community. Some people are able to receive all their healthcare at home and are not admitted to the acute-care hospital. Others spend a short time in the hospital and then return home to recover.

Home care continues to be the fastest-growing field of nursing today. In 1996, the annual employment growth rate of home care was 16.4%, compared with 4.3% for the healthcare industry overall, and 2.8% in hospitals. Many extended care facilities offer home care as one of their services.

The National Association for Home Care (**NAHC**) defines home care as:

. . . a simple phrase that encompasses a wide range of health and social services. These services are delivered at home to recovering, disabled, chronically or terminally ill persons in need of medical, nursing, social, or therapeutic treatment and/or assistance with the essential activities of daily living. Generally, home care is appropriate whenever a person prefers to stay at home but needs ongoing care that cannot easily or effectively be provided solely by family and friends.[1]

ABLECare Home Services in Minnesota states, "Our wide range of services includes skilled nursing visits, private duty nursing, home health aides, and high tech pediatrics and respite services. In addition . . . we offer specialized group living environments for medically fragile individuals, persons with traumatic brain injury and seniors." (For more information, write: 11801 Xeon Boulevard, NW, Coon Rapids, MN 55448.)

HOME CARE

Reasons for Home Care

Fewer people are being admitted to hospitals, and those who are, are going home sooner, with more needs for special care. People are discharged from hospitals with drainage tubes, heparin locks, IVs with pumps, patient-controlled analgesia (PCA) pumps, catheters, and other complicated equipment. Some ventilator-dependent children live at home. Home care nurses teach clients and families how to operate all types of equipment. They reinforce teaching given in hospitals and supervise the documentation of procedures.

The range of home care services is great. In some cases, home care nurses and assistants provide 24-hour nursing care in the client's home. In other cases, clients receive assisted living services, which allows them to live independently (see Chap. 95). Home care may be given on a long-term basis, on an intermittent basis, or on a short-term basis, for just a few visits. Box 98-1 lists some of the characteristics and advantages of home care.

Types of Agencies and Services

Several types of agencies provide home care services. These include hospital-based agencies, nursing registries, temporary staffing companies, and hospice programs. If an agency is called a "home health agency" or a "visiting nurse service," it has usually been certified by Medicare as a Community

➤➤ BOX 98-1

CHARACTERISTICS OF HOME CARE

- Third-party payers now force early discharge from hospitals. Therefore, clients leave hospitals while they are still ill or recovering. This differs from in the past. Today's clients need more total care and assistance with postoperative care and self-care activities.
- Unlike in the past, some people are not admitted to the hospital, but receive their entire care at home. This includes surgical clients.
- The aging population is increasing. As people age, they tend to have more physical disorders. Society needs a higher level of management and assistance for chronic illness and *comorbidity* (coexisting disorders).
- Family structures have changed. Clients may not have family caregivers available to provide care, requiring more healthcare attention from nurses, aides, and volunteers.
- Sophisticated electronic equipment allows clients to receive care at home. The equipment is self-contained and electronically controlled. Nearly all of this equipment can be managed by non-professionals, after receiving adequate instruction. The nurse is available to supervise and to answer questions.
- Nurses and clients can transmit information about procedures (such as electroencephalograms and ECGs) by telephone or computer to hospitals or physician offices for interpretation. Other client conditions can also be monitored electronically.
- Nurses learn to use a digital camera to record information such as the condition of a wound. This image can be transmitted to the physician for evaluation. It can also be saved on a computer disk and used to compare to past and future photos, to evaluate healing (or lack of healing) of the wound.

Advantages of Home Care
- Home care is less expensive than hospital or nursing-home care.
- Nurses, support personnel, and primary caregivers can provide continuous care from hospital to home, and until the client's recovery or death.
- Many people are more comfortable receiving care in their own home. Here, they are surrounded by their loved ones, friends, and pets. The surroundings are familiar and comfortable. Familiar food is available.
- Many clients prefer to die at home. Home care agencies often provide hospice care (see Chap. 99).
- Many clients and families experience less emotional strain at home, because they avoid separation.

Nursing Organization (**CNO**). Some agencies maintain certification by the Joint Commission on Accreditation of Healthcare Organizations (JCAHO). Other agencies are licensed by the health department of the state or territory in which they are located.

Specialized agencies often provide equipment as well as home care. Examples of these agencies include some ventilator and IV infusion companies. Many home care agencies also have access to rental equipment, such as hospital beds or wheelchairs.

The services provided by individual agencies vary. Services range from total physical care to homemaking or shopping assistance only. Other services include mental health counseling; social work; hospice care; occupational, physical, and speech therapy; companions; and the administration of IV medications or drawing blood. Some agencies also provide respite care for family caregivers.

Long-Term Home Care.   Older clients or people with chronic, disabling conditions may require long-term care. Long-term services include periodic nursing assessment, with homemaking and personal care services provided by agency staff. Nurses may assist with "restorative nursing," such as assisting in rehabilitation procedures and exercises to maintain muscle integrity (see Chap. 96). Clients with cardiac disorders continue to constitute the highest percentage of the caseload in many comprehensive home care agencies.

Some clients requiring long-term services receive care 24 hours a day or for 8- or 12-hour shifts. In some cases, families participate by providing care during the day, with nurses on duty at night so the family can rest.

Hospice care is often delivered in the client's home. Hospice care assists the terminally ill person and their family (see Chap. 99). In addition to the client's home, hospice care may be delivered in a nursing home, a shelter, or in another facility, such as a jail. Third-party payers often pay for hospice care.

Children with Special Needs.   Some families have in-home care for children with special needs. This care may be around the clock or for part of the day. The child with severe disabilities will usually need an attendant to assist him or her in school as well. The field of assisting children with special needs provides an increasing employment opportunity for LPNs.

☛ Key Concept

In some situations, a member of the home care nursing staff is in the client's home 24 hours a day. In the case of a child with special needs or an adult with a disabling injury or degenerative disorder, care continues for months or years. Unique adjustments are required for this family who is never alone.

Intermittent or Short-term Home Care.   When a client receives short-term services or intermittent care, the nurse provides care in the home for a short period of time or provides care at specific intervals. Examples include:

- Home visits two to three times a week for assessment or administration of special medications or treatments
- A home visit once a week to assist a client or family to set up medications for the next week (Fig. 98-1)
- A home visit every 2 to 3 weeks to administer a long-acting (*decanoate*) injection of a psychotropic drug

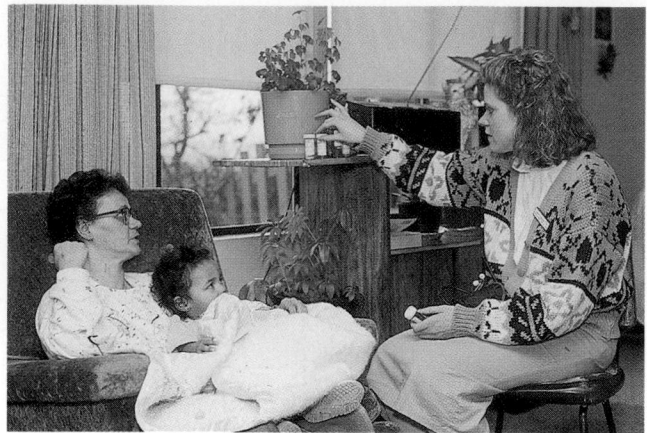

FIGURE 98-1. Many clients with chronic illnesses can manage in their own home with only a weekly visit from the nurse to help set up medications. Often, each day's medications are placed into a marked box, so the client knows which medications to take each day. One of the functions of the home care nurse is to check the box, to make sure medications have been taken each day as ordered. Here, the home care nurse teaches about medications with their desired and undesired effects, another important nursing role.

- A very limited number of home visits to assist a new mother
- Dressing changes once or twice a day postoperatively, for 1 to 2 weeks
- Administration of IV medications
- Drawing blood for various tests
- Administering and reading PPD tests (for tuberculosis)
- Administering immunizations, such as flu shots to senior citizens
- Administering a periodic electrocardiogram (ECG)
- A periodic home visit to assess care being given by family caregivers

Centers of Excellence.   The Centers of Excellence concept has been briefly described in connection with rehabilitation. This concept also functions in home care. A team of nurses with specific expertise is in place to assist local home care nurses.

The expertise of a Center of Excellence team may include:

- Wound care
- Continence care and bowel/bladder retraining
- IV and other high-technology care
- Psychiatric home care and crisis intervention
- Maternal–child healthcare or maternity consultation
- Pediatric high-technology, including care of ventilator-dependent children

The Centers of Excellence nurses may make the actual home visits or may serve as consultants to the staff nurse from the local home care agency. The local nurse then makes future home visits.

Payment for Home Care

A prospective payment system (**PPS**)[2] for home care was instituted by Medicare in October of 2000, in response to the

Balanced Budget Act of 1997. This PPS was patterned after the system used in hospitals and represented a major change in home care reimbursement. This system is an attempt by third party payers to control medical costs and to improve efficiency in delivery of home care. For 2 years prior to the implementation of PPS for home care, statistics were collected and a data bank was developed. This data bank was used to determine future reimbursement rates. During these 2 years, an interim payment system was instituted. Unfortunately, a number of home care agencies closed in response to the PPS system.

☛ KEY CONCEPT

It is important for the nurse to understand the role of client/members' rights in the provision of primary care under the auspices of managed care.

The first step in the PPS process is to assess the case mix, according to clinical, functional, and service needs. To do this, a standardized data collection tool called the Outcome and Assessment Information Set (**OASIS**) is used.[3] This data collection is performed by a RN, or in the case of therapy, only by a registered physical therapist. The client is then assigned to a Home Health Resource Group (**HHRG**) for a given episode of care, which is usually a 60-day period.

Predetermined and standardized reimbursement rates are set up, based on the client's diagnosis, using the data from the OASIS. The OASIS also allows consideration of the client's functional ability and available support systems (service needs). It looks at the total client.

Another factor in the development of the PPS was the realization that the nurse cannot do everything for the client. It is the role of the nurse to educate and prepare the family to understand, learn about, and manage their loved one's care. The family is included in the system, rather than the nursing staff trying "to do it all."

The PPS system provides an increasing employment opportunity for LPN/LVNs in home care.

Members of the Home Care Team

In addition to physicians, RNs, and LPN/LVNs, many other members make up the home care team. They include physical, occupational, and speech therapists; social workers; dietitians; chaplains; health care assistants (**HCA**s) or personal care attendants (PCAs); home health aides (**HHA**s) or certified home health aides (**CHHA**s); homemakers or chore workers; companions; and volunteers. All these individuals make visits to clients.

☛ KEY CONCEPT

Various disciplines are involved in home care. All team members plan and carry out care. They hold regular team meetings to discuss each client's case. (Not all members serve on all cases.)

Case Management.   Each home care client has a case manager. In many states, this must be an RN. In some cases,

the case manager is a social worker. The nurse makes an initial assessment visit to the home and evaluates the safety of the home and the adequacy of available family caregivers. An intake assessment is made of the client's nursing care needs. The case manager then meets with the home care team to determine what services are necessary and available for that particular client. The home care team assists the family to obtain needed equipment and makes suggestions about the setup of the home for optimum client care.

The case manager is required to visit the client at certain intervals to determine if the client's healthcare goals are being met and if the requirements of the funding agency are being satisfied.

The Role of the LPN/LVN.   Federal Medicare regulations identify the following standard duties of the LPN/LVN in home care:

- Furnish services in accordance with agency policies.
- Prepare clinical and progress notes.
- Assist physicians and RNs to perform specialized procedures.
- Prepare equipment and materials for treatments, observing aseptic technique as required.
- Assist clients in learning appropriate self-care techniques.

State guidelines dictate that LPNs practice within the guidelines of the state's nursing practice legislation and according to specified agency policies. LPNs or HHAs serve as team members, under the supervision of the case manager. The standards of the agency's accrediting body will guide LPNs by defining their role in accordance with state regulations and local policies.

The Nurse in Home Care

The nurse working in home care will be required to perform many of the skills learned in the basic nursing program. However, the home care nurse functions independently and must possess a high level of independence, as well as sound judgment.

☛ KEY CONCEPT

In the home setting, the nurse works in a more independent and isolated situation than in the hospital or extended-care facility. Therefore, it is important that you, as the nurse, have a good knowledge of state and agency policies.

Functions of the Home Care Nurse.   Nursing activities and skills commonly used in home care include:

- Coordinate care with hospital and medical staff and agency resource people.
- Provide client and family teaching about procedures, recognition of symptoms, and how and when to report to a physician. Evaluate and document teaching on an ongoing basis.
- Complete and submit the required forms and records to the reimbursement agency.

- Counsel the client. The nurse is the liaison between the client and the healthcare system.
- Accurately assess the client. Report untoward symptoms to the physician or other primary healthcare provider.
- Evaluate the client's total home situation. Assess care being given; the safety, cleanliness, and appropriateness of the home; the adequacy of the client's food and fluid intake; the administration of medications; and diversionary activities. It is important to assess the ongoing relationships between the client and the primary caregivers.
- Evaluate the home's safety for the client. Falls in the home are common and are often preventable. Suggest necessary equipment or changes to be made to help improve the safety of the home.
- Assist primary caregivers to prepare the home for the client's arrival.
- Assess for possible client abuse.
- Reassure the client on the telephone. On days when visits are not scheduled, call and give support or answer questions as necessary.
- Determine how the primary caregivers are doing. Are they performing nursing skills correctly? Are they suffering emotionally or physically from the strain of caring for a loved one 24 hours a day? Do they need to obtain some respite care for the client so they get a break?
- Have a knowledge of, and be able to suggest, community resources. Social workers often can make referrals. In some cases, a physician's order is required for a referral.

☛ KEY CONCEPT

In some cases, the client pays for a home nursing visit. However, in most cases, a third-party payer is involved. If this is the case, the number and length of visits will be limited and will be strictly regulated by the funding agency. The nurse will be expected to document the exact length of each visit and what procedures were performed.

Box 98-2 lists additional community services available to home care clients.

☛ KEY CONCEPT

The nurse may need to make adjustments in procedures when caring for a client at home. However, it is important to remember the underlying rationales behind procedures learned in the basic nursing program. Even though the nurse may need to adjust the way a procedure is performed in the home, it is vital not to jeopardize the client's safety. Do not ever be afraid to consult the client's case manager or the supervisor if you have a question.

Choosing Home Care as a Career.   There are many reasons for a nurse to choose to work in home healthcare. There are many opportunities for employment here, because acute-care hospitals are cutting the numbers of available beds. In addition, clients in the hospital are often critically ill and may require the services of an RN.

➤ ➤ BOX 98-2

COMMUNITY SERVICES AVAILABLE TO HOME CARE CLIENTS

- Meals on Wheels
- Transportation (specially equipped vans and buses)
- Escort services to appointments or errands
- Grocery shopping and delivery
- Homemaking services
- Visiting pet therapy
- Telephone safety; electronic alert equipment (eg, "Lifeline")
- Adult daycare
- Respite care
- Senior centers
- Public clinics
- Support groups
- Low-cost medical and continence-care supplies
- Rental or loaned equipment
- Volunteer services
- Ombudsperson services
- Payee services, to help manage money

The advantages of working in home care include:

- The unique opportunity to care for only one or two clients. In the home, the nurse can get to know the client better.
- The opportunity to get to know the client's family.
- Greater flexibility in planning the work day.
- Being able to assist the client to remain at home, where he or she is most comfortable.

Requirements for Home Nursing.   The nurse must furnish transportation to and from clients' homes. In most cases, this will require a car, but in some cities, it is possible to travel to worksites by public transportation.

The home care nurse is required to work alone much of the time. It is important to consult the case manager or supervisor if there are any questions or concerns.

The home care nurse must use good judgment when delivering care. This nurse needs to make independent decisions, but it is vital to base these decisions on sound nursing practice.

Protocols and Procedures.   Nurses in home care perform many of the same procedures used in other healthcare settings. They have learned these procedures throughout their nursing program. It may be necessary to make adaptations to some procedures when they are performed in the home. Home care agencies have guidelines or nursing protocols for specific procedures. A number of reference books are also available that can assist the nurse to adapt nursing care to the home setting.

Safety for the Home Care Team

Preventing injury to healthcare workers is pivotal. When going into a home, maintaining personal safety is important, because the nurse is usually going in alone. Often, an agency performs a telephone risk assessment before sending a nurse into a home. In some cases, two healthcare workers visit a home together. Most home care nurses carry cellular phones for emergencies. The rule of thumb is "trust your instincts." If you are to visit a home and it does not look safe or feel right, check it out before going in. You always have the right to maintain your own safety. Box 98-3 lists further safety tips for nurses making home visits.

➤➤ BOX 98-3

SAFETY GUIDELINES FOR HOME CARE NURSES

- Wear a name badge that clearly identifies your name and your employer. Dress professionally.
- Telephone clients in advance, alerting them to the approximate time of your home care visit. Obtain directions to the residence if necessary.
- Escort services are available.
- If a client owns a pet known to be menacing, ask the client to properly secure the animal before you come to the home. If you are confronted with an aggressive dog, back away, but do not turn around and do not run.
- Be alert to your surroundings, including other people in the home.
- Carry a cell phone. Make sure it is charged at all times.
- Keep your vehicle in good working order, with plenty of gas.
- Lock your car at all times, with windows rolled up, both when driving and when parking.
- Look into your car before getting in. Make sure the back seat is empty.
- Park your car in full view of the client's residence. Avoid parking in alleys or on deserted side streets if at all possible. Park in a well-lighted place.
- Be aware of your surroundings and of other people at all times while traveling in the community.
- Look before entering an elevator.
- When exiting the car, have the equipment you will need during the visit ready to go.
- Walk in a professional, businesslike manner directly to the client's residence.
- When passing a group of strangers, cross to the other side of the street, as appropriate, and keep eye contact with those in the group.
- In buildings, use common walkways, avoiding isolated stairs.
- Always knock on the door before entering a client's home.
- Check your agency's guidelines before giving a ride to a client or to a family member. Your insurance might not be valid.
- Take a self-defense class. Learn to protect yourself.

Adapted From: Green, K. (1998). *Home care survival guide.* Philadelphia: Lippincott Williams & Wilkins.

Respite for Primary Caregivers

Many people care for their loved ones at home (Fig. 98-2). Often, the client has a long-standing physical or mental disorder. The person may have been paralyzed in an accident or may have Alzheimer's disease. Caring for someone at home is exhausting for primary caregivers, who are responsible for the client 24 hours a day. Caregivers need support and reassurance. In addition, caregivers often need a *respite* (break) to maintain their own physical and emotional health.

The following are suggestions to assist caregivers to fulfill their own needs:

- Manage stress. Plan some recreational activity each day. If it is not possible to leave the client, the caregiver can do something such as read, knit, work puzzles, or call a friend while at the client's bedside.
- Maintain emotional balance. Seek outside counseling, if necessary.
- Maintain a sense of humor. It is often helpful to read cartoons or joke books, or to watch comedies.
- Get plenty of exercise and as much fresh air as possible.
- Stretch and relax at intervals.
- Listen to soothing music while at the bedside. The client will also enjoy this.
- Eat a well-balanced diet.
- A physician may prescribe a vitamin or mineral supplement.
- Maintain energy by eating several small meals daily.
- Use a minimum of salt and sugar.
- Avoid noticeable weight gain or loss.
- Drink plenty of liquids. Vary the liquids; do not drink just plain water. Try to avoid caffeine as much as possible.
- Avoid smoking.
- Protect the back by using good body mechanics.
- Get plenty of rest and take naps.

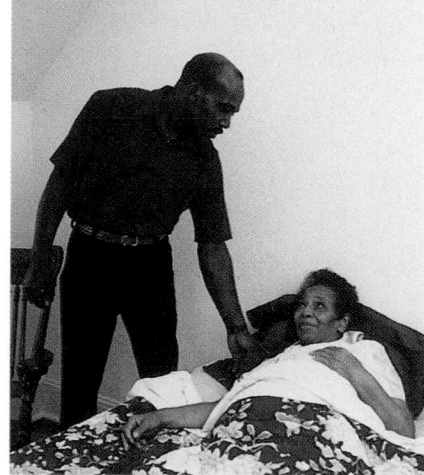

FIGURE 98-2. The role of family caregiver is vital in managing chronic illness at home. Many clients would not be able to live at home if a family caregiver were not available. The role of caregiver can be rewarding, but also can be very challenging. Caregivers need a *respite* or break from the constant demands of in-home care to maintain their own health.

- Get a checkup for physical complaints. Maintain immunizations, including a flu shot.
- Encourage the client's friends and family to visit. This provides a break for the caregiver and is enjoyable for the client.
- Take an occasional respite or time away. Hire someone to come in and help, if necessary. In some cases, volunteers are available to help.
- Keep a journal. Writing one's feelings and thoughts often helps to relieve tension.
- Attend a support group. It is often very helpful to share one's feelings with others and learn that you are not alone.

Chapter 99 further discusses the concept of respite care. Always remember that primary caregivers are vital members of the healthcare team. In order to safely and comfortably continue caring for their family member, they must be able to maintain their own physical and emotional health.

Community-based healthcare has become the largest segment of healthcare and continues to grow. Many people receive all of their primary healthcare in an ambulatory setting, particularly in the community health center. Many more people are able to live at home by taking advantage of available home care services. Home care provides employment for large numbers of nurses and other health personnel.

➤ STUDENT SYNTHESIS

Key Points

- Home care nursing is the fastest-growing segment of the healthcare delivery system, employing increasing numbers of nurses.
- Clients are being discharged from acute-care facilities with complex nursing needs, which home care workers and family caregivers must meet.
- Home care nurses have the opportunity to schedule hours and to structure their own time.
- Home care nurses must be alert to untoward signs and symptoms and report them to the appropriate person.
- Many clients opt for home care because it is cost effective and often more comfortable than hospital care.
- Home care nurses are ultimately responsible for their own personal safety.

Critical Thinking Exercises

1. Mrs. L., an 82-year-old woman, lives alone in a senior apartment complex. You are assigned to visit her once a week for a medication setup. Her prescribed medications include glipizide (Glucotrol), lisinopril (Zestril), furosemide (Lasix), KCl (Kay Ciel), thiamine, folate, and a multivitamin. When you stop by her home on Tuesday, you find that the medications for two of the days last week are still in their daily containers. Her main supply of lisino-

pril and furosemide are gone. She says she went home with her son "for a few days to visit," but cannot remember when she returned. She says she is "worried about money." She has very little food in the refrigerator. She is not wearing her TED socks. Her vision is quite poor and she does not like to wear her hearing aid. She says her dentures "hurt her mouth." Her blood pressure is 210/148.
   a. What actions would you take? In what order? What client teaching is needed?
   b. List nursing procedures that need to be performed.
   c. What items might be on the agenda for a team meeting about Mrs. L.? Who is likely to be invited to the meeting? What suggestions would you have? What possible outcomes can you envision for the meeting?
   d. What medical conditions do you think Mrs. L. is likely to have, based on the medications she is receiving? What signs and symptoms should you particularly look for?
2. Describe ways to adapt a client's home to maximize the safety and independence of clients.

NCLEX-Style Review Questions

1. Which of the following is an advantage of home care?
   a. Clients are more comfortable in their own home.
   b. Cost is more expensive than nursing-home care.
   c. Third-party payers will not pay for extended hospital care.
   d. There is no risk of infection when in the home setting.
2. A role of the LPN/LVN in home care is to:
   a. Assist client in learning appropriate self-care techniques.
   b. Assist physician in surgery.
   c. Complete complicated procedures.
   d. Complete initial client assessment and evaluation.
3. Which measure, if instituted by the nurse, would help to ensure safety during home visits?
   a. Avoid wearing a name tag.
   b. Be alert to the surroundings.
   c. Walk in a relaxed, unhurried manner.
   d. Wear clothes that are casual in appearance.

References

1. National Association for Home Care. (Undated). *How to choose a home care provider: A consumer's guide* (p. 2). Washington, DC: Author.
2. Includes information from Patricia Rusca, RN, Visiting Nurse Association of Central Jersey.
3. Utterbach, K. (2001). Prospective payment comes to Medicare home health. *American Journal of Nursing, 101*(7), 59.

CHAPTER

99

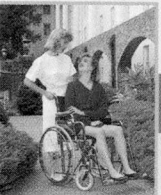

Hospice Nursing

LEARNING OBJECTIVES

1. Discuss the evolution of the hospice movement.
2. Name the four areas of human needs upon which the hospice concept focuses.
3. List at least six characteristics a program must meet to be officially classified as a hospice.
4. Explain the criteria for a person's admission to a hospice program.
5. Define the term respite care and explain its purpose.
6. Define interdisciplinary care as it applies to hospice; identify the major disciplines involved.
7. Differentiate among the functions of the case manager, the hospice nurse, and other members of the healthcare team.
8. Discuss the role of primary caregivers in hospice.
9. Describe emotional and spiritual support for the client and family.
10. Identify measures used for odor management and measures used to treat anorexia, nausea and vomiting, constipation, diarrhea, respiratory distress, and skin breakdown for hospice clients.
11. Discuss threats to mental health, such as depression and anxiety, that can occur in hospice clients and caregivers.
12. Identify medications used for pain management in hospice.
13. List and briefly describe three psychosocial modalities used in pain management.
14. List and describe at least two physical modalities used in pain management.
15. Discuss important considerations when caring for children in hospice programs.
16. Explain the nurse's role after the client dies.

NEW TERMINOLOGY

ablative surgery
adjuvant
bereavement
debulking
hospice
interdisciplinary care

palliative care
primary caregivers
respite
somnolent
titration

ACRONYMS

BSC	DNI	OTFC
CA	DNR	PCA
COP	IDG	POC
CRNH	IDT	PSDA
DME	NHPCO	TENS
DNH	OBT	

The term **hospice** does not signify a specific care setting, but rather a philosophy of care. Hospice is based on the concept that most people want to die at home, free of pain, and among their loved ones. Physical and emotional comfort and the quality of life are the primary concerns of hospice; not cure. Hospice programs care for terminally ill persons, while treating them with dignity. The goal of hospice care is to provide as much pain relief as possible, with control of other physical symptoms and emotional suffering. Hospice care promotes the idea that by controlling the client's disease symptoms, the client becomes emotionally and spiritually at peace and is free to search for meaning in life. In this way, clients can move toward self-actualization on Maslow's hierarchy of human needs. Nurses who work with hospice clients and their families will use all the skills they learned during their entire nursing program. As a nurse, you must examine your own values and feelings about death before making a decision to work in hospice with dying people.

EVOLUTION OF THE HOSPICE MOVEMENT

The term *hospice* derives from a medieval word meaning "to provide shelter for travelers on difficult journeys." In early times, little was known about how to cure diseases. People treated symptoms instead, to help provide comfort until death. As modern cures evolved, healthcare providers began to place less emphasis on comfort and more emphasis on cure. The hospice movement acknowledges that not all illnesses are curable and emphasizes the management of uncomfortable symptoms.

The primary force behind the modern hospice movement was Dame Cicely Saunders, who founded St. Christopher's Hospice in London in 1967. She believed that people and their feelings are important up to the last moment of life. Healthcare providers should do everything possible not only to help people die peacefully, but also to help them live until they die.

In 1974, Florence Wald initiated the first U.S. hospice as a home care program in New Haven, Connecticut. It was later called the Connecticut Hospice. Other early hospice projects were located in Boonton, New Jersey and Tucson, Arizona.

Legislation has greatly influenced the U.S. hospice movement. For example, in 1983, a bill involved Medicare, Medicaid, and private insurance in payment for hospice care. In 1991, Congress passed the Patient Self-Determination Act (**PSDA**) (see Chap. 4), allowing people more say regarding their end-of-life care. For example, clients can request that no heroic treatments or resuscitation be instituted to prolong their life.

The National Hospice and Palliative Care Organization (**NHPCO**), founded in 1978, establishes criteria for hospices and offers information and education to healthcare professionals and the public. According to NHPCO, there were 3,139 operational or planned hospices existing in all 50 states, the District of Columbia, and Puerto Rico by the end of 1999. U.S. hospices served more than 600,000 clients in 1999. A high percentage of managed care plans cover hospice services.

THE HOSPICE CONCEPT

Most U.S. hospice programs are either independent and community based, or they are divisions of hospitals. Others are divisions of home health agencies, nursing homes, or independent hospice corporations.

Most hospices admit people with cancer (**CA**), as well as other diagnoses. Many of them admit persons with acquired immunodeficiency syndrome (AIDS). Almost 90% of U.S. hospices admit terminally ill children. Many hospices require clients to have primary caregivers at home; other programs consider cases individually. About half of U.S. hospices admit people who need high-tech therapies, such as intravenous (IV) medications or oxygen therapy. Most hospice clients are over age 65.

Goals of Hospice

Hospice care focuses on four areas of human needs:

- Physical
- Psychological/emotional
- Social/cultural
- Spiritual

Hospice programs eliminate the emphasis on "saving lives" that permeates acute-care settings. Gone are most machines and high-tech equipment commonly found in acute-care units. Hospice programs emphasize physical and emotional comfort instead. Figure 99-1 depicts a client spending quality time with his granddaughter while in hospice care.

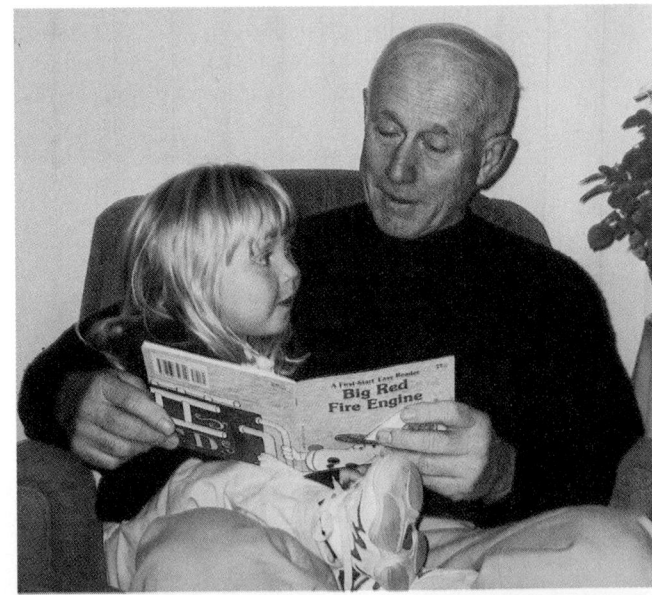

FIGURE 99-1. The support of family members is essential in hospice. Here, the hospice client is able to spend some quality time with his granddaughter. Children and pets are excellent therapy for all shut-ins, providing companionship and relief. Clients are encouraged to talk about their life and about family history, and to write it out or put it on tape for family members, if possible.

According to Buckingham[1], the goals of hospice are:

- Relief of distressing symptoms of disease
- Provision of sustained expert care
- Security of a protective environment
- Assurance that the client and family will not be abandoned

Characteristics of a Hospice

To be legitimately called a hospice, an agency must meet the following criteria:

- The hospice must be a centrally administered, autonomous program. Staff members primarily provide care in the home, with backup inpatient services.
- The goal should be symptom control (intensive **palliative care**), not curative measures. Clients should remain as alert and comfortable as possible.
- The major unit of care should be the client and his or her family. The term "family" refers to a client's significant others, whether related by blood or not. The significant others are designated as *primary caregivers*.
- Team members should practice interdisciplinary care, under a qualified physician's direction. Specially trained volunteers must be available to provide a multitude of services. Services are available on call 24 hours a day, 7 days a week.
- Support should be available for hospice staff, as well as for the client's caregivers.
- Hospice services must be extended to the family during the time of bereavement.
- Hospice services should be based on a client's physical needs, not financial resources.
- To qualify for Medicare reimbursement, the hospice must follow up with the primary (family) caregivers for 1 year following the death of their loved one.

Box 99-1 lists criteria for a person's admission to a hospice.

☛ KEY CONCEPT

The hospice concept incorporates control of physical and psychological symptoms, continuous access to medical and nursing services, trained caregivers, and bereavement support for survivors. Cure is not the goal—the focus is on relief and comfort. Hospice attempts to make the dying process an experience of coming together for clients and families.

If a client experiences a remission, the hospice program will discharge the client to resume aggressive medical treatment. If another exacerbation occurs, the client can reenter the hospice program.

Service Coordination

In most cases, hospice staff members coordinate a client's care in the client's home for as long as possible. Many clients choose to die at home; staff members help clients and families make this decision. Primary caregivers (in most cases) must be willing to assume responsibility for home care. Staff

---

➤➤ BOX 99-1

SAMPLE CRITERIA FOR ADMISSION TO A HOSPICE*

- A diagnosis of progressive, terminal illness is confirmed. The physician, client, and family agree that control of symptoms is the primary goal, after determining that no curative treatment is available or desirable.
- Life expectancy is usually no more than 6 months from date of admission.
- A person (people) agrees to be primary caregiver(s) (responsible for care 24 hours a day).
- In most cases, the patient and family have agreed on DNR/DNI status.
- Hospice care can be discontinued with the agreement of the client, family, and attending physician.
- Admission can be directed primarily toward meeting the needs of the family.

———
*Courtesy of Good Samaritan Hospice Care, Kellogg Community College, Battle Creek, Michigan and Abbott-Northwestern Home Care, Hospice Unit, St. Louis Park, Minnesota.

---

members meet with clients and primary caregivers to determine if this is feasible, and alert them to the many available supplementary services.

☛ KEY CONCEPT

Hospice care does not speed death, nor does it unduly prolong life. Team members assist clients and their primary caregivers to manage pain and other symptoms. Hospice's goal is a safe passage through terminal illness, while maintaining self-esteem. (Assisted suicide and euthanasia are not components of hospice.)

Funding. Funding is available to provide hospice care. Some clients have private insurance. In addition, the federal Social Security Act provides Medicare and Medicaid assistance to specific clients. These clients must meet requirements called conditions of participation (**COP**), which are set out in Title XXII of the Act. Services are usually covered on a per-diem (by the day) basis. This payment covers various levels of client services, including home care, SNF (skilled nursing facility, nursing home) and hospital care, as well as respite care to assist the family.

Equipment. Durable medical equipment (**DME**) is also covered by third-party payers. DME could include a hospital bed, bedside commode (**BSC**), overbed table (**OBT**) or trapeze, as well as high-tech equipment such as an IV pump or oxygen concentrator.

Symptom Management

The dying person often has many physical symptoms that require nursing management. Some are discussed in Chapter 59; however, symptoms related to hospice care often require longer periods of management or different management than in other settings. The client, the family caregivers, and the hospice team plan together to manage pain and other symptoms. Specific aspects of symptom control in hospice will be discussed as a separate section later in this chapter.

Usually, clients discontinue radiation therapy or chemotherapy before admission to a hospice. As per the PSDA of 1991, hospice clients are often encouraged to designate Do Not Resuscitate (**DNR**) and Do Not Intubate (**DNI**) status. Clients often choose to be on Do Not Hospitalize (**DNH**) status as well.

☛ KEY CONCEPT

One philosophy of hospice is that suffering is not prolonged, while not extending hope. Symptoms are managed as non-invasively as possible.

Client and Family as Care Unit

The client and his or her family, along with hospice team members, decide what type of care is most appropriate. A specially trained nurse makes an initial home visit to assess the home's physical setup and the family dynamics. This assessment includes an evaluation of the willingness, ability, and motivation of primary caregivers and the client to participate. The client is particularly encouraged to use medications and other modalities for pain control.

After the initial visit by the nurse, other hospice team members make most of the home visits. These team members assist family members to prepare for their loved one's death. They help with matters such as funeral planning and plans for the future. They can also refer clients for services such as writing a will and financial planning. Clients and family members are encouraged to join support groups. Usually, if a client has a peaceful terminal phase of life, family members feel less guilt and grief. (Staff members also observe and report on family members who experience unhealthy grieving, so they can receive assistance.)

Respite Care

Caring for a dying person is exhausting and frustrating and may cause financial hardships. A primary caregiver may be required to take excessive time away from work; the client may have been the primary breadwinner of the family. The term **respite** means that caregivers occasionally "take a break." Respite care is accomplished by admitting clients to inpatient hospices, hospitals, or nursing homes or by arranging for supplemental home care for a few days. Some hospices have contracts with inpatient facilities for family respite. The cost of respite care is often covered by third-party payers.

☛ KEY CONCEPT

Family caregivers should be encouraged to take advantage of respite services. By doing this, they will be physically and emotionally more able to continue with the difficult task of caring for their loved one.

Interdisciplinary Care

The interdisciplinary team or group (**IDT** or **IDG**) consists of physicians, nurses, medical social workers, therapists (occupational, physical, speech, respiratory), clergy, bereavement coordinators, dietitians, pharmacologists, home health aides, homemakers, and volunteers. Community agencies, such as the American Cancer Society, often have hospital beds and other DME to loan to families, or the cost of DME may be covered by a third-party payer. Figure 99-2 depicts examples of **interdisciplinary care** in hospice.

Although physician-directed services are required, the client is the center of care; the interdisciplinary team responds to each individual's needs. A plan of care (**POC**) is established for each client; input is obtained from the client, the primary caregivers, and members of the IDT.

The physician establishes the diagnosis, signs the initial certification of terminal illness, performs the admission history and physical examination, and orders required tests and medications. The physician follows up with the client throughout the illness and certifies death. (Often the physician is the first person to suggest to the client and family that hospice would be appropriate.)

Role of the Nurse.   An RN does the initial admission and evaluation of the client and the home. A nationally certified RN is entitled to use the initials **CRNH** (Certified RN, Hospice). The case manager is usually an RN. All hospice workers observe the client's ongoing condition and discuss findings with other team members.

Nurses set up medications as ordered and evaluate the client's compliance. Determining the effects of the medication regimen is essential. Questions such as the following must be answered: Are the medications effectively controlling pain? Are they causing unwanted side effects?

Hospice nurses answer caregivers' questions and assist other team members as needed. They may perform functions such as drawing blood or teaching caregivers to use specialized equipment. They function as client advocates, ensuring that each client's care is maximized.

Role of Home Health Aides and Homemakers. These team members work under the guidance of the case manager/hospice nurse. They assist primary caregivers to meet the daily needs of the client, such as cleanliness and nutrition. For example, the client may receive a bed bath three times a week, given by a home health aide.

Role of Primary Caregivers.   **Primary caregivers** are vital to the client's care. They can identify changes in the client's condition that might not be noticeable to others. They can suggest approaches to care that meet with everyone's approval. They provide a constant liaison between the client and the hospice team.

Some functions of daily care are performed by the primary caregivers. For example, after medications are set up by the nurse, their administration is supervised by the client and the caregivers.

Role of Volunteers.   Integral to any hospice program are specially trained volunteers, mostly lay people, who constitute more than 80% of all people involved in hospice. Volunteers donate over 5 million hours per year to hospice programs in

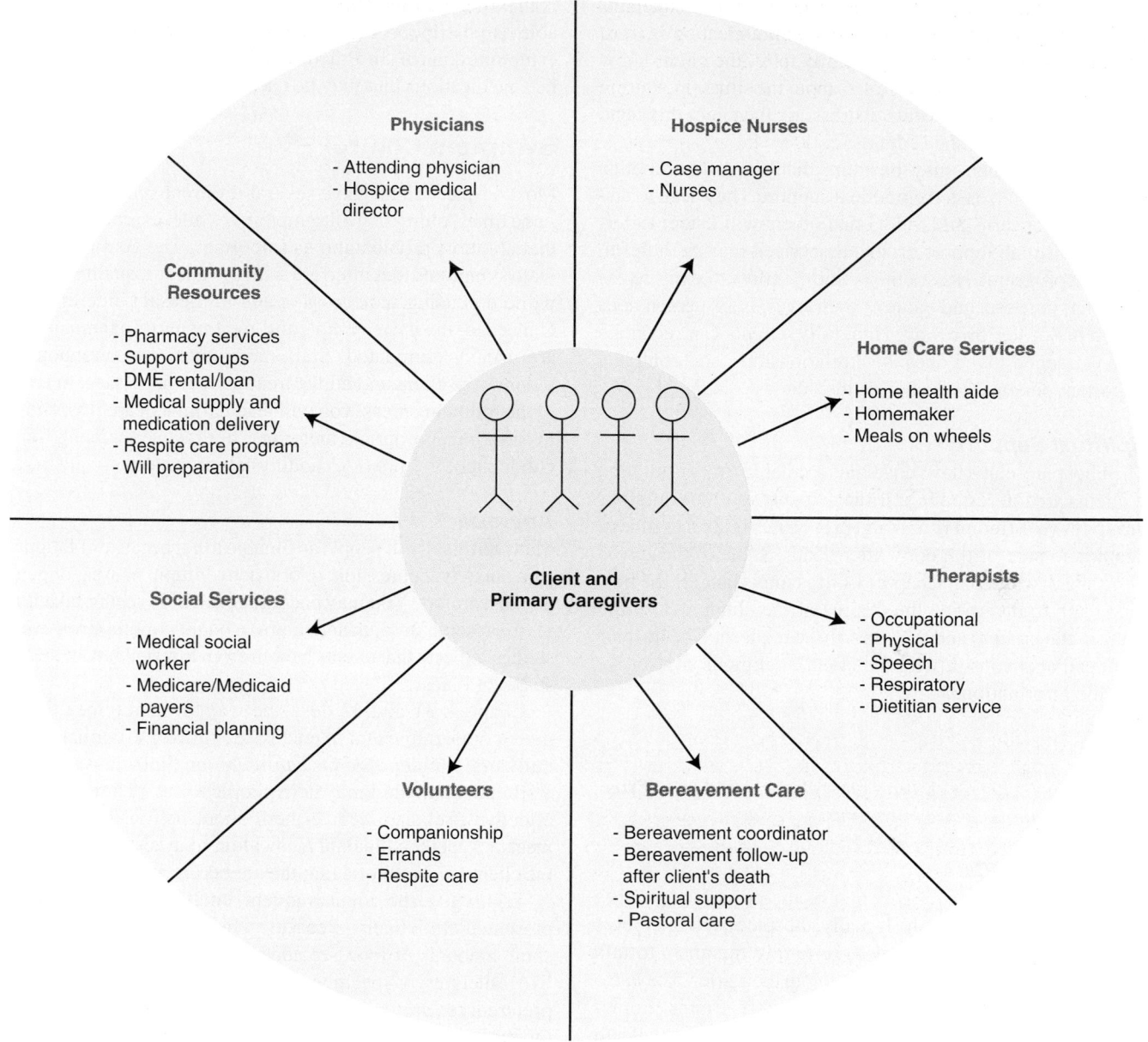

FIGURE 99-2. Interdisciplinary care in hospice. Note that the client, along with the primary care-givers, is the center of all hospice care. The care is under the direction of a physician and is carried out by nurses, volunteers, and other members of the hospice team.

the United States alone. They perform many tasks that assist and support clients and families. They provide emotional support, run errands, assist with physical care, provide short periods of respite, and help with child care and household tasks. Volunteers are often the "unconditional presence" needed to assist families to share their feelings.

☛ KEY CONCEPT

Many volunteers in hospice programs have been primary caregivers in their own families. Therefore, they can provide particular empathy and understanding.

Role of On-Call Services. Services of hospice staff are available 24 hours a day. Staff members answer questions or concerns with reassurance and assistance. They may make home visits at any time to help families deal with physical or emotional problems, and they come when the client dies. If families know on-call services are available, they usually can keep clients at home longer. In many cases, hospice clients are able to die at home, with the on-call assistance of hospice staff.

Emotional Support

The greatest fear of most clients is that they will be left alone to die. Caregivers need to be alert to this fear and provide more support as the illness progresses. Volunteers can assist by staying with clients to give respite to the family. The second greatest fear of most clients is that of having uncontrolled pain. This pain can usually be managed successfully.

Kind and thoughtful communication with hospice clients is essential. Many times, nonverbal communication is most helpful. It is important for the family to let the client know that they care and that they are sad about the situation. Putting on a "stiff upper lip" is often distressing: the client thinks no one cares that he or she is dying.

Family members may be more distressed than clients; therefore, they also need emotional support. They need to discuss their concerns and to feel that others will listen. Referrals to spiritual support or social services may be helpful. Hospice programs assist clients and families to explore the meaning, purpose, and value of their lives. Each person does this in his or her own way. Hopefully, clients can reconcile with estranged loved ones, heal relationships, and complete important personal tasks before they die.

Spiritual Support

Most hospice teams have chaplains available for consultation if clients are interested in spiritual support. Various religious groups have different rituals and procedures related to illness, death, and care of the body after death. Some of these religions are discussed in Chapter 14. It is important for the hospice team to determine the desires of the client and family early in the process and to follow these requests. The hospice team can also consult with the client's religious advisor for specific information.

☛ KEY CONCEPT

Respect each client's cultural and religious customs. If you are unsure about desired procedures, be sure to ask.

Bereavement Care

Bereavement (grieving) is part of the process of dealing with a loved one's death. Usually, hospice staff members attend funeral services. They urge family members to talk about their feelings and to work through their grief. They also encourage families to attend grief support groups. Sometimes, staff members make home visits after a client's death to evaluate family members and to assist in their adjustment. Hospice protocol includes bereavement followup for 1 year after a client's death.

Support for Hospice Staff

Hospice staff members need emotional support when they regularly work with dying people. Support groups or other outlets must be available for team members to deal with the loss of people for whom they have cared. Grieving when clients die is normal and acceptable. Family members often appreciate staff members who express their grief.

ASSISTING IN SYMPTOM CONTROL

The hospice nurse usually does not provide a great deal of direct physical care. The focus is on identifying the needs of the client and family. The case manager coordinates the client's care with other members of the team and with the family (see Fig. 99-2). A major component of all hospice care

is that of symptom control—to make the client as comfortable as possible. As a nurse, you will play a major role in symptom control. In Practice: Important Medications 99-1 lists medications that may be used.

Symptom Control

Most hospice clients have several different symptoms at the same time. Addressing all symptoms, while determining those that are most problematic, is important. The goal is to alleviate symptoms that interfere with the client's quality of life, without causing unnecessary and unpleasant side effects. Unneeded, invasive, and painful treatments or examinations are usually eliminated. Staff members must continuously monitor the client and adjust treatment as necessary. In each of the following areas, you will teach primary caregivers how to carry out appropriate measures. In Practice: Nursing Care Guidelines 99-1 provides additional information.

Anorexia

Many terminally ill people are unable to eat because of fatigue, pain, anxiety, depression, odors, dehydration, nausea, or general discomfort. You may encourage clients to eat or take fluids to preserve strength and improve quality of life. (However, studies indicate that clients benefit from low oral intake in late stages of illness.)

Chapters 31 and 32 describe ways to make mealtimes more comfortable and to encourage intake. Vitamins, tranquilizers, antidepressants, *antiemetics* (anti-nausea medications), or alcohol may help people to eat. (They are most effective if clients receive them about half an hour before meals.) Appetite-stimulant medications may also help. Be sure the client receives good mouth care before and after meals.

Try to give the client frequent, small meals and snacks, presented attractively. Reassure clients and caregivers that small amounts of food are adequate. Ask clients about dislikes, allergies, or specific food difficulties, and consider their preferences. Soft, easily swallowed foods are usually best. Often, fluids are most easily tolerated and should be varied to maintain interest. High-protein, high-calorie supplements, such as Ensure or Resource, are often ordered to provide nourishment without great volume. Clients often enjoy cold drinks, such as iced tea and lemonade. Clear liquids are usually more appealing than creamed milk products or sweetened items. Offer clients ice pops, sherbet, and ice chips.

Mealtimes can be made enjoyable by eliminating unpleasant odors (including cooking odors, perfumes, and malodorous drainage) and by providing fresh air. Other measures include providing music, television, or mail, and socializing when food is served. Bright lights, loud noises, and stuffy room air may be annoying. Teach caregivers, volunteers, and aides ways to encourage clients to eat. Dietitians can also provide suggestions.

In rare cases, nasogastric tube feedings are given. They are uncommon, however, because hospice does not encourage artificial means to prolong life.

Sometimes, clients do not eat or drink. They only receive mouth care. These clients may enjoy sucking on prepared

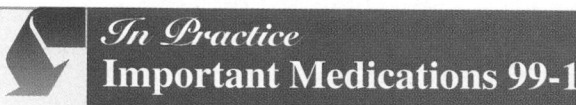

In Practice
Important Medications 99-1

SYMPTOM CONTROL IN HOSPICE CARE

Nausea
ABHR (combination of Ativan, Benadryl, Haldol, Reglan); chlorpromazine HCl (Ormazine, Thorazine); cyclizine (Marezine); dronabinol (Marinol); meclizine (Bonine); metoclopramide HCl (Reglan); ondansetron HCl (Zofran); perphenazine (Trilafon); prochlorperazine (Compazine); thiethylperazine maleate (Torecan); trimethobenzamide (Tigan). Antispasmodics, such as loperamide (Imodium) and transdermal scopolamine, are also used.

Diarrhea
bismuth subsalicylate (Pepto-Bismol); diphenoxylate and atropine sulfate (Lomotil, Lonox); kaolin and pectin mixtures (Kaopectate, Donnagel-MB); loperamide (Imodium); octreotide acetate (Sandostatin); opium tincture, camphorated opium (Paregoric)

Constipation
bisacodyl (Dulcolax, Feen-a-Mint); calcium polycarbophil (Fiberall, FiberCon); cascara sagrada and docusate calcium (Pro-Cal-Sof, Surfak); docusate sodium (Colace); docusate sodium and senna concentrate (Senokot); docusate sodium and casanthranol (Peri-Colace); glycerin (Fleet); lactulose (Cephulac, Duphalac); magnesium hydroxide–milk of magnesia (MOM); magnesium sulfate (Epsom salts); methylcellulose (Citrucel); psyllium (Metamucil, Reguloid); senna (Black-Draught, Fletcher's Castoria); sodium phosphate (Fleet Phospho-Soda)

Bladder Spasm
Belladonna or opium suppositories

Seizures
carbamazepine (Tegretol); clonazepam (Klonopin); lorazepam (Ativan); phenobarbital (Barbita, Solfotron); phenytoin (Dilantin); valproate sodium (Depakote—also for anxiety)

Depression
amitriptyline (Elavil); amoxapine (Asendin); bupropion (Wellbutrin); buspirone (BuSpar); citalopram (Celexa); desipramine (Norpramin); doxepin (Sinequan); fluoxetine (Prozac); fluvoxamine (LuVox); imipramine (Tofranil); mirtazapine (Remeron); nefazodone (Serzone); nortriptyline (Pamelor); paroxetine (Paxil); sertraline (Zoloft); tranylcypromine sulfate (Parnate); trazodone (Desyrel); trimipramine maleate (Surmontil); venlafaxine (Effexor)

Anxiety
alprazolam (Xanax); buspirone (BuSpar); carbemazapine (Tegretol); chlordiazepoxide (Librium); chlorpromazine (Thorazine); diazepam (Valium); doxepin (Sinequan); hydroxyzine HCl (Atarax, Vistaril); lorazepam (Ativan); meprobamate (Equanil, Miltown); mesoridazine (Serentil); oxazepam (Serax); prazepam (Centrax); prochlorperazine (Compazine); thioridazine (Mellaril); trifluoperazine (Stelazine)

Insomnia
amobarbital (Amytal); amobarbital and secobarbital (Tuinal); aprobarbital (Alurate); butabarbital (Butisol); chloral hydrate; diphenhydramine (Benadryl); estazolam (ProSom); ethchlorvynol (Placidyl); flurazepam (Dalmane); glutethimide; hydroxyzine (Atarax, Vistaril); lorazepam (Ativan); pentobarbital (Nembutal); quazepam (Doral); temazepam (Restoril); trazodone (Desyrel); zolpidem (Ambien)

Edema
furosemide (Lasix); metolazone (Zaroxolyn); spironolactone (Aldactone)

---

mouth swabs, a wet washcloth, or ice chips. These items provide liquid and numb the mouth. Hard candy may also be enjoyed.

Nausea and Vomiting
Hospice clients often experience nausea and vomiting caused by anorexia, tumor invasion, pain, inner ear involvement, reaction to narcotics, or increased intracranial pressure. Previous radiation or chemotherapy may also contribute to this condition. Many of the procedures suggested to treat anorexia also apply to nausea. Evaluate nausea for patterns and remove causes whenever possible. Nauseated clients should lie on their right side. Relaxation techniques are effective, as are companionship, music, meditation, backrubs, mouth breath-

ing, and cool cloths on the forehead. Antiemetics and other medications are helpful; clients should receive them approximately one-half hour before meals (see In Practice: Important Medications 99-1). Clients may drink carbonated beverages and eat dry foods, such as popcorn or soda crackers. Ice chips may be soothing. Teach all caregivers to wear gloves when caring for the client who is vomiting.

Diarrhea
Clients may develop diarrhea from lesion involvement, inadequate intake, bowel obstruction, fecal impaction, or infection. Diarrhea may also be a side effect of previous chemotherapy, radiation therapy, or current medications. After determining the cause, follow the physician's order for specific treatment.

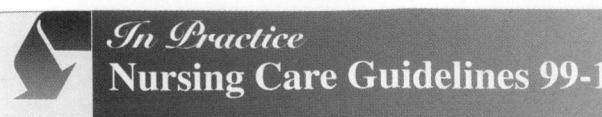

In Practice
Nursing Care Guidelines 99-1

PROVIDING CARE IN HOSPICE NURSING

- Emphasize the positive. Focus on what *can* be done, not on problems.
- Provide practical solutions.
- Control the client's symptoms.
- Do not try to predict the exact time of death.
- Do not get involved in family disputes.
- Allow the client and family to express their spiritual feelings in the way they desire.
- Respect the client's cultural customs and beliefs.
- Maintain your sense of humor.
- Allow the client to be alone or stay with the client, depending on what he or she desires.
- Realize that irrational behavior on the part of the family and the hospice client is a normal part of grieving.
- Be honest. Explain what is happening.
- When in doubt, be quiet.
- Allow the client and family to maintain hope, at whatever level.
- Remember: *comfort* is the goal of all therapy (physical and emotional).

A low-residue diet lessens stimulation. Specific foods causing gas or cramps should be eliminated. (Clients often know what foods bother them.) Encourage clients to drink a variety of fluids (not just water), to prevent electrolyte imbalance. Good skin care around the rectum is necessary. Remind caregivers to wear gloves when giving care.

Constipation

Many clients are constipated because of inactivity, low food/fluid intake, dehydration, a low-residue diet, or tumor invasion. Constipation is a common and troubling side effect of narcotics, especially morphine and codeine. Before constipation is treated, it is necessary to determine if a bowel obstruction exists. Treatment for constipation includes a high-residue diet, as long as it can be tolerated by the client. Many hospice clients routinely receive mild laxatives (eg, Milk of Magnesia), dietary fiber (eg, Metamucil), and/or stool softeners (eg, Colace). Suppositories also encourage peristalsis. If constipation is severe, cathartics and hyperosmotic agents may be necessary. In severe cases, the client may require an enema or manual disimpaction of stool.

Most hospices routinely use a bowel regime, sometimes called a "colon cocktail." A good example of this is the mixture of one cup of applesauce, one cup of prune juice, and one cup of miller's bran. The client takes 1 tablespoon twice daily. This cocktail is usually very effective and provides relief without the use of harsh laxatives and cathartics.

☛ KEY CONCEPT

Sometimes, clients think they are constipated because they are not having daily bowel movements. Teach them that a bowel movement every 2 to 3 days is common, because of physical inactivity and low intake.

Dehydration

Many clients become dehydrated shortly before death. Studies indicate that these clients do not feel hunger or thirst. Dehydration is often unavoidable. Studies have also shown that some dehydration can be beneficial because it dries secretions and reduces choking, nausea, ascites, pulmonary edema, and breathing difficulties. When clients retain fluid, however, feces may become hard and impacted, causing bowel obstruction. Assess for and report dehydration and complications. The physician, together with the client and family, can determine appropriate treatment (if any) for dehydration or electrolyte imbalance. The major area of discomfort for the dehydrated client is a dry mouth. This can be alleviated by ice pops, ice chips, drops of water, or sucking on a wet washcloth or a piece of hard candy.

Skin Breakdown

A major challenge in the physical care of hospice clients is preventing skin breakdown and pressure areas. Non-intact skin can be a source of infection and pain. Clients with terminal illnesses are often too uncomfortable or weak to move and may remain in one position. Their nutritional status and hydration may be inadequate to maintain skin integrity. The disease process may have made their skin *friable* (fragile). Stress the importance of frequent position changes and protecting pressure points when teaching caregivers. Chapter 50 discusses skin care in detail.

Caregivers should wear gloves when treating skin that is not intact. They should keep the client's skin clean and dry. If possible, clients should occasionally leave the bed to relieve pressure. Special mattresses may help prevent skin breakdown; some special beds allow clients to remain in bed continually without sacrificing skin integrity. Regular pain medications provide maximum comfort.

Respiratory Distress

Many clients have lung involvement and dyspnea. Stress reduction and position changes provide maximum comfort. Using a fan to circulate air or an air conditioner to cool the room, and elevating the head of the bed, may help. Assess the client's vital signs and level of consciousness. Some clients need supplemental oxygen because of fever, anxiety, infection, or fluid collection. Oxygen concentrators, rather than tanks, are commonly used in the home (see Chap. 86). Thoracentesis may relieve pressure, and medications may decrease secretions and improve respiration. Postural drainage and nebulizer treatments help eliminate secretions from the lungs; surgery may help relieve obstructions. The client may be able to breathe only when in a sitting position (orthopnea). Clients also may benefit from aerosolized inhalers, cough medicines, decongestants, or low doses of morphine. Hospice programs rarely use heroic measures such as mechanical ventilators.

Seizures

Clients may be at risk for seizures, secondary to lesion involvement or brain metastases. They are treated with anti-seizure medications, such as phenytoin (Dilantin) or valproate sodium (Depakote), both of which are available in tablet, liquid, and injectable forms.

Management of Odor

A problem in caring for some clients who have cancer or other disorders is a disagreeable odor that may embarrass clients and upset their families. Chapter 59 presents suggestions for controlling odor. Aerosolized sprays are available to help cover or eliminate odor; a few drops of wintergreen oil on a cotton ball may also be used. Another device for odor management is the charcoal filter dressing. Odors pass through the filter before they enter the atmosphere. These dressings are expensive and are usually only used when odors are very disturbing.

Depression

Clients or family members may need treatment for depression. You can intervene by listening with empathy and validating feelings. Clinical depression, with or without suicidal ideation (SI), may require antidepressant medication. Death is often a sad situation and may cause some level of depression. Continuing clinical depression, however, is usually treated and should be prevented as much as possible (Fig. 99-3). The hospice social worker is a good resource and is available to work with clients and families as needed. A referral to a psychologist or psychiatrist may be necessary.

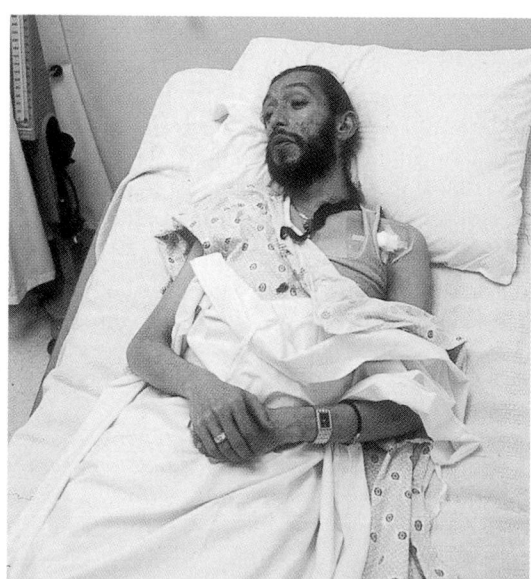

FIGURE 99-3. The person with a terminal illness, such as AIDS, may be very depressed and may feel that no one cares. It is important for hospice staff and primary caregivers to be available, to allow this person to express feelings, and to refer the client to professional counseling if necessary.

Anxiety

Major causes of anxiety include fear of severe pain and fear of being alone. Some clients are afraid of dying or are concerned about the future for their loved ones. Anxious clients sometimes become agitated or paranoid. Listen and offer reassurance. Sometimes clients need anti-anxiety medications. Some of these medications help to control other symptoms as well.

Insomnia and Hypersomnia

Sleep disturbances are common in hospice care. Insomnia includes difficulty in falling asleep or in staying asleep for an adequate length of time. Insomnia may be a result of anxiety or pain. Sleep deprivation can be serious. It may lead to further agitation and discomfort, as well as acceleration of the disease process. Extreme sleep deprivation can also lead to paranoia, hallucinations, and other mental disorders. Assist the client to sleep by providing comfort measures, such as fresh bedding or a backrub. Soft music and relaxation tapes, as well as self-hypnosis and guided imagery, may help. Medications are often prescribed to help clients fall asleep and remain asleep.

Depressed clients often sleep too much (*hypersomnia*). The goal of hospice care, especially early on in the process, is for clients to sleep adequately at night, while maintaining normal activity and as much mobility as possible during the day.

Pain Management

Often, clients experience chronic, severe, and unremitting pain that differs from the occasional and temporary pain caused by other conditions. (See Chap. 55 for general pain management considerations.) Aggressive pain management is a primary goal of hospice nursing. The hospice concept encourages clients to take advantage of available pain control measures, but this is not required. Morphine is very commonly used and works well, although a number of other modalities are available to assist in pain control. Addiction is not a concern.

Pain Assessment

The client's pain and its level of interference with activities, rest, and general comfort is evaluated. The most important factor in this assessment is the client's own description; only the client knows how the pain feels and what measures offer relief. Ask clients what makes pain worse or better. Classify pain as to its location, intensity, and severity (see Chap. 55).

☛ KEY CONCEPT

Sometimes clients want to experience pain because the pain reminds them that they are still alive. They may refuse adequate pain-control measures.

Pharmacologic Therapy

In 1986, the World Health Organization issued guidelines for managing cancer pain. Medications and other modalities are generally used. The three-step analgesic ladder (Table 99-1) suggests nonopioids, weak opioids, and strong opioids for mild, intermediate, and severe pain, respectively. **Adjuvant**

▪▪▪ TABLE 99-1 *An* ANALGESIC LADDER*

	Medication	Pain Continues	Comments
Severe Pain ↑	Strong opioid	Add stronger opioid	Client may now be NPO; use sublingual, rectal, or transdermal fentanyl, subQ morphine, etc.
Moderate Pain ↑	Weak opioid	Add strong opioid, increase dose, shorten interval between doses	
Mild to Moderate Pain	Nonopioid	Add aspirin, acetaminophen, or nonsteroidal anti-inflammatory drug (NSAID)	Opioid-sparing effect—less opioid needed

Nursing Considerations
• Other medications are often combined with the above.
• Use the least-invasive management and the mildest medications first.
• Rectal suppositories or parenteral medications are usually given if the client is nauseated.

*Based on the WHO Analgesic Ladder and other information in *Management of Cancer Pain: Adults, Quick Reference for Clinicians, Number 9,* 1994.

(assisting) medications may be added to *potentiate* (enhance) the opioid's effects or for other symptoms. The goal is to manage pain with the least amount and potency of medication and the highest possible level of client consciousness. Medications are increased as pain intensity increases. A recent American Family Physician Journal study found that "using progressive therapies demonstrates safety and effectiveness of the WHO three-tiered approach to pain management." The University of Wisconsin Pain and Policy Study Group has also endorsed this approach. Lesser amounts of medication are often needed if clients self-administer their medications (PCA) and if medications are taken around the clock.

In 1994, the World Health Organization (WHO) estimated the prevalence of use of progressive therapies as follows:

• Oral, transdermal, and rectal drugs: 75% to 85%
• IV and subcutaneous drugs: 5% to 20%
• Epidural and intrathecal analgesics: 2% to 6%
• Nerve blocks, palliative surgery, and *ablative surgery* (eg, severing nerves; see p. 1688): 1% to 5%

In Practice: Important Medications 99-2 lists medications used in pain management. Consider several points when administering medications to hospice clients:

• Gradually increase a narcotic's dose (this is called **titration** of the dose).
• Also decrease dosages ("titrate down") gradually, to prevent withdrawal symptoms if the drug is discontinued.
• When routes change (eg, from oral to rectal or intramuscular [IM]), dosages usually change as well.
• Consider the client's tolerance to other medications, as well as previous use of alcohol and street drugs. Tolerance may cause clients to require higher or lower doses.

Administration Routes. Oral medications are the first choice for pharmacologic pain management. Clients are usually involved in self-medication. Caregivers help clients to assess and evaluate severity of pain for adequate manage-

ment. Some oral medications are very effective for mild pain; oral codeine and oxycodone with aspirin (Percodan) are commonly used. Clients usually prefer liquid medications to tablets. In some cases, medications are administered by the *sublingual* (under the tongue), *buccal* (inside the cheek), or rectal route. Some drugs, such as fentanyl (Duragesic, Sublimaze), are administered *transdermally,* by use of a skin patch or oral lozenge.

When oral, rectal, or transdermal medications no longer control pain, subcutaneous or IV medications are often initiated. In the case of IV medication administration, a heparin lock is routinely placed to preclude repeated venipuncture. In this case, caregivers and clients learn to administer medications via the lock and to flush it (see Chap. 63). In some cases, clients receive subcutaneous injections, either self-administered or administered by caregivers. (The IM route is usually not used because absorption is variable, due to deterioration of muscle tissue and circulation. It is also painful and inconvenient.)

Patient-controlled anesthesia (**PCA**) pumps allow clients to control their own IV medication administration. Some clients have implanted, preprogrammed pumps that continuously dispense medications to provide constant blood levels. Routes of administration (oral, IV, and so forth) may also be combined.

☛ KEY CONCEPT

Clients who can regulate their own medication usually use less. Allowing the person to have this control also increases self-esteem.

Some clients receive IV fluids. Infusions may contain dextrose (sugar), electrolytes (eg, potassium), or medications (eg, morphine). With a continuous drip, an IV pump or controller is often used. Clients or caregivers regulate the equipment and the flow of medication, and know when to call for assistance and what to do in case of an alarm. The medical

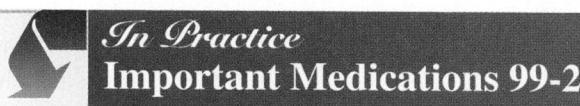

In Practice
Important Medications 99-2

MEDICATIONS USED IN PAIN MANAGEMENT

Acetaminophen and NSAIDs (Non-opioids)

acetaminophen (Mapap, Anacin Aspirin Free, Panadol, Tylenol)—because it is not an anti-inflammatory, it is not as effective; chewable aspirin (ASA); carboprofen (Rimadyl); choline magnesium trisalicylate (Trilisate); choline salicylate (Arthropan); diflunisal (Dolobid); etodolac, ultradol (Lodine); fenoprofen calcium (Nalfon); ibuprofen (Advil, Excedrin, Motrin, Nuprin, Rufen); indomethacin (Indocin); ketoprofen (Orudis); ketorolac tromethamine (Toradol); meclofenamate (Meclofen, Meclomen); mefenamic acid (Ponstel); naproxen (Naprosyn); naproxen sodium (Anaprox); sodium salicylate

Opioids

Mild opioids include: codeine, hydrocodone, and propoxyphene. They are often added to NSAIDs. Codeine is not often used because of undesirable side effects.

Mid-range opioid is oxycodone.

Strong opioids include: morphine (the most commonly used), hydro-morphone, levorphenol, and transdermal fentanyl.

(Opioid side effects include respiratory depression, sedation, nausea and vomiting, constipation, confusion, urinary problems, dry mouth, and pruritus.)

Full Morphine-Like Agonists

codeine often combined with ASA or acetaminophen (such as Amaphen—acetaminophen, butabarbital, caffeine, and codeine); fentanyl citrate (Sublimaze liquid); transdermal fentanyl (Duragesic patch); transmucosal fentanyl (Oralet); hydromorphone (Dilaudid); levorphanol (Levo-Dromoran); meperidine (Demerol); morphine in various forms, including controlled-release (MS Contin, Roxanol); oxycodone (Roxicodone); oxymorphone (Numorphan); propoxyphene (Darvon)

Partial Morphine-Like Agonists

buprenorphine HCl (Buprenex)

Mixed Agonist/Antagonists

butorphanol tartrate (Stadol); dezocine (Dalgan); nalbuphine (Nubain); pentazocine (Talwin); pentazocine and naloxone (Talwin NX)

Combination Opioid/NSAIDs

codeine with aspirin (Empirin with codeine); codeine with acetaminophen (Tylenol with codeine); hydrocodone with acetaminophen (Vicodin); fiorinal with codeine; oxycodone and ASA (Percodan); oxycodone and acetaminophen (Percocet)

Adjuvant Drugs Used for Pain Management

anticonvulsants: manage neuropathic pain—include: carbemazepine (Tegretol); clonazepam (Klonopin); gabapentin (Neurontin); phenytoin (Dilantin); valproate (Depakote)

antidepressants: manage neuropathic pain, may potentiate effects of opioids (amitriptyline first choice). Others include: desipramine (Norpramin); doxepin (Sinequan); imipramine (Tofranil); nortriptylene (Pamelor); paroxetine (Paxil)

corticosteroids: mood elevation, anti-inflammatory, antiemetic, appetite stimulation, reduce spinal cord edema, and help manage bone pain and arthralgia. Commonly used: prednisolone (Delta-Cortef); prednisone (Deltasone, Meticorten)

muscle relaxants: carisoprodol (Soma, Soridol); chlorzoxazone (Paraflex); cyclobenzaprine (Flexeril); methocarbamol (Robaxin); orphenadrine citrate (Banflex, Norflex)

neuroleptics and others: methotrimeprazine (Levoprome); hydroxyzine (Atarax, Vistaril)—also for anxiety, insomnia, nausea, itching

anesthetics: used as secondary treatment for neuropathic pain. Include: calcitonin (Cibacalcin); capsaicin cream (Zostrix); clonazepam (Klonopin); clonidine (Catapres); ketamine (Ketular); lidocaine; methotrimeprazine (Levoprome)

adjuvant medications used for deep bone pain include the biphosphonates (such as pamidronate [Aredia], which is given IV, and etidronate [Didronel], which is given orally or IV)

supply company delivers IV bags to the client's home. Nurses or pharmacists add medications and electrolytes to the solution as needed. The family hangs the bags, adjusts the pump or controller, and troubleshoots the machine.

Around-the-Clock Medication Administration. Many people survive longer and require lower medication doses when they receive medications around the clock, instead of after pain occurs. Twelve-hour pain medication taken regularly, PCA pumps, or continuous-administration

pumps are usually most effective and easiest to manage for pain control. Teach caregivers the value of administering pain medications through these methods. They should give clients medications before pain occurs or before it increases. Allay their fears about the client's addiction to narcotics or other medications.

Management of Side Effects. A major adverse side effect of opiates is sedation, sometimes with respiratory depression and dangerous lowering of blood pressure. When administering morphine or other opiates, assess the client's respiratory status and level of consciousness. Sedation precedes dangerous drug-induced respiratory depression. Evaluate the client's sedation as follows (required nursing actions are presented in parentheses):

- Awake, alert
- Drowsy, easily aroused
- Asleep, easily aroused
- Drowsy most of the time, may go to sleep during conversation (give less medication)
- **Somnolent:** very difficult or impossible to arouse; shallow respirations of fewer than 10 to 12 breaths per minute; pinpoint pupils (discontinue medication and consult physician—an antidote, such as naloxone [Narcan], may be needed if client does not respond when told to breathe deeply)

Another common side effect of opioids is constipation, which can be uncomfortable and can result in bowel impaction and obstruction. Usually, clients receive laxatives or stool softeners when taking opioids. (Remember that hospice clients have lowered intake and activity and often have a bowel movement only every 2 to 3 days.)

Long-term treatment with opiates can cause other undesirable side effects, such as nausea and vomiting, dry mouth, itching, difficulty in voiding, and sleep disturbances. Treat these side effects symptomatically.

☛ KEY CONCEPT

People who smoke, abuse drugs and other substances, or have been very athletic often require more medication to achieve comfort. Endorphin production decreases as clients become less active, which may necessitate more medication. People with severe liver or kidney damage usually metabolize medications more slowly and not as completely and may also require higher dosages.

Psychosocial Modalities for Pain Management

Cognitive and behavioral interventions may help in pain management. Clients may benefit from psychotherapy, support groups, or pastoral counseling. Education is important. Clients should visit with family and friends, play with pets, read, sew, or watch television. These activities can help to distract clients from pain. Listening to music can be soothing, particularly if clients learn to increase their level of distraction by keeping time to the music or turning up the volume. Exercise, if possible, can relieve pain by releasing endorphins into the system.

Great benefits have been achieved by many clients through the use of guided imagery, self-hypnosis, guided relaxation, and visualization. Relaxation and visualization tapes are available, which help the client to visualize a peaceful, restful place and to relax all the muscles in the body. Visualization and self-healing techniques assist the client to view the illness or the CA cells as small and weak, and his or her body as strong and viable. Self-hypnosis can assist the client to gradually "move pain out of the body." By using these and other techniques, anxiety and discomfort can be alleviated without medication. Some of these techniques can also promote sleep.

The technique of *biofeedback* allows the client to anticipate pain and to deliver an impulse that will help to alleviate the pain. This strategy can also assist the client to assess intensity of pain and to determine how much medication, if any, to use.

Physical Modalities for Pain Management

Encourage clients to maintain physical activity and to exercise for as long as possible. Movement prevents stiffness and other problems related to immobility. Immobilizing an affected part or repositioning the body is often helpful. Cutaneous stimulation modalities such as heat, massage, ultrasound, and vibration promote exercise and relieve pain. Sometimes applying ice on the *contralateral* side (side opposite from pain) helps. Acupuncture and acupressure can provide *counterstimulation* (against the pain), and can also directly interfere with pain transmission.

The transcutaneous electrical nerve stimulation (**TENS**) unit applies electrical stimulation directly to nerves and interrupts transmission of pain sensations. This unit is activated by the client. It should be activated at the first hint of discomfort, for maximum effectiveness.

Palliative Radiation, Medications, and Surgery

Palliative radiation may reduce tumor size or arrest growth. It is usually aimed at a specific area. IV injection of radioactive materials can help relieve severe pain of widespread bony metastases. In specific cases, medications, such as hormones, are given to reduce the size of a tumor and thereby relieve pain related to that tumor (usually a tumor in the reproductive system).

Surgical interventions to control intractable pain include nerve block and neurosurgery. A temporary nerve block is applied with a local anesthetic (eg, lidocaine, bupivacaine). Permanent nerve block is achieved with a neurolytic agent (eg, ethanol, phenol), which "kills" the nerve. Both types of medications are injected directly into nerves carrying pain sensations. If all else fails, neurosurgery may be performed to *sever* (cut) the pain pathway—this procedure is called **ablative surgery** or *surgical ablation*. Palliative surgery may also be performed in any body part to relieve pressure or obstruction by removing part of a tumor (**debulking**). *Hypophysectomy* (pituitary gland removal) may relieve deep bone pain.

CHILDREN IN HOSPICE PROGRAMS

Staff members must consider dying children in terms of their developmental levels and levels of understanding (see Unit III). Flexibility is essential to evaluate each child individually. Very young children may be unable to differentiate death from other types of separation (eg, sleep). As children get older, their understanding of death's permanence evolves. Children often respond to nonverbal cues such as play, drama, art, music, other children, pets, or stuffed toys more easily than they respond to adults. Children and their families need to communicate and to enjoy every chance they have to be together. Children should be involved as much as possible in decisions regarding their own care.

Children usually know what is happening. They may try to talk about death. If others discourage their questions, children may not bring up the subject again. When working with dying children, be specific when explaining death. For example, talking about "going to sleep" can be confusing and frightening. Help children to understand that they have contributed to the world and to their family, even though they have lived a short time. Let them know that they will be greatly missed. The family should be encouraged to explain death to the child in terms of their religious beliefs.

☞ KEY CONCEPT

Approach dying children at their appropriate developmental level. Children usually understand what is happening, but need their questions answered. They need to discuss their feelings, perhaps more so than do adults. Allow children to see your feelings about them and the situation. Let them know you care. Remember to adjust medication doses according to a child's size and reactions.

Family members are naturally devastated by a child's illness. They need a great deal of support and reassurance. Let them know that crying is acceptable. When family members do not show their emotions, children may mistakenly believe that others do not care. The entire family needs a great deal of support. Make sure they are referred to a support group. One such support group is "The Compassionate Friends," which has chapters in many cities. This group is particularly targeted toward families who have lost a child.

When the Client Dies

Many hospice clients choose to die at home. Assisting loved ones with end-of-life work is a special privilege and a great challenge for nurses and primary caregivers. Your nursing responsibility is to assist in this process and to make sure that caregivers know what to expect and what to do when death occurs. Encourage caregivers to participate in the process as much as possible.

When a client dies, the caregivers have been instructed to call the hospice nurse (see In Practice: Educating the Client 99-1). If you are working with the family, go to the home to assist with postmortem care (Chap. 59). Caregivers may wish to assist. Encourage them to do as much as is comfortable for them. They may wish to wash the client's hands and face, comb the hair, or more. Support the family's wishes and assist with technical details.

The following are nursing functions performed for a client who dies at home:

- Remove all equipment.
- Allow the family time alone with their deceased family member.
- Encourage the family to do as much postmortem care as they wish.
- Prepare the body for transportation to the funeral home. Assist in notifying the funeral home, if needed.

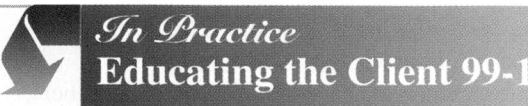

In Practice
Educating the Client 99-1

WHEN THE CLIENT DIES AT HOME

Family teaching *in preparation for the client's death* at home includes the following:

- Call the hospice nurse.
- Keep the telephone number handy.
- Provide the following information:
  - Time of death
  - Last medications administered, dosage, time given
  - Client's condition during last 8 hours
  - Name, address, and phone number of funeral home
  - Name, address, and phone number of next of kin
  - When client was last seen by a registered nurse and/or the case manager

- Count narcotics and dispose of them, per agency policy.
- Listen to and validate the family's need to talk about the loved one's final moments.
- Document all information.
- Make sure the physician and coroner have been notified. (The coroner is not required to come to the home of a registered hospice client.)
- Assist the family, as needed, to make arrangements for the body's transfer.
- Assist the family to make arrangements for the return of rented or borrowed medical equipment.
- Refer the family to a bereavement support group.
- Make sure the family knows that you wish to be notified of the time and date of the funeral and that someone from the hospice will probably attend.
- Let the family know that they will continue to be involved in the hospice program for the next year.

☞ KEY CONCEPT

Remember that grief is natural when a loved one dies, even if the death was anticipated. Allow the family to express their grief. It is appropriate for you to show your grief as well. It is also important to remember that the hospice staff needs time to "debrief" and grieve together following the death of a client.

✄ STUDENT SYNTHESIS

Key Points

- Hospice care is designed for terminally ill people. Its focus is providing aggressive, intensive palliative care and assisting with physical, psychological, social, and spiritual needs.

Upon completing a basic nursing program, the student nurse is eligible to sit for the licensing examination and obtain a nursing license. This chapter describes the licensure examination, the procedure for obtaining the initial nursing license, and the responsibilities involved in maintaining this license. In addition, this chapter discusses the change in role from that of a student nurse to that of a graduate nurse who functions as an entry-level nurse within the nursing and healthcare team. This chapter also presents information related to professional activities, along with a discussion of ways to balance work and personal responsibilities and activities.

NURSING LICENSURE

Chapters 2 and 4 of this book introduced the topics of nursing licensure, differences in licensing laws, and legal aspects of licensure. When a nursing student completes an approved nursing program, he or she is eligible to apply to "sit for" (take) the licensure examination. Upon passing this examination, the individual is licensed as an LPN/LVN or RN in that state or territory. The nursing license is one's passport to employment. It is vital for each nurse to obtain a license and to maintain it if he or she plans to work as a nurse.

☛ KEY CONCEPT

In nearly all states and territories, it is illegal *to perform certain nursing functions without a license, even if the person does not call himself or herself a nurse.*

Permit to Practice

In many states, new graduates are issued a "permit" to practice and are usually called "graduate nurses" or "graduate practical nurses" until they receive a license. Other states require new graduates to practice as nursing assistants until they are licensed. In most cases, nurses are paid less until they have taken the licensure examination or until they receive notification that they have passed the examination. If a nurse does not pass the examination on the first writing, often he or she is not allowed to practice as a nurse until fully licensed, even though a permit was issued previously. Procedures vary among states. In some states, this person can practice as a "graduate nurse"; in other states the person must now practice as a "nursing assistant" until fully licensed.

Probationary Status

In many hospitals and in some nursing homes, new graduates are required to practice for a period, often 6 months, as an intern or "nurse resident." This type of employment is considered probationary, and full employment status begins after the person satisfactorily completes the probationary requirement.

Each facility specifies the criteria for removing probationary status. Many facilities require the new graduate to pass a written and skills test in medication administration. In addition, facilities sometimes require a mentor or orientation instructor to evaluate the nurse on commonly performed nursing skills.

The probationary period gives both the employer and the employee an opportunity to determine if this job placement is appropriate. Such factors as punctuality, dependability, minimal use of sick leave, and ability to get along with co-workers and clients are also considered. An employee in the probationary period can be terminated without due process.

After the person has successfully passed probation, he or she is usually eligible to use vacation time and cannot be terminated without cause and without due process.

☛ KEY CONCEPT

If a new graduate has not become licensed during the probationary period, many facilities will terminate the person's employment.

Licensure Examination (NCLEX)

To become licensed as an RN, LPN, or LVN, a student is required to pass the National Council Licensure Examination (**NCLEX**) after graduation. This test is a computer adaptive test (**CAT**) rather than a paper-and-pencil test. It is based on a job analysis of tasks that actual nurses perform in the course of their employment.

Application to Sit for NCLEX Examination

To be eligible to apply to take the licensure examination the first time, the student must be reasonably expected to graduate from an approved nursing program. A completed application, a transcript of the student's records, and the required fee must be sent from the school to the State Board of Nursing, or the authority responsible for issuing licenses. The school must certify the applicant's expected graduation date.

If the graduate must repeat the examination, he or she is usually responsible for submitting the necessary information. The application to retake the exam is less complicated, because the licensing authority already has the pertinent information.

Because the NCLEX examination is now given via computer, it is available several times a year and in a number of sites. The applicant specifies preferences for time and location of the exam, choosing from a list prepared by the licensing agency.

Components of the NCLEX Examination

The NCLEX examination measures entry-level competencies in nursing. The NCLEX-PN must be passed in order to be licensed as an LPN/LVN; the NCLEX-RN leads to RN licensure. Having passed the test verifies that a nurse possesses the minimum competencies for practice. The examination includes questions that measure knowledge, comprehension, and application. Each examination question represents a phase of the nursing process, as it relates to a client need. The preface of this book contains an in-depth description of the components of the NCLEX-PN examination, as well as the locations of related content in this book (all components of the NCLEX-PN examination are addressed in this book).

The *four phases of the nursing process* (see Unit 6) associated with the NCLEX examination include:

- Data collection (establishing a database)
- Planning (setting goals for meeting client needs, and designing strategies to meet these goals)
- Implementation (actions necessary to achieve goals)
- Evaluation (determining the extent to which goals have been achieved)

The following are the *categories of client need* addressed by the NCLEX examination:

1. Safe, effective care environment (coordinated care, safety and infection control, safe delivery of care)
2. Health promotion and maintenance (growth and development through the life span, prevention and early detection of disease)
3. Psychosocial integrity (coping and adaptation)
4. Physiologic integrity (basic care and comfort, pharmacologic therapies, reduction of risk potential, physiologic adaptation)

The NCLEX licensing examination requires a knowledge of all the courses studied while in the nursing program. It also requires the application of knowledge by using critical thinking skills to make nursing judgments.

When taking the licensure examination, the computer selects individual test items from a large test pool. Each examination measures knowledge and skills pertaining to the phases of the nursing process and categories of client needs listed above. A candidate completes items until the computer determines that the person has either passed the exam or statistically cannot pass. The computer then terminates the exam. Therefore, each candidate receives different questions and a different number of questions.

Preparation for the NCLEX Examination

The best way to ensure success on the examination is to study throughout the entire time spent in the basic nursing program. If the material is mastered as the student goes along, the student should have little difficulty passing the examination. Try not to "cram" for the examination.

If desired, numerous types of material are available for information review and practice. These may include outline review books, review books with practice questions (and answer explanations, describing why an answer is correct or not correct), or computerized test banks with questions (and their accompanying answers) that actually simulate the test-taking experience.

On the night before the test, relax and get plenty of sleep. On the morning of the test, eat a good breakfast, and dress comfortably. Make sure to have the agency-issued identification information and photo identification for admittance to the examination. Know how to get to the examination site and where to park, and allow ample travel time.

If the person does not pass the examination the first time, several options are available. First of all, try to maintain a positive attitude. The individual is eligible to repeat the examination. Think about taking a review course before repeating the exam—helping to build skills in areas that may be weak and also helping to build self-confidence. Most review courses include practice tests. These tests help in overcoming "test anxiety" and in making the person more comfortable when retaking the exam. (In some instances, a review or preparation course is required before the candidate can retake the exam. This varies among states, but is usually required if the candidate needs a third attempt.)

The Nursing License

Upon passing the NCLEX examination, the individual will receive notification from the State Board of Nursing or agency responsible for nursing licensure and will receive the first license. After this person is notified, he or she can use the appropriate title: LPN, LVN, or RN. After receiving the license, the nurse is responsible for renewing it, according to regulations, and for keeping the state board informed about any changes in name, address, or employment status.

☛ KEY CONCEPT

It is each nurse's responsibility to present the license to the employer. The employer must keep the license on file.

In rare cases, nursing licensure may have been obtained by waiver, or "grandfather clause." Waivered nurses may have been licensed in another country or may have been licensed many years ago without formal graduation from a nursing program. These people could not be newly licensed today, but are "grandfathered in" and can keep the license for their lifetime. The waivered license is usually not transferable to another state.

Maintenance of the Nursing License

Each individual is responsible for keeping his or her nursing license current when practicing nursing.

License Renewal.   Most states require renewal of a nursing license every 1 or 2 years. Always be sure to inform the state board of changes in name, address, or employment status. Usually, any license renewal application cannot be forwarded, per Board of Nursing stipulation. If a nursing license lapses, the requirements for re-licensure are usually more stringent than are the renewal requirements. This often includes a refresher course and supervised clinical experience, as well as an additional fee.

Continuing Education Requirements.   Many states require a certain number of hours of continuing education units (**CEUs**) for renewal of a nursing license. Usually, the nurse must have a record of the presenter's name and professional credentials, and the objectives and length of the course. This information, along with a certificate of completion, may be required at the time of license renewal, or may only be needed in the event of an audit. View the CEU requirement as an opportunity and a challenge. It was implemented to improve the quality of nursing care. Take advantage of these courses to improve skills. Many healthcare facilities offer these educational opportunities free or at a low cost.

Today, the Internet offers a wide variety of continuing education courses for nurses. In addition, articles that provide CEUs are found in many nursing journals, such as the *American Journal of Nursing* (AJN) and other periodicals. Many private companies offer continuing education courses for a fee. Satisfactory completion of a test is necessary to obtain CEUs if the course was taken by correspondence or on the Internet. In many cases, CEUs can be awarded immediately upon completion of the course, and the person can print out a certificate online or receive a certificate of completion. Two examples of Internet websites that offer continuing education opportunities are http://www.springnet.com and http://nursingcenter.com.

☛ KEY CONCEPT

Each nurse must keep CEU information on file in case it is requested by the licensing agency.

License Revocation.   Every licensed nurse is responsible for practicing within the rules and regulations of the nurse practice act of the state or territory in which the nurse works. In most U.S. states and territories and in Canada, the Board of Nursing or another authority has the right to revoke or suspend a nurse's license for just cause. The following are examples of just causes:

- Conviction of a felony
- Conviction of other crimes, such as child abuse
- Chemical dependency or other addictive behavior (until it is controlled)
- Stealing of medications
- Mental incompetence
- Fraudulent acquisition of a nursing license
- Violation of the state nurse practice act (such as practicing medicine or prescribing medications without a license)
- Suspended or revoked license in another state
- Willful neglect or abuse of a client
- Sexual activity with or sexual harassment of a vulnerable client
- Proven negligence in nursing practice

The state board must notify the nurse before it takes action to suspend or revoke a license. The nurse will have the opportunity to present his or her case at a formal hearing. Actions that may be taken include denial of license renewal, denial of first license, letter of reprimand, suspension of license, or placement of the nurse on formal probation with specific conditions for full reinstatement. If a license is revoked or suspended, the licensing agency specifies exactly what the requirements are for reinstatement. In some cases of serious misconduct, willful negligence, or a felony related to nursing care, the license may be permanently revoked. However, this is rare.

License Transfer Between States.   After becoming licensed, a nurse may wish to move and transfer his or her licensure to another state. This procedure is known by several terms, depending on the state, including *interstate endorsement*, *reciprocity*, or *licensure without examination*. To become

licensed in another state, a request must be made to the new state's licensing and regulating agency. The nurse is required to complete an application and pay a fee. Because the NCLEX exam is used in nearly all states and territories, the transfer of a license has become much easier. The new state knows that the same exam was used because it is a national test. If the nursing program from which the nurse has graduated meets the new state's educational requirements, and the nurse's scores on the NCLEX examination meet its criteria, the new state will provide the nurse with a license. Because the NCLEX examination is developed nationally, most states do not require retaking the examination or taking additional courses. Plan ahead, because it may take 4 to 6 weeks to receive the new license.

To locate the proper agency to contact about transferring a license, look in the telephone book of the state or territory's capital city. Also try accessing the appropriate agency via the Internet. The current state's licensing agency can also provide the name and address for most other licensing agencies. In addition, many textbooks list all state licensing agencies. In Canada, contact the Canadian Nurses' Association in Ottawa. In many cases, the application to transfer a license can be obtained via the Internet and printed out on one's computer.

In many states, the licensing agency for nurses is called the *State Board of Nursing*. Other names may include:

- State Board of Nurse Examiners
- Department of Professional Regulation (and Licensing) (Florida, Illinois, Wisconsin)
- Bureau of Professional and Occupational Regulations (Michigan)
- Board of Examiners (Connecticut, Guam, Louisiana, Maritime Provinces, Puerto Rico, Texas)
- Board of Registration in Nursing (Massachusetts, Rhode Island)
- Bureau of Examining Boards (Nebraska)
- Board of Nurse Licensure (Virgin Islands)
- Nursing Care Quality Assurance Commission (Washington)

ROLE TRANSITION

According to the National League for Nursing (NLN), "LPNs/LVNs are concerned with basic therapeutic rehabilitative and preventive care for people of all ages and diverse cultures in various stages of dependency . . . The primary role of the licensed practical/vocational nurse is to provide nursing care for clients experiencing common, well-defined health problems in structured healthcare settings."[1] The LPN/LVN needs to demonstrate the following entry-level skills (*competencies*):

Assessment: Collects data about basic physical, emotional, spiritual, and sociocultural needs of clients; uses knowledge of normal values to identify deviations; documents data collection; communicates findings

Planning: Contributes to the development of nursing care plans; prioritizes nursing care needs; assists in review and revision of nursing care plans

Implementation: Provides nursing care; communicates effectively; collaborates with team members; instructs clients

Evaluation: Seeks guidance as needed; modifies nursing approaches based on evaluation of nursing care

Member of the discipline: Complies with the standards of practice outlined in the nurse practice act of the state in which licensed; describes the role of the LPN/LVN to others; maximizes educational opportunities; identifies personal potential and considers **career mobility** (additional education, responsibility, and status); identifies personal strengths and weaknesses; adheres to a nursing code of ethics; functions as a client advocate

Managing/supervising: Appropriately manages own actions when providing nursing care; assumes responsibility for nursing care delegated to unlicensed healthcare providers

Political activism: Is aware that as a nurse he or she affects nursing and healthcare through political, economic, and societal activities

The graduate nurse is expected to perform these skills. However, these skills are not isolated to one client or one situation. Rather, they are intertwined, requiring the graduate nurse to be focused, adaptable, flexible, and organized.

Role as a Member of the Healthcare Team

No matter what the setting, several types of nurses and many other workers make up the total healthcare team. All members work together, under the direction of the physician, advanced practice nurse, or other primary care provider to help clients return to optimum functioning as soon as possible.

The RN has more formal education than the LPN/LVN. Therefore, he or she is more likely to be a nurse manager, team leader, or charge nurse in an acute-care setting. In home care, the case manager is usually an RN. In addition, many RNs give direct client care, as do LPNs. In complex nursing situations, the LPN is expected to assist the RN. Unlicensed assistive personnel (UAP) are also valuable members of the nursing team, particularly in long-term care and community settings.

Organizing Workload
Typically, a new graduate nurse will provide care for more clients for more hours at a time than he or she did as a student. Whatever the situation, organization is key to providing efficient and safe care for all clients. Organizational skills come with experience and practice, but supervisors can provide helpful hints and guidelines. Box 100-1 highlights some key aspects for organizing the workload and practicing safely.

Maintaining Confidentiality
Maintaining client confidentiality is a must when working with any client. The licensed nurse is not only responsible for maintaining confidentiality personally, but should also be aware of the actions of the unlicensed personnel with whom he or she works. It may be necessary to teach others the importance of safeguarding the client's privacy.

➤➤ **BOX 100-1**

ORGANIZING THE WORKLOAD

Organization requires preparation and effective use of time. Use the following guidelines to help organize the workload:

- Establish goals, plans, and priorities; be aware of the "what," "how," and "when" for each.
- Set up a "to do" list of what to accomplish, in order of importance or need, and check off each task as it is completed.
- Stay focused and avoid procrastinating.
- When in doubt about a technique or procedure, *ask questions.* Know where the healthcare facility keeps the nursing protocols to follow when performing treatments. Review the protocol in advance if a specific treatment is ordered and then refer to it as needed. Know when and to whom to report significant symptoms or medication side effects.
- Know where to find information about medications.
- Be thoroughly knowledgeable about the institution's emergency, fire, and disaster regulations and procedures.
- Use the agency's protocols for disposing of hazardous wastes, cleaning up spills, reporting defective equipment, and so forth.

☛ KEY CONCEPT

Always remember to safeguard the client's confidentiality. When documenting client information on the computer, do not leave client information on the screen. "Exit" or clear the screen when finished using information. Keep the password confidential, so that unauthorized people cannot access information. (Be aware that communication via the Internet is generally not secure.)

Taking and Transcribing Orders
The licensed nurse needs to know how to check and check off orders in all situations. Some healthcare facilities require physicians to enter orders directly into a computer. In the computerized system, an order for a medication is transmitted directly to the pharmacy, for example. An order for a laboratory test is sent directly to the laboratory. Some computer programs determine client allergies, inappropriate medication dosages, or incompatible medications. These important safeguards are becoming more prevalent as computerized ordering and documentation becomes more commonplace. However, any physician's order must be communicated to the nursing staff in some way. The computer may automatically print a duplicate order or may make an electronic entry on the client's care plan. It is each nurse's responsibility to know how to check initial orders and to be aware of how new orders are updated and communicated.

If the primary healthcare provider's orders are handwritten, the nurse may be expected to transcribe orders or double-check them for accuracy. The client's nurse often cosigns orders to verify that they have been noted. **Transcribing orders** involves reading the physician's order sheet and carrying out necessary actions, so the client receives ordered treatment. Orders for medications and treatments are written on the Kardex or medication administration record (MAR) or both. Requisitions for procedures, special equipment, and tests are processed appropriately per agency protocol. Nursing staff then carries out the orders.

In some facilities, a non-nurse such as the unit manager, unit coordinator, or unit or station secretary does the initial transcription of orders. In this case, the charge nurse or the nurse caring for the client must double-check to ensure that the orders have been transcribed accurately. Usually, this nurse cosigns each order and assumes responsibility for transcription accuracy. If any question about an order exists, the nurse is responsible for clarifying the information with the primary healthcare provider. The procedure of transcribing or checking orders is briefly described here. When the nurse is expected to perform this function, the healthcare facility will need to provide specific in-service education about the facility's protocols to the individual nurse. Box 100-2 provides an example of guidelines when transcribing medication orders. Other types of orders are transcribed in much the same way.

☛ KEY CONCEPT

The nurse working in a nursing home, ambulatory, long-term, or home care setting is more likely to see handwritten orders. In many cases, standing orders are augmented by handwritten orders for the individual client.

Telephone or Verbal Orders.   Healthcare facilities vary in their policies regarding who may take telephone orders. The LPN may take telephone or verbal orders only if it is clearly defined in the institution's policies. (Verbal or telephone orders are subject to errors and disagreement.) The nurse taking a verbal order must be sure that he or she understands it, and should question anything that is unclear.

Ideally, all orders are in writing. In emergencies, verbal orders often must be taken because the primary healthcare provider has no time to write the order. Each nurse is responsible for his or her own actions, and if an error occurs, that individual is legally liable.

☛ KEY CONCEPT

If a nurse takes a verbal order, it is written in the client's chart immediately. The nurse notes "T.O." for telephone order and "V.O." for an in-person verbal order. The nurse then writes the ordering person's name and title and cosigns the order.

Telephone or verbal orders are potentially dangerous because no evidence exists that the order was given by the physician. Verbal orders are legal, however. All telephone or

> ➤➤ BOX 100-2

TRANSCRIBING MEDICATION ORDERS

To ensure the client's safety, follow these guidelines when transcribing medication orders, whether written or verbal:

- Read all orders. Always do "stat" orders first. (Note when stat meds are given and chart them immediately.)
- Make sure the medication is ordered from the pharmacy. The order should contain the name of the medication, dose, route, and frequency of administration.
- Transcribe the information on the Kardex, med card (if used), and MAR, giving times of administration. Note the date of a medication's discontinuation. Many medications must be reordered every 48 hours.
- Notify the person giving medications, or flag the order, to make sure it is seen.
- Note on the order sheet that the order has been transcribed and checked.
- When the client's medications arrive, check them against the physician's orders.
- If there are any questions, always ask.

When a medication is discontinued:

- Cross out the item on the Kardex or MAR, following your agency's protocol. The information should still be readable on the Kardex.
- Notify the nurse involved.
- Make out a drug credit if medications are remaining. Send leftover medications back to the pharmacy.
- Mark "D/C" (for discontinued) on the medication sheet or MAR. If using a med card, tear it or write "D/C" on it.
- Note completion of the order on the order sheet.

verbal orders are to be signed by the physician at the first possible opportunity, within 24 hours. Certain orders, such as those for leather restraints, must be cosigned by the physician within 1 hour. The nursing student or other unlicensed person never takes verbal or telephone orders.

Using Technology

Today's nurse must interact comfortably with various kinds of computerized and electronic equipment. Some of these items are probably familiar by now, including the electronic thermometer, ultrasound, the computed tomography scan, the computerized infusion pump, and the apnea monitor.

As technology advances, many new pieces of electronic equipment will become available for use. Do not be overwhelmed. Do not hesitate to look up information, or ask questions about how a particular piece of equipment operates. Scientific advances improve client care by ensuring greater accuracy of diagnoses and treatment and greater efficiency and safety in care delivery.

Computers.   Computers serve many purposes in health-care facilities. Examples include:

- Monitor the client's condition
- Store medical records
- Quickly call up pertinent information about clients (eg, Social Security number, allergies, previous illnesses)
- Maintain bookkeeping and business records
- Regulate specialized machines
- Assist physicians in initial assessment and diagnosis of disease
- Generate primary healthcare provider's orders and forward them to the pharmacy, laboratory, and elsewhere
- Renew clients' prescriptions from home
- Conduct quality assurance research
- Teach medical and nursing students
- Conduct literature searches
- Assist in developing a nursing care plan
- Document care given
- Order supplies
- Supply information on medication dosages, side effects, times of administration, and potential drug incompatibilities
- Generate advance directives and other forms, such as the living will
- Make appointments for x-ray examinations and diagnostic tests
- Order laboratory tests and call up results
- Schedule the operating room and other specialized areas
- Schedule nursing staff
- Generate paychecks
- Send messages via e-mail or fax
- Send and receive client records between healthcare facilities and insurance providers
- Assist in telephone triage of clients
- Transmit pertinent client information from client to physician
- Obtain consultations about a particular client with specialists from distant locations
- Assist in obtaining authorization for insurance payments
- Conduct in-service seminars, via distance education

Most communities offer courses for those who are new to or unfamiliar with computers. In addition, numerous self-help books and aids are available. Specific instructions about how to use a facility's computer system are usually provided during the nurse's orientation to the facility. Also, remember that the operation manuals for computers and new computerized equipment are usually kept on file.

The Internet.   The **Internet** (World Wide Web [**WWW**]) is an enormous source of information. Information varies across websites, but information about medications, diseases, legislation, or new nursing procedures is available from many sources. Continuing education programs are offered—sometimes, an entire continuing education course can be taken via the Internet. Application forms for advanced practice credentials, continuing education courses, or employment can be obtained. In some cases, the application can be submitted directly via the Internet. The certificate of completion can also be printed out at the end of the class.

Chat rooms, online chats, and bulletin boards allow communication with experts who will answer questions and give additional information on a wide variety of topics. (These experts may be in countries other than the United States, thereby providing an international perspective on the topic.) Interactive forums relating to many nursing and medical topics are offered regularly. Most nursing organizations, state boards of nursing, voluntary health agencies, and health promotion agencies have websites. Health maintenance organizations often have websites for their subscribers that offer a wide range of health information.

The Internet also lists many employment opportunities ("electronic classifieds"). In many cases, a person can submit a resume and application via the Internet.

Internet "browser" programs such as Netscape Navigator or Microsoft Internet Explorer, or "search engines" such as Yahoo!, AltaVista, Excite, or Infoseek (many of which are free) can be used to scan the WWW for research related to a specific disease, symptom, or medication. A search engine that specializes in health and medicine is HealthAtoZ. Surfing the Internet will often yield "links" to related websites to aid in locating the most useful information.

☛ KEY CONCEPT

A great deal of client teaching information can be downloaded from the Internet. The nurse must screen this material before giving it to the client, to make sure it is not too overwhelming or too technical. Be sure to be available to answer questions.

Some websites in healthcare provide abstracts of journal articles, entire articles, bibliography lists, clinical updates, and speeches from medical conferences. Some entire journals are available online. Reviews of new books also are available. The nurse can also access mailing lists of agencies and experts for further information. Many useful websites are listed throughout this book.

Signing up to be on a specialty mailing list via a list server ("listserv") allows one to send and receive information related to that specialty group. The participant also can communicate with individuals in the group via e-mail. Nursing listservs include those about home care, IV therapy, maternal–child, surgery, psychiatry, neurology, nursing education, research, and many other subjects.

The Internet is particularly valuable to students, people in rural areas, and those who do not have access to a large library. Remember too that websites are usually updated regularly, so information is often more up-to-date than printed material.

Maintaining a Current Knowledge Base

Although the graduate has completed the general nursing program, his or her education in healthcare is just beginning. Continuing to learn throughout one's entire nursing career is essential to be able to deliver safe and up-to-date care to clients.

Sources of information with which to stay current are everywhere. Books and magazine articles provide information about scientific discoveries that are improving the treatment of disease. Nursing journals, new textbooks, and radio and television programs discuss health problems and new procedures and equipment. Workshops, conferences, and conventions are available in many general and specialty areas to provide information on the latest advances and findings. Healthcare facilities maintain ongoing in-service education programs and libraries for their employees. The Internet is a vast resource for up-to-date, easily accessible information. Take advantage of these information sources to stay current.

Adjusting to the Workplace

The clinical arena often presents the graduate with unexpected challenges. Nursing goes on around the clock, to ensure continuity of care for all clients. However, as a student, being in the clinical facility during evening or night hours or having clinical experience for a full 8- or 12-hour shift may not have been a requirement. A new graduate may be expected to begin working during times other than the day shift. He or she may be required to work only evenings, nights, or *rotating shifts*— that is, to work days, evenings ("relief," "swing shift"), and nights ("graveyard shift") on a rotating (alternating) basis. Many acute-care facilities and extended-care facilities (ECFs) require nurses to work weekends, often every other weekend. A new graduate's first job may be totally on weekends or during "off hours." The new graduate may also be required to work on holidays, giving nurses with seniority the time off.

Work Schedules

Today's nursing shortage offers nearly any nurse the opportunity to work. Employers have offered a number of incentives to encourage nurses to work. Nursing offers unique scheduling opportunities.

Flexible Schedules. Many nurses find working flexible hours fits well into a family schedule. A number of scheduling options are available. Examples include:

Part-time or *full-time*

Straight evenings or *straight nights*

Weekends only. Variations of a scheduling plan called the *Baylor Plan* exist at many facilities. The nurse usually works 3 days of every weekend. In most cases, either a large bonus is paid or the nurse working part-time is paid a full-time wage. This allows the nurse time off during the week.

Twelve-hour shifts. Three 12-hours shifts per week is nearly full-time. Adding one 8-hour shift every two weeks is full-time. The nurse working 12-hour shifts is usually required to work every third weekend instead of every other weekend. This plan gives the nurse more days off. Twelve-hour shifts are usually from 7 to 7 and two nurses are partners, one working the days and one working the nights.

Much less common in inpatient facilities are *10-hour shifts*. However, clinics, home care, and industries often allow 10-hour shifts.

Shared jobs. Two nurses can share a single full-time position, allowing each to have more free time.

Flex time. In some situations, the nurse is allowed to set his or her own hours, fitting the work schedule around family responsibilities.

The nursing shortage also presents unique challenges. A growing concern is *mandatory overtime*. Because clients need 24-hour care, if no nurses are available for a shift, nurses from the preceding shift must stay and cover. This has become such a concern that hospitals have been forced to turn away clients if they do not have adequate staffing. Nurses have negotiated and in some cases have gone on strike to ensure competent and safe nursing care for clients. Working conditions and salaries continue to improve as nurses express their concerns and negotiate to improve client care.

The 24-Hour Day

Because nursing occurs around the clock, working in a facility during the evening or night hours is somewhat different than working during the daytime hours. When working in the evening or at night, keep in mind the following:

- Clients often exhibit different behavior compared with that during the day. For example, the person with dementia or paranoia is often more confused or afraid after dark (the "sundowner" phenomenon).
- Many clients are more anxious or worried at night when it is quiet and they are alone. Help to reassure them.
- Psychotic clients may be more likely to act out at night.
- Many clients experience an elevation of fever and exacerbation of illness in the evening.
- Pain may be accentuated by fear or by being alone in the evening or night.
- Many visitors come in the evenings, providing an excellent opportunity to meet clients' loved ones.
- Fewer staff are on duty. Accessing security assistance or a specialized physician may be more difficult.
- It is quieter. There is less confusion and hubbub on the unit. Fewer orders are written and fewer special tests and procedures performed.
- In rare cases, clients come into the hospital to be prepared for surgery or another procedure the next morning.
- Hospitalized clients may be nothing by mouth (NPO) after midnight for procedures such as electroconvulsive therapy, surgery, or various diagnostic tests.
- Assisting clients to sleep at night is important. Sometimes, a warm shower or soothing backrub helps; medications may be necessary. (Remember that noises, including conversations, seem louder at night and may keep clients awake.) Some people fall asleep more easily if soft music is playing in the background.
- Some medications, such as sedating psychotropic medications, laxatives, and vaginal suppositories, are routinely given in the evening.
- In most facilities, the night nurse performs routine daily paperwork. Intake and output sheets, IV fluids, and caloric

intakes are totaled and entered on the health records. The physician's orders for the day are double-checked and signed off. Laboratory procedures may be ordered or vital signs documented.

- The night nurse often orders medications, replenishes supplies for the unit, and checks the crash cart.

☞ KEY CONCEPT

Remember nurses are only in the healthcare facility for a work shift. The client is there 24 hours a day, and the environment is different in the evening or night.

Working the Night Shift. In some instances, new graduate nurses may be required to work the night shift as part of their orientation or because they are the "new nurses." However, some individuals may find that working the night shift fits their lifestyle. Regardless of the reason, Box 100-3 highlights some general suggestions to aid in the transition to working the night shift.

Working at night can be advantageous to the nurse. The shift is often less stressful, with fewer interruptions. The pay is usually higher, there is less traffic, and parking is easier and less expensive. Days and evenings are free for other activities, for example attending school or a child's activities during the day, shopping when stores are less crowded, or walking and exercising during safer daytime hours. It is possible to make daytime appointments for services such as dental care and car repair. Access to child care services may not be necessary. The work is often less physically demanding. Although fewer medications and treatments typically are given, more time may be available to talk with clients. If a nurse is taking classes, there may be time to study.

There are also disadvantages to working nights. Some clients are more confused or fearful at night. Fewer staff members are available to handle emergencies. The work may be less interesting along with the possibility that the nurse may not be able to interact with some clients because they are sleeping. Family members may have difficulty adjusting to the routine. Plus adjusting one's sleep schedule may be challenging, possibly with the individual getting less total sleep. Nurses with certain health problems (ie, diabetes, seizure disorders, gastrointestinal disorders, bipolar disorder, chronic obstructive pulmonary disease, and heart disorders) are at risk when they work nights. However, many nurses work permanent nights by choice.

Professional Activities

A graduate nurse is responsible for keeping up with current trends in nursing. In addition, knowledge about employment practices and reimbursement for nursing services will be beneficial. By being an active member of a nursing organization, a graduate nurse will be able to keep in touch with current trends and new advancements in nursing.

➤ ➤ **BOX 100-3**

WORKING THE NIGHT SHIFT

To help in adjusting to working the night shift, keep in mind the following:

- Eat healthy meals. Get plenty of exercise. Plan recreational time. Drink plenty of fluids, varying the types of fluids.
- Eat a snack or meal during the shift. Limit caffeine intake after about 3 AM.
- Eat a light, non-fat meal before going to bed during the day.
- Be sure to allow adequate time for sleep during the day.
- Take medications at the prescribed times. Adjust personal medications, such as insulin, psychotropics, and antiseizure medications, as appropriate for the individual schedule.
- Plan a suitable sleep schedule; for example, it may be easiest to sleep immediately after work, stay up for a few hours, and go to bed about midday; or sleep a few hours in the morning and take a nap before returning to work. Try to get your usual amount of total sleep daily.
- Sleep days when possible, even when off duty. Maintain a steady biorhythm.
- Involve family members when planning the schedule. Make sure they understand.
- Make the bedroom as dark as possible or wear an eye mask. While at work, keep the area well lighted. (The body's biorhythms are based in large part on light and darkness.)
- Keep the bedroom quiet. Turn off the telephone and doorbell. Use a fan or music to provide "sound-masking."
- Make sure friends and relatives know about the night shifts and do not call or visit during sleep time.
- Bring a sweater to work; most people get chilly in the middle of the night because of normal body cycles.
- If there is a choice between 8-hour and 12-hour shifts, choose the 8-hour shift. It is less exhausting and usually begins about 11 PM, allowing for participation in evening activities and being with one's children.
- Bring something interesting to do if any time becomes available. It will help in maintaining alertness.
- If there is a break during the night, take a nap. A short nap can help greatly in staying awake all night. Bring an alarm clock so that sleep will be relaxed without worrying about waking up on time.
- If possible, arrange to work straight nights, which is possibly easier for the body to adjust to than rotating shifts.
- Make sure to be safe during the drive home. Listen to the radio or books on tape, sing, or eat popcorn or peanuts to remain alert. Stop and rest for a few minutes if becoming too tired.

State and National Nursing Organizations

Chapter 2 provided an introduction to several state and national nursing associations. It is important for all nurses to support and participate in the activities of nursing associations. Nursing organizations publish journals that offer updated information and often offer opportunities for continuing education by correspondence. In addition, they may sponsor local continuing education activities. The local association may be the bargaining unit for a group. By working collectively, a group can get things done that one person could not accomplish alone. A representative of the local association may come to the school or place of employment and speak about the association's function and activities and how graduates can join. (Often, students join nursing organizations as student affiliates.) Instructors also will have information.

Alumni Associations

Many schools have alumni associations. Among their activities are student recruitment programs, scholarships and loans, and fund-raising events to purchase educational equipment for the school. Attending reunions provides graduates with a chance to have fun and to renew friendships with classmates. Classmates and instructors are also valuable networking resources, possibly providing information about employment or advancement opportunities.

Personal Nursing File

Keeping nursing records organized is important when making the transition from graduate to licensed nurse. Start a personal nursing file immediately on graduation and keep it updated. This information will be needed when applying for the initial license, renewing the license, and seeking employment. This file will also be needed if the nurse's CEUs are audited by the Board of Nursing. Have the following materials readily available in the personal nursing file:

- A copy of the original nursing license and of each renewed license, as well as the NCLEX test score. (These documents are particularly important when seeking licensure in more than one state. Each state may require a copy of the license or license number.) Keep track of the license's expiration date.
- A record of all continuing education courses; in some cases, a copy of completion certificates must be submitted with the license renewal application. States often require a record of each course, with its objectives, the qualifications of the instructor, the length of the course, and the completion certificate, to be kept on file and presented if an audit is done.
- A copy of any advanced or specialized certification received.
- Copies of immunization records, and most recent tuberculin testing (or negative chest x-ray study) and rubella titer information. (Some employers require or strongly recommend hepatitis immunization, in addition to regular immunizations.)
- A copy of a current cardiopulmonary resuscitation (CPR) certification card.

- Copies of all high school, college, and nursing school transcripts, as well as any additional education received.
- A complete record of previous work experience, with dates of employment, copies of written evaluations, and name, address, and telephone number of immediate supervisor(s), and other references.
- A copy of the personal resume (keep it updated).
- A list of references, with the address and telephone number of each—make sure they have agreed to be listed as a reference.
- A copy of the professional liability insurance policy.
- Birth certificate and passport, or resident alien card (green card). (These documents are required for employment in the United States.)
- Social Security card (required for employment).
- Any other pertinent information, such as volunteer work, organizational offices held, and pertinent community activities.

Be sure to maintain records of income and job-related professional expenses for tax purposes. Professional expenses include malpractice insurance premium, fees and expenses for continuing education, licensure renewal fee, and costs of required uniforms and pertinent professional journals and books.

Nursing Alert

Many states require continuing education for renewal of a nursing license. If this is the case, random audits of the documentation are done. An audit may also be done for just cause. If an audit is called, the nurse will greatly benefit from having an organized professional file.

Networking: Personal and Professional Contacts

The term *networking* refers to a person's personal and professional connectedness. The electronic address book or rolodex is an invaluable tool in finding employment, learning about new opportunities and classes, and learning about new developments in medicine and nursing. This is a person's *professional network,* which usually contains many contacts, many of which are superficial. This type of network usually is marked by minimal interdependence; the individual is self-directed. Some of this type of networking is also done by e-mail, chat rooms, and other computer-based activities.

A person's *personal network,* which includes family and close friends, is usually much more close-knit. The personal network involves interdependence with a small number of people and is marked by much closer interaction. Both types of networking involve contact with other people, either in person, by mail, or electronically. The difference lies in the depth and intimacy of the contacts. The new nurse will find that keeping track of contacts throughout a career can prove very beneficial—to both the nurse and the other people. It is impossible to predict when a question or concern will surface that can be addressed by one of the people in one's network of contacts.

PERSONAL LIFE

One's work life is interrelated with one's personal life. Be sure to have a health examination once a year. Dental insurance is also a good idea. (Most employers have such plans available at low cost to the employee and his or her family.) Get hospitalization and medical insurance with a reliable group plan. All these measures help to ensure a safer and happier life.

Balancing of Work and Personal Responsibilities and Activities

Although an individual will spend a great deal of time at work or thinking about work, it is important to have outside interests and hobbies. The new nurse, particularly one who has not worked before, will find that it is important to be able to relax and have fun after the busy day at work. There are many low-cost ways to do this for the person striking out on his or her own, establishing a place to live, buying a car, and so forth. The new graduate with a family will find that the flexibility of scheduling in nursing can fit very well into family life. Often, the new income as a nurse helps to enhance the quality of family life as well.

Financial Planning and Retirement

Financial security is important, so plan a personal budget. Be realistic: money never goes as far as one thinks it will. Although it is difficult for a new graduate to think of retirement, early planning is essential. Be aware that to receive Social Security payments and Medicare at retirement, a certain number of eligible quarters must be worked and entered into the system. Even if the employer has a private retirement plan, it is a good idea for the employee to pay into Social Security as well, if possible.

Many nurses are women and may be taking time away from work to raise children. Therefore, it is important to build up as much retirement security as possible. Invest in some sort of retirement and/or annuity plan. These funds can grow quickly when an amount from each paycheck is set aside to be put into the fund. Many employers provide access to funds such as 401k or tax-sheltered annuities. These provide a low-cost way to build a growing fund. In addition, many nurses have access to a credit union through their employer. Credit unions provide a number of benefits to their members, including automatic payroll savings account deductions, free checking accounts, and low-interest car loans. Today's nursing shortage drives a number of incentives for nurses. Some employers offer a sign-on bonus if the nurse stays for a certain length of time. In addition, nurses often receive a referral bonus if they recruit another nurse to the facility or agency. Some employers are willing to help new graduates pay off student loans, as well as paying for additional education for employees. (Many LPN/LVNs are able to go back to school and become RNs in this way.) Many employers offer a low-cost disability plan, as well as health insurance. Health insur-

ance is a must. The disability plan is a good idea, because it provides some income if the nurse becomes disabled.

Self-Fulfillment

Several factors contribute to the nurse's feelings of satisfaction and fulfillment, both professionally and personally. These factors include the following:[2]

- Knowing one's self
- Living in the present
- Reviewing the past, but not dwelling on it
- Avoiding complaining and blaming others
- Concentrating on helping
- Seeking solutions to challenges
- Being responsible for one's self: self-leadership
- Being aware of and constantly revising one's personal mission statement
- Clarifying personal values
- Having a strategic plan
- Managing one's self and one's life
- Continuing to learn
- Maintaining the ability to change
- Being positive about the future

➵ STUDENT SYNTHESIS

Key Points

- Nurses must pass the NCLEX examination to obtain nursing licensure and to practice nursing.
- The NCLEX examination, a CAT rather than a paper-and-pencil test, is based on a job analysis of tasks that actual nurses perform in the course of their employment.
- A person must be licensed to perform certain nursing tasks or to be known as a "nurse".
- Most states require renewal of a nursing license every 1 or 2 years along with evidence of continuing education.
- After becoming licensed, a nurse may wish to move and transfer his or her licensure to another state.
- Entry-level skills of the LPN/LVN include: data collection, planning, implementation, evaluation, being a member of the discipline, managing/supervising, and political activism.
- Maintaining client confidentiality, organizing workload, taking and transcribing orders, using technology, and maintaining a current knowledge base are important for the graduate LPN/LVN.
- Nurses are responsible for continuity of client care 24 hours a day; the atmosphere and some activities in the healthcare facility during the evening and night hours may differ from those during day hours.
- A graduate nurse is responsible for keeping up with current trends in nursing. By being an active member of a nursing organization, a graduate nurse will be

able to keep in touch with current trends and new advancements in nursing.
- The graduate nurse must learn to balance the demands of work with his or her personal responsibilities and activities.

Critical Thinking Exercises

1. Talk to three recently licensed nurses about the licensing examination. What were their reactions to the exam? What suggestions do they have for students who are preparing to take the exam? What are your feelings about taking the exam?
2. As a new nursing graduate, you have not yet received your license. On your fourth day of employment in a local skilled nursing facility, the evening charge nurse, who is the only licensed person on duty, calls in sick. The administrator asks you to be in charge in her place. Describe what you would say and do and why.

NCLEX-Style Review Questions

1. The NCLEX examination measures:
   a. Entry-level competencies
   b. Graduate's ability to compete in the job market
   c. Proficiency-level competencies
   d. Success of the nursing program

2. NCLEX examination questions about handwashing would fit under which category of client need?
   a. Health promotion and maintenance
   b. Physiologic integrity
   c. Psychosocial integrity
   d. Safe, effective care environment

3. A nurse's license was revoked in another state. What action could the state in which the nurse currently works take against the nurse?
   a. No action could be taken because the revocation is in another state.
   b. Place the nurse in Federal prison.
   c. Revoke or suspend the nurse's license.
   d. Take action against the nurse's employer.

4. Which of the following is an advantage for nurses working the night shift?
   a. Clients possibly more confused or fearful
   b. Fewer staff to handle emergencies
   c. Increased interaction with clients
   d. Less physically demanding work

References

1. National League for Nursing Council of Practical Nursing Programs (2001). *Nursing practice standards for the licensed practical/vocational nurse*. (Rev.). Raleigh, NC: Author.
2. Kenney, E. (1998). Creating fulfillment in today's workplace: A guide for nurses. *American Journal of Nursing, 98*(5), 44–48.

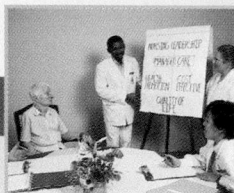

Career Opportunities and Job-Seeking Skills

LEARNING OBJECTIVES

1. List at least six types of healthcare facilities or related agencies in which LPN/LVNs might seek employment, other than the hospital or long-term care facility.
2. List at least five specialized areas of nursing available to the LPN/LVN.
3. Name at least four sources of employment information for nurses.
4. Explain how a nurse might conduct a job search or apply for a position using the Internet.
5. Describe the function of a placement service, nursing pool, or registry.
6. Identify at least six important personal considerations and six professional considerations when choosing a place of employment.
7. List items to include in a resume. Demonstrate the ability to prepare a personal resume.
8. Describe the letter of application and procedures for filling out the application form. Demonstrate the ability to correctly fill out an application for a position.
9. Describe preparation for and protocols during a job interview.
10. Identify the proper protocol for resigning from a position.

NEW TERMINOLOGY

nurses' registry   telehealth

ACRONYMS

EHS   HBO

As graduation approaches, decisions about future career plans must be made. This chapter describes employment opportunities available to LPN/LVNs and measures needed to secure desired employment.

EMPLOYMENT OPPORTUNITIES

Most graduates of nursing programs seek employment soon after graduation. This is either the first step in a career or a means to earn money for additional education. After graduating from an approved nursing program, arrangements are made to take the NCLEX licensing examination to practice as an RN or LPN/LVN. According to NFLPN (2002), average salaries for LPN/LVNs range from $30,000 to $40,000 per year in the United States and the average age is "late 30s." Licensing procedures are discussed in Chapter 100.

Entry Level Role

The LPN/LVN's role differs slightly in each state and in every facility. Currently, most LPN/LVNs are still traditionally employed as members of the healthcare team who work with RNs, physicians, and other primary care providers. Some LPN/LVNs are also receiving advanced preparation to assume positions in areas such as intravenous (IV) therapy, emergency medicine, *phlebotomy* (drawing blood), or dialysis. Many are practicing in diverse acute-care settings, including intensive care units, coronary care units, and operating rooms. Work in such settings requires specific in-service education or a specialized advanced course. It also requires an understanding of electrocardiograms (ECGs), emergency drugs, cardiac or other specialized medications, and advanced assessment skills.

Numbers of Nurses

In 1995, the National Association for Practical Nurse Education and Service (NAPNES) stated that in response to the growing needs of the aging population, LPN/LVN employment was expected to increase faster than the average rate for all occupations. This remains true today, and with the shortage of registered nurses, the demand for LPN/LVNs is ever great. Although there are currently 1,800 LPN/LVN education programs in the United States, there are waiting lists for admission. Virtually all graduates can find jobs if they want to work, according to NFLPN (2002). In 2000, there were 902,154 LPN/LVNs licensed in the United States, according to the National Council of State Boards of Nursing. In 2002, NFLPN states that there are 1.2 million LPN/LVN licenses held in the United States, although some may be counted in more than one state. (There are more than 3 million RN licenses held, but many of these people are not actively employed in nursing.)

Extended-care facilities (ECFs) are a major source of new jobs for LPN/LVNs. Continued and rapid growth is expected in nursing homes, board-and-care homes, and group homes. A survey of 98% of the nursing homes in the United States published in the *American Journal of Nursing* showed that in 1998, the following staff people were working in nursing homes:

- 103,028 RNs (full-time equivalents)
- 113,514 LPN/LVNs (full-time equivalents)
- 364,382 nursing assistants (full-time equivalents)

Home care, community health centers, and positions in physicians' offices are also expected to provide LPN/LVNs with expanded employment opportunities. Hospitals are also increasing their employment of LPN/LVNs.

☛ KEY CONCEPT

Employment opportunities for nurses outside the hospital are growing at the highest rates in community health care, ambulatory surgery, home care, and extended care for seniors and people with disabilities.

General Employment Opportunities

Many general opportunities are available for nursing employment, and most areas have current needs for nurses. Many sites of employment have been discussed in detail elsewhere in this text.

Hospitals

Many RNs and LPN/LVNs find positions in hospitals as staff nurses who give bedside care and supervise various nursing services. The employment of LPN/LVNs by hospitals is currently increasing, according to NFLPN (2002). When hiring nurses, hospitals may give consideration to a nurse's preference for a specific service, such as pediatrics, or for a specific shift. However, in many cases, the graduate will not have priority and may not be able to work immediately in the preferred area or at the preferred time of day. Presently, hospital nursing is the slowest-growing segment of the healthcare field.

Elder Care and Rehabilitation

Because of continued growth of the older adult population, the various segments of elder care are rapidly expanding. These services have been discussed elsewhere in this book. They include ECFs (including nursing homes) and assisted living. Many older citizens, as well as younger people, also receive rehabilitation services, either in their own home or in a rehabilitation center. Many staff positions for RNs and LPN/LVNs are available in all of these ambulatory and home care services and ECFs. As the level of client acuity in these facilities increases, nurses will have many opportunities to use their medical-surgical and advanced nursing skills.

Public Health and Home Care

A growing number of nurses, both RNs and LPN/LVNs, are finding employment in home care. The Certified Public Health Nurse (PHN) is an RN with a bachelor's degree. PHNs supervise other nurses and unlicensed assistive personnel (UAP) such as home health aides and homemakers. Each client must have a designated case manager. Most funding agencies require that this case manager be an RN. The RN makes the initial evaluation visit, admits clients to the services, and writes a nursing care plan. The RN then assists other nurses and UAP and makes regular assessment visits to evaluate client progress, supervise other caregivers, and update nursing care plans.

The LPN/LVN may be employed in home care to deliver routine daily care. In some cases, the LPN/LVN supervises UAP and volunteer caregivers.

Home health nursing requires high-level skills and a sense of professionalism, because these nurses usually work alone. Other qualifications include the ability to get along with people, self-motivation, independence, the ability to make sound decisions, and maturity (Fig. 101-1). The home care nurse also must know when to ask questions or to request assistance and must be familiar with community and medical resources. Home care nurses may visit clients in their homes, ECFs, or other facilities (eg, jails, homeless shelters, or schools).

Home care nurses perform nursing treatments, draw blood for routine tests, supervise medication setup, document care, evaluate client progress, and teach clients and family members. All caregivers, including physicians, therapists, volunteers, and home care nurses, participate in team conferences regarding their clients on a regular basis. Some nurses work in psychiatric outreach, visiting clients in the community and recommending hospitalization when necessary.

Home care has many employment advantages. Home care nurses care for clients individually and have the opportunity to meet family members. They often have more independence than nurses who work directly within a healthcare facility. Most agencies provide employees with insurance and paid vacation; salaries are competitive.

There are also some disadvantages in home nursing. Agencies may require nurses to work holidays and weekends and to be on call. Those who work in home care must consider safety issues when moving about the community alone. The home care nurse provides his or her own transportation to and from clients' homes (see Chap. 98). Some nurses object to the amount of paperwork required in home care. Most of this involves documentation for funding agencies.

Community Health Centers

More and more healthcare is being provided to Americans in community health centers. In many cases, these centers provide all the primary healthcare for a family or for most of the residents of a neighborhood. Although this has not been a primary source of employment for LPN/LVNs in the past, opportunities are expanding as the centers are growing in number and importance (see Chap. 97).

Private Duty and Travel Nursing

A *private duty nurse* cares for one client in his or her home, an institution, or during travel, but rarely in a hospital. This nurse is often paid directly by the client or family; insurance often does not cover this service. Working in private duty gives a nurse the opportunity to practice basic bedside and teaching skills and to meet one client's total needs. Because this practice area often includes care for clients with long-term illnesses or who are physically or emotionally challenged to some degree, private duty offers nurses steady employment on a long-term basis.

There are a number of agencies that recruit nurses as private duty nurses or travel companions for elderly or disabled clients. The nurse working as a travel companion may be "on duty" all the time. In addition, "travel nurse" agencies recruit nurses to work in understaffed parts of the country. In this case, a bonus is often paid, as well as moving expenses and

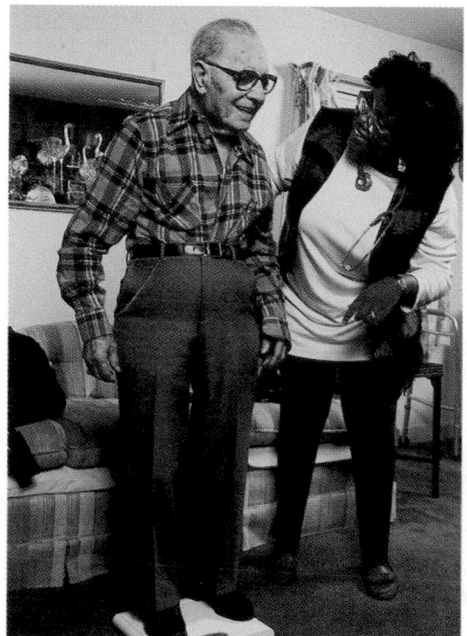
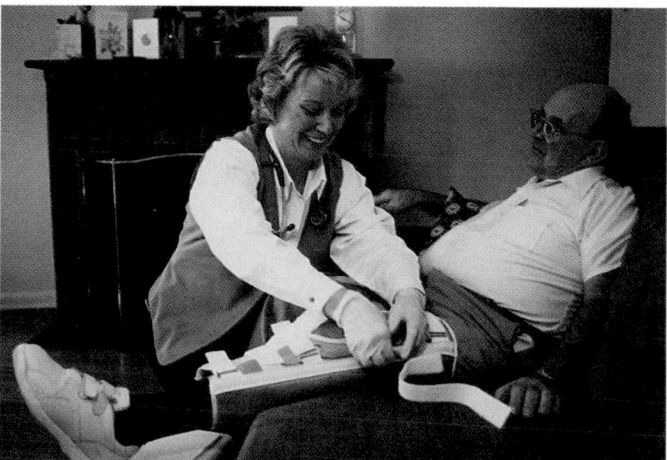

FIGURE 101-1. Home health nurses combine effective communication skills with a sound clinical knowledge base when caring for clients.

a monthly housing allowance. In some cases, nurses are re-cruited to follow the "snow birds" when they go south for the winter. This gives the nurse an opportunity to travel and to earn money at the same time; employment may be contracted for 2 to 5 months, sometimes longer. The travel nurse may work with an individual client or in a healthcare facility.

Hospice Care

Hospice nursing involves caring for terminally ill clients in hospitals, long-term care facilities, other facilities (such as hotels, shelters, or jails), or the client's own home. In rare cases, a hospice client is in a hospital. Hospice nurses help clients and their families work through the last stages of life. The goal of hospice nursing is to help clients die with dignity and to assist family members in the loss of their loved one (see Chap. 99). The nurse working in a home care agency may encounter hospice clients as part of a case load. In some agencies, the hospice program is separate and employs its own staff; in other agencies, hospice clients are integrated with other home care clients.

Substance Abuse Programs

Substance abuse (chemical dependency [CD]) nursing in-volves assisting with the rehabilitation of clients who abuse drugs, alcohol, and other substances (see Chap. 94). Nurses employed in CD may work in hospitals, private treatment cen-ters, or detoxification (detox) centers. Remember that detoxi-fication, especially from alcohol, can be life threatening and requires a high degree of nursing competence. All these areas employ RNs and LPN/LVNs as nurses, group leaders, and CD counselors. In many cases, a majority of the employees are themselves recovering alcoholics or substance abusers.

Mental Healthcare and Children with Disabilities

Mental health and psychiatric settings provide many opportu-nities for employment of both RNs and LPN/LVNs. These settings include state-run institutions, psychiatric units housed in acute-care facilities, free-standing psychiatric hospitals and clinics, and community mental health centers (see Chap. 93). Some long-term care facilities also have specialized units for adults with mental health concerns, including dementia.

In some facilities, such as long-term or state treatment centers, the length of stay may be several months or longer. This gives the nurse the opportunity to work with clients on a long-term basis.

Community mental health is a growing field. Some com-munity mental health centers are designed to treat clients with the dual diagnosis of mental illness and chemical dependency (MI/CD). This topic is discussed in Chapter 93. In some cities, crisis nurses make home visits to clients with mental health and psychiatric problems.

Nurses also have many opportunities for employment with developmentally delayed and intellectually impaired chil-dren and adults in institutions, group homes, and schools. The employment of nurses to work with "mainstreamed" children in schools is a fast-growing field. In many cases, a child with severe disabilities requires medications and treatments such as oxygen, ventilator care, or chest physiotherapy. Some of

these children are funded for a 1-to-1 nurse while at school. In some cases, nursing care is funded 24 hours a day.

Residential Treatment Centers

Nurses may find employment in specialized residential treat-ment centers that serve specific client populations. In addition to CD programs, the nurse might be employed in a group home for persons who are developmentally delayed or intellectually challenged, or people who have a chronic and persistent men-tal illness. Employment is also available at halfway houses for clients who are discharged from psychiatric hospitals or who are unable to care for themselves independently. Many of these facilities have a licensed nurse on duty for at least part of the day. One of the functions of the nurse in such a setting is to supervise the administration of medications.

Correctional Facilities

Prisons and many large jails employ nurses (RNs and LPN/LVNs) who monitor inmates with special needs, such as those who may be contemplating suicide. These nurses also give medications, assist with diabetic management and teaching, perform routine health screenings, and provide health-related counseling. If an inmate appears too physically or mentally ill to be managed in jail, the nurse consults a physician for referral to a hospital. Nurses may teach classes on topics such as sex education and healthy lifestyles.

Physicians' Offices

Nurses are often employed in a physician's office to assist with physical examinations, dressings, minor surgical proce-dures, and medication and lifestyle counseling. In addition to nursing skills, duties may include answering telephones, mak-ing appointments with clients, assisting clients into examina-tion rooms, performing some lab tests, processing items for billing, and serving as a receptionist. Office nurses must be skilled in triage, so that clients receive necessary care in a timely manner. Many office and clinic nurses are LPN/LVNs. Work is usually during daytime hours and may include part of the weekend, but usually does not involve evenings, nights, Sundays, or holidays (see Chap. 97).

Ambulatory/Day-Surgery Clinics

Many clients go to ambulatory/day-surgery clinics for surgical procedures. Some of these procedures are extensive and require the nurse to be skilled in pre- and postoperative care and in client and family teaching. In addition, the nurse in ambulatory/day surgery assists the surgeon during the procedure.

The nurse calls the client before the procedure to make sure he or she is properly prepared and does not have additional questions. In addition, this nurse performs telephone followup after clients return home. Many nurses in day surgery are LPN/LVNs. Hours are usually Monday through Friday.

Health Maintenance Organizations/ Third-Party Payers

A growing field of employment for LPN/LVNs exists in the area of pre-approval or reimbursement for healthcare. Health maintenance organizations, insurance companies, and other third-party payers train these nurses to research each client's healthcare needs to determine if the cost of a particular surgical or diagnostic test can be paid by their company. This claims analyst works with physicians and other healthcare professionals to ensure that quality care is given in the most cost-effective manner. This is a primarily sedentary position, involving extensive use of the computer, telephone, fax, and e-mail communications. In some cases, the person will visit the healthcare facility to interview healthcare personnel or clients or to review client records. Hours are most often during the day, Monday through Friday, not including holidays.

Telehealth

"Telephone nursing" or **telehealth** is a growing area of nursing employment for RNs and LPN/LVNs. Third-party payers and health maintenance organizations often provide this service in the form of "Nurse Lines" or "Dial-a-Nurse," using computerized triage systems. Clients call with symptoms and questions and nurses perform assessments over the phone, following carefully prescribed computerized protocols.

Many telehealth systems include a medical information library, with materials available for members. (Often, members can access such services via the Internet as well.) In addition, nurses make appropriate referrals to physicians and may schedule appointments for clients with primary care providers. In rare cases, these nurses may pre-approve care.

Telehealth provides healthcare facilities and third-party payers with a cost-effective way to manage clients. It also helps to increase medication compliance, decrease physician and emergency room visits, and prevent re-hospitalizations. Nurses require specialized in-service education before they can perform telehealth services.

As stated before, many day-surgery centers use telehealth systems. Nurses call clients the day before surgery to answer questions and to conduct preoperative teaching. They call clients again the day after surgery to ensure that recovery is progressing without complications. Family members and clients also have the opportunity to ask questions, and they are instructed to call if any problems arise later.

Telehealth is particularly valuable in remote areas where residents have limited access to primary healthcare services. Nurses manage as much care as possible via telephone, to avoid difficult and expensive transportation to hospitals. In some cases, telephone transmission of important data, such as ECG results, is also done. Crisis lines and suicide prevention lines are other examples of telehealth systems. Many of these services are available 24 hours a day.

The nurse in telehealth must be able to make decisions, particularly about which clients need to be seen immediately, which clients need to be seen the next day, and which clients can safely make an appointment in the future. This person may be working alone.

Occupational Health

Positive health maintenance is a goal of many companies, hospitals, and industries. These industries are interested in the welfare of their employees, as well as promoting minimal absenteeism. Nurses often act as wellness coordinators for such industries, teaching preventive care and health maintenance to employees. In many situations, nurses are responsible for enforcing safety measures and Occupational Safety and Health Act (OSHA) regulations, as well managing worker's compensation claims. These nurses are knowledgeable in first aid. They often chair safety committees and may manage employee-assistance programs, including CD education and prevention. In rare cases, the industrial nurse may perform home visits to employees.

Both RNs and LPN/LVNs are employed in occupational health, although the team leader is usually an RN. As a nursing student, you may have come in contact with the employee health service (**EHS**) of the facilities where clinical experience is gained. Employees of healthcare facilities usually are seen by the EHS for various reasons, including the initial physical examination, yearly tuberculin (PPD) testing, routine immunizations and other routine screenings, and return-to-work permits after illness or injury. EHS personnel in the healthcare facility are responsible for investigating any reports of unusual or unexpected exposure of employees to communicable disease, including needlestick incidents or cases of the assault of a nurse by a client. Nurses who develop latex sensitivity would also be assisted by the EHS, to ensure a safe environment for them. The EHS is usually only open during daytime and early evening hours, and may be closed on weekends.

Armed Forces

The active Armed Forces and the Reserves offer employment opportunities for LPN/LVNs and RNs. After basic training, licensed nurses may enter the Armed Forces at a level higher than that of other enlisted persons. Usually, they are assigned to hospitals or clinics and may be assigned to duty in another country. In many cases, qualified individuals receive salary and expenses while attending nursing programs, in exchange for enlistment during school or upon graduation. Nurses, while in service, can often earn "credits" to help pay for additional education after leaving the service and can also take college courses free of charge while on active duty.

Schools

In addition to nurses employed to assist students with disabilities, school systems and colleges usually employ nurses and other healthcare personnel to work with their students. LPN/LVNs may be employed as assistants or school health aides. Schools often have PHNs on staff as well. Duties are varied and interesting. Assistant nurses help with vision and hearing screening, immunization clinics, and athlete physical examinations. The nurse or assistant nurse in a school also performs routine first aid and assists with recordkeeping. He or she may help teach nursing assistants or other students on work-release programs, and may assist with student support groups regarding weight loss, eating disorders, CD, smoking cessation, and related topics. The nurse may help students to deal with violence in school or the death of a classmate. This nurse may be called upon to teach topics such as sex education to young students, and safer sex and pregnancy prevention to older students. The nurse works with teen parents and their children. Home visits may also be one of this nurse's assignments.

Parish Nursing

Many large churches and synagogues have *parish nurses,* who may be paid employees or volunteers. These nurses facilitate a congregation's holistic health, combining physical, emotional, and spiritual dimensions. A local hospital or public health agency may provide a case manager or nurse coordinator to help develop the concept, support the parish, and provide in-service education to the nurse. Specific training courses are available for the parish nurse, who is usually an RN. The LPN/LVN usually functions as an assistant to the parish nurse.

The functions of the parish nurse and assistants may include performing health screenings, educating individuals or groups on health and wellness topics, writing newsletter articles, and visiting parishioners in hospitals and nursing homes (and sometimes performing home visits). Parish nurses provide counseling, make referrals, serve as client advocates, and may provide hands-on nursing care, although they are more likely to assist in training family caregivers. They often accompany congregation members to physicians' offices or hospitals for test results or surgery. Parish nurses provide support to terminally ill clients and their families. They often participate in funerals for deceased parishioners. They sometimes facilitate bereavement support groups.

Occasionally, churches sponsor healthcare clinics for parishioners and the local community. Services may be limited, or the clinic may be a community health center. Parish nurses may oversee such programs and coordinate volunteers helping in the clinic. The parish nurse may also oversee a program in the community, such as Meals-on-Wheels. These programs provide volunteer opportunities as well as paid employment.

Nursing in Unique Locales

Employment is available for a limited number of nurses, both RNs and LPN/LVNs, in such unique locations as cruise ships or large resorts, particularly those catering to older people. In these positions, the nurse is often functioning under "standing orders" from a physician, who may not be on site. In the case of any emergency, the nurse must be able to contact a physician, but must be able to perform first-aid or life-support measures to stabilize the person for transport or until a physician can arrive.

Working Overseas.   In many foreign countries, nurses educated in the United States or Canada are in great demand. Sometimes, the host country's government will pay moving and living expenses, as well as a high salary. The American nursing license is often sufficient, although a local license may be required as well. Nurses who anticipate seeking employment in other countries would benefit from learning languages other than English. Understanding the customs of the host country is also essential preparation for correct personal and professional behavior. (For example, there are strict taboos and protocols of behavior for women in many developing countries.)

Volunteer Service

Nurses can help in their communities by teaching others about healthcare or by assisting in times of disaster. The events of September 11, 2001, serve to emphasize the need for first-aid volunteers in every community.

Nurses may become involved in helping teach first-aid, babysitting, or expectant parents' classes at local hospitals, or in teaching adult or community education classes. Some positions are volunteer and some are paid.

The American Red Cross is a large national program that uses nurse volunteers to assist with well-baby and immunization clinics, as well as to provide first-aid services for community events and during disasters. Red Cross nurse volunteers also teach CPR, first-aid, and other classes. The Red Cross often uses volunteer nurses during blood collection days. A small number of nurses, often RNs, are employed by the Red Cross to set up and manage blood drives, and to supervise the volunteers. All major- and minor-league stadiums have a cadre of first-aid volunteers and paid rescue personnel who work during games. Nurses can receive special training to serve in either a paid or volunteer capacity at these events.

Volunteers in Service to America (VISTA) provides care and education to people in need in the United States, especially those in medically underserved areas. To nurses who qualify, the Peace Corps offers an opportunity to volunteer for needed human services in many parts of the world. Other programs include Habitat for Humanity, and teams providing surgery or eye care in underserved areas, both in the United States and in other countries. Churches often sponsor mission trips to assist with delivering healthcare in underserved areas. Most of these programs welcome RNs and LPN/LVNs as volunteers.

☛ KEY CONCEPT

The nurse is a member of the larger community. Opportunities exist for volunteer service, in order to give back to that community.

Other Opportunities

Other potential employment opportunities may include:

   Head Start programs: Head Start employs LPNs and RNs in schools as assistant instructors in their programs for very young children.

   Weight-loss clinics: Weight-loss clinics employ nurses as support persons or counselors. These nurses are often LPN/LVNs. The nurses weigh clients, measure skinfold thickness, take blood pressure, teach classes, and perform other functions.

   Camp programs: Most camps are required to employ nurses. The lead nurse may be an RN, but LPN/LVNs are often on the staff. These nurses share many functions with school nurses, although many of the illnesses and disorders they encounter are different. Campers may have poison ivy or poison oak, insect or snake bites, fractures, lacerations, and various infections. They may be sunburned, wind-burned, or burned in connection with campfire. A near drowning may occur, or a child may be thrown from a horse. Camp nurses also must assist homesick children. They often teach wilderness safety, survival, and first-aid measures. This is typically a summer position, allowing the nurse ample time to further his or her education during the school year.

Specialized Employment Opportunities

Some positions are available for LPN/LVNs or RNs who have special qualifications and the ability to meet the demands of a particular job. Most of these positions require further education or training beyond the basic nursing program.

Practical Nursing Programs

Some *practical nursing programs* employ LPN/LVNs or non–bachelor's degree RNs to assist with clinical or laboratory supervision of practical nursing students. (In some states, this is illegal.) Qualifications include a sound educational background, clinical nursing experience, proficiency in nursing skills, patience, and the ability to work with people. Previous teaching experience is an asset. Hours are usually days, Monday through Friday.

Operating Rooms

Many hospitals now employ LPN/LVNs and newly graduated RNs in operating rooms. LPN/LVNs or RNs with postgraduate surgical and technical training assist surgeons as *scrub nurses*. In most cases, the lead *circulating nurse* must be an RN. The hours are usually Monday through Friday during the day, often starting at 4 or 5 AM. Operating-room staff members are also on call for emergencies in most facilities.

Dialysis Centers

Nurses may be specifically trained to work in hospital dialysis units, ambulatory dialysis centers, or on mobile teams that administer dialysis to clients in their homes. Some clients have their own in-home dialysis units. Nurses teach clients and family members how to operate machines; in some cases, nurses themselves operate the machines. Dialysis nurses must have a thorough understanding of the complications and emergency measures associated with this treatment.

Hyperbaric Medicine

The *hyperbaric chamber* provides oxygen under pressure to special clients. These clients include those with anaerobic diseases, such as gas gangrene or tetanus. In addition, hyperbaric oxygenation (**HBO**) is often helpful in cases of carbon monoxide poisoning; in conjunction with some types of cancer chemotherapy; in cases of near drowning; and in cases of rapid re-entry into the earth's atmosphere, such as with a fighter pilot or balloonist who crashes from a high altitude. Some types of surgery are also performed under HBO. The nurse, either RN or LPN/LVN, will require special instruction to work in hyperbaric chambers or with the supporting team outside the chamber. Because the oxygen delivered is very concentrated, special safety measures must be carefully observed. People working in the chamber must have patent auditory tubes, to adequately equalize the pressure in the middle ear with the surrounding atmosphere and thereby avoid severe discomfort. Former Navy

divers also have found hyperbaric medicine to be a good career opportunity.

Pharmaceutical Sales

Pharmaceutical companies sometimes employ RNs and LPN/LVNs in sales and marketing positions. Nurses working in these companies have an advantage over other salespeople because they understand the actions and side effects of medications, and may be able to better communicate information with physicians. The salesperson is often required to travel and must provide a professional wardrobe and a car. Hours can be long and the salesperson often works on commission, with the potential for high earnings.

Veterinary Clinics

More veterinarians are hiring nurses as assistants. Many nursing techniques for humans are useful in veterinary medicine and surgery as well. The anatomy and physiology of many animals closely parallels that of the human.

Chiropractic Clinics and Acupuncture Centers

These areas often employ nurses as assistants. In some cases, nurses receive instruction to perform some treatments, such as diathermy and ultrasound. Nurses may also return to school to receive advanced training to perform therapies such as homeopathy, flower essence therapy, acupressure/acupuncture, and other complementary therapies.

Dental, Ophthalmology, and Other Specialty Clinics

Nurses may be employed by dentists or eye specialists, particularly those who perform surgery. These nurses are often LPN/LVNs, and assist with procedures such as colonoscopy, prostate biopsy, and other biopsies. These nurses are often trained on the job by the practitioner. Functions include pre-procedure teaching, administration of medications before and during the procedure, handling of instruments and supplies during the procedure to the practitioner, monitoring of client vital signs, and emotional support of the client. The nurse also monitors the client after the procedure until he or she is stable, and makes sure the client is safe to return home. The nurse carries out postoperative instruction, including signs of complications. This nurse usually works daytime hours during the week, but may be on call for emergencies.

Emergency Rescue

Some nurses wish to work with injured clients or clients who suddenly become ill. An additional paramedic or emergency medical technician (EMT) course is often required to be employed in ground- or air-rescue services. Employment in this area requires calmness under pressure, quick thinking, and accurate decision-making. Emergency rescue personnel regularly use medical-surgical equipment and must be familiar with a variety of high-tech equipment. Other opportunities for nurses with paramedic or EMT training include park ranger rescue services and ski-patrol programs. EMTs and paramedics may be employed or may be volunteers at parades, races, sports events, concerts, and other large gatherings, and may provide rescuer services in the event of a disaster.

Self-Employment

Some nurses are entrepreneurs and are self-employed. Examples of self-employed healthcare-related businesses include running a shop that sells or rents medical equipment or uniforms, contracting individually or with other nurses to provide home care, developing and marketing a specialty health-related product, or operating a health-food or herbal-medicine store. Nurses might work from home doing medical transcription, or medical literature searches and research on the Internet for others. Some nurses, often RNs, perform chart review and do research for attorneys, in preparation for court cases. To become a medical-legal consultant, particularly if court testimony or depositions will be required, advanced specialized training is usually required.

A nurse (RN or LPN/LVN) might contract with a city or county to provide testing services for contaminants such as radon or lead. Many large cities have such programs. Some nurses write books, chapters, continuing education courses, or journal articles for which they are paid. Nurses also review and teach continuing education courses and are paid directly by the participants or by a school.

Nurses serve as item writers for the NCLEX and other examinations, and as site visitors for accreditation agencies. They may be paid a small amount or may volunteer for these duties, but their expenses are reimbursed.

☞ KEY CONCEPT

The possibilities for entrepreneurship and related volunteer activities are limited only by an individual nurse's imagination, available time, and personal energy.

OBTAINING EMPLOYMENT INFORMATION

As described in Chapter 100, nursing provides a unique opportunity for employees to choose work schedules and locations that best suit their lifestyle. Examine personal and family needs to choose the most suitable work situation.

A very large percentage of jobs are never advertised or are filled by the time an advertisement publishes. Be sure to build networks to learn about positions as they become available. If an internship, student-learning experience, or volunteer opportunity is available, take it. Future employees are often chosen from those who have had some exposure to the facility and are known to the staff.

☞ KEY CONCEPT

Remember that approximately 90% of all positions are filled based on personal contacts. Many positions are not advertised. Doing homework and expanding one's professional network increases the chances of landing the position that is desired.

Medical Pool or Personnel Service

A medical pool/**nurses' registry** recruits nurses to work in facilities that need extra help for special duty clients, vacation coverage, or during busy periods, maternity, or illness. A nurse registers with the agency, which calls when a job is available. The nurse has the option of declining, which is an advantage for those who do not wish to work full-time. Nurses who decline too often, however, run the risk of losing future opportunities with the agency. Agencies often offer insurance, vacation pay, and free in-service education to nurses who accept the required number of shifts. Many agencies have regular posts to fill in healthcare facilities, home care, and schools, and can provide nurses with full-time employment.

There are advantages and disadvantages to working for a pool. The nurse is often paid a higher hourly wage, though often without benefits. The nurse has more choice as to when and where to work. Disadvantages include not knowing if one will be working or not; unpaid time off; and difficulty in establishing strong bonds with co-workers, unless the nurse is assigned to the same location. Often the pool nurse is assigned to a very busy area, which may be a positive challenge or may be very difficult.

Some hospitals and long-term care facilities have their own internal nursing pool. This has the advantage of continuity and stability, as well as being familiar with the physical setup, nursing protocols, and staff at the facility.

State JOBS Service

Each state's JOBS or employment service is affiliated with the local government. This agency provides free job information, both in private industry and government positions. Employment opportunities are located on a computer, so positions in many areas are accessible. State JOBS services are usually accessible via the Internet. Call a local courthouse to find out how to access the state's JOBS service.

Many large organizations, counties, or states maintain a phone or Internet job hotline. A person can call or access the service 24 hours a day, usually free of charge. Many of these entities are required by law to post all positions, so the person accessing the service can peruse all available positions. In many cases, an application for employment can be obtained and submitted on the Internet.

Nursing Journals

Many nursing journals advertise positions. Some positions are in specialty areas; others are for general staff nurses, including new graduates. Specific positions advertised in a journal may be filled by the time they are actually published. However, the ads can provide some insight into which healthcare facilities are currently hiring and the geographical areas that seem to have the most available positions. Nursing journals list facility addresses, e-mail addresses, and websites for obtaining further information.

Newspapers, Bulletin Boards, and Other Sources

Newspapers publish many available positions. These positions often fill quickly, so it is important to apply promptly after seeing an ad. Even if a particular position is filled by the time an application is filed, related positions may be available. Don't forget to look on bulletin boards, either paper postings or Internet bulletin boards. The yellow pages provide names and addresses of potential employers as well.

Internet

With today's technology, locating employment sites has become faster and easier. Several national employment websites are available, some of which are specific to healthcare careers. State JOBS listings also can be accessed through the Internet. The Internet provides information about online job fairs, with information about many employers. Many hospitals and other facilities have websites with employment information. Often, major newspapers and journals post their classified advertisements directly on the Internet. In many cases, applications for employment can be obtained directly via the Internet. This service is particularly useful if the plan is to work in a part of the country different from the current residence. Sites like Monster.com also exist, where an individual can post his or her resume for potential employers to review.

In addition to individual websites, online versions of several journals' "Career Directory" are available. These directories typically include a large number of positions, as well as articles related to job-seeking. (They are also available in printed form.) The *American Journal of Nursing* publishes a career issue yearly. Although most of the positions advertised are for RNs, pertinent articles give hints on job seeking. The LPN/LVN can also get a good feeling for where jobs are located by reading this issue.

Websites that are devoted to writing resumes and cover letters, job interviewing, and other pertinent topics for employment seekers also are available. Many websites link to other helpful sites.

When searching for employment, the World Wide Web offers several advantages. For example, an individual can search for opportunities in a particular part of the country. Plus, Internet information and hints are usually helpful, providing access to a wide range of potential employers. One of the most important advantages of using the Internet is that all searching can be completed from home. In addition, communicating with potential employers via the Internet demonstrates one's experience and proficiency with this technology. To help focus and narrow the search, numerous books are also available, which list specific websites and helpful suggestions to guide the electronic job search.

JOB-SEEKING SKILLS

Before deciding on the type of employment to seek, individual personal requirements must be evaluated. Consider such factors as geographic location, shift rotation, child care, transportation, and housing in the decision-making process. An unwillingness to compromise about where to work or desired hours of work may lead to difficulty in obtaining a job. Develop a job-search plan that includes the following:

- Decide on the types of jobs desired in relation to what is available.
- Complete a self-evaluation: What are the individual's greatest skills and assets? Where is the best fit? Consider factors such as desire to work alone or with others, freedom and flexibility versus structure, and desire to be a leader or a member of the team.
- Spend at least 5 hours a day in the job search. Finding a job is the "job" now.
- Set a goal for the number of contacts per day.
- Be sure the resume and cover letter are neatly printed and error-free.
- Prepare for interviews with appropriate dress and a plan for answering difficult questions.
- Emphasize the positive: self, education, and all former positions, paid or volunteered.
- Use networking skills to find unadvertised positions.
- Arrange issues such as transportation and daycare ahead of time.

The first job is important. It forms the basis for future opportunities. Performing well the first time provides a sound basis and good references that will help in acquiring future positions.

☛ Key Concept

Consider yourself and your strengths. Then, analyze available jobs. Attempt to match the two for your greatest personal satisfaction.

Choosing a Place of Employment

Many factors need to be considered when choosing possible places of employment. The first job may not be the perfect job. Consider what is most important and choose the best job available. Box 101-1 lists specific items to consider when choosing where to work. Try to match skills, needs, and personal goals as much as possible with available positions.

Applying For a Position

After targeting the positions of interest, the next step is to apply. Because competition may be fierce for the most desirable jobs, how the application process is completed can greatly affect an employer's decision about who to hire.

Letter of Application

The value of the letter of application, sometimes referred to as the "cover letter" (if it accompanies a resume), cannot be overestimated. The letter is usually the first thing employers see. The application may not be considered if the letter fails to have a positive effect. Remember that the focus is on convincing employers that you are the best candidate. The letter should be informative and concise. First, the letter should state the position for which the person is applying and how the person found out about it. Next, the letter should explain briefly why the person feels he or she is qualified. Describe applicable job experience, skills, and education. Conclude the letter by informing the employer of availability for a personal

➤➤ BOX 101-1

FACTORS TO CONSIDER WHEN LOOKING FOR A PLACE OF EMPLOYMENT

- Personal factors: child care, hours, personal career and educational goals, distance from home
- Quality of care: client safety, means of quality assessment, legal support, average daily client load per nurse, non-nursing duties expected of nurses
- Teamwork: collegiality, general work climate, respect among coworkers, participation in quality improvement
- Type of facility: client care, research, teaching; nonprofit, proprietary; small, large; presence or absence of nursing and other students
- Available shifts: day, evening, night; full-time, part-time; permanent shift assignment or rotating shifts; flexibility of honoring special hours requests; mandatory double shifts
- Length of shifts: choices of 8-, 10-, and 12-hour shifts; special incentives, such as Baylor Plan or weekend-contract (If longer shifts are chosen, the nurse may have more days off; however, working longer shifts may be difficult to arrange for the nurse and the family.)
- Chances for advancement and leadership opportunities; available teaching and committee opportunities; use of computers in daily care: documentation, ordering treatments and medications, calling up information, e-mail
- Educational opportunities and professional growth: internships, in-service education, continuing education courses, library facilities, computer availability, pay or reimbursement for advanced education and continuing education courses, training in use of new equipment
- Salary: opportunities and requirements for moving up the salary scale; shift/weekend differential; charge nurse pay, overtime pay, holiday pay, range of holiday hours to be paid, "holiday back" policies, job stability, financial security

- Benefits: insurance (health, dental, disability, life, individual, and family), sick leave, vacation time, holidays, on-site child care (including the availability of care for ill children), adult daycare, parking, food service, worker's compensation, 401k, tax-sheltered annuities, profit sharing, optional assignment of benefits. (*Optional assignment of benefits* allows the employee to set aside a dollar amount to be used for non-covered benefits, such as insurance co-pays and deductibles, complementary health care, glasses, elective surgery, and so forth. If the total amount is not used, the employee usually loses the unused portion at the end of the year.)
- Professional feedback and evaluation: periodic review, peer review, status of facility accreditation, participation of nurses in accreditation process, praise and recognition
- Safety and security for staff: parking lot, assistance with assaultive clients, security in home care, providing nurse with beeper or phone for home care, "panic button" on dangerous unit
- Extra "perks": payment of professional dues, subscription to nursing journal, choir, theater group, discount tickets, group travel, Weight Watchers, gift shop, staff tournaments, holiday teas, retirement parties, recognition for years of service, use of gym or health club or swimming pool, pharmacy, credit union, payment for preventive healthcare or health club membership, free or reduced-rate parking or bus passes, housing allowance or nurses' residence, Internet access, payment for unused sick leave or option to convert to vacation
- Professional association membership: required or voluntary; bargaining agent, contract for nurses

---

interview and the easiest method for contact. Print out the letter neatly on conservative stationery, and enclose it along with an up-to-date personal resume. Some facilities accept applications via the Internet or by fax as well. Do not submit a handwritten letter.

☛ KEY CONCEPT

If access to a high-quality printer is not available or knowledge about composing an appropriate resume is lacking, make use of professional resume services. They can help compose and print a professional-looking resume at a relatively low cost.

Resume

There are two types of resumes: one type emphasizes strengths and abilities, the other lists experience chronologically. When seeking a first nursing position, usually the second type of resume is used. List education, previous employment, and relevant experience. In stating information about education, list

schools, their addresses, diplomas or degrees received (most recent first), and licenses and certificates held (and in what states). Dates can be omitted. List work experience, with the most recent position first (name of facility; dates employed; title of position; and supervisor's name, address, and telephone number). Identify any special skills, training, honors, or volunteer positions, and be sure to provide references. Many nursing programs offer guidelines as to what to include in a good resume. They also may have keyboarding and printing services available to new graduates. Box 101-2 gives further tips for composing a resume.

Interview

Routine procedure usually includes a personal interview with a prospective employer. When going to an interview, wear tailored, conservative clothes (a suit is usually best) and simple jewelry. Be sure shoes are neat and clean, and polished if necessary. Avoid extremes in makeup and nail polish. Clean and neatly styled hair and clean, short fingernails are essential. Men

➤➤ BOX 101-2

GUIDELINES FOR WRITING A RESUME

- Clearly list name, mailing address, phone number; include e-mail address, fax number, and cell phone number if available.
- Be positive. Don't mention shortcomings.
- Be specific.
- Be accurate. Make sure no errors exist in dates of employment or school; make sure there are no "typos" or spelling errors. Use a "spell-checker."
- Be creative.
- Be brief. Keep to one page, if possible.
- *Print out* neatly. A handwritten resume may eliminate an individual from consideration. Space the resume so it looks attractive. Use a high-quality printer. Print as many originals as necessary. Do not make carbon copies or photocopies. Use white bond paper.

Special Tips
- State the career objective.
- Briefly state special circumstances while in school (worked 20 hours a week, commuted 50 miles, perfect attendance, grade point average, special awards, activities).
- Emphasize the past 5 years.
- Include non-nursing and related volunteer positions.
- If a veteran, list branch of service and rank; be sure to indicate health-related experience.
- List memberships in organizations and offices held; include nursing and community organizations (a limited number).
- List special interests and skills.
- List references on a separate sheet. References are not always sent with the resume.
- Do not list personal data, such as married or single, number of children, age, sex, religion. (A professional-looking photograph may be included but is usually not recommended. It is illegal for prospective employers to require a photo or to ask personal questions.)
- Have another person read and react to the resume before sending it.
- If necessary, rearrange the resume or emphasize specific factors, to fit the needs of different employers.

should be sure that moustaches or beards are clean and neatly trimmed. A short haircut and a minimum of facial hair and jewelry are recommended. Practice giving a firm handshake. Remember: The first impression is made in just a few seconds.

☞ KEY CONCEPT

Arrive at least 5 minutes early for the interview. Make a practice run the day before or be sure to have good directions. Arriving late to an interview leaves the prospective employer with a negative impression.

The nursing transcript can be brought with the person to the interview. If it is in narrative form, the interviewee may need to interpret it for the interviewer if asked. Commonly, the interviewee will be asked to sign a release that permits the potential employer to contact your references. (It is illegal for schools or people to release information about an individual without that person's written consent.) Proof of citizenship or legal residence in the country is necessary in the United States. The nurse should also bring a photo identification, the school transcript, the social security card, the CPR card, evidence of a negative PPD or chest x-ray examination, and the nursing license, if received.

A prospective employer is interested in past employment, school record, punctuality, attendance records, ability to work with others (teamwork), willingness to accept assignments, and reactions in emergencies. Box 101-3 lists guidelines for the job interview. Be prepared to answer the following questions:

- What shift will you work?
- Will you work part-time?
- What are your rotation choices (eg, day–night, day–afternoon)?

Remember that most beginning nursing positions require rotating or night shifts, and often working every other weekend. Many facilities require medical-surgical nursing experience before being assigned to a specialty area such as obstetrics or psychiatry.

Informational Interview. Even if a facility has no positions available, a member of the human resources department may be willing to conduct an informational interview. In this case, the interviewee is not applying for a position, but simply finding out information about the facility. Informational interviews allow an individual to practice the interview process, get an idea what job interviews are like, and meet the interviewers for future reference. Interviewers may provide feedback on how they felt the individual handled the interview and may be willing to give suggestions for improvement. If a position becomes available in that facility later, an interviewer may consider the interviewee over other candidates, just because he or she has met with that person. In addition, the interviewee will be better prepared when participating in other interviews.

Application Forms. As part of the job-seeking process, a prospective employee is almost always required to fill out an application form. When filling out a standard application form, have Social Security number, resume, and nursing license (if received) available. Properly worded responses and careful, neat handwriting or printing in ink make a favorable impression.

Employers often use the way in which an individual completes an application as one of the criteria for evaluating him or her as a prospective employee. Think before writing. Be neat.

☞ KEY CONCEPT

How an individual writes or prints often indicates to a potential employer how that person might document care in the future.

➤➤ **BOX 101-3**

GUIDELINES FOR THE JOB INTERVIEW

- Prepare for the interview: practice to gain self-confidence. Find out who will be doing the interviewing and memorize the lead person's name. Get plenty of sleep the night before, and have tissues or cough drops available if needed.
- Dress neatly and conservatively to project a professional image. If a smoker, be sure your clothes do not smell of smoke—ask someone else to check. Wear a minimum of jewelry. Make sure fingernails are clean and shoes are clean and, if necessary, polished.
- Write down questions, and review them ahead of time. Take notes during the interview.
- Be sure to arrive a few minutes *early*.
- Do homework on the agency before going. Be able to ask intelligent questions.
- Know in advance how to handle difficult questions, such as "Why do you want to work here?" "What can you offer us?" "What are your strengths?" "What is unique about you?" "What are your weaknesses?" "What was your biggest mistake?" "What are your long-term career goals?" "What was the last book you read (or your favorite book)?"
- Be prepared to answer questions about technical competence. The employer may ask about experience with specific nursing procedures or with particular types of clients.
- Be aware that most interviewers will offer to shake hands. Make sure the handshake is *firm* but not crushing. Use the whole hand, *not* just the fingertips.
- Let the person indicate where to sit. Wait to sit until the interviewer has been seated.
- Put purse or briefcase on the floor—not on the interviewer's desk. (Do *not* bring both purse and briefcase; this is too burdensome.)
- Sit up straight. Keep hands folded on the lap or in front on the table.
- If possible, leave a coat outside the interview room to avoid having to take it off and then find a place to put it during the interview.
- Do not smoke or chew gum. Make sure not to have bad breath or "smoker's breath."
- Do not accept coffee or food.
- Look at the person when speaking, but do not stare.
- Listen carefully to the questions, and *think* before talking.
- Do not act as though getting this job is absolutely critical.
- Inform the interviewer of any special skills and preferences, but do not exaggerate. Let the employer know about any computer expertise or experience.
- Do not talk too much; give concise answers and, when finished with an answer, stop and let the interviewer resume with further questioning.
- Be prepared to ask pertinent questions, for example about the specific job description as well as about opportunities for advancement, evaluation policies, and available in-service education or tuition reimbursement. Ask if there is a formal employment contract.
- If the salary and benefits are not known, ask these questions *last*.
- Do not complain about previous employers. Speak of any previous positions in the most positive way possible.
- Avoid the use of negative terms in responses. Speak of "challenges" and "opportunities" instead of problems.
- Thank the interviewer for his or her time. Use the person's name, with Mr. or Ms. *Never* use the interviewer's first name.
- Bring the nursing license, school transcript, record of tuberculin test, driver's license, birth certificate (or passport or resident alien card), CPR card, and Social Security card, in case any are needed.
- If written evaluations from previous employment (even if not nursing-related) are available, bring *copies* of them to leave with the interviewer. It is good to show a good previous work history, whether in nursing-related jobs or not.
- If possible, have letters of reference already written to leave with the interviewer. This will save them the time of contacting the references.
- If letters of reference are not available, have a neat list of names, addresses, professional positions, and telephone numbers of references readily available to leave with the interviewer. Be sure that these references have been contacted ahead of time.
- Be prepared to be interviewed by a committee, or to have the interview tape-recorded. Look at all members of the interview team. Shake hands with each and use their names.
- If currently employed, be prepared to tell the interviewer if it is acceptable to call the current employer. (Be sure to ask the current employer ahead of time.)
- Ask the interviewer when notification about the position will be made.

Be prepared to give references to potential employers. Have the addresses and telephone numbers of the individuals acting as references neatly printed. Always contact these references in advance to ask permission before listing them. ("May I list your name on my resume for a positive reference?")

Testing.   In some instances, the prospective applicant may be asked to take aptitude tests or baseline tests in medication administration or mathematics. Relax and try not to be anxious. Generally, it is best not to change an answer after it is written. If taking a timed test, go through the entire test as quickly as possible, answering the questions known. Then, go back and work on the other questions. Do not spend too much time on any one item.

   Followup After the Interview.   After the interview is completed, follow up with a letter thanking the person for his or her time and stating interest in the position. Restate qualifications briefly. Be sure that this letter is just as neat as was the letter of application. Be sure to write the thank-you letter within 24 hours.

Accepting the Position

When an individual accepts a position, he or she is entering into an agreement. Be familiar with the pertinent personnel policies. Every institution establishes its own personnel policies, though there are many commonalities. Salaries usually vary according to a facility's size, type, and location. Salaries are usually higher in large cities and in certain areas of the country. Government hospitals (such as Veterans Administration, county, state, and university hospitals) may offer higher salaries than do private hospitals or ECFs. Clinics and home care tend to have lower salaries than hospitals, but often have the advantage of daytime hours and minimal weekend assignments. Larger facilities may offer more compensation to nurses who have additional education. Additional responsibility and higher pay may be available, based on a nurse's education level and length of service. Some hospitals pay a bonus for years of service there. Many facilities give initial credit on the salary schedule for previous experience gained in other locations.

   When offered a position, the nurse is usually given a day or two to make a decision. If offered more than one position, it is important to notify each employer of the final decision, including positions declined.

Contracts and Agreements

When accepting a position, the nurse should notify the employer as soon as possible. Make sure there is agreement on working conditions, hours, salary, and benefits. Sometimes this information is presented to the nurse in the form of a contract or letter of agreement to be signed.

   It is a good idea to write a letter of acceptance to the employer. Verify the start date, shifts to be worked, salary, benefits, and other pertinent information in the letter. Some hospitals and cities have a standard working agreement or nurses' contract, which is renegotiated on a regular basis, and which covers a number of hospitals and facilities. The terms and conditions are written and can be reviewed. There is minimal room for negotiation, however.

   Recently, more nurses are negotiating working conditions and client safety. Some nurses' contracts allow nurses to determine when a unit or hospital can no longer accept new clients because of staff shortage.

   Some hospitals and facilities are considered "union." Often a branch of the American Nurses Association (ANA) serves as the negotiating agent.

   Employer Responsibilities.   The employer is responsible for providing a safe working environment, which:

- Is free from unusual dangers and follows such factors as OSHA guidelines
- Is not discriminatory
- Negotiates in good faith
- Does not allow sexual harassment or other forms of harassment
- Does not interfere with the legal rights of employees
- Provides regular employee evaluations
- Follows federal guidelines on pay, hours worked, break time, and time off
- Provides a grievance, mediation, and arbitration process for disputes
- Offers assistance and guidance in the case of unfounded legal action against the nurse
- Provides a health service or some means for employees to obtain minimum healthcare and screening

   Employee Responsibilities.   It is important to know what is expected of employees before accepting a position. All employers have the right to expect that employees will:

- Work on assigned days and report on time
- Call in sick only when truly ill
- Maintain client confidentiality
- Practice within the parameters of the license (RN, LPN/LVN) and within the limits of individual training and experience
- Seek help at the appropriate time
- Practice with integrity: honest documentation, observation of appropriate client–nurse boundaries, proper care of medications, immediate reporting of medication errors or incidents, and so forth
- Observe the regulations of the individual facility in regard to continuing education, participation in committees, and so forth
- Maintain the nursing license and other required certificates, such as PPD testing and CPR certification
- Practice as a collaborative member of the healthcare team
- Follow rules and guidelines of the facility

After Obtaining the Position

How an individual functions after being hired will affect his or her professional status and references for the future. Having good references increases the chances that the individual will be more likely to obtain future positions. Chances are also greater that this individual will be recommended for leadership positions, salary advancement, and further education.

   Upon being hired, typically the new employee will participate in an orientation program.

Orientation

Facilities almost always provide orientation programs for new employees. Discuss with instructors any procedures that may require additional practice. The instructor can help provide extra knowledge and experience. Also, many facilities require newly graduated nurses to take medication tests and math tests.

A part of any orientation program includes learning about disaster, fire, and emergency code procedures. Other topics include personnel policies, evaluation procedures, nursing protocols, facility organizational charts, and safety and security procedures.

Internship

As stated in Chapter 100, recent graduates are often required to serve a period of internship or residency before being considered full-fledged LPN/LVNs or RNs or benefit-earning members of the staff. Ask about these probationary policies when discussing salary and benefits.

An internship helps with the transition from student to graduate nurse. Many facilities provide a mentor or preceptor to assist the new graduate during the internship or probationary period.

Resigning From a Position

If the situation arises in which the nurse is going to leave his or her position, the employer should be given written advance notice—at least 2 weeks and preferably a month. Notice gives the agency adequate time to find a replacement. Advance-notice requirements are sometimes stated in personnel policies. A letter of resignation should be just as neat and professional as was the letter of application.

Customarily, if an individual leaves before the designated time or without notice, that person will be paid up to the time of departure only. The person most likely will not receive a good reference if he or she leaves a job without giving proper notice. Try not to "burn bridges." Leave all posts in a professional and positive way. One never knows when a reference might be needed or when one might wish to return.

✎ STUDENT SYNTHESIS

Key Points

- Multiple employment opportunities exist in nursing and in other healthcare fields.
- The graduate nurse can choose employment to fit his or her personal needs—different practice areas, structured or less-structured settings, self-employment, and different parts of the country or world.
- The Internet provides a means of conducting a job search, applying for a position, and taking continuing education courses.
- Completing and updating the professional resume is an integral component of the job search.
- People form their first impressions in a matter of seconds; a positive first impression is important in obtaining employment.

- The personal interview offers both the applicant and the potential employer the opportunity to learn about each other. Always follow up an interview with a thank-you letter.
- Employers provide an orientation for new employees. A part of any orientation program includes learning about disaster, fire, and emergency code procedures. Other topics include personnel policies, evaluation procedures, nursing protocols, facility organizational charts, and safety and security procedures.
- A written advance notice of at least 2 weeks should be given to an employer when resigning from a position.

Critical Thinking Exercises

1. Conduct informational interviews in two different healthcare facilities or other occupational areas near the geographic area in which you plan to work after graduation. Make a list of factors that are important to you. How many of these factors relate to compensation? How many to other benefits? How many relate to personal and professional growth? Compare and contrast the conditions of employment in the two places.
2. Survey your local area and identify as many "non-traditional" positions for nurses as possible. What are your feelings about nursing in these areas?

NCLEX-Style Review Questions

1. LVN/LPNs are able to work in specialized areas such as:
   a. Community health centers
   b. Dialysis centers
   c. Home care
   d. Rehabilitation centers
2. Which of the following strategies will be useful for the new graduate in obtaining a job?
   a. Avoid networking for unadvertised positions.
   b. Be flexible regarding number of contacts seen per day.
   c. Prepare for the interview by dressing appropriately.
   d. Spend at least 1 to 2 hours per day in the job search.
3. What information should the new graduate include on a resume?
   a. Education history
   b. Grade transcripts from nursing school
   c. Only current work experience
   d. Persons to notify in an emergency

CHAPTER

102

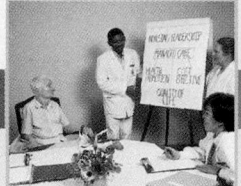

Advancement and Leadership in Nursing

LEARNING OBJECTIVES

1. Describe how an LPN/LVN can become nationally certified in long-term care.
2. Compare and contrast the terms leader and manager.
3. Discuss the characteristics of a good manager.
4. Describe leadership roles available to the LPN/LVN.
5. State at least four duties of the team leader/charge nurse.
6. List at least three characteristics of an effective manager.
7. Describe four different leadership styles.

NEW TERMINOLOGY

autocratic leadership
bureaucratic leadership
democratic leadership
due process
laissez-faire leadership
leader

manager
oral reprimand
performance review
plan of assistance
written reprimand

ACRONYMS

CLTC   CMMS   OBRA

Graduation and employment are just the beginning steps of a nursing career. Opportunities are available for advancement if the individual nurse wishes to further his or her career. Opportunities include national certification and further education. Nearly all states require nurses to take continuing education courses to maintain the license, as well. As the nurse advances in his or her career, opportunities arise for assuming positions of leadership. This chapter briefly addresses the areas of advancement and leadership in nursing.

ADVANCEMENT IN NURSING

Some nurses choose to advance their careers in various ways. Other nurses wish to continue delivering competent, caring, and safe bedside care without added responsibilities. Some career paths lead to higher salaries, while other activities enhance the nurse's professional recognition or personal satisfaction.

National Certification

The National Association for Practical Nurse Education and Services (NAPNES) has developed a certification for LPNs in long-term care. The LPN who qualifies for and passes this examination is then eligible to use the initials "**CLTC**" after his or her name, in addition to LPN. This certification, developed specifically for LPN/LVNs, offers the opportunity for recognition as a provider of quality care. Most importantly, however, obtaining this certification lets clients know that the nurse is committed and qualified to provide them with the best possible care.[1]

To qualify to take this examination, the nurse must hold an active LPN/LVN license in the United States or its territories and must have practiced in long-term care for 2,000 hours (full-time equivalent of 1 year) within the past 3 years. Many sites across the United States give the computerized examination, which consists of 150 multiple-choice questions (similar to the NCLEX examination). Three hours are allotted for completion of the test. The certification period lasts for 5 years and can be renewed by meeting specific requirements. Nurses who receive certification also receive free membership in NAPNES.

Content of the examination includes questions about the following issues as they relate to long-term care residents:

- *Physiologic integrity* (eg, dehydration, cardiovascular status, potential for aspiration, respiratory status, range of motion, functional ability, skin integrity, pain, gastrointestinal function, sleep)
- *Psychosocial integrity* (eg, lifestyle changes, independence, potential for violence, adjustment to change in body image, suspected abuse, sexuality)
- *Specialty practice issues* (eg, teaching and learning, communication, nursing process, ethics, resident rights—Omnibus Budget Reconciliation Act)
- *Leadership and management* (eg, resident care plans, collaboration with other staff, evaluation of unlicensed assistive personnel [UAP], stress reduction, care conference participation, quality assurance, cost containment, community resources)

Nurse Mobility Programs

A number of programs throughout the country offer an accelerated route to nursing. In some cases, the programs give credits for previous nursing education and experience. In some cases, they give credits for life experiences. A number of LPN/LVNs continue their education to become RNs. According to NFLPN (in 2002), currently about 10% of LPN/LVNs become RNs.

Numerous opportunities exist for further education. Opportunities are also available for specialized training for related positions, such as emergency rescue or surgical technician. Employers may provide tuition reimbursement to help cover the cost of further education. However, in some cases, in return for this reimbursement, the employee agrees to continue to work for the employer for a specified time period after completion of the education. This time period is often dependent on the amount of the reimbursement.

Information about special courses may be obtained from local and national nursing organizations or healthcare facilities. In addition, many nursing journals and the Internet provide information.

LPN/LVN to RN Programs

Many community colleges and private schools have programs that enroll LPN/LVNs and offer them a specialized program that leads to RN licensure. These programs usually last about 1 year and build on the education the student received in the practical nursing program.

In other cases, LPNs can enroll in generic RN programs, but may be exempted from taking some courses or may "test out" of certain courses. The "test out" usually includes both written and clinical demonstration components, and is designed to establish that the student is able to meet the objectives of the original course.

Associate's Degree to Bachelor's Degree RN Programs

The associate's-degree RN or LPN with an associate's degree in another field can often obtain a bachelor's degree in nursing in less time than the usual required 4 years. Local 4-year colleges vary in their admission requirements, and offer differing credits for previous education.

Bachelor's Degree to RN Programs

Some nursing programs enroll students who have a bachelor's degree in a major other than nursing. In these programs, graduates are eligible to take the RN licensure examination after a shorter period of time, because they have already taken their general liberal arts courses. Therefore, the student is not required to repeat many of the courses typically offered in the first 2 years of study, and can focus primarily on the clinical courses needed. These accelerated RN courses last about 2 years.

Refresher Courses

Many reasons exist for taking "nurse refresher" courses. The nurse may have stopped working for some time to pursue further education, travel, or raise a family. Refresher courses are a good idea when nurses have not been actively employed in nursing for several years. In addition, the nurse whose license lapses or is revoked, or who is on inactive licensure status for some time, may be required to take a refresher course to be licensed again. In addition, new graduates who do not pass the licensure examination in two or three attempts are often required to take refresher courses to take the exam again.

Practicing nurses teach refresher courses, which include overviews of several nursing areas, such as medical-surgical, pediatrics, and obstetrics. These courses may review basic sciences, such as body structure and function, nutrition, microbiology, and child development. Other topics may include new medications, equipment, and nursing procedures. A refresher course often includes several hours of clinical experience in addition to theory classes.

LEADERSHIP

In this new millennium, the LPN/LVN is expected to assume a leadership role in some healthcare settings. The NFLPN in 1996 stated that this increased responsibility is most evident in long-term or extended-care facilities (ECFs).[2] Remember that client acuity in extended care is steadily increasing. Therefore, nurses working in this area must continuously upgrade their skills and competencies to meet these growing responsibilities.

As the need for nurses to function as leaders increases, effective leadership skills become more important. A competent leader must be able to effectively direct and influence the actions of others. This section of the chapter addresses leadership styles and some basic management skills.

Effective Leadership and Management

In addition to postgraduate training in skills that leadership positions require, nurses also need other knowledge and attributes. A nurse being asked to work as a charge nurse or to assume another leadership position must decide if he or she is ready for this responsibility. The nurse may need assistance in planning and implementing client care and in coordinating and directing the activities of other staff members. The leader must be able to evaluate nursing care given and his or her personal leadership abilities. It is often helpful to consult another person who is trusted, honest, and qualified when assistance is needed. In most cases, nurses in leadership positions are responsible to a higher authority, for example, a department supervisor or Director of Nursing.

In a nursing home, the nurse in a leadership position needs information about legislation, such as Medicare, Medicaid, and the Omnibus Budget Reconciliation Act (**OBRA**). In addition, other information about third-party reimbursement policies, such as regulations of the Centers for Medicare and Medicaid Services (**CMMS**) (formerly Health Care Financing Administration [HCFA]), will be necessary.

Leader vs. Manager

The terms *leader* and *manager* refer to two distinct roles. However, these terms are commonly used interchangeably.

A leader is not necessarily a manager, but a leader can be a manager. The same is true of managers. A manager is not necessarily a leader, but a manager can be a leader.

A **leader** is a person who uses specific skills, such as role modeling, to influence others to accomplish a task or do the work. A **manager** coordinates and controls the work of others. A manager is involved with organizing, planning, directing, and controlling.

☛ KEY CONCEPT

- *The leader* influences *others.*
- *The manager* controls *others.*

Although the roles of a leader and a manager are typically separate, they often overlap. These roles may include:

- Role model
- Educator
- Advocate
- Decision-maker
- Planner
- Counselor
- Change agent

Characteristics of an Effective Manager

Being a good manager requires sound communication, decision-making, and problem-solving skills (Fig. 102-1). To be an effective manager, the following are necessary:

- A desire to manage—Comfort with the position is important
- Trust in one's own judgment—Ability to work without constant guidance from others
- Skills in stress management—To assist yourself and others
- Motivation to guide and to work with people, not just to attain power
- Ability to handle different situations

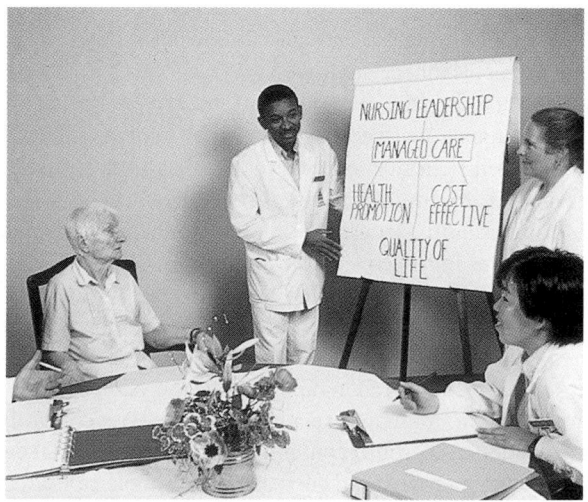

FIGURE 102-1. An effective leader communicates on a regular, consistent basis with other members of the staff.

- Ability to make competent decisions, especially in emergencies
- Ability to channel others' feelings and hostility into constructive problem-solving

Effective Leadership

One needs to develop leadership skills to supervise others effectively. Nurses develop organizational skills in daily client care; as a new graduate, additional leadership skills may need to be developed.

To be an effective leader, the following qualities or attributes are necessary:

- Self-confidence
- Self-awareness
- Strong personal values
- Skills of *value clarification* (choosing freely from alternatives, prizing the choice, and acting consistently on that choice)
- *Advocacy* (providing information and support to those being led)
- *Accountability* (taking responsibility for values and actions)

Leadership Styles

Leadership style refers to the behavior used by a leader in a specific situation. Various situations in healthcare will dictate the most appropriate leadership style, but a strong knowledge base is essential to all styles. The most effective leader often blends leadership styles. A successful leader can move from one style to another as the situation dictates.

Autocratic Leadership. **Autocratic leadership** is self-directed; this style calls for little or no input from staff. In its extreme form, autocratic leadership may be compared with a dictatorship, in which the leader makes decisions and the group is expected to carry out orders. In certain situations, such as a code or other life-threatening emergency, this style is effective in nursing. New graduates may feel more comfortable with an autocratic leader until they gain the necessary self-confidence.

Bureaucratic Leadership. **Bureaucratic leadership** is policy-minded. Bureaucratic leaders rely on established protocols for decision-making. The policy and procedure manual of the healthcare facility offers step-by-step instructions; a bureaucratic leader will consider them as rules. This style is often helpful for new graduates who need detailed instructions. In addition, some procedures, such as sterile technique, require strict guidelines and make no allowance for deviations in basic principles.

Democratic Leadership. **Democratic leadership** is people-oriented and tries to guide staff in the right direction. Some nursing approaches, such as team nursing, benefit from democratic leadership by fostering team spirit in an atmosphere of mutual respect and shared responsibility. These leaders use group input but are able to make final decisions themselves when no consensus is achieved. This style allows for a free flow of ideas, plans, and information between leader and followers.

Laissez-faire Leadership. The leadership style with the least structure is **laissez-faire leadership.** This leader has loosely structured goals, with no firm guidelines. He or she encourages followers to choose their own goals and plans for implementation. Although leaders who continuously use this style may be well liked, their team may not readily accomplish goals. However, laissez-faire leadership encourages creativity and independence and allows people to try new things without fear of mistakes.

Team Leader/Charge Nurse Role

In ECFs such as nursing homes, many LPNs "are now in leadership or charge positions, with the certified nursing assistant as the primary caregiver."[3] LPNs also function in leadership positions in other areas, such as clinics, insurance companies, and in some cases, hospitals.

The role of the *team leader/charge nurse* has many facets, those of both a leader and manager. A charge nurse is responsible for getting shift reports, assigning clients to staff members, determining client acuity, and handling emergencies. Coordinating the unit's activities by assigning staff breaks, coverage for breaks, attendance at special meetings, and client tests and procedures, as well as ensuring availability of needed supplies and equipment, are other responsibilities. The team leader or charge nurse usually performs activities such as counting narcotics at the beginning and end of the shift, checking the crash cart, reporting to the nursing supervisor, checking staffing for the next shift, and sending client acuity reports to administration.

The charge nurse must have leadership and administrative abilities, a thorough knowledge of nursing, and an intuitive understanding of people's behaviors. The LPN or new RN should not attempt to assume this role without further in-service education and experience beyond the basic nursing program.

The Practical/Vocational Nurse as Leader

LPN/LVNs can function as leaders and managers in various practice areas. The two most common areas are clinics and long-term care facilities.

The NFLPN (1996) states that LPNs, with additional preparation in specialty areas and under the direction of autonomous health professionals, are qualified to do the following:[2]

- Supervise other nursing and health-related personnel
- Coordinate and make assignments of clients to other nursing and health-related personnel
- Serve as team leaders
- Serve as charge nurses

NFLPN recommends that LPN/LVNs meet the following requirements to serve as leaders in specialty areas:

- Have at least 1 year of experience as a staff nurse in the specialty area
- Present personal qualifications that indicate potential abilities for practice in the chosen specialized nursing area

- Demonstrate evidence of completion of a program of in-service education, or a formal course approved by an appropriate agency to provide knowledge and skills necessary for effective nursing services in the specialized field
- Meet all standards of nursing practice as set forth by NFLPN

Clinics. In addition to the many previously listed functions (see Chap. 97), the nurse working in a leadership position in a medical clinic is expected to:

- Follow up on quality assurance
- Train other staff
- Attend team-leader meetings
- Write policies
- Assist in conflict resolution between staff members
- Assist in hiring new staff, ongoing evaluation, and dismissal from positions
- Establish and update nursing procedures
- Establish training protocols and programs

The nurse in the clinic often receives telephone calls and must determine what action to take first. *Telephone triage* involves sorting calls to decide which are life-threatening situations that must be referred to 911 or other emergency services. The nurse refers less-urgent calls to the appropriate physician or other healthcare provider. The nurse doing triage often must differentiate between clients who require immediate care and those who can make future appointments.

Long-Term Care. The U.S. government has established a standard for a charge nurse in the skilled nursing facility (SNF). This standard states that at least one RN or LPN must be on duty and in charge at all times. In some subacute-care facilities, a licensed nurse is not required to be on duty 24 hours a day. These facilities may have a licensed nurse on call at night.

It is desirable that the nurse in charge of each tour of duty be trained or experienced in areas such as nursing administration and supervision, rehabilitation, and psychiatric or geriatric nursing. The charge nurse must be able to recognize significant changes in the condition of clients and take necessary action. The charge nurse is ultimately responsible for the total nursing care of clients during the tour of duty.

Additional duties of the team leader/charge nurse in ECFs include:

- Receiving reports on assigned clients
- Making rounds and assessing clients
- Making client assignments to team members
- Reporting to team members on assigned clients
- Directing administration of medications and treatments
- Supervising nursing care given by UAP
- Conferring with team members regularly throughout the shift
- Communicating with the physician or primary caregiver when necessary

Box 102-1 lists the role and functions of the charge nurse in the long-term care facility. A number of books are avail-

> ➢ BOX 102-1

FUNCTIONS OF THE CHARGE NURSE

Plans Client Care
- Demonstrates awareness of the comprehensive nature of long-term care.
- Exhibits understanding of the condition, needs, and therapeutic goals of each client.
- Receives and interprets verbal and written reports about client care.
- Makes nursing rounds to observe and determine client needs.
- Assists the physician with examinations and treatments.
- Discusses client care goals with physician, nursing supervisor, and staff.
- Develops or assists other nurses to develop nursing care plans for individual clients.
- May triage to determine which unit or which bed a new client will occupy.

Coordinates Staff Activities
- Exhibits an understanding of basic human behavior.
- Demonstrates fundamental leadership techniques.
- Uses management principles and procedures.
- Communicates; listens, speaks, reads, writes, gestures effectively.
- Motivates staff to give skilled nursing care to all clients.

Implements Client Care
- Develops plans to meet needs of all clients.
- Develops plans for common types of emergencies.
- Assigns personnel in terms of client needs and staff proficiencies.
- Helps staff care for the client with special needs, the client with mental illness, the dying person.
- Coordinates work with that of other departments, such as dietary, housekeeping, physical and occupational therapy, social service.
- Seeks guidance and assistance when problems are beyond the scope of practice.
- Prepares and gives verbal and written reports about clients: conferences, nurses' notes, tour of duty and special reports.

Evaluates Client Care
- Applies basic principles of evaluation.
- Makes nursing rounds to observe and assess client care and needs.
- Assesses client care plans and modifies as necessary.
- Assesses client care given by staff and guides appropriate changes.
- Appraises self-performance and plans improvement.
- Follows through on quality assurance plans.

Source: NFLPN. (1996).

able that can be helpful when assuming leadership positions. Many of these functions also have been discussed elsewhere in this book.

☛ KEY CONCEPT

Note that the role of the team leader or charge nurse parallels the steps in the nursing process (see Box 102-1).

Staff Assignments

The charge nurse will probably be expected to assign duties to other members of the nursing team. He or she should know the clients; making rounds is usually the first thing to do, either immediately before or after the change-of-shift report. The charge nurse should also know the staff members; each person has special abilities that can be used to a specific client's greatest advantage.

The team leader/charge nurse is responsible for explaining and demonstrating procedures to staff members and assisting them in planning their workload so that all clients receive optimum care. The charge nurse also checks periodically with the staff to make sure they have no problems with their assignments.

☛ KEY CONCEPT

Not every LPN or RN has the ability to be a charge nurse or team leader. Do not feel inadequate if you are unable or unwilling to assume this role.

Performance Reviews of Staff

The charge nurse is often responsible for writing summary evaluations or **performance reviews** of staff members and for going over this information with them. This is a challenging function for those in leadership. Steps in the evaluation process include:

- Let the staff person know observations will be done.
- Observe the staff person in a number of different situations and delivering care to a variety of clients.
- Each observation should be dated—include the client's initials and a brief description of care.
- Write a few notes immediately after each observation. Describe what was observed. Identify both positive and negative observations and suggestions.
- After each observation, hold a very short, informal "debriefing" session with the staff person. If concerns were noted, let the person know this, so that hopefully they will not be repeated.
- After the interval designated by the facility, write a summary evaluation/performance review of the employee. Many facilities use a specific format for these reviews.
- Schedule a time to meet alone with the staff person and go over the evaluation with him or her, asking for his or her input. The employee may write comments if he or she does not agree with the evaluation. Notes about this meeting, and the evaluation document itself, must be dated and signed by both evaluator and staff person. A

copy is given to the staff person for his or her files. The original must be kept on file by the facility.

If an employee is showing deficiencies, the first step in *due process* is an **oral reprimand.** If the deficiency continues, a **written reprimand** is given to the employee. **Due process** procedures ensure fair labor practices and prevent frivolous or punitive actions against employees by employers.

☛ KEY CONCEPT

The due process procedures described here apply to employees in most facilities. This includes RNs, LPN/LVNs, nursing assistants, and others. After the probationary period, due process must be followed to terminate employment, except in very special circumstances. In general, employees cannot be terminated without just cause.

Plan of Assistance.   If, after an oral and written reprimand, serious deficiencies are still noted, the evaluator/supervisor writes a **plan of assistance** for the employee. The plan of assistance is dated and signed by the evaluator/supervisor.

A plan of assistance includes:

- Statement of deficiency, noting potential consequences to clients
- Employee actions needed to correct the deficiency
- Timeline for improvement to be apparent
- Consequences to employee if plan of assistance is not followed and improvement is not shown

The evaluator presents the plan of assistance to the employee and discusses it with him or her. The employee is given a copy and is asked to sign the original, to signify that he or she has read it and received a copy. The signature does not imply agreement, but simply acknowledges receipt of the information.

✚👁 Nursing Alert

If the charge nurse notes life-threatening or illegal deficiencies on the part of an employee, the Director of Nursing should be notified at once. The employee should be suspended, pending investigation. During suspension, retraining may occur. However, if the employee's act was very serious, termination of employment is often the only legal option open to the facility.

As an evaluator, it is important to continue to observe the employee to determine if the conditions set out were met by the timeline. If so, the plan of assistance is ended. If not, further actions, as set out in the plan, are taken. The nurse evaluating the work of others has an awesome responsibility. The evaluator needs to be mature, observant, fair, and tactful.

Decision-Making

The nurse in a leadership position is required to make many decisions, ranging from assigning staff to manage an assaultive client to calling a code on a lifeless client. Whatever leadership style is being used, be able to make and to communicate competent decisions. In life-and-death situations, decisions must be made quickly. The client and other team members depend on the team leader/charge nurse to determine what to do. In non–life-threatening situations, team members can give input and take part in the decision-making process. However, remember that the leader takes ultimate responsibility for any decision.

Follow basic problem-solving steps to work toward decisions (see Chap. 33). Determine the problem, set goals, gather relevant information, and determine what action to take. In an emergency, act quickly and communicate the situation's urgency. Seek advice or assistance from others when necessary; remember to follow the "chain of command" in the facility. Follow personal intuition; if the situation seems critical, act accordingly. After a decision is made, follow through, and make sure the situation is safely resolved. Evaluate the situation as it evolves, keeping in mind that revisions may need to be made continuously. After a crisis, such as a code, debrief the entire team, to allow venting of feelings and to determine the best action to take in the event of another similar emergency.

Summary

The nurse is a leader, not only in the healthcare facility, but also in the community. Take this responsibility seriously. Other people look up to nurses. The nurse continues to learn throughout the career and throughout life.

Best wishes for a successful nursing career!

➤ STUDENT SYNTHESIS

Key Points

- The role of all nurses, including LPNs, is expanding.
- LPNs can be nationally certified in long-term care.
- Many LPN/LVNs work as charge nurses or team leaders, especially in ECFs.
- As a new graduate of a nursing program, additional education and experience are needed before assuming a leadership role.
- Several different leadership styles exist. There is no right or wrong style; any of them can be effective.

- Specific evaluation procedures must be followed to ensure due process for employees.

Critical Thinking Exercises

1. Do a survey in your local area. What leadership or management opportunities exist for LPN/LVNs in sites other than hospitals and nursing homes? (Examples include home care, third-party payers, various types of clinics, Armed Forces, industry, schools.) Investigate nursing journals and the Internet for courses related to nursing leadership, and develop a list of these opportunities.

NCLEX-Style Review Questions

1. The LPN/LVN can become certified in long-term care by:
   a. Petitioning the State Board of Nursing for certification
   b. Qualifying for and passing an examination
   c. Working in long-term care for 5 years
   d. Working in long-term care for 2,000 hours in the past 3 years
2. A person who uses specific skills, such as role modeling, to influence others to accomplish a task or do the work is a(n):
   a. Autocrat
   b. Democrat
   c. Leader
   d. Manager
3. Which of the following is a quality of an effective leader?
   a. Advocacy
   b. Aggressive
   c. Inconsistent
   d. Unaccountable

References

1. NAPNES. (1996). *LPNs and LVNs—Doesn't your career deserve the same dedication you give your residents?* (Examination for Practical and Vocational Nurses Registration Information and Candidate bulletin). Chicago: Author.
2. NFLPN. (1996). *Nursing practice standards for the licensed practical/vocational nurse.* (Rev). Raleigh, NC: Author.
3. Hunt, B., James, M., & National Federation of LPNs Inc. (1997). Tomorrow's LPN: Understanding the role. *Nursing 97, 97*(3), 52–53.

Bibliography

Unit I The Nature of Nursing

Anderson, M. A. (2001). *Nursing leadership, management, and professional practice for the LPN/LVN* (2nd ed.). Philadelphia: Davis.

Auel, J. (1981). *The clan of the cave bear.* Toronto: Bantam.

Baker, J., & Baker, R. (2000). *Health care finance.* Gaithersburg, MD: Aspen.

Berger, K., & Williams, M. (1998). *Fundamentals of nursing* (2nd ed.). Englewood Cliffs, NJ: Prentice-Hall.

Bullough, V. (1990). *Florence Nightingale and her era: A collection of new scholarship.* New York: Garland Press.

Burkhardt, M. (1998). *Issues, trends and ethics in contemporary nursing.* Albany, NY: Delmar.

Burton, S. (1998). *Community-based nursing.* St. Louis: Mosby–Year Book.

Catalano, J. (1997). *Contemporary professional nursing* (rev. ed.). Philadelphia: Davis.

Colbert, B. J. (1997). *An integrated approach to health sciences.* Albany, NY: Delmar.

Daniel, E. L. (1998). *Taking sides: Clashing views on controversial issues in health and society* (3rd ed.). Guilford, CT: Dushkin/McGraw-Hill.

Delougbery, G. (1998). *Issues and trends in nursing* (3rd ed.). St. Louis: Mosby–Year Book.

Donahue, P. (1995). *Nursing, the fine art: An illustrated history* (2nd ed.). St. Louis: Mosby–Year Book.

Ellis, J. R., & Hartley, C. L. (1997). *Nursing in today's world: Challenges, issues, and trends* (6th ed.). Philadelphia: Lippincott-Raven.

Giuliana, K. (1997). Organ transplants: Tackling the tough ethical questions. *Nursing 97, 27*(5), 34–40.

Hill, S., & Howlett, H. (1997). *Success in practical nursing: Personal and vocational issues* (3rd ed.). Philadelphia: Saunders.

Hosley, J., Jones, S., & Molle-Matthews, E. (1997). *Textbook for medical assistants.* Philadelphia: Lippincott-Raven.

Katz, J. (1997). Back to basics: Providing effective patient teaching. *American Journal of Nursing, 97*(5), 33–36.

Kurzen, C. R. (2000). *Contemporary practical/vocational nursing* (4th ed.). Philadelphia: Lippincott Williams & Wilkins.

Leahy, J. (1998). *Foundations of nursing.* Philadelphia: Saunders.

Lindberg, J. (1998). *Introduction to nursing* (3rd ed.). Philadelphia: Lippincott Williams & Wilkins.

Lindeman, C. A. (1999). *Fundamentals of contemporary nursing practice.* Philadelphia: Saunders.

Mellish, J. (1990). *Basic history of nursing.* Newton, MA: Butterworth-Heinemann.

Morehead, S. (Ed.). (1997). *Nursing roles: Evolving or recycled?* Thousand Oaks, CA: Sage.

National Association for Practical Nurse Education and Service. (1993). *Standards of practice and code of ethics for licensed practical/vocational nurses.* Silver Spring, MD: Author.

Smeltzer, S., & Bare, B. (1999). *Brunner and Suddarth's textbook of medical-surgical nursing* (9th ed.). Philadelphia: Lippincott Williams & Wilkins.

Smith, S. F. (1997). *Content review for the NCLEX-PN, computerized adaptive testing* (6th ed.). Stamford, CT: Appleton & Lange.

Taylor, C., Lillis, C., & LeMone, P. (2001). *Fundamentals of nursing: The art and science of nursing care* (4th ed.). Philadelphia: Lippincott Williams & Wilkins.

Timby, B. K., Scherer, J. C., & Smith, N. E. (1999). *Introductory medical-surgical nursing* (7th ed.). Philadelphia: Lippincott Williams & Wilkins.

Whitelaw, N. (1997). *Clara Barton: Civil War nurse.* Springfield, NJ: Enslow.

Unit II Personal and Environmental Health

American Nurses Association. (1991). *Position statement on cultural diversity in nursing care.* Washington, DC: Author.

American Public Health Association: http://www.apha.org/

American Red Cross: http://www.redcross.org/

Burton, S. (1998). *Community-based nursing.* St. Louis: Mosby–Year Book.

Census 2000. http://www.census.gov/population/www/socdemo/race.html.

Centers for Disease Control and Prevention: http://www.cdc.gov/

Daniel, E. L. (1988). *Taking sides: Clashing views on controversial issues in health and society* (3rd ed.). Guilford, CT: Dushkin/McGraw-Hill.

Delougbery, G. (1998). *Issues and trends in nursing* (3rd ed.). St. Louis: Mosby–Year Book.

Ellis, J., & Hartley, C. (1997). *Nursing in today's world: Challenges, issues, and trends* (6th ed.). Philadelphia: Lippincott-Raven.

FirstGov: http://www.firstgov.gov/

Hill, S., & Howlett, H. (1997). *Success in practical nursing: Personal and vocational issues* (3rd ed.). Philadelphia: Saunders.

Hosley, J. B., Jones, S. A., & Molle-Matthews E. A. (1997). *Lippincott's textbook for medical assistants.* Philadelphia: Lippincott-Raven.

Kurzen, C. R. (2000). *Contemporary practical/vocational nursing* (4th ed.). Philadelphia: Lippincott Williams & Wilkins.

Leahy, J. (1998). *Foundations of nursing.* Philadelphia: Saunders.

Leininger, M. (1995). *Transcultural nursing.* New York: McGraw-Hill.

Lindberg, J. (1998). *Introduction to nursing* (3rd ed.). Philadelphia: Lippincott Williams & Wilkins.

Lindeman, C. A. (1999). *Fundamentals of contemporary nursing practice.* Philadelphia: Saunders.

Maslow, A. (1970). *Motivation and personality* (2nd ed.). New York: Harper.

National Center for Health Statistics. http://www.cdc.gov/nchs/

National Health Information Center: http://www.health.gov/nhic/

National Institutes of Health: http://www.nih.gov/

National Safety Council: http://www.nsc.org/

Occupational Safety and Health Administration: http://www.osha-slc.gov/index.html.

Office of Public Health and Science: http://www.surgeongeneral.gov/ophs/

Sizer, F., & Whitney, E. (1997). *Making life choices: Health skills and concepts* (11th ed.). Cincinnati: Southwest.

Smeltzer, S., & Bare, B. (1999). *Brunner and Suddarth's textbook of medical-surgical Nursing* (9th ed.). Philadelphia: Lippincott Williams & Wilkins.

Spector, R. (1996). *Cultural diversity in health and illness* (4th ed.). East Norwalk, CT: Appleton & Lange.

Taylor, C., Lillis, C., & LeMone, P. (2001). *Fundamentals of nursing: The art and science of nursing care* (4th ed.). Philadelphia: Lippincott Williams & Wilkins

Timby, B., K., Scherer, J., C., & Smith, N., E. (1999). *Introductory medical-surgical nursing* (7th ed.). Philadelphia: Lippincott Williams & Wilkins.

U.S. Public Health Service: http://www.hhs.gov/phs.

U.S. Bureau of the Census. (2000). *Current population reports.* Washington, DC: Author.

U.S. Department of Health and Human Services: http://www.dhhs.gov/ *or* http://www.hhs.gov/

U.S. Department of Labor: http://www.dol.gov/

U.S. Food and Drug Administration: http://www.fda.gov/

Visiting Nurse Association: http://www.vnahc.org/

Women, Infants, and Children: http://www.fns.usda.gov/wic/

World Health Organization: http://www.who.int/

Unit III Development Throughout the Life Cycle

Ashwill, J. W., & Droske, S. C. (1997). *Nursing care of children: Principles and practice.* Philadelphia: Saunders.

Berger, K. S. (1994). *The developing person through the life span* (3rd ed.). New York: Worth.

Craven, R. F., & Hirnle, C. J. (2000). *Fundamentals of nursing: Human health and function* (3rd ed.). Philadelphia: Lippincott Williams & Wilkins.

Eliopoulos, C. (2001). *Gerontological nursing* (5th ed.). Philadelphia: Lippincott Williams & Wilkins.

Erikson, E. (1963). *Childhood and society* (2nd ed.) New York: Norton.

Erikson, E. (1980). *Identity and the life cycle.* New York: Norton.

Goetschius, S. (1997). Families and end-of-life care: How do we meet their needs? *Journal of Gerontological Nursing, 23*(3), 43–49.

Green, K. (1998). *Home care survival guide.* Philadelphia: Lippincott Williams & Wilkins.

Havighurst, R. J. (1972). *Developmental tasks and education* (3rd ed.). New York: David McKay.

Kübler-Ross, E. (1969). *On death and dying.* New York: Macmillan.

Kübler-Ross, E. (1986). *The final stage of growth.* New York: Touchstone.

Levinson, D. J., et al. (1986). *The seasons of a man's life.* New York: Ballantine.

Marks, M. G. (1998). *Broadribb's introductory pediatric nursing* (5th ed.). Philadelphia: Lippincott Williams & Wilkins.

Matteson, M. A., McConnell, E. S., & Linton, A. D. (1997). *Gerontological nursing: Concepts and practice* (2nd ed.). Philadelphia: Saunders.

Perrin, K. (1997). Giving voice to the wishes of elders for end-of-life care. *Journal of Gerontological Nursing, 23*(3), 18–27.

Pillitteri, A. (1998). *Maternal & child health nursing: Care of the childbearing and childrearing family* (3rd ed.). Philadelphia: Lippincott Williams & Wilkins.

Reeder, S. J., Martin, L. L., & Koniak-Griffin, D. (1997). *Maternity nursing: Family, newborn, and women's health care* (18th ed.). Philadelphia: Lippincott-Raven.

Santo-Novak, D. (1997). Older adults' descriptions of their role expectations of nursing. *Journal of Gerontological Nursing, 23*(1), 32–40.

Sheehy, G. (1982). *Pathfinders: Overcoming the crises of adult life and finding your own path to well-being.* New York: Bantam.

Sheehy, G. (1984). *Passages: Predictable crises of adult life.* New York: Bantam.

Sheehy, G. (1992). *The silent passage: Menopause.* New York: Random House.

Spector, R. E. (1996). *Cultural diversity in health and illness* (4th ed.). New York: Appleton & Lange.

Spradley, B. W., & Allender, J. A. (1996). *Community health nursing: Concepts and practice* (4th ed.). Philadelphia: Lippincott-Raven.

Stanley, M., & Beare, P. G. (1999). *Gerontological nursing* (2nd ed.). Philadelphia: Davis.

Taylor, C., Lillis, C., & LeMone, P. (2001). *Fundamentals of nursing: The art and science of nursing care* (4th ed.). Philadelphia: Lippincott Williams & Wilkins.

Troiano, R., et al. (1995). Overweight prevalence and trends for children and adolescents. *Archives of Pediatric and Adolescent Medicine, 149*(10), 1085–1091.

Wadsworth, B. (1989). *Piaget's theory of cognitive and affective development* (4th ed.). New York: Longman.

Wong, D. (1995). *Whalley and Wong's nursing care of infants and children* (5th ed.). St. Louis: Mosby.

Wong, D. L., & Perry, S. E. (1998). *Maternal child nursing care.* St. Louis: Mosby.

Unit IV Structure and Function

Abrams, A. (2001). *Clinical drug therapy: Rationales for nursing practice* (6th ed.). Philadelphia: Lippincott Williams & Wilkins.

Berkow R., Beers, M., & Fletcher, A. (Eds.) (1997). *Merck manual of medical information: Home edition.* New York: Pocket Books.

Burrell, L. O., & Gerlach, M. I. (1997). *Adult nursing: Acute and community care* (2nd ed.). Stamford, CT: Appleton & Lange.

Cohen, B. J., & Wood, D. L. (2000). *Memmler's structure & function of the human body* (7th ed.). Philadelphia: Lippincott Williams & Wilkins.

Cohen, B., & Wood, D. (1996). *The human body in health and disease* (8th ed.). Philadelphia: Lippincott-Raven.

Eliopoulos, C. (1997). *Gerontological nursing* (4th ed.). Philadelphia: Lippincott-Raven.

Hays, W. H., Groothuis, J. R., Hayward, A. R., et. al. (1997). *Current pediatric diagnosis and treatment* (13th ed.). Stamford: Appleton & Lange.

Jarvis, C. (1996). *Physical examination and health assessment* (2nd ed.). Philadelphia: Saunders.

Kee, J., & Paulanka, B. (2000). *Handbook of fluid and electrolyte and acid base imbalances.* Albany: Delmar.

Lewis, S. M., Collier, I. C., & Heitkemper, M. M. (1996). *Medical-surgical nursing: Assessment and management of clinical problems* (4th ed.). St. Louis: Mosby–Year Book.

McKinney, E. S., Ashwill, J. W., Murray, S. S., et. al. (2000). *Maternal-child nursing.* Philadelphia: Saunders.

Pillitteri, A. (1998). *Maternal and newborn nursing: Care of the childbearing and childrearing family* (3rd ed.). Philadelphia: Lippincott Williams & Wilkins.

Porth, C. (2002). *Pathophysiology: Concepts of altered health states* (6th ed.). Philadelphia: Lippincott Williams & Wilkins.

Smeltzer, S. C., & Bare, B. G. (2000). *Brunner and Suddarth's textbook of medical-surgical Nursing* (9th ed.). Philadelphia: Lippincott Williams & Wilkins.

Staab, A. S., & Hodges, L. C. (1996). *Essentials of gerontological nursing: Adaptation to the aging process.* Philadelphia: Lippincott-Raven.

Swartz, M. (1998). *Textbook of physical diagnosis, history and examination* (3rd ed.). Philadelphia: Saunders.

Taylor, C, Lillis, C, & LeMone, P. (2001). *Fundamentals of nursing: The art and science of nursing care* (4th ed.). Philadelphia: Lippincott Williams & Wilkins.

Tortora, G. J., & Grabowski, S. R. (1996). *Principles of anatomy and physiology* (8th ed.). New York: HarperCollins.

Unit V Nutrition and Diet Therapy

Dudek, S. (2001). *Nutrition essentials for nursing practice* (4th ed.). Philadelphia: Lippincott Williams & Wilkins.

Lutz, C., & Przytulski, K. (1997). *Nutrition & diet therapy* (2nd ed.). Philadelphia: Davis.

Russell, R. (1997). New views on the RDAs for older adults. *Journal of the American Dietetic Association, 97*(5), 515–518.

Smeltzer, S. C., & Bare, B. G. (2000). *Brunner and Suddarth's textbook of medical-surgical nursing* (9th ed.). Philadelphia: Lippincott Williams & Wilkins.

U.S. Department of Agriculture and U.S. Department of Health and Human Services. (2000). *Nutrition and your health: Dietary guidelines for Americans* (5th ed.). http://www.health.gov/dietaryguidelines/dga2000.

U.S. Department of Agriculture, Center for Nutrition Policy and Promotion. (1996). *The Food Guide Pyramid.* Home and Garden Bulletin No. 252. Author.

Williams, S. R. (2001). *Basic nutrition and diet therapy* (11th ed.). St. Louis: Mosby.

Unit VI The Nursing Process

Ackley, B. J., & Ladwig, G. B. (1999). *Nursing diagnosis handbook: A guide to planning care* (4th ed.). St. Louis: Mosby.

Alfaro-LeFevre, R. (1998). *Applying nursing process: A step-by-step guide* (4th ed.). Philadelphia: Lippincott Williams & Wilkins.

Carpenito, L. J. (1999). *Nursing diagnosis: Application to clinical practice* (8th ed.). Philadelphia: Lippincott Williams & Wilkins.

Christensen, B. L., & Kockrow, E. O. (1999). *Foundations of nursing* (3rd ed.). St. Louis: Mosby.

Craven, R. F., & Hirnle, C. J. (2000). *Fundamentals of nursing: Human health and function* (3rd ed.). Philadelphia: Lippincott Williams & Wilkins.

deWit, S. C. (2001). *Fundamental concepts and skills for nursing.* Philadelphia: Saunders.

Doenges, M., Moorhouse, M., & Burley, J. (2000). *Application of nursing process and nursing diagnosis: An interactive text for diagnostic reasoning* (3rd ed.). Philadelphia: Davis.

Eggland, E. T. (1998). Charting tips: Avoiding generalizations. *Nursing 98, 28*(3), 18.

Eggland, E. T. (1998). Charting tips: Correcting charting errors. *Nursing 98, 28*(4), 65.

Gordon, M. (1976). Nursing diagnosis and the diagnostic process. *American Journal of Nursing, 76,* 1298–1300.

Iyer, P. W., & Camp, N. H. (1999). *Nursing documentation: A nursing process approach* (3rd ed.). St. Louis: Mosby.

Jenkins, J. E. (1997). The health care delivery system. In K. K. Chitty (Ed.), *Professional nursing: Concept and challenges* (2nd ed.). Philadelphia: Saunders.

Johnson, M., Maas, M., & Moorhead, S. (2000). *Nursing outcomes classifications* (2nd ed.). St. Louis: Mosby.

Joint Commission on Accreditation of Healthcare Organizations. (1997). *Comprehensive accreditation manual for hospitals: The official handbook.* Oakbrook, IL: Author.

Marelli, T. M., & Harper, D. S. (2000). *Nursing documentation handbook* (3rd ed.). St. Louis: Mosby.

McCloskey, J., & Bulechek, G. (2000). *Nursing interventions classifications* (3rd ed.). St. Louis: Mosby.

North American Nursing Diagnosis Association. (2001). *NANDA nursing diagnoses: Definitions and classifications 2001–2002.* Philadelphia: Author.

Potter, P., & Perry, A. (1997). *Fundamentals of nursing: Concepts, process & practice* (4th ed., pp. 136–153, 154–164). St. Louis: Mosby.

Rubenfeld, M. G., & Scheffer, B. K. (1999). *Critical thinking in nursing: An interactive approach* (2nd ed.). Philadelphia: Lippincott Williams & Wilkins.

Shuel, P. (1997). *Assessment made incredibly easy.* Springhouse, PA: Springhouse.

Springhouse Corporation (1999). Charting tips: Using SOAP, SOAPIE, and SOAPIER formats. *Nursing 99, 29*(9), 75.

Surefire documentation: How, what and when nurses need to document. (1998). St. Louis: Mosby.

Taylor, C. (1997). Problem solving in nursing practice. *Journal of Advanced Nursing, 26*(2), 329–336.

Taylor, C., Lillis, C., & LeMone, P. (2001). *Fundamentals of nursing: The art and science of nursing care* (4th ed.). Philadelphia: Lippincott Williams & Wilkins.

Wilkinson, J. M. (1997). *Nursing process: A critical thinking approach.* Menlo Park, CA: Addison-Wesley Nursing.

Unit VII Safety in the Healthcare Facility

Albrecht, H., et al. (1999). Team approach to infection prevention and control in the nursing home setting. *American Journal of Infection Control, 27*(1), 64–70.

American Heart Association. (1999). *Basic life support for healthcare providers.* Dallas: Author.

American Red Cross. (1999). *Standard first aid.* New York: Author.

Bartley, J. M. (2000). APIC State-of-the-art report: The role of infection control during construction in health care facilities. *American Journal of Infection Control, 28*(2), 159–169.

Benson, R. (2000). *The survival nurse: Turning an emergency nursing station under adverse conditions.* New York: Paladin.

Bickley, L. S., & Hoekelman, R. A. (1999). *Bates' guide to physical examination and history taking* (7th ed.). Philadelphia: Lippincott Williams & Wilkins.

Bower, F. (2000). Restraint use in acute care settings: Can it be reduced? *Journal of Nursing Administration, 30*(12), 592–598.

Briggs, J. (2001). *Telephone triage protocols for nurses* (2nd ed.). Philadelphia: Lippincott Williams & Wilkins.

Brown, S. M. (1999). Good Samaritan laws: Protection and limits. *RN, 62*(11), 65–66, 68.

Burr, J. M. (2000). Sailing through a managed care review. *RN, 63*(10), 50N–70N.

Burton, G. R. W., & Engelkirk, P. G. (1999). *Microbiology for the health sciences* (6th ed.). Philadelphia: Lippincott Williams & Wilkins.

Christensen, B. L., & Kockrow, E. O. (1999). *Foundations of nursing* (3rd ed). St. Louis: Mosby.

Cohen, S. (2000). Patient confidentiality. *American Journal of Nursing, 100*(9), 24HH–24JJ.

Collins, T. (2000). Understanding shock. *Nursing Standard, 14*(49), 35–41.

Craven, R. F., & Hirnle, C. J. (2000). *Fundamentals of nursing: Human health and function* (3rd ed.). Philadelphia: Lippincott Williams & Wilkins.

deWit, S. C. (2001). *Fundamental concepts and skills for nursing.* Philadelphia: Saunders.

Dorland's Illustrated Medical Dictionary (29th ed.) (2001). Philadelphia: Saunders.

Editors of American Health Consultants. (1997). *Disaster planning source book.* Atlanta: American Health Consultants.

Emergency Nurses Association. (1999). *Emergency nursing core curriculum* (5th ed.). Philadelphia: Saunders.

Ernst, D. (2001). The right way to do blood cultures. *RN, 64*(3), 28–32.

Flurer, N. (2000). Providing mandatory safety information to hospital employees: Finding a way that is fast, fun, and effective. *Journal for Nurses in Staff Development, 16*(1), 17–22.

Fottler, M. (2000). Creating a healing environment: The importance of the service setting in the new consumer-oriented healthcare system. *Journal of Healthcare Management, 45*(2), 91–106.

Gladwin, M., & Tratler, B. (1999). *Clinical microbiology made ridiculously simple* (2nd ed.). London: OSL.

Good role model for handwashing needed. (2000). *Nursing Standard, 14*(23), 4.

Green, K. (1998). *Home care survival guide.* Philadelphia: Lippincott Williams & Wilkins.

Gustafson, D., et al. (2000). Effects on 4 hand-drying methods for removing bacteria from washed hands: A randomized trial. *Mayo Clinic Proceedings, 75*(7), 705–708.

Hennepin County Medical Center (1999). *Frostbite: The big chill.* Minneapolis: Hennepin County Medical Center Burn Center.

Higginbotham, E. (2000). The liability risks when students practice nursing. *RN, 63*(9), 90.

Hospital Focus. (2000). Survey: Healthcare workers fear infection with super bugs. *RN, 63*(10), 24hf2–28hf8.

Jackson, M., et al. (2000). Emerging infectious diseases. *American Journal of Nursing, 100*(10), 66–71.

Landesman, L. Y. (Ed.). *Emergency preparedness in health care organizations.* Oakbrook Terrace, IL: Joint Commission on Accreditation of Healthcare Organizations.

Letizia, B. (1999). Kill germs and protect skin with these hand wipes. *RN, 62*(4), 24BB.

Letizia, B. (1999). Sterilize equipment in a flash. *RN, 62*(4), 24BB.

Letizia, B. (1999). This hand cleaner kills germs, but is gentle on skin. *RN, 62*(3), 30N.

McGwin, G., et al. (1999). Fire fatalities in older people. *Journal of the American Geriatrics Society, 47*(11), 1307–1311.

Miller-Keane (1997). *Encyclopedia and dictionary of medicine, nursing and allied health* (6th ed.). Philadelphia: Saunders.

Murphy, R., et al. (2000). Achieving department safety: A team approach to development of a department safety plan template. *Journal for Nurses in Staff Development, 16*(5), 209–215.

Musso, S. (2000). Should hospitals worry about visitors or not? *RN, 63*(9), 9.

Nicol, M., et al. (2001). Prevention of cross infection: Handwashing and use of aprons. *Nursing Standard, 15*(21), 56–57.

Pope, A., et al. (1999). Handwashing: Back to basics. *American Journal of Infection Control, 27*(2), 210–211.

Pritchard, V. (1999). Joint Commission standards for long-term care infection control: Putting together the process elements. *American Journal of Infection Control, 27*(1), 27–34.

Professional Safeguard Resources. (2001). *Workplace safety training: Special emphasis programs: Ergonomics–body mechanics.* http://www.psrcorp.com/

Richter, P. (1997). *Hospital disaster preparedness: Meeting a requirement or preparing for the worst? Healthcare Facilities Management Series.* Chicago: American Society for Healthcare Engineering of the American Hospital Association.

Scott, D. (2000). Preventing medical mistakes. *RN, 63*(8), 60–64.

Selfridge-Thomas, J., et al. (1999). *Challenges in emergency nursing: A self-study certification review with diskette for Windows.* Philadelphia: Saunders.

Shellenbarger, T. (2000). Nosebleeds: Not just kids' stuff. *RN, 63*(2), 50–54.

Smeltzer, S. C., & Bare, B. G. (2000). *Brunner and Suddarth's textbook of medical-surgical nursing* (9th ed.). Philadelphia: Lippincott Williams & Wilkins.

Taber's cyclopedic medical dictionary (19th ed.). (2001). Philadelphia: Davis.

Taylor, C., Lillis, C., & LeMone, P. (2001). *Fundamentals of nursing: The art and science of nursing care* (4th ed.). Philadelphia: Lippincott Williams & Wilkins.

Timby, B. K. (2001). *Fundamental skills and concepts in patient care* (7th ed.). Philadelphia: Lippincott Williams & Wilkins.

Travers, D. (1999). Triage: How long does it take? How long should it take? *Journal of Emergency Nursing, 25*(3), 238–240.

U.S. Occupational Safety and Health Administration. (2000). *Guidelines for workplace violence prevention programs for health care workers in institutional and community settings.* Washington, DC: Author.

Wade, C. F. (2000). Keeping Lyme disease at bay: An integrated approach to prevention. *American Journal of Nursing, 100*(7), 26–31; quiz 2.

Winslow, E., & Jacobson, A. (2000). Can a fashion statement harm the patient? *American Journal of Nursing, 100*(9), 63–65.

World Health Organization. (1999). *Containing antimicrobial resistance: Review of the literature and report of a WHO workshop on the development of a global strategy for the containment of antimicrobial resistance.* Geneva: Author. http://www.who.int/emc-documents.antimicrobial_resistance/whocdscsrdrs992c.html

Unit VIII Client Care

Acello, B. (2000). Meeting JCAHO standards for pain control. *Nursing Library,* March 2000. http://findarticles.com/m3231/3_30/60130346/pl/article.jhtml.

Agency for Health Care Policy and Research. http://www.ahcpr.gov/clinic.

Ball, E. (2000). A teaching guide for continent ileostomy. *RN, 63*(12), 35–36, 38, 40, 42.

Baranoski, S. (2000). Skin tears: Staying on guard against the enemy of frail skin. *Nursing 2000,* September 2000. http://www.springnet.com.ce/p009b.htm

Bower, F. L., & McCullough, C. S. (2000). Restraint use in acute care settings: Can it be reduced? *Journal of Nursing Administration, 30*(12), 592–598.

Briggs, J. K. (2001). *Telephone triage* (2nd ed.). Philadelphia: Lippincott Williams & Wilkins.

Brownson, D. (2001). Brownson's Nursing Notes. http://members.tripod.com/~DianneBrownson/wound-skin.html.

Bryant, G. (2000). When spinal cord injury affects the bowel. *RN, 63*(2), 26–30.

Bush, K. (2001). Do you really listen to patients? *RN, 64*(30), 35–37.

CE Connection. (1999). Table 2: Accurate blood pressure measurement for evaluating mild to moderate hypertension. *The Nurse Practitioner,* May.

Calloway, S. D. (2001). Preventing communication breakdowns. *RN, 64*(1), 71–72, 74.

Carroll, P. (1999). Monitoring the gut to prevent MODS. *RN, 62*(10), 34–38.

Centers for Disease Control and Prevention. http://www.cdc.gov/

Christensen, B., & Kockrow, E. (1999). *Foundations of nursing* (3rd ed.). St. Louis: Mosby.

Craven, R. F., & Hirnle, C. J. (2003). *Fundamentals of nursing: Human health and function* (4th ed.). Philadelphia: Lippincott Williams & Wilkins.

D'Arcy, Y. (1999). Managing postoperative CABG pain. *Nursing Library,* September 1999. http://www.findarticles.com/m32319_29/55806888/pl/article.jhtml.

deWit, S. C. (1999). *Fundamental concepts and skills for nursing.* Philadelphia: Saunders.

Educational Resource Page for Nursing Students, Nurses and Residents. http://www.mrgizmo.tripod.com/EDUCATION.html.

Effective Communication Skills. http://www.nurs.utexas.edu/n310/unit4.html.

Electronic Doctor. (2000). *Guidelines for personal hygiene.* March 2000. http://www.edoc.co.za/homehygiene/personal.html.

Elkin, M. K., Potter, P. A., & Perry, A. G. (2000). *Nursing interventions and clinical skills* (2nd ed.). St. Louis: Mosby.

Ernst, D. J. (1999). Collecting blood culture specimens. *Nursing Library,* July 1999. http://www.findarticles.com/m3231/7_29/55175734/p1/article.jhtml.

Erwin, J. (1999, June 28). A simple plan: Discharge planning improves the odds. *Nurseweek.* http://www.nurseweek.com/features/99-6/discharg.html.

Gale Group. (1999). Writing a narrative discharge summary. *Nursing Library,* January 1999.

Grandinetti, D. (2000). Patients are putting their records on line. *RN, 63*(11), 20N, 40N–50N.

Gray, M. (2000). Urinary retention: Management in the acute care setting. *American Journal of Nursing, 7*(100), 40.

Gunningberg, L., et al. (1999). Implementation of risk assessment and classification of pressure ulcers as quality indicators for patients with hip fractures. *Journal of Clinical Nursing, 8*(4), 396–406.

Gunningberg, L., et al. (1999). Implementation of risk assessment and classification of pressure ulcers as quality indicators for patients with hip fractures. *Journal of Clinical Nursing, 8*(4), 396–406.

Haddad, A. (2000). Ethics in action. *RN, 63*(9), 25–26, 28.

Hellwig, K. (2000). A family lesson in dying. *RN, 63*(12), 32–33.

Hess, C. (1999). Preventing skin breakdown. (wound care). *Nursing Library,* July 1999. http://www.findarticles.com/cf_0/m3231/n7_v28/20938130/pl/article.jhtml.

Hodge, P., & Ullrich, S. (1999). Does your assessment include alternative therapies? *RN, 62*(6), 47–49.

Hospice sites. (2002). http://www.cp-tel.net/pamnorth/hospice1.htm.

Kettelman, K. (2000). Taking the sting out of painful procedures. *Nursing Library,* June 2000. http://www.findarticles.com/m3231/6_30/62799635/pl/article.jhtml.

Kübler-Ross, E. (1997). On death and dying (reprint ed.). New York: Scribner. http://growthhouse.org.books.kubler1.htm.

Lippincott Williams & Wilkins. (2000). Mild handwashing regimen improves skin health. *American Journal of Nursing, 100*(8), 17.

McCaffery, M. (1968). *Cognition, bodily pain and man–environment interactions.* Los Angeles: University of California.

McCaffery, M. (1999). Opioids and pain management. *Nursing Library,* March 1999. http://www.findarticles.com/m3231/3_29/54153646/pl/article.jhtml.

Nguyen, B-Q. (2000). When care is needed at home. *American Journal of Nursing, 100*(10), 107.

North American Nursing Diagnosis Association. (2001–2002). *Nursing diagnoses: Definitions and classifications 2001–2002.* Philadelphia: Author.

Pasero, C., & McCaffery, M. (2000). When patients can't report pain. *American Journal of Nursing, 100*(9), 22–23.

Rice, K. L. (1999). Measuring thigh BP. *Nursing Library,* August 1999. http://www.findarticles.com/m3231/8_29/55450461/pl/article.jhtml.

Rose, B. (2000). End-of-life choices can be confusing when wording is vague. *RN, 63*(11), 10.

Ross, E. (2000). What is it like to be dying? *American Journal of Nursing, 100*(10), 96AA, 96CC, 96EE, 96GG–96II.

Sachs, P. R. (1999). Deflecting harsh words when tempers flare. *Nursing Library,* March 1999. http://www.findarticles.com.

Scott, E., et al. (1999). Understanding perioperative nursing. *Nursing Standard, 13*(49), 49–54.

Severine, J. E., & McKenzie, N. E. (1999). Advances in temperature monitoring: A far cry from shake and take. *Nursing 99,* May 1999. http://www.springnet.com/ce/temp.htm.

Smeltzer, S. C., & Bare, B. G. (1999). *Brunner and Suddarth's textbook of medical-surgical nursing* (9th ed.) Philadelphia: Lippincott Williams & Wilkins.

Talmasca. The dying person's bill of rights. (2002). http://talmasca.org/avatar/death-rights.html.

Tate, J. (2000). Using pulse oximetry. *Nursing Library,* September 2000. http://www.findarticles.com/m3231/9_30/65801763/pl/article.jhtml.

Taylor, C., Lillis, C., & LeMone, P. (2001). *Fundamentals of nursing: The art and science of nursing care* (4th ed.). Philadelphia: Lippincott Williams & Wilkins.

Timby, B. K. (2001). *Fundamental skills and concepts in patient care* (7th ed.). Philadelphia: Lippincott Williams & Wilkins.

Tupper, S. Z. (1999). When the inner ear is out of balance. *RN, 62*(11), 36–40.

Ufema, J. (2000). Death & dying: Pain control [Letter to the editor]. http://www.findarticles.com/m3231/1_30/58916389/pl/article.jhtm.

Ufema, J. (2000). Pain control. *Nursing Library,* January 2000. http://www.findarticles.com/m3231/1_30/58916389/pl/article.jhtml.

Unkle, D. (2000). Why monitor intra-abdominal pressure? *RN, 63*(6), 85–86.

Weber, J., & Kelley, J. (2003). *Health assessment in nursing* (2nd ed.). Philadelphia: Lippincott Williams & Wilkins.

Woodrow, P. (1999). Pulse oximetry. *Nursing Standard, 13*(42), 42–46.

Unit IX Pharmacology and Administration of Medications

Abrams, A. (2001). *Clinical drug therapy: Rationales for nursing practice* (6th ed.). Philadelphia: Lippincott Williams & Wilkins.

Anonymous. (2000). Drug watch. *American Journal of Nursing, 100*(12), 79.

Billups, N. (Ed.). (1999). *American drug index* (43rd ed.). St. Louis: Wolters Kluwer.

Boyer, M. (2001). *Math for nurses: A pocket guide to dosage calculation and drug preparation* (5th ed.). Philadelphia: Lippincott Williams & Wilkins.

Cohen, M. (2001). Medication errors. *Nursing, 31*(1), 14.

Compton, P., & McCaffery, M. (2001). Controlling pain: Treating acute pain in addicted patient. *Nursing, 31*(1), 17.

Craven, R., & Hirnle, C. (2000). *Fundamentals of nursing: Human health and function* (3rd ed.). Philadelphia: Lippincott Williams & Wilkins.

Eisenhauer, L., Nichols, L., Spencer, R., & Bergan, F. (1998). *Clinical pharmacology and nursing management* (5th ed.). Philadelphia: Lippincott Williams & Wilkins.

Guttadore, D. (1999). A quick way to identify compatible drugs. *RN, 62*(9), 53–55.

Henke, G. (1998). *Med-math: Dosage calculation, preparation, and administration* (3rd ed). Philadelphia: Lippincott Williams & Wilkins.

Kany, K. (2000). The rising tide of health care errors. *American Journal of Nursing, 100*(2), 86.

Karch, A. (2003). *2003 Lippincott's nursing drug guide.* Philadelphia: Lippincott Williams & Wilkins.

Karch, A. M., & Karch, F. E. (2000). Practice errors: A spoonful of medicine. *American Journal of Nursing, 100*(11), 24.

King, B. (2000). Meds and the dialysis patient. *RN, 63*(7), 55–60.

Koschel, M. (2001). Question of practice: Filter needles. *American Journal of Nursing, 101*(1; part 1), 75.

Kudzma, E. (1999). Culturally competent drug administration. *American Journal of Nursing, 99*(8), 46–52.

Lehne, R. (2000). *Pharmacology for nursing care* (4th ed.). Philadelphia: Saunders.

O'Shea, E. (1999). Factors contributing to medication errors: A literature review. *Journal of Clinical Nursing, 8*(5), 496–504.

Pisano, R. (2000). "Five rights" prevents multiple wrongs: Asking the right questions about medication safety. *Nursing, 31*(1), 10.

Sears, J., & Granger, P. (1999). Antibiotics to treat RA. *RN, 63*(1), 41–42.

Shirrell, D., et al. (1999). Therapeutic drug monitoring. *American Journal of Nursing, 99*(1), 42.

Skokal, W. (2000). IV push at home? *RN, 63*(10), 26–30.

Slugg Moore, A. (1999). High blood levels of this antibiotic can damage hearing. *RN, 62*(6), 68.

Sullivan, G. (2000). Reporting another nurse's medication error. *RN, 63*(10), 66.

Taylor, C., Lillis, C., & LeMone, P. (2001). *Fundamentals of nursing: The art and science of nursing care* (4th ed.). Philadelphia: Lippincott Williams & Wilkins

Walker, M. K., & Foreman, M. D. (1999). Medication safety: A protocol for nursing action. *Geriatric Nursing, 20*(1), 34–39.

Unit X Maternal and Newborn Nursing

AWHONN. (2000). *Every woman: The essential guide for healthy living.* New York: Profile Pursuit.

Burroughs, A. (1997). *Maternity nursing* (7th ed.). Philadelphia: Saunders.

Buschbach, D., & Bordeaux, M. S. (2001, June). Shake, rattle, and roll. Pre-conference workshop conducted at the 2001 AWHONN Convention, Charlotte, NC.

California Department of Health Services, Office of AIDS. (2002). www.dhs.ca.gov/AIDS/Statistics/

Centers for Disease Control and Prevention www.cdc.gov/hiv/stats/ *or* www.cdc.gov/nchstp/dstd/dstdp.html *or* www.cdc.gov/nchs/products/pubs/pubd/hus/adheal.htm *or* www.cdc.gov/nchs/releases/97facts/95natrel.htm.

Cunningham, F. G., et al. (1997). *Williams obstetrics* (20th ed.). Stamford, CT: Appleton & Lange.

Karch, A. M. (2003). *2003 Lippincott's nursing drug guide.* Philadelphia: Lippincott Williams & Wilkins.

Lipson, J. G., Dibble, S. L., & Minarik, P. A. (1996). *Culture & nursing care.* San Francisco: University of San Francisco Nursing Press.

Marks, M. G. (1998). *Broadribb's introductory pediatric nursing* (5th ed.). Philadelphia: Lippincott Williams & Wilkins.

Masters, V. H., & Johnson, V. E. (1966). *Human sexual response.* Boston: Little, Brown.

McFarlan, J., Parker, B., & Soekin, K. (1996). Physical abuse, smoking, and substance abuse during pregnancy: Prevalence, relationships, and effects on birth weight. *Journal of Obstetric, Gynecologic, and Neonatal Nursing, 25*(4), 313.

McHugh, M. K. (1997). Newborn care. In H. Varney (Ed.), *Varney's midwifery* (3rd ed., pp. 551–608). Sudbury, MA: Jones & Bartlett.

Miller, D., Rabello, Y., & Paul, R. (1996). The modified biophysical profile: Antepartum testing in the 1990's. *American Journal of Obstetrics and Gynecology, 174*(3), 812.

Mosby's medical nursing, allied health dictionary (6th ed.) (2002). St. Louis: Mosby.

Oehler, J., et al. (1996). Behavioral characteristics of very low birth weight infants of varying biologic risk at 6, 15, and 24 months of age. *Journal of Obstetric, Gynecologic and Neonatal Nursing, 25*(3), 233.

Pillitteri, A. (1998). *Maternal and child health nursing: Care of the childbearing and childrearing family* (3rd ed.). Philadelphia: Lippincott Williams & Wilkins.

Pillitteri, A. (1999). *Maternal and child health nursing: Care of the childbearing and childraising family* (3rd ed.). Philadelphia: Lippincott Williams & Wilkins.

Planned Parenthood. www.plannedparenthood.org/articles/bcfuture_w.html *or* http://www.ippf.org

Porth, C. (2002). *Pathophysiology: Concepts of altered health states* (6th ed.). Philadelphia: Lippincott Williams & Wilkins.

Ratcliffe, S., Baxley, E. G., Byrd, J. E., & Sakornbut, E. L. (2001). Family practice obstetrics (2nd ed.). Philadelphia: Hanley & Belfus.

Reeder, S. J., Martin, L. L., & Koniak-Griffin, D. (1997). *Maternity nursing: Family, newborn, and women's health care* (18th ed.). Philadelphia: Lippincott-Raven.

Reifsnider, E. (2000). Nutrition for the childbearing years. *Journal of Obstetric, Gynecologic, and Neonatal Nursing, 29,* 43–53.

Simpson, K. R., & Creehan, P. A. (2001). *Perinatal nursing* (2nd ed.). Philadelphia: Lippincott Williams & Wilkins.

Simpson, K. R., & Creehan, P. A. (2001). *AWHONN perinatal nursing* (2nd ed.). Philadelphia: Lippincott Williams & Wilkins.

Sloane, E. (2002). *Biology of women* (4th ed.). Albany, NY: Delmar/Thomson.

Smeltzer, S. G., & Bare, B. G. (2000). *Brunner and Suddarth's medical-surgical nursing* (9th ed.). Philadelphia: Lippincott Williams & Wilkins.

Star, W. L., Shannon, M. T., Lommel, L. L., & Gutierrez, Y. M. (1999). *Ambulatory obstetrics* (3rd ed.). San Francisco: University of San Francisco Nursing Press.

Varney, H. (1997). *Varney's midwifery* (3rd ed.). Sudbury, MA: Jones & Bartlett.

Wheeler, L. (1997). *Nurse-midwifery handbook: A practical guide to prenatal and postpartum care.* Philadelphia: Lippincott-Raven.

Wong, D. L., & Perry, S. E. (1998). *Maternal child nursing care.* St. Louis: Mosby.

Unit XI Pediatric Nursing

Aldous, M. B. (1999). Nutritional issues for infants and children. *Pediatric Annals, 28*(2), 129–135.

Behrman, R. E., & Kliegman, R. M. (1998). *Nelson essentials of pediatrics* (3rd ed.). Philadelphia: Saunders.

Bolyard, D. R. (2001). Sexuality and cystic fibrosis. *American Journal of Maternal Child Nursing, 26*(1), 39–41.

Centers for Disease Control and Prevention. (2002). Epstein-Barr virus, infections, mononucleosis. http://www.cdc.gov/ncidod/diseases/ebv.htm.

Cohen, S. M. (2001). Lead poisoning: A summary of treatment and prevention. *Pediatric Nursing, 27*(2), 32–36.

Demi, A. S., Brown, J. V. & Jones, K. D. (1998). Promoting asthma self-management skills in young children through a home-based nursing intervention: A pilot study. *American Journal for Nurse Practitioners, 2*(10), 15–30.

Droogan, J. (1999). Treatment and prevention of head lice and scabies. *Nursing Times, 95*(29), 44–45.

Enns, S. M. (1999, October). Outpatient pediatric asthma therapy. *Clinical Advisor,* 30–37.

Erdman, S. H. (1999). Nutritional imperatives in cystic fibrosis therapy. *Pediatric Annals, 28*(2), 129–135.

Fox, J. (1997). *Primary health care of children.* St. Louis: Mosby.

Gardner, J. (2000). Living with a child with fetal alcohol syndrome. *American Journal of Maternal Child Nursing, 25*(5), 252–257.

Green-Herandez, C., Singleton, J. K., & Avonzon, D. Z. (2001). *Primary care pediatrics.* Philadelphia: Lippincott Williams & Wilkins.

Hellerstein, S. (1998). Urinary tract infections in children: Why they occur and how to prevent them. *American Family Physician, 57*(10), 2440.

Hosley, J., Jones, S., & Molle-Matthews, E. (1997). *Textbook for medical assistants.* Philadelphia: Lippincott-Raven.

Huther, S. E., & McCance, K. L. (2000). *Understanding pathophysiology* (2nd ed.). St. Louis: Mosby.

Johnson, B. S. (2000). Mother's perceptions of parenting children with disabilities. *American Journal of Maternal Child Nursing, 25*(3), 127–132.

Kerney, K. (2001). Emergency: Epiglottitis. *American Journal of Nursing, 101*(8), 37–38.

Karch, A. M. (2003). *2003 Lippincott's nursing drug guide.* Philadelphia: Lippincott Williams & Wilkins.

Marks, M. G. (1998). *Introductory pediatric nursing* (5th ed.). Philadelphia: Lippincott Williams & Wilkins.

Moran, R. (1999). Evaluation and treatment of childhood obesity. *American Family Physician, 59*(4), 861—868.

Mosier, W. A. (1998, April). Update on childhood enuresis. *Clinical Advisor,* 32–34.

Muscari, M. E. (1998). Adolescent health: Screening for anorexia and bulimia. *American Journal of Nursing, 98*(11), 22, 24.

National Association of Rare Diseases. http://www.raredisease.org.

Nettina, S. M. (2001). *The Lippincott manual of nursing practice* (7th ed.). Philadelphia: Lippincott Williams & Wilkins.

Newcheck, P. W., & Hafton, N. (1998). Prevalence and impact of disabling conditions in childhood. *American Journal of Public Health, 145*(12), 1367–1373.

Newcom, K. D. (2001). Infectious mononucleosis: A clinical review. *Advances for Nurse Practitioners, 9*(9), 37–41.

Nicholson, H., & Preston, D. (1999). More than just skin deep. *Nursing Times,* 10–12.

North American Nursing Diagnosis Association. (2001). *NANDA nursing diagnoses: Definitions and classifications 2000–2001.* Philadelphia: Author.

Orbanic, S. (2001). Understanding bulimia: Signs, symptoms, and human experience. *American Journal of Nursing, 101*(3), 35–41.

Owen, C. (1999). New directions in asthma management. *American Journal of Nursing, 99*(3), 26–33.

Pillitteri, A. (1998). *Maternal & child health nursing* (3rd ed.). Philadelphia: Lippincott Williams & Wilkins.

Rennert, O. M., & Francis, G. L. (1999). Update on the genetics and pathophysiology of type I diabetes mellitus. *Pediatric Annals, 28*(9), 570–575.

Rippe, J. M., & Yanovski, S. Z. (1998, October). Obesity: A chronic disease. *Patient Care Nurse Practitioner, 8,* 33–43.

Robie, D., Edgemon-Hill, E., Phelps, B., Schmitz, C., & Laughlin, J. (1999). Suicide prevention protocol. *American Journal of Nursing, 99*(12), 53–57.

Stephens, M. B. (2000, September). Controlling head lice. *Patient Care for the Nurse Practitioner,* 37–48.

Steward, D. K. (2001). Behavioral characteristics of infants with nonorganic failure to thrive during a play interaction. *American Journal of Maternal Child Nursing, 26*(2), 79–85.

Weber, J., & Kelley, J. (2003). *Health assessment in nursing* (2nd ed.). Philadelphia: Lippincott Williams & Wilkins.

Whaley, L. F. (1995). *Nursing care of infants and children* (5th ed.). St. Louis: Mosby.

Wong, D. L., Perry, S. E., & Hockenberry, M. J. (2002). *Maternal child nursing care* (2nd ed.). St. Louis: Mosby.

Worf, N. (2000). Tetanus. *RN, 63*(6), 44–48.

Unit XII Adult Care Nursing

Abrams, A. C. (2001). *Clinical drug therapy: Rationales for nursing Practice* (6th ed). Philadelphia: Lippincott Williams & Wilkins.

American Burn Association. http://ameriburn.org.

American Cancer Society. www.ca.cancer.org.

American Cancer Society, Inc. (2002). *Cancer Facts & Figures 2002,* Atlanta: American Cancer Society.

American College of Chest Physicians. (2001). *Mechanical ventilation: Beyond the intensive care unit.* http://www.chestnet.org.

American Diabetes Association. (1997). Position statement: Diabetes mellitus and exercise. *Diabetes Care, 20*(12), 1908–1912.

American Diabetes Association. (1997). Committee report: Report of the expert committee on the diagnosis and classification of diabetes mellitus. *Diabetes Care, 20*(7), 1183–1197.

American Diabetes Association. (2000). Committee report: Report of the expert committee on the diagnosis and classification of diabetes mellitus. *Diabetes Care, 23*(1).

American Heart Association. (2002). 2002 Heart and stroke statistical update. www.americanheart.org/statistics.

American Heart Association. (2000). Heart and stroke A–Z guide. www.americanheart.org/Heart_and_Stroke_A_Z_Guide.

American Lung Association. (2000). Diseases A to Z. www.lungusa.org/diseases.

Arnold, S. (1997). Cardiac stress testing. *American Journal of Nursing, 97*(5), 58–61.

Atassi, K, & Harris, M. (2000) Action stat: Subarachnoid hemorrhage. *Nursing, 30*(1), 33.

Aucker, L. (1999). *Pharmacology and the nursing process* (2nd ed., pp. 415–416). St. Louis: Mosby.

Baird, C. (2000). Living with hurting and difficulty doing: Older women with osteoarthritis. *Clinical Excellence for Nurse Practitioners, 4*(4), 231–237.

Barton, W. (1998). Role of ophthalmic nurses with visually impaired patients. *Insight, 23*(1), 5–10.

Baumgart, C., & Hendricks, P. (1997). Long QT syndrome: A silent killer. *American Journal of Nursing, 97*(5), 9–13.

Belcher, A. (1993). *Blood disorders.* St. Louis: Mosby.

Benter, S., & Norris, S. (1997). Atrial fibrillation: Regarding atrial kick. *American Journal of Nursing, 97*(5), 21–25.

Bernie, J. E., Kambo, A. P., & Monga, M. (2000). Lithiasis: diagnostic strategies. *Consultant, 40*(14), 2313–2321.

Bickley, L., & Hoekelman, R. (2003). *Bates' guide to physical examination and history taking* (7th ed.). Philadelphia: Lippincott Williams & Wilkins.

Black, J., Hawks, J., & Keene, A. (2001). *Medical-surgical nursing: Clinical management for positive outcomes* (6th ed.). Philadelphia: Saunders.

Branson, J., & Goldstein, W. (2001). Sequential bilateral total knee arthroplasty. *AORN Journal, 73*(3), 610–635.

Briggs, F. (1996). Newly diagnosed women with breast cancer: The nurse's role. *Nurse Practitioner: American Journal of Primary Health Care, 21*(4), 153–155.

Brubaker, L. T., & Saclarides, T. J. (1998). *The female pelvic floor: Disorders of function and support.* Philadelphia: Davis.

Bryant, G. (2000). When spinal cord injury affects the bowel. *RN, 63*(2), 26–29.

Bryant, G. (2001). Stump care. *American Journal of Nursing, 100*(2), 67–71.

Cahill, M. (1996). Hematologic problems in pediatric patients. *Seminars in Oncology Nursing, 12,* 1.

Cancer Care, Inc., and Oncology Nursing Society. (2001). Lung cancer campaign shows human dimension of deadliest and most neglected cancer. www.lungcancer.org.

Cardio Info Innovations. (2001, January 27). www.cardio-info.com.

Cardiovascular Consultants Medical Group (2002, March 20). www.healthyhearts.com.

Care of a ventilator patient. (2000). http:www.rnbob.tripod.com/ventcare.

Carlson, K., Eisenstat, S., & Ziporyn, T. (1996). *The Harvard guide to women's health.* Cambridge: Harvard University Press.

Casciato, D. A., & Lowitz, B. B. (2000). *Manual of clinical oncology* (4th ed). Philadelphia: Lippincott Williams & Wilkins.

Centers for Disease Control and Prevention. (2001, March). Health topics A to Z. http://www.cdc.gov/ncidod/dbmd/diseaseinfo/

Centers for Disease Control and Prevention (1998). Diagnosis and reporting of HIV and AIDS. *Morbidity and Mortality Weekly Report, 47*(15), 312–314.

Chabner, D. (2001) *The language of medicine* (6th ed) Philadelphia: Saunders.

Chin, J. (2001). *Urology.* New York: McGraw-Hill.

Corbett, C. F. (1999). Research-based practice implications for patients with diabetes: Part 1. Diabetes knowledge. *Home Healthcare Nurse, 17*(8), 511.

Costa, M. E. (1998). Trigeminal neuralgia. *American Journal of Nursing, 98*(6), 42–43.

Craven, R., & Hirnle, C. (2003). *Fundamentals of nursing: Human health and function* (4th ed.). Philadelphia: Lippincott Williams & Wilkins.

Curran, C., & Murray, B. (1997). Dysrhythmia management: When the primary cause isn't cardiac. *American Journal of Nursing, 97*(5), 41–46.

Dangerfield, L., & Paul, S. (1997). Calcium channel blockers: An update. *American Journal of Nursing, 97*(5), 14–19.

Dee, R., Hurst, L., Gruber, M., & Kottmeier, S. (1997). *Principles of orthopaedic practice* (2nd ed.). New York: McGraw-Hill.

DeVita, V. T., Hellman, S., & Rosenberg, S. A. (2000). *Cancer principles & practice of oncology* (6th ed) Philadelphia: Lippincott Williams & Wilkins.

Dierich, M. T., & Froe, F. (2000). *Overcoming incontinence.* New York: Wiley.

Elliot, D. S., & Barrett, D. M. (2000). Artificial urinary sphincter implantation using a bulbous urethral cuff: Perioperative care. *Urologic Nursing, 20*(2), 89–98.

Fineberg, S. (1997). Insulin analogs and human insulin lispro (Humalog). *Practical Diabetology, 16*(2), 16–23.

Fischbach, F. (1999). *A manual of laboratory and diagnostic tests* (4th ed.). Philadelphia: Lippincott Williams & Wilkins.

Flannery, J., & Faria, S. (1999). Limb loss: Alterations in body image. *Journal of Vascular Nursing, 17*(4), 100–106.

Fleming, D. R. (1999). Challenging tradition in insulin injection practices. *American Journal of Nursing, 99*(2), 72–74.

Fleming, D. R. (2000). Mightier than the syringe. *American Journal of Nursing, 100*(11), 44–48.

Funnell, M. M., & Barladge, D. L. (2000). Saying a mouthful about oral diabetes drugs. *Nursing 2000, 30*(11), 34–39.

Gale Encyclopedia of Medicine. Magnetic resonance imaging. http://www.findarticles.com.

George, W., & McClurg, P. (1997). PVCs: Benign or worrisome? *American Journal of Nursing, 97*(5), 2–4.

Gillum, R. (1996). Epidemiology of hypertension in African American women. *American Heart Journal, 131,* 385–395.

Goldsmith, C. (1999). Hypothyroidism. *American Journal of Nursing, 99*(6), 42–43.

Green, K. (1998). *Home care survival guide.* Philadelphia: Lippincott Williams & Wilkins.

Groenwald, S., Hansen-Frogge, M., Goodman, M., & Yarbro, C. (1997). *Cancer nursing: Principles and practice* (4th ed.). Sudbury, MA: Jones & Bartlett.

Grubb, R. (2001). Evaluation of current AUA prostate cancer screening. www.auanet.org.

Gutowski, C. (1999). Understanding new pharmacologic therapy for type 2 diabetes. *Nurse Practitioner,* (246), 15–18, 24–25.

Hanifen, J. M., & Tofte, S. J. (1999). Patient education in the long-term management of atopic dermatitis. *Dermatological Nursing, 11*(4), 284–289.

Hanson, M. J. (1994). Modifiable risk factors for coronary heart disease in women. *American Journal of Critical Care, 3*(3), 177–186.

Harkness, G., & Dincher, J. (1999). *Medical-surgical nursing: Total patient care* (10th ed.). St. Louis: Mosby.

Heart Center Online for Patients. (2000–2001). EA Web Holdings Inc. www.heartcenteronline.com/myheartdr.

Hess, C. T. (2000). Managing a diabetic foot ulcer. *Nursing 2000, 30*(11), 87.

Hilton, G, & Kearney, K. (2001) Emergency: Acute head injury. *American Journal of Nursing, 101*(9), 51–2.

Hosley, J. B., Jones, S. A., & Molle-Matthews E., A. (1997). *Textbook for medical assistants.* Philadelphia: Lippincott-Raven.

Hudak, C. M., Gallo, B. M., & Morton, P. G. (1998). *Critical care nursing: A holistic approach* (7th ed.). Philadelphia: Lippincott Williams & Wilkins.

Hughes, K., & Hagler, D. (1997). Friend or foe? When noncardiac drugs cause cardiac dysrhythmias. *American Journal of Nursing, 97*(5), 31–33.

Ignatavicius, D. (2001). Rheumatoid arthritis and the older adult. *Geriatric Nursing, 22*(3), 139–142.

Jain, S., & Bandi, V. (1999). Electrical and lightning injuries. *Critical Care Clinics, 15*(2), 319–331.

Kane, A. M. (2000). Criteria for successful neobladder surgery: Patient selection and surgical construction. *Urologic Nursing, 20*(3), 182–200.

Karch, A. M. (2003). *2003 Lippincott's nursing drug guide.* Philadelphia: Lippincott Williams & Wilkins.

Karsch, A. M., & Karsch, F. E. (2000). Trouble shooting insulin self-administration. *American Journal of Nursing, 100*(7), 24.

Kee, C., Harris, S., Booth, L., Rouser, G., & McCoy, S. (1998). Perspectives on the nursing management of osteoarthritis. *Geriatric Nursing, 19*(1), 19–26.

Kee, J. L., (1999). *Laboratory & diagnostic tests with nursing implications* (5th ed). Stamford, CT: Appleton & Lange.

Klein, N. J. (2001). Management of primary nocturnal enuresis. *Urologic Nursing, 21*(2), 71–76.

Knutsson, S., & Engberg, I. (1999). An evaluation of patients' qualify of life before, 6 weeks and 6 months after total hip replacement surgery. *Journal of Advanced Nursing, 30*(6), 1349–1359.

Konick-McMahan, J. (1999). Riding out a diabetic emergency. *Nursing 1999, 29*(9), 34–39.

Kuebler, K. K. (2001). Palliative nursing care for the patient experiencing end-stage renal failure. *Urologic Nursing, 21*(3), 167–178.

Lewis, S., Collier, I., & Heitkemper, J. (1996). *Medical-surgical nursing assessment and management of clinical problems: Cardiovascular system.* St. Louis: Mosby.

Lewis, S., Heitkemper, M., Dirksen, S. (2000). *Medical-surgical nursing: Assessment and management of clinical problems* (5th ed). St. Louis: Mosby.

Linton, A. D., Matteson, M. A., & Maebius, N. K. (2000). *Introductory nursing care of adults* (2nd ed.). Philadelphia: Saunders.

Lipschultz, L., & Howards, S. (1997). *Infertility in the male* (3rd ed.). St. Louis: Mosby.

Lorber, D. (1997). Nutrition guidelines for people with diabetes. *Practical Diabetology, 15*(1), 9–15.

Love, S. M., & Lindsey, K. (2000). *Dr. Susan Love's breast book* (3rd ed.). Cambridge, MA: Perseus.

Lucas, L., & Mathews-Flint, L. (2001). Sound advice about hearing aids. *Nursing 2001, 31*(2), 59–61.

Lueckenotte, A. G. (2000). *Gerontologic nursing* (2nd ed). St. Louis: Mosby.

Mahoney, C. (2001). Non-invasive evaluation and treatment of bladder control problems in the primary care setting. *American Journal for Nurse Practitioners, 5*(5), 42–54.

McCain, D., & Sutherland, S. (1998). Nursing essentials: Skin grafts for patients with burns. *American Journal of Nursing, 98*(7), 34–38.

McCance, K. & Huether, S. (1998). *Pathophysiology: The biologic basis for disease in adults and children* (3rd ed.). St. Louis: Mosby.

McConnell, E. (1996). The future of technology in critical care. *Critical Care Nurse, 16*(Suppl.), 3–16.

McCreedy, T., & Johnson-Sasso, D. (1997). Treating cardiomyopathy-induced dysrhythmias: A fine line. *American Journal of Nursing, 97*(5), 26–30.

McLeskey, S., & Korniewicz, D. (1998). Understanding latex allergy. *Seminars in Perioperative Nursing, 7*(4), 206–215.

McMorrow, M. (1996). Myxedema coma: Do you recognize the clues to this rare complication of hypothyroidism? *American Journal of Nursing, 96*(10), 55.

Metheny, N., (2000). *Fluid and electrolyte balance: Nursing considerations* (4th ed.) Philadelphia: Lippincott Williams & Wilkins.

Mobley, D. F., & Baum, N. (1997). *Male infertility and sexual dysfunction.* New York: Springer-Verlag.

Moore, G. J. (Ed.) (1997). Women and cancer: A gynecologic oncology nursing perspective. Sudbury, MA: Jones & Bartlett.

Morgan, E., Bledsoe, S., & Barker, J. (2000). Ambulatory management of burns. *American Family Physician, 62*(9), 2015–2026.

Moriarty, K., & Apple, S. (1997). Understanding the impact of sudden cardiac death. *American Journal of Nursing, 97*(5), 38–40.

Mosby's medical, nursing, & allied health dictionary (6th ed.) (2002). St. Louis: Mosby.

Moyad, M. (2000). *The ABC's of advanced prostate cancer.* Chelsea: Sleeping Bear Press.

Mrowietz, U. (2001) Advances in systemic therapy for psoriasis. *Clinical Experiments in Dermatology, 26*(4), 362–367.

Nath, C., & Ponte, C. D. (2000). Lessons learned about insulin therapy. *Nursing 2000, 30*(11), 40–45.

National Institute of Neurological Disorders and Strokes. http://www.ninds.nih.gov/health_and_medical/disorders.

National Jewish Medical and Research Center. www.njc.org/medfacts.

National Multiple Sclerosis Society. http://www.nmss.org.

Naybak, A. M. (2000). Hyponatremia as a consequence of acute adrenal insufficiency and hypothyroidism. *Journal of Emergency Nursing, 26*(2), 130–133.

Neil, J. A. (2000). The stigma scale: Measuring body image and the skin. *Dermatological Nursing, 12*(1), 32–36.

Nettina, S. (Ed.). (2000, January-February). HIV-related illness. *Lippincott's Primary Care Practice, 4*(1).

O'Hanlon-Nichols, T. (1999). Neurologic assessment. *American Journal of Nursing, 99*(6), 44–50.

O'Neil, B., Forsythe, M., & Stanish, W. (2001). Chronic occupational repetitive strain injury. *Canadian Family Physician, 47*(2), 311–316.

Oncology Nursing Society. (2000). *Stem cell transplantation: A clinical textbook.* Pittsburgh: Oncology Nursing Press.

Patterson, R. (2001). *Urology.* New York: McGraw-Hill.

Pestana, C. (2000). *Fluids and electrolytes in the surgical patient* (5th ed.). Philadelphia: Lippincott Williams & Wilkins.

Peters, K. M. (2000). The diagnosis and treatment of interstitial cystitis. *Urologic Nursing, 20*(2), 101–107.

Phillips, L. L. (2000). Putting a damper on cellulites. *Nursing 2000, 12*(1), 17–18, 21–28.

Porth, C. (2002). *Pathophysiology: Concepts of altered health states* (6th ed.). Philadelphia: Lippincott Williams & Wilkins.

Portman, D., & Barden, C. (1997). Implantable cardioverter-defibrillators: Now and in the future. *American Journal of Nursing, 97*(5), 38–40.

Potter, P. A., & Perry, A. G. (2001). *Fundamentals of nursing* (5th ed). St. Louis: Mosby.

Prostate cancer overview. www.cancer.org.

Ramsey, P. I., Barret, J. P., & Herndon, D. N. (1999). Thermal injury. *Critical Care Clinics, 15*(2), 333–352.

Redfield, D., & Hayes, T. (1998). Orthopaedic infections. *Critical Care Nursing Quarterly, 21*(20), 24–35.

Rieger, P. T. (1999). *Clinical handbook for biotherapy.* Sudbury, MA: Jones & Bartlett.

Robertson, C. (2001). Diabetes update: The untold story of disease progression. *RN, 64*(3), 60–64.

Rous, S. (1996). *Urology: A core textbook* (2nd ed.). Cambridge, MA: Blackwell Science.

Rouston, J. (1999). Recognizing aneurysmal subarachnoid hemorrhage. *Nurse Practitioner, 24*(4), 19–20.

Sande, M. A., & Volberding, P. A. (1999). *The medical management of AIDS* (6th ed). Philadelphia: Saunders.

Saranath, D. (2000) *Contemporary issues in oral cancer.* Oxford: Oxford University Press.

Schilling, J. (1997). Hyperthyroidism: Diagnosis and management of Graves' disease. *Nurse Practitioner, 22*(6), 72–97.

Sheridan, R. L. (2000). Evaluating and managing burn wounds. *Dermatological Nurse, 12*(1), 17–18, 21–28.

Skidmore-Roth, L. (2001). *Drug guide for nurses* (4th ed.). St. Louis: Mosby.

Smeltzer, S. C., & Bare, B. G. (2000). *Brunner and Suddarth's textbook of medical-surgical nursing* (9th ed.). Philadelphia: Lippincott Williams & Wilkins.

Smith, R. A., et al. (2001). American Cancer Society guidelines for the early detection of cancer. *CA: A Cancer Journal for Clinicians, 51*(1), 38–75.

Smith-Temple, J., & Johnson, J. Y. (1998). *Nurses' guide to clinical procedures.* Philadelphia: Lippincott Williams & Wilkins.

Spratto, G. R., & Woods, A. L. (2000). *PDR nurses' drug handbook.* Albany, NY: Delmar.

Stern, M. (1995). Epidemiology of obesity and its link to heart disease. *Metabolism: Clinical and Experimental, 44*(9, Suppl. 3), 1–3.

Taber's cyclopedic medical dictionary (19th ed.) (2001). Philadelphia: Davis.

Tate, J., & Tasota, F. J. (2001). Assessing thyroid function with screen tests. *Nursing 2001, 31*(1), 22.

Taylor, C., Lillis, C., & LeMone, P. (2001). Fundamentals of nursing: *The art and science of nursing care* (4th ed.). Philadelphia: Lippincott Williams & Wilkins.

Thelan, L. A., Urden, L. D., Lough, M. E., & Stacy, K. M. (1998). *Critical care nursing: Diagnosis and management* (3rd ed.) St. Louis: Mosby.

Thobaben, M. (1998). Helping client with presbycusis. *Home Care Provider, 3*(4), 186–188.

Thomasson, S. (2000). Promoting outcomes for patients with spinal cord impairments and ostomies. *Medical Surgical Nursing, 9*(2), 77–82.

Timby, B. K., & Smith, N. E. (2003). *Introductory medical-surgical nursing* (8th ed). Philadelphia: Lippincott Williams & Wilkins.

Tupper, S. (1999). When the inner ear is out of balance. *RN, 62*(11), 36–39.

Turkoski, B. (2000). Glaucoma and glaucoma medications. *Orthopedic Nurse, 19*(5), 71–76.

U.S. Department of Health and Human Services. (1995). Acute low back problems in adults: Assessment and treatment. *Orthopaedic Nursing,* (14), 37–52.

U.S. Department of Health and Human Services/Henry J. Kaiser Family Foundation. (2001, February). Guidelines for the use of antiretroviral agents in HIV-infected adults and adolescents. http://www.dhhs.gov.

Varricchio, C. (Ed.). (1997). *A cancer sourcebook for nurses* (7th ed.). Atlanta: American Cancer Society.

Warren-Boulton, E., Greenberg, R., Lusing, M, & Gallivan, J. (1999). An update of primary care management of type 2 diabetes. *Nurse Practitioner, 24*(12), 14–16, 19–20, 23–24.

Weber, J., & Kelley, J. (2003). *Health assessment in nursing* (2nd ed.). Philadelphia: Lippincott Williams & Wilkins.

Wiebelhaus, P., & Hansen, S. L (1999). Burns: Handle with care. *RN, 62*(11), 52–57.

Wiebelhaus, P., & Hansen, S. L. (2001). What you should know about managing burn emergencies. *Nursing 2001, 31*(1), 36–41.

Wieland, S. (1998). Promoting health in children with atopic dermatitis. *Nurse Practitioner, 3*(4), 86–90, 96–97.

Wilson, D. D., (1999). *Nurses' guide to understanding laboratory and diagnostic tests.* Philadelphia: Lippincott Williams & Wilkins.

Winkelman, C. (1999) A review of pharmacodynamics and pharmacokinetics in seizure management. *Journal of Neuroscience Nursing, 31*(1), 50–53.

Woodhead, G., & Moss, M. (1998). Osteoporosis: diagnosis and prevention. *Nurse Practitioner, 23*(11), 18, 23–27, 31–32.

Woodruff, D. W. (1999). How to ward off complications of mechanical ventilation. *Nursing, 29*(11).

Wulf, J. (2000). Evaluation of seizure observation and documentation. *Journal of Neuroscience Nursing, 32*(1), 27–36.

Young, J. (1999). Action state: Thyroid storm. *Nursing 1999, 29*(8), 33.

Unit XIII Gerontological Nursing

Adams, T., & Page, S. (2000) New pharmacological treatments for Alzheimer's disease: Implications for dementia care nursing. *Journal of Advanced Nursing, 31*(5), 1183–1188.

Akin, C. (2000). The long road called goodbye: Tracing the course of Alzheimer's. Omaha: Creighton University Press.

Allen, M. (1998). Elder abuse: A challenge for home care nurses. *Home Healthcare Nurse, 16*(2), 103–110.

Barry, P. (2002). *Mental health and mental illness* (7th ed.). Philadelphia: Lippincott Williams & Wilkins.

Boss, P. (1988). Alzheimer's and the family: Scientist studies how people cope with "loss" of living loved-one. *News* (pp. 1–3). Minneapolis: University of Minnesota, College of Home Economics.

Brenner, Z., & Durry-Durnin, K. (1998) Toward restraint-free care. *American Journal of Nursing, 98*(12), 16F–16I.

Butler, R. (1999). Warning signs of elder abuse. *Journal of Gerontological Nursing, 23*(7), 24–32.

Castleman, M. (1999). *There's still a person in there: The complete guide to treating and coping with Alzheimer's.* New York: Putnam.

Combs, L. (1998). *A long goodbye and beyond: Coping with Alzheimer's.* Wilsonville, OR: Book Partners.

Dawbarn, D., & Allen, S. (Eds.) (2001). *Neurobiology of Alzheimer's disease* (2nd ed.). New York: Oxford University Press.

Eliopoulos, C. (2001). *Gerontological nursing* (5th ed.). Philadelphia: Lippincott Williams & Wilkins.

Glaser, V. (1998). Providing quality care in the nursing home. *Patient Care, 32*(9), 132.

Gray-Vickrey, P. (2000). Protecting the older adult. *Nursing 2000, 30*(7), 34.

Green, J. (2000). *Neuropsychological evaluation of the older adult: A clinician's guidebook.* San Diego: Academic Press.

Jaffe, M. (1999). *Geriatric long-term procedures and treatments: A problem solving approach* (2nd ed.). Englewood, CO: Skidmore-Roth.

Katzman, R., & Bick, K. (2000). Alzheimer's disease: The changing view. San Diego: Academic Press.

Khachaturian, Z., & Mesulam, M. (Eds.) (2000). *Concepts of Alzheimer's disease: Biological, clinical, and cultural perspectives.* Baltimore: Johns Hopkins University Press.

Maddox, G. (Ed.) (2001). *The encyclopedia of aging: A comprehensive resource in gerontology and geriatrics* (3rd ed.). New York: Springer.

Megly, M., & Berkman, B. (Eds.) (2000). *The encyclopedia of elder care: The comprehensive resource for geriatric and social care.* New York: Springer.

Middleton, H., Keen, R., Johnson, C., Elkins, A., & Lee, A. (1999). Physical and pharmacologic restraints in long term care facilities. *Journal of Gerontological Nursing, 25*(7), 26–33.

Molony, S., Waszynski, C., & Lyder, C. (1999). *Gerontological nursing: An advanced practice approach.* Stamford, CT: Appleton & Lange.

Schultz, R. (Ed.) (2000). *Handbook on dementia care-giving: Evidence-based interventions in family care-giving.* New York: Springer.

Schweiger, J., & Huey, R. (1999). Alzheimer's disease: Your role in the caregiving equation. *Nursing 1999, 29*(6), 34–41.

Shives, L. (2002). *Basic concepts of psychiatric–mental health nursing* (5th ed.). Philadelphia: Lippincott Williams & Wilkins.

Smyer, M. A., & Qualls, S. H. (1999). *Aging and mental health.* Malden, MA: Blackwell.

Stanley, M., & Beare, P. G. (1999). *Gerontological nursing: A health promotion approach* (2nd ed.). Philadelphia: Davis.

Tanzi, R., & Parsons, A. (2000). *Decoding darkness: The search for genetic causes of Alzheimer's disease.* Cambridge, MA: Perseus.

Unit XIV Mental Health Nursing

Adatsi, G. (1999). Health going up in smoke: How can you prevent it? *American Journal of Nursing, 99*(3), 63–69.

Allen, L. (1999). Treating agitation without drugs. *American Journal of Nursing, 99*(4), 36–41.

American Psychiatric Association. (2000). *Diagnostic and statistical manual of mental disorders* (4th ed., text rev.). Washington, DC: Author.

Amitriptyline use in geriatric care. (1999). *American Journal of Nursing, 99*(5), 16.

Andrews, M., & Boyle, J. (1999). *Transcultural concepts in nursing care* (3rd ed.). Philadelphia: Lippincott Williams & Wilkins.

Anonymous. (1996). Psychiatric nursing: Relaxation exercises reduce inpatients' anxiety. *American Journal of Nursing, 96*(11), 10.

Anonymous. (1996). Psychiatric nursing: When words fail, violence may follow. *American Journal of Nursing, 96*(5), 9–10.

Anonymous. (1999). Antipsychotics: the next generation. *Nursing 1999, 29*(4), 68.

Barry, P. (1998). *Mental health and mental illness* (6th ed.). Philadelphia: Lippincott Williams & Wilkins.

Bauer, B., & Hill, S. (2000). *Mental health nursing: An introductory text.* Philadelphia: Saunders.

Boyd, M., & Nihart, M. (1998). *Psychiatric nursing: Contemporary practice.* Philadelphia: Lippincott Williams & Wilkins.

Brent, M. (1997). Unexpected alcohol withdrawal. *American Journal of Nursing, 97*(6), 52–53.

Burke, R. (1995). *When the music's over: My journey into schizophrenia.* New York: Basic Books.

Bush, C. (2000). Cultural competence: Implications of the Surgeon General's report on mental health. *Journal of Child and Adolescent Psychiatric Nursing, 13*(4), 177–178.

Calfee, B. (1996). Documenting suicide risk: Charting tips. *Nursing 1996, 26*(7), 17.

Cardwell, T. (2001). Out of control. *Nursing 2001, 31*(5), 53.

Carson, V. (2000). *Mental health nursing: The nurse-patient journey.* Philadelphia: Saunders.

Clark, C. (1997). Posttraumatic stress disorder: How to support healing. *American Journal of Nursing, 97*(8), 27–32.

Dayer, L. (2001). Polypharmacy in the elderly. *Nursing Spectrum, 2*(4), 29–31.

Deering, C. (1999). To speak or not to speak: Self-disclosure with patients. *American Journal of Nursing, 99*(1), 34–38.

Dixon, E. (1997). *I'm free! Reaching for your inner desire to free yourself from tobacco, drugs and alcohol addictions forever.* Pittsburgh: Dorrance Publishing.

Fluegelman, A. (1981). *More new games.* Garden City, NY: Doubleday.

Fontaine, K, & Fletcher, J., et al. (1999). *Mental health nursing.* Menlo Park, CA: Addison-Wesley.

Fortinash, K., & Holoday-Worret, P. (2000). *Psychiatric mental health nursing.* St. Louis: Mosby.

Frisch, N., Frisch, L., Keegan, L., et al. (1998). *Psychiatric mental health nursing: Understanding the client as well as the condition.* Albany: Delmar.

Gorman, M. (Coordinator). (1997). When alcoholism hits home. *American Journal of Nursing, 97*(7), 68–69.

Haber, J., Krainovich-Miller, B., McMaon, A., & Prive-Hoskins, P. (1977). *Comprehensive psychiatric nursing* (5th ed.). St. Louis: Mosby.

Hatcher, T. (2001). The proverbial herb. *American Journal of Nursing, 101*(2), 36–43.

Hazelden Staff. (1966). *Alcoholism.* Center City, MN: Hazelden Foundation.

Hazelden Staff. (1996). *Managing cocaine craving.* Center City, MN: Hazelden Foundation.

Horsfall, J., Stuhlmiller, C., Champ, S., et al. (2001). *Interpersonal nursing for mental health.* New York: Springer.

Hurlburt, J. (1999). Abuse of faith [letter]. *American Journal of Nursing, 99*(9), 19.

Isaacs, A. (2000). *Mental health and psychiatric nursing.* Philadelphia: Lippincott Williams & Wilkins.

Johnson, B. (1997). *Psychiatric–mental health nursing: Adaptation and growth* (4th ed.). Philadelphia: Lippincott-Raven.

Kaplan, H., & Sadock, B. (2000). *Comprehensive textbook of psychiatry* (7th ed.). Philadelphia: Lippincott Williams & Wilkins.

Kearney, K. (2000). Delirium tremens. *American Journal of Nursing, 100*(1), 41–42.

Lego, S. (1996). *Psychiatric nursing: A comprehensive reference* (2nd ed.). Philadelphia: Lippincott-Raven.

Lerner-Durjawa, L. (1999). The truth about cats and dogs: Here's how to keep a visit from a house pet safe for your patient. *Nursing 1999, 29*(7), 73.

Lindsay, C. (2001). Unfair fight. *Nursing Spectrum, 2*(3), 34.

Karch, A. M. (2003). *2003 Lippincott's nursing drug guide.* Philadelphia: Lippincott Williams & Wilkins.

Marundla, T. (2000). Professional nurses' perception of nursing mentally ill people in a general hospital setting. *Journal of Advanced Nursing, 32*(6), 1569–1578.

Mathre, M. (2001). Therapeutic cannibis: A patient advocacy issue. *American Journal of Nursing, 101*(4), 61–68.

McCaffery, M. (1999). Opioids and pain management: What do nurses know? *Nursing 1999, 29*(3), 48–52.

McFarland, R. (1997). Cocaine. Center City, MN: Hazelden Foundation.

Miller, J., & Conner, K. (2000). Going to the dogs . . . for help. *Nursing 2000, 30*(11), 65–67.

Morrison, C. (2000). Fear of addiction: Balancing the facts and concerns about opioid use. *American Journal of Nursing, 100*(7), 81.

Navarra, T. (1995). Enabling behavior: The tender trap. *American Journal of Nursing, 95*(1), 50–52.

O'Neil, C., Avila, J., & Fetrow, C. (1999). Herbal medicines: Getting beyond the hype. *Nursing 1999, 29*(4), 58–61.

Orbanic, S. (2001). Understanding bulimia: Signs, symptoms, and the human experience. *American Journal of Nursing, 101*(3), 35–41.

Pasero, C. (Coordinator). (1997). Managing pain in addicted patients. *American Journal of Nursing, 97*(4), 17–18.

Porth, C. (2002). *Pathophysiology: Concepts of altered health states* (6th ed.). Philadelphia: Lippincott Williams & Wilkins.

Poster, E. (1999). Psychiatric nursing. *American Journal of Nursing, 99*(4), 24C–24D.

Powter, S. (1997). *Dance with the devil: A lifesaving treatment for overcoming the addiction to alcohol.* New York: Simon & Schuster.

Rimer, S. (1999, September 5). Gaps seen in treating depression in the elderly. *The New York Times*, p. 1.1.

Rivera, B. (1999). Dan and me, taking care of ourselves. *American Journal of Nursing, 99*(6), 56–58.

Rother, L. (2001). Action STAT: Neuroleptic malignant syndrome. *Nursing 2001, 31*(1), 43.

Sachse, D. (2000). Emergency: Delirium tremens. *American Journal of Nursing, 100*(5), 41–42.

Salladay, S. (2000). Psychiatric advance directive? *Nursing 2000, 30*(7), 65–66.

Schwarz, T. (2000). Do you smoke? If so, stop. *American Journal of Nursing, 100*(11), 11.

Schwarz, T. (2001). Smoking cessation online. *American Journal of Nursing, 101*(3), 87.

Shea, C., Mahoney, M., & Lacey, J. (1997). Breaking through the barriers to domestic violence intervention. *American Journal of Nursing, 97*(6), 26–33.

Shives, L. (2002). *Basic concepts of psychiatric–mental health nursing* (5th ed.). Philadelphia: Lippincott Williams & Wilkins.

Shuster, J. (1999). Psychiatric complications of corticosteroids. *Nursing 1999, 29*(6), 31.

Sizemore, S. (1999). The truth about Harry. *American Journal of Nursing, 99*(9), 25.

Sofer, D. (1999). Restraint use in psychiatric settings. *American Journal of Nursing, 99*(10), 32.

Townsend, M. (2000). *Psychiatric mental health nursing: Concepts of care.* Philadelphia: Davis.

Trimpey, J. (1996). *Rational recovery: The new cure for substance addiction.* New York: Pocket Books.

Twenge, J., et al. (2000). Anxiety is increasing in children. *Journal of Personal and Social Psychology, 79*(6), 1007–1021. (Summary in *American Journal of Nursing* [2001], *101*(3), 18).

Varcarolis, E. (2002). *Foundations of psychiatric–mental health nursing* (4th ed.). Philadelphia: Saunders.

Videbeck, S. (2001). *Psychiatric mental health nursing.* Philadelphia: Lippincott Williams & Wilkins.

Waddell, D., Hummel, E., & Sumners, A. (2001). Three herbs you should get to know. *American Journal of Nursing, 101*(4), 48–53.

Walker, T. (1999). Chronic fatigue syndrome: Do you know what it means? *American Journal of Nursing, 99*(3), 70–76.

Wallis, M. (2000). Looking at depression through bifocal lenses: How to help older adults recover from depression. *Nursing 2000, 30*(9), 58–61.

Wichowski, H. (2001). Unforgettable patient: The woman inside (schizophrenia). *Nursing 2001, 31*(3), 51.

Zollo, M., & Derse, A. (1997). The abusive patient: Where do you draw the line? *American Journal of Nursing, 97*(2), 31.

Unit XV Nursing in a Variety of Settings

Adkins, S. (1999). Teaching and grieving. *American Journal of Nursing, 99*(8), 88.

Allender J., & Spradley, B. (2001). *Community health nursing: Concepts and practice.* Philadelphia: Lippincott Williams & Wilkins.

American Nurses Association. (1997). *The acute care nurse in transition.* Waldorf, MD: American Nurses Publishing.

American Nurses Association. (1999). *Scope and standards of home health nursing practice.* Washington, DC: American Nurses Publishing.

American Public Health Association. (2000). *Healthy people 2010: National health promotion and disease prevention objectives.* Washington, DC: Author.

Anaemaet, W., & Trotter, M. (1999). *Handbook of home health therapy: Standards and guidelines for rehabilitation practice.* St. Louis: Mosby.

Anderson, E., & McFarlane, J. (2000). *Community as partner: Theory and practice in nursing* (3rd ed.). Philadelphia: Lippincott Williams & Wilkins.

Androwich, I., & Burkhart, L. (1996). *Community and home health nursing.* Albany, NY: Delmar.

Anonymous. (1999). Why I became a nurse. *RN, 62*(1), 61.

Anonymous. (2000). Hospice care: Who's eligible? *Nursing 2000, 30*(2), HH8.

Armentrout, G. (1998). *Community-based nursing: Foundations for practice.* Stamford, CT: Appleton & Lange.

Baggerly, J., & DiBlasi, M. (1996). Pressure sores and pressure sore prevention in a rehabilitation setting. *Rehabilitation Nursing, 21*(6), 321–325.

Barry, P. (1996). *Psychosocial nursing: Care of physically ill patients and their families* (3rd ed.). Philadelphia: Lippincott-Raven.

Beck, R., & Franke, D. (1996). Rehabilitation of victims of natural disasters. *Journal of Rehabilitation, 62*(4), 28–32.

Benefield, L. (1996). Making the transition to home care nursing. *American Journal of Nursing, 96*(10), 47–49.

Blastic, L. (1996). Short-stay unit emphasizes the personal touch. *Inside Ambulatory Care, 3,* 5–7.

Bowen, R. (1996). Practicing what we preach: Embracing the independent living movement. *Occupational Therapy Practice, 1*(5), 20–24.

Brimhall, N. (1998). Reflections: One hundred candles. *American Journal of Nursing, 98*(3), 53.

Brookes, T. (1997). *Signs of life: A memoir of hospice, home and hope.* New York: Random House.

Buckingham, R. (1996). *The handbook of hospice care.* Amherst, NY: Prometheus.

Buhler-Wilkerson, K. (2001). *No place like home: A history of nursing and home care in the United States.* Baltimore: Johns Hopkins.

Burden, N., Quinn, D., et al. (2000). *Ambulatory surgical nursing.* Philadelphia: Saunders.

Burke, J. (1997). Death with dignity. *Wisconsin Medical Journal, 96*(2), 23–26.

Burke, M., & Walsh, M. (1996). *Gerontologic nursing: Wholistic care of the older adult* (2nd ed.). St. Louis: Mosby.

Burton, S. (1998). *Community-based nursing.* St. Louis: Mosby–Yearbook.

Byock, I. (1997). *Dying well: The prospect for growth at the end of life.* New York: Putnam.

Cesta, T. & Falter, E. (1999). Case management: Its value for staff nurses. *American Journal of Nursing, 99*(5), 48–51.

Chabriel, J., & Rissuto, M. (1999). *Delmar's CD-ROM . . . Acute care, home care, long-term care.* Albany, NY: Delmar.

Chadderton, H. (1998). Thinking . . . about nursing homes. *Journal of Nursing Management, 6*(4), 191–192.

Chaffee, M. (1999). A telehealth odyssey. *American Journal of Nursing, 99*(7), 26–32.

Chin, P., Finocchiaro, D., & Rosebrough, A., (1997). *Comprehensive rehabilitation nursing.* New York: McGraw-Hill.

Coates, C. (1997). Finding the will and the way. *Nursing 1997, 27*(9), 32.

Cohn, S. (1997). *Do it one-handed: A manual of daily living skills for stroke rehabilitation.* South Orange, NJ: Lenox House.

Conn, D. (2000). *Practical psychiatry in the long-term care facility: A handbook for staff.* Toronto: Hogrefe & Huber.

Dahl, R. (1997). Demonstrating nursing's value in community health. *American Journal of Nursing, 97*(2), 72.

Davidhizer, R., & Shearer, R. (1997). Helping the client with chronic disability achieve high-level wellness. *Rehabilitation Nursing, 22*(3), 131–134.

Dell'Orto, A. (Ed.) (1995). *Encyclopedia of disabilities and rehabilitation.* New York: Macmillan.

Donofrio, J. (2000). Making a difference in end-of-life care. *Nursing Homes, 49*(9), 47–48.

Dougherty, M, Dwyer, J., et al. (1998). Community-based nursing: Continence care for older rural women. *Nursing Outlook, 46*(5), 233–234.

Dubuisson, W. (2001). *Hospital to home: A pocket guide.* Sudbury, MA: Jones & Bartlett.

Durning, F. (1999). *Accident and emergency nursing: A practical introduction for junior nurses.* Plymouth, UK: Studymates. http://www.studymates.com.uk.

Elhilali, M. (1997). Early hospital discharge and home care. *Canadian Journal of Surgery, 40*(1), 10–11, 39–43.

Ellis J., & Hartley, C. (1998). *Nursing in today's world: Challenges, issues and trends* (6th ed.). Philadelphia: Lippincott Williams & Wilkins.

Ellner, L. (1997). What Grandma Clara wanted. *American Journal of Nursing, 97*(8), 51.

Fanslow-Brunjes, C., Schneider, P., & Kimmel, L. (1997). Hope: Offering comfort and support for dying patients. *Nursing 1997, 27*(3), 54–57.

Faulkner, K. (1997). Talking about death with a dying child. *American Journal of Nursing, 97*(6), 64–69.

Feldman, G. (2001, January 9). Life's end: Little help, no dignity. *The New York Times*, p. F-7.

Ferrell, B. (1997). Controlling pain (managing chronic cancer pain). *Nursing 1997, 27*(4), 74.

Ferrell, B., Virani, R., Grant, M., Coyne, P., & Uman, G. (2000). End-of-life care: Nurses speak out. *Nursing 2000, 30*(7), 54–57.

Fischer, C., & Hegge, M. (2000). The elderly woman at risk. *American Journal of Nursing, 100*(6), 54–59.

Fourth, M. (1995). Home health care: Making a smooth transition. *Nursing 1995, 25*(3), 79–80.

Furman, J. (2000). Taking a holistic approach to the dying time. *Nursing 2000, 30*(6), 46–49.

Furman, J. (2001). Living and dying: How to help the family caregiver. *Nursing 2001, 31*(4), 36–41.

Fuzy, J. (1999). *Home care for the client needing rehabilitation.* Albany, NY: Delmar.

Gaguski, M. (1999). A private place: Consolation for grieving families. *American Journal of Nursing, 99*(4), 18–19.

Gallagher, R. (2000). How long-term care is changing. *American Journal of Nursing, 100*(2), 65–67.

Galvan, T. (2001). Dysphagia: Going down and staying down. *American Journal of Nursing, 101*(1), 37–42.

Goldberg, J., et al. (1996). Sponsored by Corcoran Gallery of Art and National Hospice Foundation. *Hospice: A photographic inquiry.* New York: Little, Brown.

Gorney-Moreno, M., & Faherty, B. (2000). *Introduction to home health nursing: An interactive CD-ROM.* St. Louis: Mosby.

Green, K. (1998). *Home care survival guide.* Philadelphia: Lippincott Williams & Wilkins.

Green, K., & Lydon, S. (1998). Continuing care extra: The continuum of patient care. *American Journal of Nursing, 98*(10), 16BBB–16DDD.

Gresham, G. (1997). *Post-stroke rehabilitation: Clinical practice guidelines.* Upland, PA: Diane.

Guidry, M. (2001). *Healthy people in healthy communities: A community planning guide.* Washington, DC: U.S. Superintendent of Documents.

Guzetta, C. (1998). Reflections: Healing and wholeness in chronic illness. *Journal of Holistic Nursing, 16*(2), 197–201.

Hallper, J., & Holland, N. (1998). Meeting the challenge of multiple sclerosis. *American Journal of Nursing, 98*(10), 26–32.

Harper, D. (1996). Emerging rehabilitation needs of adults with developmental disabilities. *Journal of Rehabilitation, 62*(1), 7–10.

Hart, S. (1997). A gift disguised. *American Journal of Nursing, 97*(6), 54.

Harwell, A. (1995). *Ready to live: Prepared to die: A provocative guide to the rest of your life.* Wheaton, IL: Harold Shaw.

Hayn, M., & Fisher, T. (1997). Stroke rehabilitation: Salvaging ability after the storm. *Nursing 1997, 27*(3), 40–48.

Haynor, P. (1998). Meeting the challenge of advance directives. *American Journal of Nursing, 98*(3), 26–32.

Henderson-Martin, B. (2000). No more surprises: Screening patients for alcohol abuse (in home care). *American Journal of Nursing, 100*(9), 26–32.

Hinshaw, S. (1999). All in good time. *Nursing 1999, 29*(10), 88.

Hoban, S. (2000). Emergency: Elder abuse and neglect. *American Journal of Nursing, 100*(11), 49–50.

Hoeman, S. (1996). *Rehabilitation nursing: Process and practice* (2nd ed.). St. Louis: Mosby–Yearbook.

The home health nursing audio set. (2000). Memphis, TN: Consultants in Care.

Hooks, F. and Daly B. (2000). Hastening death. *American Journal of Nursing, 100*(5), 56–63.

Horgan, K. (1997). Pants not required. *American Journal of Nursing, 97*(5), 50.

Hunt, B. (1996). Rehabilitation counseling for people with HIV disease. *Journal of Rehabilitation, 62*(3), 68–74.

Hunt, R. (1998). Community-based nursing, philosophy or setting? *American Journal of Nursing, 98*(10), 44–48.

Infeld, D., Gordon, A., & Harper, B. (Eds.) (1995). *Hospice care and cultural diversity.* Binghamton, NY: Haworth.

Jacobson, J. (1996). Rehabilitation services for people with mental retardation and psychiatric disabilities. *Journal of Rehabilitation, 62*(1), 11–22.

Jaffe, C. (1997). *All kinds of love: Experiencing hospice.* Amityville, NY: Baywood.

Johnson, J., Smith-Temple, J., & Carr, P. (1998). *Nurses' guide to home health procedures.* Philadelphia: Lippincott Williams & Wilkins.

Johnson, S. (2000). From incontinence to confidence. *American Journal of Nursing, 100*(2), 69–76.

Joseph, I., & Reele, B. (1995). Respite for the caregiver. *American Journal of Nursing, 95*(5), 55.

Kane, R., Chen, Q., et al. (1996). Do rehabilitative nursing homes improve the outcomes of care? *Journal of the American Geriatrics Society, 44*(5), 545–554.

Keay, T. (1999). Palliative care in the nursing home. *Generations, 23*(1), 96–98.

Kennedy-Schwerz, J. (2001). The visit: Whispered advice at the end of life. *American Journal of Nursing, 101*(5), 23.

Kifer, B. (2000). Death comes to visit. *Nursing 2000, 30*(10), 48–49.

Kinsella, L. (2001). Walking the hundred-mile road: A parable for someone who's nearing the end of life. *Nursing 2001, 31*(3), 62–63.

Koch, M. (1997). Going home: Is home health care for you? *Nursing 1997, 27*(10), 49.

Kovner, C., & Harrington, C. (2001). Counting nurses: What is community health-public health nursing? *American Journal of Nursing, 101*(1), 59–60.

Lai, S. (1998). Promoting lifestyle changes (cardiac rehabilitation). *American Journal of Nursing, 99*(4), 63–67.

Leverence, K. (2000). Helping Gina find the light. *Nursing 2000, 30*(12), HH4–5.

Levine, C. (2000). *Always on call: Family caregivers.* New York: United Hospital Fund.

Loeb, J. (1999). Pain management in long term care. *American Journal of Nursing, 99*(2), 48–52.

Lynch, S. (1997). Elder abuse: What to look for, how to intervene. *American Journal of Nursing, 97*(1), 26–32.

Lynn, J. (2000). After aging. *Journal of the American Geriatrics Society, 48*(8), 1017.

Marrelli, T. (2001). *Handbook of home health standards.* St. Louis: Mosby.

Marrelli, T., & Hilliard, L. (1998). *Manual of home health nursing practice.* St. Louis: Mosby.

Martin, K. (1997). *The home health client.* St. Louis: Mosby–Yearbook.

Masson, V. (2001). The underserved. *American Journal of Nursing, 101*(7), 25.

Mayer, D., Torma, L., Byock, I., & Norris, K. (2001). Speaking the language of pain. *American Journal of Nursing, 101*(2), 44–49.

McAweeney, M., Forchheimer, M., & Tate, D. (1996). Identifying the unmet independent living needs of persons with spinal cord injury. *Journal of Rehabilitation, 62*(3), 29–34.

McCaffery, M. (1997). Pain management handbook. *Nursing 1997, 27*(4), 42–45.

McCaffery, M. (1999). (Culturally sensitive) pain control. *American Journal of Nursing, 99*(8), 18.

McCaffery, M. (1999). Opioids and pain management: What do nurses know? *Nursing 1999, 29*(3), 48–52.

McCaffery, M. (2000). How to choose the best route for an opioid. *Nursing 2000, 30*(12), 34–39.

McCaffery, M., & Pasero, C. (2001). Pain control: Assessment and reactions of patients with myocardial infarction. *American Journal of Nursing, 101*(7), 69–70.

McConnell, E. (1997). Medical devices and medical futility: When is enough enough? *Nursing 1997, 27*(8), 32HN1–4.

McConnell, E. (2000). Myths and facts . . . about hospice. *Nursing 2000, 30*(11), 81.

McEwen, M. (1998). *Community-based nursing: An introduction.* Philadelphia: Saunders.

McGinley, L. (2000, September 18). Terminal patients stay at hospice for shorter period. *Wall Street Journal,* p. B-2.

McKee, R. (1999). Clarifying advance directives. *Nursing 1999, 29*(5), 52–53.

McKeon, E. (2001). Nursing home staffing crisis: The ANA responds. *American Journal of Nursing, 101*(5), 25.

Medical Tribune. (1997). AIDS file: Older adults overlooked. Quoted in *American Journal of Nursing, 98*(3), 25.

Meier, D. (2000, September 7). Fear, pain burden seriously ill, those who love them. *USA Today,* p. 27-A.

Menikoff, A. (1999). *Psychiatric home care: Clinical and economic dimensions.* San Diego: Academic Press.

Minnesota Hospice Organization. (1996). *Hospice care: A physician's guide.* St. Paul: Author.

Monks, K. (2000). *Pocket guide to home health nursing.* Philadelphia: Saunders.

Morrison, C. (2000). Fear of addiction: Balancing the facts and concerns about opioid use. *American Journal of Nursing, 100*(7), 81.

Murphy, P. (1997). Nursing's role in the assisted suicide debate. *American Journal of Nursing, 97*(6), 80.

National Association for Home Care. (Undated). How to choose a home care provider: A consumer's guide. Washington, DC: Author.

Nevil, N. (1997). *Socialization games for persons with disabilities: Structured group activities for social and interpersonal development.* Springfield, IL: Charles C Thomas.

Nguyen, B. (1999). Workplace protection: When are you protected under the Americans with Disabilities Act? *American Journal of Nursing, 99*(6), 70.

Nicholls, B. (1996). Rainbows. *Geriatric Nursing, 17*(2), 93.

Nuland, S. (2000, September 10). A witness to the final journey. *The New York Times,* p. 2.27.

Oncology Nursing Update 2001. (2001). *American Journal of Nursing* (Suppl, April), 1–52.

O'Neill, D., & Kenny, E. (1998). State of the science: Spirituality and chronic illness. *Image—the Journal of Nursing Scholarship, 30*(3), 275–280.

Parkman, C., & Calfee, B. (1997). Advance directives: Honoring your patient's end-of-life wishes. *Nursing 1997, 27*(4), 48–54.

Pasero, C., & McCaffery, M. (1999). Pain control: Managing breakthrough pain with OTFC (oral transmucosal fentanyl citrate). *American Journal of Nursing, 99*(4), 20.

Pasero, C. & McCaffery, M. (2001). Pain control: Hydromorphone. *American Journal of Nursing, 101*(2), 22–23.

Pasero, C., & McCaffery, M. (2001). Pain control: The lidocaine patch. *American Journal of Nursing, 101*(3), 22–23.

Perkins, E. (2000). Hospice comes to Blackberry Farm. *Nursing 2000, 30*(2), 53.

Pessagno, R. (1997). Postmortem care: Healing's first step. *Nursing 1997, 27*(4), 32a–b.

Phear, D. (1996). A study of animal companionship in a day hospice. *Journal of Palliative Medicine, 10*(4), 335–338.

Plaisance, L. (1997). The litany of the last meal. *American Journal of Nursing, 97*(3), 60–61.

Powers, P., Goldstein, C., et al. (2000). The value of patient and family-centered care. *American Journal of Nursing, 100*(5), 84–88.

Puopolo, A. (1999). Gaining confidence to talk about end-of-life care. *Nursing 1999, 29*(7), 49–51.

Quinn, P. (1997). *Understanding disability: A lifespan approach.* Thousand Oaks, CA: Sage.

Radcliffe, J., Webb, M., & Wood, B. (1997). Hospice nursing: A special calling. *Nursing 1997, 27*(1), 52–57.

Ray, M. (1997). *I'm here to help: A guide for caregivers, hospice workers and volunteers.* New York: Bantam.

Resnick, B. (2001). The restoration of independence. *American Journal of Nursing, 101*(10), 11.

Rice, R. (1999). *Handbook of home health nursing procedures.* St. Louis: Mosby.

Rice, R. (Ed.) (2001). *Home health nursing practice: Concepts and application* (3rd ed.). St. Louis: Mosby.

Saladay, S. (2000). Ask, don't tell. *Nursing 2000, 30*(8), 66–67.

Sauer, C. (2001). Death in the family. *Nursing Spectrum, 2*(1), 5.

Scholler-Jaquish, A. (1999). Palliating the pain of dying. *American Journal of Nursing, 99*(8), 15.

Schrader, C., et al. (1997). Community nursing organizations: A new frontier. *American Journal of Nursing, 97*(1), 63.

Sendor, V. (1997). *Hospice and palliative care: Questions and answers.* Lanham, MD: Scarecrow.

Sharp, A. (1996). *Gifts: Two hospice professionals reveal messages from those passing on.* Far Hills, NJ: New Horizon.

Sharp, A. (1999). Amanda's choice. *Nursing 1999, 29*(8), 48–52.

Silliman, S. (1997). *Medical management of stroke: A guide for rehabilitation specialists.* Gaithersburg, MD: Aspen.

Simon, S. (1999). Rachel's legacy. *Nursing 1999, 29*(4), 64.

Springhouse Corporation. (1997). *Pocket companion for home health nurses.* Springhouse, PA: Author.

Squires, A. (Ed.) (1996). *Rehabilitation of older people: A handbook for the multidisciplinary team* (2nd ed.). San Diego: Singular.

Stackhouse, J. (1998). *Into the community: Nursing in ambulatory and home care.* Philadelphia: Lippincott Williams & Wilkins.

Stalow, W. (1997). *Handbook of severe disability: A text for rehabilitation counselors, other vocational practitioners and allied health professionals.* New York: Gordon.

Stanhope, M., & Knollmueller, R. (2000). *Handbook of community-based home health nursing practice.* St. Louis: Mosby.

Steinke, E. (2000). Sexual counseling after myocardial infarction. *American Journal of Nursing, 100*(12), 38–43.

Sweeney, J. (1996). Nurses in home care: A success story. *Geriatric Nursing, 17*(4), 187–190.

Taylor, P. (2001). The trip of a lifetime. *Nursing 2001, 31*(4), 60–61.

Tesselaar, H. (1999). Joe wanted to die alone . . . or so he said. *Nursing 1999, 29*(5), 54–55.

Tully, J. (1999). Goodbye, old friend: A pet's death. *American Journal of Nursing, 99*(8), 24DDDD–24FFFF.

Tutka, M. (2001). Near-death experiences: Seeing the light. *Nursing 2001, 31*(5), 62–64.

U.S. Department of Health and Human Services. (2000). *Healthy people 2010.* McLean, VA: International Medical Publishing.

U.S. Department of Health and Human Services. (1996). Urinary incontinence in adults: Acute and chronic management. U.S. Public Health Service, (Agency for Health Care Policy and Research). Publication #96-0682. http://www.dhhs.gov.

Ufema, J. (1999) Grieving mother: Listen with your hospice heart. *Nursing 1999, 29*(3), 26.

Ufema, J. (1999). Comfort measures: Struggling with dyspnea. *Nursing 1999, 29*(8), 30.

Ufema, J. (1999). Reflections on death and dying. *Nursing 1999, 29*(6), 56–59.

Ufema, J. (1999). Talking trash: The abusive patient. *Nursing 1999, 29*(7), 22–23.

Ufema, J. (2000). When to clam up. *Nursing 2000, 30*(5), 22–23.

Ufema, J. (2001). Hospice volunteers: Top 10 tips. *Nursing 2001, 31*(4), 68–69.

Utterbach, K. (2001). Prospective payment comes to Medicare home health. *American Journal of Nursing, 101*(7), 59.

Vanderbeck, J. (2000). Till death do us part: A firsthand account of family presence. *American Journal of Nursing, 100*(2), 44.

Walsh, G. (1996). How subacute care fills the gap. *Nursing 1996,* Career Directory, 17.

Wells, S. (1996). Adding an "at home" path to your discharge plan. *American Journal of Nursing, 96*(10), 73–75.

Wheeler, S. (1996). Helping families cope with death and dying. *Nursing 1996, 26*(7), 25–31.

Wheeler, S. (2000). Telephone triage: Saved by the form. *Nursing 2000, 30*(11), 54–55.

Wheeler, S., & Siebelt, B. (1997). Calling all nurses: How to perform telephone triage. *Nursing 1997, 27*(7), 37–42.

Winslow, E. (2001). Patient education materials: Can patients read them? *American Journal of Nursing, 101*(10), 33–38.

Zang, S., & Allender, J. (1999). *Home care of the elderly.* Philadelphia: Lippincott Williams & Wilkins.

Zerwekh, J. (1997). Death, but little dignity. *American Journal of Nursing, 97*(3), 9–10.

Zerwekh, J. (1997). Do dying patients really need IV fluids? *American Journal of Nursing, 97*(3), 26–31.

Zerwekh, J. (1997). End of life care. *Nursing 1997, 27*(8), 55.

Zerwekh, J. (1997). Myths and facts: About medications for chronic cancer pain. *Nursing 1997, 27*(1), 25.

Zerzan, J. (2000). Access to palliative care and hospice in nursing homes. *Journal of the American Medical Association, 284*(19), 2489.

Zimmerman, K. (2001). Working in an underserved area? Federal program helps nurses repay student loans. *American Journal of Nursing, 101*(10), 24.

Unit XVI The Transition to Practicing Nurse

A career as a licensed practical nurse: Improving the lives of the ill, injured and elderly. (2000). Chicago, Institute for Research.

Alfaro-LeFevre, R. (1999). *Critical thinking in nursing: A practical approach.* Philadelphia: Saunders.

Allen, J. (1997). Are you ready for nursing in a developing country? *American Journal of Nursing, 97*(7), 36–38.

Anderson, M. (1997). *Nursing leadership, management and professional practice for the LPN/LVN.* Philadelphia: Davis.

Bagley, E. (1997). *Inside a job interview: Answers to the 15 most frequently asked questions* (4th ed.). Lacey, WA: Northwest Marketing.

Baxter, B. (1997). Nursing the net: Using the net to search for a job. *Nursing 1997, 27*(7), 26–27.

Beare, P. (1999). *Davis' NCLEX-PN review* (2nd ed.). Philadelphia: Davis.

Beatty, R. (1997). *The five-minute interview* (2nd ed.). New York: Wiley.

Bloch, D. (1997). *Have a winning job interview.* Lincolnwood, IL: NTC Contemporary Publishing (Here's How Series).

Bloch, D. (1997). *Write a winning resume.* Lincolnwood, IL: NTC Contemporary Publishing (Here's How Series).

Bolles, R. (1997). *The 1998 what color is your parachute? A practical manual for job-hunters and career changers* (rev. ed.). Berkeley, CA: Ten Speed Press.

Bradley, C. (2001). Your role in your annual performance evaluation. *American Journal of Nursing, 101*(7), 71–74.

Bromley, P., & Ehrenreich, D. (2001). Professional development: The journey of lifelong learning. *American Journal of Nursing, 101*(1), 73–74.

Cardillo, D. (2001). Myths about networking. *Nursing Spectrum, 2*(a), 28–29.

Cardillo, D. (2001). Job-hunting challenges take some trouble shooting. *Nursing Spectrum, 2*(8), 25.

Curtin, L., & the Editors of *Nursing 1996* (1996). Dispelling the myths about job security. *Nursing 1996,* Career Directory, 18–19.

Dheel, K. (2000). A spoonful of nursing. *Nursing 2000, 30*(6), 65.

Educational opportunities, 2001. (2001). *American Journal of Nursing,* Career Guide 2001, 132–133.

Eggland, E. (1997). Using computers to document. *Nursing 1997, 27*(1), 17.

Ellis, J., & Hartley, C. (1997). *Nursing in today's world: Challenges, issues, and trends* (6th ed.). Philadelphia: Lippincott-Raven.

Eyles, M. (2001). *Mosby's comprehensive review of practical nursing.* (1999). St. Louis: Mosby.

Farella, C. (2001) The secret to working happily ever after. *Nursing Spectrum, 2*(3), 20MW–21MW.

Filipovich, C. (1999). Dealing with the issue of inadequate staffing. *Nursing 1999, 29*(8), 54–56.

Five tips to manage your stress, faith, and your health. (1999). *Nursing 1999, 29*(3), 53. (Quoted from *Leading the way: Personal management skills for the long-term care nurse.* Cambridge, MA: Frontline, 1999.)

Grensing-Pophal, L. (1999). Multitasking made easy. *Nursing 1999, 19*(2), 55–56.

Hill, S., & Howlett, H. (1997). *Success in practical nursing: Personal and vocational issues* (3rd ed.). Philadelphia: Saunders.

Hill, S., & Howlett, H., et al. (2001). *Success in practical/vocational nursing: From student to leader* (4th ed.). Philadelphia: Saunders.

How to get a license. (2001). *American Journal of Nursing,* Career Guide 2001, 30–39.

Humphreys, K. (2000). Guide to nursing organizations 2001. *Nursing 2000, 30*(5), 46–48.

Hunt, B., James, M., & National Federation of LPNs Inc. (1997). Tomorrow's LPN: Understanding the role. *Nursing 1997, 97*(3), 52–53.

Kaltreider, N. (Ed.) (1998). *Dilemmas of a double life: Women balancing careers and relationships.* Northvale, NJ: Jason Aronson.

Kennedy, M. (2001). Nurses, and the nation, respond to disasters. *American Journal of Nursing, 101*(10), 18–19.

Kenney, E., (1998). Creating fulfillment in today's workplace. American Journal of Nursing, 98 (5), 44–48.

King, M., & Weston, L. (1995). How to organize a nursing portfolio. *Nursing 1995, 25*(8), 79, 82.

Kulig, N. (2001). Interstate licensure: Nursing beyond your state's borders. *Nursing 2001, 31*(2), 51.

Kurzen, C. (1996). *Contemporary practical/vocational nursing* (3rd ed.). Philadelphia: Lippincott-Raven.

McKeon, E. (2001). Nursing home staffing crisis. *American Journal of Nursing, 101*(5), 25.

Pronitis-Ruotolo, D. (2001). Surviving the night shift. *American Journal of Nursing, 101*(7), 63–68.

Ringsven, M. (1997). *Gerontology: Leadership skills for nurses* (2nd ed.) (LPN/LVN Nursing Series). Albany, NY: Delmar.

Rocchiccioli, J., Tilbury, M., & Eoyang, T. (1998). *Clinical leadership in nursing.* Philadelphia: Saunders.

Rubenfeld M., & Scheffer, B. (1999). *Critical thinking in nursing* (2nd ed.). Philadelphia: Lippincott Williams & Wilkins.

Russo, C. (2001). How to interview on your terms. *American Journal of Nursing,* Career Guide 2001, 17–18.

Schank, M., Weis, D., & Matheus, R. (1996). Parish nursing: Ministry of healing. *Geriatric Nursing, 17*(1), 11–13.

Smith, W. (2000). Setting up a home-based business. *American Journal of Nursing, 100*(2), 22.

Sofer, D., (1999). On the battleground. *American Journal of Nursing, 99*(9), 33–35.

Steinhauer, R. (2001). International nursing. *American Journal of Nursing,* Career Guide 2001, 12–15.

Symanski, M. (2000). A nurse on Mars? Why not? *American Journal of Nursing, 100*(10), 57–61.

Tappen, R., Weiss, S., & Whitehead, D. (1997). *Essentials of nursing leadership.* Philadelphia: Davis.

Thieman, L. (2001). Chicken soup for the nurse's soul. *Nursing 2001, 31*(5), 45.

Zerwekh, J., & Claborn, J. (2000). *NCLEX-PN: A study guide for practical nursing.* Dallas: Nursing Education Consultants.

Zimmermann, P. (1997). Advice PRN: Burning bridges. *Nursing 1997, 27*(11), 12.

Zimmermann, P. (1997). Getting a job: Dress rehearsals. *Nursing 1997, 27*(5), 12.

Zimmermann, P. (1997). *The complete idiot's guide to cover letters.* New York: Macmillan.

Zolot, J. (1999). Computer-based patient records. *American Journal of Nursing, 99*(12), 64–69.

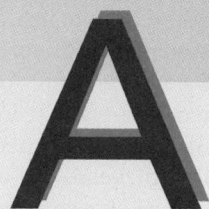

Key English-to-Spanish Healthcare Phrases

Although English is the primary language spoken in North America, a variety of languages are heard. Prominent among them is Spanish. According to the U.S. Census Bureau, Hispanics are the second largest minority group in the United States. Their number is projected to more than double in the next 50 years.

The client and family can be at ease and feel more relaxed if someone on the staff speaks their language. Some healthcare facilities, especially in areas with a large population of Spanish-speaking people, provide interpreters. In smaller communities, this may not be possible. For this reason, the following table of English-to-Spanish phrases has been prepared. Keep in mind that this is not a complete list. Rather, it contains key words and simple phrases that the nurse can use to communicate with a Spanish-speaking individual.

Here's how to use this table: Look for the word or phrase in English in the first column. Then look across to the second column for the word or phrase in Spanish. Use the third column, which contains the phonetic pronunciation, as a guide to speaking the word or phrase. The syllable in each word to be accented is printed in italic type.

Even if proficiency in English-to-Spanish is lacking, Spanish-speaking clients will appreciate the attempt to converse in their language. Begin with "Buenos días. ¿Cómo se siente?" And remember "por favor."*

INTRODUCTORY PHRASES

English	Spanish	Pronunciation
Please*	Por favor	Por fah-*vor*
Yes/No	Si/No	See/No
Thank you	Gracias	*Grah*-see-ahs
Good morning	Buenos dias	*Bway*-nos *dee*-ahs
Good afternoon	Buenas tardes	*Bway*-nas *tar*-days
Good evening	Buenas noches	*Bway*-nas *noh*-chays
My name is	Mi nombre es	Me *nohm*-bray ays
I am a student nurse.	Soy estudiante enfermera.	Soy ays-stoo-dee-*ayn*-tay ayn-fay-*may*-rah
What is your name?	¿Cómo se llama?	Koh-moh say *yah*-mah
How old are you?	¿Cuántos años tiene?	*Kwan*-tohs ahn-yos tee-*ayn*-ays
Do you understand me?	¿Me entiende?	Me ayn-tee-*ayn*-day
Speak slower.	Hable más despacio.	*Ah*-blah mahs days-*pah*-see-oh
How do you feel?	¿Cómo se siente?	*Koh*-moh say see-*ayn*-tay

NUMBERS

English	Spanish	Pronunciation
Zero	Cero	*Se*-roh
One	Uno	*Oo*-noh
Two	Dos	Dohs
Three	Tres	Trays
Four	Cuatro	*Kwah*-troh
Five	Cinco	*Sin*-koh
Six	Seis	Says
Seven	Siete	See-*ay*-tay
Eight	Ocho	Oh-choh
Nine	Nueve	New-*ay*-vay
Ten	Diez	*Dee*-ays

DAYS OF THE WEEK

English	Spanish	Pronunciation
Sunday	Domingo	Doh-*ming*-goh
Monday	Lunes	*Loo*-nays
Tuesday	Martes	*Mar*-tays
Wednesday	Miércoles	Mee-*er*-cohl-ays
Thursday	Jueves	*Hway*-vays
Friday	Viernes	Vee-*ayr*-nays
Saturday	Sábado	*Sah*-bah-doh

GENERAL TERMS

English	Spanish	Pronunciation
Good	Bien	Bee-ayn
Bad	Mal	Mahl
Physician	Médico	*May*-dee-koh
Hospital	Hospital	*Ooh*-spee-tall
Midwife	Comadre	Koh-*mah*-dray
Native Healer	Curandero	Ku-ren-*day*-roh
Right	Derecha	Day-*ray*-chah
Left	Izquierda	Ees-kee-*ayr*-dah
Week	Semana	Say-*mah*-nah
Month	Mes	Mace
A prescription	Una receta	*Oo*-na ray-*say*-tah
Pulse	Tomar su pulso	*Pool*-soh
Temperature	Temperatura	Taym-pay-rah-*too*-rah
Blood pressure	Presión	Pray-see-*ohn*
IV line	Intravenosa	Een-trah-vayn-*oh*-sah
Pain medicine	Medicación para dolor	May-dee-kah-see-*ohn* pah-rah doh-*lohr*
Enema	Lavado	Lah-*vah*-doh
Unusual vaginal bleeding?	¿Hemorragia vaginal fuera de los periodos?	Ay-moh-*rah*-hee-ah *vah*-hee-nahl foo-*ay*-rah day lohs pay-ree-*oh*-dohs
Hoarseness?	¿Ronquera?	Rohn-*kay*-rah
A sore throat?	¿Le duele la garganta?	Lay doo-*ay*-lay lah gahr-gahn-tah
Does it hurt to swallow?	¿Le duele al tragar?	Lay doo-ay-lay ahl trah-gar
Difficulty in breathing?	¿Dificultad al respirar?	Dee-fee-kool-*tahd* ahl rays-*pee*-rahr
Is your memory good?	¿Es buena su memoria?	Ays *bway*-nah soo may-moh-*ree*-ah
Have you any pain in the head?	¿Le duele la cabeza?	Lay doo-*ay*-lay lah kah-*bay*-sah
Do you feel dizzy?	¿Tiene usted vértigo?	Tee-*ay*-nay ood-stayd *vehr*-tee-goh

* Begin or end any request with the word PLEASE (POR FAVOR).

Are you tired?	¿Está usted cansado?	Ay-*stah* ood-*stayd* kahn-*sah*-doh
Can you eat?	¿Puede comer?	*Pway*-day koh-*mer*
Are you constipated?	¿Está estreñido?	Ay-*stah* ays-trayn-*yee*-do
Do you have diarrhea?	¿Tiene diarrea?	Tee-*ay*-nay dee-ah-*ray*-ah
Have you any difficulty passing water?	¿Tiene dificultad en orinar?	Tee-*ay*-nay dee-fee-kool-*tahd* ayn oh-ree-*nahr*
Do you hear voices?	¿Oye los voces?	Oy-eh los *vo*-ses

BEDSIDE CARE

Warm	Calor	Kahl-*or*
Cold	Frío	*Free*-oh
Milk	Leche	*Leh*-chay
Tea	Té	Tay
Coffee	Café	Kah-*fay*

TIMES OF THE DAY

Early in the morning	Temprano por la mañana	Tehm-*prah*-noh por lah mah-*nyah*-na
In the daytime	En el día	Ayn el *dee*-ah
At noon	A mediodía	Ah meh-dee-oh-*dee*-ah
At bedtime	Al acostarse	Al ah-kos-*tar*-say
At night	Por la noche	Por la *noh*-chay
Today	Hoy	Oy
Tomorrow	Mañana	Mah-*nyah*-nah
Yesterday	Ayer	Ai-*yer*
Before meals	Antes de las comidas	*Ahn*-tays day lahs koh-*mee*-dahs
After meals	Después de las comidas	*Days*-poo-ehs day lahs koh-mee-dahs
Every day	Todos los días	*Toh*-dohs lohs *dee*-ah
Every hour	Cada hora	*Kah*-dah *oh*-rah

QUESTIONS TO BEGIN PHRASES

Do you have . . .?	¿Tiene . . .?	Tee-*ay*-nay
Are you . . .?	¿Tiene . . .?	Tee-*ay*-nay
How long . . .?	¿Hace cúanto . . .?	*Ah*-say *kwahn*-toh
How much . . .?	¿Cuánto . . .?	*Kwahn*-toh
How . . .?	¿Cómo . . .?	*Ko*-mo

SIGNS AND SYMPTOMS

Pain?	¿Dolor?	Doh-*lorh*
Stomach cramps?	¿Calambres en el estómago?	Kah-*lahm*-brays ayn el ays-*toh*-mah-goh
Chills?	¿Escalofrios?	Ays-kah-loh-*free*-ohs
Hemorrhage?	¿Hemorragia?	Ay-moh-*rah*-hee-ah
Nosebleeds?	¿Hemorragia por la nariz?	Ay-moh-*rah*-hee-ah por-lah nah-*rees*
Where is the pain?	¿Donde está el dolor?	*Dohn*-day ay-*stah* ayl doh-*lorh*
Do you want medication for your pain?	¿Quire medicación para su dolor?	Key-*ay*-ray may-dee-kah-see-*ohn* *pa*-rah soo doh-*lorh*
Are you comfortable?	¿Está comfortable?	Ay-*stah* kohm-for-*tah*-blay
Are you hungry?	¿Tiene hambre?	Tee-*ay*-nay ahm-bray
Are you thirsty?	¿Tiene sed?	Tee-*ay*-nay sayd
You may not eat/drink.	No coma/beba.	Noh *koh*-mah/bay-*bah*
You can drink only water.	Sólo puede tomar agua.	Soh-loh *pway*-day toh-mar *ah*-gwah
You can take only ice chips.	Solo puéde tomár pedacitos de hiélo.	Soh-loh *pway*-day toh-*marh* pay-da-*zee*-tohs day eee-*ay*-loh
Keep very quiet.	Estése muy quieto.	Ays-*tay*-say moo-ay key-*ay*-toh

B

Key Abbreviations and Acronyms Used in Healthcare

↑ICP	Increased intracranial pressure
2hPP	2-hour postprandial
4P	Passage, passenger, powers, psyche
5-FU	5-Fluorouracil
A & O × 3	Alert and oriented to person, place, time
AAFP	American Academy of Family Physicians
AALPN	American Association of Licensed Practical Nurses
AAMI	Age-associated memory impairment
AAP	American Academy of Pediatricians
AARP	American Association of Retired Persons
AB	Abortion
Ab	Antibody
ABCDE	Airway, breathing, circulation, disability, expose, and examine
ABG	Arterial blood gas
ABP	Acute bacterial prostatitis
ABR	Auditory brain response
AC	Adriamycin and Cytoxan
ACE	All cotton elastic; angiotensin-converting enzyme
ACIP	Advisory Committee on Immunization Practices
ACLS	Advanced Cardiac Life Support
ACS	American Cancer Society; Ambulatory Care Sensitive
ACDA	Adult children of alcoholics
ACTH	Adrenocorticotrophic hormone
AD	Advance directive; Alzheimer's disease
ADA	American Diabetes Association
ADAMHA	Alcohol, Drug Abuse, and Mental Health Administration
ADC	AIDS dementia complex
ADDH	Attention deficit disorder with hyperactivity
ADH	Antidiuretic hormone
ADHD	Attention deficit hyperactivity disorder
ADL	Activities of daily living
AEA	Above-the-elbow amputation
AEB	As Evidenced By
AED	Automated External Defibrillator
AER	Auditory evoked response
AFP	Alpha fetoprotein; α-fetoprotein
Ag	Antigen
AGA	Appropriate-for-gestational age
AH	Auditory hallucination
AHA	American Hospital Association
AHCPR	Agency for Health Care Policy and Research
AI	Adequate intake
AICD	Automatic implantable cardioverter-defibrillator
AIDS	Acquired immunodeficiency syndrome
AIMS	Abnormal involuntary movement scale
AJN	American Journal of Nursing
AKA	Above-the-knee amputation; also known as
ALC	Acute lethal catatonia
ALL	Acute lymphocytic leukemia
ALS	Amyotrophic lateral sclerosis
ALT	Alanine aminotransferase (formerly SGPT)
AMA	American Medical Association or Against medical advice
AML	Acute myelogenous leukemia
AMSIT	Appearance, mood, sensorium, intelligence, thought process
ANA	American Nurses Association
ANCC	American Nurses Credentialing Center
ANP	Atrial natriuretic peptide
ANS	Autonomic Nervous System
AOB	Alcohol on breath
AP	Apical pulse or anteroposterior; anterior-posterior (repair); assault precautions (attack)
APA	American Psychiatric Association
APE	Acute psychotic episode
APGAR	A = appearance (color) P = pulse (heart rate) G = grimace or reflexes (irritability) A = activity (muscle tone) R = respiratory effort
APHA	American Public Health Association
APIE	Assessment, Plan, Intervention, Evaluation
APTT	Activated partial thromboplastin time
A-R	Apical radial (pulse)
ARC	American Red Cross
ARDD	Alcohol-related developmental disability
ARDS	Adult respiratory distress syndrome
ARND	Alcohol-related neurodevelopmental disorder
AROM	Active range of motion; artificial rupture of the membranes
ARRP	Anatomic retropubic radical prostatectomy
ART	Accredited record technician
AS	Aortic stenosis
ASA	Acetylsalicyclic acid (aspirin)
ASD	Atrial septal defect; autism spectrum disorders
ASO	Antistreptolysin-O titer
AST	Aspartate aminotransferase
ASU	Ambulatory Surgery Unit
ATF	Alcohol, Tobacco, and Firearms
ATLS	Advanced Trauma Life Support
ATN	Acute tubular necrosis
ATP	Adenosine triphosphate
AV (node)	Atrioventricular (node)
AV valves	Atrioventricular valves
AVPU	Alert, verbal, pain response, unresponsive
AWOL	Absent without leave

Note: These are examples and may differ slightly from facility to facility.

Ax	Axillary
BAL in oil	Dimercaprol
BBB	Blood–brain barrier
BBP	Blood-borne pathogens
BBT	Basal body temperature
BCG	Bacille Calmette-Guérin
BCLS	Basic Cardiac Life Support
BCP	Birth control pill
BDI	Beck depression inventory
BE	Barium enema x-ray
BEA	Below-the-elbow amputation
BIDS	Bedtime insulin and daytime sulfonylureas
BKA	Below-the-knee amputation
BLL	Blood lead level
BLS, BCLS	Basic (Cardiac) Life Support
BM	Bowel movement
BMI	Body mass index
BMT	Bone marrow transplantation
BOA	Born out of asepsis
BOH	Board of Health
BP	Blood pressure
BPAD	Bipolar affective disorder
BPD	Bipolar disorder
BPH	Benign prostatic hyperplasia
BPM	Beats per minute
BPRS	Brief Psychiatric Rating Scale
BRAT	Bananas, rice, applesauce, toast
BRM	Biological response modifiers
BRP	Bathroom privileges
BS	Bowel sounds
BSC	Bedside commode
BSE	Breast self-examination
BUN	Blood urea nitrogen
C	Celsius or centigrade
C-2, C-3, etc.	Refers to level of injury in the cervical section of the spinal cord
CA	Cancer
Ca^{++}	Calcium
$Ca_3[PO_4]_2$	Calcium phosphate
CABG	Coronary artery bypass grafting
$CaCl_2$	Calcium chloride
$CaCO_3$	Calcium carbonate
CAD	Coronary artery disease
CAF	Cytoxan, Adriamycin, fluorouracil
CAM	Complementary and alternative medicine
CAPD	Continuous ambulatory peritoneal dialysis
CAT	Computerized adaptive testing
CBC	Complete blood count
CBE	Charting by exception
CBP	Chronic bacterial prostatitis
cc	cubic centimeter
CC	Chief complaint
CCP	Clinical care pathway
CCU/CICU	Coronary care unit/coronary intensive care unit
CD	Chemical dependency
CD4	Helper T lymphocytes
CDC	Centers for Disease Control and Prevention
CDU	Chemical dependency unit, clinical decision unit
CEA	Carcinoembryonic antigen; cultured epithelial autografts
CEH	Continuing education hour
CF	Cystic fibrosis
CHAP	Community Health Accreditation Program
CHC	Community Health Center
CHD	Coronary heart disease
CHF	Congestive heart failure
CHHA	Certified Home Health Aide
CHI	Closed head injury
CHO	Carbohydrates
CHT	Closed head trauma
CIC	Crisis Intervention Center
CICU	Coronary intensive care unit
CJD	Creutzfeldt-Jacob disease
CK	Creatine kinase
Cl	Chloride
CLL	Chronic lymphocytic leukemia
CLTC	Citizens for Long-Term Care
CM	Case/care manager
CMF	Cyclophosphamide, methotrexate, and fluorouracil
CMG	Cystometrogram
CMHC	Community mental health center
CML	Chronic myelogenous leukemia
CMMS	Medicare and Medicaid Services
CMS	Color, motion, sensitivity (circulation, mobility, sensation)
CMV	Cytomegalovirus
CNM	Certified Nurse Midwife
CNO	Community Nursing Organization
CNS	Central nervous system
CO	Cardiac output
CO2	Carbon dioxide
COA	Children of alcoholics
COA	Coarctation of the aorta
COLD	Chronic obstructive lung disease
COPD	Chronic obstructive pulmonary disease
COP	Conditions of participation (Medicare)
COTA	Certified occupational therapy assistant
CP	Cardiopulmonary
CP	Cerebral palsy
CPAP	Continuous positive airway pressure
CPD	Cephalopelvic disproportion
CPK	Creatinine phosphokinase
CPM	Continuous passive motion
CPMI	Chronic and persistent mental illness
CPR	Cardiopulmonary resuscitation
CPT	Chest physiotherapy
CQI	Contiguous (or continuous) quality improvement
CRH	Corticotropin-releasing hormone

CRNA	Certified Registered Nurse Anesthetist	DSM-IV	Diagnostic and Statistical Manual of Mental Disorders, Revision IV
CRNH	Certified Registered Nurse—Hospice	DT	Diphtheria and tetanus toxoids
CRP	C-reactive protein	DTAD	Drain tube attachment device
CRU	Coronary rehabilitation unit	DTaP	Diphtheria, tetanus, acellular pertussis
Cryo	Cryoprecipitate		
CS	Complete stroke	DTP	Diphtheria and tetanus toxoids and pertussis vaccine
CS	Cardiac sphincter		
C & S	(Blood) culture and sensitivity	DUI	Driving under the influence
C&S	Culture and sensitivity	DVR	Division of Vocational Rehabilitation
CSF	Cerebrospinal spinal fluid; colony-stimulating factors	DVT	Deep-vein thrombosis
		EAR	Estimated average requirement
CSR, CSS	Central supply room, central service supply	EBV	Epstein-Barr virus
CT	Computed tomography	EC	Emergency contraception
CUC	Chronic ulcerative colitis	ECF	Extended-care facility or extracellular fluid
CVA	Cerebrovascular accident		
CVP	Central venous pressure	ECG (EKG)	Electrocardiogram
CVS	Chorionic villus sampling	ECR	Emergency chemical restraints
CXR	Chest x-ray	ECT	Electroconvulsive therapy
$D_5\frac{1}{2}NS$	Dextrose in half-normal saline (0.45% NS)	ED	Emergency Department; erectile dysfunction
D_5NS	Dextrose in normal saline (0.9% NS)	EDC	Estimated date of confinement
D_5W	Dextrose in sterile water	EDD	Estimated date of delivery
DAPE	Data, assessment, plan, evaluation	EDTA	Edetate calcium disodium
DARE	Data, action, response, education	EEG	Electroencephalogram or electroencephalography
DAT	Diet as tolerated		
Db	Decibel	EGD	Esophagogastroduodenoscopy
DBP	Diastolic blood pressure	EHS	Employee Health Service
D/C	Discontinue	e-IPV	Enhanced potency inactivated poliovirus vaccine
D&C	Dilation and curettage		
DCH	District court hold	ELISA	Enzyme-linked immunosorbent assay
DCT	Distal convoluted tubule	EMB	Ethambutol
DDST	Denver Developmental Screening Test	EMG	Electromyogram
DEA	Drug Enforcement Agency	EMS	Emergency Medical Services
DEP	Department of Environmental Protection	EMT	Emergency Medical Technician
		ENG	Electronystagmography
DERM	Dermatology	EP	Escape (elopement) precautions
DES	Diethylstilbestrol	EPA	Environmental Protection Agency
DIC	Disseminated intravascular coagulation	EPO	Erythropoietin
DISCUS	Dyskinesia Identification System-Condensed User Scale	EPR	Emergency physical restraints
		EPS	Electrophysiologic study
DJD	Degenerative joint disease	EPSE	Extrapyramidal side effects
DKA	Diabetic ketoacidosis	ER	Emergency room
dL	Deciliter	ERCP	Endoscopic retrograde cholangiopancreatography
DM	Dextromethorphan		
DMAT	Disaster Medical Assistance Team	ERG	Electroretinogram
DMD	Duchenne muscular dystrophy	ERT	Estrogen replacement therapy
DME	Durable medical equipment	ERV	Expiratory reserve volume
DMSA	2, 3-dimercaptosuccinic acid	ESR	Erythrocyte sedimentation rate (also see Sed Rate)
DNA	Deoxyribonucleic acid		
DNH	Do not hospitalize	ESRD	End-stage renal disease
DNI	Do not intubate	ESWL	Extracorporeal shock wave lithotripsy
DNR	Do not resuscitate	ET	Enterostomal therapist
DOA	Department of Agriculture	ETOH (EtOH) W/D	Alcohol withdrawal
DOH	Department of Health		
DOL	Department of Labor		
DRF	Drip rate factor	F	Fahrenheit
DRG	Diagnosis-related groups	FADL	Functional activities of daily living
DRI	Dietary reference intake		

FAI	Functional assessment inventory
FAM	Fertility awareness method
FAS	Fetal alcohol syndrome
FBP	Fetal biophysical profile
FBS/FBG	Fasting blood sugar (fasting blood glucose)
FDA	Food and Drug Administration
Fe^{++}	Iron
FES	Functional electrical stimulation
FFP	Fresh frozen plasma
FHC	Family Health Center
FHR	Fetal heart rate
FHT	Fetal heart tones
FOI	Flight of ideas
FPG	Fasting plasma glucose
FQHC	Federally Qualified Healthcare
FRC	Functional residual capacity
FRV	Functional residual volume
FSH	Follicle-stimulating hormone
FTT	Failure to thrive
FVD	Fluid volume deficit
FVE	Fluid volume excess
G$_6$PD	Glucose 6-phosphodehydrogenase
G	Gauge
GABHS	Group A beta-hemolytic streptococcus
GCS	Glasgow Coma Scale
GDM	Gestational diabetes mellitus
GERD	Gastroesophageal reflux disease
GERI	Geriatrics
GFR	Glomerular filtration rate
GH	Growth hormone
GHB	Gamma hydroxybutyrate
GHIH	Growth hormone-inhibiting hormone
GI (tract)	Gastrointestinal (tract)
GnRH	Gonadotropin-releasing hormone
GRH, GHRH	Growth hormone-releasing hormone
GP	General precautions
GTT	Glucose tolerance test
G-tube	Gastrostomy tube
GU	Genitourinary
GYN	Gynecology
H$^+$	Hydrogen ion
H$_2$CO$_3$	Carbonic acid
H$_2$O, HOH	Water
HAV	Hepatitis A virus
Hazmat	Hazardous materials
Hb	Hemoglobin
Hb A$_{1c}$	Glycosylated hemoglobin
HBD	Hydroxybutyric dehydrogenase
HBO	Hyperbaric oxygenation
HBV	Hepatitis B virus
HCA	Health care assistant
HCFA	Health Care Financing Administration (payor source)
HCG	Human chorionic gonadotropin
HCl	Hydrochloric acid

HCO$_3^-$	Bicarbonate ion
H$_2$CO$_3$	Carbonic acid
Hct	Hematocrit
HCTZ	Hydrochlorothiazide
HCV	Hepatitis C virus
HD	Hodgkin's disease
HD	Huntington's disease
HDL	High-density lipoprotein
HDRS	Hamilton depression rating scale
HDV	Hepatitis D virus
HEV	Hepatitis E virus
H flu	*Hemophilus influenzae*
HFCS	High-fructose corn syrup
Hgb or Hb	Hemoglobin
HGF	Hematopoietic factor
hGH	Human growth factor
HGV	Hepatitis G virus
HHA	Home health aide
HHRG	Home Health Resource Group
HHS	Department of Health and Human Services
HI	Homicidal ideation
Hib	*Haemophilus influenzae* type-B conjugate vaccine
HICPAC	Hospital Infection Control Practices Advisory Committee
HIS	Indian Health Service
HIV	Human immunodeficiency virus
HIV-RNA	Viral load of HIV
HMO	Health maintenance organization
HNP	Herniated nucleus pulposus
HOSA	Health Occupations Students of America
hPL	Human placental lactogen
H$_3$PO$_4$	Phosphoric acid
HPV	Human papilloma virus
HR	Heart rate
HRT	Hormone replacement therapy
HS	Hour of sleep
HSA	Health Services Administration
HSV-1	Herpes simplex virus type 1
HSV-2	Herpes simplex virus type 2
HTN	hypertension
HUS	hemolytic uremic syndrome
I&O	Intake and output
IADL	Instrumental activities of daily living
IBD	Inflammatory bowel disease
IBS	Irritable bowel syndrome
IBW	Ideal body weight
IC	Inspiratory capacity; interstitial cystitis
ICD	Implantable cardioverter-defibrillator
ICF	Intermediate care facility
ICN	International Council of Nurses
ICP	Intracranial pressure
ICSH	Interstitial cell-stimulating hormone
ICU	Intensive care unit
ID	Identification
IDDM	Insulin-dependent diabetes mellitus

IDG	Interdisciplinary group	LBW	Low birth weight
IDT	Interdisciplinary team	LCA	Left coronary artery
IFG	Impaired fasting glucose	LCX	Left circumflex
IFN	Interferon	LDH	Lactic dehydrogenase
IG	Immune globulins	LDL	Low-density lipoprotein
Ig	immunoglobulin	LDRP	Labor/delivery/recovery/postpartum room
IgE	Immunoglobulin E		
IgG	Gamma immunoglobulin (gamma globulin)	LEEP	Loop electrosurgical excision procedure
		LEP	Laparascopic extraperitonal approach
IGH	Impaired glucose homeostasis	LES	Lower esophageal sphincter
IGT	Impaired glucose tolerance	LFT	Liver function tests
IHS	Indian Health Service	LGA	Large for gestational age
II	Intellectual impairment	LH	Luteinizing hormone
IICP	Increased intracranial pressure	LITT	Laser-induced interstitial thermotherapy
IL	Interleukin	LLQ	Left lower quadrant
InFeD	Iron dextran	LMCA	Left main coronary artery
INH	Isoniazid	LMP	Last menstrual period
INR	International normalized ratio	LNMP	Last normal menstrual period
IOL implant	Intraocular lens implant	LOC	Level of consciousness
IOL	Intraocular lens	LOP	Left occiput posterior
IOP	Intraocular pressure	LP	Lumbar puncture
IPPB	Intermittent positive pressure breathing	LPM, L/min	Liters per minute
IPV	Inactive polio vaccine	LPN/LVN	Licensed Practical Nurse/Licensed Vocational Nurse
IQ	Intelligence quotient		
IR	Infrared (rays)	LQR/LSR	Locked quiet room/locked seclusion room
IRV	Inspiratory reserve volume		
ITP	Idiopathic thrombocytopenic purpura	LS ratio	Lecithin-sphingomyelin ratio
IUD	intrauterine device	LSD	Lysergic acid diethylamide
IV	Intravenous	LT	Leukotriene
IVC	Inferior vena cava	LTB	Laryngotracheobronchitis
IVD	Intervertebral disk disease	LTC	Long-term care
IVF	In vitro fertilization	LUQ	Left upper quadrant
IVIG	Intravenous immune globulin	MADD	Mothers Against Drunk Driving
IVP	Intravenous pyelogram	MABP	Mean arterial blood pressure
IVPB	Intravenous piggyback	MAC	Mycobacterium avium complex
JCAHO	Joint Commission on Accreditation of Healthcare Organizations	MAOI	Monoamine oxidase inhibitor
		MAP	Mean arterial pressure
JGA, JG apparatus	Juxtaglomerular apparatus	MAR	Medication administration record
		MAST	Military antishock trousers
JP	Jackson-Pratt (drains)	MCHB	Maternal Child Health Bureau
JRA	Juvenile rheumatoid arthritis	MD	Muscular dystrophy; Medical Doctor
J-tube	Jejunostomy tube	MDD	Major depressive disorder
K+	Potassium	MDI	Metered dose inhaler
kcal or C	Kilocalorie	MDS	Minimum data set
KCl	Potassium chloride	mEq	Milliequivalents
KELS	Kohlman evaluation of living skills	mEq/L	Milliequivalents per liter
KOH	Potassium hydroxide	Mg++	Magnesium
KUB	Kidney-ureters-bladder x-ray	MG	Myasthenia gravis
L-1, L-2, etc.	Refers to level of injury in the lumbar area of the spinal cord	mg/dL	Milligrams per deciliter
		MgSO4	Magnesium sulfate
LAD	Left anterior descending	MH, MHU	Mental health unit
LASIK	Laser in situ keratomileusis	MI	Myocardial infarction; mental illness
LATCH	L = Latch	MI & D	Mentally ill and dangerous
	A = Audible swallowing	MI-CD	Mentally ill and chemically dependent
	T = Type of nipple	MICU	Medical intensive care unit
	C = Comfort (breast/nipple)	MID	Multi-infarct dementia
	H = Hold (positioning)	MIF	Melanocyte inhibiting

MIS	Management information services/ systems	NIH	National Institutes of Health
mL	Milliliters	NINR	National Institute of Nursing Research
MMI	Methimazole	NIOSH	National Institute of Occupational Safety and Health
MMPI	Minnesota Multiphasic Personality Inventory	NLN	National League for Nursing
MMR	Measles, mumps, and rubella	NMR	Nuclear magnetic resonance
MMSE	Mini mental status exam	NMS	Neuroleptic malignant syndrome
MOAB	Monoclonal antibodies	NOS	Not otherwise specified
MOM	Milk of magnesia	NP	Nurse Practitioner
MPD	Multiple personality disorder	NPO	Nothing by mouth
MRI	Magnetic resonance imaging	NPT	Nocturnal penile tumescence
MRSA	Methicillin-resistant *Staphylococcus aureus*	NRM	Non-rebreathing mask
MS	Morphine sulfate	NS	Normal saline or 0.9% sodium chloride
MS	Multiple sclerosis	NSAID	Nonsteroidal anti-inflammatory drug
MSAFP	Maternal serum alpha-fetoprotein	NSC	National Safety Council
MSDS	Material Safety Data Sheet	NST	Nonstress test
MSH	melanocyte-stimulating hormone	NTG	Nitroglycerin
MSW	Medical social worker	O & P	Ova (eggs) and parasites
MUA	Medically underserved areas	O_2	Oxygen
MVA	Motor vehicle accident	O_2Sat	Percent oxygen saturation
Na^+	Sodium	OA	Osteoarthritis
Na_2SO_4	Sodium sulfate	OASIS	Outcome and Assessment Information Set
NACHC	National Association of Community Health Centers	OB	Obstetrics
NaCl	Sodium chloride	OB/GYN	Obstetrician/gynecologist
NAHC	National Association for Home Care	OBRA	Omnibus Budget Reconciliation Act
NAHCC	National Association of Health Care Centers	OBS/OBD	Organic brain syndrome/organic brain disorder
NANDA	North American Nursing Diagnosis Association	OBT	Over-bed table
NaOH	Sodium hydroxide	OCD	Obsessive-compulsive disorder
NAPNES	National Association of Practical Nurse Education and Services	OCT	Oxytocin challenge test
		OD	Overdose; right eye (oculus dexter)
NCHS	National Center for Health Statistics	OFC	Occipital-frontal circumference
NCI	National Cancer Institute	OH^-	hydroxyl ion
NCLEX-PN	National Council Licensure Examination for Practical Nurses	OMH	Office for Migrant Health
		ONS	Oncology Nursing Society
NCLEX-RN	National Council Licensure Examination for Registered Nurses	OOB	Out of bed
		OP	Occiput posterior, direct
NCP	Nursing care plan	OPD	Outpatient department
NCSBN	National Council of State Boards of Nursing	OPHS	Office of Public Health and Science
		OPV	Oral poliovirus vaccine (Live)
NEC	Necrotizing enterocolitis	OR	Operating room
NEURO	Neurology	ORIF	Open reduction and internal fixation
NF	National Formulary	ORS	Oral rehydration solution
NFLPN	National Federation of Licensed Practical Nurses	ORTHO	Orthopedics
		OS	Left eye (oculus sinister)
NG (tube)	Nasogastric (tube)	OSHA	Occupational Safety and Health Administration
NHIC	National Health Information Center	OT	Occupational therapy
NHL	Non-Hodgkin's lymphoma	OTC	Over the counter
NHP	Nursing Home Placement	OTFC	Oral transmucosal fentanyl citrate
NHPCO	National Hospice and Palliative Care Organization	OTR	Occupational Therapist, Registered
		OU	Both eyes (oculi unitas)
NICU	Neonatal Intensive Care Unit	P	Phosphorus
NIDDM	Non–insulin-dependent diabetes mellitus	PA	Physician Assistant
		PACE	Pre-Admission and Classification Examination

paCO₂ or pCO₂	Partial pressure (p) of carbon dioxide (CO_2) in arterial blood (a)	PPN	Peripheral parenteral nutrition
PACU	Postanesthesia care unit	PPO	Preferred provider organization
PADS	Preventive aggression device system	PPS	Prospective payment system
paO₂ or pO₂	Oxygen content of arterial blood	PR/R	Per rectum/rectal
Pap test	Papanicolaou test (smear)	PRH	Prolactin-releasing hormone
PAR	Postanesthesia recovery (room)	PRK	Photorefractive keratotomy
PBI	Protein-bound iodine	PRL	Prolactin
PBSC	Peripheral blood stem cell	PRM	Partial-rebreathing mask
PCA	Patient-controlled analgesia; personal care attendant	PRN	As needed
		PROM	Passive range of motion; premature rupture of membranes
PCM	Protein-calorie malnutrition	PSA	Prostate-specific antigen
PCN	Penicillin	PSDA	Patient Self-Determination Act
PCP	*Pneumocystis carinii* pneumonia; primary care provider	psi	Per square inch
		PSV	Pressure support ventilation
PCT	Proximal convoluted tubule	PSYCH	Psychiatry, represented by the Greek psi (Ψ)
PD	Provisional discharge	PT	Prothrombin time
PDA	Patent ductus arteriosus	PT	Physical therapy
PDA	Posterior descending artery	PTA	Physical therapist assistant
PDR	Physician's Desk Reference	PTCA	Percutaneous transluminal coronary angioplasty
PDT	Photodynamic therapy		
PE	Physical examination	PTH	Parathyroid hormone; parathormone
PE tubes	Polyethylene tubes	PTL	Preterm labor
PEDS	Pediatrics	PTSD	Post-traumatic stress disorder
PEG tube	Percutaneous endoscopic gastrostomy tube	PTT	Partial thromboplastin time
PEP	Postexposure prophylaxis	PTU	Propylthiouracil
PERRLA+C	Pupils equal, round, react to light, accommodation OK, and coordinated	PUBS	Percutaneous umbilical blood sampling
		PUS	Prostate ultrasound
PET	Positron emission tomography scan	PVC	Premature ventricular contraction
PFT	Pulmonary function test	PZA	Pyrazinamide
pH	Potential of hydrogen or power of hydrogen (hydrogen ion concentration)	QA	Quality assurance
		QI	Quality improvement
PIA	Prolonged infantile apnea	R/T	Related to
PIC	Peripheral indwelling catheter	RA	Rheumatoid arthritis
PICC	Peripherally inserted central catheter	RAA system	Renin-angiotensin-aldosterone system
PICU	Pediatric Intensive Care Unit	RACE	Rescue, alarm, confine, extinguish
PID	Pelvic inflammatory disease	RAI/RAIU	Radioactive iodine (uptake)
PIE	Plan, Intervention, Evaluation	RAP	Resident assessment protocol
PIH	Pregnancy-induced hypertension, prolactin-inhibiting hormone	RAS	Reticular activating system
		RBC	Red blood cell
PKR	Photorefractive keratotomy	RCA	Right coronary artery
PKU	Phenylketonuria	RDA	Recommended dietary allowance
PM&R	Physical Medicine and Rehabilitation	RDS	Respiratory distress syndrome
PMI	Point of maximal impulse	REE	Resting energy expenditure
PMP	Previous menstrual period	REHAB	Rehabilitation unit
PMS	Premenstrual syndrome	REM	Rapid eye movement
PNS	Peripheral nervous system	RET	Rational emotive therapy
PO	By mouth (per os)	RF	Rheumatoid factor
PO₄⁻	Phosphate	RGP	Rigid gas-permeable plastic
POC	Plan of care	RGP lens	Rigid gas-permeable lens
POS	Point of service	Rh+	Rh positive
PPD	Purified protein derivative	Rh−	Rh negative
PPE	Personal protective equipment	RhoGAM®	Rh immune globulin
PPF	Plasma protein fraction	RICE	Rest, ice, compression, elevation
PPG	Postprandial glucose	RIE	Recorded in error
PPI	Proton pump inhibitor	RIND	Reversible ischemic neurologic deficit
PPIP	Put prevention into practice	RK	Radial keratotomy

RLQ	Right lower quadrant	SOBOE	Short of breath on exertion
RMP	Rifampin	SP	Suprapubic (catheter)
RN	Registered Nurse	SP/GP	Suicide precautions/general precautions
RNA	Ribonucleic acid	SPECT	Single photon emission computed
ROI	Release of information		tomography
ROM	Range of motion	SPF	Sun protective factor
ROP	Retinopathy of prematurity; right occiput	SR	Sustained release
	posterior	SRO	Single room occupancy
RP	Retinitis pigmentosa	SROM	Spontaneous rupture of the membranes
RPh	Registered Pharmacist	SSA	Social Security Administration
RPT	Registered Physical Therapist	SSDI	Social Security Disability Insurance
RR	Recovery room	SSE	Soap suds enema
RRA	Registered Record Administrator	SSRI	Selective serotonin reuptake inhibitor
RSV	Respiratory syncytial virus	START	Simple triage and rapid treatment
RT	Respiratory therapy; related to	STAT	At once, immediately
RUG	Resource utilization group	STD	Sexually transmitted disease
RUQ	Right upper quadrant	STH	Somatotrophic hormone (somatotropin)
RV	Residual volume	STI	Sexually transmitted infection
S_1	The first heart sound	SV	Stroke volume
S_2	The second heart sound	SVC	Superior vena cava
SA	Status asthmaticus	SVE	Sterile vaginal examination
SA node	Sinoatrial node; sinus node	SVR	Systemic vascular resistance
SBE	Subacute bacterial endocarditis	SX P	Sexual precautions
SBFT	Small bowel follow-through (x-ray)	SZ P	Seizure precautions
SBP	Systolic blood pressure	T&A	Tonsillectomy and adenoidectomy
sBP	Systolic blood pressure	T&X	Type and crossmatch
SDSU	Same-day surgery unit	T-1, T-2, etc.	Refers to level of injury in the thoracic area
Sed rate	Erythrocyte sedimentation rate		of the spinal cord
	(also see ESR)	T_3	Triiodothyronine
SG	Suicide gesture	T_4	Thyroxine
SGA	Small for gestational age	TA	Transactional analysis
SI units	International System of Units	TAC	Time, amount, character
	(Systeme International D'Unites)	TAT	Thematic apperception test
SI	Suicidal ideation	TB	Tuberculosis
SIADH	Syndrome of inappropriate antidiuretic	TBI	Traumatic brain injury
	hormone	TBW	Total body water
SIB	Self-injurious behavior	TCA	Trycyclic antidepression
SICU	Surgical intensive care unit	TCD	Transcranial doppler
SIDS	Sudden infant death syndrome	TCDB	Turning, coughing, deep breathing
SIE	Stroke in evolution	TCN	Tetracycline
SIMV	Synchronized intermittent mandatory	TD	Tardive dyskinesia
	ventilation	TED	Thromboembolytic disease
SIRES	Stabilize, identify toxin, reverse effect,	TEE	Transesophageal echocardiography
	eliminate toxin, support	TENS	Transcutaneous electrical nerve
SIRS	Systemic inflammatory response syndrome		stimulation
SL	Sublingual	TFT	Thyroid function test
SLD	Specific learning disabilities	TGV	Transposition of the great vessels
SLE	Systemic lupus erythematosus	THA	Total hip arthroplasty
SMBG	Self-monitoring of blood glucose	THC	Cannabis (marijuana and related drugs)
SNF	Skilled nursing facility	T-hold	Transportation hold (police)
SNS	Sympathetic nervous system	TIA	Transient ischemic attack
SO	Significant other	TICU	Trauma intensive care unit
SO_4^{--}	sulfate	Title XIX	Medicaid section of the Social
SOAP	Subjective, objective, assessment, plan		Security Act
SOAPIER	Subjective, objective, assessment, plan,	Title XVIII	Medicare section of the Social
	intervention, evaluation, response		Security Act
SOB	Short of breath	Title XXII	Source of COPs

TKA	Total knee arthroplasty		UROL	Urology
TKO	To keep open (IV)		US	Ultrasound
TLC	Total lung capacity		USD	United States Dispensatory
TLSO	Thoracolumbar sacroorthosis		USDA	United States Department of Agriculture
TM	Transport maximum		USDHHS	United States Department of Health and Human Services
TMJ	Temporomandibular joint			
TMR	Transmyocardial revascularization		USP	United States Pharmacopeia
TNM	Tumor, node metastasis		USPHS	United States Public Health Service
TO	Telephone order		UTI	Urinary tract infection
TOF	Tetralogy of Fallot		UTox	Urine toxicology screen (for drugs)
TORCH	Toxoplasmosis, other, rubella, cytomegalovirus, herpes simplex		UV	Ultraviolet (rays)
			V & S (vol. and spec.)	Volume and specific gravity (urine)
t-PA	Tissue plasminogen activator			
TPA	Total parenteral alimentation			
TPN	Total parenteral nutrition		VC	Vital capacity
TPR	Temperature, pulse, and respiration		VCUG	Voiding cystourethrogram
TR	Therapeutic recreation		VDRL	Venereal Disease Research Laboratory
TRH	Thyrotropin-releasing hormone		VH	Visual hallucinations
TS	Tourette's syndrome		VLBW	Very low birth weight
TSE	Testicular self-examination		VMA	Vanillylmandelic acid
TSH	Thyroid-stimulating hormone		VNA	Visiting Nurse Association
TSLO	Thoracic-lumbar-sacral orthosis		VO	Verbal order
TSS	Toxic shock syndrome		Vol	Voluntarily admitted
TURBT	Transurethral resection of a bladder tumor		VRE	Vancomycin-resistant enterococci
TURP	Transurethral resection of the prostate		VS	Vital signs
TV	Tidal volume		VSD	Ventricular septal defect
TWE	Tap water enema		W/C	Wheelchair
U-100	100 units per milliliter		WA	While awake
UA	Urinalysis		WBC	White blood cell
UAP	Unlicensed Assistive Personnel		W/D	Withdrawal
UL	Tolerable upper intake level		WHO	World Health Organization
ULBW	Ultra low birth weight		WKS	Wernicke-Korsakoff syndrome
UN	United Nations		WIC	Women, infants, and children
UNICEF	United Nations Children's Fund		WISC-R	Weschler Intelligence Scale for Children–Revised
UNOS	United Network of Organ Sharing			
UPP	Urethral pressure profile		WNL	Within normal limits
UPT	Urine pregnancy test		WNWD	Well-nourished, well-developed
URI	Upper respiratory infection		WWW	World Wide Web

Normal Values and Reference Tables

▪▪▪ ℬLOOD CHEMISTRIES

Determination	Specimen	Age/Sex	Normal Value	
Albumin (see Protein, electrophoresis)				
Aldolase	Serum	Newborn	4 × adult value	
		Adult	<11 IU/L	
Amylase	Serum	Newborn	5–65 U/L	
		> 1 y	25–125 U/L	
Ascorbic acid	Serum		0.6–2.0 mg/dL	
Bicarbonate	Serum	Arterial	21–28 mmol/dL	
		Venous	22–29	

			Premature (mg/dL)	*Full-term (mg/dL)*
Bilirubin, total	Serum	Cord	<2	<2
		0–1 d	<8	<6
		1–2 d	<12	<8
		2–5 d	<16	<12
		Adult		0.2–1.0
		Pregnancy	Unchanged	

Determination	Specimen	Age/Sex	Normal Value
Bilirubin, direct (conjugated)	Serum		0.8–0.4 mg/dL
Calcium, ionized	Serum, plasma, whole blood	Cord, newborn	5.5 ± 0.3 mg/dL
		Infant	4.0–5.1
		Adult	4.48–5.25
Calcium, total	Serum	Cord, newborn	9–11.5 mg/dL
		Infant	9–10.9
		Adult	8.4–10.2
		Pregnancy	7.8–9.3
Carbon dioxide, partial pressure (PaCO$_2$)	Whole blood, arterial	Newborn	27–40 mm Hg
		Infant	27–40
		Pregnancy	27–32
		Female adult	32–45
Carbon monoxide	Whole blood		0.5–1.5% saturation of Hgb (children and nonsmokers); symptoms >20%
Chloride	Serum or plasma	Cord	96–104 mmol/L
		Newborn	97–110
		Adult	98–106
		Pregnancy	Slight elevation
	Sweat	Normal	0–35 mmol/L
		Marginal	30–60
		Cystic fibrosis	60–200
Cholesterol, total	Serum	Adult	140–200
Creatinine kinase, CK (creatine phosphokinase, CPK; 30°C)	Serum	Adult: M	12–70
		F	10–55 (higher after exercise)
Creatinine	Serum or plasma	Infant	0.2–0.4 mg/dL
		Adult: M	0.6–1.2
		F	0.5–1.0
		Pregnancy	(0.47–0.7)

(continued)

■■■ *B*LOOD CHEMISTRIES (CONTINUED)

Determination	Specimen	Age/Sex	Normal Value

Creatinine clearance (endogenous)	Serum or plasma and timed urine	Newborn
		Under 40 y
		    M
		    F
			$40–65 \text{ mL/min/1.73 m}^2$
			
			97–137
			88–128 (decreases 6.5 mL/min/decade)

Ethanol	Blood		0.0% Toxic: 50–100 mg/dL; CNS depression: >100 mg/dL
Fatty acids, free	Serum or plasma	Adults Children and obese adults	8–25 mg/dL <31
Fibrinogen	Whole blood	Newborn Adult Pregnancy	125–300 mg/dL 200–400 450
Folate	Serum	Newborn Adult Pregnancy	7–32 ng/mL 1.8–9 1.9–14
Glucose	Serum Blood Urine	Adult Adult	70–105 (fasting) 65–95 70–125 (non-fasting) Negative

Glucose tolerance	Serum		Time	Normal	Diabetic
Dosages: Child, 1.75 g/kg of ideal weight (maximum 75 g) Adult, 75 g total dose			Fasting 60 min 90 min 120 min	70–105 120–170 100–140 70–120	>115 ≥200 ≥200 ≥140

Determination	Specimen	Age/Sex	Normal Value
Insulin (12 h, fasting)	Serum, plasma	Newborn Adult	3–20 mcIU/mL 7–24
Iron-binding capacity (TIBC)	Serum	Infant Adult Pregnancy	100–400 µg/dL 250–400 300–450
Iron	Serum	Newborn Infant Adult: M F Pregnancy	100–250 µg/dL 40–100 50–160 40–150 Decreased
Lactate	Whole blood, venous		4.5–19.8 mg/dL
Lactate dehydrogenase (LDH)	Serum	Newborn Infant Adult	160–450 U/L 100–250 60–170
Lead	Whole blood	Child Adult Acceptable for industrial exposure Toxic	<30 µg/dL <40 <60 ≥100

Lipase (Tietz method; 37°C)	Serum	
		Child
		Adult:
		  F, premenopause
		  F, midcycle
		  F, postmenopause
			0.1–1.0 U/mL
			1–6 mIU/mL
			4–14
			4–25
			25–250
			25–200

▪▪▪ 𝓑LOOD CHEMISTRIES (CONTINUED)

Determination	Specimen	Age/Sex	Normal Value
Magnesium	Serum	Newborn	1.2–1.8 mEq/L
Oxygen capacity		Adult	1.3–2.1
Oxygen, partial pressure	Whole blood, arterial Whole blood, arterial	 Birth 5–10 min 30 min >1 h 1 d Adult	1.34 mL/g hemoglobin 8–24 mm Hg 33–75 31–85 55–80 54–95 83–108 decreases with age
Oxygen, % saturation	Whole blood, arterial	Newborn Thereafter	40–90% 95–99%
Phenylalanine	Serum	Full-term newborn Adult	1.2–3.4 mg/dL 0.8–1.8
Phosphatase, acid prostatic, 37°C	Serum		<3.0 ng/mL 0.11–0.60 U/L
Phosphatase, alkaline SKI method		Adult Pregnancy >50% rise	20–70 U/L
Phospholipids (lipids P × 25)	Serum and plasma	Adult	125–275 mg/dL
Phosphorus, inorganic	Serum	Adult Pregnancy	3.0–4.5 mg/dL Unchanged
Potassium	Serum	Infant Adult	4.1–5.3 mEq/L 3.5–5.1
Protein, total	Serum	Adult, recumbent—0.5 g higher in ambulatory patients	6.0–7.8 g/dL
Protein, electrophoresis (cellulose acetate)	Serum	Total	
Salicylates	Serum, plasma		Negative: <2.0 mg/dL Therapeutic: 15–30 Toxic: >30
Sodium	Serum	Adult	136–146 mEq/L
Testosterone	Serum	Adult: M F	572 ± 135 ng/dL 37 ± 10 ng/dL
Thiamine (vitamin B_1)	Serum		2.0 µg/dL

			(mg/dL)	
			Male	**Female**
Triglycerides (TG)	Serum, after 12-h fast	12–15 y 16–19 y 20–29 y Recommended (desirable) levels for adults:	36–138 40–163 44–185 Male, 40–160 Female, 35–135	41–138 40–128 40–128

Determination	Specimen	Age/Sex	Normal Value
Urea nitrogen	Serum/plasma	Cord Newborn Adult	21–40 mg/dL 3–12 7–18

(continued)

▪▪▪ ℬLOOD CHEMISTRIES (CONTINUED)

Determination	Specimen	Age/Sex	Normal Value
Uric acid	Serum	Child	2.0–5.5 mg/dL
		Adult: M	3.5–7.2
		F	2.6–6.0
Vitamin A	Serum	Adult	30–65 µg/dL
Vitamin B_{12}	Serum	Newborn	175–800 pg/mL
		Adult	140–700
Vitamin C	Plasma		0.6–2.0 mg/mL
Vitamin E	Serum		5–20 µg/mL
Volume	Whole blood	Adult	72–100 mL/kg
	Plasma	Adult	49–59

These values may vary slightly, depending on the particular laboratory performing the tests.

The figures stated here are considered to be "within normal range" values.

◾◾◾ 𝒰RINE CHEMISTRIES

Determination	Age/Sex	Normal Value
Catecholamines (24 h)	Infant	0–10 µg/dL
	Norepinephrine	0–2.5
	Epinephrine	
	Adult	
	Norepinephrine	15–80
	Epinephrine	0.5–20
Chloride (24 h)	Infant	2–10 mmol/d
	Adult (varies greatly with Cl intake)	110–250
Creatinine	Infant	8–20 mg/kg/d
	Adult	14–26
	Pregnancy	Elevated
Lead (24 h)		<80 µg/L
Osmolality (random)		50–1400 mOsmol/kg H_2O depending on fluid intake. After 12 h fluid restriction >850 mOsmol/kg H_2O
Protein, total 24 h		50–80 mg/dL (at rest) <250 mg/dL after intense exercise <150 mg/dL (as glucose)
Reducing substances Specific gravity		
Random void		1.002–1.030
After 12-h fluid restriction		>1.025
24 h		1.015–1.025
Vanillylmandelic acid (VMA) (24 h)	Newborn	>1.0 mg/d
	Infant	>2.0
	Adult	2–7

Source: Adapted from Fischbach F. A Manual of Laboratory and Diagnostic Tests, Ed 5. Philadelphia, J.B. Lippincott, 1996.

g/dL = grams per deciliter.

$10^3/mm^3$ = thousand per cubic meter.

IU = International Unit.

mmol/L = millimole per liter.

mL/min/1.73 m^2 = milliliter per minute per 1.73 square meter of body surface area.

(mEq) µg/dL = micrograms per deciliter.

mEq = milliequivalents.

ng/mL = nanogram per milliliter.

D

Medical Terminology

MEDICAL TERMINOLOGY: PREFIXES, ROOTS, AND SUFFIXES COMMONLY USED IN MEDICAL TERMS

Prefix/Root	Meaning/Example	Prefix/Root	Meaning/Example
A- or AB-	*Away, lack of:* abnormal, departing from normal	CIRCUM-	*Around:* circumocular, around the eyes
A- or AN-	~~*From,*~~ *without:* asepsis, without infection	CLEID-	*Clavicle:* cleidocostal, pertaining to clavicle and ribs
ACR-	*An extremity:* acrodermatitis, a dermatitis of the limbs	COLP-	*Vagina:* colporrhagia, vaginal hemorrhage
AD-	*To, toward, near:* adrenal, near the kidney	CONTRA-	~~*Against,*~~ *opposed:* contraindication, indication opposing usually indicated treatment
ADEN-	*Gland:* adenitis, inflammation of a gland	COST-	*Rib:* intercostal, between the ribs
ALG-	*Pain:* Neuralgia, pain extending along nerves	COUNTER-	*Against:* counterirritation, an irritation to relieve some other irritation (e.g., a liniment)
AMBI-	*Both:* ambidextrous, referring to both hands	CRANI-	*Skull:* craniotomy, surgical opening in skull
ANTE-	*Before:* antenatal, occurring or having been formed before birth	CRYPT-	*Hidden:* cryptogenic, of hidden or unknown origin
ANTI-	*Against:* antiseptic, against or preventing sepsis	CUT-	*Skin:* subcutaneous, under the skin
ARTH-	*Joint:* arthritis, inflammation of a joint	CYST-	*Sac or bladder:* cystitis, inflammation of any bladder
AUTO-	*Self:* autointoxication, poisoning by toxin generated in the body	CYTO-	*Cell:* cytology, scientific study of cells; cytometer, a device for counting and measuring cells
BI- or BIN-	*Two:* binocular, pertaining to both eyes	DACRY-	*Lacrimal glands:* dacryocyst, tear-sac
BIO-	*Life:* biopsy, inspection of living organism (or tissue)	DERM- or DERMAT-	*Skin:* dermatoid, skinlike
BLAST-	*Bud, a growing thing in early stages:* blastocyte, beginning cell not yet differentiated	DI-	*Two:* diphasic, occurring in two stages or phases
BLEPH-	*Eyelids:* blepharitis, inflammation of an eyelid	DIS-	*Apart:* disarticulation, taking a joint apart
BRACHI-	*Arm:* brachialis, muscle for flexing forearm	DYS-	*Pain or difficulty:* dyspepsia, impairment of digestion
BRACHY-	*Short:* brachydactylia, abnormal shortness of fingers and toes	ECTO-	*Outside:* ectoretina, outermost layer of retina
BRADY-	*Slow:* bradycardia, abnormal slowness of heartbeat	EM- or EN-	*In:* encapsulated, enclosed in a capsule
BRONCH-	*Windpipe:* bronchiectasis, dilation of bronchial tubes	ENCEPHAL-	*Brain:* encephalitis, inflammation of the brain
BUCC-	*Cheek:* buccally, toward the cheek	END-	*Within:* endothelium, layer of cells lining heart, and blood and lymph vessels
CARCIN-	*Cancer:* carcinogenic, producing cancer	ENTERO-	*Intestine:* enterosis, falling of intestine
CARDI-	*Heart:* cardialgia, pain in the heart	EPI-	*Above or on:* epidermis, outermost layer of skin
CEPHAL- or CEPHALO-	*Head:* cephalic measurements	ERYTHRO-	*Red:* erythrocyte, red blood cell
CHEIL-	*Lip:* cheilitis, inflammation of the lip	EU-	*Well:* euphoria, well feeling, feeling of good health
CHOLE-	*Bile:* cholecyst, the gallbladder	EX- or E-	*Out:* excretion, material thrown out of the body or the organ
CHONDR-	*Cartilage:* chondrectomy, removal of a cartilage		

Definitions are in italic. Example terms with their definitions follow colons.

(continued)

▪▪▪ $\mathcal{M}$EDICAL TERMINOLOGY: PREFIXES, ROOTS, AND SUFFIXES COMMONLY USED IN MEDICAL TERMS (CONTINUED)

Prefix/Root	Meaning/Example	Prefix/Root	Meaning/Example
EXO-	*Outside:* exocrine, excreting outwardly (opposite of endocrine)	KERAT-	*Horn, cornea:* keratitis, inflammation of the cornea
EXTRA-	*Outside:* extramural, situated or occurring outside a wall	LACT-	*Milk:* lactation, secretion of milk
FEBRI-	*Fever:* febrile, feverish	LEUK-	*White:* leukocyte, white cell
GALACTO-	*Milk:* galactose, a milk sugar	MACRO-	*Large:* macroblast, abnormally large red cell
GASTR-	*Stomach:* gastrectomy, excision of the stomach	MAST-	*Breast:* mastectomy, excision of the breast
GLOSS-	*Tongue:* glossectomy, surgical removal of tongue	MEG- or MEGAL-	*Great:* megacolon, abnormally large colon
GLYCO-	*Sugar:* glycosuria, sugar in the urine	MENT-	*Mind:* dementia, deterioration of the mind
GYNEC-	*Women:* gynecology, science of diseases pertaining to women	MER-	*Part:* merotomy, division into segments
HEM- or HEMAT-	*Blood:* hematopoiesis, forming blood	MESA-	*Middle:* mesaortitis, inflammation of the middle coat of the aorta
HEMI-	*Half:* heminephrectomy, excision of half the kidney	META-	*Beyond, over, change:* metastasis, change in the site of a disease, spreading (often refers to cancer)
HEPAT-	*Liver:* hepatitis, inflammation of the liver	MICRO-	*Small:* microplasia, dwarfism
HETERO-	*Other* (opposite of homo): heterotransplant, using skin from a member of another species	MY-	*Muscle:* myoma, tumor made of muscular elements
HIST-	*Tissue:* histology, science of minute structure and function of tissues	MYC-	*Fungi:* mycology, science and study of fungi
HOMO-	*Same:* homotransplant, skin grafting by using skin from a member of the same species	NECRO-	*Corpse, dead:* necrosis, death of cells adjoining living tissue
HYDR-	*Water:* hydrocephalus, abnormal accumulation of fluid in cranium (skull)	NEO-	*New:* neoplasm, any new growth or formation
HYPER-	*Above, excess of:* hyperglycemia, excess of sugar in blood	NEPH-	*Kidney:* nephrectomy, surgical excision of kidney
HYPO-	*Under, deficiency of:* hypoglycemia, deficiency of sugar in blood	NEURO-	*Nerve:* neuron, nerve cell
HYSTER-	*Uterus:* hysterectomy, excision of uterus	ODONT-	*Tooth:* odontology, dentistry
IDIO-	*Self or separate:* idiopathic, a disease self-originated (of unknown cause)	OLIG-	*Little:* oligemia, deficiency in volume of blood
IM- or IN-	*In:* infiltration, accumulation in tissue of abnormal substances (such as an IV)	OO-	*Egg:* oocyte, original cell of egg
IM- or IN-	*Not:* immature, not mature	OOPHOR-	*Ovary:* oophorectomy, removal of an ovary
INFRA-	*Below:* infraorbital, below the orbit	OPHTHALM-	*Eye:* ophthalmometer, an instrument for measuring the eye
INTER-	*Between:* intermuscular, between the muscles	ORTHO-	*Straight, normal:* orthograde, walk straight (upright)
INTRA-	*Within:* intramuscular, within the muscle	OSS-	*Bone:* osseous, bony
		OSTE-	*Bone:* osteitis, inflammation of a bone
		OT-	*Ear:* otorrhea, discharge from ear

◼◼◼ MEDICAL TERMINOLOGY: PREFIXES, ROOTS, AND SUFFIXES COMMONLY USED IN MEDICAL TERMS (CONTINUED)

Prefix/Root	Meaning/Example	Prefix/Root	Meaning/Example
OVAR-	*Ovary:* ovariorrhexis, rupture of an ovary	RETRO-	*Backward:* retroversion, turned backward (usually applies to the uterus)
PARA-	*Irregular, around, wrong:* paracystic, situated near the bladder	RHIN-	*Nose:* rhinology, knowledge concerning noses
PATH-	*Disease:* pathology, science of disease	SALPING-	*A tube:* salpingitis, inflammation of tube
PED-	*Children:* pediatrician, child specialist	SEMI-	*Half:* semilunar, half moon-shaped valve
PED-	*Feet:* pedograph, imprint of the foot	SEPTIC-	*Poison:* septicemia, poisoned condition of blood
PER-	*Through, excessively:* percutaneous, through the skin	SOMAT-	*Body:* psychosomatic, having bodily symptoms of mental origin
PERI-	*Around, immediately around* (in contradistinction to *para*): periosteum, sheath around bone	STA-	*Make stand:* stasis, stoppage of flow of fluid, as in blood (hemostasis)
PHIL-	*Love:* hemophilic, fond of blood (as bacteria that grow well in presence of hemoglobin)	STEN-	*Narrow:* stenosis, narrowing of duct or canal
PHLEB-	*Vein:* phlebotomy, opening of vein for bloodletting	SUB-	*Under:* subdiaphragmatic, under the diaphragm
PHOB-	*Fear:* hydrophobic, reluctant to associate with water	SUPER-	*Above, excessively:* superacute, excessively acute
PNEUM- or PNEUMON-	*Lung* (pneum–air): pneumococcus, organism causing lobar pneumonia	SUPRA-	*Above, on:* suprarenal, above or on the kidney
POLIO-	*Gray:* poliomyelitis, inflammation of gray substance of spinal cord	SYM- or SYN-	*With, together:* symphysis, a growing together, as symphysis pubis
POLY-	*Many:* polyarthritis, inflammation of several joints	TACHY-	*Fast:* tachycardia, fast-beating heart
POST-	*After:* postpartum, after delivery	TENS-	*Stretch:* extensor, a muscle extending or stretching a limb
PRE-	*Before:* prenatal, occurring before birth	THERM-	*Heat:* diathermy, therapeutic production of heat in tissues
PRO-	*Before:* prognosis, forecast as to result of disease	TOX- or TOXIC-	*Poison:* toxemia, poisoned condition of blood
PROCT-	*Rectum:* proctectomy, surgical removal of rectum	TRACHE-	*Trachea:* tracheitis, inflammation of the trachea
PSEUDO-	*False:* pseudoangina, false angina	TRANS-	*Across:* transplant, transfer tissue from one place to another
PSYCH-	*Soul or mind:* psychiatry, treatment of mental disorders	TRI-	*Three:* triceps, three-headed muscle
PY-	*Pus:* pyorrhea, discharge of pus	TRICH-	*Hair:* trichosis, any disease of the hair
PYEL-	*Pelvis:* pyelitis, inflammation of pelvis or the kidney	UNI-	*One:* unilateral, affecting one side
RACH-	*Spine:* rachicentesis, puncture into vertebral canal	VAS-	*Vessel:* vasoconstrictor, nerve or drug that narrows blood vessel
REN-	*Kidney:* adrenal, near the kidney	ZOO-	*Animal:* zooblast, an animal cell

(continued)

MEDICAL TERMINOLOGY: PREFIXES, ROOTS, AND SUFFIXES COMMONLY USED IN MEDICAL TERMS (CONTINUED)

Suffix	Meaning/Example	Suffix	Meaning/Example
-ALGIA	*Pain:* cardialgia, pain in the heart	-OSIS (-ASIS)	*Being affected with:* arteriosclerosis, thickening and "hardening" of arteries
-ASIS or -OSIS	*Affected with, condition or state of:* leukocytosis, excess number of leukocytes	-(O)STOMY	*Creation of an opening:* gastrostomy, creation of an artificial gastric fistula
-ASTHENIA	*Weakness:* neurasthenia, nerve weakness	-(O)TOMY	*Cutting into:* laparotomy, surgical incision into abdomen
-BLAST	*Germ:* myeloblast, immature bone marrow cell	-PATHY	*Disease:* myopathy, disease of muscle
-CELE	*Tumor, hernia:* enterocele, any hernia of intestine	-PENIA	*Decrease or deficiency of:* leukopenia, lack of white blood cells
-CID	*Cut, kill:* germicidal, destructive to germs	-PEXY	*To fix:* proctopexy, fixation of rectum by suture
-CLYSIS	*Injection:* hypodermoclysis, injection under the skin	-PHAGIA	*Eating:* polyphagia, excessive eating
-COCCUS	*Round bacterium:* pneumococcus, bacterium of pneumonia	-PHASIA	*Speech:* aphasia, loss of power of speech
-CYTE	*Cell:* leukocyte, white cell	-PHOBIA	*Fear:* hydrophobia, fear of water
-ECTASIS	*Dilation, stretching:* angiectasis, dilatation of a blood vessel	-PLASTY	*Molding:* gastroplasty, molding or reforming stomach
-ECTOMY	*Excision:* adenectomy, excision of adenoids	-PNEA	*Air or breathing:* dyspnea, difficult breathing
-EMIA	*Blood:* glycemia, sugar in blood	-POIESIS	*Making, forming:* hematopoiesis, forming blood
-ESTHESIA	*Relating to sensation:* anesthesia, absence of feeling	-PTOSIS	*Falling:* enteroptosis, falling of intestine
-FERENT	*Bear, carry:* efferent, carry out to periphery	-RHYTHMIA	*Rhythm:* arrhythmia, variation from normal rhythm of heart
-GENIC	*Producing:* pyogenic, producing pus	-RRHAGIA	*Flowing or bursting forth:* otorrhagia, hemorrhage from ear
-IATRICS	*Pertaining to a physician or the practice of healing* (medicine): pediatrics, science of medicine for children	-RRHAPHY	*Suture of:* enterorrhaphy, act of sewing up a gap in intestine
-ITIS	*Inflammation:* tonsillitis, inflammation of tonsils	-RRHEA	*Discharge:* otorrhea, discharge from ear
-LOGY	*Science of:* pathology, science of disease	-STHEN	*Pertaining to strength:* asthenia, loss of strength
-LYSIS	*Losing, flowing, dissolution:* autolysis, dissolution of tissue cells	-TAXIA or -TAXIS	*Order, arrangement of:* ataxia, failure of muscular coordination
-MALACIA	*Softening:* osteomalacia, softening of bone	-TROPHIA or -TROPHY	*Nourishment:* atrophy, wasting, or diminution
-OMA	*Tumor:* myoma, tumor made up of muscle elements	-URIA	*To do with urine:* polyuria, excessive secretion of urine

E

Standard Precautions

The Hospital Infection Control Practices Advisory Committee (HICPAC) recommends two tiers of precautions to prevent cross-examination in healthcare facilities: Standard Precautions *and* Transmission-Based Precautions. *These precautions are discussed in detail at the Centers for Disease Control and Prevention Website* www.cdc.gov/ncidod/hip/isolat/isopart2.htm. *(Refer to Chap. 42 for more detail concerning infection control.)*

Use Standard Precautions, or the equivalent, for the care of all patients. *Category IB**

A. Handwashing

(1) Wash hands after touching blood, body fluids, secretions, excretions, and contaminated items, whether or not gloves are worn. Wash hands immediately after gloves are removed, between patient contacts, and when otherwise indicated to avoid transfer of microorganisms to other patients or environments. It may be necessary to wash hands between tasks and procedures on the same patient to prevent cross-contamination of different body sites. *Category IB*

(2) Use a plain (nonantimicrobial) soap for routine handwashing. *Category IB*

(3) Use an antimicrobial agent or a waterless antiseptic agent for specific circumstances (e.g., control of outbreaks or hyperendemic infections), as defined by the infection control program. *Category IB* (See Contact Precautions for additional recommendations on using antimicrobial and antiseptic agents.)

B. Gloves

Wear gloves (clean, nonsterile gloves are adequate) when touching blood, body fluids, secretions, excretions, or contaminated items. Put on clean gloves just before touching mucous membranes and nonintact skin. Change gloves between tasks and procedures on the same patient after contact with material that may contain a high concentration of microorganisms. Remove gloves promptly after use, before touching noncontaminated items and environmental surfaces, and before going to another patient, and wash hands immediately to avoid transfer of microorganisms to other patients or environments. *Category IB*

C. Mask, Eye Protection, Face Shield

Wear a mask and eye protection or a face shield to protect mucous membranes of the eyes, nose, and mouth during procedures and patient-care activities that are likely to generate splashes or sprays of blood, body fluids, secretions, or excretions. *Category IB*

D. Gown

Wear a gown (a clean, nonsterile gown is adequate) to protect skin and to prevent soiling of clothing during procedures and patient-care activities that are likely to generate splashes or sprays of blood, body fluids, secretions, or excretions. Select a gown that is appropriate for the activity and the amount of fluid likely to be encountered. Remove a soiled gown as promptly as possible, and wash hands to avoid transfer of microorganisms to other patients or environments. *Category IB*

E. Patient-Care Equipment

Handle used patient-care equipment soiled with blood, body fluids, secretions, or excretions in a manner that prevents skin and mucous membrane exposure, contamination of clothing, and transfer of microorganisms to other patients and environments. Ensure that reusable equipment is not used for the care of another patient until it has been cleaned and reprocessed appropriately. Ensure that single-use items are discarded properly. *Category IB*

F. Environmental Control

Ensure that the hospital has adequate procedures for the routine care, cleaning, and disinfection of environmental surfaces, beds, bedrails, bedside equipment, and other frequently touched surfaces, and ensure that these procedures are being followed. *Category IB*

G. Linen

Handle, transport, and process used linen soiled with blood, body fluids, secretions, or excretions in a manner that prevents skin and mucous membrane exposure, contamination of clothing, and that avoids transfer of microorganisms to other patients and environments. *Category IB*

H. Occupational Health and Blood-borne Pathogens

(1) Take care to prevent injuries when using needles, scalpels, and other sharp instruments or devices; when handling sharp instruments after procedures; when cleaning used instruments; and when disposing of used needles. Never recap used needles, or otherwise manipulate them using both hands, or use any other technique that involves directing the point of a needle toward any part of the body; rather, use either a one-handed "scoop" technique or a mechanical device designed for holding the needle sheath. Do not remove

---

**Category IB.* Strongly recommended for all hospitals and reviewed as effective by experts in the field and a consensus of HICPAC members on the basis of strong rationale and suggestive evidence, even though definitive studies have not been done.

(From *Recommendations for Isolation Precautions in Hospitals* developed by the Centers for Disease Control and Prevention and the Hospital Infection Control Practices Advisory Committee [HICPAC], February 18, 1997.)

CHAPTER 1

1. c
2. a
3. b

CHAPTER 2

1. c
2. b
3. d

CHAPTER 3

1. a
2. c
3. b

CHAPTER 4

1. a
2. b
3. c

CHAPTER 5

1. c
2. d
3. b

CHAPTER 6

1. b
2. a
3. b

CHAPTER 7

1. b
2. d
3. b

CHAPTER 8

1. d
2. a
3. d

CHAPTER 9

1. c
2. d
3. a

CHAPTER 10

1. a
2. b
3. d

CHAPTER 11

1. d
2. a
3. c

CHAPTER 12

1. d
2. a
3. b

CHAPTER 13

1. b
2. a
3. c

CHAPTER 14

1. b
2. c
3. a

CHAPTER 15

1. b
2. c
3. d
4. a
5. b

CHAPTER 16

1. a
2. b
3. d
4. c
5. a

CHAPTER 17

1. c
2. b
3. d
4. c
5. a

CHAPTER 18

1. a
2. d
3. c
4. c
5. b

CHAPTER 19

1. b
2. a
3. d
4. a
5. c

CHAPTER 20

1. a
2. d
3. b
4. a
5. c

CHAPTER 21

1. b
2. c
3. d
4. a
5. a

CHAPTER 22

1. c
2. a
3. d

CHAPTER 23

1. a
2. d
3. b

CHAPTER 24

1. b
2. c
3. a

CHAPTER 25

1. a
2. d
3. b

CHAPTER 26

1. b
2. c
3. d

CHAPTER 27

1. d
2. c
3. b

CHAPTER 28

1. d
2. a
3. b

CHAPTER 29

1. c
2. b
3. a

CHAPTER 30

1. c
2. a
3. d
4. a
5. b

CHAPTER 31

1. a
2. c
3. b
4. b
5. d

CHAPTER 32

1. b
2. a
3. b
4. d
5. c

CHAPTER 33

1. c
2. d
3. b
4. a
5. a

CHAPTER 34

1. b
2. a
3. a
4. d
5. c

CHAPTER 35

1. b
2. b
3. a
4. d
5. c

CHAPTER 36

1. c
2. a
3. d
4. d
5. b
6. c

CHAPTER 37

1. a
2. d
3. c
4. a
5. d
6. b

CHAPTER 38

1. a
2. b
3. d
4. c
5. b

CHAPTER 39

1. d
2. d
3. c
4. a
5. c

CHAPTER 40

1. b
2. c
3. b
4. d
5. a

CHAPTER 41

1. d
2. d
3. c
4. a
5. b

CHAPTER 42

1. d
2. b
3. d
4. c
5. a

CHAPTER 43

1. a
2. b
3. a
4. c

CHAPTER 44

1. a
2. c
3. d
4. a
5. b

CHAPTER 45

1. d
2. a
3. b
4. b
5. c

CHAPTER 46

1. b
2. d
3. b
4. c
5. a

CHAPTER 47

1. b
2. b
3. c
4. a
5. d

CHAPTER 48

1. a
2. b
3. c
4. b
5. d

CHAPTER 49

1. d
2. a
3. d
4. c
5. b

CHAPTER 50

1. d
2. c
3. b
4. c
5. a

CHAPTER 51

1. a
2. c
3. c
4. d
5. b

CHAPTER 52

1. b
2. d
3. a
4. c
5. d

CHAPTER 53

1. d
2. b
3. a
4. c
5. c

CHAPTER 54

1. c
2. a
3. b
4. c
5. d

CHAPTER 55

1. a
2. d
3. b
4. b
5. c

CHAPTER 56

1. b
2. d
3. d
4. b
5. a

CHAPTER 57

1. d
2. c
3. b
4. a
5. d

CHAPTER 58

1. b
2. a
3. c
4. d
5. a

CHAPTER 59

1. a
2. b
3. b
4. c
5. c

CHAPTER 60

1. c
2. d
3. b
4. c
5. a

CHAPTER 61

1. d
2. b
3. c
4. a
5. d

CHAPTER 62

1. b
2. c
3. d
4. d
5. a

CHAPTER 63

1. d
2. b
3. b
4. c
5. d

CHAPTER 64

1. d
2. b
3. c
4. d
5. b

CHAPTER 65

1. d
2. d
3. c
4. d
5. d

CHAPTER 66

1. b
2. b
3. d
4. d
5. b
6. d

CHAPTER 67

1. c
2. c
3. a
4. b
5. d

CHAPTER 68

1. c
2. c
3. d
4. a
5. c

CHAPTER 69

1. a
2. d
3. a
4. d
5. a

CHAPTER 70

1. d
2. c
3. b
4. d

CHAPTER 71

1. c
2. d
3. d
4. a
5. d

CHAPTER 72

1. c
2. d
3. a
4. c
5. b

CHAPTER 73

1. a
2. c
3. b
4. d
5. b

CHAPTER 74

1. c
2. c
3. a
4. d
5. b

CHAPTER 75

1. c
2. a
3. b
4. d
5. d

CHAPTER 76

1. c
2. b
3. a
4. b
5. a

CHAPTER 77

1. d
2. c
3. d
4. b
5. a

CHAPTER 78

1. d
2. b
3. c
4. a
5. c

CHAPTER 79

1. c
2. d
3. a
4. d
5. c

CHAPTER 80

1. b
2. d
3. a
4. d
5. b
6. c
7. b
8. a

CHAPTER 81

1. c
2. d
3. a
4. a
5. b

CHAPTER 82

1. b
2. c
3. d
4. b
5. a

CHAPTER 83

1. d
2. a
3. b
4. b
5. c

CHAPTER 84

1. b
2. c
3. d
4. a
5. d

CHAPTER 85

1. c
2. a
3. b
4. b
5. d
6. d

CHAPTER 86

1. b
2. c
3. d
4. d
5. a

CHAPTER 87

1. a
2. c
3. c
4. b
5. d

CHAPTER 88

1. a
2. b
3. b
4. d
5. c

CHAPTER 89

1. b
2. c
3. d
4. a
5. a

CHAPTER 90

1. a
2. a
3. b
4. b
5. c
6. c
7. d

CHAPTER 91

1. b
2. c
3. d

CHAPTER 92

1. a
2. b
3. a

CHAPTER 93

1. c
2. b
3. a

CHAPTER 94

1. c
2. b
3. a
4. d
5. b

CHAPTER 95

1. b
2. a
3. c

CHAPTER 96

1. d
2. b
3. a

CHAPTER 97

1. d
2. b
3. a

CHAPTER 98

1. a
2. a
3. b

CHAPTER 99

1. b
2. d
3. a
4. a

CHAPTER 100

1. a
2. d
3. c
4. d

CHAPTER 101

1. b
2. c
3. a

CHAPTER 102

1. b
2. c
3. a

Glossary

A

abdominal thrust: force a rescuer exerts when treating obstructed airway (Heimlich maneuver).

abduct: to move away from the center line, as to *abduct* the arm.

ablative surgery: neurosurgery performed to sever or cut pain pathways.

ABO incompatibility: condition in pregnancy in which mother and baby have incompatible blood types.

abort: to prematurely halt a developmental process, as to *abort* a pregnancy.

abrasion: a scraping or rubbing off of the skin.

abruptio placentae: condition in which the placenta tears abruptly and prematurely from the uterus.

abruptio: separation, as *abruptio placentae*.

abscess: collection of pus in a localized area.

absorption: transfer of food into the circulation for transport.

accommodation: adjustment, as the *accommodation* of the lens of the eye.

accountability: responsibility for all actions that one performs.

accreditation: status given to a program that meets approved standards.

acetabulum: the depression into which the rounded head of the femur fits; also known as the hip socket.

achalasia: failure of the smooth muscles of the gastrointestinal tract to relax, especially in the lower esophagus.

acid: chemical compound with a pH below 7.

acidosis: pathology resulting from acid accumulation or alkali depletion.

acne: skin disorder characterized by papules or pustules; also called acne vulgaris.

acquired immunity: immunity that one obtains through natural or artificial sources.

acrocyanosis: newborn condition in which the extremities appear cyanotic.

acromegaly: condition resulting from overproduction of a pituitary hormone.

acronym: word formed by combining the letters of a word or phrase.

acrosclerosis: scleroderma of the distal extremities and face.

action potential: state that results when a stimulus causes an organized, rapid exchange of sodium and potassium ions across a cell membrane, which spreads like an electric current along the membrane.

active range of motion: exercises in which the client is able to move without assistance.

activities of daily living (ADLs): normal activities, such as eating, dressing, walking, bathing.

acuity: clearness; or a disorder's level of severity.

acute disease: disease that develops suddenly and runs its course in days or weeks.

acute pain: (see nociceptive pain).

acute: of short duration, but with severe symptoms; sharp.

Addison's disease: a condition caused by the destruction or degeneration of the adrenal cortex. Symptoms include a darkening of the skin and oral mucous membranes, dehydration, anemia, weight loss, low blood pressure, and thinning hair.

adduct: to draw toward the center, as to *adduct* the arm.

adenohypophysis: the anterior lobe of the pituitary gland.

adhesion: abnormal joining of tissues by a fibrous band, usually resulting from inflammation, injury, or surgery.

adjuvant: assisting or enhancing therapy given, especially in cancer, to prevent further growth.

adolescence: time between puberty's onset and cessation of physical growth, ages 11–19.

adrenal glands: two glands, each consisting of an adrenal medulla and a cortex, of which one sits atop each kidney. The adrenal medulla secretes catecholamines, including epinephrine and norepinephrine, which mimic the action of the sympathetic nervous system and help stimulate the "fight or flight" reaction. The adrenal cortex secretes corticosteroids.

adrenal: near or above the kidney.

advance directive: written instructions clients give in advance about the types of healthcare they desire should they become unable to decide for themselves.

advanced cardiac life support: techniques that include starting IV lines, administering fluids and medications, using defibrillation and cardiac monitoring, administering oxygen, and opening and maintaining the airway.

advance practice nurse: sometimes called a "nurse practitioner," an RN who is specialized in a particular field and has additional education and experience.

adverse effect: a response to a medication that is not intended or desired; a side effect.

advocate: a person who works to gain or preserve the rights of others; a defender (as in client *advocate*). (verb: to work for the rights of others, to assist)

aerobe: microorganism that requires oxygen for growth; also called obligate aerobe.

aesthetic needs: needs more complex than simply physical needs necessary for survival, needs met to give quality to life.

affect: emotional tone, feeling, or the outward manifestation of subjective emotions; also called affectivity.

afferent: sensory neurons that receive messages from all parts of the body and transmit them by way of sensory nerves to the central nervous system; conducting toward the center, as *afferent* nerves.

after-care: continued follow-up and therapy after discharge, especially from chemical dependency treatment or psychiatric hospitalization.

afterload: the amount of pressure or resistance the ventricles of the heart must overcome to empty their contents.

afterpains: abdominal discomfort or cramping after delivery caused by uterine contractions.

ageism: prejudice against people based on age.

agglutination: clumping of blood cells.

agonist therapy: drug therapy that uses specific agents to occupy opioid receptors, blocking the opioid effects.

agonist: a muscle that contracts to move a body part and is opposed by another muscle (the antagonist); a medication that produces a desired response.

agoraphobia: fear of being in a place from which escape may be difficult or embarrassing.

agranulocytosis: an acute disorder, often caused by drug toxicity, in which granulocyte production greatly decreases, causing neutropenia and rendering the body defenseless against bacterial infections. (Also called malignant neutropenia.)

AIDS: acronym for acquired immunodeficiency syndrome.

airborne precautions: precautions taken when a person has an illness that can be carried in the air or on dust particles. Common measures include special air handling and ventilation.

akathisia: constant motor activity, inability to sit down or relax, twitching (a common side effect of neuroleptic medications).

albumin: a protein substance found in animal and vegetable tissues.

alcohol hallucinosis: vivid and terrifying auditory, visual, and tactile hallucinations a person may experience during alcohol withdrawal.

alias: an assigned name under which certain clients are admitted to (and records kept in) a healthcare facility in order to maintain anonymity.

alimentary canal: tube-like structure responsible for digestion and absorption of food, also known as the digestive tract.

alkalosis: serious condition caused by accumulation of bases or loss of acids; a decrease in hydrogen ion concentration (pH) (opposite of acidosis).

allergen: a substance capable of producing hypersensitivity (allergy).

allergy: a state in which the body is hypersensitive to a substance, usually a protein.

allogeneic: persons who are not genetically related (see allograft).

allograft: a graft between individuals of the same species (as in two unrelated persons).

alopecia: abnormal hair loss, or baldness.

alveolar duct: place in the bronchi where the bronchioles first branch.

alveolar sac: grape-like clusters in the bronchi where the bronchioles end.

alveoli: the lung sacs where gas exchange takes place.

Alzheimer's disease: a common form of dementia, most often occurring in older adults.

ambiguous loss: the debilitating confusion a family may experience when a living loved one is still physically present but psychologically absent, as in dementia or psychological disorders.

Ambu bag: (see manual breathing bag).

ambulatory: walking or able to walk. (noun: ambulation)

ambylopia: subnormal vision in one eye which may fail to develop due to lack of stimulation as a child continues to use the stronger eye for vision; also called lazy eye.

amenorrhea: absence or abnormal stoppage of menses (menstruation).

amino acids: building blocks of proteins, comprised mainly of carbon, hydrogen, oxygen, and nitrogen.

amnihook: special sterile hook used to artificially rupture membranes to stimulate the beginning of true labor or to speed up the active labor process.

amniocentesis: perforation of the amniotic sac through a pregnant woman's abdomen to obtain a sample of amniotic fluid.

amnion: the inner membrane and fluid surrounding a fetus ("bag of waters").

amniotic fluid: fluid that suspends the fetus within the amnion, cushioning the fetus from injury, regulating temperature, and allowing the fetus to move freely.

amniotomy: surgical rupture of fetal membranes; artificial rupture of membranes (AROM).

ampule: small, glass-sealed flask, often containing medication.

amputation: removal of a limb or other body part.

anabolism: the constructive phase of metabolism, which involves synthesis of substances to form new, larger substances.

anaerobe: microorganism that cannot survive in the presence of oxygen; also called obligate anaerobe.

analgesic: an agent that relieves pain without causing unconsciousness.

anaphylaxis: serious state of shock resulting from hypersensitivity to an allergen; also called anaphylactic effect.

anaplastic cell: cell which lacks orderly growth, arrangement, and does not function normally; these cells are found in malignant tumors.

anasarca: severe generalized edema, a result of abnormal fluid shifts.

anastamose: communication between two blood vessels.

anastomosis: the joining together of two normally distinct spaces or organs.

anatomic position: a standard reference point used by medical texts to present the body—in which the model stands erect with the arms at the sides and the palms turned forward.

anatomy: science dealing with body structure.

androgen: a hormone that stimulates male characteristics (steroid).

anemia: a blood deficiency in quality or quantity; reduction in hemoglobin.

anencephaly: congenital disorder in which the skull and brain are absent.

anergic: unable to respond to antigens by producing antibodies; weak, lacking energy.

anesthesia: complete or partial loss of sensation.

anesthetic: a substance that produces loss of feeling or sensation.

aneurysm: a dilation of the wall of a vessel that causes the formation of a sac; a life-threatening situation, as an aortic *aneurysm.*

angina pectoris: literally "pain in the chest;" occurs when extra exertion calls for the arteries to increase blood supply to the heart and narrow or obstructed arteries are unable to provide the necessary supply and the heart muscle suffers.

angina: a spasmodic, severe attack or pain, as *angina* pectoris.

angiocardiogram: an x-ray of the heart and major vessels.

angioedema: localized edema deep within or under the skin, producing giant wheals (lumps).

angiogram: a radiograph of any blood vessel.

angioma: birthmark.

angioplasty: surgical repair of a blood or lymph vessel; often refers to repair of coronary vessels.

anhedonia: markedly diminished or lost interest or pleasure in all or most activities.

anion: a negatively charged ion.

ankylosis: abnormal consolidation of a joint, causing immobility.

anorexia nervosa: a condition in which a person refuses to eat because he or she wants to be thin, although he or she is already very thin.

anorexia: lack or loss of appetite for food, refusal to eat.

antagonist: a muscle that exerts an action opposite that of another muscle; a medication that blocks or reverses the action of another medication.

antepartal: occurring before childbirth (in reference to the pregnant woman); antepartum.

antiarrhythmic: a medication that helps regulate the heart's rhythm.

antibiotic: substance produced by a living organism that can destroy or weaken other organisms.

antibody mediated immunity: immunity that results when an antibody changes an antigen, making it harmless to the body.

antibody: a specific protein that neutralizes foreign antigens (essential to the immune response).

anticipatory guidance: education about expected changes prior to them happening.

anticonvulsant: a medication that reduces, controls, or stops seizure activity.

antidote: an agent that counteracts the effects of a poison.

antiembolism stockings: also called TED socks; elastic stockings that cover the foot (not the toes) and the leg, up to the knee or mid-thigh.

antigen: a substance that stimulates the production of antibodies.

antihypertensives: medications that reduce blood pressure.

antimicrobial agent: a chemical that decreases the number of pathogens in an area by suppressing and destroying their growth.

antineoplastic: an agent that inhibits the growth of malignant cells.

antiretroviral therapy: medications to specifically combat the retrovirus.

antitussive: an agent that reduces coughing.

anuria: complete suppression of urine secretion in the kidney.

anxiety: apprehensive uneasiness or dread (may be marked by physiologic signs, such as sweating, tension, or increased pulse).

aorta: the largest artery of the body.

aortic valve: valve which separates the left ventricle from the aorta.

apex: lower point of the heart, formed by the tip of the left ventricle.

Apgar score: a method of determining a newborn's condition at birth by rating the baby's respiration and responses.

aphasia: condition in which a person is unable to express oneself through speech or writing.

apical pulse: pulse normally heard at the heart's apex, which usually gives the most accurate assessment of pulse rate.

apical-radial pulse: reading done by measuring both the apical and radial pulses simultaneously, used when it is suspected that the heart is not effectively pumping blood.

apnea: cessation of breathing.

apoptosis: cell self-destruction.

apothecary: one of the oldest measurement systems, based on volume and weight.

appendicitis: inflammation of the appendix.

appendix: small finger-like projection of the cecum which has no known function; also called vermiform appendix.

approval: status given to a program that allows its graduates to obtain a license.

apraxia: difficulty carrying out purposeful movements.

aquathermia pad: pad which produces a dry heat by the use of temperature-controlled water flowing through a waterproof shell.

aqueous humor: liquid that flows through the anterior and posterior eye chambers in the space between the cornea and the lens.

architectural barriers: building structures that make certain areas inaccessible to individuals with physical disabilities.

arrhythmia: technically means "without a heartbeat;" cardiac standstill.

arterial blood gases: the levels of oxygen and carbon dioxide in the blood.

arteriogram: an x-ray of any artery.

arteriosclerosis: a condition of the arteries that produces abnormal loss of elasticity and hardening of the walls, especially in the middle layer; also called hardening of the arteries.

artery: any vessel through which blood passes from the heart to all body parts.

arthritis: joint inflammation.

arthrogram: x-ray of a joint.

arthroplasty: joint repair.

arthrosclerosis: stiffening of the joints.

arthroscope: an endoscope used to examine or do surgery within a joint (arthroscopy).

arthrostomy: creation of an opening drain.

articular: pertaining to a joint.

articulation: point at which bones attach; also known as a joint.

artificial insemination: process in which male sperm is artificially implanted into a woman's cervix or into an egg.

artificial sphincter: cuff placed around the bladder neck and connected to a reservoir bulb implanted in individuals with a non-functioning urethra.

artificially acquired immunity: immunity that occurs when a person is deliberately exposed to a causative agent, such as during vaccination.

ascites: abnormal fluid collection in the peritoneal cavity.

asepsis: practices that minimize or eliminate organisms that cause infections or disease.

aseptic: free from germs that cause infection or disease.

asexual: without sex; a person who has no interest in sex.

asphyxia: suffocation; deficiency of oxygen.

aspiration: withdrawal of fluid or gas from a cavity by means of suction; the act of inhaling (pathologic drawing of fluids into the lungs), often causing aspiration pneumonia.

assault: a violent act, either physical or verbal.

assaultive: threatening to hurt others or actually striking someone.

assertiveness: confidence without aggression or passivity, an important skill for a nurse to possess in interpersonal communication.

assessment: phase of the nursing process in which the nurse systematically and continuously collects and analyzes data about a client.

assisted living: programs that allow older adults to age in place, maintain independence, and choose services they want and need.

assisted suicide: helping an individual who wants to end his or her life to do so.

asthma: a disease marked by breathing difficulty, caused by spasmodic contractions of the bronchial tubes; bronchial *asthma.*

astigmatism: condition in which the eye cannot bring horizontal and vertical lines into focus at the same time, causing blurry vision, as a result of irregularities in the curvature of the cornea and lens.

ataxia: failure or irregularity of muscle coordination, often a chronic condition; inability to walk.

ataxic cerebral palsy: type of cerebral palsy that results in tremors, unsteady gait, lack of coordination and balance, rapid repeated movements of the eyeball, muscle weakness, and lack of leg movement during infancy.

atelectasis: collapse of all or part of a lung.

atherectomy: type of angioplasty in which a sharp device is used to shave away plaque from the coronary or other artery.

atherosclerosis: arteriosclerosis characterized by deposits of cholesterol, fatty acids, or plaques on the inner wall of the artery.

athetoid: involuntary writing movements of fingers, toes, or extremities.

athetosis: slow, repetitive, involuntary writhing movements.

atom: the smallest particle of an element that retains the original properties of that element.

atony: lack of firmness, as in the uterus.

atrial ablation: procedure which uses a catheter to determine the location of the abnormality within the heart and

using radiofrequency energy, destroys the diseased tissue.

atrioventricular valves: valves that lie between the atria and the ventricles.

atrium: entrance (usually refers to upper chambers of the heart). (pl: atria)

atrophy: to waste away.

auditory tube: (see Eustachian tube).

aura: a subjective sensation prior to a seizure, such as before an epileptic attack or a migraine headache; a warning.

aural: pertaining to the ear (otic).

auricle: flap of cartilage and skin that comprises the outer ear; a portion of the atrium of the heart. (Sometimes used to refer to entire atrium.) External ear, pinna.

auscultation: externally listening to sounds from within the body to determine abnormal conditions, as *auscultation* of blood pressure with a stethoscope.

autism: condition marked by preoccupation with inner thoughts and withdrawal from the outside world.

autoclave: a pressure steam sterilizer.

autocratic leadership: leadership style that is self directed and calls for little input from others.

autograft: a graft that is transplanted from one place to another on the same person's body.

autoimmune disorder: disorder in which the body fails to recognize its own cells as "self" and begins to destroy them.

autoimmune: allergic response of one's own body to cells or organs within the body; inability of the body to differentiate between "self" and "nonself."

autologous: related to self, pertaining to the same person or organism, as an *autologous* skin graft from another place on one's own body.

automated external defibrillator: a portable unit that analyzes the heart's rhythm and indicates when an electric shock is necessary; considered definitive treatment for those in cardiac arrest.

autonomic dysreflexia (AD): hyperreflexia or exaggerated autonomic nervous system reflexes occurring, for example, in clients with a spinal cord injury, especially injury above T-6.

autonomic: not subject to voluntary control, as the *autonomic* nervous system, "automatic."

autopsy: examination of the body after death; postmortem.

aversion therapy: a psychological treatment that uses adverse conditioning to prevent a person from repeating bad or destructive behaviors.

avulsion: the tearing away of a structure or part, as an *avulsion injury* when a tooth is knocked out.

axilla: the armpit.

axon: outgrowth of the body of a nerve cell that conducts impulses away from the cell body.

B

B cells: lymphocytes that originate in the bone marrow.

Babinski reflex: a reflex caused by scraping the sole of the foot (normal in a newborn; a sign of neurologic damage in an adult).

bacillus: a rod shaped bacterium (plural: bacilli).

bacteremia: presence of bacteria in the blood.

bacteria: microorganisms, some of which are disease-causing; common forms are staphylococci, streptococci, bacilli, and spirochetes.

bacteriology: the study of bacteria, commonly used to denote the study of all organisms.

bacterial vaginosis: infection of the vagina caused by a gram-negative bacteria, *Gardnerella vaginalis;* also called nonspecific vaginitis; formerly known as *Hemophilus vaginalis.*

bactericidal: a substance that kills bacteria.

bacteriophage: virus that destroys bacteria by lysis.

bacteriostatic: a substance that arrests bacterial growth.

bacteriuria: bacteria in urine.

balking: refusing to do something.

ballottement: a specific palpation to test for a floating object, such as a fetus.

bandage: a strip of material (gauze, tape, cloth, etc.) used to cover a wound or to hold a dressing in place, in order to give support or to apply pressure. (verb: to apply a bandage, to bandage)

Bartholin's glands: glands in the vagina that provide it with lubrication.

basal metabolism: minimum amount of energy the body uses at rest.

base: also called an alkali, a compound that contains the hydroxyl ion (OH-).

base of support: balance or stability provided by the feet and their positioning.

basic cardiac life support: life-saving measures such as rapid entry into emergency medical services, performance of CPR, and use of techniques to clear obstructed airway.

battery: physical striking or beating, as assault and *battery*.

bed cradle: a frame used to prevent bedclothes from touching all or part of a person's body.

beliefs: concepts that a person or group thinks are true.

benign: harmless, not malignant.

benign prostatic hyperplasia (BPH): narrowing of the urethra which results as the prostate continues to grow throughout a man's life.

benzodiazepine: class of common antianxiety medication.

bereavement: normal period of mourning or grieving following the death of a loved one.

beriberi: disease of the nervous system that can lead to paralysis and death from heart failure, caused by a severe thiamine deficiency.

beta (β) endorphins: hormones that have the same effect as opiate drugs, whose release is stimulated by stress and exercise.

bicuspid (mitral) valve: valve between the left atrium and left ventricle formed of two tissue flaps.

bile: fluid produced by the liver and stored in the gallbladder that aids in fat digestion.

biliary atresia: defect in the bile ducts that prevents bile from escaping the liver.

binuclear family: a family in which a separation or divorce of the adult partners occurs, but both adults continue to assume a high level of childrearing responsibilities.

biofeedback: using an electronic device to measure the effectiveness of inter-

nal exercises, such as Kegel's, or to expand one's ability to control the autonomic nervous system.

biohazardous: harmful to humans or animals; infectious.

biologic death: permanent and irreversible cessation of the body's physical and chemical processes and failure of body cells.

bionomics: study of the environment and its relationship to living things.

biopsy: removal of a piece of body tissue for diagnostic examination, usually microscopic; most often used to detect the presence of cancer.

biotherapy: the use of biologic response modifiers (BRM) in cancer treatment.

bipolar disorder: severe disorder in which behavior alternates between overactivity and depression.

birth plan: written document in which the expectant mother expresses her desires for labor and birth.

birthing room: room in a hospital in which both labor and delivery take place; also called labor/delivery/recovery/postpartum (LDRP) rooms.

bisexual: sexual attraction to persons of both sexes; exhibiting both heterosexuality and homosexuality.

blackout: temporary loss of vision and consciousness due to lack of blood supply to the brain and retina; sometimes refers to fainting.

bladder: a membranous muscular sac, as the gall- or urinary *bladder*.

bland diet: diet that is limited in gastric acid stimulants.

blended family: family that results when two people who already have children marry, blending two families into one.

blepharitis: inflammation of the eyelid.

blood pressure: pressure of the blood on the walls of the blood vessels, expressed as systolic (contraction phase) over diastolic (relaxation phase).

body cavity: a space within the body that contains internal organs.

body cue: personal feelings that place emphasis on self-care.

body language: impressions one conveys through body movements and posture, eye contact, and other nonverbal means.

body mass index: weight in kilograms divided by height in meters squared.

body mechanics: use of safe and efficient methods of moving and lifting.

body temperature: measure of heat inside a person's body; balance between heat produced and heat lost.

bolus: a rounded mass, as an amount of food in the intestine, a pill, or a rounded pad. A dose of IV medication given quickly, as a *bolus* dose.

bonding: the development of a close emotional tie, as between parent and child.

bore: a needle's inner diameter.

Bowman's capsule: funnel-shaped structure that encloses the glomerulus of the kidney.

bradycardia: abnormally slow heart action; slow pulse.

bradykinesia: slowness of movement.

bradypnea: condition in which breaths are abnormally slow and fall below ten per minute.

braille: an alphabet system for the nonsighted, with raised dots that one can feel with the fingers.

brain death: irreversible cessation of brain and brain stem function to the extent that cardiopulmonary function must be mechanically maintained. Criteria for determination vary between states. (Also called cerebral death, irreversible coma, and persistent vegetative state.)

brain stem: part of the brain that connects the cerebral hemispheres and the spinal cord.

brand name: copyrighted name assigned by a company that makes a medication; also called trade name.

Braxton-Hicks contractions: during pregnancy, naturally occurring tightening and relaxing of uterine muscles in preparation for labor and delivery; usually irregular and painless.

breech: positioning of the fetus in which the buttocks or either or both feet present rather than the head.

broad spectrum: classification of an antibiotic that is effective against many different organisms.

bronchi: tubular-shaped air passages that connect the trachea and lungs. (sing: bronchus)

bronchiectasis: chronic dilation of the bronchi, with large amounts of sputum production.

bronchioles: smaller bronchi.

bronchiolitis: inflammation of the bronchioles.

bronchitis: inflammation of the bronchi.

bronchodilator: a medication that causes the bronchioles to expand (dilate), thus improving respiration.

bronchoscope: a lighted instrument used to examine the interior of the bronchi (bronchoscopy).

brown fat: stored fat occurring only in infants born at term, used to produce heat; once it is used, the baby cannot create more.

bruxism: grinding of the teeth during sleep.

buccal: pertaining to the cheek or mouth.

buffer: a chemical system set up to resist changes, particularly in the level of hydrogen ions.

bulbourethral glands: glands that secrete an alkaline mucus that lubricates the penis and neutralizes the pH of urine residue, also known as Cowper's gland.

bulimia: a condition in which a person eats huge amounts of food and then self-induces vomiting or uses large amounts of laxatives (binge–purge syndrome); also called bulimia nervosa.

bureaucratic leadership: leadership style that is policy minded and relies on established protocols for decision making.

bursa: a small, fluid-filled sac that prevents friction, as in *bursae* of the shoulder. (pl: bursae)

bursitis: inflammation of a bursa.

C

cachexia: severe ill health and malnutrition; debilitated state.

Caduceus: modern symbols of medicine, two sets of wings atop two serpents twined around a staff, based on mythical figures (also known as the staff of Aesculapius).

cafe coronary: slang term for a person who dies by choking while eating, often after rushing from a restaurant to avoid embarrassment.

calcaneous: the largest tarsal bone, located in the heel (os calcis).

calcium: most abundant mineral element in the body; found especially in bones and teeth.

calculus: an abnormal concretion usually composed of mineral salts, occurring in the hollow body organs; a "stone," as a *calculus* in the kidney (pl: calculi); deposit on the teeth (tartar).

calices: (see calyces).

calyces: cuplike extensions of the renal pelvis into which urine flows from the collecting tubules (singular: calyx).

cancer: a malignant growth, neoplasm, carcinoma.

candidiasis: most common cause of vaginitis, resulting primarily by an overgrowth of the normal population of the fungus *Candida albicans;* also known as moniliasis, thrush, fungal infection, and yeast infection.

canthus (inner and outer): angle at either side of the corners of the eye.

capitation fee: a monthly or yearly payment made by a participant in an HMO.

caplet: a tablet in the shape of a capsule, making it easier to swallow.

capsule: a small gelatinous case for holding a dose of medicine; a membranous structure enclosing another body structure, as the articular *capsule* in a joint.

caput succedaneum: accumulation of fluid within the newborn's scalp caused by pressure to the head during delivery.

caput: pertaining to the head, as *caput succedaneum.*

carbohydrate: most widely used energy source in the world; found mostly in sugars and starches. (Made of carbon, hydrogen, and oxygen [CHO].)

carbohydrate-controlled diet: approach to eating which focuses on consistency in the amount of carbohydrates consumed, especially useful in maintaining healthy blood sugar and fat levels for diabetics.

carbuncle: a cluster of boils (furuncles).

carcinogen: an agent that causes cancer.

carcinogenesis: transformation of a normal cell into a malignant cell.

carcinoma: cancer, a malignant neoplasm (new growth).

cardiac: pertaining to the heart.

cardiac catheterization: procedure in which a catheter is passed into the heart through a large blood vessel to assess its structures or output.

cardiac sphincter: muscle that guards the stomach opening.

cardinal symptoms: functions necessary to life; vital signs (temperature, pulse, respiration, and blood pressure).

cardiology: field of medicine that examines the cardiovascular system and its disorders.

cardiopulmonary resuscitation (CPR): a combination of external cardiac massage and artificial ventilation.

cardioversion: delivery of an electric shock to the heart to restore normal rhythm; countershock; precordial shock; sometimes called defibrillation.

care map: plan that outlines protocols for the management of a specific disorder.

career mobility: ability of a person to advance or diversify within his or her profession.

caregiver stress: overwhelming exhaustion and frustration experienced by persons who must continually care for someone who is old or ill.

caries: decay, as in dental *caries.*

carotene: yellow or red pigment contained in many foods such as squash, carrots, and green, leafy vegetables; converted to vitamin A in the body.

carotid pulse: pulse felt on either side of the neck, over the carotid artery.

carpal: pertaining to the wrist (carpus).

cartilage: fibrous connective tissue in joints.

case management: providing high quality care while effectively using healthcare resources and controlling costs.

case manager: a person who plans and directs all necessary activities to coordinate a client's care.

cast: an appliance used to immobilize displaced or injured parts; a fatty, waxy, or epithelial substance formed in the urinary system and found (abnormally) in urine; a mold or impression, as of the jaw, used to make braces or dentures.

catabolism: the destructive phase of metabolism; breaking down.

catalepsy: state in which a person maintains the body position in which he or she is placed.

cataplexy: abrupt attacks of muscular weakness and decreased strength.

cataract: an opacity of the lens of the eye or its capsule.

catastrophic reaction: display of agitation that a person with dementia may experience when confronted with a difficult or overwhelming situation.

catatonia: stupor and muscle rigidity common in schizophrenia.

catecholamines: neurotransmitters that increase cardiac output, constrict peripheral blood vessels, increase blood pressure, and cause bronchodilation in response to stress.

cathartic: a medicine that causes bowel evacuation, laxative, purgative.

catheter: a flexible tube that is passed into the body, usually through body channels, for the withdrawal or instillation of fluids; most often refers to urinary catheter.

catheterization: procedure to insert a catheter into the client's body.

cation: an ion that carries a positive electrical charge.

caustic: burning; destructive to tissues.

cavity: a hollow space within the body or one of its organs.

cecum: a pouch 2–3 inches long that forms the first portion of the large intestine.

celiac disease: chronic intestinal disorder which involves small bowel inflammation and is the most common nutrient malabsorption syndrome in children of European descent.

cell: the minute protoplasmic building unit of living matter; the body's basic structural unit.

cell membrane: surface layer that surround the cells' outer boundary and regulates what enters and leaves the cell, also known as the plasma membrane.

cell-mediated immunity: type of immunity in which T cells have proliferated and become capable of combining with specific foreign antigens.

cellular respiration: exchange of oxygen for carbon dioxide within the cells.

center of gravity: the center of one's weight; half of one's body weight is below and half above, and half to the left and half to the right of the center of gravity. This concept is important in body mechanics.

central nervous system: brain and spinal cord.

cephalalgia: head pain.

cephalhematoma: newborn condition in which blood accumulates between the bones of the skull and the periosteum.

cephalocaudal: literally, "head to toe" (used to denote developmental progression in infants).

cerclage: nonabsorbable suture placed around an incompetent cervix to hold it closed for the duration of pregnancy.

cerebellum: part of the brain located on the back of the brain stem. It has three lobes, one median (*vermis*), and two laterals (hemispheres).

cerebral cortex: outside of the brain made of soft gray matter containing mostly nerve cell bodies.

cerebral lobes: four lobes of the brain that enable humans to associate impressions and information, which becomes knowledge.

cerebrospinal fluid: a lymphlike fluid that forms a protective cushion around and within the central nervous system.

cerebrum: the major portion of the brain, comprising 80% of its volume.

cerumen: waxy substance that collects in the outer ear canal; ear wax.

ceruminal glands: specialized glands found only in the passage that leads into the ear that function to protect the eardrum by producing cerumen.

cervical os: mouth or opening of the cervix.

cervicitis: inflammation of the uterine cervix.

cervix: the narrow lower end of the uterus, which opens into the vagina.

cesarean delivery: surgical procedure to deliver a baby through an incision in the abdomen and uterus.

Chadwick's sign: a cervix that looks blue or purple which may occur as early as the sixth week of pregnancy.

chain-of-command: hierarchy of an organizational structure.

chalazion: a small mass on the eyelid caused by inflammation of a meibomian gland.

chancre: hard, primary lesion which is the first sign of syphilis.

chancroid: soft sore caused by *Haemophilus ducreyi* and generally spread by sexual contact.

change-of-shift reporting: a means of exchanging information between outgoing and incoming staff on each shift.

chart audit: an evaluation of outcomes of care from the client's point of view.

chelation: a process for treating poisoning with a metal such as lead (plumbism), in which the chelating agent and the metal combine, become soluble and can be eliminated. (Also used to remove excess iron in sickle cell anemia.)

chemical change: a change that alters a substance's chemical composition.

chemical dependency: substance abuse, with tolerance, withdrawal, and other indicative symptoms.

chemical name: medication name that describes its chemical composition (often same as generic name).

chemical restraint: medications that are given to control behavior.

chemotherapy: use of chemical agents to destroy cancerous cells.

chest: the thorax; the part of the body that lies between the neck and the abdominal cavity.

Cheyne-Stokes respiration: breathing characterized by deep breathing alternating with very slow breathing or apnea; indicative of brain damage; often precedes death.

chlamydia: sexually transmitted disease caused by the bacteria *Chlamydia trachomatis* that is the leading cause of preventable infertility in women and the most common STD in the United States.

chloasma: hyperpigmentation (darker coloration) in particular skin areas, such as the "mask of pregnancy" or the linea nigra in pregnancy (*chloasma gravidarum*). (Also called melasma.)

chloride: elemental ion needed for the production of stomach acid and the body's complex buffering system.

choanal atresia: condition in which the newborn's nostrils are closed at the entrance to the throat so that air cannot pass through to the lungs.

cholecystic: pertaining to the gallbladder.

cholelithiasis: gallstones.

cholesterol: a steroid alcohol found only in animal tissues, needed to produce hormones, vitamin D, and bile acids; has been connected with atherosclerotic disease.

chorea: nervous condition characterized by twitching in the limbs or face, as in Huntington's chorea (also known as Huntington's disease).

choriocarcinoma: type of cancer of the uterus or at the site of an ectopic pregnancy that may develop as the result of hydatidiform mole.

chorion: the outermost fetal membrane.

chromosome: body in the nucleus of the cell that carries genetic factors.

chronic: a condition that remains for a length of time, may be progressive.

chronic illness: a disease of long duration that generally manifests itself in an individual as recurring problems that tend to worsen in severity over time.

chronic pain: pain that lasts more than six months; neuropathic pain.

chronic ulcerative colitis: relatively common disorder in adolescents and young adults characterized by inflammation of the colon and rectum.

Chvostek's sign: abnormal spasms of the facial muscles in response to light taps on the facial nerve; indicative of tetany following thyroidectomy.

chyme: partially digested food as it enters the duodenum.

cilia: hairlike threads that sweep materials across a cell.

circumcise: usually refers to surgical removal of the foreskin (prepuce) of the penis.

circumduction: circular movement of a limb or the eye.

circumoral cyanosis: darkening of skin color, particularly around the eyes, nose, and mouth due to poor oxygenation.

cirrhosis: chronic inflammation and degeneration of an organ, especially *cirrhosis* of the liver.

claudication: cramps that occur because of an insufficient supply of oxygen, as in intermittent *claudication.*

clavicle: the collar bone.

clean: in medical asepsis, devoid of all gross contamination and free of many microorganisms.

cleft lip: vertical opening in the upper lip.

cleft palate: congenital split in the roof of the mouth.

client: a person who is a participant in his or her healthcare.

client unit: area where most client care is provided.

client-oriented: focused on meeting individualized needs.

client reminder/safety device: (see protective device)

climacteric: cessation of reproductive function in the female (menopause), and decreased testicular activity in the male.

clinical breast exam: a breast examination conducted by a healthcare provider.

clinical care path: planning method that identifies the optimal sequencing and timing of healthcare interventions; designates interventions for all members of a healthcare team, not just nurses.

clinical death: absence of heartbeat and cessation of breathing.

clitoris: small structure of erectile tissue in the female at the anterior junction of the labia that is stimulated by sexual excitement.

closed bed: bed used when preparing a unit for a new client—an unoccupied bed.

closed questions: questions that can usually be answered by one word, such as "yes" or "no;" also called close-ended questions.

coagulation: the changing of a liquid to thickened, curdlike form.

coccus: a round or spherical bacterium (plural: cocci).

coccyx: tailbone.

cochlea: snail-shaped organ of the inner ear; the essential organ of hearing.

code: predetermined phrase or term used by healthcare professionals in an emergency situation that is activated to alert all necessary personnel to action.

codependent: in substance abuse, one who has let the abuser's behavior affect him or her and is now obsessed with controlling the

abuser's behavior; may also be used to refer to an alcoholic or chemically dependent person who is living with another person who is also an abuser of drugs or alcohol.

cognitive function: ability to think and reason.

cognitive: involving knowledge, understanding, and perception; in the mind.

cogwheeling movements: abnormal muscular rigor that manifests as jerky movements when the muscle is passively stretched; can be a side effect of psychotropic medications.

cohabitation: unmarried individuals in a committed partnership living together, with or without children.

coitus interruptus: withdrawal of the penis from the vagina before ejaculation.

colic: paroxysmal abdominal pain, most commonly occurring in the first three months of an infant's life; or severe, penetrating lower back pain, caused by a stone becoming lodged in the ureter (renal colic).

collaborative problem: problem in which nurses work with physicians or other healthcare providers.

collagen diseases: diseases of the connective tissue.

collagen: white, fibrous structural protein found in tendons, bone cartilage, skin, and other connective tissues, as well as in the vitreous humor of the eye.

collateral circulation: circulation that occurs when one blood vessel is plugged and another evolves to take over its function, usually in the heart.

colloid solutions: solutions used to replace circulating blood volume; also called plasma expanders.

colon: a continuous tube divided into three parts that forms the longest portion of the large intestine.

colonization: microorganisms present in a person, who shows no signs or symptoms of illness.

colonoscopy: procedure in which a scope is passed into the rectum to allow visualization of the colon.

colostomy: an artificial opening from the colon to outside the body by way of a stoma.

colostrum: the first fluid secreted by the mammary (breast) glands just before or after childbirth.

command center: place that provides overall direction of a facility's activities in a disaster.

commitment: involuntary admittance to a mental healthcare facility.

commode: toilet; bedside toilet.

communal family: family where many people live together, strive to be self-sufficient, and minimize contact with the outside society.

communicable disease: a disease that can be transmitted from one person to another.

communication: giving, receiving, and interpreting information (may be verbal or nonverbal).

community: a collection of people who interact with one another and whose common interests or characteristics form the basis for a sense of unity or belonging.

community health: aggregate health of a population.

commuter family: a family in which both adults are usually professionals, one of whom lives in another city because of employment, and the partners must travel a long distance, usually on weekends, to be together.

comorbidity: coexisting disorders.

compartment syndrome: disorder that results from inadequate or obstructed blood flow to muscles, nerves, and tissue; may also stem from compression of the muscle compartment or from an increase in contents related to edema, hemorrhage, fracture, or soft tissue injury.

complement fixation: mechanism for antigen destruction by which activated complements destroy invaders.

complement: a group of proteins normally present but inactive in the blood.

complementary healthcare: methods and beliefs other than traditional Western medicine.

compliance: muscle activity and stretch of the bladder wall; also known as accommodation.

complication: an unexpected event in a disease's course that delays a person's recovery.

compound: substance composed of two or more elements united according to chemical weights; they undergo chemical change (elements lose their original characteristics).

compulsion: a repetitive behavior or mental act that a person feels driven to perform, sometimes constantly.

conception: union of two sex cells: the ovum (female) and the sperm (male).

concussion: violent jar or shock, or the injury that results.

condom: latex, plastic, or animal sheath applied to the erect penis before sexual intercourse and used as a barrier method.

conduction: carrying or conveying energy, such as heat, electricity, or sound.

condylomata acuminata: venereal warts that grow in warm, moist body areas and are often spread by sexual contact.

cones: specialized neurons concentrated in the retina's center that receive color, add visual acuity, and require a significant amount of light to function.

confabulation: unconsciously filling in memory gaps with made-up information, often seen in organic dementias and psychoses.

confidentiality: information a client shares with a professional, expecting the information to remain with that person alone.

confusion: impairment of mental function that causes poor judgment, memory loss, and disorientation.

congenital: existing at birth (may be genetic/inherited or acquired), as in *congenital disorders.*

congregate housing: a special high rise or other building designated for a specific group.

conization: removal of a cone-shaped portion of the cervix.

conjunctiva: transparent mucous membrane covering the anterior eye (front).

conjunctivitis: commonly called pink eye; inflammation of the conjunctiva.

conscious sedation: condition in which internal sedative medications are used alone or in conjunction with local anesthetics and the client has a depressed level of consciousness but is still able to breathe and respond to verbal stimuli.

consortium: public and private organizations who share data and workers to provide more cost-efficient healthcare.

constipation: difficult or infrequent and hardened bowel movements.

consumer fraud: misleading the public.

contact precautions: precautions taken against diseases that can be transmitted through direct contact between a susceptible host's body surface and an infected or colonized person. Common measures include use of personal protective equipment.

contagious: able to be transmitted from one person to another, infectious.

contaminate: to make unsterile or unclean.

contaminated: anything that is not sterile.

continuous passive motion (CPM): machine that provides exercise for a limb without active participation by client or nurse.

contraceptive: an agent that diminishes the likelihood of pregnancy.

contractility: ability to shorten and become thicker.

contracture: abnormal shortening of muscles with resultant deformity.

contralateral: the opposite side.

contusion: injury without breaking the skin; a bruise.

convection: spread/transmission of heat in a liquid or gas by circulation of heated particles.

convoluted tubule: long, twisted tube extending from Bowman's capsule, through which water travels in the kidneys.

co-pay: predetermined fee that is charged to HMO clients at the time of an office visit.

copulation: sexual intercourse between male and female.

corium: the dermis, "true skin," the fibrous inner layer of skin just under the epidermis.

cornea: the transparent front covering of the eye, as in corneal transplant.

coronary sinus: opening in the heart which returns blood to the right atrium.

corprolalia: continuous uttering of obscenities.

corpus callosum: a band of approximately 200 million neurons connecting the brain's right and left hemi-spheres.

cortex: outer layer (see renal cortex).

corticosteroids: compounds secreted by the outer part of the adrenal glands.

crackle: an abnormal respiratory sound heard on auscultation; also called rale.

cranial nerves: one of two sets of nerve groups that comprise the peripheral nervous system; these nerves originate in the brain.

cranial: pertaining to the skull, as *cranial* nerves.

craniotomy: any operation into the cranium (skull), "brain surgery."

crash cart: a cart or rolling chest containing emergency medications and equipment.

Credé's maneuver: a technique used in bladder rehabilitation (retraining) in which the hands are held flat against the abdomen just below the umbilicus, with firm downward strokes applied toward the bladder, followed by pressure on the bladder itself, to manually express urine.

cretinism: arrested development resulting from congenital thyroid hormone deficiency.

crime: an illegal act; a felony or misdemeanor; an offense which is against the law.

crisis: the turning point of a disease; sudden intensification of symptoms.

critical thinking: mix of inquiry, knowledge, intuition, logic, experience, and common sense.

cross-sensitivity: the characteristic of a medication that reacts similarly to a related drug; common adverse effects.

crossmatch: testing of donor blood against a recipient's blood to determine compatibility.

crowning: in childbirth, the appearance of the top of the baby's head at the vaginal opening.

cryosurgery: removal of tissue by destroying it through freezing.

cryptorchidism: undescended testicles.

crystalluria: crystals in the urine.

cue: feeling that one experiences by listening to one's body rhythms.

culdoscopy: examination of the (internal) female viscera by means of an endoscope inserted through the posterior vaginal fornix.

cultural competence: sensitivity to cultural factors involved in a person's health or illness.

cultural diversity: state in which a group has members from many different cultural, ethnic, and religious backgrounds.

cultural sensitivity: understanding and tolerating all cultures and lifestyles.

culture: growing of microorganisms in specific media; the product of culture growth; the concepts, habits, skills, and institutions of a given group of people (civilization).

cultured epithelial autograft: grafts made from a biopsy of unburned skin and grown on new skin; useful in covering extensive burns.

curandero: a lay person, in Latino cultures, who assists a client with herbs and counseling during an illness.

Cushing's syndrome: condition that results from overproduction of hormones secreted by the adrenal gland. Signs and symptoms include a rounded face, heavy abdomen, thin arms and legs, weakness, soft bones, edema, hypokalemia, and urinary retention.

cyanosis: blueness or duskiness of the skin caused by oxygen deficiency and excess carbon dioxide in the blood.

cyclothymic: mild form of bipolar disorder (ie, characterized by less extreme periods of overactivity and depression).

cylindruria: cylinders (casts) in the urine.

cystic fibrosis: congenital multisystem chronic and incurable condition characterized by the dysfunction of the exocrine glands. Mucus producing glands secrete abnormal quantities of thick mucus which collect in the lungs, pancreas, and liver, disrupting their normal functioning.

cystitis: inflammation of any bladder (most often refers to urinary bladder).

cystocele: herniation of the urinary bladder into the vagina.

cystogram: a radiograph of the bladder and urethra.

cystometrogram: measurement of bladder pressure during filling.

cystoscopy: examination of the inside of the bladder.

cytokine: proteins that act as messengers to help regulate some of the functions of the lymphocytes and macrophages during the immune response.

cytology: the study of cells.

cytomegalovirus, CMV: a group of host-specific herpesviruses, causing many different symptoms.

cytoplasm: area of the cell not located in the nucleus.

D

dangling: positioning of a client so that he or she is sitting on the edge of the bed with legs down and feet supported by a footstool or the floor. This is an exercise in preparation for sitting in a chair and/or walking.

data analysis: analyzing each piece of information to determine its relevance to a client's health problems and its relationship to other pieces of information.

debridement: removal of foreign, dead, and contaminated material from a wound, so as to expose healthy underlying tissue.

debulking: removing part of a tumor.

decanoate: injectable long-lasting psychotropic medications.

decidua: the endometrium during pregnancy.

decimal fraction: fraction in which ten is always the denominator.

decubitis ulcer: (see pressure ulcer).

decussation: crossing.

defecation: discharge of solid waste matter (feces) from the intestines.

defense mechanisms: reactions to stress that help individuals resolve mental conflicts, reduce anxiety, protect self-esteem, and maintain a sense of security.

deglutition: swallowing.

dehiscence: opening or separation of the surgical incision.

dehumanize: to make a person/client feel like an object, to remove one's dignity.

dehydration: removal of water; lack of fluid/water in the body.

delirium tremens: symptoms that appear in the third stage of alcohol withdrawal that include delusions, vivid hallucinations, along with severe physical effects.

delirium: a mental disturbance, usually temporary, marked by wandering speech, delusions, excitement, and at times, hallucinations.

delivery forceps: double-bladed curved instruments that fit around the fetal head and are used to increase traction and assist in rotating the fetus during delivery.

delusion: a false belief that cannot be corrected by reason.

dementia: organic loss of intellectual function; formerly referred to as organic brain syndrome or senility.

democratic leadership: leadership style that is people oriented and tries to guide others in the right direction.

demography: study of population trends, including births, deaths, and diseases.

dendrite: nerve branch that conducts impulses toward the cell body.

denominator: bottom number in a fraction.

dentin: bonelike substance which is the bulk of tooth material.

deoxyribonucleic acid (DNA): a complex acid occurring in the nucleus of all cells, which is the basic structure of genes and carries the genetic code.

dependent actions: actions that nurses must follow explicitly according to physician's orders.

depressant: medication that slows down certain mental and physical processes.

dermabrasion: surgical means of smoothing the skin, used to minimize scarring.

dermatitis: inflammation of the skin; rash.

dermatology: study of the skin and its diseases.

dermis: the true skin.

desquamation: the shedding or scaling of the skin or cuticle; peeling.

detachment: the final stage of dying when an individual gradually separates from the world, so that a two-way communication no longer exists with those around them; becoming disconnected.

detoxification: process of removing a toxin (e.g., alcohol) or its effects.

detrusor: muscle of the bladder that pushes urine out.

development: change in body function.

developmental disability: assorted physical, cognitive, psychological, sensory, and speech impairments

that affect about 17% of children under 18 years of age.

diabetes: a disease characterized by great increase in urinary discharge and increased blood glucose; usually refers to *diabetes* mellitus; may also refer to *diabetes insipidus.*

diabetes insipidus: disease that results from an underproduction of antidiuretic hormone.

diabetes mellitus: metabolic condition involving elevated levels of glucose in the blood.

diagnosis: recognition of a disease by its signs and symptoms, made by a physician.

diagnosis-related group (DRG): grouping of medical diagnoses to determine level of payment by an agency such as Medicare.

dialysis: diffusion of dissolved molecules through a semipermeable membrane (most often refers to treatment given to remove waste products from the blood of a client who suffers from renal failure).

diaphoresis: perspiration or sweating, particularly profuse perspiration.

diaphragm: the muscular partition between the thoracic and abdominal cavities, important in breathing; a type of female contraceptive device; a part of a stethoscope.

diaphysis: shaft of a long bone.

diarrhea: abnormal frequency and fluidity of discharge from the bowels.

diastole: atrial and ventricular relaxation which allows the chambers of the heart to fill with blood.

diastolic: pressure of the blood against the arterial walls when the heart is at rest between beats (the bottom number recorded in a blood pressure reading).

diffusion: state of being widely spaced; the process whereby molecules move in an effort to equalize the concentration of a liquid or gas.

digestion: process of converting food into chemical substances for assimilation and absorption by body tissues.

dilation and curettage: expansion of the cervix and scraping of the walls of the uterus to remove material such as polyps or as in an abortion.

dilation: action of expanding, as in *dilation* and curettage or *dilation* of blood vessels, vasodilation. (Dilation and dilatation are often used interchangeably.)

diluent: liquid solution used to reconstitute injectable medications that have been prepared as powders.

diphtheria: contagious infection characterized by sore throat, fever, and malaise. Manifestations also include throat inflammation followed by formation of a whitish gray membrane that cannot be removed without causing bleeding and a possible weakening of cardiac muscles.

diplopia: double vision.

dirty: any object or person that has not been cleaned or sterilized for removal of microorganisms.

disaccharide: a double sugar molecule.

disaster medical assistance team (DMAT): team that provides assistance and support in emergencies both inside and outside healthcare facilities.

discharge planning: process by which a client is prepared for continued care after discharge from a healthcare facility.

disease management program: plan that outlines protocols for the management of a specific disorder.

disease: a deviation or departure from normal body structure or function that is characterized by certain signs and symptoms; cause and prognosis may be known or unknown.

disinfection: cleaning process that destroys most pathogens but not necessarily their spores.

dislocation: displacement of a bone from a joint.

diuresis: increased urinary output.

diuretic: medication that increases the amount of urine excreted by the kidneys.

diverticulitis: inflammation of a diverticulum (outpouching or sac in a mucous membrane), often referring to the colon. (pl: diverticula)

diverticulosis: the condition of having diverticula, without inflammation.

domestic violence: abuse or violence that occurs within the home.

Doppler: electronic stethoscope which converts ultrasonic frequencies into either audible frequencies or projects them onto a video monitor, used to detect fetal heart tones as early as the tenth week of pregnancy.

dorsal: posterior or back side.

dorsal lithotomy: examination position in which the client is lying on his or her back with the feet in stirrups.

dorsal recumbent: lying on the back with knees flexed.

dosage: an amount in a prescription that contains the dose and the scheduled time.

dose: a single amount of a medication administered to achieve a therapeutic effect.

Down syndrome: congenital abnormality characterized by specific physical defects and by varying degrees of intellectual impairment; also called trisomy 21.

droplet precautions: precautions taken to prevent the spread of diseases transmitted by microorganisms propelled through the air from an infected person and deposited on the host's eyes, nose, or mouth.

drowning: suffocation from submersion in liquid.

drug: substance other than food used to prevent disease, to aid in the diagnosis and treatment of disease, and to restore or maintain functions in body tissues. Also called medication.

dual diagnosis: two separate chronic conditions at the same time; has commonly come to mean mental illness, combined with chemical dependency.

dual-career (worker) family: nuclear family in which both parents work outside the home.

Duchenne muscular dystrophy: most common degenerative muscle disorder in children; symptoms include developmental delay, using upper extremities to compensate for weak hip muscles, walking on the toes, or falling frequently.

ductus arteriosus: connection between the pulmonary artery and aorta that allows for shunting of blood around the fetal lungs.

ductus deferens: tubes that transport sperm from the epididymis to the ejaculatory ducts.

due process: procedures that ensure fair labor practices and prevent frivolous or punitive actions against employees by employers.

dumping syndrome: immediate discomfort caused by overeating or eating foods that are not recommended after surgery.

duodenum: proximal (first) portion of the small intestine.

duration: spanning a length of time, as in *duration* of a contraction during labor.

dysfluency: interruption in the natural flow of speaking.

dysfunction: functioning or operating improperly.

dysfunctional family: family whose coping systems disintegrate as stressors build.

dyskinesia: involuntary, coordinated rhythmic movements.

dyskinetic cerebral palsy: type of cerebral palsy characterized by abnormal involuntary movements and difficulty with speech caused by involuntary facial movements; also called athetoid cerebral palsy.

dyslexia: disorder in which one has difficulty reading, spelling, or writing words and often reverses letters or numbers.

dysmenorrhea: difficult or painful menstruation.

dyspareunia: pain upon sexual intercourse.

dyspepsia: indigestion.

dysphagia: difficulty in swallowing.

dysphasia: difficulty in understanding or expressing language.

dysphonia: difficulty speaking.

dysplasia: abnormal development; alteration in shape.

dyspnea: difficulty in breathing.

dysrhythmia: lacking rhythm, without rhythm, as in an irregular heartbeat.

dysthymia: depressive disorder; chronic clinical depression over a long period.

dystocia: difficult labor.

dystonia: difficulty in speaking.

dysuria: difficult or painful urination or voiding.

E

ecchymosis: bleeding into the tissues under the skin, leaving small bruises.

echocardiography: recording of activity and location of the heart by means of ultrasound.

echolalia: automatic repeating of what has been said.

echopraxia: involuntary imitation of the movements of other people.

eclampsia: seizure disorder with high blood pressure, usually related to a complication of pregnancy, pregnancy-induced hypertension (PIH).

ecology: study of the interrelationship of organisms and their environment.

ectopic: situated in other than the normal location, as *ectopic* pregnancy.

ectropion: turning outward (eversion) of an edge.

eczema: an inflammatory skin rash, characterized by itching, redness, weeping, oozing, and crusting, and later by scaling.

edema: abnormal fluid accumulation in the intercellular tissue spaces of the body; puffiness.

edentia: absence of teeth. (adj: edentulous)

effacement: thinning of the cervix in preparation for delivery.

effectors: neurons that carry out activity in response to messages relayed by sensory neurons.

efferent: conducting away from the center, as an *efferent* nerve.

egg-crate mattress: a foam pad, shaped like an egg carton, which is used on top of a regular bed mattress to provide comfort and to prevent pressure areas.

ejaculation: forceful expulsion of semen from the ejaculatory ducts to the urethra during sexual excitement.

elasticity: ability to return to normal length after stretching.

elder abuse: emotional, physical, and sexual abuse, financial exploitation, or neglect of older adults.

elective (surgery): case in which the client's condition is not life-threatening and may choose whether or not to have surgery; also called optional surgery.

electrical stimulation: use of an electrical impulse to strengthen pelvic muscles and decrease bladder activity that causes urge incontinence.

electrocardiogram (ECG, EKG): recording of electrical activity of heartbeats for baseline or pathology readings.

electrocauterization: destruction of malignant tissues by burning.

electroconvulsive therapy (ECT): administration of an electric shock to induce convulsions (seizures) as a treatment, usually for clinical depression.

electrodesiccation: removal of tissue using intermittent electric sparks.

electroencephalogram (EEG): recording of the brain's electrical activity.

electrolyte: a chemical substance that dissociates into electrically charged ions (positive ions are called *cations;* negative ions are called *anions*) when melted or in solution (becomes capable of conducting electricity).

electromyogram (EMG): recording of electrical activity of muscles.

element: a chemical substance made of atoms that cannot be further divided without losing the characteristics of the substance; the physical and chemical properties of a particular element are always the same.

elimination: the act of expelling wastes from the body, voiding and defecation.

emaciation: a wasting away of the flesh, causing extreme leanness, starvation. (adj: emaciated)

embolus: a foreign substance, blood clot, fat globule, piece of tissue, or air bubble carried in a blood vessel, which partially or completely obstructs blood flow (embolism; pl. emboli).

embryo: a new organism in the first stage of development.

emergency medical service: service to contact in life-threatening situations.

emergi-center: free-standing facility that provides urgent care for clients with non-critical conditions.

emesis: the act of vomiting; the product of vomiting, vomitus.

emetic: an agent that causes vomiting.

emission: accumulation of sperm cells and secretions in the male urethra.

emphysema: inflation or swelling of tissues due to the presence of air; usually refers to chronic pulmonary *emphysema,* a severe lung disorder.

employee right-to-know laws: laws that state that employees have the right to be aware of dangers associated with

hazardous substances or harmful physical or infectious agents they might encounter in the workplace.

empty calories: foods that supply calories with few or no nutrients.

empyema: accumulation of pus in a body cavity, often the pleural (lung) cavity.

en face **position:** two individuals with heads aligning as they look at one another, as in a mother and baby in the beginning stages of bonding.

enabler: a person who covers for and, often unknowingly, assists another to continue chemical abuse, codependent.

encephalalgia: pain in the head; headache, cephalalgia.

encephalitis: inflammation of the brain.

encephalocele: condition in which the bones of the fetal skull do not close correctly.

encopresis: incontinence of feces not caused by age, disease, or physical disorder.

endemic: microorganisms that do not produce disease under normal conditions or are not present most or all of the time in the environment or the body.

endocarditis: inflammation of the endocardium.

endocardium: the inner lining of the heart and connective tissue bed around it.

endocrine: pertaining to internal secretions (not into ducts or tubes); applies to organs.

endocrinologist: physician who specializes in the treatment of disorders of the endocrine system.

endocytosis: the first line of defense against bacteria in which neutrophils increase in number, engulf, and devour invaders; also known as phagocytosis.

endogenous: normally occurring or existing within the body or in the community.

endometriosis: presence of endometrial tissue in places where it is not normally found.

endometrium: mucous layer of the uterus, which forms the maternal portion of the placenta during pregnancy.

endorphin: a naturally occurring analgesic that the body produces in response to exercise and other stimuli.

endorsement: process by which a licensed nurse in one state may receive a license in another state, without re-taking the licensing exam.

endoscope: a tube-shaped, lighted device used to visualize or operate on hollow organs or within body cavities. Specialized endoscopes include the gastroscope, bronchoscope, and proctoscope. (Process of visualization using this tool is called endoscopy.)

endotoxin: a heat-stable toxin (poison) that is released when a bacterial cell is disrupted (less potent than exotoxins).

enema: an injection of fluid or medication into the rectum, usually to induce evacuation of the bowel.

engagement: state in which the presenting part of the fetus has moved downward so that it cannot be pushed up and out of the pelvis.

engorgement: local congestion or distention with fluids, as in *engorgement* of the breasts during pregnancy and lactation.

enteral: within the intestine.

enteric: pertaining to the small intestine. *Enteric-coated* tablets are covered with a substance that prevents their digestion in the stomach.

entitled: psychological condition in which an individual feels that everyone should wait on him or her and often makes other unreasonable demands.

entropion: inversion, turning inward, as the turning under of the eyelid.

entry-level skills: basic competencies.

enucleate: to remove whole and clean; often refers to removal of an eye.

enuresis: involuntary urine discharge, usually occurring during sleep; bed-wetting.

environment: one's surroundings, the situation in which a person lives (as opposed to heredity).

enzyme: a protein produced in a cell that activates or speeds up a chemical reaction.

epicardium: the inner layer of the pericardium, which is in contact with the heart.

epidemic: widespread disease in a certain geographical region.

epidermis: the outermost layer of the skin.

epididymitis: inflammation of the epididymis (coiled, cordlike structures in the testes through which spermatozoa are carried).

epidural: common method of anesthesia during labor and delivery in which a small catheter is inserted into the epidural space within the spinal column and anesthesia is administered via this route.

epiglottis: cartilage that covers the entrance to the larynx.

epilepsy: a chronic disease marked by attacks of convulsions; a convulsive or seizure disorder.

epiphysis: the end of a long bone.

episiotomy: surgical incision into the perineum and vagina, usually during childbirth.

epispadias: absence of the upper wall of the urethra resulting in an abnormal location of the urethral opening, usually occurring in the male.

epistaxis: nosebleed.

eponym: a word or term based on the name of a person, such as Parkinson's disease.

Epstein's pearls: white or grayish bumps found on the mouth's hard and soft palate in newborns.

eradicated: eliminated.

erectile dysfunction: inability to achieve or maintain erection sufficient to complete sexual intercourse.

erection: process of the penis becoming engorged with blood and firm.

erythema: skin redness produced by capillary congestion, as may follow a tuberculin test; bright red color associated with capillary dilation, can indicate fever or infection.

erythema toxicum: red, raised rash that appears on the skin of some sensitive newborns.

erythroblastosis fetalis: condition in which Rh positive red blood cells from the fetus have crossed the placental barrier into an Rh negative woman, causing the woman to form antibodies which return to the fetus, destroying fetal erythrocytes. *Erythroblastosis fetailis* is this condition as it manifests itself in the newborn.

erythrocyte: red blood cell.

erythropoietin: glycoprotein hormone produced in the adult's kidney and in the child's liver which stimulates red blood cell production; also known as renal erythropoietic factor.

eschar: dead skin and tissue that slough off after a chemical or thermal burn.

esophageal atresia: newborn abnormality in which the upper end of the esophagus ends in a blind pouch, making it impossible for the baby to obtain food.

esophagoscopy: visualization of the esophagus through the intestinal tract using a specialized instrument.

esophagus: passageway for digestion that extends from pharynx to stomach.

essential nutrients: nutrients a person must obtain through food because the body cannot make them in sufficient quantities to meet its needs.

estrogens: female hormones.

ethics: code or rules of behavior.

ethnicity: sense of identification of a collective cultural group, based on common heritage.

ethnocentrism: belief that one's own culture is the best and only acceptable way.

ethnonursing: an approach to nursing that considers a client's religious and socio-cultural backgrounds during treatment, also known as ethnic sensitive nursing.

etiology: specific cause of a disease.

eupnea: normal respiration.

eustachian tube: the passage from the throat to the middle ear; auditory tube.

euthanasia: an easy or painless death (may be induced), often referred to as mercy death or mercy killing; deliberate ending of life of a person who has an incurable or painful disease.

euthymia: normal mood.

evaluation: in nursing process, measuring the effectiveness of the other steps.

evaporation: process of changing a liquid or solid into a vapor (gas); to give off moisture.

eversion: turning inside out; turning outward, as *eversion* of the foot.

evisceration: the protrusion of the intestines through an abdominal wound; removal of the internal body contents.

exocrine: secreting externally through a duct (as opposed to endocrine).

exogenous: referring to organisms that enter from outside the body and cause infection.

exophthalmos: abnormal protrusion of the eyes, most often caused by hyperthyroidism.

exoskeleton: type of inflatable trousers used to help an individual maintain an upright position and prevent vascular collapse.

exotoxin: a potent toxin (poison) formed by a bacteria, which can cause severe illness.

expected outcome: measurable behavior that indicates whether a person has achieved the expected benefit of nursing care.

expectorant: medication that liquefies secretions in the bronchi, making it easier to cough up and expel mucus.

expectoration: spitting out and coughing up mucus or other fluid from the lungs and the throat.

expiration: exhalation of air from the lungs; sometimes used to refer to death.

exstrophy: congenital defect in which an organ is turned "inside out;" a result of abnormal development causing exposure of the urinary bladder to the abdominal wall.

extended care: facilities that extend or continue care that begins in a hospital.

extended family: one's family beyond that of parents and siblings.

extensibility: ability to stretch.

extension: the straightening of a flexed limb (opposite of flexion).

external chest compressions: measures to resume the heart's action.

external disaster: a disaster occurring outside a healthcare facility that impairs normal operation.

external respiration: lung breathing.

extracellular: outside the cell wall, as *extracellular* fluid.

extracorporeal: outside the body.

extrapyramidal: causing adverse neurological side effects.

extrication: emergency removal of a victim, performed only when the danger of injury by remaining in the same place is greater than the risk of aggravating existing injuries by moving.

exudate: material that escapes from blood vessels and is deposited in tissues or on tissue surfaces; usually contains protein substances.

eye contact: looking another person in the eye, as in "making eye contact."

F

failure to thrive (FTT): a condition in which an infant or young child demonstrates inadequate physical growth and other symptoms; can result from neglect or physical disorders; marasmus.

fallopian tube: (see oviducts).

family: two or more persons who are joined together by bonds of sharing and emotional closeness and who identify themselves as being part of that family.

fasciotomy: excision of the fibrous membranes that cover and support muscles (fascia).

fat: a component of foods that is composed of fatty or greasy material and that yields the highest caloric value per gram; lipid material; adipose tissue.

fat-controlled diet: approach to eating which focuses on altering both the total amount and type of fat consumed in order to lower elevated levels of blood lipids.

fatigue: weariness resulting from overexertion; extreme tiredness.

febrile: pertaining to a fever.

fecal impaction: accumulation of hardened stool in the rectum.

feces: the residue, consisting of bacteria, secretions (chiefly of the liver), and a small amount of food residue which is discharged from the intestines; stool, bowel movement.

feedback: the receipt of external stimuli as a result of output (can be verbal, nonverbal, and emotional). Physical feedback is involved in the self-regulation of hormones and electrolytes within the body.

felony: a crime more serious than a misdemeanor, usually punishable by imprisonment for more than a year. Felonies include murder, euthanasia, kidnaping, and blackmail.

femoral pulse: pulse felt in the groin over the femoral artery.

femur: thigh bone.

fetal alcohol syndrome (FAS): a severe physical and mental birth defect caused by a woman's alcohol consumption during pregnancy.

fetal monitor: electronic device that monitors the rate and quality of the fetal heartbeat during labor.

fetoscope: special manual stethoscope used to detect fetal heart tones around the eighteenth to twentieth week of pregnancy.

fetus: the unborn offspring in the postembryonic period (7–8 weeks after fertilization), which develops in the uterus.

fever: abnormally high body temperature.

fiber: group name for the portion of plants resistant to digestion by human enzymes.

fibrillation: a quivering of muscle fibers.

fibrin: insoluble threads created by the thrombin conversion of fibrin, which form a net to entrap RBCs and platelets to form a blood clot.

fibrinogen: a protein in blood plasma that is converted into fibrin by the action of thrombin. (Also called clotting factor I.)

fibula: bone in the lower leg which is not weight bearing.

filtration: the passage or nonpassage of molecules through a filter (sieve), depending on the size of each molecule.

fimbriae: fringe-like ends of the oviducts that catch the ovum as it bursts from the ovary into the pelvic cavity.

fissure: type of skin lesion resembling a slit or furrow.

fistula: an abnormal tubelike passage, as an anal *fistula*.

flaccidity: brief loss of muscle tone, as in a seizure.

flagellum: cellular organelle resembling a long whip which can propel bacteria in different directions in response to chemical changes in the environment (plural: flagella).

flatulence: condition of having intestinal gas.

flatus: gas in the intestines or stomach; gas expelled through the anus.

flex: to bend, as to *flex* the leg. (noun: flexion)

flotation mattress: mattress or pad filled with a gel-type material which

supports the body in a way to provide comfort and avoid creating pressure points, thereby helping to prevent skin breakdown.

flow sheet: a form used to document client care (often contains check-off spaces for assessments/review of systems and nursing care items, as well as spaces to record items such as IV fluids, vital signs and weight, fluid intake, and client teaching).

fluid volume deficit: a deficiency of fluid and electrolytes in the ECF.

fluid volume excess: excessive retention of water and sodium in the ECF.

focal point: specific location, as in the certain place in the brain where a seizure originates.

focus: point of origin.

folliculitis: staphylococcal infection starting around the hair follicle.

fontanel: a soft spot in a baby's skull.

footdrop: contracture deformity that prevents the client from putting the heel on the floor; results from improper positioning or anterior leg muscle paralysis.

foramen ovale: opening between the right and left atria in the fetal heart which permits most blood to bypass the right ventricle since the fetus' lungs are not yet functioning.

foramen: a natural opening or passage, as the *foramen ovale* in the fetal heart.

forceps: a two-pronged surgical instrument for grasping or clamping tissues.

foremilk: milk produced at the beginning of a nursing session which is relatively low in fat.

forensic: pertaining to legal matters.

foreskin: a loose fold of skin covering the glans penis (removed in circumcision), also called prepuce.

foster family: family in which children live with paid caregivers.

Fowler's: examination position in which the client is lying on his or her back with the head elevated.

fracture: a break, as in a bone.

fragile X syndrome: genetic sex-linked abnormality of the X chromosome resulting in cognitive impairment and distinct physical features; the most common form of inherited mental retardation.

fraud: dishonesty, cheating, deceit, misrepresentation.

freckle: brown or tan macule-type spot on sun-exposed skin.

frequency: number of occurrences within a defined time period, as in *frequency* of contractions during labor.

friable: fragile, easily broken, as *friable* skin.

frontal: pertaining to the forehead or the front, anterior, or ventral portion of the body when divided longitudinally from side to side.

frontal lobe: cerebral lobe that is larger in humans than in all other animals and allows for higher levels of mental functioning, including conceptualization, judgement, communication, and body movements.

frostbite: freezing of tissue caused by exposure to cold.

fulguration: destruction of malignant tissues using a high-frequency current.

functional disease: disorder in which a structural cause cannot be identified.

functional disorder: type of mental illness that has no organic cause.

functional family: a family that uses its resources to cope and become stronger under stress.

functional: affecting body function, but not structure; also called idiopathic.

fundal height: measurement of the size of the uterus.

fundus: upper curve of the uterus.

furuncle: a painful, localized, pus-filled skin infection originating in a gland or hair follicle (boil).

G

gait: manner or style of walking.

gait belt: (see transfer belt).

galactosemia: genetic absence of the enzyme necessary for metabolizing galactose.

gallbladder: muscular sac on the liver's undersurface which stores and releases bile.

gamete: one of two mature reproductive cells necessary for fertilization to occur; in males the spermatozoa, in females the ova.

gamma globulin: a type of immunization given after disease exposure that results in only short-term immunity,

not specific for a certain disease; also known as immunoglobulin IgG.

gangrene: necrosis of tissue due to insufficient blood supply.

gastrectomy: surgical procedure to remove the entire stomach.

gastric lavage: pumping out the stomach.

gastroscopy: endoscopy of the stomach.

gastrostomy: creation of an artificial opening into the stomach for the instillation of food and fluids.

gavage: passing food into the stomach through a tube; forced feeding.

gay or lesbian family: partners of the same sex who live or own property together, with or without children.

gay: homosexual; sexually attracted to the same sex.

gene: a unit of heredity within a chromosome.

generalized: existing throughout a system (as opposed to localized).

generativity: passing on and sharing skills with younger generations.

generic name: name assigned by a drug's first manufacturer (often the chemical name).

genetics: the study of *heredity* or inherited characteristics.

genital herpes: viral infection caused by Herpes simplex virus type 2 (HSV-2) is characterized by recurrent episodes of painful genital sores and systemic flu-like symptoms.

geriatrics: branch of medicine that deals with aging and its related disorders.

gerontology: study of aging.

gestation: period of development from fertilization to birth.

gestational diabetes: diabetes that a woman develops for the first time during pregnancy.

giantism: excessive bone growth, resulting from overproduction of somatotropin (growth hormone).

giardiasis: illness caused by ingesting water contaminated by human excrement.

gingival: pertaining to the gum.

gland: an organ that secretes or excretes hormones and other substances.

glans penis: smooth cap of the penis.

glaucoma: eye disease characterized by increased intraocular pressure.

glial cells: (see neuroglia).

globulin: proteins that are insoluble in water or highly concentrated saline solution, but which dissolve in isotonic (normal) saline.

glomerular filtration rate: amount of filtrate formed in all glomeruli of both kidneys per minute.

glomerulonephritis: a group of diseases in which the kidneys are damaged and partly destroyed by inflammation of the glomeruli.

glomerulus: small, twisted mass of capillaries, as the *glomerulus* of the kidney (plural, glomeruli).

glucagon: hormone secreted by the alpha cells, which raises blood sugar.

glucocorticoid: corticosteroid that has an important influence on the synthesis of glucose, amino acids, and fats during metabolism and depresses immune response and decreases inflammatory response.

glucose: simple sugar, dextrose; it is the end product of carbohydrate metabolism and the primary energy source for living organisms, found in the normal blood of all animals.

glycogen: a multiple sugar (polysaccharide) that is stored in the body; animal starch.

goiter: an enlargement of the thyroid gland, causing a swelling in the front part of the neck.

gonad: a sex gland or organ.

gonadotropic hormones: hormones secreted by the gonads, which provide males and females with secondary sex characteristics and enable reproduction; also known as gonadotropins.

gonorrhea: sexually transmitted disease that generally affects the genital area and urinary function of either sex and, if left untreated, can spread to bones, joints, or the bloodstream.

Good Samaritan Act: law in effect in most states that protects health care providers from liability when performing emergency care within the limits of first aid if they act in a "reasonable and prudent manner."

Goodell's sign: softening of the cervix at about the eighth week of gestation.

gout: arthritic condition caused when the body is unable to metabolize purines and uric acid accumulates in the bloodstream and forms crystal deposits in the joints.

Gowers' sign: positive sign of muscular dystrophy exhibited by a child's need to use upper extremity muscles to compensate for weak hip muscles.

graft: transplant of skin placed on clean viable tissue.

gram: metric system measurement of weight.

Gram's stain: series of dyes used to stain a microorganism so that its features become more clearly visible and is able to be classified as either "gram negative" or "gram positive."

grand multipara: pregnant woman who has given birth at least five times.

grandiose: having delusions of grandeur.

granulation tissue: new tissue that forms when old destroyed tissue is sloughed off.

Graves' disease: a condition that includes goiter, thyrotoxicosis, exophthalmos, and sometimes skin changes.

gravida: a pregnant woman.

gravital plane: (see line of gravity).

growth: change in body structure or size; formation of abnormal tissue, such as a tumor.

guaiac: stool examination for blood; also known as Hemoccult.

guided imagery: a process through which the client receives a suggestion that helps control his or her pain or disease. The person learns to visualize himself or herself as powerful and able to conquer pain or disease.

gurney: (see litter).

gustation: sense of taste.

gynecology: the branch of medicine that treats diseases of the genital tract in women.

H

Hagar's sign: softening of the lower uterine segment that occurs at about the sixth week of pregnancy.

halitosis: bad breath.

hallucination: seeing, hearing, smelling, tasting, or feeling something that has no objective stimulus.

halo device: form of skeletal traction applied to the skull that allows the client to ambulate and perform self-care activities.

Hashimoto's thyroiditis: hypothyroidism believed to be autoimmune in origin.

health interview: way of soliciting information from the client; may also be called a nursing history.

health maintenance organization (HMO): an agency that provides prepaid healthcare, as needed, to members (as opposed to fee paid as service is given). The emphasis is on prevention.

health maintenance: approach to healthcare in which disease prevention is emphasized; also called health supervision.

health record: manual or electronic (computer) account of a client's relationship with a healthcare facility.

health supervision: (see health maintenance).

health: optimum functioning of body, mind, and spirit; absence of disease.

heart block: condition associated with diseases of the coronary arteries and rheumatic heart disease in which heart contractions are weak and lack sufficient force to effectively pump blood.

heat cramps: cramps that may occur after hard exertion when a person sweats profusely; usually located in the legs, arms, or abdomen.

heat exhaustion: a serious blood flow disturbance similar to shock that results from not taking in enough water and sodium to replace lost fluids and electrolytes.

heat stroke: classic *heat stroke* occurs when the body's heat-regulating mechanisms fail and core temperature soars; exertional *heat stroke* develops from an increased internal heat load due to muscular exertion, along with high external temperatures and humidity.

hemangiomas: overgrowths of blood vessels.

hematemesis: vomiting of blood.

hematest: a test for occult (hidden) blood in stool or body secretions.

hematologist: a physician educated in the hematologic and lymphatic systems.

hematology: study of blood and blood-forming tissues.

hematoma: a mass of coagulated blood (internal or under the skin) due to a break in the wall of a blood vessel; a mild form is a black eye or a bruise.

hematopoiesis: process of manufacturing blood cells, mostly occurring in the bone marrow.

hematuria: blood in the urine.

hemianopsia: blindness in half the visual field of one or both eyes.

hemiplegia: paralysis on one side of the body.

Hemoccult: a test for occult (hidden) blood in stool or body secretions.

hemodialysis: dialysis by way of an arterial shunt and using an artificial kidney; used to remove toxic wastes from the blood in kidney disorders.

hemodynamic monitoring: specialized device used to evaluate the pressure in the heart chambers.

hemofiltration: slow continuous renal replacement therapy that is effective in removing solutes and fluids in unstable newborns; also called hemodiafiltration.

hemoglobin: the oxygen-carrying pigment in blood that gives blood its red color.

hemophilia: a congenital condition in males characterized by spontaneous or traumatic bleeding and very slow clotting.

hemorrhage: excessive bleeding (internal or external).

hemorrhoid: a dilation of the veins (varicose veins) of the anal region (may be internal or external).

hemostasis: stoppage of bleeding (naturally or artificially).

hemothorax: fluid or blood pooling in the pleural cavity; also called pleural effusion.

heparin (hep) lock: IV catheter that is inserted into a vein and left in place for intermittent administration of medicine or as an open line in case of emergencies. Similar to a saline lock, which is flushed with saline, versus heparin.

hepatitis: inflammation of the liver. Types include A, B, C, D, and E, some of which are transmitted via blood or body secretions.

hereditary: genetically determined, transmitted from parent to child, inherited (not acquired).

heredity: the genetic transmission of physical or mental characteristics from parent to offspring.

hernia: abnormal protrusion of an organ or tissue through the structure usually containing it, as an inguinal *hernia* or hiatal *hernia;* rupture; condition is called herniation.

herpes: an inflammatory skin disease characterized by the formation of small vesicles in clusters (caused by a virus). (*Herpes simplex virus type I* causes fever blisters and canker sores in the mouth; *herpesvirus II* [herpesvirus genitalis] causes genital lesions; *herpes zoster* is also known as shingles.)

herpes zoster: condition in adults caused by the same varicella virus that causes chickenpox in children; commonly known as shingles.

hesitancy: inability to start the stream of urine.

heterograft: a graft obtained from an animal and received by a person; also called xenograft.

heterosexual: pertaining to different sexes; sexually attracted to the opposite sex.

hiatal: pertaining to an opening or gap, as a *hiatal* hernia.

hierarchy of needs: established by Maslow, the hierarchy categorizes human needs from the most basic vital needs, survival needs (necessary to life), up through higher-level needs such as beauty, love, and learning.

high-risk newborn: newborn with special problems related to maturity, hemolytic conditions, birth injuries, alterations in structure and function, infections, or chemical dependency.

high-risk pregnancy: pregnancy that is statistically more likely to have complications including prolonged, multiple, and adolescent pregnancies, and those in women over age 40.

hindmilk: milk produced near the end of a nursing session which is higher in fat and calories than the milk produced in the beginning.

Hippocratic oath: pledge based on the principles of Hippocrates repeated by physicians when they enter the field of medicine.

Hirschsprung's disease: condition in which a child's colon lacks para-sympathetic nerve supply and the abdomen becomes enlarged with stool and flatus due to lack of peristalsis; also called megacolon or *aganglionic megacolon.*

hirsutism: abnormal hairiness, particularly in women.

histamine: an amine found in all body tissues that stimulates dilation of small blood vessels and production of gastric juice. It is involved in inflammation and allergic reactions.

histology: study of tissues.

histoplasmosis: specific fungal infection.

hives: swollen patches on the skin as a result of an allergic reaction.

HIV-related-encephalopathy: dysfunction of the brain as a result of HIV infection; also known as AIDS dementia complex.

holistic healthcare: healthcare that emphasizes care of the whole person.

Homans' sign: a test for thrombophlebitis in which pain occurs behind the knee when the foot is hyperflexed upward (dorsiflexion).

home healthcare: a nurse monitoring a client in his or her home, often after being discharged while completing recovery from surgery or an illness.

homeostasis: stability, balance, or equilibrium in normal body states.

homograft: a graft from one person to another; also called allograft.

homosexual: a person who is sexually attracted to members of the same sex, gay.

hookworm: type of roundworm that usually enters the host through bare feet, migrating through the body to the mouth and throat, destroying red blood cells and causing anemia.

hormone: chemical substance secreted, usually from a ductless gland, that regulates body processes.

hospice: a facility or program of care that is specifically designed to provide emotional and physical support to terminally ill clients and their families.

human immunodeficiency virus (HIV): virus that lowers normal immune response, rendering the person susceptible to otherwise harmless (opportunistic) organisms.

humerus: single long bone found in each upper arm.

humoral immunity: immunity created by the B lymphocytes and is the body's resistance to circulating disease-producing antigens and bacteria.

hydatidiform mole: disease in which the embryo dies in utero and chorionic villi degenerate, forming grape-like clusters of vesicles and abnormal enlargement of the uterus.

hydramnios: excessive amniotic fluid surrounding a fetus. Polyhydramnios.

hydrocele: painless swelling of the scrotum caused by fluid collection.

hydrocephalus: fluid accumulation in the skull; it is typically characterized by enlargement of the head if a shunt is not successful; also called water on the brain.

hydrodistension: bladder that is stretched out with fluid.

hydrogenated: a liquid oil to which hydrogen has been added to make it more stable and decrease the chance of rancidity.

hydrometer: urinometer (used to measure specific gravity of a liquid, such as urine).

hydronephrosis: distention of the pelvis and calices of the kidney with urine as a result of obstruction of the ureter or other urinary structure.

hydrospadia: condition in which the urinary meatus is located on the bottom of the penis.

hymen: a fold of membrane sometimes found at the vagina's external opening.

hyperbaric: high-pressure; as in hyperbaric oxygenation (HBO).

hyperbilirubinemia: condition that results from elevated bilirubin levels in a newborn.

hyperemesis: excessive vomiting.

hyperemesis gravidarum: pernicious vomiting in pregnancy.

hyperglycemia: abnormally high blood sugar.

hyperlipidemia: excess fat in the blood.

hyperopia: condition in which light rays focus behind the retina; farsightedness.

hyperparathyroidism: condition that stems from an excess of parathormone, causing elevated blood calcium levels, resulting in calcium depletion in the bones.

hyperplasia: enlargement, as in benign prostatic *hyperplasia.*

hyperpnea: abnormal increase in rate and depth of respirations.

hypersomnia: excessive sleep.

hypertension: elevated blood pressure; also called high blood pressure.

hyperthyroidism: excessive functioning of the thyroid gland, causing excessive thyroid hormone in the body.

hypertonic: a solution that is stronger than what is found on the opposite side of a membrane.

hypertrophy: enlargement.

hyperventilation: abnormally fast and deep breathing, usually caused by anxiety, resulting in reduction of carbon dioxide and an increase in oxygen.

hypervigilance: state of increased watchfulness.

hyphema: hemorrhage into the anterior chamber of the eye.

hypnotic: a drug or agent that induces sleep.

hypodermis: also called subcutaneous tissue, a single layer of fat below the dermis that cushions, supports, nourishes, and insulates the skin.

hypoglycemia: abnormally low blood sugar.

hypomanic: hyperactive individual who has not reached the level of mania; usually does not require hospitalization.

hypoparathyroidism: condition that stems from parathormone deficiency, with a consequent reduction in the amount of calcium available in the body and an accumulation of phosphorus in the blood.

hypophysectomy: surgical removal of the pituitary gland.

hypospadias: abnormal male condition in which the urethra opens on the underside of the penis or onto the perineum.

hypotension: chronic depression in blood pressure; abnormally low blood pressure.

hypothalamus: a tiny but complex portion of the brain believed to be the "master controller" of the hormones.

hypothermia: low body temperature; also a syndrome (accidental *hypothermia*), caused by exposure to

cold, which may be fatal. Hypothermia may also be induced for therapeutic purposes such as surgery, or pathologic as a result of faulty thermoregulation (temperature control).

hypothermic blanket: cooling blanket; also called hypothermia blanket.

hypothyroidism: condition that occurs as a result of a deficiency in thyroid secretion which lowers metabolism.

hypotonic: a solution that is less concentrated than that found on the opposite side of a membrane.

hypoxia: reduction of oxygen in the tissues; also called hypoxemia.

hysterectomy: surgical removal of the uterus.

I

iatrogenic incontinence: urinary leakage caused by medical interventions or treatments.

ice cap: a flat, oval, bag with a leakproof, screw-in top.

ileal diversion: urinary diversion.

ileostomy: surgical opening of the ileum onto the abdomen by means of a stoma.

ileum: distal portion of the small intestine. (adj: ileal)

ileus: intestinal obstruction, usually as a result of inadequate peristalsis.

ilium: upper flaring portion of the bones that form the pelvis, usually identified as the hip bone.

illness: pronounced deviation from normal health.

immunity: condition of being nonsusceptible to a certain disease.

immunization: the process of providing protection against infection from a particular disease; vaccination, inoculation.

immunogen: a substance capable of initiating or stimulating an immune response.

immunoglobulins: antibodies.

immunosuppressive: referring to deliberate suppression of the natural immune system, as in chemotherapy for cancer. (adj: immunosuppression)

immunotherapy: administering minute doses of allergens subcutaneously to help a client slowly develop a tolerance to an allergen; also called desensitization or hyposensitization.

imperforate anus: congenital defect in which the newborn's rectum ends in a blind pouch, obstructing the normal passage of feces.

impetigo: bacterial infection of the skin; also called impetigo contagiosa.

implant: burrowing of the future embryo into the endometrium.

implementation: in nursing process, the carrying out of nursing care plans; also called interventions.

impotence: a male's inability to achieve or sustain an adequate erection for sexual intercourse.

inborn immunity: immunity that is inherited or genetic.

incentive programs: rewards given to employees by their employers for practicing healthy habits such as smoking cessation, weight loss, and having regular physical examinations.

incentive spirometer: a device used to promote full inflation and oxygenation of the lungs, used particularly after surgery and in lung disorders such as pneumonia.

incise: to cut; to make a surgical incision. (noun: incision)

incontinence: inability to control urination or defecation (adj: incontinent).

incubation: disease period between exposure to a pathogen and manifestation of clinical symptoms.

incus: the "anvil," one of three tiny bones within the middle ear which are set in motion by sound waves.

independent actions: nursing actions that do not require a physician's order.

induction: stimulating the beginning of labor by using a medication such as pitocin; beginning stage of anesthesia.

induration: a hardened place, a lump, as in the skin in a positive reaction to a tuberculin test.

infancy: a child from one to twelve months of age.

infection: the invasion and multiplication of infective agents in body tissues with a resultant reaction to their presence and their toxins.

infertility: inability to produce offspring; lack of fertility or productivity; barren.

infiltration: the diffusion or accumulation in the tissues or cells of substances not normally present or found in those amounts.

inflammation: a condition resulting from irritation in any body part, marked by pain, heat, redness, and swelling.

inflammatory bowel disease: general term for ulcerative colitis and Crohn's disease.

informed consent: giving full information and making sure the client understands before the client consents to surgery or other medical procedures.

infrared rays: rays that relax muscles, stimulate circulation, and relieve pain.

infusion: slow induction of fluids (not blood) into a vein, as an intravenous (IV) *infusion.*

ingestion: to take a material into the digestive tract.

inhalant: medications that are inhaled or breathed in.

injectable: medications that are administered via a needle into the subcutaneous tissues, muscles, or blood vessels.

insensible: not perceptible to the senses.

insignia: a distinguishing badge of authority or honor.

insomnia: sleeplessness; chronic inability to sleep.

inspection: careful, close, and detailed visual examination of a body part.

inspiration: inhalation; drawing air into the lungs.

insulin: a hormone which is vital in carbohydrate metabolism and is secreted by the islets of Langerhans of the pancreas.

insulin resistance: a decreased tissue sensitivity to insulin that occurs in people who have type 2 diabetes mellitus.

integument: the skin, the integumentary system.

intellectual impairment: demonstrating below average intellectual abilities accompanied by difficulty functioning independently; also called cognitive impairment.

intellectual skills: knowing and understanding essential information.

intercom: system that allows clients in their rooms to communicate directly with healthcare providers at the nursing station; also known as an intercommunication system.

intercostal muscles: muscles located between the ribs.

interdependent: depending on one another; one action occurs because of another. Activities of various organ systems (for example, the nerves, muscles, and bones) are *interdependent.*

interdependent actions: nursing actions that occur in cooperation with physicians and other team members.

interdisciplinary care: team of individuals from different disciplines acting together to care for a client under a physician's direction.

intermediate care facilities: facilities that provide room, board, and nursing care.

intermittent positive pressure breathing: treatment method that assists a person to breathe more easily by liquefying mucus.

internal disaster: a disaster in which a healthcare facility itself is in danger or damaged and its function is impaired.

internal respiration: cellular breathing.

Internet: an enormous online source of information; also called the World Wide Web (WWW).

interneuron: a neuron between the first afferent neuron and the last motor neuron; neurons whose processes are all in a specific area, such as the olfactory lobe.

interpersonal skills: believing, behaving, and relating.

interstate endorsement: procedure in which a nurse transfers licensure from one state to another.

interstitial: situated in the interspaces of tissue, as in interstitial or extracellular fluid (not blood or lymph).

interstitial cells: small clusters of specialized endocrine cells which secrete testosterone and other androgens.

interstitial cystitis: disease in which the bladder's lining allows for irritants from the urine to contact the bladder wall, causing extreme irritation.

interval: in labor, the time from the start of one contraction to the start of the next.

interview: a goal-directed conversation in which one person seeks information from the other.

intimacy: establishing relationships with others.

intracellular: within the cells, as in *intracellular* fluid.

intracranial pressure (ICP): the pressure of subarachnoidal fluid in the space between the skull and the brain and around the spinal cord. Elevated, increased intracranial pressure (IICP) is a significant sign in determining neurologic disorders.

intractable: that which cannot be relieved; continuous, relentless, as in *intractable* pain.

intradermal: within the substance of the skin (dermis); intracutaneous, as an *intradermal* tuberculin or allergy test.

intramuscular: within the muscle substance, as an *intramuscular* injection.

intraoperative: occurring during a surgical operation.

intrapartum: occurring during childbirth.

intravascular: within the blood vessels.

intravenous: within a vein, as *intravenous* infusion.

intravenous therapy: injecting into a vein any number of sterile solutions that the body needs, including medications and electrolytes.

intrusion injury: an injury in which a structure or part is pushed out of place into the body.

intrusive: in psychiatry, a client who interrupts or constantly interferes with others or who invades their personal space.

intubation: the insertion of a tube, as into the larynx for breathing.

intussusception: the telescoping or prolapsing of one part of the intestine into an adjacent part.

in utero: within the uterus.

invasive: term used to describe surgery and some diagnostic tests that involve an incision or puncture through the skin, insertion of an instrument (such as an endoscope), or injection of a foreign substance (such as dye) into the body; quickly spread widely throughout the body, such as *invasive* cancer.

inversion: turning inside out; reversing.

involution: turning inward; a retrograde change of the entire body or in a particular organ, as *involution* of the uterus after childbirth.

ion: an atom with an electrical charge; positive (cation), negative (anion). Substances forming ions are called electrolytes.

iris: pigmented section over the front of the eyeball that gives the eye its color.

iron: an essential part of every body cell and a constituent of hemoglobin, which carries oxygen.

irritability: ability to respond to a stimulus.

ischemia: decrease or lack of blood supply to a body part as a result of the obstruction or constriction of blood vessels.

islets of Langerhans: 500,000–1,000,000 small islands of cells scattered throughout the endocrine portion of the pancreas that secrete the pancreatic hormones.

isolation: separation from others; separation of people with infectious diseases from others.

isometric: having the same length or dimensions, as isometric exercises (pushing against stable resistance); also called muscle setting.

isotonic: of equal tension; normal, as *isotonic* saline that is the same tonicity as body fluids; exercise that shortens the muscle but does not change the force of contraction.

J

jaundice: yellowish skin discoloration due to excess bile.

jejunum: portion of the small intestine.

joint: point at which bones attach to one another.

K

Kaposi's sarcoma: opportunistic malignancy associated with AIDS that primarily affects the skin.

kardex: a flip-file with card slots or a notebook for each client on a unit or nursing care team; a system for recording background information and care related to a client's treatment.

karma: Buddhist/Hindu belief that reincarnation depends on behavior in life; karma is also significant in promoting health and causing disease.

Kawasaki disease: febrile, multisystem disorder in which platelets in the blood tend to be caught in the vessels and can develop into serious cardiac problems; also called mucocutaneous lymph node syndrome.

Kegel exercises: exercises designed to increase sphincter tone by tightening, holding, and releasing the muscles of the pelvic floor and sphincter, used to improve incontinence.

keloid: scar or scar tissue.

keratin: protein that is a major component of hair, nails, and the epidermis and is the organic matrix of tooth enamel. (Keratin is sometimes used as the coating for enteric-coated tablets.)

keratoplasty: plastic surgery of the cornea of the eye, corneal grafting, corneal transplantation.

Kerlix: type of stretchy gauze used to hold dressings in place.

ketoacidosis: (see ketosis).

ketogenic diet: approach to eating that is extremely low in carbohydrates and very high in fat, aimed at controlling seizures, especially in children.

ketosis: an increase in ketone bodies in the body tissues and fluids; also called ketoacidosis, a complication of diabetes mellitus.

kidneys: two bean-shaped organs located at the small of the back at the lower edge of the ribs on either side of the vertebral column. Urine is formed in the kidneys and levels of many electrolytes are regulated by the kidneys. Blood pressure is greatly influenced by the kidneys.

kilocalorie: unit of measurement that specifies the heat energy in a particular amount of food (1 kilocalorie = 1000 calories).

Koplik's spots: bluish white pinpoint spots with a red rim that appear around the mouth about day 2 or 3 after being infected with rubella.

Korotkoff's sounds: sounds heard when measuring blood pressure with a stethoscope (auscultation).

kosher: food that has been ritually prepared and served according to Jewish law.

Kussmaul's respiration: severe paroxysmal dyspnea, as in diabetic acidosis and coma.

kwashiorkor: condition caused by a severe protein deficiency.

kyphosis: an abnormal increase in the thoracic curvature of the spine, giving a hunchback appearance, commonly as a result of osteoporosis.

L

labia: literally means lip, as the *labia* minora and *labia* majora of the external female genitalia.

labia majora: two rounded folds of skin of the female genitals, posterior to the mons pubis.

labia minora: thin pair of skin folds of the female genitals, medial to the labia majora.

labile: unstable; fluctuating, as a labile fever. In psychiatry: rapid mood swings and marked behavior changes (lability).

labor: the process by which the uterus contracts and expels the fetus.

labor contractions: rhythmic contracting and relaxing of the uterus during the four stages of labor; also called uterine contractions.

labyrinth: the inner ear, including the vestibule, cochlea, and semicircular canals.

laceration: a wound produced by tearing or ripping (as opposed to an incision made in surgery).

lacrimal: pertaining to tears, as the *lacrimal* glands of the eyes.

lacrimation: tearing of the eyes.

lactation: milk secretion by the mammary glands (breasts).

lacteal: dead-end lymph capillaries within each villus that absorbs fat-soluble nutrients.

lacto-ovo vegetarian: a person who eats plant foods, dairy products, and eggs.

lactose: sugar found in milk; commonly called milk sugar.

lactose intolerance: genetic absence of the enzyme necessary for metabolizing lactose in milk and dairy products (lactase).

laissez-faire: leadership style that has loosely structured goals and no firm guidelines.

laminectomy: type of lumbar decompression that exposes the spinal canal and allows for relief of compression of the spinal cord and spinal nerve roots.

lanugo: fine, downy hair covering the body of a fetus.

laparoscope: endoscope used to examine the peritoneal cavity (laparoscopy).

laryngectomy: surgical removal of the larynx; the person is then called a laryngectomee.

laryngopharynx: lowest portion of the pharynx, extending from the epiglottis to the opening of the larynx and esophagus. It is divided to provide separate passages for food and air.

larynx: boxlike structure of cartilage in the midline of the neck; also called voice box.

lavage: washing out of an organ, such as the stomach or bowel; irrigation.

leader: individual who is able to effectively direct and influence the actions of others.

leak point pressure: pressure at which one can no longer hold one's urine, used to assess continence status.

learning disability: disorder in one or more of the processes involved in understanding or using language.

lens: a transparent, crystalline eye structure that converges or scatters light rays before they focus as images on the retina.

lesbian: a female homosexual.

let-down: sensation in the breasts of a lactating woman when she hears or thinks about her baby. *Let-down* reflex: flowing of milk into the breasts when the mother begins to nurse (milk-ejection reflex).

leukemia: malignant disease of blood-forming organs; may be classified as acute or chronic and also in relationship to the specific blood cell affected, as acute lymphoid (lymphocytic), myelocytic, or granulocytic *leukemia.*

leukocyte: white blood cell (WBC).

leukocytosis: condition in which white blood cells increase in number.

leukopenia: condition in which white blood cells decrease in number.

leukoplakia: disorder characterized by white patches on the mucous membrane of the cheeks, gums, or tongue that cannot be rubbed off, as *leukoplakia buccalis.*

leukorrhea: whitish vaginal discharge which is a symptom of vaginitis.

levator: pelvic muscle.

liability: something one is required to do, an obligation, often financial; being found guilty of inappropriate or illegal acts.

libel: a false or damaging written statement or photograph.

licensure: status that says a nurse has the minimum requirements for competence and practice.

lie: term used to compare the position of the fetal spinal cord to that of the woman.

lifestyle factor: one of many patterns of living one follows, including levels of exercise, nutrition, smoking, substance abuse, stress, and violence.

ligament: fibrous band connecting bones or cartilages.

lightening: feeling of decreased abdominal distention caused by the descent of the pregnant uterus deeper into the pelvis, usually 2–3 weeks before delivery.

limbic system: part of the brain largely responsible for maintaining a person's level of awareness.

line of gravity: direction of gravitation pull; an imaginary vertical line through the top of the head, center of gravity, and base of support.

linea: narrow ridge or line. *Linea alba:* a white line, the vertical line in the center of the abdomen. *Linea nigra:* black line, the linea alba when it is darkly pigmented during pregnancy.

lipid: fat.

lipoma: benign tumor composed of fatty tissues.

liquid diet: approach to eating that consists entirely of liquids, used mostly during acute illnesses or certain body disturbances such as gastrointestinal irritation.

liter: metric system measurement of liquid volume.

lithiasis: condition of having stones (calculi), as in *cholelithiasis* (stones in the gallbladder).

lithotripsy: crushing or breaking up of stones (calculi) in the urinary tract or gallbladder. Extracorporeal shock wave *lithotripsy* (ESWL): noninvasive breaking up of stones by means

of shock waves directed onto the outside of the body.

litter: four-wheeled cart; also called gurney, wheeled stretcher. A *litter* scale is used to weigh clients who cannot stand.

liver: largest glandular organ in the body; plays an important part in many bodily functions.

living will: legal form a person signs requesting no extraordinary measures to be taken to save his or her life in terminal illness; a form of advance directive.

lobectomy: removal of a lobe of the lung.

local: limited to one part or place; not general, as *local* anesthesia or *localized* pain.

lochia: vaginal discharge that occurs for 1–2 weeks following childbirth.

lochia alba: white or yellow discharge that begins about the tenth day after delivery.

lochia serosa: pink or brown-tinged discharge that begins after bleeding diminishes, around the second through the ninth day after delivery.

logroll turn: method of turning a client that keeps the body in straight alignment, used for clients with injuries to the back and/or spinal cord.

long-term objective: an outcome or goal that a client hopes to achieve but may require an extended amount of time to do so.

loop of Henle: middle portion of the convoluted tubule, with ascending and descending loops.

lordosis: an abnormal increase in the lumbar curvature of the spine; sometimes called swayback.

lower tract: division of the urinary tract that includes the bladder and urethra.

low-residue diet: approach to eating composed of foods that the body can absorb completely so that little residue is left over for the formation of feces and is prescribed for severe diarrhea, colitis, diverticulitis, other gastrointestinal disorders, intestinal obstruction, and before and after intestinal surgery; also known as a fiber-controlled diet.

lumpectomy: removal of a node or lump from the breast, without removing the breast.

lung: one of two cone-shaped organs that fills the chest cavity; the organ of respiration.

Lyme disease: bacterial illness carried by the deer tick and transferred to humans through its bite.

lymph: transparent fluid that circulates throughout the body tissues to filter wastes; can be a means by which a malignancy spreads.

lymph nodes: small bundles of special lymphoid tissue that remove bacteria and toxins from the blood and may assist in the formation of antibodies.

lymphangiomas: overgrowths of lymph vessels.

lymphocyte: particular type of leukocyte that is formed in lymphoid tissue and participates in cell-mediated immunity, as in T cells or T *lymphocytes.*

lymphoma: a malignant condition of lymphoid tissue.

lysis: destruction due to a specific agent, as *lysis* of red blood cells; also a gradual recovery from disease (as opposed to crisis); or an elevated temperature that gradually returns to normal.

M

maceration: softening of a solid due to soaking, until connective tissue fibers are dissolved, such as *maceration* of the skin under a cast or bandage.

macronutrients: carbohydrates, fats, and proteins.

macrophage: large cell derived from a monocyte.

macropsia: objects appearing larger than normal.

macrosomia: condition in which a newborn is born large-for-gestational age; may also refer to an oversized fetus.

macula: a flat discolored spot on the skin (also, macule); a dense scar of the cornea that can be seen without optical aids.

magnesium: mineral found in the bones of the body.

mainstreaming: bringing physically and intellectually challenged people into school or activities involving nonchallenged people their own age.

malaise: feeling of illness; general bodily discomfort.

malignant: deadly; tending to become progressively worse.

malingering: faking illness to stay in the hospital or otherwise receive desired attention.

malleolus: protrusions where the lower ends of the tibia and fibula meet the ankle bones.

malleus: the "hammer," one of three tiny bones within the middle ear which are set in motion by sound waves.

malnutrition: poor intake or inadequate use of food by the body; faulty nourishment.

malocclusion: incorrect tooth positioning, often corrected by orthodontia.

malpractice: injurious or faulty treatment; professional misconduct.

mammary glands: glands within the female breast that are stimulated by hormones after childbirth to release milk.

mammary: pertaining to the mammary gland (breast).

mammography: x-ray examination of the breasts, capable of detecting some breast cancers.

mammoplasty: plastic surgery of the breast. Augmentation mammoplasty: enlarging or lifting of the breast. Reconstruction mammoplasty: repair following mastectomy or injury. Reduction mammoplasty: decreasing the size of the breast.

managed care protocol: formally established guidelines based on national criteria that detail the required management of specific disorders.

manager: individual who coordinates and controls the work of others.

mandatory licensure: regulation that makes it illegal for any nurse to practice nursing for pay without a license.

mandible: lower jaw bone.

mania: disordered mental state of extreme excitement; extreme and exaggerated hyperactivity as a phase of bipolar disorder; expansiveness, increased speed of speech and thoughts, grandiosity.

manual breathing bag (Ambu bag): bag that affords high oxygen concentrations and effective and sanitary resuscitation.

marasmus: particular form of malnutrition usually seen in infants; also called failure to thrive, often due to a protein deficiency.

marrow: spongelike material in the hollow cavities in bones. (The red bone marrow produces many blood cells.)

mastalgia: breast pain.

mastectomy: surgical removal of all or part of the breast. (Removal of a lump only is called lumpectomy.)

masticate: to chew.

mastitis: inflammation of the breast.

masturbation: handling one's own genitals for erotic stimulation.

maxilla: two bones that fuse to create the upper jaw bone.

mayo stand: stand that holds equipment used in examination or surgery.

mean arterial pressure: approximately the value of the diastolic blood pressure plus one third of the pulse pressure.

meatus: opening, as in the urinary meatus.

mechanical ventilation: device that moves air in and out of the lungs.

Meckel's diverticulum: congenital disorder in which a small portion of the ileum ends in a blind pouch just before its junction with the colon.

meconium: dark green or black fecal substance in the intestines of the fully grown fetus or newborn, passed as the first one or two stools after birth.

mediastinal shift: during a traumatic injury, shift of the heart, great vessels, and trachea to the side opposite the injury.

mediastinum: area lying between the lungs and thorax.

Medicaid: public, tax-supported health insurance program for which people must qualify, a joint effort of federal and state governments.

medical asepsis: practice of reducing the number of microorganisms or preventing and reducing transmission of microorganisms from one person (source) to another; also referred to as "clean technique."

medical diagnosis: statement formulated by a primary healthcare provider that identifies the disease a person is believed to have, which provides a basis for prognosis and treatment decisions.

medical terminology: vocabulary used in the healthcare field.

medically-complex nursing unit: unit that cares for clients who require specialized care but who do not require hospitalization or care in subacute units.

Medicare: federal health insurance program available to nearly everyone over the age of 65, regardless of financial status, and to younger people who qualify.

medication: substance other than food used to prevent disease, to aid in diagnosis and treatment of disease, and to restore or maintain functions in body tissues; also called drug.

medication administration record (MAR): document that lists all medications that a physician orders for a client with spaces for marking when medications are given.

medulla: inner portion of an organ, as the *medulla* oblongata (a center portion of the hindbrain) or the renal *medulla.*

megacolon: (see Hirschsprung's disease).

meiosis: cell division that produces eggs or sperm containing half the number of needed chromosomes.

melanin: dark pigment that may be present in a tumor (melanoma) or may be excreted in the urine (melanuria).

melasma: a "sun-tanned" or bronze-like masking across the face that may occur during pregnancy; also called *chloasma gravidarum* or the "mask of pregnancy."

melena: passage of dark-colored stools containing partially or fully digested blood; also used to mean abnormal blood in the stool or vomitus.

membrane: a thin layer of tissue covering a surface (as cell or plasma *membrane*), covering a body part or lining a body cavity (as mucous *membrane*). Drum membrane: tympanic membrane (ear drum). Fetal membranes: membranes that protect the embryo, "bag of waters."

membranous labyrinth: set of tunnels and chambers in the inner ear.

menarche: establishment of menstruation; the first menses.

Ménière's disease: a disorder of the labyrinth of the inner ear, causing vertigo, headache, tinnitus, and hearing loss.

meninges: membranes that cover the brain and spinal cord (dura mater, arachnoid, pia mater).

meningitis: inflammation of the meninges.

meningocele: condition in which one or more layers of the meninges (spinal cord covering) protrude through an opening in the vertebral column.

meningomyelocele: herniation of a portion of the spinal cord, meninges, spinal fluid, and nerves through a defect in the spinal column.

menopause: cessation of menstruation; also called climacteric, change of life.

menorrhagia: abnormally profuse menstrual flow.

menstrual cycle: two interrelated cycles (ovarian and uterine) that cause the flow of blood and other materials approximately every 28 days in the nonpregnant woman.

menstruation: periodic vaginal discharge of blood and tissues from the nonpregnant uterus; also called period, menses.

metabolic acidosis: a condition that results from a deficit in bicarbonate ions or an excess of hydrogen ions.

metabolic alkalosis: condition that results from an excess of bicarbonate, often due to excess administration, or a loss of acids.

metabolism: ability to process, obtain energy from, and create new products using the chemicals found in foods.

metastasis: transfer of disease organisms or cells from one organ or body part to another not directly connected with it; often refers to cancer cells or tuberculosis.

meter: metric system measurement of length.

metric: measurement system based on the number ten.

metrorrhagia: uterine bleeding at irregular intervals and sometimes for a prolonged time.

micelles: glue-like particles that transport digested fats to the intestinal villi for absorption.

microbiology: study of microorganisms.

microcirculation: blood flow through the capillaries.

microencephaly: congenital condition characterized by a small skull and small amount of brain tissue.

micronutrients: water, minerals, and vitamins.

microorganisms: minute living cells not visible to the human eye but found most everywhere in the environment.

micropsia: objects appearing smaller than normal.

micturition: passage of urine from the urinary bladder; also called voiding, urinating.

midbrain: brain area that functions as an important reflex center.

midlife transition: sense that arises in middle adulthood that others of the same age have achieved more and that one must contribute to society before it is too late.

midline: an imaginary line dividing the body into right and left halves, as a *midline* incision.

midwife: a person (not a physician) who is specially trained to assist in prenatal care and the delivery of babies, usually a registered nurse.

milia: pinhead sized white spots that may appear on the nose and cheeks of a newborn, caused by unopened sweat and oil glands.

milieu: environment, surroundings.

milieu therapy: therapy in a comfortable, therapeutic environment.

mineral: a nonorganic chemical element or compound vital for building bones and teeth, maintaining muscle tone, regulating body processes, and maintaining acid–base balance. Common minerals in the body include calcium and iron.

mineralocorticoid: corticosteroid that regulates the amount of electrolytes in the body.

minim: apothecary system unit of measurement of liquid, approximately equal to one drop.

minimum data set: a form that measures a client's ability to perform activities of daily living and identifies functional losses that affect this ability.

minority: the smaller in number of groups in a certain population; or, segment(s) of population having different characteristics or backgrounds than the majority.

misdemeanor: a crime less serious than a felony, usually punishable by a fine or imprisonment for less than a year.

mitered: the type of beveled corners used when making a hospital bed.

mitosis: cell division.

mitral valve: (see bicuspid valve).

mittelschmerz: "middle pain" a woman may experience during ovulation or midway between menstrual periods.

mixture: a blend of two or more substances that have been brought together without forming a new compound.

modified diet: approach to eating that has been specifically altered (whether in vitamins, nutrients, serving size, etc.) to meet the individual needs of a client.

molding: temporary elongation of the head of a newborn, caused by the overlap of skull bones due to the pressure of traveling through the birth canal.

molecule: the smallest division of a substance that still possesses the characteristics of that substance; if divided further, it breaks down into its individual chemical elements (atoms).

Mongolian spots: dark blue areas of discoloration that may appear on the buttocks, lower back, and upper legs of nonwhite babies which usually disappear by early childhood.

monocyte: a particular type of white blood cell that has one nucleus.

mononucleosis: contagious infection characterized by flu-like symptoms and often an enlarged liver or spleen.

monosaccharide: a single sugar molecule.

mons: a raised area, prominence, as the *mons* pubis.

mons pubis: fatty pad overlying the pubic area.

Montgomery straps: easily removable straps that stay in place to facilitate dressing removal.

mood: internal, subjective emotional state.

morbid: inducing disease or having a disease; thoughts of death or severe disease, as *morbid* thoughts.

morbidity: illness.

morgue: a place for keeping dead bodies temporarily until they are identified or claimed by relatives or until an autopsy is done.

mortal: terminating in death, as a *mortal* wound.

mortality: death, or rate of death per certain number of population.

morula: the fertilized zygote when it has divided rapidly and formed a ball of about 16 identical cells.

multifetal: pregnancy of twins or more.

multigravida: pregnant woman who has given birth at least once.

mumps: viral disease that affects the salivary glands, especially the parotids; also called *epidemic parotitis.*

muscle tone: state of slight contraction with the ability to spring into action.

mutism: refusal or inability to speak.

mycosis: disease caused by a fungus.

myelin: fatty covering of some nerve fibers, as the *myelin* sheath; electrically insulate one nerve call from another.

myelogram: a radiograph showing the differential count of various cells in the bone marrow.

myelosuppression: reduction in bone marrow function.

myocardial: pertaining to the myocardium, as in *myocardial* infarction ("heart attack").

myocarditis: inflammation of the heart's muscular walls.

myocardium: middle and thickest layer of the heart wall, the muscular layer.

myopia: nearsightedness; light rays focus in front of the retina.

myringotomy: surgical incision into the eardrum.

myxedema: condition that results from hypothyroidism (lack of the hormone thyroxine). (The adult form is cretinism.)

N

narcolepsy: a condition characterized by uncontrollable sleep.

nares: nostrils.

narrow spectrum: classification of antibiotics that are specific, or effective in fighting only a few microorganisms.

nasal cannula: a device used to administer small to moderate increases in oxygen concentration.

nasopharynx: section of the pharynx that extends from the nares to the uvula that is used for air passage only.

naturally acquired immunity: immunity that occurs when a person is accidentally exposed to a causative agent.

near drowning: recovery that occurs after submersion in liquid and apparent cessation of body processes.

necrosis: tissue death.

negative feedback system: a system by which once a gland stimulates another gland to produce a hormone and the hormone level rises highly enough, the first gland stops stimulating the target gland and stops the hormone release.

negligence: harm done to a person because of failure to do something that a responsible person would do; doing something a responsible person would not do; irresponsible care.

neologism: new word created by an individual that is not actually a word.

neonate: a newborn during the first 28 days of life.

neoplasm: tumor, new growth (may be benign or malignant); often refers to cancer. (adj: neoplastic)

nephrectomy: kidney removal.

nephrolithiasis: kidney stones (calculi).

nephrologist: a physician who specializes in medical aspects of kidney disease.

nephroma: cancer of the kidney.

nephron: the functional unit of the kidney.

nephropathy: nerve damage.

nephrotic syndrome: condition in which changes in the basement membrane of the glomeruli cause the kidneys to excrete massive amounts of protein.

nephrotoxicity: kidney damage, which can be caused by aminoglycosides and manifested by blood and protein in the urine.

nerve: a macroscopic cordlike structure that contains individual nerve fibers that carry impulses within the body. Sensory (afferent) nerves carry information to the brain; motor (efferent) nerves carry impulses from the brain to muscles. Some nerves are mixed sensory and motor.

neuralgia: pain that extends along one or more nerves, as trigeminal *neuralgia* (tic douloureux).

neurodiagnostic: hospital department that performs and records "brain wave" tests, administers evoked potential examinations, does specialized sleep studies, and monitors clients who have seizures; also called the electroencephalography (EEG) department.

neurogenic: originating in the nervous system.

neuroglia: supporting structure of nerve tissue; also called glial cells.

neurohypophysis: the posterior lobe of the pituitary gland.

neuroleptic: an agent that modifies psychotic behavior.

neuroleptic malignant syndrome (NMS): rare, life-threatening complication of neuroleptic medications; a medical emergency.

neurology: medical specialty related to the nervous system.

neurons: cells that make up nervous tissue.

neuropathic pain: chronic pain or discomfort that continues for six months or longer and interferes with normal functioning.

neurotransmitter: a chemical that an axon releases to allow nerve impulses to cross the synapse and reach the dendrites.

neutropenia: decreased neutrophils in the blood. Malignant neutropenia is called agranulocytosis.

neutropenic isolation: (see protective isolation).

newborn: a human being in the first four weeks of life.

Nightingale lamp: a standard in nursing insignia (also known as the *Lamp of Nursing*).

nirvana: Buddhist/Hindu state of enlightenment in which the soul no longer lives in the body and is free from desire and pain.

nits: lice eggs.

nociception: normal pain transmission.

nociceptive pain: acute pain; a pain sensation that results abruptly.

nocturia: excessive voiding (urination) during the night.

nocturnal emission: involuntary discharge of semen while sleeping.

nodule: type of skin lesion appearing as a small knot or protuberance.

non-pitting edema: observable edema that does not indent when slight pressure is applied.

non seminoma: a type of testicular tumor.

non–organ specific: a disease that affects one or more organs.

nonproductive: term used to describe a dry cough in which the person does not cough up any sputum or other material.

nonrebreathing mask: device that can deliver high doses of oxygen.

nonspecific immunity: immunity that helps fight against a variety of foreign invaders; also known as nonspecific defense systems which include the skin, tears, neutrophils and monocytes, etc.

nonverbal communication: conveying information or messages without speaking or writing. Components include items such as therapeutic touch, gestures, body language, facial expression, and eye contact.

norms: "rules" for behavior in a group.

nosocomial: originating in a hospital, as a *nosocomial* infection.

nuchal cord: loops of umbilical cord that may have become wrapped around a baby's neck during delivery.

nuchal rigidity: stiff neck.

nuclear dyad: a married couple who live together without children.

nuclear family: a two-generation unit consisting of a husband, wife, and their immediate children—biologic, adopted, or both—living within one household.

nuclear medicine: diagnosis and treatment of body disorders using radioactivity (includes x-ray, scintillation scan, and radiation therapy).

nucleus: body within the cell that contains chromosomes (sometimes referred to as the regulator).

numerator: top number of a fraction.

Nurse Practice Act: the law governing nursing practice in a state or territory.

nurses' registry: central location to place nurses for full- or part-time work, either locally or nationally.

nursing assessment: systematic and continuous collection and analysis of information about the client.

nursing bottle mouth: a serious dental condition resulting from regularly placing an infant in bed with a bottle of breast milk, formula, or juice propped on a blanket or towel.

nursing care plans: guidelines used by healthcare facilities to plan the care for clients.

nursing diagnosis: a statement about the client's actual or potential health concerns that can be managed through independent nursing intervention.

nursing history: way of soliciting information from the client; may also be called a health interview.

nursing peer review: an evaluation of nursing activities and client outcomes as demonstrated in the nursing documentation.

nursing process: systematic method in which the nurse and client work together to plan and carry out effective nursing care. (The steps include assessment, nursing diagnosis, planning, implementation, and evaluation.)

nursing unit: hospital area that contains several client units.

nutrient: substances needed for growth, maintenance, and repair of the body.

nutrient density: significant amounts of key nutrients per volume consumed.

nutrition: body process of using food for growth and development; the study of foods, nutrients, and diet.

nystagmus: rapid, repetitive involuntary movement of the eyeball; may be horizontal, rotating, vertical, or a combination of these.

O

obese: overweight; morbid obesity or gross obesity is usually considered to be more than 100 pounds overweight or twice normal weight.

object permanence: the knowledge that an object seen in a particular spot but temporarily hidden from view continues to exist and will return to view.

objective: able to be perceived by another person by means of the senses (a rash is an *objective* sign, as opposed to subjective); a goal or criterion (as *objectives* for each book chapter); a test item that has a definite answer (open to only one interpretation).

objective data: all measurable and observable pieces of information about a client and his or her overall state of health.

observation: assessment tool that relies on the use of the five senses to discover objective information about the client.

obsession: a recurrent, persistent, intrusive thought or belief that the person cannot ignore.

obstetrics: branch of medicine that deals with pregnancy, labor, delivery, and the puerperium. (An obstetrician is a physician who specializes in this field.)

occipital lobe: cerebral lobe that directs visual experiences.

occult: hidden.

occupational therapy (OT): department that rehabilitates clients so they can perform activities of daily living (ADLs) and return to work and leisure following an injury or illness.

occupied bed: bed holding a client that is unable to get up as a result of his or her condition or generalized weakness.

oculogyric crisis: involuntary backward rolling of the eyes.

official name: a medication's name as identified in the United States Pharmacopeia and the National Formulary.

olfaction: sense of smell.

oliguria: deficient urinary secretion or infrequent urination.

ombudsperson: state required representative who provides assistance and information to residents of long-care facilities and their families.

oncogene: a cancer-causing gene.

oncologist: cancer specialist.

oncology: study of tumors; the study of cancer, as *oncologic* nursing.

oocyte: ova at a female baby's birth.

open bed: bed that allows linens to be turned down, making it easier for a person to get into or out of.

open-ended questions: questions used in therapeutic communication and interviews that promote in-depth answers and encourage clients to talk about themselves and their concerns.

ophthalmia neonatorum: blindness in the neonate.

ophthalmic: medications that are instilled or administered directly into the eye.

ophthalmoscope: a lighted instrument used to inspect the eye.

opiate: analgesic derived from the seeds of a certain species of poppy plant or a synthetic derivative with similar pain-blocking effects.

opisthotonos: a spasm in which the head and heels are close together and the body is bowed forward.

opportunistic: causing disease under certain circumstances.

opportunistic infections: invasions by microorganisms that proliferate widely when the immune system is defective.

optic disk: eye region that is not light sensitive.

oral: of or pertaining to the mouth, as in the *oral cavity*.

oral/written reprimand: respectively, the first and second steps in due process informing an employee of deficiencies.

orbit: ball-shaped cavity in the skull that contains the eye.

orchiectomy: removal of one or both testes.

orchiopexy: corrective surgery in which undescended testes are sutured, so they remain in the scrotum.

orchitis: inflammation of the testicles.

organ: a group of body tissues having a particular function.

organ of Corti: small but intricate organ in the inner ear where the transmission of nerve stimuli begins.

organic: pertaining to an organ.

organic brain syndrome: irreversible condition that affects cognitive function; now called dementia, formerly called senility.

organic disease: a disorder in which a detectable structural change has occurred in one or more organs, also alters usual function (as opposed to a functional disease).

organic disorder: mental illness that is caused by an actual physical disorder.

organ-specific: having an effect only on a particular organ.

orgasm: climax of sexual excitement.

oropharynx: part of the pharynx extending from the uvula to the epiglottis that carries food to the esophagus and air to the trachea; commonly called the throat.

orthodontia: branch of dentistry that deals with malocclusion (misplaced teeth) and other jaw and facial deformities.

orthopedic: pertaining to the correction of deformities of the musculoskeletal system.

orthopnea: difficult breathing, relieved by sitting or standing erect.

orthostatic hypotension: drop in blood pressure upon standing, often causing dizziness.

orthotics: the practice that deals with the application of braces or appliances to the body; closely related to prosthetics (the science that deals with the fabrication of braces and other orthopedic devices).

os: opening; any body orifice. Specifically refers to the mouth and the cervical opening (cervical *os*).

osmosis: passage of a solvent from one side of a selectively permeable membrane to the other, due to the relative pressures on both sides.

ossicle: collectively, the three tiny bones in the middle ear (the malleus, incus, and the stapes) which are set in motion by sound waves.

ossify: to change or develop into bone, sometimes an abnormal situation. (noun: ossification—the process of bone formation.)

osteoblast: a cell that is associated with bone production; a "bone cell."

osteoclast: large multinuclear bone cells that assist in the resorption or breakdown of bone.

osteocyte: hardened, mature muscle cell.

osteomalacia: adult form of vitamin D deficiency which results in a softening of the bones.

osteomyelitis: bone inflammation caused by a pyogenic (pus-forming) infection.

osteoporosis: a chronic bone disorder caused by mineral loss, especially of calcium, in the bone (often occurs in aging).

ostomate: one who has a stoma outside the abdomen to drain feces or urine.

ostomy: an opening.

otic: pertaining to the ear.

otitis externa: inflammation of the external ear; also called swimmer's ear.

otitis media: acute infection of the middle ear.

otology: study of the anatomy and physiology of the ear and related disorders.

otosclerosis: abnormal spongy bone formation in the labyrinth of the ear (often causes hearing loss because the ossicles become fixed and unable to transmit sound waves).

otoscope: a lighted instrument used to inspect the ear.

ototoxic: drugs used to treat conditions unrelated to the ear that may harm the inner ear.

ototoxicity: damage to the eighth cranial nerve which can be caused by aminoglycosides and manifested by dizziness, tinnitis, and gradual hearing loss.

outcome-based care: quality management in which delivery of care is judged by results achieved.

ova: female gametes (eggs).

ovaries: female gonads.

overflow: incontinence that occurs when the bladder overfills with urine but is not able to release it; also called paradoxical incontinence.

overhydration: excess water in the extracellular spaces.

overweight: ten percent over the desirable weight for the body's frame.

oviducts: passageways for ova between the ovaries and the uterus. Also called ovarian tubes, uterine tubes (formerly called fallopian tubes).

ovulation: process by which an ovum (egg cell) ruptures the ovary's surface and is expelled into the pelvic cavity.

P

pain threshold: lowest intensity of a stimulus that causes a subject to recognize pain.

pain tolerance: point at which a person can no longer tolerate pain.

palliative: measures that give relief, but are not curative (as chemotherapy is palliative for some types of advanced cancer).

pallor: absence of skin pigment; paleness.

palpation: the act of feeling with the hand, placing the fingers on the skin to determine the condition of underlying parts.

pancarditis: widespread, general inflammation of the heart.

pancytopenia: having a decreased number of platelets.

pandemic: widespread epidemic of disease.

Pap test: a method of examining body secretions from the cervical area for malignant cells; also called Pap smear or Papanicolaou's test.

papule: a small, solid, circumscribed skin elevation, less than 0.5–1.0 cm in diameter.

paracentesis: surgical puncture of a body cavity for the aspiration of fluid (often refers to abdominal paracentesis). (Removal of fluid from the thoracic cavity is called thoracentesis.)

paradoxical: opposite reaction.

paralysis: motion loss or impairment of sensation in a body part.

paralytic ileus: intestinal paralysis.

paranoia: mental disorder in which one has delusions of persecution or thinks others will harm him/her.

paraplegia: paralysis of the legs and sometimes the lower part of the body; a person with this condition is called a paraplegic.

parasites: plants or animals that live on or within another organism, taking something from that other organism.

parasympathetic: division of the autonomic nervous system that produces body responses that are normal while at rest or under normal conditions.

parathyroid: small glands lying on either side of the undersurface of the thyroid gland.

parenteral: administered into the body in a way other than through the alimentary canal (subcutaneous, intravenous, intramuscular), as *parenteral* medications.

paresis: slight or incomplete paralysis or loss of sensation.

parietal pleura: outer layer of pleura that lines the chest cavity.

parietal lobe: cerebral lobe responsible for sensations of touch, spatial ability, speech, and communication.

Parkinsonism: chronic progressive neurological disease affecting the dopamine producing cells in the brain; also called Parkinson's disease; symptoms similar to Parkinson's disease caused by some medications.

partial rebreathing mask: a low-flow oxygen device.

passive immunity: immunity that occurs during pregnancy and lactation, when a woman passes protection to the baby through the placenta or breast milk.

passive: submissive, or not produced by active efforts, as *passive* range of motion exercises.

passive range of motion: range of motion exercises with which the client may need physical assistance.

patella: kneecap.

patent: unobstructed, open, as a *patent* drainage tube or *patent* airway.

pathogen: a disease-producing agent or organism. (adj: pathogenic)

pathology: study of changes in body tissues or organs as a result of disease; also used to mean a disease process. (The physician who specializes in this field is a pathologist.)

pathophysiology: study of disorders in functioning.

patient: individual being treated by a healthcare provider, now called a "client."

payee: person designated to receive a client's monthly check and disburse funds appropriately if the client is unable to do so for him- or herself

pedal pulse: pulse in the foot felt over the dorsalis pedis artery or the posterial tibial artery, used to determine status of circulation in the lower extremities.

pediatrics: branch of medicine concerned with disorders of children. (Pediatrician: physician who treats children.)

pediculi: lice.

pediculosis pubis: pubic lice or parasites that attach themselves to pubic hair follicles and cause intense itching.

pediculosis: infested with lice.

peer group: contemporaries, friends, group of people with whom one is associated.

pellagra: disease in which the mucous membranes of the mouth and digestive tract become red and inflamed, and lesions appear on the skin (in severe cases can lead to dermatitis, diarrhea, dementia, and even death) due to a marked niacin deficiency.

pelvic exenteration: surgical procedure in which the entire contents of the pelvis are removed.

pelvis: the pelvic girdle.

penis: the male sex organ.

percussion: tapping a body part with short sharp blows to elicit sounds or vibrations that aid in diagnosis; often refers to the use of a percussion hammer to elicit a reflex.

performance review: written evaluation of an employee's work performance which is discussed in an interview between the individual and his or her supervisor.

pericardial fluid: small amount of fluid contained in the space between the visceral and parietal layers in the pericardium that acts as a lubricant and reduces friction between the layers as the heart contracts and relaxes.

pericarditis: inflammation of the pericardium.

pericardium: the sac enclosing the heart and the roots of some of the great vessels.

perineal care: bathing the genitalia and surrounding area.

perineum: the pelvic floor and associated structures (from the symphysis pubis to the coccyx).

perioperative: the period surrounding surgery; includes the preoperative, intraoperative, and postoperative periods.

periosteum: the specialized connective tissue that covers all bones. Periosteum is able to form bone in some cases.

peripheral: pertaining to the outward part of surface; further from the center, as *peripheral* nervous system.

peristalsis: wavelike contractions of the intestines by which they propel their contents through the GI tract.

peritoneum: serous membrane that lines walls of body cavities and encloses viscera.

peritonitis: inflammation of the peritoneum.

permeable: allowing passage of a substance, as a *permeable* membrane.

permissive licensure: regulation that forbids a nurse from using the title RN or LPN without a license.

pernicious: tending to be fatal unless treated, as *pernicious* anemia.

perseverate: to dwell on one subject.

personal protective equipment: pieces of equipment that serve as barriers against organisms from entering or leaving the respiratory tract: gloves, eye protection, gowns, and masks.

personal space: an invisible, mutually understood area or zone around a person that is considered inappropriate for strangers to violate (varies between cultures). If a person invades another's personal space (comes too close), it may cause discomfort. Much nursing care must occur within the client's personal space.

pertussis: highly contagious respiratory disease; also known as whooping cough.

pessary: device inserted into the vagina to support the organs of the pelvis.

pH: symbol for hydrogen ion concentration (use of the symbol with a number denotes whether a substance is acidic [below 7.0] or basic [above 7.0]).

phagocyte: a cell that ingests or engulfs other cells, microorganisms, or foreign particles. This process is called phagocytosis.

phalanges: bones of the fingers and toes (singular: phalanx).

pharmacokinetics: actions of drugs.

pharmacology: the study of chemicals (drugs, medications) and their effects.

pharynx: tube-shaped passage for food and air.

phenylketonuria (PKU): a congenital disease caused by a defect in metabolism of phenylalanine (an essential amino acid) that, if not treated, leads to intellectual impairment.

pheochromocytoma: a catecholamine-secreting tumor.

phimosis: constriction in the foreskin or prepuce so that it cannot be drawn back over the glans penis.

phlebitis: inflammation of a vein. (Thrombophlebitis is inflammation *and* blood clots.)

phobia: a persistent, abnormal fear or dread. (Claustrophobia is fear of small, enclosed places.)

phoropter: instrument that simulates different corrective lenses during an eye examination in order to better test vision and select glasses.

phosphorus: an important mineral found in every body cell.

photophobia: intolerance to light.

photosensitivity: sensitivity to light.

phototherapy: treatment with light, as in physiologic, nonhemolytic jaundice of the newborn.

physiatrics: branch of medicine involved with physical medicine, physical therapy, and rehabilitation.

physical change: a change in a substance's outward properties (e.g., ice into water).

physical therapy (PT): department that rehabilitates clients with limited physical mobility, using physical modalities, exercises, and assistive devices. Chest physiotherapy is a form of respiratory therapy that uses percussion and postural drainage to loosen and drain secretions from the lungs.

physiologic jaundice: newborn condition in which the baby's immature liver cannot handle bilirubin, and thus bilirubin levels increase in the body.

physiologic needs: needs required to sustain life such as oxygen, food, water, and elimination; survival needs.

physiologic: pertaining to physiology, the function of the body; normal.

physiology: science that deals with body functions.

phytochemical: previously unidentified naturally occurring components in plant foods that may help protect against disease.

pica: a craving to eat inedible items or unnatural food items, such as *pica* in pregnancy.

pilonidal cyst: cyst above the anus, often believed to result from an infolding of skin in which hair continues to grow.

pilonidal: having a group of hairs, as in *pilonidal* cyst or sinus tract.

pineal: shaped like a pine cone, as the *pineal* body within the brain, or the *pineal* gland.

pineal gland: small cone-shaped structure located at the top portion of the brain's third ventricle that produces melatonin.

pinna: external ear; auricle.

pinworms: a common parasitic infestation in children causing anal and perineal itching.

pitting edema: observable edema that dents under slight finger pressure.

pituitary: a tiny gland located at the base of the brain that secretes or releases several hormones, including growth hormone; called the master gland.

placenta accreta: condition in which a placenta fails to separate and be expelled within 20–30 minutes after delivery or leaves remnants in the uterus; also called retained placenta.

placenta previa: low implantation of the placenta so that it partially or completely covers the cervical os.

placenta: an organ joining woman and fetus during pregnancy in human beings and other mammals. The placental blood furnishes nutrients, oxygen, hormones, and other substances to the fetus and carries away wastes. (Also called afterbirth.)

plan of assistance: third step in due process in which a supervisor writes a statement describing a deficiency, employee actions needed to correct it, timeline for improvements, and consequences to employee if the plan is not followed and improvement is not shown.

plane: an imaginary flat surface that divides the body into sections.

planning: in nursing process, developing goals to prevent, reduce, or eliminate problems and identifying nursing interventions that will assist in meeting these goals.

plasma membrane: (see cell membrane).

plasma: the fluid portion of the blood.

platelet: type of blood cell composed of cell fragments that provide a major step in the blood clotting process.

pleura: membrane covering the lungs and lining the walls of the chest cavity, as the parietal *pleura.*

pleural cavity: space between the two layers of the pleura; also called pleural space.

pleurisy: inflammation of the pleura.

plexus: a network or tangle, as of veins or nerves.

plication: surgical pleating or taking of tucks to shorten a structure, as in treatment of retinal detachment.

plumbism: chronic lead poisoning.

Pneumocystis carinii pneumonia: an interstitial plasma cell pneumonia, one of the most common opportunistic diseases of AIDS.

pneumonectomy: removal of an entire lung.

pneumonia: lung inflammation, with consolidation and drainage.

pneumothorax: collapse of a lung, due to air or gas in the chest cavity.

poison: any substance that affects health or threatens life when absorbed into the body or when in contact with the body surface.

poliomyelitis: contagious viral disease that attacks the CNS and can cause temporary or permanent paralysis or weakness; commonly known as "polio."

pollution: act of contamination or making impure by noxious substances; may refer to air, food, water, or noise contamination.

polycythemia vera: disorder in which the total number of RBCs, WBCs, and platelets are increased; also called primary polycythemia.

polydactylism: condition in which an individual is born with an extra finger or toe.

polydipsia: excessive thirst.

polyhydramnios: excessive amniotic fluid.

polyneuritis: inflammation of many nerves.

polypectomy: removal of polyps from the lower bowel.

polyphagia: an abnormal craving for all kinds of food.

polysaccharide: long chain of many sugar molecules; a complex carbohydrate.

polysubstance abuse: abuse of two or more substances.

polysubstance dependent: individual who is dependent on several drugs.

polyuria: voiding an excessive amount of urine.

pons: brain area that contains nerve tracts that carry messages between the cerebrum and medulla.

popliteal pulse: pulse located posteriorly to the knee, sometimes used as an alternative means of assessing blood pressure with a large leg cuff.

ports: entry or exit points.

port-wine stain: a permanent birthmark consisting of a flat, purple-red area with sharp borders.

positive Homans' sign: pain that occurs on the knee upon dorsiflexion, which is indicative of thrombophlebitis.

postmortem: after death, as *postmortem* examination (autopsy); "post."

postoperative: after surgery.

postoperative bed: bed prepared for a client who is returning from surgery or another procedure that requires transfer into the bed from a stretcher or wheelchair.

postpartum: after childbirth or delivery (refers to the mother).

postpartum hematoma: bleeding into the subcutaneous tissue in the perineal area after delivery.

postpartum hemorrhage: any blood loss from the uterus after delivery in the amount of 500 mL–1000 mL within 24 hours.

postterm: fetus remaining in the uterus beyond 42 weeks.

postural drainage: method of drainage that uses position and gravity to drain secretions and mucus from a person's lungs.

potassium: chemical element that plays a major role in the acid–base and water balance in the body; a major ion in the intracellular fluid, symbol is K^+.

potentiation: enhancement of one agent by another, so that the combined action is greater than the sum of the two (e.g., alcohol and Valium *potentiate* each other); synergism.

practical nurse: nurse who cares for the sick, injured, convalescent and handicapped under the direction of physicians and registered nurses.

preadolescence: early adolescence (approximately ages 11–14).

preconception: period in time before the woman is pregnant, as in *preconceptional* care.

preeclampsia: condition in which a woman whose pregnancy was previously progressing normally develops hypertension with either edema, proteinuria, or both, usually after the 20th week of gestation.

pregnancy: the state of having a developing embryo or fetus within the uterus; being with child; gravid.

pregnancy-induced hypertension (PIH): an abnormal complication of pregnancy, and for a short time following delivery, characterized by hypertension (high blood pressure), edema, and proteinuria. Seizures may occur if not successfully treated. Also called gestosis, toxemia of pregnancy, and preeclampsia–eclampsia syndrome. May be fatal to woman and/or fetus.

prejudice: an opinion formed without knowing the facts.

preload: the amount of pressure, or "stretching force" against the ventricular wall at end diastole.

premature cervical dilation: condition in which the cervix is unable to support a pregnancy and the weight of the fetus is enough to force it to dilate, causing a spontaneous abortion.

preoperative: before surgery.

preparatory depression: depression that occurs when a person realizes the impact of a loss before it happens.

prepuce: foreskin of the penis.

presbycusis: hearing loss that occurs with aging.

presbyopia: farsightedness that occurs with aging.

prescription: written formula for preparing and administering medication.

presentation: part of the fetus that lies closest to the pelvis and will first enter the birth canal, usually the head.

pressure ulcer, pressure sore (pressure area): ulcerated sore often caused by prolonged pressure on a bony prominence or other area, especially if the client is allowed to lie in one position for an extended period. Also called decubitus ulcer, (formerly called "bedsore").

preterm birth: born early, prior to the end of the 37th week of gestation.

priapism: persistent, painful, abnormal penile erection.

primary caregivers: a client's significant others, whether blood-related or not.

primary disease: a disease that occurs independently, not related to another disease.

primary healthcare: family-focused healthcare that emphasizes health education and wellness to promote healthy lifestyles and decrease the potential for illness.

primary needs: needs that must be satisfied before attempting to meet other needs (such as oxygen, food, water, and elimination).

primigravida: a woman pregnant for the first time.

primipara: a woman who has had one live birth (often used interchangeably with primigravida).

probationary: an internship period a recent graduate nurse is required to serve before becoming a full-fledged RN or LPN/LVN.

prodromal: the period before actual symptoms occur; may involve a premonition that a disease is about to occur. Some disorders, such as genital herpesvirus, are more contagious during the prodromal period.

products of conception: the placenta and fetus.

progesterone: female hormone that functions primarily during pregnancy.

prognosis: projected client outcome.

progress note: form nurses fill out at regular intervals to summarize a client's condition or response to treatment.

projectile vomiting: emesis expelled with great force.

prolapse: condition in which an organ or internal part drops or sags.

prolapsed cord: umbilical cord that precedes the baby in delivery.

pronation: turning the hand so that the palm faces downward or backward.

prone: positioning a client so that he or she is lying on the stomach.

prophylaxis: medications given to prevent infections.

proportion: two ratios separated by an equal sign.

proprioception: the sensation of body position in space. (Older people often lose proprioception.)

prospective: predetermined, before the fact.

prospective payment: reimbursement for health care made by third-party payers according to a formula or average reimbursement of actual costs per case.

prostaglandins: fatty acids that are widespread in body tissues and that generally stimulate contraction or relaxation of smooth muscles.

prostate: a doughnut-shaped gland lying just below the bladder in the male.

prostate specific antigen (PSA): a glycoprotein found only in the tissue of the prostate gland; elevated PSA level is indicative of a prostate disorder.

prostatectomy: removal of the prostate.

prostatitis: inflammation of the prostate gland.

prosthesis: the replacement of a missing part by an artificial substitute (e.g., an artificial eye, arm, or leg is a prosthesis).

prosthetics: the manufacture of prostheses, splints, and braces for limbs and the back.

protective device: piece of equipment, most often a vest or a belt, used to ensure the safety of the client (ie, helping client to remain in a chair without falling); also called a client reminder device.

protective isolation: attempts to prevent harmful microorganisms from coming into contact with the client; also called reverse or neutropenic isolation.

protein: groups of amino acids in complex compounds that are vital to life. Protein-rich foods are essential to building and repairing all body tissues and include meat, eggs, fish, legumes, and dairy products.

prothrombin: a plasma protein that is converted to thrombin during blood clotting. (Also called clotting factor II).

protocol: specific policies outlining a healthcare facility's standards for care.

protoplasm: the essential component of the living cell.

proximodistal: from the center or core outward. (Refers to the pattern of development and achievement of motor control of the infant.)

pruritus: itching.

pseudodementia: a condition in which a person appears to have dementia but is actually suffering from depression.

pseudomenstruation: small amount of vaginal bleeding in newborns, caused by maternal hormones.

psoriasis: a chronic skin disorder that involves red macules and patches covered with flakes or silvery scales. It is believed to have a hereditary or autoimmune origin in some cases.

psyche: the mind.

psychiatrist: a physician who specializes in the treatment of mental disorders.

psychological: pertaining to the mind, behavior, or thoughts, rather than to the physical body.

psychological needs: those human needs related to safety and security.

psychometric: type of testing for mental disorders that includes an in-depth interview and various other tests; also called neuropsychiatric testing.

psychosis: a mental disturbance in which personality disintegrates and the person escapes into unreality (more serious than neurosis).

psychotropic: types of medications that modify moods.

ptosis: drooping or sagging of an organ or part from its normal position (usually refers to eyelid).

ptyalism: increase in salivation during pregnancy.

puberty: period in life when a person becomes sexually able to reproduce.

pubic arch: opening of the pelvis.

pubococcygeal: pelvic muscles.

puerperal: complication occurring following the birth of a baby.

puerperium: period immediately after childbirth, continuing through involution (return of the uterus to its non-pregnant state).

pulmonary emphysema: abnormal, permanent enlargement of the alveoli and alveolar ducts with destruction of the alveolar walls.

pulmonic valve: valve that separates the right ventricle from the pulmonary aorta, also called the pulmonary semilunar valve.

pulse: the heartbeat as felt through the walls of the arteries and the skin or as heard at the apex of the heart with a stethoscope.

pulse deficit: a difference that exists between the apical and the radial pulse.

pulse oximeter: a convenient monitor that measures the amount (percentage) of oxygen saturation in the blood.

pulse pressure: difference of systolic pressure minus diastolic pressure.

pulse rate: measure of how often a person's heart beats.

pulse rhythm: spacing between heart beats.

puncture: a hole made by a pointed object; penetration.

pupil: black center of the eye that regulates the amount of light that enters it.

purulent: consisting of or secreting pus.

pus: the liquid product of inflammation made up of leukocytes, liquid, and cellular debris.

pustule: a small elevation of the skin filled with pus or lymph.

pyelonephritis: potentially dangerous infection of the kidney and renal pelvis.

pyloric sphincter: circular muscle that controls the opening between the stomach and the duodenal portion of the small intestine.

pyloric stenosis: a congenital anomaly in which an increase in the size of the musculature at the junction of the stomach and small intestine occurs, causing the pyloric opening to constrict and block food passage.

pylorus: lower narrow portion of the stomach which attaches to the small intestine.

pyorrhea: copious discharge of pus. *Pyorrhea* alveolaris, a purulent mouth infection.

pyrexia: fever.

pyuria: pus in the urine.

Q

quadrant: one of four corresponding quarters, as of the abdomen or buttock. For example, the appendix is in the lower right abdominal *quadrant*.

quadriplegia: paralysis of both arms and both legs; also called tetraplegia.

quality assurance: standards of care that represent acceptable, expected levels of performance by nursing staff and other staff members. (The Quality Assurance Committee sets these standards.)

quickening: first fetal movements a woman feels in pregnancy; signs of life.

R

rabies: an acute infectious disease of the central nervous system that can be transmitted by an animal bite.

race: term used to differentiate large groups of humankind that share common genetic characteristics associated with having ancestors from a specific part of the world.

radial pulse: pulse measured above the radial artery on the inside of the wrist.

radiation: giving off infrared heat rays; radioactive energy.

radius: the small bone of the forearm.

radon: a by-product of the disintegration of radium that contributes to diseases.

rale: an abnormal respiratory sound more descriptively called crackle (see description of crackle).

range of motion: ability to move various joints and structures of the body.

rape: violent crime in which an individual is sexually assaulted without his or her consent.

rapport: a state of harmony or good relationship between two individuals, particularly emphasized in mental health.

ratio: relationship of one quantity to another; may be written as a fraction or separated by a colon.

rationale: reason or underlying principle behind every nursing procedure.

reabsorption: the process of absorbing again.

reactive depression: depression that results when an individual concentrates on past losses.

receptor: a sensory nerve ending that responds to stimuli.

reciprocity: procedure in which a person transfers licensure from one state to another.

Recommended Dietary Allowance: recommendations for average daily amounts of nutrients considered adequate in meeting the nutritional needs of all healthy people.

reconstituted family: a family that consists of a couple who both have custody of their children from previous relationships and any new children from this arrangement.

recovery position: used in emergency rescue, in which the person is rolled to the side so the head, shoulders, and torso move simultaneously, without twisting.

rectocele: herniation of part of the rectum into the vagina.

rectum: distal portion of the large intestine between the sigmoid colon and the anal canal. (adj: rectal. Temperature is taken and some medications are administered rectally.)

recumbent: lying down.

refeeding syndrome: illness that results when a starving person receives carbohydrates too quickly, overstimulating insulin production and seriously upsetting electrolyte balance; can be fatal.

referred: (referring to pain) pain that is felt at a location other than its origination; when one physician sends (refers) a client to another physician or specialist.

reflex: an automatic movement in response to a particular stimulus, as the knee jerk in response to a tap below the kneecap.

reflex arc: circle in the spinal cord that receives and sends messages through nerve fibers.

reflex incontinence: urinary leakage due to bladder instability as a result of upper motor lesions or neuropathies.

reflux: backing up of urine into the kidneys as a result of a bladder obstruction.

refraction: determination of refractive errors of the eye and their correction.

registered nurse: nurse who spends 2–4 years learning the profession.

registered pharmacist: a healthcare professional who is licensed to prepare and to dispense medications upon the order of a licensed practitioner of medicine.

registry: a service that recruits nurses to work in facilities that need extra help for special duty clients, during busy periods, or for vacation coverage.

regression: return to a former state, as a child *regresses* when ill. Regression of a disease process refers to its relief or subsiding.

rehabilitation: restoration of a person to as normal as possible body structure and/or function after an injury or illness.

reminder device: (see protective device).

reminiscence: remembering past joys and successes.

remission: period in which symptoms of a disease or disorder lessen or abate.

renal: pertaining to the kidney, as *renal* failure.

renal colic: severe, penetrating lower back pain, caused by a stone becoming lodged in the ureter.

renal cortex: outer portion of the kidney.

renal erythropoietic factor: (see erythropoietin).

renal failure: disorder in which the kidneys can no longer meet everyday demands.

renal medulla: kidney portion that contains the renal tubules, loops of Henle, and collecting tubules.

renal pelvis: end of the ureter that receives urine from the calyces.

renal threshold: maximum amount of a substance that the renal tubules can reabsorb back into the body before the excess is excreted into the urine.

renin: hormone that is important in blood pressure regulation.

replantation: reattachment of a completely severed body part back to the body.

replication: reproduction of cancer cells.

rescue breathing: one component of CPR, that of blowing breaths into the victim who has stopped breathing.

research laboratory: laboratory where studies and experiments on animals are conducted to understand, cure, or prevent human disease.

resection: excision of a portion of an organ or structure, as a gastric (stomach) *resection*.

reservoir: any place where a microorganism can multiply or survive before moving to a place where it can multiply.

resident assessment protocol: form that aids the nursing care team to create an individualized plan of care for every client.

resident: term used to refer to the client, particularly in a nursing home or other long-term facility; term used to refer to a physician who is studying in a medical specialty.

residual: amount remaining or left behind, as *residual* urine.

residual urine volume: amount of urine that remains in the bladder after voiding at least once.

respiration: the total process of the exchange of oxygen and carbon dioxide between the air and body cells. (External respiration denotes the exchange of gases in the lungs; internal respiration denotes exchange of gases between the blood and body cells.)

respirator: a machine that forces air into the lungs; also called a ventilator.

respiratory acidosis: condition that stems from an increase in carbon dioxide in the blood.

respiratory alkalosis: condition that stems from a deficit of plasma CO_2 or carbonic acid.

respiratory distress syndrome (RDS): leading cause of death in premature newborns in whom the lungs have not fully developed and do not expand for adequate breathing. Also called hyaline membrane disease.

respiratory therapy (RT) (respiratory care): department concerned with treatment, management, and care of clients with respiratory disorders through use of oxygen and other gases and assistive devices for breathing and maintenance of ventilation.

respite: rest; care provided for long-term or chronic clients so family members can have some time off (a respite).

resting energy expenditure: total calories a person needs to maintain his or her body processes.

resume: document that emphasizes a person's strengths and abilities and/or that lists a person's employment and educational experiences and achievements.

retention: holding or keeping within the body something that is usually expelled, as *retention* of urine.

retina: the innermost tunic of the eyeball that contains rods and cones and is the origin of the optic nerve. Light rays focus at the retina in normal vision.

retinitis: inflammation of the retina, as *retinitis* pigmentosa.

retinopathy: any noninflammatory disorder of the retina of the eye, as diabetic *retinopathy* (which may lead to blindness).

retrovirus: one of a large group of RNA-based viruses that tend to infect immunocompromised persons.

reverse isolation: (see protective isolation).

Reye's syndrome: acute and potentially fatal childhood disease which often follows a viral illness and may be related to aspirin use during that time.

Rh factor: inherited antigens present in blood that can cause severe reactions during blood transfusions if not compatible, named for the Rhesus monkey in which it was first identified.

Rh sensitization: condition in which a pregnant Rh negative woman has had Rh positive RBCs from the fetus cross the placental barrier, stimulating the formation of antibodies within her circulatory system which then return to the fetus and destroy fetal erythrocytes. This condition is prompted by, but does not occur, during the first pregnancy but does so with increasing sensitivity in subsequent pregnancies.

rheumatic carditis: complication of rheumatic fever in which valvular lesions impair valve efficiency and increase the heart's workload.

rheumatic fever: autoimmune reaction to group A beta-hemolytic *Streptococcus*, believed to develop as a result of continued streptococcal infections.

rhinitis: inflammation of the mucous membrane lining the nasal cavity.

rhinoplasty: plastic surgery/repair of the nose.

rhinorrhea: a runny rose.

rhonchi: rattling sounds in the throat that resemble snoring (singular, rhoncus).

ribonucleic acid: genetic material responsible for taking messages from DNA and transporting them to the ribosomes in the cytoplasm.

rickets: a condition in children caused by lack of vitamin D.

risk factors: factors that increase a person's likelihood of developing a certain disease.

rituals: practices that provide a group with comfort, acceptance, and inclusion.

rods: specialized neurons dispersed throughout the retina, suited to dim light and especially useful in night vision.

roseola: rose-colored rash. *Roseola infantum,* an acute viral disease that usually occurs in children under age 2 and disappears suddenly; *exanthem subitum.*

rotation: process of turning about an axis, as *rotation* of the hand or of the fetus in preparation for delivery.

roundworm: intestinal parasite common to warm climates and unsanitary conditions, which mature in the intestines and can cause diarrhea, intestinal obstruction, and sometimes intestinal rupture.

rubella: mild disease with fever and a mild rash; German measles (in English); 3-day measles.

rubeola: measles (in English); German measles (in French and Spanish). Preventable by immunization.

rugae (sing. ruga): folds of the stomach when it is empty (they allow the stomach to distend when food is eaten).

S

sacrum: solid bone in the spinal column of adults that anchors the pelvis.

sagittal: an imaginary vertical plane that divides the body into right and left sides, from top to bottom. The midsagittal plane divides the body into equal, symmetrical halves. (Also means shaped like an arrow, as the coccyx or xiphoid process of the sternum.)

saline lock: (see heparin lock).

saliva: thin, watery fluid secreted into the mouth which moistens food particles and begins the digestive process by breaking down starch into smaller sugar molecules.

salivation: secretion of saliva.

sally port: a system of two doors, only one of which can be opened at a time, used to prevent escape of disturbed or incarcerated clients.

salt: any compound of a base or an acid; table salt (sodium chloride); a purgative, as Epsom salt.

sarcoma: connective tissue tumor, often malignant, as Kaposi's *sarcoma.*

saturated fat: a fat, such as an animal fat, which already contains its full complement of hydrogen.

scabies: contagious skin disorder caused by the itch mite. Often sexually transmitted.

scapula: shoulder blade.

schizophrenia: psychological condition in which the person loses contact with reality.

scientific problem solving: precise method of investigating problems and arriving at solutions.

sclera: outer coating of the eyeball.

sclerodactyly: scleroderma of the fingers and toes.

scleroderma: chronic hardening and shrinking of the connective tissues of any body organ; often refers to thickened, hard, and darkened skin.

scoliosis: lateral curvature of the normally straight, vertical line of the spine, sometimes is S-shaped ("curvature of the spine").

scrotum: saclike structure that encloses the testes.

scurvy: disease caused by a vitamin C deficiency. Lesser deficiencies cause listlessness, irritability, and lowered resistance to disease; greater deficiencies cause bleeding gums, loose teeth, sore and stiff joints, tiny hemorrhages, and great weight loss.

sebaceous: pertaining to sebum (the oily, fatty secretion of the sebaceous gland).

sebaceous glands: oil secreting glands located close to the hair follicles into which they usually drain.

sebum: oily secretion of the sebaceous (oil) glands composed of fat and dead skin and released into the hair follicles.

secondary disease: a disease that directly results from or depends on another disease.

secondary needs: needs, according to Maslow, that don't sustain life, but enhance quality of life (such as beauty, learning, and love). A person must meet primary needs before attempting to meet secondary needs.

sedative: a remedy that has a quieting effect, sometimes enabling sleep.

seizure: a sudden attack or recurrence of a disease, as in epilepsy (cerebral seizure), formerly called convulsion.

self-actualized: according to Maslow, state of being fulfilled, complete, and reaching full potential.

self-esteem: how one feels about oneself; self-respect, self-worth, self-image.

semen: fluid that carries spermatozoa which are manufactured in the male's testes.

semicircular canals: section of the inner ear that contains hairlike nerve endings that respond to movement and control the sense of balance.

semilunar valves: heart valves with three crescent (half-moon) shaped cusps.

seminal vesicles: convoluted, sac shaped glands that store semen.

seminiferous tubules: the functional units of the testes, where sperm cells are produced and mature.

seminoma: malignancy of the testis.

senility: (see dementia).

sensitivity: test performed on a culture to discern which medication is most effective in treating an organism; also called a culture and sensitivity (C & S) test.

sentinel lymph node: node that drains the area of a breast involved by tumor.

septicemia: generalized infection (sepsis) throughout the body.

septum: dividing wall between two cavities, as the nasal *septum* or the *septa* (pl.) between the chambers of the heart.

sequela: an illness or injury that follows as a direct result of a previous condition or event.

sequestration: abnormal separation of a part from the whole, as a part of a bone.

serosanguinous: fluid composed of serum and blood.

serous: containing clear fluid.

sexual dysfunction: the inability to enjoy or to engage in sexual activity.

sexual orientation: term referring to which gender a person finds sexually desirable.

sexuality: the way in which individuals physically, mentally, emotionally, and socially experience and express themselves as sexual beings.

sexually transmitted disease (STD): a disease that can be (and most often is) transmitted by sexual intercourse or other intimate contact, formerly known as venereal disease.

shaman: a Native American medicine man or woman.

shingles: (see herpes zoster).

shock: depression of body functions due to the failure of the circulation or loss of blood.

shock wave: treatment used to blast stones in the kidney into small gravel-like fragments that are more easily passed from the body.

short-term objective: an expected outcome or goal that a client can reasonably meet in a matter of hours or days.

show: discharge of blood, usually as a beginning sign of labor (bloody show).

shunt: a bypass; u-shaped tube inserted into blood vessels to facilitate repeated hemodialysis; also called a fistula.

siblings: two or more people having at least one parent in common.

sickle cell: an abnormal crescent-shaped erythrocyte. (*Sickle-cell anemia* is a genetic blood defect that is most commonly found in African Americans, also known as sicklemia.)

sickle cell crisis: severe, painful episodes of sickle cell anemia due to clumping and occlusion of blood vessels.

sickle cell disease: genetic disorder characterized by the formation of abnormally curved RBCs which are ineffective as oxygen-carriers (thereby causing anemia) and because of their shape are able to clump together (causing further anemia and circulatory occlusion).

side effect: a result from a therapeutic agent other than originally intended (often refers to the result of a prescribed medication).

sign: objective evidence of disease that another person can note (as opposed to symptom, which only the client can describe).

significant figure: term used to refer to numbers that have practical meaning; in determining doses, rounding up or down to a certain decimal place.

simian line: abnormal crease appearing straight across the palms in the hands of children with Down syndrome.

simple mask: a transparent green mask with a simple nipple adapter that fits over a client's nose, mouth, and chin, which provides low-flow oxygen.

simple triage and rapid treatment (START): system that identifies people who will die quickly if they don't receive immediate medical care.

Sims' position: examination position in which the client is lying on his or her left side with right knee flexed.

single adult household: adults who live alone in their own apartments or houses with no children.

single-parent family: a family in which one adult is head of household with dependent children. The adult who is single may be single by choice or as a result of separation, divorce, or death.

sinus: a cavity or channel, often refers to the paranasal *sinuses;* may also refer to fistula (a sinus tract).

sinusitis: inflammation of the sinuses.

sitz bath: a bath used to apply heat to the pelvic area.

Sjögren's syndrome: a complex combination of symptoms that usually occurs in middle-aged women. Symptoms include dry eyes and mucous membranes, conjunctivitis, and connective tissue disorders such as rheumatoid arthritis, systemic lupus erythematosus, or scleroderma.

skeletal traction: form of directly applying traction to a client's bones by surgically inserting metal pins or wires into the bones.

skilled nursing facility: facility that provides 24-hour care to clients who live there or stay there temporarily to recover from injury or severe illness.

skin traction: traction applied to the skin which transmits the pull to the musculoskeletal system.

skin turgor: skin tone.

slander: malicious and false verbal statements.

slough: to shed; to cast off (noun: slough—a mass of dead tissue).

smegma: sebaceous gland secretion found under the foreskin of the penis.

social needs: needs for love and belonging.

sodium: a chemical element that is a major ion in extracellular fluids (common table salt is composed of sodium [Na$^+$] and chloride).

soft diet: a nutritionally adequate diet that is low in fiber, connective tissue, and fat.

solute: a substance dissolved in a solvent.

solvent: a liquid that dissolves a solute.

somnambulism: sleepwalking.

somniloquism: sleeptalking.

somnolent: state in which a person is very difficult or impossible to rouse.

Somogyi phenomenon: condition in diabetes mellitus in which overtreatment with insulin causes hypoglycemia. This is followed by a compensatory period of rebound hyperglycemia as the body tries to correct the initial problem by increasing glucose production.

sordes: foul, dark matter that collects around the teeth and lips in low-grade fevers.

soul food: cooking style and particular foods commonly eaten by people in the southeastern United States.

spastic cerebral palsy: most common type of cerebral palsy, characterized by increased muscle tone or spasticity, partial or full paralysis, and sensory abnormalities.

specific gravity: a substance's weight, as compared with another. Fluids,

such as urine, are compared to pure water, which has a specific gravity of 1.000.

specific immunity: immunity in which specific defense mechanisms are able to recognize and act against particular harmful substances.

spermatozoa: sperm cells; male reproductive cells.

sphincter: circular muscle that guards an opening.

sphygmomanometer: device used in conjunction with a stethoscope to measure blood pressure, consisting of an inflatable bladder attached to a bulb or pump, enclosed in a cuff, with a deflating mechanism.

spina bifida: congenital anomaly in which the vertebral spaces fail to close.

spinal bifida oculta: an opening in a child's vertebral column with no apparent symptoms.

spinal cord: a long mass of nerve cells and fibers extending though a central canal from the brain's medulla to the approximate level of the first or second lumbar vertebra.

spinal nerves: nerves that originate in the spinal cord.

spinal stenosis: narrowing of the intervertebral space.

spirillum: spiral shaped bacteria (plural: spirilla).

spleen: an organ containing lymphoid tissue that is designed to filter blood. Its functions in an adult include destroying old RBCs, forming bilirubin, producing lymphocytes and monocytes, and acting as a reservoir for blood.

splint: an appliance, either rigid or flexible, that holds body parts in place, as an arm *splint*. (verb: splint—to provide firm support as postoperative splinting or a splint to immobilize a fracture.

splinting (incision): use of a pillow or large towel to provide support along a suture line.

spore: protective capsule formed by some microorganisms to safeguard themselves.

sprain: twisting a joint with rupture of ligaments (not a fracture) and possibly other damage to blood vessels, tendons, or nerves.

squamous: scaly, platelike, as *squamous* epithelium.

stabilization (stābe) room: room in an emergency facility in which clients are triaged and stabilized for transfer to an operating room or other area.

stages of labor: process of delivery that spans from the onset of true labor to the stabilization of the mother afterwards; the four stages are, specifically: dilation, expulsion, placental, and recovery.

standard precautions: precautions designed for the care of all clients regardless of diagnosis or infection status.

stapes: the "stirrup," one of three tiny bones within the middle ear which are set in motion by sound waves.

stasis: standstill, stationary or not moving.

station: level of descent of the fetal presenting part into the birth canal.

status asthmaticus: dangerous condition that exists when medications do not relieve an acute episode of asthma.

steatorrhea: excess fecal fat; occurs in malabsorption syndromes or deficiencies of pancreatic enzymes.

stenosis: narrowing or constriction of an opening or tube, as aortic *stenosis* or pyloric *stenosis*.

stent: a wire coil similar to the coil in a ball point pen used to keep open an artery.

stereotype: classifying or categorizing people; believing that all those who belong to a certain group are alike.

sterile technique: surgical asepsis.

sterile: free of microorganisms, aseptic; unable to bear children, infertile, barren.

sterilization: process that destroys all microorganisms and spores.

sternal: pertaining to the sternum, as a *sternal* puncture.

sternum: breast bone

steroid: adrenocortical hormone produced by the adrenal glands or a synthetic derivative that mimics its action.

stertorous breathing: breathing that occurs when air travels through secretions in the air passage; snoring.

stethoscope: instrument used to amplify internal body sounds, especially heartbeat.

stimulant: any agent that increases activity in the body or one of its parts (stimulus).

stoma: an opening on a free surface, such as a pore; an artificially created opening between a body cavity and the body's surface, such as the stoma of a colostomy, ileostomy, or tracheostomy.

stool: feces, discharge from the bowels.

stork bite: birthmark that appears on the newborn's eyelid or forehead that usually fades during infancy.

strabismus: a deviation of the eye; squint. (Convergent strabismus is called cross-eye; divergent strabismus is called exotropia or walleye. Other types include cyclotropia, esotropia, hypertropia, and hypotropia.)

strain: overextension of a muscle.

stranger anxiety: condition seen in infants and children, in which unfamiliar people, places, and events upset them.

strangulated: closed because of constriction, as a *strangulated* hernia.

strangulation: suffocation resulting from externally applied pressure to the throat.

streptococcal (strep) throat: viral infection caused by the *streptococcus* bacterium that is common in children and responds well to antibiotic therapy if treated promptly; otherwise, it may develop more serious complications such as rheumatic fever, rheumatic heart disease, and nephritis.

stress: pressure; reaction to adverse stimulus, as emotional stress or as physical stress placed upon the body by injury, pregnancy, chemicals, or disease, as a *stress* fracture.

stress incontinence: urinary leakage following a sudden increase in intra-abdominal pressure such as coughing or sneezing.

stress test: (1) method of evaluating the response of the fetal heart to contractions and providing information as to how well the placenta is supplying oxygen to the fetus; also known as the oxytocin challenge test (OCT). (2) method of evaluating the severity of heart disease by measuring the heart's response to physical activity and/or medication.

stressor: an agent that produces stress and disrupts homeostasis.

striae: stretch marks.

stricture: fibrous band that can form along the ureters or urethra, narrowing it, and interfering with urine passage.

stridor: a shrill and harsh sound (usually refers to the inspiratory sound that occurs when the larynx is obstructed).

subacute: between an acute or chronic state, with some acute features.

subacute care: facilities that provide an "in-between" level of care for a client for approximately two to four weeks between hospitalization and return to independent living or a long-term care facility; also called transitional or continual care.

subculture: groups within a dominant culture who share a characteristic such as profession, religion, geographical origin, age, etc.

subcutaneous: beneath the skin.

subcutaneous tissue: tissue that lies below the dermis and binds the skin to the underlying muscle tissue.

subdural hematosis: slow-forming clot in the skull, below the dura, caused by an accumulation of blood, usually from a torn vein on the brain's surface.

subjective: perceived only by the affected individual (pain is a subjective sign); also refers to a test item that requires judgment and interpretation as to the correct answer, open to more than one interpretation.

subjective data: information that consists of the client's opinions and feeling about what is happening, conveyed to the nurse either directly or through body language.

sublingual: under the tongue; (nitroglycerin is administered sublingually).

substance abuse: a maladaptive pattern of substance use leading to clinically significant impairment or distress.

sudden death: a situation in which breathing and heartbeat stop; also called cardiopulmonary arrest.

sudden infant death syndrome (SIDS): crib death, cot death, infantile apnea syndrome. Thought to be a result of untreated prolonged infantile apnea (PIA) or "near miss."

sudoriferous: conveying or transmitting sweat.

suffocation: stoppage of breathing; asphyxia.

suicidal ideation: thoughts or ideas of killing oneself, which usually precede an actual suicide attempt.

supination: act of turning to the supine position; turning the hand so the palm is upward.

supine: lying on the back.

suppository: a conical mass to be introduced into the vagina, rectum, or urethra, usually containing medication (easily melted).

suppuration: formation or discharge of pus (adj: suppurative).

suprapubic: above the pubic arch.

surfactant: surface-active agent, such as soap; a mixture of phospholipids (mostly lecithin and sphingomyelin) in the respiratory passages, used as a test for fetal maturity.

surgical asepsis: destruction of all pathogens, "sterile technique."

survival needs: according to Maslow, those needs that are vital to sustain life, primary needs.

suture: thread used to hold an incision together while it heals; also called stitches.

sympathetic: division of the autonomic nervous system that responds to emergencies, pressure, danger, or extreme stress.

symphysis pubis: juncture where the pubic bones meet in front and are joined by a pad of cartilage.

symptom: functional evidence of a disease or condition that a client perceives subjectively (as opposed to signs, which the examiner or others perceive).

symptomatic: treating symptoms as they occur, rather that treating an underlying condition.

synapse: the functional junction between two neurons (nerve cells) at which point the impulse is transmitted.

syncope: fainting, caused by an insufficient supply of blood and oxygen to the brain.

syndactylism: condition in which an infant is born with two or more digits fused together.

synergism: joint action of agents in which the combined effect is greater than the sum of the individual parts (synergistic medications enhance the action of each other); potentiation.

synovectomy: excision of the synovial membrane.

syringectomy: surgical removal of a fistula.

system: group of organs.

systemic: pertaining to the entire body, general, total (as opposed to local).

systole: contraction of the heart; systolic blood pressure is the pressure of the blood against the walls of the arteries when the heart beats (the top number in the blood pressure reading).

T

T cells: lymphocytes that mature in the thymus.

tablet: a compressed, spherical form of a medication.

taboos: practices or beliefs that a group's members cannot violate without discomfort and risk of exclusion.

tachycardia: abnormally fast heart rate.

tachypnea: condition in which breaths are abnormally rapid, more than 20 per minute.

tactile sense: sense of touch.

talipes: condition in which one or both feet turn out of the normal position; commonly known as "club foot."

tardive dyskinesia: a condition that results from long-term use of neuroleptics. A common symptom is obvious mouth and tongue movements.

target population: subgroups in the community with unique or special healthcare needs.

T-binder: a binder made of two strips of material, 3–4 inches wide, which are fastened together, forming a T. This device is used to hold rectal or perineal dressings in place.

technical skills: skills used to perform interventions, such as changing a sterile dressing or administering injections.

TED socks: (see antiembolism stockings).

telecommunications: system that enables healthcare providers to communicate with clients in different locations using a telephone and a computer.

telehealth: telephone nursing.

telephone triage: system of sorting calls to determine which need immediate attention.

temporal lobe: cerebral lobe that controls hearing, auditory interpretation, and smell.

tendon: tough cords that attach muscle to bone.

tenesmus: painful abdominal cramps or spasms.

tenosynovitis: inflammation of a tendon sheath.

tension pneumothorax: occurs when air leaks out of the lung into the chest cavity and cannot escape, causing pressure to build in the chest and the lung on the side of the leak to collapse.

tepid sponge bath: bath with water below body temperature, 70 to 85 degrees, used to reduce fever.

teratogen: an agent or factor that causes defects in a developing embryo, such as a medication a woman takes during pregnancy.

terminal illness: a state in which an individual faces a medical condition that will end in death within a limited period.

testes: the male gonad. (sing: testis)

testosterone: major male hormone.

tetanic contractions: irregular, uncoordinated uterine contractions; also called tonic contractions.

tetanus: a highly fatal disease characterized by muscle spasms and seizures ("lock-jaw"). Can be prevented by immunization.

thalamus: relay station between the cutaneous receptors and the cerebral cortex for all sensory impulses except smell.

theoretical framework: skeleton on which to base knowledge.

therapeutic communication: communication (usually verbal) with a client that is helpful and beneficial; creating a healing, curative, and safe milieu by using communication.

therapeutic diet: approach to eating that is prescribed as part of the treatment of more than one disease or condition.

therapeutic effect: a medication's desired effect; produces the result for which it was given.

therapy: treatment of disease (therapeutic).

thermoregulation: heat regulation, heat control.

third-party payment: system developed to help individuals pay for the cost of medical bills, usually a health insurance plan.

third-space (fluid): fluid found in the interstitial tissue spaces.

thoracentesis: surgical puncture and drainage of the thoracic (chest) cavity.

thoracotomy: incision into the thorax or chest cavity.

thorax: the chest.

thrill: a vibration felt upon palpation.

thrombin: clotting agent created by the reaction of prothrombin activator and calcium ions, which converts fibrinogen into threads of fibrin.

thrombocytes: blood platelets, which are essential for clotting.

thrombocytopenia: platelet disorder characterized by too few thrombocytes.

thrombocytosis: condition marked by an increased number of platelets.

thrombolytic: type of medication designed to dissolve a clot and clear a blocked blood vessel.

thrombophlebitis: formation of a blood clot in a vein, with inflammation.

thrombus: a stationary blood clot.

thrush: fungal infection of the oral mucous membrane.

thymus: small gland in the upper chest that functions as an endocrine gland.

thyroid: resembling a shield. The thyroid gland, located in the neck, is the largest endocrine gland. It secretes hormones vital to growth and metabolism.

thyroidectomy: surgical removal of the thyroid gland.

tibia: shin bone, which is the long, weight-bearing bone of the lower leg.

tidal volume: amount of gas passing into and out of the lungs during each respiratory cycle.

tinnitus: ringing in the ears.

tissue: a group of similar, specialized cells united to perform a specific function, as epithelial *tissue*.

titration: gradually increasing a medication's dose.

tocodynamometer: pressure sensitive device used to monitor the frequency of uterine contractions.

toddler: a child from one to three years in age.

tofu: soybean curd.

toileting: various nursing interventions to assist the client with either bowel or bladder elimination.

tolerance: ability to endure a substance's continued use, such as of a medication or illegal drug; sometimes refers to increased dosage needed to achieve the desired effect.

tongue: tough skeletal muscle covered with mucous membrane whose function include sensing temperature and texture of food, mixing food with saliva, and moving food into position to be chewed and swallowed.

tonometer: instrument which can indirectly measure intraocular pressure.

tonsil: a ring of lymphatic tissue around the pharynx forming a protective barrier for infectious substances entering the oral and respiratory passages.

tonsillitis: inflammation of the tonsils caused by a virus or bacteria.

topical: medications that are applied directly to the skin or mucous membranes.

tort: a wrong or injury committed against a person or property for which the injured person has the right to sue.

torticollis: torsion (twisting) of the neck; "wry neck."

tortillas: round, flat bread made from unleavened flour or cornmeal.

total incontinence: nearly continuous urinary leakage.

total parenteral nutrition (TPN): method of nutrition in which a catheter is inserted into a large blood vessel and nutrient solution is administered by continuous drip.

tourniquet: a device used to inhibit bleeding.

toxic: pertaining to a poison or toxin.

toxic shock syndrome: bacterial infection characterized by fever, vomiting, and/or diarrhea, believed to be facilitated by the use of tampons, especially those with plastic inserters.

toxicity: undesired, harmful effect of medication that results from an increased blood level of the agent beyond its therapeutic level.

toxin: poison; especially refers to protein poisons produced by pathogenic bacteria and some animals and plants.

toxoplasmosis: a congenital or acquired disease that can cause lesions in most body systems. It is particularly dangerous to pregnant women and can be prevented by careful cooking of meat and by avoiding the handling of cat litter.

trachea: the windpipe, through which food and air pass.

tracheotomy: incision into the trachea.

traction: exertion of a pulling force; an apparatus attached to the client to maintain stability of a joint or aligned fracture or to exert a pulling force elsewhere, as in the lower back, to relieve pressure.

trade name: the copyrighted brand name of a medication assigned by its manufacturer. (A medication with the same generic/chemical name can have several trade or proprietary names.)

transcribing orders: reading of a physician's order sheet and carrying out of necessary actions.

transcultural nursing: unbiased care of persons from all races, religions, and ethnic groups.

transdermal: through the skin, a substance absorbed into the body after being placed on the skin, as *transdermal* administration of medication by ointment or patch; transcutaneous.

trans-fat: process in which a polyunsaturated fatty acid is hydrogenated to make it solid at room temperature. These have fewer essential fatty acids than the original oil because unsaturated fat content is lowered.

transfer belt: sturdy webbed belt used by the nurse to help provide support to the weak or unsteady person.

transfer board: board made of hard plastic used to move patients who are unable to stand from the side of the bed to a chair.

transfusion: injection of blood or blood components or substitutes into a person's circulation.

transmission-based precautions: precautions designed for clients with specific infections or diagnoses.

transverse: from side to side; crosswise.

transverse lie: positioning in which the fetus lies across the woman's abdomen in the uterus.

trapeze: horizontal bar suspended above and attached to the bed, which is used to pull up to a sitting position or to lift the shoulders and hips off the bed.

trauma: a wound or injury from an external source.

triage: sorting out of victims of disaster to determine the priority of treatment.

trial and error: experimental problem solving that tests ideas to decide which methods work and which do not.

trichomoniasis: second most common type of vaginitis; symptoms include itching and burning of the vulva and a foul-smelling greenish-yellow or gray bubbly discharge; usually sexually transmitted.

tricuspid: with three cusps or points, as the *tricuspid* valve of the heart, between the right atrium and ventricle.

triglyceride: a compound consisting of three molecules of fatty acids and one molecule of glycerol, which is the usual form of fat storage in the body.

trimester: 3 months, as a *trimester* in pregnancy.

trisomy 21: (see Down syndrome).

Trousseau's sign: an abnormal carpal spasm induced by inflating a sphygmomanometer cuff on the upper arm to a pressure exceeding systolic blood pressure for 3 minutes; indicative of tetany following accidental removal of the parathyroid glands during thyroidectomy, hypocalcemia, or hypomagnesemia.

tubal ligation: most common and effective procedure for permanent sterilization in women; ligation of the oviducts.

tube feeding: providing liquid nourishment through a tube into the intestinal tract.

tuberculosis (TB): a communicable disease caused by the tubercle bacillus (any organ may be affected, but it primarily affects the lung in human beings).

tumor: an abnormal new tissue growth that has no physiologic use and grows independent of its surrounding structures. May be benign or malignant.

turgor: skin resiliency and plumpness; also called skin turgor.

tympanic membrane: eardrum.

tympanoplasty: plastic reconstruction of the ossicles of the middle ear.

Tzanck's smear: examination of cells and fluids from vesicles, which are applied to a glass slide, stained, and examined under a microscope.

U

ulcer: open sore on an external or internal body surface that causes gradual disintegration of tissues, often an ulcer of the stomach (peptic *ulcer*) or a pressure sore (decubitus *ulcer*).

ulna: large bone of the forearm.

ultrasound: a method of applying deep, penetrating heat to muscles and tissues.

ultraviolet rays: rays used to treat skin infections and wounds.

umbilicus: the navel, or site where the umbilical cord is joined to the fetus.

units: specific measurements used for certain nutrients and drugs.

unoccupied bed: bed that is empty at the time it is made up.

upper tract: division of the urinary tract that includes the kidneys and ureters.

ureter: narrow tube that carries urine from the kidney to the urinary bladder.

urethra: tube through which urine passes from the urinary bladder to outside the body.

urethral pressure profile: technique used to evaluate smooth muscle activity along the urethra.

uretolithotomy: surgical removal of a stone blocking a ureter.

urge incontinence: urinary leakage due to irritation of the bladder wall or from urine components.

urgency: desire or sensation of needing to void immediately.

urinalysis: examination of urine.

urinary catheter: tube inserted into the bladder through the urethra to remove urine.

urinary frequency: voiding more often than usual without an increase in total urine volume.

urinary incontinence: involuntary voiding or urine loss.

urinary retention: inability to empty the bladder of urine.

urination: passing urine from the urinary bladder to outside; voiding; micturition.

urine: fluid output of waste projects from the kidneys.

urinometer: an instrument that determines urine's specific gravity; also called urometer, hydrometer.

urodynamics: series of urination tests that best determines the actual level of functioning of the detrusor muscle, external sphincter muscle, and pubococcygeal muscles; also called urodynamic testing.

uroflowmetry: noninvasive assessment of the status of voiding.

urology: the study of urinary disorders in the female and genitourinary disorders in the male. A urologist is the physician who specializes in this area.

urticaria: an allergic skin reaction characterized by superficial wheals and often accompanied by severe itching; also called hives.

uterine inertia: insufficient, uncoordinated contractions that do not produce effective dilation for delivery.

uterine tubes: (see oviducts).

uterus: hollow, pear-shaped organ in the female pelvis where the fetus develops and grows; also called womb.

V

vaccine: an injection of a disease-causing agent into a person to induce immunity to the agent.

vacuum extraction: method of delivery in which a round soft plastic cup is gently suctioned to the fetal head and traction exerted to ease the fetus out of the birth canal.

vagina: the female sex organ.

vaginismus: involuntary contraction of the vaginal outlet muscles, preventing penetration during sexual intercourse.

vaginitis: vaginal inflammation.

vagus nerve: cranial nerve X (ten)—affects many body functions beyond conscious control.

values: a person's or group's "rights" and "wrongs" or what is considered desirable or important.

values clarification: examining values, beliefs, and feelings about life and healthcare issues.

variance: an actual outcome that differs from an expected outcome.

varicella: viral infection in children, which is characterized by an outbreak of rash that progresses into papules, vesicles, then pustules; also called chickenpox.

varices: outpouching blood vessels.

varicocele: scrotal swelling caused by varicosities in the spermatic blood vessels (described as feeling like a "bag of worms").

vasectomy: excision of the vas deferens that renders a male sterile.

vasoconstriction: lessening a blood vessel's circumference.

vasoconstrictor: medication that raises blood pressure by constricting or narrowing the blood vessels.

vasodilator: medication that lowers blood pressure by causing dilation (enlargement of lumina) of blood vessels, used to treat hypertension (high blood pressure).

vector: carrier, especially of a disease organism.

vegan: a vegetarian who eats no animal-originated foods. (A lacto-vegetarian eats milk and dairy products; an ovo-vegetarian eats eggs.)

vegetarian: diet based mainly on plant foods. Some vegetarians exclude all animal products from their diet (vegans); others vary on what animal products they consume.

vein: blood vessel that returns blood from the body to the heart (in most cases, deoxygenated blood).

venipuncture: puncture of a vein, usually with a needle. May be used to obtain a blood specimen or to start an intravenous infusion (IV).

venous access lock: catheter used to maintain an open route to a client's venous system to give fluids and/or medications.

ventilation: supplying oxygen to the body through the lungs; breathing.

ventilator: a machine that supplies oxygen and forces breathing; also called a respirator.

ventilatory failure: state of being unable to breathe adequately alone.

ventral: anterior or front.

ventricles: two lower chambers of heart (pump blood to the body and lungs).

Venturi mask: mask with a hard plastic adapter, with large "windows" on the sides; this device provides the most reliable and consistent oxygen enrichment.

verbal communication: giving information, news, or messages by speaking or writing.

vermiform appendix: (see appendix).

vernix caseosa: substance covering the fetus before and at birth.

vernix: (Latin) varnish.

version: turning, as of the fetus during normal delivery.

vertebral column: the spine.

vertex: normal, head-first presentation.

vertical client: a client who has a non-critical condition; ambulatory care client.

vertigo: sensation of rotation or movement of self (subjective *vertigo*) or surroundings (objective *vertigo*). (Not all dizziness is true vertigo.)

vesicle: small sac containing liquid; small blister.

viability: state in which a fetus is mature enough to survive outside the woman's uterus (usually 24 weeks' gestation).

vial: glass container equipped with a self-sealing rubber stopper that contains either a single or multiple dose of a medication.

villi: fingerlike projections in the small intestine that provide greater absorption area for nutrients to enter into the bloodstream (sing: villus).

viral load: amount and strength of the HIV virus in an individual; also called HIV-RNA.

virulence: ability of a microorganism to cause disease; strength, potency.

virus: protein-covered sac containing genetic or other organic materials, which enters a living organism and uses the host cell for viral reproduction to cause an illness or disease.

viscera: internal organs contained within a body cavity.

visceral pleura: layer of the pleura that covers the lungs.

vital signs: measurements of temperature, pulse, respiration, and blood pressure.

vitamin: various organic substances essential to life (includes fat-soluble vitamins [A, D, E, and K] and water-soluble vitamins [B-complex, C, and others]).

vitiligo: skin condition characterized by white patches that often become larger.

vitreous humor: a transparent, gelatin-like material that fills the space behind the lens of the eye.

vocal cords: two triangular-shaped membranous folds that extend from the front to back of the larynx that vibrate and produce sound as air passes over them.

void: to cast out wastes, as to urinate, micturate.

voiding study: use of sensors to measure detrusor pressure when voiding.

voluntary: controlled by the will, as a *voluntary* muscle.

volvulus: twisting of a loop of intestine; may or may not strangulate.

vomitus: stomach contents expelled by vomitus.

vulnerable adult: an adult who is intellectually impaired, mentally ill, or otherwise unable to protect himself or herself.

vulva: the external parts of the female genital organs.

vulvitis: inflammation of the vulva.

W

walking rounds: caregivers move from client to client, discussing pertinent information.

wart: a skin tumor caused by a virus; verruca.

wellness: state of physical and emotional well-being; optimum health.

Wernicke-Korsakoff syndrome: disorder caused by a chronic deficiency of thiamine, often related to malnutrition due to chemical dependence.

wet-to-dry dressing: saturated dressing that is wrapped around a wound and left to dry. Upon removal, the dressing pulls away tissue debris and drainage, making it a useful tool in debridement.

Wharton's jelly: soft jelly-like substance that protects the umbilical cord.

wheal: a smooth, slightly elevated skin area, usually pale in the center with a reddened periphery, often accompanied by severe itching.

wheeze: a whistling respiratory sound, typical of asthma.

Wilms' tumor: malignant adenosarcoma and common neoplasm of childhood, which usually affects only one kidney; also called nephroblastoma.

wind chill factor: mathematical calculation of temperature and wind speed.

withdrawal: discontinuance of use of a drug.

Wood's light: special high-pressure mercury lamp that produces long-wave UV rays used to diagnose abnormalities and infections of the skin.

worker's compensation: program that provides financial compensation to a person who has been injured at work or who has contracted a disease that can be directly related to his or her job.

wound: injury to any body structure caused by physical means.

wound sinus: canal or passage leading to an abscess.

X

xenograft: graft of tissue between animals of different species, as in the grafting of pigskin onto a human in burn treatment; also called heterograft.

Y

Yin-Yang: belief system that emphasizes balance and its influence on illness and health.

Z

z-track: "zig-zag" method of injecting caustic medications deep into muscle tissue.

zydis: solid instantly dissolving medication that is placed on the tongue.

zygote: cell that results from the fusion of two mature germ cells.

Note: Page numbers followed by f indicate figures; those followed by t indicate tables; and those followed by b indicate boxes.

Dating, 131
Daycare, 119
Day-surgery center, 1666–1669, 1708
DDAVP. *see* Desmopressin acetate
Death
  biologic, 509
  brain, 46, 796
  caring for body after, 797, 798b
  caring for client's body after, 499, 499b
  clinical, 509, 796
  coping with, 797, 799
  cultural influences, 94, 149
  definition of, 46
  determination of, 46
  exceptions in determining, 46–47
  family impact of, 151–152
  hospice care, 1689, 1689b
  leading causes of, 62, 365
  newborn, 1001
  postmortem examination, 797
  religious beliefs and practices, 149t
  signs of approaching, 795, 795b
  spirituality and, 149–150
Debridement
  burn wound, 1159
  description of, 526, 781, 1146
Deciduous teeth, 117
Decimal fractions, 807–808
Decongestants, 848, 849
Decubitus ulcers. *see* Pressure ulcers
Decussation, 218
Deep, 161t
Deep relaxation, 741
Deep venous thrombosis, 1202, 1306
Deep-tendon reflexes, 228
Defamation, 41
Defecation, 311, 680
Defecation reflex, 311
Defense mechanisms, 68, 285–286, 1570, 1571t,
  1612
Defibrillation, 1298–1299
Deficiency disease, 73
Deglutition, 303
Dehiscence, 763, 764f
Dehumanization, 550–551
Dehydration
  description of, 182–183, 1007–1008, 1168
  hospice care, 1684
Delirium, 1553
Delirium tremens, 1623
Delsym. *see* Dextromethorphan
Delta cells, 239
Deltoid
  anatomy of, 208t
  injections in, 885
Delusional disorder, 1575
Delusions, 1602, 1604b
Dementia
  activities of daily living assessments,
    1560–1561
  advance directives, 1565
  aggression, 1560, 1565
  AIDS-related, 1557
  Alzheimer's disease
    causes of, 1554
    description of, 1553–1554, 1555–1556
    physiologic changes of, 1554–1555
    risk factors, 1554b

  stages of, 1555b, 1555–1556
    treatment of, 1556
  bathing concerns, 1562
  behavior management, 1564–1565
  caregiver assistance, 1565
  communication assistance, 1564, 1564b
  crack-related, 1558
  Creutzfeldt-Jakob disease, 1557
  definition of, 1553
  diagnosis of, 1554b, 1558–1559
  laboratory tests, 1559t
  multi-infarct, 1553, 1556
  nursing process for, 1559–1566
  Parkinson's disease, 1557
  physical assessment of, 1559–1560
  Pick's disease, 1557
  psychological assessment of, 1560
  support systems, 1561–1562
  Wernicke-Korsakoff syndrome, 1557
Demerol. *see* Meperidine
Democratic leadership, 1722
Demographics, 146
Demography, 76
Dendrites, 216
Denial, 1570, 1571t, 1612
Denominator, 807
Dental health, 66b
Dental hygienist, 13t
Dental injuries, 518
Dentin, 303
Dentures, 656, 657b–658b, 1437
Denver-II Developmental Screening Test, 1037
Deoxyribonucleic acid, 161, 163, 471
Depakote. *see* Valproic acid
Department of Health and Human Services
  agencies in, 77
  description of, 76–77
Dependent actions, 429
Dependent personality disorder, 1574
Depo-Provera, 1022
Depressants, 829
Depressed fracture, 1190f
Depression
  childhood, 1132–1133
  description of, 369–370
  diagnosis of, 1572–1573
  dying-related, 150
  epidemiology of, 1572
  hospice care, 1684
  mental health nursing considerations,
    1605b–1606b
  in older adults, 1545
  postpartum, 1000–1001
  preparatory, 150
  prevention of, 1545b
  reactive, 150
  situational, 1573
Dermabrasion, 1108
Dermatitis
  atopic. *see* Eczema
  contact, 1149, 1354, 1355b
  description of, 1145
  seborrheic, 1153–1154
Dermatologic nurse, 1144
Dermatologist, 1144
Dermatology, 1144
Dermis, 171
Desipramine, 1585t
Desmopressin acetate, 856

Desquamate, 961
Desquamation, 171
Desyrel. *see* Trazodone
Detachment, 150–151
Detoxification
  description of, 1615
  immediate treatment, 1616, 1620
  long-term followup, 1621
  medications for, 1617b
  motivation for, 1615–1616
  refeeding syndrome, 1616, 1620
  therapeutic community, 1616
  withdrawal symptoms, 1616, 1618t–1619t,
    1620
Detoxification center, 1616
Developmental disabilities, 1126–1127
Dexedrine. *see* Dextroamphetamine
Dexpanthenol, 852t
Dextrin, 348
Dextroamphetamine, 833t
Dextromethorphan, 847t, 849
Diabeta. *see* Glyburide
Diabetes insipidus, 1242
Diabetes mellitus
  in children, 1113–1114
  classification of, 1248, 1248t
  client teaching regarding, 1259–1264
  complications of
    hyperglycemia, 1256–1258, 1257t
    hypoglycemic reaction, 1256, 1257t
    infections, 1258
    macrovascular, 1258–1259
    microvascular, 1259
    nephropathy, 1259
    neuropathy, 1259
    nonketotic hyperosmolar state, 1258
    retinopathy, 1259
    ulcers, 789, 1259, 1259f
  definition of, 1248
  description of, 71
  diagnostic tests for
    blood tests, 1239–1240
    description of, 1249b
    urine tests, 1240
  dietary guidelines, 389–390, 1117
  during pregnancy, 988–989, 989b
  foot care in, 1263, 1264b
  gestational, 989, 1251
  glucose monitoring, 1260, 1261b–1262b,
    1263b
  health promotion for, 66b
  insulin-dependent, 1113
  meal planning for, 1262
  non-insulin-dependent, 1113
  pediatric, 1113–1114
  signs and symptoms of, 1248–1249
  treatment of
    exercise, 1252
    goals, 1251
    insulin, 1252–1254
    nutrition, 1251–1252
    oral medications, 1254–1256, 1255t
    pancreatic transplantation, 1256
  type 1, 1248t, 1249, 1250b–1251b
  type 2, 1248t, 1249
Diabetic ketoacidosis, 1256–1258, 1257t
Diabinese. *see* Chlorpropamide
Diagnosis-related groups, 34, 431
Diagnostic statements, 423

shampoo, 662, 663b–664b
  special situations, 662
  melanin in, 172
Hair covering, 768
Halcion. *see* Triazolam
Halfway house, 1577
Halitosis, 654, 1543
Hallucinations, 1560, 1602–1603, 1604b
Hallucinogens, 1628–1629
Halo device, 1194b, 1194–1195
Haloperidol (Haldol), 1584t
Hand
  bones of, 201f, 205
  muscles of, 209
Hand massage, 666, 667b
Handwashing, 483, 484b, 485f–486f
Hard palate, 302
Hashimoto's thyroiditis, 1244
Havighurst, Robert, 115, 116b, 128, 135, 142
Hazardous substances
  disposal of, 488–489
  exposure to, 526–527
  safety concerns, 462–463
  spills, 488
Head
  assessment of, 609b
  circumference measurements, 1043
  molding of, 958
  newborn assessments, 958–960
  traumatic injuries to
    concussion, 1229–1230
    contusion, 1230
    description of, 222, 1228
    hematoma, 1230, 1232, 1232f
    intracranial pressure increases, 1228–1229, 1229b
    laceration, 1230
    nursing considerations, 1232
    penetrating, 1232
    skull fractures, 1230, 1231f
    treatment for, 1232
Headaches, 1210–1211
Healers, 90b
Healing of wound, 781
Health
  age-related concerns, 69–72
  components of, 61
  definition of, 61
  education benefits for, 69
  environmental, 61
  lifestyle factors that affect, 65–69
  risk factors that affect, 65–69
  websites for, 62
Healthcare
  acute care facilities, 26–27
  ambulatory. *see* Ambulatory healthcare
  community health services, 28
  computer use in, 543
  contemporary view of, 14f
  cost-effective, 430–431
  expenditures for, 62, 63t
  extended care facilities, 26, 28
  financing of, 31–34, 62–63, 63t
  fraud in, 36
  home. *see* Home care
  hospice care. *see* Hospice care
  local-level, 81–82
  managed. *see* Managed care
  multidisciplinary approach, 13–14

prevention and, 63–64
quality assurance of, 28–29
in schools, 28
settings and services, 26–28
state-level, 81
telehealth, 27–28
traditional view of, 14f
21st-century trends in, 25b, 25–26
websites, 62b
worldwide, 76
Healthcare team
  communication in, 542–545
  cultural diversity in, 99
  nurse's role in, 1697–1700
Health departments, 81
Health interview, 416–418, 417b–418b
Health maintenance organizations, 26, 32–33, 1708–1709
Health Occupations Students of America, 22
Health record
  contents of
    assessment documents, 437
    plans for care and treatment, 437
    plans for continuity of care, 440
    progress records, 437–438
    summary overview of, 438t
  definition of, 436
  documentation systems for, 436–437
  educational uses of, 436
  electronic, 437
  flow sheet, 439
  legal requirements and protection, 436
  manual, 437
  newborn, 956–957
  note formats for, 438–439, 439t
  purposes of, 436
  regulatory requirements, 436
  research uses of, 436
Health Resources and Services Administration, 77, 77b
Healthy People 2000, 64
Healthy People 2010, 64
Hearing
  aging effects, 252–253, 253t
  assessment of, 1273b
  description of, 249–250
  loss of, 1281–1282, 1657
  tests of, 1268
Hearing aid, 656, 659, 1274
Hearing impairment
  description of, 1132
  nursing considerations for, 1274–1275, 1275b–1276b
Heart
  apex of, 256
  blood flow through, 257, 258f
  blood vessels of, 258–259
  chambers of, 256
  circulation by, 277f
  conduction of, 262–263, 264f
  disorders of
    arrhythmias, 1297
    atrial fibrillation, 1298
    bacterial endocarditis, 1301
    cardiomyopathy, 1300–1301
    congestive heart failure, 1299–1300
    coronary artery disease, 1301–1302
    dysrhythmias, 1297
    fibrillation, 1298–1299

rheumatic heart disease, 1301
    ventricular fibrillation, 1298
  health promotion for, 66b
  hormones produced by, 240
  layers of, 256
  valves of, 256–257
Heart attack, 520, 522, 522b
Heart block, 1297–1298
Heart disease, 71
Heart rate, 265
Heart sounds, 264–265, 605f
Heart transplantation, 1293
Heart valve replacement, 1293
Heartburn, 304, 921t, 1440
Heat
  application of, 723, 723b
  dry, 723–725
  moist, 725–727
  pain management using, 740
  uses of, 723
Heat cradle, 724
Heat cramps, 514
Heat exhaustion, 514–515, 515t
Heat lamps, 724
Heat production and conservation, 175
Heat receptors, 251
Heat stroke, 515, 515t
Heat transfer, 174, 175t
Heat-related injuries, 514–516
Heberden's nodes, 1184
Heelstick procedure, 969b
Hegar's sign, 907
Height of client
  assessment of, 554
  child, 1042
Heimlich maneuver, 520
Helicobacter pylori, 1441
Hemangiomas, 1075
Hematemesis, 1453
Hematest, 706
Hematologic system
  aging effects, 279t
  blood. *see* Blood
  components of, 167t
  functions of, 269t
Hematoma
  characteristics of, 1230, 1232, 1232f
  ocular, 1279–1280
  postpartum, 998–999
Hematopoiesis, 196, 269
Hemianopsia, 1312
Hemiarthroplasty, 1198
Hemiplegia, 1311, 1649
Hemiplegic, 636
Hemoccult testing, 706, 710f
Hemoglobin
  description of, 172, 271
  glycosylated, 1240
Hemolytic anemia, 1323
Hemolytic uremic syndrome, 1101
Hemophilia, 1092–1093, 1328
Hemoptysis, 1400
Hemorrhage
  controlling of, 508–509
  description of, 272
  diseases and, 585t
  first aid, 523
  fracture-related, 1202
  internal, 524–525

PROGRAM LICENSE AGREEMENT

Read carefully the following terms and conditions before using the Software. Use of the Software indicates you and, if applicable, your Institution's acceptance of the terms and conditions of this License Agreement.

If you do not agree with the terms and conditions, you should promptly return this package to the place you purchased it and your payment will be refunded.

Definitions

As used herein, the following terms shall have the following meanings:

"Software" means the software program contained on the diskette(s) or CD-ROM or preloaded on a workstation and the user documentation, which includes all accompanying printed material.

"Institution" means a nursing or professional school, a single academic organization that does not provide patient care and is located in a single city and has one geographic location/address.

"Geographic location" means a facility at a specific location; geographic locations do not provide for satellite or remote locations that are considered a separate facility.

"Facility" means a health care facility at a specific location that provides patient care and is located in a single city and has one geographic location/address.

"Publisher" means Lippincott Williams & Wilkins, Inc., with its principal office in Philadelphia, Pennsylvania.

"Developer" means the company responsible for developing the software as noted on the product.

License

You are hereby granted a nonexclusive license to use the Software in the United States. This license is not transferable and does not authorize resale or sublicensing without the written approval or an authorized officer of Publisher.

The Publisher retains all rights and title to all copyrights, patents, trademarks, trade secrets, and other proprietary rights in the Software. You may not remove or obscure the copyright notices in or on the Software. You agree to use reasonable efforts to protect the Software from unauthorized use, reproduction, distribution or publication.

Single-User license

If you purchased this Software program at the Single-User License price or a discount of that price, you may use this program on one single-user computer. You may not use the Software in a time-sharing environment or otherwise to provide multiple, simultaneous access. You may not provide or permit access to this program to anyone other than yourself.

Institutional/Facility license

If you purchased the Software at the Institutional or Facility License Price or at a discount of that price, you have purchased the Software for use within your Institution/Facility on a single workstation/computer. You may not provide copies of or remote access to the Software. You may not modify or translate the program or related documentation. You agree to instruct the individuals in your Institution/Facility who will have access to the Software to abide by the terms of this License Agreement. If you or any member of your Institution fail to comply with any of the terms of this License Agreement, this license shall terminate automatically.

Network license

If you purchased the Software at the Network License Price, you may copy the Software for use within your Institution/Facility on an unlimited number of computers within one geographic location/address. You may not provide remote access to the Software over a value-added network or otherwise. You may not provide copies of or remote access to the Software to individuals or entities who are not members of your Institution/Facility. You may not modify or translate the program or related documentation. You agree to instruct the individuals in your Institution/Facility who will have access to the Software to abide by the terms of this License Agreement. If you or any member of your Institution/Facility fail to comply with any of the terms of this License Agreement, this license shall terminate automatically.

Limited warranty

The Publisher warrants that the media on which the Software is furnished shall be free from defects in materials and workmanship under normal use for a period of 90 days from the date of delivery to you, as evidenced by your receipt of purchase.

The Software is sold on a 30-day trial basis. If, for whatever reason, you decide not to keep the software, you may return it for a full refund within 30 days of the invoice date or purchase, as evidenced by your receipt of purchase by returning all parts of the Software and packaging in saleable condition with the original invoice, to the place you purchased it. If the Software is not returned in such condition, you will not be entitled to a refund. When returning the Software, we suggest that you insure all packages for their retail value and mail them by a traceable method.

The Software is a computer assisted instruction (CAI) program that is not intended to provide medical consultation regarding the diagnosis or treatment of any specific patient.

The Software is provided without warranty of any kind, either expressed or implied, including but not limited to any implied warranty of fitness for a particular purpose of merchantability. Neither Publisher nor Developer warrants that the Software will satisfy your requirements or that the Software is free of program or content errors. Neither Publisher nor Developer warrants, guarantees, or makes any representation regarding the use of the Software in terms of accuracy, reliability or completeness, and you rely on the content of the programs solely at your own risk.

The Publisher is not responsible (as a matter of products liability, negligence or otherwise) for any injury resulting from any material contained herein. This Software contains information relating to general principles of patient care that should not be construed as specific instructions for individual patients.

Manufacturers' product information and package inserts should be reviewed for current information, including contraindications, dosages and precautions.

Some states do not allow the exclusion of implied warranties, so the above exclusion may not apply to you. This warranty gives you specific legal rights and you may also have other rights that vary from state to state.

Limitation of remedies

The entire liability of Publisher and Developer and your exclusive remedy shall be: (1) the replacement of any CD which does not meet the limited warranty stated above which is returned to the place you purchased it with your purchase receipt; or (2) if the Publisher or the wholesaler or retailer from whom you purchased the Software is unable to deliver a replacement CD free from defects in material and workmanship, you may terminate this License Agreement by returning the CD, and your money will be refunded.

profits, event will Publisher or Developer be liable for any ages arising including any damages for personal injury, lost any error or defect or other incidental or consequential damor in the programming, Software whether in the database an authorized wholesaler or retailer Publisher, Developer, or possibility of such damage. as been advised of the

Some states do not allow the limitation or exclusion of liability for incidental or consequential images. The above limitations and exclusions may not apply to you.

General

This License Agreement shall be governed by the laws of the State of Pennsylvania without reference the conflict of laws provisions thereof, and may only be modified in a written statement signed by an authorized officer of the Publisher. By opening and using the Software, you acknowledge that you have read this License Agreement, understand it, and agree to be bound by its terms and conditions. You further agree that it is a complete and exclusive statement of the agreement between the Institution/Facility and the Publisher, which supersedes any proposal or prior agreement, oral or written, and any other communication between you and Publisher or Developer relative to the subject matter of the License Agreement.

Note

Attach a paid invoice to the License Agreement as proof of purchase.

AUDIO PRONUNCIATON CD-ROM

Running the Program

To start the program:
1. View the contents f the C...
2. Double-click the e...lossary.exe.

Note: In order to r this program, you must have Macromedia Flash Player installed on your PC. If you do not currently have th program installed, it can be downloaded free of charge at: http://www.macromedia.com/software/flashplaer/.

Using the Program

Access the pron...ciation glossary by clicking on the (+) button next to your choice, either by chapter, or alphabetically.
  Then, choos the chapter or letter containing the words you want to hear pronounced by clicking on the button or name.
Listen to th pronunciations simply by clicking once on each word you wish to hear.
To go to different section, click the "Menu" button to return to view the chapters or letters.
If you want to listen by a different order, click the (–) button to close either "Terms by Chapter" or "Terms Aphabetically," and then click the (+) button for the other choice.
To completely exit the program, click the Exit button.

CASE STUDY IN DIABETIC FOOT WOUND CARE: A CLINICAL SIMULATION

Installation Instructions

The installation program should automatically start a few seconds after you have inserted the CD-ROM into your CD-ROM drive. Follow the directions on the screen to complete the installation. If the installation program does *not* automatically start, follow these steps:

1. Open the "Start" menu and select "Run…".
2. In Open box, type "d:\setup", where d is the letter representing your CD-ROM drive, and press Enter. (If your CD-ROM drive is a letter other than d, substitute that letter.)
3. Follow the directions on the screen to complete the installation.

Note: This product requires Internet Explorer 5.0 or higher. The complete installation for IE 5.0 is included on this CD-ROM. The installation requires 36–66 MB of hard disk space.

Running the Program

Open the "Start" menu, go to "Programs", and select the "Lippincott Williams & Wilkins" group created by the installation program. Then select "Diabetic Foot Wound Care" to run the program.

Technical Support

Our technical support staff is available to answer your questions and provide information about other Lippncott Williams & Wilkins software. Call toll free Monday through Friday during normal business hours in the Estern Time Zone 800-638-3030, 410-528-4532, or fax 410-528-4422. You may also write to Technical Support t this address: Lippincott Williams & Wilkins Technical Support, 351 W. Camden Street, Baltimore, Maryland 21201-2436, or e-mail at techsupp@lww.com.